PHYSICAL
MEDICINE &
REHABILITATION

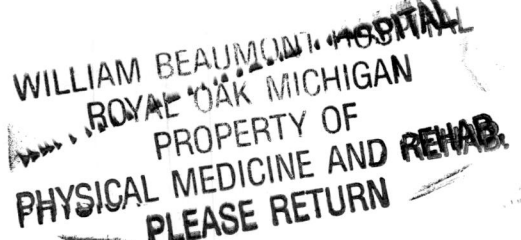
Commissioning Editor: **Dolores Meloni**
Development Editors: **Tim Kimber/Karen Carter**
Editorial Assistant: **Nani Clansey**
Project Manager: **Rory MacDonald**
Designer: **Andy Chapman**
Illustration Buyer: **Gillian Murray**
Illustrations: **Cactus**
Marketing Manager(s) (UK/USA): **Verity Kerkhoff/Matt Latuchie**

PHYSICAL MEDICINE & REHABILITATION

THIRD EDITION

Edited by

RANDALL L. BRADDOM MD MS

Clinical Professor
University of Medicine and Dentistry of New Jersey Medical School
and Clinical Professor
Robert Wood Johnson Medical Schools
New Brunswick, New Jersey

Associate Editors

Ralph M. Buschbacher MD
Professor and Chairman
Department of Physical Medicine and
  Rehabilitation
Indiana University Medical Center
Indianapolis, Indiana

Leighton Chan MD MPH MS
Associate Professor
Department of Rehabilitation Medicine
University of Washington School of Medicine
Seattle, Washington

Karen J. Kowalske MD
Associate Professor and Chairman
Department of Physical Medicine and
  Rehabilitation
University of Texas, Southwestern Medical
  Center
Dallas, Texas

Edward R. Laskowski MD
Professor of Physical Medicine and
  Rehabilitation
Mayo Clinic College of Medicine
Co-Director, Mayo Clinical Sports Medicine
  Center
Rochester, Minnesota

Dennis J. Matthews MD
Professor and Chairman
Department of Physical Medicine and
  Rehabilitation
University of Colorado School of Medicine
Denver, Colorado

Kristjan T. Ragnarsson MD
Lucy G. Moses Professor and Chairman
Department of Rehabilitation Medicine
Mount Sinai Medical Center
New York, New York

SAUNDERS

ELSEVIER

SAUNDERS
ELSEVIER

An imprint of Elsevier Inc

© 2000, 1996 by W.B. Saunders Company
© 2007, Elsevier Inc. All rights reserved.

First edition 1996
Second edition 2000
Third edition 2007

ISBN-13 978-1-4160-2610-5
ISBN-10 1-4160-2610-X

This book is also available as an **edition** package, including access to online updates:
ISBN-13 978-1-4160-3138-3
ISBN-10 1-4160-3138-3

British Library Cataloguing in Publication Data
A catalogue record for this book is available from the British Library

Library of Congress Cataloging in Publication Data
A catalog record for this book is available from the Library of Congress

Notice
Medical knowledge is constantly changing. Standard safety precautions must be followed, but as new research and clinical experience broaden our knowledge, changes in treatment and drug therapy may become necessary or appropriate. Readers are advised to check the most current product information provided by the manufacturer of each drug to be administered to verify the recommended dose, the method and duration of administration, and contraindications. It is the responsibility of the practitioner, relying on experience and knowledge of the patient, to determine dosages and the best treatment for each individual patient. Neither the Publisher nor the author assume any liability for any injury and/or damage to persons or property arising from this publication.

The Publisher

Printed in China
Last digit is the print number: 9   8   7   6   5   4   3

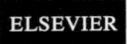 your source for books,
journals and multimedia
in the health sciences
www.elsevierhealth.com

Working together to grow
libraries in developing countries

www.elsevier.com | www.bookaid.org | www.sabre.org

ELSEVIER   BOOK AID International   Sabre Foundation

The
Publisher's
policy is to use
**paper manufactured
from sustainable forests**

Contents

Section 1 Evaluation

Section 2 Treatment Techniques and Special Equipment

Section 3 Common Clinical Problems

Section 4 Issues in Specific Diagnoses

Contributors

Richard T. Abresch MS
Research Director
Department of Physical Medicine & Rehabilitation
Davis School of Medicine
University of California
Davis, CA

Augusta Alba MD
Associate Professor, Clinical Rehabilitation Medicine, NYU Medical Center
Chief, Department of Rehabilitation Medicine
Coler-Goldwater Speciality Hospital and Nursing Facility
Roosevelt Island, NY

Susan D. Apkon MD
Assistant Professor of Physical Medicine and Rehabilitation
University of Colorado School of Medicine
Department of Rehabilitation Medicine
The Children's Hospital
Denver, CO

Lars Arendt-Nielsen Dr Med Sci PhD
Director of the International Doctorate School in Biomedical Science and Engineering
Center for Sensory-Motor Interaction
Aalborg University
Aalborg, Denmark

Jan R. Avent PhD
Professor of Communicative Sciences and Disorders
Department of Communication Sciences and Disorders
California State University, East Bay
Hayward, CA

Karen P. Barr MD
Assistant Professor
Department of Rehabilitation Medicine
University of Washington School of Medicine
Seattle, WA

Brent A. Bauer MD
Associate Professor of Medicine
Mayo Clinic College of Medicine
Director, Complementary and Integrative Medicine Program
Mayo Clinic
Rochester, MN

Terrie Black MBA BSN RN BC CRRN
UDS-PRO® Product Manager
Manager of Consultation, Education and Training
Uniform Data System for Medical Rehabilitation
Amherst, NY

Donna Jo Blake MD
Chief, Physical Medicine & Rehabilitation Service
Denver VA Medical Center
Eastern Colorado Health System
Denver, CO

Rina M. Bloch MD
Associate Professor
Department of Rehabilitation Medicine
Tufts University School of Medicine
New England Medical Center
Boston, MA

Cathy Bodine PhD CCC-SLP
Associate Professor/Director
Assistive Technology Partners
Department of Physical Medicine and Rehabilitation
University of Colorado Denver and Health Sciences Center
Denver, CO

Randall L. Braddom MD MS
Clinical Professor
University of Medicine and Dentistry of New Jersey Medical School
Clinical Professor
Robert Wood Johnson Medical Schools
New Brunswick, NJ

Fernando Branco MD
Assistant Professor
Department of Clinical Rehabilitation Medicine
University of Miami School of Medicine
Miami, FL

Jeffrey S. Brault DO PT
Assistant Professor
Department of Physical Medicine & Rehabilitation
Mayo Clinic College of Medicine
Mayo Clinic
Rochester, MN

Susan L. Braun MLS OTR
WeeFIM® Product Manager
Uniform Data System for Medical Rehabilitation
Amherst, NY

Andrew D. Bronstein MD
Clinical Assistant Professor
Department of Radiology
University of Washington
Radiology Consultants of Washington
Bellevue, WA

Theodore Brown MD MPH
Director of Rehabilitation Medicine
MS Hub Medical Group
Seattle, WA

Thomas N. Bryce MD
Assistant Professor
Department of Rehabilitation Medicine
Mount Sinai Medical Center
New York, NY

Mary Ellen Buning OTR PhD
Assistant Professor
Assistive Technology Partners
University of Colorado Health Sciences Center
Denver, CO

Ralph M. Buschbacher MD
Professor and Chairman
Department of Physical Medicine & Rehabilitation
Indiana University Medical Center
Indianapolis, IN

Diana D. Cardenas MD MHA
Professor and Chair
Department of Rehabilitation Medicine
University of Washington School of Medicine
Seattle, WA

Gregory T. Carter MD
Clinical Professor of Rehabilitation Medicine
Department of Rehabilitation Medicine
University of Washington School of Medicine
Seattle, WA

Leighton Chan MD MPH MS
Associate Professor
Department of Rehabilitation Medicine
University of Washington School of Medicine
Seattle, WA

Andrea Cheville MD
Assistant Professor
Department of Rehabilitation Medicine
Abramson Family Cancer Research Institute
Philadelphia, PA

David X. Cifu MD
Herman J Flax, MD Professor & Chairman
Department of Physical Medicine & Rehabilitation
Virginia Commonwealth University School of Medicine
Department of PM&R
Richmond, VA

Albert Clairmont MD
Associate Professor—Clinical
Department of Physical Medicine & Rehabilitation
The Ohio State University
College of Medicine & Public Health
Columbus, OH

Andrew J. Cole MD
Physiatrist
Physical Medicine and Rehabilitation
Northwest Spine & Sports Physicians
Bellevue, WA

Rory A. Cooper PhD
Distinguished Professor & FISA IPVA Endowed
    Chair
Department of Rehabilitation Science and
    Technology
University of Pittsburgh
Director, Human Engineering Research
    Laboratories
VA Pittsburgh Healthcare System
Pittsburgh, PA

Richard Drew Davis MD
Assistant Professor
Department of Pediatrics
University of Alabama at Birmingham
Birmingham, AL

Michael J. DePalma MD
Physiatrist
Sheltering Arms Spine & Sport Center
Richmond, VA

Timothy R. Dillingham MD MS
Professor and Chairman
Department of Physical Medicine and
    Rehabilitation
The Medical College of Wisconsin
Brookfield, WI

Jeanne Doherty MD
Assistant Professor of Rehabilitation Medicine
Magee Rehabilitation Hospital
Philadelphia, PA

Daniel Dumitru MD
Professor and Deputy Chairman
Department of Rehabilitation Medicine
The University of Texas—HSC at San Antonio
San Antonio, TX

Alberto Esquenazi MD
Chair, Department of PM&R & Chief Medical
    Officer
MossRehab
Albert Einstein Medical Center
Elkins Park, PA

Peter C. Esselman MD
Associate Professor
Department of Rehabilitation Medicine
University of Washington School of Medicine
Harborview Medical Center
Seattle, WA

Frank J.E. Falco MD
Director, PM&R Pain Medicine Fellowship
Clinical Assistant Professor
Temple University Medical School, Philadelphia
Mid Atlantic Spine
Newark, DE

Jonathan T. Finnoff DO
Physiatrist
Department of Physical Medicine &
    Rehabilitation
Utah State University
Logan, UT

Brian S. Foley MD
Assistant Professor
Medical Director of Occupational Health
Department of Physical Medicine &
    Rehabilitation
Indiana University School of Medicine
Indianapolis, IN

Guy Fried MD
Associate Professor of Rehabilitation Medicine
Magee Rehabilitation Hospital
Philadelphia, PA

Nancy Q. Fung MD
Assistant Attending Physiatrist, New York
    Presbyterian Hospital
Instructor of Physical Medicine & Rehabilitation
Department of Rehabilitation Medicine
Weill Medical College
Cornell University
New York, NY

Deborah J. Gaebler-Spira MD
Associate Professor
Pediatric Rehabilitation Medicine
Rehabilitation Institute of Chicago
Chicago, IL

Laura M. Garber
Certified Hand Therapist
Saint Luke's East
Rehabilitation and Wellness Center
Lee's Summit, MO

Ralph E. Gay MD DC
Assistant Professor
Department of Physical Medicine &
    Rehabilitation
Mayo Clinic
Rochester, MN

Robert Goldman MD
Visiting Clinical Associate Professor
Hyperbaric, Wound Care and Lymphedema
    Center
Memorial Hermann Hospital
Department of Anesthesiology
University of Texas
Houston, TX

Carl V. Granger MD
Executive Director, Uniform Data System for
    Medical Rehabilitation
Professor, Department of Rehabilitation
    Medicine
School of Medicine and Biomedical Sciences
University at Buffalo
The State University of New York
Buffalo, NY

Brian E. Grogg MD
Instructor, Physical Medicine & Rehabilitation
Mayo Clinic College of Medicine
Rochester, MN

Jaime Guzman MD
Assistant Professor of Medicine, University of
    Toronto
Clinician Investigator, Toronto Rehabilitation
    Institute
Associate Scientist
Institute for Work and Health
Toronto, ON, Canada

Jay J. Han MD
Assistant Professor
Department of Physical Medicine &
    Rehabilitation
Davis School of Medicine
University of California
Davis, CA

Pamela A. Hansen MD
Physician
Department of Physical Medicine &
    Rehabilitation
University of Utah School of Medicine
Salt Lake City, UT

R. Norman Harden MD
Director, Center for Pain Studies
Rehabilitation Institute of Chicago
Chicago, IL

Mark A. Harrast MD
Assistant Professor of Rehabilitation Medicine
    and Orthopedics and Sports Medicine
Department of Rehabilitation Medicine
University of Washington School of Medicine
Seattle, WA

Richard L. Harvey MD
Medical Director, Stroke Program
Rehabilitation Institute of Chicago
Chicago, IL

Peter Kerr Henke MD
Associate Professor of Surgery
Department of Vascular Surgery
University of Michigan Health System
Ann Arbor, MI

William J. Hennessey MD
Medical Director
Rehabilitation Services
Latrobe Area Hospital
Greensburg, PA

Cathy Thomas Hess BSN RN CWOCN
President and Director
Clinical Operations
Wound Care Strategies, Inc
Harrisburg, PA

Felicia Hill-Briggs PhD ABPP
Assistant Professor
Department of Physical Medicine &
    Rehabilitation
Johns Hopkins School of Medicine
Welch Center for Prevention, Epidemiology &
    Clinical Research
Baltimore, MD

Kurtis M. Hoppe MD
Consultant, Mayo Clinic
Instructor
Department of Physical Medicine &
    Rehabilitation
Mayo Clinic College of Medicine
Rochester, MN

Mark E. Huang MD
Assistant Professor of PM&R
Neural Engineering Center for Artificial Limbs
Rehabilitation Institute of Chicago
Chicago, IL

Franklin Lee Irwin Jr. MD
Attending Physician
Mid Atlantic Spine & Pain Specialists, P.A.
Newark, DE

Rebecca D. Jackson MD
Professor of Internal Medicine
Division of Endocrinology, Diabetes and
    Metabolism
The Ohio State University
Columbus, OH

Jeffrey Jenkins MD
Assistant Professor
Department of Physical Medicine &
    Rehabilitation
University of Virginia School of Medicine
Charlottesville, VA

Douglas Johnson-Greene PhD ABPP
Associate Professor
Department of Physical Medicine and
    Rehabilitation
Johns Hopkins University of Medicine
Baltimore, MD

Robert E. Kappler DO FAAO
Professor of Osteopathic Manipulative Medicine
Osteopathic Manipulative Medicine Department
Midwestern University
Downer's Grove, IL

Priti Khanna MD
Assistant Professor
Department of Physical Medicine &
    Rehabilitation
University of Texas Southwestern Medical
    Center
Dallas, TX

Daniel W. Kim MD
Attending Physician
Mid Atlantic Spine & Pain Specialists, P.A.
Newark, DE

John C. Kincaid MD
Department of Physical Medicine &
    Rehabilitation
Indiana University School of Medicine
Indianapolis, IN

John C. King MD
Professor of Rehabilitation Medicine and
    Director, Reeves Rehabilitation Center
Department of Rehabilitation Medicine
University of Texas—HSC at San Antonio
San Antonio, TX

Heidi Klingbeil MD
Chief of Geriatric Rehabilitation
Kessler Institute for Rehabilitation
Clinical Assistant Professor
University of Medicine & Dentistry of
    New Jersey
East Orange, NJ

Alicia M. Koontz PhD RET ATP
Research Health Scientist
Center of Excellence in Wheelchairs and
    Associated Rehabilitation Engineering
Human Engineering Research Laboratories
VA Pittsburgh Healthcare System
Pittsburgh, PA

Kathleen Bechtold Kortte PhD
Assistant Professor
Department of Physical Medicine &
    Rehabilitation
Johns Hopkins University School of Medicine
Baltimore, MD

Karen J. Kowalske MD
Associate Professor and Chairman
Department of Physical Medicine and
    Rehabilitation
University of Texas, Southwestern Medical
    Center
Dallas, TX

George H. Kraft MD MS
Professor of Rehabilitation Medicine
Adjunct Professor of Neurology
Department of Neurology
University of Washington School of Medicine
Seattle, WA

Jeffrey S. Kreutzer PhD ABPP
Professor, Director of Rehabilitation and
    Neuropsychological
Department of Physical Medicine &
    Rehabilitation
Virginia Commonwealth University
Richmond, VA

Todd A. Kuiken MD PhD
Associate Professor of PM&R
Neural Engineering Center for Artificial Limbs
Rehabilitation Institute of Chicago
Chicago, IL

Alison E. Lane MD
Lecturer in Occupational Therapy
School of Health Sciences
University of South Australia
Adelaide, Australia

Edward R. Laskowski MD
Professor of Physical Medicine and
    Rehabilitation
Mayo Clinic College of Medicine
Co-Director, Mayo Clinical Sports Medicine
    Center
Rochester, MN

Charles Law MD
Assistant Professor, Medical Director
Department of Pediatrics
The Children's Hospital of Alabama
Birmingham, AL

C. David Lin MD
Assistant Attending Physiatrist, New York
    Presbyterian Hospital
Assistant Professor of Rehabilitation Medicine
Department of Rehabilitation Medicine
Weill Medical College
Cornell University
New York, NY

Robert Lipschutz BSME CP
Director
Prosthetics & Orthotics Clinical Center
Rehabilitation Institute of Chicago
Chicago, IL

Shane E. Macaulay MD
Clinical Assistant Professor
Department of Radiology
University of Washington School of Medicine
Radiology Consultants of Washington
Bellevue, WA

Koichiro Matsuo DDS PhD
Assistant Professor of Physical Medicine and
    Rehabilitation
Department of Physical Medicine and
    Rehabilitation
Johns Hopkins University School of Medicine
Baltimore, MD

Dennis J. Matthews MD
Professor and Chairman
Department of Physical Medicine and
    Rehabilitation
University of Colorado School of Medicine
Denver, CO

Michael E. Mayo MD MBBS
Professor Emeritus
Department of Urology
University of Washington School of Medicine
Seattle, WA

Craig M. McDonald MD
Professor
Department of Physical Medicine &
  Rehabilitation
University of California Davis School of
  Medicine
Lawrence J. Ellison Ambulatory Care Center
Sacramento, CA

Jay M. Meythaler MD JD
Professor-Chair
Department of Physical Medicine and
  Rehabilitation
Wayne State University School of Medicine
Specialist in Chief for PM&R
The Detroit Medical Center
Rehabilitation Institute of Michigan
Detroit, MI

William F. Micheo MD
Chairman & Professor
Department of Physical Medicine, Rehabilitation
  & Sports Medicine
University of Puerto Rico School of Medicine
San Juan, Puerto Rico

Laura Miller PhD CP
Assistant Professor
Department of Physical Medicine and
  Rehabilitation
Northwestern University and the Rehabilitation
  Institute of Chicago
Chicago, IL

Yousef M. Mohammad MD MSc
Assistant Professor of Neurology
Department of Neurology
Ohio State University Medical Center
University Hospital
Columbus, OH

Denise M. Monahan MS CCC-SLP
Senior Speech Language Pathologist
Department of Rehabilitation
The Good Samaritan Hospital
Baltimore, MD

Daniel P. Moore MD
Professor of Physical Medicine & Rehabilitation
  and Pediatrics
Department of Physical Medicine &
  Rehabilitation
Brody School of Medicine
East Carolina University
Greenville, NC

Merilyn L. Moore PT
Rehabilitation Therapies Manager
Harborview Medical Center
Seattle, WA

Shubhra Mukherjee MD
Instructor in Physical Medicine and
  Rehabilitation
Northwestern University
Pediatric Rehabilitation
Rehabilitation Institute of Chicago
Attending Physician
Children's Memorial Hospital
Chicago, IL

W. Jerry Mysiw MD
Bert C. Wiley Chair and Associate
Professor of Physical Medicine & Rehabilitation
Department of Physical Medicine &
  Rehabilitation
The Ohio State University
Columbus, OH

Patricia W. Nance MD
Chief, Rehabilitation Service and Professor
Department of Physical Medicine and
  Rehabilitation
VA Long Beach Healthcare System
University of California Irvine
Long Beach, CA

Steven M. Nash MD
Assistant Professor of Clinical Neurology
Department of Neurology
Ohio State University Medical Center
University Hospital
Columbus, OH

Sharon P. Nations MD
Assistant Professor
Department of Physical Medicine &
  Rehabilitation
University of Texas Southwestern Medical
  Center
Dallas, TX

Michael W. O'Dell MD
Associate Chief and Attending Physiatrist,
  New York-Presbyterian Hospital
Professor of Clinical Rehabilitation Medicine
Department of Rehabilitation Medicine
Weill Medical College
Cornell University
New York, NY

C. Obi Onyewu MD
Attending Physician
Mid Atlantic Spine & Pain Specialists, P.A.
Newark, DE

Jeffrey B. Palmer MD
Lawrence Cardinal Shehan Professor of
  Physical Medicine and Rehabilitation
Professor of Otolaryngology and Functional
  Anatomy & Evolution
Department of Physical Medicine &
  Rehabilitation
Johns Hopkins University
Johns Hopkins Hospital
Baltimore, MD

Sara Palmer PhD
Assistant Professor
Department of Physical Medicine and
  Rehabilitation
Johns Hopkins University
Baltimore, MD

André Panagos MD
Assistant Professor, Weill Medical College of
  Cornell University
Assistant Attending Physiatrist
Department of Rehabilitation Medicine
New York Presbyterian Hospital
Weill Cornell Medical Center
New York, NY

Atul T. Patel MD MHSA
Medical Director, Rehabilitation Unit
Research Medical Center
Kansas City Bone & Joint Clinic, Inc
Kansas City, MO

Andrea Peterson DO
Practising Physiatrist
Department of Physical Medicine
Marshfield Clinic
Marshfield, WI

Adrian Popescu MD
Research Associate
Department of Physical Medicine and
  Rehabilitation
University of Pennsylvania School of Medicine
Philadelphia, PA

Kristjan T. Ragnarsson MD
Lucy G. Moses Professor & Chairman
Department of Rehabilitation Medicine
Mount Sinai Medical Center
New York, NY

James P. Robinson MD PhD
Clinical Associate Professor
Department of Rehabilitation Medicine
University of Washington School of Medicine
Seattle, WA

Elliot J. Roth MD
The Paul B. Magnuson Professor & Chairman
Department of Physical Medicine &
  Rehabilitation
Northwestern University Feinberg School of
  Medicine
The Donnelley Senior Vice President & Medical
  Director
Rehabilitation Institute of Chicago
Chicago, IL

Richard Salcido MD
Chairman
Rehabilitation Medicine Department
Hospital of the University of Pennsylvania
Philadelphia, PA

Cynthia Salorio PhD
Pediatric Neurophysiologist/Assistant Professor
Department of Physical Medicine &
   Rehabilitation
Johns Hopkins School of Medicine
Kennedy Krieger Institute
Baltimore, MD

Michael Saulino MD PhD
Assistant Professor of Rehabilitation Medicine
MossRehab
Elkins Park, PA

Mark R. Schmeler MS OTR/L ATP
Instructor, Department of Rehabilitation Science
   & Technology
Senior Clinician, Center for Assistive
   Technology
University of Pittsburgh
Pittsburgh, PA

Dan D. Scott MD
Associate Professor
Department of Physical Medicine and
   Rehabilitation, University of Colorado Health
   Sciences Center
Physical Medicine & Rehabilitation Service
Denver VA Medical Center
Denver, CO

Richard E. Seroussi MD MSc
Clinical Assistant Professor
Department of Rehabilitation Medicine,
   University of Washington
Seattle Spine & Rehabilitation Medicine
Seattle, WA

Craig Seto MD
Assistant Professor
Department of Family Medicine
University of Virginia School of Medicine
Charlottesville, VA

Andrew Sherman MD
Assistant Professor
Department of Clinical Rehabilitation Medicine
University of Miami
Miami, FL

Hilary C. Siebens MD
Adjunct Professor of Clinical Physical Medicine
   & Rehabilitation
Department of Physical Medicine &
   Rehabilitation
University of Virginia
Seal Beach, CA

Mehrsheed Sinaki MD MS
Professor of Physical Medicine and
   Rehabilitation
Department of Physical Medicine &
   Rehabilitation
Mayo Clinic
Rochester, MN

Ranjeet B. Singh MD
Clinical Assistant Professor
Department of Radiology
University of Washington
Radiology Consultants of Washington
Bellevue, WA

Marca Lee Sipski MD
Professor of Physical Medicine & Rehabilitation
Department of Physical Medicine &
   Rehabilitation
University of Alabama at Birmingham
Spain Rehabilitation Center
Birmingham, AL

Daniel N. Slater MD
Assistant Professor
Department of Physical Medicine &
   Rehabilitation
Virginia Commonwealth University
Richmond, VA

Curtis W. Slipman MD
Director, Penn Spine Center
Chief, Division of Musculoskeletal Rehabilitation
Associate Professor of Physical Medicine and
   Rehabilitation
University of Pennsylvania Health System
Philadelphia, PA

Donald M. Spaeth PhD RET ATP
Associate Director of Engineering
Human Engineering Research Laboratories
VA Pittsburgh Healthcare System
Pittsburgh, PA

Mary Catherine Spires MD
Associate Professor
Department of Physical Medicine &
   Rehabilitation
University of Michigan Health System
Ann Arbor, MI

Steven P. Stanos DO
Medical Director
Chronic Pain Care Center
Rehabilitation Institute of Chicago
Chicago, IL

Adam B. Stein MD
Associate Professor of Rehabilitation Medicine
Department of Rehabilitation Medicine
Mount Sinai School of Medicine
New York, NY

Steven A. Stiens MD MS
Associate Professor, Department of
   Rehabilitation Medicine, University of
   Washington
Attending Physician
VA Puget Sound Health Care System
Seattle, WA

Paul Sugg CP FAAOP
Clinical Manager
Hanger Prosthetics and Orthotics
Greenville, SC

Mukul Talaty PhD
Research Engineer
Gait & Motion Analysis Laboratory
MossRehab
Albert Einstein Medical Center
Elkins Park, PA

Laura Taylor PhD
Assistant Professor
Department of Physical Medicine &
   Rehabilitation
Virginia Commonwealth University
Richmond, VA

Edward Tilley CO
Manager, Orthotics Services
University Health Systems of Eastern North
   Carolina
Pitt County Memorial Hospital
Greenville, NC

Jaya R. Trivedi MD
Assistant Professor of Neurology
Department of Neurology
University of Texas Southwestern Medical
   Center
Dallas, TX

Mark D. Tyburski MD
Physician
Rehabilitation Institute of Chicago
Chicago, IL

Delaina Walker-Batson PhD
Director, The Stroke Center—Dallas
Professor, Department of Communication
   Sciences and Disorders
Texas Woman's University—Dallas
Dallas, TX

David C. Weber MD
Assistant Professor
Department of Physical Medicine &
   Rehabilitation
Mayo Clinic College of Medicine
Rochester, MN

Stephen T. Wegener PhD ABPP
Associate Professor & Director of Rehabilitation
   Psychology
Department of Physical Medicine &
   Rehabilitation
Johns Hopkins University
Baltimore, MD

Jonathan H. Whiteson MD BSc
Assistant Professor of Rehabilitation Medicine
Co-Director, Cardiovascular and Pulmonary
    Rehabilitation
Rusk Institute of Rehabilitation Medicine
New York, NY

Robert P. Wilder MD
Associate Professor
Department of Physical Medicine and
    Rehabilitation
University of Virginia Health System
Charlottesville, VA

Stuart E. Willick MD
Associate Professor
University of Utah Orthopedic Center
Salt Lake City, UT

Pamela Wilson MD
Assistant Professor of Physical Medicine and
    Rehabilitation
Department of Rehabilitation Medicine
University of Colorado School of Medicine
The Children's Hospital
Denver, CO

Robert K. Yang MD
Assistant Professor
Department of Physical Medicine &
    Rehabilitation
Mayo Clinic
Rochester, MN

Mark A. Young MD MBA FACP
Chair
Physical Medicine & Rehabilitation Department
The Maryland Rehabilitation Center/WTC
The University of Maryland
Baltimore, MD

David Yu MD
Assistant Professor & Rehabilitation Physician
Department of Rehabilitation Medicine
University of Washington School of Medicine
Seattle, WA

Jie Zhu MD
Attending Physician
Mid Atlantic Spine & Pain Specialists, P.A.
Newark, DE

Preface to the third edition

The Third Edition of the textbook is written and edited to expand the goals of the First and Second Editions, which were to create a practical, clinically useful, and user friendly textbook that covered the breadth of the field of Physical Medicine & Rehabilitation (PM&R). Feedback from our readers indicated that one of the reasons the first two editions were so popular was because of their readability. In this edition, additional emphasis has been placed on maximizing 'reader efficiency'. The text, figures and tables have been designed to let the reader learn the 'most per minute' of reading.

Since the first two editions were very popular in the PM&R community outside the USA, another goal of the Third Edition was to intentionally make it more international in scope. We established an Advisory Board of senior physiatrists from around the world, who guided us to some outstanding authors outside the USA. They also provided feedback about the selection of chapters to make sure the book was relevant not only to clinical practice in the USA but also throughout the world.

The Third Edition also represents a marked change in authorship, as the majority of the chapters are brand new with new authors. The few chapters that are continued from the second edition have been radically updated.

The field of PM&R is a dynamic one that continually changes in scope and practice. One of the additions to the field over the last decade has been spinal procedures and injections for both diagnosis and treatment. This change is now reflected in new content for a number of chapters including Chapter 25 on injection techniques, Chapter 38 on the treatment of neck problems, and Chapter 41 on low back pain. In addition, a brand new chapter (26) on interventional pain procedures has been included.

Thanks to our friends at Elsevier, the Third Edition represents a marked upgrade in production values. Most illustrations are now in color, and a color theme runs throughout the book. For the first time the book also has a website that has additional information that would not fit in the book, including 20 multiple choice questions on each chapter to help readers determine how well they have mastered the material. The website will also include important updates over the course of time. These features are state of the art in medical textbooks and unique among PM&R textbooks.

It is true that one could write an entire book about the topic of each of the chapters in this text. One of the tasks of the authors and editors was to take the huge body of information that now comprises the field of PM&R and condense it into a textbook of reasonable size. The length of each chapter in this edition again reflects the editors' feelings about the current importance of that topic relative to others. Since some details had to be left out, the authors have prepared an extensive alphabetized reference list at the end of each chapter for readers wanting to explore a subject in greater depth. The advantage of each chapter's reference list is that it is prepared by an expert in the field, and is not just a cold computer search that results in a polyglot of references that might or might not be clinically useful. In this edition we have also listed suggested internet web sites at the end of some chapters.

The book is again divided into four major sections. Section 1 deals with the evaluation of patients typically seen in the practice of PM&R (Chapters 1–12). Section 2 deals with treatment techniques and special equipment used in the field of PM&R (Chapters 13–26). Section 3 discusses the therapeutic issues and problems that are commonly seen the practice of PM&R (Chapters 27–36). Section 4 deals with specific diagnoses faced by the physiatrist, both in Physical Medicine and in Rehabilitation (Chapters 37–61).

We are happy to report that the Third Edition is still in one volume rather than two, and that we have been able to use the massive publishing resources and efficiencies of Elsevier to hold the line on price. As with the first two editions, we welcome comments, suggestions and constructive criticism from members of the PM&R community and from all readers.

Randall L. Braddom MD MS

Dedication

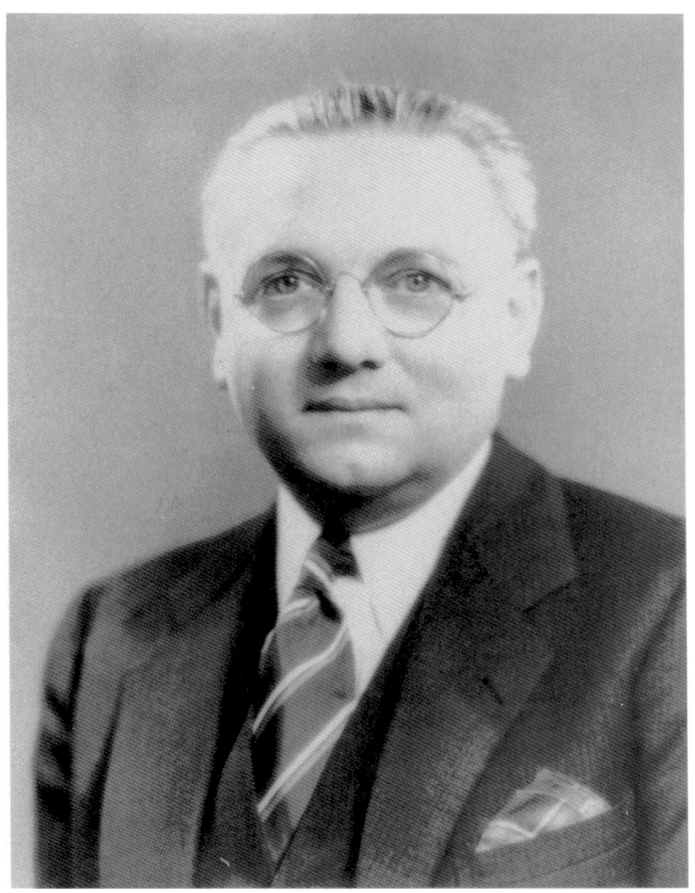

The third edition is dedicated to the memory of Dr. Frank Hammond Krusen. Dr. Krusen wrote the first widely used textbook of physical medicine in 1941, entitled Physical Medicine, The Employment of Physical Agents for Diagnosis and Therapy. At that time Dr. Krusen was an Associate Professor of Physical Medicine at the Mayo Foundation and the University of Minnesota, and he dedicated the book to the memory of William James Mayo and Charles Horace Mayo.

Dr. Krusen's book was instrumental in garnering the respect of our peers in the medical community that was essential for the early development of the field as a medical specialty. He also coined the word physiatrist, which has been used by Physical Medicine & Rehabilitation practitioners since (although we can't quite agree how to pronounce it). This book is a direct descendent of and successor to the Krusen textbook series.

Although I never had the opportunity to meet Dr. Krusen personally, I am proud to be able to consider him my physiatric great-grandfather. He was responsible for the training of Dr. Ralph Worden, who trained Dr. Ernest W. Johnson, who was responsible for my training at The Ohio State University Department of Physical Medicine from 1969–1972.

Randall L. Braddom MD MS

Acknowledgments

My sincerest thanks to:

Over one hundred contributors, our Advisory Board members, the Associate Editors, and many others, without whom this textbook could not have been completed.

My wife Diana Verdun Braddom, whose constant encouragement and support made this undertaking a labor of love.

The excellent staff of Elsevier, especially Dolores Meloni and Tim Kimber.

Advisory Editorial Board
Barbara deLateur, MD
Martin Grabois, MD
Ernest W. Johnson, MD
Chang Il Park, MD
Haim Ring, MD
Thomas Strax, MD
Daniel Wever, MD

Associate Editorial Board
Ralph M. Buschbacher, MD
Leighton Chan, MD, MPH
Karen J. Kowalske, MD
Edward R. Laskowski, MD
Dennis J. Matthews, MD
Kristjan Ragnarsson, MD

Question Editor
Ernest W. Johnson, M.D
(Assisted by Justin Collier, MD)

Randall L. Braddom MD MS

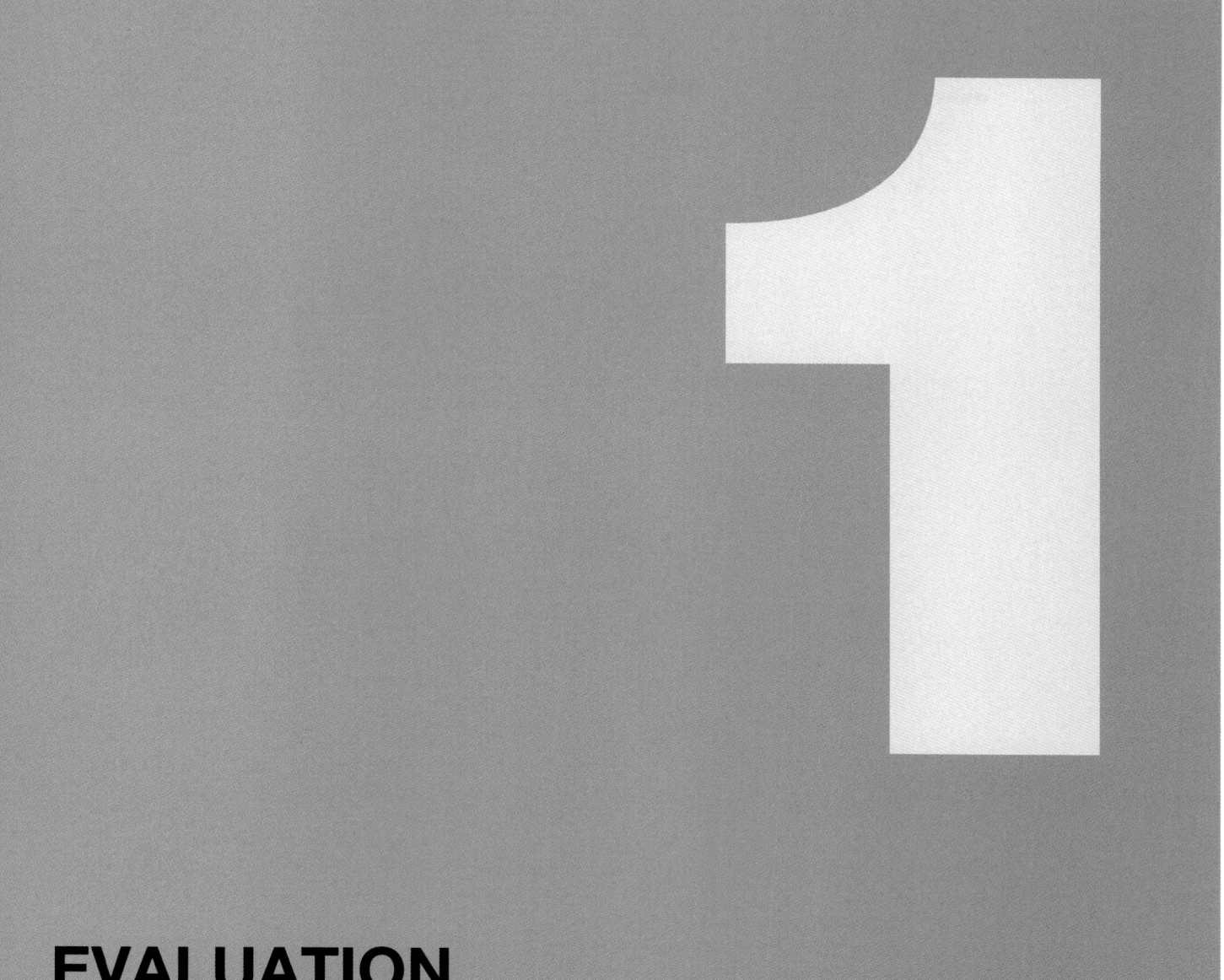

EVALUATION

The Physiatric History and Physical Examination

Michael W. O'Dell, C. David Lin, André Panagos and Nancy Q. Fung

The physiatric history and physical examination (H&P) serves several purposes. It is the data platform from which a treatment plan is developed. It also serves as a written record that communicates to other rehabilitation and non-rehabilitation healthcare professionals. Finally, the H&P provides the basis for physician billing[12] and serves as a medicolegal document. Physician documentation has become the critical component in inpatient rehabilitation reimbursement under prospective payment, as well as proof for continued coverage by private insurers. The scope of the physiatric H&P varies enormously depending on the setting, from the focused assessment of an isolated knee injury in an outpatient setting, to the comprehensive evaluation of a patient with traumatic brain or spinal cord injury admitted for inpatient rehabilitation. An initial evaluation is almost always more detailed and comprehensive than subsequent or follow-up evaluations. Physicians in training tend to over-assess, but with time the experienced physiatrist develops an intuition for how much detail is needed for each patient given a certain presentation and setting.

The physiatric H&P resembles the traditional format taught in medical school but with an additional emphasis on history, signs, and symptoms that impact function (performance). The physiatric H&P also identifies those systems *not* affected that might be used for compensation.[18] Familiarity with the 1980 and 1997 World Health Organization classifications is invaluable in understanding the philosophic framework for viewing the evaluation of persons with physical and cognitive disabilities (see Table 1-1).[63,64] Identifying and treating the primary *impairments* to maximize *performance* becomes the primary thrust of the physiatric evaluation.

Because patients cared for in rehabilitation medicine can be extremely complicated, the H&P is many times a work in progress. Confirmation of historical and functional items by other team members, healthcare professionals, and family members can take several days. Many of the functional items discussed in this chapter can actually be assessed and explored more fully by other interdisciplinary team members during the course of inpatient or outpatient treatment. It is imperative that the physiatrist stays abreast of additional information and findings as they become available, and that lines of verbal or written communication be directed through the medical leadership of the team.

The exact structure of the physiatric assessment is determined in part by personal preference, training background, and institutional requirements (physician billing compliance expectations, forms committees, and regulatory oversight). The use of templates can be invaluable in maximizing the thoroughness of data collection and minimizing documentation time. Pertinent radiologic and laboratory findings should be clearly documented. The essential elements of the physiatric H&P are summarized in Table 1-2. Assessment of some or all of these elements is required for a complete understanding of the patient's state of health and the illness for which he or she is being seen. These elements also form the basis for how to treat the patient.

THE PHYSIATRIC HISTORY

History-taking skills are part of the art of medicine and are required to fully assess a patient's presentation. One of the unique aspects of physiatry is the recognition of functional deficits caused by illness or injury. Identification of these deficits allows for the design of a treatment program to restore performance. In a person with stroke, for example, the most important questions for the physiatrist are not just the etiology or location of the lesion but also 'What functional deficits are present as a result of the stroke?' The answer could include deficits in swallowing, communication, mobility, cognition, activities of daily living (ADL), or a combination of these.

The time spent in taking a history also allows the patient to become familiar with the physician, establishing rapport and trust. This initial rapport is critical for a constructive and productive doctor–patient–family relationship, and can also help the physician learn about such sensitive areas as the sexual history and substance abuse. It can also have an impact on outcome, as a trusting patient tends to be a more compliant patient.[53] Assessing the tone of the patient and/or family (such as anger, frustration, resolve, and determination), understanding of the illness, insight into disability, and coping skills are also gleaned during history taking. In most cases, the patient leads the physician to a diagnosis and conclusion. In other cases, such as when the patient is rambling and disorganized, frequent redirection and refocus are required.

Table 1-1 World Health Organization definitions	
Term	**Definition**
1980	
Impairment	Any loss or abnormality of psychologic, physiologic, or anatomic structure or function
Disability	Any restriction or lack resulting from an impairment of the ability to perform an activity in the manner or within the range considered normal for a human being
Handicap	A disadvantage for a given individual, resulting from an impairment or a disability, that limits or prevents the fulfillment of a role that is normal for that individual
1997	
Impairment	Any loss or abnormality of body structure or of a physiologic or psychologic function (essentially unchanged from the 1980 definition)
Activity	The nature and extent of functioning at the level of the person
Participation	The nature and extent of a person's involvement in life situations in relationship to impairments, activities, health conditions, and contextual factors

(From World Health Organization 1980[63] and 1997,[64] with permission of the World Health Organization.)

Patients are generally the primary source of information. However, patients with cognitive or mood deficits (denial or decreased insight) or with communication problems, as well as small children, might not be able to fully express themselves. In these cases, the history taker might rely on other sources, such as family members; friends; other physicians, nurses, and medical professionals; or previous medical records. Caution must be exercised in using previous medical records, as inaccuracies are sometimes promulgated from provider to provider, sometimes referred to as 'chart lore'.

Chief complaint

The chief complaint is the symptom(s) that caused the patient to seek medical treatment. The most common chief complaints seen in an outpatient physiatric practice are pain or weakness of various musculoskeletal or neurologic origins. On a physiatric consultation on an inpatient rehabilitation service, the predominant chief complaints are related to mobility, ADL, communication, or cognitive deficits. Unlike the relatively objective physical examination, the chief complaint is a subjective measure and, when possible, the physician should use the patient's own words. A patient can present with several related or unrelated complaints, in which case it is helpful to have the patient rank problems from 'most bothersome' to 'least bothersome'.

The specific circumstance of a patient offering a chief complaint can also allude to a degree of disability or handicap. For example, knowing that an obese mail carrier presents with the chief complaint of difficulty in walking because of knee pain could suggest not only the impairment, but also that he might no longer be able to perform his duties as a mail carrier.

History of the present illness

The HPI details the chief complaint(s) for which the patient is seeking medical attention, as well as any related or unrelated functional deficits. It should also explore other information relating to the chief complaint, such as recent and past medical or surgical procedures, complications of treatment, and potential restrictions or precautions. The HPI should include some or all of eight components related to the chief complaint: location, time of onset, quality, context, severity, duration, modifying factors, and associated signs and symptoms (see Table 1-2).

In this case example, the patient is a 70-year-old man referred by his neurologist for physical therapy because the patient cannot walk properly (chief complaint). Over the past few months (duration), he has noted slowly progressive weakness of his left leg (location). Subsequent work-up by his neurologist suggested amyotrophic lateral sclerosis (context). The patient was active in his life and working up until a few months previously, ambulating without an assistive device (context). Now he uses a straight cane for fear of falling (modifying factor). Besides difficulty with walking, the patient also has some trouble swallowing foods (associated signs and symptoms).

Functional status

Detailing the patient's current and prior functional status is an essential aspect of the physiatric HPI. This generally entails better understanding the issues surrounding mobility, ADL, instrumental activities of daily living (I-ADL), communication, and cognition, among others. The data should be as accurate and detailed as possible in order to guide the physical examination and develop a treatment plan with reasonable short- and long-term goals.

Assessing the potential for functional gain or deterioration requires an understanding of the natural history, cause, and time of onset of the functional problems. For example, most motor recovery following stroke occurs within 3–6 months of the event.[34] For a recent stroke patient with considerable motor impairments, there is a greater expectation for functional gain than in a patient with minor deficits related to a stroke 2 years ago. On the other hand, functional gains in speech deficits can still be seen beyond 1 year post stroke.[52]

It is sometimes helpful to assess functional status using a standardized scale. No single scale is appropriate for all patients, but the Functional Independence Measure (FIM) is the most commonly used in the inpatient rehabilitation setting (see Table 1-3 and Ch. 8).[3] Measuring only disability or performance, each of 18 different activities is scored on a scale of 1–7, with a score of 7 indicating complete independence. Intermediate scores indicate varying levels of assistance from very little (from an assistive device, to supervision, to hands-on assistance). A score

Table 1-2 Essential elements of the physiatric history and physical examination

Chief complaint	
History of present illness	Exploring location, onset, quality, context, severity, duration, modifying factors, and associated signs and symptoms
Functional history	Mobility: bed mobility, transfers, wheelchair mobility, ambulation, driving, and devices required Activities of daily living: bathing, toileting, dressing, eating, hygiene and grooming, etc. Instrumental activities of daily living: meal preparation, laundry, telephone use, home maintenance, pet care, etc. Cognition Communication
Past medical and surgical history	Specific conditions: cardiopulmonary, musculoskeletal, neurologic, and rheumatologic Medications
Social history	Home environment and living circumstances, family and friends support system, substance abuse, sexual history, vocation activities, finances, recreational activities, psychosocial history (mood disorders), spirituality, and litigation
Family history	
Review of systems	
General medical physical examination	Cardiac Pulmonary Abdominal Other
Neurologic physical examination	Level of consciousness Attention Orientation Memory General fund of knowledge Abstract thinking Insight and judgment Mood and affect
Communication Cranial nerve examination Sensation Motor control	Strength Coordination Apraxia Involuntary movements Tone
Reflexes	Superficial Deep Primitive
Musculoskeletal physical examination Inspection	Behavior Physical symmetry, joint deformity, etc.
Palpation	Joint stability Range of motion (active and passive) Strength testing (see above) Painful joints and muscles
Joint-specific provocative maneuvers	

Table 1-3 Levels of function on the functional independence measure		
Level of function	Score	Definition
Independent		Another person is not required for the activity (*no helper*)
	7	Complete independence: all the tasks described as making up the activity are performed safely; without modification, assistive devices, or aids; and within a reasonable amount of time
	6	Modified independence: one or more of the following can be true. • The activity requires an assistive device • The activity takes more than a reasonable time • There are safety considerations
Dependent		The patient requires another person for either supervision or physical assistance for the activity to be performed (*requires helper*)
	5	Supervision or set-up: the patient requires no more help than stand-up or cueing without physical contact, or the helper sets up needed items
	4	Minimal contact assistance: the patient requires no more help than touching and expends 75% or more of the effort
	3	Moderate assistance: the patient requires more help than touching and expends 50–75% of the effort
	2	Maximal assistance: the patient expends 25–50% of the effort
	1	Total assistance: the patient expends less than 25% of the effort

(From Anonymous 1997,[3] with permission of the State University of New York at Buffalo.)

of 1 indicates complete dependence on caregiver assistance. FIM scores also serve as a kind of rehabilitation shorthand among team members to quickly and accurately describe functional deficits.

Mobility

Mobility is the ability to move about in one's environment and is taken for granted by most healthy people. Because it plays such a vital role in society, any impairment related to mobility can have major consequences for a patient's quality of life. A clear understanding of the patient's functional mobility is needed to determine independence and safety, including the use of, or need for, mobility assistive devices. There is a range of mobility assistive devices that patients can use, such as crutches, canes, walkers, orthoses, and manual and electric wheelchairs, among others (see Table 1-4, and Chs 15 and 18).

Bed mobility includes turning from side to side, going from the prone to supine positions, sitting up, and lying down. A lack of bed mobility puts the patient at greater risk for skin ulcers, deep vein thrombosis, and pneumonia. In severe cases, bed mobility can be so poor as to require a caregiver. In other cases, bed rails might be appropriate to facilitate movement. Transfer mobility includes getting in and out of bed, standing from the sitting position (whether from a chair or toilet), and moving between a wheelchair and another seat (car seat or shower seat). Once again, the history taker should assess the level of independence, safety, and any changes in functional ability.

Wheelchair mobility can be assessed by asking if patients can propel the wheelchair independently, how far or how long they can go without resting, and whether they need assistance with managing the wheelchair parts. It is also important to assess the extent to which they can move about at home, in the commu-

Table 1-4 Commonly used mobility assistive devices	
Crutches	Axillary crutches Forearm crutches Platform crutches
Canes	Straight cane Wide- or narrow-based quad cane Hemiwalker or pyramid cane
Walkers	Standard or pick-up walker Rolling walker Platform walker
Wheelchairs Types	Manual Powered
Common modifications or specifications	Lightweight Folding or solid frame Elevated or removable leg rests Removable armrests Reclining
Off the shelf ankle foot orthoses Common custom orthoses	Plastic ankle–foot orthosis Metal ankle–foot orthosis Knee orthosis Knee–ankle–foot orthosis

nity, and up and down ramps. Whether the home is potentially wheelchair-accessible is particularly important in cases of new onset having severe disability.

Ambulation can be assessed by how far or for how long patients can walk, whether they require assistive devices, and their need for rest breaks. It is also important to know if any symptoms are associated with ambulation, such as chest pain, shortness of breath, pain, or dizziness. Patients should be asked about any history of falling or instability while walking, and their ability to navigate uneven surfaces. Stair mobility, along with the number of stairs the patient must routinely climb and descend at home or in the community, and the presence or absence of handrails should also be determined.

Driving is a critically important activity for many people, not only as a means of transportation but also as an indication and facilitator of independence. For example, elders who stop driving have an increase in depressive symptoms.[43] It is important to identify factors that might prevent driving, such as decreased cognitive function and safety awareness, and decreased vision or reaction time. Other factors affecting driving can include lower limb weakness, contracture, tone, or dyscoordination. Some of these conditions might require use of adaptive hand controls for driving. Cognitive impairment sufficient to affect the ability to drive can be due to medications or organic disease (dementia, brain injury, stroke, or severe mood disturbance). Ultimately, the risks of driving are weighed against the consequences of not being able to drive. If the patient is no longer able to drive, alternatives to driving should be explored, such as the use of public or assisted transportation. Laws differ widely from state to state on the return to driving after a neurologic impairment develops.

Activities of daily living and instrumental activities of daily living

Activities of daily living encompass activities required for personal care, including feeding, dressing, grooming, bathing, and toileting. I-ADL encompass more complex tasks required for independent living in the immediate environment, such as care of others in the household, telephone use, meal preparation, house cleaning, laundry, and in some cases use of public transportation. In the Occupational Therapy Practice Framework, there are 11 activities for both ADL and I-ADL (see Box 1-1).[4]

The clinician should identify and document ADL the patient can and cannot perform, and determine the causes of limitation. For example, a woman with a stroke might state that she cannot put on her pants. This could be due to a combination of factors such as a visual field cut, balance problems, weakness, pain, contracture, tone, or deficits in motor planning. Some of these factors can be confirmed later in the physical examination. A more detailed follow-up to a positive response to the question is frequently needed. For example, a patient might say 'yes' to the question 'Can you eat by yourself?' On further questioning, it might be learned that she cannot prepare the food by herself or cut the food independently. The most accurate assessment of ADL and mobility deficits often comes from the hands-on assessment by other members of the rehabilitation team.

Cognition

Cognition is the mental process of knowing (see Chs 3 and 4). Although objective assessment of cognition comes under physical examination (memory, orientation, and the ability to assimi-

---

Box 1-1 Activities of daily living and instrumental activities of daily living

ADL
- Bathing and showering
- Bowel and bladder management
- Dressing
- Eating
- Feeding
- Functional mobility
- Personal device care
- Personal hygiene and grooming
- Sexual activity
- Sleep and rest
- Toilet hygiene

I-ADL
- Care of others (including selecting and supervising caregivers)
- Care of pets
- Child rearing
- Communication device use
- Community mobility
- Financial management
- Health management and maintenance
- Home establishment and management
- Meal preparation and clean-up
- Safety procedures and emergency responses
- Shopping

(After Anonymous 2002,[4] with permission.)

---

late and manipulate information), impairments in cognition can also become apparent during the course of the history taking. Because persons with cognitive deficits often cannot recognize their own impairments (deficits in insight), it is important to gather information from family members and others familiar with the patient. Cognitive deficits and limited awareness of these deficits are likely to interfere with the patient's rehabilitation program unless specifically addressed. These deficits can pose a safety risk as well. For example, a man with a previous stroke who falls, sustaining a hip fracture, might not be able to follow hip precautions, resulting in possible refracture or hip dislocation. Executive functioning is another aspect of cognition, which includes the mental functions required for planning, problem solving, and self-awareness. Executive functioning correlates with functional outcome because it is required in many real world situations.[39]

Communication

Communication skills are used to convey information, including thoughts, needs, and emotions. Verbal expression deficits can be very subtle and might not be noticed in a first encounter. If there is a reason to think that speech or communication has been affected by a recent event, it is advisable to ask family members if they have noticed recent changes. Patients who cannot communicate through speech might or might not be able to communicate through other means, known as augmentative communication, depending on the type of communication dysfunction and other physical and cognitive limitations. This can include writing and physicality (such as sign language, gestures, and body language). They can also utilize a variety of augmentative communication aids ranging from simple picture, letter, and word boards to electronic devices.

Past medical and surgical history

The physiatrist needs to understand the patient's past medical and surgical history. This knowledge allows the physiatrist to review and address functional deficits caused by preexisting illnesses, and to tailor the rehabilitation program for precautions and limitations. The patient's past medical history can also have a major impact on rehabilitation outcome.

Cardiopulmonary

Mobility, ADL, I-ADL, work, and leisure can be severely compromised by cardiopulmonary deficits. The patient should be asked about any history of congestive heart failure, recent and distant myocardial infarction, arrhythmias, and coronary artery disease. Past surgical procedures such as bypass surgery, heart transplantation, stent placement, and recent diagnostic testing (stress test or echocardiogram) should be ascertained. This information is important to ensure that exercise prescriptions do not exceed cardiovascular activity limitations. Patients should also be asked about their activity tolerance, surgery such as lung volume reduction or lung transplant, and whether they require home oxygen. Dyspnea from chronic obstructive pulmonary disease can be a significant contributor to functional limitations. It is also important to identify modifiable risk factors for cardiac disease, such as smoking, hypertension, and obesity.

Musculoskeletal

There can be a wide range of musculoskeletal disorders from acute traumatic injuries to gradual functional decline with chronic osteoarthritis. The patient should be asked about any history of trauma, arthritis, amputation, joint contractures, musculoskeletal pain, congenital or acquired muscular problems, weakness, or instability. It is important to understand the functional impact of such impairments or disabilities. Patients with chronic physical disability often develop overuse musculoskeletal syndromes, such as the development of shoulder pain secondary to chronically propelling a wheelchair.[28]

Neurologic disorders

Preexisting congenital or acquired neurologic disorders can have a profound impact on the patient's function and recovery from both neurologic and non-neurologic illness. It is helpful to know whether a neurologic disorder is congenital versus acquired, progressive versus non-progressive, central versus peripheral, demyelinating versus axonal, or sensory versus motor. This information can be helpful in understanding the pathophysiology, location, severity, prognosis, and implications for management. The interviewer must assess the premorbid need for assistive devices, orthoses, and the degree of speech, swallowing, and cognitive impairments.

Rheumatologic

The history should assess the type of rheumatologic disorder, time of onset, number of joints affected, pain level, current disease activity, and past orthopedic procedures (see Ch. 37). Discussions with the patient's rheumatologist might address whether medication changes could improve activity tolerance in a rehabilitation program.

Medications

All medications should be documented, including prescription and over the counter drugs as well as nutraceuticals, supplements, herbs, and vitamins. Patients typically do not mention medications that they do not think are relevant to their current problem, unless asked about them in detail. Drug and food allergies should be noted. It is especially important to gather the complete list of medications being used in patients who are seeing multiple physicians. Particular attention should be paid to non-steroidal antiinflammatory agents, because these are commonly prescribed by physiatrists for musculoskeletal disorders and care must be taken not to double-dose the patient.[22,27] The indications, precautions, and side effects of all drugs prescribed should be explained to the patient.

Social history

Home environment and living situation

Understanding the patient's home environment and living situation includes asking if the patient lives in a house or an apartment, if there is elevator access, whether it is wheelchair-accessible, if there are stairs, whether the bathroom is accessible from the bedroom, and whether the bathroom has grab bars or handrails (and on which side). A home visit might be required to gain the best assessment. If there is no caregiver at home, the patient could require a home health aide. These factors help determine many aspects of the discharge plan.

Family and friends support

Patients who have lost function might require supervision, emotional support, or actual physical assistance. Family, friends, and neighbors who can provide such assistance should be identified. The clinician should discuss the level of assistance they are willing and able to provide. The assistance provided by caregivers can be limited if they are elderly, have some type of impairment, work, or are not willing to assist with bowel or bladder hygiene.

Substance abuse

Patients should be asked about their history of smoking, alcohol use or abuse, and drug abuse. Because patients often deny substance abuse, this topic should be discussed in a non-judgmental manner. Patients frequently feel embarrassment or guilt in admitting substance abuse, and also fear the legal consequences of such admission. Substance abuse can be a direct and an indirect cause of disability, and is often a contributing factor in traumatic brain injury.[15] It can also have an impact on community reintegration, because patients with pain and/or depression are at risk of further abuse. Patients who are at risk should be referred to social work to explore options for further assistance, either during the acute rehabilitation or later in the community.

Sexual history

Patients and healthcare practitioners alike are often uncomfortable discussing the topic of sexuality, so developing a good rapport during history taking can help. Discussion of this topic is made easier if the healthcare practitioner has a good knowledge of how sexual function can be changed by illness or injury (see Ch. 32). Sexuality is particularly important to patients in their reproductive years (such as most spinal cord and brain-injured persons), but the physician should enquire about sexuality in adolescents and adults of all ages. Sexual orientation and safer sex practices should be addressed when appropriate.

Vocational activities

Vocation is not only a source of financial security; it also significantly relates to self-confidence and even identity. The history should include the patient's educational level, recent work history, and the ability to fulfill job requirements subsequent to the injury or illness. If an individual cannot fully regain the previous function level, the vocational options available should be explored. It is possible that the work environment can be modified to compensate for a functional loss. An example of this might be as simple as installing a wheelchair ramp.

Finances and income maintenance

Patients can have financial concerns that are due to or exacerbated by their illness or injury. These concerns can also be addressed by the rehabilitation team social worker. Whether a patient has the financial resources or insurance to pay for adaptive devices such as a ramp or mobility equipment can significantly impact discharge planning. If patients cannot safely be discharged home, skilled nursing facility placement might need to be explored, at least on a temporary basis.

Recreation

The ability to engage in hobbies and recreational activities is important to most people, and any loss or limitation of the ability to perform these activities can be stressful. The recreational activity affected can involve physical exercise, such as a sporting activity, or can be more sedentary, for example playing cards. The team recreational therapist can be helpful in helping to restore the patient's favorite recreations and offer new ones.

Psychosocial history

The history taker must recognize the psychosocial impact of impairment. Beyond the loss of function, the patient can also feel a loss of overall health, body image, mobility, or independence. The loss of function, and possibly of income as well, can place great stress on the family unit and caregivers. The treatment plan should recognize the patient's psychosocial context and provide assistance in developing coping strategies, espe-

cially for depression and anxiety. This can help accelerate the patient's process of adjusting to a new disability.

Spirituality and belief

Spirituality is an important part of the lives of many patients, and some preliminary studies indicate that it can have positive effects on rehabilitation, life satisfaction, and quality of life.[13] Healthcare providers should be sensitive to the patient's spiritual needs, and appropriate referral or counseling should be provided.

Pending litigation

Patients should be asked, in a non-judgmental way, if they are involved in litigation related to their illness, injuries, or functional impairment. The answer should not change your treatment plan, but litigation can be a source of anxiety, depression, or guilt. In some cases, the patient's legal representation can play an important role in obtaining needed services and equipment.

Family history

Patients should be asked about the health, or cause and age of death, of parents and siblings. It is always important to know whether any family members have a similar condition. They should also be asked about any family history of heart disease, diabetes, cancer, stroke, arthritis, hypertension, or neurologic illness. This will help to identify genetic disorders within the family. A knowledge of the general health of family members can also provide insight into their ability to provide functional assistance to the patient.

Review of systems

A detailed review of organ systems should be done in order to discover any problems or diseases not previously identified during the course of the history taking. Table 1-5 lists some questions that can be asked about each system.[19] Note that this list is not comprehensive, and more detailed questioning might be necessary.

PHYSIATRIC PHYSICAL EXAMINATION

The general medical physical examination is a key component of the physiatric examination, especially since more medically complicated patients are being admitted for inpatient rehabilitation. A full evaluation of heart, lungs, and abdomen could be required to determine the impact of underlying medical conditions on the mobilization or physical management of the patient.

Neurologic examination

Neurologic problems are very common in the setting of inpatient and outpatient rehabilitation, including functional deficits in persons with such conditions as stroke, multiple sclerosis, peripheral neuropathy, spinal cord injury, and brain injury. The neurologic examination should be conducted in an

Table 1-5 Sample questions for the review of systems

System	Questions
Systemic	Any general symptoms such as fever, weight loss, fatigue, nausea, and poor appetite?
Skin	Any skin problems? Sores? Rashes? Growths? Itching? Changes in the hair or nails? Dryness?
Eyes	Any changes in vision? Pain? Redness? Discharge? Double vision? Watery eyes?
Ears	How are the ears and hearing? Running ears? Poor hearing? Ringing ears?
Nose	How are your nose and sinuses? Stuffy nose? Discharge? Bleeding? Unusual odors?
Mouth	Any problems with your mouth? Sores? Bad taste? Sore tongue? Gum trouble?
Throat and neck	Any problems with your throat and neck? Sore throat? Hoarseness? Swelling? Swallowing?
Breasts	Any problems with your breasts? Lumps? Nipple discharge? Bleeding? Swelling? Tenderness?
Pulmonary	Any problems with your lungs or breathing? Cough? Sputum? Bloody sputum? Pain in the chest on taking a deep breath? Shortness of breath?
Cardiovascular	Do you have any problems with your heart? Chest pain? Shortness of breath? Palpitations? Cough? Swelling of your ankles? Trouble lying flat in bed at night? Fatigue?
Gastrointestinal	How is your digestion? Any changes in your appetite? Nausea? Vomiting? Diarrhea? Constipation? Changes in your bowel habits? Bleeding from the rectum? Hemorrhoids?
Genitourinary	Male: Any problems with your kidneys or urination? Painful urination? Frequency? Urgency? Nocturia? Bloody or cloudy urine? Trouble starting or stopping? Female: Number of pregnancies? Abortions? Miscarriages? Any menstrual problems? Last menstrual period? Vaginal bleeding? Vaginal discharge? Cessation of periods? Hot flashes? Vaginal itching?
Endocrine	Any problems with your endocrine glands? Feeling hot or cold? Fatigue? Changes in the skin or hair? Frequent urination? Fatigue?
Musculoskeletal	Do you have any problems with your bones or joints? Joint or muscle pain? Stiffness? Limitation of motion?
Nervous system	Numbness? Weakness? Pins and needles sensation?

(From Eneleow et al. 1996,[19] with permission of Oxford University Press.)

organized fashion to confirm the neurologic disorder, and subsequently to identify which components of the nervous system are the most and the least affected. The precise location of the lesion should be identified, if possible, and the impact of the neurologic deficits on the overall function and mobility of the patient should be noted. If a cause of the patient's condition has not been identified at presentation to the rehabilitation service, a differential diagnosis list should be developed and the neurologic examination tailored appropriately. An accurate and efficient neurologic examination requires that the examiner have a thorough knowledge of both central and peripheral neuroanatomy prior to the examination.

Weakness is a common sign in neurologic disorders and is seen in both upper motor neuron (UMN) and lower motor neuron (LMN) disorders. UMN lesions involving the central nervous system (CNS) are typically characterized by spastic weakness and hyperreflexia without significant muscle atrophy, fasciculation, or fibrillation (on electromyography). They *tend* to occur in a hemiparetic, paraparetic, and tetraparetic pattern. UMN lesions include stroke, multiple sclerosis, and traumatic and non-traumatic brain and spinal cord injuries, among others. LMN defects are characterized by flaccid weakness, hypo-

reflexia, significant muscle atrophy, fasciculations, and electromyographic changes. They occur in the distribution of the affected nerve root, peripheral nerve, or muscle. UMN and LMN lesions often coexist; however, the LMN system is the final common pathway of the nervous system. An example of this is amyotrophic lateral sclerosis, which is characterized by both UMN and LMN signs.[44]

Similar to physical examination in other organ systems, testing of one neurologic system is often predicated by the normal functioning of other systems. For example, severe visual impairment can be confused with cerebellar dysfunction, as many cerebellar tests have a visual component. The integrated functions of all organ systems should be considered in order to provide an accurate clinical assessment, and potential limitations of the examination should be considered.

Mental status examination

The MSE should be performed in a comfortable setting where the patient is not likely to be disturbed by external stimuli such as televisions, telephones, or pagers. The bedside MSE is often limited secondary to distractions from within the room. Having a familiar person such as a spouse or relative in the room can often help reassure the patient. The bedside MSE might need to be supplemented by far more detailed and standardized evaluations performed by neuropsychologists (see Ch. 4).

Level of consciousness   Consciousness is the state of awareness of one's surroundings. A functioning pontine reticular activating system is necessary for normal conscious functioning. The conscious patient is awake and responds directly and appropriately to varying stimuli. Decreased consciousness can significantly limit the MSE and the general physical examination.

The examiner should understand the various levels of consciousness. Lethargy is the general slowing of motor processes (such as speech and movement), in which the patient can easily fall asleep if not stimulated, but is easily aroused. Obtundation is a dulled or blunted sensitivity in which the patient is difficult to arouse, and once aroused is still confused. Stupor is a state of semiconsciousness characterized by arousal only by intense stimuli such as sharp pressure over bony prominence (i.e. sternal rub), and the patient has few or even no voluntary motor responses.[48] The American Congress of Rehabilitation Medicine has recently used three terms to describe severe alterations in consciousness.[61] In *coma*, the eyes are closed with absence of sleep–wake cycles and no evidence of a contingent relationship between the patient's behavior and the environment.[24,61] *Vegetative state* is characterized by presence of sleep–wake cycles but no contingent relationship. *Minimally conscious state* indicates a patient who remains severely disabled but demonstrates visual fixation and/or tracking. The patient with minimally conscious state also has inconsistent non-reflexive behaviors, which occur in response to a specific environmental stimulation. In the acute settings, the Glasgow Coma Scale is the most often used objective measure to document level of consciousness, assessing eye opening, motor response, and verbal response (see Table 1-6).[33]

Attention   Attention is the ability to address a specific stimulus for a short period of time without being distracted by internal or external stimuli.[56] Vigilance is the ability to hold attention over longer periods of time. For example, with inadequate vigilance a patient can begin a complex task but be unable to sustain performance to completion. Attention is tested by digit recall, where the examiner reads a list of random numbers and the patient is asked to repeat those numbers. The patient should repeat digits both forward and backward. A normal performance is repeating seven numbers in the forward direction, with less than five indicating significant attention deficits.[45,56]

Orientation   Orientation is necessary for basic cognition. Orientation is comprised of four parts: person, place, time, and situation. After asking the patient's name, place can be determined by asking the location the patient is currently in or her or his home address. Time is assessed by asking the patient the time of day, the date, the day of the week, or the year. Situation refers to why the patient is in the hospital or clinic. Time sense is usually the first component lost, and person is typically the

last to be lost. Temporary stress can account for a minor loss of orientation; however, major disorientation usually suggests an organic brain syndrome.[59]

Memory   The components of memory include learning, retention, and recall. During the bedside examination, the patient is typically asked to remember three or four objects or words. The patient is then asked to repeat the items immediately to assess immediate acquisition (encoding) of the information. Retention is assessed by recall after a delayed interval, usually 5–10 min. If the patient is unable to recall the words or objects, the examiner can provide a prompt (i.e. 'It is a type of flower' for the word 'tulip'). If the patient still cannot recall the words or objects, the examiner can provide a list from which the patient can choose (i.e. 'Was it a rose, a tulip, or a mum?'). Although abnormal scores must be interpreted within the context of the remaining neurologic examination, normal individuals under 60 should recall three of four items.[56]

Recent memory can also be tested by asking questions about the past 24 hours, such as 'How did you travel here?' or 'What did you eat for breakfast this morning?' Assuming the information can be confirmed, remote memory is tested by asking where the patient was born or the school or college attended.[40]

Table 1-6 Glasgow Coma Scale

Function	Rating
Eye opening	**E**
Spontaneous	4
To speech	3
To pain	2
Nil	1
Best motor response	**M**
Obeys	6
Localizes	5
Withdraws	4
Abnormal flexion	3
Extensor response	2
Nil	1
Verbal response	**V**
Oriented	5
Confused conversation	4
Inappropriate words	3
Incomprehensible sounds	2
Nil	1
Coma score (E + M + V)	**3–15**

(From Jennett and Teasdace 1981,[33] with permission.)

Visual memory can be tested by having the patient identify four or five objects hidden in clear view.

General fundamentals of knowledge   Intelligence is a global function derived from the general tone and content of the examination and encompasses both basic intellect and remote memory. The examiner should note the patient's educational level and highest grade completed during the history. Examples of questions that can be asked include names of important elected officials, such as the current president of the USA or recent past presidents. It can be very difficult to identify when a patient with a very high intelligence premorbidly drops to a more average level after injury or illness. The history of memory or intellectual decline from a family member or close friend should prompt further evaluation of the patient.

Abstract thinking   Abstraction is a higher cortical function and can be tested by the interpretation of common proverbs such as 'a stitch in time saves nine' or 'when the cat's away the mice will play', or by asking similarities, such as 'How are an apple and an orange alike?' A concrete explanation for the first proverb would be 'You should sew a rip before it becomes bigger', whereas an abstract explanation would be 'Quick attention to a given problem would prevent bigger troubles later'. An abstract response to the similarity would be 'They are both kinds of fruit', and a concrete response would be 'They are both round' or 'You can eat them both'. Most normal individuals should be able to provide abstract responses. Concrete responses are given by persons with dementia, mental retardation, or limited education. Abstract thinking should always be considered in the context of intelligence and cultural differences.[59]

Insight and judgment   Insight has been conceptualized into three components: awareness of impairment, need for treatment, and attribution of symptoms. Insight can be ascertained by asking what brought the patient into the hospital or clinic.[8] Recognizing that one has an impairment is the initial step for recovery. A lack of insight can severely hamper a patient's progress in rehabilitation and is a major consideration in developing a safe discharge plan.

Judgment is an estimate of a person's ability to solve real life problems. The best indicator is usually just observing the patient's behavior. Judgment can also be assessed by noting the patient's responses to hypothetical situations in relation to family, employment, or personal life. Hypothetical examples of judgment that reflect societal norms include 'What should you do if you find a stamped, addressed envelope?' or 'How are you going to get around the house if you have trouble walking?' Judgment is a complex function that is part of the maturational process and is consequently unreliable in children and variable in the adolescent years.[59] Assessment of judgment is important to assess the patient's capacity for independent functioning.

Mood and affect   Mood is assessed by asking 'How do you feel most days?' Establishing accurate information pertaining to the length of a particular mood is important. The examiner should document if the mood has been reactive (i.e. sadness in response to a recent disabling event or loss of independence), and whether the mood has been stable or unstable. Mood can be described in terms of being, including happy, sad, euphoric, blue, depressed, angry, or anxious.

Affect describes how a patient feels at a given moment, which can be described by terms such as blunted, flat, inappropriate, labile, optimistic, or pessimistic. A patient's affect is determined by the observations made by the examiner during the course of the interview.[9]

General mental status assessment   The Folstein Mini Mental Status Examination is a brief and convenient tool to test general cognitive function. It is useful for screening patients for dementia and brain injuries. Of a maximum 30 points, a score 24 or above is considered within the normal range.[20] The clock drawing test is another quick test sensitive to cognitive impairment. The patient is instructed to 'Without looking at your watch, draw the face of a clock, and mark the hands to show 10 minutes to 11 o'clock'. This task utilizes memory, visual spatial skills, and executive functioning. The drawing is scored on the basis of whether the clock numbers are generally intact or not intact out of a maximum score of 10.[57] The use of the three-word recall test in addition to the clock drawing test, which is known collectively as the Mini-Cog Test, has recently gained popularity in screening for dementia. The Mini-Cog can usually be completed within 2–3 min.[51] The reader is referred to other excellent descriptions of the MSE for further reading.[56]

Communication

Aphasia   Aphasia involves the *loss of production or comprehension of language*. The cortical center for language resides in the dominant hemisphere. The examiner should listen to the content and fluency of speech. Testing of comprehension of spoken language should begin with single words, progress to sentences that require only yes–no responses, and then progress to complex commands. The examiner should also assess visual naming, repetition of single words and sentences, word-finding abilities, and reading and writing from dictation and then spontaneously. Circumlocutions are phrases or sentences substituted for a word the person cannot express, such as responding 'What you tell time with on your wrist' when asked to name a watch. Alexia without agraphia is seen in dominant occipital lobe injury. Here the patient is able to write letters and words from a spoken command but is unable to read the information after dictation.[10] Some commonly used aphasia measures include the Boston Diagnostic Aphasia Examination and the Western Aphasia Battery (see Ch. 3).[58]

Dysarthria   Dysarthria refers to *defective articulation*, but with the content of speech unaffected. The examiner should listen to spontaneous speech and then ask the patient to read aloud. Key sounds that can be tested include 'ta ta ta', which is made by the tongue (lingual consonants); 'mm mm mm', which is made by the lips (labial consonants); and 'ga ga ga', which is made by the larynx, pharynx, and palate.[40] There are several subtypes of dysarthria, including spastic, ataxic, hypokinetic, hyperkinetic, and flaccid.[45]

Dysphonia   Dysphonia is a deficit in sound production and can be secondary to respiratory disease, fatigue, or vocal cord paralysis. The best method to examine the vocal cords is by indirect laryngoscopy. Asking the patient to say 'ah' while viewing the vocal cords is used to assess vocal cord abduction. When the patient says 'e', the vocal cords will adduct. Patients with weakness of both vocal cords will speak in whispers with the presence of inspiratory stridors.[40]

Verbal apraxia   Apraxia of speech involves a deficit in motor planning, i.e. awkward and imprecise articulation in the *absence* of impaired strength or coordination of the motor system. It is characterized by inconsistent errors when speaking. A difficult word might be spoken correctly, but trouble is experienced when repeating it. People with verbal apraxia of speech often appear to be 'groping' for the right sound or word, and might try to speak a word several times before saying it correctly. Apraxia is tested by asking the patient to repeat words with an increasing number of syllables. Oromotor apraxia is seen in patients with difficulty organizing non-speech, oral motor activity. This can adversely impact swallowing. Tests for oromotor apraxia include asking patients to stick out their tongue, show their teeth, blow out their cheeks, or pretend to blow out a match.[1]

Cognitive linguistic deficits   Cognitive linguistic deficits involve the pragmatics and context of communication. Examples can include confabulation after a ruptured aneurysm of the anterior communicating artery, or disinhibited or sexually inappropriate comments from a patient with frontal lobe damage after a traumatic brain injury. Cognitive linguistic deficits are distinguished from fluent aphasias by the presence of relatively normal syntax and grammar.

Cranial nerve examination

CNI: olfactory nerve   The examiner should test both perception and identification of smell using aromatic non-irritating materials that avoid stimulation of the trigeminal nerve fibers in the nasal mucosa. Irritant substances such as ammonia should be avoided. The patient is asked to close the eyes while the opposite nostril is compressed separately. The patient should identify the smell in a test tube containing a common substance with a characteristic odor, such as coffee, peppermint, or soap. The olfactory nerve is the most commonly injured cranial nerve in head trauma due to shearing injuries that can be associated with fractures of the cribiform plate.[5]

CNII: optic nerve   The optic nerve is assessed by testing for visual acuity and visual fields, and by performing an ophthalmologic examination. Visual acuity refers to central vision, while visual field testing assesses the integrity of the optic pathway as it travels from the retina to the primary visual cortex. Testing visual field by confrontation is most commonly performed. The patient faces the examiner while covering one eye so the other eye fixates on the opposite eye of the examiner directly in front. The examiner wiggles a finger at the outer boundaries of the four quadrants of vision while the patient points to the quadrant where he or she senses movement. More accurately, a red 5-mm pin can be used to map out the visual field.[5]

CNIII, IV, and VI: oculomotor, trochlear, and abducens nerves   These three cranial nerves are best tested together, as they are all involved in ocular motility. The oculomotor nerve (III) provides innervation to all the extraocular muscles except the superior oblique and lateral rectus, which are innervated by the trochlear (IV) and abducens nerves (VI), respectively. The oculomotor nerve also innervates the levator palpebrae muscle, which elevates the eyelid, the pupilloconstrictor muscle that constricts the pupil, and the ciliary muscle that controls the thickness of the lens in visual accommodation.

The primary action of the medial rectus is adduction (looking in) and that of the lateral rectus is abduction (looking out). The superior rectus and inferior oblique primarily elevate the eye, whereas the inferior rectus and superior oblique depress the eye. The superior oblique muscle controls gaze, looking down and in.[40]

Examination of the extraocular muscles involves assessing the alignment of the patient's eyes while at rest and when following an object or finger held at an arm's length. The examiner should observe the full range of horizontal and vertical eye movements in the six cardinal directions.[5] The optic (afferent) and oculomotor (efferent) nerves are involved with the pupillary light reflex. A normal pupillary light reflex (CNII and III) should result in constriction of *both* pupils when a light stimulus is present to either eye separately. A characteristic head tilt when looking down is sometimes seen in CNIV lesions.[62]

CNV: trigeminal nerve   The trigeminal nerve provides sensation to the face and mucous membranes of the nose, mouth, and tongue. There are three sensory divisions of the trigeminal nerve: the ophthalmic, maxillary, and mandibular branches. These branches can be tested by pinprick sensation, light touch, or temperature along the forehead, cheeks, and jaw on each side of the face. The motor branch of the trigeminal nerve also innervates the muscles of mastication, which include the masseters, the pterygoids, and the temporalis. The patient is asked to clamp the jaws together, and then the examiner will try to open the patient's jaw by pulling down on the lower mandible. Observe and palpate for contraction of both the temporalis and the masseter muscles. The pterygoids are tested by asking the patient to open the mouth. If one side is weak, the intact pterygoid muscles will push the weak muscles, resulting in a deviation toward the weak side. The corneal reflex tests the ophthalmic division of the trigeminal nerve (afferent) and the facial nerve (efferent).

CNVII: facial nerve   The facial nerve provides motor innervation to all muscles of facial expression; provides sensation to the anterior two-thirds of the tongue and the outer ear; innervates the stapedius muscle, which helps dampen loud sounds by decreasing excessive movements of the ossicles in the inner ear; and provides secretomotor fibers to the lacrimal and salivary glands.

The facial nerve is first examined by watching the patient as she or he talks and smiles, watching specifically for eye closure, flattening of the nasolabial fold, and asymmetric elevation of one corner of the mouth. The patient is then asked to wrinkle the forehead (frontalis), close the eyes while the examiner attempts to open them (orbicularis oculi), puff out both cheeks while the examiner presses on the cheeks (buccinator), and show the teeth (orbicularis oris). A peripheral injury to the facial nerve, such as Bell palsy, affects both the upper and the lower face, whereas a central lesion typically affects mainly the lower face.

CNVIII: vestibulocochlear nerve

The vestibulocochlear nerve, also known as the auditory nerve, comprises two divisions. The cochlear nerve is the part of the auditory nerve responsible for hearing, while the vestibular nerve is related to balance. The cochlear division can be tested by checking gross hearing. A rapid screen can be done if the examiner rubs the thumb and index fingers near each ear of the patient. Patients with normal hearing usually have no difficulty hearing this.

The vestibular division is seldom included in the routine neurologic examination. Patients with dizziness or vertigo associated with changes in head position or suspected of having benign paroxysmal positional vertigo should be assessed with the Dix–Hallpike maneuver (Fig. 1-1). The absence of nystag-

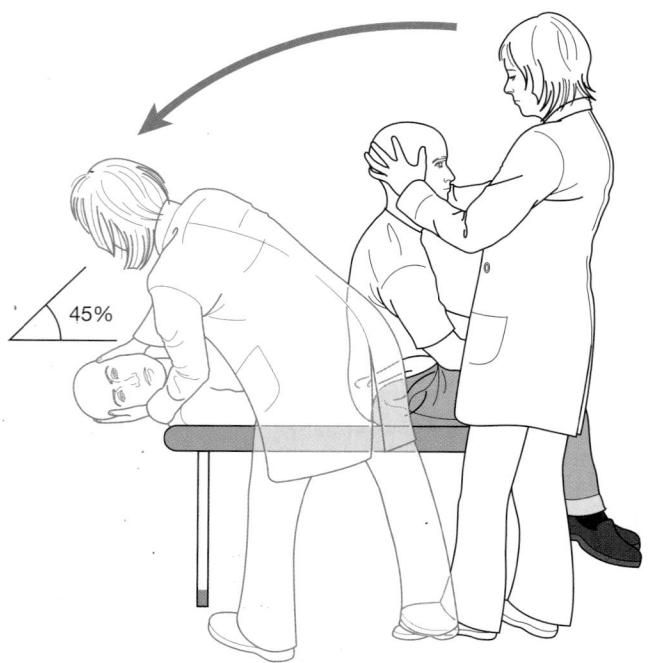

Figure 1-1 The Dix–Hallpike maneuver is performed with the patient initially seated upright. The patient is asked to fall backward so that the head is below the plane of his or her trunk. The examiner then turns the patient's head to one side and asks the patient to look in the direction to which the head is turned.

mus indicates normal vestibular nerve function. With peripheral vestibular nerve dysfunction, however, the patient complains of vertigo and rotary nystagmus appears, after an approximately 2- to 5-s latency, toward the direction in which the eyes are deviated. With repetition of maneuvers, the nystagmus and sensation of vertigo fatigue and ultimately disappear. In central vestibular disease, such as from a stroke, the nystagmus has latency and is non-fatigable.[21]

CNIX and X: glossopharyngeal nerve and vagus nerve

The glossopharyngeal nerve supplies taste to the posterior one-third of the tongue, along with sensation to the pharynx and the middle ear. The glossopharyngeal nerve and vagus nerve are usually examined together. The patient's voice quality should be noted, as hoarseness is usually associated with a lesion of the recurrent laryngeal nerve, a branch of the vagus nerve. The patient is asked to open the mouth and say 'ah'. The examiner should inspect the soft palate, which should elevate symmetrically with the uvula in midline. In an LMN vagus nerve lesion, the uvula will deviate to the side that is contralateral to the lesion. A UMN lesion presents with the uvula deviating toward the side of the lesion.[26]

The gag reflex can be tested by depressing the patient's tongue with a tongue depressor and touching the pharyngeal wall with a cotton tip applicator until the patient gags. The examiner should compare the sensitivity of each side (afferent: glossopharyngeal nerve) and observe the symmetry of the palatal contraction (efferent: vagus nerve). The absence of a gag reflex indicates loss of sensation and/or loss of motor contraction. The presence of a gag reflex does not imply the ability to swallow without risk of aspiration (see Ch. 28).[49]

CNXI: accessory nerve

The accessory nerve innervates the trapezius and sternocleidomastoid muscles. While standing behind the patient, the examiner should look for atrophy or spasm in the trapezius and compare the symmetry of both sides. To test the strength of the trapezius, the patient is asked to shrug the shoulders and hold them in this position against resistance. To test the strength of the sternocleidomastoid muscle, ask the patient to rotate the head against resistance. The ipsilateral sternocleidomastoid muscle turns the head to the contralateral side. The ipsilateral muscle brings the ear to the shoulder.

CNXII: hypoglossal nerve

The hypoglossal nerve is a pure motor nerve innervating the muscles of the tongue. It is tested by asking the patient to protrude the tongue, noting evidence of atrophy, fasciculation, or deviation. Fibrillations in the tongue are common in patients with amyotrophic lateral sclerosis.[25] The tongue typically points to the side of the lesion in peripheral hypoglossal nerve lesions, but toward the opposite side of the lesion in UMN lesions such as stroke

Sensory examination

The examiner should be familiar with the normal dermatomal and peripheral nerve sensory distribution (see Fig. 1-2). Evaluation of the sensory system requires testing of both super-

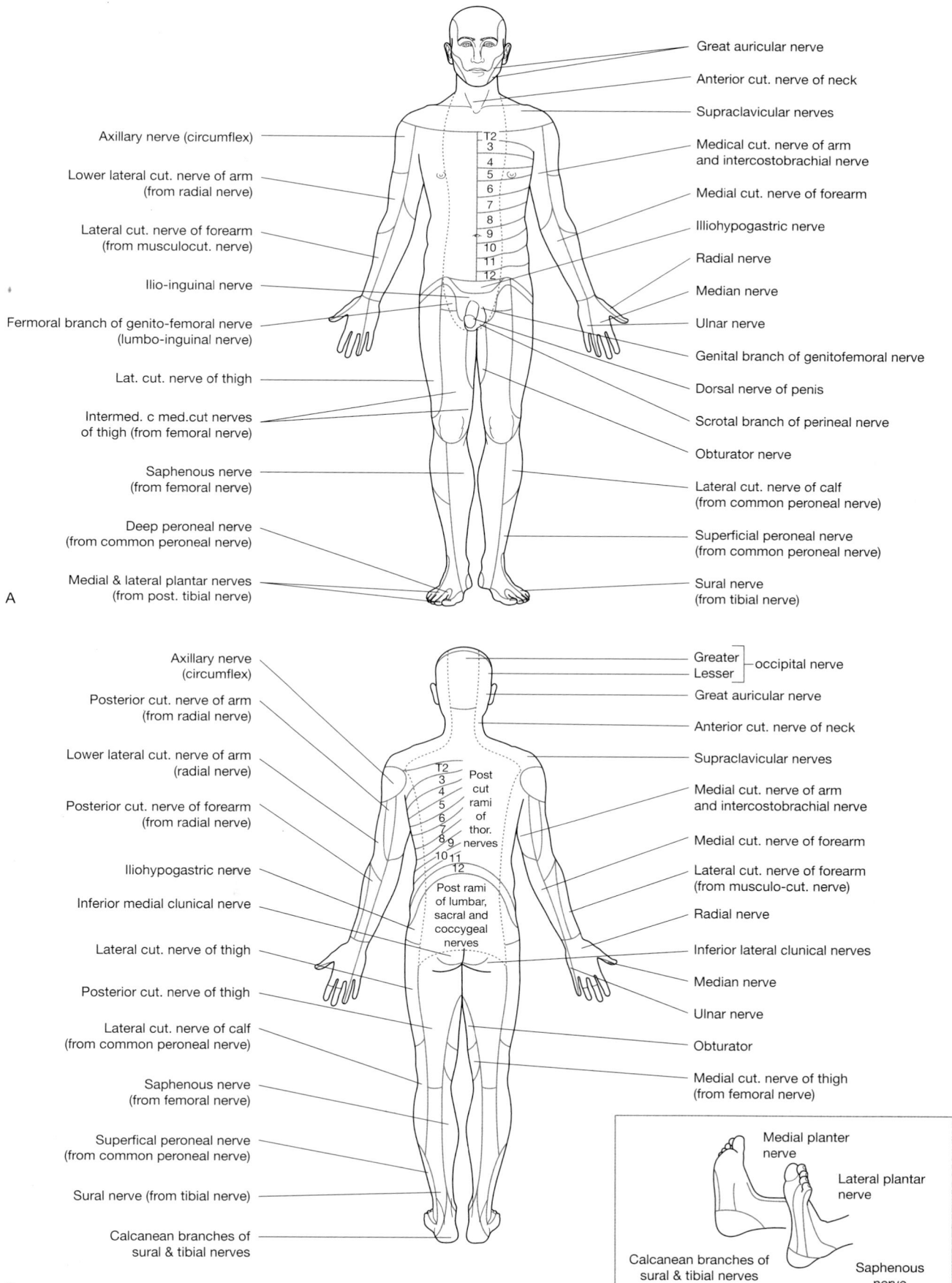

Figure 1-2 Distribution of peripheral nerves and dermatomes. (From Haymaker and Woodhall 1953,[29] with permission.)

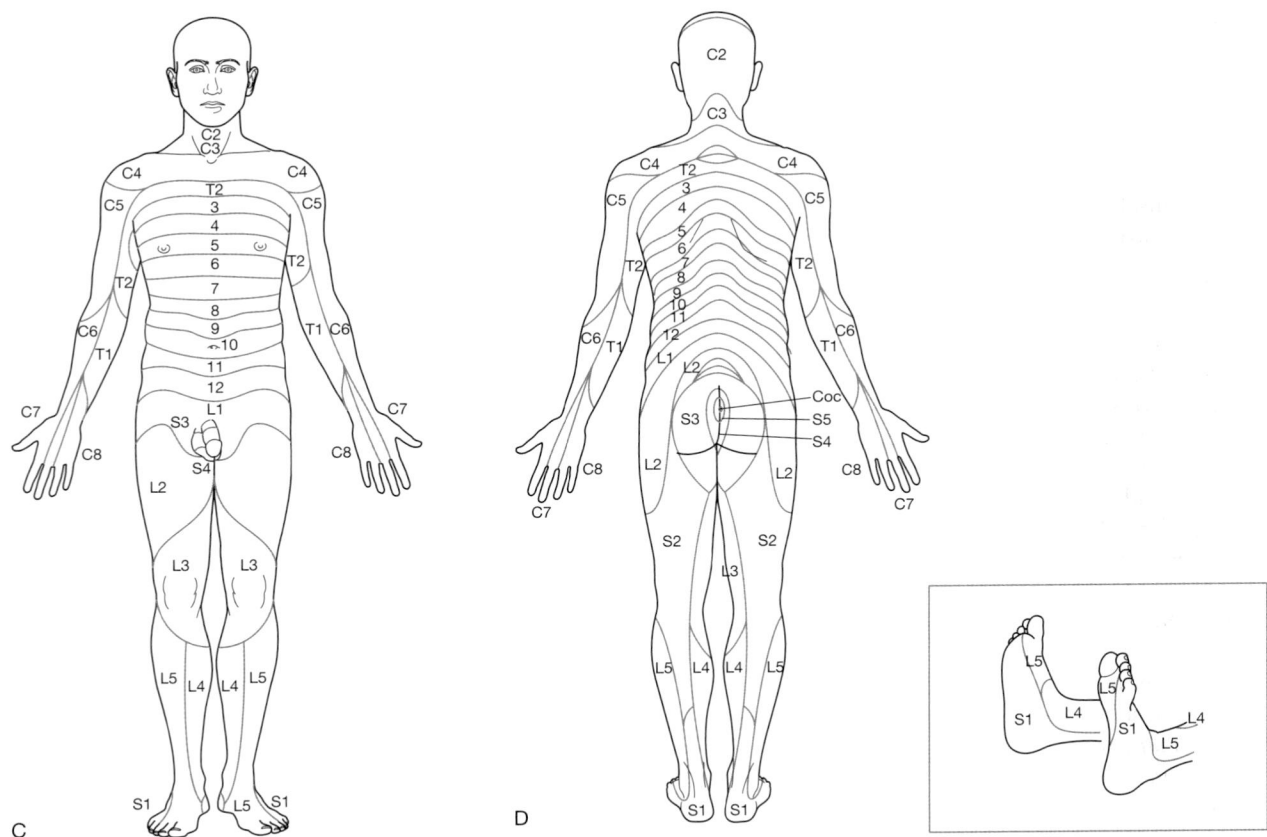

C   D

Figure 1-2 Continued.

ficial sensation (light touch, pain, and temperature) and deep sensation (involves the perception of position and vibration from deep structures such as muscle, ligaments, and bone).

Light touch can be assessed with a fine wisp of cotton or a cotton tip applicator. The examiner should touch the skin lightly, avoiding excessive pressure. The patient is asked to respond when a touch is felt, and to say whether there is a difference between the two sides. Pain and temperature both travel via the spinothalamic tracts and are assessed using a safety pin or other sharp sanitary object, while occasionally interspersing the examination with a blunt object. Patients with peripheral neuropathy might have a delayed pain appreciation and often change their minds a few seconds after the initial stimuli. Some examiners use the single or double pinprick of brief duration to test for pain, while others use a continuous sustained pinprick to better test for delayed pain.[45] Temperature testing is not often used and rarely provides additional information, but it is sometimes easier for patients to delineate insensate areas. Thermal sensation can be checked by using two different test tubes, one filled with hot water (not hot enough to burn) and one filled with cold water and ice chips.

Joint position sense or proprioception travel via the dorsal columns along with vibration sense. Proprioception is easily tested by vertical passive movement of the toes or fingers. The examiner holds the sides of the patient's finger or toes and asks the patient if the digits are in the upward or downward direc-

tion. It is important to grasp the sides rather than the nail bed, as the patient might be able to perceive pressure in these areas, reducing the accuracy of the examination. Most normal persons make no errors on these maneuvers.

Vibration is tested in the limbs with a 128-Hz tuning fork. The tuning fork is placed on a bony prominence such as the dorsal aspect of the terminal phalange of the great toe, the malleoli, or the olecranon. The patient is asked to indicate when the vibration ceases. The vibration stimulus can be controlled by changing the force used to set the tuning fork in motion, or by noting the amount of time that a vibration is felt as the stimulus dissipates. Assuming the examiner is normal, both patient and examiner should feel the vibration cease at approximately the same time.

Two-point discrimination is most commonly tested using calipers with blunt ends. The patient is asked to close the eyes and indicate if one or two stimulation points are felt. The normal distance of separation that can be felt as two distinct points depends on the area of body being tested. For example, the lips are sensitive to point separation of 2–3 mm, normally identified as two points. Commonly tested normal two-point discrimination areas include the fingertips (3–5 mm), the dorsum of the hand (20–30 mm), and the palms (8–15 mm).[40]

Graphesthesia is the ability to recognize numbers, letters, or symbols traced on to the palm. It is performed by writing recognizable numbers on to the patient's palm with his or her eyes closed. Stereognosis is the ability to recognize common objects placed in the hand, such as keys or coins. This requires normal peripheral sensation as well as cortical sensation.

Motor control

Strength   Manual muscle testing provides an important method of quantifying strength and is outlined below.

Coordination   The cerebellum controls movement by comparing the intended activity with actual activity that is achieved. The cerebellum smoothes motor movements and is intimately involved with coordination. Ataxia or motor coordination can be secondary to deficits of sensory, motor, or cerebellar connections. Ataxic patients who have intact function of the sensory and motor pathways usually have cerebellar compromise.

The cerebellum is divided into three areas: the midline, the anterior lobe, and the lateral hemisphere. Lesions affecting the midline usually produce truncal ataxia in which the patient cannot sit or stand unsupported. This can be tested by asking the patient to sit at the edge of the bed with the arms folded so they cannot be used for support. Lesions that affect the anterior lobe usually result in gait ataxia. In this case, the patient is able to sit or stand unsupported but has noticeable balance deficits on walking. Lateral hemisphere lesions produce loss of ability to coordinate movement, which can be described as limb ataxia. The affected limb usually has diminished ability to correct and change direction rapidly. Tests that are typically used to test for limb coordination include the finger to nose test and the heel to shin test.[44]

Rapid alternating movements can be tested by observing the amplitude, rhythm, and precision of movement. The patient is asked to place the hands on the thighs, and then rapidly turn the hands over and lift them off the thighs for 10 s. Normal individuals can do this without difficulty. Dysdiadochokinesis is the clinical term for an inability to perform rapidly alternating movements.

The Romberg test can be used to differentiate a cerebellar deficit from a proprioceptive one. The patient is asked to stand with the heels together. The examiner notes any excessive postural swaying or loss of balance. If loss of balance is present when the eyes are open and closed, the examination is consistent with cerebellar ataxia. If the loss of balance occurs only when the eyes are closed, this is classically known as a positive Romberg sign indicating a proprioceptive deficit.[40]

Apraxia   Apraxia is the loss of the ability to carry out programmed or planned movements despite adequate understanding of the tasks. This deficit is present even though the patient has no weakness or sensory loss. In order to accomplish a complex act, there first must be an idea or a formulation of a plan. The formulation of the plan then must be transferred into the motor system where it is executed. The examiner should watch the patient for motor-planning problems during the physical examination. For example, a patient might be unable to perform transfers and other mobility tasks but has adequate strength on formal manual muscle testing.

Ideomotor apraxia associated with a lesion of the dominant parietal lobe occurs when a patient cannot carry out motor commands but can perform the required movements under different circumstances. These patients usually can perform many complex acts automatically but cannot carry out the same acts on command. Ideational apraxia refers to the inability to carry out sequences of acts, although each component can be performed separately. Other forms of apraxia are constructional, dressing, oculomotor, and gait apraxia. Dressing and constructional apraxia are often related to impairments of the non-dominant parietal lobe, which is typically due more to neglect than to actual deficit in motor planning.[40]

Involuntary movements   Documenting involuntary movements is important in the overall neurologic examination. A careful survey of the patient usually shows the presence or absence of voluntary motor control. Tremor is the most common type of involuntary movement and is a rhythmic movement of a body part. Lesions in the basal ganglia produce characteristic movement disorders. Chorea describes movements that consist of brief, random, non-repetitive movements in a fidgety patient unable to sit still. Athetosis consists of twisting and writhing movements and is commonly seen in cerebral palsy. Dystonia is a sustained posturing that can affect small or large muscle groups. An example is torticollis, in which dystonic neck muscles pull the head to one side. Hemiballismus occurs when there are repetitive violent flailing movements that are usually caused by deficits in the subthalamic nucleus.[45]

Tone   Tone is the resistance of muscle to stretch or passive elongation (see Ch. 31). Spasticity is a velocity-dependent increase in the stretch reflex, whereas rigidity is the resistance of the limb to passive movement in the relaxed state. Variability in tone is common, as patients with spasticity can vary in their presentation throughout the day and with positional changes. Accurate assessment of tone requires repeated examinations.[48]

Initial observation of the patient usually shows abnormal posturing of the limbs or trunk. Palpation of the muscle also provides clues, because hypotonic muscles feel soft and flaccid on palpation, whereas hypertonic muscles feel firm and tight. Passive range of motion (ROM) provides information about the muscle in response to stretch. The examiner provides firm and constant contact while moving the limbs in all directions. The limb should move easily and without resistance when altering the direction and speed of movement. Hypertonic limbs feel stiff and resist movement, while flaccid limbs are unresponsive. The patient should be told to relax, because these responses should be examined without any voluntary control. Clonus is a cyclic alternation of muscular contraction in response to a sustained stretch, and is assessed using a quick stretch stimulus that is then maintained. Myoclonus refers to sudden, involuntary jerking of a muscle or group of muscles. Myoclonic jerks can be normal, because it occasionally happens in normal individuals and is typically part of the normal sleep cycle.

Tone can be quantified by the modified Ashworth scale, a six-point ordinal scale. A pendulum test can also be used to

Table 1-7 Important normal superficial reflexes

Reflex	Elicited by	Response	Segmental level
Corneal	Touching cornea with hair	Contraction of orbicularis oculi	Pons
Pharyngeal	Touching posterior wall of pharynx	Contraction of pharynx	Medulla
Palatal	Touching soft palate	Elevation of palate	Medulla
Scapular	Stroking skin between scapulae	Contraction of scapular muscles	C5–T1
Epigastric	Stroking downward from nipples	Dimpling of epigastrium ipsilaterally	T7–9
Abdominal	Stroking beneath costal margins and above inguinal ligament	Contraction of abdominal muscles in quadrant stimulated	T8–12
Cremasteric	Stroking medial surface of upper thigh	Ipsilateral elevation of testicle	L1, L2
Gluteal	Stroking skin of buttock	Contraction of glutei	L4, L5
Bulbocavernous (male)	Pinching dorsum of glans	Insert gloved finger to palpate anal contraction	S3, S4
Clitorocavernous (female)	Pinching clitoris	Insert gloved finger to palpate anal contraction	S3, S4
Superficial anal	Pricking perineum	Contraction of rectal sphincters	S5, coccygeal

(After Mancall 1993,[42] with permission of FA Davis.)

quantify spasticity. While in the supine position, the patient is asked to fully extend the knee and then allow the leg to drop and swing like a pendulum. A normal limb swings freely for several cycles, whereas a hypertonic limb quickly returns to the initial dependent starting position.[58]

Reflexes

Superficial reflexes   The plantar reflex is the most common superficial reflex examined. A stimulus (usually by the handle end of a reflex hammer) is applied on the sole of the foot from the lateral border to up and across the ball of the foot. A normal reaction consists of flexion of the great toe or no response. An abnormal response consists of dorsiflexion of the great toe with an associated fanning of the other toes. This response is the Babinski sign and indicates dysfunction of the corticospinal tract. Stroking from the lateral ankle to the lateral dorsal foot can also produce dorsiflexion of the great toe (Chaddock sign). Flipping the little toe outward can produce the up-going great toe also, and is called the Stransky sign. Other superficial reflexes include the abdominal, cremasteric, bulbocavernous, and superficial anal reflexes (see Table 1-7).[45]

Muscle stretch reflexes   Muscle stretch reflexes (which in the past were called deep tendon reflexes) are assessed by tapping over the muscle tendon with a reflex hammer (see Table 1-8). In order to elicit a response, the patient is positioned into the midrange of the arc of joint motion and instructed to relax. Tapping of the tendon results in visible movement of the joint. The response is assessed as 0, no response; 1+, diminished but present and might require facilitation; 2+, usual response;

Table 1-8 Muscle stretch reflexes

Muscle	Peripheral nerve	Root level
Biceps	Musculocutaneous nerve	C5, C6
Brachioradialis	Radial nerve	C5, C6
Triceps	Radial nerve	C7, C8
Pronator teres	Median nerve	C6, C7
Patella (quadriceps)	Femoral nerve	L2–L4
Medial hamstrings	Sciatic (tibial portion) nerve	L5–S1
Achilles	Tibial nerve	S1, S2

3+, more brisk than usual; and 4+, hyperactive with clonus. If muscle stretch reflexes are difficult to elicit, the response can be enhanced by reinforcement maneuvers such as hooking together the fingers of both hands while attempting to pull them apart (Jendrassik maneuver.) While pressure is still maintained, the lower limb reflexes can be tested. Squeezing the knees together and clenching the teeth can reinforce responses to the upper extremities.[40]

Primitive reflexes   Primitive reflexes are abnormal adult reflexes that represent a regression to a more infantile level of reflex activity. Redevelopment of an infantile reflex in an adult suggests significant neurologic abnormalities.

Examples of primitive reflexes include the sucking reflex, in which the patient sucks the area around which the mouth is stimulated. The rooting reflex is elicited by stroking the cheek, resulting in the patient turning toward that side and making sucking motions with the mouth. The grasp reflex occurs when the examiner places a finger on the patient's open palm. Attempting to remove the finger causes the grip to tighten. The snout reflex occurs when a lip-pursing movement occurs when there is a tap just above or below the mouth. The palmomental response is elicited by quickly scratching the palm of the hand. A positive reflex is indicated by sudden contraction of the mentalis (chin) muscle. It arises from unilateral damage of the prefrontal area of the brain.[46]

Musculoskeletal examination
Caveats
The musculoskeletal examination (MSK exam) confirms the diagnostic impression and lays the foundation for the physiatric treatment plan. It incorporates inspection, palpation, passive and active ROM, assessment of joint stability, manual muscle testing and joint-specific provocative maneuvers, or special tests.[23,29] The functional unit of the musculoskeletal system is the joint. The comprehensive examination of a joint includes related structures such as muscles, ligaments, and the synovial membrane and capsule.[55] The physiatric MSK exam also indirectly tests coordination, sensation, and endurance.[23,38] There is overlap between the examination (and clinical presentation) of the neurologic and musculoskeletal systems. The primary impairment in many cases in neurologic disease is the secondary musculoskeletal complications of immobility and suboptimal movement (in which the concept of the kinetic chain is important for evaluation). The MSK exam should be performed in a routine sequence for efficiency and consistency, and must be approached with a solid knowledge of the anatomy. The reader is referred to several excellent references that provide in-depth reviews of the MSK exam.[17,29,30,35,41,45]

Inspection and palpation
Inspection of the musculoskeletal system begins during the history. Attention to subtle cues and behaviors can guide the approach to the examination. Inspection includes observing mood, signs of pain or discomfort, functional impairments, or evidence of malingering. The spine should be specifically inspected for scoliosis, kyphosis, and lordosis. Extremities should be examined for limb symmetry, circumference, and contour. In persons with amputation, the level, length, and shape of the residual limb should be noted. Depending on the clinical situation, it can be important to assess for muscle atrophy, masses, edema, scars, and fasciculations.[55] Joints should be inspected for abnormal positions, swelling, fullness, and redness.

These isolated findings can coalesce to influence global movement patterns that affect the kinetic chain. The term *kinetic chain* refers to the fact that the joints of the human body are not isolated but instead are linked in a series. Joint motion is always accompanied by motion at adjacent as well as distal joints, resulting in asymmetric patterns causing pathology of seemingly unrelated sites. This is especially true with a fixed distal limb. For example, very tight hamstring muscles decrease the lumbar lordosis, resulting in an increased risk of lower back pain. It is important to include this concept in any musculoskeletal assessment.

Palpation is used to confirm initial impressions from inspection, helping to determine the structural origins of soft tissue or bony pain and localize trigger points, muscle guarding, or spasm and referred pain.[55] Joints and muscles should be assessed for swelling, warmth, masses, tight muscle bands, tone, and crepitus.[30] Tone is typically determined while assessing the ROM. It is important to palpate the limbs and cranium for evidence of fracture in patients with a change in mental status following a fall or trauma.[45]

Assessment of joint stability   The assessment of joint stability judges the capacity of structural elements to resist forces in non-anatomic directions.[45,55] Stability is determined by several factors, including bony congruity, capsular and cartilaginous integrity, and the strength of ligaments and muscles.[45] Assessing the 'normal' side establishes a patient's unique biomechanics. The examiner first identifies pain and resistance in the affected joint, followed by an evaluation of joint play to assess 'end feel', capsular patterns, and hypomobility or hypermobility. Radiographic imaging can be helpful in cases of suspected instability, for example flexion–extension spine films to assess vertebral column instability or magnetic resonance imaging to visualize the degree of anterior cruciate ligament rupture.

Joint play or capsular patterns assess the integrity of the capsule in an open-packed position. *Open-packed* refers to positions in which there is minimal bony contact with maximum capsular laxity.[50] Voluntary movement of a joint (active ROM) does not generally exploit the fullest range of that joint. Extreme end ranges of joint movements not under voluntary control must be assessed by passive ROM. There are several types of end feels (see Table 1-9). Soft tissue compression is normal in extreme elbow flexion, yet if felt sooner than expected can indicate inflammation or edema. Tissue stretch is usually firm yet slightly forgiving, such as in hip flexion. However, firmness that occurs prior to the end point of range can be a sign of increased tone and/or capsular tightening. A hard end feel is normally seen with elbow extension, but in an arthritic joint it can occur before full range is achieved. An 'empty' feel suggests an absence of mechanical restriction due to muscle contraction caused by pain. With muscle involuntary guarding or spasm, one notes an abrupt stop associated with pain.

It is important to differentiate between hypomobile and hypermobile joints. The former increase the risk for muscle strains, tendonitis, and nerve entrapments, while the latter increase the risk for joint sprains and degenerative joint disease.[50] An inflammatory synovitis, for example, can increase joint mobility and weaken the capsule. In the setting of decreased muscle strength, the risk of trauma and joint instability is increased.[45] If joint instability is suspected, confirmatory diagnostic testing can be done (i.e. radiography).[17,31,35,41] The

Table 1-9 Types of 'end feels' in range of motion testing

End feel	Normal	Example(s)	Abnormal	Example(s)
Soft	Soft tissue approximation	Knee flexion	Tissue change occurring sooner or later than expected A change in a joint that normally has a firm or hard end feel	Soft tissue edema Synovitis
Firm	Muscular stretch Capsular stretch Ligamentous stretch	Hip flexion Metacarpophalangeal extension Forearm supination	Tissue change occurring sooner or later than expected A change in a joint that normally has a soft or hard end feel	Increased muscular tonus Contracture of capsular, muscular, or ligamentous structures
Hard	Bone contacting bone	Elbow extension	Tissue change occurring sooner or later than expected A change in a joint that normally has a soft or firm end feel	Osteoarthritis Loose bodies in the joint Fracture
Empty	Abnormal joint end feel	–	No end feel noted due to resistance caused by pain	Acute joint inflammation Bursitis Abscess Fracture Psychogenic disorder

(After Norkin and White 2003, with permission of FA Davis.)

temporal relationship between pain and resistance on examination actually changes from acute to chronic injury. An acute joint demonstrates pain *before* resistance to passive ROM. In a subacute joint, there is pain *at the same time* as resistance to passive ROM. In a chronic joint, pain occurs *after* resistance to ROM is noted.[50]

Assessment of range of motion

General principles   Range of motion testing is used to document the integrity of a joint, to assess the efficacy of treatment regimens, and to determine the mechanical cause of an impairment.[37] Limitations not only affect ambulation and mobility, but also ADL. Normal ROM varies based on age, gender, conditioning, obesity, and genetics.[45] Males have a more limited range when compared with females, depending on age and specific joint action.[7] Occupational patterns of activity also potentially alter ROM. For example, gymnasts generally have increased ROM at the hips and lower trunk.[50] Passive ROM should be performed through all planes of motion by the examiner in a relaxed patient to thoroughly assess end feel.[50] Active ROM performed by the patient through all planes of motion without assistance from the examiner simultaneously evaluates muscle strength, coordination of movement, and functional ability.

Contractures are often obvious simply from visual inspection. Contractures impact the true, full ROM of a joint via either soft tissue or bony changes. A soft tissue or muscle contracture decreases with a prolonged stretch, whereas a bony contracture does not. It can be difficult or impossible to differentiate a contracture from severe hypertonia in CNS diseases. A diag-nostic peripheral nerve block can eliminate the hypertonia for a few hours to determine the etiology of the contracture and guide the correct treatment for impaired mobility or ADL.

Assessment techniques   Range of motion should be performed prior to strength testing. ROM is a function of joint morphology, capsule and ligament integrity, and muscle and tendon strength.[50,55] Range is measured with a universal goniometer, a device that has a pivoting arm attached to a stationary arm divided into 1° intervals (see Fig. 1-3). Regardless of the type of goniometer used, reliability is increased by knowing and using consistent surface landmarks and test positions.[23] Joints are measured in their plane of movement with the stationary arm parallel to the long axis of the proximal body segment or bony landmark.[50] The moving arm of the goniometer should also be aligned with a bony landmark or parallel to the moving body segment. The impaired joint should always be compared with the contralateral unimpaired joint, if possible.

Sagittal, frontal, and coronal planes divide the body into three cardinal planes of motion (see Fig. 1-4). The sagittal plane divides the body into left and right halves, while the frontal (coronal) plane into anterior and posterior halves. The transverse plane divides the body into superior and inferior parts.[23] For sagittal plane measurements, the goniometer is placed on the lateral side of the joint, except for a few joint motions such as forearm supination and pronation. Frontal planes are measured anteriorly or posteriorly, with the axis coinciding with the axis of the joint.

The 360° system was first proposed by Knapp and West[36] and denotes 0° directly overhead and 180° at the feet. In the 360°

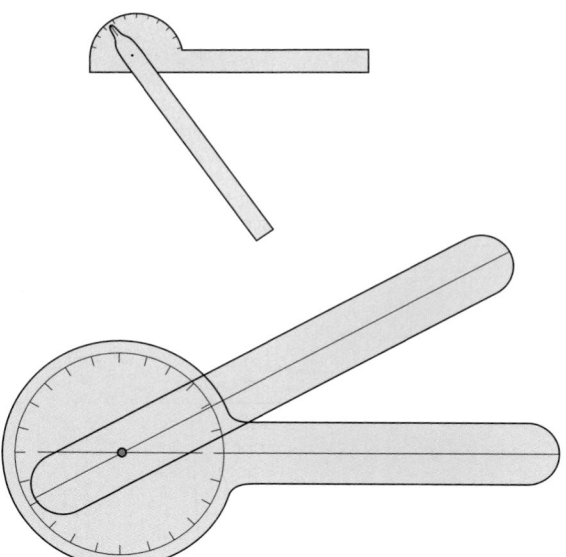

Figure 1-3 Universal goniometer. (From Kottke and Lehman 1990,[38] with permission.)

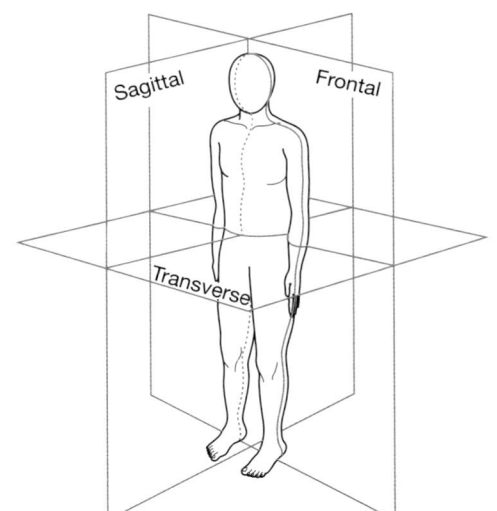

Figure 1-4
Cardinal planes of motion.

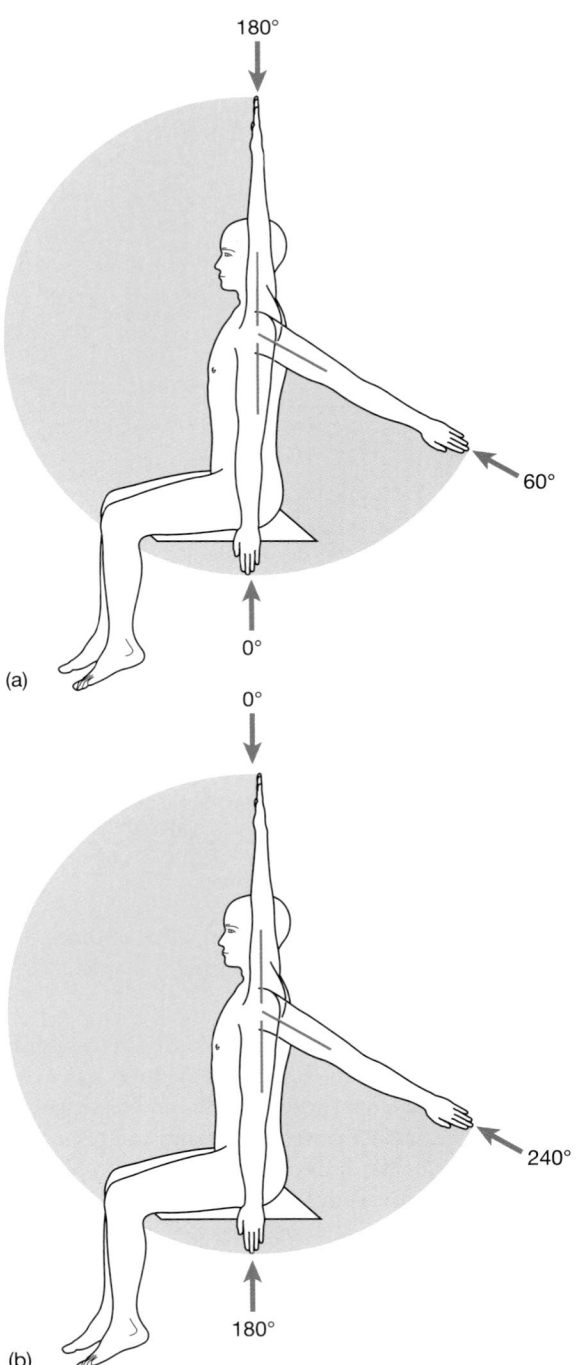

Figure 1-5 Comparison of two range of motion systems.

system, shoulder forward flexion and extension ranges from 0 to 240° (see Fig. 1-5b). The American Academy of Orthopedic Surgeons uses a 180° system.[47] The standard anatomic position[11] is described as an upright position with the feet facing forward, the arms at the side with the palms facing anterior.[23] A joint at 0° is in the anatomic position, with movement occurring up to 180° away from 0° in either direction.[23] Using shoulder forward flexion as an example, the normal range for flexion in the 180° system is 0–180°, and for extension is 0–60° (see Fig. 1-5a). These standardized techniques have been well described.[2,14,23,30,31,47,50]

Figures 1-6 to 1-21 outline the correct patient positioning and plane of motion for the joint and goniometer placement. To increase accuracy, many practitioners recommend taking several measurements and recording a mean value.[50] Measurement inaccuracy can be as high as 10–30% in the limbs and can

be without value in the spine if based on visual assessment alone.[2,60] In joint deformity, the starting position is the actual starting position of joint motion. Spinal ROM is more difficult to measure, and its reliability has been debated.[23,30] The most accurate method of measuring spinal motion is with radiographs. Because this is not practical in most clinical scenarios, the next most accurate system is based on inclinometers. These are fluid-filled instruments with a 180 or 360° scale. One or two devices are required.[2,30] The American Medical Association

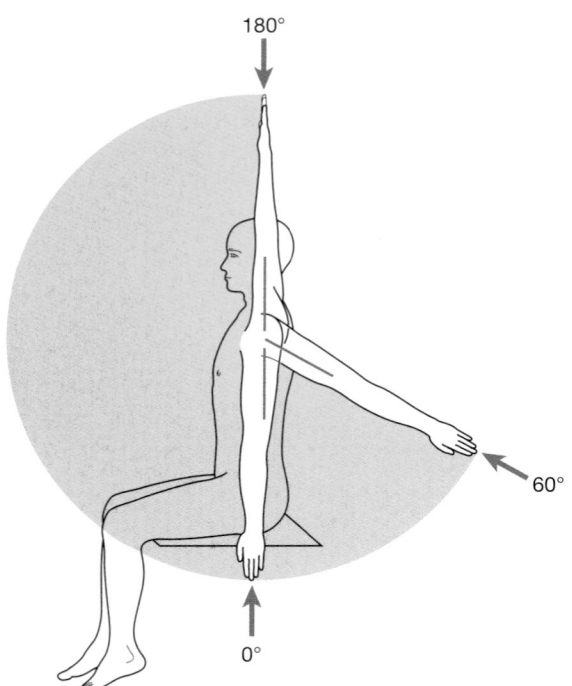

Figure 1-6 Shoulder flexion and extension. Patient position: supine or sitting, arm at side, elbow extended. Plane of motion: sagittal. Normal range of motion: flexion, 0–180°; extension, 0–60°. Movements the patient should avoid: arching back, trunk rotation. Goniometer placement: axis is centered on the lateral shoulder, stationary arm remains at 0°, movement arm remains parallel to humerus.

Guides to the Evaluation of Permanent Impairment[2] outlines the specific inclinometer techniques for measuring spinal ROM.

Assessment of muscle strength

General principles   Manual muscle testing is used to establish baseline strength, to determine the functional abilities of or need for adaptive equipment, to confirm a diagnosis, and to suggest a prognosis.[50] *Strength* is a rather generic term and can refer to a wide variety of assessments and testing situations.[6] Manual muscle testing specifically measures the ability to voluntary contract a muscle or muscle group at a specific joint. It is quantified using a system first described by Robert Lovett, M.D., an orthopedic surgeon, in the early twentieth century.[16] Isolated muscles can be difficult to assess. For example, elbow flexion strength depends not only on the biceps muscle but also on the brachialis and brachioradialis muscles. Strength is affected by many factors, including the number of motor units firing, functional excursion, cross-sectional area of the muscle, line of pull of the muscle fibers, number of joints crossed, sensory receptors, attachments to bone, age, sex, pain, fatigue, fear, motivational level, and misunderstanding.[6,45,50] Pain can result in breakaway weakness due to pain inhibition of function and should be documented as such. It is important to recognize the presence of substitution when muscles are weak or movement is uncoordinated. Females increase strength up to age 20, plateau through their twenties, and gradually decline in strength after age 30. Males increase strength up to age 20 years and then plateau until somewhat older than 30 years before declining.[50] Muscles that are predomi-

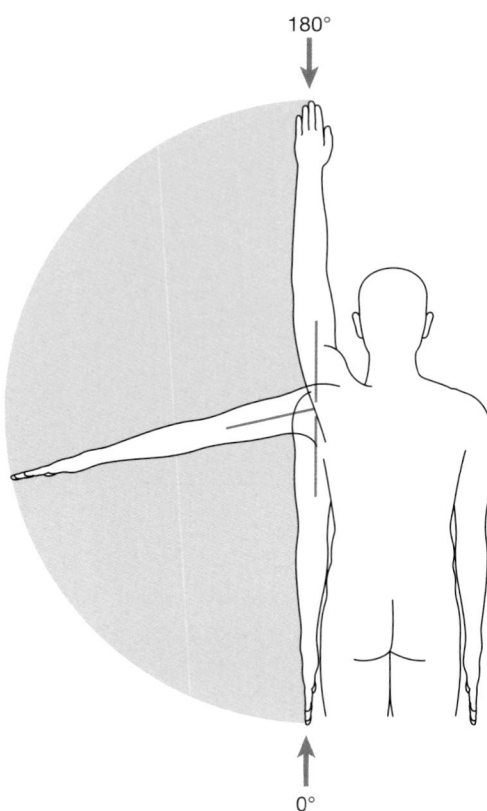

Figure 1-7 Shoulder abduction. Patient position: supine or sitting, arm at side, elbow extended. Plane of motion: frontal. Normal range of motion: 0–180°. Movements the patient should avoid: trunk rotation or lateral movement. Goniometer placement: axis is centered on posterior or anterior shoulder, stationary arm remains at 0°, movement arm remains parallel to humerus.

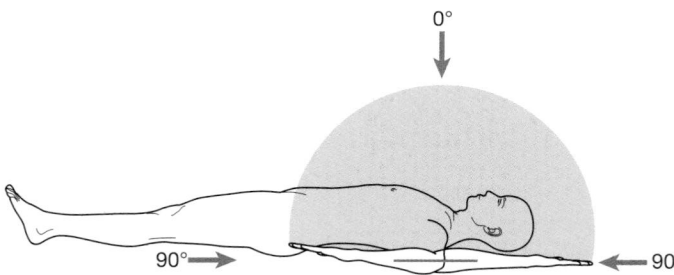

Figure 1-8 Shoulder internal and external rotation. Patient position: supine, shoulder at 90° of abduction, elbow at 90° of flexion, radioulnar joint pronated. Plane of motion: transverse. Normal range of motion: internal rotation, 0–90°; external rotation, 0–90°. Movements the patient should avoid: arching back, trunk rotation, elbow movement. Goniometer placement: axis on elbow joint through longitudinal axis of humerus, stationary arm remains at 0°, movement arm remains parallel to forearm.

nantly Type 1 or slow-twitch fibers (e.g. soleus muscle) tend to be fatigue-resistant and can require extended stress on testing (such as several standing toe raises) to uncover weakness.[50] Type 2 or fast-twitch fibers (e.g. sternocleidomastoid) fatigue quickly, and weakness can be more straightforward to uncover abnormalities. Patients who cannot actively control muscle tension (e.g. those with spasticity from CNS disease) are not appropriate for standard manual muscle testing methods.[50]

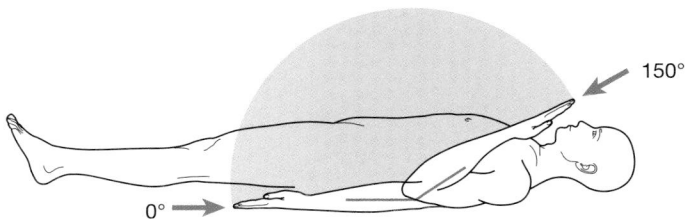

Figure 1-9 Elbow flexion. Patient position: supine or sitting, radioulnar joint supinated. Plane of motion: sagittal. Normal range of motion: 0–150°. Goniometer placement: axis is centered on lateral elbow, stationary arm remains at 0°, movement arm remains parallel to forearm.

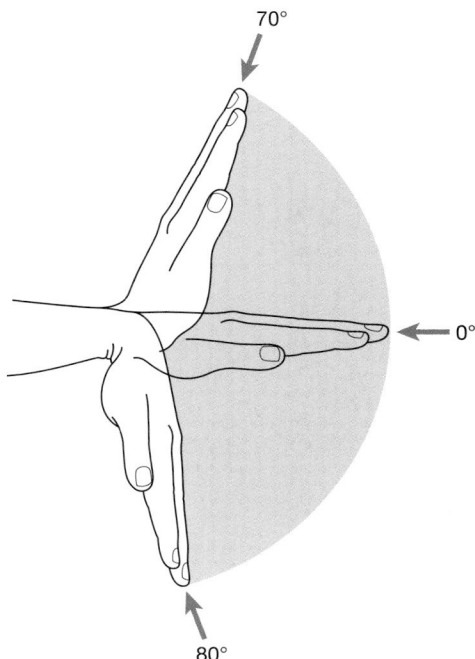

Figure 1-11 Wrist flexion and extension. Patient position: elbow flexed, radioulnar pronated. Plane of motion: Sagittal. Normal range of motion: flexion, 0–80°; extension, 0–70°. Goniometer placement: axis is centered on lateral wrist over ulnar styloid, stationary arm remains at 0°, movement arm remains parallel to fifth metacarpal.

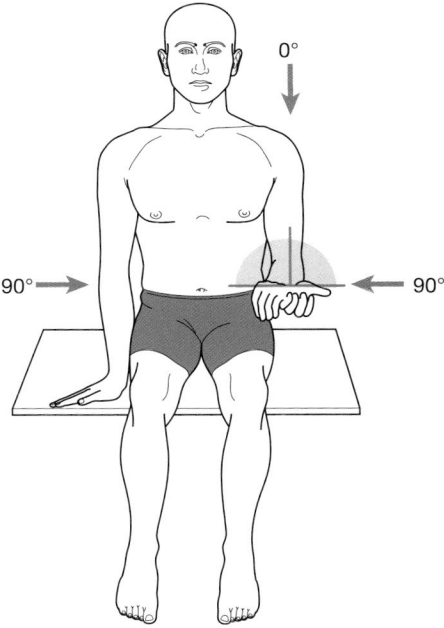

Figure 1-10 Radioulnar pronation and supination. Patient position: sitting or standing, elbow at 90°, wrist in neutral, pencil held in palm of hand. Plane of motion: transverse. Normal range of motion: pronation, 0–90°; supination, 0–90°. Movements the patient should avoid: arm, elbow, and wrist movements. Goniometer placement: axis through longitudinal axis of forearm, stationary arm remains at 0°, movement arm remains parallel to pencil held in patient's hand.

Assessment techniques Manual muscle testing takes into account the weight of the limb without gravity, with gravity, and with gravity plus additional manual resistance.[50] Most examiners use the Medical Research Council scale, where grades of 0–2 indicate gravity-minimized positions and grades 3–5 indicate increasing degrees of resistance applied as an isometric hold at the end of the test range (see Table 1-10).[50] A muscle grade of 3 is functionally important, as antigravity strength implies that a limb can be used for activity, whereas a grade of < 3 implies that the limb will require external support and is prone to contracture.[55] A 1- or 2-grade intertester difference is acceptable,[50] but poor intertester reliability can be a problem with grades below 3.[6] Other pitfalls encountered in testing strength are outlined in Table 1-11. To reduce measurement errors, one hand should be placed above and one below the joint being tested. As detailed in extended Tables 1-12 and

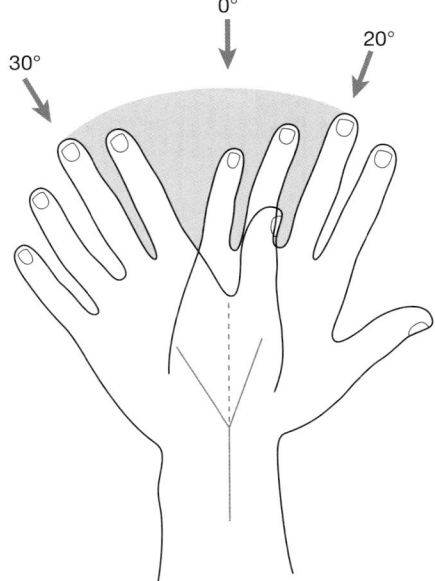

Figure 1-12 Wrist radial and ulnar deviation. Patient position: elbow flexed, radioulnar joint pronated, wrist in neutral flexion and extension. Plane of motion: frontal. Normal range of motion: radial, 0–20°; ulnar, 0–30°. Goniometer placement: axis is centered over dorsal wrist midway between distal radius and ulna, stationary arm remains at 0°, movement arm remains parallel to third metacarpal.

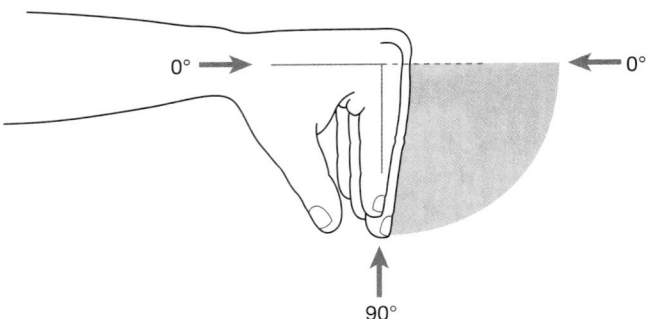

Figure 1-13 Second to fifth metacarpophalangeal flexion. Patient position: elbow flexed, radioulnar joint pronated, wrist in neutral, fingers extended. Plane of motion: sagittal. Normal range of motion: 0–90°. Goniometer placement: axis on dorsum of each metacarpophalangeal joint, stationary arm remains at 0°, movement arm remains on dorsum of each proximal phalanx.

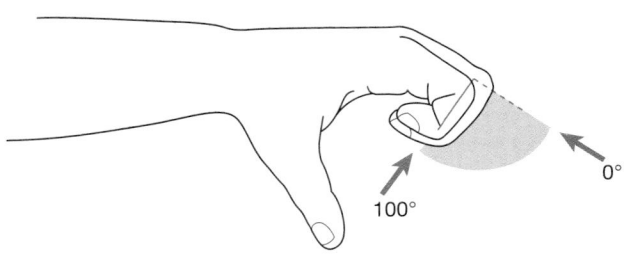

Figure 1-14 Second to fifth proximal interphalangeal flexion. Patient position: elbow flexed, radioulnar pronated, wrist in neutral, metacarpophalangeal joints in slight flexion. Plane of motion: sagittal. Normal range of motion: 0–100°. Goniometer placement: axis on dorsum of each interphalangeal joint, stationary arm remains at 0°, movement arm remains on dorsum of each middle phalanx.

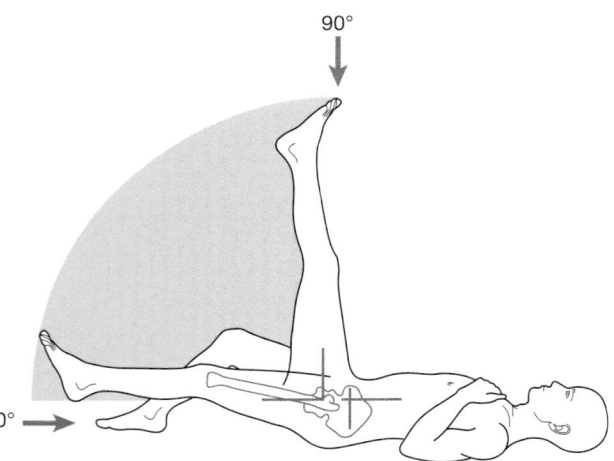

Figure 1-15 Hip flexion, knee extension. Patient position: supine or lying on side, knee extended. Plane of motion: sagittal. Normal range of motion: 0–90°. Movements the patient should avoid: arching back. Goniometer placement: axis is centered on lateral leg over greater trochanter, stationary arm remains at 0°. (This is found by drawing a line from the anterior superior iliac spine to the posterior superior iliac spine, and then drawing another line, perpendicular to the first, that goes through the greater trochanter. The last line is 0°.) Movement arm remains parallel to lateral femur.

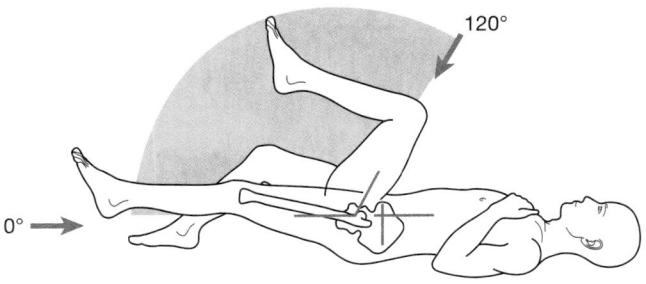

Figure 1-16 Hip flexion, knee flexion. Patient position: supine or lying on side, knee flexed. Plane of motion: sagittal. Normal range of motion: 0–120°. Movements the patient should avoid: arching back. Goniometer placement: axis centered over greater trochanter, stationary arm is parallel to and below a line on patient drawn through both anterior superior iliac spines (this is perpendicular to 0°), movement arm remains parallel to anterior femur.

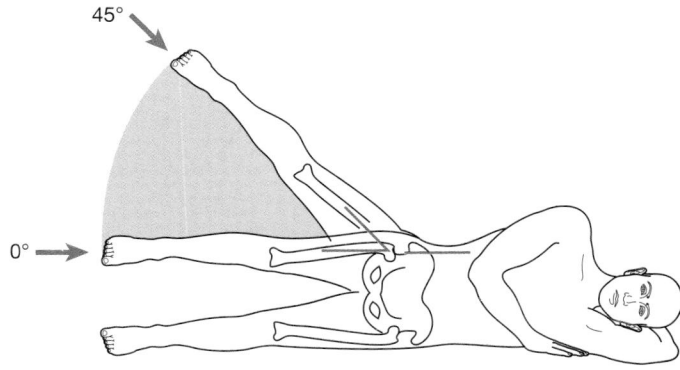

Figure 1-17 Hip abduction. Patient position: supine or lying on side, knee extended. Plane of motion: frontal. Normal range of motion: 0–45°. Movements the patient should avoid: trunk rotation. Goniometer placement: axis centered over greater trochanter, stationary arm is parallel to and below a line on patient drawn through both anterior superior iliac spines (this is perpendicular to 0°), movement arm remains parallel to anterior femur.

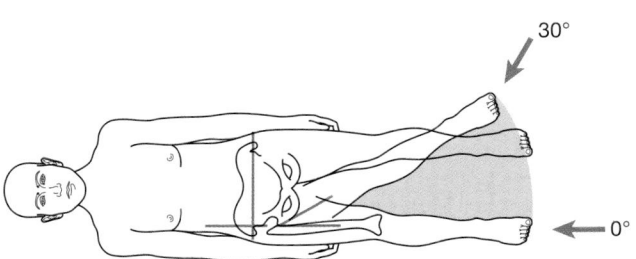

Figure 1-18 Hip adduction. Patient position: supine, knee extended. Plane of motion: frontal. Normal range of motion: 0–30°. Movements the patient should avoid: trunk rotation. Goniometer placement: axis over knee joint through longitudinal axis of femur, stationary arm remains at 0°, movement arm remains parallel to anterior tibia.

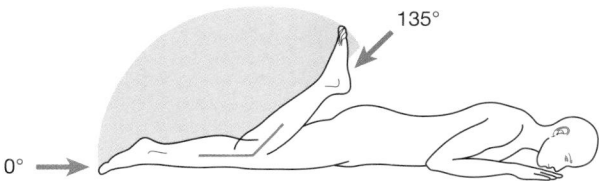

Figure 1-19 Knee flexion. Patient position: prone or sitting, hip in neutral. Plane of motion: sagittal. Normal range of motion: 0–135°. Goniometer placement: axis on lateral knee joint, stationary arm remains at 0°, movement arm remains parallel to fibula laterally.

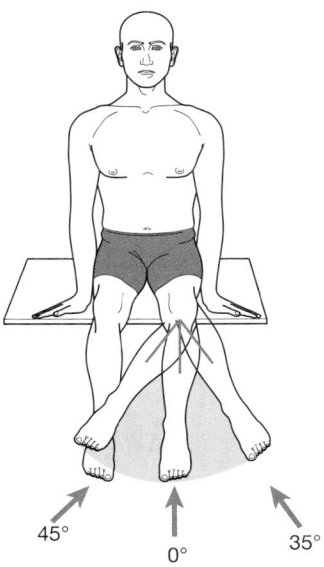

Figure 1-20 Hip internal and external rotation. Patient position: supine or sitting, hip at 90° flexion, knee at 90° flexion. Plane of motion: transverse. Normal range of motion: internal, 0–35°; external, 0–45°. Movements the patient should avoid: hip flexion movement, knee movement. Goniometer placement: axis over knee joint through longitudinal axis of femur, stationary arm remains at 0°, movement arm remains parallel to anterior tibia.

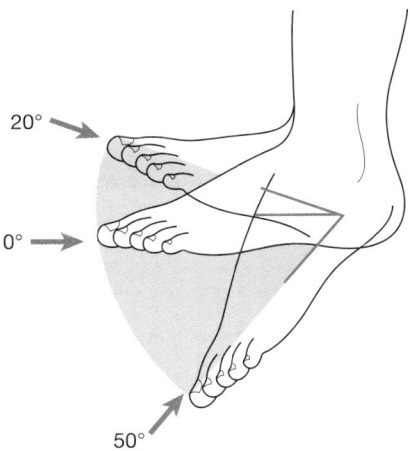

Figure 1-21 Ankle dorsiflexion and plantar flexion. Patient position: sitting or supine with knee flexed to 90°. Plane of motion: sagittal. Normal range of motion: dorsiflexion, 0–20°; plantar flexion, 0–50°. Goniometer placement: axis is on sole of foot below lateral malleolus, stationary arm remains along shaft of fibula (this is perpendicular to 0°), movement arm remains parallel to fifth metatarsal.

Table 1-10 Manual muscle testing

Grade	Term	Description
5	Normal	Full available range of motion (ROM) is achieved against gravity and is able to demonstrate maximal resistance
4	Good	Full available ROM is achieved against gravity and is able to demonstrate moderate resistance
3	Fair	Full available ROM is achieved against gravity *but* is not able to demonstrate resistance
2	Poor	Full available ROM is achieved only with gravity eliminated
1	Trace	A visible or palpable contraction is noted, with no joint movement
0	Zero	No contraction is identified

(After Cutter and Kevorkian 1999,[16] with permission of McGraw-Hill.)

Table 1-11 Caveats in manual muscle testing

Caveat	Rationale
Isolation	It is important to isolate individual muscles with similar functions instead of testing the entire muscle group
Substitution patterns	It is important to be aware of basic substitution patterns (e.g. elbow flexion)
Suboptimal testing conditions	These occur when determining patients' muscle strength when they are under the influence of, for example, sedation, significant pain, positioning, language or cultural barriers, spasticity, and hypertonicity
Over-grading	This occurs when the practitioner applies increased force when the patient is unable to achieve the full available range of motion (ROM) yet is able to demonstrate a muscle grade of 3 or more in a lengthened position
Under-grading	This occurs when the examiner is not aware of the effects of muscle contracture on ROM, and the muscle appears to lack full ROM when it has achieved its full available ROM

(After Cutter and Kevorkian 1999,[16] with permission of McGraw-Hill.)

Table 1-12 Upper limb muscle testing

Upper extremity chart	Muscle[a]	Nerve, roots	Plexus	Manual muscle testing technique	Figure
Shoulder flexion	*Deltoid, anterior portion*	Axillary, C5, C6	Posterior cord	• The shoulder is flexed to 90° with the elbow flexed at 90°. • The practitioner should attempt to force the arm into extension, with force applied over the distal humerus.	
	Pectoralis major, clavicular portion	Medial or lateral pectoral, C5 to T1	–		
	Biceps brachii	Musculocutaneous, C5, C6	Lateral cord		
	Coracobrachialis	Musculocutaneous, C5-7			
Extension	*Deltoid, posterior portion*	Axillary, C5, C6	Posterior cord	• The shoulder is extended to 45° with the elbow extended. • The practitioner attempts to force the arm into flexion, with force applied over the distal humerus.	
	Latissimus dorsi	Thoracodorsal, C6-8			
	Teres major	Lower subscapular, C5, C6			
Abduction	*Deltoid, middle portion*	Axillary, C5, C6	Posterior cord	• The shoulder is placed in 90° of abduction. • The practitioner attempts to adduct the arm, with force applied over the distal humerus.	
	Supraspinatus	Suprascapular, C5, C6	Upper trunk		
Adduction	*Pectoralis major*	Medial or lateral pectoral, C5 to T1	–	• The patient is supine with the shoulder in 120° of abduction and the elbow flexed. • The practitioner resists adduction of the arm.	
	Latissimus dorsi	Thoracodorsal, C6-8	Posterior cord		
	Teres major	Lower subscapular, C5, C6			
Internal rotation	*Subscapularis*	Upper or lower subscapular, C5, C6	Posterior cord	• The patient is prone and the shoulder is abducted to 90° with full internal rotation and the elbow at 90° of flexion. • The practitioner attempts to externally rotate the arm, applying force over the distal forearm.	
	Pectoralis major	Medial or lateral pectoral, C5 to T1	–		
	Latissimus dorsi	Thoracodorsal, C6-8	Posterior cord		
	Deltoid, anterior portion	Axillary, C5, C6			
	Teres major	Lower subscapular, C5, C6			

Continued on page 27

Continued from page 26 Table 1-12 Upper limb muscle testing

Upper extremity chart	Muscle[a]	Nerve, roots	Plexus	Manual muscle testing technique	Figure
External rotation	*Infraspinatus* Teres minor Deltoid, posterior portion	Suprascapular, C5, C6 Axillary, C5, C6	Upper trunk Posterior cord	• The patient is prone and the shoulder is placed in 90° of abduction with full external rotation and the elbow at 90° of flexion. • The practitioner attempts to internally rotate the arm, applying force over the distal forearm.	
Elbow flexion	*Biceps brachii* Brachialis Brachioradialis	Musculocutaneous, C5, C6 Radial, C5, C6	Lateral cord Posterior cord	• The elbow is positioned in 90° of flexion. • The practitioner attempts to extend the elbow, applying force over the distal forearm. • The biceps muscle is the primary elbow flexor, with full forearm supination. • The brachialis is the primary flexor, with full forearm pronation. • The brachioradialis is the primary elbow flexor when the forearm is in a thumbs-up position.	
Extension	*Triceps*	Radial, C6–8	Posterior cord	• The elbow is placed into flexion to prevent stabilization and to detect subtle weakness. • The practitioner attempts to flex the elbow, applying force over the distal forearm.	
Forearm pronation	*Pronator quadratus* Pronator teres	Anterior interosseus branch of median, C8, T1 Median, C6, C7	– Lateral cord	• The forearm is placed in full pronation. • The practitioner attempts to supinate the forearm, applying force to the distal forearm. • The pronator teres is tested when the elbow is at 90°. • The pronator quadratus is tested when the elbow is in full flexion.	
Forearm supination	*Supinator* Biceps brachii	Radial (posterior interosseus nerve), C5, C6 Musculocutaneous, C5, C6	Posterior cord Lateral cord	• The elbow is extended with the forearm in full supination. This position inhibits assistance from the biceps. • The practitioner attempts to pronate the forearm, applying force to the distal forearm.	

Continued on page 28

Continued from page 26 Table 1-12 Upper limb muscle testing

Upper extremity chart	Muscle[a]	Nerve, roots	Plexus	Manual muscle testing technique	Figure
Wrist flexion	*Flexor carpi radialis* Flexor carpi ulnaris	Median, C6–8 Ulnar, C6–8	Lateral cord Medial cord	• The wrist is placed in neutral position in full flexion, with the fingers extended. • The practitioner attempts to extend the wrist, applying force at the midpalm level. • The flexor carpi radialis is tested by placing the wrist in radial deviation and full flexion. The practitioner force the wrist into extension and ulnar deviation. • To test the flexor carpi ulnaris, the wrist is placed in ulnar deviation and full flexion. The practitioner attempts to force the wrist into extension and radial deviation.	
Wrist extension	*Extensor carpi radialis longus* Extensor carpi radialis brevis Extensor carpi ulnaris	Radial, C6, C7 Radial, C7, C8	Posterior cord	• The wrist is fully extended in a neutral position. • The practitioner attempts to flex the wrist, applying pressure over the dorsum of the hand. • To test the extensor carpi radialis longus, the patient's wrist is placed into radial deviation and full extension. The practitioner attempts to force the wrist into flexion and ulnar deviation. • To test the extensor carpi ulnaris, the wrist is placed in ulnar deviation and full extension. The practitioner attempts to force the wrist into flexion and radial deviation.	
Thumb abduction	*Abductor pollicis brevis* Abductor pollicis longus Extensor pollicis brevis	Median, C8, T1 Radial, C7, C8	Lateral or medial cord Posterior cord	• The thumb is abducted perpendicular to the plane of the palm. • The practitioner attempts to adduct the thumb (toward the palm), applying pressure just above the first metacarpophalangeal joint.	
Thumb opposition	*Opponens pollicis* Flexor pollicis brevis Abductor pollicis brevis	Median, C8, T1 Median: superficial head Ulnar: deep head, C8, T1 Median, C8, T1	Lateral or medial cord	• The thumb is placed in opposition. • The practitioner attempts to return the thumb into anatomic position, applying force above the first metacarpophalangeal joint.	

Continued on page 29

Upper extremity chart	Muscle[a]	Nerve, roots	Plexus	Manual muscle testing technique	Figure
Second to fifth digit flexion	*Flexor digitorum superficialis* Flexor digitorum profundus Lumbricals Interossei	Median, C7, C8, T1 Lateral portion: median Medial portion: ulnar, C7, C8, T1 Lateral two: median Medial two: ulnar, C8, T1 Ulnar, C8, T1	Lateral or medial cord	• The flexor digitorum superficialis extends to the proximal phalanx. • The practitioner attempts to force each proximal phalangeal joint into extension from a position of flexion. • The flexor digitorum profundus extends to the distal phalanx. • The practitioner tests both superficialis and profundus by forcing each middle phalangeal joint into extension from flexion. • The primary flexors of the metacarpophalangeal joints of the second to fourth digits are the lumbricals and the interossei. The practitioner tests these muscles by forcing each metacarpophalangeal joint into extension from a position of flexion. • The primary flexors of the fifth digit metacarpophalangeal joint are the flexor and abductor digiti minimi muscles. • The practitioner can test for fifth digit abduction.	– –
Second to fifth digit extension	*Extensor digitorum communis* Extensor indicis Extensor digiti minimi	Radial, C6–8 Radial, C7, C8	Posterior cord	• The second to fifth digits are placed in extension with the wrist at neutral position. • The practitioner attempts to force each finger into flexion by applying force over each proximal phalanx.	
Second to fourth digit abduction, first to fifth digit adduction	*Dorsal* or palmar interossei	Ulnar, C8, T1	Medial cord	• Abduction is tested by placing each digit in abduction and attempting to force the digit into adduction. • The third digit cannot adduct, as movement of this digit to either side is abduction.	
Fifth digit abduction	*Abductor digiti minimi* Flexor digiti minimi			• The patient's fifth digit is placed in abduction. • The practitioner attempts to force the digit into adduction by applying force above the metacarpophalangeal joint.	

Continued from page 26 Table 1-12 Upper limb muscle testing

[a]The primary muscles tested in the figures are in italics.
(After Jenkins 1998,[32] with permission, and Cutter and Kevorkian 1999,[16] with permission of McGraw-Hill.)

Table 1-13 Lower limb muscle testing

Lower extremity chart	Muscle(s)[a]	Nerve, roots	Testing	Figure(s)
Hip flexion	Iliacus Psoas Tensor fascia lata Rectus femoris Pectineus Adductor longus, brevis, anterior portion of magnus	Femoral, L2–4 Lumbar plexus, L1–4 Superior gluteal, L4, L5, S1 Femoral, L2–4 Femoral or obturator, L2, L3 Obturator, L2–4	• Hip flexion can be tested with the patient in a seated or supine position. • With the patient in the supine position, the practitioner forces the hip into extension, applying force over the distal anterior thigh. • With the patient in a sitting position, the hip is flexed while the practitioner attempts to extend the knee.	
Hip extension	Gluteus maximus	Inferior gluteal, L5, S1, S2	• With the patient in a prone position, the hip is extended with the knee flexed to 90°. • The practitioner attempts to flex the hip, applying force over the distal posterior thigh.	
Hip abduction	Gluteus medius Gluteus minimus Tensor fascia lata	Superior gluteal, L4, L5, S1	• The patient is placed in a side-lying position with the hip abducted. • The practitioner attempts to adduct the hip, applying force over the distal lateral thigh. • The test can also be performed with the patient seated. With the patient seated, the hips are abducted. The practitioner adducts the hips, applying force over the distal lateral thighs.	
Hip adduction	Adductor brevis Adductor longus Adductor magnus, anterior portion Pectineus	Obturator, L2–4 Obturator, L3, L4 Femoral or obturator, L2, L3	• With the patient in a side-lying position, the practitioner positions the top leg in abduction and the patient is asked to bring the bottom leg up into adduction to meet the top leg. • The practitioner attempts to abduct the bottom leg, applying pressure over the distal medial thigh. • The test can also be performed with the patient seated. With the patient seated, the hips are adducted. The practitioner abducts the hips, applying force over the distal medial thighs.	
Hip internal rotation	Tensor fascia lata Pectineus Gluteus minimus, anterior portion	Superior gluteal, L4, L5, S1 Femoral or obturator, L2, L3 Superior gluteal, L4, L5, S1	• The patient is seated with knees flexed at 90° and the hip is internally rotated. • The practitioner uses one hand to externally rotate the leg, applying lateral force just above the ankle, while stabilizing the knee with the other hand.	

Continued on page 31

Continued from page 30 Table 1-13 Lower limb muscle testing				
Lower extremity chart	Muscle(s)[a]	Nerve, roots	Testing	Figure(s)
Hip external rotation	*Piriformis* Gluteus maximus Superior gemelli or obturator internus Inferior gemelli or quadratus femoris	Nerve to piriformis, S1, S2 Inferior gluteal, L5, S1, S2 Nerve to obturator internus, L5, S1, S2 Nerve to quadratus femoris, L4, L5, S1	• The patient is seated with knees flexed at 90° and the hip is externally rotated. • The practitioner uses one hand to internally rotate the leg, applying medial force just above the ankle, while stabilizing the knee with the other hand.	
Knee flexion	*Semitendinosus* *Semimembranosus* *Biceps femoris*	Tibial portion of sciatic, L5, S1 Tibial portion of sciatic, L5, S1, S2	• The patient's knee is flexed at 90° while the patient is prone. • The practitioner attempts to force the leg into extension, applying pressure over the posterior tibial surface.	
Knee extension	*Quadriceps femoris*	Femoral, L2–4	• The knee is placed at 30° of flexion while the patient is seated or supine. Try to avoid full knee extension because the patient can stabilize the knee, allowing minor weakness to be missed. • The practitioner attempts to force the leg into flexion, applying pressure over the anterior tibial surface.	
Ankle dorsiflexion	*Tibialis anterior* Extensor digitorum longus Extensor hallucis longus	Deep peroneal, L4, L5, S1	• The ankle is placed in dorsiflexion. • The practitioner attempts to force the ankle into plantar flexion, applying force over the dorsum of the foot. • To test the anterior tibialis, the ankle is inverted and fully dorsiflexed. The practitioner attempts to plantar flex and evert the ankle. • To test the extensor digitorum longus, the ankle is everted and fully dorsiflexed. The practitioner attempts to plantar flex and invert the ankle.	
Plantar flexion	*Gastrocnemius* Soleus	Tibial, S1, S2	• The ankle is placed in plantar flexion. • The practitioner attempts to dorsiflex the foot, applying pressure over the plantar surface of the foot. • To test the gastrocnemius, the knee is extended. • To test the soleus, the knee is flexed at 90°. • More functional tests such as standing or walking on toes can show weakness missed during manual muscle testing.	

Continued on page 32

Table 1-13 Lower limb muscle testing

Lower extremity chart	Muscle(s)[a]	Nerve, roots	Testing	Figure(s)
Inversion	Tibialis anterior *Tibialis posterior* Flexor digitorum longus Flexor hallucis longus	Deep peroneal, L4, L5, S1 Tibial, L5, S1 Tibial, L5, S1, S2	• The tibialis anterior is tested in a position of inversion and dorsiflexion. The practitioner attempts to evert and plantar flex the foot, applying pressure on the medial surface of the foot. • The other three muscles produce plantar flexion and inversion. They are more selectively tested with placement of the foot in inversion and plantar flexion. The practitioner attempts to evert and dorsiflex the foot, applying pressure on the medial surface of the foot.	
Eversion	Extensor digitorum longus *Peroneus longus* *Peroneus brevis*	Deep peroneal, L4, L5, S1 Superficial peroneal, L4, L5, S1	• The extensor digitorum longus is tested in the position of eversion and dorsiflexion. • The practitioner attempts to invert and plantar flex the foot, applying pressure over the lateral surface of the foot. • The peroneus longus and brevis produce plantar flexion and eversion. They are more selectively tested with the foot everted and plantar flexed. The practitioner attempts to invert and dorsiflex the foot, applying pressure over the lateral surface of the foot.	
First digit extension	Extensor hallucis longus	Deep peroneal, L4, L5, S1	• The first toe is placed in full extension. • The practitioner attempts to flex the toe, applying pressure over the dorsum of the first toe.	
Second to fifth digit extension	*Extensor digitorum longus* Extensor digitorum brevis	Deep peroneal, L4, L5, S1 Deep peroneal, L5, S1	• The second and fifth toes are fully extended. • The practitioner attempts to flex them, applying pressure over the dorsum of the toes.	
First digit flexion	*Flexor hallucis longus* Flexor hallucis brevis	Tibial, L5, S1, S2 Medial plantar, L5, S1	• The first toe is placed in full flexion. • The practitioner attempts to extend the toe, applying pressure over the plantar surface of the first toe.	
Second to fifth digit flexion	*Flexor digitorum longus* Flexor digitorum brevis	Tibial, L5, S1 Medial plantar, L5, S1	• The second to fifth toes are placed in full flexion. • The practitioner attempts to extend them, applying pressure over the plantar surface of the toes.	

[a]The primary muscles tested in the figures are in italics.
(After Jenkins 1998,[32] with permission, and Cutter and Kevorkian 1999,[16] with permission of McGraw-Hill.)

1-13, the examiner's hands should not cross two joints, if possible. Placing a muscle at a mechanical disadvantage, such as flexing the elbow beyond 90° to assess triceps strength, can help demonstrate mild weakness.[30] Extended Tables 1-12 and 1-13 summarize the joint movement, innervation, and manual strength testing techniques for all major upper and lower extremity muscle groups, respectively. The use of a dynamometer can add a degree of objectivity to measurements for pinch and grip.

Dynamic screening tests of strength can also be done. A quick screen for the upper extremity strength is to have the patient grasp two of the examiner's fingers while the examiner attempts to free the fingers by pulling in all directions. For a proximal lower limb screen, the patient can demonstrate a deep knee bend (squat and rise), and for the distal lower extremity can walk on heels and toes. To make gait abnormalities more evident, patients can be asked to increase the speed of their cadence, and walk sideways and backward. Abdominal strength can be screened by observing the patient's ability to go from supine to sitting with the hips and knees bent. If the hips and knees are extended, the iliopsoas is tested as well.[30]

ASSESSMENT, SUMMARY, AND PLAN

Only after completing a thorough H&P is the physiatrist able to develop a comprehensive treatment plan. The organization of the initial treatment plan and goals can vary from setting to setting but should clearly state impairments, performance deficits (disability), community or role dysfunction (handicap), medical conditions that can impact achieving the functional goals, and goals for the interdisciplinary rehabilitation team (if other disciplines are involved in the patient's care). Follow-up treatment plans and notes are likely be shorter and less detailed, but they *must* address important interval changes since the last documentation and any significant changes in treatment or goals. This documentation is often used to justify continued payment for third-party payers. Noting whether problems are new, stable, improving, or worsening can be critical for accurate physician billing compliance documentation. Accurate identification and documentation of the etiologic cause of the impairment and disability can be required for hospital payment.

A summary statement of no more than a few to several sentences is helpful to medical consultants and other team members. Although development of a separate medical and functional problems list is acceptable and often recommended, the physiatrist should make very clear how those medical issues alter the approach to treatment (i.e. how either brittle diabetes, activity-induced angina, or pain issues might impact mobilization).

With a medical and functional problem list at hand, the management plan can be developed. Considering six broad interventional categories as originally outlined by Stolov et al.[54] is very helpful, particularly with complex patients in an inpatient rehabilitation setting. These six categories include prevention or correction of additional disability, enhancement

of affected systems, enhancement of unaffected systems, use of adaptive equipment, use of environmental modification, and use of psychologic techniques to enhance patient performance and education. The physician should clearly delineate the therapeutic precautions for the other team members. Goals, both short and longer term, should be outlined, as well as estimated timeframes for achieving those goals. Box 1-2 is an example of a rehabilitation plan for a patient following subarachnoid hemorrhage.

SUMMARY

Physiatrists pride themselves in their ability to do a complete physiatric H&P. The physiatric H&P begins with the standard medical H&P but goes beyond that to assess impairment,

---

Box 1-2 Rehabilitation plan

Summary statement
Ms. Jones is a right-handed, divorced, 69-year-old woman with a past medical history of hypertension, coronary artery disease (CAD), and depression, with recent rupture of a left middle cerebral artery (MCA) aneurysm, now 9 days post craniotomy for clipping. She currently is slightly lethargic and has moderately severe right hemiparesis, mild aphasia, right shoulder pain, and possible exacerbation of her underlying depression. She is on a regular diet with thickened liquids and is continent of bladder but has experienced some constipation. She is participating well in therapies, walking 15 ft with a wide-based quad cane, transferring with minimal assistance, and requiring moderate assistance in virtually all activities of daily living (ADL). Ms. Jones lived alone in an elevator-accessible apartment building where two of her daughters also live with their families.

Rehabilitation problem list and management plan
- Ambulatory dysfunction due to right hemiparesis: initiate neurodevelopmental techniques, forced-use paradigms, hold off on ankle–foot orthosis for now, evaluate for best assistive device, narrow-based quad cane, tone not a limitation at present.
- ADL dysfunction due to right hemiparesis: use neurodevelopmental techniques and encourage weight bearing on right upper extremity. Defer nighttime splint unless substantial increase in tone. See shoulder pain below. Tone not a limitation at present.
- Mild expressive aphasia: speech language pathology to evaluate, focus on higher level communication, especially in home setting.
- Dysphagia: swallowing evaluation per speech, proceed to modified barium swallow if needed.
- Shoulder pain: use of glass lap tray for constant support of right arm, will speak with physiotherapist regarding use of sling only with ambulation, to consider trial of non-opiate analgesic (watch for sedation), or diagnostic or therapeutic shoulder injection.
- Bowel and bladder: bladder fine, initiate oral stimulant to facilitate regular bowel habits.

Medical problem list and management plan
- Ruptured left MCA aneurysm: discontinue nimodipine 21 day post op, check phenytoin level as possible cause of slight lethargy, check with neurosurgery about changing

> **Box 1-2** Rehabilitation plan—cont'd
>
> or stopping antiepileptic as she has remained seizure-free, to consider repeat brain computerized tomography to rule out hydrocephalus as cause of lethargy.
> - Hypertension: stable in 140/90 range, monitor vitals closely in physiotherapy and occupational therapy, continue beta-blocker and diuretic.
> - CAD: no angina currently; monitor for shortness of breath, chest pain, and lightheadedness in therapies.
> - Depression: continue trazodone 300 mg at bedtime, doubt a cause of sleepiness as has been on this dose for many years. Monitor for mood disturbance, as a limitation in therapy participation.
> - Precautions: cardiac precaution, frequent vital sign monitoring during initial therapy sessions.
>
> **Goals**
> - Independent ambulation for household distances with assistive device (to be determined).
> - Independent in all transfers.
> - Supervision with assistive device for short-distance community ambulation, even surfaces.
> - Independent in ADL, except shoes, with assistive devices (to be determined); minimal assist for shoes.
> - Independent in all instrumental ADL, except meal preparation, supervision for meal preparation.
> - Independent in home exercise program, including passive range of motion to right hand or wrist and ankle.
> - Identify family members to provide supervision after discharge and complete hands-on teaching.
> - Maintain mood to participate fully in therapy.

disability, and handicap. The H&P is critical in gathering the information needed to formulate a treatment plan that can help the patient achieve the appropriate goals in the most efficient, least dangerous, and most cost-effective way possible.

REFERENCES

1. Adams RD, Victor M. Principles of neurology. 7th edn. New York: McGraw-Hill; 2001.
2. American Medical Association. Guides to the evaluation of permanent impairment. 4th edn. Chicago: American Medical Association; 1993.
3. [Anonymous]. Guide for the uniform data set for medical rehabilitation, version 5.1. Buffalo: State University of New York at Buffalo; 1997.
4. [Anonymous]. Occupational Therapy Practice Framework: domain and process. Am J Occup Ther 2002; 56:609–639 (Erratum in: Am J Occup Ther 2003; 57:115).
5. Bates BA. Guide to physical examination and history taking. 7th edn. Philadelphia: Lippincott; 1998.
6. Beasley WC. Quantitative muscle testing: principles and application to research and clinical services. Arch Phys Med Rehabil 1961; 42:398–425.
7. Bell BD, Hoshizak TB. Relationships of age and sex with range of motion of seventeen joint actions in humans. Can J Appl Sport Sci 1981; 6(4):202–206.
8. Birchwood M, Smith J, Drury V, et al. A self-report insight scale for psychosis: reliability, validity, and sensitivity to change. Acta Psychiatr Scand 1994; 89(1):62–67.
9. Brannon GE. History and mental status examination, 2002. Online. Available: http://www.emedicine.com
10. Caffarra P. Alexia without agraphia or hemianopia. Eur Neurol 1987; 27:65–71.
11. Cave EF, Roberts SM. A method of measuring and recording joint function. J Bone Joint Surg 1936; 18:455–466.
12. Centers for Medicare and Medicaid Services. Online. Available: http://www.cms.hhs.gov/
13. Chally PS, Carlson JM. Spirituality, rehabilitation, and aging: a literature review. Arch Phys Med Rehabil 2004; 85(suppl 3):S60–S65.
14. Cole TM, Tobis JS. Measurement of musculoskeletal function. In: Kottke FJ, Stillwell GK, Lehmann JF, eds. Handbook of physical medicine and rehabilitation. 3rd edn. Philadelphia: Saunders; 1982:20–72.
15. Corrigan JD. Substance abuse as a mediating factor in outcome from traumatic brain injury. Arch Phys Med Rehabil 1995; 76:302.
16. Cutter NC, Kevorkian CG. Handbook of manual muscle testing. New York: McGraw-Hill; 1999.
17. DeGowin RL. DeGowin's diagnostic examination. 6th edn. New York: McGraw-Hill; 1994.
18. DeLisa JA, Currie DM, Martin GM. Rehabilitation medicine: past, present and future. In: DeLisa JA, Gans BM, eds. Rehabilitation medicine: principles and practice. 3rd edn. Philadelphia: Lippincott; 1998:3–32.
19. Enelow AJ, Forde DL, Brummel-Smith K. Interviewing and patient care. 4th edn. New York: Oxford University Press; 1996:69–70.
20. Folstein MF, Folstein SE, McHugh PR. Mini-Mental State: a practical method for grading the cognitive state of patients for the clinician. J Psychiatr Res 1975; 12:189–198.
21. Froehling DA, Bowen JM, Mohr DN, et al. The canalith repositioning procedure for the treatment of benign paroxysmal positional vertigo: a randomized controlled trial. Cano Clin Proc 2000; 75:695–700.
22. Gabriel SE, Jaakkimainen L, Bombardier C. Risk for serious gastrointestinal complications related to use of nonsteroidal anti-inflammatory drugs. A meta-analysis. Ann Intern Med 1991; 115:787–796.
23. Gerhardt JJ, Rondinelli RD. Goniometric techniques for range-of-motion assessment. Phys Med Rehabil Clin N Am 2001; 12(3):507–527.
24. Giacino JT, Zasler ND, Katz DI, et al. Development of practice guidelines for assessment and management of the vegetative and minimally conscious states. J Head Trauma Rehabil 1997; 12(4):79–89.
25. Gilman S, Newman SW. Manter and Gatz's essentials of clinical neuroanatomy and neurophysiology. 8th edn. Philadelphia: FA Davis; 1992.
26. Goldberg S. The four-minute neurologic exam. Miami: Medmaster; 1999.
27. Griffin MR, Yared A, Ray WA. Nonsteroidal anti-inflammatory drugs and acute renal failure in elderly persons. Am J Epidemiol 2000; 151:488–496.
28. Groah SL, Lanig IS. Neuromusculoskeletal syndromes in wheelchair athletes. Semin Neurol 2000; 20:201–208.
29. Haymaker W, Woodhall B. Peripheral nerve injuries. Philadelphia: Saunders; 1953.
30. Hislop HJ. Daniels and Worthingham's muscle testing: techniques of manual examination. 6th edn. Philadelphia: Saunders; 1995.
31. Hoppenfeld S. Physical examination of the spine and extremities. Norwalk: Appleton & Lange; 1976.
32. Jenkins DB. Hollinshead's functional anatomy of the limbs and back. 7th edn. Philadelphia: Saunders; 1998.
33. Jennett B, Teasdale G. Assessment of impaired consciousness. Contemp Neurol 1981; 20:78.
34. Kelly-Hayes M, Wolf PA, Kase CS, et al. Time course of functional recovery after stroke: the Framingham Study. J Neurol Rehabil 1989; 3:65–70.
35. Kendall FP, McCreary EK, Provance PG. Muscles: testing and function. Baltimore: Williams & Wilkins; 1993.
36. Knapp ME, West CC. Measurement of joint motion. Univ Minn Med Bull 1944; 15:405–412.
37. Knapp ME. Measuring range of motion. Postgrad Med 1967; 42: A123–A127.
38. Kottke FJ, Lehman JF, eds. Krusen's handbook of physical medicine. 4th edn. Philadelphia: Saunders; 1990:21.
39. Lezak MD, Howieson DB, Loring DW. Neurological assessment. 4th edn. New York: Oxford University Press; 2004.
40. Lindsay KW, Bone I, Callander R. Neurology and neurosurgery illustrated. 3rd edn. New York: Churchill Livingstone; 1997.
41. Magee DJ. Orthopedic physical assessment, 3rd edn. Philadelphia: Saunders; 1997.

42. Mancall EL. Examination of the nervous system. In: Alpers and Mancall's essentials of the neurologic examination. 2nd edn. Philadelphia: FA Davis; 1993: 25.

43. Marottoli RA, et al. Driving cessation and increased depressive symptoms: prospective evidence from the New Haven EPESE. Established Populations for Epidemiologic Studies of the Elderly. J Am Geriatr Soc 1997: 45(2):202–206.

44. Martin RA, Lee EK, Langston EL. The neurologic examination: the family practice curriculum in neurology, 2001. Online. Available: http://www.aan.com/familypractice

45. Members of the Department of Neurology. Cano Clinic examination in neurology. 7th edn. Rochester: Cano Clinic and Cano Foundation; 1998.

46. Molnar GE, Alexander MA, eds. Pediatric rehabilitation. 3rd edn. Philadelphia: Hanley and Belfus; 1999.

47. Norkin CC, White J. Measurement of joint motion: a guide to goniometry. 3rd edn. Philadelphia: FA Davis; 2003.

48. O'Sullivan SB. Assessment of motor function. In: O'Sullivan SB, Schmitz TJ, eds. Physical rehabilitation: assessment and treatment. 4th edn. Philadelphia: FA Davis; 2001:177–212

49. Palmer JB, Drennan JC, Baba M. Evaluation and treatment of swallowing impairments. Am Fam Physician 2000; 61(8):2453–2462.

50. Palmer ML, Epler ME. Fundamentals of musculoskeletal assessment techniques. 2nd edn. New York: Lippincott; 1998.

51. Scalan J, Borson S. The Mini-Cog: receiver operating characteristics with expert and naive raters. Int J Geriatr Psychiatr 2001; 16:216–222.

52. Skilbeck CE, Wade DT, Langton Hewer R, et al. Recovery after stroke. J Neurol Neurosurg Psychiatr 1983; 46:5–8.

53. Stewart MA. Effective physician–patient communication and health outcomes: a review. CMAJ 1995; 152:1423–1433.

54. Stolov WC, Hayes RM, Kraft GH. In: Hayes RM, Kraft GH, Stolov WC, eds. Treatment strategies in chronic disease and disability: a contemporary approach to medical practice. New York: Demos; 1994:27–31.

55. Stolov WC. Evaluation of the patient. In: Kottke FJ, Stillwell GK, Lehmann JF, eds. Handbook of physical medicine and rehabilitation. 3rd edn. Philadelphia: Saunders; 1982:1–18.

56. Strub RL, Black FW. The mental status examination in neurology. 4th edn. Philadelphia: FA Davis; 2000.

57. Sunderland T, Hill JL, Mellow AM, et al. Clock drawing in Alzheimer's disease: a novel measure of dementia severity. J Am Geriatr Soc 1989; 37(8):725–729.

58. Tan JC. Practical manual of physical medicine and rehabilitation. St. Louis: Mosby; 1998.

59. Tomb D. House officer series: psychiatry. 5th edn. Baltimore: Williams & Wilkins; 1995.

60. Waddell G, Somerville D, Henderson I, et al. Objective clinical evaluation of physical impairment in chronic low back pain. Spine 1992; 17:617–628.

61. Whyte J, Laborde A, DiPasquale M. Assessment and treatment of the minimally conscious state. In: Rosenthal M, Griffith ER, Kreutzer JS, et al. Rehabilitation of the adult and child with traumatic brain injury. 3rd edn. Philadelphia: FA Davis; 1999:435–452.

62. Woo BH, Nesathurai S. The rehabilitation of people with traumatic brain injury. Malden: Blackwell Science; 2000.

63. World Heath Organization. International classification of impairments, disabilities, and handicaps. Geneva: World Health Organization; 1980.

64. World Heath Organization. International classification of impairments, activities, and participation. Geneva: World Health Organization; 1997.

Examination of the Pediatric Patient
Pamela Wilson and Susan D. Apkon

Assessment of an infant or a child requires that the examiner has the ability to attain a complete medical, developmental, and family history; has a flexible approach to the physical examination; and understands the unique interaction between a child and that child's physical and psychosocial environment. Establishing a diagnostic label is important, but determining the child's functional status is also important for the rehabilitation management of the child. Although the evaluation of children has many similarities to that of adults (see Ch. 1), it also has many distinctive features, as highlighted in this chapter.

DIAGNOSTIC EVALUATIONS

History

The clinical and developmental history is the basis of an accurate medical and rehabilitation diagnosis. The history is typically obtained from the parent, but children are generally able to participate in the diagnostic interview by the time they reach school age. Obtaining a medical history can be facilitated by having the parent fill out a new patient questionnaire before the clinical examination is started. Identification of the chief complaint focuses the history and the physical examination.

Many childhood disabilities reflect prenatal or perinatal problems. A history of maternal disease or acute illnesses, or pregnancy or labor abnormalities, can help guide the examination and diagnostic studies. The duration of the pregnancy, description of fetal movements, the ease or difficulty of labor, and complications during labor and delivery should be included in the history. Decreased fetal movement can be an indicator of a primary neuromuscular disorder such as spinal muscular atrophy.

Events during the newborn period might retrospectively shed light on a current disorder. The examiner should record any unusual episodes of cyanosis or respiratory distress, seizures, and other physical symptoms such as jaundice or anemia. The Apgar score is an important piece of information about the infant in the immediate perinatal period. The Apgar score is usually recorded at 1 min and 5 min after birth. When problems are apparent or the Apgar score is less than 7 after 5 min, the infant is reevaluated every 5 min up to 20 min. A score of 7–10 is considered normal. Five factors are used to evaluate the baby's condition, and each factor is scored on a scale of 0–2. The five factors are heart rate, respiratory effort, muscle tone, reflex response, and color.

The feeding history can also suggest potential neurologic abnormalities. The examiner should ask about and record any difficulties with sucking or swallowing, whether the baby is or was breast-fed or bottle-fed, and the volume and frequency of feedings. If feeding difficulties are present, obtaining growth records from the primary care provider is important to determine the impact on height and weight.

The medical history in all children should include chronic medical problems, hospitalizations, procedures, and surgeries. A list of medications and allergies should be documented as well as the status of the child's immunizations.

A history should include a determination of the ages at which major developmental milestones were met, as this aids in assessing deviations from normal (Table 2-1). The achievement of major landmarks in gross motor, fine motor, and adaptive skills; in speech and language; and in personal and social behavior should clarify whether the disability is confined primarily to the neuromuscular system or involves deficits in other areas as well. The coexistence of multiple problems influences the rehabilitation program, interventional methods, and ultimate outcome.

A psychosocial history contributes to the understanding and management of able-bodied as well as disabled children. It is important to determine how the child interacts with family and friends. A child with an autistic spectrum disorder such as Asperger syndrome has a difficult time interacting with both adults and peers.[46] Another example is that children with significant behavioral problems can have learning problems in the school setting.

A family history can assist in the identification of inherited or congenital problems. Formal genetic counseling and evaluation is required whenever an inherited disease is suspected or known to exist. It frequently is helpful to briefly examine a family member if a genetic disorder is suspected. For example, assessing a parent for grip myotonia or the inability to release and quickly open up the hand can be done with a simple handshake. Examination of the parent's foot can demonstrate a pes cavus or high-arched foot, which when present in the child is suggestive of the autosomal dominant form of Charcot–Marie–Tooth disease (see Ch. 48).

Physical examination

There is no standardized approach to the physical examination of infants and children.[1,5,21,22,29] Pediatric examinations are

Table 2-1 Developmental milestones

Age (months)	Milestone(s)
1	Lifts head (prone), vocalizes
3	Follows, laughs, smiles, has good head control
5	Plays with feet, reaches for and grasps objects
6	Sits with support
8	Sits without support, equilibrium reflexes present, looks for objects
9	Plays peek-a-boo, gets to sitting position, parachute reflex present, stranger anxiety
10	Pulls to stand, cruises, babbles
12–14	First words, walks
18	Multiple single words, uses spoon, removes clothes
24	Uses two-word phrases, throws overhand, 'terrible twos'
30	Knows full name, puts on clothing
36	Jumps, pedals tricycle, learns nursery rhymes
48	Hops, plays with others

tailored to the individual child, based on age and developmental stage. Knowledge of developmental stages is key in evaluating both acute and chronic diseases. Young children should be examined with the parents present, but the parents' presence is optional for adolescents.

It is critical to develop rapport with the child before performing a hands-on examination. This can be achieved by playing with and talking to the child. During this time, the examiner carefully observes the child's every movement and interaction. Observation is a primary tool used by a skilled practitioner. Even before touching the child, the clinician typically has gained a wealth of information.

The actual hands-on approach varies from child to child. A flexible approach that capitalizes on opportunities to evaluate different systems as they present themselves is recommended. Young children often are best examined while sitting on a parent's lap, while the older child can be examined on the table. The child's clothing should be removed for a complete examination. Removing clothing from very young children can be very stressful to the child and should be done gradually. The modesty of older children must be respected.

Growth

Growth during infancy occurs at a very rapid rate, slows during early childhood, and increases once again during adolescence. Routine healthcare visits should emphasize the evaluation of growth parameters for every child, including height, weight, and head circumference. It is critical for a child's growth to be plotted on age- and gender-appropriate charts.[9] Growth is influenced not only by genetic programming but also by medical conditions and nutrition. The onset of organic or psychosocial illness might be accompanied by a sudden acceleration or cessation of growth. The rate of growth is more important than the absolute values, as evidenced by a child whose head circumference increases from the 5th percentile to the 50th percentile in a 2-month period, representing untreated hydrocephalus. Growth charts are now available for specific genetic syndromes, including Turner and Down syndromes, and for specific disabilities such as quadriplegic cerebral palsy.

Head circumference is measured serially using the occipitofrontal circumference. The average head circumference at birth is 35 cm and increases to 47 cm by 1 year of age.[25] Microcephaly is defined by a head circumference that falls below two standard deviations from the mean, and is suggestive of central nervous system abnormalities including congenital infections, anoxic encephalopathy, or a degenerative disorder. Macrocephaly, defined as a head circumference greater than two standard deviations above the mean, can be associated with hydrocephalus, a metabolic disease, or presence of a mass and requires further evaluation. Approximately 50% of macrocephaly in children is familial in nature. Parental head size should be plotted on adult growth charts. A child with an isolated large head, no developmental delays, and a parent with a large head is probably normal.

The average height of a newborn is 50 cm, increasing by 50% at 1 year of age, and doubling by age 4 (100 cm).[25] An estimate of adult height is obtained by doubling the child's height at age 2 years. Many genetic syndromes are associated with short stature, including Down and Turner syndromes. Guidelines for predicting the weight gain of young children include doubling birth weight by 6 months and tripling that weight by 1 year of age.

Adolescents pass through a predictable sequence of pubertal events as they mature. The Tanner stages of sexual maturity describe the secondary sexual characteristics of teenage girls and boys.[32,33] Assessment of breast development and pubic hair in girls, and genital size and pubic hair in boys, is the basis for assigning a Tanner stage to an adolescent. The average age of menarche in girls is typically around 12 years. Precocious puberty is diagnosed if there is a premature development of secondary sexual characteristics. It is present when there are findings of puberty in girls under 8 years of age and in boys under 9 years of age.[53] The etiology can be either peripheral or within the central nervous system, such as a hypothalamic–pituitary abnormality. Precocious puberty is well documented in children with spina bifida and brain injuries.[50] Tanner staging is useful in evaluating musculoskeletal issues such as leg length discrepancies and scoliosis, as treatment options can vary depending on the pubertal stage of the child.

General inspection

Visual inspection is critical in the examination of a child. It begins with a general assessment of the child's appearance. This gives the examiner a sense of how the infant or child interacts

Table 2-2 Common syndromes and the associated abnormal features

Syndrome	Abnormalities
Angelman syndrome	Severe mental retardation, delay in attainment of motor milestones, microbrachycephaly, maxillary hypoplasia, deep-set eyes, blond hair (65%), ataxia and jerky arm movements resembling a puppet gait (100%), seizures
Hunter syndrome	Growth deficiency, coarsening of facial features, full lips, macrocephaly, macroglossia, contractures of joints, broadening of bones, hepatosplenomegaly, delayed tooth eruption
Marfan syndrome	Tall stature with long slim limbs, little subcutaneous fat, arachnodactyly, joint laxity, scoliosis (60%), retinal detachment, upward lens subluxation, dilatation of ascending aorta
Neurofibromatosis syndrome	Areas of hyper- or hypopigmentation with café au lait spots (94%); 'freckling' of axilla, inguinal folds, and perineum; cutaneous neurofibromas that are small, soft, pigmented nodules; plexiform neurofibromas; Lisch nodules

with the parents as well as information about the child's general movements, abnormal physical features, and overall general health. The presence of abnormal physical features can be helpful in identifying common syndromes (Table 2-2). The examiner should pay specific attention to facial abnormalities such as abnormal spacing of the eyes, position and size of the ears, philtrum, and size of the upper and lower jaws. Normal measurements can be referenced when attempting to distinguish specific features such as ocular hypertelorism or small-appearing ears.[26]

The assessment of the head and neck includes inspection of shape and symmetry. Since the American Academy of Pediatrics initiated the *Back to Sleep* program in 1992, the recommendation for newborns and infants to sleep in the supine position, more infants are presenting to their primary care providers with the presence of plagiocephaly, primarily observed as a unilateral flattening of the occiput.[40] Examination of the head and neck can also identify the presence of torticollis involving tightness of the sternocleidomastoid muscle. Children with torticollis have a head tilt to the involved side, and the chin will be turned to the contralateral side. Children with a short, broad neck with webbing can represent Klippel–Feil syndrome or Turner syndrome in girls.

Abnormalities of the chest wall shape often signify a specific disease such as the bell-shaped chest in an infant with spinal muscular atrophy Type 1. Inspection of the genitalia can be useful in characterizing certain syndromes. Boys with fragile X syndrome typically have large testes, while boys with Prader–Willi syndrome classically have a small penis. Visual inspection of the extremities might reveal pseudohypertrophy of the calves, as seen in boys with Duchenne muscular dystrophy. Children with hemiplegic cerebral palsy often have asymmetries in the girth of the arm or leg, with the affected side being visibly smaller.

Evaluation of the skin includes an assessment of the nails and hair. The examiner looks for neurocutaneous lesions and other skin abnormalities. Café au lait spots in the axilla or inguinal regions can be an indication of neurofibromatosis, while white ash leaf spots can point toward a diagnosis of tuberous sclerosis. Port wine stains (flat hemangiomas) that involve the first branch of the trigeminal nerve are associated with Sturge–Weber syndrome. The presence of calluses and abrasions on the feet are often indicators of abnormal weight bearing or insensate skin, as seen in a child with a spinal cord injury or peripheral neuropathy.

Musculoskeletal assessment

The pediatric musculoskeletal evaluation includes observation, palpation, range of motion determination, and functional assessment. Observation focuses on posture, body symmetry, and movement. Palpation should include the skin, muscles, and joints. The muscle examination should focus on size, bulk, and tone. The joints are palpated to detect tenderness, swelling, synovial thickening, and warmth. Range of motion should be assessed for all major joints.

The spine and back examination includes an assessment of the bones and muscular elements, as well as a postural assessment. Evaluation includes having the child stand or sit while the back is examined. The height of the shoulders, position of scapula, and height of the pelvis should be assessed. The child is asked to bend forward so the examiner can look for rib and back asymmetries indicating scoliosis (Fig. 2-1). Radiographs of the spine help define the severity of kyphotic and scoliotic curves. Scoliosis is categorized as infantile, juvenile, adolescent, or neuromuscular. The most common form is adolescent idiopathic scoliosis seen in pubertal girls with a right thoracic curve.[34] Children should also be evaluated for other spinal pathology (Table 2-3).

Examination of the lower limbs includes an evaluation of joint range of motion and torsional forces. Most torsional deformities tend to correct spontaneously as children grow and develop. Evaluation of the foot includes the toes and the three parts of the foot: forefoot, midfoot, and hind foot. The shoes should be assessed for patterns of wear. The most common foot deformity is metatarsus adductus, which is medial deviation of the metatarsal bones (Fig. 2-2). It is usually caused by intra-uterine position, and the severity of the deformity can be classified according to the flexibility of the foot. Mild anomalies are easily corrected, while moderate cases require that some force be applied to the foot. Severe abnormalities cannot be corrected by conservative means and should be referred to an orthopedic surgeon.

Pes planus, or flatfoot, is a normal variant seen in children up to the age of 3–5 years.[48] It occurs when the medial longitudinal arch is not well developed or there is underlying ligamentous laxity. Flexible flatfeet can also be a normal variant into adulthood, as long as an arch forms when the individual stands on their toes. Rigid or painful feet with reduced subtalar joint motion are often associated with tarsal coalition. This is an abnormal fusion of two or more bones in the midfoot or hind foot that restricts motion. The two most common joints involved are the talocalcaneal and calcaneonavicular. Congenital vertical talus is a rigid flatfoot deformity with a rocker bottom and a dorsal dislocation of the navicular on the talus. It is associated with the genetic syndromes myelodysplasia and arthrogryposis.

Pes cavus is a high-arched foot that does not flatten with weight bearing. It is often associated with clawing of the toes, hind foot varus, plantar fascia contractures, and great toe cock-up deformities. It can be a normal variant or might indicate a neuromuscular disorder such as Charcot–Marie–Tooth (Fig. 2-3).

Congenital talipes equinovarus, or the classic clubfoot, is a complex deformity characterized by a small foot with a medial border crease, hind foot equinus, and forefoot and hind foot

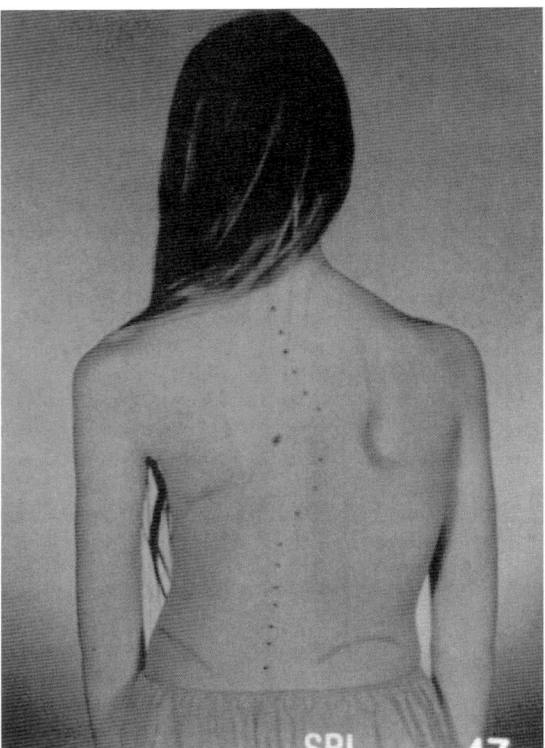

Figure 2-1 The evaluation of scoliosis includes an assessment of the spine with the child sitting or standing. This adolescent girl has an obvious curve in the standing position. She also has a rotational component.

Table 2-3 Spinal abnormalities	
Spine abnormality	Clinical findings
Scoliosis (idiopathic, congenital, neuromuscular)	Curvature of spine on forward bending Rib humping Shoulder asymmetry Pelvic obliquity
Kyphosis (congenital, Scheuermann, neuromuscular)	Abnormal posture increases with flexion
Spondylolisthesis	Loss of lordosis, reduced range of motion Step-off back deformity Gait abnormalities Transverse abdominal creases

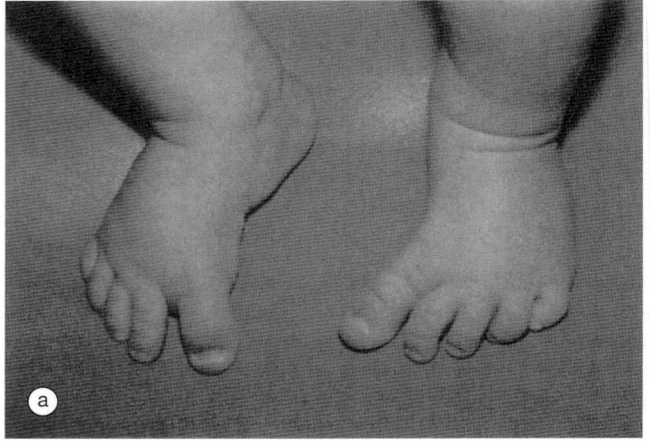

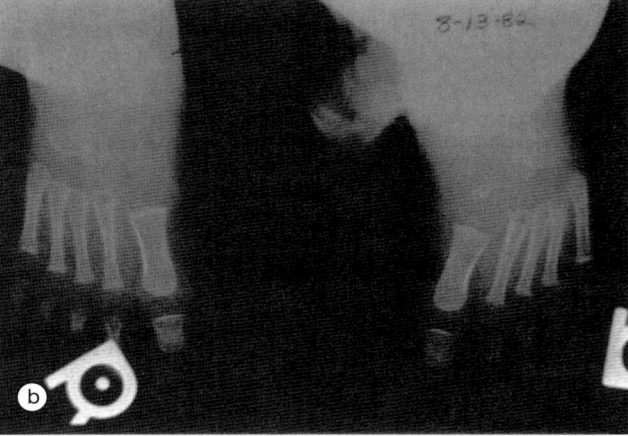

Figure 2-2 A child with bilateral metatarsus adductus (**a**). X-rays showing medial deviation of the metatarsal bones (**b**).

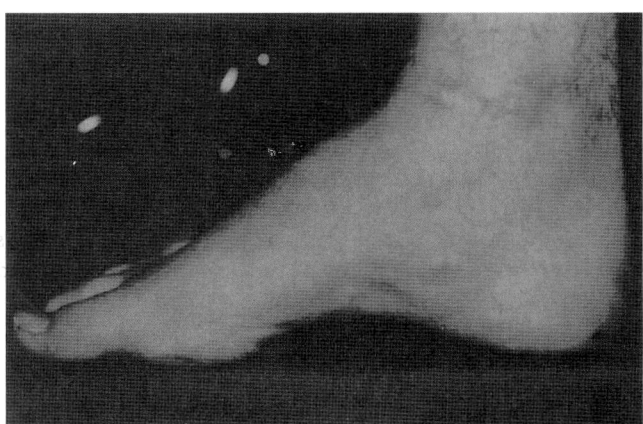

Figure 2-3 High-arched foot, or pes cavus, is seen in neuromuscular disorders.

varus, along with forefoot adductus.[42] The etiology remains controversial, as several theories have been proposed including intrauterine position, primary germ cell defect in the talus causing persistent plantar flexion and inversion, and soft tissue abnormalities impacting the neuromuscular units. There is an association with other disorders such as cerebral palsy, arthrogryposis, chromosomal abnormalities, spina bifida, and neuromuscular diseases.

The knee should be evaluated for mobility and stability. The child should be assessed for genu varum and genu valgum. The lower extremities progress through predictable changes over the course of development. Initially, children are bowlegged (genu varus position) until about age 2 years. Knee growth is rapid, and the lower limbs shift to a valgus or knock-kneed position until 5–7 years, at which time they tend to straighten out into a more adult-type position. If excessive bowing persists, the child might have Blount disease. This condition refers to disordered growth of the proximal medial physis, epiphysis, and metaphysis, which causes varus angulation and internal rotation of the tibia. It is more common in females of African-American descent who are early walkers. It is generally progressive and requires lower leg radiographs for diagnosis. The normal metaphyseal–diaphyseal angle is less than 11° and the tibial–femoral angle should be less than 15°.

Tibial torsion is a twisting of the distal tibia in relationship to the proximal segment.[31] It can result in either internal or external rotation of the tibia and can cause an abnormal-appearing gait pattern. Children have approximately 5° of internal tibial torsion at birth, which progresses to 10–15° in the adult. It is the most common reason for in-toeing in the toddler age range. The evaluation includes assessment of the position of the patella during gait, along with the thigh–foot angle (Fig. 2-4). Thigh–foot angle is assessed in the prone position with the knee flexed to 90°. Two bisecting lines are drawn: one along the femur and the other through the heel and third web space. The angle should be −10° to +10°.

The hip should be evaluated for torsional forces, including femoral anteversion and retroversion, along with routine range

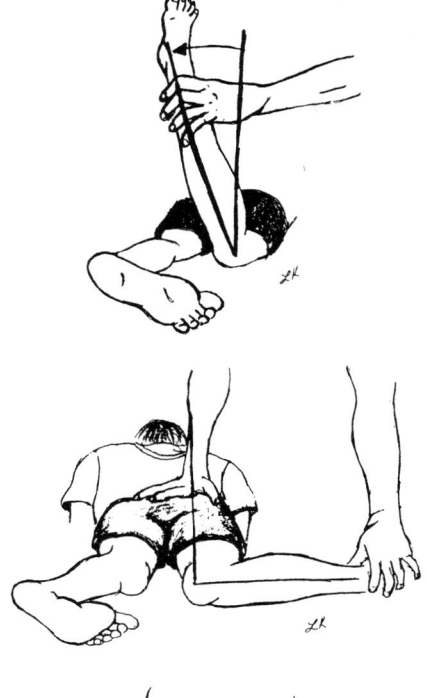

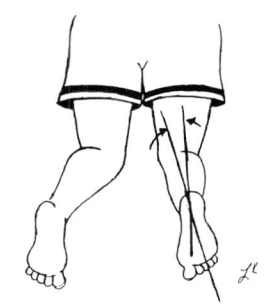

Figure 2-4 Evaluation of a child in the prone position allows assessment of the thigh–foot angle, and internal and external rotation of the hip. The thigh–foot angle is demonstrated in the lower diagram and ranges from −3° to +20°.

of motion including assessment of both internal and external rotation. Femoral anteversion is a twisting of the femur between the femoral neck and the femoral condyles. The femoral neck moves forward in relation to the rest of the femur. The result is increased internal rotation at the hip. Infants normally have 30–40° of anteversion at birth, which shifts to around 15–25° when full grown. Femoral anteversion is the most common cause of in-toeing in the older child up to age 10 years. Children with excessive femoral anteversion often present as clumsy, pigeon-toed walkers whose patella are rotated medially. Femoral retroversion can cause out-toeing, clinically opposite to anteversion and less likely to correct with growth, as the forces tend to rotate the femur outward. Evaluation of hip rotation measurements are done with the child in the prone position (Fig. 2-4). Hip abduction should be assessed with the child supine (Fig. 2-5). Asymmetry of the range of motion can indicate hip subluxation, dislocation, contracture, or spasticity.

All newborns should be screened for developmental dysplasia of the hip (DDH) at birth and during subsequent evaluations. DDH is a common disorder that has a higher incidence in firstborn children, females, and infants with a family history of DDH. A complete examination includes evaluating skin folds, leg lengths (Galeazzi sign), range of motion, and provocative tests. The provocative maneuvers are referred to as the Ortolani and Barlow tests. Both tests are done with the infant supine and the hips flexed to 90°. In the Ortolani test, the examiner attempts to relocate a dislocated hip. With the fingers placed over the greater trochanter, the examiner gently abducts the hips and lifts up on the trochanter. A click or a clunk suggests a hip instability. In the Barlow method, the examiner attempts to dislocate the infant's hips. Holding the hips in the same manner as in the Ortolani examination, the hips are adducted and a downward force is applied, causing a click or clunk in a dislocated hip. Early diagnosis of DDH is critical for achieving the best long-term outcome.

The musculoskeletal assessment is not complete without a thorough evaluation of the upper limbs. A routine examination should include traditional observation, palpation, range of motion, and functional assessment. In newborns and infants, reflexive patterns can be used to grossly evaluate the shoulder

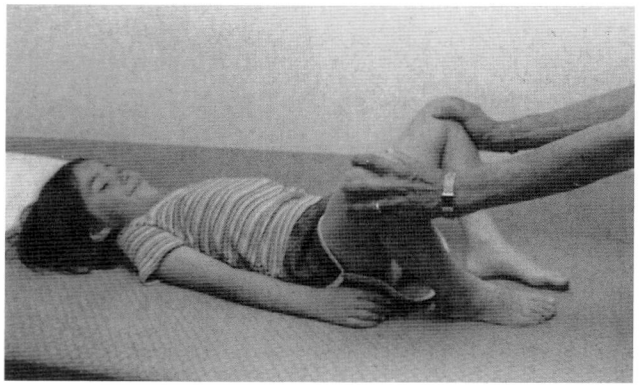

Figure 2-5 Examination of the hips should include passive range of motion, such as hip abduction, along with assessment of tone and spasticity.

and elbow. An asymmetric Moro reflex can be the first indicator of a brachial plexus lesion. These are fairly common. Most are neurapraxic nerve injury due to stretch and typically spontaneously resolve. Brachial plexus injuries referred to as an Erb palsy are located in the upper trunk and diagnosed when children present with the classic waiter tip posture (adducted, internally rotated shoulders, extended elbow, and flexed wrist). Less commonly observed is the Klumpke palsy or lower trunk injury. These children have a normal shoulder examination but have hand involvement. Other problems encountered at the shoulder include clavicular fractures, shoulder dislocations, and overuse injuries. The most common congenital shoulder abnormality is a Sprengel deformity. It is a failure of the scapula to descend, causing it to be abnormally placed too high. This results in asymmetry of the shoulder, a short-appearing neck, and limited range of motion.

The hand is critical in a child's ability to develop play skills. Hand movement progresses from a very primitive grasp and release pattern to a sophisticated ability to manipulate objects. Many classic pathologic processes are reflected in the position and appearance of the hand. Palmar creases are an indication of fetal movement and genetic syndromes. Individuals with Down syndrome often have a transverse or simian palmar crease. The shape and size of the fingers can indicate genetic disorders. Developmental skills can be noted by observing the function of the hand and fingers. Absent or delayed skills can indicate a focal or global process. Development of dominant handedness prior to 18 months is abnormal and can be the first indicator of hemiplegic cerebral palsy.

The child's gait should be carefully analyzed and evaluated. Components of the gait cycle including the stance and swing phases are evaluated. Young children typically have progressive changes in gait characteristics, but generally the patterns mature by 7 years of age.[28] Understanding normal and abnormal gait patterns helps the practitioner make diagnostic and functional decisions (Table 2-4).

Table 2-4 Gait abnormalities		
Gait	Characteristic(s)	Clinical association
Spastic	Adducted hips Internal rotation of hips Toe walking	Cerebral palsy
Crouched	Weak quadriceps Weak hip extensors Excessive dorsiflexion Hip or knee contractures	Neuromuscular disease Cerebral palsy
Hemiparetic	Posturing of upper extremity Circumduction of hip Inversion of foot	Cerebral palsy Cerebral vascular accident
Waddling (Trendelenburg) Ataxic	Weakness of hip girdle Wide-based gait Coordination problems Poor tandem walking	Neuromuscular disease Cerebellar ataxia Friedreich ataxia

Neurologic assessment

Examination of the neuromuscular system includes assessment of muscle strength, a mental status examination, cranial nerve evaluation, assessment of reflexes, observation of coordination and balance, and assessment of the sensory system. The examiner must be flexible, as these components might have to be done simultaneously instead of sequentially. The evaluation of normal and abnormal primitive reflexes and postural responses is a critical part of the assessment.

Developmental reflex assessment is a critical tool in evaluating a typical infant or an infant or child with a disability. Motor behaviors in newborns are dominated by primitive reflexes that are controlled at the level of the brain stem and spinal cord.[16] These reflexes develop during gestation and disappear between the third and sixth month of life. Primitive reflexes are a predictable, involuntary response to a specific sensory stimulus (Table 2-5). Suppression of primitive reflexes reflects central nervous system maturation. Persistence or reoccurrence of abnormal reflexes is a strong indicator of neurologic dysfunction. The presence of an obligatory primitive reflex, one that a child cannot volitionally get out of, is always abnormal and suggests a central nervous system disorder. Primitive reflexes are precursors to volitional motor skills. Developmentally, primitive

reflexes are replaced by postural reactions, which are involuntary postural patterns that enable righting, equilibrium, or protective movements (Table 2-6). Postural reactions appear in an organized fashion after 2–3 months of age and allow an infant to predictably progress with motor development, including rolling, sitting, and walking. Head righting is one of the automatic postural responses, elicited by sensory input that signals when the head or trunk is not in the midline. The parachute reaction, a protective extension of limbs to prevent or break a fall, is elicited by vestibular input signaling a change in head position. With few exceptions, postural reactions persist throughout life. Delays in the appearance of postural reactions are often detrimental to acquiring new voluntary motor skills.

Muscle tone refers to the amount of resistance present in muscles through passive range of motion. Muscle tone changes during development and can be affected by activity, alertness, and comfort. Flexor tone predominates in the first several months of infancy. A newborn infant is more hypotonic than a toddler. If true hypotonia persists, it generally points to an abnormality in the central nervous system, peripheral nervous system, or muscle. Hypertonia indicates an abnormality within the central nervous system that can be further defined as spas-

Table 2-5 Common primitive reflexes and the time period they typically disappear

Reflex	Stimulus	Response	Disappears by
Moro	Sudden neck extension	Shoulder abduction, elbow and finger extension followed by shoulder adduction and elbow flexion	4–6 months
Rooting	Stroking area around mouth	Head and mouth move toward stimulus	4 months
Asymmetric tonic neck	Head turned to side	Arm or leg extend on face side and flex on occipital side	6–7 months
Symmetric tonic neck	Neck flexion, neck extension	Arms flex, legs extend; arms extend, legs flex	6–7 months
Palmar grasp	Touch palm	Flexion of all fingers	5–6 months

Table 2-6 Postural reactions and the time period they typically occur

Postural reaction	Stimulus	Response	Age of emergence
Head righting	Vestibular or visual	Head and face aligned vertical and mouth aligned horizontal	Prone 2 months, supine 3–4 months
Protective extension	Center of gravity displaced outside base of support in sitting	Abduction of upper extremity toward displacement to prevent falling	Sitting anterior, 5–7 months; lateral, 6–8 months; posterior, 7–8 months
Parachute reaction	Center of gravity displaced outside base of support in standing	Extension of upper extremities toward displacement to prevent falling	Standing, 12–14 months

ticity, rigidity, or dystonia.[45] Spasticity is velocity-dependent and results in resistance to muscle stretch, while dystonia is an involuntary pattern of muscle contractions and posture causing twisting and abnormal postures. Rigidity is present when resistance to movement is not influenced by the speed or position of the limb. An individual with a disability can have an isolated movement disorder or a combination of patterns. Muscle stretch reflexes are easily elicited in children of all ages. Absent or reduced reflexes can indicate an anterior horn cell disease, a peripheral neuropathy, or a myopathy. An increase in reflexes is often associated with an upper motor neuron process, suggesting central nervous system involvement.

Strength testing or manual muscle testing can be formally examined in the schoolage child, utilizing the same scoring system as in adults (see Ch. 1). Young children can present a challenge to the examiner as a result of a short attention span or a lack of understanding or cooperation, depending on their age and developmental level. A modified scale must be used in this situation. Use of a 0- to 4-point scale is recommended, with 0 indicating no movement; 1, trace movement; 2, movement with gravity eliminated; 3, movement against gravity; and 4, the child can take resistance. (This is the same as the adult scale except for combining grades 4 and 5 into one grade.) In testing the strength of infants and very young children, helpful techniques include checking for age-appropriate head and trunk control. This can be done by holding the child under the arms and lifting him or her into the air, placing in ventral suspension, and observing the child sitting and standing. Muscle strength in the older child can be evaluated through observation of simple activities such as rising from the floor, walking, reaching overhead, or throwing or kicking a ball. Quantitative measurements are generally not required unless specific therapeutic interventions are contemplated.

Coordination is best assessed by evaluating gross motor and fine motor skills. Impaired coordination is a common sign of a central movement disorder. Specific tests can be done in the older child. Most children are able to walk a straight line, although unsteadily, by age 3 years. Tandem walking is a 5-year-old skill. Schoolage children can be more formally tested. Subtle symptoms can be seen by evaluating handwriting, drawing, and other higher level physical skills. The child's avoidance of organized sports or physical activity can be a clue that coordination problems exist. Ataxia is evaluated by having the child reach for an object, do the finger to nose test, sit or stand, and do tandem walking.

Sensory evaluation is difficult in young or uncooperative children and must be age-adjusted to obtain information that is useful. A child of 4–5 years can interpret joint position, vibration, light touch, temperature, and pain. In the very young child, behavioral responses are the best indicator of sensory awareness. These responses include withdrawing and stopping the activity, as well as looking, crying, or squirming.

The vision examination also must be adapted to the child's ability to cooperate. An infant is able to follow a stimulus with the eyes to midline by 1 month and through 180° by 3 months. Perception of color develops by approximately 8 weeks and binocular depth perception by 3–5 months of age. Central nervous system dysfunction frequently presents with ocular motor imbalance.

STANDARDIZED ASSESSMENT TOOLS

Familiarity with the normal landmarks of early child development is essential to the developmental assessment of the infant and toddler. The assessment includes observing and describing the child's gross motor and fine motor responses, verbal and non-verbal language, personal and social behavior, emotional characteristics, and adaptive skills. A formal assessment of the child's developmental status requires the use of a standardized examination. An interdisciplinary evaluation is particularly helpful when the initial diagnosis is being established or when interventions are being planned for a young child. It can also be used for periodic assessment of developmental progress throughout childhood and adolescence, especially for appropriate educational planning. Formal assessments of schoolaged children often focus on academic skills. A diagnostic assessment relies on normed reference instruments that convey the child's developmental standing relative to a normal peer group. It provides valuable information on the assessment and formulation of the child's strengths and weaknesses for the purpose of individual program planning.

A formal developmental assessment of an infant and a young child can be accomplished with the use of standardized developmental evaluations (Table 2-7). Use of the Denver Developmental Screening Test (DDST-II)[17] by primary care providers can identify a child who requires a further evaluation. This standardized screening tool can be used with children from birth to 6 years in an office setting. The four domains in the DDST-II that are assessed include gross motor, fine motor, language, and personal–social behavior. Direct observation and parent report compose this screening test. A child who fails the DDST-II can be further evaluated by a specialist using either the Bayley Scale of Infant Development,[3] which provides separate mental and motor scores, or the Gesell Developmental Schedule.[20] These tests are easy to administer but require some test familiarity and the cooperation of the child. The appropriate interpretation of the information obtained is most important. Many infant evaluation measures rely heavily on motor responses to assess the child's interest in learning.[12] If a child has major physical disabilities, drawing correct inferences about the child's current or future intellectual abilities can be difficult. Repeated studies have found a low correlation between abilities measured on infant tests and later childhood intelligence quotients.[2,8,10] Infant test results must be considered provisional and should be followed by periodic reevaluation for further diagnostic and prognostic clarification.

The assessment of preschool and schoolage children includes assessment of both physical and intellectual abilities (Table 2-8). The chief strength of intelligence tests lies in their correlation with school performance. If the results are appropriately interpreted, the tests reflect the probability of standard aca-

Table 2-7 Developmental evaluation and screening tests

Test	Age range	Scope and value
Denver Developmental Screening Test[17]	Birth to 6 years	Quick screen for deviations from normal development of normal and near-normal children; pattern of functional deviations guides further evaluation
Bayley Scale of Infant Development[3]	Birth to 30 months	Separate mental and motor scales; well-standardized; heavily weighted with motor-based items, which limits predictive value in physically handicapped children
Gesell Developmental Schedule[20]	4 weeks to 6 years	Indicator of current developmental level

Table 2-8 Intellectual evaluations

Test	Age range	Scope and value
Stanford–Binet Intelligence Scale[49]	2 years to adult	Detailed diagnostic assessment (mental age and IQ); guidelines for hearing, visual, and motor handicaps
Wechsler Preschool and Primary Scale of Intelligence—Revised (WPPSI-R)[52]	3–6½ years	Verbal, performance, and full-scale scores; delineates strengths and weaknesses; not appropriate for children with severe developmental delays
Wechsler Intelligence Scale for Children—Revised (WISC-R)[51]	6–16 years	Verbal, performance, and full-scale scores; subtests point to specific areas of strength or dysfunction
Kaufman Assessment Battery for Children[27]	2½–12 years	Measures mental processes independent of the content of acquired knowledge; useful for children from disadvantaged backgrounds

demic achievement. It is important to note both the overall score and the subscores to assess whether a child's abilities are evenly developed, or whether there are patterns of strengths and weaknesses that are relevant to learning and general adaptation.[10]

Most of the standardized intelligence tests rely heavily on language and motor performance. For some disabled children, such as those with central language impairments, significant motor difficulties, or sensory deficits, alternative non-verbal and motor-eliminated assessments might be needed (Table 2-9). Vocabulary tests typically show the strongest correlation with overall intellectual ability and school success.

The test composite scores, or full-scale scores (IQs), are used to designate a child's overall level of intellectual functioning.[10] This is derived by comparing an individual child's performance with the performance of hundreds of children in a representative age-stratified norm group. On most of these tests, the mean score is 100, representing average or normal intelligence. Classifications as superior or subaverage typically refer to scores that fall two standard deviations above or below the mean.

A definition of mental retardation includes three components: subaverage general intelligence, concurrent deficits in adaptive behavior, and developmental delay. Generally, all three criteria must be present to make a formal diagnosis of mental retardation.

The classification of mild mental retardation (IQ of 55–69) encompasses the largest number of children with mental retardation. Generally, they show delayed language development as toddlers and weakness in the acquisition of preacademic writing skills. These children generally reach the third- to fifth-grade level academically. If the associated physical handicaps are mild, they can be independent in activities of daily living and achieve relative independence in adulthood.

Children with moderate mental retardation (IQ of 40–54) have a slower rate of developmental attainment. There is also a higher incidence of neurologic and physical disabilities. These children are frequently in special classes and are primarily taught self-care and practical daily living skills. As adults, many are able to achieve some independence in self-care skills, but they usually continue to need supervision either at home or in group homes. Vocationally, they function primarily in sheltered workshops or protected employment.

Children with severe mental retardation (IQ of 25–39) develop some functional language skills but no formal academic skills. They require intensive programming to master independence in activities of daily living. They need close

Table 2-9 Alternative non-verbal and motor-eliminated tests

Test	Age range	Scope and value
Peabody Picture Vocabulary Test (PPVT)[15]	2½–18 years	Effective test of language, especially in children with speech and motor impairments
Leiter International Performance Scale[30]	2–18 years	Measures non-verbal problem-solving abilities in deaf and in speech- and motor-handicapped children
Pictorial Test of Intelligence[18]	3–8 years	Measures intellectual ability of multiply handicapped children; requires receptive language
Raven's Progressive Matrices[41]	6 years to adult	Measures non-verbal intelligence and concept formation

Table 2-10 Perceptual evaluations

Test	Age range	Scope and value
Beery–Buktenica Development Test of Visual Motor Integration[4]	2–16 years	Assesses visual motor performance, ability to copy geometric shapes, age equivalence
Bender Visual Motor Gestalt Test[7]	5 years to adult	Assesses visual motor performance; easy to administer; nine geometric designs

supervision and supportive care as adults. Profoundly retarded children (IQ less than 25) have limited language ability and limited potential for acquiring self-care skills. There is also a very high association with severe motor handicaps.

Several tests have been designed to evaluate visual motor maturity in children, and to detect delays or impairment in visual perceptual skills and eye–hand coordination (Table 2-10). Children with neurologic and developmental disabilities sometimes exhibit difficulties in visual perceptual, perceptual motor, auditory, kinesthetic, and tactile functioning. A wide variety of instruments are available to test for these impairments. Achievement tests are designed specifically to evaluate the child's performance in school subject areas, such as reading and mathematics (Table 2-11). Scores are typically given in terms of school grade equivalence, which can provide an estimate of the child's level of academic skill, as well as standard scores based on age norms. Many are paper and pencil tests that penalize handicapped children for their slower pace, poor attention, or difficulty keeping track of their place on the page. It is important that a skilled observer administer the test, because observation of task approach can be used to adjust quantitative results.

Assessment tools for the child with a disability

Formal assessment tools identify those children who do not achieve expected motor milestones, but the quality of a child's movement is not taken into consideration in the typical standardized tool. Children with disabilities benefit from use of assessment tools that evaluate the quality of their movements and changes in performance over time.

The Gross Motor Function Measure (GMFM) is a reliable and valid measure of motor function designed for quantifying change in the gross motor abilities of children with cerebral palsy.[44] The GMFM-88 consists of 88 items that have been grouped into five different dimensions of gross motor function: lying and rolling; sitting, crawling and kneeling; standing; and walking, running, and jumping. Scoring is based on a four-point scale for each item, using the following key: 0, does not initiate; 1, initiates; 2, partially completes; and 3, completes. All items are attainable by 5-year-old children with normal motor development. A newer version, GMFM-66, comprises a subset of the original GMFM-88.[43] The GMFM-88 version is also valid for use with children who have Down syndrome.[19,39]

The Quality of Upper Extremity Skills Test (QUEST) is an outcome measure designed to evaluate movement patterns and hand function in children with cerebral palsy.[11] The QUEST is both reliable and valid.

The Pediatric Evaluation of Disability Inventory (PEDI) was developed to provide a comprehensive clinical assessment of key functional capabilities and performance in children between the ages of 6 months and 7 years.[23] The PEDI can also be used for the evaluation of older children if their functional abilities fall below that expected of 7-year-old children without disabilities. The assessment was designed to serve as a descriptive measure of the child's current functional performance, as well as a method for tracking change across time. The PEDI measures both capability and performance of functional activities in three content domains: self-care, mobility, and social function. Capability is measured by the identification of functional skills for which the child has demonstrated mastery and competence. Functional performance is measured by the level of assistance a caregiver must provide in order for the child to accomplish major functional activities such as eating or outdoor mobility.

Table 2-11 Academic achievement tests

Test	Grade level or age range	Scope and value
Wide Range Achievement Test—Revised (WRAT)[24]	Kindergarten to 12th grade	Yields academic achievement level in reading, spelling, arithmetic; can measure programs
Woodcock–Johnson Psychoeducational Battery: Test of Achievement[54]	3 years to adult	Yields age and grade level, percentiles, and standard scores in reading, mathematics, written language, and general tasks
Peabody Individual Achievement Test[14]	Kindergarten to 12th grade	Only pointing response for overview of achievement; useful for handicapped

Table 2-12 Social and adaptive skills

Test	Age range	Scope and value
Vineland Adaptive Behavior Scale[47]	1 month to adult	Questionnaire of social competence in communication, socialization, daily living skills, and motor skills; adjusted for handicapped
American Association of Mental Deficiency Adaptive Behavior Scale[35]	3 years to adult	Activities of daily living; adaptive and maladaptive behaviors; assists in program planning

A modifications scale provides a measure of environmental modifications and assistive devices used by the child in routine daily activities.

The WeeFIM is a tool to assess a child's function in the domains of mobility, locomotion, self-care, sphincter control, communication, and social cognition.[36,37] It measures the level of independence and degree of caregiver assistance that is necessary to accomplish daily activities. The WeeFIM can be used to track outpatients over time, as well as the changes within an inpatient rehabilitation program. There are other disability-specific evaluation tools, such as the spina bifida neurologic scale[38] and the prosthetic upper extremity functional index,[55,56] which can be used when evaluating special populations in the outpatient clinic setting.

A complete assessment of the disabled child should include a description of social and adaptive abilities (Table 2-12). It is important to establish the level of achievement in locomotion, communication, and self-care activities such as feeding, dressing, and toileting. It is also important to assess the mode and methods of interaction with family members and peers, and the child's ability to assume increasing levels of responsibility. A number of social adaptive scales have been developed to look at the ages at which children usually achieve such competencies, along with emotional adjustment (Table 2-13).

Care must be taken when arriving at a specific diagnosis on the basis of developmental testing performed early in a child's life, due to the inherent limitations of the tests. In addition, central nervous system dysfunction is not incompatible with normal intelligence, and the degree to which a child might be

Table 2-13 Emotional adjustment

Test	Age range	Scope and value
Manual Children's Apperception Test[6]	3–10 years	Pictures of animals and humans in various situations; assesses adjustment patterns
Figure drawings[13]	4 years to adult	Self-image and interpersonal relationships

intellectually impaired cannot be predicted solely from physical or motor deficits. Familiarity with the tests being utilized is essential when interpreting this information.

SUMMARY

The pediatric physical examination is unique in its need to focus on the developmental skills of the infant and child. The examiner must understand the predictable sequence of physical development in the child and adolescent. Finally, comprehension of the sizeable battery of developmental, intelligence, academic, and social adaptive assessment tools can allow for a thorough evaluation of the infant, child, and adolescent in order to develop a comprehensive rehabilitation program.

REFERENCES

1. Barness CA. Manual of pediatric physical diagnosis. St. Louis: Mosby-Year Book; 1991.

2. Barness CA. Principles and practice of pediatrics. Philadelphia: Lippincott; 1994:29–34.

3. Bayley N. Bayley Scale of Infant Development. New York: Psychological Corp.; 1969.

4. Beery K, Buktenica N. Developmental Test of Visual-Motor Integration. Chicago: Follett; 1967.

5. Behrman RE, Vaughan VC, eds. Nelson's textbook of pediatrics. Philadelphia: Saunders; 1987.

6. Bellak L. Manual Children's Apperception Test. New York: Grune & Stratton; 1961.

7. Bender L. The Bender Visual-Motor Gestalt Test. New York: Orthopsychiatric Association; 1946.

8. Capute AJ, Accardo PF, Vining EPG. Primitive reflex profile. Baltimore: University Park Press; 1977.

9. Centers for Disease Control and Prevention. 2000 CDC growth charts: United States. National Center for Health Statistics. Online. Available: http://www.cdc.gov/growthcharts/ 20 May 2004

10. Chinitz SP, Feder CZ. Psychological assessment. In: Molnar GE, ed. Pediatric rehabilitation. Baltimore: Williams & Wilkins; 1992.

11. DeMatteo C. QUEST: Quality of Upper Extremity Skills Test. In: Law M, Russell D, Pollock N, et al, eds. Hamilton: McMaster University; 1992.

12. DiBose R. Predictive value of infant intelligence scales with multiply handicapped children. Am J Ment Defic 1977; 81:388–390.

13. DiLeo J. Children's drawings as diagnostic aides. New York: Brunner–Mazel; 1973.

14. Dunn L, Markwardt F. Manual: Peabody Individual Achievement Test. Circle Pines: American Guidance Service; 1970.

15. Dunn LM. Peabody Picture Vocabulary Test—Revised. Circle Pines: American Guidance Service; 1970.

16. Fiorentino MR. Normal and abnormal development. Springfield: Charles C Thomas; 1972.

17. Frakenburg WC, Dodds J, Archer P. Denver II technical manual. Denver: Denver Developmental Materials; 1990.

18. French J. Manual: Pictorial Test of Intelligence. Boston: Houghton Mifflin; 1964.

19. Gemus M, Palisano R, Russell D, et al. Using the Gross Motor Function Measure to evaluate motor development in children with Down syndrome. Phys Occup Ther Pediatr 2001; 21(2-3):69–79.

20. Gesell A. Gesell Developmental Schedule. New York: Psychological Corp.; 140.

21. Green M. Pediatric diagnosis: interpretation of symptoms and signs in different age periods. Philadelphia: Saunders; 1985.

22. Gundy JH. The pediatric physical examination. In: Hoekelman RA, ed. Primary pediatric care. St. Louis: Mosby-Year Book; 1992.

23. Haley SM. Pediatric Evaluation of Disability Inventory. In: Coster WJL, Larry H, eds. Boston: Boston University; 1992.

24. Jastak S, Wilkinson GS. The Wide Range Achievement Test—Revised. Wilmington: Jastak Associates; 1984.

25. Johnson CP, Blasco PA. Infant growth and development. Pediatr Rev 1997; 18(7):224–242.

26. Jones KL. Smith's recognizable patterns of human malformation. 5th edn. Philadelphia: Saunders; 1997.

27. Kaufman A, Kaufman N. Kaufman Assessment Battery for Children. Circle Pines: American Guidance Service; 1983.

28. Keen M. Early development and attainment of normal mature gait. J Prosthet Orthot 1993; 5(2):35–38.

29. Kottke FJ, Lehman JF, eds. Krusen's handbook of physical medicine and rehabilitation. Philadelphia: Saunders; 1990.

30. Leiter R. The Leiter International Performance Scale. Chicago: Stoelting; 1969.

31. Lincoln TL, Suen PW. Common rotational variations in children. J Am Acad Orthop Surg 2003; 11(5):312–320.

32. Marshall WA, Tanner JM. Variations in pattern of pubertal changes in girls. Arch Dis Child 1969; 44(235):291–303.

33. Marshall WA, Tanner JM. Variations in the pattern of pubertal changes in boys. Arch Dis Child 1970; 45(239):13–23.

34. Mehlman CT. Idiopathic scoliosis. Online. Available: http://www.emedicine.com/orthoped/topic504.htm 30 Jun 2004

35. Mihira K, Foster R, Shellhaas M. AAMD adaptive behavior scales. Washington: American Association of Mental Deficiency; 1974.

36. Msall ME, DiGaudio K, Duffy LC, et al. WeeFIM. Normative sample of an instrument for tracking functional independence in children. Clin Pediatr (Phila) 1994; 33(7):431–438.

37. Msall ME, DiGaudio K, Rogers BT, et al. The functional independence measure for children (WeeFIM). Conceptual basis and pilot use in children with developmental disabilities. Clin Pediatr (Phila) 1994; 33(7):421–430.

38. Oi S, Matsumoto S. A proposed grading and scoring system for spina bifida: Spina Bifida Neurological Scale (SBNS). Childs Nerv Syst 1992; 8(6):337–342.

39. Palisano RJ, Walter SD, Russell DJ, et al. Gross motor function of children with Down syndrome: creation of motor growth curves. Arch Phys Med Rehabil 2001; 82(4):494–500.

40. Persing J, James H, Swanson J, et al. Prevention and management of positional skull deformities in infants. American Academy of Pediatrics Committee on Practice and Ambulatory Medicine, Section on Plastic Surgery and Section on Neurological Surgery. Pediatrics 2003; 112(1 part 1):199–202.

41. Raven J. Raven's Progressive Matrices. Dumfries: Crichton Royal; 1958.

42. Roye DP, Jr., Roye BD. Idiopathic congenital talipes equinovarus. J Am Acad Orthop Surg 2002; 10(4):239–248.

43. Russell DJ, Avery LM, Rosenbaum PL, et al. Improved scaling of the Gross Motor Function Measure for children with cerebral palsy: evidence of reliability and validity. Phys Ther 2000; 80(9):873–885.

44. Russell DJ, Rosenbaum PL, Cadman DT, et al. The Gross Motor Function Measure: a means to evaluate the effects of physical therapy. Dev Med Child Neurol 1989; 31(3):341–352.

45. Sanger TD, Delgado MR, Gaebler-Spira D, et al. Classification and definition of disorders causing hypertonia in childhood. Pediatrics 2003; 111(1): e89–e97.

46. Simms MD, Schum RL. Preschool children who have atypical patterns of development. Pediatr Rev 2000; 21(5):147–158.

47. Sparrow SS, Balla DA, Cicchetti DV. Vineland Adaptive Behavior Scale. Circle Pines: American Guidance Service; 1984.

48. Sullivan JA. Pediatric flatfoot: evaluation and management. J Am Acad Orthop Surg 1999; 7(1):44–53.

49. Thorndike RL, Hagen EP, Sattler JM. The Stanford–Binet Intelligence Scale. 4th edn. Chicago: Riverside; 1986.

50. Trollmann R, Dorr HG, Strehl E, et al. Growth and pubertal development in patients with meningomyelocele: a retrospective analysis. Acta Paediatr 1996; 85(1):76–80.

51. Wechsler D. Wechsler Intelligence Scale for Children—Revised. New York: Psychological Corp.; 1974.

52. Wechsler D. Wechsler Preschool and Primary Scales of Intelligence—Revised. San Antonio: Psychological Corp; 1989.

53. Wheeler MD, Styne DM. Diagnosis and management of precocious puberty. Pediatr Clin North Am 1990; 37(6):1255–1271.

54. Woodcock R, Johnson MD. Woodcock–Johnson Psychoeducational Battery: Tests of Achievement. Allen: DLM Teaching Resources; 1989.

55. Wright FV, Hubbard S, Jutai J, et al. The prosthetic upper extremity functional index: development and reliability testing of a new functional status questionnaire for children who use upper extremity prostheses. J Hand Ther 2001; 14(2):91–104.

56. Wright FV, Hubbard S, Naumann S, et al. Evaluation of the validity of the prosthetic upper extremity functional index for children. Arch Phys Med Rehabil 2003; 84(4):518–527.

Chapter

3

Adult Neurogenic Communication Disorders

Delaina Walker-Batson and Jan R. Avent

The various physical and sensory deficits following many neurologic disorders seen by the physiatrist are accompanied by an array of communication disorders. This chapter reviews the major acquired communication disorders seen in adults as a result of a disturbance of the neurologic system. As noted by Brookshire,[9] the prefix *neuro* means 'related to the nervous system', while the suffix *genic* means 'resulting from' or 'caused by'. Combining the two yields *neurogenic* communication disorders.

HANDEDNESS AND LANGUAGE

The human brain is highly specialized regarding language and cognitive functions. In addition to the complexities of site, magnitude, and type of neurologic insult, the relationship between handedness and the side of the brain that is injured determines the characteristics of the communication disorder. For the majority of right-handed and left-handed individuals, the language association areas are in the left hemisphere. In a small percentage of left-handed individuals, the language centers might be in the right hemisphere or bilaterally represented. The left hemisphere is specialized for speech and language functions in the vast majority of people (approximately 96%), regardless of handedness. The right hemisphere is specialized for constructional, visual spatial, and attentional functions.

TYPES OF COMMUNICATION DISORDERS CAUSED BY NERVOUS SYSTEM PATHOLOGY

A wide variety of speech and language disorders result from neurologic injury or pathology. These include aphasia and related neurobehavioral disorders, communicative cognitive disorders secondary to right hemisphere stroke, traumatic brain injury (TBI), dementia, and the motor speech disorders including the dysarthrias and apraxia of speech. Table 3-1 presents the major neurogenic communication disorders, neurologic diagnosis or disease, and salient speech, language and cognitive characteristics.

BRAIN PLASTICITY AND NEUROREHABILITATION

Over the past 25 years, there has been increasing evidence from animal studies regarding brain plasticity and recovery of function that has application to human rehabilitation. It is now recognized that administration of drugs and/or direct manipulation of motor and sensory experience can modify brain plasticity and functional outcome after experimental cortical injuries. A large body of research demonstrates that the type of input affects brain reorganization.[27,36,40] This has been termed *use-dependent*,[36] or more recently *learning-dependent*, activity.[40] This refers to the specificity of the experience following brain injury being critical in determining what brain and behavioral changes will occur. Nudo and colleagues found that motor maps are altered by motor skill acquisition and not by repetitive use alone.[40] Brain topographic plasticity coincided with the reacquisition of motor skills in lesioned animals and the acquisition of new motor skills in intact animals. These data imply that, at critical recovery periods, the restorative treatments should target the most complex behaviors that a patient can produce. It could be that focusing only on compensatory activities rather than on restorative functions has costs in terms of ultimate recovery of function.

Neuromodulation can be done with certain pharmacologic agents, particularly those known to affect the catecholamine system. When paired with behavioral treatment, some agents (dextroamphetamine, methylphenidate, levodopa) have also been found to enhance outcome after both focal[16,25,26,49] and diffuse[34,51] cortical experimental injury. It should be noted that this does not extend to all behaviors.[47] Explorations of pharmacologic modulation have been done in humans to facilitate recovery from post-stroke deficits such as aphasia and hemiplegia,[21,46,56,57] and to enhance recovery of cognitive deficits subsequent to TBI.[29,60] Physiologic events following brain injury can complicate the timing for administration of various agents. Drugs that are effective in the very acute or subacute period following injury might be ineffective or even detrimental at later recovery periods.[19] Our research group has explored the use of paced low-dose dextroamphetamine administration paired with focused behavioral treatment to enhance recovery from aphasia and hemiplegia subsequent to stroke.[56,57] Our experience, and that of others,[21,46] is encouraging regarding the use of certain agents to accelerate recovery. A number of questions still need to be explored before rehabilitation pharmacology becomes a standard of care.[58]

- What is the amount of time post onset that neuromodulation can have an effect?
- What is the amount of learning-dependent practice that must be paired with the pharmacologic intervention for optimal recovery?
- What are the optimal drug combinations and dosages?

Table 3-1 Major neurogenic communication disorders, neurologic diagnosis, and language and cognitive characteristics

Communication substrate	Disorder(s)	Neurologic diagnosis, disease	Salient speech, language, and cognition characteristics
Language and cognition	Aphasia	Unilateral cortical or subcortical stroke	Language impairment affecting speaking, listening, reading, and writing
	Right hemisphere communication disorders	Unilateral cortical or subcortical stroke	Processing deficits resulting in impaired attention, visual spatial, cognition, and communication skills; communication deficits might include anomia, higher order discourse expression, and comprehension skills
	Traumatic brain injury	Penetrating or non-penetrating head injury; coup and contrecoup damage	Impaired cognition, memory, and executive functioning; anomia; disorganized language skills; socially inappropriate
	Dementia	Progressive	Progressively severe loss of memory and cognition
Motor planning	Apraxia of speech	Unilateral cortical or subcortical stroke	Articulatory errors, impaired initiation of oral movement, reduced speaking rate, impaired articulatory sequencing
Speech execution	Dysarthrias	Degenerative disease such as Parkinson disease, multiple sclerosis, amyotrophic lateral sclerosis; unilateral, bilateral, or brain stem strokes	Impaired articulatory, respiratory, laryngeal, and resonance abilities

APHASIA AND RELATED NEUROBEHAVIORAL DISORDERS

Aphasia

Aphasia in adults occurs as a result of acquired brain damage to the language-dominant hemisphere, usually the left, and shares common neurophysiologic features with other stroke consequences. Chapey provides a straightforward definition: 'Aphasia is an acquired communication disorder caused by brain damage, characterized by an impairment of language modalities, speaking, listening, reading and writing, it is not the result of a sensory deficit, a general intellectual deficit or a psychiatric disorder' (p. 3).[12]

Since the time of Broca,[8] aphasia has probably been the most studied neurogenic communication disorder. Because of the nature of the injury and the critical left hemisphere language association areas (Fig. 3-1), aphasia has been classified in terms of the characteristics of the linguistic deficits and the location of the lesion.

The traditional aphasia classification system[7,32] is based on clusters of language symptoms and contrasts the characteristics of verbal output, auditory comprehension, and repetition ability (Table 3-2). This framework forms the basis for two of the most frequently employed formal assessments used by speech-language pathologists: the Boston Diagnostic Aphasia Examination[20] and the Western Aphasia Battery.[31]

Modern imaging studies and research in psycholinguistics have shown limitations with the traditional classification scheme. In particular, the roles of Wernicke's and Broca's area are not as clear as they first appeared.[13] A variety of other left

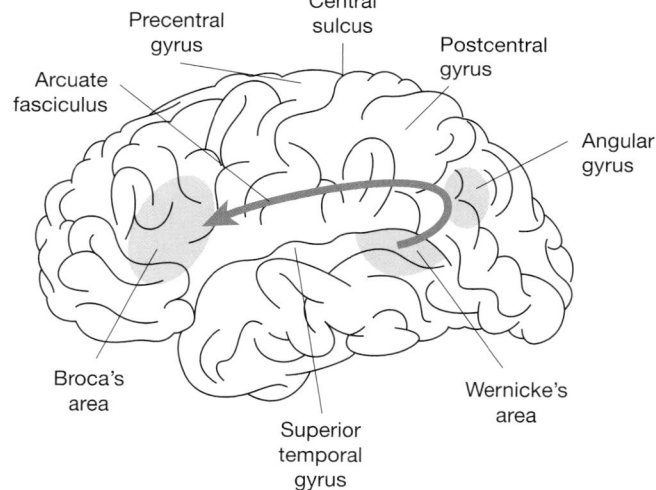

Figure 3-1 Language-related areas in the brain: a simplified lateral view of the left hemisphere, showing primary language areas of the brain. The central sulcus provides an arbitrary division between anterior and posterior brain regions. Broca's area is adjacent to the precentral gyrus (motor strip) that controls the movements of facial expression, articulation, and phonation. Wernicke's area is in the posterior part of the superior temporal gyrus adjacent to the primary auditory cortex (superior temporal gyrus). The arcuate fasciculus is a pathway that connects Broca's and Wernicke's areas. Many of the cortical language association areas lie close to the sylvian fissure and participate in a complex network of areas that contribute to language processing.

Table 3-2 The aphasias: comparisons of verbal output, repetition, auditory comprehension, associated signs, and region affected

Type of aphasia	Verbal output	Repetition	Comprehension	Associated signs	Region affected
Broca's aphasia	Non-fluent, effortful	Impaired	Relatively intact, difficulty with complex syntax	Right hemiparesis, right hemisensory loss; ±apraxia of left limbs	Left inferior frontal, subcortical white matter
Wernicke's aphasia	Fluent, paraphasic errors; ±logorrhea	Impaired	Impaired	±Right hemianopsia	Left posterior superior temporal; ±inferior parietal
Conduction	Fluent, some paraphasias	Impaired	Intact	±Right hemiparesis, sensory loss, hemianopsia; ±apraxia	Left superior temporal and supramarginal gyrus
Global	Non-fluent, mute initially	Impaired	Impaired	Right hemiparesis, right hemisensory, right hemianopsia	Major occlusion of the middle cerebral artery: frontotemporoparietal
Transcortical motor	Non-fluent, dysarthric	Intact	Relatively preserved	±Right hemiparesis	Left medial frontal or anterior border zone
Transcortical sensory	Fluent	Intact	Impaired	±Right hemianopsia	Left medial parietal or posterior border zone
Anomic	Fluent, word-finding pauses	Intact	Relatively preserved	Variable	Left temporal, left angular gyrus

hemisphere regions, both cortical and subcortical, have been found to be involved in language processing. While it is now recognized that the processing of language requires a large network of interacting brain areas,[13] it is also the case that certain linguistic behaviors group together and are often predictable depending on the anterior or posterior location of the lesion. Anterior aphasias include Broca's and transcortical motor aphasia. Posterior aphasias include Wernicke's, conduction, and transcortical sensory aphasias. Global and anomic aphasias are not as localized. Whether speech output is non-fluent versus fluent, the degree of auditory comprehension deficit, and the ability to repeat can be checked by the physiatrist at the bedside (see Fig. 3-2) to get an estimate of the type of aphasia.

Broca's aphasia

This is the classic type of non-fluent aphasia. The patient's speech is effortful, and articulation is often impaired (see Table 3-3 for speech samples of the primary aphasia types). There is restricted vocabulary and problems with syntax. Auditory comprehension is relatively better than speech production. The reading deficit in Broca's aphasia is variable. An acquired reading disorder resulting from frontal pathology has been well described.[7] Writing is usually as severely impaired as speech. Lesions causing Broca's aphasia are most often in the left posterior inferior frontal cortex and underlying structures.

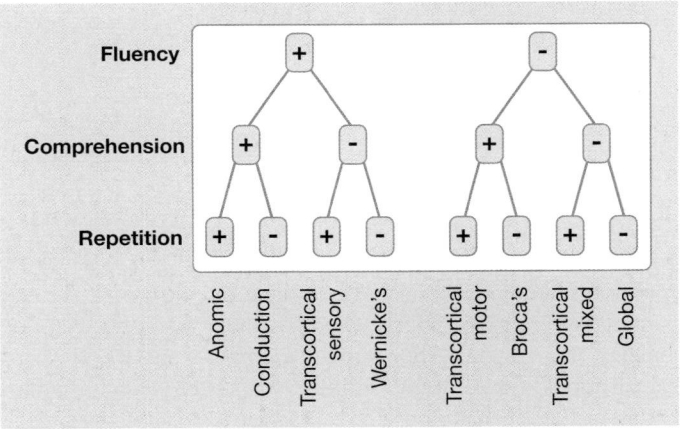

Figure 3-2 Flow chart to assess aphasia types: a flow chart to characterize fluency of speech output, auditory comprehension, and repetition ability for brief bedside screening of patients with aphasia. The plus symbol (+) indicates that the specific function is intact or at least fairly good. The minus symbol (−) indicates that the specific function is relatively impaired, i.e. a plus does not necessarily indicate that the function is normal or a minus does not necessarily indicate that a function is completely defective. (From Canter 1979,[11] with permission.)

Wernicke's aphasia

In 1874, Karl Wernicke described an aphasia syndrome very different from Broca's aphasia.[13] Patients with Wernicke's aphasia have fluent speech output with normal prosody (vocal pitch and stress) and close to normal grammar. However, their

Table 3-3 Spontaneous speech samples, auditory comprehension, and repetition for the four primary aphasia types

Type of aphasia	Verbal output *Stimulus: cookie theft picture*[a]	Auditory comprehension *Stimulus: What seems to be the trouble?*[b]	Repetition *Stimulus: The telephone is ringing*[b]
Broca's	'The . . . dishes' 'This . . .' 'The tookie' 'Fall . . .'	'I can read'	'De telephone is ringing'
Wernicke's	'She could have been' 'Looking toward her face with a hand' 'Possibly to a choice or she really could' 'Have been laughing' 'The other one fell into the stell step bane bant it fell' 'It fell over' 'The other one person has a stair stuffy . . .' 'Into reaching toward the other girl'	'Problem with my spayter hearing, speaking'	'Telephone is fogging'
Conduction	'Uh there's a boy on a uh . . . uh . . . stole . . . stool' 'He's getting cookies from a jar' 'The woman uh . . . uh . . . is wasing the dishes' 'And uh water . . . um . . . running over' 'She's . . . drying some dishes and' 'The girl is uh, uh, ready'	'I need help with my . . . uh . . . peech [speech]'	'The telephone uh . . . uh the telephone is binging'
Global	'Looky, looky, looky' 'Okay' 'Looky, looky' 'No, looky, looky' 'Yeah, looky, looky'	[No response]	'Looky' [preservations]

[a]Stimuli for picture description from the *Boston Diagnostic Aphasia Examination*.[20]
[b]Stimuli for repetition and auditory comprehension from the *Western Aphasia Battery*.[31]

speech is filled with literal and verbal paraphasic errors. (Literal paraphasias are sound substitutions within a word, for example 'binging' for 'ringing'. Semantic paraphasias are whole word substitutions, for example 'mother' for 'sister'.) These paraphasias and other made-up words (*neologisms*) cause the speech of the Wernicke's patient to be empty, although the sentence length can be normal. Another characteristic of speech output in Wernicke's aphasia can be an inability to stop speaking (logorrhea) and press of speech (rapid, compressed utterances). Patients with Wernicke's aphasia have severely impaired auditory comprehension, sometimes to the point of understanding no spoken language, and are often unaware of their own deficits.[32]

To be classified as Wernicke's aphasia, there must be a repetition deficit. Wernicke's aphasia usually occurs from damage to the left superior temporal region. It might also occur following damage in the inferior parietal cortex involving the supramarginal and angular gyri.[32]

Conduction aphasia

Conduction aphasia is relatively uncommon and occurs in only about 10% of patients with aphasia. In this type of aphasia, the speech output is fluent but with considerable word-finding difficulties (*anomia*), preserved auditory comprehension, and significant difficulty with repetition. The speech of patients with conduction aphasia is characterized by literal paraphasias and numerous self-corrections as they search for the right word. This self-correction can cause the speech of the individual with conduction aphasia to have numerous pauses and filled pauses ('ah . . . a . . . ah . . . ah'). Reading and writing deficits are variable depending on the specific site of the lesion. Brain damage in conduction aphasia is in the left superior temporal area and/or supramarginal gyrus of the parietal lobe.

Global aphasia

Patients with global aphasia have severe impairments in all language modalities (speaking, listening, reading, and writing).

Global aphasia is characterized by severely impaired auditory comprehension and very limited speech output. Individuals with global aphasia produce few understandable utterances, and their speech is marked by perseverative utterances used repeatedly. It should not be overlooked, however, that many patients with global aphasia have some islands of spared intact function, and these must be found to utilize for communication. A type of global aphasia has been described with severe communication deficits but absence of hemiplegia.[55] Brain damage causing global aphasia is usually massive (fronto-temporoparietal), caused by complete occlusion of the middle cerebral artery with dense right hemiplegia of both arm and leg.

Transcortical motor aphasia

Patients with transcortical motor aphasia have some similarities to those with Broca's aphasia but with intact repetition. The transcortical aphasias refer to aphasias occurring from lesions in the border zone outside the perisylvian language areas. Individuals with transcortical motor aphasia have non-fluent, limited speech output that sometimes has a dysarthric quality. There are often long pauses between utterances. The patient with transcortical motor aphasia does not have as much difficulty with syntax as one with Broca-type aphasia.[13] Auditory comprehension and reading comprehension are generally well preserved. Writing deficits can mirror those seen in spoken language.[13] Transcortical motor aphasias occur as a result of occlusion of the anterior cerebral artery or damage to border zone areas in the frontal lobe superior or anterior to Broca's area.[32]

Transcortical sensory aphasia

Individuals with the relatively rare syndrome of transcortical sensory aphasia have shared linguistic profiles to those with Wernicke's aphasia, but with preserved repetition ability. There are also deficits in all language modalities. Patients with transcortical sensory aphasia speak fluently but have *echolalia* (repeating a phrase over and over). Although these patients can repeat, they do not recognize what they say and have much difficulty communicating in any modality. Lesions in transcortical sensory aphasia are usually posterior or inferior to Wernicke's area.

Anomic aphasia

Anomic aphasia can often be the residual of a good recovery from other aphasia syndromes. Patients in the acute stage who are classified as having anomic aphasia have the best prognosis for recovery of any of the aphasias. The primary difficulty in anomic aphasia is word finding and naming. Speech output is fluent, with numerous pauses, filled pauses, and *circumlocutions* (describing and/or defining a function of an object for which a name cannot be retrieved, e.g. 'You brush your teeth with it'). Repetition is intact. Auditory comprehension, reading, and writing are generally intact. Although anomic aphasia is the least localized of all the aphasias, it often occurs from focal damage to left temporal and parietal areas.[32]

Crossed aphasia

Rarely (incidence between 1 and 11%), a classic aphasia occurs in a strongly right-handed person from a lesion on the right side of the brain. When this occurs, it is referred to as a crossed aphasia. The language characteristics in this case can be classic, paralleling the types of aphasias seen from left hemisphere lesions, with almost reversed mirror image specialization of the two hemispheres.[59] Other patients have anomalous hemispheric specialization with both language functions and visual spatial functions in the right hemisphere.[3]

Management of aphasia

All aphasias evolve over time, allowing probable prognoses to be made based on careful baseline assessment (3–4 weeks post onset). For example, the condition of a patient with severe non-fluent (global) aphasia at baseline with adequate speech and language treatment is likely to evolve to a chronic Broca-type aphasia. The condition of a patient who has severe fluent (Wernicke's) aphasia at baseline with adequate treatment has a good probability of evolving to a conduction or anomic aphasia (see Table 3-4).

Treatment by the speech-language pathologist is based on a careful assessment of all communication modalities: speaking, listening, reading, and writing. The patient's deficit areas and his or her relative strengths and weaknesses are determined. Both impairment and disability level assessments are ideally done, as defined by the World Health Organization.[61,62] The focus of treatment in the acute and subacute recovery period is restoration of speech and language abilities, and treatment is individualized.

Numerous therapy approaches specific to the complex of speech and language behaviors exhibited by patients with aphasia are available and have been demonstrated to be effective. Metaanalysis of the efficacy of therapy for aphasia has shown that language therapy for aphasia has a significant positive impact on recovery in the acute phase, and to a lesser

Table 3-4 Patterns of evolution in aphasia	
Aphasia at onset	Potential end point
Non-fluent Broca's aphasia	Non-fluent anomic
Global	Chronic Broca's aphasia
Transcortical motor	Non-fluent anomic
Fluent Wernicke's aphasia Conduction	Conduction or anomic Anomic
Transcortical sensory	Anomic
Anomic	Mild residual anomic or complete Recovery (common end stage for many aphasias, fluent or non-fluent)

extent during the chronic phase.[44] Outcome data from randomized clinical trials on the efficacy of aphasia therapy revealed that more intensive aphasia therapy (on average 108 h) appeared to be a requirement for positive outcomes.[52] Twice a week outpatient treatment over a long period was not efficacious.[53] Evidence-based practice is not the least expensive use of rehabilitation dollars, but it is the better investment of resources if significant improvement is expected.

How should information from neuroscience and evidence-based practice influence the way that aphasia treatment is delivered? The science suggests that aphasia treatment might best be administered in at least three phases that are qualitatively distinct in rationales and approaches. During phase 1 (between 3 and 4 weeks post onset), family and staff are educated about communication. Baselines are obtained to determine a probable prognosis. Phase 2 (roughly 21 days to 180 days post onset) is the period of impairment level individualized treatment. Impairment refers to the World Health Organization framework[61,62] and is defined as loss or abnormality of underlying physiologic or psychologic processes, i.e. disruption of phonologic or grammatical systems, hemiplegia, etc. This phase might include administration of specific drugs known to enhance brain plasticity for learning, speech and language recovery. Phase 3 (after intensive individualized treatment is concluded or paralleling individual treatment) includes group treatment with opportunities to practice in real life contexts and transition for community reentry, including vocational and psychosocial counseling.

Related neurobehavioral disorders

Often co-occurring with aphasia are a number of related neurobehavioral disorders, and it is important to differentiate them from the communication disorder. Only apraxia and agnosia are reviewed here. The physiatrist should consult a more detailed mental status examination such as Strub and Black[50] and/or a neuropsychologist for differential diagnosis of these higher order motor and sensory processing disorders.

Apraxia

Apraxia is an acquired disorder of learned skilled, sequential motor movements that cannot be accounted for by elementary disturbances of strength, coordination, sensation, or lack of comprehension or attention.[18] Apraxia is not a low-level motor disturbance but a deficit in motor planning that involves the integrative steps that precede skilled or learned movements.[50] Apraxias occur more often as a result of left hemisphere lesions. Because adequate verbal comprehension is a prerequisite to valid praxis (motor integration needed for execution of complex learned movements) testing, it is important for the speech language-pathologist to be consulted regarding auditory comprehension abilities when a motor planning problem is suspected. It is also important that patients with motor planning deficit are not diagnosed with comprehension difficulties because the motor planning disorder prevents their making an adequate response to comprehension testing.

Ideamotor apraxia is the most common type of apraxia. Patients with this form of apraxia fail to perform previously learned motor acts accurately. Impairments can be seen in buccofacial, limb, or whole body musculature. Ideational apraxia is a disturbance of complex motor planning of a higher order than is seen in ideamotor apraxia. It is a breakdown in the performance of a task that involves a series of related steps.[50] Brief screening by commands can help the physiatrist to differentiate a motor planning disorder from a true language disorder (Table 3-5).

Agnosia

Agnosias are acquired complex disorders of recognition in some sensory modality, i.e. visual, auditory, and tactile. Agnosia can also be specific for a particular class within a modality, such as agnosia for objects, agnosia for pictures, agnosia for faces (prosopagnosia), or agnosia for colors.[50] Most agnosias are caused by bilateral lesions, although there are exceptions to this.

Just as in the case of the apraxias, it is important to differentiate agnosia from aphasia. Visual agnosia is a complex disorder in which the patient is unable to recognize objects or pictures of objects presented visually, even though visual acuity is adequate. Patients with auditory agnosia can have complete cortical deafness to partial deficits of recognition of specific types of sound.[50] Differentiating auditory agnosia from aphasia is complex and requires assessment by a speech-language pathologist and neuropsychologist. Patients with auditory agnosia can hear noises, for example a vacuum cleaner or a doorbell ring, but not recognize their meanings. Many patients with auditory agnosia cannot recognize any speech but can respond to the same questions in written form. Tactile agnosias occur from parietal lesions and contribute to a range of sensory disorders. These include astereognosis (inability to identify objects palpated by the opposite hand) or agraphesthesia (inability to recognize numbers or letters written on the opposite side of the body).[50] Some consider these deficits part of cortical sensory loss rather than a true agnosia; others call them apperceptive tactile agnosias.[50]

RIGHT HEMISPHERE COMMUNICATION DISORDERS

Patients suffering from stroke of the non-dominant or right hemisphere present a very different profile from those with left hemisphere lesions and aphasia (Table 3-6). In the right hemisphere patient, the communication disorder is often a secondary consequence of significant cognitive or neurobehavioral deficits. Mesulem provided one of the earliest descriptions of the complex deficits resulting from right hemisphere damage.[37] He suggested four cardinal signs of right hemisphere involvement: constructional deficits, left-sided unilateral or hemispatial neglect, dressing apraxia, and denial or indifference. Numerous studies of non-brain-damaged as well as brain-damaged adults show the right hemisphere to be specialized for certain aspects of attention and visual spatial skills, sensory integration, face recognition, memory, affective (emotional) expression or interpretation, non-verbal expression or interpre-

Table 3-5 Evaluation of ideomotor apraxia

Commands	Errors
Buccofacial 'Show me how to . . . . . . blow out a match'	Difficulty giving short, controlled exhalation; saying 'blow'; inhaling; difficulty maintaining appropriate mouth posture
. . . protrude your tongue'	Inability to stick out tongue; tongue moving in mouth but tending to push against front teeth and not protruding
. . . drink through a straw'	Inability to sustain a pucker; blowing instead of drawing through the straw; random mouthing movements
Limb 'Show me how to . . . . . . salute'	Hand over head; hand waving; improper position of hand
. . . use a toothbrush'	Failure to show any proper grip; failure to open mouth; grossly missing the mouth; using finger to pick teeth; not allowing adequate distance for shaft of toothbrush; using the finger as a toothbrush
. . . flip a coin'	Movements miming tossing the coin into the air with an open hand; supinating or pronating the hand as though turning a doorknob; flexing the arm without flipping thumb against finger
. . . hammer a nail'	Moving hand back and forth horizontally; pounding with fist
. . . comb your hair'	Using fingers as teeth of comb; smoothing the hair; making inexact hand movements
. . . snap your fingers'	Extension of fingers with patting movements; tapping of finger on thumb; sliding finger off thumb with insufficient force
. . . kick a ball'	Stamping foot; pushing foot along floor; moving foot laterally
. . . crush out a cigarette'	Stamping foot; kicking foot on floor
Whole body 'Show me how to . . . . . . stand like a boxer'	Awkard arm position; hands at side
. . . swing a baseball bat'	Difficulty in placing both hands together; chopping movements
. . . bow' (for a man) or '. . . curtsy' (for a woman)	Any inappropriate truncal movement

(After Strub and Black 2000,[50] with permission of FA Davis.)

tation, and problem solving. Because of the complexities of the neurobehavioral deficits, right hemisphere-damaged patients might have a few or many of the salient features.

There is currently little information about lesion localization and a specific type of right hemisphere communication disorder. This is due no doubt to the fact that many of the neurobehavioral abilities of the right hemisphere, which can affect communication, are more diffusely organized. Not all individuals with right hemisphere damage have communication deficits.[38] The attentional deficits seen in right hemisphere patients either as a primary deficit or as a consequence of left-sided hemispatial neglect can impact reading and writing ability. Patients with right hemisphere communication disorders miss the gist in a communication message due to difficulties in processing emotional and prosodic input. This can impact their ability to interpret implied meanings, non-verbal signals, and/or intonation patterns that signal a question or sarcasm. Individuals with right hemisphere communication disorders often have difficulty conversing with others, because they tend to be verbose, digressive, tangential, and convey little relevant information.[39,54]

Management of right hemisphere communication deficits

Patients with right hemisphere communication disorders should have both a neuropsychologic assessment and an evaluation by the speech-language pathologist to assess the cognitive communicative profile. Several screening and diagnostic tests have been developed to assist the speech-language pathologist in determining a plan of treatment. These include the Mini Inventory of Right Brain Injury[41] and the Burns Brief Inventory of Communication and Cognition[10] for screening. The Rehabilitation Institute of Chicago's *Clinical Management of Right Hemisphere Dysfunction*[23] can be used for more in-depth evaluation and treatment planning. Current practice suggests that treatments for right hemisphere communication disorders should be designed to compensate for deficits. This is accomplished by improving underlying attention deficits, targeting

Table 3-6 Comparison of communication and neurobehavioral deficits between aphasia and right hemisphere communication disorders

Aphasia	Right hemisphere disorder
Pure linguistic deficits are dominant	Linguistic deficits not dominant
More severe problems in naming, fluency, auditory and comprehension, reading, and writing	Only mild problems
No left-sided neglect	Left-sided neglect
No denial of illness	Denial of illness
Speech is generally relevant	Speech is often irrelevant, rambling
Generally normal affect	Often lack affect
Recognizes familiar faces	May not recognize familiar faces
Simplification of drawings	Rotation and left-sided neglect of drawings
No significant prosodic defect	Significant prosodic defect
Appropriate humor	Inappropriate humor
May retell the essence of a story	May retell only non-essential, isolated details
May understand implied meanings	Understands only literal meanings

tasks to improve problem-solving abilities, improving task-oriented functional communication, and referring for counseling as needed.

Like patients with aphasia, patients with right hemisphere communication disorders and co-occurring neurobehavioral deficits typically improve over time. Recovery is obviously on a continuum depending on the extent of the brain damage. In general, often there is faster recovery for those functions mediated diffusely than for those mediated in a more localized way. There is fairly rapid recovery in a matter of weeks to months of left-sided hemispatial neglect and facial recognition. A somewhat slower recovery occurs for constructional and dressing apraxia deficits, and a much slower recovery occurs for hemiparesis and attentional deficits. Those communication disorders affected by these neurobehavioral problems likewise follow a similar recovery course.

COGNITIVE COMMUNICATION DISORDERS OF TRAUMATIC BRAIN INJURY

There are multiple neurobehavioral and cognitive disorders and stages of recovery resulting from TBI that either directly or indirectly affect communicative function. The primary causes of TBI are vehicular and pedestrian accidents, falls, assaults, and alcohol use.[2] There are two main types of TBI: penetrating and closed head injuries. Penetrating injuries, such as a gunshot wound, usually result in focal damage. Closed head injuries generally result in diffuse, bilateral damage as a result of several co-occurring factors. These factors include the following.

- The impact force (site of impact: *coup effect*).
- The translational pressure force (*contrecoup effect*, opposite from site of impact, and shearing strains from friction that might involve a wide range of brain areas, including the cingulate, midbrain, anterior temporal lobes, basal frontal, and frontal poles).
- The rotational force (which causes shearing strains from friction as well as shearing strains of long fiber tracts in regions where white and gray matter join, such as the basal ganglia, hypothalamus, superior cerebellar peduncles, corpus callosum, and fiber tracts of the brain stem).

The result to brain tissue can be diffuse axonal damage, loss of myelin, and small hemorrhages.

Speech and language disorders typically associated with TBI include dysarthria, deficits in naming, auditory and reading comprehension, writing, discourse cohesion, social language skills, non-verbal communication, and impaired attention and information processing.[2,63] Focal deficits can have communication deficits similar to those of stroke, depending on the site of the damage, with the added burden of problems with memory. Diffuse brain injury results in communication deficits caused by general attention, information-processing, cognition and memory deficits.[63] Individuals who sustain TBI can have severe attention deficits characterized by perseveration, distractibility, impulsivity, and disinhibition.[48]

Management of communication disorders due to traumatic brain injury

The young age of the typical patient with TBI (15–24 years) presents a societal problem, requiring the expertise of all members of the rehabilitation team. Obviously, the stage of recovery of a TBI patient determines the targeted intervention goals set by the speech-language pathologist. Numerous scales to assess cognitive functioning[22] and to rate the disability[28,43] have been developed. The Rancho Los Amigos Scale of Cognitive Levels[22] provides a set of eight categories to assess TBI according to the cognitive and behavioral characteristics, and is widely used by speech-language pathologists (Table 3-7). After a patient has entered a focused rehabilitation program, intervention is usually geared toward community reentry.[63] The speech-language pathologist can use a variety of screening tools, such as the Scales of Cognitive Ability for Traumatic Brain Injury[1] or Brief Test of Head Injury,[15] and/or more detailed tests such as the Ross Information Processing Assessment,[45] to determine current cognitive communicative function. Treatment programs for patients with TBI can include a wide range of targets, including attention training, management of memory impairments, social skills and behavior regulation management, and executive function deficits, as well as the use of amplifiers and

Table 3-7 The Rancho Los Amigos Scale of Cognitive Levels

Level	Definition
1. No response	No response to pain, touch, sound, or sight.
2. Generalized response	Inconsistent, non-purposeful, non-specific responses to intense stimuli. Responds to pain, but response might be delayed.
3. Localized response	Blinks to strong light, turns toward or away from sound, responds to physical discomfort. Inconsistent responses to some commands.
4. Confused agitated	Alert, very active, with aggressive and/or bizarre behaviors. Attention span is short. Behavior is non-purposeful, and patient is disoriented and unaware of present events.
5. Confused non-agitated	Exhibits gross attention to environment. Is highly distractible, requires continual redirection to keep on task. Is alert and responds to simple commands. Performs previously learned tasks but has great difficulty learning new ones. Becomes agitated by too much stimulation. Might engage in social conversation but with inappropriate verbalizations.
6. Confused appropriate	Behavior is goal-directed, with assistance. Inconsistent orientation to time and place. Retention span and recent memory are impaired. Consistently follows simple directions.
7. Automatic appropriate	Performs daily routine in highly familiar environments without confusion but in an automatic, robot-like manner. Is oriented to setting; insight, judgment, and problem solving are poor.
8. Purposeful appropriate	Responds appropriately in most situations. Can generalize new learning across situations. Does not require daily supervision. Might have poor tolerance for stress and might exhibit some abstract reasoning disabilities.

(From Hagen and Malkamus 1979,[22] with permission.)

vocal programs. (See Ch. 50 for additional information on TBI.)

COMMUNICATIVE COGNITIVE DEFICITS ASSOCIATED WITH DEMENTIA

While the physiatrist might not associate language as a major aspect of the early cognitive deficit of the dementias, the original case described by Alzheimer revealed a clear description of a fluent aphasia.[4] The communicative cognitive difficulties associated with dementia are multifaceted depending on the etiology of the disease, for example Alzheimer, vascular disease, Lewy body disease, or Parkinson disease. *The Diagnostic and Statistical Manual of Mental Disorders* (4th edition) specifies the criteria required for a diagnosis of dementia.[5] A patient must have multiple cognitive deficits that include both of the following.

- Evidence of short- and long-term memory impairment.
- At least one of the following conditions: aphasia, apraxia, agnosia, or impaired executive functioning.

Bayles describes the complexity of separating the cognitive problems from language difficulties in dementia.[6] Patients might fail a naming task not because of a language deficit but because the demands on attention or other cognitive processes are too great. The memory deficits that define the syndrome of dementia devastate the patient's ability to communicate normally.[6] Patients can also present with serious memory problems because of depression. One of the first screens for the physician who works with the elderly patient is to distinguish dementia from pseudodementia (which is really depression). Table 3-8 shows the clear contrasts between these two disorders.

A very specific primary progressive aphasia, in reality also a dementia, has now been recognized.[33] This disorder blurs the lines between focal and diffuse disease.[33] During the first 2 years, the patient with primary progressive aphasia has symptoms that appear to be localized like the aphasia subsequent to stroke. After the early course of the disease, primary progressive aphasia usually progresses to dementia, with the characteristic cognitive disorders of other dementias.

Management of communicative cognitive disorders resulting from dementia

Treatment for speech and language deficits subsequent to dementia obviously is determined by the cause and course of the disease. Early in the disease course, maintenance and compensatory activities for speech and cognitive problems are merited. Treatment of the dysarthrias for many of the progressive neurologic motor diseases focuses on compensatory speech and voice techniques and the administration of drugs. Treatments for the cognitive deficits focuses on reducing demands on memory.[24] This type of treatment would capitalize on preserved recognition memory and avoid free recall situations. Quayhagen and associates have shown preliminary evidence that intensive cognitive therapy can slow the general cognitive and behavioral decline associated with dementia.[42] A major role of the speech-language pathologist is to work with the families of dementia

Table 3-8 Differential features of pseudodementia and dementia

	Pseudodementia	Dementia
Clinical course and history	Onset fairly well demarcated, history short	Onset indistinct, history quite long before consultation
	Rapidly progressive	Early deficits that often go unnoticed
	History of previous psychiatric difficulty or recent life crisis	Uncommon occurrence of previous psychiatric problems or emotional crisis
Clinical behavior	Detailed, elaborate complaints of cognitive dysfunction	Little complaint of cognitive loss
	Little effort expended on examination items	Struggles with cognitive tasks
	Affective change often present	Usually apathetic, with shallow emotions
	Behavior does not reflect cognitive loss	Behavior compatible with cognitive loss
	Nocturnal exacerbation rare	Nocturnal accentuation of dysfunction common
Examination findings	Frequently answers 'I don't know' before even trying	Usually tries items
	Inconsistent memory loss for both recent and remote items	Memory loss for recent items worse than for remote items
	May have particular memory gaps	No specific memory gaps exist
	Generally inconsistent performance	Rather consistently impaired performance

(From Strub and Black 2000,[50] with permission of FA Davis.)

patients in terms of education, behavioral management, and approaches that might ease frustration and enhance communication with their family member(s).

MOTOR SPEECH DISORDERS

Apraxia of speech and dysarthria are motor speech disorders associated with both acute and progressive neurologic disease. The differential diagnosis of motor speech disorders is based on a motor speech assessment that includes a medical history, an oral mechanism examination, perceptual speech characteristics assessment, speech intelligibility rating, and acoustic and physiologic analyses.[14]

Apraxia of speech is a motor planning and programming disorder. It is characterized by articulation errors, impaired initiation of oral movement, reduced speaking rate, and prosodic errors.[14,35] Automatic speech (reciting the days of the week) can be relatively unimpaired compared with purposeful, propositional speech (describing an illness). Apraxia of speech often results from damage to the dominant hemisphere, usually the left, in the perisylvian and insular areas and subcortical structures. The typical neurologic diagnosis of disease is a unilateral cortical or subcortical stroke.

Dysarthria is a collective term for a variety of distinct sensorimotor speech execution disorders.[14] Overall, dysarthria is characterized by impairments to the articulatory, respiratory, laryngeal, and resonance subsystems of speech.[14] It results from damage to the central and/or peripheral nervous system, including the cerebrum, cerebellum, basal ganglia, brain stem, and cranial nerves. Depending on the underlying neurologic disease, its onset can be sudden or gradual and evolve in a recovering, stable, degenerative, or exacerbating–remitting course.[14,30]

The more common causes of dysarthria include unilateral, bilateral, or brain stem stroke; Parkinson disease; multiple sclerosis; and amyotrophic lateral sclerosis. Accurate diagnosis of type of dysarthria is crucial to adequate management and treatment. Table 3-9 outlines the defining characteristics of each type of dysarthria and the typical neurologic diagnoses.

Flaccid dysarthria results from lower motor neuron lesions. The salient speech characteristics include breathy vocal quality, short phrase length, hypernasality, imprecise articulation, monopitch, and monoloudness. The presence of these characteristics depends on the site of damage, for example Bell palsy can cause imprecise articulation but vocal quality and prosody is unimpaired. The confirming signs of flaccid damage are hypotonic muscles, hyporeflexia, diminished reflexes, muscle atrophy, and fasciculations.[14]

Spastic dysarthria results from upper motor neuron lesions. The salient speech characteristics are a strained–strangled voice quality, slow speaking rate, and imprecise articulation.[14]

Ataxic dysarthria results from damage to the cerebellum. It is characterized by imprecise and irregular articulation breakdown, distorted vowels, excess and equal prosodic stress, prolonged phonemes, slow speaking rate, harsh voice quality, monopitch, and monoloudness quality. Confirming signs of ataxic dysarthria include ataxia, dysmetria, disordered stance and gait, and ocular motor abnormalities.[14]

Hypokinetic dysarthria is associated with damage to the basal ganglia. The salient speech characteristics include monopitch and monoloudness, reduced prosodic stress, short rushes of speech or fast speaking rate, variable speaking rates, and imprecise articulation. Confirming signs of hypokinetic damage are tremor, rigidity, bradykinesia or hypokinesia, and postural abnormalities. Hyperkinetic dysarthria is also associated with damage to the basal ganglia. The salient speech characteristics

Table 3-9 Various types of dysarthria; neurologic diagnosis; onset and course; salient speech, language, cognition characteristics

Type of dysarthria	Neurologic diagnosis or disease	Onset and course	Salient speech, language, and cognition characteristics
Flaccid	Myasthenia gravis, Wallenberg lateral medullary syndrome, Guillain–Barré syndrome, muscular dystrophy, progressive bulbar palsy, Bell palsy	Acute or progressive and recovering; stable, degenerative, or exacerbating–remitting	Breathy, short phrases; hypernasality; imprecise articulation; monopitch and monoloudness
Spastic	Bilateral cortical stroke, unilateral brain stem stroke, primary lateral sclerosis, leukoencephalitis	Acute or progressive and recovering; stable, degenerative	Strained–strangled voice quality, slow rate, imprecise articulation, dysphagia
Ataxic	Stroke, tumors, trauma, Friedreich ataxia, olivopontocerebellar atrophy, multiple sclerosis, acute and chronic alcohol abuse, hypothyroidism	Acute or progressive and recovering; stable, degenerative, or exacerbating–remitting	Imprecise and irregular articulation, distorted vowels, excess and equal prosodic stress, prolonged phonemes, slow rate, harsh voice, monopitch, monoloudness
Hypokinetic	Parkinson disease, progressive multiple or bilateral strokes, repeated head trauma	Acute or progressive and degenerative, or exacerbating–remitting	Monopitch, monoloudness, rushes of speech, variable rate, imprecise articulation
Hyperkinetic	Huntington disease, orofacial dyskinesia, tardive dyskinesia, stroke, Tourette syndrome	Acute or progressive, and recovering, stable, degenerative, or exacerbating–remitting	Imprecise articulation, variable rate, prolonged intervals, inappropriate silences, excess loudness variations, prolonged phonemes, sudden forced inspiration or expiration
Unilateral upper motor neuron	Unilateral stroke, tumor	Acute or progressive	Imprecise articulation
Mixed	Amyotrophic lateral sclerosis, multiple sclerosis, Friedreich ataxia, progressive supranuclear palsy, Shy–Drager syndrome, Wilson disease, multiple strokes, trauma, tumor, AIDS, encephalitis, meningitis	Acute or progressive, and recovering, stable, degenerative, or exacerbating–remitting	Imprecise articulation, impaired resonance, prosody, vocal quality, and respiration
	Traumatic brain injury	Penetrating or non-penetrating head injury; coup and contrecoup damage	Impaired cognition, memory, and executive functioning; anomia; disorganized language skills; socially inappropriate
	Dementia	Progressive	Progressively severe loss of memory and cognition
Motor planning	Apraxia of speech	Unilateral cortical or subcortical stroke	Articulatory errors, impaired initiation of oral movement, reduced speaking rate, impaired articulatory sequencing
Speech execution	Dysarthrias	Degenerative disease such as Parkinson disease, multiple sclerosis, amyotrophic lateral sclerosis; unilateral, bilateral, or brain stem strokes	Impaired articulatory, respiratory, laryngeal, and resonance abilities

differ from those of hypokinetic dysarthria, and include imprecise articulation, variable speaking rate, inappropriate silences, excess loudness variations, prolonged phonemes, and sudden forced inspiration or expiration. Confirming signs of hyperkinetic damage are dyskinesia, tics, chorea, ballism, athetosis, dystonia, spasm, and essential tremor.[14]

Unilateral upper motor neuron dysarthria is a relatively new diagnostic subtype. It is characterized by a primary articulatory disorder and is caused by a unilateral stroke or tumor affecting the upper motor neuron system.[14] It differs from spastic dysarthria due to its lack of respiratory, laryngeal, and resonance impairments. It differs from apraxia of speech due to its lack of initiation and sequencing error.

Mixed dysarthrias result from multiple motor system damage that can occur in the central and peripheral nervous system. These mixed dysarthrias are characterized by imprecise articulation and impaired resonance (hyponasal or hypernasal quality), prosody (fast or slow speaking rate), vocal quality (breathy, or strained–strangled or harsh), and respiration (short rushes of speech or excessive loudness).[14] The specific characteristics depend on which motor systems are damaged, but the most common types of mixed dysarthria are spastic flaccid resulting from amyotrophic lateral sclerosis, and spastic ataxic resulting from stroke.

Management of motor speech disorders

Management of motor speech disorders can include medical (e.g. pharmacologic), prosthetic (e.g. augmentative device), and/or behavioral interventions (e.g. improving speech intelligibility).[64] Effective treatments for respiratory and phonatory impairments resulting from dysarthria include biofeedback and augmentative devices such as delayed auditory feedback.[65] Defining evidence-based practice for motor speech disorders is in process.[17]

ACKNOWLEDGMENTS

This work was supported in part by a gift from Mylo and Jesse Kirk. The authors thank Dr. Sharon Parsons, Dr. Mitchell Jones, and Sandra Curtis, M.A., for helpful comments on an earlier draft of this chapter, and Tracy Lindsay and Deby Miller for manuscript preparation.

REFERENCES

1. Adamovich B, Henderson H. Scales of Cognitive Ability for Traumatic Brain Injury. Austin: Pro-Ed.

2. Adamovich BLB. Traumatic brain injury. In: LaPointe LL, ed. Aphasia and related neurogenic language disorders 2nd edn. New York: Thieme; 1997:226–237.

3. Alexander MP, Fischette MR, Fischer RS. Crossed aphasias can be mirror image or anomalous. Brain 1989; 112:953–973.

4. Alzheimer A. Uber eine eigenartige erkrankung der kirnrinde. Allg Z Psychiatr Psych-Gerich Med 1907; 64:146–148. In: Rottenberg DA, Hochberg FH, eds. Neurological classics in modern translation. New York: Hafner Press; 1977:41–43.

5. American Psychiatric Association. Diagnostic and statistical manual of mental disorders. 4th edn. Washington: APA; 1994.

6. Bayles KA. Language in aging and dementia. In: Kirshner HS, ed. Handbook of neurological speech and language disorders. New York: Marcel Dekker; 1995:351–372.

7. Benson DF. Aphasia, alexia and agraphia. New York: Churchill Livingstone; 1979.

8. Broca P. Remarques sur le siege de la faculte du langage articule, suivies d'une observation d'aphemie (perte de la parole). Bull Soc Anat Paris 1861:6330–6357. In: Rottenberg DA, Hochberg FH, eds. Neurological classics in modern translation. New York: Hafner Press; 1977:136–149.

9. Brookshire RH. Introduction to neurogenic communication disorders. St. Louis: Mosby; 2003.

10. Burns MS. Burns Brief Inventory of Communication and Cognition. San Antonio: Psychological Corp.; 1997.

11. Canter GJ. Syndromes of aphasia in relation to cerebral connectionism. Short course presented to the Indiana Speech and Hearing Association. South Bend; 1979.

12. Chapey R, Hallowell B. Introduction to language intervention strategies in adult aphasia. In: Chapey R, ed. Language intervention strategies in aphasia and related neurogenic communication disorders. 4th edn. Philadelphia: Lippincott Williams & Wilkins; 2001.

13. Dronkers NF, Pinker S, Damasio A. Language and the aphasias. In: Kandel ER, Schwartz JH, Jessel TM, eds. Principles of neural science. 4th edn. New York: McGraw-Hill; 2000:1169–1187.

14. Duffy JR. Motor speech disorders. St. Louis: Mosby; 1995.

15. Helm-Esterbrooks N, Hotz G. Brief Test of Head Injury. Pro-Ed; 1991.

16. Feeney DM, Gonzales A, Law W. Amphetamine, haloperidol and experience interact to affect rate of recovery after motor cortex injury. Science 1982; 217:855–857.

17. Frattali C, Bayles K, Beeson P, et al. Development of evidence-based practice guidelines: committee update. J Med Speech-Lang Pathol 2003; 11(3): ix–xviii.

18. Geschwind N. The apraxias: neural mechanisms of disorders of learned movement. Am Sci 1975; 63:188.

19. Goldstein LB. Potential impact of drugs on post stroke motor recovery. In: Goldstein LB, ed. Restorative neurology: advances in pharmacotherapy for recovery after stroke. Armonk: Futura; 1998:241–256.

20. Goodglass H, Kaplan E. The Boston Diagnostic Aphasia Examination. 3rd edn. Philadelphia: Lippincott Williams & Wilkins; 2001.

21. Grade C, Redford B, Chrostowski J, et al. Methylphenidate in early post stroke recovery: a double-blind, placebo controlled study. Arch Phys Med Rehabil 1999; 79:1047–1050.

22. Hagen C, Malkamus D. Interaction strategies for language disorders secondary to head trauma. Paper presented at the Annual Convention of the American Speech-Language-Hearing Association. Atlanta; 1979.

23. Halper AS, Cherney LR, Burns MS. Clinical management of right hemisphere dysfunction. 2nd edn. Gaithersburg: Aspen; 1996.

24. Hopper R, Bayles KA. Management of neurogenic communication disorders associated with dementia. In: Chapey R, ed. Language intervention strategies in aphasia and related neurogenic communication disorders. 4th edn. Philadelphia: Lippincott Williams & Wilkins; 2001:829–246.

25. Hovda DA, Feeney DM. Amphetamine and experience promote recovery of locomotor function after unilateral frontal cortex injury in the cat. Brain Res 1984; 298:358–361.

26. Hurwitz BE, Dietrich WD, McCabe PM, et al. Amphetamine promotes recovery from sensory-motor integration deficit after thrombotic infarction of the primary somatosensory rat cortex. Stroke 1991; 22: 648–654.

27. Jenkins WM, Merzenich MM, Ochs MT, et al. Functional reorganization of primary somatosensory cortex in adult owl monkeys after behaviorally controlled tactile stimulation. J Neurophysiol 1990; 63:82–104.

28. Jennett B, Bond M. Assessment of outcome after severe brain damage: a practical scale. Lancet 1972; 1:480–484.

29. Karli DC, Burke DT, Kim HJ, et al. Effects of dopaminergic combination therapy for frontal lobe dysfunction in traumatic brain injury rehabilitation. Brain Inj 1999; 13:63–68.

30. Kent RD. Models of speech motor control: implications from recent developments in neurophysiological and neurobehavioral science. In: Maassen B, Kent R, Peters H, et al, eds. Speech motor control in normal and disordered speech. Oxford: Oxford University Press; 2004:3–28.

31. Kertesz A. The Western Aphasia Battery. Orlando: Grune & Stratton; 1982.

32. Kirshner HS. Classical aphasia syndromes. In: Kirshner HS, ed. Handbook of neurological speech and language disorders. New York: Marcel Dekker; 1995:57–89.

33. Kirshner HS. Primary progressive aphasia syndrome. In: Kirshner HS, ed. Handbook of neurological speech and language disorders. New York: Marcel Dekker; 1995:373–386.

34. Kline AE, Yan HQ, Bao J, et al. Chronic methylphenidate treatment enhances water maze performance following traumatic brain injury in rats. Neurosci Lett 2000; 280:163–166.

35. McNeil MR, Pratt SR, Fossett TRD. The differential diagnosis of apraxia of speech. In: Maassen B, Kent R, Peters H, et al, eds. Speech motor control in normal and disordered speech. Oxford: Oxford University Press; 2004:389–413.

36. Merzenich MM, Kaas JH, Wall J. Topographic reorganization of somatosensory cortical areas 3B and 1 in adult monkeys following restricted deafferentation. Neuroscience 1983; 8:33–55.

37. Mesalum MM. A cortical network for directed attention and unilateral neglect. Ann Neurol 1981; 10:307–325.

38. Myers PS. Right hemisphere syndrome. In: LaPointe LL, ed. Aphasia and related neurogenic language disorders. 2nd edn. New York: Thieme, 1997:201–225.

39. Myers PS. Toward a definition of RHD syndrome. Aphasiology 2001; 15(10–11):913–918.

40. Nudo RJ, Plautz EJ, Milliken GW. Adaptive plasticity in primate motor cortex as a consequence of behavioral experience and neuronal injury. Semin Neurosci 1997; 9:13–23.

41. Pimental PA, Kingsbury NA. Mini Inventory of Right Brain Injury. Austin: Pro-Ed; 1989.

42. Quayhagen MP, Quayhagen M, Corbeil RR, et al. A dyadic remediation program for care recipients with dementia. Nurs Res 1995; 44:153–159.

43. Rappaport M, Hall KM, Hopkins K, et al. Disability rating scale for severe head trauma: coma to community. Arch Phys Med Rehabil 1982; 63:118–123.

44. Robey RR. A meta-analysis of clinical outcomes in the treatment of aphasia. J Speech Lang Hear Res 1998; 41:172–187.

45. Ross-Swain D. Ross Information Processing Assessment. 2nd edn. Austin: Pro-Ed; 1996.

46. Scheidtmann K, Fries W, Muller F, et al. Effect of levodopa in combination with physiotherapy on functional motor recovery after stroke: a prospective, randomized, double-blind study. Lancet 2001; 358:787–790.

47. Schmanke TD, Avery RA, Barth TM. The effects of amphetamine on recovery of function after cortical damage in the rat depend on the behavioral requirement of the task. J Neurotrauma 1996; 13:293.

48. Sohlberg MM, Avery J, Kennedy M, et al. Practice guidelines for direct attention training. J Med Speech-Lang Pathol 2003; 11(3):xix–xxxix.

49. Stroemer RP, Kent TA, Hulsebosch CE. Enhanced neocortical neural sprouting, synaptogenesis and behavioral recovery with D-amphetamine therapy after neocortical infarction in rats. Stroke 1998; 29:2381–2395.

50. Strub RL, Black FW. The mental status examination in neurology. 4th edn. Philadelphia: FA Davis; 2000.

51. Sutton RL, Feeney DM. α-Noradrenergic agonists and antagonists affect recovery and maintenance of beam-walking ability after sensorimotor cortex ablation in the rat. Restor Neurol Neurosci 1992; 4:1–11.

52. Teasell RW, Foley NC, Bhogal SK, et al. An evidence-based review of stroke rehabilitation. Top Stroke Rehabil 2003; 10:29–58.

53. Teasell RW, Jutai JW, Bhogal SK, et al. Research gaps in stroke rehabilitation. Top Stroke Rehabil 2003; 10:59–70.

54. Tompkins CA. Right hemisphere communication disorders: theory and management. San Diego: Singular; 1995.

55. Tranel D, Biller J, Damasio H, et al. Global aphasia without hemiparesis. Arch Neurol 1987; 44:304–308.

56. Walker-Batson D, Curtis S, Rajeshwari N, et al. A double-blind, placebo-controlled study of the use of amphetamine in the treatment of aphasia. Stroke 2001; 32(9):2093–2097.

57. Walker-Batson D, Smith P, Curtis S, et al. Amphetamine paired with physical therapy accelerates recovery from stroke: further evidence. Stroke 1995; 26:2254–2259.

58. Walker-Batson D, Smith P, Curtis S, et al. Neuromodulation paired with learning dependent practice to enhance post stroke recovery? Restor Neurol Neurosci 2004; 22:387–392.

59. Walker-Batson D, Wendt JS, Devous M, et al. A long-term follow-up case study of crossed aphasia assessed by single-photon emission tomography (SPECT), language, and neuropsychological testing. Brain Lang 1988; 33:311–322.

60. Whyte J, Hart T, Schuster K, et al. Effects of methylphenidate on attentional function after traumatic brain injury. A randomized, placebo-controlled trial. Am J Phys Med Rehabil 1997; 76:440–450.

61. World Health Organization. International classification of impairments, disability and handicaps—prefinal draft. Geneva: World Health Organization; 2000.

62. World Health Organization. International classification of impairments, disability and handicaps. Geneva: World Health Organization; 1980.

63. Ylvisaker M, Szekeres SF, Fenney T. Communication disorders associated with traumatic brain injury. In: Chapey R, ed. Language intervention strategies in aphasia and related neurogenic communication disorders. 4th edn. Philadelphia: Lippincott, Williams and Wilkins; 2001:745–808.

64. Yorkson KM, Beukelman DR, Strand EA, et al. Management of motor speech disorders in children and adults. 2nd edn. Austin: Pro-Ed; 1999.

65. Yorkston KM, Spencer KA, Duffy JR. Behavioral management of respiratory/phonatory dysfunction from dysarthria: a systematic review of the evidence. J Med Speech-Lang Pathol 2003; 11(2):xiii–xxxviii.

Chapter 4

Psychologic Assessment and Intervention in Rehabilitation

Stephen T. Wegener, Kathleen Bechtold Korrte, Felicia Hill-Briggs, Douglas Johnson-Greene, Sara Palmer and Cynthia Salorio

Care more particularly for the individual patient than for the special features of the disease

Sir William Osler

FOUNDATIONS OF REHABILITATION PSYCHOLOGY

Sir William Osler, the noted physician and teacher, in his quote often paraphrased as 'The type of man who has the disease is more important than the type of disease the man has', recognized the importance of understanding and focusing on the person in maximizing health and function. The field of physical medicine and rehabilitation has also recognized and included psychologic assessment and intervention as an integral and critical component in the rehabilitation process. The purpose of these activities is to assist the individual with a chronic, traumatic, or congenital injury or illness in achieving optimal physical, psychologic, and social functioning. This chapter provides an overview of the scientific basis and applied practice of rehabilitation psychology. We begin by reviewing the foundations of rehabilitation psychology, describe intervention and assessment techniques, and conclude by addressing special topics regarding psychologic aspects of rehabilitation.

Rehabilitation psychology practice is influenced by the history and scientific literature of diverse fields, including neuroscience, vocational rehabilitation, social psychology, behavioral psychology, counseling, and clinical psychology. The rehabilitation psychology assessment and intervention process is guided by several key principles.

- The process is *person-centered*, as services are provided based on the preferences, needs, and resources of the individual.
- Theory and practice are grounded in the *biopsychosocial model*, which recognizes the need to address the multidimensional nature of impairments and disability.[69]
- Recognition that the *disablement process* is determined by both personal and environmental factors.
- The *interdisciplinary team*, which includes the person served, is the key component in the rehabilitation enterprise. Rehabilitation psychologists consistently involve the interdisciplinary team, including the person served in their practice, to achieve optimal rehabilitation outcomes.

Psychologists contribute to the rehabilitation process through assessment of multiple domains (cognitive, neuropsychologic, academic or vocational, emotional, coping processes, behavioral, and policy). This assessment shapes rehabilitation care and subsequent intervention, which can occur at multiple levels: individual, family, rehabilitation team, healthcare organization, or society. A variety of interventions and methods are used, including psychotherapy, counseling, behavior management, cognitive rehabilitation, consultation, and advocacy. The goal of all the interventions and methods used is to improve outcomes for persons with impairments.

Rehabilitation psychology is rooted in both basic psychologic science and applied practice. Rehabilitation psychologists have completed doctoral degrees in psychology, and extensive predoctoral and postdoctoral training in healthcare settings. The American Board of Professional Psychology recognizes rehabilitation psychology as a specialty area of practice within psychology (http://www.abrp.org). While rehabilitation psychologists belong to many professional organizations relevant to their area of practice and specialization, the major organization representing rehabilitation psychology is the American Psychological Association, Division of Rehabilitation Psychology (http://www.apa.org/divisions/div22/). The Commission on the Accreditation of Rehabilitation Facilities recognizes rehabilitation psychology services as critical to the rehabilitation process, and rehabilitation psychology is a required component of the rehabilitation team in acute and subacute programs.

Adaptation and coping

It is useful to examine the underlying theoretic models of responses to impairments and disability that guide assessment and intervention. Two points are key to understanding the individual's responses and adaptation. First, these responses need to be understood in light of the biopsychosocial model.[69] It is likely that biologic, psychologic, and social or environmental variables are involved in determining a particular individual's responses and level of adaptation. Individuals arrive at the onset of injury or illness with preexisting biologic, psychologic, or social diatheses or strengths for a particular response (e.g. depression or resilience). These preexisting factors interact with the stressors associated with impairments and disability to shape the individual's responses and ultimate adaptation trajectory. Unfortunately, outside specific diseases such as depression, the literature is not well developed regarding the role of these biopsychosocial diatheses in the adaptation process. Second, historically, adaptation models have emphasized the role of the individual in determining outcomes, the universality of responses to crises, and acceptance as an end point. Further, the focus has been on pathologic responses and outcomes following illness or trauma and the development of disability. Existing research indicates these models and their major tenets either are not supported by the data or are not adequate to understand individual outcomes or to plan interventions. While individual characteristics contribute to our reactions to trauma or illness and subsequent outcomes, early rehabilitation psychologists demonstrated the importance of the physical environment and societal responses in the shaping of the individual's response and outcome.[51,231]

The assumption of the universality of responses to crises has not been supported by the data. This concept of universality of responses is also most clearly exemplified by stage theory. Stage theory predicts individuals will respond to crises or loss in specific and predictable ways over time and eventually accept or resolve the emotional crises. While stage theory has some attraction as a heuristic device and as a convenient tool to explain emotional responses for patients and their families, it is not supported by the literature.[230] Following impairment, there is little evidence of specific and predictable reactions,[230] predictable stages over time,[64] or universal resolution of the emotional crises.[230] Finally, there is a need to adopt models and practice patterns to accommodate data indicating that, following physical trauma or illness, individuals can identify benefits and experience positive growth.[65]

More recently, the literature has emphasized models that:

- conceptualize coping as a transactional process where the individual's cognitive and behavioral responses interact with external factors;
- recognize the importance of social and environmental factors; and
- provide a theoretic basis for understanding the positive growth that can occur following trauma or illness.

Four specific models will be discussed: the crises coping model, behavioral model, social model, and resilience and growth models. This is followed by an overview of factors associated with positive and negative adaptation.

Crises coping model

The crises coping model was originally based on observations of individual's responses to loss and grief.[138] The model incorporates the individual's premorbid functioning and potential cognitive and behavioral responses, is predicated on individual's desire to achieve psychologic and social balance, and allows for the option of growth following crises. The model posits that, following a crisis, effective coping is characterized by:

- initially minimizing the seriousness of crises;
- obtaining relevant information;
- seeking emotional reassurance and support;

- learning tasks relevant to the crises;
- setting specific, limited goals;
- considering alternative outcomes; and
- finding purpose and meaning in the crises and subsequent events.

While the entire model lacks empiric support, research indicates that specific components of the model are associated with better outcomes. The model fits well with the rehabilitation process, and provides a useful tool to organize interventions as the individual moves through this process.

Behavioral model

Behavioral models emphasize the importance of attending to observable events and applying behavioral principles to modify behavior.[117] Fordyce, as a leading proponent of this model, stressed that behavioral principles and techniques are useful in achieving the primary tasks faced by persons with impairments. These tasks include increasing participation in the rehabilitation process, shaping and increasing adaptive behaviors, reducing maladaptive responses, and maintaining behaviors that minimize disability over time.[80] This model has several advantages. It recognizes the importance of social and contextual cues in shaping an individual's response to the process of rehabilitation and disability. It provides for specific interventions, using established techniques, to shape and maintain adaptive responses. The process is data-driven, because self-monitoring and observable results are a key component of the behavioral model. Finally, the behavioral model does not assume a pathologic focus, but can be applied equally to development and maintenance of adaptive responses and reduction of maladaptive behaviors. Particular examples of the behavior model are skill models that emphasize skill deficits and acquisition in adaptation to impairments. Successful coping with disability requires numerous skills, including self-care skills, social skills, assertiveness, communication, and self-advocacy.[59] Skills can be enhanced and are associated with positive outcomes.[58,67] (See the intervention section that follows for a detailed discussion of behavioral principles and methods.)

Social model

The social model of disability departs from the medical model, and conceptualizes the individual's responses and emotional distress associated with disability as a product of social and environmental conditions rather than individual traits, problems, or deficits.[163] This model states that the social and environmental context in which impairment occurs is a major determinant of whether that impairment will become a disability, and any resulting emotional distress. For example, if the environment were more accessible, mobility impairments and wheelchair use would be less disabling. Further, if discriminatory barriers in hiring people with disabilities were reduced and equal access to social interaction was available, there would be less disability and related psychosocial distress. The social model stresses the social barriers to participation (stigma, discrimination, lack of resources, and inaccessible environments) as the primary factor in poor adaptation to impairments and increased disability. The minority model defines problems in responding to disability as a function of the negative attitudes of people without disabilities (the majority) toward those with disabilities (the minority), and a social environment that fails to accommodate the needs of persons with disabilities.[163] Persons with disabilities are viewed as a minority group that has been denied civil rights, protection, and equal access, with related social isolation and inferior treatment. Major impediments to successful coping and solutions to psychosocial difficulties for people with disabilities require changes in social, political, environmental, and economic spheres. In this model, psychologic intervention to assist people in their response to disability includes education; empowerment; and strategies for assertiveness, self-advocacy, and social support.

Resilience and growth models

There is a long history in psychology recognizing the human potential to cope effectively, find meaning, and grow when confronted with adversity.[84] This early work and more recent theory and data[65] indicate that, following a crisis such as trauma or illness, a number of potential outcomes are possible. These potential courses and outcomes are depicted in Figure 4-1. Clinically and in research, we primarily focus attention on individuals who have maladaptive responses or poor outcomes. We devote less attention to understanding those individuals who demonstrate resilience with return to baseline functioning or demonstrate resilience with growth. Resilience generally refers to patterns of positive adaptation in the face of significant adversity or risk. Several constructs have been postulated as

mechanisms to account for the positive variations in individuals' responses following illness or trauma. Overarching constructs such as hope[192] have limited but growing support. However, the research has focused on largely specific behavioral, cognitive, or affective coping strategies rather than demonstrating the validity of one overarching construct.

Coping theory argues that the emotional response to any adverse event depends largely on the individual's appraisal of the event in terms of its meaning, opportunities for control, available support, and past experience. Coping involves dynamic cognitive and behavioral efforts to manage stressors that are appraised as challenging or threatening. These efforts to contain the resulting emotional distress were initially conceptualized as falling into problem-focused or emotion-focused domains.[131] Emotion-focused strategies focused on managing undesirable feelings, while problem-focused strategies focused on managing the stressful situations that were perceived as controllable. Carver and Scheier argued that it is more accurate to classify coping strategies into emotion-focused (e.g. seeking emotional social support, positive reinterpretation, denial), problem-focused (active coping, planning, seeking instrumental social support), and avoidance (venting emotions, behavioral disengagement, mental disengagement).[35] Subsequent research has identified coping strategies and patterns associated with positive and negative adaptation.

Factors associated with positive adaptation

While both individual and environmental factors have been associated with positive adaptation, the majority of the research has focused on individual and negative factors. Enduring demographic characteristics such as race, gender, and age generally account for a limited amount of variance in adaptation following injury or illness. Socioeconomic status, which is related to the social and environmental context, appears to have a larger impact on adaptation than other demographic variables.[49,68,85] Aspects of injury (e.g. duration and severity) do not reliably predict within a given injury group long-term adaptation, although differences between different types of injuries or illness are evident. Enduring personality characteristics of the individual, such as greater levels of hope,[63] lower levels of neuroticism,[126] higher levels of agreeableness,[65] and internal locus of control,[82] are associated with better adaptation as reflected in mood and life satisfaction ratings.

Positive adaptation appears related to various cognitive styles and coping strategies. Individuals who report less stress and better adaptation are those who initially seek to establish control over their responses rather than external events,[103] look to find meaning and positive aspects of the experience,[57,205] and positively reinterpret the experience and seek growth.[121] Denial bears special consideration, as it is often misunderstood in the rehabilitation setting. Denial falls into the category of emotion-focused coping. Denial was previously conceived to be a maladaptive response, whereas realistic appraisal of deficits and limitations were thought to be the hallmarks of psychologic adjustment after injury or disability. More recent research suggests that denial is a complex phenomenon that can be

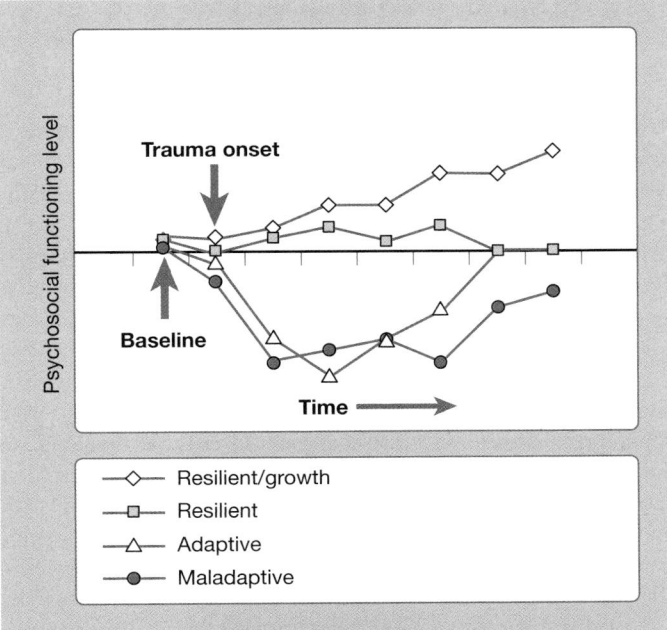

Figure 4-1 Potential responses to trauma or illness. (After Sherman and Rambaldo 2002,[188] with permission.)

maladaptive or adaptive, depending on when in the course of illness or recovery it is employed, and whether or not there is a neurologic component.[124] 'Positive illusions' and related cognitive beliefs such as optimism and positive appraisal of seemingly negative events have been linked with better health outcomes and improved mood in individuals under stress.[204] While it appears clear that certain coping responses are related to positive adaptation, it is not well established whether these responses can be taught to individuals who do not spontaneously use them. Finally, while additional work is necessary regarding the role of policy (e.g. the Americans with Disabilities Act) and increased physical and social accessibility, environment factors of higher levels of social support[85] and family problem-solving[66] are both associated with better adaptation.

Factors associated with negative adaptation

While it is expeditious to assume that the opposite levels of personality characteristics that are associated with better adaptation would be associated with poor adaptation, this might not be true. It has been observed that higher levels of neuroticism, specifically an affinity for negative emotions, have been associated with poor adaptation.[126] The use of avoidance coping strategies has been associated with poor outcomes across a number of populations, and is one of the most robust findings in the literature.[97,121] The use of avoidance might prevent individuals from engaging in cognitions or behaviors that minimize the impact of the disability and prevent identification of potential growth opportunities.

One coping strategy that appears to be particularly destructive in the adaptation process is catastrophizing. This is a cognitive response to an event that is marked by exaggerated negative expectations and focus. Catastrophizing has been reliably and repeatedly associated with poor adaptation in a number of health conditions, particularly in the area of pain.[28,212] In contrast to other factors, it has been demonstrated that catastrophizing is an important intervening variable that can be modified through cognitive behavior theory interventions. This makes it a critical target of assessment and intervention.[29] Finally, individuals who are below the poverty level are at greater risk for poor adaptation, potentially due to the social and material disadvantages associated with this condition.[49,68]

Given the prevalence of depression and anxiety in rehabilitation populations, some additional points are warranted. In addition to the psychologic and social factors discussed above, biologic diatheses (e.g. genetic predisposition) are associated with increased risk for mood disorders in the general population, and this is likely to be true in rehabilitation populations. Depression is a common response to overwhelming loss, and new physical impairments can be associated with a host of losses: loss of body parts or functions, loss of social functions including decreased participation in work and social status, and separation from family and friends during hospitalization. Loss and grief can be better thought of as predisposing factors for depression, rather than its cause. In those who become depressed after an injury, illness, or other loss, other factors can also play a role. These factors include biologic predisposition,

personality, cognitive schemas or belief systems, and social supports. Preinjury belief systems marked by negative expectations or external locus of control are risk factors for depression. Locus of control refers to a person's beliefs regarding their ability to affect events and control outcomes. Those with an internal locus of control see themselves controlling events and outcomes through their own actions, whereas those with an external locus of control see others as controlling events or outcomes. Internal locus of control is associated with a more hopeful and positive outlook, and lower depression scores.[83] A related concept from cognitive psychology is learned helplessness,[186] which occurs when a person's attempts to change events or create positive experiences have been repeatedly thwarted, and the person comes to believe that future efforts are futile.

Anxiety is not necessarily a maladaptive emotion. Anxiety is a normal response to stress or threat, and can be highly adaptive as a signal for needed action. Impairment, hospitalization, and disability-related events can increase anxiety and might lead to the development of maladaptive anxiety disorders. Sensory deprivation and lack of orienting stimuli are inherent to the experience of the intensive care unit. The sensory deficits associated with neurologic conditions such as tetraplegia or stroke contribute to sensory deprivation and can have disorienting and anxiety-provoking effects. Loss of control over bodily functions and mobility, personal routines, and decision making also contribute to anxiety in the rehabilitation setting. Over the longer term, an illness or disability whose symptoms and progression are unpredictable leads to anticipation of aversive experiences, which in turn increase anxiety. When anxiety or negative events reoccur, anticipatory anxiety[41,116] can develop. This creates a situation in which one is anxious about potential negative events or anxiety. This can result in a maladaptive cycle, in which any stimuli or behaviors associated with the anticipated event or anxiety are avoided. As a result, behavior becomes increasingly restricted. Anxiety can further impair rehabilitation through interference of concentration, memory, and learning.

Prevalence of mood and cognitive impairment in rehabilitation populations

While the prevalence of mood, cognitive morbidities, and substance use in rehabilitation populations is often advanced as the rationale for inclusion of psychologic care in rehabilitation, many individuals with physical impairments do not develop mood disturbances or other psychologic symptoms, most do not develop major psychiatric disorders, and professionals are likely to overestimate the level of mood disturbances in persons with disability.[82,175] The rates of these symptoms and conditions vary depending on the sample and diagnostic criteria used and on the point in time of evaluation. They are higher in rehabilitation populations than in the general population,[224] but are similar to those found in other medical populations.[176] Common symptoms include poststroke depression (10–61%) and anxiety (5–30%);[33,221] post-spinal cord injury (SCI) depression (22–40%) and anxiety disorders (25–60%);[64,86,120] post-lower limb amputation depression (20–35%);[115,184] and post-traumatic brain injury (TBI) psychiatric symptomatology including depression, anxiety, and behavioral disturbance (30–80%).[74,114] These rates reflect a range of psychologic distress responses and are not indicative of the percentage of individuals who would meet the diagnostic criteria for the formal disorder. Substance abuse has been identified as a significant problem in persons with TBI and SCI.[74,104] Comorbid cognitive impairments of varying degrees of severity occur, for example in 24–60% of stroke patients[54,203,221] and 25–60% of acute traumatic SCI patients.[50,180] Cognitive impairment can significantly impact the rehabilitation process and functional outcomes, and is common in rehabilitation populations. Cognitive impairment characterizes the clinical presentation of most patients with moderate to severe TBI, and cognitive dysfunction associated with vascular disease is detectable in many lower limb amputees.[168] While recognizing that psychologic distress is not a universal response, psychologic evaluation and intervention can improve mood, increase adaptive behaviors, reduce cognitive dysfunction, and facilitate the rehabilitation process.

Behavioral and learning principles

Behavioral and learning theorists define behavior as everything an individual says or does. Behaviors can be adaptive or maladaptive in nature, and can help individuals achieve a goal or hinder their ability to be successful in that goal. Theories of behavior and learning were influenced by early studies of classical and operant conditioning procedures in animals. Ivan Pavlov noted that a specific stimulus (i.e. food placed in a dog's mouth) would lead to a predictable and consistent biologic reflex (i.e. salivation).[167] He also noted that the pairing of the biologic stimulus (i.e. food) with other things in the environment (i.e. a technician in a white lab coat) would eventually lead to the response on presentation of the 'paired stimulus' alone. This reflexive or biologic response to a neutral object is a phenomenon that has been termed Pavlovian conditioning, respondent conditioning, or classical conditioning. Other concepts stemming from this work include habituation (in which a response becomes less intense with repeated exposure to the stimulus), generalization (in which other similar stimuli begin to elicit the response), and discrimination (in which the response is elicited by a particular stimulus but not to other similar stimuli). This methodology has been used in humans to treat cigarette addiction, for example by pairing an unpleasant stimulus with the act of smoking. This leads to a negative reaction to the act of smoking itself.[48] Systematic desensitization[229] also relies on classical conditioning principles, in that it strives to 'unpair' a conditioned response from the stimulus that elicits it (e.g. a physiologic anxiety response to a feared stimulus).

Other theorists sought to explain how a new behavior could develop, and noted that a behavior can be impacted by the consequences that follow. Thorndike[207] and Skinner[189,190] noted that animals (and humans) increase the frequency of behaviors that lead to positive consequences, and decrease behaviors that lead to negative consequences. The increase or decrease of a behavior in response to consequences is termed operant conditioning. This methodology has been used to increase desirable behaviors and decrease undesirable behaviors in both children and adults through the behavior modification techniques described below. In general, operant conditioning and its clinical application, behavior modification, assume that all behavior is maintained, changed, or shaped by the consequences of that behavior. *Reinforcers* are consequences that strengthen behavior. *Punishments* are consequences that weaken behavior.[171]

Other early learning theorists elaborated on how new behaviors are developed or learned by imitation of others and by observation of positive consequences received by the model.[13,14] Learning by observation, often referred to as latent learning, can occur without the presence of an observable reward.[208] Behavioral techniques such as modeling and shaping use these principles and serve as the fundamental principles behind milieu treatments.[16]

ASSESSMENT

Clinical interview

Information about the patient's medical, psychiatric, and social history is a key component in the treatment and discharge planning of individuals participating in rehabilitation services. Understanding premorbid functioning provides a context for current functioning. Knowledge of a patient's history can assist the rehabilitation psychologist in identifying potential areas of intervention, to reduce the risk of behavioral or emotional issues becoming barriers to the rehabilitation process. Understanding the patient's history is critical for a clear interpretation of observations and diagnosis of current condition.

Background information can be collected from a number of sources. The patient's medical chart provides important information about past medical history and the current medical condition. Certain aspects of the patient's history, however, are best collected from the patient through a well-directed interview. The interview includes specific questions regarding understanding of the current situation and how it has affected functioning. It is also important to learn the current emotional, behavioral, and cognitive symptoms; past history of psychiatric or adjustment difficulties; and social history. The quality of the information collected from the patient is dependent on the nature and severity of the medical condition, whether cognitive impairment is present, and whether the patient is motivated to participate in the interview. Given that there are many factors that could affect the patient's ability to convey accurate history, the family is another important source of information regarding social history, past psychiatric or medical problems, and level of functioning. Additionally, their observations and insights about changes in the patient's functioning can clarify whether certain impairments in functioning represent an acute change or a preexisting condition. Box 4-1 provides a description of the key elements typically reviewed during a clinical interview.

Behavioral observations

Important information about a patient's functioning can be gleaned by observing the behavior exhibited. Indicators of mood, neurologic functioning, and discomfort are evident in a person's facial expressions, speech patterns, interaction style,

---

Box 4-1 Key concepts addressed in the psychologic interview

History
- Genesis of current condition and symptoms
- Medical history: trauma, chronic conditions
- Social history: family of origin, physical or sexual abuse, current living situation, primary relationship status and quality, educational and vocational background, military service, legal involvement, religious or spiritual life, interactions with persons with disability
- Self-care history: health behaviors, assistance needs, difficulty with self-care
- Significant stressors in life, coping style and effectiveness
- Psychiatric history: illness, treatment
- Substance use

Current status
- Mental status: alertness, orientation, attention, reality testing
- Affect: range, lability, stability, appropriateness
- Mood: dysthemic, euthymic, euphoric
- Vegetative function: sleep, appetite, energy, libido
- Threat of harm to self or others
- Understanding of medical condition and illness
- Level of awareness of, and concerns, regarding current situation
- Level and quality of social support

Pain
- Immediate concerns, goals for rehabilitation, expectations for recovery, impact of residual impairments on lifestyle and relationships

---

Box 4-2 Behavioral observations

- Arousal level: alert, drowsy, stuporous, comatose
- Affect: broad, restricted, flat, dysphoric
- Psychopathology: paranoia, delusional thinking
- Speech: fluent, intelligible, dysarthric
- Language:
  expressive (evidence of paraphasic errors, word-finding problems)
  receptive (difficulty following commands, needs repetition of information presented)
- Thinking: focused, tangential, goal-directed, perseverative
- Self-monitoring: disinhibited, impulsive, awareness of impairments
- Motor functioning:
  tone and spasticity
  coordination (ataxia)
  tremor, reflexes (Babinski, frontal release signs)
- Memory functioning: carryover of information during session
- Attention skills: distractible, focused
- Level of effort, motivation, resistance
- Pain: facial grimacing, muscle tension, bracing during movement

---

motor behavior, and the content of information presented. Behavioral data provide the context for objective measures of emotional and cognitive functioning, as well as a basis for differential diagnosis, by providing qualitative information about a person's functioning. Box 4-2 provides a summary of areas of behavior that are important to observe within the rehabilitation setting.

Neuropsychologic assessment
Goals and purpose
Patients can be quite diverse in terms of the severity of their cognitive deficits and the quality of their behavior. Neuropsychologic assessment is important in understanding the nature and severity of the central nervous system impairments presumed to underlie cognitive and behavioral disturbances. There has been a gradual shift in the role of neuropsychology from one of primarily differential diagnosis to a relatively greater emphasis on interventions. Increasingly, information from neuropsychologic evaluations is used in planning and implementing rehabilitation treatments.[195]

A neuropsychologic evaluation is concerned with the functional integrity of the brain. A neuropsychologic evaluation allows for the quantitative measurement of brain function in terms of cognitive strengths and weaknesses by an expert in brain–behavior relationships. Objective observations are made using standardized tests of cognitive ability across a variety of domains, and are interpreted in light of the contextual variables associated with each patient's unique history.

Accurate interpretation of standardized test results requires contextual information that begins with a review of the patient's case history, hospital records, and interviews with patients and their family members. While accurate background information is important in all major life domains, it is of particular significance in patients with central nervous system impairments in the areas of educational attainment, previous neurologic risk factors such as history of head trauma and learning disabilities, and premorbid substance abuse. Neuropsychologists commonly seek consistency of information in terms of patients presenting complaints and the following:

- performance on cognitive tests;
- observations from family members and employers;
- injury characteristics as identified in medical records;
- impairment in activities of daily living; and
- presentation over time.

Emotional states can influence test results and should be assessed as part of any neuropsychologic evaluation. Assessment of behavior and mood can be problematic in patients with central nervous system impairment, because many depression inventories have physical and cognitive items that are not specific to depression in this population. This can result in artificially inflated estimates of depression incidence and severity.[162] Assessment of premorbid emotional disorders allows one to consider their impact on test interpretation.

The specific goals of neuropsychologic services vary, but there are several goals common to all patients.

tion: http://tbims.org/combi/list.html.) The choice of tests is based on several factors, including the referral question, patient's medical diagnosis, stability or instability of cognitive impairment, rehabilitation goals, and patient characteristics such as age or years of education. In settings in which a brief determination of whether a patient probably has cognitive impairment, a cognitive screening measure could be used. These cognitive screening measures generally sample multiple cognitive domains (e.g. orientation, language, immediate and brief delay recall), perhaps with one or a few items. However, cognitive screenings are not designed for diagnostic purposes. Screenings can be used to determine whether further evaluation, for diagnostic purposes, is warranted.

A comprehensive evaluation should focus on all major cognitive domains to make a definitive determination regarding the cognitive integrity. This includes evaluating the sensory and perceptual processes, verbal and non-verbal intelligence, simple and complex attention, processing speed, learning and memory, language, motor functions, and executive functions. A comprehensive approach takes considerable time, and it is not unusual for evaluation to take 6–8 h of direct face to face testing time and additional time for test scoring, interpretation, and report preparation. The alternative is to focus primarily on areas that are commonly associated with the presumed etiologic entity, although there would be a greater likelihood that significant impairments would be missed. An appropriate neuropsychologic evaluation strikes a balance between comprehensiveness and adequately sampling areas commonly impaired. Preferably, two or more instruments that measure the same domain are used to show consistency across the same cognitive construct.

A neuropsychologic evaluation is often utilized when a diagnosis regarding cognitive impairment is desired. This can help determine whether the patient is cognitively intact (no cognitive impairment), exhibits cognitive dysfunction (subclinical), exhibits cognitive impairment (clinical: mild, moderate, or severe), exhibits a focal cognitive disorder (e.g. aphasia, amnestic disorder), or has dementia (e.g. vascular, probable Alzheimer disease, frontotemporal). An evaluation can also be conducted to identify relative cognitive strengths to aid in the rehabilitation process. From the neuropsychologic evaluation, specific treatment recommendations can be made to guide the rehabilitation team in designing and conducting cognitive rehabilitation and intervening on functional tasks impeded by cognition. A brief description of the primary cognitive domains and common neuropsychologic measures can be found in Table 4-1.

Box 4-3 Common reasons for neuropsychologic referral

Diagnosis
- Identifying central nervous system impairments and their likely neuroanatomic correlates
- Differentiating between psychiatric and neurologic conditions
- Describing relationships between neurologic symptoms and behavior
- Determining prognosis and course of illness
- Screening for further work-up

Evaluating cognitive and emotional strengths and weaknesses
- Placement and supervision needs
- Goals for post-discharge planning and self-care
- Determining emotional adjustment to neurologic illness
- Identification of positive coping strategies
- Identification of cognitive abilities and strengths

Specific assessment needs
- Disability determination and vocational planning
- Forensic issues
- Competency (trial or decision making)

Intervention and treatment
- Developing appropriate cognitive remediation or treatment plans
- Determining efficacy and response to psychotropic medication
- Design of behavioral programs within the scope of patient's capabilities

Research

- Providing recommendations that will facilitate rehabilitation efforts, including illumination of potential assets and obstacles for acute and long-term recovery.
- Outlining functional impairments that can be reasonably inferred from neuropsychologic data (e.g. inability to drive), safety issues associated with cognitive impairments (e.g. problem solving), or lack of awareness of impairments.
- Addressing motivational and emotional issues that could adversely affect quality of life.
- Indicating strategies for treatment intervention and adaptation to disability.

Implicit in these goals is the diversity of patients' needs, the multifactorial nature of their impairments, and the need to provide interventions that will improve the person's quality of life. Potential reasons for referral for neuropsychologic services can be found in Box 4-3.

Primary measurement domains and common measures

There are a few hundred cognitive and neuropsychologic tests available, although fewer have acceptable reliability and validity.[135] A list of selected, commonly used tests in adult rehabilitation is provided in Table 4-1 (see Lezak et al 2004[135] for references on individual measures). In addition to those cited in this table, scales have been developed and validated specifically for the TBI population by the TBI Model Systems program's Center for Outcome Measurement in Brain Injury (COMBI). (See the COMBI web site for additional informa-

Fixed versus flexible battery approach

One area of controversy in neuropsychology, particularly in the area of forensic assessment in TBI populations, has to do with the clinician's decision whether to use a fixed or flexible battery for their assessment. In a flexible battery approach, sometimes referred to as a hypothesis-driven approach, a group of individual tests are selected based on the patient's presenting problems, each test having established validity for assessing a particular domain. In a fixed battery approach, tests are selected prior to learning of the patient's presenting complaints that as

Table 4-1 Examples of neuropsychologic tests in adult rehabilitation[135]

Type or focus of assessment	Common neuropsychologic measures
Academic achievement and premorbid functioning	Wide Range Achievement Test, 3rd revision (WRAT-3) National American Adult Reading Test (NAART) Wechsler Individualized Achievement Test (WIAT)
Attention	Connor's Continuous Performance Test—II (CPT-II) Paced Auditory Serial Addition Test (PASAT) Trail Making Test (TMT) Auditory Consonant Trigrams (ACT) Line bisection Behavioral Inattention Test
Cognitive screenings	Mini Mental-State Examination (MMSE) Repeatable Battery for the Assessment of Neuropsychological Status (RBANS) Neurobehavioral Cognitive Status Examination (COGNISTAT)
Dementia scales	Mattis Dementia Rating Scale (DRS-3) Consortium to Establish a Registry for Alzheimer's Disease (CERAD)
Executive functions (planning, mental flexibility)	Wisconsin Card Sorting Test (WCST) Booklet Category Test (BCT) Delis–Kaplan Executive Function System (D-KEFS)
Fixed neuropsychologic batteries	Halsted–Reitan Neuropsychological Battery (HRNB) Luria–Nebraska Neuropsychological Battery (LNNB)
Intelligence	Wechsler Adult Intelligence Scale—III (WAIS-III) Test of Non-verbal Intelligence (TONI), 2nd edn
Language	Boston Diagnostic Aphasia Examination (BDAE) Controlled Oral Word Association Test (COWAT) Multilingual Aphasia Examination—III (MAE-III)
Learning and memory	Wechsler Memory Scales (WMS-III) California Verbal Learning Test—II (CVLT-II) Rey Complex Figure Test (RCFT)
Processing speed	Symbol Digit Modalities Test (SDMT) Stroop Neuropsychological Screening Test
Psychomotor	Finger tapping test Grooved pegboard Grip strength
Sensory, visual perceptual, visuospatial, and visuomotor	Clock drawing Hooper Visual Organization Test (HVOT) Judgment of Line Orientation (JLO) Reitan–Klove Sensory Perceptual Examination

a group have been shown to validly detect brain impairment across a number of domains. There are several advantages and disadvantages of each approach. For example, the Halstead–Reitan Neuropsychological Test Battery (HRNTB) has been extensively researched and has been used in the current format for nearly five decades. When given as a complete battery, it provides relatively broad examination across most cognitive domains. The problems include the fact that the tests in the HRNTB rely on multiple cognitive domains, complicating interpretation of impaired test performance. There is inadequate normative data for some HRNTB tests and summary scores, and some domains (e.g. intelligence and memory) have either cursory assessment or are not assessed at all. In contrast, the flexible battery approach has the potential for fine-grain analysis

of the patient's presenting problems. Perhaps more importantly, it can identify the underlying cognitive processes that might suggest effective treatment interventions. For these reasons, many neuropsychologists use a hybrid approach in which the fixed battery HRNTB is supplemented with additional flexible battery tests.

Factors that influence test performance

Accurate and valid neuropsychologic evaluation requires certain prerequisites to permit attribution of impaired performance to brain dysfunction and not to extraneous factors. First and foremost, patients must be able to sustain sufficient arousal to attempt completion of cognitive tasks. They must have adequate integrity of sensory functions to utilize and interact with test stimulus materials. For tests that require manipulation of test materials or writing, they must have adequate function of the upper limbs. Last, they must have adequate attention to attend to test instructions, changing contingencies, and task demands. The presence of one or more of these problems has the potential to inhibit or impair performance on many neuropsychologic tests. When these prerequisites are not met, decreased performance can be unrelated to the patient's cognitive state. At a minimum, this diminishes the psychologist's ability to differentiate the contribution of cognitive impairments to the patient's test performance. Later in this chapter, we will discuss how tests can be adapted to account for some situations.

Another prerequisite for obtaining valid test data is having a high degree of confidence that the patients are attempting to put forth their best effort, because impaired performance can look quite similar to unmotivated performance. Several standardized instruments that have been designed specifically for examining motivational issues, which are now routinely administered by psychologists, include the Test of Memory Malingering and the Validity Indicator Profile.[135] It is also common to look for signs of diminished motivation on neuropsychologic tests by examining 1) the degree of consistency across tests that measure the same cognitive domains, 2) level of test performance impairment and severity of the injury or illness, 3) pattern of test performance and typical pattern of deficits for the presumed underlying disorder, 4) test performance and reported functional impairments, and 5) test administrations. For example, a patient might have severe impairments across multiple cognitive domains that are inconsistent with the presumed diagnostic etiology and are at odds with their relatively intact functional skills. These inconsistencies are a possible indicator of diminished motivation in the absence of other explanatory factors. It is important to note that diminished motivation does not necessarily reflect intentional misrepresentation. The reasons for decreased motivation vary, and can range from mild detriments secondary to emotional states such as depression to more pervasive detriments associated with malingering.

Premorbid estimation and the deficit assessment approach

In 1937, the British neurologist Sir Charles Symonds, commenting on TBI outcome, stated, 'It is not only the kind of injury that matters, but the kind of head'. Having a full understanding of factors that can impact premorbid brain functioning and intellectual ability is essential for understanding central nervous system impairments. It is the nature of neuropsychologic assessment to compare current performance with an estimate of the patient's premorbid level of functioning as a means of defining deficits and retained abilities.[137] While it is sometimes possible to obtain information on specific premorbid cognitive impairments, such as reading impairment in an adult with well-documented childhood dyslexia, it is most common to estimate premorbid abilities using premorbid intelligence as a proxy. Cognitive deficits and retained strengths are highlighted in the typical neuropsychologic report within

a context of a specified range of premorbid intellectual ability.

As preinjury intellectual measurement scores are typically not available, there are several approaches to determine an estimated premorbid intelligence.

- Obtaining educational records of academic attainment and achievement, particularly those that contain results of achievement test scores.
- The use of demographic regression equations that use patient characteristics (e.g. attained educational level) to estimate intelligence.
- The use of 'hold' measures that are thought to be resistant to brain insults and injuries (vocabulary subtest from the Wechsler Adult Intelligence Scale—III and tests of sight-reading ability).
- 'Best performance' approaches in which premorbid functioning is estimated based on the best level of performance on several measures from among a battery of tests.

It is not unusual to use several of these approaches to provide a likely range of premorbid functioning. Performance on cognitive tests can then be compared with a patient's estimated premorbid intellectual level. Estimates of premorbid ability are generally the most accurate when the actual ability is within the average range, and become less accurate with departures from the average range.[200]

Test interpretation and use of normative data

Test interpretation is only as good as the normative information used to interpret the test performance. The closer a normative sample is to the examinee's characteristics, the more confidence one can have that the test interpretation was valid. This would be a problem, for example, if the patient was an 85-year-old African-American man with recent TBI. This results from the fact that the normative sample contained relatively few ethnic minority persons, and none who were over 80 years of age. It would not be possible to accurately interpret the patient's test results, because we would not know the performance of the average 85-year-old African-American man without TBI.

The most common demographic variables considered in compiling normative data are age and education, because these have been shown to be highly correlated with performance on cognitive tests.[135] Gender and ethnicity are also sometimes available in normative samples, and can increase the accuracy of interpretation for some types of tests. In general, neuropsychologic tests that have a large normative sample (e.g. several hundred or more) and sampling of diverse cultural, ethnic, gender, educational, intellectual, and age strata are the most likely to promote good inferences about test performance.

Adaptation of tests and methods for specific populations

While nearly all psychometric tests of cognitive abilities have procedures for standardized administration, there are variations in standard administration throughout clinical practices. Variation of standardized procedures may be for appropriate rationale, such as a desire to test the limits of the individual's abilities by modifying procedures, as well as for inappropriate reasons such as improper administration, convenience, or personal preference. It is also sometimes necessary to adopt special strategies for gaining maximal test performance when working with persons with impairments. Although not specifically addressed in most test manuals, clinicians might need to work harder at developing appropriate patient–provider rapport. This includes providing encouragement for patients to remain task-oriented, assisting with managing frustration associated with poor test performance, providing frequent repetition of test stimuli and instructions, or choosing alternate measures to accommodate physical limitations. When the purpose of the evaluation is to obtain the individual's best performance, it can be appropriate to modify standardized test procedures for persons with disabilities while still preserving important aspects of the standardized administration.[102,107]

Modification of test procedures is most commonly done when a patient has physical or sensory limitations. Careful test selection should be the first choice when confronted with these limitations, and can obviate the need for any test modification. For example, in patients with upper limb motor problems (e.g. SCI, stroke, or Parkinson disease), it may be wise to select tests that do not require manipulation of objects or writing.[179] For persons with visual impairment, it might be possible to use tests with auditory stimuli, or to use visually mediated tests for those with impaired hearing.

A second-tier choice is actual modification of test procedures and stimuli. Rephrasing questions or elaborating on instructions can allow the patient to complete the tests while still preserving test validity. Stimuli for some tests can be enlarged for those who have visual impairments. Psychologists might need to enlarge the materials themselves, although for some tests enlarged print or stimuli can be purchased. For those with unilateral visual field inattention, stimuli can be placed in the intact visual field instead of the patient's midline. For some verbally mediated tests, recognition items have been developed for those who have expressive communication deficits.[22] A number of modifications of various tests have been reported in the literature for other specific populations. For a comprehensive list of tests that have had published modifications, the reader is referred to Caplan and Scherer (1995).[31]

Psychologists have an ethical responsibility to use tests that are appropriate and meaningful for the population being assessed, and to draw valid inferences from the tests they administer. It can be appropriate to judiciously modify standardized tests in certain situations. Indeed, psychologists might have an affirmative need to modify tests as part of a legal requirement for reasonable accommodations under the Americans with Disabilities Act.[62] Modifications to standardized test administration should be noted in any subsequent report, along with any interpretative caveats. This requires a more cautious interpretation, or at least a broader-defined range of performance. When possible, psychologists can provide both modified and unmodified scores, assuming that both versions can be administered, and provide explanations for any score discrepancies.

Integrating neuropsychologic assessment and functional evaluations

The neuropsychologic evaluation aims to assess brain and behavior relationships through assessment of specific neurocognitive domains using standardized, usually novel, testing stimuli.[135] Functional evaluations identify cognitive deficits in the context of performing everyday tasks and activities.[151] These include scanning the environment for obstacles while ambulating, sequencing steps while dressing or preparing a meal, or remembering therapy activities performed during the day. The neuropsychologic evaluation and the functional evaluation each contribute important, independent information to the overall formulation of the patient's cognitive functioning. This formulation guides the rehabilitation treatment planning with regard to rehabilitation goals, cognitive interventions, and need for supervision.

Emphasis is increasingly being placed on the functional implications of cognitive assessment. Inferences are now routinely made about functional skills based on cognitive test results. Reasonably intact cognitive skills are arguably a prerequisite for most functional activities, although there tends to be more preserved performance on tasks that were previously learned and had been performed often compared with novel task performance following brain injury or illness. Neuropsychology has made considerable strides in the past decade in demonstrating the functional implications of cognitive deficits. While it is clear that most indices of brain injury and illness correlate well with the severity of both cognitive and functional impairments, additional work needs to be done to demonstrate more fully the ecologic validity of neuropsychologic tests.[105]

Not infrequently, rehabilitation teams find that the results of a patient's neuropsychologic evaluation and the results of the patient's functional assessment by other members of the rehabilitation team can differ regarding the absence or presence of cognitive impairment.[39] When this occurs, understanding the nature of the patient's cognitive presentation (and how to intervene) requires that the psychologist consider several factors. These factors include the circumstances under which the neuropsychologic and functional evaluations occurred (environment, context, cues), novelty or familiarity of the cognitive tasks presented, amount of structure provided during the evaluations, and ecologic validity of the evaluation methods used.

When a neuropsychologic evaluation finds that cognition is impaired, but a functional evaluation finds that cognition is intact, considerations include the following. First, although neurocognitive skills are impaired, the patient might be able to perform tasks that rely on routines, familiarity, and previously over-learned or automatic behaviors. In this case, the patient is likely to exhibit vulnerability to functional impairment when confronted with complicated or new functional tasks. Second, the patient's individual cognitive skills might be impaired when examined in isolation but, when aided by cues provided by the context in which an activity takes place, is able to function better than expected. For example, the patient might be able to function in a kitchen when asked to begin to prepare a meal, versus a novel neurocognitive test of planning and organization. The development of cognitive skills in a case like this might benefit from use of environmental context to trigger a specific functional activity or chain of behaviors.

At times, a neuropsychologic evaluation finds cognition is intact, but a functional assessment finds cognition is impaired. One reason may be the testing environment, which for a neuropsychologic evaluation is highly structured and designed to minimize distractions. However, the environment in which functional activity takes place has more stimulation, with multiple activities, sounds, and people. Environmental factors can impede the patient's ability to utilize intact cognitive skills adequately. A second potential reason deals with the threshold for use of the clinical term *impairment* in cognition. Neuropsychologic scores are generally standardized and take into account normal changes or differences in cognitive performance due to age, education, and/or gender. In the case of an elderly patient, for example, a diagnosis of cognitive impairment requires that the patient perform below what is expected for normal (healthy or typical) persons of similar age or below the patient's baseline. This same elderly patient might demonstrate significant difficulty preparing a meal in an unfamiliar environment (e.g. kitchen in the occupational therapy treatment room), resulting in a conclusion of cognitive impairment. When this seeming disagreement in testing occurs, it is important to distinguish between clinical impairment and the need for functional assistance.

Academic or vocational assessment

Research has shown that people with disabilities are often under-employed or unemployed compared with their non-disabled peers. This occurs despite developments in assistive technologies and innovations in rehabilitation approaches.[27] Understanding the legal rights under the Americans with Disabilities Act of individuals with disabilities, and the legal responsibilities of their employers, can facilitate rehabilitation specialists' abilities to assist their clients in achieving better vocational outcomes. This is needed to make sure that return to work can be fully supported by the legal provisions available.[27] See Box 4-4 for a brief description of the Americans with Disabilities Act and the particular requirements under the employment section of the Act (see Ch. 36).[8]

The accommodation needs vary for each person with a disability. It is crucial that a thorough assessment of the individual's needs is completed. This process includes assessing the person's aptitudes and interests, exploring job opportunities, seeking out further training or educational opportunities when needed, and advocating for accommodations.[182] When the goal is to return a client with a cognitive impairment to the educational or vocational setting, the process must include assessment of achievement, intellectual, and neuropsychologic functioning.

Box 4-4 The Americans with Disabilities Act

A law enacted on July 26, 1990 that:

- provides civil rights protection to individuals with disabilities;
- applies to physical, sensory, cognitive, and psychiatric disabilities; and
- guarantees equal opportunities in five areas.
  1. Employment
  2. State and local government services
  3. Transportation (public and privately operated transportation available to the public)
  4. Places of public accommodation
  5. Telecommunication services offered to the general public

Requirements under the employment portion of the Act

- Equal opportunities for jobs for which an individual with a disability is qualified.
- Accessibility of prescreening and hiring practices.
- Reasonable accommodations to permit qualified individuals with disabilities to perform the essential functions of their jobs.

One of the most commonly used tests of achievement is the Woodcock–Johnson Psychoeducational Battery.[135] It tests a variety of academic skills and can be administered to individuals aged 2 through 65. Intellectual functioning is assessed most commonly with the Wechsler Adult Intelligence Test, 3rd edition.[135] This instrument consists of 11 subtests that can be administered to persons 16–74 years of age. Full administration of all subtests allows for calculation of a verbal intelligence quotient and performance intelligence quotient (non-verbal intelligence), as well as an overall or full-scale intelligence quotient. Supplementary scores can also be calculated that provide information regarding the person's processing speed, verbal processing, perceptual organizational skills, and working memory. See Table 4-1 for examples and descriptions of measures of neuropsychologic functioning. A comprehensive assessment that includes evaluation of achievement, intellectual, and neuropsychologic functioning allows for identification of learning, cognitive, emotional, and behavioral strengths and weaknesses, as well as general aptitude. This information can be used in conjunction with recommendations regarding accommodations for any physical or sensory disabilities to provide the basis for a comprehensive educational plan.

When the results of the comprehensive assessment reveal that return to work is a reasonable goal and further education or training is not needed, then the focus shifts to identification of a specific job. The rehabilitation psychologist can assist with identifying vocational interests for career change. Such instruments as the Self-Directed Search[109] or the Strong Interest Inventory[98] are tools for identifying interests that can coincide with specific jobs. When the goal is to return the individual back to the job held prior to the onset of the disability, the psychologist can assist in identifying potential barriers and assets for performing job duties. The goal is to outline accommodations and compensatory strategies that can assist the individual in being successful in the workplace.

Personality, adaptation, and mood assessment
Personality and adaptation
Assessment of premorbid adaptation and personality can assist the clinician in identifying an individual's level of risk for psychosocial problems and poor health outcomes. Premorbid psychosocial adaptation is assessed primarily through a clinical interview, as described above. There are a range of factors, including cognitive belief systems and coping mechanisms, that are important in the clinical picture. Instruments have been developed to assess these factors, but these instruments do not have normative data and are not suitable for clinical interpretation. The discussion here emphasizes instruments with established psychometric properties and normative data critical for interpretation. Table 4-2 provides examples of commonly used measures for personality and mood assessment.

Personality assessment
The Millon Clinical Multiaxial Inventory (MCMI-III)[123] provides an assessment of personality disorders, i.e. maladaptive patterns of personality traits and behavior. The MCMI-III is primarily used to identify psychopathology but is not as useful for identifying adaptive patterns of coping.

Table 4-2 Common assessment measures for personality, mood, and psychologic distress

Type or focus of assessment	Common psychologic measures
Personality or psychopathology	Minnesota Multiphasic Personality Inventory (MMPI) Millon Clinical Multiaxial Inventory (MCMI-III) Neuroticism, Extroversion and Openness Personality Inventory (NEO-PI) Sixteen Personality Factor Questionnaire (16-PF) Personality Assessment Inventory (PAI)[158]
Depression	Beck Depression Inventory—II (BDI-II) Center for Epidemiological Studies Depression Scale (CES-D)[174] Geriatric Depression Scale (GDS) Inventory to Diagnose Depression (IDD) Zung Depression Scale[237]
Anxiety	Beck Anxiety Inventory (BAI)
Psychologic distress	Symptom Check List 90—Revised (SCL-90-R) Brief Symptom Inventory (BSI)

The Minnesota Multiphasic Personality Inventory (MMPI)-2 is also used primarily for the identification of psychopathology. It has also been used in the analysis of normal personality patterns, as well as patterns of behavior and coping relevant to specific conditions such as chronic pain.[79] The MMPI is well established, but at 567 items (370 on the short form) has some utility problems in the rehabilitation setting due to length of administration. There can also be significant difficulty adapting the MMPI for people with physical or sensory impairments.

The Sixteen Personality Factor Questionnaire[36] and the Neuroticism, Extroversion and Openness Personality Inventory[46] measure both maladaptive and adaptive personality traits, which have particular relevance to rehabilitation. The Ways of Coping Questionnaire[77,78] identifies various coping strategies individuals employ to manage adverse events. These coping strategies include, for example, escape–avoidance, positive reappraisal, and seeking social support. While normative data do not allow for a data-driven interpretation, this measure can be used for providing feedback to clients about their preferred coping strategies. It can also be used to help them explore alternative strategies that might be more effective. In combination with a clinical interview, these tests of personality and adaptation can be useful in identifying individual strengths and coping styles as well as areas of pathology.

Mood and adjustment
Depression is an important clinical problem in rehabilitation, and is associated with decreased participation in rehabilitation therapies,[90] disruption in family relationships,[7] and increased risk for comorbid conditions. It is important for the psychologist to evaluate patients for the presence of clinically significant depression. If found, depression can warrant treatment with medications or psychotherapy. Depression should be distinguished from feelings of sadness and grief, which if situation-appropriate do not necessarily require intervention. Several tests are commonly used in addition to the clinical interview to assist in the diagnosis of depression. These include the Beck Depression Inventory;[19] the Center for Epidemiological Studies Depression Scale;[174] and the Geriatric Depression Scale,[113] which is designed specifically for older adults. The Stroke Inpatient Depression Inventory[183] is designed specifically to assess depressive symptoms in stroke patients. All these depression instruments are paper and pencil tests. They can be self-administered or presented by an examiner. They are brief tests that can easily be included in a standard clinical evaluation, and provide valuable information on both the presence and the severity of depressive symptoms.

Anxiety in the rehabilitation setting is a common reaction to circumstances of new-onset impairments and hospitalization. Early identification and treatment of anxiety syndromes and disorders are important for ensuring maximal benefit from rehabilitation efforts, and avoiding unnecessary suffering. Several brief tests for assessing anxiety include the Beck Anxiety Inventory[18] and the anxiety subscales of the Symptom Check List 90—Revised (SCL-90-R) and Brief Symptom Inventory (BSI) (see below).

There are measures that assess psychologic distress across a variety of dimensions. The SCL-90-R[53] has 90 items and 9 clinical scales. These measure a variety of symptom clusters, including somatization, obsessive-compulsive, interpersonal sensitivity, depression, anxiety, hostility, phobic anxiety, paranoid ideation, and psychoticism. There are three measures of global distress, based on overall item responses reflecting the depth and severity of the problems reported. The BSI[52] is an abbreviated version of the SCL-90, and measures the same nine subscales as the SCL-90-R with 53 items. BSI norms for persons with SCI have been developed.[45] An even shorter version of the BSI, with only 18 items,[235] has recently been used to measure distress in medical patients.

Pain assessment

There is extensive literature on the psychosocial impact of chronic pain in persons with disabling conditions such as low back pain, osteoarthritis, and rheumatoid arthritis. There is also a growing body of research on the impact of pain in neuro-rehabilitation populations.[20] Independent findings suggest that many patients in these populations experience chronic pain and sequelae similar to those reported in the general chronic pain literature.[20] Clinicians must avoid discounting the problem of pain in persons with other, more obvious impairments. Optimizing function requires effective pain management. Assessment of pain should be a basic component of a comprehensive psychologic evaluation, because pain can impact function, cognitive abilities, and emotional status. Due to the subjective nature of the pain, the individual's self-report is a central and valid measure of the pain experience (see Ch. 43).

Standardized measures for assessing pain have been developed for use in both clinical and research settings. Key dimensions and established measures are presented in Table 4-3. While comprehensive pain assessment is not a component of every psychologic evaluation, basic pain assessment is essential in every case. The importance of pain assessment is recognized by recent recognition of pain as the 'fifth vital sign'.

Table 4-3 Key dimensions and measures for pain assessment

Dimension	Tool
Pain intensity or severity	Visual analog scale[215] Numeric rating scale[215] Graded chronic pain scale[214] Multidimensional Pain Inventory[122]
Pain interference	Multidimensional Pain Inventory[122] Graded chronic pain scale[214] Pain Disability Index[201]
Pain affect	McGill Pain Questionnaire,[152] short-form McGill Pain Questionnaire[153]
Pain behavior	Behavioral observation[118]

Substance abuse

One in 10 Americans has significant problems with alcohol.[155] The relationship between alcohol and traumatic injuries resulting in disability has been well documented. The rates of abuse of other substances in patients with traumatic injuries have not been as carefully studied. The rate of alcohol problems in consecutive trauma admissions has been documented to be as high as 44%.[193] Acquired conditions such as TBI have long been associated with a high rate of premorbid and postinjury alcohol-related problems.[45,108] The prevalence of problem drinking in persons with chronic disabling conditions is higher than in the general population. This has led to concern that alcohol might not only contribute to the development of a number of chronic conditions, but also slow the rate of recovery and produce secondary complications. This is a particular concern in the elderly, as the prevalence of chronic disease increases with age.

While there is general agreement that the incidence of alcohol abuse and dependence decreases with age, recent epidemiologic studies suggest that the extent of alcohol abuse in the elderly is significantly greater than previously reported.[3] It has been estimated that up to 10% of the elderly population are 'problem' drinkers. For large numbers of the elderly, alcohol abuse goes undiagnosed and untreated because of difficulties with recognition of the problem and attitudes about the elderly. There is also a general reluctance to report problem drinking in this cohort by both the problem drinkers themselves and those with whom they interact. Problem drinking in the elderly can mimic other medical and behavioral disorders common in this population. Somatic complaints, apathy, and emotional dysphoria are symptoms that are often erroneously associated with normal aging. Increased efforts to educate health practitioners about common signs of alcohol misuse in the elderly have resulted in increased identification of problem drinking, particularly in general medical settings and emergency departments.[3] Some common screening instruments—CAGE,[73] the Alcohol Use Disorders Identification Test,[12] and the Michigan Alcohol Screening Test—Geriatric Version[23]—are listed in Table 4-4.

Rates of illicit substance abuse are highest in individuals aged 18–25, and tend to decrease steadily across age groups. Utilization of prescription and over the counter medications, however, increases dramatically with age.[2] A number of factors combine to increase the risk of medication mistakes, misuse, and adverse events in persons with disabilities.

- The number of medications taken might be very high.
- The types of medications prescribed can often be habit-forming and are associated with greater impairment of alertness and cognition.
- Pharmacokinetic changes are known to occur with age.

In addition to increased use of medication and physiologic changes that can predispose patients to adverse drug reactions, the increased incidence of cognitive impairment in patients with disabilities heightens their risk for medication misuse. This can lead to neurotoxicity and adverse drug reactions, and can precipitate or worsen cognitive impairments.

Table 4-4 Screening instruments for the assessment of problem drinking

Measure	No. of items	Maximum score	Impaired range	Format
CAGE	4	4	≥2	Yes or no
Alcohol Use Disorders Identification Test (AUDIT)	10	40	≥8	Five-point description
Michigan Alcohol Screening Test—Geriatric Version (MAST-G)	24	24	≥5	Yes or no

INTERVENTION

The large majority of psychologic interventions have traditionally taken the form of direct services provided to individuals and their families in an individual or a group format. This intervention pattern is based on:

- theoretic models that have guided medical and psychologic practice, and that focus on individual factors as primary determinants of functioning and quality of life;
- diagnostic classifications and reimbursement systems that support this class of interventions; and
- research efforts and training programs that focus on direct interventions.

The impact of social and environmental factors in determining individual behavior and rehabilitation outcomes has long been recognized in rehabilitation psychology. Lewin demonstrated the importance of social and environmental factors in determining behavior.[134] Wright, Dembo, and others applied this work to the area of physical disability, recognizing the importance of these external factors in understanding the individual's reaction to impairment and level of disability.[51,231] This concept is represented in the formula $B = f(P \times O \times E)$, indicating that behavior (B) is a function of the person (P), the organic (O, biologic), and environmental factors (E).[209] Adopting this theoretic model requires clinicians, consumers, and advocates to intervene at multiple levels to achieve optimal outcomes. The model moves the sole source of the target problem from the individual with the impairment to the interface of the individual and the social environment. Psychotherapeutic interventions should be targeted at individual, group, family, team, and societal levels. These interventions can take the form of services directly provided to the patient and family, or applying psychologic theory and knowledge for the provision of indirect services. We will first focus on direct services (psychotherapy in its various forms, psychoeducation, and cognitive rehabilitation). Later, we will review other techniques and interventions that rely on psychologic theory that have special utility in the rehabilitation setting (consultation, self-management, peer modeling, and advocacy).

Psychotherapy

Psychotherapy can take many forms and utilize a variety of techniques. All successful forms of psychotherapy provide for:

- a caring, competent therapist, whom the patient believes can help;
- an opportunity for cognitive, emotional, and experiential learning;
- instillation and revitalization of hope;
- success experiences that increase the sense of mastery over oneself and the environment; and
- alleviation of negative or dysphoric feelings.[81]

The beneficial effects of psychotherapy for the typical mental health patient are well established.[119] Recently, there has been growing emphasis on evidence-based therapies to allow for matching of interventions to specific problems. Most, but not all, of the evidence-based treatments use cognitive behavioral, behavioral, or interpersonal techniques.[37] For some clinical problems (e.g. depression, anxiety, substance abuse, and pain), treatment protocols are available, although these are not widely used.[128]

Along with the data that support specific treatment approaches, there is also strong documentation in the literature of aspects of the therapeutic relationship that contribute to positive treatment outcome. The therapy relationship appears to account for as much of the treatment outcome as the specific treatment technique used.[220] There is as much need to attend to the quality of the therapeutic relationship as there is to choosing empirically supported interventions. Qualities of the relationship that are related to clinical effectiveness are a positive therapeutic alliance, therapist empathy, consensus and collaboration on goals, and cohesiveness in group therapy.[161] It is likely these same qualities are critical in the provider–consumer relationships of all members of the rehabilitation team. It is well established that individuals vary in their preparedness to engage in behavior change.[150] Matching the therapeutic technique to the individual's stage of change is probably an effective means of customizing psychotherapy. Techniques that emphasize cognitive and emotional components might be more effective with patients in the precontemplation and contemplation stages. Behavioral approaches might be more effective in the action and maintenance stages.[161]

Behavior modification targets behaviors that are observable and measurable. Behavior modification principles assume that all behavior follows a set of consistent rules. Thus methods can be developed for defining, observing, and measuring behaviors. Methods can also be developed to design specific effective interventions for changing, increasing, or decreasing target behaviors (for detailed descriptions and techniques, see Clark and Robb 1996,[42] Kazdin 2000,[117] Martin and Pear 2002,[148] and Mitenberger 2003,[157]). In many cases, the environmental consequences maintaining a behavior are not immediately obvious. For example, several studies have shown that a child's tantrums or isolated play can increase or be maintained by attention from adults.[100,236] The behavior and consequences need to be carefully examined before an intervention is designed. This is sometimes called the experimental analysis of behavior.[189]

Behavior modification does not require that the person whose behavior is being targeted is aware of the behavior or the intervention. This makes it possible to use these principles in young children and in individuals with cognitive impairments. The use of these principles, in conjunction with the individual's efforts to modify their own behaviors or cognitive responses to stimuli, is the basis for cognitive behavioral therapy (CBT) techniques and cognitive rehabilitation.

For interventions to have the most impact, the consequences of the 'target' behavior should be directly related to preceding behavior, and should be applied quickly, consistently, and at maximum intensity.[154,227] Although not necessary, it is helpful to include an explanation to the individual as to why the behavior was reinforced or punished. There has been a significant amount of research on schedules of reinforcement, or how often to provide the consequence to maximize behavior change and minimize the risk of the individual getting bored or satiated with the reinforcer.

Techniques used clinically to *increase desired behaviors* include positive reinforcement (presenting something positive in response to the behavior), negative reinforcement (removing something negative in response to the behavior), and token economy (presenting 'points' or small tokens in response to the behavior that can be exchanged for rewards). Techniques used clinically to *develop a new desired behavior* include shaping (waiting for the appropriate target behavior or something close to that behavior to occur before reinforcing the behavior) and modeling (demonstration of the target behavior via a model; the model can be a therapist, another patient, a peer, or a family member). Techniques used clinically to *decrease undesired behaviors* include punishment (presenting something negative in response to the behavior), extinction (removing the reinforcement of the behavior or ignoring), time out (removing all positive environmental stimuli in response to the undesired behavior), response cost (requiring the individual to give up something positive when the undesired behavior occurs), and differential reinforcement of other or incompatible behaviors (providing positive reinforcement of other behaviors and ignoring the undesired behavior, or reinforcing behaviors that are incompatible with the undesired behavior).

Applied behavior analysis is a set of techniques used to eliminate very problematic or dangerous behaviors (such as head banging). This method focuses more on the antecedents than the consequences of the behaviors, so as to predict when the behavior will occur and eliminate the behavior quickly.[44]

Interpersonal psychotherapy (IPT) is a time-limited, structured psychotherapy that addresses interpersonal dimensions to provide symptom relief.[223] Originally developed for the treatment of depression, recent studies indicate it might have utility in the treatment of various anxiety disorders and social phobia.[141] Because interpersonal and social factors play an important role in the lives of persons with impairments, IPT might be useful in traditional rehabilitation populations. IPT can be adapted to target specific issues in the interpersonal life of the individual.

Cognitive behavioral therapy uses a structured psychotherapeutic approach to develop beliefs, attitudes, thoughts, and skills that modify various components of the target problem. (For detailed descriptions of cognitive behavioral principles and techniques in the area of behavioral medicine and rehabilitation, see Turk et al. 1983.[211]) The cognitive component focuses on modification of the individual's thoughts and feelings through examination of the cognitions that arise in response to stressors. It also looks at how these thoughts influence emotional responses. The behavioral component focuses on activation programs, modification of environmental contingencies, and development of coping skills such as relaxation or assertiveness. Learning procedures such as rehearsal, graded practice, training in self-control techniques, and homework are a key component of CBT.

Motivational interviewing is a specific cognitive technique first utilized in the addictions field. It uses active listening and open-ended questions to understand the individual's perspective and strategically elicit commitment and motivation to change. This is achieved through creating a discrepancy between the individual's behavior and their desired goals or values. Patients are actively engaged in the process and are encouraged to think out loud about changes they want to occur and their confidence in achieving these changes.[178] This technique has been found to be effective in engaging patients in health behavior change. Due to its brief duration and focus on specific health behaviors, the technique can be especially useful in the rehabilitation setting, where time for intervention is limited.

Crisis intervention is a model for brief, focused treatment designed to reduce emotional distress associated with an emotionally overwhelming event. Crisis intervention develops solutions for coping and problem solving in traumatic or natural disasters.[4] Crisis intervention techniques have been used in patients with head injury,[194] breast cancer,[234] and stroke.[165] Patients with significant impairments are being admitted to inpatient rehabilitation units more acutely, and length of stay is typically shorter than in the past. Inpatient rehabilitation is a time of intense pressure for patients and families to solve a myriad of practical problems (home accessibility, caregiver arrangements, etc.), while simultaneously experiencing emotional upheaval. This makes crisis intervention appropriate and potentially effective in the inpatient rehabilitation setting. Both patients and their families can be included in this brief, solution-focused treatment, which combines supportive, psychoeducational, and cognitive behavioral techniques.

Skill training utilizes behavioral principles to teach patients specific skills to manage behavioral and emotional symptoms. The application of skills by the patient to manage symptoms has been shown to increase a patient's sense of control and self-esteem, reduce symptoms of depression and anxiety, and reduce reliance on others or medication for symptom management.[160,210] The skills typically used in the rehabilitation setting are for managing the social interactions, pain, and anxiety. Patients are taught to use techniques such as diaphragmatic breathing, progressive muscle relaxation, and visual imagery to help during their therapies when pain and anxiety might be exacerbated.

Social skills training is another application of skill training that is useful in rehabilitation populations. Following an injury or illness that results in changes in daily functioning, the individual is faced with interacting in a social environment with impaired abilities and with others who have little understanding of disability. The rehabilitation psychologist can assist the individual in gaining the skills to manage the more challenging social ramifications of physical and/or cognitive behavioral issues specific to the disability (i.e. assisted mobility, forgetfulness, disinhibition, incontinence). The individual can also gain experience in managing anxiety and uncertainty, while communicating with others about disability-related issues. Practicing such skills within the rehabilitation setting has been shown to promote more successful social interactions and adaptation.[24]

Psychoeducation refers to efforts to teach people about the psychologic aspects of disability or illness, and adaptive coping and social skills. This can include information presented under the broad heading of patient education. Patients can be provided with educational materials to read and discuss with the psychologist. This bibliotherapy can provide vicarious role modeling or answer questions that patients might not raise in a face to face session. Education of patients and their family members regarding psychologic aspects of specific conditions, along with strategies for coping with and compensating for such changes, is a key component of a comprehensive rehabilitation program.

Cognitive impairment following stroke or TBI can lead to significant disability. Effective rehabilitation of these patients must include goals, treatment planning, and interventions that specifically address cognition.[40,55] Recovery of function theories provide the basis for strategies aimed at improving or restoring cognitive abilities.[133] Other *cognitive rehabilitation* interventions can focus on compensatory training or environmental change. Evidence-based cognitive rehabilitation methods compiled by the Brain Injury Special Interest Group of the American Congress of Rehabilitation Medicine's Cognitive Rehabilitation Committee include recommendations regarding strategies to address visuospatial skills, cognitive linguistic and specific functional communication deficits, compensatory memory training, attention skills, visual scanning, and comprehensive holistic neuropsychologic rehabilitation.[40]

A cognitive or neuropsychologic evaluation is necessary to begin the cognitive rehabilitation process.[92] The neuropsychologic evaluation provides information on both the patient's cognitive strengths (preserved abilities or relative assets) and cognitive weaknesses (impairments). This information is used to identify specific cognitive goals for the rehabilitation process,

and to identify specific methods of meeting the cognitive goals. The rehabilitation neuropsychologist can provide knowledge of the patient's neuropsychologic functioning, and knowledge of evidence-based cognitive rehabilitation strategies. This helps guide the rehabilitation treatment team in addressing the functional tasks that are impacted by cognitive impairment, as well intervening directly through cognitive rehabilitation services.[32,151]

Psychologic and behavioral interventions are critical components of comprehensive *pain management*. Patients undergoing comprehensive pain treatment rate educational and psychologic therapies higher than physical therapy and medical modalities both at posttreatment and at follow-up evaluations.[38] Patients having these interventions typically have a positive cost–benefit ratio, with the patient reporting relatively significant levels of improvement at a relatively low cost.[38]

A number of psychologic treatments for chronic pain are currently available. Two important treatment modalities include CBT[211] and hypnosis.[166] CBT uses a structured psychotherapeutic approach to develop individuals' beliefs, attitudes, thoughts, and skills to modify various components of the pain experience. Although there are variations in the specific pain management strategies taught to individuals, all CBT programs utilize a similar process. This process includes:

- an initial assessment of pain, mood, behavior, cognition, and environmental variables;
- patient education regarding the interaction of the variables assessed;
- training in behavioral and cognitive strategies;
- graded increase in activity levels;
- practice and reinforcement of pain management strategies; and
- self-monitoring of measurable outcomes.

The process requires an active collaboration between the individual and a clinician with training in CBT pain management skills. The efficacy of CBT interventions for modification of pain and related disturbances is well established.[159] CBT is often underutilized in persons with disability-related pain who are highly willing to try it.[222]

Hypnotic analgesia is a form of pain treatment that has been receiving more recent attention.[166] Hypnosis involves techniques for using enhanced imagery to induce states of selective attentional focusing or diffusion. There is a presuggestion component that includes introduction of goals (e.g. a suggestion for analgesia for pain control), and a postsuggestion component that emphasizes maintenance of the behavior following hypnosis. A recent comprehensive review indicates that there is growing evidence for positive effects of hypnosis in both laboratory and clinical acute and chronic pain populations.[166]

There are several treatment options that have been shown to be effective in the treatment of *substance abuse*. Drinkers who are at risk might benefit from simple, brief interventions that focus on education, assessment, and feedback on the potential for future alcohol-related consequences. Problem drinkers, on the other hand, might benefit from the use of contracting, goal setting, and other behavior modification techniques to help curtail drinking. Brief interventions have been successful in reducing consumption in 10–30% of non-dependent problem drinkers.[76] Motivational interviewing techniques have also been shown to be effective with problem drinkers.[156] The underlying premise for all intervention strategies is to avoid approaches that blame or punish the drinker, and focus more on education and mutual exploration of behavior change options. There remains an ongoing debate over the goal of alcohol interventions, with some clinicians promoting abstinence and others focusing on harm reduction as a means of reducing alcohol-related consequences.

Medication use and abuse assessment in persons with disabilities should begin with a thorough clinical interview. Special emphasis should be given to specific medications being taken, medication compliance, number of medical providers prescribing medication, and past history of substance abuse. Potential concerns in the interview include polypharmacy, lack of an organized system to track medication administration, use of medications with potential for addiction, use of multiple medical providers, or positive history of past substance abuse. Treatment of substance abuse can vary widely depending on patient characteristics and circumstances. Recommendations might include consultation with medical providers to minimize the potential for polypharmacy, reduction in number of providers prescribing medications, or appointment of one physician as a coordinator to enhance medication monitoring. Other recommendations include the use of a pillbox or other aide in medication administration to strengthen compliance and ensure proper dosing of medications. It is important to note that most individuals who abuse prescription medications do not intend to abuse medications from the outset. Open discussion and education are initial steps, followed by treatment modalities similar to those utilized in the treatment of alcohol abuse, when indicated.

Team consultation

In addition to working directly with individuals with the impairments, psychologists consult with the rehabilitation team to improve rehabilitation process and outcomes. Team treatment characterizes the rehabilitation process, and is viewed as a useful tool to improve the quality of medical care.[112] Selected characteristics of team functioning have been associated with enhanced rehabilitation outcomes, including organization, task orientation, and communication clarity.[198] Psychologists can often assist the team in improving these factors. As rehabilitation is based on principles of learning, psychologists consult with team members to solve problems associated with learning, participation in treatment, and maintenance of treatment gains. Cotreatment with other members of the team can be an effective method to assist therapists and patients in improving interaction and outcomes.

The nature of the rehabilitation enterprise creates a high degree of intensity and intimacy in the relationship between the patient and the rehabilitation staff. The emotional reactions of staff can be based on their own difficulty coping with strong emotions, their belief systems and biases about how patients should respond to impairments, or their individual professional role concept. Staff can minimize a patient's emotional distress, but more often overestimate the degree of patient distress or psychopathology.[87] Psychologists on the rehabilitation team can assist other staff members in understanding and coping more effectively with these reactions.[88]

Consultation with psychiatry

Psychiatric consultation can be very useful in the management of psychiatric conditions encountered in the rehabilitation process. There can be overlap roles of the psychiatrist and psychologist, which can create confusion for the rehabilitation staff. The concept of a psychosocial team[164] has been proposed as a means of clarifying roles and responsibilities, and integrating the unique contributions of psychology and psychiatry into the rehabilitation setting. Psychiatric consultation in rehabilitation contributes to the proper treatment of patients requiring pharmacologic management, and those with substance abuse that complicates pain management, or mental status changes with unclear etiology. Medically complex patients on multiple medications who also require treatment for psychiatric disorders can also benefit from psychiatric consultation with regard to medication effects on mental status and medication interactions. Psychologists can be instrumental in suggesting referral in these situations, after initial assessment of the patient. The psychologist might have more regular contact with the patient and can provide feedback on the patient's response to a particular medication, as well as providing psychotherapy in concert with pharmacologic treatment. Communication between these disciplines is important in achieving the maximal therapeutic effect for the patient.

Peer interactions, self-management, and advocacy

In addition to working directly with individuals with the impairments, psychologists use psychologic theory to assist the efforts of others to improve rehabilitation outcomes. Peer counseling or support groups are grounded in modeling theory, which states that individuals are likely to learn best from those whom they identify as being most like themselves. Wright has long advocated the importance of the 'insider perspective' when interacting with persons with disabilities.[231] It is believed that, through exposure to successful individuals with similar disabilities, less experienced persons can develop hope, learn and adopt more effective behaviors, and have increased social support. Peer role models or support groups are sometimes part of formal rehabilitation programs,[202] and in other cases are part of consumer organizations. For example, one national consumer program is the peer visitor program offered by the Amputee Coalition of America (http://www.amputee-coalition.org). The timing and benefits of these peer interventions has yet to be empirically established.

Interventions for disabling impairments and related secondary conditions have traditionally focused on standard medical treatments such as medication, surgery, or rehabilitative therapies. Self-management interventions, on the other hand, have been found to be effective in reducing secondary conditions and disability associated with some chronic conditions using individual and group-based delivery methods.[146] Key elements in self-management include knowledge, self-monitoring, skills acquisition, and problem solving.[146] Self-management interventions can be provided by professionals, lay persons, or peers. More recently, self-management interventions using Internet and distance technologies have achieved successful outcomes in persons with chronic impairments.[145] Self-management interventions appear to achieve long-term reductions in pain and disability primarily through increases in self-efficacy.[144] This class of interventions has not been widely used in traditional rehabilitation populations. Using new technologies, self-management interventions have the potential to improve outcomes for individuals who do not have ready access to other psychosocial or peer support interventions.

Advocacy to modify public policy is indicated due to recognition that behavior, function, and quality of life are due to interaction of the individual and the environment. Advocacy efforts through professional organizations, in concert with consumers, are a key component of comprehensive rehabilitation efforts. Changes in public policy that have resulted from advocacy include the American with Disabilities Act, which has the potential to benefit those with impairments

SPECIAL TOPICS

Denial of illness and anosognosia

It has been well established that many individuals following onset of a disability or a disease process have difficulty recognizing and/or accepting the existence, nature, degree, and/or impact of their condition.[124] In the face of medical evidence, rehabilitation patients can report, behave, and cope in ways that indicate they do not believe the medical condition is present. It appears that they do not feel that their medical condition will impact their lives in any tangible way. This reduced awareness might be rooted in neurologic dysfunction (anosognosia) and/or might reflect psychologic processes (denial) to preserve self-image and prevent psychologic distress.[173]

Unawareness has generally been thought of as a negative construct that forms a barrier to active participation in rehabilitation.[106] However, research has demonstrated that the effect of anosognosia and denial of illness on rehabilitation participation and outcomes is not always negative. Anosognosia typically leads to difficulty because the individual does not have the ability to assess the changes in physical, cognitive, or behavioral functioning. This leads to a lack of knowledge that changes have even occurred. Although patients with anosognosia lack this knowledge and appear perplexed by feedback that their abilities have changed, they also show a cautious willingness or indifference when asked to perform tasks with this new information about themselves.[172] Interventions for anosognosia are aimed at providing the patient with examples of impairment during daily activities. When difficulty secondary to impairments is encountered, the patient is provided with feedback regarding the

potential role of the impairment. Repeated exposure to such information in the face of difficulties in functioning is presumed to result in improved awareness of the impairment. There has been very little empiric research on the effectiveness of specific interventions for reduced awareness.

A review of the medical rehabilitation literature over the past century reveals that denial of illness can be associated with maladaptive behavior. This includes delays in seeking treatment, poorer compliance with treatment regimens, and poorer emotional adjustment. There also is evidence of denial of illness being related to better emotional adjustment, fewer medical complications, and better recovery.[124] The key to whether denial of illness leads to positive or negative outcomes appears to be how the patient uses the denial. If the patient uses the denial to *reinterpret* the meaning of the event to reduce personal threat ('I will walk again, so I need to work extra hard in therapy to make that happen'), then the research supports that denial of illness is related to more positive outcomes and is adaptive. Patients who use denial to *avoid* the reality of their illness or injury ('My memory problem is not that bad. I don't need speech therapy') tend to have poorer outcomes.

Interventions for denial of illness need to take a different slant than the interventions for anosognosia. First, the type of denial of illness needs to be identified. If patients are actively participating in the rehabilitation program despite repeated denial of the permanency of the injury or the seriousness of the diagnosis, then the denial might not be maladaptive. If patients are refusing to participate actively in the rehabilitation program or are engaging in activities that put them at safety risk because impairments are not being considered, then the denial is a barrier to the patient benefiting from rehabilitation and adapting. The typical approach of pushing individuals to acknowledge impairments by simply reinforcing and repeating a list of their impairments might be detrimental.[129] Assisting the individual in understanding the resistance and the nature of the threat, however, might soften denial, reduce reliance on avoidance strategies, and aid the individual in tolerating awareness of the impairments.[129] Clinical research on avoidance in other psychologic populations suggests that focusing treatment on adaptation by helping the individual actively experience psychologic reactions directly, fully, and without needless defense helps the individual behave more effectively.[101] Overall, the key in managing anosognosia and denial of illness is correct identification of the type of unawareness syndrome so that the appropriate intervention can be applied.

Determining supervision needs

The amount and type of supervision required by a person with disabilities has important implications for their living arrangements. Surprisingly little research has been done regarding prediction of supervision needs based on cognitive or physical impairments. The severity of cognitive impairments is often used as a guide for determining the patient's supervision needs, with patients whose cognitive impairments are more severe receiving recommendations for more intensive supervision. Because rehabilitation professionals see a cautious approach as desirable, there is a tendency to recommend the most intensive level of supervision a patient might possibly need rather than the minimal amount required. This can lead to increased care cost related to hiring aides, adult day care, or assisted living arrangements if a patient's supervision needs exceed family resources. For family members who decide to provide supervision, there is a high likelihood of caregiver burden.[197]

There are few standardized instruments for classifying or predicting the level of supervision required based on current functioning. The Supervision Rating Scale classifies the amount of supervision being received on a 13-point ordinal scale ranging from independent to full direct supervision.[25] The scale correlates with measures of global cognition as well as independence in self-care.

Driving

Driving ability can play a major role in maintaining an individual's ability to remain independent. Loss of driving privileges can result in major detriments to self-esteem and image, as well as representing a financial and functional hardship. The decision to recommend driving resumption or cessation should be empirically based using adequate off- and on-road assessment. While some rehabilitation programs have comprehensive driving evaluation programs, many do not. On the road evaluations represent the best indicator of actual performance, although the costs for these programs are not typically covered by insurance. Only a small number of those who could benefit from these services ever receive on the road tests.[75] In addition to on road testing of driving ability by a specially trained professional, the rehabilitation psychologist can play a crucial role in making recommendations about a patient's driving ability and can communicate driving recommendations to the patient, their family members, and regulatory agencies. Neuropsychologic tests are often used to provide an indication of driving ability, although literature on the utility of these tests to predict driving ability has been rather disappointing.[26] Cognitive domains such as attention, memory, visual perception, judgment, and reaction time are relevant to driving and appropriate targets of assessment in determining driving ability. Psychologists should thoroughly familiarize themselves with the state laws regarding driving regulations, including mandatory reporting requirements. In most instances, it is also advisable to inform family members, with the patient's permission, of all driving recommendations.

Decision-making capacity

Within the rehabilitation setting, there are many instances in which patients must make key decisions about their treatment and discharge plan. The patient's capacity must be established so the rehabilitation team knows whether to rely on the patient's decisions or to identify a representative for the patient to make these decisions.

Capacity is a medicolegal construct referring to an individual's ability to make adequate judgments as determined by clinicians. This is contrasted with *competency*, which denotes a legal status determined by a judge, which involves consideration of non-clinical factors. Within the rehabilitation setting, the treatment team must consider whether a patient has the capacity to make decisions.

Over the past decade or so, researchers have attempted to identify the key activities of daily living for which intact decision-making capacity is critical. Guidelines and methodology for assessing capacity related to a patient's ability to consent to medical treatment, manage finances, return to driving, and perform other daily functioning tasks have been developed.[15,60,95] The common thread among all types of capacity is that individuals have the ability to rationally understand the process affecting their functioning. This includes understanding the medical condition, injury, and impairments. It also includes understanding the pertinent facts (i.e. impact on daily life functioning, need for assistance), and communicating with others regarding the situation and the facts to make an informed decision.

Following injury or illness, capacity is typically questioned when a patient demonstrates changes in mental status. Additional factors that could affect an individual's comprehension, reasoning and judgment, and expression abilities include impaired hearing, impaired eyesight, comprehension of dominant language, denial of illness, psychiatric comorbidities (e.g. depression, anxiety), cognitive impairments, aphasia, and inadequate information regarding the medical condition. A comprehensive interview and neuropsychologic examination is indicated to evaluate the presence and potential impact of the cognitive and emotional factors.

Comorbid psychopathology

Major psychiatric illness complicates patients' response to physical disability, as well as influencing their ability to cope with psychosocial and physical changes and new self-care requirements. Schizophrenia and other psychotic disorders impair insight, judgment, perception, and awareness of reality. Persons with psychotic disorders might not fully understand the limitations or new needs imposed by a physical illness or disability, and are therefore at greater risk for non-compliance, unsafe behavior, and medical complications. Abnormal affective expression and thought distortions associated with psychotic disorders impact communication with staff, impair concentration and new learning, and can result in rejection of rehabilitation therapies. Psychiatric consultation should be sought if there is any doubt regarding the diagnosis or proper medication management. Psychologists play an important role in developing behavior management programs, providing psychotherapeutic interventions, and assisting team members in communicating with patients with preexisting psychotic disorders.

Somatization is the psychologic mechanism whereby psychologic distress is expressed in the form of physical symptoms.[140] Somatoform disorders all present with an alteration or loss of a physical function suggestive of a medical disorder but, by definition, the symptoms cannot be fully explained physiologically or traced to a specific physical cause.[5] Conversion disorder is a specific form of somatization in which the patient presents with symptoms and signs that are confined to the central nervous system, and thus can be seen in rehabilitation settings.[130] Conversion disorder can present at any age, but is rare in children younger than 10 years or in persons older than 35 years. The incidence has been estimated to be about 15–20 cases per 100 000 people. Data suggest that women with conversion disorder outnumber men by 6:1.[5] Symptoms in a conversion reaction are related to severe stress, emotional conflict, or an associated psychiatric disorder. There is a high incidence of depression and anxiety in patients with conversion disorder, and as many as half of these patients have comorbid personality disorders.[96,111,139]

The presence of conversion symptoms, in isolation or in conjunction with other medical conditions, can make rehabilitation challenging, in that psychologic issues can serve to produce, exacerbate, or maintain physical symptoms.[34] The degree of impairment seen in these disorders is often significant and interferes with daily activities. Prolonged loss of function can produce complications such as muscle atrophy or joint contractures.[147] Patients are not typically aware of the psychologic underpinnings of the symptoms, and are not thought to be intentionally producing the symptoms. This is in contrast to factitious disorders, in which the symptoms are intentionally feigned for some kind of secondary gain (i.e. avoidance of an activity or social attention), or malingering, in which symptoms are intentionally feigned for monetary gain.[143,228]

Treatment for conversion disorders frequently uses a combination of rehabilitation and psychiatric models. This includes active physical rehabilitation for the physical manifestations or symptoms, combined with psychologic treatment to help reduce stress and learn more healthy coping strategies (e.g. Abbey and Lipowski 1987,[1] Hughes and Alltree 1990,[110] and Speed 1996[196]). Theoretic frameworks and treatment approaches that incorporate the biopsychosocial framework, recognizing the interaction of mind and body in determining behavior rather than dichotomous thinking (e.g. 'Is the symptom physical or psychologic?'), are key in treating conversion disorders.[142]

In pediatric patients, the incidence of conversion is higher after physical or sexual abuse.[127] Incidence also increases in children whose family members have chronic medical conditions or chronic pain.[181,213] Children and adolescents with conversion symptoms are often described as 'high achievers', and several authors suggest that the manifestation of physical symptoms might provide relief from achievement pressures without the need for rebellion or the risk of family disappointment.[89,94] Treatment in children is often complicated by family response to the symptoms (e.g. Seltzer 1985[187]). Parental anxiety can increase the child's anxiety, or symptoms might lead to a decrease in parental pressure for academic success in the child. The shift of the family focus on the 'affected' child, as opposed to other stressors in the household, can also lead to familial secondary gain that serves to maintain symptoms.[125] Family therapy is almost always necessary in the successful treatment of children with conversion symptoms.[132]

Family and support systems

Social support is strongly associated with positive rehabilitation and health outcomes.[21,91] Social support in this context is mainly emotional support, as distinguished from instrumental or practical support. Families form the core of the social support network and are the major providers of care for people living with disability. These tasks require skills in communication, cooperation, management of affect, and ability to access resources in the larger social network and community. Better family function in the areas of communication, problem solving, and affective involvement is associated with improved treatment adherence after discharge from inpatient rehabilitation.[61] Better family function is also positively associated with increased participation in social and leisure activities, and increased performance of activities of daily living after stroke.[191] Conversely, family dysfunction reduces the family's ability to cope with a serious illness.[177,199] Stressful life transitions that coincide with rehabilitation (e.g. head injury of a young adult who has just started college) affect the family's response to the injury and the extent to which they can provide appropriate support for rehabilitation efforts. More chaotic and disengaged families, families where there is active substance abuse, and families who are isolated from larger social networks have more difficulty providing social and emotional support for an ill family member.[177] They can also be more vulnerable to the stresses associated with caring for a family member, such as depression and social isolation.[93]

For these reasons, assessment of family dynamics and function is important in the rehabilitation setting. While assessment of family function, resources, and adaptability is often conducted through clinical interview, several assessment tools for quantifying family function (most notably the McMaster Family Assessment Device[70]) have been used in rehabilitation research and clinical settings.[43,61,72]

PEDIATRIC REHABILITATION PSYCHOLOGY

Several additional issues must be kept in mind regarding cognitive and psychologic assessment and treatment in the pediatric population. Pediatric rehabilitation strives to help a child regain functional skill and return to 'baseline' status, as well as to promote continued successful growth and development in the future. It is important to view children as changing and developing, rather than viewing their ability level as static. To this end, rehabilitation psychologists must be ever mindful of typical child development. Assessment tools and intervention strategies have to be modified depending on both the chronologic age and the developmental stage of the child.

Cognitive and psychologic developmental milestones are rooted in central nervous system maturation[199] and generally occur in a predictable sequence. Rehabilitation psychologists in a pediatric setting are often confronted with medical conditions and diagnostic groups in addition to those previously listed, including developmental disorders such as spina bifida, cerebral palsy, genetic disorders, autism spectrum disorders, and attention deficit hyperactivity disorder. These conditions can present with abnormal developmental patterns as well as psychologic and neuropsychologic sequelae. In addition, extended hospitalization or illness can interfere with a child's development due to missed school and decreased opportunities for socialization.

Undiagnosed visual or hearing impairments are more likely in pediatric populations, and are more frequent in childhood disabilities, therefore hearing and vision checks should be a prerequisite to assessment and treatment of a child's cognitive abilities or emotional status.

There are many theoretic models of cognitive and emotional development, and a thorough review of these frameworks and concepts is beyond the scope of this chapter. Some of the classic developmental psychology concepts include Piaget's model of cognitive states of development;[169] Erikson's stages of emotional and personality development;[71] Selman's phases of peer interaction and friendships;[195] and theories of temperament, coping, and personality style (see Bates and Wachs 1994[17] and Thomas and Chess 1977[206]).

Assessment and treatment of children raises several ethical issues that need to be considered. Issues related to consent for treatment, assent to treatment, and confidentiality arise when the parent or guardian has legal authority but the child is the individual being evaluated or treated.[6]

In order to evaluate and treat a child, especially a young child, the environment must be adapted to be child-friendly. Familiar toys, pictures, or family members should be present in the rehabilitation environment whenever possible. Behavioral or observational assessment tools are often helpful, because children often are unable to express symptoms, pain, or emotional distress verbally, whether because of age or developmental status. Observation of play and play therapies are helpful in the evaluation and treatment of younger children.

In addition, there is often a greater focus on the family as a whole, and family-level or parent–child interventions are common. Psychologic adjustment in the child is often closely tied with family factors such as cohesiveness, resilience, family support, maternal stress and coping, and parental reactions to injury or illness.[99,218,225,226] Yeates and colleagues reported that good preinjury family environment, particularly regarding social support and financial resources, was associated with a faster rate of recovery and better outcome 1 year after TBI in children.[232] Positive family coping and supportive family environment were also associated with better recovery and lower rates of depression and other psychiatric disorders in children after TBI.[216] The family environment and parental coping style have been shown to impact functional status and social adjustment in a variety of developmental conditions and illness.[217,218]

Children in need of rehabilitation have a greater risk for adjustment problems,[219] and children with disabilities have been shown to have more social and behavioral problems than children without disabilities.[30,226] Pless and Roghmann reported that 30% of children with chronic illness developed secondary psychosocial maladjustment.[170]

Assessment of children uses a different set of assessment tools depending on the age and developmental status of the child. Sattler notes that assessment of children frequently makes use of individually administered tests, behavioral observations, caregiver and teacher reports and checklists, and structured interviews.[185] (See Table 4-5 for a list of assessment tools for use with children.) With the exception of children with significant development delays, tests of infant abilities are felt to be most useful to describe the child's current status, rather than having predictive validity for a child's future cognitive abilities.[56,149] Research has suggested that overall intellectual functioning (e.g. IQ) does not stabilize until 4 years of age.[185]

In children with medical conditions impacting development, assessments that provide general developmental quotients or overall IQ might not be the most useful in describing a child's abilities and impairments. This is due to confounding factors, such as a child's language or motor deficits, differentially impacting the overall score.[136] Therefore careful and comprehensive assessment of the child's neuropsychologic strengths and weaknesses, academic status, adaptive skills, motor skills, and psychologic status might be more useful in educational and treatment planning for children with medical conditions.[16,233]

One of the primary tasks for children and adolescents is attending school. Psychologists in the rehabilitation setting frequently assist with the integration or reintegration of a child into a school setting. Careful evaluation of the psychologic and cognitive factors that can impact the success of the transition back to school is important. Psychologists also can assist with recommendations for accommodations to minimize the impact of psychologic and cognitive factors impeding a child's success in school.

The Education for All Handicapped Children Act[9] (PL 94-142, now called the Individuals with Disabilities Act), passed in 1976, mandated that a 'free and appropriate' education be provided in the least restrictive environment for children with handicapping conditions. This law requires the development of an individualized education plan for those between 3 and 21 to address needs and modifications required to ensure that the student will succeed in the educational environment. In 1986, this was expanded to include early intervention services for infants and toddlers.[10] In addition, section 504 of the Rehabilitation Act of 1973[11] states that it is illegal to discriminate against a person with a disability solely because of the disability, and that individuals with disabilities must have equal access to programs and services. These and other federal laws provide mechanisms by which children can be provided with school services and accommodations.

SUMMARY

Rehabilitation psychology is a key component of the rehabilitation enterprise. The underlying theory is based in the biopsychosocial model and recognizes that disability is determined by both personal and environmental factors. The practice of rehabilitation psychology is based on the empiric literature and

Text continued on p. 88

Table 4-5 Common tests used in pediatric rehabilitation assessment and appropriate age ranges

Test	Age range(s)[a]
Infant development tests	
Batelle Developmental Inventory	Birth to 7:11
Bayley	1–42 months
Brazelton Neonatal Assessment Scale	3 days–4 weeks
McCarthy Scales of Children's Abilities	2:5–8:5
Mullen Scales of Early Learning	Birth to 68 months
Rossetti Infant–Toddler Language Scale	Birth to 3
Receptive Expressive Emergent Language Test (REEL-3)	Birth to 3
General abilities test	
Kaufman Assessment Battery for Children (K ABC)	2:6–12:5
Differential Abilities Scales (DAS)	2:6–17:11
Das Naglieri Cognitive Assessment System (CAS)	5–17
Comprehensive Test of Non-verbal Intelligence (CTONI)	6+
Hiskey–Nebraska	3–17
Universal Non-verbal Intelligence Test (UNIT)	5:0–17:11
Wide Range Intelligence Test (WRIT)	4–85
Leiter-R (attention and memory, growth scales, visualization and reasoning)	2:0–22:11
Test of Non-verbal Intelligence (TONI)-3	5:0–85:11
Woodcock–Johnson III Cognitive	2–80+
IQ	
Standford–Binet IV	–
Wechsler Adult Intelligence Scale—III (WAIS-III)	16:0–89:0
Wechsler Abbreviated Scale of Intelligence (WASI)	6–89
Wechsler Intelligence Scale for Children, 3rd edn (WISC-III)	6:6–16:11
Wechsler Intelligence Scale for Children, 4th edn (WISC-IV)	6:0–16:11
Wechsler Intelligence Scale for Children—Integrated (WISC-IV-I)	6:0–16:11
Wechsler Preschool and Primary Scale of Intelligence, 3rd edn (WPPSI-III)	2:6–7:3
Multiple domains	
NEPSY	(2–5), (5–12)
Luria–Nebraska Neuropsychological Battery, Children's Revisions	8–12
Halstead–Reitan Neuropsychological Test Battery for Children	9–14
Reitan–Indiana Neuropsychological Test Battery	5–8
General behavior rating scales	
Behavior Assessment System for Children (BASC): parent	(2½–5), (6–11), (12–18)
BASC: teacher	(2½–5), (6–11), (12–18)
BASC: self	(8–11), (12–18)
Child Behavior Check List (CBCL): parent	(1½–5), (6–18)
CBCL: teacher	(1½–5), (6–18)
CBCL: youth self-report	11–18

Continued on page 85

Continued from page 84 Table 4-5 Common tests used in pediatric rehabilitation assessment and appropriate age ranges	
Test	Age range(s)[a]
Attention deficit–hyperactivity disorder rating scales Attention Deficit Disorders Evaluation Scale (ADDES): home	4:5–18
ADDES: school	4:5–18
ADDES: secondary-age student	–
Adult ADDES: self report	–
Brown Attention Deficit Disorder Scales	(3–12), (12–18)
ECADDES: home	24–84 months
ECADDES: school	24–84 months
CPRS-S/L	3–17
CTRS-S/L	3–17
DuPaul ADHD: home or school	5–17
Adaptive behavior rating scales ABAS—Parent/Teacher/Adult	Birth to 89
Scales of Independent Behavior (SIB-R)	Birth to adult
Vineland	Birth to 19
Autism spectrum rating scales and diagnostic tests Asperger's Syndrome Diagnostic Scale (ASDS)	–
Autism Behavior Checklist	–
Childhood Autism Rating Scale	2:5–12
Gilliam Autism Rating Scale (GARS)	–
Attention Auditory CPT	–
Brief Test of Attention (BTA)	–
Conners' CPT-II	4–18
Gordon Diagnostic System	(4–5), (6–16)
Test of Variables of Attention (TOVA)	4–80
Test of Everyday Attention for Children (TEA-CH)	6–16
Paced Auditory Serial Addition Test	16+
Language Boston Aphasia Examination	–
Boston Naming	(6–14), (18+)
Clinical Evaluation of Language Fundamentals, 3rd edn (CELF-3)	3:6–6:6
Comprehensive Test of Phonological Processing (CTOPP)	5–6, 7–24
Expressive One Word Picture Vocabulary Test (EOWPVT)	2:0–18:11
Peabody Picture Vocabulary Test (PPVT)	2:0+
Rapid Automatized Naming Test (RAN)	5:0–18:11
Test of Language Competence (TLC)	5:0–18:11
Test of Language Development—Primary, 3rd edn (TOLD-P: 3)	4:0–8:11
Test of Language Development—Intermediate, 3rd edn (TOLD-I: 3)	8:0–12:11
Preschool Language Scale	Birth to 6:11

Continued on page 86

Continued from page 85 Table 4-5 Common tests used in pediatric rehabilitation assessment and appropriate age ranges

Test	Age range(s)[a]
Test of Auditory Perceptual Skills, Revised (TAPS-R)	4:0–12:11
Test of Auditory Reasoning and Processing Skills (TARPS)	5–14
Test for Auditory Comprehension of Language (TACL-3)	3:0–9:11
Test of Early Language Development (TELD-3)	2:0–7:11
Test of Adolescent and Adult Language (TOAL-3)	12:0–24:9
Token tests	–
Token Test for Children	3:0–12:5
Test of Phonological Awareness (TOPA)	5–10
Word Fluency (FAS)	–
Executive function Behavior Rating Inventory of Executive Function (BRIEF)—Parent/Teacher	5–18
Behavior Rating Inventory of Executive Function (BRIEF)—Preschool	2:0–5:11
Children's Category Test	5–8
Intermediate Booklet Category Test	9–14
Booklet category test, 2nd edn	15+
Delis Kaplan Executive Function System (DKEFS)	8–89
Stroop Color Word Test (Children's version, Adult)	(5–14), (15+)
Knox Cubes	3+
Ravens Colored Progressive Matrices	5–11
Ravens Standard Progressive Matrices	6–17
Ravens Advanced Progressive Matrices	13+
TRAILS A and B	15+
TRAILS A and B Children	9–14
Wisconsin Card Sorting Test (WCST)	6:5–89:0
Motor Grooved pegboard	–
Finger tapper	–
Purdue pegboard	–
Visuospatial, visuomotor, and visuoconstructional Benton Facial Recognition	–
Benton Visual Form Discrimination	–
Benton Visual Retention	–
Bender Visual Motor Gestalt Test	3+
HOOPER	(5–13)
Judgment of Line Orientation (JLO)	–
Mesulam Cancellation Tests	–
Test of Visual-Motor Skills—Revised	5–14

Continued on page 87

Continued from page 86 Table 4-5 Common tests used in pediatric rehabilitation assessment and appropriate age ranges	
Test	Age range(s)[a]
VMI, VMI-Motor, VMI-Visual Perception	2:0–15:11
Visual Object and Space Perception (VOSP)	–
Test of Visual Perceptual Skills (TVPS-Rev)	4:0–12:11
Memory and learning California Verbal Learning Test (CVLT-I/II)	16+
CVLT-C	3:5–16:11
Children's Memory Scale (CMS)	(5–8), (9–16)
Rey Auditory Verbal Learning Test	7–89
Rey–Osterrieth Complex Figure	6+
Rivermead Behavioral Memory Test	(5–10), (11–95)
Wechsler Memory Scale, 3rd edn (WMS-III)	16–89
Wide Range Assessment of Memory and Language (WRAML)	5:0–17:0
Test of Memory and Learning (TOMAL)	5:0–19:11
Academic skill Bracken Basic Concept Scale—Revised	2:6–7:11
Diagnostic Achievement Battery (DAB-2)	6:0–14:11
Diagnostic Achievement Test for Adolescents (DATA-2)	Grades 7–12
Durrell Analysis of Reading Difficulty	Kindergarten to 12
Nelson Denny Reading Test	High school +
Gates–MacGinitie Reading Test	Kindergarten to 12
Gray Oral Reading Test (GORT-4) (III)/(IV)	6:0–18:11
Key math Kaufman Test of Educational Achievement (KTEA)	6:0–22:11
Woodcock–Johnson—III Achievement	2–80+
Wide Range Achievement Test, 3rd revision (WRAT-3)	5:0–75:0
Wechsler Individual Achievement Test, 2nd edn (WIAT-II)	4:0–85:0 (prekindergarten to 16)
Peabody Individual Achievement Tests (PIAT)	5:0–22:11
Process Assessment of Learner (PAL)	Kindergarten to 6th grade
Test of Early Mathematics Ability (TEMA-2)	3:0–8:11
Test of Early Reading Ability, 2nd edn (TERA-2)	3:6–8:6
Test of Written Language, 3rd edn (TOWL-3)	8–17
Test of Reading Comprehension, III (TORC-3)	7:0–17:11
Test of Early Written Language (TEWL-2)	3:0–10:11
Woodcock Reading Mastery Tests—Revised	5–75
Test of Word Reading Efficiency (TOWRE)	6:0–24:11
Personality Minnesota Multiphasic Personality Inventory—A	14–18
Minnesota Multiphasic Personality Inventory—2	–

Continued on page 88

Continued from page 87 Table 4-5 Common tests used in pediatric rehabilitation assessment and appropriate age ranges

Test	Age range(s)[a]
Children's Apperception Test (CAT)	3–10
Million Adolescent Clinical Inventory (MACI)	–
Piers–Harris Children's Self Concept	7:0–18:11
Personality Inventory for Children (PIC)	3–5, 6–16
Roberts Apperception Test for Children	6–15
RISB (Rotter)—Sentence Completion: elementary, high school, adult	–
Rorschach	2+
Thematic Apperception Test (TAT)	4+
Mood Beck Depression Inventory—II (BDI-II)	13+
Children's Depression Inventory (CDI)	7–17
Goodenough–Harris Draw a Person	6+
Guess Why Game	–
Reynolds Child Depression Scale (RCDS)	Grades 3–6
Revised Children's Manifest Anxiety Scale (RCMAS): 'What I think and feel'	6–19
Reynolds Adolescent Depression Scale (RADS)	11–20
Other	
Children's Orientation and Amnesia Scale (COAS)	–
Pediatric Pain Questionnaire	–
Family Environment Scale	–
Stress Index for Parents of Adolescents (SIPA)	–
Parenting Stress Index (PSI)	–

[a]*In years unless otherwise stated.*

driven by the needs of the person being served. Psychologists contribute to the rehabilitation process through assessment and intervention, which can occur at multiple levels: individual, family, rehabilitation team, healthcare organization, or society.

REFERENCES

1. Abbey SE, Lipowski ZJ. Comprehensive management of persistent somatization: an innovative inpatient program. Psychother Psychosom 1987; 48:110–115.

2. Abrams RC, Alexopoulos GS. Substance abuse in the elderly: over-the-counter and illegal drugs. Hosp Community Psychiatry 1988; 39:822–829.

3. Adams WL, Barry KL, Fleming MF. Screening for problem drinking in older primary care patients. JAMA 1996; 276:1964–1967.

4. Aguilera D. Crisis intervention: theory and methodology. 8th edn. St. Louis: Mosby; 1998:335.

5. American Psychiatric Association. Diagnostic and statistical manual of mental disorders. 4th edn. Washington: American Psychiatric Association; 1994.

6. American Psychiatric Association. Ethical principles of psychologists and code of conduct. Am Psychol 2002; 57:1060–1073.

7. Angeleri F, Angeleri VA, Foschi N, et al. The influence of depression, social activity, and family stress on functional outcome after stroke. Stroke 1993; 24(10):1478–1483.

8. [Anonymous]. Americans with Disabilities Act. 1990:101–336.

9. [Anonymous]. The Education for All Handicapped Children Act. 1976.

10. [Anonymous]. The Education of the Handicapped Act, Amendments. 1986.

11. [Anonymous]. The Rehabilitation Act. 1973.

12. Babor TF, de la Fuenta JR, Saunders J, et al. AUDIT: the Alcohol Use Disorders Identification Test: guidelines for its use in primary health care. Geneva: World Health Organization; 1992.

13. Bandura A. Influence of models' reinforcement contingencies in the acquisition of imitative responses. J Pers Soc Psychol 1965; 1:589–595.

14. Bandura A. Principles of behavior modification. New York: Holt, Rinehart and Winston; 1969.

15. Barbas NRW. Competency issues in dementia: medical decision making, driving, and independent living. J Geriatr Psychiatry Neurol 2001; 14:199–212.

16. Barlow DH. Clinical handbook of psychological disorders: a step-by-step treatment manual. 3rd edn. New York: Guilford; 2001.

17. Bates JE, Wachs TD, eds. Temperament. Washington: American Psychological Association; 1994.

18. Beck AT, et al. An inventory for measuring clinical anxiety: psychometric properties. J Consult Clin Psychol 1988; 56(6):893–897.

19. Beck AT, et al. An inventory for measuring depression. Arch Gen Psychiatry 1961; 4:51–571.

20. Benrud-Larson LM, Wegener ST. Chronic pain in neurorehabilitation populations: prevalence, severity and impact. NeuroRehabilitation 2000; 14(3):127–137.

21. Berkman LF, Leo-Summers L, Horwitz RI. Emotional support and survival after myocardial infarction: a prospective, population-based study of the elderly. Ann Intern Med 1992; 117(12):1003–1009.

22. Berninger V, Robinson R, Price T, et al. Modified WAIS-R for patients with speech and/or hand dysfunction. Arch Phys Med Rehabil 1988; 69:250–255.

23. Blow FC, Brower KJ, Schulenberg JE, et al. The Michigan Alcohol Screening Test—Geriatric Version (MAST-G): a newly elderly-specific screening instrument. Alcohol Clin Exp Res 1992; 16:372.

24. Boake C. Social skills training following head injury. In: Kreutzer JS, Wehman PH, eds. Cognitive rehabilitation for persons with traumatic brain injury: a functional approach. Baltimore: Brookes Publishing; 1991: 181–189.

25. Boake C. Supervision Rating Scale: a measure of functional outcome from injury. Arch Phys Med Rehabil 1996; 77:765–772.

26. Brooke M, Questad K, Patterson D, et al. Driving evaluation after traumatic brain injury. Am J Phys Med Rehabil 1992; 71:177–182.

27. Bruyere SM, Erickson WA, VanLooy S. Comparative study of workplace policy and practices contributing to disability nondiscrimination. Rehabil Psychol 2004; 49:28–38.

28. Buer N, Linton SJ. Fear-avoidance beliefs and catastrophizing: occurrence and risk factor in back pain and ADL in the general population. Pain 2002; 99(3):485–491.

29. Burns JW, et al. Do changes in cognitive factors influence outcome following multidisciplinary treatment for chronic pain? A cross-lagged panel analysis. J Consult Clin Psychol 2003; 71(1):81–91.

30. Cadman D, et al. Chronic illness, disability and mental and social well-being: findings of the Ontario Child Heath Study. Pediatrics 1987; 79(5):805–813.

31. Caplan BS, Scherer LCM. The role of nonstandard neuropsychological assessment in rehabilitation: history, rationale, and examples. In: Scherer LCM, ed. Psychological assessment in medical rehabilitation. Washington: American Psychological Association; 1995:359–391.

32. Carlson CC, et al. Association between executive attention and physical functional performance in community-dwelling older women. J Gerontol 1999; 54B:S262–S270.

33. Carson AJ, et al. Depression after stroke and lesion location: a systematic review. Lancet 2000; 356(9224):122–126.

34. Carter AB. The functional overlay. Lancet 1967; 2(7527):1196–1200.

35. Carver CS, Scheier MF. On the self-regulation of behavior. New York: Cambridge University Press; 1998.

36. Castillo CS, et al. Generalized anxiety disorder after stroke. J Nerv Ment Dis 1993; 181(2):100–106.

37. Chambless DL. Compendium of empirically supported therapies. In: Koocher GP, Norcross JC, Hill SS, eds. Psychologists' desk reference. 2nd edn. Oxford: Oxford University Press; 2005.

38. Chapman SL, et al. Perceived treatment helpfulness and cost in chronic pain rehabilitation. Clin J Pain 2000; 16(2):169–177.

39. Chaytor N, Schmitter-Edgecombe M. The ecological validity of neuropsychological tests: a review of the literature on everyday cognitive skills. Neuropsychol Rev 2003; 13(4):181–197.

40. Cicerone KD, et al. Evidence-based cognitive rehabilitation: recommendations for clinical practice. Arch Phys Med Rehabil 2000; 81(12): 1596–1615.

41. Clark DB, et al. Motor activity and tonic heart rate in panic disorder. Psychiatry Res 1990; 32(1):45–53.

42. Clark L, Robb J. SOS: help for parents. 2nd edn. Berkeley: Parents' Press; 1996.

43. Clark MS, Smith DS. Psychological correlates of outcome following rehabilitation from stroke. Clin Rehabil 1999; 13(2):129–140.

44. Cooper JO, Heron TE, Heward WL. Applied behavior analysis. Upper Saddle River: Pearson Education; 1987.

45. Corrigan JD. Substance abuse as a mediating factor in outcome from traumatic brain injury. Arch Phys Med Rehabil 1995; 76:302–309.

46. Costa PT, McCrae R. The NEO Personality Inventory: manual. Odessa: Psychological Assessment Resources; 1985.

47. Cushman LA, Scherer MJ. Psychological assessment in medical rehabilitation. Washington: American Psychological Association; 1995.

48. Danaher BF. Research on rapid smoking: interim summary and recommendations. Addict Behav 1977; 2:151–166.

49. Darnall BD, et al. Depressive symptoms and mental health service utilization among persons with limb loss: results of a national survey. Arch Phys Med Rehabil 2005; 86(4):650–658.

50. Davidoff GN, Roth EJ, Richards JS. Cognitive deficits in spinal cord injury: epidemiology and outcome. Arch Phys Med Rehabil 1992; 73(3): 275–284.

51. Dembo T, Leviton GL, Wright BA. Adjustment to misfortune: a problem of social-psychological rehabilitation. Artif Limbs 1956; 3(2):4–62.

52. Derogatis LR, Melisaratos N. The Brief Symptom Inventory: an introductory report. Psychol Med 1983; 13(3):595–605.

53. Derogatis LR. Symptom checklist-90R administration, scoring, and procedures manual. Towson: Clinical and Psychometric Research; 1977.

54. Desmond DW, et al. Incidence of dementia after ischemic stroke: results of a longitudinal study. Stroke 2002; 33(9):2254–2260.

55. Diller LD. Poststroke rehabilitation practice guidelines. In: Christensen AL, Uzzell BP, eds. International handbook of neuropsychological rehabilitation. New York: Kluwer Academic; 2000.

56. DuBose RF. Predictive value of infant intelligence scales with multiply handicapped children. Am J Ment Defic 1977; 81:388–390.

57. Dunn DS. Well-being following amputation: salutory effects of positive meaning, optimism and control. Rehabil Psychol 1996; 41:285–302.

58. Dunn M, Van Horn E, Herman S. Social skills and spinal cord injury: a comparison of three training procedures. Behav Ther 1981; 12: 153–164.

59. Dunn M. Social discomfort in the patient with SCI. Arch Phys Med Rehabil 1977; 58:257–260.

60. Dymek MP, et al. Competency to consent to medical treatment in cognitively impaired patients with Parkinson's disease. Neurology 2001; 56(1):17–24.

61. Eans RL, et al. Family interaction and treatment adherence after stroke. Arch Phys Med Rehabil 1987; 68(8):513–517.

62. Ebener DJ, Burkhead EJ, Merydith SP. The Americans with Disabilities Act: implications for vocational assessment. Assess Rehabil Exceptionality 1994; 1:91–97.

63. Elliott TR, et al. Negotiating reality after physical loss: hope, depression, and disability. J Pers Soc Psychol 1991; 61(4):608–613.

64. Elliott TR, Frank RG. Depression following spinal cord injury. Arch Phys Med Rehabil 1996; 77(8):816–823.

65. Elliott TR, Kurylo M, Rivera P. Positive growth following acquired physical disability. In: Snyder CR, Lopez SJ, eds. Handbook of positive psychology. Oxford: Oxford University Press; 2002:687–699.

66. Elliott TR, Shewchuk R, Richards JS. Caregiver social problem solving abilities and family member adjustment to recent-onset physical disability. Rehabil Psychol 1999; 44:104–123.

67. Elliott TR, Shewchuk RM. Social problem-solving abilities and distress among family members assuming a caregiving role. Br J Health Psychol 2003; 8(part 2):149–163.

68. Elliott TR, Uswatte G. Ethnic and minority issues in physical medicine and rehabilitation. In: Grabois M, et al, eds. Physical medicine and rehabilitation: the complete approach. Franklin: Blackwell Science; 2000: 1820–1828.

69. Engel GL. The need for a new medical model: a challenge for biomedicine. Science 1977; 196(4286):129–136.

70. Epstein NB, Baldwin LM, Bishop DS. The McMaster Family Assessment Device. J Marital Fam Ther 1983; 9(2):171–180.

71. Erikson EH. Insight and responsibility. New York: Norton; 1964.

72. Evans RL, et al. Family intervention after stroke: does counseling or education help? Stroke 1988; 19(10):1243–1249.

73. Ewing JA. Detecting alcoholism: the CAGE questionnaire. JAMA 1984; 252:1905–1907.

74. Fann JR, et al. Psychiatric illness following traumatic brain injury in an adult health maintenance organization population. Arch Gen Psychiatry 2004; 61(1):53–61.

75. Fisk GD, Owsley C, Pulley LV. Driving after stroke: driving exposure, advice, and evaluations. Arch Phys Med Rehabil 1997; 78:1338–1345.

76. Fleming MF, Barry KL, Manwell LB, et al. Brief physician advice for problem alcohol drinkers: a randomized controlled trial in community-based primary care practices. JAMA 1997; 277:1039–1045.

77. Folkman S, Lazarus RS. Coping as a mediator of emotion. J Pers Soc Psychol 1988; 54(3):466–475.

78. Folkman S, Lazarus RS. The relationship between coping and emotion: implications for theory and research. Soc Sci Med 1988; 26(3):309–317.

79. Fordyce WE, et al. MMPI scale 3 as a predictor of back injury report: what does it tell us? Clin J Pain 1992; 8(3):222–226.

80. Fordyce WE. Behavioral methods for chronic pain and illness. St. Louis: Mosby; 1976.

81. Frank JD. Persuasion and healing. Baltimore: Johns Hopkins University Press; 1973.

82. Frank RG, et al. Depression after spinal cord injury: is it necessary? Clin Psychol Rev 1987; 7:611–630.

83. Frank RG, et al. Differences in coping styles among persons with spinal cord injury: a cluster-analytic approach. J Consult Clin Psychol 1987; 55(5):727–731.

84. Frankl VE. Man's search for meaning. Boston: Beacon; 1959.

85. Fuhrer MJ, et al. Relationship of life satisfaction to impairment, disability, and handicap among persons with spinal cord injury living in the community. Arch Phys Med Rehabil 1992; 73(6):552–557.

86. Fullerton DT, et al. Psychiatric disorders in patients with spinal cord injuries. Arch Gen Psychiatry 1981; 38(12):1369–1371.

87. Gans JS. Depression diagnosis in a rehabilitation hospital. Arch Phys Med Rehabil 1981; 62(8):386–389.

88. Gans JS. Hate in the rehabilitation setting. Arch Phys Med Rehabil 1983; 64(4):176–179.

89. Garrada ME. A selective review of child psychiatric syndromes with a somatic presentation. Br J Psychiatry 1992; 161:759–773.

90. Gillen R, et al. Depressive symptoms and history of depression predict rehabilitation efficiency in stroke patients. Arch Phys Med Rehabil 2001; 82(12):1645–1649.

91. Glass TA, Maddox GL. The quality and quantity of social support: stroke recovery as psycho-social transition. Soc Science Med 1992; 34(11):1249–1261.

92. Gouvier WD, O'Jile JR, Ryan LM. Neuropsychological assessment for planning cognitive interventions. In: Goldstein G, Beers SR, eds. Rehabilitation. New York: Plenum Press; 1998:181–199.

93. Grant JS, et al. Social problem-solving abilities, social support, and adjustment among family caregivers of individuals with a stroke. Rehabil Psychol 2001; 46(1):44–57.

94. Grattan-Smith P, Fairley M, Procopis P. Clinical features of conversion disorder. Arch Dis Child 1988; 63:408–414.

95. Griffith HR, et al. Impaired financial abilities in mild cognitive impairment: a direct assessment approach. Neurology 2003; 60(3):449–457.

96. Guze S, Woodruff R, Clayton P. A study of conversion symptoms in psychiatric outpatients. Am J Psychiatry 1971; 128:643–646.

97. Hanson S, et al. The relationship between coping and adjustment after spinal cord injury: a 5-year follow-up study. Rehabil Psychol 1993; 7(1):41–52.

98. Harmon LW, et al. Strong Interest Inventory: applications and technical guide. Stanford: Stanford University Press; 1994.

99. Harper DC. Child behavior toward the parent: a factor analysis of mothers' reports of disabled children. J Autism Dev Disord 1984; 14:165–182.

100. Harris FR, Wolf MM, Baer DM. Effects of adult social reinforcement on child behavior. In: Ulrich R, Stachnik T, Mabry J, eds. Control of human behavior. Glenview: Scott Foresman; 1966:130–137.

101. Hayes SC, et al. Experiential avoidance and behavioral disorders: a functional dimensional approach to diagnosis and treatment. J Consult Clin Psychol 1996; 64(6):1152–1168.

102. Heaton SRH. Testing the impaired patient. In: Filskov SB, ed. Handbook of clinical neuropsychology. New York: Wiley; 1981:526–544.

103. Heckhausen J, Schulz R. A life-span theory of control. Psychol Rev 1995; 102(2):284–304.

104. Heinemann AW, et al. Toxicology screening in acute spinal cord injury. Alcohol Clin Exp Res 1988; 12(6):815–819.

105. Heinrichs RW. Current and emergent applications of neuropsychological assessment: problems of validity and utility. Prof Psychol Res Pract 1990; 21:171–176.

106. Herbert CM. Insight and progress in rehabilitation. Clin Rehabil 1989; 3:125–130.

107. Hibbard MRG. The comprehensive psychological assessment of individuals with stroke. NeuroRehabilitation 1992; 2:9–20.

108. Higgins JP, Wright SW, Wrenn KD. Alcohol, the elderly, and motor vehicle crashes. Am J Emerg Med 1996; 14:265–267.

109. Holland JL. Making vocational choices: a theory of vocational personalities and work environments. Englewood Cliffs: Prentice-Hall; 1985.

110. Hughes S, Alltree J. A behavioral approach to the management of functional disorders. Physiotherapy 1990; 6:255–258.

111. Hurwitz T, Kosaka B. Primary psychiatric disorders in patients with conversion reactions. J Depress Anxiety 2001; 4:4–10.

112. Institute of Medicine. Crossing the quality chasm. Washington: National Academy of Medicine; 2001.

113. Jamison C, Scogin F. Development of an interview-based geriatric depression rating scale. Int J Aging Hum Dev 1992; 35(3):193–204.

114. Jorge RE, et al. Major depression following traumatic brain injury. Arch Gen Psychiatry 2004; 61(1):42–50.

115. Kashani JH, et al. Depression among amputees. J Clin Psychiatry 1983; 44(7):256–258.

116. Katerndahl DA. Natural history of phobic anxiety. Fam Pract Res J 1992; 12(4):401–409.

117. Kazdin AE. Behavior modification. In: Applied Settings. 6th edn. Wadsworth Publishing; 2000.

118. Keefe FJ. Pain behavior observation: current status and future directions. Curr Rev Pain 2000; 4(1):12–17.

119. Kendall PC, Chambless DL. Empirically supported psychological therapies. J Consult Clin Psychol 1998; 66(1):3–6.

120. Kennedy P, Rogers BA. Anxiety and depression after spinal cord injury: a longitudinal analysis. Arch Phys Med Rehabil 2000; 81(7):932–937.

121. Kennedy PC, et al. A longitudinal analysis of psychological impact and coping strategies following spinal cord injury. Br J Health Psychol 2000; 34:627–639.

122. Kerns RD, Turk DC, Rudy TE. The West Haven–Yale Multidimensional Pain Inventory (WHYMPI). Pain 1985; 23(4):345–356.

123. Koocher GP, Norcross JC, Hill SS, eds. Psychologists' desk reference. 2nd edn. Oxford: Oxford University Press; 2005:735.

124. Kortte KB, Wegener ST. Denial of illness in medical rehabilitation populations: theory, research, and definition. Rehabil Psychol 2004; 49(3):187–199.

125. Kozlowska K. Good children presenting with conversion disorder. Clin Child Psychol Psychiatry 2001; 6(4):575–591.

126. Krause J, Rohe D. Personality and life adjustment after spinal cord injury: an exploratory study. Rehabil Psychol 1998; 43:118–130.

127. LaBarbera JD, Dozier E. Hysterical seizures: the role of sexual exploitation. Psychosomatics 1980; 21:897–903.

128. Lambert MJ, et al. Compendium of treatment manuals. In: Koocher GP, Norcross JC, Hill SS, eds. Psychologists' desk reference. Oxford: Oxford University Press; 2005.

129. Langer K, Pandrone F. Psychotherapeutic treatment of awareness of acute rehabilitation of traumatic brain injury. Neuropsychol Rehabil 1992; 2:59–70.

130. Lazare A. Current concepts in psychiatry: conversion symptoms. N Engl J Med 1981; 305:745–748.

131. Lazarus RS. Progress on a cognitive-motivational-relational theory of emotion. Am Psychol 1991; 46(8):819–834.

132. Leslie SA. Diagnosis and treatment of hysterical conversion reactions. Arch Dis Child 1988; 63:506–511.

133. Levin HS, Grafman J. Cerebral organization of function after brain damage. Oxford: Oxford University Press; 2000.

134. Lewin K. Field theory and experiment in social psychology. Am J Sociol 1939; 44:868–896.

135. Lezak MD, Howieson DB, Loring DW, et al, eds. Neuropsychological assessment. New York: Oxford University Press; 2004.

136. Lezak MD. Neuropsychological assessment. 3rd edn. New York: Oxford University Press; 1995.

137. Lezak MD. The rationale of deficit measurement. 3rd edn. In: Lezak MD. Neuropsychological assessment. 3rd edn. New York: Oxford University Press; 1995:97–109.

138. Lindemann E. Symptomatology and management of acute grief. Am J Psychiatry 1994; 151(6 suppl):155–160.

139. Lipowski ZJ. Somatization and depression. Psychosomatics 1990; 31:13–21.

140. Lipowski ZJ. Somatization: medicine's unsolved problem. Psychosomatics 1987; 28(6):296–297.

141. Lipsitz JD, et al. Open trial of interpersonal psychotherapy for the treatment of social phobia. Am J Psychiatry 1999; 156(11):1814–1816.

142. Loeser JD, Turk DC. Multidisciplinary pain management. Semin Neurosurg 2004; 15(1):13–29.

143. LoPiccolo C. Current issues in the diagnosis and management of malingering. Ann Med 1999; 31:166–174.

144. Lorig K, Holman H. Arthritis self-management studies: a twelve-year review. Health Educ Q 1993; 20(1):17–28.

145. Lorig KR, et al. Can a back pain e-mail discussion group improve health status and lower health care costs? A randomized study. Arch Intern Med 2002; 162(7):792–796.

146. Lorig KR, Holman H. Self-management education: history, definition, outcomes, and mechanisms. Ann Behav Med 2003; 26(1):1–7.

147. Mace CJ, Trimble MR. Ten-year prognosis of conversion disorder. Br J Psychiatry 1996; 169:282–288.

148. Martin GL, Pear J. Behavior modification: what it is and how to do it. 7th edn. New Jersey: Prentice Hall; 2002.

149. McCall RB, Hogarty PS, Hurlburt N. Transitions in infant sensorimotor development and the prediction of childhood IQ. Am Psychol 1972; 27:728–748.

150. McConnnaughy E, Prochaska J, Velicer W. Stages of change in psychotherapy: measurement and sample profiles. Psychother Theory Res Pract 1983; 20.

151. McCue M, Pramuka M. Functional assessment. In: Goldstein G, Beers SR, eds. Rehabilitation. New York: Plenum Press; 1998:113–129.

152. Melzack R. The McGill Pain Questionnaire: major properties and scoring methods. Pain 1975; 1(3):277–299.

153. Melzack R. The short-form McGill Pain Questionnaire. Pain 1987; 30(2):191–197.

154. Michael J. Repertoire-altering effects of remote contingencies. Anal Verbal Behav 1986; 4:10–18.

155. Miller WRB. Why psychologists should treat alcohol and drug problems. Am Psychol 1997; 52:1269–1279.

156. Miller WRR. Motivational interviewing. New York: Guilford Press; 1991.

157. Mitenberger RG. Behavior modification: principles and procedures. 3rd edn. Wadsworth Publishing; 2003.

158. Morley LC. Essentials of PAI assessment. New York: John Wiley; 2003:255.

159. Morley S, Eccleston C, Williams A. Systematic review and meta-analysis of randomized controlled trials of cognitive behaviour therapy and behaviour therapy for chronic pain in adults, excluding headache. Pain 1999; 80(1–2):1–13.

160. Mostofsky DI, Barlow DH, eds. The management of stress and anxiety in medical disorders. Needham Heights: Allyn & Bacon; 2000.

161. Norcross JC, Hill CE. Compendium of empirically supported therapy relationships. In: Koocher GP, Norcross JC, Hill SS, eds. Psychologists' desk reference. Oxford: Oxford University Press; 2005.

162. Nyenhuis DL, Rao SM, Zajecka JM, et al. Mood disturbance versus other symptoms of depression in multiple sclerosis. J Int Neuropsychol Soc 1995; 36:390–395.

163. Olkin R. What psychotherapists should know about disability. New York: Guilford Press; 1999:368.

164. Palmer S, et al. Psychosocial services in rehabilitation medicine: an interdisciplinary approach. Arch Phys Med Rehabil 1985; 66(10):690–692.

165. Palmer S, Glass TA, Palmer JB, et al. Crisis intervention with individuals and their families following stroke: a model for psychosocial service during inpatient rehabilitation. Rehabil Psychol (in press).

166. Patterson DR, Jensen MP. Hypnosis and clinical pain. Psychol Bull 2003; 129(4):495–521.

167. Pavlov I. Conditioned reflexes. Oxford: Oxford University Press; 1927.

168. Phillips NA, Mate-Kole CC, Kirby RL. Neuropsychological function in peripheral vascular disease amputee patients. Arch Phys Med Rehabil 1993; 74(12):1309–1314.

169. Piaget JP. The origins of intelligence in children. New York: International Universities Press; 1952.

170. Pless IB, Roghmann KJ. Chronic illness and its consequences: observations based on three epidemiological studies. J Pediatrics 1971; 79(3):351–359.

171. Premack D. Toward empirical behavioral laws. I. Positive reinforcement. Psychol Rev 1959; 66:219–233.

172. Prigatano GP, Klonoff PS. A clinician's rating scale for evaluating impaired self-awareness and denial of disability after brain injury. Clin Neuropsychol 1998; 12:56–67.

173. Prigatano GP. Principles of neuropsychological rehabilitation. New York: Oxford University Press; 1999:356.

174. Radloff LS. The CES-D scale: a self-report depression scale for research in the general population. Appl Psychol Meas 1977; 1(3):385–401.

175. Richards JS. Psychologic adjustment to spinal cord injury during first postdischarge year. Arch Phys Med Rehabil 1986; 67(6):362–365.

176. Rodin G, Voshart K. Depression in the medically ill: an overview. Am J Psychiatry 1986; 143(6):696–705.

177. Rolland J. Families, illness and disability: an integrative treatment model. New York: Basic Books; 1994.

178. Rollnick S, Mason P, Butler C. Health behavior change. New York: Churchill Livingstone; 1999.

179. Roth E, Davidoff G, Thomas P, et al. A controlled study of neuropsychological deficits in acute spinal cord injury patients. Paraplegia 1989; 27:480–489.

180. Roth E, et al. A controlled study of neuropsychological deficits in acute spinal cord injury patients. Paraplegia 1989; 27(6):480–489.

181. Routh DK, Ernst AR. Somatization disorder in relatives of children and adolescents with functional abdominal pain. J Pediatr Psychol 1984; 9:427–437.

182. Rubin SE, Roessler IS. Foundations of the vocational rehabilitation process. 4th edn. Austin: Pro-Ed; 1995.

183. Rybarcyk B, et al. Validation of a screening measure for depression in stroke inpatients. Am J Geriatr Psychiatry 1996; 4(2):131–139.

184. Rybarczyk BD, et al. Social discomfort and depression in a sample of adults with leg amputations. Arch Phys Med Rehabil 1992; 73(12):1169–1173.

185. Sattler JM. Assessment of children. 3rd edn. San Diego: Jerome M. Sattler; 1992.

186. Seligman ME. Learned helplessness as a model of depression. Comment and integration. J Abnorm Psychol 1978; 87(1):165–179.

187. Seltzer WJ. Conversion disorder in childhood and adolescence: a familial cultural approach, part I. Fam Syst Med 1985; 3:261–280.

188. Sherman JE, Rambaldo L. Coping with the trauma of spinal cord injury: a model of resiliency. Paper presented to Wisconsin Psychological Association, Madison, WI, 2002.

189. Skinner BF. Science and human behavior. New York: Macmillan; 1953.

190. Skinner BF. The behavior or organisms. New York: Appleton-Century-Crofts; 1938.

191. Smith DS, Clark MS. Competence and performance in activities of daily living of patients following rehabilitation from stroke. Disabil Rehabil 1995; 17(1):15–23.

192. Snyder CR, Irving LM, Anderson JR. Hope and health: measuring the will and the way. In: The handbook of social and clinical psychology: the health perspective. Elmsford: Pergamon Press; 1991.

193. Soderstrom C, Smith G, Dischinger P, et al. Psychoactive substance abuse disorders among seriously injured trauma center patients. JAMA 1997; 277:1769–1774.

194. Soderstrom S, et al. A program for crisis-intervention after traumatic brain injury. Scand J Rehabil Med Suppl 1988; 17:47–49.

195. Sohlberg MM, Mateer CA. Introduction to cognitive rehabilitation. New York: Guilford Press; 1989.

196. Speed J. Behavioral management for conversion disorder: retrospective study. Arch Phys Med Rehabil 1996; 63:148–153.

197. Stein P, Berger A, Hibbard M, et al. Interventions with the spouses of stroke survivors. In: Gordon W, ed. Advances in stroke rehabilitation. Andover: Andover Medical; 1993:242–257.

198. Strasser DC, et al. Team functioning and patient outcomes in stroke rehabilitation. Arch Phys Med Rehabil 2005; 86(3):403–409.

199. Swaiman KF, Ashwal S. Pediatric neurology: principles and practice. 3rd edn. St. Louis: Mosby; 1999.

200. Sweet JJ, Moberg PJ, Tovian SM. Evaluation of Wechsler Adult Intelligence Scale—Revised premorbid IQ formulas in clinical populations. Psychol Assessment 1990; 2:41–44.

201. Tait RC, et al. The Pain Disability Index: psychometric and validity data. Arch Phys Med Rehabil 1987; 68(7):438–441.

202. Tate DG, Rasmussen L, Maynard F. Hospital to community: a collaborative medical rehabilitation and independent living program. J Appl Rehabil Couns 1992; 23(spring):18–21.

203. Tatemichi TK, et al. Cognitive impairment after stroke: frequency, patterns, and relationship to functional abilities. J Neurol Neurosurg Psychiatry 1994; 57(2):202–207.

204. Taylor SE, Armor DA. Positive illusions and coping with adversity. J Pers 1996; 64(4):873–898.

205. Tennen H, Affleck G. Benefit finding and benefit reminding. In: Snyder CR, Lopez SJ, eds. Handbook of positive psychology. Oxford: Oxford University Press; 2002:584–597.

206. Thomas A, Chess S. Temperament and development. New York: Bruner/Mazel; 1977.

207. Thorndike EL. Animal intelligence: experimental studies. New York: MacMillan; 1911.

208. Tolman EC. Purposive behavior in animals and men. New York: Appleton-Century-Crofts; 1932.

209. Trieschmann RB. Spinal cord injuries: psychological, social, and vocational rehabilitation. 2nd edn. New York: Demos; 1988.

210. Turk DC, Gatchel RJ, eds. Psychological approaches to pain management: a practitioner's handbook. 2nd edn. New York: Guilford Press; 2002.

211. Turk DC, Meichenbaum D, Genest M. Pain and behavioral medicine. New York: Guilford Press; 1983.

212. Turner JA, et al. Catastrophizing is associated with pain intensity, psychological distress, and pain-related disability among individuals with chronic pain after spinal cord injury. Pain 2002; 98(1–2):127–134.

213. Volkmar FR, Poll J, Lewis M. Conversion reactions in childhood and adolescence. J Am Acad Child Psychiatry 1984; 23:424–430.

214. Von Korff M, et al. Grading the severity of chronic pain. Pain 1992; 50(2):133–149.

215. Von Korff M, Jensen MP, Karoly P. Assessing global pain severity by self-report in clinical and health services research. Spine 2000; 25(24): 3140–3151.

216. Wade SL, et al. The relationship of caregiver coping to family outcomes during the initial year following pediatric traumatic injury. J Consult Clin Psychol 2001; 69(3):406–415.

217. Wallander JL, et al. Disability parameters, chronic strain, and adaptation of physically handicapped children and their mother. J Pediatric Psychiatry 1989; 14:23–42.

218. Wallander JL, et al. Family resources as resistance factors for psychological maladjustment in chronically ill and handicapped children. J Pediatric Psychiatry 1989; 14:157–173.

219. Wallender JL, Thompson RJ. Psychosocial adjustment of children with chronic physical conditions. In: Roberts MC, ed. Handbook of pediatric psychology. New York: Guilford Press; 1995.

220. Wampold BE. The great psychotherapy debate: models, methods, and findings. Mahwah: Erlbaum; 2001.

221. Warlow CP, et al. Stroke: a practical guide to management. 2nd edn. London: Blackwell Science; 2001.

222. Wegener ST, et al. Spinal cord injury related pain: treatments used and perceived barriers to opioid treatment. Paper presented to the American Pain Society, Atlanta, 2000.

223. Weissman MM, Markowitz JC, Klerman GL. Comprehensive guide to interpersonal psychotherapy. New York: Basic Books; 2000.

224. Weissman MM, Myers JK. Affective disorders in a US urban community: the use of research diagnostic criteria in an epidemiological survey. Arch Gen Psychiatry 1978; 35(11):1304–1311.

225. Wells RD, Scwebel A. Chronically ill children and their mothers: predictors of resilience and vulnerability to hospitalization and surgical stress. J Dev Behav Pediatr 1987; 8:83–89.

226. Werner E, Smith R. Overcoming the odds: high-risk children from birth to adulthood. New York: Cornell University; 1992.

227. Williams JA, Koegel RL, Egel AL. Response–reinforcer relationships and improved learning in autistic children. J Appl Behav Anal 1981; 14:53–60.

228. Wise MG, Ford C. Factitious disorders. Prim Care 1999; 26:315–326.

229. Wolpe J. Psychotherapy by reciprocal inhibition. Stanford: Stanford University Press; 1958.

230. Wortman CB, Silver RC. The myths of coping with loss. J Consult Clin Psychol 1989; 57(3):349–357.

231. Wright BA. Physical disability: a psychological approach. New York: Harper & Row; 1983.

232. Yeates KO, et al. Pre-injury family environment as a predictor of neurobehavioral outcomes following pediatric traumatic brain injury. J Int Neuropsychol Soc 1997; 3:617–630.

233. Yeates KO, Ris MD, Taylor HG, eds. Pediatric neuropsychology: research, theory and practice. New York: Guilford Press; 1999.

234. Youssef FA. Crisis intervention: a group-therapy approach for hospitalized breast cancer patients. J Adv Nurs 1984; 9(3):307–313.

235. Zabora J, et al. A new psychosocial screening instrument for use with cancer patients. Psychosomatics 2001; 42(3):241–246.

236. Zimmerman EH, Zimmerman J. The alteration of behavior in a special classroom situation. J Exp Anal Behav 1962; 5:59–60.

237. Zung WW. A self-rating depression scale. Arch Gen Psychiatry 1965; 12:63–70.

Chapter

5

Gait Analysis: Technology and Clinical Applications

Alberto Esquenazi and Mukul Talaty

For over 25 years, gait analysis has been a useful clinical tool in the management of walking and movement problems. Technology related to gait analysis and our understanding of the role of gait analysis in clinical application have improved significantly in recent years. Gait analysis was initially used as an investigational technique starting in the last decade of the nineteenth century, first by the Weber brothers. Muybridge contributed to the understanding of movement with his famous sequential photographs, first of horses and later of walking and running men.[17] (There are World Wide Web sites that have compiled some of Muybridge's original work into animated sequences—point your browser to http://photo.ucr.edu/photographers/muybridge/contents.html# for a series of animations as well as many additional links to Muybridge photo sequences.) Later, Marey used light-colored marking strips on dark-clad subjects for the analysis of body movements.[15] Bernstein initiated the formal study of kinematics with his detailed photographic studies of normal human locomotion movement.[2] In 1947, Schwartz made the first quantitative studies of the forces generated at the floor–foot interface during walking.[20] Later, electromyography (EMG) recordings were possible. Inman's group at the University of California Biomechanics Laboratory refined the simultaneous recording of multiple muscle group activity during normal ambulation.[10]

Gait analysis has evolved into a recognized objective evaluation that is important in surgical planning and in the planning of other therapeutic interventions, such as botulinum toxin injection in the management of spasticity and the prescription and optimization of lower extremity orthotic and prosthetic devices. Other applications include sport movement analysis, analysis of other musculoskeletal conditions, and outcomes measurement. The most important contribution of gait analysis may be as a quantitative assessment tool for movement generally and walking specifically. In some centers, computer models of walking are used to drive simulation models that are then modified with the proposed interventions to determine if the treatment will achieve the desired goal.

These advances have been possible because of the improvement in technology related to the recording of movement and forces, and the use of dynamic EMG. Computer technology can be used to analyze large amounts of data obtained simultaneously from a variety of sources (force transducers, foot switches, EMG electrodes, motion analysis systems, etc.). Specialized transducers are used to record a physiologic quantity, such as movement or muscle potentials, and then transform it into a digital signal that can be captured on to almost any standard computer. Information can easily be saved and retrieved for future reference. These data can then be analyzed for information such as body segment velocities, accelerations, joint moments, powers, and mechanical energy, and under certain conditions internal joint forces can be estimated. Our desire to quantify neurophysiologic function, combined with the progress in computer technology, has promoted the proliferation of gait analysis laboratories.

A clear understanding of gait analysis data and the ability to perform a meaningful interpretation that is clinically applicable and relevant remain a challenge for many physicians. The goal of this chapter is to introduce and familiarize the clinician with the terminology, the biomechanics, and the complex interaction that exists between the body and the physical factors that impact human gait. For gait analysis to be useful in the clinical evaluation of patients, certain criteria must be fulfilled. The measured parameters should:

- supply additional and more pertinent information than that of the clinical examination;
- correlate with the functional capacity of the patient;
- be accurate and repeatable;
- result from a test that does not or only minimally alters the natural performance of the patient; and
- be interpreted by experienced clinicians familiar with the scope of the test protocol, instrumentation, and limitations of the equipment.

These criteria require that the clinician be familiar with the complex physiologic interactions of normal gait biomechanics, with normal and abnormal patterns of motor control, and with the technology used for its assessment. In addition, the clinician must possess the ability to relate these features to the pathologic motion that is observed during walking to effectively diagnose and address the problems of abnormal gait. In order to properly identify and evaluate the gait problems of the patient, the clinician must be able to produce a hypothesis and then attempt to understand *what* the problem is, *where* and *when* it is present, and *why* it occurs. Knowledge of appropriate available interventions, as well as a thorough medical history and examination, is needed to determine the most appropriate treatment interventions.[6]

NORMAL LOCOMOTION

Humans are the only animals who characteristically have upright walking. The fundamental goal of ambulation is to move from one place to another and to do so in a safe and efficient manner.[3] Because of the complex interaction of both lower limbs, the head, the trunk, and the arms during gait, a series of time-based descriptors have evolved to better describe normal and pathologic gait. Gait is cyclic and can be characterized by the timing of foot contact with the ground; an entire sequence of functions by one limb is identified as a *gait cycle* (Fig. 5-1).[3,10] Each gait cycle has two basic components: *stance phase*, which designates the duration of foot contact with the ground, and *swing phase*, the period during which the foot is in the air for the purpose of limb advancement. The swing phase can be further divided into three functional subphases: *initial swing*, *mid swing*, and *terminal swing*. In the same manner, the stance phase can be partitioned into five subphases: *initial contact*, *loading response*, *midstance*, *terminal stance*, and *preswing*.[1,5]

The stance phase can alternatively be subdivided into three periods according to foot–floor contact patterns. The beginning and the end of the stance phase mark the period of *double support*, during which both feet are in contact with the floor, allowing the weight of the body to be transferred from one limb to the other. When double support is absent, the motion is, by one definition, running. *Single limb support* begins when the opposite foot is lifted from the ground for the swing phase. For normal subjects walking at self-selected comfortable speeds, the normal distribution of the floor contact period during the gait cycle is broadly divided into 60% for the stance phase and 40% for the swing phase, with approximately 10% overlap for each double support time. These ratios vary greatly with changes in walking velocity (Fig. 5-2).

The *step* period is the time measured from an event in one foot to the subsequent occurrence of the same event in the other foot. There are two steps in each stride or gait cycle. The step period is useful for identifying and measuring asymmetry between the two sides of the body in pathologic conditions. *Step length* is the distance between the feet in the direction of progression during one step. The *stride* period is defined as the time from an event of one foot until the recurrence of the same event for the same foot; most often, initial contact to initial contact is used to define the stride period. *Stride length* is the distance between the same foot in the direction of progression during one stride. In most conditions for normal and pathologic ambulators, left and right strides are equal. The stride period is often time-normalized for the purpose of averaging gait parameters over several strides both between and within subjects (i.e. the absolute time is transformed to 100%). *Cadence* refers to the number of steps in a period of time (commonly expressed as steps/minute). The step length, step time, and cadence are fairly symmetric for both legs in normal individuals.

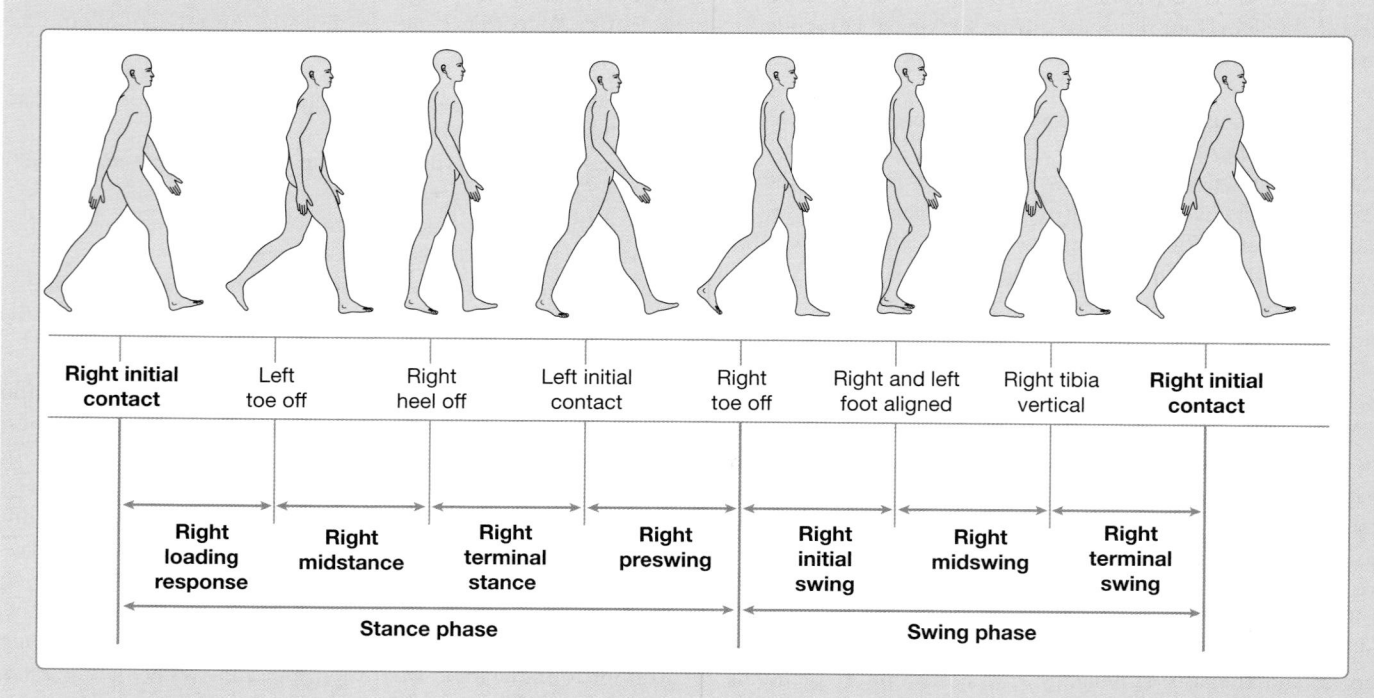

Figure 5-1 Gait cycle.

Chapter 5

Gait Analysis: Technology and Clinical Applications   95

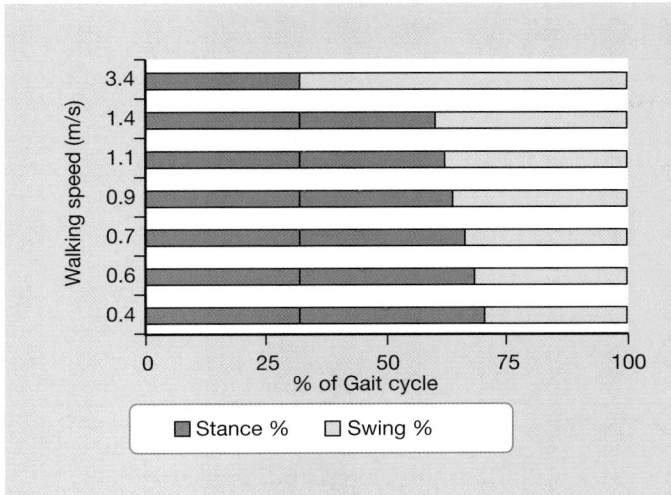

Figure 5-2 Stance:swing ratio as a function of walking speed. As walking speed increases, the stance phase comprises a relatively shorter portion of the total gait cycle. Thus the subject spends a larger fraction of time in swing phase. In the example shown, the subject spends more time in swing than in stance when running at 3.4 m/s. ª Running (no double support).

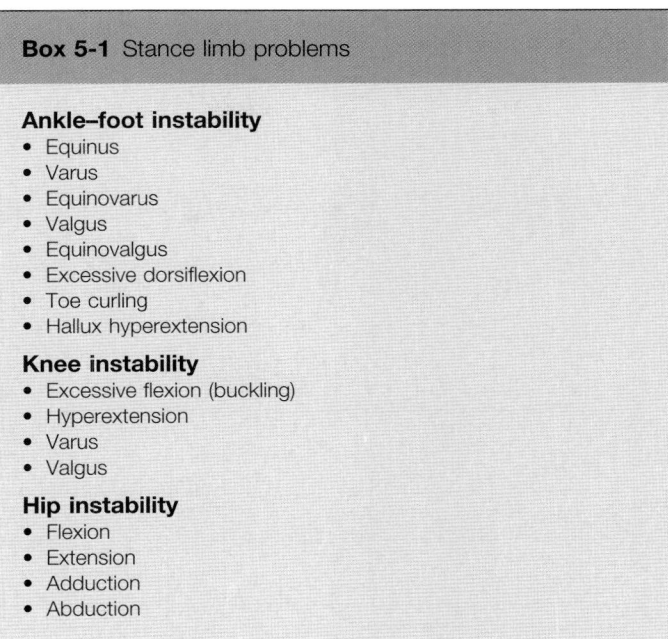

These are all useful parameters when evaluating pathologic gait. The base of support refers to the lateral distance between the feet. This is usually measured as the perpendicular distance between the medial borders or centerlines of the left and right feet.

GAIT DYSFUNCTION

Because of the complex relationship of multiple body segments, it is difficult to clearly identify the primary cause and compensation (substitution) in a gait deviation. One approach is to look at the different phases of locomotion and identify factors that affect the particular expected functional component when attempting to understand pathologic gait. Following this functional approach, the stance phase dysfunctions can be categorized into three groups, as shown in Box 5-1.

Ankle–foot instability
The foot interaction with the ground is inadequate, interfering with its inherent weight-bearing function. This can be exemplified as an abnormal posture of the foot present in the form of equinus, equinovarus, ankle valgus with or without equinus, toe flexion, hallux extension (hitchhiker's great toe),[16] and/or excessive ankle dorsiflexion as seen with insufficient plantar flexor strength. This is commonly seen in the patient with neurologic sequelae after central nervous system injuries.

Knee instability
This problem refers to flexed, hyperextended, varus, or valgus knee posture. In the sagittal plane, it may be a compensatory response to avoid limb instability such as that seen secondary

to knee extensor or ankle plantar flexor weakness. Cases of excessive knee hyperextension, or valgus or varus knee, can also be the result of an inherently unstable joint. Problems with adducted hip and flexed hip may also impact knee stability.

Hip instability
Hip abductor or extensor weakness, or limited hip extension range of motion, characterize this problem (i.e. Trendelenburg gait). Abnormal hip posture can also be a compensation for an abnormal base of support or limb instability. As an example, the patient with knee extensor weakness and an equinus deformity (which negatively affects balance) leans forward to improve or promote knee stability by moving the center of mass (CoM) anterior to the knee joint.

Swing phase deviations can be divided into impaired limb clearance and impaired limb advancement. Impaired limb clearance results from a drop foot, stiff knee, limited hip flexion, excessive or untimely hip adduction, and/or pelvic drop. Impaired limb advancement can be the result of a flexed knee, limited hip flexion or contralateral extension, and adducted hips. Ultimately, it is the interaction of a multijoint system that will determine the degree of gait impairment that will be present. Compensation for the lack of foot dorsiflexion during the swing phase can occur if the patient can generate sufficient timely hip and knee flexion during this phase of gait. If the patient has involvement of the hip or knee, or insufficient pelvic control, the foot will inevitably drag.

QUANTITATIVE GAIT ANALYSIS

Informal visual analysis of gait is routinely performed by clinicians and used as the basis to develop the initial questioning and examination of a patient (Table 5.1). This sometimes casual

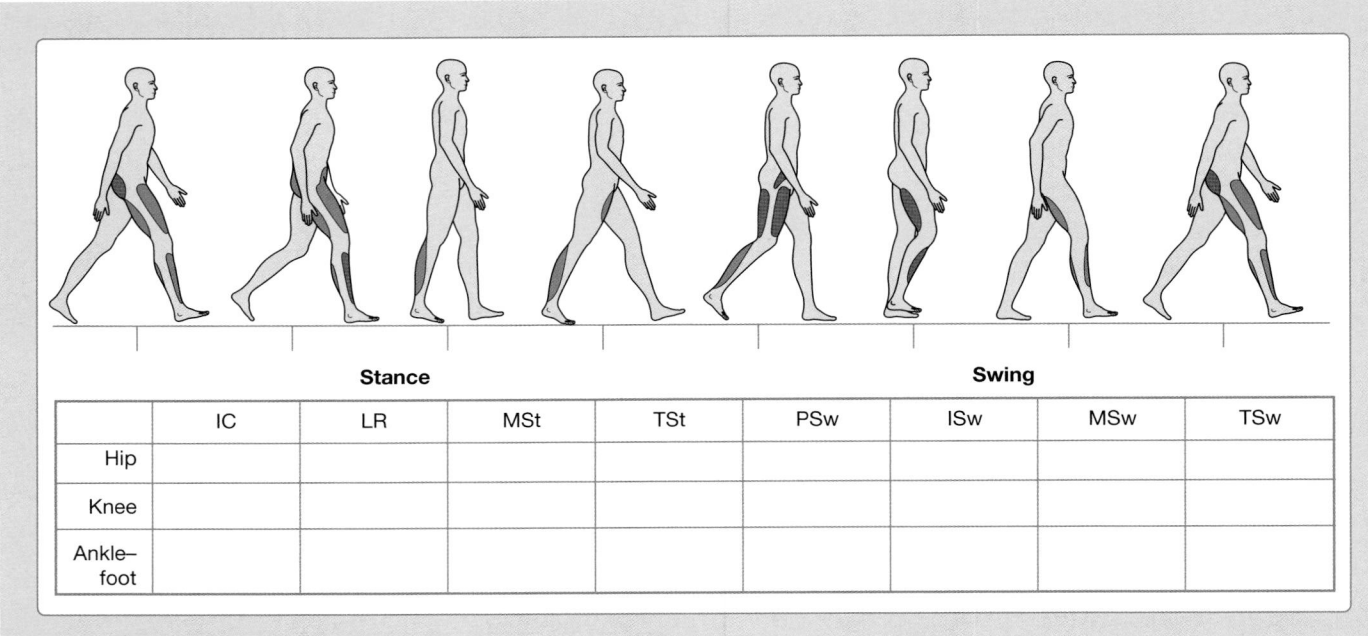

	IC	LR	MSt	TSt	PSw	ISw	MSw	TSw
Hip								
Knee								
Ankle–foot								

Figure 5-3 Sample form to systematize observational gait analysis findings.

Box 5-2 Components of gait analysis

- Video
- Kinetics
- Dynamic polyelectromyography
- Kinematics
- Energetics

Table 5-1 Phases of the gait cycle

Phase of gait cycle	Description
Stance phase	
Initial contact	The instant the foot contacts the ground
Loading response	From flat foot position until the opposite foot is off the ground for swing
Mid-stance	From the time the opposite foot is lifted until the ipsilateral tibia is vertical
Terminal stance	From heel rise until the opposite foot contacts the ground (contralateral initial contact)
Pre-swing	From initial contact of the opposite foot and ends with ipsilateral toe-off
Swing phase	
Initial swing	Begins with lift-off of the foot from the floor and ends when the foot is aligned with the opposite foot
Mid swing	Begins when the foot is aligned with the opposite foot and ends when the tibia is vertical
Terminal swing	Begins when the tibia is vertical and ends when the foot contacts the ground (initial contact)

observation can be more useful, albeit with many limitations, if performed in a careful, systematic manner. This can be done using a simple form that guides the clinician on documenting the findings (Fig. 5-3). This type of analysis can yield good descriptive information, especially when slow-motion video technology is used. The complexity and speed of events that occur during walking, coupled with deviations and possible compensations that occur in pathologic gait, define the limitations of a visual-based qualitative analysis of locomotion.[3] Fortunately, there are a great many tools available to increase our ability to observe and quantify gait.

In the laboratory, gait can be studied through the collection of a wide range of information. Four primary components of *quantitative* gait analysis (Box 5-2) that can be recorded are:

1. kinetics (analysis of forces that produce motion);
2. poly-EMG or dynamic EMG (analysis of muscle activity);
3. kinematics (analysis of motion and resulting temporal and stride measures); and
4. energetics (analysis of metabolic or mechanical energy).

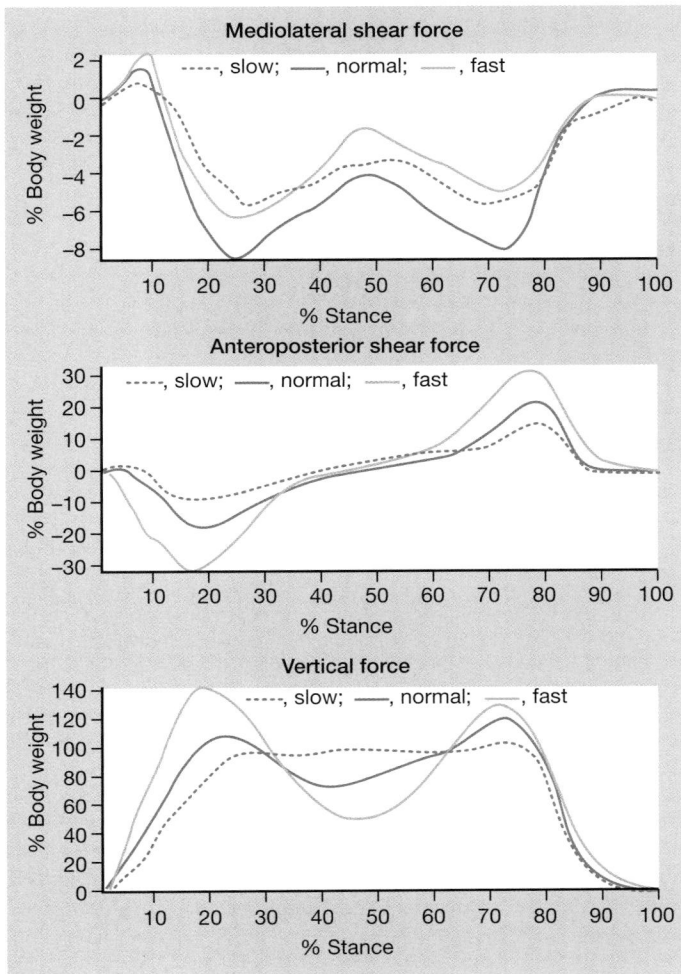

Figure 5-4 The effect of walking speed on force plate data (vertical, anterior–posterior, and mediolateral at slow, normal, and fast walking speeds). As walking speed increases, the peak forces of all components become more pronounced. Note at the fast speed, vertical force peaks at 140% of body weight. The reaction forces are often time-normalized (transformed to a percentage of the stride or cycle time, as shown) or could be plotted as a function of absolute time (in seconds or milliseconds). For comparison across subjects, the measured ground reaction forces may be amplitude-normalized as well. In this case, they may be reported as a percent of body mass or body weight.

Kinetics

Kinetic analysis deals with the forces that are produced during walking. Sir Isaac Newton described basic but critical concepts that are useful in understanding the effect of gravity on gait. He stated in his third law of motion that 'for every action there is an equal and opposite reaction'. This concept indicates that, as long as gravity is present, there is a reaction force where the body interacts with the ground. The ground reaction force is a reflection of the body weight and the acceleration of our body. This force can be resolved into a convenient set of directions, such as vertical, anterior–posterior, and mediolateral (Fig. 5-4). The anterior–posterior shear forces are sometimes referred to as propulsion and breaking forces. Friction is responsible for the generation of shear forces. Together, the forces in all three

directions measured by the force plates comprise the total force.

A force plate is a 'sophisticated scale' that can measure vertical (downward force similar to the body weight registered on a scale) as well as shear forces, which are those acting in the plane of the floor due to friction. Triaxial force plates measure the total force (a vector summation of all three components) acting on the center of pressure (a focal point under the foot at which the force is idealized to be concentrated). Preferably two platforms placed adjacent to each other are used, so that the total force under each foot can be recorded independently and simultaneously. In most instances, the force platforms are placed in the midpoint of the walkway and concealed in the floor so that steady-state, natural walking parameters are measured.

The components of the total force can be measured using two triaxial force platforms. An innovation, however, is that the force is superimposed in real time as a visible line on an image of the walking subject at the location at which the force acts. This is accomplished using laser optics[4] or computer processing in a specialized system (Digivec, BTS, Italy). This force line visualization system has a significant clinical utility, as it provides visual information regarding the effects of gravity on joint rotation without the need to instrument the patient.

A force is transmitted from the floor to the foot, and it is literally 'passed on up' to all other body segments. The product of the magnitude of the ground reaction force under each foot and its location with respect to a given joint center (ankle, knee, hip, etc.) are major factors that determine the torque or moments produced by the external force about that joint. This moment is a measure of the joint rotational tendency (flexion or extension, abduction or adduction, internal or external rotation) produced by the external force. Internal forces—generated primarily by muscles, ligaments, and the geometry of the joint articulation (bony contact)—act to control the rotation of the joints caused by this external force. For example, the ground reaction force, when positioned anterior to the knee (Fig. 5-5), produces a moment that tends to drive the knee into extension, and must be countered and controlled by muscle force (knee flexors, extensors, etc.).

Other components that contribute to the total joint moment are the products of the accelerations and masses of individual lower limb segments. It is important to note that the product of force and distance and the product of mass and acceleration quantities comprise the total joint moment. The product of force and distance provides only an estimate of the total joint moment. The product of mass and acceleration (inertial effects) contributes a relatively small component to this total. Error caused by omitting inertial effects increases the further away the given joint is from the point of contact with the floor (1% at the ankle, 5% at the knee, and 8% at the hip).

The relative motion of body segments produces forces that affect the motion of the entire body. The inertial effects error noted above is in part a reflection of the fact that all body segments are connected. This brings to light an important but not commonly considered concept (which is currently an area of

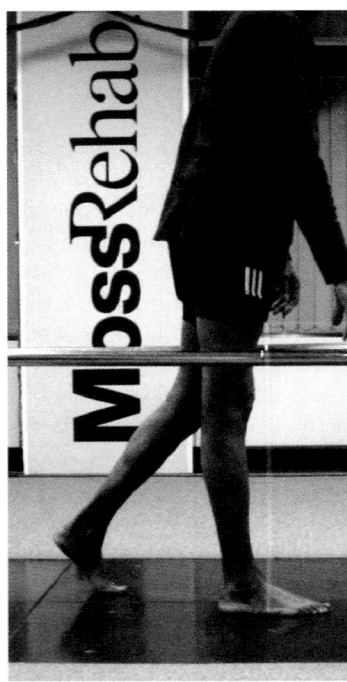

Figure 5-5 Visualization of a ground reaction force that passes anterior to the knee joint, and its association with knee extension.

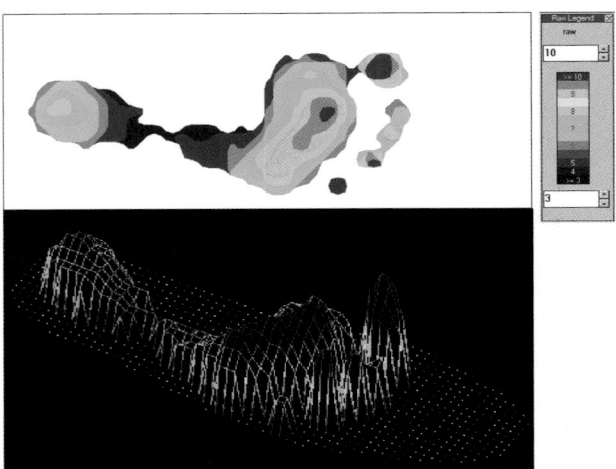

Figure 5-6 Graphic map of foot pressures obtained by the F-scan system. The top image shows a two-dimensional map of pressure at the foot–shoe interface. Shade intensity (normally shown in color) indicates variations in pressure under the foot. The lower figure is a three-dimensional contour plot of the same foot shown in the top trace. Note the shade intensity pressure key to the right of the top figure. A horizontal line through the middle of the foot map (not shown) can track the path of the center of pressure as the subject moves over the foot in the stance phase of gait cycle.

research in a few laboratories): that the acceleration of *each* body segment affects the acceleration of *all* other segments in the body.[22] A fairly involved engineering analysis is necessary to understand these interactions, but these effects should further our understanding of whole body mechanics and interactions, and ultimately have the potential to reshape some of the traditional lines of thinking in gait biomechanics.[12]

While force plates measure the sum or total force acting under the entire foot, it is sometimes useful to measure discrete components of that force acting over specific areas of the foot, or the distribution of pressure. Mathematically, *pressure = force/area*. Pressure is defined as a force acting over a certain area. A given force acting over an area produces larger pressures than the same force distributed over a large area. The pressure–time characteristics of the contact surface may have profound effects on the gait pattern. The forces generated at the point of contact with the floor can be measured with force platforms, as described above. Measuring the force distribution, for example as it occurs inside the shoe, necessitates the use of devices that can be placed inside the footwear and in direct contact with the foot without disturbing the foot–shoe interface. Ultrathin Mylar pressure-resistive sensors and specialized software permit collection of multiple gait cycles. Analysis of these data is done by calibrated color pressure grids. Software allows evaluation of force and pressure, as well as integrals of these measures. These systems are produced by Tekscan in the USA and others in Europe and Japan, and are useful for this purpose. Floor-embedded pressure sensor mats are also available to measure discrete pressures (Fig. 5-6). One disadvantage is that only one step at a time can be captured, and frequent guidance to capture

a complete step may be necessary due to the size of the mat sensor. Pressure measurement devices have clinical value particularly in the assessment of the deformed, insensate, or painful foot, and in the evaluation and fitting of customized foot or ankle–foot orthoses.

Dynamic polyelectromyography

In normal locomotion (Fig. 5-7), forces are elicited from 28 muscles in each lower limb to carefully control the gravitational forces, yielding a smooth, coordinated, and energy-efficient movement pattern. Redundancy exists in the relationship between muscles and the joints on which they act; in other words, the association between a particular movement and the muscle forces producing the movement is not unique. The cause of a particular movement cannot be specifically assigned to a muscle based on the observed movement. Persons with spastic paraparesis secondary to brain or spinal cord injuries present the greater diagnostic challenge, as muscle function is disrupted at many levels and the overlay of spasticity often causes the clinical evaluation during an examination to differ significantly from the muscle pattern used during walking and standing.

The electrical activity of all the muscles (EMG) that are capable of producing the target movement—which is not limited to a muscle directly spanning a particular segment or joint—needs to be evaluated. EMG recordings provide information about the timing and duration of muscle activation and, under certain conditions, relative strength can also be ascertained. The EMG signal is an accurate indicator of muscle activation and can be used to infer neurologic control informa-

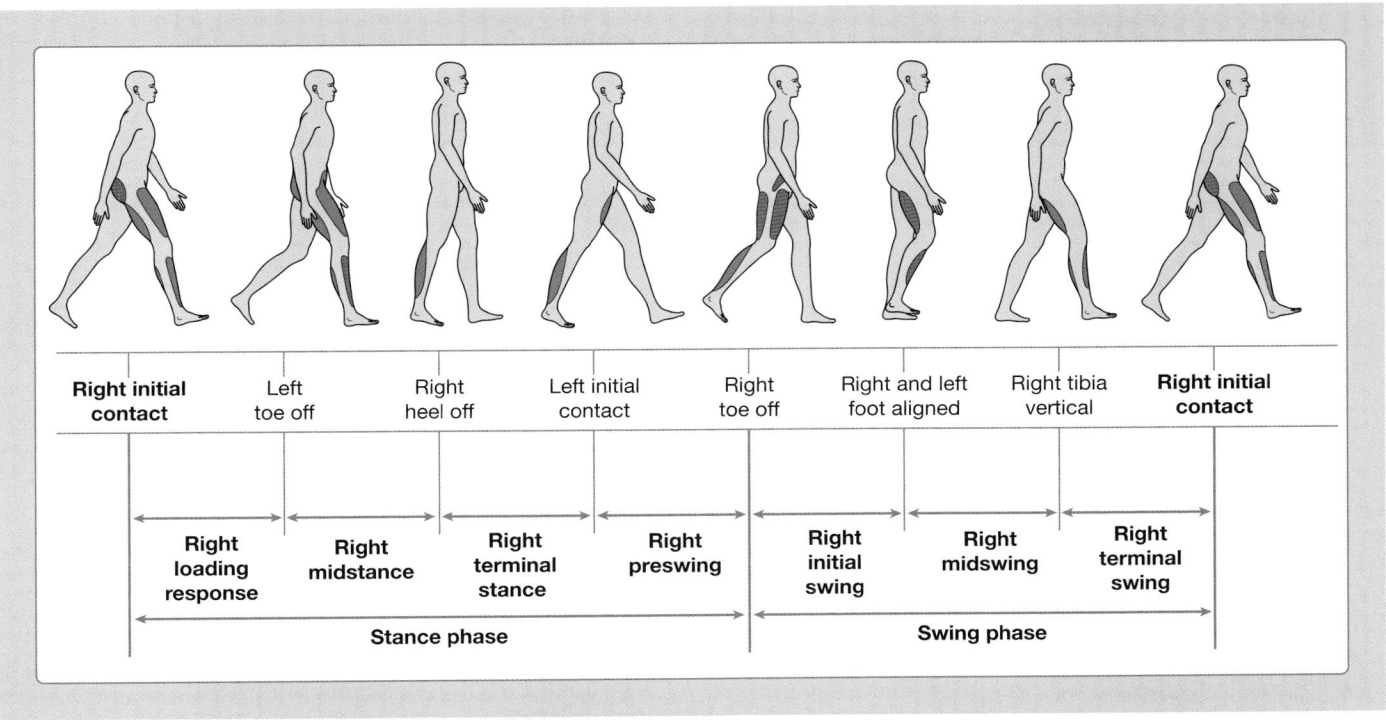

| Right initial contact | Left toe off | Right heel off | Left initial contact | Right toe off | Right and left foot aligned | Right tibia vertical | Right initial contact |

| Right loading response | Right midstance | Right terminal stance | Right preswing | Right initial swing | Right midswing | Right terminal swing |

Stance phase | Swing phase

Figure 5-7 Normal walking gait cycle terminology with selected lower limb electromyography representation. Human figures in the different phases of gait with superimposed primary gait muscles. Muscle shade intensity is roughly proportional to strength of muscle contraction.

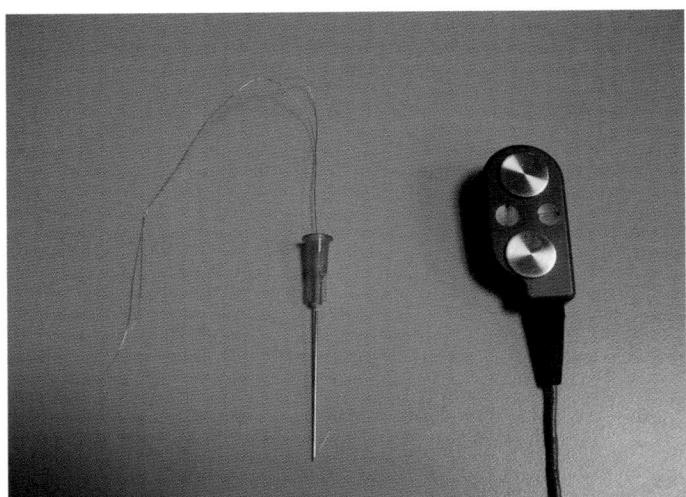

Figure 5-8 A wire electromyography electrode. The needle shown is 25 gauge and 1.5 inches long. A standard surface electrode is shown for reference.

tion. Superficial muscles are preferentially studied using surface bipolar electrodes secured to the skin with double-sided tape after the skin has been prepared. For deep muscles, or to differentiate between adjacent muscles when cross talk can be of concern, a pair of indwelling fine wire electrodes (Fig. 5-8) are inserted through a 25-gauge hypodermic needle, which is immediately removed, leaving only the wires behind. The thin wires measure 50 μm and are coated with Teflon or nylon except at the tips, where the muscle electrical potentials are recorded.

It is critical to note that EMG patterns are highly sensitive to walking speed. It is incorrect and potentially misleading to compare the recording of a patient with a slow gait to that of an able-bodied control population walking at a higher speed with a natural cadence. In addition to timing, amplitude of the EMG signal may provide valuable information for clinical decision making. A particular muscle may be over- or underactive during a given portion of the cycle. Such deviations should be carefully correlated with patient kinematics. When interpreting dynamic EMG data, it is important to distinguish cause and effect.

Patient EMG profiles can be compared with the mean and standard deviations of tabulated normative data, if speed-matched, to identify how the timing deviates from the normal. The timing classification scheme for EMG activity shown in Table 5-2 was devised in an attempt to standardize terminology.[11]

Kinematics

A kinematic analysis refers to the patterns of motion, regardless of what forces (external or internal) are required to produce those motions, and the resulting temporal and spatial parameters.

Temporal and spatial descriptive measures

This is a relatively simple and integrated method of quantifying some useful gait parameters. Temporal-spatial footfall patterns

Table 5-2 Classification of dynamic electromyographic activity	
Class	Definition
1	Premature
2	Premature prolonged
3	Out of phase
4	Normal

are the end product of the total integrated locomotor movement. Because gait is periodic in nature, data from a single cycle, or better yet an average of several cycles, can be used to partially characterize a gait pattern. Measurement of basic temporal-spatial variables of stance and swing phases is often used. These data can be obtained by measuring the distances and timing that characterize the foot–floor contact patterns.

Available techniques include use of ink and paper, foot switches, and instrumented walkways to the most sophisticated systems that require the patient to be more instrumented (which may provide considerable additional data). One example of a system that requires no patient instrumentation is the Electronic Gait Mat II. This instrumented walkway measures 3.8 m in length, and contains approximately 10 000 electronic switches, scanned at 100 Hz. Patients can use gait aids or shoes and braces, if necessary, as they walk over the mat, which is mounted flush with the laboratory floor. A recording of foot contact generates a timed 'electronic footprint'. A printout that provides calculated data about walking speed, cadence, stance, and swing times for each foot, as well as stride lengths, step lengths, and the width of the base of support, is generated.[5,21] The data can be easily stored for future reference or to perform other data analysis.[7] Comparing left- and right-side data from one subject can be used to determine the extent of unilateral impairment. Comparisons can also be made with normative gender, age, and walking speed-matched data. This allows inference of the level of dysfunction.

Motion analysis

Motion analysis refers to a quantitative description of the motion of body segments, without regard to the forces that are responsible for generating this motion. It is preferred to measure this in three dimensions, although it is sometimes done in two dimensions only. Early techniques included photographic and cinematographic analysis. Other techniques include the use of accelerometers and electrogoniometers. Most modern systems involve the use of specialized optoelectronic apparatus. For the optoelectronic system, passive or active optical sources (e.g. infrared-reflecting markers or self-powered light-emitting diodes, respectively) are attached to the subject and serve as markers. Calibrated cameras or detectors track each marker as it moves with the subject. When two or more cameras or detec-

tors identify the same marker, three-dimensional coordinates can be generated by mathematic triangulation, in a manner similar to the way in which we see an object with both eyes in order to be able to gauge its depth (the third dimension).

Video and passive optoelectronic systems utilize retroreflective markers applied to the subject. The markers are 'illuminated' by an external power source, and are tracked by the detectors (camera). Near-automatic marker identification and digitization are reliable if marker paths do not cross, as can usually be expected for standard marker placements in normal walking. However, conversion into quantitative data can require some manual intervention for marker identification in pathologic gait, where increased limb rotation, sudden motions, or crossover of segment paths may occur. Manual digitization and tracking of the raw data can be error-prone and in some instances time-consuming.[5,18] With active optoelectronic systems, each marker is self-illuminated (hence the designation 'active'). No postcollection marker identification is needed, as time sequencing between marker illumination and detector reception uniquely identify each light-emitting diode.[5] Each marker is activated at a slightly different (in the order of microseconds) instant in time. Telemetry (via infrared transmitters) in newer active systems such as the CODA MX1 (Charnwood Dynamics Ltd, England) have eliminated the use of long wires or 'umbilical cords' to power each marker. The advantage of not having to manually identify or track markers is still preserved.

Once the marker trajectories are available as three-dimensional data, they can be processed and displayed as a function of time or as a percent of the gait cycle (normalized). Joint angles, linear and angular velocities, and accelerations are some of the commonly calculated measures. When combined with anthropometric and kinetic (force) data, joint moments and powers as well as mechanical energy can be calculated. The physical meaning behind these quantities must be clearly understood if they are to provide any useful diagnostic information about the cause(s) of dysfunction.

Energetics

Normal walking requires a relatively low level of metabolic energy consumption during steady state at comfortable walking speeds. Normal gait on level surfaces is most efficient at a waking speed of 1–1.3 m/s, which is equivalent to 60–80 m/min or 3 miles/h. Comfortable walking speed for an individual usually corresponds to minimum energy cost per unit distance. The CoM is a point where all the mass of the body is idealized to be concentrated. In a homogeneous object, the CoM is simply the geometric center of the object. For a symmetric object, like a sphere or cube, the CoM is the center of the object. For the human body, the CoM has been experimentally found to be located 2 cm in front of the second sacral vertebra (in anatomic position). It has a dynamic nature (meaning that its location changes as the orientation of the body changes) and under certain conditions may even be located outside the body. The position of the CoM is intimately related to the location of the ground reaction force; simply put, they move in tandem. During walking, the CoM moves in a sinusoidal path with an

1. Pelvic rotation in the horizontal plane: the swinging hip moves forward faster than the stance hip.
2. Pelvic tilt in the frontal plane: the pelvis on the side of the swinging leg is lowered; this is controlled by activity in the hip abductors of the stance limb.
3. Early knee flexion (15°) during the first part of stance.
4. Weight transfer from the heel to flat foot, associated with controlled plantar flexion during the first part of stance.
5. Late knee flexion (30–40°) during the last part of the stance phase.
6. Lateral displacement of the pelvis toward the stance limb: the aim of this determinant is to reduce the displacement of the center of mass.

average of 5 cm vertical and horizontal displacement. This displacement of the CoM requires work, which in turn has an energy cost. In fact, the six determinants of gait, as described by Inman and his colleagues (Box 5-3), were identified as the strategies necessary to produce forward progression with the least energy expenditure by minimizing the excursion of the CoM.[19] While regarded as true for many years, recently the effect of the determinants on energy expenditure during gait have come under closer scrutiny, and researchers have begun to challenge some of the original precepts.[8,9,13,14]

There is a link between motion of the CoM and energy expended during walking. Sudden acceleration or deceleration of the CoM will increase energy consumption. The three main events that consume energy during walking are controlled deceleration toward the end of swing phase, shock absorption at heel strike, and forward propulsion of the CoM at push-off. Running is more efficient than walking faster than 2 m/s. Walking on a 10–12% incline will double energy expenditure.

There are several methods of metabolic energy measurement. Indirect calorimetry, expired air collection, and heart rate monitoring are all useful techniques. This last method can be used to calculate the energy expenditure index by subtracting the resting heart rate from the walking heart rate and dividing by the walking speed. This technique may be prone to have an error of 10–15% compared with the other methods.

PATHOLOGIC GAIT

This section begins a clinically oriented look at gait disorders and methods to diagnose and treat them. In the beginning of this chapter, an anatomic approach was used to list the gait deviations. In this section, we use a more functional and perhaps more useful method to describe the various gait deviations. Scenarios provided below illustrate some common problems with base of support, limb and trunk instability, and limb clearance and advancement. These scenarios outline possible bio-

mechanical implications and manifestations of each disorder, and provide strategies to properly diagnose them. It should be noted that the biomechanics described are often similar, if not identical, for different base of support problems, as well as those for other gait dysfunctions such as limb instability or impaired clearance. This suggests that biomechanics are not unique within a particular dysfunction or across dysfunction modalities. More importantly, this redundancy emphasizes the need to properly understand, diagnose, and treat the *primary* cause of the overall gait problem first. In some instances, the additional abnormalities or deficiencies (compensations) in the gait pattern will remedy themselves, or, oftentimes, will at least change in character once the patient has had a chance to come to a new plateau. Remaining deficiencies in the gait pattern can be addressed utilizing the same approach as indicated above.

Abnormal base of support

Base of support is presented first, because it is literally the foundation on which a stable gait pattern is built. The base of support is critical to all aspects of gait but particularly safety and comfort, as it is the foot–floor interaction that transmits the entire weight of the body to the ground and consequently characterizes the ground reaction force interaction with the body. The rate and magnitude of the loading (i.e. the gradual increasing of force under the stance leg) and unloading (the gradual decreasing of force as the leg prepares for swing) responses are shaped in large part by the interaction of the foot or feet with the ground. In addition, the location and magnitude of the ground reaction force in relation to the joints—which ultimately largely determine the joint moments that the muscles will have to stabilize and counteract—are affected by this foot–ground interaction as well.

Equinus foot deformity

Equinus foot deformity is frequently seen after an upper or lower motor neuron injury. This deformity can also be the result of ankle immobilization, fractures, and surgery. The foot and ankle are in a toe-down and frequently turned-in position (varus); toe curling may coexist. In this pathologic gait, limb contact with the ground occurs first with the forefoot; weight is borne primarily on the anterior and lateral border of the foot and may be concentrated in the area of the fifth metatarsal, resulting in an antalgic gait. Toe flexion can be present, particularly in neurologic injuries or cases where a plantar flexion contracture is present. Limited ankle dorsiflexion during midstance prevents forward progression of the tibia over the stationary foot, increasing pressure over the metatarsals, promoting ankle instability, and causing knee hyperextension. During the swing phase, sustained plantar flexion of the foot may result in a limb clearance problem unless proximal mechanisms of compensation such as increased hip and knee flexion are used.

A prosthesis set in excessive plantar flexion or set anterior to the trochanter–knee–ankle line, or in the case of an articulated foot-limited dorsiflexion, can result in the same abnormal gait pattern. An ankle–foot orthosis that limits dorsiflexion beyond 5° of equinus can impose the same gait deviation (Fig. 5-9).

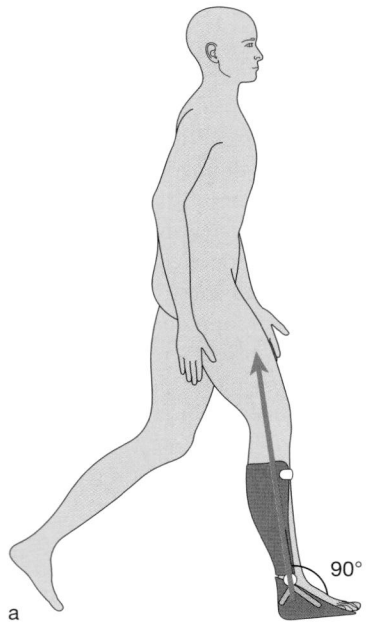 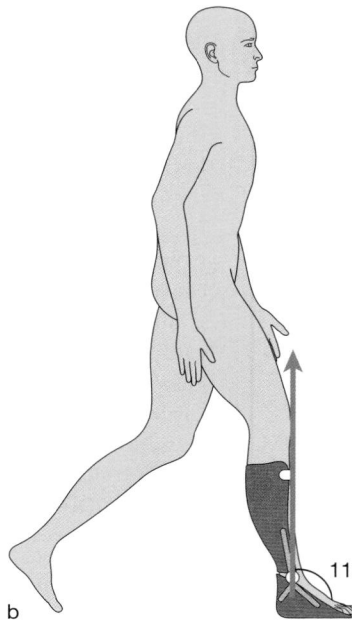

90°

110°

a

b

Figure 5-9 The effect of a plantar-flexed brace on the position of force line. Note the position of the ground reaction force, depicted by an arrow from the floor through the leg. In the relatively dorsiflexed brace (**a**), the force vector passes slightly posterior to the knee joint center, indicating that the body must stabilize a knee flexion moment to maintain stability. In (**b**), the brace is more plantar flexed and the force vector passes anterior to the knee joint, indicating that an extensor moment is now present at the knee. The brace can directly provide a force on the tibia and directly modify the knee moment.

Ankle equinus posture during late stance and preswing interferes with rollover, push-off, and forward propulsion. This can be seen in the configuration of the vertical and anterior–posterior ground reaction forces.

Clinical examination, combined with kinetics, kinematics, and dynamic EMG recordings, will elucidate the cause of the deformity. Over-activation of ankle plantar flexors during swing and/or stance phase, or under-activation of ankle dorsiflexors during swing phase, can lead to inadequate position of the foot during the stance phase. This can be seen in dynamic EMG as well as reduced or inadequate ankle range of motion, and also may be reflected in abnormal power generation or absorption. When it is difficult to differentiate between the muscular contribution of tibialis anterior and tibialis posterior to a varus deformity, a diagnostic tibial nerve block with lidocaine (lignocaine) can be performed. If the deformity is corrected, then the tibialis posterior is the offending muscle.

Following is a clinical case presentation to exemplify the use of the described methodology and technology for the evaluation of gait disorders and formulation of a treatment plan.

Clinical case presentation   The patient is a 52-year-old man who was involved in an automobile collision against a truck 26 months ago. He sustained a severe craniocerebral trauma with residual spastic right hemiparesis. No pelvic or lower limb fractures were evident. He presents with difficulty ambulating, with complaints of right ankle and knee pain aggravated by walking, as well as reduced balance. He drags his right toes against the ground when not paying attention to his walking. He uses a right ankle–foot orthosis (plastic, moderate resistance set in neutral) and straight cane for walking outdoors; he walks without a cane at home. Past medical history is non-contributory.

Clinical features of problem   The clinical features are:

- equinovarus right ankle–foot in terminal swing and stance phases;
- right knee hyperextension in stance phase;
- right stiff knee gait and occasional right toe drag; and
- poor balance, with unstable gait.

Differential diagnosis and analysis   The differential diagnoses are R/O ankle ligamentous instability or peripheral neuropathy; and R/O soft tissue contracture (static), dynamic deformity, or both.

Determine the specific muscle causing the ankle–foot deformity, i.e. gastrocnemius, soleus, tibialis anterior, tibialis posterior, extensor hallucis longus, flexor digitorum longus, or peroneus longus.

Diagnostic work-up   In the examination, the patient is an alert, pleasant, cooperative, moderately obese man who is in no acute distress. His body weight is 105 kg. Passive range of motion and manual muscle testing are as shown in Table 5-3.

Expected functional penalties   These are as follow.

- Impaired right limb weight bearing; decreased balance and right leg weight acceptance.
- Increased right loading phase time and decreased unloading phase time.
- Increased pressure over the lateral portion of the right foot, with decreased heel weight bearing and resulting ankle inversion instability.
- Right forefoot and ankle pain during the loading phase, prolonged right stance time, and shortened right step length.
- Right genu recurvatum with pain and hip flexion during stance phase.

Table 5-3 Clinical case presentation: clinical examination

	Right	Left	Normal
Ankle			
Dorsiflexion/plantar flexion	−15/50	0/50	0–20/0–50
Strength	Unable/3+	4+/5	5/5
Inversion/eversion	30/20	30/20	0–30/0–20
Strength	3+/unable	5/5	5/5
Knee			
Extension/flexion	−5/130	0/130	0/135
Strength	4+/4+	5/5	5/5
Hip			
Extension/flexion	−10/120	0/120	0/120
Strength	4+/4+	5/4+	5/5
Abduction/adduction	25/30	25/30	0–50/0–30
Strength	4+/5	5/5	5/5
IR/ER	30/50	30/50	30/50
Scoliosis	−		
Flexibility	−		
Ely's test	+	−	
SLR	−		
LE Ashworth[a]	2	1	
Ankle-selective control	Impaired	Normal	
Knee-selective control	Impaired	Normal	
Hip-selective control	Normal	Normal	
Ankle joint instability or effusion	−	−	
Knee joint instability or effusion	+	−	
Clonus			
Ankle	+ sustained	+ unsustained	
Patellar	−	−	
Light touch sensation	+	+	
Proprioception	+	+	
Leg length (cm)	95.5	96	

[a]Ashworth scale: 0, none; 1, slight increase ½ range of motion; 2, increase all range of motion; 3, difficult passive range of motion; 4, rigid.

- Impaired smooth, forward progression of the center of gravity, increased vertical displacement of center of gravity, functional leg length discrepancy (ankle equinus), and increased energy consumption.

Instrumented gait analysis   Analysis includes the following.

- Video with slow motion and superimposed force line visualization.
- Temporospatial parameters of locomotion.
- Poly-EMG of gastrocnemius, soleus, tibialis anterior, tibialis posterior, extensor hallucis longus, flexor digitorum longus, and peroneus longus. We will not evaluate hip or knee muscles at this time to simplify the analysis.

- Kinematic data to quantify ankle equinus and varus, as well as the effect of this deformity on other joints and temporal-spatial parameters of locomotion.
- Kinetic analysis to quantify joint moments and powers.

Findings   Figure 5.10 summarizes the findings. Video frame by frame analysis demonstrates evidence of abnormal right ankle–foot posture, with equinus, varus, and toe flexion in swing phase. Ankle equinus and varus as well as toe curling are evident in stance phase. Abnormal force line location in front of the right knee is noted.

Kinematic data demonstrate limitation in right hip range of motion. The right hip is abducted and slightly externally rotated.

The right knee demonstrates reduced flexion with valgus in late stance phase. Increased internal rotation of the knee is evident. The right ankle demonstrates marked increased inversion and limited dorsiflexion. Slight limitation in left ankle dorsiflexion is also evident. Other parameters appear to be within normal limits. Kinetic data demonstrate reduction in the right hip and knee extensor moment, and reduced power generation. The right ankle also demonstrates reduction in power generation.

Poly-EMG demonstrates gastrocnemius more than soleus to have abnormal activation (out of phase) in swing phase and premature activation in stance phase. The peroneus longus has premature prolonged activation in stance, with abnormal activity in swing phase—a compensation in an attempt to control ankle posture.

The tibialis posterior demonstrates no significantly abnormal activation in swing phase but appears to activate prematurely in stance phase. The tibialis anterior demonstrates premature activation in swing phase and abnormal activation in late stance phase. This muscle appears to be the primary cause of ankle inversion during swing phase.

The flexor digitorum longus demonstrates increased activation in stance phase. The extensor hallucis longus demonstrates increased activation in swing phase and abnormal low-level activation in stance phase, likely to supplement tibialis anterior and/or because of spastic response.

Impression The right equinus posture appears to be caused by over-activation of the gastrocnemius more than the soleus. The ankle varus results from out of phase activation of the tibialis anterior and extensor hallucis longus. No abnormal activation of the tibialis posterior is evident in the swing phase of this evaluation. The reduction in right hip, knee, and ankle power are probably related to the abnormal ankle–foot posture. Spastic right 'stiff knee' cannot be ruled out. There is no evidence of right knee hyperextension on the kinematic data, but this may be related to mechanical joint limitation in extension (see above). Stretching of hamstrings during stance might be the cause of pain.

Possible treatment interventions The clinician should x-ray the right knee to rule out bony block or foreign intraarticular body.

Consider the use of botulinum toxin type A (Botox) or other focal antispasticity intervention to right ankle plantar flexors (gastrocnemius more than soleus) and tibialis anterior (for this muscle, avoid overdose), followed by rehabilitation interventions to stretch the Achilles tendon and strengthen ankle dorsiflexors as well as for gait retraining.

Because Botox requires repeated injections and the patient is more than 2 years post injury, surgical intervention in the form of Achilles tendon lengthening, split tibialis anterior tendon transfer, and myotendinous lengthening of the extensor hallucis longus may be considered. To supplement the weak ankle plantar flexors and avoid toe curling when the ankle dorsiflexion range of motion is increased, a release and transfer of the long toe flexors to the os calcis can be considered. Rehabilitation interventions to strengthen ankle plantar flexors and dorsi-

flexors are appropriate. Gait retraining followed by reevaluation for stiff knee is recommended if gait deviation continues.

Equinovalgus foot

The equinovalgus foot can be caused by a number of different problems, including limited ankle dorsiflexion, particularly in the child or young adult in whom the subtalar joint can accommodate limited dorsiflexion with valgus posture. Upper or lower motor neuron injury, bony and ligamentous injuries, surgery, and prolonged immobilization with loss of ankle range of motion can all contribute to this deformity. During gait, contact with the ground occurs with the forefoot, and weight is borne primarily on the medial aspect of the foot. This position is maintained or worsened during the stance phase and interferes with weight bearing. Antalgic gait may be present if the navicula is overloaded. During the swing phase, sustained plantar flexion of the foot may result in a limb clearance problem unless proximal mechanisms of compensation such as increased hip and knee flexion are used.

Combined with clinical and radiographic examination, dynamic EMG recordings provide greater detail in understanding the cause of the deformity. If the deformity is muscular in nature and due to an upper motor neuron injury, it may be difficult to differentiate between the valgus contribution of peroneus longus and peroneus brevis; for this, a diagnostic lidocaine motor point block to one of them could be performed.

Flexion deformity of the toes

The toes may be held in flexion during the swing and stance phases. When wearing shoes, the patient complains of pain at the tip of the toes and also over the dorsum of the phalangeal joints, which is worsened by weight bearing. Callus formation in these areas is frequently seen. The gait pattern will demonstrate gradual loading of the affected limb and shortening of the step length and stance time. Likely causes are neurologic injuries, reflex sympathetic dystrophy, prolonged immobilization, and contractures. Clinical examination combined with kinetics and dynamic EMG recordings can be helpful in sorting out the cause of the deformity. In patients with spasticity, the recordings probably will demonstrate prolonged or out of phase activation of the flexor digitorum longus and flexor hallucis longus, and may demonstrate abnormal coactivation of gastrocnemius–soleus or lack of activation of the toe extensors.

Hitchhiker's great toe

This deformity is a notable problem in patients with upper motor neuron problems. The great toe is held in extension during stance and frequently during swing phases. Equinus and varus posture of the ankle may accompany this deformity. When wearing shoes, the patient frequently complains of pain at the dorsum and the tip of the big toe and, during the weight-bearing phase of the gait cycle, under the first metatarsal head. During gait, big toe extension can interfere with the weight-bearing phase of locomotion. Over-activation of the extensor hallucis longus and reduction or lack of activation of flexor hallucis longus frequently contribute to this deformity. Clinical

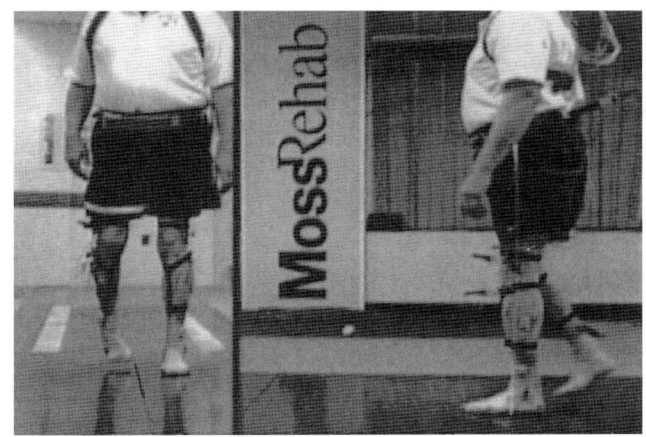

Gait Analysis Report MossRehab Hospital

Patient Data:

Sex	Age	Date of Birth	Height (m)	Weight (kg)
Male	52	07/46	1.899	105

Gait Parameters	Left	Right	Joint Angles (deg)	Left	Right	Normal
Velocity (m/s)	1.15	1.19	Hip Range	38.80	25.40	35.43
Stride Length (m)	1.19	1.20	Hip Max	32.30	24.50	32.71
Stride Time (s)	1.03	1.01	Hip Min	−6.50	−0.90	−2.72
Step Length (m)	0.64	0.57	Knee Range	42.50	30.80	54.86
Step Time (s)	0.48	0.53	Knee Max	42.40	26.60	58.23
Cadence	126.05	112.57	Knee Min	−0.10	−4.20	3.37
Percent Stance	75.07	68.42				
Swing Time (s)	03.32	0.26	Ankle Range	23.40	23.40	24.01
			Ankle Max	15.70	12.30	14.40
Double Support (s)	0.22	0.21	Ankle Min	−7.70	−11.10	−9.61

Figure 5-10 Patient data generated by CODA mpx30.

examination, in combination with dynamic EMG recordings, is helpful to elucidate the source of the deformity and whether it is obligatory or compensatory in nature.

Joint instability

Ankle instability
This deviation is caused by excessive untimely forward progression of the tibia in mid to late stance phase. This is usually the result of insufficient calf musculature, which is intended to provide control for the forward progression of the tibia over the stationary foot. Manual muscle testing of the ankle plantar flexors can be performed by having patients walk on their toes. Obtaining kinetic, kinematic data, and dynamic EMG recordings might be necessary to understand the biomechanical causes of the problem.

Knee instability
This refers to either knee buckling or hyperextension, and can occur when the expected early stance–phase knee flexion is combined with quadriceps weakness, as may be seen in persons with lower motor neuron syndrome, knee extensor weakness, quadriceps tendon rupture, or tears of the cruciate ligaments. It can also be observed in the early phase of recovery after upper motor neuron injury, when flaccidity and weakness affect the involved limb. A knee flexion deformity would further complicate this problem. If knee buckling occurs, the patient can require the use of the upper extremity for support. The patient may not produce the normally expected full knee extension in late swing phase and/or stance phase, further compromising limb stability. Bilateral knee and hip flexion might be present, which can result in a crouched gait. This results in a marked increase in energy consumption, and muscle fatigue and

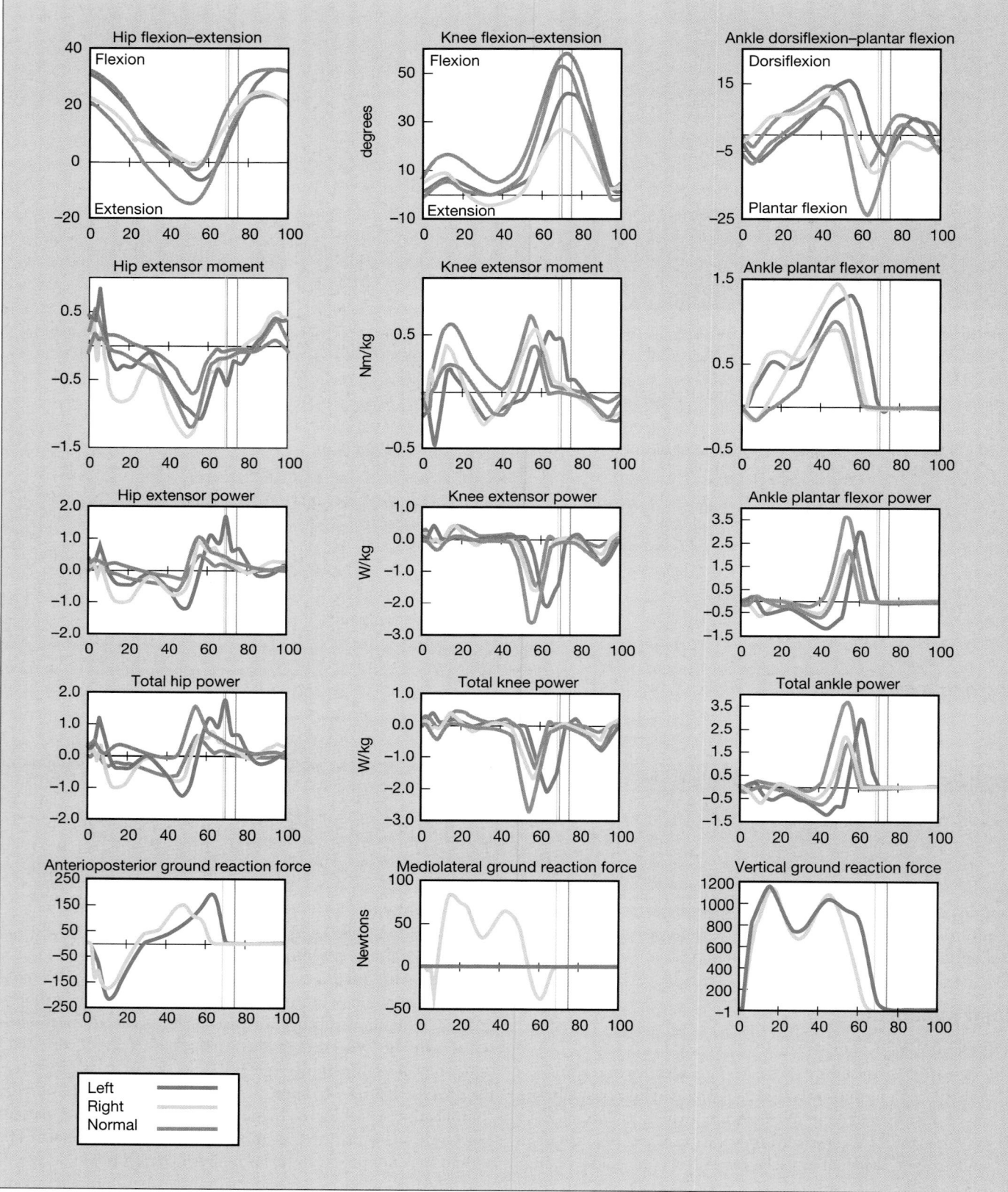

Figure 5-10 Continued

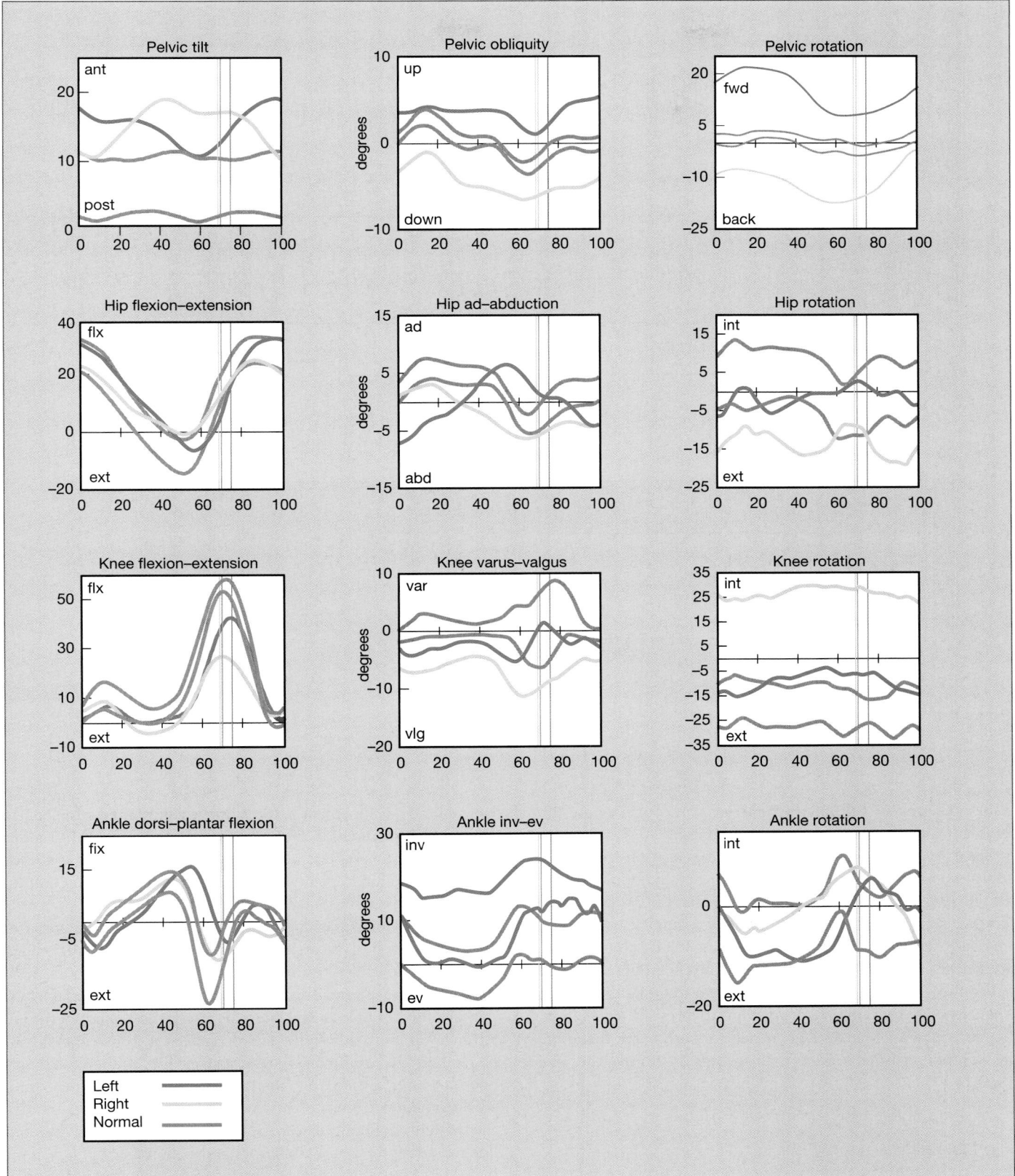

Figure 5-10 Continued

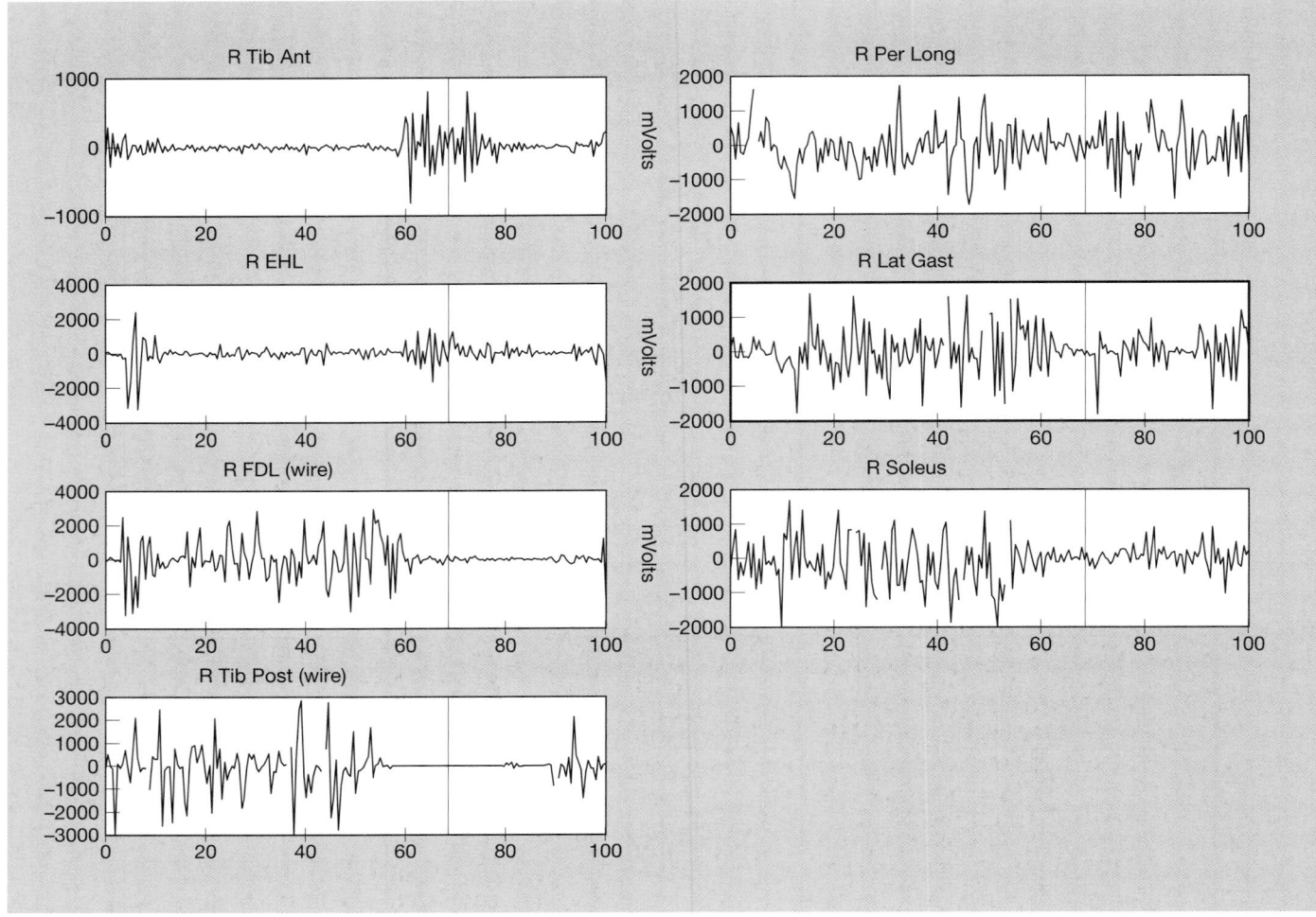

Figure 5-10 Continued

pain. The lack of full knee extension in terminal swing limits limb advancement and reduces step length.

Knee hyperextension may be a compensation for knee extensor weakness during stance phase. Knee hyperextension can also be present in this phase of gait as a result of an ankle plantar flexion contracture, or spastic ankle equinus produced by increased activity of the gastrocnemius–soleus group. Marked weakness of the ankle plantar flexor muscle group can produce a 'drop-off' gait, for which the patient may compensate through knee hyperextension in an attempt to prevent knee flexion. Spasticity of the knee extensors and forward trunk flexion may be another cause for knee hyperextension during the stance phase.

Hip instability

Excessive hip flexion during stance phase is a less common gait deviation. This deformity is characterized by sustained hip flexion that interferes with limb positioning during gait. During the stance phase, excessive hip flexion interferes with contra-lateral limb advancement and results in a shortened step length. Possible causes include degenerative changes of the hip joint, bony deformities such as heterotopic ossification, knee extensor weakness and ankle plantar flexor posture, hip flexion contractures, and flexor spasticity.

Hip adduction can occur during the swing phase, and this can interfere with limb clearance and advancement. During stance phase, this deviation results in a narrow base of support, with potential balance impairment. Because many patients may compensate for hip flexion weakness by using the hip adductors to advance the limb during the swing phase, the clinician needs to be certain that reducing or eliminating hip adductor activity does not interfere with hip flexion, which can compromise limb advancement, increase effort required to walk, or even render the patient non-ambulatory. Dynamic poly-EMG of the hip flexors, adductors, and abductors and in some patients a temporary diagnostic obturator nerve block may provide critical information on this issue. Severe hip adduction can interfere with a patient's hygiene, dressing, toileting, and sexuality in addition to imposing a gait problem.

Trunk instability

Trunk instability is an abnormal anterior or lateral lean of the trunk during walking, when it is normally mostly upright. Trunk instability can result from hip extensor weakness, limited hip extension, compensation for knee extensor weakness and ankle plantar flexor posture, and hip flexor spasticity. Hip hiking and contralateral trunk lean may be used to compensate for decreased limb advancement and swing phase clearance problems.

Limb clearance and advancement

Limb clearance and advancement occur during the swing phase of gait, and are vital precursors for proper limb positioning in order for the leg to accept the body weight during the ensuing stance phase. When limb clearance is inadequate, limb advancement is usually compromised. Impaired limb clearance may cause a patient to trip and fall, particularly when walking on uneven, inclined, or carpeted surfaces. Reduction of limb advancement produces shortening of step length and reduction in walking speed.

Stiff knee gait

Stiff knee gait is most commonly seen in the patient with spastic hemiplegia. The use of a locked knee prosthesis for the transfemoral amputee, or a locked knee brace in a patient who requires a knee ankle–foot orthosis, can be the cause of this gait deviation. Other pathologies, such as degenerative joint diseases of the knee or a failed joint replacement, may reduce the arc of motion of the joint. In stiff knee gait, the knee and hip maintain an extended attitude in the swing phase instead of flexing up to the average normal 60° for the knee and 30° for the hip. Even if the ankle–foot system has an appropriate dorsiflexed position, the lack of adequate limb clearance can result in a foot drag. At times, only a mild reduction in the range of motion for the knee and hip may be present, but it may be delayed in relationship to the gait cycle. The patient's inability to flex the knee in an appropriate manner results in an increased moment of inertia, which requires more hip flexion activity to advance the leg during the swing phase. The patient will utilize compensatory mechanisms for limb clearance; these can include trunk and ipsilateral hip mechanisms. Contralateral limb compensatory motions such as vaulting (early heel rise) may also be present.

Excessive pelvic obliquity (pelvic drop)

Increased hip adduction can interfere with limb advancement by contacting the contralateral stance leg. In contrast to ipsilateral swing phase hip adductor activity, overactive stance phase hip abductor weakness can compromise limb clearance and advancement also. Normally, hip abductors help to counter gravity's pull in the swing side pelvis by producing an abductor moment to help keep the pelvis level. Weakness may allow the pelvis to sag (more obliquity). Imbalance of the abductor and adductor muscle groups is the main cause. Because many hemiplegic patients use the adductors to compensate for reduced hip flexion in limb advancement, the clinician needs to be certain that elimination or reduction of adductor activities does not render the patient non-ambulatory.

Inadequate hip flexion

Inadequate hip flexion is another cause of abnormal limb clearance. This problem effectively prevents physiologic 'shortening' of the limb, producing a swing phase toe drag or early foot contact. The use of compensatory techniques, such as hip external rotation or circumduction, to promote the use of the adductors to advance the limb should be attempted. The use of a shoe lift to cause functional lengthening of the contralateral limb can be attempted.

Drop foot

Drop foot refers to the lack of ankle dorsiflexion during the swing phase. This can result in impairment of limb clearance unless appropriate compensation is afforded in other anatomic segments such as the knee and hip (steppage gait) or by the contralateral limb (vaulting). The frequent cause of this problem is lack of activation of the tibiales anterior. This may be secondary to a peroneal nerve injury, loss of strength such as that seen residual of polio, spastic imbalance between ankle plantar flexors and dorsiflexors, or out of phase activation of the tibiales anterior in the swing phase of locomotion.

SUMMARY

Gait analysis should be seen as a key adjuvant to clinical examination and other appropriate diagnostic studies in the management of walking and mobility problems. When used appropriately by a clinician who can adequately interpret the data, these tools and methodologies can provide direct evidence of cause and effect in an otherwise redundant physiologic system that may produce a deformity or deviation based on many different muscle–joint interactions or adaptive mechanisms. Gait analysis can also help differentiate primary problems from those that may be compensatory in nature. Gait analysis should be seen as a necessary diagnostic test to guide the development of a rational treatment intervention strategy in patients with moderate to severe gait dysfunction, particularly when surgery is to be considered, and as a helpful aid in those patients with mild problems. Computerized gait analysis also can be used as an outcome assessment tool to determine the effects of therapeutic interventions or to assess progression of conditions affecting gait. Interventions that can be used to address gait dysfunctions include the prescription of therapeutic exercises, use of orthotic devices and their alignment optimization, use of pharmacology (systemic, local, or intrathecal), prosthetic alignment optimization, and surgical planning. A clinical case presentation has been included to illustrate its use in one particular gait problem. A clear understanding of the biomechanics of normal locomotion, pathologic gait, and the potential pitfalls of gait analysis are necessary to appropriately use this technique for the benefit of our patients.

REFERENCES

1. Bampton S. A guide to the visual examination of pathological gait. Philadelphia: Temple University–Moss Rehabilitation Hospital; 1979.

2. Bernstein N. The technique of the study of movements. In: Slonim A, ed. Textbook of the physiology of work. Moscow; 1934.

3. Cappozzo A. Gait analysis methodology. Hum Mov Sci 1984; 3:27–50.

4. Cook TM, Cozzens BA, Kenosian H. A technique for force-line visualization. Philadelphia: Moss Rehabilitation Hospital; 1979.

5. Esquenazi A, Hirai B. Assessment of gait and orthotic prescription. Phys Med Rehabil Clin North Am 1991; 2:473–485.

6. Esquenazi A, Keenan M. Gait analysis. In: Gans B, ed. Rehabilitation medicine: principles and practice. 2nd edn. Philadelphia: Lippincott; 1993: 122–130.

7. Esquenazi A, Talaty M. Normal and pathological gait analysis. In: Lehmkuhl LD, ed. Physical medicine and rehabilitation: the complete approach. Malden: Blackwell Science; 2000:2002.

8. Gard S, Childress D. The effect of pelvic list on the vertical displacement of the trunk during normal walking. Gait Posture 1997; 5:233–238.

9. Gard S, Childress D. The influence of stance-phase knee flexion on the vertical displacement of the trunk during normal walking. Arch Phys Med Rehabil 1999; 80:26–32.

10. Inman V, Ralston H, Todd F. Human walking. Baltimore: Williams & Wilkins; 1981.

11. Keenan MAE, Haider T, Stone LR. Dynamic electromyography to assess elbow spasticity. J Hand Surg 1990; 15A:607–614.

12. Kepple TM, Siegel KL, Stanhope SJ. Relative contributions of the lower extremity joint moments to forward progression and support during gait. Gait Posture 1997; 6:1–8.

13. Kerrigan D, Della Croce U, Marciello M, et al. A refined view of the determinants of gait: significance of heel rise. Arch Phys Med Rehabil 2000; 81:1077–1080.

14. Kerrigan D, Riley P, Lelas J, et al. Quantification of pelvic rotation as a determinant of gait. Arch Phys Med Rehabil 2001; 82:217–220.

15. Marey E. La methode graphique dans les sciences experimentales et particularierement en physiologie et en medicine. In: Masson G, ed. Deuxieme tirage augmente d'un supplement sur le development de le methode graphique par l'emploi de la photographie. Paris; 1885.

16. Mayer N, Keenan M, Esquenazi A. Limbs with restricted or excessive motion after traumatic brain injury. In: Rosenthal M, Griffith ER, Kreutzer GS, eds. Rehabilitation of the adult and child with traumatic brain injury. 3rd edn. Philadelphia: FA Davis; 1999:503–535.

17. Muybridge E. Animal locomotion: an electro-photographic investigation of consecutive phases of animal movements. Philadelphia: University of Pennsylvania; 1887.

18. Rowell D, Mann R. Human movement analysis. Soma 1989; 3:13–20.

19. Saunders JB, Inman VT, Eberhart HD. The major determinants in normal and pathological gait. J Bone Joint Surg Am 1953; 35-A:544–553.

20. Schwartz R, Heath A, Misiek W, et al. Kinetics of human gait: the making and interpretation of electrobasographic records of gait. J Bone Joint Surg 1934; 16:343–350.

21. Taylor D. An instrumented gait mat. The International Conference on Rehabilitation Engineering, Toronto, 1980.

22. Zajac FE, Gordon ME. Determining muscle's force and action in multiarticular movement. Exerc Sport Sci Rev 1989; 17:187–230.

Chapter

6

Impairment Rating and Disability Determination

James P. Robinson and Richard E. Seroussi

The purpose of this chapter is to provide basic information about disability and impairment evaluations. It covers four main topics:

1. the types of agencies that administer impairment and disability programs;
2. the concepts central to this area of medicine;
3. the physician's role in performing these evaluations, highlighting ethical and clinical challenges; and
4. practical strategies for disability evaluation.

While physicians of many different specialties are actively involved in disability and impairment evaluation, physiatrists have skills that are central to understanding disability and impairment evaluation. The physiatric emphasis on assessing and restoring function among the severely ill or injured provides a key component of what is typically needed by agencies requesting disability evaluations.

This chapter is not intended to be used to determine impairment or disability for a specific patient. The reader is referred in this regard to the American Medical Association (AMA) *Guides to the Evaluation of Permanent Impairment*, fifth edition.[9] The AMA Guides outline a method for rating impairment for virtually every organ system. In practical terms, however, the great majority of impairment and disability evaluations are directed toward musculoskeletal disorders (AMA Guides, Chs 15–17), neurologic disorders (AMA Guides, Ch. 13), and psychiatric disorders (AMA Guides, Ch. 14). Because chronic pain (AMA Guides, Ch. 18) cuts across all these disorders, it is often the focus of impairment and disability evaluations.

DISABILITY AGENCIES

Communities frequently provide assistance to individuals who are incapacitated. This type of helping behavior can be seen not only in modern societies, but also in primitive ones and even in communities of primates.[15] During the past 100 years, the informal understandings that have existed in communities regarding help for the infirm have been supplemented or replaced by formal disability programs. The development of such programs—for example, the Social Security Disability Insurance (SSDI) and the Supplemental Security Income (SSI) programs run by the Social Security Administration (SSA)—has changed

the dynamics of disability. In order to receive benefits, an individual having a medical problem that produces activity limitations must submit an application to an agency that administers a disability program. Adjudicators from the agency then determine whether the applicant meets eligibility criteria for benefits. In order to make this determination, the adjudicators typically request medical information from the applicant's treating physicians. Because of this need for pertinent medical information, physicians are routinely drawn into the disability determination process. This is true not only for SSI and SSDI, but also for other disability systems such as workers' compensation, Veterans Administration, and private disability insurance programs.

Impairment and disability are not absolutely defined and rated within a single system, but are dependent on particular administrative systems. For example, workers' compensation systems in the USA are 'no fault' insurance programs that are regulated at the state level and vary considerably from one state to the other. Coverage is available for workers who have documented occupational injuries or 'occupational exposures' (such as cumulative trauma disorders). Benefits can include medical care, time loss benefit payments, vocational retraining if needed, and payment for impairment at the time of claim closure.

When you are assessing impairment or disability, you must do so within the guidelines of an individual system. In the present chapter, the term *disability agency* is used to refer to any organization that evaluates disability applications or dispenses disability benefits. Private disability agencies, depending on the individual disability policy, can award compensation for claimants who are no longer able to perform their profession, without a requirement that the claimant be completely unemployable. There is often a requirement of continuous disability of at least 6 months, and there can be an additional requirement that the claimant apply for and be eligible for Social Security Disability.

Social Security Administration

The SSA has its own set of guidelines for determining disability. If claimants are found eligible, they are awarded disability payments on an ongoing basis, as well as eligibility for Medicare or Medicaid. For claimants to be considered eligible for social security, they must be totally disabled from any gainful employment, and they must have an impairment that is considered 'disabling' and likely to last or have lasted at least 12 months.

Veterans Administration

The Veterans Administration has its own disability benefits program, described as follows.

> Disability compensation is a monetary benefit paid to veterans who are disabled by injury or disease incurred or aggravated during active military service. The service of the veteran must have been terminated through separation or discharge under conditions that were other than dishonorable. Disability compensation varies with the degree of disability and the number of dependants, and is paid monthly.
>
> US Department of Veterans Affairs 2004[56]

DEFINITIONS: DISABILITY AND IMPAIRMENT

The concepts of disability and impairment are fundamental to understanding disability programs. There is no unique formal definition of disability, because various disability programs define the term differently.

Agencies have different definitions of disability, because they have different mandates and different eligibility criteria. For example, the SSA defines disability as 'the inability to engage in any substantial gainful activity . . . by reason of any medically determinable physical or mental impairment that can be expected to result in death or that has lasted or can be expected to last for a continuous period of not less than 12 months'.[53] This definition reflects three facts about eligibility criteria for the SSDI and SSI programs:

1. applicants must be totally disabled from work;
2. the work disability must be 'permanent' (or at least long term); and
3. causation is irrelevant—that is, individuals are eligible for benefits regardless of how or why they became disabled.

In contrast, the AMA Guides define disability as 'an alteration of an individual's capacity to meet personal, social, or occupational demands or statutory or regulatory requirements because of an impairment'.[9] The AMA Guides are based on an evaluation system that assumes impairment to be the cause for gradations of disability, rather than on the binary concept of an inability to engage in 'any substantial gainful activity'.

The definition of impairment is fairly uniform from one agency to another. As an example, the AMA Guides define impairment as 'a loss, loss of use, or derangement of any body part, organ system, or organ function' (p. 2). Impairment is conceptualized as existing at the level of organs or body parts. Using this system, one might say 'Mr. Jones's heart has been impaired since he suffered a myocardial infarction' or 'Mrs. Brown's right hand is impaired because of her carpal tunnel syndrome'.

Disability agencies typically assume a strong linkage between impairment and disability. First, they construe impairment as a necessary condition for disability. The logic underlying this requirement is simple. Disability programs are designed to assist individuals who are unable to compete in the workplace because of a medical condition. In essence, disability programs attempt to partition individuals who fail in the workplace into two large groups: those who fail because of a medical condition, and those who fail for other, non-medical reasons. There are many potential non-medical reasons, including a lack of demand for their skills, or a lack of motivation. Disability programs require evidence that applicants have a medical problem underlying their workplace failure. Impairment provides the needed evidence, because it can be viewed as a marker that individuals have a medical problem that diminishes their capability. Conversely, if individuals have no identifiable impairment, this implies that they do not have limitations due to a medical condition.

Second, disability agencies typically assume that the severity of patients' impairment correlates with the degree and/or probability of their being disabled from work. Even when an agency compensates for work disability and not for impairment, it will often seek information about a patient's impairment to rationalize its decision about whether or not to award disability benefits. As will be discussed, the assumption that increasing impairment leads to increased disability can be challenged both conceptually and at a practical level when quantifying impairment.

In practice, disability agencies typically ask physicians to make judgments about both impairment and disability for the patients they evaluate. In some instances, the agency operates under a mandate to compensate patients for impairment. The physician's impairment rating typically has a direct bearing on the award that a patient receives, because the amount awarded is keyed to the severity of the patient's impairment. Alternatively, some agencies make payments only if a patient is judged to be disabled from work. In this setting, an impairment rating might well be performed, but it serves only as an intervening step in the broader task of determining whether or not the patient warrants a disability award.

It should be noted that, while it is possible to distinguish conceptually between impairment (meaning dysfunction of an organ or a body part) and disability (meaning an activity limitation secondary to an impairment), the distinction is not always clear in many practical situations. For example, the notion of a measurably dysfunctional organ does not readily apply to psychiatric impairments. While the distinction between impairment and disability is easy to make in some medical conditions, it is difficult to make in others.

Another problem is that the correlation between severity of impairment and severity of disability (in the sense of limitation in work ability) is far from perfect, as illustrated in the following examples.

- A patient might have serious impairment yet very little apparent vocational disability. The most striking example would be the world-famous physics professor Dr. Stephen Hawking. He is incapacitated from the most basic activities of daily living because of motor neuron disease, and would qualify for a very high total body impairment according to the AMA Guides. However, he is not work-disabled. In fact, he remains active as a theoretic physicist of international acclaim.

- A patient might have very mild ratable impairment, as measured through the AMA Guides, for example from a lumbar or cervical facet injury as a result of a motor vehicle crash. However, such an injury can cause devastating vocational consequences if the patient has a job that requires constant heavy physical labor. Such a patient may even be rated as having 'no impairment' according to some examiners, because of a lack of a demonstrable disk herniation with advanced imaging and/or radicular findings on examination. When subjected to a functional capacity evaluation, the patient might be shown to be truly incapable of doing heavy physical labor. Consequently, they could be considered 100% disabled from such labor, and yet they might have little or no ratable impairment according to some examiners' interpretations of impairment rating guidelines.

- A patient might have had a demonstrable disk herniation with radiculopathy, and has responded well to spinal surgery. According to both the AMA Guides and a number of workers' compensation guidelines, this patient would have significant whole body impairment, typically between 10 and 25% of whole body impairment, depending on whether she or he received spinal fusion or laminectomy. Despite this impressive level of impairment, they might have little or no disability, given a good surgical outcome, in terms of their profession and activities of daily living.

- As a final example, the patient could have a well-defined impairment, for example amputation of the fifth digit of the non-dominant hand. This type of amputation is very well described in the AMA Guides, but the patient's disability, if any, will be strongly dependent on their profession. If he or she is a concert pianist, the disability might be 100%. If the patient is a psychiatrist, there will probably be no disability. If the patient is a construction worker, she or he will probably have minimal, mild, or possibly moderate disability, depending on the individual tasks performed.

ROLES OF PHYSICIANS IN DISABILITY EVALUATION

Some physicians become expert in disability evaluation, and make disability evaluation a central part of their clinical practices. Some function as consultants to other physicians when they perform disability evaluations. For example, many Kaiser Permanente centers include occupational medicine clinics, where physicians provide disability management services for injured workers who have been referred from other providers, and perform disability evaluations when the workers' claims are ready for closure.

Other physicians with an interest in disability evaluation perform independent medical examinations (IMEs) that are commissioned by insurance carriers, disability agencies, or attorneys. Still others work as employees of disability agencies or insurance companies. As part of this work, they may perform disability evaluations by directly examining claimants. More typically though, such consultants play a variety of indirect roles, for example advising claims managers when to order IMEs, or reviewing IMEs that have been performed.

Many physicians do not seek opportunities to perform disability evaluations. Such physicians often feel uncomfortable when they are called on to evaluate disability in patients whom they are treating. They correctly perceive that the process of disability evaluation places physicians between the interests of their patient and those of an insurance company or disability agency. In the best of circumstances, this can be seen to the physician like trying to fit a round peg into a square hole, because the categories of disability established by such agencies often do not match the clinical realities of patients.

In the worst case, clinicians end up feeling caught in the cross fire between adversaries. They may perceive employees of disability agencies as unenlightened bureaucrats who make excessive demands for documentation and seem to lose the forest for the trees. At the same time, they may perceive their patients as reporting excessive incapacitation and trying to enlist physicians as allies in their battle to legitimize their disability.

The concerns that treating physicians have about doing disability evaluations appear to fall into two categories: knowledge deficits and ethical concerns. Physicians who work primarily as clinicians are likely to be unfamiliar with the disability laws and regulations relevant to their patients, and the disability agencies that administer them. They are also likely to lack expertise in the mechanics of rating impairment, such as those detailed in the AMA Guides,[9] and in the methods that can be used to assess work ability.[30,32,48] Treating physicians may be concerned about conflicts between the clinical role they normally play when they treat patients, and the adjudicative role that is required during a disability evaluation. Informal observation, as well as examination of the limited literature on these roles,[27,43,55,60] suggests several differences between the two roles. For example, whereas physicians performing disability evaluations are expected to focus on objective findings and legal responsibility (including causation) for an examinee's disorder, these are not the main concern of physicians when they provide clinical treatment.[47] As Sullivan and Loeser have noted, significant ethical issues arise when physicians switch back and forth between these two roles.[55]

Assessing self-reports of patients regarding physical capacity

A key challenge for any disability evaluator is to combine examinees' self-reports regarding their incapacitation with objective medical information regarding the severity of their incapacitation.[44] As a starting point in addressing this difficult area, it is worth noting that the definition of 'objective medical information' is not entirely clear. One problem is that the existence of objective medical findings in various disorders depends on the degree to which technologies have advanced. For example, before myelography became available, radiographic studies (i.e.

x-rays) did not demonstrate objective findings for patients with radiculopathies. A second problem is that a high level of inter-rater reliability is a necessary condition for objectivity in any endeavor. However, in the arena of impairment and disability evaluation, it is common for different examiners—many of whom consider themselves to be 'forensic experts'—to generate disparate conclusions about the same patient.[10]

One way for a physician to resolve potential discrepancies between self-report data and objective findings is to accept at face value what patients say about their physical capacities. A physician who adopted this strategy would run the risk of underestimating the rehabilitation potential of individuals who overstate their incapacitation, either deliberately (as in the case of malingerers) or as a result of genuine misperceptions regarding their abilities. At the opposite extreme, a physician might try to make decisions about the disability status of patients strictly on the basis of what they perceive to be 'objective findings', and react skeptically to reports of incapacitation that are not closely linked to these findings.

A position somewhere between these two extremes is probably most appropriate. The perceptions that patients have about their abilities certainly should not be ignored or discounted. As a practical matter, research demonstrates that these self-appraisals are important predictors of whether or not patients with pain problems will perform well on physical tests and/or succeed in getting off disability.[18,20,24–26,29] Consequently, physicians who make disability decisions without considering patients' appraisals are discarding valuable data. As a result, their decisions can go awry in two ways. First, they can pressure patients to return to work in jobs that the patients are realistically not capable of performing. Second, they may be completely ineffective in resolving disability issues. Consider, for example, patients who are released to work by their treating physician or by an independent medical examiner, even though they are convinced that they are unable to work. Such patients are likely to retain an attorney and start a protracted legal battle regarding their work status.

But the fact that patients' perceptions are important does not mean that they are valid or immutable. In fact, research on patients with disability related to chronic pain suggests the opposite: some have distorted views of their capabilities, and these views are modifiable.[1,14,28,33] These results indicate that, when performing a disability evaluation, a physician needs to consider the validity of a patient's stated activity limitations in light of the biomedical information available and their assessment of the patient's credibility. They should reserve the right to challenge the patient's self-assessments and to make decisions that are discordant with these assessments.

In summary, the treating physician should carefully assess examinees' perceptions regarding their ability to perform various tasks and, whenever feasible, should take them into account when rendering judgments about their ability to work. But this does not mean that the physician should let examinees control the discussion about disability. Instead, physicians should be ready to challenge the appraisals of examinees when they believe them to be inaccurate.

Blending administrative imperatives with patient realities

Disability agencies and insurance companies follow what might be called an administrative imperative as they adjudicate disability claims. The imperative is to reach decisions about disability benefits for applicants on the basis of procedures that are objective, consistent, and efficient. These goals are reasonable, but they may lead agencies to oversimplify the process. The 'administrative model' of injury and disability is most apparent in workers' compensation systems. It typically assumes the following.

- That incapacitation following an injury should be 'transparent' to a physician, i.e. activity limitations described by patients should be highly correlated with evidence of tissue damage or organ dysfunction objectively assessed by a physician.
- That recovery after trauma follows a fairly predictable course, such that an injured worker initially shows progressive improvement and then reaches a plateau or fully recovers (see Fig. 6-1). In compensation law, workers are said to be 'fixed and stable' or to have reached 'maximal medical improvement (MMI)' when they reach this plateau. At this juncture, compensation law generally dictates that medical treatment be terminated and, if patients are not able to return fully to their job of injury, either a definitive vocational plan needs to be developed or the patient should be pensioned.
- That work injuries typically occur when a previously healthy individual is exposed to an obvious and overwhelming source of trauma, such as a fall from a height, or a crush injury from a heavy object.

The assumption of transparency is notably problematic. This assumption is so pervasive that most physicians, and essentially all disability adjudicators, accept it without question. However, with historical perspective, it is apparent that physicians have not always believed that incapacitation from trauma should be transparent. In fact, when the SSDI program was being

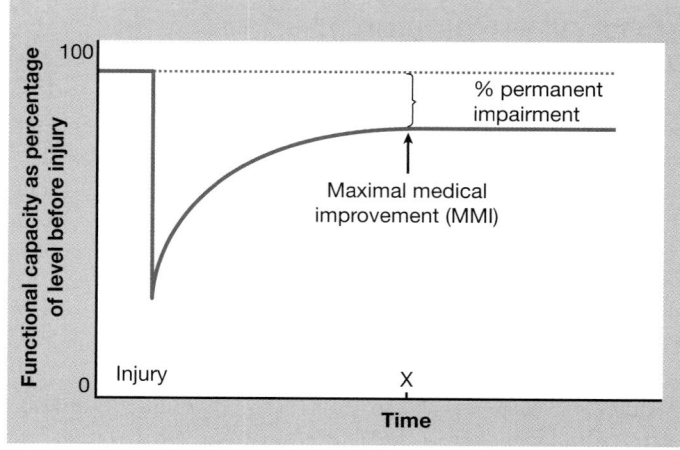

Figure 6-1 Hypothetical recovery curve following an injury.

considered by Congress during the 1950s, physician groups almost uniformly protested that they would not be able to do the assessments that were envisaged in the SSDI legislation.[42]

For some impairments, objective criteria can be utilized in a transparent manner. For example, physicians have straightforward tools to quantify impairment stemming from amputations, complete spinal cord injuries, or clear cases of radiculopathy supported by magnetic resonance imaging (MRI) evidence of a focal disk herniation. However, in many medical conditions—including many of the musculoskeletal and neurologic disorders that physiatrists often evaluate—physicians cannot easily identify injury to organs or body parts that lead inevitably to the activity limitations that examinees report. Again, the example of spinal facet joint injuries is given. Carefully controlled studies have documented that cervical facet joint injury is the probable primary pain generator for 50% of whiplash patients with non-radicular neck pain.[3,4,35] However, although cervical facet joints show up on MRI scanning, injury to them, or pain stemming from them, is generally not detected. Facet arthropathy, when viewed on advanced imaging studies, can be seen among asymptomatic patients and cannot be taken as a reliable physical sign of facet joint injury.[51,52]

In addition, there is increasing evidence that patients with chronic whiplash develop changes in central nervous system functioning that may greatly augment the severity of their chronic pain.[11,31,54] These changes are also difficult to quantify but can become the basis for significant loss of function, and vocational disability. Thus disability evaluators cannot easily rate impairment for this common clinical scenario. More importantly, they cannot offer a clear correlation between severity of impairment and severity of disability, even utilizing the latest edition of the AMA Guides.[9]

Even for radiculopathy, a condition thought to be fairly well assessed within the AMA Guides, there are pitfalls for assessing spinal impairment. Research has shown that most lumbar MRI findings among patients with radiculopathy do not correlate well with their pain diagrams and physical examination findings, except in the rare case of a disk extrusion and/or severe spinal stenosis.[5] In practice, most MRI findings do not demonstrate such severe pathology.

Topics addressed in disability evaluations

Physicians are typically asked to address the following when they conduct disability evaluations:

- diagnosis;
- causation;
- need for further treatment;
- impairment;
- activity limitations and functional capacity; and
- ability to work (i.e. work disability).

A fundamental goal of the disability evaluation process is to determine whether a patient can work. From this perspective, the first five items above can be viewed as preliminary items that set the stage for addressing the sixth and crucial question.

PRACTICAL STRATEGIES FOR DISABILITY EVALUATION

The discussion below is largely based on our experiences treating patients in clinical settings, performing IMEs, and consulting with the Washington State Department of Labor and Industries. It cannot be based on a recognized body of scientific data, because no such data exist. For example, information on the reliability of disability evaluations is scanty,[7,8,10] and there are virtually no credible scientific data on the predictive or concurrent validity of the evaluations. In the absence of scientific data, it is impossible to say what decision-making strategies are appropriate when performing disability evaluations. In this ambiguous situation, it is easy for practitioners to fall into the trap of believing they are making valid judgments, when in fact their judgments are based on a variety of biases.[22,47]

Before the disability form arrives

You will do a better job of responding to disability requests if you have thought about the disability issues that might arise for a particular patient. The material below gives basic information about the types of questions you are likely to be asked during disability evaluations, and issues that you should take into account as you develop answers to these questions. However, in addition to considering specific questions that you might be asked, it is important to gain an overall understanding of the disability agency with which you are interacting. Unfortunately, this understanding is difficult to achieve, in part because of the heterogeneity of disability agencies and the programs they administer. The policies and practices that a disability agency follows when it determines eligibility for benefits are generally also not available to physicians. In this ambiguous situation, you can increase your understanding substantially by reviewing monographs that deal with disability agencies and disability evaluation.[12,13,42,48] Also, if you are observant as you perform disability evaluations on your patients, you can learn a lot about the disability agencies with which you interact.

Addressing the main questions
Diagnosis
Of the issues commonly addressed in a disability evaluation, diagnosis is the only one that you routinely consider in a clinical evaluation of a patient. But even here, complications arise when disability evaluations are performed. For example, adjudicators sometimes make inferences about causation on the basis of a diagnosis. For example, if you diagnose a patient as having lumbar degenerative disk disease (International Classifications of Diseases 722.52), an adjudicator might take the position that the patient's back pain was not caused by a specific injury.

Causation and apportionment
The issue of causation is important, because many disability agencies will give benefits only for medical conditions that arise from specific causes. For example, workers' compensation carriers are responsible only for work-related medical conditions, and automobile insurance carriers are responsible only for

injuries that occur in motor vehicle accidents. Although causation is straightforward for many injuries, a number of pitfalls can arise.

First, patients might have cumulative trauma disorders, which would be the result of an 'occupational exposure' rather than a specific injury. In this setting, especially if the injured worker has had multiple employers over the time interval when the exposure appears relevant, the issue of how to distribute liability becomes critical. In this case, there is a need for apportionment. Apportionment is an attempt to distribute causation among multiple possible sources. In the fifth edition of the AMA Guides,[9] this is defined as follows.

> Apportionment analysis in workers' compensation represents a distribution or allocation of causation among multiple factors that caused or significantly contributed to the injury or disease and resulting impairment.
> Cocchiarella and Andersson 2001[9]

Second, the claimant might have a preexisting condition. In this case, the issue of apportionment of liability again becomes critical. Medical experts and treating physicians often disagree about the magnitude and nature of a preexisting condition, despite administrative guidelines regarding this issue. For example, a patient who has undergone a lumbar diskectomy in the remote past might report a return of radicular symptoms after a fall. In this kind of setting, a disability agency could ask you to apportion causation of the patient's impairment between the index injury and the patient's preexisting lumbar disk condition.

Third, an examiner might support causation for an index injury but state that a patient should have recovered from this injury. In this case, the examiner does not believe that the patient's ongoing symptoms—and possibly signs measured during physical examination or with diagnostic studies—are causally related to the index injury. This can lead to controversy. This situation is most often encountered when injuries are subtle, such that pain and disability outweigh obvious objective findings.

It is worth noting that disability agencies differ significantly in the standard they set for establishing causation. Some agencies follow the principle that, in order for an index injury to be accepted as the cause of a patient's impairment, the injury must be the major factor contributing to the impairment. Others adopt a much lower standard of causation that has been described as 'lighting up'. When this standard applies, an index injury can be viewed as the cause of increased impairment even when the injury is minor and when preexisting impairment is severe. For example, consider an individual with a multiply operated knee who falls at work, develops an effusion in the knee, and is told by an orthopedist that she or he needs a total knee replacement. If the individual's workers' compensation carrier operated under the 'lighting up' standard of causation, this person's knee symptoms and need for a total knee replacement would be viewed as caused by the fall at work.

The physician should ideally apportion, in the setting of a preexisting condition, in at least three areas when doing a forensic evaluation regarding impairment and disability.

1. Apportionment for the need for care. This attempts to answer whether, on a more probable than not basis, the claimant would have required treatment (often already paid within a claim) if the index injury had not occurred. In other words, in the absence of the index injury, how much care, if any at all, would the claimant have required for the treatment of an active or inactive preexisting condition?
2. Apportionment for impairment. This attempts to split the total current impairment between a preexisting component and that which has been created by an index injury. In the example of the patient with a multiply operated knee, there might be significant preexisting impairment—although the need for care for the preexisting condition may be minimal or zero, were it not for the index injury.
3. Apportionment for disability. This is usually taken to mean work disability, which is generally compensable, but can also be extended to disability from activities of daily living. This again draws a distinction between the effects of an injury on the level of impairment versus one's ability to function in everyday life. In the setting of a significant preexisting impairment, marginally increased impairment from a new injury may cause, or may be alleged to cause, significant work disability.

The determination of apportionment is at best an imprecise process. Apportionment analysis is most commonly described for impairment only,[9] and is determined by subtracting preexisting impairment, with respect to an index injury, from the current impairment. However, it is clear that apportionment analyses for the cost of care and for disability are critical to the successful adjudication of claims.

Take the example of an actual patient who has had three previous neck surgeries, including two fusions, who is undergoing active conservative pain management, and then is involved in a motor vehicle crash. The patient subsequently had some of the hardware from a previous fusion removed. A careful analysis revealed that, on a more probable than not basis, this hardware removal would not have been necessary were it not for the motor vehicle crash. This cost of care was therefore covered by the motor vehicle claim, but it was clear that the patient had majority preexisting cervical impairment, as compared with her overall impairment after she reached maximum medical improvement from the effects of the crash. She also had neck care costs that were independent of the motor vehicle crash history.

Some of the factors that help with a credible apportionment analysis include the following.

• Obtaining a functional history from patients, which includes understanding their ability to perform activities of daily living, vocational activities, and recreational activities prior to an index injury.

- Judging the credibility of this functional history. Does the medical record support the patient's contention that there has been a loss of function? Some patients might not consciously fabricate their stated loss of function, but they could be mistaken, given that years have passed since the index injury. For example, a patient might state that, due to inactivity from the index injury, they may have gained 40 lbs. The medical record, however, might reflect otherwise, and there might be only a few pounds gained. Ideally, the patient should be directly confronted with these data, and the examiner should try to gauge whether they appear truly mistaken or are being consciously deceptive in their history.
- Related to this is a careful examination of preexisting medical records, including a time line for the need for care, work restrictions, and (if applicable) preexisting impairment ratings.
- The willingness to ask, as an examiner, the critical question of were it not for the index injury, on a more probable than not basis, what would be the patient's current impairment, ability to function (i.e. disability in the broad sense of the word), and need for medical care since the date of the index injury?

All three concepts of apportionment are critical to examine.

Need for further treatment

Disability agencies generally adopt an idealized model of the course of recovery following an injury. This model is shown in Figure 6-1. It embodies the assumption that people show rapid improvement following injury but then reach a plateau. Before patients reach this hypothetical plateau, they presumably can benefit from further treatment. When they reach the plateau, they are considered to have achieved MMI. When a patient has reached MMI, insurance companies and disability agencies typically refuse to pay for additional medical care, and attempt to make a final determination regarding a patient's impairment and work capacity. From an administrative perspective, the model is convenient because it provides guidelines for intervention and decision making. For example, when a patient has reached point X on the graph, curative treatment should be abandoned, and a permanent partial impairment rating should be made.

Unfortunately, patients frequently present with clinical problems that are hard to conceptualize in terms of the idealized recovery shown in Figure 6-1. The difficulties in this area are myriad. First, it is not clear that patients with repetitive strain injuries or chronic spinal pain[39] should be expected to follow the trajectory shown in Figure 6-1. Second, patients can have comorbidities that complicate recovery and make it difficult to determine when they have reached MMI. An example is a patient with diabetes who has a work-related carpal tunnel syndrome in addition to a peripheral polyneuropathy. Third, many who utilize the MMI concept fail to remember that a

patient who has reached maximal benefit from a particular kind of treatment might not have reached maximal benefit from treatment in general. For example, consider a patient who is examined 6 months after a low back injury. Assume that her or his treatment has consisted entirely of chiropractic care during the 6-month interval, and that she or he has not shown any measurable improvement during the past 2 months. This patient might be judged to have reached maximal medical benefit from chiropractic care, but an examining physician would understandably be uncertain about whether the patient could benefit from physical therapy, epidural steroids, lumbar surgery, aggressive use of various medications, or other therapies that might not be offered by the chiropractor. This problem is not just a hypothetical one, because examiners routinely find that some patients with chronic conditions have not had exposure to all reasonable treatments for their condition.

At times, it is more sensible to state that the patient has reached MMI, with respect to specific care. For example, the statement 'the patient has reached maximal medical improvement with respect to conservative care options' would probably be more accurate than simply stating that the patient is at MMI. If interventional care options are not appropriate, then the patient may truly be at MMI with respect to all reasonable care options.

Finally, disability and health insurance companies typically take the position that no more medical treatment should be authorized after a patient has reached MMI. This administrative perspective frequently does not match the clinical needs of patients. For example, a patient may have reached MMI from a low back injury in the sense that a significant period of time has elapsed since injury, and no further curative treatment is available. However, individuals might still need maintenance treatment for their condition, such as ongoing medication. This issue is often ignored by agencies that administer benefits.

A workers' compensation company might state that such maintenance treatment is 'palliative' and not curative, and therefore not covered within the claim. One interpretation of this distinction might view dialysis as 'palliative' and not curative, because it does not cure the patient from the loss of kidney function. And yet dialysis would probably be covered indefinitely within a claim. Might one also argue that long-term medication or massage, although probably palliative, should be covered for chronic spinal pain if dialysis is covered for renal failure? These are ethical issues that raise more questions than they answer.

Impairment

Physicians need to use careful clinical judgment in deciding when to perform an impairment rating. For example, an impairment rating would not be appropriate for a patient who has not reached MMI, or (at least in workers' compensation cases) for a patient whose injury was not causally related to a work exposure.

Once you decide that an impairment rating is appropriate for a patient, the rating itself is a fairly mechanical task that is based on formulas and procedures described in various texts, or in manuals published by disability agencies. The agency that requests an impairment rating typically specifies the system that physicians are required to use. For example, the AMA *Guides to the Evaluation of Permanent Impairment* describe an impairment rating system that is used by multiple jurisdictions.[9] Some states have their own impairment rating systems. In order to perform an impairment evaluation according to the rules of a jurisdiction, you need to be familiar with the system used by that jurisdiction.

Physical capacities assessment

The assessment of physical capacities is a precursor to the determination of a patient's ability to work. Disability agencies typically request detailed physical capacities data, and usually provide supplementary forms for this purpose. In general, a clinical evaluation in your office will not provide detailed physical capacities information. You can supplement information gleaned from your clinical evaluation in a variety of ways.

The simplest way is to ask patients to estimate their capacities. You should consider filling out a physical capacities form on the basis of a patient's reports if you judge the patient to be highly credible, or if you do not have access to objective data regarding the patient's capacities. If you follow this approach, you should indicate this on the form.

Another way to obtain physical capacities data is to refer a patient for a functional capacities evaluation (FCE), also called a performance-based physical capacities evaluation.[30,32,48] FCEs are formal, standardized assessments typically performed by physical therapists. They typically last from 2 to 5 h. The therapist gathers information about a patient's strength, mobility, and endurance in various tasks, preferably ones that simulate the type of work that the patient is expected to do. As noted by King et al.,[30] FCEs are popular with insurance carriers and attorneys, because they provide objective performance data. However, in their comprehensive review, King et al. also note that there is a paucity of data that validate FCEs against actual job performance. A more recent review identifies evidence supporting the predictive validity of one FCE system (the Isernhagen work system), but the reviewers conclude that 'More rigorous studies are needed to demonstrate the reliability and the validity of FCE methods'.[23]

Finally, you can get physical capacities data on patients by referring them to a functional restoration program, a pain center, or a work-hardening program.[26,37,38,41] A common feature of these programs is that they both assess physical capacities and provide treatment designed to improve those capacities. The performance data from one of these programs might have more validity than performance data from a FCE, because these programs typically observe performance over a few weeks, and indicate what patients can do after they have completed rehabilitative treatment.

If you have assessed a patient's physical capacities, you are in a position to make statements about the activity limitations imposed by his or her medical condition. The summary sections of most FCE reports contain such information.

Ability to work

The ability of a patient to work is the key issue in most disability evaluations. The reason for this is that disability agencies are often required to make wage compensation payments to patients if, and only if, the patients are judged not to be employable because of a medical condition. Unfortunately, assessing employability is difficult, and there is no simple set of techniques to apply when a decision about employability is requested. Box 6-1 outlines issues that you should consider when you judge a patient's employability.

A physician makes a judgment about a patient's employability by balancing the patient's functional capacities (or limitations) against the functional demands of jobs for which the patient is being considered.

Concerning job demands, the physician usually has to rely on information provided by vocational rehabilitation counselors or employers. In workers' compensation claims, vocational rehabilitation counselors often prepare formal job analyses. Figure 6-2 gives a sample job analysis. Note that the job analysis form includes a section in which the evaluating physician is asked to

---

Box 6-1 Issues to consider in determining employability

- What specific questions about employability are you being asked to address?
  Can the patient work at a specified job?
  What general category of work can the patient perform (sedentary, light, medium, heavy, or very heavy)?
  Is the patient employable in any capacity?
- For work in a specific job:
  Is there a job analysis?
  Does the patient agree with the demands stated on the job analysis?
  Are there any collateral sources of information about the job (e.g. information from the employer)?
  Do you believe the patient can perform the job with modifications?
  Do you believe the patient needs assistance in transitioning to the job (e.g. a graduated reentry or a work-hardening program)?
- Do you have reliable physical capacities data that permit you to determine the appropriateness of a specific job or the appropriateness of a general work category?
- Are there any 'trick questions'?
  Description of a job with minimal physical requirements (e.g. phone solicitor).
  Description of a job that seems inappropriate for the patient from an economic and a career standpoint (e.g. a description of a cashiering job for a person who has spent the past 20 years working as an electrician).
- Based on the questions addressed to you, does it seem that the disability agency is making a sincere attempt to find a place in the workforce for the patient, as opposed to trying to 'set the patient up' (i.e. contrive vocational options that will maneuver him or her out of the disability system)?
- Does it appear that the patient is making a sincere effort to return to work, or is she or he exaggerating pain complaints and/or maneuvering in some way to get long-term disability?

Job title	Taxi dispatcher
DOT	913.367-010
GOE	07.04.05
SVP	3

Job description Dispatches taxicabs in response to telephone requests for service by entering client name and pickup and drop-off locations into the computer. Direct calls to dispatch supervisor if needed.

Job qualifications Good customer service skills; ability to type and learn computer program.

Types of machines, tools, special equipment used Telephone with headset, computer.

Materials, products, subject matter, services Local and suburban transit and interurban buses.

Work schedule Full time, 8-h shifts

Physical demands

1. Stand	Occasionally. Daily total 0.5 h.
2. Walk	Occasionally. Daily total 0.5 h.
3. Sit	Constantly, with option to stand. Daily total 7 h.
4. Lift/carry	Occasionally lift/carry ounces.
5. Push/pull	Occasionally with minimum force to open file drawers and keyboard trays.
6. Controls	Frequently use controls on telephone. Most calls incoming.
7. Climb	Not required.
8. Balance	Not required.
9. Bend/stoop	Not required.
10. Crouch	Not required.
11. Twist	Occasionally at the neck while answering the phones.
12. Kneel	Not required.
13. Crawl	Not required.
14. Handle/grasp	Occasionally handle/grasp office supplies and handset.
15. Fine manipulation fingering	Frequent to constant typing is involved during workday. Fingering to dial telephone.
16. Feeling	Not required.
17. Reach	Occasionally at midwaist level, three-quarters to full arm extension.
18. Vision	Correctable vision is desirable.
19. Talk/hear	Speech and hearing are mandatory.
20. Taste/smell	Not required.
21. Environmental factors	Office environment. Floors are carpeted.
22. Work environment access	On-site parking available.

Physician's judgment

☐ The injured worker can perform this job without restrictions and can return work on

☐ The injured worker can perform this job without restrictions, but only on a part-time basis for ____ h per day

____ days per week. The worker can be expected to return to full-time in ____ days/weeks.

☐ The injured worker can perform this job, but only with the following modifications: _____

_____

Modifications are needed on a ☐ permanent/ ☐ temporary basis.

☐ The injured worker temporarily cannot perform this job based on the following physical limitations: _____

_____

Anticipated release date: _____

☐ The injured worker permanently cannot perform this job based on the following physical limitations:

Comments

_____

_____

_____

_____

Signature of physician _____ **Date** _____

Figure 6-2 A sample job analysis.

give their opinion about whether or not the worker can perform the job.

A detailed job analysis can be extremely helpful in the assessment of the work demands that a patient is likely to face. However, you need to check with patients to see if they agree with the physical requirements listed in a job analysis. If the patient vigorously disputes the job analysis, you should attempt to reconcile the discrepancy.

Several problems involving employability determinations occur frequently enough to warrant further discussion.

- Sometimes you will be asked whether your patient can do a specific job, and you will be provided with a job analysis. In other situations, you will be asked much broader questions. For example, you might be asked to rate the general 'category' of work for which the patient is suited. Broad work categories are defined in the *Dictionary of Occupational Titles* and a supplementary publication by Field and Field.[16,32,57] Typical categories are sedentary, light, medium, heavy, and very heavy. The problem with these work categories is that they might not capture specific activity limitations of your patient. When you are asked to place your patient in a general work category, probably the best approach is to get physical capacities data and use these data to assign the patient.
- Sometimes you will be presented with 'trick' questions dealing with employability. As an example, imagine that you are treating a patient with chronic low back pain who has failed multiple spine surgeries, and continues to complain of relentless pain despite the implantation of an intrathecal opiate delivery system. Imagine that you do not believe it is realistic for this patient to return to competitive employment. Suppose that a disability agency asks you whether your patient can work as a telephone solicitor. This question poses a dilemma. If you indicate 'Yes', your patient will probably have his or her disability benefits terminated. If you say 'No', you are implicitly saying that the patient's low back pain prevents him or her from doing a job that has essentially no physical demands. This can represent an ethical dilemma, and you ultimately have to use your own clinical judgment, at the same time addressing guidelines within the disability system.
- Some patients 'drag their feet' and emphasize the severity of their incapacitation. These behaviors should make you suspicious of their agendas. In such a situation, it is reasonable to stick closely to objective data regarding the patient's capacities, rather than to be influenced strongly by the patient's subjective assessments.

FURTHER SPECIAL ISSUES IN DISABILITY EVALUATIONS

Possibility of deception

You need to be aware of the possibility that any of the participants in a disability claim can have a hidden agenda. Opportunities for deception are particularly notable in workers' compensation claims. An extensive medical literature on secondary gain, compensation neurosis, and malingering has dealt with hidden agendas of patients.[6,21,34,40,58]

Of note, behavioral signs associated with psychologic distress and observed among patients with chronic pain might be inappropriately used within a medicolegal setting as evidence for malingering. The most famous example are the Waddell signs, developed by the well-known spinal surgeon Dr. Gordon Waddell, who urged his fellow surgeons 'to operate on a patient, not a spine', as this 'may save years of coping with the human wreckage caused by ill-considered surgery on the lumbar disks'.[59] There have been numerous papers reappraising the Waddell signs, one of which has been coauthored by Dr. Waddell himself,[36] making clear that these behavioral signs do not have a role in the detection of malingering.[17,19]

In summary, most experts in disability believe that frank malingering or deception is uncommon among patients who seem to report 'excessive' disability. However, you should be alert to the following.

- Is there any evidence that a patient who claims to be disabled is 'double dipping', i.e. working at the same time he or she is getting disability benefits?
- Is there evidence from surveillance tapes or other collateral sources that a patient's physical capabilities are far greater than he or she claims?

Other parties to a workers' compensation claims, including employers and adjudicators for disability agencies, can have hidden agendas. Their agendas have been ignored almost completely in research on disability, so you need to use clinical judgment in deciding whether participants in a disability claim are behaving in a deceptive manner. You should consider the following.

- Is there evidence that the disability system is 'playing hardball' with the patient? For example, does it appear that the patient has had her or his claim closed arbitrarily?
- Has the compensation carrier refused to authorize services requested by the attending physician?
- Does it appear that the patient's claims manager is requesting multiple evaluations in order to maneuver the patient out of the compensable claim on the basis of 'preponderance of evidence'?
- Is there any indication that the patient's (former) employer has created misleading job descriptions?
- Have they put pressure on the patient not to file a workers' compensation claim?
- Have they fired the patient in apparent response to the patient's report of injury?

Objective findings

The request for objective findings can create at least two kinds of problems for an examining physician. First, some patients, for example those with fibromyalgia or chronic headaches, might not have any unequivocally objective findings. Second, and far more importantly, even when some patients have objective findings, the findings might not explain the extent of the self-reported incapacitation.

As noted earlier, the term *objective findings* is not precisely defined.[44] Some examiners believe that objective data refer to laboratory or physical findings that are measurable, valid, and reliable, and are not subject to voluntary control or manipulation by a patient. Objective findings can be contrasted with 'subjective findings' such as patients' reports of activity restrictions caused by pain. However, a lot of clinically important examination findings—including range of motion (ROM), tested strength, and some muscle stretch reflex findings—might be described as 'semiobjective'. They are objective in the sense that they can be observed and measured. But they might not be completely reliable, because patients can voluntarily modify them. Most adjudicators who request objective findings are not aware of these subtleties.

The AMA Guides generally accept physical examination findings as objective data, even if they are able to be voluntarily manipulated by the patient. For example, on p. 593 of the fifth edition of the AMA Guides,[9] in an appendix addressing ROM measurements, the following is stated:

> Physicians have questioned the reproducibility of ROM measurements, as well as their ability to predict aspects of function. Reproducibility may be improved with the use of standardized measurement techniques, proper equipment, trained evaluators, adequate designated warm-up exercises, and uniform recording . . . Active movements are recommended since they may be more consistent than passive movements, less of a risk to individual injury, and a better approximation of the individual's function.
>
> Cocchiarella and Andersson 2001[9]

As with so many dilemmas in medicine, your clinical judgment becomes paramount in sorting out 'non-organic' responses from patients during physical examination. Take the example of a schoolage child who does not want to go to school because of abdominal pain. During a medical examination, you might take this child in your lap and distract her or him with something fun to play with, at the same time palpating around the abdomen. If you do not get a palpation response consistent with your official 'physical examination' when they were not distracted, you would take this discrepancy into account when deciding the severity or even presence of your patient's illness.

When you perform a disability evaluation on one of your patients, you can finesse the objective findings issue within the assessment and discussion portions of your report. If you do not find your patient credible, it would be perfectly reasonable to indicate that there are no reliable objective findings to support his or her claimed incapacitation. However, you should provide documentation of why you believe there are no reliable objective findings. For example, you might state that, with the patient distracted, there was no significant tenderness noted in the upper trapezius region, and yet there was a very severe pain response from the patient when she or he was conscious of your palpating this region. If your patient has consistent physical findings that you find credible, you can simply list them in the space where you are requested to give objective findings. If your findings are challenged, you can indicate that, in your clinical judgment, they represent valid indices of the patient's condition.

Practical applications of principles

Regarding impairment rating, one of the best available resources is the AMA Guides,[9] which give dozens of clinical case examples illustrating this process. A smaller number of detailed case histories can also be found in a text titled *Writing and Defending your IME Report*.[2] In contrast to examples in the AMA Guides, which only address impairment, these case histories cover a broader range of issues challenging the physician performing impairment and disability evaluations.

While performing your own evaluations, you will discover that the AMA Guides and other systems have struggled with the problem of integrating objective and subjective data for determining impairment and disability. You will also find that no system has produced a completely satisfactory integration.[45]

As an example of this problem, you will find marked inconsistencies in the manner in which painful conditions are handled in different chapters of the AMA Guides.[9] For example, if an individual with upper limb complex regional pain syndrome were evaluated according to the system described in Chapter 18 of the AMA Guides, he or she would receive no more than 3% whole person impairment. If that same individual were evaluated on the basis of Table 13-22 in Chapter 13 of the AMA Guides, he or she might receive as much as 60% whole person impairment!

CONCLUSION

This chapter can only point out some of the challenges associated with disability evaluation. It by no means gives you all the information you need to conduct disability evaluations on your patients. Unfortunately, there is no cookbook for doing disability evaluations. One reason for this is that there is enormous variation from one disability evaluation to another. Busy physicians might want a simple answer to the question 'How should I fill out Mr. Smith's disability form?' In reality, this is akin to asking the question 'What medical or surgical treatment should I provide for Mr. Smith?' In both instances, it is necessary to answer the question based on factors that are specific to Mr. Smith.

Another reason is that there is strikingly little published information on the subject of disability evaluation, despite the fact that millions of evaluations are done each year in the USA. At a very basic level, we have very little evidence about whether the decisions made by large agencies such as the SSA are, on the whole, good or bad, i.e. whether the SSA is awarding benefits to individuals who are truly disabled, or are withholding them from individuals who are truly unable to work.[46,49,50]

In the face of this large-scale uncertainty, it is difficult for individual physicians to know if they are rendering appropriate judgments regarding their patients. This is particularly the case for disability evaluation in the context of chronic pain, or in other settings where it is difficult to correlate the subjective complaints of patients with objective findings of tissue pathology. As noted earlier, chronic pain challenges the assumption of administrative agencies that impairments should be objectively observable. At this point, no disability agency has resolved this challenge.

Some of you will understandably be tempted to ask 'Why bother?' That is, why should a physiatrist take the extra time to learn about disability agencies, disability evaluation methods, the ethics of disability evaluation, etc.? To some extent, the answer to this question is 'Because you have no choice'. Society forces physicians to make judgments about the capacities of their patients. Physicians can do disability evaluations thoughtfully or thoughtlessly, but they do not have the option of simply not doing them.

Another answer to the 'Why bother?' question is that disability evaluation is important. In an ideal world, we would completely cure all patients and would not have to worry about disability. In reality, our interventions might only partially resolve our patients' inability to work and function in the community. Consequently, we have to be concerned about residual impairment and workplace incapacity after treatment has been optimized. Once we have done what we can to help our patients return to economic productivity, we need to avoid doing them a disservice by either grossly overstating or understating their capacities to disability adjudicators.

REFERENCES

1. Alaranta H, Rytokoski U, Rissanen A, et al. Intensive physical and psychosocial training program for patients with chronic low back pain. A controlled clinical trial. Spine 1994; 19(12):1339–1349.
2. Babitsky S, Mangraviti JJ, Melhorn JM. Writing and defending your IME report: the comprehensive guide. Falmouth: SEAK; 2004.
3. Barnsley L, Lord S, Wallis B, et al. False-positive rates of cervical zygapophysial joint blocks. Clin J Pain 1993; 9(2):124–130.
4. Barnsley L, Lord SM, Wallis BJ, et al. The prevalence of chronic cervical zygapophysial joint pain after whiplash. Spine 1995; 20(1):20–25, discussion 26.
5. Beattie PF, Meyers SP, Stratford P, et al. Associations between patient report of symptoms and anatomic impairment visible on lumbar magnetic resonance imaging. Spine 2000; 25(7):819–828.
6. Bellamy R. Compensation neurosis: financial reward for illness as nocebo. Clin Orthop 1997; 336:94–106.
7. Clark W, Haldeman S. The development of guideline factors for the evaluation of disability in neck and back injuries. Division of Industrial Accidents, State of California. Spine 1993; 18(13):1736–1745.
8. Clark WL, Haldeman S, Johnson P, et al. Back impairment and disability determination. Another attempt at objective, reliable rating. Spine 1988; 13(3):332–341.
9. Cocchiarella L, Andersson GBJ, eds. Guides to the evaluation of permanent impairment. 5th edn. Chicago: American Medical Association Press; 2001.
10. Colledge A, Krohm G. Impairment rating—ambiguity, part 1. In: Schmidt RF, Willis WD, eds. Encyclopedia of pain. Heidelberg: Springer; 2006.
11. Curatolo M, Petersen-Felix S, Arendt-Nielsen L, et al. Central hypersensitivity in chronic pain after whiplash injury. Clin J Pain 2001; 17(4):306–315.
12. Demeter SL, Andersson G, Smith GM. Disability evaluation. 1st edn. Chicago: American Medical Association; 1996.
13. Demeter SL, Andersson G. Disability evaluation. 2nd edn. St. Louis: Mosby; 2003.
14. Estlander AM, Mellin G, Vanharanta H, et al. Effects and follow-up of a multimodal treatment program including intensive physical training for low back pain patients. Scand J Rehabil Med 1991; 23(2):97–102.
15. Fabrega H. Evolution of sickness and healing. Berkeley: University of California Press; 1997.
16. Field JE, Field TF. Classification of jobs. Athens: Elliott & Fitzpatrick; 1992.
17. Fishbain DA, Cole B, Cutler RB, et al. A structured evidence-based review on the meaning of nonorganic physical signs: Waddell signs. Pain Med 2003; 4(2):141–181.
18. Fishbain DA, Cutler RB, Rosomoff HL, et al. Impact of chronic pain patients' job perception variables on actual return to work. Clin J Pain 1997; 13(3):197–206.
19. Fishbain DA, Cutler RB, Rosomoff HL, et al. Is there a relationship between nonorganic physical findings (Waddell signs) and secondary gain/malingering? Clin J Pain 2004; 20(6):399–408.
20. Fishbain DA, Cutler RB, Rosomoff HL, et al. Prediction of 'intent', 'discrepancy with intent', and 'discrepancy with nonintent' for the patient with chronic pain to return to work after treatment at a pain facility. Clin J Pain 1999; 15(2):141–150.
21. Fishbain DA, Rosomoff HL, Cutler RB, et al. Secondary gain concept: a review of the scientific evidence. Clin J Pain 1995; 11(1):6–21.
22. Gilovich T. How we know what isn't so: the fallibility of human reason in everyday life. New York: Free Press; 1991.
23. Gouttebarge V, Wind H, Kuijer PP, et al. Reliability and validity of Functional Capacity Evaluation methods: a systematic review with reference to Blankenship system, Ergos work simulator, Ergo-Kit and Isernhagen work system. Int Arch Occup Environ Health 2004; 77(8):527–537.
24. Hazard RG, Bendix A, Fenwick JW. Disability exaggeration as a predictor of functional restoration outcomes for patients with chronic low-back pain. Spine 1991; 16(9):1062–1067.
25. Hidding A, van Santen M, De Klerk E, et al. Comparison between self-report measures and clinical observations of functional disability in ankylosing spondylitis, rheumatoid arthritis and fibromyalgia. J Rheumatol 1994; 21(5):818–823.
26. Hildebrandt J, Pfingsten M, Saur P, et al. Prediction of success from a multidisciplinary treatment program for chronic low back pain. Spine 1997; 22(9):990–1001.
27. Holleman WL, Holleman MC. School and work release evaluations. JAMA 1988; 260(24):3629–3634.
28. Jensen MP, Turner JA, Romano JM. Correlates of improvement in multidisciplinary treatment of chronic pain. J Consult Clin Psychol 1994; 62(1):172–179.
29. Kaplan GM, Wurtele SK, Gillis D. Maximal effort during functional capacity evaluations: an examination of psychological factors. Arch Phys Med Rehabil 1996; 77(1):161–164.
30. King PM, Tuckwell N, Barrett TE. A critical review of functional capacity evaluations. Phys Ther 1998; 78(8):852–866.
31. Koelbaek Johansen M, Graven-Nielsen T, Schou Olesen A, et al. Generalised muscular hyperalgesia in chronic whiplash syndrome. Pain 1999; 83(2):229–234.
32. Lechner DE. Functional capacity evaluation. In: King PM, ed. Sourcebook of occupational rehabilitation. New York: Plenum Press; 1998.
33. Lipchik GL, Milles K, Covington EC. The effects of multidisciplinary pain management treatment on locus of control and pain beliefs in chronic nonterminal pain. Clin J Pain 1993; 9(1):49–57.
34. Loeser JD, Henderlite SE, Conrad DA. Incentive effects of workers' compensation benefits: a literature synthesis. Med Care Res Rev 1995; 52(1):34–59.
35. Lord SM, Barnsley L, Wallis BJ, et al. Chronic cervical zygapophysial joint pain after whiplash. A placebo-controlled prevalence study. Spine 1996; 21(15):1737–1744, discussion 1744–1745 (see comments).
36. Main CJ, Waddell G. Behavioral responses to examination. A reappraisal of the interpretation of 'nonorganic signs'. Spine 1998; 23(21):2367–2371.
37. Mayer TG, Gatchel RJ. Functional restoration for spinal disorders: the sports medicine approach. Philadelphia: Lea & Febiger; 1988.

38. Mayer TG, Polatin P, Smith B, et al. Spine rehabilitation. Secondary and tertiary nonoperative care. Spine 1995; 20(18):2060–2066.

39. McGorry RW, Webster BS, Snook SH, et al. The relation between pain intensity, disability, and the episodic nature of chronic and recurrent low back pain. Spine 2000; 25(7):834–841.

40. Mendelson G. Psychiatric aspects of personal injury claims. Springfield: Thomas; 1988.

41. Niemeyer LO, Jacobs K, Reynolds-Lynch K, et al. Work hardening: past, present, and future—the Work Programs Special Interest Section National Work-hardening Outcome Study. Am J Occup Ther 1994; 48(4): 327–339.

42. Osterweis M, Kleinman A, Mechanic D. Pain and disability: clinical, behavioral, and public policy perspectives. Washington: National Academy Press; 1987.

43. Peterson KW, Babitsky S, Beller TA, et al. The American Board of Independent Medical Examiners. J Occup Environ Med 1997; 39(6): 509–514.

44. Robinson JP, Turk DC, Loeser JD. Pain, impairment, and disability in the AMA Guides. J Law Med Ethics 2004; 32(2):191, 315–326.

45. Robinson JP, Turk DC. Introductory essay. In: Schmidt RF, Willis WD, eds. Encyclopedia of pain. Heidelberg: Springer; 2006.

46. Robinson JP. Evaluation of function and disability. In: Loeser JD, ed. Bonica's management of pain. 3rd edn. Philadelphia: Lippincott Williams & Wilkins; 2001.

47. Robinson JP. Pain and disability. In: Jensen TS, Wilson P, Rice A, eds. Chronic pain. London: Edward Arnold; 2002.

48. Rondinelli RD, Katz RT. Impairment rating and disability evaluation. Philadelphia: Saunders; 2000.

49. Rucker KS, Metzler HM, Kregel J. Standardization of chronic pain assessment: a multiperspective approach. Clin J Pain 1996; 12(2):94–110.

50. Rucker KS, Metzler HM. Predicting subsequent employment status of SSA disability applicants with chronic pain. Clin J Pain 1995; 11(1):22–35.

51. Saal JS. General principles of diagnostic testing as related to painful lumbar spine disorders: a critical appraisal of current diagnostic techniques. Spine 2002; 27(22):2538–2545, discussion 2546.

52. Schwarzer AC, Wang SC, O'Driscoll D, et al. The ability of computed tomography to identify a painful zygapophysial joint in patients with chronic low back pain. Spine 1995; 20(8):907–912.

53. Social Security Administration. Disability evaluation under social security. Washington: US Government Printing Office; 1994.

54. Sterling M, Jull G, Vicenzino B, et al. Sensory hypersensitivity occurs soon after whiplash injury and is associated with poor recovery. Pain 2003; 104(3):509–517.

55. Sullivan MD, Loeser JD. The diagnosis of disability. Treating and rating disability in a pain clinic. Arch Intern Med 1992; 152(9):1829–1835.

56. US Department of Veterans Affairs. Federal benefits for veterans and dependents. Washington: Department of Veterans Affairs; 2004.

57. US Employment and Training Administration. Dictionary of occupational titles. 4th edn. Lanham: Bernan Press; 1991.

58. Voiss DV. Occupational injury. Fact, fantasy, or fraud? Neurol Clin 1995; 13(2):431–446.

59. Waddell G, McCulloch JA, Kummel E, et al. Nonorganic physical signs in low-back pain. Spine 1980; 5(2):117–125.

60. Ziporyn T. Disability evaluation: a fledgling science? JAMA 1983; 250(7): 873–874, 879–880.

Chapter

7

Neurologic and Musculoskeletal Imaging Studies

Andrew D. Bronstein, Shane E. Macaulay, Ranjeet B. Singh and Andrew J. Cole

Multiple imaging modalities are available to help in making a neurologic or musculoskeletal diagnosis. This chapter describes imaging methods, indications, contraindications, and artifacts specific to various types of imaging methods. The chapter also presents the preferred imaging methods for specific anatomic areas and tissues. The purpose of the discussion is to help the physiatrist, in concert with the consulting radiologist, choose the most appropriate imaging study or studies for a patient.

The American College of Radiology (ACR) has developed appropriateness criteria for various imaging modalities for specific clinical indications.[1] As of 2004, musculoskeletal and spinal clinical indications pertinent to the physiatrist that have appropriateness criteria include imaging evaluation of suspected ankle fractures, cervical spine trauma, avascular necrosis (AVN) of the hip, soft tissue mass, bone tumors, stress or insufficiency fractures (excluding vertebral), metastatic bone disease, painful hip or knee arthroplasty, shoulder trauma, non-traumatic knee pain, chronic ankle pain, chronic wrist pain, chronic elbow pain, chronic neck pain, chronic foot pain, acute knee trauma, acute hand and wrist trauma, chronic hip pain, acute low back pain and radiculopathy, myelopathy, and spine trauma. The appropriateness of a given imaging study on a scale of 1–9 is tallied for each clinical situation by expert panels. Ratings of the appropriateness criteria are presented under the specific anatomic discussions later in this chapter.

IMAGING MODALITIES

Plain radiography and its variants (stress radiography, arthrography, myelography, diskography, fluoroscopy, and videofluoroscopy)

Plain radiographs are obtained when an x-ray beam is directed through the body part being imaged to a sensitized plate; part of the beam is absorbed by the body, producing a shadow image on the plate. Five different types of tissues can be imaged with plain radiography: gas, fat, soft tissue and water, bone, and metal (metals, barium, and iodinated contrast material). The differentiation of tissue within each of these five groups is limited, however, which makes it difficult to differentiate entities such as edema from blood, or muscle from tumor. Nevertheless, plain radiographs are a relatively inexpensive way to assess fractures or bony abnormalities.

It is crucial to have plain radiograph protocols for each body part. The protocols should specify the number of views, technique, and film–screen combination. To exclude a fracture, at least two orthogonal views perpendicular to each other are necessary, and often three or more are needed, depending on the body part. Patient history and skin markers placed on the region of interest can help identify abnormalities and might alter the patient positioning or imaging technique.

Stress radiography is a procedure in which stress is placed on a given joint to assess for any change in joint width or alignment caused by ligamentous laxity or disruption, usually in comparison with the asymptomatic normal side. Acromioclavicular joint views holding weights, Telos stress examination of the ankles with varus or posterior stresses,[20] and valgus stress on the elbow[86] are examples of stress radiography. Flexion and extension views of the cervical spine can also be considered stress views, although the stress is achieved passively using the weight of the head and the tension of the cervical muscles.

Arthrography is a procedure in which iodinated contrast material or air (or both) is instilled into a joint before plain radiographs are obtained. This outlines the joint space as well as structures within or surrounding the joint. Arthrography can be performed on virtually any synovial joint, but at present it is used less often than in the past because of the development of newer, non-invasive modalities. The risks of arthrography are those of a needle puncture, including hemorrhage, infection, and drug reaction. Tenography involves injection of iodinated contrast material into a tendon sheath to assess for tendon pathology or rupture of a ligament and abnormal communication with an adjacent joint space.

Myelography is plain radiography performed after instillation of iodinated contrast material into the thecal sac. Non-ionic iodinated contrast material can be injected via a lateral C1–C2 approach or posterior upper lumbar approach. Although myelography has largely been supplanted by magnetic resonance imaging (MRI), there are some advantages of myelography over MRI. Myelography and postmyelography computed tomography (CT) better show bony detail and subtle impressions on the nerve roots. Myelography also allows imaging of the lumbar spine in the upright weight-bearing position as well as in flexion and extension. The risks of myelography include hemorrhage, infection or meningitis, drug reaction, nerve damage, and cerebrospinal fluid (CSF) leak or spinal headache. These risks can be minimized with careful technique.

Diskography is a procedure in which plain radiography is performed after instillation of iodinated contrast material into the intervertebral disk spaces. Suspected symptomatic disks are injected, along with a 'control' disk. The most important aspect of diskography is whether pressurization of the disk space during injection reproduces the location and quality of the patient's symptoms.[53,73] Unequivocal concordant symptoms during the injection correlate with that disk being the pain generator. The risks of diskography are similar to those of myelography, except for a slightly higher risk of infection due to the low vascularity of the intervertebral disk space.

Fluoroscopy is the real time x-ray visualization of structures, and is used during spinal diagnostic and therapeutic procedures and in the instillation of contrast medium for arthrography, myelography, and diskography. Fluoroscopy might or might not involve obtaining plain radiographs.

Videofluoroscopy entails recording fluoroscopic images to study the motion of joints. It can demonstrate dynamic abnormalities during motion, such as in the cervical spine and especially in the atlantoaxial occipital region. When there is a question of vertebral fusion in a postoperative patient, dynamic videofluoroscopy can sometimes be helpful.

Computed tomography

Computed tomography is the production of cross-sectional images of the body by selective absorption of a traveling x-ray or electron beam. Multiple detectors measure the transmission of the beam at multiple angles, and computer algorithms are used to form images from the data. Contrast between different tissue types is significantly higher with CT than with plain radiography, and there is more precise localization of structures on the cross-sectional imaging. The imaging plane is usually axial or axial oblique, although coronal images of the foot and ankle and sagittal or coronal images of the wrist and elbow can be obtained with variations in patient positioning. CT has a definite advantage over MRI in the imaging of cortical bone. CT can also better image chondroid and osteoid matrices. The detection of fractures and delineation of positioning of fracture fragments are achieved well with CT, but a fracture tangential to the imaging plane can be missed, in part due to partial voluming artifact (see explanation below).

Axial images can be reformatted into sagittal, coronal, oblique, or complex planes,[84] but the resolution depends on the section thickness of the original images and is degraded if there is patient motion during the scan. Three-dimensional reformatted images can also be obtained and are occasionally helpful for surgical reconstruction of complex fractures.[59]

CT with contrast agent enhancement

Computed tomography with intravenous contrast agent enhancement is more commonly used for imaging the brain, neck, chest, abdomen, and pelvis. Intravenous contrast medium is rarely used to image the spine or extremities, except in the detection of soft tissue tumors or in the evaluation of post-

operative spine patients, especially when MRI cannot be performed because of contraindications or artifacts from metal internal fixation devices.

Postarthrography CT delineates well the joint space as well as surrounding bony structures. Postarthrography CT of the shoulder is good at delineating the glenoid labrum but is limited to the axial plane. Air and a low volume of contrast agent are injected into a joint if CT is to be performed.

CT myelography and postdiskography CT

Postmyelography CT is a requisite adjunct to myelography. The bony intervertebral foramina and spondylosis are best seen on axial CT images. Intraforaminal or far lateral disk abnormalities can be invisible on the plain film myelogram and are best shown on CT. Disk abnormalities at L5–S1 might be invisible on myelography (because of the ample ventral epidural fat at this level) but visible on CT. The postmyelography CT levels should include any levels with abnormality detected on myelography, as well as any levels of clinical abnormality. The L5–S1 level should be included on all lumbar CT myelograms because of the insensitivity of myelography due to the ventral epidural fat at this level.

Postdiskography CT is an adjunct to diskography to better demonstrate the anatomy of an annular tear (Fig. 7-1).

Magnetic resonance imaging

Magnetic resonance imaging is the production of cross-sectional images of the body through placement of the imaged body part in a large static magnetic field with a varying magnetic gradient pulsed in such a way as to allow the resonance of hydrogen to

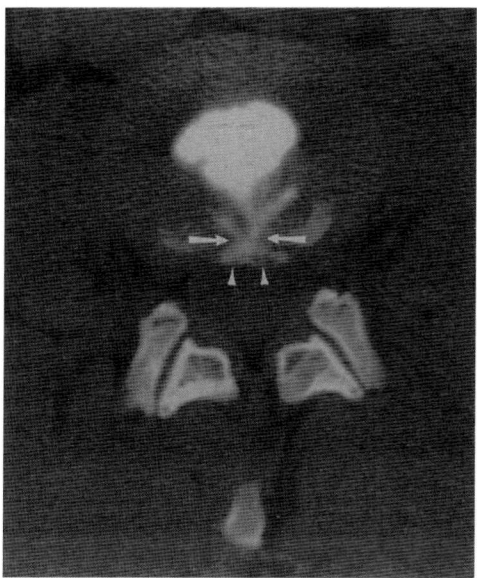

Figure 7-1 Postdiskography computed tomography (CT) scan of a posterior central annular tear, demonstrating iodinated contrast material extending from the nucleus through a midline tear (arrows) to a subannular location posteriorly (arrowheads). No focal convexity to the posterior disk margin is present; this abnormality would not be seen on plain CT or postmyelography CT.

Table 7-1 Relative advantages and disadvantages of magnetic resonance imaging and computed tomography

	Computed tomography	Magnetic resonance imaging

Advantages	Rapid acquisition time
	Less sensitive to motion than MRI
	Detection of calcification and ossification
	Less artifact from metallic foreign bodies
	   or prostheses than MRI
	Good patient tolerance
		Anatomic and pathologic information (proton density, T1, T2, chemical
		   shift)
		Better tissue contrast than CT
		Direct multiplanar imaging
		No ionizing radiation

Disadvantages	Anatomic information predominantly; less
	   pathologic information than with MRI
	Ionizing radiation
	Limited imaging planes
		More sensitive to motion than CT
		Longer acquisition time than CT
		Lower resolution for cortical bone or calcification than CT
		Considerable signal loss from metallic foreign bodies or prostheses
		Some problems with claustrophobia, although lessened with large-bore
		   or open MRI scanners

be detected.[82] The data obtained are then converted by computer algorithms into cross-sectional images. These images depend on the number of mobile hydrogen atoms and specific tissue characteristics of the hydrogen. Pulse sequence parameters can be adjusted to accentuate certain inherent qualities of tissues, allowing for much higher contrast between different types of tissue (Table 7-1). For example, fat-containing tissues can be accentuated or suppressed, and water-containing tissues can be accentuated or suppressed.

Because the patient is placed in proximity to a large magnetic field, there are contraindications to MRI. Patients with pacemakers, pacemaker wires, implanted electronic devices, ferromagnetic cerebral aneurysm clips, and metal around or within the orbits should not be scanned. Some other metallic devices are contraindications to MRI and, if there is a question of compatibility with the scanner, the consulting radiologist should be contacted prior to the examination.

Magnetic resonance imaging has multiple available imaging planes, including complex imaging planes. Multiple magnetic gradient pulse sequences are also available to accentuate different characteristics of tissues (Table 7-2). Standard pulse sequences include T1-weighting, proton density, T2-weighting, short inversion time–inversion recovery (STIR), and fat suppression imaging. Numerous pulse sequences are available on any given magnetic resonance scanner, and different manufacturers typically use different abbreviations for the sequences. The advent of fast spin-echo sequences has shortened imaging times. However, the natural fat signal suppression on T2-weighted spin-echo images is partially lost on fast spin-echo T2-weighted images unless additional fat suppression techniques are included.

The signal to noise ratio and image quality of a magnetic resonance image depend on multiple factors, including magnetic field strength, surface coil design, field of view, matrix size, number of repetitions of the pulse sequences, other pulse sequence parameters, patient size, and body habitus.

Short inversion time–inversion recovery imaging shows additive T1 and T2 characteristics and has a high sensitivity for

Table 7-2 Magnetic resonance signal characteristics of different tissues

Tissue	T1-weighted images	T2-weighted images
Fat	High	Low[a]
Cortical bone	Low	Low
Fatty bone marrow	High	Low[a]
Red bone marrow	Intermediate	Intermediate
Muscle	Low to intermediate	Low to intermediate
Tendon	Low	Low
Ligament	Low	Low
Fluid	Low	High
Intervertebral disk	Low	High
Desiccated disk	Low	Low

[a]Low signal with routine spin-echo imaging. Fast spin-echo T2-weighted images do not show as much loss of fat signal.

edema and many types of tumors. There is also suppression of the signal from fat, which causes the fat to appear dark, although some non-fat tissues can be suppressed if they have a short T1.[51] Magnetic resonance myelography is a more recent magnetic resonance technique that preferentially images CSF and eliminates the potential risks of contrast myelography, but lacks the information about bony detail and upright weight bearing with flexion and extension that can be obtained with contrast myelography.

Kinematic magnetic resonance images are obtained as a joint is moved stepwise through a range of motion. This is useful to assess patellar tracking abnormalities.[100] Kinematic imaging of the temporomandibular joint and shoulder[94] can also be performed for specific clinical indications.

MRI with contrast agent enhancement

Intravenous gadolinium contrast agents have several specific indications when used in conjunction with MRI. In spine imaging, intravenous contrast material is useful for assessing for postoperative scar versus recurrent or residual disk extrusion. Gadolinium contrast agents can show a breakdown of the blood–brain barrier with intramedullary or extramedullary intradural tumors. Musculoskeletal tumor detection can also be improved with intravenous contrast, although additional fat suppression techniques accentuate this enhancement.

Dilute gadolinium contrast material injected into joints significantly improves the delineation of many intraarticular and periarticular structures,[45] including the glenoid labrum and glenohumeral ligaments,[7,76] the acetabular labrum,[27] a post-operative meniscus,[4] and the articular cartilage. Intraarticular gadolinium can also improve differentiation of partial-thickness from full-thickness tears of the rotator cuff. Non-enhanced bursal fluid has a different signal characteristic than intraarticular gadolinium. The risks of intraarticular injection of gadolinium are the same as for arthrography, and include hemorrhage, infection, and rare anaphylactic reactions.

Nuclear medicine studies

Radionuclide bone scintigraphy is performed after intravenous injection of a bone-seeking isotope such as technetium-99m–methylene diphosphonate to detect areas of increased bone turnover. Multiple lesions throughout the skeleton can be demonstrated in a single study, but radionuclide scintigraphy often has a low specificity. It can be useful for whole body screening for bony metastases, but bony metastases in a given area can also be detected with MRI, which has a higher specificity and spatial resolution. A bone scan of the foot and ankle for chronic foot pain can help isolate the location of the abnormality, which might then be studied with MRI or CT. In the patient with mechanical back pain, a bone scan can help show the level of facet joint abnormality, although the facet joint with abnormal activity might not necessarily be the one that is painful. Often, the contralateral facet is painful from abnormal stresses caused by the 'hot' facet joint. Bone scanning is often used to detect stress or insufficiency fractures, but MRI might actually show these lesions earlier and provide better spatial resolution and specificity.

Single-photon emission computed tomography (SPECT) is an adjunct to the planar bone scan. It provides cross-sectional images of the body (axial, coronal, sagittal) using the same radioisotope emissions as a bone scan, but with a moving gamma camera. This is especially useful in the spine to show whether activity is greatest at the vertebrae anteriorly or around the facet joints or other posterior elements. The signal to background ratio is also improved with SPECT imaging. However, SPECT imaging takes additional time and adds expense, so it is used only for specific indications.

Radiolabeled white blood cell imaging is sometimes used to identify areas of osteomyelitis or infection. However, some non-infected areas such as around the tip of an orthopedic prosthesis or an amputated bone end can show increased activity.

Ultrasound

Shoulder ultrasound for rotator cuff pathology was initially popular, but has become less utilized with the advent of improved shoulder MRI. Ultrasound does not provide information about bone, the supraspinatus outlet anatomy, the glenoid labrum, or the glenohumeral ligaments. Shoulder ultrasound is very operator-dependent, with the attendant variation in sensitivity and specificity.

High-resolution ultrasound allows targeted assessment of tendons and muscles for higher grade tears, hematomas, and calcification, and can be used to guide aspiration and injection of cysts or hematomas. MRI is much more sensitive in the detection and grading of muscle and tendon pathology.

IMAGING ARTIFACTS

Imaging artifacts exist in great variety. Some of the most common artifacts are discussed here, as they are routinely seen on image interpretation.

Plain radiography artifacts

On plain radiographs, a common artifact is the Mach line, which occurs when a bony edge overlaps another bone. A thin dark line appears just adjacent to the overlapping bone and can be mistaken for a fracture (Fig. 7-2).

CT artifacts

The three artifacts seen most commonly with CT are those of partial voluming, streak, and beam hardening. A partial voluming artifact occurs because a CT section has a finite thickness (1, 3, 5, or 10 mm). If a structure extends only through a portion of the section, the attenuation is averaged with that of the structure beside it in the section. For this reason, partial voluming is more likely to occur with thicker sections. Partial voluming can result in missing a fracture in the axial plane, where it is averaged with the solid bone on either side of the fracture. Use of a thinner section thickness minimizes this artifact, which is why cervical spine CT images are obtained with a 1- or 1.5-mm section thickness. CT of ankle or foot fractures is performed with a relatively thin section thickness of 3 mm in both the coronal and the axial planes, which minimizes the likelihood of missing a fracture from partial voluming. Helical volumetric CT imaging can also reduce partial voluming.

Reconstruction of the CT data to form an image assumes a constant energy of the x-ray beam as it circles around the patient. An area of increased density, such as thick bone, can attenuate the lower energy portion of the x-ray spectrum and cause a relatively higher energy beam to pass through. This difference in energy over a portion of the data stream can result in beam-hardening artifact, with variable attenuation central to the high-density bone (Fig. 7-3).

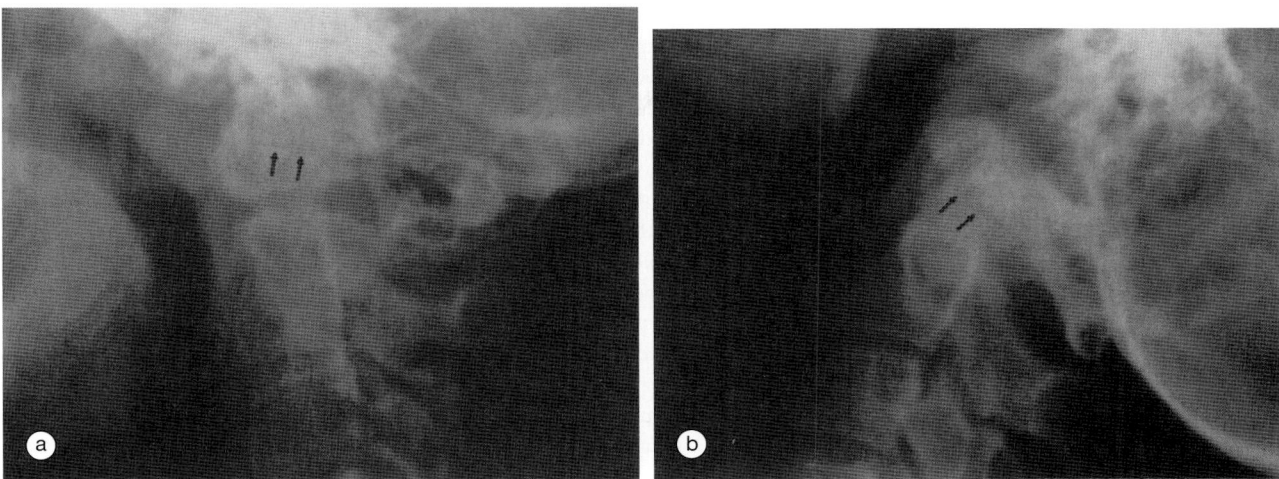

Figure 7-2 Mach line simulating a dens fracture. (**a**) Lateral plain film of the cervical spine demonstrates a curvilinear lucency traversing the dens (arrows), but this parallels the undersurface of the C1 ring and mastoid bones as well as extending past the margins of the dens. (**b**) Repeat extension lateral view of the same patient demonstrates no fracture line at the same site, and there is a fainter Mach line, now located more caudad (arrows).

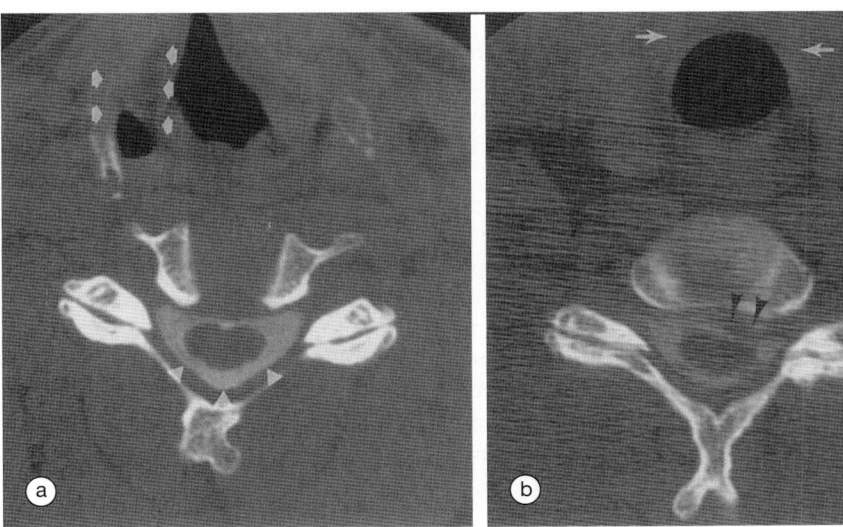

Figure 7-3 Streak and beam-hardening artifact on computed tomography (CT). (**a**) Postmyelography CT demonstrates low- and high-attenuation anteroposterior streaks at the air–soft tissue interfaces of the piriform sinuses (arrows). This image, obtained at the midcervical level, does not show beam-hardening artifact from the shoulders, and the spinal cord cross-section is well delineated, surrounded by intrathecal iodinated contrast material (arrowheads). (**b**) A more caudal image in the same patient shows beam-hardening artifact from the shoulders, with multiple transverse lines degrading the image and making it more difficult to detect the left posterior extrusion tilting the cord (arrowheads). Streak artifact is seen at the air–soft tissue interface of the trachea (arrows).

Streak artifact occurs where there is an interface between tissues of very different attenuation, such as bone and air, resulting in linear streaks extending along the plane of the interface. This can be seen at the bone–air interface of sinuses or at the interface of a metal prosthesis and bone. A metal prosthesis can result in both beam-hardening and streak artifacts. Certain CT reconstruction algorithms can reduce these artifacts but not totally eliminate them. Newer CT scanners with multirow detector arrays can significantly reduce or eliminate artifact from internal fixation hardware or prostheses in concert with improved reconstruction algorithms.

MRI artifacts

Partial voluming can occur with MRI, in that there is a finite thickness of tissue sample to make an image, and there can be averaging of signal from tissue components within the thickness of the section. This effect can be reduced with thinner section thickness.[110] Partial voluming is routinely seen on sagittal images obtained through the spine at the lateral edge of the thecal sac, where there is partial voluming of the CSF with the epidural fat. Partial voluming of the edge of the spinal cord with the adjacent CSF on sagittal images can artifactually increase the signal intensity of the cord on the most lateral images of the cord.

Magic angle artifact is a phenomenon seen on imaging of anisotropic structures that course 55° (the 'magic angle') relative to the main magnetic field in the magnetic resonance scanner.[33,34] There is an artifactually increased signal within the structure at this angle. This artifact most commonly occurs during imaging of tendons that are anisotropic and course at a 55° angle to the main magnetic field, such as in the rotator cuff supraspinatus tendon[113] or the ankle tendons as they course around the malleoli. The artifact is especially problematic in the rotator cuff, where increased T1 and proton density signal in the critical zone (which may course 55° relative to the main magnetic field) can represent tendinopathy. A partial-thickness or full-thickness tear of the supraspinatus should not be confused with the increased signal intensity arising from imaging at the magic angle, as T2-weighted images show more signal abnormality with tears and less magic angle effect. Signal intensity of peripheral nerves on magnetic resonance neurography can increase as the nerve courses at the magic angle.[22]

Chemical shift artifact is seen because the resonance frequency of hydrogen varies with the structure that the hydrogen is within.[110] The resonance frequency of fat is slightly different from that of water because of the different hydrogen bonds. Consequently, the reconstruction algorithm can position fat slightly differently than water-containing structures, leading to artifacts in the frequency encoding direction. This can cause misregistration of fatty bone marrow in relation to soft tissues adjacent to the bone, giving an asymmetry and inaccuracy of cortical bone thickness in the extremities[30] or at the vertebral end plate or cortex.

Motion artifact is usually visible on magnetic resonance images as blurring or double images.[110] Flow artifact from vessels or CSF can cause artifacts, usually in a line in the phase encoding direction. These artifacts can often be minimized with flow compensation or saturation bands in the imaging protocol. However, if there is an unusual round focus of signal not expected within a structure, it is worth checking to see if it lies in a horizontal or vertical line with a blood vessel and if it is of the same caliber.

Metal artifact occurs when either microscopic or macroscopic metal fragments cause a localized change in the homogeneity of the magnetic field. This can result in a focus of signal void with an adjacent high signal intensity ring.[110] These artifacts are dramatically evident when a prosthesis or internal fixation device is present, and they appear as small foci in the postoperative patient if microscopic fragments of metal break off the drills or other instruments during surgery. The small high-signal ring or partial ring near the signal void helps differentiate this artifact from a calcification or hemosiderin. Artifact from metal can be reduced by using T2-weighted fast spin-echo techniques rather than conventional spin-echo techniques.[111]

IMAGING OF THE SPINE

Trauma

Imaging for spinal trauma depends on the clinical situation and presence of symptoms, neurologic deficit, and sensorium of the patient. Plain radiography is usually the best initial screening procedure to use in assessing for fracture. In the cervical spine, a minimum three-view examination (lateral, anteroposterior, and open mouth odontoid) should be obtained. All of C7 and the C7–T1 interspace should be visualized. If a fracture is seen or suspected, thin-section CT with reformatting or helical CT can better delineate that fracture, and can also disclose other associated vertebral fractures not seen on the plain radio-graphs.[74] Some authors advocate helical CT in the initial assessment for cervical fracture.[10] MRI can best show any traumatic disk extrusion or spinal cord abnormality if the patient has myelopathic symptoms.[32] Fast spin-echo T2-weighted images with fat suppression can show soft tissue edema or hemorrhage associated with ligamentous tearing in whiplash injuries in the acute setting, but this study is not routinely done in patients without myelopathy or neurologic deficit.

For cervical spine trauma, the ACR appropriateness criteria have many clinical scenarios depending on patient sensorium, pain, neurologic deficit, and plain film findings. The panel gives a lower appropriateness rating to plain radiographs in the asymptomatic and alert patient with normal physical examination findings, with or without a cervical collar. If the patient is symptomatic or has neurologic signs or symptoms of cervical injury, then a minimal screening examination of three-view plain radiographs is given a high appropriateness rating. If the patient has normal plain radiographs but neurologic signs or symptoms are present, MRI is given a higher appropriateness rating, with CT myelography as an alternative if MRI is not possible. CT is given a high appropriateness rating in many clinical settings, including paresthesias of the hands or feet, unconsciousness, impaired sensorium, and neurologic findings.

Magnetic resonance imaging performed before and after intravenous gadolinium instillation can help differentiate vertebral collapse due to osteoporosis from that due to malignancy.[26]

Intramedullary abnormalities

Magnetic resonance imaging is the procedure of choice for assessing the intramedullary spinal cord. Six MRI patterns have been defined by their appearance on T1-weighted images, before and after contrast injection, and on T2-weighted images, with a short differential diagnosis for each.[13]

American College of Radiology appropriateness criteria are available for different types of myelopathy, including traumatic, painful, sudden onset, stepwise progressive, slowly progressive, seen in an infectious disease patient, and seen in an oncology patient. All these earn high ratings for MRI and predominantly high ratings for plain radiography. The addition of postcontrast enhancement MRI is considered appropriate in several of the situations, such as in the infectious disease patient or with a stepwise progressive condition. It is also appropriate if the non-contrast-enhanced MRI is negative or symptoms are not explained in an oncology patient. If the myelopathy is painful, of sudden onset, or of slow progression, contrast studies might be appropriate if MRI is negative. This can be done to find the abnormality or to better characterize a known abnormality.

Intramedullary primary and metastatic neoplasms are well shown on magnetic resonance T2-weighted images. Most intramedullary spinal tumors enhance with gadolinium contrast agents.[78] Contrast-enhanced MRI can help differentiate enhancing tumor from non-enhancing demyelination or a non-enhancing myelitis. Metastatic tumors can show a very focal enlargement of the cord as opposed to the more diffuse enlargement with primary gliomas.

The abnormalities of multiple sclerosis can be located entirely in the cervical spinal cord without brain involvement. Spinal cord multiple sclerosis plaques are characteristically peripherally located, are less than two vertebral segments in length, and occupy less than half the cross-sectional area of the cord.[112] If a cord lesion is suspicious for multiple sclerosis, either by imaging or by clinical criteria, MRI of the head should be performed to look for additional lesions and to strengthen the putative diagnosis.

Magnetic resonance imaging can well demonstrate enlargement of the cord from syringomyelia and can demonstrate an associated Chiari 1 malformation. If a syrinx involves the entire cervical region with no Chiari malformation to explain it, consideration should be given to imaging the rest of the cord. Cord tumors located more caudally can be associated with a holocord syrinx.

Increased T2 signal within the cord can be seen in areas of chronic compression from degenerative disk disease and from spondylosis. The likelihood of detecting increased cord signal is proportional to the severity of the clinical myelopathy and the degree of spinal canal compression. The response to surgery is less favorable in patients with intense, well-defined, increased cord signal than in those with a faint, poorly defined signal or those with normal signal.[23]

Intradural extramedullary abnormalities

Magnetic resonance imaging with intravenous gadolinium contrast is the most sensitive imaging study for assessing abnormalities within the dural sac, including drop metastases, hematogenous leptomeningeal metastases, meningitis, and arachnoiditis (Fig. 7-4).[40] T2-weighted axial images without contrast can well demonstrate the three different types of arachnoiditis seen on MRI. These include nerve clumping,

tumefactive masslike arachnoiditis, and the 'empty sac' sign of the roots being attached to the thecal sac.[91] Residual Pantopaque, a possible cause for arachnoiditis, can be seen as fat signal on MRI due to its oily base.

Nerve root tumors such as schwannomas or neurofibromas can actually be shown on myelography, as they may move with the roots with upright and prone positioning, indicating their origin. MRI with contrast agent enhancement, however, increases the conspicuity of intradural or intradural–extradural root sheath tumors and their relation to the nerve root.

Extradural abnormalities
Degenerative disk disease and spondylosis

Magnetic resonance imaging is probably the single best examination to assess the intervertebral disk and surrounding structures. However, plain CT and postmyelography CT can both also demonstrate any morphologic abnormalities of the disk. Plain CT or postmyelography CT can show gas within the epidural space from extension through a full-thickness annular tear when the degenerated disk space contains gas, the 'vacuum phenomenon' (Fig. 7-5). There is little correlation between plain radiograph findings and the presence or absence of a disk extrusion.

The high incidence of asymptomatic imaging abnormalities in the general population makes it difficult to prove that an imaged abnormality is the pain generator. Diskography with pressurization of the disk space might be the most accurate method of determining whether an abnormal-appearing disk is a generator of lower back pain,[73] or a generator of pain radiating to the lower extremities, in a patient with no MRI evidence of

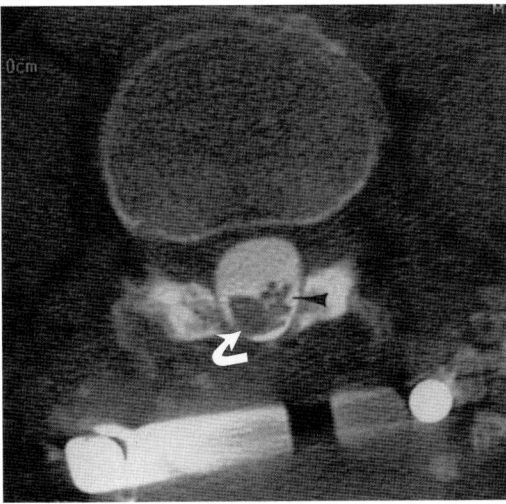

Figure 7-4 Postmyelography computed tomography of arachnoiditis following laminectomy, fusion, and dural tear demonstrates clumping of the right-sided roots (arrow), with more evenly spaced left-sided roots (arrowhead). This clumping was seen just cephalad to the site of dural repair and dural surgical clips.

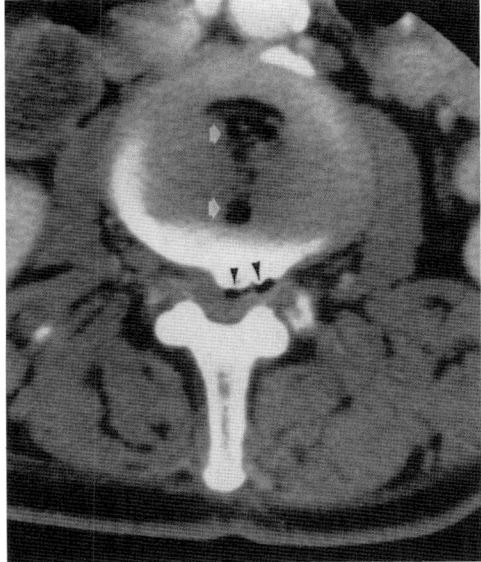

Figure 7-5 Non-contrast-enhanced CT of the spine, demonstrating 'vacuum' phenomenon, with gas in the disk space (arrows) and extension of gas into the left ventral epidural space (arrowheads), indirect evidence of an annular tear. The ventral epidural gas is just posterior to the left paracentral end plate osteophyte contributing to acquired spinal stenosis.

nerve root compression,[53,65] if the patient has unequivocal concordant symptoms during pressurization different from a control disk level. Controversy remains regarding the utility of diskography.[70,73]

The ACR appropriateness criteria for lower back pain include ratings for variants of uncomplicated lower back pain with no red flags; acute lower back pain in the setting of trauma, steroid use, osteoporosis, or age over 70; acute lower back pain with suspicion of cancer or infection; acute lower back pain with radiculopathy; acute lower back pain with prior lumbar surgery; and acute lower back pain with cauda equina syndrome. For uncomplicated lower back pain with no red flags, all imaging modalities are assigned a low appropriateness rating. MRI becomes more appropriate in the other clinical settings, and is rated more appropriate than plain lumbar radiography in all the different variants of lower back pain except for that seen with trauma, steroid use, osteoporosis, and age over 70. Postcontrast magnetic resonance is given a higher appropriateness rating in the setting of cancer, infection, previous surgery, and cauda equina syndrome.

The normal intervertebral disk has a low T1 and high T2 signal, with a lower T2 signal cleft centrally and a surrounding low-signal annulus. With disk degeneration, the T2 signal of the nucleus begins to decrease as the nucleus dehydrates. Once the disk has lost T2 signal, the signal does not return. Loss of the T2 signal can be seen with either intervertebral disk space narrowing or normal disk height, but more commonly with the former.

Combined task forces of the North American Spine Society, American Society of Spine Radiology, and American Society of Neuroradiology have developed a standardized nomenclature and classification of lumbar disk pathology.[2] Other than normal and disk desiccation, there are four general descriptions of disk disease (Fig. 7-6).[15]

1. Circumferential bulging of the disk, suggesting laxity of the annulus fibrosus.
2. Protrusion of the disk, in which a focal convexity has a width wider than depth, consistent with a partial-thickness tear through the annulus fibrosus. Protrusions can be described as focal, less than 25% of the circumference, and broad-based, between 25 and 50% of the circumference. These partial tears can also show a focus of increased T2 signal that represents fluid or granulation tissue extending through the annular tear. These annular lesions can sometimes appear more like a radial tear, and in some cases more like a partially concentric tear, shaped like a bucket handle tear.
3. Extrusion of the disk, in which a focal convexity has a depth greater than the width, consistent with the nucleus extending through a full-thickness tear of the annulus and extending extraannularly. Other criteria for extrusion that can be used are extension of the nuclear material cephalad and caudad past the levels of the end plates, or visible extension through the annulus and posterior longitudinal ligament.

4. Sequestered or free fragment, in which the extruded disk material is not connected with the native nucleus pulposus. These fragments can be located well cephalad or caudad from the donor site, and can extend into the intervertebral foramen. Often, these sequestered fragments have different signal characteristics than the native disk.

Imaging findings of degenerative disk disease must be correlated with clinical history, physical examination findings, and possibly diagnostic injection results. Many abnormal imaging findings can be asymptomatic. In 60 asymptomatic patients 20–50 years old, the prevalence of lumbar disk bulge was 20–28%. For protrusion, it was 38–42%; for annular tears, 32–33%; for extrusion, 18%; and there were no disk sequestrations.[120] Disk extrusion, sequestration, nerve root compression, end plate abnormalities, and moderate to severe facet joint osteoarthritis were rare in asymptomatic patients younger than 50 years when the prevalence among all 300 lumbar intervertebral disk levels in the study was considered.[120] In 36 patients (17–71 years old) without lower back pain or sciatica, the prevalence of disk bulge was 81%, protrusion 33%, and annular tears 56%, with no extrusions noted.[109] Annular tears showed contrast enhancement in 96%. However, assessment of T2 high-intensity zones in the disk (annular tears) by other authors in other studies showed a high correlation with pain at diskography and a low prevalence in asymptomatic patients.[5,95] A high prevalence of abnormal findings on cervical MRI of asymptomatic individuals, increasing with age, is also seen.[11]

Intervertebral disk contour abnormalities can occur anywhere along the circumference of the disk, and can be described by location as central zone, subarticular zone (posterolateral), foraminal zone, and extraforaminal (far lateral). Foraminal zone disk abnormalities can be further described as occurring at the entrance zone, within the foramen, or at the exit zone of the foramen. The level of a herniation can be described as disk level, suprapedicle level, pedicle level, and infrapedicle level.[2,123] MRI criteria to differentiate subligamentous from transligamentous disk extrusion, such as the presence of a continuous low signal intensity line posterior to the extrusion, disk extrusion size less than 50% of the size of the spinal canal, and absence of disk fragments, are unreliable.[101]

Small epidural hematomas can be associated with disk extrusions[42] and cause a larger mass effect than can be accounted for by the extrusion itself. If the extradural mass effect trails along a root sheath toward the foramen, or has signal characteristics more like those of fluid or hemorrhage, then a small epidural hematoma should be considered.

End plate degenerative changes associated with disk degeneration have been classified into type 1 (low T1 and high T2 signal), edema or fibrovascular signal; type 2 (high T1 and high T2 signal), fat signal; and type 3 (low T1 and low T2 signal), consistent with diskogenic sclerosis. Some of these end plate abnormalities can be associated with painful disks at diskography in patients with low back pain.[121]

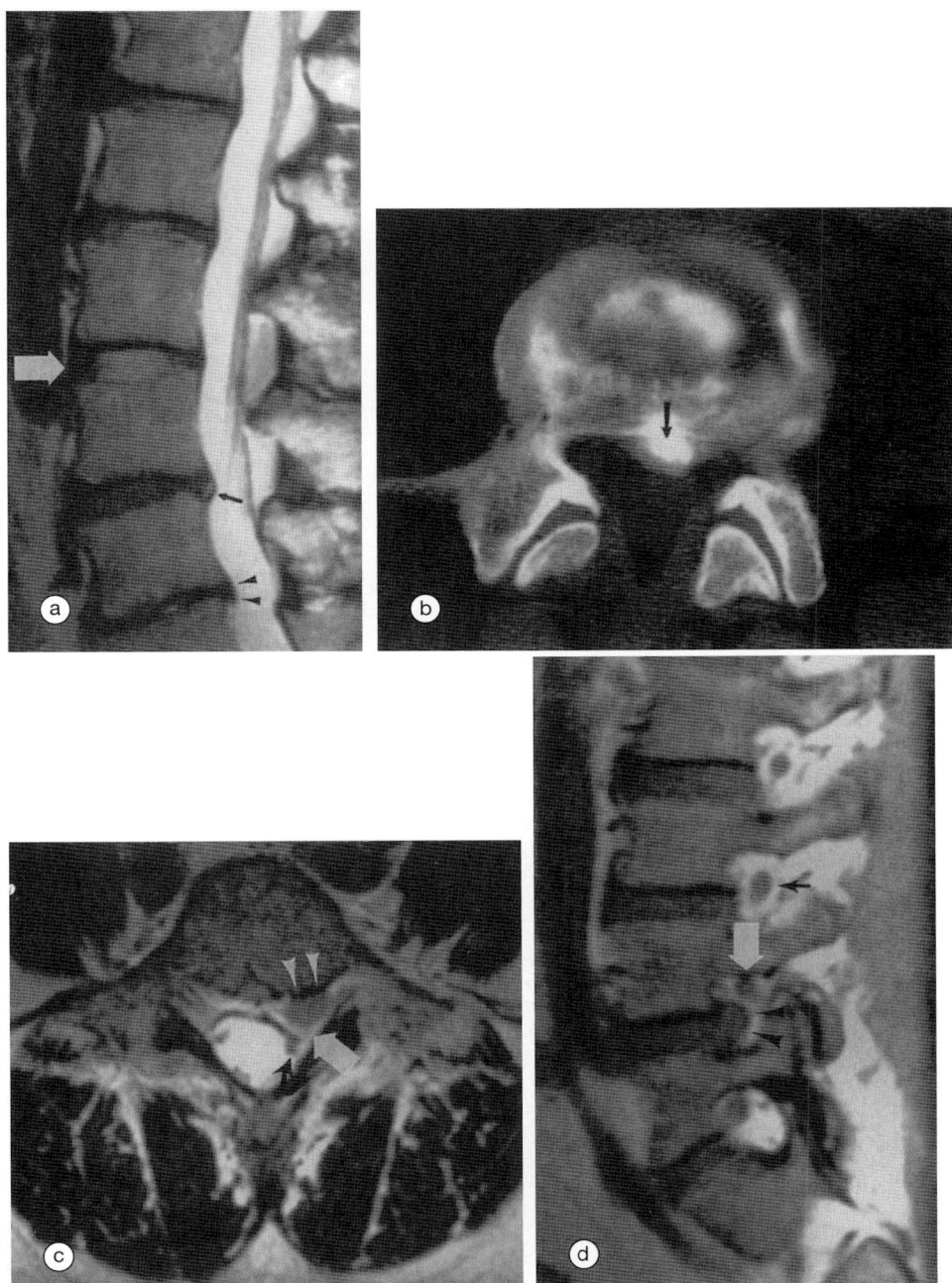

Figure 7-6 Various disk abnormalities. (**a**) T2-weighted sagittal magnetic resonance imaging (MRI) of the lumbar spine demonstrates normal height and hydration of the L3–L4 disk (thick arrow). The L5–S1 disk space is severely narrowed, with loss of hydration and low T2 signal intensity as well as a circumferential bulging of the disk (arrowheads). The L4–L5 disk space shows moderate loss of height and hydration, with a focal convexity to the posterior disk having a focus of increased T2 signal intensity (thin arrow), consistent with annular tear and protrusion. (**b**) Postdiskography computed tomography demonstrates extension of contrast material into a left central subannular region (arrow), consistent with an annular tear and protrusion. This disk lesion is similar to that seen at L4–L5 in (a). (**c**) Axial T2-weighted MRI of the lumbar spine demonstrates a focal convexity to the disk extending caudad from the left posterior aspect of the disk, consistent with a focal extrusion, as the depth is greater than the width (arrowheads). This extrusion impinges on the exiting left root just posterior (thick arrow) and deviates the descending root within the thecal sac just adjacent (arrow). (**d**). Sagittal T1-weighted MRI obtained more laterally at the intervertebral foramina shows a focal convexity to the L4–L5 disk, which extends cephalad into the intervertebral foramen (arrowheads) and deviates the exiting L4 root superiorly (thick white arrow), representing an intraforaminal extrusion. The adjacent normal intervertebral foramen shows a low-signal exiting root (black arrow) surrounded by high T1 signal foraminal fat.

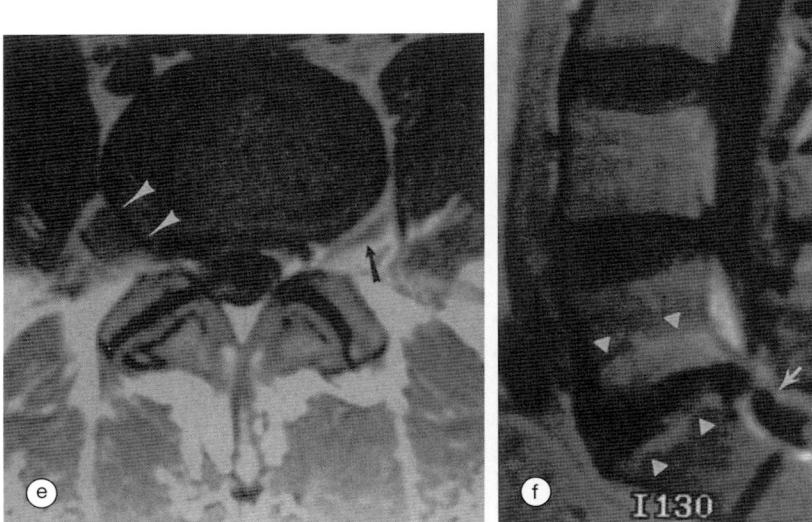

Figure 7-6 Continued. (**e**) Axial T1-weighted image of the lumbar spine demonstrates a focal convexity to the right far lateral disk (arrowheads) deviating the exited nerve root in comparison with the normally exiting root on the contralateral side (arrow). The disk abnormality has a depth similar to width, best described as an extrusion. (**f**) Sagittal T1-weighted image of the lumbar spine after intravenous injection of gadolinium contrast agent demonstrates narrowing of the L5–S1 disk space and degenerative changes of the adjacent end plate (arrowheads). Just caudad to the posterior aspect of the disk space is a non-enhancing mass (arrows) that is separate from the native disk space and best described as a free fragment or sequestered disk.

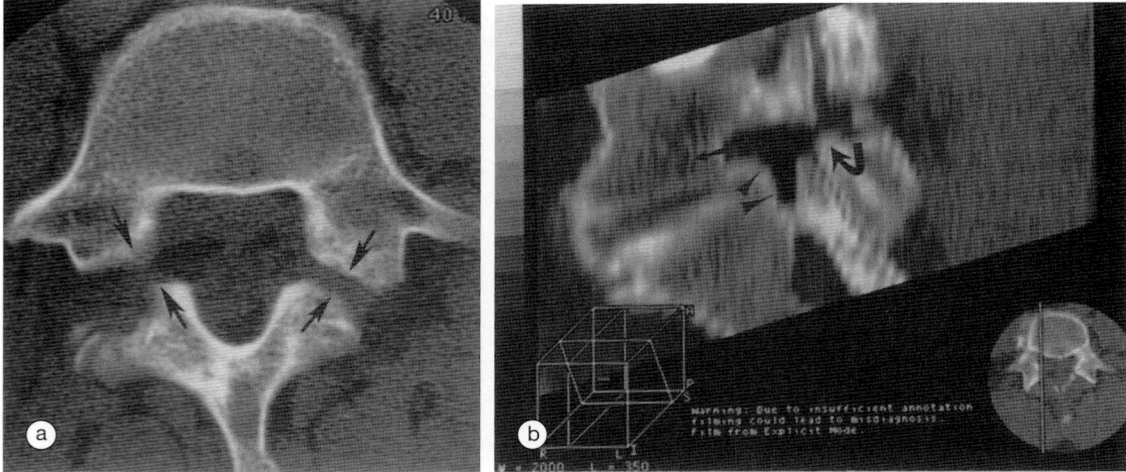

Figure 7-7 Computed tomography (CT) of pars interarticularis defects. (**a**) Axial CT scan demonstrates discontinuity of the lumbar vertebral ring (arrows). (**b**) Sagittal reformation of axial CT images obtained at a plane through the facet joints and pars interarticularis demonstrates the pars defects (curved arrow) as well as a grade 1 spondylolisthesis (straight arrow). The combination of disk space narrowing and anterolisthesis contributes to bony foraminal narrowing (arrowheads).

Facet joint abnormalities

Facet and pars interarticularis abnormalities can often be seen with plain radiography. Oblique views are necessary to assess for a pars defect (spondylolysis). Thin-section CT with bone detail is the most accurate means of assessing for a pars defect, and can demonstrate any hypertrophic bone formation at the facet or pars contributing to foraminal narrowing (Fig. 7-7). MRI is relatively insensitive to cortical bone defects, and so 30% of cases of lumbar spondylolysis might be undiagnosed if the physician relies on direct visualization of pars interarticularis defects.[116] However, 97% of levels of spondylolysis have been shown to yield one or more secondary MRI signs, including increased sagittal diameter of the spinal canal, wedging of the posterior aspect of the vertebral body, and reactive marrow changes in the pedicle distinct from normal adjacent levels.[116] Spondylolysis without spondylolisthesis can appear as widening of the sagittal dimension of the spinal canal because of dorsal subluxation of the posterior elements.[115] Fluoroscopy during

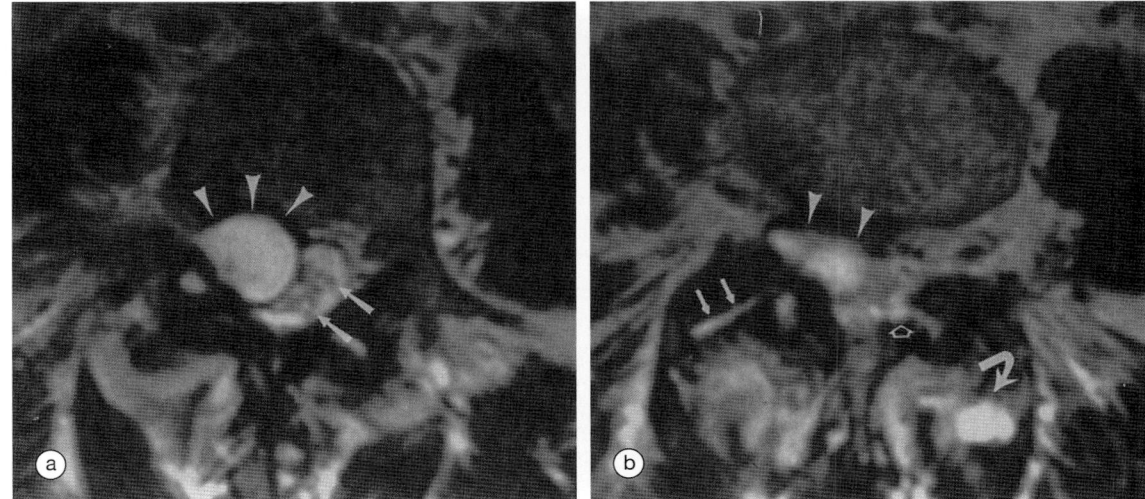

Figure 7-8 Magnetic resonance imaging of a large synovial cyst associated with facet degenerative joint disease. (**a**) Axial T2-weighted image of the lumbar spine demonstrates a right lateral extradural mass with high T2 signal (arrowheads) impinging on the thecal sac containing the descending roots (arrows). (**b**) An image obtained just inferior to that in (a) again shows the high T2 signal mass (arrowheads) as well as its association with a narrowed and sclerotic facet joint (arrows). On the left are two additional synovial cysts, with the smaller just medial to the facet joint (open arrow) and another just posterior to the facet joint (curved arrow).

facet joint injection below a pars defect shows flow of the contrast agent into the pars defect and often then to the facet joint above the pars defect.

Facet degenerative changes of sclerosis, joint space narrowing, and marginal osteophytosis can be shown on oblique plain radiographs but are optimally demonstrated with CT. MRI is relatively insensitive for demonstrating cortical bone or osteophyte, and shows foraminal narrowing indirectly by effacement of fat around the exiting root. Cartilage degeneration and sclerosis are related to age, lumbar spinal level, and overall facet joint angle, while tropism at the facet joints may result in slightly more sclerosis but not cartilage degeneration.[41]

Synovial cysts are best demonstrated on MRI, where the signal characteristics of the lateral extradural mass are usually those of fluid, with low T1 and high T2 signal (Fig. 7-8). This will also demonstrate the associated lateral recess stenosis. Postmyelography CT can also be diagnostic if the cyst is large enough to show water attenuation and the adjacent bony facet joint abnormalities are also shown.

Spinal stenosis

Spinal stenosis can be described as congenital–developmental or acquired. Acquired spinal stenosis can be further classified as central, lateral recess, and foraminal. Central and lateral recess stenosis is usually caused by a combination of disk degeneration, facet hypertrophic change, and ligamentum flavum enlargement. While MRI and CT myelography can both demonstrate narrowing of the spinal canal, myelography and postmyelographic CT have the additional benefit of showing facet bony detail and end plate osteophytosis, and allow upright weight-bearing views with flexion and extension, which often accentuate the stenosis. Symptoms of spinal stenosis are usually worse with standing or walking, and there is often a discrepancy in the imaging appearance when the patient is imaged standing

versus supine or prone. Foraminal narrowing is often well demonstrated on sagittal MRI images, where there is normally an exiting root surrounded by epiradicular fat. Disk space narrowing and consequent craniocaudal foraminal narrowing, any anterolisthesis, and facet hypertrophic change can be well shown on MRI. The cross-sectional measurement of the spinal canal and intervertebral foramina has been shown to change significantly with body position on a magnetic resonance scanner allowing upright and flexion–extension positioning, but few magnetic resonance scanners allow this positioning.[96]

Nerve roots

Visualization of the nerve roots is excellent on MRI, especially on sagittal images of the lumbar region and thin-section axial images of the cervical region. However, cervical myelography can be better at showing subtle impressions on the root sleeves that are difficult to discern on MRI. Furthermore, postmyelography CT affords a more accurate measurement of the foraminal caliber than MRI, for cervical foraminal narrowing is often accentuated by the pulse sequences used with MRI. Magnetic resonance neurography using high-resolution surface coils may show some correlation between abnormal increased T2 signal of a cervical root and associated radiculopathic symptoms.

Lumbar nerve root enhancement can correlate with root compression and radicular symptoms,[40,47] but transient enhancement at the affected level can be seen in asymptomatic patients in the first 6 months following surgery.[31] Indentation and swelling of the dorsal root ganglion may correlate with clinical symptoms.[125]

Postoperative spine imaging

Postoperative spine patients with residual or recurrent symptoms have special imaging considerations. Plain radiographs can often demonstrate any hardware malpositioning or failed

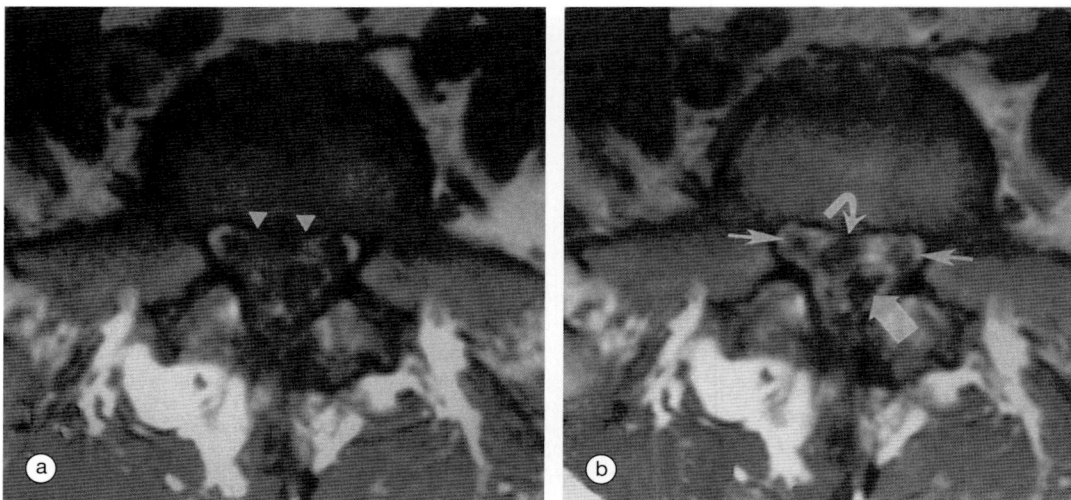

Figure 7-9 Magnetic resonance imaging of a recurrent disk extrusion after previous diskectomy. (**a**) Axial T1-weighted image obtained without contrast enhancement demonstrates low T1 signal material within the spinal canal and poor delineation of the thecal sac and nerve roots (arrowheads). (**b**) Postcontrast axial T1-weighted image obtained at the same level as that in (a) shows enhancement of epidural fibrosis and better delineation of the thecal sac (thick arrow), descending nerve roots (thin arrows), and recurrent disk extrusion (curved arrow).

fusion.[103] If hardware is present, both CT and MRI have some limitations,[111] as described previously. Flexion and extension plain radiographs can show motion at a failed fusion site. CT can show gas within the disk space (vacuum phenomenon), which is an indicator of movement. If the patient is asked to fully flex and then fully extend prior to CT, the vacuum phenomenon can develop and can be utilized as a sign of non-fusion. With posterior fusions, if the facet joint remains visible and there is resorption of fusion bone, this is an indicator of non-fusion. Persistent lucency above or below a bone plug or anterior fusion cage also suggests non-fusion if enough time has elapsed since the surgery.

Recurrent or residual disk extrusion is best assessed with MRI before and after intravenous contrast agent injection to differentiate extruded disk material from epidural scar or fibrosis (Fig. 7-9).[31] Extruded disk material does not show central enhancement during the first 15 min following intravenous gadolinium administration but may show some central enhancement later.[46] An extruded disk can exhibit superficial enhancement due to an inflammatory component or surrounding scar (the 'wrapped disk'). It might be reasonable to perform both MRI and CT myelography in problematic diagnoses, because some end plate osteophytes, calcified disk fragments, or facet osteophytes can be relatively invisible on MRI. Spearlike osteophytes impinging on the spinal cord or nerve roots might also be invisible on MRI.

The postoperative disk can show linear enhancement—two thin bands paralleling the end plates, sometimes with end plate enhancement—as well as enhancement at the curettage site in asymptomatic patients.[92]

Non-contrast-enhanced MRI, or myelography or postmyelography CT, is usually sufficient for imaging the cervical postoperative patient. Contrast-enhanced MRI sequences are not usually indicated in a cervical postoperative patient, as most operations are performed by the anterior approach and there is rarely scar formation in the cervical epidural space. If the patient has had a foraminotomy or surgical complication, then cervical spine MRI with contrast agent enhancement might be a consideration.

Infection

Classic plain radiographic findings of diskitis or osteomyelitis can clinch the diagnosis if disk space narrowing and end plate loss are shown. However, MRI can demonstrate the disk space narrowing, abnormal disk space signal, end plate loss, and adjacent changes in the vertebral marrow (Fig. 7-10).[54] There is a decrease in the normal high T1 signal from fatty marrow as well as increased T2 signal in the marrow. Most narrowed disk spaces exhibit low T2 signal from desiccation. If the T2 signal within the narrowed disk is increased, diskitis is a consideration. Vertebral end plate degenerative changes with low T1 and high T2 signal can mimic the marrow changes of osteomyelitis but are usually not associated with high disk T2 signal.

Postoperative diskitis or osteomyelitis can sometimes be problematic in that a postoperative disk can exhibit increased T2 signal from scar, and there might be degenerative marrow changes showing low T1 and high T2 signal edema. However, the end plates usually remain sharp and intact in the postoperative patient as opposed to in patients with osteomyelitis or diskitis. In the patient with infection, contrast-enhanced MRI is the best means of assessing for any epidural spread or paravertebral abscess.

Tumors and extraspinal abnormalities

Non-contrast-enhanced MRI is more sensitive in demonstrating vertebral metastatic disease than is radionuclide bone scan. MRI is especially sensitive (relative to radionuclide bone scan or plain radiography) in demonstrating myeloma involvement.[28] Bone

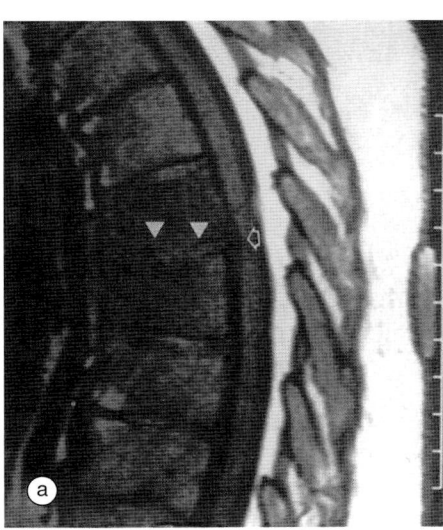
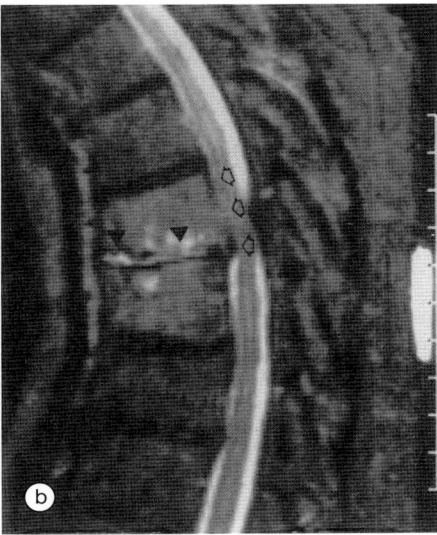

Figure 7-10 Magnetic resonance imaging of diskitis and osteomyelitis. (**a**) Sagittal T1-weighted image at the midline shows decreased signal within the thoracic vertebral bodies adjacent to a narrowed disk space with an irregular end plate (arrowheads). The spinal cord is indented ventrally at the disk level (open arrow). (**b**) Sagittal T2-weighted image obtained through the same area as (a) demonstrates increased T2 signal within the vertebral marrow and disk space with irregular end plates (arrowheads). There is a ventral extradural mass effect on the cord at the disk level and posterior to the vertebral body (open arrows), consistent with epidural extension of the infection.

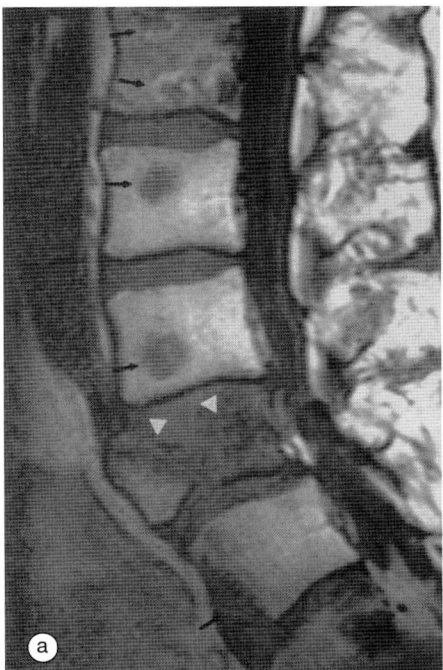
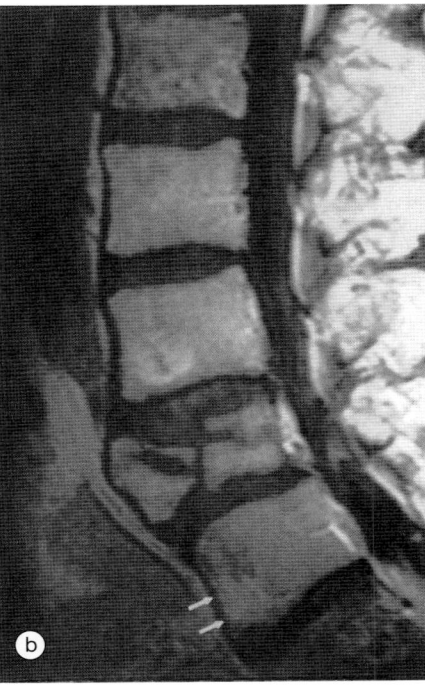

Figure 7-11 Magnetic resonance imaging of vertebral metastases before and after intravenous injection of gadolinium contrast. (**a**) Sagittal T1-weighted image of the lumbar spine obtained without contrast enhancement in a patient with multiple vertebral metastases (arrows) and L4 pathologic vertebral compression fracture (arrowheads) demonstrates predominantly low T1 signal of the lesions against the higher signal fatty marrow. (**b**) After intravenous injection of gadolinium contrast, the metastases enhance and become less conspicuous. The lesion involving the anterior aspect of the L5 vertebral body has become much less apparent (arrows). The tumor involving the L4 compressed vertebral body enhances to demonstrate the bony fragments.

scintigraphy, however, has the advantage of being able to survey the whole body for metastases. If the only area of interest is the vertebrae, then MRI can be both more sensitive and more specific. MRI also shows any extradural mass effect on the thecal sac, spinal cord, or nerve roots. STIR images are most sensitive for marrow-replacing tumors.[64] Intravenous gadolinium administration can actually make MRI less sensitive for vertebral metastases, as the usual appearance—low T1 signal metastases on a bed of high T1 signal fatty marrow—becomes less conspicuous with enhancement and increased T1 signal of the metastases (Fig. 7-11).

In the setting of a primary vertebral tumor, it is imperative to obtain plain radiographs and possibly CT scans as well to assess for chondroid or osteoid matrix. Radionuclide bone scan can be helpful in determining whether the tumor is monostotic or polyostotic.

Magnetic resonance imaging, with its multiplanar capabilities, can demonstrate extraspinal abnormalities,[75] but the field of view might be limited, as the images are usually tailored (and filmed) to the spinal structures. Coronal images of the spine can show causative paraspinal abnormalities in patients with scoliosis.

MUSCLE IMAGING

Muscle is seen as soft tissue attenuation on plain radiographs, demarcated by adjacent fat planes. Differentiation of the separate muscles and muscular abnormalities is usually not possible with plain radiography.

Imaging assessment of muscles includes assessment of position, size, and magnetic resonance signal intensity. CT can be used to assess for position and often for the size of the muscles. Except for hemorrhage within a muscle, there is little CT attenuation difference between normal and abnormal muscle. MRI is best for assessing muscle position, size, and pathologic changes.

Muscle position is assessed for evidence of retraction, as with a full-thickness muscle or tendon tear, such as with the supraspinatus tendon in rotator cuff injury. Anomalous muscles should not be confused with a tumor, such as an accessory soleus muscle causing an asymmetry between the calf muscles.

Muscle size can vary over a wide range of normal, but a large asymmetry can be indicative of muscle atrophy if there is volume loss, such as can be seen in the paraspinal muscles with previous poliomyelitis. Increased muscle size can be seen with weight training, but the muscles retain their normal magnetic resonance signal. Increased muscle size with abnormal signal intensity can be seen with muscle inflammation, edema, or contusion. Increased muscle size and abnormal signal can be seen with delayed-onset muscle soreness or rhabdomyolysis from exercise-induced injury.

Normal muscle has a low T1 and low to intermediate T2 signal. Increased T1 signal can be seen with old intramuscular hemorrhage or chronic fatty atrophy. On STIR sequences, an increased T2 signal within the muscle can be seen with trauma, inflammation, and acute to subacute denervation.

Muscle trauma can be graded on a spectrum from strain (grade 1) to partial tear (grade 2) to full-thickness tear (grade 3). Muscle strain is characterized by a mild, poorly circumscribed, increased T2 signal and greater increased STIR signal, with an intact muscle and no discrete fluid collections within the muscle. There can be some fluid collection in the fascial planes between muscles or beneath the muscle capsule.[14] A partial tear is characterized by a more discrete focus of increased T2 signal intensity, with possibly some disrupted muscle fibers or fluid tracking longitudinally between muscle fibers. There should be no retraction of the muscle. A full-thickness tear is characterized by retraction of the muscle and free edges, usually with material of increased T2 signal intensity in the gap.

Muscle strains are an indirect injury to muscle caused by excessive stretch. The muscles most commonly involved are those that contain the highest proportion of fast-twitch (type 2) muscle fibers: the hamstrings, quadriceps, adductors of the hip, medial gastrocnemius, triceps, biceps brachialis, and abdominal wall muscles. Muscles involved in eccentric action (lengthening), such as in the case of the hamstrings, are the most likely to be strained. Clinical grading can be difficult due

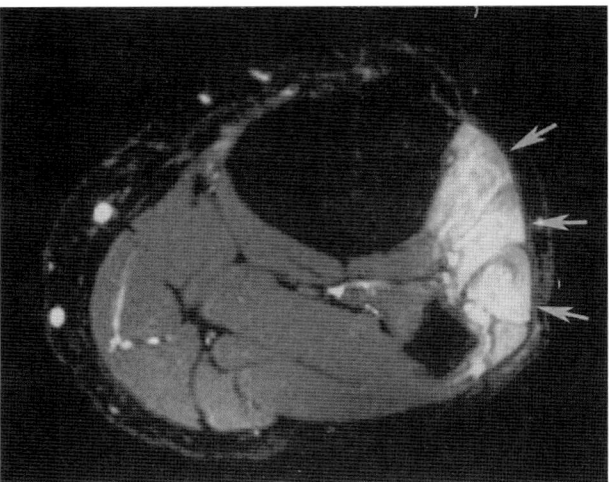

Figure 7-12 Axial short inversion time–inversion recovery image of the proximal leg demonstrates markedly increased signal in the tibialis anterior, extensor digitorum longus, and peroneus longus muscles (arrows) in a patient with peroneal nerve palsy clinically. These signal abnormalities resolved over a time course similar to that of the clinical improvement.

to swelling and pain. MRI allows detection and grading of complications such as hematoma or muscle herniation.

Acute to subacute denervation of muscle results in a mildly increased T2 signal and more prominently increased STIR signal.[93,122] Increased muscle signal in the acute to subacute stage changes to fatty atrophy with increased T1 signal, and loss of muscle mass in the chronic stage. Idiopathic peroneal nerve palsy can result in early changes of abnormal increased T2–STIR signal within the extensor digitorum longus and tibialis anterior muscle (Fig. 7-12). Acute to subacute denervation changes can be seen in the infraspinatus and supraspinatus muscles with impingement on the suprascapular nerve by a paralabral ('ganglion') cyst.[114] Transection of a muscle with proximal innervation can result in denervation changes distal to the transection or partial transection. Neurotoxic chemotherapy can result in a patchwork appearance of muscle signal changes.

NERVE IMAGING

The larger peripheral nerves can be imaged in cross-section on CT when they are surrounded by fat. They are better imaged with MRI, where they have a low T1 signal surrounded by high-signal fat, or with STIR sequences, where they have an intermediate to high signal surrounded by low-signal fat. MRI is excellent for assessing an extrinsic mass effect on nerves, such as in the spinoglenoid notch from a suprascapular paralabral cyst, or in the brachial plexus from a tumor. Intrinsic abnormalities of the nerves are more difficult to assess on routine MRI unless there is an enlargement of the nerve to indicate the level of abnormality. However, high-resolution experimental phased array surface coil imaging can show areas of intrinsic nerve abnormality.[60] The field of view can be relatively small with high-resolution scans, so the site of suspected abnormality needs to be established as accurately as possible prior to the scan.

TENDON IMAGING

As with muscle, CT can demonstrate tendon position and (to an extent) size but is unable to show intrinsic abnormalities. It is also sometimes limited by the fact that adjacent muscle, ligament, and tendon can have a similar CT attenuation. Tendons can be assessed in imaging studies for position, size, and magnetic resonance signal intensity.[9,35,49,98,126] The multiplanar capabilities and tissue discrimination available with MRI make it the best imaging modality to assess tendons.

Tendon position is assessed and shows retraction in the case of a complete rupture. Subluxation or dislocation of an intact tendon can be seen with the biceps tendon in a subscapularis tendon tear or transverse ligament tear.

Tendon caliber is best assessed in a true cross-section, which in some cases can require an oblique plane, as with curving of the peroneal tendons behind the lateral malleolus.[49] Imaging in planes tangential to the tendon can be compromised by partial voluming with adjacent fat. Assessment of tendons should include the musculotendinous junction, where many of the traumatic injuries occur.

Tendon size is easily comparable between extremities as well as between adjacent tendons (Fig. 7-13). Tibialis posterior tendon tears are graded as from 1 to 3. Grade 1 is a partial tear

with enlargement of the tendon and longitudinal split. Grade 2 is a partial tendon tear with attenuation of size and disruption of some of the tendon fibers. Grade 3 is a full-thickness tendon tear with retraction of the tendon.[90] Enlargement of a tendon can be seen with an acute partial tear, and longitudinal split with fluid between the tendon fibers, with a chronic tendon tear and scar tissue increasing the girth of the tendon, as well as with acute or chronic tendinitis. The signal characteristics of the enlarged tendon help to differentiate these entities.[126]

The normal tendon is of very low, homogeneous T1 and T2 signal intensity. The magic angle phenomenon can artifactually increase signal intensity within the tendon when it is coursing at a 55° angle to the main magnetic field. The problem is greatest at the supraspinatus tendon in the rotator cuff[113] and at the ankle tendons as they course around the malleoli. In these two cases, the region of artifactually increased signal is unfortunately also that where pathology is most likely to be seen.

Increased T1 and proton density signal in tendons can be seen with tendinosis (degeneration) or with tendinitis. Tendinosis usually becomes less evident with increasing T2 weighting, whereas tendinitis might or might not. Fluid or hemorrhage within the tendon becomes increasingly evident with increased T2 weighting. Chronic scarring of the tendon is usually of low signal intensity on all sequences, similar to the native tendon, and may appear as an enlargement of the tendon.

Fluid within the tendon sheath can be a normal finding in specific tendons, such as tendons of the biceps, or flexor hallucis longus. This is due to both of them being in communication with the joint space. Fluid within other tendon sheaths, such as in the peroneus longus tendon sheath, can be indicative of a calcaneofibular ligament tear with fluid extending from the mortise joint. Synovitis is also a consideration when fluid is seen between the tendon sheath and a normal tendon. Tenosynovitis is suspected when fluid is seen between the tendon sheath and an enlarged tendon. Fluid surrounding a tendon that has no tendon sheath, such as the Achilles tendon, is consistent with a peritendonitis, shown best on T2-weighted images with fat saturation.

LIGAMENT IMAGING

Ligaments can be indirectly assessed on plain radiographs by the presence of subluxation or dislocation, or movement with stress maneuvers. The Telos stress examination is used to assess the ankle ligaments with posteriorly directed and varus stress.[20] Three-compartment arthrography is utilized to indirectly assess the carpal ligaments for rupture.[124]

Direct visualization of ligaments is best performed with MRI.[20,50,80,87,99,107,117] Ligaments are assessed for continuity, size, and signal intensity.

A ligament should be continuous between insertions, with a smooth linear or curvilinear contour. Waviness of the ligament is consistent with a tear and partial retraction. Some ligaments will have a normal curvature in certain joint positions, and this should be taken into account during assessment. For example,

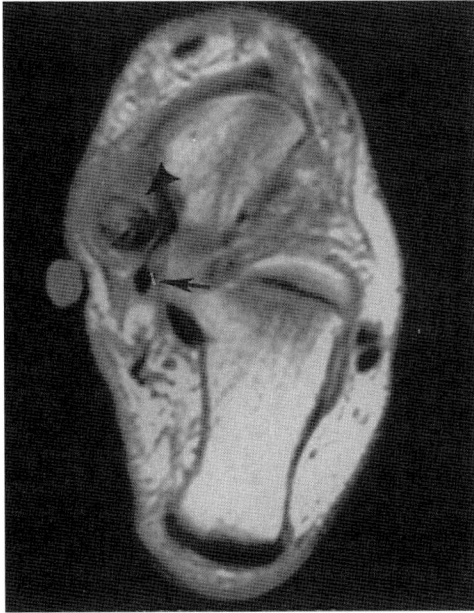

Figure 7-13 Axial T1-weighted image of the hind foot demonstrates a grade 1 partial tear and longitudinal split with enlargement and increased signal in the tibialis posterior tendon (arrowhead) and lower signal surrounding the tendon, consistent with soft tissue edema. The tendon is markedly enlarged in comparison with the adjacent flexor digitorum longus tendon (arrow), which shows a uniform low signal intensity and normal caliber.

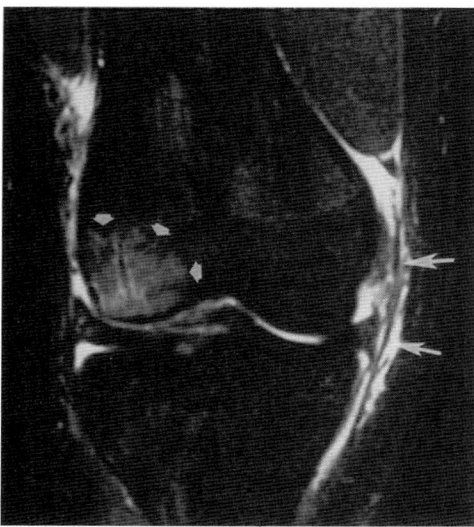

Figure 7-14 Coronal short inversion time–inversion recovery image of the knee demonstrates high-signal fluid deep and superficial to the medial collateral ligament (arrows), which is avulsed from its femoral attachment, indicating grade 3 (complete) tear. Increased signal intensity within the lateral femoral condyle (short arrows) is consistent with a bone bruise, as may be seen with a varus injury at the knee.

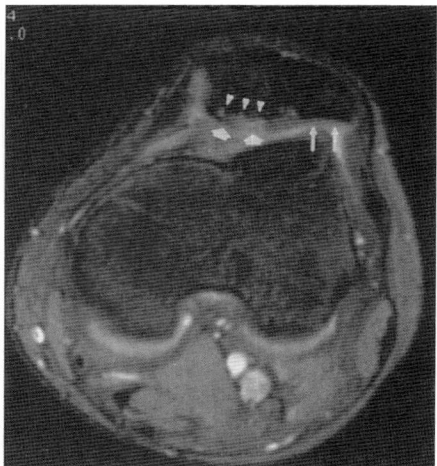

Figure 7-15 Axial proton density fat-suppressed image of the knee demonstrates grade 3 and grade 4 chondromalacia of the patellar cartilage. Focal loss of cartilage to the bone (short arrows) is accompanied by abnormal signal within the adjacent marrow (arrowheads). A small area of normal cartilage shows intermediate signal intensity and normal underlying cortex (thin arrows).

the posterior cruciate ligament (PCL) takes a more curvilinear course with the knee in extension and a more linear course with the knee in flexion. The course of the ligament must also be assessed, in that some complete ligament tears can heal in an abnormal position, such as a chronic anterior cruciate ligament (ACL) tear that has healed in a more horizontal position.[117]

Knowledge of the range of normal ligament calibers is helpful during assessment. Many ligaments, such as the anterior talofibular ligament, are uniform in thickness along their lengths. Others, however, comprise multiple smaller fascicles and can assume a more fan-shaped appearance, such as the posterior inferior tibiofibular ligament. Thickening or thinning of the ligament can occur with an acute or a chronic partial tear.

Ligaments have homogeneous, low T1 and low T2 signal intensity on MRI. Increased T1 and T2–STIR signal intensity within or around the ligament is suggestive of a sprain or partial tear. A complete tear disrupts the ligament, usually with intervening high T2 signal intensity in the acute stage (Fig. 7-14). A healing or healed full-thickness ligament tear might show low T2 signal material at the site of the tear, making it more difficult to delineate the location or even the presence of a tear.[117]

CARTILAGE IMAGING

Cartilage thickness cannot be directly seen on plain radiographs, although secondary changes of severe chondromalacia—such as joint space narrowing, subcortical sclerosis, and cyst formation—can be seen.[44] Chondrocalcinosis is probably best detected on plain radiographs. Arthrography can demonstrate the thickness and surface contour of hyaline cartilage, as can postarthrography CT.[44] MRI and magnetic resonance arthrography best demonstrate cartilage thickness, contour, and any intrinsic signal abnormalities.[44,88] Fat-suppressed proton density images show excellent contrast between bone, cartilage, and intraarticular fluid (Fig. 7-15).[88]

There are four arthroscopic stages of chondromalacia. The earliest chondromalacia appears as a small focus of softening. This grade of chondromalacia might not be visible on MRI, but with probing it can be identified as a focal soft area on arthroscopy. Grade 2 chondromalacia is a focally increased thickness, with the cartilage showing some increased T2 signal, like a small blister or edema. Grade 3 chondromalacia is a thinning and focal irregularity of cartilage. Grade 4 chondromalacia is loss of cartilage down to the bone, possibly with additional cortical sclerosis and/or cystic changes.

Magnetic resonance arthrography is superior to CT arthrography for demonstrating osseous and cartilaginous intraarticular bodies.[17] MRI and CT without intraarticular contrast are less accurate than either magnetic resonance arthrography or CT arthrography.

BONE IMAGING

Plain radiography is the initial screening procedure for assessing fractures throughout the body, except in the skull, where head CT is the initial procedure of choice. Orthogonal views of the body part of interest are mandatory to exclude a fracture. Some regions require a special view, such as a mortise view in the ankle; an oblique view in the hand, wrist, and foot; and an axillary or transscapular view in the shoulder.

Non-contrast-enhanced CT with or without multiplanar reformatting is utilized to assess the position of fracture fragments in more complex fractures, such as those involving the wrist or ankle–foot. Preoperative assessment of highly comminuted fractures can include CT.[59]

Magnetic resonance imaging is insensitive in assessing cortical bone. MRI images mobile hydrogen, and cortical bone has very little mobile hydrogen. MRI does well in assessing bone marrow, as well as bone marrow edema, making it quite sensitive to any fractures or processes that change the normal bone marrow signal. Fat within the bone marrow gives marrow a high T1 signal, depending on the degree of fatty versus red marrow, and a lower T2 signal. Consequently, any process that decreases the T1 signal and increases the T2 signal, such as edema or intratrabecular hemorrhage, might be quite conspicuous on MRI. The high sensitivity of MRI to bone marrow signal changes is best shown on non-contrast-enhanced T1-weighted images and highly T2-weighted or STIR images. Intravenous contrast enhancement of marrow processes can decrease the conspicuity of the abnormality in relation to the high T1 signal intensity of marrow.

Magnetic resonance imaging is highly sensitive in the detection of reticular infractions (bone bruises), geographic infractions, stress or insufficiency fractures (Fig. 7-16), osteochondral fractures, and (indirectly) macrofractures.[16,77,118] Bone bruises can occur in typical locations for a given injury, such as lateral knee bone bruises with the 'terrible triad of O'Donohue', the medial patellar facet and lateral femoral condyle with a patellar dislocation, and anteroinferior glenoid with an anteroinferior humeral dislocation. These bone bruises can be the only sign of a previous dislocation if there has been spontaneous reduction. Some authors have thought that osteochondral defects can be a sequela of certain geographic infractions.[118]

Palmer et al. showed in 78 fractures of the knee and shoulder that MRI demonstrates prominent marrow edema with impaction fractures, and minimal edema with distraction fractures.[77] Impaction fractures are more often missed on plain radiographs,

while distraction fractures (such as Segond fractures) are more often missed on MRI.

The ACR has appropriateness criteria for imaging of suspected stress or insufficiency fractures (excluding vertebral fractures). Eleven different clinical scenarios are presented, each with recommended imaging studies. The first imaging study should be plain radiography.

Assessment for AVN should initially be performed with plain radiography. If the study is negative, then MRI imaging is highly sensitive and specific for AVN.[25] Bone scintigraphy might be able to demonstrate AVN in earlier stages as 'cold spots'. However, there is a crossover period when AVN might not be detected by bone scan, between when the bone scan is 'cold' and when it becomes 'hot'.[25] Even if a hip radiograph indicates AVN, MRI can be considered to assess for asymptomatic AVN in the contralateral hip. MRI is useful in assessing the percent involvement of the femoral head, as well as in characterizing the marrow signal within the avascular region. The 'double-line sign' of low and high T2 signal intensity at the margin of AVN is a relatively specific finding seen in 80% of cases.[67]

Osteochondritis dissecans in its intermediate to severe stages can be well shown on plain radiographs and non-contrast-enhanced CT scans. The earliest phase of geographic marrow edema is not visible on plain radiographs, but it is well shown on magnetic resonance, especially STIR sequences (Fig. 7-17). Magnetic resonance further shows the condition of the cartilage overlying the bony defect and can show if there is loosening, indicated by high T2 signal fluid extending around the lesion or displacement of the osteochondral fragment.[44]

BONE AND SOFT TISSUE TUMORS

The ACR appropriateness criteria for suspected primary bone tumors list routine radiography as an absolute requirement in a patient with a suspected bone lesion. If the radiograph is normal and there is focal pain, then MRI is the second imaging study. If the radiograph shows a lesion suspicious for malignancy, MRI is indicated, and if the lesion appears benign on radiographs, CT or MRI is indicated only for preoperative planning. If the lesion is a suspected osteoid osteoma, CT is recommended.

Non-contrast-enhanced CT can be considered for more accurate localization of bone lesions or assessment of any cartilaginous or osteoid matrix or cortical involvement. A whole body bone scan is useful to assess the entire skeleton to determine whether the lesion is single or multiple. Sometimes, bone tumor magnetic resonance signal can be pathognomonic, such as with an intraosseous lipoma with uniform high T1 fatty signal, or an aneurysmal bone cyst with blood product layering. However, a significant percentage of lesions cannot be accurately categorized as benign or malignant with MRI, even with plain radiographic correlation.[57] MRI is effective at demonstrating origin, margins, and extension into bone marrow or adjacent soft tissue structures, as well as subperiosteal tracking and marrow 'skip' lesions.

The ACR has appropriateness criteria ratings for imaging metastatic bone disease in 15 different clinical scenarios. In

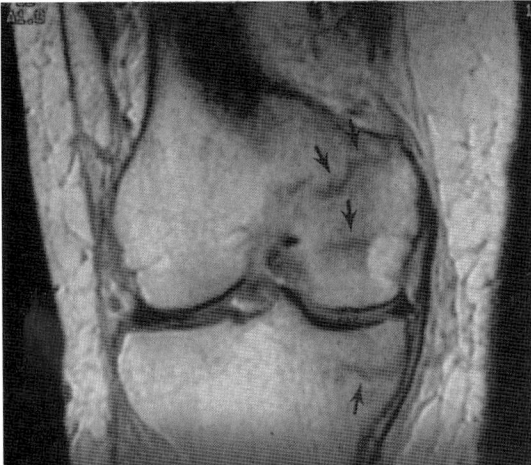

Figure 7-16 Coronal T1-weighted magnetic resonance imaging of the knee demonstrates stress fractures of the medial femoral condyle and medial tibial plateau with serpentine linear low T1 signal (arrows) on a background of high T1 signal fatty marrow.

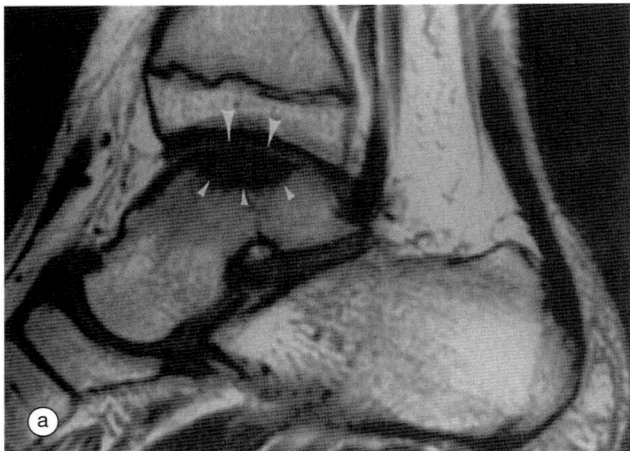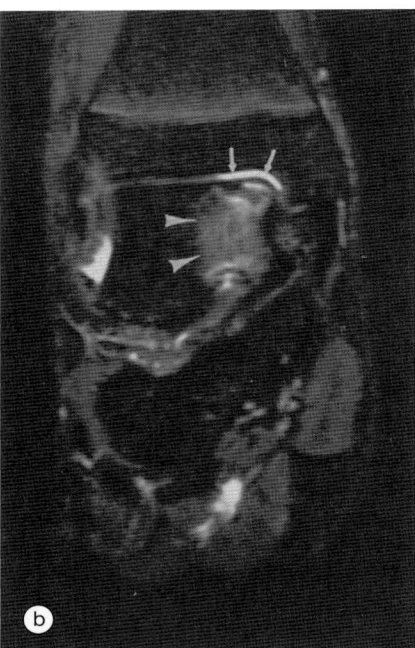

Figure 7-17 Magnetic resonance imaging appearance of talar dome osteochondritis dissecans. (**a**) Sagittal T1-weighted image of the hind foot demonstrates a geographic focus of decreased T1 signal within the talar dome (small arrowheads). There is irregularity to the cortex overlying this lesion (large arrowheads). (**b**) Coronal short inversion time–inversion recovery (STIR) image in the same patient demonstrates increased signal at the medial talar dome, with at least a portion of the lesion having intact overlying cortex (arrows). The signal abnormality from bone marrow edema is more conspicuous on the STIR sequence (arrowheads) than on the T1-weighted sequence.

some scenarios, no imaging is recommended, and in others a different combination of plain radiography, bone scan, MRI, and/or CT is considered most appropriate.

The ACR appropriateness criteria indicate routine radiography as the first imaging study for suspected soft tissue mass. MRI is usually the second imaging examination recommended, except that CT can be useful for characterizing types of calcification and assessing myositis ossificans. It can possibly be more useful than MRI in areas with motion artifact. MRI is thought to be the most useful study to assess extension into bone marrow and adjacent soft tissues, while also providing multiplanar delineation of the tumor.

Certain magnetic resonance signal characteristics can be helpful in characterizing soft tissue masses, such as high T1 signal fat with a lipoma or liposarcoma, or low-signal hemosiderin with pigmented villonodular synovitis. MRI is useful for primary subjective identification of some benign lesions (lipoma, superficial and deep skeletal muscle hemangiomas, arteriovenous malformations, periarticular cysts, hematomas), but for tumors with a non-specific imaging appearance MRI is not reliable for distinguishing benign from malignant tumors.[57,69]

To be considered benign, cystic lesions must meet three MRI criteria.

1. Signal intensities that are homogeneous and lower than those of muscle on T1-weighted images.
2. T2 signal intensities homogeneously bright and similar to those of fluid.
3. A uniformly thin rim, which may or may not enhance.[58]

A thick rim, a multiseptated thick rim, or nodular components suggest that a simple cyst is not present.

IMAGING OF SPECIFIC BODY REGIONS
Shoulder imaging
In the trauma setting, plain radiography is the initial imaging study of choice for the shoulder. Internal rotation and external rotation views, as well as an orthogonal view such as axillary or transscapular view, should be obtained. A posterior dislocation could theoretically be missed if only internal and external rotation views are obtained, unless one recognizes that there is limited rotation between the views because of the dislocation.

The ACR appropriateness criteria for imaging in the setting of acute shoulder trauma to rule out fracture or dislocation recommend an anteroposterior view and an axillary lateral or scapular Y view as most appropriate. If a patient has persistent shoulder pain and has had normal radiographs within the preceding 2 weeks, there is no consensus as to the most appropriate study. Some experts say that MRI is indicated, and some recommend repeating plain radiography. In the patient with subacute shoulder pain and a question of bursitis or calcific tendinitis of approximately 3 months' duration, the first study recommended is radiography with internal and external rotation views.

Impingement and rotator cuff tears
The ACR appropriateness criteria indicate routine MRI for suspected rotator cuff tear or impingement in patients over the

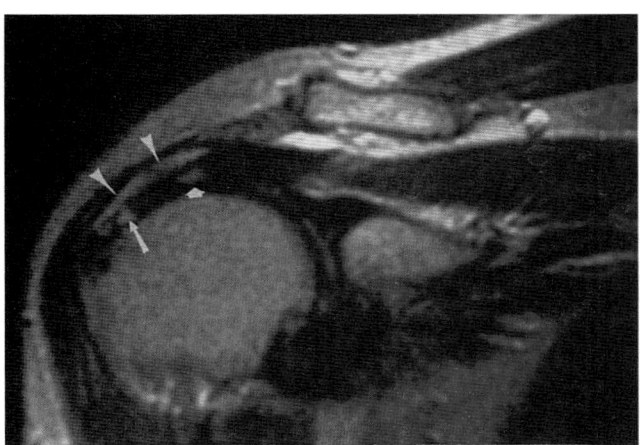

Figure 7-18 Coronal oblique T2-weighted image of the shoulder demonstrates a full-thickness tear of the distal supraspinatus tendon (arrow), with high T2 signal extending through the thickness of the tendon and increased T2 signal fluid within the subacromial–subdeltoid bursa (arrowheads). Increased T2 signal from a partial-thickness tear does not completely extend through the tendon (short arrow).

age of 40 with normal plain radiographs. Direct visualization of the tendons and muscles, as well as detection of indirect evidence of rotator cuff tear, is available with MRI (Fig. 7-18).[36,83,102] Coronal oblique and sagittal oblique planes of imaging (perpendicular and tangential to the plane of the glenoid) are utilized to obtain images parallel or perpendicular to the muscles and tendons of the rotator cuff.

Assessment of rotator cuff tendon position, thickness, and signal intensity is optimal with MRI. Early impingement results in thickening of the tendon, usually of the supraspinatus. More advanced tendinopathy results in thinning of the tendon. When the rotator cuff abnormality progresses to a partial-thickness tear, there is increased T1, proton density, and T2 signal intensity within the tendon that reflects a morphologic thinning. A full-thickness tear shows through and through increased signal. The position of the musculotendinous junction can be identified to determine whether there is any retraction from a full-thickness rotator cuff tear. The proximodistal and anteroposterior dimensions of a rotator cuff tear can be estimated. Unenhanced MRI is much less sensitive for partial tears than for full-thickness tears.[6]

Partial and complete rotator cuff tears can be seen on MRI in a significant percentage of asymptomatic individuals, the percentage increasing with age.[72] MRI-evident bone and peritendinous shoulder abnormalities are highly prevalent among asymptomatic individuals, but the prevalence of subacromial spurs, humeral head cysts, subacromial–subdeltoid bursal fluid, and disruption of the peribursal fat plane in each case is closely associated with an increasing severity of MRI-evident rotator cuff abnormalities.[72]

Contrast-enhanced arthrography with plain radiographs might demonstrate only articular side partial tears and not bursal side tears. Full-thickness tears can be shown with contrast-enhanced arthrography, but the size of the tear and the condition of the torn edges are poorly defined. Plain radiographs are useful for assessing for undersurface osteophytes at the acromion and acromioclavicular joint. They can also reveal the calcification of calcific tendinitis. Factors predisposing to impingement, such as undersurface osteophytes or a laterally down-sloping acromion, can be detected using either arthrography or MRI. Ultrasound is sometimes used to assess for rotator cuff tear, but it is highly operator-dependent and provides less information than MRI does.

In the postoperative rotator cuff repair patient with a question of complication or recurrent tear, MRI is the best imaging technique. However, scar tissue in the rotator cuff can sometimes be associated with an abnormal signal intensity pattern mimicking that of a recurrent tear. Arthrography or MRI with intraarticular contrast agent instillation can be helpful to assess for a recurrent tear and passage of fluid through the tendon, and to differentiate the condition from the abnormal signal in the tendon from scar.[68] Postarthrography CT is useful to assess for dislodgement of Mitek anchors used for rotator cuff repair.

Glenoid labral lesions and instability

The ACR appropriateness criteria committee could not reach a consensus on a recommended imaging study when there is a suspicion of instability or labral tear, but listed CT arthrography, MRI, or magnetic resonance arthrography as all being appropriate. CT can better show fractures of the bony glenoid. CT arthrography yields high-definition images of the labrum, but the study is limited in its multiplanar capabilities and gives less information about any other possible causes of shoulder pain.[21] Unenhanced MRI[43] and magnetic resonance arthrography[7,8] allow multiplanar imaging, which can be useful for assessing superior labral tears on coronal oblique images (Fig. 7-19), the inferior glenohumeral ligament on sagittal oblique and axial images, and the biceps tendon and rotator cuff. Non-enhanced MRI does not outline the labral structures as well as magnetic resonance arthrography if there is no significant effusion present, but some researchers have shown a high accuracy with unenhanced MRI.[43] Some experts prefer to use magnetic resonance arthrography to assess the labrum and biceps–labral complex. The glenohumeral ligaments are best shown with postarthrography MRI.[8] The abduction–external rotation position has been shown to best demonstrate the inferior glenohumeral ligaments,[52] but this position requires a longer imaging time and repositioning of the patient during the examination.

The labrum is evaluated for morphology, signal intensity, and position. There is variability in labral morphology, especially at the superior aspect of the anterior labrum.[56] Superior labral anterior to posterior lesions and involvement of the biceps–labral complex are ideally shown following intraarticular contrast agent injection, where there is insinuation of the contrast agent between the cartilage and the superior labrum. The axial images can show a Hill–Sachs lesion or Bankhardt lesion of the bony glenoid or labrum if the patient has had a previous anteroinferior humeral dislocation.

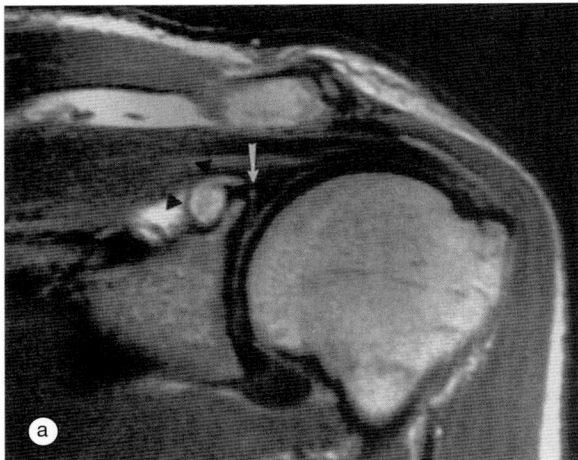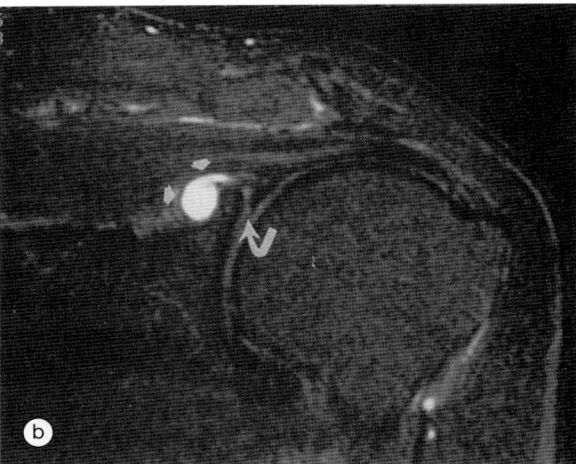

Figure 7-19 Magnetic resonance imaging appearance of a superior labral anterior to posterior lesion and paralabral cyst. (**a**) Proton density coronal oblique image of the shoulder demonstrates a superior labral tear with increased signal intensity between the superior labrum and the bony glenoid (arrow). Just adjacent to this is a comma-shaped paralabral cyst (arrowheads). (**b**) Coronal oblique T2-weighted fat-suppressed image demonstrates the labral tear (curved arrow), as well as the high-signal cyst (short arrows), more conspicuously. Denervation changes are not seen in the supraspinatus muscle, which is located just superior to the paralabral cyst and is innervated by the suprascapular nerve, which courses near the cyst.

Impingement on the suprascapular nerve, the first takeoff of the brachial plexus, is relatively common and can cause denervation of the infraspinatus and possibly supraspinatus muscles.[93] Suprascapular ganglion cysts (paralabral cysts) are well demonstrated on MRI, with high T2–STIR signal intensity. It is thought that most, if not all, suprascapular ganglion cysts are associated with labral tears,[114] but labral tears are often not demonstrated on MRI in these patients.

Elbow imaging

Plain radiography in orthogonal planes is the first imaging study that should be obtained in the trauma setting. The posterior fat pad sign or anterior 'sail' sign is indirect evidence of a fracture. Fractures in a child's elbow can be more difficult to assess on plain radiographs because of incomplete ossification, and MRI can be helpful in these cases.

Because of its multiplanar capabilities and excellent contrast resolution, MRI is the best modality for assessing the elbow for muscular, ligamentous, or tendinous injuries; bone marrow edema; or osteochondral injury (Fig. 7-20).[37,79,108] Coronal imaging ideally assesses the collateral ligaments, and the extensor and flexor tendons. The annular ligament and the distal biceps tendon are best assessed on axial images.[35] Magnetic resonance arthrography can better show partial tears of the ulnar collateral ligament than unenhanced MRI can.[71,97]

Lateral epicondylitis ('tennis elbow') can manifest with increased T2 signal intensity and thickening of the common extensor tendon. Medial epicondylitis ('Little Leaguer's elbow' in children, medial tendinosis or 'golfer's elbow' in adults) can manifest with bone marrow edema and medial epicondyle apophyseal separation in children, and with increased T2–STIR signal intensity and thickening of the common flexor pronator tendons and muscles in adults. Valgus stress on the ulnar collateral ligament can result in traction osteophytes if chronic,

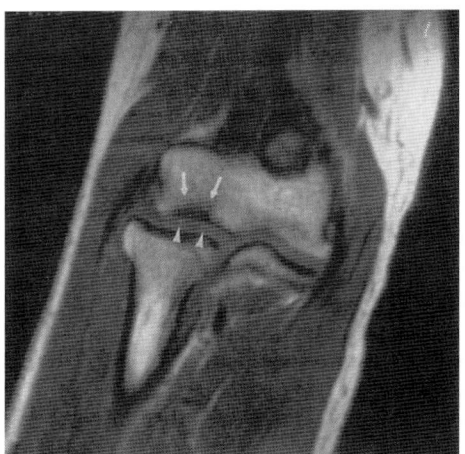

Figure 7-20 Coronal T1-weighted image of the elbow demonstrates osteochondritis dissecans of the capitellum (arrows) as a low T1 signal abnormality against normal fatty marrow. The overlying cartilage (arrowheads) appears intact.

while acute trauma can result in a sprain, a partial tear, or a full-thickness tear, with imaging characteristics similar to those of ligament injuries elsewhere in the body.[38,66]

Magnetic resonance imaging can be useful for assessing ulnar nerve abnormalities at the elbow if there is an abnormality of size, signal, or position.[89,108]

Wrist and hand imaging

In the setting of suspected wrist or hand fracture, preferably at least three radiographic views should be obtained: orthogonal anteroposterior, lateral views, and an oblique view. If a scaphoid fracture is suspected, an additional scaphoid view can be obtained that lays out the length of the scaphoid. A carpal tunnel view can be useful in a suspected fracture of the hook of the hamate. Knowledge of the clinical history and examination findings is helpful in determining which additional views are necessary to exclude a fracture. Some scaphoid fractures are occult and should be reimaged 7–10 days following the initial injury if there is a high suspicion of scaphoid fracture and snuffbox tenderness. The patient should be splinted until the follow-up radiograph. Alternatively, MRI is quite sensitive for occult fractures of the scaphoid and distal radius[16] where there is bone marrow edema and/or intratrabecular hemorrhage early after fracture.[105] ACR appropriateness criteria for chronic wrist pain include 12 clinical settings with initial imaging being plain radiographs. Some of the clinical scenarios then list magnetic resonance, CT, or arthrography as the next step in the imaging work-up.

Sacroiliac joint imaging

Anteroposterior angled and bilateral oblique views of the sacroiliac joints are the standard initial work-up. Limited sacroiliac joint CT has proved to be a cost-competitive screening examination that has higher sensitivity for subtle erosive changes of the sacroiliac joints and in the detection of subtle sclerosis.

Hip and pelvis imaging

In the trauma setting, orthogonal plain radiography is the initial imaging study. CT can be considered in the setting of more complex acetabular and pelvic fractures to aid in surgical planning.[25,81] Fractures, muscle injuries, and soft tissue injuries can be detected with MRI of the pelvis in patients with non-revealing radiographs after acute trauma.[12,62] CT is the preferred modality for assessment of osseous-based abnormalities of the hip, and MRI is the preferred modality, following plain radiography, to image AVN, marrow replacement processes, musculoskeletal tumors, and osteomyelitis.[25] Magnetic resonance arthrography has a much higher accuracy than non-enhanced MRI in the detection and staging of acetabular labral lesions when the labrum is being assessed for abnormalities of morphology, signal intensity, the presence or absence of a tear, and attachment to the acetabulum.[27]

Avascular necrosis

In the setting of unilateral or bilateral hip pain when AVN is suspected clinically, anteroposterior pelvis and frog leg lateral views of the hip or hips are the most appropriate initially, according to the ACR appropriateness criteria. If there is evidence of AVN on plain films, MRI can be considered to assess for occult AVN in the contralateral hip. If plain radiographs are suspicious but not definite for AVN, or if there is a high clinical suspicion of AVN with normal plain radiographs, then MRI is the most sensitive and specific imaging study to assess for AVN.

Painful prostheses

In the patient with a painful hip or knee prosthesis and a clinical suspicion of loosening or infection, the ACR appropriateness criteria give a most appropriate rating to plain radiography with comparison with prior studies, as the first imaging study. If the initial plain radiographs are normal but there is clinical suspicion of loosening or infection, then joint aspiration with or without arthrography is considered the most appropriate study. If the plain radiographs are abnormal and consistent with loosening but infection is suspected, then aspiration, possibly with arthrography, is considered most appropriate. If aspiration is purulent, arthrography is contraindicated because increased pressure within the joint can lead to intravasation and hematogenous seeding of the infection.

Knee imaging

In the trauma setting, the minimum initial examination includes orthogonal anteroposterior and lateral views. If there is a high clinical suspicion of fracture or lipohemarthrosis, then further views, such as bilateral oblique, sunrise, and/or tunnel notch, should be considered.[19] Bone bruise or occult stress fracture are best shown with MRI. MRI in a study of 84 patients with acute knee injury was shown to decrease the number of arthroscopic procedures, improve clinician diagnostic certainty, and change the management proposed prior to MRI.[61] MRI prior to arthroscopy in 50 patients who met clinical criteria for knee arthroscopy showed that 42% of the arthroscopies were unnecessary.[18]

The ACR appropriateness criteria recommend imaging studies for 12 variants of non-traumatic knee pain. The mandatory minimum initial study consists of anteroposterior and lateral plain radiographs, with an axial patellar view added if there are anterior patellofemoral symptoms. If the initial radiographs are normal or show joint effusion, then MRI is considered the next appropriate study. When the initial plain radiographs are abnormal, then other additional studies might or might not be considered appropriate.

Meniscal injuries

Magnetic resonance imaging is the best method of assessing the meniscus in a patient who has not previously undergone surgery.[24,48] MRI is non-invasive and multiplanar, allowing assessment of the meniscus. Radial imaging planes can be obtained that give similar views to those seen with knee arthrography.

Menisci are described according to the following scheme.

- Normal, with homogeneous low signal intensity on all sequences and normal morphology.
- Grade 1: degenerative change manifesting as poorly circumscribed, increased T1 or proton density signal intensity within the meniscus not contacting an articular surface.
- Grade 2: degenerative change manifesting as a horizontal line of increased T1 or proton density signal intensity within the meniscus that does not contact an articular surface.
- Grade 3: torn, manifesting as abnormal signal intensity extending from the meniscus to an articular surface, or

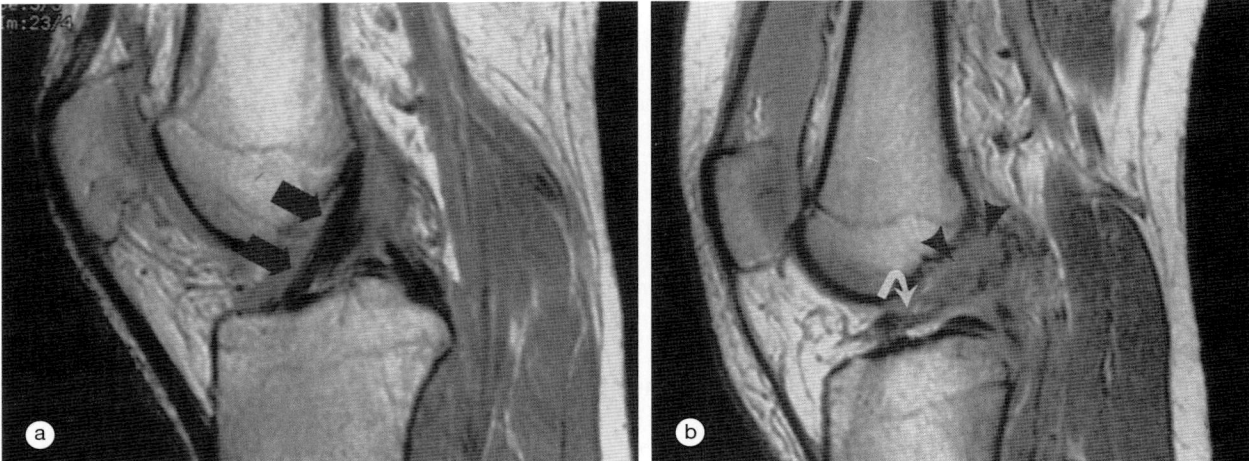

Figure 7-21 Magnetic resonance imaging appearance of an anterior cruciate ligament (ACL) tear. (**a**) Sagittal proton density image of the knee demonstrates a normal intact ACL (arrows) with uniform low signal, sharp linear contour anteriorly, and continuous extension from the femur to the tibia. (**b**) Sagittal proton density image demonstrates disruption of the ACL with loss of the normal low-signal fascicles and intermediate-signal material in the expected location of the ligament (arrowheads). The distal stump of the ligament is folded downward (curved arrow).

when the morphology is definitely abnormal, possibly with a displaced bucket handle fragment.

In a series of 400 knee MRI studies with 333 meniscal tears, 6% of tears found on arthroscopy could not be identified on routine MRI, even in retrospect.[29] False positive diagnoses in the 400 patients occurred in 1.5% due to healed tears or tears missed at arthroscopy.

In the setting of an operated meniscus where the morphology can be abnormal and inherent degenerative change extends to the articular surface, knee arthrography or MRI with intra-articular contrast agent injection[4] can be considered to determine whether the fluid extends into a tear in the meniscus. Comparison with previous studies can be helpful in assessing for recurrent tear versus postoperative change. The two best signs of recurrent tear of the postoperative meniscus on routine MRI are:

1. a line of abnormal meniscal signal intensity extending to an articular surface on proton density-weighted images; and
2. fluid extending into a linear area on T2-weighted images.[55]

Knee ligament injuries

The cruciate ligaments,[87,107,117] medial collateral ligament,[99] and lateral collateral ligament complex are best shown with multiplanar MRI. Again, the ligaments are assessed for continuity, caliber, and signal intensity. There is a continuum of sprain, partial tear, and full-thickness tear in the setting of ligamentous injury, similar to what is seen in ligaments elsewhere in the body.

Discontinuity of the ACL on sagittal and axial MRI planes and failure of the fascicles to parallel Blumensaat's line are the most accurate MRI signs of ACL tear (Fig. 7-21).[87] Multiple other indirect signs are good predictors of ACL tear, including disruption of the fascicles, a posterolateral tibial bruise, a

buckled PCL, a positive PCL line sign, a positive posterior femoral line sign, displacement of the lateral meniscus more than 3.5 mm posteriorly, displacement of the tibia more than 7 mm anteriorly, and a lateral femoral sulcus deeper than 1.5 mm.[39,87] In 20 patients with two different sagittal MRI sequences of the ACL showing intact fibers on one sequence and disrupted or poorly seen fibers on the other sequence (discordant findings), the ACL fibers were found to be intact on arthroscopy.[104] A combination of plain radiography and MRI best assesses for complications after ACL repair.[85]

Patellofemoral abnormalities

Patellofemoral abnormalities are best assessed in the axial and sagittal planes on MRI.[106] Fat-suppressed proton density MRI shows excellent contrast between the articular cartilage, bone, and any joint fluid.[63,88] Grading of chondromalacia is most accurate on axial MRI. Additionally, MRI can demonstrate patella baja or alta and the patellar position within the trochlear groove. Kinematic MRI studies are available to assess patellar tracking[100] and can show subluxation in certain positions. This can decrease or increase with knee flexion, depending on the cause of the tracking abnormality. Plain radiographs might or might not show patellar subluxation, depending on the degree of knee flexion utilized to obtain the axial patellar (sunrise) view.

Ankle and foot imaging

A three-view plain radiography that includes anteroposterior, lateral, and mortise views is considered the most appropriate by the ACR in patients with suspected ankle injury meeting Ottawa rules. Fluoroscopy with stress views can be necessary to assess for Lisfranc fracture dislocations. CT with reformations is often useful for preoperative planning in patients with complex comminuted fractures of the foot and ankle, and can alter clinical management.[59]

Chronic ankle instability can be detected with a Telos stress examination using posteriorly directed or varus stress, although magnetic resonance arthrography is more accurate and sensitive in the detection of anterior talofibular ligament tears.[20] In the patient with more diffuse foot pain of no definite cause, a radionuclide bone scan can often localize the abnormality to a specific joint or joints. In nine clinical scenarios of chronic ankle pain, the ACR appropriateness criteria list plain radiographs as the initial imaging study, with magnetic resonance second for several.

Magnetic resonance imaging of the ankle or foot provides excellent delineation of ligaments,[20,50] tendons,[49,90,98] and any abnormal bone marrow signal to indicate AVN or a bone bruise or stress fracture. In 81 patients referred for MRI of the foot and ankle by a group of four orthopedic surgeons and podiatrists, the post-MRI diagnosis differed from the pre-MRI diagnosis in 47%, and treatment plans were changed in 34%.[3] ACR appropriateness criteria for chronic foot pain list plain radiographs as the most appropriate initial imaging study, and then magnetic resonance as highly appropriate in many of the nine clinical scenarios listed. Bone scan is considered highly appropriate to assess for complex regional pain syndrome if plain radiographs are not diagnostic. The Achilles tendon is ideally shown with MRI in the sagittal and axial planes. MRI can be helpful in differentiating partial tears from tendinitis or peritenonitis. The tendon is assessed for continuity, caliber, and signal intensity, as elsewhere in the body.

Tarsal coalition can be evident on plain radiographs and is clearly shown on CT if it is a bony coalition. Sometimes MRI will more effectively show a fibrous coalition.[119]

SUMMARY

Knowledge of the strengths and weaknesses of the multiple imaging modalities available can help the treating physician decide on the optimal imaging study in a given clinical situation for a specific anatomic site. Good communication between the referring physician and the consulting radiologist aids in selecting the most appropriate imaging study or studies and additionally helps in the interpretation of the study. Sometimes a single study is sufficient, but in other clinical situations more than one study might be necessary. Furthermore, treatment plans can dictate whether additional studies are required, in that some imaging is more for an interventional procedure or surgical planning than for simple diagnosis.

REFERENCES

1. American College of Radiology. ACR appropriateness criteria™. Online. Available: http://www.acr.org/dyna/?doc=departments/appropriateness_criteria/text.html 2004.
2. American Society of Neuroradiology. Nomenclature and classification of lumbar disc pathology. Online. Available: http://www.asnr.org/spine_nomenclature/ 2004.
3. Anzilotti K Jr, Schweitzer ME, Hecht P, et al. Effect of foot and ankle MR imaging on clinical decision making. Radiology 1996; 201:515–517.
4. Applegate GR, Flannigan BD, Tolin BS, et al. MR diagnosis of recurrent tears in the knee: value of intraarticular contrast material. Am J Roentgenol 1993; 161:821–825.
5. Aprill C, Bogduk N. High intensity zone: a diagnostic sign of painful lumbar disc on magnetic resonance imaging. Br J Radiol 1992; 65:361–369.
6. Balich SM, Sheley RC, Brown TR, et al. MR imaging of the rotator cuff tendon: interobserver agreement and analysis of interpretive errors. Radiology 1997; 204:191–194.
7. Beltran J, Bencardino J, Mellado J, et al. MR arthrography of the shoulder: variants and pitfalls. Radiographics 1997; 17:1403–1412.
8. Beltran J, Rosenberg ZS, Chandnani VP, et al. Glenohumeral instability: evaluation with MR arthrography. Radiographics 1997; 17:657–673.
9. Bencardino J. MR imaging of tendon lesions of the hand and wrist. Magn Reson Imaging Clin North Am 2004; 12:333–347.
10. Berlin L. CT versus radiography for initial evaluation of cervical spine trauma: what is the standard of care? Am J Roentgenol 2002; 180:911–915.
11. Boden SD, McCowin PR, Davis DO, et al. Abnormal magnetic resonance scans of the cervical spine in asymptomatic subjects. J Bone Joint Surg 1990; 72:1178–1183.
12. Bogost GA, Lizerbram EK, Crues JV III. MR imaging in evaluation of suspected hip fracture: frequency of unsuspected bone and soft-tissue injury. Radiology 1995; 197:263–267.
13. Bourgouin PM, Lesage J, Fontaine S, et al. Pattern approach to the differential diagnosis of intramedullary spinal cord lesions on MR imaging. Am J Roentgenol 1998; 170:1645–1649.
14. Brandser EA, El-Khoury GY, Kathol MH, et al. Hamstring injuries: radiographic, conventional tomographic, CT, and MR imaging characteristics. Radiology 1995; 197:257–262.
15. Brant-Zawadski MN, Jensen MC, Obuchowski N, et al. Interobserver and intraobserver variability in interpretation of lumbar disc abnormalities: a comparison of two nomenclatures. Spine 1995; 20:1257–1264.
16. Breitenseher MJ, Metz VM, Gilula LA, et al. Radiographically occult scaphoid fractures: value of MR imaging in detection. Radiology 1997; 203:245–250.
17. Brossman J, Preidler KW, Daenen B, et al. Imaging of osseous and cartilaginous intraarticular bodies in the knee: comparison of MR imaging and MR arthrography with CT and CT arthrography in cadavers. Radiology 1996; 200:509–517.
18. Bui-Mansfield LT, Youngberg RA, Warme W, et al. Potential cost savings of MR imaging obtained before arthroscopy of the knee: evaluation of 50 consecutive patients. Am J Roentgenol 1997; 168:913–918.
19. Capps GW, Hayes CW. Easily missed injuries around the knee. Radiographics 1994; 14:1191–1210.
20. Chandnani VP, Harper MT, Ficke JR, et al. Chronic ankle instability: evaluation with MR arthrography, MR imaging, and stress radiography. Radiology 1994; 192:189–194.
21. Chandnani VP, Yeager TD, DeBerardino T, et al. Glenoid labral tears: prospective evaluation with MR imaging, MR arthrography, and CT arthrography. Am J Roentgenol 1993; 161:1229–1235.
22. Chappell KE, Robson MD, Stonebridge-Foster A, et al. Magic angle effects in MR neurography. Am J Neuroradiol 2004; 25:431–440.
23. Chen CJ, Lyu RK, Lee ST, et al. Intramedullary high signal intensity on T2-weighted MR images in cervical spondylotic myelopathy: prediction of prognosis with type of intensity. Radiology 2001; 221:789–794.
24. Cheung LP, Li KCP, Hollett MD, et al. Meniscal tears of the knee: accuracy of detection with fast spin-echo MR imaging and arthroscopic correlation in 293 patients. Radiology 1997; 203:508–512.
25. Conway WF, Totty WG, McEnery KW. CT and MR imaging of the hip. Radiology 1996; 198:297–307.
26. Cuenod CA, Laredo JD, Chevret S, et al. Acute vertebral collapse due to osteoporosis or malignancy: appearance on unenhanced and gadolinium-enhanced MR images. Radiology 1996; 199:541–549.
27. Czerny C, Hofmann S, Neuhold A, et al. Lesions of the acetabular labrum: accuracy of MR imaging and MR arthrography in detection and staging. Radiology 1996; 200:225–230.
28. Daffner RH, Lupetin AR, Dash N, et al. MRI in the detection of malignant infiltration of bone marrow. Am J Roentgenol 1986; 146:353–358.
29. De Smet AA, Tuite MJ, Norris MA, et al. MR diagnosis of meniscal tears: analysis of causes of errors. Am J Roentgenol 1994; 163:1419–1423.
30. Dick BW, Mitchell DG, Burk DL, et al. The effect of chemical shift misrepresentation on cortical bone thickness on MR imaging. Am J Roentgenol 1988; 15:537–538.

31. Dina TS, Boden SD, Davis DO. Lumbar spine after surgery for herniated disk: imaging findings in the early postoperative period. Am J Roentgenol 1995; 164:665–671.

32. El-Khoury GY, Kathol MH, Daniel WW. Imaging of acute injuries of the cervical spine: value of plain radiography, CT, and MR imaging. Am J Roentgenol 1995; 164:43–50.

33. Erickson SJ, Cox IH, Hyde JS, et al. Effect of tendon orientation on MR imaging signal intensity: a manifestation of the 'magic angle' phenomenon. Radiology 1991; 181:389–392.

34. Erickson SJ, Prost RW, Timins ME. The 'magic angle' effect: background physics and clinical relevance. Radiology 1993; 188:23–25.

35. Fitzgerald SW, Curry DR, Erickson SJ, et al. Distal biceps tendon injury: MR imaging diagnosis. Radiology 1994; 191:203–206.

36. Fritz RC et al. MR imaging of the rotator cuff. Magn Reson Imaging Clin North Am 1997; 5(4):735–754.

37. Fritz RC, Steinbach LS, Tirman PFJ, et al. MR imaging of the elbow. An update. Radiol Clin North Am 1997; 35:117–144.

38. Gaary EA, Potter HG, Altcheck DW. Medial elbow pain in the throwing athlete: MR imaging evaluation. Am J Roentgenol 1997; 168(3):795–800.

39. Gentili A, Seeger LL, Yao L, et al. Anterior cruciate ligament tear: indirect signs at MR imaging. Radiology 1994; 193:835–840.

40. Georgy BA, Snow RD, Hesselink JR. MR imaging of spinal nerve roots: techniques, enhancement patterns, and imaging findings. Am J Roentgenol 1996; 166:173–179.

41. Grogan J, Nowicki BH, Schmidt TA, et al. Lumbar facet joint tropism does not accelerate degeneration of the facet joints. Am J Neuroradiol 1997; 18:1325–1329.

42. Gundry CR, Heithoff KB. Epidural hematoma of the lumbar spine: 18 surgically confirmed cases. Radiology 1993; 187:427–431.

43. Gusmer PB, Potter HG, Schatz JA, et al. Labral injuries: accuracy of detection with unenhanced MR imaging of the shoulder. Radiology 1996; 200:519–524.

44. Hayes CW, Conway WF. Evaluation of articular cartilage: radiographic and cross-sectional imaging techniques. Radiographics 1992; 12:409–428.

45. Helgason JW, Chandnani VP, Yu JS. MR arthrography: a review of current technique and applications. Am J Roentgenol 1997; 168:1473–1480.

46. Hueftle MG, Modic MT, Ross JS, et al. Lumbar spine: postoperative MR imaging with Gd-DTPA. Radiology 1988; 167:817–824.

47. Itoh R, Murata K, Kamata M, et al. Lumbosacral nerve root enhancement with disk herniation on contrast-enhanced MR. Am J Neuroradiol 1996; 17:1619–1625.

48. Jee WH et al. Meniscal tear configurations: categorization with MR imaging. Am J Roentgenol 2003; 180(1):92–97.

49. Khoury NJ, El-Khoury GY, Saltzman CL, et al. Peroneus longus and brevis tendon tears: MR imaging evaluation. Radiology 1996; 200:833–841.

50. Klein MA. MR imaging of the ankle: normal and abnormal findings in the medial collateral ligament. Am J Roentgenol 1994; 162:377–383.

51. Krinsky G, Rofsky NM, Weinreb JC. Nonspecificity of short inversion time inversion recovery (STIR) as a technique of fat suppression: pitfalls in image interpretation. Am J Roentgenol 1996; 166:523–526.

52. Kwak SM, Brown RR, Trudell D, et al. Glenohumeral joint: comparison of shoulder positions at MR arthrography. Radiology 1998; 208:375–380.

53. Lebwohl NH. Diskography for the diagnosis of radiculopathy without nerve root compression. Am J Neuroradiol 1995; 16:1614–1615.

54. Ledermann HP, Schweitzer ME, Morrison WB, et al. MR imaging findings in spinal infections: rules or myths? Radiology 2003; 228:506–514.

55. Lim PS, Schweitzer ME, Bhatia M, et al. Repeat tear of postoperative meniscus: potential MR imaging signs. Radiology 1999; 210:183–188.

56. Liou JTS, Wilson AJ, Totty WG, et al. The normal shoulder: common variations that simulate pathologic conditions at MR imaging. Radiology 1993; 186:435–441.

57. Ma LD, Frassica FJ, Scott WW Jr, et al. Differentiation of benign and malignant musculoskeletal tumors: potential pitfalls with MR imaging. Radiographics 1995; 15:349–366.

58. Ma LD, McCarthy EF, Bluemke DA, et al. Differentiation of benign from malignant musculoskeletal lesions using MR imaging: pitfalls in MR evaluation of lesions with a cystic appearance. Am J Roentgenol 1998; 170: 1251–1258.

59. Magid D, Michelson JD, Ney DR, et al. Adult ankle fractures: comparison of plain films and interactive two- and three-dimensional CT scans. Am J Roentgenol 1990; 154:1017–1023.

60. Maravilla KR, Bowen BC. Imaging of the peripheral nervous system: evaluation of peripheral neuropathy and plexopathy. Am J Neuroradiol 1998; 19:1011–1023.

61. Maurer EJ, Kaplan PA, Dussault RG, et al. Acutely injured knee: effect of MR imaging on diagnostic and therapeutic decisions. Radiology 1997; 204:799–805.

62. May DA, Purins JL, Smith DK. MR imaging of occult traumatic fractures and muscular injuries of the hip and pelvis in elderly patients. Am J Roentgenol 1996; 166:1075–1078.

63. McCauley TR. MR imaging of chondral and osteochondral injuries of the knee. Radiol Clin North Am 2002; 40(5):1095–1107.

64. Mehta RC, Marks MP, Hinks RS, et al. MR evaluation of vertebral metastases: T1-weighted, short-inversion-time inversion recovery, fast spin-echo, and inversion-recovery fast spin-echo sequences. Am J Neuroradiol 1995; 16:281–288.

65. Milette PC, Fontaine S, Lepanto L, et al. Radiating pain to the lower extremities caused by lumbar disk rupture without spinal nerve root involvement. Am J Neuroradiol 1995; 16:1605–1613.

66. Mirowitz SA, London SL. Ulnar collateral ligament injury in baseball pitchers: MR imaging evaluation. Radiology 1992; 185(2):573–576.

67. Mitchell DG, Rao VM, Dalinka MK, et al. Femoral head avascular necrosis: correlation of MR imaging, radiographic staging, radionuclide imaging, and clinical findings. Radiology 1987; 162:709–715.

68. Mohana-Borges AVR, Chung CB, Resnick D. MR imaging and MR arthrography of the postoperative shoulder: spectrum of normal and abnormal findings. Radiographics 2004; 24:69–85.

69. Moulton JS, Blebea JS, Dunco DM, et al. MR imaging of soft-tissue masses: diagnostic efficacy and value of distinguishing between benign and malignant lesions. Am J Roentgenol 1995; 164:1191–1199.

70. Nachemson A. Lumbar discography: where are we today? [editorial]. Spine 1989; 14:555–557.

71. Nakanishi K, Masatomi T, Ochi T, et al. MR arthrography of the elbow: evaluation of the ulnar collateral ligament of the elbow. Skeletal Radiol 1996; 25(7):629–634.

72. Needell SD, Zlatkin MB, Sher JS, et al. MR imaging of the rotator cuff: peritendinous and bone abnormalities in an asymptomatic population. Am J Roentgenol 1996; 166:863–867.

73. North American Spine Society. Position statement on discography. Spine 1988; 13:1343.

74. Nunez DB, Zuluaga A, Fuentes-Bernardo DA, et al. Cervical spine trauma: how much more do we learn by routinely using helical CT? Radiographics 1996; 16:1307–1318.

75. Olson EM, Wong WHM, Hesselink JR. Extraspinal abnormalities detected on MR images of the spine. Am J Roentgenol 1994; 162:679–684.

76. Palmer WE, Caslowitz PL. Anterior shoulder instability: diagnostic criteria determined from prospective analysis of 121 MR arthrograms. Radiology 1995; 197:819–825.

77. Palmer WE, Levine SM, Dupuy DE. Knee and shoulder fractures: association of fracture detection and marrow edema on MR images with mechanism of injury. Radiology 1997; 204:395–401.

78. Parizel PM, Baleriaux D, Rodesch G, et al. Gd-DTPA-enhanced MR imaging of spinal tumors. Am J Neuroradiol 1989; 10:249–258.

79. Patten RM. Overuse syndromes and injuries involving the elbow: MR imaging findings. Am J Roentgenol 1995; 164:1205–1211.

80. Plancher KD, Ho CP, Cofield SS, et al. Role of MR imaging in the management of skier's thumb injuries. MRI Clin North Am 1999; 7:73–84.

81. Potok PS, Hopper KD, Umlauf MJ. Fractures of the acetabulum: imaging, classification, and understanding. Radiographics 1995; 15:7–23.

82. Prost R, Czervionke LF. How does an MR scanner operate? Am J Neuroradiol 1994; 15:1383–1386.

83. Quinn SF, Sheley RC, Demlow TA, et al. Rotator cuff tendon tears: evaluation with fat-suppressed MR imaging with arthroscopic correlation in 100 patients. Radiology 1995; 195:497–501.

84. Rabassa AE, Guinto FC Jr, Crow WN, et al. CT of the spine: value of reformatted images. Am J Roentgenol 1993; 161:1223–1227.

85. Recht MP, Piraino DW, Applegate G, et al. Complications after anterior cruciate ligament reconstruction: radiographic and MR findings. Am J Roentgenol 1996; 167:705–710.

86. Rijke AM, Goitz HT, McCue FC, et al. Stress radiography of the medial elbow ligaments. Radiology 1994; 191:213–216.

87. Robertson PL, Schweitzer ME, Bartolozzi AR, et al. Anterior cruciate ligament tears: evaluation of multiple signs with MR imaging. Radiology 1994; 193:829–834.

88. Rose PM, Demlow TA, Szumowski J, et al. Chondromalacia patellae: fat-suppressed MR imaging. Radiology 1994; 193: 437–440.

89. Rosenberg ZS, Beltran J, Cheung YY, et al. The elbow: MR features of nerve disorders. Radiology 1993; 188:235–240.

90. Rosenberg ZS, Cheung Y, Jahss MH, et al. Rupture of the posterior tibial tendon: CT and MR imaging with surgical correlation. Radiology 1988; 169:229–235.

91. Ross JS, Masaryk TJ, Modic MT, et al. MR imaging of lumbar arachnoiditis. Am J Neuroradiol 1987; 8:885–892.

92. Ross JS, Zepp R, Modic MT. The postoperative lumbar spine: enhanced MR evaluation of the intervertebral disk. AJNR Am J Neuroradiol 1996; 17:323–331.

93. Sallomi D, Janzen DL, Munk PL, et al. Muscle denervation patterns in upper limb nerve injuries: MR imaging findings and anatomic basis. Am J Roentgenol 1998; 171:779–784.

94. Sans N, Richardi G, Railhac JJ, et al. Kinematic MR imaging of the shoulder: normal patterns. Am J Roentgenol 1996; 167:1517–1522.

95. Schelhaus KP, Pollei SR, Gundry CR, et al. Lumbar disc high-intensity zone: correlation of magnetic resonance imaging and discography. Spine 1996; 21:79–86.

96. Schmid MR, Stucki G, Duewell S, et al. Changes in cross-sectional measurement of the spinal canal and intervertebral foramina as a function of body position: in vivo studies on an open-configuration MR system. Am J Roentgenol 1999; 172:1095–1102.

97. Schwartz ML, Al-Zahrani S, Morwessel RM, et al. Ulnar collateral ligament injury in the throwing athlete: evaluation with saline-enhanced MR arthrography. Radiology 1995; 197:297–299.

98. Schweitzer ME, Caccese R, Karasick D, et al. Posterior tibial tendon tears: utility of secondary signs for MR imaging diagnosis. Radiology 1993; 188:655–659.

99. Schweitzer ME, Tran D, Deely DM, et al. Medial collateral ligament injuries: evaluation of multiple signs, prevalence and location of associated bone bruises and assessment with MR imaging. Radiology 1995; 194: 825–829.

100. Shellock FG, Mink JH, Deutsch AL, et al. Patellofemoral joint: identification of abnormalities with active-movement, 'unloaded' versus 'loaded' kinematic MR imaging techniques. Radiology 1993; 188: 575–578.

101. Silverman CS, Lenchik L, Shimkin PM, et al. The value of MR in differentiating subligamentous from supraligamentous lumbar disk herniations. Am J Neuroradiol 1995; 16:571–579.

102. Singson RD, Hoang T, Dan S, et al. MR evaluation of rotator cuff pathology using T2-weighted fast spin-echo technique with and without fat suppression. Am J Roentgenol 1996; 166:1061–1065.

103. Slone RM, MacMillan M, Montgomery WJ. Spinal fixation: part 3. Complications of spinal instrumentation. Radiographics 1993; 13:797–816.

104. Smith DK, May DA, Phillips P. MR imaging of the anterior cruciate ligament: frequency of discordant findings on sagittal-oblique images and correlation with arthroscopic findings. Am J Roentgenol 1996; 166:411–413.

105. Sofka CM, Potter HG. Magnetic resonance imaging of the wrist. Semin Musculoskelet Radiol 2001; 5(3):217–226.

106. Sonin AH, Fitzgerald SW, Bresler ME, et al. MR imaging appearance of the extensor mechanism of the knee: functional anatomy and injury patterns. Radiographics 1995: 15:367–382.

107. Sonin AH, Fitzgerald SW, Hoff FL, et al. MR imaging of the posterior cruciate ligament: normal, abnormal, and associated injury patterns. Radiographics 1995; 15:551–561.

108. Sonin AH, Fitzgerald SW. MR imaging of sports injuries in the adult elbow: a tailored approach. Am J Roentgenol 1996; 167:325–331.

109. Stadnik TW, Lee RR, Coen HL, et al. Annular tears and disk herniation: prevalence and contrast enhancement on MR images in the absence of low back pain or sciatica. Radiology 1998; 206:49–55.

110. Taber KH, Herrick RC, Weathers SW, et al. Pitfalls and artifacts encountered in clinical MR imaging of the spine. Radiographics 1998; 18: 1499–1521.

111. Tartaglino LM, Flanders AE, Vinitski S, et al. Metallic artifacts on MR images of the postoperative spine: reduction with fast spin-echo techniques. Radiology 1994; 190:565–569.

112. Tartaglino LM, Friedman DP, Flanders AE, et al. Multiple sclerosis in the spinal cord: MR appearance and correlation with clinical parameters. Radiology 1995; 195:725–732.

113. Timins ME, Erickson SJ, Estkowski LD, et al. Increased signal in the normal supraspinatus tendon on MR imaging: diagnostic pitfall caused by the magic-angle effect. Am J Roentgenol 1995; 164:109–114.

114. Tirman PFJ, Feller JF, Janzen DL, et al. Association of glenoid labral cysts with labral tears and glenohumeral instability: radiologic findings and clinical significance. Radiology 1994; 190: 653–658.

115. Ulmer JL, Matthews VP, Elster AD, et al. Lumbar spondylolysis without spondylolisthesis: recognition of isolated posterior element subluxation on sagittal MR. Am J Neuroradiol 1995; 16:1393–1398.

116. Ulmer JL, Matthews VP, Elster AD, et al. MR imaging of lumbar spondylolysis: the importance of ancillary observations. Am J Roentgenol 1997; 169:233–239.

117. Vahey TN, Broome DR, Kayes KJ, et al. Acute and chronic tears of the anterior cruciate ligament: differential features at MR imaging. Radiology 1991; 181:251–253.

118. Vellet AD, Marks PH, Fowler PJ, et al. Occult posttraumatic osteochondral lesions of the knee: prevalence, classification, and short-term sequelae evaluated with MR imaging. Radiology 1991; 178:271–276.

119. Wechsler RJ, Schweitzer ME, Deely DM, et al. Tarsal coalition: depiction and characterization with CT and MR imaging. Radiology 1994; 193: 447–452.

120. Weishaupt D, Zanetti M, Hodler J, et al. MR imaging of the lumbar spine: prevalence of intervertebral disk extrusion and sequestration, nerve root compression, end plate abnormalities, and osteoarthritis of the facet joints in asymptomatic volunteers. Radiology 1998; 209:661–666.

121. Weishaupt D, Zanetti M, Hodler J, et al. Painful lumbar disk derangement: relevance of endplate abnormalities at MR imaging. Radiology 2001; 218:420–427.

122. West GA, Haynor DR, Goodkin R, et al. Magnetic resonance imaging signal changes in denervated muscles after peripheral nerve injury. Neurosurgery 1994; 35:1077–1085.

123. Wiltse LL, Berger PE, McCulloch JA. A system for reporting the size and location of lesions of the spine. Spine 1997; 22:1534–1537.

124. Yin Y, Evanoff BA, Gilula LA, et al. Surgeons' decision making in patients with chronic wrist pain: role of bilateral three compartment wrist arthrography. Prospective study. Radiology 1996; 200:829–832.

125. Yohichi A, Katsuhiro O, Howard A, et al. Dorsal root ganglia morphological features in patients with herniation of the nucleus pulposus: assessment using magnetic resonance myelography and clinical correlation. Spine 2001; 26:2125–2132.

126. Zanetti M, Weishaupt D, Gerber C, et al. Tendinopathy and rupture of the tendon of the long head of the biceps brachii muscle: evaluation with MR arthrography. Am J Roentgenol 1998; 170:1557–1561.

Chapter

8

Quality and Outcome Measures for Medical Rehabilitation

Carl V. Granger, Terrie Black and Susan L. Braun

The quality of healthcare services has moved from being primarily an issue for regulating and accreditation agencies to a concern of clinicians, administrators, researchers, and consumers. The Institute of Medicine has defined quality of care as 'the degree to which health services for individuals and populations increase the likelihood of desired health outcomes and are consistent with current professional knowledge'.[39] Because an important purpose of medical rehabilitation is to improve the functional status of patients, reliable and valid methods of performing functional assessment are necessary.

DEFINITION OF FUNCTIONAL ASSESSMENT

In medical rehabilitation, the term *function* usually refers to the use of skills included in performing tasks necessary to daily living, leisure activities, vocational pursuits, social interactions, and other required behaviors. The goals of medical rehabilitation are to monitor, support, and facilitate human performance and behavior, while considering environmental, structural, physiological, and psychological limitations. Measurement of function is essential to its goals.

M. Powell Lawton first defined *functional assessment* as any systematic attempt to objectively measure the level at which a person is functioning in a variety of domains.[36] Functional assessment requires measurement of an individual's abilities and limitations, often for the purpose of describing the outcomes of a single or a series of interventions. Measurement begins with understanding what is to be measured. This understanding must be grounded in theory, and must be connected to a comprehensive model for identifying and then meeting the needs of the person being assessed. Each tool used in measurement must be designed and tested, ideally over a period of time, with respect to its reliability, validity, responsiveness to change, feasibility for use, and meaningfulness in the clinical setting. The technique includes coding the component skills and tasks according to categories of activities required to support quality

of daily living. The data help to formulate judgments as to how well these essential skills are used, and to gauge the degree to which tasks are accomplished and social role expectations are met.

Figure 8-1 proposes that an individual's fulfillment and quality of daily living are a result of balancing functional opportunities and functional requirements or demands. We have chosen the term *quality of daily living* in preference to the more common term *quality of life* because it is less expansive, more subject to empirical investigation, and analogous to another commonly used term, *activities of daily living (ADL)*. Functional opportunities are expressed as an individual's choices, options, and expectations. Functional requirements are expressed in physical, cognitive, and emotional terms. In order to achieve fulfillment and to maximize the quality of daily living, there must be a balance between improved opportunities through individual health and functioning, and the reduction or removal of life's barriers causing constraints.

A clinician who is proficient in using functional assessment can obtain performance-oriented data that can be analyzed in conjunction with diagnostic descriptors of pathologic conditions and impairment states. This integration of medical status with status in performance of tasks and fulfillment of social roles, together with knowledge of the individual's level of social supports, allows the construction of a set of data that profiles the whole person. Given this profile, problems can be identified more accurately and reviewed in an orderly manner. Interventions and coordination strategies (e.g. care management, chronic disease management, and critical pathways) can be developed after this analysis.

It is possible to compare the changes in status over time for an individual by assessing function at appropriate intervals. In this manner, outcomes of professional interventions of healthcare, rehabilitation, education, or psychological and social counseling can be described and monitored. Outcomes that are measurable are manageable.

The objectives of a functional assessment instrument, which Donaldson and coauthors summarized in 1973,[11] still hold today. They are:

- objective description of functional status at a given point in time;
- serial repetition, allowing detection of changed functional status;

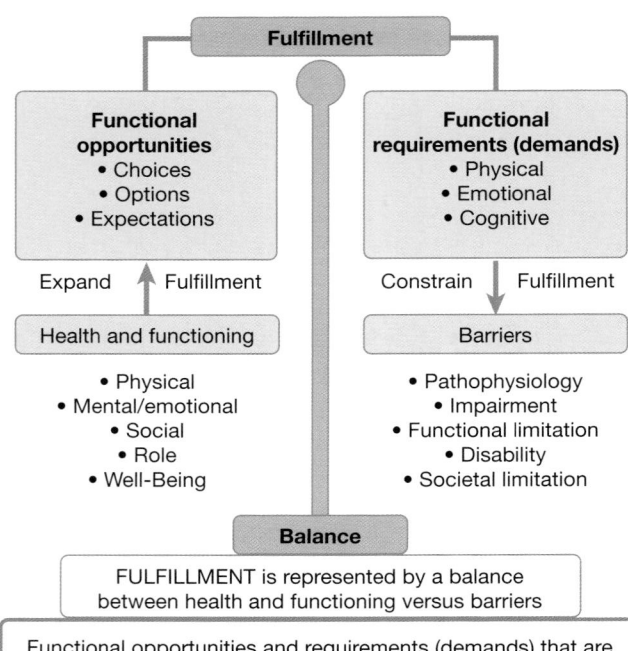

Figure 8-1 Challenges to quality of daily living.

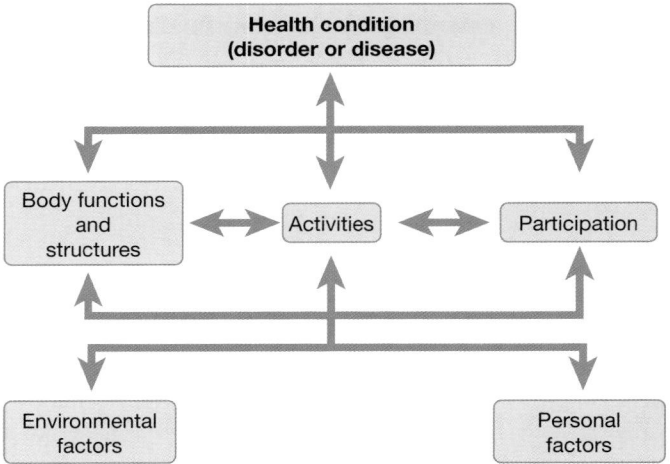

Figure 8-2 The World Health Organization published a revised model referred to as the *International Classification of Functioning, Disability and Health*. The components of this model and their interactions are presented in this diagram.

Table 8-1 Disablement model definitions	
Term	**Definition**
Pathophysiology	Any interruption of, or interference with, normal physiological and developmental processes or structures
Impairment	Any loss or abnormality at the organ or organ system level of the body
Functional limitation	Any restriction or lack of ability to perform an action in the manner or within a range consistent with the purpose of an organ or organ system
Disability	Any limitation in performing tasks, activities, and roles to levels expected within physical and social contexts
Societal limitation	Any restriction attributable to social policy or barriers (structural or attitudinal) that limits fulfillment of roles or denies access to services and opportunities associated with full participation in society
(After National Institutes of Health, National Institute of Child Health and Human Development 1993,[45] with permission.)	

- data collected through observation relevant to and useful in monitoring the treatment program;
- enhancement of communication among treatment team members and between referral agencies; and
- comparable clinical observations compatible with research questions.

The conceptual underpinnings for functional assessment are provided by disablement models proposed by Nagi[44] and Wood for the World Health Organization (WHO)[62] and the National Center for Medical Rehabilitation Research (NCMRR).[45] The model of the NCMRR is intended to facilitate research efforts that probe how persons with a disability might interact with the rehabilitation process to achieve optimal accommodation in the environment. The terms specific to the NCMRR[45] model are listed in Table 8-1. In the 1980 WHO document,[62] social norms are defined within six key roles or dimensions of experiences in which competence is expected of the individual for survival: orientation, physical independence, mobility, occupation, social integration, and economic self-sufficiency. To satisfy these social roles, the individual employs a variety of functional skills that result in complex behaviors and in performance of tasks. WHO, in 2001, published a revision called the International Classification of Functioning, Disability and Health[61] to represent concepts of health and disease as interactions (Fig. 8-2).

MEASUREMENT STANDARDS AND PRINCIPLES OF SCALING

There have been many attempts to improve the quality of measurement in rehabilitation for 30 or more years.[16,23,32–34,42] Experts repeatedly warned that functional assessment scales and procedures in common use had distinct failings. The empirical properties of scales—including basic validity, reliability, scaling characteristics, and standardization—had been insufficiently developed. The domains of functional assessment scaling sometimes have been stated in global, indistinct terms, such as *quality of life* or *function*, without specification of the exact meaning of these terms. Rehabilitation facilities have commonly relied on locally developed scales and documentation procedures that lack formal study or development. Even simple clinical terms such as *mild*, *moderate*, and *severe*, when applied without specific or objective reference, are used inconsistently.[56] All the disciplines involved in medical rehabilitation face similar technical problems in the assessment of human function and performance.

Attempts to write specific measurement standards applicable to rehabilitation did not coalesce until the end of the 1980s, when the American Congress of Rehabilitation Medicine formed the Task Force on Measurement and Evaluation. This interdisciplinary task force included members of the American Congress of Rehabilitation Medicine and the American Academy of Physical Medicine and Rehabilitation. Disciplines represented in the task force included physiatry, psychology, physical therapy, occupational therapy, rehabilitation nursing, rehabilitation counseling, and others. After several years of work, *Measurement Standards for Interdisciplinary Medical Rehabilitation* was published in December 1992 in a special issue of the *Archives of Physical Medicine and Rehabilitation.*[25]

The interdisciplinary standards document presents guidelines for the development and use of assessment procedures for measurement for the several disciplines involved in medical rehabilitation. Its purpose is to facilitate improved assessment in all the disciplines. The interdisciplinary standards were designed to serve as a resource in courses and to guide the development, choice, use, and interpretation of assessments, both in research and in clinical practice.[24]

The relationship between pathophysiological processes and wider life issues is crucial to medical rehabilitation, both in research and in practice. Interdisciplinary measurement standards are intended to apply to the assessment of impairment (specific anatomic, physiological, and psychological functional limitations) as well as to the assessment of broader domains, such as disability, societal limitations, and quality of daily living. Similar measurement standards have been developed for psychology[2] and physical therapy.[54]

There are many difficulties in applying measurement principles to function and outcomes because the concepts to be evaluated relate to whole person perceptions, attitudes, knowledge, or behaviors. These often are intangible and are the so-called latent traits. For example, physical performance measured in terms of muscle strength, power, endurance, velocity of contraction, oxygen uptake, or even timed ambulation are much more tangible than measuring the ease or difficulty that a person as a whole experiences in the tasks of daily living. Another example is the longstanding difficulty in measuring pain. Pain is a factor that often limits a person's ability to complete daily living activities, social interactions, and role participation. Current scientific understanding requires empirical testing of the reliability and validity of disablement and health-related scales.[1,22,24,25,35,37,63]

Validity and related guidelines

Validity is the paramount criterion for choice and use of a measure. Validity is commonly regarded as the extent to which a test measures what it is intended to measure.

(Johnston et al. 1992)[25]

Validation involves linking a concept with specific operations involved in the assessment procedure, and accumulating evidence that supports the logical inferences from the measurement procedure.

Scales of human function or performance can be quite broad or robust across diagnoses,[21,38,41] but they still cannot be assumed to have universal or unlimited validity. Validity is delimited by a particular construct, setting, and population or problem. Validity always relates to a specified use. Measurement standards are based on scientific validity principles. The initial standard (1.1)[25] in the interdisciplinary standards states that a measure should have evidence of validity that is appropriate to its intended use. Content validity, predictive validity, concurrent validity, and construct validity are four types of validity that have stood the test of time.

Content validity is the extent to which a test contains items critical or appropriate to a domain. The content of a functional assessment domain must be examined to choose a scale that has items that are appropriate to the clinical problem. For example, an item addressing indoor mobility should be included in a basic functional assessment tool that measures independence in ADL. However, it is not an item that is sufficient to measure the abilities of persons who need speed and endurance in moving about in the community. A knowledge of pathophysiology is also helpful in analyzing functional assessment scales logically. Careful analysis of the sensibility of scales is essential in medical applications.[14] Even though content validity is often established by a panel of experts representing experience and authority, only empirical evidence will resolve the many disputes about the validity and uses of functional assessment scales.

Predictive (or criterion-referenced) validity is the extent to which a scale is related to some outcome or external criterion. A truly useful assessment procedure should predict something outside itself in the future. This is an acid test of the information provided by functional assessment scales. For example, a Barthel Index[40] or FIM™ instrument[20] rating can help to predict the likelihood of a patient's returning to the community versus going to a nursing home after discharge from a stroke rehabilitation program.[19]

Concurrent validity—the ability to predict something that occurs at the same point in time—occasionally is of interest. For instance, one might be interested in patient performance at home, but it is impractical to leave the outpatient clinic to observe actual home performance. The outpatient clinic assessment should then be shown to correlate with home performance.

Construct validity is the extent to which a scale behaves as it should according to a theory. It involves study of the interactions of theoretically important constructs. A well-developed theory typically states that a construct should converge toward certain empirical criteria (convergent validity) on the one hand, but, on the other hand, the construct should be distinguishable by diverging from different criteria (divergent validity). For a given scale, there should be an accumulation of evidence of convergent and divergent relationships.[1,22,25] Construct validation involves study of the interactions of parameters that are theoretically important. For instance, one expects certain disease processes to affect related aspects of function, while unrelated aspects of function are not affected. This is an example of the dynamic logic by which rehabilitation is developing as a science. Tools that measure a physical quantity often can be validated against a single gold standard criterion. An inexpensive way to measure efficiency of ambulation can, for instance, be validated against an expensive and cumbersome laboratory measure of oxygen uptake. However, scales of complex concepts such as disability and societal limitation cannot be fully validated against a single ideal criterion. More complex construct validation analyses are required.

Guidelines for reliability and scaling

Functional assessment tools must have more than external validity characteristics such as predictive validity. They also must have internal validity characteristics such as reliability and internal homogeneity of the dimensional structure. Rehabilitation measurement standards require that adequate scales have numeric estimates of reliability (standard 2.1).[25]

Reliability is usually defined as freedom from random error.[1,35] Because freedom from error is theoretic but not practical, error should be at least minimal. It can be thought of as the extent to which the data contain relevant information with a high signal-to-noise ratio, having minimal irrelevant static and confusion. Reliability is a necessary but not sufficient condition for validity. Although assessment tools of narrow physical quantities or impairments can attain high reliability coefficients, one cannot assume that such tools are more reliable or more valid than assessment tools of the wider and more complex behaviors, which often reveal much more about daily life and the priority needs of persons with disabilities.

Empirical testing of reliability begins with computation of the degree of agreement when a test is administered more than once under similar circumstances.[22] Agreement is not precisely the same as reliability, however. Agreement means that the results of testing are similar despite variances in raters, time, or subjects tested. Percent of agreement is affected by population base rates, number of categories in the rating scale, and other factors that are not relevant to the balance between information and error in the measurement procedure. Several texts discuss the statistics that are used to estimate underlying reliability from surface-level agreement data.[13,22,35]

There are several ways of estimating reliability. Interrater reliability is crucial for rating scales that can be applied differently by various observers. Ratings of physical independence in basic ADL have shown high reliability coefficients, in the range of 0.89 to 0.95.[41] (The coefficients are Pearson correlations, which are acceptable summaries of reliability only if there are no significant differences in rater means or variabilities, i.e. a normal distribution of the values.) Test–retest reliability is a critical form of reliability when results of the measurement procedure fluctuate over short periods of time, such that the ability to measure gain in basic status or ability is unlikely.

A great deal hinges on the internal structure of tests involving multiple items. Internal consistency is essential to a scale formed by adding ratings from a series of items. Statistics such as split-half correlations and Cronbach's alpha have been used to estimate internal consistency.[1,13,22,47] Factor analysis is used to identify latent factors or dimensions (items that fit together).[1,46]

In contrast to continuous linear measures (such as those for length, weight, etc.), item-response scales are most commonly used for functional assessment and outcome analysis. Scales are typically discontinuous-ordinal. The raw scores they provide are neither linear nor equal-interval, so they should not be used in parametric statistical analyses. Interval measurement derived from raw scores through Rasch-based transformation improves functional status analysis by providing unidimensionality and additivity.[37] Unidimensionality means that items cooperate with each other as they progress in difficulty across a common range of performance, with each item adding a level of difficulty for the subjects. Unidimensionality also means that the abilities of the subjects can be located along the continuum defined by the items, according to common standard units. Additivity means that adding one more unit always increases the pool by the same amount whatever the overall level of the measure. Together, these two concepts of item difficulty and person ability being measured on the same linear metric are referred to as conjoint additivity. Conjoint additivity is achieved only if the measure is independent of the particular sample being tested, and of the particular set of items adopted. Therefore Rasch-transformed measures, complying with the requirement of conjoint additivity, permit statistical validity and generalizability in comparing individuals on the basis of results using an aggregate rating, and in comparing changes in ratings over time. The Rasch measurement model offers opportunities for comparing standardized expected values for both aggregate ratings and item responses when persons have problems that are relevant to the latent trait being measured.

The degree of ability or disability can be gauged by relating a person's performance to that of a wider age or gender severity-adjusted comparison group. Explicit norms enhance the value of a test. Whenever possible, the characteristics of the comparison group used for evaluating patient performance should be explicitly stated (standard 3.1).[25]

Guidelines for clinical application of scales

Although measurement standards are based in science and apply most directly to researchers and developers of scales, they also have important implications for clinical practice. Simply stated, the idea is that scientific findings, when they exist and are relevant, should be applied to clinical assessment procedures. The first standard for use of measures is that 'Users of measures should read the technical manual or relevant available documentation . . .' (standard 6.1).[25] Users need to understand the scientific basis for the inferences they make from their clinical assessments (standard 6.2)[25] and the boundaries of this knowledge (standards 6.3–6.6).[25]

Scales used in rehabilitation often need to be altered to fit unusual impairments or problems, and these modifications ought to be made within bounds understood by the user (standards 6.22–6.25).[25] Additionally, it must be kept in mind that persons being assessed have rights that must be respected (standards 7.1–7.4).[25]

Guidelines for outcomes management, quality improvement, and group applications

Formal measures are frequently applied at a group or systems level rather than at the level of individual patients. Group applications include outcome management, quality improvement, ongoing utilization review, and policy making by government and managed-care organizations. Evidence of validity and reliability should be provided for measures used in all group applications, and the measures used should be shown to be relevant to the populations involved (standard 8.1).[25]

The most respected scientific methodologies are based and validated on group rather than on single-subject studies. Usually, individual outcomes are aggregated into some form of an average. When individual function varies greatly from the average, however, knowledge of the average might tell little about the individual. Standard 8.2 provides a caution, stating that comparisons of an individual with a group average need explicit justification.[25]

Outcomes are affected by many factors other than the effectiveness of treatment. One can rarely infer effective treatment from outcomes alone. The effectiveness of rehabilitative interventions is based instead on a pattern of input, process, and outcome measures compared with some measured or assumed comparison.[27] One must adjust for case severity. Although severity adjustment is important everywhere in outcomes research, nowhere is it more critical than in rehabilitation, which specializes in treatment of persons with severe, permanent impairment. Standard 8.3 warns against evaluation of service providers on the basis of outcome scores alone in the absence of any other data.[25]

A challenge that remains for the medical rehabilitation field to solve is the predictable relationship between the dose of rehabilitative services and the response of the person. Depending on the problem and the treatment, rehabilitation outcomes follow teaching-learning paradigms (e.g. in therapeutic exercises) in the same way as chemical dose-response dynamics (e.g. in chemical treatments for pain or spasticity) do. A related need is for a 'dashboard' approach to managing treatment by being able to gauge the rate of change that the patient is undergoing while the treatment is in progress. This is the same way that the dashboard speedometer informs the driver of the rate of speed at which the destination is being approached.

The movement to improve and standardize measurement in rehabilitation should result in a smaller number of better-developed scales and measures. Quality and outcome monitoring will be facilitated by large sample sizes and valid comparisons.

CHARACTERISTICS OF FUNCTIONAL ASSESSMENT INSTRUMENTS

Functional assessment methods have been influenced by changes in the concept of rehabilitation and technologic advances. With the expanded scope of rehabilitation, there has been an increase in the number of domains routinely assessed as part of the rehabilitation process. Historically, it was common practice in rehabilitation services to utilize a large number of assessment instruments to document impairments, the ability to complete basic and more complex daily living skills, and perceptions of quality of daily living. The combination of these instruments provides the evaluation of the critical components that make up independent or interdependent active life. Although the assessment instruments can be either generic to rehabilitation patients or disease-specific, most documentation of functional abilities is determined using generic tools.

Comprehensive functional assessment is an essential clinical management component. It goes beyond disease categories and physical impairments to address the resultant disability that is targeted by the rehabilitation. Information from assessment instruments can be utilized for descriptive, evaluative, or predictive purposes. The use of functional assessment for descriptive purposes is a common screening method in rehabilitation and chronic illness, documenting the type and severity of disabilities at a given point in time. Assessment instruments are also used to set therapeutic goals and to monitor the clinical course of the disease, while measuring clinical changes over time. The predictive use of assessment instruments provides objective criteria to plan the treatment and evaluate the goals that have been set. Regardless of the instrument chosen, it should be practical, simple to administer, and yield meaningful results that can direct the rehabilitation process. The guiding principles in choosing a functional assessment scale are that the scale be a valid measure of the function being tested, that previous studies document validity and adequate reliability, and that the measurement be sensitive enough to document clinically important change.[29]

The ability to distinguish between the concepts of functional capacity and functional performance is an important consideration for test administration. Methodological differences in obtaining the assessment measures and the type of populations being assessed are two sources of discrepancies. Often measures do not clearly differentiate between the presence of a functional impairment that makes an activity impossible to carry out and the actual performance of an activity. As a simple example, a low score in locomotion could mean either that the subject had severe paralysis of limbs or else lacked the will or ability to use limbs that were otherwise intact. Performance ADL was shown to have an integral cognitive component in the Framingham study of non-institutionalized persons with strokes, and in patients after traumatic brain injury.[30,33] This factor is a major consideration in rehabilitation. In addition, Nagi also has documented that disability, unlike functional limitation, has a major social component.[44] Because disability reflects performance within a sociocultural context, one could expect that daily performance would be strongly influenced by social as well as physical factors. The goals of and rationale for choosing a specific functional assessment instrument need to take these considerations into account. One needs to be aware that performance-based functional assessment takes the social and physical contexts into account.

The functional assessment scale employed should be able to measure disability, monitor progress, enhance communications, measure the effectiveness of treatment, and document the benefits of rehabilitation interventions. Because assessment instruments are used repeatedly during the course of rehabilitation, the results should be reliable and valid measures for the disabilities being treated.

FUNCTIONAL ASSESSMENT SCALES

Activities of daily living scales

Activities of daily living refer to those basic skills that one must possess in order to care for oneself independently. Instruments that assess ADL usually assess abilities in self-care (eating, bathing, grooming, dressing, etc.), transfers, continence, and in most cases, locomotion. ADL scales are usually hierarchic in arrangement. They include easier activities, such as eating, and more difficult tasks, such as climbing stairs. The FIM™ instrument[20] and the Patient Evaluation and Conference System[49] are examples of scales that include the domains of functional communication and social cognition. Information is collected by observing actual performance rather than capacity as demonstrated in an artificial setting, such as during therapy. There are a number of valid and reliable scales that document ADL. Most are administered by trained clinicians, although there are some that are based on subjective judgment. The utility of these instruments is that they provide a minimum number of items for describing physical functioning, and can be used to track a clinical course of treatment. Selected ADL scales that have met adequate validity and reliability standards include the Barthel Index,[40] Index of Independence in Activities of Daily Living,[31] Kenny Self-Care Evaluation,[52] FIM™ instrument,[20] WeeFIM® instrument,[58,59] Level of Rehabilitation Scale (LORS) and LORS American Data System (LADS) (LORS/LADS),[6] and the Patient Evaluation and Conference System.[49]

Instrumental activities of daily living scales

Instrumental activities of daily living (IADL) scales can be used to measure the ability to accomplish activities related to maintaining one's living environment. These tasks can include using a telephone, shopping, preparing meals, and managing money. Developing and restoring these skills are often part of a rehabilitation program, but the skills are difficult to evaluate until the individual returns home. IADL scales can be rated either by an interviewer or by the individual, depending on the disability and circumstances. A limitation of this type of scale is that not all activities are pertinent to everyone. They also do not take safety into account as a feature of performance. Three IADL scales utilized in rehabilitation services are the Functional

Health Status,[51] the Older Americans Resources and Services Multidimensional Functional Assessment Questionnaire,[12] and the Philadelphia Geriatric Center Instrumental Activities of Daily Living.[36]

Quality of life scales

Quality of life scales denote a wide range of capabilities, symptoms, and psychosocial characteristics that describe functional ability and satisfaction with life. Components of quality of life include social roles and interactions, functional performance, intellectual functioning, perceptions, and subjective health. Indicators can include standards of living and general satisfaction with life. Although there is controversy over the measurement of quality of life, it is a powerful indicator of successful rehabilitation. The relevance of these types of scales to populations with permanent disability has not yet been established. Rather than being criterion-referenced, these scales generally ask subjects to compare themselves with a prior healthy state. Three quality of life scales that have met criteria for reliability, validity, and sensitivity are the MOS 36-Item Short Form Survey,[57] Sickness Impact Profile,[7] and the LIFEware^{SM} System.[3]

OUTCOMES MANAGEMENT AND CONTINUOUS QUALITY IMPROVEMENT

Definition

The Commission on Accreditation of Rehabilitation Facilities (CARF) defines outcomes measurement and outcomes management as a systematic procedure for measuring the effectiveness and efficiency of outcomes of care.[9] An outcomes management system measures outcomes by obtaining, aggregating, and analyzing data. Quality assessment and quality improvement are 'ongoing activities designed to objectively and systematically evaluate the quality of patient care and services, pursue opportunities to improve patient care and services, and resolve identified problems'.[28] Gonnella described program evaluation as a branch of quality assessment and improvement, and also stated that program evaluation in rehabilitation has come to mean the measurement of outcomes.[17] Other branches include utilization review, risk management, infection control, and documentation. The directives for achieving quality healthcare through outcomes management from CARF, the Joint Commission on Accreditation of Healthcare Organizations (Joint Commission),[28] state health departments, and other agencies have been a major stimulus for documentation of outcomes in medical rehabilitation.

Outcomes management is one way to measure the effectiveness and efficiency of rehabilitation services. Structure, process, outcome, or a combination of these factors can be addressed in the evaluation. Structural evaluation data include information about certification of professional healthcare providers. Process evaluation data include information about the provision of treatment in terms of number and type. Outcome evaluation data include information about the level of functional independence achieved or the level of patient satisfaction. Good patient outcomes are the culmination of the combined effects of structure and process. For practical purposes then, outcomes management in medical rehabilitation has come to mean a comparison of the measurement of the functional performance of patients, as well as related variables, at the beginning of rehabilitation and after care has been completed. Use of benchmarks from data aggregated from other facilities with similar treatment programs is advantageous when available.

Elements of outcomes management

The elements of an outcomes management system can include a description of the purpose of the program (mission statement), program structure, program goals, program objectives, methods of applying measures, and utilization of outcome data in various reports and communications.[9] The outcome measures should be related to the overall goals of the rehabilitation service.

The program mission statement is a broad summary of the rehabilitation program, the patients served, and the treatments provided. The program structure describes the organizational framework. This includes the type of facility, admission criteria, patients served, and services provided.[9] The program goals are derived from the mission statement and are written for each rehabilitation program (e.g. the stroke program). The goal statements are expressed in achievable terms.

Program objectives follow the program goals and are stated in terms that are measurable according to expected results. Achievement of objectives should relate to effectiveness and efficiency of the program and to satisfaction of the individuals served. Effectiveness objectives address the extent to which outcomes are attained. Efficiency objectives indicate the quantity of resources used to attain program goals. For example, program objectives of a stroke program might be to:

- optimize self-care skills;
- optimize sphincter management;
- optimize transfer skills;
- optimize locomotion skills;
- optimize communication skills;
- optimize social cognition skills;
- return patients to the community;
- optimize vocational independence;
- ensure appropriate length of stay;
- optimize the average cost per unit of improvement (gain in function); and
- ensure patient satisfaction.

Functional assessment scales are used to determine whether these objectives have been achieved. They might reflect improvement from admission to discharge, or else they might represent criterion levels to be matched or exceeded. This information typically is derived from using a functional assessment instrument that compares admission and discharge levels of independence. On the other hand, criterion measures indicate improvement to a predetermined level. An example of criterion measures might be a facility's objective to achieve a certain percentage of community discharges. From past per-

formance, a facility might choose a level of 72% as minimally acceptable, 80% as a goal, and 88% as an optimal level. A facility with less severely affected or younger patients might choose as optimal a level that is closer to 100%. Some facilities choose a criterion based on case-mix-adjusted (expected) data that are based on national data and the facility case mix.[9]

Additional data to be collected and analyzed for the program evaluation reports include demographic data and descriptors of the problems or barriers to individual success. Typically, demographic data include:

- average age and age distribution;
- sex distribution;
- average time from onset of impairment to admission to rehabilitation;
- frequency of program interruptions;
- vocational status prior to impairment; and
- payment sources.

Having collected and aggregated the outcome data, feedback reports must be compiled to summarize the findings. The data are then used for management reports, quality improvement and research, and communications to the community and third-party payers.

Rationale and usefulness

Forer succinctly described the benefits of outcomes management (Box 8-1).[15] Outcomes reports form the basis for monitoring the rehabilitation program. For example, they can be used to identify patients whose outcomes did not meet previously established goals and expectations. Identification of these patients can lead the quality improvement committee to suggest revision of existing programs, treatments, or interventions. By following certain indicators over time, administrators and clinicians can monitor the impact of those revisions and make further adjustments. It is important to establish a baseline of values with which results can be compared before and after a change of program is implemented.

Using outcome data to understand and improve the results of patient care is the most significant reason for doing program

---

Box 8-1 Benefits of outcomes management

- Ensure that a program is functioning within predetermined standards
- Provide guidance for alignment of program goals and objectives with patient needs
- Facilitate collecting outcome data systematically for research purposes
- Make information available for evaluation of cost-effectiveness
- Plan for the future with the help of informed decision making
- Support marketing efforts with objective data
- Promote understanding and acceptance of the rehabilitation program by the community

---

> **Box 8-2** Using data to monitor for change
>
> - Distribution of patient characteristics such as age and sex
> - Diagnostic mix
> - Case severity
> - Number of patients treated
> - Length of stay
> - Costs per patient
> - Frequency of program interruptions
> - Discharge patterns
> - Intensity, modalities, and types of clinicians involved in treatment

evaluation. Outcome data can identify those patients who fail to attain maximal benefits from the program as well as those patients who exceed expectations. Patients who could have had adjustment problems or medical complications, or who have deteriorated in functional status, can be identified and the program improved to serve them better.[15]

Outcome data from several facilities can be pooled to support research studies. For example, Granger et al.[19] and Johnston et al.[26] studied characteristics that predict outcomes for stroke patients in rehabilitation. The existence of a large and current data pool, such as that of the Uniform Data System for Medical Rehabilitation (UDSMR), allows investigators to study the interactions of many different factors in order to identify characteristics of patients with selected outcomes such as functional status, placement at discharge, and estimated length of stay.[53]

Outcome data can also be used to address a facility's operational issues, such as the effectiveness and efficiency with which care is provided, in relation to outcomes. The average cost per patient, the average length of stay, and the average cost per unit of improvement are important parameters for managing a facility. In these days of rapid changes in the manner of providing and paying for healthcare, planning for future program needs is another critical use of outcome data. Data should be used to monitor for changes in certain factors (Box 8-2).[15]

Performance measurement systems

The medical rehabilitation industry has been interested in comparing facility data with national comparison data since the 1980s, and many programs subscribe to national performance measurement systems.

The largest measurement system for medical rehabilitation is the UDSMR,[20] described below. Other systems had performed similar services. Medirisk, which became Care Data, offered the Formations Clinical Outcomes System, which maintained a database for inpatient medical rehabilitation programs. The Patient Evaluation and Conference System,[49] developed by Richard Harvey and associates at Marianjoy Hospital, had been used by dozens of rehabilitation programs. The Patient Evaluation and Conference System[49] provided comprehensive assessment and was used to organize communication and set goals in the rehabilitation team conference, as well as to evaluate the rehabilitation program.

The Joint Commission on Accreditation of Healthcare Organizations' ORYX® initiative

The Joint Commission on Accreditation of Healthcare Organizations requires that facilities adhere to standards of patient care, staff education, and organizational performance.[28] In 1987, the Joint Commission initiated its Agenda for Change, which emphasized the use of process and outcome measures to improve performance and quality of care.

In 1998, under its ORYX® initiative, hospitals and long-term care facilities accredited by the Joint Commission began working with performance measurement systems to collect and report performance measurement data in a standardized manner. The performance measurement systems then transmit a report summarizing the facility data, as well as case-mix-adjusted comparison (e.g. national) data to the Joint Commission.[28]

Beginning in 2000, the Joint Commission moved to the use of core measures so that data reported from different performance measurement systems could be compared.[28]

Uniform Data Set for Medical Rehabilitation and the Uniform Data System for Medical Rehabilitation

A national task force was established in 1983 to develop a uniform data set for medical rehabilitation that could be used to document the outcomes and costs of inpatient medical rehabilitation. The task force recognized the need for the creation of a tool that could be used uniformly to measure the functional status of the person with long-term needs.[20] The work of the task force, supported by a grant from the US Department of Education's National Institute on Disability and Rehabilitation Research, resulted in the development of the FIM™ instrument.[20] Demographic, diagnostic, and other variables were added to form the Uniform Data Set for Medical Rehabilitation.[20] The FIM™ instrument is composed of 18 items that assess performance of basic daily living skills (13 motor, 5 cognition), using a seven-level scale that measures major gradations in function from complete independence to total assistance (Fig. 8-3).[20] It can be administered by a trained clinician within 15–20 min. Inpatient admission, discharge, and follow-up ratings are collected for analysis and comparison with data from comparable facilities across the nation. This represented the next step in uniform use of a measure applied to persons with disability. Since 1987, more than 5 million records have been collected on medical rehabilitation patients with a variety of diagnoses.

The UDSMR was founded in 1987 on the campus of the University at Buffalo, The State University of New York, Buffalo, New York, to serve as a repository and provide data management functions for information about medical rehabilitation. UDSMR is a division of UB Foundation Activities, Inc., which owns the FIM™ instrument,[20] the WeeFIM® instrument,[58,59] and the LIFEware℠ System.[3] Subscribers to UDSMR sign license agreements in order to use these systems and to receive UDSMR®-produced reports. The data are downloaded to disk and returned to UDSMR, or transmitted via the Internet,

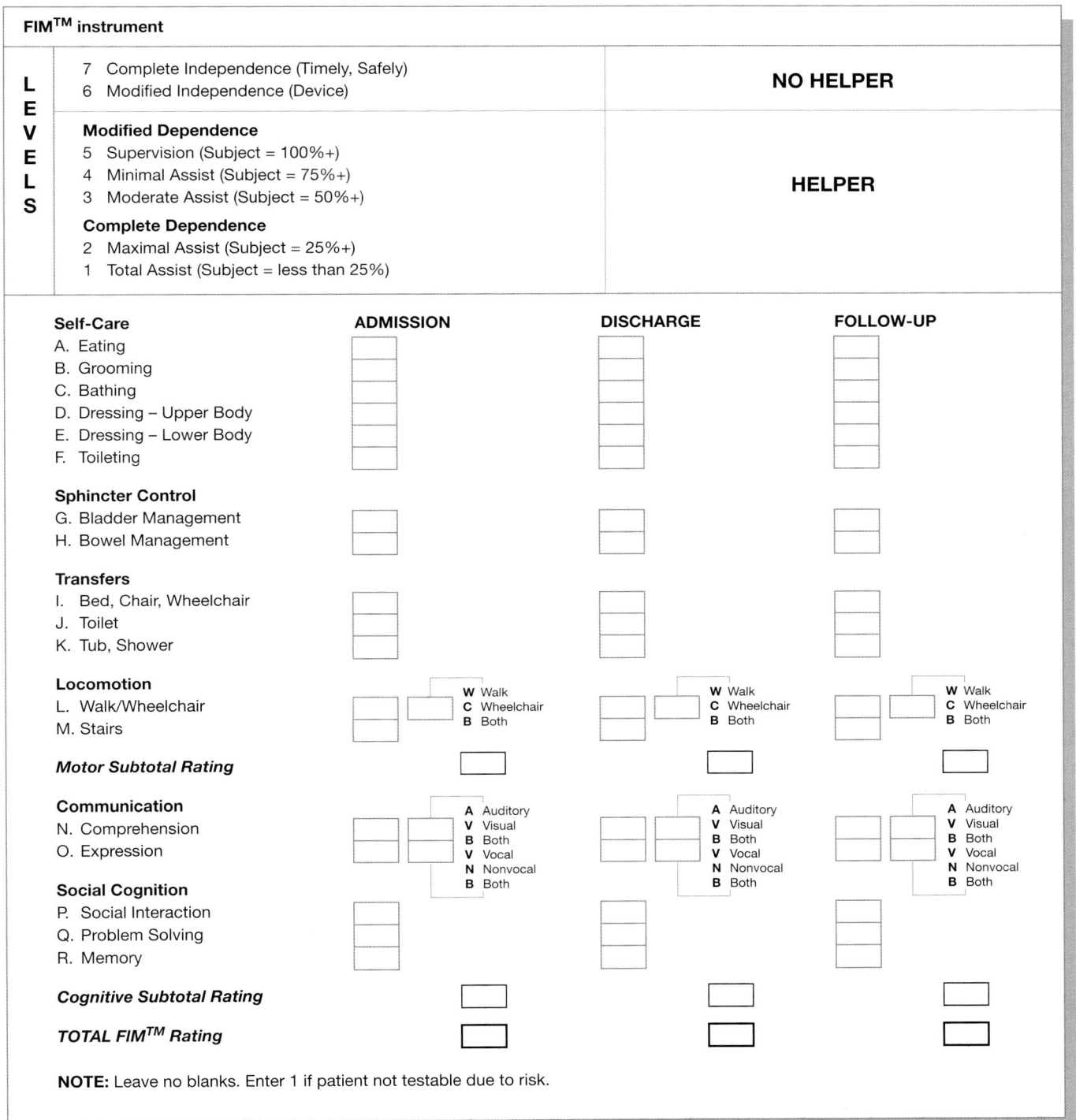

Figure 8-3 FIM™ instrument.[20] Uniform Data System for Medical Rehabilitation, a division of UB Foundation Activities Inc. (UBFA). Reprinted with the permission of the UDSMR. All marks associated with FIM and UDSMR are owned by UBFA.

on a quarterly basis, for aggregation into large national databases. UDSMR uses the data to prepare standard and special reports that each subscriber can then use to examine the outcomes of its medical rehabilitation services, and for a variety of other purposes. These include program evaluation, the ORYX®[28] initiative, and marketing. This data set is required for use by US inpatient medical rehabilitation facilities for Medicare Part A payment. It also is licensed for use in 14 additional countries around the world.

The FIM™ instrument[20] was adapted for use in pediatrics in 1987 by a multidisciplinary team of physicians, nurses, and therapists.[4,5,43] The resulting scale, known as the WeeFIM®

instrument,[58,59] is a measure of functional abilities and the need for assistance that are associated with levels of disability in children 6 months to 7 years of age. It can also be used with children well beyond the age of 7 years when delays in functional performance are evident. The WeeFIM® instrument measures functional status within a developmental framework.[58,59] Function is measured by determining a child's ability to perform basic daily living skills at specific assessment points. Development is measured by determining gross and fine motor, adaptive, personal-social, and cognitive skills over a span of time. Although the WeeFIM® instrument[58,59] utilizes the same items and rating scale as its parent, the definitions have been modified and the 18 items have been reorganized into three subscales: self-care, mobility, and cognition. Age-based norms were developed in order to compare children under age 7 years with disabilities to children under age 7 years without disabilities. An Internet-based WeeFIM II® System,[59] using the same instrument, was introduced in 2004.

The data sets for adult and pediatric inpatients include admission, discharge, and follow-up FIM™ instrument[20] ratings (Fig. 8-3) or WeeFIM® instrument[58,59] ratings. The data sets also include demographic, diagnostic, financial, and length-of-stay variables. The UDSMR data management services provide subscribing adult facilities with quarterly reports on such variables as FIM™ instrument[20] item rating levels; subscale, domain, and total raw scores; demographics; charges; and length of stay. The report data are arranged in three columns, allowing direct comparisons of the clinical site with the appropriate regional data and national data. Because the data set is uniform across clinical sites, these comparisons provide critical evaluation and planning data for any one site at any single point in time, and across time from admission to discharge to follow-up. UDSMR also provides severity-adjusted data reports that use the national data and the facility case mix to calculate expected values.

The WeeFIM II® System[59] can be used in inpatient and outpatient settings. Subscribing pediatric facilities receive quarterly inpatient reports containing three columns that permit comparisons of facility data with aggregate data from similar facilities and national data. Subscribers also receive outpatient reports that compare facility data with national aggregate data. Separate outpatient reports are provided for children who receive ongoing therapy services, children who are seen for evaluation only, and children who undergo day treatment.

The adult and pediatric databases also can be used as tracking devices by examining trends across reporting periods. The adult data revealed in a study in 2004 that a reduction in treatment days in medical rehabilitation hospitals did not diminish treatment effectiveness, but mortality increased after discharge.[48] Comparisons within sites allow clinicians and administrators to determine patterns of care within their facilities. The tracking of regional, similar facility (pediatric only), and national data across reports allows the same staff to be aware of changes in either regional or national medical rehabilitation policies and procedures. Because of the unique reporting by type of impairment across all diagnoses, the facilities can use the data to focus, with considerable detail, on their individual patient groups, and

---

Box 8-3 LIFEware℠ System[3] domains and purposes

Domains
- Physical functioning
- Pain experience
- Emotional and mood status
- Cognitive status
- Degree of social interaction
- Degree of selected role participation
- Satisfaction with the treatment process

Purposes
- Determine functional status and monitor changes in patients
- Evaluate the effectiveness and efficiency of the outpatient rehabilitation process
- Generate data to facilitate communication with patients healthcare providers, and third parties
- Provide continuity of assessment and tracking of outcomes in the transition from hospital inpatient to outpatient status

---

to make comparisons within impairment types with regional and national trends.

The LIFEware℠ System[3] was launched in 1998 for adult outpatients via the Internet to provide flexibility and comprehensiveness in assessing functional status and in measuring outcomes of persons with musculoskeletal, neurologic, and other conditions involving disability or chronic health problems. Domains and purposes appear in Box 8-3.

A key advantage of a large national data repository or registry is that it allows for site-specific, multiple-site, regional, state, national, and international comparisons. Another advantage is the ability to study patterns of care and monitor trends over time. Statistical research often depends on the availability of large sample sizes to reach substantive conclusions about healthcare outcomes. A third advantage is that clinical sites can contribute to the national databases, while at the same time keeping their own data in a readily accessible form for in-house data analysis and research efforts. This allows for improvements at both the local and national level, and for comparisons of the trends at each clinical site with regional and national trends. These comparisons can be made on a quarterly basis or can be examined in trend form over periods of time.

Perhaps most importantly, large ongoing databases, such as those maintained by UDSMR, can provide national data of sufficient sample size that key indicators at admission can be incorporated into statistical models to predict more precisely the course of medical rehabilitation and the outcomes at discharge and follow-up. This predictive power of the FIM™ instrument[20] ratings has been developed into models of Function-Related Groups (FIM-FRGs) through the work of Stineman and colleagues.[53] (The FRG system was developed at and is owned by Penn Ability Systems® [PAS™] at the University of Pennsylvania.) The appearance of FIM-FRGs[53] signaled the next step in putting the national database to work for improving rehabilitative care. The database currently provides

Box 8-4 Modification of the FIM™ instrument[20] for incorporation into the Inpatient Rehabilitation Facility–Patient Assessment Instrument

- A code of zero has been added to cover an activity that did not occur during the admission assessment period.
- Time frames for admission and discharge assessments have been changed: to the first 3 days of the hospital stay for admission assessment, and to one 24-h period within the last 3 days of the hospital stay for discharge assessment.
- A period of program interruption has been changed from 30 days to 3 days.
- Function modifiers have been added to the rating of certain items, namely bowel, bladder, locomotion, and tub or shower transfer.
- Item level definitions were modified for bladder and bowel.

Table 8-2 Overview of the Centers for Medicare & Medicaid Services Inpatient Rehabilitation Facility–Patient Assessment Instrument rehabilitation impairment categories

Code	Definition
01	Stroke
02	Traumatic brain injury
03	Non-traumatic brain injury
04	Traumatic spinal cord injury
05	Non-traumatic spinal cord injury
06	Neurological
07	Fracture of lower extremity
08	Replacement of lower extremity joint
09	Other orthopedic
10	Amputation, lower extremity
11	Amputation, other
12	Osteoarthritis
13	Arthritis, rheumatoid and other
14	Cardiac
15	Pulmonary
16	Pain syndrome
17	Major multiple trauma without brain injury or spinal cord injury
18	Major multiple trauma with brain injury or spinal cord injury
19	Guillain-Barré
20	Miscellaneous
21	Burns

the data for prediction models, with enough data left over for cross-validation studies of the predictive models to verify their accuracy and report their confidence limits.

On January 1, 2002, the US Centers for Medicare & Medicaid Services (CMS) initiated the Inpatient Rehabilitation Facility Prospective Payment System, which was substituted for the prior cost-based system for reimbursement for Medicare Part A services. The FIM™ instrument[20] is the major component of the Inpatient Rehabilitation Facility-Patient Assessment Instrument (IRF-PAI),[55] which is the assessment tool used by adult medical rehabilitation programs to collect the data for submission to CMS for reimbursement. To be incorporated into the IRF-PAI,[55] the FIM™ instrument[20] was modified in several ways (Box 8-4). It remains to be determined whether these changes enhance or detract from use of the FIM™ instrument.[20]

Payment for Medicare Part A inpatient rehabilitation services is tied now for the first time to the level of severity of the patient's functional status at the time of admission. The classification of patients into payment groups on admission is patterned after the FIM-FRG system.[53] The Inpatient Rehabilitation Facility Prospective Payment System requires that there be documentation of the medical condition for which the patient is admitted to the inpatient rehabilitation program. The reason for rehabilitation admission need not necessarily be the same as the reason for prior admission to the acute care hospital. Each patient must be assigned to one of 85 impairment group codes (IGCs)[20] that fall under 17 impairment groups. For example, a stroke with left body involvement would be coded as IGC 01.1 under the stroke impairment group.[20] In addition, the etiology must be identified in terms of an ICD-9-CM code.[60] Each IGC[20] falls into one of 21 general diagnostic categories called rehabilitation impairment categories (RICs; see Table 8-2).[55] For example, all types of stroke are assigned to the 01 Stroke RIC.[55] The case mix group (CMG),[55] similar to the FRG,[53] is assigned based on the IGC admission-FIM™ instrument motor rating,[20] and in some cases, admission-FIM™ instrument cognition rating[20] and age. The intent is to group

patients with similar use of resources and likely lengths of stay. It is the CMG[55] designation, along with appropriate comorbid conditions and/or complications, that determine the payment. This system requires that the patient be 'typical', meaning that the patient is returned to the community at discharge, has a length of stay greater than three days, and completes a full course of rehabilitation. A comorbid condition is a specific medical condition that affects a patient in addition to the principal diagnosis or impairment. Complications are conditions that occur after admission to the rehabilitation unit but not on the day of or day prior to discharge.

The physician has added responsibilities to:

- understand the coding conventions;
- provide clear documentation that assists team members in accurate coding;
- facilitate open communication between rehabilitation team members to assure that supportive documentation is accurate; and

- maintain the medical record such that diagnostic and treatment procedures are documented, as well as the presence of actual and suspected conditions.

Although comparative follow-up assessments are available through UDSMR, more attention needs to be given to the follow-up of patients to study the impact of medical rehabilitation after discharge. Examination of both the short- and long-term impacts of medical rehabilitation on its patients becomes even more valuable when considering linkages of databases. When connections can be made between the UDSMR and other national data sets, then increasingly more detailed studies will become available. This already has been done with a study that showed enhanced evaluation of the trauma system by incorporating the rehabilitation component.[10] The development of UDSMR databases for skilled nursing facilities, outpatients, and children allows for a broad perspective on patients from birth through old age. The advantages of uniformity and matching measuring tools (FIM[TM] instrument,[20] WeeFIM® instrument,[58,59] and LIFEware[SM] System[3]) allow for a unique opportunity to develop secondary prevention models by linking pediatric databases to adult databases to study lifetime outcomes.

The measurement of functional changes over time has received considerable attention in the statistical literature[8,50] due to the complicated nature of repeated measures statistics. The application of good measurement principles to the FIM[TM] instrument,[20] WeeFIM® instrument,[58,59] and LIFEware[SM] System[3] has resulted in tools that investigators can have confidence in using over time with little measurement error. UDSMR can be used with considerable statistical power and measurement confidence to provide unique insights into long-term care of patients in medical rehabilitation. The advantages of uniformity and large numbers of patients allow a broad range of clinical research to be applicable across the lifespan, from childhood to old age. This unique uniformity of measurement across time will provide an important key to understanding and meeting the needs of a diverse population with disabilities.

SUMMARY

Reviewing and assuring quality of healthcare delivery are daunting issues for all providers of healthcare. Almost two decades ago, the field of medical rehabilitation adopted a model of program evaluation that is facility-based, with certain common elements. Reliable and valid methods of functional assessment are necessary, because an important purpose of medical rehabilitation is to improve the functional status of patients.

Functional assessment is a method for describing a person's abilities and limitations. The essence of functional assessment is the measurement of a person's use of the variety of skills included in performing tasks necessary to daily living, leisure activities, vocational pursuits, social interactions, and other required behaviors. The data are used to help formulate judgments as to how well these essential skills are being used, and

to gauge the degree to which tasks are accomplished and social role expectations are being met. Performance-based functional assessments take the social and physical contexts of the person into account.

It is possible to compare changes in status over periods of time for an individual or a group of individuals by assessing function at appropriate intervals. In this manner, outcomes of professional interventions of healthcare, rehabilitation, education, or psychologic and social counseling can be described and monitored. Once outcomes become measurable, they become manageable. Care must be exercised, however, in applying standards derived from group studies to the management of an individual. Factors that are unique to a particular case must be taken into account.

There have been many attempts to improve the quality of measurement in rehabilitation over the past 30 or more years. Validity is the paramount criterion for choice and use of a measure. Reliability is usually defined as freedom from random error and is necessary but not sufficient. The acid test of the utility of a functional assessment tool is that it predicts something in the future that is outside itself.

Development of a sound functional assessment instrument involves having a good idea that is conceptually clear and feasible, operationalizing the idea in the form of a stable instrument with logical procedures, tedious testing, and finally dissemination, with opportunities to follow the consequences of use of the instrument.

The design of an effective program evaluation system involves many ingredients. Program evaluation data must be presented in a clear, concise, and timely manner. The information must be relevant and understandable to those reviewing the information. Some form of the information should be shared with managers, clinical staff, and others. Presentation can take a variety of formats, including statistics, graphs, matrices, and narrative descriptions. This information should be used by providers to solve problems and improve the quality of care delivered to patients. The results of program evaluation could prove useful for evaluating alternative treatment modalities within a rehabilitation facility, but will become crucial for evaluating outcomes among different types of rehabilitation settings.

In 1985, Granger predicted that, by the year 2000,

... all healthcare workers will be using standardized terminology to describe the problems consequent to chronic disease and we will be employing systematic computerized methods for tracking individuals' functional abilities and their unmet needs over time. Medical rehabilitation programs will be mandated into the healthcare plans of individuals disabled by accident or disease. However, authorization for payment by third parties will entail requirements for (a) an organized system of care with a comprehensive plan of management, (b) a functional prognosis in terms of probabilities for therapeutic gains in terms of quality of life, (c) efficient delivery of services, and (d) documentation of outcomes through periodic assessments of functional status in order to determine the most favorable benefit/cost ratios.

(Granger 1985)[18]

As standardized functional assessment measures are developed that closely approximate the clinical situation, they will be used to predict the outcomes of care. They also will be a part of the cost-benefit analysis that will be integral to decision making in the health and rehabilitative care systems. Functional assessment will allow comparison of the effectiveness and efficiency of alternative therapeutic interventions and settings. Predictable relationships will emerge between the dose of rehabilitative services and the response of the patient. Finally, the wedding of functional assessment with prospective payment validates the importance of functional assessment and measurement of outcomes to provide necessary services effectively and efficiently to persons with disabilities, and also validates that there is a science behind the use of functional assessment.

ACKNOWLEDGMENT

We acknowledge the contributions of the authors of the 2nd edition: Carl V. Granger, M.D., Margaret Kelly-Hayes, Ed.D., R.N., C.R.R.N., Mark Johnston, Ph.D., Anne Deutsch, Ph.D., M.S., R.N., C.R.R.N., Susan Braun, M.L.S., O.T.R., and Roger C. Fiedler, Ph.D.

REFERENCES

1. Allen MJ, Yen WM. Introduction to measurement theory. Monterey: Brooks–Cole; 1979.

2. American Educational Research Association, American Psychological Association, National Council on Measurement in Education. Standards for educational and psychological testing. Washington: American Psychological Association; 1985.

3. Baker JG, Granger CV, Fiedler RC. A brief outpatient functional assessment measure: validity using Rasch measures. Am J Phys Med Rehabil 1997; 76:8–13.

4. Braun S. The Functional Independence Measure for Children (WeeFIM instrument): gateway to the WeeFIM System. J Rehabil Outcomes Meas 1998; 2:63–68.

5. Braun SL, Granger CV. A practical approach to functional assessment in pediatrics. Occup Ther Pract 1991; 2:46–51.

6. Carey RG, Posavac EJ. Program evaluation of a physical medicine and rehabilitation unit: a new approach. Arch Phys Med Rehabil 1978; 59:330–337.

7. Carter WB, Bobbitt RA, Bergner M, et al. Validation of an interval scaling: the Sickness Impact Profile. Health Serv Res 1976; 11:515–528.

8. Collins LM, Horn JL, eds. Best methods for the analysis of change. Washington: American Psychological Association; 1991.

9. Commission on Accreditation of Rehabilitation Facilities. Standards manual. Tucson: Commission on Accreditation of Rehabilitation Facilities; 2004.

10. Copes WS, Stark MM, Lawnick MM, et al. Linking data from national trauma and rehabilitation registries. J Trauma 1996; 40:428–436.

11. Donaldson SW, Wagner CC, Gresham GE. A unified ADL form. Arch Phys Med Rehabil 1973; 54:175–179.

12. Duke University Center for the Study of Aging and Human Development. Multidimensional Functional Assessment: the OARS methodology. Durham: Duke University; 1978.

13. Dunn G. Design and analysis of reliability studies. New York: Oxford University Press; 1989.

14. Feinstein AR. Clinimetrics. New Haven: Yale University Press; 1987.

15. Forer S. How to make program evaluation work for you. Neurorehabilitation 1992; 2:52–71.

16. Frey WD. Functional assessment in the '80s: a conceptual enigma, a technical challenge. In: Halpern AS, Fuhrer MJ, eds. Functional assessment in rehabilitation. Baltimore: Paul H Brookes; 1984: 11–43.

17. Gonnella C. Program evaluation. In: Fletcher GF, Banja JD, Jann BB, et al, eds. Rehabilitation medicine: contemporary clinical perspectives. Philadelphia: Lea & Febiger; 1992: 243–268.

18. Granger CV. Medical rehabilitation: predicting needs and measuring outcomes for quality of life. In: Gaitz CM, Niederehe G, Wilson NL, eds. Aging 2000: our health care destiny, vol 2. Psychosocial and policy issues. New York: Springer-Verlag; 1985: 255.

19. Granger CV, Hamilton BB, Fiedler RC. Discharge outcome after stroke rehabilitation. Stroke 1992; 23:978–982.

20. Guide for the Uniform Data Set for Medical Rehabilitation (including the FIM™ instrument), version 5.1. Buffalo: Uniform Data System for Medical Rehabilitation; 1997.

21. Heinemann AW, Linacre JM, Wright BD, et al. Relationships between impairment and physical disability as measured by the Functional Independence Measure. Arch Phys Med Rehabil 1993; 74:566–573.

22. Hinderer SR, Hinderer KA. Objective measurement in rehabilitation: theory and application. In: DeLisa J, Gans BM, Currie DM, eds. Rehabilitation medicine: principles and practices. 2nd ed. Philadelphia: Lippincott; 1993.

23. Johnston MV, Findley TW, deLuca J, et al. Research in physical medicine and rehabilitation: XII. Measurement tools with application to brain injury. Am J Phys Med Rehabil 1991; 70:40–56.

24. Johnston MV, Keith RA. Measurement standards for medical rehabilitation and clinical applications. Phys Med Rehabil Clin North Am 1993; 4:425–449.

25. Johnston MV, Keith RA, Hinderer S. Measurement standards for interdisciplinary medical rehabilitation. Arch Phys Med Rehabil 1992; 73(suppl): S3–S23.

26. Johnston MV, Kirshblum S, Zorowitz R, et al. Prediction of outcomes following rehabilitation of stroke patients. Neurorehabilitation 1992;2: 72–97.

27. Johnston MV, Wilkerson DL, Maney M. Evaluation of the quality and outcomes of medical rehabilitation programs. In: DeLisa J, Gans BM, Currie DM, eds. Rehabilitation medicine: principles and practices. Philadelphia: Lippincott; 1993.

28. Joint Commission on Accreditation of Healthcare Organizations. 1993 accreditation manual for hospitals. Oakbrook Terrace: Joint Commission on Accreditation of Healthcare Organizations; 1992.

29. Kane RA, Kane RL. Assessing the elderly: a practical guide to measurement. Lexington: Lexington Books; 1981.

30. Kaplan CP, Corrigan JD. The relationship between cognition and functional independence in adults with traumatic brain injury. Arch Phys Med Rehabil 1994; 75:643–647.

31. Katz S, Ford AB, Moskowitz RW, et al. Studies of illness in the aged: the index of ADL: a standardized measure of biological and psychological function. JAMA 1963; 185:914–919.

32. Keith RA. Functional assessment measures in medical rehabilitation: current status. Arch Phys Med Rehabil 1984; 65:74–78.

33. Kelly-Hayes M, Jette A, Wolf PA, et al. Functional limitations and disability among elders in the Framingham Study. Am J Public Health 1992; 82:841–845.

34. Kelman HR, Willner A. Problems in measurement and evaluation of rehabilitation. Arch Phys Med Rehabil 1962; 63:172–181.

35. Kraemer HC. Evaluating medical tests: qualitative and objective guidelines. Newbury Park: Sage; 1992.

36. Lawton MP. The functional assessment of elderly people. J Am Geriatr Soc 1971; 19(6):465–481.

37. Linacre JM. A user's guide to WINSTEPS. Ministep Rasch-model computer programs. Chicago:Winsteps; 1991–2000.

38. Linacre JM, Heinemann AW, Wright BD, et al. The structure and stability of the Functional Independence Measure. Arch Phys Med Rehabil 1994; 75:127–132.

39. Lohr KN, Donaldson MS, Harris-Wehling J. Medicare: a strategy for quality assurance. Quality of care in a changing health care environment. Qual Rev Bull 1992; 18:120–126.

40. Mahoney FI, Barthel D. Functional evaluation: the Barthel Index. Md Med J 1965; 14:61–65.

41. McDowell I, Newell C. Measuring health: a guide to rating scales and questionnaires. New York: Oxford University Press; 1987.

42. Merbitz C, Morris J, Grip JC. Ordinal scales and foundations of misinference. Arch Phys Med Rehabil 1989; 70:308–312.

43. Msall ME, DiGaudio K, Duffy LC, et al. WeeFIM: normative sample of an instrument for tracking functional independence in children. Clin Pediatr 1994; 33:431–438.

44. Nagi S. Disability concepts revisited. In: Sussman MB, ed. Sociology and rehabilitation. Washington: American Sociological Association; 1965: 100–113.

45. National Institutes of Health, National Institute of Child Health and Human Development. Research plan for the National Center for Medical Rehabilitation Research. US Department of Health and Human Services, Public Health Service (NIH) publication no 93-3509. Rockville: National Institutes of Health; 1993.

46. Norusis MJ, ed. SPSS guide to data analysis for SPSS-X. Chicago: SPSS; 1988.

47. Nunnally J. Psychometric theory. New York: McGraw-Hill; 1978.

48. Ottenbacher KJ, Smith PM, Illig SB, et al. Trends in length of stay, living setting, functional outcome, and mortality following medical rehabilitation. JAMA 2004; 292(14):1687–1695.

49. Patient Evaluation and Conference System (PECS). Wheaton (PO Box 795, Wheaton, IL 60189, USA): Marianjoy Rehabilitation Hospital and Clinics.

50. Rogosa DR, Willett JB. Understanding correlates of change by modelling individual differences in growth. Psychometrica 1985; 50:203–228.

51. Rosow I, Breslau N. A Guttman health scale for the aged. J Gerontol 1966; 21:556–559.

52. Schoening HA, Iversen IA. Numerical scoring of self-care status: a study of the Kenny Self-Care Evaluation. Arch Phys Med Rehabil 1968; 49:221–229.

53. Stineman MG, Escarce JJ, Goin JE, et al. A case mix classification system for medical rehabilitation. Med Care 1994; 32:366–379.

54. Task Force on Standards for Measurement in Physical Therapy. Standards for tests and measurements in physical therapy practice. Phys Ther 1991; 71:589–622.

55. US Department of Health and Human Services, Centers for Medicare & Medicaid Services, Baltimore, Maryland. Inpatient Rehabilitation Facility—Patient Assessment Instrument (IRF-PAI). OMB-0938-0842. 2002.

56. Wanlass RL, Reutter SL, Kline AE. Communication among rehabilitation staff: 'Mild', 'moderate', or 'severe' deficits? Arch Phys Med Rehabil 1992; 73:477–481.

57. Ware JE, Sherbourne CD. The MOS 36-item short form survey (SF-36): conceptual framework and item selection. Med Care 1992; 30:473–483.

58. WeeFIM System® clinical guide, version 5.01. Buffalo Uniform Data System for Medical Rehabilitation; 1998, 2002.

59. WeeFIM II® System clinical guide. Buffalo: Uniform Data System for Medical Rehabilitation; 2004.

60. World Health Organization. International classification of disease, ninth revision, clinical modification (ICD-9-CM). Geneva: WHO; 2004.

61. World Health Organization. International classification of functioning, disability and health. Geneva: WHO; 2001.

62. World Health Organization. International classification of impairments, disabilities, and handicaps. Geneva: WHO; 1980.

63. Wright BD, Masters GN. Rating scale analysis. Chicago: Mesa; 1982.

Evidence-based Medicine in Physical Medicine and Rehabilitation

Hilary C. Siebens

INTRODUCTION

Evidence-based medicine (EBM) is a major and somewhat controversial new theme in the evolving history of medical practice and rehabilitation. Only one Medline citation included this term in 1992.[49] A letter to the editor in 1997 encouraged the field of physical medicine and rehabilitation (PM&R) to pay more attention to EBM if 'the general consensus within medicine—that EBM is the right path into the future—is correct'.[37] From 1990 to 1997, only one citation in PM&R addressed the topic, compared with 250 in the rest of Medline's biomedical literature. In 1999, Joel DeLisa highlighted the growing importance of EBM in the Zeiter Lecture at the annual meeting of the American Academy of Physical Medicine and Rehabilitation.[12] He also identified some of its limitations. That same year, an academic PM&R department did a survey of its faculty, fellows, and residents.[11] The group agreed that physicians needed to use current information from medical articles for clinical decision making. They recognized that EBM techniques for reviewing articles were important, but many felt they didn't have the necessary skill set to use the techniques correctly. Recent letters to the editor discuss the absolute and relative frequency of EBM articles in the rehabilitation literature.[36,44] A 2004 search of PubMed's Clinical Query identified 4439 citations having a significant content about rehabilitation and good-quality evidence. A search of the entire Medline biomedical literature yielded over 13 000 EBM citations. Courses have addressed the use of EBM in rehabilitation, EBM web sites exist, and now EBM textbooks are available. The interest in EBM in the medical community continues to grow. Patients and families are also more interested in health information and are getting educated through print information and the Internet. They expect clinical practice to be based on current research evidence.[14] The interest in EBM is further documented by this chapter, which is one of the first devoted to the topic in a major rehabilitation textbook.

Definition and rationale

The term *evidence-based medicine* came from McMaster Medical School in Canada in the 1980s, and was used to label a clinical teaching and learning strategy that had been evolving over a decade.[14] The seminal text on the subject, *Evidence-based Medicine: How to Practice and Teach EBM*, is described by its authors as 'short, lean, and highly practical'. It defines the topic: 'Evidence-based medicine (EBM) is the integration of best research evidence with clinical expertise and patient values'.[46] Its core technique includes clear identification of questions about a patient's care and structured review of the literature using basic biostatistics and clinical epidemiology. The literature can be used to answer either:

- 'background' questions or general knowledge about a condition (textbooks can be adequate for this type of information); or
- 'foreground' questions about a specific patient's clinical situation. These questions focus on prevention, diagnosis, prognosis, and management.

This process involves four steps (Table 9-1). First, the clinician asks a question about the specific patient problem. It can include several parts. Second, the clinician searches the medical literature for relevant articles. Special search engines and databases are available that index articles that use rigorous research methods. Third, the facts or evidence in these articles is critically appraised or evaluated. Fourth, useful findings are implemented after discussion with the patient. A fifth step (not shown) includes evaluating the effectiveness and efficiency in executing the first four steps in the practice setting in order to improve the entire process. Anyone reading or skimming the brief text will quickly appreciate the general concepts and required skills.

The EBM approach addresses four problems:

1. the daily need in clinical practice for more information;
2. inadequacy of usual sources of information (out of date or inaccessible at time of need);
3. the disparity as time passes between physicians' increasing diagnostic skills and clinical judgment but potential decrease in up-to-date knowledge; and
4. most physicians have only a few seconds per patient to assimilate relevant evidence, and generally only 30 min per week for general reading and study.[46]

(In a PM&R residency survey of 30 residents or fellows and 49 faculty staff, average time spent reading per week was 4 h.)[11]

Evidence-based medicine uses five recent developments:

1. effective strategies for efficiently tracking down and appraising evidence;

Table 9-1 Core steps in practicing evidence-based medicine

Step	Action
1	Formulation of a clear single or multipart question on a patient's condition
2	Search medical literature for relevant articles
3	Appraise critically the literature using simple biostatistics
4	Apply findings as appropriate after discussion with the patient

2. new systematic reviews and concise summaries about healthcare;
3. evidence-based journals of secondary publication (that publish, according to EBM developers, 2% of clinical articles that are both valid and of immediate clinical use);
4. information systems like the Internet that bring the evidence to the clinician in seconds; and
5. effective strategies that clinicians can use for lifelong learning and improving clinical practice.[46]

Evidence-based medicine directly addresses two significant problems in clinical practice:

1. sound decision making to reduce idiosyncratic variations in clinical practice; and
2. the gap between knowledge and practice that result in ineffective, expensive, or even harmful decision making.[6,48]

In the initial description of these practices, the developers of EBM called the approach a paradigm shift. It represents a significant change in the way medicine is practiced and in how the literature is used.[14] However, the EBM approach is best viewed as another step in the evolution of the longstanding goal that medical practice should be based on scientific evidence whenever possible.

Medical statistics probably started being used in practice in the first third of the nineteenth century in Paris. The word comes from *statistik*, derived from *staat* or 'state', in the eighteenth-century Enlightenment. Statistik described how numbers could be used to help the state, or rulers, know about population sizes, natural resources, trade, etc.[40] A little later, Florence Nightingale believed in the value of facts and described statistics as 'the most important science in the world'.[39] The correlation of pathologic and clinical findings to alter practice patterns, in a reproducible and numerically meaningful fashion, also started at this time. The German revolution in laboratory-based medicine and the change in medical practice occurred in the mid to late nineteenth century. Clinicians used biostatistical models in British medical practice in the early twentieth century. By the end of the twentieth century, rapid electronic communication through the Internet brought evidence that was based

on statistical evaluations directly to clinicians. The ongoing challenge for busy clinicians with limited time is how to couple the tremendous volume of available information into the clinical decision-making process for the care of individual patients.

A fundamental challenge of evidence-based medicine

There are two steps in orderly medical decision making:

1. recalling and processing information in order to identify options for the problem at hand and their pros and cons; and
2. choosing among the options through reasoned judgment and the values of the clinician and patient.[55]

Any assistance with the first part of this clinical decision making must help clinicians make correct diagnostic and treatment decisions, in real time, and discuss the options with patients.

> It is widely recognized that accessing and processing medical information in libraries and patient records is a burden beyond the capacities of the physician's unaided mind in the conditions of medical practice. Physicians are quite capable of tremendous intellectual feats but cannot possibly do it all.
>
> (Weed 1999)[56]

Any busy clinician acknowledges how difficult, if not impossible, it is in the hectic course of clinical care to have access to all the valid information for a particular patient's condition.*

> Upon this gifted age, in its dark hour,
> Rains from the sky a meteoric shower
> Of facts . . . they lie unquestioned, uncombined.
> Wisdom enough to leech us of our ill
> Is daily spun, but there exists no loom
> To weave it into fabric . . .
> (Edna St. Vincent Millay, 1892–1950)[34]

An example of the clinical challenge involves a 15-year-old teenager who had been unable to attend school for 3 months due to fatigue.[23] She had lost 6.8 kg over the prior 7 months, had amenorrhea, and had shortness of breath on exertion. She was mildly hypotensive on examination and had multiple normal-looking nevi. It took several weeks and three hospitalizations for nausea, epigastric pain, and emesis before her Addison disease was diagnosed. During the course of the illness, the possibility of contacting child-protective services was considered. Her group of conscientious, caring physicians missed putting together, in a combined way, the multiple presenting

---

*Many of the following points have been expressed by Lawrence Weed, M.D., who is currently president of PKC Corp. (PKC stands for problem–knowledge couplers.) He developed in the late 1960s the well-known concept of the problem-oriented medical record. This included the subjective, objective, assessment, plan (SOAP) note format (see Weed 1968[53,54]). His keen interest was in the use of computers to improve healthcare. Structured notes and organizing patients' problems were an essential first step.

symptoms and signs accurately in order to make the correct diagnosis quickly. When the patient's presenting symptoms and signs were entered into a PKC software module[2] ('coupler'), Addison disease, a less common cause of the teenager's initial mild hypotension and fatigue, became the first cause listed in the differential diagnosis.[55] Many of the teenager's illness features when she first presented matched that diagnosis, including her multiple skin moles. If her doctors had had access to this type of information tool, Addison disease could have been tested for much sooner. It might have shortened the patient's course of illness significantly and avoided three hospitalizations, colonoscopy, gastric biopsies, and other tests. Instead, the diagnosis was delayed until the eventual electrolyte abnormality and hyponatremia of 128 mmol/L occurred. While this diagnostic task didn't require new research evidence, such evidence is included in other couplers, such as those for AIDS and congestive heart failure management.

New tools such as couplers are needed that help clinicians retrieve and process information. New technologies allow researchers to make major advances in medicine as well as other fields. The human genome was mapped when plate track machines and computerized sequencers became available. Powerful informational tools are needed in medicine to collect systematic data from a patient's history, physical examination, and laboratory results. This information, when combined or coupled with the evidence in the literature, presents clinicians with diagnostic and treatment options that can then be discussed with patients. Valid evidence from the medical literature is programmed into the process, with citations available to the clinician and patient as needed.[52,57,58] This type of information tool has already been created and is used by some physicians.[4] Tools like this are desperately needed for busy clinicians. Until such tools are accepted and widely available, EBM is the currently available approach to improving decision making by incorporating evidence more systematically into clinical practice.

COMPLEXITIES OF CLINICAL PRACTICE AND THE NATURE OF EVIDENCE

Medical practice in general

There are inherent realities of clinical practice that are sometimes viewed as shortcomings of the EBM process. These include the lack of evidence, difficulties in applying any evidence to an individual patient, and the barriers to practicing high-quality medicine in general (time, etc.). These perennial challenges in clinical medicine point out that EBM is not, nor even claims to be, a cure-all for inherent challenges in medical practice.[45] EBM also calls for using both 'hard', objective evidence and evidence about the 'soft' or subjective side of medicine. The emphasis in EBM to date has stressed evidence regarding screening and prevention, disease etiology, diagnosis, therapeutics, and prognosis. However, EBM includes the need for other types of knowledge and clinician skills for healing. Good clinicians identify patients' emotional needs, understand their suffering, and relieve this suffering. New research information supports improved ways of accomplishing these clinical goals.[14] For example, studies in the behavioral sciences have evaluated clinician–patient interactions. A randomized controlled trial demonstrated better outcomes when patients were involved more in their care compared with when provided with routine care.[20] This 'hard' evidence supports ways to improve the 'softer' side of medicine through greater patient involvement.

Another fundamental controversy exists about the nature of the evidence on which the entire EBM process depends.[1,15,58] EBM emphasizes a hierarchy of evidence, with primary value placed on systematic reviews and metaanalyses, followed by (in order) randomized controlled trials with definitive results, randomized controlled trials with non-definitive results, cohort studies, case control studies, cross-sectional surveys, and case reports.[25] The major sources of data—systematic reviews, metaanalyses, and randomized controlled trials—base conclusions on a large number of patients and a necessarily limited number of patient characteristics. This methodology can produce conclusions that might not be correct for individual patients.[1] A specific example relevant to PM&R follows.

> . . . one EBM synopsis review of studies on treatment of lateral ankle sprains concludes that "functional treatment" is likely to be beneficial.[50] The authors define "functional treatment" to include a variety of ankle supports as well as propriocepsis training. By arbitrarily combining these treatments under the single heading "functional treatment" the authors of the systematic review come to a particular conclusion. However, the conclusion reached is entirely dependent on the question asked. If the treatment in question is more specific (for example, is the Air-Stirrup ankle brace effective in treating lateral ankle sprains, or are balance board exercises effective in treating lateral ankle sprains?) the authors' conclusions and the subsequent choices made by a patient and provider may be significantly different'.[1]

Stated differently, a problem arises in the application of information learned from studying large, homogeneous population. With specific patients, it is often not clear if their clinical situation really fits the knowledge gained statistically. One excellent example comes from biologist Steven J. Gould's own experience. He wrote:

> Our culture encodes a strong bias either to neglect or ignore variation. We tend to focus instead on measures of central tendency, and as a result we make some terrible mistakes, often of considerable practical import.
>
> (Gould 1996)[19]

Figure 9-1 graphically shows how statistical measurement of central tendency, emphasizing the mean and median results, does not communicate well the range of clinical possibilities for individual patients. This dramatic example deals with prediction of death, but the principle applies to any other outcome

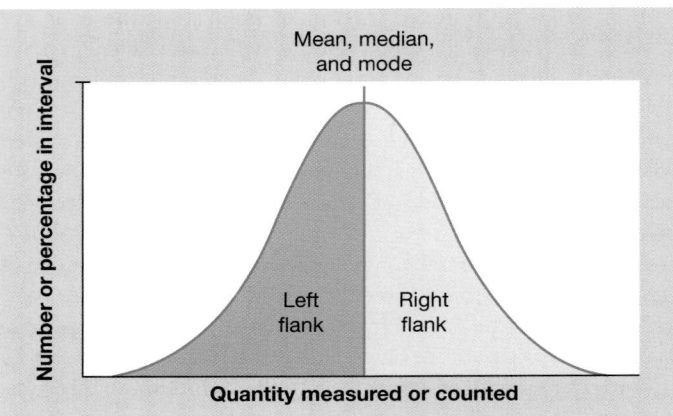

Figure 9-1 An idealized bell curve or normal frequency distribution, showing that all measures of central tendency (mean, median, and mode) coincide. (From Gould 1996,[18] with permission of Harmony Books.)

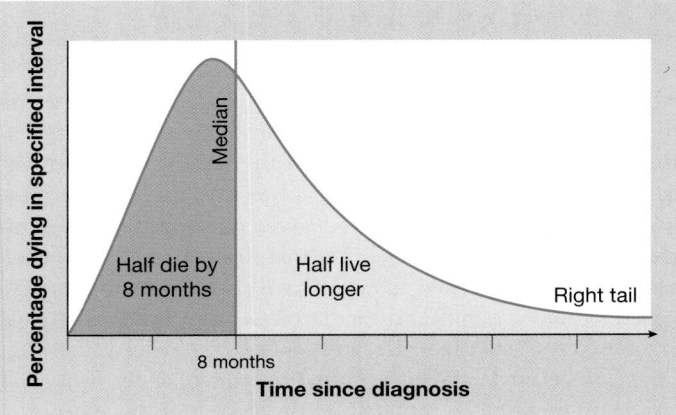

Figure 9-2 A right-skewed distribution for time of death for an illness with a medical mortality of 8 months. Each individual must be considered as a separate entity, and the entire distribution cannot be characterized by its median value. (From Gould 1996,[17] with permission of Harmony Books.)

or characteristic described by a distribution curve. Gould went on to discuss his personal experience with mesothelioma.

> Central tendency is an abstraction, variation the reality . . . I am not a measure of central tendency, either mean or median. I am one single human being with mesothelioma, and I want a best assessment of *my own* chances—for I have personal decisions to make, and my business cannot be dictated by abstract averages. I need to place myself in the most probable region of the variation based upon particulars of my own case; I must not simply assume that my personal fate will correspond to some measure of central tendency.
>
> (Gould 1996)[16]

The median survival for his diagnosis was 8 months, and he survived 20 years. Figure 9-2 shows the graphic representation of this wide range of clinical possibility.

These points identify the considerable complexities involved in the whole area of defining valid knowledge and applying it to treat individual patients and to improve clinical outcomes.[15,45,58] In October 2004, the *British Medical Journal* was devoted to the theme 'What's the evidence that evidence-based medicine changes anything?'[49]

In physical medicine and rehabilitation

Special considerations about the evidence in PM&R include the tremendous number of variables involved in the patient population receiving rehabilitation. At the patient level, risk adjustment is required in observational studies about rehabilitation outcomes, because patients vary across clinicians and institutions. No study can account for all possible factors. Risk adjustment is more difficult in rehabilitation than in other clinical services.[22] At the intervention level, characterizing rehabilitation interventions is difficult and outcomes are diverse. Multiple factors contribute to these outcomes: medical, mental, emotional, social supports, and financial resources, to name just a few.[10,21,22,24] Subpopulations of rehabilitation patients can have

multiple underlying diagnoses, comorbid conditions, or complications. These can vary among providers and treatments. The challenge in measuring rehabilitation outcomes is 'to distinguish immutable patient and system characteristics from those aspects of patient care that are amenable to intervention and improvement.'[43]

One approach to the problem of having appropriate evidence has been to develop a topic list of important questions through discussions with clinicians, patients, and carers.[24] Then this clinically relevant list is matched with the available trials and systematic reviews to make the best evidence available to clinicians. A recent review found 600 trials potentially relevant to stroke rehabilitation, for example, and these trials can be matched to clinical questions. This process then clarifies what topics require more reliable research.

EVIDENCE-BASED MEDICINE: THE PRACTICE

Teaching evidence-based medicine

Medical students, residents, and clinicians in practice need to learn EBM through specific study and practice. It restructures clinical decision making and therefore requires behavioral change by clinicians untrained in the practice. Specific skills are required to practice EBM as described by its developers. These include learning how to identify and ask the clinical question about a patient's clinical situation. This is harder than one might expect and includes defining four elements of the question: patient, intervention (test, therapeutics, etc.), comparison (gold standard, other treatment, etc.), and outcome.[46] This is referred to as the PICO format. From this specific question, electronic searching of information sources is required—either original studies or systematic reviews. Assessing the literature requires a working knowledge of some basic key criteria to be included in any study about particular areas: diagnostic tests, disease prognosis, therapeutic interventions, and systematic reviews.

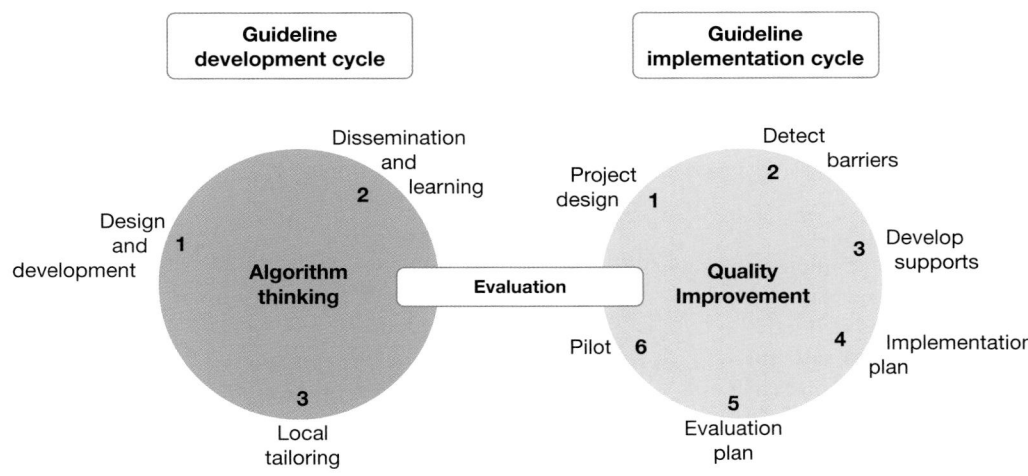

Figure 9-3 The guidelines bi-cycle: process steps in guideline development and implementation. (From Margolis and Cretin 1999,[31] with permission of the American Hospital Association Press.)

Clinicians need to understand some basic statistical terms in order to assess numeric conclusions from the studies. These statistics are either descriptive, about the patient sample, or inferential, testing for significance of differences between groups of patients.[30] For example, understanding the value of diagnostic or screening tests requires knowing the tests' sensitivity and specificity. Additional calculations from these basic values clarify the tests' value: likelihood ratios, positive predictive value, negative predictive value, prevalence, pretest and posttest odds, and posttest probability. Evidence on prognosis requires knowing confidence intervals and the 1-year survival, medical survival, and inspection of the actual survival curves. Evidence on therapy requires understanding relative risk ratios, absolute risk reduction, number needed to treat (NNT), and number needed to harm. In evaluating systematic reviews, odds ratios, patient expected event rates, and NNTs quantify the significance of the reviews (see Sackett et al 2000[46] for definitions and examples).

These skills of question formulation and reviewing the literature have not been routinely taught in, or at least remembered from, medical schools or residency programs in the past. Only 34% of residents and faculty in one PM&R residency program felt they had received adequate training in appraising the medical literature.[11] Students may lack support from peers and from clinical teachers who are themselves unfamiliar with EBM. They might be unable to use the skills efficiently in actual practice.[51] Complexities in teaching EBM include the detection of 'maybe' disease (abnormalities that may not ever be overtly expressed in the patient's lifetime), preparing students for situations when data is absent, and guidelines for when evidence needs to be sought to help with treatment decisions (knowing that one doesn't know).[58] Despite these challenges, clinical educators are creating educational assessment tools and EBM curricula for undergraduate and postgraduate students.

Guidelines

Clinical guideline development and implementation is similar to EBM in that evidence is reviewed and specific recommenda-

tions are made to help guide clinical care. Guidelines were believed to be one means, like EBM, to close the gap between known evidence and lack of its use in clinical practice, and to help decrease geographic variation in practice patterns. Guidelines generally have two components: the evidence summary and the specific recommended actions in patient care. The levels of evidence vary for different types of specific recommendations. Some recommendations are completely supported with quality information, while other recommendations depend on expert consensus due to the lack of good data.

Guidelines, even those with excellent supporting evidence, frequently are not implemented. Barriers to specific guidelines occur and are independent of the level of evidence.[46] The *burden* of illness of the particular guideline might not be high enough to warrant the effort required. Patients' and communities' *beliefs* might not agree or value the guideline. The cost of implementation could be a bad *bargain* for the organization. Other *barriers* that can be too high to overcome include the unavailability of a treatment in the geographic area.

Further evaluation of some of these 'killer bees', a term used to describe the above barriers, reveals the multiple, complicated steps in moving from a guideline to actual improvement in patient care.[31] Implementation of any guideline requires a cycle of process (or performance or quality) improvement:

- project design;
- detection of barriers;
- development of supports;
- implementation plan;
- evaluation of plan; and
- piloting of the plan (Fig. 9-3).

This cycle can be simple (as in a small office practice implementing a better fall flu vaccination process) or complex (a hospital establishing a stroke unit because patient outcomes are better with this type of organized care). These process steps are essential and are not always easily implemented. To date, many professionals in healthcare remain 'process-illiterate' unless they have specific training or have actively participated in performance improvement projects. This situation is changing gradually, however.[†] Guideline adherence in stroke care is associated with better patient outcomes. For example, functional outcomes in stroke rehabilitation were better in those care systems that followed many of the national post-stroke rehabilitation guidelines.[13] Patient satisfaction was greater as well when many of these guidelines were followed.[42]

Barriers for clinicians

Changing clinician behavior to follow guidelines or implement EBM approaches requires specific knowledge and supportive attitudes.[5] One systematic review of 76 studies divided the reasons physicians are unable to follow guidelines into three categories.[5] As indicated in Box 9-1, multiple reasons exist. Physicians and others who work in implementing EBM identify similar barriers.[46] Individual studies have evaluated physicians' experiences when they try to modify their practice patterns.

In a randomized trial, two physician groups received clinical information about cardiovascular risk factors in a traditional continuing medical education format.[32] The intervention group also received information about barriers to implementation. On a survey 4–5 weeks later, those who had changed their behavior were those who immediately after the continuing medical education course indicated an intent to change. Simply learning about barriers made no difference.

Clinical educators in rehabilitation who attended a 2-day course on evidence-based rehabilitation reported on their level of readiness to change their practice to a more evidence-based approach.[47] The 21 clinicians had a combined clinical experience of 350 years in physical therapy, occupational therapy, and rehabilitation counseling. The Model of Behavioral Change was used as a framework to identify readiness to implement evidence-based practice (EBP) in the clinical setting.[‡] Response categories included:

- no thought about changing;
- thinking about changing;
- making a plan to change;
- implementing a specific action plan; and
- continuing to implement a plan of action.

The majority (76%) did not use an EBP approach for a sustained period of time. Twelve of the participants increased in their readiness to use an EBP approach by at least one stage after having taken the course.

Participants identified barriers and facilitators to EBP, and the authors analyzed these using a constant comparative method. Four recurring themes classified barriers and facilitators: self-reflection, EBP knowledge, practice management, and peers. In

---

Box 9-1 Barriers to physician adherence to practice guidelines in relation to behavior change

Knowledge
- Lack of awareness or familiarity
- Volume of information
- Time needed to stay informed
- Guideline accessibility

Attitudes
- Lack of agreement with guideline
- Interpretation of evidence
- Applicability to patient
- Not cost-beneficial
- Lack of confidence in guideline developer
- Lack of agreement with guidelines in general
- 'Too cookbook'
- Too rigid to apply
- Biased synthesis
- Challenge to autonomy
- Not practical
- Lack of outcome
- Expectancy
- Lack of self-efficacy
- Physician believes that she or he cannot perform recommendation
- Lack of motivation or inertia of previous practice

Behavior
- External barriers
- Patient factors
- Guideline factors
- Guideline characteristics
- Presence of contradictory guidelines
- Environmental factors
- Lack of time
- Lack of resources
- Organizational constraints
- Lack of reimbursement
- Perceived increase in malpractice liability

---

each theme, barriers and facilitators were either internal (to the participant) or external (in the participant's work environment). Barriers were similar to those listed in Box 9-1. Participants identified feasible facilitators such as 'coworkers who value intellectual exchanges' and 'EBP incorporation into scheduled activities'. Both of these studies highlight that a first step in actual change in practice performance could be a clinician's increased readiness or an intention to change practice.

Another study evaluated barriers to EBP using focus groups of non-physician stroke rehabilitation professionals.[38] Ninety-two percent ($n = 79$) agreed that keeping up to date with research findings was important to them. They were motivated to practice according to guidelines or an EBM approach. However, 92% also cited lack of time to do the tasks, 67% ($n = 58$) perceived a need for further training, and 95% ($n = 101$) acknowledged difficulty in transferring research findings into their daily practice. Other therapists note these challenges as well.[29]

Porzsolt and colleagues creatively modified the EBM technique for asking questions to overcome some of the resistance

---

[†]An excellent quick read, even if skimmed, is *Curing Health Care* by D. Berwick, D. Godfrey, and J. Roessner (San Francisco: Jossey-Bass; 1990). Clinicians will be able to get 'the big picture' of what is occurring with quality improvement from the personal stories of the several early efforts made in several healthcare organizations. Spending some time browsing the Institute for Healthcare Improvement's web site is edifying as well (http://www.ihi.org).

[‡]Non-physician rehabilitation professionals use the term *evidence-based practice* to encompass additional knowledge that is not traditionally included in medicine.

that clinicians expressed.[41] Clinical decisions synthesize internal and external evidence. Experienced clinicians have their own internal knowledge gained from daily practice experience. They have trouble differentiating between actual scientific evidence and what seems obvious (because 'that's the way we've always done it and it seems to work'). It isn't clear to them when and if they need to find new information. To overcome this hurdle, after formulating the clinical question, clinicians record their own answer to the clinical question based on their experience and knowledge. This answer is compared with the new evidence, found in steps 3 and 4 (acquiring or finding evidence, assessing or critically appraising the evidence). The clinician then learns whether his or her knowledge was correct in the first place. If the internal and external information conflict, clinicians can:

- change their mind and align their internal knowledge with the new information;
- decide the external evidence isn't convincing enough and stick with their internal information; or
- discuss the conflict between the internal and external evidence with the patient and have the patient help make the clinical decision.

This approach values the clinician's own, often hard-earned, knowledge and judgment by explicitly comparing the clinician's internal knowledge with the new external evidence.

The current climate in healthcare in the USA and the rapid pace of change might make it particularly difficult for clinicians to change practice patterns. Some physicians have expressed an increasing dissatisfaction with medical practice.[33,59] Similar complaints are voiced in other non-medical professional groups. There are no 'magic bullets' available to help physicians, specifically, improve professional practice.[8,35] However, short term, some practical EBM approaches might be feasible, not overly burdensome, and could lead to improved clinical outcomes.

PRACTICAL APPROACHES FOR REHABILITATION PHYSICIANS, THERAPISTS, AND MANAGERS

Facilitating evidence-based medicine for clinicians

If clinicians remain unconvinced or confused about the benefits of some of the EBM techniques, reading more about EBM and discussing questions with experienced colleagues can be helpful.[9] Once practitioners decide to change some of their prior practice habits, external supports help. A starting place can include open discussions with colleagues. Next, clinicians can start practicing seven basic steps with the patients they treat.

1. Admit there may be some new information one doesn't know.
2. Assess the patient using excellent history and physical examination skills.
3. Ask a focused question using the structured PICO format: patient issue, intervention (therapy or test), comparison intervention (therapy or gold standard test), and outcome (clinical or test accuracy).
4. Acknowledge (by writing down) what one believes to be the answer (internal knowledge).
5. Acquire the best evidence using electronic sources (see Table 9-2).
6. Assess the validity of the evidence and compare to one's own understanding.
7. Apply to the patient's specific situation based on the patient's perspective and wishes.

This process requires practice. Peer support and collaboration is very helpful. The range of resources to support this EBM approach, some of which are listed in Table 9-2, continue to grow.

Another very helpful EBM technique includes written critically appraised topics (CATs).[27,46] These document the seven-step process described above and make the clinical reasoning and evidence available for sharing and debate (Table 9-3). Different formats exist, and their essential characteristic is that they are simultaneously brief, informative, and useful. A free downloadable program, the CATmaker, is available through http://www.cebm.utoronto.ca/ (select CATmaker in EBM Toolbox). The virtue of documenting a question and the evidence in writing, in a format like the CATs, is that it clarifies the thought process. In a given practice setting, this disciplined process can review patient care decisions for the most frequent clinical conditions. For example, in an outpatient musculoskeletal physiatry practice, the role of non-steroidal anti-inflammatory medication versus acetaminophen for pain associated with osteoarthritis can be evaluated using the CAT format. This single CAT will apply to many patients, because this question arises frequently. These CATs can be kept in their own notebook to organize the collective work of a single practitioner or a group practice. The information remains easily available for quick reference if the clinician forgets or if someone else needs the same information. The CAT can also communicate the clinical approach to others in the clinical practice, such as office staff, so that they can help implement a particular strategy when necessary.

Additional strategies for implementation of EBM practices are listed in Box 9-2 for those specifically seeking approaches at their work sites.[11,28,48] Some of the suggestions identify changes in activities that may be ongoing and require no additional time, but others might include adding new activities not yet scheduled into the work routine. In this case, the unproductive and less worthwhile work routines need to be eliminated first. More effective practices can replace these without any additional expenditure of time.

Introducing some fun into this process is essential. For example, one group of residents did an inventory on a group of patients and the clinical decisions their care involved.[46] Decisions were classified as being based on sound evidence (randomized controlled trials or systematic trial reviews), based on

Table 9-2 Evidence-based medicine resources

Resource	Details	Notes
Books *Evidence-based Medicine: How to Practice and Teach EBM* *Evidence-based Rehabilitation*	Sackett DL et al. Edinburgh: Churchill Livingston; 2000 Law M, ed. Thorofare: Slack; 2002	Comprehensive, brief, practical guide Excellent discussion of concepts and related relevant topics
Evidence-based medicine databases PubMed: Clinical Queries	National Library of Medicine search site; each article under *Clinical Queries* has been individually reviewed and rated as meeting standards for good evidence (http://www.ncbi.nlm.nih.gov/entrez/query.fcgi)	–
Netting the Evidence	The University of Sheffield, UK; has links to evidence-based medicine (EBM) resources, along with databases, summary articles from major medical journals (http://www.shef.ac.uk/scharr/ir/netting/)	Quick, easy to use
Cochrane Reviews	From the Cochrane Collaboration, an international EBM group with multiple activities including conducting systematic reviews (http://www.cochrane.org/reviews)	–
Database of Abstracts of Reviews of Effects (DARE)	University of York, UK (http://www.york.ac.uk/inst/crd/darehp.htm)	A look in *Databases, Best Evidence, Top 10 Articles* in 2003 led to excellent commentary on study of treatment of cervicogenic headache; structured reviews; abstracts for secondary reviews; free
Pedro	University of Sydney, Australia (http://www.fhs.usyd.edu.au/index.htm)	Reviews of physical therapy evidence
SumSearch	University of Texas Health Science Center at San Antonio; online screen prompts guide search strategy (http://sumsearch.uthscsa.edu/)	Metasearch engine of all databases
Journals American College of Physicians Journal Club	Summary of research study, with commentary of implications in the context of current practice (http://www.acponline.org/)	Survey of three issues in past 24 months revealed about 20–25% of reviews relevant to physical medicine and rehabilitation practice
Bandolier	Summaries of systematic reviews and metaanalyses from PubMed and Cochrane Library, as well as their own systematic reviews (http://www.jr2.ox.ac.uk/bandolier/)	–
Web sites Centre for Evidence-based Medicine	University Health Network and University of Toronto libraries (http://www.cebm.utoronto.ca)	Much free information, with sample critically appraised topics on many EBM topics
The Cochrane Collaboration	Not for profit organization with network of reviewers writing evidence summaries (http://www.cochrane.org)	–
Clinical Evidence	British Medical Journal Publishing Group's site for best evidence (http://www.clinicalevidence.org)	Pay per view charges or free if other print products purchased
Patient or Consumer Web Site Informed Health Online	http://www.informedhealthonline.org/item.aspx	Lay summaries of Cochrane Collaboration systematic reviews

Table 9-3 Critically appraised topic format with comments that suggest potential modifications

Critically appraised topic component	Content	Comment
Title	Name of topic	–
Clinical bottom line	The summary conclusion from all the information	What does the evidence mean clinically?
Clinical scenario	Brief summary of case's facts	–
Question: two or three parts	–	–
Clinician's answer	Clinician's preevidence answer to the question	Step developed by Porzsolt (see text) to help incorporate clinicians' internal evidence in this process
Search terms		Can list database used
Critically appraised topic (CAT) author and date		–
The study	Review of reference, including key factors of study design	Can combine study or results into a single category labeled *the evidence* (findings and their validity)
Results	Summary of evidence results	–
The patient		This does *not* appear in traditional CAT formats to date but could be added; documents the patient's concerns (financial, fear of complications, etc.) and preferences that need to be considered along with the clinical evidence in making a final decision
Management decision	The clinical decision for a particular patient by the CAT developer (note: the decision may be to not do what evidence supports, due to the patient's choice or other factors after discussion with the patient)	Again, this section does *not* appear in a traditional CAT; clarifies decision given research evidence, patient's perspective, and clinician's judgment and expertise
Comments	Any useful commentary, including practical implementation information, etc.	–

convincing non-experimental evidence, or based on no current evidence. It is likely that a greater number of decisions in rehabilitation practice will be based on no evidence as compared with some other fields. This survey could be a stimulating way to review how frequently clinicians are using good evidence. Group debate can then focus on the results and what, if anything, needs to change.

Organizational perspectives

The ultimate goal of incorporating evidence into clinical problem solving is to improve patients' health and clinical outcomes. When done well, EBM has the potential to also improve the health of the health system that is treating the patients.[26] Ideally, EBM is a shared goal for both practitioners and the systems in which they work. Multiple external factors and constraints influence actual patient care, such as payment mechanisms, limitations of time, attitudes of colleagues, and availability of Internet and electronic database access. Davis studied continuing medical education and its impact on physi-

cian behaviors extensively, and has proposed *knowledge translation* to encompass the other disciplines and processes required to close the gap between evidence and practice.[7,8,26] Berwick categorized four environment levels of processes responsible for improving the quality of care.[2]

1. Level A: the experience of patients and communities (i.e. patients and frontline caregivers).
2. Level B: microsystems of care (i.e. hospital unit, outpatient office practices).
3. Level C: healthcare organizations.
4. Level D: environment external to healthcare (i.e. financing, accreditation).

Clinicians know that various factors in large medical systems can support, or discourage, EBP. What and when system changes are needed, and when, are complex issues. Innovation and organizational change are difficult.[3] Despite this, however, clinicians have always known that they do have control over some important components of their own practice environments.

Box 9-2 Evidence-based practice implementation strategies

- Develop a system to track clinical questions.
- Work evidence-based practice (EBP) into current scheduled activities, replacing current, less effective approaches (rounds, journal clubs, in-services).
- For academic institutions, incorporate EBP into clinical education and have students assist with searches and critically appraised topic (CAT) development.
- Establish or join an EBP working group.
- Make use of online EBP resources.
- Discuss evidence with patients as a component of patient education.
- Develop an EBP folder with CATs.
- Include some evidence-based medicine competencies and include in staff assessments and performance evaluations.
- Be creative: 'write your own textbook' using CATs, etc.
- Review journal articles from evidence-based sites using a few simple review criteria until more familiar with the process.
- Establish protected reading time.
- Establish a standard search routine for common practice topics.
- Meet with a medical librarian for training in searching techniques.

They control their collaborations with peers, their own personal education about topics such as EBM, and much of their own decision making with their patients. Clinicians can strive to improve the care of their patients through these types of choices.

CONCLUSION

Evidence-based medicine is an evolving clinical approach that incorporates scientific evidence more systematically into the care of individual patients. It can help with problems of rapid growth in the medical literature and the need for improved quality and best possible patient outcomes. Detailed explanations of EBM exist, and the strengths and weaknesses of EBM are increasingly acknowledged. Special challenges exist for the use of EBM in PM&R practice. The rehabilitation patient population experiences a large variety of medical problems and disabilities. Rehabilitation outcomes depend on multiple variables. Despite the complexity of PM&R practice, however, no one can argue against the goals of working toward better inclusion of valid evidence in clinical decision making. Clinical decisions will always be based on a two-step process:

1. retrieving and processing available information; and
2. decision making based on this information, clinician judgment, and patients' values.

Evidence will range from rigorous research, to accepted practice, to experience and instincts. EBM challenges clinicians and others in healthcare to use quality evidence, when it exists, in the first step, and to share it explicitly with patients in the second step. The goal of EBM might not be fully achievable in routine clinical practice until better information tools are available.

ACKNOWLEDGMENTS

I want to thank Mary Slavin, Ph.D., P.T., and Carole Warde, M.D., for their insights and resources for teaching and practicing EBM, and Lawrence L. Weed, M.D. and David Harr for generosity in answering multiple queries.

REFERENCES

1. [Anonymous]. Problem-knowledge couplers® and evidence-based medicine. Online. Available: http://www.pkc.com/papers/ebm.pdf 2004 14 Sep 2004
2. Berwick D. A user's manual for the IOM's 'Quality chasm' report. Health Aff 2002; 21:80–90.
3. Berwick DM. Disseminating innovations in health care. JAMA 2003; 289:1969–1975.
4. Burger CS. The use of problem knowledge couplers in a primary care practice. Healthc Inf Manage 1997; 11:13–26.
5. Cabana MD, Rand CS, Powe NR, et al. Why don't physicians follow clinical practice guidelines? JAMA 1999; 282:1458–1465.
6. Chalmers I, Dickersin Chalmers K TC. Getting to grips with Archie Cochrane's agenda. Br Med J 1992; 305:786–787.
7. Davis D, Evans M, Jadad A, et al. The case for knowledge translation: shortening the journey from evidence to effect. Br Med J 2003; 327: 33–35.
8. Davis D, O'Brien MA, Freemantle N, et al. Impact of formal continuing medical education. JAMA 1999; 282:867–874.
9. Dean-Baar S, Pakieser-Reed K. Closing the gap between research and clinical practice. Top Stroke Rehabil 2004; 11:60–68.
10. Dejong G, Horn SD, Gassawy JA, et al. Toward a taxonomy of rehabilitation interventions: using an inductive approach to examine the 'black box' of rehabilitation. Arch Phys Med Rehabil 2004; 85:678–686.
11. DeLisa JA, Jain SS, Kirshblum S, et al. Evidence-based medicine in physiatry. Am J Phys Med Rehabil 1999; 78:228–232.
12. DeLisa JA. Issues and challenges for physiatry in the coming decade. Arch Phys Med Rehabil 1999; 80:1–12.
13. Duncan PW, Horner RD, Reker DM, et al. Adherence to postacute rehabilitation guidelines is associated with functional recovery in stroke. Stroke 2002; 33:167–178.
14. Evidence-based Medicine Working Group. Evidence-based medicine: a new approach to teaching the practice of medicine. JAMA 1992; 268: 2420–2425.
15. Feinstein AR, Horwitz RI. Problems in the 'evidence' of 'evidence-based medicine'. Am J Med 1997; 103:529–535.
16. Gould S. Full house: the spread of excellence from Plato to Darwin. New York: Harmony Books; 1996:1–244, 48–49.
17. Gould S. Full house: the spread of excellence from Plato to Darwin. New York: Harmony Books; 1996:51.
18. Gould S. Full house: the spread of excellence from Plato to Darwin. New York: Harmony Books; 1996:52.
19. Gould S. Full house: the spread of excellence from Plato to Darwin. New York: Harmony Books; 1996:1–244, 44.
20. Greenfield S, Kaplan S, Ware JE Jr. Expanding patient involvement in care: effects on patient outcomes. Ann Intern Med 1985; 102:520–528.
21. Hoenig H, Sloane R, Horner RD. A taxonomy for classification of stroke rehabilitation services. Arch Phys Med Rehabil 2000; 81:853–862.
22. Iezzoni LI. Risk adjusting rehabilitation outcomes: an overview of methodologic issues. Am J Phys Med Rehabil 2004; 83:316–326.
23. Keljo D, Squires R. Clinical problem-solving: just in time. N Engl J Med 1996; 334:46–48.

24. Langhorne P, Legg L, Pollock A, et al. Evidence-based stroke rehabilitation. Age Ageing 2002; 31(suppl 3):17–20.

25. Law M, Philp I. Evaluating the evidence. In: Law M, ed. Evidence-based rehabilitation. Thorofare: Slack; 2002:97–108.

26. Law M, Philp I. Research dissemination and transfer of knowledge. In: Law M, ed. Evidence-based rehabilitation: a guide to practice. Thorofare: Slack; 2002:255–268.

27. Law M. Evidence-based rehabilitation. Thorofare: Slack; 2002:1–364.

28. Law M. Introduction to evidence-based practice. In: Law M, ed. Evidence-based rehabilitation: a guide to practice. Thorofare: Slack; 2002:1–12.

29. Maher CG, Sherrington C, Elkins M. Challenges for evidence-based physical therapy: accessing and interpreting high-quality data on therapy. Phys Ther 2004; 84:644–654.

30. Mandich A, Miller L, Law M. Outcomes in evidence-based practice. In: Law M, ed. Evidence-based rehabilitation. Thorofare: Slack; 2002:49–70.

31. Margolis CZ, Cretin A. Implementing clinical practice guidelines. Chicago: American Hospital Association Press; 1999:xxi, 1–223.

32. Mazmanian PE, Daffron SR, Johnson RE, et al. Information about barriers to planned change: a randomized controlled trial involving continuing medical education lectures and commitment to change. Acad Med 1998; 73:882–886.

33. Mechanic D. Physician discontent: challenges and opportunities. JAMA 2003; 290:941–946.

34. Millay ES. Collected sonnets. New York: Harper and Row; 1988:140.

35. Oxman AD, Thomson MA, Davis DA, et al. No magic bullets: a systematic review of 102 trials of interventions to improve professional practice. Can Med Assoc J 1995; 153:1423–1431.

36. Pittler MH, Ernst E. Author reply. Arch Phys Med Rehabil 2004; 85:1561–1562.

37. Pittler MH, Ernst E. Letter to the editor. Arch Phys Med Rehabil 1997; 78:1281.

38. Pollock AS, Legg L, Langhorne P, et al. Barriers to achieving evidence-based stroke rehabilitation. Clin Rehabil 2000; 14:611–617.

39. Porter R. The greatest benefit to mankind. London: HarperCollins; 1997:378.

40. Porter R. The greatest benefit to mankind. London: HarperCollins; 1997:1–831.

41. Porzsolt F, Ahletz A, Thim A, et al. Evidence-based decision making—the 6-step approach. ACP J Club 2003; 139:A11.

42. Reker DM, Duncan PW, Horner RD, et al. Postacute stroke guideline compliance is associated with greater patient satisfaction. Arch Phys Med Rehabil 2002; 83:750–756.

43. Reker DM, O'Donnell JC, Hamilton BB. Stroke rehabilitation outcome variation in Veterans Affairs rehabilitation units: accounting for case-mix. Arch Phys Med Rehabil 1998; 79:751–757.

44. Rocha AP, Beraldo PS. Evidence-based PM&R? Yes! Arch Phys Med Rehabil 2004; 85:1561–1562.

45. Sackett DL, Rosenberg WMC, Gray JAM, et al. Evidence based medicine: what it is and what it isn't. Br Med J 1996; 312:71–72.

46. Sackett DL, Straus SE, Richardson WS, et al. Evidence-based medicine: how to practice and teach EBM. Edinburgh: Churchill Livingstone; 2000: 1–261.

47. Slavin MD, Siebens HC, Keysor JJ. Change in readiness toward using an evidence-based approach in the clinical setting. APTA Comb Sect Meet Proc 2003.

48. Slavin MD. Teaching evidence-based practice in physical therapy: critical competencies and necessary conditions. J Phys Ther Education 2004; in press.

49. Straus SE. What's the E for EBM? Br Med J 2004; 328:535–536.

50. Struijis P, Kerkhoffs G. Ankle sprain. Clin Evid 2001; 6:798–806

51. Taylor R, Reeves B, Mears R, et al. Development and validation of a questionnaire to evaluate the effectiveness of evidence-based practice teaching. Med Educ 2001; 35:544–547.

52. Weaver RR. Resistance to computer innovation: knowledge coupling in clinical practice. Comput Soc 2002:16–21.

53. Weed LL. Medical records that guide and teach. N Engl J Med 1968; 278:593–600

54. Weed LL. What physicians worry about: how to organize care of multiple-problem patients. Mod Hosp 1968; June:90–94

55. Weed LL, Weed L. Opening the black box of clinical judgment. eBMJ 1999.

56. Weed LL. Clinical judgment revisited. Methods Inf Med 1999; 38:279–286.

57. Weed LL. New connections between medical knowledge and patient care. Br Med J 1997; 315:231–235.

58. Weed LL. Shedding our illusions: a better way of medicine. Fertil Steril 2004; 81:45–52.

58. Welch HG, Lurie JD. Teaching evidence-based medicine: caveats and challenges. Acad Med 2000; 75:235–240.

59. Zuger A. Dissatisfaction with medical practice. N Engl J Med 2004; 350:69–75.

Chapter

10

Electrodiagnostic Medicine I: Fundamental Principles

Daniel Dumitru

Performing an electrodiagnostic medicine consultation requires a thorough understanding of nerve and muscle physiology and pathophysiology. Of equal importance is knowing the manner in which the electrodiagnostic instrument processes and displays the various electrical signals generated during the examination. Mastering this information and acquiring the manual skill necessary to record the electrophysiologic data allows the practitioner to accurately diagnose various disorders affecting the neuromuscular system.

ACTION POTENTIAL GENERATION

Nerve and muscle tissues are capable of generating an electrical difference across their cellular membranes, as well as generate and sustain a propagating action potential. Interestingly, action potential generation is relatively similar between these two dramatically different tissues. The reader is strongly encouraged to read basic physiology texts[22,25] to gain a more complete appreciation of the intricate relationship between excitable cells and their associated action potentials.

Resting membrane potential

All living cells generate an electrical potential across their membranes, with the intracellular region relatively negative compared with the extracellular environment.[25] This potential difference across the cell membrane is referred to as the resting membrane potential. The development and maintenance of the resting membrane potential can be explained by a simple model.

We can partition a beaker into right and left halves with an impermeable membrane containing multiple closed potassium channels. This membrane separates two different concentrations of a potassium chloride (KCl) solution (left, 10 mM, and right, 100 mM potassium chloride; Fig. 10-1).[14] Potassium chloride in solution exists as positive potassium (K^+) ions (cations) and negative chloride (Cl^-) ions (anions). A voltmeter (a device that detects potential differences) measuring the two solutions fails to detect a potential difference, because there is a lack of physical continuity between the left and right halves of the beaker when the partition's potassium channels are closed. In other words, the two solutions are electrically independent.

If we now open the membrane's potassium channels, K^+ cations will flow 'down' their concentration gradient from the high (100 mM) to low (10 mM) ion concentration side of the beaker (Fig. 10-1). The potassium ions will continue this directional flow until there is a balance between:

- the forces of the physical concentration gradient difference driving potassium to the lower-concentration region; and
- the electrical gradient opposing this directional ion flow.

Because there are only potassium channels, the negative chloride ions cannot pass through the membrane and remain on their respective sides of the beaker. As more and more positive potassium ions leave one side of the beaker, there begins to develop an unbalanced or 'excess' amount of negative charges (Cl^-) on the high-concentration side of the beaker, with an equal buildup of 'excess' positive charges (K^+) on the other side of the beaker. The increasing net negative charge of the beaker half with the increasing number of unbalanced chloride ions begins to make it increasingly difficult for the positive potassium charges to leave the high-concentration side of the beaker. This is because the progressively building net negative charge increasingly attracts those remaining positive potassium ions. Similarly, a growing amount of positive potassium ions on the formerly low potassium concentration side of the beaker begin to increasingly repel additional potassium ions attempting to enter this side of the beaker.

At some point, the opposing electrical charges on the two sides of the beaker prevent any more potassium from leaving the beaker's high-concentration side, even though there is still a higher potassium concentration on this side compared with the other. A balance is established between the ionic concentration forces driving potassium ions from the high- to low-concentration regions, and the electrical forces (positive repelling and negative attracting) tending to keep potassium ions in the more concentrated portion of the beaker. Any potassium ions that randomly enter the lower-concentration side of the beaker are balanced by other potassium ions similarly crossing in the opposite direction. The situation where balance between electrical and concentration forces exists is said to be a dynamic equilibrium. Placing a voltmeter across the partition measures a negative potential difference, as electrical continuity is now present between the two halves of the beaker through the open potassium ion channels.

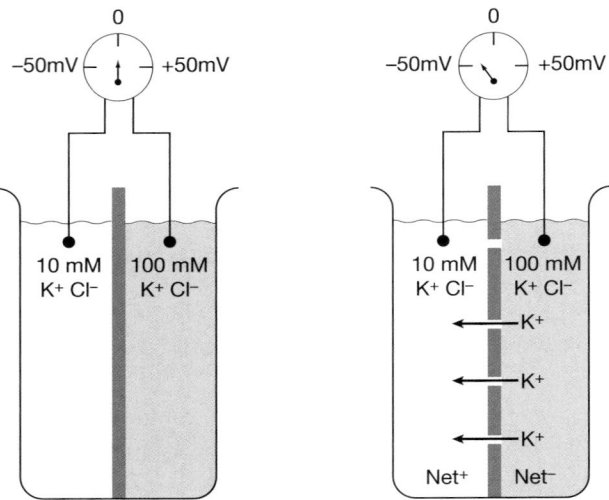

Figure 10-1 A beaker containing two different concentrations (10 mM and 100 mM) of a potassium chloride (KCl) solution existing as potassium (K^+) and chloride (Cl^-) ions. An impermeable partition containing closed potassium channels separates the two different concentration solutions. A voltmeter placed across the partition fails to register any voltage difference. If the partition is now made selectively permeable to just the potassium ions (potassium channels are opened), the concentration gradient difference will drive potassium ions into the lower-concentration side of the beaker until the electrical attraction from the accumulating negatively charged chloride ions prevent any further net K^+ ion movement, thus establishing a dynamic equilibrium. At this point, a potential difference exists across the partition and represents the equilibrium potential. (From Dumitru et al. 2002,[12] with permission of Hanley & Belfus.)

The above simple example can be applied to all cells in the body, and in particular to nerve and muscle cells. A nerve's axon will be used as a prototypical example, although the same principles apply to muscle cells. The nerve cell is known to have a specialized cell membrane permeable primarily to potassium and chloride ions in the resting state, because of proteinaceous transmembranous ion channels rendering the membrane selectively permeable, i.e. semipermeable.[28] The potassium channels are referred to as passive, because they are always open and permit the free flow of this ion. Contained within the axon but incapable of crossing the cell membrane are large, negatively charged protein molecules. This negative charge attracts potassium ions from outside the cell to enter through the passive potassium channels, resulting in a buildup of potassium ions within the axon. This process continues until there is so much potassium within the axon that the continued entry of more potassium ions is prevented by the high intracellular potassium concentration, even though all the negative charges have not yet been electrically balanced. This is because the force of the accumulated potassium ions' concentration gradient now attempting to drive potassium out of the cell is just large enough to balance the intracellular anions electrical attractive force attracting potassium ions into the cell.

Similar to the above beaker example, a dynamic equilibrium eventually develops between:

- intracellular negative charges attracting potassium ions; and
- high intracellular potassium concentration impeding further potassium ion entry.

This dynamic equilibrium occurs at a point when the intracellular negative potential is reduced by the inflowing potassium ions to a value approximating a negative 80–90 mV compared with the extracellular environment.

Nernst equation

The above examples of beakers and cells can be expressed mathematically by simply stating that the net 'work' of both the electrical gradient work (W_{elec}) and the concentration gradient work (W_{con}) is zero in the resting state ($W_{con} + W_{con} = 0$). This means that the work, or energy, of developing the concentration gradient (W_{con}) is balanced by, or equal but opposite to, that developed by the electrical gradient (W_{elec}) during the resting state: $W_{elec} = -W_{con}$. The negative sign is present to denote the 'opposite' or balanced aspect of the work. The electrical work is expressed as $W_{elec} = Z_iFE_m$. The symbols designate specific aspects defining electrical ion work: Z_i is the ion's charge, F is Faraday's constant, and E_m is the transmembrane potential. The work required to move ions across the membrane can be expressed as the natural logarithm of the ionic concentration differences between the intracellular ($[I]_i$) and extracellular ($[I]_e$) ions. Universal gas (R) and temperature (T) constants are conversion factors necessary to balance units between all the variables. Substituting the above-noted variables into the balanced work equation results in the following equations.

$$W_{elec} = -W_{con}$$
$$Z_iFE_m = -RT\{Ln[I]_i - Ln[I]_e\}$$

This formula can be rearranged to find the potential at which the electrical work just balances the concentration work, i.e. the dynamic equilibrium or resting membrane potential, by solving the above equation for E_m.

$$E_m = -\frac{RT\ Ln[I]_i}{Z_iF\ [I]_e}$$

The above equation is more commonly known as the Nernst equation, and is a mathematical statement of the potential at which all the electrical and concentration forces are balanced in the cell's resting state, i.e. the resting membrane potential.[25,28] By substituting the actual values for the different variables and using the more familiar base 10 logarithm, the equation converts to the more recognizable form. Also, the approximate concentration ratio of intracellular to extracellular potassium is 20:1. The Nernst equation then becomes:

$$E_m = -(26\ mV)2.3\log_{10}[20 \div 1]$$
$$E_m = -75\ mV$$

Sodium pump

Experimentation has shown that the Nernst equation predicts the resting membrane potential quite well with different extracellular potassium concentrations, as long as the potassium concentration is relatively high. When the extracellular potassium concentration is low, there is a deviation of the resting membrane potential from that predicted, with a less-negative potential achieved. This finding suggests that another ion (sodium: Na^+) has some influence on the resting membrane potential. It turns out that sodium has a very high extracellular compared with intracellular ion concentration, which results in small quantities of sodium ions leaking into the membrane through a few passive sodium channels present in the cell's membrane. This relative impermeability of positive sodium ions, combined with a high extracellular but low intracellular sodium ion concentration, and the resulting electrical drive to enter the cell (negative inside), would tend to 'run down' the cell resting membrane potential over time. Fortunately, the cell has developed a mechanism whereby this run down is prevented. Located within the cell membrane is an energy-dependent sodium-potassium pump, which pumps in potassium ions and pumps out sodium ions in just the right ratio to match the sodium ions entering and the compensatory potassium ions exiting the cell. This ratio is two sodium ions being extruded for every three potassium ions taken into the cell. The sodium–potassium pump maintains the exact ionic balance necessary to sustain a stable resting membrane potential.

Goldman–Hodgkin–Katz equation

An important modification of the Nernst equation is the inclusion of ion permeability as being the primary influence on the cell's transmembrane voltage. The greater an ion's permeability, the more likely it is to influence the transmembrane potential. This is due to the fact that the equilibrium potential of the most permeable ion in effect becomes the cell's resting membrane potential. The equation accounting for the different permeability (designated as 'p' in the equation below) factors is known as the Goldman–Hodgkin–Katz equation:[25,27,28]

$$E_m = -2.3\left(\frac{RT}{F}\right)\left(log_{10}\frac{pK[K^+]_i + pNa[Na^+]_i + pCl[Cl^-]_e}{pK[K^+]_e + pNa[Na^+]_e + pCl[Cl^-]_i}\right)$$

In this equation, it can be seen that the cell's transmembrane voltage (E_m) is primarily dependent on which ion has the greatest permeability. For example, in the resting state, we know that the permeability of potassium is relatively high due to non-voltage-gated potassium passive leak channels, while the permeability of sodium ions is very low. Chloride ions are distributed through chloride channels that are always open at the resting membrane voltage, and thus adjust to whichever ion's permeability predominates between potassium and sodium as dictated by the net transmembrane potential. With a high potassium and low sodium permeability, the above equation simplifies to the Nernst equation, i.e. potassium is the predominant ionic species and E_m becomes −75 mV. If sodium permeability were to increase dramatically, then E_m would approach the sodium ion equilibrium potential of +55 mV. It would not quite reach this value, because potassium and chloride ions continue to have some influence and would hold the maximum

potential to a less positive (more negative) value of about +40 mV.

Action potential generation

In addition to the passive (always open) potassium ion channels and relatively few passive sodium ion channels, there are also sodium and potassium ion channels within nerve and muscle cell membranes modulated by transmembrane voltage differences. These channels are *voltage-gated*, because they open and close depending on the transmembrane voltage.[22] Muscle and unmyelinated nerve contain both sodium and potassium voltage-gated channels. These voltage-gated sodium and potassium ion channels are closed at the resting membrane potential. If the transmembrane voltage changes toward a more depolarized direction (less negative) and reaches about 15–20 mV less negative than the resting membrane potential, the voltage-gated sodium channels open. This results in an increased permeability of the sodium ion, a process known as sodium activation. As noted above, the Goldman–Hodgkin–Katz equation predicts that the transmembrane potential shifts toward the sodium ion equilibrium potential. This massive shift in transmembrane potential is referred to as depolarization. After staying open for a short period of time, the sodium gates automatically close (sodium inactivation), with a return of the resting membrane potential again dictated by the resting state ion permeabilities (repolarization). In muscle and unmyelinated nerve membranes, a delayed opening of potassium voltage-gated channels occurs secondary to the depolarization and assists in repolarization.

Very few ions actually cross the membrane for sodium-induced depolarization or potassium-mediated repolarization. The region of membrane where there are large numbers of voltage-gated sodium channels in the open conformation acts as a so-called current sink for sodium ions to 'sink', or enter, the cell's interior. This implies that a nearby source for the sodium ions must be present. The surrounding extracellular membrane region acts as the current source, thus permitting an ionic flow from the region surrounding the current sink. Sodium ions are thereby removed from the outside of the membrane surrounding the sink (making this region relatively more negative) and deposited on the inside of the cell (Fig. 10-2). The newly introduced intracellular ions migrate to help neutralize some of the cell's interior negative charges. This current flow, or charge transfer, from the extracellular to intracellular space is referred to as a *local circuit current*.[14] The net effect of charge transfer is to make the cell's interior less negative and exterior more negative, thereby shifting the transmembrane voltage in the more depolarized direction about the current sink. If the charge transfer is sufficient to depolarize the cell by approximately 15–20 mV, the membrane surrounding the sink is induced to permit sodium activation and hence undergo a significant depolarization. This process can then continue along the length of the cell.

The above process creates an action potential spike at the original site of sodium activation. A mechanical, chemical, or electrical stimulus that causes the membrane potential to reach threshold over a localized region is all that is required to serve

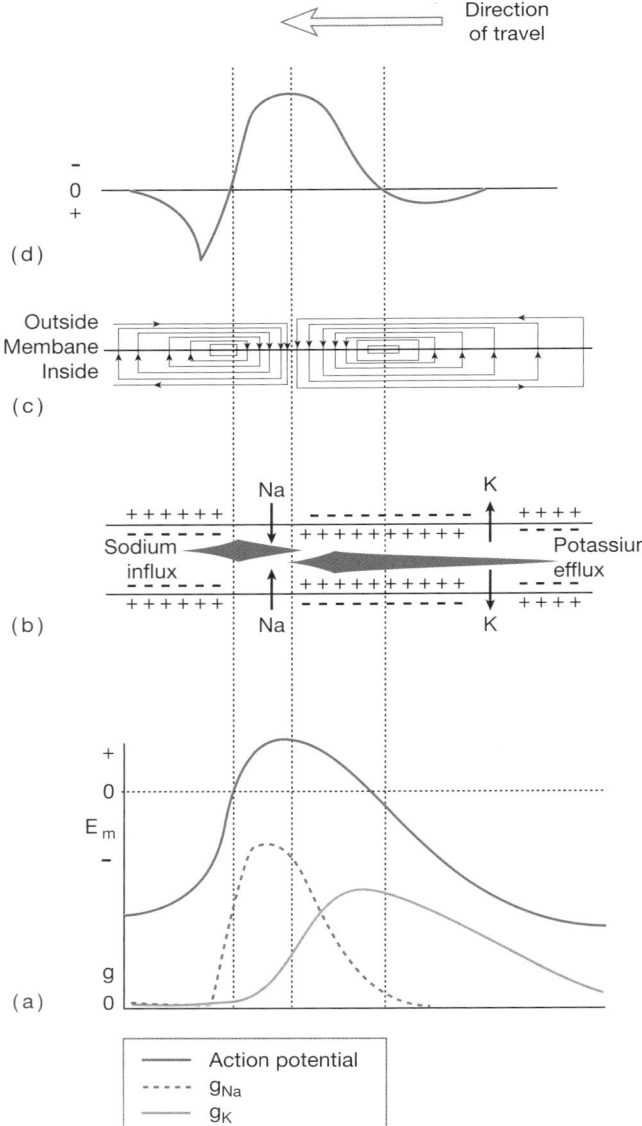

Figure 10-2 (**a**) Sodium (g_{Na}) and potassium (g_K) ion conductances are depicted over time resulting in an alteration of the transmembrane potential, creating an action potential. (**b**) The spatial relationship of the sodium and potassium ion flux during an action potential is schematically depicted. Note the alteration of the transmembrane ionic potential differences corresponding to the depolarization and repolarization. (**c**) Local circuit currents described the pathways of extracellular sodium ions entering the cell and then migrating longitudinally within the cell. (**d**) Triphasic extracellular waveform associated with the intracellular monophasic action potential. (From Dumitru et al. 2002,[12] with permission of Hanley & Belfus.)

as the initiating stimulus of action potential generation. Once the process begins, it is self-sustaining as long as there are sufficient ion channels to repeat the depolarization process. The intracellular action potential is essentially a monophasic positive spike: −75 mV resting potential; +40 mV spike; return to resting −75 mV with sodium inactivation and potassium activation (Fig. 10-2). The membrane's threshold value must be reached in order to generate the self-sustaining action potential

that is the same at all regions of the membrane. This concept is referred to as the *all or none phenomenon*.

It should be noted that the nodes of Ranvier in myelinated nerves lack voltage-gated potassium channels and contain only voltage-gated sodium channels.[42,43] The action potential actually 'jumps' from one node to the next, creating an efficient means of action potential propagation that is referred to as saltatory conduction. Repolarization in myelinated nerve does not require a delayed potassium current. As noted above, the resting membrane potential is restored once the permeability of sodium is reduced. Passive 'back-leak' sodium and potassium currents are believed to mediate the discharge of the membrane's capacitance, which accumulates over time with multiple action potential discharges.

PHYSIOLOGIC FACTORS AFFECTING ACTION POTENTIAL PROPAGATION

There are a number of physiologic factors that have a direct effect on action potential propagation. These factors can be divided into those that can be altered by the practitioner and those intrinsic to the subject and beyond control. The most important factor that is readily amenable to change is the limb's surface temperature. Physiologic variables beyond the control of the clinician include gender, age, height, and digit circumference.

Gender
Only a few studies have attempted to investigate the difference in nerve conduction studies between males and females.[3] There is noted to be a slight increase in the antidromic sensory nerve amplitudes for both the median and ulnar nerves recorded from the digits in women. Also, women demonstrate a greater nerve conduction velocity (NCV) for upper and lower limb nerves compared with men. Both of these differences, however, are eliminated when one considers limb length and digit circumference (see below).[35]

Aging
Several generalizations can be made regarding peripheral evoked sensory nerve action potentials (SNAPs) and aging. The conduction velocity demonstrates a consistent decline approximating 1–2 m/s per decade.[32] The SNAP's duration is about 10–15% longer in 40–60-year-old persons, and 20% longer in 70–88-year-old individuals, compared with persons 18–25 years old.[7] Compared with the 18–25-year-old group, the SNAP amplitude is one-half and one-third, respectively, for the 40–60 and 70–88-year-old groups. The distal sensory latencies reveal a similar prolongation with age. There is a suggestion that the median and radial nerves do not demonstrate considerable alteration with age.[16] At present, there is disagreement as to the magnitude of change in SNAP parameters induced by the aging process.

The results of aging on conduction velocity have been examined in a number of upper and lower limb nerves. Motor NCVs reveal similar changes to those described for sensory nerves. The newborn's motor NCVs are about half of adult values that are reached by 3–5 years of age.[2] After the age of 50 years, there is a progressive decline in the conduction velocity of the fastest motor fibers, approximating 1–2 m/s per decade. There is a concurrent increase in the distal motor latency and decrease in the motor response's amplitude with advancing age. H-reflex latency demonstrates little alteration with aging in the healthy elderly.[17] The decrease in amplitude is difficult to ascertain clinically due to the wide range of normal H-reflex amplitudes and the central effects on amplitude that are difficult to control and quantify.

Digit circumference

Females consistently demonstrate significantly higher antidromic SNAP amplitudes for the median and ulnar nerves recorded from the second and fifth digits.[3] A negative linear correlation exists between finger circumference and amplitude for these two nerves. It is known that, as the distance between the recording electrode and neural generator increases, the amplitude precipitously declines. Increasing the circumference of the finger displaces the electrode further from the nerve. Because men have significantly larger finger circumferences than women, this appears to explain the difference in SNAP amplitudes. There is no evidence that this difference is due to an intrinsic neural difference between male and female nerves.

Height

Several investigations have documented slower lower limb NCVs in taller compared with shorter individuals.[9,29] This difference is independent of the limb's temperature or subject's age. The etiology of this finding is unknown. Distal nerve tapering or an abrupt change in axon diameter has been speculated to account for this finding, but the exact etiology has not been definitively identified.[12]

Temperature

Temperature is one of the most important factors influencing nerve conduction studies. As the temperature of the nerve is lowered, the amount of current required to generate an action potential increases. Neural excitability is lowered with a reduction in temperature. This decreased excitability is a direct temperature effect on the nerve's action potential-generating mechanism at the nodes of Ranvier, and not a result of membrane resistance changes, i.e. the transmembrane resistance is not increased by a drop in temperature.[23,24] In addition to excitability, the configuration of an action potential is profoundly affected by a drop in temperature.

The action potential's amplitude, rise time, and fall time all increase as the nerve's temperature declines. The time required for the action potential of a cold nerve to reach its peak depolarization from the resting membrane level increases approximately 33%.[33] Similarly, the time necessary for the action potential to return to its resting level is also increased, but much more so than the rise time (69%). Because both the SNAP's

duration and the spike height increase, the area of the SNAP increases dramatically at lower temperatures.

The compound muscle action potential (CMAP) arising from cooled muscle tissue demonstrates similar changes as those noted for SNAPs. The CMAP amplitude, duration, rise time, and area all increase as the muscle's temperature is reduced. Intramuscular recordings also reveal that those motor units in close proximity to the recording electrode are also increased in the same parameters noted above.

Temperature also has an impact on NCVs. Based on the prolongation of the rise and fall time noted above, we should be able to infer the nerve's response to cooling with respect to NCV. Because propagation is saltatory in myelinated nerves, decreased temperature results in an increase in the amount of time necessary to reach the action potential's peak at each node of Ranvier, thereby slowing action potential propagation and reducing conduction velocity.

The first detailed investigation of temperature effects on NCV in human nerves revealed an NCV to temperature correlation of 2.4 m/s per °C for median and ulnar motor conduction.[21] With every one degree drop in temperature, there was a 2.4 m/s decrease in the conduction velocity. Reductions in conduction velocity for upper limb motor nerve fibers have also been found to approximate a decrease of 4 or 5% per °C.[10,26] Correction factors utilizing subcutaneous and intramuscular readings are equally correct, but it is more convenient and less painful to use surface measurements.[18]

In the upper limb, the relationship between temperature and NCV has been investigated for the surface temperature range of 26–33°C, measured at the midline of the distal wrist crease. Calculations reveal that, for median motor and sensory nerves, NCV is altered 1.5 and 1.4 m/s per °C, respectively, while the distal latency for both nerves change 0.2 ms/°C.[18–20] The ulnar nerve demonstrated motor and sensory temperature relationships of 2.1 and 1.6 m/s per °C, respectively, and a distal motor and sensory latency correlation of 0.2 ms/°C.

Because of the profound effects of temperature on NCV, it is clear that reliable nerve studies require temperature control. A cool limb, irrespective of the ambient room temperature, can result in latencies, NCVs, and amplitudes that are not in the 'normal' range. A normal limb study can yield results that are spuriously thought to be abnormal, but that are due only to the low temperature. This is an especially important issue when an abnormal nerve is being studied. Correction factors are well known for normal nerve, but serious questions remain about how abnormal nerves respond to temperature variations. Although applying a correction factor is less time-consuming than heating the limb, it is doubtful how accurately correction factors can be applied to abnormal nerves. Until more data are available regarding the best correction factor for diseased nerves, warming of the limb should be considered superior to using correction factors. The surface temperature approximating the recording electrodes should be at least 32°C in the upper limbs, and 30°C in lower limbs. Caution must be exercised when attempting to warm the limbs of patients with ischemic limbs, or those with altered sensation, to avoid injury.

WAVEFORM CONFIGURATION GENERATION

The current flow created by a depolarized region of membrane (current sink) is associated with a specific pattern of voltages known as isopotential lines (Figs 10-2 and 10-3).[12] Recording a voltage at any point in space along an isopotential line results in the same voltage being recorded. As one moves further from the current sink, the corresponding voltage and the current density also decrease. The pattern of isopotential lines in space creates three distinct voltage regions. The current sink is associated with a negative voltage, while the two surrounding (leading and trailing) current sources are considered zones of relative positive voltage. Separating the current sink zone from the current sources are zero isopotential lines. These lines correspond to regions of zero voltage associated with that portion of the recorded waveform crossing the baseline (Fig. 10-3).

An action potential with its local circuit current and associated isopotential lines propagating past an electrode can be considered essentially equivalent to a stationary action potential sequentially sampled by a recording electrode passing through its electrical field (Fig. 10-3). The latter situation is used as an example for discussion purposes because it is easier to visualize the ensuing action potential waveform.

Suppose a propagating nerve or muscle action potential is frozen for an instant in time. A characteristic pattern of isopotential voltage lines are described in the region surrounding the nerve or muscle. We can then move a recording electrode through the activated tissue's electrical field to simulate a propagating action potential (Fig. 10-3). The final waveform configuration associated with an action potential propagating along a straight portion of nerve or muscle is a triphasic waveform with a large negative spike flanked by an initial large and subsequent small terminal positive phase. For discussion purposes, positive is denoted by a downward cathode ray tube (CRT) deflection, while an upward CRT deflection designates a net negative potential difference between the two recording electrodes. This example implies that for both nerve and muscle, when an action potential approaches, reaches, and then travels past a recording electrode, the fundamental waveform configuration is triphasic. These same simple principles can be applied to understand the generation of all waveforms observed during the electrodiagnostic medicine examination.

NERVE AND MUSCLE WAVEFORM CONFIGURATIONS AND CHARACTERISTICS
Nerve potentials
Sensory nerve action potentials
Clinical recordings   Sensory nerve action potentials can be obtained with either antidromic or orthodromic techniques.[7] The term *antidromic* implies that the induced neural impulse propagates along the nerve in a direction opposite to its physiologic direction; for example, stimulating the median nerve at the wrist and recording the ensuing response from the second or third digit. A nerve will conduct an impulse proximally and distally from the point of stimulation by a depolarizing current. On the other hand, stimulating the median sensory fibers on the second digit and recording from the wrist is an example of

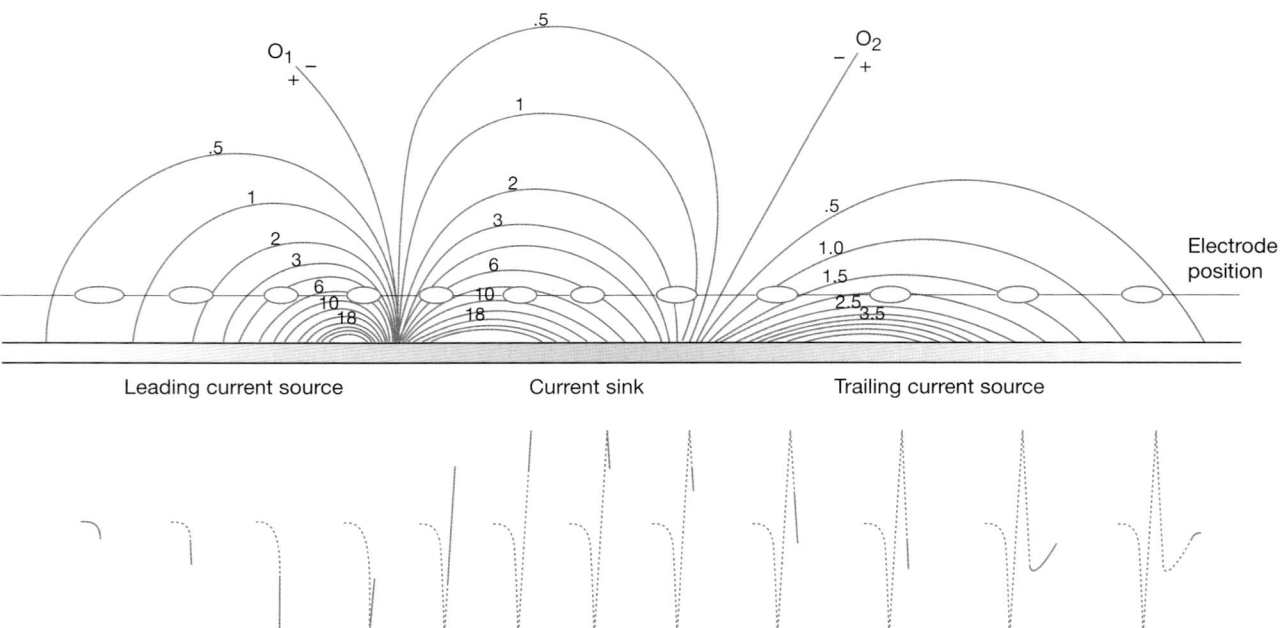

Figure 10-3 A propagating nerve or muscle action potential generates a characteristic pattern of voltages associated with the corresponding current flows. Passing an electrode through a hypothetically stationary action potential (open ovals) results in the recording of a triphasic extracellular waveform. This basic conceptualization of extracellular waveforms applies equally to nerve and muscle tissue. (From Dumitru et al. 2002,[12] with permission of Hanley & Belfus.)

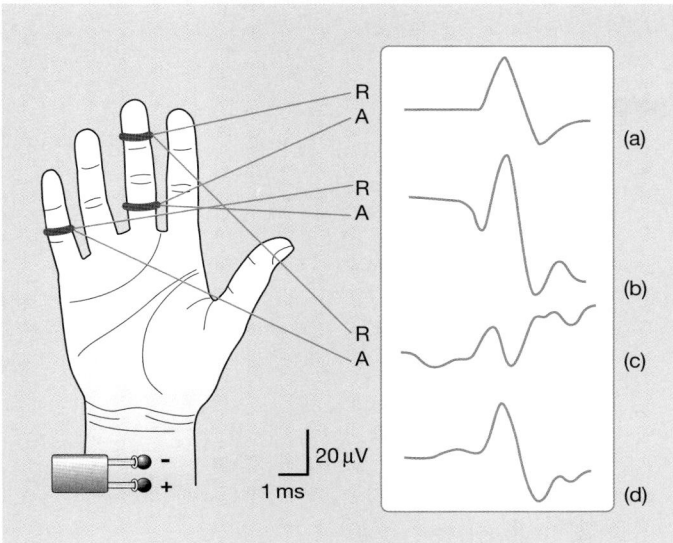

Figure 10-4 The median nerve is stimulated at the wrist with an antidromic sensory recording montage. Active (A) and reference (R) are located on fingers as designated above. (**a**) Bipolar recording with the commonly observed biphasic median nerve sensory nerve action potential (SNAP). (**b**) The same active electrode location in (a) is referenced to the fifth digit, resulting in a triphasic SNAP. (**c**) An active electrode placed on the fifth digit but referenced to the third digit permits one to observe what this electrode records when the median nerve is stimulated. An inverted triphasic potential of small magnitude is detected. It is inverted because of its connection to the inverting amplifier port. (**d**) Electronically summating the potential recorded in (b) and (c) yields that recorded with a bipolar montage in (a). (From Dumitru 1989,[15] with permission of Hanley & Belfus.)

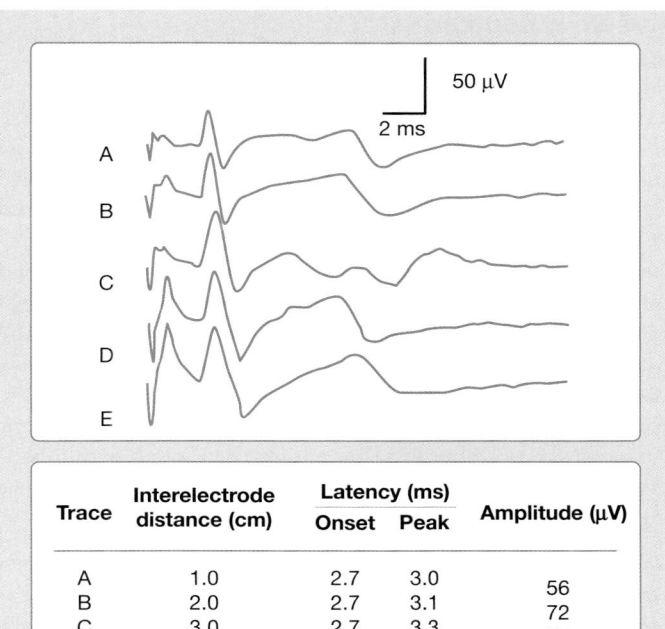

Trace	Interelectrode distance (cm)	Latency (ms) Onset	Latency (ms) Peak	Amplitude (μV)
A	1.0	2.7	3.0	56
B	2.0	2.7	3.1	72
C	3.0	2.7	3.3	77
D	4.0	2.7	3.3	86
E	5.0	2.7	3.3	86

Figure 10-5 The effect of interelectrode separation can be easily demonstrated by evoking an antidromic median sensory nerve action potential (SNAP) and progressively increasing the interelectrode separation between the active and reference electrode. The active electrode remains in the same location, while the reference electrode is sequentially displaced more distal on the digit. As can be seen, the SNAP amplitude increases, peak latency increases, and the onset latency remains the same. (From Dumitru and Walsh 1988,[14] with permission of Hanley & Belfus.)

an orthodromic technique. In orthodromic recordings, the sensory fiber impulses are detected at a site proximal to the stimulus as they travel physiologically from a distal to a more proximal region. Antidromically obtained SNAPs are usually larger and hence easier to assess, because the recording electrodes are in close proximity to the proper digital nerves than when a recording electrode is placed over the median nerve at the wrist for orthodromic techniques.

SNAP configuration Antidromic and orthodromic bipolar SNAP waveform recordings are typically biphasic rather than triphasic. The biphasic, negative–positive potential is a result of the bipolar recording technique and not a violation of volume conductor theory. Biphasic SNAP waveforms can best be understood by use of bipolar and referential recording montages for median nerve stimulation at the wrist (Fig. 10-4).[15] The median SNAP is indeed a triphasic waveform and conforms to the principles of volume conduction but only appears biphasic because of the recording montage used.

It is also possible to predict the optimal interelectrode separation to maximize the biphasic potential's amplitude in the bipolar recording.[14] The critical factor in this instance is the rise time, baseline to negative peak, of the biphasic potential, because it is this parameter that defines the waveform's maximum amplitude. The recording electrodes must be located

at a distance greater than the action potentials' spatial extent, represented by the rise time duration. The rise time of most SNAPs approaches 0.8 ms, which represents a longitudinal extent of 40 mm for an action potential conducting at 50 m/s (50 000 mm/1000 ms = D/0.8 ms; D = 40 mm). If the two recording electrodes are separated by a distance less than 40 mm, some similar information regarding the main peaks of the waveforms recorded by both recording electrodes (active and reference) results in mutual cancellation of data, producing a potential with a smaller amplitude. A portion of the nerve will be depolarizing under the reference electrode while still in some degree of depolarization under the active electrode. At interelectrode separations greater then 40 mm, the biphasic potential's negative peak amplitude will no longer grow, but the terminal positive phase will enlarge slightly and may change its configuration. These findings can be demonstrated by varying the distance between recording electrodes and observing the ensuing results (Fig. 10-5). In effect, as the recording distance decreases below 40 mm, the amplitude of the recorded waveform declines and the peak latency shortens.

Muscle potentials

Needle insertional activity

Normal insertional activity Placing a needle (monopolar or standard concentric) recording electrode into healthy muscle tissue and advancing it in quick but short intervals results in brief bursts of electrical potentials referred to as insertional activity (Fig. 10-6a).[12] The observed electrical activity is believed to result from the needle electrode mechanically depolarizing the muscle fibers surrounding its leading edge as it pierces and deforms the tissue. Minimal and localized muscle tissue damage may occur from direct needle trauma and is the basis for the synonymous term of *injury potentials*. The purpose of including insertional activity analysis as part of the electromyographic examination is that the probing needle may provoke transient and/or sustained abnormal potentials associated with membrane instability prior to this abnormal activity being present with the muscle at rest.

Decreased insertional activity Muscle that has been replaced by fibrous tissue, or that is otherwise electrically inexcitable, can no longer generate electrical activity. Consequently, the needle electrode is incapable of mechanically depolarizing this tissue. The result is that few, if any, electrical waveforms will be detected following needle movement (Fig. 10-6b).

Increased insertional activity Practitioners have noted that insertional activity may appear to persist following needle movement cessation. This finding has led to the term *increased insertional activity*. In disease states where the muscle is no longer connected to its nerve or the muscle membrane is inherently unstable from primary muscle pathology or abnormal ion channels, the increased insertional activity completes a temporal continuum from the previously normal insertional activity to the development of sustained membrane instability (Fig. 10-6c).

End-plate potentials

Miniature end-plate potentials An active needle electrode located in the end-plate region can record two distinct waveforms. One of the waveforms is a short duration (0.5–2 ms), small (10–50 µV), irregularly occurring (once every 5 s per axon terminal), monophasic negative waveform.[12] These potentials represent the random release of acetylcholine vesicles. Volume conduction theory would suggest that, for a potential to be monophasic and negative, the current sink would have to start and finish within the active electrode's recording region (Fig. 10-7a). Clinically, multiple miniature end-plate potentials (MEPPs) are usually observed with an intramuscular recording electrode, and the sound is referred to an end-plate noise or 'seashell murmur' (Fig. 10.7b).

End-plate spikes A second waveform that can be detected with an active needle electrode placed in the end-plate region is relatively short in duration (3–4 ms), of moderate amplitude (100–200 µV), irregularly firing, and biphasic with an initial negative deflection.[12] The biphasic potential has an initial negative phase, produced when a current sink originates in the

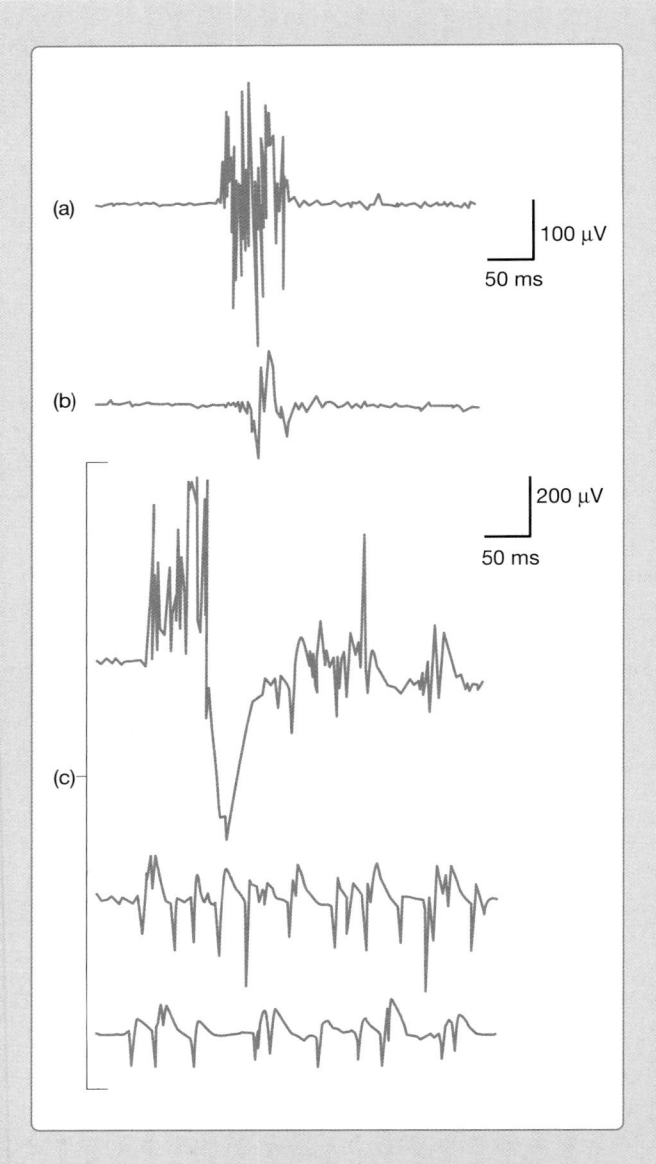

Figure 10-6 (**a**) Inserting a monopolar needle into healthy muscle tissue results in mechanical depolarization of muscle tissue, which generates a brief burst of electrical activity designated as insertional activity. (**b**) Inserting the same needle into fibrotic muscle or subcutaneous fatty tissue results in decreased insertional activity. (**c**) Inserting a monopolar needle into denervated muscle tissue produced not only the initial burst of electrical activity but also associated positive sharp waves and fibrillation potentials that abate over several hundred milliseconds. (From Dumitru et al. 2002,[12] with permission of Hanley & Belfus.)

vicinity of the active electrode and then propagates away (Fig. 10-8). Triphasic end-plate spikes may also occur if the active electrode induces an action potential in the terminal axon but the electrode's recording surface is some distance from the end plate. End-plate spikes and MEPPs are frequently observed together, as they arise from the same region (Fig. 10-9).

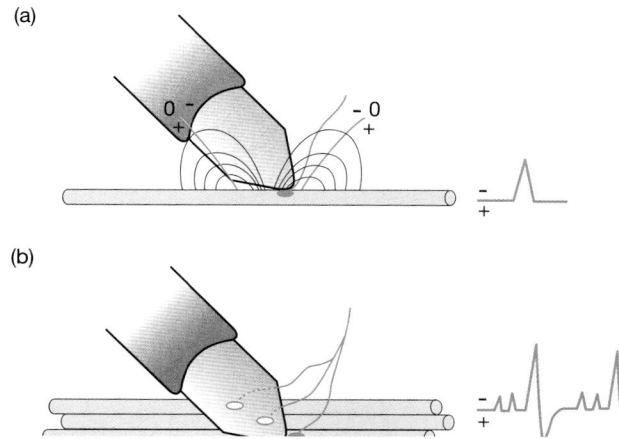

Figure 10-7 (a) Monopolar needle electrode located over a muscle's end plate records the spontaneous depolarization of a miniature end-plate potential (MEPP). As the electrode is located over this potential's subthreshold central current sink, and hence does not propagate, a monophasic negative potential is recorded. (b) The large recording electrode is usually positioned over several end plates, thus recording multiple MEPPs and end-plate spikes. (From Dumitru et al. 2002,[12] with permission of Hanley & Belfus.)

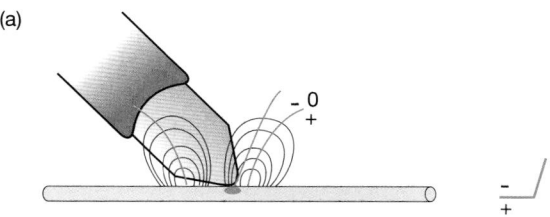

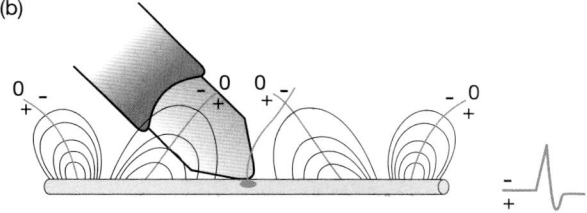

Figure 10-8 (a) Irritation of the terminal axon results in a suprathreshold end-plate depolarization, thus generating a single muscle fiber potential. Because the electrode is located over the end-plate zone, an initial negative deflection is recorded. (b) The terminal positive current sources are then recorded, with action potential propagation thereby generating a biphasic, initially negative potential referred to as an end-plate spike. (From Dumitru et al. 2002,[12] with permission of Hanley & Belfus.)

Single muscle fiber

The single muscle fiber's extracellular waveform configuration, like nerve tissue, depends on the characteristics of the muscle's intracellular action potential. A muscle's action potential is approximately 4–20 times longer than a nerve's, due to the prolonged repolarization process.[12] Aside from the longer duration of local circuit currents compared with neural tissue, the concept of a current sink surrounded by two source currents (source–sink–source) remains unchanged. A triphasic waveform

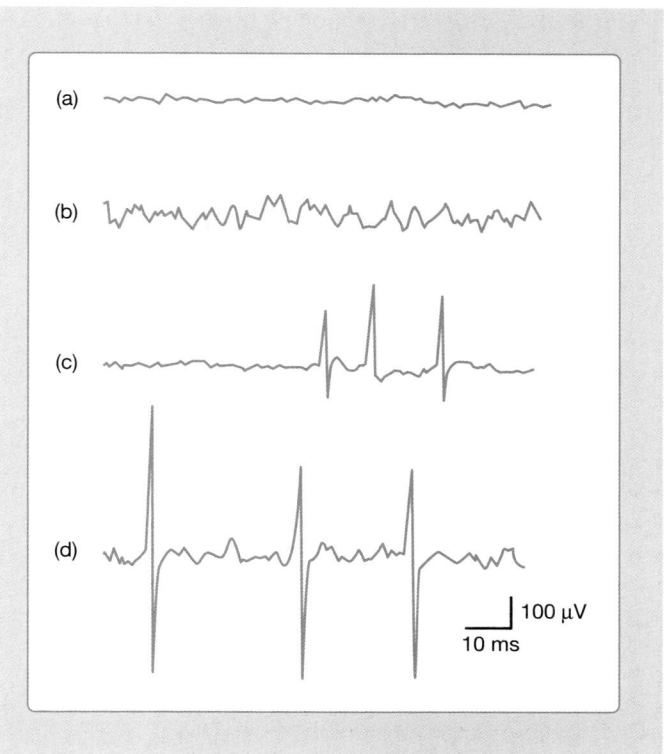

Figure 10-9 (a) Monopolar needle located in a healthy muscle at rest. (b) Slight needle movement positions the electrode in an end-plate region with the recording of multiple miniature end-plate potentials of a negative spike configuration. (c) Repositioning the needle electrode to a slightly different region primarily records biphasic, initially negative end-plate spikes. (d) Advancing the needle electrode slightly permits the simultaneous recording of both potentials noted individually in (b) and (c). (From Dumitru et al. 2002,[12] with permission of Hanley & Belfus.)

with a small terminal phase should then be recorded from an extracellular active electrode placed adjacent to a propagating single muscle fiber action potential at some distance from the end-plate region (Fig. 10-10).

Motor unit potential configuration

Anatomy One anterior horn cell gives rise to a peripheral axon that splits into multiple terminal axons, each of which innervates a single muscle fiber. One anterior horn cell, its axon, and all the single muscle fibers supplied by that nerve are referred to as a motor unit. The electrical activity from all these muscle fibers summates to produce a motor unit action potential (MUAP).

Amplitude and rise time The MUAP configuration can be described in terms of its *amplitude* (maximum peak to peak CRT trace displacement), *rise time* (temporal aspect of a potential's peak), *duration* (departure from and return to baseline), and number of *phases* (baseline crossings plus one) (Fig. 10-11). The amplitude of potentials declines exponentially with increases in distance from the current generator. This occurs because the surrounding muscle and its supportive tissues act

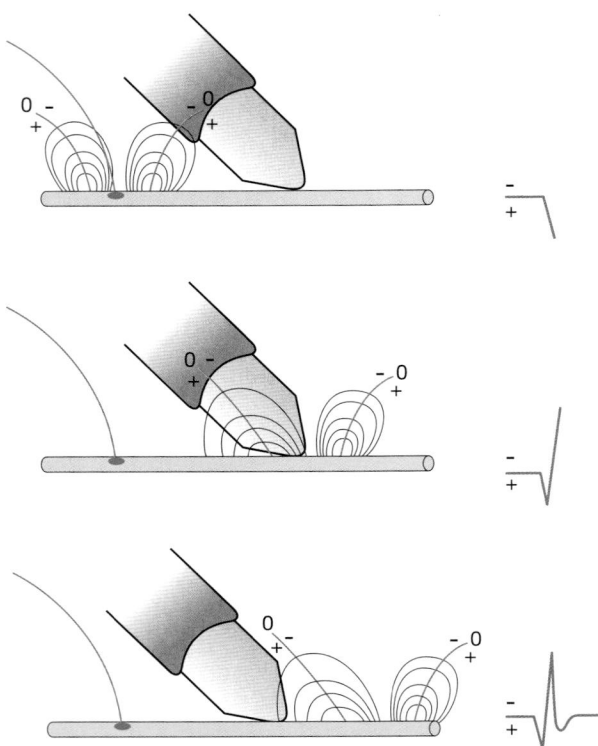

Figure 10-10 A single muscle fiber action potential propagating past a needle recording electrode results in a triphasic waveform. This is because the voltage distribution creates an initial and terminal positive voltage source surrounding a negative current sink zone. (From Dumitru et al. 2002,[12] with permission of Hanley & Belfus.)

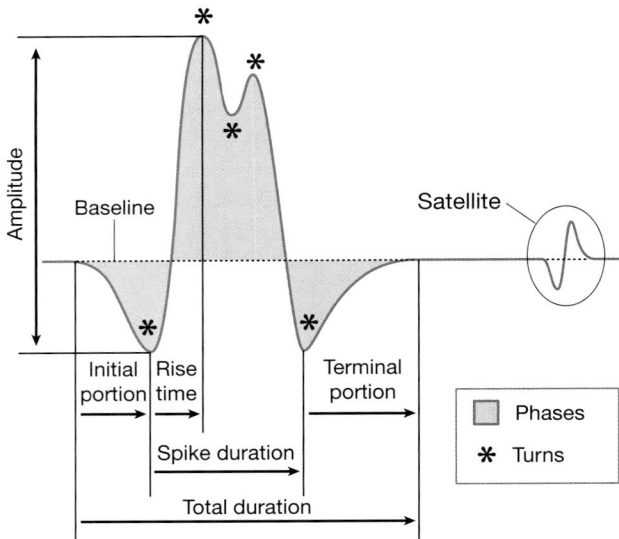

Figure 10-11 A motor unit action potential is depicted, with various morphologic aspects measured. (From Dumitru et al. 2002,[12] with permission of Hanley & Belfus.)

as a high frequency filter to impede potentials that change rapidly over a short period of time. As a result, the peak-to-peak MUAP's amplitude is believed to arise from fewer than 12, and possibly just one or two, single muscle fibers located within 0.5 mm of the electrode's recording surface.

Duration   The MUAP's duration depends on the shortest and longest lengths of terminal axons from the point they separate from the parent nerve to the end plate. The duration of the MUAP also depends on the conduction velocities of the terminal axons and individual muscle fibers with respect to the recording electrode, and the muscle fiber length (Fig. 10-11).[5,6] A MUAP's duration is the most sensitive clinical parameter that can be routinely quantified to diagnosing disease.

Phases   As previously stated, the single muscle fiber usually has a triphasic appearance when recorded outside the end-plate zone and away from the tendinous insertion. The voltages from all the single muscle fibers belonging to one motor unit summate to yield a MUAP that is also usually triphasic: positive–negative–positive. This voltage summation does not always produce a smooth result, and small serrations, or *turns*, can occasionally be seen as part of a MUAP's major phase (Fig. 10-11). The number of *phases* is defined as the number of CRT trace baseline crossings plus one. Normal MUAPs are consid-

ered to have four or fewer phases. MUAPs with five or more phases are called *polyphasic potentials*. Recordings of multiple MUAPs from normal muscle tissue can have between 12% (concentric needle) and 35% (monopolar needle) polyphasic potentials, depending on the type of recording electrode used.[12] Slightly different MUAP configurations can be expected, depending on the exact location of the recording electrode with respect to different single muscle fibers within the motor unit territory (Fig. 10-12).

Pathology can also alter the number of phases a MUAP waveform can have. The motor unit can be affected in two general ways following injury or disease: a pathologic condition may affect either the anterior horn cell or peripheral nerve (including the neuromuscular junction), or the muscle fibers comprising the motor unit. If the neural component of a motor unit is compromised severely enough to experience degeneration, all the muscle fibers innervated by the parent nerve will become denervated. These denervated muscle fibers somehow induce nearby terminal axons of intact nerves to send out neural projections to reinnervate the orphaned muscle fibers. Through collateral sprouting, the total number of muscle fibers belonging to a specific motor unit may increase dramatically (Fig. 10-13). Neurogenic diseases can lead over a period of time to larger amplitude, longer duration, and highly polyphasic MUAPs.

If the muscle fibers comprising a motor unit undergo random degeneration, such as occurs in some myopathies, there is a decrease in the total number of fibers belonging to that motor unit (Fig. 10-14). A decrease in muscle fiber numbers would result in a reduction of the overall MUAP's amplitude, including its initial baseline departure and subsequent return. If the original MUAP's initial baseline departure and subsequent return to baseline decline in magnitude, this portion of the

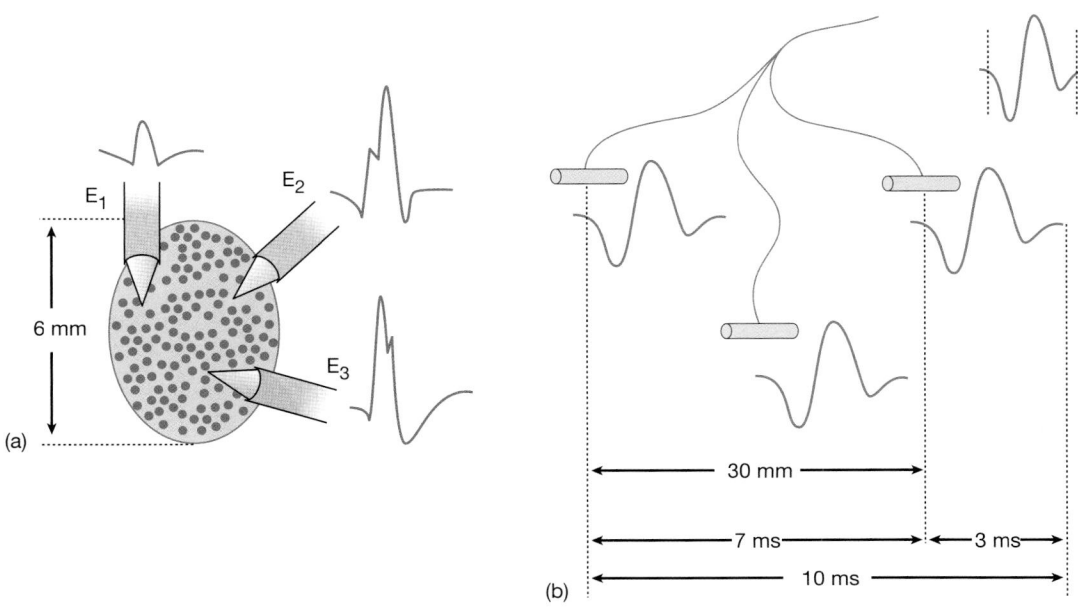

Figure 10-12 Muscle fibers belonging to a single motor unit are randomly distributed within an approximately 6-mm oval territory. Four individual motor unit action potential waveforms are recorded from the same motor unit, and depend on the location of the recording electrode with respect to different muscle fibers within that motor unit's spatial territory. (From Dumitru et al. 2002,[12] with permission of Hanley & Belfus.)

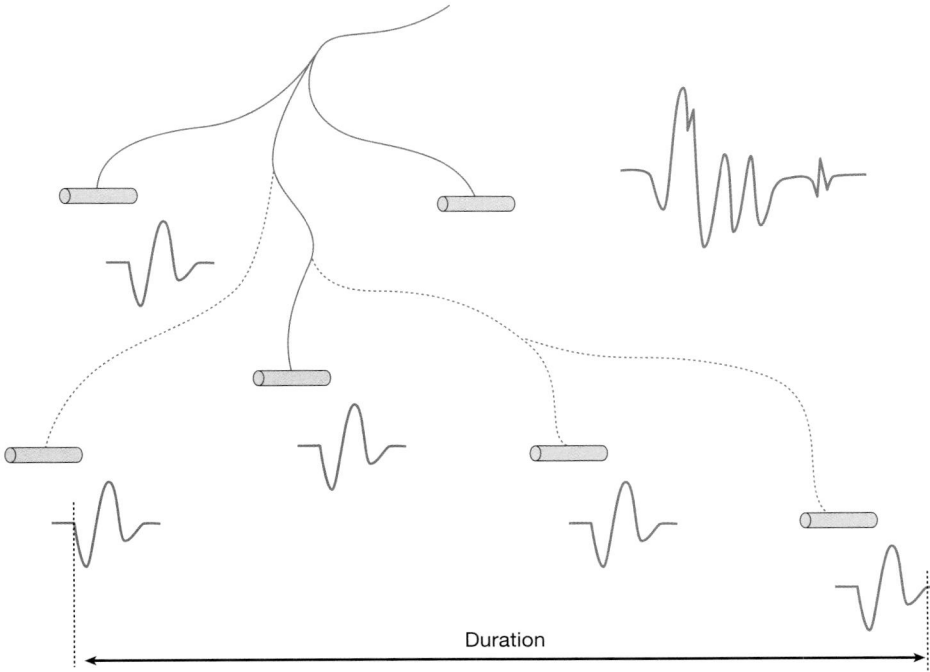

Figure 10-13 Several muscle fibers are denervated in the above example. Collateral terminal nerve sprouts from an intact motor unit (dotted lines) grow to reinnervate those denervated muscle fibers. The end result is a large amplitude, long duration potential with more phases. (From Dumitru et al. 2002,[12] with permission of Hanley & Belfus.)

waveform can no longer be observed (assuming the amplifier's gain is not increased). As a result, the MUAP's total duration would correspondingly appear to decrease. Finally, the dropout of single muscle fiber waveforms would produce less voltage with respect to the spatial summation of single fiber potentials. Fewer muscle fibers could lead to 'gaps' in the MUAP waveform, causing an increase in the number of phases. Conse-

quently, a primary myopathic process tends yield a shorter duration, highly polyphasic, low-amplitude MUAPs.

Compound muscle action potential

To elicit a CMAP from a particular muscle, the active electrode is located on the skin's surface directly over the muscle's motor point (end-plate region).[12] The end-plate region typically lies

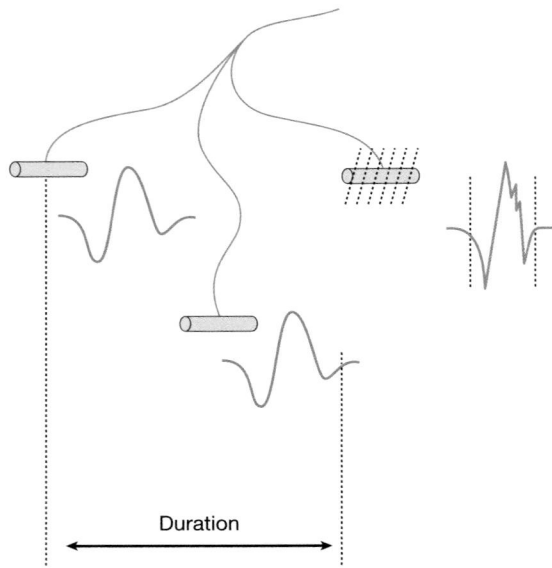

Figure 10-14 Loss of single muscle fibers from a motor unit results in the generation of motor unit action potentials with smaller amplitude, shorter durations, and possibly more phases. (From Dumitru et al. 2002,[12] with permission of Hanley & Belfus.)

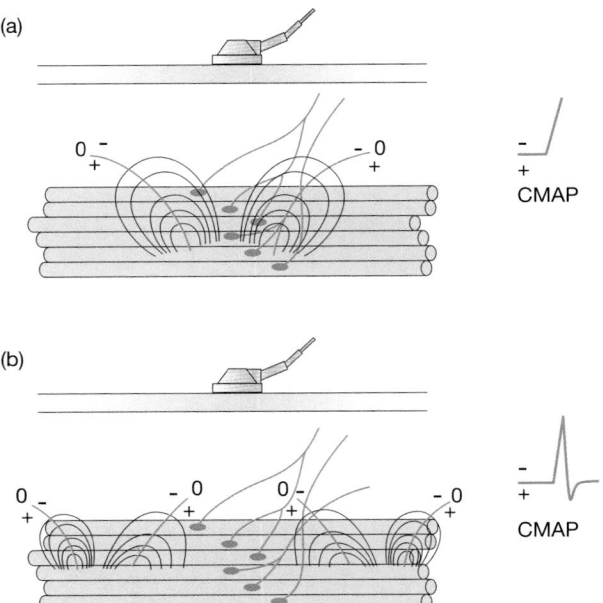

Figure 10-15 (**a**) Locating an active recording electrode over the motor point of a muscle places this electrode over the central region of the negative current sink generating all the muscle's action potentials. An initial negative deflection is recorded because of this location, thereby producing the compound muscle action potential's characteristic morphology. (**b**) A terminal positive phase is then recorded as the action potential propagates away from the electrode. (From Dumitru et al. 2002,[12] with permission of Hanley & Belfus.)

midway between the muscle's origin and insertion. The reference electrode is usually placed on or distal to the tendinous insertion of the muscle, so as not to record electrical activity from the activated muscle. Stimulating the peripheral nerve innervating the muscle under investigation will result in a relatively large, biphasic waveform with an initial negative deflection (Fig. 10-15).

Occasionally, a positive deflection can precede the CMAP's negative phase. Volume conductor theory can explain this observation (Fig. 10-16). The active electrode may not be located directly over the motor point but displaced longitudinally away from it. An active electrode located off the motor point will first record some portion of one of the source currents 'feeding' the current sink. Recall that the leading portion of the source current will result in a positive deflection of the CRT trace. As propagation ensues in the muscle, the current sink will eventually reach the active electrode, resulting in a negative deflection. Finally, the terminal source current is detected, producing a positive deflection. Instead of the anticipated biphasic potential, a triphasic positive–negative–positive waveform is recorded. Relocating the active electrode over the anticipated motor point region will usually remedy the situation.

This situation is complicated by the interaction of near-field and far-field waveforms. At times, a far-field waveform may predominate, depending on the active and reference electrodes' respective locations. This can lead to a waveform with an initial positive deflection or a varying negative waveform onset (so called false motor points). The interested reader is encouraged to explore these fascinating concepts of near-field and far-field waveform interactions.[12]

MUSCLE GENERATORS OF ABNORMAL SPONTANEOUS POTENTIALS

Fibrillation potentials

In vitro observations have shown that, approximately 6 days following denervation, a skeletal muscle fiber's resting membrane potential decreases to a less negative level of −60 mV compared with the normal value of −80 mV.[8,40] Additionally, the resting membrane potential begins to oscillate. Because the threshold level for initiating the all or none action potential is now closer to the new resting membrane potential, an oscillating membrane potential will eventually reach the threshold level. Once threshold is achieved, a propagating action potential is induced (referred to as a fibrillation potential). The repolarization phase of denervated muscle results in a temporarily more hyperpolarized (−75 mV or more) level than the newly established resting membrane potential of −60 mV. When the hyperpolarized membrane level (−75 mV or more) returns to its resting membrane level of −60 mV, an action potential is again produced. This process regularly repeats, resulting in the commonly observed spontaneous and regularly repetitive discharge of fibrillation potentials. Irregularly firing fibrillation potentials occur at times, and are less well understood but thought to arise from spontaneous depolarizations within the transverse tubule system.

Fibrillation potentials are simply spontaneous depolarizations of a single muscle fiber, and demonstrate waveform configurations similar to those of single muscle fibers that are voluntarily

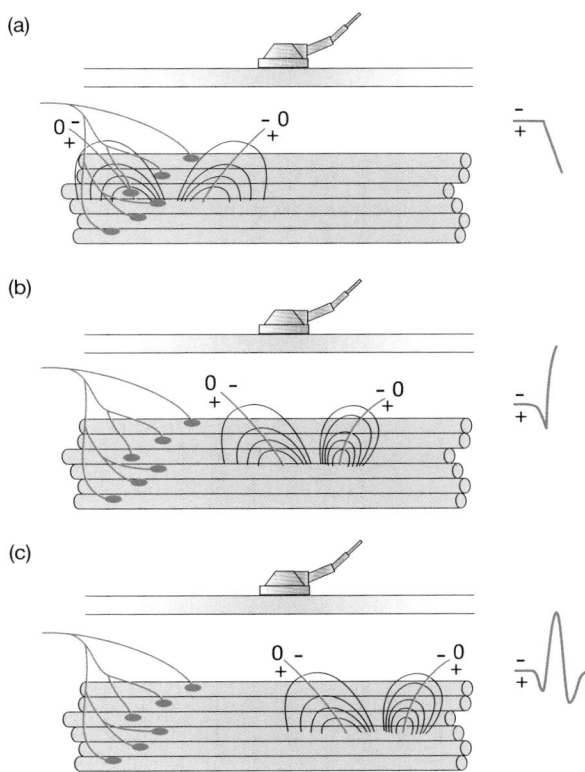

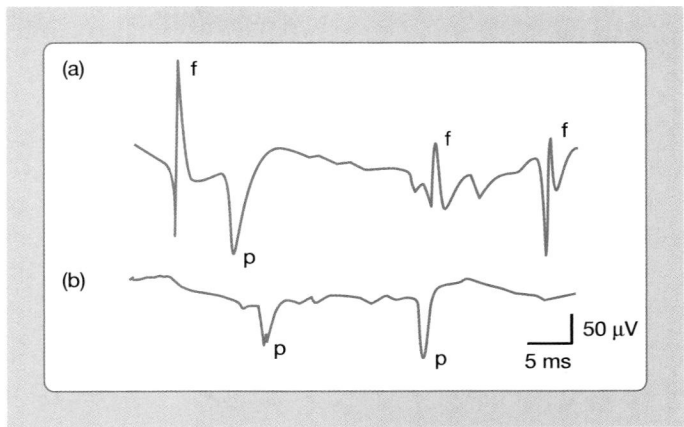

Figure 10-17 (**a**) Monopolar needle recording of positive sharp waves (PSWs) (p) and fibrillation potentials (f). (**b**) Only PSWs are depicted. (From Dumitru et al. 2002,[12] with permission of Hanley & Belfus.)

Figure 10-16 (**a**) Relocating the active electrode in Figure 10-15 off the motor point results in a compound muscle action potential with an initial positive deflection, as some of the muscle's action potentials no longer originate under the electrode but propagate toward it. (**b**) When the main negative sink reaches the electrode, the potential's main negative spike is detected. (**c**) Finally, the terminal positive source currents are recorded, generating the potential's terminal positive phase. (From Dumitru et al. 2002,[12] with permission of Hanley & Belfus.)

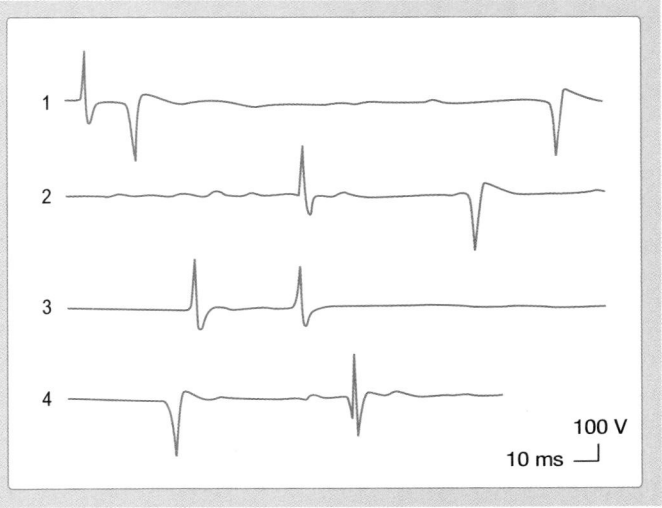

Figure 10-18 A needle electrode is purposefully located in an end-plate region where prototypical as well as atypical end-plate spikes are evoked. Note that end-plate spikes may appear biphasic, initially negative, as anticipated, as well as triphasic and biphasic, initially positive, resembling fibrillation potentials and positive sharp waves, respectively. The important distinction between normal and abnormal waveforms in this case is not waveform configuration but rather firing rate (highly irregular for end-plate spikes). (From Dumitru et al. 2002,[12] with permission of Hanley & Belfus.)

activated (Fig. 10-17). Fibrillation potentials are typically short in duration (less than 5 ms), less than 1 mV in amplitude, and fire at rates between 1 and 15 Hz. They have a typical sound, likened to a high-pitched tick like 'rain on a tin roof', when amplified through a loudspeaker. When the recording electrode is located in the previous end-plate zone of a denervated muscle, fibrillation potentials can be biphasic with an initial negative deflection. A recording electrode outside the end-plate zone, but far from the tendinous region, will detect fibrillation potentials that are triphasic (positive–negative–positive).

It is possible to generate waveforms with similar configurations to fibrillation potentials while examining healthy muscle tissue. Specifically, inadvertently irritating the terminal axon or end-plate zone with the electrode's shaft, and evoking end-plate potentials while simultaneously recording at some distance from the end-plate zone, will generate triphasic end-plate spikes that are identical in appearance to fibrillation potentials (Fig. 10-18).[12] This is understandable, because both waveforms are single muscle fiber discharges. The key to identification is the rapid and irregular discharge of end-plate spikes, while fibrillation potentials fire much slower and very regularly.

Positive sharp waves

These are waveforms that can be recorded from a single muscle fiber having an unstable resting membrane potential secondary to denervation or intrinsic muscle disease. Typically, it has a large primary sharp positive deflection followed by a small negative potential. These potentials are called positive sharp waves (PSWs; Fig. 10-17). This waveform is believed to have the same clinical significance as a fibrillation potential, in that it is a single muscle fiber discharge. Amplified through a loudspeaker, PSWs have a regularly firing rate (1–15 Hz) and a dull

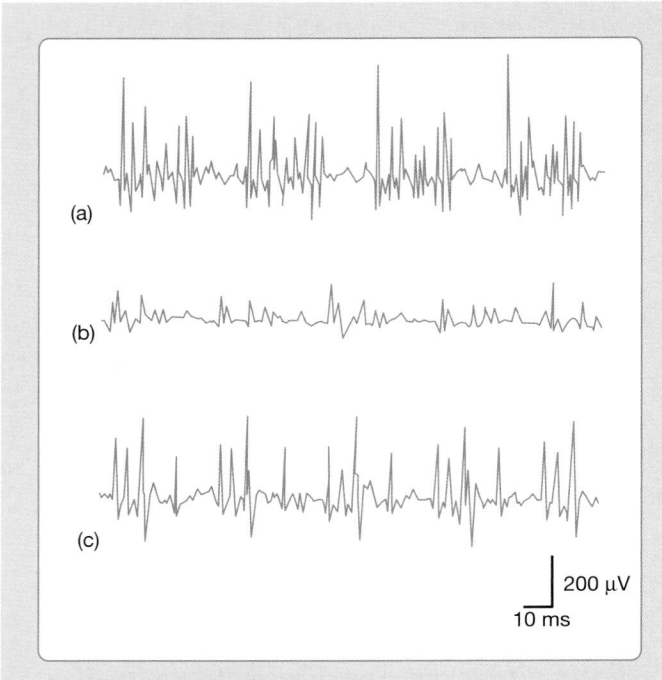

(a)

(b)

(c)

200 µV

10 ms

Figure 10-19 Several examples of complex repetitive discharges. Note how the same pattern of potentials repeats. The sound is like that of heavy machinery, and they start and stop abruptly. (From Dumitru et al. 2002,[12] with permission of Hanley & Belfus.)

thud sound. Their durations are from several milliseconds to 100 ms or longer. Although commonly observed to fire spontaneously, PSWs can be provoked by electrode movement, as can fibrillation potentials.

A number of other waveforms can be observed that have the configurations resembling a PSW. A MUAP recorded from the tendinous region can also have an initial positive deflection followed by a negative potential, because the current sink cannot pass beyond the recording electrode.[12] It is also possible for the recording electrode to damage a number of muscle fibers in close proximity to the recording surface, again preventing an action potential from passing its recording surface, resulting in a primarily positive potential. These two potentials can be distinguished from a PSW in that they are MUAPs and subject to voluntary control, whereas a PSW is not. Asking the individual to contract and relax the muscle under investigation should demonstrate that the waveform has a variable firing rate. A PSW typically fires at a regular rate and is not under voluntary control. If any doubt remains, the electrode should be repositioned until successful recordings are obtained.

Transient runs of 'PSW-appearing potentials' may be seen in healthy skeletal muscle, particularly in the paraspinal and hand or foot intrinsic muscles. The 'non-pathologic' PSWs are believed to arise because the needle electrode is oriented in such a manner as to irritate an end plate's terminal axon, but extend along the muscle fiber while compressing the tissue and preventing action potential conduction.[12] The induced end-

plate spike appears like a PSW, but it displays a relatively rapid and irregularly firing rate characteristic of end-plate spikes (Fig. 10-18).

Complex repetitive discharge (CRD)

A CRD is a spontaneously firing group of action potentials (formerly called bizarre high-frequency discharges or pseudo-myotonic discharges) and require a needle recording electrode for detection.[12] The configuration of these waveforms is that they are continuous runs of simple or complex spike patterns (fibrillation potentials or PSWs) that regularly repeat at 0.3–150 Hz. The repetitive pattern of spike potentials has the same appearance with each firing, and bears the same relationship with its neighboring spikes (Fig. 10-19). A distinct sound, likened to that of heavy machinery or an idling motorcycle, is produced by the firing of CRDs. In addition to the sound and repetitive pattern, a hallmark of these waveforms is that they start and stop abruptly. CRDs may begin spontaneously or be induced by needle movement, muscle percussion, or muscle contraction. Nerve block and curare do not abolish CRDs, suggesting that the origin of these potentials is within the muscle tissue. Detection of these waveforms usually suggests that a chronic process has resulted in a group of muscle fibers becoming separated from their neuromuscular junctions. They may be associated with a currently active disease, or be the residua of a past disorder.

Myotonic discharges

The phenomenon of delayed muscle relaxation following muscle contraction is referred to as myotonia or action myotonia.[12] The finding of delayed muscle relaxation after reflex activation, or induced by striking the muscle belly with a reflex hammer, is called percussion myotonia. Clinical myotonia is usually accentuated by energetic muscle activity following a rest period. Continued muscle contraction lessens the myotonia and is known as the 'warm up'. It is believed that cooling the muscle accentuates myotonia, but this finding has only been objectively documented in paramyotonia congenita.

Myotonic discharges can present in one of two waveform types (Fig. 10-20). The myotonic potential induced by needle electrode insertion usually assumes a morphology similar to that of a PSW or a fibrillation potential. It is believed that the needle movement induces a repetitive firing of the unstable membranes of multiple single muscle fibers. This is because the recording needle is thought to have damaged that portion of the muscle fiber with which it is in contact. Regardless of the waveform type, the hallmark of myotonia is the waxing and waning in both frequency and amplitude. The myotonic discharge has a characteristic sound, likened to that of a dive-bomber and easily recognized. Amplitudes range from 10 µV to 1 mV, and firing rates from 20 to 100 Hz.[37]

Myotonic discharges can occur with or without clinical myotonia. The observation of these potentials requires needle movement or muscle contraction. These waveforms persist after nerve block, neuromuscular block, or frank denervation.

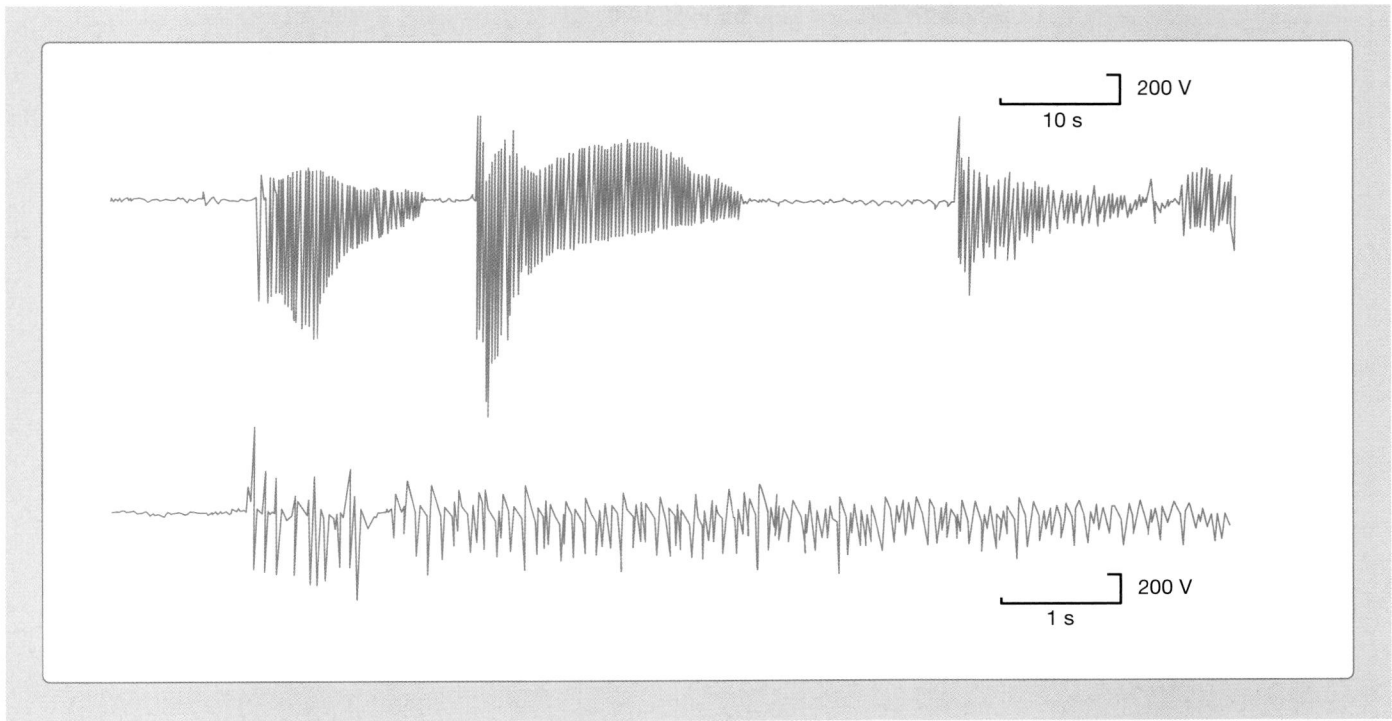

Figure 10-20 A run of myotonic potentials demonstrating the waxing and waning nature of the discharge.

This suggests that their site of origin is the muscle membrane itself, and they appear to be due to a channelopathy. Although the exact mechanism of myotonic discharge production remains unclear, it is proposed that decreased chloride conductance is responsible at least in part for the findings in myotonia congenita.[12] In addition to the syndromes noted above, myotonic discharges can also be detected at times in acid maltase deficiency, polymyositis, and other disorders.

NEURAL GENERATORS OF ABNORMAL SPONTANEOUS POTENTIALS

Fasciculation potentials

The visible spontaneous contraction of a portion of muscle is referred to as a fasciculation. When these contractions are observed with an intramuscular needle recording electrode, they are called fasciculation potentials.[4,12] A fasciculation potential is the electrically summated voltage of depolarizing muscle fibers belonging to all or part of one motor unit. Occasionally, fasciculation potentials can be documented only with needle electromyography, because they lie too deep in muscle to be seen.

Fasciculation waveforms can be characterized with respect to phasicity, amplitude, and duration (Fig. 10-21). Their discharge rate (1 Hz to many per minute) is irregular. They are not under voluntary control, nor are they influenced by mild contraction of the agonist or antagonist muscles. The site of origin of fasciculation potentials remains unclear, although it appears that

there are three possible sites: the spontaneous discharge may arise from the anterior horn cell, or along the entire peripheral nerve (particularly the terminal portion), or at times within the muscle itself.

Fasciculation potentials occur in almost all normal persons in the foot intrinsic or gastrocsoleus muscles, and in patients with a variety of diseases. Typical diseases in which fasciculation potentials can be found include motor neuron disorders, radiculopathies, entrapment neuropathies, and cervical spondylotic myelopathy. Fasciculation potentials have also been described in metabolic disturbances, including tetany, thyrotoxicosis, and anticholinesterase overdoses. Studies have unsuccessfully attempted to distinguish between benign (normal) and pathologic fasciculation potentials. There is no reliable way to categorize whether fasciculation potentials indicate a disease state just by considering their inherent characteristics based on routine needle electromyography. Perhaps the best way to evaluate fasciculation potentials is to analyze the 'company they keep'. A careful analysis of voluntary MUAP morphology, combined with a search for abnormal spontaneous potentials, is required prior to concluding that fasciculation potentials are either a normal or an abnormal finding.

Myokymic discharge

Myokymia is readily observable as vermicular (bag of live worms) or rippling movement of the skin. It is usually associated with myokymic discharges.[12] The myokymic discharge

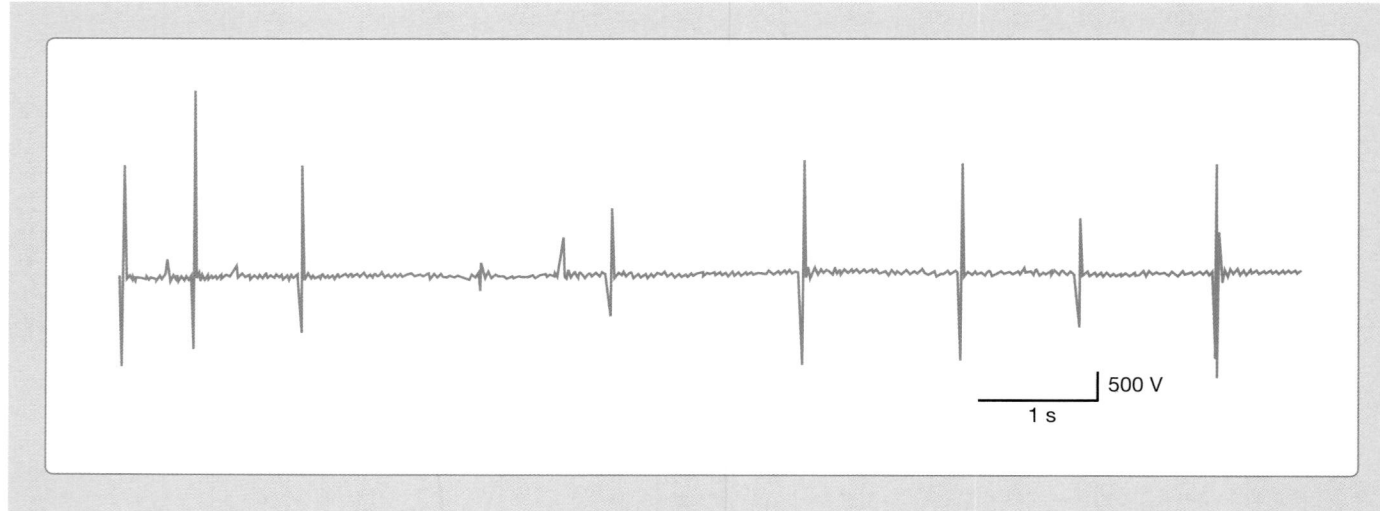

Figure 10-21 Fasciculation potentials recorded from a healthy individual's abductor hallucis.

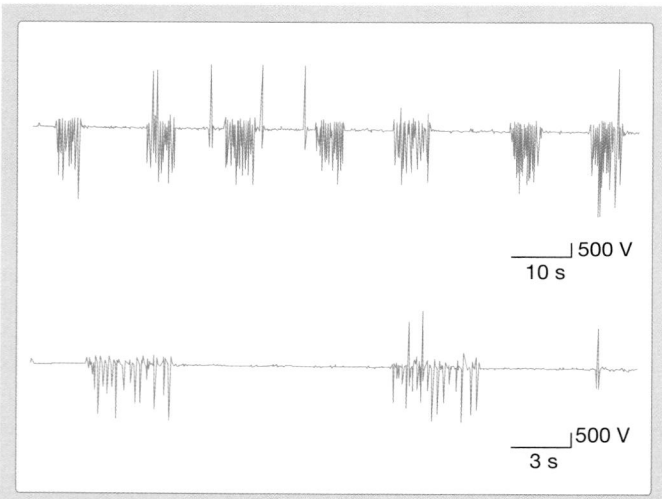

Figure 10-22 Myokymic discharge from a person with radiation plexopathy. Note the bursts of motor unit activity with electrical silence between bursts.

consists of bursts of normal-appearing motor units, with interburst intervals of electrical silence. Typically, the firing rate is 0.1–10 Hz in a semirhythmic pattern. Two to 10 potentials within a single burst may fire at 20–150 Hz. These potentials are not affected by voluntary contraction (Fig. 10-22). The sound associated with these potentials is a type of sputtering often heard with a low-powered motorboat engine. The actual discharge may be distinguished from CRDs in that myokymic discharges do not display a regular pattern of spikes from one burst to the next, nor do they typically start and stop abruptly. Myokymic discharges are groups of motor units, while CRDs

represent groups of single muscle fibers. The groups of motor units within a burst may fire only once or possibly several times. The sputtering bursts of myokymic discharges sound quite different than the continuous drone of a CRD.

Myokymic potentials can be observed in the face (facial myokymia), arising from multiple sclerosis or a brain stem neoplasm. Segmental myokymic discharges can be noted in syringomyelia or radiculopathies. Generalized myokymic discharges have been detected in uremia, thyrotoxicosis, and inflammatory polyradiculoneuropathy. Limb myokymic discharges have also been described associated with radiation plexopathy.

Continuous muscle fiber activity

A number of relatively rare syndromes producing continuous muscle fiber activity associated with muscle stiffness have been reported.[12] Portions of both the central and the peripheral nervous system have been implicated in generating the sustained firing of motor units. One syndrome with continuous muscle fiber activity is known as 'stiff man syndrome'. The motor unit discharges in this condition are believed to have a central origin, as they are abolished or attenuated by peripheral nerve block, neuromuscular block, spinal block, general anesthesia, and sleep. The continuous motor unit firing is diminished by diazepam but not by phenytoin or carbamazepine. The patient can voluntarily control motor unit activity, but the overriding involuntary firing returns when the patient relaxes. Progressive muscle stiffness involving all muscles (including the chest wall and pharynx) eventually occurs, resulting in contractures and profound impairment. A needle electrode recording reveals normal motor unit potentials producing a sustained discharge pattern in both the agonists and the antagonists.

A 'peripheral' form originating in the peripheral motor axon is referred to as Isaac syndrome. The continuous motor unit activity is eliminated by neuromuscular block but not peripheral nerve block, spinal or general anesthesia, or sleep. The motor unit activity usually begins in the lower limbs in the late teens and progresses to all skeletal muscles. Needle recordings demonstrate motor unit discharges with frequencies up to 300 Hz, including doublets, triplets, and multiplets (see below).

Cramps

A sustained and possibly painful muscle contraction of multiple motor units, lasting seconds or minutes, may appear in normal individuals or specific disease states.[30] In healthy subjects, a cramp usually occurs in the calf muscles or other lower limb muscles following exercise, abnormal positioning, or maintaining a fixed position for a prolonged period of time. Cramps may also be induced by hyponatremia, hypocalcemia, vitamin deficiency, or ischemia. They also occur in early motor neuron disease and peripheral neuropathies. Familial syndromes have been reported that involve fasciculations and cramps; alopecia, diarrhea, and cramps; and simply an autosomal dominantly inherited cramp syndrome.

A needle recording electrode placed into a cramping muscle shows multiple motor units firing synchronously between 40 and 60 Hz, and occasionally reaching 200–300 Hz (Fig. 10-23). A large portion of the muscle is simultaneously involved in a cramp, as opposed to the asynchronous excitation of motor units during voluntary activation. Cramps are believed to arise from a peripheral portion of the motor unit. A cramp that results in a taut muscle with electrical silence is the physiologic contracture seen in McArdle disease.

Multiplet discharges

A clinical syndrome manifested by spontaneous muscle twitching, cramps, and carpopedal spasm is known as tetany.[12] This entity usually results from peripheral and/or central nervous system irritability associated with systemic alkalosis, hypocalcemia, hyperkalemia, hypomagnesemia, or local ischemia. Clinically, one may induce tetany by tapping the facial nerve (Chvostek's sign), the peroneal nerve at the fibular head (peroneal sign), and inducing limb ischemia (Trousseau's sign).

In the above conditions, characteristic motor unit potentials may be observed. A single motor unit potential may fire rather rapidly, with an interdischarge interval of 2–20 ms. If the motor unit fires twice, it is referred to as a doublet; three times denotes a triplet; and more than three firings is called a multiplet (Fig. 10-24). These potentials can be seen following voluntary contraction, or can be observed spontaneously from the induction maneuvers noted above (Chvostek's sign or Trousseau's sign), in which MUAPs may fire in long trains or short bursts of 5–30 Hz (tetany). Motor units with an interdischarge interval of 20–80 ms are called 'paired discharges' but can arise in similar states, as previously described.

NERVE INJURY CLASSIFICATION

Peripheral nerve injury is one of the most common types of pathology likely to be encountered during an electrodiagnostic medicine evaluation. It is necessary to be familiar with the various classification systems available to categorize an insult to neural tissue.

Seddon's classification

The degree to which a nerve is damaged has obvious implications with respect to its present function and potential for recovery. There are essentially two general classification systems.[34,38] One classification is that of Seddon, and considers neural injury from the perspective of a combination of functional status and histologic appearance. In Seddon's scheme, there are three degrees or stages of injury to consider: neurapraxia, axonotmesis, and neurotmesis (Table 10-1).

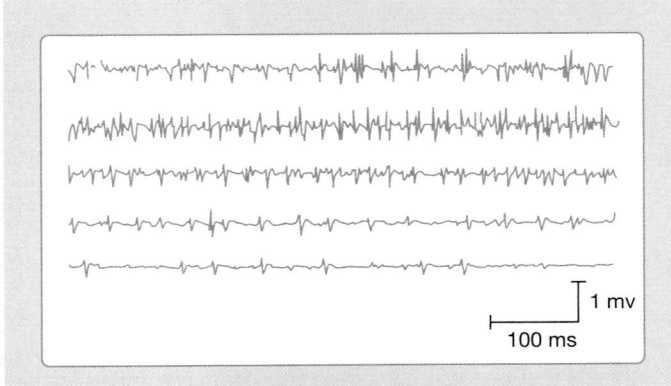

Figure 10-23 A characteristic muscle cramp as recorded with an intramuscular needle electrode. There is an initial burst of motor unit activity that eventually subsides as the cramp dissipates. (From Daube 1979,[11] with permission of the AAEM.)

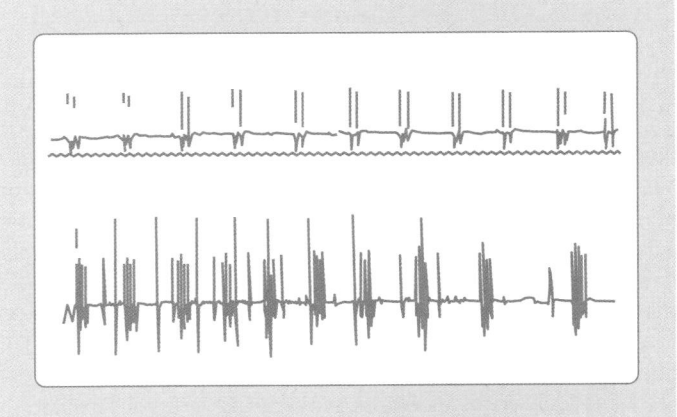

Figure 10-24 Doublets (upper trace) and multiplets (lower trace), motor unit action potentials resulting from voluntary contraction. (From Daube 1979,[11] with permission of the AAEM.)

Table 10-1 Nerve injury classification

Type	Function	Pathologic basis	Prognosis
Lundborg Physiologic conduction block Type a	Focal conduction block	Intraneural ischemia; metabolic (ionic) block; no nerve fiber changes	Excellent; immediately reversible
Type b	Focal conduction block	Intraneural edema; increased endoneurial fluid pressure; metabolic block; little or no fiber changes	Recovery in days or weeks
Seddon–Sunderland Neurapraxia Type 1	Focal conduction block; primarily motor function and proprioception affected; some sensation and sympathetic function may be present	Local myelin injury, primarily larger fibers; axonal continuity; no Wallerian degeneration	Recovery in weeks to months
Axonotmesis Type 2	Loss of nerve conduction at injury site and distally	Disruption of axonal continuity with Wallerian degeneration; endoneurial tubes, perineurium, and epineurium intact	Axonal regeneration required for recovery; good prognosis, because original end organs reached
Type 3	Loss of nerve conduction at injury site and distally	Loss of axonal continuity and endoneurial tubes; perineurium and epineurium preserved	Disruption of endoneurial tubes, hemorrhage, and edema produce scarring; axonal misdirection; poor prognosis; surgery may be required
Type 4	Loss of nerve conduction at injury site and distally	Loss of axonal continuity, endoneurial tubes, and perineurium; epineurium intact	Total disorganization of guiding elements; intraneural scarring and axonal misdirection; poor prognosis; surgery necessary
Neurotmesis Type 5	Loss of nerve conduction at injury site and distally	Severance of entire nerve	Surgical modification of nerve ends required; prognosis guarded and dependent on nature of injury and local factors

(After Lundborg 1988,[31] with permission.)

Neurapraxia

The term *neurapraxia* is used to designate a mild degree of neural insult that results in blockage of impulse conduction across the affected segment. It is also acceptable to simply designate this type of neural insult as *conduction block*. The most important aspect of conduction block is its reversibility. Muscle wasting usually does not occur in conduction block because muscle innervation is maintained and, secondly, recovery is typically rapid enough to avoid disuse atrophy. Fibrillation potentials should not be observed in conduction block, because the axon is not disrupted. Keep in mind that some nerve injuries can be mixed lesions in which some fibers have conduction block and some have axonal loss. In this case, it is certainly possible to observe fibrillation potentials.

Axonotmesis

The second degree of neural insult in Seddon's classification is *axonotmesis*, which is a specific type of nerve injury where only the axon is physically disrupted, with preservation of the enveloping endoneurial and other supporting connective tissue structures (perineurium and epineurium). Compression of a profound nature or traction on the nerve are typical lesion etiologies. Once the axon has been disrupted, the characteristic changes of Wallerian degeneration occur. The fact that the endoneurium remains intact is a very important aspect of this type of injury. A preserved endoneurium implies that once the remnants of the degenerated nerve have been removed by phagocytosis, the regenerating axon simply has to follow its original course directly back to the appropriate end organ. A good prognosis can be expected when neural damage results only in axonotmesis.

Neurotmesis

The greatest degree of nerve disruption is designated in Seddon's system as *neurotmesis*. This is complete disruption of the axon and all supporting connective tissue structures, whereby the endoneurium, perineurium, and epineurium are no longer in continuity. A neurotmetic lesion has a poor prognosis for complete functional recovery. Surgical reapproximation of the nerve ends will probably be required. Surgery does not guarantee proper endoneurial tube alignment, but at least it improves the chances that axonal growth will occur across the injury site.

Sunderland's classification

A second popular and somewhat more detailed classification is that proposed and subsequently modified by Sunderland. This classification of nerve injury is based on the results of trauma with respect to the axon and its supporting connective tissue structures. Basically, Sunderland's classification is divided into five types of injury, based exclusively on which connective tissue components are disrupted (Fig. 10-25). Type 1 injury corresponds to Seddon's designation of neurapraxia. Seddon's axonotmesis is subdivided by Sunderland into three forms of neural insult (types 2–4). A Type 2 injury involves loss of axonal continuity with preservation of all supporting neural structures, including the endoneurium (this closely corresponds to Seddon's axonotmesis). Type 3 and 4 injuries result in progressively more neural disruption. Sunderland's Type 5 injury corresponds to Seddon's neurotmesis (complete neural disruption).

INSTRUMENTATION

An electrodiagnostic instrument actually comprises many separate components, of which the electrodes, amplifier, filters, sound, and stimulator are discussed in this chapter. Practitioners of electrodiagnostic medicine are urged to gain a thorough understanding of instrumentation principles and all the instrument's subcomponents (Fig. 10-26).[13,14,36]

Electrodes

The two types of electrodes are surface and needle. Surface electrodes are manufactured in various sizes and shapes so as to best conform to the body part under investigation. The electrode must be firmly secured to the patient to preclude any movement. Well-secured electrodes minimize movement artifact that could contaminate the desired signal.

Two commonly used needle recording electrodes are monopolar and concentric (Fig. 10-27). The monopolar needle is a solid, stainless steel shaft coated completely with Teflon except for the bare metal tip. It is this bare metal tip that acts as the

recording surface. The needle is typically 12–75 mm in length and 0.3–0.5 mm in diameter, with a recording surface of 0.15–0.6 mm^2. Separate reference and ground electrodes are required. The concentric needle electrode is a hollow, stainless steel hypodermic needle with a central platinum or nichrome–silver wire about 0.1 mm in diameter, surrounded by epoxy resin acting as an insulating material from the surrounding cannula. The cannula has a similar length and diameter to that of the monopolar needle. A separate ground is required, but the cannula serves as the reference electrode.

There has been considerable discussion about the merits of each of these electrodes compared with the other. Both electrodes have advantages and disadvantages depending on the clinical circumstances. Monopolar needle electrodes have a wider recording territory and a distant reference, which makes the recording 'noisier' with respect to distant activity and interference. On the other hand, the Teflon coating reduces patient discomfort. The concentric needle electrode has the active and reference electrodes close together, making them electrically quieter than monopolar needles. Concentric electrodes typically cause more patient discomfort in this practitioner's opinion. Concentric needle electrodes yield the following as compared with monopolar needle electrodes: smaller potential amplitudes, possibly fewer phases, comparable durations, and less distant motor unit activity. The introduction of commercially available disposable monopolar and concentric needle electrodes has eliminated such worries as Teflon peeling back on the monopolar needles, and hook formation on the tip of the concentric needle electrodes. The quality of disposable needle electrodes has improved, eliminating the need to use non-disposable needle electrodes. If electrodes are reused, they should be properly sterilized with presoaking in sodium hypochlorite and steam autoclaving.[12]

Single-fiber electrodes are essentially modified concentric needle electrodes. A small, 25-μm recording port is placed opposite the electrode's bevel and several millimeters from the tip. This makes this special electrode capable of recording the electrical activity from a single muscle fiber. The uptake area for this electrode is approximately 300 μm (Fig. 10-27).

Amplifier

Biologic signals range in size from microvolts to millivolts, thereby requiring significant amplification prior to being analyzed. An amplifier is simply a device with the ability to magnify the desired signals and minimize unwanted signals or noise. Amplification is expressed as gain or sensitivity. Gain is a ratio of the signal's output divided by the input. For example, an output of 1 V for an input of 10 mV implies that the amplifier has a gain factor of 100 000 (output − input = 1 V $\sqrt{}$ 0.00001 V = 100 000). Sensitivity is the ratio of the input voltage to the size of deflection on the CRT, and is usually measured in centimeters. For example, an amplifier that produces a 1-cm deflection for an input of 10 mV has a sensitivity of 10 mV/cm or 10 mV/division. The sensitivity or gain setting used is important, because it can influence the onset latency. Increasing the sensitivity for a given waveform results in the instrument

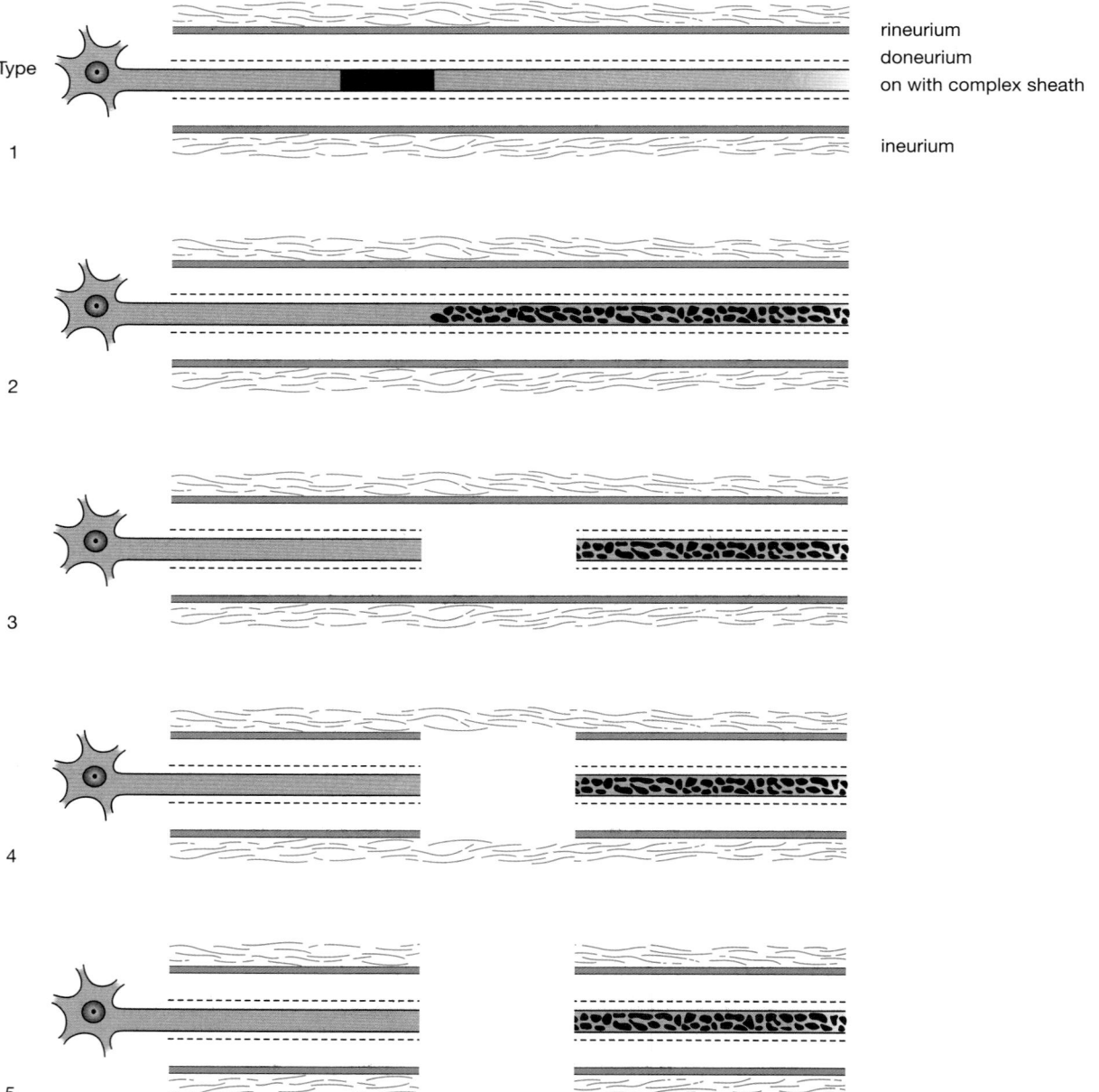

Figure 10-25 The five degrees of neural injury as classified by Sunderland. Type 1, conduction block; 2, Wallerian degeneration occurring secondary to a lesion confined to the axon, with preservation of the endoneurial sheath; 3, there is noted to be disruption of the axon and endoneurial tube, within an intact perineurium; 4, disruption of all neural elements except the epineurium; and 5, complete discontinuity of the entire nerve trunk. (From Sunderland 1991,[39] with permission.)

displaying the potential's initial departure from baseline earlier in time, because progressively earlier and hence smaller baseline deviations can now be observed.

The standard electromyograph has two amplifiers. The amplifier connected to the active electrode is known as the non-inverting amplifier, while the reference electrode is connected to the inverting amplifier. The inverting amplifier magnifies the signal presented to it in essentially the same manner as the non-inverting amplifier, with the exception of inverting the signal. Both amplified signals (inverted and non-inverted) are then electronically summated, and like signals are canceled. This is the concept of differential amplification, i.e. different signals are amplified while common signals are eliminated. When an identical signal is presented to both amplifiers, theoretically there should be no output from the instrument because there is elimination of the same or so-called common signals. For example, 60-Hz interference recorded by the active and reference electrodes is eliminated as a common mode signal. It is impossible to build two amplifiers with identical properties, so common mode rejection can never be perfect. The ratio of the

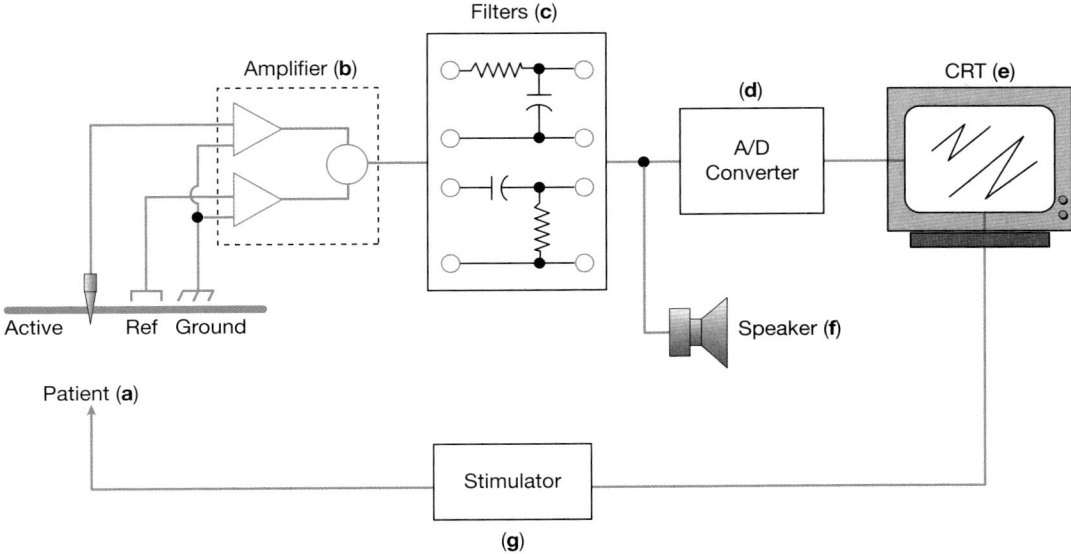

Figure 10-26 The subcomponents of the electrophysiologic instrument are depicted. Electrodes on or in the patient (**a**) detect bioelectric changes, which are transmitted to a differential amplifier (**b**). This signal is filtered (**c**), undergoes analog to digital conversion (**d**), and is displayed on the cathode ray tube (**e**) as well as the sound being presented through a loudspeaker (**f**). Time-locked evoked potentials can be generated with the stimulator (**g**). (From Dumitru and Walsh 1989,[13] with permission of Hanley & Belfus.)

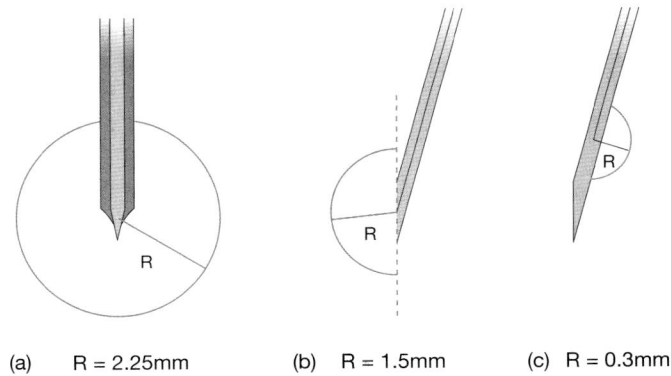

(a)   R = 2.25mm   (b)   R = 1.5mm   (c)   R = 0.3mm

Figure 10-27 Three needle electrodes and their recording areas. (**a**) A monopolar needle electrode requires a separate reference and ground electrode. (**b**) The concentric needle electrode uses the cannula as the reference, while a separate ground is required. (**c**) The single-fiber electrode is essentially a modified concentric needle electrode. (From Dumitru and Walsh 1989,[13] with permission of Hanley & Belfus.)

instrument's differential to common output (common mode rejection ratio) should exceed 100 000:1. For example, suppose the non-inverting amplifier is set with a gain of 100 and the inverting amplifier is also set with a gain of 100 but in reality has a gain of 99.9 (remember, the two amplifiers can be very similar but not identical). A 100-μV signal of interest is presented to our non-inverting amplifier as recorded by the active recording electrode. The reference electrode presents no signal to the inverting amplifier, because it is located in an 'electrically silent' area compared with the signal of interest. The result is a signal that has been magnified to 10 000 μV. Additionally, there is a 1-μV noise signal present that is detected by both the active and the reference electrodes, resulting in this signal amplified to 100

μV and 99.9 μV for the non-inverting and inverting amplifiers, respectively. The difference between these two signals, as electrically subtracted from each other by the two amplifiers, is 0.1 μV. The common mode rejection ratio is then the difference signal (10 000 μV) divided by the common mode signal (noise presented to both amplifiers) of 0.1 μV (10 000 μV/0.1 μV), yielding the anticipated ratio of 100 000:1.

Filters

Perhaps the most misunderstood and ignored aspects of the electrodiagnostic instrument are the filters. The main purpose of filters is to form a window or bandwidth of frequencies containing the desired waveform, but excluding those frequencies not comprising the signal of interest ('noise'). Low- and high-frequency filters are used to prevent those frequencies below and above the respective filter settings from being amplified and subsequently interfering with the signal of interest. A high-frequency filter eliminates those frequencies higher than its numeric designation, and permits frequencies lower than its numeric designation to pass. This is why a high-frequency filter is also known as a low-pass filter: it permits low frequencies to pass through and be displayed. Similarly, a low-frequency filter extracts low frequencies from the total recorded signal below its numeric designation. A low-frequency filter permits frequencies greater than its numeric designation to pass.

Any biologic signal can be conceptualized as a series of sine waves of various frequencies and amplitudes. The combination of 'appropriate' sine wave amplitudes and frequencies can result in the formation of essentially any waveform. In this way, the biologic signal recorded by the instrument consists of multiple subcomponent waveforms with specific frequency and amplitude characteristics. Eliminating any of these subcomponent waveforms results in a distortion of the waveform's appearance.

This is exactly what can happen if the high- or low-frequency filters are set such that the desired biologic waveform has various subcomponent frequencies eliminated. The examples provided below apply equally well to nerve and muscle potentials.

In our example, a recorded median SNAP and CMAP are sequentially distorted by altering the low- and high-frequency filter settings. Let us begin with an arbitrary low-frequency filter setting of 1 Hz and a high-frequency filter cutoff of 10 000 Hz. Sequentially elevating the low-frequency filter from 1 to 10 Hz, 100 Hz, and finally 300 Hz, while maintaining a high-frequency filter at 10 000 Hz, results in characteristic waveform distortions (Fig. 10-28). The onset latency does not change, the peak latency decreases, amplitude is serially reduced, and the total potential duration decreases. Also, an additional phase is created. The use of sequentially higher low-frequency filter settings removes progressively more low frequencies from the SNAP. In other words, the remaining potential now has a predominance of high frequencies in it as compared with the original potential. The onset of the potential remains unaltered, because it is a quick departure from baseline and is not influenced by an alteration in the low-frequency content of the waveform. The remainder of the potential, however, is influenced by the now predominant high-frequency subcomponent waveforms. By taking out the low frequencies, the amplitude declines as subcomponent waveforms are removed. Clearly, the waveform's magnitude could not possibly increase, because we are taking out part of its content. Further, the remainder of the waveform is shifted to an earlier time of occurrence because of the high frequencies remaining in the SNAP. Because comparatively high frequencies occur sooner in time, it is logical that all the waveform shifts toward the potential's stationary onset, producing decreases in its peak latency, negative spike duration, and total duration. A third phase is created as the potential begins to appear more like a sine wave as the higher frequencies begin to emerge. Remember, high frequencies have more phases per unit time. A similar but more dramatic occurrence is noted for the CMAP, because it comprises comparatively more low frequencies than a SNAP does.

Eliminating high frequencies results in a somewhat different set of alterations. Because we are removing waveforms from the total potential, a reduction in amplitude can be anticipated. Because the SNAP is now biased toward a potential with more low frequencies, it takes longer to occur in time. This results in a delay of both the onset and the peak latencies (Fig. 10-29). Lowering the high-frequency filter while maintaining a constant low-frequency filter results in a waveform with a comparatively smaller amplitude, longer onset latency, and longer peak latency, as well as longer overall duration. Similar findings can be observed for a CMAP.

There are no universally agreed filter settings for any electrodiagnostic medicine procedure. Arriving at optimal filter settings is highly empiric. The high- and low-frequency filters are lowered and raised respectively until waveform distortions are observed. The filters are then expanded until no waveform changes are noted. The goal is to include the major components

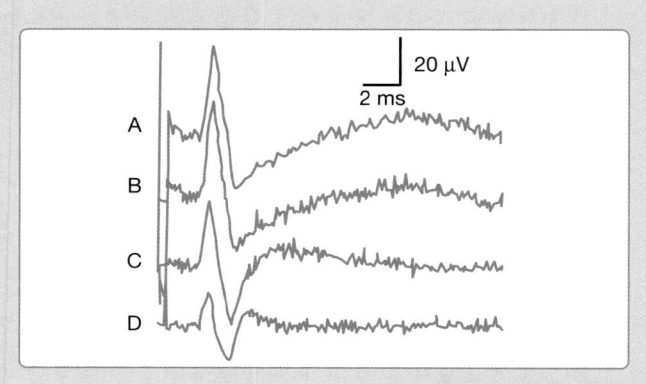

Trace	Low frequency (Hz)	Latency (ms) Onset	Peak	Duration negative spike (ms)	Amplitude (μV)
A	1	2.6	3.3	1.4	65
B	10	2.6	3.3	1.4	65
C	100	2.6	3.1	1.0	54
D	300	2.6	3.0	0.8	30

Figure 10-28 An antidromic median sensory nerve action potential is evoked from the third digit while the low-frequency filter is sequentially elevated with a constant high-frequency filter of 10 000 Hz. Note how the onset latency does not change; however, the peak latency decreases, as does the potential's amplitude. A third phase is also produced at the low-frequency filter setting of 300 Hz. (From Dumitru and Walsh 1988,[14] with permission.)

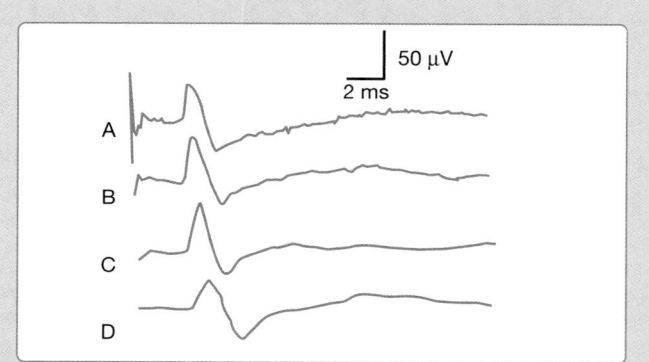

Trace	High frequency filter (Hz)	Latency (ms) Onset	Peak	Amplitude (μV)
A	10 000	2.7	3.3	76
B	2 000	2.8	3.4	76
C	1 000	2.8	3.8	75
D	500	3.0	4.2	64

Figure 10-29 An antidromic median sensory nerve action potential is recorded from the third digit while a constant low-frequency filter of 10 Hz but different high-frequency filters are employed. Note how the onset and peak latencies are sequentially delayed with decreasing high-frequency filter settings. The potential's amplitude also decreases. (From Dumitru and Walsh 1988,[14] with permission.)

Table 10-2 Recommended filter settings

Procedure	Low frequency (Hz)	High frequency (Hz)
Nerve conduction velocity (motor)	2–10	10 000
Nerve conduction velocity (sensory)	2–10	2 000
Needle electromyography (routine)	20–30	10 000
Needle electromyography (quantitative)	2–5	10 000
Single-fiber electromyography	500–1000	10 000–20 000
Somatosensory evoked potential	1–10	500–3 000

(From Dumitru and Walsh 1988,[14] with permission.)

of the waveforms while eliminating undesired signals or noise. The most important factor is to reproduce all filter settings originally described by those investigators whose reference data is being used (Table 10-2).

Sound

After the biologic signal is filtered, it is fed to a loudspeaker. The acoustic analysis of both normal and abnormal potentials is extremely important. It is not uncommon for practitioners to 'hear' an abnormality prior to viewing it on the CRT. The instrument must have a relatively good speaker so as to accurately present the sounds associated with the biologic signals.

Stimulator

Two different types of stimulators are commercially available: constant current and constant voltage. For both types of devices, neural tissue is activated under the cathode (negative pole) while the anode (positive pole) completes the stimulating circuit. A constant current stimulator effectively delivers the desired current output for each stimulus irrespective of the resistance between the skin and cathode or anode. This is accomplished by varying the voltage or current driving force as is necessitated by any alterations in the skin–stimulator interface's resistance. Similarly, a constant voltage stimulator is designed to deliver the same voltage with each stimulus, even if the resistance between the skin and stimulator changes. A compensatory increase or decrease in current is provided so as to maintain the same voltage level. In short, a constant current stimulator is effectively a variable voltage stimulator, while a constant voltage stimulator is a variable current stimulator. Both stimulators are acceptable for most purposes. The constant current stimulator is preferred when the same current must be delivered for each stimulus in clinical situations requiring quantification of current delivery, such as in somatosensory evoked potentials, research, or evaluating side to side stimulation thresholds during facial nerve excitability testing.

An important problem associated with stimulators is the stimulus artifact. It is commonly a large potential recorded during the delivery of the stimulus. At times, the magnitude of the potential is large enough to compromise the desired neural or muscular response. In such situations, it is necessary to minimize the shock artifact. An effective method of reducing the shock artifact is to employ fast recovery amplifiers that act to suppress this artifact by quickly recovering from the overwhelming voltage delivered. These amplifiers are not available on all instruments, and so other means must be found to deal with the artifact. The skin surface must be dry, and any perspiration, body lotion, makeup, or other surface conductors should be removed. Wiping a large portion of the body segment under investigation with an alcohol pad usually removes all surface conducting films. A ground electrode is best placed between the stimulus site and the active recording electrode. Wire leads between the patient and stimulator should be separated to avoid any type of capacitive interaction. The stimulator circuit should be isolated from the instrument's ground circuit, which is true of virtually all commercially manufactured instruments. Perhaps the most effective method of reducing stimulus artifact, once all the above have been addressed, is to rotate the anode about the cathode. This optimizes the stimulator's voltage output, as recorded by the active and reference electrode, to take advantage of differential amplification and the elimination of the shock artifact as a common mode signal. An attempt is made to have both the active and the reference electrodes record similar voltages, thereby minimizing the stimulator's signal from being amplified and displayed along with the signal.

Anodal block is an interesting concept that has been widely discussed but that has little supporting experimental data. Theoretically, the anode hyperpolarizes the neural tissue in its immediate vicinity and should result in an action potential failing to conduct past the anode. In humans, investigations employing bipolar and monopolar anodal current stimulation at the highest current outputs failed to document any type of anodal block. Because the anode is capable of stimulating neural tissue and not blocking it, at this time it appears that anodal block does not occur during the routine electrodiagnostic medicine consultation.

CONCLUSION

Mastering the above information gives the practitioner a firm grasp of the fundamental principles that underpin the electrodiagnostic medicine consultation. Appreciating the formation and generation of an action potential is not a trivial matter. Of equal importance is the manner in which the electrophysiologic instrument processes the biologic signal of interest. A less than functional understanding of how the instrument can potentially distort the biologic signal can predispose the practitioner to errors in diagnosis.

REFERENCES

1. Albers JW, Allen AA, Bastron JD, et al. Limb myokymia. Muscle Nerve 1981; 4:494–504.

2. Baer RD, Johnson EW. Motor nerve conduction velocities in normal children. Arch Phys Med Rehabil 1965; 46:698–704.

3. Bolton CF, Carter KM. Human sensory nerve compound action potential amplitude: variation with sex and finger circumference. J Neurol Neurosurg Psychiatr 1980; 43:925–928.

4. Brown WF. The physiological and technical basis of electromyography. Boston: Butterworth; 1984:317–368.

5. Buchthal F, Guld C, Rosenfalck P. Multielectrode study of the territory of a motor unit. Acta Physiol Scand 1957; 39:83–104.

6. Buchthal F, Guld C, Rosenfalck P. Volume conduction of the spike of the motor unit potential investigated with a new type of multielectrode. Acta Physiol Scand 1957; 38:331–354.

7. Buchthal F, Rosenfalck A. Evoked action potentials and conduction velocity in human sensory nerves. Brain Res 1966; 3:1–122.

8. Buchthal F. Fibrillations: clinical electrophysiology. In: Culp WJ, Ochoa J, eds. Abnormal nerves and muscle generators. New York: Oxford University Press; 1982:632–662.

9. Campbell WW, Ward LC, Swift TR. Nerve conduction velocity varies inversely with height. Muscle Nerve 1981; 4:520–523.

10. Cummins KL, Dorfman LJ. Nerve fiber conduction velocity distributions: studies of normal and diabetic human nerves. Ann Neurol 1981; 9:67–74.

11. Daube JA. AAEM minimonograph #11: needle examination in electromyography. Rochester: AAEM; 1979.

12. Dumitru D, Amato AA, Zwarts MJ. Electrodiagnostic medicine. 2nd edn. Philadelphia: Hanley & Belfus; 2002.

13. Dumitru D, Walsh NE. Electrophysiologic instrumentation. In: Dumitru D, ed. Physical medicine and rehabilitation state of the art reviews: clinical electrophysiology. Philadelphia: Hanley & Belfus; 1989:684–699.

14. Dumitru D, Walsh NE. Practical instrumentation and common sources of error. Am J Phys Med Rehabil 1988; 67:55–65.

15. Dumitru D. Volume conduction: theory and application. In: Dumitru D, ed. Physical medicine and rehabilitation state of the art reviews: clinical electrophysiology. Philadelphia: Hanley & Belfus; 1989:665–682.

16. Falco FJE, Hennessey WJ, Braddom RL, et al. Standardized nerve conduction studies in the upper limb of the healthy elderly. Am J Phys Med Rehabil 1992; 71:263–271.

17. Falco FJE, Hennessey WJ, Goldberg G, et al. H reflex latency in the healthy elderly. Muscle Nerve 1994; 17:161–167.

18. Halar EM, DeLisa JA, Brozovich FV. Nerve conduction velocity: relationship of skin, subcutaneous and intramuscular temperatures. Arch Phys Med Rehabil 1980; 61:199–203.

19. Halar EM, DeLisa JA, Soine TL. Nerve conduction studies in upper extremities: skin temperature corrections. Arch Phys Med Rehabil 1983; 64:412–416.

20. Halar EM, DeLisa JA. Peroneal nerve conduction velocity: the importance of temperature control. Arch Phys Med Rehabil 1981; 62:439–443.

21. Henrikson JD. Conduction velocity of motor nerves in normal subjects and patients with neuromuscular disorders. Thesis, University of Minnesota, Minneapolis; 1956.

22. Hille B. Introduction to physiology of excitable cells. In: Patton HD, Fuchs AF, Hille B, et al, eds. Textbook of physiology. 21st edn. Philadelphia: Saunders; 1989:1–80.

23. Hodgkin AL, Huxley AF. A quantitative description of membrane current and its application to conduction and excitation in nerve. J Physiol 1952; 117:500–544.

24. Hodgkin AL, Katz B. The effect of temperature on the electrical activity of the giant axon of the squid. J Physiol 1949; 109:240–249.

25. Jewett DL, Rayner MD. Basic concepts of neuronal function. Boston: Little, Brown and Co.; 1984.

26. Johnson EW, Olsen KJ. Clinical value of motor nerve conduction velocity determination. JAMA 1960; 172:2030–2035.

27. Katz B. Nerve, muscle, and synapse. New York: McGraw-Hill; 1966.

28. Koester J. Resting membrane potential and action potential. In: Kandel ER, Schwartz JH, ed. Principles of neural science. 2nd edn. New York: Elsevier; 1985:49–57.

29. Lang AH, Forsstrom J, Bjorkqvist SE, et al. Statistical variation of nerve conduction velocity: an analysis in normal subjects and uraemic patients. J Neurol Sci 1977; 33:229–241.

30. Layzer RB, Rowland LP. Cramps. N Engl J Med 1971; 285:30–31.

31. Lundborg G: Nerve injury and repair. Edinburgh: Churchill Livingstone; 1988.

32. Oh SJ. Clinical electromyography: nerve conduction studies. 2nd edn. Baltimore: Williams & Wilkins; 1993.

33. Schoepfle GM, Erlanger J. The action of temperature on the excitability, spike height and configuration, and the refractory period observed in the responses of single medullated nerve fibers. Am J Physiol 1941; 134:694–704.

34. Seddon H. Three types of nerve injury. Brain 1943; 66:237–288.

35. Soudmand R, Ward LC, Swift TR. Effect of height on nerve conduction velocity. Neurology 1982; 32:407–410.

36. Stolov W. Instrumentation and measurement in electrodiagnosis. Minimonograph #16. Rochester: American Association of Electrodiagnostic Medicine; 1981.

37. Streib EW. AAEM minimonograph #27: differential diagnosis of myotonic syndromes. Muscle Nerve 1987; 10:603–615.

38. Sunderland S. A classification of peripheral nerve injuries producing loss of function. Brain 1951; 74:491–516.

39. Sunderland S. Nerve injuries and their repair: a critical appraisal. Edinburgh: Churchill Livingstone; 1991.

40. Thesleff S. Fibrillation in denervated mammalian muscle. In: Culp WJ, Ochoa J, eds. Abnormal nerve and muscle as impulse generators. New York: Oxford University Press; 1982:678–694.

41. Trojaborg W. Motor nerve conduction velocities in normal subjects with particular reference to the conduction in proximal and distal segments of median and ulnar nerve. Electroencephalogr Clin Neurophysiol 1964; 17:314–321.

42. Waxman SG, Foster RE. Ionic channel distribution and heterogeneity of the axon membrane in myelinated fibers. Brain Res Rev 1980; 2:205–34.

43. Waxman SG. Action potential propagation and conduction velocity—new perspectives and questions. Trends Neurosci 1983; 6:157–161.

Chapter

11

Electrodiagnostic Medicine II: Clinical Evaluation and Findings

Timothy R. Dillingham

Electrodiagnostic medicine is a unique area of medicine that differs from other medical and surgical consultations in many important ways. Electrophysiologic testing is an extension of the history and physical examination, and is tailored to the clinical scenario. There are a variety of tests that can be performed, and it is incumbent on the electrodiagnostician to select those relevant to the clinical circumstances. Unlike other tests, such as an electrocardiogram, the testing procedure may change as data are acquired and new findings interpreted. Like any other clinical area of medicine, high-quality consultations are rendered by physicians with experience and technical competence coupled with an understanding of the peripheral nervous system.

Consultants in electrodiagnostic medicine provide referring physicians with critical information regarding neuromuscular disorders. Such conclusions are often a crucial part of the complex decision-making process that influences subsequent diagnostic and surgical interventions.

This chapter provides an overview of electrodiagnostic tests, the extent of such testing for different clinical scenarios based on recent guidelines, and the types of abnormalities one can expect to find with different neuromuscular disorders.

CLINICAL ASSESSMENT: HISTORY AND PHYSICAL EXAMINATION

History

A directed history enables the electrodiagnostician to develop a conceptual framework for subsequent testing. The history should include information as to whether symptoms are confined to a single limb or more than one limb is involved. The character and nature of symptoms, as well as their duration and time of onset, are important to elicit. Pain and numbness indicate that the sensory system is involved. Motor weakness without pain and numbness indicates primarily involvement of the motor system, motor axons, neuromuscular junction, or muscles. For patients with more generalized symptoms, meaning symptoms in more than one limb, the electrodiagnostician should inquire about other neurologic complaints, such as dyspnea, bladder urgency, dysphagia, dysphonia, and visual changes. Previous cervical or lumbar spine conditions such as spinal stenosis or surgical interventions should be noted.

Activities that aggravate or relieve a patient's symptoms can often help differentiate musculoskeletal problems from entrapments, plexopathies, and radiculopathies.

Diabetes and alcohol are common causes of polyneuropathy in the USA, and an appropriate history would include questioning about such issues. Any family history of neurologic disorders is important to elicit for persons with generalized or unexplained symptoms. A brief recording of the person's vocation is often helpful to identify persons at risk for overuse syndromes.

Important past medical history to elicit includes any history of malignancy, chemotherapy, or radiation, as such conditions and treatments can have peripheral neurologic implications. Previous surgeries for entrapment neuropathies, such as ulnar transposition or carpal tunnel release, are important as well. For instance, a transposed ulnar nerve complicates nerve conduction calculations for the segment across the elbow, as measurement is less precise, and stimulus sites above and below the elbow can be more difficult to find. Whether or not a person is thrombocytopenic, has bleeding disorders, or is on anticoagulants should be noted. In one case series, minor paraspinal muscle hematomas were noted on magnetic resonance imaging (MRI) performed shortly after needle electromyography (EMG) examination in 4 of 17 patients who were not anticoagulated. These hematomas were small and of no clinical significance.[18] In this report, the authors state that, in their review of the literature, there has *never been* a case report of paraspinal hematoma compressing the spinal roots or the epidural space.[18] Although clinicians should always weigh carefully the risk to benefit ratio of testing, a person with appropriate levels of anticoagulation for venous thromboembolism can be safely studied with little risk of neurologic complications. Appropriate pressure should be applied to the area after testing to prevent intramuscular hematoma. The paraspinal muscles are such an important region to study, not only for persons suspected of radiculopathy but in neuromuscular evaluations as well, that electrodiagnosticians should examine them whenever reasonably possible.

Implantable pacemakers are not a contraindication to nerve conduction testing, but proximal stimulations near the chest site should be avoided, and patients should be appropriately grounded.[6] For patients with implanted defibrillators, caution should be used with distal stimulation as well.[6] No stimulus

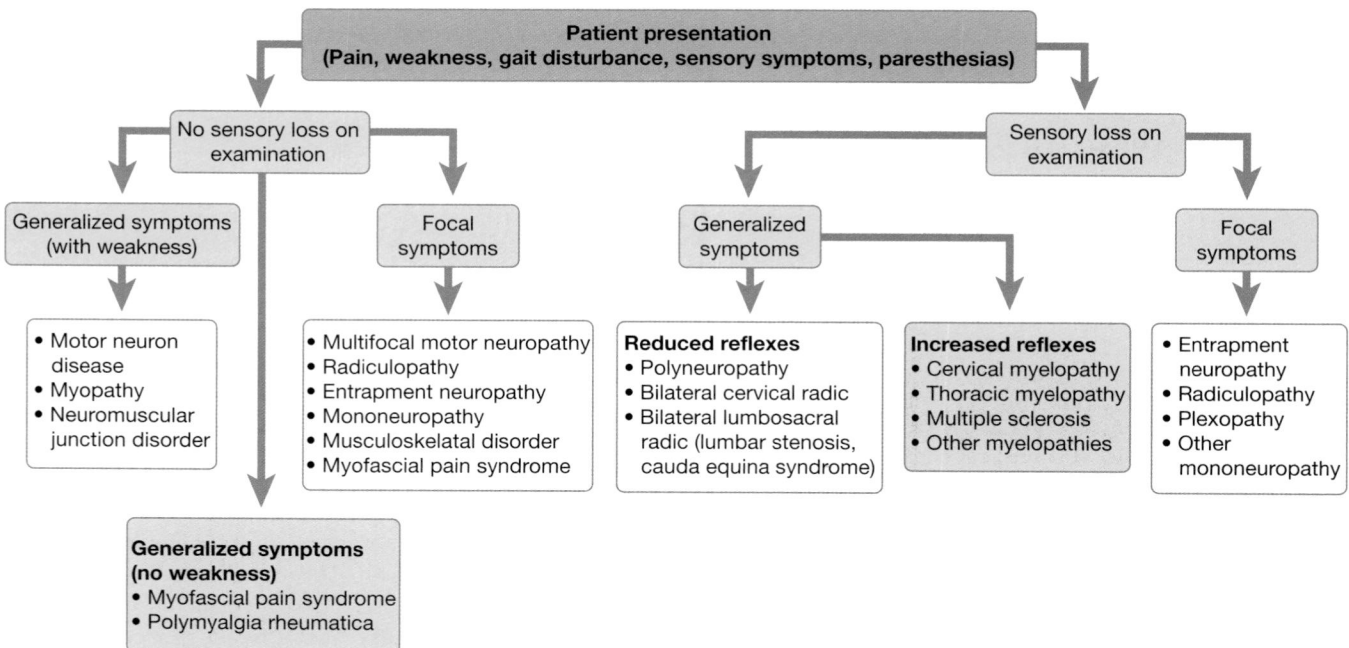

Figure 11-1 An algorithmic approach to using physical examination and symptom information to tailor the electrodiagnostic evaluation.

should be performed faster than 1 Hz, and the stimulus duration should be no more than 0.2 ms in duration.[6]

Physical examination

Strength, sensation, and reflex testing are the most important aspects of the physical examination. Motor weakness is often seen in neuromuscular disorders. Subtle motor weakness can be elucidated by comparing sides and examining smaller muscles such as the extensor hallucis longus or the hand intrinsic muscles. Reduced reflexes indicate peripheral nervous system problems, whereas increased reflexes suggest a central nervous system disorder, particularly when seen in combination with spasticity and increased tone. An important caveat is the fact that, in acute spinal cord injury, there can be an initial reduction in reflexes due to spinal shock. Cranial nerve examination can identify weakness, and should be performed if stroke or another generalized condition is suspected. Neck flexor or extensor weakness can be somewhat harder to grade.

In many cases, these signs can, when combined with the history, point to the correct condition. There are other tests that can further clarify the clinical picture. These include Phalen's test for carpal tunnel syndrome. Palpation over the elbow to reproduce symptoms in someone with suspected ulnar neuropathy can be helpful. Straight leg raise testing for persons with suspected lumbosacral radiculopathy is useful when clearly positive. For persons with less clear conditions, palpation over the site of discomfort can help define trigger points or tendinopathies. Shoulder impingement signs can identify bursitis and bicipital tendonitis to help the electrodiagnostician in assessment for suspected C5 or C6 radiculopathy. Finklestein's test for de Quervains tenosynovitis is useful for persons presenting

with wrist pain. Lateral epicondylitis can mimic C6 radiculopathy. Lateral epicondylitis is characterized by reproduction of pain with palpation over the extensor forearm muscles and with resisted wrist extension. These examinations put the clinical scenario in the proper context.

An algorithmic approach to utilizing physical examination and symptom information to tailor the electrodiagnostic evaluation is shown in Figure 11-1. In this approach, the patient's physical examination signs of sensory loss and weakness create a conceptual framework for approaching these sometimes daunting problems. For the purposes of this discussion, generalized findings are defined as being present in two or more limbs. While helpful, there are many exceptions to this taxonomy. The electrodiagnostician must refocus the diagnostic effort as data are acquired. Sensory loss is a key finding on examination for someone presenting with generalized symptoms, and provides a branch point in the algorithmic approach to tailoring the electrodiagnostic study (Fig. 11-1). Myopathies, neuromuscular junction disorders, motor neuron disease, and multifocal motor neuropathy are all characterized by preservation of the sensory system. In contrast, polyneuropathies, bilateral radiculopathies, myelopathies, and central nervous system disorders frequently result in reduced sensation. In persons with no sensory loss or weakness on examination, the electrodiagnostician should maintain a heightened suspicion for myofascial pain syndrome or fibromyalgia, polymyalgia rheumatica, or multiple musculoskeletal disorders.[9]

PURPOSE OF ELECTRODIAGNOSTIC TESTING

Electrodiagnostic testing excludes conditions in the differential diagnosis and alters the referring diagnostic impression 42% of the time.[55] Electrodiagnostic testing can to some extent suggest severity, or extent of the disorder beyond the clinical symptoms. Involvement of other extremities can be delineated, or the involvement of multiple roots can be demonstrated, such as in the case of lumbosacral spinal stenosis. Finally, there is utility in solidifying a diagnosis. An unequivocal radiculopathy on EMG or median nerve entrapment provides greater diagnostic certainty and identifies avenues of management.

The value of any test depends on the a priori certainty of the diagnosis in question. For a condition or diagnosis for which there is great certainty before additional testing, the results of the subsequent tests are of limited value. For instance, in a patient with acute-onset sciatica while lifting, L5 muscle weakness, a positive straight leg raise, and an MRI showing a large extruded L4–L5 nucleus pulposus, an EMG test will be of limited value in confirming the diagnosis of radiculopathy because the clinical picture is so convincing. In contrast, an elderly diabetic patient with sciatica, having limited physical examination findings and equivocal or age-related MRI changes, presents an unclear picture. In this case, electrodiagnostic testing is of high value, placing in perspective the imaging findings and excluding diabetic polyneuropathy as a confounding condition.

TYPES OF ELECTRODIAGNOSTIC TESTS

Motor and sensory nerve conduction studies

Electrodiagnostic testing consists of EMG and nerve conductions. Standard nerve conduction studies that are utilized in the evaluation of patients typically include motor nerve conductions, sensory nerve conductions, F-waves, and H-reflexes. It is important to properly perform these tests and compare the data to well-derived normative values. Enough testing should be performed to properly delineate the conditions being sought and eliminate other conditions in the differential diagnosis.

Sensory nerve conductions should always be incorporated when assessing a patient.[7] In the upper limb, there are multiple sensory nerves that are easily accessible and allow assessment for both entrapments and polyneuropathies. In the lower limbs, perhaps the most readily accessible is the sural nerve. Indeed, in the recent position paper on polyneuropathies, this nerve was felt to be an excellent nerve for screening a patient for distal symmetric polyneuropathy.[47]

Motor nerve conduction studies should be performed in almost all situations.[7] Examiners should assess the morphology of the waveform, its latency, amplitude, and conduction velocity. Conduction should be performed across any suspected sites of entrapment or injury. Enough nerves should be studied in order to determine if a generalized condition is present.

H-reflexes

The H-reflex is an electrophysiologically recorded Achilles muscle stretch reflex. It is generated by recording over the gastrocnemius and soleus muscles, and stimulating the tibial nerve in the popliteal fossa. Care must be taken to perform this test correctly. It is a submaximally elicited reflex. The stimulus

duration is 1 ms, and the stimulus should be slowly increased by 3- to 5-mA increments. The patient should be relaxed, and the stimulus frequency should be less than once per second. The H-reflex is consistent in latency and morphology, and occurs when the motor response over the gastrosoleus is submaximal. As the stimulus current is gradually increased, the H-reflex will reach its maximum amplitude then extinguish as the motor response becomes maximal. Many researchers have evaluated its sensitivity and specificity with respect to lumbosacral radiculopathies, and generally found a range of sensitivities from 32% to 88%.[77,80,82,96,110] The specificity, however, has been reported at 91% for H-reflexes in lumbosacral S1 radiculopathy.[82] The H-reflex can also help discern S1 radiculopathy from L5 radiculopathy, the latter being more likely to have a normal reflex.[82]

H-reflexes are most helpful for assessing for polyneuropathy or confirming sciatic neuropathy. It is important to remember that delay in the H-reflex can occur with lesions of the sciatic nerve, the lumbosacral plexus, or the S1 root, and does not distinguish between these clinical entities.

F-waves

F-waves are late responses involving the motor axons and axonal pool at the spinal cord level. They can be elicited in most upper and lower limb muscles, and are typically tested by stimulating the median, ulnar, peroneal, or tibial nerves when recording from muscles they innervate. In contrast to H-reflexes, they are elicited by maximal stimulation of the nerve. They vary in morphology and latency, although when recording multiple F-waves they should fall roughly within the same latency period. When responses that look like F-waves are seen across the screen at widely varying latencies, the examiner should turn up the machine sound and determine whether or not background motor unit firing due to poor relaxation is responsible for these responses. F-waves demonstrate low sensitivities for radiculopathy, and so have a limited role in such evaluations.[77,98,101] However, they are quite useful for assessing persons for whom polyneuropathy is suspected (see below).

NEEDLE ELECTROMYOGRAPHY

Electromyographic testing, a vital part of electrodiagnostic evaluations, provides highly useful information and, although somewhat uncomfortable, poses minimal risks to the patient. The American Association of Neuromuscular and Electrodiagnostic Medicine supports the Occupational Health and Safety Administration rule that mandates the use of gloves and universal precautions. Disposable needles are now readily available and are sufficiently inexpensive that they should be used. It is recommended that surface electrodes should be cleaned with a 1 : 10 dilution of household bleach or 70% isopropyl alcohol solution between patients. Disposable surface electrodes are inexpensive, widely available, and easy to use.[6]

In the vast majority of cases, it makes no difference if the skin is prepared prior to needle insertion.[6] Some examiners use alcohol as an antiseptic, and certainly if the skin is not clean then alcohol represents a useful skin preparation. The needle should not penetrate infected skin or open ulcerations or wounds. Needle EMG is not listed by the American Heart Association as a procedure requiring prophylactic antibiotic treatment to prevent endocarditis.[4,6]

Electrodes for standard EMG generally fall into two categories. Monopolar needles are those in which the needle is coated with Teflon except for the tip, and the differences in potential from the tip of the electrode to a nearby surface electrode are recorded. Concentric needles are those with a fine wire running through the center of an insulated shaft that is electrically referenced to an outer metal shaft. Concentric needles are most useful for quantitative motor unit analysis, and are now commercially available in disposable form. Background interference is minimized with concentric needles, and the ground electrode can remain in one place for a given limb.

It is important that the examiner use a one-handed technique when resheathing needles. The plastic sheath should be held by a clip or taped to some part of the electrodiagnostic instrumentation such that one hand can replace the needle, thereby preventing needlestick injuries to providers.

The needle examination consists of four separate types of evaluations, which assess for:

1. insertional activity;
2. spontaneous activity;
3. morphology and size of motor units; and
4. motor unit recruitment.

Insertional activity is examined by moving the needle through the muscle briefly, and observing the amount and duration of electrical noise produced. This sound is mechanically evoked muscle depolarizations due to the advancement of the needle. Usually, insertional activity and spontaneous activity are examined using three or four insertions in each of four muscle quadrants. Smaller muscles, such as the abductor pollicis brevis, can be adequately assessed with fewer needle movements. After brief small movement of the needle, insertional activity usually persists for no more than a few hundred milliseconds.[68] Insertional activity can be decreased in the case of atrophied muscle or placement of the needle into fatty tissue. Increased insertional activity is activity that lasts for more than about 300 ms after the needle stops advancing. It is sometimes difficult to sort this out from spontaneous activity, and such determination is a qualitative assessment. Diffuse abnormal insertional activity with prolonged trains of positive sharp waves (PSWs) in essentially every muscle, yet without any symptoms or disability, has been described as 'EMG disease'.[109]

Spontaneous activity consists of electrical discharges occurring after the needle movement has stopped. A variety of potentials can be seen when the needle is not moving. If the needle is in an end-plate region, then end-plate noise can be heard. This noise is generated from miniature end-plate potentials, which sound like noise generated by a seashell held close to the ear. End-plate spikes are fully propagated action potentials from the end-plate region. These are typically biphasic potentials

with an initially negative (upward) deflection. They can be mistaken for fibrillation potentials, but they fire irregularly, a distinction easily made visually on the display screen as well as by listening carefully. They tend to have a sputtering sound, and are associated with excessive pain. The needle should be moved to a new location after it enters an end-plate region, to reduce pain and enter muscle more conducive to assessment for fibrillation potentials.

Fibrillation potentials represent spontaneous discharges of single muscle fibers, and are the most important EMG finding in clinical EMG. They are usually of short duration, and they can be biphasic (PSWs) or triphasic (fibrillation potentials).[27,45,68] They represent individual muscle fiber depolarizations. Such muscle membrane irritability can be caused by the mechanical stimulation of the needle but persist after needle movement has stopped. Fibrillations result from motor axonal loss that is not balanced by reinnervation. They are seen in inflammatory myopathies and in direct muscle trauma as well.[90] It is an interesting phenomenon that, in persons with complete spinal cord injury, muscles innervated by roots below the level of the lesion demonstrate fibrillation potentials.[69,103] Such prevalence of these findings in the legs of spinal cord-injured individuals with complete myelopathies makes electrodiagnostic testing for such patients indeterminate. Similar fibrillations and positive waves can be seen in stroke patients as well, and such findings should be interpreted with caution in the hemiplegic limb.[52,61]

Fibrillation potentials as well as PSWs are graded using a 0–4 grading scheme.[68] This grading scale is described as follows.

- 1+: transient but reproducible trains of discharges (fibrillations or PSWs) after moving the needle, in more than one site or quadrant.
- 2+: occasional spontaneous potentials in more than two different quadrants.
- 3+: spontaneous potentials are present in all quadrants.
- 4+: abundant spontaneous potentials nearly filling the screen in all four quadrants.

The finding of a fibrillation or PSW in only one area of the muscle that is not easily reproducible is probably of uncertain significance and can represent an end-plate spike. The density of fibrillation potentials does not necessarily correlate with the degree of nerve damage and loss of axons. The compound muscle action potential (CMAP) gives a better estimate of the proportion of axons remaining. The innervation ratio is the average size of the motor unit expressed as a ratio between the total number of extrafusal muscle fibers and the number of innervating motor axons. For small extraocular muscles, this ratio is 1 to 3. For large muscles such as the gastrocnemius, this ratio increases to 1934 muscle fibers per motor axon. This means that the loss of relatively few motor axons results in many fibrillating muscle fibers.[68]

Motor unit morphology involves placing the needle near a group of muscle fibers such that the rise time of the motor unit action potential (MUAP) is sharp (less than 300 μs). At this location, a proper quantification of the MUAP can be made. Polyphasic potentials are those with greater than four phases.[68]

Serrated potentials have the same clinical relevance, but the turns do not cross the baseline. Polyphasic potentials are associated with reinnervation of denervated motor units when the duration of these MUAPs is increased. This is seen in chronic motor axonal loss from an entrapment, radiculopathy, or other axonal polyneuropathy. If the polyphasic potentials are short in duration, they can be associated with myopathies or neuromuscular junction disorders. If profound axonal loss has occurred and the remaining axons are reinnervating many muscle fibers, polyphasic satellite potentials can be seen that are of short duration and appear myopathic. Large motor units, recruited with low force and greater than 6 mV in amplitude, are seen in chronic or old axonal loss conditions where there has been substantial reinnervation and reorganization of the motor unit. Remember that motor unit morphology assessment is generally a qualitative statement and less clear than the presence or absence of fibrillations, particularly for less skilled electrodiagnosticians. Such motor unit changes, however, when quite clear and profound can be very helpful, particularly in the proper clinical context. Quantitative EMG is necessary to precisely characterize motor unit morphology but is rarely necessary in clinical EMG testing.

Recruitment is another important parameter to assess. For this evaluation, it is most important to examine low to moderate levels of muscle contractions. Full-force contractions fill the screen with overlapping motor unit potentials, rendering assessment of individual motor units impossible. At low force levels, there should be one or two firing units at about 10 Hz. As greater force is generated, more units will be recruited, and the firing rates for those already recruited increase. In normal situations, the ratio of highest firing rate to the number of units seen on a 100-ms display screen is less than five. This means that, if the firing rate is 20 Hz, there should be about four distinct motor units seen.[68] When this firing ratio is increased to over 10, it indicates dropout of motor units and is termed *reduced recruitment*.

Reduced recruitment with a high firing ratio represents one end of a spectrum of recruitment findings, strongly suggestive of motor axonal loss or functional dropout due to conduction block. At the other end of a spectrum of recruitment findings is a situation in which many units are recruited to generate a low level of force. This is termed *early* or *myopathic recruitment*, and is seen in myopathies and neuromuscular junction disorders. Such recruitment is often seen with small, short-duration MUAPs that are characteristic for myopathies. At these two extremes of recruitment, findings are relatively specific for the underlying types of neuromuscular pathology. Beyond this, there are many recruitment findings that are less clear. In the case of pain, poor cooperation, or upper motor neuron disorders, there can be slow firing rates with few units activated.

Other spontaneous discharges can be seen beyond fibrillations and positive waves that are more continuous and unique. One such discharge is the complex repetitive discharge (CRD). This machine-like discharge is of constant firing frequency and demonstrates consistent morphology with abrupt starts and

Table 11-1 Complex repetitive discharge characteristics

Characteristic	Details
Appearance	May take any form, but this form is constant from one potential complex to the next
Rhythm	Regular
Frequency	10–100 Hz
Amplitude	50–1000 μV
Stability	Abrupt onset and cessation
Observed in	Myopathies: polymyositis, limb girdle dystrophy, myxedema, Schwartz–Jampel syndrome Neuropathies: poliomyelitis, spinal muscular atrophy, amyotrophic lateral sclerosis, hereditary neuropathies, chronic neuropathies, carpal tunnel syndrome 'Normal': iliopsoas, biceps brachii

Adapted from Dumitru, 1995.[45]

Table 11-2 Characteristics of myokymic discharges

Characteristic	Details
Appearance	Normal motor unit action potentials
Rhythm	Regular
Frequency	0.1–10 Hz
Burst frequency	20–250 Hz
Stability	Persistent firing or occasional abrupt cessation
Observed in	Facial: multiple sclerosis, brain stem neoplasm, polyradiculopathy, Bell palsy, normal Extremity: radiation plexopathy, chronic nerve compression (carpal tunnel syndrome, radiculopathy), rattlesnake venom

Adapted from Dumitru, 1995.[45]

stops. In Table 11-1, the firing characteristics are shown, along with some of the conditions in which they can be found. They are seen in conditions with chronic denervation, as well as in inflammatory myopathies. They are thought to be generated by a pacemaker muscle fiber with ephaptic conduction to other muscle fibers.

Myokymic potentials are grouped potentials that fire at regular rates. They have the characteristic sound of marching soldiers and are often seen in radiation plexopathies (Table 11-2). Myotonic discharges are fast firing with waxing and waning sounds somewhat like a dive-bomber. The characteristics and conditions in which they are found are shown in Table 11-3.

Table 11-3 Characteristics of myotonic discharges	
Characteristic	Details
Appearance	Brief spikes, positive waveform
Rhythm	Wax and wane
Frequency	20–100 Hz
Amplitude	Variable (20–300 µV)
Stability	Firing rate alterations
Observed in	Myopathies: myotonic dystrophy, myotonia congenita, paramyotonia, polymyositis, acid maltase deficiency, hyperkalemic periodic paralysis Other: chronic radiculopathy, chronic peripheral neuropathy

Adapted from Dumitru. 1995[45]

EXTENT OF ELECTRODIAGNOSTIC TESTING

Guidelines from the American Association of Neuromuscular and Electrodiagnostic Medicine (AANEM), published in 1999,[5] provide valuable guidance regarding the extent of appropriate electrodiagnostic testing. The guidelines and recommendations are summarized in Table 11-4.[5] Electrodiagnostic testing is uncomfortable for patients, and for this reason the assessment is a balance between performing excessive studies and examining a sufficient number of nerves and muscles to confidently recognize the target disorder if it is present and can be confirmed electrodiagnostically. Guidelines in electrodiagnostic medicine provide parameters for testing, and give clinicians and insurers critical information regarding how many tests should be conducted, for example what is enough and what is excessive. The AANEM guidelines, synthesized from the scientific literature as well as expert clinical opinions, provide an important framework for establishing consistency in judging what

Table 11-4 Recommendations representing minimum study for addressing a target disorder

Suspected condition	Sensory testing	Motor testing	Electromyography	Proximal conductions	Other special tests
Radiculopathy	One sensory nerve conduction study (NCS) to exclude polyneuropathy	One motor nerve conduction study (NCS) to exclude polyneuropathy	Sufficient number of muscles representing all myotomes with paraspinal muscles	None	None
Carpal tunnel syndrome	Median sensory NCS and another for comparison	Median motor NCS and another for comparison	Optional, although useful to determine severity CTS and exclude concomitant C8 radiculopathy	None	None
Ulnar neuropathy	Ulnar sensory NCS and another for comparison	Ulnar motor NCS and another for comparison; need to examine conduction velocity across the elbow	Several ulnar-innervated muscles, always the first dorsal interosseous, as it is most frequently abnormal, plus median muscles for comparison to exclude C8 radiculopathy	None	Inching motor NCS across the elbow
Peroneal neuropathy	Superficial peroneal sensory NCS and another for comparison	Peroneal motor with stimulation below and above the fibular head, assessing for conduction velocity and amplitude changes; test another for comparison	Peroneal nerve-innervated muscles and tibial nerve muscles for comparison; suggest paraspinal and L4–L5 muscles to assess for radiculopathy	None	None
Entrapment neuropathies	Two sensory NCSs, one in the distribution and a comparison	Two motor NCSs, one in the distribution and a comparison	Muscles in the involved distribution and comparison muscles	None	None

Continued on page 207

Continued from page 206 Table 11-4 Recommendations representing minimum study for addressing a target disorder					
Suspected condition	Sensory testing	Motor testing	Electromyography	Proximal conductions	Other special tests
Myopathy	One or two sensory NCSs in a clinically involved limb	One or two motor NCSs in a clinically involved limb	Two muscles (proximal and distal) in two limbs, one of which is symptomatic	—	Consider repetitive nerve stimulation
Neuromuscular junction disorders	One sensory NCS in a clinically involved limb	One motor NCS in a clinically involved limb	One proximal and one distal muscle in clinically involved limbs	—	Repetitive nerve stimulation at 2–3 Hz in clinically weak muscle and, if normal, other weak muscles; single-fiber electromyography if high suspicion and repetitive nerve stimulation is negative—can be first test in ocular myasthenia gravis
Polyneuropathy	Sensory NCS in at least two extremities: if abnormalities in one limb, study the contralateral limb; four or more may be necessary to classify the polyneuropathy	Motor NCS in at least two extremities; if abnormalities in one limb, study contralateral limb; four or more may be necessary to classify the polyneuropathy	One distal muscle in both legs and a distal muscle in one arm	Consider proximal NCSs (H-reflexes, F-waves, and blink reflexes) to assess demyelination	—
Motor neuron diseases	One sensory NCS in at least two clinically involved limbs	One motor NCS in at least two clinically involved limbs; proximal stimulation sites to exclude conduction block in the case of multifocal motor neuropathy	Several muscles in three extremities, *or* two extremities and cranial nerve-innervated muscles as well as lumbar or cervical paraspinal muscles; thoracic paraspinal muscles may be considered an extremity; sample distal and proximal muscles	Consider F-waves	Consider repetitive nerve stimulation

(Adapted from American Association of Electrodiagnostic Medicine 1999,[5] with permission.)

constitutes sufficient testing. From time to time, cases occur for which these guidelines are inadequate, and additional testing is needed; however, for the vast majority of cases these guidelines are entirely applicable. These guidelines were developed to improve electrodiagnostic patient care, as well as to combat unscrupulous providers of electrodiagnostic services in the USA who perform excessive studies far beyond what is necessary to make a diagnosis, simply for the purpose of increasing the electrodiagnostic fee.

LIMITATIONS OF ELECTRODIAGNOSIS

Unfortunately, there are very few electrodiagnostic findings that are clearly specific for any single diagnostic entity.

Repetitive nerve stimulation at 2 or 3 Hz can reveal decrements in motor neuron disease, myopathies, peripheral neuropathies, and myotonic disorders, as well as in neuromuscular junction disorders.[64] Fibrillations and PSWs are seen in polyneuropathies, motor neuron disease, inflammatory myopathies, radiculopathies, and entrapment neuropathies. Marked facilitation of the CMAP to over 400% of the baseline amplitude after a brief contraction in persons with Eaton–Lambert myasthenic syndrome is one finding that is unique to this rare disease.[59,64,97,106]

The time course over which a disease process progresses and the time at which electrodiagnostic testing is conducted both play major roles in determining whether or not the electrodiagnostic testing can provide a reasonably certain diagnosis. It is frequently necessary to repeat the study if the diagnosis remains in question or if the clinical situation changes.

One important issue related to electrodiagnostic medicine is the possibility of false positive results. In Table 11-5, the probabilities of finding false positive results on the basis of chance alone are shown according to the number of independent measures.[39] It is important to realize that, if five measurements are performed, there will be a 12% chance of having one false positive. If nine measurements are made, there is a 20% chance of a spuriously false positive result. However, if there are two abnormal results when six or more tests are conducted, the likelihood that they are false positive tests is quite low, less than about 1%. This underscores the need for electrodiagnosticians to critically examine their findings and not over-diagnose a disorder based on one subtle abnormality. If one electrodiagnostic parameter is markedly abnormal, far beyond the upper limit of normal, this can be compelling, particularly when that abnormality is consistent with the clinical impression. This study should be repeated to make certain of its validity. Two abnormalities, however, indicating the same diagnosis, are far more likely to represent true findings and a clear underlying disorder.

Other common conditions, such as diabetes and its corresponding polyneuropathy, can make electrodiagnostic testing more difficult to interpret. With a diffuse polyneuropathy, the consultant is often unable to identify focal lesions against the backdrop of this disorder. In this scenario, the electrodiagnostician must assess the magnitude of the background polyneuropathy, and make a judgment as to whether or not findings for the nerve in question are out of proportion to the background

polyneuropathy. Caution is urged in this scenario to avoid overcalling entrapment neuropathies when a generalized polyneuropathy is present.

These issues are another reason why it is critically important that the electrodiagnostician have sufficient training to be able to interpret the findings appropriately in the clinical context of the patient.

Nerve conduction and needle EMG studies: proper technique accounts for temperature, age, and height

The well-known effects of temperature on nerve conduction velocity, distal latency, amplitude, and neuromuscular transmission should be prevented by maintaining the upper limbs at 35°C and the lower limbs at 32°C.[28] Normative reference values provide the electrodiagnostician with information that allows a determination as to whether a particular nerve conduction parameter is significantly different from a person without symptoms or known neurologic disorders. Besides temperature, it has been demonstrated that age and height influence electrodiagnostic findings, and that these factors must be taken into consideration. Buschbacher published extensive normative information derived from large samples, which account for height and age.[12-16]

Anatomic variations in muscle and nerve pathways can confound electrodiagnostic interpretation as well. Two well-described variants are important for the electrodiagnostician. The Martin–Gruber anastomosis is formed by a branch from the median nerve, usually the anterior interosseus nerve, joining the ulnar nerve in the forearm. In this situation, the median CMAP with wrist stimulation is smaller than that with proximal stimulation. The ulnar nerve demonstrates a larger amplitude with wrist stimulation than with below-elbow or above-elbow stimulation. If a suspected conduction block is found in the forearm when testing the ulnar nerve, then median nerve conduction should be performed to exclude a Martin–Gruber anastomosis as the cause of CMAP reduction with proximal stimulation.

An accessory deep peroneal nerve is a part of the deep peroneal nerve that remains with the superficial peroneal nerve and innervates the extensor digitorum brevis after passing around the lateral malleolus. It should be suspected if stimulation at the fibular head yields a larger CMAP than ankle stimulation when recorded over the extensor digitorum brevis. Stimulation of the accessory deep peroneal nerve behind the lateral malleolus will confirm the presence of such an anatomic variant.

PEDIATRIC ELECTRODIAGNOSIS

The pediatric examination poses challenges for even the most experienced electrodiagnostic physician. Diagnosis of pediatric neuromuscular disorders is a specialized and rapidly evolving area of medicine in which genetic testing plays an ever greater role in diagnosis. Interested readers are encouraged to examine specialized textbooks and recent articles, as much of this material is beyond the scope of this chapter.

Table 11-5 Probability (percent) of finding false positive 'abnormal' results, on the basis of chance, according to the number of independent measurements made[a]

No. of measurements	No. of 'abnormalities'				
	1+	2+	3+	4+	5+
1	2.5				
2	4.9	0.1			
3	7.3	0.2	<0.1		
4	9.6	0.4	<0.1	<0.1	
5	11.9	0.6	<0.1	<0.1	<0
6	14.0	0.9	<0.1	<0.1	<0
7	16.2	1.2	<0.1	<0.1	<0
8	18.3	1.6	0.1	<0.1	<0
9	20.4	2.0	0.1	<0.1	<0
10	22.4	2.5	0.2	<0.1	<0
15	31.5	5.2	0.5	<0.1	<0
20	39.5	8.5	1.3	0.1	<0

[a]Each measurement has a 2.5% false positive rate (mean ±2 standard deviations for a Gaussian distribution).
Adapted from Dorfman, Robinson, 1997.[39]

In terms of equipment required for pediatric electrodiagnosis, a pediatric bipolar stimulating probe is available and is useful for small children.[105] Monopolar needles are generally used due to smaller diameter and less insertional resistance due to the Teflon coating. It is critically important to maintain a skin surface temperature of 36–37°C to avoid spurious results.[105] There are strong advocates for and against the use of sedation and analgesia during electrodiagnostic examination.[105] Performance of all conscious sedation and anesthesia should be done by specialists in pediatric anesthesia. When general anesthetic is required, children with possible neuromuscular diseases should not be given halogenated inhalation agents such as halothane due to the risks of malignant hyperthermia.[100] Nerve conduction testing should include both sensory and motor studies. The needle examination, although difficult, should always be part of the diagnostic evaluation. Despite the challenging nature of the needle examination, a complete needle EMG is necessary to reach appropriate conclusions. A single muscle exploration is insufficient for diagnosis in a child.[105]

The conduction velocities in newborns are about half of those found in adults. There is a rapid increase in values during the first year of life. Median values for conduction velocities in children and adults are equalized by age 5.[105] Tables 11-6 and 11-7 show values for infants and newborns.[87] Motor conduction velocities in full-term infants should be no less than 20 m/s.[105] Clinicians who examine newborns, infants, and children should have this information readily available in their laboratories.

Late responses evaluate an infant's proximal peripheral nervous system. They offer several advantages, including reduced problems with temperature control, longer conduction distance, reduced measurement error, and a single stimulation site. In contrast to in adults, the H-reflex can be elicited from any muscle during infancy, but most responses are gradually suppressed by the age of 1 year.[65,105] The tibial nerve, however, retains its electrophysiologic H-reflex through life.

The needle EMG examination in infants is challenging, and should begin with the muscles of highest diagnostic yield such as those in a weak limb. Needle manipulation and repositioning is often necessary because of the greater relative amount of adipose tissue and reduced muscle activation. Muscle relaxation to examine for spontaneous or normal insertional activities is best obtained by placing the muscle at its shortest length from origin to insertion.[105] The neonate's foot and hand intrinsic muscles can best be used to study insertional and spontaneous activity, as they are usually not very active.[105] These distal muscles, however, exhibit high levels of end-plate noise, because of the relatively larger end-plate regions, which may be confused with fibrillation potentials.[105] Extensor muscles are not activated as often by the neonate, and therefore are good choices as well for evaluation of spontaneous and insertional activity.[105]

Assessment of motor unit morphology and recruitment is difficult. Motor unit potentials in the pediatric population differ from those in the adult. Motor unit potentials in the newborn are usually biphasic or triphasic, their amplitudes range from 100 to 700 µV, and they are shorter in duration at 5–9 ms.[65,105] Recruitment of motor units is often difficult to interpret, as there is typically no voluntary control. When looking for motor unit morphology and recruitment, it is advisable to examine flexor muscles, because there is usually strong flexor tone and muscle activation. It is important to remember that this is a difficult examination, and over-interpretation is common for the inexperienced practitioner.

Repetitive nerve stimulation is used to evaluate presynaptic and postsynaptic neuromuscular disorders.[19,24] Immobilization of the arm or leg and maintenance of warm body and limb temperatures are critical for optimizing sensitivity for this

Table 11-6 Motor conduction studies in 155 children[a]

Age (n)	Median nerve[b]				Peroneal nerve[c]			
	Distal motor latency (ms)	Conduction velocity (m/s)	F-latency (ms)	Amplitude (mV)	Distal motor latency (ms)	Conduction velocity (m/s)	F-latency (ms)	Amplitude (mV)
7 days to 1 month (20)	2.23 (0.29)	25.43 (3.84)	16.12 (1.50)	3.00 (0.31)	2.43 (0.48)	22.43 (1.22)	22.07 (1.46)	3.06 (1.26)
1–6 months (23)	2.21 (0.34)	34.35 (6.61)	16.89 (1.65)	7.37 (3.24)	2.25 (0.48)	35.18 (3.96)	23.11 (1.89)	5.23 (2.37)
6–12 months (25)	2.13 (0.19)	43.57 (4.78)	17.31 (1.77)	7.67 (4.45)	2.31 (0.62)	43.55 (3.77)	25.86 (1.35)	5.41 (2.01)
1–2 years (24)	2.04 (0.18)	48.23 (4.58)	17.44 (1.29)	8.90 (3.61)	2.29 (0.43)	51.42 (3.02)	25.98 (1.95)	5.80 (2.48)
2–4 years (22)	2.18 (0.43)	53.59 (5.29)	17.91 (1.11)	9.55 (4.34)	2.62 (0.75)	55.73 (4.45)	29.52 (2.15)	6.10 (2.99)
4–6 years (20)	2.27 (0.45)	56.26 (4.61)	19.44 (1.51)	10.37 (3.66)	3.01 (0.43)	56.14 (4.96)	29.98 (2.68)	7.10 (4.76)
6–14 years (21)	2.73 (0.44)	57.32 (3.35)	23.23 (2.57)	12.37 (4.79)	3.25 (0.51)	57.05 (4.54)	34.27 (4.29)	8.15 (4.19)

[a]Mean (standard deviation).
[b]Median motor recorded from APB and stimulated at wrist.
[c]Median motor recorded over EDB and stimulated at ankle.
Adapted from Parano, Uncini, DeVivo, et al. 1993.[87]

Table 11-7 Sensory conduction studies in 155 children[a]

Age (n)	Median nerve[b]		Sural nerve	
	Conduction velocity (m/s)	Amplitude (μV)	Conduction velocity (m/s)	Amplitude (μV)
7 days to 1 month (20)	22.31 (2.16)	6.22 (1.30)	20.26 (1.55)	9.12 (3.02)
1–6 months (23)	35.52 (6.59)	15.86 (5.18)	34.63 (5.43)	11.66 (3.57)
6–12 months (25)	40.31 (5.23)	16.00 (5.18)	38.18 (5.00)	15.10 (8.22)
1–2 years (24)	46.93 (5.03)	24.00 (7.36)	49.73 (5.53)	15.41 (9.98)
2–4 years (22)	49.51 (3.34)	24.28 (5.49)	52.63 (2.96)	23.27 (6.84)
4–6 years (20)	51.71 (5.16)	25.12 (5.22)	53.83 (4.34)	22.66 (5.42)
6–14 years (21)	53.84 (3.26)	26.72 (9.43)	53.85 (4.19)	26.75 (6.59)

[a]Mean (standard deviation).
[b]Median sensory recorded at wrist with stimulation of index fingers.
Adapted from Parano, Uncini, DeVivo, et al. 1993.[87]

testing. Use of 20-Hz stimulation to assess for postactivation decrement repair or to look for postexercise facilitation is necessary. This is painful, and an anesthetized immobile infant is optimal to derive a meaningful study. Stimulated single-fiber EMG can be performed, and is an ideal, sensitive means of testing for neuromuscular junction disorders.[19,24]

The hypotonic infant poses diagnostic challenges and is the most common referral for electrodiagnostic examination in the infant. Within this category, the most common etiology for generalized hypotonia is central nervous system causes.[105] In fact, only 10–20% of hypotonic infants and children with hypotonia have a neuromuscular etiology.[105] Probably the most common neuromuscular diagnosis in hypotonic infants is spinal muscular atrophy.

Several peripheral nerve entities occur in the newborn. Partial facial paralysis or asymmetric faces might occur, and motor nerve conduction studies and needle EMG of the facial nerve and its corresponding innervated muscles are useful to clarify the mononeuropathy. Side to side comparisons of the CMAPs can give a rough idea of the degree of axonal loss and some prognostic information. Brachial plexopathies at birth are rare, occurring in 1.5 per 1000 live births.[37] These brachial plexus palsies are difficult to predict, and are unrelated to identifiable obstetric characteristics such as gestational age, oxytocin augmentation, delivery mode (forceps, spontaneous, breech, or caesarean), or birthweight.[37] However, the duration of labor and presence of shoulder dystocia were significantly related to the occurrence of brachial plexus palsy.[37] Erb palsy involves the upper plexus and C5 or C6 roots. A Klumpkes, lower plexus palsy primarily demonstrates C8 or T1, lower trunk involvement. The needle EMG will help confirm the site of pathology and location of primary involvement.[105] In one series, supra-costoclavical space narrowing due to anatomic variations such as cervical ribs or fibrous bands were identified as predisposing factors that render the brachial plexus more prone to injury.[8]

A particularly interesting case report discussed the intrauterine onset of a peroneal neuropathy with fibrillations found within 20 h of birth in the affected muscles, underscoring the onset prior to delivery and arguing against obstetric trauma as the cause.[62] In this case report, the authors discuss other cases in which onset pre-dated the delivery, as evidenced by fibrillations in clinically affected muscles shortly after birth. These findings have profound implications for medicolegal issues surrounding brachial plexus palsies and other mononeuropathies in newborns. For situations in which a neurologic deficit is found at the time of delivery, an electrodiagnostic study shortly afterward (within 24 h) can help elucidate whether such a deficit developed intrauterine or during delivery. Intrauterine onset of a focal neuropathy or plexopathy will demonstrate fibrillation potentials in the weak muscles if tested by EMG shortly after delivery.[62]

MONONEUROPATHIES AND ENTRAPMENT NEUROPATHIES

Suspected mononeuropathies are the most common reasons for electrodiagnostic laboratory referral. Top among these conditions is median neuropathy at the wrist or carpal tunnel syndrome. Other entrapments include ulnar neuropathy at the elbow, common peroneal neuropathy at the fibular head, and tibial nerve entrapment at the ankle (tarsal tunnel syndrome). In addition to these entrapments, focal nerve injuries can occur with penetrating trauma and fractures. The common entrapments and nerve injuries, their anatomic causes, and their electrodiagnostic correlates are given in Table 11-8.

The approach to assessing for mononeuropathies is to fully test the nerve in question and another nerve in the affected limb for comparison. Stimulation both below and above the suspected site of injury is imperative to assess for conduction block or conduction slowing. EMG of selected muscles

Table 11-8 Entrapment neuropathies

Nerve	Causes	Clinical features	Suggested electrodiagnostic evaluation	Potential EMG findings
MEDIAN NEUROPATHIES				
Carpal Tunnel Syndrome (CTS): Median entrapment at wrist	The most common entrapment neuropathy Incidence: 55–125 cases/100 000 Causes: Repetitive trauma, obesity, pregnency, lupus, etc[42]	Aching pain in forearm and wrist with insidious onset, tingling, paresthesias of thumb, index and long finger, thenar weakness, nocturnal pain	Sensory NCS across the wrist and another sensory nerve in the affected limb to compare Motor NCS of median nerve and another motor nerve (usually ulnar) Needle EMG is optional[5]	Mild CTS: prolonged SNAP, and/or slightly reduced SNAP amplitued Moderate CTS: Abnormal median SNAP as above, plus prolonged median motor latency Severe CTS: prolonged motor and sensory distal latencies, plus either an absent SNAP or a low amplitude or absent CMAP. The EMG often shows fibrillations in thenar (median) muscles if severe[99a]
Pronator syndrome: Entrapment of median nerve between heads of the pronator teres and beneath FDS arch at forearm	Trauma from repetitive overuse, tight casting, penetrating injuries such as intravenous catheter, carrying a bag with the arm flexed "grocery bag neuropathy"[42]	Aching pain in the volar forearm, hand numbness, worsened by repeated pronation, clumsiness, loss of dexterity, weakness, flexor muscle and thenar muscle wasting if severe, tender pronator muscle	Motor nerve conduction across this area Median sensory study distally EMG of median muscles Evaluation of ulnar nerve for comparison Radiculopathy screen to exclude this condition EMG findings should be confined to median distribution	SNAP: Normal unless axonal loss CMAP: normal or reduced if motor axonal loss present. NCV slowed across the pronator area or conduction block across this site EMG: reduced recruitment in median innervated muscles, fibrillations and motor unit changes if there is motor axonal loss Pronator teres usually spared
Anterior interosseous: Entrapment at forearm (Kiloh-Nevin syndrome)	Direct trauma, inflammation, strenuous exercise, fractures, variant of brachial neuritis, compression by anomalous fibrous bands in this region[42]	Acute pure motor syndrome with pain in forearm and elbow, weak flexor pollicis longus and flexor digitorum profundus of index and long finger, weak pronator quadratus. "OK" sign No sensory complaints	Motor nerve conduction across this area Median sensory study distally EMG of median muscles Evaluation of ulnar nerve for comparison Radiculopathy screen to exclude this condition EMG findings should be confined to anterior interosseus nerve distribution.	Median SNAPs are normal Normal median nerve conduction studies to the APB With surface or needle recordings from the pronator quadratus, there may be slowed median nerve conduction velocity On EMG findings will be limited to FPL, PQ and FDP (index and long)
Median nerve entrapment beneath the ligament of Struthers	Caused by trauma or inflammation Seen in 0.7–2.7% population[42] Associated with fibrous band from supra condylar process to medial epicondyle (Supracondylar process 5 cm above medial epicondyle on X-ray is noted)	Weak grip, weakness in flexion of wrist, deep aching pain in forearm, numbness of 1–3 digits, weak hand pronation, second and third digit flexion, wasting of APB	Motor nerve conduction across this area Median sensory study distally EMG of median muscles Evaluation of ulnar nerve for comparison Radiculopathy screen to exclude this condition EMG findings should be confined to median distribution Pronator teres often involved	Decreased or absent SNAP amplitude Reduced motor NCV or conduction block across this segment Decreased CMAP from APB EMG findings in Median nerve distribution including pronator teres[42]
RADIAL NEUROPATHIES				
Radial nerve entrapment at axilla	Improper use of crutches, falling asleep with arm over a sharp chairback or edge	Weakness in all radial nerve innervated muscles including triceps, decreased sensation in posterior arm and forearm	Superficial radial sensory Radial motor testing with recording from EIP with either surface or needle electrodes. Should stimulate at Erb's point Testing at least one additional motor and sensory nerve in the involved limb EMG of radial innervated muscles EMG screen for radiculopathy, eg; other non-radial muscles	Reduced or absent SNAP if axonal loss Normal or reduced motor CMAP if axonal loss occurred Conduction block across the axilla EMG findings in radial innervated muscles including triceps when motor axonal loss is present
Radial Nerve entrapment at spiral groove (Saturday Night palsy, or Honeymooner's palsy)	Acute prolonged compression of the nerve in the humeral region due to a person sleeping on the arm or falling asleep in an improper position Frequently associated with alcohol use Other causes include an injection or compression with a tournquet	Involves all radial innervated muscles except *Triceps brachii* and *Anconeus*. Wrist extension weakness and finger extension weakness. Sensory loss over dorsal hand and posterior forearm	Same as above	Reduced or absent SNAP if axonal loss. Normal or reduced motor CMAP if axonal loss occurred. Conduction block across the spiral groove region EMG findings in radial innervated muscles excluding triceps and anconeus when motor axonal loss is present
Radial nerve with posterior interosseous nerve compression	Radial tunnel syndrome encompasses entrapment by fibrous bands at the radial head, or the sharp tendinous margin of the ECRB Posterior interosseus syndrome or Supinator syndrome is where the PIN is entrapped at the fibrous band at the origin of supinator muscle called the *Arcade of Frohse*[42] Other causes include, dislocation of elbow, Monteggia fracture, fall on outstretched hand, surgical resection of radial head, mass lesions	Deep pain at elbow Weakness with wrist extension Weakness of MCP extension yet preserved ability to extend IP joints due to interrossei No loss of sensation	Same as above	Normal superficial radial sensory response Slowed motor conduction across the elbow. Low CMAP over EIP EMG findings in PIN innervated muscles. Brachioradialus and ECRL are usually spared

Continued on page 212

Continued from page 211 Table 11-8 Entrapment neuropathies

Nerve	Causes	Clinical features	Suggested electrodiagnostic evaluation	Potential EMG findings
Radial nerve entrapment at the wrist (Wartenberg syndrome or handcuff neuropathy)	Bracelets and handcuff neuropathy Ganglions, overuse syndrome	Numbness, paresthesias of dorso-radial aspect of hand and dorsum of first three digits, tender to palpation in this area No motor weakness	Same as above In certain compelling clinical circumstances the exam can be abbreviated and focused on the superficial radial nerve with another nerve for comparison	Superfical radial sensory response delayed in latency or low in amplitude

ULNAR NEUROPATHIES

Nerve	Causes	Clinical features	Suggested electrodiagnostic evaluation	Potential EMG findings
Ulnar nerve compression at Guyon's canal at wrist	Chronic pressure from using tools, bicycle riding, ganglion, rheumatoid arthritis	Type 1: Hypothenar and deep ulnar branch Type 2: Deep ulnar branch Type 3: Superficial ulnar sensory branch. Numbness, paresthesias, weakness, intrinsic muscle atrophy, nocturnal pain Painless wasting of hand intrinsics	Ulnar sensory testing Ulnar motor testing with recording electrodes over ADM and FDI and conduction across the elbow Dorsal ulnar cutaneous Another motor and sensory nerve in the affected limb for comparison EMG ulnar muscles	Prolonged motor latency Dorsal ulnar cutaneous nerve is spared Ulnar sensory response to fifth digit is prolonged in latency or normal if mostly motor fibers are involved CMAP is decreased if axonal loss is present EMG demonstrates fibrillations or motor unit changes in hand intrisics, but not in thenar (median innervated) muscles
Ulnar nerve compression at the elbow	Trauma, cubitus valgus, bony spurs, tumours, overuse, previous fracture Proximal to elbow the nerve may be entrapped by the, Arcade of Struthers, a fibrous structure associated with the medial triceps muscle Cubital tunnel made of the fibrous entrance to the FCU is the most common site	Vague dull aching forearm, intermittent parasthesia, hypoasthesia on ulnar side of hand, weakness of abduction of little finger, ulnar clawing in severe cases, wasting of 1st dorsal interosseus and hypothenar eminence, wasting ulnar border of forearm	Ulnar motor conduction across the elbow and in forearm. If abnormal additional motor and sensory to exclude diffuse process Consider an inching study across elbows[5,17] Ulnar sensory Dorsal ulnar cutaneous EMG ulnar muscles	The ulnar sensory nerve may be reduced in amplitude or absent The dorsal ulnar cutaneous nerve may be reduced or absent Ulnar motor amplitude might be reduced Conduction block across the elbow can occur Nerve conduction velocity is more than 10 m/s slower across the elbow than in the forearm segment Short segmental inching at 1 cm intervals can reveal greater than 0.4 ms segmental change, or a clear discontinuity[17]

LOWER LIMB MONONEUROPATHIES

Nerve	Causes	Clinical features	Suggested electrodiagnostic evaluation	Potential EMG findings
Femoral neuropathy	Trauma, retroperitoneal hematoma due to anticoagulation cardiac catheterizations[5]	Weak quadriceps muscle, weakness of knee extension, absent knee jerk, groin pain and decreased sensation over medial and anterior thigh and lower leg in the saphenous nerve distribution	Motor nerve conduction to quadriceps Saphenous sensory study EMG of quadriceps as well as other L3 and L4 muscles, e.g.; the adductor muscles Consider an EMG screen for radiculopathy	Reduced amplitude or absent saphaneous nerve response Reduced CMAP over rectus femoris On EMG fibrillations in the femoral nerve innervated muscles
Lateral femoral cutaneous nerve entrapment at thigh (Meralgia paresthetica)	Repeated low grade trauma, obesity, pregnancy, tight clothing most commonly under the lateral end of the ilioinguinal ligament	Pure sensory syndrome at the lateral thigh including unplesant paresthesias, burning or a dull ache. No motor symptoms Can be aggravated by prolonged standing or walking	Lateral femoral cutaneous study Femoral evaluation as above should be considered	Reduced amplitude in lateral femoral cutaneous nerve
Peroneal nerve entrapment at the head of the fibula	Fractures, plaster casts, tight stockings, improper positioning, excessive weight loss, farm work, tumors, crossing legs for a long time	Foot drop, weakness of eversion, numbness on the dorsum of the foot, pain	Superficial peroneal sensory (SPS) testing Motor nerve conduction below and across the fibular head recorded from EDB or Tibialis ant. if EDB is atrophied. Exclude L5 radiculopathy by EMG Test and additional motor and sensory in the same leg	Reduced or absent SPS response Conduction block across the fibular head Conduction velocity reduced in fibular head segment by >10 m/s Fibrillations in muscles innervated by peroneal nerve
Tibial nerve entrapment at tarsal tunnel under flexor retinaculum of medial malleolus	Compression from shoes, casting, post-traumatic fibrosis, overuse ganglion cysts	Pain in foot and ankle, wasting and weakness in feet, sensory impairment at toes and sole of the foot	Plantar sensory (mixed) nerve conductions Tibial motor to AH muscle Another motor and sensory in the same limb to exclude polyneuropathy EMG of intrinsic foot muscles Consider EMG screen for radiculopathy or sciatic neuropthy	Prolonged latencies or low amplitudes in plantar nerves. Prolonged tibial motor latency across tarsal tunnel Fibrillations in the flexor digitorum brevis, AH, or other tested foot muscle

innervated by the particular nerve is mandatory. If these muscles are abnormal, the study should be expanded to ensure that these EMG findings are confined to a single peripheral nerve distribution and that they are not due to a radiculopathy, plexopathy, or polyneuropathy. The electrodiagnostician should have a low threshold for testing the same nerves in the opposite limb. Sorting out a focal process versus a generalized process such as polyneuropathy is imperative.

BRACHIAL PLEXOPATHIES

Brachial plexopathies are important causes of shoulder and neck region pain.[21,22,111] The EMG examination is critical and should be extensive and detailed, particularly for proximal muscles and muscles in which there is clinical weakness.[89] Sensory nerve action potentials (SNAPs) are a key part of the evaluation. SNAPs are readily available for C6 (radial to the thumb), C7 (median to digit 2), and C8 (ulnar to digit 5) root levels in the hand, and L5 (superficial peroneal sensory) and S1 (sural sensory) in the leg. Other SNAPs, such as the lateral antebrachial cutaneous (C5, C6) or the medial antebrachial cutaneous (C8, T1), can provide additional information to the study. SNAPs are generally low in amplitude or absent with postganglionic plexopathies, and help differentiate between radiculopathies and plexopathies. The exception to this rule is in the case of traumatic plexopathy when a root is avulsed. This severe injury with little chance of recovery should be recognized. In this case, the patient's weakness is profound and the CMAPs are low or absent, but the SNAPs are preserved. A myelogram or MRI often reveals a traumatic meningocele associated with such root avulsions.

The amplitudes of CMAPs should be elicited when possible in the weak muscles and compared with the uninvolved side. After Wallerian degeneration has occurred, this gives a rough estimate of the amount of axonal loss. It is thought that CMAPs less than 10–20% of the uninvolved side portend poor prognosis; however, the literature supporting this statement is weak and in large measure derived from Bells palsy experience.[36] The presence of an elicitable CMAP over involved muscles indicates, with an 88% certainty, that the strength will improve to a grade 4 are greater.[24a]

Electrodiagnosticians should understand the peripheral neuroanatomy of both the lumbosacral and the brachial plexus. A thorough appreciation for muscular anatomy, root innervations, and needle localization is a prerequisite. The consultant should specify, with as much precision as the study will allow, the location of the lesion, the magnitude (severity), and whenever possible rough estimates of probable outcomes. It is important to also appreciate that different parts of the brachial plexus may be involved with differing severities. The electrodiagnostician should elucidate when possible these differential injuries, as such information can help surgeons who contemplate tendon transfers.

RADICULOPATHIES

Cervical and lumbosacral radiculopathies are conditions involving a pathologic process affecting the spinal nerve root. Commonly, this is a herniated nucleus pulposus that anatomically compresses a nerve root within the spinal canal. Another common etiology for radiculopathy is spinal stenosis resulting from a combination of degenerative spondylosis, ligament hypertrophy, and spondylolisthesis. Inflammatory radiculitis is another pathophysiologic process that can cause radiculopathy. It is important to remember, however, that other more ominous processes, such as malignancy and infection, can manifest the same symptoms and signs of radiculopathy as those of the more common causes.

The dorsal root ganglion lies in the intervertebral foramen. This anatomic arrangement has implications for the clinical electrodiagnosis of radiculopathy, namely that SNAPs are preserved in most radiculopathies. This is due to the fact that the nerve root is affected proximal to the dorsal root ganglion.

In the lumbar spine, the dorsal and ventral lumbar roots exit the spinal cord at about the T11–L1 bony level and travel in the lumbar canal as a group of nerve roots in the dural sac. This is termed the 'horse's tail' or cauda equina. This poses challenges and limitations to the EMG examination. A destructive intramedullary (spinal cord) lesion at T11 can produce EMG findings in muscles innervated by any of the lumbosacral nerve roots, and manifest the precise findings on needle EMG as those seen with a herniated nucleus pulposus at any of the lumbar disk levels. For this reason, the electromyographer cannot determine for certain the anatomic location of the lumbar intraspinal lesion producing distal muscle EMG findings in the lower limbs. The needle EMG examination can identify only the root or roots that are physiologically involved, but not the precise anatomic site of pathology in the lumbar spinal canal. This is an important limitation requiring correlation with imaging findings to determine which anatomic location is most probably the offending site. These findings underscore the limitations of precise localization for root lesions by EMG.

By far the most useful test for confirming the presence of a radiculopathy is needle EMG. Needle EMG testing with a sufficient number of muscles and at least one motor and one sensory nerve conduction study should be performed in the involved limb.[7] The nerve conduction studies are necessary to exclude polyneuropathy. An EMG study is considered diagnostic for radiculopathy if EMG abnormalities are found in two or more muscles innervated by the same nerve root and different peripheral nerves, yet muscles innervated by adjacent nerve roots are normal.[110] This assumes that other generalized conditions such as polyneuropathy are not present. The need for EMG, particularly in relationship to imaging of the spine, has been highlighted.[94] Needle EMG is particularly helpful in view of the fact that the false positive rates for MRI of the lumbar spine are high, with 27% of normal subjects having a disk protrusion.[60] For the cervical spine, the false positive rate for MRI is lower, with 19% of subjects demonstrating an abnormality but only 10% showing a herniated or bulging disk.[10] Radiculopathies can occur without structural findings on MRI, and likewise without EMG findings. The EMG evaluates only motor axonal loss or motor axon conduction block (reduced recruitment is seen), and for these reasons a radiculopathy affecting the sensory root will not yield abnormalities by EMG. If the rate of denervation is balanced by reinnervation in the muscle, then spontaneous activity is less likely to be seen with EMG. The sensitivity for EMG ranges from 49% to 92%.[58,66,73,104,107] While EMG is not a highly sensitive test, it has a higher level of specificity.

Cervical and lumbar paraspinal muscles are important to examine with EMG when assessing for radiculopathy. If positive, they localize the site of pathology to the spine or root level. When assessing paraspinal muscles, only fibrillations, PSWs, CRDs, or myotonic discharges have clinical relevance. Recruitment findings and motor unit morphology for these muscles have not been well established. There are no normative data regarding motor unit morphology in either the cervical or lumbar paraspinal muscles to which precise comparisons can be made. Likewise, it requires quantitative EMG to accurately assess motor unit size, duration, and polyphasicity—time-consuming tasks. Examiners should not overcall radiculopathies based on 'reduced recruitment' or 'increased polyphasicity' of the paraspinal muscles. Paraspinal muscles show either spontaneous activity or other abnormal discharges (CRDs), and therefore they localize the lesion to the root level or they do not. It is important that the electrodiagnostician not overcall paraspinal fibrillations (see below). There is considerable overlap in paraspinal muscles, with single roots innervating muscle fibers above and below their anatomic levels. For this reason, the level of radiculopathy cannot be delineated by paraspinal EMG alone, but rather is based on the root level that best explains the distribution of limb muscles with fibrillations.

The lumbar paraspinal muscle examination can be easily performed and should be studied in persons with suspected radiculopathies. Haig and colleagues derived a means of quantifying the degree of findings in the paraspinals by means of an index derived by adding the fibrillations found in a standard set of muscle insertions.[53,54,56] Such quantitative assessment distinguishes patients with radiculopathies and spinal stenosis with greater precision.

Dumitru, Diaz, and King examined the lumbosacral paraspinal muscles and intrinsic foot muscles with monopolar EMG.[41] These investigators recorded potentials, and found that there were irregularly firing potentials with similar waveform characteristics as fibrillations and PSWs. By excluding irregularly firing potentials (atypical end-plate spikes) and considering only regularly firing potentials with appropriate morphology consistent with fibrillations, they found that only 4% of these subjects had false positive paraspinal EMG findings. This well-designed quantitative study underscores the need to assess both firing rate and rhythm as well as discharge morphology when evaluating for fibrillations and positive waves in the lumbar paraspinal muscles. Fibrillations fire regularly, and this should be confirmed by listening carefully and seeing consistent intervals between fibrillations on the display screen. Electrodiagnosticians should take care not to overcall paraspinal muscle EMG findings by mistaking irregularly firing end-plate spikes for regularly firing fibrillations.

How many and which muscles to study

A screening EMG study involves determining whether or not the radiculopathy can be confirmed by EMG. The concept of a screening EMG encompasses identifying the possibility of an electrodiagnostically confirmable radiculopathy. If one of the muscles in the screen is abnormal, the screen must be expanded to exclude other diagnoses and to fully delineate the radiculopathy level. Because of the screening nature of the EMG examination, electrodiagnosticians with experience should look for more subtle signs of denervation and, if present in the screening muscles, then expand the study to determine if these findings are limited to a single myotome or peripheral nerve distribution. If they are limited to a single muscle, their clinical significance is uncertain.

A prospective multicenter study evaluating patients referred to participating electrodiagnostic laboratories with suspected cervical radiculopathy was conducted to address the issue regarding how many muscles are sufficient to confidently identify an electrodiagnostically confirmable cervical radiculopathy.[29] There were 101 patients with electrodiagnostically confirmed cervical radiculopathies representing all cervical root levels. When paraspinal muscles were one of the screening muscles, five muscle screens identified 90–98% of radiculopathies, six muscle screens identified 94–99%, and seven muscle screens identified 96–100% (Table 11-9). When paraspinal muscles were not part of the screen, eight distal limb muscles recognized 92–95% of radiculopathies. Six muscle screens including paraspinal muscles yielded consistently high identification rates, and studying additional muscles led to marginal increases in identification. Individual screens useful to the elec-

Table 11-9 Six-muscle screen identifications of patients with cervical radiculopathies

Muscle screen	Neuropathic (%)	Spontaneous activity (%)
Six muscles without paraspinals		
Deltoid, APB, FCU, triceps, PT, FCR	93	66
Biceps, triceps, FCU, EDC, FCR, FDI	87	55
Deltoid, triceps, EDC, FDI, FCR, PT	89	64
Biceps, triceps, EDC, PT, APB, FCU	94	64
Six muscles with paraspinals		
Deltoid, triceps, PT, APB, EDC, PSM	99	83
Biceps, triceps, EDC, FDI, FCU, PSM	96	75
Deltoid, EDC, FDI, PSM, FCU, triceps	94	77
Biceps, FCR, APB, PT, PSM, triceps	98	79

Adapted from Dillingham, Lauder, Andary, et al. 2000.[29]

Table 11-10 Six-muscle screen identifications of patients with lumbosacral radiculopathies

Muscle screen	Neuropathic (%)	Spontaneous activity (%)
Six muscles without paraspinals		
ATIB, PTIB, MGAS, RFEM, SHBF, LGAS	89	78
VMED, TFL, LGAS, PTIB, ADD, MGAS	83	70
VLAT, SHBF, LGAS, ADD, TFL, PTIB	79	62
ADD, TFL, MGAS, PTIB, ATIB, LGAS	88	79
Six muscles with paraspinals		
ATIB, PTIB, MGAS, PSM, VMED, TFL	99	93
VMED, LGAS, PTIB, PSM, SHBF, MGAS	99	87
VLAT, TFL, LGAS, PSM, ATIB, SHBF	98	87
ADD, MGAS, PTIB, PSM, VLAT, SHBF	99	89
VMED, ATIB, PTIB, PSM, SHBF, MGAS	100	92
VMED, TFL, LGAS, PSM, ATIB, PTIB	99	91
ADD, MGAS, PTIB, PSM, ATIB, SHBF	100	93

Adapted from Dillinghem, Lauder, Andary, et al. 2000.[30]

tromyographer are listed in Table 11-9. These findings were consistent with those derived from a large retrospective study.[79]

A similar prospective multicenter study was conducted to assess the optimal screening electrodiagnostic assessment for persons with suspected lumbosacral radiculopathy.[30,31] In this study, there were 102 patients with electrodiagnostically confirmed lumbosacral radiculopathies representing all lumbosacral root levels. When paraspinal muscles were one of the screening muscles, four muscle screens identified 88–97%, five muscle screens identified 94–98%, and six muscle screens identified 98–100% (Table 11-10). When paraspinal muscles were not part of the screen, identification rates were lower for all screens, and eight distal muscles were necessary to identify 90%. Other retrospective studies are consistent with these findings.[25,78,79]

In summary, for both cervical and lumbosacral radiculopathy screens, the optimal number of muscles appears to be six muscles, which include the paraspinal muscles and muscles that represent all root level innervations. When paraspinal muscles are not reliable, then eight non-paraspinal muscles must be examined. Another way to think of this is: 'to minimize harm, six in the leg and six in the arm'.

If one of the six muscles studied in the screen is positive, there is the possibility of confirming electrodiagnostically that a radiculopathy is present. In this case, the examiner must study additional muscles to determine the radiculopathy level and to exclude a mononeuropathy. If the findings are found in only a single muscle, they remain inconclusive and of uncertain clinical relevance. If none of the six muscles are abnormal, the examiner can be confident of not missing the opportunity to confirm electrodiagnostically that a radiculopathy is present, and the examiner can curtail the needle examination. The patient might still have a radiculopathy, but other tests such as MRI will be necessary to confirm this clinical suspicion. This logic is illustrated in Figure 11-2.

In the past, a well-defined temporal course of events was thought to occur with radiculopathies, despite the absence of studies supporting such a relationship. It was a commonly held notion that, in acute lumbosacral radiculopathies, the paraspinal muscles denervated first, followed by distal muscles, and that reinnervation started with paraspinal muscles and then with distal muscles. This paradigm was addressed with a series of investigations.[31–33, 92a] For both lumbosacral and cervical radiculopathies, symptom duration had no significant relationship to the probability of finding spontaneous activity in paraspinal or limb muscles. This simplistic explanation, although widely quoted in the older literature, does not explain the complex pathophysiology of radiculopathies. Electrodiagnosticians should not invoke this relationship to explain the absence or presence of fibrillations in a particular muscle.

TRAUMATIC NERVE INJURIES

Trauma to the peripheral nervous system often accompanies other traumatic injuries. Electrodiagnosis is a valuable means of identifying the location of a peripheral nerve lesion, and can to some extent assess the magnitude of the nerve injury.[46] Electrodiagnostic testing has important implications but also clear limitations regarding precise nerve injury classification.[11] Recovery can be expected to be days to weeks in the case of

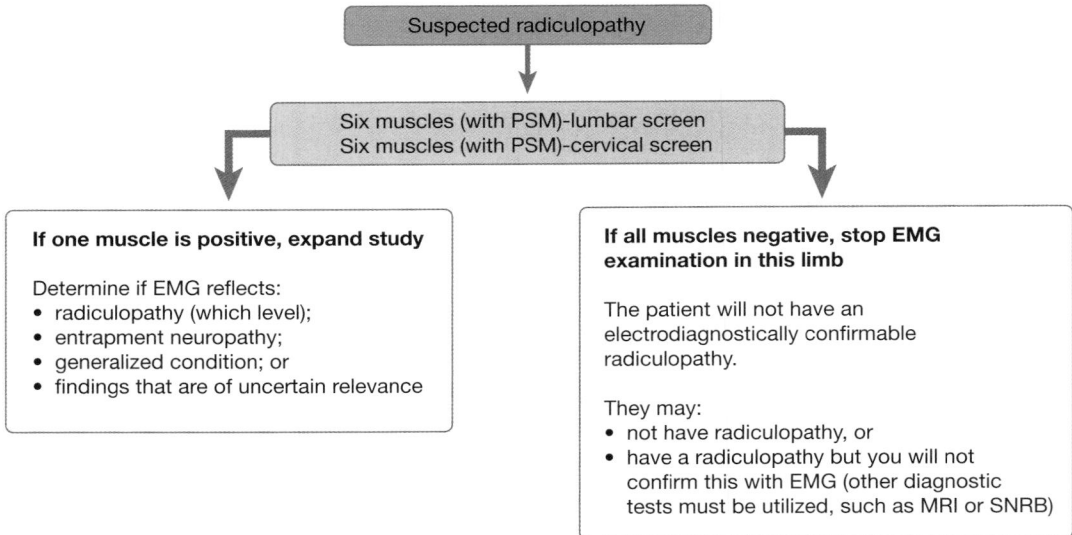

Figure 11-2 Algorithm for suspected radiculopathy. SNRB, sensory nerve root block.

an injury resulting only in neurapraxia. Months may be required for peripheral nerve injuries showing substantial axonal loss. Nerve conduction studies distal to the site of the lesion after Wallerian degeneration has taken place can help delineate the degree of axonal loss. Here, the side to side amplitudes are compared, yielding a semiquantitative means of determining the degree of axonal loss. What must be appreciated is the considerable variability in side to side motor and sensory amplitudes. Intraoperative nerve action potential assessment across individual fascicles is a very important assessment that further defines whether or not a fascicle has axons in continuity.[63,70–72]

A major use of electrodiagnosis is to identify electrophysiologic evidence of spontaneous regeneration that precedes clinical findings of recovery.[81] In the case of a traumatically injured limb, the electrodiagnostician can probably elucidate the general location of the lesion and delineate if axonal loss has occurred. The electrodiagnostic examination can determine with certainty that there is not complete neurotmesis (section of the nerve). If there are any voluntarily controlled MUAPs in muscles distal to and innervated by the injured nerve, then there is some nerve continuity remaining.

Following complete nerve section, failure at the neuromuscular junction occurs in 2–5 days in animals.[51,83,85] Regeneration occurs through axonal sprouting from undamaged axons in proximity to denervated muscle fibers in the case of partial nerve injuries. Axonal sprouting can reinnervate muscle fibers within days. Axonal regeneration occurring at the site of injury, on the other hand, requires months to reinnervate the denervated muscle fibers.[85]

Chaudhry and Cornblath studied Wallerian degeneration in humans.[20] They found that motor-evoked responses were absent in 9 days, sensory responses were absent by 11 days, and denervation potentials were seen 10–14 days after injury. These results indicate that the motor and sensory responses reliably

assess the status of the nerve after 11 days. Clinically, it takes 3 weeks for fibrillations to fully develop and be consistently recorded by needle EMG.

Kraft studied fibrillation potential amplitudes and their relationship to time following injury.[74] The mean fibrillation amplitude in the first 2 months post injury was 612 μV. This important study showed that 1 year following traumatic nerve injury, no population of fibrillation potentials were greater than 100 μV in amplitude. These findings enable some differentiation of more recent denervation from older denervation.

An informative study regarding fibrillation potential generation resulting from direct muscle injury was reported by Partanen and Danner.[90] They studied 43 patients after muscle biopsy. At 6–7 days after biopsy, about half the subjects showed fibrillations on needle EMG testing. At 16 days, all subjects revealed fibrillation potentials in the biopsied muscles, and these fibrillations persisted for up to 8 months. These findings suggest that direct muscle trauma can result in denervation potentials, and can occur in the absence of any nerve injury.[85,90] Such information is important when evaluating traumatically injured limbs. Areas of muscle damage or surgical scars should be avoided, as fibrillation potentials in these areas are uninterpretable.

Electrodiagnostic assessment of nerve injuries

The pertinent issues in electrodiagnosis of peripheral nerve injuries are localization of the injury, pathophysiology of the lesion, severity of the dysfunction, and progress of reinnervation.[40] Frykman, Wolf, and Coyle presented an algorithmic approach to the assessment and management of traumatic peripheral nerve injuries based on the clinical examination and electrodiagnostic findings (Fig. 11-3).[50] In those patients for whom little or no recovery is evident at 3 weeks by clinical examination, electrodiagnostic studies are performed. If no voluntary motor units and no motor or sensory responses are

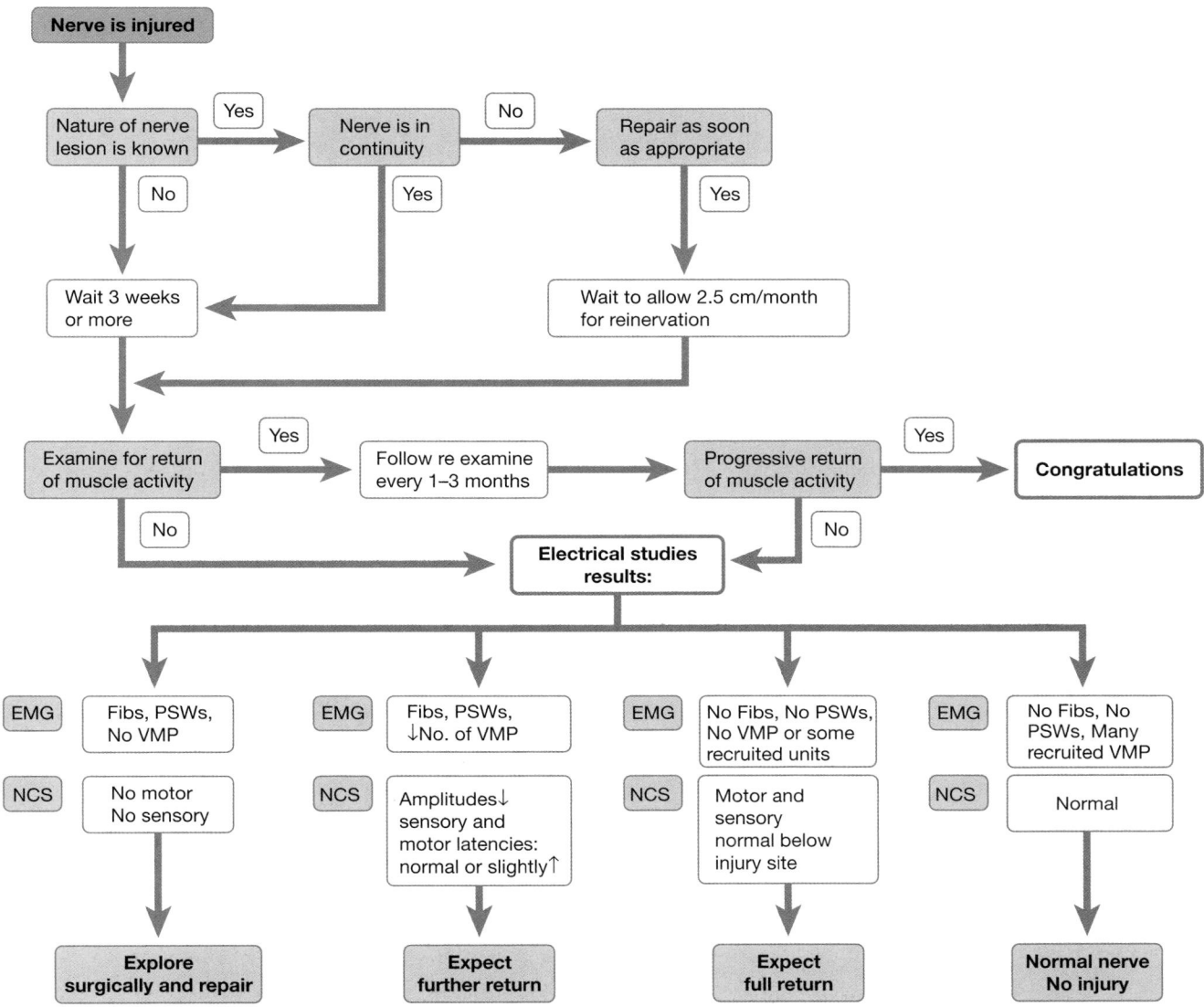

Figure 11-3 Algorithm for management of peripheral nerve injuries. EMG, electromyography; Fibs, fibrillation potentials; NCS, nerve conduction study; PSWs, positive sharp waves; VMP, voluntary motor unit potentials (interference pattern). (Adapted from Frykman et al. 1981,[50] with permission.)

elicited, then surgical exploration is considered. If fibrillations are present, yet some voluntary units are noted along with reduced but present sensory or motor responses, then one can reasonably expect further recovery. If there are no fibrillations and normal sensory and motor amplitudes, then one can expect full recovery.[50] Although somewhat simplistic, this approach provides a conceptual framework for consolidating electrodiagnostic and clinical information into a treatment plan. The algorithm by Frykman is somewhat dated and was slightly modified regarding the presence of voluntary MUAP's.[50] It might not hold up to newer surgical approaches to peripheral nerve surgery that utilize intraoperative nerve conduction studies. Information derived from peripheral nerve imaging techniques may well play an important role. However, it is a reasonable conceptual framework for managing nerve injuries.

GENERALIZED DISORDERS

Electrodiagnostic testing is an extension of the physical examination, and as such should be placed within a conceptual framework of physical findings and patient symptoms. Figure 11-1 provides a conceptual framework for utilizing the clinical scenario and examination findings to address the highest probability disorders. For the purposes of this discussion, generalized disorders are those affecting more than one limb. The guidelines in Table 11-4 provide a framework for structuring the examination to evaluate for these disorders.

Polyneuropathy

Evaluation for polyneuropathy involves identifying peripheral nervous system involvement. Further, the electrodiagnostician should strive to categorize the type of neuropathy based on its electrodiagnostic features. Donofrio and Albers compiled a comprehensive list of polyneuropathies classified by their characteristic electrodiagnostic findings.[38] Determining whether sensory, motor, or both types of nerves are involved, and whether the primary type of pathology is demyelination or axonal loss, allows the electrodiagnostician to narrow the list of potential etiologies for the polyneuropathy (Box 11-1).

The electrodiagnostic changes seen with demyelinating and axonal neuropathies are shown in Table 11-11. Persons with polyneuropathies involving acute or recent motor axonal loss show fibrillations and PSWs in predominantly distal muscles. The distribution of EMG findings in polyneuropathies is such that distal lower limb muscles often demonstrate the greatest involvement. In persons with a more chronic process with either old axonal loss or slow axonal loss that is balanced with reinnervation and reorganization of the motor unit, large amplitude, long duration MUAPs can be seen.[67,75]

Absent SNAPs and CMAPs can reflect either axonal loss or conduction block. EMG can provide supporting information about motor axonal loss. Nerve conduction velocity is an important parameter to measure from multiple nerves. Temporal dispersion suggests an acquired demyelinating polyneuropathy. Care must be taken to study enough nerves to confidently

determine if a diffuse process is present rather than a single entrapment neuropathy. If one extremity is affected, the electrodiagnostician should study the contralateral limb. If this is abnormal, then another limb should be examined.

F-waves measure longer neurologic pathways and are important in screening for polyneuropathies. They are helpful in identifying diabetic polyneuropathy, acute inflammatory demyelinating polyneuropathy (AIDP), and chronic inflammatory demyelinating polyradiculoneuropathy (CIDP).[49,86] F-waves and H-reflexes are important tests for assessing proximal segments of the peripheral nervous system, and are recommended for peripheral neuropathy evaluations.

Acute inflammatory demyelinating polyneuropathy, or Guillain–Barré syndrome, the most common and important acute rapidly progressive polyneuropathy in clinical practice, must be recognized when present.[3] Patients present with sensory symptoms and weakness, with disease progression over 2–4 weeks. Sensory nerve conduction abnormalities, reduced amplitude or prolonged distal latency, particularly in the median nerve, are observed but may take 4–6 weeks to peak.[42,43] Motor nerve conduction studies reveal prolonged distal latencies, temporal dispersion and conduction block, or slowed velocities in 80–90% of these patients. Reduced CMAPs in ulnar and median nerve-innervated muscles that are 10–20% of normal values

Table 11-11 Electrodiagnostic findings in peripheral neuropathies

Parameter	Early demyelinating	Chronic demyelinating	Acute axonal	Chronic axonal
Distal latency	Increased	Increased	Normal or slightly increased	Normal or slightly increased
Nerve conduction velocity	Decreased	Decreased	Normal or slightly decreased	Normal or slightly decreased
F-latency	Increased or absent	Increased or absent	Normal or absent	Normal or absent
H-reflex	Increased latency or absent	Increased latency or absent	Absent	Absent
Sensory nerve action potential amplitude	Decreased or absent	Decreased or absent	Decreased or absent	Decreased or absent
Compound motor action potential amplitude	Normal or decreased	Normal or decreased	Decreased	Decreased
Motor unit action potential duration	Normal	Normal (hereditary) or increased (acquired)	Normal	Increased
Motor unit action potential amplitude	Normal	Normal or increased	Normal	Increased
Polyphasics	Normal	Increased	Normal	Increased
Recruitment	Normal or decreased	Decreased, rapid	Decreased, rapid	Decreased, rapid
Abnormal spontaneous activity	None	None, or fibrillations, positive sharp waves, complex repetitive discharges	Fibrillations, positive sharp waves, complex repetitive discharges	None, or fibrillations, positive sharp waves, complex repetitive discharges

Adapted from Krivickas, 1998.[75]

Box 11-1 Classification of polyneuropathies by their electrodiagnostic characteristics

Uniform, demyelinating, mixed sensorimotor polyneuropathy
- Hereditary motor sensory neuropathy types 1, 3, and 4
- Metachromatic leukodystrophy
- Krabbe globoid leukodystrophy
- Adrenomyeloneuropathy
- Congenital hypomyelinating neuropathy
- Tangier disease
- Cockayne's syndrome
- Cerebrotendinous xanthomatosis

Segmental, demyelinating, motor greater than sensory polyneuropathy
- Acute inflammatory demyelinating polyneuropathy (AIDP)
- Chronic inflammatory demyelinating polyneuropathy (CIDP)
- Multifocal demyelinating neuropathy with persistent conduction block
- Osteosclerotic myeloma
- Waldenstrom macroglobulinemia
- Monoclonal gammopathy of undetermined significance
- Gamma heavy chain disease
- Angiofollicular lymph node hyperplasia
- Hypothyroidism
- Leprosy
- Diphtheria
- Acute arsenic polyneuropathy
- Pharmaceuticals: amiodarone, perhexilene, high-dose cytarabine (Ara-c)
- Lymphoma
- Carcinoma
- AIDS
- Lyme disease
- Acromegaly
- Hereditary neuropathy with susceptibility to pressure palsies
- Systemic lupus erythematosus
- Glue-sniffing neuropathy
- Post portocaval anastomosis
- Neuropathy associated with progressive external ophthalmoplegia
- Ulcerative colitis
- Marinesco–Sjögren syndrome
- Cryoglobulinemia

Axon loss, motor greater than sensory polyneuropathy
- Porphyria
- Axonal Guillain–Barré syndrome
- Hereditary motor sensory neuropathy types 2 and 5
- Lead neuropathy
- Dapsone neuropathy
- Vincristine neuropathy
- Remote effect motor neuronopathy associated with lymphoma
- Remote effect motor neuronopathy associated with carcinoma
- Hypoglycemia or hyperinsulinemia

Axon loss sensory neuronopathy or neuropathy
- Hereditary sensory neuropathy types 1–4
- Friedreich ataxia
- Spinocerebellar degeneration
- Abetalipoproteinemia (Bassen–Kornzweig disease)
- Primary biliary cirrhosis
- Acute sensory neuronopathy
- Cis-platinum toxicity
- Carcinomatous sensory neuronopathy
- Lymphomatous sensory neuronopathy

- Chronic idiopathic ataxic neuropathy
- Sjögren syndrome
- Fisher variant Guillain–Barré syndrome
- Paraproteinemias
- Pyridoxine toxicity
- Idiopathic sensory neuronopathy
- Styrene-induced peripheral neuropathy
- Crohn disease
- Thalidomide toxicity
- Non-systemic vasculitic neuropathy
- Chronic gluten enteropathy
- Vitamin E deficiency

Axon loss, mixed sensorimotor polyneuropathy
- Amyloidosis
- Chronic liver disease
- Nutritional disease
  Vitamin's B_{12} deficiency
  Folate deficiency
  Whipple disease
  Postgastrectomy syndrome
  Gastric restriction surgery for obesity
  Thiamine deficiency
- Alcoholism
- Sarcoidosis
- Connective tissue diseases
  Rheumatoid arthritis
  Periarteritis nodosa
  Systemic lupus erythematosus
  Churg–Strauss vasculitis
  Temporal arteritis
  Scleroderma
  Behçet disease
  Hypereosinophilia syndrome
  Cryoglobulinemia
- Toxic neuropathy
  Acrylamide
  Carbon disulfide
  Dichlorophenoxyacetic acid
  Ethylene oxide
  Hexacarbons
  Carbon monoxide
  Organophosphorus esters
  Glue sniffing
- Mental neuropathy
  Chronic arsenic intoxication
  Mercury
  Thallium
  Gold
- Pharmaceuticals
  Colchicine
  Phenytoin
  Ethambutol
  Amitriptyline
  Metronidazole
  Misonidazole
  Nitrofurantoin
  Chloroquine
  Disulfiram
  Glutethimide
  Nitrous oxide
  Lithium
- Carcinomatous axonal sensorimotor polyneuropathy

Box 11-1 Classification of polyneuropathies by their electrodiagnostic characteristics—cont'd

Axon loss, mixed sensorimotor polyneuropathy—con'd
- Chronic obstructive pulmonary disease
- Giant axonal dystrophy
- Olivopontocerebellar atrophy
- Neuropathy of chronic illness
- Acromegaly
- Hypophosphatemia
- Lymphomatous axonal sensorimotor polyneuropathy
- Hypothyroidism
- Myotonic dystrophy
- Necrotizing angiopathy

- Lyme disease
- AIDS, ARC
- Jamaican neuropathy
- Tangier disease
- Gouty neuropathy
- Polycythemia vera
- Typical multiple myeloma

Mixed axon loss, demyelinating sensorimotor polyneuropathy
- Diabetes mellitus
- Uremia

(After Donofrio and Albers 1990,[38] with permission.)

signify a poor prognosis and can provide early information to guide clinical management.[84] In severe cases, EMG findings of fibrillations and PSWs can be seen if motor axonal loss has occurred. Facial muscle weakness and bulbar muscle involvement are commonly found in patients with AIDP.[108] Nerve conduction findings of slowed conduction velocity, temporal dispersion, prolonged distal latencies, or prolonged F-waves should be found in two or more nerves to support a diagnosis of AIDP.[2,108] In some cases, late responses (F-waves and H-reflexes) are the only findings noted on electrodiagnostic testing early on in persons with AIDP.

Chronic inflammatory demyelinating polyradiculoneuropathy represents a demyelinating polyneuropathy of chronic nature with fluctuating weakness and stepwise progression. Weakness and sensory symptoms similar to those of AIDP are found, but the chronicity is longer. In CIDP, sensory responses are usually absent in both upper and lower limbs, and the nerve conduction velocities are reduced.[84] EMG findings depend on the rate of disease progression and can reveal reduced recruitment, fibrillation potentials, polyphasic potentials, and reorganized MUAPs with large amplitudes and increased durations.

Multifocal motor neuropathy is a disorder that is sometimes confused with motor neuron disease. Patients present with asymmetric weakness in a single body region, frequently the hand, but without sensory symptoms. Progression is slow and spans many years.[20,88,92,102] Sensory nerves are usually normal on electrodiagnostic testing. Motor nerve testing reveals conduction block in multiple nerves at sites not prone to focal entrapments: midforearm, midleg, arm, and brachial plexus. Distal motor latencies and amplitudes are usually normal. Proximal motor nerve stimulations at Erb's point are important to exclude conduction block over proximal nerve segments.

Diabetes is on the rise in the USA, with increasing prevalence and incidence.[57] Diabetes often confounds the accurate diagnosis of radiculopathy and spinal stenosis.[1,23] Inaccurate recognition of sensory polyneuropathy, diabetic amyotrophy, or mononeuropathy can lead to unnecessary surgical interventions.

The pattern of involvement can take the form of symmetric polyneuropathies, or focal and multifocal patterns of mononeuropathies. The proximal lower limb can be involved, with pain and weakness in patients with diabetic amyotrophy. The sensory nerve involvement, particularly in the legs, often results in complaints of numbness, tingling, burning, ache, and pain. Up to 80% of patients with diabetes having clinical polyneuropathies will demonstrate an abnormality of the SNAP.[91,95] Sensory findings usually precede motor findings. Motor nerve conduction is 15–30% below normal. EMG can show fibrillations and motor unit changes along with reduced recruitment.[42,43]

Accurate assessment for polyneuropathy requires heightened suspicion coupled with sufficient testing. Unfortunately, non-physicians perform 17% of studies in the USA.[34] In a sample of 6381 diabetic patients undergoing electrodiagnostic testing in 1998, it was demonstrated that polyneuropathy identification rates were highest for physiatrists, osteopathic physicians, and neurologists (12.5%, 12.2%, and 11.9%, respectively).[35] Podiatrists and physical therapists identified 2.4% and 2.1%, respectively, as having polyneuropathy—rates about one-sixth that of physiatrists and neurologists, despite controlling for case mix differences. Non-physician providers who did not recognize polyneuropathy in this group of patients with diabetes performed almost exclusively EMG testing (>90%) at the expense of nerve conduction studies. These findings underscore the need for high-quality consultations of sufficient scope by well-trained physicians to accurately diagnose patients with complex disorders.[35]

Alcoholic polyneuropathy is a common peripheral nerve disease accounting for almost 30% of all cases of generalized polyneuropathy.[99] This clinical entity usually occurs in the setting of longstanding alcoholism and nutritional deficiency. Substantial weight loss often occurs before or concurrent with the development of polyneuropathy. Presenting symptoms are pain, dysesthesias, and weakness in the feet and legs. Alcoholic polyneuropathy is an axonal loss sensory and motor nerve disorder (Box 11-1).[38] Low SNAP amplitudes are seen in the legs, and EMG reveals fibrillations and positive waves in distal muscles.

Hereditary sensory and motor neuropathies (HSMNs) are a diverse group of polyneuropathies that are rapidly becoming better characterized through genetic studies, and are beyond the scope of this chapter (see Ch. 48).[42,43] From an electrophysiologic standpoint, they are distinctly different from acquired polyneuropathies due to the relative lack of temporal dispersion and conduction block. HSMN type 1 is the hypertrophic variety with onion bulb formation and axonal atrophy.[67] Symptoms begin in the first two decades, and reduced nerve conduction velocities (25 m/s) are seen but without substantial temporal dispersion. HSMN type 2 presents in adult life or later. Patients have severe distal muscle atrophy and weakness. Nerve conduction studies show mild slowing, but EMG reveals large, reorganized MUAPs with fibrillations and PSWs. Dejerine–Sottas HSMN type 3 is a severe type of neuropathy appearing in infancy with delayed motor development, and reveals the slowest nerve conduction velocities—less than 10 m/s and often as low as 2–3 m/s.[67,75]

The AANEM, in conjunction with the American Academy of Neurology and the American Academy of Physical Medicine and Rehabilitation, determined that there was a need for a formal case definition for polyneuropathy.[47] The results of their recommendations were recently published. They described that no single reference standard was most appropriate for distal symmetric polyneuropathy. The most accurate diagnosis comprised a combination of clinical signs, symptoms, and electrodiagnostic findings. Electrodiagnostic findings should be included as part of the case definition because of their higher level of specificity. Electrodiagnostic studies are sensitive and specific validated measures for the presence of polyneuropathy.

This panel recommended a simplified nerve conduction study protocol for screening for the presence of distal symmetric polyneuropathy.[47] *Sural sensory* and *peroneal motor* nerve conductions performed in one lower extremity, taken together, were thought by this group to be the most sensitive tests for detecting a distal symmetric polyneuropathy. If both studies are normal, there is no evidence of typical distal symmetric polyneuropathy, and in such a situation no further nerve conduction studies are necessary. If, however, one of these tests is abnormal, then additional nerve conduction studies are recommended. This would include at least the ulnar sensory, median sensory, and ulnar motor nerves in one upper limb. A contralateral sural sensory and one tibial motor nerve conduction study can also be performed at the discretion of the examiner. These experts recommended caution when interpreting median and ulnar studies, because of the possibility of an abnormality due to compression at the wrist or elbow.[47] They further recommended that, if a response is absent for any of the nerves studied, nerve conduction studies of the contralateral nerve should be performed. In addition, if a peroneal motor response is absent, an ipsilateral tibial motor nerve conduction should be performed. These tests (sural sensory and peroneal motor) do not exclude all acquired (e.g. AIDP) or hereditary polyneuropa-

thies; they only exclude distal symmetric polyneuropathies. The electrodiagnostician should structure evaluation for these other suspected conditions with examination of weak muscles and involved nerve distributions.

Myopathies

Myopathic disorders include acquired inflammatory types such as polymyositis and dermatomyositis, as well as congenital myopathies, metabolic myopathies, muscular dystrophies, and mitochondrial myopathies. A detailed discussion is beyond the scope of this treatise, and the interested reader is directed to other specialized references for a complete description of the rarer forms of myopathy (see Ch. 49). Unfortunately, the electrodiagnostic examination is less sensitive or specific for detecting myopathies than for any other group of neuromuscular diseases.[75] Myopathies are one of the most challenging disorders to identify and classify by electrodiagnosis, because there are no characteristic findings specific for myopathy. There is often patchy involvement of proximal muscles, and the EMG findings can vary depending on the severity and duration of the myopathy. Characteristic findings on EMG can indicate myopathy, yet the precise etiology of the myopathy requires other testing, such as muscle biopsy and chromosome analyses. The electromyographic findings for myopathies are shown in Table 11-12. Nerve conduction studies are usually normal except when a muscle is atrophic, and then the CMAP can be reduced. Sensory nerve conduction studies are normal unless a concomitant polyneuropathy exists.

Needle EMG is the most helpful part of the examination. In the acute inflammatory myopathies polymyositis and dermatomyositis, the characteristic findings are fibrillations and PSWs, CRDs, and early or increased recruitment of short duration, polyphasic, low amplitude MUAPs.[93] Early recruitment or increased recruitment refers to the case in which more motor units are recruited than would be expected to generate a low muscular force. This is because, in myopathies, more diseased muscle fibers are necessary to generate force than in the normal situation. At low force levels, many units are present on the display screen. Proximal limb girdle and paraspinal muscles are frequently involved. In progressive muscular dystrophies such as Duchenne and Becker, fibrillations and PSWs are widespread, with occasional CRDs and myotonic discharges.[75] Inclusion body myositis accounts for 30% of all inflammatory myopathies and requires muscle biopsy to diagnose the condition. The findings are similar to those seen in polymyositis, with fibrillations and PSWs more widespread and prominent.[75]

Neuromuscular junction disorders

Disorders of the neuromuscular junction can be classified as either presynaptic or postsynaptic. The presynaptic disorders are Lambert–Eaton myasthenic syndrome and botulism. Myasthenia gravis is a postsynaptic disorder.[59,64,97] These rare causes of generalized weakness demonstrate characteristic electrodiagnostic features (Table 11-13), making them readily identifiable to the electrodiagnostician with a heightened suspicion for these entities.

Table 11-12 Electrodiagnostic findings in myopathies

Parameter	Muscular dystrophy	Congenital	Mitochondrial	Metabolic	Inflammatory	Channelopathy
Distal latency	Normal	Normal	Normal	Normal	Normal	Normal
Nerve conduction velocity	Normal	Normal	Normal	Normal	Normal	Normal
H-reflex	Normal or absent	Normal or absent	Normal	Normal	Normal or absent	Normal
Sensory nerve action potential amplitude	Normal	Normal	Normal	Normal	Normal	Normal
Compound motor action potential amplitude	Normal or decreased	Normal or decreased	Normal or decreased	Normal or decreased	Normal or decreased	Normal
Motor unit action potential duration	Decreased and/or increased	Decreased or normal	Decreased or normal	Decreased or normal	Decreased and/or increased (inclusion body myositis)	Decreased or normal
Motor unit action potential amplitude	Decreased and/or increased	Decreased or normal	Decreased or normal	Decreased or normal	Decreased and/or increased (inclusion body myositis)	Decreased or normal
Polyphasics	Increased	Increased or normal	Increased or normal	Increased or normal	Increased	Increased or normal
Recruitment	Increased	Increased or normal	Increased or normal	Increased or normal	Increased	Increased or normal
Fibrillations and positive sharp waves	Yes	Centronuclear myopathy	No	Yes	Yes	Occasionally
Complex repetitive discharges	Yes	Centronuclear myopathy	No	Yes	Yes	Occasionally
Myotonic potentials	Myotonic dystrophy	Centronuclear myopathy	No	Acid maltase deficiency	No	Yes
Electrical silence	No	No	No	Contractures in McArdle disease	No	During attacks of paralysis

Adapted from Krivickas, 1998.[75]

Myasthenia gravis is an autoimmune disorder caused by antibodies directed at the acetylcholine receptors of skeletal muscle. Electrodiagnostic techniques most useful for identifying this disorder are repetitive nerve stimulation and single-fiber EMG.[59] Elevated acetylcholine receptor antibodies have been demonstrated in patients with generalized and ocular myasthenia gravis in 81% and 51%, respectively. Elevated acetylcholine receptor antibody levels can be seen in those with penicillamine-induced myasthenia, in some elderly patients with autoimmune diseases, and in first-degree relatives of patients with myasthenia gravis. Decrementing responses in a distal hand muscle on repetitive nerve stimulation at 2 or 3 Hz are seen in 68% of persons with definite generalized myasthenia gravis, and in 31% with mild myasthenia gravis.[64] Repetitive nerve stimulation of a proximal muscle increases the sensitivity to 89% for definite and 68% for mild myasthenia gravis. Single-fiber EMG is the most sensitive test for myasthenia gravis. In persons with gen-eralized myasthenia gravis, the sensitivity of single-fiber EMG performed on the extensor digitorum communis muscle was 92%. In patients with ocular myasthenia gravis, 78% had abnormal jitter in the extensor digitorum communis, and 92% had increased jitter with a facial muscle study (frontalis). Single-fiber EMG is a non-specific test, unfortunately, and increased jitter can be seen in amyotrophic lateral sclerosis, peripheral neuropathies, and some myopathies.

Lambert–Eaton myasthenic syndrome is a unique condition characterized by weakness and fatigability of proximal limb muscles with sparing of ocular muscles. Dry mouth is often reported, and the patients demonstrate hyporeflexia and normal sensation.[64] There is a strong association with malignancy, most commonly oat cell carcinoma of the lung. There is reduced release of acetylcholine quanta from the presynaptic nerve terminal. A unique feature of this disorder is that, with rapid repetitive nerve stimulation (20 Hz) or a brief voluntary

Table 11-13 Electrodiagnostic findings in neuromuscular junction transmission disorders

Parameter	Myasthenia gravis	Lambert–Eaton myasthenic syndrome	Botulism
Distal latency	Normal	Normal	Normal
Nerve conduction velocity	Normal	Normal	Normal
Sensory nerve action potential amplitude	Normal	Normal	Normal
Compound motor action potential amplitude	Usually normal	Decreased	Normal or decreased
Slow repetitive stimulation	Decrement	Decrement	± decrement
Fast repetitive stimulation or brief exercise	± mild increment	Large increment (lasting 20–30 s)	Intermediate increment (lasting up to 4 min)
Postactivation exhaustion	Yes	Yes	No
Motor unit action potential configuration	Moment to moment amplitude variation (weak muscles) ± decreased amplitude and duration	Moment to moment amplitude variation (all muscles), decreased amplitude and duration, increased polyphasics	Moment to moment amplitude variation (weak muscles), decreased amplitude and duration, increased polyphasics
Recruitment	Normal or increased	Increased	Increased
Spontaneous activity	Fibrillation in severe disease	None	Fibrillation in severe disease
Single-fiber electromyography	Increased jitter and blocking (increases with increased firing rate)	Increased jitter and blocking (decreased with increased firing rate)	Increased jitter and blocking (decreased with increased firing rate)

(From Krivickas 1998,[75] with permission.)

maximal contraction, a postactivation increase in CMAP of over 200% is seen. Although such potentiation can be seen in myasthenia gravis and botulism, it is usually to a much lesser degree than that seen in Lambert–Eaton myasthenic syndrome. This profound potentiation is the hallmark electrodiagnostic finding in Lambert–Eaton myasthenic syndrome. Other features of Lambert–Eaton myasthenic syndrome—normal sensory conductions, decrementing response to 2-Hz stimulation, and increased jitter on single-fiber EMG—are similar to those found in myasthenia gravis.[75]

Botulism is a rare disorder caused by the potent toxin of the bacterium *Clostridium botulinum*, through both oral ingestion or wound infection.[64] A rapid onset paralysis of the eye muscles, followed by rapid spread to other parts of the body, is seen. The toxin irreversibly blocks acetylcholine release from presynaptic nerve terminals. Electrodiagnostic findings reveal low CMAPs, with decrementing responses on 2-Hz repetitive nerve stimulation. The incremental increase in CMAP amplitude with exercise is less dramatic than in Lambert–Eaton myasthenic syndrome but should be over 40%.[75] With severe involvement, the neuromuscular junction is completely blocked and no facilitation with rapid stimulation is seen. In these cases, the end plates break down and fibrillation potentials are seen.

In this group of disorders, the SNAPs are normal. The CMAPs are normal or of low amplitude, particularly in Lambert–Eaton myasthenic syndrome and botulism. Needle EMG reveals normal or polyphasic MUAPs with low amplitudes and short durations, similar to those found in myopathies. With EMG, MUAP variation in size can be seen as well. Fibrillation potentials are seen only in severe disease with complete disintegration of the neuromuscular junction (Table 11-13). Stimulated single-fiber EMG offers advantages over conventional single-fiber EMG. Stimulated single-fiber EMG can be performed in patients who cannot maintain a voluntary contraction or in children and infants.[19] It is less time-consuming and, by controlling the rate of stimulation, better quantification of the neuromuscular junction disorder can be obtained.[19]

Ertas et al. reported the use of concentric needle electrodes for single-fiber EMG.[48] They showed that, when the low-frequency filter is set at 2 kHz, concentric needle electrodes are comparable with single-fiber EMG electrodes and yield the same jitter values for normal individuals and for persons with myasthenia gravis. Additional advantages include the fact that they are disposable. Because of a larger recording area, somewhat more single muscle fiber discharges were identified than with standard single-fiber EMG electrodes.[48]

Motor neuron disease

Motor neuron disease will be discussed in the context of the most common type in adults: amyotrophic lateral sclerosis. This is a progressive motor system disease with upper motor neuron findings from spinal white matter involvement, and lower motor neuron findings on EMG from anterior horn cell loss.[44,76] There are different classifications based on the predominance of these characteristics. From an electrodiagnostic standpoint, EMG is the most helpful part of the study. In order to electrodiagnostically confirm amyotrophic lateral sclerosis in the appropriate clinical circumstances, the patient must demonstrate the following findings:

1. PSWs and/or fibrillation potentials in three limbs or two limbs and bulbar muscles;
2. normal sensory nerve conduction studies;
3. normal motor conduction velocities, except if the CMAP is <30% of the mean, in which case the conduction velocities may not be less than 70% of normal; and
4. needle examination demonstrates a reduced recruitment, with altered MUAP duration and amplitude.[75]

Motor unit morphology depends on the rate of denervation and reinnervation. In a rapidly progressive amyotrophic lateral sclerosis, there might be little motor unit remodeling. Reduced recruitment of MUAPs is the primary EMG finding in ALS (see Ch. 47).[26]

FINAL ELECTRODIAGNOSTIC CONCLUSIONS AND REPORT

The electrodiagnostic report is a critical document that conveys the findings and conclusions derived from testing. The electrodiagnostic report should include a brief history regarding the presenting complaint, a focused physical examination, the tabulated electrodiagnostic findings, and the final assessment and conclusions. There should be internal consistency within the report, such that the conclusions are supported by the electrophysiologic data, independent of the investigator's clinical impression. The electrodiagnostician can then comment on how these electrodiagnostic findings correlate with the clinical impression, the limitations of the test, and any other observations made. This then gives a more complete clinical picture. In electrodiagnostic reports, the referring question(s) should be addressed. In addition, conditions that were excluded can be listed. It is best to state that there is 'no electrodiagnostic evidence of' a particular disorder if the testing for that disorder was normal. This reflects that fact that electrodiagnostic testing can be normal in persons with the particular condition that the referring physicians suspect. Electrodiagnostic testing is not as sensitive, yet more specific, for many conditions, and for this reason quite helpful when positive.

It is often useful to the referring physician if the electrodiagnostician comments on other clinical conditions that were identified during the work-up, such as shoulder impingement syndrome or lateral epicondylitis. Such observations can reveal other treatment alternatives in addition to addressing the electrodiagnostically confirmed disorders.

The limitations of a particular study, as well as confounding issues, should be clearly stated. One such issue is pedal edema, which can make it difficult to obtain normal sural sensory responses. Morbid obesity can impede adequate stimulus of a peripheral nerve or accurate measurement of conduction distance. Previous ulnar nerve transpositions can complicate calculation of conduction velocity across the elbow. Limited patient tolerance for testing can compromise the completeness of testing. These statements can alert the referring physician or other provider of the limitations of the study and better place into context the strength of the results.

SUMMARY

Electrodiagnostic medicine is a complex consultation that relies on clinical insights, technical skills, solid normative data, and sound clinical judgment. Such consultations frequently influence surgical decision making and can have profound influence on subsequent diagnostic and therapeutic interventions. Only experienced and well-trained physicians should perform such diagnostic procedures. A healthy appreciation for the spectrum of normal values seen in people of different ages and heights should be maintained. Normative values should be well derived and interpreted correctly by electrodiagnosticians to avoid overcalling common disorders. Sufficient testing should be performed to confidently identify the suspected disorder and eliminate from the differential other confounding conditions.

REFERENCES

1. Adamova B, Vohanka S, Dusek L. Differential diagnostics in patients with mild lumbar spinal stenosis: the contributions and limits of various tests. Eur Spine J 2003; 12:190–196.
2. Alan TA, Chaudhry V, Cornblath DR. Electrophysiological studies in the Guillain–Barré syndrome: distinguishing subtypes by published criteria. Muscle Nerve 1998; 21:1275–1279.
3. Albers JW, Kelly JJ Jr. Acquired inflammatory demyelinating polyneuropathies: clinical and electrodiagnostic features. Muscle Nerve 1989; 12:435–451.
4. American Association of Electrodiagnostic Medicine. Guidelines for establishing a quality assurance program in an electrodiagnostic laboratory. Muscle Nerve 1999; suppl 8:S33–S39.
5. American Association of Electrodiagnostic Medicine. Guidelines in electrodiagnostic medicine. Muscle Nerve 1999: S1–S300.
6. American Association of Electrodiagnostic Medicine. Guidelines in electrodiagnostic medicine. Risks in electrodiagnostic medicine. Muscle Nerve 1999; suppl 8:S53–S58.
7. American Association of Electrodiagnostic Medicine. Guidelines in electrodiagnostic medicine. The electrodiagnostic medicine consultation. Muscle Nerve 1999; 8:S73–S90.
8. Becker MH, Lassner F, Bahm J, et al. The cervical rib. A predisposing factor for obstetric brachial plexus lesions. J Bone Joint Surg Br 2002; 84(5):740–743.
9. Bennett R. The fibrositis–fibromyalgia syndrome. In: Schumacher R, Klippel J, Robinson J, eds. Primer on the rheumatic diseases. Atlanta: Arthritis Foundation; 1988:227–229.
10. Boden SD, McCowin PR, Davis DO, et al. Abnormal magnetic-resonance scans of the cervical spine in asymptomatic subjects. A prospective investigation. J Bone Joint Surg Am 1990; 72(8):1178–1184.
11. Bralliar F. Electromyography: its use and misuse in peripheral nerve injuries. Orthop Clin North Am 1981; 12(2):229–238.
12. Buschbacher RM. Median nerve F-wave latencies recorded from the abductor pollicis brevis. Am J Phys Med Rehabil 1999; 78:S32–S37.
13. Buschbacher RM. Normal range for H-reflex recording from the calf muscles. Am J Phys Med Rehabil 1999; 78:S75–S79.

14. Buschbacher RM. Peroneal nerve F-wave latencies recorded from the extensor digitorum brevis. Am J Phys Med Rehabil 1999; 78: S48–S52.

15. Buschbacher RM. Tibial nerve F-waves recorded from the abductor hallucis. Am J Phys Med Rehabil 1999; 78:S43–S47.

16. Buschbacher RM. Ulnar nerve F-wave latencies recorded from the abductor digiti minimi. Am J Phys Med Rehabil 1999; 78:S38–S42.

17. Campbell WW, Pridgeon RM, Singh Sahni K. Short segment incremental studies in the evaluation of the ulnar neuropathy at the elbow. Muscle Nerve 1992; 15(9):1050–1054.

18. Caress JB, Rutkove SB, Carlin M, et al. Paraspinal muscle hematoma after electromyography. Neurology 1996; 47(1):269–272.

19. Chaudhry V, Crawford TO. Stimulation single-fiber EMG in infant botulism. Muscle Nerve 1999; 22:1698–1703.

20. Chaudhry V, Cornblath DR. Wallerian degeneration in human nerves: serial electrophysiological studies. Muscle Nerve 1992; 15(6):687–693.

21. Chiou-Tan FY, Kemp K Jr, Elfenbaum M, et al. Lumbosacral plexopathy in gunshot wounds and motor vehicle accidents: comparison of electrophysiologic findings. Am J Phys Med Rehabil 2001; 80(4):280–285.

22. Chuang TY, Chiou-Tan FY, Vennix MJ. Brachial plexopathy in gunshot wounds and motor vehicle accidents: comparison of electrophysiologic findings. Arch Phys Med Rehabil 1998; 79(2):201–204.

23. Cinotti G, Postacchini F, Weinstein JN. Lumbar spinal stenosis and diabetes. Outcome of surgical decompression. J Bone Joint Surg Br 1994; 76(2):215–219.

24. Cornblath DR, Sladky JT, Sumner AJ. Clinical electrophysiology of infantile botulism. Muscle Nerve 1983; 6:448–452.

24a. Cupka B, Zaza D, Dillingham TR. Traumatic nerve injuries: outcome prediction using clinical and diagnostic findings. Muscle Nerve 2006 (in review).

25. Dasher KJ, Dillingham TR. The lumbosacral electromyographic screen: revisiting a classic paper. Clin Neurophysiol 2000; 111(12):2219–2222.

26. Daube JR. AAEE minimonograph #18: EMG in motor neuron diseases. Rochester: American Association of Electrodiagnostic Medicine; 1982: 3–11.

27. Daube JR. AAEM mini-monograph #11: needle examination in clinical electromyography. Rochester: American Association of Electrodiagnostic Medicine; 1991.

28. Denys EH. AAEM minimonograph #14: the influence of temperature in clinical neurophysiology. Rochester: American Association of Electrodiagnostic Medicine; 1991:3–19.

29. Dillingham TR, Lauder TD, Andary M, et al. Identification of cervical radiculopathies: optimizing the electromyographic screen. Am J Phys Med Rehabil 2001; 80(2):84–91.

30. Dillingham TR, Lauder TD, Andary M, et al. Identifying lumbosacral radiculopathies: an optimal electromyographic screen. Am J Phys Med Rehabil 2000; 79(6):496–503.

31. Dillingham TR, Pezzin LE, Lauder TD, et al. Symptom duration and spontaneous activity in lumbosacral radiculopathy. Am J Phys Med Rehabil 2000; 79(2):124–132.

32. Dillingham TR, Pezzin LE, Lauder TD. Cervical paraspinal muscle abnormalities and symptom duration: a multivariate analysis. Muscle Nerve 1998; 21(5):640–642.

33. Dillingham TR, Pezzin LE, Lauder TD. Relationship between muscle abnormalities and symptom duration in lumbosacral radiculopathies. Am J Phys Med Rehabil 1998; 77(2):103–107.

34. Dillingham TR, Pezzin LE, Rice B. Electrodiagnostic services in the United States. Muscle Nerve 2004; 29(2):198–204.

35. Dillingham TR, Pezzin LE. Under-recognition of polyneuropathy in persons with diabetes by non-physician electrodiagnostic services providers. Am J Phys Med Rehabil 2005; 84(6):339–406.

36. Dillingham TR. Approach to trauma of the peripheral nerves. American Association of Electrodiagnostic Medicine Course Proceedings, AAEM Annual Scientific Meeting, 1998, Orlando, Florida.

37. Donnelly V, Foran A, Murphy J, et al. Neonatal brachial plexus palsy: an unpredictable injury. Am J Obstet Gynecol 2002; 187(5):1209–1212.

38. Donofrio P, Albers J. AAEM minimonograph #34: polyneuropathy: classification by nerve conduction studies and electromyography. Muscle Nerve 1990; 13:889–903.

39. Dorfman LJ, Robinson LR. AAEM minimonograph #47: normative data in electrodiagnostic medicine. Muscle Nerve 1997; 20:4–14.

40. Dorfman LJ. Quantitative clinical electrophysiology in the evaluation of nerve injury and regeneration. Muscle Nerve 1990; 13(9):822–828.

41. Dumitru D, Diaz CAJ, King JC. Prevalence of denervation in paraspinal and foot intrinsic musculature. Am J Phys Med Rehabil 2001; 80(7): 482–490.

42. Dumitru D. Focal peripheral neuropathies. In: Dumitru D, ed. Electrodiagnostic medicine. 2nd edn. Philadelphia: Hanley & Belfus; 2002.

43. Dumitru D. Generalized peripheral neuropathies. In: Dumitru D, ed. Electrodiagnostic medicine. Philadelphia: Hanley & Belfus; 1995: 741–850.

44. Dumitru D. Myopathies. In: Dumitru D, ed. Electrodiagnostic medicine. Philadelphia: Hanley & Belfus; 1995:1031–1129.

45. Dumitru D. Needle electromyography. In: Dumitru D, ed. Electrodiagnostic medicine. Philadelphia: Hanley & Belfus; 1995.

46. Dumitru D. Reaction of the peripheral nervous system to injury. In: Dumitru D, ed. Electrodiagnostic medicine. Philadelphia: Hanley & Belfus; 1995.

47. England JD, Gronseth GS, Franklin G, et al. Distal symmetrical polyneuropathy: definition for clinical research. Muscle Nerve 2005; 31: 113–123.

48. Ertas M, Baslo MB, Yildiz N, et al. Concentric needle electrode for neuromuscular jitter analysis. Muscle Nerve 2000; 23:715–719.

49. Fraser JL, Olney RK. The relative diagnostic sensitivity of different F-wave parameters in various polyneuropathies. Muscle Nerve 1992; 15:912–918 (see comments).

50. Frykman GK, Wolf A, Coyle T. An algorithm for management of peripheral nerve injuries. Orthop Clin North Am 1981; 12(2):239–244.

51. Gilliatt RW, Hjorth RJ. Nerve conduction during Wallerian degeneration in the baboon. J Neurol Neurosurg Psychiatry 1972; 35:335–341.

52. Goldkamp O. Electromyography and nerve conduction studies in 116 patients with hemiplegia. Arch Phys Med Rehabil 1967; 48:59–63.

53. Haig AJ, LeBreck DB, Powley SG. Paraspinal mapping. Quantified needle electromyography of the paraspinal muscles in persons without low back pain. Spine 1995; 20(6):715–721.

54. Haig AJ, Talley C, Grobler LJ, et al. Paraspinal mapping: quantified needle electromyography in lumbar radiculopathy. Muscle Nerve 1993; 16(5): 477–484.

55. Haig AJ, Tzeng HM, LeBreck DB. The value of electrodiagnostic consultation for patients with upper extremity nerve complaints: a prospective comparison with the history and physical examination. Arch Phys Med Rehabil 1999; 80(10):1273–1281.

56. Haig AJ. Clinical experience with paraspinal mapping. II: A simplified technique that eliminates three-fourths of needle insertions. Arch Phys Med Rehabil 1997; 78(11):1185–1190.

57. Harris MI. Diabetes in America: epidemiology and scope of the problem. Diabetes Care 1998; 21(suppl 3):C11-4–C11-14.

58. Hong CZ, Lee S, Lum P. Cervical radiculopathy. Clinical, radiographic and EMG findings. Orthop Rev 1986; 15(7):433–439.

59. Jablecki CK. AAEM case report #3: myasthenia gravis. Rochester: American Association of Electrodiagnostic Medicine; 1981:3–14.

60. Jensen MC, Brant-Zawadzki MN, Obuchowski N, et al. Magnetic resonance imaging of the lumbar spine in people without back pain. N Engl J Med 1994; 331(2):69–73.

61. Johnson EW, Denny ST, Kelley JP. Sequence of electromyographic abnormalities in stroke syndrome. Arch Phys Med Rehabil 1975; 56:468–473.

62. Jones HR Jr, Herbison GJ, Jacobs SR, et al. Intrauterine onset of a mononeuropathy: peroneal neuropathy in a newborn with electromyographic findings at age one day compatible with prenatal onset. Muscle Nerve 1996; 19(1):88–91.

63. Kaplan BJ, Gravenstein D, Friedman WA. Intraoperative electrophysiology in treatment of peripheral nerve injuries. J Fla Med Assoc 1984; 71(6): 400–403.

64. Keesey J. AAEM minimonograph #33: electrodiagnostic approach to defects of neuromuscular transmission. Muscle Nerve 1989; 12:613–626.

65. Kerman K, Shahani B. Pediatric electromyography. Indian J Pediatr 1990; 57:469–479.

66. Khatri BO, Baruah J, McQuillen MP. Correlation of electromyography with computed tomography in evaluation of lower back pain. Arch Neurol 1984; 41(6):594–597.

67. Kimura J. Polyneuropathies. In: Kimura J, ed. Electrodiagnosis in diseases of nerve and muscle: principles and practice. Philadelphia: FA Davis; 1989:462–494.

68. Kimura J. Techniques in normal findings. In: Kimura J, ed. Electrodiagnosis in diseases of nerve and muscle: principles and practice. 2nd edn. Philadelphia: FA Davis; 1989.

69. Kirshblum S, Lim S, Garstang S, et al. Electrodiagnostic changes of the lower limbs in subjects with chronic complete cervical spinal cord injury. Arch Phys Med Rehabil 2001; 82:604–607.

70. Kline DG, Hackett ER, Happel LH. Surgery for lesions of the brachial plexus. Arch Neurol 1986; 43(2):170–181.

71. Kline DG. Physiological and clinical factors contributing to the timing of nerve repair. Clin Neurosurg 1977; 24:425–455.

72. Kline DG. Surgical repair of peripheral nerve injury. Muscle Nerve 1990; 13(9):843–852.

73. Knutsson B. Comparative value of electromyographic, myelographic, and clinical-neurological examinations in diagnosis of lumbar root compression syndrome. Acta Orthop Scand 1961; suppl 49:1–123.

74. Kraft GH. Fibrillation potential amplitude and muscle atrophy following peripheral nerve injury. Muscle Nerve 1990; 13:814–821.

75. Krivickas L. Electrodiagnosis in neuromuscular diseases. Phys Med Rehabil Clin North Am 1998; 9(1):83–114.

76. Kuncl RW, Cornblath DR, Griffin JW. Assessment of thoracic paraspinal muscles in the diagnosis of ALS. Muscle Nerve 1988; 11:484–492.

77. Kuruoglu R, Oh SJ, Thompson B. Clinical and electromyographic correlations of lumbosacral radiculopathy. Muscle Nerve 1994; 17(2): 250–251.

78. Lauder TD, Dillingham TR, Huston CW, et al. Lumbosacral radiculopathy screen. Optimizing the number of muscles studied. Am J Phys Med Rehabil 1994; 73(6):394–402.

79. Lauder TD, Dillingham TR. The cervical radiculopathy screen: optimizing the number of muscles studied. Muscle Nerve 1996; 19(5):662–665.

80. Linden D, Berlit P. Comparison of late responses, EMG studies, and motor evoked potentials (MEPs) in acute lumbosacral radiculopathies. Muscle Nerve 1995; 18:1205–1207.

81. MacKinnon SE, Dellon AL. Surgery of the peripheral nerve. New York: Thieme Medical Publishers; 1988.

82. Marin R, Dillingham TR, Chang A, et al. Extensor digitorum brevis reflex in normals and patients with L5 and S1 radiculopathies. Muscle Nerve 1995; 18(1):52–59.

83. Miledi R, Slater CR. On the degeneration of rat neuromuscular junctions after nerve section. J Physiol 1970; 207:507–528.

84. Miller RG, Peterson GW, Daube JR, et al. Prognostic value of electrodiagnosis in Guillain-Barré syndrome. Muscle Nerve 1988; 11:769–774.

85. Miller RG. AAEE minimonograph #28: injury to peripheral motor nerves. Muscle Nerve 1987; 10:698–710.

86. Olney RK, Aminoff MJ. Electrodiagnostic features of the Guillain–Barré syndrome: the relative sensitivity of different techniques. Neurology 1990; 40:471–475.

87. Parano E, Uncini A, DeVivo DC, et al. Electrophysiologic correlates of peripheral nervous system maturation in infancy and childhood. J Child Neurol 1993; 8-4:336–338.

88. Parry GJ. AAEM case report #30: multifocal motor neuropathy. Muscle Nerve 1996; 19:269–276.

89. Parry GJ. Electrodiagnostic studies in the evaluation of peripheral nerve and brachial plexus injuries. Neurol Clin 1992; 10(4):921–934.

90. Partanen JV, Danner R. Fibrillation potentials after muscle injury in humans. Muscle Nerve 1982; 5(9S):S70–S73.

91. Pastore C, Izura V, Geijo-Barrientos E, et al. A comparison of electrophysiological tests for the early diagnosis of diabetic neuropathy. Muscle Nerve 1999; 22:1667–1673.

92. Pestronk A. Multifocal motor neuropathy: diagnosis and treatment. Neurology 1998; 51:S22–S24.

92a. Pezzin LE, Dillingham TR, Lauder TD, et al. Cervical radiculopathies: relationship between symptom duration and spontments EMS activity. Muscle Nerve 1999; 22(10):1412–1418.

93. Robinson L. AAEM case report #22: polymyositis. Muscle Nerve 1991; 14:310–315.

94. Robinson LR. Electromyography, magnetic resonance imaging, and radiculopathy: it's time to focus on specificity. Muscle Nerve 1999; 22(2): 149–150.

95. Rondinelli RD, Robinson LR, Hassanein KM, et al. Further studies on the electrodiagnosis of diabetic peripheral polyneuropathy using discriminant function analysis. Am J Phys Med Rehabil 1994; 73:116–123.

96. Sabbahi MA, Khalil M. Segmental H-reflex studies in upper and lower limbs of patients with radiculopathy. Arch Phys Med Rehabil 1990; 71(3):223–227.

97. Sanders D, Stalberg E. AAEM minimonograph #25: single fiber electromyography. Muscle Nerve 1996; 19:1069–1083.

98. Scelsa SN, Herskovitz S, Berger AR. The diagnostic utility of F waves in L5/S1 radiculopathy. Muscle Nerve 1995; 18(12):1496–1497.

99. Shields R. AAEE case report #10: alcoholic polyneuropathy. Muscle Nerve 1985; 8:183–187.

99a. Stevens JC. AAEM Minimonograph 26: The electrodiagnosis of carpol tunnel syndrome. Miscle Nerve 1997; 20:1977–1986.

100. Swoboda KJ, Edelbol-eeg-olofsson K, Harmon RL, et al. Pediatric electromyography. In: Jones H, et al, eds. Neuromuscular disorders of infancy, childhood and adolescence. Oxford: Butterworth-Heinemann; 2002.

101. Tackmann W, Radu EW. Observations of the application of electrophysiological methods in the diagnosis of cervical root compressions. Eur Neurol 1983; 22(6):397–404.

102. Taylor BV, Wright RA, Harper CM, et al. Natural history of 46 patients with multifocal motor neuropathy with conduction block. Muscle Nerve 2000; 23:900–908.

103. Taylor RG, Kewalramani LS, Fowler WM Jr. Electromyographic findings in lower extremities of patients with high spinal cord injury. Arch Phys Med Rehabil 1974; 55:16–23.

104. Tullberg T, Svanborg E, Isacsson J, et al. A preoperative and postoperative study of the accuracy and value of electrodiagnosis in patients with lumbosacral disc herniation. Spine 1993; 18(7):837–842.

105. Turk MA. Pediatric electrodiagnostic medicine. In: Dumitru D, ed. Electrodiagnostic medicine. 2nd edn. Philadelphia: Hanley & Belfus; 1995.

106. Valls-Canals J, Montero J, Pradas J. Stimulated single fiber EMG of the frontalis muscle in the diagnosis of ocular myasthenia. Muscle Nerve 2000; 23:779–783.

107. Weber F, Albert U. Electrodiagnostic examination of lumbosacral radiculopathies. Electromyogr Clin Neurophysiol 2000; 40(4):231–236.

108. Weinberg DH. AAEM case report 4: Guillain–Barré syndrome. American Association of Electrodiagnostic Medicine. Muscle Nerve 1999; 22:271–281.

109. Wiechers DO, Johnson EW. Diffuse abnormal electromyographic insertional activity: a preliminary report. Arch Phys Med Rehabil 1979; 60: 419–422.

110. Wilbourn AJ, Aminoff MJ. AAEM minimonograph 32: the electrodiagnostic examination in patients with radiculopathies. Muscle Nerve 1998; 21:1612–1631.

111. Wilbourn AJ. Electrodiagnostic testing of neurologic injuries in athletes. Clin Sports Med 1990; 9(2):229–245.

Chapter

12

Electrodiagnostic Medicine III: Case Studies

Albert Clairmont, Steven M. Nash and Yousef M. Mohammad

The electrodiagnostic (EDX) medicine consultant plays a pivotal role in the diagnosis and management of persons having a range of diseases affecting nerve and muscle. Clinical neurophysiology is essentially an extension of the physical examination, and provides an additional tool to help confirm the clinical impression formed from completing the history and physical examination. Nerve conduction studies (NCS) and needle electromyography (EMG) provide direct information about the functional aspects of nerve and muscle.

The EDX study begins with a thorough history and physical examination that leads to a clinical impression. Results of the physical examination guide the EDX study.

The cases presented in this chapter build on the information presented in Chapters 10 and 11. They show clinical neurophysiologic approaches to evaluating the person with nerve or muscle disease. Some cases reflect commonly and easily diagnosed pathology, while others are very complicated or represent coexistent problems. Sequencing of the tests and details of testing can vary with the individual EDX consultant, but the general approach would be similar.

UPPER LIMB CASES

A wide range of problems affecting nerve and muscle in the upper limb are routinely diagnosed by the clinical neurophysiologist. Some of the commonest problems evaluated include median mononeuropathy (e.g. carpal tunnel syndrome), cervical radiculopathy, ulnar neuropathy, brachial plexus injury, long thoracic nerve injury, and superficial radial and dorsal ulnar sensory and other isolated motor or sensory neuropathies. Some conditions affecting the upper limbs can do so as part of more general disease, such as motor neuron disease, polyradiculopathy, neuromuscular junction disease, hereditary or acquired polyneuropathy, metabolic disease, and primary disease of muscle.

Case 1

A 26-year-old man presented to his primary care physician complaining of right shoulder weakness of 3 weeks duration. Six weeks ago, he had noticed right shoulder and paraspinal neck pain, but that had dissipated. This new onset of weakness was accompanied by a feeling of numbness over the lateral right deltoid area. The patient realized while playing basketball that he was having difficulty taking shots because of right shoulder weakness. One week ago, he also noticed that extending the neck caused right shoulder pain, but that had improved. The past medical history was negative except for an episode of numbness in the lateral left deltoid area 3 years previously that had spontaneously resolved. Physical examination of the left upper limb was normal. The right upper limb showed no atrophy, but there was weakness of shoulder abduction, external rotation of the shoulder, and elbow flexion. There was a sensory deficit along the lateral right shoulder down to his thumb.

Thought process

The history and physical examination strongly suggested cervical radiculopathy at C6, but other root levels could be involved, such as C5 or C7. A brachial plexus problem such as injury to the upper trunk was also noted as a possibility. The sensory deficit was dermatomal in distribution, making it unlikely that it was due to radial, lateral antebrachial cutaneous, median, or other peripheral nerve etiology. Spinal cord injury or myelopathy is possible, but the history here is not compatible with spinal cord injury. Metastatic brain disease should always be considered in the differential diagnosis of a patient with numbness, but the time course of the disease and distribution of symptoms and signs in this patient indicated otherwise.

Based on the differential diagnosis, needle EMG was the most appropriate diagnostic test to accurately identify the location of the lesion causing the clinical presentation in this case. NCS can help evaluate for conduction block, mononeuropathy, brachial plexopathy, and degree of axonal loss (Table 12-1).

Discussion

A needle EMG examination of the right upper limb should be performed. This approach can accurately identify the anatomic level of the lesion. A needle EMG study is considered positive for radiculopathy if abnormalities are present in two or more muscles innervated by the same nerve root but different peripheral nerves, and abnormal findings are not detected in muscles innervated by unaffected roots above or below the abnormal root.[83]

Table 12-1 Shoulder weakness, numbness, and neck pain (case 1)

MONOPOLAR NEEDLE ELECTROMYOGRAPHY

Muscle		Spontaneous				MUAP			Recruitment pattern
	PSW	Fib	Fasc	HF	Amplitude	Duration	Poly	
R rhomboid major	None	None	None	None	N	N	N	N
R deltoid	2+	1+	None	None	N	N	N	1–
R biceps	2+	1+	None	None	N	N	N	1–
R brachioradialis	1+	None	None	None	N	N	N	1–
R triceps	None	None	None	None	N	N	N	N
R extensor carpi radialis longus	1+	None	None	None	N	N	N	N
R extensor digitorum communis	None	None	None	None	N	N	N	N
R pronator teres	1+	None	None	None	N	N	N	N
R 1st dorsal interosseus	None	None	None	None	N	N	N	N
R cervical spinal	1+	1+	None	None	N	N	N	1–

NERVE CONDUCTION STUDIES

Sensory nerve	Site	Recording site	Peak latency (ms)	Peak amplitude (μV)	Distance (cm)	Velocity (m/s)
R median: CTS screen	Median wrist	Digit 1	2.45	28.2	10	51.3
	Radial wrist	Digit 1	2.35	5.6	10	66.7
	Median wrist	Digit 3	3.05	35.1	14	54.9
	Median palm	Digit 3	1.85	38.5	7	63.6
	Ulnar wrist	Digit 5	3.35	26.4	14	53.8

Motor nerve	Site	Latency (ms)	Amplitude (mV)	Distance (cm)	Velocity (m/s)
R median: APB	Wrist	3.45	15.7	8	–
	Elbow	7.85	15.3	28	63.6
	Palm	2.15	15.0	–	–
R ulnar: ADM	Wrist	2.90	11.8	8	–
	Below elbow	6.95	11.3	24	59.3
	Above elbow	9.15	12.0	14	63.6

Fib, Fibrillation potentials; Fasc, fasciculation potentials; HF, complex repetitive discharges; MUAP, motor unit action potential; N, normal; Poly, polyphasic motor unit potentials; PSW, positive sharp waves.

The cervical paraspinal EMG findings indicated that the lesion was proximal to the brachial plexus. Normal sensory and motor NCS were also compatible with radiculopathy, because NCS tend to be normal except in some cases of severe radiculopathy. Positive waves and fibrillation potentials were found most prominently in the biceps and deltoids, as well as in other C6 spinal-innervated muscles and cervical paraspinals. The triceps (C7 and C8) and rhomboids (C5) were normal. There was also decreased recruitment in a C6 spinal nerve distribution, plus a 3-week history of right shoulder weakness. These findings are most compatible with an active right C6 radiculopathy.

Case 2

A 62-year-old man complained of having numbness of digits 4 and 5 of the right hand for 2 months. Recently, he had noted similar numbness in the left hand. Five years previously, he had developed pain and tingling across the dorsum of the entire right hand, especially digits 4 and 5. At that time, EDX studies showed evidence of C7 radiculopathy with no evidence of ulnar neuropathy. He responded well to cervical epidural steroid injections for 1 year, then noted that his symptoms were returning. He has had three courses of cervical epidural steroids in the past 3 years, the last one having been done 11 months ago. His physician is curious to better define the reason for the patient's now refractory upper limb symptoms.

Physical examination showed bilateral weakness of elbow flexion and external rotation of the shoulder. The remainder of upper limb manual muscle testing was normal. Muscle stretch reflexes showed that the right biceps brachii and triceps were 1+, with the brachioradialis being absent. The left biceps and triceps reflexes were absent, and there was a trace response of the brachioradialis. There was an ulnar distribution of sensory deficit on the left hand, and median sensory deficit on the right. It was not possible to further characterize the additional sensory dysfunction in the upper limbs, except to note that it was patchy in distribution.

Thought process

The initial clinical impression was that the patient had recurrent cervical radiculopathy at C7, because the clinical presentation was similar to his initial presentation 5 years ago of proven C7 radiculopathy. He had also had intermittent complaints or flare-ups that suggested an ongoing, low-grade process. Note the many incongruent sensory and motor findings that involve several spinal nerve levels.

In view of these findings, C7 radiculopathy is unlikely to be the only cause of his symptoms. The possibility of multilevel cervical radiculopathy has to considered, even though it is an uncommon occurrence. One should also consider problems involving the spinal cord. Cervical myelopathy and cervical stenosis causing cord compromise, with or without myelomalacia, were noted as possibilities. Considering the time course of the disease process and the patchy distribution of abnormal physical examination and EDX findings, a cervical syrinx or spinal tumor could also be involved.

Neural problems above the level of the spinal cord should always be kept in mind, but are not high on the list of differential diagnoses, given the past medical history. Ulnar and median nerve entrapment could explain some of the distal sensory findings, but not the muscle weakness proximal to the distribution of these nerves. F-wave studies of the bilateral median and ulnar nerves showed prolonged latencies, suggesting some degree of proximal conduction slowing.[22] Selected studies performed on this patient are listed in Table 12-2.

Discussion

The median sensory distal latency to digit 3 was marginally delayed bilaterally, and the right median motor distal latency was slightly delayed. The median motor nerve conduction velocity was borderline slow bilaterally. Taking the left median nerve sensory conduction studies into account, the patient had mild bilateral median mononeuropathy that explained only some of his findings. Ulnar NCS were normal bilaterally, excluding ulnar mononeuropathy. Needle EMG showed decreased recruitment and motor units of abnormally large amplitude and duration in muscles innervated from C5 through T1 bilaterally. Many unstable motor unit action potentials (MUAPs) were also recorded diffusely. The presence of unstable MUAPs in this scenario was best explained by ongoing or incomplete reinner-

vation. Chronic low-grade axonal degeneration and regeneration explained the decreased recruitment and the motor units of abnormally large amplitude and duration. Fasciculation potentials were recorded in many muscles explored. Fasciculations are generally absent in myopathy, but are frequently present in radiculopathy or myelopathy.[42]

The absence of abnormal membrane irritability can be explained by the very low-grade clinical process in this patient, or to the effect of cervical epidural steroids acting as membrane stabilizers. Absence of abnormal membrane irritability essentially removes motor neuron disease from consideration. The best explanation of the clinical and EDX findings in this case is multilevel cervical spinal stenosis. A magnetic resonance imaging (MRI) scan of the cervical spine prior to surgery showed multilevel spinal stenosis, moderate to severe at C5–C6 and C6–C7. At C4–C5, a large midline disk protrusion causing compression and flattening of the cord with edema, and myelomalacia was also noted.

Case 3

A 50-year-old woman complained of numbness of the right thumb that had been present for 3 or 4 months. She had also noted tingling if she applied the distal pad of her thumb to the index finger. There were no complaints of pain. Further questioning showed that she had right hand weakness and had been requesting others to open jars for her. She had been dropping things and reported that her handwriting now 'looked like chicken scratching'. Past medical history was positive for hydrocephalus, severe unremitting headache, and difficulty walking, for which a shunt that drained into her peritoneum had been placed several years ago. She had recovered completely and been essentially asymptomatic.

Physical examination showed a right median nerve pattern of sensory deficit to light touch. There was a sensory deficit to pinprick on digit 1 of the right hand, but hyperesthesia on digit 2. There was no reliable pattern of sensory deficit on testing the remaining digits of the right hand, forearm, and arm. Sensory examination of the left upper limb was normal. Muscle stretch reflexes of the biceps and brachioradialis were normal bilaterally, and the triceps reflex was absent bilaterally. Manual muscle testing showed weakness of thumb abductors on the right, but strength was otherwise normal in all other major muscle groups in the upper limbs.

Thought process

The most probable etiology of this lady's complaints was at the spinal cord level. Cervical spine canal stenosis was a consideration. Cervical syrinx, although not common, was higher on the list of possibilities because of the history of shunt placement for hydrocephalus in the remote past. A lesion or mass impinging on the spinal cord was also considered. A supraspinal etiology should also be included in the differential diagnosis of diffuse or incongruent neurologic findings in a limb.

Further questioning showed that she was also experiencing hand weakness on the symptomatic side sufficient to interfere with some aspects of activities of daily living. There were a

Table 12-2 Numbness of the hand (case 2)

MONOPOLAR NEEDLE ELECTROMYOGRAPHY

| | | Spontaneous | | | | MUAP | | Recruitment pattern |
	PSW	Fib	Fasc	HF	Amplitude	Duration	Poly	
R deltoid	None	None	None	None	1+	1+	N	1−
R biceps	None	None	1+	None	N	1+	3+	2−
R brachioradialis	None	None	None	None	N	N	1+	N
R triceps	None	None	None	None	1+	2+	2+	2−
R extensor carpi radialis longus	None	None	2+ (slow)	None	N	1+	N	1−
R extensor digitorum communis	None	None	1+	None	1+	1+	1+	Discrete
R flexor carpi ulnaris	None	None	None	None	N	N	1+	1−
R flexor carpi radialis	None	None	None	None	N	N	1+	1−
R extensor carpi ulnaris	None	None	None	None	N	1+	1+	2−
R 1st dorsal interosseus	None	None	None	None	N	1+	N	2−
L deltoid	None	None	None	None	1+	1+	1+	1−
L biceps	None	None	None	None	1+	1+	N	1−
L triceps	None	None	None	None	2+	2+	N	Discrete
L brachioradialis	None	None	1+	None	N	N	1+	2−
L extensor digitorum communis	None	None	None	None	2+	N	N	2−
L 1st dorsal interosseus	None	None	2+ (slow)	None	2+	2+	N	Discrete
L extensor carpi radialis longus	None	None	1+	None	1+	1+	N	1−
L cervical paraspinal	None	None	None	None	N	N	N	N

NERVE CONDUCTION STUDIES

Sensory nerve	Site	Recording site	Peak latency (ms)	Peak amplitude (μV)	Distance (cm)	Velocity (m/s)
L median: CTS screen	Median wrist	Digit 1	3.15	11.3	10	42.6
	Radial wrist	Digit 1	2.90	3.0	10	42.6
	Median wrist	Digit 3	4.35	7.2	14	40.6
	Median palm	Digit 3	2.45	8.4	7	43.8
	Ulnar wrist	Digit 5	3.80	11.0	14	48.3
R median: CTS screen	Median wrist	Digit 1	3.45	7.0	10	37.0
	Radial wrist	Digit 1	3.10	3.3	10	45.5
	Median wrist	Digit 3	4.25	9.6	14	41.8
	Median palm	Digit 3	2.35	5.6	7	38.9
	Ulnar wrist	Digit 5	3.95	10.3	14	45.2

Motor nerve	Site	Latency (ms)	Amplitude (mV)	Distance (cm)	Velocity (m/s)
L median: APB	Wrist	4.20	10.5	8	–
	Elbow	8.10	10.9	20	51.2
	Axilla	–	–	–	–
	Palm	2.05	12.4	–	–
L ulnar: ADM	Wrist	3.35	8.9	8	–
	Below elbow	6.80	8.6	20	58.0
	Above elbow	8.70	8.2	12	63.2
R median: APB	Wrist	4.45	7.3	8	–
	Elbow	8.90	6.9	22	50.0
	Axilla	2.20	8.6	–	–
R ulnar: ADM	Wrist	3.20	11.3	8	–
	Below elbow	7.05	10.8	23	59.7
	Above elbow	8.85	10.4	11	61.1

Fib, Fibrillation potentials; Fasc, fasciculation potentials; HF, complex repetitive discharges; MUAP, motor unit action potential; N, normal; Poly, polyphasic motor unit potentials; PSW, positive sharp waves.

number of diagnostic possibilities, because there was no clear distribution of sensory dysfunction. An individual peripheral nerve lesion was unlikely, because neurologic findings were noted across peripheral nerve territories. A brachial plexus problem should be considered, but normal motor and nearly normal sensory nerve conductions made brachial plexopathy less likely. It was felt that the pathology was most probably at the spinal cord level. Results of EDX studies done on this patient are listed in Table 12-3.

Discussion

The needle EMG findings were comparatively few in relation to the patient's complaints and physical findings. There are no clinical or EDX findings known to be typical or pathognomic of syrinx, posttraumatic or otherwise. A wide range of findings are possible, including involuntary movements, respiratory synkinesis, continuous motor unit activity, myokymic discharges, ulnar neuropathy at the elbow, dissociated sensory loss, and muscle atrophy. Therefore the electromyographer must have a high level of suspicion regarding the possibility that a syrinx could be the cause of the patient's complaints.[4,57,58,75] In this case, abnormal muscle membrane irritability was not elicited, making motor neuron disease unlikely. There was decreased recruitment, and also motor units of abnormally large amplitude in the hand muscles and in the lateral triceps. Motor NCS were essentially normal. The plan to return for additional EDX studies never materialized. F-wave studies would probably have been abnormal, and would have suggested a proximal conduction problem, but were not done per patient preference. Multifocal mononeuropathy with conduction block was excluded by normal motor NCS. Bilateral median sensory NCS were normal. Needle EMG abnormalities were limited mostly to the hand, suggesting C8 or T1 pathology. In the absence of isolated peripheral nerve pathology, no clear evidence of brachial plexus involvement, needle EMG findings that were outside a single peripheral nerve territory, and incongruous sensory deficit, a central or spinal cord etiology was the most likely diagnosis.

Presurgical MRI showed abnormal signal intensity from C4–C5 through T7–T8, with a suggestion of underlying syrinx. Neurosurgical intervention confirmed syrinx from C5–T8.

Case 4

A 64-year-old woman was referred to the EDX laboratory with complaints of pain and numbness of the hands and feet, worse at night, present for 5 years. The symptoms have been worsening recently. She also reported experiencing total body pain, worse in the extremities, and morning stiffness lasting 3 h. The patient reported joint swelling, especially of the fingers and ankles. Past medical history was positive for osteoarthritis, adult-onset diabetes mellitus, hypertension, and fibromyalgia.

Physical examination showed a stocking and glove distribution of sensory deficit to pinprick and light touch bilaterally. Muscle stretch reflexes in the upper limbs were somewhat asymmetric. The biceps was absent on the left and trace on the right. The left brachioradialis and triceps were trace, while the right side showed trace biceps and absent brachioradialis and triceps. Muscle stretch reflexes were absent at the knees and ankles. Manual muscle testing was normal, except for slightly decreased grip strength and moderately decreased thumb abduction strength bilaterally.

Thought process

Bilateral carpal tunnel syndrome in the presence of polyneuropathy secondary to diabetes mellitus is the best explanation for the clinical presentation in this patient. Progressive pain and numbness of the extremities over a period of years, worse at night, is a characteristic feature of diabetic polyneuropathy.[39] The timing of the disease process here would not support the diagnosis of a more acute acquired polyneuropathy. Arthritis could be a contributory factor causing pain but would not explain the sensory findings. There was no history of alcohol intake or abuse, heavy metal contamination, or other obvious causes of polyneuropathy. Isolated or multiple mononeuropathy might be present, but the symptoms of a motor and sensory polyneuropathy would make it difficult to identify multiple mononeuropathy without the benefit of EDX studies.

Multifocal mononeuropathy with conduction block is highly unlikely, because the slight weakness of the upper extremities observed on physical examination is symmetric, unlike the asymmetric focal weakness noted in multifocal mononeuropathy.[2] Sensory symptoms would be unusual in multifocal mononeuropathy. Weakness of the abductor pollicis brevis bilaterally suggests bilateral carpal tunnel syndrome coexisting with diabetic polyneuropathy. Results of EDX studies done on this patient are listed in Table 12-4. In the interest of brevity, only EDX findings from the upper limbs are presented and discussed.

Discussion

There are a range of abnormal findings in diabetic neuropathy, and symptomatic patients are more likely to show EDX abnormalities than asymptomatic patients are.[39] Patients with diabetic neuropathy and more likely to have slower nerve conduction velocity and diminished sensory nerve action potentials (SNAPs) and compound muscle action potentials (CMAPs) than those without symptoms.[39] The radial SNAPs are of normal latency but abnormally low in amplitude, with near-normal conduction velocity, compatible with an axonal problem. The median and ulnar SNAPs are absent bilaterally. However, the ulnar motor distal latencies are normal bilaterally, and amplitudes of the ulnar compound motor action potentials are normal. In the presence of abnormally slow conduction velocity, this would indicate a problem with myelin. Finally, the median motor distal latency across the carpal ligament was tremendously delayed bilaterally, the median CMAP is severely reduced in amplitude, and median nerve conduction velocity is abnormally slow bilaterally.

Needle EMG showed mildly decreased recruitment and an increased percentage of motor units high in amplitude in a few muscles of the upper limbs. This is compatible with chronic low-grade polyneuropathy. There is also evidence of severe

Table 12-3 Numbness of the thumb (case 3)

MONOPOLAR NEEDLE ELECTROMYOGRAPHY

	I activity	Spontaneous Fib	PSW	Fasc	HF	Amplitude	MUAP Duration	Poly	Recruitment pattern[a]
R triceps	N	None	None	None	None	1+	N	N	–
R 1st dorsal interosseus	N	None	None	None	None	1+	N	N	– –
R abductor pollicis brevis	N	None	None	None	None	1+	N	N	– –
R biceps	N	None	None	None	None	N	N	N	N
R deltoid	N	None	None	None	None	N	N	N	N
R brachioradialis	N	None	None	None	None	N	N	N	N
R pronator teres	N	None	None	None	None	N	N	N	N
R extensor digitorum communis	N	None	None	None	None	N	N	N	N
R extensor carpi radialis brevis	N	None	None	None	None	N	N	N	N
R abductor digiti minimi	N	None	None	None	None	1+	N	N	–
R cervical paraspinal (low)	N	None	None	None	None	1+	N	N	
R cervical paraspinal (mid)	N	None	None	None	None	N	N	N	
R cervical paraspinal (upper)	N	None	None	None	None	N	N	N	
R thoracic paraspinal (upper)	N	None	None	None	None	N	N	N	

NERVE CONDUCTION STUDIES

Sensory nerve	Site	Recording site	Peak latency (ms)	Peak amplitude (µV)	Distance (cm)	Velocity (m/s)
R median: CTS screen	Median wrist	Digit 1	2.65	15.8	10	60.6
	Radial wrist	Digit 1	2.60	17.7	10	51.3
	Median wrist	Digit 3	3.25	28.8	14	59.6
	Median palm	Digit 3	1.95	11.0	7	48.3
L median: CTS screen	Median wrist	Digit 1	2.40	33.3	10	66.7
	Radial wrist	Digit 1	2.65	13.6	10	47.6
	Median wrist	Digit 3	3.45	33.7	14	54.9
	Median palm	Digit 3	–	–	7	–

Motor nerve	Site	Latency (ms)	Amplitude (mV)	Distance (cm)	Velocity (m/s)
R median: APB	Wrist	3.10	12.4	8	–
	Elbow	6.55	12.9	21	60.9
	Palm	–	–	–	–
	EP	2.00	12.4	–	–
R ulnar: ADM	Wrist	3.05	13.9	–	–
	Below elbow	6.35	13.0	19.5	59.1
	Above elbow	8.40	12.1	13	63.4

Fib, Fibrillation potentials; Fasc, fasciculation potentials; HF, complex repetitive discharges; MUAP, motor unit action potential; N, normal; Poly, polyphasic motor unit potentials; PSW, positive sharp waves.
[a]Monopolar needle electromyography: –, reduced; – –, significantly reduced.

Table 12-4 Pain and numbness of hands and feet (case 4)

NERVE CONDUCTION STUDIES

Sensory nerve	Site	Recording site	Peak latency (ms)	Peak amplitude (μV)	Distance (cm)	Velocity (m/s)
L median: CTS screen	Median wrist	Digit 1	No response	–	10	–
	Radial wrist	Digit 1	2.60	1.6	10	48.8
	Median wrist	Digit 3	No response	–	14	–
	Median palm	Digit 3	No response	–	7	–
	Ulnar wrist	Digit 5	No response	–	14	–
R median: CTS screen	Median wrist	Digit 1	No response	–	10	–
	Radial wrist	Digit 1	2.80	1.7	10	47.6
	Median wrist	Digit 3	No response	–	14	–
	Median palm	Digit 3	No response	–	7	–
	Ulnar wrist	Digit 5	No response	–	14	–

Motor nerve	Site	Latency (ms)	Amplitude (mV)	Distance (cm)	Velocity (m/s)
R median: APB	Wrist	13.00	3.8	8	–
	Elbow	19.05	2.5	21.5	35.5
	Palm	2.75	3.3	–	–
L ulnar: ADM	Wrist	3.65	10.5	–	–
	Below elbow	7.85	9.7	20	47.6
	Above elbow	10.60	9.5	14	50.9
R ulnar: ADM	Wrist	3.35	11.6	8	–
	Below elbow	7.90	10.9	22	48.4
	Above elbow	10.55	9.9	13	49.1
L median: APB	Wrist	12.00	4.7	8	–
	Elbow	17.45	4.0	23.5	43.1
	Palm	3.25	3.6	–	–

bilateral carpal tunnel syndrome superimposed on diabetic polyneuropathy with mixed axonal sensory and motor features. The evidence for this includes the absent ulnar and median SNAPs; the abnormally low-amplitude radial SNAPs with normal distal latency; the great disparity in median and ulnar motor latency, with ulnar being normal and median very significantly delayed; the normal ulnar CMAPs; the abnormally small median CMAPs; and the abnormally slow ulnar and median motor conduction velocity.

Case 5

A 36-year-old, right-handed truck driver developed pain and numbness in his right hand after starting a new job that required long hours of driving. He described the sensory changes as a feeling of numbness that at times became painful and affected the whole hand. When the pain was at its worst, his forearm and shoulder also became uncomfortable. In retrospect, he had experienced similar symptoms but to a milder degree over the past few years, especially at times when his work schedule kept him busier than usual. Holding a tight grip on the steering wheel for hours at a time made the sensory changes worse, and he frequently would shake his hand to try to relieve the symptoms. He occasionally experienced a similar discomfort on awakening

in the morning. Recently, he had been dropping things from the right hand without warning. He had not experienced sensory changes in the left hand. He sought medical attention when he noticed that he was having a harder time gripping the steering wheel.

Clinical examination demonstrated normal strength in all muscle groups of both upper limbs, as well as normal, symmetric muscle stretch reflexes. The sensory symptoms were reproduced on the right by tapping the anterior wrist (Tinel's sign) and by holding the wrist in flexion (Phalen's sign). Careful sensory examination using a safety pin showed slightly diminished sensation distributed mainly over the second and third digits and part of the palm of the hand.

Thought process

The most likely cause for the symptoms in this patient would be median nerve compression at the wrist, typical of carpal tunnel syndrome. The worsening of symptoms with repeated use of the hands and the presence of symptoms in the dominant hand[68] are supportive of that diagnosis. The presence of Tinel's and Phalen's sign on physical examination also supports the diagnosis of carpal tunnel syndrome, but neither of these signs is perfectly sensitive or specific. His description of frequently shaking the hand (flick sign)[67] is commonly described in the carpal tunnel syndrome. Although occurrence of pain in the forearm and shoulder is often seen in carpal tunnel syndrome,[45] a more proximal injury to the median nerve and an injury to the C6 or C7 nerve root must also be considered in the differential diagnosis. A 'double-crush' injury,[82] in this case a median nerve injury at the wrist plus an additional injury more proximally, should also be considered as a diagnostic possibility.

Because a median nerve injury at the carpal tunnel is the most likely diagnosis, median nerve conductions should be performed. Slowing of the median sensory conduction across the wrist is the most common abnormality on the EDX examination.[13,41,43,76] The sensory conduction velocity should be compared with that of the ulnar nerve to distinguish a median mononeuropathy from a length-dependent polyneuropathy, or from slowing due to cooling of the limb. In moderately severe median nerve injuries at the wrist, the distal latency of the median motor conduction is delayed. In more proximal median nerve injuries, the conduction velocity across the injury might be slowed,[78,79] as can the F wave. However, mild slowing of the conduction velocity in the forearm can also be seen in carpal tunnel syndrome, especially if the distal latency is prolonged.

In severe median nerve injuries at the carpal tunnel, there is denervation (i.e. axonal loss) of median-supplied muscles of the hand, causing changes on needle electrode examination (e.g. positive sharp waves, fibrillation potentials). In the case of a cervical nerve root injury, muscles supplied by the involved nerve root would be expected to show similar changes. Results of EDX studies done on this patient are listed in Table 12-5.

Discussion

As is the case with almost all median nerve injuries in the carpal tunnel, the median sensory conduction is slowed across the right wrist—both when compared with the laboratory's normal values and when compared with the velocity of the ulnar nerve conduction in the same segment. The slowing of the velocity from the palm to the wrist compared with the velocity from the second digit to the wrist further supports the wrist (carpal tunnel) as the site of injury. The additional finding of a delayed distal latency of the right median motor conduction (the segment of the nerve that passes through the carpal tunnel) indicates that this is at least a moderately severe injury. The slight slowing of the conduction velocity in the forearm is often associated with moderate to severe median nerve injuries at the carpal tunnel but, without comparison with the motor conduction velocity in another nerve, a polyneuropathy cannot be excluded as a cause for these changes. The normal ulnar NCS and the normal F-wave latencies support the theory that this patient has a focal abnormality of the median nerve rather than a more diffuse polyneuropathy.

Patients with carpal tunnel syndrome who have significant findings on NCS of the more symptomatic limb often have milder or even subclinical changes in the opposite limb. Left median NCS were also performed, and showed that the left median sensory conductions were slowed across the wrist. The motor conductions were entirely normal, however, suggesting a relatively mild injury of the left median nerve at the carpal tunnel.

The needle electrode examination of the right upper limb muscles selected to evaluate the C5–T1 nerve roots and the major motor nerves of the right upper limb was entirely normal, making a superimposed nerve root injury or brachial plexopathy very unlikely. The absence of signs of active denervation (i.e. fibrillation potentials, positive sharp waves) in the abductor pollicis brevis muscle indicated that the axons supplying the muscle were intact. The same muscle was examined during a limited needle electrode study of the left hand to evaluate further the severity of the left median nerve injury, and was found to be normal. The patient was diagnosed with a moderately severe right median neuropathy at the carpal tunnel and a mild left median neuropathy at the carpal tunnel.

Case 6

A 33-year-old man presented with complaints of numbness along the ulnar border of the hand bilaterally, and also of cold intolerance. About 9 months previously, he had fallen on his right elbow while playing volleyball, and 8 days later presented with pain and swelling, numbness, and tingling of digits 2 through 4 of the right hand. There was purple discoloration of the right hand but strength was normal. The right hand was objectively warmer than the left. He was diagnosed with complex regional pain syndrome of the right upper limb and treated aggressively. He also reported that the swelling of the right hand was gone, but he still had cold intolerance of the right hand, and numbness and tingling of digits 4 and 5 of the hand bilaterally, right more than left. Note that the left hand was not initially involved when he was injured 9 months ago. He admitted to habitually leaning on the elbows.

Physical examination showed normal grip strength bilaterally. There was a positive Tinel's sign at the right ulnar groove. There was decreased appreciation to light touch and pinprick involving digits 4 and 5 of the left hand. There was no consistent pattern of sensory deficit when testing the right hand.

Thought process

There appears to be a number of processes occurring concurrently. There is good clinical evidence for a partially resolved complex regional pain syndrome of the right upper limb, with possible mirror imaging on the left. The history of trauma to the right elbow, followed by subsequent hand discoloration, temperature differential, cold intolerance pain, and sensory dysfunction not fitting a specific peripheral nerve territory confirmed the clinical impression of a complex regional pain syndrome. The inconsistent right sensory evaluation caused some difficulty in identifying a possible right ulnar neuropathy at the elbow. The physical examination on the left side, however, supported an ulnar nerve distribution of sensory deficit. Because the patient admitted to habitually leaning on the elbows, it was felt that a diagnosis of bilateral ulnar neuropathy at the elbows was justified. Chronic manifestations of complex regional pain syndrome Type 1 of the right upper limb were also in evidence.

Table 12-5 Pain and numbness in the hand (case 5)

NERVE CONDUCTION STUDIES

Sensory nerve	Stimulation site	Recording site	Amplitude (μV)	Conduction velocity (m/s)
R median	Digit 2	Wrist	14 (N > 10)	42 (N > 50)
	Palm	Wrist	32	38 (N ≥ 50)
R ulnar	Digit 5	Wrist	16 (N ≥ 10)	56 (N ≥ 50)
L median	Digit 2	Wrist	17 (N ≥ 10)	49 (N ≥ 50)
	Palm	Wrist	62	45 (N ≥ 50)
L ulnar	Digit 5	Wrist	15 (N≥ 10)	58 (N ≥ 50)

Motor nerve	Stimulation site	Latency (ms)	Conduction velocity (m/s)	Amplitude (mV)
R median (record thenar)	Wrist	4.6 (N < 4.3)	–	4.3
	Elbow	–	49 (N > 50)	4.0
R median F wave	–	29 (N < 32)	–	–
R ulnar (record hypothenar)	Wrist	3.3 (N < 3.5)	–	5.2
	Below elbow	–	54 (N > 50)	5.0
	Above elbow	–	51 (N > 50)	5.0
R ulnar F wave	–	28 (N <32)	–	–
L median (record thenar)	Wrist	4.0 (N < 4.3)	–	4.9
	Elbow	–	53 (N > 50)	4.7
R median F wave	–	27 (N < 32)	–	–

CONCENTRIC NEEDLE ELECTROMYOGRAPHY STUDIES

Muscle	Spontaneous activity		Recruitment	Motor unit potentials	
	Positive waves	Fibrillation potentials		Amplitude	Duration
R deltoid	0	0	N	N	N
R biceps	0	0	N	N	N
R triceps	0	0	N	N	N
R 1st dorsal interosseus	0	0	N	N	N
R abductor pollicis brevis	0	0	N	N	N
L abductor pollicis brevis	0	0	N	N	N

Results of EDX studies done on this patient are listed in Table 12-6.

Discussion

The ulnar sensory nerve distal latencies were normal bilaterally; but the left ulnar distal latency was slightly slower than the corresponding median sensory distal latency to digit 3 at 14 cm. There was slowing of the ulnar motor conduction velocity across the elbow bilaterally, 5% on the right and 20% on the left. There was a corresponding 20% drop in amplitude of the right ulnar CMAP across the elbow, and a 23% drop in ulnar CMAP across the elbow on the left. A drop in amplitude and conduction velocity stimulating across the elbow are commonly accepted criteria for diagnosing ulnar neuropathy at the elbow.[33,38] A slight difference in waveform morphology was noted when stimulating distal versus proximal to the elbows. Changes in waveforms are thought to be more sensitive than a 10% drop in motor conduction velocity across the elbow.[38] It is recommended that ulnar NCS be performed with the elbow in the flexed position, as this position has been shown to render more accurate results.[44] Bilateral median motor and sensory, and bilateral radial sensory NCS were normal. Needle EMG of the upper limbs was normal. The final diagnosis was bilateral ulnar mononeuropathy across the elbow in the presence of complex regional pain syndrome of the right upper limb.

Table 12-6 Bilateral numbness of digits 4 and 5 of the hand (case 6)

NERVE CONDUCTION STUDIES						
Sensory nerve	Site	Recording site	Peak latency (ms)	Peak amplitude (μV)	Distance (cm)	Velocity (m/s)
R median: CTS screen	Median wrist	Digit 1	2.60	18.5	10	58.8
	Radial wrist	Digit 1	3.05	6.2	10	40.0
	Median wrist	Digit 3	3.45	16.5	14	51.9
	Median palm	Digit 3	2.15	15.8	7	46.7
	Ulnar wrist	Digit 5	3.45	14.7	14	53.8
L median: CTS screen	Median wrist	Digit 1	3.10	15.8	10	43.5
	Radial wrist	Digit 1	2.95	4.8	10	45.5
	Median wrist	Digit 3	Normal	Normal	14	–
	Median palm	Digit 3	Normal	Normal	7	–
	Ulnar wrist	Digit 5	3.85	20.9	14	47.5

Motor nerve	Site	Latency (ms)	Amplitude	Distance (cm)	Velocity (m/s)
R median: APB	Wrist	3.85	13.7	8	–
	Elbow	7.45	13.3	26	72.2
	Palm	2.15	11.6	–	–
L median: APB	Wrist	3.95	9.2	8	–
	Elbow	8.60	8.9	27	58.1
	Palm	2.25	9.5	–	–
R ulnar: ADM	Wrist	3.15	11.4	–	–
	Below elbow	7.05	10.5	25	64.1
	Above elbow	9.25	9.0	13	59.0
L ulnar: ADM	Wrist	3.35	11.3	–	–
	Below elbow	7.65	10.3	27	62.8
	Above elbow	10.45	8.7	14.5	51.8

Case 7

A 52-year-old, right-handed man was noted to have weakness of his left arm during recovery from abdominal surgery. The postoperative course was complicated by slightly delayed weaning from the ventilator, and he was not able to get up in a chair until the third postoperative day. By the fifth postoperative day, it was noted that he had diminished movement of his left arm. He denied feeling pain in the neck, shoulder, or arm but did report a feeling of 'numbness' over the left shoulder and lateral arm that 'comes and goes'. There was no history of previous neck pain or trauma, nor was there history of shoulder trauma or weakness.

Examination showed that the patient held the limb adducted and internally rotated at the shoulder. He was unable to abduct the shoulder or flex the elbow against gravity. Wrist flexion and elbow extension were also weak, but less so than shoulder abduction and elbow flexion. The biceps and brachioradialis reflexes were absent on the left but normal on the right. Sensation was slightly diminished to pinprick over the lateral shoulder, arm, and forearm down to the base of the thumb.

The weakness improved somewhat during the second postoperative week. Elbow extension and wrist flexion strength returned to normal. Shoulder abduction and elbow flexion improved to the point that they slightly better than antigravity.

Thought process

The best explanations for the distribution of weakness were injuries to the C5, C6, and C7 nerve roots or to the upper and middle trunks of the brachial plexus. Injuries to the upper trunk or C5–C6 would better explain the sensory changes. The return to normal of strength in the C7–middle trunk-innervated muscles suggested that part of the injury was less severe than the C5 and C6–upper trunk lesion.

The occurrence of focal paralysis such as seen in this case in the postoperative setting is usually attributed to poor positioning of the patient on the operating table, leading to traction on the brachial plexus and/or the cervical nerve roots.[36] In those cases, a stretch injury is thought to result in focal demyelination, and good recovery occurs within a few weeks. If the traction is sustained, however, a more severe nerve injury can occur, leading to some degree of axonal degeneration. Another cause of brachial plexopathy in the postoperative setting is neuralgic amyotrophy (Parsonage–Turner syndrome).[61] The cause of the condition is unknown but thought to be autoimmune-mediated. However, this syndrome is typically accompanied by severe pain with sudden onset.

The EDX examination provided useful information to help localize the lesion (cervical nerve root(s) versus brachial plexus versus both) and predict severity (focal demyelination versus axonal degeneration). Changes on sensory studies of reduced amplitudes of the sensory responses indicated that the lesion was located distally to the dorsal root ganglion, i.e. at the level of the brachial plexus or nerve trunk. Abnormal findings on needle electrode examination can help localize the lesion, but might not distinguish plexus from root lesion very early in the process. All the EDX changes resulting from the lesion might not yet be present, assuming the injury occurred at the time of surgery some 12 days earlier. Reduced recruitment of motor

unit potentials could be due to either demyelinating or axonal injuries. It might be too early to see fibrillation potentials, because the effects of Wallerian degeneration can take up to 3 weeks to show up as abnormal membrane irritability on needle EMG. However, needle EMG of the paraspinal muscles can show abnormal membrane irritability as early as 7–8 days after the onset of radicular symptoms.[16] Results of EDX studies done on this patient are listed in Table 12-7.

Discussion

Several abnormal findings were seen on this study. Side to side comparison of the superficial radial SNAP showed that the amplitude of the response on the affected left side was very abnormal, because it was less than 50% of the amplitude of the response on the unaffected right side. The superficial radial

Table 12-7 Left upper limb weakness (case 7)

NERVE CONDUCTION STUDIES

Sensory nerve	Stimulation site	Recording site	Amplitude (µV)	Conduction velocity (m/s)
L median	Digit 2	Wrist	19 (N > 10)	55 (N > 50)
	Palm	Wrist	76	57 (N > 50)
L ulnar	Digit 5	Wrist	15 (N > 10)	58 (N > 50)
L superficial radial	Forearm	Wrist	16	56
R superficial radial	Forearm	Wrist	36	61

Motor nerve	Stimulation site	Latency (ms)	Conduction velocity (m/s)	Amplitude (mV)
L median (record thenar)	Wrist	4.1 (N < 4.3)	–	5.1 (N > 4.0)
	Elbow	–	52 (N > 50)	4.8
L median F wave	–	31 (N < 32)	–	–
L ulnar (record hypothenar)	Wrist	3.3 (N < 3.5)	–	4.8 (N > 4.0)
	Below elbow	–	54 (N > 50)	4.2
	Above elbow	–	52 (N > 50)	4.2
L ulnar F wave	–	30 (N < 32)	–	–

CONCENTRIC NEEDLE ELECTROMYOGRAPHY STUDIES

| Muscle | Spontaneous activity | | Recruitment | Motor unit potentials | |
	Positive waves	Fibrillation potentials		Amplitude	Duration
L deltoid	2+	2+	Decreased	N	N
L biceps	2+	2+	Decreased	N	N
L triceps	1+	0	Decreased	N	N
L flexor carpi radialis	1+	0	Decreased	N	N
L extensor digitorum communis	0	0	N	N	N
L 1st dorsal interosseus	0	0	N	N	N
L abductor pollicis brevis	0	0	N	N	N
L midcervical paraspinal	0	0	–	–	–

sensory nerve is composed mainly of fibers from the upper trunk of the brachial plexus. The median and ulnar sensory amplitudes were within normal limits, and a side to side comparison was not made, because the distribution of the patient's clinical symptoms was less suggestive of a lower trunk (ulnar sensory) or middle trunk (median sensory) injury. The findings on sensory conductions suggested a significant upper trunk injury in this clinical setting, but a more peripheral injury to either the radial nerve or the superficial radial branch could not be excluded as a diagnostic possibility by these findings alone.

The findings on needle electrode examination were indicative of active denervation (i.e. axonal degeneration) affecting primarily the deltoid and biceps (innervated by C5 and C6 roots and the upper trunk of the brachial plexus), with less severe involvement of the triceps and flexor carpi ulnaris (innervated by C6 and C7 roots and a combination of the middle and upper trunks). The normal findings on examination of the paraspinal muscles were more suggestive of a plexopathy than a radiculopathy.

The absence of changes in the extensor digitorum communis muscle made lesions of the radial nerve, C7 and C8 nerve roots, and lower and middle trunks of the brachial plexus very unlikely, given the severity of changes in affected muscles. If the needle electrode examination had been normal, or if the only abnormalities had been reduced recruitment of motor unit potentials, a follow-up study would have been recommended in 2 weeks to look for signs of active denervation after Wallerian degeneration would be complete. But, in this case, a follow-up study was not needed to make the diagnosis.

The patient was diagnosed with an injury to the upper trunk of the left brachial plexus, presumed to be due to positioning during surgery. The presence of motor unit potentials in the affected muscles, although with reduced recruitment, indicated the nerve injury was incomplete, so surgical treatment was not appropriate. Reinnervation after such proximal nerve injuries with significant axonal degeneration is a very slow process that can take many months. However, significant gains in function can occur within a few weeks, due to repair of the demyelinating component of the injury.

Case 8

A 58-year-old man presented with a 6-week history of constant bilateral hand and wrist pain. Digits 2–5 were primarily affected. If he were to accidentally strike a finger, he experienced a much higher level of pain than would be anticipated. There was stiffness of the fingers, causing difficulty when making a fist. Making a fist induced pain in the finger joints. He reported swelling of the finger joints and random bilateral intense shooting pain on the ulnar border of the forearm when the hand was in the anatomic position. No particular triggers were recorded for his pain. The patient reported constantly experiencing the perception of having the skin being scraped off the distal ulnar border of the forearm bilaterally. He was extremely sensitive and responded with pain to a number of usually innocuous stimuli. Past medical history was significant for hypertension and polymyalgia rheumatica. At the time of the EDX studies, he had been treated with methotrexate for 1 week and reported much improvement in his symptoms.

Physical examination showed muscle stretch reflexes that were generally 3+ and symmetric, except that the triceps were 2+ and symmetric. Despite the history of hyperesthesia, sensory responses to light touch and pinprick were normal. Grip strength was weak bilaterally, the right more affected than the left. Generally, he showed some degree of pain inhibition weakness of the upper limbs and normal strength in the lower. An accurate quantification of the upper limb strength deficit was not obvious clinically. There was tenderness on using moderately firm pressure on palpation of the right finger joints, but no complaints on the left. He verbalized increased strength and decreased symptoms since starting methotrexate a few days earlier.

Thought process

A rheumatic process would be high on the list of differential diagnoses for this patient. He had painful, stiff joints and bilateral hand weakness that responded to a disease-modifying, antirheumatic, antiinflammatory agent within a matter of days. The history and physical findings were compatible with a systemic vasculitis associated with giant cell arteritis affecting large- and medium-sized vessels.[6,24] Inflammatory disease of muscle had to be considered, but weakness was not the presenting symptom, and he seemed to be experiencing neuropathic pain. The patient is unlikely to have one of the common inflammatory myopathies, including polymyositis, dermatomyositis, or inclusion body myositis, as neuropathic pain is not typical of these conditions. The most probable diagnosis in this patient is neuropathy secondary to polymyalgia rheumatica.[24] Systemic vasculitides such as polyarteritis nodosa must also be kept in mind. Bilateral ulnar mononeuropathy is possible and could be superimposed on a primary disease process, as the patient's symptoms are clearly more involved than would be expected with isolated ulnar mononeuropathy. Results of EDX studies done on this patient are listed in Table 12-8.

Discussion

Sensory NCS in the upper limbs reveal a general pattern of delayed distal latency, abnormally small amplitudes, and slowed conduction velocity. SNAPs are not recordable in the left lower limb. Motor conduction studies of the upper limbs show essentially normal distal latencies but slowed conduction velocities. There is bilateral slowing of the ulnar nerve conduction velocity across the elbow, with decreased CMAP amplitude, compatible with bilateral ulnar neuropathy across the elbow. The median nerve CMAP is severely reduced bilaterally, and conduction velocity is slowed. However, there is no matching delay in distal latency that would normally accompany carpal tunnel syndrome. The median nerve findings are not on the basis of carpal tunnel syndrome. Motor NCS in the lower limbs show delayed distal latency, abnormally small CMAPs, and slowed conduction velocity. There is decreased F-wave persistence of the left tibial nerve, because there is an F wave in only 2 out of 10 responses. The onset of the shortest F-wave latency is at 70 ms.[22] Needle

Table 12-8 Bilateral wrist and hand pain (case 8)

NERVE CONDUCTION STUDIES

Sensory nerve	Site	Recording site	Peak latitude (ms)	Peak amplitude (µV)	Distance (cm)	Velocity (m/s)
R median: CTS screen	Median wrist	Digit 1	3.20	12.1	10	38.5
	Radial wrist	Digit 1	3.45	5.5	10	34.5
	Median wrist	Digit 3	4.50	12.8	14	38.9
	Median palm	Digit 3	2.40	4.3	7	35.9
	Ulnar wrist	Digit 5	4.15	6.4	14	41.2
L median: CTS screen	Median wrist	Digit 1	3.55	21.3	10	35.7
	Radial wrist	Digit 1	3.70	5.8	10	32.3
	Median wrist	Digit 3	4.45	18.9	14	39.4
	Median palm	Digit 4	2.75	21.5	7	36.8
	Ulnar wrist	Digit 5	4.80	12.8	14	36.8
L sural: lat malleolus	Calf	Lat malleolus	No response	No response		
L sup peroneal: foot	Lateral leg	Foot	No response	No response		
R sural: lat malleolus	Calf	Lat malleolus	No response	No response		
R sup peroneal: foot	Lateral leg	Foot	No response	No response		

Motor nerve	Site	Latency (ms)	Amplitude (mV)	Distance (cm)	Velocity (m/s)
R median: APB	Wrist	4.35	2.7	8	–
	Elbow	9.65	3.0	25	47.2
	Palm	2.65	3.0	–	–
R ulnar: ADM	Wrist	3.75	8.7	–	–
	Below elbow	7.55	6.9	21	55.3
	Above elbow	9.65	7.0	10	47.6
L ulnar: ADM	Wrist	3.75	10.2	8	–
	Below elbow	7.65	9.5	20.5	52.6
	Above elbow	9.30	9.1	8	48.5
L median: APB	Wrist	3.70	4.6	8	–
	Elbow	10.05	5.1	27	42.5
	Axilla	–	–	–	–
	Palm	2.15	6.2	–	–
L comm peroneal: EDB	Ankle	6.25	2.4	8	–
	Fib head	16.15	2.0	37	37.4
L tib malleolus: 2 ch AH-ADM (1)	Malleolus	4.95	4.2	8	–
	Malleolus	–	–	–	–
	Knee	17.10	2.6	44.5	36.6

MONOPOLAR NEEDLE ELECTROMYOGRAPHY STUDIES

	Spontaneous				MUAP			Recruitment
	PSW	Fib	Fasc	HF	Amplitude	Duration	Poly	pattern
L deltoid	None	None	None	None	N	N	N	1–
L triceps	None	None	None	None	N	N	N	1–
L biceps	None	None	None	None	N	N	N	1–

Continued on page 240

| MONOPOLAR NEEDLE ELECTROMYOGRAPHY STUDIES | | Spontaneous | | | | MUAP | | Recruitment |
	PSW	Fib	Fasc	HF	Amplitude	Duration	Poly	pattern
L brachioradialis	None	None	None	None	1–	N	N	N
L extensor digitorum communis	None	None	None	None	N	N	N	1–
L abductor digiti minimi (ul)	None	None	None	None	1+	N	N	1–
L 1st dorsal interosseus	None	None	None	None	2+	N	N	1–
R deltoid	None	None	None	None	N	N	N	N
R biceps	None	None	None	None	N	N	N	1–
R triceps	None	None	None	None	N	N	N	1–
R extensor carpi radialis longus	None	None	None	None	N	N	N	1–
R brachioradialis	None	None	None	None	N	N	N	N
R extensor digitorum communis	None	None	None	None	N	N	N	1–
R 1st dorsal interosseus	None	None	None	None	2+	N	N	1–
R abductor digiti minimi (ul)	None	None	None	None	1+	N	N	1–
R cervical P spinal	None	None	None	None	N	N	N	N
L cervical P spinal	None	None	None	None	N	N	N	N
L gastrocnemius (med)	None	None	2+ (slow)	None	N	N	N	1–
L semimembran	None	None	None	None	N	N	N	1–
L semitendin	None	None	2+ (slow)	None	N	N	N	2–
L adductor magnus	None	None	2+ (slow)	None	N	N	N	1–
L tibialis anterior	None	None	2+ (slow)	None	N	1+	N	2–
L peroneus longus	None	None	1+	None	N	N	N	1–
L vastus lateralis	None	None	1+	None	N	N	N	1–
L lumbar PSP (L)	None	None	1+	None	N	N	N	N
L lumbar PSP (M)	None	None	1+	None	N	N	N	N
L lumbar PSP (U)	None	None	1+	None	N	N	N	N

EDB, Extensor digitorum brevis; Fib, fibrillation potentials; Fasc, fasciculation potentials; HF, complex repetitive discharges; MUAP, motor unit action potential; N, normal; Poly, polyphasic motor unit potentials; PSW, positive sharp waves.

Continued from page 239 Table 12-8 Bilateral wrist and hand pain (case 8)

EMG shows generally decreased recruitment in upper and lower limbs, and MUAPs of abnormally large amplitude in ulnar-innervated muscles and the tibialis anterior. Fasciculation potentials are also present in all muscles examined in the lower limb. Low-amplitude, short-duration, polyphasic MUAPs are not seen. The findings are compatible with an acquired sensory and motor polyneuropathy, primarily axonal, related to polymyalgia rheumatica.

Polymyalgia rheumatica is a systemic vasculitis affecting large- and medium-sized vessels. The disease process is global, and a number of different clinical presentations are possible. Polymyalgia rheumatica can present with symmetric proximal weakness, and the usual high erythrocyte sedimentation rate and high C-reactive protein, which can cause some difficulty in differentiating it from polymyositis. Polymyositis symptomatic enough to cause severe weakness is usually accompanied by very high creatine phosphokinase. Creatine phosphokinase is often normal in polymyalgia rheumatica, even in the presence of significant weakness.[24] The EDX consultant must remain aware of the potential for neuropathy in the person with giant cell arteritis or polymyalgia rheumatica referred for evaluation.

LOWER LIMB PROBLEMS

Problems that manifest in the lower limbs can be local, regional, or global in scope or importance, and present with weakness, numbness, and pain (alone or in combination). Possible conditions include myopathies, peripheral neuropathies and poly-neuropathies, motor neuron diseases, neuromuscular junction disorders, and metabolic diseases. Lumbar and sacral radiculopathies, plexopathies, spinal stenosis, and paraspinal mass or abscesses can also occur. Entrapment neuropathies of the lower limbs occur less frequently than in the upper limbs, the commonest being peroneal neuropathy at the fibular head. Other possible entrapment mononeuropathies of the lower limb include femoral, lateral femoral cutaneous, sciatic, tibial, saphenous, and medial and lateral plantar nerve entrapment syndromes. Some illustrative case presentations follow.

Case 9

An 18-year-old man presented with a complaint of having difficulty walking among the campus buildings during his first year of college. He described difficulty making it to classes on time because he could not walk fast enough. When he tried to walk faster, he would sometimes trip and fall. Although he had not recognized the problem until the beginning of the school year, he admits that he had never considered himself athletic and had occasionally found it difficult to physically keep up with friends when he was younger. He denied experiencing pain or sensory loss and had not noticed any changes in his upper limb strength.

The patient had no other significant medical problems. His mother told him her pregnancy was uncomplicated and his delivery went smoothly. Growing up, he was an above-average student. He was raised by his mother and had no contact with his father or his father's family from a very young age. The patient's mother had told him that his father had problems with his legs, but no other information was available about the father's medical history.

On physical examination, the patient was noted to have high-arched feet and hammertoes. Muscle bulk in both legs appeared to be diminished, but he had normal muscle bulk in the thighs. Although he had denied experiencing sensory changes, he was found to have loss of vibratory sensation in the lower limbs to a level above the knees, and in the upper limbs to the wrists. Position sensation was poor in the toes. Sensitivity to pinprick was diminished in a stocking distribution to the mid shins. Manual muscle testing showed mild weakness of bilateral ankle dorsiflexors. There was also slight intrinsic hand muscle weakness and little movement at all of the toes. He had diminished reflexes in the upper limbs and at the knees. Ankle jerk reflexes were absent. Toes were down going to plantar stimulation. He walked with a slightly broad-based gait.

Thought process

The occurrence of sensory loss in a stocking and glove distribution, combined with distal muscle loss and weakness, are compatible with the presence of a length-dependent sensorimotor polyneuropathy. Several features of the patient's history and examination are suggestive of a longstanding, probably hereditary, etiology. The high-arched feet and hammertoes and the diminished muscle bulk in the legs compared with the thighs are typical of Charcot–Marie–Tooth disease (CMT) and other hereditary neuropathies.[28] His unawareness of his substantial sensory deficits was more compatible with a longstanding neuropathy than a recently acquired one.

Charcot–Marie–Tooth disease is a hereditary polyneuropathy associated with several different genetic defects, usually transmitted in an autosomal dominant pattern.[27] The EDX examination can help subdivide the condition into Type 1, with predominantly demyelinating characteristics, and Type 2, with chronic denervation (axonal loss) and reinnervation.[12,21,77] CMT Type 1 nerve conductions are characterized by marked, fairly uniform slowing. On the other hand, CMT Type 2 conductions have normal velocities or only slight slowing, but significantly reduced amplitudes of the sensory and motor responses.

Another hereditary neuropathy that should be considered is hereditary neuropathy with susceptibility to pressure palsies (HNPP), characterized by multiple mononeuropathies affecting nerves at common points of injury due to compression or entrapment.[26,59,60] Typical findings in patients with HNPP include evidence of median neuropathies at the carpal tunnel, ulnar neuropathies at the elbow, and peroneal neuropathies at the fibular head. In this case, the patient's ankle dorsiflexor weakness could potentially be explained by peroneal nerve injuries, and his intrinsic hand muscle weakness could be explained by ulnar and median nerve injuries.

Because the father's medical history is unobtainable and the mother is apparently unaffected, acquired neuropathies such as those associated with endocrine diseases and other systemic diseases should also be considered. Although such neuropathies are usually indistinguishable from each other by EDX examination, acquired autoimmune neuropathies such as chronic inflammatory demyelinating polyradiculoneuropathy (CIDP) and vasculitic neuropathies do have distinctive characteristics. CIDP, like CMT Type 1, is characterized by marked slowing of NCS, but the slowing is generally less uniform.[49] Areas of focal conduction block are also seen in CIDP and other acquired demyelinating neuropathies, but not typically with a hereditary etiology.

Vasculitic neuropathies (previously known as mononeuritis multiplex) are characterized by an asymmetric, primarily axonal process. EDX studies demonstrate a marked asymmetry of motor amplitudes when comparing the same nerve from one side with the other.[8] Focal areas of conduction block at locations other than common sites of nerve compression or entrapments can also be seen.[32,53,69]

Distinguishing among the differential diagnoses requires studies of multiple sensory and motor nerve conductions, as well as a needle electrode examination of carefully selected muscles. In order to look for asymmetry, studies of nerves on both sides of the body should be compared. Conductions should be performed across common sites of nerve compression or entrapment. F-wave latencies should be evaluated to look for more proximal slowing than can be seen with routine sensory and motor studies.[37] Results for this patient are listed in Table 12-9.

Table 12-9 Trouble walking (case 9)

NERVE CONDUCTION STUDIES

Sensory nerve	Stimulation site	Recording site	Amplitude (µV)	Conduction velocity (m/s)
R sural	Calf	Ankle	No response	–
L sural	Calf	Ankle	No response	–
R median	Digit 2	Wrist	4 (N > 10)	24 (N > 50)
	Palm	Wrist	18	29 (N > 50)
R ulnar	Digit 5	Wrist	3 (N > 10)	22 (N > 50)

Motor nerve	Stimulation site	Latency (ms)	Conduction velocity (m/s)	Amplitude (mV)
R peroneal (record EDB)	Ankle	8.3 (N < 5/5)	–	1.4 (N > 2.0)
	Below knee	–	17 (N > 40)	1.2
	Above knee	–	19 (N > 40)	1.2
R peroneal F wave	–	78 (N < 55)	–	–
L peroneal (record EDB)	Ankle	7.9 (N < 5.5)	–	1.8 (N > 2.0)
	Below knee	–	18 (N > 40)	1.4
	Above knee	–	19 (N > 40)	1.3
L peroneal F wave	–	82 (N < 55)	–	–
R median (record thenar)	Wrist	6.6 (N < 4.3)	–	4.1 (N > 4.0)
	Elbow	–	20 (N > 50)	4.0
R median F wave	–	48 (N < 32)	–	–
R ulnar (record hypothenar)	Wrist	5.0 (N < 3.5)	–	4.3 (N > 4.0)
	Below elbow	–	23 (N > 50)	4.1
	Above elbow	–	26 (N > 50)	4.1
R ulnar F wave	–	50 (N < 32)	–	–

CONCENTRIC NEEDLE EMG STUDIES

Muscle	Spontaneous activity		Motor unit potentials		
	Positive waves	Fibrillation potentials	Recruitment	Amplitude	Duration
R tibialis anterior	0	0	Decreased	N	N
R extensor hallucis longus	0	0	Decreased	Few large	Few long
R medial gastrocnemius	0	0	N	N	N
R vastus medialis	0	0	N	N	N
R gluteus medius	0	0	N	N	N

EDB, Extensor digitorum brevis.

Discussion

The absent sural responses and the abnormal median and ulnar conductions (slowed velocities and reduced amplitudes of the responses) are typical of polyneuropathies. The abnormalities on motor conductions, however, are more useful for distinguishing the types of neuropathy in the differential diagnosis. Although the peroneal motor responses have reduced amplitudes, the degree of slowing of latencies and velocities is disproportionate. The slowing is also uniform (distal latency is slowed, F-wave latency is slowed, and conduction velocity across the knee varies little from that below the knee), and fairly symmetric from side to side. The median and ulnar motor responses have normal amplitudes, but the latencies and velocities are markedly slowed. There is no disproportionate slowing at common sites of compression or entrapment that would suggest peroneal nerve at the knee, ulnar nerve at the elbow, or median nerve at the wrist. There are no foci of significant motor amplitude reduction that would indicate conduction block. The findings on needle electrode examination suggest there has been some degree of denervation followed by reinnervation of distal muscles.

All the abnormalities in this case point to a hereditary, symmetric, predominantly demyelinating sensorimotor polyneuropathy, most probably CMT Type 1. The mild chronic changes on needle electrode examination indicate there has been some axonal involvement as well, but the findings are mostly indicative of demyelination. CIDP is a less likely cause for the changes because of the uniformity of the slowing, but it cannot be entirely excluded by these findings alone. In fact, in some cases evidence for an acquired neuropathy such as CIDP is seen superimposed on an underlying hereditary neuropathy. The absence of focal changes at common sites of nerve compression or entrapment argues against a diagnosis of HNPP. The symmetry of the findings also argues against a vasculitic neuropathy.

Because of the incomplete family history, the patient was given a presumed diagnosis of CMT Type 1. He subsequently underwent genetic testing, which was positive for CMT Type 1A, the most common genetic abnormality associated with CMT Type 1.

Case 10

The patient is a 54-year-old man with the primary complaint of numbness of the left thigh that began 1 year ago. The numbness recently extended to include the ball of his left foot. He has noticed tingling of the left lower limb within 5–10 min of standing. The tingling is relieved by sitting. There is no history of left lower limb pain, but he has experienced right lower limb pain that is not temporally related to the left-sided dysesthesias. Adult-onset diabetes mellitus was diagnosed 2–3 years ago and is under good control. There is a history of controlled hypertension. Physical examination showed sensory deficit to pinprick or light touch in the lower limbs, both proximally and distally. Muscle stretch reflexes were brisk and symmetric in all limbs. No atrophy was seen, and the patient could walk on his heels and toes, and could squat and rise without difficulty. Strength testing was normal except for single-sided toe raises, where the rate and amplitude of his movements on the left were, respectively, slower and lower than those on the corresponding right.

Thought process

The patient most probably has radiculopathy at S1. Although sensory symptoms are present, sensory testing is clinically normal. However, motor function is mildly but obviously impaired for toe raising on the left, suggesting a probable compromise or irritation of the S1 spinal nerve. The sensory pattern does not fit with meralgia paraesthetica, and a motor deficit is present. The history is incompatible with diabetic amyotrophy, because the diabetes is well controlled, pain is not an issue, and there is no atrophy. Diabetic peripheral neuropathy tends to be present symmetrically. Diabetic polyneuropathy is not the

probable cause of the complaints of numbness, because there was no distal to proximal gradient of sensory deficit, the onset of diabetes was relatively recent, muscle stretch reflexes were brisk, and motor function of the lower limbs was asymmetric. Spinal stenosis is a possibility, because sensory dysesthesia is precipitated by weight bearing and improved by sitting. However, persons with symptomatic lumbar spinal stenosis usually complain of pain as a prominent feature. Results of EDX studies done on this patient are listed in Table 12-10.

Discussion

Sensory NCS were normal, suggesting that diabetic polyneuropathy is not the main source of the patient's complaints. The amplitude of the left tibial CMAP was 40% smaller than the normal right tibial CMAP, and tibial motor conduction velocities were normal bilaterally. The differential amplitude is probably due to axonal loss.[17] There is abnormal membrane irritability in muscles supplied by three different peripheral nerves, in turn supplied by the left S1 spinal nerve. The paraspinal muscles supplied by the posterior primary rami of S1 also show abnormal membrane irritability. The left soleus H reflex is delayed 2 ms when compared with the right H reflex. A greater than 1.5-ms side to side difference in soleus H-reflex latencies is indicative of S1 radiculopathy in the appropriate clinical setting.[9,22] The constellation of findings provides incontrovertible evidence of left S1 radiculopathy.

Case 11

A 78-year-old woman presented with a 5-month history of bilateral foot, leg, and thigh pain. The posterior and posterolateral thigh and leg bilaterally, and the right heel, were the most troublesome for her. There was also a complaint of right anterior hip pain referred to the inguinal region. The pain tended to present when walking, and would quickly resolve whenever she sat down to rest. No other aggravating or alleviating factors for her pain were identified, except pain-induced limitation of stair climbing. She had been losing her balance. She experienced multiple joint pains and morning stiffness. Past medical history was positive for Type 2 diabetes, hypertension, asthma, and some difficulty with memory. She also complained of numbness and tingling of the hands. She had been diagnosed with bilaterally severe carpal tunnel syndrome 4 years previously, but it was unclear how this had been treated. In an effort to keep the emphasis on the lower limb complaints, carpal tunnel syndrome in this patient will not be discussed further. There is no history of weight loss.

Physical examination showed a person whose ability to cooperate was limited. Sensory examination showed a short stocking gradient distribution of deficit to pinprick and light touch bilaterally that was a bit asymmetric, but it could not be characterized further. Muscle stretch reflexes were 2+ for biceps brachii bilaterally, but all other muscle stretch reflexes were absent in all limbs. Toe position sense was erratic. There was weakness of big toe extension bilaterally. However, the patient could walk on heels and toes, complete a full squat and return, and perform tandem walking without difficulty.

Table 12-10 Numbness of the lower limb (case 10)

NERVE CONDUCTION STUDIES

Sensory nerve	Site	Recording site	Peak latency (ms)	Peak amplitude (μV)
L sural: lat malleolus	Calf	Lat malleolus	4.20	11.8
R sural: lat malleolus	Calf	Lat malleolus	3.95	12.9

Motor nerve	Site	Latency (ms)	Amplitude (mV)	Distance (cm)	Velocity (m/s)
L tib (knee): AH	Ankle	5.75	5.2	–	–
	Knee	14.75	3.4	36.5	40.0
R tib (knee): AH	Ankle	6.35	8.7	–	–
	Knee	15.25	6.7	39.5	44.4

Soleus H reflex

Nerve	H latency (ms)
R tib (knee): soleus	32.45
L tib (knee): soleus	34.50

MONOPOLAR NEEDLE ELECTROMYOGRAPHY STUDIES

Muscle	I activity	Spontaneous Fib	PSW	Fasc	HF	MUAP Amplitude	Duration	PPP	Recruitment pattern
L gastrocnemius (med)	–	1+	1+	None	None	N	N	N	N
L gastrocnemius (lat)	–	1+	1+	None	None	N	N	N	N
L semitendin	–	None	1+	1+	None	N	N	N	N
L lumbar PSP (L)	–	1+	1+	1+	1+	N	N	N	N
L lumbar PSP (M)	–	1+	1+	1+	None	N	N	N	N
L lumbar PSP (U)	–	None	None	None	None	N	N	N	N
R lumbar PSP (L)	–	None	None	None	None	N	N	N	N
R lumbar PSP (M)	–	None	None	None	None	N	N	N	N
R lumbar PSP (U)	–	None	None	None	None	N	N	N	N
L tibialis anterior	–	None	None	None	None	N	N	N	N
L peroneus longus	–	None	None	1+	None	N	N	N	N
L vastus medialis	–	None	None	None	None	N	N	N	N
L rect femoris	–	None	None	None	None	N	N	N	N
R rect femoris	–	None	None	None	None	N	N	N	N
R vastus medialis	–	None	None	None	None	N	N	N	N
R peroneus longus	–	None	None	None	None	N	N	N	N
R semitendin	–	None	None	None	None	N	N	N	N
R semimembran	–	None	None	None	None	N	N	N	N
R gastrocnemius (lat)	–	None	None	None	None	N	N	N	N
L gastrocnemius (med)	–	None	None	None	None	N	N	N	N

Fib, Fibrillation potentials; Fasc, fasciculation potentials; HF, complex repetitive discharges; MUAP, motor unit action potential; N, normal; Poly, polyphasic motor unit potentials; PSW, positive sharp waves.

Thought process

The history of neurogenic claudication, plus the patient's age and findings on physical examination, are very suggestive of lumbar spinal stenosis or other compressive spinal etiology. Type 2 diabetes mellitus complicates the picture. However, there is no evidence for diabetic amyotrophy to explain the limb pain. The pain associated with diabetic amyotrophy is usually limited to the proximal lower limb.[15] The patient is usually an older man with a history of recent significant weight loss and weakness of proximal lower limb muscle, with sparing of the more distal muscles. This woman is experiencing right proximal lower limb pain in addition to distal or extremity pain. There is no history of weight loss. She has a stocking distribution of sensory deficit that is probably due to diabetic neuropathy but could also be related to spinal stenosis. The impaired balance could be a feature of spinal stenosis, diabetes, or both. Multilevel lumbar radiculopathy is possible but is unlikely to occur as an individual event; however, multilevel radiculopathy would more often be related to spinal stenosis. Results of EDX studies done on this patient are listed in Table 12-11.

Discussion

The sural and superficial sensory distal latencies are normal, but the SNAPS are abnormally small in amplitude. Note that the sural SNAP is often absent in normal persons over 60 years old, so results of sensory NCS might be normal in this patient. An axonal neuropathy could account for the findings of normal sensory latency and conduction velocity with decreased SNAP amplitude. Motor NCS reveal severely reduced CMAP amplitude in the lower limbs, with normal distal latency. Tibial motor conduction velocity was slowed bilaterally, but the peroneal motor conduction velocity was normal bilaterally. The tibial F waves were temporally dispersed and delayed in latency, suggesting central slowing.[22] The picture becomes better defined with the needle EMG examination. There is abnormal membrane irritability demonstrated in muscles supplied by the posterior primary rami, and diffuse chronic neurogenic changes recorded in muscles supplied by the anterior rami of the spinal nerves. The lumbar paraspinal findings localize the problem at the spinal level. Lumbar spinal stenosis would best explain the apparent multiple level spinal nerve involvement, low-amplitude tibial CMAPs, F-wave abnormalities, and decreased conduction velocity. The peroneal motor conduction velocity remained within normal limits because not all of the fastest conducting motor fibers traveling in the peroneal nerve had been compromised.

There is an established relationship between multiradicular findings on EMG and clinical or operative findings of spinal stenosis or spondylosis. Multiradicular findings in a person presenting with radicular pain and neurogenic claudication would suggest lumbar spinal stenosis.[31] After EDX was completed in this patient, MRI was ordered to evaluate the anatomic extent of spinal stenosis as a presurgical necessity. The MRI showed grade 1 anterolisthesis of L4 on L5, and L5 on S1, and moderately severe spinal stenosis at L4–L5, less severe at L5–S1. Additionally, there was bilateral foraminal encroachment at L4–L5 and, to a lesser degree, at L5–S1. The possible contribution of diabetic neuropathy to the clinical picture in this patient is difficult to quantify.

Case 12

A 31-year-old man presented to the emergency department complaining of numbness of the legs. He had a history of polysubstance abuse documented by laboratory studies on admission. The friends who accompanied him verified that he had lost consciousness for a number of hours. On awakening, the patient had summoned emergency medical services from his hotel room. Apparently, emergency medical services personnel found him lying, unable to get up, with the right leg doubled underneath him. Although he could ambulate at the scene, he was unsteady and the right ankle 'kept rolling'. There was an unresolved question of whether or not he had been physically assaulted. The emergency department physician reported that the patient had significant ecchymoses and small bruises on all limbs, no edema, symmetric four-fifths strength in the lower limbs, normal strength in the upper limbs, a question of decreased sensation below the knees, normal peripheral arterial pulses, and rhabdomyolysis and renal insufficiency that required dialysis. Spine films were obtained and were read as negative. The patient was admitted to the general medical service for further evaluation and treatment.

Nine days later, the patient was referred to the EDX consultant for evaluation of right foot drop, with the presumptive diagnosis of peroneal neuropathy at the fibular head. He was somewhat confused and minimally cooperative with the history, physical examination, and EDX studies. He did not seem to understand why EDX was necessary, or the potential seriousness of his situation. There was generalized edema, marked in the lower limbs, right more than left. Muscle stretch reflexes were brisk at the knees and left ankle, but 1+ at the right ankle. Sensory function testing was not completely reliable, secondary to poor compliance and easy distractibility. Sensory deficit to light touch and pinprick was noted in a long stocking distribution starting just below the knee. Although sensory function improved as one proceeded proximally from the knee, sensory function was not normal in the lower limbs. The patient gave a history of severe spontaneous bilateral foot pain with hyperpathia and hyperesthesia, but examination showed the dorsum and soles of his feet to be completely insensate to pinprick. Manual muscle testing was normal in the upper limbs, but showed only one-fifth strength of right ankle dorsiflexion, and three-fifths on the left. Hip flexors and knee extensors were three-fifths bilaterally. Strength in the lower limbs appeared otherwise functional within the limits of his compliance with the physical examination.

Thought process

The most likely diagnosis was spinal or perispinal pathology leading to bilateral lower limb problems, right more than left. The clinical picture was somewhat confusing, especially in view of having a non-compliant patient with impaired memory, gross edema, renal failure, and polysubstance abuse. Although the

Table 12-11 Bilateral thigh, leg, and foot pain (case 11)

NERVE CONDUCTION STUDIES

Sensory nerve	Site	Recording site	Peak latency (ms)	Peak amplitude (μV)	Distance (cm)	Velocity (m/s)
L sural: lat malleolus	Calf	Lat malleolus	3.75	4.8	14	49.1
L sup peroneal: foot	Lateral leg	Foot	3.80	2.5	14	46.7
R sural: lat malleolus	Calf	Lat malleolus	3.85	8.0	14	44.4
R sup peroneal: foot	Lateral leg	Foot	4.00	2.8	14	38.9

Motor nerve	Site	Latency (ms)	Amplitude (mV)	Distance (cm)	Velocity (m/s)
L comm peroneal: EDB	Ankle	4.65	3.1	8	–
	Fib head	11.05	2.7	28	43.8
R comm peroneal: EDB	Ankle	4.25	0.9	8	–
	Fib head	10.65	0.8	29	45.3
R tib malleolus: 2 ch AH-ADM (1)	Malleolus	6.00	1.1	8	–
	Malleolus	–	–	–	–
	Knee	15.70	0.8	34	35.1
	Knee	–	–	–	–
L tib malleolus: 2 ch AH-ADM (1)	Malleolus	6.15	1.8	8	–
	Malleolus	1.95	0.4	–	–
	Knee	6.20	2.1	–	–
	Knee	11.50	0.7	34	35.6

MONOPOLAR NEEDLE ELECTROMYOGRAPHY STUDIES

| | Spontaneous | | | | MUAP | | | Recruitment |
	PSW	Fib	Fasc	HF	Amplitude	Duration	Poly	pattern
L bic fem (L head)	None	None	None	None	N	N	1+	1–
L gastrocnemius (lat)	None	None	None	None	N	N	N	N
R semimembran	None	None	None	None	N	N	1+	2–
L semimembran	None	None	None	None	N	N	1+	1–
R gastrocnemius (lat)	None	None	None	None	N	N	N	N
R lumbar PSP (L)	1+	1+	None	None	N	N	N	N
L tibialis anterior	None	None	None	None	1+	1+	1+	1–
R tibialis anterior	None	None	None	None	1+	1+	N	1–
R peroneus longus	None	None	None	None	N	N	N	1–
L peroneus longus	None	None	None	None	N	1+	1+	2–
L rect femoris	None	None	None	None	2+	2+	1+	1–
R rect femoris	None	None	None	None	N	N	N	1–
L lumbar PSP (U)	None	None	None	None	N	N	N	N
R lumbar PSP (U)	None	None	None	None	N	N	N	N
R lumbar PSP (M)	1+	1+	None	None	N	N	N	N
L lumbar PSP (M)	1+	1+	None	None	N	N	N	N
L lumbar PSP (L)	1+	1+	None	None	N	N	N	N

EDB, Extensor digitorum brevis; Fib, fibrillation potentials; Fasc, fasciculation potentials; HF, complex repetitive discharges; MUAP, motor unit action potential; N, normal; Poly, polyphasic motor unit potentials; PSW, positive sharp waves.

patient seemed more confused now than reported on admission, he did complain of back pain, right hip pain, weakness of both lower limbs, rolling of the right ankle, and numbness of both legs when examined in the emergency department. The history that he was found with the right leg doubled under him might be significant, but could be a 'red herring' in terms of right peroneal mononeuropathy.

The initial examination showed symmetric lower limb weakness, but he now had unequivocal right foot drop and apparently functional strength of the left lower limb. It was felt that a central or spinal problem would best explain the clinical findings during the EDX consultation. There could be superimposed focal nerve injury at the fibular head, but this would be extremely difficult to define in the present clinical situation. A paraspinal or epidural abscess should be suspected in the multidrug abuser. Normal upper limb strength would not support a myopathic or generalized neuropathic picture. Guillain–Barré type polyneuritis was a possibility and had to be ruled out. Although lumbar plexopathy was worth considering, the history of back pain lessened the possibility of lumbar plexopathy and increased the chances of a central or spinal problem. Results of EDX studies done on this patient are listed in Table 12-12.

Discussion

Bilateral sural and right superficial peroneal SNAPs were absent. The left superficial peroneal SNAP was of normal latency but abnormally small amplitude. The tibial and peroneal motor conduction studies were grossly abnormal. There was no response to stimulating the right peroneal nerve below the fibular head or at the ankle. Distal motor latencies were abnormally delayed, and CMAPs were abnormally small in amplitude bilaterally. Needle EMG showed abnormal membrane irritability in right-side muscles innervated by different peripheral nerves and supplied by more than one spinal nerve (L4–S2). Similarly, on the right-side, motor unit recruitment was severely reduced or absent in the L4 to S2 distribution. On the left side, there was decreased recruitment in muscles supplied from L4 to S2, but no abnormal membrane irritability. The patient did not cooperate for satisfactory evaluation of lumbar paraspinal muscles, making it difficult to rule in or out lumbosacral plexus involvement based solely on needle EMG.

The initial symptoms included bilateral lower limb numbness and weakness, and back pain. EDX of both lower limbs proved the etiology of his complaints to be more centrally located than previously thought. The EMG can identify abnormal neurophysiology but not abnormal gross anatomy. In the present clinical situation, the EDX consultant recommended an MRI of the lumbar spine. An enhancing mass interpreted as a right paraspinal muscle abscess was identified on MRI, and appropriate treatment measures were instituted.

Case 13

The patient is a 38-year-old white female recreational runner with the primary complaint of right leg and foot pain. She had noticed atrophy of the leg, and gave a history of vasomotor instability and discoloration of the right leg and foot. The problem began 8 weeks prior to EDX consultation, when she noticed discomfort below the right patella, referred to the medial knee. Within 1 week, the discomfort had progressed to the right ankle and developed into severe pain that interfered with her ability to run. The pain was particularly severe between the metatarsal heads of the right foot. One week later, she developed numbness of the right foot and observed the foot to have a blanched discoloration. She noted that the right foot color changed with position; for example, it would blanch if she transferred from sitting to standing, but the left foot remained normal. Past medical history was positive for a 2-year history of Crohn disease in this very active recreational multiathlete. Her Crohn disease was thought to be inactive. She gave a 2-year history of right back and buttock pain that had not been addressed. There was no history of unexplained weight loss, and no family history of rheumatologic or neurologic disease. A number of specialists had evaluated the patient, including vascular surgery, pain management, orthopedics, and rheumatology, without reaching a definitive diagnosis. Nuclear medicine scans; MRI scans including abdomen, lumbosacral spine, and foot; CT scans of the right knee; and blood serologies were not diagnostic. She had EDX studies by two consultants. One study was reported as normal, and the second study was judged non-specific.

Physical examination showed obvious atrophy of the right leg affecting the anterior and posterior compartment muscles. There was livedo reticularis of all limbs, with all extremities abnormally cold to touch subjectively. This coldness was confirmed objectively by liquid crystal thermometry. Atrophy of right foot muscles was noted, and foot bones were easily palpated, especially when compared with the left. The right foot was smaller than the left in circumference, when measured across the metatarsal heads in this right-footed patient. Heel, toe, and tandem walking were completed without difficulty. Squatting and return were difficult, and returning to the upright position was accomplished with obvious weight shifting toward the left side. She had decreased appreciation of pinprick along the medial and dorsal right hallux that reverted to normal above the medial malleolus. Muscle stretch reflexes were brisk at knees and ankles, but the right ankle jerk was less active than the left. At the beginning of the examination, the left foot appeared dusky and the right pale in color. As the examination proceeded, the right foot attained normal color, but the left remained dusky.

Thought process

This patient is experiencing extraintestinal manifestations of Crohn disease. A variety of neurologic problems have been described in inflammatory bowel disease including Crohn disease and ulcerative colitis. Acute peripheral neuropathy, multiple mononeuropathy, and small fiber neuropathy have been described.[23,25,30,55] Vasculitis with circulating immune complexes was postulated to be a possible mechanism to explain cutaneous vasculitis and other evidence of vasculitis noted in Crohn disease. Myositis has been described as a manifestation of Crohn disease.[1] This patient has a 2-year history of Crohn

Table 12-12 Right foot drop (case 12)

NERVE CONDUCTION STUDIES

Sensory nerve	Site	Recording site	Peak latency (ms)	Peak amplitude (μV)
L sural: lat malleolus	Calf	Lat malleolus	No response	No response
L sup peroneal: foot	Lateral leg	Foot	3.90	2.0
R sural: lat malleolus	Calf	Lat malleolus	No response	No response
R sup peroneal: foot	Lateral leg	Foot	No response	No response

Motor nerve	Site	Latency (ms)	Amplitude (mV)	Distance (cm)	Velocity (m/s)
L comm peroneal: EDB	Ankle / Fib head	6.70 / 14.85	0.2 / 0.2	8 / 35	– / 42.9
R comm peroneal: EDB	Ankle / Fib head	No response / No response	– / –	– / –	– / –
R tib malleolus: 2 ch AH-ADM (1)	Malleolus / Knee	6.05 / No response	6.6 / –	8 / –	– / –
L tib malleolus: 2 ch AH-ADM (1)	Malleolus / Knee	7.15 / No response	1.9 / –	8 / –	– / –

MONOPOLAR NEEDLE ELECTROMYOGRAPHY STUDIES

Muscle	Spontaneous PSW	Fib	Fasc	HF	Amplitude	MUAP Duration	Poly	Recruitment pattern
R bic fem (L head)	None	None	None	None	N	N	N	N
R dorsal interosseus (LL)	1+	1+	None	1+	N	N	N	2–
R abductor hallucis	1+	1+	None	None	N	N	N	Discrete
R tibialis anterior	1+	1+	None	None	1–	1+	1+	Discrete
R peroneus longus	2+	2+	None	None	N	N	N	No activity
R gastrocnemius (med)	None	None	None	None	1+	1+	N	1–
R adductor longus	None	None	None	None	N	N	N	N
R vastus medialis	None	None	None	None	N	N	N	1–
L bic fem (L head)	None	None	None	None	N	N	N	N
L gastrocnemius (med)	None	None	None	None	N	N	N	1–
L semimembran	None	None	None	None	N	N	N	N
L tibialis anterior	None	None	None	None	N	N	N	1–
L peroneus longus	None	None	None	None	N	N	N	1–
L vastus medialis	None	None	None	None	N	N	N	N

EDB, Extensor digitorum brevis; Fib, fibrillation potentials; Fasc, fasciculation potentials; HF, complex repetitive discharges; MUAP, motor unit action potential; N, normal; Poly, polyphasic motor unit potentials; PSW, positive sharp waves.

disease, a 2-year history of back pain and right buttock pain, an 8-week history of right leg and foot pain and atrophy, vasomotor instability, functional weakness of right hip extension, and limited sensory deficit of the right foot. She has been in good health and was exceptionally active prior to the new symptoms that developed 8 weeks earlier.

Raynaud disease had been disproved clinically, and complex regional pain syndrome was felt to be unlikely. Laboratory studies were negative for rheumatic illnesses, including lupus. Single level lumbar or sacral radiculopathy was not supported by the physical examination, as both anterior and posterior leg muscles were involved. The pattern of sensory deficit was nonspecific for peripheral nerve or radiculopathy. Lumbar plexopathy was possible but usually does not present with vasomotor instability, foot pain, and narrowly restricted sensory findings. Results of EDX studies done on this patient by the second EDX

Table 12-13 Right leg and foot pain (case 13)

NERVE CONDUCTION STUDIES

Sensory nerve	Site	Recording site	Peak latitude (ms)	Peak amplitude (μV)	Distance (cm)	Velocity (m/s)
L sural: lat malleolus	Calf	Lat malleolus	3.2	22.6	12	46.8
R sural: lat malleolus	Calf	Lat malleolus	3.1	20.3	12	44.4

Motor nerve	Site	Latency (ms)	Amplitude (mV)	Distance (cm)	Velocity (m/s)
L comm peroneal: EDB	Ankle	3.8	4.7	–	–
	Fib head	9.6	4.4	27.5	47.1
R comm peroneal: EDB	Ankle	3.8	2.3	–	–
	Fib head	9.0	2.2	26	49.5
R tib malleolus: 2 ch AH-ADM (1)	Malleolus	6.6	3.6	–	–
	Knee	14.5	2.8	35	44.2
L tib malleolus: 2 ch AH-ADM (1)	Malleolus	4.4	6.5	–	–
	Knee	12.2	5.9	35.5	45.8

CONCENTRIC NEEDLE ELECTROMYOGRAPHY STUDIES

Muscle	I activity	Spontaneous Fib	PSW	Fasc	HF	Amplitude	MUAP Duration	Poly	Recruitment pattern
L soleus	–	None	None	None	None	N	N	N	N
L extensor dig brevis	–	None	None	None	None	N	N	N	N
L lumbar PSP	–	None	None	None	None	N	N	N	N
R lumbar PSP	–	None	None	None	None	N	N	N	N
L tibialis anterior	–	None	None	None	None	N	N	N	N
L peroneus longus	–	None	None	None	None	N	N	N	N
L vastus lateralis	–	None	None	None	None	N	N	N	N
R vastus lateralis	–	None	None	None	None	N	N	N	N
R peroneus longus	–	None	None	None	None	1+	N	N	1–
R extensor dig brevis	–	None	None	None	None	1+	N	1+	1–
R tibialis anterior	–	None	None	None	None	1+	N	1+	2–
R soleus	–	None	None	None	None	1+	N	N	1–

EDB, Extensor digitorum brevis; Fib, fibrillation potentials; Fasc, fasciculation potentials; HF, complex repetitive discharges; MUAP, motor unit action potential; N, normal; Poly, polyphasic motor unit potentials; PSW, positive sharp waves.

consultant are listed in Table 12-13. At the patient's request, the EDX examination was not repeated for a third time.

Discussion

Right lower limb motor NCS showed that the right peroneal CMAP amplitude was reduced by 50% when compared with that of the left. The right tibial CMAP was almost 50% smaller in amplitude, and the distal motor latency was significantly delayed compared with the left. Needle EMG was remarkable only for decreased recruitment, increased percentage of polyphasic MUAPs, and increased amplitude of MUAPs. Needle electrode exploration of hip and posterior thigh muscles would

have improved the accuracy in determining the exact anatomic distribution of the problem. For example, was this an isolated sciatic nerve problem or tibial and peroneal mononeuropathy? Normal paraspinal needle examination and normal MRI suggested that radiculopathy was not likely but could not be completely discounted. Bilateral superficial peroneal sensory NCS were normal per the first EDX consultant, and bilateral sural sensory NCS were documented normal per the second EDX consultant. Note that, on physical examination, there was only a very small area of numbness affecting the hallux and medial ankle. Some of the sensory dysfunction and the vasomotor features were probably related to small fiber activity and autonomic dysfunction that are not measured by traditional EDX. The findings were most compatible with multiple mono-neuropathy involving the right tibial and peroneal nerves.[2]

Case 14

A 62-year-old man sought medical attention for a tingling sensation in his feet and hands. The symptoms started 1 year ago in the feet and recently spread to the hands. The tingling sensation was initially mild but progressively intensified. He is now unable to tolerate the bed sheets touching his feet at night. He also recently noted mild difficulty with hand dexterity. His past medical history was significant for a 12-year history of diabetes mellitus, for which he was taking insulin and oral hypoglycemic agents. There was no family history of similar problems. The patient denied alcohol abuse, illicit drug abuse, or chemical exposure. However, review of systems was positive for impotence for 5 years and occasional light-headedness when he would stand up quickly.

Physical examination was significant for a drop in systolic blood pressure on assuming the upright position, from 160 mmHg to 110 mmHg. The neurologic examination was significant for minimal weakness in the bilateral hand muscles. Pinprick and light touch sensation was reduced in a stocking distribution to below the knees, and in a glove distribution to the wrists. Vibration sensation was also impaired below the knees bilaterally. The muscle stretch reflexes were diffusely hypoactive and were absent at the ankles.

Thought process

Tingling sensations in the feet and hands can occur in spinal cord injury, but the stocking and glove distribution is more typical of length-dependent sensory neuropathies. The absence of urinary or bowel incontinence and the hypoactive reflexes also argue against a spinal cord lesion. A myopathy or a defect of neuromuscular transmission would be unlikely to explain the predominantly sensory findings, with only mild distal weakness.[65] From the history and examination, this appeared to be neuropathic process, which involved sensory, motor, and autonomic nerve fibers. Given the patient's longstanding diabetes, a diabetic polyneuropathy was most likely.[11]

The EDX findings vary widely among different patients with diabetes. Most commonly, there is a length-dependent, symmetric, axonal more than demyelinating, sensorimotor polyneuropathy. In those patients, the longest nerves (i.e. those supplying the feet) are the earliest and most severely affected, and the changes are fairly symmetric from side to side. Typically, the sensory responses have reduced amplitudes, and the motor studies might have reduced amplitudes and/or slowing of conduction velocities.

In other cases, there is a length-dependent neuropathy, but the abnormalities are limited to the smallest diameter nerve fibers, the unmyelinated and lightly myelinated fibers that carry information about pain and temperature sensation and about autonomic function. In those patients, the NCS and needle electrode examination (both of which evaluate only function of large diameter, myelinated fibers) might be completely normal.

Further, patients with diabetes are more prone to mononeuropathies at common sites of compression or entrapment. Diabetic patients can present with a multiple mononeuropathy picture similar to that seen with vasculitic neuropathies. And proximal diabetic neuropathies can affect the lumbosacral plexus and nerve roots.

The EDX examination is useful to determine the distribution, type, severity, and chronicity of the neuropathy. Usually, the examination is started with nerves considered most likely to be affected, i.e. those in the lower limbs. An upper limb study is often done to prove that the problem is global and not caused by spinal or other etiology. Results for this patient are listed in Table 12-14.

Discussion

Bilateral sural sensory NCS showed normal velocities with reduced amplitudes of the SNAP. Bilateral peroneal motor NCS showed slightly slowed conduction velocity, and F-wave latencies less in severity than one would anticipate in predominantly demyelinating neuropathies. These findings are suggestive of a symmetric, sensorimotor polyneuropathy with axonal more than demyelinating features. NCS in the upper limb were normal except for slightly reduced ulnar SNAP amplitude. The relatively normal findings in the upper limbs, along with symmetric abnormalities in the lower limbs, suggested this was a length-dependent process.

The distribution of the abnormalities on needle electrode examination supported length-dependent neuropathy. Fibrillation potentials and positive sharp waves recorded in the leg muscles indicated active axonal involvement. The presence of abnormal MUAPs in the most distal muscles indicated a chronic process, with evidence of denervation followed by some reinnervation.[63] In this patient, the history, physical examination, and EDX studies were diagnostic of a chronic, length-dependent, symmetric, predominantly axonal, sensorimotor polyneuropathy, compatible with longstanding diabetes mellitus.

Case 15

A 24-year-old male postal worker presented to the emergency room with a complaint of generalized weakness and difficulty walking. His symptoms started 4 days earlier, when he noted a painful tingling sensation at the tips of his fingers and toes. The next day, he noticed difficulty climbing the stairs and standing from a seated position. Two days later, he was unable to carry heavy mailbags. These problems rapidly progressed to difficulty walking on flat surfaces, prompting his visit to the emergency room. The patient's past medical history was essentially unremarkable, except for 4–5 days of diarrhea 2 weeks prior to the onset of his current symptoms.

General physical examination was significant only for mild tachycardia. Cranial nerve examination was normal. Muscle tone was decreased and strength was mildly reduced in all limbs, slightly worse proximally than distally. Position and vibration sensation were slightly impaired in the feet. Muscle stretch reflexes were diffusely absent except at the biceps, where reflexes were present but diminished.

Table 12-14 Worsening tingling sensations in feet and hands (case 14)

NERVE CONDUCTION STUDIES Sensory nerve	Stimulation site	Recording site	Amplitude (µV)	Conduction velocity (m/s)
R sural	Ankle	Foot	6 (N > 10)	42 (N > 40)
L sural	Ankle	Foot	4 (N > 10)	41 (N > 40)
R median	Digit 2	Wrist	15 (N > 10)	52 (N > 50)
	Palm	Wrist	–	50 (N > 50)
R ulnar	Digit 5	Wrist	9 (N > 10)	59 (N > 50)

Motor nerve	Stimulation site	Latency (ms)	Conduction velocity (m/s)	Amplitude (mV)
R peroneal (record EDB)	Ankle	5.3 (N < 5.5)	–	2.1 (N > 2.0)
	Below knee	–	37 (N > 40)	1.9
	Above knee	–	41 (N > 40)	1.8
R peroneal F wave	–	56 (N < 55)	–	–
L peroneal (record EDB)	Ankle	5.2 (N < 5.5)	–	2.2 (N > 2.0)
	Below knee	–	38 (N > 40)	2.0
	Above knee	–	43 (N > 40)	1.9
L peroneal F wave	–	58 (N < 55)	–	–
R median (record thenar)	Wrist	4.2 (N < 4.3)	–	4.3 (N > 4.0)
	Elbow	–	51 (N > 50)	4.0
R median F wave	–	31 (N < 32)	–	–
R ulnar (record hypothenar)	Wrist	3.3 (N < 3.5)	–	4.4 (N > 4.0)
	Below elbow	–	55 (N > 50)	4.2
	Above elbow	–	51 (N > 50)	4.2
R ulnar F wave	–	30 (N < 32)	–	–

CONCENTRIC NEEDLE ELECTROMYOGRAPHY STUDIES Muscle	Spontaneous activity		Motor unit potentials		
	Positive waves	Fibrillation potentials	Recruitment	Amplitude	Duration
R extensor hallucis longus	2+	2+	Decreased	Few large	Few long
R tibialis anterior	1+	1+	N	N	N
R gastrocnemius	1+	0	N	N	N
R vastus medialis	0	0	N	N	N
R gluteus medius	0	0	N	N	N
R 1st dorsal interosseus	0	0	N	N	N

EDB, Extensor digitorum brevis.

Thought process

The reduced tone and depressed reflexes were suggestive of a condition affecting part of the motor unit (motor nerve, axon, neuromuscular junction, or muscle). The bilateral, symmetric reflex loss was a characteristic feature of peripheral neuropathy but could also occur in patients with muscle disease. However, in myopathies, the mildly impaired muscle strength usually leads to hypoactive reflexes rather than total abolition. More importantly, the sensory signs and symptoms were not typical of a myopathic process. A neuromuscular junction disorder was also unlikely, both because of the sensory impairment and also the absence of a fluctuating pattern of weakness.

The findings of both sensory and motor signs and symptoms, the autonomic dysfunction (tachycardia),[81] and the depressed tone and reflexes all support the presence of a neuropathic process. In general, the distal muscles are more severely affected in peripheral neuropathies. One of the exceptions to that rule occurs in the Guillain–Barré syndrome, in which the proximal muscles can be more severely affected.[70] The preceding viral illness (diarrhea);[84] the acute onset of an ascending, symmetric

Table 12-15a Acute ascending progressive weakness: 5 days after onset

NERVE CONDUCTION STUDIES

Sensory nerve	Stimulation site	Recording site	Amplitude (μV)	Conduction velocity (m/s)
R median	Digit 2	Wrist	16 (N > 10)	55 (N > 50)
	Palm	Wrist	32	51 (N > 50)
R ulnar	Digit 5	Wrist	16 (N > 10)	56 (N > 50)
R sural	Ankle	Foot	17 (N > 10)	43 (N > 40)
L sural	Ankle	Foot	16 (N > 10)	42 (N > 40)

Motor nerve	Stimulation site	Latency (ms)	Conduction velocity (m/s)	Amplitude (mV)
R median (record thenar)	Wrist	4.2 (N < 4.3)	–	4.0 (N > 4)
	Elbow	–	51 (N > 50)	3.9
R median F wave	–	36 (N < 32)	–	–
R ulnar (record hypothenar)	Wrist	3.3 (N < 3.5)	–	4.1 (N > 4)
	Below elbow	–	54 (N > 50)	4.0
	Above elbow	–	51 (N > 50)	4.0
R ulnar F wave	–	37 (N < 32)	–	–
R peroneal (record EDB)	Ankle	5.0 (N < 5.5)	–	1.8 (N > 2)
	Below knee	–	43 (N > 40)	1.6
	Above knee	61 (N <55)	44 (N > 40)	1.6
R peroneal F wave	–	–	–	–
L peroneal (record EDB)	Ankle	5.3 (N < 5.5)	–	1.9 (N > 2)
	Below knee	–	41 (N > 40)	1.7
	Above knee	–	46 (N > 40)	1.7
L peroneal F wave	–	63 (N < 55)	–	–

CONCENTRIC NEEDLE ELECTROMYOGRAPHY STUDIES

Muscle	Spontaneous activity		Motor unit potentials		
	Positive waves	Fibrillation potentials	Recruitment	Amplitude	Duration
R vastus medialis	0	0	Decreased	N	N
R tibialis anterior	0	0	Decreased	N	N
R peroneus longus	0	0	Decreased	N	N
R medial gastrocnemius	0	0	Decreased	N	N
R extensor hallucis longus	0	0	Decreased	N	N

EDB, Extensor digitorum brevis.

weakness; the predominantly motor impairment; and early loss of reflexes are all suggestive of Guillain–Barré syndrome. Results of EDX studies done on this patient are listed in Table 12-15.

Discussion

The NCS performed approximately 5 days into the illness were remarkable for delayed F-wave latencies, slightly low CMAP amplitudes, and slightly decreased recruitment of MUAPs. In many cases of the Guillain–Barré syndrome, NCS are normal or only slightly abnormal during the first week of the illness.

The potentially life-threatening nature of Guillain–Barré syndrome, the delayed F-wave latencies, diminished amplitude of CMAP, reduced recruitment, and clinical suspicion prompted admission to hospital for aggressive treatment and serial examinations, spinal fluid analysis, serial pulmonary function tests, and treatment with intravenous immunoglobulin. The patient stabilized clinically by the middle of the following week.

A follow up EDX study 2 weeks later was clearly abnormal. Results of motor conduction studies of the right median and

Table 12-15b Acute ascending progressive weakness: follow-up study 2 weeks later

NERVE CONDUCTION STUDIES

Sensory nerve	Stimulation site	Recording site	Amplitude (µV)	Conduction velocity (m/s)
R median	Digit 2	Wrist	13 (N > 10)	50 (N > 50)
	Palm	Wrist	32	51 (N > 50)
R ulnar	Digit 5	Wrist	12 (N > 10)	51 (N > 50)
R sural	Ankle	Foot	11 (N > 10)	40 (N > 40)
L sural	Ankle	Foot	10 (N > 10)	40 (N > 40)

Motor nerve	Stimulation site	Latency (ms)	Conduction velocity (m/s)	Amplitude (mV)
R median (record thenar)	Wrist	4.9 (N < 4.3)	–	3.7 (N > 4)
	Elbow	–	38 (N > 50)	1.7
R median F wave	–	44 (N < 32)	–	–
R ulnar (record hypothenar)	Wrist	4.2 (N < 3.5)	–	3.6 (N > 4)
	Below elbow	–	34 (N > 50)	2.5
	Above elbow	–	35 (N > 50)	2.5
R ulnar F wave	–	47 (N < 32)	–	–
R peroneal (record EDB)	Ankle	5.8 (N < 5.5)	–	1.6 (N > 2)
	Below knee	–	29 (N > 40)	0.8
	Above knee	61 (N < 55)	33 (N > 40)	0.8
R peroneal F wave	–	–	–	–
L peroneal (record EDB)	Ankle	5.6 (N < 5.5)	–	1.7 (N > 2)
	Below knee	–	31 (N > 40)	0.8
	Above knee	–	34 (N > 40)	0.8
L peroneal F wave	–	63 (N < 55)	–	–

CONCENTRIC NEEDLE ELECTROMYOGRAPHY STUDIES

Muscle	Spontaneous activity		Motor unit potentials		
	Positive waves	Fibrillation potentials	Recruitment	Amplitude	Duration
R vastus medialis	0	0	Decreased	N	N
R tibialis anterior	0	0	Decreased	N	N
R peroneus longus	0	0	Decreased	N	N
R medial gastrocnemius	0	0	Decreased	N	N
R extensor hallucis longus	0	0	Decreased	N	N

EDB, Extensor digitorum brevis.

ulnar nerves, and of bilateral peroneal nerves, showed that distal latencies, conduction velocities, and F-wave latencies were markedly slowed when compared with the laboratory's normal values and with the values from the patient's earlier study. In addition, the right median nerve CMAP amplitude with proximal stimulation was less than 50% of that of the distal CMAP, suggesting the presence of conduction block between the proximal and distal sites.[64] Evidence for conduction block was also present in the right peroneal nerve. The needle electrode examination continued to show decreased recruitment.

All the abnormal findings were suggestive of a demyelinating process. The presence of conduction block was supportive of an acquired demyelinating process, for example Guillain–Barré syndrome, rather than a longstanding or hereditary process, for example CMT Type 1. The acute onset of ascending weakness and loss of reflexes, the preceding viral illness, and the spinal fluid finding of elevated protein and normal cells all supported the diagnosis of Guillain–Barré syndrome. The most important diagnostic test to confirm the clinical diagnosis was the nerve conduction study.[18]

Case 16

A previously healthy 51-year-old woman presented with a 3- to 4-month history of difficulty walking and doing her usual tasks at home and work. The patient first noticed a reduction in stamina and difficulty climbing the stairs at home. She has a sedentary job working at a desk, but finds that, by the end of a workday, she is much more fatigued than usual. She has difficulty standing up from a low chair. She has also noticed that she has to stop to rest when she is drying her hair before work in the morning. On further questioning, she might have some difficulty swallowing and has had a decreased appetite lately. She denies shortness of breath. The patient is currently taking no medications and has had no significant medical problems except for an attack of cholecystitis at age 43, for which she underwent a cholecystectomy. There is no family history of nerve or muscle diseases.

On physical examination, the patient was a slightly overweight, middle-aged woman in no acute distress. Extraocular muscles were conjugate. She had normal facial strength and normal movement of her palate. Her tongue had normal bulk and protrudes in the midline. Manual muscle testing showed mild weakness of neck flexors. Shoulder abductors, elbow flexors, and hip flexors were antigravity but could be easily overcome by the examiner. Elbow extensors and knee extensors were also slightly weak. Strength in the wrist flexors and extensors, and the ankle dorsiflexors and plantar flexors, was within normal limits. Reflexes were normal to slightly hypoactive, jaw jerk was absent, and she had no Babinski's, Hoffmann's, or palmomental signs. Sensation was normal. The patient had difficulty standing up from a chair and walked slowly, but appeared to have a normal gait once she was upright. No skin changes were noted. The patient was sent to the phlebotomy laboratory for some initial testing and scheduled for EDX testing. Her serum creatine kinase level was elevated to more than three times the upper limit of normal.

Thought process

Symmetric, predominantly proximal weakness, along with a significantly elevated creatine kinase level, in this age group is most suggestive of an acquired myopathic process. The most common of the acquired myopathies in adults over the age of 50 are the idiopathic inflammatory myopathies (i.e. polymyositis, dermatomyositis, or inclusion body myositis).[51] These three conditions have distinctive pathologic findings but have inflammation of the muscles in common.[54]

New-onset weakness from hereditary myopathies including muscular dystrophies would be uncommon in this age group, especially in the absence of a family history, but these muscle disorders remain in the differential diagnosis. The symmetry of the weakness and the proximal muscle involvement in all limbs would be atypical for a lower motor neuron disease, but this condition would also be in the differential diagnosis. An abnormality of neuromuscular transmission such as systemic myasthenia gravis can present with predominantly proximal weakness. Most patients with myasthenia have prominent involvement of the extraocular muscles and/or bulbar muscle function as well.[74]

Electrodiagnostic distinction of myopathies and lower motor neuron diseases requires a careful needle electrode examination. In myopathies, motor unit potentials are short in duration, low in amplitude, and polyphasic. The recruitment pattern is increased in myopathies. In other words, the oscilloscope screen is filled with motor unit potentials even when the patient provides weak contraction of the affected muscle. The only way to make a definitive distinction between inflammatory and non-inflammatory myopathies, or for that matter to distinguish among the three idiopathic inflammatory myopathies, is to look at a biopsy specimen. But generally, signs of abnormal membrane irritability including fibrillation potentials, positive sharp waves, and complex repetitive discharges, might be seen on needle electrode examination of a muscle affected by an inflammatory myopathy.

Lower motor neuron diseases are also characterized by fibrillation potentials and positive sharp waves in the affected muscles, but motor unit potentials tend to be normal in size or enlarged as a result of ongoing reinnervation of denervated muscle fibers. The recruitment pattern is reduced, meaning that, instead of recruiting an increasing number of motor unit potentials with increased strength of contraction, a limited number of motor unit potentials fire at abnormally fast rates. In patients with myasthenia gravis, significant decrement can be seen on repetitive stimulation of affected muscles at slow rates (2–3 Hz) in the majority of patients. Results of EDX studies done on this patient are listed in Table 12-16.

Discussion

The NCS were performed to look for other potential abnormalities of the motor unit and, as expected, these were all normal. The findings on needle electrode examination of motor unit potentials with decreased amplitude and duration and with increased recruitment pattern were strongly suggestive of a primary myopathic process. Furthermore, the presence of fibrillation potentials in several proximal muscles was suggestive of an inflammatory etiology. In less severe cases, a more extensive needle electrode examination is often required in order to find fibrillation potentials and positive sharp waves, and the likelihood of finding these changes increases when muscles that are clinically weak—especially proximal muscles—are tested. Abnormalities are seen in the paraspinal muscles of this patient, as they are in many patients with inflammatory myopathy.

The findings were not likely due to a lower motor neuron disease because of the morphology and recruitment of the motor unit potentials. Because the clinical and EDX findings were so suggestive of a myopathy, repetitive nerve stimulation studies to look for evidence of myasthenia gravis were not performed. The clinical and EDX picture gave clues to help distinguish among the idiopathic inflammatory myopathies. In the vast majority of dermatomyositis cases, characteristic skin changes accompany the weakness. Inclusion body myositis is characterized by disproportionate weakness and EDX changes in the finger flexors and knee extensors.[3,50]

This patient's clinical and EDX picture were most compatible with a diagnosis of polymyositis, but the definitive diagnosis of one of the idiopathic inflammatory myopathies requires

Table 12-16 Weakness (case 16)

NERVE CONDUCTION STUDIES				
Sensory nerve	Stimulation site	Recording site	Amplitude (µV)	Conduction velocity (m/s)
R median	Digit 2	Wrist	28 (N > 10)	56 (N > 50)
	Palm	Wrist	92	58 (N > 50)
R ulnar	Digit 5	Wrist	19 (N > 10)	61 (N > 50)

Motor nerve	Stimulation site	Latency (ms)	Conduction velocity (m/s)	Amplitude (mV)
R median (record thenar)	Wrist	3.9 (N < 4.3)	–	6.1 (N > 4.0)
	Elbow	–	55 (N > 50)	5.8
R ulnar (record hypothenar)	Wrist	3.0 (N < 3.5)	–	5.9 (N > 4.0)
	Below elbow	–	57 (N > 50)	5.6
	Above elbow	–	54 (N > 50)	5.6

CONCENTRIC NEEDLE ELECTROMYOGRAPHY STUDIES						
Muscle	Spontaneous activity		Polyphasics	Motor unit potential		
	Positive waves	Fibrillation potentials		Recruitment	Amplitude	Duration
R deltoid	2+	2+	3+	Increased	Decreased	Decreased
R biceps	2+	1+	2+	Increased	Decreased	Decreased
R triceps	1+	1+	1+	Increased	Decreased	Decreased
R pronator teres	1+	0	1+	N	Decreased	Decreased
R iliopsoas	2+	1+	3+	Increased	Decreased	Decreased
R adductor longus	2+	1+	3+	Increased	Decreased	Decreased
R 1st dorsal interosseus pedis	0	0	Occasional	N	N	N
R 1st dorsal interosseus manus	0	0	Occasional	N	N	N
R extensor indicis	0	0	1+	N	N	N
R midcervical paraspinal	2+	2+	3+	Increased	Decreased	Decreased

muscle biopsy, which should be performed prior to starting immunosuppressive therapy when possible.[54] The biopsy is most likely to be diagnostic if taken from a muscle with significant abnormalities on needle electrode examination, so the EDX consultant should provide the surgeon with advice when choosing a muscle.

Case 17

A 28-year-old male custodian sought medical attention for a 6-month history of difficulty holding his mop stick. Specifically, he had difficulty letting go of the mop when he was gripping it, and he experienced painful cramps in his hands. There were no associated swallowing or ocular symptoms and no sensory symptoms besides the painful muscle cramps. On further questioning, he noted that during adolescence he frequently tripped and fell. Later he developed slowly progressive weakness of the hand muscles. Neither hot nor cold temperatures influenced his symptoms. He did not seek medical attention until recently, when the symptoms started to interfere with his job. His family

history was significant for similar complaints in his father and one of his three sisters.

General physical examination was significant for frontal balding and early bilateral cataracts.

Cranial examination showed bitemporal muscle atrophy, mild bilateral ptosis, and bilateral facial weakness. There was evidence of slight muscle atrophy and mild weakness in proximal and distal limb muscles. He demonstrated bilateral grip myotonia, in that he could not quickly release an object from the hand after gripping it tightly. He also had percussion myotonia at the thenar eminence (the muscle contracted after being struck by a reflex hammer, then released slowly) and eyelid myotonia (he could not quickly open his eyes after tightly closing them). Sensory examination was entirely normal. Reflexes were only minimally depressed and were symmetric.

Thought process

The bilateral ptosis and facial weakness might be seen in conditions causing multiple cranial neuropathies, or in disorders of neuromuscular transmission such as myasthenia gravis. However, the other findings on examination, including myotonia and mild diffuse weakness, would indicate the problem was more likely one of the myotonic myopathies. The facial features and family history (probably autosomal dominant transmission) were typical of myotonic dystrophy.[35,62,80] Myotonia congenita and paramyotonia congenita are less common and are characterized by myotonia in association with extremes of temperatures.

The EDX work-up in this patient should include NCS to evaluate for mononeuropathies that would contribute to muscle cramps in the hands. A patient who develops hand pain after repetitive use should always be evaluated for a median neuropathy at the carpal tunnel. The needle electrode examination should include some of the weak proximal and distal muscles to identify the presence of a myopathy. It would be especially useful to explore muscles in the thenar eminence affected by percussion myotonia. Results of EDX studies done on this patient are listed in Table 12-17.

Discussion

In this patient, whose occupation requires repetitive use of the hands, it is not surprising that there is mild slowing of the median sensory conductions across the carpal tunnel. While this is compatible with a mild right carpal tunnel syndrome, it does not explain the majority of his complaints or his findings on physical examination. Needle electrode examination was remarkable for profuse electrical myotonia in all muscles tested. Myotonia potentials are spontaneously discharges of single muscle fiber action potentials that wax and wane in frequency and amplitude,[5,64] providing a characteristic audio cue that has been described as the sound of a dive bomber or accelerating and decelerating motorcycle. There are changes in motor unit morphology, recording short duration, low-amplitude MUAPs and increased recruitment suggestive of a myopathic process.[14] The clinical presentation, family history, and EDX studies are all supportive of a diagnosis of myotonic dystrophy. Genetic testing is available to distinguish myotonic dystrophy from other myotonic disorders, and to screen family members.

Case 18

A 54-year-old man presented with complaints of 6 months of progressive weakness in the right hand. The patient was an accountant whose occupation required some repetitive use of the hands. His doctor referred him to the EDX laboratory to have an evaluation for carpal tunnel syndrome.

Table 12-17 Longstanding weakness and clumsiness (case 12–17)

NERVE CONDUCTION STUDIES

Sensory nerve	Stimulation site	Recording site	Amplitude (µV)	Conduction velocity (m/s)
R median	Digit 2	Wrist	16 (N > 10)	49 (N > 50)
	Palm	Wrist	48	41 (N > 50)
R ulnar	Digit 5	Wrist	15 (N > 10)	57 (N > 50)

Motor nerve	Stimulation site	Latency (ms)	Conduction velocity (m/s)	Amplitude (mV)
R median (record thenar)	Wrist	4.1 (N < 4.3)	–	4.8 (N > 4.0)
	Elbow	–	51 (N > 50)	4.3
R median F wave	–	28 (N < 32)	–	–
R ulnar (record hypothenar)	Wrist	3.0 (N < 3.5)	–	5.7 (N > 4.0)
	Below elbow	–	58 (N > 50)	5.2
	Above elbow	–	56 (N > 50)	5.2
R ulnar F wave	–	29 (N < 32)	–	–

CONCENTRIC NEEDLE ELECTROMYOGRAPHIC STUDIES

Muscle	Potentials	Spontaneous activity		Motor unit potentials		
		Positive waves	Fibrillation potentials	Recruitment	Amplitude	Duration
R deltoid	Myotonic	0	0	Increased	Few short	Few small
R biceps	Myotonic	0	0	N	Few short	Few small
R triceps	Myotonic	0	0	N	N	N
R 1st dorsal interosseus	Myotonic	0	0	N	N	N
R abductor pollicis brevis	Myotonic	0	0	N	N	N

At the time of the evaluation, the patient reported that his hand was clumsy and that he kept dropping things. He denied pain or numbness in the hand but did note occasional cramping, especially with repeated use of the hand. He denied similar symptoms on the left. The past medical history and family history were unremarkable. A focused examination of the right upper limb showed weakness of wrist extensors and weakness and atrophy of the intrinsic hand muscles, both the thenar and hypothenar groups. There was also mild weakness of elbow flexors and extensors as well as shoulder abductors.

These examination findings led to the conclusion that this was a case of more than simple carpal tunnel syndrome. On further questioning, the patient denied problems with speech, swallowing, breathing, and walking. He denied vision changes. He denied changes in bowel or bladder control.

A more detailed neurologic examination demonstrated some weakness of muscles in the left upper limb, although less severe than the weakness on the right. Cranial nerve examination was normal except that he could not hold air in his cheeks against resistance. He appeared to have mild weakness of the right ankle dorsiflexor muscles. His muscle stretch reflexes were brisk in all limbs, and he had a few beats of clonus at the ankles and bilateral Hoffmann's signs. There was a normal jaw jerk reflex. Gait was normal except that he held his right wrist in a flexed position and did not move that limb as much as the left upper limb when he walked.

Thought process

The distribution of weakness in the right upper limb includes multiple nerves and/or nerve roots, made a simple mononeuropathy such as a median neuropathy at the carpal tunnel an unlikely explanation. A painless right brachial plexopathy would explain the right upper limb weakness, but would not explain the hyperreflexia and weakness in other limbs. An asymmetric neuropathy (multiple mononeuropathies) could cause weakness and atrophy in this distribution, but then significant sensory complaints would be expected.

Cervical spine disease could cause this combination of diffuse weakness and hyperreflexia from cord compression, along with more severe focal right upper limb weakness and atrophy from compression of multiple right-sided cervical nerve roots. The inability of the patient to hold air in his cheeks against resistance, while suggestive of mild facial weakness, could also be within normal limits. Cervical spine disease would not explain facial weakness.

A motor neuron disease, specifically amyotrophic lateral sclerosis (ALS), would explain all the findings, including the facial weakness and hyperreflexia. One other diagnosis in the differential was multifocal motor neuropathy with conduction block, a potentially treatable, autoimmune motor neuropathy.

The right upper limb was examined first, because it was the most affected limb. Sensory conductions were performed to look for evidence of a brachial plexopathy or multiple mononeuropathies. Motor conductions were performed to assess for asymmetry, conduction block, and abnormalities affecting the motor unit (anterior horn cell, nerve root, nerve trunk,

neuromuscular junction, and muscle cell). The needle electrode examination was the most important to look for signs of active and chronic denervation. The presence and distribution of these abnormalities helps to distinguish the diagnostic possibilities. Results of EDX studies done on this patient are listed in Table 12-18.

Discussion

The motor conductions in the right median and ulnar nerves had normal latencies and velocities with reduced amplitudes of the CMAP responses. The motor conductions in the left median nerve were entirely normal. No evidence was seen for conduction block, making multifocal motor neuropathy with conduction block an unlikely diagnostic possibility. Motor responses could be affected by pathology at the level of the anterior horn cell, the motor root, the nerve trunk, and even the neuromuscular junction and muscle. The normal sensory conductions in the right median, ulnar, and radial nerves make injuries at the level of the brachial plexus or nerve trunks unlikely and suggest that the injury to the motor unit is proximal to the dorsal root ganglion (i.e. nerve root or anterior horn cell).

The abnormal findings on needle electrode examination also implicate active injury to the motor unit at multiple spinal levels.

Because of these abnormalities on needle electrode examination of right upper limb muscles, muscles in other regions of the body were also examined and found to be abnormal. Had the needle electrode examination of the right upper limb muscles (where clinical weakness and atrophy were greatest) been normal, examination of these other regions would not likely have been useful. The thoracic paraspinal muscles were evaluated after abnormalities were discovered in the cervical and lumbosacral regions. Because normal values for MUAP size and morphology are not well established in the paraspinal muscles, only resting activity was evaluated in those muscles.

The presence of signs of active denervation (i.e. fibrillation potentials, positive sharp waves) in multiple muscles with different nerve supply in the cervical, thoracic, and lumbosacral regions was most suggestive of a lower motor neuron disease. Multiple nerve root injuries due to degenerative spine disease could also explain the findings. But such spinal abnormalities are quite rare in the thoracic region, and the patient would be expected to have significant pain complaints.

A systematic EDX approach should be employed in the work-up of motor neuron diseases. Using such an approach, Lambert used EDX criteria for ALS, including signs of active (fibrillation potentials, positive sharp waves) and chronic (enlarged, polyphasic motor unit potentials) denervation in multiple muscles with different nerve supply (different nerve root and nerve trunk) in three limbs, along with normal sensory conductions.[47,48] The criteria have since been modified. The El Escorial criteria for diagnosis of ALS, which uses mainly clinical criteria to establish degree of certainty of the diagnosis, include the category probable ALS, laboratory-supported.[10] A patient who has one definite upper motor neuron sign on physical

Table 12-18 Progressive hand weakness (case 18)

NERVE CONDUCTION STUDIES

Sensory nerve	Stimulation site	Recording site	Amplitude (μV)	Conduction velocity (m/s)
R median	Digit 2	Wrist	22 (N > 10)	55 (N > 50)
	Palm	Wrist	84	59 (N > 50)
R ulnar	Digit 5	Wrist	19 (N > 10)	56 (N > 50)
R radial	Forearm	Wrist	37 (N > 10)	61 (N > 50)

Motor nerve	Stimulation site	Latency (ms)	Conduction velocity (m/s)	Amplitude (mV)
R median (record thenar)	Wrist	4.2 (N < 4.3)	–	2.1 (N > 4.0)
	Elbow	–	50 (N > 50)	1.9
R median F wave	–	31 (N < 32)	–	–
R ulnar (record hypothenar)	Wrist	3.4 (N < 3.5)	–	3.2 (N > 4.0)
	Below elbow	–	50 (N > 50)	2.8
	Above elbow	–	51 (N > 50)	2.8
R ulnar F wave	–	30 (N < 32)	–	–
L median (record thenar)	Wrist	4.0 (N < 32)	–	5.2 (N > 4.0)
	Elbow	–	53 (N > 50)	4.9
L median F wave	–	27 (N < 32)	–	–

CONCENTRIC NEEDLE ELECTROMYOGRAPHY STUDIES

Muscle	Spontaneous activity		Recruitment	Motor unit potentials	
	Positive waves	Fibrillation potentials		Amplitude	Duration
R deltoid	2+	2+	Decreased	Few large	Few long
R biceps	2+	2+	N	N	N
R triceps	2+	2+	Decreased	Few large	Few long
R 1st dorsal interosseus	4+	4+	Markedly decreased	Most large	Most long
R pronator teres	3+	3+	Decreased	Few large	Few long
R iliopsoas	2+	1+	N	N	N
R vastus medialis	1+	1+	N	N	N
R tibialis anterior	2+	2+	Decreased	N	N
R gastrocnemius	1+	1+	N	N	N
R gluteus medius	1+	1+	N	N	N
R midthoracic paraspinal	2+	2+	–	–	–
R low thoracic paraspinal	2+	2+	–	–	–

examination and EDX signs of active denervation affecting at least two regions (i.e. cranial, cervical, thoracic, lumbosacral) can be given this classification. It is worth noting that the EDX evaluation can only give supportive evidence for lower motor neuron component in ALS.

When a patient with motor neuron disease presented with predominantly bulbar symptoms and signs (unlike this patient, who had limb onset), myasthenia gravis might be considered in the differential diagnosis. In those patients, repetitive nerve stimulation is often performed as part of the work-up. It should be noted that significant decrement sometimes occurs with repetitive stimulation at slow rates in patients with lower motor neuron diseases.[7,19]

Case 19

A 43-year-old woman sought medical attention because of a 6-month history of episodic double vision, drooping of the eyelids, slurred speech, and difficulty chewing. She described the symptoms as usually mild in the morning but worsening by the end of the day. She also complained of arm weakness during physical activity, which quickly resolved with rest. She denied any associated sensory symptoms. The past medical history was significant only for hypothyroidism, which was well controlled with medication. Clinical examination was significant for ptosis, worse on the right than on the left. Ptosis worsened after 25 s of sustained upward gaze. Right eye abduction was limited. Limb strength was normal at rest, but mild proximal weakness was detected after brief exercise. The remainder of the neurologic examination was normal.

Thought process

Both the history and physical examination were consistent with weakness of bilateral eye opening (levator plapebrae superior muscle) and right eye abduction (lateral rectus muscle). These muscles are innervated by cranial nuclei at different levels of the brain stem. Because the patient is fully awake and alert, a brain stem lesion is not implicated. More likely would be a disorder of the peripheral nervous system, i.e. nerve, neuromuscular junction, or muscle. The distribution of weakness, normal muscle stretch reflexes, and normal sensory examination essentially precluded a generalized peripheral neuropathy, but multiple mononeuropathies as seen in association with diabetes and vasculitis remain diagnostic possibilities. Myopathy was an unlikely explanation given the distribution of weakness.[46]

The fluctuating nature of the patient's voluntary muscle weakness, which worsens with exercise and improves with rest, was consistent with a disorder of neuromuscular transmission such as myasthenia gravis.[72] The involvement of cranial-innervated muscles and relative sparing of the limb muscles make the Lambert–Eaton myasthenic syndrome, another disorder of neuromuscular transmission, unlikely as well. Ocular symptoms such as ptosis and diplopia are the most common presenting symptoms in myasthenia gravis and are almost always involved in this disorder.[20,52]

Nerve conduction studies were performed to evaluate for mononeuropathy, multiple mononeuropathies, or polyneuropathy. Because myasthenia gravis was the most likely explanation based on the clinical findings, repetitive nerve stimulation at 3 Hz was also performed. Finally, the needle electrode examination was performed to rule in or rule out an 'irritable' myopathic process, occasionally seen in association with myasthenia gravis. Results of EDX studies done on this patient are listed in Table 12-19.

Discussion

Nerve conduction studies showed normal latencies, normal amplitudes of motor and sensory responses, and normal sensory and motor conduction velocities. These findings are incompatible with an axonal or demyelinating neuropathy.[40] Myopathic injury is also unlikely, because needle EMG showed normal motor unit potential amplitude, duration, complexity, and recruitment. Moreover, fibrillation potentials and positive sharp waves were not present.

Repetitive nerve stimulation at 3 Hz produced a significant decremental response (>10% decrement from first to fourth

stimulus is considered significant) of the CMAP amplitude in one of three nerves tested at baseline. In all three nerves, there was no significant decrement following 20 s of isometric contraction, proving postexercise potentiation. Significant decrement was recorded in all nerves tested 1 min after ceasing isometric contraction, demonstrating postexercise exhaustion. A decremental response to low rates of repetitive stimulation is seen in disorders of neuromuscular transmission, including myasthenia gravis, Lambert–Eaton myasthenic syndrome, and botulism. In addition, a significant incremental response (>100%) of the CMAP to high-frequency (20–50 Hz) repetitive nerve stimulation is seen in presynaptic neuromuscular transmission defects such as Lambert–Eaton myasthenic syndrome or botulism.[29,66,73] Repetitive stimulation at 50 Hz was not performed in this case, because 50-Hz stimulation is painful, and the clinical findings and neurographic findings of postexercise facilitation and exhaustion strongly support the diagnosis of myasthenia gravis.

In selected patients, the diagnosis of myasthenia gravis can be further clarified by single-fiber EMG, which would be expected to show increased dispersion of latencies of muscle fiber potentials within a motor unit (jitter) in patients with myasthenia gravis[71] as well as in those with other conditions. The history, neurologic examination, and EDX studies were all consistent with myasthenia gravis.

Case 20

A 57-year-old man was referred for EDX consultation to evaluate progressive shortness of breath. He had an extremely complicated past medical history that included a 25-year history of Wegener granulomatosis, chronic renal failure, status post renal transplant with failed transplant, removal of the kidney and continuing renal dialysis, coronary artery disease, cardiomyopathy, status post coronary artery bypass graft (CABG), posttransplant lymphoproliferative disorder, and hyperhomocysteinemia. He was status post CABG and his ejection fraction was 40%. He was readmitted a few weeks prior to EDX consultation because of orthopnea, progressive dyspnea, and ejection fraction of 20%. His respiratory symptoms were thought to be secondary to volume overload because of cardiomyopathy. Aggressive dialysis was successfully instituted, resulting in weight loss and appropriate fluid loss, but right pleural effusion and respiratory difficulties persisted. Significant medications include chronic steroids and atorvastatin. A previous EDX consultant had established the presence of unspecified peripheral polyneuropathy secondary to Wegener granulomatosis, although the exact details were not available. Wegener granulomatosis is a rare disorder wherein necrotizing granulomas affect the respiratory tract and the kidneys, and cause systemic small vessel disease.[34] In the present case, Wegener granulomatosis did not involve the lung tissue per referral source evaluation. There were no other respiratory symptoms reported, other than shortness of breath. Given the patient's clinical condition and reported poor tolerance to testing of any type, the consultation is limited mostly to evaluation of the diaphragm as requested.

Table 12-19 Fluctuating diplopia and ptosis (case 19)

NERVE CONDUCTION STUDIES				
Sensory nerve	Stimulation site	Recording site	Amplitude (μV)	Conduction velocity (m/s)
R median	Digit 2	Wrist	24 (N > 10)	61 (N > 50)
	Palm	Wrist	78	62 (N > 50)
R ulnar	Digit 5	Wrist	22 (N > 10)	59 (N > 50)

Motor nerve	Stimulation site	Latency (ms)	Conduction velocity (m/s)	Amplitude (mV)
R median (record thenar)	Wrist	3.9 (N < 4.3)	–	5.4
	Elbow	–	58 (N > 50)	5.1
R median F wave	–	27 (N < 32)	–	–
R ulnar (record hypothenar)	Wrist	3.0 (N < 3.5)	–	6.3
	Below elbow	–	59 (N > 50)	6.1
	Above elbow	–	61 (N > 50)	6.1
R ulnar F wave	–	28 (N < 32)	–	–

REPETITIVE NERVE STIMULATION			
Muscle/nerve		Stimulation site	Percentage difference amplitude 1–4
R trapezius/spinal accessory	Neck	Baseline	–9
		Immediately post exercise	+1
		1 min post exercise	–15
R orbicularis oris/facial	Mandible	Baseline	–12
		Immediately post exercise	–4
		1 min post exercise	–25
R biceps/musculocutaneous	Axilla	Baseline	–2
		Immediately post exercise	+3
		1 min post exercise	–12

CONCENTRIC NEEDLE ELECTROMYOGRAPHY STUDIES					
Muscle	Spontaneous activity *Positive waves*	Motor unit potentials *Fibrillation potentials*	*Recruitment*	*Amplitude*	*Duration*
R deltoid	0	0	N	N	N
R biceps	0	0	N	N	N
R triceps	0	0	N	N	N

Physical examination showed a man who was not in significant respiratory distress. Muscle stretch reflexes were normal at the biceps but absent at brachioradialis and triceps bilaterally. Knee jerks were 1+ and ankle jerks absent bilaterally. There was an easily elicited stocking distribution to pinprick bilaterally, but pinprick to the upper limbs appeared intact. Light touch was decreased in a glove distribution bilaterally. Strength was normal in the upper limbs. Gait and station were normal. Chest expansion was less than 2 cm at maximum inspiration.

Thought process

Wegener granulomatosis has a number of presentations, including peripheral neuropathy, mononeuropathy multiplex, distal symmetric polyneuropathy, and unclassified.[56] Given that the patient's volume overload problem was corrected by aggressive dialysis, and considering that he had a known progressive polyneuropathy, the highest likelihood is of polyneuropathy affecting the respiratory muscles.

Previous EDX did not include diaphragm or intercostal muscles, so comparative studies cannot be done in this case. Current studies would serve as baseline and give information that could help the referral source manage this patient's problems. The patient has continued right pleural effusion, which could be a source of his ongoing respiratory distress. EDX evaluation of respiratory muscle function should help define the contribution of various pathologies to the clinical picture. New-onset Guillain–Barré syndrome was possible but unlikely. The

Table 12-20 Progressive shortness of breath (case 20)

NERVE CONDUCTION STUDIES Motor nerve		Site			Latency (ms)			Amplitude (mV)
L phrenic		SCM			Absent			Absent
R phrenic		SCM			Absent			Absent

MONOPOLAR NEEDLE ELECTROMYOGRAPHY STUDIES Muscle	Spontaneous					MUAP		Recruitment
	PSW	Fib	Fasc	HF	Amplitude	Duration	Poly	pattern
L diaphragm	None	None	None	None	N	N	N	2−
R diaphragm	None	None	None	None	N	N	N	1−
L intercostals	None	None	None	None	N	N	N	2−
R intercostals	None	None	None	None	N	N	N	2−

Fib, Fibrillation potentials; Fasc, fasciculation potentials; HF, complex repetitive discharges; MUAP, motor unit action potential; N, normal; Poly, polyphasic motor unit potentials; PSW, positive sharp waves.

patient has had increasing respiratory distress over several weeks, and no other symptoms or signs, making Guillain–Barré a more remote possibility. Results of limited EDX studies done on this patient are listed in Table 12-20.

Discussion

The phrenic nerve CMAP was absent bilaterally. Needle EMG exploration of the diaphragm and intercostal muscles bilaterally show significantly decreased recruitment. The findings were compatible with polyneuropathy, with partial conduction block of the phrenic nerves bilaterally. There was no evidence for acute denervation. The possibility that the phrenic nerve might be hyporesponsive to electrical stimulation must be considered. The referral source now has information that can guide the management process for this very complicated clinical situation.

REFERENCES

1. Al-Kawas FH. Myositis associated with Crohn's colitis. Am J Gastroenterol 1986; 81:583–585.

2. Amato AA, Dumitru D. Acquired neuropathies. In: Zwarts MJ, ed. Electrodiagnostic medicine. 2nd edn. Philadelphia: Hanley & Belfus; 2002:956–959.

3. Amato AA, Gronseth GS, Jackson CE, et al. Inclusion body myositis: clinical and pathological boundaries. Ann Neurol 1996; 40:581–586.

4. Bagnato S, Rizzo V, Quartarone A, et al. Segmental myoclonus in a patient affected by syringomyelia. Neurol Sci 2001; 22:27–29.

5. Barchi RL. A mechanistic approach to the myotonic syndromes. Muscle Nerve 1982; 5:S60–S63.

6. Berlit P. Clinical and laboratory findings with giant cell arteritis. J Neurol Sci 1992; 111:1–12.

7. Bernstein LP, Antel JP. Motor neuron disease: decremental responses to repetitive nerve stimulation. Neurology 1981; 31:204–207.

8. Bouche P, Leger JM, Travers MA, et al. Peripheral neuropathy in systemic vasculitis: clinical and electrophysiologic study of 22 patients. Neurology 1986; 36:1598–1602.

9. Braddom RI, Johnson EW. Standardization of H reflex and diagnostic use in Sl radiculopathy. Arch Phys Med Rehabil 1974; 55:161–166.

10. Brooks BR. El Escorial World Federation of Neurology criteria for the diagnosis of amyotrophic lateral sclerosis. Subcommittee on Motor Neuron Diseases/Amyotrophic Lateral Sclerosis of the World Federation of Neurology Research Group on Neuromuscular Diseases and the El Escorial 'Clinical limits of amyotrophic lateral sclerosis' workshop contributors. J Neurol Sci 1994; 124(suppl):96–107.

11. Brown MJ, Asbury AK. Diabetic neuropathy. Ann Neurol 1984; 15: 2–12.

12. Buchthal F, Behse F. Peroneal muscular atrophy (PMA) and related disorders. I. Clinical manifestations as related to biopsy findings, nerve conduction and electromyography. Brain 1977; 100(part 1):41–66.

13. Buchthal F, Rosenfalck A. Sensory conduction from digit to palm and from palm to wrist in the carpal tunnel syndrome. J Neurol Neurosurg Psychiatry 1971; 34: 243–252.

14. Buchthal F. Electromyography in the evaluation of muscle diseases. Neurol Clin 1985; 3:573–598.

15. Chokroverty S. AAEE case report #13: diabetic amyotrophy. Muscle Nerve 1987; 10:679–684.

16. Clairmont AC, Johnson EW. Evaluation of the patient with possible radiculopathy. In: Pease WS, ed. Practical electromyography. 3rd edn. Baltimore: Williams & Wilkins; 1997:123–124.

17. Colachis SC III, Klejka JP, Shamir DY, et al. Amplitude of M responses. Side to side comparability. Am J Phys Med Rehabil 1993; 72:19–22.

18. Cornblath DR. Electrophysiology in Guillain–Barré syndrome. Ann Neurol 1990; 27(suppl):S17–S20.

19. Denys EH, Norris FH Jr. Amyotrophic lateral sclerosis. Impairment of neuromuscular transmission. Arch Neurol 1979; 36:202–205.

20. Drachman DB. Myasthenia gravis (first of two parts). N Engl J Med 1978; 298:136–142.

21. Dyck PJ, Lambert EH. Lower motor and primary sensory neuron diseases with peroneal muscular atrophy. I. Neurologic, genetic, and electrophysiologic findings in hereditary polyneuropathies. Arch Neurol 1968; 18:603–618.

22. Fisher MA. AAEM minimonograph #13: H reflexes and F waves: physiology and clinical indications. Muscle Nerve 1992; 15:1223–1233.

23. Gariballa SE, Gunasekera NP. Bilateral foot drop, weight loss and rectal bleeding as an acute presentation of Crohn's disease. Postgrad Med J 1994; 70:762–763.

24. Golbus J, McCune WJ. Giant cell arteritis and peripheral neuropathy: a report of 2 cases and review of the literature. J Rheumatol 1987; 14:129–134.

25. Gondim FA, Brannagan TH III, Sander HW, et al. Peripheral neuropathy in patients with inflammatory bowel disease. Brain 2005; 128(part 4): 867–879.

26. Gouider R, LeGuern E, Gugenheim M, et al. Clinical, electrophysiologic, and molecular correlations in 13 families with hereditary neuropathy with liability to pressure palsies and a chromosome 17p11.2 deletion. Neurology 1995; 45:2018–2023.

27. Harding AE, Thomas PK. Genetic aspects of hereditary motor and sensory neuropathy (types I and II). J Med Genet 1980; 17:329–336.

28. Harding AE, Thomas PK. The clinical features of hereditary motor and sensory neuropathy types I and II. Brain 1980; 103:259–280.

29. Howard JF Jr, Sanders DB, Massey JM. The electrodiagnosis of myasthenia gravis and the Lambert–Eaton myasthenic syndrome. Neurol Clin 1994; 12:305–330.

30. Humbert P, Monnier G, Billerey C, et al. Polyneuropathy: an unusual extraintestinal manifestation of Crohn's disease. Acta Neurol Scand 1989; 80:301–306.

31. Jacobson RE. Lumbar stenosis. An electromyographic evaluation. Clin Orthop Relat Res 1976: Mar–Apr(115):68–71.

32. Jamieson PW, Giuliani MJ, Martinez AJ. Necrotizing angiopathy presenting with multifocal conduction blocks. Neurology 1991; 41:442–444.

33. Jia ZR, Shi X, Sun XR. Pathogenesis and electrodiagnosis of cubital tunnel syndrome. Chin Med J (Engl) 2004; 117:1313–1316.

34. Jimenez-Medina HJ, Yablon SA. Electrodiagnostic characteristics of Wegener's granulomatosis-associated peripheral neuropathy. Am J Phys Med Rehabil 1992; 71:6–11.

35. Jozefowicz RF, Griggs RC. Myotonic dystrophy. Neurol Clin 1988; 6:455–472.

36. Kiloh LG. Brachial plexus lesions after cholecystectomy. Lancet 1950; 1:103–105.

37. Kimura J. F-wave velocity in the central segment of the median and ulnar nerves. A study in normal subjects and in patients with Charcot–Marie–Tooth disease. Neurology 1974; 24:539–546.

38. Kimura J. Mononeuropathies and entrapment syndromes. In: Kimura J, ed. Electrodiagnosis in diseases of nerve and muscle: principles and practice. 3rd edn. New York: Oxford University Press; 2001:724–726.

39. Kimura J. Polyneuropathies. In: Kimura J, ed. Electrodiagnosis in diseases of nerve and muscle: principles and practice. 3rd edn. New York: Oxford University Press; 2001:652–654.

40. Kimura J. Principles and pitfalls of nerve conduction studies. Ann Neurol 1984; 16:415–429.

41. Kimura J. The carpal tunnel syndrome: localization of conduction abnormalities within the distal segment of the median nerve. Brain 1979; 102:619–635.

42. Kimura J. Types of electromyographic abnormalities. In: Kimura J, ed. Electrodiagnosis in diseases of nerve and muscle: principles and practice. 3rd edn. New York: Oxford University Press; 2001:352–356.

43. Kopell HP, Goodgold J. Clinical and electrodiagnostic features of carpal tunnel syndrome. Arch Phys Med Rehabil 1968; 49:371–375.

44. Kothari MJ, Preston DC. Comparison of the flexed and extended elbow positions in localizing ulnar neuropathy at the elbow. Muscle Nerve 1995; 18:336–340.

45. Kummel BM, Zazanis GA. Shoulder pain as the presenting complaint in carpal tunnel syndrome. Clin Orthop Relat Res 1973; 92:227–230.

46. Kuncl R, Hoffman P. Myopathies and disorders of neuromuscular transmission. In: Newman N, ed. Walsh and Hoyt's clinical neuro-ophthalmology. 5th edn. Baltimore: Williams & Wilkins; 1998:1351–1460.

47. Lambert EH, Mulder DW. Electromyographic studies in amyotrophic lateral sclerosis. Mayo Clin Proc 1957; 32:441–446.

48. Lambert EH. Electromyography in amyotrophic lateral sclerosis. In: Kurland LT, ed. Motor neuron diseases: research on amyotrophic lateral sclerosis and related disorders. New York: Grune & Stratton; 1969.

49. Lewis RA, Sumner AJ. The electrodiagnostic distinctions between chronic familial and acquired demyelinative neuropathies. Neurology 1982; 32:592–596.

50. Lotz BP, Engel AG, Nishino H, et al. Inclusion body myositis. Observations in 40 patients. Brain 1989; 112(part 3):727–747.

51. Maat-Schieman ML, Macfarlane JD, Bots GT, et al. Inclusion body myositis: its relative frequency in elderly people. Clin Neurol Neurosurg 1992; 94(suppl):S118–S120.

52. Meriggioli MN, Sanders DB. Myasthenia gravis: diagnosis. Semin Neurol 2004; 24:31–39.

53. Mohamed A, Davies L, Pollard JD. Conduction block in vasculitic neuropathy. Muscle Nerve 1998; 21:1084–1088.

54. Nash SM, Kissel JT. Idiopathic inflammatory myopathies. In: Pourmand R, ed. Neuromuscular diseases: expert clinicians' views. Boston: Butterworth Heinemann; 2001:199–226.

55. Nemni R, Fazio R, Corbo M, et al. Peripheral neuropathy associated with Crohn's disease. Neurology 1987; 37:1414–1417.

56. Nishino H, Rubino FA, DeRemee RA, et al. Neurological involvement in Wegener's granulomatosis: an analysis of 324 consecutive patients at the Mayo Clinic. Ann Neurol 1993; 33:4–9.

57. Nogues MA, Leiguarda RC, Rivero AD, et al. Involuntary movements and abnormal spontaneous EMG activity in syringomyelia and syringobulbia. Neurology 1999; 52:823–834.

58. Nogues MA, Stalberg E. Electrodiagnostic findings in syringomyelia. Muscle Nerve 1999; 22:1653–1659.

59. Pareyson D, Solari A, Taroni F, et al. Detection of hereditary neuropathy with liability to pressure palsies among patients with acute painless mononeuropathy or plexopathy. Muscle Nerve 1998; 21:1686–1691.

60. Pareyson D. Charcot–Marie–Tooth disease and related neuropathies: molecular basis for distinction and diagnosis. Muscle Nerve 1999; 22:1498–1509.

61. Parsonage MJ, Turner AJW. Neuralgic amyotrophy: the shoulder girdle syndrome. Lancet 1948; 1:973.

62. Perini GI, Menegazzo E, Ermani M, et al. Cognitive impairment and (CTG)n expansion in myotonic dystrophy patients. Biol Psychiatry 1999; 46:425–431.

63. Perkins BA, Bril V. Diabetic neuropathy: a review emphasizing diagnostic methods. Clin Neurophysiol 2003; 114:1167–1175.

64. Pleasure D, Shawn B, Steven S, et al. Neuromuscular disease. In: Demasio AR, ed. Atlas of clinical neurology. Philadelphia: Butterworth-Heinemann; 1998:11–16.

65. Poncelet AN. Diabetic polyneuropathy. Risk factors, patterns of presentation, diagnosis, and treatment. Geriatrics 2003; 58:16–18, 24–25, 30.

66. Preston DC, Shapiro BE. Electromyography and neuromuscular disorders: clinical electrophysiological correlations. Newton: Butterworth-Heinemann; 1998.

67. Pryse-Phillips WE. Validation of a diagnostic sign in carpal tunnel syndrome. J Neurol Neurosurg Psychiatry 1984; 47:870–872.

68. Reinstein L. Hand dominance in carpal tunnel syndrome. Arch Phys Med Rehabil 1981; 62:202–203.

69. Ropert A, Metral S. Conduction block in neuropathies with necrotizing vasculitis. Muscle Nerve 1990; 13:102–105.

70. Ropper AH. The Guillain–Barré syndrome. N Engl J Med 1992; 326:1130–1136.

71. Sanders DB. Clinical impact of single-fiber electromyography. Muscle Nerve 2002; Suppl 11:S15–S20.

72. Sanders DB. Diseases associated with neuromuscular transmission. In: Aminoff MJ, ed. Neuromuscular function and disease. Basic, clinical and electrodiagnostic aspects. Philadelphia: Saunders; 2001:1346–1347.

73. Sanders DB. The electrodiagnosis of myasthenia gravis. Ann NY Acad Sci 1987; 505:539–556.

74. Sanders DM. Myasthenia gravis and Lambert–Eaton myasthenic syndromes. In: Pourmand R, ed. Neuromuscular diseases: expert clinicians' views. Boston: Butterworth Heinemann; 2001:439–458.

75. Scelsa SN. Syringomyelia presenting as ulnar neuropathy at the elbow. Clin Neurophysiol 2000; 111:1527–1530.

76. Stevens JC. AAEE minimonograph #26: the electrodiagnosis of carpal tunnel syndrome. Muscle Nerve 1987; 10:99–113.

77. Thomas PK, Calne DB. Motor nerve conduction velocity in peroneal muscular atrophy: evidence for genetic heterogeneity. J Neurol Neurosurg Psychiatry 1974; 37:68–75.

78. Thomas PK, Sears TA, Gilliatt RW. The range of conduction velocity in normal motor nerve fibers to the small muscles of the hand and foot. J Neurol Neurosurg Psychiatry 1959; 22:175–181.

79. Thomas PK. Motor nerve conduction in the carpal tunnel syndrome. Neurology 1960; 10:1045–1050.

80. Timchenko L, Monckton DG, Caskey CT. Myotonic dystrophy: an unstable CTG repeat in a protein kinase gene. Semin Cell Biol 1995; 6:13–19.

81. Tuck RR, McLeod JG. Autonomic dysfunction in Guillain–Barré syndrome. J Neurol Neurosurg Psychiatry 1981; 44:983–990.

82. Upton AR, McComas AJ. The double crush in nerve entrapment syndromes. Lancet 1973; 2:359–362.

83. Wilbourn AJ, Aminoff MJ. AAEE minimonograph #32: the electrophysiologic examination in patients with radiculopathies. Muscle Nerve 1988; 11:1099–1114.

84. Yuki N, Taki T, Inagaki F, et al. A bacterium lipopolysaccharide that elicits Guillain–Barré syndrome has a GM1 ganglioside-like structure. J Exp Med 1993; 178:1771–1775.

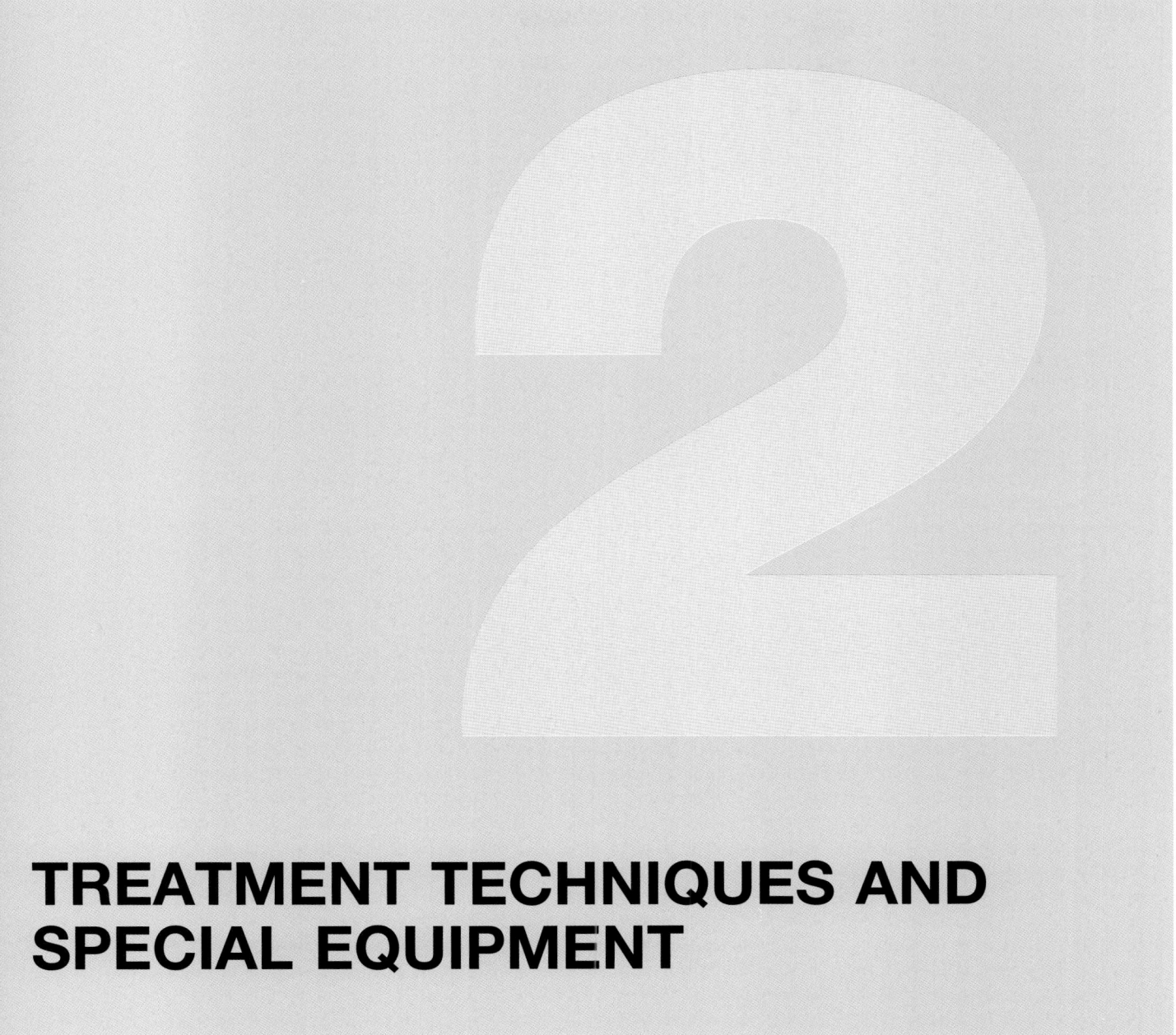

TREATMENT TECHNIQUES AND SPECIAL EQUIPMENT

Chapter

13

Upper Limb Amputee Rehabilitation and Prosthetic Restoration

Alberto Esquenazi

INCIDENCE AND DEMOGRAPHICS

Based on the most recent information available from the National Center for Health Statistics, approximately 1 230 000 amputees are living in the USA (all levels of amputation), with approximately 50 000 new amputations performed annually.[30] The ratio of upper limb to lower limb amputation estimated from this information is 1:4.9. The most frequent causes of upper limb amputation are trauma and cancer, followed by vascular complications of disease. The most common major upper limb amputation is at the transradial level, which accounts for 57% of all arm amputations. Transhumeral amputation accounts for 23% of all amputations. The right arm is more frequently involved in work-related injuries. Sixty percent of arm amputees are between the ages of 21 and 64 years, and 10% are younger than 21 years.[11,18]

Congenital upper limb deficiency has an incidence of approximately 4.1 per 10 000 live births.[30] The congenital limb deficiencies are best classified according to the International Organization for Standardization and the International Society for Prosthetics and Orthotics classifications as modified from Frantz-O'Reilly. The limb deficiencies can be transverse or longitudinal. The term *terminal* is used to describe the fact that the limb has developed normally to a particular level, beyond which no skeletal element exists. In intercalary limb deficiency, a reduction or absence of one or more elements occurs within the long axis of the limb, and in this case normal skeletal elements may be found distal to the affected segments.[18] The most common congenital limb deficiency is the left terminal transverse radial limb deficiency (Table 13-1).

LIMB SALVAGE VERSUS AMPUTATION SURGERY

Severe hand injuries frequently challenge the skills of the surgeon to the point of having to consider amputation. The absolute surgical indication for amputation in trauma is ischemia in a limb with unreconstructible vascular injury. As reconstruction techniques have improved, more attempts at limb salvage have been made, although amputation is often ultimately required after multiple surgical procedures. Such surgical procedures also represent a substantial investment of time,

money, and emotional energy. Massively crushed or burned muscle[9] and ischemic tissue release myoglobin and cell toxins, which can lead to renal failure, adult respiratory distress syndrome, and death. The risk of infection, contractures, and nerve injuries that interfere with function also need to be considered. Recent studies show the value of early amputation not only in saving lives, but also in preventing the emotional, marital, and financial disasters and opiate analgesic addictions that can follow desperate attempts at limb salvage.

In establishing guidelines for immediate or early amputation of mangled limbs, the surgeon must bear in mind that upper limb salvage should be based on providing an extremity that has sufficient sensation to provide protective feedback, has a durable soft tissue cover, and can be used to interact with the environment. An upper limb with limited motion, multiple scars, or lack of sensation functions poorly because of the constant risk of tissue injury. This type of limb often functions worse than a modern prosthetic replacement. Grading scales for mangled lower limbs have recently been developed and should serve as guidelines to help the surgeon assess the gravity of the injury and the subsequent risk of salvage.[13]

Amputation should never be viewed as surgical failure, but rather as the means to return the patient to a more functional status. The value of approaching amputation with a positive and reconstructive approach cannot be overemphasized. The decision to amputate is an emotional process for all involved, and the rehabilitation team should stand ready to respond and assist early in the process.

The selection of the surgical level of amputation is probably one of the most important decisions that must be made for the amputee. The viability of soft tissue and the amount of skin coverage with adequate sensation usually determine the most distal possible functional level for amputation. After surgery, the patient with an upper limb amputation should ideally be able to use a prosthesis (either body or externally powered) during most of the day. Bony prominences, skin scars, soft tissue traction, shear, hypersensitivity, and perspiration can complicate prosthesis use. For these reasons, the residual limb must be surgically constructed with care to optimize the intimacy of fit, maintain muscle balance, and allow assumption of stresses necessary to meet the limb's new function. New surgical techniques that permit myocutaneous transfers, skin expansion methods, and bony lengthening procedures are available to

Table 13-1 International terminology for the classification of congenital limb deficiencies[a]

Term	Definition
Terminal	The limb has developed normally to a particular level, beyond which no skeletal elements exist
Intercalary	There is a reduction or absence of one or more elements within the long axis of the limb, and normal skeletal elements may be present distal to the affected segment

[a]Derived from the International Organization for Standardization and the International Society for Prosthetics and Orthotics classifications.

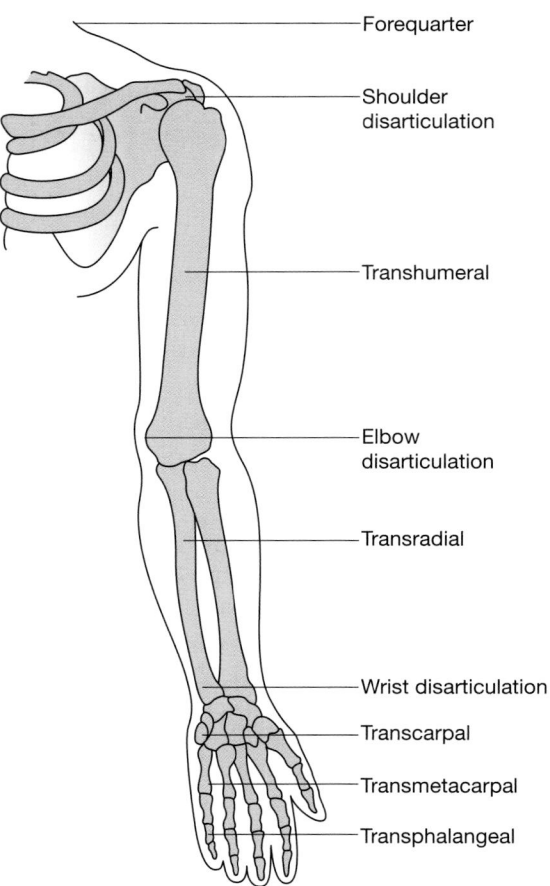

Figure 13-1 Upper limb levels of amputation and anatomic terminology.

optimize the residual limb shape, size, and function.[15] This optimization should preferably be done at the time of the amputation, but it can be done at a second stage. Using a staged approach delays prosthetic fitting and can decrease the success of prosthetic restoration. Early prosthetic fitting after arm amputation (1–4 months) is imperative if successful prosthetic restoration is to be expected.[27] During healing, prevention of scar tissue adhesion formation and joint contracture is critical.

Levels of amputation

Finger amputation can occur at the distal interphalangeal, proximal interphalangeal, and metacarpophalangeal levels (Fig. 13-1). Transcarpal amputation and wrist amputation are seen less frequently because of their limited functional outcome. Multiple finger amputations, including thumb and partial hand amputations and those through the wrist, need to be considered carefully in view of the possible functional and cosmetic implications of prosthesis fitting and restoration. Inappropriate choice of amputation site can result in a prosthesis with disproportional length or width. It can also preclude the use of externally powered devices.

The transradial amputation is preferred in most cases, and it can be performed at three levels (resulting in long, medium, and short residual limbs). The long forearm residual limb is preferred when optimal body-powered prosthetic restoration is the goal. It is the ideal level for the patient who is expected to perform physically demanding work. The medium forearm residual limb is preferred when optimal externally powered prosthetic restoration is the goal. This length typically permits good function and cosmesis. The short transradial amputation level can complicate suspension, and limit elbow flexion strength and elbow range of motion. Transradial amputation is the most common level and allows the highest level of functional recovery in the majority of cases. These three amputation levels require the same type of rehabilitation interventions and make use of similar prosthetic components. The suspension system for each one of them can be different.

The elbow disarticulation has some surgical and prosthetic advantages and disadvantages. The surgical technique permits reduction in surgery time and blood loss, provides improved

prosthetic self-suspension while permitting the use of a less encumbering socket, and reduces the rotation of the socket on the residual limb as compared with the transhumeral level of amputation.[42] Major disadvantages are the marginal cosmetic appearance caused by the required external elbow mechanism, and current limitations in technology, which impede the use of externally powered elbow mechanisms at this level of amputation. These drawbacks often outweigh the advantages in the long run. In the patient for whom bilateral transhumeral amputation is the alternative, the elbow disarticulation is a more desirable level when feasible, despite the possible cosmetic drawbacks.

The transhumeral amputation can be performed at three levels: long (three-quarters of bone length), medium, and short (one-third of bone length). The long arm residual limb (7–10 cm from the distal humeral condyle) is preferred for optimal prosthetic restoration. These three amputation levels require the same type of rehabilitation interventions and, in most cases, require similar prosthetic components. These can be externally powered, body-powered, passive, or a combination of these assembled into a hybrid system.

The shoulder disarticulation and forequarter amputations fortunately are seen less frequently than amputations at other levels. In most cases, they are made necessary as part of the surgical intervention to remove a malignant lesion or the result of severe trauma. Patients with these levels of amputation are the most difficult to fit with a functional prosthesis, due to the number of joints to be replaced, the multiple degrees of freedom available for control, and the problems related to maintaining secure suspension of the prosthesis.

In regard to surgical techniques, soft tissue handling is especially critical to wound healing and functional outcome in amputation surgery. The risk of wound failure and infection is high when tissues are excessively traumatized. Flaps should be kept thick, and unnecessary dissection between the skin, subcutaneous, fascial, and muscle planes should be avoided. All bone edges should be rounded, and prominences should be beveled for optimal force transmission during prosthetic use. Split-thickness skin grafts are generally discouraged, except as a means to save essential residual limb length (and with the understanding that future surgical revision might be necessary). Skin grafts do best with adequate soft tissue support, and are most durable when not adherent to bone. Muscle loses its contractile function when the skeletal attachments are divided during amputation. Stabilizing the distal insertion of muscle can improve residual limb function and comfort. *Myodesis* is the direct suturing of muscle or tendon to bone. This technique is most effective in stabilizing muscles that are needed to counteract strong antagonistic muscular forces. *Myoplasty* involves suturing of muscles to periosteum. Myoplasty does not provide as secure a distal stabilization of the muscle, as does myodesis. Care must be taken to prevent having a mobile sling of muscle over the distal end of the bone, which can result in formation of a painful bursa that could interfere with prosthetic fitting and use.

All transected nerves form a neuroma. Nerves should be transected cleanly, allowing the cut end to retract into the soft tissues away from the scar and prosthetic pressure points. The integrity of the peripheral nervous system should be assessed as early as feasible after traumatic amputation, because traction injuries frequently result in temporary or permanent nerve injury that has direct implications for arm function as well as for rehabilitation and prosthetic restoration programs.

The amputee rehabilitation program

The amputee rehabilitation program should ideally be designed to cover the wide spectrum of care from preamputation to reintegration into the community. The proposed stages are outlined in Table 13-2.[28]

Preamputation counseling

During this stage, it is essential to develop direct communication involving the patient, the family, and the surgeon regarding the need for amputation and the expected surgical outcome. Communication with the physiatrist, therapists, and other members of the treatment team should be facilitated. At this point, it is appropriate for the clinician to have introductory discussions about phantom limb sensation, prosthetic devices, prosthesis fitting and training, and the timing of these events. When possible, a demonstration of a prosthesis by a trained

Table 13-2 Stages of an upper limb amputation rehabilitation program

Stage	Description
1	Preamputation counseling
2	Amputation surgery
3	Acute postamputation period
4	Preprosthesis training
5	Preparatory prosthesis fitting
6	Prosthesis fitting and training
7	Reintegration into the community
8	Long-term follow-up

volunteer with a similar level of amputation and discussion of realistic expected functional outcomes should be arranged. Family involvement throughout this process should be encouraged. For all levels of amputation, a 'prehabilitation' program should include strengthening exercises for the trunk and remaining upper limb musculature and range of motion exercises for the involved glenohumeral, scapulothoracic, and elbow joints (if present).

Amputation surgery

Partial hand amputations should be carefully planned to ensure adequate residual sensation and movement. There is little point in salvaging a partial hand if no metacarpals are present to provide pinch. Prosthetic restoration of the thumb should be attempted before any pollicization procedures or toe transfers are attempted. Many patients find that a thumb prosthesis provides adequate functional restoration, and they choose to forgo further surgical reconstruction.[28] Toe transfers can also result in the partial loss of the normal foot function during walking.

Selecting a transhumeral level amputation over a transradial amputation presents a number of important dilemmas in rehabilitation. The lack of an anatomic elbow joint requires increased effort and cost for prosthetic restoration, and results in greater impairment. The selection of the level of amputation should take into consideration the amount of space necessary for the appropriate prosthetic components with adequate cosmesis. The transradial amputation has to be a minimum of 5 cm proximal to the distal radius to accommodate an externally powered terminal device. Transhumeral amputations should be performed 7–10 cm proximal to the distal humeral condyles to accommodate most of the prosthetic elbows. Longer residual limbs affect the location of the artificial elbow joint center of rotation, which can compromise cosmesis.

Transradial and transhumeral amputations

In the traumatic transradial and transhumeral amputation, it is not uncommon to find a more proximal fracture, a dislocation, or occasionally a peripheral nerve injury that can temporarily or permanently interfere with optimal prosthesis fitting and arm motion. Early diagnosis of these problems is needed to ensure inclusion of the necessary appropriate prosthetic modifications and alterations to the rehabilitation program.

Shoulder disarticulation and forequarter amputation

Shoulder disarticulation is performed in severe electrical injuries, in trauma cases, and in tumor surgery. Prosthetic replacement in these cases is more successful in those who are healthy, young, and male. In the majority of cases, the loss of the anatomic shoulder necessitates the use of an external prosthetic shoulder joint. This joint requires control mechanisms in addition to the body-powered or externally powered control mechanisms needed for the elbow, wrist, and hand.

Forequarter amputation is rarely performed, but it may be required in some cases of severe trauma or malignant lesion involving the shoulder. Functional prosthetic use is uncommon after this procedure, as suspension is difficult to maintain. Special considerations should be made for providing a shoulder cap to allow the patient to wear clothing more easily and to improve cosmesis. An ultralight passive prosthesis is usually well accepted by the patient.

Acute postamputation period

The goals of this stage include pain control, maintenance of range of motion and strength, and promotion of wound healing (Box 13-1). This stage begins with the surgical closure of the wound and culminates in wound healing. Pain control and residual limb maturation should be pursued aggressively. Immediate application of postoperative plaster of Paris rigid dressing (immediate postoperative rigid dressing, IPORD) or soft elastic bandage and subsequent pneumatic compression are indicated for edema control. An increasingly popular method of wound protection, swelling control, early shaping and soft tissue shrinking, and return to function is the immediate postoperative prosthesis, as reported by Malone and others.[26] Soft compressive dressings or Unna bandages are used in many centers.[7] The dressing should be extended to the proximal joint to better control swelling and to improve the dressing suspension. Proper postoperative positioning and rehabilitation are essential to prevent elbow flexion and shoulder adduction contractures when wounds are present over or close to the joints. This is most important if the wounds are caused by burn injuries, open reduction, or internal fixation, or if skin grafts were applied.

Acute pain management

Pain control can be best achieved initially with a patient-controlled analgesia system, followed by the use of scheduled parenteral and oral analgesia. A skin desensitization program that includes gentle tapping, massage, soft tissue and scar mobilization, and lubrication is recommended for the patient with a soft or elastic dressing.

When the patient's condition is medically stable, early mobilization, general endurance, and strengthening exercise are started. Special attention is paid to the shoulder and scapulae, and to the prevention of joint contractures. It is also important to carefully observe the remaining limbs, especially their strength and function, with attention to switching hand dominance if necessary. At this time, emotional counseling for the patient and the family should begin, with special focus on the significant other and children. Psychosocial evaluation of the patient and family should be initiated to assess and manage depression and anxiety. It is important during this phase to promote patient participation in the decision-making process to encourage independence and a sense of control.

Postoperative care

Postoperative edema is common following amputation. If soft dressings are used, they should be combined with elastic wrapping to control edema, especially if the patient is a candidate for a prosthesis. The ideal shape of the upper residual limb is cylindric, not conical. The major complication from elastic wrapping is applying the bandage too tightly at the proximal end in an attempt to improve bandage suspension. This causes congestion, worsens edema, and results in a dumbbell-shaped residual limb. The recommended elastic dressing involves the use of a figure of eight wrapping technique that extends over the proximal joint and that is reapplied every 4–6 h.

The use of an IPORD to control postoperative edema, promote healing, protect the limb from trauma, decrease postoperative pain, desensitize the limb, and allow early mobilization and rehabilitation is the preferred treatment approach for the transradial level (Box 13-2). In some centers, the rigid dressing is applied and managed by a team of specialists that includes the surgeon, the physiatrist, and the prosthetist. In other facilities, where the team approach to amputee treatment has not been implemented, a trained clinician can apply the dressing. The dressing is made out of plaster of Paris bandages that extend beyond the proximal joint for suspension. An IPORD should be replaced at 1-week intervals. By the time the

---

Box 13-1 Frequently utilized postoperative wound-dressing systems

- Immediate postoperative rigid dressing
- Immediate postoperative prosthesis
- Elastic bandage dressing
- Unna bandage
- Soft dressing

Box 13-2 Indications for immediate postoperative rigid dressing (IPORD)

- Pain control
- Promotion of wound healing
- Protection from trauma
- Edema control
- Desensitization
- Prevention of contractures

second dressing is replaced, the prosthesis can be casted, and a few days later it can be fitted. If the patient has a fever for which no other apparent cause can be determined, the IPORD should be removed and the wound inspected. The IPORD should be reapplied if the wound shows no signs of infection.

Phantom limb, phantom pain, and painful residual limb

Phantom limb sensation is the feeling that all or a part of the amputated limb is still present. This sensation is felt by nearly all 'acquired' amputees but is not always bothersome.[29] Phantom sensation usually diminishes over time, and telescoping (the sensation that the phantom hand has moved proximally) commonly occurs. Phantom sensation is not necessarily painful. As many as 70% of amputees perceive phantom pain in the first few months after amputation. Such pain usually disappears, however, or decreases sufficiently so that it does not interfere with prosthesis fitting and day to day activities.[5,20] A smaller percentage of patients experience long-term pain, whereas others have recurrent pain later in life. When pain persists for more than 6 months, the prognosis for spontaneous improvement is poor, and it can be extremely difficult to treat successfully. Perceived pain intensity is closely related to anxiety level, depression, prosthesis-fitting problems, and other personal factors.[41]

The traditional explanation for phantom sensation and pain is that the remaining nerves in the amputated limb continue to generate impulses that flow through the spinal cord and the thalamus to the somatosensory areas of the cerebral cortex. Another theory suggests that the phantom arises from excessive, spontaneous firing of spinal cord neurons that have lost their normal sensory input from the missing body part. Another suggests that the phantom sensation is caused by changes in the flow of signals through the somatosensory circuit in the brain.[8,29]

Appropriate management of phantom limb begins by preventing prolonged periods of pain before the amputation, because preamputation pain often results in postoperative phantom pain. Treatment includes prosthetic socket revisions, desensitization techniques, transcutaneous nerve stimulation, neuropharmacologic intervention, and the voluntary control of the phantom limb (mental imaging).[20,38] Robinson recently published a randomized controlled study that demonstrated the lack of effectiveness of amitriptyline in improving phantom limb pain or residual limb pain.[33] For severe cases, nerve blocks, steroid injections, and epidural blocks can be useful. Nonsurgical interventions are far more successful than surgical ones.[8] The etiology of the phantom limb phenomenon is clearly more complex than any of the theories here presented would suggest, and treatment can be complex. An important issue to discuss with the patient is normal phantom sensation, phantom pain, and the relationship between phantom pain and tension, anxiety, stress, and pain perception.[8]

Joint contractures

Joint contractures can occur between the time of amputation and prosthesis fitting. Efforts should be directed at preventing contractures with aggressive rehabilitation efforts, beginning soon after surgery. If burns, degloving injury, or severe trauma with proximal fractures are the cause of amputation, special attention should be given to the prevention of frozen shoulder and contractures induced by scar tissue formation. In the case of peripheral nerve or brachial plexus injury, appropriate positioning, splinting, and passive and assisted range of motion should be implemented to preserve joint mobility.

Preprosthetic rehabilitation

It is not unusual for patients with amputations to be provided with artificial limbs without much attention being paid to prosthetic training or other special needs. The outlook for the upper limb amputee has improved with the advent of specialized treatment teams, regional centers, and new prosthetic devices. A preprosthetic rehabilitation program must be initiated as soon as possible.[6] Pain control and residual limb maturation should be promoted during this phase. An IPORD or soft elastic bandages are indicated for edema control. This is also a time for the patient to initiate emotional adaptation to a body image without the artificial limb, and to learn basic skills without a prosthesis, which is essential for the times when the device is not worn. Soft tissue desensitization, early mobilization, improving general endurance, strengthening, avoidance of joint contractures, and emotional counseling are the key goals of this phase.

Limb loss is often interpreted in our society as punishment for a misdeed. An amputation typically causes patients to initiate a process of introspection and reassessment of goals. This process can result in an individual taking a more mature approach toward life goals and actively pursuing plans. Occasionally, however, a patient can become so emotionally disturbed by the limb loss that the result can be a chronic failure to cope. This can have a very negative effect on the rehabilitation outcome.[40]

The use of the first prosthesis should be implemented as soon as possible in this stage. The early fitting of the prosthetic device is intended to promote prosthesis use for bimanual activities. As reported by Malone and others,[26,27] there is a direct relationship between the time of fitting and long-term prosthetic use. There is a 3- to 6-month window of opportunity for the unilateral upper limb amputee. If a prosthesis is fitted during this period, there is a much greater rate of acceptance and integration of the artificial arm.

The first prosthesis is intended to promote residual limb maturation and desensitization, to build up wearing tolerance, and to allow the patient to become a functional user. This is commonly done with a body-powered or a switch-controlled externally powered prosthesis. Suction suspension or myoelectric control is not practical at this stage because of limb volume fluctuation, which results in the loss of the necessary intimate contact of the socket and electrodes with the soft tissues. When no significant volume fluctuation is noted in the residual limb over a period of 2 months, consideration should be given to proceeding with fitting of the first permanent prosthesis. Serial circumferential measurements of the limb at preestablished locations are the simplest clinical method of determining residual limb size stability. Volumetric measurements in a water displacement chamber or with a computer-aided design system are more precise, although more time-consuming, techniques.

Prosthesis fitting and training

Prosthesis prescription options for the amputee have changed greatly since the mid 1980s. Selecting the most appropriate componentry for prosthetic restoration of the upper limb is an extremely challenging task in view of the variety and complexity of available prosthetic components (prosthetic terminal devices, wrists, elbows, and shoulders), socket fabrication techniques, suspension systems, and sources of power and control. An expert team of professionals in close communication should accomplish this task with the patient. Members of the team ideally should include the surgeon, a physiatrist who devotes time in practice to amputee rehabilitation and prostheses a certified prosthetist, an occupational therapist, a physical therapist, a recreational therapist, a psychologist, a social worker, and the patient and family. Other specialists can be added to the team as needed. The team members can best serve the needs of the patient if they have significant experience in the specialized rehabilitation techniques for the upper limb amputee, and prosthetic fabrication and training. This typically occurs most commonly in large, specialized, regional rehabilitation centers.

Terminal devices

The functional capacity of the upper limb is determined by the development of multiple integrated spheres of action by the shoulder complex, elbow, wrist, and hand. Given the normal proportions of limb segments, this capacity is limited in relation to the surrounding space. The functional activities of the hand are extensive, but they can be grouped into non-prehensile and prehensile activities. The former include touching, feeling, pressing down with the fingers, tapping, vibrating the cord of a musical instrument, and lifting or pushing with the hand. Prehensile activities are grouped into precision and power grips. Three-jaw chuck involves grip with the thumb and the index and middle fingers. A lateral or key grip involves contact of the pulp of the thumb with the lateral aspect of the corresponding finger. These two patterns provide precision prehension. Power grip predominantly involves the ulnar aspect of the hand, with less involvement of the ring and little fingers. The hook power grip involves flexion of both interphalangeal joints and minimal participation of the metacarpophalangeal joint. This grip pattern is used in carrying a briefcase. The spherical grip is very much like the power grip but with minimal flexion of the fingers, which are abducted and rotated; the thumb is used to stabilize the object and to provide counter-pressure.

Most patients who have had an upper limb amputation and undergo prosthetic restoration require a terminal device for their prosthesis. The human hand is a very complex anatomic and physiologic structure whose functions cannot be completely replaced by the current level of prosthetic technology. A variety of prosthetic terminal devices are available, and include passive, body-powered, and externally powered hooks and hands (Fig. 13-2). They all lack sensory feedback and have limited

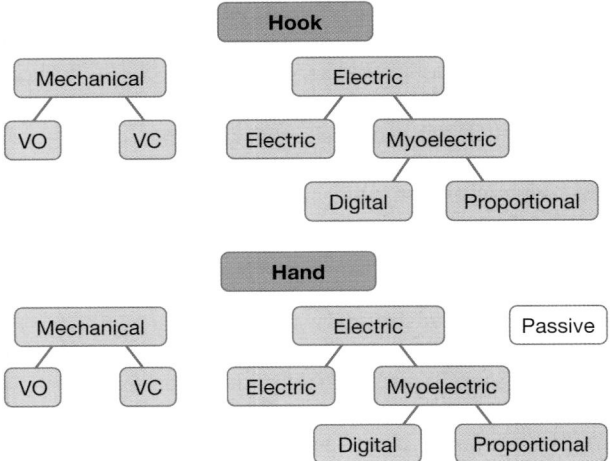

Figure 13-2 Classification and availability of terminal devices. VO, voluntary opening; VC, voluntary closing.

mobility and dexterity. Prosthetic hands provide a three-jaw chuck pinch, and hooks provide the equivalent of lateral or tip pinch. Body-powered terminal devices can be voluntary opening (most common and practical) or voluntary closing (most physiologic). The voluntary opening device is maintained in the closed position by rubber bands or tension springs. The patient can open the device by 'pulling' with the cable on the harness system in preparation to grasp. To grasp, the patient releases the opened terminal device on an object; the rubber bands or spring provide the prehensile force. The number of springs or rubber bands predetermines the maximum prehensile force possible. To control the amount of prehensile force, the patient must generate an opening force all the time.

Voluntary closing terminal devices require that the patient close the device by 'pulling' the cable with the harness system to grasp an object. To release, the patient releases the pull on the harness, and a spring in the terminal device opens it. The maximum prehensile force possible is determined by the strength of the individual. One major disadvantage of this system is that prolonged prehension requires constant pull on the harness, but it might allow improved speed of motion. The human hand normally does not reach out to grasp an object in the closed position, but rather uses the semiopen position to facilitate the interaction with the environment. This is why a VC device is said to be more physiological.

Externally powered devices can have digital (on or off) or proportional (stronger signal equals faster action) control systems. More recently, a slip control system was introduced by the Otto Bock Company to improve hand grip and increase speed of motion. The device has a sensor that maintains a constant pressure on an object to prevent slippage. If the sensor perceives that the object is slipping, it automatically slightly increases the pressure on the object.

Prosthetic wrists

The type of prosthetic wrist (Box 13-3) most commonly used allows passive pronation and supination. Spring-assisted rota-

Box 13-3 Types of prosthetic wrists

Mechanical
- Pronosupination
  - Friction
  - Quick disconnect
  - Spring-assisted
- Flexion
- Spring-assisted internal or external

Electric
- Pronosupination
  - Myoelectric
  - Switch control

Box 13-4 Classification of prosthetic elbows

Body-powered elbow
- External, with or without spring-assisted flexion
- Internal, with or without spring-assisted flexion
- Internal, with rotating turntable

Externally powered elbow
- Digital switch control
- Proportional switch control
- Digital myoelectric control
- Proportional myoelectric control

Passive elbow
- Manual lock

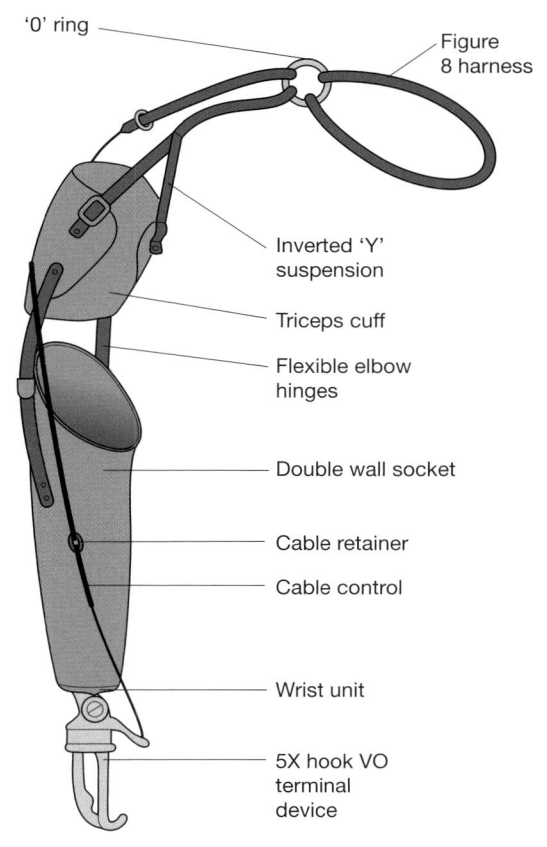

Figure 13-3 A body-powered transradial prosthesis with components identified.

tion is available for the bilateral amputee. The friction control permits ease of positioning, but it can rotate when lifting heavy objects. This is particularly problematic when the wearer is carrying a plate or tray. Quick disconnect wrists are also available, and permit rapid interchange of different terminal devices. When locked, the quick disconnect wrist also provides a secure control for wrist rotation. An externally powered switch or myoelectric control wrist pronosupination system exists, but it is prescribed primarily for bilateral transhumeral or higher level of amputation. A mechanical spring-assisted wrist flexion unit is indispensable for the bilateral upper limb amputee. This device permits the patient to reach the body's midline for grooming, feeding, hygiene activities, and buttoning of clothing.

Prosthetic elbows

The prosthetic elbows available in the treatment of transhumeral amputation have either external or internal joints. These joints can be passive, body-powered, or externally powered (Figs 13-3 and 13-4). These devices are controlled via mechanical cables, electric switches, or myoelectric signals (Box 13-4). The externally powered systems have digital or proportional control mechanisms. The mechanical elbows have a locking mechanism that is manually applied using the contra-

lateral hand, the chin, or the ipsilateral shoulder via a cable system. Electric elbows have an electromechanical brake or a switch-controlled lock mechanism to maintain the selected position. The rotation function of the arm (internal or external rotation) is provided through the use of a turntable. This device is useful to provide reach to the body midline. Electric elbows have limited active flexion force. The flexion force across a mechanical elbow is dependent on the wearer's strength, the comfort of the socket fit, and the ability to efficiently transfer the power from the residual limb to the prosthesis.

For elbow disarticulation, the external elbow joint is indicated in an attempt to maintain the optimal length of the arm. This joint is larger and protrudes medially. The problems with this type of joint include limited flexion strength and increased maintenance.

Prosthetic sockets

Socket configuration and materials have improved greatly since the mid 1980s. The key functions of a prosthetic socket include comfortable total contact interface with the residual limb, efficient energy transfer from the residual limb to the prosthetic device, secure suspension, and cosmetic appearance (Box 13-5). A patient often fails to accept the prosthesis if the socket does not provide most of these characteristics.

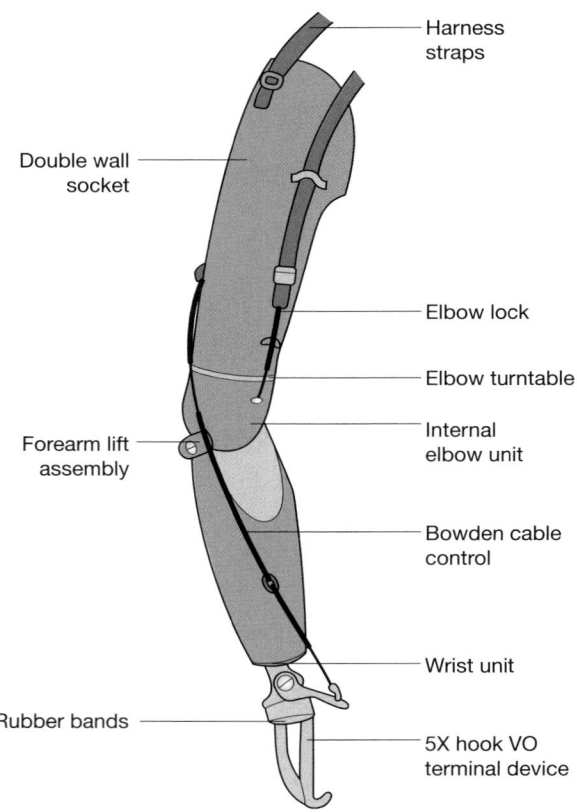

Harness
straps

Double wall
socket

Elbow lock

Elbow turntable

Internal
elbow unit

Forearm lift
assembly

Bowden cable
control

Wrist unit

Rubber bands

5X hook VO
terminal device

Figure 13-4 A body-powered transhumeral prosthesis with components identified.

Box 13-5 Key functions of the prosthetic socket

- Comfortable residual limb–prosthesis interface
- Efficient energy transference to the prosthesis
- Secure suspension of the prosthesis
- Adequate cosmesis

Sockets used in the past were carved out of wood. These sockets had the disadvantage of being open-ended, which promoted distal residual limb swelling with potential development of chronic edema and trophic skin changes. With the development of high-temperature rigid plastic materials such as polyester resin, sockets with decreased weight and increased durability can be molded to have total contact. More recently, acrylic lamination, the use of carbon graphite, and the introduction of flexible thermoplastics have permitted the design of sockets with windows that are lined with flexible materials and are more comfortable, lighter, and durable.[16] Most upper limb prosthetic sockets have two layers. The first one is closely contoured to the residual limb, and the external layer gives the necessary length and shape to the socket. It is to this external layer that the necessary prosthetic components (e.g. elbow and wrist) are attached.

Sockets are custom-made by obtaining a negative impression of the residual limb by plaster of Paris wrap. This is then converted to a positive mold that can be modified by the prosthetist to appropriately distribute pressure throughout the entire surface of the residual limb. Typically, a transparent plastic socket is first manufactured to permit direct visualization of the soft tissues. The transparent socket can be modified to ensure comfortable total contact. Eventually, a final socket is fabricated. The concepts of computer-assisted design and computer-assisted manufacturing have been adapted to prosthesis fabrication. Direct surface video imaging of the residual limb, ultrasound and/or magnetic resonance imaging, and direct digitization from a plaster of Paris mold are being used in some centers as sources of digital data to be manipulated in a computer environment. A computer-controlled carver can then create a positive mold of wax or plaster from which a socket can be manufactured from vacuum-formed thermoplastics.[1]

New flexible plastic materials have made sockets lighter and more comfortable.[11] The use of these new materials in prosthetics has resulted in the development of improved socket construction techniques.[20,37] The inner socket provides total contact with the residual limb, and is the interface that provides suction suspension if desired. The outer socket or frame is made of a more rigid material, thermoplastic or resin, and provides the structural integrity of the socket. When double sockets are used, windows can be cut in the exterior frame to allow muscles to expand during contraction and to improve comfort and sensory feedback. The elasticity of the thermoplastic material results in a more comfortable fit. Although more costly and time-consuming to fabricate initially, the frame socket design has the added advantage of allowing replacement of the inner socket to accommodate small residual limb changes without changing the external frame to which the other prosthetic components are attached. It is a fairly simple process to pull out the old liner and slip in a new one. Velcro or another removable fastener usually holds the inner socket in place. The frame socket design is particularly appealing for externally powered prostheses and self-suspended ones (wrist and elbow disarticulation and Muenster sockets). One disadvantage of these materials is their poor temperature insulation characteristics, which make them uncomfortable during cold weather. This can be partially corrected by using clothing layers to cover the arm.

Suspension systems

The suspension and control system of a body-powered prosthesis needs to provide two distinct important functions to make the prosthetic device work. One of these is suspension, which is the means of securing the prosthetic device to the body. The other is to permit control of the prosthesis, including the terminal device. The more secure the suspension system, the more likely the patient can experience optimal prosthetic control and comfort. The upper limb amputee has traditionally been provided with suspension systems that are uncomfortable and that limit mobility. They consist mostly of straps with metal and

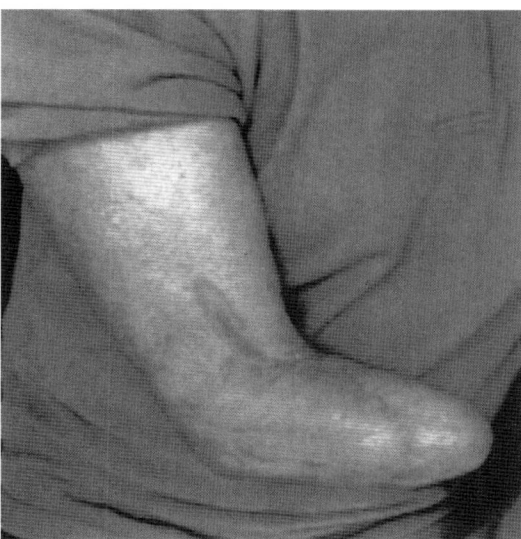

Figure 13-5 Transradial amputation with significant scar tissue that would benefit from silicone sleeve suspension.

plastic attachments. The traditional suspension mechanisms (Box 13-6) for the upper limb sockets include a strap that suspends the prosthesis over the shoulder (a figure of eight harness). The harness is used as a control mechanism to transmit body power to the terminal device and elbow. For the more proximal level amputation, a chest strap or shoulder saddle can be used to further improve suspension. Patients with wrist or elbow disarticulation or transradial amputations can use bony prominences for suspension. The Muenster[14] or condylar suspension is perhaps the best of these. When this type of suspension is used, a figure of nine harness can be used for control purposes only.

The transradial Muenster socket design was developed in Germany in the early 1950s,[14] and was later modified at Northwestern University. This socket configuration provides excellent suspension by encasing the elbow condyles. The main disadvantage is the loss of terminal elbow extension and flexion range of motion. This can prevent its use as the preferred type of suspension for the patient with bilateral transradial amputations. This type of suspension works extremely well with externally powered, myoelectric control prostheses, as the patient can be completely free of straps.

In most cases, a sock is used as an interface between the residual limb and the socket. Using different numbers of sock layers can adjust for the physiologic volume changes that occur from day to day. Socks also protect the skin and improve hygiene. The only exceptions are suction sockets, for which direct skin to socket contact is required, and socks cannot be used.

Hypobaric and semisuction suspension is best thought of as a transition between non-suction and full-suction suspension. This suspension system utilizes socks that have a special silicone band in them, and the socket is provided with a one-way valve that permits the expulsion of air during donning. The band creates a seal between the socket and the skin of the residual limb, and permits the development of partial suction that can be used for suspension. The advantage of this suspension system

is that the changes in residual limb volume that typically occur early in the rehabilitation process can be accommodated simply by altering the number of plies (thicknesses) of socks used.

Silicone suction suspension application to upper limb body and externally powered prostheses

Since 1986, the Icelandic roll or silicone sleeve, invented by Kristinsson,[20] has been in use as a suspension system for the transtibial amputee, with consistent improvement in the suspension of the prosthesis. More recently, its use has been extended to suspend the upper limb prosthesis while protecting the skin. It has also been applied more recently for upper limb myoelectric prostheses.[34]

The silicone liner provides improved suspension function by creating a negative atmospheric pressure and an adhesive bond to the skin.[25] The silicone sleeve also improves the socket–residual limb interface by protecting the skin through significant reduction of shear forces and added cushioning. The silicone sleeve provides improved suspension by reducing pistoning and shear, allows for volume adjustment with residual limb girth changes, and improves cosmesis, as it reduces or eliminates the need for harness suspension.[14]

Donning of the prosthesis is simplified and can be done with one hand. Silicone sleeve systems do not interfere with elbow range of motion, unlike other types of self-suspension systems such as supracondylar sockets. Patients perceive the prosthesis to be lighter and more comfortable when silicone suspension is used, due to the improved suspension.

The system consists of a silicone sleeve with a distal attachment pin that interfaces with a shuttle lock mechanism built into the prosthetic socket (Figs 13-5 through 13-7). The patient rolls on the silicone liner directly over the skin after spraying the external surface of the liner with alcohol (or, in the case of

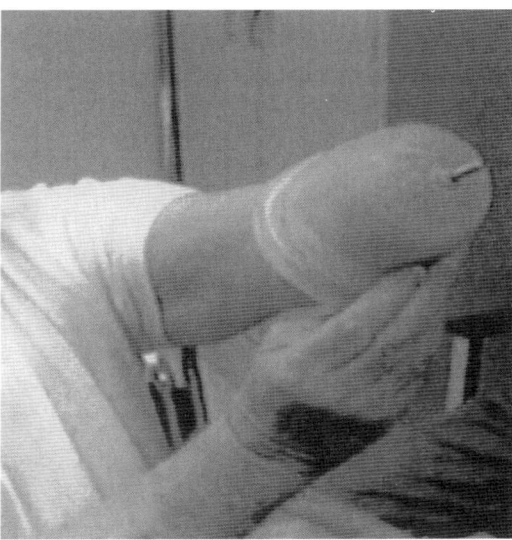

Figure 13-6 Patient demonstrating one-handed application of a silicone sleeve suspension system.

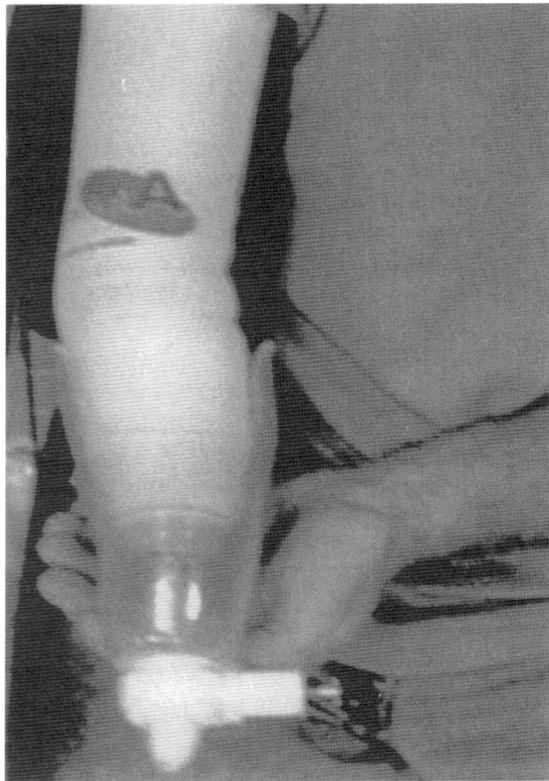

Figure 13-7 Patient demonstrating application of transradial check socket prosthesis over silicone sleeve suspension. Note the suspension pin, which will connect with the shuttle lock system.

a prelined liner, just pulling it on). This results in a suspension system that makes use of negative pressure on the distal third of the residual limb, and of friction and pressure between the sleeve and the skin in the upper two-thirds portion of the limb. Once in place, one or more socks can be applied over the sili-

cone liner to improve fit, adjust for changes in the limb girth, and reduce friction between the silicone material and the prosthesis. Some systems rely on this friction to suspend the prosthesis if no pin mechanism is used. If a high degree of cushioning and pressure distribution is desirable, a thicker liner system can be used. Liner thickness ranges from 3 to 9 mm to provide optimal suspension and cushioning. More recently available are silicone liners that have a variable thickness, and a distal silicone pad can be added to protect sensitive areas.

Excessive perspiration and irritation can occur with roll-on silicone sleeve use. Excessive perspiration can be controlled with antiperspirant lotions or Botox® injections of the affected skin area to control the focal hyperhidrosis.[31] A contact dermatitis-like reaction can also occur, even though silicone is a hypoallergenic material. Commonly, this problem occurs only in the first weeks of use and when the weather is very warm. It affects primarily the edge of the sleeve where the transition of pressure gradients and the free edge of the silicone can trigger this dermatologic reaction. A period of increased skin and sleeve hygiene and protecting the skin from direct contact by using a partial sock are recommended. A bland skin protectant agent such as zinc oxide or petrolatum paste (Desitin®) can rapidly resolve the problem.[22]

Silicone sleeves are best used by patients who are likely to have problems with skin integrity, such as patients who have undergone skin grafting for burns or degloving injuries; those with delicate, insensate skin (such as patients with diabetes and scleroderma); or those with adhesive scar tissue. We have applied this type of suspension to the upper limb amputee (transradial and transhumeral) and expanded its use to externally powered prosthesis (myoelectric control), with excellent results.

Silicone sleeves afford excellent skin protection and are a good prosthetic suspension system for patients who are very active users, play sports, or have short, very sensitive, or delicate residual limbs. Patients with skin grafts after burns, trauma, or degloving injuries or those with areas of reduced sensitivity are also prime candidates for this type of suspension system.

In the upper limb externally powered socket design, silicone suspension can be implemented and can permit the use of myoelectric controls if the residual limb is not extremely short and if other selection characteristics are met.

Individuals who live in areas of the world with warm and humid weather are more likely to develop dermatologic problems. These can be minimized by strict hygienic care of the skin and the insert.

Suction suspension

For the transhumeral amputee, suction suspension (negative pressure) without the use of straps is the preferred type of suspension. For this system to work well, and to be able to don the prosthesis independently, the patient should have good contralateral upper limb strength, endurance, and coordination. The socket is made small enough and provided with a one-way valve that permits the expulsion of air during donning. The amputee dons the socket using a pull sock or elastic (such as Ace) bandage, or with a wet fit (using a lubricant liquid or powder). The intimate fit between the socket and the skin of the residual limb, especially distally, results in a tight seal between the socket and skin. Doffing requires breaking the vacuum seal. To maintain proper suspension over time, the residual limb must be mature and volume stable.[7]

Control mechanisms

When a body harness is used as a control mechanism for a body-powered prosthesis, the patient needs to be able to produce movements that generate the power requirements to activate the terminal device or elbow. These movements include scapular abduction; chest expansion; shoulder depression, extension, and abduction and humeral flexion; and elbow flexion and extension. These movements can be difficult to perform if the residual limb is short, painful, or has limited motion, or if the prosthetic socket does not fit well. A poorly adjusted harness decreases the power transmission of the movements.[6]

Electric switch control mechanisms can be activated with residual limb movements that depress a switch inside the socket. For other cases, a chest strap, waist belt, or figure of nine harness can be used. Servo controls that sense tension have been introduced into clinical use.

Myoelectric controls use the electrical activity generated during a muscle contraction to control the flow of energy from a battery to a motor in the prosthetic device. The control signals come from muscle sites in the amputated limb that still have normal innervation and voluntary control.[35] Ideally, muscles in the more distal portion of the residual limb should be used. Antagonistic muscles are best for this function (i.e. wrist or elbow flexor or extensor). This ensures that the control is easy to use, physiologic, consistent, and precise. At times, more proximal muscles or muscles in the trunk or other limb can be used. Systems that use single-channel control mechanisms use two electrode sites, one to trigger hand closure or elbow flexion and the other to trigger hand opening or elbow extension. Multichannel systems permit the use of one muscle to control two different functions. This requires that the patient be able to produce a slow, gentle muscle contraction for one function and a strong, faster one for the other function. Myoelectronic prosthetic components, such as the Boston or Utah arms, use an 'electronic switch' to alternate between the hand and the elbow function. Some systems also include proportional controls, which respond to the speed and strength of the muscle contraction by correspondingly producing a faster or slower movement of the hand or elbow. A very snug fit of the socket is required to avoid shift of the muscles in reference to the electrodes for proper function. Hybrid systems combine two or more of the available control mechanisms, either electric or body-powered (Fig. 13-8). Recently, experimental targeted muscle reinnervation allowed simultaneous multifunction myoelectric control in one subject with shoulder disarticulation.[21]

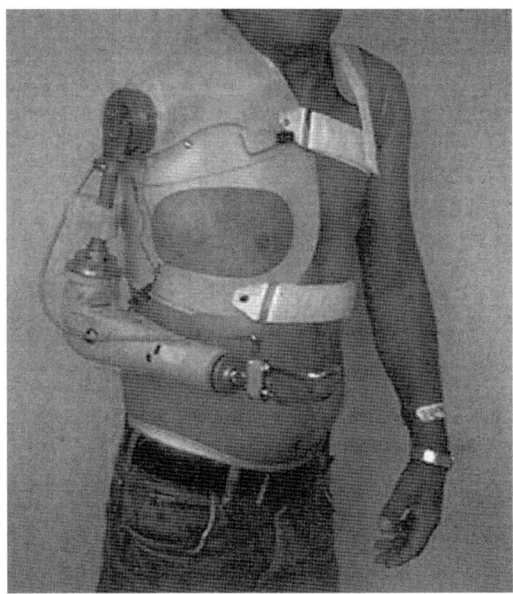

Figure 13-8 Hybrid forequarter amputation prosthesis. The device uses a MICA shoulder with chin control locks, Utah myoelectronic elbow, and interchangeable 5X voluntary opening hook or myoelectric hand.

Shoulder disarticulation and forequarter amputation

There has been little change in the basic socket design for shoulder disarticulation or forequarter amputation since it was designed. The main changes have been modification of the socket trim lines and suspension, and use of lighter materials to construct the socket. As in sockets for other levels of amputation, thermoplastic and silicone materials are being used to provide lighter, more secure, and more comfortable sockets at these proximal levels of amputation. Most of the advances in prosthetic design for these levels have occurred with externally powered components, which are described elsewhere in this chapter. A shoulder joint with an electric lock that provides improvement in the arm control and position is now available.

Cosmetic covers

Cosmetic covers can be manufactured for a single digit, for the hand, or to extend to the elbow. They should be considered an integral part of the prosthesis, because for many patients the cover is the factor that determines success or failure of prosthetic restoration. Custom-made silicone cosmetic covers can provide excellent cosmetic results, but they can be very expensive and difficult to maintain, and they deteriorate over time. Intrinsic coloration is a newer technique that provides a more realistic look. The colors are integrated at the time of fabrication instead of coloring the cover after it has been applied to the arm.

Activity-specific devices

To optimally perform at work, sports, or recreational activities, it might be necessary to provide the patient with a specially designed terminal device. Many devices are commercially available that are designed for participation in sports (e.g. golf, fishing, and skiing). Many more have been designed by the users for activities such as construction, cooking, archery, and photography.

Prosthetic prescription
The prosthetic prescription should be carefully prepared to satisfy the needs and desires of the patient. A team approach to prescription writing should be used. The prescription should clearly spell out the components, control system, suspension, materials, and any special features that might be required. The prescription should serve to clearly communicate with the prosthetist and the insurance company. A clear, well thought out, organized prescription should achieve this (Fig. 13-9).

Prosthetic training
Training is integral to the rehabilitation process. A new amputee or an experienced one who receives a prosthetic device that has different components should participate in such training. This program in most cases should be a coordinated effort among the occupational, physical, and recreational therapists and the prosthetist, with frequent physiatric input (kinesiotherapists are also used at some centers). Each of the team members uses different techniques to teach what needs to be learned by the amputee. Before initiating a program of upper limb prosthetic training, one must realistically orient the patient to what the prosthesis can and cannot do.[2] The patient should learn prosthetic management, including the basic principles behind the function, care, and maintenance of each of the components in the prosthesis. The patient should practice independently donning and doffing the prosthesis. Skin care and inspection techniques are also reviewed. For the body-powered devices, dismounting the harness for washing and replacing it should be practiced. Written instructions are useful for explaining the care and maintenance of the batteries used in externally powered devices. A review and practice of the use of the prosthesis for bimanual activities, such as grooming, dressing, feeding, driving, sports, work, and recreation activities, should always be included in the training process.

Special considerations for the bilateral upper limb amputee
For the bilateral upper limb amputee, training should promote the development of a dominant prosthesis and skills for independent donning. Alternative techniques for putting on the prosthesis are frequently required. This might include using the bed for set-up and suspending the prosthetic devices from special wall hooks or frames. The prosthesis should have a wrist rotation and flexion device that permits access to the body midline.

For bathing activities, the patient with bilateral upper limb amputations ideally should have a modified shower with wall brushes and liquid soap dispensers. In some cases, simplified shower prostheses (devices that are waterproof) are a medical

necessity, because they allow the patient to perform this activity independently (Fig. 13-10).

Brachial plexus and other nerve injuries
Brachial plexus injuries can be the result of many different causes, which can be divided into two main categories: closed injuries and open penetrating trauma. The majority of cases are caused by closed injuries. Traction on the upper plexus and the C5 and C6 roots occurs when the head and neck are stretched away from the shoulder. When the arm is stretched overhead, traction to the lower plexus and the C8 and T1 roots occurs most frequently. The injuries can be preganglionic (indicating injury or avulsion of the nerve root proximal to the spinal ganglion), with resulting severe or even complete motor and sensory loss. This can also be accompanied by Horner syndrome. Postganglionic injuries occur distal to the spinal ganglion and tend to have a more favorable prognosis (Box 13-7).

Reintegration into the community
Reintegration into the community is best done gradually over a few weeks or months. This process can be initiated early in the rehabilitation program with the supervision of the team members during organized trips for shopping, recreation, and part-time work or school. When possible, the use of 'day' rehabilitation programs, in which the patient participates in rehabilitation 6 h a day, 5 days a week (with return to home every evening and weekend), is a good system to foster community reintegration.

The patient can return to work when safety concerns are met.[19,28] Modified or restricted work should be provided initially, but the patient should not be discouraged from returning to the premorbid work level if it is safe to do so. Work simulation or supervised return to work is a good technique to reintroduce patients to their work environment. The use of a partial 'day program' rehabilitation program in which the patient participates in rehabilitation for 3 h a day, 5 days a week, or for 6 h a day, 2 or 3 days a week, also encourages and allows time for the return to part-time work in the community. The availability of psychologic counseling or assistance from the team members during each of these steps is important for the smooth transition of patients and their families to independent functioning.

Box 13-7 Types and common causes of brachial plexus injuries

Closed injuries
- Traction
- Compression
- Combined
- Radiation

Penetrating injuries
- Gunshot
- Fracture
- Knife wound

MossRehab   Upper Limb Prosthetic Prescription

Name: _____   **Age:** _____   **Date:** _____

Diagnosis: _____   **Patient ready:** yes   no   **Room #** _____

Prosthetist: _____   **Third Party Coverage:** _____

Preparatory Prosthesis   **Permanent Prosthesis**

Circle and complete as necessary

Side: Right   Left   Bilateral

Site: Partial Hand   Wrist   Transradial   Transhumeral   Shoulder or Forequarter Disarticulation

Socket configuration: Frame   Single wall   Double wall   Pre-flexed   Silicone sleeve

Socket construction: Hard   Flexible   Suction   Expandable Shuttle

Suspension: Biceps cuff   Triceps cuff   Muenster   Suction   Chest strap

Structure: Endoskeletal   Exoskeletal   Hybrid

Control: Myoelectric   Procontrol   Body powered   External powered

Harness: Figure 8   Double "O" ring   Figure 9   Chest strap   Shoulder saddle   None

Shoulder: Manual lock   Friction   Heavy duty

Elbow: Internal   External   Spring flexion   Balanced forearm   Electric   Myoelectric

Lock: Manual   Friction   Cable Control   Electronic   Switch control (rocker/pull/push)

Wrist: Oval   Round   Friction   Quick disconnect   Flexion unit

                       Spring prono/supination   Electric prono/supination

Terminal device: Hand   Hook   VO   VC   Passive   Myoelectric   Electric (rocker/pull/push)

Cover: Cosmetic glove   Semi custom glove   Intrinsic colration   Custom

Power supply: Batteries # _____   Chargers # _____   110 or 220 V _____

Socks: Nylon # _____   1 Ply # _____   3 Ply # _____   Sillpos # _____   Pull socks #

Special instructions: _____

_____

_____

                                        Signature _____ **M.D./D.O.**

Figure 13-9 Sample of an upper limb prosthetic prescription developed at the MossRehab Regional Amputee Center.

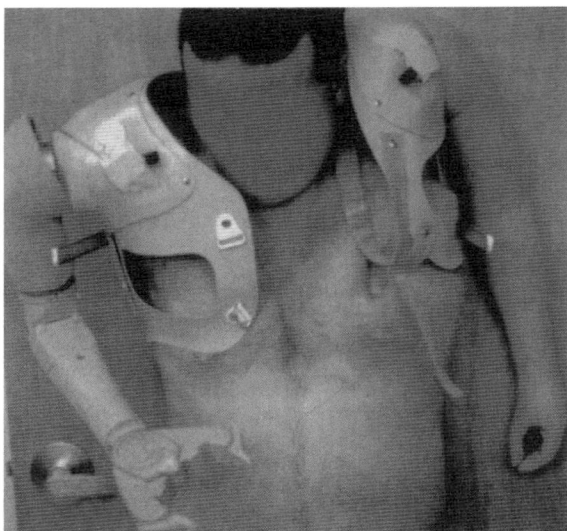

Figure 13-10 Patient demonstrating donning of a bilateral shoulder disarticulation myoelectric prosthesis. Note the right-sided Greifer terminal device, left-sided hand.

Table 13-3 Typical functional outcomes for upper limb amputation with prosthesis	
Type of amputation	Functional outcomes
Unilateral transradial or transhumeral	Independent activities of daily living, household activities, driving, and work, with some limitations
Bilateral	After assisted donning of prosthesis, independent activities of daily living, household activities, driving, and work, with many limitations

Functional outcomes

Realistic goals for the majority of unilateral transradial or transhumeral amputees include independence in all activities of daily living, most household activities, driving, and work (Table 13-3). Some restrictions should be imposed in relationship to handling delicate, heavy, or voluminous objects. The typical patient with a transradial amputation can be expected to lift 20–30 lbs, unless the residual limb is very short or sensitive. The typical patient with a transhumeral amputation can be expected to lift 10–15 lbs, unless the residual limb is very short or sensitive. This is also affected by the type of elbow used.

Realistic goals for the bilateral transhumeral amputee include independence in most activities of daily living (in some cases after assisted donning), some household activities, driving with a spin ring, and most types of sedentary work with environmental modifications. Restrictions should be imposed in relationship to handling delicate, heavy objects (up to 20 lbs), unless the residual limb is very short or sensitive, or voluminous objects are involved.

If work is to take place where magnetic fields or large electrical currents are present, myoelectric prostheses might not work well unless special shielding materials are used during fabrication to prevent electronic interference. In very cold environments, battery power can drain more quickly.

Psychosocial issues

To truly capitalize on the current rate of advancement in the development of limb prostheses, it is important to attend not only to the physical and technologic factors that play a fundamental role, but also the social and psychologic issues facing people who will ultimately be using the prescribed technology. There have been recent attempts to relate psychosocial variables to the adjustment process.[10] Psychosocial perspectives are very significant to the individual's response, which is an inevitable and integral part of adjustment to disability and to a prosthesis, and ultimately to the overall outcomes. As a result, the need to measure the results of treatment has been the catalyst for steady progress in the development of outcomes tools appropriate for patients using prosthetic services, such as the Trinity Amputation and Prosthesis Experience Scales.[10,28] This is a brief, multidimensional, self-administered assessment tool that comprises psychosocial adjustment (general, social, and adjustment to limitation), activity restriction (athletic, social, and functional), and prosthetic satisfaction (functional, aesthetic, and weight) domains. It also explores the experience of residual limb pain, phantom limb pain, and other medical problems, thereby incorporating both the physical and psychosocial aspects of adjustment.

Long-term follow-up

The patient who has successfully completed a rehabilitation program should be seen for follow-up by a minimum of two of the team members at least every 3 months for the first 18 months. These visits might need to be more frequent and include other members of the team if the patient is having difficulties with prosthesis fitting, the residual limb, specific activities, or psychosocial adjustment. After this critical period, the patient should be seen at least every 6 months to ensure adequate prosthetic fit and function, and to assess the need for maintenance and the overall medical condition and functional level of the patient. When the patient's condition is stable, it might be necessary to replace a prosthesis or parts of it every 18 months to 3 years for body-powered devices and every 2–4 years for myoelectric prostheses.[28]

Neuromas

Neuroma is the formation of scar tissue around the distal end of the severed nerve. As previously mentioned, every time a nerve is cut it forms a neuroma. Good surgical technique results in the neuroma being buried under large soft tissue masses that serve to protect it from irritation. Because of limited soft tissue coverage or very large neuroma formation with compression of the nerve, at times adhesion of the tissues, or complications from the surgical technique, a neuroma, can become symptomatic. This results in pain that can be perceived at the site of the neuroma and that radiates distally to the end of the residual limb (or, at times, into the phantom limb). A painful neuroma is palpable most of the time, and pressure over it reproduces the symptoms. Desensitization techniques, prosthetic modifications, and, at times, use of flexible materials with windowed frame construction to decrease pressure over the neuroma can help.[8] Injection of the neuroma with a mixture of long- and short-acting local anesthetics and a corticosteroid should reduce the scar tissue pressure on the nerve and produce symptomatic improvement. When correctly performed, this technique reproduces the presenting symptoms with increasing severity as the needle is advanced. The injection can be repeated several times at 6- to 8-week intervals. Surgical removal of the neuroma with careful retraction of the nerve prior to cutting it should be reserved for those cases in which all other interventions have failed, and in which the tissues allow repositioning of the neuroma to a less pressure-exposed location.

Dermatologic problems

The skin of a patient who wears a prosthesis is subject to much abuse. Most prosthetic sockets prevent appropriate air circulation, thereby trapping perspiration moisture. This can result in a variety of problems such as hyperhidrosis, folliculitis, allergic dermatitis, and even skin breakdown where adherent scars are present. Poor hygiene is frequently the cause of some of these problems, and for this reason the patient should be trained in the proper washing technique of the residual limb, silicone liners, socks, and the socket and its interfaces. A daily routine of washing the skin and the internal wall of the socket with a mild soap might suffice. It can be necessary at times to use concentrated antiperspirants, bacteriostatic or bactericidal soaps, and even antibiotics in some cases. Topical antibiotics or steroids should not generally be used if the prosthesis has silicone components, because part of the socket materials has direct contact with the skin. Contact dermatitis can frequently occur because of this.[24]

Support groups

Support groups are a source of information, peer counseling, and motivation for many patients. These groups ideally should constitute one more component of the comprehensive rehabilitation approach to the patient with an amputation. Patients who have recently sustained an amputation benefit from contact with experienced amputees; at the same time, the veteran amputee enjoys serving as a resource. This forum can also be used effectively as a resource for the family of the patient with an amputation.

Care of the non-amputated upper limb

Jones and Davidson reported the first study of problems related to overuse in the remaining arm of the unilateral upper limb amputee.[17] There is a high incidence of overuse injuries to the soft tissues, tendon–muscle complex, and the joint itself. In order of frequency, elbow, shoulder, and wrist injuries were reported. The more proximal the amputation, the more prevalent were the problems. A program of education to avoid

overuse and promote habilitation, aggressive early management of injuries, and preventive care of the limb, with avoidance of potentially injurious activities, should be implemented.

PEDIATRIC LIMB DEFICIENCY AND AMPUTATION REHABILITATION

The pediatric patient can have an acquired or a congenital limb deficiency. The child with a congenital limb deficiency has no sense of loss and does not have to go through the psychologic adjustment process. The prosthesis is perceived as an aid rather than as a replacement. If the device cannot serve in this role, it will be discarded. These children try to engage in the same types of activities as other children. Their only limitations are usually those imposed by adults. In contrast, the child with an acquired limb deficiency goes through the natural readjustment process of limb loss. How well they are able to adjust has a direct impact on their acceptance of an artificial limb.[41]

Some special considerations should be made for the pediatric patient with upper limb deficiency or amputation.[12] Three specific points to consider in this population are:

1. normal growth and development, which will necessitate frequent prosthetic adjustments or replacements;
2. bony overgrowth; and
3. the more rigorous use to which the device will be subjected.[36]

It can be expected that a prosthesis (socket only, or all of it) will need to be replaced yearly in the first 5 years of life, every 18 months from 5 to 12 years of age, and every 2 years until age 21 years.[3] To address growth problems, multilayered sockets (onion sockets) for body-powered devices can be used. These allow removal of one layer at a time to accommodate growth. This results in gradual enlargement of the socket to coincide with periods of growth. The socket made in this fashion increases the lifespan of the prosthesis from 6 months to as much as 18 months. Length adjustment is also important, although it is not as critical as with lower limb prostheses. This can be adjusted by adding material at the wrist or elbow sites when necessary. Harnesses and cables need to be adjusted for length and replaced more frequently.[4] For bony overgrowth, surgery with bony capping can be necessary.[23] For myoelectric devices, two problems are noted: the limitation imposed by the weight and size of the components,[32] and the necessary frequent alterations to the socket to maintain optimal electrode contact as the residual limb size changes.[39] Frequently required socket replacements can make myoelectric devices less practical for this population due to their cost. Terminal devices and elbows might need to be replaced frequently. Prosthetic component banks are available in some countries, which make myoelectric prosthetic component replacement less expensive.

Parental counseling and support are integral components in the rehabilitation of the pediatric amputee. The prosthetic fitting for the pediatric patient with upper limb deficiency or the pediatric amputee should be initiated at 3–9 months of age.

This should coincide with sitting and the initiation of bimanual activities. The use of a passive mitten, hand, or inactive hook or California Amputee Pediatric Project terminal device and a preflexed fixed elbow is indicated at this stage. The terminal device can be activated at ages 18–24 months and the elbow at ages 36–48 months.[36] Myoelectric devices have been used at these young ages, with good results.[38] For very proximal upper limb deficiency, use of the feet should be encouraged.

SUMMARY

The rehabilitation process for the patient with an upper limb amputation is a complex one, and it is best accomplished by the patient who is able to work in a close cooperative relationship with a comprehensive, interdisciplinary, specialized treatment team. The team members should be ready and able to assist the patient throughout the rehabilitation program, from preamputation to community reintegration. The availability of psychologic counseling and/or assistance from the team members during each one of these steps is very important for the smooth transition of the patient back into the community.

REFERENCES

1. [Anonymous]. AD-CAM special issue. J Prosthet Orthot 1989; 1:116–190.
2. Atkins D. Adult upper-limb prosthetic training in rehabilitation planning for the upper extremity amputee. In: Meier RH, Atkins DJ, eds. Functional restoration of adults and children with upper extremity amputation. New York: Demos Medical Publishing; 2004.
3. Challenor Y. Limb deficiencies in children. In: Molnar G, ed. Pediatric rehabilitation. Baltimore: Williams & Wilkins; 1992:400–424.
4. Curran B, Hambrey R. The prosthetic treatment of upper limb deficiency. Prosthet Orthot Int 1991; 15:82–87.
5. Davis RW. Phantom sensation, phantom pain and stump pain. Arch Phys Med Rehabil 1993; 74:79–91.
6. Edelstein JE. Preprosthetic management of patients with lower or upper limb amputation. Phys Med Rehabil Clin North Am 1991; 2:285–297.
7. Esquenazi A. Amputation rehabilitation and prosthetic restoration. From surgery to community reintegration. Disabil Rehabil 2004; 26(14–15):831–836.
8. Esquenazi A. Pain management post amputation. In: Monga TN, Grabois M, eds. Pain management in rehabilitation. New York: Demos Medical Publishing; 2003:191–202.
9. Fletchall S, Hickerson WL. Early upper-extremity prosthetic fit in patients with burns. J Burn Care Rehabil 1991; 12:234–236.
10. Gallagher P, Maclachlan M. The Trinity Amputation and Prosthesis Experience Scales and quality of life in people with lower-limb amputation. Arch Phys Med Rehabil 2004; 85(5):730–736.
11. Glatly HW. A statistical study of 12,000 new amputees. South Med J 1964; 57:1373–1378.
12. Gover AM, McIvor J. Upper limb deficiencies in infants and young. Infant Young Child 1992; 5:58–72.
13. Gregory RT, Gould RJ, Peclet M, et al. The mangled extremity syndrome (MES): a severity grading system for multisystem injury of the extremity. J Trauma 1985; 25:1147–1150.
14. Heim M, et al. Silicone suspension of external prostheses: a new era in artificial limb usage. J Bone Joint Surg Br 1997; 79:638–640.
15. Illizarov GA. Possibilities offered by our method for lengthening various segments in upper and lower limbs. Basic Life Sci 1988; 48:323.
16. Jendrzejczyk D. Flexible socket systems. Clin Prosthet Orthot 1985; 9:27–31.
17. Jones LE, Davidson JH. Save that arm: a study of problems in the remaining arm of unilateral upper limb amputees. Prosthet Orthot Int 1999; 23:55–58.
18. Kay HW, Newman JD. Relative incidence of new amputations: statistical comparisons of 6,000 new amputees. Orthot Prosthet 1975; 29:3–16.
19. Kejlaa GH. The social and economic outcome after upper limb amputation. Prosthet Orthot Int 1992; 16:25–31.
20. Kristinsson O. Flexible above-knee socket made from low density polyethylene suspended by a weight-transmitting frame. Orthot Prosthet 1983; 37:25–27.
21. Kuiken TA, Dumanian GA, Lipschutz RD, et al. Prost Orthot Int 2004; 28:245–253.
22. Lake C, Sopan T. The incidence of dermatological problems in the silicone suspension sleeve user. J Prosthet Orthot 1997; 9:97–104.
23. Lambert C. Amputation surgery in the child. Orthop Clin North Am 1972; 3:473–482.
24. Levy WS. Skin problems of the amputee. In: Bowker JH, Michael JW, eds. Atlas of limb prosthetics. 2nd edn. St. Louis: Mosby-Year Book; 1992:681–688.
25. Madigan RR, Fillauer KD. 3-S prosthesis: a preliminary report. J Pediatr Orthop 1991; 11:112–117.
26. Malone JM, Childers SJ, Underwood J, et al. Immediate postsurgical management of upper extremity amputation: conventional, electric and myoelectric prosthesis. Orthot Prosthet 1981; 35:1.
27. Malone JM, Fleming LL, Roberson J, et al. Immediate, early and late postsurgical management of upper limb amputation. J Rehabil Res Dev 1984; 21:33.
28. Meier R, Esquenazi A. Rehabilitation planning for the upper extremity amputee. In: Meier RH, Atkins DJ, eds. Functional restoration of adults and children with upper extremity amputation. New York: Demos Medical Publishing; 2004:55–61.
29. Melzack R. Phantom limbs. Sci Am 1992; April:120–126.
30. National Center for Health Statistics. Current estimates from the National Health Interview Survey. US Department of Health and Human Services; 1994.
31. Neumann M, Bergmann I, Hoffmann U, et al. Botulinum toxin for focal hyperhidrosis: technical considerations and improvements in application. Br J Dermatol 1998; 139:1123–1124.
32. Patton J, Shida-Tokeshi J, Setoguchi Y. Prosthetic components for children. Phys Med Rehabil 1991; 5:2.
33. Robinson LR, Czerniecki JM, Ehde DM, et al. Trial of amitriptyline for relief of pain in amputees: results of a randomized controlled study. Arch Phys Med Rehabil 2004; 85(1):1–6.
34. Salem Y. The use of silicone suspension sleeves with myoelectric fittings. J Prosthet Orthot 1994; 6(4):119–120.
35. Scott RN. Biomedical engineering in upper-extremity prosthetics. In: Atkins DJ, Meier RH III, eds. Comprehensive management of the upper-limb amputee. New York: Springer-Verlag; 1989:173–189.
36. Setoguchi Y, LeBlanc M. Upper limb strength of young limb deficient children as a factor in using body powered terminal devices: a pilot study. J Assoc Child Prosthet Orthot Clin 1992; 27:89–96.
37. Setoguchi Y, Rosenfelder R, eds. The limb deficient child. Springfield: Charles C Thomas; 1982.
38. Sherman AR, Sherman JC, Gall GN. A survey of current phantom limb pain treatment in the United States. Pain 1980; 8:85–99.
39. Sorbye R. Myoelectric prosthetic fitting in young children. Clin Orthop 1980; 148:34–40.
40. Van Dorsten B. Integrating psychological and medical care: practice recommendations for amputation. In: Meier RH, Atkins DJ, eds. Functional restoration of adults and children with upper extremity amputation. New York: Demos Medical Publishing; 2004:73–88.
41. Varni JW, Setoguchi Y. Effects of parental adjustment on the adaptation of children with congenital or acquired limb deficiencies. J Dev Behav Pediatr 1993; 14:13–20.
42. Wilson AB Jr. Limb prosthetics. 6th edn. New York: Demos; 1989:69–90.

Chapter

14

Rehabilitation of People with Lower Limb Amputation

Todd A. Kuiken, Laura Miller, Robert Lipschutz and Mark E. Huang

Lower limb amputation remains one of the classic rehabilitation diagnoses amenable to intervention by a physiatrist. Rehabilitation and prosthetic interventions offer tremendous potential for improvement of amputee physical functioning, emotional well-being, and quality of life. Administering treatment to this population is profoundly rewarding.

Despite advances in medicine, industry, and technology, amputation remains a leading source of disability. Approximately 130 000 lower limb amputations are performed each year,[19] and peripheral vascular disease accounts for the vast majority of lower limb amputations. Amputations due to vascular conditions accounted for 82% of limb loss discharges, with incidence increasing by 27% from 1988 to 1996. Trauma-related amputations accounted for 16% of amputations, while those due to malignancy or congenital deformity were 0.9% and 0.8%, respectively. The incidence of amputations is not expected to subside anytime soon, for a number of reasons, including the aging of the population and the increased incidence of diabetes in the USA. As the population ages, the number of amputations in persons older than 65 is expected to double.[32] Diabetes creates the greatest risk of amputation, surpassing the risks created by both smoking and hypertension. Diabetes is related to 67% of all amputations.[67] The age-adjusted amputation rate for persons with diabetes is as high as 18 to 28 times more than that of persons without diabetes.[78]

In terms of level of amputation, Dillingham et al. reported that lower limb amputation accounted for 97% of all amputations between 1988 and 1996, with the following distributions: 31.5% toes, 10.5% midfoot, 0.8% ankle disarticulation, 27.6% transtibial, 0.4% knee disarticulation, 25.8% transfemoral, and 0.4% hip disarticulation. Other sources report that 64–73% of amputations were transtibial, 26–31% transfemoral, and 4.5% knee disarticulation.[5,31] Older studies have shown that patients with diabetes are at greater risk for a second amputation, with rates as high as 18% at 2 years and 45% at 4 years.[23] The second operation is shown by more recent studies to be a conversion to a more proximal amputation level in 9%, with amputation of the contralateral limb in 11–20% of the general amputee population.[5,31,42]

Survival rates after amputation vary based on a variety of factors. Those who have amputations from trauma tend to have good long-term survival, but those who have amputations from vascular etiology face sobering survival statistics. After a vascular amputation, the 30-day mortality rate is reported to be from 9 to 16%,[1,5,25,42] and long-term survival has recently been found to be 69% at 1 year, 42% at 3 years, and 35–45% at 5 years.[5,15,25,66] More proximal levels of amputation have also been associated with decreased survival rates.[5,15,32,66] Diabetes and end-stage renal disease have been shown to negatively impact survival, with 5-year survival rates as low as 30.9% and 14.4%, respectively.[5]

The chances of prosthetic fitting vary depending on etiology of amputation, level of amputation, and age. Patients with amputations due to trauma or tumor have high success rates of prosthetic fitting. MacKenzie found that 97% of all traumatic amputees were ambulating with a prosthesis at 3 months.[50] Success rates are lower for people with amputation due to vascular disease and diabetes. Overall success rates for prosthetic fitting in dysvascular patients have been reported to be over 80%.[36,61] Fletcher reported a 78% success rate in transtibial patients and a 57% success rate in transfemoral patients for functional prosthetic use among people over 65 who were referred to an amputee clinic.[32] He noted that success of fitting diminished with age and level of amputation. Patients with transtibial amputation older than 85 years of age had less than a 2% chance of successful prosthetic fitting. Johannesson reported that 43% of all patients received a prosthesis after primary amputation.[42] Multiple limb amputees can also be successful ambulators. Two studies have reported that 70% of bilateral transtibial amputees were able to use their prostheses for ambulation.[13,77]

Regardless of its etiology, amputation remains a source of significant physical and psychologic trauma in individuals facing limb loss. Although many patients and physicians alike might consider it to be a failure of medical and surgical management, amputation is a reconstructive surgery that maximizes the patient's function and quality of life. Most patients have the potential for a successful outcome following amputation. Although elderly vascular amputees might never run or participate in competitive sports, they can still have the potential for improved function with a prosthesis. For the young amputee, an active lifestyle with a prosthesis is expected. To illustrate the functional potential of a patient with amputation, Marlon Shirley holds the men's amputee record for the 100-m sprint at 10.97 s. That is only a short step behind the able-bodied time of 9.78 s by Tim Montgomery in 2004.[20]

PRESURGICAL MANAGEMENT

Rehabilitation of the lower limb amputee should begin as soon as amputation is considered. The primary goals of the presurgical period are medical stabilization, patient assessment for amputation level, pain control, psychologic support, and initiation of a functional rehabilitation program. Whenever possible, the physiatrist should see the patient prior to surgery in order to conduct a patient evaluation, begin patient education about the rehabilitation process, and offer the patient emotional support.

Selection of amputation level

The quality and type of amputation performed greatly affects the overall outcome for the patient. When determining amputation level, all the factors affecting the patient's function must be considered. These factors include not only tissue viability, but also prosthetic options, gait dynamics, cosmesis, and the biomechanics of the residual limb. The objective of preoperative evaluation is to determine the level at which healing will occur, and at which maximal function will be restored after removal of all compromised or infected tissue. Preservation of tissue is balanced with restoration of function, as higher amputations result in increased morbidity and decreased rehabilitation potential. Prediction of healing requires careful evaluation of surgical technique, postoperative care, nutritional status, and arterial circulation—particularly tissue perfusion.

The earliest attempts to judge the appropriate level of amputation focused on the presence of palpable pulses, angiographic findings, skin color and temperature, character and location of pain, and, most notably, the presence of incisional skin bleeding at the time of surgery. Various diagnostic methods exist to help determine the level at which healing will occur. These include Doppler pressure measurements, pulse volume recordings, photoplethysmographic pressures, laser Doppler blood flow studies, xenon skin blood flow studies, arterial angiography, and transcutaneous oxygen determinations (see Ch. 57). However, these tests have not been more consistently reliable than clinical judgment in predicting wound healing at a given level.[6,22] Most surgeons use a combination of objective data and assessment of the appearance of the tissues at the time of surgery, particularly bleeding, to decide on the site of amputation.

Several other factors that influence the patient's prosthetic function need to be considered when determining amputation level. For example, Chopart and Lisfranc amputations might allow some ambulation for short distances without a device, but they have a short forefoot lever arm, and they are difficult to fit with an adequate prosthesis biomechanically. They also have a high rate of equinovarus deformity. Alternatively, higher levels of amputation, such as a Symes or transtibial amputation, allow for better gait with a prosthesis and superior performance in more demanding activities. Cosmesis is also an important consideration. Ankle and knee disarticulations have the advantage of long lever arms for prosthesis control and end weight bearing, but the prostheses have considerably poorer appearance than

that of transtibial or transfemoral prostheses. This can be a determining factor for some patients.

Amputations are classified into three categories: closed, open, and guillotine. Closed amputation is the most commonly used technique for amputations necessitated by arterial disease. For this procedure, an incision is made through presumably healthy tissues, and skin flaps are shaped for primary (sutured) closure. In contrast, open amputations are performed only in instances of severe trauma or overwhelming infection. This type of intervention allows for appropriate drainage and observation of the wound. Finally, guillotine amputation is an open procedure in which all the tissues are cut at the same level by a circular incision. This type of amputation eventually requires a closed amputation performed at a higher level. Guillotine amputation is rarely necessary today, and is reserved for extremely ill patients who require quick control of rapidly spreading infection (such as gas gangrene).

Pain control

Good perioperative pain control is essential for the patient facing limb loss. Beyond patient comfort, adequate pain control minimizes the patient's stress, allows the patient to participate more fully in a rehabilitation program, and aids in preventing central nervous system 'wind-up' and chronic pain syndromes.[51] Uncontrolled pain also impairs postoperative healing and immune functions.[9,18]

The mainstay of perioperative pain control treatment is opioid therapy. Oral opiates are usually sufficient, but there should be no hesitation to use more aggressive pain control measures including transdermal, subcutaneous, intramuscular, or intravenous routes. A scheduled dose of a long-acting agent is recommended so that the patient has consistent pain relief. This should be with 'as needed' shorter acting 'rescue' medicine. A sufficient dose of analgesia just prior to therapies often helps the patient fully participate.

Patient-controlled analgesia systems are useful for patients having severe pain in the perioperative period. They provide a continuous infusion of analgesic, with the ability of the patient to employ a supplemental dose as needed. Patient-controlled analgesia systems provide excellent analgesia and can reduce some of the patient's stress or fear related to pain. Continuous regional nerve blocks and epidural anesthesia can also be used for perioperative pain control.[52]

Psychologic support

Psychologic assessment and support for the patient facing limb loss should be a high priority. Assessment of the patient's expectations and goals is important. Frequently, patients fear that they will never be able to walk again after amputation, and might not expect to be able to accomplish more demanding occupational or recreational tasks. These perceptions are often unfounded, because most amputees can do very well functionally. As noted above, several studies indicate that over 80% of amputees at all levels will be able to successfully walk with a prosthesis,[36,55,61] and this is consistent with our experience. Each patient's specific long-term goals should be identified before surgery, and a comprehensive rehabilitation program should be outlined to achieve these goals. Patients feel empowered and reassured when higher functions (such as sports) are recognized as legitimate goals and the rehabilitation team helps them achieve these goals.

Describing the rehabilitation process in detail to patients and educating them about prosthetics can help to allay their fear of the unknown. Providing educational literature and web site addresses can be a valuable and calming service to patients and their families (see Box 14-1). Some programs utilize a peer counseling program in which patients who are successful prosthetic users visit patients with new amputations on request. Finally, it is important to discuss phantom limb sensation and phantom limb pain with patients prior to surgery. Phantom limb sensation is the temporary non-painful feeling that the amputated limb is still present. This feeling typically fades away over a period of weeks. Phantom pain is the usually temporary pain that can occur in a limb after its amputation, especially in a patient with a long history of preamputation limb pain. All patients need to be told to expect these sensations in the missing limb after surgery and to realize that they are normal.

Functional rehabilitation

There are often a few days or even weeks from the time a decision is made to do an amputation until it actually occurs. This time can be used to initiate a functional rehabilitation program

---

Box 14-1 Educational resources available for amputees

Booklets
- Broyles N. *For the New Amputee*. Amputee Coalition of America, National Limb Loss Information Center; 1991.
- *First Step: a Guide for Adapting to Limb Loss*. Amputee Coalition of America, National Limb Loss Information Center; 2000.
- Helminski JO. *Pre-Prosthetic Care for Above-Knee Amputees*. Rehabilitation Institute of Chicago; 1993.
- Helminski JO. *Pre-Prosthetic Care for Below-Knee Amputees*. Rehabilitation Institute of Chicago; 1993.
- Kuiken T, Edwards M, Micelli N. *Below-Knee Amputation: a Guide for Rehabilitation*. Rehabilitation Institute of Chicago; 2002.
- Kuiken T, Edwards M, Soltys N. *Above-Knee Amputation: a Guide for Rehabilitation*. Rehabilitation Institute of Chicago; 2003.
- Novotny MP, Michael JW. *You Have a Choice: Improving Outcomes in O&P*. Amputee Coalition of America, National Limb Loss Information Center.
- Shurr DG. *Patient Care Booklet for Above-Knee Amputees*. American Academy of Orthotists and Prosthetists; 1999.
- Uellendahl JE. *Patient Care Booklet for Below-Knee Amputees*. American Academy of Orthotists and Prosthetists; 1999.
- United Amputee Services Association, Inc. *Survivor's Guide*. Amputee Coalition of America, National Limb Loss Information Center; 1992.

Books
- Dravecky D, Dravecky J, Gire K. *When You Can't Come Back*. Zondervan Publishing House; 1992.
- Le Ratto L, ed. *Coping with Being Physically Challenged*. Rosen Publishing Group; 1991.
- Lockette KF, Keyes AM. *Conditioning with Physical Disabilities*. Human Kinetics Europe; 1994.
- Madruga L. *One Step at a Time: A Young Woman's Struggle to Walk Again*. McGraw-Hill; 1979.
- Maxfield G, Williams A, Toner F. *The Novel Approach to Sexuality and Disability*. Northern Nevada Amputee Support Group; 1996.
- Sabolich J. *You're Not Alone*. Sabolich Prosthetic & Research Center; 1993.
- Wallace CS. *Challenged by Amputation: Embracing a New Life*. Inclusion Concepts Publishing House; 1995.
- Winchell E. *Coping with Limb Loss*. Avery Publishing Group; 1995.

Web sites
- Active Amputee Lifestyle: http://www.activeamp.org
- American Academy of Orthotists and Prosthetists: http://www.oandp.org
- American Amputee Soccer Association: http://www.ampsoccer.org
- American Orthotic and Prosthetic Association: http://www.aopanet.org
- Amputee Coalition of America: http://www.amputee-coalition.org
- Amputee-Online.com: http://www.amputee-online.com
- Challenged Athletes Foundation: http://www.challengedathletes.org
- Diabetes Resource Center: http://www.diabetesresource.com
- Disabled Sports USA: http://www.dsusa.org
- Hemipelvectomy and hip disarticulation information: http://www.hphdhelp.org
- Limbless Association: http://www.limbless-association.org
- Limbs for Life Foundation: http://www.limbsforlife.org
- National Amputee Golf Association: http://www.nagagolf.org
- National Center on Physical Activity and Disability: http://www.ncpad.org
- Orthotic and Prosthetic Assistance Fund: http://www.opfund.org
- Orthotics and Prosthetics careers: http://www.opcareers.org
- Rehabilitation Institute of Chicago LIFE Center for people with disabilities: http://lifecenter.ric.org
- Stumps R Us (an amputee support group): http://www.stumps.org
- Surviving Limb Loss: http://www.survivinglimbloss.org
- The Global Resource for Orthotics and Prosthetics Information: http://www.oandp.com
- US Paralympics: http://www.usparalympics.org

prior to the amputation. It is easier to stretch out a tight or contracted joint using the entire limb length before the amputation, than it is after surgery, when the limb is shortened and tender. Preoperative rehabilitation should emphasize range of motion, conditioning remaining limb segments, increasing endurance, improving transfers, and training the patient in one-legged gait with an assistive device. This can reduce or even eliminate the need for inpatient rehabilitation after the amputation.

POSTSURGICAL MANAGEMENT

Wound care

Wound healing is dependent on adequate tissue perfusion, good wound care, and adequate nutrition. Care for primary surgical wounds is straightforward. The limb should be washed on a daily basis with either normal saline or simple soap and water; antiseptic agents such as iodine solutions or hydrogen peroxide inhibit wound healing and should be avoided unless there are signs of infection. Dressings should be kept clean and changed daily.

In traumatic amputations, there are often large open wounds that could have been contaminated in the trauma, and additional coverage procedures such as flaps and grafts might have been performed. These wounds require close observation and meticulous wound care. They often cause a delay in the fitting of the initial lower limb prosthesis. Wounds do not need to be completely healed for the fitting of the prosthesis, but the viability of flaps and grafts needs to be established and monitored carefully.

In patients with vascular compromise, wound margin necrosis can develop. The limb should be monitored closely in these cases, kept clean, and protected from any trauma that could cause a dehiscence in such a fragile wound. Once the non-viable tissue is clearly demarcated, debridement can be considered.

Good nutrition must be encouraged, and supported with supplements when necessary. Eneroth found that, when supplementary nutrition was given to malnourished patients, twice as many adequately nourished patients healed their residual limb wound when compared with control subjects.[27]

Edema control

Reducing postsurgical edema is important to promote wound healing, minimize postoperative pain, and shape the limb for prosthetic fitting. Postsurgical edema stretches a surgical wound, which stretches nerve endings and causes pain. Edema puts tension on the wound, compromising healing. Swelling gives a bulbous shape to the residual limb, which interferes with prosthetic fitting and can slow the patient's functional recovery. An effective compressive dressing can minimize these problems.

Several different edema control systems are available. The most commonly used treatment is elastic wraps on the residual limb (e.g. Ace bandages). Although elastic wraps can provide effective compression, they are high-maintenance items that must be properly applied and changed about every 4–6 hours to maintain consistent compression.[53] This can be difficult and time-consuming for a patient, or even the healthcare team, to accomplish. Elastic wraps that are improperly applied or displaced in the normal course of regular movement can turn into tourniquets causing pressure wounds and even limb ischemia. Consequently, the use of elastic wrapping is not recommended.

The use of elastic socks or elastic stockinet provides a better alternative to elastic wraps. Elastic stockinet (e.g. Compressigrip and Tubigrip) can be applied in multiple layers to give graded and increasing compression toward the end of the residual limb (Fig. 14-1). They are inexpensive and easily applied. Premanufactured residual limb shrinkers can also be used. For transfemoral amputees, a residual limb shrinker with a waist belt must be used, because otherwise the dressing tends to slide off the conical-shaped residual limb. The waist belt should be attached to the elastic dressing at the *side* of the limb. If the attachment is worn in front, the shrinker will slide off during sitting.

Prosthetic elastomeric liners can also be used as compression socks for edema reduction in amputees.[42,44] They can provide compression and also lend some degree of protection to the residual limb. Due to their suction fit, they can be used on the transfemoral amputee without a waist belt. When using any elastic dressing, bony prominences should be closely monitored, because pressure can concentrate at protruding bony areas and lead to skin breakdown.

Rigid dressings provide additional benefits over soft dressings alone for transtibial amputees (Fig. 14-2). Rigid dressings help protect the residual limb from any inadvertent trauma, such as a fall.[28] They provide good compression to minimize edema, and the cast can be conformed to minimize pressure over bony prominences. Weight bearing can also be started through the rigid dressing to help desensitize the limb and build tolerance to pressure.

A non-removable rigid dressing is a cast that is applied over the fully extended residual limb up to the midthigh (Fig. 14-2a). This type of cast is helpful in preventing knee flexion contractures and can be used as an immediate postoperative prosthesis (IPOP, as discussed below). A non-removable cast does not allow for wound inspection, except at cast changes. It also does not allow patients to massage their residual limbs, an important part of the desensitization program.

A removable rigid dressing (RRD)[86,87] is a custom-made cast that covers the residual limb up to the knee (Fig. 14-2b). It is

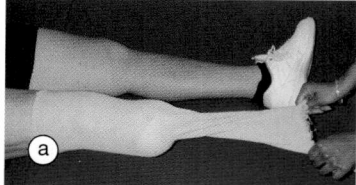
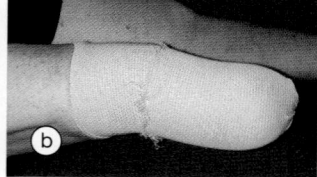

Figure 14-1 Use of an elastic stockinet for edema control. (**a**) Place just over half of the length on the limb and twist a half turn. (**b**) Pull second half over leg to provide two layers of compression.

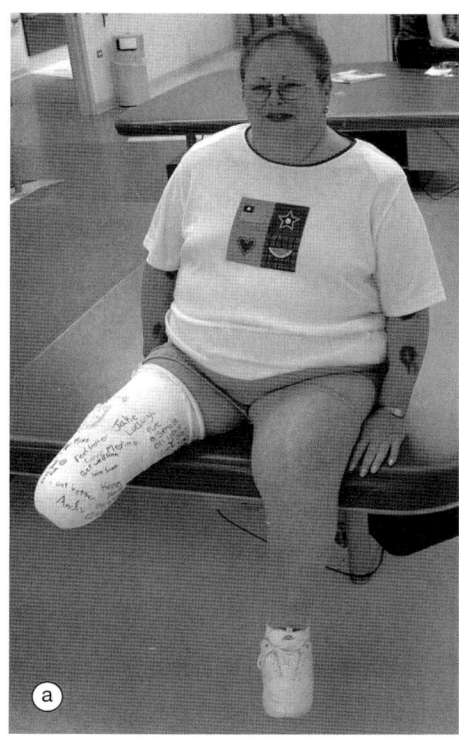

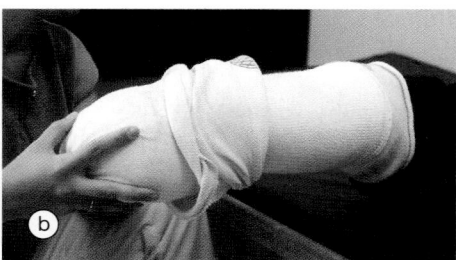

Figure 14-2 Rigid dressings for a transtibial amputee. (**a**) Rigid dressing. (**b**) Rigid removable dressing.

held in place with either elastic stockinet or a thigh cuff. As the limb shrinks, socks, shrinker socks, and elastic stockinet are added underneath the RRD to keep it snug. The RRD allows for frequent wound inspection and massage of the residual limb. It also helps to teach patients how to adjust sock ply, a necessary skill for using most types of prostheses. A suggested protocol is to start with a non-rigid removable dressing applied immediately after surgery. After the first 3–6 days, the cast should be changed to an RRD, which should be used until most of the edema is resolved and the wound is well healed. If more than 12–18 ply of sock is required to keep the RRD snug, a new RRD is recommended.

Postoperative pain issues

Identifying the etiology of postoperative limb pain is important for successful control of the pain. Because of nerve fiber damage and ongoing stimulation of the nerves in the residual limb, a generalized residual limb pain is initially expected secondary to surgical incision and postoperative edema. Ectopic activity at the cut end of nerves is expected and can be due to 'leaky sodium channels' or the uncovering of new pathologic receptors.[7,8] Ephaptic transmission, which is the stimulation of afferent fibers (nociceptors) by efferent neurons (motor or sympathetic), can also contribute to limb pain.[41,64] This acute pain responds well to intravenous or intramuscular opiates. It subsides fairly rapidly, and the parenteral opiates can usually be discontinued within 2–3 days. Scheduled doses of oral opiates with rescue medications as needed should be continued beyond this period, and weaned slowly so that the patient continues to receive adequate pain control.

Desensitization techniques should be added to the treatment plan within a few days of surgery. The patient should be instructed to start massaging and tapping the residual limb, which can be performed through any soft dressing. This gentle stimulation can help to reduce residual limb pain by closing the 'pain gate',[51] and gives the patient a technique for controlling the pain independently. Self-massage also forces patients to attend to their amputation; this can help with their new body image and psychologic adjustment to limb loss.

When generalized residual limb pain does not subside as expected, the patient should be reevaluated. Wound infection and abscess must be excluded, and reevaluation of the arterial system needs to be considered. Patients with peripheral vascular disease and/or diabetes can have continued limb ischemia that is a form of claudication. This claudication can be constant or intermittent due to activity. Patients with residual limb ischemia often exhibit poor skin color, and the residual limb pain is frequently dependent on the limb's position. Over the course of weeks, ischemic pain often resolves as the swelling goes down, the circulation remodels with the decreased distal tissue load, and the limb heals. Sometimes reamputation to a higher level is required if the wound fails to heal, tissue necrosis progresses, or ischemic pain persists. During the interim, the patient needs to continue to receive adequate analgesia, although giving adequate pain relief without excessively sedating the patient can be difficult. When ischemic limb pain does not quickly subside, the patient, the family, and the entire rehabilitation team need to be made aware of the plan to wait and see whether the residual limb is salvageable or if reamputation is necessary.

Functional rehabilitation

Early rehabilitation management is critical in the postoperative period. It is hoped that the team has been involved already but, if not, consultation with physiatry and involvement of physical therapy and occupational therapy should begin as soon as possible. Therapy staff work on a variety of areas, such as self-care, bed mobility, transfers, wheelchair skills, ambulation, and patient and family teaching. Amputee rehabilitation principles include proper positioning, initiation of range of motion, early mobilization, and evaluation for durable medical equipment and adaptive devices.

Patients should be educated in proper positioning. Prevention of hip and knee contractures is critical in this period. Patients should not have pillows placed under the knee, as this can lead to knee flexion contracture. To prevent hip abduction contractures, pillows should not be placed between the legs. Dangling the residual limb over the side of the bed or wheelchair should be avoided. A knee extension board (Fig. 14-3) can be fitted underneath the wheelchair or chair to promote knee extension and help prevent dependent edema. Wheelchair elevating leg rests are generally less effective and more expensive than these boards. If knee flexion contractures are of great concern, a knee immobilizer can be used while the patient is in bed to maintain knee extension. Patients should be instructed to lie prone several times a day for 10–15 min at a time to prevent hip flexion contractures. Individuals who cannot tolerate prone positioning can lie supine on a mat while performing hip extension exercises of their affected limb.

Range of motion and strengthening exercises of the affected limb are important adjuncts to positioning. Muscles that oppose the common sites of contraction must be strengthened, especially knee and hip extensors. Other important muscle groups that should be strengthened include the hip adductors and abductors. Because patients are increasingly reliant on their arms to assist with mobility, arm strengthening and conditioning is needed. Specific exercises include strengthening of the wrist, elbow extensors, and scapular stabilizers. This training prepares patients to properly execute transfers and to correctly use crutches or a walker. Initiation of aerobic exercise is needed to increase endurance and cardiovascular fitness but, given the high incidence of concomitant cardiovascular disease in individuals with vascular etiology of amputation, adherence to cardiac precautions is important.

Early mobilization facilitates early functional improvements. Usually the first activities include bed mobility, transfers, and mobilization to a chair or wheelchair. As the patient progresses, the activities should increasingly focus on standing and balance exercises in the parallel bars, and hopping. The use of a walker or crutches is the next step in mobilization.

Early partial weight bearing can begin in the first few days if there are no wound complications. For transtibial amputees with rigid dressings, limited weight bearing can be performed through their cast using a strap across their wheelchair (Fig. 14-4). When the patient is up in the parallel bars, weight bearing can be done via a tire jack or adjustable footstool. Immediate postoperative prostheses can also be used for early weight bearing, as described below. Inspection after weight bearing is important in monitoring wound tolerance of pressure. This is especially important in individuals with amputation from vascular disease or in patients with impaired sensation.

Evaluation for appropriate adaptive equipment and durable medical equipment is important. Adaptive devices such as reachers, long handles, sponges, shoehorns, dressing sticks, and sock aids can be issued as needed to assist with activities of daily living. Long-handled mirrors can also be helpful to allow patients to monitor the status of their residual limb easily.

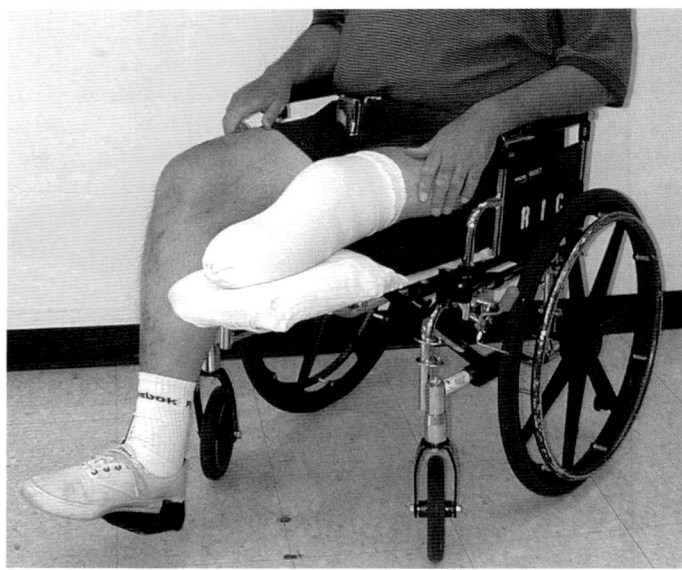

Figure 14-3 Knee extension board to prevent flexion contracture in a transtibial amputee.

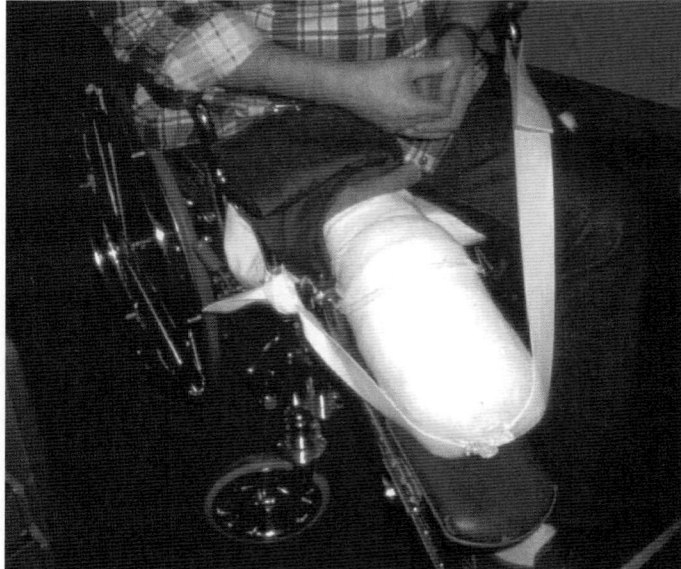

Figure 14-4 Partial weight bearing with rigid dressing through strap on wheelchair armrests.

Because sitting in a wheelchair makes the amputee's center of gravity higher and more posterior, rear wheels should be set posterior to the chair back and antitippers should be placed to minimize the risk of tipping backward and suffering head injury. This is particularly important for transfemoral and bilateral amputees.

A plan for ongoing rehabilitation services needs to be made during the early postoperative period. Younger patients with unilateral amputations can usually be discharged home as crutch ambulators with ongoing outpatient rehabilitation. Older and marginally functioning patients and multilimb amputees usually need acute inpatient rehabilitation before they can safely return home. These patients can generally be admitted to a rehabilitation unit between postoperative days 3–7, after any drains are removed, pain is under control with oral medications, and they have the endurance to participate in a comprehensive rehabilitation program. The acute postoperative period prepares the patient for a safe return home with the temporary assistance of a wheelchair, walker, or crutches, or with an early-fitted prosthesis.

Patients need to be observed closely for the first 12–18 months. Early on, the key issues remain wound healing, edema control, psychologic adjustment, and pain control. Prosthetic fitting and prosthetic gait training can usually be started within 3–6 weeks of surgery, and patients are usually able to ambulate independently (perhaps with an assistive device) within 1 month of starting therapy with their prosthesis. The residual limb continues to shrink during the first 6–12 months. This requires constant monitoring to assure an adequate fit of the device by both the patient and the rehabilitation team. After shrinkage abates in 6–12 months, the patient can then be fitted with a new, definitive prosthesis (or at least a new socket).

Most amputees need a full year to completely adjust to their limb loss. Regular physician visits during this time are needed. Follow-up should be done, if possible, in multidisciplinary amputee clinics by a physiatrist, prosthetist, nurse, and a physical therapist. A multidisciplinary clinic also gives amputees the opportunity to visit with others being seen in the clinic. This provides a peer support or 'milieu therapy' that is very beneficial.

Prosthetic considerations

Prosthetic sponsorship must be considered as soon as possible, even before the patient is ready to be fitted with an artificial limb. Many insurers require preapproval before the patient can be fitted with a prosthesis. Such authorization can sometimes take weeks (or even months) to obtain and cause detrimental delays in the rehabilitation of the amputee. Starting the required paperwork as soon as possible can minimize these delays. Some providers also have copayment restrictions in coverage that affect prosthetic prescription (preferred providers, component limitations, even a restriction of one prosthesis per lifetime!). These restrictions need to be determined, considered, and discussed with the patient when designing a treatment plan.

Determining when to fit the lower limb amputee with a prosthesis and what kind of prosthesis to use are issues open to considerable debate. One option for transtibial amputees is to use an IPOP. IPOPs traditionally have been thigh-high casts with a pylon and foot attached (Fig. 14-5a). Prefabricated devices are also now available (Fig. 14-5b,c). These devices allow for earlier bipedal ambulation. Although many claims have been made for the advantages of IPOPs over soft dressing management (including improved psychologic acceptance, reduction in pain, accelerated rehabilitation times, reduced revision rates, and reduced time to healing), these claims have rarely been evaluated with controlled studies.[76] A review of 10 controlled studies yielded only two proven claims for the IPOP:

1. that rigid plaster casts result in accelerated rehabilitation times and significantly less edema compared with soft dressings; and
2. that prefabricated pneumatic prostheses were found to have significantly fewer postsurgical complications and fewer higher level revisions compared with soft gauze dressings.

Only limited weight bearing can take place with an IPOP, and patient compliance is important for such success.[76] Although weight bearing is limited through IPOPs, patients clearly have greater stability in standing and walking with the bipedal support. Some studies have shown an increase in wound dehiscence and infection with these devices.[16] Frequently, the residual limb is too tender and painful to allow early weight bearing to take full advantage of these devices. With the non-removable IPOPs, the patients are unable to inspect or massage their residual limbs, which can interfere with desensitization and emotional adjustment to their amputation.

Another option is early fitting of a custom prosthesis, which requires a delay of 3–6 weeks until much of the surgical swelling is down and the wound has started to heal. Ideally, the limb has also become cylindrically shaped (i.e. the circumference of the distal residual limb is equal to or less than the proximal size). It is preferable that the wound has also attained some integrity (although it need not be completely healed and sutures or staples do not need to be removed). Because most of the postsurgical pain has subsided by the time of early prosthetic fitting, patients are better able to tolerate weight bearing. Much of the postoperative edema is gone, so the residual limb has a better shape for fitting with a prosthesis. A custom device is used so there is a more intimate and secure fit with the prosthesis, and full weight bearing is allowed. However, patients have only one leg for any support until the prosthesis is made, and they are less stable for transfers and gait as compared with when using an IPOP.

The most conservative option is to wait until the wound on the residual limb is completely healed and surgical edema has resolved. Then the patient is fitted with a custom prosthesis. This generally takes 3–6 months with dysvascular amputees. Although this approach can minimize wound problems related to early weight bearing, there is a higher risk of complications

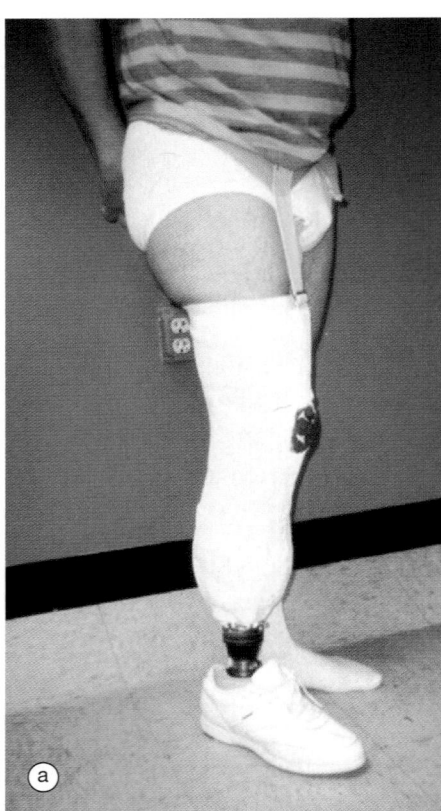
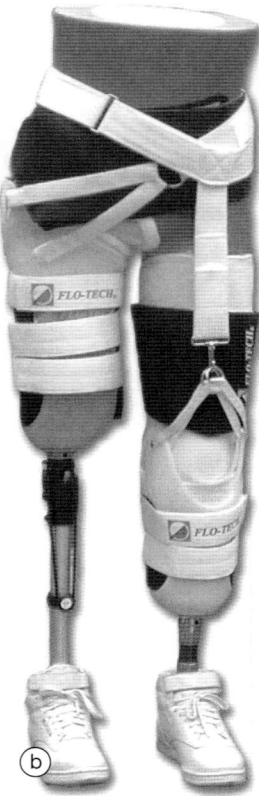
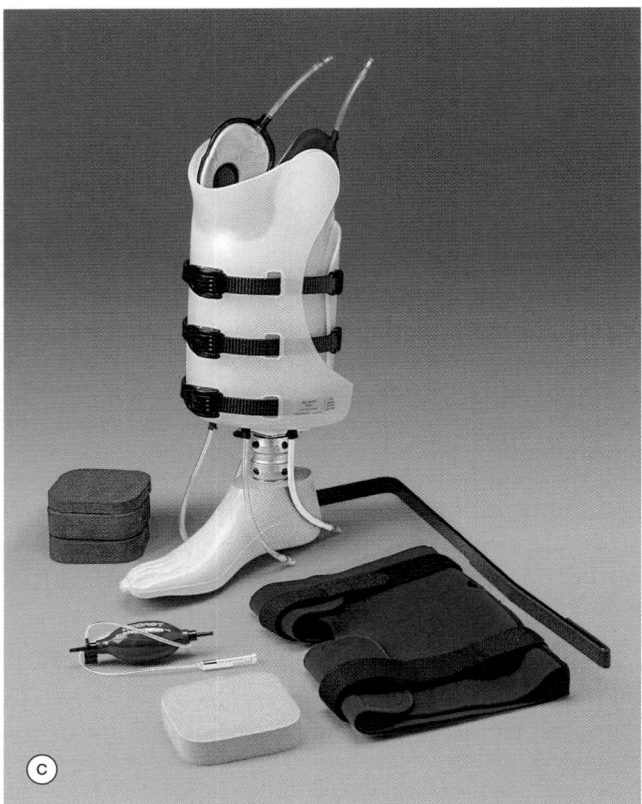

Figure 14-5 Examples of immediate postoperative prostheses (IPOPs) for transtibial amputees. (**b**) Custom-made full-length cast IPOP. (**b**) Prefabricated adjustable socket IPOPs. (**c**) Prefabricated IPOP with air–cell interface. (a, Photo courtesy of Prosthetic Research Study; b, photo courtesy of Flo-Tech O&P Systems; c, photo courtesy of Aircast.)

such as joint contracture, deconditioning, pressure ulcers, and an unnecessarily long delay in returning to functional ambulation.

After 6–12 months, when the residual limb volume stabilizes, a new prosthesis, or at least a new socket, is recommended. At this point, different componentry can be reconsidered. If a new prosthesis is made, the preparatory prosthesis can serve as a back-up prosthesis.

All new amputees require prosthetic gait training from an experienced physical therapist. The therapist initially trains the patient to independently don and doff the prosthesis, monitor skin tolerance, and adjust sock ply fitting as the residual limb shrinks. The training maximizes the patient's function. The level of performance will vary with each patient, but community ambulation and the negotiation of stairs and curbs are goals for most patients. A floor to sit transfer should also be a goal for most patients and is frequently overlooked. Therapy does not need to stop with this level of performance. For more active amputees, continuing to work in therapy on vocational activities, running, bike riding, or other sports are legitimate therapeutic goals.

Psychologic adjustment

The emotional impact of limb loss is devastating and is frequently underestimated by the rehabilitation team. Grieving over the loss of one's limb is necessary, and a brief exogenous (reactive) depression is expected. Amputees are at high risk of developing more severe psychologic problems. The incidence of persistent clinical depression is estimated to be 21–35% for people with limb loss.[69] Posttraumatic stress disorder is a recognized complication after traumatic amputation but frequently goes untreated. Non-traumatic amputees can also develop anxiety disorders from the stress related to limb loss.

The rehabilitation team should assist patients with their psychologic adjustment by giving encouragement about prognosis, providing educational materials, and incorporating the patient's specific goals into the rehabilitation plan. Team members can also reassure their patients by emphasizing gains made in therapy. They should also initiate discussion about prosthetic options with patients early on, and impress on patients that their input in the decision-making process is necessary. This not only educates patients and optimizes their prosthetic prescriptions, but it also helps to empower them and give them a sense of control.

Peer counseling and amputee support groups are another important emotional support mechanism. The opportunity to talk to someone who has been through a similar amputation, and to see how well they are doing, can be very valuable to the patient. The Amputee Coalition of America (see Box 14-1) has a national peer network that provides peer counselor training sessions and lists amputee support groups by region.

The physician should regularly monitor the patient's emotional adjustment to amputation by assessing mood, appetite, weight changes, quality of sleep, and the occurrence of nightmares. Any correlation between the patient's perceived stress level and pain should be explored. Sometimes, adjustment issues will not become problematic until shock and denial wear off and time passes. Because studies have shown that the incidence of depression in younger amputees increases with time,[34] continued monitoring by the rehabilitation team is necessary. The whole team, not just the physician, must be involved in monitoring the patient's emotional state. In most cases, the therapists and prosthetists will spend much more time with the patient and might have better insight regarding a patient's emotional status.

Each patient should be encouraged to have an evaluation by an experienced psychologist. This evaluation should include an assessment of mood, pain, other stressors, coping skills, past psychologic problems, alcohol or drug use, body image issues, and sexuality. When clinical depression, anxiety disorders, or adjustment disorders are identified, a comprehensive treatment plan should be initiated, and it should include cognitive behavioral psychotherapy and pharmacotherapy as needed.

Pain issues

Postamputation pain requires special attention to optimize the patient's quality of life and maximize the success of rehabilitation. The differential diagnoses for pain in an amputated lower limb are diverse, and treatment options differ significantly based on the etiology of pain. Consequently, the source and mechanism of the pain must be investigated and identified so that an optimal treatment plan can be implemented.

Prosthesis use is a common cause of pain in amputee patients. They report pain to be worse while wearing their prostheses and during ambulation. There is usually skin irritation that correlates with the area of the prosthesis causing the pain. Many things can contribute to prosthetic pain, including socket fit, suspension, alignment, and gait pathology. Consideration must be given to all these areas when an amputee complains of pain in the residual limb during prosthetic use. As an example, Table 14-1 lists some of the common causes of distal tibial pain, a very common site for prosthesis-related pain in transtibial amputees.

Phantom limb sensation, phantom limb pain, and generalized residual limb pain are complicated feelings, probably maintained by afferent, central, and efferent (sympathetic) dysfunction.[48] Phantom limb sensation and pain are neuropathic perceptions in a portion of the limb that was amputated. Most amputees experience some degree of phantom limb sensation and pain, but the natural history is for these feelings to diminish in both frequency and intensity over the first few weeks to months following the amputation.[26] These sensations are highly variable in character. Phantom limb sensations are frequently described as numbness, tingling, pins and needles, or itching. Some amputees report the sensation of the phantom limb

Table 14-1 Prosthetic adjustments for distal tibial pain in the transtibial amputee

Contributing factor	Treatment
Excessive socket pressure	Socket relief Remove sock ply
Pistoning in the socket	Add socks to tighten fit Build up the liner Tighten socket Tighten suspension system
Excessive pressure from liner	Change suspension system
Excessive early knee flexion	Move foot forward Plantar flex foot Decrease socket flexion Soften heel of foot or shoe Add anteroposterior ankle motion Round heel of shoe or change shoe Quadriceps or hamstring muscle strengthening

becoming shorter, known as 'telescoping'. The patients can also complain that the missing limb feels like it is moving or is in a cramped or awkward position. It is important to explain that these are normal sensations that will probably diminish with time. Sometimes patients do not consider the sensation to be 'painful', but 'uncomfortable' or 'bothersome'. These sensations can be severe enough to interfere with sleep, impair the patients' function, or significantly reduce their quality of life. At this point, the phantom limb sensation should be treated as neuropathic pain.

The character of phantom limb pain is often described as sharp, burning, stabbing, tingling, shooting, electric, or cramping. Patients frequently perceive the same type of pain that they had prior to the amputation. For example, they might feel like they still have a painful foot ulcer.

Residual limb pain, previously referred to as stump pain, is another manifestation of central sensitization. Preliminary work in the area suggests that it is a form of allodynia or hyperpathia (i.e. pain evoked by previously innocuous stimuli), or a spontaneous pain of peripheral and/or central neuropathic origin. Spontaneous residual limb pain is usually described as aching, burning, or throbbing, while evoked pain can be electric or shooting (which can easily be confused with a clinically significant neuroma).[79] The pain is localized in the residual limb and can be associated with phantom limb pain. Ehde et al. reported residual limb pain to be as common as phantom limb pain in lower limb amputees, and often more distressing.[26] In another study of 188 lower limb amputees, 22% of patients reported residual limb pain at 6 months and 21% at 2 years post amputation.[75]

The first line of treatment for bothersome phantom limb sensation, phantom limb pain, and residual limb pain is desensitization techniques. Massaging, tapping, slapping, wrapping, and friction rubbing of the residual limb often diminish such sensations. Patients frequently find that their phantom limb pain diminishes with the stimulation of using a prosthesis. Anecdotally, many patients find that for a phantom itch, scratching the remaining leg in the same spot is helpful. For cramped or malpositioned limb sensations, hypnosis can be helpful.[24,57,74] Under hypnosis, the patient can be able to alleviate a cramped phantom hand, or move an awkwardly positioned phantom limb to a more comfortable position.

If desensitization techniques are insufficient and these pains are significantly interfering with quality of life, pharmacologic treatment should be considered. The two primary categories of medicines used to treat chronic phantom limb phenomenon are antidepressants and anticonvulsants (see Table 14-2). Antidepressants have several advantages in addition to pain control. They can also treat depression, which is a common problem in new amputees. They generally have anxiolytic effects and, some being sedative, can improve sleep. They are convenient because they are usually taken just once a day, and they are generally less expensive than the newer antiseizure medications. Analgesic antidepressants apparently need to have both noradrenergic and serotonergic receptor activity in order to effectively treat neuropathic pain,[29] which explains why the selective serotonin reuptake inhibitors do not help with the treatment of phantom limb pain. Tricyclic antidepressants have the most anecdotal and empiric support for treating pain, but they also have undesirable anticholinergic side effects.[45,68] Trazodone, an atypical quadracyclic, has also been used with success (anecdotally). Several newer antidepressants have both serotinergic and noradrenergic activity without the anticholinergic activity, and might help in treating neuropathic pain. Mirtazapine can be useful for the treatment of phantom limb pain, because it has no anticholinergic side effects and it enhances sleep (night is often the time that phantom limb pain is most problematic). It is an effective antidepressant and an anxiolytic, although weight gain can be a significant side effect.[71] Bupropion and venlafaxine might also have some value for the treatment of neuropathic pain.

A number of anticonvulsants have been used to treat neuropathic pain syndromes.[7] At present, gabapentin is probably the most widely prescribed neuropathic pain medicine in the USA. Despite its name, gabapentin's mechanism of action is unknown. Nevertheless, gabapentin has demonstrated efficacy with neuropathic pain, has minimal side effects, and has been shown in a small study to have efficacy in phantom pain.[10,39] However, it usually requires frequent dosing (generally three to four times a day) and is expensive. Traditional anticonvulsants such as carbamazepine and phenytoin are 'membrane-stabilizing' agents (sodium channel blockers) that have the widest historical use for the treatment of neuropathic pain syndromes.[17,60] However, they have a high incidence of significant side effects (Table 14-2). Other newer anticonvulsants that are being used to treat neuropathic pain include oxcarbazepine, topiramate, levetiracetam, and zonisamide, but little data exist yet concerning their efficacy. Anticonvulsants can also be used in combination with antidepressants or with each other to maximize relief from phantom limb pain. This must be done in a thoughtful fashion that employs complementary mechanisms.

Some success has been reported with topical anesthetic agents such as various analgesic balms, sprays, and patches. Capsaicin, a substance P inhibitor, has been anecdotally reported to be effective for phantom limb pain and residual limb pain.[45] Lidocaine (lignocaine) cream, ointment, and patches have also been used with some success.

Other non-pharmacologic modalities exist for the treatment of phantom limb pain,[73] such as stress relaxation techniques and biofeedback.[33,43,74] Transcutaneous electrical nerve stimulation has also been shown to give temporary pain relief.[30,49]

If these measures are unsuccessful or inadequate, then a judicious use of opioids can significantly improve the amputee's quality of life. Care must be taken in prescription, with consideration of addiction, tolerance, and side effects.

Neuromas are bundles of nerve endings that form after a nerve is cut, as is done during an amputation. They can produce sharp, focal pain under pressure or on palpation (i.e. Tinel's sign).[18] If a neuroma is superficial, then a small, tender mass can be palpated. It can cause significant pain and can preclude use of a prosthesis. Initially, prosthetic socket adjustments are used to relieve pressure over a neuroma. If this is unsuccessful, neuropathic pain medication; intralesional steroid and anesthetic injection; or neuroma ablation with phenol, alcohol, or cryoablation can provide pain relief. There are no studies of these treatments, and the outcome results for these procedures are purely anecdotal. If these interventions are all ineffective, the neuroma can be surgically excised and the nerve endings buried deep in the soft tissue to protect them from mechanical pressures. However, satisfactory results after surgery rarely exceed 80%.[12,38]

While the causal relationship between amputation and phantom limb pain or residual limb pain is obvious, other conditions can also cause pain in a phantom limb. In trauma, referred pain can be generated down the leg by a proximal nerve injury, plexopathy, radiculopathy, or occult fractures—even if the leg has been amputated. Referred leg pain from spinal stenosis or arthritis at the knee or hip can also be mistaken for phantom limb pain. These alternative diagnoses must be considered and clearly require different treatment plans.

Skin complications
Pressure or shear ulcerations
A frequent skin disorder in the residual limbs of lower limb amputees is ulceration due to excessive pressure and/or shear. The most common places for pressure sores are over bony prominences and at the brim of the socket. Problematic bony prominences include the anterior surface of midfoot amputations; the malleoli of ankle disarticulations; the distal tibia, fibular head, and tibial crest of transtibial amputees; and the distal femur of transfemoral amputees (especially when myodesis and myoplasty have not been performed to stabilize the femur).

These wounds can be caused by a variety of things. Patients might not be donning their prostheses correctly. Wrinkles in

Table 14-2 Pharmacotherapy for neuropathic pain including phantom limb pain and residual limb pain

Drug	Mechanism of action[a]	Primary side effects[a]	Cost[b]
Antidepressants			
Amitriptyline	++ adrenergic +++ serotonergic +++ sodium channel blocker	+++ weight gain +++ drowsiness +++ dry mouth	$
Nortriptyline	+++ adrenergic ++ serotonergic +++ sodium channel blocker	+ weight gain + drowsiness ++ dry mouth	$
Desipramine	+++ adrenergic +++ sodium channel blocker	+ insomnia + agitation	$$
Doxepin	+ adrenergic +++ serotonergic +++ sodium channel blocker	++ weight gain +++ drowsiness +++ dry mouth	$
Trazodone	++ serotonergic	++ drowsiness	$$
Mirtazapine	++ adrenergic ++ serotonergic	+++ weight gain ++ drowsiness	$$$
Venlafaxine (Effexor)	+ adrenergic + serotonergic + dopaminergic	+++ weight gain ++ drowsiness	$$$$
Bupropion (Wellbutrin)	++ adrenergic ++ serotonergic	+ headache + dry mouth + nausea	$$$$
Anticonvulsants			
Gabapentin	? GABAergic ? Calcium channel blocker	+ drowsiness + ataxia + edema	$$$$
Topiramate (Topamax)	++ GABAergic + sodium channel blocker + non-NMDA antagonist ? calcium channel blocker	++ drowsiness ++ cognitive changes ++ weight loss	$$$$$
Oxcarbazepine (Trileptal)	++ sodium channel blocker	+ hyponatremia	$$$$
Levetiracetam (Keppra)	Unknown	+ drowsiness + asthenia	$$$$$
Zonisamide (Zonegran)	++ calcium channel blocker + sodium channel blocker	+ weight loss ++ drowsiness + dizziness	$$$$
Carbamazepine	+++ sodium channel blocker	++ drowsiness Aplastic anemia (rare) Agranulocytosis (rare)	$
Phenytoin	+++ sodium channel blocker	+ drowsiness + ataxia + gingival hyperplasia Agranulocytosis (rare) Hepatotoxicity (rare)	$

[a]The primary reference for mechanisms of action and side effects is Murray 2004.[54] Degree of effect is approximately +, mild; ++, moderate; and +++, pronounced. GABA, γ-aminobutyric acid; NMDA, N-methyl-D-aspartate.
[b]From Anonymous 2005.[4] Cost 'per month of maintenance therapy': $, less than $25; $$, $25–49; $$$, $50–99; $$$$, $100–199; $$$$$, $200 or more.

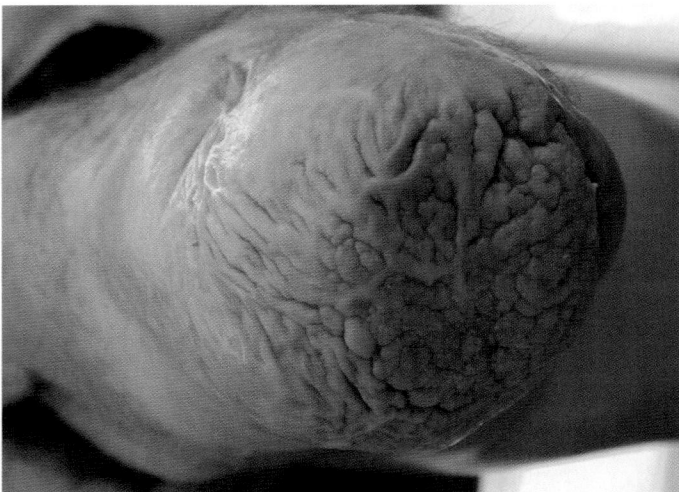

Figure 14-6 Severe verrucose hyperplasia.

socks and liners, as well as too many sock plies, can cause excessive pressure. Insufficient sock plies can lead to pistoning (up and down movement in the socket), with bottoming out on the bone as well as excessive shear. Socket fit is clearly important, and pressure-sensitive areas need to have adequate 'reliefs' in the socket. The suspension system must be adequate to prevent pistoning and rotational shear. Socket brims must not dig into soft tissues and need to be rounded adequately in problematic areas. Finally, the patient's biomechanics must be examined, because poor gait mechanics can lead to excessive pressures and shear, causing skin ulceration.

Bulky wound dressings should be avoided, because they can put additional pressure on the ulcer when the limb is in the prosthesis. Transparent film dressing and elastomeric liners can reduce shear. If wounds are large or do not respond to initial treatments, then a decrease in wear time for the prosthesis is indicated. In refractory cases, a change to a different type of socket or suspension system should be considered.

Verrucose hyperplasia

Verrucose hyperplasia is the development of a wart-like lesion on the end of the residual limb (Fig. 14-6). Cracks in the skin and even infection can occur in severe cases. Verrucose hyperplasia is most common in the transtibial amputee, but it can occur with other levels of amputation. This dysplastic skin condition is thought to be due to 'choking' of the residual limb. It is hypothesized that if the prosthesis fits tightly around the limb (circumferentially) and there is a lack of distal pressure, then vascular congestion can occur that somehow leads to verrucose hyperplasia. Although the pathophysiology of the condition is uncertain, treatment is clear. Adjusting the prosthesis to create adequate distal pressure usually resolves the verrucose hyperplasia within a few weeks or months. Adjustments such as simply adding an end pad to the socket can be sufficient, otherwise a new total contact socket is recommended.

Contact dermatitis

Contact dermatitis is inflammation of the skin manifested by erythema and sometimes mild edema. It can be due to an irritant that causes scaling, or it can be an allergic reaction that induces vesiculation. Contact dermatitis is a common problem with prostheses, especially with the increased use of elastomeric liners. It is treated by locating the causative agent and preventing it from contacting the residual limb. Hygiene of the residual limb and its prosthetic components must be considered first, because poor hygiene can allow the accumulation of allergens on the residual limb. Soaps can also be the causative agent, and the patient should wash the residual limb each night with a mild or hypoallergenic soap and then rinse the limb well. Similarly, the skin interface system (e.g. socks, liners, or the socket itself) should be washed daily per the manufacturer's recommendations, rinsed well, and allowed to dry before donning. If these simple measures fail, then a change in the skin interface system is needed. Wool socks can be changed to cotton or acrylic. Elastomeric liners made of a different material can be tried. If the contact dermatitis persists, then a change to a different interface system must be considered. For acute contact dermatitis, a short course of topical steroids can decrease inflammation and discomfort. Because the use of topical steroids cannot be considered a long-term plan, the causative agent must be identified and eliminated.

Infections

Bacterial or fungal infection can affect the residual limb at any point in the postoperative period. A superficial cellulitis can be seen in the early postoperative period. This can present as erythema, persistent or new drainage at the incision line, or increased incisional tenderness. In most cases, these can be treated with oral antibiotics. A boil or abscess can form near the surgical incision site. In these cases, an incision is necessary to allow the purulent material to drain. Most cases require parenteral antibiotics for treatment, in addition to local wound care. Fungal infections, such as candida, can accompany a local cellulitis and might be seen early or late. These infections usually develop in moist areas, making it advisable to air out the limb when possible. Topical antifungal and moisture barrier combination agents are useful for treatment.

Once the residual limb is healed, other infections can arise. Aeration of the residual limb, good limb hygiene, good prosthetic hygiene, and proper prosthetic fitting can all prevent and treat such infections. Residual limbs tend to harbor more abundant bacterial flora than unaffected limbs.[3] Folliculitis is a hair root infection that can occur in limbs with excessive perspiration and oily skin. This is aggravated by sweating and is worse in warmer, humid months. Skin maceration and moisture can allow bacterial invasion of the hair follicles. This can eventually lead to cellulitis.[47] Treatment consists of warm compresses and topical antimicrobials. More severe cases warrant the use of oral or parenteral antibiotics, and incision and drainage of boils.

Other fungal infections such as tinea corporis and cruris can occur, especially in patients with a tendency to perspire. Treat-

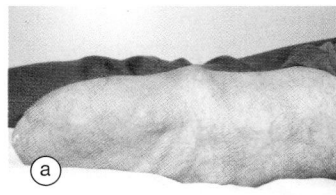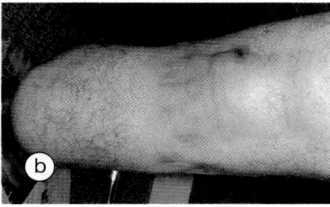

Figure 14-7 Epidermoid cysts. (**a**) Early cyst. (**b**) Epidermoid cyst with hemorrhage. (a, Photo courtesy of James Leonard, M.D.)

ment consists of topical agents such as ketoconazole and terbinafine, with the latter preferred because of the shorter treatment duration. Once the infection is resolved, cornstarch, unscented talc, and antiperspirant agents (without a deodorant) can be useful in prevention of recurrence. Prescription-strength antiperspirants (Drysol) are available when needed. Limiting prosthetic use until the infections are resolved or stop draining will facilitate recovery.

Epidermoid cysts

Epidermoid cysts occur when sebaceous glands are plugged. These cysts are firm, round, mobile, subcutaneous nodules of variable size that are most commonly found in the popliteal fossa of transtibial amputees and the upper thigh of transfemoral amputees (Fig. 14-7). They can be quite tender and can become inflamed by the pressure of the prosthesis. Sometimes, bleeding into the cyst makes them appear dark. Ruptured epidermoid cysts have a purulent or serosanguinous discharge. Treatment with topical or oral antifungal and/or antibacterial agents has been recommended.[46] Treatment should also include minimizing pressure over the cysts by adjusting the prosthesis and ensuring an optimal fit. Sometimes, larger inflamed cysts can require incision and drainage. However, recurrences are frequent because incision and draining does not remove the keratin-producing lining of the cyst. A more definitive treatment consists of surgical excision, but even this intervention cannot completely eliminate the possibility of recurrence.

Other complications

Joint contractures are frequent complications in the rehabilitation of people with limb loss. Initial treatment consists of a stretching program both in therapy and at home. For knee contractures, extension devices such as knee immobilizers can provide relief. For hip flexion contractures, prone lying on a daily basis is helpful. Ultrasound heating can also be an effective therapy when combined with aggressive stretching, provided the patient's vasculature is adequate for vigorous heating. For transtibial patients who are expected to ambulate, the knee flexion contracture is initially accommodated in the prosthetic alignment. Once the patient is ambulating adequately, flexion is gradually taken out of the socket. This causes an extension stretch when the patient walks, and progressively reduces the contracture. In severe cases that do not respond to the above treatment, surgical release can be considered.

Bony growths at the end of the amputated bone are called bone spurs. They occur frequently and are usually asymptomatic. Similarly, heterotopic ossification is a spontaneous development of bone in soft tissue, usually occurring after traumatic amputations. If a bone spur or heterotopic ossification protrudes distally and is not covered by adequate soft tissue, it can become painful and cause skin breakdown. Accommodating the spur or heterotopic ossification with a relief and/or padding in the socket might solve the problem. If this fails, surgical excision can be required.

PROSTHESES

Factors affecting prosthetic prescription

Prostheses are made up of several different components. Many factors determine which components should be used for each individual patient. Residual limb length and strength affect inherent limb stability, and can inversely affect the need for added stability in the prosthesis. The quality of the residual limb tissue must be considered in selecting a residual limb interface system. Anatomic stability of joints is a further issue central to selecting socket types and suspension systems. Hand function can be an issue for donning and doffing the prosthesis. Additionally, an amputee's weight can limit component options, because many components are limited to a weight of 250–300 lbs. The desired activities of the amputee are clearly important in component selection: both work and leisure activities must be considered. A prosthesis with low maintenance might be necessary if the user lives in a rural area with poor access to a prosthetist. The relative importance of cosmesis is an issue, as some components have more natural contours and others project out regardless of any coverings. Good compliance is essential for using some systems such as gel liners that require daily care for hygiene. Cognitive function can be an important factor. Cognitively impaired people might require the use of simple donning and doffing systems, and family or caregiver support can be necessary for the successful use of a prosthesis. Additionally, there are financial restrictions that are sometimes placed on the availability for individuals to obtain their desired prosthetic components.

In 1994, the federal government attempted to clarify which knee, ankle, and foot components should be used for patients with particular functional abilities or *functional levels*. The functional level is 'a measurement of the capacity and potential of the patient to accomplish his/her expected postrehabilitation, daily function'. This functional classification was designed to assist the Durable Medical Equipment Regional Committees in determining appropriate reimbursement for prosthetic components.[21] It limits patients with lower functional abilities to simpler prosthetic components, while allowing more active people to use more advanced (and expensive) devices. It should be pointed out that the determination of these levels is for individuals with unilateral lower limb amputations, and is at the discretion of the prescribing physician. Items to take into consideration are past history of the patient, his or her present condition or functional status, and future goals and expectations for this person to ambulate with a prosthesis. The prescribing physician should keep an open mind regarding the potential or expected functional level, focusing on the current status of patients and their functional abilities. Documentation of functional level determination should be maintained in the patient's records.

The functional levels (often referred to as the K modifiers) are listed in Table 14-3. It is worth emphasizing that these levels are based on the patient's *potential*, not on the current level of function; even deconditioned patients can reach a higher level of function than anticipated with appropriate rehabilitation. Also, the K1 level includes the use of a prosthesis for assisting with transfers. Many low-functioning people with amputations below the knee or lower benefit from the use of a prosthesis. For higher levels of amputation, a prosthesis does not generally assist with transferring; instead, it often gets in the way.

The final determination of prosthetic components should be a team decision involving the physician, the prosthetist and, most importantly, the patient. The real goal is to educate patients and their families about reasonable, available options and their advantages and disadvantages. The decision should then be based primarily on what the patient desires.

Prosthesis construction

Prosthesis design encompasses socket design, suspension, and construction. The socket, or interface, of a prosthesis is typically custom-made for the user. The socket can be constructed using a cast of the residual limb. The residual limb shape can

Table 14-3 K-level descriptors of a patient's functional level[a]

K level	Description
K0	Does not have the ability or potential to ambulate or transfer safely with or without assistance, and a prosthesis does not enhance quality of life or mobility.
K1	Has the ability or potential to use a prosthesis for transfers or ambulation on level surfaces at fixed cadence. Typical of the limited and unlimited household ambulator.
K2	Has the ability or potential for ambulation with low-level environmental barriers such as curbs, stairs, and uneven surfaces. Typical of the limited community ambulator.
K3	Has the ability or potential for ambulation with variable cadence. Typical of the community ambulator who can traverse most environmental barriers and has vocational, therapeutic, or exercise activity that demands prosthetic utilization beyond simple locomotion.
K4	Has the ability or potential for prosthetic ambulation that exceeds basic ambulation skills, exhibiting high-impact, stress, or energy levels. Typical of the prosthetic demands of the child, active adult, or athlete.

[a]*Based on the patient's* potential, *not on the current level of function.*

also be recorded via manual measurements only or by digital measurements that track the outer shape of the limb. This shape is then used to create the socket interface. In most sockets, the goal is to achieve total contact with the residual limb. Total contact does not necessarily imply equal pressure distribution. Pressure-tolerant areas can receive higher pressures, and pressure-sensitive areas can receive lower pressures. Total contact helps decrease edema, increase proprioception, and increase the overall weight-bearing surface. Open-ended, or plug fit, sockets have no distal contact and are no longer used. The exception to this is the individual who has traditionally had one and wants to continue to use this type of socket. With many socket designs, socks are worn over the residual limb to allow for adjustments to fit with small volume changes.

The interface of the residual limb with the socket can be through either a hard interface or a soft interface. Examples of soft interface materials are foam inserts, silicone liners, or other gel materials. Soft interface materials are indicated for most amputees. They provide cushion to the residual limb, and allow for adjustment and comfort if the volume of the residual limb changes. Soft inserts are often necessary for individuals with bilateral limb loss, who cannot transfer weight to a non-prosthetic limb, and for individuals with bony or scarred residual limbs. Vascular amputees can also benefit from soft liners, because sensitive tissue needs extra cushion. Individuals with neuropathy, who are unable to know when an extra sock should be added, can benefit as well. The disadvantage of soft inserts is that they are susceptible to wear and tear. They add bulk, and they can also absorb odors. A hard interface, on the other hand, consists of just the socket. These are most commonly used with transfemoral suction suspension, yet they can also be appropriate for other individuals where damage of the liner could occur.

Suspension is the method by which the prosthesis is held on to a person's residual limb. It can be provided through the anatomic shape of the limb, by a liner, by a sleeve, or with suction. An auxiliary suspension is often used, depending on the individuals' activities. For example, a transfemoral amputee with suction suspension might still wear a belt to provide suspension in activities where suction can be lost or where residual limb volume changes are possible.

The prosthetic socket is connected to the remaining components in two ways: through exoskeletal or endoskeletal construction (Fig. 14-8). In the more common endoskeletal construction (Fig. 14-8b), the socket connects to the remaining components through pipes called pylons. The modularity of these components allows for angular and linear changes in both the sagittal and coronal planes, and makes it easy to adjust the height of the prosthesis if necessary. An important benefit of this modularity includes the ability to utilize many different components (e.g. adapters and feet). At higher levels (transfemoral and higher) the endoskeletal design is also lighter in weight. Many endoskeletal systems have carbon fiber or titanium pylons, which are even lighter in weight than standard steel components. Endoskeletal pylons also allow the ability to finish the prosthesis with softer, more realistic covers.

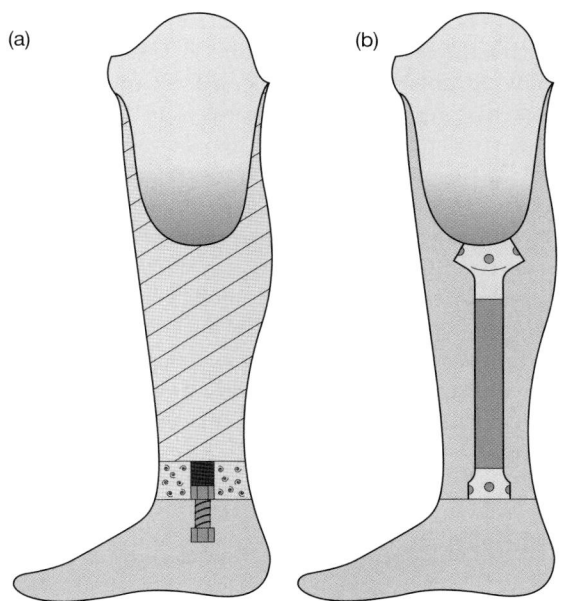

(a)   (b)

Figure 14-8 Prosthesis construction. (**a**) Exoskeletal prosthesis. Strength is provided through the outer lamination. This design is more durable and often prescribed for heavy-duty use. (**b**) Endoskeletal prosthesis. This design has an inner pylon covered by a soft foam cover. It allows for changes to components and adjustability, and at higher levels it is a lighter prosthesis.

Exoskeletal construction (Fig. 14-8a) uses a rigid exterior lamination from the socket down and has a lightweight filler inside. This rigid lamination gives the device strength. Because exoskeletal designs do not have a soft foam cosmesis, they are more durable and can be indicated for heavy-duty use and for children. Fewer components are designed for exoskeletal construction, so this construction can limit foot and knee options, as well as long-term adjustability.

There are a plethora of prosthetic feet available to prosthetists. Feet can be made out of many different materials, including wood, plastic, foam, and carbon fiber. All the feet can be classified into four different categories: solid ankle, cushion heel (SACH), single-axis, multiaxis, and dynamic response. Activity, weight, level of amputation, prosthesis construction, and foot size can all influence the choice of prosthetic foot for an amputee. These various choices are discussed in the section on transtibial amputation.

Prosthetic knee selection is also based on patient activity, weight, level of amputation, prosthesis construction, and the strength and ability of the patient to voluntarily control the knee. The five major classifications for the joint design are outside hinges, single-axis, weight-activated stance control, polycentric, and manual locking. In addition to the joint design, prosthetic knees are designed to provide resistance to knee flexion through either mechanical friction or fluid friction. This resistance helps to limit heel rise and the rate of knee extension. At higher speeds, the fluid friction provides cadence responsive-

ness by increasing resistance with increasing speed. Mechanical friction is constant for all speeds.

Additional add-on components designed to provide movement in specific ways can also benefit the amputee, such as shock absorbers for higher impact activities and rotation units for activities such as golf.

Fitting considerations

Socks are a common interface material, and they are frequently used to adjust for limb volume. They are made of wool, cotton, and synthetic materials, and are also available with a soft gel layer similar to gel liners. Socks come in various thicknesses called ply, and it is useful to keep track of how many ply of sock the patient is using. Socks are very helpful when a patient is adjusting to changes in residual limb size. Many amputees add a sock part way through the day when their limb has reduced in volume with walking. Socks can also be added to keep a snug fit as the residual limb shrinks with time. It is important that amputees learn how to appropriately manage the use of socks. They must use clean socks only, avoid wrinkles when donning their prostheses, and use the correct number of sock ply.

Shoes affect the dynamics of prosthetic gait, and users need to be instructed in wearing appropriate footwear. A new amputee should begin with a good walking shoe (either a casual shoe or tennis shoe). Special attention should be paid to a patient's heel height. Prosthetic feet are generally aligned for an average heel height of about half an inch. If the amputee then uses a shoe with less heel (or walks with no shoe), the foot experiences too much plantar flexion and the knee is pushed back. This can be compensated for by giving the user a heel lift. Conversely, a higher heel puts the foot into too much dorsiflexion, pushing the knee forward. A toe lift for this generally will not fit into a shoe. If variable heel height is important to the amputee (e.g. for wearing dress high heels or cowboy boots), variable heel height feet are available. Another option is to set the amputee's backup leg to a different heel height than the primary prosthesis.

Shoe characteristics also affect gait. A tennis shoe with a rounded heel has less of a knee flexion moment at heel strike than a stiffer dress shoe has. The tightness of the shoe also affects gait mechanics, and should fit securely but not so tight as to cause compression of the soft cover or heel of the foot within the shoe.[62] The prosthetic foot size should allow for easy donning of shoes.

PARTIAL FOOT AMPUTATIONS

There are various levels of partial foot amputations, including toe amputations, ray amputations, transmetatarsal amputations, the tarsometatarsal disarticulation (Lisfranc) amputation, and the transtarsal disarticulation (Chopart) amputations (Fig. 14-9). For many partial foot amputations, it is necessary to fit orthopedic shoes, or shoes with a large toe box, to allow for the extra material of the prosthesis.

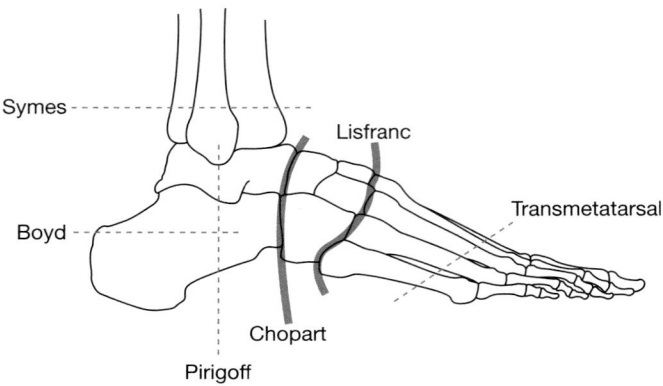

Figure 14-9 Levels of partial foot amputation.

For toe and ray amputations, a custom foot orthosis with a toe filler is usually needed to load the remaining foot in an acceptable manner. The orthosis should distribute the pressure more evenly under the foot, with relatively less pressure under vulnerable bony prominences (e.g. the end of the amputated toes, rays, or remaining prominent distal metatarsal heads), while relatively more pressure should be placed under the arch of the foot. The toe filler will also prevent movement of the remaining foot inside the shoe, reducing the possibility of frictional sores (blisters) occurring. A carbon fiber footplate is often added to the insert, or a steel shank is built into the shoe to lengthen the foot's lever arm. The longer lever arm prevents collapse of the shoe at the end of the amputation, and promotes a more even step length. Ray amputations are generally more successful with amputation of the fourth or fifth rays than with the first or second.

The transmetatarsal amputation is a very successful amputation level. In this case, the forefoot is transversely amputated through the shaft of the metatarsals. The remaining portions are usually beveled inferiorly, with a predominantly plantar skin flap. For transmetatarsal amputations, a custom-molded foot orthosis is essential. It should have good arch support to distribute pressure, and a carbon fiber footplate or steel shank. A rocker bottom shoe can be used to aid in rollover and to unweight the metatarsal ends.

More proximal foot amputations include the tarsometatarsal disarticulation (Lisfranc amputation) and the transtarsal disarticulation (Chopart amputation). These are problematic amputations for several reasons. First, the remaining foot is so short that there is no effective lever arm, and the remaining ankle motion is essentially non-functional. These levels of amputation lead to equinovarus deformities and anterior bony prominences that are painful and prone to skin breakdown. Finally, these amputations are difficult to fit with an adequate prosthesis. Due to these difficulties, midfoot amputations are not recommended.

The Lisfranc is the highest level for which a shoe filler can be adequate. It often requires high-top shoes or a boot-type prosthesis to provide suspension, and it can require an ankle–foot orthosis with a filler to provide stability and functional length.

At the higher Chopart level of amputation, an ankle–foot orthosis–style prosthesis is usually required. The ankle–foot orthosis extends up to the patellar tendon level to distribute the high forces that result from the torques in late stance. Lower trim lines with an active patient will result in breakdown along the crest of the tibia. With the Chopart amputation, a boot-type device can occasionally be used if ankle range of motion and anterior tissues are good. Prosthetic fittings at both the Lisfranc and the Chopart levels can result in the need for a lift on the contralateral side to accommodate the height of the prosthesis.

As with all vascular and diabetic patients, the contralateral foot should be consistently monitored. Early treatment of foot wounds and pressure sores is essential to successfully prevent another amputation.

SYME'S AMPUTATION

The Syme's amputation is an ankle disarticulation amputation in which the foot is removed and the calcaneal fat pad is anchored to the distal fibula or tibia. The medial and lateral malleoli are shaved down to reduce the bulbous nature of the residual limb. This has been described as a single-stage or two-stage amputation. The single stage is currently the most frequently used. The main advantages of the Syme's are that there is a long residual limb and that it is an end weight-bearing amputation. However, many Syme's amputees cannot tolerate much full distal end weight bearing. They either do not ambulate without a prosthesis or weight bearing is limited to transfers and walking short distances. The main disadvantages of the Syme's amputation are the poor prosthetic cosmesis (because the distal residual limb is quite bulbous with a socket), and prosthetic foot options are also limited.

Although the goal of the Syme's is to have significant distal loading bearing available, the amount of distal loading that is available is dependent on the individual. The Syme's level prosthesis trim lines should extend to the patellar tendon to increase the loading surface. Moments created by the lever of the foot can result in significant anterior loading. If the trim lines do not extend proximally enough, they can dig into the crest of the tibia.

There are three conventional socket designs for the Syme's level: posterior opening socket, medial opening socket, and a stovepipe construction (Fig. 14-10). For the posterior opening socket, the posterior opening is cut down to the level of the malleoli and is constructed as a removable section that is held with Velcro. This is used for the more bulbous residual limbs. This is the weakest of the three designs, due to the limited material in the sagittal plane. The medial opening design has a window cut out to allow the malleoli to pass. Because of the increased material in the sagittal plane, the bending resistance is increased, and this is a stronger design than the posterior opening. The strongest design is the stovepipe design. With the stovepipe design, no flaps or windows are cut in the socket. Instead, a soft insert is built up into a tapered cylinder to slide

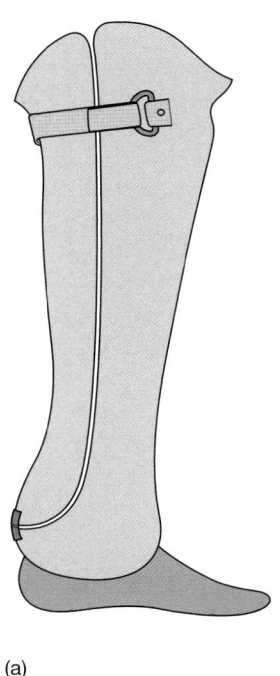
(a)

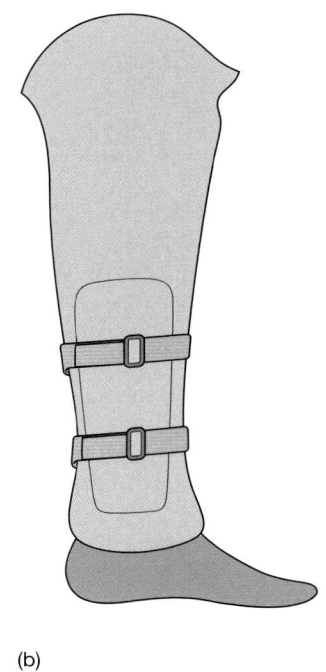
(b)

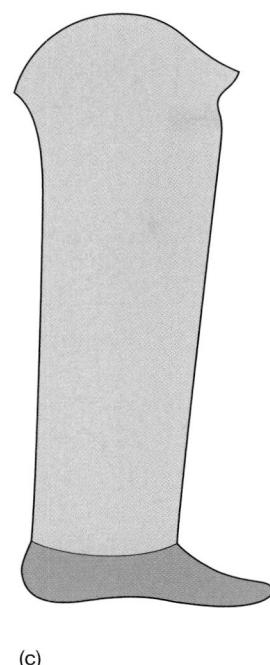
(c)

Figure 14-10 Three common Syme's-style prostheses: (**a**) posterior opening, (**b**) medial opening, and (**c**) stovepipe.

into a cylindric socket, or an expandable wall is built into a cylindric socket to allow passage of the malleoli. If the malleoli are not prominent, suspension is similar to in transtibial prostheses.

Because of the limited space available distally, foot selection is limited for Syme's-level amputations. The two most common designs are specially designed low-profile dynamic response feet and specially designed SACH feet. Both of these are made to bolt or bond directly to the bottom of the socket.

The Boyd and Pirigoff amputations are variations of the Syme's where part of the calcaneus is arthrodesed to the bottom of the tibia to lengthen the limb further and reduce limb length discrepancy. The Boyd uses the inferior half of the calcaneus, while the Pirigoff uses the posterior half. These amputations also allow distal weight bearing, but the minimal limb shortening makes prosthetic fitting very challenging in adults. They can be useful in pediatric amputees when there is a desire to maintain length, or in situations where no prosthetic care would be available (e.g. in developing countries).

TRANSTIBIAL (BELOW-KNEE) AMPUTATION

A standard transtibial amputation, as advocated by Burgess, is performed one-third of the way down the tibia, and a posterior myocutaneous flap is used to cover the residual tibia.[14] At this length, the bulk of the posterior compartment muscles are available for a flap; they provide good soft tissue coverage over the distal tibia, and the primary vascular structures for the lower limb are preserved in the flap.

Long transtibial amputations are sometimes performed to give patients a longer lever arm and more surface area for load distribution.[84] However, no functional muscle attachments are saved with a long transtibial amputation, and it is associated with multiple complications and poorer cosmesis.[59,72] A standard-length transtibial amputation (from 35 to 50% of tibial length) is strongly recommended as the procedure of choice at this level. The fibula should be cut approximately 1 cm shorter than the tibia, and both bones should be beveled to eliminate sharp ends. Other suggested procedures, including skewed flaps and the Ertl procedure (a bone bridge between the tibia and fibula), have not gained widespread support.

Formulation of a prosthetic prescription for an individual with a transtibial amputation is dependent on many factors, some of which have been previously discussed. The four main aspects of a transtibial prosthesis that need to be determined are the socket construction, the suspension design, endoskeletal versus exoskeletal construction, and the foot–ankle mechanisms. The first two items are not mutually exclusive, in that the design of the socket can influence or contribute to the means by which the prosthesis is suspended.

Socket designs

The transtibial socket designs available are intended to provide a means of comfortable weight acceptance of the residual limb during stance on the prosthetic side. These have evolved from plug fit through patellar tendon-bearing (PTB), and now include total surface-bearing (TSB) and hydrostatic designs. Each of these designs, with the exception of the plug fit design, is intended to create a total contact environment between the residual limb and the socket. Some of the socket designs also have features added to them that enable the socket to act as both a weight acceptance and a suspension mechanism.

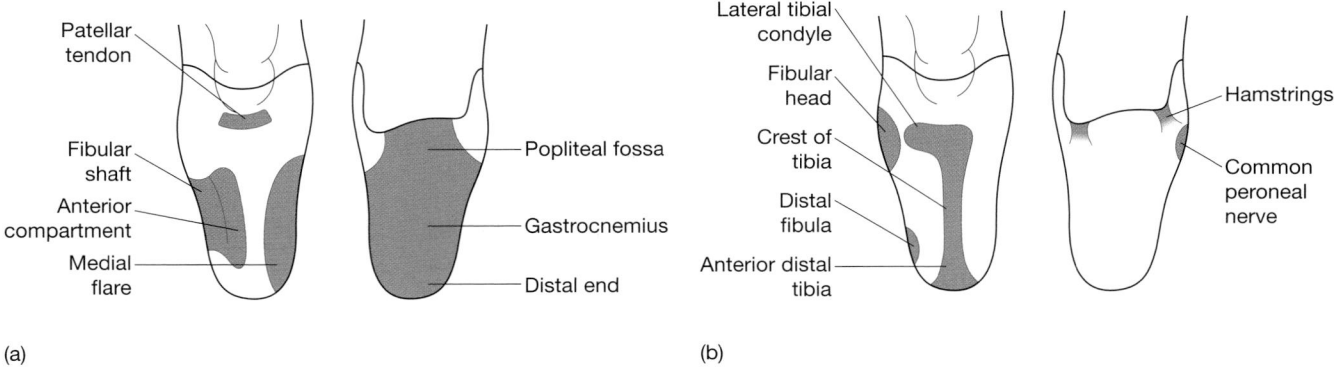

(a)   (b)

Figure 14-11 (**a**) 'Pressure-tolerant' and (**b**) 'pressure-sensitive' areas for the patellar tendon–bearing socket.

Plug fit

The plug fit design is not used anymore in the USA, but it is still used in developing countries. Wood is hollowed out to approximate the shape of the transtibial limb, and the end of the socket is left open. The limb is then inserted into the socket to plug up the hole that was created. Much of the weight bearing is distributed through a thigh lacer, which can be attached to the prosthesis with metal uprights and a single-axis hinge. With an open-ended socket design, distal contact is obviously not achieved and many problems can arise.

Patellar tendon-bearing

The PTB design focuses on specific weight-bearing areas. Although the socket has total contact with the residual limb, it concentrates force in 'pressure-tolerant' areas and relieves force in 'pressure-sensitive' areas (Fig. 14-11). The PTB design gets its name from the amount of force that is borne on the patellar ligament. The socket is designed with an anteriorly directed force, from pressure in the popliteal area, pushing the residual limb on to a 'bar' that is created between the distal pole of the patella and the tibial tubercle. Other regions of the residual limb that are used for distribution of forces (pressure-tolerant areas) include pretibial and gastrocnemius musculature, medial tibial flare, and fibular shaft. Pressure-sensitive areas include the patella, hamstring tendons, fibular head, femoral epicondyles, tibial shaft, distal tibia, and distal fibula. An essential part of the PTB design is the alignment of the socket and prosthesis. The PTB design was created to take advantage of normal, or perpendicular, forces on the patellar ligament. This is done by adding initial flexion of the socket to that which is present on the individual's residual limb. This increased socket flexion loads pressure-tolerant areas of the anterior surface by allowing the patellar ligament to be more parallel with the ground. This provides a surface that is more perpendicular to the ground reaction forces during stance phase. The foot is also aligned medially relative to the socket in order for the individual wearing the prosthesis to experience an external knee varus moment. This moment, in the coronal plane, simulates normal human locomotion and ensures that forces are distributed on the medial tibial flare and the fibular shaft, two of the pressure-tolerant areas on the transtibial limb.

Total surface-bearing

Total surface-bearing designs are intended to utilize the total contact of the limb to more evenly distribute the forces that occur during weight bearing. Unlike the PTB design, the TSB design attempts to globally apply forces throughout the residual limb. Although there is some controversy regarding the 'even distribution' of pressure throughout the limb, it is clear that the design varies from previous designs in that reliefs are not provided in the aforementioned pressure-sensitive areas. Many of the TSB designs are those utilizing gel-type interfaces. These interfaces enhance the prosthetist's ability to design the socket to utilize both the shear and parallel forces being applied to the entire residual limb. The magnitude of these individual forces is then much smaller than that of the PTB design, because of the increased area about which these forces are being applied. Another differentiation between the TSB and the PTB design is the initial prosthetic bench alignment. The TSB socket is often set in less initial flexion in the sagittal plane, and the foot is less inset in the coronal plane. These two changes are directly related to the fact that the socket forces in the TSB design are not focused on specific pressure-tolerant areas.

Hydrostatic

Hydrostatic socket designs are similar to the TSB designs in that they attempt to utilize shear forces more than normal forces. Although the differences are somewhat ambiguous, even to prosthetists, the major difference in the hydrostatic design is the attempt to create an environment that does not permit translation of the bony anatomy within the soft tissue. Many of the prosthetists who are designing hydrostatic sockets take an impression of the residual limb under vacuum. This procedure is done in order to elongate the tissue surrounding the tibia and fibula distally, while theoretically increasing the pressure in the residual limb. This increased pressure is designed to provide a hydrostatic environment where the movement of tibial and soft tissue should be in unison. In order for wearers to create this hydrostatic environment in their sockets, they must don the socket in such a manner that their limb becomes elongated, similar to that of the casting technique.

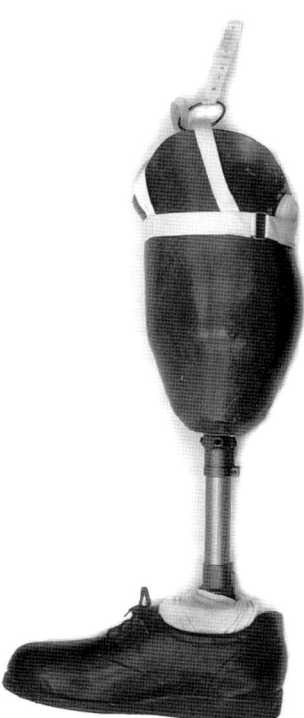

Figure 14-12 Example of a fork strap and waist belt suspension for a transtibial prosthesis.

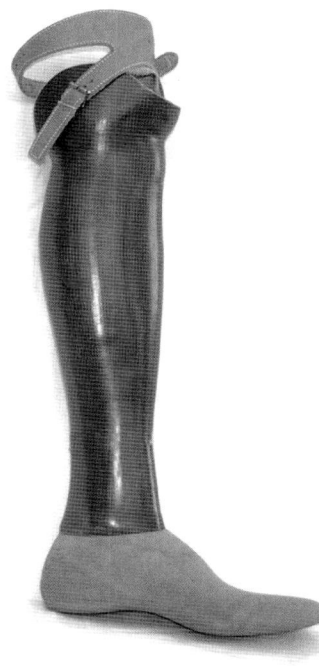

Figure 14-13 Example of a supracondylar cuff suspension for a transtibial prosthesis. Despite the name, the cuff suspends over the patella.

Suspension

There are several means of suspending transtibial prostheses. Suspension mechanisms can be external to the socket (e.g. a fork strap, cuff, or sleeve), integral with the socket (e.g. supracondylar or supracondylar–suprapatellar suspension), or part of a system in which a locking mechanism is incorporated into a prosthesis containing a pin or other attachment. Although one of the designs can create a more positive seal than another, the 'better' design is that which works best for the particular patient being fit.

Fork strap with waist belt

A fork strap combined with a waist belt is a very simple suspension technique (Fig. 14-12). The fork strap, sometimes referred to as a Y strap, is attached to the medial and lateral aspects of the socket with the junction proximal to the patella. The upper portion of the strap often has some elastic component inherent in its design to permit freedom of knee flexion and extension throughout ambulation and sitting. There is no medial–lateral or anterior–posterior support provided by the fork strap. Its sole purpose is to suspend the prosthesis securely to the waist belt attachment. Due to the bulk and cosmesis of this suspension, it is typically used only when maximum security is required and no other suspension technique is viable (e.g. in obese patients).

The fork strap can be combined with a PTB socket design, thigh lacer, and joints and rigid sidebars called a joint and corset. This design has the maximum medial–lateral and anterior–posterior stability, provided through the rigid sidebars and mechanical stop of the joints, respectively. The joints and corset are required for an unstable knee associated with a traumatic amputation. The joint and corset can also be cinched tightly to provide significant weight bearing. This can be useful in difficult cases where off-loading of the end of the residual limb is needed to help heal a problematic wound that has failed other measures, or to relieve a hyperpathic residual limb. However, the joint and corset is very heavy and often not tolerated well by patients.

Cuff

Cuff suspension (Fig. 14-13) has been used successfully for centuries for individuals with transtibial amputations. Although it is sometimes referred to as a supracondylar cuff or strap, the suspension is provided on the proximal border of the patella and not over the femoral epicondyles. The cuff is attached to the medial and lateral aspects of the socket, over the proximal aspect of the patella, and encircles the distal thigh at a level just proximal to the femoral epicondyles. A prominent patella is required, making this design contraindicated for the obese or those with excessive thigh musculature. When appropriately applied, the cuff provides an adequate means of suspension between 0 and 60° of knee flexion, and loosens up after 60° of knee flexion to permit comfortable sitting. Similar to the fork strap, the supracondylar cuff provides minimal, if any, medial–lateral or anterior–posterior stability to the knee, and has considerable pistoning in the socket. The tightness and width of the circumferential strap can contraindicate the cuff for individuals with vascular compromise.

Sleeve

Suspension provided by a sleeve (Fig. 14-14) is done with elastic and sometimes tacky material. The distal aspect of the sleeve is stretched over the proximal portion of the prosthesis,

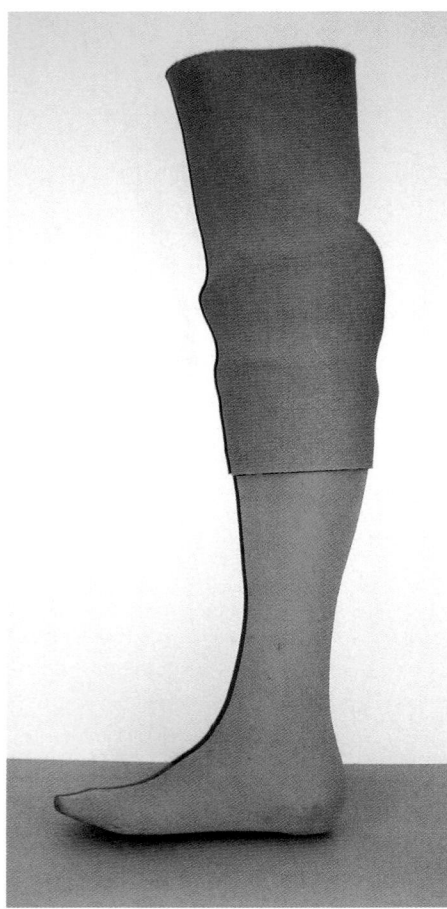

Figure 14-14 Example of sleeve suspension for a transtibial prosthesis.

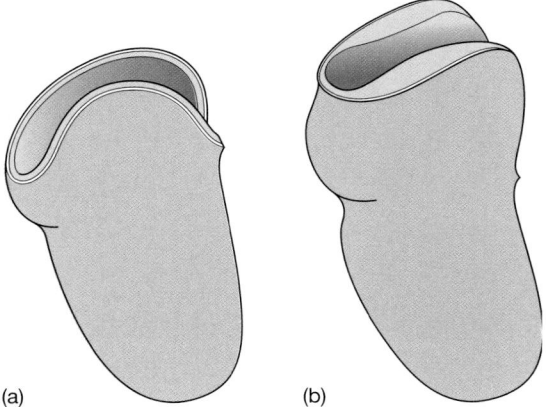

(a)   (b)

Figure 14-15 Example of trim lines for (**a**) the patellar tendon supracondylar and (**b**) the supracondylar-suprapatellar socket suspension designs.

limb and foam liner are inserted into the hard socket. The hard socket keeps the wedge compressed against the medial distal thigh, thereby preventing the prosthesis from falling off.

The two other forms of supracondylar suspension are constructed with removable medial wedges or removable medial brims. Removable medial wedges are placed between the outer hard socket and inner socket or limb. The user must push this wedge into place after the limb is inserted into the socket. Removable medial brims are fabricated by creating a medial wall that can be quickly disconnected from the remainder of the socket. This wedge-shaped brim is removed to facilitate donning and is pushed into place once the limb is appropriately seated into the socket. Both of these latter designs are used when a large difference between the measured medial–lateral dimensions of the epicondyles and the area proximal to the epicondyle exists, or when a 'hard socket' fit is desired. With this type of anatomic presentation, it would be very difficult to don supracondylar suspension with the wedge incorporated into the insert.

Supracondylar suspension is a very popular design, because it is easily donned and provides good medial–lateral stability. It must be noted, however, that problems can arise due to a tight lateral grasp, as the iliotibial band does not lend itself to pressure like the medial thigh does. Pressure and skin breakdown over and on the medial epicondyle can occur if insufficient or excessive sock ply, respectively, are worn. Supracondylar suspension is contraindicated for obese patients and those who have thigh musculature that would prevent the wedge from grasping above the femoral epicondyles.

Supracondylar-suprapatellar suspension

Supracondylar-suprapatellar suspension (Fig. 14-15b) is similar to the supracondylar design, with one major addition. The suprapatellar socket addition provides added suspension over the proximal aspect of the patella and can provide a 'stop' to help prevent hyperextension of the knee. This stop is accomplished by cupping in over the patella and creating a 'quadriceps bar', which comes into contact with the distal quadriceps during

and is held in place by the compression of the sleeve against the outer wall of the prosthesis. The proximal aspect of the sleeve is folded inside out and is reflected down beyond the trim lines of the socket to facilitate donning. Once the individual has seated the residual limb appropriately inside the socket, the sleeve can be pulled up or rolled up on to their distal thigh to create a bond with the person's skin and body. These sleeves come in a variety of materials and fabrics, including neoprene, latex, silicone, and urethane. Some of these sleeves can provide a vacuum seal inside the socket to provide enhanced suspension via suction. Although most sleeves provide an excellent means of suspension, they are often difficult to don, retain heat, and provide minimal to no stability about the knee. They are relatively inexpensive but require frequent replacement.

Supracondylar suspension

Supracondylar suspension (Fig. 14-15a) is designed to use the anatomy as a means of suspension. A compression of medial–lateral dimensions of the prosthesis above the femoral epicondyles differentiates this design from those previously mentioned. A supracondylar wedge, mostly on the medial aspect of the prosthesis, is used to create this suspension. The wedge can be incorporated into the prosthesis in three ways. First, it can be incorporated into a soft insert made from a material such as foam. The foam liner is donned on the limb first, and then the

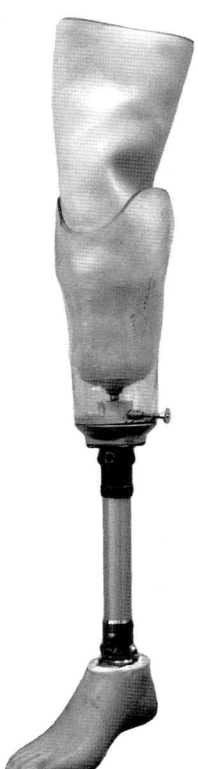

Figure 14-16 Example of suction sock suspension: a gel liner and pin-locking suspension mechanism.

With the gel liner donned on the limb in a suction design, the limb and liner then must be connected to the socket and prosthesis. There are a few methods of providing this connection. The most popular means of joining liner and socket is by means of a pin (stepped or smooth) attached to the distal end of the liner and a locking mechanism built into the distal socket. As the limb and liner are inserted into the socket, the pin engages into the locking mechanism to create this mechanical bond. Most stepped pins create an audible click, which is necessary for some individuals wearing prostheses, while the smooth pin enters the locking mechanism quietly. When the prosthesis has been donned completely and the individual wearing the prosthesis feels that she or he is completely in the socket, the pin should be fully engaged into the locking mechanism, ensuring a total contact fit. This should not occur abruptly, but the limb should gradually work its way into the socket, creating a series of clicks in the stepped pin design. If the limb enters the socket too quickly, sock ply management needs to be addressed. When these pin locks are being used with a hydrostatic design, the wearer is encouraged to engage the pin into the lock and to step on and off the prosthesis until the limb becomes fully seated inside the socket. This creates an elongated residual limb and approximates a hydrostatic environment where the bone is less apt to move within the surrounding soft tissue. Another way of elongating this tissue is with the use of a clutch-type mechanism. The pin need only be engaged slightly into the lock, and the user, with the assistance of a key, can twist the locking mechanism to further seat the limb and locking pin into the prosthesis. This procedure also acts to elongate the limb. To remove the prosthesis, a release button is pushed that is built into the side of the prosthesis.

If there are space limitations for the locking mechanism, or when engaging the pin proves difficult for the user, suspension can also be achieved with a lanyard at the end of the liner. A lanyard is a cord or strap that is fed through the distal socket and attached to the exterior of the prosthesis. The user can pull the lanyard through the hole while sitting, than tighten it when standing. For some elderly or obese people, the lanyard system proves easier than the pin system.

Gel liner suspension provides an excellent means of suspension, transmits great control of the prosthesis, offers better cushioning of the residual limb, decreases shear forces on the residual limb, and provides a low-profile appearance, as they are inside the socket walls. There are a number of difficulties with liner use that must be considered. They can prove challenging to don and doff. In some cases, individuals have difficulty donning the liners appropriately. The pin can pierce the liner during donning, or the angle at which the pin is canted off of the distal liner can make it difficult to engage the locking mechanism properly. The liners also retain heat, and people often experience excessive sweating when first using gel liners. Fortunately, the limb usually accommodates in the first few weeks and sweating declines. Antiperspirants can be used if needed. Good hygiene is imperative, or skin problems such as rash or infection can occur. If there is concern that a patient can have poor compliance with residual limb and liner care,

knee extension. Supracondylar-suprapatellar designs are a good choice for individuals with short residual limbs, because the forces are distributed over as large a surface area as possible. This encapsulation of the limb can restrict some range of motion and is designed to restrict excessive extension.

Gel or elastomeric liner suspension

Suction sock suspension is a very popular design of recent times that provides both suspension and weight distribution through the use of a gel liner and pin-locking mechanism (Fig. 14-16). The gel liners that are available, like the sleeves, are fabricated from various materials such as silicone, urethane, and mineral oil gel. The liners come in different thicknesses, and some provide more padding in different areas than others. In addition to cushioning and suspension, these liners minimize shear on the limb. Custom-made liners are also available for use with residual limbs that have a complex shape (such as crevices from traumatic amputation) or other skin problems.

Appropriate donning of these gel liners is crucial to the comfort and maintenance of good skin integrity. Most of the liners need to be turned inside out so that the distal end of the inside of the liner is flat when it is applied to the distal residual limb. This is done so that no air becomes trapped between the distal limb and liner, creating a negative pressure within the suction liner that can cause erythema and capillary rupture. A well-fitting, appropriately donned gel liner provides a barrier of comfort and creates a suction environment between the limb and liner.

then gel liners should be avoided. It should also be noted that liner suspension systems are expensive, and the liners require frequent replacement.

Suction suspension

Suction can be achieved with the use of a one-way expulsion valve placed in the distal aspect of the socket. These allow air to escape from the socket but not enter into it. Some of these expulsion valves are used in conjunction with gel liners only, while others require both the liner and an outer sleeve. As with gel liners, these are used when there are space limitations for the locking mechanism or when engaging the pin proves difficult for the user.

Vacuum-Assisted Suction Suspension

Lastly, and fairly new to the market, are systems that provide an active means of expelling air from the inner socket. These designs require the user to wear a gel liner and a sealing sleeve, and they have a valve at the distal end of the socket through which air is drawn. The Vacuum-Assisted Suction Suspension (VASS) provides this active removal of air with a telescoping vertical compression unit (a vacuum pump) built into the pylon section of the prosthesis. As the vertical compression pylon deforms, air is pumped out of the area between the liner and socket. This method has proven to be beneficial in the suspension of prostheses, while also maintaining limb volume throughout the course of daily use. The downside of this suspension is that if a hole forms in the outer sleeve, the suction is lost. These systems are also expensive.

Foot–ankle assemblies

The number of prosthetic feet available on the market today has grown dramatically since the early 1980s. The introduction of the dynamic response (at that time called 'energy-storing') foot started a revolution of prosthetic feet, because they could provide users the ability to more easily return to their desired functional ability. The means by which feet are categorized is almost as vast as the number of feet themselves. For the purpose of this text, the feet have been divided into four categories: SACH feet, single-axis feet, multiaxial feet, and dynamic response feet. Because of the advancements in prosthetic component designs, these categories, although differing in their basic descriptions, are not mutually exclusive of each other. Combinations of categories will be described in further detail.

SACH feet

The SACH feet, introduced in 1956 by Foort and Radcliffe, are one of the most basic and widely used feet in prosthetics. The acronym SACH stands for solid ankle, cushion heel (Fig. 14-17). SACH feet have 'solid ankles' in that there is no articulation within the foot. They attach to the distal aspect of the shank (endoskeletal pylon–ankle adapter or ankle block) in a way that permits no motion. It is important to understand that motion in all planes is arrested. No plantar flexion, dorsiflexion, inversion, eversion, or transverse plane motion is allowed during gait. The 'cushion heel' aspect of the foot allows for a 'simulated

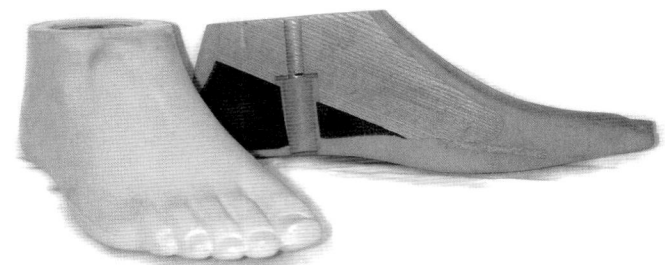

Figure 14-17 Cutaway of a solid ankle, cushion heel foot.

plantar flexion' during initial contact-loading response by means of compression underloading. This compression lowers the forefoot to the ground and brings the ground reaction force anterior, thus simulating the function of true plantar flexion. Heel compression also acts to absorb shock during loading response. With correct heel stiffness, shock absorption benefits all the lower limb, especially the reduction of external knee flexion moment that would be caused by a stiffer heeled foot. External knee flexion moments directly correlate to increased quadriceps activity and decreased stability in individuals with transtibial and transfemoral amputations, respectively. A drawback of SACH feet is that most are designed with keels (the main inner structure of the foot) that are not flexible or are non-responsive to the typical loads that they will encounter. These keels are usually made of wood or hard plastic. However, these feet are very durable and inexpensive (as compared with other designs). They can vary in heel height and stiffness, and they come in Syme's varieties. For these reasons, they are still widely used.

Single-axis feet

Single-axis feet are named very appropriately, because a single mechanical axis runs through the foot from medial to lateral, allowing motion in the sagittal plane. The sagittal plane motion that is observed is mostly plantar flexion; however, some of the single-axis feet permit graded dorsiflexion as well.

The motion of ankle plantar flexion is very important to the stability of ambulation, especially for individuals with lower limb amputations. As the foot begins to plantar flex, the ground reaction force moves forward under the foot. It then moves from posterior to the knee to anterior to the knee, providing for an external knee extension moment. This is good for individuals with transtibial prostheses that can have weak quadriceps, or for individuals with transfemoral amputations who do not have adequate control of the prosthetic knee joint (usually controlled via hip extensor muscles). Ankle plantar flexion can also aid an individual when walking down an incline. The rapid shifting anteriorly of the ground reaction force greatly reduces the external knee flexion moment. This allows an individual to descend the decline without the knee flexing as abruptly as it would with a non-articulating foot. This allows the prosthetic user to descend ramps directly, rather than having to walk down hills sideways.

Ankle dorsiflexion is also permitted by some single-axis feet. This motion is not as crucial as the aforementioned plantar flexion, but it permits the individuals with lower limb amputations to walk more comfortably. Ankle dorsiflexion is usually permitted in mid to late stance as the ground reaction forces begin to move anteriorly to the ankle. This permits the individual with a lower limb prosthesis to 'roll over' the keel of the foot more readily. If this motion of dorsiflexion were not permitted, the individual would experience an excessive external knee extension moment and would have difficulty progressing into terminal stance and preswing.

The usual method by which the ankle motion, in a single-axis foot, is permitted is by bumpers that are installed anteriorly and posteriorly to the ankle (Fig. 14-18). These bumpers regulate the amount and speed of motion in which the foot can rotate about the mechanical axis. The plantar flexion bumper

is posterior to the ankle axis. As the bumper is compressed, the foot is permitted to slowly or quickly rotate about the axis, depending on whether the bumper is firm or soft, respectively. If the bumper is too stiff, the external knee flexion moment will be great, and vice versa. The dorsiflexion bumper is mounted anterior to the ankle. As the ground reaction force moves anterior to the ankle, the bumper begins to compress to permit graded ankle dorsiflexion. The speed and degree of this motion can be varied as well with the stiffness of these dorsiflexion bumpers.

Multiaxial feet

Multiaxial feet are designed to replicate the actions of the anatomic foot. Multiaxial motion can be obtained either with a foot that has a 'flexible keel' or one that has true mechanical joint axes. A flexible keel foot allows the motion to occur within the keel itself as the ground reaction forces cause deformation of the foot, especially on uneven terrain. This deformation is expected and is an inherent design of the foot. As the foot deforms, it maintains contact with the ground, therefore providing a stable base of support for the individual wearing the prosthesis.

True multiarticular feet allow motion in all three planes: plantar flexion–dorsiflexion, inversion–eversion, and transverse plane motion. This is accomplished with the aid of adjustable bumpers. These bumpers are relatively durable and are designed to control similar motions to those of single-axis feet.

Multiaxial feet have now been fabricated with the materials necessary to enhance their energy return as well (Fig. 14-19).

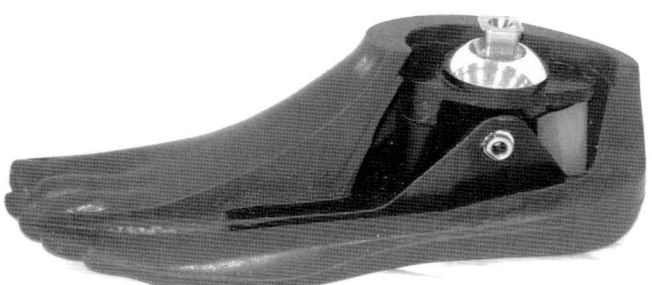

Figure 14-18 Single-axis foot. The bumpers allow plantar flexion and dorsiflexion movement.

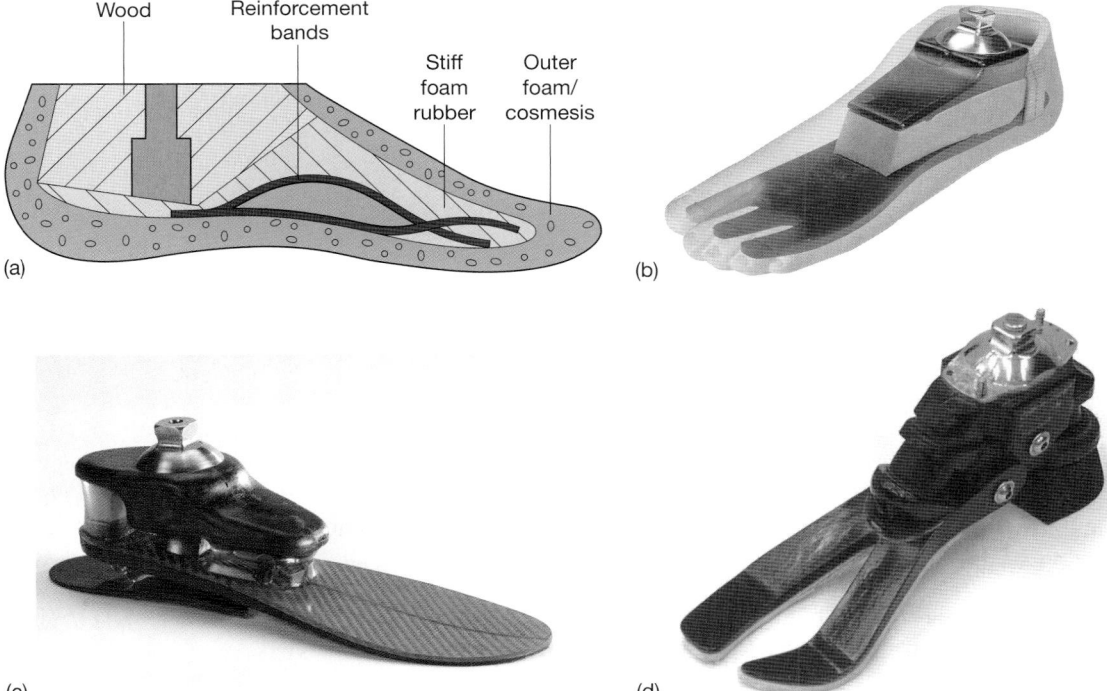

Figure 14-19 Various flexible keel or multiaxial feet: (**a**) SAFE, (**b**) K2, (**c**) Journey, and (**d**) Trustep. These feet allow plantar flexion and dorsiflexion as well as inversion and eversion. This movement makes them better for walking on uneven terrain. (Photo (b) courtesy of Ossur International; photo (c) courtesy of OttoBock Health Care)

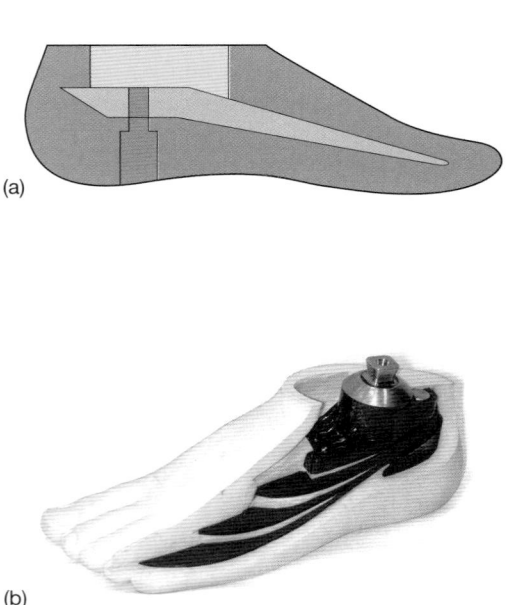

(a)

(b)

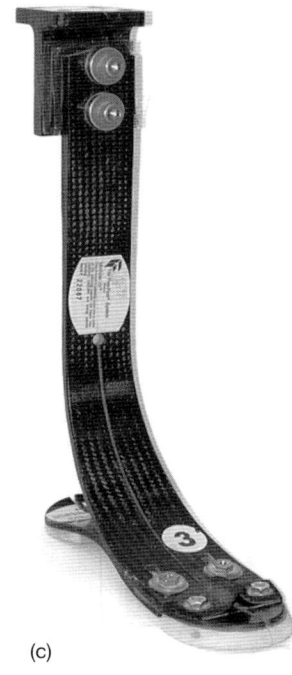

(c)

Figure 14-20 Various dynamic response feet: (**a**) Seattle Lite Foot, (**b**) Carbon Copy Foot, (**c**) Modular 3 Flex Foot. These feet are designed to store and release energy, and are indicated for variable cadence ambulators.

These multiaxial, dynamic response feet can give an individual the benefits of compensating for uneven ground, absorbing shock, and providing some responsiveness to reduce energy expenditure during ambulation.

Dynamic response feet

Dynamic response feet enhance the mobility of the user by using materials that are 'energy storing'. Materials in the keel of these feet are required to deflect under load and return to their original shape. This return, while being unloaded, is what propels the foot and leg forward. In doing so, the foot is providing the response to the user that lessens their energy expenditure.[56] Single-speed, low-activity (often elderly) individuals do not have the ability to load the foot enough to warrant their use.

There are various types of dynamic response feet (Fig. 14-20). Some low-profile feet simply have a dynamic keel inside a foot shell providing a smaller spring. Other feet incorporate the pylon and keel as one flexible larger spring. These feet are indicated for variable cadence ambulators, and are much better for high-level activities such as running and jumping.

Ankles

As mentioned previously, the feet can be designed to accommodate for motions that have been lost by the absence of the anatomic ankle. Stand-alone ankles have also been designed to replicate these lost motions. Ankle units (Fig. 14-21) can be added to most solid keel feet (SACH or low-profile dynamic response feet) that can provide the user with multiaxial motion in addition to the functions provided by the foot itself. This addition allows the user to more easily traverse inclines, declines, and uneven terrain.

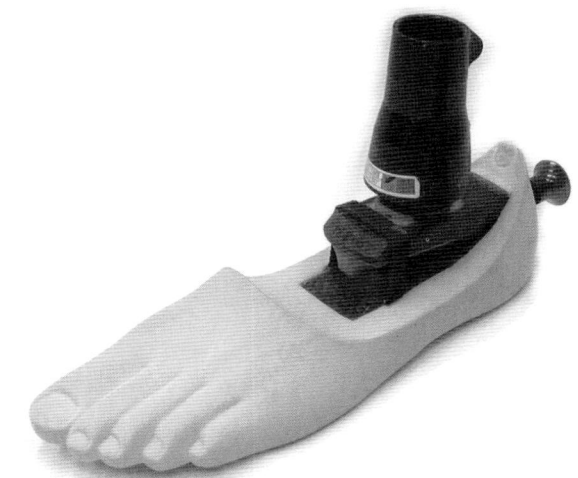

Figure 14-21 Example of an additional multiaxial ankle unit, the Endolite Multiflex Ankle with the Endolite Dynamic Response Foot.

Pylon components

Other components are available for absorbing vertical shock or transverse plane motion, or to perform a combination of both (Fig. 14-22). Torsion adapters are incorporated into pylons or are stand-alone components. These allow transverse plane rotation that simulates tibial rotation. The stiffness of the devices is adjustable based on the user's size and activity level. They are particularly useful for people who do a lot of twisting motion (e.g. manual laborers) and for some sports, especially golf.

Vertical compression units (or vertical shock pylons) are pylon-integrated systems that incorporate vertical compression

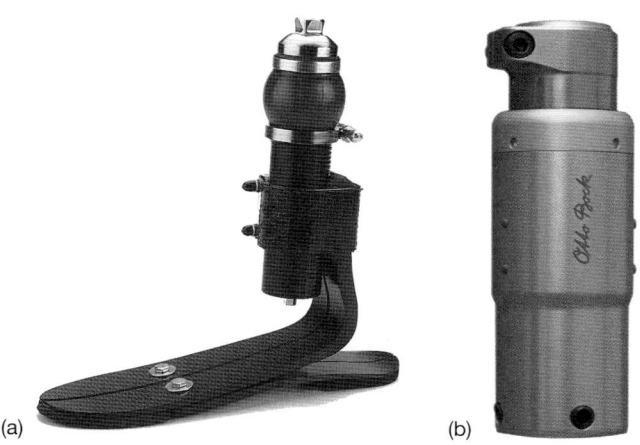

(a)   (b)

Figure 14-22 Rotation and shock components. (**a**) Example of a shock absorber pylon incorporated into a foot, Ceterus, and (**b**) separate, Delta Twist. (Photos courtesy of Ossur International and Otto Bock Health Care.)

resistance. They serve as shock absorbers to decrease the impact of initial contact, and work much like the shock absorbers of an automobile. Some units combine torsional adaptation with vertical shock absorption. In other designs, the foot is integrated with a vertical shock pylon and/or tibial rotation capability.

Gait analysis

Gait patterns for individuals with transtibial amputations vary greatly from person to person. Many factors influence the way amputees walk. Physiologic factors include limb length, knee and hip muscle strength, range of motion, and presence of contractures. Socket design, suspension, and foot selection are a few prosthetic factors that can greatly influence the way in which an individual with a transtibial amputation can walk. The amputee must also be trained how to condition their bodies and how to use their prosthesis appropriately. The timing, quality, and quantity of physical therapy are very important. The clinic team attempts to minimize gait deviations by selecting the most appropriate designs and components for each individual, assuring optimal alignment of the prosthesis and effectively training the amputee.

There are many deviations that occur secondary to muscle weakness and prosthetic alignment, and they vary greatly from person to person. Gait deviations based on sound mechanical principles have been described in Table 14-4. These gait deviations are primarily due to an incorrect placement of the foot with relationship to the socket, or vice versa. Other factors in this table include component selection. Although it can be easy to decipher these deviations, it might not be consistent in the gait pattern of the user. For example, an amputee might have presented with a wonderful gait pattern at one point of rehabilitation, only to present later with a dramatically changed gait pattern. Changes can be due to decreased or increased function by the user, a change in fit, or a change in shoe wear. The wearer might have had a contracture that has been reduced through use of the prosthesis and daily ambulation. This is an example where an increased function can lead to problems with the

prosthesis. However; if the alignment of the prosthesis were rectified, the prosthesis would accommodate this improved range of motion and greatly improve the gait and overall function of the user.

Knee disarticulation and transcondylar or supracondylar amputation

The knee disarticulation amputation is a procedure that preserves the femoral condyles, either with or without the patella. This leaves a residual limb that is a long lever arm, and provides for a stronger residual limb than a transfemoral amputation because the muscular attachments to the condyles are preserved as well. Knee disarticulation amputation is an end weight-bearing amputation and this, combined with the length, allows for significantly lower trim lines than a transfemoral amputation, often resulting in more comfort and greater range of motion in the hip. The bulbous nature of the limb has a poorer cosmesis but can be helpful in using supracondylar suspension of the prosthesis. Variations of knee disarticulation amputations have been described in which the condyles are partially resected to reduce bulk of the residual limb, but this can interfere with supracondylar suspension. The primary problem with the knee disarticulation is the length at the knee. When a socket and prosthetic knee are added, the functional thigh length is too long. This mandates a poor appearance when sitting, because the leg lengths are uneven; sitting in tight places such as church pews and public transportation is difficult, and kneeling is problematic. For these reasons, the knee disarticulation amputation is rarely performed.

Socket designs

The socket designs for the knee disarticulation limb are highly dependent on the musculature present and the size of the condyles. In designs similar to the transtibial supracondylar suspension, the knee disarticulation socket can be created with an insert to provide both cushioning and suspension. This insert has a thickness of padding, or wedge, incorporated proximal to the femoral epicondyles that provides suspension when donned into a hard socket. As is the case for a Syme's prosthesis, a door can be cut out of the hard socket or femoral section to permit donning, and then a strap or elastic webbing can close the door to provide suspension of the prosthesis. If no large discrepancy exists between the femoral epicondyles and the region proximal to them, hard sockets can be utilized with socks over the residual limbs to facilitate donning through the narrowing distal socket. Gel or foam liners have also been used to suspend the knee disarticulation prosthesis. When donning the hard socket, the liner displaces over the condyles to allow the residual limb to slip past the narrowing socket and then rebounds when the limb is fully seated into the socket.

Individuals with long transfemoral limbs (e.g. transcondylar or supracondylar) have the advantage of a more cylindric limb. Without the presence of the femoral epicondyles, donning the prosthesis can be easier, and more traditional designs such as pull-in suction sockets can be utilized. However, these levels might sacrifice the adductor longus insertion and the associated

Table 14-4 Gait analysis of the transtibial amputee

Gait deviation	Prosthetic causes	Solutions
Delayed, abrupt, and limited knee flexion after heel strike	Heel wedge is too soft Foot is too far anterior Foot keel is too stiff	Stiffen heel wedge Move foot posterior Use more flexible keel foot
Extended knee throughout stance phase	Too much plantar flexion	Dorsiflex foot
Toe stays off floor after heel strike	Heel wedge too stiff Foot too anterior Too much dorsiflexion	Soften heel wedge Move foot posterior Plantar flex foot
'Hill-climbing' sensation toward end of stance phase	Heel wedge is too soft Foot is too far anterior Foot keel is too stiff Too much plantar flexion	Stiffen heel wedge Move foot posterior Use more flexible keel foot Dorsiflex foot
High pressure against patella throughout most of the stance phase; heel is off floor when patient stands	Too much plantar flexion	Dorsiflex foot
Knee too forcefully and rapidly flexes after heel strike; high pressure against anterior-distal tibia and heel strike, and/or prolonged discomfort at this point	Heel wedge too stiff Foot too far posterior Foot too dorsiflexed Keel too soft	Soften heel Move foot anterior Plantar flex foot Use stiffer keel foot
Hips level, but prosthesis seems short	Foot too far posterior Foot too dorsiflexed	Move foot anterior Plantar flex foot
Drop off at end of stance phase	Foot too far posterior Foot too dorsiflexed Keel too soft	Move foot anterior Plantar flex foot Use stiffer keel foot
Toe off of floor as patients stand or knee flexed too much	Foot too dorsiflexed	Plantar flex foot
Valgus moment at knee during stance; excessive pressure on distal-medial limb and/or proximal-lateral surface of knee	Foot too outset	Inset foot
Excessive varus moment at knee during stance (a varus moment at the knee should occur in stance phase but should never be excessive); the distal-lateral and or proximal-medial residual limb is painful	Foot too inset Medial-lateral dimension of socket is too large	Reduce inset of foot Fit of socket should be evaluated

(Courtesy of the Northwestern University Prosthetic–Orthotic Center.)

stability that it offers. A gel liner can be used in these levels as well; however, there still might not be room for a locking mechanism. In these cases, a lanyard system can be used in order to provide the mechanical connection between the gel liner and prosthesis.

Component selection

Knee components are selected for the longer residual limb based on muscular control, limb length, and cosmesis. Most individuals with long transfemoral limbs or knee disarticulation limbs have excellent control of their limbs in all planes and, when trained appropriately, can walk with a variety of component designs. The components for knee disarticulation prostheses are chosen to minimize hardware distally, enhancing its esthetics. Outside (single pivot) hinges (Fig. 14-23) are often used in the exoskeletal-style knee disarticulation prosthesis. This offers the best opportunity to equalize femoral segment lengths, but the joints offer no resistance to flexion and exten-

sion. Low-profile polycentric joints are very popular for this level of amputation, as they provide for a more natural-looking femoral section during sitting, due to the fact that the linkages allow the knee unit to fold under the femoral section. It must be noted, however, that many polycentric knee units offer little stability, which may be necessary for the individual with this residual limb length. Care must be taken to appropriately align the prosthesis to readily permit knee flexion during the pre-swing and swing phases.

TRANSFEMORAL (ABOVE-KNEE) AMPUTATION

The primary surgical goal of a transfemoral amputation is to stabilize the femur while retaining maximal femur length. During this procedure, the adductor magnus is pulled over the end of the femur, with myodesis (suturing muscle to bone) to the lateral femur. Myoplasty (suturing of muscle to muscle) of the quadriceps and the hamstrings is recommended.[37] This

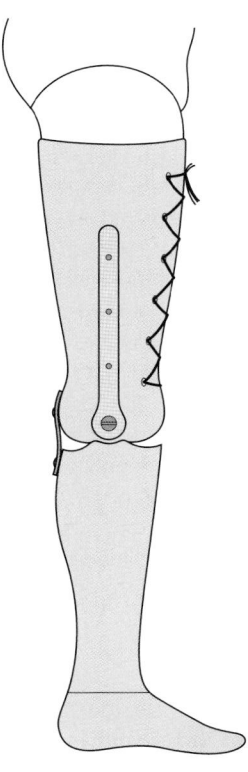

Figure 14-23 Outside hinges for a knee disarticulation-level prosthesis.

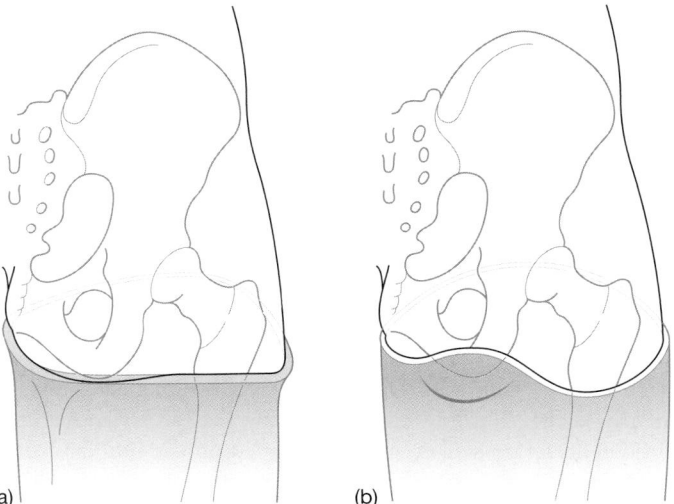

(a)   (b)

Figure 14-24 Location of ischium and pelvis for the quadrilateral and ischial containment-style transfemoral sockets.

procedure provides optimal adductor magnus function and padding of the distal femur. Myoplasty alone is inadequate, because it does not optimize muscle length. It also does not allow for adequate control of the femur. If the femur is too mobile within the residual limb, the lateral distal femur can be a focus of excessive pressure, causing pain, and the transfer of energy into the prosthesis is probably compromised.

Prosthetic prescription

There are two standard socket designs for transfemoral prostheses: the quadrilateral design and the ischial containment design (Fig. 14-24). The quadrilateral socket, described in 1955 by Charles Radcliffe,[63] is designed to allow for muscle function and to provide a seat for the ischium. The quadrilateral socket has four distinct walls with specific biomechanical objectives. The lateral wall supports the femur and provides a surface for the abductor muscles to fire against. The medial wall is in the line of progression and supports the adductor region. The posterior wall is angled away from the medial wall to allow for function of the gluteal tissue, which is critical for knee stability. The anterior wall is contoured to compress the Scarpa's triangle bounded by the inguinal ligament, the adductor tendon, and the sartorius. There is also relief built into the shape for function of the rectus femoris. Compression of the anterior surface provides the counterforce that maintains the ischium on the posterior shelf.

The ischial containment design was first described as the Normal Shape Normal Alignment socket by Ivan Long in 1975. There are now multiple variations in the socket design for ischial containment sockets.[40,58,70,80] However, the main biome-

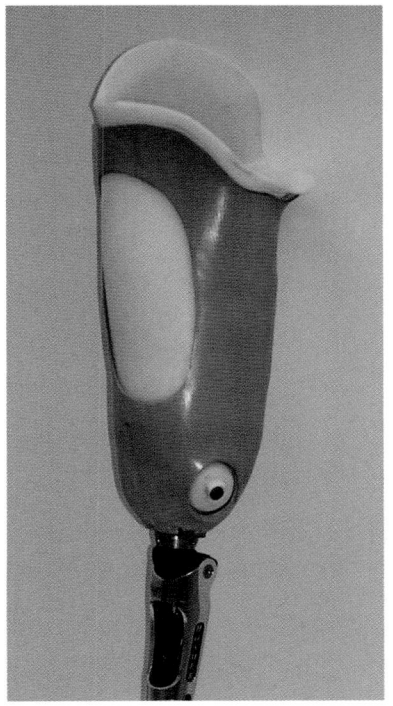

Figure 14-25 Example of a flexible inner socket and rigid frame construction for the transfemoral level prosthesis. This design provides comfort for the more aggressive ischial containment socket designs.

chanical principle of this design is to provide for a bony lock of the ischium in the prosthetic socket. Preventing lateral movement of the socket through containment of the ischium increases medial lateral stability during the stance phase and allows better adduction. This is helpful for all amputees, but is even more important for individuals with shorter residual limbs and for those with mild hip abductor weakness. The ischial containment socket is now the most commonly used design.

Ischial containment sockets are often made with a flexible inner socket and external frame (Fig. 14-25). The flexible socket can be made out of a variety of thermoplastic materials.

It provides for increased comfort proximally, which is important with the more aggressive ischial containment designs. The frame can be made out of stiffer thermoplastic or laminated materials. Cutouts can be made in the frame posteriorly to provide increased sitting comfort, and along the anterior surface to provide freedom of movement for rectus femoris contraction.

Suspension
Suction suspension
There are various methods for suspending a prosthesis, including suction, liners, and belts. Suction suspension is the most secure suspension method. A one-way valve is placed distally in the socket to allow air to exit the socket but not enter. To don a suction socket, a sock is placed on the limb and then the limb is slid into the socket. The sock is then pulled out of the valve opening, pulling the tissue into the socket. Variations on the sock donning method include the use of a special nylon sock, which makes donning easier by reducing friction; the use of an elastic bandage spirally wrapped on the limb and then pulled out through the opening; and the 'wet fit' method, in which lotion is placed on the limb before it is slid down into the socket. Although wet fit is an easier donning technique, if a large amount of soft tissue is present, it can be pushed up and out of the socket rather than being contained in the socket. This can result in a medial adductor roll, which can be a long-term fitting obstacle. The advantage of suction suspension is that it is the most secure suspension available and provides for the greatest control of the prosthesis. The disadvantage of suction is that it can be difficult to don and also that volume stability is critical for suspension. Volume loss can result in loss of suspension and volume (weight) gain can result in an adductor roll, lack of distal contact, and/or erythema.

Gel or elastomeric liner suspension
As with transtibial prostheses, liners with pins or lanyards can be used to suspend a transfemoral prosthesis, and can be a useful alternative for those with volume fluctuations. If the socket is loose, socks can be added over the liner to make an appropriately snug fit. The advantage of the lanyard over the pin is that donning can be easier. Engaging a pin into a lock with the presence of more mobile tissue of the thigh can be difficult. Additionally, the lock mechanism for the pin adds length to the femoral section. For longer limbs, the lanyard can decrease the added length, possibly increasing cosmesis. However, lanyards add bulk around the outside of the limb and disrupt the smoothness of the thigh section. For both the pin and the lanyard, the advantages of liners are the same as for transtibial, in that they provide increased shear control, increased cushioning, and good suspension. The disadvantages are that they require increased maintenance and replacement of liners, increase bulk, and pose significant hygiene issues. They also potentially decrease rotational control, because the covered liners have little friction against the socket wall.

Belt suspension
Belts can be used to suspend a transfemoral prosthesis or provide increased medial–lateral stability. There are three main types of belt: a total elastic suspension belt, a Silesian belt, and a hip joint and pelvic band (Fig. 14-26). Total elastic suspension (TES) belts, because they are elastic, provide less secure suspension and medial–lateral control. They are typically used more for auxiliary suspension and rotational control. The Silesian belt is made of Dacron webbing and can also be used for auxiliary suspension. When this belt is used alone for suspension, the socket is often worn with a sock ply fit. When better medial–lateral control is needed (for a short limb or for someone with mild hip abductor weakness), a Silesian belt should be used. A high lateral wall also increases the effectiveness of the belt in these cases. A hip joint and pelvic band should be worn for severe hip abductor weakness or by active individuals with a very short limb. The metal hip joint connects the socket to a metal pelvic band and leather belt. This provides the maximum medial–lateral stability; however, it also increases bulk and weight.

Prosthetic knees
Knee units can be organized into five classes: outside hinges, single axis, polycentric, weight-activated stance, and locking. The designs vary in the amount of voluntary control required and the amount of inherent stability. Voluntary control refers to the ability of the hip extensors to actively pull the thigh into extension prior to and during stance phase. Voluntary control stabilizes the prosthetic knee unit. The more voluntary control that is available, the less inherent stability is required, and vice versa. Outside hinges were described in the previous section on knee disarticulation prostheses.

Knee mechanisms also have friction to provide resistance to excessive knee flexion (heel rise) in swing. Mechanical friction is constant and independent of speed, making it appropriate for single-speed ambulators. Younger individuals tend to walk at variable speeds, while older individuals tend to adopt a single speed for the great majority of their walking. For more active variable cadence ambulators, mechanical friction does not adapt and provide enough resistance as the walking speed is increased or for running. Fluid friction is used to provide friction proportionate to the velocity of movement. The fluid used can be air (pneumatic systems) or liquid (hydraulic systems). Pneumatic systems are lighter and do not need to be sealed, but they can seem 'bouncy' for the more aggressive walkers because of the compressibility of air. Both pneumatic and hydraulic systems are more expensive and require more maintenance than mechanical friction units.

Some knee units also include an extension assist (Fig. 14-27). An extension assist acts to help limit heel rise (similar to friction), and it also helps to initiate and ensure full extension. The extension assist can be built into the knee or in some cases be a optional feature. Not all knee units can have an extension assist. They are more common on knees designed for individuals with less voluntary control.

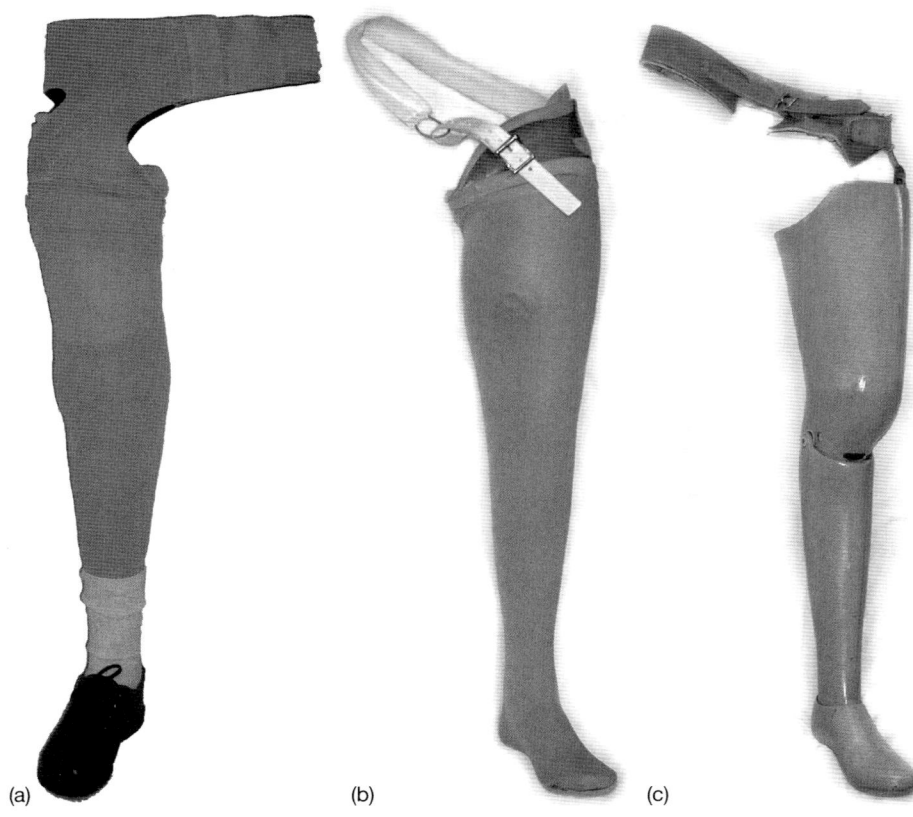

(a)   (b)   (c)

Figure 14-26 Three transfemoral belts:
(**a**) total elastic suspension belt, (**b**) Silesian
belt, and (**c**) hip joint with pelvic band.

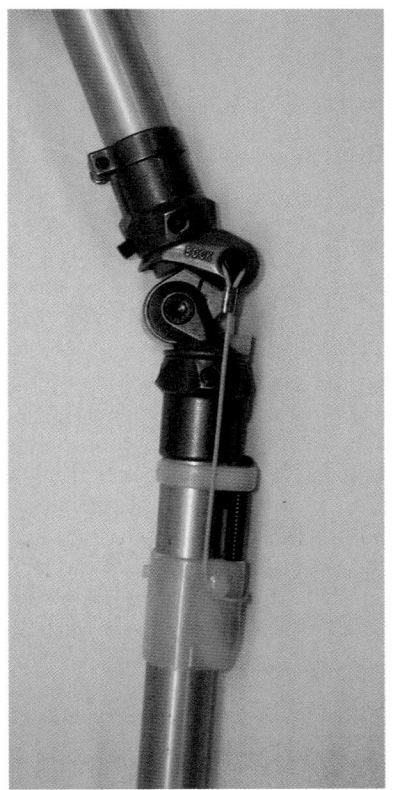

Figure 14-27 Example of
stance control single-axis
knee with extension assist
(the wire and springs in front
of the knee).

Single-axis knees

Single-axis knees have a single axis of rotation similar to that
of a basic door or hinge joint. Stability is achieved only through
alignment and voluntary control. A single-axis knee is typically
aligned with the weight line slightly in front of the knee axis.
As the voluntary control increases, the knee can be moved
further anterior to the zero mark, where the weight line passes
through the knee axis, often referred to as 'trigger'. The knee
should not be moved ahead of this point or instability can occur
when the user is momentarily distracted.

Polycentric knees

Polycentric knees (*poly*, many; *centric*, centers) (Fig. 14-28)
have more than one axis of rotation. Four-bar knees are a sub-
class of polycentric knees. Many polycentric knees have more
than four axes. The advantages of polycentric knees are that
they have a mobile center of rotation, provide an effective
shortening of the prosthesis in swing phase, and fold under
themselves for increased cosmesis in sitting. Polycentric knees
can be designed for individuals with short residual limbs by
having a center of rotation that is proximal and posterior to
the mechanical joint axes. This allows for increased stability
(because the center is posterior) and more voluntary control
(because the center is proximal and closer to the residual limb).
They can also be designed for long limbs or knee disarticulation

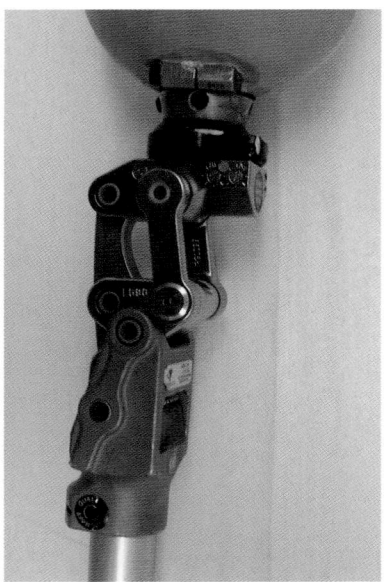

Figure 14-28 Example of a polycentric knee.

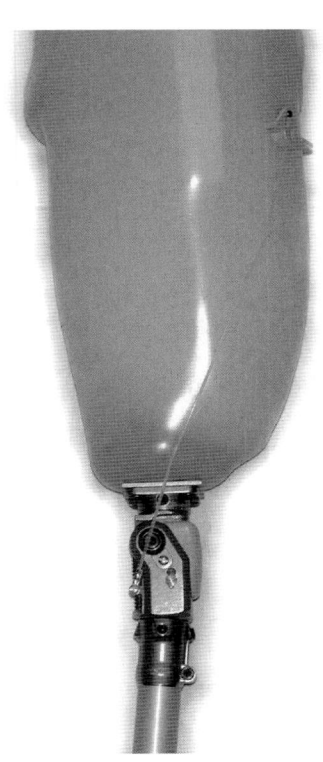

Figure 14-29 Example of a manual locking knee.

amputees, where the center of rotation is close to the knee joint but the knee is designed to fold under the thigh, leaving a lower sitting profile and improving cosmesis.

Weight-activated stance control knees

Weight-activated stance control knees have a braking mechanism that prevents further flexion when weight is applied (Fig. 14-27). In this figure, the extension assist is external to the knee along the anterior aspect of the brace. The braking mechanism is located internally, and can be adjusted to be more or less sensitive to the weight required to engage the stance control. These knees have occasionally been referred to as 'safety knees', but because the possibility of knee flexion remains, this is an inappropriate term and should not be used. The braking mechanism of these knees functions when weight is applied and the knee is flexed less than approximately 20°. The sensitivity of this adjustment can be set for each individual user, allowing for momentary stability and stumble recovery for those with poor balance. The knee should not be aligned or used in a manner where every step relies on the breaking mechanism to prevent knee flexion, because the wear of the mechanism can cause premature failure and falls.

Manual locking knees

Manual locking knees (Fig. 14-29) are the most stable of the knee designs. These knees have a switch release for sitting and snap into place at full extension. They cannot be flexed again until the switch release is engaged. Manual locking knees compromise gait mechanics because the patient must walk with a straight leg. The leg should be shorter than the contralateral side to allow clearance. This design is used only for those for whom maximal stability is the main goal: those with significant weakness or instability, some bilateral amputees, and/or those using the prosthesis primarily for transfers.

Microprocessor-controlled knees

New microprocessor-controlled hydraulic knee systems are also available. One example, the C-leg by Otto Bock (Fig. 14-30a), measures the knee joint angle and the forces in the pylon to determine the phase of the gait cycle and the speed at which the user is ambulating. The microprocessor then adjusts valves to control fluid flow within the unit. Another computerized knee, the Rheo Knee by Ossur (Fig. 14-30b), is filled with a magnetorheologic fluid that changes flow characteristics when a magnetic field is applied. This knee also uses measured force and position data to determine how to adjust friction for speed or stumbling. Instead of controlling valves, however, the microprocessor controls resistance by adjusting the magnetic field around the fluid. The advantage of computerized knee systems is that they allow knee friction to be varied based on knee angle, forces, speed, and type of activity. When the microprocessor determines that the user is walking faster, it increases friction in swing phase, eliminating excessive knee flexion. If the microprocessor determines that the user has stumbled or is not in a phase of the gait cycle where the knee should bend, it can lock the knee (or increase friction substantially) to allow for recovery and improved stability. These knees can also be set to allow an appropriate friction for easier descent of stairs. As microprocessor computing power evolves, computer-controlled components will continue to allow for a more dynamic responsiveness and make inadvertent flexion of the knee less likely. The primary disadvantage of these microprocessor control knees is that they are very expensive.

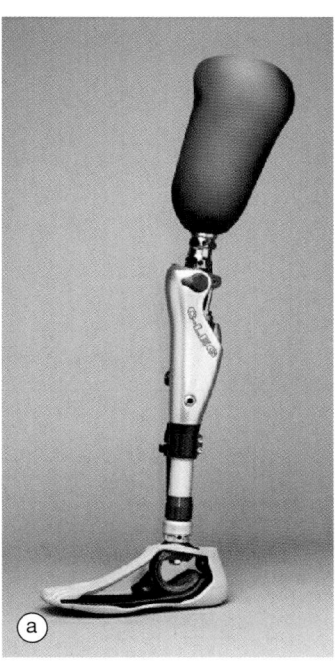 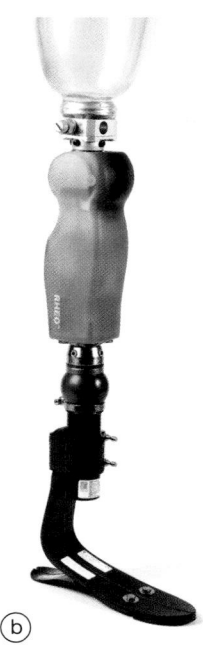

Figure 14-30 Examples of computer controlled prosthetic knee joints: (**a**) The C-leg, (**b**) the Rheo. (a, Photo courtesy of Otto Bock Health Care; b, photo courtesy of Ossur International.)

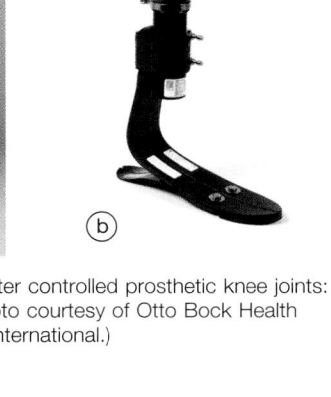

Figure 14-31 The trochanter–knee–ankle (TKA) alignment. For the knee to be stable, the line between the trochanter mark and the ankle must pass in front of the knee axis.

Considerations for other component selection

Prosthetic feet and ankle assemblies are the same as for transtibial amputation. When additional components such as rotators and shock absorbers are used, they should be placed distal to the knee, but as proximal as possible to reduce the apparent weight. An additional component available for transfemoral prostheses is a positional rotator, which is added distal to the socket and proximal to the knee. By depressing a button, the lower leg can be rotated, permitting the legs to be crossed and increasing the ease of donning pants and of entering and exiting tight spaces such as vehicles. Because it adds length to the proximal segment, however, it cannot be used for the longest residual limbs.

Transfemoral prosthesis alignment

Alignment of the transfemoral prosthesis depends on component selection and user strength and range of motion. The foot and knee are usually aligned outset with respect to the ischium in the coronal plane. The foot should be further outset (up to approximately the middle of the socket) for those with shorter residual limbs or mild abductor weakness. For those with moderate abductor weakness or for those with a very short limb, however, a Silesian belt or hip joint and pelvic band must be used. In the sagittal plane, the socket should be preflexed 5° from vertical beyond the amputee's hip flexion range. For example, if the amputee has a 5° flexion contracture, the prosthesis should be aligned with 10° of flexion in the socket. This accommodates the loss of knee flexion in late stance at opposite heel contact, and allows the user to take a normal sound side step. If this alignment is not made, the prosthetic user might take a short step and, if a flexion contracture is not accommodated, can also result in an unstable knee. For knee alignment with the quadrilateral socket fitting, the trochanter–knee–ankle (TKA) line is used (Fig. 14-31). For this alignment, a single-axis knee should fall 6 mm posterior to a line connecting the greater trochanter and ankle. For ischial containment sockets, a weight line is typically used. The starting point for alignment is a plumb line from the bisection of the socket at ischial level. Each knee design has a manufacturer-suggested alignment, but generally the knee axis should be posterior to this line. Moving the knee axis further posterior increases the stability. A knee positioned closer to the weight line requires more voluntary control, but allows easier knee flexion in late stance phase and a more normal-appearing gait. During dynamic alignment, the goal is to have a knee that is stable but easy to control. The foot should progress from heel to toe smoothly and, in the coronal plane, the pelvis should be maintained close to level and the foot should be flat on the floor. A list of common gait deviations is presented in Table 14-5.

HIP DISARTICULATION AND TRANSPELVIC AMPUTATION (HEMIPELVECTOMY)

Hip disarticulation and hemipelvectomy amputations are usually performed on patients with femoral malignancy or severe trauma. The basic technique for hip disarticulation was described by Boyd.[11] The wound is generally closed, with the gluteus maximus being sutured to remnant of the adductor muscles to provide padding to the residual tissue.

Table 14-5 Gait analysis of the transfemoral amputee

Gait deviation	Prosthetic causes	Amputee causes
Lateral trunk bending: excessive bending occurs laterally away from midline toward prosthetic side	Prosthesis too short Improperly shaped lateral wall fails to support femur Lack of ischial support (high medial wall can cause amputee to hold prosthesis away to avoid ramus pressure) Prosthesis aligned in abduction, causing a wide-based gait	Inadequate balance Abduction contracture Residual limb painful Short limb can fail to provide sufficient lever arm for the pelvis Poor gait habit
Abducted gait: wide-based gait with prosthesis held away from body at all time (stance and swing)	Prosthesis too long Too much abduction built into prosthesis Lack of ischial support (high medial wall can cause amputee to hold prosthesis away to avoid ramus pressure) Improperly shaped lateral wall fails to support femur Pelvic band can be positioned too far away from the body	Abduction contracture Poor gait habit
Circumducted gait: the swinging of the prosthesis laterally in a wide arc, returning to vertical for stance phase	Prosthesis too long Too much alignment stability or friction in the knee, making it difficult to bend in swing phase Extension aid too strong	Abduction contracture Lack of confidence for flexing the knee because of muscle weakness or fear of stubbing the toe Poor gait habit
Vaulting	Prosthesis too long Inadequate suspension Excessive knee stability due to alignment, excessive knee friction, or an excessive extension assist	Poor gait habit Fear of stubbing the toe Residual limb pain
Rotation of the prosthetic foot at heel strike	Heel too firm Too much toe out Loose socket fit Posterior socket tightness	User can extend limb too vigorously at heel strike Poor muscle control of the limb
Uneven arm swing, with arm on prosthetic side held close to the body	Improperly fitting socket Poor suspension	Poor balance Fear and insecurity accompanied by uneven timing Poor gait habit
Uneven timing, characterized by a short stance phase on the prosthetic side	Improperly fitting socket Weak extension aid or insufficient friction can cause excessive heel rise and result in a longer amount of time spent on the sound side Knee instability	Weak residual limb User cannot have developed good balance Fear and insecurity Pain
Uneven heel rise	Knee joint can have insufficient friction Inadequate extension aid	User can be using more power than necessary to force the knee into flexion
Terminal swing impact, characterized by rapid forward movement of the shin allowing the knee to reach maximum extension with too much force before heel strike	Insufficient knee friction Knee extension aid can be too strong	User can deliberately and forcibly extend residual limb to ensure full extension of knee
Instability of the prosthetic knee, which creates a danger of falling	Knee joint can be aligned anterior to weight line or trochanter–knee–ankle (TKA) line Insufficient initial flexion can have been built into the socket Heel can be too firm, causing the knee to buckle at heel strike Foot keel can be too soft, allowing knee flexion to occur late in stance	User can have weak hip extensors Severe flexion contracture can cause instability

Continued on page 315

Continued from page 314 Table 14-5 Gait analysis of the transfemoral amputee

Gait deviation	Prosthetic causes	Amputee causes
Medial or lateral whip: these are best observed as the user walks away A medial whip is present when the heel travels medially on initial flexion at the beginning of swing phase, and a lateral whip exists when the heel moves laterally	Lateral whips occur from excessive internal rotation of the knee with respect to the socket Medial whips can result from excessive external rotation of the knee Socket can fit too tightly, reflecting limb rotation Excessive valgus in the prosthesis can contribute The socket can have been donned improperly	Faulty gait habits can result in whips
Foot slap: a rapid descent of the anterior of the foot at heel strike	Plantar flexion resistance is too soft (heel too soft)	User can be driving the prosthesis into the ground at heel strike to ensure knee stability
Drop-off at the end of stance: downward movement of the trunk as the body moves forward over the prosthesis	Inadequate limitation of dorsiflexion of the foot Keel of the foot can be too short or too soft Socket can have been placed to far anterior with respect to the foot	None
Long prosthetic step (or short sound side step): the user takes a longer step with the prosthesis than with the sound leg	Insufficient flexion included in the socket	A flexion contracture that cannot be accommodated prosthetically
Excessive trunk extension: during stance phase the user creates excessive active lumbar lordosis	Improperly shaped posterior wall causing forward rotation of the pelvis to avoid full weight bearing on the ischium Insufficient initial flexion built into the socket	Hip flexor tightness Weak hip extensors, substituted for by lumbar erector spinae Weak abdominal muscles Poor gait habit Poor balance
External rotation of the foot at heel off: viewed from posterior, the heel is seen to rotate internally prior to swing phase	Insufficient flexion included in the socket	Hip flexor tightness

(Courtesy of the Northwestern University Prosthetic–Orthotic Center.)

Hemipelvectomies vary greatly in the amount of bone removed. They range from focal osteotomy to a complete transaction of the pelvis that spares only the sacrum. Pelvic x-rays to determine which bony structures are missing and which remain for weight bearing can be helpful for the prosthetic socket design.

For the hip disarticulation level of amputation, the pelvis should be intact. In some cases, those with short transfemoral amputation (when there is not enough femur length to control a transfemoral prosthesis) can be fitted with a hip disarticulation prosthesis. The hip disarticulation and hemipelvectomy socket must allow for weight bearing during stance phase, provide coronal plane stability during stance phase, and provide suspension during swing phase. When the ischium is present (for the hip disarticulation and some hemipelvectomy cases), it can provide a loading surface and increase medial–lateral stabil-

ity. Some weight must also be applied along the lateral surface of the torso. Typically, the socket wraps around the pelvis (Fig. 14-32), with loading occurring above the iliac crest, and medial–lateral stability occurring through loading of the iliac fossa. For hemipelvectomy fittings where a significant portion of the pelvis has been removed, the trim lines should continue to just below the costal margin and further include the abdominal tissue. The higher trim lines ensure more area for weight bearing.

The hip joint is mounted anteriorly on the socket and the thigh, then folds forward for sitting. For ambulation, the prosthesis length should be at least one-half to one inch shorter than the sound side to permit swing phase clearance. This is necessary, since knee flexion timing may not assist with foot clearance. At heel contact, the knee should be fully extended and a soft heel should be used to further ensure knee stability. When the hip extension stop has been engaged and after opposite heel

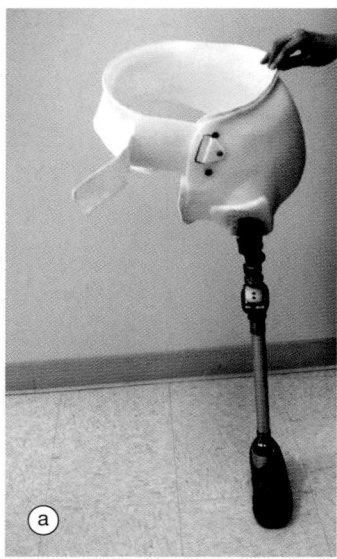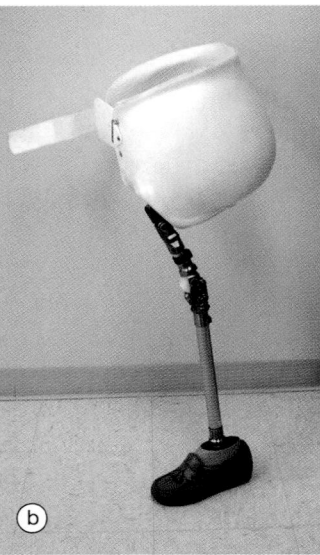

(a) (b)

Figure 14-32 Hip disarticulation–level prosthesis. (**a**) Front view. (**b**) Side view.

contact, the user pushes into the back of the socket to provide a knee flexion moment and allow knee flexion to be initiated. If the hip extension stop engages too early (prior to midstance), the knee can buckle. If it engages too late (after midstance), initiation of knee flexion can be difficult. During swing phase, the knee has to fully extend before momentum can be transferred to the hip flexion. For this reason, the leg should be initially set shorter than the sound side for clearance.

TRANSLUMBAR AMPUTATION (HEMICORPORECTOMY)

The translumbar amputation is essentially an ablation of the caudal 50% of the human body, including the legs, pelvis, and genitourinary and reproductive organs. It is also termed the hemicorpectomy, although in this case the 'hemi' refers to this lower half of the body as opposed to half of one side being amputated. The lower half of the body with pelvis is removed, with creation of colostomy and urinary diversion stoma for bowel and bladder elimination.[82]

Individuals with a hemicorpectomy level of amputation typically do not ambulate as a primary means of transportation. However, they can be fitted with a prosthetic socket to increase loading surface area for wheelchair sitting. This can help prevent the occurrence of decubitus ulceration, and can also assist with upright posture. Some individuals can be fitted with prosthetic components, including hip joints and manual locking knees, so that they can ambulate with a walker and a swing-to gait pattern.

BILATERAL AMPUTEE CONSIDERATIONS

The occurrence of bilateral transtibial amputations unfortunately is becoming increasingly common. Literature shows that

between 28 and 51% of individuals with diabetic amputations lose their contralateral limb within 5 years of their first limb amputation.[65] This population of patients require that attention be paid to techniques that preserve the alternate limb (see Ch. 57). Bilateral amputees do not have a non-involved or 'sound side' to compensate for the limitations of a prosthesis, especially the loss of ankle motion. A torsion pylon or foot with ankle motion in various planes is often recommended, because it assists the patient in attempting to compensate for these lost motions. Multiaxial feet or ankles used to be thought of as being contraindicated for bilateral lower limb amputees, because it was felt that solid ankle systems were necessary for the amputee to be able to stand stably within a secure base of support. However, with proper fitting and training, they have proven to be a beneficial addition. Without the sensory feedback, however, some individuals feel unsteady and prefer solid ankle systems.

Prosthetic alignment can enhance stability in the bilateral amputee. Prosthetic feet can be placed further posterior and in initial dorsiflexion to shift the individual's center of mass forward during quiet standing. When fitting ankles to this patient population, the component that contributes toward ankle plantar flexion should be soft to enable the foot to easily plantar flex. If the bumper is stiff, the foot will not plantar flex as easily, and the forces will be transmitted to the posterior aspect of the prosthetic knee. These forces will tend to create an external knee flexion moment that must be controlled by the wearer. Conversely, the dorsiflexion bumper can be softer to allow the person to lean into the prostheses during ambulation. This also enables them to traverse inclines easier, as they can 'roll over' the foot more easily. For all levels of bilateral lower limb loss, it is often recommended that the prostheses be set with less initial inset of the prosthetic feet with respect to the sockets. This allows individuals to maintain a wider base of support, and thus create better stability while wearing their prostheses. Going from sit to stand is one of the most demanding tasks for a bilateral amputee. It is obvious that bilateral lower limb amputees can choose their height, and being willing to be a few inches shorter can be helpful in allowing for an easier sit to stand transition. This also lowers the center of gravity a little, adding to stability in gait.

When a patient has had one transtibial and one transfemoral amputation, concerns with transfemoral fittings (such as control of the knee during initial contact or loading response) are even more problematic. Balance and stumble recovery are more difficult. The major difference in this type of fitting is the length of the prostheses. The user can have difficulty initiating knee flexion on the prosthetic knee. Therefore the transfemoral prosthesis should be made slightly shorter than the transtibial side so that there are no issues with swing phase clearance of the transfemoral prosthesis.

Although gait with bilateral transfemoral prostheses can be difficult, younger, stronger people with long residual limbs can walk surprisingly well and become unlimited community ambulators without the use of a gait aid (although most use a cane outdoors). With shorter residual limbs, a more supportive gait aid is generally needed, such as crutches or a walker. It is very difficult for bilateral transfemoral amputees secondary to vascular disease to ambulate with prostheses. Older amputees generally have less strength and more comorbidities (such as impaired cardiac function) that further impair their ability to use prostheses. Nevertheless, appropriate patients (those who are not obese, have reasonable residual limb length, and have fair strength), who are very motivated and understand the potential risks of bilateral transfemoral amputee gait, should be given the opportunity to attempt ambulation. Most of these patients will be successful, at least to some degree.

One way to facilitate a successful bilateral transfemoral prosthetic gait is to start with very short prostheses call 'stubbies' (Fig. 14-33). Stubbies are prostheses that are close to the ground, with the foot component attached directly to the distal end of the transfemoral socket (or close enough to make the height of the prosthesis even with the contralateral side). These 'training prostheses' bring the center of mass closer to the ground, providing more stability for ambulation. The feet are initially mounted in reverse to keep the center of mass farther back in the user's base of support and to minimize risk of falling backward. There are no knees in stubbies. Thus the user does not have to concentrate on controlling the prosthetic knee and preventing the knee from flexing. Patients begin by focusing on socket fit and basic ambulation skills. As progress is made, the devices are raised to greater height, the feet are reversed to a forward-pointing direction, and knee units are added one at a time (usually on the longer residual limb first). Eventually, the devices are raised to the desired final height, and the amputee can progress to using knees with less inherent stability, as well as using less restrictive gait aids. This is a long and time-consuming process that demands commitment from both the patient and the rehabilitation team.

Energy expenditure

The effect of amputation on the energy cost of ambulation is significant. Typically, the 'cost' of gait is measured in oxygen consumption. Although various measurement techniques exist, usually the volume of air inhaled and the amount of carbon dioxide exhaled is used to calculate energy expenditure, and is subsequently scaled as a function of body mass. The results can be reported as a function of distance or as a rate. Oxygen rate, which is dependent on velocity, is often reported as well. In addition to oxygen consumption and rate, maximal aerobic capacity influences an individual's ability to perform with a prosthesis. This capacity decreases with both age and vascular involvement.[84]

Individuals with an amputation typically walk slower than non-amputees in order to keep the oxygen consumption rate within a tolerable aerobic range. If transtibial amputees walk with their speed reduced, they incur a larger oxygen cost per distance than non-amputees walking at the same speed. Vascular amputees also have higher oxygen consumption per distance than traumatic amputees.[84]

When using oxygen consumption per unit distance measurements, unilateral traumatic transtibial amputees use approximately 7% more energy to walk the same distance as non-amputees. This increases to 25% for traumatic transfemoral amputees. Vascular transtibial and transfemoral amputees use 25% and 87% more energy, respectively.[83] Bilateral amputation increases the cost even further.[85] A bilateral vascular transtibial amputee has a walking speed of 40 m/min at an oxygen cost 107% greater than normal. This study had only a small number of subjects, but showed that a bilateral traumatic transfemoral amputee walking at a reduced speed of 54 m/min had a reported oxygen cost that was 120% greater than normal.

Recreational activities

People with lower limb loss can enjoy most recreational activities with conventional prostheses, but some components are better suited than others for different activities. High-level activity functions require very secure suspension for safe participation. Suction-type suspension systems are generally preferred. Sports involving running and jumping are best served by high-profile dynamic response feet. For transfemoral amputees, running requires a high performance variable cadence (hydraulic) knee. Competitive running is a sport where a dedicated prosthetic foot is seen. These feet are custom-made to provide the correct energy return for the individual's weight and running style. Most designs lack a heel because, during short runs, force is applied only to the toes (Fig. 14-34). This makes stopping and standing difficult, especially for bilateral amputees. Insurance companies rarely fund these dedicated devices, and cost can make personal purchase prohibitive. Competitive athletes who require dedicated devices like a running foot are often sponsored by companies that supply the componentry.

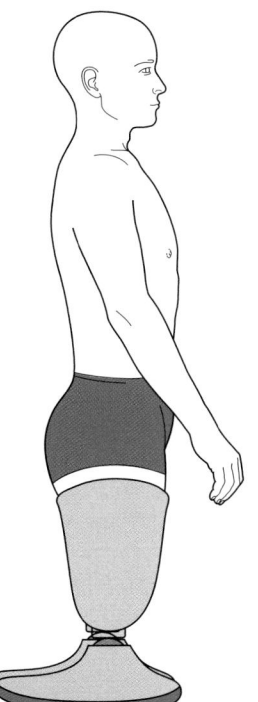

Figure 14-33 Example of 'stubbies', bilateral transfemoral prosthesis with no knees and the feet mounted backward.

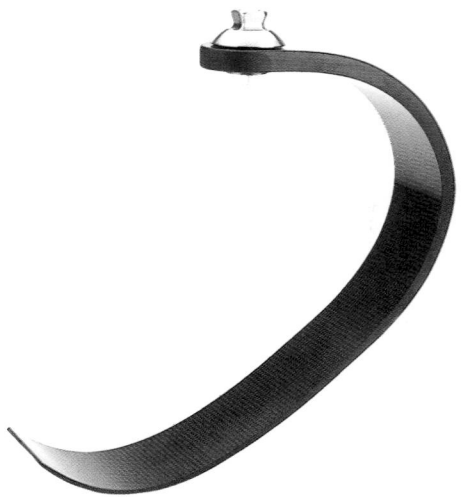

Figure 14-34
Example of a
sprinting foot
(Cheetah Foot).
(Photo courtesy of
Ossur International.)

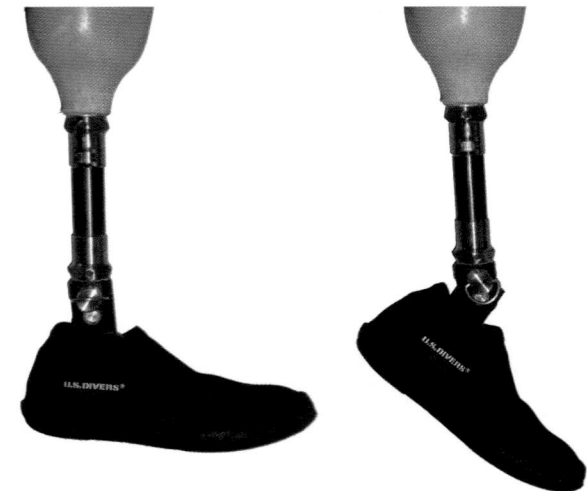

Figure 14-35 The Leisure Activity Ankle. This unit allows for locking in plantar flexion for swimming.

Golf is a very popular sport for amputees, including dysvascular amputees. The National Amputee Golf Association (see Box 14-1) exists to assist people with this sport and sponsors many events. While golfing can be done with most prostheses, the addition of a tibial rotation unit can be helpful, as it allows the necessary tibial rotation to occur during the swing of the golf club.

Racket sports are demanding, and the use of dynamic response feet is recommended. Amputees must decide which type of dynamic response foot works better for them. They can use the multiaxial dynamic response foot that allows medial–lateral motion for aggressive lateral motions, or the high-profile dynamic response foot that is better for running and jumping.

Although most amputees enjoy swimming without the use of a prosthesis, a 'water leg' is useful for the beach or being around water. This can be a prosthesis with water-resistant components or even just a pull-up covering that keeps the prosthesis reasonably dry. Prostheses for use with swimming are also made, and include ankles that allow the foot to be plantar flexed for a 'kicking' position. The Leisure Activity Ankle (Fig. 14-35) has a design that can be incorporated into modular prostheses. The design permits the ankle to be locked in a neutral or plantar flexed posture with the turn of a lever. The neutral position is used for limited ambulation, while the plantar flexed position is designed to be used in water activities such as scuba diving. Because most prosthetic devices are not waterproof, dedicated sockets and attachments are required. Often hollow exoskeletal designs are used, which eliminate most of the metal components. It is also necessary to design a construction that can fill with water and drain easily to limit the effects of buoyancy or 'weighting down' of the limb. Some swimmers attach a fin directly to the end of their residual limb, eliminating the need for a dedicated prosthesis. All these components are typically used by recreational swimmers and scuba divers, because competitive swimmers are not allowed to use assistive devices.

Individuals with a prosthesis sometimes struggle with bike riding, because the prosthetic foot is difficult to keep on the pedal, especially for transfemoral amputees. Recreational bikers can either use cages to help keep the foot from sliding off the pedal, or use biking shoes with cleats that lock on to the pedal. This creates a safety concern, however, because the lock can be difficult to disengage. Sometimes, an old prosthesis can be dedicated to bike riding and aligned in a more advantageous position. Competitive cyclists are usually fitted with extremely rigid feet (to better transfer forces to the pedals) and shoe cleats that are built directly into the bottom of the foot.

Recreational activities should always be kept in mind when determining the functional level of the amputee and the recommended components. Although not all things can be done for all people due to limb length, weight, financial considerations, etc., an effort should be made to recommend a device that allows the amputee to return to as many activities as possible. Additional therapy should also be considered to assist the amputee with sport and leisure activities as needed (see Box 14-1, Disabled Sports USA).

PEDIATRIC AMPUTATION
General

Differences between fitting adults and fitting children with prostheses truly exist. Although it is important to involve family members of adults who have had amputations, it is imperative that the family, more specifically the parents, be involved in the decision making and fitting of their child's prosthesis. These decisions will surround not only the prosthetic intervention but, in many limb anomalies, will involve potential surgical intervention. The various limb anomalies and configurations without or following surgery create challenges to the prosthetist. Additionally, the unpredictable growth of the child must be factored into the decision making of the design. In most instances, in pediatric fittings, some type of growth compensation is made (e.g. growth liners, distal end pads, and modular fittings).

The etiology behind pediatric amputations is much different than that of the adult population. Most of the pediatric amputations and/or prosthetic fittings are made for children with congenital anomalies. The most common limb deficiencies will be defined later in this section. Trauma and tumors also present themselves to the pediatric clinics, but do so at a smaller percentage.

Classifications of limb deficiencies

There have been many ways of describing limb deficiencies in the past, but currently there are two main headings for these classifications under the International Organization for Standardization and the International Society for Prosthetics and Orthotics classification of congenital limb deficiency: transverse and longitudinal. Transverse deficiencies are defined as 'normal development until the point of the deficiency, beyond which the normal anatomy does not exist'. These transverse deficiencies present themselves as guillotine-type amputations, in the fact that no segments distal to the 'amputation' site exist. Most of the causes for these are unknown, and they are thought to have resulted from vascular disruptions in utero. Transverse deficiency can also result from amniotic band syndrome, where the limb bud is caught in a 'band' that constricts it and prevents normal development. Other regions of the body can experience this banding as well.

Longitudinal deficiencies are defined as 'absence of skeletal anatomy within the long axis of a limb, sometimes includes normal anatomy distal to the affected bone/bones'. As described, the longitudinal deficiencies are a random absence of bony structures. These types of deficiencies are usually of unknown origin and are commonly treated with some type of surgical correction. Longitudinal deficiencies are more common than transverse lower limb amputations and prosthetic fittings, and are described below in order of their frequency of occurrence.

Common lower limb deficiencies
Longitudinal deficiency of the fibula

Longitudinal deficiency of the fibula is the most common long bone absence (Fig. 14-36).[35] It is often associated with other anomalies present, including a deformed foot, usually with absent lateral ray(s); valgus angulation at the knee; anterior (kyphoscoliotic) bowing of the tibia; a subcutaneous dimple over the apex of the tibia; ipsilateral femoral shortening; and limited hip internal rotation. The two most common treatments for this anomaly are some form of ankle disarticulation amputation, or lengthening with an external fixator and often subsequent ankle arthrodesis (fusion). There are conflicting opinions regarding the outcome of these two interventions. If the family elects to proceed with the ankle disarticulation, the child can be fitted with a prosthesis shortly thereafter. The more traditional Syme's amputation for children with fibular deficiencies has proven to be very beneficial. Migration of the heel pad posterior-proximally has sometimes led surgeons to perform Boyd procedures in order to ensure the centralization of the heel pad. Once fitted with a prosthesis, the child is able to walk

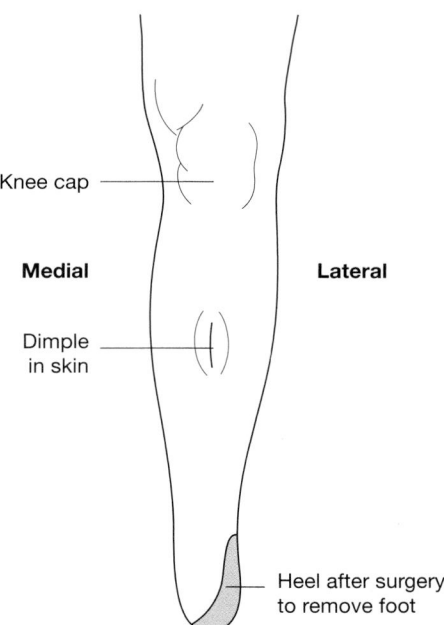

Knee cap

Medial   **Lateral**

Dimple
in skin

Heel after surgery
to remove foot

Figure 14-36 Amputation level commonly seen for a fibular deficiency.

with a relatively normal gait. Although there are space limitations for prosthetic feet while the child is very young, the natural occurrence of ipsilateral femoral shortening or the use of an epiphysiodesis can lead to adequate room for most prosthetic foot designs as the child matures. Other factors that can compromise the prosthetic fittings are the lack of ability to end bear as the child gets larger, and the increased genu valgum due to the absence of a lateral stabilizer. This valgus attitude, combined with a long residual limb and an appropriate prosthetic alignment, creates a large bump on the lateral aspect of the prosthesis, compromising cosmesis.

Longitudinal deficiency of the femur (proximal femoral focal deficiency)

Proximal femoral focal deficiency (PFFD), the second most common congenital deficiency of the lower limb, is a prosthetic, surgical, and rehabilitative challenge. PFFD is a congenital deficiency that can present itself in a large variety of ways, primarily as a clinical presentation of hip flexion, abduction, and external rotation. Several methods of classifications for femoral malformation or PFFD have been described. Aitken's method is the most broadly accepted (Fig. 14-37).[2] Aitken classified the PFFD levels according to acetabular and femoral involvement. This classification of A through D is designed with class A being the least involved and class D being the most severely involved. In addition to the femoral and acetabular involvement, the aforementioned longitudinal deficiency of the fibula is present in a large percentage of individuals with PFFD. Due to this severe instability and proximal position of the foot, surgical intervention is often recommended to reshape the acetabulum, disarticulate the foot, fuse the knee, and/or rotate the foot

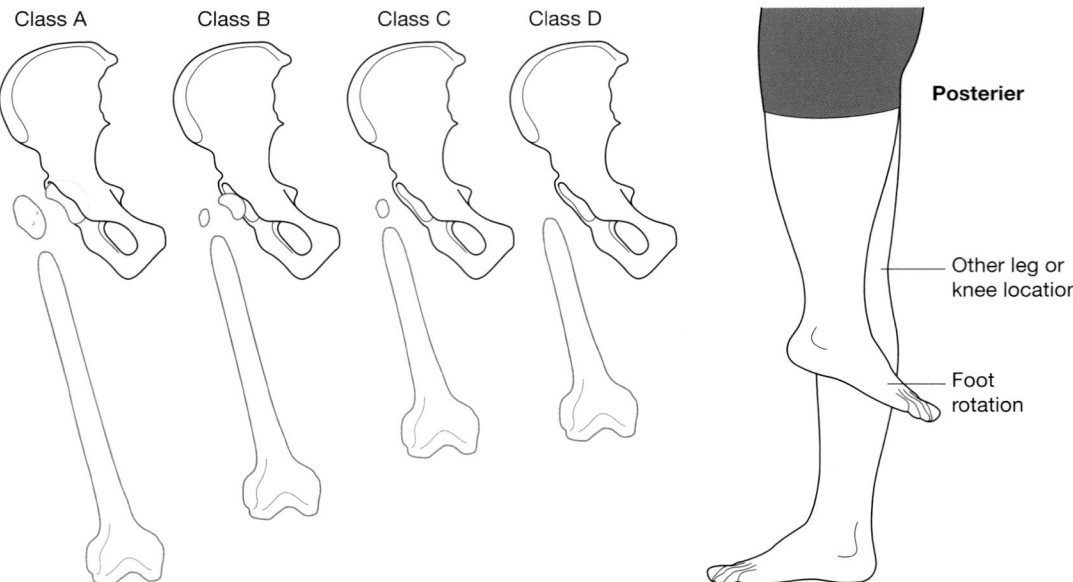

Class A   Class B   Class C   Class D

Figure 14-37 The classification levels for proximal femoral focal deficiency.

Posterier

Other leg or knee location

Foot rotation

Figure 14-38 Example of the Van Nes rotationplasty technique that is performed on individuals with a proximal femoral focal deficiency. This technique uses the ankle to function as the knee

posteriorly. These interventions vary based on clinical setting, geographic location, cultural issues related to body image, and parental wishes.

If no surgical intervention is performed, the prosthesis will be fitted around the involved hip and encompass the affected foot. This 'foot in foot' prosthesis will require an ankle-foot-type socket and have a prosthetic foot distal to the socket. Many of these first fittings involve a shoe lift due to the lack of space distally, and will later progress into an 'extension prosthesis' with prosthetic foot distal to the socket. In early fittings, articulated joints can be added to provide a knee joint. This can be accomplished by using outside hinges, as an endoskeletal prosthetic knee will create a femoral length discrepancy. If the femoral length is short enough, there might eventually be space for an endoskeletal knee beneath the footplate.

Syme's amputation is commonly performed on the PFFD limb to ablate the foot and provide a bulbous residual end for end bearing and suspension. This is performed at approximately 1 year of age to prevent the child's dependence on her or his foot and allow early prosthetic fitting. The same prosthetic designs are used when fitting a child with the Syme's amputation, as there was when no surgical intervention was performed. Fitting without and with knee units progresses as the child grows and length permits. Subsequent surgeries are often performed in addition to the Syme's amputation, including hip reconstruction, knee fusion to create a singular lever arm inside the prosthetic socket, and possibly epiphysiodeses to equalize femoral lengths at full maturity.

The third most common intervention for PFFD is to perform a rotationplasty of the foot 180° (Fig. 14-38). This procedure, popularized by Van Nes,[81] allows the child to use his or her ankle as a knee unit. To ensure success of a rotationplasty, the

hip joint and ankle joint integrity must not be compromised. The ankle dorsiflexors will be used as knee flexors, while the ankle plantar flexors will be used as knee extensors. It is critically important for these individuals to maintain ankle strength and range of motion in order for this procedure to be a success. Once again, the individual can be successfully fitted with a prosthesis that has outside hinges. They can also need an endoskeletal knee below the foot complex to provide increased knee flexion in order to enter tight spaces such as cars.

Longitudinal deficiency of the tibia

A longitudinal deficiency of the tibia is the last of the three more common lower limb deficiencies. Tibial deficiencies also present in many different forms, but are defined primarily by whether or not the tibia is completely or partially absent. This distinction, however, cannot be possible until the child is approximately 2 years of age, because of the slow ossification rate of the proximal tibial.

Partial longitudinal deficiency of the tibia has a variety of recommended surgical interventions, most of which result in amputation surgery below the knee. If the fibular section is much longer than the tibial section, a surgical synostosis (bone fusion) can be performed between the tibia and fibula, along with ablation of the foot, to create an ankle disarticulation-style limb. After osseous stabilization, these individuals would then require an ankle disarticulation prosthesis, with the benefit of having room at the distal end of their residual limb to incorporate a full-size prosthetic foot. If the fibula is approximately the same length as the tibia, the non-functional foot is usually amputated and the heel pad retained to provide a transtibial length residual limb with end-bearing capabilities. The outcomes of this level of amputation can be quite good, with a few minor complications. Often the tibia and fibula syndesmose (form a union between bones with fibrous connective tissue) distally, creating a union that grows medially. The proximal fibula then begins to grow proximally and laterally, creating a lateral projection of the fibular head and a 'varus-like' curvature to the limb.

A complete longitudinal deficiency of the tibia provides the clinic team with one of the most obvious surgical recommendations. A knee disarticulation amputation is almost always recommended for these children, as the fibular segment will not be able to sustain the weight of the individual at full maturity. The child is then be fitted with a knee disarticulation-style prosthesis following the amputation. These knee disarticulation fittings and components are similar to those described in the previous section on knee disarticulations. The one difference is that, early on in the fittings, the child will not have room for a knee, and smaller joints (e.g. upper limb single-pivot hinges) will be used for the child's articulation.

Hip disarticulation and hemipelvectomy
It is rare to see a child with a congenital hip disarticulation or hemipelvectomy. Many times, these anomalies are associated with other involvements, such as sacral agenesis. The selection of components for these younger children is quite limited, as is their ability to ambulate with the prostheses. It is essential for these children to remain well fitted, as any significant weight gain greatly decreases their ability to fit well into and ambulate with their prosthesis.

Acquired amputations
Trauma
There are many ways a child can receive a traumatic amputation; however, there are a few that occur more frequently than others. Accidents involving lawn mowers occur quite frequently and often psychologically involve additional family members in the trauma. Usually the child was invited to assist with or ride on a lawn mower, and a partial foot amputation was the unfortunate result. These levels of partial feet vary, and treatment is similar to that of adult partial foot amputations. Trains are also a source of traumatic amputations in children. There still exists a fairly large appeal for adolescents and teens to try and 'jump' on to trains. Transfemoral and bilateral transfemoral amputations often result from these failed attempts. These limbs are also fitted similar to those of the adult population.

Tumors
The two most common tumor-related reasons for amputation in children are osteogenic sarcoma and Ewing sarcoma. Osteogenic sarcoma can appear at any level, but is typically seen at or around the knee. The more common treatment for this malignancy is a transfemoral amputation above the site of the tumor. Ewing sarcoma traditionally is found higher in the lower limb. If individuals survive the treatment, they often must undergo a hip disarticulation amputation as part of the life-saving process.

Training and treatment goals
Training for children is, in most cases, playing outside and participating in daily activities. The initial training for children requiring prostheses below the knee is minimal. They will begin with a very abducted 'diaper gait' at first, and then progress to a more normal gait as they mature. Children with amputations above the knee, at various PFFD levels or hip disarticulation, require more formalized gait training. All these children are encouraged to use the prostheses for 'pull to stand' activities, which occur anywhere from 8 months to 18 months. The children's progress will be based on their limb lengths, strength, and range of motion in their affected limb.

The goal for children with ankle disarticulation and transtibial fittings is to ambulate with a 'normal gait'. Many of these children learn to walk very well and their gait goes unnoticed by the general population by the time they reach adolescence. The children with PFFD limbs and prostheses often have to sacrifice their gait earlier in life in order for their bones to grow to further lengths. When the timing is appropriate, epiphysiodeses and fusions can be performed to create singular limb segments inside the prosthesis. This affords the child better leverage and control of the prosthesis. Children with transfemoral and hip disarticulation levels are encouraged to achieve as normal a gait as possible. Many of the children with transfemoral amputations from a congenital deficiency, trauma, or tumor can achieve a fairly normal gait pattern. Children with hip disarticulations are not as successful, relying on assistive devices such as canes, crutches, and wheelchairs.

Psychosocial issues
The family
A child under the care of a family member or guardian creates situations outside the prosthetic fitting that directly affect what transpires during the fitting. The guilt of giving birth to a child with a congenital limb deficiency weighs heavily on many of the parents. Parents need frequent reassurance that they did nothing wrong during pregnancy to cause the deformity; indeed, the causative agent is rarely ever known. Involvement in support groups and larger clinical settings is strongly encouraged so that families realize the benefits of prosthetic fitting and their successful outcomes. If these groups or larger clinics do not exist in their area, contact with other families via telephone or in person can prove very beneficial to a parent or expecting parent of a child with a limb deficiency. Professional family or psychologic counseling should be recommended when needed, and genetic counseling can be reassuring to families, especially if more children are desired.

The child
The psychosocial adjustment of children with limb deficiencies varies greatly from child to child and from anomaly to anomaly. Some children are able to accept themselves as they are, and function in society regardless of what others might think or say.

Other children with congenital deficiencies or acquired amputations who become adults might attempt to hide their amputation and prosthetic fitting. This deception can drive some amputees to miss school or work, because they do not want their fellow classmates or coworkers to know about their need for a prosthesis. As with all amputees, the emotional well-being of the amputee should be closely monitored by the rehabilitation team. When problems occur, counseling, peer counseling, support groups, and even pharmacologic therapy should be initiated as needed.

REFERENCES

1. Adunsky A, Wershawski M, Arad M, et al. Non-traumatic lower limb older amputees: a database survey from a geriatric centre. Disabil Rehabil 2001; 23(2):80–84.

2. Aitken G. Proximal femoral focal deficiency: a congenital anomaly. Natl Acad Sci 1969: 1734.

3. Allende MF, Barnes GH, Levy SW, et al. The bacterial flora of the skin of amputation stumps. J Invest Dermatol 1961; 36:165–166.

4. [Anonymous]. Tarscon pocket pharmacopoeia. Lompoc: Tarascon Publishing; 2005.

5. Aulivola B, Hile CN, Hamdan AD, et al. Major lower limb amputation: outcome of a modern series. Arch Surg 2004; 139(4):395–399; discussion 399.

6. Bacharach JM, Rooke TW, Osmundson PJ, et al. Predictive value of transcutaneous oxygen pressure and amputation success by use of supine and elevation measurements. J Vasc Surg 1992; 15(3):558–563.

7. Backonja MM. Anticonvulsants (antineuropathics) for neuropathic pain syndromes. Clin J Pain 2000; 16(2 suppl):S67–S72.

8. Baron R. Peripheral neuropathic pain: from mechanisms to symptoms. Clin J Pain 2000; 16(2 suppl):S12–S20.

9. Bennett GJ. Neuropathic pain. In: Wall PD, Melzack R, eds. Textbook of pain. Edinburgh: Churchill Livingstone; 1994:201–224.

10. Bone M, Critchley P, Buggy DJ. Gabapentin in postamputation phantom limb pain: a randomized, double-blind, placebo-controlled, cross-over study. Reg Anesth Pain Med 2002; 27(5):481–486.

11. Boyd H. Anatomic disarticulation of the hip. Surg Gynecol Obstet 1947; 84:346–349.

12. Bradley N, Miller WA, Evans JP. Plantar neuroma: analysis of results following surgical excision in 145 patients. South Med J 1976; 69(7):853–854.

13. Brodzka WK, Thornhill HL, Zarapkar SE, et al. Long-term function of persons with atherosclerotic bilateral below-knee amputation living in the inner city. Arch Phys Med Rehabil 1990; 71(11):895–900.

14. Burgess EM, Romano RL. The management of lower limb amputees using immediate postsurgical prostheses. Clin Orthop 1968; 57:137–146.

15. Canfield JA, Reiber GE, Cannard C, et al. Survival following lower-limb amputation in a veteran population. J Rehabil Res Dev 2001; 38(3): 341–345.

16. Cohen SI, Goldman LD, Salzman EW, et al. The deleterious effect of immediate postoperative prosthesis in below-knee amputation for ischemic disease. Surgery 1974; 76(6):992–1001.

17. Davis RW. Phantom sensation, phantom pain, and stump pain. Arch Phys Med Rehabil 1993; 74(1):79–91.

18. Devor M. The pathophysiology of damaged peripheral nerves. In: Wall PD, Melzack R, eds. Textbook of pain. Edinburgh: Churchill Livingstone; 1994:79–100.

19. Dillingham TR, Pezzin LE, MacKenzie EJ. Limb amputation and limb deficiency: epidemiology and recent trends in the United States. South Med J 2002; 95(8):875–883.

20. Disabled Sports USA. Blazing Marlon Shirley beats 11-second barrier. Challenge 2003; summer:16.

21. Durable Medical Equipment Regional Committees. Region A Medicare News 1994; Dec(14).

22. Dwars BJ, van den Broek TA, Rauwerda JA, et al. Criteria for reliable selection of the lowest level of amputation in peripheral vascular disease. J Vasc Surg 1992; 15(3):536–542.

23. Ebskov B, Josephsen P. Incidence of reamputation and death after gangrene of the lower limb. Prosthet Orthot Int 1980; 4(2):77–80.

24. Edelson J, Fitzpatrick JL. A comparison of cognitive-behavioral and hypnotic treatments of chronic pain. J Clin Psychol 1989; 45(2):316–323.

25. Eggers PW, Gohdes D, Pugh J. Nontraumatic lower limb amputations in the medicare end-stage renal disease population. Kidney Int 1999; 56(4): 1524–1533.

26. Ehde DM, Czerniecki JM, Smith DG, et al. Chronic phantom sensations, phantom pain, residual limb pain, and other regional pain after lower limb amputation. Arch Phys Med Rehabil 2000; 81(8):1039–1044.

27. Eneroth M. Improved wound healing in transtibial amputees receiving supplementary nutrition. Paper presented at the Xth World Congress of the International Society for Prosthetics and Orthotics, Amsterdam, 28 June–3 July 1998.

28. English R. Removable rigid dressing for transtibial amputees: a randomized study. Paper presented at the Xth World Congress of the International Society for Prosthetics and Orthotics, Glasgow, 1–6 July 2001.

29. Fields HL, Heinricher MM, Mason P. Neurotransmitters in nociceptive modulatory circuits. Ann Rev Neurosci 1991; 14:219–245.

30. Finsen V, Persen L, Lovlien M, et al. Transcutaneous electrical nerve stimulation after major amputation. J Bone Joint Surg Br 1988; 70(1):109–112.

31. Fletcher DD, Andrews KL, Butters MA, et al. Rehabilitation of the geriatric vascular amputee patient: a population-based study. Arch Phys Med Rehabil 2001; 82(6):776–779.

32. Fletcher DD, Andrews KL, Hallett JW Jr, et al. Trends in rehabilitation after amputation for geriatric patients with vascular disease: implications for future health resource allocation. Arch Phys Med Rehabil 2002; 83(10):1389–1393.

33. Flor H. Cortical reorganisation and chronic pain: implications for rehabilitation. J Rehabil Med 2003; 41(suppl):66–72.

34. Frank RG, Kashani JH, Kashani SR, et al. Psychological response to amputation as a function of age and time since amputation. Br J Psychiatry 1984; 144:493–497.

35. Froster UG, Baird PA. Congenital defects of lower limbs and associated malformations: a population based study. Am J Med Genet 1993; 45(1): 60–64.

36. Gauthier-Gagnon C, Grise MC, Potvin D. Enabling factors related to prosthetic use by people with transtibial and transfemoral amputation. Arch Phys Med Rehabil 1999; 80(6):706–713.

37. Gottschalk F. Transfemoral amputation. In: Bowker J, Michael J, eds. The atlas of limb prosthetics: surgical, prosthetic, and rehabilitation principle. 2nd edn. St. Louis: Mosby; 1992:509–533.

38. Greenfield J, Rea J Jr, Ilfeld FW. Morton's interdigital neuroma. Indications for treatment by local injections versus surgery. Clin Orthop 1984; May(185):142–144.

39. Harden RN. Gabapentin: a new tool in the treatment of neuropathic pain. Acta Neurol Scand 1999; 173(suppl):43–47.

40. Hoyt C, Littig D, Lundt J, et al. The UCLA CAT-CAM above-knee socket. Los Angeles: UCLA Prosthetics Education and Research Program; 1987.

41. Jänig W. Pathophysiology of nerve following mechanical injury in man. In: Dubner R, Gebhart GF, Bond M, eds. Pain research and clinical management. Amsterdam: Elsevier; 1988:89–108.

42. Johannesson A, Larsson GU, Oberg T. From major amputation to prosthetic outcome: a prospective study of 190 patients in a defined population. Prosthet Orthot Int 2004; 28(1):9–21.

43. Kuiken T, Huang M, Harden N. Peri-operative rehabilitation of the transtibial and transfemoral amputee. Phys Med Rehabil: State Art Rev 2002; 16(3):521–537.

44. Larsson G. Post-operative treatment with silicone liner in 176 amputees. Paper presented at the Xth World Congress of the International Society for Prosthetics and Orthotics, Glasgow, 1–6 July 2001.

45. Levy CE, Bryant PR, Spires MC, et al. Acquired limb deficiencies. 4. Troubleshooting. Arch Phys Med Rehabil 2001; 82(3 suppl 1):S25–S30.

46. Levy S. Skin problems in the amputee. In: Smith DG, Michael J, Bowker JH, eds. Atlas of amputations and limb deficiencies. Rosemont: American Academy of Orthopaedic Surgeons; 2004:701–710.

47. Levy S. Skin problems of the amputee. In: Bowker JH, ed. Atlas of limb prosthetics: surgical, prosthetic, and rehabilitation principles. St. Louis: Mosby; 1992.

48. Loeser J. Pain after amputation: phantom limb and stump pain. In: Bonica J, ed. The management of pain. London: Churchill Livingstone; 1994: 244–256.

49. Loeser JD, Black RG, Christman A. Relief of pain by transcutaneous stimulation. J Neurosurg 1975; 42(3):308–314.

50. MacKenzie EJ, Bosse MJ, Castillo RC, et al. Functional outcomes following trauma-related lower-limb amputation. J Bone Joint Surg Am 2004; 86A(8):1636–1645.

51. Melzack R, Wall PD. Pain mechanisms: a new theory. Science 1965; 150:971–979.

52. Melzack R. The tragedy of needless pain. Science 1990; 262:27–33.

53. Muilenberg AC, Wilson AB. A manual for above-knee amputees. Alexandria: American Academy of Orthotists and Prosthetists; 1989:6.

54. Murray L, ed. Physician's desk reference 2004. 58th edn. Montvale: Thompson PDR; 2004.

55. Ng D, Berbrayer E, Hunter G, et al. Transtibial amputation: preoperative vascular assessment and functional outcome. J Prosthet Orthot 1996; 8(4):123–129.

56. Nielsen D, Shurr D, Golden J, et al. Comparison of energy cost and gait efficiency during ambulation in below-knee amputees using different prosthetic feet—a preliminary report. J Prosthet Orthot 1988; 1(1): 24–31.

57. Oakley DA, Whitman LG, Halligan PW. Hypnotic imagery as a treatment for phantom limb pain: two case reports and a review. Clin Rehabil 2002; 16(4):368–377.

58. Ortiz M. Medical ramus containment socket design for transfemoral prosthesis. Paper presented at the American Academy of Orthotists and Prosthetists Annual Meeting and Scientific Symposium, 2004.

59. Ouriel K, Green R. Arterial disease. In: Shires EA, ed. Principles of surgery. 7th edn. New York: McGraw Hill; 1999:931–1003.

60. Patterson JF. Carbamazepine in the treatment of phantom limb pain. South Med J 1988; 81(9):1100–1102.

61. Pinzur MS, Littooy F, Daniels J, et al. Multidisciplinary preoperative assessment and late function in dysvascular amputees. Clin Orthop Relat Res 1992; Aug(281):239–243.

62. Radcliffe C, Foort J. The patellar-tendon-bearing below-knee prosthesis. San Francisco–Berkeley: University of California Biomechanics Laboratory; 1961.

63. Radcliffe C. Functional considerations in the fitting of above-knee prostheses. Artif Limbs 1955; 1:35–60.

64. Raymond S, Rocco A. Ephaptic coupling of large fibers as a clue to mechanisms in chronic neuropathic allodynia following damage to dorsal roots. Pain 1990; 5:S276.

65. Reiber G, Boyko E, Smith D. Lower limb foot ulcers and amputations in diabetes. In: Harris M, Cowie C, et al, eds. Diabetes in America. 2nd edn. Washington: National Institutes of Health; 1995:409–428.

66. Reiber GE, Smith DG, Carter J, et al. A comparison of diabetic foot ulcer patients managed in VHA and non-VHA settings. J Rehabil Res Dev 2001; 38(3):309–317.

67. Resnick HE, Valsania P, Phillips CL. Diabetes mellitus and nontraumatic lower limb amputation in black and white Americans: the National Health and Nutrition Examination Survey epidemiologic follow-up study, 1971–1992. Arch Intern Med 1999; 159(20):2470–2475.

68. Robinson LR, Czerniecki JM, Ehde DM, et al. Trial of amitriptyline for relief of pain in amputees: results of a randomized controlled study. Arch Phys Med Rehabil 2004; 85(1):1–6.

69. Rybarczyk B, Nicholas J, Nyenhuis D. Coping with a leg amputation: integrating research and clinical practice. Rehabil Psychol 1997; 42(3): 241–256.

70. Sabolich J. Contoured adducted trochanteric-controlled alignment method (CAT-CAM): introduction and basic principles. Clin Prosthet Orthot 1985; 9:15–26.

71. Schechtman L, Kuiken T, Harden N. Phantom limb pain treatment with mirtazapine: a case series. Arch Phys Med Rehabil 2002; 83:1668.

72. Scully S, Harrelson J. Amputation and limb substitution. In: Sabiston D, ed. Textbook of surgery: the biological basis of modern surgical practice. 15th edn. Philadelphia: Saunders; 1997:1452–1458.

73. Sherman RA, Gall N, Gormly J. Treatment of phantom limb pain with muscular relaxation training to disrupt the pain–anxiety–tension cycle. Pain 1979; 6(1):47–55.

74. Siegel EF. Control of phantom limb pain by hypnosis. Am J Clin Hypn 1979; 21(4):285–286.

75. Smith DG, Ehde DM, Legro MW, et al. Phantom limb, residual limb, and back pain after lower limb amputations. Clin Orthop 1999; 361:29–38.

76. Smith DG, McFarland LV, Sangeorzan BJ, et al. Postoperative dressing and management strategies for transtibial amputations: a critical review. J Rehabil Res Dev 2003; 40(3):213–224.

77. Thornhill HL, Jones GD, Brodzka W, et al. Bilateral below-knee amputations: experience with 80 patients. Arch Phys Med Rehabil 1986; 67(3): 159–163.

78. Trautner C, Haastert B, Giani G, et al. Amputations and diabetes: a case-control study. Diabet Med 2002; 19(1):35–40.

79. Tremont-Lukats IW, Megeff C, Backonja MM. Anticonvulsants for neuropathic pain syndromes: mechanisms of action and place in therapy. Drugs 2000; 60(5):1029–1052.

80. Uellendahl J, Edwards M, Uellendahl E. Northwestern University transfemoral fitting manual: ischial containment above-knee prosthesis. Chicago: Northwestern University Prosthetic Certification Program; 1998.

81. Van Nes C. Rotation-plasty for congenital defects of the femur: making use of the ankle shortened limb to control the knee joint of a prosthesis. J Bone Joint Surg 1950; 32B:12–16.

82. Wagman L, Terz J. Translumbar amputation (hemicorpectomy). In: Bowker J, Michael J, eds. Atlas of limb prosthetics: surgical, prosthetic, and rehabilitation principles. St. Louis: Mosby; 1992:553–562.

83. Waters RL, Mulroy S. The energy expenditure of normal and pathologic gait. Gait Posture 1999; 9(3):207–231.

84. Waters RL, Perry J, Antonelli D, et al. Energy cost of walking of amputees: the influence of level of amputation. J Bone Joint Surg Am 1976; 58(1): 42–46.

85. Waters RL, Perry J, Chambers R. Energy expenditure of amputee gait. In: Moore W, Malone JM, eds. Lower limb amputation. Philadelphia: Saunders; 1989:250–260.

86. Wu Y, Brncick MD, Krick HJ, et al. Interim prosthesis for below-knee amputees. Bull Prosthet Res 1981; 10–36,40–45.

87. Wu Y, Keagy RD, Krick HJ, et al. An innovative removable rigid dressing technique for below-the-knee amputation. J Bone Joint Surg Am 1979; 61(5):724–729.w

Chapter

15

Upper Limb Orthotic Devices

Atul T. Patel and Laura M. Garber

This chapter provides a guide for prescribing and the basic principles for using upper limb orthotic devices, commonly known as splints or braces. The word *orthosis* (derived from the Greek *orthos*, meaning to correct or make straight) encompasses the full spectrum of devices currently fabricated by therapists and orthotists. As defined by the International Standards Organization of the International Society for Prosthetics and Orthotics, an orthosis is any externally applied device used to modify structural and functional characteristics of the neuromuscular skeletal system.[18] *Orthosis*—or, alternatively, *orthotic device*[12]—is the preferred term. The terms *splint* and *brace* are less preferred because they imply mere immobilization, and do not suggest either improved function or restoration of mobility. But these terms remain common, and in this chapter we use the terms orthotic device and splint interchangeably.

PRINCIPLES AND INDICATIONS

The objectives of upper limb orthotic applications can be classified into three major areas: protection, correction, and assistance with function.

- Protection: orthotic devices can provide compressive forces and traction in a controlled manner, protecting the impaired joint or body part. Restricting or preventing joint motion allows for corrective alignment and serves to prevent deformity. Protective orthoses can also stabilize unstable bony components and promote healing of soft tissues and bones. Traction forces can permit joint motion, with decreased compressive forces applied to the joint cartilage and maintain soft tissue length.
- Correction: orthoses help in correcting joint contractures and subluxation of joints or tendons, thus preventing or reducing joint deformities.
- Assistance with function: orthoses can assist function by compensating for deformity, muscle weakness, or increased muscle tone.

Physicians prescribe orthotic devices based on their knowledge of diagnosis and preferred treatment. Other health professionals, including occupational therapists and orthotists, are involved in the design and application of these devices.

CLASSIFICATION

We use many different terms to describe upper limb orthotic devices. We call them by the joint they cover, the function they provide (e.g. immobilization), or the condition they treat. Some are named by their appearance (e.g. banjo or sugar tong), and still others bear the name of the person who designed them (e.g. Kleinert).[17]

Most splints are known by their common names (see Table 15-1)—names that have evolved over time. But such names are not fully informative, are not systematic, and are not even universally accepted. And this lack of a universally accepted terminology often presents a communication barrier between the physician and other health professionals. Consequently, more systematic naming systems have been developed—naming systems that classify orthotic devices according to anatomic region or to purpose and function. Table 15-1 compares the common names of several orthotic devices with those in three other naming systems.

The simplest naming system is that developed by the International Organization for Standards (ISO). It reports the anatomic region the orthotic device encompasses. A wrist–hand orthosis, for example, is called a WHO.[19] This system, however, fails to define the purpose or function of the orthosis.

In 1992, the American Society of Hand Therapists (ASHT) published the ASHT *Splint Classification System* (SCS).[1] This system provides standard nomenclature for splints based on function. It classifies splints by characteristics (e.g. articular or non-articular) and location of the body part covered. A humeral fracture brace, for example, is identified as a non-articular splint—humerus (see Table 15-1). It also identifies the direction of the force applied, and whether the splint is for mobilization, immobilization, or restriction. In this system, a long arm splint (Fig. 15-1) is characterized as a 45° elbow flexion immobilization. In addition, this system provides a way to indicate the number of primary and secondary joints. A primary joint is the anatomic joint affected by a splint, while a secondary joint is a joint included in a splint to provide counterforce control, position, or stabilization of joint(s) immediately adjacent to primary articular structures. The numbering system is indicated by the word 'type'. The number that follows the word 'type' indicates the number of secondary joints involved, while the number in brackets is the total number of joints included in the

Table 15-1 Nomenclature systems in current use

Common name	American Society of Hand Therapists *Splint Classification System*[1]	International Organization for Standards[19]	McKee and Morgan[17]
Humeral fracture brace	Non-articular splint—humerus	Not applicable	Circumferential non-articular humerus-stabilizing
Tennis elbow splint or brace	Non-articular splint—proximal forearm	Elbow orthosis (EO)	Circumferential non-articular proximal forearm strap
Long arm splint	45° elbow flexion immobilization; type 1[1]	Shoulder–elbow–wrist–hand orthosis (SEWHO)	Posterior static elbow–wrist orthosis
Resting hand splint	Index through small finger proximal interphalangeal (PIP) extension, thumb carpometacarpal (CMC) palmar abduction mobilization; type 3[16]	Wrist–hand orthosis (WHO)	Volar forearm-based static (or serial static) wrist–hand orthosis
Ulnar deviation splint	Index through small finger metacarpophalangeal (MCP) extension–radial deviation mobilization; type 0[4]	Hand orthosis (HO)	Circumferential hand-based dynamic traction D2–5 MCP corrective radial deviation orthosis
Kleinert splint, modified Kleinert splint, postoperative flexor tendon splint	Wrist, MCP, PIP, distal interphalangeal (DIP) flexion immobilization–extension restriction; type 0[13]	WHO	Dorsal forearm-based dynamic MCP–interphalangeal (IP) protective flexion and MCP extension-blocking orthosis
Duran splint, postoperative flexor tendon splint	Wrist and finger flexion immobilization; type 0[4]	WHO	Dorsal forearm-based static MCP–IP protective flexion and MCP extension-blocking orthosis
Postoperative dynamic extensor tendon splint	Wrist, MCP, PIP, DIP extension immobilization–flexion restriction; type 0[13]	WHO	Volar–dorsal forearm-based dynamic MCP–IP protective extension and flexion-blocking orthosis
Swan neck splint	Index finger PIP extension restriction; type 0[1]	Finger orthosis (FO)	Finger-based static PIP extension-blocking orthosis
Postoperative MCP arthroplasty splint, Swanson splint	Index through small finger MCP extension–radial deviation mobilization; type 1[5]	Wrist–hand–finger orthosis (WHFO)	Dorsal forearm-based dynamic D2–5 MCP assisted extension–radial deviation orthosis
Radial nerve palsy splint	Wrist extension, MCP flexion mobilization or MCP flexion, wrist extension mobilization; type 0[5]	WHFO	Dorsal forearm-based dynamic low-profile wrist and D1–5 MCP assistive extension orthosis
Ulnar nerve palsy splint	Ring though small finger MCP extension restriction; type 0[2]	Hand-finger orthosis (HFO)	Circumferential hand-based dynamic joint-aligned coil spring D4–5 MCP assistive flexion orthosis
Median nerve palsy splint	Index through small finger MCP flexion mobilization and thumb CMC opposition mobilization; type 0[5]	HFO	Circumferential hand-based dynamic joint-aligned coil spring D2–5 MCP assistive flexion and thumb assistive opposition orthosis
Flail arm splint	Not classified	SEWHO	Not classified
Dynamic finger flexion splint, forearm-based	Index through small finger MCP flexion mobilization; type 3[7]	WHFO	Volar hand-based dynamic MCP corrective-flexion orthosis
Dynamic finger final flexion splint, hand-based	Index through small finger flexion mobilization; type 0[12]	WHFO	Volar forearm-based dynamic MCP, PIP, DIP corrective-flexion orthosis

Continued on page 327

Continued from page 326 Table 15-1	Nomenclature systems in current use		
Common name	American Society of Hand Therapists *Splint Classification System*[1]	International Organization for Standards[19]	McKee and Morgan[17]
Dynamic finger extension splint, forearm-based	Index through small PIP and DIP extension mobilization; type 2[13]	WHFO	Volar forearm-based dynamic MCP, PIP, DIP corrective-extension orthosis
Dynamic finger extension splint, hand-based	Index through small finger extension mobilization; type 0[12]	WHFO	Circumferential hand-based dynamic D4–5 MCP, PIP, DIP assistive flexion orthosis
Static progressive splint	Index finger MCP flexion mobilization; type 1[4]	WHFO	Volar forearm-based static progressive MERiT screw MCP flexion orthosis
Dynamic wrist flexion splint	Wrist flexion mobilization; type 0[1]	WHO	Dorsal forearm-based dynamic joint-aligned wrist assistive flexion orthosis
Dynamic wrist extension splint	Wrist extension mobilization; type 0[1]	WHO	Dorsal forearm-based dynamic joint-aligned wrist assistive extension orthosis
Rehabilitation Institute of Chicago tenodesis splint	Not classified	Functional orthosis	Volar forearm-based tenodesis WHO
Elbow flexion splint	Elbow flexion mobilization; type 0[1]	Elbow–wrist orthosis (EWO)	Posterior dynamic elbow corrective flexion orthosis
Elbow extension splint	Elbow extension mobilization; type 0[1]	EWO	Anterior serial static elbow corrective extension orthosis
Dynamic pronation–supination splint	Forearm pronation–supination mobilization; type 2[3]	Elbow–wrist–hand orthosis (EWHO)	Posterior forearm-based dynamic radius–ulna corrective pronation–supination orthosis
Wrist splint, carpal tunnel splint	Wrist extension immobilization; type 0[1]	Wrist orthosis (WO)	Volar forearm-based static wrist orthosis
Thumb spica splint	Thumb MCP extension immobilization; type 2[3]	Wrist–thumb orthosis (WHFO)	Volar forearm-based static wrist–thumb orthosis
Mallet finger splint, DIP extension splint, Stax splint	Index finger DIP extension immobilization; type 0[3]	FO	Volar finger-based static DIP flexion-blocking orthosis
Capener splint	PIP extension mobilization; type 0[1]	FO	Three-point finger-based dynamic joint-aligned coil spring PIP corrective extension orthosis
Figure of eight harness	Non-articular splint—axilla	Shoulder orthosis (SO)	Figure of eight non-articular axilla orthosis
Airplane splint, gunslinger splint	Shoulder abduction immobilization; type 3[4]	SEWHO	Lateral trunk-based static shoulder–elbow–wrist orthosis
Mobile arm support	Not classified	SEWHO	Not classified
Orthosis sugar tong	Elbow extension immobilization; type 3[4]	SEWHO	Bivalved static elbow orthosis

splint—the sum of the primary joints plus the secondary joints. Consider, for example, a thumb spica splint, forearm-based (Fig. 15-2), which is commonly used for de Quervain's stenosing tenosynovitis. In the ASHT *Splint Classification System*, this splint is known as a thumb metacarpophalangeal (MCP) extension immobilization; type 2[3]. *Type 2* refers to the two secondary joints covered, i.e. the wrist and thumb carpometacarpal (CMC) joint. The number in brackets, *[3]*, refers to the total number of joints covered: the thumb MCP joint, plus the wrist, plus the thumb CMC joint).

DESIGN CATEGORIES

Orthotic devices can be classified by the support or forces provided to improve motion or function. Categories of splint design are as follow.[17]

Non-articular

This type of splint provides support to a body part without crossing any joints, and protects a bone or body part. For example, a humeral fracture splint provides circumferential

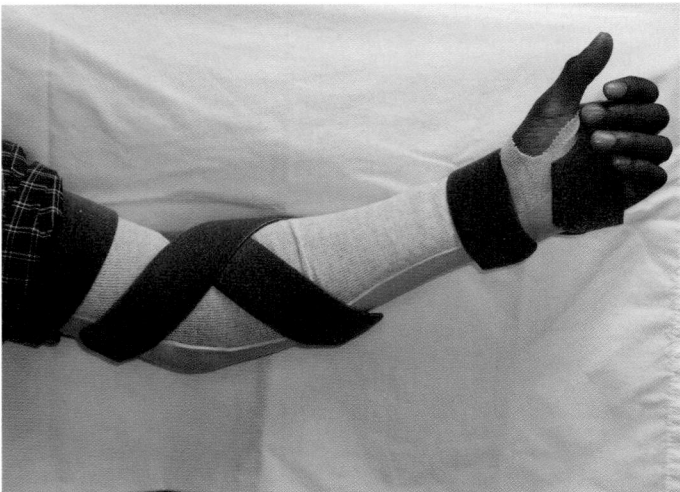

Figure 15-1 Long arm splint used for cubital tunnel syndrome.

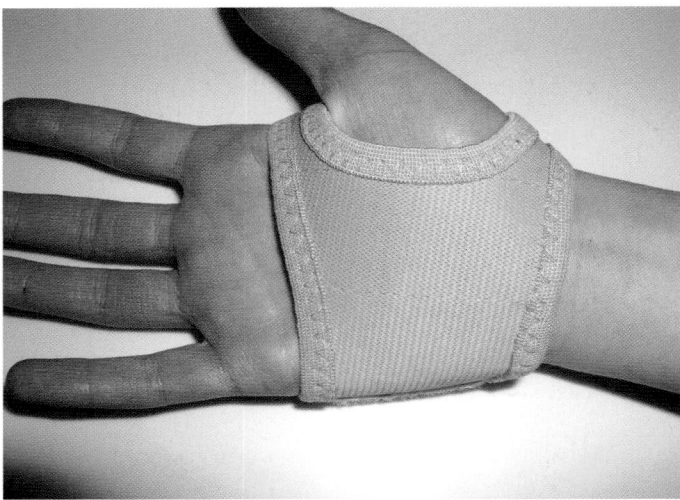

Figure 15-3 Gel shell splint.

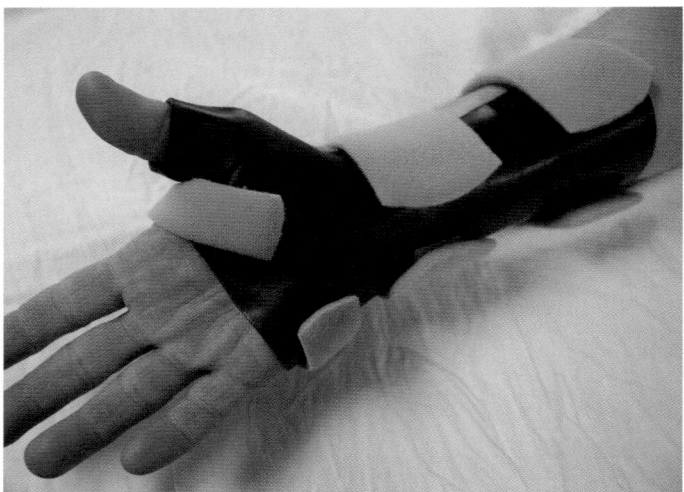

Figure 15-2 Forearm-based thumb spica splint used for de Quervain's stenosing tenosynovitis.

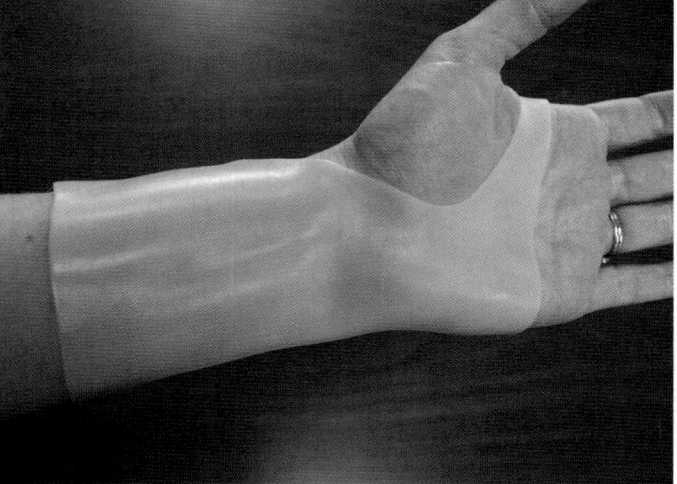

Figure 15-4 Wrist splint for carpal tunnel syndrome, with the wrist in a position of 0–5° of extension; distal palmar crease free to allow for full metacarpophalangeal motion.

support to the upper arm during fracture healing. Other examples are a sugar tong splint to immobilize a proximal radius fracture, or a gel shell splint (Fig. 15-3) to exert pressure over a healing scar to prevent hypertrophic scarring.

Static

This type of splint provides static support to hold a joint or joints stationary. For example, a volar wrist splint for acute carpal tunnel syndrome reduces motion and rests injured tissues (Fig. 15-4). Static splints can be used to protect healing structures (Fig. 15-5), to decrease or prevent deformity, and to reduce tone in spastic muscles.

Serial static

This splint is also static but is periodically changed to alter the joint angle at which the splint is positioned. For example, a wrist splint is changed periodically to increase extension in a

wrist with a flexion contracture after a wrist fracture. This serial repositioning provides a prolonged gentle stretch to involved structures, permitting a stiff joint to regain motion.

Static motion-blocking

This type of splint permits motion in one direction but blocks motion in another. For example, a swan neck splint (Figs 15-6 and 15-7) is designed to allow flexion but to block hyperextension of the proximal interphalangeal (PIP) joint. (See the section on *Rheumatoid arthritis*.)

Static progressive

This type of splinting is the one most commonly used for regaining joint motion. Unlike the serial static splint, the orthosis is not remolded to increase joint motion. Instead, it uses a static (non-elastic) line of pull that is tightened periodically to

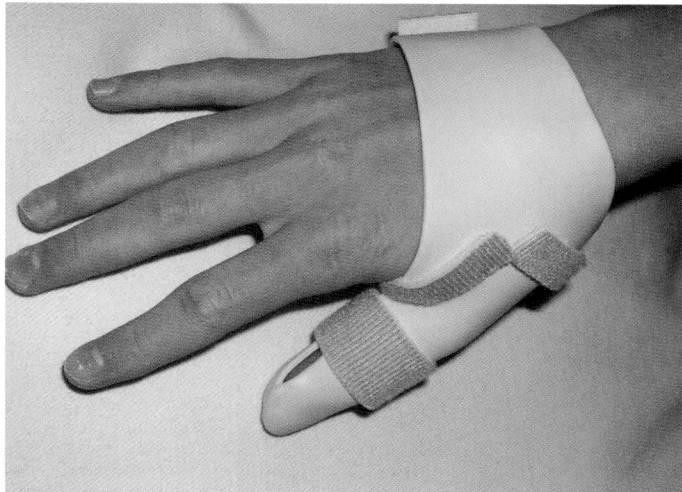

Figure 15-5 Hand-based static thumb splint with interphalangeal included for immobilization of a distal phalanx fracture.

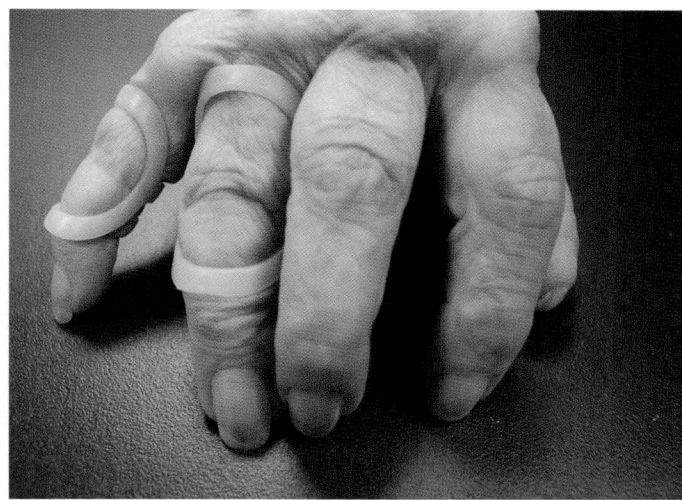

Figure 15-7 Swan neck splint: Oval 8 product of 3-Point Products; note that the deformity reduced.

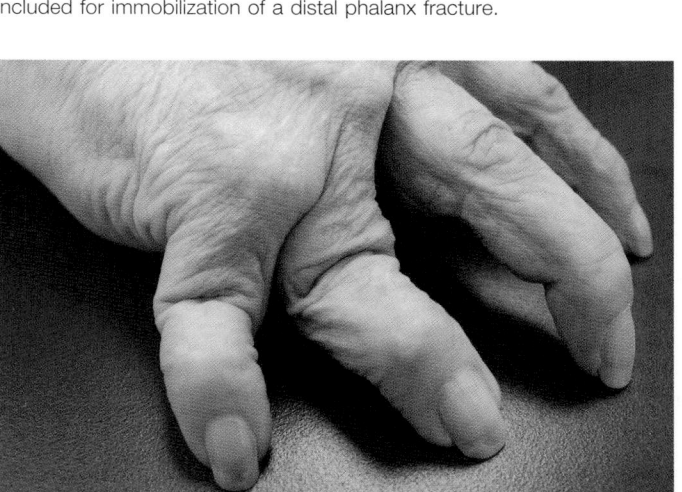

Figure 15-6 Swan neck deformity with no splint support on.

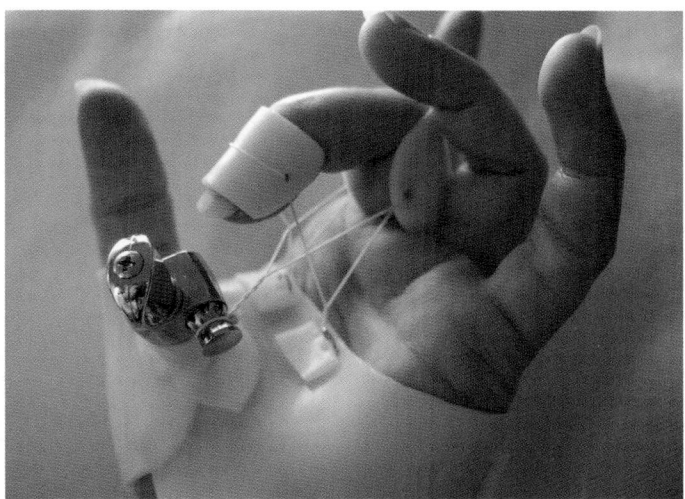

Figure 15-8 Static progressive flexion splint using a MERiT component.

increase tissue length. One such device is similar in principle to a tuning screw on a guitar. The MERiT static progressive component[2] (available commercially) decreases the static line length as it is turned, thereby increasing the range of joint motion (Fig. 15-8). This type of splinting uses the principle advocated by Kenneth Flowers and Paul LaStayo,[10] placing the joint in a position of stretch to regain motion. As the joint begins to regain motion, the wearer can then increase the tension on the line (Fig. 15-9). The joint is then statically held in this position using the principle of total end-range time (TERT), the length of time the joint is held at the end of its range. The longer the TERT, the more quickly a contracture resolves.[11] This type of pull has been extremely effective in regaining joint motion, particularly in very stiff joints.

Dynamic

This type of splint provides an elastic force to regain motion. An example of such an orthosis is a Capener splint, which uses

a spring coil assist to increase extension in a PIP joint with a mild contracture (Fig. 15-10).

Dynamic motion-blocking

This type of splint allows certain motions but blocks others. It utilizes a passive, elastic line of pull in the desired direction but permits active motion in the opposite direction. An example is a Kleinert postoperative splint for flexor tendon repairs (Fig. 15-11). It passively pulls the finger into flexion with an elastic thread or rubber band. It allows active digital extension, while parts of the splint block full extension of the MCP joint and the wrist.

Dynamic traction splints

This type of splint offers traction to a joint while allowing controlled motion. An example is a splint for an intraarticular fracture, often called a Schenck splint (Fig. 15-12), which gives

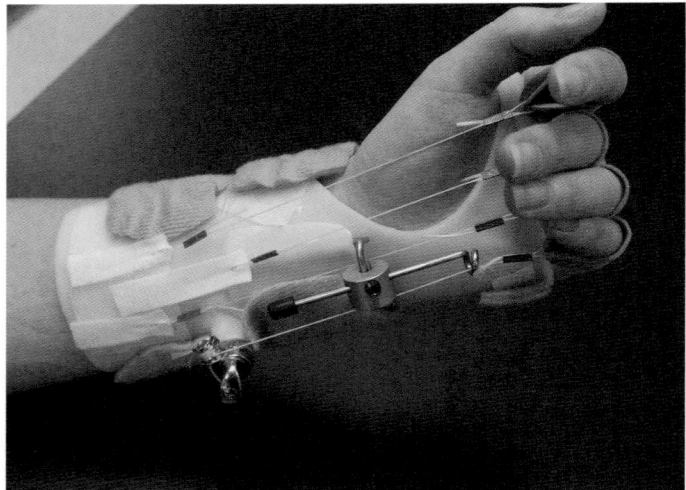

Figure 15-9 Forearm-based splint with both static line pull and MERiT component for increasing metacarpophalangeal flexion.

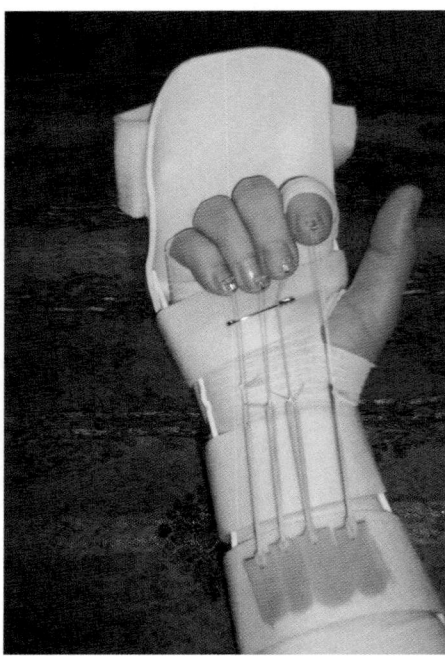

Figure 15-11 Kleinert splint used for postoperative care for patients with flexor tendon injuries. It allows for passive flexion, holding digits flexed at rest.

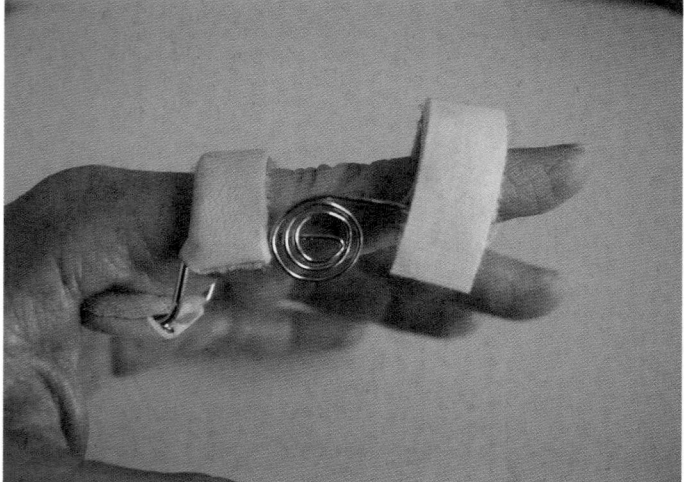

Figure 15-10 Capener splint for increasing joint extension in the proximal interphalangeal joint of the finger.

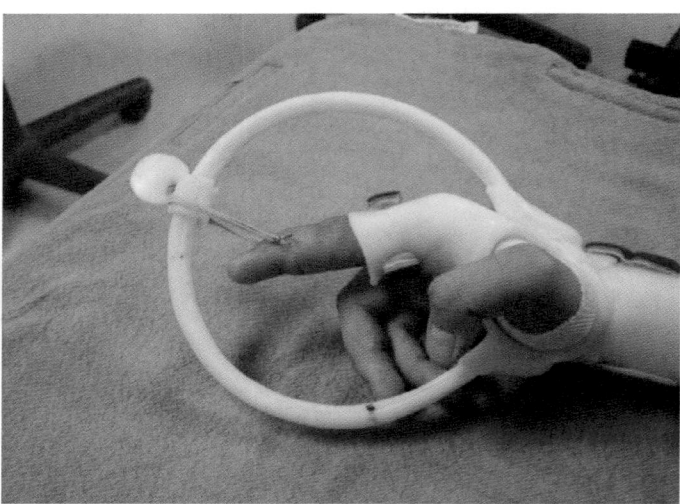

Figure 15-12 Schenck design splint used for intraarticular fracture, placing dynamic traction on the digits while allowing for passive range of motion. (Courtesy of Kelly Mikle, O.T.R./L., C.H.T.)

constant longitudinal traction while the joint is gently flexed and extended.

Tenodesis

This type of splint facilitates function in a hand that has lost motion due to nervous system injury. An example is the Rehabilitation Institute of Chicago tenodesis splint (Figs 15-13 and 15-14), which assists the patient with a C6 spinal cord injury to achieve a functional pinch. Active extension of the wrist produces, through tenodesis action, controlled passive flexion of the fingers against a static thumb post.

Continuous passive motion orthoses

These are electrically powered devices that mechanically move joints through a desired range of motion. This keeps the joints supple and maintains articular, ligamentous, and tendinous structure mobility during the healing phases following injury or surgery.

Adaptive or functional usage

These devices promote functional use of the upper limb with impairment due to weakness, paralysis, or loss of a body part. An example is the universal cuff, which encompasses the hand and holds various small items, such as a fork, a pen, or a toothbrush. This cuff allows patients to manipulate these items, known as activities of daily living tools, and enhances their degree of independence.

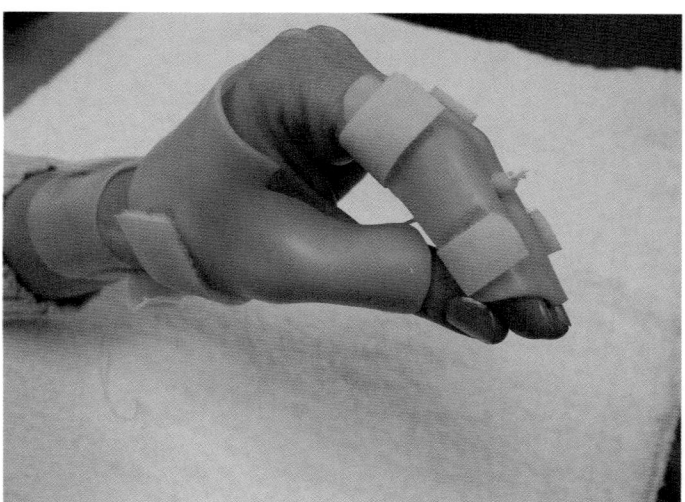

Figure 15-13 Rehabilitation Institute of Chicago tenodesis splint, used for functional pinch during activities of daily living; pinching to thumb post.

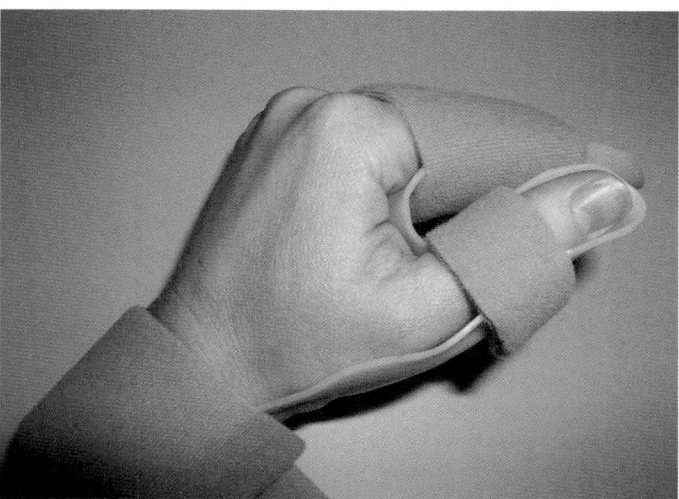

Figure 15-15 Splint often used with burn patients, used to position the hand and wrist, keeping the metacarpophalangeal joints flexed and the interphalangeal joint extended with the wrist in slight extension.

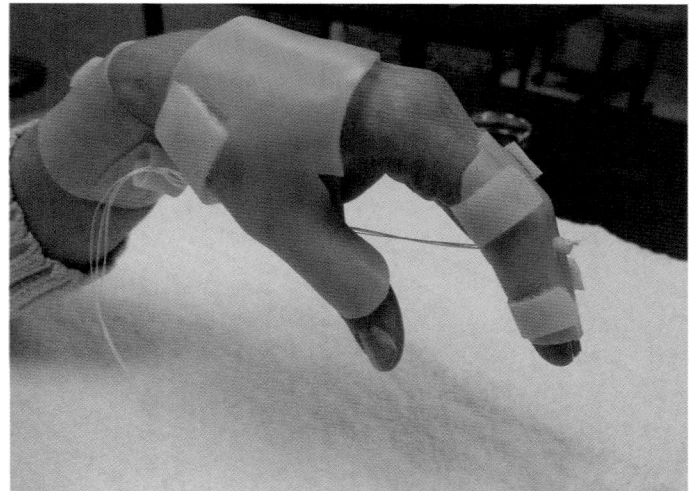

Figure 15-14 Rehabilitation Institute of Chicago tenodesis splint, used for functional pinch during activities of daily living; relaxation, allowing hand to fall into flexion, opens fingers through tenodesis action.

BIOMECHANICAL CONSIDERATIONS

Healthcare personnel involved in the fabrication and application of an orthotic device need a good understanding of biomechanics and anatomy as well as the physiologic response to tissue healing. They also need technical and creative skills that allow them to design and fabricate orthotic devices that win patient acceptance and meet treatment goals. In the USA, upper limb splinting is performed by occupational therapists, certified hand therapists, orthotists, and some physical therapists. The physician ordering these devices needs to understand the technical factors involved in fabrication and fitting. Some of these are listed here.

- When increasing joint range of motion with splinting, the angle of pull needs to be perpendicular to the bony axis that is being mobilized.[6] If this is not taken into account, forces on the skin and underlying structures can be sufficient to cause injury through excessive pressure on the skin and deforming stresses on the underlying healing structures.
- Wrist position is an important consideration in the design of a splint.[17] Power grasp is most effectively achieved when the wrist is extended and radially deviated slightly. When writing, most right-handed individuals extend the wrist; however, many left-handed individuals place their wrists in slight flexion. All these examples indicate that individual considerations of wrist position can be paramount in fabricating a wrist orthosis.
- To maintain tissue length through static positioning, one needs to consider the ligamentous structures involved, the anatomic angle of pull on structures, and the positions that may produce deformity. For example, when the hand is made non-functional after a dorsal burn, the MCP joints tend toward hyperextension. This position alters the tension on the collateral ligaments of the MCP joints and puts them at risk of shortening, with subsequent loss of full flexion. In such a case, it is imperative to place the MCP joints in full flexion and the interphalangeal (IP) joints in extension. The wrist should also be placed in slight extension to maintain flexor tendon length and to improve hand function (Fig. 15-15).
- A study by Flowers and LaStayo demonstrated the TERT principle: that is, the improvement in range of motion is directly proportional to the length of time a joint is held at its end range.[10] This principle is used with static progressive splinting, as noted previously. They also emphasize that the clinically safe amount of force covers a very narrow range.

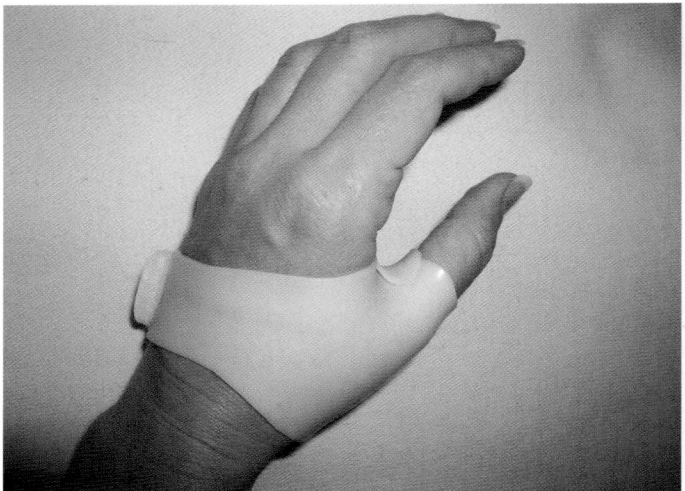

Figure 15-16 Hand-based thumb spica splint used to limit motion in the metacarpophalangeal and carpometacarpal joint of the thumb.

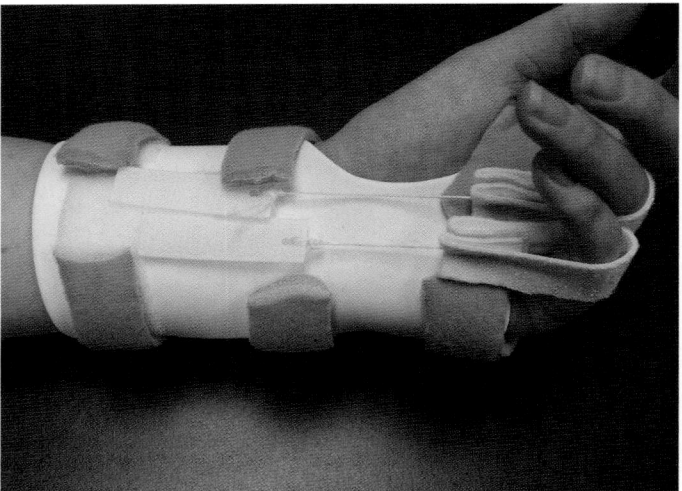

Figure 15-18 Static progressive splint with static pull; note that the angle is toward the scaphoid.

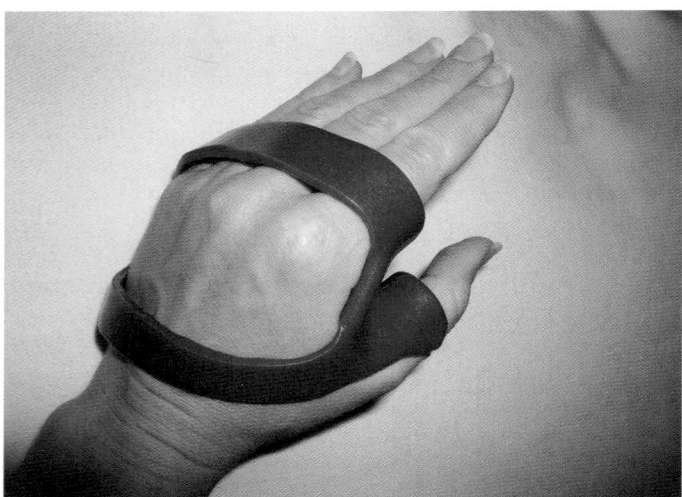

Figure 15-17 Combined median and ulnar nerve palsy splint blocking the metacarpophalangeal into slight flexion.

- When making a splint, the therapist should fabricate it in a position that enhances prehension, and that does not force the thumb into a position of extension and radial abduction. This position causes the rest of the arm to compensate for poor thumb positioning. To decrease the stresses on the hand and thumb, built-up pens and pencils can be used for improved function, especially with a thumb spica splint (Fig. 15-16). Thumb position is most often compromised in low median and ulnar nerve injuries, which leave the patient with no or weakened ability to place the thumb in opposition and palmar abduction (Fig. 15-17).
- Splints designed to encompass the hand must preserve both longitudinal and transverse arches. The distal palmar crease must not be blocked if full MCP flexion is desired (Figs 15-4, 15-18).

- In designing dynamic or static progressive hand splints to improve digital flexion, the direction of pull should be toward the scaphoid bone on the palmar surface to mimic the angle noted in the healthy hand.[16] The angle of pull across the palm is oblique, not straight down toward the wrist. This is most apparent when the fingers are flexed individually, and less pronounced when flexed all at once.
- The mobility of digits 4 and 5 is critical to the power grasp of the hand. The radial three digits (1, 2, and 3) are used for pinch and prehension. This has to be accommodated in splint design and fabrication.
- Active and passive range of motion measurements need to be assessed to determine the mechanics of the joint. Joint torque angle measurements can be used to determine whether or not a splint is needed, whether or not conservative treatment would be beneficial, and whether or not surgery is indicated. Torque angle measurement assesses what occurs at the joint as the force is applied at a given distance from the joint axis. This measurement gives the examiner an understanding of whether the joint has a 'soft end feel' (more motion with a given force) or a 'hard end feel' (little or no motion with the same force).

DIAGNOSTIC CATEGORIES AND SPLINT EXAMPLES

There are many common clinical conditions for which orthotic intervention is appropriate. This section gives a brief overview of the features of specific diagnoses, followed by the type of splint(s) commonly indicated for each diagnosis. This is not an all-inclusive list, and the reader is referred to comprehensive overviews of upper limb orthotic devices in splinting texts and other references.[1,8,9,14–18]

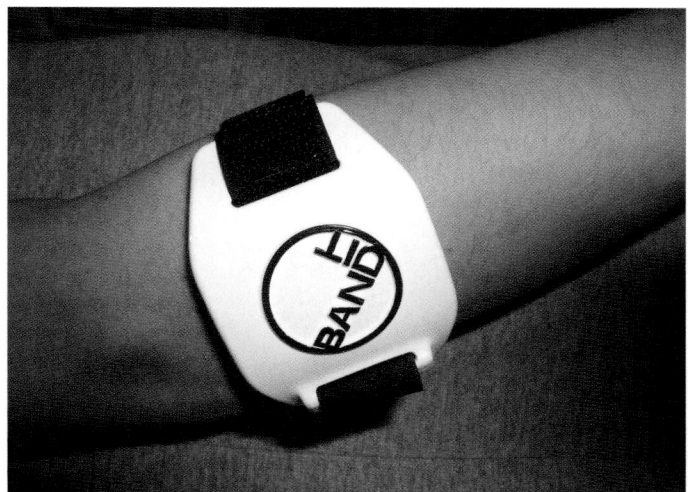

Figure 15-19 BAND-IT brace by Pro Band Sports Industries, Inc. Used for lateral epicondylitis.

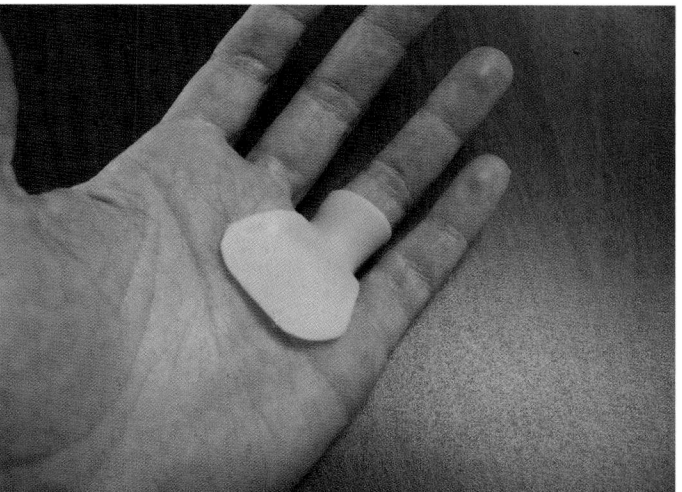

Figure 15-20 Trigger finger splint used for conservative treatment.

Musculoskeletal conditions

Tendinitis, tenosynovitis, and enthesopathy

Tendinitis (inflammation of the tendon), tenosynovitis (inflammation of the tendon sheaths), and enthesopathy (inflammation at a muscle or tendon origin or insertion) can all result from excessive repetitive movement or external stressors. The upper limb tendons most commonly involved are the wrist extensors or the abductor pollicis longus and extensor pollicis brevis muscles of the thumb, commonly called de Quervain's stenosing tenosynovitis. The goal of splints for these conditions is to immobilize the affected structures in order to facilitate healing and decrease inflammation. The thumb spica splint, forearm-based, immobilizes the wrist, the CMC joint, and the MCP joint of the thumb. The IP joint of the thumb does not need fixation because the affected tendons do not move this joint (see Fig. 15-2).

Lateral epicondylitis is the most common enthesopathy of the upper limb. It can be treated by a tennis elbow orthosis (Fig. 15-19). This is a forearm band that changes the lever arm against which the wrist extensors pull. In essence, it puts the origin of the extensor muscles at rest and decreases the micro-trauma from overuse. This orthotic device is placed approximately two fingerbreadths distal to the lateral epicondyle, and is a firm strap against which the extensors press against when contracting. A similar brace is used for medial epicondylitis (also known as golfer's elbow; see Ch. 39).

Trigger finger causes a snapping sensation in the volar surface of the digits on release of grasp. It is usually a result of trauma to the flexor tendon sheath of the fingers or thumb, producing thickened tendinous sheaths and restriction of motion. In advanced trigger finger, the digit can become 'locked' in flexion. This can be due to an intense acute episode or repetitive trauma. The goal in this condition is to halt the repetitive motion temporarily to allow for healing. This is usually achieved by immobilization, but patients should have functional use of the hand while the affected digit is immobilized (Fig. 15-20). The splint for trigger finger covers the proximal phalanx and the MCP joint of the involved digit. This splint decreases the tendinous excursion through the first annular pulley, at the base of the MCP joint, and allows the inflamed structures to rest.

Sprains

Sprains are defined as momentary subluxations with spontaneous reduction that result in torn ligamentous structures. Patients experience pain, swelling, and decreased function. Sprains require joint immobilization in a position of function to allow for healing as well as functional use. Common sprains include dislocation of the IP and MCP joints caused by hyperextension injuries—often seen in sports injuries (see Ch. 45). For a first- or second-degree ligamentous tear, the goal is to protect and rest the area by applying functional splinting. The goal for a third-degree tear is to fully immobilize and approximate the ligaments.

Common splints used for digital sprains are finger extension splints that hold the PIP joint in extension but allow flexion of the distal interphalangeal (DIP) joint. This action keeps the oblique retinacular ligament and the terminal extensor tendon lengthened, preventing boutonnière deformities during healing. Ulnar collateral ligamentous injuries at the MCP joint of the thumb are treated with a hand-based thumb spica splint, producing immobilization during the healing phase (see Fig. 15-16). Wrist splints that place the wrist in slight extension are used for wrist sprains. For mild sprains, splints with no spline (metal bar insert) permit some motion but avoid creating significant stiffness. They also keep available range to about 40° of total motion (Fig. 15-21). Elbow neoprene sleeves are helpful for mild sprains at the elbow, because they limit the extremes of range but permit limited function.

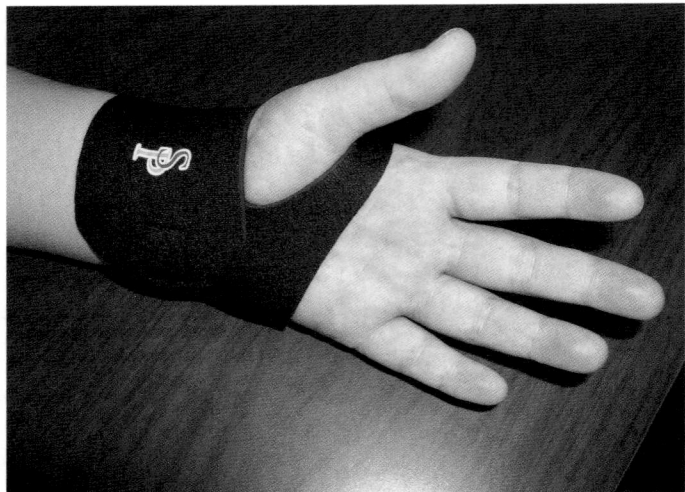

Figure 15-21 Neoprene wrist wrap used for wrist sprains and arthritis, providing neutral warmth and light support.

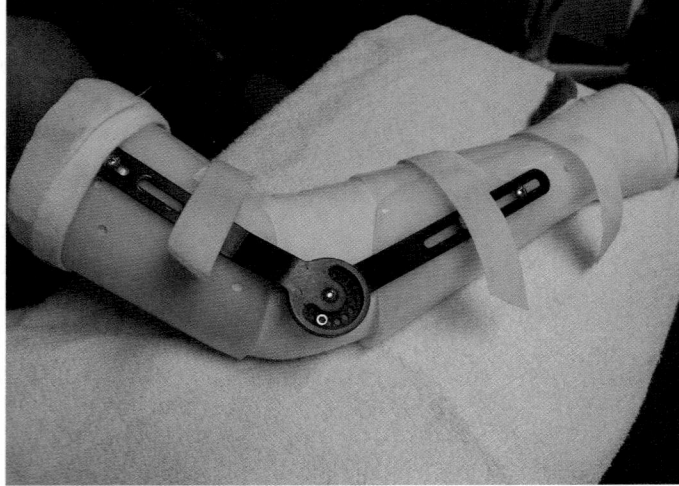

Figure 15-22 Hinged elbow splint with stops to limit extremes of motion during the rehabilitation phase after a fracture.

Fractures

Most major fractures need total immobilization, requiring casting and/or surgical intervention. Some fractures, however, do not need total limb immobilization and can be treated with orthotic devices (Fig. 15-22). These devices should immobilize the body part or the joint sufficient to promote healing, while also optimizing function. An example of such an orthotic device is the humeral fracture brace, which has a circumferential design to hold healing bony parts in alignment. This orthosis permits motion of the elbow, forearm, and hand, which is desirable because rigid arm immobilization can lead to the development of edema and resultant joint stiffness. Other examples are the traction-type splints that allow for very controlled motion during the healing phase of intraarticular finger fractures treated with pinning. Joint movement has been credited with

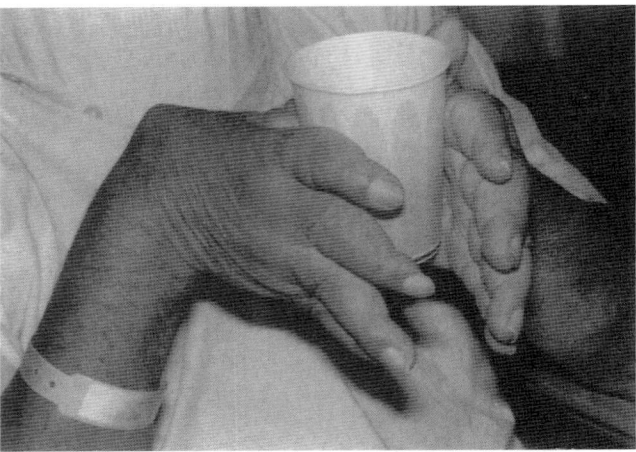

Figure 15-23 Swan neck deformities at the proximal interphalangeal joints. The patient is holding a cup without the aid of splints. (Courtesy of the Silver Ring Splint Company.)

enhancing cartilage nutrition and preventing intraarticular adhesions (see Fig. 15-12).[10]

Arthritis

Osteoarthritis is the most common disease affecting the joints in the upper limb. Joint diseases of the hand and wrist have the most significant impact on function. Chronic inflammation often exposes these digital joints to further risk of deformity and injury. Orthotic devices can provide functional positioning to prevent further deformity and loss of use in arthritic diseases, as well as protecting the joints from further injury.[1]

Rheumatoid arthritis Rheumatoid arthritis is a chronic inflammatory disease that primarily affects synovial joints. The joints most frequently affected in the upper limb are the wrist, MCP joint, and PIP joint. Deformities include subluxation and ulnar deviation at the MCP joints, subluxation and radial deviation at the wrist, and swan neck deformity and boutonnière deformity of the fingers. These deformities usually progress, especially if no attempt is made to rest and protect the affected joints from overuse (see Ch. 37).

Several options are available for splinting the rheumatoid hand. Ulnar deviation splints that pull the MCP joints toward radial deviation and increase the functional use of the hand are now lightweight and permit full MCP joint motion in flexion and extension. Wrist splints that provide light support for the wrist are usually tolerated very well (see Fig. 15-21). Swan neck and boutonnière splints can be made from thermoplastics but are often bulky and cosmetically unpleasing. Very thin Siris Silver Ring Splints[4] are now available for digital deformities (Figs 15-23 and 15-24). Made of sterling silver, these splints are cosmetically similar to jewelry; they provide excellent improvement in function and are well tolerated. The Silver Ring Splint Company[4] makes a wide variety of splints for the finger and thumb joints; each is individually tailored to exact specifications and reasonably priced. The swan neck splint allows for flexion of the digit but blocks hyperextension. The boutonnière splint holds the DIP or PIP joint in extension.

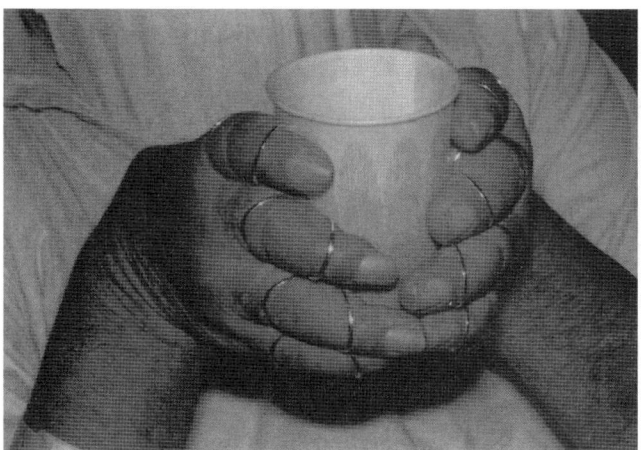

Figure 15-24 Siris Swan Neck Splints, which greatly enhance function of the digits for activities of daily living. The patient is holding a cup with the aid of these splints. (Courtesy of the Silver Ring Splint Company.)

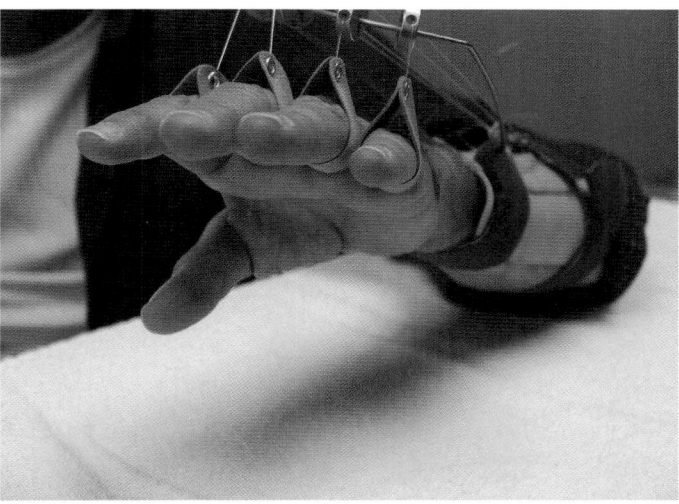

Figure 15-26 The radial nerve palsy splint assists with wrist and digit extension to improve functional use of the hand.

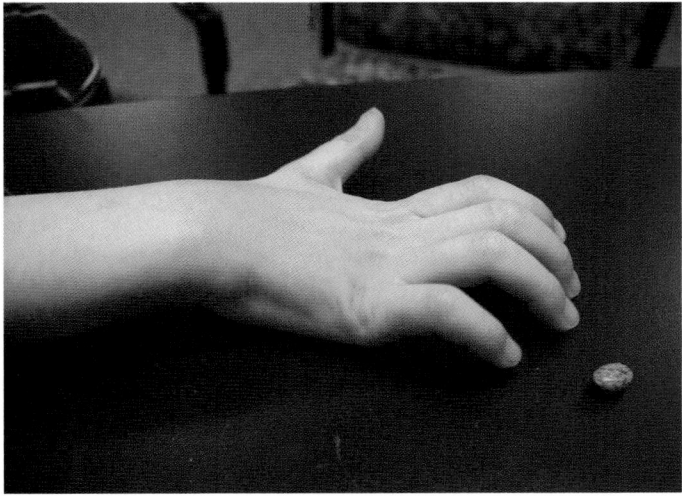

Figure 15-25 Simian hand, as seen in low median and ulnar nerve injuries.

Osteoarthritis Osteoarthritis, the most common form of arthritis, is primarily a disease of cartilage, not of the synovium. In the upper limb, it most commonly involves the CMC joint of the thumb. A thumb spica hand-based (see Fig. 15-16) or forearm-based (see Fig. 15-2) splint can be prescribed for CMC joint osteoarthritis. By limiting motion at the base of the thumb, the splint decreases pain, especially with pinching-type activities.

Neuromuscular conditions
Nerve injuries
In a peripheral nerve injury, which can affect a nerve anywhere along its course, the level of injury determines the extent of deficit incurred. For example, in a distal median nerve injury, the type of deformity incurred is usually described as a simian hand, and the function most affected is thumb palmar abduction and opposition (Fig. 15-25). The goal of an orthotic device

is to help restore this function. The splint usually has a spring coil design holding the MCP joints in slight flexion but permitting MCP extension. This splint also has a portion to position the thumb in palmar abduction.

With radial nerve injuries distal to the humeral spiral groove, the most common presenting condition is wrist drop and finger drop. The goal of an orthotic device is to enhance wrist and finger extension. A radial nerve palsy splint (Fig. 15-26) is forearm-based with an outrigger that holds the wrist, fingers, and thumb in extension and allows for flexion of the digits.[12]

With a proximal ulnar nerve injury, the patient has what is called a 'benediction hand', featuring hyperextension of the fourth and fifth MCP joints and flexion of the PIP joints due to the loss of balance between the extrinsic and intrinsic hand muscles. The goal of the orthotic device is to prevent fixed deformity of the fourth and fifth MCP joints and improve function. An ulnar nerve palsy splint holds the MCP joints of the fourth and fifth fingers in slight flexion by a spring coil or figure of eight splint design. The spring coil design assists MCP flexion and permits extension of the MCP joints but blocks hyperextension (Fig. 15-27). This can also be accomplished by using a static splint that prevents hyperextension of the MCP joints of the fourth and fifth digits with the use of a 'lumbrical bar'.

Incomplete nerve injuries can be caused by compression without producing complete paralysis as, for example, in median nerve injury from carpal tunnel syndrome. One cause of this is an overuse syndrome that produces an inflammatory response in the synovium surrounding the flexor tendons at the wrist, causing decreased blood supply to the median nerve. The purpose of the splint is to immobilize the wrist to minimize swelling from overuse of the tendons. Complete resolution of this syndrome can occur if wrist orthoses are applied early, when symptoms first appear. The splint is molded to the patient from a thermoplastic that offers excellent conformity to hold

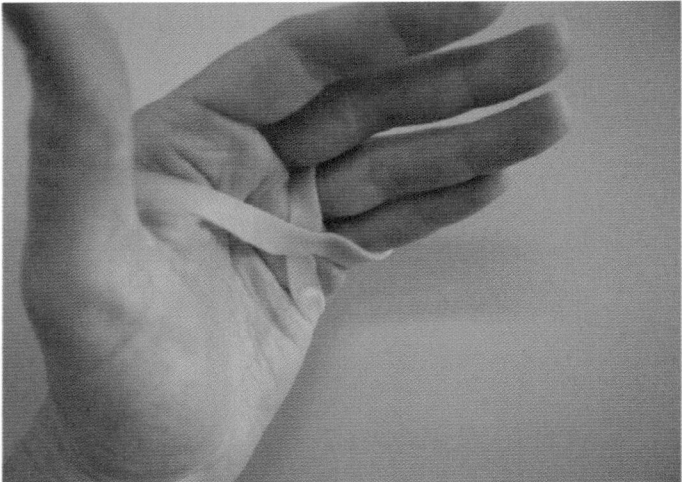

Figure 15-27 Ulnar nerve palsy. Allows extension but blocks hyperextension of the metacarpophalangeal joints of the ring and small fingers.

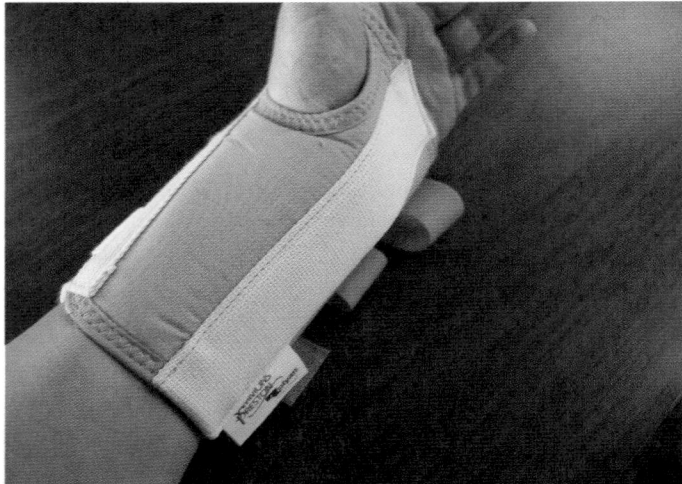

Figure 15-28 Commercially available wrist splint. The preset angle, which may be appropriate in some patients with wrist sprains, far exceeds that recommended for the treatment of acute carpal tunnel syndrome.

the wrist in 0–5° of extension. Its common name, wrist cock-up splint, is misleading and should be avoided because this name implies that the wrist should be placed in extension (see Fig. 15-4). The patient should be instructed to reduce stresses at the wrist, and to wear the splint all night.

A word of caution is in order in using prefabricated wrist splints for carpal tunnel syndrome. Many of these splints have a metal spline formed to hold the wrist at a 45° angle of extension (Fig. 15-28). This angle far exceeds the recommended 0–5° of extension needed to decrease pressure in the carpal tunnel. Patients need to be instructed to remove the metal spline, flatten it, and then replace it in the fabric covering. Usually, this splint should be worn for 4–6 weeks, with a gradual weaning

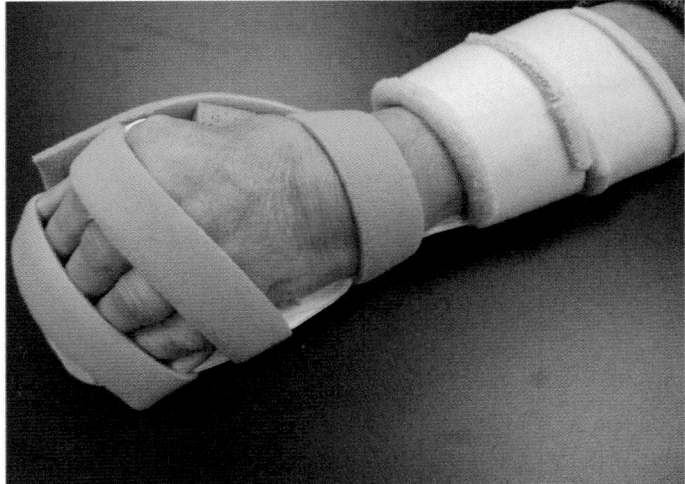

Figure 15-29 Resting hand splint.

from the splint, as well as a gradual return to activity with workstation modifications.

Cubital tunnel syndrome (compression of the ulnar nerve at the elbow) can be treated with long arm splints (see Fig. 15-1) that hold the elbow in 45° of flexion, the forearm in neutral, and the wrist in 0–5° of extension with thumb and fingers free.

In patients with multiple nerve injuries or brachial plexopathy with essentially a flail arm, the goal with orthotic devices is to provide some functional use. One type of orthosis is in the form of an exoskeleton on the arm, similar to a prosthesis; this device uses a shoulder harness with scapular activation to produce elbow function, similar to scapular action in an above-elbow prosthesis.[14]

Brain injury and stroke

Depending on the area of brain injury and ensuing deficits, particularly if there is a change in muscle tone, orthotic devices should be designed to prevent deformities and to help adjust muscle tone. Resting and positioning orthotic devices are also necessary to prevent such complications as distal edema, joint subluxation, and contracture formation. In upper limb paralysis, a resting hand splint is commonly used to position the wrist in slight extension, the MCP joints in slight flexion, and the IP joints in extension. The thumb is supported in a position between palmar and radial abduction. Full support of the first CMC joint prevents ligamentous stresses on the thumb, especially in the insensate hand. This thumb position also utilizes the reflex inhibiting posture, which decreases tone in the hand (Fig. 15-29). Botulinum toxin is now being used to decrease the tone in patients with focal spasticity, followed by serial splinting to regain normal posture or position (Fig. 15-30).[13]

A mobile arm support can be used to enhance function for patients with proximal upper limb weakness, especially when the weakness is profound and the outlook for recovery is guarded. A mobile arm support is particularly helpful when performing such activities of daily living tasks as eating and

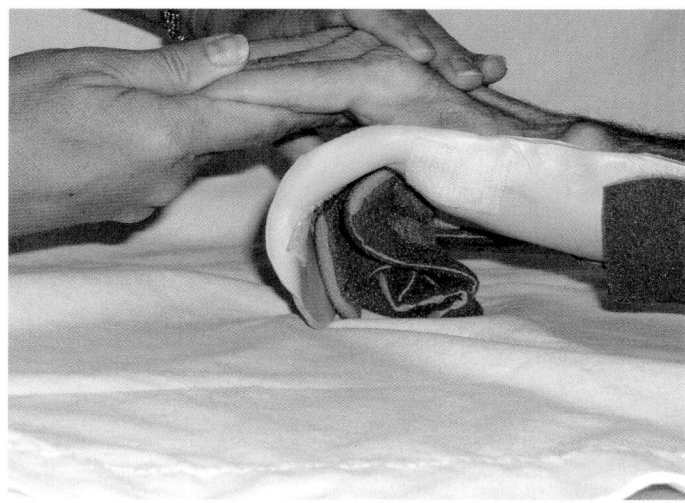

Figure 15-30 Improved passive range of motion after botulinum toxin injection to reduce spasticity; splint is preinjection level for passive range of motion.

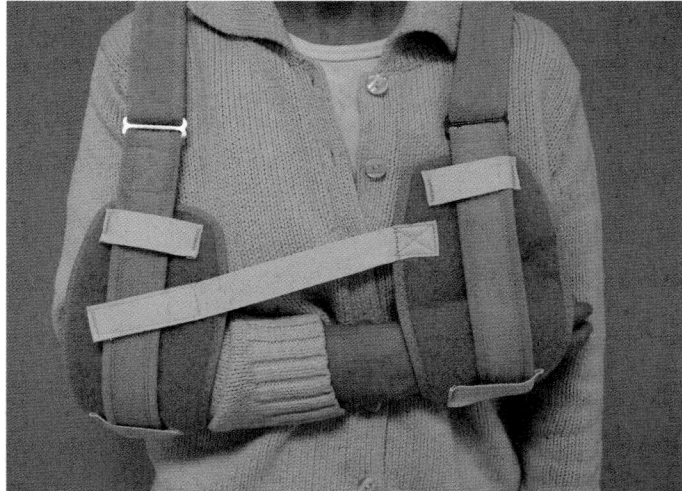

Figure 15-31 Rolyan figure of eight sling used for reducing subluxation of the shoulder joint in a patient with hemiplegia.

grooming. When attached to a wheelchair with a swivel joint, this is often also called a balanced forearm orthosis.

Many types of slings are available for patients with decreased tone of the upper limb (Fig. 15-31). Decreased tone can result in shoulder subluxation, and these slings can help reduce the degree of this deformity. Unfortunately, nothing—no sling or arm tray attached to a wheelchair—has been found to correct shoulder subluxation completely. An overhead sling device can help increase the function of weakened shoulder and scapular musculature.

Spinal cord injury

In patients with spinal cord injury, orthotic devices are needed to enhance function and/or help with positioning. The type of such devices depends on the level of injury and the extent of

neurologic compromise. With spinal cord injury at the C1–C3 level, the goal is to prevent contractures and to hold the wrist and digits in a position of function with a resting hand splint (see Fig. 15-29). In a C4-level injury, the goal is to use the available shoulder strength, providing a mobile arm support to enhance function as previously described. In a C5-level injury, the goal is to statically position the wrist in extension with a ratchet-type hinged orthotic device to hold devices and utilize the shoulder musculature for function. An orthotic device for a C6 tetraplegic patient can enhance finger flexion using a tenodesis flexion effect from wrist extension. For example, a Rehabilitation Institute of Chicago tenodesis splint molded from thermoplastic materials has several positioning components (see Figs 15-13 and 15-14). A thumb post component positions the thumb in palmar abduction. A dorsal finger piece component, which is attached with a static line to a volar forearm component, holds the PIP joints of the index and long fingers in slight flexion. When the patient extends the wrist, the static line pulls the fingers toward the thumb post. This produces a three-point pinch, allowing the patient to grasp an object. When the patient flexes the wrist, the fingers extend passively, releasing the object. The degree of pinch varies depending on the strength of the wrist extensors and the degree of finger flexion, extension, and opposition. This custom-made thermoplastic tenodesis device is mainly used in training and practice. If a patient finds the device useful, a light metal custom-made tenodesis orthosis achieves better functional restoration.

Orthoses for other injuries

Postsurgical and postinjury orthoses
Many types of splints have been developed to help regain motion in stiff joints. Examples of such splints include dynamic elbow flexion and extension splints during rehabilitation after upper arm or elbow fracture (see Fig. 15-22), dynamic wrist flexion and extension after a Colles fracture, and dynamic finger flexion (Fig. 15-32) and extension splints for stiffness after crush injuries to the hand. Similar splints can be fabricated using a static progressive approach. Joints that have soft end feel do well with dynamic splints. Those with a hard end feel typically respond better to a static progressive approach. Examples of static progressive splints are the Joint Jack (Fig. 15-33) or cinch straps and splints for PIP and DIP joint contractures using the MERiT components (Fig. 15-8).[7] Selection of forearm- or hand-based splints is determined by the need for stabilization. Generally, the goal is to immobilize as few joints as feasible. Forearm pronation–supination splints using both dynamic and static features, such as the Collelo splint and Joint Active Systems splint (Fig. 15-34), are very helpful in regaining motion after fractures of the radius and ulna.[15]

Several splint designs are currently employed following repair of tendon injuries. Often, the type of surgical procedure or injury level dictates the type of splint used, so that the splints cannot be used interchangeably. For flexor tendon repair, the Kleinert and Duran are commonly used. The Kleinert splint

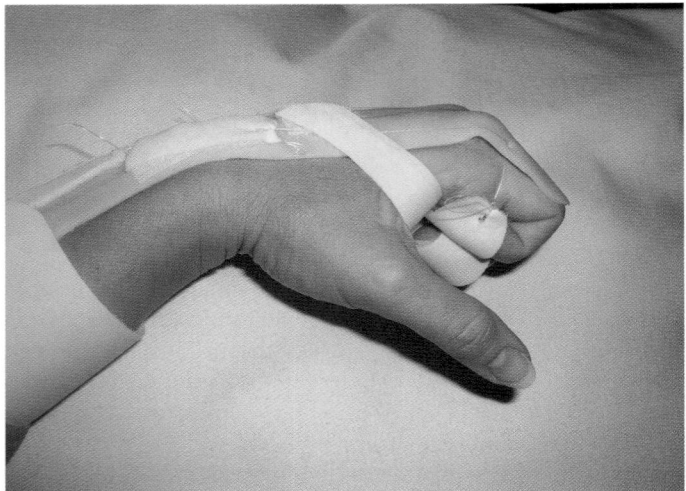

Figure 15-32 Extrinsic extensor stretching splint to increase finger flexion in combination with increasing increments of wrist flexion.

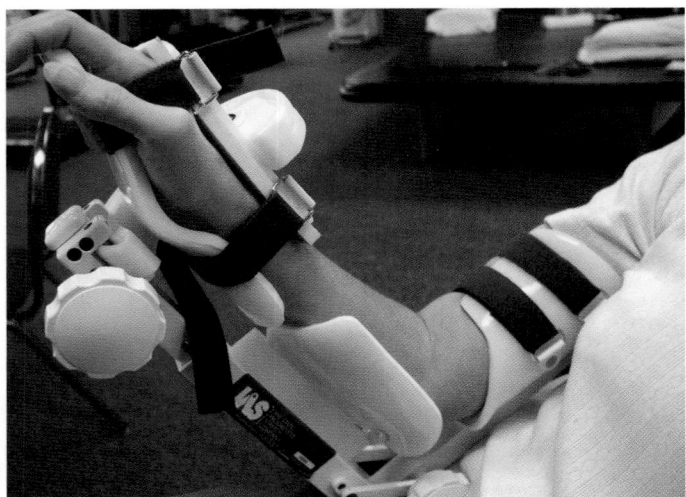

Figure 15-34 Static progressive pronation–supination splint, by Joint Active Systems, used to increase motion in the forearm.

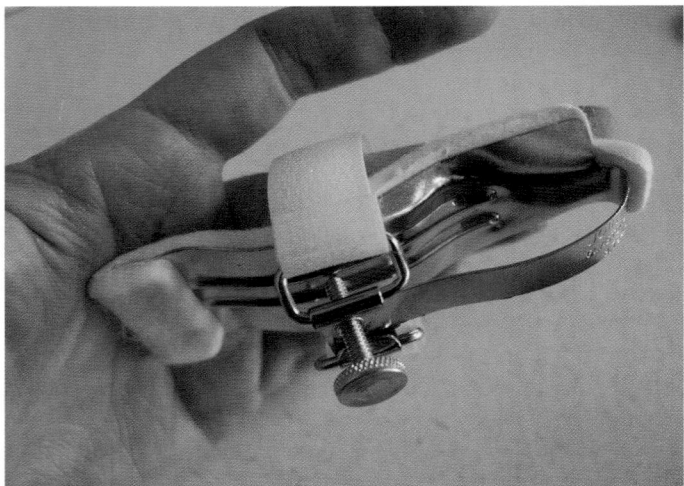

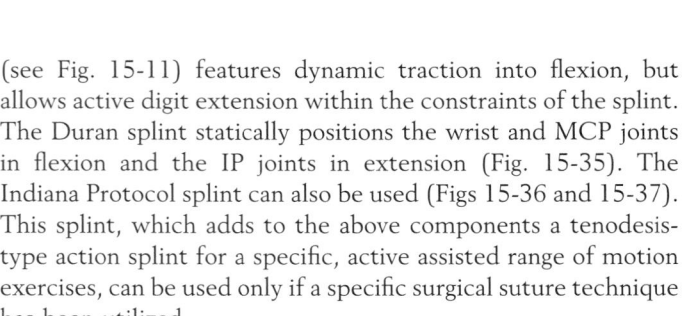

Figure 15-33 Joint Jack is a static progressive splint used to increase extension in the proximal interphalangeal joint.

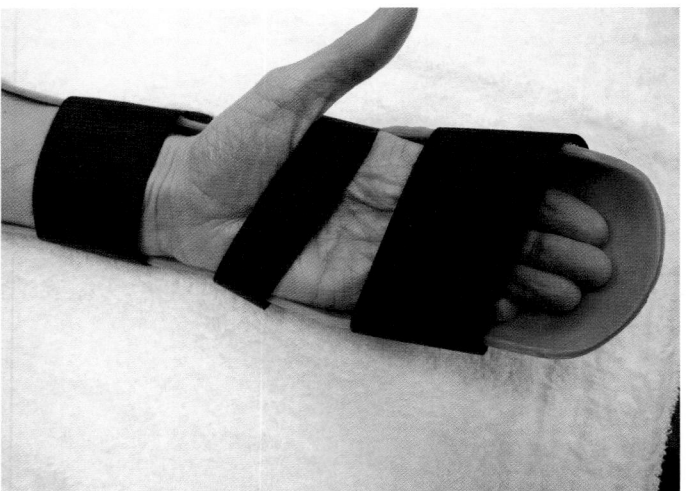

Figure 15-35 Duran flexor tendon repair splint used for postoperative care.

(see Fig. 15-11) features dynamic traction into flexion, but allows active digit extension within the constraints of the splint. The Duran splint statically positions the wrist and MCP joints in flexion and the IP joints in extension (Fig. 15-35). The Indiana Protocol splint can also be used (Figs 15-36 and 15-37). This splint, which adds to the above components a tenodesis-type action splint for a specific, active assisted range of motion exercises, can be used only if a specific surgical suture technique has been utilized.

The form of extensor tendon repair splints depends on the level of injury. A mallet finger injury can require only a Stax splint, which is a static splint holding the DIP joint in full extension. A more proximal injury, however, needs a splint that holds the wrist statically in extension with dynamic extension of MCP and IP joints (Fig. 15-38). Such a splint permits active flexion of the MCP joints within the constraints of the splint

to an angle of approximately 30°. Injuries to the thumb flexor or extensor tendons require more specific splinting (Fig. 15-39), again dependent on the level of the injury.

Postoperative joint replacements for the PIP, DIP, or MCP joints of the hand require specific splints that promote healing or encapsulation of the joints while preserving range of motion during the healing phases (Fig. 15-40).

Return to play splints are often fabricated for high-level athletes. These splints are made from a silicone 'cast' material called RTV-11. Indications include metacarpal fractures and dislocations, carpal fractures (scaphoid is most common), and select stable distal radius and ulna fractures. RTV-11 is a soft pliable material accepted by officials for wear during play.[15]

Orthoses for burns
Burn patients typically prefer an adducted and flexed position of the upper limbs to maintain comfort, but this preference can

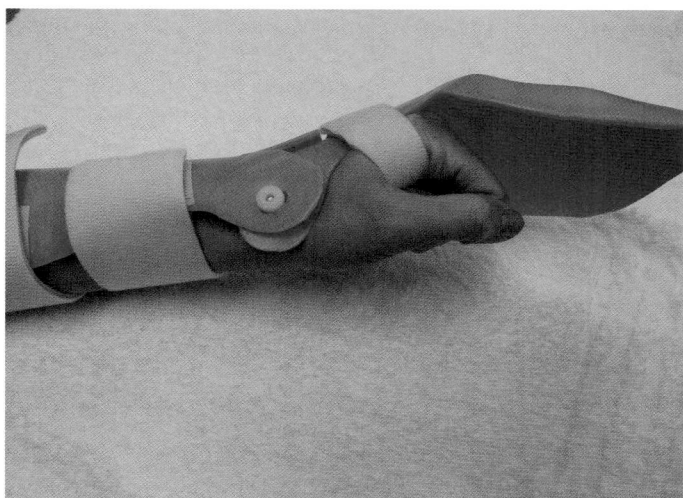

Figure 15-36 Indiana Protocol postoperative flexor tendon splint: tenodesis flexion exercises.

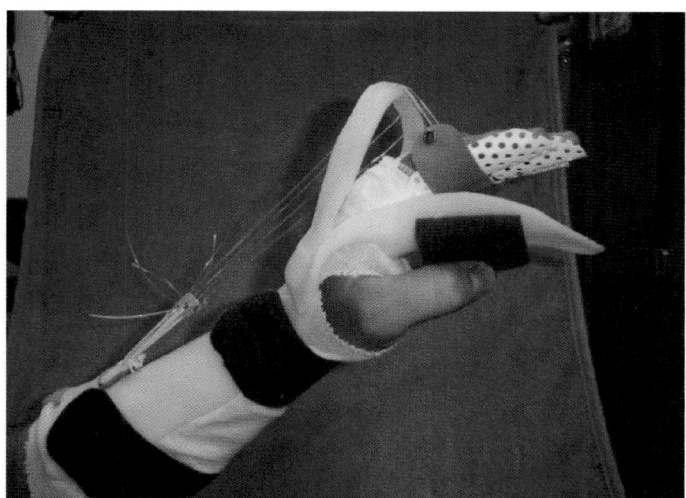

Figure 15-38 Extensor tendon splint used for postoperative care, allowing protected motion during the healing phase. (Courtesy of Kelly Mikle, O.T.R./L., C.H.T.)

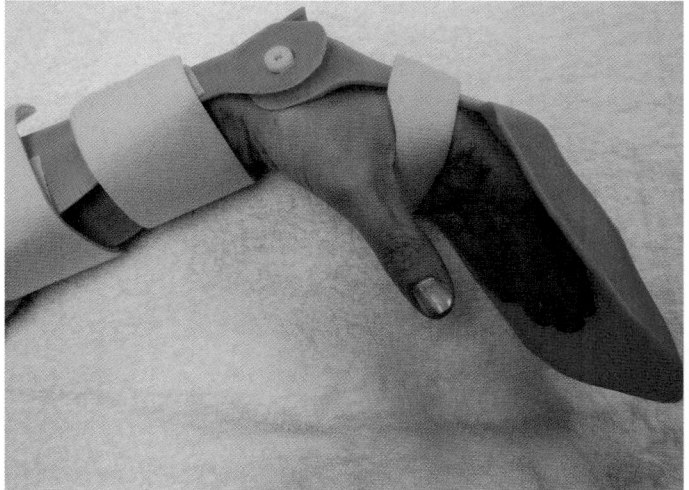

Figure 15-37 Indiana Protocol postoperative flexor tendon splint: tenodesis extension exercises.

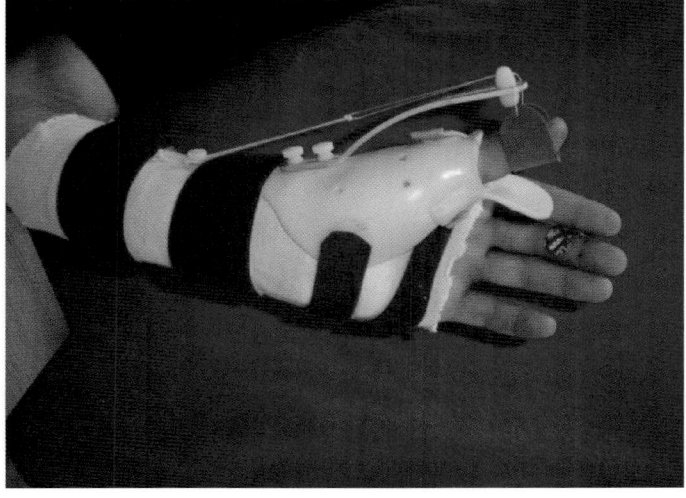

Figure 15-39 Postoperative splint for a patient with an extensor tendon pollicis longus repair. (Courtesy of Kelly Mikle, O.T.R./L., C.H.T.)

lead to loss of functional range of motion. In this case, the splint acts to prevent contractures and deformities from developing. This is especially important when the patient cannot voluntarily maintain the range or when soft tissues underlying the skin are exposed. With tendon exposure, the splint plays a more protective role. It is important to monitor these patients frequently and reassess the needs for splinting.

After burn injuries, body parts should be positioned to prevent the development of expected deformities. For example, in burns of the dorsal surface of the hand, the wrist is kept in slight extension, the MCP joints in 60–70° of flexion, the PIP and DIP joints in full extension, and the thumb between radial abduction and palmar abduction (see Fig. 15-15). To combat a tendency for shoulder adduction deformity after axillary burns, the shoulder should be held in abduction with an airplane splint. The tendency toward hypertrophic scarring after a burn is

addressed with a selection of compression garments, elastomer molds, facial splints, gel shell splints, and silicone gel sheeting.

SPECIAL CONSIDERATIONS

Splints can be perfectly designed and skillfully fabricated but are useless if not worn. The more choice and input patients have in splint design, the more compliant they are likely to be with splint wear. It is important to ask the patient about goals, likes, and dislikes before choosing a splint design (see Table 15-2 for a list of points to consider for optimization of splint use).

Cosmesis is often a problem for patients, because they care about the way splints look. To assure splint wear, the splint has

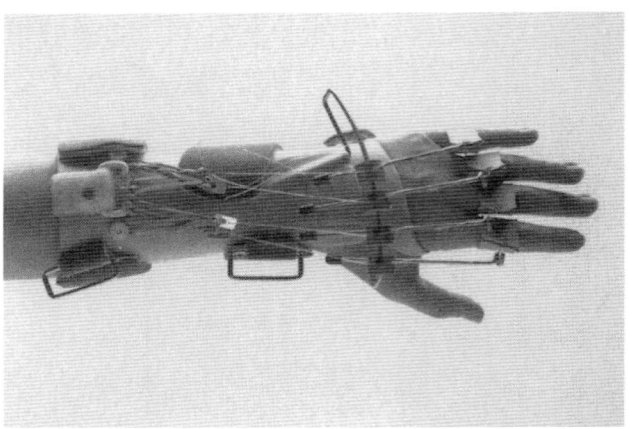

Figure 15-40 The metacarpophalangeal arthroplasty postoperative splint positions fingers in extension with slight radial pull.

Table 15-2	Points to consider for optimization of splint use
Factor	Comments
Material thickness	Use thinner materials for finger splints, and thicker materials for forearm and elbow splints.[a]
Function	Consider patient's goals and functional needs.
Patient input	Elicit patient's ideas, preferences, and goals.
Cosmesis	Consider patient's age, occupation, and other factors.
Color	Allow color choices to improve compliance.
Wearing schedule	Tailor wearing schedule to meet the goals of the splint.
Design	Consider goals as well as biomechanics when choosing whether a splint should be static, static progressive, dynamic, etc.

[a]*Thinner materials cool faster, decreasing working time.*

to be as cosmetically acceptable as possible. Patients should have every opportunity to assist in choosing design and appearance. Patients often have very good ideas about the design of a splint and suggest good ways to strap it into place. They might also have color preferences. Low-temperature thermoplastic materials are now available in a wide range of colors. The person's age or occupation can also be factors. For example, a young patient who works in an amusement park might like a hot pink splint, while an older autoworker might prefer a black one. Adolescents should be given as much freedom as possible and encouraged to 'decorate' their splints if they so desire, as long as the splint mechanics are not altered.

Comfort is also important. The thinner the materials used and the more care the therapist takes in making a close, com-

fortable fit, the better the acceptance of the splint. For example, areas around bony prominences need to be 'popped' out to prevent pressure, while edges and joints frequently need to be padded to reduce skin irritation. Arthritic patients who have been taking corticosteroids for long periods of time often have fragile skin, so their splints should be padded throughout. Stockinet worn under splints also helps, particularly with perspiration in warmer weather.

The wearing schedule depends on the goals you have for the splint and the patient's tolerance for wear. For example, you have a patient with head injury who is 'storming'; that is, sweating excessively and being combative. In this case, a resting hand splint for positioning might be worn just 30 min on and 3 h off. In contrast, a patient with stroke and with mild spasticity could wear a resting hand splint 2 h on and 2 h off during the day and keep it on all night. Static progressive splint wear depends on tissue response to gentle stretching. The stretch should be perceived as mild, and it should never awaken the patient at night. In a patient with both flexion and extension splinting needs, the flexion splint can be worn 1 h on, 2 h off during the day, and the extension splint can be worn at night. Patients tolerate the splint better and spend more daytime with the splint off so they can do hand exercises and incorporate use.

A resting hand splint for positioning is often indicated when edema is present. But a splint can also induce edema because of an inflammatory response due to an overly aggressive stretch, particularly in a patient with increased tone. Splint design should address this possibility. Often, special strapping techniques can lessen the response. Other tissue responses are also possible. Blueness or redness of the digits when wearing a splint tells the observer that an overly aggressive stretch is being applied to the shortened neurovascular bundles. These structures sometimes change in length due to the joint contracture, in which case splint tension must be decreased and the contracture stretch should be less aggressive.

Splint prescriptions should explain the diagnosis or problem to be addressed. A description of the function or motion desired helps to alleviate confusion. It can also facilitate discussion with the therapist, physician, and patient regarding the best design to meet mutually agreed goals. A good description can also help clarify misunderstandings arising from conflicting naming systems (see Table 15-1).

ORTHOTIC MATERIALS

Most splinting materials are low-temperature thermoplastics, some of which are listed in Table 15-3. Many are known by their trademark names, such as Orthoplast, Aquaplast, and Orfit.[3,5] Low-temperature thermoplastics become soft and pliable when exposed to relatively low temperatures, and can be shaped in a water bath at 150–180°F. High-temperature thermoplastics are more durable but require oven heating (up to 350°F) and placement over a mold to achieve the desired shape. All splinting materials have certain characteristics determined by the temperature and material properties. Some, like

Table 15-3 Commonly used low-temperature thermoplastic materials for splint fabrication

Material name	Resistance to stretch	Memory	Rigidity	Surface finish	Typical splint uses
Aquaplast	Minimal	100%	Moderate	Marks with firm pressure	Wrist splint, thumb spica splint, finger splints
Ezeform	Maximal	Moderate	Maximal	Resists fingerprints	Resting hand splint, pronation–supination splint
Orfit	Moderate	100%	Moderate	Resists fingerprints	Thumb spica splints
Prism	Minimal	100%	Moderate; withstands application of dynamic components	Resists fingerprints	Wrist splint, thumb spica splint, flexor tendon splints (e.g. Duran and Kleinert)
Orthoplast	Moderate	Poor	Maximal	Resists fingerprints	Resting hand splint, humeral fracture brace
Polyform	Minimal	Maximal	Poor	Marks easily	Mallet finger splints, dynamic finger splints

Ezeform,[5] are very rigid when cool. Others, such as Polyform,[5] are very drapeable when warm. Firm materials can be desirable for patients with increased tone, whereas drapeable materials can be desirable when conformability is needed, as when splinting a finger. Some plastic materials have a great deal of 'memory'. This means they return to their original shape when reheated. This characteristic can help control costs, especially those incurred when providing serial static splinting.

Therapists use heat guns and water baths to heat thermoplastic materials to mold them for splint fabrication. Velcro[3] straps are almost universally used to hold orthotic devices in place. There are multiple attachments available to add to the splint base to achieve particular goals; these include outriggers from wire, line guides to position the line of pull, and loops or slings to pull a digit into the desired position. Most often, the choices of attachments are based on the therapist's experience with the materials and their previous training.

SUMMARY

This chapter has provided guidelines concerning the principles for upper limb orthotic devices, as well as various classification systems and descriptions of design categories. To fabricate an orthosis, a sound understanding of the anatomy, biomechanics, and tissue physiology of the upper limb is required. Persons prescribing upper limb orthotic devices should have a thorough knowledge of the musculoskeletal and neurologic conditions amenable to treatment by orthoses. They must also understand other avenues of treatment, such as exercise therapy, and be alert to surgical indications.

The most important principle in prescription of orthotic devices is gaining the cooperation of the patient. Through attention and concern by the physician and therapist, the patient must be able to see the benefit of the orthosis. It also must fit comfortably and be cosmetically appealing. Everyone involved must have the same goals and purpose for the device, or it will end up being abandoned soon after it has been fitted.

As we continue to learn more about the biomechanics of the hand, we better understand how to redress externally the internal imbalance caused by disease and injury. Keeping the internal dynamics of the hand in mind, we find that splinting is the most efficient and effective way to affect this mechanical rebalance.[14]

REFERENCES

1. American Society of Hand Therapists, Splint Nomenclature Task Force. Splint Classification System. Garner: ASHT; 1991.
2. [Anonymous]. MERiT static progressive component product catalog, 1998. UE Tech; 1998.
3. [Anonymous]. North Coast Medical Company hand therapy catalog, 1998. North Coast Medical Company; 1998.
4. [Anonymous]. Silver Ring Splint Company catalog, 1994. Silver Ring Splint Company; 1994.
5. [Anonymous]. Smith & Nephew Inc. Rehabilitation Division catalog, 1997. Smith & Nephew; 1997.
6. Austin GP, Slamet M, Cameron D, et al. A comparison of high-profile and low-profile dynamic mobilization splint designs. J Hand Ther 2004; 15(3):335–343.
7. Bash DS, Spur ME. An alternate to Turnbuckle splinting for elbow flexion. J Hand Ther 2000; 13(3):237–240.
8. Coppard BM, Lohman H. Introduction to splinting, a critical-thinking and problem-solving approach. 2nd edn. St. Louis: Mosby; 2001.
9. Falkenstein N, Weiss S. Hand rehabilitation: a quick reference guide and review. St. Louis: Mosby; 2004.
10. Flowers KR, LaStayo P. Effect of total end range time. J Hand Ther 1989; 2:71.
11. Glasgow C, Wilton J, Tooth L. Optimal daily total end range time for contracture: resolution in hand splinting. J Hand Ther 2003; 16(3):207–218.
12. Hannah SD, Hudak PL. Splinting and radial nerve palsy: a single subject experiment. J Hand Ther 2001; 14(3):195–201.
13. Hesse S, Brandi-Hesse B, Bardeleben A, et al. Botulinum toxin A treatment of adult upper and lower limb spasticity. Drugs Aging 2001; 18(4):255–262.
14. Hunter JM, Mackin EJ, Callahan AD. Rehabilitation of the hand: surgery and therapy. 4th edn. St. Louis: Mosby; 1995.

15. Mackin EJ, Callahan AD, Skirven TM. Rehabilitation of the hand and upper extremity. 5th edn. St. Louis: Mosby; 2002.

16. Malick MH. Manual on dynamic hand splinting with thermoplastic materials. 2nd edn. Pittsburg: Harmarville Rehabilitation Center; 1982.

17. McKee P, Morgan L. Orthotics in rehabilitation, splinting the hand and body. Philadelphia: FA Davis; 1998.

18. Redford JB, Basmajian JV, Trautman P. Orthotics: clinical practice and rehabilitation technology. New York: Churchill Livingstone; 1995.

19. Schuch CM, Pritham CH. International Standards Organization terminology: application to prosthetics and orthotics. J Prosthet Orthot 1994; 6(1):29–48.

Chapter

16

Lower Limb Orthoses

William J. Hennessey

An orthosis is defined as a device attached or applied to the external surface of the body to improve function, restrict or enforce motion, or support a body segment.[35] Lower limb orthoses are indicated to assist gait, reduce pain, decrease weight bearing, control movement, and minimize progression of a deformity. Lower limb orthoses assist non-ambulatory patients with transfer and mobility skills, and assist ambulatory patients in becoming safe walkers. Ambulation aids can be used in combination with lower limb orthoses to help patients ambulate more safely. Ambulation aids represent extensions of the upper limb but are discussed in this chapter because of their importance in gait.

PRINCIPLES OF LOWER LIMB ORTHOSES

Orthoses should be used for the specific management of selected disorders. As in all fields of medicine, specific treatment should be based on a specific medical diagnosis with an established goal of treatment.[51] Placement of orthotic joints should approximate anatomic joints. Box 16-1 outlines this principle as well as other common lower limb orthotic principles. Most orthoses utilize a three-point system to ensure proper positioning of the limb within the orthosis.[24] For example, a knee that has a tendency to hyperextend, or 'back knee', can be treated with a knee orthosis that applies force posterior to the knee but also applies forces anteriorly along the leg and the thigh. Such an orthosis ensures adequate control of the knee by exerting these forces proximal to, distal to, and at the knee joint.

TERMINOLOGY FOR LOWER LIMB ORTHOSES

Orthoses are frequently and incorrectly referred to as orthotics. Words ending in *-ic* are typically adjectives. *Orthotic* is the adjective derived from the noun *orthosis*. An orthosis can be referred to as an orthotic device. An orthosis is also made in an orthotic laboratory.

Terminology pertinent to the anatomy of the lower limb is also frequently used incorrectly. The term *lower extremity* specifically refers to the foot. The term *leg* should be used to refer to the portion of the lower limb between the knee and ankle joints. The *thigh* is located between the hip and knee joints. *Lower limb* refers to the thigh, leg, and foot.

Pathologic abnormalities regarding angulation have also been referred to incorrectly as varus and valgus deformities at the knee and hip. Correct use of the Latin-derived terminology for these deformities requires the suffix of *-us* at the ankle, *-um* at the knee, and *-a* at the hip. Varus and valgus deformities of the foot are described for both the hind foot and forefoot (i.e. hind foot valgus or forefoot varus). A bow-legged condition is correctly referred to as genu varum. Deformity at the hip is referred to as coxa valga and coxa vara.

Lower limb orthoses are frequently referred to with abbreviations. Standard orthotic nomenclature uses the first letter of each joint the orthosis crosses from proximal to distal. It then lists the first letter of the limb to which it is affixed (i.e. 'F' for foot). Lastly, the letter 'O' is used to signify it is an orthosis. Thus AFO designates an ankle–foot orthosis. KAFO means knee–ankle–foot orthosis. HKAFO means hip–knee–ankle–foot orthosis.

The orthotic literature uses variable medical terminology. The calcaneus is frequently referred to as the os calcis. A plantar flexion deformity is referred to as an equinus deformity. Torsion and rotation have incorrectly been used interchangeably. *Torsion* refers to twisting of a portion of a limb. *Rotation* of a limb occurs only at a joint. Pronation has been referred to as *inrolling*, whereas supination has been referred to as *outrolling*. An orthosis is not put on and taken off but rather *donned* and *doffed*. *Checkout* means an examination of the patient after the orthosis is fitted.

SHOES

The purpose of wearing shoes is to protect the feet. The normal foot does not require support from shoes. The sole should be pliable, so as not to interfere with the normal biomechanics of the foot. A practical way of ensuring that a shoe is of adequate length is to determine whether the index finger can be placed between the tip of the great toe and the toe box.[54] The presence of calluses indicates areas of friction from poorly fitting (loose) shoes. The presence of corns indicates areas of friction over bony prominences, most often due to tight-fitting shoes. Leather shoes are good choices for all types of activity. They are durable, allow ventilation, and mold to the feet with time. A good pair of shoes can often eliminate the need for foot orthoses and should be considered before orthotic prescription.

Box 16-1 Principles of lower limb orthoses

- Use only as indicated and for as long as necessary.
- Allow joint movement wherever possible and appropriate.
- Orthoses should be functional throughout all phases of gait.
- An orthotic ankle joint should be centered over the tip of the medial malleolus.
- An orthotic knee joint should be centered over the prominence of the medial femoral condyle.
- An orthotic hip joint should be in a position that allows the patient to sit upright at 90°.
- Patient compliance will be enhanced if the orthosis is comfortable, cosmetic, and functional.

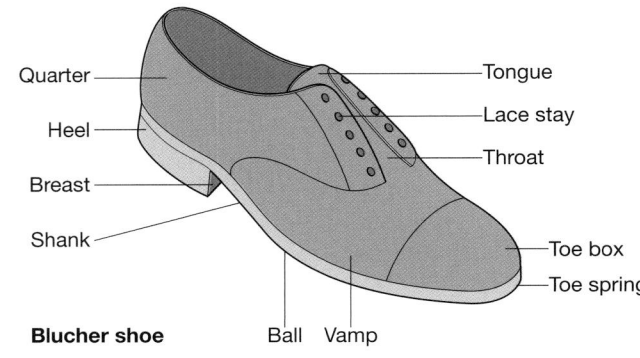

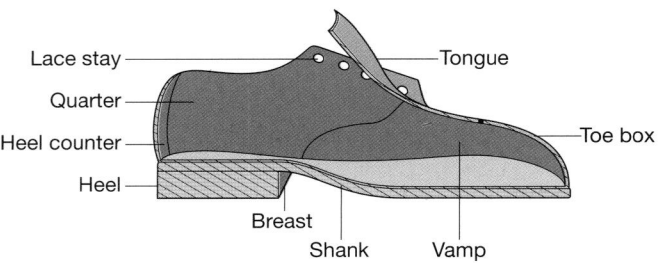

SHOE PARTS

Two types of dress shoes are commonly worn: the Blucher and the Bal (Fig. 16-1). The tongue is part of the vamp in the Blucher shoe. The quarters overlap the vamp. A Blucher shoe is recommended for patients requiring an orthosis, because there is more room to don and doff the shoe and the orthosis due to the open throat.[57] In the Bal shoe style, the quarters meet at the throat. The vamp is stitched over the quarters at the throat, thereby limiting the ability of the shoe to open and accommodate an orthosis.

FOOT ORTHOSES

Foot orthoses range from arch supports found at a local pharmacy or athletic store to customized orthoses fabricated by an orthotist. The effectiveness of an orthosis depends on proper diagnosis of the foot condition, the appropriate selection of orthotic material, and proper molding. Foot orthoses affect the ground reactive forces acting on the joints of the lower limb. They also have an effect on the rotational components of gait (Fig. 16-2).

Mild conditions can be treated with over the counter orthoses. More severe problems and chronic medical conditions require customized orthoses.[56] These are available in three types. A soft type is most commonly used in over the counter orthoses. Orthotists usually provide semirigid orthoses, which provide more support than the soft type but are still shock absorbing. A rigid orthosis is indicated only for a problem that requires aggressive bracing to control a deformity.

To make a custom foot orthosis, the subtalar joint should be placed in a neutral position prior to casting. This position minimizes abnormalities related to foot and ankle rotation, such as hyperpronation, and it is also the position in which the foot functions best.[38] The subtalar neutral position is utilized to treat conditions associated with hyperpronation, including pes planus, patellofemoral pain, and even patients with painful rheumatoid arthritis affecting the first metatarsophalangeal.[7,44] The foot is then covered with a parting agent, such as stockinet or a clear plastic wrap. The foot is then wrapped in either plaster of Paris

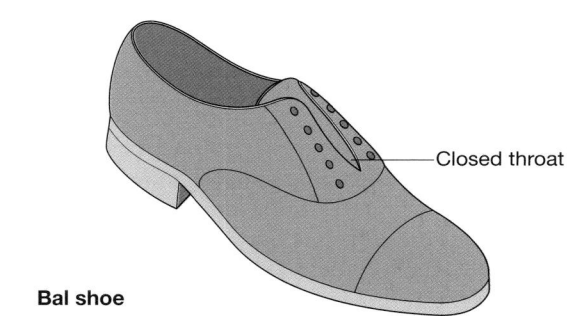

Figure 16-1 Shoe types and components. The open throat of the Blucher shoe accommodates an orthosis better than the Bal shoe does.

strips or fiberglass tape and allowed to harden. Fiberglass casting is also used for difficult orthotic cases, where the fiberglass casting itself can be used as a temporary orthosis to determine whether the mold properly controls the deformity. This negative mold is then removed to allow a positive mold to be made from the negative mold. The positive mold can be modified to increase the effectiveness of the orthosis. The custom orthosis is obtained by heating and form fitting (often by use of a vacuum) the plastic to the positive mold.

It should be noted that research has not determined the length of time an orthosis remains effective. The orthosis should be examined at each follow-up visit to determine when a new one is necessary.

Common foot conditions
Pes planus (flatfoot)
Symptomatic relief of pain is obtained by controlling excess pronation of the foot. Pronation of the foot can be defined as

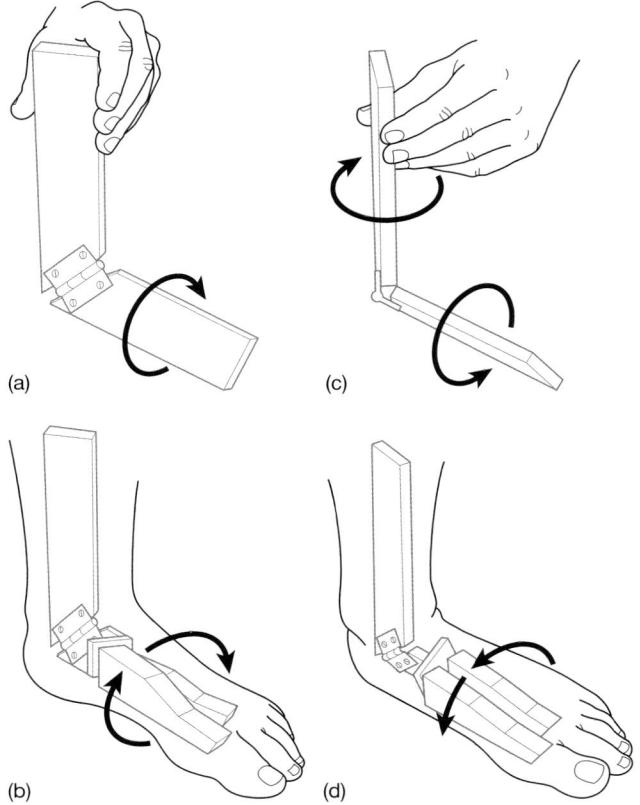

(a)

(b)

(c)

(d)

Figure 16-2 Analogy of subtalar axes to an oblique hinge. (**a** and **b**). Outward rotation of the upper stick (tibia) results in inward rotation of the lower stick (calcaneus). This results in elevation of the medial border of the foot and depression of the lateral border. (**c** and **d**). Inward rotation of the upper stick (tibia) results in outward rotation of the lower stick (calcaneus). This results in depression of the medial side of the foot with elevation of the lateral side. (After Mann 1985,[26] with permission.)

a rotation of the foot in the longitudinal axis, resulting in a lowering of the medial aspect of the foot. Pronation occurs at the subtalar joint; it is also referred to as inrolling. Foot pronation is a component of eversion. Eversion involves pronation at the subtalar joint, dorsiflexion at the ankle joint, and abduction of the forefoot at the tarsometatarsal joints. The key to controlling excess pronation is controlling the calcaneus to keep the subtalar joint in a neutral position.

Pes planus can be due to abnormalities such as excessive internal torsion of the tibia (which results in pronation of the foot) or malalignment of the calcaneus. It is the interaction between the tibia and the foot at the subtalar joint that allows pathology outside the foot to cause inrolling of the foot (Fig. 16-2).

The reduction of pronation is accomplished by maintaining the calcaneus and the subtalar joint in correct alignment. The subtalar joint should be in a neutral position during the custom molding process. The subtalar joint neutral position prevents rotational deformities associated with excessive supination or pronation from occurring (panels b and d of Fig. 16-2). Elevation of the anteromedial calcaneus exerts an upward thrust against the sustentaculum tali to help prevent inrolling.[5] The

orthosis should extend beyond the metatarsal heads to provide better leverage for control of the deformity. A custom-made foot orthosis designed to prevent hyperpronation is also referred to as a UCBL orthosis (or UCB), denoting the University of California Biomechanics Laboratory, where the original work regarding this type of orthosis was performed in the 1940s.

Some cases of pes planus are due to ligamentous laxity within the foot. For these cases, a medial longitudinal arch support can be helpful for alleviating pain. Initial use of an arch that is too high can cause discomfort. The height of the arch can be increased as necessary as the foot develops a tolerance for the inlay. A Thomas heel extension (term for increased medial length to heel) can also offer medial support, particularly for heavier individuals. A most practical piece of advice for runners who have hyperpronation or pes planus is to purchase a pair of running shoes with a firm medial heel counter as well as shoes with a wide last at the shank (Fig. 16-1). Each of these applications helps prevent pronation at the subtalar joint.

Pes cavus (high-arched foot)

A typical complication of pes cavus is excess pressure along the heel and metatarsal head areas, which can lead to pain. This can be prevented by making the height of the longitudinal support just high enough to fill in the space between the shank of the shoe and the arch of the foot, to distribute weight more effectively. Weight should also be evenly distributed over the metatarsal heads. The lift is extended just to the metatarsal head area to help distribute and alleviate pressure over the metatarsal weight-bearing area. Because there is no tendency to pronate, as in pes planus, the high point of the arch is located at the talonavicular joint. If the tibia is externally rotated (Fig. 16-2), this can give the appearance of an elevated arch as the foot supinates and the lateral aspect of the foot assumes additional weight-bearing responsibility. In these cases, a foot orthosis is custom molded with the subtalar joint in a neutral position to prevent excess supination from occurring.

Forefoot pain (metatarsalgia)

Relief of pain in the forefoot is accomplished by distributing the weight-bearing forces to an area proximal to the metatarsal heads. This can be done by either internal or external modification. A metatarsal pad (also referred to as a 'cookie') can be placed inside the shoe just proximal to the second, third, and fourth metatarsal heads. It should also be just proximal to the lateral aspect of the first metatarsal head and medial to the fifth metatarsal head (Fig. 16-3). A metatarsal bar (Fig. 16-4) is recommended for cases in which the foot is too sensitive to tolerate a pad inside the shoe. The metatarsal bar is typically a quarter of an inch thick and tapers distally. The distal edge should be proximal to the metatarsal heads. It is often applied to a leather or neoprene sole.[31] The metatarsal bar can also be used for forefoot pain associated with pes cavus (Fig. 16-4).

Prevention of forefoot pain should also be emphasized to patients. Patients should avoid shoes with high heels or pointed toes, which place excess stress on the metatarsal heads.[3]

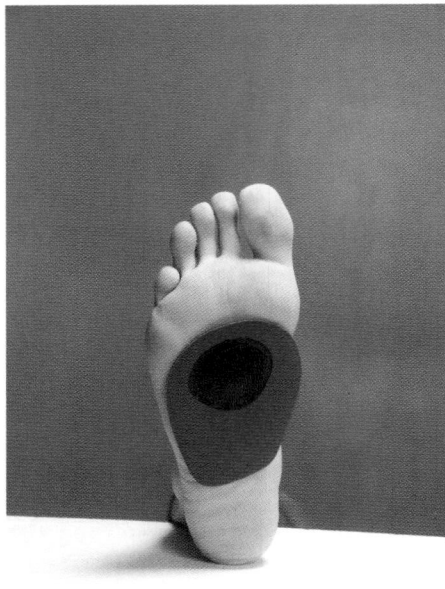

Figure 16-3
Metatarsal pad for forefoot pain. This should be placed proximal to the metatarsal heads in order to reduce weight distribution on the metatarsal heads.

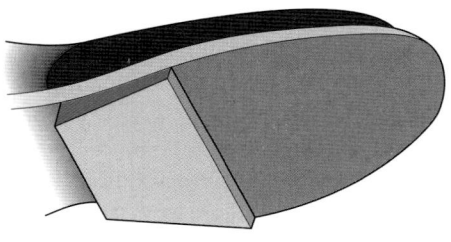

Figure 16-4
Metatarsal bar. (After Pfeffinger 1985,[33] with permission.)

Heel pain

The painful area can be alleviated by using an orthosis to help distribute weight. Rubber heel pads can be applied inside the shoe to offer relief in cases of minor discomfort. A calcaneal bar is recommended for cases in which the foot is too sensitive to tolerate a pad inside the shoe and the heel pain is associated with a chronic condition. The calcaneal bar is placed distal to the painful area to prevent the calcaneus from assuming full weight-bearing status.

A common cause of heel pain along the anteromedial calcaneus is plantar fasciitis. Pain occurs at the attachment site of the fascia along the medial aspect of the heel. Point tenderness is located over the anteromedial calcaneus. It is common in people who hyperpronate their feet, thereby placing excess stress on the medial longitudinal arch. A custom-made orthosis with the subtalar joint in a neutral position (such as that described for pes planus) helps prevent excessive inrolling from occurring and reduces the stress placed along the proximal arch. A custom-made orthosis is indicated for cases in which conservative treatment has failed. From an orthotic standpoint,

conservative treatment should include the use of a pair of shoes with a firm medial heel counter and a wide shank.

Plantar fasciitis is also common in patients with high arches. For these patients, the medial longitudinal arch undergoes marked stress during weight bearing. This can be treated with either an elevated arch support or a heel well that helps distribute pressure along the medial longitudinal arch.

Heel spurs are frequently mistaken as the source of heel pain. Heel spurs related to plantar fasciitis are the result of mechanical stress acting through the plantar fascia on to its origin at the calcaneus and are not the source of the pain.[36] Inferior heel spurs are related to advancing age and are not painful in nature.

Heel lifts help some causes of Achilles pain by decreasing the amount of stretch placed on the Achilles tendon (by keeping the ankle joint plantar flexed). A heel lift can be used to treat Achilles enthesitis, an inflammatory reaction at the insertion of the tendon into the periosteum of the calcaneus. A heel lift can also be helpful for treating plantar flexion spasticity or contracture by increasing the total heel height to help ensure that the patient has a heel strike prior to toe touch during gait.

Toe pain

The goal of orthotic intervention in toe pain is to decrease pain by immobilization. This is done by incorporating a full-length carbon insert along the sole of the shoe. Alternatively, a steel shank can be extended forward to reduce the mobility of the distal joints, particularly if metal AFO componentry is being utilized. Alternatively, a metatarsal bar can also be used for partial immobilization. Common conditions associated with toe pain include hallux rigidus, gout, and arthritis.

Leg length discrepancy

A symptomatic leg length discrepancy should first be evaluated with proper measurement. True leg length is measured from the distal tip of the anterior superior iliac spine to the distal tip of the medial malleolus. Apparent leg length is measured from a midline point, such as the pubic symphysis or umbilicus, to the distal tip of each malleolus. This can be abnormal in cases in which the true leg length is normal but pelvic obliquity is present secondary to conditions such as scoliosis, pelvic fracture, or muscle imbalance. There is no support in the medical literature for treating low back pain associated with an alleged leg length discrepancy. It is not advised unless there is a traumatic event, such as a femur fracture, resulting in a significant acute-onset 'leg' (lower limb) length discrepancy.

Leg length discrepancies of less than one-half an inch do not need correction. The total discrepancy is never corrected. At most, 75% of the leg length discrepancy should be corrected. The first one-half inch of the discrepancy can be managed with a heel pad. Additional correction requires the heel to be built up externally. The sole should also be built up proportionally when the heel is built up externally, in order to provide a comfortable, stable gait. A taller sole should have a rocker bottom to help normalize the gait pattern at toe-off (Fig. 16-5).

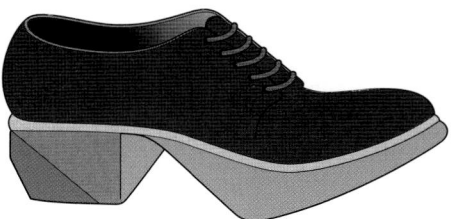

Figure 16-5 Solid ankle cushion heel and rocker bottom. Note that the elevated heel requires an elevated sole with rocker bottom to facilitate gait. The heel must also slant inward to prevent an excessive flexion moment at the knee at heel strike. (After Pfeffinger 1985,[33] with permission.)

Osteoarthritis of the knee

Although osteoarthritis of the knee is not a foot condition, it is mentioned here because pain related to it can be alleviated with foot orthoses. Foot orthoses alter the ground reaction forces affecting the more proximal joints, such as the knee, and this relationship should be considered when prescribing a foot orthosis. Lateral heel wedges can be used for conservative treatment of osteoarthritis when medial compartment narrowing is present. The heel wedges used are a quarter of an inch thick along the lateral border and taper medially. Relief was obtained with heel wedges in 74 of 121 knees from 85 patients in one study.[13] Relief of pain was most frequently obtained in patients with mild osteoarthritis, but it was also documented in some patients with complete obliteration of the medial joint space. Wedge use widened the gait pattern. This orthosis has not been studied in patients with medial meniscus injuries, but it may afford some pain relief with medial compartment unloading.

Pediatric shoes

Children's shoes should have a simple design. To facilitate gait, a heel should not be present. Soft soles are recommended to permit the natural development of feet. Tennis shoes are adequate for most children. A high quarter or three-quarter shoe will stay on a child's foot better than a low-cut shoe, and is recommended during the first few years of life.

It is a common misconception that all flatfeet need to be treated in children. Flatfeet are usual in infants, common in children, and occur occasionally in adults.[46] Flatfeet improve over time, in part because of the loss of subcutaneous fat and the reduction of laxity of the joints that occur with growth[46] and the maturation of the gait pattern. Intensive treatment with corrective shoes or inserts for a 3-year period did not alter the natural history of flatfeet in 129 children who were 1–6 years of age.[53] One cannot make the asymptomatic person feel any better. Frequent shoe size change is necessary in the first few years of life.[54]

ANKLE–FOOT ORTHOSES

Ankle–foot orthoses are the most commonly prescribed lower limb orthoses. They were formerly known as short leg braces.

Metal or plastic AFOs can be used effectively to control ankle motion. Metal AFOs are relatively contraindicated in children, because the weight of the brace can cause external tibial rotation. Plastic AFOs are now more common in all age groups.

Ankle–foot orthoses should provide mediolateral stability as a safety feature.[22] Although much emphasis with AFOs is placed on controlling the amount of dorsiflexion and plantar flexion, movements at the subtalar joint also significantly influence the biomechanics of gait. Inversion includes supination at the subtalar joint, adduction at the tarsometatarsal joints, and plantar flexion at the ankle joint, which results in the foot being in an equinovarus position. Eversion includes pronation at the subtalar joint, abduction of the forefoot at the tarsometatarsal joints, and dorsiflexion at the ankle joint, resulting in the foot being in a valgus position. Rotation at the subtalar joint is also accompanied by rotation of the tibia (Fig. 16-2).

Ankle–foot orthoses can also stabilize the knee during gait.[18] They are prescribed for conditions affecting knee stability, such as genu recurvatum. An AFO should be considered for conditions affecting the knee, particularly when a concurrent problem exists at the ankle or subtalar joints. A proper AFO prescription considers the biomechanical influence of the orthosis at the foot, ankle, and knee in all planes of movement. *It should be remembered that plantar flexion creates a knee extension moment and dorsiflexion creates a knee flexion moment.*

Metal ankle–foot orthoses

Metal AFOs are now used much less commonly than the plastic type. They will be discussed for the following four reasons.

1. Much of the research regarding the biomechanical influence of AFOs on gait was performed with metal AFOs. These principles also apply to plastic orthoses.
2. Metal components (especially joints) are frequently used in combination with plastic orthoses.
3. Some older patients wish to continue to use the metal orthoses to which they have become accustomed.
4. Morbidly obese patients may require more if not all metal componentry for durability and subtalar joint stability.

Recent research has offered support that metal AFOs provide better stabilization of the ankle during the gait cycle.[6]

The metal AFO consists of a proximal calf band, two uprights, ankle joints, and an attachment to the shoe to anchor the AFO (Fig. 16-6). The posterior metal portion of the calf band should be 1.5–3 inches wide in order to adequately distribute pressure.[9] The calf band should be 1 inch below the fibular neck to prevent a compressive common peroneal palsy. A leather strap with Velcro is used to close the calf band, because it provides ease of closure for patients with only one functional upper limb.

Ankle joint motion is controlled by pins or springs inserted into channels (Figs 16-7 through 16-10). The pins are adjusted with a screwdriver to set the desired amount of plantar flexion and dorsiflexion. The spring is also adjusted with a screwdriver to provide the proper amount of tension necessary to aid motion at the ankle joint (used to assist dorsiflexion). Longer channels

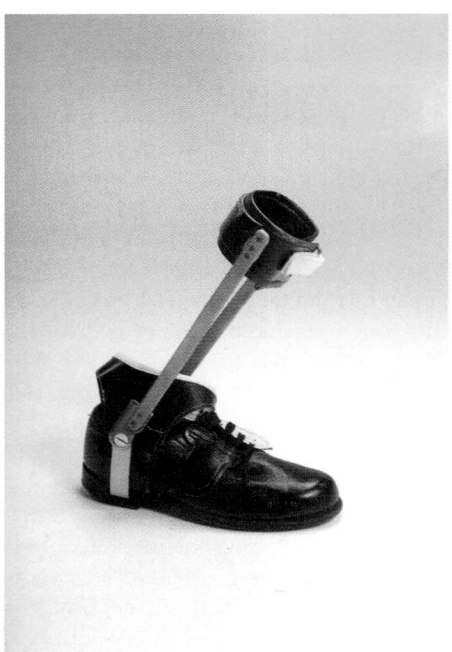

Figure 16-6 Metal double-upright dorsiflexion assist ankle–foot orthosis on right shoe with lateral T strap for control of varus deformity. The metal dorsiflexion assist ankle joint has also been referred to as a Klenzak ankle joint. Note the split stirrup in the heel that allows the wearing of the orthosis with other shoes.

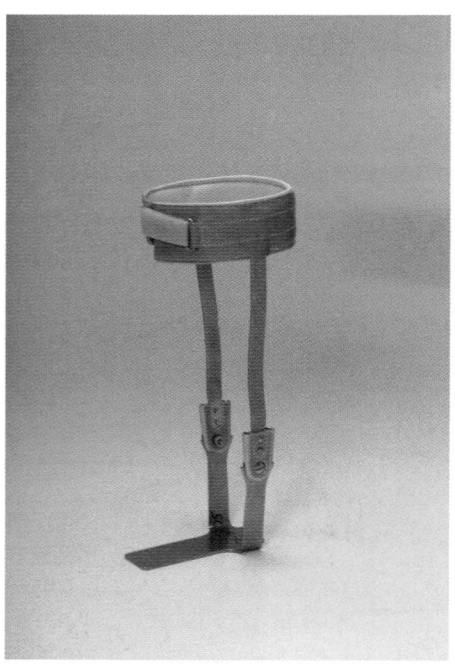

Figure 16-7 Double-action metal ankle joint with solid stirrup.

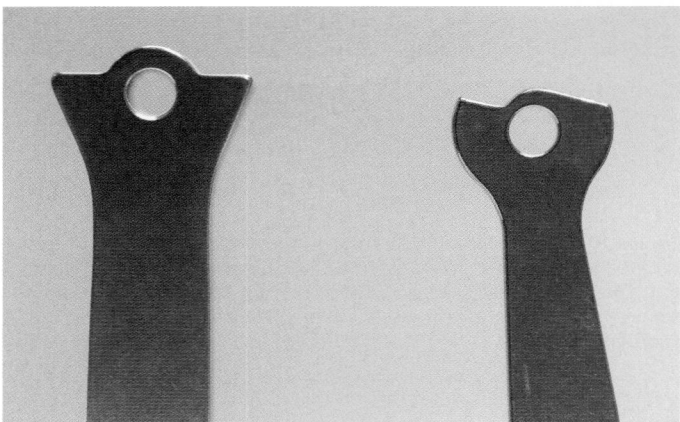

Figure 16-8 Double-action stirrup and dorsiflexion assist stirrup, used with the ankle joints shown in Figures 16-7 and 16-6, respectively. (Courtesy of USMC, Pasadena.)

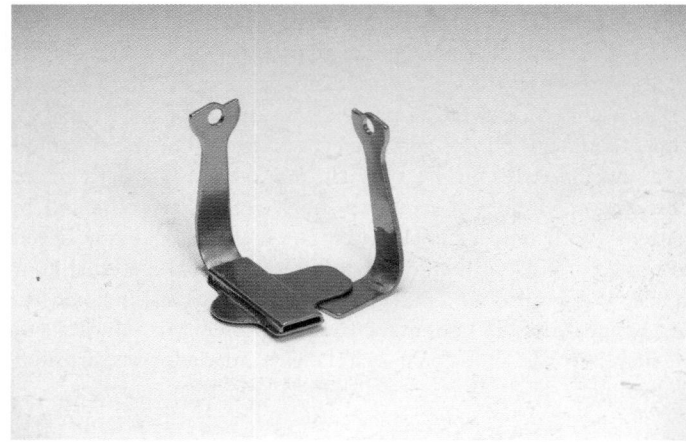

Figure 16-9 Split stirrup. The stirrup extends anteriorly to attach at the shank area of a shoe for stability.

help prevent the spring mechanism from 'bottoming out', and provide for more precise control of ankle motion.

A solid stirrup is a U-shaped metal piece permanently attached to the shoe. Its two ends are bent upward to articulate with the medial and lateral ankle joints (Fig. 16-7). The proximal stirrup attachment sites are shaped to enforce the desired movements at the ankle joint (Fig. 16-8). The sole plate can be extended beyond the metatarsal head area for conditions requiring a longer lever arm for better control of plantar flexion (e.g. plantar spasticity).

A split stirrup can be used instead of a solid stirrup (Figs 16-6 and 16-9). The split stirrup has a sole plate with two flat channels for insertion of the uprights. The two uprights are now called calipers, as they can open and close distally to allow donning and doffing of the AFO. A split stirrup allows removal of the uprights from the shoes so that the AFO can be worn with other shoes (Fig. 16-6). Other pairs of shoes should also have the sole plate with channels for calipers incorporated into the heel area. The split stirrup is not as stable as the solid stirrup.

Ankle stops and assists

The ankle joint can be positioned so that it is in a neutral, dorsiflexed, or plantar-flexed position, depending on the gait disturbance. It can be set to permit a partial range of motion or to eliminate a certain motion. An understanding of the effect on the placement of pins and screws into the two channels of an ankle joint (Fig. 16-10) facilitates the proper orthotic prescription for the patient. This section reviews the common uses of the posterior stop, anterior stop, and posterior dorsiflexion assist. A spring in the anterior channel has not been demonstrated to be of clinical value.

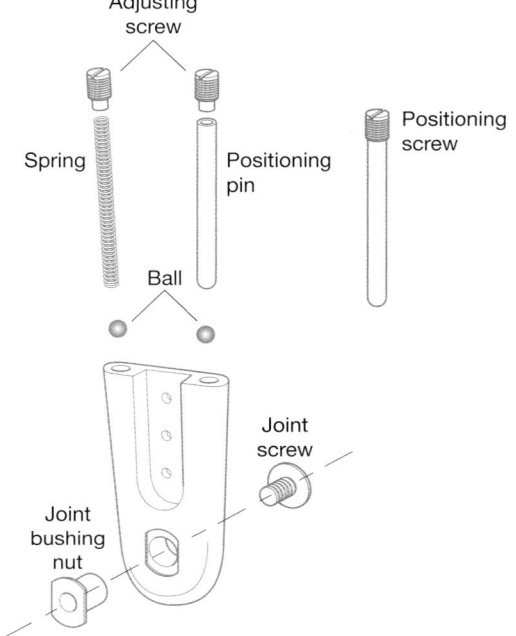

Figure 16-10 Metal ankle joint components. This type of ankle joint has also been referred to as a double-action ankle joint, a double Klenzak ankle joint, and a bichannel adjustable ankle locking (BiCAAL) joint. (Courtesy of USMC, Pasadena.)

Plantar stop (posterior stop) The plantar stop is used to control plantar spasticity or help incrementally stretch plantar contractures. The plantar stop is most commonly set at 90°. A pin is inserted into the posterior channel of an ankle joint, such as that in Figure 16-10, to limit plantar flexion. An AFO with a plantar stop at 90° produces a flexion moment at the knee during heel strike. Because the dorsiflexors cannot eccentrically activate to permit the foot to make contact with the ground, the ground reactive force remains posterior to the knee after heel strike, which creates a flexion moment at the knee (and possibly an unstable gait). The proximal portion of the AFO also has an effect on knee stability. The posterior portion of the proximal AFO exerts a forward push on the proximal leg to increase the knee flexion moment after heel strike (Fig. 16-11). The opposite occurs at toe-off, with an extension moment created at the knee. This concept has been used to develop what has been referred to as a plastic ground reaction AFO, with a solid proximal anterior tibial closing that provides a greater influence on the knee. This device will be discussed in more detail later. The greater the plantar flexion resistance, the greater the flexion moment at the knee at heel strike, and the greater the need for active hip extensors to prevent the body from collapsing forward on a buckling knee.

A solid ankle cushion heel (SACH) heel wedge (see Fig. 16-5) can be used to reduce the flexion moment at the knee. The term SACH is a misnomer borrowed from the prosthetic literature. The 'SA' (solid ankle) refers to the type of prosthetic ankle joint. The SACH heel wedge in this case should be referred to only as a cushioned heel. A cushioned heel serves as a shock absorber at heel strike, and is able to partially substitute for the dorsiflexors, which cannot be activated when an AFO's ankle plantar stops are set at 90°. A cushioned heel also

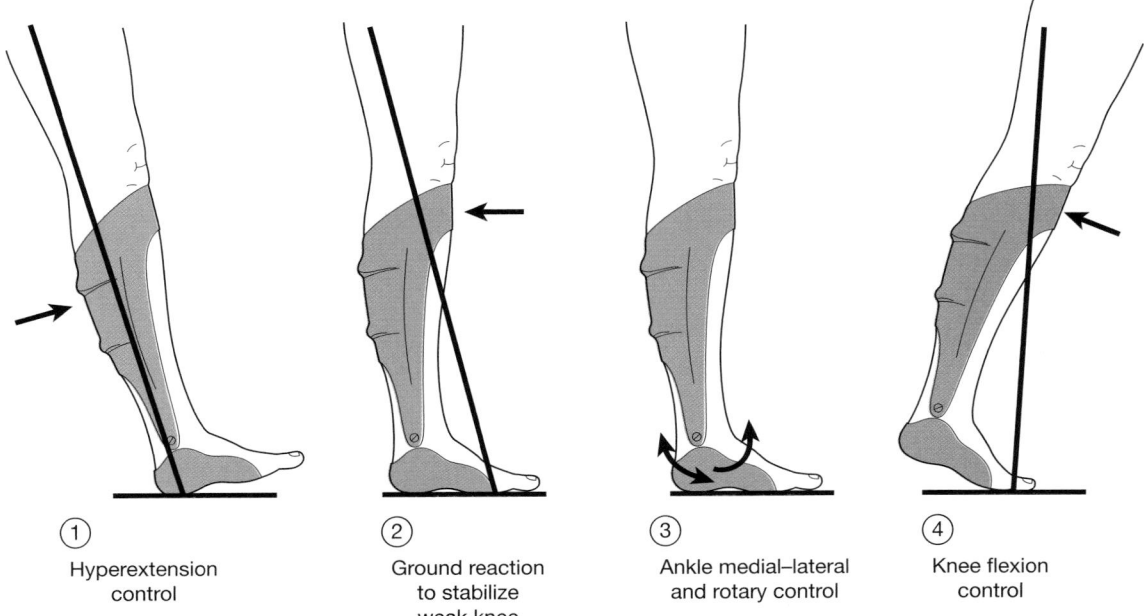

① Hyperextension control

② Ground reaction to stabilize weak knee

③ Ankle medial–lateral and rotary control

④ Knee flexion control

Figure 16-11 Ground reaction–ankle–foot (AFO) orthosis dynamic. Note the effect of the proximal portion of the AFO on the knee throughout gait. (Courtesy of Oregon Orthotic System, Albany.)

helps move the ground reactive force more anteriorly at the foot and subsequently at the knee. In essence, a soft heel helps stabilize the knee. It helps keep the ground reaction force anterior to the knee joint. A firm heel decreases knee stability via a knee flexion moment while moving the ground reaction force posterior to the knee joint. A cushioned heel can also be used with an AFO to minimize the amount of plantar flexion spasticity present after heel strike.

The posterior stop should be set at the minimal amount of plantar flexion required to clear the foot during swing-through.[14] Remember, plantar flexion creates a knee extension moment at the knee after heel strike. This provides a more stable knee during gait than when the ankle plantar stops are set in any degree of dorsiflexion.

A balanced decision should be made between providing resistance to plantar flexion to clear the foot during the swing phase of gait, and the amount of instability at the knee during the stance phase of gait. No AFO is effective in reducing the amount of knee flexion to 'normal' levels during the stance phase of gait.[16]

Dorsiflexion stop (anterior stop)

An anterior stop is used to substitute for the function of the gastrocnemius–soleus complex (Fig. 16-12). It is used in conditions with weak calf muscles or weak quadriceps (because of its effect on the knee). Weak calf musculature allows the ankle to enter dorsiflexion. The

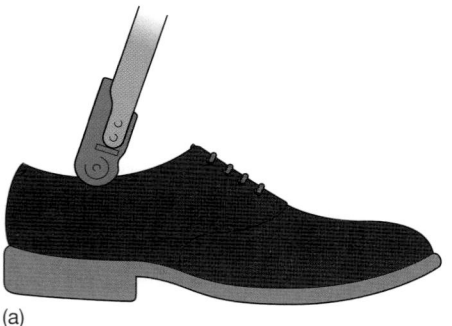

(a)

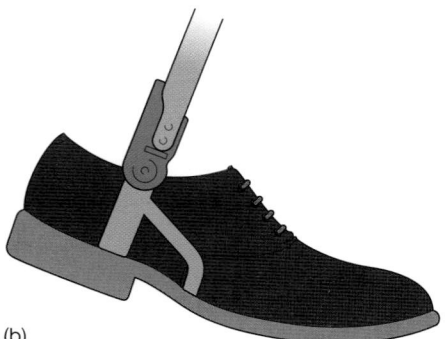

(b)

Figure 16-12 Anterior pin stop simulating plantar flexion. (**a**) Anterior channels of the ankle–foot orthosis component of a knee–ankle–foot orthosis left open in a spinal cord-injured patient. Note that the heel does not lift up (i.e. no plantar flexion). (**b**) Anterior channels of the same orthosis with anterior pins in place set at 5° of dorsiflexion and with metal sole plate. Note that the heel does lift up (i.e. plantar flexion) as momentum causes the lower limb to 'pole-vault' over the anterior pin setting.

anterior stop set at 5° of dorsiflexion best substitutes for gastrocnemius–soleus function.[14,16]

The anterior stop assists with push-off and assists the knee joint into extension. It should be used in combination with a stirrup with a sole extension to the metatarsal heads, to simulate the action of the calf muscles. The dorsiflexion stop simulates the gastrocnemius–soleus function by causing the heel to rise during the latter part of stance rather than remaining flat on the ground. The shoe pivots over the metatarsal heads, creating an extension moment at the knee that helps stabilize the knee from midstance to toe-off.

The earlier the dorsiflexion stop occurs during the stance phase, the greater the extension moment at the knee. This is useful in clinical situations where quadriceps weakness is also present. If the extension moment at the knee is too great for too long, then genu recurvatum (back knee) can occur. A balance should be obtained such that the extension at the knee is sufficient to stabilize the knee in extension yet prevent genu recurvatum. If too much dorsiflexion is permitted by the anterior stop, there will be too much knee flexion during gait from midstance to toe-off.

Dorsiflexion assist (posterior spring)

The posterior spring serves two purposes. It substitutes for concentric contraction of dorsiflexors to prevent flaccid foot drop after toe-off. It also substitutes (inadequately) for the eccentric activation of the dorsiflexors after heel strike. The metal dorsiflexion assist ankle joint has also been known as a Klenzak ankle joint (see Fig. 16-6).

The posterior spring prevents rapid plantar flexion at heel strike during its compression in the posterior channel. The posterior spring is again compressed during plantar flexion during late stance prior to toe-off. The posterior spring assists with toe clearance during the swing phase of gait by providing a downward thrust posterior to the ankle joint at toe-off, which results in dorsiflexion anterior to the ankle joint. The longer the channel, the greater the ability to control dorsiflexion.

A summary of some of the common indications for the various channel components is found in Table 16-1.

Metal AFO varus–valgus control

Varus and valgus deformities are associated with rotation at the subtalar joint. A T strap is attached along the side of the shoe distal to the subtalar joint to help minimize the deformity (Fig. 16-6). T straps are also used to help prevent worsening of the deformity. T straps also help distribute pressure properly along the foot during weight bearing.

T straps are referred to as being either medial or lateral. A lateral T strap is sewn to the lateral aspect of the shoe, and the belt is cinched around the medial upright of the AFO (Fig. 16-6). A lateral T strap is used to control a varus deformity. The belt is secured with a buckle around the medial upright. This helps create a force directing the subtalar joint outward, which counteracts the supination and adduction tendency that would result in excess varus. The opposite is true for a valgus deformity with the T strap being medially located. A pressure ulcer can develop over the malleolus if the T strap is buckled too tightly.

Table 16-1 Clinical indications for various metal ankle channel components

Channel	Pin or spring	Function	Clinical indications
Posterior	Pin	Limits plantar flexion	Plantar spasticity, toe drag, pain with ankle motion
Posterior	Spring	Assists dorsiflexion	Flaccid foot drop, knee hyperextension
Anterior[a]	Pin	Limits dorsiflexion	Weak plantar flexors, weak knee extensors, pain with ankle motion
Anterior	Spring	Assists plantar flexion	None

[a]*Used in combination with an extended sole plate to the metatarsal head area to help compensate for weak plantar flexors.*

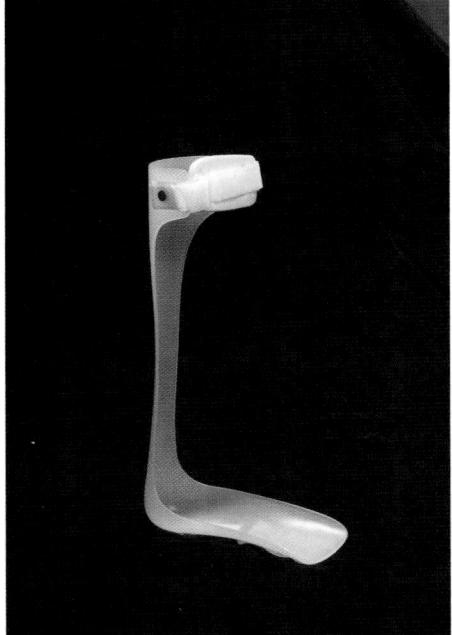

Figure 16-13
Custom plastic solid (means no ankle joint, although still flexible) ankle–foot orthosis (AFO) with posterior trim line to allow some flexibility with plantar flexion. This is the most commonly prescribed AFO for foot drop. It is also referred to as a posterior leaf spring AFO.

The T strap inadequately substitutes for the foot pronators, supinators, abductors, and adductors, because it does not have an attachment on the plantar surface of the foot to create the mechanical advantage offered by the plantar-attached muscles and tendons.

Plastic ankle–foot orthoses

Plastic AFOs are the most commonly used AFOs because of their cost, cosmesis, light weight, interchangeability with shoes, ability to control varus and valgus deformities, provision of better foot support with the customized foot portion, and ability to achieve what is offered by the metal AFO (Fig. 16-13). Energy consumption is equal with a plastic solid AFO or a metal double-upright AFO.[2] Although a plastic orthosis weighs less than its metal counterpart, the weight of the orthosis is not as important as the influence of the ground reactive force created by the presence of the orthosis. The same orthotic principles apply to orthoses made of plastic or metal. The plastic AFO's effect on knee stability should be recognized. The plastic AFO prescribed for toe clearance should be just rigid enough to provide resistance for toe clearance. Excessive resistance to plantar flexion can make the knee unstable (create a flexion moment) after heel strike.[17]

Plastic AFOs can be prefabricated or custom made. The reasons for prescribing a custom-molded orthosis include long-term need, conformed molding for comfort or insensate feet, placement of the orthosis in a fixed amount of plantar or dorsi-flexion, better control of rotational deformities, and further reduction of weight bearing for a tibial fracture or diabetic plantar ulcer. The custom process is similar to that previously described in this chapter for foot orthoses, with the positive mold serving as the model for the orthosis.

Some practical advice should be offered to the patient regarding the use of a plastic AFO. If changing shoes, it is best to have another pair with a similar heel height, to prevent altering the biomechanical effects at the foot, ankle, and knee. Tennis shoes are most accommodating for donning and doffing of the AFO. However, if dress shoes are to be worn, patients should also be told that their shoe size might need to be one-half size greater and the next width larger to accommodate the orthosis. A Blucher-style dress shoe helps accommodate the orthosis (Fig. 16-1).

Plastic AFO components

The foot component of the AFO should extend beyond the metatarsal heads. The footplate can be extended beyond the toes to reduce spasticity aggravated by toe flexion. The shape and molding of the foot portion influence the biomechanics of more proximal joints.

The ankle and subtalar joints can be made more stable under four circumstances.

1. The trim line extends more anteriorly at the ankle level (a trim line is the anterior border of the plastic AFO).
2. The plastic material is thicker.
3. Carbon inserts are placed along the medial and lateral aspects of the ankle joint.
4. Corrugations are made within the posterior leaf of the AFO.

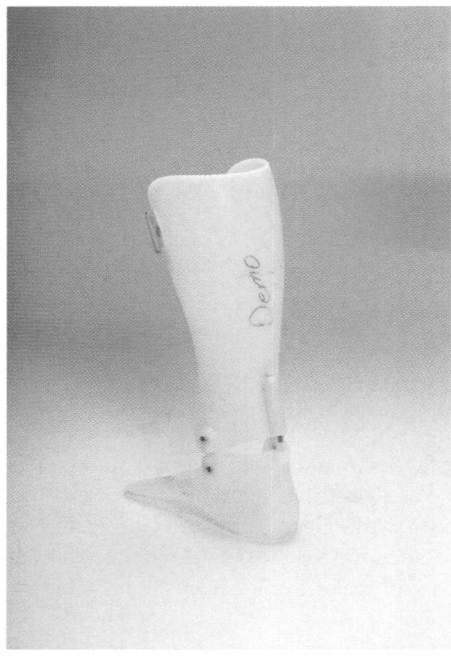

Figure 16-14 Midline posterior stop articulated ankle–foot orthosis. Note the use of a plastic ankle joint to further decrease weight. Plastic ankle joints are more commonly used by children (lightweight individuals). The use of a plantar stop with ankle joints is recommended for an active lightweight patient with plantar spasticity (e.g. a child with cerebral palsy).

Table 16-2 Orthotic componentry with knee flexion and exxtension moments		
Orthotic factor	Knee extension moment–stability	Knee flexion moment–instability
Heel	Cushioned	Solid
Ankle–foot orthosis fixed in:	Plantar flexion	Dorsiflexion
Trim line on ankle–foot orthosis	Posterior (flexible)	Anterior
Knee joint	Posterior offset	—

The strength of the AFO should be matched to the patient's weight and activity level.

Plastic AFOs can also be hinged at the ankle. Ankle hinges allow full or partial ankle motion, which can permit a more natural gait. They should be considered when complete restriction of ankle motion is not required. Plastic ankle joints are light and are a good choice for children. Metal ankle joints are preferred for adults, particularly heavy adults. Newer designs have a single midline posterior pin–spring mechanism (Fig. 16-14). This midline spring functions like the more traditional medial and lateral dual posterior spring assist mechanism (Figs 16-8 and 16-9). This makes the AFO narrower in the mediolateral direction and slightly longer in the anterior posterior direction, which better conforms to the design of most trousers.

The leg component should encompass three-quarters of the leg and should be padded along its internal surface.[9] The proximal extent should end 1 inch below the fibular neck to prevent a compressive common peroneal nerve palsy.

The solid plastic ankle–foot orthosis The solid plastic AFO is the most commonly prescribed plastic AFO (Fig. 16-13). It can be made to serve several purposes. The term *solid* refers to an AFO that is made of a single piece of plastic. It does not have ankle joints. A solid AFO can still be flexible enough to allow some ankle motion, and it should be flexible with a posterior trim line for the treatment of foot drop without mediolateral instability. A solid AFO should be truly solid (not flexible) for the treatment of plantar spasticity.

Solid AFOs set at 90° are commonly used for foot drop. Less obvious but equally important is the solid AFO's ability to treat conditions affecting the knee. Again, it should be remembered that plantar flexion creates knee extension and dorsiflexion creates knee flexion at heel strike. The AFO can be fixed in a

few degrees of plantar flexion to provide stability at the knee during the stance phase of gait. Genu recurvatum can also be treated with a solid AFO. The more rigid the AFO, the greater the flexion moment at the knee at heel strike, which helps reverse the extension moment at the knee associated with genu recurvatum. The flexion moment at the knee also becomes greater during midstance if the ankle is placed in a few degrees of dorsiflexion. Table 16-2 summarizes the important orthotic factors involved in creating knee extension and flexion moments throughout the gait cycle.

Plastic AFO varus–valgus control The goal of orthotic intervention is to alter the ground reactive forces with custom molding to help maintain proper alignment of the lower limb by 'building up' selected portions of the AFO. A three-point system is used to provide the counterforces necessary to oppose the forces of the deformity (Fig. 16-15).[24,27] Some orthotists believe that an orthosis should be firm ('not conforming') in order to control a deformity. Pressure points should be present in expected areas at follow-up visits if the orthosis is serving its purpose. A custom ground reaction orthosis provides appropriate foot support that influences the rotation of more proximal joints (Fig. 16-16). The anterior tibial shell closing helps stabilize the knee during gait (Fig. 16-11).

An equinovarus (or inversion) deformity is controlled by applying forces medially at the metatarsal head area and calcaneus. The next force is applied more proximally along the lateral aspect of the fibula. This helps prevent inversion at the subtalar and ankle joints. A more proximal medial tibial force is applied to provide stabilization of the leg portion of the plastic AFO by providing an opposing force to the fibular area (Fig. 16-15). A three-point system also exists at the foot level to help prevent supination of the foot related to the equinovarus deformity (Fig. 16-15). A three-point system is again applied to control the plantar flexion deformity associated with equinovarus (Fig. 16-15).

The reverse of the above-described three-point system to control varus can be used to control valgus at the foot. Movements in all joints should be considered when prescribing an orthosis.

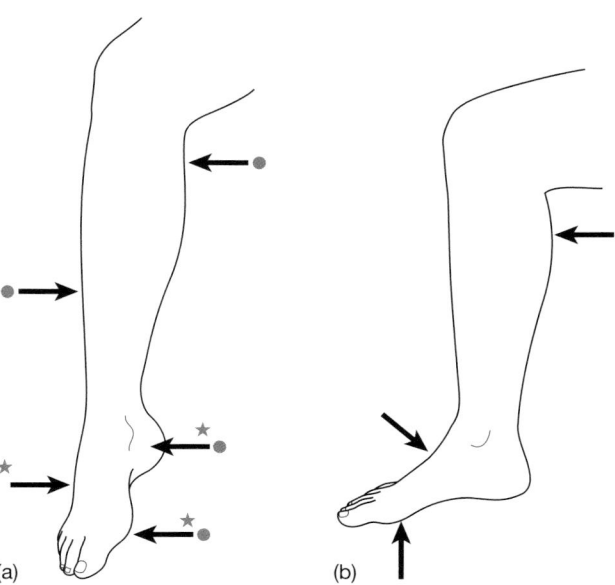

Figure 16-15 Three-point system control of equinovarus deformity.
(**a**) Control of varus rotational component at the foot (stars) and subtalar
joint (dots). (**b**) Control of equinus deformity. (After Marx 1974,[27] with
permission.)

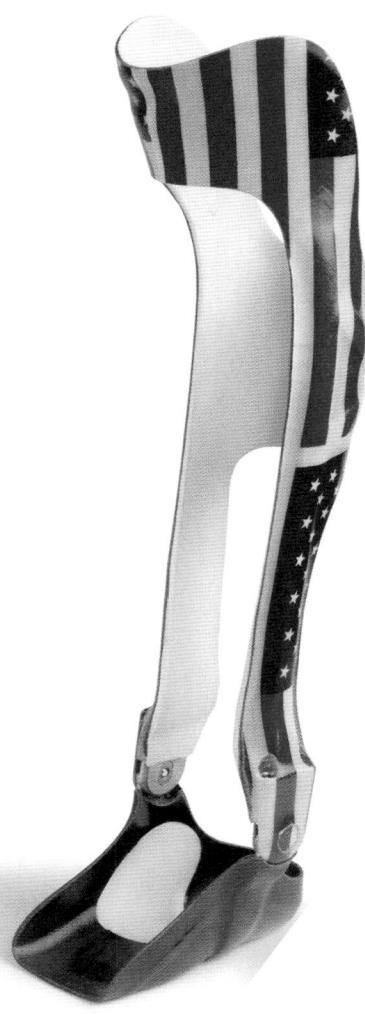

Figure 16-16
Oregon Orthotic System
rotational control ankle–foot
orthosis. Note the
corrugations that add
strength to the orthosis.
Also note the metal ankle
joint that is similar to those
in Figures 16-9 and 16-10.
(Courtesy of Oregon
Orthotic System, Albany.)

Patellar tendon-bearing AFOs

A patellar tendon-bearing (PTB) AFO uses the patellar tendon
and the tibial condyles to partially relieve weight-bearing stress
on skeletal structures distally, with more weight bearing distributed along the medial tibial condyle.[20] PTB is a misnomer for
this orthosis, because only about 10% of the weight is distributed along the patellar tendon and the medial tibial condyle.
Most of the weight bearing is distributed throughout the soft
tissues of the leg that are compressed by an appropriately fitted
orthosis. Compression of the soft tissues of the leg is also
responsible for maintaining alignment and length of the tibia
after a fracture.[41,42]

Patellar tendon-bearing AFOs are often prescribed for
diabetic ulcerations of the foot, tibial fractures, relief of the
weight-bearing surface in painful heel conditions such as calcaneal fractures, postoperative ankle fusions, and avascular necrosis of the foot or ankle. The orthoses are made of plastic and
are bivalved. They fit snugly with the use of Velcro straps (Fig.
16-17) or buckles similar to those of ski boots. A custom-
molded PTB AFO can reduce weight bearing in the affected
foot by up to 50%.

Custom-made PTB AFOs are indicated when maximum
weight-bearing reduction is necessary to ensure proper healing
(such as in a debrided diabetic heel ulcer) and reduction of pain.
It should first be determined that the painful condition is associated with weight bearing rather than with range of motion. If
pain occurs with range of motion, then the pain-producing
range of motion should be eliminated.

The solid plastic orthosis makes contact with the ground
before the reactive force is absorbed significantly by the foot,
and then distributes this force more proximally along the leg.
Compared with a prefabricated AFO, a custom-made PTB AFO

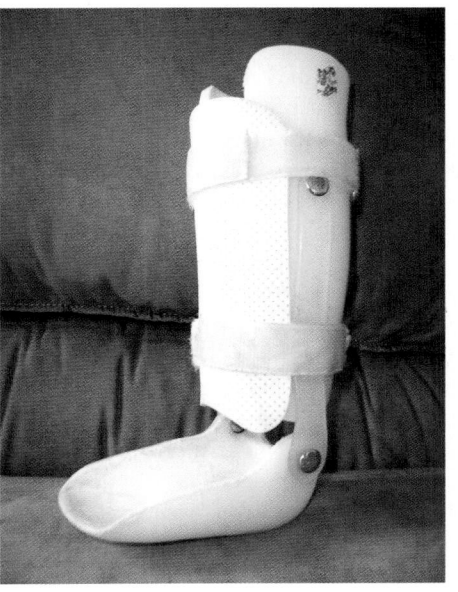

Figure 16-17
Custom bivalved
patellar tendon-
bearing ankle–foot
orthosis. Ten percent
of the weight is
transferred to the
patellar tendon. Fifty
percent weight-
bearing reduction
is achieved by
custom-fitted contact
distributed throughout
the leg. This was
prescribed for a
young girl with a
large benign left leg
tibia tumor resection.

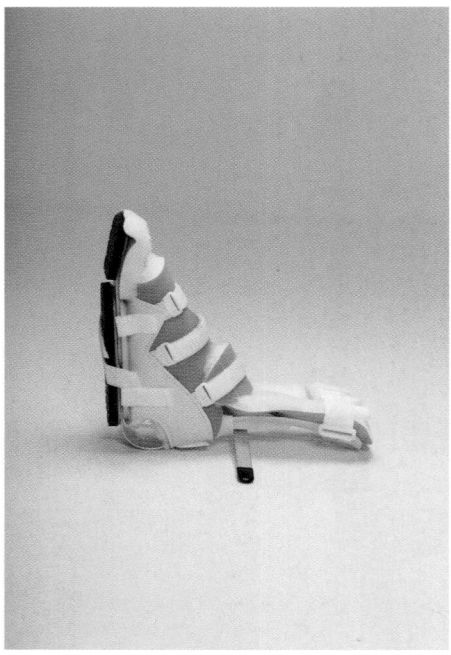

Figure 16-18
Pressure relief ankle–foot orthosis. The heel cutout provides complete heel pressure relief. The hinged posterior lever arm prevents ankle pressure sore development either medially or laterally, and can be adjusted as necessary to prevent medial or lateral malleolar pressure.

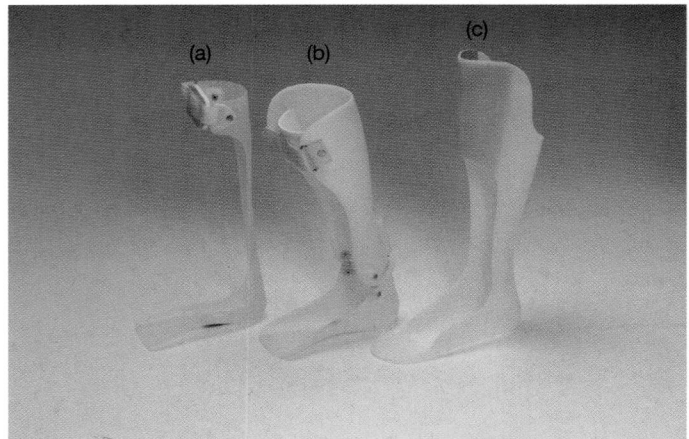

Figure 16-19 Common ankle–foot orthosis (AFO) prescriptions. (**a**) Foot drop AFO. (**b**) Plantar spasticity AFO. (**c**) Lumbar spinal cord injury AFO.

more effectively distributes pressure over a greater surface contact area for maximal weight-bearing reduction. Additional weight-bearing reduction is obtained by eliminating ankle movement via carbon graphite inserts and/or the use of a rocker bottom (Fig. 16-5), which eliminates active push-off.[23] A rocker bottom is directly incorporated into the plastic orthosis.

Pressure relief AFOs

A pressure relief AFO is also known by its acronym: PRAFO (Fig. 16-18). This type of AFO has different brand names depending on the company who furnished it, including PRAFO, multipodus AFO, and Lennard AFO. This orthosis serves two purposes: pressure relief and contracture prevention. Pressure relief is achieved at the heel by completely eliminating weight bearing with the heel cutout, and also by using a hinged lever arm posteriorly that can be adjusted medially or laterally to prevent medial or lateral malleolar pressure sore development. This should be applied on the immobilized or motionless affected lower limb at all times while in bed. A PRAFO is frequently utilized in dementia patients with hip fractures who do not have much lower limb mobility. Plantar flexion contracture prevention occurs by keeping the ankle joint in a neutral position while the AFO is donned.

Common AFO prescriptions

The three most common physiatric AFO prescriptions are those for foot drop, plantar spasticity, and lumbar spinal cord injury (Fig. 16-19). The most common AFO prescription for foot drop is a custom non-hinged plastic AFO set in a few degrees of dorsiflexion with a posterior trim line. This is also referred to as a posterior leaf spring AFO. The few degrees of dorsiflexion assure foot clearance during the swing phase of gait. It helps

the ankle 'spring' into dorsiflexion after the foot is lifted off the ground in a plantar-flexed position from push-off. The minimal weight and bulk of this AFO are highly desired by the patient with foot drop. The avoidance of hingeing not only minimizes bulk, but from a practical standpoint it keeps the mediolateral dimension of the AFO narrow to best accommodate a variety of shoes and pants. If there is significant subtalar joint instability, a metal double-upright AFO with springs in the posterior channels (dorsiassist) would provide mediolateral stability yet also permit plantar flexion.

The most common AFO prescription for plantar spasticity is either a hinged custom plastic AFO with a single midline posterior stop or a hinged custom plastic AFO with pins in the posterior channels to provide plantar stop at 90°. The former is more likely to be considered in milder cases of spasticity without a significant inversion deformity. The latter is more likely to be considered if there is a significant inversion deformity still present after all other medical treatment measures to manage the spasticity have been exhausted. Metal ankle joints with posterior pins in this case would provide better mediolateral support yet still permit some dorsiflexion with the anterior channels left open. Recent research studies support the use of hinged AFOs with plantar stops at neutral (90°) as a preferred AFO for an active pediatric population with lower limb spasticity.[34,37,45,48,49]

The most common lumbar spinal cord injury AFO prescription is bilateral custom plastic ground reaction (anterior tibial shell closing) AFOs fixed in 10° of plantar flexion. The anterior tibial shell closing and 10° of plantar flexion both help create knee extension moments with weight bearing to add stability to the knees during ambulation. A walker or bilateral Lofstrand forearm orthoses are still needed to permit ambulation.

Checkout

The patient should be examined after fitting and use of the orthosis. The first and most obvious form of a checkout is to verify that the gait pattern is improved with the orthosis in comparison to without the orthosis. The orthotic ankle joint should coincide with the tip of the medial malleolus. The patient is to be checked for ease of donning and doffing the orthosis and, while it is off, observed for areas of skin breakdown. If the AFO was prescribed to control spasticity, the orthotic evaluation should include determining its effectiveness in a dynamic setting, because spasticity can worsen with ambulation. In cases where significant deformity is being addressed with orthotic intervention, some redness can and should be present if the orthosis is doing its job. Some redness is acceptable, as long as it is dispersed in as large an area as possible and as long as there is no skin breakdown.

KNEE–ANKLE–FOOT ORTHOSES

Knee–ankle–foot orthoses were formerly referred to as long leg braces. The components are the same as those of an AFO but also include knee joints, thigh uprights, and a proximal thigh band. Various knee joints and knee locks are available for a variety of conditions. KAFOs are used in patients with severe knee extensor and hamstring weakness, structural knee instability, and knee flexion spasticity. The purpose of the KAFO is to provide stability at the knee, ankle, and subtalar joints during ambulation. They are most commonly prescribed bilaterally for patients with spinal cord injuries, and unilaterally for patients with poliomyelitis. There is a common misconception that patients with a complete femoral neuropathy (i.e. no quadriceps function) should have their knees braced. From a functional anatomic standpoint, it should be kept in mind that there are three stabilizers to the knee: the quadriceps, the hamstrings (via eccentric activation at heel strike), and the plantar flexors (plantar flexion creates a knee extension moment). These stabilizers should all be evaluated carefully by physical examination before a KAFO is prescribed.

Knee–ankle–foot orthoses can be prescribed for functional ambulation or exercise (or both). The benefits of exercise to the patient requiring bilateral KAFOs include preventing lower limb contractures, enhancing cardiovascular fitness, maintaining upper body strength for activities of daily living, delaying the development of osteoporosis, and fewer medical complications such as deep venous thromboses.

The use of KAFOs often complements the use of a wheelchair for ambulation. The proprioceptive level is a reliable indicator of which spinal cord-injured patients can achieve ambulation status.[52] It is helpful to have sensation and proprioception in the lower limbs in order to ambulate safely with KAFOs. The level of the spinal cord injury is also important in predicting the ability to ambulate. Adult spinal cord-injured patients with lesions at or above T12 generally are not functional ambulators because of the metabolic cost involved.[29] Children have a higher center of gravity and can have a functional gait with a higher spinal cord lesion. Muscle function is a predictor of the quality of ambulation. Good trunk control and upper body strength are needed in order to ambulate with KAFOs, because these devices are used in combination with ambulation aids such as walkers and Lofstrand forearm orthoses.

Some patients with paraplegia, such as those with lower lumbar lesions with some knee extensor strength, are able to ambulate without KAFOs. Ambulation in these patients can often be accomplished with the use of bilateral plastic ground reaction AFOs (Figs 16-11 and 16-16) with the ankles fixed in 10–15° of plantar flexion. The plantar flexion provides an extension moment at the knee during gait for stability with ambulation. The proximal anterior tibial shell closing provides further stability at the knee from midstance to toe-off (see part 4 of Fig. 16-11). A walker or two Lofstrand forearm orthoses can be used for additional support and balance.

Knee joints

There are three basic types of knee joints. The straight-set knee joint provides rotation about a single axis (Fig. 16-20). It allows free flexion but prevents hyperextension. It is often used in combination with a drop lock, which keeps the knee in extension throughout all phases of gait for further stability.

The polycentric knee joint uses a double-axis system to simulate the flexion–extension movements of the femur and tibia at the knee joint (Fig. 16-21). Although this concept is theoretically sound, the polycentric knee joint has not proved to be advantageous over the straight-set knee joint, and it is less commonly used. It also adds bulk to the orthosis. It is most frequently used in sport knee orthoses.

The third type of knee joint is the posterior offset knee joint (Table 16-2, Figs 16-22 and 16-23). It is prescribed for patients with weak knee extensors and some hip extensor strength. It allows free flexion and extension of the knee during the swing phase of gait, and helps keep the *orthotic* ground reactive force in front of the knee axis for stability during stance. The center of gravity is normally posterior to the knee at heel strike, creating a flexion moment at the knee, which requires knee extensor

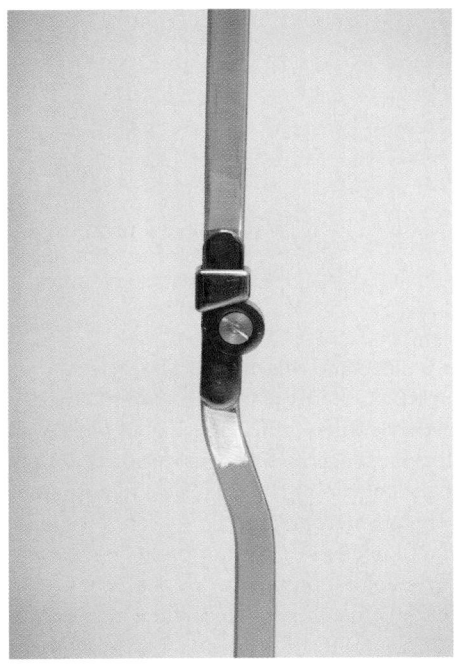

Figure 16-20
Straight-set knee with drop lock.

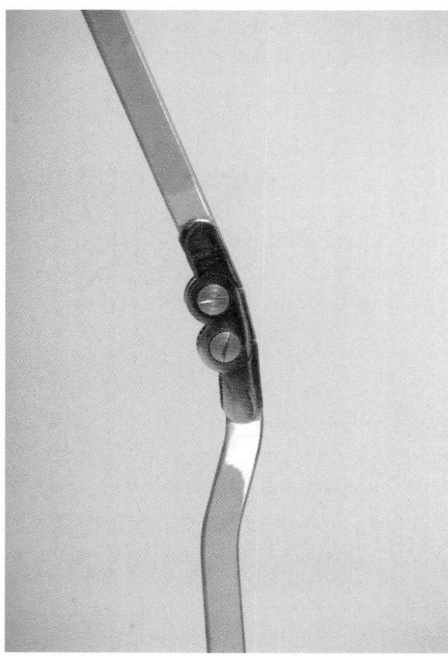

Figure 16-21
Polycentric knee joint.

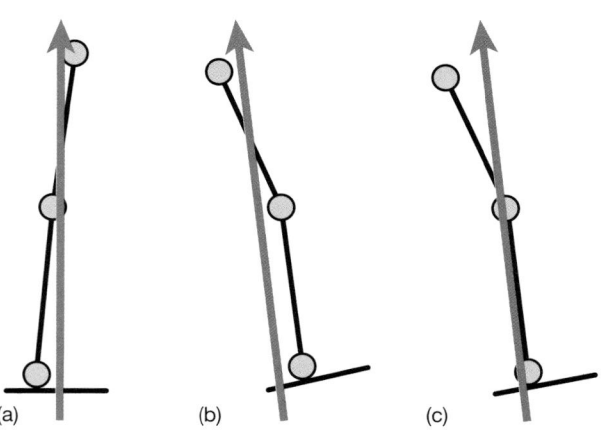

Figure 16-23 Ground reaction force (GRF). The line depicted pointed upward from the ground is representative of the GRF. The knee joint remains extended (e.g. stable) if the GRF is anterior to the knee. A knee flexion moment is created if the GRF is posterior to the knee. (**a**) GRF at stance. (**b**) GRF at heel strike. (**c**) Orthotic GRF at heel strike with posterior offset orthotic knee joint. A solid heel also moves the GRF posteriorly (i.e. knee flexion moment–instability), and a soft heel moves the GRF anteriorly (i.e. knee extension moment–stability).

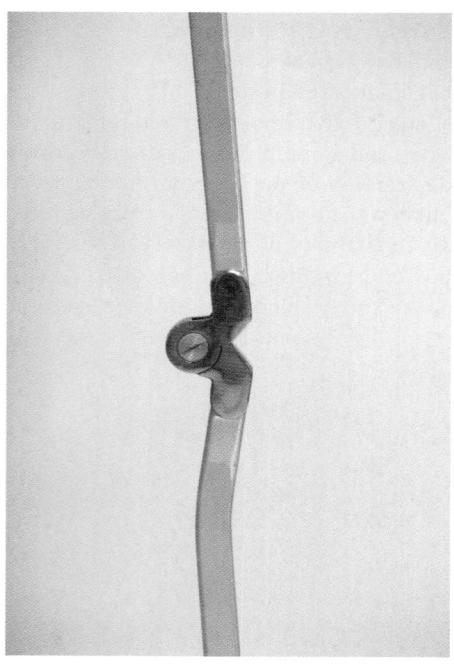

Figure 16-22
Posterior offset knee joint with drop lock.

measures are insufficient at providing knee stability, the posterior offset knee joints can be locked in extension.

Knee locks

Knee locks are used to provide complete stability at the knee. There are four common types of knee locks; these are discussed in order of their frequency of use, beginning with the most commonly used.

The ratchet lock (Fig. 16-24) has recently become the most commonly prescribed knee lock. The ratchet lock has a catching mechanism that operates in 12° increments. As the user rises from a seated to a standing position, if there is a tendency for the knee to become unstable and flex, the ratchet lock prevents that movement and keeps the gains made toward extension. Once the patient is standing with the knees extended, knee flexion is achieved by either pressing down on a release lever or by sliding the locking mechanism.

Prior to the development of the ratchet lock, the drop lock (ring lock) was used most commonly in both the medial and the lateral uprights of the KAFO (Fig. 16-20). Its advantage is simplicity of design without bulk. However, fine motor coordination skills are needed to lock the knee in complete extension. In addition, there are two locks per side yet only two hands. The drop lock also can 'settle' after ambulation and might be difficult to pull up to unlock the knee. The disadvantage of the drop lock in comparison with the ratchet lock is that there is no locking mechanism until full knee extension is obtained. Consequently, a patient's knee can collapse into flexion when not sufficiently extended to activate the drop lock. A collapse into flexion does not occur with the ratchet lock, and so the patient is less likely to fall. A drop lock can be used unilaterally along the lateral upright if the patient is relatively lightweight and has a low activity level.

muscle contraction to counteract this force. The offset knee joint component of the KAFO helps place the ground reactive force anterior to the orthotic knee joint, creating an extension moment at the knee during stance to compensate for the weak knee extensors. The offset knee joint should have a hyperextension stop to help prevent genu recurvatum.

Occasionally, the offset knee joint does not provide adequate stability at the knee. The ankle component of the KAFO can then be set in 10–15° of plantar flexion to further help create an extension moment at the knee for stability. Lastly, if these

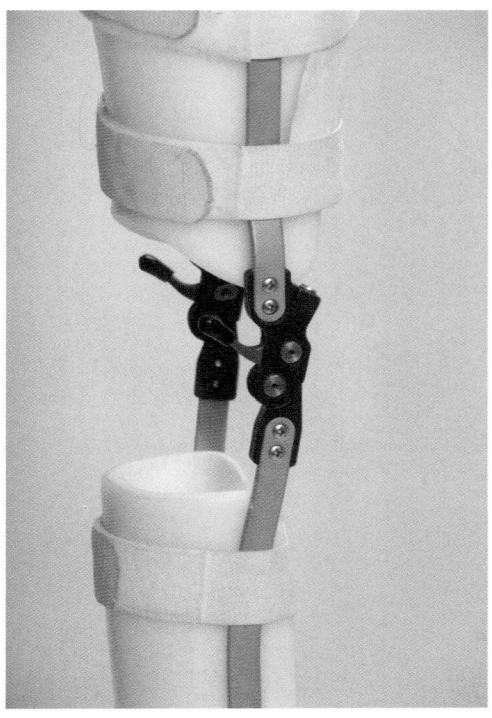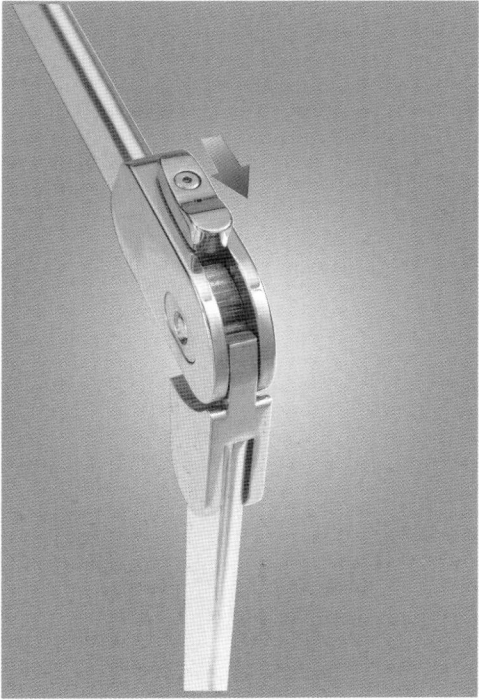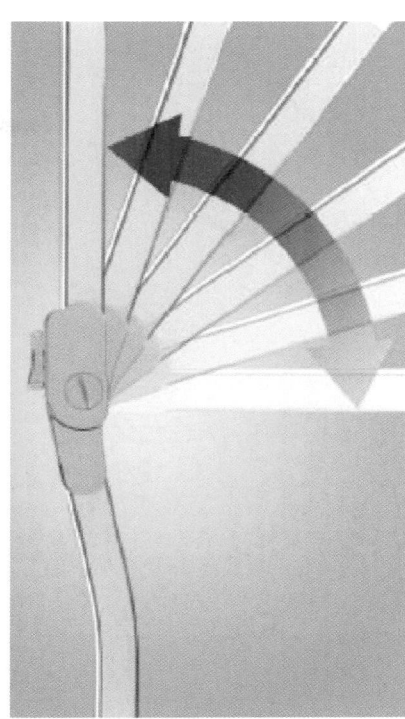

Figure 16-24 Ratchet lock. The 12° increments gained with knee extension prevent the knee from going into flexion, thereby adding stability and a safety factor as one rises from a seated to a standing position. The mechanism is released by using the lever arm to allow one to resume a seated position. (Illustrations courtesy of Becker Orthopedic Co., Troy.)

The bail lock (Swiss, French, Schweitzer, or pawl lock) provides the easiest method of simultaneously unlocking the medial and lateral knee joints of a KAFO (Figs 16-25 and 16-26). Two hands can be used for two bail locks, whereas there are a total of four ratchet locks or four drop locks with other bilateral KAFOs. Lifting up the bail posteriorly releases the knee joint to permit flexion, allowing the patient to sit down. The patient can also alternatively catch the bail on the edge of a chair to release the lock mechanism to permit sitting. The locking mechanism is often spring-loaded to assist locking the knee into extension (Fig. 16-26). The bail is often padded with rubber to protect the clothing from being torn or soiled. The KAFO with a bail lock can be worn over or under clothes, depending on the size of the bail lock and the size of the clothing.

The dial lock (formerly known as a turn buckle) is used to stabilize the knee in varying amounts of flexion (Fig. 16-27). It can be adjusted in 6° increments and is more precise for the management of a knee with a flexion contracture than a KAFO with ratchet locks. Its uses include helping prevent progression of a flexion contracture or assisting with the gradual reduction of a flexion contracture.

The thigh component of a KAFO

The thigh band needs to be wide enough to adequately distribute the pressure of the ground reactive force transmitted through the knee axis. A partial plastic thigh shell can provide a greater contact area and decrease high-pressure areas if properly fitted. Plastic–metal combination KAFOs also decrease the

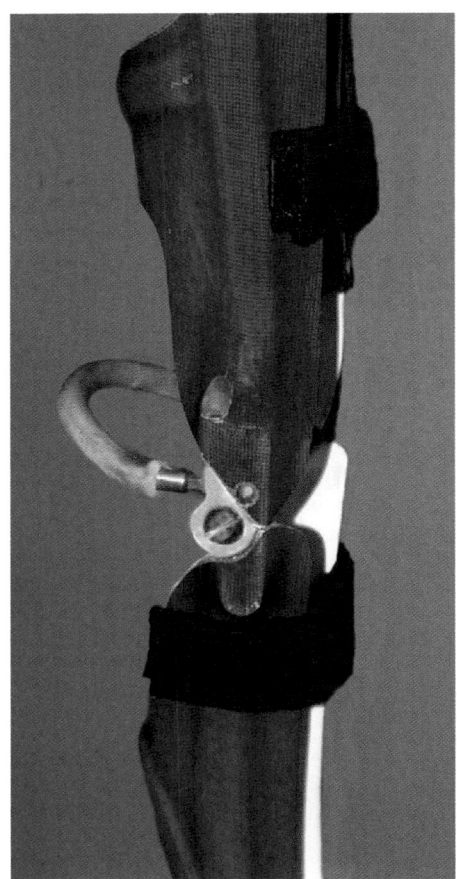

Figure 16-25
Padded spring-loaded bail lock. (Courtesy of Becker Orthopedic Co., Troy.)

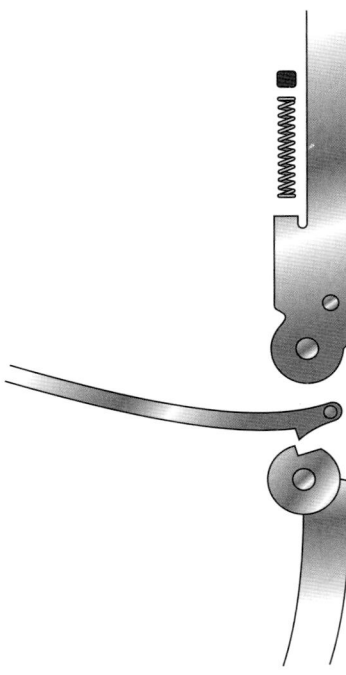

Figure 16-26 Spring-loaded bail lock mechanism. Lifting the bail permits free flexion for sitting, and the spring mechanism helps lock the knee joint into extension.

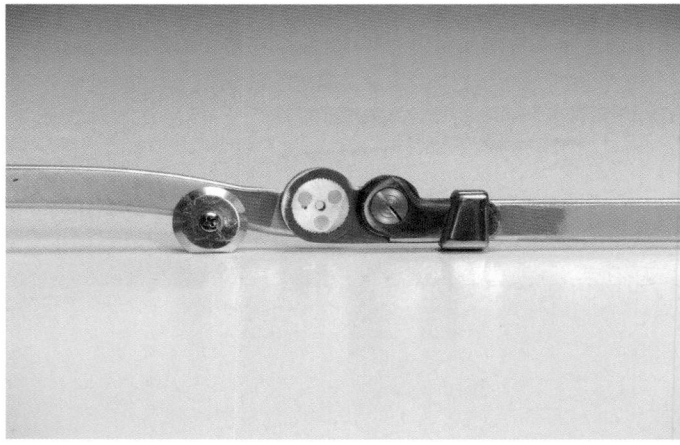

Figure 16-27 The dial lock can be adjusted every 6° for precise control of knee flexion.

weight of the KAFO, which can increase patient comfort and usage. A low thigh band is used to prevent genu recurvatum.

Scott–Craig orthosis

The Scott–Craig orthosis (Fig. 16-28) was designed to provide the patient with paraplegia having a complete lesion at L1 or higher with a more functional and comfortable gait.[43] It was also designed to reduce unnecessary hardware, to be a KAFO of lighter weight, and to be easy to don and doff.

The orthotic design consists of an ankle joint with anterior and posterior pin stops, a soleplate extending to the metatarsal heads, a crossbar added to the metatarsal head area for mediolateral stabilization, and an offset knee joint with a bail

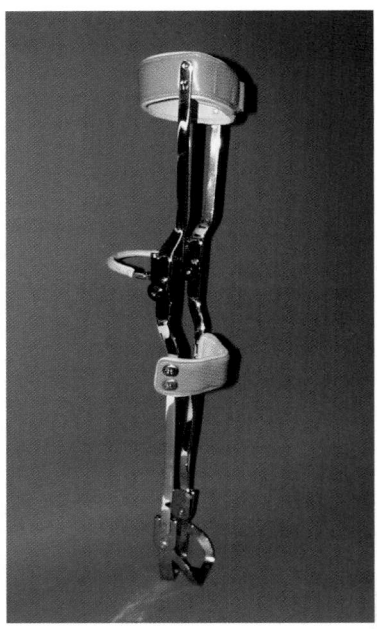

Figure 16-28 Scott–Craig knee–ankle–foot orthosis. (Courtesy of Becker Orthopedic Co., Troy.)

lock.[43] A rigid anterior tibial band is positioned directly below the tibial tubercle. A rigid proximal thigh band is positioned posteriorly and is closed anteriorly with a soft strap secured with Velcro. These two bands should be shallow enough to hold the knee in extension. A three-point system helps keep the knee in extension by applying pressure at the proximal thigh posteriorly, at the proximal tibia anteriorly, and at the calcaneus posteriorly.[21] The ankle joint functions with a dorsiflexion stop used to simulate the triceps surae function as previously described, and with a posterior stop set at 90° to prevent toe drag.

A group headed by Lehmann analyzed the Scott–Craig orthosis and found that it was the easiest of the KAFOs tested to don and doff.[19] The original design of this orthosis is still being prescribed for patients with paraplegia.

KNEE ORTHOSES

Swedish knee cage

The knee orthosis known as a Swedish knee cage (Fig. 16-29) is used to control minor to moderate genu recurvatum due to ligamentous or capsular laxity. This articulated knee orthosis permits full knee flexion and prevents hyperextension. The Swedish knee cage uses a classic three-point orthotic system with two bands placed anterior to the knee axis (one above and one below the knee) and a third band posterior to the knee joint in the popliteal area. It also has an additional thigh band with longer uprights to obtain better leverage at the knee joint. Severe genu recurvatum might need to be controlled with longer lever arms, such as that offered by a KAFO.

Genu recurvatum can also be controlled through additional orthotic measures, including a solid plastic AFO that resists plantar flexion. This can be used in cases where pathology also affects the ankle or subtalar joints. The more rigid the AFO, the greater the flexion moment at the knee during heel strike

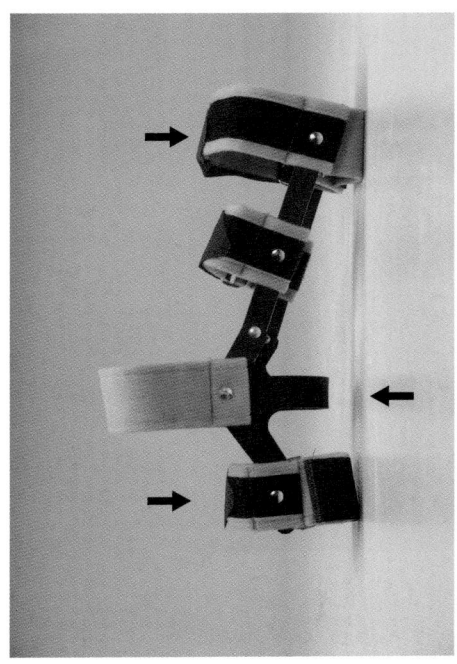

Figure 16-29 The articulated Swedish knee cage, which uses a three-point system to control genu recurvatum.

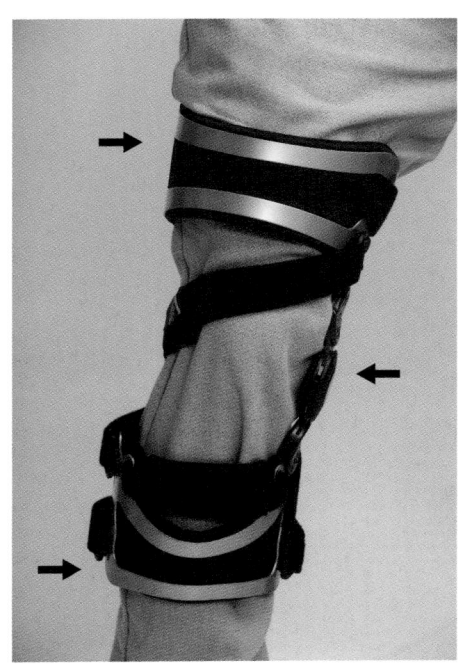

Figure 16-30 The Generation II knee orthosis for tricompartmental osteoarthritis of the knee. This utilizes the standard orthotic three-point distribution system in a medial–lateral distribution rather than in an anterior–posterior distribution, as was noted with the Swedish knee cage (Fig. 16-29).

(which counters the extension moment of the recurvatum). A shoe with a solid heel also helps create a greater knee flexion moment, which is preferred in this case over a shoe with a cushioned heel (which would facilitate a knee flexion moment). An additional flexion moment at the knee during midstance can be obtained by fixing the AFO in a few degrees of dorsiflexion.

Osteoarthritis knee orthoses

The same orthotic three-point principle that has been applied for years in the Swedish knee cage for genu recurvatum has recently also been applied to osteoarthritis of the knee, more commonly with medial compartment narrowing (Fig. 16-30). The three-point system distribution is achieved by a strap that is applied across the knee joint. In one study, 19 of 20 patients with varying degrees of osteoarthritis experienced significant relief of knee pain.[28] Radiographic improvement in joint alignment was also noted. The limiting factor regarding this knee orthotic prescription is the patient's weight. A morbidly obese patient with an abundance of fatty tissue around the knee will not support the knee orthosis adequately. In such cases where this knee orthosis and surgery are precluded, the foot orthoses with lateral buildup as described earlier in this chapter should be considered. The foot orthosis with a lateral buildup is considered the preferred first-line orthotic treatment for osteoarthritis of the knee (see *Osteoarthritis of the knee* in the *Foot orthoses* section).

Sport knee orthoses

There is an increasing abundance of sport orthoses on the market. There is also a lack of definitive research regarding their role in sports. This can lead to much confusion regarding their prescription, unless the knee orthosis is reviewed systemati-cally. Sport knee orthoses can be divided into prophylactic, rehabilitative, and functional categories.[32]

Prophylactic knee bracing attempts to prevent or reduce the severity of knee injuries. There is currently no evidence to support the use or cost benefit of these orthoses. Some studies have found that the use of these orthoses actually increased the number of athletes with knee injuries.[40,47] It is theorized that knee-braced players can put themselves in compromising positions because of over-reliance on the orthosis, and that this can contribute directly to the increasing injury rates observed. The use of prophylactic knee bracing has also been associated with increased energy consumption, which can impair athletic performance.[11]

Rehabilitative knee bracing is used to allow protected motion within defined limits.[32] It is useful for postoperative and conservative management of knee injuries.

Functional knee bracing is designed to assist or provide stability for the unstable knee. Functional knee bracing does not replace the need for rehabilitation of the knee. Knee braces are used most commonly to stabilize a laterally subluxing patella or an anterior cruciate ligament-deficient knee. Their use has been shown to be effective only at loads much lower than those placed on the knee during athletic participation. In summary, functional knee bracing can possibly play a role in the treatment of pathologic laxity by possibly decreasing the frequency of unstable episodes.[32]

PEDIATRIC ORTHOSES

Caster cart

The disabled child should identify early with motion so that ambulatory skills can progress naturally.[1] Without familiarity with motion, disabled children lack the desire to ambulate

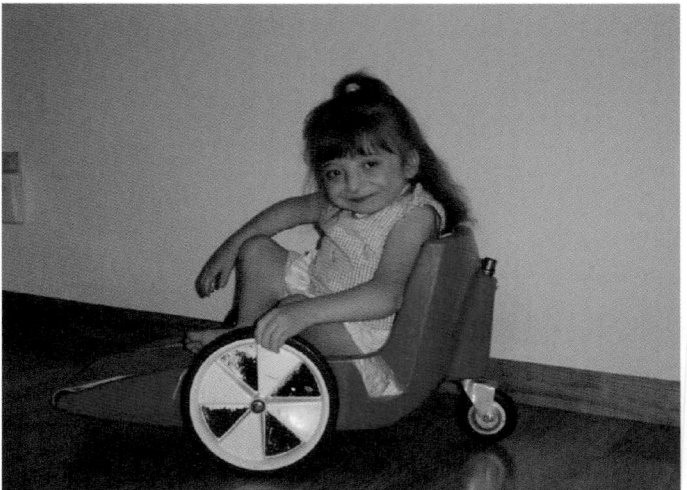

Figure 16-31 Caster cart. This is an initial mobility aid for the disabled child. The child uses it as a 'prewheelchair device' for mobility.

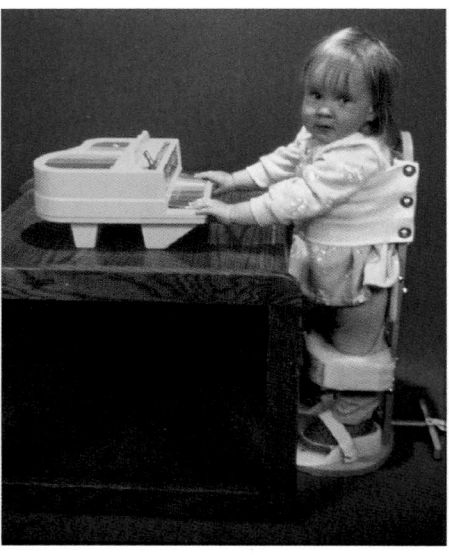

Figure 16-32 A standing frame for initial upright activities. Used by children who desire to stand, as determined by attempts to pull themselves upright.

once placed in a parapodium or reciprocating gait orthosis (RGO).

The caster cart (Fig. 16-31) is used for children with a developmental delay in ambulatory skills, and it serves as an initial mobility aid. It is most often prescribed for children with spina bifida. Most children are upright and cruising by 10 months.[12] Children with paraplegia should be fitted for a caster cart once they have obtained enough upper limb strength and trunk balance to propel themselves. If balance is a problem for the child, a deep seat bucket can be prescribed to help provide balance so that the child can use the upper limbs for propulsion.

The caster wheel at the back of the cart facilitates multidirectional movement. Initially, the child can be pushed around in the cart with a handle attached posteriorly so that the cart serves as a stroller.

Standing frame

The use of a standing frame (Fig. 16-32) typically follows successful use of a caster cart. The age range for initial use is usually 8–15 months. Children can continue to use their caster carts during this time. Children who are pulling themselves up along furniture are typically ready for a standing frame. This is the first sign that they are interested in standing and moving.[12]

The standing frame helps balance the body in space and allows free use of the upper limbs for participation in activities. Children with thoracic-level lesions need AFOs to provide good ankle and foot support in the standing frame or parapodium. Initial gait training can occur with the use of the standing frame via a swing-through gait with the assistance of parallel bars.

Parapodium

The parapodium (Fig. 16-33) was also referred to in the past as a swivel orthosis. Before children are given a parapodium, they should first demonstrate adequate use of a standing frame

and exhibit a desire to ambulate. A child's standing frame can be evaluated for wear and tear to determine whether it has been used sufficiently so that the child can advance to a parapodium. A frequently used standing frame (or any orthosis) will show evidence of wear and tear that includes soiling and scratches. It is important to note this, because parents frequently set expectations too high for the disabled child. A child who has not used a standing frame will probably be unable or unwilling to ambulate with a parapodium.

A parapodium is an appropriate prescription for children who are unlikely to become functional walkers due to the severity of their impairment. It often complements wheelchair use.[23] It is most commonly prescribed for children between 2.5 and 5 years of age.

A parapodium allows crutchless gait. Ambulation occurs by the child pivoting the hips and using 'body English' to swivel one side of the oval-based stand forward and then repeating the same event for the other side. Its design is similar to the standing frame, but it has hip and knee joints. The hip and knee joints remain locked in extension to permit ambulation in the upright position but can be unlocked (simultaneously in some models) to permit sitting. The difficulties experienced with the use of this orthosis include donning and doffing, and rising from a seated position to a standing position.

Reciprocating gait orthosis

The RGO (Fig. 16-34) was formerly known as a hip-guided orthosis. It can also be referred to as a bilateral hip–knee–ankle–foot orthosis. The purpose of the RGO is to provide contralateral hip extension with ipsilateral hip flexion. The RGO is appropriate for children who have used the standing frame, developed good trunk control and coordination, can safely stand, and are mentally prepared for ambulation. Good upper limb strength, trunk balance, and active hip flexion are important positive variables for ambulation.[8] Obesity, advanced age,

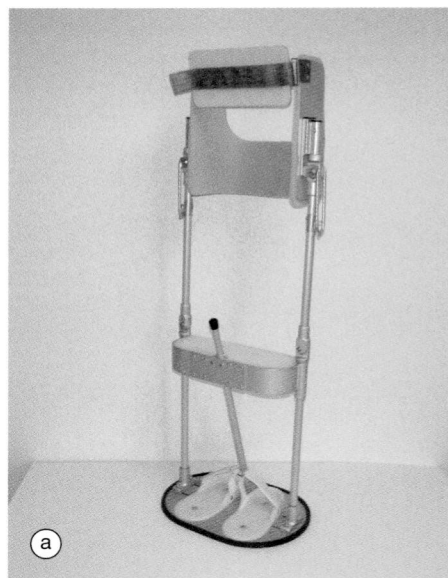
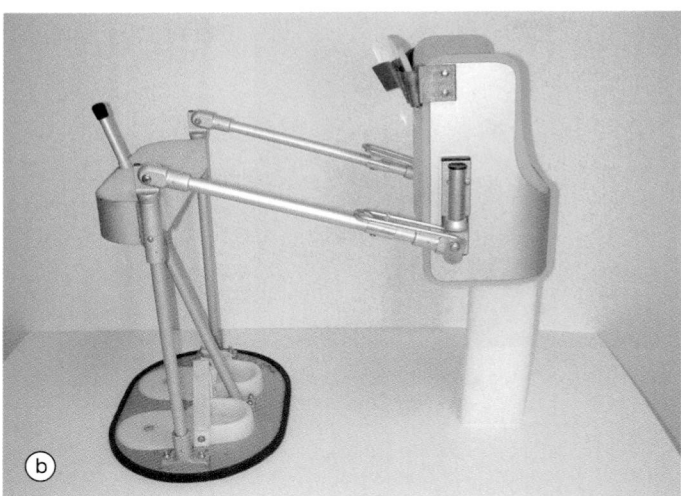

Figure 16-33 (a) Parapodium with hip and knee joints locked in extension. **(b)** Parapodium with hip and knee joints unlocked and in a flexed position. (Courtesy of Variety Ability Systems, Inc., Toronto, Ontario, Canada.)

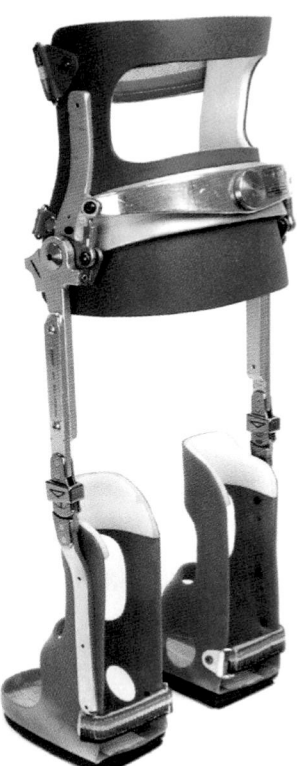

Figure 16-34 Isocentric reciprocating gait orthosis. (Courtesy of the Center for Orthotic Design, Redwood City, and Fillauer Companies, Inc., Chattanooga.)

lack of patient or family motivation, scoliosis, spasticity,[8] and contractures are significant negative factors in the long-term use of the RGO. This type of orthosis clearly only complements the use of a wheelchair for mobility purposes and serves therapeutic purposes of exercise and upright activities. One newer type of spinal cord injury orthosis is the Walkabout, which has

a scissoring mechanism in the groin area attaching two KAFOs via a hinge. The trade-off with this device is a lack of contralateral hip extension with ipsilateral hip flexion for a less bulky orthosis to don and doff.[10,30]

Spinal cord injury level is not a very reliable predictor of ambulation capability for children. As children with spinal cord injuries grow taller, they might experience more difficulty walking as their center of gravity becomes lower.

The RGO is prescribed most commonly for children aged 3–6 years. The concept of the RGO was developed by researchers working with a patient who had active hip flexion and no hip extension. Gait is initiated with unilateral hip flexion and can be assisted by swaying the trunk when hip flexion is inadequate. This type of gait pattern can also be considered to be a form of physical therapy, because hip extension occurs passively with each step, helping to reduce flexion contractures. Cables were initially used to provide the necessary hip motion, but newer mechanical methods of reciprocal gait employ a 'teeter totter' concept (Fig. 16-34). This type of RGO has been reported to be more energy-efficient than an RGO with cables.[55]

Crutches are used with the RGO to provide a control mechanism, taking advantage of the forward momentum to produce small propulsive forces when needed.[25] This also is a disadvantage of this orthosis (compared with the parapodium), because the upper limbs are not free for other activities. The patient with an RGO is able to negotiate a greater variety of surfaces than would be possible with the parapodium.[39]

The hip joints of the RGO have hip flexion and abduction capabilities on release of the locking mechanisms (Fig. 16-35). It is recommended that one hip joint has abduction capability to permit catheterization and to allow sitting in a hip-flexed and abducted position.

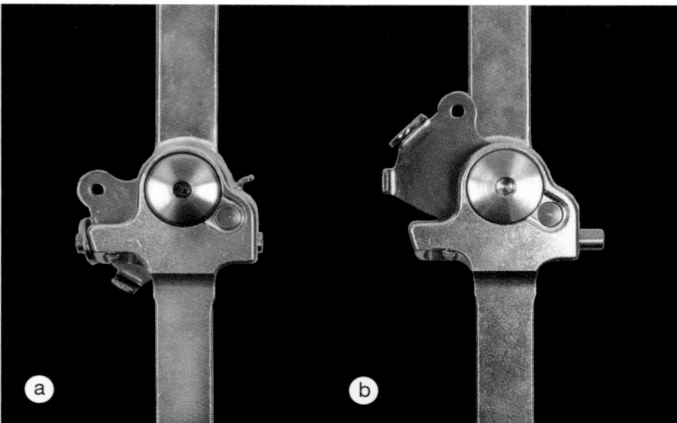

Figure 16-35 Unique hip joints for use with the isocentric reciprocating gait orthosis. (**a**) Hip joint locked in the extended and adducted position. (**b**) Hip joint unlocked and capable of abduction for easy catheterization without removal of the brace. (Courtesy of the Center for Orthotic Design, Redwood City, and Fillauer Companies, Inc., Chattanooga.)

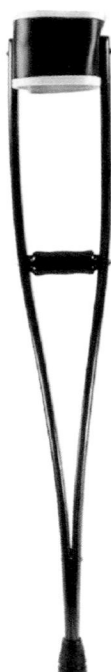

Figure 16-37 Wooden forearm orthosis (Kenny stick). The leather band encloses the proximal forearm. (Courtesy of Thomas Fetterman, Inc., Southampton, PA.)

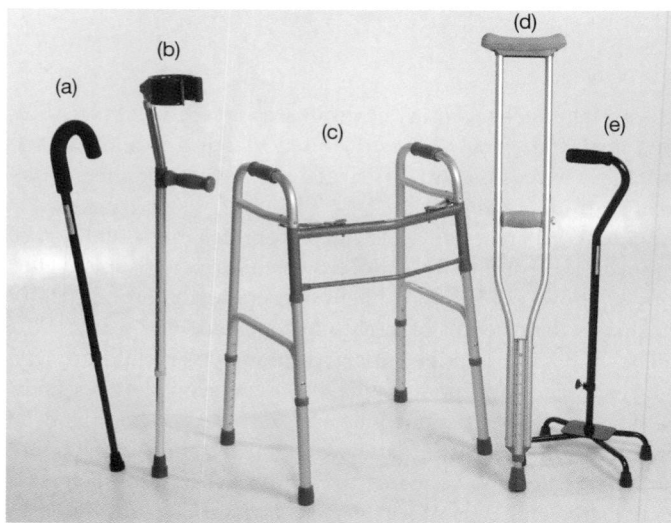

Figure 16-36 Ambulation aids: (**a**) C cane, (**b**) Lofstrand forearm orthosis, (**c**) walker, (**d**) crutch, and (**e**) quad cane.

AMBULATION AIDS

The purpose of using ambulation aids (Figs 16-36 and 16-37) is to increase the area of support for patients who have difficulty maintaining their center of gravity safely over their own support area. A variety of aids are available for the individual needs of patients. Ambulation aids improve balance, redistribute and extend the weight-bearing area, reduce lower limb pain, provide small propulsive forces, and provide sensory feedback. They should be considered an extension of the upper limb. Their proper use requires adequate upper limb strength and coordination. An exercise program for the upper limbs is useful and can complement ambulation with the aid by increasing endurance and stability. A supervised period of training is recommended after prescription of an aid.

The type of aid needed depends on how much balance and weight-bearing assistance is needed. The body weight transmission for a unilateral cane opposite the affected side is 20–25%.[4] It is 40–50% with the use of a forearm cane or an arm cane.[4] Body weight transmission with bilateral crutches is estimated at up to 80%.[4]

Canes

When prescribing a cane:

- measure the tip of the cane to the level of the greater trochanter with the patient in an upright position to determine the proper cane length.[50]

The elbow should be flexed approximately 20°, which is a desirable elbow position for all ambulation aids. Canes are made of wood or aluminum, with the aluminum alloy cane having adjustable notches so that 'one cane fits all'.

There are three common types of cane (see Fig. 16-36). The C cane is most commonly used. It is also known as a crook top cane or a J cane. A functional grip cane offers the patient a grip that can be more comfortable than with the C cane. A quad cane provides an increased area of support compared with the other canes. Quad canes also come in narrow- and wide-based forms for different degrees of support. The lateral two legs are directed away from the body.

A cane is used on the side opposite the supporting lower limb. It is advanced with the opposite lower limb. It is usually held on the patient's unaffected side. This can be done to lessen the force exerted on a hip with pathology. The load is increased by four times the body weight on the stance side during gait, due to the gravitational forces and the gluteus medius–minimus force exerted across the weight-bearing hip.[4] The cane helps decrease the force generated across the affected hip joint by decreasing the work of the gluteus medius–minimus complex. This occurs when the upper limb exerts force on the cane to help minimize pelvic drop on the side opposite the weight-bearing lower limb.

Patients should be instructed on how to ascend and descend stairs. The pneumonic 'up with the good and down with the bad' serves as an easy reminder. The patient should always have the 'good' lower limb assume the first full weight-bearing step on level surfaces.

Walker

Prescribing a walker involves the following.

- Place the front of the walker 12 inches in front of the patient (the walker should partially surround the patient).
- Determine the proper height of the walker by having the patient stand upright with the shoulders relaxed and the elbows flexed 20°.[50]

A walker provides maximum support for the patient but also necessitates a slow gait. It is useful for hemiplegic and ataxic patients. Wheels can be added to the front legs to facilitate movement of the walker for those who lack coordination in the upper limbs. Patients using wheeled models should be supervised initially to ensure safety. Some walkers also have a front U-shaped extension with extra supports to provide stability for stair climbing. A patient needs to be motivated and have good strength and coordination to use this model of walker.

Visual impairment cane

Prescription of a visual impairment cane involves the following.

- Instruct the patient to flex the shoulder until the upper limb is parallel with the floor.
- Measure the distance from the hand to the floor. That is the proper length.

A visual impairment cane should be lightweight, flexible, and easily collapsible. The distal inches of the cane are red.

Crutches

The steps in crutch prescription are as follow.

- Crutch length: measure the distance from the anterior axillary fold to a point 6 inches lateral to the fifth toe with the patient standing with the shoulders relaxed.
- Handpiece: measure with the patient's elbow flexed 30°, the wrist in maximal extension, and the fingers forming a fist. This is measured *after* the total crutch height is determined with the crutch 3 inches lateral to the foot.[50]

A crutch is defined as a device that provides support from the axilla to the floor. Although there are different types of crutches and canes, they can all be referred to as orthoses because they are applied to the external surface of the body to improve function.

The patient should be able to raise the body 1–2 inches by complete elbow extension. Despite the popularity of padding the axillary area of the crutch, this should not be done. It needs to be emphasized to the patient that crutches are not designed to be rests for body support. This point should be made to the patient in order to reduce the incidence of compressive radial neuropathies or plexopathies.

Non-axillary crutches

Non-axillary crutches are more appropriately called forearm or arm canes, or forearm or arm orthoses. The Lofstrand forearm orthosis, Kenny sticks, the Everett or Warm Spring orthosis, the Canadian crutch, and the platform forearm orthosis will be discussed (Figs 16-36 and 16-37).

FOREARM ORTHOSES

Lofstrand forearm orthosis

To prescribe a Lofstrand forearm orthosis:

- measure the handpiece as described above for crutches, with the patient standing upright and the elbow in 20° of flexion.

The proximal portion of the orthosis is also angled at 20° to provide for a comfortable, stable fit. It is often made of tubular aluminum. It provides less support than crutches for ambulation but is sufficient for many patients. Lofstrand forearm orthoses are most often used bilaterally. The open end of the cuff is placed on the lateral aspect of the forearm to permit elbow flexion and grasping without dropping the orthoses. The advantages of this orthosis are that it is shorter than an axillary crutch, and the forearm cuff pivots to allow the patient to lean on the crutch for hand activities.

Wooden forearm orthosis (Kenny stick)

Another forearm orthosis option is the Kenny stick (Fig. 16-37). It was named after Sister Kenny, who sawed off the top half of wooden crutches and placed a leather band around the proximal portion of the forearm. It was designed for poliomyelitis patients who had satisfactory proximal upper limb musculature but were weak distally and unable to effectively hold and control the orthosis. Its advantage over the Lofstrand orthosis is the presence of a closed leather band. This assures patients (more so than the Lofstrand forearm orthosis does) that they will not drop the ambulation aid.

Platform forearm orthosis

To prescribe a platform forearm orthosis:

- have the patient stand upright with the shoulders relaxed and the elbows flexed 90°. The distance from the ground to the forearm rest is the proper length.

This orthosis is helpful for patients with painful wrist and hand conditions, as well as for those with elbow contractures. Velcro straps are applied around the forearm, especially for patients with weak hand grips.

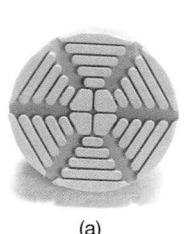
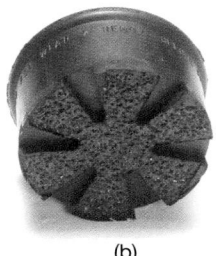

(a)   (b)

Figure 16-38 (**a**) Snow Boot crutch tip for use in snowy and icy conditions. (**b**) Rain Guard crutch tip for use in wet conditions. (Courtesy of Hi-Trac Industries, Holley.)

Triceps weakness orthoses (arm orthoses)

These orthoses, also known as triceps weakness crutches, were originally developed for patients with poliomyelitis. The metal version is known as a Warm Spring crutch or Everett crutch. The wooden version is known as a Canadian crutch. These crutches resemble the 'axillary' crutches in style, but end proximally with a cuff at the midarm level. These ambulation aids help prevent flexion (buckling) of the elbow during gait.

Crutch tips and hand grips

The purpose of crutch tips is to absorb shock and prevent slippage. Crutches are only as safe as the quality of their crutch tips. Special crutch tips are available for rainy and icy conditions (Fig. 16-38). At each checkup, the physician should make sure that the crutch tips are not worn out. Hand grips are used to reduce pressure on the hands and are also safety features because they help prevent slippage.

PRESCRIPTION

A medical diagnosis with delineation of the impairment and any resulting disability should be made before an orthotic prescription is written. The orthotic goals should be documented for the orthotist. An AFO prescription should include the type of ankle (rigid, flexible, or jointed) and the position of the ankle (neutral, dorsiflexed, or plantar flexed). If the ankle is jointed, the range of motion should be specified. In the case of a compressive peroneal nerve palsy, for example, the physical impairment would be a flaccid foot drop. The ankle should be flexible and held in a neutral position with a plastic AFO set in a few degrees of dorsiflexion. The goals include toe clearance during swing-through and prevention of foot slap during early stance.[15]

From an orthotic prescription standpoint, most of this chapter is concisely summarized in Figure 16-39, a full-size prescription pad with convenient check boxes and room at the top of the page to copy this on to a letterhead for clinical use. Adjacent to this sheet is a quick summary reference that can be copied on to the back of the prescription sheets (Box 16-2).

Box 16-2 Summary reference for prescription pad

Foot orthosis
- University of California Biomechanics Laboratory (UCBL): hyperpronating 'flat' foot.
- Metatarsal pad: temporary mild to moderate metatarsalgia.
- Metatarsal bar to shoe: severe metatarsalgia (cannot stand something in shoe) or permanent metatarsalgia (e.g. arthritis).
- Heel lift: temporary use for Achilles tendinitis or plantar fasciitis.
- Heel cup: fat pad syndrome (heel bruise).
- Lateral heel wedge: osteoarthritis with medial compartment narrowing.

Ankle–foot orthosis
- Over the counter: for a trial basis only
- Custom: for long-term use
- Plastic: for almost everyone
- Metal: for the patient > 250# with a hinged AFO

Common types
- Custom solid (flexible) AFO set at 90°: foot drop
- Custom solid (rigid) AFO set at 90°: plantar spasticity

Hinge indications
- Significant mediolateral instability at subtalar joint but patient with ankle dorsi- and plantar flexion (rare).
- Tight plantar flexors in spastic patients with improving lower limb function (they can take advantage of a more 'normal' gait via dorsiflexion from midstance to toe-off, and plantar stretching is therapeutic over this part of the gait cycle).
- An active patient with foot drop or plantar flexor spasticity can take advantage of the hinged feature during stair climbing, rising from sit to stand, frequent walking, etc.

Knee–ankle–foot orthosis

Knee type
- Straight set: most common; always used unless posterior offset is indicated.
- Posterior offset: patient with weak knee extensor triad (quads, plantar flexors, and hamstrings).
- Polycentric: a two-joint system that theoretically simulates femur–tibia translation. Standard on most sport orthoses for the above marketing purpose. No clear-cut indications.

Knee locks
- Ratchet lock: most common.
- Drop lock: can be difficult to pull up after 'settling in' from walking.
- Bail lock: bulkier and less desirable than the drop locks for most patients but necessary for those without fine hand control.
- Dial lock: used to lock an unstable knee in extension, but they are adjusted to account for knee flexion contractures.

Hip joints (common to prescribe one of each of the below)
- Standard: allows flexion and extension.
- Abduction: permits flexion and extension but also permits abduction to allow self-urinary bladder straight catheterization and seating in a hip-flexed and abducted position.

Lower limb orthotic prescription

Name: _____   Age _____

Diagnosis: _____

Orthotic goals: _____

Justification: _____

Orthotic company: _____

Referring physician: _____

☐ FO   ☐ AFO   ☐ KAFO   ☐ HKAFO   ☐ KO

☐ Right   ☐ Left   ☐ Bilateral

☐ Custom

☐ Plastic   ☐ Metal   ☐ Combination

Ankle type: ☐ Solid (flexible)   ☐ Solid (rigid)   ☐ Hinged: — dorsiassist
                                                                                                      — dorsistop
                                                                                                      — plantar stop

Ankle ROM: ☐ Plantar flexion — degrees
                                 ☐ Dorsiflexion — degrees
                                 ☐ Neutral (90°)

Knee type: ☐ Straight set   ☐ Posterior offset   ☐ Polycentric

Knee locks: ☐ Two per knee joint   ☐ One per knee joint

Knee lock type: ☐ Ratchet lock   ☐ Drop lock   ☐ Bail lock   ☐ Dial lock

Hip joints with drop locks   ☐ Standard   ☐ Abduction

Miscellaneous _____

Physician name _____   **Date** _____

Figure 16-39 Lower limb orthotic prescription sheet.

SUMMARY

An appropriate lower limb orthotic prescription requires a thorough biomechanical analysis of gait and knowledge of the available orthotic components available to treat specific conditions. The prescribing physician should maintain a close working relationship with the certified orthotist to make cer-tain that the patient is receiving the best orthotic options available.

Patient complaints about orthoses usually are related to cosmesis, comfort, clothing soiling or damage, weight, and difficulty with donning and doffing. All practitioners should work toward the goal of achieving the ideal orthosis for the patient that enhances comfort, cosmesis, and function. Accomplishing this will in turn enhance compliance. The ideal orthosis would be weightless, invisible, without cost, maintenance-free, comfortable, and strong, and would normalize the gait pattern while simultaneously reducing energy consumption to within normal limits.

Acknowledgments

A special thanks to Gene Flenner, C.P.O., and Jan Lewandowski, C.P.O., of Union Orthotic and Prosthetic Company; Bradd L. Rosenquist, C.P.O., of Columbus Orthopaedic Prosthetic and Orthotic Center, Inc.; Mike Russell, C.P.O., and colleagues of Hanger Orthopedics; and also Rosalind Batley, M.D., Kurt Kuhlman, D.O., and Richard Kozakiewicz, M.D., for reviewing this chapter. I also thank R. Douglas Turner of Becker Orthopedic; Wally Motloch, C.O., and Carla David of Fillauer Companies, Inc.; Robert Evans of High-Trac Industries, Inc.; Martin Mifsud of Variety Ability Systems, Inc. and Thomas Fetterman, Inc. for providing photographs of their products for this chapter. Lastly, I thank Dennis Pushkar, owner, Impressions Studio, Jeannette, PA for his time, expertise and assistance with many of the high quality color orthotic images in this chapter.

REFERENCES

1. Bleck EE. Developmental orthopaedics: III. Toddlers. Dev Med Child Neurol 1982; 24:533–555.
2. Corcoran PJ, Jebsen RH, Brengelmann GL, et al. Effects of plastic and metal leg braces on speed and energy cost of hemiparetic ambulation. Arch Phys Med Rehabil 1970; 51:69–77.
3. D'Ambrosia RD. Conservative management of metatarsal and heel pain in the adult foot. Orthopedics 1987; 10:137–142.
4. Deathe AB, Hayes KC, Winter DA. The biomechanics of canes, crutches, and walkers. Crit Rev Phys Rehabil Med 1993; 5:15–29.
5. Diveley RL. Foot appliances and alterations. In: American Academy of Orthopaedic Surgeons, eds. Orthopaedic Appliances Atlas, vol 1. Ann Arbor: JW Edwards; 1952:463–464.
6. Gok H, Kucukdeveci A, Yavuzer G, et al. Effects of ankle–foot orthoses on hemiparetic gait. Clin Rehabil 2003; 17:137–139.
7. Gross MT, Foxworth JL. The role of foot orthoses as an intervention for patellofemoral pain. J Orthop Sports Phys Ther 2003; 33:661–670.
8. Guidera KJ, Smith S, Raney E, et al. Use of the reciprocating gait orthosis in myelodysplasia. J Pediatr Orthop 1993; 13:341–348.
9. Halar E, Cardenas D. Ankle–foot orthoses: clinical implications. Phys Med Rehabil State Art Rev 1987; 1:45–66.
10. Harvey LA, et al. Functional outcomes attained by T9–12 paraplegic patients with the Walkabout and the Isocentric reciprocal gait orthoses. Arch Phys Med Rehabil 1997; 78:706–711.
11. Houston ME, Goemans PH. Leg muscle performance of athletes with and without knee support braces. Arch Phys Med Rehabil 1982; 63:431–432.
12. Johnson EW, Spiegel MH. Ambulation problems in very young children. JAMA 1961; 175:858–863.
13. Keating EM, Faris PM, Ritter MA, et al. Use of lateral heel and sole wedges in the treatment of medial osteoarthritis of the knee. Orthop Rev 1993; 22:921–924.
14. Lehmann JF, Condon SM, de Lateur BJ, et al. Ankle–foot orthoses: effect on gait abnormalities in tibial nerve paralysis. Arch Phys Med Rehabil 1985; 66:212–218.
15. Lehmann JF, Condon SM, de Lateur BJ, et al. Gait abnormalities in peroneal nerve paralysis and their correlation by orthoses: a biomechanical study. Arch Phys Med Rehabil 1986; 67:380–386.
16. Lehmann JF, de Lateur BJ, Warren CG, et al. Biomechanical evaluation of braces for paraplegics. Arch Phys Med Rehabil 1969; 50:179–188.
17. Lehmann JF, Esselman P, Ko MJ, et al. Plastic ankle foot orthoses: evaluation of function. Arch Phys Med Rehabil 1983; 64:402–407.
18. Lehmann JF, Warren CG, de Lateur BJ. A biomechanical evaluation of knee stability in below knee braces. Arch Phys Med Rehabil 1970; 51:687–695.
19. Lehmann JF, Warren CG, Hertling D, et al. Craig Scott orthosis: a biomechanical and functional evaluation. Arch Phys Med Rehabil 1976; 57:438–442.
20. Lehmann JF, Warren CG, Pemberton DR, et al. Load bearing function of patellar tendon bearing braces of various designs. Arch Phys Med Rehabil 1971; 52:367–370.
21. Lehmann JF, Warren CG. Restraining forces in various designs of knee ankle orthoses: their placement and effect on anatomical knee joint. Arch Phys Med Rehabil 1976; 57:430–437.
22. Lehmann JF. The biomechanics of ankle foot orthoses: prescription and design. Arch Phys Med Rehabil 1979; 60:200–207.
23. Liptak GS, Shurtleff DB, Bloss JW, et al. Mobility aids for children with high-level myelomeningocele: parapodium versus wheelchair. Dev Med Child Neurol 1992; 34:787–796.
24. Loke M. New concepts in lower limb orthotics. Phys Med Rehabil Clin North Am 2000; 11:477–496.
25. Major RE, Stallard J, Rose GK. The dynamics of walking using the hip guidance orthosis (HGO) with crutches. Prosthet Orthot Int 1981; 5:19–22.
26. Mann RA. Biomechanics of the foot. In: American Academy of Orthopaedic Surgeons, eds. Atlas of Orthotics. St. Louis: Mosby-Year Book; 1985:118.
27. Marx HW. Lower limb orthotic designs for the spastic hemiplegic patient. Orthot Prosthet 1974; 28:14-20.
28. Matsuno H, Kadowaki, Tsjui H. Generation II knee bracing for severe medial compartment osteoarthritis of the knee. Arch Phys Med Rehabil 1997; 78:745–749.
29. Merritt JL. Knee–ankle–foot orthotics: long leg braces and their practical applications. Phys Med Rehabil State Art Rev 1987; 1:67–82.
30. Middleton JW, Yeo JD, Blanch L, et al. Clinical evaluation of a new orthosis, the 'Walkabout', for restoration of functional standing and short distance mobility in spinal paralysed individuals. Spinal Cord 1997; 35:574–579.
31. Milgram JE, Jacobson MA. Footgear: therapeutic modifications of sole and heel. Orthop Rev 1978; 7:57–61.
32. Millet C, Drez D Jr. Knee braces. Orthopedics 1987; 10:1777–1780.
33. Pfeffinger LL. Foot orthoses. In: American Academy of Orthopaedic Surgeons, eds. Atlas of Orthotics. St. Louis: Mosby-Year Book; 1985:350.
34. Radtka SA, Skinner SR, Dixon DM, et al. A comparison of gait with solid, dynamic and no ankle–foot orthoses in children with spastic cerebral palsy. Phys Ther 1997; 77:395–409.
35. Redford JB. Orthoses. In: Basmajian JV, Kirby RL, eds. Medical rehabilitation. Baltimore: Williams & Wilkins; 1984:101.
36. Reid DC. Heel pain and problems of the hindfoot. In: Reid DC, ed. Sports injury assessment and rehabilitation. New York: Churchill Livingstone; 1992:196–212.
37. Rethlefsen S, Kay R, Dennis S, et al. The effects of fixed and articulated ankle–foot orthoses on gait patterns in subjects with cerebral palsy. J Pediatr Orthop 1999; 19:470–474.
38. Riegler HF. Orthotic devices for the foot. Orthop Rev 1987; 16:293–303.
39. Rose GK, Stallard J, Sankarankutty M. Clinical evaluation of spina bifida patients using hip guidance orthoses. Dev Med Child Neurol 1981; 23:30–40.
40. Rovere GD, Haupt HA, Yates CS. Prophylactic knee bracing in college football. Am J Sports Med 1987; 15:111–116.

41. Sarmiento A, Gersten LM, Sobol JA, et al. Tibial shaft fractures treated with functional braces: experience with 780 fractures. J Bone Joint Surg Br 1989; 71:602–609.

42. Sarmiento A. A functional below the knee brace for tibial fractures: a report of its use in 135 cases. J Bone Joint Surg Am 1970; 52:295–311.

43. Scott BA. Engineering principles and fabrication techniques for Scott-Craig: long leg brace for paraplegics. Orthop Prosthet 1974; 28:14–19.

44. Shrader JA, Siegel KL. Nonoperative management of functional hallux limitus in a patient with rheumatoid arthritis. Phys Ther 2003; 83:831–843.

45. Smiley SJ, Jacobsen FS, Mielke C, et al. A comparison of the effects of solid, articulated, and posterior leaf-spring ankle–foot orthoses and shoes alone on gait and energy expenditure in children with spastic diplegic cerebral palsy. Ortho 2002; 25:411–415.

46. Staheli LT, Chew DE, Corbett M. The longitudinal arch. J Bone Joint Surg Am 1987; 69:426–428.

47. Teitz CC, Hermanson B, Kronmal RA, et al. Evaluation of the use of braces to prevent injury to the knee in collegiate football players. J Bone Joint Surg Am 1987; 69:2–9.

48. Thomas SS, Buckon CE, Jakobson-Huston SJ, et al. Comparison of three ankle–foot orthosis configurations for children with spastic hemiplegia. Dev Med Child Neurol 2001; 43:371–78.

49. Thomas SS, Buckon CE, Jakobson-Huston SJ, et al. Stair locomotion in children with spastic hemiplegia: the impact of three different ankle foot orthosis (AFOs) configurations. Gait Posture 2002; 16:180–187.

50. Varghese G. Crutches, canes, and walkers. In: Redford JB, ed. Orthotics etcetera. 2nd edn. Baltimore: Williams & Wilkins; 1980:453–463.

51. Von Werssowetz OF. Basic principles of lower extremity bracing. Orthot Prosthet Appl J 1962; 323–350.

52. Waters RL, Miller L. A physiologic rationale for orthotic prescription in paraplegia. Clin Prosthet Orthot 1987; 11:66–73.

53. Wenger DR, Mauldin D, Morgan D, et al. Foot growth rate in children age one to six years. Foot Ankle 1983; 3:207–210.

54. Wenger DR, Mauldin D, Speck G, et al. Corrective shoes and inserts as treatment for flexible flatfoot in infants and children. J Bone Joint Surg Am 1989; 71:800–810.

55. Winchester PK, Carollo JJ, Parekh RN, et al. A comparison of paraplegic gait performance using two types of reciprocating gait orthoses. Prosthet Orthot Int 1993; 17:101–106.

56. Woodburn J, Barker S, Helliwell PS. A randomized control trial of foot orthoses in rheumatoid arthritis. J Rheumatol 2002; 29:1377–1383.

57. Zamosky I, Redford JB. Shoes and their modifications. In: Redford JB, ed. Orthotics etcetera. 2nd edn. Baltimore: Williams & Wilkins; 1980:388–452.

Spinal Orthoses in Rehabilitation
Daniel P. Moore, Edward Tilley and Paul Sugg

HISTORY OF ORTHOTIC MANAGEMENT

The first evidence of the use of spinal orthoses can be traced back to Galen in approximately 131–201 AD. Primitive orthotic devices were made of items that were readily available during their time period (Fig. 17-1). These items consisted of leather, whalebone, and tree bark. Spinal orthoses, although crude in their construction, have been recovered by archeologists from the cliff dwellings of pre-Columbian Indians. The word *orthosis* is Greek and means 'to make straight'.[2] Ambroise Paré (1510–1590) wrote about bracing and spinal supports, and Nicholas Andry (1658–1742) coined the term *orthopaedia* pertaining to the straightening of children.[4] Unstable areas such as fractures were often held in a corrected position with an orthosis, to allow for healing to occur. Normally fixed deformities were accommodated while flexible deformities were corrected. Orthopedia was the predecessor to the field of orthotics.[1]

In the past, there were no organized training programs in the fabrication and application of orthoses, and an orthotist began as an apprentice, much like the village blacksmith. The training process for orthotists is now well defined and rigorous, with a certification process in the USA. Orthotists are now required to have extensive knowledge of pathologies and the proper fabrication and use of orthotic devices. Technology has revamped the field of orthotics, with new stronger and lighter materials. Although materials available for orthotic construction have changed, the types of pathologic conditions treated have remained virtually constant for years.

The primary goal of modern orthoses is to aid a weakened muscle group or correct a deformed body part. The orthosis can protect a body part to prevent further injury, or can correct the position (immediate or long term) of the body part. The same approach is true for spinal orthoses. The clinician's priority should be to determine which spinal motion to control. Good clinical outcomes can be maximized through the proper selection, use, and application of the orthosis. (See Chs 15 and 16 for further information on orthoses.)

TERMINOLOGY

Terminology is currently often misused in the field of orthotics. Definitions of some terms commonly used in the field are listed below.

- Orthosis: a singular device used to aid or align a weakened body part.
- Orthoses: two or more devices used to aid or align a weakened body part.
- Orthotics: the field of study of orthoses and their management.
- Orthotic: an adjective used to describe a device (e.g. an orthotic knee immobilizer); this term is improperly used as a noun (e.g. 'the patient was fit with a foot orthotic').
- Orthotist: a person trained in the proper fit and fabrication of orthoses.
- Certified orthotist (e.g. ABC). In the USA, academic requirements can be fulfilled by a baccalaureate degree in orthotics or a 4-year science degree followed by a postbaccalaureate certificate program in orthotics. A 1-year residency program is required after the academic program. Extensive training in the proper fit and fabrication of orthoses is required. After the education and residency is completed, a national examination for certification can be taken in the USA by the American Board for Certification (ABC) in Prosthetics and Orthotics.

Acronyms are frequently used to describe orthoses. They are named for the parts of the body where they are located and have some influence on the motion in that body region. Some examples of spinal orthoses follow.

- CO: cervical orthosis.
- CTO: cervical–thoracic orthosis.
- CTLSO: cervical–thoracic–lumbar–sacral orthosis.
- TLSO: thoracic–lumbar–sacral orthosis.
- LSO: lumbar–sacral orthosis.
- SO: sacral orthosis.

PREFABRICATED VERSUS CUSTOM ORTHOSES

The availability of prefabricated orthoses today presents the rehabilitation team with a variety of choices and some challenges. Many of the prefabricated orthoses come in various sizes and can be fitted to patients often with little or no adjustments. While this can be a benefit to the patient and the team in terms of time, care should be taken to ensure that the design and function of these orthoses is appropriate for the patient's condition and not used purely for convenience. Custom orthoses, in

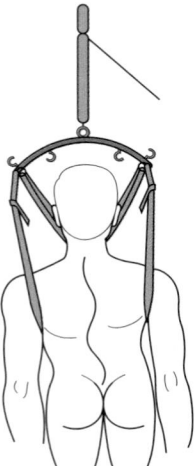

Figure 17-1 Traction device, 1889.

most cases, provide a more comfortable fit with a higher degree of control, and can be designed to accommodate a patient's unique body shape or deformities. Recognition of the time needed to fabricate the orthosis, the experience of the fabricator, the patient's specific condition, and the expectations of the patient are all factors that should be considered when ordering a custom orthosis.

ORTHOTIC PRESCRIPTION

The orthotic prescription allows for improved communication between clinicians, and it serves as a source to justify funding of the orthosis. Insurer-requested justification for the orthosis is becoming more common as medical costs have increased. Insurer approval of the prescription can be more successful if it clearly increases independence or helps prevent detrimental outcomes such as a fall. The prescribing rehabilitation physician is responsible for the final order. The prescription should be accurate and descriptive, but not limit the orthotic team's independent ability to maximize functionality and patient acceptance.

Prescriptions should include the following items:

- patient's name, age, and gender;
- current date;
- date the orthosis is needed;
- vendor's name;
- diagnosis;
- functional goal;
- orthosis description;
- precautions;
- physician's name and unique physician identifier number; and
- physician's signature with office address and contact phone number.

Prescriptions should include a justification, such as the correction of alignment, to decrease pain, or to improve function. Brand names and eponyms for the orthosis should be avoided.

Established acronyms are acceptable, for example TLSO. Detailed descriptions of the orthosis, the joints involved, and the functional goals are important. For a non-articulated orthosis, the fixed angle should be indicated. For an orthosis with a moveable joint, the range of motion desired, end limitations of range, and assistance (or resistance) through the range should be specified. Before the prescription is finalized, input from the patient, physician, therapist, and orthotist are needed. It is especially important to review the use, or lack of use, of past orthoses, as this will help guide your new prescription. If a patient discontinues the use of an orthosis prematurely, the reason why this occurred should be investigated by the provider before additional resources are expended. Knowledge of the patient's medical condition(s) is essential for a number of reasons. For example, the disease might be progressive, with further expected functional loss. On the other hand, the disease might be expected to improve partially or completely in the future.

SPINAL ANATOMY

The vertebral column is composed of 33 vertebrae, including 7 cervical, 12 thoracic, 5 lumbar, 5 inferiorly fused vertebrae that form the sacrum, and 5 coccygeal. The spinal column not only bears the weight of the body, but it also allows motion between body parts and serves to protect the spinal cord from injury. Prior to birth, there is a single C-shaped concave curve anteriorly. At birth, infants have only a small angle at the lumbosacral junction. As a child learns to stand and walk, lordotic curves develop in the cervical and lumbar region (age 2 years). These changes can be attributed to the increase in weight bearing and differences in the depth of the anterior and posterior regions of the vertebrae and disks.[29,33]

The cervical vertebrae are small and quadrangular, except for C1 and C2, which have some unique features. The cervical articular processes face upward and backward, or downward and forward. The orientation of the facet joints is important to note, as it relates to limitations of movement of the vertebral column. The thoracic vertebrae have heart-shaped bodies. The thoracic vertebrae are intermittent in size but increase in size caudally. This is related to the increased weight-bearing requirements. The ventral length of the thoracic vertebrae is approximately 2 mm more than the dorsal side, which could account for the thoracic curve. Their superior articular processes face backward and outward, and the inferior ones face forward and inward. The lumbar vertebrae have a large, kidney-shaped body. Their upper articular processes face medially and slightly posteriorly, and the lower ones face laterally and slightly anteriorly. The five sacral vertebrae are fused in a solid mass and do not contain intervertebral disks. The sacral bony structure acts as a keystone, and weight bearing increases the forces that maintain the sacrum as an integral part of the spinal pelvic complex.

The spine is composed of more than vertebral bodies. The intervertebral disk is composed of a nucleus pulposus, annulus fibrosus, and cartilaginous end plate. Disks make up approximately one-third of the entire height of the vertebral column. The nucleus contains a matrix of collagen fibers, mucoprotein, and mucopolysaccharides. They have hydrophilic properties, with a very high water content (90%) that decreases with age.[28] The nucleus is centrally located in the cervical thoracic spine, but more posteriorly located in the lumbar spine. The annulus fibrosus has bands of fibrous laminated tissue in concentric directions, and the vertebral end plate is composed of hyaline cartilage.

NORMAL SPINE BIOMECHANICS

Movement of the vertebral column occurs as a combination of small movements between vertebrae. The mobility occurs between the cartilaginous joints at the vertebral bodies and between the articular facets on the vertebral arches. Range of motion is determined by muscle location, tendon insertion, ligamentous limitations, and bony prominences. In the cervical region, axial rotation occurs at the specialized atlantoaxial joint. At the lower cervical levels, flexion, extension, and lateral

flexion occur freely. In these areas, however, the articular processes, which face anteriorly or posteriorly, limit rotation. In the thoracic region, movement in all planes is possible, although to a lesser degree. In the lumbar region, flexion, extension, and lateral flexion occur, but rotation is limited due to the inwardly facing articular facets.[11]

Spine motion can be classified with reference to the horizontal, frontal, and sagittal planes. Spinal motion can shift the center of gravity, which is normally located approximately 2–3 cm anterior to the S1 vertebral body. White and Panjabi provided a summary of the current literature revealing motion in flexion and extension, laterally and axially (Fig. 17-2).[34] In the cervical spine, extension occurs predominantly at the occipital C1 junction. Lateral bending occurs mainly at the C3, C4 and C4, C5 levels. Axial rotation occurs mostly at the C1, C2 levels. In the thoracic spine, flexion and extension occur primarily at the T11, T12 and T12–L1 levels. Lateral bending is fairly evenly distributed throughout the thoracic levels. Axial rotation occurs mostly at the T1, T2 level, with a gradual decrease toward the lumbar spine. The thoracic spine is the least mobile due to the restrictive nature of the rib cage. In the lumbar spinal segment, movement in the sagittal plane occurs more at the distal

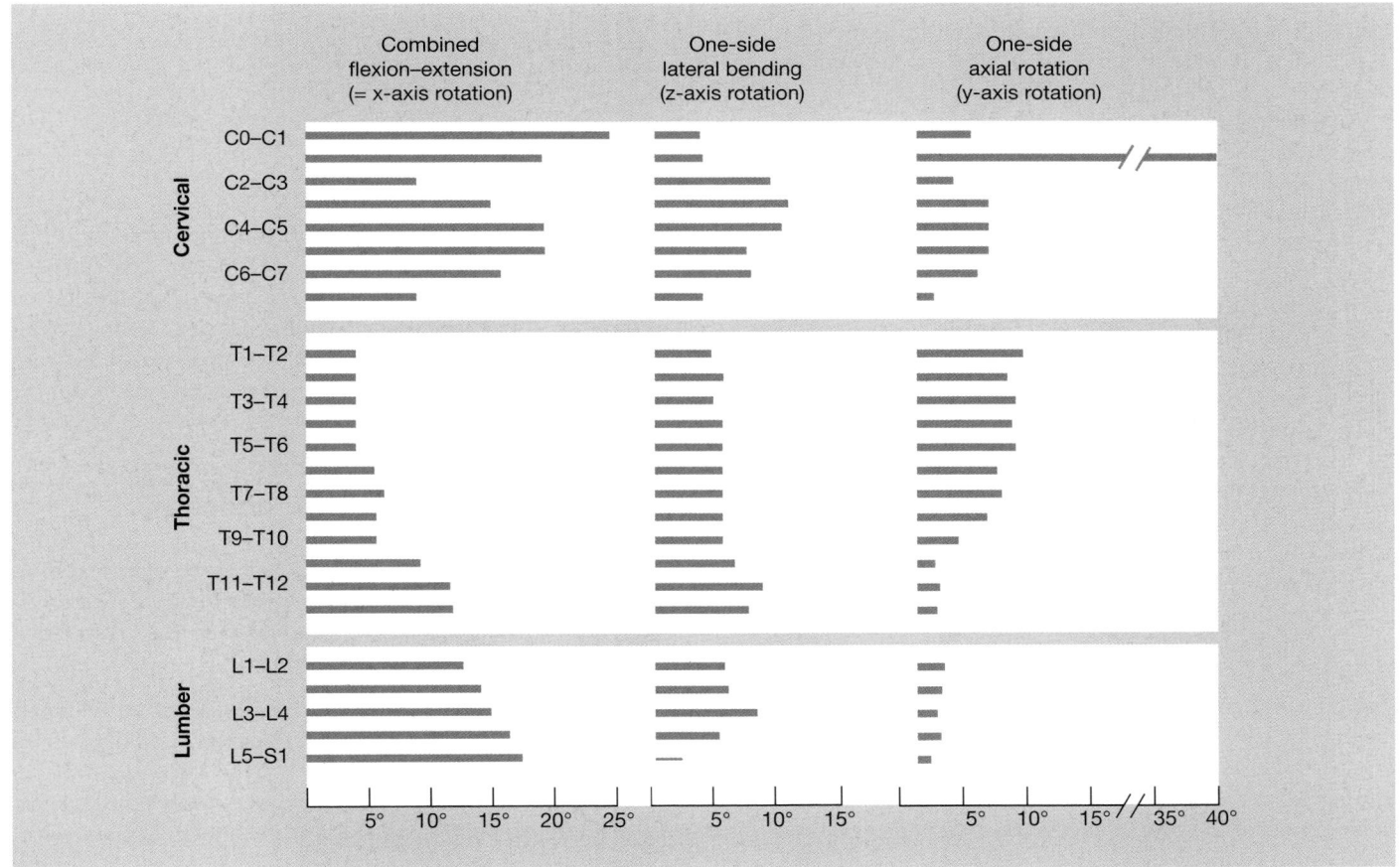

Figure 17-2 Representative values for range of motion of the cervical, thoracic, and lumbar spine as summarized from the literature. (From White and Panjabi 1990,[34] with permission of Lippincott.)

Table 17-1 Normal cervical motion from occiput to first thoracic vertebra and the effects of cervical orthoses			
Orthosis	Mean of normal motion (%)		
	Flexion or extension	Lateral bending	Rotation
Normal[a]	100.0	100.0	100.0
Soft collar[a]	74.2	92.3	82.6
Philadelphia collar	28.9	66.4	43.7
Sternal occipital mandibular immobilizer brace	27.7	65.6	33.6
Four-poster brace	20.6	45.9	27.1
Yale cervicothoracic brace	12.8	50.5	18.2
Halo device[a]	4.0	4.0	1.0
Halo device[b]	11.7	8.4	2.4
Minerva body jacket[c]	14.0	15.5	0

[a]Data from Johnson et al. (1977).[13]
[b]Data from Lysell (1969).[17]
[c]Data from Maiman et al. (1989).[18]

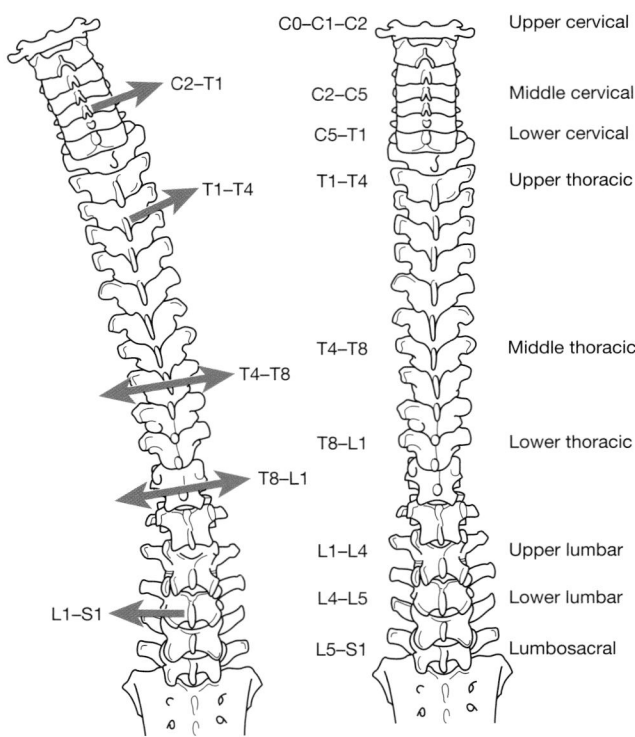

Figure 17-3 Regional coupling patterns. Summary of the coupling of lateral bending and axial rotation in various subdivisions of the spine. In the middle and lower cervical spine as well as the upper thoracic spine, the same coupling pattern exists. In the middle and lower thoracic spine, the axial rotation, which is coupled with lateral bending, can be in either direction. In the lumbar spine, the spinous processes go to the *left* with *left* lateral bending. (From White and Panjabi 1990,[34] with permission of Lippincott.)

segment, with lateral bending predominantly at the L3, L4 level. There is insignificant axial rotation in the lumbar spinal segment.

Knowledge of the normal spinal range of motion helps in understanding how the various cervical orthoses can limit that range (Table 17-1). Soft collars provide very little restriction in any plane. The Philadelphia-type collar mostly limits flexion and extension. The four-poster brace and Yale orthosis have better restriction, especially with flexion–extension and rotation. The halo brace and Minerva body jacket have the most restriction in all planes of motion.

An interesting phenomenon related to movement in the spine occurs during motion. If the movement along one axis is consistently associated with movement around another axis, *coupling* is occurring. For example, if a patient performs left *lateral movement* (frontal plane) motion, the middle and lower cervical and upper thoracic spine rotate to the left in the *axial* plane (Fig. 17-3). This causes the spinous processes (posterior side of the body) to move to the *right*. In the lower thoracic spinal segment, left lateral movement in the frontal plane can cause rotation in the axial plane, with the spinal processes moving in either direction. The lumbar area has a contradictory movement pattern when compared with the cervical spine. With left lateral bending of the lumbar spine, the spinous processes move to the *left*. A three-dimensional perspective is important to maintain during examination. Patients with scoliosis and patients who undergo radiologic testing would benefit from an evaluation for the normal coupling patterns noted.

Nachemson performed the classic studies on normal adults, and measured intradiskal pressures during a variety of activities

and positions.[22,23,26] Standing pressure was referenced as 100 in the lumbar disk. Lowest pressure measurements were noted in the supine position, with progressively higher pressures in the following positions: side lying, standing, sitting, standing with hip flexion, sitting with forward flexion, standing with forward flexion, and lifting a load while sitting with forward flexion.[25]

DESCRIPTION OF ORTHOSES

Cervical and cervicothoracic orthoses
Type: halo (Fig. 17-4)

Biomechanics The halo provides flexion, extension, and rotational control of the cervical region. Pressure systems are utilized for control of motion, as well as to provide slight distraction for immobilization of the cervical spine.

Design and fabrication The halo has prefabricated halo pins, ring, superstructure, and vest. On the typical adult patient, the ring is attached to the skull pins around the equator of the skull, leaving approximately 1 inch of clearance for the superior border of the ear and proximal to the eyebrows. The pin placement is usually at the lateral third of the eyebrows (anteriorly), while avoiding the sinuses. Posteriorly, pin placement is 1 inch posterior and proximal to the ear. The pins should oppose each

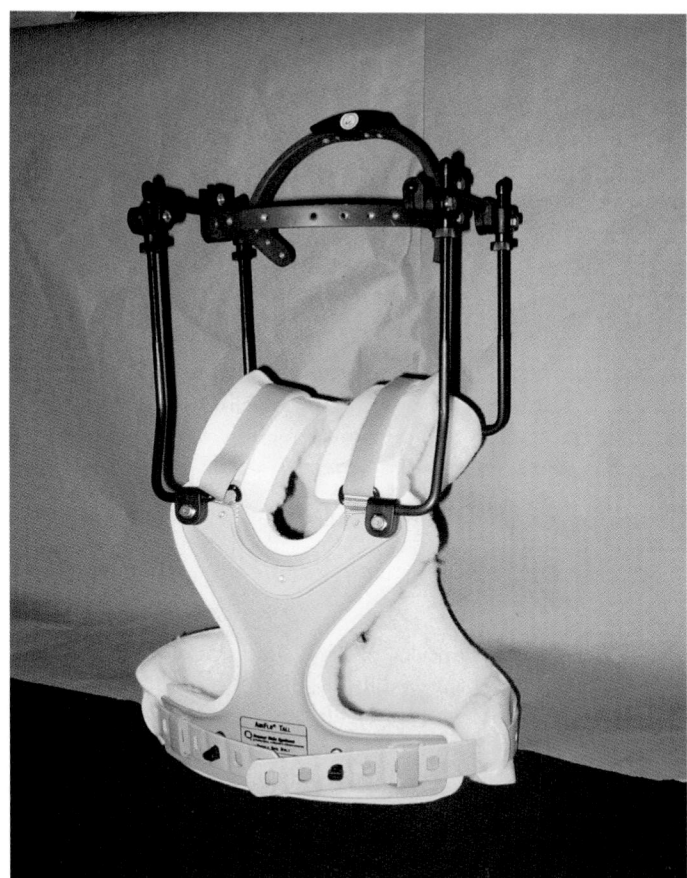

Figure 17-4 Halo.

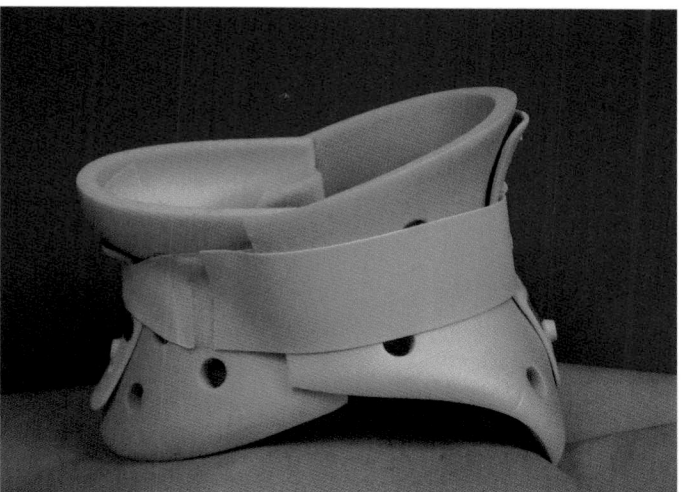

Figure 17-5 Philadelphia.

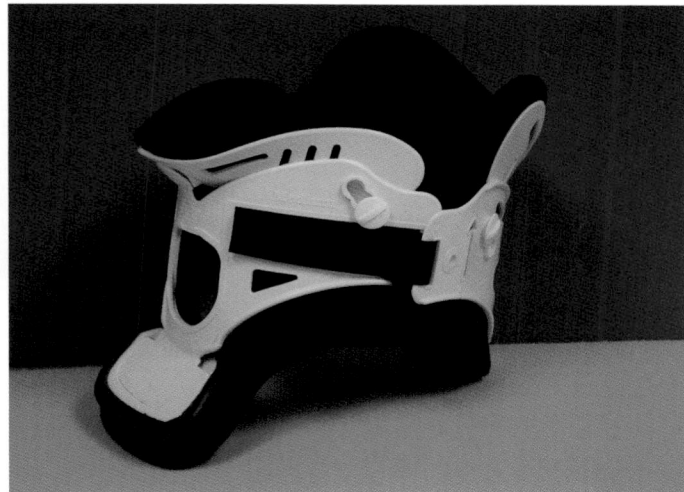

Figure 17-6 Miami J.

other. The halo pins are torqued into the outer table of the skull through the halo ring that supports the pins. The ring is attached to the superstructure that is attached to the vest. The superstructure allows for the ring to be held in position by use of the attachment to the vest or anchor point of the halo. The halo is adjustable for flexion, extension, anterior and posterior translation, rotation, and distraction. The vest wraps around the thoracic region of the spine, and is lined with lamb's wool and fastened laterally, usually by buckles. The design is used to effectively immobilize the cervical spine.

This orthosis provides maximum restriction in motion of all the cervical orthoses. It is the most stable orthosis, especially in the superior cervical spine segment. A halo is used for approximately 3 months to ensure healing. Usually, a cervical collar is indicated after the halo is removed, as the muscles and ligaments supporting the head become weak after disuse. All pins on the halo ring should be checked to ensure tightness 24–48 h after application, and retorqued if necessary.

Indications   The halo is generally used for unstable cervical fractures or postoperative management.

Contraindications   Contraindications are stable fractures or when other, less invasive management could be used. Patients

with an extremely soft skull might not tolerate the pin placement.

Special considerations   Skull density determines halo pin placement as well as the number of halo pins to be used. While four pins are used on average, more can be necessary in soft skulls (e.g. osteoporotic, fractured, or in an infant) to distribute the force over a broader area of the skull.

Type: Miami J or Philadelphia (Figs 17-5 and 17-6)
Biomechanics   This type of orthosis provides some control of flexion, extension, and lateral bending, and minimal rotational control of the cervical region. Pressure systems are utilized for control of motion, as well as to provide slight distraction for immobilization of the cervical spine. Circumferential pressure is also intended to provide warmth and as a kinesthetic reminder for the patient.

Design and fabrication   These orthoses are prefabricated, consisting of one or two pieces that are usually attached with Velcro straps. Two-piece designs have an anterior and posterior section. The anterior section supports the mandible and rests on the superior edge of the sternum. The posterior aspect of the collar supports the head at the occipital level.

Indications   They are used primarily for cervical sprains, strains, or stable fractures. They can also be used for protection and to limit mobility after surgery to allow healing.

Contraindications   These orthoses are not indicated for unstable fractures.

Type: sternal occipital mandibular immobilizer (SOMI; Fig. 17-7)

Biomechanics   The SOMI provides control of flexion, extension, lateral bending, and rotation of the cervical spine. Pressure systems are utilized for control of motion, as well as to provide slight distraction for immobilization of the spine. A benefit of the SOMI orthosis is that it can be donned while the patient is in the supine position. The SOMI is a good choice for patients who are restricted to bed, because there are no posterior rods to interfere with comfort of the patient. A headband can be added so that the chin piece can be removed. This maintains

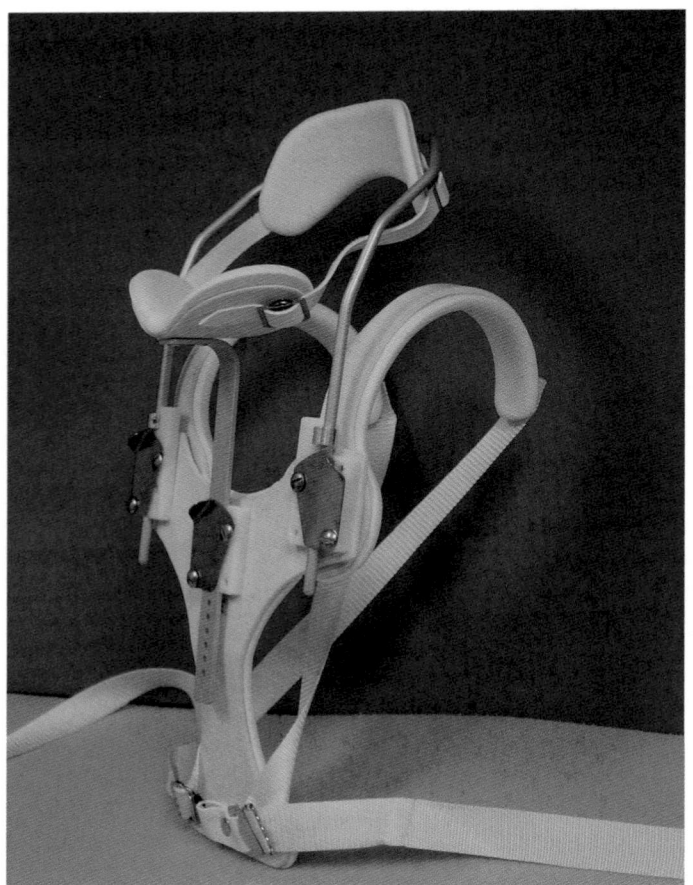

Figure 17-7 Sternal occipital mandibular immobilizer.

stability but improves accessibility for daily hygiene and eating.

Design and fabrication   The SOMI is prefabricated, consisting of a cervical portion with removable chin piece and bars that curve over the shoulders. Also utilized are posts that fixate the cervical portion to the sternal portion of the orthosis. The anterior section supports the mandible and rests on the superior edge of the sternum, with the inferior anterior edge terminating at the level of xiphoid. The posterior aspect of the orthosis supports the head at the occipital level.

Indications   The SOMI is used primarily for cervical sprains, strains, or stable fractures with intact ligaments. It can also be used for protection and to limit mobility during the healing process in the postoperative patient.

Contraindications   This orthosis is not indicated for unstable fractures with ligament instability.

Yale

The Yale orthosis consists of chin and occipital pieces that extend higher on the skull in the posterior region; this increases comfort. The Yale orthosis is a modified Philadelphia collar with a thoracic extension. The extension consists of fiberglass that extends both anteriorly and posteriorly, and has thoracic straps that hold the sections together. The thoracic extension to the orthosis helps to stabilize injuries at the vertebral levels of C6–T2.

Four-poster

The four-poster is a rigid cervical orthosis with anterior and posterior sections consisting of pads that lie on the chest and are connected by leather straps. The struts on the anterior and posterior sections are adjustable in height. Straps are used to connect the occipital and mandibular support pieces by way of the over the shoulder method.

Type: TLSO (prefabricated, Fig. 17-8)
Biomechanics   This provides control of flexion, extension, lateral bending, and rotation using three-point pressure systems and circumferential compression.

Design and fabrication   This orthosis can be designed in modular forms, with anterior and posterior sections connected by padded lateral panels and fastened with Velcro straps or pulley systems. Many of these are covered in breathable fabric and have a variety of different shapes and options, such as sternal pads or shoulder straps.

Indications   They can be used for treatment of traumatic or pathologic spinal fractures in the mid to lower thoracic region or lumbar region.

Contraindications   These include a body habitus that is obese with a pendulous abdomen, excessive lordosis, or a need for increased lateral stability.

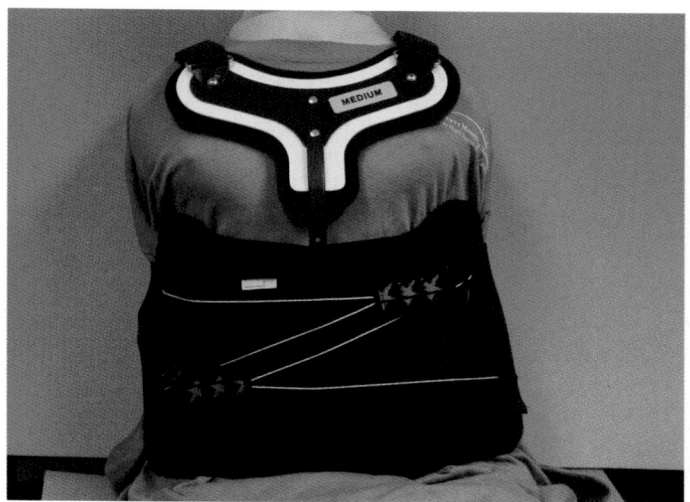

Figure 17-8 Thoracic–lumbar–sacral orthosis (prefabricated).

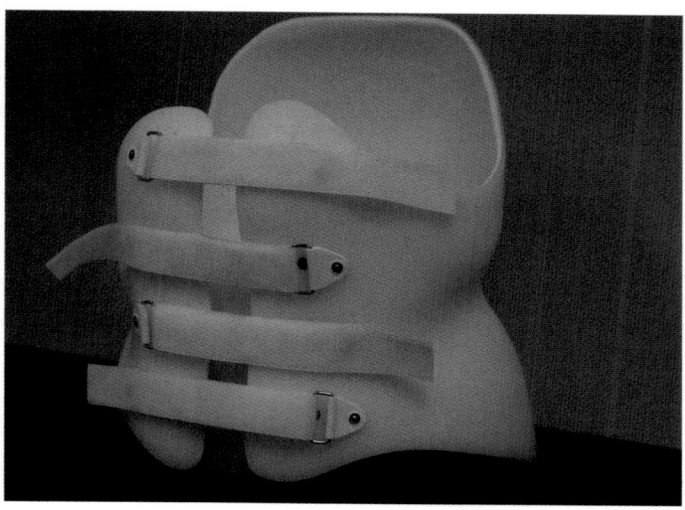

Figure 17-9 Thoracic–lumbar–sacral orthosis (custom-fabricated body jacket).

Special considerations Cost is reduced in some models due to the mass production of prefabricated modules. The use of breathable material can increase compliance with wearing.

Type: TLSO (custom-fabricated body jacket; Fig. 17-9)

Biomechanics The body jacket provides control of flexion, extension, lateral bending, and rotation. It uses three-point pressure systems and circumferential compression.

Design and fabrication It is molded to fit the patient and designed for patient needs. Anterior trim lines are usually located inferior to the sternal notch and superior to the pubic symphysis. The posterior trim lines have a superior border at the spine of the scapula, and an inferior border at the level of the coccyx. These trim lines are adjusted during fitting to allow patients to sit comfortably and to use their arms as much as possible without compromising the function of the orthosis.

Indications This orthosis can be used for treatment of traumatic or pathologic spinal fractures in the mid to lower thoracic region or lumbar region. Most are used for postsurgical management of fractures, such as compression, chance, or burst. The brace is also used after surgical correction spondylolisthesis, scoliosis, spinal stenosis, herniated disks, and disk infections.

Contraindications Complications include application of the orthosis over a chest tube, colostomy, or large dressings.

Special considerations Care must be taken to ensure that contact is maximized to decrease the pressure in any one area. Trim line changes must be made in small increments to prevent loss of control in terms of both leverage and tissue control. Ventilating holes are often made to improve airflow. Other factors to be considered when making the design include patients who might attempt to remove the orthosis when out of bed. The orthosis can be made with a posterior opening to reduce the risk.

Type: cruciform anterior spinal hyperextension (CASH) TLSO (Fig. 17-10)

Biomechanics The CASH provides flexion control for the lower thoracic and lumbar regions. It accomplishes this by way of a three-point pressure system. The system consists of posteriorly directed forces through a sternal and suprapubic pad, and an anteriorly directed force applied through a thoracolumbar pad attached to a strap that extends to the horizontal anterior bar.

Design and fabrication It is prefabricated, consisting of an anterior frame in the form of a cross, from which pads are attached laterally on a horizontal bar and at the sternal and suprapubic areas. A thoracolumbar pad is attached to a strap that extends to the lateral sections of the horizontal bar and adjusts the tension on the body. When properly fitted, the sternal pad is one-half an inch below the sternal notch, and the suprapubic pad is half an inch above the symphysis pubis.

Indications This orthosis is used primarily for the treatment of mild compression fracture of the lower thoracic and thoracolumbar regions.

Contraindications The CASH is not indicated for unstable fractures or burst fractures.

Special considerations Excessive pressure on the sternum can result in poor compliance with wearing schedule. Subclavicular pads may be added to help distribute this pressure.

Type: Jewett hyperextension TLSO (Fig. 17-11)

Biomechanics This orthosis provides flexion control for the lower thoracic and lumbar regions. This is done with a three-point pressure system consisting of posteriorly directed forces through a sternal and suprapubic pad, and an anteriorly directed

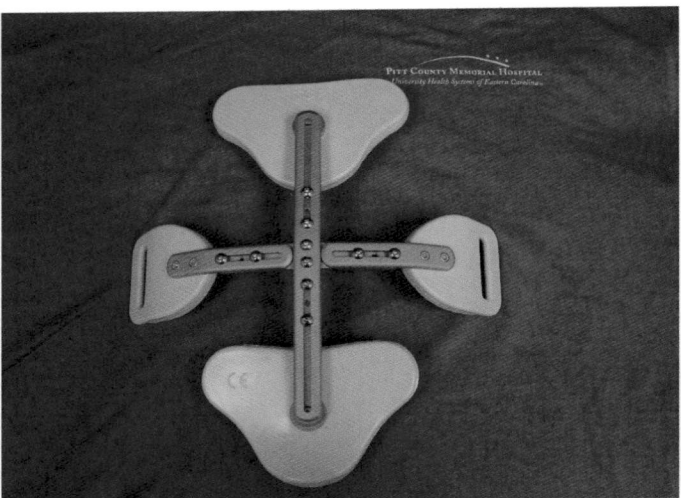

Figure 17-10 Cruciform anterior spinal hyperextension thoracic–lumbar–sacral orthosis.

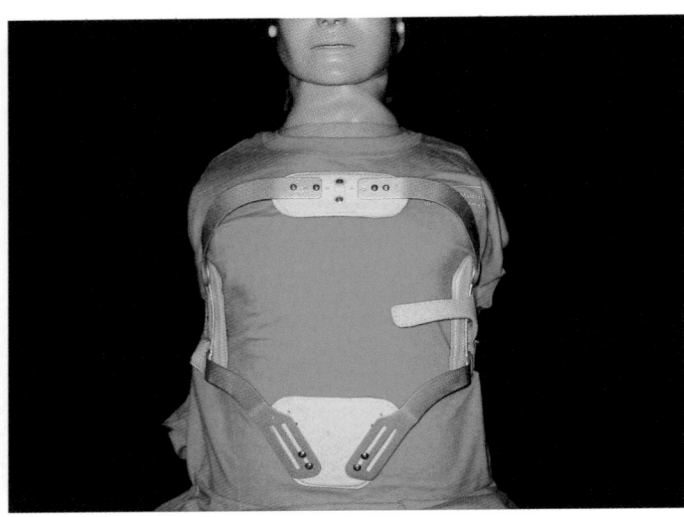

Figure 17-11 Jewett hyperextension thoracic–lumbar–sacral orthosis.

force applied through a thoracolumbar pad attached to a strap that extends to the lateral uprights.

Design and fabrication   It is prefabricated, consisting of an anterior and lateral frame to which pads are attached laterally on and at the sternal and suprapubic areas. A thoracolumbar pad is attached to a strap that extends to the lateral uprights and adjusts the tension on the body. When properly fit, the sternal pad will be one-half inch below the sternal notch, and the suprapubic pad will be one-half inch above the symphysis pubis.

Indications   The Jewett hyperextension TLSO is used primarily for the treatment of mild compression fractures of the lower thoracic and thoracolumbar regions. The Jewett has a little more lateral support than the CASH does.

Contraindications   It is not indicated for unstable fractures or burst fractures.

Special considerations   Excessive pressure on the sternum might result in poor compliance with wearing schedule. Subclavicular pads can be added to help distribute this pressure.

Type: Taylor and Knight–Taylor
Biomechanics   This orthosis provides control of flexion, extension, and a minimal axial rotation via the three-point pressure systems for each direction of motion. For example, flexion is controlled by the posteriorly directed forces applied through the axillary straps and the abdominal apron, and an anteriorly directed force through the paraspinal uprights.

Design and fabrication   The design of the Taylor consists of a posterior pelvic band extending past the mid-sagittal plane and across the sacral area. Two paraspinal uprights extend to the spine of the scapula. An apron front extends from the xiphoid to just above the pubic area. There are straps extending

from the top of the posterior uprights around the posterior axillary to the scapular bar and forward to the apron. Other straps extend from the paraspinal uprights to the apron.

The Knight–Taylor has an additional thoracic band that extends from the uprights just below the inferior angle of the scapula to the mid-sagittal plane, and a lateral upright on each side that connects the pelvic band and the thoracic band. These bands provide additional lateral support and motion control to the trunk.

Indications   These orthoses have been used for years for post-surgical support of traumatic fractures, spondylolisthesis, scoliosis, spinal stenosis, herniated disks, and disk infections. However, clinicians typically prefer the custom-molded TLSO body jackets, because better control of position is obtained.

Contraindications   Contraindications are unstable fractures that require maximum stabilization.

Special considerations   Pressure per square inch is higher, due to the width of the bands and uprights.

Type: lumbosacral corset (Fig. 17-12)
Biomechanics   The lumbosacral corset provides anterior and lateral trunk containment, and assists in the elevation of intra-abdominal pressure. Restriction of flexion and extension can be achieved with the addition of steel stays posteriorly.

Design and fabrication   This orthosis is usually made from cloth that wraps around the torso and hips. Adjustments are done with laces on the sides, back, or front. Closure can be with hook and loop (Velcro) or hook and eye fasteners or snaps. Many different styles are available in prefabricated sizes, usually in 2-inch increments, and are designed to fit the circumference of the hip. The orthosis can be adjusted for body type and proper fit by taking tucks in the cloth, as needed. Steel stays must be contoured to the body shape to encourage a reduction of lordosis or to accommodate a deformity. Custom corsets can

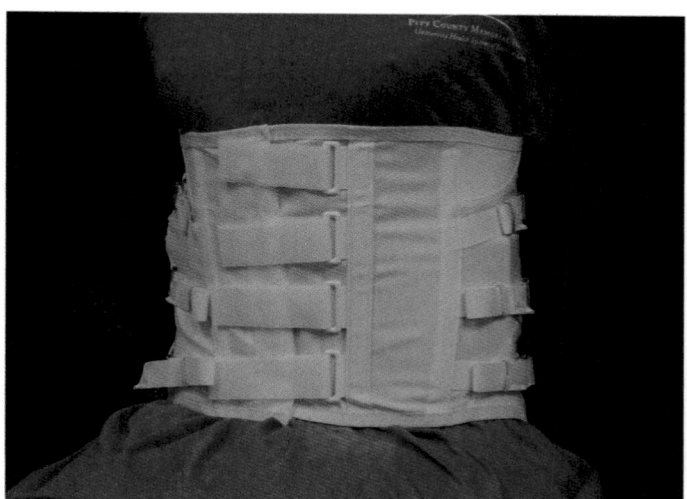

Figure 17-12 Lumbosacral corset.

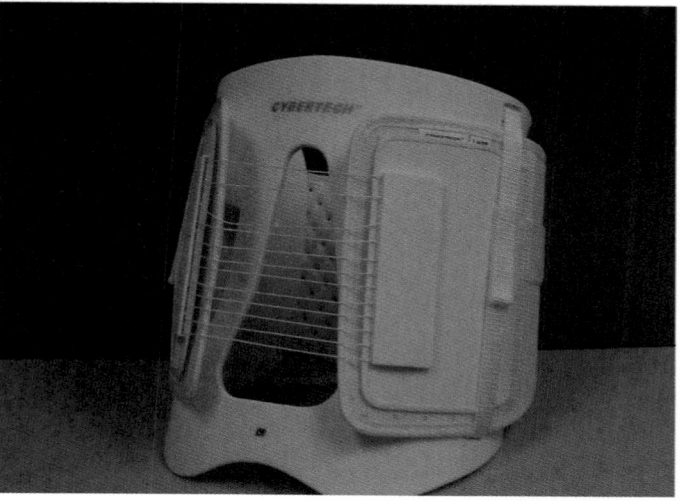

Figure 17-13 Lumbar–sacral orthosis Knight and chair back brace.

be fabricated based on careful measurements of the individual patient.

Indications This orthosis is the most frequently prescribed support for patients with low back pain.[30] It has been used for herniated disks and lumbar muscle strain, and to control gross trunk motion for pain control following single-column compression fractures with one-third or less anterior height loss.[35]

Contraindications The orthosis should not be used for unstable fractures, as well as fractures or conditions above the lower lumbar region.

Special considerations Long-term use of a lumbosacral corset can cause an increase in motion in the segments above or below the area controlled by the orthosis.[27] Muscle atrophy can also potentially occur after long-term use, causing an increased risk of reinjury. Patients can also develop a psychologic dependence on the support following injury.[16]

Type: LSO Knight and chair back orthoses (Fig. 17-13)

Biomechanics This brace provides limitation of flexion, extension, and lateral flexion. It also provides elevation of intraabdominal pressure.

Design and fabrication This orthosis has a pelvic band that lies posteriorly and extends laterally to just anterior to the mid-sagittal line. Laterally, the ends fall midway between the iliac crest and the greater trochanter. The superior edge of the thoracic band is at the level of T9–T10 or just distal to the inferior angle of the scapulae. The pelvic and thoracic bands are connected by two paraspinal uprights posteriorly and a lateral upright on each side at the mid-sagittal line. Orthoses can be fabricated from a traditional aluminum frame covered in leather, or thermoplastic material molded into the same shape. Straps are connected in a variety of ways to the frame, providing attachment to the anterior apron front.

Indications This brace is often used for lower lumbar pathologies, including degenerative disk disease, herniated disk, spondylolisthesis, and mechanical low back pain, and for post-surgical supports for lumbar laminectomies, fusions, or diskectomies.[24]

Contraindications These are unstable fractures, or conditions in the upper lumbar or thoracic area.

Special considerations Adequate clearance of the paraspinal uprights is required to allow for some reduction of lumbar lordosis when the anterior apron is tightened and while sitting. Clearance on the lateral uprights over the iliac crests are also areas to be monitored.

SCOLIOSIS

Idiopathic (infantile, juvenile, adolescent), congenital, and neuromuscular scoliosis have different etiologies, treatment approaches, and outcomes. Idiopathic scoliosis is the most common form.[31] Idiopathic infantile scoliosis is typically described from birth to 3 years of age, juvenile from 4 years until the onset of puberty, and the adolescent type from puberty to closure of the facets.

With idiopathic scoliosis, the evaluation should reveal no anomalous vertebrae, spinal tumor, or other neurologic abnormality. The majority spontaneously resolve, but progressive curves need to be treated.

Juvenile idiopathic scoliosis is more likely to be associated with adult cor pulmonale and death. Treatment should begin when curves reach approximately 25°. As thoracic curves predominate, the Milwaukee brace might be more effective than the TLSO.

The adolescent idiopathic scoliosis is the most common type for which an orthosis is indicated, usually between curves of 25 and 45°. Curves with an apex at T9 or lower can be managed with a TLSO. Curves with a higher apex require a Milwaukee brace. Single lumbar curves are treated with an LSO.[8]

Congenital scoliosis is secondary to a vertebral anomaly that is present at birth. Failure of part of the vertebrae to form (e.g. hemivertebrae) or failure of the vertebrae to properly segment (block vertebrae), or a combination of both, can occur. Congenital scoliosis is associated with abnormal development in the embryo, and associated developmental abnormalities in other organ systems should be considered, especially in the renal, urinary, and cardiac systems.[20]

Neuromuscular diseases are also associated with scoliosis. The prevalence of scoliosis in this population is much higher than with idiopathic scoliosis, from 25–100%. In general, there is a greater chance of progression in the presence of severe neurologic disease. Atypical for scoliosis in general, progression of the curve can occur in adulthood, and spasticity or flaccidity can be present, depending on upper versus motor neuron involvement. Multisystem involvement is more common in this group, as these diseases are not isolated to the spinal column alone. Consideration should also be made for presence of contraction, hip dislocations, sensory abnormities, mental retardation, and pressure ulcers.[15]

Scoliosis might continue to progress despite the proper use of an orthosis, and appropriate surgical referrals should be made. An important factor to consider prior to surgery is the pulmonary function in a patient with neuromuscular disease. Before surgery is considered, the forced vital capacity and forced expiratory volume in 1 s should be at least 40% of that predicted for the patient's age. Fusions are delayed as long as possible in an attempt to achieve maximal spinal growth (> 10 years of age). Declining pulmonary function, however, is a consideration for performing surgery earlier.[21]

Duval-Beaupere followed the long-term progression of idiopathic scoliosis, and noted that curve progression accelerated during growth spurts, and that the younger the child the higher the risk of curve progression, due to a greater amount of growth that remained.[7] It has also been shown that the greater the curve, the more likely the curve will increase.[14] Curves measured from 5 to 29°, and the curves from 20 to 29°, progressed in almost 100% of the patients. Approximately 50% of the curves from 5 to 19° appeared to progress.

Curve progression has been explained using Euler's theory of elastic buckling of a slender column.[32] Axial compressive forces evidently cause a column to buckle. This is associated with height growth and weight gain, especially increased upper limb weight during growth spurts. An increase in height and weight commonly occur together and might synergistically promote curve progression. It has been noted by these authors and others that the condition of a child with a large curve is more likely to progress than that of a child with a small curve.

Type: TLSO low-profile scoliosis orthosis
(Fig. 17-14)
Boston brace, Miami orthosis, Wilmington brace
Biomechanics These braces provide dynamic action using three principles (end-point control, transverse loading, and

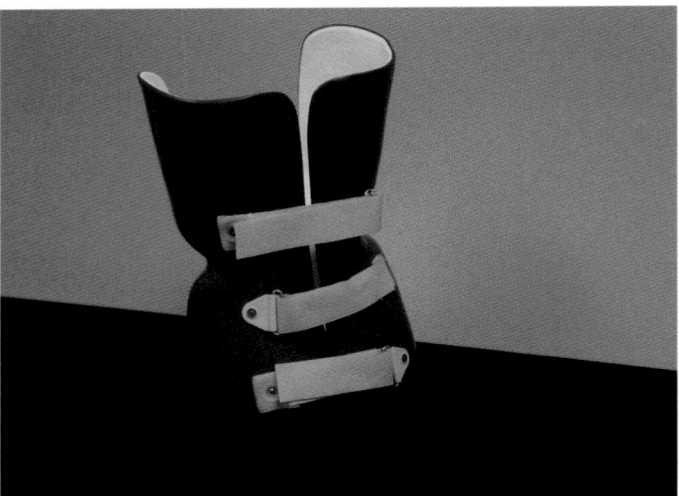

Figure 17-14 Thoracic–lumbar–sacral orthosis low-profile scoliosis orthosis.

curve correction) to prevent curve progression and to stabilize the spine.

Design and fabrication The use of orthoses or other devices to halt the curve progression of structural scoliosis has been reported as far back as Hippocrites.[19] Many different types of braces have been described in the literature. The one that stands out as being the most successful is the Milwaukee brace, which was described previously.

The effective non-operative treatment of idiopathic scoliosis using a low-profile TLSO has been demonstrated over the past 30 years. The most common of these braces is the Boston brace, introduced by J.E. Hall and M.E. Miller in 1971.[3,10] This system is available in prefabricated modules that are available in 30 sizes and can be ordered by measurement; they are then custom-fit to the patient. Modules can be used to fit approximately 85% of patients. Six of these sizes will fit approximately 60% of patients requiring an orthosis.[9] The orthosis can also be custom-fabricated from a mold of the patient's body. Trim lines are established based on the patient's curve; they are designed to provide pressure in specified areas to maximize corrective forces, and at the same time be less visible under the patient's clothing.

Indications This orthosis is indicated in patients with an immature skeleton and documented progression of a thoracic or thoracolumbar idiopathic scoliosis that measures 25 to 35° (measured by the Cobb method) and has an apex of T7 or lower.[5]

Contraindications The orthosis is contraindicated in patients with curves that measure greater than 40° and who are skeletally immature, or with curves in excess of 50° after the end of growth. Both these types of patients are typically candidates for surgery.[6]

Special considerations Idiopathic scoliosis occurs mostly in adolescent females. Treatment regimens, both non-operative and operative, are major events for the patients and their families. To be successful, the treatment team must be sensitive, supportive, honest, and communicate accurate information to patients and their families.

The effectiveness of any orthotic system depends on compliance with the wearing schedule. Most patients should wear the orthosis 23–24 h per day for it to be effective. Some physicians allow time out of the orthosis to participate in athletic activities or swimming and some special occasions, and this seems to improve acceptance and compliance.

FUTURE TECHNOLOGY, AVAILABLE NOW

Technology is available to help the practitioner improve efficiency in design and fabrication, as well as reducing the invasiveness of orthotic measurement of the patients. The development of computer-aided design (CAD) and computer-aided manufacturing (CAM) have allowed the fabrication of orthoses today in less time than it took only a few years ago. Insignia is one of the CAD–CAM systems available (Hanger Prosthetics and Orthotics; Fig. 17-15).[12] It combines CAD, laser scanning,

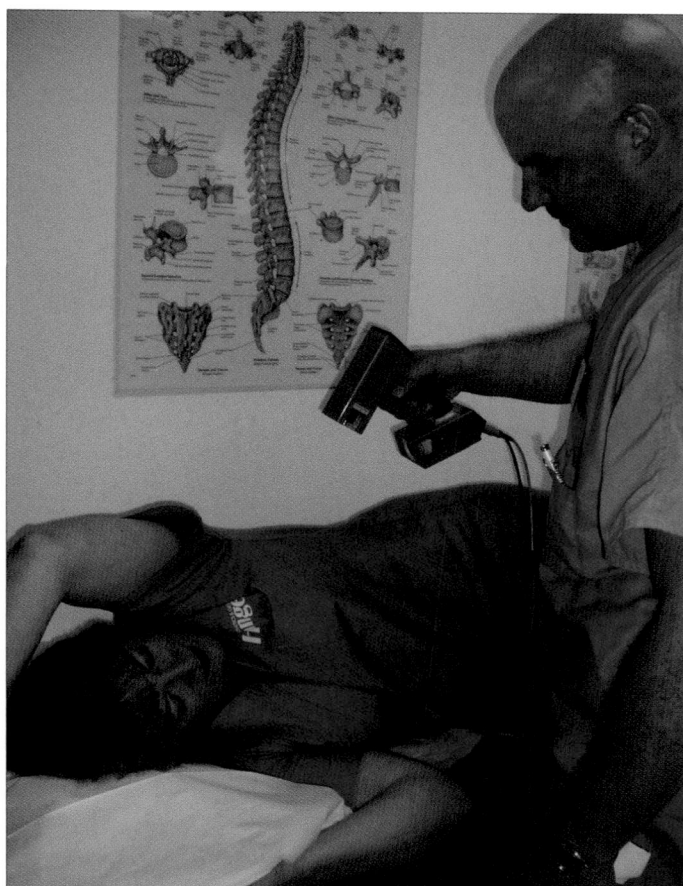

Figure 17-15 Insignia computer-aided design–computer-aided manufacturing system.

three-dimensional imagery, and motion-tracking technology to design orthotic and prosthetic devices. This is an alternative to traditional casting methods. The body part involved is scanned via a handheld scanning wand, which utilizes a motion-tracking device embedded in the scanner. A small receiver is attached to the area to be scanned. The wand is passed over the body part. A three-dimensional image of the body part is transmitted to the computer, and the software interprets the data. It provides the clinician with detailed and accurate three-dimensional measurements. Patients can be scanned for spinal jackets without movement from supine to prone positions. An option in the computer software allows one hemisphere to be scanned and then the computer develops the other hemisphere to form a complete image. The older plaster cast methods are becoming obsolete, due to the fact that the scanning system is not messy, can be done quickly, minimizes pain for the patient, and is more accurate. Modifications to these scanned computerized models can then be made before fabrication of the device begins.

Accuracy of measurement is within 1 mm, and the three-dimensional feature gives detailed surface information often lost with a cast or mechanical digitizer. A unique feature is the motion-tracking capability. If the patient moves during the scan, the movement is tracked and the final image is not distorted. The patient's scan is maintained in the computer database, allowing for rapid refitting and medical justification of new devices by showing volumetric changes.

SUMMARY

The proper prescription, construction, and fitting of a spinal orthosis is a complicated process. It is important that a complete, clear, and agreed plan of care is constructed. Success is likely to be limited if there is no agreement or understanding of the process and goals. The typical orthotic team in the USA includes the patient, orthotist, rehabilitation physician, and therapist. Experienced and knowledgeable providers working in a team approach provide the maximum likelihood that the orthosis will contribute to the overall therapeutic goals for the patient.

REFERENCES

1. Andry N. Orthopaedia [facsimile reproduction of the first edition in English, London, 1743]. Philadelphia: Lippincott; 1961.
2. [Anonymous]. Dorland's medical dictionary. 24th edn. Philadelphia: Saunders; 1989:438.
3. Boston Brace International. Online. Available: http://www.bostonbrace.com
4. Bunch WH, Keagy R. Principles of orthotic treatment. St. Louis: Mosby; 1975:1–5.
5. Carr WA, Moe JH, Winter RB, et al. Treatment of idiopathic scoliosis in the Milwaukee brace: long term results. J Bone Joint Surg (Am) 1980; 62:599–612.
6. Cassella MC, Hall JE. Current treatment approaches in the nonoperative and operative management of adolescent idiopathic scoliosis. Phys Ther 1991; 71:897–909.
7. Duval-Beaupere G. Pathogenic relationship between scoliosis and growth. In: Zorab BA, ed. Proceedings of the Third Symposiums on Scoliosis and Growth. Edinburgh: Churchill Livingstone; 1971.

8. Fisher SV, Winter RB. Spinal orthosis in rehabilitation. In: Braddom RL, ed. Physical medicine and rehabilitation. Philadelphia: Saunders; 1996:364–366.

9. Hall JE, Miller ME, Cassella MC, et al. Manual for the Boston brace workshop. Boston: Children's Hospital; 1976.

10. Hall JE, Miller W, Shuman W, et al. A refined concept in the orthotic management of idiopathic scoliosis. Prosthet Orthot Int 1975; 29:7–13.

11. Hall-Craggs ECB. The back and spinal cord. In: Tyler NC, ed. Anatomy as a basis for clinical medicine. Baltimore: Urban and Schwarzenberg; 1985:37–39.

12. Hanger Orthopedic Group. Insignia information. Online. Available: http://www.hanger.com

13. Johnson RM, Hart DL, Simmons EF, et al. Cervical orthoses: a study comparing their effectiveness in restricting cervical motion in normal subjects. J Bone Joint Surg (Am) 1977; 59:332

14. Lonstein JE, Carlson M. The prediction of curve progression in untreated idiopathic scoliosis during growth. J Bone Joint Surg 1984; 66A:1061–1071.

15. Lonstein JE. Orthoses for spinal deformities. In: Goldberg B, Hsu JD, ed. Atlas of orthoses and assistive devices. 3rd edn. St. Louis: Mosby-Year Book; 1985:271–274.

16. Luskin R, Berger N. Atlas of orthotics: biomechanical principles and application. American Academy of Orthopaedic Surgeons. St. Louis: Mosby; 1975:364–366.

17. Lysell E. Motion in the cervical spine, thesis. Acta Orthop Scand Suppl 1969; 123.

18. Maiman D, Millington P, Novak S, et al. The effects of the thermoplastic Minerva body jacket on cervical spine motion. Neurosurgery 1989; 25:363–368.

19. Moe JH, Bradford DS, Winter RB, et al. Scoliosis and other spinal deformities. Philadelphia: Saunders; 1978.

20. Monstein, JKE. Orthosis for spinal deformities. In: Goldberg B, Hsu JD, eds. Atlas of orthosis and assistive devices. St. Louis: Mosby-Year Book; 1997:259–278.

21. Murphy KP, Steele BM. Musculoskeletal conditions and trauma in children. In: Molnar DE, Alexander MA, eds. Pediatric rehabilitation. 3rd edn. Philadelphia: Hanley & Belfus; 1999:398–402.

22. Nachemson AL. A critical look at the treatment for low back pain: the research status of spinal manipulative therapy. DHEW publication no. (NIH) 76-998:21B. Bethesda: DHEW; 1975.

23. Nachemson AL. In vivo discometry in lumbar discs with irregular radiograms. Acta Orthop Scand 1965; 36:418.

24. Nachemson AL. Orthotic treatment for injuries and diseases of the spinal column. Phys Med Rehabil 1987; 1:22–24.

25. Nachemson AL. The lumbar spine: an orthopedic challenge. Spine 1976; 1:59–71.

26. Nachemson AL. The influence of spinal movement on the lumbar intradiscal pressure and on the tensile stresses in the annulus fibrosus. Acta Orthop Scand 1963; 33:183.

27. Norton P, Brown T. The immobilization efficiency of back braces: the effect on the posture and motion of the lumbosacral spine. J Bone Joint Surg 1957; 39A(1):111–139.

28. Panagiotacopulos ND, et al. Water content in human intervertebral discs: part II. Viscoelastic behavior. Spine 1987; 12:918.

29. Panjabi MM, et al. Thoracic human vertebrae, quantitative three-dimensional anatomy. Spine 1991; 16:888–901.

30. Perry J. The use of external support in the treatment of low back pain. J Bone Joint Surg (Am) 1970; 52:1440–1442.

31. Tachdejian MO. Pediatric orthopedics. 2nd edn. Philadelphia: Saunders; 1990.

32. Timoshenko S, Gere J. Theory of elastic stability. 2nd edn. New York: McGraw-Hill; 1961.

33. Wambolt A, Spencer DL. A segmental analysis of the distribution of lumbar lordosis in the normal spine. Orthop Trans 1987; 11:92–93.

34. White AA, Panjabi MM, eds. Clinical biomechanics of the spine. 2nd edn. Philadelphia: Lippincott; 1990:107.

35. White AA, Panjabi MM, eds. Clinical biomechanics of the spine. 2nd edn. Philadelphia: Lippincott; 1990:235–255.

Prescription of Wheelchairs and Seating Systems

Alicia M. Koontz, Donald M. Spaeth, Mark R. Schmeler and Rory A. Cooper

There are a wide range of choices in wheelchairs. One can choose a wheelchair that is manual, fully powered, hybrid (manual wheelchair with supplemental power), standing, multifunctional, and three- and four-wheeled scooters. There is also an abundance of seating and postural support hardware that can be used to correct or accommodate a wide range of orthopedic deformities and conditions. These include contoured cushions and backrests, tilt in space, recline, and custom-molded seating systems.

The goals for a wheelchair or seating system are listed in Box 18-1.

MAXIMIZE FUNCTIONAL INDEPENDENCE WITH ACTIVITIES OF DAILY LIVING

The wheelchair or seating system should enable individuals to perform the activities of daily living (ADL) that are important to them, with minimal to no assistance and with the least amount of energy expenditure. Types of activities can include transfers, personal needs (e.g. bathing and toileting), working, preparing meals, cleaning, and shopping.

MINIMIZE THE RISK OF SECONDARY INJURIES

Tips and falls account for over 70% of wheelchair-related accidents.[37] It is imperative that individuals be provided with mobility devices that comply with internationally recognized wheelchair standards, and can be safely operated (as determined by a skilled therapist or assistive technology practitioner). Seat belts, wheel locks, and a properly adjusted wheelchair can prevent serious wheelchair-related injuries. Pressure ulcers are a significant risk for those who use wheelchairs. Advanced cushion designs and seat functions can provide adequate pressure relief for persons who cannot independently off-load the buttocks. Shoulder pathology and nerve compression injuries at the wrist are common among wheelchair users.[35] Using proper wheelchair propulsion biomechanics and an optimal wheelchair set-up can help delay the onset of overuse injuries.

CORRECT OR ACCOMMODATE SKELETAL DEFORMITIES

When the skeletal deformity is 'flexible', the seating system should correct the deformity, and when the skeletal deformity is 'fixed', the seating system should accommodate the deformity.

The seating system should not create a 'new' deformity such as a sacral posture (posteriorly tilted pelvis), which results from sitting in a seat that is too long or using footrests that do not account for tight hamstrings.

ASSURE COMFORT

Along with mobility, comfort has been reported as the most important attribute or function of a wheelchair.[16] Research has shown that a majority of wheelchair users experience regular discomfort. Many either ignore it, or seek relief by getting out of the wheelchair, using pain medications, or doing weight shifting (either manually or with tilt and recline).[16] A wheelchair that allows for 'fine tuning' of the adjustments provides greater options for achieving comfort, as well as meeting the individual's postural and pressure needs.

PROMOTE POSITIVE AND UNOBTRUSIVE SELF-IMAGE

Because a wheelchair is often considered as an extension of one's body, it should be as aesthetically appealing as possible. Wheelchair designers and manufacturers are using materials that not only have high-strength mechanical properties, but also have finishes that are smooth, polished, sleek, and attractive. Power base systems are more compact than ever, with colorful and contoured plastic shrouds that cover the hardware and ergonomic seating systems. These look similar to the seats found in sports cars.

MANUAL WHEELCHAIRS

Persons with good upper body function and stamina might well be able to use a manual wheelchair for mobility. Manual wheelchairs for daily use are often categorized by their design features and costs. Table 18-1 provides an overview of each adult wheelchair category as defined by the Centers for Medicare and Medicaid Services, the leading third-party payer for wheelchairs. The dimensions contained in Table 18-1 describe most models of wheelchair within each category. The categories are

Table 18-1 Types of adult manual wheelchairs for daily mobility

Class[a]	Weight (lbs)	Seat width(s) (inches)	Seat heights (inches)	Seat depth(s) (inches)	Back heights (inches)
Standard	>36	16, 18	>19 and <21	16	16, 17
Standard 'hemi'	>36	16, 18	>15 and <17	16	16, 17
Lightweight	<36	16, 18	>17 and <21	16	16–18
High-strength lightweight	<34	14, 16, 18	>17 and <21	14, 16	15–19
Ultralightweight	<30	14, 16, 18	>17 and ≤21	12–20	>8 and <21
Heavy duty	Supports person weighing >250 lbs	≥18	>19 and <21	16, 17	16, 17
Extra–heavy duty	Supports person weighing >300 lbs	≥18	>19 and <21	16, 17	16, 17

[a]*Manual wheelchair classes as defined by the Centers for Medicare and Medicaid Services (http://www.cignamedicare.com/dmerc/lmrp_lcd/index.html).*

Box 18-1 Goals for a wheelchair and seating system

- Maximize functional independence with activities of daily living
- Minimize the risk of secondary injuries
- Correct or accommodate skeletal deformities
- Assure comfort
- Promote positive and unobtrusive self-image

---

somewhat outdated, however, as some ultralightweight (ultralight) wheelchairs are now less than 25 lbs. This is due to using higher strength, lighter weight materials to construct the frames and components. Manufacturers have also added features to lower end wheelchairs to meet provider and consumer needs without adding cost. For example, many standard and lightweight wheelchairs are available with larger seat widths (>18 inches), and high-strength lightweight wheelchairs are available with lower seat to floor heights (13- to 15-inch superhemi models).

The standard wheelchair (Fig. 18-1) is designed for short-term, hospital or institutional use and should not be recommended for the patient to use as a personal wheelchair. As noted in Table 18-1, these can be rather heavy, with limited sizes available. Figure 18-1 also illustrates the basic components of a wheelchair. The standard wheelchair folds for easy storage and transportability. A 'hemi' wheelchair is essentially a standard wheelchair with a lower seat to floor height for persons of shorter stature or who use one or both feet for propulsion. A lightweight wheelchair is slightly lighter in weight but with limited sizes. The first three models have few adjustable parts (some models have no adjustable parts) and generally have sling-type upholstery. Sling upholstery has no capacity to provide pressure relief, and the hammock effect that occurs from wear causes uncomfortable or unstable inward rotation of the hips. However, many users have been sitting in a sling

seating system for years, and have become accustomed to the hammock effect for comfort. Making the switch to a seating system that supports their posture better can be both frustrating and uncomfortable for these users.

The high-strength lightweight and ultralight wheelchairs are designed for long-term use by individuals who spend more than a couple of hours each day in a wheelchair. They have adjustable features, especially the ultralights. There are many advantages to using ultralight wheelchairs over the other wheelchair types. These are highlighted in the following sections that discuss selecting the appropriate seat dimensions, setting up the wheelchair, propulsion mechanics, and transportability. An ultralight wheelchair is depicted in Figure 18-2.

The last two classes of manual wheelchair listed in Table 18-1 pertain to persons who weigh over 250 lbs. These wheelchairs are heavier than the wheelchairs in the other classes in order to support more body weight. These categories are also outdated, due to the increasing number of persons with disabilities who are overweight or obese and need wheelchairs. This trend has resulted in an expanded class of extra-heavy-duty wheelchairs, referred to as bariatric wheelchairs, which are built to support individuals who weigh between 300 and 1000 lbs.

Pediatric manual wheelchairs are similar to the adult wheelchairs, but are smaller (seat width or depth <14 inches). Many of these wheelchairs have adjustable frames or kits for accommodating the growth of the child (Fig. 18-3). If the child is unable to self-propel the chair, a powered mobility device might provide independent mobility. Strollers equipped with a wide range of seating options (Fig. 18-4) can also be used to transport children with orthopedic deformities.

Sports wheelchairs are designed specifically for participating in such athletic endeavors as racing, rugby, tennis, and basketball. These wheelchairs are made of lightweight materials, and usually have very aggressive axle positions and camber. Some of the sport wheelchairs have only one wheel in the front, which allows quick turns and enhanced maneuverability (Fig. 18-5).

- Plastic mag wheels
- Sling seating
- Folding frame
- Non-streamlined appearance

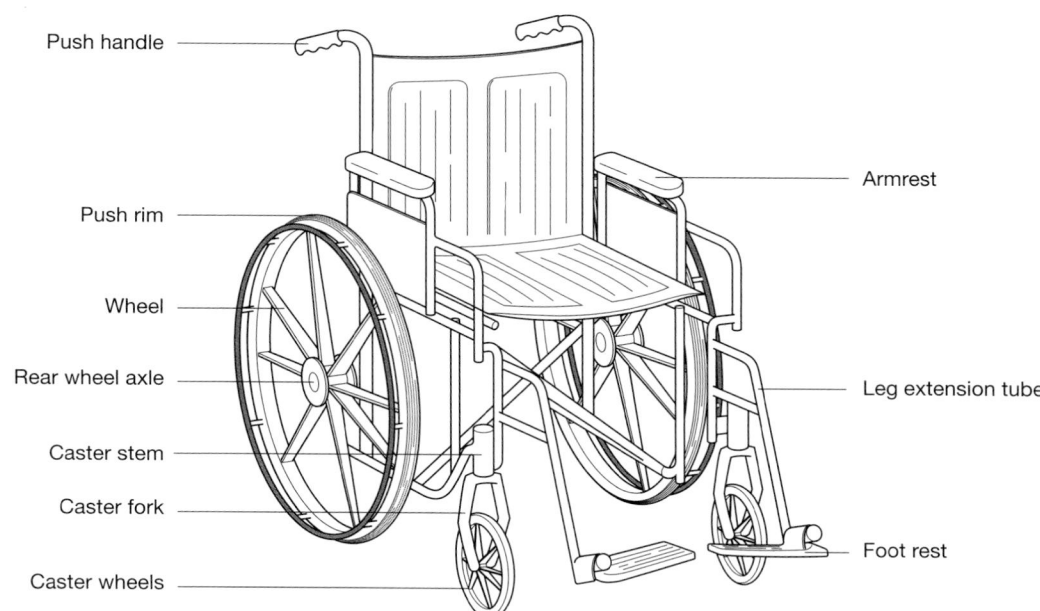

Push handle

Push rim

Wheel

Rear wheel axle

Caster stem

Caster fork

Caster wheels

Armrest

Leg extension tube

Foot rest

Figure 18-1 Standard manual wheelchair and components, including plastic mag wheels, sling seating, folding frame, and non-streamlined appearance.

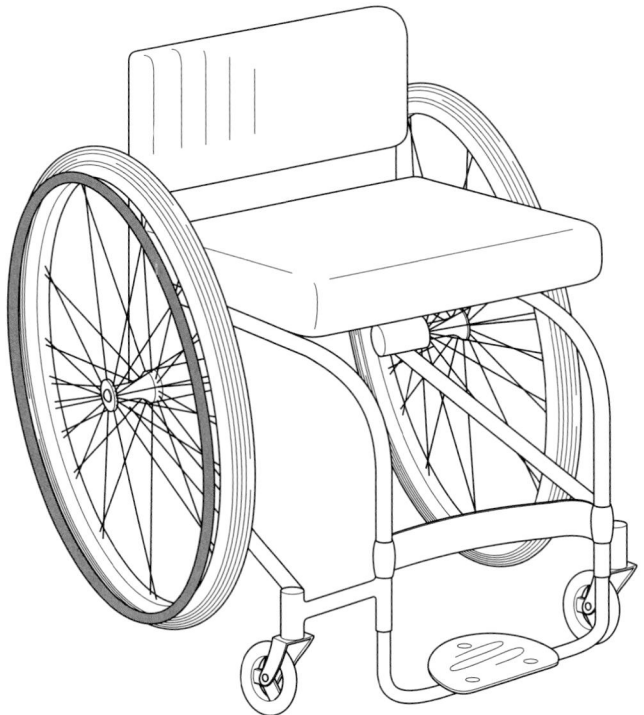

Figure 18-2 Ultralight manual wheelchair with a rigid frame, a fixed footrest, an adjustable camber, and caster housing built into the frame.

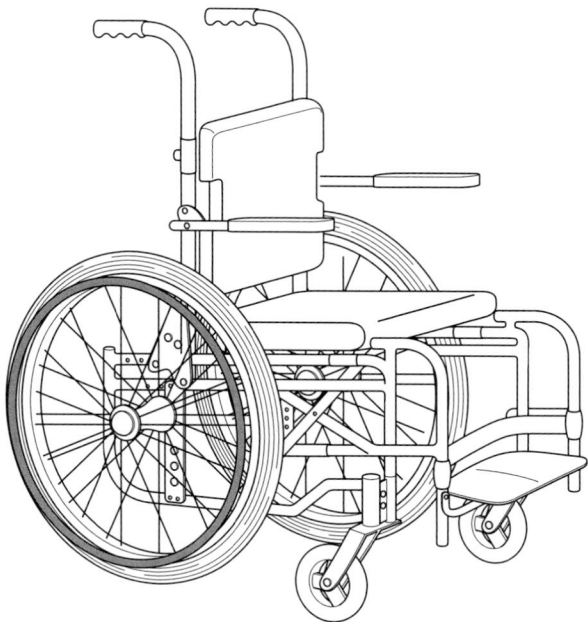

Figure 18-3 Pediatric manual wheelchair. Note the growth-adjustable frame, push handle canes that are high relative to the seat, and the footrest hangers at 90° to the seat.

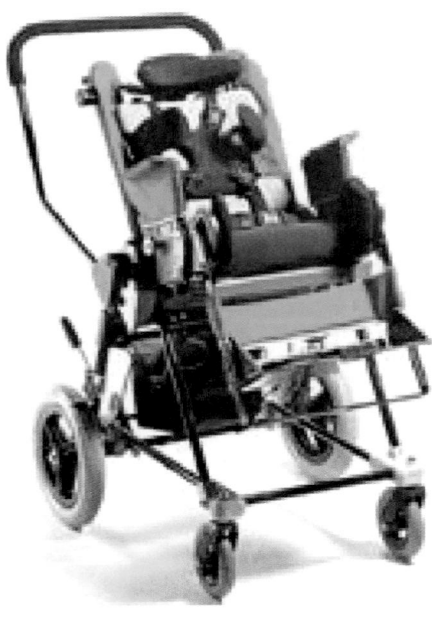

Figure 18-4 Pediatric adaptive stroller. (Reproduced by courtesy of the manufacturer.)

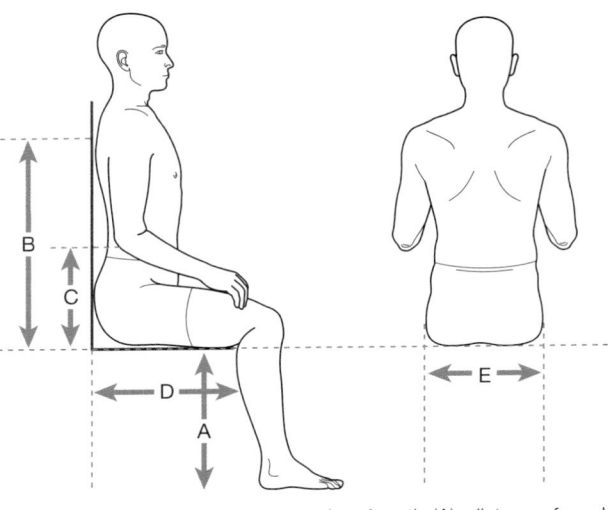

Figure 18-6 Body measurements. Leg length (A): distance from bottom of heel to popliteal area. Back height (B): distance from buttocks to the inferior angle of the scapula. Armrest height (C): distance from buttocks to forearm with elbow at 90°. Seat depth (D): distance from back of buttocks to popliteal area. Seat width (E): distance between the widest parts of the buttocks.

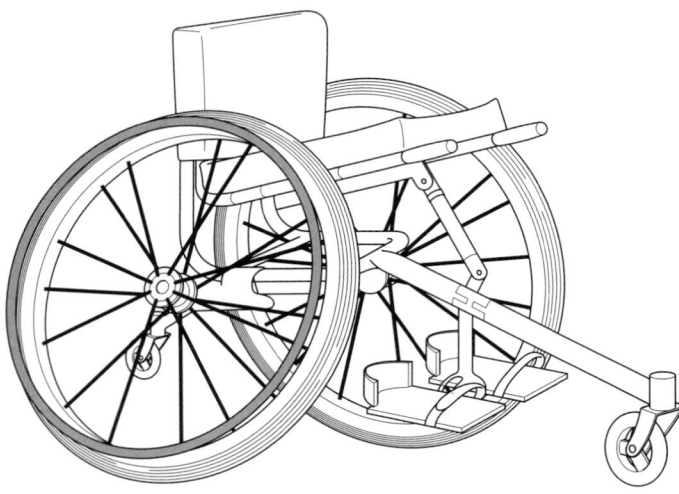

Figure 18-5 Tennis sport wheelchair. This has a high degree of camber, extreme seat dump (adjustable), footrests tucked out of the way, and a single caster in front for ground access.

Arm crank exercise has emerged as a possible solution to improving cardiovascular fitness, with research showing that arm cranking is more efficient and less of a physical strain than conventional wheelchair propulsion.[28] Wheelchairs equipped with arm crank mechanisms (called hand cycles) for exercise are available from many manufacturers.

Basic wheelchair dimensions

Figure 18-6 shows the measurements that should be taken of the patient's body for determining wheelchair dimensions.

These dimensions are required not only for determining the correct manual (or power) wheelchair size, but also for determining seating system sizes (e.g. cushion, back supports, and leg rest lengths).

Seat height

The seat should be just high enough to accommodate leg length while leaving enough space under the footrests (about 2 inches or so) to clear obstacles.[2] Persons with longer legs often need angled or elevating leg rests that extend the legs slightly outward instead of straight down (knee angle of 90°). This is needed to allow them to get their knees underneath tables. It is more difficult to do if the patient has tight hamstrings. The height of the seat should be adjusted so that the person has enough knee clearance to fit under tables, counters, and sinks at home, at work, at school, and in the community (the Americans with Disabilities Act mandates at least 27-inch high knee clearance under tables and surfaces). Seat height is also an important consideration for persons who drive while seated in the wheelchair and need to be able to access the steering wheel or hand controls.

Seat depth

The depth of the seat provides support for the thighs. A seat that is too shallow causes higher sitting pressures because less of the seat is in contact with the thighs. A seat that is too deep can cause excess pressure behind the knees and calves. There can also be a tendency for the pelvis to slide into a posterior tilt so that the back can be adequately supported by the backrest. A 1- to 2-inch gap between the popliteal area and the front edge of the cushion is recommended, but it might need to be more if the person propels with their feet.[2]

Seat width

The wheelchair seat width should be about 1 inch wider than the width of the widest part of the buttocks. When sitting on the seat, the individual's hips should be at or close to the edge of the cushion. If the seat is too narrow, the individual might develop pressure sores on the pelvic bony prominences. If the seat is too wide, the individual is forced to abduct their shoulders excessively, making it more difficult to push the chair.

Back height

The height of the back is determined by the amount of postural support the person needs. The backrest should be low enough to provide adequate support, but still allow the upper limbs access to as much of the push rims as possible. Many practitioners use the inferior angle of the scapula as a basis for determining backrest height. The backrest height should be below the inferior angle so that it does not impede arm movements. There are various kinds of back support (Table 18-2), and some have a tapered area that allows for greater freedom of scapular movement. Only the high-strength lightweight and ultralight wheelchairs permit the attachment of different kinds of back support.

Armrest height

The armrest height should be determined by measuring the distance between the forearm and the buttocks. The forearm should be parallel to the ground when positioned on the armrest.

Manual wheelchair set-up

Ultralight wheelchairs provide the highest degree of adjustability. This makes it possible to optimize the fit of the wheelchair to the user, which is likely to have a positive impact on propulsion mechanics. In addition to the basic adjustments that can be made on most other wheelchairs (e.g. footrests and armrests), ultralight wheelchair adjustments also allow for adjusting the seat and back angle, rear wheel camber, and rear axle position.

Seat and back angle adjustments

The angle that the seat makes relative to the horizontal plane can be adjusted, as can the angle the back makes relative to the vertical plane. The adjustments separately or together are done to provide the best postural support and comfort for the wheelchair user. Adjusting the seat so that it slopes downward toward the rear of the wheelchair can be done, and is referred to as seat dump. This can assist persons who have limited trunk control by stabilizing their pelvis and spine, making it easier to propel the wheelchair. Too much dump, however, can cause the pelvis to rotate backward and the lumbar spine to flatten. Increased dump also increases pressure on the sacrum and increases the risk of skin breakdown. Increased dump can also make it more difficult to transfer into and out of the wheelchair. An increased back angle or reclined back might be needed when the person's hips do not flex well or gravity is needed to assist with balancing the trunk. Using a combination of seat and back

---

Box 18-2 Advantages and disadvantages of camber

Advantages
- Brings wheels inward and closer to the body, which enables the arms to access more of the push rim
- Reduces shoulder abduction, because the wheels are closer to the body
- Increases lateral stability
- Protects the hand when pushing in tight areas, because the wheels make contact first with walls and doorframes

Disadvantages
- Wider wheelchair, which can be problematic in tight areas
- Diminished traction and uneven tire wear on a conventional tire (some tires have offset treads that accommodate for camber)

---

angle adjustments increases the number of possible postural accommodations.

Rear wheel camber

Camber is the angle of rear wheel tilt. Zero degrees of camber imply that the rear wheels line up vertically and with the side of the wheelchair. Angling the rear wheels so the top is tilted inward and the bottom outward (Fig. 18-5) results in increased camber and distance between the rear wheels. Most wheelchairs generally have up to 8° of camber. While more camber is usually possible, it can impede the ability to enter and exit doors and openings. Box 18-2 lists the advantages and disadvantages of camber.

Rear axle position

Ultralight wheelchairs allow for customizing the rear axle position both vertically and horizontally. Selecting the rear axle allows for optimal positioning of the rear wheels relative to the body and arms. Raising the axle has the effect of lowering the seat, while lowering the axle raises the seat. Moving the axle forward moves the seat back relative to the wheels, and moving the axle rearward brings the seat forward. Both kinds of adjustments can have a dramatic influence on propulsion biomechanics. Adjusting the axle position can also affect wheel alignment and seat angle. Keeping the chair in good alignment might require other adjustments, such as to the brakes or to caster alignment or height. Axle tubes on rigid ultralight frames can eliminate many of these problems.

Horizontal axle position

Rolling resistance is lower when more of the individual's weight is centered over or slightly behind the rear wheels.[8] This can be achieved by moving the axle forward. A more forward axle position requires less muscle effort and fewer strokes to push the wheelchair.[27] In a study of 40 individuals with paraplegia using their own manual wheelchairs, a more forward axle position was associated with lower peak forces, less rapid loading

Table 18-2 Back supports

Back support type	Image	Application	Benefits	Limitations
Basic upholstery fabric (vinyl or nylon) sling back found on standard wheelchairs		Casual transport for multiple patient	Inexpensive, easy to fold	Non-adjustable in either height or width, 'hammock'-quality support
Fabric back with tension ties		For consumers needing moderate customization	Relatively inexpensive, easy to adjust without tools and readjust as needed	Limited support; still a suspension back
Firm back, minimum contour		Consumers with moderate trunk support needs	Remains firm longer than suspension systems, option to choose height	More cost and weight than suspension support
Contour-molded foam over hard back		For persons with unstable trunks or back curvatures needing support	Provides a more rigid support, and can include lateral trunk as well as back support; different size options	Higher cost and weight, cannot be resized, more effort to break down chair for travel
Hardback with softer foam or gel central region		For consumers with asymmetries or prone to pain	Higher comfort, option to remove foam to obtain custom fit	Higher cost and more skill required of the fitting therapist, thicker foam requires a larger size and a wider seat frame

of the push rim, fewer strokes to go the same speed, and greater hand contact with the push rim.[4] Two of these parameters, stroke frequency and rate of loading the push rim, have been associated with carpal tunnel syndrome, a repetitive strain disorder affecting manual wheelchair users.[5] Lower stroke frequency and rate of loading might help protect the median nerve from injury. When more weight is centered over the larger wheels, it is easier to 'pop a wheelie', negotiate obstacles, and ascend or descend curbs. In contrast, moving the axle forward can make the wheelchair more 'tippy' and difficult to push up a ramp because of the tendency to tip backward. For this reason, wheelchairs are usually delivered with the axle in the most rearward position possible. This position usually needs to be changed, based on input from the patient and the practitioner. An antitipper (Fig. 18-7) can help prevent rearward falls but might also make it more difficult to negotiate a curb and pop a wheelie. Because of the effects on stability, the axle should be moved forward incrementally, provided the wheelchair user feels stable. Adding weight to the chair can also affect stability.[23] This is why packages or backpacks should ideally be located underneath the seat of the chair.

Vertical axle position

Research studies have shown that a lower seat position improves propulsion biomechanics. A lower seat position has been associated with greater upper limb motions,[21,40] greater hand contact with the push rim,[4,40] lower stroke frequency, and higher mechanical efficiency.[40] Lowering the seat height also increases the stability of the wheelchair. If the seat height is too low, however, the patient has to push with the arm abducted. This can increase the risk of shoulder impingement, another upper limb injury common among manual wheelchair users. The ideal seat height is the point at which the angle between the upper arm and forearm is between 100° and 120° when the hand is resting on the top and center of the push rim (Fig. 18-8a).[4,40] An alternative method that can be used to approximate the same position and angle is to have the individual rest with their arms hanging at the side. The fingertips should be at the same level as the axle of the wheel. If the seat height is too high, less of the push rim can be accessed and more strokes are needed to go the desired speed (Fig. 18-8b).

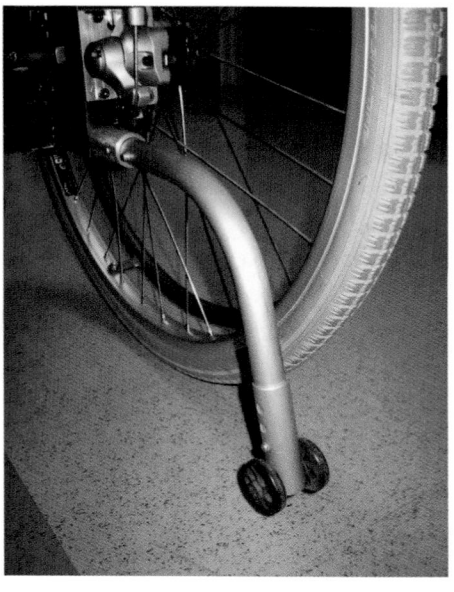

Figure 18-7 An antitipper.

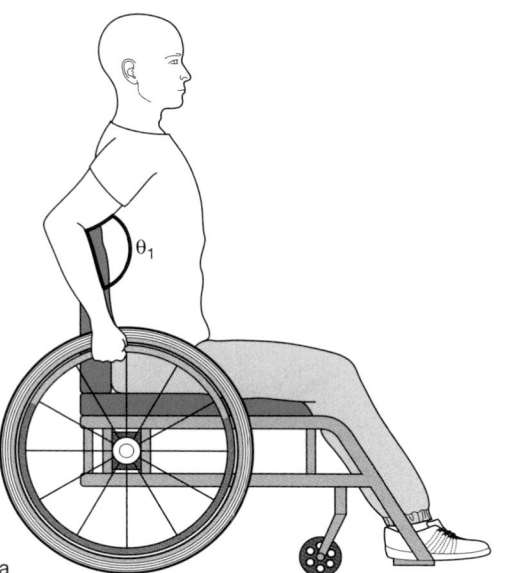
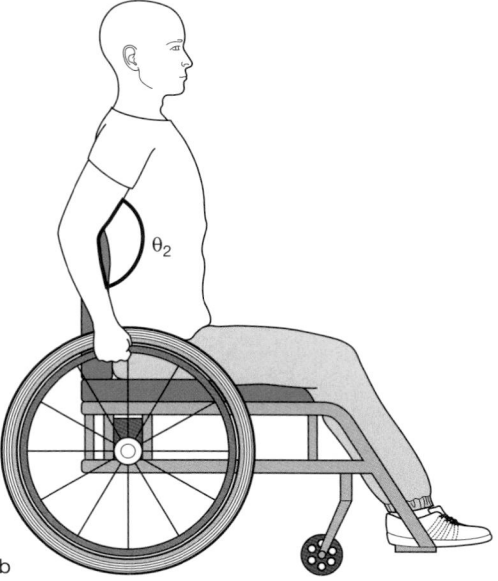

Figure 18-8 Differences in the elbow flexion angle (θ) and hand contact with the push rim after adjusting the height of the axle. (**a**) The recommended elbow angle ($\theta_1 = 100-120°$). (**b**) Angle θ_2 is larger because the seat is too high (axle too low), resulting in less hand contact with the push rim.

Amputee axle

Persons with lower limb amputations might need to have their axles adjusted further back than those without amputations to increase stability of the wheelchair. This is due to the loss of the counterbalancing weight of the lower limbs. Amputee axle adapters can be attached to the wheelchair frame to add additional rearward axle positions.

Wheelchair propulsion

The ability to effectively propel the wheelchair not only depends on the individual's physical capabilities (e.g. strength, stamina, spasticity, and fatigue), but also on such factors as the weight of the wheelchair, quality of the wheelchair, set-up, and technique. These factors are discussed in more detail below.

Wheelchair weight

The weight of the wheelchair is an important consideration, especially when prescribing manual wheelchairs. Rolling resistance is related to body weight and the weight of the wheelchair.[5] Less propulsive force is needed to push a lighter wheelchair. Ultralight wheelchairs have frames and components made with materials having high strength to weight ratios, so less material is needed. One study directly compared ultralight and standard wheelchairs, and found that ultralight wheelchair users pushed at faster speeds, traveled further distances, and used less energy.[3] The reduction of force is even more important on inclines, where gravitational forces add to the rolling resistance. A light wheelchair will also be easier to load into and out of a vehicle.

More manufacturers are starting to use titanium metal for the frame and parts. Titanium is very strong and somewhat flexible, providing a smoother ride while reducing harmful whole body vibration exposure.[26] Titanium wheelchairs tend to be more expensive but have many beneficial features, including increased durability and anticorrosive properties.

Quality of the wheelchair and set-up

Ultralight wheelchairs have better components and are less likely to become malaligned with use, which helps minimize rolling resistance. As discussed previously, a wheelchair that fits the user and is optimized for propulsion by adjusting the axle position makes it easier to push the wheelchair.

Propulsion technique

The propulsion techniques of manual wheelchair users have been examined in detail.[6,33,34,38] Propulsive strokes are generally described in two phases: when the hand is in contact with the push rim applying forces (push phase), and when the hand is off the rim and preparing for the next stroke (recovery phase). Four distinct propulsion patterns have been identified, which are defined by the path the hand takes during the recovery phase: arc, semicircular, single looping over, and double looping over (Fig. 18-9). The single looping over form of propulsion, which consists of having the hand above the push rim during recovery, is the most prevalent pattern in individuals with paraplegia.[6] However, the semicircular pattern, in which the user's hand drops below the push rim during recovery, has better biomechanics (Fig. 18-9a). The semicircular pattern has been associated with lower stroke frequency and greater time spent in the push phase relative to the recovery phase.[6] The semicircular pattern is preferred because the hand follows an elliptic pattern, with no abrupt changes in direction and no extra hand movements. By applying forces to the push rim in smooth, long strokes, the same amount of energy is imparted to the rim without high peak forces or a high rate of force loading. For example, a long stroke (Fig. 18-9a), as opposed to a short stroke (Fig. 18-9b), is likely to minimize the number of strokes needed to push at a desired speed.

Manual wheelchair transportability

There are basically two types of manual wheelchair frames: folding and rigid. Folding frames have a cross-brace under the seat that allows the wheelchair to collapse for storage (Fig. 18-1). Rigid frames are mainly available for high-performance (ultralight) wheelchairs (Fig. 18-2) and wheelchairs with special positioning aids (e.g. tilt or custom seating systems). Rigid frames tend to be more durable than folding, because there are fewer moving parts. Fewer parts also means that rigid frame

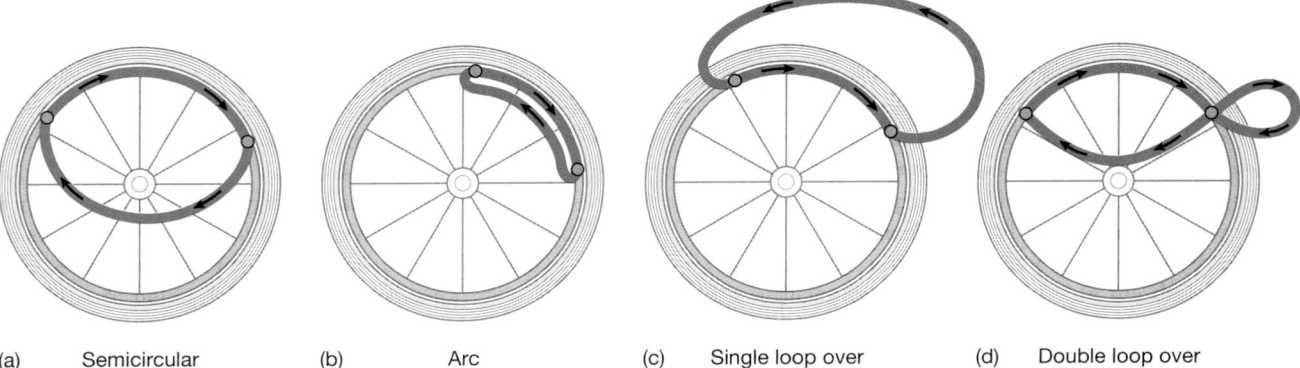

| (a) | Semicircular | (b) | Arc | (c) | Single loop over | (d) | Double loop over |

Figure 18-9 The four propulsion patterns identified from the hand motions of manual wheelchair users. The thick black line on the wheel is the path followed by the hand, and the arrows indicate the direction the hand moves. The circles indicate hand–push rim contact and hand release.

wheelchairs tend to be lighter. The backrests on rigid frames are designed to fold down for improved compactness. A 'quick-release' axle allows for easy removal of the wheels on rigid frames and certain folding frames. This option is not available on standard and some lightweight wheelchair models.

Manual wheelchair components and accessories (also see *Seating and positioning*)

Wheels and tires

There are several factors to consider when choosing the most suitable wheel and tire configuration for a wheelchair, including type of indoor or outdoor terrain, activity level, maintenance, weight, and cost. Many standard and lightweight wheelchairs come equipped with either mag-style or spoked wheels (Fig. 18-10). Mag wheels are made from composite plastics or metal (initially they were made from magnesium, hence the term *mag*). They are usually heavier than spoked wheels but are more durable and require less maintenance. Newer types of mag wheels comprise high-strength lightweight materials and can even be lighter than spoked wheels, but are more costly. Spoked wheels have a tendency to get out of alignment (wheel wobbles when spun), requiring a trip to a bicycle shop or a wheelchair dealer for the wheels to be trued.

Wheels are available in many different sizes. The most common rear tire diameters for manual wheelchairs are 22, 24, and 26 inches. Smaller tires can be found on pediatric manual wheelchairs and wheelchairs that are foot-propelled to keep the seat to floor height at a minimum.

Tires are available in many different tread designs and widths to accommodate almost any type of terrain, as well as the individual's mobility needs. Treads range from very smooth to extremely knobby, such as those typically seen on high-performance mountain bikes. Smoother tread and skinnier tires result in lower rolling resistance. If the wheelchair is primarily used indoors, a smooth to lightly treaded skinny tire is most desirable. However, if the wheelchair will be used outdoors, a wider tire with a medium knobby tread provides increased traction on rougher surfaces. The inner part of the tire or insert can either be air-filled (pneumatic) or solid foam. A pneumatic tire makes for a smoother ride for indoor or outdoor propulsion,

but rolling resistance is greater and more maintenance is required (e.g. the need to be able to repair a flat). Many standard and lightweight wheelchairs are equipped with solid plastic or foam tires, which require less maintenance than air-filled tires but tend to be heavier than pneumatic wheels.

Caster wheels also come in various sizes and configurations. Smaller casters provide for greater foot clearance and agility, but they are more apt to get stuck in cracks and at bumps, or cause forward falls. They are often found on high-performance, ultralight, and sports wheelchairs. The smallest casters available for manual wheelchairs are approximately 2 inches in diameter and are the same kind used on most 'in-line' skates. Casters are found to be as large as 8 inches in wheelchairs designed for daily use. The larger casters can provide the user with more security, because they roll over changes in surface height more easily. Like the rear tires, casters can be either pneumatic or solid (usually made of polyurethane). The polyurethane casters are very durable but do not offer the user as much comfort as the pneumatic tires.

Wheel locks

Wheel locks are also commonly referred to as brakes. They come in various styles but basically consist of two levers hinged together. When one is lever is pulled (or pushed), the other presses against the wheel and holds it in place. Sometimes the levers are difficult for persons to reach, and devices called wheel lock extensions can be added to essentially lengthen the lever. Wheel locks are essential for safety; however, some wheelchair users opt not to have them on their wheelchair. This is usually because the user's hands interfere with the braking levers or parts when propelling the wheelchair. Not having wheel locks requires that users be able to stabilize themselves well enough with the upper body, either by grasping the tires and/or nearby surfaces. This unfortunately can result in awkward postures and excessive strain on the upper body and back. A wheelchair without wheel locks also makes it more difficult to keep stable when transferring to and from the wheelchair.

Grade aids

Grade aids are devices that attach to the frame and are used for persons who have difficulty with slopes and have a tendency to roll down hills. These devices only prevent the wheelchair from rolling backward, and forward motion is unimpeded.

Push rims

Push rims are available in different sizes, shapes, and surface finishes. The push rim most commonly found on wheelchairs is about half an inch in diameter, with a smooth surface finish and round cross-sectional area (Fig. 18-1). Persons who have limited gripping ability (e.g. those with low-level cervical injuries) might need a larger diameter push rim and/or a high-friction surface finish (e.g. vinyl or foam). Sometimes these individuals need a push rim with vertical, horizontal, or angled projections (Fig. 18-11a) to be able to effectively propel their wheelchairs. New designs provide for greater surface area (Fig. 18-11b) that is also contoured for a more natural hand grip.

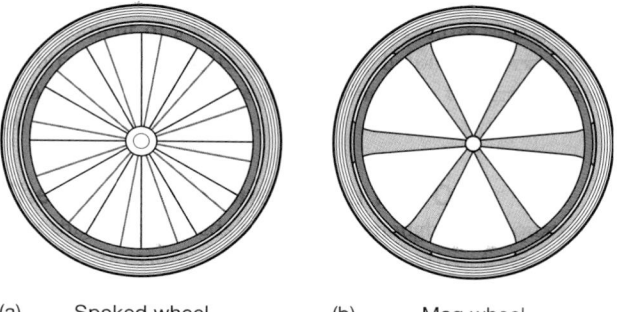

(a)   Spoked wheel   (b)   Mag wheel

Figure 18-10 Mag and spoked wheels.

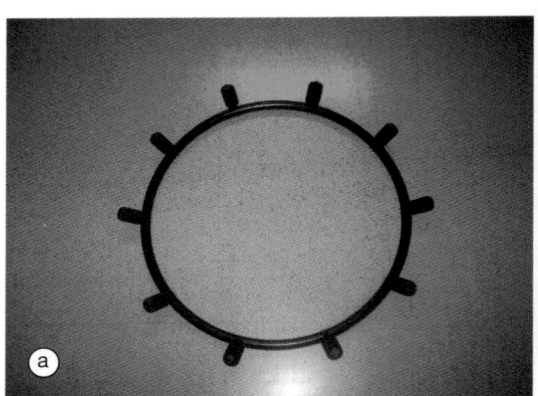
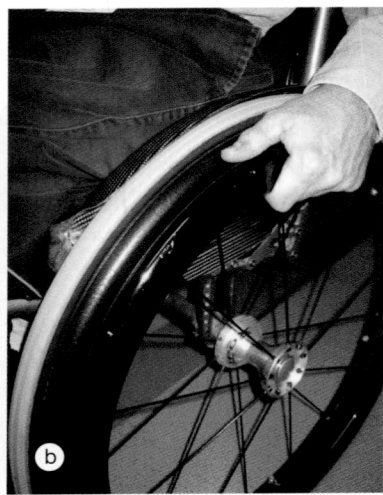

Figure 18-11 (**a**) Push rim with angled projections. (**b**) Contoured push rim with large surface area for gripping.

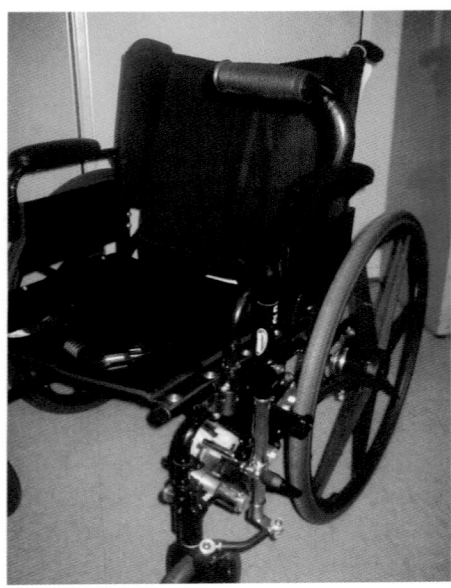

Figure 18-12 One-arm lever drive system.

Lever drives

Propelling the wheelchair using levers versus push rims has proven to be more mechanically efficient. Dual-lever drive wheelchairs are more common in Europe, China, and other countries of the Far East. They are well suited for persons who frequently propel long distances and over outdoor terrain (e.g. dirt roadways). The drawbacks of using a lever drive system include difficulties with maneuvering in tight places, transfers, and transportability. Single-lever drive systems are quite popular in the USA and allow for the wheelchair to be propelled using one arm (Fig. 18-12).

Antitippers

Antitippers are devices that attach to the rear of the wheelchair frame and usually have adjustable length tubes with small wheels at the end (Fig. 18-7). These devices protect the user from tipping the wheelchair backward, but can make it difficult for the user to ascend a curb or pop a wheelie. The tube length can be adjusted to allow the user to traverse over small obstacles, while still providing some stability. All new manual wheelchairs generally come equipped with antitippers; however, high-end users often remove them after receiving the wheelchair.

POWER-ASSISTED WHEELCHAIRS

Power-assist devices are appropriate for individuals who use or prefer their manual wheelchairs for mobility, but who need some assistance to reduce the physical effort required to self-propel. These devices are particularly likely to help those with muscle paralysis or weakness, overuse, and fatigue. They are also ideal for individuals who are apprehensive about transitioning to a fully powered wheelchair. This can be due to not wanting to be viewed by peers as being 'more disabled', having homes that do not accommodate the increased size, lacking the financial resources, or having difficulties with transportation. Power-assist devices include stand-alone powered units that are external to the wheelchair, and that the wheelchair user holds on to. Another is a power add-on device that attaches to the wheelchair and has a steering mechanism or input device for controlling the wheelchair. Figure 18-13 shows a push rim-activated system with motors in the wheelchair hubs. Power-assist devices cost less than a fully powered wheelchair system, but require that the individual have a manual wheelchair that is compatible with the power-assist device.

Some physical effort is needed to move the wheelchair with a push rim-activated system, but to a much lesser extent than that required for operating a manual wheelchair. Applying torque to the push rims sets the wheelchair in motion. Research has shown that using a push rim-activated wheelchair results in significant reductions in the physiologic demand of propulsion compared with using a manual wheelchair.[10] Using a power-assist wheelchair also reduces upper limb range of movement required at the wrist and shoulder, which might help reduce

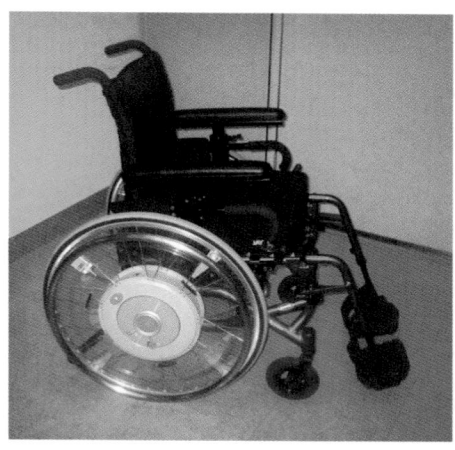

Figure 18-13 Push rim-activated power-assist wheelchair.

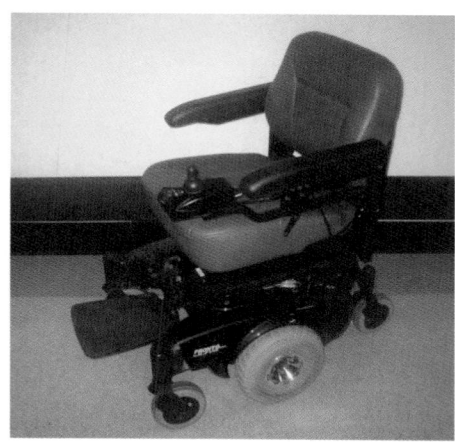

Figure 18-14 Conventional power wheelchair.

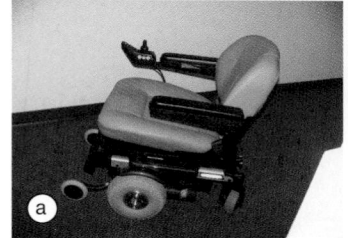 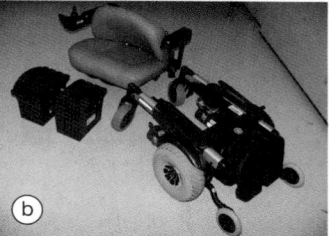

Figure 18-15 Transportable, lightweight power wheelchair.

the incidence of soft tissue injuries.[14] Power-assist devices can increase the width or length of the manual wheelchair base a few inches. They are more difficult to transport than manual wheelchairs, mainly because the equipment adds about 40–50 lbs to the wheelchair. This is still considerably lighter, however, than a fully powered wheelchair.

POWER WHEELCHAIRS

People who do not have the strength and/or stamina to propel manual wheelchairs typically need power wheelchairs for mobility independence. The origins of commercial power wheelchairs can be traced to the 1950s,[39] when the power wheelchair with twin internal motors and joystick control[24] became the model for commercial production. The advent of single-board microprocessors in the mid 1970s allowed controllers to be improved, enhancing drivability and safety.[1]

Power wheelchairs can be grouped into four categories based on the functions provided by the wheelchair and the intended use: low-cost standard folding or lightweight, indoor, outdoor, and heavy-duty indoor or outdoor wheelchairs.

Conventional power wheelchairs

These wheelchairs are not programmable (e.g. no adjustments in acceleration or deceleration, turning speed, or joystick sensitivity), and have very basic seating with limited sizes available (Fig. 18-14). They are low cost and low quality (see *Wheelchair standards* section below). They are appropriate for higher functioning individuals with good trunk control who do not need specialized seating and plan to use the device indoors.

Folding and transport power wheelchairs

Folding and transport power wheelchair models are designed to be broken down into pieces to facilitate transport (Fig. 18-15). They are usually compact for indoor use and have a small footprint (i.e. the area connecting the wheels). This allows them to be maneuverable in confined spaces. However, they might not have the stability or power to negotiate obstacles outdoors, and are typically used by individuals with reasonably good trunk

and upper body control. The batteries are often housed in separate boxes having easy to separate electrical connectors, which facilitate dismantling the wheelchair. These wheelchairs are not designed to be durable, and users need to consider the trade-off of car transportation and their power mobility driving needs.

Combination indoor–outdoor power wheelchairs

Combination indoor–outdoor power wheelchair models (Fig. 18-16) are often purchased by people who wish to have mobility at home, at school, at work, and in the community, but who stay on finished surfaces (e.g. sidewalks, driveways, and flooring). These wheelchairs are usually equipped with standard proportional joysticks and standard programmable electronics. They come with either standard seating (such as that shown in Fig. 18-17) or rehabilitation seating (Fig. 18-16). Rehabilitation seating allows for the attachment of modular seating hardware (e.g. backrests, cushions, laterals, hip guides, and headrests).

Heavy-duty indoor–outdoor power wheelchairs

Heavy-duty indoor–outdoor power wheelchair models (see Fig. 18-18) are for use by people who live in mostly rural areas or who enjoy outdoor activities, but who also need to use the wheelchair indoors. These wheelchairs usually have large-diameter drive wheels with heavily treaded tires or four-drive wheels for climbing obstacles and traversing rough terrains. These wheelchairs are generally designed to support persons who weigh more than 250 lbs, and have greater power output for handling the extra weight and rough terrain. These wheelchairs usually weigh as much as 300–500 lbs.

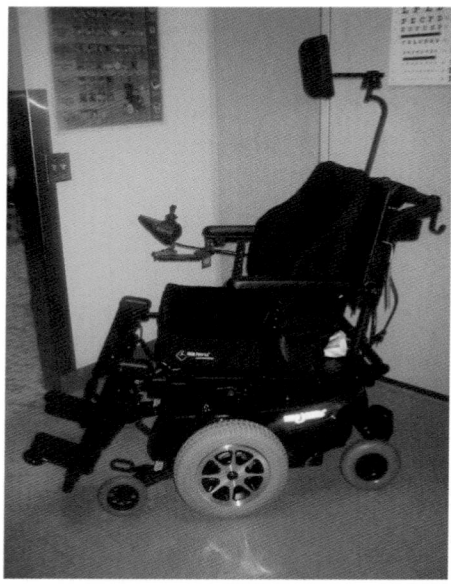

Figure 18-16 Indoor–outdoor power wheelchair shown with rehabilitation seating, a power tilt in space and recline seating system, headrest, and power-elevating leg rests.

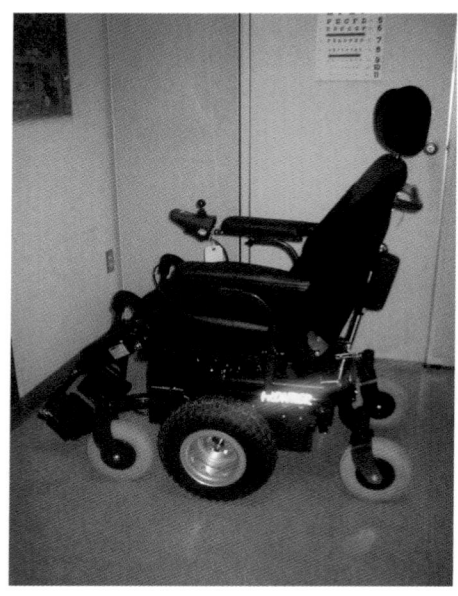

Figure 18-18 Heavy-duty indoor–outdoor power wheelchair.

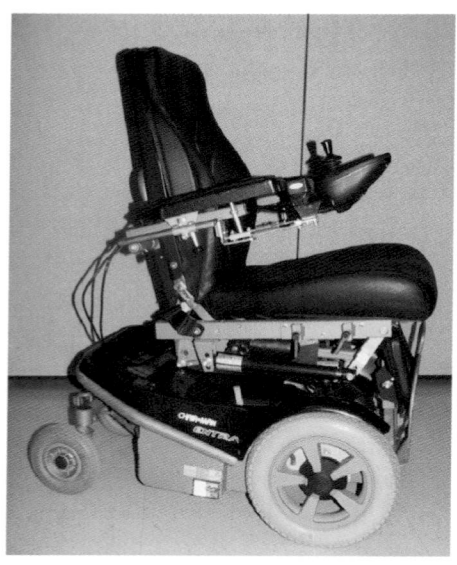

Figure 18-17 Front-wheel drive power wheelchair.

The latter two categories are power base wheelchairs, where the main chassis consists of motors, drive wheels, casters, controllers, batteries, and the frame. The seating system (e.g. seat, backrest, armrests, leg rests, and footrests) is a separate integrated unit. These wheelchairs usually have programmable control parameters including speed adjustment, tremor dampening, acceleration control, and breaking. Power bases tend to offer higher performance than conventional power wheelchairs (i.e. higher speeds and more torque). Power seating options, such as tilt in space, power recline, and seat elevation, can be integrated with the power bases to adapt for progressive disease or severe disability. A significant advantage of some power bases is that the position of the wheels with respect to the seat can be changed.

Power wheelchairs typically use two deep-cycle lead–acid batteries in series, each producing 12 V, for a total of 24 V. There are two types of lead–acid batteries, i.e. wet cell batteries and gel cell batteries. Gel cell lead–acid batteries are generally recommended, because there is no potential for chemical spills and they are maintenance-free.

Power wheelchair base selection
Power wheelchair choices have increased dramatically in the past decade. It is important to consider the lifestyle and functional ADL prior to making a final choice on a power wheelchair. There are three basic drive configurations for power wheelchair bases: front-wheel, mid-wheel, and rear-wheel drive. The drive configuration of a power wheelchair plays an important role in how well a chosen power wheelchair fits the user's lifestyle and environment.

Rear-wheel drive
Rear-wheel drive is a common drive configuration, characterized by large drive wheels in the rear and small pivoting casters in the front (Fig. 18-19). The rear-wheel drive power wheelchair steers and handles predictably, and naturally tracks straight, making it is the most appropriate drive configuration for high-speed applications. Additionally, due to its consistent tracking, the rear-wheel drive wheelchair is preferred by people who drive with special input devices or have reduced coordination. The disadvantages of this configuration include limited obstacle climbing by the small front casters, as well as sinking into soft surfaces more readily than larger wheels. It also has the largest turning radius among the three configurations.

Front-wheel drive
The front-wheel drive power wheelchair features large drive wheels in the front and small pivoting casters in the rear (Fig. 18-17). It is a very stable set-up for uneven terrain and hills.

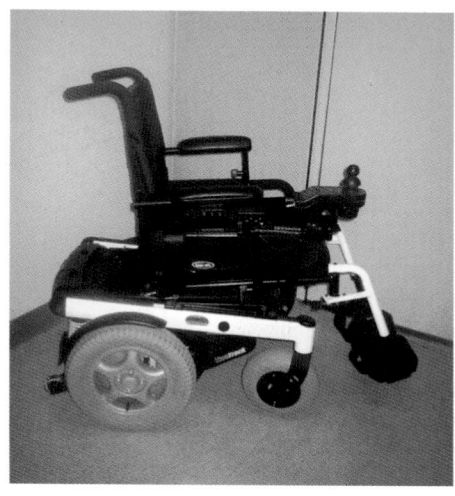

Figure 18-19
Rear-wheel drive
power wheelchair.

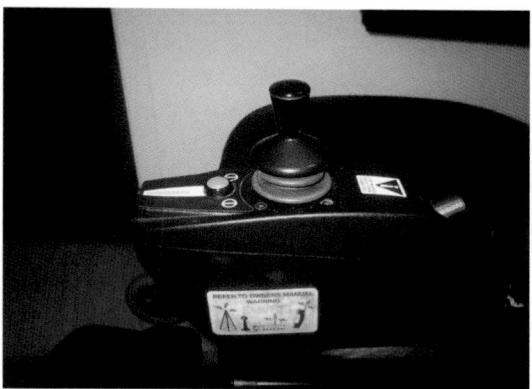

Figure 18-20 Conventional position-sensing joystick.

Out of the three configurations, it has the best capability to climb forward over small obstacles. The overall turning radius is medium. On the less favorable side for some users, the front-wheel drive power wheelchair has a tendency for the back of the chair to wander side to side (commonly called 'fishtailing'), especially as speeds increase. This directional instability requires steering corrections, and this might make the wheelchair difficult for some users to steer. The front-wheel drive has one of the slowest top speeds.

Mid-wheel drive

The mid-wheel drive power wheelchair (Fig. 18-16) has been one of the fastest growing in the wheelchair industry. In this configuration, the drive wheels are located near the center of the power wheelchair, allowing the user to seemingly turn on center, dramatically increasing indoor maneuverability. With the drive wheels directly under the user, traction is increased, and with the use of suspended front antitip wheels, the mid-wheel drive can be among the most effective at both ascending and descending obstacles for skilled, practiced users. However, one of the concerns is that, when riding on uneven terrain or up and down curb cuts with a steep transition, there is a possibility of getting stuck on the front or rear casters, suspending the drive wheel in mid air with no contact with the ground.

The drive tires for power wheelchairs come in many different sizes (9- to 17-inch diameter). Larger drive tires are generally found on heavy-duty outdoor power wheelchairs. The casters on power wheelchairs are larger than those found on manual wheelchairs, and are either air-filled or have solid foam inserts or tires.

Overall, there is no perfect drive configuration for a power wheelchair, as all have their benefits and drawbacks. By aligning a user's needs with the benefits and disadvantages of each configuration, and testing models within the categories, mobility can be optimized.

Input methods

The interface between the wheelchair user and the wheelchair itself is often the most critical component of a powered wheel-

chair. A safe, consistent, and reliable method of accessing powered mobility can sometimes be the most difficult step of the evaluation.[7] It is important to try different input devices during the evaluation, because of the plug and play technology. This technology allows the input device to be changed as the patient's condition changes, without having to replace the electronics or wheelchair. This improves control and safety, and helps reduce costs.

There are different types of input method for operating a power wheelchair. The most common commercially available control interface between the user and the wheelchair is a joystick (Fig. 18-20).

Proportional control versus switched control

A joystick can be either proportional control or switched control. Proportional control is usually the optimum solution for wheelchair control, because it provides continuously variable adjustment of speed and direction. If the user does not have the fine motor skills necessary for reliable control of a proportional joystick, however, a switched joystick should be chosen. Switched joysticks respond to discrete positions of the joystick, and usually have eight driving directions. These directions typically are forward, reverse, left and right, and the four diagonal directions. Being a switched device, speed is not directly controllable by joystick position. For users without appropriate hand control, the joystick can be mounted on the wheelchair and positioned for operation by the chin, head, shoulder, elbow, arm, knee, foot, tongue, mouth, etc. Joysticks can be ordered in various sizes (e.g. 'mini' for small movements) and with different handles (e.g. round, oblong, goalpost-shaped).

Position-sensing versus force-sensing

For proportional control, a joystick can use either the position-sensing or force-sensing method. The control output from a position-sensing joystick is proportional to the deflection of the joystick from a neutral position. A change in electrical resistance or inductance can be used to signal the position of the joystick. The control output from a force-sensing joystick is proportional to the force exerted on the stick by the user.[13] A strain gauge bridge is usually instrumented to the joystick shaft to measure forces. Force-sensing joysticks are effective in some conditions, for example tremors, spasms, weakness, and inadequate range of motion. However, they are difficult to use in rough terrains.

Sip and puff switches, head array switches, and voice command are types of digitally controlled input devices. The user provides a command to activate the input device by a breath, tapping a switch or moving near a proximity switch, or using their voice to move the wheelchair in the desired direction. The wheelchair moves at a predetermined speed until a reverse command is given or the input to the switch is removed.

Sip and puff   A sip and puff input device is a type of switch that allows input of data by sipping and puffing on a straw located near the mouth (Fig. 18-21). Generally, a user will sip a specific number of times to indicate a direction, and puff to confirm the choice and activate the movement of the wheelchair.

Head array   The head array device usually has a three-piece headrest with proximity switches built into each pad. By being in proximity to the switch embedded in the center pad, the client moves the wheelchair forward. Activating the side pads moves the chair in the corresponding direction. A reset switch toggles between the forward and reverse functions.

Voice control   A throat microphone picks up the vibrations of the vocal cords when the user speaks the commands. In some cases, a headset microphone can also be used. The wheelchair can be driven with several distinct sounds to emulate the movements of a switched joystick.

The placement site of the input device is crucial in getting the accuracy and consistency needed to use the device safely for safe and functional power wheelchair negotiation. Hand-operated joysticks with proportional control are the conventional method of interface for most wheelchair users. For those who are unable to access a joystick by hand, the joystick can be placed around other body parts. Although chin or head control joysticks can be effective, they are visually intrusive, and obstruct feeding and wheelchair transfers. They are also difficult to use to steer accurately over rough surfaces, because of the relative movements of joystick and head. The control method of the input device is also an important factor in determining the right device for a wheelchair user. For example, a head control device can use either proportional or switched control methods. With the proportional head control, full directional and proportional speed control can be achieved. If the client does not have refined head control, however, their speed might be erratic. Users also tend to forcefully extend the neck and sustain pressure on the headrest to move the wheelchair forward, which increases muscle tone. With the switched head control, the proximity switches do not require any pressure to activate, preventing further increases in muscle tone. The head array does not offer full directional control, however, but only four or eight directional controls.

Integrated controls

Wheelchair input devices are not only used for controlling the wheelchair, but also to access environmental control systems and computers. When a single control interface (e.g. joystick, head switches, voice recognition system, and keypad) is used to operate two or more assistive devices, the system is called an integrated control system (Fig. 18-22).[17] The advantages of

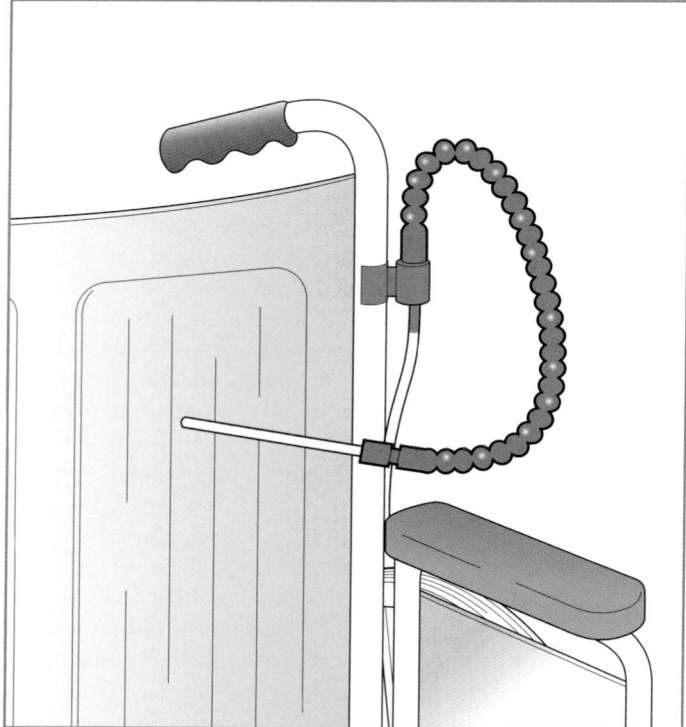

Figure 18-21 Sip and puff input device. (Reproduced by courtesy of the manufacturer.)

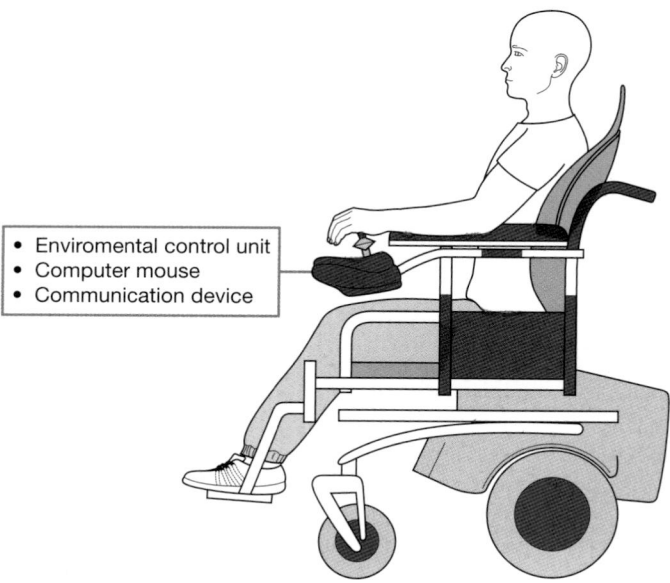

- Enviromental control unit
- Computer mouse
- Communication device

Figure 18-22 An integrated control system.

integrated control include access to several devices with one access site, without requiring assistance. This provides increased opportunities and convenience to function as independently as possible. Often, one switch is used to toggle between the functions of computer access and powered wheelchair control.

While integrated control is beneficial, if the input device is broken, users can lose access to every operation mode. In addition, to use an integrated controller the user must understand modes of operation and must be able to sequence commands. It is cognitively more demanding to use an integrated controller than to use separate input devices for each piece of equipment. The use of one input device (e.g. wheelchair joystick) to operate various equipment (e.g. wheelchair and computer) is often not as straightforward as using separate input devices and might require additional learning capabilities.

Programmability

Performance of a power wheelchair also depends on how the wheelchair control module has been adjusted. Not all power wheelchairs are programmable; however, programming or fine tuning the wheelchair to meet the needs of the individual can improve control, safety, and general satisfaction. Fast and simple adjustments can be made to set forward, reverse, and turning speeds; acceleration and deceleration; and sensitivity of the joystick. These basic adjustments affect how the wheelchair responds to different commands.

Maximum speed varies significantly among different manufacturers and models. Some power wheelchairs are capable of going two to three times faster than other models. Wheelchairs are usually tuned to higher speeds when they are used outdoors. A slow mode of operation is needed for maneuvering indoors or on to a van lift. Braking or deceleration is another critical adjustment. Too hard a setting can cause patients to be thrown forward when they release the joystick. Too soft a setting can cause the wheelchair to coast, and not stop in time to avoid an obstacle. Sudden braking by pulling back on the joystick, or accidentally turning the wheelchair off, can cause a patient to be thrown from the chair. Sensitivity of an input device also needs to be finely tuned. For example, adjusting the joystick throw for wheelchair users with limited arm movement allows them to have access to full control with smaller motion of their arms. For users with static hand tremors, the joystick threshold should be raised to eliminate unintended motion.

SCOOTERS

A scooter is designed to increase mobility for those who have good arm strength and upper body balance, and only need mobility assistance occasionally. Scooters are also popular with elderly users, and people whose walking abilities are limited by medical problems such as chronic obstructive pulmonary disease or arthritis.

Scooters typically have motors in the back and are steered with a tiller (which looks and acts like the handlebar on a bicycle). This tiller can be tilted forward or back and locked at

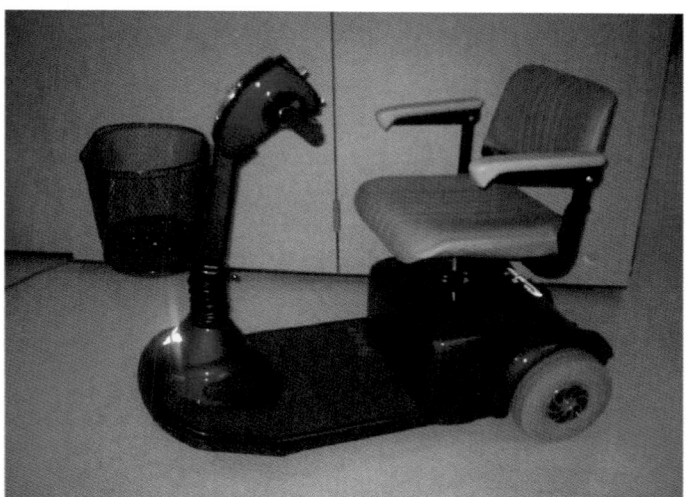

Figure 18-23 Three-wheeled scooter.

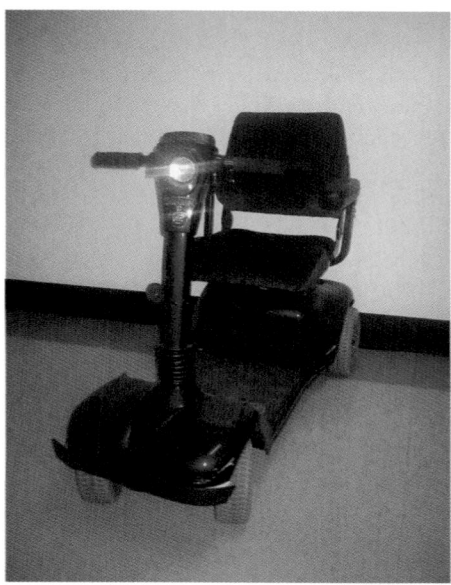

Figure 18-24 Four-wheeled scooter.

any desired position. Thumb levers are used to drive the scooter, usually pressing with the right thumb to go forward, the left to reverse. Scooters are usually equipped with automatic braking and are not able to coast. Controls have to be pressed and released gently to modulate acceleration and deceleration. Three-wheeled scooters are most common (Fig. 18-23). Four-wheeled scooters can traverse more rugged terrain, but are so large that they are impractical in most indoor settings (Fig. 18-24). Compared with power wheelchairs, many scooters are relatively easy to disassemble for storage in a car or trunk. Scooters can also cost less than a typical power chair.

Scooters usually have a relatively wide turning radius. This means that they require more room and effort to maneuver in closed or tight environments. Scooters also require some level of upper limb strength, dexterity, and range of motion to drive and steer. In addition, they are difficult to sit down in and rise from if the user cannot stand and transfer independently. They lack the capacity to allow modification of seating to accommodate postural deformities, and have limited control options. They cannot accommodate for changes as the user's needs change, and are not recommended for persons with progressive diseases such as multiple sclerosis, muscular dystrophy, and amyotrophic lateral sclerosis.

STAND-UP WHEELCHAIRS

Stand-up wheelchairs have been developed and tested over the past 30 years. The developers and manufacturers have generally been unable to obtain insurance coverage, and as a result few stand-up wheelchairs are available on the market. Stand-up wheelchairs offer a variety of advantages over standard wheelchairs. The fact that a person is able to adopt an almost vertical position has a practical advantage (i.e. reaching into high cupboards) (Fig. 18-25) and psychologic advantage (i.e. interacting with colleagues face to face). Physically, it is also useful for pressure relief and to improve circulation and digestion. It provides weight bearing, which is good for bone density.

Stand-up wheelchairs are more complex than most manual or power wheelchairs. A stand-up wheelchair can either have an electric-powered base or can be manually propelled. All power wheelchairs with a stand-up feature use a separate electric drive system for the stand-up mechanism. Manually powered stand-up wheelchairs use a manual lifting mechanism or an electric-powered lifting mechanism. When in the elevated position, this type of wheelchair has a very high center of gravity and can easily topple over. For this reason, the user of a stand-up wheelchair should never transition into a stand-up position when outdoors or when on cracked, rough, or broken floor indoors. Stand-up wheelchairs are safe only on perfectly flat and smooth flooring, and only if the user is properly strapped to the seat and seat back. People who have not stood for a long time might not have the hip, knee, or ankle range of motion to accommodate standing, and can experience orthostatic hypotension. The stand-up mechanism also adds weight to the wheelchair, making it more difficult to lift and transport.

STAIR-CLIMBING WHEELCHAIRS

Stairs present a formidable obstacle to wheelchair users. Climbing a set of stairs presents two central issues. First, there is the actual climbing or negotiating of each single step. Second, there must be stability for the overall mechanism while on the stairs. Stair-climbing mobility devices are currently rated by the US Food and Drug Administration as 'class 3' high-risk devices, defined as 'life-sustaining or life-supporting, implanted in the body, or present an unreasonable risk of illness or injury'.[30] The provision of acceptable stability at all times for a stair-climbing mobility device is essential for safety during stair climbing.

Stair-climbing wheelchairs come in two basic types: the articulated wheel clusters and track-based mechanisms. The Independence 3000 IBOT Transporter is a powered, multifunctional, wheeled mobility system that features a two-wheel cluster design and can climb stairs.[9] Stair climbing is achieved by controlling the cluster rotation on the basis of the position of the center of gravity. The device strives to keep the system center of gravity above the ground-contacting wheels and between the front and rear wheels at all times, regardless of disturbances and forces operating on the system. Users can initiate the function on their own and maintain stability by holding the stair handrails, or assistants can control the rate of climbing through the assist handle. Besides stair climbing, the system performs well in other functional modes, including balancing on two wheels for an elevated seat height (Fig. 18-26) and climbing or

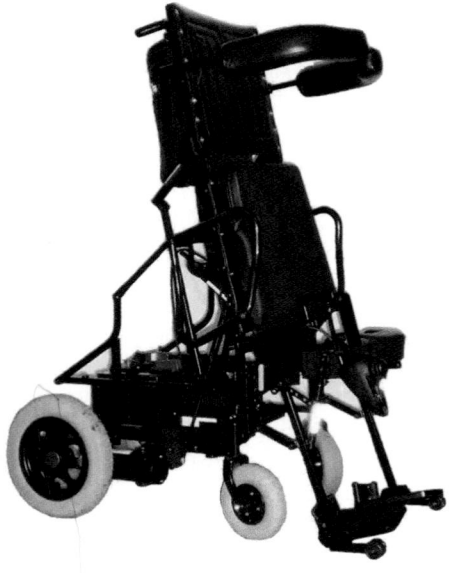

Figure 18-25 Stand-up wheelchair. (Reproduced by courtesy of the manufacturer.)

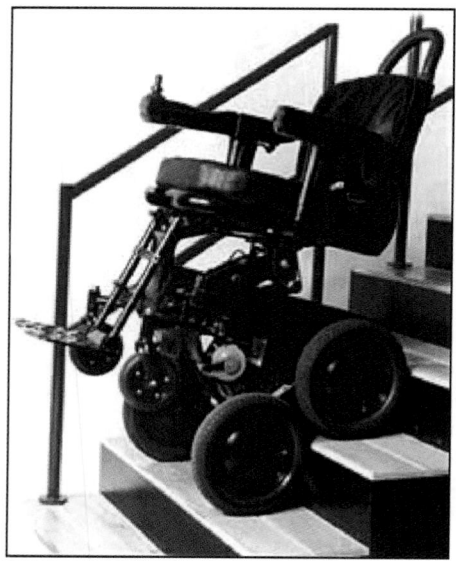

Figure 18-26 The IBOT 3000 transportation system on the stairs. (Reproduced by courtesy of the manufacturer.)

descending up to 6-inch curbs. The major advantage of track-based stair-climbing wheelchairs is simple control and robustness in operation on irregular stairs. A disadvantage is the high pressure exerted on the stair edges.

POWER WHEELCHAIR TRANSPORTATION

The number of people with disabilities who remain in their wheelchairs to travel in vehicles has increased in recent years. Adequate access to transportation is a key issue to wheelchair users. The ability to travel outside the home allows increased opportunities for employment, recreation, and fulfillment of needs.

Wheelchair transportation issues involve how to transport a wheelchair or rider system on to a vehicle, and how to secure the system while the vehicle is moving. The two ways to get wheelchair users on to or out of vehicles are ramps and lift systems.

Ramps

Ramps are the inexpensive alternative to vehicle lifts.[36] They can be portable or mounted inside the vehicle (non-powered or powered), or integrated into the frame of the vehicle. They are usually installed on the side or at the rear of the vehicle, and have either single track or double track with a non-slip surface. With powered ramps, a remote entry button opens the door and extends the ramp. Vehicles having powered ramps (Fig. 18-27) can also have a 'kneeling' feature that lowers the vehicle before extending the ramp to accommodate for ramp slope needs. A ramp should support the size and weight of the user and wheelchair. The user's ability to push or drive up a ramp is usually a concern when choosing between ramps and lifts.

Lifts

For wheelchair users who can drive private vehicles, a vehicle equipped with an automatic lift can eliminate difficult or awkward transfers and problems loading and unloading the wheelchair. Lifts also provide easy transportation for non-folding wheelchairs and heavy powered wheelchairs.

There are many variables and optional features to consider when choosing a vehicle lift. There are several different types, including the platform, rotary, and overhead strap lift.

A platform lift (see Fig. 18-28a) folds out from the van similar to a drawbridge, and requires perpendicular access to load or unload a wheelchair. It also uses minimal storage space within the van, folding upright against the door. When using a pull-in type of parking space, the equivalent of two parking spaces (8–10 ft.) is needed to lower the platform lift and load or unload a wheelchair. This is a problem if other drivers park cars too close to the side of the van. A platform lift can also be installed on the rear door of the van, but this often requires loading or unloading the wheelchair in a traffic lane. Rear door mounting also eliminates the use of space for extra passenger seats.

A rotary lift (see Fig. 18-28b) is mounted to a vertical post and rotates outward from the side door on its vertical axis. It uses access parallel to the van to load or unload a wheelchair. It usually operates within the width of the open front door or approximately 3 ft. When using pull-in parking spaces, operation requires enough room to open the front passenger door completely. If the spaces are narrow or other cars are parked too closely to open the passenger door fully, there will not be enough space to operate the lift. Parallel parking by curbs presents some difficulty for rotary van lifts. The van must either be as close as possible to the curb to lower the lift on the grass or

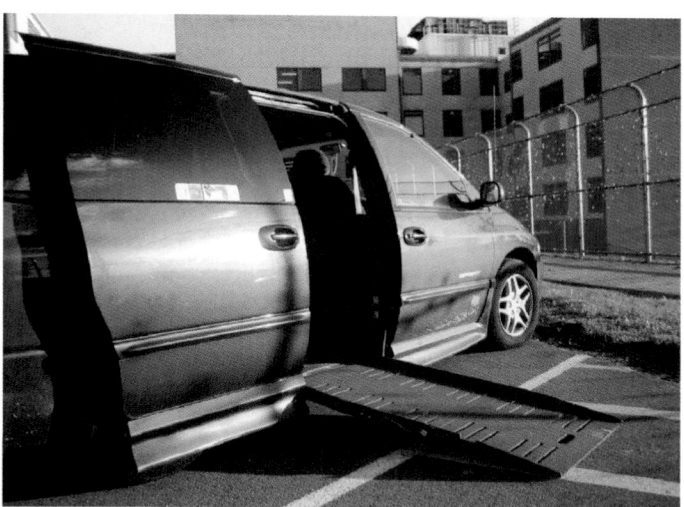

Figure 18-27 Modified minivan with a powered ramp system.

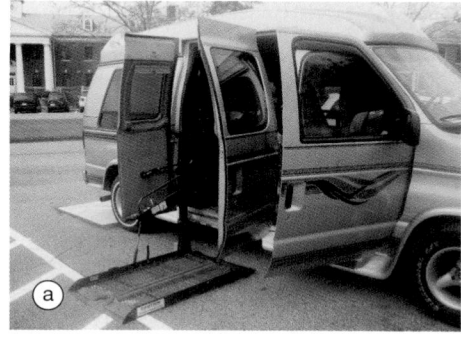
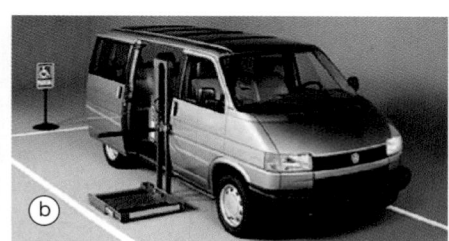
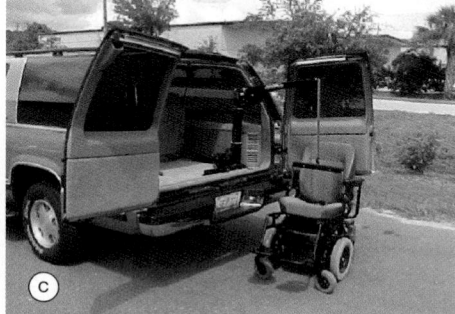

Figure 18-28 Vehicle lift systems: (**a**) platform lift, (**b**) rotary lift, (**c**) overhead strap lift. (Reproduced by courtesy of the manufacturer.)

sidewalk, or far enough away from the curb to lower the lift completely on to the street. If the platform of the lift is partly over the curb, it is impossible to load or unload a wheelchair. The rotary-style lift can be used only with side doors, and some models do not fold for storage and use much more space within the van. This can interfere with rear passenger seating. These lifts might also block normal use of the side door by ambulatory passengers.

An overhead strap lift (see Fig. 18-28c) uses an arm with nylon straps that attach to several points on the wheelchair and hook on to the arm of the lift. The lift has no platform and uses little storage space in the van. The wheelchair is loaded and unloaded perpendicular to the van, but less space is required because there is no platform to lower.

Compatibility is often an issue when selecting a proper lift system, as not all van lifts fit all models of vans. The type of operation, such as electric or hydraulic, can also be an important decision in extreme climates and temperatures.

To secure a wheelchair and its occupant in a moving vehicle, both the occupant restraint and the wheelchair securement must act together as an integral crash protection system. There are essentially two basic approaches to secure wheelchairs that are in common use today: attendant-operated securement systems and mechanical latching or docking devices. The attendant-operated type is the recognized industry standard, dominated by the four strap-type system that attaches to the wheelchair frame. Use of docking securement devices is currently limited mainly to private vehicle applications, due primarily to the need to match wheelchair securement geometry with vehicle anchorage geometry.[32]

Occupant orientation in a vehicle is also important, and usually front facing is most practical and safe. Wherever possible, it is recommended that wheelchair occupants transfer to a vehicle seat during a journey, with the wheelchair securely stored separately in a purpose-made storage area.

Tie-downs and securement

If a wheelchair user is going to remain in a wheelchair while riding in a vehicle, special tie-down or restraint systems for the wheelchair and the occupant must be used for safety. Wheelchairs are not designed to withstand crash-level forces like an automobile seat is, and can be tipped over easily by even a minor collision or sudden braking. A tie-down system with an occupant restraint as well as wheelchair anchorage provides the best protection (see Fig. 18-29a). A typical four-point restraint system has four webbing straps that are secured to the main frame of the chair. The preferred angles for rear wheelchair tie-down are between 30° and 45° to the horizontal plane. The preferred angles for front tie-down are between 40° and 60° to the horizontal plane. The wheelchair tie-down system only stops the chair from tipping or moving; it does not stop the person from being thrown out of the wheelchair in a collision. In addition to the four-point wheelchair restraint system, a pelvis belt is usually used as the occupant restraint. A properly positioned pelvis belt can prevent an occupant from being ejected from the vehicle. Sometimes, a shoulder belt fixed to the side wall of a vehicle can provide an upper torso restraint. It can reduce chest and head excursions in a crash environment. While the four-point, strap-type securement system has been shown to be one of the most effective and versatile methods for securing a wide range of wheelchairs, it is also a system that is difficult and time-consuming to use.

A docking system (see Fig. 18-29b) is another type of wheelchair restraint system. For example, the EZ Lock wheelchair restraint system is a simple and effective docking system to secure an occupied wheelchair in a moving vehicle. The automatic locking mechanism simply requires that the occupant guides the wheelchair over the top of the lock until the interface on the wheelchair is fully engaged. A conveniently located push button switch is used to release the wheelchair from the system. A dock-type restraint system requires matching components, one attached to the wheelchair frame and the other to the vehicle. The advantages are that it is quick and easy to operate, and offers increased user independence. However, it relies on having a location on the wheelchair frame to which one component of the securement system can be attached, and it is two to five times as expensive as belt restraint systems. Docking devices have been shown to work reasonably well for

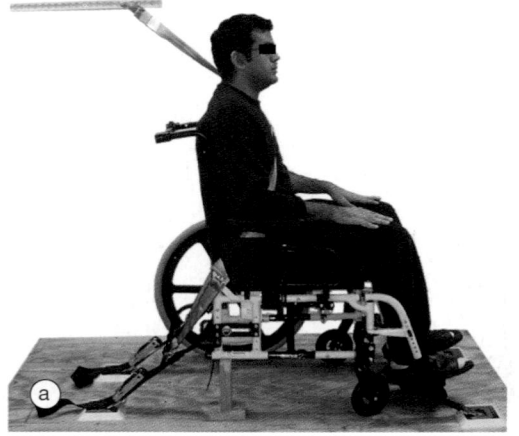

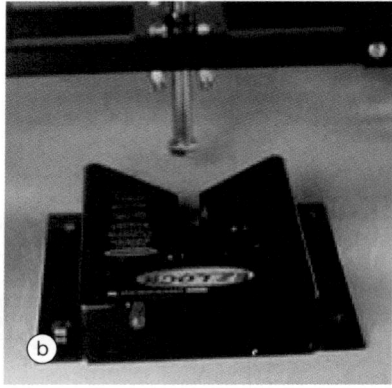

Figure 18-29 Wheelchair tie-downs and securement: (**a**) wheelchair and occupant restraint system, (**b**) wheelchair docking system. (Reproduced by courtesy of the manufacturer.)

private vehicles in which the matching components can be individually configured to the specific wheelchair and vehicle. This has yet to happen in public vehicles that must be able to accept any wheelchair in order to be universally applicable.

WHEELCHAIR STANDARDS

Wheelchair standards were developed to provide a means to objectively compare the durability, strength, stability, and cost-effectiveness of commercial products. Wheelchair standards were developed as a result of consumer demand, increased competition among manufacturers, and pressure by the payers. They comprise test methods developed through years of laboratory validation and arbitration. Wheelchair standards are voluntary in the USA, but the test results are accepted by the US Food and Drug Administration, which approves commercial marketability of the device. Most countries have adopted the International Organization for Standardization (ISO), which acts to continually develop and refine wheelchair standards. The American National Standards Institute (ANSI) and Rehabilitation Engineering and Assistive Technology Society of North America (RESNA) are member organizations of ISO for the USA.

The standards are currently being used by researchers to test and compare wheelchair characteristics, and to develop databases containing wheelchairs that meet the minimum performance standards. However, many wheelchair manufacturers conduct their own evaluations of competitive products and do not follow ANSI–RESNA testing standards. Unfortunately, the manufacturers tend to use the test results for their own benefit, and few choose to disclose the information to the public. Even if this information were available, it would be difficult to compare the test results due to differences in evaluation (non-standardized) procedures. Wheelchair standards provide a solution to the problem by providing a specific protocol and equipment to be used when testing a product. In this manner, the results of the standardized tests, whether performed at manufacturers' test facilities or ANSI–RESNA wheelchair testing laboratories, can be used to accurately compare hundreds of products.

The ANSI–RESNA Wheelchair Standards Committee has produced test procedures that evaluate the strength and stability of the wheelchair. Fatigue testing is one of the procedures used to assess the strength and durability of a wheelchair and its components. This test involves subjecting the wheelchair to a large number of low-level stresses, similar to stresses experienced during daily use of the wheelchair. This is accomplished with two machines: a double-drum tester and a curb drop tester. The double-drum tester consists of two rollers with 12-mm high, 30-mm wide slats attached to each drum to simulate bumps and small obstacles. The wheelchair or scooter is positioned over the rollers, which turn at 1 m/s for 200 000 cycles. If the wheelchair completes this part of the test without sustaining permanent damage, deformation, or failure that significantly affects the operability of the wheelchair, it is then transferred to the curb drop tester for 6666 drops. The curb drop tester lifts the wheelchair 5 cm and allows it to free-fall to a hard surface. This protocol simulates 3–5 years of wheelchair use. Some wheelchairs and scooters are tested until failure as opposed to stopping at the minimum number of cycles or drops. This information is used to calculate the operational cost of the wheelchair by taking the initial purchase price and dividing it by the combined number of cycles or drops until a failure occurred. Other tests include testing the durability and strength of wheelchair components (e.g. armrests, footrests, seat, backrest, wheels, casters, and push rims), as well as static and dynamic stability (how stable the wheelchair or user is on various slopes).

Manual wheelchair performance
Ultralight wheelchairs have been shown to last about 13 times longer than standard wheelchairs, and cost about three and a half times less to operate.[12] Ultralights lasted about five times longer and cost approximately two times less to operate than lightweight wheelchairs.[11] When tested to failure, ultralight wheelchairs had the longest survival rate and fewer catastrophic failures in comparison with standard and lightweight wheelchairs.[19] Premature failures of wheelchairs can place the user at risk for injury.[22,37] Using ultralight wheelchairs that are durable and cost-effective is also safer for individuals. Wheelchair standard test results of ultralight models with suspension elements incorporated into the frame and/or casters show that they perform similarly to lightweight wheelchairs with respect to wheelchair durability and cost-effectiveness.[25]

Power wheelchair performance
Component failures and engineering factors are responsible for 40–60% of the injuries to power wheelchair users.[20,22] Wheelchair standards test results can help with the selection of better engineered power wheelchairs for individuals who need them. Power wheelchairs undergo all the same tests as manual wheelchairs, and also have a series of tests on the power and control systems and batteries. These include testing the battery life and distance traveled on a full charge, electric circuit connections, automatic braking system operation, and climatic effects on the controllers. As with manual wheelchairs, power wheelchairs are separated into classes according to the Centers for Medicare and Medicaid Services (see Table 18-3).

While differences between wheelchair makes and models within the classifications have been reported, overall, class C power wheelchairs outperform the other classes in terms of durability (total equivalent cycles on the double-drum machine).[18] Class A power wheelchairs perform the worst in several areas (poorer durability and reliability, dynamically unstable, and prone to wiring failures).[29] It is important to look at the test results in each area in relation to what is important to the individual. For instance, a wheelchair might outperform others in terms of durability but have poor static and dynamic stability results. If durability is an important factor (most health insurance companies limit the patient to one wheelchair per 5 years), the user might choose to sacrifice the wheelchair's

Table 18-3 Three classifications of power wheelchairs evaluated using wheelchair test standards

Class	Description
A	Conventional power wheelchair, low-cost power wheelchair, basic seating, non-programmable
B	Indoor or outdoor power wheelchair with a programmable controller for adjusting the wheelchair's acceleration, deceleration, turning speed, braking, and tremor dampening according to the individual's function and needs
C	Heavy-duty power wheelchair with 'specialized' features for individuals who weigh over 250 lbs, need seat functions (e.g. tilt, recline, elevation), are active outdoors, or need a ventilator tray

performance concerning stability. Stability for certain individuals can be a more important factor than durability if the patient has a high risk for falling from the wheelchair or frequently traverses up or down steep ramps. Power wheelchairs perform similar to ultralight wheelchairs in terms of their durability.[18] If the power wheelchairs experienced failures during testing, this typically did not interfere with the wheelchair's operability during the required number of cycles on fatigue test machines. In contrast, manual wheelchair failure can affect the user's operation or safety, including broken casters, cracked seat and frame, and other difficult to repair faults. In regard to value, power wheelchairs are more costly than ultralight and lightweight manual wheelchairs. They are, however, more economical than standard wheelchairs, considering how long they last, number of repairs, cost of repairs, and initial cost of the device. Very little test data have been reported on scooter performance. Three-wheel scooters are reportedly less stable than power and manual wheelchairs in the lateral direction.[31]

SEATING AND POSITIONING

Proper seating and positioning are a medical necessity and essential to daily living. Almost any disability that requires the use of a wheelchair for mobility imposes seating and positioning needs. A seating system should assure a comfortable, healthy, and functional sitting posture for work, study, and leisure. Disability can significantly affect the integrity or stability of the muscle–skeletal system, putting the individual at risk for a number of secondary injuries. Failure to provide adequate seating can cause serious secondary injuries, which can require hospitalization or surgery to correct.

In general, commercial off the shelf seating and positioning components are the simplest but tend to have generic sizes and contours. They work well for people with less complex needs and with little to no postural deformities. Other seating systems are more modular, and components including trunk lateral supports and pelvic obliquity pads can be added to accommodate

mild to moderate fixed and semiflexible postural deformities. Custom-contoured seating systems are available, and are based on negative molds of the body's seated surfaces taken through a variety of methods including a seating simulator. The molds are then utilized to custom-carve the seat and back support. This process is more involved and requires clinicians, engineers, and suppliers with specific expertise in this area. Positioning systems, such as tilt and recline, are useful for handling complex seating needs and pressure distribution management. The following sections outline the commercial seating and positioning technologies available and their indications.

Seat cushions
Table 18-4 provides an overview of the types of cushions that are commercially available. Commercial cushions comprise foam, air, gel, or a combination of these materials. If pressure sores remain a problem with these cushions, more aggressive measures must be taken. Alternating pressure cushions are one alternative. These products have a small, battery-powered air compressor and an embedded microprocessor chip that directs the compressed air, alternately inflating multiple air bladders and providing rolling pressure reduction at variable time intervals. Tilt in space and/or recline can also be used to redistribute weight for more effective pressure relief.

Back cushions
A well-chosen back cushion should meet several criteria.

- For folding chairs, the backrest must be easily removable from the frame with hand-operated fasteners or be collapsible.
- The backrest must be the proper width and contour to support the back for extended activities without discomfort.
- For manual wheelchairs, the backrest must not impose any unnecessary weight burden.
- Backrest height is a crucial feature, and should be just high enough to maintain trunk stability. Unneeded extra height adds weight, blocks the ability to look over the shoulder during backing, and increases the perception of medical frailty.

Table 18-2 reviews various types of back support.

Custom-molded seating systems
Certain disabilities resulting in complex and fixed orthopedic deformities and/or conditions (e.g. spasticity, high tone) might need to be supported with a custom-fabricated or custom-fitted seating system. The approach to custom molding seating was borrowed from the prosthetics industry, where molds are obtained from the residual limb to create a socket that is custom-fitted to the patient. This process involves taking a plaster impression of the patient and making a positive model. This can then be sculpted and covered with foam and fiberglass to create the final seating system. After hardening, the 'shell' is pulled off the positive model and mounted on a manual or power base wheelchair.

Table 18-4 Seat cushions

Cushion type	Image	Application	Benefits	Limitations
Plain rectangular foam		Low-risk patients	Inexpensive	No pressure relief regions, typically wears out in 6 months to a year, low maintenance
Contoured foam with skin		Provides cutaway regions to relieve pressure on bony prominences	Reduces risk of pressure ulcers, less expensive than custom-made cushion	Application limited to individuals without asymmetries, cushion has limited life expectancy
Carve and assemble foam		For patient with asymmetries needing custom cutouts	Low-cost method of custom fabrication, lightweight	Custom-fitted, hard to replicate
Contour-molded with gel-filled inserts		Higher risk patients prone to ulcers	Semiliquid gel will mold to body contours	Heavier than regular foam cushions, uncomfortable when cold
Air cushion with insert padding		For patients with asymmetries; the air-filled tetrahedron 'balloons' can be nested together to build shape	Lightweight, personalized fit; no special tools required	Moderate cost, lower life expectancy, customization harder to replicate
Matrix of air-filled elastic capsules		High-risk patents who cannot maintain skin integrity with foam products	Improved pressure relief; bladders can be tied off to create pressure relief regions	More expensive than foam cushion, loss of trunk stability, bladders can be punctured, high maintenance
Alternating air cell inflation		Very high-risk patients with intractable ulcers	Battery-powered air compressor sequentially inflates and deflates cells	Cost >$2000, requires charging, electronics add complexity

A newer system known as the bead seat is a faster and cleaner method of fabrication. For the fitting, the consumer sits on a large rubber 'balloon' filled with tiny foam pellets similar to a bean bag chair. The therapist can freely push and shape the pellets or 'beads' around the consumer through the rubber balloon skin to obtain a comfortable, close-fitting contour. When the molding is completed, a vacuum pump is used to draw the balloon tightly against the foam pellets. This locks the shape and captures the contour of the consumer's body. Often, the patient sits on the bead seat for a while to see if any discomfort develops. The vacuum can be released and the beads repositioned several times if needed. When the seat is perfected, an adhesive is drawn between the beads with a vacuum pump, making the shape permanent. This lightweight seat is finished with waterproof upholstery.

Laterals

Laterals are frame-mounted pads used to stabilize the trunk and accommodate or correct asymmetric deformity. Fitting laterals requires good communication skills with the client and knowledge of how gravity and other forces act on the trunk. Laterals that encircle the trunk should be equipped with mechanical releases so that they pivot out of the way during transfers. Laterals should be firm enough to provide trunk control but should not cause undue pressure or tissue compression.

Armrests and troughs

Standard wheelchairs have narrow armrests covered with fairly firm upholstery. The armrests on standard wheelchairs are integrated with the side frames and cannot be adjusted or removed. A wheelchair for long-term use should provide height-adjustable armrests and the ability to remove them for side transfers. Armrests can be ordered with conventional mounting hardware (Fig. 18-30a) or 'space-saving' hardware (Fig. 18-30b), which reduces the overall wheelchair width. Users of ultralight wheelchairs often choose not to have armrests in order to improve access to the push rims for propulsion. Another option found on high-strength or ultralight wheelchairs are tubular armrests that pivot at the rear. These are lightweight and easy to swivel out of the way for desk access and transfers. Individuals using manual and power wheelchairs who need access to desks can order desk-style armrests, which are a few inches shorter in the front section to fit under a table or desk. Arm troughs are available for individuals who cannot lift or self-stabilize the arm. They are available molded out of polyurethane foam, with a water-resistant 'skin' or vinyl cover. These can be lined with natural or artificial fleece for additional comfort. The trough contains a hollow cavity that captures the forearm in a level position, and protects the arm from drifting into the wheels or being sideswiped by walls. Arm troughs can also improve joystick control by eliminating the need to elevate the arm against gravity while grasping the handle.

Footrests, leg rests, and footplates

Also referred to collectively as front rigging, these components provide support for the legs and feet. If an individual has remaining leg function that can be used to assist the arms in propulsion, the front riggings might need to be removed on one or both sides. For the majority of wheelchairs, the front rigging must be fully and quickly detachable to facilitate transfers and transportability.

Footrests have length adjustments and sometimes angular adjustments. These allow fitting the footrests to the individual with comfortable support. Individuals with impaired lower limb circulation and those having a powered recliner often use powered elevating leg rests with calf supports. It is important to consider the tightness of hamstring muscles when evaluating for foot leg rest type. Overextending the legs in this case can lead to sacral sitting. Table 18-5 shows examples of various types of front rigging.

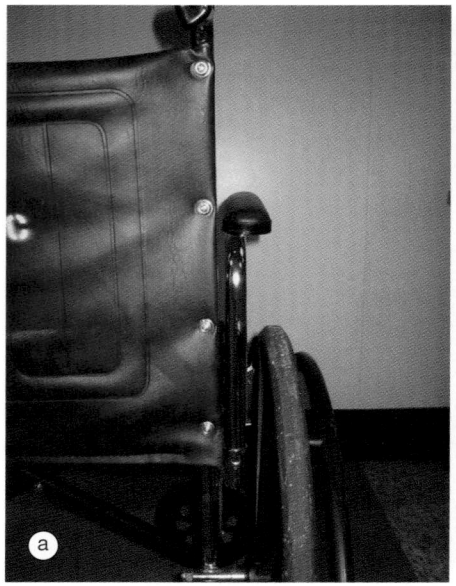
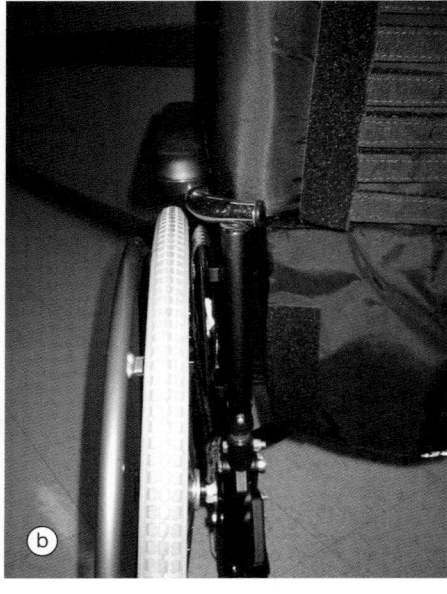

Figure 18-30 (**a**) Traditional armrest attachment and (**b**) space-saver armrest attachment.

Table 18-5 Front riggings

Description	Image	Application	Benefits	Limitations
Fixed frame integrated		Used on ultralights and sport frame chairs	Lightweight, no detachable parts	Limited to no adjustability, minimal foot stabilization provided
Swing away tubular footrests with folding footplates and heel loops		Standard hardware on most manual used wheelchairs, tube lengths can be adjusted	Easy removal for transfers, footplates typically fold, convenient for travel	Additional weight, no footplate angle adjustments, fixed angle tubing
Higher adjustability footrests and calf supports		Elevating footrest provides leg and footplate angle adjustability	Better foot support for individuals with lower limb abnormalities, permits leg elevation for comfort	More expensive, more weight and complexity
Power-elevating leg rests		Accessory for power chairs, provides appropriate leg support for power tilt and recline users	Allows for independent positioning through joystick or other input method, typically removable or swing away	Extra cost; additional complexities of motor drive, and requires power supply cable
Flip-up, flip-down footplate for power chairs		Unimpaired lower extremity posture	Less stigmatizing, easier to operate, improved driving clearances	Transfers may be more difficult

Headrests

Individuals with unstable neck posture or with tilt and recline seat function benefit from a headrest. Several factors should be considered when choosing a headrest.

- It adds additional weight and can restrict rear vision.
- It increases the perception of medical frailty and disability.

- It must be well anchored and offer accurate positioning. A headrest mounted on a flexible surface offers little benefit.
- Headrests sometimes form the foundation for a 'head array', which is a driving control system for individuals who cannot use joysticks.

Seat belts

Seat belts are typically in the form of a lap belt with a latch similar to those found in motor vehicles. They can help keep the buttocks back in the seat and keep the individual from sliding forward. A seat belt or postural strap, if improperly used, can cause choking. Although many wheelchair users choose not to wear a seat belt, it can help prevent serious wheelchair-related injuries.[15]

Postural straps, harnesses, and belts

These items fit around the torso, and are sometimes used by persons with poor trunk control and balance to keep the trunk in a more upright position in the wheelchair for performing ADL. Different styles are available based on the person's needs and preferences. Postural straps, harnesses, and belts should not be used as a safety restraint.

SEAT FUNCTIONS: TILT, RECLINE, AND ELEVATION

Pressure ulcers are a significant health risk for individuals who use wheelchairs, especially those with loss of sensation. The five vulnerable areas for patients in wheelchairs are the coccyx, ischial tuberosities, and greater trochanters. Other locations include areas around the knees and torso, in which ulcers occur in ill-fit seating systems. Regular pressure relief through redistribution of body mass reduces the risk of pressure ulcers. If the individual has upper limb weakness or pain that limits independent weight relief (e.g. 'push up' or leaning to the side or forward), a wheelchair equipped with tilt and/or recline might be needed. Table 18-6 provides an overview of the seating configurations possible with tilt and recline.

Tilt

This is also called tilt in space, and refers to rotating the person's entire body, the seat base, and back and front rigging as a single unit in the sagittal plane. The traditional rocking chair provides an example of the tilt in space maneuver. Both manual and power wheelchairs can be ordered with a tilt in space feature. Tilt provides weight relief for the sitting surface by redistributing the effects of gravity away from the buttocks and on to the back. Tilt can also provide a position of rest and relaxation. A wheelchair that tilts is less stressful to the body than a reclining wheelchair, because shear forces to the skin are almost negligible.

Recline

Recline refers to a means of increasing the angle between the seat base and back, typically between 90 and 180°. Because the hinge between the chair seat and back and the natural folding of the human frame do not match completely, reclining forces some parts of the consumer's body to slide as well. This is a risk factor for skin injury in some individuals. Many modern power chairs have special linkages or mechanical compensation to minimize skin shear during recline. Recline is less frequently prescribed for this reason, but is often required for self-catheterization.

Seat elevation

Power-elevating seats can be ordered to improve the wheelchair user's ability to reach. These seats provide 6–9 inches of additional height. A seat elevator can also make transfers easier, because the wheelchair seat can be adjusted to the same height as the target surface. A seat elevator adds additional weight to the wheelchair, and can increase the seat to floor height in some models.

SEATING AND MOBILITY ASSESSMENT

Optimal wheelchair prescription is most likely to occur when done by an interdisciplinary team that includes the physiatrist as well as occupational and/or physical therapists with specialty training and certification and a good working knowledge of wheelchair seating and mobility needs. A rehabilitation engineer also plays an important role in understanding and assessing the capabilities and application of various technologies. A qualified equipment supplier is another important team member to include early in the process, as such suppliers are well versed in available devices and how they can be applied to solve problems and address needs. The supplier is also the team member who will order, assemble, and deliver the equipment, and consult with the team regarding securing funding. RESNA offers certifications for assistive technology practitioner, assistive technology supplier, and rehabilitation engineering technologist. These certifications are for clinicians and engineers who meet certain qualifications and who pass an examination. RESNA provides a directory of certified professionals (http://www.resna.org).

The end user of the equipment, the family, and/or caregivers are key members of the team. A proper assessment begins with listening to their needs, concerns, and goals for a device. Realistic goal setting fosters discussion about the actual capacity of different types of wheelchair technologies. The following sections describe and discuss the key elements of a wheelchair and seating system assessment, as well as the major variables that need to be considered.

Initial interview

Selecting the most appropriate wheelchair and seating system requires obtaining information about type of disability, prognosis, physical capacity and limitations, involvement in work or related activities, physical and social environment, and means of transportation. Questioning about prior history with wheelchair and seating technology can also provide an indication of what has and has not worked for the person in the past.

Medical variables

It is the role of the physiatrist to assess and share with the team the underlying medical conditions that require prescription of a wheelchair. The prognoses for certain conditions need to be

Table 18-6 Seating configurations possible with tilt in space, recline, and leg rest elevation

Position	Image	Use
Normal driving position		Travel position
Leg elevation		Comfort and improved circulation
Recline		Rest, pressure relief, self-catheterization
Recline plus leg elevation		Rest, pressure relief, self-catheterization
Tilt in space		Rest, comfort, pressure relief
All combined, tilt in space, recline, leg elevation		Rest, comfort, sleep

considered in the prescription decision, especially if a condition is progressive in nature. Equipment should ideally address current and future needs based on the anticipated natural progression of a disease or condition. In addition to age, other factors that need to be factored in include pain, obesity, cardiopulmonary or musculoskeletal problems, and risk for falls. Potential risks and secondary injuries such as pressure sores, postural deformities, or upper extremity repetitive strain injuries associated with the use of equipment need to be assessed and considered.

Physical and functional variables

Therapists and rehabilitation engineers assist the team in assessing the wheelchair user's physical capacities and limitations, especially as they affect mobility. They can also provide an assessment of functional capacity and deficits in basic and instrumental ADL. It is important to know how the wheelchair user performs tasks, where the deficits are, and how wheelchairs and seating systems can compensate for deficits to augment task performance.

Obtaining a basic understanding of the wheelchair user's capacities is an important step in considering equipment needs. This includes a physical–motor assessment of strength, range of motion, coordination, balance, posture, tone, contractures, endurance, sitting posture, cognition, perception, and use of external orthoses. Capacity assessments do not necessarily indicate conclusively whether a person will be able to perform tasks with the equipment. This is best assessed by giving the user an opportunity to try the equipment to determine how they perform. For example, persons with low vision are often capable of using powered mobility devices under appropriate interventions, just as people with low vision are able to ambulate with the use of a navigation cane.

Physical assessments should be followed by observation of performance in ADL that are reported by the person or their family or caregiver as being essential. These include self-care, reaching, accessing various height surfaces, transferring to various surfaces, and functional mobility. Functional mobility should be assessed in the user's home and community. Ambulation should be assessed from the perspective of the surfaces and distances encountered in a routine day, and whether walking or pushing a manual wheelchair is safe and efficient. When considering wheelchair propulsion, stress applied to the upper limbs needs to be considered for manual wheelchair users, because this has been associated with repetitive strain injuries. There is no evidence that upper limb strength correlates with the ability to propel manual wheelchairs, especially when one considers people with cardiac or pulmonary impairments, arthritis, multiple sclerosis, or cerebral palsy.

Obtaining proper seating includes observation of posture in a seat and on a therapy mat table to assess postural alignment and joint range of motion. This can determine what limitations are present and whether they are fixed or flexible. Assessment of pelvic alignment is critical, because the pelvis becomes the base of seating support. An obliquity of the pelvis to one side needs to be accommodated or corrected (if possible) to prevent leaning or development of spinal deformities. Likewise, spinal deformities need to accommodated in the design of the backrest, to allow the user to tolerate sitting. The amount of available hip flexion determines what seat to back angle can be tolerated. The degree of knee extension with the hips flexed is important, because the hamstrings cross both these joints. Tight hamstrings (common in many wheelchair users) significantly affect the positioning of foot supports. It is important that excessive tension not be placed on the hamstrings, because this can be painful and pull the pelvis into a posterior tilt. It is necessary also to respect a person's preference for different seated postures, even if these postures do not appear appropriate. Humans automatically find different alternative positions to sit to be comfortable, functional, and stable.

Following the physical motor assessment, measurements of the body are taken (discussed earlier under *Basic wheelchair dimensions*). The various seating system options can then be considered. As described in the section *Seating and positioning*, there are a wide variety of cushions, back supports, and custom seating systems available.

Environmental variables

It is important to assess both the physical and social environments. Physical accessibility to the home and within the home often has a major impact on the choices and feasibility of wheelchair and seating system options. A thorough assessment and survey of the home is almost always warranted when considering various options. A home assessment is often needed to ensure that the device will be compatible, especially when there are stairs, narrow doorways and hallways, or other tight spaces to be negotiated. The assessment involves taking devices to the home, surveying the environment for accessibility, and having the user get into the device and maneuver it in the spaces used in a typical day. The home assessment should also involve having the wheelchair user complete specific tasks such as transferring to various surfaces, reaching for objects, cooking, pulling up to tables or work surfaces, and completing any other vital activity. The surfaces, terrains, and distances the user will encounter daily also need to be factored into the prescription and decision-making process.

The social environmental assessment includes the roles, interests, responsibilities, and occupation important to the user. The roles include being a parent, spouse, worker, homemaker, or community volunteer. The level of available assistance from others needs to be assessed from the perspective of ability to maintain and troubleshoot complex equipment. The physical capacity and health of caregivers needs to be assessed. Family, social, and cultural values can be barriers or can facilitate a person's inclusion in the community.

Aesthetics

Aesthetics is an increasingly important factor in wheelchair prescription. This is because a wheelchair is such a personal and intimate product (both for children and adults). The appearance of the wheelchair is mainly a function of the frame design and materials. For example, titanium metal has a satin, polished finish and maintains a new, fresh look. Some users also choose to decorate the tires or casters. It is important that wheelchairs have as attractive an appearance as possible so that the user is pleased with using it and gains the most positive attention possible from peers and from the community.

Transportation variables

We live in a society that requires access to transportation resources. In the past, the portability of wheelchairs and seating systems was limited to folding frame manual wheelchairs. The modularity of powered mobility devices, including scooters and portable power wheelchairs, now permits greater transportability in a car. However, the feasibility of assembling and disassembling equipment by the user or caregiver needs to be carefully assessed. The portable design can compromise durability as well as the capabilities of the device to negotiate uneven and soft surfaces. If transporting the wheelchair and seating system is an essential goal, the person who will be stowing the device should get an opportunity to try it prior to the final prescription being written.

If wheelchair users plan to be transported by an accessible vehicle such as a van with a lift or ramp, they should have a trial at driving the device into the vehicle, maneuvering it into an appropriate position for securement or transfer to another seat, and then exiting the vehicle. It is critical to make certain that the wheelchair and the vehicle have the appropriate attachment points to ensure optimal safety during transportation.

SEATING PRINCIPLES

What is traditionally known to be an ideal sitting position (knees at 90°, hips at 90°, and elbows at 90°) might not be functional or comfortable for many users. It might even be impossible for some, due to skeletal deformity or physical limitation. Proper positioning of the pelvis and trunk provides a stable base for the upper limbs. Without this base of support, the arms might be at risk for injury from the extra work necessary to compensate for instability. The head and neck will also not be aligned with the spine. The pelvis should be stabilized on a cushion that provides postural support as well as pressure distribution. The cushion should be mounted on to a hard surface that maintains its position, as opposed to placing it directly on to a sling upholstery seat. Solid seat inserts (thin wood boards) are often inserted into the cushion cover to provide a solid base for sitting. For flexible deformities, the pelvis should sit in as neutral a position as possible, with the trunk having normal lumbar and cervical lordosis. The seating system needs to accommodate a pelvis and trunk in positions other than neutral. Proper positioning support of the head and neck facilitates breathing and swallowing, and might prevent muscle pain due to strained neck muscles. Tilt and recline systems should always be equipped with a headrest to support the head when adjusting the seat orientation and back angles. Additional considerations include the items explained below.

Loss of sensation
When unimpaired persons sit on hard or irregular surfaces, they rapidly feel discomfort and alter their position to relieve the pressure or get up and stretch. If sensation is impaired, the patient can be unaware that a particular contact area is being injured. An inadequate pressure-relieving seating system or technique ultimately leads to ulcer formation.

Paralysis and paresis
Paralysis and paresis prevent an individual from easily changing position and limit the increase in circulation normally stimulated by movement. Paralysis destabilizes body segments (trunk, legs, arms, and head). Unless these segments are supported and protected, they can collapse to a 'gravity position'. This might lead to increased pressures on bony prominences, joint subluxations, and other secondary skeletal and joint deformities. Paralysis and paresis can also lead to entanglement of the limbs in the wheelchair if they are not properly supported.

Contractures
Contractures are best supported by adjustable hardware, such as adjustable-angle leg rests to support knee flexion contractures, and seating systems that recline to open up the seat to back angle for those with hip extension contractures.

Spasticity and high tone
Persons with spasticity and high tone usually require very aggressive and sturdy seating systems. It is not uncommon for the forces generated during extensor thrusts over time to damage the seat back. It is possible to manage spasticity and high tone in a seating system using custom-contoured seating systems. These provide total contact support, as well as dynamic seating components such as back support attachments that 'give' and bounce back into place during and after an extensor thrust.

PRESSURE MAPPING AS AN ASSESSMENT TOOL

A pressure-mapping device is often used to supplement clinical observations and impressions. This is a thin mat with pressure sensors that can be placed over a surface where the person sits to determine interface pressures. The mat is connected to a computer that produces the topography of pressure, which can then be displayed on a monitor (Fig. 18-31). This can be helpful in comparing the pressure-relieving qualities of various cushions, or to verify the effectiveness of a custom-molded system. Pressure mapping alone should not be the sole determinant for selecting a specific cushion, because there are performance trade-offs with different designs and materials. Other factors need to weigh in the decision, especially user preference. For example, fluid- or air-filled cushions can provide optimal pressure distribution, but might be difficult to slide across for transfers, give the user a sense of instability, or require significant maintenance. Pressure mapping can also serve as a biofeedback method to show the wheelchair user effective weight-shifting techniques.

MANUAL WHEELCHAIR VERSUS POWER WHEELCHAIR DEBATE

For some people who have been long-term users of manual wheelchairs, there comes a point when there is a need to transition to powered mobility because of upper limb repetitive strain injuries or the onset of comorbidities such as cardiopulmonary conditions. The same can occur with people who have progressive conditions. This can be a very difficult situation from both a psychologic and a feasibility perspective. It can be difficult for a person with an existing impairment to emotionally deal with the onset of new impairments later in life. People with static disabilities (such as spinal cord injury) experience the same conditions associated with aging as those of able-bodied people. Wheelchair users typically find these aging changes to be more debilitating, because they had decreased functional capacity

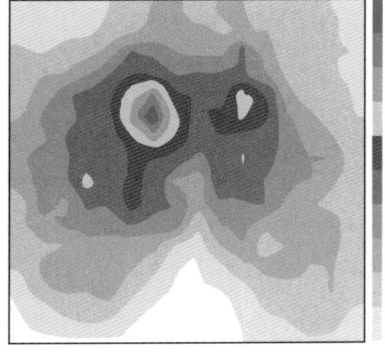
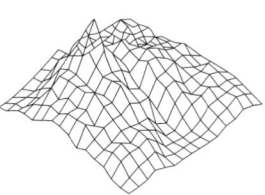

a

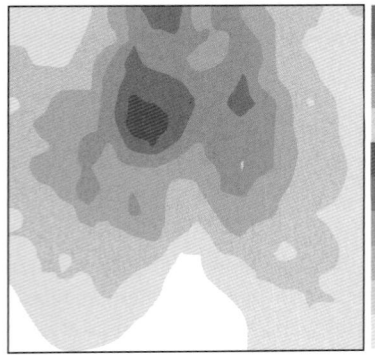
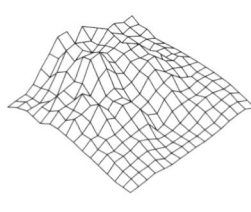

b

Figure 18-31 Pressure mapping of the wheelchair seat–buttocks interface. (**a**) The backrest was in an upright position. (**b**) The backrest was reclined 24°. Areas of high pressure are denoted in yellow, orange, and red. Areas of low pressure are denoted in gray, blue, and green.

already. Some people with progressive conditions have a tendency to 'fight' the disease, and view having to use a wheelchair as giving into the disease. They might use a manual wheelchair out of necessity, but refuse to go on to a powered chair as they feel it represents giving in to the disease process.

The feasibility of transitioning from a manual wheelchair to powered mobility is often a significant issue. Manual wheelchair users typically adapt their environment and daily routine around a manual wheelchair. This might include the type of vehicle they use, home and work site accessibility, transfer methods, or popping wheelies to negotiate curbs. The use of a powered mobility device often requires a significant change in the way ADL are performed, as well as the need to learn new skills. Other changes include procuring alternative transportation resources, such as using a ramp-equipped van or accessible public transportation, and modifying the home or relocating to a completely barrier-free living arrangement. Clinicians need to recognize these issues and address them appropriately on a case by case basis.

REIMBURSEMENT

Wheelchairs and seating systems are reimbursed in a variety of ways, with health insurance the most common means of funding. The Medicare program is the largest payer of this equipment, and sets the standard for coverage policies. These policies are currently undergoing a significant overhaul, due to increased utilization of these benefits associated with an aging population.

Wheelchairs and seating systems are considered a durable medical equipment benefit. Durable medical equipment is defined within the Social Security Act of 1965, section 1862(a)(1)(A), as a device that can withstand repeated use, is primarily used to serve a medical purpose, is not useful to a person in the absence of illness or injury, and is appropriate for use in the home. In order for a wheelchair or seating system to be covered under health insurance, it must be well documented as being medically necessary. Medical necessity is defined by the Social Security Act as a service or intervention that is reasonable and necessary for the diagnosis or treatment of illness or injury, or improves the functioning of a malformed body member. Definitions of medical necessity vary across payers and state Medicaid programs, but tend to follow this basic theme. It is important for the physiatrist and therapists to document well the need for wheelchair and seating system interventions in clinic notes and in letters of medical necessity. A few basic strategies to follow in the letters of medical necessity are to describe in detail the person's medical condition and contextual situation, why the equipment is needed to compensate for functional deficits or address medical needs, and why lower cost alternatives are not appropriate. Describing the potential ramifications if the wheelchair equipment is not funded, such as loss of further function and the onset of secondary medical problems, is important and helps to justify funding by third-party payers.

FITTING AND DELIVERY

When the wheelchair is delivered and is ready for use by the patient, the fitting should ideally take place in the presence of key team members. At a minimum, this should include the therapist and supplier. During the fitting session, the goals established during the initial assessment should be reviewed, because a significant amount of time might have lapsed. The person using the equipment needs to feel comfortable, knowing adjustments can be made to optimize fit and address functional needs. The equipment will often need to go back to the supplier's shop for alteration prior to final fit. During the final fitting, the person and any caregivers need to be fully trained in and demonstrate the proper use and maintenance of the equipment. The person should be advised of parties to contact in case of equipment failure. Training by a therapist might be necessary to ensure the safe and effective operation of a device. Follow-up appointments should be scheduled on a set basis to ensure the equipment is meeting the person's needs and to identify any need for modification, preventive maintenance, or replacement.

CONSIDERATIONS FOR SELECT POPULATIONS

Pediatric

Children have special mobility needs. Childhood years are formative years in which every child is learning, growing, and acquiring a positive self-image. Early disability impacts multiple spheres of living, including the ability to attend school, interact with peers, and access learning materials.

In terms of wheelchair and seating selection, children need the following.

- Wheeled mobility that can be adjusted to accommodate growth.
- Mobility that can be managed by parents, i.e. wheelchairs that can be readily disassembled for car transport.
- Special technology to complete school assignments, such as augmentative communication aids, alternative computer access, and sensory aids. These devices are often mounted on the wheelchair so they can travel with the child to and from school.
- Wheelchairs that facilitate interaction with other children. One example is a power wheelchair that lowers the seating surface to the floor, so that the child is at eye level with peers and can participate in exploratory activities that unimpaired children carry out while seated on the floor (Fig. 18-32).

Progressive disorders

Progressive disorders such as amyotrophic lateral sclerosis, multiple sclerosis, or Parkinson disease require special consideration when prescribing a wheelchair and seating system. While many individuals with these disorders begin with manual wheelchairs, they might have trouble at times due to fatigue, tremors, weakness, etc. Power wheelchairs with programmable functions are good choices, because they can be tailored to the individual's driving abilities as the disease progresses, and can accept multiple inputs (e.g. joystick, head array, sip and puff). From a seating perspective, these patients will need periodic seating updates as the disease progresses. Power base or power wheelchairs allow for interchanging seating and positioning hardware, or adding a tilt and/or recline system. It is important to think about power wheelchair use early and the funding source. For example, because of the type of funding they have, some patients wait 6 months before receiving their wheelchairs.

Vision impairments

Individuals with poor vision have an additional challenge when using wheeled mobility. When individuals with poor vision walk, they typically use the upper extremities haptically to scan for hazards, either with hands outstretched or with a long cane. When using wheeled mobility, the arms can no longer explore ahead of the body and are partly occupied either with propulsion or using a joystick to drive. Driving safety with wheeled mobility has to be assessed on a case by case basis.

Weight disparity

Individuals with chronic disabilities who use wheeled mobility are at risk for weight problems. Individuals with cerebral palsy who have athetoid movements and difficulty with mastication, for example, can end up chronically underweight. Reduced tissue thickness across bony prominences increases the risk of pressure sores. On the other end of the weight disparity spectrum, the sedentary lifestyle of wheeled mobility can result in poor fitness and obesity. In addition to the regular health risks, obesity has an impact on wheeled mobility by the following.

- Requiring a wider, heavier wheelchair. This can impose navigation limits on access through narrow doorways and small rooms.

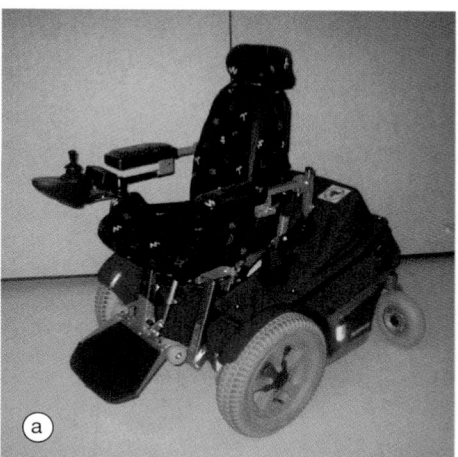 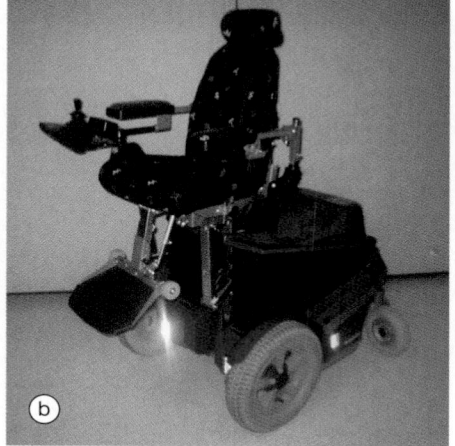 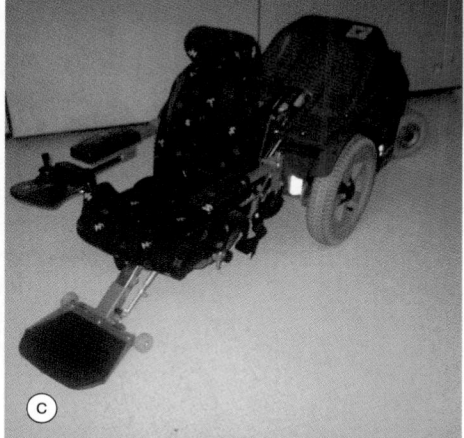

Figure 18-32 Pediatric power wheelchair with a seat that can be raised or lowered to the floor for play.

- Interfering with propulsion of manual wheelchairs, requiring more force to overcome the increased rolling resistance.
- Makes transfers, pressure relief, and personal care substantially more difficult, leading to increased risk of skin breakdown and pressure ulcers.
- It has been known to delay third-party funding, as some funding sources believe obesity to be a preventable complication.

Older adults

Aging can be thought of as a collection of progressive disorders that can complicate wheelchair prescription and seating. Affects of aging vary widely, but pertinent problems include the following.

- Osteoporosis, stress fractures, and arthritis. These can increase pain, limit range of motion, and reduce sitting tolerance.
- Impaired circulation due to coronary artery disease and diabetes, which can increase the risk of pressure ulcers.
- Sedentary lifestyle, with weight gain and reduced muscular strength.
- Cognitive impairments and depression.
- If an older patient relies on a partner for personal care, aging of the partner can limit this assistance and result in a caregiver injury during a strenuous procedure such as a transfer.
- Older patients are often on fixed incomes and might not be able to absorb the cost of chair accessories not covered by Medicare.

In general, the older patient is more frail and requires extra diligence by the clinician. The partner should be included in the clinical decision making, and it is often necessary to have a home assessment made to determine additional hazards or accommodations required.

WHEELCHAIR-MOUNTED ACCESSORIES: ASSISTIVE TECHNOLOGY

In addition to mobility, wheelchairs serve as a platform for assistive technology devices for many daily activities. They are often equipped with lap trays, tote bags, cell phones, portable entertainment devices, and even cup holders. In addition to these common accessories, wheelchairs frequently carry advanced electronic assistive technology to enhance communication or provide medical care. Categories of communication devices include environmental control systems, computer access products, and electronic voice output communication aids. Medical assistive technology can include auxiliary oxygen and ventilators.

Environmental control systems

Due to the postural restrictions imposed by wheelchairs, consumers often have difficulty reaching standard doorknobs, switches, appliances, and home entertainment systems, even if they have unimpaired arm function. Seat elevators and stand-up wheelchairs are one solution, but are costly and not always funded by third-party payers. One way to gain increased access to items in the environment is to use wireless environmental control units (ECUs). These units operate by transmitting ultrasound, radiofrequency, or infrared signals to receivers that are connected to the appliance or device to be controlled. Examples of devices include door openers, and controls for lights, television, radio, fan, and thermostat. Some power wheelchairs are equipped with an ECU mode so that the individual can operate items directly from their wheelchair see Ch. 24).

Electronic voice communication aids

Voice output communication aids are computer-based devices that provide an electronic voice for individuals unable to speak. These can be accessed by keypads of various sizes, with optical pointers, or with single-switch scanning strategies. To keep the device in reach, they are typically mounted on a swing-away arm that attaches to the wheelchair frame. The control input method must be positioned so that the user can readily reach it, which can require additional wheelchair-mounting hardware.

SUMMARY

The past decade has seen vast improvements in wheelchair design, fabrication, and innovative seating technologies. What used to be considered 'environmentally inaccessible' (e.g. curbs, rough and uneven terrain, stairs, and high cabinets) is now 'accessible' with the use of advanced wheelchair technology. Successful wheelchair prescription requires current knowledge about the equipment available, the intended application, and the seating and positioning parameters. It also requires an interdisciplinary team to execute a systematic approach to wheelchair assessment. The team should consider the persons' mobility goals; their medical, physical, and functional variables; environments where the device will be used; transportation needs; past experience with wheelchair or seating technology; and reimbursement. Ideally, the individual should try various technologies in the actual environments where the device will be used before making the final decision. Adequate fitting, training, and follow-up are key in ensuring comfort, satisfaction, and a successful match between the individual and mobility device.

REFERENCES

1. Attali X, Pelisse F. Looking back on the evolution of electric wheelchairs. Med Eng Phys 2001; 23:735–743.
2. Axelson PW, Yamada Chesney D, Minkel J, et al. The manual wheelchair training guide. Minden: PAX Press, Beneficial Designs; 1998.
3. Beekman CE, Miller-Porter L, Schoneberger M. Energy cost of propulsion in standard and ultralight wheelchairs in people with spinal cord injuries. Phys Ther 1999; 79:146–158.
4. Boninger ML, Baldwin MA, Cooper RA, et al. Manual wheelchair pushrim biomechanics and axle position. Arch Phys Med Rehabil 2000; 81: 608–613.

5. Boninger ML, Cooper RA, Baldwin MA, et al. Wheelchair pushrim kinetics: body weight and median nerve function. Arch Phys Med Rehabil 1999; 80:910–915.

6. Boninger ML, Souza AL, Cooper RA, et al. Propulsion patterns and pushrim biomechanics in manual wheelchair propulsion. Arch Phys Med Rehabil 2002; 83:718–723.

7. Brienza DM, Angelo J, Henry K. Consumer participation in identifying research and development priorities for power wheelchairs input devices and controllers. Assist Technol 1995; 7:55–62.

8. Brubaker CE. Wheelchair prescription: an analysis of factors that affect mobility and performance. J Rehabil Res Dev 1986; 23:19–26.

9. Cooper RA, Boninger ML, Cooper R, et al. Use of the Independence™ 3000 IBOT™ Transporter at home and in the community. J Spinal Cord Med 2003; 26:79–85.

10. Cooper RA, Fitzgerald SG, Boninger ML, et al. Evaluation of a pushrim-activated, power-assisted wheelchair. Arch Phys Med Rehabil 2001; 82: 702–708.

11. Cooper RA, Gonzalez J, Lawrence B, et al. Performance of selected light-weight wheelchairs on ANSI/RESNA tests. American National Standards Institute–Rehabilitation Engineering and Assistive Technology Society of North America. Arch Phys Med Rehabil 1997; 78:1138–1144.

12. Cooper RA, Robertson RN, Lawrence B, et al. Life-cycle analysis of depot versus rehabilitation manual wheelchairs. J Rehabil Res Dev 1996; 33:45–55.

13. Cooper RA, Widman LM, Jones DK, et al. Force sensing control for electric powered wheelchairs. IEEE Trans Control Syst Technol 2000; 8:112–117.

14. Corfman TA, Cooper RA, Boninger ML, et al. Range of motion and stroke frequency differences between manual wheelchair propulsion and pushrim-activated power-assisted wheelchair propulsion. J Spinal Cord Med 2003; 26:135–140.

15. Corfman TA, Cooper RA, Fitzgerald SG, et al. Tips and falls during electric powered wheelchair driving: effects of seatbelt use, legrests, and driving speed. Arch Phys Med Rehabil 2003; 84:1797–1802.

16. Crane B, Hobson D. No room for discomfort. Rehabil Manage 2003; 16:30–35.

17. Ding D, Cooper RA, Kaminski BA, et al. Integrated control and related technology of assistive devices. Assist Technol 2003; 15:89–97.

18. Fass MV, Cooper RA, Fitzgerald SG, et al. Durability, value, and reliability of selected electric powered wheelchairs. Arch Phys Med Rehabil 2004; 85:805–814.

19. Fitzgerald SG, Cooper RA, Boninger ML, et al. Comparison of fatigue life for 3 types of manual wheelchairs. Arch Phys Med Rehabil 2001: 82(10): 1484–1488.

20. Gaal RP, Rebholtz N, Hotchkiss RD, et al. Wheelchair rider injuries: causes and consequences for wheelchair design and selection [see comments]. J Rehabil Res Dev 1997; 34:58–71.

21. Hughes CJ, Weimar WH, Sheth PN, et al. Biomechanics of wheelchair propulsion as a function of seat position and user-to-chair interface. Arch Phys Med Rehabil 1992; 73:263–269.

22. Kirby RL, Ackroyd-Stolarz SA. Wheelchair safety—adverse reports to the United States Food and Drug Administration. Am J Phys Med Rehabil 1995; 74:308–312.

23. Kirby RL, Ashton BD, Ackroyd-Stolarz SA, et al. Adding loads to occupied wheelchairs: effect on static rear and forward stability. Arch Phys Med Rehabil 1996; 77:183–186.

24. Klein GJ. A wheelchair electric drive designed for the use of quadriplegics. Ottawa: National Research Council of Canada; 1953.

25. Kwarciak AM, Cooper RA, Ammer WA, et al. Fatigue testing of selected suspension manual wheelchairs using ANSI/RESNA standards. Arch Phys Med Rehabil 2005; 86(1):123–129.

26. Kwarciak AM. Performance analysis of suspension manual wheelchairs. Pittsburgh: University of Pittsburgh; 2003.

27. Masse LC, Lamontagne M, O'Riain MD. Biomechanical analysis of wheelchair propulsion for various seating positions. J Rehabil Res Dev 1992; 29:12–28.

28. Mukherjee G, Samanta A. Physiological response to the ambulatory performance of hand-rim and arm-crank propulsion systems. J Rehabil Res Dev 2001; 38:391–399.

29. Pearlman J, Cooper RA, Karnawat J, et al. Economical (K0010) power wheelchairs have poor reliability and important safety problems: an ANSI/RESNA wheelchair standards comparison study. Proceedings of the RESNA 2005 Annual Conference, Atlanta, Georgia, 18–22 June 2004.CD-ROM.

30. Rados C. FDA works to reduce preventable medical device injuries. FDA Consum 2003; 37:29–33.

31. Rentschler AJ, Cooper RA. A comparison of the dynamic and static stability of power wheelchairs versus scooters. Proceedings of the First Joint BMS/EMBS Conference, 13–16 October 1999. CD-ROM.

32. van Roosmalen L, Bertocci GE, Hobson D, et al. Preliminary evaluation of wheelchair occupant restraint system usage in motor vehicles. J Rehabil Res Dev 2002; 39:83–93.

33. Sanderson DJ, Sommer HJ. Kinematic features of wheelchair propulsion. J Biomech 1985; 18:423–429.

34. Shimada SD, Robertson RN, Bonninger ML, et al. Kinematic characterization of wheelchair propulsion. J Rehabil Res Dev 1998; 35:210–218.

35. Sie IH, Waters RL, Adkins RH, et al. Upper extremity pain in the post-rehabilitation spinal cord injured patient. Arch Phys Med Rehabil 1992; 73:44–48.

36. Storr T, Spicer J, Frost P, et al. Design features of portable wheelchair ramps and their implications for curb and vehicle access. J Rehabil Res Dev 2004; 41:443–452.

37. Ummat S, Kirby RL. Nonfatal wheelchair-related accidents reported to the National Electronic Injury Surveillance System. Am J Phys Med Rehabil 1994; 73:163–167.

38. Veeger HEJ, van der Woude LHV, Rozendal RH. Wheelchair propulsion technique at different speeds. Scand J Rehabil Med 1989; 21:197–203.

39. Woods B, Watson N. A short history of powered wheelchairs. Assist Technol 2003; 15:164–180.

40. van der Woude LHV, Veeger DJ, Rozendal RH, et al. Seat height in handrim wheelchair propulsion. J Rehabil Res Dev 1989; 26:31–50.

Chapter

19

Therapeutic Exercise

Robert P. Wilder, Jeffrey Jenkins and Craig Seto

I repeat my advice to take a great deal of exercise on foot. Health is the first requisite after morality.

> Thomas Jefferson, author of the Declaration of American Independence and the Statute of Virginia for Religious Freedom, and Father of the University of Virginia

GENERAL PRINCIPLES

Introduction

Regular physical activity is an important component of a healthy lifestyle. Increases in physical activity and cardiorespiratory fitness have been shown to reduce the risk of death from coronary heart disease as well as from all causes. The primary focus on achieving these health-related goals in the past has been on prescribing exercise to improve cardiorespiratory fitness, body composition, and strength. More recently, the Centers for Disease Control and Prevention (CDC) and the American College of Sports Medicine (ACSM) suggested that the focus be broadened to address the needs of more sedentary individuals, especially those who cannot or will not engage in structured exercise programs. There is increasing evidence showing that regular participation in moderate-intensity physical activity is associated with health benefits, even when aerobic fitness remains unchanged. To reflect this evidence, the CDC and ACSM are now recommending that every US adult accumulate 30 min or more of moderate-intensity physical activity on most, and preferably all, days of the week. Those who follow these recommendations can experience many of the health-related benefits of physical activity, and if they are interested are ready to achieve higher levels of fitness.[35,36,91,108]

Important in prescribing exercise is an understanding of the principles of specificity and periodization. The principle of specificity states that metabolic responses to exercise occur most specifically in those muscle groups being used. Furthermore, the types of adaptation will be reflective of the mode and intensity of exercise. The principle of periodization reflects the importance of incorporating adequate rest to accompany harder training bouts. Overall training programs (macrocycles) are divided into phases (microcycles), each with specific desired effects (i.e. enhancing a particular energy system or sport-specific goal).

This chapter provides a brief overview of the basic fundamentals of exercise physiology, including the metabolic energy systems, and the basic muscle and cardiorespiratory physiology associated with exercise. It will then provide an overview of the exercise prescription according to the current ACSM guidelines, and the fundamentals of exercise programming, including preexercise screening.

Energy systems

A 70-kg human has an energy expenditure at rest of about 1.2 kcal/min, with less than 20% of the resting energy expenditure attributed to skeletal muscle. During intense exercise, however, total energy expenditure can increase 15–25 times above resting values, resulting in a caloric expenditure between 18 and 30 kcal/min. Most of this increase is used to provide energy to the exercising muscles that can increase energy requirements by a factor of 200.[23,87]

The energy used to fuel biologic processes comes from the breakdown of ATP, specifically from the chemical energy stored in the bonds of the last two phosphates of the ATP molecules. When work is performed, the bond between the last two phosphates is broken, producing energy and heat:

$$\text{ATP} \xrightarrow{\text{ATPase}} \text{ADP} + \text{Pi} + \text{energy}.$$

The limited stores of ATP in skeletal muscles can fuel approximately 5–10 s of high-intensity work (Fig. 19-1). ATP must be continuously resynthesized from ADP to allow exercise to continue.[61,96] Muscle fibers contain three metabolic pathways for producing ATP: the creatine phosphate system, rapid glycolysis, and aerobic oxidation.[23,87,91]

Creatine phosphate system

When limited stores of ATP are nearly depleted during high-intensity exercise (5–10 s), the creatine phosphate system transfers a high-energy phosphate from creatine phosphate to rephosphorylate ATP from ADP:

$$\text{ADP} + \text{creatine phosphate} \xrightarrow{\text{creatine kinase}} \text{ATP} + \text{creatine}.$$

Because it involves a single reaction, this system can provide ATP at a very rapid rate. Because there is a limited supply of creatine phosphate in the muscle, however, the amount of ATP that can be produced is also limited.

There is enough creatine phosphate stored in skeletal muscle for approximately 25 s of high-intensity work (Fig. 19-1). The ATP–creatine phosphate system lasts for about 30 s (5 s for the

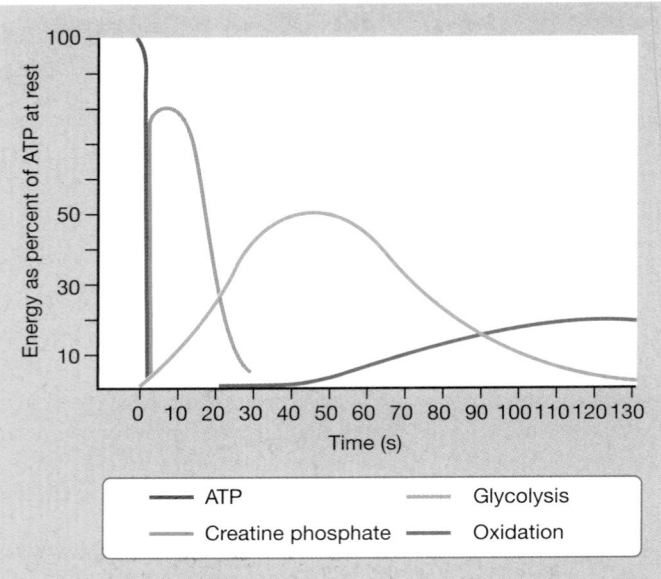

Figure 19-1 Energy sources in relation to duration of contraction. Muscular metabolism available from the various substrates participating in supplying energy during the first 2 min of an attempted maximal contraction. The relative contribution of each substrate at any moment is indicated. The intensity of metabolic activity over the 2-min period is adjusted to the change of the isometric tension produced during a sustained voluntary maximal contraction. (From DeLateur 1982,[22] with permission.)

stored ATP, and 25 s for creatine phosphate). This provides energy for activities such as sprinting and weightlifting. The creatine phosphate system is considered an anaerobic system, because oxygen is not required.[23,87,91]

Rapid glycolysis (lactic acid system)
Glycolysis uses carbohydrate, primarily in the form of muscle glycogen, as a fuel source. When glycolysis is rapid, it is capable of producing only a small amount of ATP without the involvement of oxygen (anaerobically). Lactic acid is also produced as a by-product of this reaction. The accumulation of excessive amounts of lactic acid in muscle tissue is associated with fatigue. The lactic acid system produces enough energy to last approximately 1–2 min before the accumulation of excessive lactic acid produce fatigue (Fig. 19-1). It would fuel activities such as middle-distance sprints (400, 600, and 800-m runs). Although glycolysis is considered an anaerobic pathway, it can readily participate in the aerobic metabolism when oxygen is available, and is considered the first step in the aerobic metabolism of carbohydrate.[23,87,91]

Aerobic oxidation system
The final metabolic pathway for ATP production combines two complex metabolic processes: the Krebs cycle and the electron transport chain. This system resides in the mitochondria. It is capable of using carbohydrates, fat, and small amounts of protein to produce energy (ATP) during exercise, through a process called oxidative phosphorylation. During exercise, this pathway uses oxygen to completely metabolize the carbohydrates to produce energy (ATP), leaving only carbon dioxide and water as by-products. The aerobic oxidation system is complex, and requires 2–3 min to adjust to a change in exercise intensity (Fig. 19-1). It has an almost unlimited ability to regenerate ATP, however, limited only by the amount of fuel and oxygen that is available to the cell. Maximal oxygen consumption, also known as $\dot{V}O_{2max}$, is a measure of the power of the aerobic energy system, and is generally regarded as the best indicator of aerobic fitness.[23,87,91]

All the energy-producing pathways are active during most types of exercise, but different exercise types place greater demands on different pathways. The contribution of the anaerobic pathways (creatine phosphate system and glycolysis) to exercise energy metabolism is inversely related to the duration and intensity of the activity. The shorter and more intense the activity, the greater the contribution of anaerobic energy production, whereas the longer the activity and the lower the intensity, the greater the contribution of aerobic energy production. In general, carbohydrates are used as the primary fuel at the onset of exercise and during high-intensity work. But during prolonged exercise of low to moderate intensity (longer than 30 min), a gradual shift from carbohydrate toward an increasing reliance on fat as a substrate occurs. The greatest amount of fat use occurs at about 60% of maximal aerobic capacity ($\dot{V}O_{2max}$).[23,87,91]

CARDIOVASCULAR EXERCISE
Cardiorespiratory physiology
The cardiorespiratory system consists of the heart, lungs, and blood vessels. The purpose of this system is the delivery of oxygen and nutrients to the cells, as well as the removal of metabolic waste products in order to maintain the internal equilibrium.[61,87,91]

Cardiac function
Heart rate
Normal resting HR is approximately 60–80 beats per minute. HR increases in a linear fashion with the work rate and oxygen uptake during exercise. The magnitude of HR response is related to age, body position, fitness, type of activity, the presence of heart disease, medications, blood volume, and environmental factors such as temperature and humidity. HR during maximal exercise can exceed 200 beats per minute, depending on the person's age and training state. With the onset of dynamic exercise, HR increases in proportion to the relative workload. The maximal HR (HR_{max}) decreases with age, and can be estimated in healthy men and women by using the formula $HR_{max} = 220 - age$. There is considerable variability in this estimation for any fixed age, with a standard deviation of ±10 beats per minute.[61,87,91]

Stroke volume
Stroke volume is the amount of blood ejected from the left ventricle in a single beat. SV is equal to the difference between

end diastolic volume and end systolic volume. Greater diastolic filling (preload) will increase SV. Factors that resist ventricular outflow (after-load) will result in a reduced SV.

Stroke volume is greater in males than in females. At rest in the upright position, it generally ranges from 60 to 100 mL/beat, while maximum SV approximates 100–120 mL/beat. During exercise, SV increases curvilinearly with the work rate until it reaches near maximum at a level equivalent to approximately 50% of aerobic capacity. SV starts to plateau, and further increases in workload do not result in increased SV, primarily due to reduced filling time during diastole.

Stroke volume is also affected by body position, with SV being greater in the supine or prone position and lower in the upright position. Static exercise (weight training) can also cause a slight decrease in SV due to increased intrathoracic pressure.[61,87,91]

Cardiac output

Cardiac output (Q) is the amount of blood pumped by the heart each minute. It is calculated by the formula

$$Q \text{ (L/min)} = HR \text{ (beats/min)} \times SV \text{ (mL/beat)}.$$

Resting cardiac output in both trained and sedentary individuals is approximately 4–5 L/min, but during exercise the maximal cardiac output can reach 20 L/min. Maximal cardiac output in an individual depends on many factors, including age, posture, body size, presence of cardiac disease, and physical conditioning. During dynamic exercise, cardiac output initially increases with increasing exercise intensity by increases in SV and HR. Increases in cardiac output initially beyond 40–50% of $V_{O_{2max}}$, however, are accounted for only by increases in HR.[61,87,91]

Blood flow

At rest, 15–20% of the cardiac output is distributed to the skeletal muscles, with the remainder going to visceral organs, the brain, and the heart. During exercise, 85–90% of the cardiac output is selectively delivered to working muscles and shunted away from the skin and splanchnic vasculature. Myocardial blood flow can increase four to five times with exercise, whereas blood supply to the brain is maintained at resting levels. The difference between the oxygen content of arterial blood and the oxygen content of venous blood is termed the *arteriovenous oxygen difference*. It reflects the oxygen extracted from arterial blood by the tissues. The oxygen extraction at rest is approximately 25%, but at maximal exercise the oxygen extraction can reach 75%.[61,87,91]

Venous return

Venous return is maintained and/or increased during exercise by the following mechanisms:[61,87,91]

- Contracting skeletal muscle acts as a 'pump' against the various structures that surround it, including deep veins, forcing blood back toward the heart.
- Smooth muscle around the venules contracts, causing venoconstriction. This increases the pressure on the venous side, maintaining blood flow toward the heart.

- Diaphragmatic contraction during exercise creates lowered intrathoracic pressure, facilitating blood flow from the abdominal area and lower extremities.

Blood pressure

Blood pressure is the driving force behind blood flow. Systolic blood pressure (SBP) is the maximal force of the blood against the walls of the arteries when cardiac muscle is contracting (systole). Normal resting SBP is <130 mmHg. Diastolic blood pressure (DBP) is the force of the blood against the walls of the arteries when the heart is relaxing (diastole). Normal resting DBP is <85 mmHg.[87]

Systolic blood pressure increases linearly with increasing work intensity, at 8–12 mmHg per metabolic equivalent (MET) (where 1 MET = 3.5 mL of O_2 per kg per min). Maximal values typically reach 190–220 mmHg. Maximal SBP should not be greater than 260 mmHg. DBP remains unchanged or only slightly increases with exercise.[61,87]

Because blood pressure is directly related to cardiac output and peripheral vascular resistance, it provides a non-invasive way to monitor the inotropic performance (pumping capacity) of the heart. Failure of SBP to rise, decreased SBP with increasing work rates, or a significant increase in DBP are all abnormal responses to exercise, and indicate either severe exercise intolerance or underlying cardiovascular disease.[61,87,91]

Postural considerations

In the supine position, gravity has less effect on return of blood to the heart, so the SBP is lower. When the body is upright, gravity works against the return of blood to the heart, so SBP increases. DBP does not change significantly with body position in healthy individuals.[39,91]

Effects of arm versus leg exercise

At similar oxygen consumptions, HR, SBP, and DBP are higher during arm work than during leg work. This is primarily because the total muscle mass in the arms is smaller, and consequently a greater percentage of the available mass is recruited to perform the work. In addition, arm work is less mechanically efficient than leg work.[61,87,91]

Pulmonary ventilation

Pulmonary ventilation (Ve) is the volume of air exchanged per minute, and generally is approximately 6 L/min at rest in an average sedentary adult man. However, at maximal exercise, Ve increases 15- to 25-fold over resting values. During mild to moderate exercise, Ve increases primarily by increasing tidal volume, but during vigorous activity it increases by increasing the respiratory rate.[39]

Increases in Ve are generally directly proportional to an increase in oxygen consumption ($\dot{V}_{O_2}$) and carbon dioxide that is produced ($\dot{V}_{CO_2}$). At a critical exercise intensity (usually 47–64% of the $\dot{V}_{O_{2max}}$ in healthy untrained individuals and 70–90% $\dot{V}_{O_{2max}}$ in highly trained individuals), however, Ve increases disproportionately relative to the $\dot{V}_{O_2}$ (paralleling an abrupt increase in serum lactate and $\dot{V}CO_2$). This is called the anaerobic (ventilatory) threshold.[39,91]

The anaerobic threshold

The anaerobic threshold signifies the onset of metabolic acidosis during exercise, and traditionally has been determined by serial measurements of blood lactate. It can be non-invasively determined by assessment of expired gases during exercise testing, specifically Ve and carbon dioxide production ($\dot{V}CO_2$). The anaerobic threshold signifies the peak work rate or oxygen consumption at which the energy demands exceed circulatory ability to sustain aerobic metabolism.[39,91]

Maximal oxygen consumption

The most widely recognized measure of cardiopulmonary fitness is the aerobic capacity, or $\dot{V}O_{2max}$. This variable is defined physiologically as the highest rate of oxygen transport and use that can be achieved at maximal physical exertion.

The resting oxygen consumption of an individual (250 mL/min) divided by body weight (70 kg) give the resting energy requirement, 1 MET (about 3.5 mL/kg per min). Multiples of this value are used to quantify levels of energy expenditure. For example, running a 6-mph pace requires 10 times the resting energy expenditure, giving an aerobic cost of 10 METs, or 35 mL/kg per min. Because there is little variation in maximal HR and maximal systemic arteriovenous oxygen difference with physical training, $\dot{V}O_{2max}$ virtually defines the pumping capacity of the heart. When expressed as milliliters of oxygen per kilogram of body weight per minute (mL/kg per min) or in METs, it is considered the best index of physical work capacity or cardiorespiratory fitness.[39,91]

Oxygen pulse

The oxygen pulse (mL/beat) is the ratio of $\dot{V}O_2$ (mL/min) to HR (beats/min), when both measures are obtained simultaneously. Oxygen pulse increases with increasing work effort. A low value during exercise indicates an excessive HR for workload and can be an indicator of heart disease.[25]

Respiratory quotient and respiratory exchange ratio

The respiratory quotient (RQ) is the ratio of CO_2 produced by cellular metabolism to O_2 used by tissues. It quantifies the relative amounts of carbohydrate and fatty acids being oxidized for energy. An RQ of 0.7 implies dependence on free fatty acids. An RQ of 1.0 indicates dependence on carbohydrate. The RQ does not exceed 1.0.

The respiratory exchange ratio (RER) reflects pulmonary exchange of CO_2 and O_2 at rest and during exercise. The RER also ranges between 0.7 and 1.0 during rest, and can also reflect substrate preference. During strenuous exercise, however, the RER can exceed 1.0 because of increasing metabolic activity not matched by $\dot{V}O_2$ and additional CO_2 derived from bicarbonate buffering of lactic acid. The terms RQ and RER are often used interchangeably, but their distinction is important.[25]

Effects of exercise training

Cardiovascular system

The effects of regular exercise on cardiovascular activity can be grouped into changes that occur at rest, during submaximal exercise, and during maximal work (Box 19-1).[87,91] Regular exercise may also impact a number of physiologic parameters (Box 19-2).

Detraining

The changes induced by regular exercise training generally are lost after 4–8 weeks of detraining. If training is reestablished, the rate at which the training effects occur do not appear to be faster.[87,91]

Overtraining

Overtraining fatigue syndrome presents as a prolonged decreased sport-specific performance, usually lasting greater than 2 weeks. It is characterized by premature fatigability, emotional and

---

Box 19-1 The effects of regular exercise on cardiovascular activity

Changes at rest
- Heart rate decreases, probably secondary to decreased sympathetic tone, increased parasympathetic tone, and a decreased intrinsic firing rate of the sinoatrial node.
- Stroke volume increases secondary to increased myocardial contractility.
- Cardiac output is unchanged at rest.
- Oxygen consumption does not change at rest.[87,91]

Changes at submaximal work[a]
- Heart rate decreases, at any given workload, due to the increased stroke volume and decreased sympathetic drive.
- Stroke volume increases due to increased myocardial contractility.
- Cardiac output does not change significantly, because the oxygen requirements for a fixed workload are similar. The same cardiac output is generated, however, with a lower heart rate and higher stroke volume.
- Submaximal oxygen consumption does not change significantly, because oxygen requirement is similar for a fixed workload.
- Arteriovenous oxygen difference increases during submaximal work.
- Lactate levels are decreased due to metabolic efficiency and increased lactate clearance rates.[87,91]

Changes at maximal work
- Maximal heart rate does not change with exercise training.
- Stroke volume increases due to increased contractility and/or increased heart size.
- Maximal cardiac output increases due to increased stroke volume.
- Maximal oxygen consumption ($\dot{V}O_{2max}$) increases primarily due to increased stroke volume.
- Improved ability of the local mitochondria to utilize oxygen.[87,91] (Since measured avO_2 difference represents whole body avO_2 difference, there is generally little change in the measured avO_2 difference)

[a]Submaximal work is defined as a workload during which a steady state is achieved.

Box 19-2 Physiologic changes following a regular exercise program

Blood pressure
- In normotensive individuals, regular exercise does not appear to have a significant impact on resting or exercising blood pressure. In hypertensive individuals, there can be a modest reduction in resting blood pressure as a result of regular exercise.[87,91]

Blood volume changes
- Total blood volume increases due to an increased number of red blood cells and expansion of the plasma volume.[87,91]

Blood lipids
- Total cholesterol can be decreased in individuals with hypercholesterolemia.
- High-density lipoprotein cholesterol increases with exercise training.
- Low-density lipoprotein cholesterol can remain the same or decrease with regular exercise.
- Triglycerides can decrease in those with elevated triglycerides initially. This change is facilitated by weight loss.[87,91]

Body composition
- Total body weight usually decreases with regular exercise.
- Fat-free weight does not normally change.
- Percent body fat declines.[87,91]

Biochemical changes
- Stored muscle glycogen increases.
- The percentage of fast- and slow-twitch fibers does not change, but the cross-sectional area occupied by these fibers may change due to selective hypertrophy of either fast- or slow-twitch fibers.[87,91]

Energy system changes
- Specificity of training refers to the fact that the changes that occur are specific to the muscles and energy systems that are being used.
- Chronic anaerobic training using the ATP–creatine phosphate system results in improved capacity and power of this system due to enhancement of enzyme activity and increases in the amount of ATP and creatine phosphate in the muscle.
- Anaerobic glycolysis is improved if the training program utilizes this system, resulting in increased stores of muscle glycogen and improved ability of enzymes in the system.
- Regular aerobic training improves $\dot{V}O_{2max}$. It increases muscle glycogen and triglyceride stores, as well as the rate at which it metabolizes carbohydrates and fat.[87,91]

Box 19-3 Symptoms of overtraining syndrome

- Sudden decline in quality of work or exercise performance
- Extreme fatigue
- Elevated resting heart rate
- Early onset of blood lactate accumulation
- Altered mood states
- Unexplained weight loss
- Insomnia
- Injuries related to overuse

---

from an objective evaluation of that individual's response to exercise, including observations of HR, blood pressure, rating of perceived exertion (RPE) to exercise, electrocardiogram when appropriate, and $\dot{V}O_{2max}$ measured directly or estimated during a graded exercise test.

The exercise prescription should be developed with careful consideration of the individual's health status, medications, risk factor profile, behavioral characteristics, personal goals, and exercise preferences.[36,91]

Components of an exercise prescription

- *Mode* is the particular form or type of exercise. The selection of mode should be based on the desired outcomes, focusing on exercises that are most likely to sustain participation and enjoyment.
- *Intensity* is the relative physiologic difficulty of the exercise. Intensity and duration of exercise interact and are inversely related.
- *Duration* or *time* is the length of an exercise session.
- *Frequency* refers to the number of exercise sessions per day and per week.
- *Progression* (*overload*) is the increase in activity during exercise training, which, over time, stimulates adaptation.[36,87,91]

These five essential components apply when developing an exercise prescription for persons of all ages and fitness levels. Each component of fitness (e.g. cardiorespiratory endurance, muscular strength and endurance, and flexibility) has its own specific exercise prescription associated with it. The following section reviews the ACSM guidelines for each component of fitness.

Exercise prescription for cardiorespiratory endurance

Cardiorespiratory endurance is the ability to take in, deliver, and utilize oxygen. It is dependent on the function of the cardiorespiratory system (heart and lungs) and the cellular metabolic capacities. The degree of improvement that can be expected in cardiorespiratory fitness is directly related to the frequency, intensity, duration, and mode of exercise. Maximal oxygen uptake ($\dot{V}O_{2max}$) can increase between 5% and

---

mood changes, lack of motivation, infections, and overuse injuries. Recovery is markedly longer and variable among affected athletes, sometimes taking months before the athlete returns to baseline performance (Box 19-3).[87,91]

Exercise prescriptions

Exercise prescriptions are designed to enhance physical fitness, promote health by reducing risk factors for chronic disease, and ensure safety during exercise participation. The fundamental objective of the prescription is to bring about a change in personal health behavior to include habitual physical activity. The optimal exercise prescription for an individual is determined

30% with training. It has become apparent recently, however, that the level of physical activity necessary to achieve the majority of health benefits is less than that needed to attain a high level of cardiorespiratory fitness.[36,91]

ACSM recommendations for cardiorespiratory endurance training

Mode

- The best improvements in cardiorespiratory endurance occur when large muscle groups are engaged in rhythmic aerobic activity.
- Various activities can be incorporated into an exercise program to increase enjoyment and improve compliance.
- Appropriate activities include walking, jogging, cycling, rowing, stair climbing, aerobic dance ('aerobics'), water exercise, and cross-country skiing.[36,91]

Intensity

- The ACSM recommends that exercise intensity be prescribed within a range of 70–85% of maximum HR, 50–85% of $\dot{V}O_{2max}$, or 60–80% of maximum METs or HR reserve.
- Because of the variability in estimating maximal HR from age, whenever possible use an actual maximal HR from a graded exercise test.
- Lower intensities (40–50% of $\dot{V}O_{2max}$) elicit a favorable response in individuals with very low fitness levels.[36,91]

Rating of perceived exertion   The RPE may be used with HR for regulating intensity.

- The ACSM recommends an intensity that will elicit an RPE within a range of 12–16 on the original 6–20 Borg Scale (Table 19-1).
- The RPE is considered a reliable indicator of exercise intensity, and is particularly useful when participants are unable to monitor their pulse or when HR response to exercise has been altered by medications.[36,91]

Calculating intensity   Because of limitations in using VO_2 calculations for prescribing intensity, the most common methods of setting the intensity of exercise to improve or maintain cardiorespiratory fitness use HR and RPE.[36,85,91]

Heart rate methods   Heart rate is used as a guide to set exercise intensity, because of the relatively linear relationship between HR and percentage of VO_{2max}. It is best to measure maximal HR (HR_{max}) during a progressive exercise test whenever possible, because HR_{max} declines with age. HR_{max} can be estimated by using the equation $HR_{max} = 220 -$ age. This estimation has significant variance, with a standard deviation of 10–12 beats per minute.[36,85,91]

HR_{max} method   One of the oldest methods of setting the target HR range uses a straight percentage of the HR_{max} Using 70–85% of an individual's HR_{max} approximates 55–75% of

Table 19-1 Borg Scale of Perceived Exertion[81]

Level	Perceived exertion
6	—
7	Very, very light
8	
9	Fairly light
10	
11	
12	
13	Somewhat hard
14	
15	Hard
16	
17	Very hard
18	
19	Very, very hard
20	

$\dot{V}O_{2max}$ and provides the stimulus needed to improve or maintain cardiorespiratory fitness.[36,85,91] For example, if HR_{max} is 180 beats per minute, then target HR (70–85% of HR_{max}) would range 126–152 beats per minute.

Heart rate reserve method   The HR reserve method is also known as the Karvonen method. In this method, the target range is calculated as follows: subtract standing resting HR (HR_{rest}) from maximal HR (HR_{max}) to obtain HR reserve. Calculate 50% and 85% of the HR reserve. Add each of these values to the resting HR to obtain the target range. Therefore the target range is

$$[(HR_{max} - HR_{rest}) \times 0.50 - 0.85] + HR_{rest}.$$

The small but systematic differences between the two HR methods are due to the fact that the percentage HR_{max} is 55–75% of $\dot{V}O_{2max}$ and the percentage HRR_{max} is 60–80% of $\dot{V}O_{2max}$. Either method can be used to approximate the range of exercise intensities known to increase or maintain cardiorespiratory fitness or $\dot{V}O_{2max}$.[36,91]

Rating of perceived exertion   The RPE is a subjective grading of how hard individuals feel they are exercising. Use of RPE is considered an adjunct to monitoring HR. It has proven to be a valuable aid in prescribing exercise for individuals who have difficulty with HR palpation, and in cases where the HR response to exercise may have been altered due to a change in medication. The most commonly used scale of perceived exertion is the Borg Scale (Table 19-1). The average RPE range associated with physiologic adaptation to exercise is 13–16 ('somewhat hard' to 'hard') on the Borg Scale category. One should suit the RPE to the individual on a specific mode of exercise, and not expect an exact matching of the RPE to a percentage HR_{max} or percentage HR reserve. It should be used only as a guideline in setting the exercise intensity.[36,81,85,91]

The appropriate exercise intensity is one that is safe and compatible with a long-term active lifestyle for that individual and achieves the desired outcome given the time constraints of the exercise session.

Duration

- The ACSM recommends 20–60 min of continuous aerobic activity.
- Deconditioned individuals, however, can benefit from multiple, short-duration exercise sessions of less than 10 min with frequent interspersed rest periods.
- An inverse relationship exists between the intensity and duration of training.
- There might be greater musculoskeletal and cardiovascular risk with exercise performed at high intensities for short durations as compared with lower intensity exercise for a longer duration.[36,85,91]

Frequency

- The ACSM recommends that aerobic exercise be performed 3–5 days per week for most individuals.
- Less conditioned people can benefit from lower intensity, shorter duration exercise performed at higher frequencies per day and/or per week.[36,91]

Progression (overload)

- The rate of progression depends on health and fitness status, individual goals, and compliance rate.
- Frequency, intensity, and/or duration can be increased to provide overload.
- The goal for most healthy individuals is 30 min, 3–4 days per week, at 85% of HR reserve.[36,91]

Medical clearance

Exercise training might not be appropriate for everyone. Patients whose adaptive reserves are severely limited by disease processes might not be able to adapt to or benefit from exercise. In this small subpopulation of people with severe or unstable cardiac, respiratory, metabolic, systemic, or musculoskeletal disease, exercise programming can be fatal, injurious, or simply not beneficial, depending on the clinical status and condition of the individual.[37]

The recommended level of screening prior to beginning or increasing an exercise program depends on the risk of the individual and the intensity of the planned physical activity. For individuals planning to engage in low- to moderate-intensity activities, the Physical Activities Readiness Questionnaire (PAR-Q) (Box 19-4) should be considered the minimal level of screening. The PAR-Q was designed to identify the small number of adults for whom physical activity might be inappro-

---

Box 19-4 Physical activity readiness questionnaire[a]

- Has your doctor ever said that you have a heart condition and that you should only do physical activity recommended by a doctor?
- Do you feel pain in your chest when you do physical activity?
- In the past month, have you had chest pain when you were not doing physical activity?
- Do you lose your balance because of dizziness or do you ever lose consciousness?
- Do you have a bone or joint problem that could be made worse by a change in your physical activity?
- Is your doctor currently prescribing drugs (for example water pills) for your blood pressure or heart condition?
- Do you know of any other reason why you should not do physical activity?

[a]A 'yes' answer to any of the questions indicates the necessity of a physician's referral for a preexercise evaluation before the person begins or increases physical activity.[37]

---

priate or those who should receive medical advice concerning the most suitable type of activity.[37,91]

The preexercise evaluation

A preexercise evaluation by a physician will be more comprehensive and should include the following.

Patient history

- Current and previous exercise patterns.
- Discussion of motivations and barriers to exercise.
- Beliefs regarding risks and benefits of exercise.
- Preferred types of exercise activity.
- Review of heart disease risk factors: family history of heart disease before age 50; diabetes, hypertension, smoking, hyperlipidemia; and sedentary lifestyle and obesity.
- Physical limitations.
- Current medical problems (cardiac, pulmonary, and musculoskeletal).
- History of exercise-induced symptoms (chest pain, shortness of breath, and hives).
- Time and scheduling considerations.
- Social support for exercise.
- Current medications.[38]

Identification of those who need an exercise stress test
Indications for an exercise stress test according to the American College of Cardiology and American Heart Association are as follow.[96]

- To evaluate patients for suspected coronary artery disease (typical and atypical angina pectoris).
- To evaluate patients with known coronary artery disease after myocardial infarction or intervention.
- To evaluate healthy asymptomatic individuals in the following categories:

Table 19-2 American College of Sports Medicine recommendations for medical examination and exercise testing prior to participation and for physician supervision of exercise tests

Guideline		Apparently healthy		Increased risk[a]		Known disease[b]
		Younger[c]	Older	No symptoms	Symptoms	
Medical examination and clinical exercise test recommended prior to participation	Moderate exercise[d]	No[e]	No	No	Yes	Yes
	Vigorous exercise[f]	No	Yes[g]	Yes	Yes	Yes
Physician supervision recommended during exercise test	Submaximal testing	No[e]	No	No	Yes	Yes
	Maximal testing	No	Yes[g]	Yes	Yes	Yes

[a]*Persons with two or more risk factors (see Table 19-3) or one or more signs or symptoms (see Box 19-5).*
[b]*Persons with known cardiac, pulmonary, or metabolic disease.*
[c]*Younger implies ≤40 years for men, ≤50 years for women.*
[d]*Moderate exercise as defined by an intensity of 40–60% of VO_{2max}; if intensity is uncertain, moderate exercise may alternatively be defined as one that has an intensity well within the individual's current capacity, that can be comfortably sustained for a prolonged period of time (that is, 60 min), that has a gradual initiation and progression, and that is generally non-competitive.*
[e]*A 'No' response means that an item is deemed not necessary, and is generally non-competitive.*
[f]*Vigorous exercise is defined by an exercise intensity >60% of VO_{2max}; if intensity is uncertain, vigorous exercise may alternatively be defined as exercise intense enough to represent a substantial cardiorespiratory challenge or if it results in fatigue within 20 min.*
[g]*A 'Yes' response means that an item is recommended. For physician supervision, this suggests that a physician is in close proximity and readily available should there be an emergent need.*
(From Kenny et al. 1995,[70] with permission of Williams & Wilkins.)

Box 19-5 Major symptoms or signs suggestive of cardiopulmonary disease

- Pain and discomfort (or other anginal equivalent) in the chest, neck, jaw, arms, or other areas that may be ischemic in nature
- Shortness of breath at rest or with mild exertion
- Dizziness or syncope
- Orthopnea or paroxysmal nocturnal dyspnea
- Ankle edema
- Palpitations or tachycardia
- Intermittent claudication
- Known heart murmur
- Unusual fatigue or shortness of breath with usual activities

(From Kenny et al. 1995,[70] with permission of Williams & Wilkins.)

Box 19-6 Contraindications to exercise testing

Absolute[38]
- Recent acute myocardial infarction
- Unstable angina
- Ventricular tachycardia or other dangerous arrhythmias
- Severe aortic stenosis
- Acute infection and/or fever
- Recent systemic or pulmonary embolus
- Thrombophlebitis or intracardiac thrombi
- Active or suspected myocarditis or pericarditis
- Acute congestive heart failure
- Dissecting aortic aneurysm

Relative[38]
- Severe hypertension (uncontrolled or untreated)
- Complicated pregnancy
- Moderate aortic stenosis
- Severe subaortic stenosis
- Supraventricular dysrhythmias
- Ventricular aneurysm
- Frequent or complex ventricular ectopy
- Cardiomyopathy
- Uncontrolled metabolic disease (thyroid or diabetes) or electrolyte abnormality
- Chronic or recurrent infectious disease (malaria, hepatitis, etc.)
- Neuromuscular, musculoskeletal, or rheumatoid diseases exacerbated by exercise

high-risk occupations such as pilot, firefighter, law enforcement officer, and mass transit operator; men over age 40 and women over age 50 who are sedentary and plan to start vigorous exercise; and individuals with multiple cardiac risk factors or concurrent chronic diseases.

- To evaluate exercise capacity in patients with valvular heart disease (except severe aortic stenosis).
- Individuals with cardiac rhythm disorders for the following reasons:
  to evaluate response to treatment of exercise-induced arrhythmia; and
  to evaluate response of rate-adaptive pacemaker setting.

The ACSM guidelines are summarized in Box 19-5, and Tables 19-2 and 19-3.[70] Contraindications to exercise testing are listed in Box 19-6.

MUSCLE PHYSIOLOGY

Each skeletal muscle is made of many muscle fibers, which range in diameter between 10 and 80 µm. Each muscle fiber, in turn, contains hundreds to thousands of myofibrils. Each

Table 19-3 Coronary artery disease risk factors[a]

Risk factor	Defining criteria
Positive risk factors	
Age	Men >45 years, women >55 or with premature menopause without estrogen replacement therapy.
Family history	Myocardial infarction or sudden death before 55 years of age in father or other male first-degree relative, or before 65 years of age in mother or other female first-degree relative.
Current cigarette smoking	—
Hypertension	Blood pressure ≥140/90 mmHg, confirmed by measurements on at least two separate occasions, or on antihypertensive medication. Total serum cholesterol >200 mg/dL (5.2 mmol/L) (if lipoprotein profile is unavailable) or high-density lipoprotein (HDL) <35 mg/dL (0.9 mmol/L).
Diabetes mellitus	Persons with insulin-dependent diabetes mellitus (IDDM) who are >30 years of age or have had IDDM for >15 years, and persons with non-insulin-dependent diabetes mellitus who are >35 years of age and should be classified as patients with known disease.
Sedentary lifestyle or physical inactivity	Persons comprising the least active 25% of the population, as defined by the combination of secondary jobs involving sitting for a large part of the day and no regular exercise or active recreational pursuits.
Negative risk factor	
High serum HDL cholesterol	>60 mg/dL (1.6 mmol/L)

[a]It is common to sum risk factors in making clinical judgments. If HDL is high, subtract one risk factor from the sum of positive risk factors, because high HDL decreases coronary artery disease risk. Obesity is not listed as an independent positive risk factor, because its effects are exerted through other risk factors (e.g. hypertension, hyperlipidemia, and diabetes). Obesity should be considered as an independent target for intervention. (After Anonymous 1993,[3] with permission.)

myofibril comprises about 1500 myosin (thick) filaments and 3000 actin (thin) filaments, which are responsible for muscle contraction (Fig. 19-2).[52]

Myosin and actin filaments partially interdigitate, causing myofibrils to have alternate light and dark bands. The light bands contain only actin filaments and are called I bands (as they are isotropic to polarized light). Dark bands contain myosin as well as the ends of the actin filaments where they overlap the myosin, and are called A bands (because they are anisotropic to polarized light). Small projections, called cross-bridges, protrude from the surface of myosin filaments along their entire length, except in the very center. The interaction between the myosin cross-bridge and the actin filaments results in contraction.[52]

The ends of actin filaments are attached to Z disks. From the Z disk, actin filaments extend in either direction, interdigitating with the myosin filaments. The Z disk passes from myofibril to myofibril, attaching the myofibrils across the muscle fiber, thus the entire muscle fiber has light and dark bands, as do individual myofibrils, and thus its striated appearance.[52]

The portion of a myofibril or the whole muscle fiber between two Z disks is called a sarcomere. The myofibrils within the muscle fibers are suspended in a matrix called sarcoplasm. The sarcoplasm contains potassium, magnesium, phosphate, enzymes, and mitochondria. The sarcoplasm also contains the sarcoplasmic reticulum, an extensive endoplasmic reticulum important in the control of muscle contraction.[52]

Physiology of muscle contraction
Sliding filament mechanism
Muscle contraction occurs by a sliding filament mechanism. In the relaxed state, the ends of actin filaments derived from two successive Z disks barely overlap each other, while at the same time completely overlapping the myosin filaments. In the contracted state, the actin filaments overlap each other to a great extent, and the Z disks are pulled up to the end of the myosin filaments (Fig. 19-3).

The muscle contraction is initiated by the release of acetylcholine from the motor nerve. Acetylcholine opens protein channels in the muscle fiber membrane, allowing sodium to flow into the muscle fiber membrane and initiating a muscle action potential. The action potential depolarizes the muscle fiber membrane, causing the sarcoplasmic reticulum to release calcium. Calcium, in turn, generates attraction between actin and myosin cross-bridges, causing them to slide together.[52]

Molecular characteristics of the contractile filaments
Each myosin filament is composed of 200 or more myosin molecules. Each myosin molecule is composed of six polypeptide chains: two heavy chains and four light chains. The two heavy chains are wrapped around each other to form a double helix, the tail and arm of the myosin molecule. One end of each of the chains is folded into a globular mass called the myosin head. There are, therefore, two myosin heads lying side by side.

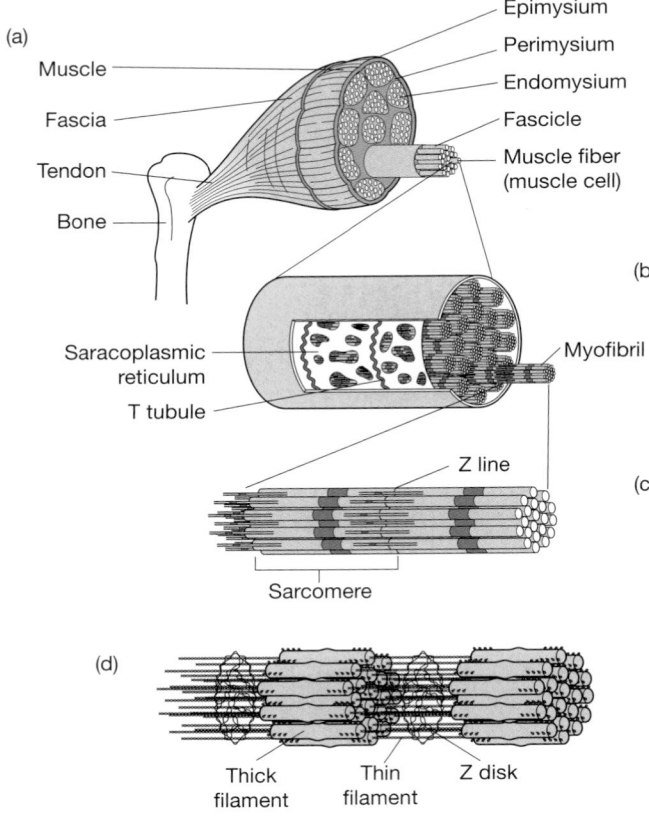

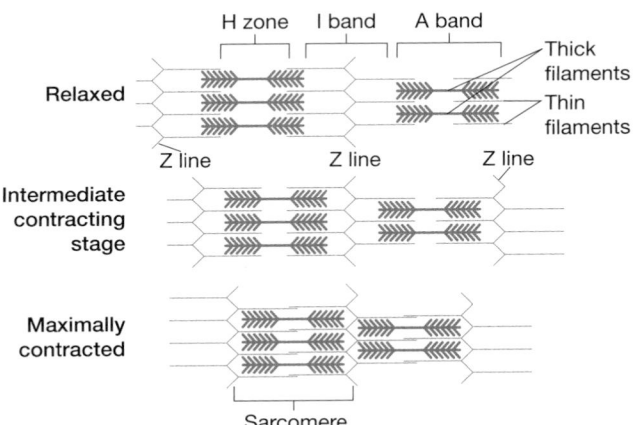

Figure 19-3 Sliding filament theory. During contraction, myosin cross-bridges pull the thin filaments toward the center of each sarcomere, thus shortening the myofibril and the entire muscle fiber. (From Thibodeau and Patton 1999,[101] with permission.)

Figure 19-2 Structure of skeletal muscle. (**a**) Skeletal muscle organ, composed of bundles of contractile muscle fibers held together by connective tissue. (**b**) Greater magnification of a single fiber, showing smaller fibers, myofibrils, in the sarcoplasm. Note the sarcoplasmic reticulum and T tubules forming a three-part structure called a triad. (**c**) A myofibril magnified further to show sarcomere between successive Z lines. Cross-striae are visible. (**d**) Molecular structure of a myofibril, showing thick myofilaments and thin myofilaments. (From Thibodeau and Patton 1999,[101] with permission.)

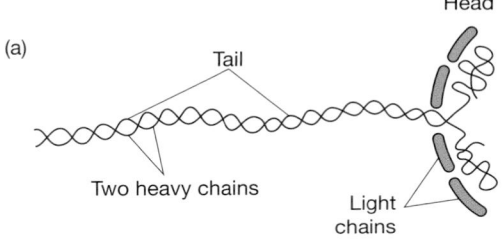

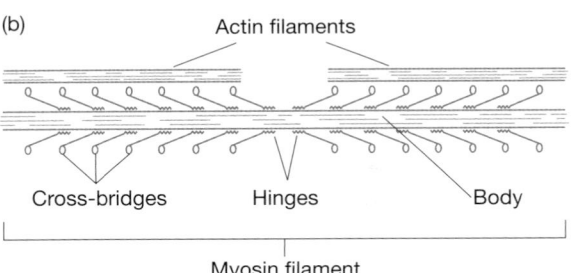

Figure 19-4 The myosin filament. (**a**) The myosin molecule. (**b**) The combination of many myosin molecules to form a myosin filament. Also shown are the cross-bridges and the interaction between the heads of the cross-bridges and adjacent actin filaments. (From Guyton 1996, with permission.)

The four light chains are also parts of the myosin heads, two to each head (Fig. 19-4).

The tails of myosin molecules are bonded together, forming the body of the myosin filament. Protruding from the body, the arm and heads of the myosin molecules are called cross-bridges, which are flexible at two points called hinges. In addition to serving as a component of the cross-bridge, the myosin head also functions as ATPase, allowing the head to cleave ATP and energize contraction (Fig. 19-5).

Actin filaments are composed of three protein components: actin, tropomyosin, and troponin (Fig. 19-6).

Several G-actin molecules form strands of F-actin. Two F-actin stands are then wound in a double helix. One molecule of ADP is attached to each G-actin molecule. These ADP molecules represent the active sites of the actin filaments with which myosin cross-bridges interact to cause muscle contraction.

Tropomyosin molecules are wrapped around the F-actin helix. In the resting state, tropomyosin covers the active sites of the actin strands, preventing contraction. Attached near one end of each tropomyosin molecule is a troponin molecule. Each troponin molecule consists of three protein subunits. Troponin I has a strong affinity for actin, troponin T for tropomyosin, and troponin C for calcium.

In the resting state, the troponin–tropomyosin complex is believed to cover the active sites of actin, providing an inhibitory effect on contraction. In the presence of calcium, this inhibitory effect is removed, allowing contraction to proceed.[52]

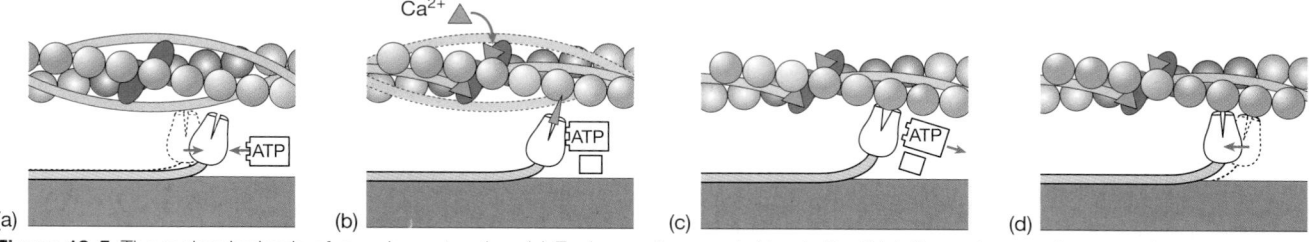

Figure 19-5 The molecular basis of muscle contraction. (**a**) Each myosin cross-bridge in the thick filament moves into a resting position after an ATP binds and transfers its energy. (**b**) Calcium ions released from the sarcoplasmic reticulum bind to troponin in the thin filament, allowing tropomyosin to shift from its position blocking the active sites of actin molecules. (**c**) Each myosin cross-bridge then binds to an active site on a thin filament, displacing the remnants of ATP hydrolysis: ADP and inorganic phosphate. (**d**) The release of stored energy from step (a) provides the force needed for each cross-bridge to move back to its original position, pulling actin along with it. Each cross-bridge will remain bound to actin until another ATP binds to it and pulls it back to its resting position (a). (From Thibodeau and Patton 1999,[101] with permission.)

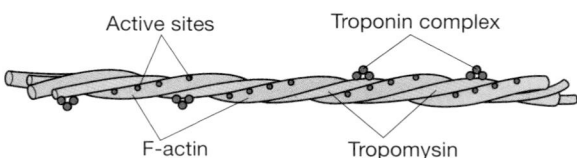

Figure 19-6 Tropomyosin molecules. The actin filament, composed of two helical strands of F-actin and tropomyosin molecules that fit loosely in the grooves between the actin strands. Attached to one end of each tropomyosin molecule is a troponin complex that initiates contraction. (From Guyton 1996, with permission.)

Muscle fiber types

Muscle fibers can be characterized based on their speed of contraction or twitch. Type 1 fibers (slow oxidative) are best suited for endurance activities requiring aerobic metabolism. Type 2 fibers (fast twitch) are most active during activities requiring strength and speed. Type 2 fibers are further categorized into type 2A (fast, oxidative glycolytic) and type 2B (fast glycolytic). Type 2A represents a type of hybrid that retains some oxidative capacity. Features of each muscle type are summarized in Table 19-4.

During anaerobic activity, slow oxidative fibers (type 1) are used almost exclusively at intensities below 70% of VO_{2max}. Beyond this intensity, anaerobic pathways are stimulated. At VO_{2max}, both type 1 and type 2 are relied on, and oxygen debt eventually occurs secondary to aerobic metabolism.

During isometric contractions, type 2 fibers are generally recruited when force exceeds 20% of the maximal voluntary contraction. If sustained for long periods of time, however, type 2 units can be recruited at thresholds below 20% of maximal voluntary contraction.[21,48]

Muscle fiber orientation

Parallel muscles have their fibers arranged parallel to the length of the muscle, and produce a greater range of motion than similar-sized muscles with pennate arrangement. Pennate muscles have shorter fibers that are arranged obliquely to their tendons (similar to the makeup of a feather), increasing cross-sectional area and the power produced.

Types of muscle contraction

Isometric contractions are contractions in which there is no change in the length of the muscle. No joint or limb motion occurs. Isotonic contractions occur when the muscle changes length, thus producing limb motion. Concentric contractions occur when the muscle shortens. Eccentric contractions occur when the muscle lengthens. More fast-twitch fibers are recruited during eccentric contractions. Isokinetic contractions occur when muscle contraction is performed at a constant velocity. This can be done only with the assistance of a preset rate-limiting device. This type of exercise does not exist in nature.

Factors affecting muscle strength and performance

Determinants of strength

A muscle's ability of produce force is directly proportional to its cross-sectional area. For parallel muscles, this corresponds to the cross-section at the bulkiest part of the muscle. For pennate muscles, multiple cross-sections are taken at right angles to each of the muscle fibers. Pennate muscles are particularly adapted to force production, as many more muscle fibers are contained in pennate muscles and these fibers are shorter.[70]

Length–tension relationship

Maximum force of contraction occurs when a muscle is at its normal resting muscle length. For the muscles, this corresponds to about midrange of joint motion or slightly longer, and is the length at which tension just begins to exceed zero. If a muscle is stretched to much greater than resting length prior to contraction, resting tension develops, and active tension (the increase in tension during contraction) decreases.

Efficiency (percentage of energy that is converted into work instead of heat) occurs at a velocity of contraction of about 30% of maximum.[21]

Torque–velocity relationship

The greatest amount of force is generated by a muscle during fast eccentric (lengthening) contractions.[21] The least amount of force is produced during fast concentric (shortening) contractions. The amount of force developed is summarized as fast

Table 19-4 Skeletal muscle fiber characteristics

	Type 1 (slow oxidative)	Type 2B (fast glycotic)	Type 2A (fast oxidative glycotic)
Major source of ATP	Oxidative phosphorylation	Glycolysis	Oxidative phosphorylation
Mitochondria	High	Low	High
Myoglobin content	High	Low	High
Capillarity	High	Low	High
Muscle color	Red	White	Red
Glycogen content	Low	High	Intermediate
Glycolytic enzyme activity	Low	High	Intermediate
Myosin ATPase activity	Low	High	High
Speed of contraction	Slow	Fast	Fast
Rate of fatigue	Slow	Fast	Intermediate
Muscle fiber diameter	Small	Large	Intermediate

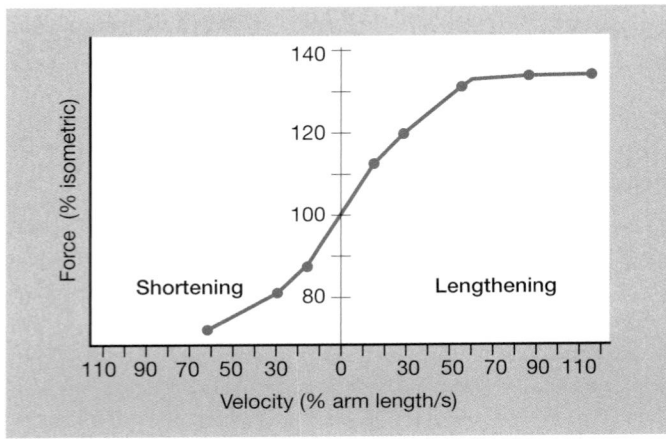

Figure 19-7 Relationship of maximal force of human elbow flexor muscles to velocity of contraction. Velocity on the abscissa is designated as a percentage of arm length per second. (From Knuttgen 1976,[74] with permission of University Park Press.)

eccentric > slow eccentric > isometric > slow concentric > fast concentric (Fig. 19-7).

Effects of exercise training

The SAID principle (specific adaptations to imposed demands) states that a muscle will adapt to a specific demand imposed on it, making it better able to handle the greater load.

Neural adaptations

Observed strength gains within the first few weeks of a weight-lifting program are mostly due to neuromuscular adaptations. The nervous system recruits larger motor units with higher frequencies of stimulation to provide the force necessary to overcome the imposed resistance. Early strength gains and increased muscle tension production from training therefore result from a more efficient neural recruitment process. This means that most of the improvement in strength-related functional activities gained on inpatient rehabilitation units are due to neural recruitment rather than muscle hypertrophy, due to the relatively short length of stays.

Muscle hypertrophy

Muscle hypertrophy represents enlargement of total muscle mass and cross-sectional area. Muscle hypertrophy is more common in fast-twitch than in slow-twitch muscles. Type 2A fibers exhibit the greatest growth, more so than type 2B and type 1 fibers. Muscle hypertrophy is typically experienced after 6–7 weeks of resistance training.[24,56] Conversely, muscle atrophy due to disuse occurs primarily in type 2 fibers.

Virtually all muscle hypertrophy occurs from hypertrophy of the individual muscle fibers. During muscle hypertrophy, the rate of muscle contractile protein synthesis is greater than decay, leading to greater numbers of actin and myosin filaments in the myofibrils. The myofibrils within each muscle fiber split, resulting in more myofibrils in each muscle fiber. Only under very rare conditions of extreme muscle force generation do the numbers of muscle fibers increase (fiber hyperplasia), and even then by only a few percent.[21,52]

Another type of muscle hypertrophy occurs when muscles are stretched to a greater than normal length, causing new sarcomeres to be added at the ends of muscle fibers where they attach to the tendons. Conversely, when a muscle remains shortened at less than its resting length, sarcomeres at the end of the muscle fibers disappear.[21]

Exercise prescription

Advancing in a training program can include increasing one's weight lifted (progressive resistive exercise), increasing repetitions, or increasing velocity of training. A commonly used term to express one's current strength level is the one-repetition maximum (RM), the most weight that a person can lift one time. The current strength fitness level for a particular exercise can be expressed in terms of one's multiple RM (i.e. the 10 RM is the amount of weight that one is capable of lifting 10 times).

Progressive resistance exercise

Popular protocols include the DeLorme, Oxford, and daily adjusted progressive resistance exercise (DAPRE) methods.

DeLorme   In the DeLorme method, three sets are performed for each exercise. Ten repetitions are performed in each set. The weight for the first set is 50% of the 10 RM, the second set 75% of the 10 RM, and the third set 100% of the 10 RM.[20] This is usually referred to clinically as progressive resistive exercise.

Oxford   In the Oxford technique, one starts with 10 repetitions at 100% of the 10 RM, then 10 repetitions at 75% of the 10 RM, then a third set of 10 repetitions at 50% of the 10 RM. This is usually referred to in the clinical setting as regressive resistive exercise.

Daily adjusted progressive resistance exercise   The DAPRE method of strength training guides the athlete through four sets of exercise per muscle group. The first set in DAPRE involves 10 repetitions at 50% of one's predetermined 6 RM. The second set consists of six repetitions at 75% of one's 6 RM. The third set consists of as many repetitions as can be performed at one's 6 RM. The number of repetitions performed in the third set determines the resistance for the fourth set. If five to seven repetitions were performed in set 3, resistance stays the same. If fewer than five repetitions were performed in set 3, the weight is lowered by 5#. If more that seven repetitions are performed in set 3, the weight is raised by 5#. Set 4 consists of as many repetitions as can be performed to fatigue. The working weight for the next day is established based on one's performance during set 4, using the same formula for determining resistance change from set 3 to 4.[56,73]

It is important to note that none of these three types of resistive training programs have been determined to be superior to the others.

Increasing number of repetitions or rate

Critical to developing muscle strength is to exercise to the point of fatigue. Both high weight–low repetition and low weight–high repetition programs can be effective in achieving strength as long as exercise proceeds to muscle fatigue. Far more repetitions must be carried out with low weights to reach this point of fatigue. In fact, the amount of mechanical work required by low weight–high repetition exercise to reach muscle fatigue might be much greater than during higher weight exercise. Although circumstances exist where low weight–high repetition exercise can be appropriate for training (such as during injury or when training for a highly repetitive task), in general the use of higher weights to fatigue is a more effective means of strength training.

Hellebrandt advocates increasing the rate of contraction (controlled by a metronome) each session while lifting the same number of repetitions (10–20).[21,58]

Effects of aging

Although it was previously believed that strength training in the elderly was due only to learning or neural factors,[79] more recent reports have demonstrated that the muscles of older persons can demonstrate hypertrophy following strength training.[40,70]

Exercise for fat reduction

The threshold for change in body weight appears to be 30 min of exercise per day, with more marked losses noted with 60 min/day. Land-based exercise such as cycling and walking appear effective choices. Swimming in the absence of caloric restriction did not appear to result in weight loss. In fact, subjects gained weight, although this appeared to be all muscle weight, thus increasing lean body mass. It stands to reason, however, that swimming can be effective in weight loss if combined with caloric restriction.[21,53]

ACSM guidelines for prescription of strength-training exercise

Muscular strength and endurance can be developed with both dynamic and static exercise. Both forms have their indications, but for most persons dynamic exercise is recommended. Strength exercise should be rhythmic, performed at low to moderate speed, and performed through a full range of motion. Normal breathing should be maintained. Heavy resistance training associated with breath holding can result in dramatic rises in SBP and DBP.

Specific technique for each exercise should be closely adhered to. Both the lifting (concentric) and lowering (eccentric) phases of resistance exercise should be performed in a controlled fashion. When possible, training with a partner can provide feedback, assistance, motivation, and safety.

Recommended guidelines for strength training are listed in Table 19-5.

FLEXIBILITY

Flexibility generally describes the range of motion commonly present in a joint or group of joints that allows normal and unimpaired function.[16] More specifically, flexibility has been defined as 'the total achievable excursion (within limits of pain) of a body part through its range of motion'.[88] With regard to flexibility, the following generalizations can be made. Flexibility is an individually variable, joint-specific, inherited characteristic that decreases with age; varies by gender and ethnic group; bears little relationship with body proportion or limb length; and, most importantly for the purposes of this chapter, can be acquired through training.[16,43,49–51]

Table 19-5 Recommended guidelines for strength training

Component	Details
Mode	Perform a minimum of 8–10 exercises that train the major muscle groups.
Intensity	One set of 8–12 repetitions resulting in volitional fatigue for each exercise[a]
Duration	The entire program should last no more that 1 h. Programs lasting greater than 1 h are associated with a higher dropout rate.
Frequency	At least 2 days per week.[a]

[a]*While more frequent training with additional sets or repetitions might elicit additional strength gains, the additional improvement is considered relatively small.*[70]

From a developmental standpoint, flexibility is greatest during infancy and early childhood. Flexibility reaches minimal levels between ages 10 and 12 years. It then improves again toward early adulthood, but not sufficiently to allow ranges of motion seen in childhood.[27] The early adolescent growth spurt results in short-term tightness of the joints, probably as a result of increased tension in connective tissue. Girls are generally more flexible than boys,[72,83,86] and this advantage probably persists into adulthood.

Achieving a maximal functional range of motion is an important goal of many therapeutic exercise regimens. Most typically, increased range of motion is achieved via the process of stretching. The term *stretching* defines an activity that applies a deforming force along the rotational or translational planes of motion of a joint.[88] Stretching should respect the lines of geometry of the joint as well as its planes of stability. In addition to stretching, mobilization is used to maintain flexibility. Mobilization moves a joint through its range of motion without applying a deforming force.

Importance of flexibility

Flexibility has only recently been identified as an important component of therapeutic exercise. Cureton emphasized flexibility as an important component of physical fitness after working with swimmers during the 1932 Olympic Games.[18] Later, Kraus stressed the importance of flexibility in preventing low back pain.[75] His work inspired much of the subsequent research on flexibility. It was not until 1964 that Fleishman proved flexibility to be an independent factor in physical fitness that was unrelated to other factors, including strength, power, endurance, and coordination.[34] During the same decade and in another landmark work, DeVries proved the value of passive stretching in improving flexibility and range of motion.[26] Subsequent study has demonstrated the value of flexibility training for patients in the industrial setting, in the athletic setting, those with back pain, and those who are status post orthopedic surgical procedures.

Subsequent to Kraus's work, biomechanical studies have shown that lower extremity flexibility is needed for the prevention of lumbar spine injuries.[32] Wyke et al. reported increased frequency of spondylolysis and spondylolisthesis in subjects with severe hamstring inflexibility.[82] Cady demonstrated an inverse relationship between flexibility and the incidence of back injuries and workers' compensation costs in a cohort study of firefighters placed on a fitness program.[11]

The work of Salter and associates has emphasized the importance of maintaining motion and flexibility postoperatively in patients who have undergone orthopedic procedures. The benefits of the mobilization of postoperative joints to the surrounding ligamentous and musculotendinous structures have been well established.[71,90,110]

In the realm of athletic training, flexibility has been both extensively applied and extensively studied. The proposed benefits of flexibility to athletes include injury prevention, reduced muscle soreness, skill enhancement, and muscle relaxation.[10,15,19,28,30,44,64,106] With regard to injury prevention, muscles possessing greater extensibility are less likely to be overstretched during athletic activity, lessening the likelihood of injury. A 1987 review of all studies of soccer injuries suggested an important role for flexibility in the prevention of injury, and attributed up to 11% of all injuries to poor flexibility.[68] A prospective study of a flexibility program in soccer players demonstrated a correlation between improvement in range of motion and reduction in incidence of muscle tears.[30] There is some evidence that delayed muscular soreness can be prevented and treated by static stretching.[104,105]

Flexibility has generally been hypothesized to improve athletic performance through skill enhancement. For example, mastery of the serve in tennis requires sufficient shoulder flexibility. Similarly, proficient golf skills require flexibility throughout the hips, trunk, and shoulders.[15] On the biomechanical level, prestretching a muscle has been shown in several studies to enhance the force of muscle contraction.[7,8,12,13]

There is, however, considerable uncertainty regarding two of the most important proposed benefits of flexibility training for athletes: prevention of injury and improvement of performance. Although currently held teaching states that stretching is a preventive measure for athletic injury, it has been pointed out that little conclusive epidemiologic evidence supports this idea.[54,57] In fact, it has been proposed that a certain degree of tightness might protect against injury by allowing load sharing when joints are stressed.[57] Hypermobility or excessive stretching could theoretically result in increased stress on the ligaments, bone, and cartilage at the joint, resulting in injury or arthritis.[50,80] In support of this is the fact that there is general agreement that the major predictive factor for joint injury is a previous joint injury or indeed the presence of excessive joint laxity, rather than inadequate flexibility.[30,31,45,67,69,92] With regard to athletic performance, several laboratories have shown that, among runners, less flexible individuals have a lower rate of oxygen consumption while covering the same distance at the same speed as their more flexible cohorts.[17]

The athletic literature seems to show in general that flexibility training, when employed appropriately, plays a positive role in sports injury and performance. However, excessive flexibility can actually be both a risk factor for injury and a detriment to performance. Stiff structures do appear to benefit from stretching, while hypermobile structures require stabilization rather than additional mobilization.

Determinants of flexibility

The determinants of joint mobility can be subdivided into static and dynamic factors.

Static factors include the types of tissues involved, the types and state of collagen subunits in the tissue, the presence or absence of inflammation, and the temperature of the tissue. Dynamic factors include neuromuscular variables such as voluntary muscle control and the length–tension 'thermostat' of the musculotendinous unit, as well as external factors such as pain associated with injury.[88]

Static factors

The most important tissue with regard to flexibility is the muscle–tendon unit, which is the primary target of flexibility training.[88] This structure includes the full length of the muscle and its supporting tissue, the musculotendinous junction, and the full length of the tendon to the tendon–bone junction. Within the muscle–tendon unit, it is the muscle that has the largest capacity for percent lengthening[63,97,98] of the tissues involved in a stretch. A ratio of 95 : 5% for muscle:tendon length change has been demonstrated.[97]

From a mechanical standpoint, muscle is composed of contractile and elastic elements arranged in parallel.[62] Muscle can respond to an applied force or stretch with permanent elongation. Animal studies have shown that this results from an increase in the number of sarcomeres, which translates to increased peak tension of a muscle at longer resting lengths. By contrast, muscle at rest has a tendency to shorten due to its contractile element. This shortening can be permanent, and is associated with a reduction in sarcomeres.[46,47,111] Tendon has a much more limited capacity for lengthening than muscle, probably due to its proteoglycan content and collagen cross-links (2–3% of its length, compared with 20% for muscle).[97,98,113] Of the external static factors, temperature has been studied the most. Warmer tissues are generally more distensible than cold ones.[29,107,109]

Dynamic factors

Perhaps the most clinically and physiologically significant dynamic determinant of flexibility is the muscle length–tension thermostat or feedback control system. Intrafusal fibers (muscle spindles), innervated by gamma motor neurons, lie in parallel with extrafusal contractile fibers. The intrafusal fibers serve the purpose of regulating the tension and length of the muscle as a whole. Muscle spindle length and tension are regulated by the gamma motor neuron, which in turn is subject to influences from the central nervous system. These include segmental input at the spinal cord level and suprasegmental input from the cerebellum and cortex. Consequently, muscle length and tension can be subject to multiple influences simultaneously.

An additional complicating factor is that receptors in the musculotendinous unit called the Golgi tendon organs act to inhibit muscle contraction at the point of critical stresses to the structure. The Golgi tendon organs allow lengthening and facilitate relaxation. When acting in conjunction, these dynamic mechanisms facilitate a response to a stretch in the following way. As the muscle spindle is initially stretched, it sends impulses to the spinal cord that result in reflex muscle contraction. If the stretch is maintained longer than 6 s, the Golgi tendon organ fires, causing relaxation.[88]

The relative contribution of static muscle factors and dynamic neural factors to flexibility remains somewhat controversial. It seems clear that the changes in flexibility noted immediately after the institution of a stretching program occur too rapidly to be attributable solely to structural alteration of the muscle and connective tissue. The consensus view is that neural factors probably play the major role in this early flexibility. After prolonged periods of training, changes in sarcomere number can play a role in the establishment of a new elongated muscle length.[88]

Assessment of flexibility

Flexibility is generally assessed in terms of joint range of motion. Joint range of motion in turn is generally assessed with a goniometer or similar device. A goniometer consists of a 180° protractor designed for easy application to joints. The methods used when employing a goniometer, as well as the normal ranges of motion encountered with these methods, are well standardized (see Ch. 1).[31,84] Inter- and intraobserver reliability are good.[31] Limitations of the standard goniometer include application to only single joints at a given time, static measurements only, and difficulty of application to certain joints (e.g. costoclavicular).

The Leighton Flexometer contains a rotating circular dial marked in degrees and a pointer counterbalanced to remain vertical. It can be strapped to a body segment, and range of motion is determined with respect to the perpendicular. Its reliability is good but is not quite equivalent to that of the standard goniometer.[55]

The electrogoniometer substitutes a potentiometer for a protractor. The potentiometer provides an electrical signal that is directly proportional to the angle of the joint. This device is able to give continuous recordings during a variety of activities, allowing a more realistic assessment of functional flexibility and dynamic range of motion during actual physical activity.

With regard to measuring trunk flexibility, goniometric devices are generally considered inadequate. The Schober test, originally designed to measure spinal flexion and extension in patients with ankylosing spondylitis, is commonly employed, as modified by Moll and Wright. Two marks are made along the ends of the lumbar spine, and tape measurements are made between them with the spine in flexion, neutral, and extension. This test has been shown to be more reliable than other methods, including fingertip to floor measurements and the Loebl inclinometer technique. 'Eyeball' measurements show marked variability. These tests of trunk flexibility are all non-specific, and each is limited to a gross measurement of compound motion of the entire thoracolumbar spine. None of these methods can assess articular mobility in the translational and rotational planes.[88] The optimal measurement of trunk flexibility is probably that obtained with plain films, but these have the obvious disadvantages of cost and radiation exposure.

Methods of stretching

It is important to take several factors into consideration when employing a stretching program. Prevention of injury and treatment of specific joint injury, as well as the presence and effects of pain or muscle spasm, require modification of the program. Stretching can be dangerous, and might result in significant injury if performed incorrectly.[89,92,93] As with any form of therapeutic exercise, flexibility training must be approached within a program aimed at addressing the specific functional needs of the individual.

Numerous options now abound for improving flexibility with stretching techniques. A distinct superiority of any one method has not been demonstrated. For the purposes of this chapter, stretching techniques are divided into the following four categories: ballistic, static, passive, and neuromuscular facilitation.

Ballistic

Ballistic stretching employs the repetitive rapid application of force in a bouncing or jerking maneuver. Momentum carries the body part through the range of motion until the muscles are stretched to the limits. This method is less efficient than other methods, due to the fact that muscle will contract under these stresses to protect itself from overstretching. Additionally, the rapid increase in force can cause injury.[92,99] An example would be the 10-count bouncing toe touches popularized in the 1970s but since abandoned due to lack of efficacy and risk of injury.

Passive

Passive stretching employs a partner or therapist who applies a stretch to a relaxed joint or extremity. This method requires excellent communication and the slow and sensitive application of force. This method is most appropriately and most safely employed in the training room or in a physical or occupational therapy context. Outside these contexts, passive stretching can be dangerous for recreational or competitive athletes due to increased risk of injury.

Static

Static stretching applies a steady force for a period of 15–60 s. This method is the easiest and probably the safest type of stretching. Static stretching seems to be particularly helpful as a warm up to any other form of therapeutic or recreational exercise, including athletic activity. Static stretching has the added advantage here of being associated with decreased muscle soreness after exercise.

Neuromuscular facilitation

The efficacy of stretching afforded by neuromuscular facilitation techniques has been documented in several studies.[89,100] These methods typically require a trained therapist, aide, or trainer. The specific activities most frequently employed include hold–relax and contract–relax techniques, characterized by an isometric or concentric contraction of the musculotendinous unit followed by a passive or static stretch. The prestretch contraction is thought to facilitate relaxation and flexibility via the muscle length–tension thermostat discussed previously in this chapter.

ACSM guidelines for prescription of exercise for musculoskeletal flexibility

Optimal musculoskeletal function requires that adequate range of motion be maintained in all joints. Particularly important is maintenance of flexibility in the low back and posterior thigh muscles. Poor flexibility in these regions can predispose to low back pain.[70]

Some common stretching exercises might not be appropriate for all people, particularly those with a prior injury, joint insufficiency, or other condition that could place them at risk for injury. Furthermore, exercises requiring substantial flexibility or skill are not recommended for older, less flexible, or less experienced persons.[70]

Recommended guidelines for flexibility training are listed in Table 19-6.[70]

Plyometrics

Plyometrics are a relatively recent addition to the panoply of therapeutic exercise. This class of exercises is employed primarily in the training of athletes. Proponents of plyometrics advocate it because of its apparent muscle-strengthening and injury prevention effects. Plyometric exercises are generally defined as brief, explosive maneuvers that consist of an eccentric muscle contraction followed immediately by a concentric contraction. An example is the action of planting and jumping during sport activity. Here, the process of planting the feet and flexing the hips, knees, and ankles while loading the lower extremities

Table 19-6 Recommended guidelines for flexibility training	
Component	Details
Mode	Static stretching of major muscle groups including the low back and posterior thigh.
Intensity	To a mild degree of discomfort.
Duration	10–30 s per stretch.
Frequency	At least three times per week.
Repetitions	Three to five for each stretch.

(eccentric contraction) is followed by a quick changeover to concentric contractions as these joints are extended to propel upward into a jump. This type of stretch-shortening cycle is analogous to a spring coiling and uncoiling.

Plyometrics allow the body to store elastic energy briefly in the muscle during the eccentric phase. This stored energy, combined with activation of the myotactic stretch reflex, results in a more powerful concentric contraction than is otherwise possible. This type of relatively complex action relies more heavily on the interplay between central nervous system and muscular system than do many other forms of exercise. Feedback from the central nervous system to the muscles influences the length of each muscle at any point during the movement, as well as the tension required for maintaining postural stability and initiating or stopping movement.[14] With training, according to plyometrics proponents, this neuromuscular interplay can be finely tuned. The widespread use of plyometric training in the athletic community suggests general acceptance of these methods by trainers, therapists, and athletes. However, many techniques in use have not been adequately studied. Results of research so far has generally been promising.

Hewett has reported that plyometric jump training improved lower body strength in high school-age girls. Specifically, hamstring isokinetic strength and vertical jump height were improved after a 6-week program. A 22% decrease in peak ground reaction forces and a 50% decrease in the abduction–adduction moments at the knee during landing were also observed.[60] In a later study employing the same plyometric program, Hewett et al. prospectively analyzed the effect of this neuromuscular training on the incidence of serious knee injuries in female athletes.[59] The authors reported a statistically significant decrease in the number of knee injuries sustained by the trained group versus matched control subjects.

Plyometric exercises vary in intensity, from simple, two-footed, in-place jumps, to hopping and bounding for maximum distance, to depth jumps from boxes of varying height. Plyometrics have been shown to result in ground reaction forces of four to seven times the body weight.[6,112] Clearly, these exercises should be approached with caution and begun at an elementary level. Progression to more advanced exercises should be based on the patient's proficiency with the basic movements, taking into account baseline levels of strength, stability, and coordination.

Proprioception

Proprioception denotes the process by which information about the position and movement of body parts is related to the central nervous system. Proprioceptive organs, including muscle (particularly intrafusal spindle fibers), skin, ligaments, and joint capsules, generate afferent information, which is crucial to the effective and safe performance of motor tasks. The process of proprioception is unfortunately subject to impairment from injury and disease. For example, knee and ankle ligament injuries have been shown to reduce proprioception. The same is true for both osteoarthritis and rheumatoid arthritis.[5,33] Neuropathies, most notably diabetic neuropathy, can also cause sig-

nificant loss of proprioception.[94] Proprioception has also been shown to decrease with age.[95]

The importance of proprioception to injury prevention and rehabilitation from injury is generally accepted. Impaired proprioception has been associated with increased risk of joint damage, athletic injury, and falls. Decreased joint proprioception is believed to influence the progressive joint deterioration associated with osteoarthritis, rheumatoid arthritis, and Charcot disease.[4,5] In a study of soccer players, a significantly greater incidence of ankle injury was observed among players with abnormal proprioceptive testing results as compared with those who tested within normal parameters.[103] Some findings suggest also that return to sport after knee injury might be more dependent on proprioception than on ligament tension.[5] It has also been demonstrated in several studies that the risk of falling in the elderly population correlates with postural sway, a variable that is determined in large part by proprioception.[76–78,102]

Proprioceptive exercise regimens, by definition, seek to improve joint and limb position sense. These exercises are typically employed after an injury has occurred to a joint, resulting in a deficit in proprioception. For example, the tilt or wobble board is commonly employed after ankle ligamentous injuries. Classically, unidirectional boards are used first, with a progression to multidirectional boards. This type of training has led to measurably improved position sense in athletes.[42] Other proprioceptive exercises include carioca (sideways running) and backward walking or running. It has also been shown that elastic bandaging improves position sense in subjects with previously impaired proprioception,[5] perhaps through stimulation of proprioceptors in the skin.

NEUROFACILITATION TECHNIQUES

Central nervous system dysfunction poses a unique set of challenges to both the patient and the treatment team. The following therapeutic exercise techniques were developed specifically for patients with central nervous system impairment, particularly impairment resulting from an acquired cortical lesion (i.e. stroke or brain injury).

Proprioceptive neuromuscular facilitation

This form of therapy employs resistance to indirectly facilitate movement. The therapist provides maximal resistance to the stronger motor components of specific spiral and diagonal movement patterns, thereby facilitating the weaker components of the patterns. Proprioceptive neuromuscular facilitation techniques are best applied to patients with hypotonia associated with supraspinal lesions to promote normalization of tone. In patients with spasticity, these techniques can actually further increase tone in a potentially detrimental fashion.[65,66]

Brunnstrom

These techniques use resistance and primitive postural reactions to facilitate gross synergistic movement patterns and increase muscle tone during early recovery from central nervous system injury.[9] During later stages, Brunnstrom techniques emphasize development of isolated movement and control. Like proprioceptive neuromuscular facilitation, this approach is felt to be effective in normalizing tone in a hypotonic or flaccid hemiplegic patient.

Bobath

The neurodevelopmental techniques (NDTs) developed by the Bobaths differ significantly from proprioceptive neuromuscular facilitation and Brunnstrom methods. Bobath techniques employ reflex inhibitory movement patterns to inhibit increased tone. These inhibitory patterns, which are generally antagonistic to the primitive synergistic patterns, are performed without resistance. NDT also incorporates advanced postural reactions to stimulate recovery. Advocates of these techniques claim reduction of hypertonicity and facilitation of motor recovery as their primary benefits.[41]

The techniques described above are all in common clinical use, with most therapists employing an eclectic approach, borrowing some from each. There is no convincing evidence, however, that any of these methods actually alter the natural history of recovery from neurologic insult. These approaches to therapy seem to be most useful in providing compensatory techniques during the course of recovery. Using these methods, patients are able to improve performance in and gain independence with such tasks as making transfers, stretching, bed mobility, and safe ambulation.[41]

EXERCISE FOR SPECIAL POPULATIONS

Pregnancy

In women who are pregnant, special considerations exist because of the possible competition between exercising maternal muscle and the fetus for blood flow, oxygen delivery, glucose availability, and heat dissipation. Metabolic and cardiorespiratory adaptations to pregnancy can alter the responses from exercise training. There are no data in humans to indicate that pregnant women should or should not limit exercise intensity and lower target HRs because of potential adverse effects.[70] For women who do not have any additional risk factors for adverse maternal or perinatal outcomes, the American College of Obstetricians and Gynecologists (ACOG) has established guidelines for the safe prescription of exercise.[1,2] Participation in a wide range of recreational activities appears to be safe during pregnancy. The safety of each sport is determined largely by the specific movements required by that sport. Participation in recreational sports with a high potential for contact, such as ice hockey, soccer, and basketball, could result in trauma to both the woman and the fetus. Recreational activities with an increased risk of falling, such as gymnastics, horseback riding, downhill skiing, and vigorous racquet sports, have an inherently high risk for trauma in pregnant and non-pregnant women. Those activities with a high risk of falling or for abdominal trauma should be avoided during pregnancy. Scuba diving should be avoided throughout pregnancy, because during this activity the fetus is at increased risk for decompression sickness secondary to the inability of the

fetal pulmonary circulation to filter bubble formation. Exertion at altitudes of up to 6000 ft. appears to be safe, but engaging in physical activities at higher altitudes carries various risks.

- During pregnancy, women can continue to exercise and derive health benefits even from mild to moderate exercise routines. Regular exercise (at least three times per week) is preferable to intermittent activity. Thirty minutes or more of moderate exercise a day on most, if not all, days is recommended.
- Women should avoid exercise in the supine position after the first trimester. Such a position is associated with decreased cardiac output in most pregnant women. Because the remaining cardiac output is preferentially distributed away from splanchnic beds (including the uterus) during vigorous exercise, such regimens are best avoided during pregnancy. Prolonged periods of motionless standing should also be avoided.
- Women should be aware of the decreased oxygen available for aerobic exercise during pregnancy. They should be encouraged to modify the intensity of their exercise according to maternal symptoms. Pregnant women should stop exercising when fatigued and not exercise to exhaustion. Weight-bearing exercises can under some circumstances be continued at intensities similar to those prior to pregnancy throughout the pregnancy. Non-weight-bearing exercises, such as stationary cycling or swimming, will minimize the risk of injury and facilitate the continuation of exercise during pregnancy.
- Morphologic changes in pregnancy should serve as a relative contraindication to types of exercise in which loss of balance could be detrimental to maternal or fetal well-being, especially in the third trimester. Any type of exercise involving the potential for even mild abdominal trauma should be avoided.
- Pregnancy requires an additional 300 kcal/day in order to maintain metabolic homeostasis. Women who exercise during pregnancy should be particularly careful to ensure an adequate diet.
- Pregnant women who exercise in the first trimester should augment heat dissipation by ensuring adequate hydration, appropriate clothing, and optimal environmental surroundings during exercise.

The American College of Obstetricians and Gynecologists recommends that women who currently participate in a regular exercise program can continue their training during pregnancy, following the above recommendations. Studies have demonstrated that women naturally decrease their exercise duration and intensity as their pregnancy advances. Those who begin an exercise program after becoming pregnant are advised to receive physician authorization and begin exercising with low-intensity, low- (or non-) impact activities, such as walking and swimming.[1,2] Contraindications for exercise during pregnancy have also been established by the ACOG (Box 19-7).[1]

Many of the physiologic and morphologic changes of pregnancy persist 4–6 weeks postpartum. Thus prepregnancy exer-

Box 19-7 Contraindications to aerobic exercise during pregnancy

Absolute contraindications
- Hemodynamically significant heart disease
- Restrictive lung disease
- Incompetent cervix or cerclage
- Multiple gestation at risk for premature labor
- Persistent second- or third-trimester bleeding
- Placenta previa after 26 weeks of gestation
- Premature labor during the current pregnancy
- Ruptured membranes
- Preeclampsia or pregnancy-induced hypertension

Relative contraindications
- Severe anemia
- Unevaluated maternal cardiac arrhythmia
- Chronic bronchitis
- Poorly controlled type 1 diabetes
- Extreme morbid obesity
- Extreme underweight (body mass index < 12)
- History of extremely sedentary lifestyle
- Intrauterine growth restriction in current pregnancy
- Poorly controlled hypertension
- Orthopedic limitations
- Poorly controlled seizure disorder
- Poorly controlled hyperthyroidism
- Heavy smoker

Further reasons to discontinue exercise and seek medical advice during pregnancy[1,70]
- Vaginal bleeding
- Dyspnea prior to exertion
- Dizziness
- Headache
- Chest pain
- Muscle weakness
- Calf pain or swelling (need to rule out thrombophlebitis)
- Preterm labor
- Decreased fetal movement
- Amniotic fluid leakage

Table 19-7 Guidelines for aerobic exercise prescription for the elderly

Component	Details
Mode	The exercise modality should be one that does not impose significant orthopedic stress. The activity should be accessible, convenient, and enjoyable to the participant—all factors directly related to exercise adherence. Consider walking, stationary cycling, water exercise, swimming, or machine-based stair climbing.
Intensity	Intensity must be sufficient to stress (overload) the cardiovascular, pulmonary, and musculoskeletal systems without overtaxing them. High variability exists for maximal heart rates in persons over 65 years of age. It is always better to use a measured maximal heart rate (HR_{max}) rather than age-predicted HR_{max} whenever possible. For similar reasons, the HR reserve method is recommended for establishing a training HR in older individuals, rather than a straight percentage of HR_{max}. The recommended intensity for older adults is 50–70% of HR reserve. Because many older persons suffer from a variety of medical conditions, a conservative approach to prescribing aerobic exercise is warranted.
Duration	During the initial stages of an exercise program, some older adults can have difficulty sustaining aerobic exercise for 20 min. One viable option can be to perform the exercise in several 10-min bouts throughout the day. To avoid injury and ensure safety, older individuals should initially increase exercise duration rather than intensity.
Frequency	Alternate between days that involve primarily weight bearing and non-weight-bearing exercise.

cise routines may be resumed gradually as soon as it is physically and medically safe. This will vary from one individual to another, with some women able to resume an exercise routine within days of delivery. There are no published studies to indicate that, in the absence of medical complications, rapid resumption of activities will result in adverse affects. Having undergone detraining, resumption of activities should be gradual. No known maternal complications are associated with resumption of training.

The elderly

The elderly can demonstrate improvements in aerobic capacity and muscle strength when given a sufficient training stimulus. Resistance training can enable elderly individuals to perform activities of daily living with greater ease, and counteract muscle loss and frailty in very 'older elderly' persons. The same general principles of exercise prescription apply to individuals of all ages. However, the wide range of health and fitness levels observed among older adults make generic exercise prescription more problematic.[70] Care must be taken in establishing the type, intensity, duration, and frequency of exercise. Specific recommendations for the elderly are outlined in Table 19-7.[70]

Individualization of resistance training prescriptions is also essential, and should be based on the health and fitness status and specific goals of the participant. Some guidelines follow, with reference to the intensity, frequency, and duration of exercise (Table 19-8).[70]

Regardless of which specific protocol is adopted, several common sense guidelines pertaining to resistance training for older adults should be followed.

- The major goal of the resistance training program is to develop sufficient muscular fitness to enhance an individual's ability to live a physically independent lifestyle.

Table 19-8 Guidelines for resistance exercise prescription for the elderly

Component	Details
Intensity	Perform one set of 8–10 exercises that train all the major muscle groups (e.g. gluteals, quadriceps, hamstrings, pectorals, latissimus dorsi, deltoids, and abdominals). Each set should involve 8–12 repetitions that elicit a perceived exertion rating of 12–13 (somewhat hard).
Frequency	Resistance training should be performed at least twice a week, with at least 48 h of rest between sessions.
Duration	Sessions lasting longer than 60 min can have a detrimental effect on exercise adherence. Following the above guidelines should permit individuals to complete total body resistance training sessions within 20–30 min.

- The first several resistance training sessions should be closely supervised and monitored by trained personnel who are sensitive to the special needs and capabilities of the elderly.
- Begin (the first 8 weeks) with minimal resistance to allow for adaptations of the connective tissue elements.
- Teach proper training techniques for all the exercises to be used in the program.
- Instruct older participants to maintain their normal breathing pattern while exercising.
- As a training effect occurs, achieve an overload initially by increasing the number of repetitions, and then by increasing the resistance.
- Never use a resistance that is so heavy that the exerciser cannot perform at least eight repetitions.
- Stress that all exercises should be performed in a manner in which the speed is controlled (no ballistic movements should be allowed).
- Perform the exercises in a range of motion that is within a 'pain-free arc' (i.e. the maximum range of motion that does not elicit pain or discomfort).
- Perform multijoint exercises (as opposed to single-joint exercises).
- Given a choice, use machines to resistance train, as opposed to free weights (machines require less skill to use, protect the back by stabilizing the user's body position, and allow the user to start with lower resistances, to increase by smaller increments, and to more easily control the exercise range on motion). Heavy free weights should be used only by those who have had special training in how to lift properly, and who have a spotter with them during the exercise.
- Do not overtrain. Two strength-training sessions per week are the minimum number required to produce positive

physiologic adaptations. Depending on the circumstances, more sessions might not be productive.
- Arthritic participants should never participate in strength-training exercises during active periods of joint pain or inflammation.
- Engage in a year-round resistance-training program on a regular basis.
- When returning from a lay-off, start with resistances <50% of the intensity at which they had been previously training (as tolerated), then gradually increase the resistance.

Children

Children tend to be more habitually active than adults, and accordingly maintain adequate levels of physical fitness. Healthy children should be encouraged, nonetheless, to engage in physical activity on a regular basis. However, because children are anatomically, physiologically, and psychologically immature, special precautions should be applied when designing exercise programs. Children can experience a higher incidence of overuse injuries, or damage the epiphyseal growth plates if endurance exercise is excessive. The risk of injury can be significantly decreased by ensuring appropriate matching of competition in terms of size, maturation or skill level, the use of properly fitted protective equipment, liberal adaptation of rules toward safety, proper conditioning, and appropriate skill development. Children have less efficient thermoregulation than that of adults, and are more prone to hyperthermia and hypothermia.[70] Specific recommendations for strength training in children are listed in Box 19-8.[70]

Hypertension

The ACSM makes the following recommendations regarding exercise testing and training of persons with hypertension.[70]

- Mass exercise testing is not advocated to determine those individuals at high risk for developing hypertension in the future as a result of an exaggerated exercise blood pressure response. However, if exercise test results are available and an individual has an exercise blood pressure response above the 85th percentile, this information does provide some indication of risk stratification for that patient and the necessity for appropriate lifestyle behavior counseling to ameliorate this increase.
- Endurance exercise training by individuals who are at high risk for developing hypertension can reduce the rise in blood pressure that occurs with time, justifying its use as a non-pharmacologic strategy to reduce the incidence of hypertension in susceptible individuals.
- Endurance exercise training elicits an average reduction of 10 mmHg for both SBPs and DBPs in individuals with mild essential hypertension (blood pressures in the range of 140/90 to 180/105 mmHg) and secondary hypertension due to renal dysfunction.
- The recommended mode, frequency, duration, and intensity of exercise are generally the same as those for apparently healthy individuals. Exercise training at

Box 19-8 Guidelines for strength training in children

- No matter how big, strong, or mature a young man or woman appears, remember that he or she is physiologically immature.
- Teach proper training techniques for all the exercise movements involved in the program and proper breathing techniques (i.e. no breath holding).
- Stress that exercises should be performed in a manner in which the speed is controlled, avoiding ballistic (fast and jerky) movements.
- Under no circumstances should a weight be used that allows less than eight repetitions to be completed per set, because heavy weights can be potentially dangerous and damaging to the developing skeletal and joint structures.
- As a training effect occurs, achieve an overload initially by increasing the number of repetitions, and then by increasing the absolute resistance.
- Perform one or two sets of 8–10 different exercises (with 8–12 repetitions per set), ensuring that all the major muscle groups are included.
- Limit strength-training sessions to twice per week, and encourage children and adolescents to seek other forms of physical activity.
- Perform full-range, multijoint exercises (as opposed to single-joint exercises).
- Do not overload the skeletal and joint structures of adolescents with maximal weights.
- Finally, and perhaps most important, all strength-training activities should be closely supervised and monitored by appropriately trained personnel.

Table 19-9 Guidelines for exercise prescription in patients with hypertension

Component	Details
Mode	Aerobic exercise preferred. High-intensity and isometric activities should be avoided. Weight training should involve low resistance with high repetitions.
Frequency	Four or five times per week.
Duration	30–60 min.
Intensity	40–70% of VO_{2max}.

Table 19-10 Guidelines for exercise prescription in patients with peripheral vascular disease

Component	Details
Mode	Weight-bearing activities are preferred, but non-weight-bearing activities may allow longer duration and higher intensity exercise.
Frequency and duration	Begin with 20 min twice daily (or less), with a goal of increasing to one 40- to 60-min session per day.
Intensity	Daily exercise to maximum tolerable pain with intermittent rest periods.

somewhat lower intensities (e.g. 40–70% of $\dot{V}O_{2max}$) appears to lower blood pressure as much, or more, than exercise at higher intensities. This can be especially important in specific hypertensive populations, such as the elderly.
- Based on the high number of exercise-related health benefits and low risk for morbidity and mortality, it seems reasonable to recommend exercise as part of the initial treatment strategy for individuals with mild to moderate essential hypertension.
- Individuals with marked elevations in blood pressure should add endurance exercise training to their treatment regimen only after initiating pharmacologic therapy. Exercise can reduce their blood pressure further, allowing them to decrease their antihypertensive medications, and attenuate their risk for premature mortality.
- Resistance training is not recommended as the primary form of exercise training for hypertensive individuals. With the exception of circuit weight training, resistance training has not consistently been shown to lower blood pressure. Resistance training is recommended as a component of a well-rounded fitness program, but it should not be the only form of exercise in the program.

Specific guidelines for exercise in patients with hypertension are as listed in Table 19-9.[70]

Peripheral vascular disease

Patients with peripheral vascular disease experience ischemic pain (claudication) during physical activity as a result of a mismatch between active muscle oxygen supply and demand. The symptoms can be described as burning, searing, aching, tightness, or cramping. Pain is most often experienced in the calf, but can begin in the buttock region and radiate down the leg. The symptoms typically disappear on cessation of exercise, although some patients can have claudication at rest in severe cases.

Severe peripheral vascular disease is treated initially with exercise and medications that decrease blood viscosity. Treatment with angioplasty or bypass grafting might also be indicated. Weight-bearing exercise is preferred to facilitate greater functional changes, but might not be well-tolerated initially. Prescription of non-weight-bearing exercise (which can permit a greater intensity or longer duration) is a suitable alternative.[70] Specific guidelines for exercise in patients with peripheral vascular disease are listed in Table 19-10.[60]

Diabetes

The response to exercise in the patient with insulin-dependent diabetes mellitus depends on a variety of factors, including the adequacy of control by exogenous insulin. If the patient is under appropriate control or only slightly hyperglycemic without ketosis, exercise can decrease blood glucose concentration and lower the insulin dosage required. Patients with insulin-dependent diabetes mellitus must be under adequate control prior to beginning an exercise program. Serum glucose concentrations in the general range of 200–400 mg% (mg/dL) require medical supervision during exercise, and exercise is contraindicated for those with fasting serum values >400 mg%. Exercised-induced hypoglycemia is the most common problem experienced by exercising patients with diabetes.

Hypoglycemia can occur not only during the exercise but for up to 4–6 h following an exercise bout.[70]

The risk of hypoglycemic events may be minimized by taking the following precautions.

- Monitor blood glucose frequently when initiating an exercise program.
- Decrease insulin dose (by 1–2 units as prescribed by the physician) or increase carbohydrate intake (10–15 g carbohydrate per 30 min of exercise) prior to an exercise bout.
- Inject insulin in an area such as the abdomen that is relatively inactive during exercise.
- Avoid exercise during periods of peak insulin activity.
- Eat carbohydrate snacks before and during prolonged exercise bouts.
- Be knowledgeable of the signs and symptoms of hypo- and hyperglycemia.
- Exercise with a partner.

Other precautions that should be taken include the following.[70]

- Use proper footwear and practice good foot hygiene.
- Be aware that beta-blockers and other medications can interfere with the patient's ability to discern hypoglycemic symptoms and/or angina.
- Be aware that exercise in excessive heat can cause problems in patients with diabetes with peripheral neuropathy.
- Patients with advanced retinopathy should not perform activities that cause excessive jarring or marked increases in blood pressure.
- Patients should have physician approval to resume exercise training following laser treatment.

Specific guidelines for exercise in patients with diabetes are listed in Table 19-11.[70]

CONCLUSION

The benefits of exercise for health and human performance are well known. Applying appropriate exercise prescriptions based on physiologic response to exercises and the principle of specificity of training will ensure appropriate training response and minimize risk for injury. Special populations, including the young, elderly, and those with disease states, may require specific modifications in exercise programs to maximize safety.

Table 19-11 Guidelines for exercise prescription in patients with diabetes

Component	Details
Frequency	Daily exercise for insulin-dependent diabetes mellitus.
Duration	Use a 20- to 30-min session to achieve glucose control. Non-insulin-dependent diabetes mellitus: maximize caloric expenditure if obese.
Intensity	Might need to use rating of perceived exertion as adjunct to heart rate for monitoring exercise intensity.

REFERENCES

1. American College of Obstetricians and Gynecologists. Exercise during pregnancy and the post partum period. Obstet Gynecol 2002; 99: 171–173.
2. American College of Obstetricians and Gynecologists. Exercise during pregnancy and the post partum period. Washington: American College of Obstetricians and Gynecologists; 1994.
3. [Anonymous]. Summary of the second report of the National Cholesterol Education Program (NCEP) Expert Panel on Detection, Evaluation, and Treatment of High Blood Cholesterol in Adults (Adult Treatment Panel II). JAMA 1993; 269(23):3015–3023.
4. Barrack RL, Skinner H, Cook S, et al. Effect of articular disease and total knee arthroplasty on knee joint-position sense. J Neurophysiol 1983; 50(3):684–687.
5. Barrett DS. Proprioception and function after anterior cruciate reconstruction. J Bone Joint Surg Br 1991; 73(5):833–837.
6. Bobbert M, Mackey M, Schenkelshoek D. Biomechanical analysis of drop and countermovement jumps. Eur J Appl Phys 1986; 54:566–573.
7. Bosco C, Komi PV. Potentiation of the mechanical behavior of the human skeletal muscle through prestretching. Acta Physiol Scand 1979; 106(4): 467–472.
8. Bosco C, Tihani J, Komi P. Store and recoil of elastic energy in slow and fast types of human skeletal muscles. Acta Physiol Scand 1982; 116: 343–349.
9. Brunnstrom S. Movement therapy in hemiplegia. New York: Harper & Row; 1971.
10. Bryant S. Flexibility and stretching. Physician Sports Med 1984; 12:171.
11. Cady LD Jr, Thomas PC, Karwasky RJ. Program for increasing health and physical fitness of fire fighters. J Occup Med 1985; 27(2):110–114.
12. Cavagna G, Dusman B, Margaria R. Positive work done by a previously stretched muscle. J Appl Physiol 1968; 24:21–32.
13. Cavagna G, Saibene F, Margaria R. Effects of negative work on the amount of positive work performed by an isolated muscle. J Appl Physiol 1965; 20:157–158.
14. Chu D. Jumping into plyometrics. Champaign: Human Kinetics; 1998.
15. Ciullo JV. Biomechanics of the musculotendinous unit. Clin Sports Med 1983; 2:71.
16. Corbin C. Flexibility. Clin Sports Med 1984; 3:101–117.
17. Craib MW, Mitchell VA, Fields KB, et al. The association between flexibility and running economy in sub-elite male distance runners. Med Sci Sports Exerc 1996; 28:737–743.
18. Cureton T. Flexibility as an aspect of physical fitness. Res Q 1951; 12:381–390.
19. D'Ambrosia R, Drez D. Prevention and treatment of running injuries. Thorofare: Charles Slack; 1982.

20. DeLateur BJ, Lehman JF, Fordyce WE. A test of the DeLorme axiom. Arch Phys Med Rehabil 1968; 49:245–248.

21. DeLateur BJ. Therapeutic exercise. In: Braddom RL, ed. Physical medicine and rehabilitation. Philadelphia: Saunders; 1996.

22. DeLateur BJ. Therapeutic exercise to develop strength and endurance. In: Kottke FJ, Stillwell GK, Lehmann JF, eds. Krusen's handbook of physical medicine and rehabilitation. Philadelphia: Saunders; 1982:427–464.

23. Demaree SR, Powers SK, Lawler JM. Fundamentals of exercise metabolism. In: Roitman JL, Haver EJ, Herridge M, et al, eds. ACSM resource manual for guidelines for exercise testing and prescription. Philadelphia: Lippincott Williams & Wilkins; 2001.

24. Deschenes M, Kraemer W. Performance and physiologic adaptations to resistance exercise. Am J Phys Med Rehabil 2002; 81(11 suppl):S3–S16.

25. Deuster P, Keyser D. Basics in exercise physiology. In: O'Connor F, Sallis R, Wilder R, et al, eds. Sports medicine: just the facts. New York: McGraw Hill; 2005.

26. DeVries H, Housh TJ. Evaluation of static stretching procedures for improvement of flexibility. Res Q 1962; 33:222–229.

27. DeVries H, Housh TJ. Physiology of exercise for physical education, athletics and exercise science. 5th edn. Dubuque: William C. Brown; 1994.

28. Doucette S, Globe E. The effect of exercise on patellar tracking in lateral patellar compression syndrome. Am J Phys Med 1992; 20:434–440.

29. East J, Smith F, Burry L. Evaluation of warm-up for improvement in flexibility. Am J Phys Med 1986; 14:316–319.

30. Ekstrand J, Gillquist J. The avoidability of soccer injuries. Int J Sports Med 1983; 4(2):124–128.

31. Ekstrand J, Gillquist J. The frequencies of muscle tightness and injuries in soccer players. Am J Phys Med 1982; 10:75–78.

32. Farfan H, Gracovetsky S. The mechanism of the lumbar spine. Spine 1989; 6:249–262.

33. Ferrell WR, Crighton A, Sturrock RD. Position sense at the proximal interphalangeal joint is distorted in patients with rheumatoid arthritis of finger joints. Exp Physiol 1992; 77(5):675–680.

34. Fleishman E. The structure and measurement of physical fitness. Englewood Cliffs: Prentice Hall; 1964.

35. Franklin B, Whaley M, Howley E. Benefits and risks associated with exercise in ACSM's guidelines for exercise testing and prescription. 6th edn. Philadelphia: Lippincott Williams & Wilkins; 2000.

36. Franklin B, Whaley M, Howley E. General principles of exercise prescription in ACSM's guidelines for exercise testing and prescription. 6th edn. Philadelphia: Lippincott Williams & Wilkins; 2000.

37. Franklin B, Whaley M, Howley E. Health screening and risk stratification in ASCM's guidelines for exercise testing and prescription. 6th edn. Philadelphia: Lippincott Williams & Wilkins; 2000.

38. Franklin B, Whaley M, Howley E. Physical fitness testing and interpretation in ACSM's guidelines for exercise testing and prescription. 6th edn. Philadelphia: Lippincott Williams & Wilkins; 2000.

39. Franklin BA. Normal cardiorespiratory response to acute aerobic exercise. In: Roitman JL, Haver EJ, Herridge M, eds. ACSM resource manual for guidelines for exercise testing and prescription. Philadelphia: Lippincott Williams & Wilkins; 2001.

40. Frontera W, Meredith CN, O'Reilly KP. Strength conditioning in older men: skeletal muscle hypertrophy and improved functioning. J Appl Physiol 1988; 64:1038–1044.

41. Frontera WR, Moldover JR, Borg-Stein J, et al. Exercise. In: Gonzalez EG, Myers SJ, eds. Downey and Darling's physiological basis of rehabilitation medicine. 3rd edn. Boston: Butterworth-Heinemann; 2001.

42. Gauffin H, Tropp H, Odenrick P. Effect of ankle disk training on postural control in patients with functional instability of the ankle joint. Int J Sports Med 1988; 9(2):141–144.

43. Gleim GW, McHugh MP. Flexibility and its effects on sports injury and performance. Sports Med 1997; 24(5):289–299.

44. Glick J. Muscle strains: prevention and treatment. Physician Sports Med 1980; 6:73–77.

45. Godshall RW. The predictability of athletic injuries: an eight-year study. J Sports Med 1975; 3(1):50–54.

46. Goldspink D. The influence of immobilization and stretch on protein turnover of rat skeletal muscle. J Physiol 1977; 264:267–282.

47. Goldspink G, Williams P. The nature of the increased passive resistance in muscle following immobilization of the mouse soleus muscle. J Physiol 1979; 289:55P.

48. Golnick P, Karlsson J, Peihl K. Selective glycogen depletion in skeletal muscle fibers of man following sustained contractions. J Physiol 1974; 241:59–67.

49. Grahame R, Jenkins JM. Joint hypermobility—asset or liability? A study of joint mobility in ballet dancers. Ann Rheum Dis 1972; 31(2):109–111.

50. Grahame R. Joint hypermobility—clinical aspects. Proc R Soc Med 1971; 64(6):692–694.

51. Grana WA, Moretz JA. Ligamentous laxity in secondary school athletes. JAMA 1978; 240(18):1975–1976.

52. Guyton A. Textbook of medical physiology. Philadelphia: Saunders; 1996.

53. Gwinup G. Weight loss without dietary restriction: efficacy of different forms of aerobic exercise. Am J Sports Med 1987; 15:275–279.

54. Halpern B, Thompson N, Curl W. High school football injuries: identifying the risk factors. Am J Sports Med 1987; 15:316–320.

55. Harris M. Flexibility. Phys Ther 1968; 49:591–601.

56. Hart J, Ingersoll C. Weightlifting. In: O'Connor F, Sallis R, Wilder R, et al, eds. Sports medicine: just the facts. New York: McGraw-Hill; 2005.

57. Hattori K, Ohta S. Ankle joint flexibility in college soccer players. J Hum Ergol 1986; 15:85–89.

58. Hellebrandt FA, Houtz SJ. Methods of muscle training: the influence of pacing. Phys Ther Rev 1958; 38:319–322.

59. Hewett T, Lindenfield T, Riccobene J. The effect of neuromuscular training on the incidence of knee injury in female athletes: a prospective study. Am J Phys Med 1999; 24:765–773.

60. Hewett TE, Stroupe AL, Nance TA, et al. Plyometric training in female athletes. Decreased impact forces and increased hamstring torques. Am J Sports Med 1996; 24(6):765–773.

61. Holly RG, Shaffrath JD. Cardiorespiratory endurance. In: Roitman JL, Haver EJ, Herridge M, et al, eds. ACSM resource manual for guidelines for exercise testing and prescription. Philadelphia: Lippincott Williams & Wilkins; 2001.

62. Huxley AF, Simmons RM. Mechanical properties of the cross-bridges of frog striated muscle. J Physiol 1971; 218(1):59P–60P.

63. Johns R, Wright V. Relative importance of various tissues in joint stiffness. J Appl Physiol 1962; 17:814–828.

64. Johnson JE, Sim FH, Scott SG. Musculoskeletal injuries in competitive swimmers. Mayo Clin Proc 1987; 62(4):289–304.

65. Kabat H. Proprioceptive facilitation in therapeutic exercise. In: Licht S, ed. Therapeutic exercise. 2nd edn. New Haven: E Licht; 1961.

66. Kabat H. Studies on neuromuscular dysfunction, XI. New principles of neuromuscular reeducation. Perm Found Med Bull 1947; 5:111.

67. Kalenak A, Morehouse CA. Knee stability and knee ligament injuries. JAMA 1975; 234(11):1143–1145.

68. Keller C, Noyes F, Buchner R. Sports traumatology series: the medical aspects of soccer injury epidemiology. Am J Phys Med 1987; 15:230–237.

69. Keller C, Noyes F, Buchner R. Sports traumatology series: the medical aspects of soccer injury epidemiology. Am J Phys Med 1987; 15:230–237.

70. Kenny W, Humphrey R, Bryant C. ACSM's guidelines for exercise testing and prescription. 5th edn. Philadelphia: Williams & Wilkins; 1995.

71. Kim H, Kerr R, Cruz T, et al. Effects of continuous passive motion and immobilization on synovitis and cartilage degradation in antigen arthritis. J Rheumatol 1995; 22:1714–1721.

72. Kirchner G, Glines D. Comparative analysis of Eugene, Oregon elementary school children using the Kraus–Weber test of minimum muscular fitness. Res Q 1957; 28:16–25.

73. Knight KL. Knee rehabilitation by the daily adjustable progressive resistive exercise technique. Am J Sports Med 1979; 7:336–337.

74. Knuttgen HG. Development of muscular strength and endurance. In: Knuttgen HG, ed. Neuromuscular mechanisms for therapeutic and conditioning exercises. Baltimore: University Park Press; 1976:97–118.

75. Kraus H. Backache, stress, and tension. Their cause, prevention and treatment. New York: Simon & Schuster; 1965.

76. Lichtenstein MJ, Shields SL, Shiavi RG, et al. Clinical determinants of biomechanics platform measures of balance in aged women. J Am Geriatr Soc 1988; 36(11):996–1002.

77. Lord SR, Sambrook PN, Gilbert C, et al. Postural stability, falls and fractures in the elderly: results from the Dubbo Osteoporosis Epidemiology Study. Med J Aust 1994; 160(11):684–685.

78. Maki BE, Holliday PJ, Fernie GR. Aging and postural control. A comparison of spontaneous and induced-sway balance tests. J Am Geriatr Soc 1990; 38(1):1–9.

79. Moritani T, de Vries H. Potential for gross muscle hypertrophy in older men. J Gerontol 1980; 35:672–682.

80. Nicholas JA. Injuries to knee ligaments. Relationship to looseness and tightness in football players. JAMA 1970; 212(13):2236–2239.

81. Noble B, Borg G, Jacobs I. A category-ratio perceived exertion scale: relationship to blood and muscle lactates and heart rate. Med Sci Sports Exerc 1983; 15:523–528.

82. Phalen G, Dickson J. Spondylolisthesis and tight hamstrings. J Bone Joint Surg Am 1961; 43:505–512.

83. Phillips M. Analysis of results from the Kraus–Weber test of minimum fitness in children. Res Q 1955; 26:314–323.

84. Polley H, Hunder G. Physical examination of the joints. 2nd edn. Philadelphia: Saunders; 1978.

85. Pollock M, Gaesser G, Butcher J. The recommended quantity and quality of exercise for developing and maintaining cardiorespiratory and muscular fitness, and flexibility in healthy adults. American College of Sports Medicine position stand. Med Sci Sports Exerc 1998; 30(6).

86. Ross J, Gilbert G. National Children and Youth Fitness Study: a summary of findings. J Phys Educ Recreation Dance 1985; 56(1):45–50.

87. Rupp JC. Exercise physiology. In: Roitman JL, Bibi KW, Thompson WR, eds. ACSM health fitness certification review. Philadelphia: Lippincott Williams & Wilkins; 2001.

88. Saal J. Flexibility training. In: Kibler W, ed. Functional rehabilitation of sports and musculoskeletal injuries. Gaithersburg: Aspen; 1998:85–97.

89. Sady SP, Wortman M, Blanke D. Flexibility training: ballistic, static or proprioceptive neuromuscular facilitation? Arch Phys Med Rehabil 1982; 63(6):261–263.

90. Salter R. History of rest and motion and the scientific basis for early continuous passive motion. Hand Clin 1996; 12:1–11.

91. Seto C. Basic principles of exercise training. In: O'Connor F, Sallis R, Wilder R, et al, eds. Sports medicine: just the facts. New York: McGraw-Hill; 2005.

92. Shellock F, Prentice W. Warming up and stretching for improved physical performance and prevention of sports-related injuries. Sports Med 1985; 2:267–278.

93. Shyne K, Dominquez R. To stretch or not to stretch? Physician Sports Med 1982; 10:137–140.

94. Simoneau GG, Derr JA, Ulbrecht JS, et al. Diabetic sensory neuropathy effect on ankle joint movement perception. Arch Phys Med Rehabil 1996; 77(5):453–460.

95. Skinner HB, Barrack RL, Cook SD. Age-related decline in proprioception. Clin Orthop Relat Res 1984; 184:208–211.

96. Stephens MB, O'Connor F, Deuster P. Exercise and nutrition. American Academy of Family Physician's home study self-assessment program, monograph 283. Leawood: American Academy of Family Physicians; 2002.

97. Stolov WC, Weilepp TG Jr, Riddell WM. Passive length–tension relationship and hydroxyproline content of chronically denervated skeletal muscle. Arch Phys Med Rehabil 1970; 51(9):517–525.

98. Stolov WC, Weilepp TG Jr. Passive length–tension relationship of intact muscle, epimysium, and tendon in normal and denervated gastrocnemius of the rat. Arch Phys Med Rehabil 1966; 47(9):612–620.

99. Surburg P. Flexibility exercises re-examined. Athl Train 1983; spring: 37040.

100. Surburg P. Neuromuscular facilitation techniques in sports medicine. Physician Sports Med 1981; 9:115–127.

101. Thibodeau GA, Patton KT. Anatomy and physiology. St. Louis: Mosby; 1999.

102. Topper AK, Maki BE, Holliday PJ. Are activity-based assessments of balance and gait in the elderly predictive of risk of falling and/or type of fall? J Am Geriatr Soc 1993; 41(5):479–487.

103. Tropp H, Ekstrand J, Gillquist J. Stabilometry in functional instability of the ankle and its value in predicting injury. Med Sci Sports Exerc 1984; 16(1):64–66.

104. de Vries H, Housh T. Prevention of muscular distress after exercise. Res Q 1960; 32:177–185.

105. de Vries H. Electromyographic observations of effects of static stretching upon muscular distress. Res Q 1960; 32:468–479.

106. de Vries HA, Whistle RA, Bulbulian R. Tranquilizer effect of exercise. Acute effects of moderate aerobic exercise on spinal reflex activation level. Am J Phys Med 1981; 60:57–66.

107. Warren C, Lehmann J, Koblanski J. Heat and stretch procedures: an evaluation using rat tail tendon. Arch Phys Med Rehabil 1976; 57:122–126.

108. Whaley MH, Kaminsky LA. Epidemiology of physical activity, physical fitness and selected chronic diseases. In: Roitman JL, Haver EJ, Herridge M et al, eds. ACSM resource manual for guidelines for exercise testing and prescription. Philadelphia: Lippincott Williams & Wilkins; 2001.

109. Wiktorsson-Moller M, Oberg B, Ekstrand J, et al. Effects of warming up, massage, and stretching on range of motion and muscle strength in the lower extremity. Am J Sports Med 1983; 11(4):249–252.

110. Williams J, Moran M, Thonar E, et al. Continuous passive motion stimulates repair of rabbit knee articular cartilage after matrix proteoglycan loss. Clin Orthop 1994; 304:252–262.

111. Williams P, Goldspink G. Changes in sarcomere length and physiological properties in immobilized muscle. J Anat 1978; 127(3):459–468.

112. Witzke KA, Snow CM. Effects of plyometric jump training on bone mass in adolescent girls. Med Sci Sports Exerc 2000; 32(6):1051–1057.

113. Zarins B. Soft tissue repair: biomechanical aspects. Int J Sports Med 1982; 3:9–11.

Chapter

20

Manipulation, Traction and Massage
Jeffrey S. Brault, Robert E. Kappler and Brian E. Grogg

The 'laying on of hands' has been a diagnostic and therapeutic modality used since antiquity, and has created a special bond between practitioner and patient. Over the millennia, a multitude of 'hands on' techniques have been employed to treat human suffering. Although they have waxed and waned in popularity, these modalities and techniques have been gaining acceptance in recent years. These methods have been utilized as an 'aggressive' non-surgical approach to the treatment of musculoskeletal disorders, particularly neck and low back pain.

Neck and low back pain have reached epidemic proportions in many industrialized nations. It has been estimated that approximately 80% of all adults will experience low back pain in their lives, and approximately 50% of individuals will experience neck pain in their lives.[51] This escalation of axial pain has created great financial ramifications for society. In recent years, there has been an attempt to reduce morbidity and improve the cost-effectiveness of therapy options.

Many physiatrists employ these modalities or lead a multidisciplinary team that does. It is imperative, as a profession, that we understand the basic principles behind manipulation, traction, and massage; their application; and their potential for complications. This chapter will address many of these issues.

MANIPULATION
Definition and goals
The International Federation of Manual Medicine[3] defines *manipulation* as 'the use of the hands in the patient management process using instructions and maneuvers to maintain maximal, painless movement of the musculoskeletal system in postural balance'. The goal of manipulation or manual medicine is to help maintain optimal body mechanics and to improve motion in restricted areas. Enhancing maximal, pain-free movement in a balanced posture and optimizing function are major goals.[39,60,112] These goals are accomplished by treatments that attempt to restore the mechanical function of a joint and normalize altered reflex patterns,[98,112] as evidenced by optimal range of motion, body symmetry, and tissue texture. The indications for successful use of manual medicine techniques are determined by structural evaluation before and after treatment.[60,94]

Manual medicine can involve manipulation of spinal and peripheral joints as well as myofascial tissues (muscles and fascia). The most fundamental use of manual medicine is to relieve motion restriction and improve motion asymmetry. Improved motion and flexibility are helpful in restoring optimal muscle function and ease of motion. A decrease in pain is often associated with restoration of normal motion. Sometimes therapy is directed at reduction of afferent (nociceptive) input to the cord. Endorphin release increases pain threshold and reduces pain severity.[59,80,98]

The ultimate goal of manipulation is to improve the function and well-being of the patient. Examples of this include reduction of pain, improved ambulatory ability, and improved efficiency of biomechanical motion. The most basic enabling objective is to improve motion. There are physiologic objectives, such as decreasing nociceptive input, decreasing gamma gain, enhancing lymphatic return, and improving circulation to the tissues.

Manual medicine continues to be widely practiced and is in high demand by patients.[40] It is estimated that 12 to 17.6 million Americans[114,118] receive manipulations each year, with a high degree of patient satisfaction.[23]

Overview of various types of manual medicine
Manual medicine techniques can be classified in different ways. Techniques may be classified as soft tissue technique, articulatory technique, or specific joint mobilization.[94] The objective to be accomplished may be used as a type of technique, such as movement of fluids. The terms 'direct' and 'indirect' are used to classify technique, with several types of technique in each category. Direct technique means that the practitioner moves the body part(s) in the direction of the restrictive barrier. Indirect technique means the practitioner moves the body part away from the restrictive barrier.

Direct techniques are as follow.

- Thrust (impulse, high velocity, low amplitude): the final activating force is operator force.
- Articulation: low velocity, high amplitude.
- Muscle energy (direct isometric types): the final activating force is a patient contraction.
- Direct myofascial release: load (stretch) tissues, hold, and wait for release.

The following are indirect techniques:

- strain–counterstrain;
- indirect balancing;
- multiple names (functional, balanced ligamentous tension);
- indirect myofascial release; and
- craniosacral.

Historical perspective and practitioners

Manual medicine has regained popularity over the past 30–40 years, but its practice dates back to the time of Hippocrates (460–377 BC) and Galen (131–202 BC).[67,68] Many other physicians (e.g. Sydenham, Hahnemann, Boerhaave, and Shultes) deviated from the traditional disease-oriented form of medicine during the sixteenth and seventeenth centuries,[68] but manual medicine fell out of favor until the nineteenth century. The pioneers of manual medicine at that time included the 'bone-setters' of England (Richard Hutton, Wharton Hood, and Sir Herbert Baker);[20,68] Andrew Taylor Still, the founder of osteopathic medicine in 1874;[60] and Daniel David Palmer, the founder of chiropractic medicine in 1895.[60,68]

Still's philosophy stressed wellness and wholeness of the body.[100] Osteopathic principles include the body is a unit, the body possesses self-healing mechanisms, and structure and function are interrelated; all these are incorporated into practice.[142] Manual medicine was an integral part of his treatment.

'Traditional' medical professionals have also shown interest in manual medicine. Mennell[101] and his son John M. Mennell,[105] as well as Edgar and James Cyriax,[33] have espoused the use of joint manipulation within the British medical community. Beginning in the 1940s, James Cyriax, a British orthopedic surgeon, published several works related to manipulation, incorporating massage, traction, and injections.[33] Travell's[138] use of manual techniques for examination purposes has been widely accepted. Today, the Fédération Internationale de Médecine Manuelle represents manual medicine practitioners throughout the world.

Barrier concept

The barrier concept recognizes limitation of motion of a normal joint in which asymmetric motion is present. Motion is relatively free in one direction, with loss of some motion in the other direction. Motion loss occurs within the normal range of motion for that joint (see Fig. 20-1).

The barrier concept implies that something is preventing a full range of motion of a joint. The term *pathologic barrier* was initially used to describe that point where normal motion is limited. The current term used is *restrictive barrier*, which means there is no organic pathology that might be seen under the microscope: these are functional restrictions. The motion restriction associated with somatic dysfunction occurs within the normal range of motion of the joint. The new neutral position has shifted in the direction of less restricted motion. This gives rise to positional asymmetry. The lay terms 'out' or 'out of place' are often used to describe this positional asymmetry. Manipulation is designed to restore normal motion. Manipula-

tion does not put the joint back in place. If a joint is dislocated, this is not somatic dysfunction. Dislocation involves movement beyond the anatomic barrier and involves associated tissue damage.

Normal and abnormal coupled spinal motion

Motion of the spine follows principles of spinal motion often attributed to Harrison H. Fryette.[50] Flexion (forward bending) and extension (backward bending) are sagittal plane motions and are not coupled. However, rotation and side bending are coupled. The amount of pure rotation or pure side bending of spinal joints is limited. Rotation and side bending occur together in normal spinal joints. Fryette stated that when there is an absence of marked flexion or extension (termed *neutral*) and side bending is introduced, a group of vertebrae rotate into the produced convexity, with maximum rotation at the apex. Rotation and side bending occur to opposite sides when compared with the original starting position. This is sometimes referred to as neutral mechanics or type 1 dysfunction. Non-neutral or type 2 mechanics involve a component of flexion or extension with rotation and side bending to the same side. This is usually single-segment motion, although several segments may be involved. The cervical spine (C2–C7) exhibits rotation and side bending to the same side, whether flexed, neutral, or extended.

Some atypical joints (occiput, atlas, and sacrum) do not have an intervertebral disk. Their motion patterns are dictated by anatomy. The major motion of the occiput is flexion and extension. Rotation and side bending occur to opposite sides because of the anatomic construction of the joint. The major motion of the atlas is rotation. The atlas rotates around the dens (odontoid process). Half the rotation of the cervical spine occurs at the atlas. Flexion and extension occurs but is not involved in motion restriction of the atlas. The atlas does not side bend as it rotates. Actually, both sides of the atlas translate inferiorly during rotation, but side bending does not occur. Trauma can produce atypical motion patterns!

Nomenclature
Somatic dysfunction

Manual medicine or manipulation involves treating motion restrictions. Nomenclature to describe this motion restriction, which is being manipulated, has changed. The term *manipulatable lesion* is a generic term to describe musculoskeletal dysfunction that might respond to manipulation. Previous terms included *osteopathic lesion*, *subluxation*, *joint blockage*, *loss of joint play*, and *joint dysfunction*.[97,98,112]

Somatic dysfunction is a diagnostic term listed in the International Classification of Diseases-9 classification of diagnoses. It is defined as impaired or altered function of related components of the somatic (body framework) system; skeletal, arthrodial, and myofascial structures; and related vascular, lymphatic, and neural elements.[60] Somatic dysfunction represents a critical concept in manipulative medicine. Somatic dysfunction is diagnosed by palpation. Dysfunctions that are palpated include changes in tissue texture, increased sensitivity to touch (hyper-

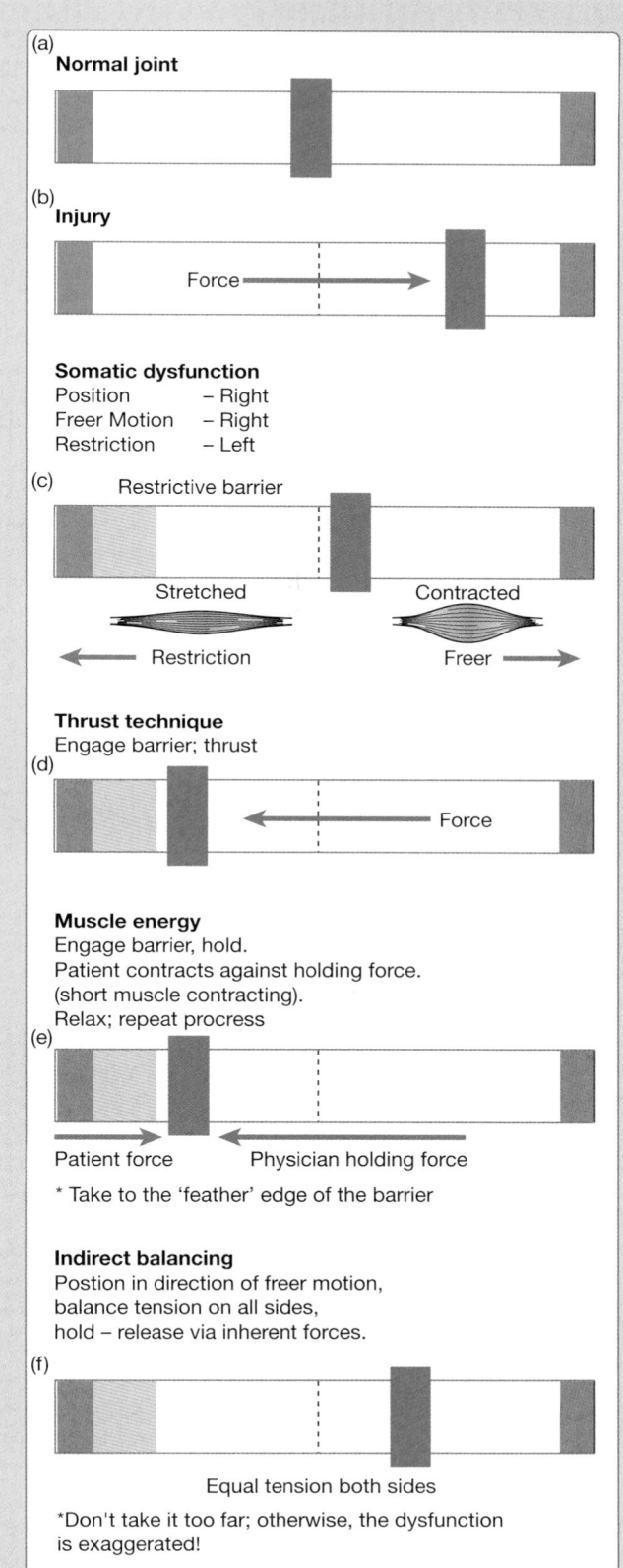

(a) Normal joint

(b) Injury

Force

Somatic dysfunction
Position   – Right
Freer Motion   – Right
Restriction   – Left

(c) Restrictive barrier

Stretched   Contracted

← Restriction   Freer →

Thrust technique
Engage barrier; thrust
(d)

Force

Muscle energy
Engage barrier, hold.
Patient contracts against holding force.
(short muscle contracting).
Relax; repeat procrress
(e)

Patient force   Physician holding force

* Take to the 'feather' edge of the barrier

Indirect balancing
Postion in direction of freer motion,
balance tension on all sides,
hold – release via inherent forces.
(f)

Equal tension both sides

*Don't take it too far; otherwise, the dysfunction
is exaggerated!

Figure 20-1 A model of somatic dysfunction. The first three panels depict production of somatic dysfunction from a mechanical cause. The last three panels depict treatment positions using thrust technique, isometric muscle energy technique, and indirect balancing. (**a**) A *normal joint* is positioned in the center, with free motion available in either direction. The shaded area at either end depicts the end of permitted motion. The outside line is termed the anatomic barrier. If joint motion goes beyond this point, structural damage will occur. The *Glossary of Osteopathic Terminology* describes the anatomic barrier as the end point of passive motion, and the physiologic barrier as the end point of active motion. (**b**) This graph, *injury*, shows a force moving the center of the joint to the right. (**c**) The third graph, *somatic dysfunction*, shows the effect of the injury. The neutral point is now positioned to the right. The muscle on the right is contracted and shortened, the muscle on the left is stretched (strained). Motion to the right is freer, motion to the left exhibits bind or restriction. This is asymmetric motion, which is typical of spinal somatic dysfunction. There is restriction of motion to the left, so that the range of motion is impaired. The end point of this restriction of motion to the left is termed the *restrictive barrier*. Think of the barrier as a series of restrainers that are preventing motion to the left, as contrasted to a brick wall preventing motion. The short, tight muscle on the right prevents full motion to the left. The last three graphs show treatment position. (**d**) Thrust technique (impulse, high velocity, low amplitude) is a direct technique. The barrier is engaged by moving the joint to the left. The final corrective force is a physician force. (**e**) Direct isometric muscle energy technique looks very similar on the graph. The barrier is engaged by moving the joint to the left. Mitchell describes this as engaging the 'feather edge' of the barrier. The physician holds, and asks the patient to contract against the holding force. The shortened contracted muscle is the one that is contracting. (**f**) Indirect balancing involves moving the joint to the right, away from the restrictive barrier. The tension should be balanced on both sides. Final corrective force is a release by inherent forces.

algesia), altered ease or range of motion, and anatomic asymmetry or positional change.[144]

Naming of a lesion (somatic dysfunction)

The *Glossary of Osteopathic Terminology*[142] describes three ways of naming somatic dysfunction.

1. Where is it or what position is it in (e.g. right rotated)?
2. What will it do or what is the direction of freer motion (e.g. right strain)?
3. What won't it do or what is the direction of restriction (e.g. restriction of left rotation)?

Segmental dysfunctions are named for the anterior superior portion of the upper vertebrae in relation to the lower, for example T3 in relation to T4. Nomenclature can be expanded to include the three planes of motion, for example T3 flexed, rotated, and side bent right. Group curves are traditionally named for the convex side. For example, a right thoracic curve is a thoracic curve convex right. It can also be termed *dextroscoliosis*.

A dysfunction should be named in three planes of motion, with the upper segment described in relation to the lower. For type 2 dysfunctions, an example of proper nomenclature would be T3 in relation to T4, flexed, rotated, and side bent right. Abbreviations are often used. An example of naming a type 1 group curve would be L1–L5 neutral, rotated right, side bent left. This would be a lateral curve convex right.

The Educational Council on Osteopathic Principles has described the point for naming vertebral motion as the most anterior superior part of the vertebral body. For flexion, this point moves forward; for extension, it moves backward. For side bending right, the point moves to the right. Naming rotation is the most common problem. Right rotation involves this point moving right. With left rotation, this point moves left. With right rotation, the right transverse process moves posteriorly. Some practitioners describe rotation using movement of the spinous process. An easy way to remember rotation is to consider riding a bicycle. The handlebars represent the transverse processes. How do you turn the handlebars to turn right? Turning right is an example of right rotation.

Physiologic rationale for manual therapies

Gamma system
Two types of motor neuron exit the spinal cord through the ventral rami to innervate skeletal muscle. Alpha motor neurons innervate large skeletal muscle fibers. A motor unit consists of a single alpha motor neuron and the skeletal muscle fibers it innervates. Gamma motor neurons innervate intrafusal fibers in the muscle spindle. These intrafusal fibers have annulospiral and flower spray endings that report information about muscle length or rate of change of muscle length. Increased gamma activity of the muscle spindles results in increased alpha motor neuron activity to extrafusal fibers of skeletal muscle. From a clinical perspective, if a muscle is too tight, the practitioner attempts to bring about muscle relaxation. Decreasing gamma gain activity is one mechanism that results in muscle relaxation.[38]

Golgi tendon reflex
Golgi tendon organs are encapsulated sensory mechanoreceptors located in tendons between the muscle and tendon insertions. These receptors report on tension, and at the spinal cord level they synapse with inhibitory interneurons. Increased tension in a skeletal muscle inhibits alpha motor neurons to that muscle, which causes decreased firing of motor units.

If the muscle spindle is stretched, increased activity of the gamma system stimulates muscle activity. This is just the opposite activity of the Golgi tendon reflex. The gamma system functions to prevent tearing or overstretching of the belly of a muscle. The Golgi apparatus serves to protect the tendon. If a muscle is shortened sufficiently, the stretch receptors cease firing and the alpha motor neurons are turned off.

Muscle stretch reflexes
Muscle stretch reflexes, such as the patellar tendon reflex, are considered to be monosynaptic. With the knee flexed to 90°, the quadriceps muscle is placed in a mild stretch. A sudden strike of a hammer against the tendon results in a dynamic stretch. This stimulates the alpha motor neurons to contract the quadriceps muscle, extending the knee.

Spinal facilitation
Spinal cord facilitation is maintenance of a pool of neurons in a state of subthreshold excitation. In this state, less afferent stimulation is required to produce a response. Consider a model of a sound system with a microphone, amplifier, and speaker. Facilitation acts as if the gain control on the amplifier is turned up. Given a normal input to the microphone, the speaker is too loud. In patients with somatic dysfunction, the muscles are hypertonic and shortened. Spinal facilitation results in hyperactivity of both the general somatic system and the sympathetic nervous systems.

Early research studies on facilitation demonstrate how behavior of the spinal cord is altered. Korr and Denslow[97] applied pressure to spinous processes and measured how much pressure was necessary to produce an electromyographic response in the muscle. A facilitated segment requires less pressure to produce a response. The sympathetic nervous system innervates sweat glands (although this is a cholinergic response). Spinal cord facilitation results in increased sweating at the segmental level. Other factors affect spinal cord behavior. Patterson demonstrated that the spinal cord has 'memory' that results in conditioned reflexes. If a stimulus is maintained for a certain period of time, then removal of the stimulus does not eliminate the response.[115] At one time, it was considered that the amount of afferent input produced facilitation. However, when the mix of afferent input is altered, it is as if the cord listens more carefully to the signals (sensitization) coming in. Afferent input from dysfunctional visceral structures produces viscerosomatic reflexes and facilitation.

What maintains facilitation? At one time, it was thought that the muscle spindle with increased gamma tone was the basic factor in maintaining facilitation. Subsequent studies have shown that nociception maintains facilitation.[140] Animal studies have been conducted in which afferent fibers from the spindle to the cord were cut, and facilitation continued. Blocking nociceptive input tends to cause facilitation to disappear.

The previous discussion of neurophysiology only scratches the surface. The spinal cord is connected to the brain. There is a vertical component to nerve conduction to and from the brain, as well as a horizontal component between dorsal and ventral roots. There is a neuroendocrine immune system at work. Neuropeptides can sensitize primary afferent fibers, as well as fibers within the central nervous system. The practitioner needs to understand the physiologic mechanisms behind muscle tightness, motion restriction, nociception, and inflammation that create dysfunction. Manipulation is one of the treatments used to decrease dysfunction and help the patient. Much of the data necessary to use manipulation effectively come from palpatory assessment rather than high-tech testing. Simple soft tissue techniques are designed to relax tight muscles and fascia. Forces applied too fast or too heavy will cause the muscle to fight back. The response to the application of force is continuously monitored to make sure the muscle is relaxing. The focus of the practitioner during treatment is to assess how the patient is responding to the treatment rather than whether or not the gamma gain has been reduced. Figure 20-1 illustrates how a shortened and contracted muscle can restrict motion.

Examination and diagnosis

An examination is a process of data gathering. Subjective data can be obtained by taking a history. Patient complaints are elicited. Sometimes, there are complaints or concerns that are held back by the patient. The practitioner should be aware of these possibilities and attempt to elicit an accurate history. Pain, discomfort, or functional loss is a frequent complaint.

Physical examination includes acquiring a sufficient physical examination database to enable appropriate diagnosis and treatment. Emergency room patients are routinely examined for head, eyes, ears, nose, and throat (HEENT), heart, lungs, and abdomen. The musculoskeletal examination goes beyond looking for problems in a system. You should look for clues about the health status and function of the patient. Is there a somatic component(s) to the patient's problem(s)? The musculoskeletal screening examination looks at gait, posture, and symmetry or asymmetry. This is ordinarily done in the standing position. A standardized 12-step biomechanical screening examination may be done,[60] or the screening examination may be non-standard, using a systematic approach to evaluate all body regions. This examination can be integrated into a comprehensive physical examination.

Experienced physicians often raise questions, and the examination is tailored to finding answers to the questions. Students ordinarily follow a standardized process when doing an examination. For efficiency, the examination should utilize multiple positions: standing, seated, supine, and prone. In order to conserve time and enhance efficiency, you should complete all tests in one position before moving the patient to the next position. The mnemonic for a musculoskeletal examination is TART: T, tenderness or sensitivity; A, asymmetry (look); R, restriction of motion (move); T, tissue texture abnormality (feel). The diagnosis of somatic dysfunction is based on a palpatory examination using TART.

Palpation for tissue texture abnormality

Tissue texture abnormality is palpable evidence of physiologic dysfunction. The approach to palpation is to compare right versus left and above versus below. When evaluating a single area without comparing with adjacent areas, it is difficult to come to a meaningful conclusion. Palpation is done in layers, projecting your sense of touch to the depth required.

Acute tissue texture change can be described and remembered by thinking of acute inflammation and the four cardinal signs: red, puffy, painful or tender, and warm. With acute tissue texture changes, sweating is increased and the skin is usually moist (increased sympathetic tone). Chronic tissue texture abnormality is associated with thin, dry, atrophic skin that is cool. The palpatory quality is firm or fibrotic. Motion testing reveals motion loss.

Paraspinal viscerosomatic reflexes have palpatory qualities that are characteristic and allow the experienced clinician to come to a conclusion that these changes are due to visceral disturbances. The maximum intensity of the findings is reported to be at the costotransverse and rib angle areas. The greatest number of findings is in the skin and subcutaneous tissue. Dr. Kimberly[94] described these findings as 'minimal motion loss lesions'. Chronic viscerosomatic findings take on the characteristics of any chronic somatic dysfunction. Clinically, findings present as an acute exacerbation of a chronic problem, with the superficial puffiness of acute change and the motion restriction of chronic somatic dysfunction. In the interscapular area, failure to move the scapula laterally to allow adequate palpation of the rib angles will result in failure to detect musculoskeletal findings.

Palpating for tissue texture abnormality can be an accurate and efficient method of identifying problem areas in the musculoskeletal system that require further examination.

Motion testing

There are multiple methods for motion testing. Because manipulative treatment has as its immediate objective the improvement of motion, motion testing skills and treatment skills become intertwined. Norman J. Larson, D.O., stated, 'Your ability to treat is directly proportional to your ability to palpate' (N.J. Larson, personal communication).

Types of motion testing include the following.

- Inspection of active motion.
- Palpation of active motion with palpating fingers over the facet area.
- Rib motion, which is often tested by palpating motion as the patient inhales and exhales.
- Active hand–passive hand, which is motion testing in which one hand does the moving and the other hand assesses motion (e.g. moving the head and neck while palpating in the upper thoracic spine).
- Direct passive motion testing in which the physician's hands provide the force and also monitor response to this force. Terms to describe the 'feel' might be ease and bind or freedom and resistance (Fig. 20-2).

The muscle energy type of motion testing looks for the most posterior transverse process. Place the palpating fingers on the transverse process area of both sides of the segment to be tested. Instruct the patient to flex and extend. For example, assume T3 is extended, rotated, and side bent right. When T3 is flexed (this is the barrier), the muscle on the right side 'balls up' under the palpating finger, and the right transverse process becomes more posterior. When T3 is extended, the findings on either side are decreased. The concept demonstrated is that positional asymmetry is increased when the barrier is engaged.

Using the same example of T3 extended, rotated, and side bent right, flex T3 by flexing the head and neck. Attempt to rotate right and left. Left rotation will be very restricted. Extend T3 and again rotate. Left rotation will be much freer. This confirms that the barrier is flexion, and the dysfunction is extended.

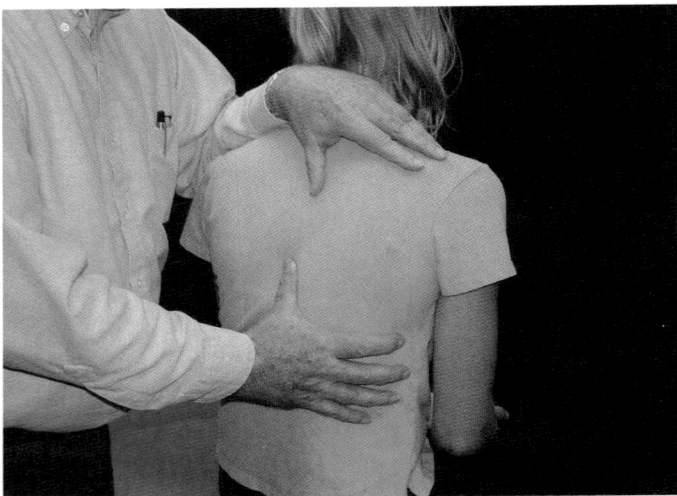

Figure 20-2 Motion testing or articulatory treatment of the thoracic spine. The patient is seated, and the physician stands behind the patient. The physician's left arm is draped over the patient's shoulder girdles. This enables the physician to introduce forces from above: rotation, side bending, lateral translation, and flexion–extension. The physician's other hand contacts the right side of the thoracic spine. This position is useful for motion evaluation with the patient seated. Articulatory treatment involving left rotation can be done with a combination of force with both the physician's arms or hands.

Functional technique assessment[16,84]

The tissues on either side of the dysfunction are palpated for tension with the joint close to the midline and not close to the barriers. Tension is evaluated in the three cardinal planes, three translations, and respiration. The position for indirect treatment involves equal tension on both sides.

Assessment of fascia

Fascia has unique features that include the formation of sheets with multidirectional fibers giving it tensile strength, and sheets with non-linear motion that allow for shortening and elongating, thus accounting for its flexibility and pliability. In contrast, there is little or no motion in scar tissue. Fascia is three-dimensional and can form sleeves to compartmentalize, act as cables, or form diaphragms. All these properties must be considered when assessing fascia.

Assessment of fascia starts with placement of the hands to perceive the combined vector force in the tissue. Hand placement varies depending on the area to be assessed and treated. Assessment of an extremity would start with hand placement proximal and distal to the area. An example of this would be the assessment of the forearm. One hand grasps the patient's hand and the other hand grasps the proximal forearm near the elbow.

In the assessment of a three-dimensional region such as the chest cage, the hands will start with one anterior and the other posterior on the thorax. The hands should be placed in such a manner that they are 180° to one another. Assessment of a large area, such as the thoracolumbar fascia, may begin with the

hands placed in the same direction, on either side of the spine, adjacent to each other.

Once the hands are placed, the fascia must be 'entered' by adding tension to the area to engage the viscoelastic property of fascia. The viscoelastic property allows fascia to deform. With tension in place, the practitioner can now 'read' the tissue and simultaneously assess and treat. One can move the fascia to a tightened position by combining multiple motion vectors (clockwise–counterclockwise rotation, anterior–posterior motion, cephalad–caudad motion, pronation–supination) as in a direct release, or follow the combined vector to a point of balance as in an indirect release. Examination of the fascia and myofascial structures may include looking for special 'points' or 'triggers'. These include counterstrain tenderpoints, the myofascial triggers of Simon and Travell, and acupuncture points.

Types of technique
Overview of various types of manual medicine
Manual medicine techniques can be classified in different ways. Techniques can be classified as soft tissue technique, articulatory technique, or specific joint mobilization. The objective to be accomplished may be used as a type of technique, such as movement of fluids. The terms *direct* and *indirect* are used to classify technique, with several types of technique in each category. Direct technique means that the operator moves the body part(s) in the direction of the restrictive barrier. Indirect technique means the operator moves the body part away from the restrictive barrier. Combined technique starts with indirect technique and, once the release has occurred, switches to a direct technique.

Direct techniques
Soft tissue technique   The purpose of soft tissue technique is to relax muscles and fascia. There are an infinite number of modifications of soft tissue technique. Usually, they involve lateral force to stretch the muscle, direct longitudinal stretching, or careful kneading. Sensitive hands and experience are necessary to assess the response of the tissues to the treatment. Apply forces slowly and release slowly. Do not allow tissues to snap back quickly, or they could go into spasm. Do not allow your fingers to slide over the skin. Avoid excess force per unit area; instead, spread the forces out. Avoid direct pressure over bony prominences. Soft tissue technique may be the primary approach. It may be used to prepare an area for specific mobilization. It may be used to facilitate movement of fluids. It may reduce or modify pain.

Articulatory treatment   Articulatory treatment, a form of direct technique, is a procedure to move a joint back and forth repeatedly in order to increase freedom of range of motion. Articulatory treatment may be classified as a low-velocity, high-amplitude approach. Sometimes articulatory treatment is a form of soft tissue treatment in which the only way to access deep muscles is to move origin and insertion (Fig. 20-2). Articulatory treatment is very useful for stiff joints and for older patients. It may be the only form of treatment applicable for some patients. There are many modifications to articulatory technique.

Mobilization with impulse (thrust; high velocity, low amplitude)   Thrust technique is often considered synonymous with manipulation. In Europe, thrust techniques are reserved for the physician, whereas other techniques are termed *mobilization*. Given an expansion of the various forms of techniques other than thrust, these techniques are sometimes termed *soft manipulation*. Thrust techniques are applicable for restriction of motion in joints. Thrust technique is often the quickest form of addressing restriction of joint motion. An audible pop may occur with application of the technique. The noise has no effect on treatment outcome. To assess the effectiveness of treatment, reevaluation is required.

A diagnosis of motion restriction is essential prior to application of thrust technique, and this diagnosis should incorporate the three planes of motion: flexion–extension, rotation, and side bending. The first principle of thrust technique is to engage the barrier. With an accurate diagnosis, engaging the barrier is specific. The barrier must feel solid, not rubbery. A thrust should not be applied if the barrier does not feel solid. Instead of addressing the restriction of motion of the joint, the force is dissipated by muscles and fascia. The thrust must be low amplitude, meaning a very short distance. The thrust should be high velocity (Figs 20-3–20-5). There is no place for high-velocity, high-amplitude technique.

The tissues should be prepared for thrusting technique. Soft tissue treatment is often a precursor to thrust technique. If the tissues are not properly prepared, it is more difficult to engage the barrier and more force is used. The dissipation of excess force may cause iatrogenic problems. The patient must be relaxed. There is no substitute for skilled hands that allow the patient to relax. Often, the thrust is given during exhalation, as the tissues are more relaxed at this time. The final activating force is operator force.

Muscle energy: direct isometric types   Muscle energy technique[56,108] was introduced by Fred Mitchell, Sr.[107] Muscle energy

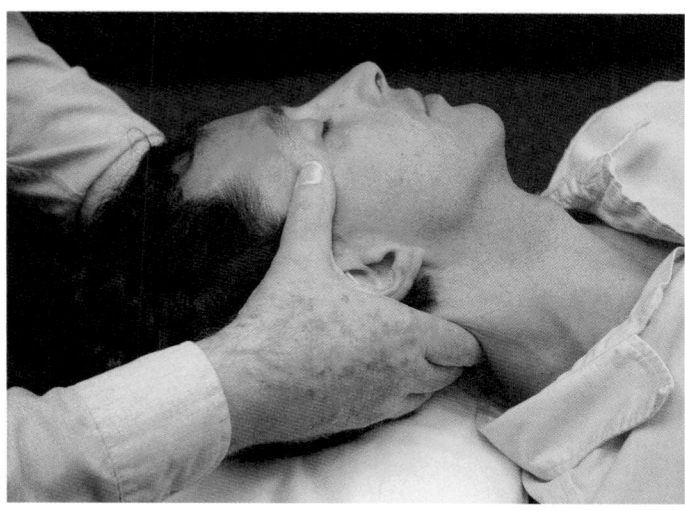

Figure 20-3 Treatment of cervical spine C2–C7. In this example, the diagnosis is C4 flexed, rotated, and side bent right. The right lateral mass of C4 is contacted with the index finger. An extension break at C4–C5 keeps force localized to the segment. The force is directed toward the patient's eye. This force is rotation left, side bending left, following the principles of physiologic motion of the cervical spine. Additionally, the plane of the facets angles up toward the eye. The force follows the plane of the facets, rather than jamming the facets, which would occur if proper side bending was not considered.

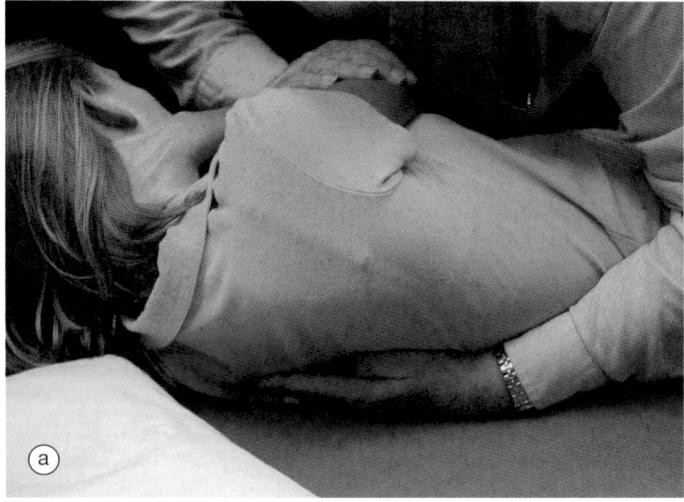
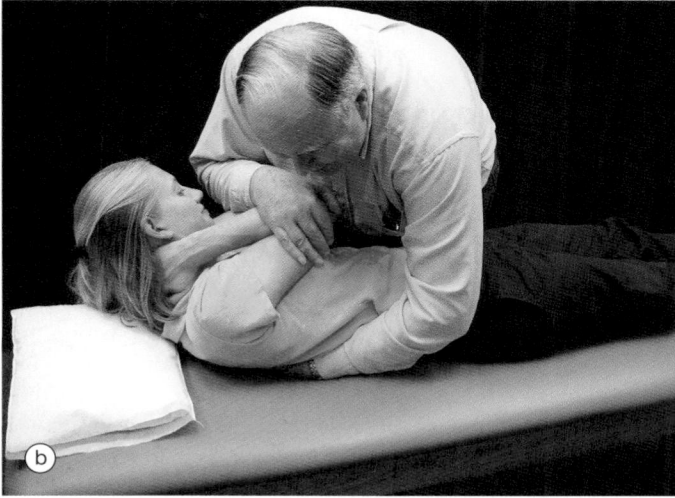

Figure 20-4 Treatment of thoracic somatic dysfunction, patient supine. There are multiple variations of this technique, sometimes referred to as the 'Kirksville krunch'. It is used for thoracic type 1 and type 2 dysfunctions, as well as ribs. The technique pictured involves T7 flexed, rotated, and side bent left. The physician stands on the left side of the supine patient. The patient's arms are folded across the chest or, as in this demonstration, the patient's hands are placed behind the neck with fingers clasped together and elbows approximated. The physician's fulcrum hand is placed over T8 right (segment below, side opposite) (**a**). The patient's torso is rolled back, and the corrective force is applied through the patient's arms (**b**). Note: many physicians place the fulcrum directly over the posterior transverse process or the posterior rib. If the thoracic dysfunction is extended, care must be given to maintain a flexed position at the site of the somatic dysfunction. The fulcrum tends to produce extension.

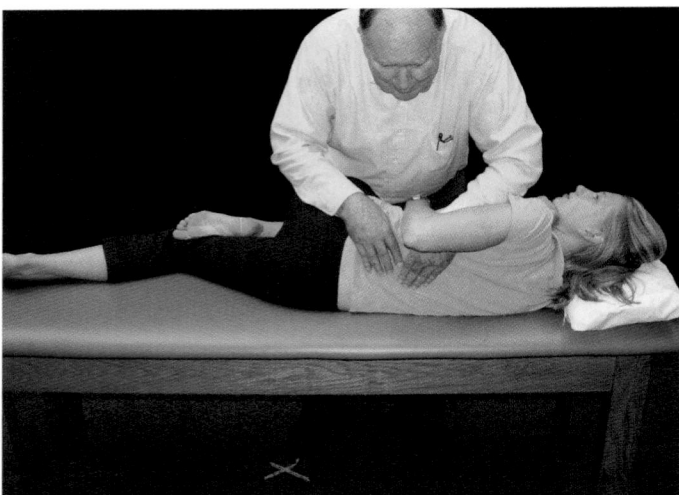

Figure 20-5 Treatment of lumbar somatic dysfunction, patient on side. The literature contains multiple approaches for side lumbar techniques. The technique being demonstrated follows principles of physiologic motion of the spine. The dysfunction is L2 flexed, rotated, and side bent right. The posterior transverse process is placed down (right side down). The patient's torso is perpendicular to the table. The patient's hips and knees are flexed, the upper leg flexed more. Extension at L2 is obtained from above. Side bending is maintained by stretching out the right side. Rotation from below is obtained by contacting the patient's iliac crest, rotating toward the operator, and applying side bending by pushing cephalad. Rotation from above is obtained by pushing the shoulder posteriorly. Additional localization is obtained by having the patient look toward the ceiling. The final corrective force on the iliac crest emphasizes side bending toward the patient's head; rotation is automatic.

technique involves the patient voluntarily moving the body as specifically directed by the physician; this directed patient action is from a precisely controlled position against a defined resistance by the physician. The initial classification of muscle energy techniques was based on whether the force was equal (isometric), greater (isotonic), or less (isolytic) than the patient force. Most muscle energy techniques used by physicians are direct isometric techniques. This technique has been utilized extensively by therapists and is often referred to as contract relax technique.

Muscle energy technique requires a specific diagnosis. The first step is moving the dysfunctional component into the restrictive barrier. Fred Mitchell, Jr.[109] emphasizes that the practitioner moves the dysfunctional component to the 'feather edge' of the barrier. The practitioner holds this position and instructs the patient to contract against the holding force. The patient controls the amount of force, so injury is not likely. Additionally, the manner in which the practitioner holds the patient position suggests the amount of force. A heavy-handed vice grip will suggest more force than a lighter touch. The muscle contraction is held for 3–5 s. Then there is a period of relaxation sometimes termed *postisometric relaxation*. The practitioner then reengages a new barrier, and the process is repeated several times. If there is no further increase in the range of motion, it is time to stop. Three repetitions are the usual number, followed by reassessment.

Most direct isometric muscle energy techniques involve the patient actively contracting the shortened (sometimes referred to as the 'sick') muscle. The usual mistakes in using muscle energy technique are failure to properly engage the barrier, application of too much force, or not allowing enough time for postisometric relaxation. While engaging the barrier involves three planes of motion, the patient contraction may be in one, two, or three planes. Often the patient contraction will be a flexion or extension. In muscle energy technique, the final activating force is a patient muscle contraction.

Direct myofascial release   The goal of myofascial technique is to identify tissue restriction and to remove the restriction. This requires sensing arms and hands. Direct myofascial technique involves loading the myofascial tissues (stretch), holding the tissues in position, and waiting for release. Release is by inherent forces. When collagen is stretched, the viscoelastic properties of collagen allow the tissues to slowly stretch. The term *creep* is applied to this phenomenon. When release occurs, there is additional lengthening of the tissues without an increase of force being applied. This phenomenon takes several seconds. This release might be described as like an ice cube melting. The release is perceived by the physician treating the patient. Reevaluation of the patient reveals a decrease of the restriction being treated, with increased freedom of range of motion.

Indirect techniques

Strain–counterstrain   Counterstrain is a type of manipulative treatment that employs spontaneous release by positioning, and utilizes tenderpoints serving as a monitor to achieve the proper position. Lawrence Jones D.O.[85] developed this method of treatment. Counterstrain is classified as indirect technique. The objective is to relieve painful dysfunction through a reduction of inappropriate afferent proprioception activity. Referring to Figure 20-1, the shortened muscle remains shortened because of inappropriate proprioceptive activity. Tenderpoints are located in the muscle belly, tendon (usually at or near the bony attachment of the tendon), or dermatome of the shortened muscle. Treatment position further shortens the short muscle, as a 'counterstrain' is applied to the originally strained muscle on the other side. The neurophysiologic mechanism is based on the fact that shortening the muscle quiets the muscle and breaks into the inappropriate strain reflex.

Tenderpoints are related to specific dysfunctions. The practitioner must know where to look for these specific points.[86] For example, if the patient has a dysfunction at L3 that is flexed, rotated, and side bent left, an anterior lumbar tenderpoint is located in the abdominal wall in the vicinity of the anterior inferior iliac spine. The use of counterstrain requires a structural evaluation and assessment for tenderpoints. Tenderpoints are tissue areas that are tender to palpation. They are sometimes described as 'pealike' areas of tension. The common denominator is the tissue change and tenderness.

Treatment involves identifying the tenderpoint, maintaining a palpating finger on the tenderpoint, and placing the patient in a position so that tenderness in this point is eliminated or

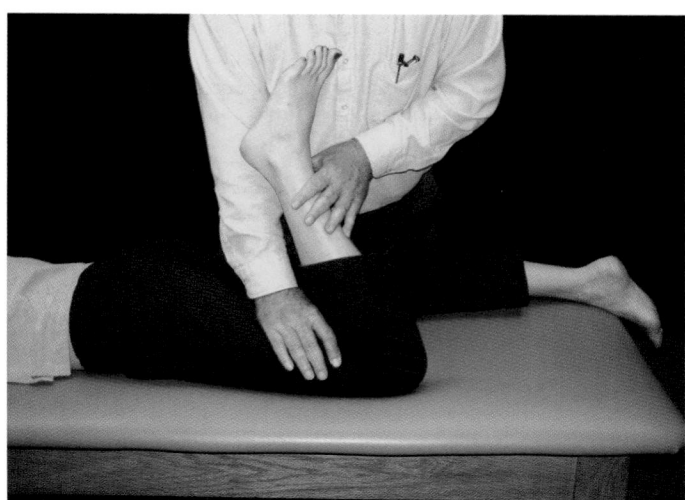

Figure 20-6 Hamstring release technique, counterstrain. The technique follows the principles of counterstrain without looking for a tenderpoint. The patient is prone, and the monitoring fingers contact the hamstring tendons close to the knee. The knee is flexed until the rectus femoris muscle is loaded, preventing increased flexion of the knee. The hamstrings are unloaded, the rectus femoris is loaded. Hold and wait for release, as monitored by contact over the hamstring tendons.

reduced significantly. This position is in a pain-free direction of ease. Also, the position places the patient in the original position of injury. Counterstrain is not a form of acupressure. The monitoring finger continues to palpate and assess the point, but pressure is not applied. The amount of time that the treatment position is held is 90 s, and for ribs 120 s. It is essential that the patient be slowly returned from the treatment position to the starting point. The patient should remain passive during the entire process. Following return, the tenderpoint is reassessed. If the physician's palpating finger stays on the tenderpoint, and tenderness is now absent, both practitioner and patient know that a change was made (Fig. 20-6).

Counterstrain is a very gentle technique with an extremely low risk of injury. However, patients can become very sore after counterstrain treatment. It is appropriate to caution patients that they might become sore after treatment. Sometimes analgesics are used to treat the soreness. Patients are often advised to drink plenty of water to maintain adequate hydration. Counterstrain can be used to treat tenderness that remains after other manual treatments have addressed motion restriction.

Indirect balancing   There are multiple names to describe types of indirect technique. These names include functional technique and balanced ligamentous tension. The common denominator in all these technique types is that they are indirect, in that the dysfunction is positioned in a direction of freer motion away from the restrictive barrier. The positioning involves achieving a balance of tension on all sides of the dysfunction. The functional technique of Johnston[84] involves balancing tension in the three translations (front–back, side to side, up–down) and respiration. The more perfect this balance, the quicker the release. Release is by inherent forces.

Indirect balance techniques are difficult for some physicians, and much easier for others. With counterstrain, a tenderpoint helps in finding the proper treatment position. Achieving the proper treatment position with other forms of indirect technique can be a challenge. Functional technique involves continuously palpating for tension on both sides. Proper position for some indirect techniques 'feels right' to the physician. The exact mechanism involved in this perception is not documented. However, when release occurs, this is very apparent to the treating clinician, as there is a decrease of overall tension surrounding the dysfunction.

Some forms of indirect technique utilize various methods to facilitate a release. Facilitated positional release, developed by Schiowitz,[38] is an indirect technique that uses a facilitating force (compression, distraction, or torque) to speed the release. Dr. Eileen DiGiovanna was once asked about the difference between counterstrain and facilitated positional release. She thought for a moment and replied, 'about 85 seconds!'

Combined technique or a combined approach is often used with indirect technique. As release is occurring, the original barrier is softening and the dysfunction is moved into the restrictive barrier. Combined technique means that one starts with indirect technique and finishes with direct technique.

Indirect myofascial release   In this case, the focus is on muscles and fascia as contrasted to a specific joint. Take the tissues in a direction of freer motion to a point of balance, hold, and wait for release. Sometimes the principle is described as 'unload and follow'. Release is by inherent forces.

Craniosacral   Craniosacral technique is applied to the bony calvarium and the sacrum. Most of the techniques are indirect. For example, if the patient has a right torsion with the right sphenoid and the left occiput high, take the cranial mechanism into right torsion, which is the freer motion. Hold, and wait for release. There are some cranial techniques that are direct, for example disengagement of sutural impaction (Fig. 20-7).

Summary of the principles of indirect technique

Strain–counterstrain   Identify a counterstrain tenderpoint. They are located in the muscle belly, tendon, or dermatome of the shortened muscle that is maintaining restriction. Move the body part(s) in a direction of freer motion (also the direction of the original injury) until tenderness in the tenderpoint is absent or minimal. Hold for 90 s. Return to the original position slowly. Recheck. (Note: the first paper by Jones was titled 'Spontaneous release by positioning'.)

Indirect balancing   Move the body part(s) away from the restrictive barrier and in a direction of freer motion. The proper position is obtained when tension is equal on all sides of the dysfunction. Hold, and wait for release. Release is described as occurring as the result of intrinsic forces.

Combined technique   Start with indirect technique and, as release occurs, move the part(s) slowly toward the original

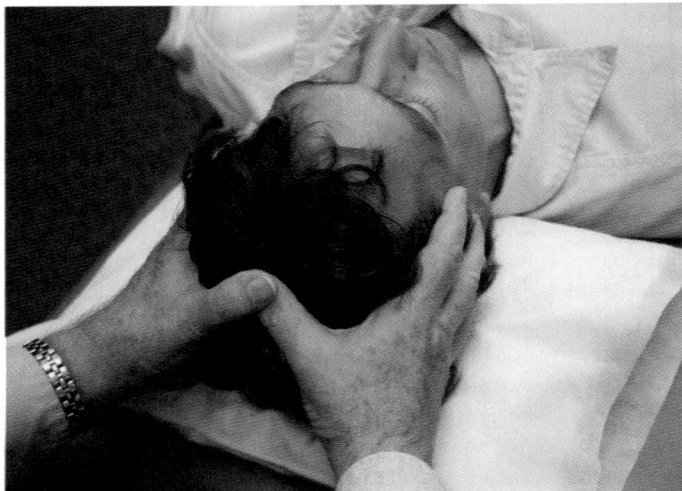

Figure 20-7 Vault hold. The vault hold is used for cranial diagnosis and treatment. The index finger contacts the great wing of the sphenoid, the middle finger is in front of the ear, the ring finger contacts the temporal bone, and the fifth digit contacts the occiput. If the physician's hands are large enough, cross the thumbs together but keep them off the skull. Pressure with the thumbs impairs cranial motion.

barrier. The combined approach can be applied to most forms of indirect technique.

Indications and goals of treatment

Somatic dysfunction is the indication for manual medicine and is diagnosed by palpatory examination. If manual medicine is being considered as a treatment option, there is an overriding question: does the patient have a significant musculoskeletal component to their problem(s)?

Somatic dysfunction can coexist with 'orthopedic disease' (e.g. osteoarthritis or disk disease). Manual medicine treatment helps the somatic dysfunction and helps the patient, but the underlying orthopedic disease process will remain. Other confounding factors are causes for the somatic dysfunction. The patient might have an anatomic short leg, which will continue to maintain sacroiliac and low back dysfunction. Certain activities might be too stressful for the musculoskeletal system. In a controlled study of low back pain, it is impossible to control for these confounding factors.

Evidence-based use of manual therapies in practice

The effectiveness as well as the risks of manual medicine continue to generate controversy. Adequate randomized controlled studies to determine long-term benefit are not available. Available studies have been limited by the heterogeneity of patients, duration of pain, variety of manual medicine techniques used, difficulty of 'blinding' patients, and lack of widely accepted or validated outcome measures.[12,48,61,75,104,133,139,148,149] Recent reviews of manual medicine studies[1,2,4,81,96] indicate effectiveness in some subpopulations, especially in persons with low back pain of 2–4 weeks' duration.[64,102] These reports contributed to the support for their use in *Guidelines for Acute*

Low Back Problems by the Agency for Health Care Policy and Research.[9] There are no current guidelines for treatment regimens for the cervical and thoracic spine. However, several studies support the use of manipulation in these areas.[6,22,61,81] A recent study by Mills supports the effectiveness of manipulation in the treatment of acute otitis media.[106]

Contraindications and side effects

Perhaps the most serious complication of cervical manipulation is stroke associated with vertebrobasilar artery dissection. Approximately 275 cases of adverse events with cervical spine manipulation have been reported in the literature since 1925.[4,66,141] It has been suggested that there may be an underreporting of adverse events.[66] The number of cervical spine manipulations is estimated to be from a low of 33 million to a high of 193 million annually in the USA and Canada.[81] The estimated risk of adverse outcome following cervical spine manipulation ranges from 1 in 400 000 manipulations to 1 in 3.85 million manipulations.[99] The risk of a vertebrobasilar accident occurring spontaneously is nearly twice the risk of a vertebrobasilar accident resulting from cervical spine manipulation.[81]

In an attempt to identify patients who might be at risk for vertebral artery injury from cervical spine manipulation, some provocative tests were developed. The DeKline test was the most popular. This test and others like it have been found to be unreliable.[30] Complications from cervical spine manipulation most often occur in patients who have had prior cervical spine manipulation uneventfully and without obvious risk factors for vertebrobasilar artery dissection.[81] The most common risk factors for vertebrobasilar artery dissection are migraine, hypertension, use of oral contraceptives, and smoking.[65] Most vertebrobasilar dissections occur in the absence of cervical manipulation, either spontaneously or after trivial trauma or common daily movements of the neck, such as backing out of a driveway, painting the ceiling, playing tennis, sneezing, or engaging in yoga.[66]

Unfortunately, accidents do occur. What can be done to minimize the occurrence of accidents from cervical spine manipulation? H.D. Wolff, president of the German Manual Medicine Society, conducted a study for the German government of 40 accidents.[3] Manipulations were done by manual medicine physicians, chiropractors, and therapists. Two problems were common to all 40 cases. At least one or both problems existed in every case. First, a diagnosis of blockage (motion restriction) was not made. Second, the barrier was not engaged prior to thrusting. Instead, a high-amplitude, high-velocity, high-force thrust was used (whipping the neck around). This study establishes two rules: never manipulate without first diagnosing and, if direct technique is used, carefully engage the barrier prior to high-velocity, low-amplitude thrust. The author proposes two more rules:

1. treat the upper thoracic upper rib area before treating the neck; and
2. use indirect technique if these skills are available to you.

Box 20-1 Contraindications for high-velocity manipulation techniques

- Unstable fractures
- Severe osteoporosis
- Multiple myeloma
- Osteomyelitis
- Primary bone tumors
- Paget disease
- Any progressive neurologic deficit
- Spinal cord tumors
- Cauda equina compression
- Central cervical intervertebral disk herniation
- Hypermobile joints
- Rheumatoid arthritis
- Inflammatory phase of ankylosing spondylitis
- Psoriatic arthritis
- Reiter syndrome
- Anticoagulant therapy
- Congenital bleeding disorder
- Acquired bleeding disorder
- Inadequate physical and spinal examination
- Poor manipulative skills

(From Haldeman 1980,[64] with permission of JB Lippincott.)

Most complications are associated with high-velocity thrusting techniques. Box 20-1 is a list of conditions that are contraindications to thrusting technique. Contraindications can arise from several causes. Practitioner errors involve diagnostic errors, lack of manual skill, and failure to obtain needed consultation. There are patient pathologies that contraindicate thrusting techniques. There are other patient-related problems of a psychologic or behavioral nature that are also contraindications to the technique.

Side effects can occur with manipulation and are not always complications. Patients sometimes experience a rebound phenomenon with a temporary increase of symptoms, which often occurs several hours after the treatment. These symptoms subside spontaneously, and the patient is usually much improved after the rebound symptoms subside. Counterstrain technique is a gentle, non-traumatic technique. Posttreatment pain can occur several hours later. Patients should be informed that they might experience this posttreatment pain, and that it will subside.

The practitioner must consider the risks versus the potential benefits whenever manipulation is considered. A comprehensive list of contraindications does not replace this assessment by the physician. Experience in treating patients with manipulation is helpful in making these judgments. There is also a possibility of an overdose of manipulative treatment. The dose must be limited by the ability of the patient to respond to the treatment.

TRACTION

Traction: definition

Traction is a technique used to stretch soft tissues and to separate joint surfaces or bone fragments by use of a pulling force.[74]

The force applied must be of sufficient magnitude and duration in the proper direction, while resisting movement of the body with an equal and opposite force.

Historical perspective

Traction dates back to the time of Hippocrates, who recommended its use for scoliosis, kyphosis, and fractures of the femur.[74,77] Throughout history, it has most commonly been used to reduce fractures and dislocations. For many centuries after Hippocrates, it was the preferred method of treating femur fractures. Over the past 150 years, traction methods have continuously been modified for the treatment of fractures.[72]

The use of traction to treat spinal disorders has become more widespread in the past 50 years, being popularized by Cyriax.[34,35] He proposed traction for the treatment of lumbar disk disorders. He hypothesized that it should be constant traction of at least 20 minutes' duration to produce stretch and decompression of spinal structures. Judovich stated that higher forces were poorly tolerated with constant traction, and that the greater forces to overcome surface resistance were best employed with intermittent traction.[88–90] He discovered that 20–25 lbs were required to produce distraction in the cervical spine. In the 1960s, Colachis and Strohm studied the biomechanics of traction and attempted to define the optimal angle of pull for cervical traction, as well as the optimal duration of traction for both the lumbar and the cervical regions.[25–28] They concluded that 24° of flexion intermittently for 25 min produced optimal distraction. Further studies regarding the optimal angle of pull, duration, and force have produced varying results.[8,32,77]

Traction continues to be used in the treatment of cervical and lumbar pain disorders. More recent advances have included inversion techniques,[53] motorized systems,[122,127,130,146] and the development of stabilizing tables.[54,122,130,136]

Types of traction

Traction can be delivered by several different methods, including manual, mechanized,[74] motorized or hydraulic,[122,127,130,146] or with the assistance of gravity via inversion.[53] Irrespective of the method, the surface resistance must be overcome. It is approximately equal to one-half the weight of the body segment.[89,90] The force can be continuous, sustained, or intermittent. *Continuous* traction uses a low force over a long period of time, such as 30–40 h.[74] Continuous traction is typically not well tolerated and is not used very commonly. *Sustained* traction uses a larger force but for a shorter period of time (typically 30–60 min).[74] Sustained traction is still difficult to tolerate, but is commonly used in the lumbar spine with a split traction or autotraction table. *Intermittent* traction utilizes greater forces over shorter periods of time.[74] The traction force can be increased or decreased during each treatment cycle, and the duration of pull can be adjusted. The cycle is usually repeated for 15–25 min, with the traction phase ranging from 5 to 60 s, and the rest phase ranging from 5 to 15 s.[26,28] The magnitude, duration, and direction of the pull can be varied.

Cervical traction is commonly performed manually, mechanically, or motorized with a head or chin sling, or with a supine posterior distraction unit.[74] The optimal angle of pull ranges between 20 and 30° of flexion,[25,32] while 25 lbs of force is required to reverse the normal cervical lordosis and bring about the earliest distraction of vertebral segments.[89] Mechanical cervical traction can be applied in the supine position, which reduces the weight of the head but increases the frictional resistance. This position also allows for better control of the

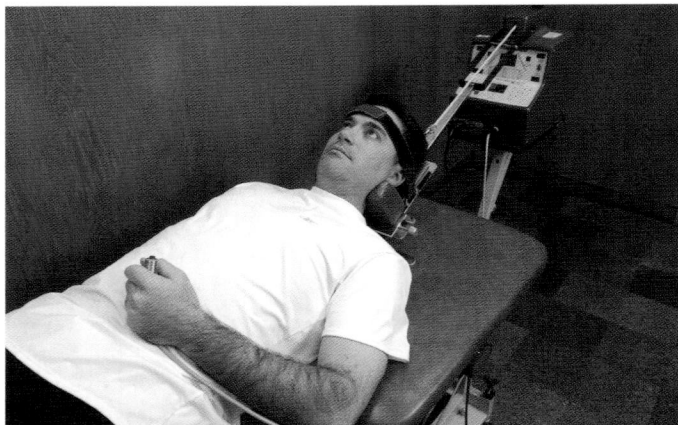

Figure 20-8 Mechanical cervical traction. Cervical traction can be performed utilizing a mechanical device. The patient is placed in a comfortable supine position with the neck flexed slightly.

head by the patient, and is typically more comfortable (Fig. 20-8).[146] Traction in the sitting position allows more accurate positioning for the correct angle of pull, but usually affords less head control and is less comfortable. Cervical traction can be utilized at home with a traditional over the door unit (Fig. 20-9) or a supine posterior distraction unit (Fig. 20-10). The posterior distraction is becoming more popular.

Lumbar traction requires significantly greater force to create distraction of the vertebral segments than cervical traction does. Common traction systems include a thoracic or chest belt with a pelvic belt (Fig. 20-11), inversion, split traction table, or autotraction table.[130] Split traction tables have a mobile and a stationary half. The lower body rests on the mobile half, which separates from the stationary portion. The force necessary to overcome resistance is reduced, and the force required for distraction is significantly less.[74,77,90,122,130] The autotraction table allows both segments of the table to move and is controlled by the patient. The patient assumes the most pain-free position and performs the active traction by pulling on an overhead bar. The patient then uses his or her feet to activate a bar, which alternates compressive and distracting forces.[136] There has been no study of lumbar traction to determine the most efficacious angle of pull, magnitude, or duration of pull.

Vertebral axial decompression (VAX-D) has been more recently advocated for lumbar pain with or without leg pain. This method of traction utilizes a split traction table with the patient lying prone. An initial study by Ramos and Martin suggested that negative intradiskal pressures in the order of

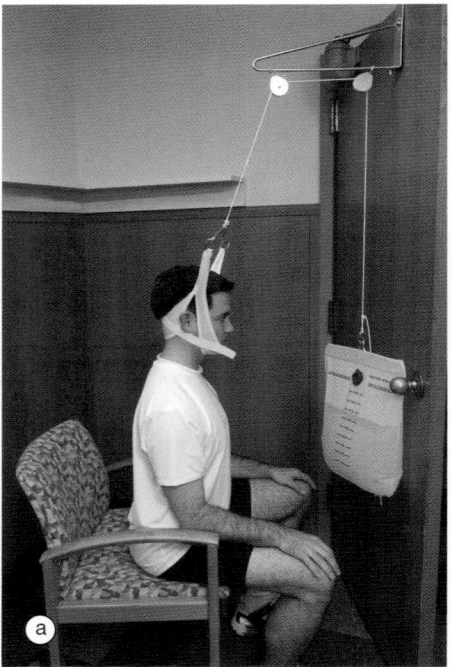
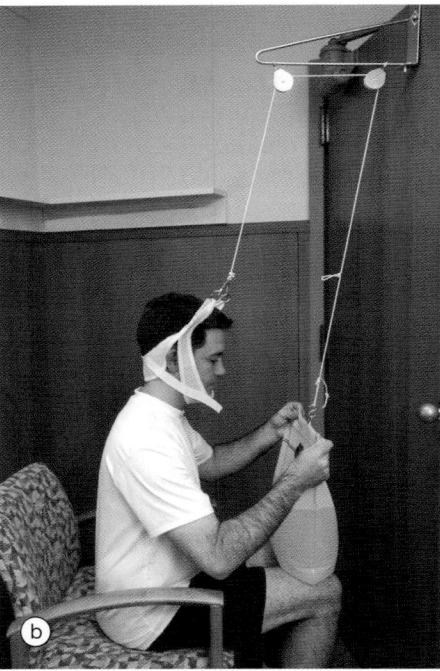
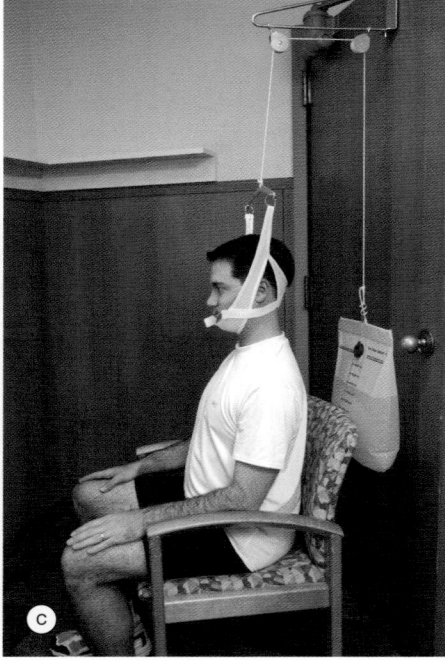

Figure 20-9 Home cervical traction. (**a**) Cervical traction performed using an over the door pulley system. This type of traction is performed with the patient facing the door to allow for the cervical spine to be slightly flexed. Movement of the door should be avoided during treatment. (**b**) Intermittent traction can be performed by resting the weight (water bag) on the patient's lap, producing a slack in the tension rope. The cervical posture is maintained throughout the course of traction. (**c**) The patient is improperly positioned, with the back to the door. This can lead to extension and possible worsening of the cervical condition.

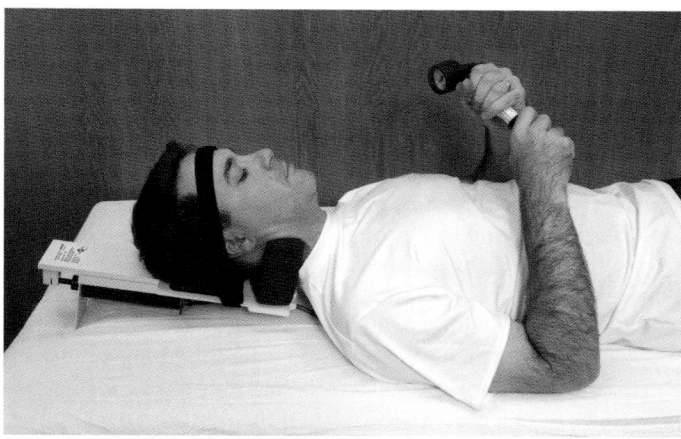

Figure 20-10 Alternative home traction device. The patient is placed in a supine position with gravity eliminated. The neck is positioned in slight flexion against a padded groove. The edges of the groove come in contact with the base of the skull. The amount of distraction pressure is controlled by the patient, utilizing a hand pump.

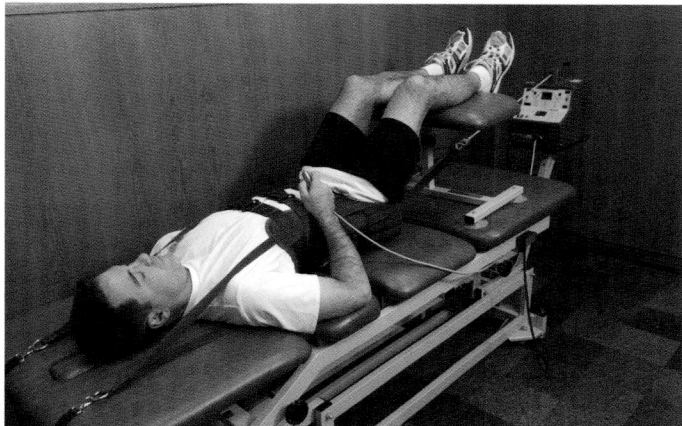

Figure 20-11 Motorized lumbar traction. The patient is placed in a supine position with the hips and knees flexed. The distraction force is mechanically created by pulling on a pelvic belt. The upper body is stabilized by another strap around the chest. Additional distraction force can be accomplished on a traction table that allows the upper and lower segments to separate.

100 mmHg could be obtained during VAX-D treatment.[122] However, Nachemson, in a letter to the editor, stated that these results were probably invalid due to improper calibration, lack of accounting for temperature, and the fact that this was not a closed system. Three clinical studies suggest clinical efficacy for back and/or leg pain, but none were blinded.[57,123,131] Only one of the studies was randomized, being compared with transcutaneous electrical stimulation. One case report of an enlarged disk herniation during VAX-D treatment has been published.[79] Despite its rising popularity, the definitive benefit is still unknown.

Physiologic effects

The physiologic effects of traction have been extensively evaluated and reported. Traction can stretch muscles and ligaments,

tighten the posterior longitudinal ligament to exert a centripetal force on the annulus fibrosis,[74] enlarge the intervertebral space,[25] enlarge the intervertebral foramina,[25–28] and separate apophyseal joints.[25–28] It naturally follows that indications for traction include conditions in which these physiologic effects would be deemed beneficial.

Indications and goals of treatment

There is no consensus on the definitive indications for traction, but the condition having the most support for its use is cervical radiculopathy. The use of traction with lumbar radiculopathy, neck pain, and low back pain is more controversial, with contradictions existing in the literature.[74] In the absence of contraindications, traction can be employed to treat any condition in which the physiologic effects of traction would theoretically be beneficial.

Efficacy

Traction is most commonly prescribed to treat cervical radiculopathies.[128] The literature supporting this practice is scant, with two case series suggesting good resolution of symptoms.[29,110] The utilization of traction for axial neck pain is even less well established. Three articles extensively reviewed this topic and concluded that the efficacy of traction in treating cervical pain is unknown.[62,79,70]

The popularity of lumbar traction in treating low back pain, with or without radicular features, has declined over the past few decades.[37] This change came about due to the lack of efficacy and an emphasis on more active treatment programs. A case series of 49 patients with sciatica of greater than 6 weeks' duration found 79% improvement with traction, but the study was uncontrolled.[54] One study compared traction with a sham treatment,[8] while another compared traction plus physical therapy with physical therapy alone.[15] Both these studies found no difference in outcome between the respective treatment groups. Gianakopoulos and colleagues found improvement in 13 of 16 patients with low back pain treated with an inversion device.[53] Side effects, however, including elevated blood pressure, headaches, and periorbital and pharyngeal petechiae, were significant. Three review articles concluded that there was not enough information to support the use of traction for lumbar spine disorders, or that there simply was no indication for its use.[69,70,103]

Contraindications

Absolute contraindications to traction include malignancy, infection such as osteomyelitis or diskitis, osteoporosis, inflammatory arthritis, fracture, pregnancy, cord compression, uncontrolled hypertension or cardiovascular disease, and in the setting of carotid or vertebral artery disease.[74,89] Caution should also be employed in the elderly, in the setting of midline disk herniations, and in the lumbar region when abdominal problems are present. Inversion traction involves more risks, as blood pressure increases and heart rate decreases are known to occur,[53] leading to headaches and periorbital petechiae. Most practitioners agree that traction should be discontinued if there is exacerbation of symptoms, discomfort from the traction device, or with production of systemic symptoms such as dizziness.

MASSAGE

Definition

The application of a 'soothing hand' to a sick person can be considered the prototype of any therapeutic treatment.[93] *Massage* is the term used to describe certain manipulations of the soft tissue of the body. Massage has further been defined as a group of procedures, which are usually done with the hands, and include friction, kneading, rolling, and percussion of the external tissues of the body. This is done in a variety of ways, with a curative, palliative, or hygienic objective in view.[58] These manipulations are most commonly and effectively performed with the hands. They are administered for the purpose of producing effects on the nervous and muscular systems, as well as the effects on local and general circulation of the blood and lymph.[7]

Massage and manipulation have common historical roots. In early descriptions of these two techniques, the words are used interchangeably. More recently, they have been separated into two distinct modalities but continue to share similar terminology, philosophy, and technique.

History

Massage has waxed and waned in popularity throughout the millennia in different cultures. Even the etymology of the term massage fosters debate.[93] The postulated origins of this word include the Arabic verb *massa*, which means 'to touch'; the Greek word *massein*, meaning 'to knead'; or the Sanskirt term *makek*, which means 'to press or condense'.[58,93] All these terms were derived at different times and in different cultures, depicting the significant role that massage played in these societies. The earliest known reference to massage is in cave paintings in the Pyrenees that date back to 15 000 BC, which depict the use of hands for therapeutic touch.[31] The ancient medical records depicting massage as a therapeutic intervention originate out of China, India, and Babylon.

In a Chinese text written on kung fu in 2700 BC, references are made on the use of massage for the relief of ailing muscles.[93] In 1000 BC, *Nei Ching*, also known as *The Yellow Emperor's Classic of Internal Medicine*, massage of the skin and flesh and breathing exercises were utilized in the treatment of complete paralysis.[93,111] The *Ayur Veda* (1500–1200 BC) is considered the oldest medical text written in India, and it makes frequent reference to massage. In Babylon of Assyria, around 900 BC, massage was prescribed to expel demons and to aid in healing.[93]

The ancient Greek and Roman medical literature makes abundant references to the use of massage as a therapeutic modality. Hippocrates (460–375 BC), who is generally considered the father of modern medicine, wrote extensively on the use of massage in his book *On Articulations*.[93] Plato (427–347 BC) and Socrates (470–399 BC) made reference to anointing with oils when performing massage. The Greek physician Asclepiades (129–40 BC), who practiced in Rome and is considered the father of physical medicine, wrote about hydrotherapy, exercise, and massage as the three most important therapeutic modalities to utilize in the treatment of patients.[93]

In the Middle Ages, the 'Church of Rome' discouraged the use of massage as a healing practice, and it fell out of favor.[119] Massage practitioners during this time were felt to be practicing quackery by the medical profession. This dealt a crushing blow to the advancement of massage as a therapeutic modality. During the Renaissance, medical scholars resurrected massage and attempted to understand the physiology and anatomy this modality affected. The French medical community embraced 'friction of the skin' and described many different techniques for providing massage. Many of the terms for these techniques, such as *effleurage*, *pétrissage*, *tapotement*, and *friction massage*, are still in use today.[93]

The roots of modern day massage are derived from the work of Per Henking Ling (1776–1839) of Sweden.[93] He was the founder of curative gymnastics, an approach that incorporated massage and exercise. Ling employed many of the previously described French techniques and nomenclature. He also used terms such as *rolling*, *sliding*, *pinching*, *shaking*, and *vibration* to define massage techniques. Ling was instrumental in establishing the Central Royal Institute for Gymnastics, which practiced, taught, and promoted what has become known as 'Swedish' massage. Several of Ling's students emigrated to New York and established the Swedish Institute of Massage in 1916.[93]

In the past century, two physicians strongly advocated the use of massage in their orthopedic practices. James Mennell wrote the book *Physical Treatment by Movements, Manipulation, and Massage* in 1917.[93] This book greatly influenced the field of physical therapy to utilize massage as a therapeutic modality. James Cyriax wrote extensively on the use of manipulation and deep friction massage, which today is used for the treatment of musculoskeletal and other sports injuries.[93,119]

The popularity of massage as a therapeutic intervention has fluctuated significantly, even over the past several decades. This fluctuation has been influenced by the medical profession, who believed that medication and surgical procedures were needed to improve disease and suffering. In recent years, however, there has been a resurgence of interest in massage that has generated scientific inquiry into its usage as a therapeutic modality.[40,114,118]

Indications and goals of treatment

Massage has multiple effects on the body, including mechanical, reflexive, neurologic, and psychologic.[20,33,147] The exact therapeutic mechanism by which massage works is not fully understood, and probably represents a combination of the above. The method and application of massage correlate with the magnitude of these effects. The goals of therapeutic massage are to produce relaxation, relieve muscle tension, reduce pain, increase mobility of soft tissues, and improve circulation. These techniques can be used on patients who would benefit from mobilization of tissues and reduction of swelling and discomfort.

Mechanical effects

The mechanical effects of massage are the most apparent and are well understood. This effect is brought on by the physical forces applied to the body tissues, such as compression, shearing, or vibration. The mechanical pressure created by massage moves fluid from areas of relative stasis (low pressure) to higher pressure areas by creating a hydrostatic pressure gradient. Once fluids leave the cells or interstitial fluid, they can enter the lymphatic or vascular system. Valves within the lymphatic and venous system prevent return of the fluid to the tissue.[21,117,145]

Massage can have an immediate effect on cutaneous blood flow, with hyperemia being noticed even with superficial techniques.[55] The mechanism of action for this is not well understood, but is most likely due to stimulation of the mast cells and release of histamines. This local histamine release causes the triple response of Lewis, including flare, redness, and wheal formation at the site of stimulation.

Deep massage has an effect on the underlying fascia and deep connective tissues.[20,147] Injury to this deeper tissue can result in restrictions, adhesions, and scarring. These fascial constrictions can potentially cause restriction of fluid movement within the vasculature, as well as reduction in muscle activity. Deep massage can help to release these restrictions, adhesions, and microscarring.[147]

Pain, inactivity, and debilitation result in insufficient muscle contraction to produce fluid immobilization.[147] This hypomobility can result in increased fluid stasis, producing a self-perpetuating feedback loop. This hypomobility can result in fluid accumulation, but just as important can result in the accumulation of metabolic by-products. These metabolic by-products can create an osmotic influence on fluid shifts and result in stimulation of pain fibers. Massage increases the mobility of these metabolic by-products and the dispersion of fluid accumulations. Once this self-perpetuating cycle of pain, stasis, and hypomobility is broken, the body can restore its normal healing mechanism.[13,63]

It has been postulated that massage results in neural reflex reactions.[97,98,116] It is felt that these reactions are what account for the global effects produced with massage techniques. Somatic afferent nerve fibers carry information from the somatic system to the spinal cord. Dysfunction within the somatic structure can result in increased afferent neural input. This increased input results in a change in the efferent activity at the same spinal cord level through interneurons. This increased efferent activity can result in muscle hypertonicity and contraction. This hypertonic region can localize to a specific spinal cord level. This has been considered by many to be called 'facilitative spinal segment' and is discussed extensively in the manipulation section.

Types of massage

There has been a vast array of techniques used to perform a therapeutic massage. These techniques can be categorized as of either classic western (European) or eastern (Asian) origin. The most common western (European) techniques are those outlined by the Swedish system. These four basic massage strokes are effleurage, pétrissage, friction massage, and tapotement (described below). There are several treatment schemes that combine massage with other techniques, such as structural reintegration, function restoration, and movement therapies (see below).

Effleurage

Effleurage involves gliding the palms, fingertips, and/or thumbs over the skin in a rhythmic circular pattern with varying degrees of pressure.[33,76,147] This stroke is performed by maintaining continuous contact with the skin, and stroking from a distal to a proximal position on the extremities, torso, or spine (Fig. 20-12). Once the proximal position is reached, the hands can be gently dragged over the skin and repositioned over the distal position and the process repeated. This technique is often used as a prelude to more aggressive massage techniques or manipulation.

Effleurage performed superficially can result in reflexive and psychologic changes. The blood flow to the area is increased, introducing relaxation when done slowly and stimulation when done more quickly. Deeper mechanical stroking can result in mechanical effects on the circulatory and deep myofascial systems. Effleurage is utilized to stimulate lymphatic drainage, and to relieve joint sprain-type pain, muscle strains, and bruising, as well as vascular congestion related to surgery, peripheral vascular disease, or complex regional pain syndrome.

Pétrissage

Pétrissage is also known as the 'kneading massage'. It involves both hands compressing the skin between the thumb and fingers.[33,60,76,147] The tissue is grasped from the underlying skeletal structures, lifted, and massaged. Both hands alternate rhythmically in a rolling motion. The depth of pétrissage can determine the mechanical effect. Superficial techniques promote relaxation, while deeper techniques increase blood

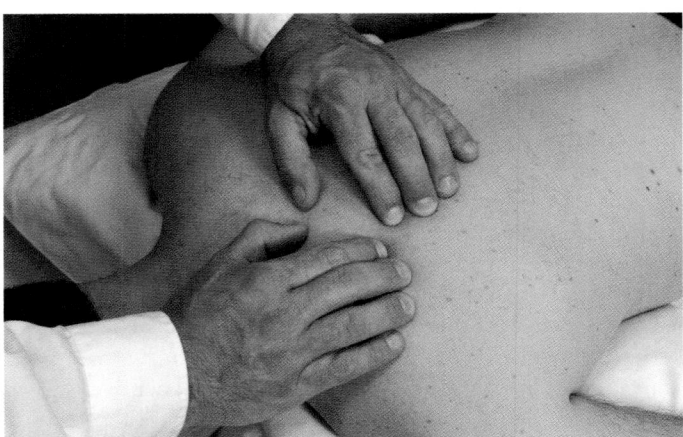

Figure 20-12 Effleurage massage. This type of massage being performed on the patient's posterior shoulder is a rhythmic circular motion with the fingertips. Pressure can be varied to massage deeper structures.

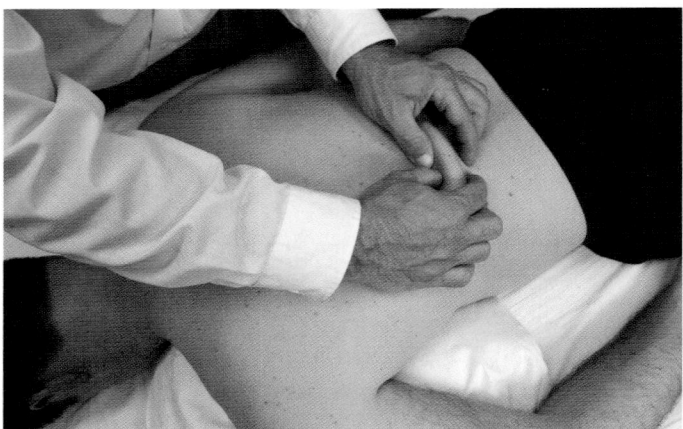

Figure 20-13 Pétrissage massage: 'rolling'. In this form of pétrissage, the skin or muscle is gathered up between the fingers and thumb, and rolled continuously, gathering new skin and muscle.

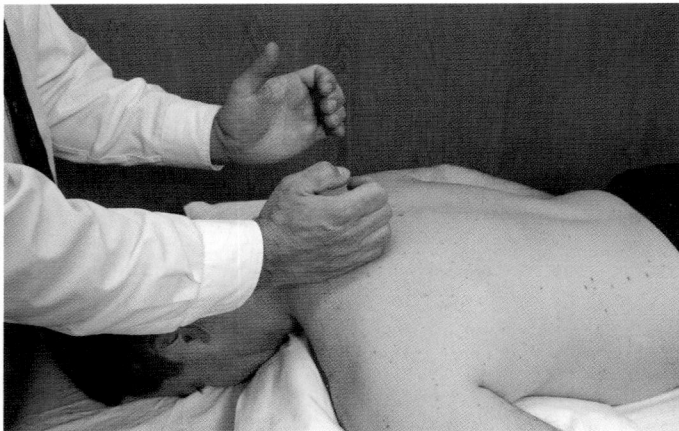

Figure 20-14 Tapotement massage: 'hacking'. Hacking involves striking the body at right angles with the ulnar aspect of the hands.

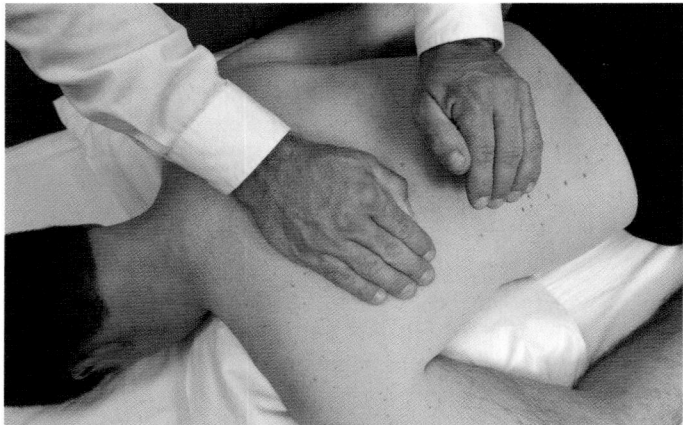

Figure 20-15 Tapotement massage: 'cupping'. Cupping is frequently performed over the rib cage to loosen secretions in the lungs.

flow, mobilize fluid and tissue deposits, decrease adhesions, and increase tissue pliability.

Pétrissage is also considered compression massage and several variations exist, including kneading or picking up, wringing, rolling, or shaking the tissue. 'Kneading' involves circular movements of one hand superimposed on the other. The finger pads and thumb compress tissue and distract it from the deeper underlying structures. 'Picking up' involves four basic steps: compression of the soft tissue against the underlying structures, grasping the soft tissue and compression, release, and repositioning the hands in a more proximal position to repeat the process. 'Wringing' resembles picking up, except that, once tissue is grasped, one hand pushes while the other one pulls, creating a shearing-type force in the tissue planes. 'Rolling' involves grabbing a small amount of tissue between the finger pads and thumb, and rolling the tissue as if moving a small object under the skin (Fig. 20-13). 'Shaking' is a technique in which the tissue is grabbed and vigorously shaken between the hands. The hands are then repositioned along the course of the muscle being treated.

Tapotement

Tapotement, or percussion massage, utilizes rhythmic alternating contact of varying pressure between the hands and the body's soft tissue.[33,76,147] Various techniques are utilized to produce this type of massage, including hacking, clapping, beating, pounding, and vibration. 'Hacking' involves using the ulnar aspect of the hands to alternate striking the body tissues. These rapid strokes (2–6 Hz) are delivered in a sequential pattern along the entire region to be treated (Fig. 20-14). 'Cupping' involves the use of a cupped palm, which is percussed against the chest wall. This technique is frequently used to loosen secretions in disease processes such as cystic fibrosis (Fig. 20-15). 'Beating' involves using a clenched fist to repetitively pummel the tissue. This is a very aggressive type of tapotement and is not frequently used. 'Tapping' uses the finger pads, typically of the index and middle fingers, to percuss. The finger

pads strike the underlying tissue in rapid succession. Frequently, this technique is used over the sinuses to loosen secretions.

Friction massage

Friction massage is a circular, longitudinal, or transverse pressure applied by the fingers, thumb, or hypothenar region of the hand to small areas.[60,76,147] Cross-friction massage is perpendicular to the fibers and was used extensively by Cyriax.[33] Very little motion occurs at the fingertips overlying the skin. The tissues are massaged from superficial to deep by increasing the pressure applied. The goal of friction massage is to break down adhesions in scar tissue, loosen ligaments, and disable trigger points. It is often uncomfortable and can even result in some bruising. Despite this, it is an effective treatment for tendonitis or tendinopathy, subacromial bursitis, plantar fascitis, and trigger points (as described by Travell) (Fig. 20-16).[138]

Other techniques that integrate massage, structure, function, and movement into a rehabilitation program include Tager psychologic integration, Alexander and Feldenkrais techniques, 'Rolfing', myofascial release, and manual lymphatic drainage

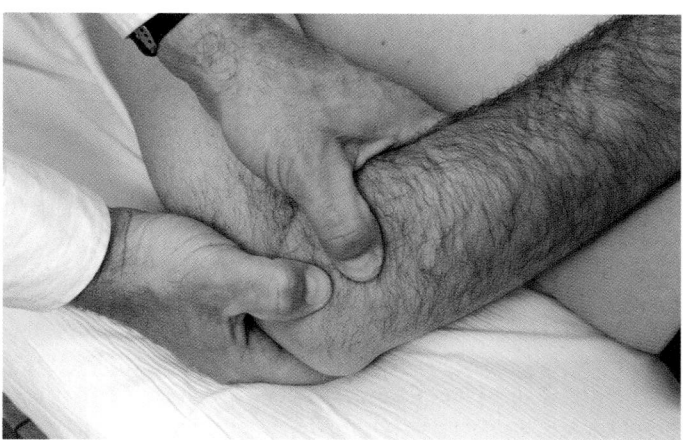

Figure 20-16 Friction massage. Friction massage being performed on the lateral epicondylitis to promote tendon healing.

(MLD). Although these techniques are not utilized as much as the common Swedish techniques, they are gaining in popularity.

Tager psychologic integration

This treatment method was developed by Milton Tager, M.D. in the 1940s. This technique combines the use of gentle hands-on tissue work and reintegration of movement through reeducation and relaxation exercises. The technique teaches patients to move with ease and efficiency. The hands-on work consists of gently rocking, stretching, or rolling movements to relax and diminish tension. The movement component of the Tager technique is coined 'mentastics', which is a combination of mental, psychologic, and gymnastic elements, and focuses on making movements lighter and easier.[31]

Tager therapists employ the use of 'hook-up', which involves the therapist attaining a calm and focused state of mind. They use this hook-up to connect with the patient's needs and how they are responding to treatment. Information is communicated from the therapist's hands to the patient's body and assists in easing movements.

Alexander technique

F.M. Alexander (1869–1955) was a Shakespearean actor who suffered from recurrent neck and vocal problems. After much self-reflection and postural reeducation, he noted that his vocal problems could be corrected by postural reeducation. He developed a series of techniques for the treatment of chronic neck and low back pain.[31]

His approach centers on balance between head and neck movement 'primary control', and a state of dynamic postures and breathing exercises. This technique teaches patients to engage their mind to understand beneficial patterns and overcome motion patterns, which are considered automatic. It is felt that these unbeneficial patterns can be broken through conscious training.

Feldenkrais pattern

Mosheid Feldenkrais, D.Sc. (1880–1967) was a physicist and mechanical engineer who suffered from a knee dysfunction and was told that he most likely would have to be a wheelchair user. Utilizing his black belt judo techniques and physics background, he studied movement and the interrelationship between muscle contraction and motion. Through self-rehabilitation of his knee problem, he developed several techniques.[31] He began teaching his students these simple exercises that could be performed during functional tasks. The goals of these techniques are to learn efficient and pain-free motion. Feldenkrais emphasizes multiple repetitions to lay down new neuromuscular engrams, and considers the entire body, even in the simplest of movements.

Rolfing structural integration

Ida Rolf (1896–1979), a chemist who had health problems of her own, was inspired by such medical philosophies as osteopathy, Alexander technique, and yoga. She viewed the body as a group of units and studied their relationship to each other. Rolf saw gravity as one of the primary causes of dysfunction. The primary tenet of her structural integration system was to help clients achieve proper vertical alignment and efficient movement.[31] The typical regimen consists of a series of ten 60- to 90-min sessions. Superficial massage is performed initially, with progression to deeper friction massage. This is in an attempt to stretch fascia and allow muscles to relax and lengthen. The sessions build on one another, and additional treatments are frequently required to accommodate for the changes promoted. The deep friction massage traditionally performed with Rolfing techniques can be painful. Newer techniques have been implemented, which are less painful and less invasive. Other practitioners have been influenced by Rolfing, including Kellerwork and Aston patterning.

Myofascial release

The term *myofascial release* was coined by Robert Ward, D.O. in the 1960s[143] and further developed by John Barnes, P.T.[5] This technique is founded on the premise that the body is encased in connective tissue (i.e. fascia). This fascia is the ground substance that interconnects all bones, muscles, nerves, and other internal organs and tissues. Injury or tension within one area of the fascia can result in pain and tenderness. Due to the interconnections, injury in one area of the fascia can result in pain and dysfunction at a distant point. Practitioners of myofascial release use gentle stretching and massage to release the fascial tension, and can often work on areas that seem unrelated to the primary pain or injury. Myofascial release is frequently used to treat chronic pain and restore normal range of motion.

Manual lymphatic drainage

Manual lymphatic drainage (MLD) was developed in Europe in the 1930s by Danish physiotherapists Estrid and Emil Vodder as a technique to control postmastectomy lymphedema. MLD is a gentle and superficially focused massage where lymph is moved from areas of lymphatic vessel damage to watershed regions.[14]

The first part of the treatment involves massage of the proximal region of the extremity to be treated. This is thought to dilate the watershed lymph vessels and allows them to accept fluid from distal areas. After proximal areas have been gently massaged, a more rhythmic massage is performed from a distal to a proximal part of the extremity. The typical session lasts 45–60 min. Complex lymphedema therapy includes MLD combined with other modalities, such as sequential pumping, low-tension wraps, skin care, compressive garments, and exercise. Long-term maintenance is required for sustained edema control. It has been demonstrated that the limb volume can be reduced by as much as 25–63% after this treatment.[14,83] MLD is quickly becoming popular in the USA, and many therapists have become trained in these techniques.

Eastern forms of massage

Acupressure

Acupressure has been defined as digital pressure performed in a circular motion to treat areas that are typically treated with acupuncture needles and for the same reason.[135] Acupuncture was developed over 3000 years ago in China. The basic philosophy behind this technique is to restore energy flow or *qi*. Qi has two basic components that flow along 12 meridians: *yin* is associated with passivity, rest, and cold, whereas *yang* is associated with activity, stimulation, and heat. Balance of these forces is thought to be associated with health, and an imbalance with disease.

The goal of treatment is to restore energy balance or homeostasis. Acupressure is performed with the patient lying on a table. Deep pressure is applied to the acupuncture points in a circular fashion without the use of lubrication. Acupressure can be used for the treatment of nausea and vomiting associated with chemotherapy, to decrease postoperative pain, for treatment of headaches, and to decrease temporomandibular joint pain. Acupressure is a technique that can easily be converted to a self-performed treatment modality.

Shiatsu

Shi (meaning finger) *atsu* (meaning pressure) is the Japanese type of body work based on acupuncture.[135] This technique was initially practiced by visually impaired clinicians. Pressure is applied in particular meridians similar to acupuncture. This type of treatment has been westernized and is being increasingly utilized in the USA.

Reflexology

Ancient medical practitioners hypothesized that there is a homuncular representation of the body on the sole of the feet.[135] This philosophy probably dates back to ancient Egypt, but the Chinese medical literature demonstrated a homunculus of the body on the ears, feet, and hands. Palpations of specific areas on the feet were thought to be tender if their corresponding body part was dysfunctional. Reflexology is the application of deep circular pressure applied to specific dysfunctional points

on the soles of the feet. This is considered a separate discipline in the USA, but is used by some Swedish massage practitioners to treat areas of extreme tenderness. It has been used to treat hypertension, stress, fatigue, and digestive complaints.

Evidence-based use of massage

Massage has been used in multiple forms for the treatment of many conditions. Traditional research is difficult to perform on these techniques due to the lack of a standardized sham treatment. Although there is a paucity of quality research on these techniques, there has been a renewed interest in establishing the efficacy of massage.

There is at least one large randomized controlled trial that supports the use of massage in the treatment of anxiety and stress;[41,43,45,49,72,87,113] arthralgias and various arthritides;[42,44] fibromyalgia;[17] lymphedema;[18] musculoskeletal disorders such as whiplash, low back pain, and sports-related injuries;[24,82,92,120] and sleep disorders.[124,125]

There are recommendations suggesting that massage therapy might be useful as an adjunct treatment or possible alternative treatment for the following conditions (research data for these are less compelling than a randomized control trial): burn care,[46,47,73] care of people with cancer,[10,18,41] chronic pain,[36,52,91] exercise-induced injury,[19,71,78,126,132,134,137] headaches,[121] and HIV and AIDS.[11,129] While massage therapy is obviously not curative in these conditions, it might enhance the effectiveness of other therapeutic interventions.

Contraindications to massage

Massage therapy is a relatively safe modality. Complications are rare and usually not serious. There are several absolute and relative contraindications to traditional Swedish massage. Potential complications for shiatsu, reflexology, and acupuncture have not been specifically delineated. Massage should not be performed over areas of malignancy, cellulitis, or lymphangitis.[95] The effect of massage on these regions can cause mobilization of tumor cells into the vascular lymphatic supply or the spread of infection.

Areas of trauma or recent bleeding should not be treated with deep tissue massage. Mobilization of these areas can increase the propensity for rebleeding. Patients who are taking anticoagulants should be treated with gentler techniques and observed for bruising and ecchymoses. Deep tissue work should be utilized with extreme caution in those on anticoagulants or who have a bleeding diathesis.

Massage should not be utilized over areas of known deep venous thrombosis or atherosclerotic plaques. This could result in dislodgement of these vascular thrombi, resulting in embolic infarcts into the pulmonary, cerebral, or peripheral systems. Special care should be observed in patients with osteoarthritis or severe osteoporosis to avoid any excess range of motion or stretching that could alter articulating surfaces. Patients with low blood pressure might experience postural hypotension after treatment and should be observed carefully. Victims of physical or sexual abuse can reexperience elements of trauma during treatment. Special care regarding touch is especially warranted with these individuals. People with edema should not undergo deep tissue massage or any other massage technique that could result in local accumulation of interstitial fluid.

CONCLUSION

Massage, traction, and manipulation have been an integral part of healthcare since ancient times. The popularity of these techniques ebbs and flows with changes in the traditional medical paradigm of the time. They have enjoyed resurgence in popularity in recent years. Research efforts, while in their infancy, have shown that a spectrum of physiologic and clinical changes can be associated with these modalities. Massage, manipulation, and traction are becoming increasingly recognized as a valuable adjunct to standard medical care.

REFERENCES

1. Abenhaim L, Bergeron AM. Twenty years of randomized clinical trials of manipulative therapy for back pain: a review. Clin Invest Med 1992; 15(6):527–535.

2. Anderson R, Meeker WC, Wirick BE. A meta-analysis of clinical trials of spinal manipulation [see comments]. J Manipulative Physiol Ther 1992; 15:181–194.

3. [Anonymous]. International Federation of Manual Medicine Workshop, Fischingen, 1983.

4. Assendelft WJ, Bouter SM, Knipschild PG. Complications of spinal manipulation: a comprehensive review of the literature. J Fam Pract 1996; 42:475–480.

5. Barnes J. Myofascial release: the missing link in traditional treatment. In: Davis C, ed. Complementary therapies in rehabilitation—holistic approaches for prevention and wellness. Thorofare: Slack; 1997:21–47.

6. Beal MC, Vorro J, Johnston WL. Chronic cervical dysfunction: correlation of myoelectric findings with clinical progress. J Am Osteopath Assoc 1989; 89(7):891–900.

7. Beard G. Massage—principles and techniques. Philadelphia: Saunders; 1964.

8. Beurskens AJ, et al. Efficacy of traction for nonspecific low back pain. 12-week and 6-month results of a randomized clinical trial. Spine 1997; 22(23):2756–2762.

9. Bigos SJ. Acute low back problems in adults. Rockville: Agency for Health Care Policy and Research; 1994.

10. Billhult A. A meaningful relief from suffering experiences of massage in cancer care. Cancer Nurs 2001; 24:180–184.

11. Birk TJ, MacArthur RD, Khuder S. The effects of massage therapy alone and in combination with other complementary therapies on immune system measures and quality of life in human immunodeficiency virus. J Altern Complement Med 2000; 6:405–414.

12. Blomberg S, Svardsudd K, Mildenberger F. A controlled, multi-centre trial of manual therapy in low-back pain. Initial status, sick-leave and pain score during follow-up. Scand J Prim Health Care 1992; 10:170–178.

13. Boone T, Thompson WR. A physiologic evaluation of sports massage. Athl Train 1991; 26:51–54.

14. Boris M, Weindorf S, Lasinksi S. Persistence of lymphedema reduction after noninvasive complex lymphedema therapy. Oncology 1997; 11(1):99–109.

15. Borman P, Bodur H. The efficacy of lumbar traction in the management of patients with low back pain. Rheumatol Int 2003; 23:82–86.

16. Bowles CH. Functional technique: a modern perspective. J Am Osteopath Assoc 1981; 80(5):326–331.

17. Brattberg G. Connective tissue massage in the treatment of fibromyalgia. Eur J Pain 1999; 3:235–244.

18. Bunce IH, Hennessy JM, Ward LC, et al. Post-mastectomy lymphoedema treatment and measurement. Med J Aust 1994; 161:125–128.

19. Cafarelli E. The role of massage in preparation for and recovery from exercise. An overview. Sports Med 1992; 14:1–9.

20. Cantu RL, Grodin AJ. Myofascial manipulation: theory and clinical application. New York: Aspen Publishers; 1992.

21. Carrier EB. Studies on physiology of capillaries: reaction of human skin capillaries to drugs and other stimuli. Am J Physiol 1992; 61:528–547.

22. Cassidy JD, Lopes AA, Yong-Hing K. The immediate effect of manipulation versus mobilization on pain and range of motion in the cervical spine: a randomized controlled trial [see comment]. J Manipulative Physiol Ther 1992; 15(9):570–575.

23. Cherkin DC, MacCornack FA. Patient evaluations of low back pain care from family physicians and chiropractors [see comment]. West J Med 1989; 150(3):351–355.

24. Cherkin DC, Sherman KJ, Barlow W, et al. Randomized trial comparing traditional Chinese medical acupuncture, therapeutic massage, and self-care education for chronic low back pain. Arch Intern Med 2001; 161:1081–1088.

25. Colachis SC Jr, Strohm BR. A study of tractive forces and angle of pull on vertebral interspaces in the cervical spine. Arch Phys Med Rehabil 1965; 46(12):820–830.

26. Colachis SC Jr, Strohm BR. Cervical traction: relationship of traction time to varied tractive force with constant angle of pull. Arch Phys Med Rehabil 1965; 46(12):815–819.

27. Colachis SC Jr, Strohm BR. Effect of duration of intermittent cervical traction on vertebral separation. Arch Phys Med Rehabil 1966; 47(6):353–359.

28. Colachis SC Jr, Strohm BR. Radiographic studies of cervical spine motion in normal subjects: flexion and hyperextension. Arch Phys Med Rehabil 1965; 46(11):753–760.

29. Constantoyannis C. Intermittent cervical traction for cervical radiculopathy caused by large-volume herniated discs. J Manipulative Physiol Ther 2002; 25:188–192.

30. Cote P, Kreitz BG, Cassidy JD. The validity of the extension–rotation test as a clinical screening procedure before neck manipulation: a secondary analysis. J Manipulative Physiol Ther 1996; 19:59–164.

31. Cotter AC, Schulman RA. An overview of massage and touch therapies. In: Manual medicine—state of the art reviews, vol 14. Philadelphia: Hanley & Belfus; 2000.

32. Crue BL, Todd EM. The importance of flexion in cervical halter traction. Bull Los Angeles Neurol Soc 1965; 30:95–98.

33. Cyriax J, Russell G. Textbook of orthopaedic medicine, vol 2: treatment by manipulation, massage and injection. London: Baillière Tindall; 1980.

34. Cyriax J. Conservative treatment of lumbar disc lesions. Physiotherapy 1964; 50:300–303.

35. Cyriax J. Discussion on the treatment of backache by traction. Proc R Soc Med 1955; 45:808.

36. Day JA, Chesrown SE. Effect of massage on serum level of beta-endorphin and beta-lipotropin in healthy adults. Phys Ther 1987; 67:926–930.

37. Deyo R. Descriptive epidemiology of low-back pain and its related medical care in the United States. Spine 1987; 12:264–268.

38. DiGiovanna EL. Osteopathic approach to diagnosis and treatment. 2nd edn. Philadelphia: Lippincott-Raven; 1997.

39. Dvorak J, Dvorak V. Manual medicine: diagnostics. Stuttgart: Thieme; 1990.

40. Eisenberg DM, Kessler RC, et al. Unconventional medicine in the United States. Prevalence, costs, and patterns of use [see comment]. N Engl J Med 1993; 328:246–252.

41. Ferrell-Tory AT. The use of therapeutic massage as a nursing intervention to modify anxiety and the perception of cancer pain. Cancer Nurs 1993; 16:93–101.

42. Fiechtner JJ. Manual and manipulation techniques for rheumatic diseases. Rheum Dis Clin North Am 2000; 26:83–96.

43. Field T, Quintino O, Henteleff T, et al. Job stress reduction therapies. Altern Ther Health Med 1997; 3(4):54–56.

44. Field T, Hernandez-Reif M, Seligman S, et al. Juvenile rheumatoid arthritis: benefits from massage therapy. J Pediatr Psychol 1997; 22(5):607–617.

45. Field T, Ironson G, Scafidi F, et al. Massage therapy reduces anxiety and enhances EEG pattern of alertness and math computations. Int J Neurosci 1996; 86(3–4):197–205.

46. Field T, Hernandez-Reif M, Krugman S, et al. Postburn itching, pain, and psychological symptoms are reduced with massage therapy. J Burn Care Rehabil 2000; 21:189–193.

47. Field T, Krugman S, Tuchel T, et al. Burn injuries benefit from massage therapy. J Burn Care Rehabil 1998; 19:241–244.

48. Fisk JW. A controlled trial of manipulation in a selected group of patients with low back pain favouring one side. NZ Med J 1979; 90(645): 288–291.

49. Fraser J. Psychophysiological effects of back massage on elderly institutionalized patients. J Adv Nurs 1993; 18:238–245.

50. Fryette HH. Principles of osteopathic technique. Kirksville: Journal Printing Company; 1980.

51. Frymoyer J. Back pain and sciatica. N Engl J Med 1988; 318(5): 291–300.

52. Furlan AD, Welch V, Wong J. Massage for low back pain. Cochrane Database Syst Rev 2000;4.

53. Gianakopoulos G, Waylonis GW, Grant PA. Inversion devices: their role in producing lumbar distraction. Arch Phys Med Rehabil 1985; 66: 100–102.

54. Gillstrom P, Ehrnberg A. Long-term results of autotraction in the treatment of lumbago and sciatica. An attempt to correlate clinical results with objective parameters. Arch Orthop Trauma Surg 1985; 104(5):294–298.

55. Goats GC. Massage—the scientific basis of an ancient art: part 1. The techniques. Br J Sports Med 1994; 28(3):149–152.

56. Goodridge JP. Muscle energy technique: definition, explanation, methods of procedure. J Am Osteopath Assoc 1981; 81(4):249–254.

57. Gose EE, Naguszewski RK. Vertebral axial decompression therapy for pain associated with herniated or degenerated discs or facet syndrome: an outcome study. Neurol Res 1998; 20:186–190.

58. Graham D. Practical treatise on massage. New York: William Wood; 1884.

59. Greenman PE. Models and mechanisms of osteopathic manipulative medicine. Osteopath Med News 1987; 4:1–20.

60. Greenman PE. Principles of manual medicine. 3rd edn. Baltimore: Williams & Wilkins; 2003.

61. Gross AR, Aker PD, Quartly C. Manual therapy in the treatment of neck pain. Rheum Dis Clin North Am 1996; 22(3):579–598.

62. Gross AR, Goldsmith CH, Penose P. Physical medicine modalities for mechanical neck disorders. Cochrane Database Syst Rev 2004:2.

63. Gupta S, Sadhukan AK, Mather DN. Comparative study of lactate removal in short term massage of extremities: active recover and passive recovery periods after submaximal exercise sessions. Int J Sports Med 1996; 17:55–59.

64. Hadler NM, Curtis P, Gillings DB, et al. A benefit of spinal manipulation as adjunctive therapy for acute low-back pain: a stratified controlled trial. Spine 1987; 12(7):702–706.

65. Haldeman S, McGregor M. Risk factors and precipitating neck movements causing vertebrobasilar artery dissection after cervical trauma and spinal manipulation. Spine 1999; 24:785–794.

66. Haldeman S, McGregor M. Unpredictability of cerebrovascular ischemia associated with cervical spine manipulation: a review of 64 cases after cervical spine manipulative therapy. Spine 2002; 27:49–55.

67. Haldeman S. Spinal manipulative therapy in the management of low back pain. In: Finneson BE, ed. Low back pain. Philadelphia: JB Lippincott; 1980:245–275.

68. Harris JD. History and development of manipulation and mobilization. In: Basmajian JV, ed. Manipulation, traction and massage. Baltimore: Williams & Wilkins; 1985:3–21.

69. Harte AA, Gracey JH. The efficacy of traction for low back pain: a systematic review of randomized controlled trials. Arch Phys Med Rehabil 2003; 84:1542–1552.

70. van der Heijden GJ, Beurskens AJ, Koes BW, et al. The efficacy of traction for back and neck pain: a systematic, blinded review of randomized clinical trial methods. Phys Ther 1995; 75(2):93–104.

71. Hemmings B, Graydon J, Dyson R. Effects of massage on physiological restoration, perceived recovery, and repeated sports performance. Br J Sports Med 2000; 34:109–114.

72. Hemphill L. Implementing a therapeutic massage program in a tertiary and ambulatory care VA setting: the healing power of touch. Nurs Clin North Am 2000; 35:489–497.

73. Hernandez-Reif M, Largie S, Hart S, et al. Childrens' distress during burn treatment is reduced by massage therapy. J Burn Care Rehabil 2001; 22:191–195.

74. Hinterbuchner C. Traction. In: Basmajian JV, ed. Manipulation, traction and massage. Baltimore: Williams & Wilkins; 1985:172–201.

75. Hoehler FK, Tobis JS, Buerger AA. Spinal manipulation for low back pain. JAMA 1981; 245:1835–1838.

76. Hofkosh JM. Classical massage. In: Basmajian JV, ed. Manipulation, traction and massage. Baltimore: Williams & Wilkins; 1985:263–269.

77. Hood LB, Chrisman D. Intermittent pelvic traction in the treatment of the ruptured intervertebral disk. Phys Ther 1968; 48(1):21–30.

78. Hovind H. Effect of massage on blood flow in skeletal muscle. Scand J Rehabil Med 1974; 6:74–77.

79. Hoving JL, Gross AR, Gasner D, et al. A critical appraisal of review articles on the effectiveness of conservative treatment for neck pain. Spine 2001; 26:196–205.

80. Hruby RJ. Pathophysiologic models and the selection of osteopathic manipulative techniques. J Osteopath Med 1992; 6:25–30.

81. Hurwitz EL, Aker PD, Adams AH. Manipulation and mobilization of the cervical spine. A systematic review of the literature [see comment]. Spine 1996; 21:1746–1759.

82. Irnich D, Molzen H, Konig A, et al. Randomized trial of acupuncture compared with conventional massage and 'sham' laser acupuncture for the treatment of chronic neck pain. Br Med J 2001; 322:1574–1578.

83. Johannson K, Lie A, Ekdah C. A randomized study comparing manual lymph drainage with sequential pneumatic compression for treatment of postoperative arm lymphedema. Lymphology 1998; 31:56–64.

84. Johnston WL. Functional method. Ann Arbor: Edwards Brothers; 1994.

85. Jones LH. Strain and counterstrain. Newark: American Academy of Osteopathy; 1992.

86. Jones LH. Strain–counterstrain. Boise: Jones Strain-Counterstrain; 1995.

87. Jones NA. Massage and music therapies attenuated frontal EEG asymmetry in depressed adolescents. Adolescence 1999; 34:529–534.

88. Judovich BD, Nobel GR. Traction therapy: a study of resistance forces. Am J Surg 1957; 93:108.

89. Judovich BD. Herniated cervical disc: a new form of traction therapy. Am J Surg 1952; 84:646–656.

90. Judovich BD. Lumbar traction therapy—elimination of physical factors that prevent lumbar stretch. JAMA 1955; 159:549–550.

91. Kaada B. Increase of plasma beta-endorphins in connective tissue massage. Gen Pharmacol 1989; 20:487–489.

92. Kalauokalani D, Sherman KJ, Koepsell TD, et al. Lessons from a trial of acupuncture and massage for low back pain: patient expectations and treatment effects. Spine 2001; 26:1418–1424.

93. Kanemetz HL. History of massage. In: Basmajian JV, ed. Manipulation, traction and massage. Baltimore: Williams & Wilkins; 1985:211–255.

94. Kimberly PE. Formulating a prescription for osteopathic manipulative treatment. J Am Osteopath Assoc 1980; 79(8):506–513.

95. Knapp ME. Massage. In: Kottke FJ, Lahman JF, eds. Krusen's handbook of physical medicine and rehabilitation. Philadelphia: Saunders; 1990: 433–435.

96. Koes BW, Assendelft WJ, Kripschild PG, et al. Spinal manipulation for low back pain. An updated systematic review of randomized clinical trials. Spine 1996; 21(24):2860–2871; discussion 2872–2873.

97. Korr IM. Proprioceptors and somatic dysfunction. J Am Osteopath Assoc 1975; 74(7):638–650.

98. Korr IM. Somatic dysfunction, osteopathic manipulative treatment, and the nervous system: a few facts, some theories, many questions. J Am Osteopath Assoc 1986; 86(2):109–114.

99. Koss R. Quality assurance monitoring of osteopathic manipulative treatment. J Am Osteopath Assoc 1990; 90(5):427–433.

100. Kuchera ML. Osteopathic principles and practice. 2nd edn. Columbus: Greyden Press; 1994.

101. Lehmann JF, Brunner GD. A device for the application of heavy lumbar traction: its mechanical effects. Arch Phys Med Rehabil 1958; 39: 696–700.

102. MacDonald RS, Bell CM. An open controlled assessment of osteopathic manipulation in nonspecific low-back pain. Spine 1991; 15:364–370. Erratum in Spine 1991; 16(1):104.

103. Malanga GA. Nonoperative treatment for low back pain. Mayo Clin Proc 1999; 74:1135–1148.

104. Meade TW, Dyer S, Browne W. Low back pain of mechanical origin: randomised comparison of chiropractic and hospital outpatient treatment. Br Med J 1990; 300:1431–1437.

105. Mennell JM. Diagnosis and treatment using manipulative techniques. London: J & A Churchill; 1964.

106. Mills MV, Barnes LLB, Carriero JE, et al. The use of osteopathic manipulative treatment as adjunct therapy in children with recurrent otitis media. Arch Pediatr Adolesc Med 2003; 157:861–866.

107. Mitchell FL. Structural pelvic function. In: AAO yearbook. Indianapolis: American Academy of Osteopathy; 1958:71–89.

108. Mitchell FLJ, Moran PS, Pruzzo NA. An evaluation and treatment manual of osteopathic muscle energy procedures. Valley Park: Mitchell, Moran, and Purzzo Associates; 1979.

109. Mitchell FL Jr. The muscle energy manual, vols 1–4. East Lansing: MET Press; 1995.

110. Moeti P. Clinical outcome from mechanical intermittent cervical traction for the treatment of cervical radiculopathy: a case series. J Orthop Sports Phys Ther 2001; 31(4):207–213.

111. Monte T. World medicine. The east west guide to healing your body. New York: Putnam; 1993.

112. Neumann H-D. Introduction to manual medicine. Berlin: Springer-Verlag; 1989.

113. Oleson T. Randomized controlled study of premenstrual symptoms treated with ear, hand, and foot reflexology. Obstet Gynecol 1993; 82:906–911.

114. Paramore LC. Use of alternative therapies: estimates from the 1994 Robert Wood Johnson Foundation National Access to Care Survey. J Pain Symptom Manage 1997; 13(2):83–89.

115. Patterson MM. Long-lasting alterations of spinal reflexes: a potential basis for somatic dysfunction. J Am Osteopath Assoc 1986; 86(2):38–42.

116. Patterson MM. Louisa Burns Memorial Lecture 1980: the spinal cord—active processor not passive transmitter. J Am Osteopath Assoc 1980; 80(3):210–216.

117. Postacchini F, Facchini M, Palieri P. Efficacy of various forms of conservative treatment in low back pain. A comparative study. Neuro-orthopedics 1988; 6:28–35.

118. Powell FC, Hanigan WC, Olivero WC. A risk/benefit analysis of spinal manipulation therapy for relief of lumbar or cervical pain. Neurosurgery 1992; 33:73–78.

119. Prentice WE. Therapeutic massage. In: Therapeutic modalities for allied health professionals. New York: McGraw-Hill; 1998.

120. Pryde M. Effectiveness of massage therapy for subacute low-back pain: a randomized control trial. CMAJ 2000; 162:1815–1820.

121. Puustjarvi K, Poltinen PJ. The effects of massage in patients with chronic tension headache. Acupunct Electrother Res 1990; 15:159–162.

122. Ramos G, Martin W. Effects of vertebral axial decompression on intradiscal pressure [see comment]. J Neurosurg 1994; 81:350–353.

123. Ramos G. Efficacy of vertebral axial decompression on chronic low back pain. Neurol Res 2004; 26:320–324.

124. Richards K. Effect of back massage and relaxation intervention on sleep in the critically ill patients. Am J Crit Care 1998; 7:288–299.

125. Richards KC, Overton-McCoy AL. Effects of a massage in acute and critical care. AACN Clin Issues 2000; 11:77–96.

126. Rodenburg JB, Schiereck P, Bar PR. Warm-up stretching and massage diminish harmful effects of eccentric exercise. Int J Sports Med 1994; 15:414–419.

127. Rogoff JB. Motorized intermittent traction. In: Basmajian JV, ed. Manipulation, traction and massage. Baltimore: Williams & Wilkins; 1985:201–207.

128. Saul JS, Yurth EF. Nonoperative treatment of herniated cervical intervertebral disc with radiculopathy. Spine 1996; 21:877–883.

129. Scafid F. Massage therapy improves behavior in neonates born to HIV-positive mothers. J Pediatr Psychol 1996; 14:176–180.

130. Shealy CN, Borgmeyer V. Emerging technologies: preliminary findings. Decompression, reduction, and stabilization of the lumbar spine: a cost-effective treatment for lumbosacral pain. Am J Phys Med 1997; 7:63–65.

131. Sherry E, Smart R. A prospective randomized control study of VAX-D and TENS for the treatment of chronic low back pain. Neurol Res 2001; 23:780–784.

132. Shoemaker JK, Mader R. Failure of manual massage to alter limb blood flow: measures by Doppler ultrasound. Med Sci Sports 1997; 29: 610–614.

133. Sims-Williams H, Jayson MIV, Young SMS. Controlled trial of mobilisation and manipulation for low back pain: hospital patients. Br Med J 1979; 2:1318–1320.

134. Smith LL, Holbert D, Spratt DJ, et al. The effects of athletic massage on delayed onset muscle soreness, creatine kinase, and neutrophil count: a preliminary report. J Orthop Sports Phys Ther 1994; 19:93–99.

135. Tappan F. Healing massage techniques: holistic, classic, and emerging methods. Norwalk: Appleton & Lange; 1988.

136. Tesio L, Merlo A. Autotraction versus passive traction: an open controlled study in lumbar discontinued herniation. Arch Phys Med Rehabil 1993; 74:871–876.

137. Tiidus PM. Manual massage and recovery of muscle function following exercise: a literature review. J Orthop Sports Phys Ther 1997; 25: 107–112.

138. Travell J. Myofascial pain and dysfunction: the trigger point manual. Baltimore: Williams & Wilkins; 1983.

139. Triano JJ, McGregor M, Hondras MA. Manipulative therapy versus education programs in chronic low back pain. Spine 1995; 20:948–955.

140. Van Buskirk R. Nociceptive reflexes and the somatic dysfunction: a model. J Am Osteopath Assoc 1990; 90(9):797–809.

141. Vick DA, Zengerle CR. The safety of manipulative treatment: review of the literature from 1925 to 1993. J Am Osteopath Assoc 1996; 96(2): 113–115.

142. Ward RC. Foundations for osteopathic medicine. 2nd edn. Philadelphia: Lippincott Williams & Wilkins; 2003.

143. Ward RC. Myofascial release concepts. In: Basmajian JV, Nyberg R. Rational manual therapies. Baltimore: Williams & Wilkins; 1993: 223–241.

144. Willard F. Nociception, the neuroendocrine immune system and osteopathic medicine. In: Ward RC, ed. Foundations for osteopathic medicine. 2nd edn. Philadelphia: Lippincott Williams & Wilkins; 2003.

145. Wolfson H. Studies on effect of physical therapeutic procedures on function and structure. JAMA 1931; 96:2020–2021.

146. Wong AM, Lee MY, Chang WH. Clinical trial of a cervical traction modality with electromyographic biofeedback. Am J Phys Med Rehabil 1997; 76:19–25.

147. Wood EC. Beard's massage: principles and techniques. Philadelphia: Saunders; 1974.

148. Wreje U, Nordgren B, Aberg H. Treatment of pelvic joint dysfunction in primary care—a controlled study. Scand J Prim Health Care 1992; 10:310–315. Erratum in Scand J Prim Health Care 1993; 11(1):25.

149. Yong HK. Sacro-iliac joint pain: etiology and conservative treatment. Chir Organi Mov 1994; 79:35–45.

Physical Agent Modalities

David C. Weber and Kurtis M. Hoppe

Modalities are physical agents that are utilized to produce a therapeutic response in tissue. They include heat, cold, water, sound, electricity, and electromagnetic waves (including infrared, visible, or ultraviolet light; shortwaves; and microwaves) (Fig. 21-1). This chapter focuses on these physical agent modalities, except for most of the therapeutic uses of electrical stimulation (which are covered in Ch. 22). These modalities are generally considered adjunctive treatments rather than primary curative interventions. This chapter reviews the physiologic effects, common uses, techniques of application, and precautions for the therapeutic use of modalities. Although there is a growing body of literature to support the use of physical agent modalities, further research is needed to more specifically define the efficacy and indications for these agents.[15,146–149]

MODALITY PRESCRIPTION

The elements of a prescription for heat or cold are listed in Box 21-1. The condition for which the modality is being used should be clearly indicated. The location to be treated influences modality selection, in that large areas can preclude the use of modalities such as ultrasound or ice massage. The surface to be treated can also influence selection. If using ultrasound over an irregular surface, degassed water might be preferred over a gel coupling agent. If using superficial heat over an irregular surface, hot packs or heating pads can result in focal heating over prominences, so radiant heat might be preferred. Intensity should be indicated where appropriate (e.g. ultrasound power output, hydrotherapy, fluidotherapy, and paraffin bath temperature). Most modalities allow only qualitative dosimetry as currently used in physical medicine, and therefore rely on patient perception of thermal intensity for safety. Duration for most modalities is 20–30 min, except for ultrasound, which is typically 5–10 min per site. Frequency is based on the severity of the condition being treated and on clinical judgment. Although information about duration and intensity of treatment is noted in this chapter, it is intended only as a guideline, and should be modified by clinical experience and the clinical condition.

Modality selection is influenced by multiple factors (Box 21-2). In selecting a modality, one should recognize that there are few well-designed clinical trials demonstrating the efficacy of *specific* modalities in *specific* conditions. There are, however,

numerous studies that review the physiologic effects of modalities. Having a firm understanding of the physiologic effects of a particular modality allows one to make an educated selection. One must understand the heating or cooling capabilities of the various modalities to ensure the selection of the proper modality for the target tissue. Body habitus influences modality selection in that subcutaneous adipose affects the depth of penetration of many modalities. Comorbid conditions should also be considered. For example, both cold and heat can have adverse effects in the patient with significant arterial insufficiency. Cold can have harmful effects via the production of arterial vasoconstriction, and heat can cause complications via the production of increased metabolic activity, which can exceed the potential increase in blood supply and produce ischemia. Age is also a factor in modality selection. In the pediatric population, ultrasound should generally be avoided near open epiphyses.[169] In the elderly population, there can be comorbidities that affect modality choice. Gender can also play a role in modality use, because fetal malformations have been reported following ultrasound near a gravid uterus.[121]

HEAT

Forms of heat can be broadly classified by depth of penetration and form of heat transfer (Table 21-1). Depth of penetration is arbitrarily divided into superficial and deep. Superficial heat includes hot packs, heating pads, paraffin baths, fluidotherapy, whirlpool baths, and radiant heat. Deep heating agents (or diathermies) include ultrasound, shortwave, and microwave. Mechanisms of heat transfer include conduction, convection, radiation, evaporation, and conversion (Fig. 21-2). *Conduction* is the transfer of thermal energy between two bodies in direct contact. *Convection* uses movement of a medium (e.g. water, air, or blood) to transport thermal energy, although the actual transfer of thermal energy is ultimately by conduction. *Radiation* refers to the thermal radiation emitted from any body whose surface temperature is above absolute zero (−273.15°C or −459.67°F). *Evaporation* involves the transformation of a liquid into a gas, a process that requires thermal energy. Evaporation is actually a process of heat dissipation, and plays a role in cooling modalities such as vapocoolant sprays. For each gram of water that evaporates from the body surface, approximately

Frequency in Hertz

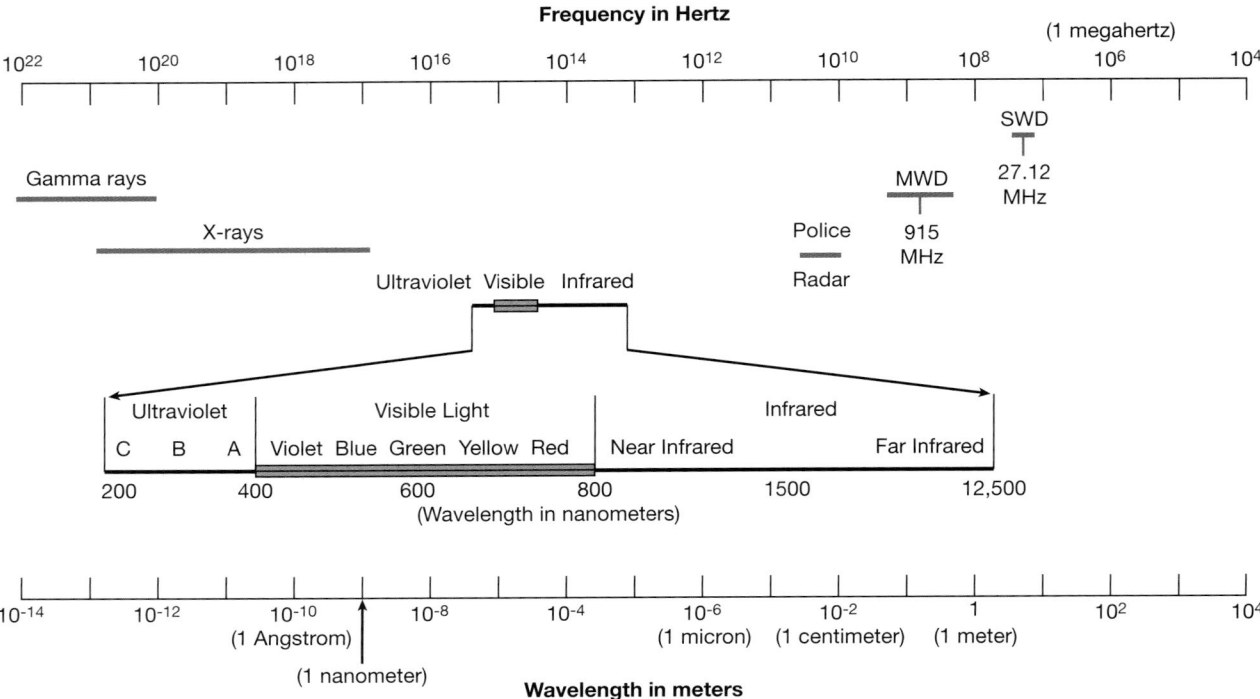

Figure 21-1 Electromagnetic spectrum.

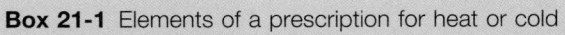

Box 21-1 Elements of a prescription for heat or cold

- Indication or diagnosis
- Modality
- Location
- Intensity
- Duration
- Frequency

Box 21-2 Factors to consider in modality selection

- Target tissue
- Depth of heating or cooling desired
- Intensity of heating or cooling desired
- Body habitus (i.e. amount of subcutaneous adipose)
- Comorbid conditions (e.g. cancer, vascular disease, neuropathy)
- Specific patient features (e.g. metal implants, pacemaker, cold allergy)
- Age (e.g. open epiphyses)
- Sex (e.g. pregnant woman)

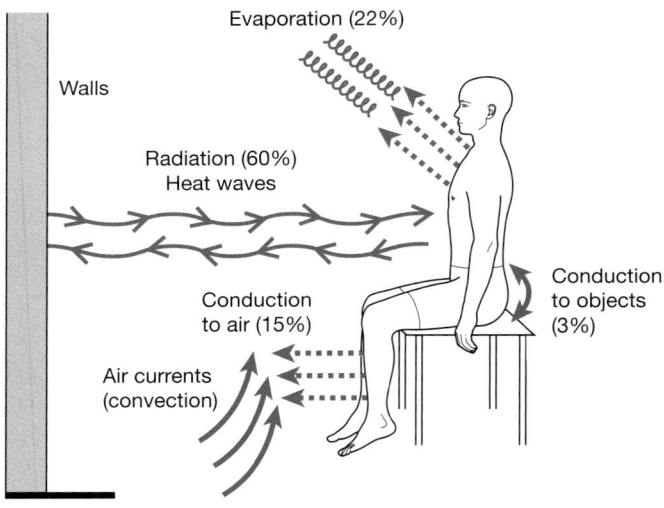

Figure 21-2 Mechanisms of heat transfer. (From Guyton 1991,[73] with permission.)

therapeutic use of heat, followed by discussions of the general uses of heat (see Box 21-4), some general precautions (see Box 21-5), and descriptions of the agents currently used in physical medicine.

Physiologic effects of heat
Hemodynamic

Localized heating produces a variety of hemodynamic effects. A two- to threefold increase in forearm blood flow has been demonstrated following hydrotherapy at 44–45°C (111.2–

0.6 cal (kilocal) of heat is lost.[73] *Conversion* refers to the transformation of energy (e.g. sound or electromagnetic) to heat. Likewise, the human body converts protein, carbohydrates, and fats to thermal energy via numerous metabolic processes. The next section reviews the physiologic effects (Box 21-3) of the

Table 21-1 Classification of various types of heating

Type of heating	Depth	Main mechanism of energy transfer
Hot packs or heating pads	Superficial	Conduction
Paraffin baths	Superficial	Conduction
Fluidotherapy	Superficial	Convection
Whirlpool baths	Superficial	Convection
Radiant heat	Superficial	Radiation
Ultrasound	Deep	Conversion
Shortwave diathermy	Deep	Conversion
Microwave	Deep	Conversion

Box 21-3 Physiologic effects of heat

Hemodynamic
- Increased blood flow
- Decreased chronic inflammation
- Increased acute inflammation
- Increased edema
- Increased bleeding

Neuromuscular
- ?Increased group 1a fiber firing rates (muscle spindle)
- ?Decreased group 2 fiber firing rates (muscle spindle)
- ?Increased group 1b fiber firing rates (Golgi tendon organ)
- Increased nerve conduction velocity

Joint and connective tissue
- Increased tendon extensibility
- Increased collagenase activity
- Decreased joint stiffness

Miscellaneous
- Decreased pain
- General relaxation

Box 21-4 General uses of heat in physical medicine

- Musculoskeletal conditions (tendinitis, tenosynovitis, bursitis, capsulitis, etc.)
- Pain (neck, low back, myofascial, neuromas, postherpetic neuralgia, etc.)
- Arthritis
- Contracture
- Muscle relaxation
- Chronic inflammation

Box 21-5 General precautions for the use of heat

- Acute trauma, inflammation
- Impaired circulation
- Bleeding diatheses
- Edema
- Large scars
- Impaired sensation
- Malignancy
- Cognitive or communication deficits that preclude reporting of pain

113°F) or shortwave diathermy (SWD).[1] This vasodilatation results in increased ingress of nutrients, leukocytes, and antibodies, and increased egress of metabolic by-products and tissue debris, and can facilitate resolution of inflammatory conditions.[72,157] Vasodilatation with heating can unfortunately also contribute to increased bleeding and increased edema formation, and can exacerbate acute inflammatory conditions.[157] There are a number of experimental animal models of acute and chronic inflammation that support the general clinical impression that acute inflammatory conditions tend to react unfavorably to heat, whereas chronic inflammatory conditions tend to benefit from heat.[157]

Neuromuscular

Animal experiments of localized heating have demonstrated increased firing rates in all group 1a fibers (muscle spindle) and many group 1b (Golgi tendon organ) fibers, and decreased firing rates in the majority of group 2 fibers (muscle spindle).[124] It should be noted that all experiments on muscle spindle and Golgi tendon organ firing rates are significantly influenced by the length and tension at which they are performed. This factor probably accounts for many of the differences among investigators.[56,124] In contrast, the effects of temperature change on nerve conduction velocity are much more consistent. Heating produces modest increases in conduction velocity, whereas cooling is capable of producing dramatic decreases in conduction velocity. Abramson et al. noted increases in conduction velocity of up to 7.5 m/s following hydrotherapy at 44–45°C (111.2–113°F) or SWD, whereas cooling produced conduction velocity decreases of up to 35.8 m/s.[1] The effects of temperature in clinical neurophysiology are succinctly summarized elsewhere.[44]

Joint and connective tissue

In vitro experiments demonstrate the importance of combined heating and stretching to maximize tendon extensibility. Lehmann et al. measured tendon extensibility under a variety of temperature and loading conditions.[106] Tendon extensibility was greater at 45°C (113°F) than at 25°C (77°F). Furthermore, simultaneous use of heating and stretching produced significantly increased tendon extensibility when compared with the isolated use of either agent. Sustaining stretching during the cool down period also facilitated tendon elongation. Other investigators have demonstrated metacarpophalangeal joint stiffness to decrease by as much as 20% at 45°C (113°F) compared with at 33°C (91.4°F).[186] Temperature also affects enzymatic activity. In vitro experiments have shown a fourfold increase in collagenase activity with a temperature increase from 33 to 36°C (91.4 to 96.8°F).[75]

Miscellaneous effects of heat

It is generally accepted that heat produces an analgesic effect. A variety of mechanisms for the analgesic effect of heat have been postulated.[57,110] These include a cutaneous counterirritant effect, vasodilatation resulting in decreased ischemic pain, vasodilatation resulting in washout of pain mediators, an endorphin-mediated response, alteration of nerve conduction, and alteration of cell membrane permeability. Elevation of pain threshold has been demonstrated following therapeutic application of ultrasound, microwave, and infrared radiation.[100] Many patients also find heat to have a general relaxation effect, although the specific mechanisms are not well defined.

General uses of heat in physical medicine

The general uses of heat are summarized in Box 21-4. These uses are based on the physiologic effects previously described. Heat is used in a variety of musculoskeletal conditions because of its potential to produce analgesia and muscle relaxation, and to facilitate resolution of inflammation. Increased soft tissue extensibility and decreased joint stiffness make heat useful in contractures and a variety of arthritides.

General precautions for the use of heat

The general precautions for the use of heat are listed in Box 21-5. As noted earlier, heat can exacerbate acute inflammation, and should generally be avoided in the acute management stage.[157] In the patient with impaired circulation, increased metabolic activity with heating can exceed the capacity of arterial supply, so heat should be used with caution in this patient population. Vasodilatation from heat can result in increased bleeding in persons with bleeding diatheses. Vasodilatation can also produce increased edema. Because scars can be relatively avascular and have reduced ability to dissipate heat, they can be selectively heated. Heat should generally be avoided in areas of impaired sensation because of the obvious potential for thermal injury, due to the lack of precise dosimetry in modality use. This same reason justifies caution in using heat in patients with impaired cognition or communication, which precludes reporting of pain. Lehmann cautioned against the use of heat over malignancies because of the potential for increased rate of tumor growth or hyperemia increasing hematogenous spread.[110] However, this should be distinguished from the use of specific local hyperthermia in the adjunctive treatment of malignancies.[142] It also does not preclude the use of heat for adjunctive analgesia in the terminally ill cancer patient.

SUPERFICIAL HEAT

Superficial heating agents achieve their maximum tissue temperatures in skin and subcutaneous fat. Deeper tissue heating is limited by vasodilatation (which dissipates heat) and the insulating properties of fat. Superficial heating agents can heat via conduction (hot packs, heating pads, and paraffin baths), radiation (heat lamps), or convection (fluidotherapy and whirlpool baths). Superficial heat is used in osteoarthritis, rheumatoid arthritis, neck pain, low back pain, muscle pain syndromes, and a variety of musculoskeletal conditions.[110]

Hot packs

Commercially available hot packs, such as Hydrocollator packs, typically contain silicon dioxide encased in a canvas pack. They come in a variety of sizes and styles for use over different areas. Hot packs are immersed in tanks at 74.5°C (166°F) and applied over several layers of insulating towels.[109] After several minutes, the skin should be inspected briefly to ensure that the heating is not excessive. Total treatment time is usually 30 min. Lehmann et al. showed that the 30-min application of a Hydrocollator pack to the posterior thigh produced approximately 3.3 and 1.3°C tissue temperature elevations at 1- and 2-cm depths, respectively.[109] Other investigators observed a 1.1°C temperature rise 4 cm deep in the brachioradialis muscle following a 30-min application of a Hydrocollator pack.[2] A 1.2°C increase in intraarticular temperature (knee) has also been demonstrated following hot pack application.[182] General heat precautions should be observed. The patient should not lie on the pack. This can squeeze water from the pack, wetting the insulating towels, thereby raising their thermal conductivity and increasing the risk of burns. The focal pressure from lying on a hot pack can also produce increased heating over bony prominences. Lying on the hot pack also puts the pressure of the weight of the body on the skin next to the pack. This pressure exceeds capillary pressure and makes it difficult for blood to come into the area to carry away the heat. Hot packs are among the more common causes of burns in physical therapy. This is because heat has sedative effects, and the patient is typically not directly supervised when this modality is used.

Heating pads

Two main types of heating pad are available: electric heating pads and circulating fluid pads. Electric heating pads usually control heat output by regulating current flow. Circulating fluid (e.g. water) heating pads usually control heat output thermostatically. Peak temperatures of nearly 52°C (125°F) were achieved with an electric heating pad set on the *lowest* setting.[45] Periodic temperature oscillations of up to 5°C were also noted.[45] General heat precautions should be observed with heating pads. There is an obvious potential for electric shock, particularly when used in conjunction with moist toweling. Many commercially available heating pads are designed to be used in conjunction with moist toweling, but caution should be taken to inspect them regularly to ensure that all insulating materials are intact.

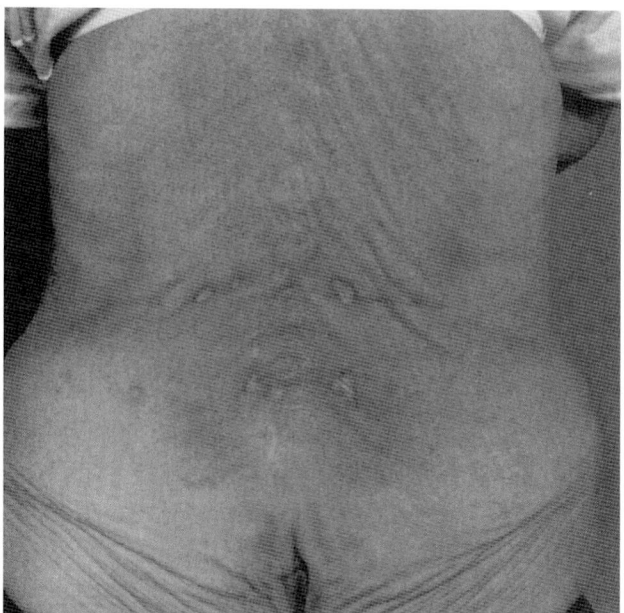

Figure 21-3 Typical heating pad burn. Note the focal hypopigmentation from burns at areas of increased pressure. Also note the more diffuse hyperpigmentation changes (erythema ab igne).

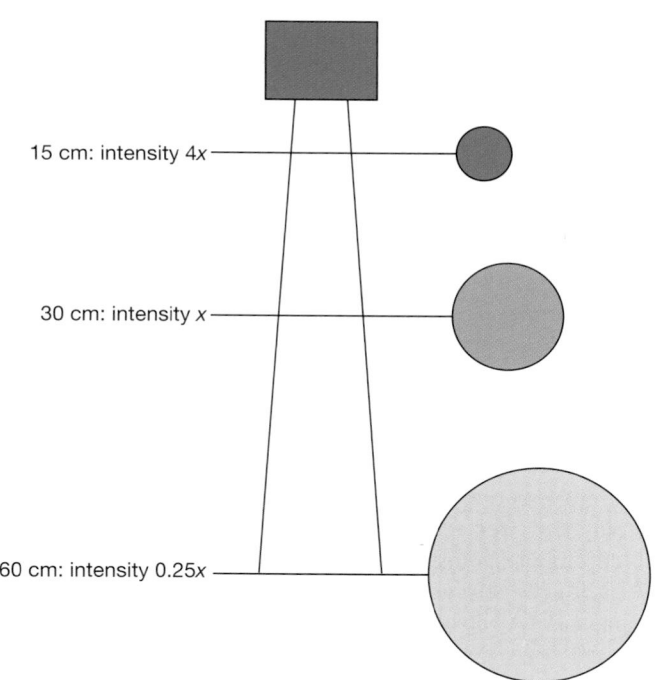

15 cm: intensity 4*x*

30 cm: intensity *x*

60 cm: intensity 0.25*x*

Figure 21-4 Example of inverse square law, with the intensity arbitrarily defined as *x* at a distance of 30 cm. With a change in distance from the heat source, the area of heating changes, and therefore the heat intensity per unit of area changes.

The patient should not lie on a heating pad, as this can result in focal temperature increases, leading to burns. This is of particular concern in the slender or cachectic patient with minimal subcutaneous adipose over bony prominences. Figure 21-3 shows a typical heating pad burn. The patient was an elderly woman who had not received adequate instruction in home use of her modalities, and had been repeatedly lying supine on an electric heating pad. Repeated and prolonged skin exposure to heat can result in erythema ab igne, a skin condition characterized by reticular pigmentation, and telangiectasia, which has been noted following the use of a variety of superficial heating modalities.[47]

Radiant heat

Radiant energy, including infrared radiation, is emitted from any substance with a temperature above absolute zero. Infrared is the portion of the electromagnetic spectrum adjacent to the long-wavelength, low-frequency (red) end of the visible spectrum. Luminous infrared heat lamps emit radiation in the near-infrared spectrum (wavelength 770–1500 nm), and non-luminous infrared heat lamps emit radiation in the far-infrared spectrum (wavelength 1500–12 500 nm).[110] Infrared produces heating by inducing molecular vibration.[47] A 1.3°C temperature rise has been noted at a depth of 2 cm following heat lamp application.[109]

The main determinants of intensity of radiant heating are distance and angle of delivery. The inverse square law states that the intensity of radiation varies inversely with the square of the distance from the source (Fig. 21-4). This means that doubling the distance from a heat lamp reduces the heating intensity by a factor of four. Conversely, decreasing the distance

from the heat lamp by half would increase the intensity fourfold. Typical distances are 30–60 cm from the patient's body, depending on heat lamp wattage.[110] The angle of delivery also affects the intensity of thermal radiation. Maximal radiation is applied when the source of radiation is perpendicular to the surface. As the angle away from perpendicular increases, the intensity of radiation decreases in proportion to the cosine of the angle.

Radiant heat is often preferable in patients who cannot tolerate the weight of hot packs. Caveats for the use of radiant heat include general heat precautions, light sensitivity, skin drying, and dermal photoaging.[47,110] Some laboratory data suggest a potential for infrared acting synergistically with ultraviolet radiation in cutaneous photocarcinogenesis, but the clinical significance of this, if any, remains to be determined.[47]

Fluidotherapy

Fluidotherapy is a superficial, dry heating modality that uses convective heating with forced hot air and a bed of finely divided solid particles.[18] This solid–gas system reportedly behaves like a heterogeneous fluid of low viscosity, a phenomenon labeled fluidization.[17] Reputed advantages include the massaging action of the highly turbulent solid–gas mixture, and the freedom to perform range of motion exercises.[17] Peak hand muscle and joint capsule temperatures of nearly 42°C (107.6°F), and peak foot muscle and joint capsule temperatures of approximately 39.5°C (103.1°F), have been achieved following 20 min of fluidotherapy at 47.8°C (118°F).[18] Both the temperature and the amount of agitation can be controlled. The typical temperature range is 46.1–48.9°C (115–120°F). Decreased degrees of agitation can be utilized for sensitive areas. Although fluidotherapy is touted for use in a variety of conditions, further study is needed to more objectively define its role in physical medicine.[82] General heat precautions should be observed, and infected wounds should probably be avoided because of the risk of cross-contamination.

Paraffin baths

A paraffin bath is a superficial heating agent that uses conduction as the primary form of heat transfer. Paraffin wax and mineral oil are mixed in a ratio of 6:1 or 7:1.[110] Treatment temperatures are 52.2–54.4°C (126–130°F). These are tolerated because of the low heat conductivity of the paraffin mixture.[110] A thermometer should be used to ensure proper temperature. A thin film of unmelted paraffin on the tank walls generally indicates a safe temperature. Methods of application include dipping, immersion, and brushing. After removing all jewelry, thoroughly wash and dry the area to be treated. The dipping method involves 7–12 dips followed by wrapping in plastic and towels or insulated mitts to retain heat.[2] The immersion method involves several dips to form a thin glove of paraffin, followed by immersion for 30 min.[2] The brushing method involves brushing on several coats of paraffin, followed by covering with towels. The brushing method is more cumbersome, and infrequently used in the adult population. However, children often find paraffin brushing to be fun, thereby improving their treatment compliance. Paraffin brushing can also be useful for areas difficult to immerse. For home treatment, patients can use a double boiler, although commercial paraffin tanks are reasonably inexpensive, probably safer, and more convenient. The equipment safety precautions should be carefully reviewed. General heat precautions apply to paraffin use. Open wounds and infected areas should be avoided.

The immersion method produces the greatest quantity and duration of temperature increase, with peak forearm subcutaneous tissue temperatures of 5.5°C over baseline, and brachioradialis temperatures of 2.4°C over baseline.[2] The dip method produces a 4.4°C peak forearm subcutaneous tissue temperature rise and a 1.0°C brachioradialis temperature rise, but these temperature rises decrease significantly by 15–20 min post dipping.[2] In a study of scleroderma patients, paraffin baths in conjunction with friction massage and active range of motion exercise resulted in statistically significant improvement in skin compliance and overall hand function.[5] In a study of rheumatoid arthritis patients, statistically significant improvements in range of motion and grip function were noted following paraffin treatment in conjunction with active range of motion exercises, whereas paraffin baths alone had no statistically significant effect.[42] This again emphasizes the importance of using exercise in combination with the modality.

DEEP HEAT

Diathermy is derived from *dia* ('through') and *therme* ('heat'), and refers to several forms of deep heating, namely shortwave,

microwave, and ultrasound. Because the target tissue in physical medicine is generally muscle, tendon, ligament, or bone (rather than skin or subcutaneous fat), the goal of early investigators was to discover a mode of heating that minimized skin and subcutaneous tissue heating but maximized heating of deeper tissues.[72] The challenge of diathermy developers was to discover a modality that could penetrate the skin and subcutaneous fat to produce a maximum temperature rise in underlying soft tissues. Conversely, the modality should not produce excessive temperatures in more superficial tissues (subcutaneous fat, being relatively avascular compared with muscle, is unable to adequately dissipate heat via vasodilatation). The therapeutic target temperature is generally considered to be 40–45°C (104–113°F).[72] Lower temperatures might not produce adequate vasodilatation and increased metabolism, whereas higher temperatures can result in tissue damage. Because the thermal pain threshold is approximately 45°C (113°F), pain perception can be used to monitor intensity of heating in the neurologically intact and alert person.[72] One gradually increases modality intensity to the earliest pain perception, then slightly decreases intensity. However, there is only a fine line between the therapeutic temperature range and potential thermal injury.

Ultrasound

Ultrasound is defined as acoustic vibration with frequencies above the audible range (i.e. greater than 20 000 Hz). Medical uses of ultrasound can be diagnostic or therapeutic. Diagnostic ultrasound is used for a variety of obstetric, urologic, cardiovascular, and other imaging studies, and is outside the scope of this chapter. Therapeutic ultrasound involves the use of high-frequency acoustic energy to produce thermal and non-thermal effects in tissue. Ultrasonic signals are typically generated using the reverse piezoelectric effect. Certain quartz crystals and synthetic ceramics have piezoelectric characteristics, such that when they vibrate they produce an electric current.[171] The reverse happens when an electric current is passed across such crystals, causing vibration at a specific frequency.

As ultrasonic waves travel through tissue, they lose a proportion of their energy, a process called *attenuation*.[187] Attenuation in tissue is produced by several mechanisms: absorption, beam divergence, and deflection.[187] *Absorption* is the major cause of ultrasound attenuation.[187] Ultrasonic energy is absorbed by the tissue, and is ultimately converted into heat.[187] For most tissues, attenuation increases as frequency increases, so a 1.0-MHz signal would penetrate deeper than a 3.0-MHz signal because of its lower attenuation by the tissue.[187] *Beam divergence* is the amount that the beam spreads out from the transducer. Beam divergence decreases as frequency increases, so a higher frequency signal has a more focused beam.

Deflection includes the processes of *reflection*, *refraction*, and *scattering*.[187] The *angle* of the reflected wave is equal to the angle of the incident wave (Fig. 21-5). The *magnitude* of the reflected wave depends on the difference in acoustic impedance between the tissues on each side of the reflecting surface.[187] Acoustic impedance is a measure of the resistance to the transmission of a sound wave, and is the product of the velocity of sound and the density of the medium.[171,187] The magnitude of the reflected wave is proportional to the following formula:[171]

$$A_2 - A_1/A_2 + A_1,$$

where A_2 is the acoustic impedance of tissue 2 and A_1 is the acoustic impedance of tissue 1. The greater the mismatch of acoustic impedance of the two tissues, the greater the magnitude of the reflected wave. Because the impedance mismatch between skin and air is extremely high, essentially all the acoustic signal is reflected if a coupling agent is not used (see below).[187] *Refraction* is a deviation of beam direction as it is transmitted between two media (see Fig. 21-5). The angle of the transmitted (refracted) wave is determined by the velocity of sound in the two media, and is given by Snell's law:[187]

$$\text{sine } 1/\text{sine } 2 = \text{velocity } 1/\text{velocity } 2,$$

where sine 1 is the sine of the incident wave, sine 2 is the sine of the transmitted wave, velocity 1 is the velocity of sound in the first tissue, and velocity 2 is the velocity of sound in the

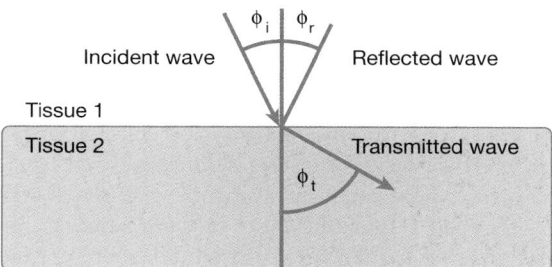

Figure 21-5 Example of reflection and refraction at a tissue interface. ϕ_i, Angle of incident wave; ϕ_r, angle of reflected wave; ϕ_t, angle of transmitted wave.

second tissue. *Scattering* is the last mechanism of beam deflection. It occurs when surface irregularities scatter the signal. Scattering is minimized when surface irregularities are small with respect to the wavelength.

Parameters for therapeutic ultrasound are noted in Table 21-2. Frequency is generally in the range of millions of cycles per second (or megahertz, MHz). The most commonly used frequencies in the USA are in the range of 0.8–1.1 MHz, although frequencies around 3.0 MHz are also fairly common. Power is total energy per unit time, whereas intensity is power per unit area. Intensity can be expressed in terms of peak or average intensity, and spatial or temporal intensity, and is indicated in units of watts per square centimeter. These different measures of intensity are defined in Table 21-2. The World Health Organization and the International Electrical Commission both recommend limiting spatial average intensity to 3 W/cm².[81] Most clinically used intensities of therapeutic ultrasound are in the 0.5–2.0 W/cm² range. Temperatures of up to 46°C (114.8°F) in deep tissues (e.g. bone–muscle interface) are easily achieved with ultrasound.[102–104] If very deep heating (e.g. of the hip joint) is the goal, ultrasound appears to be superior to microwave or SWD.[108]

Ultrasound delivery can be continuous or pulsed. Pulsed delivery involves the emission of brief bursts or pulses of ultrasound, interspersed with periods of silence (Fig. 21-6). For pulsed ultrasound delivery, additional parameters should be indicated.[171] These include pulse duration, pulse repetition period, pulse repetition frequency, and duty factor, and are defined in Table 21-2. In most machines available for use in the USA, selecting a duty factor automatically determines the other parameters. Duty factor commonly ranges from 10% to 50%. For example, a 2-ms pulse duration might be interspersed with 8 ms of silence. The pulse repetition period would be

Table 21-2 Ultrasound parameters	
Parameter	**Details**
Frequency	Millions of cycles per second (MHz)
Power	Total energy per unit time (W)
Effective radiating area	The area of the transducer that actually radiates ultrasonic waves (cm²)

Intensity
  Spatial average intensity
  Spatial peak intensity
  Temporal average intensity
  Temporal peak intensity
	May be expressed in terms of peak or average and spatial or temporal (W/cm²)
	Total power output divided by effective radiating area
	Maximal intensity anywhere within the beam
	Average intensity of 'on' and 'off' periods of a pulsed signal
	Maximal intensity of 'on' period of a pulsed signal

Duration	Generally 5–10 min per site

Additional parameters for pulsed ultrasound
  Pulse duration
  Pulse repetition period
  Pulse repetition frequency
  Duty factor
	
	Time of actual ultrasound pulse ('time on')
	Time interval from one pulse to the next ('time on' and 'time off')
	Number of pulses per second
	Fraction of total time during which ultrasound is emitted (calculated by dividing pulse duration by pulse repetition period)

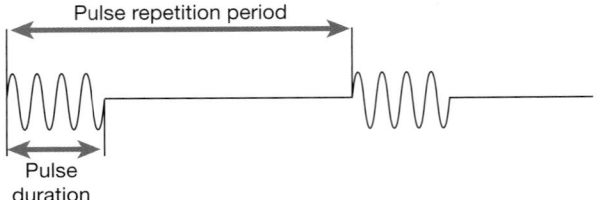

Figure 21-6 Example of a pulsed ultrasound signal.

10 ms, the pulse repetition frequency would be 100 Hz, and the duty factor would be 20%. Pulsed delivery, especially at low duty factors, results in less heating than continuous wave ultrasound, and thereby presumably emphasizes non-thermal effects.

The physiologic effects of ultrasound can be divided into thermal and non-thermal effects. Thermal effects are produced when acoustic energy is absorbed, producing molecular vibration, which results in heat production.[32] Non-thermal effects include cavitation, media motion (acoustic streaming, microstreaming), and standing waves. *Cavitation* is the production of gas bubbles in a sound field.[32] These bubbles can expand and contract with alternating compressions and rarefactions of a sound wave.[32] Stable cavitation refers to bubbles that oscillate in size within the sound field.[53] Unstable cavitation refers to bubbles that continue to grow in size and then collapse. The high temperatures and pressures generated by this can produce platelet aggregation, localized tissue damage, and cell death.[53] Both forms of cavitation are capable of mechanical distortion, movement of material, and alteration of cellular function, but their clinical significance is not yet clearly defined.[32,126]

Media motion includes acoustic streaming and microstreaming. Acoustic *streaming* is defined as unidirectional movement in an ultrasonic pressure field, and results from an ultrasonic wave traveling through a compressible medium.[53] Acoustic *microstreaming* is produced by stable cavitation. As the stable cavitation bubbles oscillate in size, the surrounding fluid is set in motion, with nearby particles being attracted to the oscillating bubble.[53] In addition to movement of material, acoustic streaming and microstreaming can result in cell membrane damage and accelerate metabolic processes.[53]

Standing waves are produced by the superimposition of incident and reflected sound waves, and can result in focal heating at tissue interfaces of different densities.[53] Stasis of red blood cells at one-half wavelength intervals in a sound field has also been demonstrated in the laboratory.[52] Although numerous subcellular, cellular, and tissue non-thermal ultrasound effects have been reported, their clinical significance remains to be elucidated.[32,38,52,53,126] Certain measures can minimize the nonthermal effects of ultrasound. Higher frequency, lower intensity, and pulsed delivery mode minimizes acoustic cavitation.[38] Stroking technique of application minimizes standing wave formation.[53]

As noted previously, the amount of ultrasound reflected at an interface between two media depends on the difference in acoustic impedance, so the ideal coupling medium is one with acoustic impedance similar to that of tissue. Three factors have an impact on the effectiveness of a coupling medium:

1. absorption by the medium, which attenuates the ultrasound power;
2. impedance match between the coupling media and the transmitter sound head, which determines the amount of power reflected into the ultrasound source; and
3. impedance match between the coupling medium and the body tissue, which determines the amount of power reflected into the medium.[6]

Degassed water is a commonly used coupling medium, and is used to prevent bubble formation on the skin surface. Allowing tap water to stand overnight typically allows for adequate gas evaporation. In tests of acoustic transmissivity, mineral oil and several commercially available coupling gels had similar transmissivities to the reference standard of distilled degassed water.[178] However, the hydrocortisone phonophoresis coupling agents tested had a significantly lower transmissivity, presumably related to microscopic air bubbles introduced into the media. Variation in transducer pressure produced dramatic differences in transmissivity, which outweighed the differences between the various coupling media. The investigators concluded that coupling media can be chosen primarily on the basis of cost and convenience, without compromising function.[178] Encased silicon gel shows promise for use as a coupling agent over irregular body surfaces, sensitive skin areas, and open wounds, if the issue of impedance mismatch with the sound head can be rectified.[6] In addition to accommodating for impedance mismatches, coupling media also lubricate to permit smooth movement of the transducer over the skin.

The most common technique of ultrasound application is the stroking technique. It allows a more even energy distribution over the site being treated. The applicator is moved slowly over an area of approximately 25 cm^2 (4 square inches) in a circular or longitudinal manner.[110] The applicator size (usually 5–10 cm^2) limits the size of the area that can be treated, so multiple fields of treatment might be needed for larger areas (i.e. shoulder and hip anterior, lateral, and posterior ports). The stationary technique generally should be avoided because of the potential for standing waves and the production of hot spots.[135] Intensity is indicated by specifying the particular watts per square centimeter or by titrating to just below pain threshold. In surveys of performance of ultrasonic therapy equipment, variations in frequency and power output were common.[81,164] Although the frequency of commercially available ultrasound applicators was typically within 5% of manufacturer's specifications, the overwhelming majority (85%) of applicators tested had power output variations of over 20%.[164] Consequently, it is important to have ultrasound applicators recalibrated regularly.

More than 35 clinical uses of ultrasound have been described, but many of these are not well supported by experimental evidence.[169] More recent systematic reviews have not conclusively shown the benefits of ultrasound in the care of a number of musculoskeletal and related conditions, for similar lack of

Box 21-6 Ultrasound precautions

- General heat precautions
- Near brain, eyes, reproductive organs
- Gravid or menstruating uterus
- Near pacemaker
- Near spine, laminectomy sites
- Malignancy
- Skeletal immaturity
- ?Arthroplasties
- ?Methyl methacrylate or high-density polyethylene

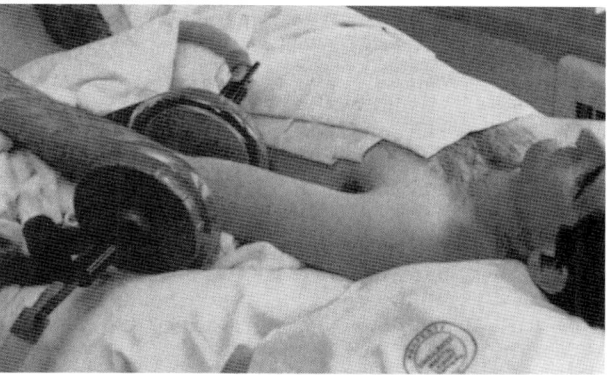

Figure 21-7 Example of shortwave diathermy application with capacitive applicator (condenser plates). (From Kotke and Lehmann 1990,[98] with permission.)

evidential support.[19,25,58,59,77,118,153,175,176] Nonetheless, the purported clinical uses of ultrasound continue to expand, as witnessed by the current clinical interest in fracture healing, especially of bony non-unions.[22,55,79,99,132]

Ultrasound precautions are summarized in Box 21-6.[121,135,169] Concern about the use of heat near malignancies was discussed previously. Deep heating over an open epiphysis could result in either increased growth (from hyperemia) or decreased growth (from thermal injury). Avoiding ultrasound near pacemakers is reasonable because of potential thermal or mechanical injury to the pacemaker. Ultrasound over laminectomy sites could theoretically result in spinal cord heating. Ultrasound at therapeutic dosage over the peroneal nerve has been shown to produce a reversible conduction block in some patients with polyneuropathy.[87] There are also case reports of increased radicular pain with ultrasound.[65] There are even case reports of patient abuse of ultrasound.[113] The concern with ultrasound use over arthroplasties and other metallic implants is the potential for focal heating. Gersten reported that temperature rises near metal were actually lower than temperature rises near bone, so metal per se should not be a contraindication to ultrasound.[64] Lehmann cautioned against the use of ultrasound near methyl methacrylate or high-density polyethylene because of their high coefficient of absorption.[110] The effect of ultrasound on bony ingrowth arthroplasties is not yet well defined. Because the effects of ultrasound on arthroplasties are not yet completely delineated, the most prudent course would be to avoid ultrasound over these areas whenever possible.

Shortwave diathermy

Shortwave diathermy is a modality that produces deep heating via conversion of electromagnetic energy to thermal energy. Oscillation of high-frequency electrical and magnetic fields produces movement of ions, rotation of polar molecules, and distortion of non-polar molecules, with resultant heat generation.[66,91] The Federal Communications Commission limits industrial, scientific, and medical (ISM) use to 13.56 MHz (22-m wavelength), 27.12 MHz (11-m wavelength), and 40.68 MHz (7.5-m wavelength).[93] The 27.12-MHz frequency is most commonly used. The heating pattern produced depends on the type of shortwave unit, and on the water content and electrical properties of the tissue. Tissues can be grossly divided into those with high water content (muscle, skin, blood, etc.) and those with low water content (bone, fat, etc.).[91]

Shortwave diathermy units can be inductive or capacitive. Inductive applicators use induction coils that apply a magnetic field to induce circular electrical fields in the tissue.[72] They achieve higher temperatures in water-rich tissues with higher conductivity.[93] These applicators typically have a cable or drum configuration.[93] Cables are semiflexible induction coils that can be formed to the contour of the area to be treated. Drum applicators consist of induction coils enclosed in a rigid housing or drum. For a capacitive applicator, the patient is placed between two metal condenser plates (Fig. 21-7). The plates and the patient's intervening tissue act as a capacitor (an object that stores electrical charge), and heat is generated by rapid oscillations in the electric field from one plate to the other.[66] Capacitive applicators might achieve higher temperatures in water-poor tissues such as subcutaneous adipose tissue.[72,93]

Currently available shortwave applicators do not allow precise dosimetry, so initial pain perception is used to monitor intensity. Terrycloth towels are used for spacing and to absorb sweat, which is highly conductive and could result in potentially severe focal heating.[110] Typical treatment time is 20–30 min. Specific applicator configuration can greatly affect the distribution of heating.[93,107] In a review of several different induction applicators, the ratio of muscle heating versus fat heating ranged from 0.39 to 2.67 for the various applicators tested.[107]

Lehmann et al. evaluated the effect of subcutaneous fat thickness and technique of SWD application.[101] In comparing distance from the applicator, 2 cm of air space between patient and applicator produced a more desirable heating pattern than did 3 mm of terrycloth between patient and applicator. Depth of subcutaneous fat also had a significant effect on temperature distribution. Muscle temperature rise in subjects with less than 1 cm of subcutaneous fat was 9.5°C, compared with 5.6°C in subjects with more than 2 cm of subcutaneous fat.[101] Following application of pulsed SWD, Draper noted mean temperature increases of 1.36°C at 5 min, 2.87°C at 10 min, 3.78°C at 15 min, and 3.49°C at 20 min, at a depth of 3 cm in the gastrocnemius muscle.[49] SWD has been purported to be useful in a

---

Box 21-7 Shortwave precautions

- General heat precautions
- Metal (jewelry, pacemakers, intrauterine devices, surgical implants, deep brain stimulators, etc.)
- Contact lenses
- Gravid or menstruating uterus
- Skeletal immaturity

Box 21-8 Physiologic effects of cold

Hemodynamic
- Immediate cutaneous vasoconstriction
- Delayed reactive vasodilatation
- Decreased acute inflammation

Neuromuscular
- Slowing of conduction velocity
- Conduction block and axonal degeneration with prolonged exposure
- Decreased group 1a fiber firing rates (muscle spindle)
- Decreased group 2 fiber firing rates (muscle spindle)
- Decreased group 1b fiber firing rates (Golgi tendon organ)
- Decreased muscle stretch reflex amplitudes
- Increased maximal isometric strength
- Decreased muscle fatigue
- Temporarily reduced spasticity

Joint and connective tissue
- Increased joint stiffness
- Decreased tendon extensibility
- Decreased collagenase activity

Miscellaneous
- Decreased pain
- General relaxation

---

variety of musculoskeletal conditions, although, as with most of the physical agent modalities, there are conflicting data regarding efficacy.[48,60,66,119,127] SWD precautions are listed in Box 21-7. Metal can result in focal heating and should be strictly avoided. All jewelry should be removed, and the treatment table ideally should not contain metal. Likewise, electromagnetic energy can seriously interfere with pacemaker function, so a pacemaker is an absolute contraindication. Severe central nervous system damage has been reported following use of SWD near a deep brain stimulator.[134] Contact lenses are a concern because of the potential for focal heating.[158] The other precautions listed are self-explanatory. Regular maintenance and calibration of equipment should be performed to ensure safe operation of SWD.[46]

Microwave diathermy

Microwave diathermy is another form of electromagnetic energy that uses conversion as its primary form of heat production. Thermal energy is produced by increased kinetic energy of molecules within the microwave field.[140] Federal Communications Commission-approved frequencies for therapeutic microwave are 915 MHz (wavelength 33 cm) and 2456 MHz (wavelength 12 cm).[110] The lower frequency has the advantage of increased depth of penetration but also the disadvantages of greater beam dispersion and the requirement of larger applicators.[140]

Temperature distribution in a particular tissue is affected largely by its water content. The fraction of power absorbed in a particular tissue depends on several factors, including the frequency of the electromagnetic wave, the dielectric constant, and the electrical conductivity of the tissue.[140] In general, tissues with high water content absorb greater amounts of energy and are selectively heated.[110] If muscle heating is a primary objective, 915-MHz applicators are preferable to 2456-MHz applicators.[105] Non-thermal effects of microwave diathermy have been documented, but Lehmann points out that there is no evidence that these are of any therapeutic significance.[110] Average temperatures of approximately 41°C (105.8°F) at a depth of 1–3 cm have been demonstrated.[41] Microwave, although once quite popular, has been largely replaced by other modalities in the USA.[167]

General heat precautions should be observed with microwave. Metal implants, pacemakers, sites of skeletal immaturity, reproductive organs and brain, and fluid-filled cavities (eye, bullae, effusions, etc.) should be avoided.[92,110]

Table 21-3 Classification of various types of cooling

Type of cooling	Depth	Main form of energy transfer
Cold packs	Superficial	Conduction
Ice massage	Superficial	Conduction
Cold water immersion	Superficial	Conduction
Cryotherapy–compression units	Superficial	Conduction
Vapocoolant spray	Superficial	Evaporation
Whirlpool baths	Superficial	Convection

CRYOTHERAPY

All forms of cryotherapy (therapeutic use of cold) are considered superficial cooling agents, usually transferring thermal energy by conduction. Exceptions include convective cooling in the whirlpool, and evaporative cooling with vapocoolant sprays (Table 21-3). This section reviews the physiologic effects (Box 21-8), general uses (Box 21-9), and general precautions (Box 21-10) for cryotherapy, followed by a discussion of the agents currently used in physical medicine.

Physiologic effects of cold
Hemodynamic

Application of cold to the skin results in immediate cutaneous vasoconstriction through sympathetically mediated reflex mechanisms and by directly stimulating smooth muscle contraction.[73,143] Lewis observed phasic oscillations of temperature in the fingers after initial vasoconstriction during cold water immersion.[115] The initial vasoconstriction is thought to be due to a cold-induced increase in the affinity of the postjunctional α-adrenergic receptors for existing norepinephrine in vascular smooth muscle.[161] Reactive vasodilatation occurs as further cooling interrupts noradrenaline release. Vasodilatation warms the tissues, again releasing norepinephrine to sensitized receptors, and the cycle repeats. This 'hunting' of temperature is believed to be a mechanism by which peripheral exposed parts of the body are protected from cold injury. Others have demonstrated vasodilatation after cooling of the hand and forearm, without the phasic oscillations observed by Lewis.[31,61] The effects of localized cooling on heart rate and blood pressure are variable, and have been summarized elsewhere.[122] Cryotherapy has also been shown to moderate inflammation, more effectively in the acute phase than in the chronic phase.[157]

Neuromuscular

The initial response of peripheral nerves to cold application is a marked slowing of conduction velocity.[1,44] With more prolonged exposure, there is conduction block, cessation of axoplasmic transport, and eventual axonal degeneration.[133] Decreased muscle spindle (both group 1a and 2 fibers) and Golgi tendon organ (group 1b fibers) firing rates have been demonstrated after local cooling in animals.[56] The clinical neuromuscular effects of cooling include a decrease in gastrocnemius muscle stretch reflex amplitude,[15,97] an increase in maximal

isometric strength,[30,120] and slowing in the rate of muscle fatigue.[30] Cold has also been shown to temporarily reduce spasticity in patients with hemiplegia and multiple sclerosis, improving exercise tolerance and enhancing function.[80,125] Other investigators, however, have noted increased spasticity after cold application in some subjects.[27,150]

Joint and connective tissue

Topical cold application (approximately 4°C) to the knee in dogs induced significant and sustained depression of intraarticular temperature without significant effect on core temperature.[16] Synovial collagenase activity also decreases with temperature. In vitro experiments demonstrate negligible synovial collagenase activity after cooling to 30°C (86°F), suggesting that therapy that decreases intraarticular temperature in inflammatory arthropathies could slow the rate of collagenolysis.[75] It should be noted, however, that in one study of the use of cryotherapy after cruciate ligament surgery, skin temperature had to be lowered to 20°C in order to produce significant intraarticular temperature declines.[36] Potentially negative effects such as decreased tendon extensibility and increased joint stiffness have also been demonstrated following cooling.[106,186]

Miscellaneous effects of cold

The analgesic effect of cold can be related to reflex muscle relaxation, cutaneous counterirritation, or its effects on nerve conduction.[122] As with heat, some patients note cold to produce a general relaxation, although the mechanisms are not well defined.

General uses of cryotherapy in physical medicine

The general uses for therapeutic cold are summarized in Box 21-9. Cryotherapy is most commonly used acutely after musculoskeletal injury to minimize formation of edema, and for symptomatic relief in painful soft tissue and articular inflammatory states.[68,85,122,123,172] Two recent reviews nicely summarize the use of modalities in arthritis.[76,138] Studies of the use of cryotherapy following orthopedic procedures have produced mixed results: some investigators report favorable effects on factors such as range of motion, pain, analgesic use, swelling, postoperative blood loss, and hospital length of stay, while others demonstrate no significant effect from cryotherapy.[8,33,37,54,78,89,112,114,154,181,184] There have also been mixed results with the use of cryotherapy in spasticity management.[27,80,125,150,179] Cryotherapy in the form of immediate ice water immersion is advocated as emergent primary treatment for minor burns.[163]

General precautions for the use of cold

The general precautions for the use of cold are outlined in Box 21-10. The most common relative contraindication to the use of cold is simple cold intolerance. A patient who does not tolerate cold application will tend to increase muscle guarding and cocontraction, which is directly counterproductive to the therapeutic goals. Simple cold intolerance should be distinguished from true cold hypersensitivity, which is discussed below. Caution should also be used when applying cold over the course of superficial nerves, as peroneal and ulnar palsies have been reported following cryotherapy.[50] Application of cold over areas of compromised arterial vascularity can theoretically produce further ischemia from local vasoconstriction and should be avoided. Likewise, because of the potential for cold injury, cryotherapy should be used with caution in areas of impaired sensation, or in patients who have cognitive or communication deficits that preclude reporting of pain.

The cryopathies are also contraindications to the use of cold.[152] Cryoglobulinemia is a condition that results in the precipitation of immune complexes at low temperatures. Paroxysmal cold hemoglobinuria is a rare disorder resulting from an antibody directed against a red blood cell surface antigen, with hemolysis precipitated by cold exposure. Cold hypersensitivity is a mast cell-mediated process producing urticaria and angioedema on exposure to cold. Raynaud *disease* is an idiopathic condition characterized by arteriolar spasm precipitated by cold exposure or stress. Raynaud *phenomenon* is secondary to other rheumatologic conditions (rheumatoid arthritis, scleroderma, systemic lupus erythematosus, etc.) and is classically manifested by digital pallor, followed by cyanosis and eventual reactive hyperemia.

Cryotherapy agents

Cold packs

Cold packs include Hydrocollator packs, endothermic chemical gel packs, and ice packs. Hydrocollator packs are cooled in a freezer to −12°C (10°F) and applied over a moist towel.[97] Endothermic chemical gel packs have separate compartments with compounds such as ammonium nitrate and water that, when mixed, undergo a heat-absorbing reaction. They are portable, pliable, and easily used in the field. Although many endothermic chemical gel packs are designed for one-time use, some have the advantage that they can be refrozen and reused as a simple cryogel pack. Ice packs are easily used at home and might be best applied by elastic bandage or tape, as external compression appears to increase their cooling effectiveness.[10] The duration of application is typically 20–30 min. With application of a cooled Hydrocollator pack, the skin is cooled immediately, subcutaneous tissues are cooled within minutes, and muscle at a depth of 2 cm is cooled by approximately 5°C after 20 min.[97] Precautions for cold packs are as listed in Box 21-10.

Ice massage

Ice massage is the direct application of ice to the skin using gentle stroking motions. It combines the therapeutic effects of cooling with the mechanical effects of massage. Water is frozen in a paper cup, with the ice being exposed by tearing the top rim of paper off as the ice melts (Fig. 21-8). Alternatively, a wooden tongue depressor can be placed in the water, to be used as a handle after the water is frozen. Ice massage is generally used for localized symptoms and applied for 5–10 min per site,

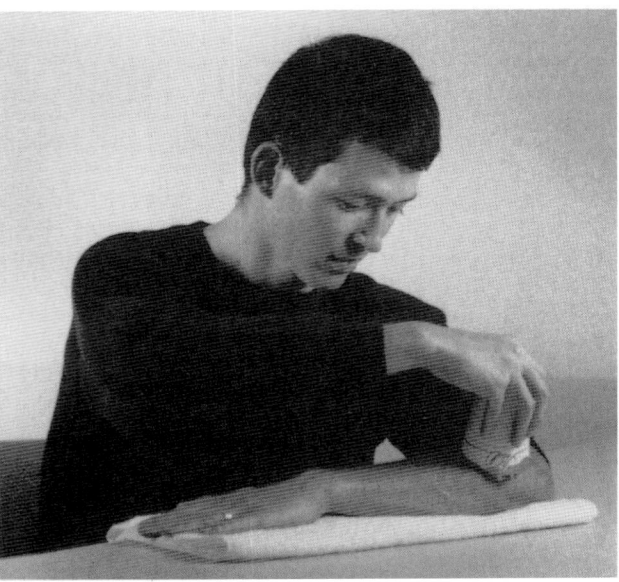

Figure 21-8 Example of ice massage.

depending on the amount of subcutaneous adipose tissue.[117] There is typically a phasic response to ice massage, beginning with an initial perception of coolness, followed by a burning or aching, then hypoesthesia and analgesia.[68] Intramuscular temperatures at a depth of 2 cm after 5 min of ice massage have been reported to be reduced by 4.1°C in the posterior thigh[180] to as much as 15.9°C in the biceps brachii muscle.[117] In his initial description of ice massage, Grant reported a 'satisfactory treatment result' in over 80% of a series of over 7000 patients with a variety of painful musculoskeletal conditions treated with ice massage and mobilization exercises, although no statistical analysis was reported.[68] Precautions for ice massage are as listed under general cold precautions.

Cold water immersion

Immersion in cold water is best suited for circumferential cooling of the limbs, usually at temperatures of 5–13°C (41–55.4°F).[163] It is often uncomfortable and poorly tolerated, although reportedly effective with localized burns, as skin temperature rapidly approaches water temperature.[163] Gastrocnemius muscle temperature decreases to approximately 6°C below baseline after 30 min of cold water immersion.[125,145] Precautions for cold water immersion are listed in Box 21-10.

Cryotherapy–compression units

Cryotherapy–compression units consist of a cuff or boot through which cold water is circulated, and can be pneumatically compressed statically or in a serial, distal to proximal pumping action. They are designed to combine the beneficial effects of cryotherapy with the advantages of pneumatic compression. They are used primarily after acute musculoskeletal injury with soft tissue swelling, and after some surgical procedures.[155] Typical temperatures of 7.2°C (45°F) and pressures up to 60 mmHg are used.

Vapocoolant spray

Vapocoolant spray and stretch methods are used by some practitioners to treat myofascial and musculoskeletal pain syndromes. The technique consists of a series of unidirectional applications of Fluori-Methane spray, which has replaced the highly flammable ethyl chloride spray in clinical usage.[172] Treatment begins in the 'trigger area' (area of deep myofascial hypersensitivity) and extends over the 'reference zone' (area of referred pain) while passively stretching the muscle.[172] The spray and stretch is performed parallel to the muscle fibers, at an approximate rate of 4 inches/s. Waiting briefly between applications helps prevent skin freezing. The therapeutic effect of spray and stretch is postulated to result from a counterirritant phenomenon.[172] Precautions include general cold precautions and avoidance of cutaneous freezing.

HYDROTHERAPY

Hydrotherapy is defined as the external application of hot or cold water, in any form, for the treatment of disease.[62] The main forms of hydrotherapy are whirlpool baths, the Hubbard tank, the shower cart, and contrast baths. Their primary uses are in arthritis and a variety of musculoskeletal conditions, and in the cleansing and debridement of burns and other dermal injuries.

Whirlpool baths and Hubbard tanks

Whirlpool baths and Hubbard tanks control water temperature and agitate it by aeration, dispersing thermal energy by convection (although, as noted previously, the actual transfer of heat to or from the body is by conduction). Whirlpool baths come in a variety of sizes, and are typically used for treatment of a limb or localized lesion. Because only a portion of the body is immersed, greater extremes of temperature can be tolerated without significant core body temperature change.[62,145] As more body surface area is immersed and the extremes of temperature increase, there is increasing potential for alteration of core body temperature. Hubbard tanks are larger tanks generally used for whole body immersion, so neutral temperatures (34–36°C, 93–97°F) should be used to prevent core temperature fluctuations.

An immersed body experiences a vertical antigravity force equal to that of the volume of the displaced water, decreasing stress on bones and joints.[62] This property, along with the therapeutic effects of the water temperature, make hydrotherapy appropriate for adjunctive treatment of degenerative arthritis, acute musculoskeletal injuries, burns, and skin ulceration[21] and infection.[62] Antiseptic conditions can be used for hydrotherapy of burns or infected areas, but truly sterile conditions are not easily achieved, necessitating provider vigilance in patient selection, given reports of *Pseudomonas* infections.[173] Sodium hypochlorite is the most commonly used antibacterial solution used in burn programs.[170] For Hubbard tank treatment of large wounds, salt can also be added to minimize fluid shifts. Isotonic saline is 0.9% sodium chloride (0.9 g of NaCl, 100 mL of H_2O), so 900 g (approximately 2 lbs) of salt should be added per 100 L (approximately 25 gallons) of water.

Shower cart

Hydrotherapy has several features that are desirable for treatment of burns or other wounds. It loosens adherent dressings to facilitate removal, allows for removal of antimicrobial cream prior to reapplication, and softens eschar to facilitate debridement.[177] There is a risk of autocontamination and cross-contamination, however, with conventional whirlpool baths or Hubbard tanks.[177] The shower cart was developed in response to this risk.[177] It allows for gentle spray or shower hydrotherapy during mechanical debridement of large surface area burns and other wounds under relatively sterile conditions.[177] Typical units have overhead retractable shower heads (Fig. 21-9), with independently adjustable water temperature and pressure. A shower cart also uses significantly less water, less space, and requires less maintenance than a Hubbard tank (see Ch. 59).

Contrast baths

Contrast baths consist of alternating immersion of the distal limbs in hot (42–45°C, 108–113°F) then cold (8.5–12.5°C, 47–55°F) water.[185] The effect is believed to be related to the cyclic vasoconstriction and vasodilatation produced by the temperature extremes. Thirty-minute treatment sessions are typical, beginning with a 10-min immersion in hot, followed by alternating immersions of 1 min cold and 4 min hot, ending the session with cold immersion to theoretically limit swelling. The technique might be beneficial in the treatment of rheumatologic disease, neuropathic pain, or other chronic pain syndromes such as complex regional pain syndrome.

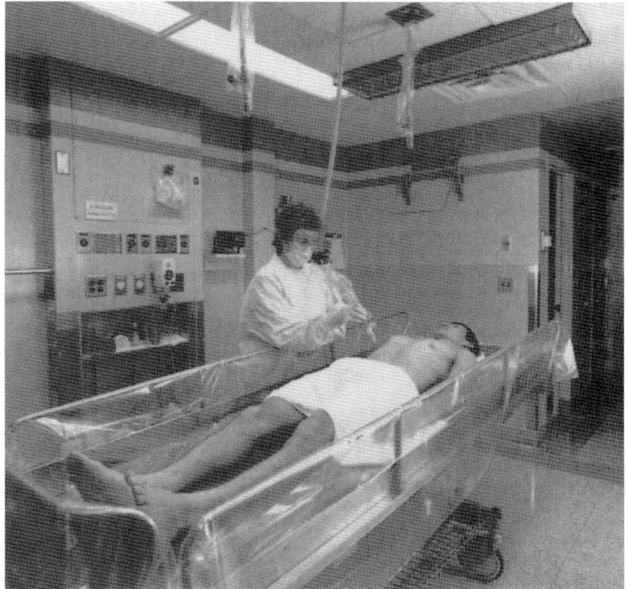

Figure 21-9 Shower cart.

OTHER MODALITIES

Ultraviolet

Ultraviolet radiation is that part of the electromagnetic spectrum adjacent to the short-wavelength, high-frequency (violet) end of the visible light spectrum. Ultraviolet radiation has historically been used in physical medicine for the treatment of skin ulcers, but now its therapeutic use is almost exclusively dermatologic.[130] Most current treatments with ultraviolet radiation utilize either ultraviolet A (wavelength 320–400 nm) or ultraviolet B (wavelength 290–320 nm) radiation.[130] The minimal erythema dose can be used to titrate intensity, and is determined by exposing small areas of skin to different durations of ultraviolet radiation. The minimal erythema dose is that duration of exposure that produces erythema. Although originally used mainly in the treatment of psoriasis, there are now more than 30 dermatologic disorders for which ultraviolet radiation could be efficacious.[130] Potential adverse effects include premature aging of the skin, non-melanoma skin cancer, and cataracts.[130]

Iontophoresis

Iontophoresis is the migration of charged particles across biologic membranes under an imposed electrical field.[111] Its primary use has been in transcutaneous systemic or local delivery of medicines. For systemic drug delivery, it avoids the problems associated with oral or intravenous routes such as gastric irritation, first-pass hepatic metabolism, and variable serum concentrations.[28,29] Iontophoresis in physical medicine is used to deliver medicines directly to soft tissues, limiting systemic absorption.[26,34,116] Ionic medications (local anesthetics, corticosteroids, analgesics, and antibiotics) or plain tap water have been used with this technique. The ionic solution to be iontophoresed is placed on the electrode of the same polarity, and then the negative, positive, and ground electrodes are applied to the skin. A direct current, typically between 10 and 30 mA, is applied to drive the solution away from the electrode and into the surrounding tissues.[162] The quantity of solution transported appears to be dependent on the local current density, the duration of treatment, and the solution concentration.[137] Although the mechanism of action and the clinical efficacy of iontophoresis continue to be debated, it is a modality commonly used by practitioners to treat a variety of conditions.[7,26,34,43,71,83,116,129,139,144,151,162,165,166] Iontophoresis is generally well tolerated, although miliariasis has been reported when treating hyperhydrosis.[162]

Phonophoresis

Phonophoresis involves the use of ultrasound to facilitate transdermal migration of topically administered medications. Corticosteroids are the most frequently used phonophoresis agents. The antiinflammatory effects of ultrasound and corticosteroids are thought to be synergistic.[131] The actual mechanism of transdermal migration has not been well defined, but could involve increased cell permeability from the thermal effects of ultrasound.[131] Ultrasonic coupling gel is mixed with various chemical substances to produce the phonophoresis coupling agent.[131] Studies have documented significant differences in acoustic transmission among different phonophoresis agents, and these differences should be considered in choosing an agent.[24] Typical phonophoresis treatment parameters are similar to those of standard ultrasound: pulsed mode, 1-MHz transducer frequency, stroking technique, at $1.0–1.5 \text{ W/cm}^2$, for approximately 5 min per site.[131] Proposed indications for phonophoresis include osteoarthritis, bursitis, capsulitis, tendinitis, strains, fasciitis, epicondylitis, tenosynovitis, contracture, scar tissue, neuromas, and adhesions.[70,131] Phonophoresis is a modality with some measure of clinical effectiveness, but there continue to be differences of opinion about its mechanism of action, clinical efficacy, and the extent of transdermal migration of agents.[9,23,39,83,86,94,141] The precautions for and contraindications to phonophoresis are listed in Box 21-6.

Low-energy laser

Laser is the acronym for light amplification by stimulated emission of radiation. It consists of a coherent (in phase), collimated (restricted in area) beam of photons of identical frequency. Low-energy lasers typically deliver less than 90 mW, and should be distinguished from the higher power (10–100+ W) lasers utilized in surgery, dermatology, and ophthalmology. Low-energy lasers deliver minimal energies (between 1 and 4 J) and can be considered a form of intense, focal light therapy.[13] They have been shown to affect many subcellular and cellular processes, although the mechanisms have not been well defined.[13] However, it is important to note that low-energy laser does not produce significant tissue temperature changes, so any potential physiologic effects appear to be non-thermal. Low-intensity laser therapy has been used experimentally to treat a wide variety of clinical conditions, but no consensus regarding indication or effectiveness has been established.[11,12,20,35,40,63,74,84,128] There is also wide variation in equipment, experimental design, and stimulation parameters reported in the low-energy laser therapy literature, and some believe this may be responsible for the conflicting results.[13,156] Low-energy laser was recently approved by the Food and Drug Administration for selected indications. Protective goggles should be worn by both the patient and the treating therapist to protect against potential retinal injury.

Interferential current therapy

Interferential current therapy (IFC) is a modality that utilizes two alternating current signals of slightly different frequency. To understand the mechanism of IFC, one must have an understanding of how waves interact. Figure 21-10 illustrates that interaction. At the intersection of two sinusoidal waveforms, the 'interference' of the two waves produces a summated wave. When the two waves are in phase, there is *constructive interference*: the summated wave has an amplitude equal to the sum of the individual wave amplitudes.[67] When the two waves are out of phase, there is *destructive interference*: the summated wave has a lower amplitude because the opposite polarities of the waves partially cancel each other.[67] When two waves of

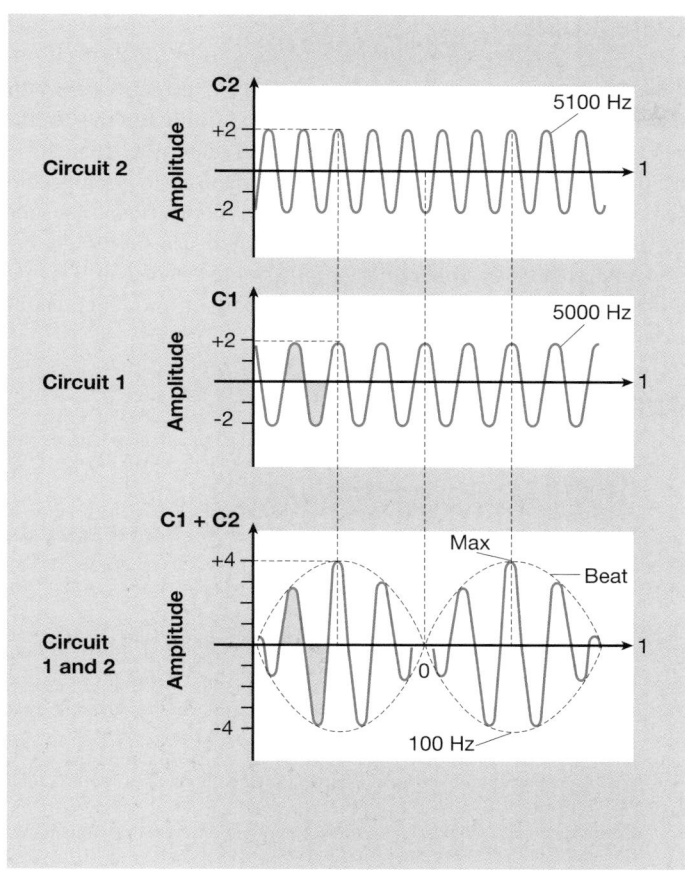

Figure 21-10 Interaction of two sinusoidal waves of slightly different frequency, demonstrating cyclic constructive and destructive interference. (From Anonymous 1984,[4] with permission of Nemectron.)

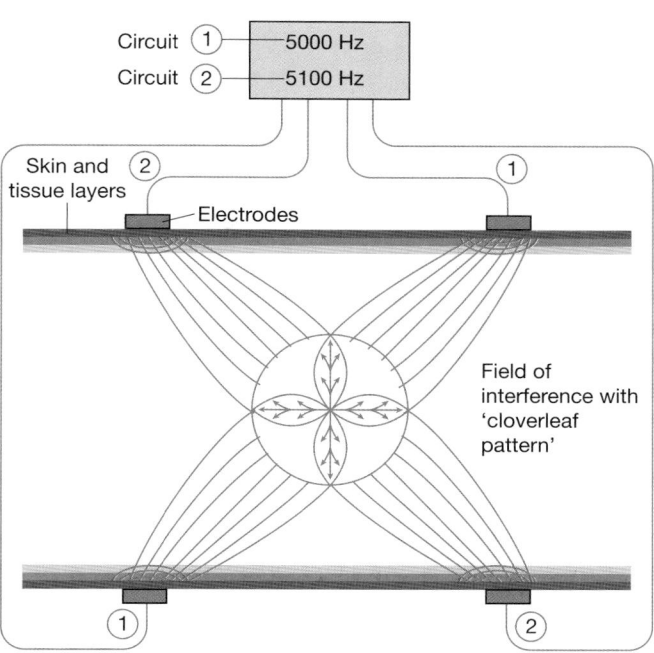

Figure 21-11 Quadripolar interferential current therapy application demonstrating classic 'cloverleaf' pattern of interference. (From Anonymous 1984,[4] with permission of Nemectron.)

equal amplitude and frequency are exactly in phase, the amplitude of the summated wave is exactly twice that of the individual waves. When two waves of equal amplitude and frequency are out of phase by exactly one-half wavelength (i.e. the peak of one wave intersects with the trough of the other wave), the amplitude of the summated wave is zero. As noted, IFC utilizes two alternating current signals of slightly different frequencies. As these two waveforms intersect, they are periodically in phase (constructive interference) and periodically out of phase (destructive interference). This periodic interference results in a new wave with cyclic modulation of amplitude, due to the cyclic constructive and destructive interference. The amplitude of the summated wave modulates at a *beat frequency*, equal to the difference in frequency between the two signals.[67] For example, if one applicator channel frequency is 5100 Hz and the other is 5000 Hz, the beat frequency would be 100 Hz (5100 − 5000 = 100).

Interferential current therapy machines typically use medium-frequency currents of approximately 4000–5000 Hz. Alternating currents of medium frequency (1000–10 000 Hz) have lower skin resistance than low-frequency currents (<1000 Hz); it is therefore postulated that they penetrate tissue more easily.[67,160] However, many factors other than signal frequency also affect skin resistance and depth of penetration.[3,95,96] Most IFC machines use two, four, or six applicators. These can be arranged in the same plane (*planar*), as in the lumbar area, or in different planes (*coplanar*), as in the shoulder. Figure 21-11 demonstrates a typical quadripolar IFC application. The classic 'cloverleaf' pattern of interference produced between two circuits in a perfectly homogeneous medium is diagrammed. However, due to the marked heterogeneity of electrical conductance of human tissues, the actual summation is unlikely to occur as precisely as in this diagrammatic representation.[3]

Interferential current therapy parameters that can be manipulated include signal frequency, beat frequency, amplitude, and cycle time. IFC machines allow for either a fixed frequency difference (most machines are capable of producing beat frequencies from 1 to 120 Hz), or for a modulated frequency difference, where the beat frequency varies over time.[96] Frequency modulation is sometimes referred to as 'sweep'.[159] In theory, the use of frequency modulation limits neural adaptation.[95] Amplitude may also be fixed or modulated. By manipulating the amplitude, the point of maximal amplitude interference changes. As Figure 21-12 shows, with equal amplitude in each circuit, the field of interference is at a 45° angle to the circuits. If the amplitude of circuit 1 is increased, the field will rotate toward circuit 1. Conversely, if the amplitude in circuit 1 is decreased, the field will rotate away from circuit 1. Amplitude modulation is sometimes referred to as 'scan'.[159] IFC scan mode might be preferable when the treatment area is large or poorly localized; theoretically, the area of tissue stimulation is larger with modulated amplitude than with fixed amplitude IFC.[159] Some IFC machines also allow for on–off cycling. IFC treatment parameters can be manipulated to produce stimulation

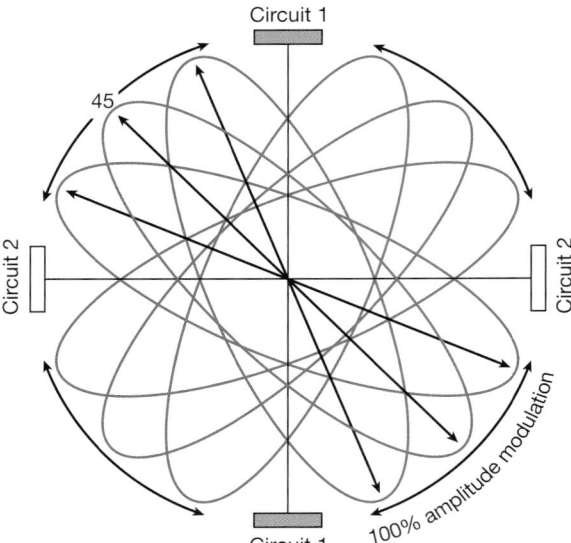

Figure 21-12 Interferential current therapy amplitude modulation or 'scanning'. If the amplitude is increased or decreased in a circuit, the zone of maximum interference rotates toward or away from that circuit, respectively. (From Kloth 1991,[96] with permission of Appleton & Lange.)

parameters similar to the different categories of transcutaneous electrical nerve stimulation (TENS) delivery: conventional, acupuncture-like, hyperstimulation, or burst modes.[95,96] But Kloth notes that a major difference between IFC and TENS might be the ability of IFC to deliver higher currents than those of TENS.[96]

Some have reported that IFC is useful in a variety of musculoskeletal conditions, in neurologic conditions, and in the management of urinary incontinence,[51,69,88,90,96,160,183] although other literature fails to demonstrate its superiority over other interventions or placebo.[136,168,174]

Precautions and contraindications for IFC are the same as those for other forms of transcutaneous electrical stimulation.[67,96] IFC should not be used near implanted stimulators (pacemakers, intrathecal pumps, spinal cord stimulators, etc.) because of the potential for interference with the function of these devices.[67,96] One should be aware of the potential for vascular responses when IFC is used near sympathetic ganglia or the carotid sinus.[96] IFC should not be used near open incisions or abrasions because of the potential for concentration of electrical current.[96] It should not be used near the gravid uterus, because of concern about potential adverse effects on fetal development or the potential for stimulating uterine contractions.[67,96] In the presence of venous thrombosis, IFC could result in mechanical stimulation of vascular smooth muscle, with the theoretic potential of precipitating emboli.[67,96] It should not be used in an insensate area or in a patient cognitively incapable of accurately reporting pain.[96] Additionally, IFC should not be used near shortwave diathermy, because of the potential for interference with resultant excessive electrical stimulation.[96]

CONCLUSION

This chapter has reviewed the physiologic effects, common uses, techniques of application, and precautions for the therapeutic use of modalities. It is important to remember that these modalities are adjunctive treatments, to be used in conjunction with appropriate therapeutic exercise and medications. Because of the potential for deleterious effects, their use should generally be preceded by appropriate professional evaluation. Having a firm understanding of the physiologic basis of modality selection is crucial to their proper use.

REFERENCES

1. Abramson DI, Chu LSW, Tuck S, et al. Effect of tissue temperatures and blood flow on motor nerve conduction velocity. JAMA 1966; 198: 1082–1088.

2. Abramson DI, Tuck S, Chu SW, et al. Effect of paraffin bath and hot fomentations on local tissue temperatures. Arch Phys Med Rehabil 1964; 45:87–94.

3. Alon G. Interferential current news [letter]. Phys Ther 1986; 66: 280–281.

4. [Anonymous]. Nemectrodyn model 7 manual. Karlsruche: Nemectron; 1984.

5. Askew LJ, Beckett VL, An K, et al. Objective evaluation of hand function in scleroderma patients to assess effectiveness of physical therapy. Br J Rheumatol 1983; 22:224–232.

6. Balmaseda MT, Fatehi MT, Koozekanani SH, et al. Ultrasound therapy: a comparative study of different coupling media. Arch Phys Med Rehabil 1986; 67:147–150.

7. Banga A, Panus P. Clinical applications of ionophoretic devices in rehabilitation medicine. Crit Rev Phys Med Rehabil 1998; 10:147–179.

8. Barber FA, McGuire DA, Click S. Continuous-flow cold therapy for outpatient anterior cruciate ligament reconstruction. Arthroscopy 1998; 14(2):130–135.

9. Bare AC, McAnaw MB, Pritchard AE, et al. Phonophoretic delivery of 10% hydrocortisone through the epidermis of humans as determined by serum cortisol concentrations. Phys Ther 1996; 76:738–745.

10. Barlas D, Homan CS, Thode HC. In vivo tissue temperature comparison of cryotherapy with and without external compression. Ann Emerg Med 1996; 28:436–439.

11. Basford JR, Malanga GA, Krause DA, et al. A randomized controlled evaluation of low-intensity laser therapy: plantar fasciitis. Arch Phys Med Rehabil 1998; 79:249–254.

12. Basford JR. Low intensity laser therapy: still not an established clinical tool. Lasers Surg Med 1995; 16:331–342.

13. Basford JR. The clinical and experimental status of low energy laser therapy. Crit Rev Phys Rehabil Med 1989; 1:1–9.

14. Belanger A. Evidence-based guide to therapeutic physical agents. Philadelphia: Lippincott Williams & Wilkins; 2002.

15. Bell KR, Lehmann JF. Effect of cooling on H- and T-reflexes in normal subjects. Arch Phys Med Rehabil 1987; 68:490–493.

16. Bocobo C, Fast A, Kingery W, et al. The effect of ice on intra-articular temperature in the knee of the dog. Am J Phys Med 1991; 70:181–185.

17. Borell RM, Henley EJ, Ho P, et al. Fluidotherapy: evaluation of a new heat modality. Arch Phys Med Rehabil 1977; 58:69–71.

18. Borell RM, Parker R, Henley EJ, et al. Comparison of in vivo temperatures produced by hydrotherapy, paraffin wax treatment, and fluidotherapy. Phys Ther 1980; 60:1273–1276.

19. Brosseau L, Casimiro L, Judd MG, et al. Therapeutic ultrasound for treating patellofemoral pain syndrome. Cochrane Database Syst Rev 2001:4.

20. Brosseau L, Welch V, Wells G, et al. Low level laser therapy for osteoarthritis and rheumatoid arthritis: a metaanalysis. J Rheumatol 2000; 27: 1961–1969.

21. Burke D, Ho C, Saucier M, et al. Effects of hydrotherapy on pressure ulcer healing. Am J Phys Med Rehabil 1998; 77:394–398.

22. Busse JW, Bhandari M, Kulkarni AV, et al. The effect of low-intensity pulsed ultrasound therapy on time to fracture healing: a meta-analysis. CMAJ 2002; 166:437–441.

23. Byl NN. The use of ultrasound as an enhancer for transcutaneous drug delivery: phonophoresis. Phys Ther 1995; 75(6):539–553.

24. Cameron M, Monroe L. Relative transmission of ultrasound by media customarily used for phonophoresis. Phys Ther 1992; 72:142–148.

25. Casimiro L, Brosseau L, Judd MG, et al. Therapeutic ultrasound for the treatment of rheumatoid arthritis. Cochrane Database Syst Rev 2002:3.

26. Chantraine A, Ludy JP, Berger D. Is cortisone iontophoresis possible? Arch Phys Med Rehabil 1986; 67:38–40.

27. Chiara T, Carlos J, Martin D, et al. Cold effect on oxygen uptake, perceived exertion, and spasticity in patients with multiple sclerosis. Arch Phys Med Rehabil 1998; 79:523–528.

28. Chien YW, Banga AK. Iontophoretic (transdermal) delivery of drugs: overview of historical development. J Pharm Sci 1989; 78:353–354.

29. Chien YW, Siddiqui O, Shi WM, et al. Direct current iontophoretic transdermal delivery of peptide and protein drugs. J Pharm Sci 1989; 78:376–383.

30. Clarke DH, Stelmach GE. Muscular fatigue and recovery curve parameters at various temperatures. Res Q 1966; 37:468–479.

31. Clarke RS, Hellon RF, Lind AR. Vascular reactions of the human forearm to cold. Clin Sci 1958; 17:165–179.

32. Coakley WT. Biophysical effects of ultrasound at therapeutic intensities. Physiotherapy 1978; 64:166–169.

33. Cohn BT, Draeger RI, Jackson DW. The effects of cold therapy in the postoperative management of pain in patients undergoing anterior cruciate ligament reconstruction. Am J Sports Med 1989; 17:344–349.

34. Costello CT, Jeske AH. Iontophoresis: application in transdermal medication delivery. Phys Ther 1995; 75(6):554–563.

35. Craig JA, Barlas P, Baxter GD, et al. Delayed-onset muscle soreness: lack of effect of combined phototherapy/low-intensity laser therapy at low pulse repetition rates. J Clin Laser Med Surg 1996; 14(6):375–380.

36. Dahlstedt L, Samuelson P, Dalen N. Cryotherapy after cruciate knee surgery. Acta Orthop Scand 1996; 67(3):255–257.

37. Daniel DM, Stone ML, Arendt DL. The effect of cold therapy on pain, swelling, and range of motion after anterior cruciate ligament reconstructive surgery. Arthroscopy 1994; 10(5):530–533.

38. Daniels S, Blondel D, Crum LA, et al. Ultrasonically induced gas bubble production in agar based gels. Part I: experimental investigation. Ultrasound Med Biol 1987; 13:527–539.

39. Darrow H, Schulthies S, Draper D, et al. Serum dexamethasone levels after decadron phonophoresis. J Athl Train 1999; 34:338–341.

40. DeBie R, deVet H, Lenssen T, et al. Low-level laser therapy in ankle sprains: a randomized clinical trial. Arch Phys Med Rehabil 1998; 79:1415–1420.

41. DeLateur BJ, Lehmann JF, Stonebridge JB, et al. Muscle heating in human subjects with 915 MHz microwave contact applicator. Arch Phys Med Rehabil 1970; 51:147–151.

42. Dellhag B, Wollersjo I, Bjelle A. Effect of active hand exercise and wax bath treatments in rheumatoid arthritis patients. Arthritis Care Res 1992; 5:87–92.

43. Demirtas R, Oner C. The treatment of lateral epicondylitis by iontophoresis of sodium salicylate and sodium diclofenac. Clin Rehabil 1998; 12:23–29.

44. Denys EH. AAEM minimonograph no. 14: the influence of temperature in clinical neurophysiology. Muscle Nerve 1991; 14:795–811.

45. Diller KR. Analysis of burns caused by long-term exposure to a heating pad. J Burn Care Rehabil 1991; 12:214–217.

46. Docker M, Bazin S, Dyson M, et al. Guidelines for the safe use of continuous shortwave therapy equipment. Physiotherapy 1992; 78:755–757.

47. Dover JS, Phillips TJ, Arndt KA. Cutaneous effects and therapeutic uses of heat with emphasis on infrared radiation. J Am Acad Dermatol 1989; 20:278–286.

48. Draper D, Castro J, Feland B, et al. Shortwave diathermy and prolonged stretching increase hamstring flexibility more than prolonged stretching alone. J Orthop Sports Phys Ther 2004; 34:13–20.

49. Draper D, Knight K, Fujiwara T, et al. Temperature change in human muscle during and after pulsed short-wave diathermy. J Orthop Sports Phys Ther 1999; 29:13–18.

50. Drez D, Faust DC, Evans JP. Cryotherapy and nerve palsy. Am J Sports Med 1981; 9:256–257.

51. Dumoulin C, Seaborne DE, Quirion-DeGirardi C, et al. Pelvic-floor rehabilitation, part 1: comparison of two surface electrode placements during stimulation of the pelvic-floor musculature in women who are continent using bipolar interferential currents. Phys Ther 1995; 75: 1067–1074.

52. Dyson M, Woodward B, Pond JB. Flow of red blood cells stopped by ultrasound. Nature 1971; 232:572–573.

53. Dyson M. Non-thermal cellular effects of ultrasound. Br J Cancer 1982; 45(suppl):165–171.

54. Edwards DJ, Rimmer M, Keene GCR. The use of cold therapy in the postoperative management of patients undergoing arthroscopic anterior cruciate ligament reconstruction. Am J Sports Med 1996; 24(2):193–195.

55. Einhorn TA. Current concepts review: enhancement of fracture-healing. J Bone Joint Surg 1995; 77A:940–956.

56. Eldred E, Lindsley DF, Buchwald JS. The effect of cooling on mammalian muscle spindles. Exp Neurol 1960; 2:144–157.

57. Falconer J, Hayes KW, Chang RW. Therapeutic ultrasound in the treatment of musculoskeletal conditions. Arthritis Care Res 1990; 3:85–91.

58. Flemming K, Cullum N. Therapeutic ultrasound for pressure sores. Cochrane Database Syst Rev 2000:4.

59. Flemming K, Cullum N. Therapeutic ultrasound for venous leg ulcers. Cochrane Database Syst Rev 2000:4.

60. Foley-Nolan D, Barry C, Coughlan R, et al. Pulsed high frequency (27MHz) electromagnetic therapy for persistent neck pain. a double blind, placebo-controlled study of 20 patients. Orthopedics 1990; 13: 445–451.

61. Folkow B, Fox RH, Krog J, et al. Studies on the reactions of the cutaneous vessels to cold exposure. Acta Physiol Scand 1963; 58:342–354.

62. Franchimont P, Juchmes J, Lecomte J. Hydrotherapy—mechanisms and indications. Pharmacol Ther 1983; 20:79–93.

63. Gam A, Thorsen H, Lonnberg F. The effect of low-level laser therapy on musculoskeletal pain: a meta-analysis. Pain 1993; 52:63–66.

64. Gersten JW. Effect of metallic objects on temperature rises produced in tissue by ultrasound. Am J Phys Med 1958; 37:75–82.

65. Gnatz SM. Increased radicular pain due to therapeutic ultrasound applied to the back. Arch Phys Med Rehabil 1989; 70:493–494.

66. Goats GC. Continuous shortwave (radiofrequency) diathermy. Br J Sports Med 1989; 23:123–127.

67. Goats GC. Interferential current therapy. Br J Sports Med 1990; 24: 87–91.

68. Grant AE. Massage with ice (cryokinetics) in the treatment of painful conditions of the musculoskeletal system. Arch Phys Med Rehabil 1964; 45:233–238.

69. Green RJ, Laycock J. Objective methods for evaluation of interferential therapy in the treatment of incontinence. IEEE Trans Biomed Eng 1990; 37:615–623.

70. Griffin JE, Echternach JL, Price RE, et al. Patients treated with ultrasonic driven hydrocortisone and with ultrasound alone. Phys Ther 1967; 47:594–601.

71. Gudeman S, Eisele S, Heidt R, et al. Treatment of plantar fasciitis by iontophoresis of 0.4% dexamethasone. A randomized, double-blind, placebo-controlled study. Am J Sports Med 1997; 25:312–316.

72. Guy AW, Lehmann JF, Stonebridge JB. Therapeutic applications of electromagnetic power. Proc IEEE 1974; 62:55–75.

73. Guyton AC. Body temperature, temperature regulation, and fever. In: Guyton AC, ed. Textbook of medical physiology. 8th edn. Philadelphia: Saunders; 1991:797–808.

74. Hansen H, Thoroe U. Low-power laser biostimulation of chronic oro-facial pain. A double-blind, placebo-controlled cross-over study in 40 patients. Pain 1990; 43:169–179.

75. Harris ED, McCroskery PA. The influence of temperature and fibril stability on degradation of cartilage collagen by rheumatoid synovial collagenase. N Engl J Med 1974; 290:1–6.

76. Hayes KW. Heat and cold in the management of rheumatoid arthritis. Arthritis Care Res 1993; 6(3):156–166.

77. Hay-Smith EJC. Therapeutic ultrasound for postpartum perineal pain and dyspareunia. Cochrane Database Syst Rev 1998:3.

78. Hecht PJ, Bachmann S, Booth RE, et al. Effects of thermal therapy on rehabilitation after total knee arthroplasty. Clin Orthop 1983; 178: 198–201.

79. Heckman JD, Ryaby JP, McCabe J, et al. Acceleration of tibial fracture-healing by non-invasive, low-intensity pulsed ultrasound. J Bone Joint Surg 1994; 76A:26–34.

80. Hedenberg L. Functional improvement of the spastic hemiplegic arm after cooling. Scand J Rehabil Med 1970; 2:154–158.

81. Hekkenberg RT, Oosterbaan WA, vanBeekum WT. Evaluation of ultrasound therapy devices. Physiotherapy 1986; 72:390–394.

82. Henley E. Fluidotherapy. Crit Rev Phys Med Rehabil 1991; 3:173–195.

83. Henley E. Transcutaneous drug delivery: iontophoresis, phonophoresis. Crit Rev Phys Med Rehabil 1991; 2:139–151.

84. Heussler H, Hinchey G, Margiotta E, et al. A double-blind, randomized trial of low-power laser treatment in rheumatoid arthritis. Ann Rheum Dis 1993; 52:703–706.

85. Hocutt JE, Jaffe R, Rylander CR, et al. Cryotherapy in ankle sprains. Am J Sports Med 1982; 10:316–319.

86. Holdsworth L, Anderson D. Effectiveness of ultrasound used with a hydrocortisone coupling medium or epicondylitis clasp to treat lateral epicondylitis: pilot study. Physiotherapy 1993; 79:19–25.

87. Hong C-Z. Reversible conduction block in patients with polyneuropathy after ultrasound thermotherapy at therapeutic dosage. Arch Phys Med Rehabil 1991; 72:132–137.

88. Hurley D, Minder P, McDonough S, et al. Interferential therapy electrode placement technique in acute low back pain: a preliminary investigation. Arch Phys Med Rehabil 2001; 82:485–493.

89. Ivey M, Johnston RV, Uchida T. Cryotherapy for postoperative pain relief following knee arthroplasty. J Arthroplasty 1994; 9(3):285–290.

90. Jarit GJ, Mohr KJ, Waller R, et al. The effects of home interferential therapy on post-operative pain, edema, and range of motion of the knee. Clin J Sport Med 2003; 13:16–20.

91. Johnson CC, Guy AW. Nonionizing electromagnetic wave effects in biological materials and systems. Proc IEEE 1972; 60:692–718.

92. Jones SL. Electromagnetic field interference and cardiac pacemakers. Phys Ther 1976; 56:1013–1018.

93. Kantor G. Evaluation and survey of microwave and radiofrequency applicators. J Microw Power 1981; 16:135–150.

94. Klaiman MD, Shrader JA, Danoff JV, et al. Phonophoresis versus ultrasound in the treatment of common musculoskeletal conditions. Med Sci Sports Exerc 1998; 30:1349–1355.

95. Kloth LC. Electrotherapeutic alternatives for the treatment of pain. In: Gersh MR, ed. Electrotherapy in rehabilitation. Philadelphia: FA Davis; 1992.

96. Kloth LC. Interference current. In: Nelson RM, Currier DP, eds. Clinical electrotherapy. 2nd edn. Norwalk: Appleton & Lange; 1991.

97. Knutsson E, Mattsson E. Effects of local cooling on monosynaptic reflexes in man. Scand J Rehabil Med 1969; 1:126–132.

98. Kotke FJ, Lehmann JF, eds. Krusen's handbook of physical medicine and rehabilitation. 4th edn. Philadelphia: Saunders; 1990:293.

99. Kristiansen TK, Ryaby JP, McCabe J, et al. Accelerated healing of distal radial fractures with the use of specific, low-intensity ultrasound. J Bone Joint Surg 1997; 79A:961–973.

100. Lehmann JF, Brunner GD, Stow RW. Pain threshold measurements after therapeutic application of ultrasound, microwaves and infrared. Arch Phys Med Rehabil 1958; 39:560–565.

101. Lehmann JF, DeLateur BJ, Stonebridge JB. Selective muscle heating by shortwave diathermy with a helical coil. Arch Phys Med Rehabil 1969; 50:117–123.

102. Lehmann JF, DeLateur BJ, Warren CG, et al. Heating of joint structures by ultrasound. Arch Phys Med Rehabil 1968; 49:28–30.

103. Lehmann JF, DeLateur BJ, Warren CG, et al. Heating produced by ultrasound in bone and soft tissue. Arch Phys Med Rehabil 1967; 48:397–401.

104. Lehmann JF, DeLateur BJ, Warren CG, et al. Therapeutic temperature distribution produced by ultrasound as modified by dosage and volume of tissue exposed. Arch Phys Med Rehabil 1967; 48:662–666.

105. Lehmann JF, Johnston VC, McMillan JA, et al. Comparison of deep heating by microwaves at frequencies 2456 and 900 megacycles. Arch Phys Med Rehabil 1965; 46:307–314.

106. Lehmann JF, Masock AJ, Warren CG, et al. Effect of therapeutic temperatures on tendon extensibility. Arch Phys Med Rehabil 1970; 51:481–487.

107. Lehmann JF, McDougall JA, Guy AW, et al. Heating patterns produced by shortwave diathermy applicators in tissue substitute models. Arch Phys Med Rehabil 1983; 64:575–577.

108. Lehmann JF, McMillan JA, Brunner GD, et al. Comparative study of the efficiency of short-wave, microwave and ultrasonic diathermy in heating the hip joint. Arch Phys Med Rehabil 1959; 40:510–512.

109. Lehmann JF, Silverman DR, Baum BA, et al. Temperature distributions in the human thigh, produced by infrared, hot pack and microwave applications. Arch Phys Med Rehabil 1966; 47:291–299.

110. Lehmann JF. Therapeutic heat and cold. 4th edn. Baltimore: Williams & Wilkins; 1990.

111. Lekas MD. Iontophoresis treatment. Otolaryngol Head Neck Surg 1979; 87:292–298.

112. Leutz DW, Harris H. Continuous cold therapy in total knee arthroplasty. Am J Knee Surg 1995; 8:121–123.

113. Levenson JL, Weissberg MP. Ultrasound abuse: case report. Arch Phys Med Rehabil 1983; 64:90–91.

114. Levy AS, Marmar E. The role of cold compressive dressings in the postoperative treatment of total knee arthroplasty. Clin Orthop Relat Res 1993; 297:174–178.

115. Lewis T. Observations upon the reactions of the vessels of the human skin to cold. Heart 1930; 15:177–208.

116. Li LC, Scudds RA. Iontophoresis: an overview of the mechanisms and clinical application. Arthritis Care Res 1995; 8(1):51–61.

117. Lowdon BJ, Moore RJ. Determinants and nature of intramuscular temperature changes during cold therapy. Am J Phys Med 1975; 54:223–233.

118. Marks R, Ghanagaraja S, Ghassemi M. Ultrasound of osteo-arthritis of the knee: a systematic review. Physiotherapy 2000; 86:452–463.

119. Marks R, Ghassemi M, Duarte R, et al. A review of the literature on shortwave diathermy as applied to osteo-arthritis of the knee. Physiotherapy 1999; 85:304–316.

120. McGown HL. Effects of cold application on maximal isometric contraction. Phys Ther 1967; 47:185–192.

121. McLeod DR, Fowlow SB. Multiple malformations and exposure to therapeutic ultrasound during organogenesis. Am J Med Genet 1989; 34:317–319.

122. Meeusen R, Lievens P. The use of cryotherapy in sports injuries. Sports Med 1986; 3:398–414.

123. Melzack R, Jeans ME, Stratford JG, et al. Ice massage and transcutaneous electrical stimulation: comparison of treatment for low-back pain. Pain 1980; 9:209–217.

124. Mense S. Effects of temperature on the discharge of muscle spindles and tendon organs. Pflugers Arch 1978; 374:159–166.

125. Miglietta O. Action of cold on spasticity. Am J Phys Med 1973; 52:198–205.

126. Miller DL. A review of the ultrasonic bioeffects of microsonation, gas-body activation, and related cavitation-like phenomena. Ultrasound Med Biol 1987; 13:443–470.

127. Moffett J, Richardson P, Frost H, et al. A placebo controlled double blind trial to evaluate the effectiveness of pulsed short wave therapy for osteo-arthritic hip and knee pain. Pain 1996; 67:121–127.

128. Mokhtar B, Baxter GD, Walsh DM, et al. Double-blind, placebo-controlled investigation of the effect of combined phototherapy/low intensity laser therapy upon experimental ischaemic pain in humans. Lasers Surg Med 1995; 17(1):74–81.

129. Montorsi F, Salonia A, Guazzoni G, et al. Transdermal electromotive multi-drug administration for Peyronie's disease: preliminary results. J Androl 2000; 21:85–90.

130. Morison WL. Phototherapy and photochemotherapy. Adv Dermatol 1992; 7:255–271.

131. Newman JT, Nellermoe MD, Carnett JL. Hydrocortisone phonophoresis. J Am Podiatr Med Assoc 1992; 82:432–435.

132. Nolte PA, Van Der Krans A, Patka P, et al. Low-intensity pulsed ultrasound in the treatment of nonunions. J Trauma 2001; 51:693–703.

133. Nukada H, Pollock M, Allpress S. Experimental cold injury to peripheral nerve. Brain 1981; 104:779–811.

134. Nutt J, Anderson V, Peacock J, et al. DBS and diathermy interaction induces severe CNS damage. Neurology 2001; 56:1384–1386.

135. Oakley EM. Dangers and contraindications of therapeutic ultrasound. Physiotherapy 1978; 64:173–174.

136. Olah KS, Bridges N, Denning J, et al. The conservative management of patients with symptoms of stress incontinence: a randomized, prospective study comparing weighted vaginal cones and interferential therapy. Am J Obstet Gynecol 1990; 162:87–92.

137. O'Malley EP, Oester YT. Influence of some physical chemical factors on iontophoresis using radio-isotopes. Arch Phys Med Rehabil 1955; 36:310–316.

138. Oosterveld FGJ, Rasker JJ. Treating arthritis with locally applied heat or cold. Semin Arthritis Rheum 1994; 24(2):82–90.

139. Ozawa A, Haruki Y, Iwashita K, et al. Follow-up of clinical efficacy of iontophoresis therapy for postherpetic neuralgia (PHN). J Dermatol 1999; 26:1–10.

140. Paliwal BR, Shrivastava PN. Microwave hyperthermia: principles and quality assurance. Radiol Clin North Am 1989; 27:489–497.

141. Penderghest C, Kimura I, Gulick D. Double-blind clinical efficacy study of pulsed phonophoresis on perceived pain associated with symptomatic tendinitis. J Sport Rehabil 1998; 7:9-19.

142. Perez CA, Emami B. Clinical trials with local (external and interstitial) irradiation and hyperthermia—current and future perspectives. Radiol Clin North Am 1989; 27:525–542.

143. Perkins JF, Li M, Nicholas CH, et al. Cooling as a stimulus to smooth muscles. Am J Physiol 1950; 163:14–26.

144. Perron M, Malouin F. Acetic acid iontophoresis and ultrasound for the treatment of calcifying tendinitis of the shoulder: a randomized control trial. Arch Phys Med Rehabil 1997; 78:379–384.

145. Petajan JH, Watts N. Effects of cooling on the triceps surae reflex. Am J Phys Med 1962; 41:240–251.

146. Philadelphia Panel. Philadelphia Panel evidence-based clinical practice guidelines on selected rehabilitation interventions for low back pain. Phys Ther 2001; 81:1641–1674.

147. Philadelphia Panel. Philadelphia Panel evidence-based clinical practice guidelines on selected rehabilitation interventions for knee pain. Phys Ther 2001; 81:1675–1700.

148. Philadelphia Panel. Philadelphia Panel evidence-based clinical practice guidelines on selected rehabilitation interventions for neck pain. Phys Ther 2001; 81:1701–1717.

149. Philadelphia Panel. Philadelphia Panel evidence-based clinical practice guidelines on selected rehabilitation interventions for shoulder pain. Phys Ther 2001; 81:1719–1730.

150. Price R, Lehmann JF, Boswell-Bessette S, et al. Influence of cryotherapy on spasticity at the human ankle. Arch Phys Med Rehabil 1993; 74:300–304.

151. Riedl C, Plas E, Engelhardt P, et al. Iontophoresis for treatment of Peyronie's disease. J Urol 2000; 163:95–99.

152. Ritzmann SE, Levin WC. Cryopathies: a review. Arch Intern Med 1961; 107:186–204.

153. Robinson VA, Brosseau L, Peterson J, et al. Therapeutic ultrasound for osteoarthritis of the knee. Cochrane Database Syst Rev 2001:3.

154. Scarcella JB, Cohn BT. The effect of cold therapy on the postoperative course of total hip and knee arthroplasty patients. Am J Orthop 1995; 24(11):847–852.

155. Scheffler N, Sheitel P, Lipton M. Use of Cryo/Cuff for the control of postoperative pain and edema. J Foot Surg 1992; 31:141–146.

156. Schindl A, Schindl M, Pernerstofer-Schon H, et al. Low-intensity laser therapy: a review. J Invest Med 2000; 48:312–326.

157. Schmidt KL, Ott VR, Rocher G, et al. Heat, cold and inflammation [review]. Z Rheumatol 1979; 38:391–404.

158. Scott BO. Effects of contact lenses on short-wave field distribution. Br J Ophthalmol 1956; 40:696–697.

159. Selkowitz DM. Electrical currents. In: Cameron MH, ed. Physical agents in rehabilitation: from research to practice. Philadelphia: Saunders; 1999.

160. Shafshak TS, El-Sheshai AM, Soltan HE. Personality traits in the mechanisms of interferential therapy for osteoarthritic knee pain. Arch Phys Med Rehabil 1991; 72:579–581.

161. Shepherd JT, Rusch NJ, Vanhoutte PM. Effect of cold on the blood vessel wall. Gen Pharmacol 1983; 14:61–64.

162. Shrivastava SN, Singh G. Tap water iontophoresis in palmo-plantar hyperhidrosis. Br J Dermatol 1977; 96:189–195.

163. Shulman AG. Ice water as primary treatment of burns. JAMA 1960; 173:96–99.

164. Stewart HF, Harris GR, Herman BA, et al. Survey of use and performance of ultrasonic therapy equipment in Pinellas County, Florida. Phys Ther 1974; 54:707–714.

165. Stolman L. Treatment of excess sweating of the palms by iontophoresis. Arch Dermatol 1987; 123:893–896.

166. Stolman L. Treatment of hyperhydrosis. Dermatol Clin 1998; 16:863–869.

167. Stuchly MA, Repacholi MH, Lecuyer DW, et al. Exposure to the operator and patient during short wave diathermy treatments. Health Phys 1982; 42:341–366.

168. Taylor K, Newton RA, Personius WJ, et al. Effects of interferential current stimulation for treatment of subjects with recurrent jaw pain. Phys Ther 1987; 67:346–350.

169. Ter Haar G, Dyson M, Oakley EM. The use of ultrasound by physiotherapists in Britain, 1985. Ultrasound Med Biol 1987; 13:659–663.

170. Thomson PD, Bowden ML, McDonald K, et al. A survey of burn hydrotherapy in the United States. J Burn Care Rehabil 1990; 11:151–155.

171. Thornton KL. Principles of ultrasound. J Reprod Med 1992; 37:27–32.

172. Travell J. Ethyl chloride spray for painful muscle spasm. Arch Phys Med 1952; 33:291–298.

173. Tredget EE, Shankowsky HA, Joffe AM, et al. Epidemiology of infections with *Pseudomonas aeruginosa* in burn patients: the role of hydrotherapy. Clin Infect Dis 1992; 15:941–949.

174. Van der Heijden G, Leffers P, Wolters P, et al. No effect of bipolar interferential electrotherapy and pulsed ultrasound for soft tissue disorders: a randomised controlled trial. Ann Rheum Dis 1999; 58:530–540.

175. Van Der Windt DAWM, Van Der Heijden GJMG, Van Den Berg SGM, et al. Ultrasound therapy for musculoskeletal disorders: a systematic review. Pain 1999; 81:257–271.

176. Van der Windt DAWM, Van der Heijden GJMG, Van den Berg SGM, et al. Therapeutic ultrasound for acute ankle sprains. Cochrane Database Syst Rev 2002;1:CD001250.

177. Walk EE, Himel HN, Batra EK, et al. Aquatic access for the disabled. J Burn Care Rehabil 1992; 13:356–363.

178. Warren CG, Koblanski JN, Sigelmann RA. Ultrasound coupling media: their relative transmissivity. Arch Phys Med Rehabil 1976; 57:218–222.

179. Watson CW. Effect of lowering of body temperature on the symptoms and signs of multiple sclerosis. N Engl J Med 1959; 261:1253–1259.

180. Waylonis GW. The physiologic effects of ice massage. Arch Phys Med Rehabil 1967; 48:37–42.

181. Webb JM, Williams D, Ivory JP, et al. The use of cold compression dressing after total knee replacement: a randomized controlled trial. Orthopedics 1998; 21(1):59–61.

182. Weinberger A, Fadilah R, Lev A, et al. Intra-articular temperature measurements after superficial heating. Scand J Rehabil Med 1989; 21:55–57.

183. Werners R, Pynsent PB, Bulstrode CJ. Randomized trial comparing interferential therapy with motorized lumbar traction and massage in the management of low back pain in a primary care setting. Spine 1999; 24:1579–1584.

184. Whitelaw GP, DeMuth KA, Demos HA, et al. The use of the Cryo/Cuff versus ice and elastic wrap in the postoperative care of knee arthroscopy patients. Am J Knee Surg 1995; 8(1):28–31.

185. Woodmansey A, Collins DH, Ernst MM. Vascular reactions to the contrast bath in health and in rheumatoid arthritis. Lancet 1938; 2:1350–1353.

186. Wright V, Johns RJ. Quantitative and qualitative analysis of joint stiffness in normal subjects and in patients with connective tissue diseases. Ann Rheum Dis 1961; 20:36–45.

187. Ziskin MC. Fundamental physics of ultrasound and its propagation in tissue. Radiographics 1993; 13:705–709.

Chapter

22

Electrical Stimulation

W. Jerry Mysiw and Rebecca D. Jackson

The history of electrical stimulation as an adjunct to traditional medicine has its roots in Greek philosophy. Although early applications with a variety of electricity-generating devices were advocated for use in the treatment of many different medical conditions, its initial association with quackery limited its general acceptance. Acceptance has gradually grown as the systematic collection and analysis of scientific and clinical data have helped to define its beneficial impact. Current clinical applications of electrical stimulation therapy have crossed the lines of many specialties, including rehabilitation medicine, neurology, urology, gynecology, orthopedics, dermatology, and pain management.

The first significant application of electrical stimulation to improve muscle function dates back to 1950, with the invention of the cardiac pacemaker.[169] Effective application of functional electrical stimulation (FES) in a rehabilitation system is generally credited to Liberson, who applied electrical stimulation to the peroneal nerve to produce ankle dorsiflexion in hemiplegic patients during the swing phase of gait.[145] This was followed by reports of the use of electrical stimulation of the quadriceps to aid in static standing following spinal cord injury (SCI).[123] Together, these are the first reports of FES utilizing electrical stimulation to serve as a neuroorthosis or external control of motor function.

Since the 1960s, advances have come rapidly. The gate theory of pain by Melzack and Wall, described in 1965,[157] provided the rationale for the development of such stimulation techniques as transcutaneous electrical nerve stimulation (TENS) and the use of both implanted dorsal column and conus medullaris root stimulators for neuropathic pain or neurogenic bladder control. Most recently, electrical stimulation has returned to its functional roots in cardiology, and has been applied to the development of latissimus dorsi cardiomyoplasty assist devices for the treatment of cardiomyopathy.

Over the past several decades, improvements in electronic technology and a better understanding of neuromuscular physiology have worked together to improve the use of electrical stimulation for functional and therapeutic purposes. Today, there is a substantial body of experimental data supporting its application in the treatment of a variety of medical conditions, based on its unique properties in modifying certain biologic and chemical aspects of biologic tissues in vivo and increasing the contractile properties of muscle.

PHYSIOLOGIC EFFECTS OF NEUROMUSCULAR ELECTRICAL STIMULATION

Normal muscle physiology

The motor unit involved in contraction consists of an alpha motor neuron, its axon, the myoneural junction, and the muscle fibers that it innervates. The alpha motor neurons differ in size and function, with the small motor neurons, which have the lowest activation frequency, innervating slow muscle fibers and the large motor neurons innervating fast fibers. Muscle fibers within the motor unit can be classified into three main categories[156] based on specific functional, metabolic, and histochemical features of the individual muscle fibers (Table 22-1). Within each motor unit, all muscle fibers are histologically identical,[33] although with any muscle, all fiber types can be present in varying amounts, resulting in unique contractile characteristics.

During normal muscle contraction, a motor unit with a low axonal conduction velocity (or activation frequency) is recruited before a unit with a higher conduction velocity.[100,101] This size principle suggests that axonal conduction of a motor unit is related to the muscle fiber parameters, such that a unit with low conduction velocity has a slow twitch force, long contraction time, and higher resistance to fatigue. This theory explains the orderly progression of fiber activation with the onset of isometric voluntary contraction. Weak, slowly conducting, fatigue-resistant motor units containing type 1 fibers are recruited first to allow for slow increases in firing rate and increasing tension in the muscle.[162,163] This is followed sequentially by the recruitment of the high conduction velocity, type 2b fibers, which can increase gain.[166]

When the motor unit is stimulated by artificial rather than voluntary action, this orderly progression of fiber activation does not always occur.[129] With functional neuromuscular stimulation, the order of recruitment is reversed because activation of motor units is dependent on the excitation current threshold, which varies inversely with the diameter of the nerve fiber.[239] This results in initial stimulation of type 2 fibers, followed by activation of the slow type 1 fibers with continued stimulation.

Response of muscle fibers to electrical stimulation

Following chronic, continuous, low-frequency (10-Hz) electrical stimulation of normal, fast-twitch skeletal muscles, a stereotypical series of events occurs, resulting in transformation of the muscle fiber from a fast-twitch type 2b fiber to a composition with slow-twitch type 1 characteristics (Table 22-2). Although most of the data come from studies in mammalian models in which different low-frequency, continuous stimulation regimens were used, the consistency of changes reported supports generalization of the results to many animals, including humans.

Within 2–4 days of the onset of stimulation, initial changes are noted in the sarcoplasmic reticulum. First, there is a decrease in the rate and capacity of ionized calcium uptake that is associated with a decrease in the activity of calcium-dependent ATPase and its phosphorylated intermediate.[98,151,216,231] There also occur an associated decrease in calsequestrine, the major calcium-binding protein in the sarcoplasmic reticulum,[99] an increase in the specific membrane proteins that are typical of the slow-twitch type 1 sarcoplasmic reticulum,[258] and a rearrangement of the membrane phospholipid matrix.[232] The transformation of the sarcoplasmic reticulum is associated with a decline in parvalbumin, the calcium-binding cytosolic protein, which almost completely disappears within 3 weeks of stimulation.[128] These histochemical changes result in both a decrease in calcium sequestration in the sarcoplasmic reticulum and a reduction in calcium-buffering capacity, which functionally affects contractile properties by increasing the time to peak velocity within the first week.[99,199] The isotonic twitch characteristics, a function of myosin heavy and light chains and other contractile proteins, are unaltered during this early stage of transformation.[3]

Ultrastructurally, there is an early decrease in T tubuli, terminal cisternae, and sarcoplasmic reticulum,[65] as well as a decrease in calcium-transporting membranes. In addition, there is a decrease in high-density intermembranous particles of the sarcoplasmic reticulum. These particles are thought to be oligomers of calcium-pumping ATPase, and their decline is associated with a reduction in the rate and capacity of calcium uptake in the sarcoplasmic reticulum.[62]

Table 22-1 Properties of muscle fiber types			
Property	Type 1	Type 2a	Type 2b
Morphologic			
Name	Red	Intermediate	White
Capillary density	↑	Intermediate	↓↓
Histochemical			
Myosin ATPase	↓	↑	↑
Mitochondria	↑	↑	↓
Glycogen	Low	Intermediate	High
Myosin heavy chain	HC_s	HCfa	HCfb
Myosin light chain	$LC_{1a,1b,2}$	$Lcf_{1,2,3}$	$Lcf_{1,2,3}$
Metabolic			
Type	Oxidative Aerobic	Oxidative–glycolytic Mixed	Glycolytic Anaerobic
Contractile			
Twitch	Slow	Fast	Fast
Fatigability	Slow	Intermediate	Rapid

Table 22-2 Chronic low-frequency stimulation of fast-twitch muscle: sequence of events in transformation		
Property	Acute (0–3 weeks)	Subacute (4–8 weeks)
Contractile	↑ resistance to fatigue ↑ time to peak twitch ↑ time to half-relaxation ↑ tetanus to twitch	↓ maximal velocity of shortening
Ultrastructural	Swelling sarcoplasmic reticulum ↑ T system ↓ particle in sarcoplasmic reticulum bilayer ↑ mitochondrial fraction ↑ Z-band width	Broad Z band Declining mitochondria
Histochemical	↑ type 2a, ↓ type 2b heavy chain	↓ type 2a → type 1 heavy chain ↓ LC_2 → ↑ LC_{2s} ↓ LC_3 then ↓ LC_1 ↓ NCH_3-histidine
Metabolic	↑ oxidative enzyme mRNA Δ α-, β-tropomysin ↓ calcium transport and calcium-active ATPase ↓ glycolytic enzymes mRNA	↑ oxidative enzyme activity ↓ glycolytic activity
Morphologic	↑ capillary density ↑ blood flow	↓ muscle fiber area ↓ muscle fiber wet weight

Although the most rapid transformation responses to electrical stimulation are centered on the sarcoplasmic reticulum, continued low-frequency stimulation can eventually affect the myosin contractile proteins to result in the ultimate transformation to a slow fiber type. Calcium-activated myosin ATPase activity begins to decline by 3 weeks, eventually reaching the low levels typical of slow type 1 muscle fibers. Concomitantly, there is an increase in the alkali lability of the myosin ATPase corresponding to changes in myosin light chain (LC) patterns.[240] Changes in LC patterns occur at the level of transcription and translation during the transformation from fast to slow fiber type. In an orderly sequence, the fast DTNB-LC chain (LC-f2) is replaced by its slow counterpart (LC-S2), followed by declines in LC-f3, then LC-f1, with replacement by the corresponding slow LC.[28,225,236] The changes in the DTNB-LC occur simultaneously with the initial changes in myosin heavy chain (MHC). MHC mRNA expressed in each muscle fiber encodes a unique myosin cross-bridge for types 1, 2a, and 2b fibers that is responsible for the characteristic intrinsic velocity of contraction and economy of force for each muscle fiber type. Within 4 days of the onset of electrical stimulation, there is a decline in the mRNA of the MHC characteristics of type 2b fibers (MHC-fb), with eventual suppression of these mRNA levels by 90% after 21 days (Fig. 22-1).[30] This is followed by a decline in MHC-fb protein within 12 days.[97] The decreasing MHC-fb is initially replaced by an MHC reflecting the type 2a fiber (MHC-fa), and only after prolonged stimulation is the phenotypic transformation completed with replacement of MHC-fa by MHC-s.[28] However, if electrical stimulation is combined with stretch, there is a synergistic effect of mechanical and electrical forces leading to a rapid (within 4 days) stimulation of MHC-s mRNA (Fig. 22-2).[84] This asynchronous transforma-

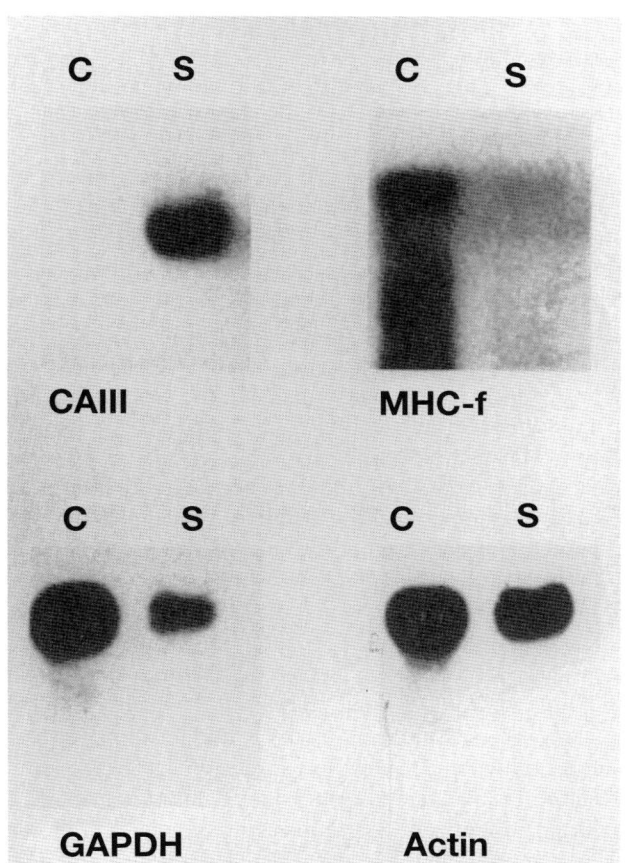

Figure 22-1 Northern blot analysis of the changes in mRNA expression of four different muscle genes in response to 21 days of electrical stimulation of the tibialis anterior muscle. There is a stimulation of carbonic anhydrase III (CAIII) expression and suppression of both glyceraldehyde-3-phosphate dehydrogenase (GAPDH) and the fast myosin heavy chain (MHC-f) with electrical stimulation-induced fast to slow transition. (From Brownson et al. 1988,[30] with permission of John Wiley.)

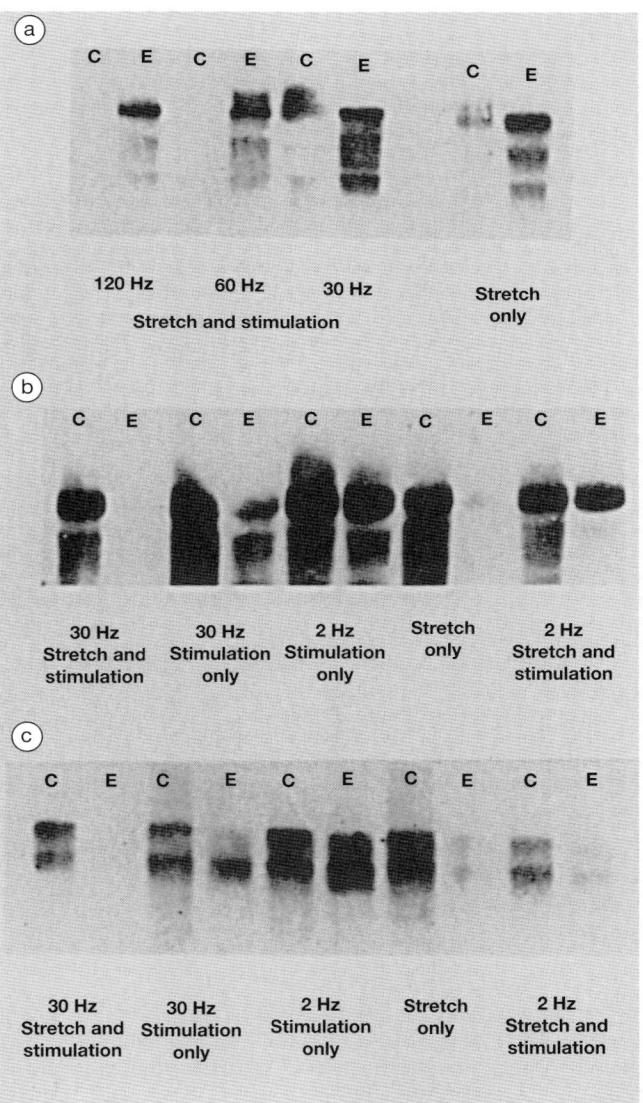

Figure 22-2 Northern blot analysis of RNA from normal (C) and electrically stimulated and stretched (E) rabbit tibialis anterior muscle after 4 days. There is activation of slow myosin heavy chain (MHC) (a) with repression of both fast type 2b MHC (b) and MHC genes detected with a myosin light chain 1 and 3 probe (c). Note that the two bands in (c) represent the two light chains encoded by the same gene. (From Goldspink et al. 1991,[85] with permission.)

tion from fast to slow type within the different myosin subunits can lead to the coexistence of both slow and fast isoforms of myosin within a single muscle fiber (type 2c fibers).[151,197,227]

By 3 weeks after the onset of stimulation, alpha and beta tropomyosin changes from fast to slow type,[226] and Z lines become evident, with a corresponding development of the M band structure. Conversion of fiber type is completed within 8 weeks of initiation of chronic, low-frequency stimulation.[195] This new type 1 muscle fiber composition is functionally associated with both an increase in resistance to fatigue and a decrease in the maximum velocity of shortening.

The changes in ultrastructural and contractile properties from a fast- to a slow-twitch muscle fiber are also associated with important changes in metabolic activity: from use of an anaerobic, glycolytic pathway in the type 2b fiber to the aerobic Krebs cycle-associated pathway of type 1 fibers. With the onset of continuous low-frequency electrical stimulation, there is an enhancement of the enzymes responsible for phosphorylation and oxidation of glucose. Within 10 days of initiation of electrical stimulation, there is a rapid rise in GLUT-4, a facilitative glucose transporter isoform present in skeletal muscle.[69] The stimulatory effect of both insulin and exercise on glucose transport is higher in the more oxidative type 1 and 2a fibers than in glycolytic type 2b fibers. However, electrical stimulation increases glucose uptake similarly in both oxidative type 1 and 2a fibers and glycolyte type 2b fibers, presumably due to the fact that electrical stimulation similarly increased the plasma membrane content of GLUT-4 in both types of fiber.[224,225] In contrast, the activity of citrate synthase (an enzyme of the Krebs cycle) increases more slowly after the onset of electrical stimulation, with rises in protein levels over 30–40 days and a plateauing of the peak effect by day 60–90, reflecting the metabolic change to an aerobic oxidative enzyme system. The mRNA of carbonic anhydrase II, an enzyme that facilitates carbon dioxide movement in muscle, is also rapidly stimulated with electrical stimulation to reach levels seen in type 1 fibers over 10–20 days (Fig. 22-1).[30] Finally, there is a pronounced increase in many other enzymes involved in terminal substrate oxidation and in fatty acid and ketone body oxidation.[32,113,128,196,198,218] These metabolic changes are also associated with pronounced increases in capillary density[29,115,218] and oxygen consumption, which in combination might be responsible for the development of increased resistance to fatigue.[114]

Recent data suggest that the adaptive response to electrical stimulation may in part be regulated by uncoupling protein (UCP)-3, a transmembrane carrier protein on the inner mitochondrial membrane that has been proposed to contribute to basal tissue metabolic rate by uncoupling mitochondrial electrochemical H^+ gradient from ADP phosphorylation. UPC-3 protein is increased in response to short-term electrical stimulation, whereas with long-duration electrical stimulation both protein and mRNA UCP-3 are down-regulated coincident with the emergence of oxidative type 2a fibers.[212]

In addition to the increase in oxidative capacity, there is a suppression of enzymes involved in anaerobic glycogenolysis. There are progressive declines in the level of phosphorylase

kinase,[142] a regulator of glycogen metabolism that promotes glycogenolysis by phosphorylating and activating phosphorylase enzyme. These changes might reflect the very early changes in metabolic activity in the sarcoplasmic reticulum in response to electrical stimulation, as this enzyme is allosterically activated by calcium through its delta subunit, calmodulin, thus providing a potential link between electrically stimulated calcium changes and glycogenolysis. There are also dramatic changes in mRNA levels of glyceraldehyde-3-phosphate dehydrogenase (GAPDH), a glycolytic enzyme abundant in fast-twitch fibers (see Fig. 22-2).[30] There are steady declines in GAPDH mRNA to the levels seen in slow-twitch fibers after 21 days of electrical stimulation, suggesting that part of the regulation of fast- to slow-twitch fiber transformation is occurring at the level of gene transcription. When temporal data of GAPDH enzyme activity are compared with the temporal data of its mRNA, it appears that the declines in mRNA concentration precede the observed protein changes.[128,201] This is similar to a pattern of events described for aldolase,[261] an enzyme adjacent to GAPDH in the glycolytic pathway. These data suggest that there is a relative delay in the turnover of the glycolytic proteins that potentially delays the rate of change observed in metabolic activity in response to electrical stimulation.

Several studies have helped to confirm the applicability of some aspects of these data derived from animal models to the effects of electrical stimulation on human muscle in vivo. After 21 days of electrical stimulation (50 Hz, alternating current) in normal muscle, there is a significant increase in total capillary length per tissue volume, a decrease in intercapillary distance, and a decrease in Krogh cylinders, leading to an improvement in capillary supply to muscle;[36] these findings are similar to those changes noted in animal models. Using intermittent electrical stimulation (square wave, 20–30 Hz, 0.003-s pulse, 33% duty cycle) with surface electrodes for 30 min twice a day for 90 days in individuals with chronic SCI, electrical stimulation of the lower extremity has resulted in an increase in the number of type 2a muscle fibers (Fig. 22-3).[87] Munsat and associates have shown more dramatic changes in fiber type in response to electrical stimulation, with type 1 muscle fibers increasing from 4% to 48% after FES of the quadriceps in patients with disuse atrophy.[170] Studies using electrical stimulation of triceps surae muscle for 20 days at medium (50 Hz) and high (2500 Hz) frequencies have also shown an increase in fiber size, mitochondrial fraction, and DNA fiber content.[34,35] Finally, similar changes have also been noted in normal muscle from subjects with scoliosis, in whom chronic, low-intensity electrical stimulation resulted in increases in type 1 and 2c muscle fiber percentages after 6 months of continuous stimulation. In addition to changes in muscle fiber types, an increase was also noted in citrate synthase activity, suggesting a move toward an oxidative metabolism[80] and a more fatigue-resistant muscle.

After discontinuation of electrical stimulation, the muscle fiber type begins to transform to its prestimulation characteristics in a time course that reflects a 'first in, last out' relationship. Within 6 weeks, the former fast-twitch muscle fiber regains its previous contractile behavior with a change in maximum

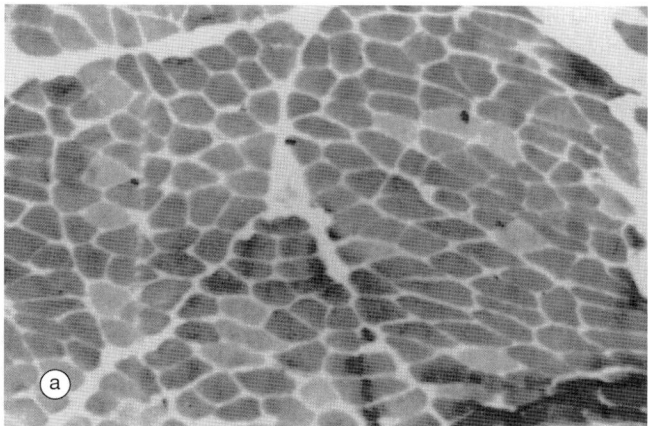

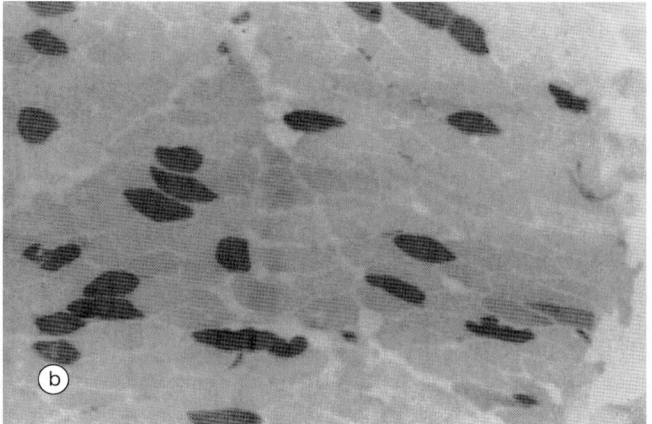

Figure 22-3 Biopsy of vastus lateralis of the quadriceps femoris muscle from a subject with a spinal cord injury before (**a**) and after (**b**) undergoing functional electrical stimulation for 90 days. The muscle biopsy was stained with a dye for ATPase myofibrillar activity. Note the increase in type 2a fibers after electrical stimulation. (From Greve et al. 1993,[87] with permission.)

velocity of contraction. This is associated with changes in *N*-methylhistidine content, myosin ATPase, and LC. Changes in oxidative and glycolytic enzymes lag behind the contractile protein changes, with a return to an anaerobic metabolic pathway by 12 weeks. Capillary density changes are one of the last features to be modified and may be present for up to several months.[230] If electrical stimulation therapy is discontinued, a series of changes occurs in the muscle fiber that depend on the length of discontinuation of therapy. This can affect the muscle response to resumption of electrical stimulation (detraining effect).

The importance of stimulation frequency for fiber transformation has also been a subject of intense investigation.[231] Application of low-frequency (10 Hz) stimulation for 8 h per day results in a delay of the acquisition of the transformation from fast- to slow-twitch muscle fiber composition when compared with a continuous (24 h per day), low-frequency (10 Hz) stimulation protocol.[196] Despite this delay, similar changes in contrac-

tile properties eventually occur with both stimulation regimens. If an equal number of stimuli are given per minute as a short burst of high-frequency (40 Hz) stimuli, versus continuous low-frequency (10 Hz) stimulation, similar histochemical changes reflecting a transition from fast- to slow-twitch muscle fiber type are noted in both groups.[116] Increases in succinate dehydrogenase activity are also seen in response to each of these stimulation patterns, although the increase in succinate dehydrogenase occurs at a slower rate when the stimulation frequency is 40 Hz.[200] Using even higher frequencies (2.5-s trains at 60 Hz delivered every 10 s), with the number of stimuli equivalent to continuous low-frequency (10 Hz) stimulation over a 5-week period, produced nearly identical changes in ATPase, fiber type, calcium uptake, and contractile properties with each regimen.[241]

The impact of a change in frequency, however, is dramatically different if there is an increase in *both* frequency and number of stimuli. In the denervated rat soleus model, intermittent high-frequency (100 Hz) electrical stimulation resulted in conversion of the muscle from a slow- to fast-twitch fiber type.[146,147] In contrast, continuous low-frequency (10 Hz) stimulation of this muscle maintained the slow-twitch characteristics of the denervated soleus muscle.[147] It appears that both the specific frequency and the number of stimuli per minute with electrical stimulation can dramatically affect the phenotypic expression of the muscle fiber in response to treatment. This switch from slow- to fast-twitch fiber type, at this point, is unique to denervated muscle and has never been reported in innervated muscle.

To exclude the influence of the release of local neurotropic factor(s) on the transformation of muscle fiber type in response to electrical stimulation, investigations have focused on the response of denervated muscle to electrical stimulation. Using a 1-s train of low-frequency (10 Hz) pulses every 2 s, electrical stimulation started within 24 h of denervation resulted in a decrease in atrophy and maintenance of oxidative enzyme levels at or above normal levels in 95% of samples.[175] Somewhat surprising, however, were findings that the late-onset initiation of electrical stimulation (28 days post denervation) using an intermediate frequency (25 Hz) stimulus with a long bidirectional impulse duration (200 μs) markedly retarded atrophy and induced a hybrid fiber type with mitochondrial changes suggestive of a type 1 fiber and type 2b myofibrillar ATPase expression.[165] These studies and other histologic and biochemical data suggest that denervated muscles exhibit some properties of plasticity independent of neurologic input.

WAVES

Therapeutic electricity is characterized according to its waveform, amplitude, duration, and frequency. Three basic types of waveform exist: direct current, alternating current, and pulsed current. Direct current involves the unidirectional flow of a charge, with no change in waveform characteristics over time. This type of uninterrupted direct current waveform is not

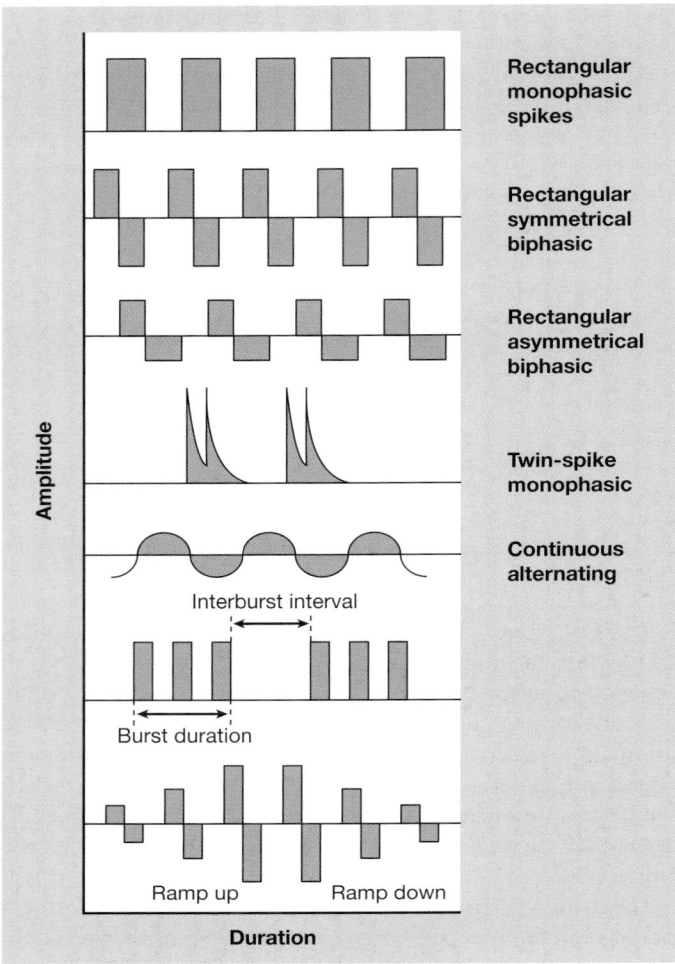

Figure 22-4 Diagrammatic representations of waveforms and modulations.

applicable to FES systems. Alternating current refers to an uninterrupted bidirectional flow of charged particles that can be symmetric or asymmetric (Fig. 22-4).[136,171] The pulsed waveforms are the most common waveforms applied for therapeutic purposes.[136] Pulsed waves can be further classified as monophasic or biphasic. The biphasic waveforms can be symmetric or asymmetric with respect to the baseline. The reference to symmetry applies to any combination of parameters, such as current intensity, duration, rise time, or decay of the waveform.[171]

Pulsed or alternating currents can be varied, or modulated, with respect to amplitude, duration, or frequency.[136,171] These modulations can be sequential, intermittent, or variable. *Ramping* refers to a form of modulation in which either the pulse amplitude or the duration is increased (ramped up) or decreased (ramped down) over time. A *burst* refers to a type of modulation in which a finite series of pulses, or an envelope of alternating current, is delivered at a specific frequency (carrier frequency) over a specified time interval (burst duration). The interval between bursts is referred to as the *interburst interval* (Fig. 22-4). The *duty cycle* is defined as the ratio between burst duration and total cycle time, where the total

cycle time equals the duration of the burst duration plus the interburst interval. The duty cycle is often expressed as a percentage, therefore a duty cycle ratio of 1:4 corresponds to a duty cycle of 20%.

A number of studies have been done to explore the impact of different waveforms and stimulation parameters on patient comfort, force of contraction, strengthening effect, and fatigue. The majority of these studies have been done in normal muscle, and these data are presumably transferable to upper motor neuron and myopathic conditions.

Both burst-modulated alternating current and asymmetric biphasic pulsed current appear to induce the most forceful contractions.[133,253] No consensus exists as to which waveform provides the greatest patient comfort. Various studies have advocated the burst-modulated alternating current, asymmetric biphasic pulsed current, symmetric biphasic pulsed current, and twin spiked monophasic pulsed currents.[8,89,260]

The relationship between current amplitude (milliamperes [mA]) and the force of muscle contraction is linear.[136] A stimulus duration in excess of 200 μs is likely to produce a more forceful muscle contraction, but waveforms with durations in excess of 60 μs are also associated with greater pain.[25,111] Stimulation frequencies of 60–100 Hz are necessary to produce the most forceful muscle contraction, but stimulation at these rates rapidly results in muscle fatigue.[21] Muscle fatigue is significantly diminished by utilizing stimulation rates of approximately 20 Hz, but this results in approximately a 35% drop in the force generated at higher stimulation frequencies.[121] Current studies are attempting to maximize the effectiveness of stimulation parameters through the manipulation of duty cycles and the development of biophysically based mathematic models of how muscle responds to electrical stimulation, in the hope that these models will optimize FES-generated movement.[57,58] In summary, data demonstrate that waveform amplitude, duration, and frequency can all be manipulated to control both the force and endurance of muscle contraction, but the optimal combinations of stimulation parameters for therapeutic or functional purposes are not identical. This area is an area of active research.

ELECTRODES

The development of neuromuscular stimulation electrodes remains problematic. A number of different types of electrode are available, including surface, epimysial, intramuscular, juxta-neural, nerve cuff, epineural, intraneural–intrafascicular, and intraspinal.[243] The choice of an electrode type is based on the goal of the electrical stimulation program and its ease of use for the patient. In addition, selection criteria for the choice of an electrode type should include general biocompatibility of the electrode and leads, electrochemistry at the electrode–tissue interface, the possibility of actively or passively induced tissue damage by the electrodes or leads, electrode invasiveness, ease of surgical placement, ease of electrode retrieval and/or replacement, electrode reliability and failure rate, selectivity of the desired elicited muscle contractions, potential for side effects,

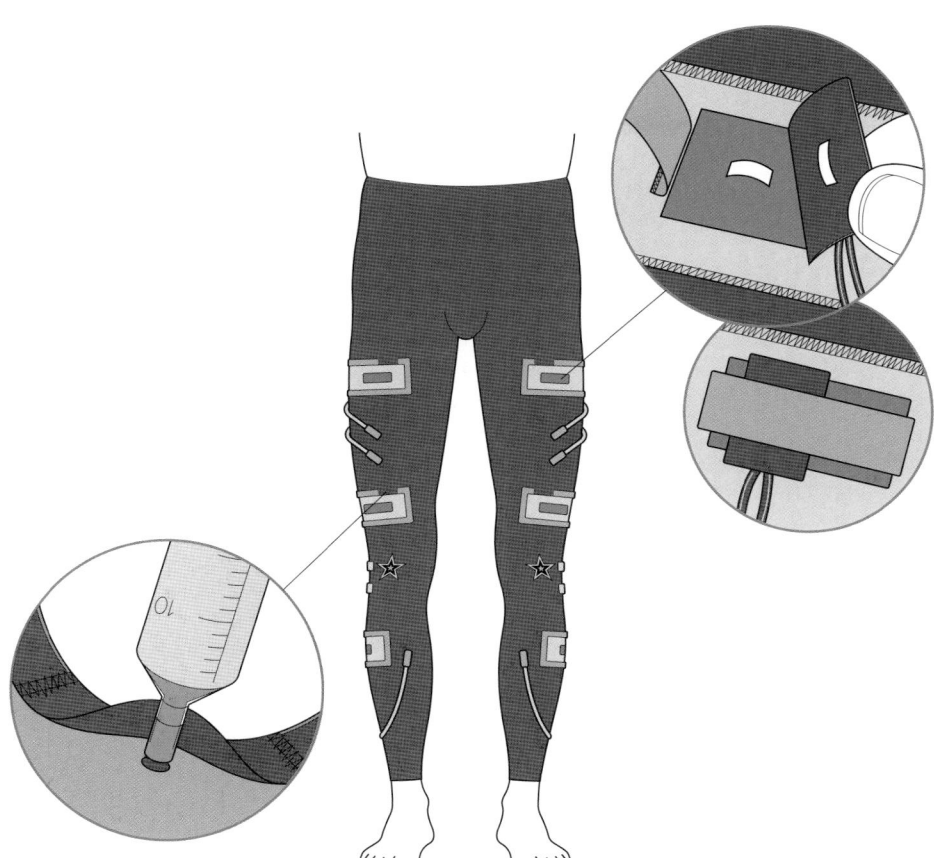

Figure 22-5 Example of a custom-made electrode garment manufactured by Bioflex, Inc. Electrodes are made of stretch materials, and conductive gel is inserted into the pocket on the side of the electrode. Velcro connectors are arranged to allow connection of all anteriorly and posteriorly placed electrodes to stimulators while the patient is seated.

repeatability and reproducibility of the muscle responses over time, dependence of contractile responses over time, dependence of contractile responses on muscle length and joint angle, and electrode system economics.[243]

Surface electrodes remain the most commonly utilized electrode type for most FES therapeutic and functional interventions. The force of muscle contractions induced with surface electrodes is influenced by electrode size and alignment. Longitudinal placement of electrodes produces as much as a 64% increase in the maximal tolerable torque when compared with a transverse placement.[136] Larger surface electrodes result in a more forceful muscle contraction and cause less discomfort than smaller surface electrodes.[136]

Electrical stimulation protocols that require multiple surface electrodes are often impractical if long-term FES utilization is anticipated. In an effort to improve the practicality of surface stimulation, a number of electrode garments have been developed (Fig. 22-5). These garments are particularly useful for FES cycle ergometry and for standing and gait protocols, in that they decrease preparation time for FES, increase patient independence, and provide more consistent electrode placement.

Patient discomfort associated with surface stimulation and the lack of precision achieved with surface stimulation are, at least in part, overcome with implanted electrode systems. Epimysial, intramuscular, and nerve cuff electrodes are the most common examples of implanted electrodes presently utilized.

A number of material science issues need to be resolved to be able to design neuromuscular stimulation electrodes that minimize tissue injury while maintaining electrode reliability. For example, failure rates of percutaneously inserted intramuscular electrodes have apparently been reduced from an early failure rate of 20% to a subsequent failure rate of approximately 1% per year.[255] However, percutaneous intramuscular electrodes resulted in local tissue injury when the voltage output that created the maximum contraction was utilized. This problem can be somewhat circumvented by inserting electrodes into multiple motor points of a muscle, with subsequent sequential or simultaneous stimulation at a lower voltage. This decreases the problems with fatigue and presumably tissue injury.[140]

Cuff electrodes, which are placed around peripheral nerves that innervate several muscles, offer the opportunity to activate numerous muscles through a single electrode, thereby diminishing the extent of required hardware. Snug-fitting cuff electrodes are available that can improve selectivity by stimulating portions of a peripheral nerve.[194] Endoscopic implantation techniques have been explored for cuff electrodes that overcome the lack of precision of surface and percutaneous electrodes while avoiding the need for surgical exposure of target nerves.[182] Problems with electrode movement continue to cause variability of the input–output properties of nerve cuff stimulating electrodes.[88] Implanting nerve cuff electrodes also results in the loss of axons during the first several weeks, but follow-up studies document considerable regeneration.[137] Stimulation techniques such as decreasing the duration of stimulation, stimulating at lower rates (20 Hz versus 50 Hz), and using a shorter duty cycle require ongoing development to minimize neural damage from cuff electrodes.[1]

THERAPEUTIC NEUROMUSCULAR ELECTRICAL STIMULATION FOR MUSCLE STRENGTHENING

Stimulation of normal muscle

Although electrical stimulation therapy has been shown to be effective in improving muscle force,[37] there are no data to suggest that the use of neuromuscular electrical stimulation (NMES) in a normal healthy human results in substantial improvement in muscle strength compared with that achieved by voluntary isometric exercise. Multiple studies comparing the efficacy of NMES with isometric voluntary contraction of the quadriceps have shown that similar gains in isometric muscle strength occur with both exercise regimens.[51,52,92,133,135,141] NMES can improve the endurance of muscle in sedentary humans trained with stimulation rates of 8 Hz, but the benefit did not exceed the endurance noted in normal active adults.[248] The lack of additional benefit from NMES in combination with voluntary contraction for strengthening probably reflects the fact that, with maximal voluntary contraction, nearly 100% of the recruitable motor units are activated. Consequently, the additional stimulation provided by NMES is unable to recruit additional motor units to result in further increments in force.

A systematic review of randomized clinical trials of NMES of the quadriceps identified 35 trials examining both unimpaired quadriceps and individuals postinjury or postoperatively.[16] NMES was compared with no exercise and with volitional (active) exercise and, based on the available evidence, NMES was shown to be effective for both impaired and non-impaired quadriceps training. However, NMES was only shown to be preferred over voluntary exercise for within cast training or in situations where subject adherence might be insufficient.

Despite the fact that NMES and voluntary exercise result in comparable increases in isometric strength, these two training regimens differ. With voluntary training, type 1 fibers are activated first, followed by the progressive recruitment of type 2 fibers with increasing force. In contrast, the NMES protocols lead to an activation of type 2 fibers to a greater extent than of type 1 fibers. As maximal force depends on type 2 fiber activation, selected augmentation of the type 2 muscle fibers by NMES might lead to greater increases in the overall strength of the muscle at submaximal training intensity. This hypothesis has been supported by data showing that voluntary exercise groups train at higher muscle contraction intensity (78–119% of initial maximal voluntary isometric contraction [MVIT]) than NMES groups do (33–68% of MVIT) to achieve an equivalent degree of strengthening.[52] In one study of isometric strength training in elderly men, these higher workloads resulted in increases in heart rate during the training sessions. Subjects

randomized to NMES, in contrast, had similar gains in strength without a change in cardiovascular work.[38] NMES strengthening might offer specific advantages in training over voluntary contraction in certain populations of individuals who have cardiovascular disease or other limitations that preclude training at higher workloads.

Studies of NMES or voluntary isometric contraction of the adductor pollicis of the non-dominant hand have shown the importance of understanding the unique contractile properties of the specific muscle involved in the training regimen. Both NMES and voluntary training result in increases in muscle force, although the observed increase in response to NMES was significantly smaller. With voluntary training, a greater increase was seen in tetanic force of contraction, speed of contraction, and speed of relaxation in comparison with NMES. Training with NMES, however, had no effect on mechanical twitch tension and resulted in no reduction in fatigue. Finally, voluntary training resulted in faster kinetics of contraction, whereas no improvements were noted with NMES. The authors concluded that, in small muscles such as the adductor pollicis,[59] all or nearly all motor units were recruited during voluntary contractions, but not during electrical stimulation. Thus the number of trained motor units was different with the two training regimens. In this specific muscle group, voluntary contraction using activation of synaptic ionic current with excitation–contraction coupling was more efficient in stimulating the smaller motor neurons with the higher input resistance that were present in the hand. In contrast, electrical stimulation affected changes in peripheral processes beyond the membrane ionic mechanisms of the muscle excitation–contraction coupling, recruiting larger cells with lower external input, which reflected a smaller population of the motor units within the hand muscle. Based on these data, it is clearly important to understand the motor unit composition of the muscle in order to determine the most appropriate therapeutic intervention and response.

Neuromuscular electrical stimulation might also have a therapeutic application in augmenting strengthening at skeletal regions in which attainment of maximal volitional contraction is difficult to achieve. NMES at both high (2000 Hz) and moderate (50 Hz) frequencies has been shown to increase maximal isometric force of the triceps surae.[37] NMES with voluntary contraction can also result in significantly higher gains in abdominal strength and endurance when compared with NMES or voluntary exercise alone.[6] Finally, biphasic NMES of the back muscles has been shown to improve isokinetic strength to a degree that is equal to voluntary exercise, with the added benefit of enhanced endurance.[122]

Not only has NMES been shown to increase muscle strength, it has also been shown to improve functional performance. NMES applied to the quadriceps femoris muscle bilaterally has been shown to improve performance on force measurements from a squat machine, the 25-yard dash time, and vertical jump.[263] Another benefit of NMES in normal muscle is in the prevention of the muscle atrophy associated with prolonged immobilization. Individuals undergoing knee immobilization following ligament reconstruction surgery experience significant muscle atrophy, as demonstrated by decreases in strength, endurance, muscle mass, and oxidative capacity.[136] Early intervention with NMES of the quadriceps femoris (Fig. 22-6) results in improved preservation of quadriceps muscle strength, muscle mass,[167] and succinate dehydrogenase activity,[136] as well as in higher isokinetic peak torque values.[96,259] In a study using NMES protocols (30 Hz, 300 μs) for isometric quadriceps contraction for a 10-min session repeated four times per day, three times per week, together with voluntary quadriceps contraction, versus exercise alone, the combination of NMES plus voluntary exercise resulted in a significant reduction in muscle wasting, a reduction in the loss of isometric torque, and preservation of oxidative enzyme activity as defined by the levels of citrate synthase and triphosphate dehydrogenase during the period of immobilization (Table 22-3).[259]

The benefit of NMES appears to be limited to the period of immobilization. In one prospective study of NMES after knee

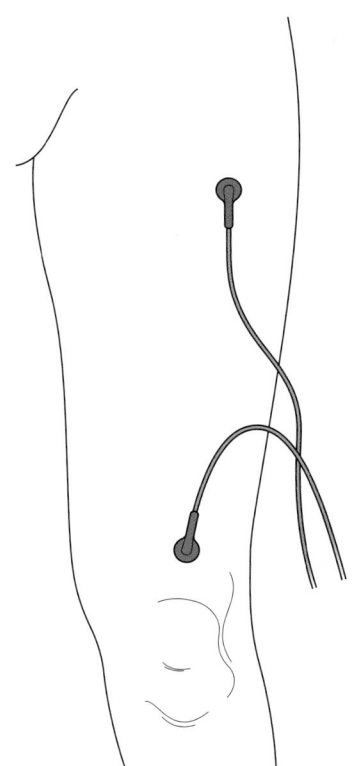

Figure 22-6 Electrode placement for isometric quadriceps femoris strengthening. The active electrode is placed proximally and the indifferent electrode is placed both laterally and distally to stimulate the vastus lateralis muscle. The lateral position is used to avoid stimulation of the rectus femoris, which if stimulated would cause knee extension and hip flexion.

immobilization, although losses of thigh girth and maximal voluntary contraction during immobilization were significantly smaller with the use of NMES, by 12 weeks post surgery (6 weeks after discontinuation of immobilization), no significant differences were seen in maximal voluntary isokinetic torque or thigh girth between patients randomized to the non-exercise control or NMES group.[55] This suggests that NMES could be of greatest benefit in the treatment of elite athletes or other individuals who desire a rapid return to maximal performance levels. It might be of little or no benefit in individuals who can afford the delay in return to peak physical activity until after the period of immobilization and reconditioning is complete.

Neuromuscular electrical stimulation (30 Hz per 18% duty cycle for 1 h per day), using surface electrodes on the quadriceps femoris, prevents the development of disuse muscle atrophy in individuals immobilized with a long leg cast for a tibial fracture. This preservation of muscle mass was associated with maintenance of muscle protein synthesis and rate of muscle protein synthesis per unit of muscle RNA (Fig. 22-7).[79] NMES of the calf muscles (7 Hz for 30 min twice a day) in patients hospitalized in the intensive care unit for postoperative ventilatory failure or cerebral infarctions decreased urinary 3-methylhistidine and creatinine excretion, reflecting a slowing of negative nitrogen balance and improved preservation of muscle mass, in contrast to non-stimulated control subjects.[24]

Recent interest has been focused on a potential role of NMES in enhancing glucose transport activity in skeletal muscle independent of insulin. In response to acute NMES, the glucose disposal rate is acutely increased and remains elevated for more than 90 min after stimulation has been discontinued. This suggests that involuntary muscle contraction can lead to enhancement of energy and glucose utilization. Thus NMES may have a future role in enhancing glucose uptake in patients with peripheral insulin resistance.[106]

One final application of NMES in normal muscle is to help in evaluating the etiology of weakness in a patient. Under conditions of normal volitional central control, a decrease occurs in electrical stimulation-induced contraction response with increasing voluntary muscle contraction at different levels (Fig. 22-8a).[221] Thus, if a subject is volitionally attempting to maximally contract muscle, leading to an optimal pattern of recruitment of all the motor units, direct electrical stimulation of the muscle will not lead to a further increment in muscle force. If, however, the subject is not maximally trying (or if other forces

Group	Isometric torque	Cross-sectional area	Citrate synthesis activity	Triphosphate dehydrogenase activity
Electrical stimulation	−39.2	−22.9	−5.8[a]	−10.1[a]
Control	−57.8	−25.9	−29.4	−16.8

Table 22-3 Effects of neuromuscular electrical stimulation on the quadriceps femoris during immobilization (% change)

[a]$P < 0.05$, electrical stimulation versus control.

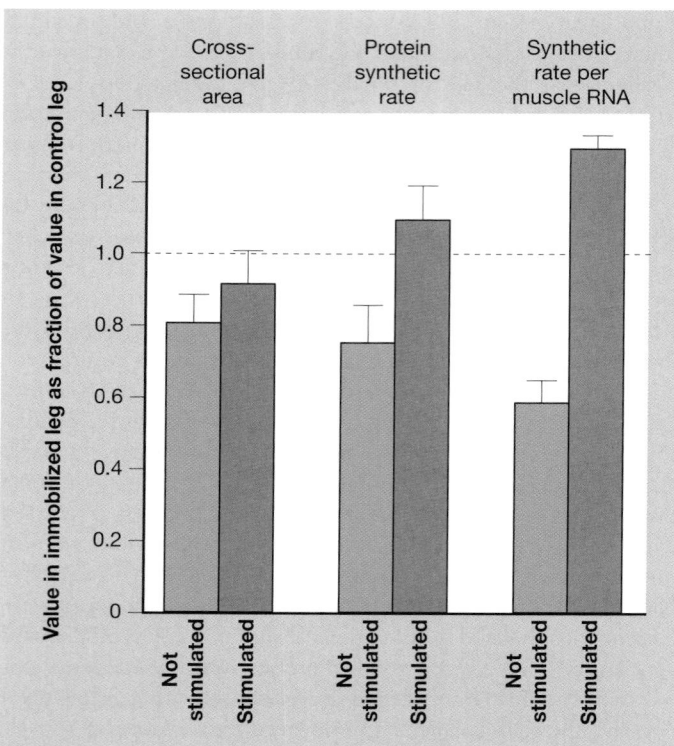

Figure 22-7 Effect of 6 weeks of electrical stimulation of the cast-immobilized quadriceps femoris muscle on muscle protein synthesis and quadriceps cross-sectional area in comparison with the same parameters in immobilized control subjects. (From Gibson et al. 1988,[79] with permission.)

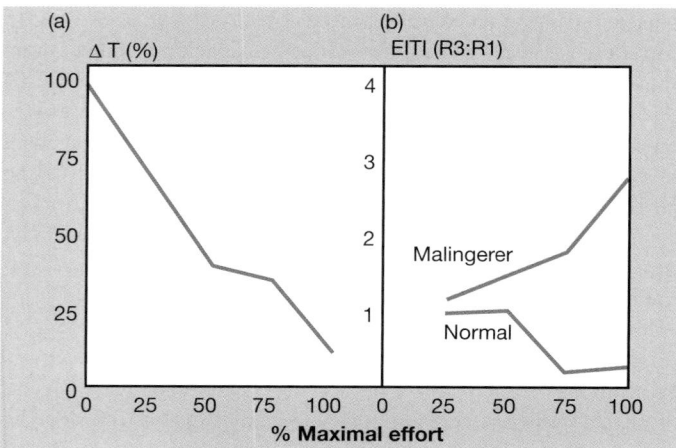

Figure 22-8 Effect of central and peripheral factors in fatigue elicited by electrical stimulation with voluntary contraction of the quadriceps femoris. (**a**) The dependence of the amplitude of electrically stimulated torque increments (T) on the percent of maximal voluntary contraction. (**b**) The utility of measuring the ratio of the electrically induced torque increments (EITI) in the third to the first trial (R3:R1) to detect malingerers. The amplitude of force at 100% maximal voluntary force drops on successive trials in normal control subjects due to fatigue, but the target torque is dramatically different in the malingerer. (Data from Latash et al. 1994,[139] with permission.)

contribute to a drop in volitional muscle force), electrical stimulation will lead to an increase in muscle force. This is best seen as a striking difference in the ratio of the electrically induced torque increment (EITI) in the fourth to first stimulation in response to increases in voluntary contraction in normal control subjects versus malingerers (Fig. 22-8b). The decrease in the fourth to first EITI ratio in normal subjects at 75% and 100% voluntary contraction reflects the effect of the development of peripheral fatigue at near-maximal contractions, which subsequently results in a reduced responsiveness of the motor unit to electrical stimulation.[52]

Stimulation of myopathic muscle

There remains considerable controversy regarding the benefit of electrical stimulation in preservation of motor function in individuals with neuromuscular disease. Previous studies have suggested that aggressive physical exercise might result in overwork weakness and a loss of physical function.[119,250] In dystrophic animal models, low-frequency electrical stimulation has been shown to improve muscle function, delay degeneration of muscle fibers, and increase the quantity of oxidative enzymes.[53,149,219,252] In the genetically dystrophic chicken, NMES applied early after hatching delayed the onset of righting disability, gradually increased muscle mass, increased dystrophic protein by 29%, and increased circulating creatine phospho-

kinase levels. Surprisingly, however, electrical stimulation in this model resulted in a discernible shift toward a glycolytic metabolism, which is the opposite of the effect seen with NMES in normal muscle.[112]

When low-frequency electrical stimulation is applied to dystrophic muscle in children with muscular dystrophy, improvements occur in maximal voluntary contraction of the stimulated muscle[161,233,234,265] and in torque, with no increase in fatigue.[265] If, however, electrical stimulation is initiated after significant strength has already been lost, there appears to be no benefit from electrical stimulation treatment. After discontinuation of NMES, strength gains are lost rapidly.[161] It appears that if NMES is to be used for strengthening in neuromuscular disease, it is of benefit only in individuals who have retained more than 15% of normal strength, and that the benefit is likely to be short-lived, resulting in only a delay of the inevitable outcome.

Stimulation of denervated muscle

The therapeutic relevance of NMES in a denervated muscle model is predicated on the ability of the technique to prevent or reduce atrophy and the ability of the technique to enhance reinnervation. Denervated muscle appears to have some plasticity, as NMES has been shown to facilitate the transformation from fast- to slow-twitch (or slow- to fast-twitch) fiber. This result has been associated with improved maintenance of muscle fiber area[81,184] and muscle girth[91,178] for a short time interval until reinnervation sets in. NMES, however, has no benefit in maintaining certain isometric contractile properties that are associated with prolongation of the action potential, including the twitch to peak time and twitch half-relaxation time.[45]

The data are mixed on the effect of initiating NMES late after denervation injury. If the electrical stimulation is initiated immediately at the time of injury, the acceleration of the half-life of the slow-degrading acetylcholine receptor can be prevented.[7] If started after the acetylcholine receptor has begun to destabilize, NMES cannot reverse the switch to a faster degrading receptor, nor can it slow the degradation of the rapid acetylcholine receptor. These data suggest that maximal maintenance of normal motor unit characteristics in a short-term stimulation program depends on very early initiation of stimulation.

In contrast, NMES using an unusually long duration (200 μs), bidirectional, rectangular impulse at a frequency of 25 Hz, begun 28 days after denervation, has been shown to preserve muscle fiber diameter and to induce a hybrid fiber type having properties of both slow- and fast-twitch muscle.[165] The authors of the study postulated that the relatively dramatic results of this late application of NMES might be due in part to the long impulse duration used in the stimulation protocol. This is consistent with data from a previous study comparing 8 Hz/1 ms with 1 Hz/7 ms stimulation regimens in the denervated rabbit fast-twitch muscle, which found that only the lower frequency stimulation pattern reduced atrophy.[177] The overall consensus of several studies on the dose–response of tetanic stimulation in prevention of muscle atrophy is that stimulation durations ranging from 5 to 45 μs are beneficial, with no utility of shorter duration impulses.[256] Although the application of NMES for muscle denervated for 4–10 months did cause some improvement in muscle tension, the resultant upper end of tension noted in the studies was only 10% of normal values.[4]

The data supporting the efficacy of NMES in human studies are less clear than noted in an animal model. For example, in humans, low-frequency NMES started within 7 weeks of injury and continued for more than 35 weeks resulted in no benefit over the long term as measured by clinical muscle force testing, dynamometry, muscle mass measurement (by computed tomography or ultrasound), or maximal amplitude or frequency of denervation activity.[23] In contrast, galvanic stimulation (30 stimulations three times per day) has been reported to maintain hand muscle bulk.[119] In other studies, the initiation of NMES in a chronic denervation state has been shown to increase both muscle mass and cross-sectional area toward normal after months of training.[228] The discrepancies among these studies, other data in the literature, and the animal models could reflect differences in stimulation parameters and muscle characteristics. Additional research is needed to resolve the conflicting recommendations as to the optimal stimulation parameters. Parameters that have been shown to be most effective to date for NMES in denervation are high voltage and short duration, or long duration and low voltage, both of which can be clinically impractical due to discomfort.[102]

There are no data to support that NMES of denervated muscle speeds the process of reinnervation.[224] In fact, a number of studies have suggested that stimulation inhibits terminal sprouting and reinnervation.[61] The discrepancies in the literature concerning the impact of NMES to effect sprouting has been due in part to methodology. Recent studies demonstrate that, in acute injuries, NMES (20 Hz, 8 h) reduced motor unit enlargement and sprouting, primarily in extensively denervated muscle where less than 20% of motor units were intact. It also appears that NMES may be more detrimental to smaller and slower motor units than to larger motor units.[246] The mechanism for this is unclear, and appears to contradict experiments that show an increase in the tropic factor neurotrophin-4 after electrical stimulation.[74] Despite this observed increase in neurotrophin-4 that has been shown in other models to promote axonal sprouting, studies have consistently shown that reinnervation is at least partially suppressed by NMES.[61]

Ultimately, the decision to use any therapeutic intervention should depend on evidence of an improved outcome. Such a benefit has been shown in an animal study comparing outcomes after nerve repair in a group receiving NMES and a second group that did not receive NMES. Both the morphology and the functional capacity of the muscle were improved in the NMES-treated group.[260] Hence, in a denervated muscle, long-term NMES might be effective in improving functional outcome by preventing atrophy when reinnervation is expected over a long period of time, such as after a surgical nerve repair or in a partial injury with greater than 20% of the motor units surviving. In chronic denervation states where NMES is unlikely to benefit reinnervation, it may still offer the prospect of improved cosmetic appearance and reduced risk of pressure sores.

Stimulation of decentralized muscle

Electrical stimulation of muscle following central nervous system injury or SCI can result in reversal of the muscular atrophy seen in association with the relative immobilization associated with these disorders. Although applications of NMES after cerebral vascular accident have, in general, been limited to use of NMES as an orthotic assist rather than as a therapeutic adjunct to strengthening, NMES has been used successfully in the small superficial muscles of the hand and wrist to improve strength and decrease atrophy.[185] Recommendations for electrical stimulation in the hand muscles suggest that strength is maintained at greater than 80% of initial value over an 8-month period at a 1:5 duty cycle, with decreases in dorsiflexion force output as duty cycle is equalized to 50%. Modification of electrical stimulation parameters to meet the fatigability of the muscles undergoing training is necessary, especially in situations in which spasticity and severe weakness can limit therapeutic gain.

Much more attention has been paid to the use of NMES as a modality for rehabilitation of paralyzed muscle following SCI. Following SCI, type 1 and type 2a fibers, myofibrillar ATPase, succinate dehydrogenase activity, and the capillary to fiber ratio are reduced in comparison with what is seen in normal control muscles.[40] In addition, loss of muscle bulk, a decrease in fiber cross-sectional area, a reduction in torque, a significant slowing of contractile speed, and increased fatigability have been noted.[220] Electrical stimulation (20 Hz for 15% of a duty cycle) of the tibialis anterior in individuals with chronic SCI resulted in an increase in the proportion of type 1 fibers from 14% ± 8%

to 25% ± 10% (although the final level was well below that of control muscles), but had no effect on the distribution of fiber sizes or mean fiber area.[155]

Biochemical changes can also occur after NMES training. Hydroxyproline content and a tissue inhibitor of metalloproteinase 1 both increase twofold over baseline levels after NMES, and are fourfold higher than seen in able-bodied control subjects.[130] In light of the lack of evidence of increased type 4 collagen with NMES training, these data suggest that NMES is associated with accelerated type 4 collagen turnover as a part of an adaptive process of the paralyzed muscle to reinstitution of muscle contraction.

Neuromuscular electrical stimulation enhances the oxidative capacity of the muscle as defined by an increase in succinate dehydrogenase activity. In response to NMES, there is a rapid rise in hexokinase, lactate dehydrogenase, citrate synthase, and 3-hydroxyacyl-coenzyme A dehydrogenase consistent with improved glycolytic and mitochondrial oxidation capacity.[126] The elevation in these enzymes persists even after NMES has been stopped, and improvements in V_{O_2} return to baseline. There are also significant increases in the expression and protein content of GLUT-1 and GLUT-4[42] with improved insulin-stimulated 3-O-methyl-1-glucose transport.[164] These changes suggest enhanced insulin sensitivity[42] in the skeletal muscle.

These histologic and biochemical responses to NMES are similar to those seen with the application of low-frequency electrical stimulation to normal muscle. Muscle strength and contractile properties also showed a positive response to NMES. Daily NMES increased endurance of the muscle to levels found in able-bodied control subjects, with a slowing of the time course of contraction and half-relaxation.[208,224] These data suggest substantial increases in fatigue resistance from characteristics of a fast-twitch, fatigable muscle (type 2b) to a fast-twitch fatigue-resistant type (type 2a). In contrast, there is also an increased speed of relaxation and altered force–frequency relationships following training that may be due to adaptations in calcium-handling processes.[78]

Despite these improvements in fatigue, there was no marked change in muscle force with a stimulation pattern. This is consistent with the reciprocal relationship between strength and endurance in normal motor units.[86] Other studies of NMES in SCI have shown that increases in force are achieved with stimulation when the stimulated muscle contracts against resistance.[86]

Although NMES-induced muscle contraction has been shown to increase certain contractile and histochemical properties of decentralized muscle, actual increases in muscle strength and endurance are most dramatically seen when NMES is combined with resistance training or functional activities. Since the mid 1980s, isometric quadriceps strengthening using NMES to move the knee through a 45° arc with increasing resistance has resulted in increases in quadriceps endurance and mass. The development of a FES hybrid cycle ergometry system (FES-CE) (Fig. 22-9) has resulted in further therapeutic benefits. The

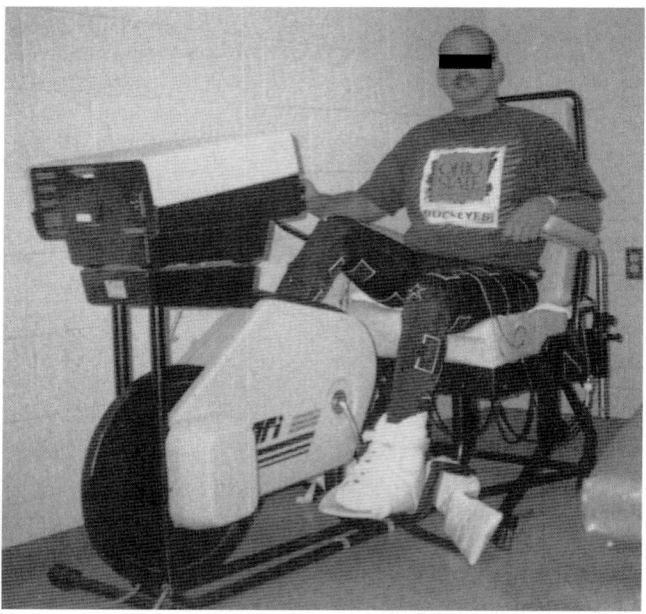

Figure 22-9 Functional electrical stimulation cycle ergometer by Therapeutic Technologies, Inc. Cycling is produced with sequential stimulation of the quadriceps femoris, hamstring, and gluteal muscles, using surface electrodes.

system uses a rectangular, monophasic waveform of 30 Hz, 0–130 mA, at 375-μs duration, to sequentially stimulate the quadriceps, hamstrings, and gluteal muscles to produce a smooth pedaling motion of a Monark lower extremity cycle ergometer. This closed loop system is set to maintain a cycling rate of 35–50 rpm, with automatic shutoff if the impedance is greater than 16 000 Ω, if the voltage exceeds 220, or if the pedaling rate is less than 35 rpm (suggesting fatigue). Using FES cycle ergometry, several investigators have shown increases in thigh circumference,[191,192,213] muscle strength and endurance,[206] quadriceps muscle area (by computed tomography),[186] and quadriceps muscle protein synthesis rates (from 0.071% to 0.0985% per hour), with no change in whole body protein turnover.[186] Changes in contractile properties include a decrease in the initial slope of quadriceps twitch, which is assumed to be compatible with a disproportionate increase in the function of slow-twitch fibers.[206]

Not only can FES result in changes in localized muscle mass, it can also affect overall body composition. Following SCI, lean body mass decreases and fat mass increases. Short-term, low-intensity NMES has suggested only modest gains in lean body mass (+1.9%).[164] However, data from our laboratory have shown that individuals with chronic SCI who were randomized to an FES-CE protocol showed gains in total body lean body mass of 7.9%, with a decrease in percent body fat of 12.1%. These gains in lean body mass were primarily attributed to gains in the lower extremity lean body mass, which increased 9.7% over baseline. FES-CE is also a promising intervention to prevent the losses in lean body mass associated with acute SCI.

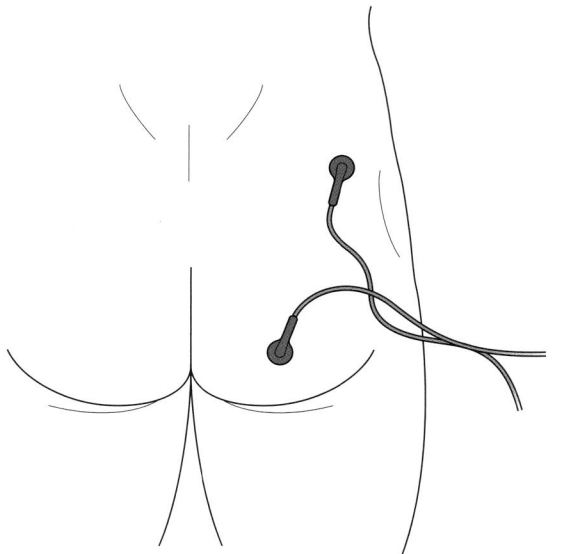

Figure 22-10 Hip extension is produced with placement of the active electrode on the gluteus maximus below the posterior superior iliac crest, and the indifferent electrode is placed inferiorly on the muscle.

Initiation of FES-CE within 3 months of acute SCI has been shown to prevent lower limb muscle atrophy after 3 months of training, and to cause muscle hypertrophy after 6 months of training.[13]

Finally, the use of NMES to stimulate muscle contraction and maintain muscle mass might be applicable to the prevention of pressure sores. In an animal model, chronic stimulation at 10 Hz for 8 h per day resulted in an increase in capillarization in as little as 7 days.[64,94] NMES (50 Hz for 33% of the duty cycle) resulted in an increase in blood flow under the ischial tuberosity of humans. During electrical stimulation in untrained SCI subjects, this change was not statistically significant. Because significant benefits were noted in able-bodied subjects, the authors postulated that fatigue might have contributed to a reduction in the increment of blood flow in the SCI subjects, and that training might improve the hemodynamic benefit. NMES has also been shown to increase resting arterial inflow and to result in a greater hyperemic response to experimental occlusion ischemia. This latter response is postulated to be due to greater endothelium-released vasodilator (nitric oxide)–altered arterial compliance and/or skeletal muscle neovascularization.[174] In addition, NMES (50 Hz) of the gluteus maximus (Fig. 22-10) in able-bodied subjects can produce appreciable changes in seating interface pressure distribution, and result in substantial shape changes of the buttocks at stimulation levels producing only a small fraction of maximum voluntary contraction.[144] The buttock shape obtained during stimulation more nearly resembles the shape of the suspended buttocks, implying a reduction in tissue distortion. If similar results could be obtained in an SCI population, NMES could have a potential application as a form of 'pressure release' to decrease the incidence of pressure sores.

ELECTRICAL STIMULATION TO PREVENT COMPLICATIONS OF DISUSE

Following a neurologic insult, a person is predisposed to a number of complications that arise over the long term due to the resultant decrease in physical activity. This is especially true in patients with SCI. With the loss of voluntary bipedal locomotion, individuals with SCI are at greater risk for cardiovascular disease, osteoporosis, pressure ulcers, and thromboembolic disease. In addition, changes in self-image can have a major influence on well-being. In an attempt to reduce these disuse-associated medical conditions, physicians have turned to NMES techniques.

Cardiovascular deconditioning

During the past few decades, with improvement in bladder and skin management, cardiovascular disease has become the primary cause of death in individuals with SCI. A body of evidence shows that SCI is associated with a decrease in cardiopulmonary performance.[204] Within the first 3 months of SCI, a significant decline occurs in aerobic capacity, with declines in maximal oxygen consumption (V_{O_2max}) of more than 40%.[66] After discharge from rehabilitation, the workload of a paraplegic individual performing independent activities of daily living is only 24% of the maximal work capacity, which is insufficient to maintain cardiovascular fitness.[108] This cardiovascular deconditioning is even more pronounced in quadriplegic persons, for whom data show a decrease in maximum heart rate, stroke volume, and cardiac output,[183] and the development of left ventricular atrophy.[173] Studies of V_{O_2max} in persons with chronic SCI reveal an inverse relationship to the level of SCI.[109]

Cardiovascular deconditioning, however, is not an inevitable consequence of SCI. Wheelchair athletes have been shown to have significantly higher V_{O_2max}, cardiac output, and stroke volume than sedentary individuals with SCI.[181,266] In addition, their lipid levels are nearly the same as those of able-bodied individuals, with the exception of a lower HDL_3 level.[27] Arm crank ergometry has been proposed as a means to improve cardiovascular training, but it is inefficient, because recruitment of small muscle mass during exercise results in a V_{O_2} level that is 15–35% lower than that which can be obtained with lower extremity exercises.[49,67,215] For quadriplegic individuals, arm crank ergometry can be impractical because of upper limb weakness. Attention has therefore turned toward the therapeutic use of NMES as an intervention to improve cardiovascular fitness. Chronic use of arm crank ergometry might also accelerate the deterioration of the shoulder joints seen in chronic SCI.

A consensus has existed since the initial studies in the late 1980s that short-term training with FES-CE can produce an increase in both endurance and V_{O_2max} when stress testing is performed with the lower limb cycle ergometer.[173,202] There is a significant widening of the mixed (arteriovenous) O_2 difference during NMES that implies increased O_2 extraction from the blood.[110] Increases in minute ventilation are observed with

NMES and have been postulated to be due to enhanced aerobic metabolism in respiratory muscles.[18] FES-CE can also result in reversal of the adaptive left ventricular atrophy seen in quadriplegic persons, with near normalization of left ventricular mass to able-bodied individuals.[173]

Lower limb training, however, has not been shown to translate to a cardiovascular improvement when exercise testing is done via arm crank ergometry stress testing.[109] This is consistent with data in able-bodied individuals that indicate that a training effect is specific to the muscle groups trained.[43]

During an acute bout of FES-CE, a relative increase occurs in VO_2, pulmonary ventilation, heart rate, and stroke volume, with greater increases noted in paraplegic versus quadriplegic persons. The increase in VO_2 is thought to be due to augmented blood flow to the exercised muscles. Work by Petrofsky and Stacy has shown that the respiratory efficiency of FES cycling is only 3.6% (3.6% of the energy of cycling is converted to energy to move the pedals),[193] which is substantially lower than the value of 20–30% for lower limb ergometry in able-bodied individuals. Despite the low respiratory efficiency, however, prolonged training with FES-CE does result in increases in blood pressure, heart rate, cardiac output, and VO_{2max} that are linear with the metabolic demand on the muscle. The increase in blood pressure during NMES has been used for clinical purposes. Portable NMES units have been used as an intervention for the orthostatic hypotension associated with SCI.[247]

In an attempt to increase the efficiency of cardiovascular training, studies have combined arm crank ergometry with lower extremity FES. Training with these hybrid systems has shown improved increments in VO_2, minute ventilation, cardiac output, and stroke volume in comparison with arm crank ergometers or FES-CE alone.[138,203] New approaches include the combination of FES quadriceps extension against 20 lbs of resistance with arm crank ergometry at 50 rpm,[63] FES-CE with voluntary arm crank ergometry,[134] or FES rowing.[138]

Increased cardiovascular risk associated with SCI could also be associated with the development of significant insulin resistance and glucose intolerance, and might be amenable to intervention with NMES. Although local increases in GLUT-1 and GLUT-4[42] suggest improved insulin sensitivity, 1-year lower extremity NMES resulted in no improvement in glucose tolerance or insulin response to an oral glucose load.[106] The increase in insulin sensitivity noted was ascribed to increased muscle mass, conversion to aerobic fibers, and improved GLUT-4. Further studies are required to determine if these modest improvements in local insulin sensitivity will substantially change cardiovascular risk.

In summary, advances in FES have resulted in the development of several systems that can increase muscle mass, reduce venous pooling, increase stroke volume and cardiac output, and improve cardiorespiratory fitness.[90] Additional long-term data analyzing the efficacy of various FES techniques and treatment protocols are necessary to determine whether the short-term improvements in cardiorespiratory fitness can be maintained over long periods of time, and whether they will have a substantial influence on cardiovascular morbidity and mortality.[90]

Osteoporosis

One prominent metabolic consequence of SCI is an acute disruption of normal calcium balance, which contributes to a rapidly evolving osteopenia that is a permanent consequence of the injury. The severe osteopenia results in an increased risk of fractures, and as many as 9% of all SCI patients present with one or more fractures within the first 10 years after injury.[214] Cross-sectional studies of regional bone mass changes have documented that bone mass loss is not uniform below the level of neurologic injury, but that the magnitude of loss is determined, at least in part, by the degree of reduction in biomechanical loading.[19] One of the mechanisms thought to contribute to this profound bone loss is the loss of muscle contraction and mechanical loading in the patient with SCI. Based on Wolff's law, which states that the form and structure of bone are organized to optimally resist perceived loads from functional demands, attention has been focused on the therapeutic use of NMES to reduce immobilization, increase biomechanical strain, and potentially improve bone mass at localized skeletal regions.

High-frequency, low-amplitude, short-duration muscle contraction that can generate 500-ue compressive loading in hind limb–suspended rats results in significantly higher bone mass in the stimulated limb, with enhanced new bone in the tibial diaphysis.[160] However, the bone mass was still less than that for control rats, suggesting that the disuse osteopenia was not completely prevented. It has therefore been hypothesized that the static load used is less effective than dynamic load at increasing bone mineral density.

In an attempt to increase the compressive load, contralateral limb NMES against an isokinetic load has been examined. Over 24 weeks, in subjects with SCI, this NMES protocol has been shown to increase distal femur and proximal tibia bone mineral density by 30% relative to control subjects, but there was no difference between sides within the subject at any level.[17]

Functional electrical stimulation cycle ergometry has also been employed as an intervention that could generate significant intermittent force across regions of the skeleton where bone loss was greatest after SCI. Initial studies by Leeds et al.[143] and Pacy and colleagues[186] showed no benefit of FES-CE on bone mass at the proximal femur or lumbar spine in individuals with SCI of long duration. More recent work has supported a positive effect of FES on bone mass. One group demonstrated a 0.2–3.3% reduction in tibial bone loss in a group of chronic SCI subjects training with FES-CE.[93] Data from our laboratory suggest that FES-CE can produce small increments in bone mass in patients with chronic SCI, but these benefits are localized to the two skeletal regions (proximal tibia and distal femur) receiving the greatest mechanical strain with the exercise regimen.[22] In addition, as seen in able-bodied individuals, these increments in bone mass are dependent on achieving a sufficient workload, with gains limited to individuals who were able to cycle at workloads of 18 W or greater.

Because interventions aimed at preventing bone loss have been more effective than reversing lost bone mass for most models of osteoporosis, investigators have also examined the efficacy of FES-CE in early SCI, when bone loss is rapid. Data from our laboratory suggest that early intervention (within 4–6 weeks post injury) with FES-CE significantly slows rates of bone loss and decreases hypercalciuria.[172] However, when FES was discontinued, bone loss recurred. Not all studies confirm a benefit, however: tibial diaphyseal cortical bone mass, as assessed by computed tomography, showed no evidence of reduced rates of loss over 6 months.[68] Longer duration studies with continued use of FES-CE will help to define whether NMES is a practical and an effective means of preventing osteopenia and of reducing the incidence of fractures.

Deep venous thrombosis

Another complication associated with the relative immobilization seen after a neurologic insult is an increase in the risk of thromboembolic disease. Following a cerebrovascular accident, there is a 23–75% incidence of deep venous thrombosis (DVT) and a 10% incidence of pulmonary emboli during the first 6 months. The role of reduced muscle activity is suggested by data that show that the DVT is most commonly localized to the paretic limb (5- to 10-fold increase). The incidence of DVT is even greater following SCI, with a reported incidence between 47% and 100% in the first year post SCI. Thromboembolic disease accounts for 37.5% of acute deaths in this population. Because some individuals have contraindications to subcutaneous heparin prophylaxis (e.g. blood in the central nervous system), there has been some exploration of the use of NMES to reduce the incidence of thromboembolic disease. NMES (10 Hz, 50-μs pulse for a 33% duty cycle) of the tibialis anterior and gastrocnemius–soleus muscle groups for 23 h per day over a 28-day period in combination with low-dose heparin in patients with acute SCI showed a significant decrease in the incidence of DVT in comparison with a group receiving low-dose heparin alone.[158] This result might be due in part to the effects of NMES in increasing plasma fibrinolytic activity.[124] Promising results from FES were also seen in a stroke population, in which FES compared favorably with adjusted dose heparin and intermittent pneumatic compression in preventing DVT.[187]

Psychologic effects

A number of psychosocial problems have been reported in patients following SCI, including mood disorders, and diminished social and vocational functioning. It has been proposed that exercise might result in some psychologic benefits, such as improved self-esteem. Utilizing FES-CE, 62% of paraplegic and 56% of quadriplegic patients reported improved self-image with participation.[238] Other benefits included increased self-esteem,[91,238] well-being,[12] and independence,[95] and diminished depression.[5] Not all changes, however, are positive: some subjects also report decreased motivation, and increased anger and tension. Expectations played an important role in resultant negativity, with individuals with unrealistic expectations (e.g. anticipation of improved neurologic function) showing the fewest psychologic benefits.[26] The positive feelings noted with FES-CE can have a physiologic explanation, as regular exercise with FES-CE has been shown to significantly increase beta-endorphin levels.[235]

THERAPEUTIC FUNCTIONAL ELECTRICAL STIMULATION

Urinary incontinence

Urinary incontinence is a significant public health problem that carries an economic burden estimated at $10 billion per year.[39] Although Kegel introduced exercises for the management of urinary incontinence in the late 1940s and early 1950s, the primary method of intervention has remained surgical intervention.[31] The conservative management of urinary incontinence is, however, considered to be the wave of the future.[31]

Caldwell was the first to report positive results after implantation of an electrical stimulation system for the correction of urinary incontinence in 1963 (reviewed in Jonasson et al.[120]). A subsequent study treated women with both stress and motor urge incontinence with intravaginal electrodes. After 12 weeks of stimulation, 20 min daily, a markedly diminished leakage of urine was noted in 35% of women with stress incontinence and in 65% of women with motor urge urinary incontinence.[120] Another study combined pelvic floor exercises with intravaginal maximal electrical stimulation. After 6 weeks of stimulation for 15 min daily, 89% of women with stress urge incontinence, 73% with motor instability, and 70% with mixed incontinence demonstrated improvement. Long-term follow-up demonstrated that 80% of women maintained the improvement.[39] Subsequent studies suggested cure rates of 30–50% and improvement rates of 67–90% for stress incontinence with FES.[264]

The mechanism for this therapeutic response is believed to be secondary to the fact that incontinence might represent a denervation injury; that is, the observed improvements could be due to the muscle-strengthening properties of electrical stimulation.[31] The validity of this hypothesis is questioned in view of the fact that many humans do not tolerate stimulation intensities sufficiently high to directly stimulate motor nerves. Therefore it is suggested that pelvic floor afferents with reflex connections to the muscle are stimulated.[72]

The stimulation systems for the management of bladder incontinence include electrodes implanted into pelvic floor muscles and external electrodes that are primarily intraanal or intravaginal.[264] The intravaginal electrodes appear to be the most commonly utilized technique. Both anal and vaginal external electrodes are recommended because of safety and ease of use. Stimulation programs typically utilize biphasic pulsed waveforms. Less than 10-Hz stimulation is optimal for bladder inhibition, whereas stimulation rates approaching 50 Hz are recommended for optimal urethral closure. Mixed stress and urge incontinence protocols utilize stimulation rates of 20 Hz.[72] Pulse duration and amplitude are adjusted to the maximal tolerable level. However, controversy continues as to the relative benefit of chronic (long-term, continuous) stimulation versus short-term stimulation.[264]

In summary, data clearly suggest that the electrical stimulation of pelvic floor muscles is an important adjunct to the conservative management of stress and motor urge urinary continence. It has been suggested that this technique is primarily suited as an adjunct to therapy for individuals who are not able to voluntarily stop urine flow and who cannot contract the pelvic floor muscles.[31]

Electrical stimulation has also been utilized extensively for the restoration of bladder function after SCI. Sphincter stimulation with an anal plug stimulator for 30 min twice daily did not improve cystometric findings in one study, and most patients in this study did not wish to continue utilizing this technique.[118] Similarly, pudendal nerve stimulation via the penis or clitoris for 20 min, five times per week for 4 weeks, did not improve bladder capacity or incontinence.[210] However, stimulation of the pudendal nerve at twice the bulbocavernosus threshold has been shown to increase bladder capacity.[209]

Implanted electrodes have been applied to the bladder wall, pelvic splanchnic nerves, conus medullaris, mixed sacral nerves, sacral anterior roots, and sacral spinal cord.[159] Electrodes implanted into the bladder have been largely abandoned due to unacceptable complication rates. The greatest attention has been directed toward stimulation of the sacral anterior roots. The procedure is, however, complicated by the reflex activation of sphincters. A number of techniques have been explored to reduce the subsequent outflow obstruction, such as pudendal neurectomy, external sphincterotomy, and the development of stimulation parameters that sufficiently maintain the peak contraction of the sphincter and bladder out of phase to produce micturition between bursts.[48] Posterior root rhizotomy has been advocated in conjunction with sacral anterior root stimulation as a means of abolishing uninhibited reflex bladder contractions, thereby increasing bladder capacity, restoring bladder compliance to normal, and abolishing reflex contraction of the sphincter.[48,123] The disadvantages of the posterior root rhizotomy include the loss of reflex erection and reflex ejaculation. The combination of these techniques is useful in that they decrease residual urine volume, improve bladder compliance, improve urinary incontinence, and decrease reflux and hydronephrosis. Additional benefits of these two interventions are restoration of full erections sufficient for coitus in 60% of patients and production of defecation with the stimulator alone in 50% of patients.[48]

Numerous other techniques have been explored to improve bladder continence using electrical stimulation technology, with results that are intriguing. These techniques include stimulation of the thigh muscles 20 min daily for 14 days, with a resulting improvement in the bladder capacity of patients with detrusor hyperreflexia or instability.[180] Additionally, neurovascularly intact gracilis muscle transposition to the proximal urethra, with subsequent stimulation of the transposed muscle using intramuscular electrodes and a subcutaneously placed pulse generator, has resulted in a decrease in urinary incontinence.[41]

The advances in FES applications to mimic bladder function have now resulted in a commercially available implantable system. Thus the major challenge in achieving effective micturition regardless of the site or stimulation technique remains the selection of parasympathetic fibers supplying the detrusor

muscle with simultaneous relaxation of the external sphincter and pelvic floor muscles.[159] Continued refinement of electrode placement and stimulation techniques are needed to improve patient continence, micturition, and satisfaction.

Ejaculatory failure

Ejaculatory failure is noted in approximately 95% of SCI survivors. Semen retrieval, however, is possible with subcutaneous physostigmine, vas aspiration, vibratory stimulation, and electrostimulation by rectal probe.[116] Ejaculation via rectal probe stimulation is apparently accomplished with either sinusoidal or pulsed waveforms utilizing a variety of stimulation parameters.[190,235] This technique does not adversely affect sperm motility.[229] One other study documented that, in a group of 25 survivors of SCI, electroejaculation resulted in bidirectional emission in 12 patients, antegrade in 9, retrograde in 1, and failure in 3.[254] Sperm quality or quantity did not correlate with SCI level, age at injury, or patient age. Ejaculation via electrostimulation appears to be well tolerated and safe, with minimal autonomic dysreflexia and mild rectal mucosal changes.[254]

Management of spasticity

Electrical stimulation has been used therapeutically for the management of spasticity since Duchenne's first use of it in 1871. Since then, electrical stimulation for the management of spasticity has been administered by epidural, implanted, subcutaneous, and surface stimulation. Most of the available information regarding the efficacy of this modality is based on observations noted during the application of electrical stimulation for functional purposes. Few studies have attempted to systematically evaluate the therapeutic efficacy of this modality in spasticity. Short-term effects of surface electrical stimulation utilizing an intensity of 100 mA, a duration of 0.5 ms, a stimulation frequency of 20 Hz, and a compensated monophasic waveform, with a duty cycle ratio of 1:1 for 20 min in 12 SCI survivors, resulted in a significant improvement in the pendulum drop test. This improvement did not persist past 24 h.[221]

In contrast, application of an 8-week electrical stimulation protocol in which subjects with SCI received 20 min of electrical stimulation twice a day, 6 days per week, demonstrated a tendency toward increasing spasticity with long-term surface electrical stimulation.[222] However, a 3-month program of FES decreased spasticity and improved both gait patterns and velocity (determined by gait analysis) in a subject with familial spastic paraplegia.[188]

Observations noted in hemiplegic individuals have been more consistently favorable for the benefits of FES in the management of spasticity. One study, for example, observed a group of hemiplegic patients receiving surface stimulation via an implanted peroneal stimulator for 12 months. The stimulation parameters were described as a pulse width of 0.5 ms and a stimulation frequency of 30–33 Hz. This group noted a significant decrease in passive resistance and tonic reflex activity. These changes were thought to result in improved voluntary control in agonist and antagonist muscle groups.[242] A second study applied electrical stimulation to wrist extensors of hemiplegic individuals with flexor spasticity. Their stimulation program involved training individuals for three 30-min periods per day, 7 days per week, with stimulation parameters described as square wave pulses at 33 Hz, a pulse width of 200 μs, and a pulse amplitude of 100 mA. The stimulation cycle was described as 7 s on followed by a 10-s rest interval. This group also demonstrated a decrease in flexor spasticity, a decrease in the contractures noted in persons with chronic hemiplegia, and a prevention of flexion contractures noted in 'subacute' hemiplegic individuals.[11]

More recent applications of FES in the management of spasticity have documented benefit when FES is used in conjunction with botulinum toxin.[103,104] One randomized, double-blind, placebo-controlled trial used FES three times, one-half hour each, for 3 days after injection, in a group of stroke survivors. Follow-up at 2, 6, and 12 weeks evaluated tone and arm function. The use of FES appeared to enhance the response to the botulinum toxin injections.[103]

In summary, these data clearly indicate that electrical stimulation results in a short-term decrease in spasticity that can persist for several hours after a treatment session. There also appears to be evidence to suggest that both short-term treatment in conjunction with botulinum toxin and long-term treatment decrease spasticity in hemiplegic individuals. However, the data are less clear regarding the impact of long-term stimulation on survivors of SCI. More information is needed to determine whether the type and completeness of the lesion affect the observed responses from long-term FES intervention.

Upper limb in hemiplegia

The most common application of electrical stimulation in the upper limb of hemiplegia is in the treatment and prevention of shoulder subluxation. Electrical stimulation is thought to be a superior option, because it does not restrict the use of the limb as physical supports do. One study demonstrated that electrical stimulation could reduce existing subluxation. The study protocol involved stimulating the supraspinatus and posterior deltoid muscles (Fig. 22-11) with an asymmetric biphasic waveform over a 6-week period.[10] The results indicated that electrical stimulation was superior to slings and wheelchair arm supports in reducing subluxation, but this apparently had no impact on reduction of shoulder pain. A subsequent controlled study evaluated the efficacy of electrical stimulation in a group of recent hemiplegic stroke patients. The goal was to evaluate the efficacy of electrical stimulation in the prevention of glenohumeral joint stretching and subsequent subluxation, and to facilitate recovery of the flaccid shoulder. The protocol also involved placing the active electrode over the posterior deltoid, and the passive electrode over the supraspinatus muscles. Stimulation frequency was set at 33 Hz, and the intensity was adjusted to elicit the desired response. The duty cycle varied throughout the duration of the study. Patients were treated for 1.5–6 h per day over a 6-week period. The results suggested that FES resulted in improvement in arm muscle tone and function, decreased shoulder subluxation, and a more rapid

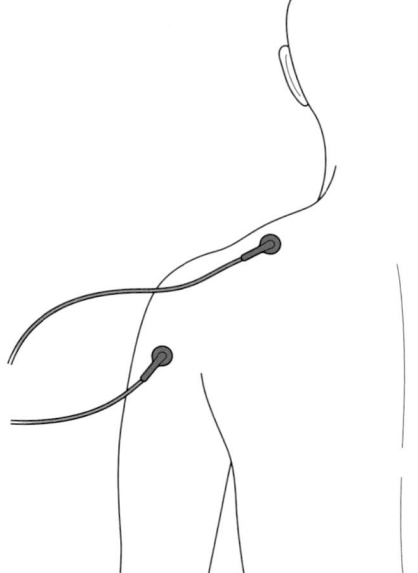

Figure 22-11 Use of electrical stimulation for treatment of shoulder subluxation involves placement of electrodes over the supraspinatus and posterior deltoid muscles.

recovery of arm function.[70] This observation was supported by a metaanalysis of randomized controlled trials of FES in stroke. These pooled data supported FES as promoting recovery of muscle strength after stroke.[82]

Another recent review of electrical stimulation for the prevention and treatment of poststroke shoulder pain concluded that there is no evidence that NMES can influence poststroke shoulder pain.[211] However, this review also concluded that NMES improved passive humeral range of motion but the impact of this range of motion on quality of life was uncertain. Additional work is needed to distinguish the effect of different types of stimulation on pain, range of motion, and subluxation.

It has also been demonstrated that electrical stimulation can improve functional use of a chronically hemiplegic upper limb (more than 6 months after cerebrovascular accident) by combining electrical stimulation techniques with voluntary effort. One of the earliest studies that demonstrated this outcome assigned subjects to four groups that received electromyographically (EMG) induced electrical stimulation of wrist extensors, low-intensity electrical stimulation of wrist extensors combined with voluntary contractions, proprioceptive neuromuscular facilitation exercises, or no treatment. The EMG-initiated electrical stimulation protocol (0.2-ms biphasic square wave, pulse at 30–90 Hz, and a constant current of 20–60 μV) utilized low-level voluntary EMG activity in target muscles to trigger electrical stimulation of forearm wrist extensor muscles to produce a joint movement. The group with low-intensity electrical stimulation of wrist extensors with combined voluntary contractions received 30 min of stimulation to the wrist extensors with a 0.3-ms square wave pulse at 30–90 Hz. The stimulation intensity was adjusted to increase voluntary range of wrist extension. The subjects were told to perform voluntary wrist extension exercises during the stimulations. The results of this study are compelling in that the electrical stimulation appeared to improve the function of chronically hemiparetic upper limbs, with subjects who received the EMG-induced electrical stimulation of wrist extensors demonstrating the greatest improvement. In addition, these gains were retained for 9 months.[131]

Phrenic nerve stimulation

Modern phrenic nerve stimulation dates to 1948.[179] Since that time, the technique has proved to be a valuable adjunct in the care of the patient with chronic ventilatory insufficiency and who has a normal phrenic nerve, diaphragm, and lungs. Specifically, this technique is useful in persons with high-level quadriplegia accompanied by respiratory paralysis and central hypoventilation syndromes.[179] It has been estimated that, nationally, 100 SCI survivors would annually meet the criteria for use of a phrenic nerve pacer.[179] The goal of this technique is to circumvent the need for mechanical ventilation. One series demonstrated that 40% of all quadriplegic patients who received the device were supported full time by the phrenic nerve pacers.

Initial protocols involved pacing a single phrenic nerve with high-frequency stimulation (25–30 Hz) at a respiratory rate of 12–17 per minute. Problems with this approach included loss of efficiency secondary to paradoxical motion of the contralateral unpaced side, and myopathic changes noted in animal diaphragms subjected to the same stimulation program.[83] In 1981, protocols evolved that utilized uninterrupted simultaneous pacing of both hemidiaphragms using low-frequency stimulation (7–8 Hz) and a respiratory rate of 5–9 per minute. This approach improved minute volumes and resulted in better air mixing.[83] In addition, it is speculated that the low-frequency stimulation converts the normal mixture of fast-twitch and slow-twitch fibers to a preponderance of fatigue-resistant type 1 fibers.[83] This speculation is supported in part by the fact that endurance and respiratory function improve slowly after initiation of phrenic nerve pacing.

Several battery-powered implanted systems exist, which differ in electrode systems and waveforms.[47] Benefits from phrenic pacing include decreased infections, the ability to speak and smell more normally, and reduced cost and time for ventilation care.[47]

THERAPEUTIC FES AS AN ORTHOTIC DEVICE

Scoliosis

The importance of bracing in the prevention of scoliosis curve progression was documented in the 1970s and 1980s. During the same period, studies were initiated that examined the efficacy of FES in the management of scoliosis. The technique involved placement of electrodes along the convex portion of the curve above and below the apex. Stimulation parameters typically approximate a stimulation rate of 35 Hz, a pulse width of 200 μs, and a pulse amplitude of 0–100 mA. In addition, the stimulation was modulated to deliver 5 s of stimulation

followed by 25 s of rest. The advantage of this technique is that the electrical stimulation was performed for only 8–10 h per night.[73]

Although the technique was typically well tolerated with few complications, the efficacy of the technique remains unclear. Some studies have documented that electrostimulation was equal in efficacy to a Milwaukee brace in the treatment of adolescents with mild curves (20–40°).[73] However, other studies documented failure rates with electrostimulation that approximated the rates of progression noted in studies examining the natural history of this disorder.[61] Moreover, patients whose curves progressed with electrostimulation then underwent bracing, with a subsequent halting of the progression of the scoliosis.[60,73]

Therefore the data examining the efficacy of electrical stimulation in the management of idiopathic scoliosis are inconclusive. Although some data indicate that electrostimulation is as effective as a Milwaukee brace in halting the progression of the disease, other data imply that electrical stimulation does not alter the natural course of the disorder.[61,73] A metaanalysis of the efficacy of non-operative treatments for idiopathic scoliosis suggested that lateral electrical surface stimulation is equal in outcome to observation only.[223] Therefore the role for electrical stimulation in the management of idiopathic scoliosis is at best limited to use in a patient who is unable to tolerate appropriate bracing.

Hemiplegic gait and foot drop

Electrical stimulation has been utilized as a neural orthosis since 1961.[145] Since that time, NMES has been an important adjunct in the rehabilitation of patients with hemiplegia. Primarily, this has involved utilizing NMES to improve the gait pattern of hemiplegic patients by increasing the torque output of the ankle dorsiflexors and reciprocally decreasing spastic reflexes in the plantar flexors (Fig. 22-12).[56]

The development of NMES systems has gone through a number of evolutionary changes, from single and multichannel surface electrode systems to completely implanted systems.[150] A limited number of patients are suitable for surface stimulation due to problems tolerating the sensation of stimulation intensity needed to achieve dorsiflexion. Problems with electrode placement have also prompted the development of implanted systems. Several implanted systems are now commercially available, but they have not yet restored gait function adequately to gain widespread utilization.

FUNCTIONAL NEUROMUSCULAR STIMULATION: CLINICAL APPLICATIONS

Standing and gait

Since the 1970s, FES for gait restoration after SCI has progressed from feasibility studies to the development of a commercially available, US Food and Drug Administration (FDA)-approved ambulation system.[132,237] Despite the considerable progress, a number of barriers remain that continue to render this a cumbersome clinical application of technology. In

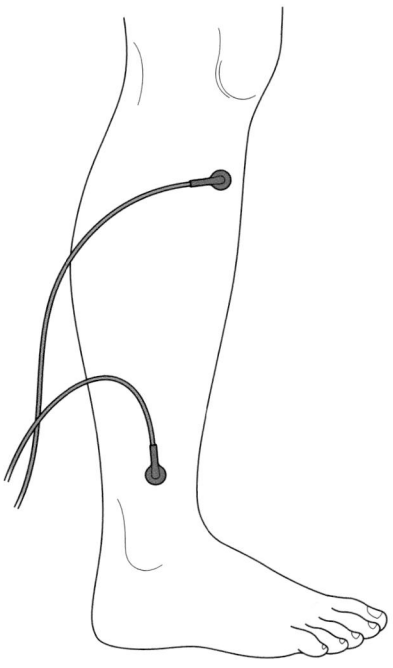

Figure 22-12 Ankle dorsiflexion is produced with placement of the active electrode proximally over the anterior tibialis and peroneal muscle groups, and placement of the indifferent electrode distally over the tendons of the peroneal muscle.

addition to requiring a user-friendly system, the ideal FES gait system should be safe (in that it does not cause additional injury, such as degenerative joint changes), reliable, sufficiently functional to provide community ambulation, and both inexpensive and cosmetically acceptable. Many of these goals have not yet been realized.

The typical components of the FES system include a power source plus cables, a control mechanism, display and ground, stimulator with cables, and electrodes.[205] Additionally, FES systems require a feedback mechanism. In open loop systems, the feedback is controlled by the patient or therapist in response to observations. More sophisticated, closed loop systems automatically incorporate feedback into the FES system. This permits the FES system to adjust to changes in muscle spasticity and fatigue. In addition, closed loop systems probably improve endurance by keeping the stimulation intensity to the minimum necessary to accomplish a given functional task. Finally, closed loop systems require less concentration on the part of the ambulator. Types of FES feedback system include input from external sensors, EMG of muscle, sensory nerve, or motor areas of the brain.[153] The most common and practical sensors are externally mounted devices that feed back information regarding limb position and movement.

There are now several major categories of FES system for ambulation: surface stimulation (Fig. 22-13), implanted electrodes attached to an external stimulator, and implanted electrodes attached to an internal generator.[20] The number of channels in FES ambulation systems varies according to the sophistication of the system. Two-channel systems typically stimulate the knee extensors, while four-channel systems typically activate knee extensors and hip flexors.[105,237] FES ambulation systems employing more than eight channels often require

implanted electrodes to provide more precise stimulation and to avoid the stimulation of adjacent muscles.

A survivor of a thoracic level SCI presently has three options for pursuing the ability to walk: utilizing a mechanical orthosis (reciprocal gait orthosis, long leg brace, etc.), an FES gait system, or a hybrid system that utilizes a mechanical orthosis with the assistance of FES. Ambulation with a mechanical orthosis alone is impractical, in part because the energy consumption is three to nine times that needed in normal control subjects.[44] However, FES gait systems also consume considerable energy, as it has been estimated that these patients utilize 59–75% of their maximum aerobic power.[152] It appears that the energy consumption of some FES systems rival, if not exceed, that required for walking with a mechanical orthosis.

Functional electrical stimulation ambulation systems are also somewhat impractical, because they permit only a limited range of activity. The typical standing time for these systems ranges from minutes to hours.[132] The speed of ambulation is slow, typically in the range of 0.1–0.4 m/s.[127] Finally, the walking distance with these devices is limited to approximately 20 m, although distances of more than 1000 m have been reported.[132,154]

The fatigue associated with FES ambulation is attributed to several factors. First, considerable energy is expended in stimulating the muscles necessary to maintain a standing position.[152] The rapid onset of FES-induced muscle fatigue is also in part caused by the preferential recruitment of rapidly fatiguing, type 2 muscle fibers.[148] In an effort to minimize this fatigue, several stimulation techniques have been developed. First, stimulation intensities are limited to the minimum necessary to achieve a desired functional response. Second, stimulation rates are kept within the physiologic ranges of 15–50 Hz.[159] Specifically, lower stimulation rates are desirable, presumably because of the greater likelihood of stimulating slow-twitch, fatigue-resistant muscle fibers.[41] The third approach to diminishing muscle fatigue involves an electrode distribution that permits the stimulation of portions of muscles or muscle groups. In this electrode distribution, muscle fatigue is diminished by sequentially activating portions of an individual muscle or muscle group, thereby producing the minimum necessary force to accomplish a functional task.[107,194]

Because the technology does not yet exist for FES to produce truly functional community ambulation, most FES systems are hybrid systems that concomitantly utilize FES with a mechanical orthosis. This combination of devices offers several advantages. First, the mechanical orthosis permits standing without considerable energy expenditure.[132] Hybrid systems also appear to use less energy than either mechanical orthoses or FES ambulation systems. One study specifically compared the energy consumption during ambulation with a reciprocating gait orthosis (RGO), RGO and FES, FES alone, long leg braces, and a hip-guided orthosis. The order of energy expenditure (from lowest to highest) was RGO with FES to the thigh muscles, hip-guided orthosis, long leg brace, and FES systems. The addition of FES to the RGO decreased energy consumption by approximately 16% in one study but increased energy

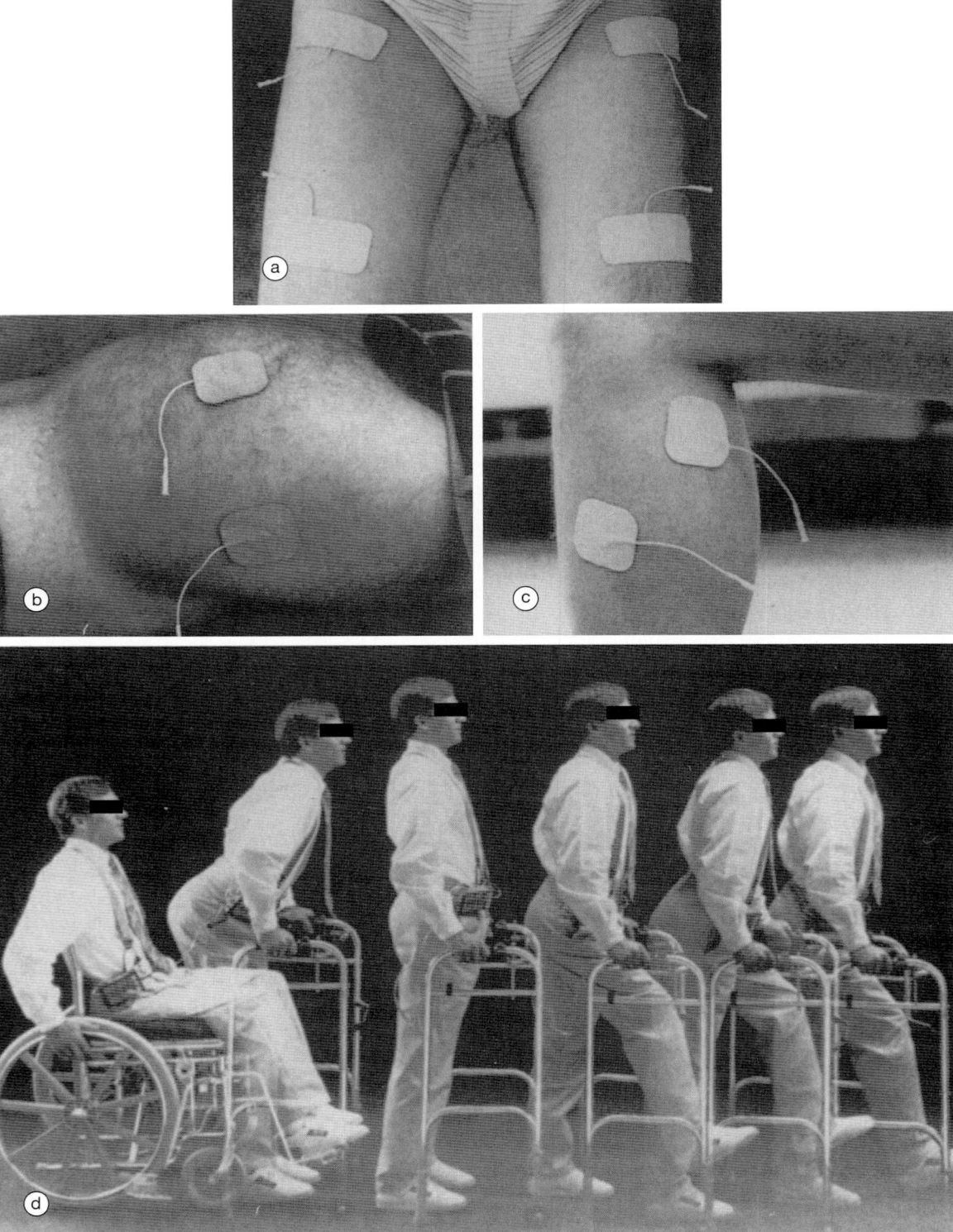

Figure 22-13 Parastep system developed by Sigmedics, Inc. These systems use surface electrodes. Both four- and six-channel systems exist that assist spinal cord injury individuals to stand and ambulate with use of a walker. Electrodes are placed over the quadriceps (**a**), peroneal nerve behind the fibula head and tibialis anterior (**c**), and gluteus medius and maximus (**b**; six-channel system only) to allow for standing and walking (**d**).

consumption in another study.[105,244] Finally, hybrid systems increase the speed of ambulation.[168,176] The addition of FES to an RGO increases the optimum speed of ambulation from 1.2 km/h with the RGO to 2.4 km/h with the hybrid system.[176] However, studies have also shown that RGO use at home is low, and that the addition of electrical stimulation does not increase RGO use.[245]

Advances in FES gait systems have extended to the commercial availability of an FDA-approved ambulation system.[237] However, the technology is still not capable of resolving or compensating for issues such as FES-induced muscle fatigue, excessive energy expenditure associated with FES ambulation, reduced FES-induced joint torques, autonomic hyperreflexia, osteoporosis, modified reflex activity, and spasticity.[154] Because FES ambulation systems to date are unable to meet many of the criteria for a truly functional system, the patients who might benefit from existing FES ambulation systems are relatively few. One study estimated that approximately 10% of patients admitted to an SCI service are candidates for an FES gait restoration program. Only half of those, or 5% of survivors in the cohort, eventually learned to walk, but fewer than 3% of those patients ultimately utilized the FES ambulation system functionally within their home.

The therapeutic benefit of FES in gait might extend beyond simply functioning as an orthotic device. The combination of FES with locomotion training in motor-incomplete SCI subjects has been shown to increase walking speed. This gain in speed is retained when the FES is temporarily not utilized. This observed therapeutic benefit suggests a potential role for FES in facilitating neural plasticity.[14]

Restoration of upper limb function

The traditional option for survivors of a high cervical SCI with loss of hand function has included functional restoration via orthotic devices or surgical procedures, such as arthrodesis and tendon transfers. The goal of FES in this population is to provide palmar and lateral prehension grasp, and to develop a means to easily change from one type of grasp to the other.[189]

A number of FES-based neural prostheses have been developed for the upper limb. Each of these systems is suited for individuals with specific impairments, therefore detailed knowledge of the upper limb's residual function is required to match the device to the individual for maximal functional benefit. Examples of available systems include the Bionic Glove, which uses a position sensor at the wrist to detect flexion and extension; this then is used to trigger the appropriate hand muscle groups.[207] Other systems, such as the Handmaster NMS-1 and Belgrade Grasping System, require switches to control the device.[207]

However, the NeuroControl Freehand System is the first implantable commercially available system for the upper limb. This system is intended for patients with C5 and C6 level SCI who have good shoulder and elbow function.[189,207] Functional activities of daily living skills achieved through this implanted system have included handling eating utensils, cups, writing instruments, books, and the telephone. More complex tasks,

such as pouring, washing, brushing teeth, and handling computer diskettes, have been demonstrated.[189] Operative procedures such as arthrodesis tenodesis and tendon transfer are available to minimize joint movement and to improve upper limb stability for FES utilization.[189]

Both the reliability of this particular implanted system and its patient satisfaction ratings have been high.[54] As the stimulation of multiple muscle groups across several segments is quite complex, the availability of multiple implanted systems appropriate for a variety of neurologic impairments is limited.

ELECTRICAL STIMULATION FOR THE TREATMENT OF SOFT AND HARD TISSUE INJURY

Wound healing

A body of scientific evidence has been accumulating to suggest that electrical stimulation can be used to promote the healing of wounds. Investigators have previously demonstrated that the surface of human skin is electronegative with respect to the inner layers. Wounded skin demonstrates the existence of a natural bioelectric current, with the ionic body fluids allowing for transmission of electricity between outer and inner layers. When electrical stimulation is applied to a wound, a number of biologic processes in the wound are modified that might lead to enhanced healing. Electrical stimulation increases the number and function of fibroblasts,[50,76] collagen, protein, and DNA synthesis,[15] and causes changes in expression of cellular receptors for transforming growth factor-β,[71] enhancing calcium uptake and neurite growth. The fibroblasts and epithelial cells move along the path of the voltage gradient (the galvanotaxic effect)[46,262] toward the cathode. Electrical stimulation has also been shown to increase the relative number of neutrophilic granulocytes while suppressing the number of mast cells.[257] This suppression of mast cells has been postulated to result in improved wound healing with a decrease in fibrotic scarring, and thus better cosmetic results. It appears that electrical stimulation can augment the endogenous chemical factors that initiate the inflammatory stage of healing. Evidence also indicates that electrical stimulation has bacteriostatic and bactericidal properties.[117] The duration of exposure and voltage shows a linear relationship with inhibition of growth of several common wound pathogens when negative polarity is used.[125]

Electrical stimulation can also improve blood flow.[117] The improved vascularity has been associated with decreased lipid peroxidation and prevention of damage to oxygen-derived free radicals. High-voltage pulsed current, however, has also been shown to have a bimodal effect on foot blood flow in humans at risk for diabetic ulcers. One study found that 27% of subjects increased transcutaneous oxygen, whereas 73% of subjects showed a decrease in transcutaneous oxygen. The mechanism for this bimodal response is not understood.[80]

Several studies published since the mid 1960s[251] have demonstrated the effectiveness of electrical stimulation to promote the healing of dermal ulcers (Table 22-4). The initial studies were non-randomized, prospective trials undertaken to

Table 22-4 Effect of electrical stimulation on wound healing

Type of trial Non-randomized	Type of ulcer	Unilateral ulcer		Bilateral ulcers (% healed)	
		No. participating	% healing	Electrical stimulation	Control
	Chronic[249]	75	13.4	27	5
	Ischemic	150	20.0	28.3	8.3
	Ischemic[75]	106	28.4	30	14.7
	Elderly	223	89.7	—	—

Randomized	Type	No.	Electrical stimulation			Control		
			% Δ ulcer size	% healed	Time to heal (days)	% Δ ulcer size	% healed	Time to heal (days)
	Pressure	8	—	100	50.1	+13.8	—	74
	Pressure[123]	16	−38[a]	100	50	+28.9	—	52
	Mixed[237]	17	—	88.9	51.2	—	37.5	77
	Pressure[86]	17	−80	—	—	−52	—	—
	Diabetic[145]	64	−61	42	84	−41	15	84

[a]Improvement in ulcer size after crossover of ulcers from sham treatment to electrical stimulation.

determine the safety and efficacy of electrical stimulation in the treatment of chronic dermal ulcers. The use of electrical stimulation to treat pressure ulcers or ischemic ulcers in a variety of patient populations showed a significant increase in ulcer healing. When patients entered into a study were found to have more than one ulcer, several trials utilized those patients to randomize one ulcer to treatment with electrical stimulation and the other to a non-electrical stimulation control group. In these substudies, significant improvements were noted in the rate of ulcer size reduction and number of healed ulcers in the ulcers receiving electrical stimulation in comparison with control ulcers. Recognizing the need for randomized trials, several studies have subsequently been published comparing electrical stimulation with sham-treated ulcers. In general, these studies have shown increased rates and percentages of healing with electrical stimulation in comparison with control populations (see Table 22-4), with no significant complications. Recent studies have focused on the use of pulsed galvanic electrical stimulation, with demonstration of similar benefits.[77]

The more effective stimulation pattern is pulsed electrical stimulation, because it allows for higher current density without tissue irritation or burning. Asymmetric biphasic waveforms have been shown to be more effective in healing diabetic ulcers than symmetric biphasic or square wave pulses are.[9] Recent studies have used alternating polarities, beginning with a negative polarity; the alternating polarity protocol is thought to have antibacterial effects and is associated with increased vascular support. When no further improvements in wound healing are noted (*plateauing*), polarity is changed. The absolute charge

density needed to cause successful wound healing is in the order of 0.1–2.0 coulombs/cm², [217] and the duration of treatment sessions can vary from 1 to 24 h per day

A recent metaanalysis of controlled clinical trials was performed to examine the effect of electrical stimulation on wound and bone healing.[2] Because of significant methodological shortcomings with most of the reported trials, the selected pool of trials did not constitute acceptable proof of benefit, yet there was a consistency of positive response noted. In summary, the data suggest that electrical stimulation might augment wound healing, and the efficacy appears to be generalizable to ischemic ulcers and pressure ulcers as well as to other types of deep wound.

SUMMARY

Electrical stimulation is a historical physiatric modality, but an explosion of new interest in this subject has occurred since the mid 1970s. In addition to rehabilitation medicine, a renewed interest in electrical stimulation has been demonstrated in various fields, such as physiology, molecular biology, engineering, neurosurgery, neurology, orthopedics, urology, and plastic surgery. The result has been a significant improvement in the technology available for functional applications. A far greater understanding has also developed of the physiologic basis for the improvements noted with therapeutic applications of electrical stimulation.

The importance of electrical stimulation as a modality in rehabilitation medicine continues to grow. There are, for example, increasing numbers of commercially available FES systems available to treat primarily paralysis-related conditions. However, their utilization remains modest, as the functional benefit of FES is apparently not sufficient to overcome the burden or complexity of these systems. Toward this end, continued advancements in technology, a better understanding of optimal stimulation parameters, and a better understanding of the physiologic changes induced by this technology are required if electrical stimulation is to achieve its potential as a therapeutic modality and neural prosthesis.

REFERENCES

1. Agnew WF, McCreery BB, Yuen TGH, et al. Histologic and physiologic evaluation of electrically stimulated peripheral nerve: considerations for the selection of parameters. Ann Biomed Eng 1993; 17:39–60.
2. Akai M, Hayashi K. Effect of electrical stimulation on musculoskeletal systems: a meta-analysis of controlled clinical trials. Bioelectromagnetics 2002; 23:132–143.
3. al-Amood WS, Buller AJ, Pope R. Long-term stimulation of cat fast-twitch skeletal muscle. Nature 1973; 244:225–227.
4. al-Amood WS, Lewis DN, Schmalbruch H. Effects of chronic electrical stimulation on contractile properties of long-term denervated rat skeletal muscle. J Physiol 1991; 441:243–256.
5. Alexander CJ, Sipski ML. Electrical stimulation bicycle ergometry with spinal cord injured patients: potential medical and physiological benefits. SCI Psychosoc Proc 1990; 3:18–20.
6. Alon G, McCombe SA, Koutsantonis S, et al. Comparison of the effects of electrical stimulation and exercise on abdominal musculature. J Orthop Sports Phys Ther 1987; 8:567–573.
7. Andreose JS, Xu R, Lomo T, et al. Degradation of two AChR populations at rat neuromuscular junctions: regulation in vivo by electrical stimulation. J Neurosci 1993; 13(8):3433–3438.
8. Baker LL, Bowman BR, McNeal DR. Effects of waveform on comfort during neuromuscular electrical stimulation. Clin Orthop Relat Res 1988; 233:75–85.
9. Baker LL, Chambers R, DeMuth SK, et al. Effect of electrical stimulation on wound healing in patients with diabetic ulcers. Diabetes Care 1997; 20:405–412.
10. Baker LL, Parker K. Neuromuscular electrical stimulation of the muscles surrounding the shoulder. Phys Ther 1986; 66:1930–1937.
11. Baker LL, Yeh C, Wilson D, et al. Electrical stimulation of wrist and fingers for hemiplegic patients. Phys Ther 1979; 59:1495–1499.
12. Baker RC, Heinemann AW, Yarkony GM, et al. Functional neuromuscular stimulation for standing and ambulation: six month evaluation of psychological effects. In: Proceedings of the RESNA 12th Annual Conference, New Orleans, 1989:401–402.
13. Baldi JC, Jackson RD, Moraille R, et al. Muscle atrophy is prevented in patients with acute spinal cord injury using functional electrical stimulation. Spinal Cord 1998; 36:463–469.
14. Barbeau H, Ladouceur M, Norman KE, et al. Walking after spinal cord injury: evaluation, treatment and function. Arch Phys Med Rehabil 1999; 80:225–235.
15. Bassett CA, Hermann I. The effect of electrostatic fields on macromolecular synthesis by fibroblast in vitro. J Cell Biol 1968; 39:9A.
16. Bax L, Staes F, Verhagen A. Does neuromuscular electrical stimulation strengthen the quadriceps femoris? A systematic review of randomized controlled trials. Sports Med 2005; 35:191–212.
17. Belanger M, Stein RB, Wheeler GD, et al. Electrical stimulation: can it increase muscle strength and reverse osteopenia in spinal cord injured individuals? Arch Phys Med Rehabil 2000; 81:1090–1098.
18. Bhambhani Y, Tuchak C, Burnham R, et al. Quadriceps muscle deoxygenation during functional electrical stimulation in adults with spinal cord injury. Spinal Cord 2000; 38:630–638.
19. Biering-Sorensen F, Bohr H, Schaadt O. Bone mineral content of the lumbar spine and lower extremities years after spinal cord lesion. Paraplegia 1988; 26:293–301.
20. Bijak M, Rakos M, Hofer C, et al. Stimulation parameter optimization for FES supported standing and walking in SCI patients. Artif Organ 2005; 29:220–223.
21. Binder-MacLeod SA, Guerin T. Preservation of force output through progressive reduction of stimulation frequency in human quadriceps femoris muscle. Phys Ther 1990; 70(10):619–625.
22. Bloomfield SA, Mysiw WJ, Jackson RD. Bone mass and endocrine adaptations to training in spinal cord injured individuals. Bone 1996; 19:61–68.
23. Boonstra AM, van Weerden TW, Eisma WH, et al. The effect of low-frequency electrical stimulation on denervation atrophy in man. Scand J Rehabil Med 1987; 19:127–134.
24. Bouletreau P, Patricot MC, Saudin F, et al. Effects of intermittent electrical stimulation on muscle metabolism in intensive care patients. J Parenter Enteral Nutr 1987; 11:552–555.
25. Bowman BR, Baker LL. Effects of waveform parameters on comfort during transcutaneous neuromuscular electrical stimulation. Ann Biomed Eng 1985; 13:59–74.
26. Bradley MB. The effect of participating in a functional electrical stimulation exercise program on affect in people with spinal cord injuries. Arch Phys Med Rehabil 1994; 75:676–679.
27. Brenes G, Dearwater S, Shapera R, et al. High density lipoprotein cholesterol concentration in physically active and sedentary spinal cord injured patients. Arch Phys Med Rehabil 1986; 67:445–450.
28. Brown MC, Holland RL. A central role for denervated tissues in causing nerve sprouting. Nature 1979; 282:724–726.
29. Brown MD, Cotter MA, Hudlicka O, et al. The effects of different patterns of muscle activity on capillary density, mechanical properties and structure of slow and fast rabbit muscles. Pflugers Arch 1976; 361: 241–250.
30. Brownson C, Isenberg H, Brown W, et al. Changes in skeletal muscle gene transcription induced by chronic stimulation. Muscle Nerve 1988; 11: 1183–1189.
31. Brubaker L, Kotarinos R. Kegel or cut? Variations on his theme. J Reprod Med 1993; 38:672–678.
32. Buchegger A, Nemeth PM, Pette D, et al. Effects of chronic stimulation on the metabolic heterogeneity of the fibre population in rabbit tibialis anterior muscle. J Physiol 1984; 350:109–119.
33. Burke RE, Levine DN, Tsairis P, et al. Physiological types and histochemical profiles of motor units of the cat gastrocnemius. J Physiol 1973; 234:723–748.
34. Cabric M, Appell HJ, Resic A. Effects of electrical stimulation of different frequencies on the myonuclei and fiber size in human muscle. Int J Sports Med 1987; 8:323–326.
35. Cabric M, Appell HJ, Resic A. Fine structural changes in electrostimulated human skeletal muscle: evidence for predominant effects on fast muscle fibers. Eur J Appl Physiol 1988; 57:1–5.
36. Cabric M, Appell HJ, Resic A. Stereological analysis of capillaries in electrostimulated human muscles. Int J Sports Med 1987; 8:327–330.
37. Cabric M, Appell HJ. Effect of electrical stimulation of high and low frequency on maximum isometric force and some morphological characteristics in man. Int J Sports Med 1987; 8:256–260.
38. Caggiano E, Emrey T, Shirley S, et al. Effects of electrical stimulation or voluntary contraction for strengthening the quadriceps femoris muscles in an aged male population. J Orthop Sports Phys Ther 1994; 20:22–28.
39. Caputo RM, Benson JT, McClellan E. Intravaginal maximal electrical stimulation in the treatment of urinary incontinence. J Reprod Med 1993; 38:667–671.
40. Castro MJ, Apple DF, Staron RS, et al. Influence of complete spinal cord injury on skeletal muscle within 6 months of injury. J Appl Physiol 1999; 86:350–358.
41. Chancellor MB, Heesakkers JP, Janknegt RA. Gracilis muscle transposition with electrical stimulation for sphincteric incontinence: a new approach. World J Urol 1997; 15:320–328.
42. Chilibeck PD, Bell G, Jeon J, et al. Functional electrical stimulation exercise increases GLUT-1 and GLUT-4 in paralyzed skeletal muscle. Metab Clin Exp 1999; 48:1409–1413.
43. Clausen JP. Circulatory adjustments to dynamic exercise and effect of physical training in normal subjects and in patients with coronary artery disease. Prog Cardiovasc Dis 1976; 18:459–495.
44. Clinkingbeard JR, Gersten JW, Hoehn D. Energy cost of ambulation in traumatic paraplegia. Am J Phys Med Rehabil 1964; 43:157–165.

45. Cole BG, Gardiner PF. Does electrical stimulation of denervated muscle, continued after reinnervation, influence recovery of contractile function? Exp Neurol 1984; 85:52–62.

46. Cooper MS, Schliwa M. Electrical and ionic controls of tissue cell locomotion in DC electric fields. J Neurosci Res 1985; 13:223–244.

47. Creasey G, Elefteriades J, DiMarco A, et al. Electrical stimulation to restore respiration. J Rehabil Res Dev 1996; 33:123–132.

48. Cresey GH. Electrical stimulation of sacral roots for micturition after spinal cord injury. Urol Clin North Am 1993; 20:505–515.

49. Crowell LL, Squires WG, Raven PB. Benefits of aerobic exercise for paraplegics: a brief review. Med Sci Sports Exerc 1982; 18:501–508.

50. Cruz NI, Bayron FE, Suarez AJ. Accelerated healing of full thickness burns by the use of high-voltage pulsed galvanic stimulation in the pig. Ann Plast Surg 1989; 23:49–55.

51. Currier DP, Lehman J, Lightfoot P. Electrical stimulation in exercise of the quadriceps femoris muscle. Phys Ther 1979; 59:1508–1512.

52. Currier DP, Mann R. Muscular strength development by electrical stimulation in normal individuals. Phys Ther 1983; 63:915–921.

53. Dangain J, Vrbova G. Effect of chronic electrical stimulation at low frequency on the passive membrane properties of muscle fiber from dystrophic mice. Exp Neurol 1983; 79:630–640.

54. Degnan GG, Wind TC, Jones EV, et al. Functional electrical stimulation in tetraplegic patients to restore hand function. J Long Term Eff Med Implants 2002; 12:175–188.

55. Delitto A, Rose SJ, McKowen JM, et al. Electrical stimulation versus voluntary exercise in strengthening thigh musculature after anterior cruciate ligament surgery. Phys Ther 1988; 68:660–663.

56. DeVahl J. NMES and rehabilitation. In: Gersh M, ed. Electrotherapy in rehabilitation. Philadelphia: FA Davis; 1992:244–245.

57. Ding J, Binder-Macleod SA, Wexler AS. Two-step, predictive, isometric force model tested on data from human and rat muscles. J Appl Physiol 1998; 85:2176–2189.

58. Dorgan JJ, O'Malley MJ. A nonlinear mathematical model of electrically stimulated skeletal muscle. IEEE Trans Rehabil Eng 1997; 5:179–194.

59. Duchateau J, Hainaut K. Training effects of sub-maximal electrostimulation in a human muscle. Med Sci Sports Exerc 1988; 20:99–104.

60. Durham JW, Moskowitz A, Whitney J. Surface electrical stimulation versus brace in treatment of idiopathic scoliosis. Spine 1990; 15:888–892.

61. Eberstein A, Eberstein S. Electrical stimulation of denervated muscle: is it worth it? Med Sci Sports Exerc 1996; 28:1463–1469.

62. Edstrom L, Grimby L. Effect of exercise on the motor unit. Muscle Nerve 1986; 9:104–126.

63. Edwards BG, Marsolais EB. Metabolic responses to arm ergometry and functional neuromuscular stimulation. J Rehabil Res Dev 1990; 27:107–113.

64. Egginton S, Hudlicka O. Early changes in performance, blood flow and capillary fine structure in rat fast muscles induced by electrical stimulation. J Physiol 1999; 515:265–275.

65. Eisenberg BR, Salmons S. The reorganization of subcellular structure in muscle undergoing fast-to-slow type transformation: a stereological study. Cell Tissue Res 1981; 220:449–471.

66. Ellenberg M, MacRitchie M, Franklin B, et al. Aerobic capacity in early paraplegia: implications for rehabilitation. Paraplegia 1989; 27:261–268.

67. Emes CG. Fitness and the physically disabled. A review. Can J Appl Sport Sci 1981; 6:176–178.

68. Eser P, de Bruin ED, Telley I, et al. Effect of electrical stimulation-induced cycling on bone mineral density in spinal cord-injured patients. Eur J Clin Invest 2003; 33:412–419.

69. Etgen GJ Jr, Farrar RP, Ivy JL. Effect of chronic electrical stimulation on GLUT-4 protein content in fast-twitch muscle. Am J Physiol 1993; 264: r816–r819.

70. Faghri PD, Rodgers MN, Glaser RM, et al. The effects of functional electrical stimulation on shoulder subluxation, arm function recovery, and shoulder pain in hemiplegic stroke patients. Arch Phys Med Rehabil 1994; 75:73–79.

71. Falanga V, Bourguignon GJ, Bourguignon LY. Electrical stimulation increases the expression of fibroblast receptors for transforming growth factor-beta. J Invest Dermatol 1987; 88:488.

72. Fall M, Lindstrom S. Electrical stimulation: a physiologic approach to the treatment of urinary incontinence. Urol Clin North Am 1991; 18:393–407.

73. Fisher DA, Rapp GF, Emkes M. Idiopathic scoliosis: transcutaneous muscle stimulation versus the Milwaukee brace. Spine 1987; 12:987–991.

74. Funakoshi H, Bellvardo N, Arenas E, et al. Muscle-derived neurotrophin-4 as an activity-dependent trophic signed for adult motor neurons. Science 1995; 268:1495–1499.

75. Gault WR, Gatens PF. Use of low intensity direct current in management of ischemic skin ulcers. Phys Ther 1976; 56:265–269.

76. Gentzkow GD, Miller KH. Electrical stimulation for dermal wound healing. Clin Podiatr Med Surg 1991; 8:827–841.

77. Gentzkow GD, Pollick SV, Kloth LC, et al. Improved healing of pressure ulcers using dermapulse, a new electrical stimulation device. Wound 1991; 3:158–170.

78. Gerritis HL, de Haan A, Sargeant AJ, et al. Altered contractile properties of the quadriceps muscle in people with spinal cord injury following functional electrical simulated cycle ergometry. Spinal Cord 2000; 38:214–223.

79. Gibson JN, Smith K, Rennie MJ. Prevention of disuse muscle atrophy by means of electrical stimulation: maintenance of protein synthesis. Lancet 1988; 2(8614):767–769.

80. Gilcreast DM, Stotts NA, Froelicher ES, et al. Effect of electrical stimulation on foot skin perfusion in persons with or at risk for diabetic foot ulcers. Wound Repair Regen 1998; 6:434–441.

81. Girlanda PR, Dattola R, Vita G, et al. Effect of electrotherapy on denervated muscles in rabbits: an electrophysiological and morphological study. Exp Neurol 1982; 77:483–491.

82. Glanz M, Klawansky S, Stason W, et al. Functional electrical stimulation in poststroke rehabilitation: a meta-analysis of the randomized controlled trials. Arch Phys Med Rehabil 1996; 77:549–553.

83. Glenn WW, Hogan JF, Loke JS, et al. Ventilatory support by pacing of the conditioned diaphragm in quadriplegia. N Engl J Med 1984; 310: 1150–1155.

84. Goldspink G, Scutt A, Loughna PT, et al. Gene expression in skeletal muscle in response stretch and force generation. Am J Physiol 1992; 262: r356–r363.

85. Goldspink G, Scutt A, Martindale J, et al. Stretch and force generation induce rapid hypertrophy and isoform gene switching in adult skeletal muscle. Biochem Trans 1991; 19:368–373.

86. Gordon T, Mao J. Muscle atrophy and procedures for training after spinal cord injury. Phys Ther 1994; 74:50–60.

87. Greve JMD, Muszkat PT, Schmidt B, et al. Functional electrical stimulation (FES): muscle histochemical analysis. Paraplegia 1993; 31:764–770.

88. Grill WM, Mortimer JT. Stability of the input–output properties of chronically implanted multiple contact nerve cuff electrodes. IEEE Trans Rehabil Eng 1998; 6:364–373.

89. Grimby G, Wigerstad-Lossing I. Comparison of high- and low-frequency muscle stimulators. Arch Phys Med Rehabil 1989; 70:835–838.

90. Gurney AB, Robergs RA, Aisenbray J, et al. Detraining from total body exercise ergometry in individuals with spinal cord injury. Spinal Cord 1998; 36:782–789.

91. Gutmann E, Gutmann L. Effects of electrotherapy on denervated and reinnervated muscles in rabbit. Lancet 1942; 1:169–170.

92. Halbach JW, Straus D. Comparison of electro-myostimulation to isokinetic power of the knee extensor mechanism. J Orthop Sports Phys Ther 1980; 2:20–24.

93. Hangartner TN, Rodgers MM, Glaser RM, et al. Tibial bone density loss in spinal cord injured patients: effects of FES exercise. J Rehabil Res Dev 1994; 31:50–61.

94. Hansen-Smith F, Egginton S, Hudlicka O. Growth of arterioles in chronically stimulated rat muscle. Microcirculation 1998; 5:49–59.

95. Harvey JR, Bradley MB. Staff perceptions of the psychological benefits of FES training: a grounded therapy approach. SCI Psychosoc Proc 1992; 5:8.

96. Haug J, Wood LT. Efficacy of neuromuscular stimulation of the quadriceps femoris during continuous passive motion following total knee arthroplasty. Arch Phys Med Rehabil 1988; 69(6):423–424.

97. Heilig A, Pette D. Changes induced in the enzyme activity pattern by electrical stimulation of fast twitch muscle. In: Pette D, ed. Plasticity of muscle. Berlin: Walter de Gruyter; 1980:409–420.

98. Heilmann C, Muller W, Pette D. Correlation between ultrastructural and functional changes in sarcoplasmic reticulum during chronic stimulation of fast muscle. J Membr Biol 1981; 59:143–149.

99. Heilmann C, Pette D. Molecular transformation in sarcoplasmic reticulum of fast-twitch muscle by electro-stimulation. Eur J Biochem 1979; 93:437–446.

100. Henneman E, Somjen G, Carpenter DO. Excitability and inhibitability of motoneurons of different sizes. J Neurophysiol 1965; 28:599–620.

101. Henneman E, Somjen G, Carpenter DO. Functional significance of cell size in spinal motoneurons. J Neurophysiol 1965; 28:560–580.

102. Herbison GJ, Jaweed MM, Ditunno JF Jr. Exercise therapies in peripheral neuropathies. Arch Phys Med Rehabil 1983; 64:201–205.

103. Hesse S, Mauritz KH. Management of spasticity. Curr Opin Neurol 1997; 10:498–501.

104. Hesse S, Reiter F, Konrad M, et al. Botulinum toxin type A and short-term electrical stimulation in the treatment of upper limb flexor spasticity after stroke: a randomized, double-blind, placebo-controlled trial. Clin Rehabil 1998; 12:381–388.

105. Hirokawa S, Grimm M, Le T, et al. Energy consumptions in paraplegic ambulation using the reciprocating gait orthosis and electric stimulation of the thigh muscles. Arch Phys Med Rehabil 1990; 71:687–694.

106. Hjeltnes N, Galuska D, Bjornholm M, et al. Exercise-induced over-expression of key regulatory proteins involved in glucose uptake and metabolism in tetraplegic persons: molecular mechanisms for improved glucose homeostasis: FASEB J 1998; 12:1701–1712.

107. Hjeltnes N, Lannem A. Functional neuromuscular stimulation in four patients with complete paraplegia. Paraplegia 1990; 28:235–243.

108. Hjeltnes N, Vokac Z. Circulatory strain in everyday life of paraplegics. Scand J Rehabil Med 1979; 11:67–73.

109. Hoffman MD. Cardiorespiratory fitness and training in quadriplegics and paraplegics. Sports Med 1986; 3:312–330.

110. Hooker SP, Figoni SF, Glaser RM, et al. Physiologic responses to prolonged electrically stimulated leg-cycle exercise in the spinal cord injured. Arch Phys Med Rehabil 1990; 71:863–869.

111. Howson DC. Peripheral neural excitability: implications for transcutaneous electrical nerve stimulation. Phys Ther 1978; 58:1467–1473.

112. Hudecki MS, Caffiero AT, Gregorio CC, et al. Effects of percutaneous electrical stimulation on functional ability, plasma creatine kinase, and pectoralis musculature of normal and genetically dystrophic chickens. Exp Neurol 1985; 90:53–72.

113. Hudlicka O, Aitman T, Heilig A, et al. Effects of different patterns of long-term stimulation on blood flow, fuel uptake and enzyme activities in rabbit fast skeletal muscles. Pflugers Arch 1984; 402:306–311.

114. Hudlicka O, Brown M, Cotter M, et al. The effect of long-term stimulation of fast-muscles on their blood flow, metabolism and ability to withstand fatigue. Pflugers Arch 1977; 369:141–149.

115. Hudlicka O, Dodd L, Renkin EM, et al. Early changes in fibre profile and capillary density in long-term stimulated muscles. Am J Physiol 1982; 243: h528–h535.

116. Hudlicka O, Tyler KR, Srihari T, et al. The effect of different patterns of long-term stimulation on contractile properties and myosin light chains in rabbit fast muscles. Pflugers Arch 1982; 393:164–170.

117. Im MJ, Lee WP, Hoopes JE. Effect of electrical stimulation on survival of skin flaps in pigs. Phys Ther 1990; 70:37–40.

118. Ishigooka M, Hashimoto T, Hayami S, et al. Electrical pelvic floor stimulation: a possible alternative treatment for reflex urinary incontinence in patients with spinal cord injury. Spinal Cord 1996; 34:411–415.

119. Johnson EW, Braddom R. Over-work weakness in fascioscapulo-humeral muscular dystrophy. Arch Phys Med Rehabil 1971; 52:333–336.

120. Jonasson I, Larsson B, Pschera H, et al. Short-term maximal electrical stimulation: a conservative treatment of urinary incontinence. Gynecol Obstet Invest 1990; 30:120–123.

121. Jones DA, Bigland-Ritchie B, Edwards RH. Excitation frequency and muscle fatigue: mechanical responses during voluntary and stimulated contractions. Exp Neurol 1979; 64(2):401–413.

122. Kahanovitz N, Nordin M, Verderame R, et al. Normal trunk muscle strength and endurance in women and the effect of exercises and electrical stimulation: 2. Comparative analysis of electrical stimulation and exercises to increase trunk muscle strength and endurance. Spine 1987; 12:112–118.

123. Kantrowitz A. Electronic physiologic aids. Brooklyn: Maimonides Hospital; 1960:4–5.

124. Katz RT, Green D, Sullivan T, et al. Functional electrical stimulation to enhance systemic fibrinolytic activity in spinal cord injury patients. Arch Phys Med Rehabil 1987; 68:423–426.

125. Kincaid CB, Lavoie KH. Inhibition of bacterial growth in vitro following stimulation with high voltage, monophasic, pulsed current. Phys Ther 1989; 69:651–655.

126. Kjaer M, Mohr T, Biering-Sorensen F, et al. Muscle enzyme adaptation to training and tapering off in spinal-cord injured humans. Eur J Applied Physiol 2001; 84:482–496.

127. Kloth LC, Feedar JA. Acceleration of wound healing with high voltage, monophasic, pulsed current. Phys Ther 1988; 68:503–508.

128. Klug G, Wiehrer W, Reichmann H, et al. Relationships between early alterations in parvalbumins, sarcoplasmic reticulum and metabolic enzymes in chronically stimulated fast twitch muscle. Pflugers Arch 1983; 399:280–284.

129. Knaflitz M, Merletti R, Deluca CJ. Inference of motor unit recruitment order in voluntary and electrically elicited contraction. J Appl Physiol 1990; 68:1657–1667.

130. Koskinen SOA, Kjaer M, Mohr T, et al. Type IV collagen and its degradation in paralyzed human muscle: effect of functional electrical stimulation. Muscle Nerve 2000; 23:580–589.

131. Kraft GH, Fitts SS, Hammond MC. Techniques to improve function of the arm and hand in chronic hemiplegia. Arch Phys Med Rehabil 1992; 73:220–227.

132. Kralj AR, Bajd P, Munih M, et al. FES gait restoration and balance control in spinal cord injured patients. Prog Brain Res 1993; 97:387–396.

133. Kramer JF, Semple JE. Comparison of selected strengthening techniques for normal quadriceps. Physiol Ther Can 1983; 35:300–304.

134. Krauss JC, Robergs RA, Depaepe JL, et al. Effects of electrical stimulation and upper body training after spinal cord injury. Med Sci Sports Exerc 1993; 25:1054–1061.

135. Kubiak RJ, Whitman KM, Johnston RM. Changes in quadriceps femoris muscle strength using isometric exercise versus electrical stimulation. J Orthop Sports Phys Ther 1987; 8:537–541.

136. Lake DA. Neuromuscular electrical stimulation: an overview and its application in the treatment of sports injuries. Sports Med 1992; 13:320–336.

137. Larsen JO, Thomsen M, Haugland M, et al. Degeneration and regeneration in rabbit peripheral nerve with long-term nerve cuff electrode implant: a stereological study of myelinated and unmyelinated axons. Acta Neuro-pathol 1998; 96:365–378.

138. Laskin JJ, Ashley EA, Olenik LM, et al. Electrical stimulation-assisted rowing exercise in spinal cord injured people: a pilot study. Paraplegia 1993; 31:534–541.

139. Latash ML, Yee MJ, Orpett C, et al. Combining electrical muscle stimulation with voluntary contraction for studying muscle fatigue. Arch Phys Med Rehabil 1994; 75:29–35.

140. Lau HK, Liu J, Pereira BP, et al. Fatigue reduction by sequential stimulation of multiple motor points in a muscle. Clin Orthop Relat Res 1995; 321:251–258.

141. Laughman RK, Youdas JW, Garrett TR, et al. Strength changes in the normal quadriceps femoris muscle as the result of electrical stimulation. Phys Ther 1983; 63:494–499.

142. Lawrence JC Jr, Krsek JA, Salsgiver WJ, et al. Phosphorylase kinase iso-zymes in normal and electrically stimulated skeletal muscles. Am J Physiol 1986; 250:c84–c89.

143. Leeds EM, Klose KJ, Ganez W, et al. Bone mineral density after bicycle ergometry training. Arch Phys Med Rehabil 1990; 71:207–209.

144. Levine SP, Kett RL, Cederna PS, et al. Electric muscle stimulation for pressure sore prevention: tissue shape variation. Arch Phys Med Rehabil 1990; 67:108–116.

145. Liberson WT, Holmquest HJ, Scot D, et al. Functional electrotherapy: stimulation of the peroneal nerve synchronized with the swing phase of gait of hemiplegic patients. Arch Phys Med Rehabil 1961; 42:101–105.

146. Lomo T, Westgaard RH, Dahl HA. Contractile properties of muscle: control by pattern of muscle activity in the rat. Proc R Soc Lond Biol 1974; 187:99–103.

147. Lomo T, Westgaard RH, Engebretsen L. Different stimulation patterns affect contractile properties of denervated rat soleus muscle. In: Pette D, ed. Plasticity of muscle. Berlin: Walter de Gruyter; 1980:297–309.

148. Lundeberg TCM, Eriksson SV, Malm M. Electrical nerve stimulation improves healing of diabetic ulcers. Ann Plast Surg 1992; 29:328–331.

149. Luthert P, Vrbovà G, Ward KM. Effects of slow frequency electrical stimulation on muscles of dystrophic mice. J Neurol Neurosurg Psychiatry 1980; 43:803–809.

150. Lyons GM, Sinkjaer T, Burridge JH, et al. A review of portable FES-based neural orthoses for correction of drop foot. IEEI Trans Neural Syst Rehabil Eng 2002; 10:260–279.

151. Mabuchi K, Szvetko D, Pinter K, et al. Type IIB to IIA fiber transformation in intermittently stimulated rabbit muscles. Am J Physiol 1982; 242: c373–c381.

152. Marsolais EB, Edwards BG. Energy costs of walking and standing with functional neuromuscular stimulation and long leg braces. Arch Phys Med Rehabil 1988; 69:243–249.

153. Marsolais EB, Kobetic R, Barnicle K, et al. FNS application for restoring function in stroke and head injury patients. J Clin Eng 1990; 15:489–496.

154. Marsolais EB. FES ambulatory assist. In: Neural Prosthesis: Motor Systems IV, Engineering Foundation Conferences, New York, 23–28 July 1994.

155. Martin TP, Stein RB, Hoeppner PH, et al. Influence of electrical stimulation or the morphological and metabolic properties of paralyzed muscle. J Appl Physiology 1992; 72:1401–1406.

156. McDonagh JC, Binder MD, Reinking RM, et al. Tetrapartite classification of motor units of cat tibialis posterior. J Neurophysiol 1980; 44:696–712.

157. Melzack R, Wall PD. Pain mechanism: a new theory. Science 1965; 150:171–179.

158. Merli GJ, Herbison GJ, Ditunno JF, et al. Deep vein thrombosis: prophylaxis in acute spinal cord injured patients. Arch Phys Med Rehabil 1988; 69:661–664.

159. Middleton JW, Keost JR. Artificial autonomic reflexes: using functional electrical stimulation to mimic bladder reflexes after injury or disease. Auton Neurosci 2004; 113:3–15.

160. Midura RJ, Dillman CJ, Grabover MD. Low amplitude, high frequency strains imposed by electrically stimulated skeletal muscle retards the development of osteopenia in the tibiae of hindlimb suspended rats. Med Eng Phys 2005; 27:285–293.

161. Milner-Brown HS, Miller RG. Muscle strengthening through electrical stimulation combined with low-resistance weights in patients with neuromuscular disorders. Arch Phys Med Rehabil 1988; 69:20–24.

162. Milner-Brown HS, Stein RB, Yemm R. The contractile properties of human motor units during voluntary isometric contractions. J Physiol 1973; 228:285–306.

163. Milner-Brown HS, Stein RB, Yemm R. The orderly recruitment of human motor units during voluntary isometric contraction. J Physiol 1973; 230:359–370.

164. Mohr T, Dela F, Handberg A, et al. Insulin action and long-term electrically induced training in individuals with spinal cord injuries. Med Sci Sports Exerc 2001; 33:1247–1252.

165. Mokrusch T, Engelhardt A, Eichorn KF, et al. Effects of long-impulse electrical stimulation on atrophy and fibre type composition of chronically denervated fast rabbit muscle. J Neurol 1990; 237:29–34.

166. Monster AW, Chan H. Isometric force production by motor units of extensor digitorum communis muscle in man. J Neurophysiol 1977; 40:1432–1443.

167. Morrissey MC, Brewster CE, Shields CL Jr, et al. The effects of electrical stimulation on the quadriceps during postoperative knee immobilization. Am J Sports Med 1985; 13:40–45.

168. Mortiemer JT. Extra neural neuromuscular stimulating electrodes. In: Neuroprosthesis: Motor Systems IV, Engineering Foundation Conferences, New York, 23–28 July 1994.

169. Mullett K. State-of-the-art in neurostimulation. PACE 1987; 10:162–175.

170. Munsat TL, McNeal D, Waters R. Effects of nerve stimulation on human muscle. Arch Neurol 1976; 33:608–617.

171. Myklebust BM, Kloth L. Electrodiagnostic and electrotherapeutic instrumentation: characteristics of recording and stimulation systems and principles of safety. In: Gersh MR, ed. Electrotherapy in rehabilitation. Philadelphia: FA Davis; 1992:51–100.

172. Mysiw WJ, Jackson RD. Hypercalciuria permitted by functional electrical stimulation [abstract]. Arch Phys Med Rehabil 1990; 71:795.

173. Nash MS, Bilsker S, Marcillo AE, et al. Reversal of adaptive left ventricular atrophy following electrically-stimulated exercise training in human tetraplegics. Paraplegia 1991; 29:590–599.

174. Nash MS, Montalvo BM, Applegate B. Lower extremity blood flow and responses to occlusion ischemia differ in exercise-trained and sedentary tetrapelgic persons. Arch Phys Med Rehabil 1996; 77:1260–1265.

175. Nemeth PM. Electrical stimulation of denervated muscle prevents decreases in oxidative enzymes. Muscle Nerve 1982; 5:134–139.

176. Nene AV, Patrick JH. Energy cost of paraplegic locomotion using the ParaWalker electrical stimulation 'hybrid' orthosis. Arch Phys Med Rehabil 1990; 71:116–120.

177. Nix W. Effect of electrical stimulation on denervated muscle. In: Nix WA, Vrbovà G, eds. Electrical stimulation and neuro-disorders. Berlin: Springer-Verlag; 1986:115–124.

178. Nix WA. The effect of low-frequency electrical stimulation on the denervated extensor digitorum longus muscle of the rabbit. Acta Neurol Scand 1982; 66:521–528.

179. Nochomovitz ML, Peterson BK, Stellato TA. Electrical activation of the diaphragm. Clin Chest Med 1988; 9:349–358.

180. Okada N, Igawa Y, Ogawa A, et al. Transcutaneous electrical stimulation of thigh muscles in the treatment of detrusor overactivity. Br J Urol 1998; 81:560–564.

181. Okuma H, Ogata H, Hatada K. Transition of physical fitness in wheelchair marathon competitors over several years. Paraplegia 1989; 27:237–243.

182. Osman SG, Marsolais EB. Endoscopic implantation of cuff electrodes on the hamstring branches of the sciatic nerve in paralyzed subjects. In: Neuroprosthesis: Motor Systems IV, Engineering Foundation Conferences, New York, 23–28 July 1994.

183. Osterman AL, Bora FW Jr. Electrical stimulation applied to bone and nerve injuries in the upper extremity. Orthop Clin North Am 1986; 17:353–364.

184. Pachter B, Eberstein A, Goodgold J. Electrical stimulation effect on denervated skeletal myofibers in rats: a light and electron microscopic study. Arch Phys Med Rehabil 1982; 63:427–430.

185. Packman-Braun R. Relationship between functional electrical stimulation duty cycle and fatigue in wrist extensor muscles of patients with hemiparesis. Phys Ther 1988; 68:51–56.

186. Pacy PJ, Hesp R, Halliday DA, et al. Muscle and bone in paraplegic patients, and the effect of functional electrical stimulation. Clin Sci 1988; 75:481–487.

187. Pambianco G, Orchard T, Landan P. Deep vein thrombosis prevention in stroke patients during rehabilitation. Arch Phys Med Rehabil 1995; 76:324–330.

188. Pease WS. Therapeutic electrical stimulation for spasticity: quantitative gait analysis. Am J Phys Med Rehabil 1998; 77:351–355.

189. Peckham PH, Keith MW, Freehafer AA. Restoration of functional control by electrical stimulation in the upper extremity of the quadriplegic patient. J Bone Joint Surg Am 1988; 70:144–148.

190. Perkash I, Martin DE, Warner H, et al. Electroejaculation in spinal cord injury patients: simplified new equipment and technique. J Urol 1990; 143:305–307.

191. Petrofsky JS, Phillips CA, Heaton HH, et al. Bicycle ergometer for paralyzed muscle. J Clin Eng 1984; 9:13–19.

192. Petrofsky JS, Phillips CA. The use of functional electrical stimulation for rehabilitation of spinal cord injured patients. Central Nerv Syst Trauma 1984; 1:57–74.

193. Petrofsky JS, Stacy R. The effect of training on endurance and the cardiovascular responses of individuals with paraplegia during dynamic exercise induced by functional electrical stimulation. Eur J Appl Physiol 1992; 64:487–492.

194. Petrofsky JS. Sequential motor unit stimulation through peripheral motor nerves in the cat. Med Biol Eng Comput 1979; 17:87–93.

195. Pette D, Müller W, Leisner E, et al. Time dependent effects on contractile properties, fibre population, myosin light chains and enzymes of energy

metabolism in intermittently and continuously stimulated fast twitch muscle. Pflugers Arch 1976; 364:103–112.

196. Pette D, Ramirez BU, Müller W, et al. Influence of intermittent long-term stimulation on contractile, histochemical and metabolic properties of fibre populations in fast and slow rabbit muscles. Pflugers Arch 1975; 361: 1–7.

197. Pette D, Schnez U. Coexistence of fast and slow type myosin light chains in single muscle fibres during transformation as induced by long-term stimulation. FEBS Lett 1977; 83:128–130.

198. Pette D, Smith ME, Staudte HW, et al. Effects of long-term electrical stimulation on some contractile and metabolic characteristics of fast rabbit muscles. Pflugers Arch 1973; 338:257–272.

199. Pette D, Staudte HW, Vrbová G. Physiological and biochemical changes induced by long-term stimulation of fast muscle. Naturwissenschaften 1972; 59:469–470.

200. Pette D, Tyler KR. Response of succinate dehydrogenase activity in fibres of rabbit tibialis anterior muscle to chronic nerve stimulation. J Physiol 1983; 338:1–9.

201. Pette D. Activity-induced fast- to slow-transition in mammalian muscle. Med Sci Sports Exerc 1984; 16:517–528.

202. Phillips CA, Petrosky JS, Hendershot DM, et al. Functional electrical exercise: comprehensive approach for physical conditioning of spinal cord injured patients. Orthopedics 1984; 7:1112–1123.

203. Phillips WT, Burkett LN. Augmented upper body contribution to oxygen uptake during upper body exercise with concurrent leg functional electrical stimulation in persons with spinal cord injury. Spinal Cord 1998; 36: 750–755.

204. Phillips WT, Kiratli BJ, Sarkarati M, et al. Effect of spinal cord injury on the heart and cardiovascular fitness. Curr Probl Cardiol 1998; 23:641–716.

205. Polando G, Schiner A, Marsolais EB. Reliability of lower extremity FES systems: analysis of a current laboratory system. In: Neuroprosthesis: Motor Systems IV, Engineering Foundation Conferences, New York, 23–28 July 1994.

206. Pollack SF, Axen K, Spielholtz N, et al. Aerobic training effects of electrically-induced lower extremity exercises in spinal cord injured people. Arch Phys Med Rehabil 1989; 70:214–219.

207. Popovic DB. Finite state model of locomotion for functional electrical stimulation systems. Prog Brain Res 1993; 97:397–407.

208. Popovic MB. Control of neural prostheses for grasping and reaching. Med Eng Phys 2003; 25:41–50.

209. Previnaire JG, Soler JM, Perrigot M, et al. Short-term effect of pudendal nerve electrical stimulation on detrusor hyperreflexia in spinal cord injury patients: importance of current strength. Paraplegia 1996; 34:95–99.

210. Previnaire JG, Soler JM, Perrigot M. Is there a place for pudendal nerve maximal electrical stimulation for the treatment of detrusor hyperreflexia in spinal cord injury patients? Spinal Cord 1998; 36:100–103.

211. Price CI, Pandyan AD. Electrical stimulation for preventing and treating post-stroke shoulder pain: a systematic Cochrane review. Clin Rehabil 2001; 15(1):5–19.

212. Putman CT, Dixon WT, Pearcey JA, et al. Chronic low-frequency stimulation upregulated uncoupling protein-3 in transforming rat fast-twitch muscle. Am J Physiol Integr Comp Physiol 2004; 287: R1419–R1426.

213. Ragnarsson KT, Pollack SF, O'Daniel W, et al. Clinical evaluation of computerized functional electrical stimulation after spinal cord injury: a multicenter pilot study. Arch Phys Med Rehabil 1988; 69:672–677.

214. Ragnarsson KT, Sell G. Lower extremity fractures after spinal cord injury: a retrospective study. Arch Phys Med Rehabil 1981; 62:418–423.

215. Ragnarsson KT. Physiologic effects of functional electrical stimulation-induced exercises in spinal cord injured individuals. Clin Orthop Relat Res 1988; 233:53–63.

216. Ramirez BU, Pette D. Effect of long-term electrical stimulation on sarcoplasmic reticulum of fast rabbit muscle. FEBS Lett 1974; 49:188–198.

217. Reich JD, Tarjan PP. Electrical stimulation of skin. Int J Dermatol 1990; 29:395–400.

218. Reichmann H, Hoppeler H, Mathieu-Costello O, et al. Biochemical and ultrastructural changes of skeletal muscle mitochondria after chronic electrical stimulation in rabbits. Pflugers Arch 1985; 404:1–9.

219. Reichmann H, Pette D, Vrbová G. Effects of low frequency electrical stimulation on enzyme and isozyme patterns of dystrophic mouse muscle. FEBS Lett 1981; 128:55–58.

220. Rijkhoft NJ, Hendrickx LB, van Verrebroeck PE, et al. Selective detrusor activation by electrical stimulation of the human sacral nerve roots. Artif Organs 1997; 21:223–226.

221. Robinson CJ, Kett NA, Bolam JM. Spasticity in spinal cord injured patients: 1. Short-term effects of surface electrical stimulation. Arch Phys Med Rehabil 1988; 69:598–604.

222. Robinson LR, Mustovic EH, Lieber PS, et al. A technique for quantifying and determining the site of isometric muscle fatigue in the clinical setting. Arch Phys Med Rehabil 1990; 71:901–904.

223. Rowe DE, Bernstein SM, Riddick MF, et al. A meta-analysis of the efficacy of non-operative treatments for idiopathic scoliosis. J Bone Joint Surg Am 1997; 79:664–674.

224. Roy D, Johannsson E, Bonen A, et al. Electrical stimulation induces fiber type-specific translocation of GLUT-4 to T tubules in skeletal muscle. Am J Physiol 1997; 273:E688–E694.

225. Roy RK, Mabuchi K, Sarkar S, et al. Changes in tropomyosin subunit pattern in chronic electrically stimulated rabbit fast muscles. Biochem Biophys Res Commun 1979; 89:181–187.

226. Rubinstein N, Mabuchi K, Pepe F, et al. Use of type-specific antimyosins to demonstrate the transformation of individual fibers in chronically stimulated rabbit fast muscles. J Cell Biol 1978; 79:252–261.

227. Saito K, Kinoshita Y, Hosaka M. Direct and indirect effects of electrical stimulation on the motility of human sperm. Int J Urol 1999; 6:196–199.

228. Salmons S, Ashley Z, Sutherland H, et al. Functional electrical stimulation of denervated muscle: basic issues. Artif Organs 2005; 29:199–207.

229. Salmons S, Henriksson J. The adaptive response of skeletal muscle to increased use. Muscle Nerve 1981; 4:94–105.

230. Salmons S, Sréter FA. Significance of impulse activity in the transformation of skeletal muscle type. Nature 1976; 263:30–34.

231. Salmons S, Vrbová G. The influence of activity on some contractile characteristics of mammalian fast and slow muscles. J Physiol 1969; 210:535–549.

232. Sarzala MG, Szymanska G, Wiehrer W, et al. Effects of chronic stimulation at low frequency on the lipid phase of sarcoplasmic reticulum in rabbit fast-twitch muscle. Eur J Biochem 1982; 123:241–245.

233. Scott OM, Hyde SA, Vrbová G, et al. Therapeutic possibilities of chronic long-frequency electrical stimulation in children with Duchenne muscular dystrophy. J Neurol Sci 1990; 95:171–182.

234. Scott OM, Vrbová G, Hyde SA, et al. Responses of muscles of patients with Duchenne muscular dystrophy to chronic electrical stimulation. J Neurol Neurosurg Psychiatry 1986; 49:1427–1434.

235. Seager SW, Halstead LS. Fertility options and success after spinal cord injury. Urol Clin North Am 1993; 20:543–548.

236. Seedorf K, Seedorf U, Pette D. Coordinate expression of alkali and DTNB myosin light chains during transformation of rabbit fast muscle by chronic stimulation. FEBS Lett 1983; 158:321–324.

237. Sigmedics. Parastep update. Northfield: Sigmedics; 1994.

238. Sipski ML, Delisa JA, Schweer S. Functional electrical stimulation bicycle ergometry: patient perceptions. Am J Phys Med Rehabil 1989; 68: 147–149.

239. Solomonow M. External control of the neuromuscular system. IEEE Trans Biomed Eng 1984; 31:752–763.

240. Sréter FA, Gergely J, Salmon S, et al. Synthesis by fast muscle of myosin light chain characteristic of slow muscle in response to long-term stimulation. Nature 1973; 241:17–19.

241. Sréter FA, Pinter K, Jolesz F, et al. Fast to slow transformation of fast muscles in response to long-term phasic stimulation. Exp Neurol 1982; 75:95–102.

242. Stefanoviska A, Gros N, Vodovnik L, et al. Chronic electrical stimulation for the modification of spasticity in hemiplegic patients. Scand J Rehabil Med 1988; 17(suppl):115–121.

243. Sweeney JD. Selection criteria for neuromuscular stimulation electrodes. In: Neuroprosthesis: Motor Systems IV, Engineering Foundation Conferences, New York, 23–28 July 1994.

244. Sykes L, Campbell IG, Powell ES, et al. Energy expenditure of walking for adults with spinal cord lesions using the reciprocating gait orthosis and functional electrical stimulation. Spinal Cord 1996; 34:659–665.

245. Sykes L, Ross ER, Powell ES, et al. Objective measurement of use of the reciprocating gait orthosis (RGO) and the electrically augmented RGO in

adult patients with spinal cord lesions. Prosthet Orthot Int 1996; 20:182–190.

246. Tan SL, Archibald V, Jessar B, et al. Increased neuromuscular activity reduces sprouting in partially denervated muscle. J Neurosci 2001; 21:654–667.

247. Taylor PN, Tromans AM, Harris KR, et al. Electrical stimulation of abdominal muscle for control of blood pressure and augmentation of cough in a C3/4 level tetraplegic. Spinal Cord 2002; 40:34–36.

248. Theriault R, Boulay MR, Theriault G, et al. Electrical stimulation-induced changes in performance and fiber type proportion of human knee extensor muscles. Eur J App Physiol Occup Physiol 1996; 74:311–317.

249. Tulgar M, McGlone F, Bowsher D, et al. Comparative effectiveness of different stimulation modes in relieving pain: II. A double blind controlled long-term clinical trial. Pain 1991; 47:157–162.

250. Vignos PJ, Watkins MP. The effect of exercise in muscular dystrophy. JAMA 1966; 197:843–848.

251. Vodovnik L, Karba R. Treatment of chronic wounds by means of electrical and electromagnetic fields: I. Literature review. Med Biol Eng Comput 1992; 30:257–266.

252. Vrbovà G, Ward K. Observations on the effects of low frequency electrical stimulation on fast muscles of dystrophic mice. J Neurol Neurosurg Psychiatry 1981; 44:1002–1006.

253. Walsfley RP, Letts G, Booyf J. A comparison of torque generated by knee extension with a maximal voluntary muscle contraction: vis-a-vis electrical stimulation. J Orthop Sports Phys Ther 1984; 6:10–17.

254. Wang YH, Chiang HS, Wu CH, et al. Electroejaculation in spinal cord injured males. J Formosa Med Assoc 1992; 91:413–418.

255. Weber RJ. Functional neuromuscular stimulation. In: DeLisa JA, Gans BM, eds. Rehabilitation medicine: principles and practice. Philadelphia: JB Lippincott; 1993:463–476.

256. Wehrmacher WH, Thomson JD, Hines HM. Effects of electrical stimulation on denervated skeletal muscle. Arch Phys Med Rehabil 1945; 26:261–266.

257. Weiss DS, Eaglstein WH, Falanga V. Pulsed electrical stimulation decreases scar thickness at split thickness graft donor sites [abstract]. J Invest Dermatol 1989; 92:3.

258. Wiehrer W, Pette D. The ratio between intrinsic 115 kDa and 30 kDa peptides as a marker of fibre type-specific sarcoplasmic reticulum in mammalian muscles. FEBS Lett 1983; 158:317–320.

259. Wigerstad-Lossing I, Grimby G, Jonnson T, et al. Effects of electrical stimulation combined with voluntary contractions after knee ligament surgery. Med Sci Sports Exerc 1988; 20:93–98.

260. William HB. The value of continuous electrical muscle stimulation using a completely implantable system in the preservation of muscle function following motor nerve injury and repair: an experimental study. Microsurgery 1996; 17:589–596.

261. Williams RS, Salmons S, Newsholme EA, et al. Regulation of nuclear and mitochondrial gene expression by contractile activity in skeletal muscle. J Biol Chem 1986; 261:376–380.

262. Winter GD. Movement of epidermal cells over the wound surface. Adv Biol Skin 1964; 5:113.

263. Wolf SL, Ariel GB, Saar D, et al. The effect of muscle stimulation during resistive training on performance parameters. Am J Sports Med 1986; 14:18–23.

264. Yamanish T, Yasuda K. Electrical stimulation for stress incontinence. Int Urogynecol J Pelvic Floor Dysfunct 1998; 9:281–290.

265. Zupan A, Gregoric M, Valencic V, et al. Effects of electrical stimulation on muscles of children with Duchenne and Becker muscular dystrophy. Neuropediatrics 1993; 24:189–192.

266. Zwiren LD, Bar-Or O. Responses to exercise of paraplegics who differ in conditioning level. Med Sci Sports 1975; 7:94–98.

Chapter

23

Integrative Medicine in Rehabilitation
Ralph E. Gay, Brent A. Bauer and Robert K. Yang

Complementary and alternative medicine (CAM) is a group of diverse medical and healthcare systems, practices, and products that are not presently considered to be part of conventional medicine. These therapies are either complementary to standard medical therapies (used with) or alternative to (used in place of) orthodox treatments. CAM is popular in both North America[41] and Europe. The US National Institutes of Health organized the National Center for Complementary and Alternative Medicine[84] (NCCAM; http://nccam.nih.gov/) in 1998 to advance the study of these therapies.

The term *integrative medicine* is now widely used to describe the practice of combining mainstream medical therapies and CAM therapies for which there is some high-quality scientific evidence of safety and effectiveness.[84] Although many CAM treatments have not been properly studied, there are many that can be safely integrated into physical medicine and rehabilitation practice.

Complementary and alternative medicine therapies have been categorized by NCCAM[84] into the following groups:

- *Alternative medical systems* that are 'built upon complete systems of theory and practice'.
- *Mind–body interventions*, which include 'a variety of techniques designed to enhance the mind's capacity to affect bodily function and symptoms'.
- *Biologically based therapies* that 'use substances found in nature, such as herbs, foods, and vitamins'.
- *Manipulative and body-based therapies*, which are treatment methods 'based on manipulation and/or movement of one or more parts of the body'.
- *Energy therapies*, which involve the use of energy fields and include both biofield therapies and bioelectromagnetic-based therapies.

ALTERNATIVE MEDICAL SYSTEMS

Alternative medical systems often incorporate concepts and ideas that are foreign or antithetic to conventional medicine. They are generally based on empiric observation, and underlying scientific principles often have yet to be verified through well-designed scientific studies. Given the empiric nature of some allopathic and osteopathic treatment, the boundary between CAM and conventional medicine is often indistinct.

Over time, many different schools of thought have developed with regard to optimal practice. As a result, there can be considerable variability between alternative medicine providers. Most systems posit an innate ability of the body to heal itself, and act to stimulate or enhance that natural ability. All the systems discussed in this chapter are holistic, created to treat the entire person rather than a single complaint. Some incorporate elements of cultures that are quite different from our own, and many have an extensive history dating back thousands of years.

Chiropractic

Chiropractic is a profession founded on the theory that minor spinal misalignments can detrimentally affect the neurologic function of spinal nerves and the organs and structures supplied by those nerves (see also Ch. 20). These misalignments are often called *subluxations*. The chiropractic use of the term subluxation is not congruent with the medical definition, which requires partial dislocation of a joint. This disparity not uncommonly leads to confusion between practitioners and patients when discussing a specific condition. Chiropractors treat subluxations with various interventions, the most common being spinal manipulation. Although much is written about subluxations, there is little agreement among chiropractors on how to define, detect, or treat them. Because these proposed lesions cannot be reliably measured or detected (and are therefore difficult to study), their effect on health is unclear. Despite this, there are many randomized, controlled studies of chiropractic treatments for various conditions, particularly musculoskeletal disorders such as back pain and neck pain. Spinal manipulation is considered to be the active intervention in most studies.

Chiropractors often incorporate other techniques, such as massage and exercise prescription, in treatment. They also utilize radiography to aid in diagnosis and treatment. Chiropractors do not dispense prescription medication or perform surgery or invasive treatments. There are approximately 50 000 chiropractors practicing in the USA, and many practicing in developed countries including Australia, the UK, and most northern European countries. A comprehensive report has detailed the chiropractic profession in the USA.[33]

Osteopathy

Osteopathic medicine was founded in the USA in the late 19th century by Dr. Andrew T. Still. The osteopathic philosophy focuses on utilizing the bones as manual levers to remove bony and myofascial entrapment of nerves and vascular structures, thus restoring normal function. These *somatic* dysfunctions within the musculoskeletal system can be addressed through manual manipulation. Today, osteopathic physicians (DOs) and allopathic physicians (MDs) are relatively indistinguishable in that both are fully licensed in all realms of medicine including surgery, obstetrics, and the prescription of medications. There is a small subgroup of osteopaths, however, who continue to use traditional manual therapies to treat disease.

Homeopathy

Homeopathy originated as a medical system in Germany in the late 1700s based on the theories of a physician, Samuel Hahnemann. Immunization against smallpox was being successfully demonstrated at about the same time, and it is likely that the theories of immunology influenced the theories underlying homeopathy. Much of the development of homeopathy occurred in Europe, and culminated in a decision in 1996 by the European Commission's Homeopathy Medicine Research Group to integrate homeopathy into medical practice.

Homeopathy's central tenets are the principle of similars and the principle of dilution. The principle of similars, or 'like begets like', can be found in many systems of magical thought. In application, the idea is that small quantities of an agent can ameliorate the same symptoms that are evoked in a healthy patient when given in larger quantities. For some practitioners, actual determination of the causative agent is as critical as matching the symptoms that are being treated (i.e. the complaint may not have been caused by a bee sting, but the patient is responding just like they were stung). The principle of dilution states that highly dilute solutions have biologic activity and the more dilute the solution, the more potent the remedy. Some remedies are diluted but still possess measurable biologic activity. Others might be diluted to the point that conventional science has difficulty explaining their efficacy (a solution could be so dilute that not every dose contains a single molecule of the active substance). While most of these remedies are safe, their potential for interaction with other ingested substances can be difficult to predict.

Homeopaths typically seek to identify substances or agents that can produce the symptoms that afflict the patient. Many substances are studied and cross-referenced in the homeopathic literature. Computerized tools are available for matching symptoms to a specific remedy to aid the homeopath in the selection of an appropriate remedy. A recent double-blind randomized controlled trial demonstrated benefit from homeopathic treatment of mild traumatic brain injury.[32] While homeopathy is rarely used by physical medicine and rehabilitation practitioners, and these results need to be verified by large-scale independent replication, this study suggests that homeopathic treatments might have a place in the treatment of brain injury.

Naturopathy

Naturopaths use a multimodal approach to health problems. Most of the principles espoused by naturopaths are familiar to physicians: do no harm, identify and treat causes of disease, disease prevention, and treatment of the whole individual. One primary difference is belief in the healing power of nature as demonstrated in the ability of living things to heal themselves. The naturopath views the physician's role as removing obstacles to health and fostering a supportive environment for healthy living. A naturopath might use many different techniques to achieve this objective. They range from the mundane, such as diet and lifestyle counseling, to more unusual modalities such as acupuncture and homeopathy. This openness to diverse approaches to healthcare is integrative and often calls for several different modes of treatment. The profession uses science to help determine which treatments to administer.

Ayurveda

Ayurvedic medicine (literally means 'the science of life') developed in India. Early ayurvedic texts date to 1500 BC. Ayurvedic philosophy describes a relationship between all the matter in the universe. There are three *doshas* (life forces or energies), which must be at equilibrium for good health. Imbalances in these doshas are responsible for disease. Both intrinsic and extrinsic factors can contribute to health problems. There is a very complex taxonomy that categorizes the organization and interaction of matter, energy, and spirit.

Ayurvedic medicine often employs multiple modalities. The ayurvedic concept of physical fitness refers as much to resistance to a hostile environment as to strength and flexibility. Diet, sleep, sexual activity, personal hygiene, and exercises such as yoga are used to increase physical fitness. Mental discipline and spirituality are also important components to maintaining good health. Ayurvedic medicines encompass a gamut of herbal and mineral preparations, and are prescribed based on the energetic qualities of the preparation.

Traditional Chinese medicine

Traditional Chinese medicine (TCM) is a system of healthcare based on traditional Chinese beliefs about the universe. One of the fundamental principles of this system is that two opposite forces (*yin* and *yang*) balance in nature. Disease states reflect a disturbance in the balance of yin and yang that can be extrinsic or intrinsic to the body.

Proper function of the human body requires proper functioning in physical, energetic, and spiritual aspects of an individual. TCM posits energy, called *qi*, that infuses living tissue. Qi is not a homogenous entity, as there are many different types of qi in the body. Each has different functions, from aiding in digestion to protecting against harmful outside agents. These energies support the material substances of the body such as blood and tissues. There is a complex interaction between the different types of qi and the symptoms that disturbances in qi produce.

Disease can manifest in a number of different ways. Sometimes disturbances have a material manifestation altering blood, tissues, or organs. At other times, they manifest as more energetic (qi) symptoms such as fatigue, anxiety, or depression. Diagnosis of disease focuses on eliciting a history to determine the underlying disturbance. The TCM examination might include determining the characteristics of pulses at specific locations on the body, the appearance of the tongue, characteristics of olfaction, and careful palpation of the body. This information aids the TCM practitioner in the diagnosis of an individual's complaint. A diagnosis in TCM (such as ascending fire of the liver or kidney qi deficiency) might have no analog in the allopathic model.

The primary goal of TCM is the restoration of the balance of these forces. This rebalancing can be achieved through a number of different therapeutic options, including diet, exercise, herbal medicines, massage, and acupuncture. While treatments are initiated to treat disease states, they are also designed to preserve health. Qi gong and t'ai chi were developed as methods of strengthening the qi or energy of the body to prevent disease and prolong life. A proper balance in diet promotes the harmonious flow of energy through the body. While acupuncture is the most well-known aspect of TCM, it is only a single aspect of it and is often used in combination with other modalities.

Mind–body therapies

The NCCAM identifies mind–body therapies as those that use 'a variety of techniques designed to enhance the mind's capacity to affect bodily function and symptoms'. Included in this group are such therapies as cognitive behavioral therapy, meditation, prayer, guided imagery, and therapies employing creative outlets (e.g. art, music, and dance therapies).

Cognitive behavioral therapy

Although included as a CAM therapy, cognitive behavioral therapy has moved into the mainstream of conventional practice. It is basically an integration of the cognitive restructuring approach of cognitive therapy, combined with the behavioral modification techniques of behavioral therapy. A therapist typically works with the patient to identify thoughts and behaviors that are maladaptive; and attempts to change the thought patterns, leading to a change in behavior. Cognitive behavioral therapy has been successfully employed for a variety of conditions, including insomnia,[105] fibromyalgia,[112] headache,[3] and pain.[39]

Meditation

The American Heritage Dictionary defines the act of meditation as 'to train, calm, or empty the mind, often by achieving an altered state, as by focusing on a single object'.[5] Meditation is also frequently described as self-regulation of attention. It is perhaps one of the most commonly employed mind–body modalities, and is a significant component in many of the world's major religions. There are numerous types of meditation (e.g. transcendental, mindfulness, and focused meditation). Much of the current interest in meditation can be traced to the 1970s work of Dr. Herbert Benson, who studied the physiologic responses to meditation. It was this early work by Benson that led to the identification of the 'relaxation response'.[19] Most patients employ meditation to help manage stress and anxiety,[15,29,96] although there are numerous specific applications such as helping deal with pain,[11] improving quality of life after

brain injury,[17] and improving irritable bowel syndrome.[60] One study of practitioners of transcendental meditation revealed that, over a span of 5 years, healthcare utilization was significantly reduced.[89]

Guided imagery

This is a technique that employs images or symbols to train the mind to create a physiologic or psychologic effect. This process, often guided by a practitioner or audiotape, has been used to reduce anxiety and pain, and to relieve physical problems caused by stress. Studies suggest it might have benefit in treating headaches,[78] recurrent abdominal pain in children,[13] depression,[103] and fibromyalgia.[46]

Spirituality

Spirituality has been described as an awareness of something greater than the individual self. Some authors have argued against the inclusion of spirituality in the CAM realm, recognizing that spirituality is a part of normal life for the majority of people, regardless of cultural origin. The mind–body–spirit emphasis frequently found in CAM disciplines, however, has usually led to its inclusion in CAM therapy discussions. While spirituality can take many forms, typically it involves prayer, either for one's self or another. It can be pursued alone or in a group (e.g. in a church or synagogue). There are many possible psychologic benefits of spiritual awareness and focus, including reduction of stress and anxiety, and the creation of a positive attitude. Rigorous scientific studies of the effect of spirituality, however, are relatively few. Some studies indicate a positive effect of prayer on illness severity ratings in AIDs patients and a positive effect of church attendance on immune function. One study reported that spirituality can play an important role in rehabilitation.[30]

Aromatherapy

This modality uses *essential oils* distilled from plants to improve mood and/or health. Scents can be inhaled or applied in oil during massage. For inhalation, a few drops of the essential oil are placed in steaming water, diffusers, or humidifiers that are used to spread the steam–oil combination throughout the room. They can be added to bathwater. For application to the skin, the oils are combined with a carrier, usually vegetable oil. Early clinical trials suggest aromatherapy might have some benefit as a complementary treatment in reducing stress, pain, and depression.[28,66]

Expression- or art-based therapies

The American Art Therapy Association defines art therapy as the 'therapeutic use of art making, within a professional relationship, by people who experience illness, trauma, or challenges in living, and by people who seek personal development'.[4] It uses creative activities to help patients with physical and emotional problems. Proponents claim that both the creative process and the final work can help express and heal trauma. Patients can create paintings, drawings, sculptures, and other types of artwork, and can work individually or in groups. Art therapists typically have a master's degree in art therapy or a related field. They help patients express themselves through the art they create. They also discuss emotions and concerns that the patient may identify as they work on their art.

Music therapy is the use of specific music (with specific vibration frequencies) to promote relaxation and healing. Although most healing music is soft and soothing, individual patient preferences (jazz, classical, etc.) can also be relaxing and healing to that individual. Music is used to help patients express deep-set emotions, both positive and negative. It is thought to be helpful in treating autism; mentally or emotionally disturbed children and adults; elderly and physically challenged people; and patients with schizophrenia, nervous disorders, or stress. Music therapists design music sessions for individuals and groups based on individual needs and tastes. Some aspects of music therapy include music improvization, receptive music listening, song writing, lyric discussion, imagery, music performance, and learning through music. Individuals can also perform their own music therapy at home by listening to music or sounds that help relieve their symptoms.[70,111]

Dance therapy is 'the psychotherapeutic use of movement as a process which furthers the emotional, cognitive, social and physical integration of the individual'.[2] It is sometimes also referred to as movement therapy. From a physical standpoint, dance therapy can provide exercise, improve mobility and muscle coordination, and reduce muscle tension. From an emotional standpoint, dance therapy has been reported to improve self-awareness, self-confidence, and interpersonal interaction, and is an outlet for communicating feelings.[56]

Biologically based therapies

Patients undergoing rehabilitative treatment are just as likely to be interested in or using dietary supplements as the rest of the population. In fact, most studies suggest that patients with chronic problems are even more likely to use CAM therapies, including herbs. Therefore it is important to have a basic understanding of herbs and dietary supplements, so that helpful information can be shared with patients to enable them to make informed decisions. Because the possible number of supplements a patient can use is practically endless, this review focuses only on the dietary supplements most likely to be encountered in a physiatry practice. Specific attention is paid to herbs and dietary supplements used for arthritis and pain.

Select dietary supplements frequently encountered in physical medicine and rehabilitation practice
Chondroitin sulfate
Evidence Numerous studies have been conducted on chondroitin, chondroitin and glucosamine, and glucosamine. The majority indicate that these two supplements, either in combination or by themselves, are modestly effective at relieving symptoms of osteoarthritis. Proponents believe that chondroitin acts as a substrate needed for joint matrix structure.[61] If this mechanism is indeed correct, the finding that it could require at least 2–4 months of therapy before significant improvement is noted is not surprising.[73] A number of studies have suggested

that adding chondroitin sulfate to conventional analgesic or non-steroidal antiinflammatory drugs (NSAIDs) is synergistic, possibly allowing reduction or elimination of those agents.[73,82]

Adverse effects Toxicity appears to be very limited. Most commonly reported side effects are generally gastrointestinal in nature, and include nausea and epigastric discomfort.

Glucosamine sulfate
Evidence Studies of efficacy have been centered on knee osteoarthritis. The majority of studies evaluating glucosamine sulfate for knee osteoarthritis have been positive.[80] Glucosamine was found to be effective for osteoarthritis of the lumbar spine in one study.[45] Some studies suggest efficacy equivalent to that of certain NSAIDs.[75] Like chondroitin, onset of relief is generally delayed, requiring up to 8 weeks for full effect. In addition to symptom control efficacy, glucosamine might also have disease-modifying properties. Long-term studies suggest that glucosamine might result in significantly less joint space narrowing and knee joint degeneration than with placebo.[95]

Adverse effects Mild gastrointestinal symptoms (e.g. nausea, heartburn, diarrhea, and constipation) are not uncommon, but are usually self-limited and rarely require discontinuation.

S-adenosyl-l-methionine
Evidence A number of clinical trials have shown that S-adenosyl-L-methionine (SAMe) is superior to placebo and comparable with NSAIDs for decreasing symptoms associated with osteoarthritis.[50,67,83] The full effect might require up to 1 month of treatment. Mechanism of action could include stimulation of articular cartilage growth and repair.[24]

Adverse effects These are gastrointestinal symptoms (e.g. flatulence, nausea, diarrhea, and constipation), dry mouth, headache, mild insomnia, and nervousness.[7]

Bromelain (Ananas comosus)
Evidence In a single study, bromelain taken in conjunction with trypsin and rutin resulted in decreased pain and improved knee function in patients with osteoarthritis.[63]

Adverse effects Gastrointestinal upset and diarrhea can occur in patients taking bromelain.

Camphor (Cinnamomum camphora)
Evidence Camphor is Food and Drug Administration-approved as a topical analgesic. A topical cream containing camphor, glucosamine sulfate, and chondroitin sulfate was found to provide reduction in pain due to osteoarthritis.[36] Because there is no evidence that glucosamine and chondroitin can be absorbed topically, the relief could have been due to the counterirritant effect of camphor.

Adverse effects These are limited to occasional contact irritation.

Cat's claw (Uncaria tomentosa)
Evidence Found in Peru, cat's claw is a large vine with curved thorns resembling the claws of a cat. It is touted as an effective remedy for a number of conditions. In the USA, many patients

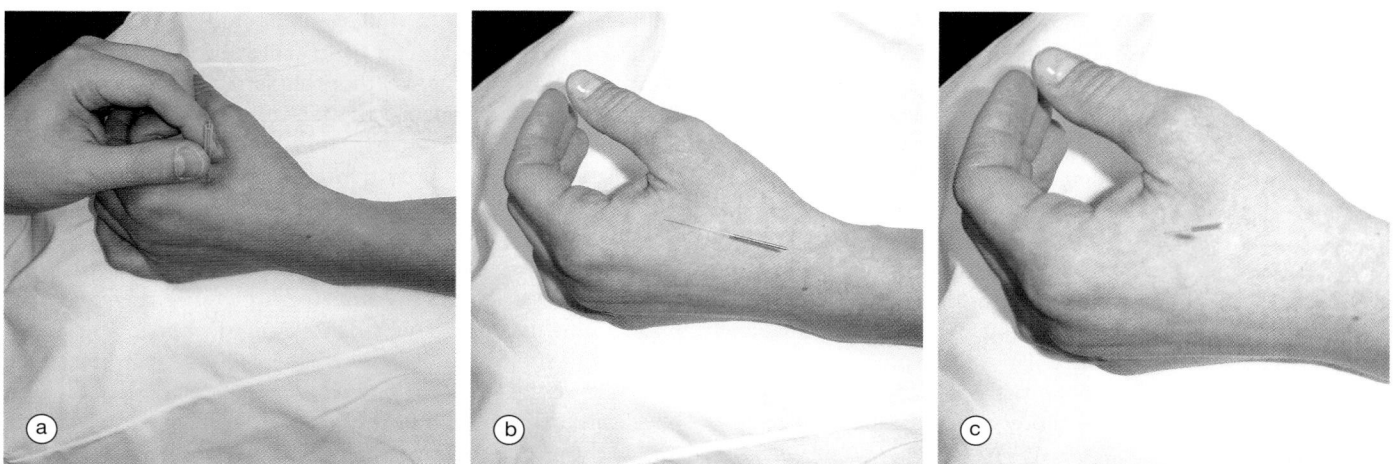

Figure 23-2 (**a**) The acupuncture needle sits in a guide tube on the patient's skin. The length of the needle is slightly longer than the guide tube. The guide tube acts to guide the needle, keep the skin taut, and, when tapped, provide a sensation that distracts from the needle insertion. (**b**) The needle has been tapped into the skin and the guide tube removed. The tip of the needle is subcutaneous but has not reached the muscle. The needle is almost parallel to the skin, as it has not been inserted deeply enough to support its weight. (**c**) The needle tip has been advanced into the first dorsal interosseous muscle. It is now able to stand perpendicular to the skin surface.

> **Box 23-3** Conditions commonly treated by acupuncturists in North America
>
> - Back pain (upper and lower)
> - Neck pain
> - Headaches
> - Perioperative pain
> - Osteoarthritic pain
> - Tennis elbow (lateral epicondylitis)
> - Fibromyalgia and myofascial pain

vidual studies demonstrate significant benefit from acupuncture for multiple conditions, these tend to be small, less rigorous, and sometimes difficult to reproduce. Larger, more rigorous trials typically demonstrate less favorable results. In addition, there is also the question of publication bias, because Asian studies tend to produce more favorable results that those studies performed in the USA. Some of the controversy with acupuncture research is the difficulty of establishing adequate sham acupuncture. There is considerable variability in the design of different studies, and often the precision of the diagnosis is lacking, as patients are classified by symptoms rather than a specific medical diagnosis.

The literature regarding acupuncture safety is quite positive, noting a low rate of complications even among acupuncture students.[6] Risks of acupuncture include bleeding, infection, and organ puncture (including pneumothorax).[71] Needle shock is a side effect that is uncommon but typically occurs during a first acupuncture treatment. The description of this event is similar to a vasovagal episode: sweating, flushing, and the sensation that the world is being seen from down a long tunnel. Treatment of this condition requires immediate removal of the needles. One technique that is particularly prone to cause complications utilizes permanent needles. These needles are inserted and then

the handles are broken off.[34] Unfortunately, these needles can migrate to regions of the body where they might result in damage to internal organs.

Acupuncture is a modality that is safe, but whose efficacy, with a few notable exceptions, still lacks the support of definitive evidence-based trials. There is considerable anecdotal evidence and a large number of clinical trials that support its use. A systematic review suggested that it is helpful for back pain, but better studies are needed.[44] Recently, the Agency for Healthcare Research and Quality issued guidelines regarding the use of acupuncture for osteoarthritis. That report recommended acupuncture as a second-line treatment for osteoarthritis. In general, the use of acupuncture as a second-line treatment has a reasonable place in the treatment algorithm (i.e. after therapies with more evidence have been tried and failed). This practice also lessens the medicolegal risk associated with the prescription of CAM treatments.

Acupressure

Acupressure is similar to acupuncture in terms of its analysis of the human body, but it utilizes pressure rather than needles to achieve changes in the human body. Acupressure is often utilized for many of the same complaints and conditions as acupuncture, and can be used to achieve many of the same effects. Acupressure practitioners might incorporate massage as part of their practice. Japanese shiatsu and Chinese tui na both utilize acupressure principles. Direct manipulation of the tissues is believed to open up channels to the flow of qi. Manual manipulation of the soft tissues, in addition to topical herbal treatments and salves, can be used as well.

Compared with acupuncture, acupressure can be applied differently, which can yield advantages depending on the patient. Most obviously, the potential complications of bleeding and infection are eliminated. This also expands the range of patients who might benefit from this treatment, including individuals on anticoagulants, the needle-phobic, or severely immunosuppressed patients. Acupressure can also be taught to the patient, who can subsequently apply treatment on a more frequent basis. This can be very helpful in the early stages of treatment when the duration of the relief from acupressure might be short-lived. Acupuncture needles are currently classified as class 2 devices by the Food and Drug Administration, limiting their sale to acupuncture practitioners. They cannot be given to patients so they can administer the treatment at home. Acupressure forces a practitioner to treat each individual area sequentially, while acupuncture allows more points to be simultaneously stimulated. This potentially allows a practitioner to determine which points are more effective in achieving the desired effect.

Studies on acupressure are limited, and the evidence is not particularly rigorous at present. There are some limited data to suggest that acupressure can be more effective than either acupuncture or physical therapy.

Reiki and healing touch

Healing touch and reiki are both energy-based methods of healing. They both posit the ability of one human being to positively influence the energy field of another individual to improve their health. This energy influence or transfer is also an intelligent one, as the specifics of this energy manipulation are automatic for the most part. Healing touch does require some specific hand positions for certain conditions, but this is not always necessary. Both disciplines also advance the practice of healing at a distance, as close physical contact is not always required to affect health.

A number of investigational protocols are currently being conducted by the National Institutes of Health in conjunction with reiki and healing touch. Completed studies suggest that both of these modalities can be effective in reducing psychologic sequelae of disease, as well as speeding healing. Methodological flaws and biases make it difficult to draw significant conclusions from the data, but there was sufficient noted positive treatment effect to merit further study.[12]

Reflexology

This is a natural healing art, based on the theory that there are reflexes in the feet and hands which correspond to every part of the body. Reflexology relies on the concept of a microsystem, with the entire body mapped out on a smaller part of the brain. This concept is seen in conventional medicine, such as the topographic mapping of the somatosenory cortex in the brain. Pressure can be applied to specific parts of the hands and feet to influence the parts of the body being treated.

Research on reflexology has produced mixed results. As with many of the other treatments listed above, methodological flaws are prevalent in a large number of studies. Large-scale systematic studies are not available to help interpret the conflicting data. Smaller scale studies suggest that it is helpful for certain conditions. One recent study found significant improvement in spasticity, paresthesias, and urinary symptoms of mul-

tiple sclerosis patients,[102] while another study found that it was not helpful in the treatment of irritable bowel syndrome.[107] It is difficult to determine whether this variability is secondary to reflexology's effectiveness, variation in how reflexology is practiced, or study design. Most studies call for further large-scale systematic studies to verify the findings.

Electromagnetic fields and magnets

Unlike the energy therapies discussed above, where many of the fields defy scientific attempts to characterize them, electromagnetic fields are very well-defined physical phenomena that are widely used in ubiquitous technologies. Electromagnetic fields are very familiar to physical medicine and rehabilitation physicians and are used in testing, such as magnetic resonance imaging scans, electromyography, and electrocardiograms.

The human body is composed of multiple structures and molecules that are highly charged, and therefore particularly sensitive to strong magnetic fields. Magnets are commonly used in the relief of pain. They are used in varying field strengths and polarity. While the theoretic framework is in place, potential clinical effects of magnetic therapy have not yet been substantiated. The data from trials on this modality are mixed, with the majority not reporting significant improvement in the condition being studied. The studies in peer-reviewed literature are generally those for limited treatment effect for specific conditions such as rotator cuff conditions[20,72] rather than for a general class of conditions. Recent radomized controlled trials showed that magnetic insoles had no significant beneficial effect in the treatment of plantar heel pain and nonspecific foot pain.[113a,113b]

In summary, the biofield CAM treatments are safe, but systematic studies regarding their efficacy are lacking, with a few notable exceptions. This would suggest that these modalities would be appropriate only as second-line therapies to be used when proven or better studied treatments have not been shown to be efficacious.

HOW TO DISCUSS INTEGRATIVE MEDICINE WITH YOUR PATIENT

Many physicians and other caregivers feel challenged by CAM topics when dealing with patients. Many physicians whose training occurred prior to the boom in interest in CAM can feel inadequately trained or educated to make sound recommendations in regard to the use or avoidance of such complicated supplements and/or interventions. At the same time, many patients feel that they have been dismissed in the past when they have raised questions regarding CAM or integrative medicine. As a result, they become 'gun-shy' about asking such questions of their current physician. Surveys have also shown that patients frequently consider therapies such as herbs 'natural', and therefore not of interest to or worth discussing with their physicians. Sometimes, it is not a matter of patients withholding information so much as it is simply a lack of recognition of the importance the usage of herbs can have in their healthcare. Either way, both physicians and patients need to

Table 23-1 Herb, dietary supplement, and complementary and alternative medicine information on the World Wide Web (selected references)

Database	URL	Cost per year	Comment(s)
Natural Medicines Comprehensive Database	http://www.naturaldatabase.com	$92	Very comprehensive (herbs and dietary supplements only) Up to date Well referenced Good patient handouts
Natural Standard	http://www.naturalstandard.com	$99	Moderately to very comprehensive (herbs, dietary supplements, and therapies) Up to date Well referenced Excellent patient handouts
Herbmed	http://www.herbmed.org	Free	Moderately comprehensive (herbs and dietary supplements only) Well referenced Not as intuitive to navigate as above databases
M.D. Anderson Complementary/ Integrative Medicine	http://www.mdanderson.org/departments/CIMER	Free	Moderately comprehensive (herbs, dietary supplements, and therapies) Cancer-specific Well referenced
Memorial Sloan-Kettering Cancer Center Integrative Medicine Service Herb and Botanical Information	http://www.mskcc.org/mskcc/html/11570.cfm	Free	Small database (herbs and dietary supplements only) Cancer-specific Brief monographs
MayoClinic.com	http://www.mayoclinic.com	Free	Small database (herbs, dietary supplements, and therapies) Patient-friendly language Not referenced
General information National Institutes of Health	http://www.healthfinder.gov/	Free	Guide to reliable consumer health information
National Center for Complementary and Alternative Medicine	http://nccam.nih.gov	Free	Growing number of articles and references Many links to other quality sites
National Cancer Institute	http://www.cancer.gov/cancerinfo	Free	Moderately comprehensive (herbs, dietary supplements, and therapies)
American Cancer Society	http://www.cancer.org	Free	Moderately comprehensive (herbs, dietary supplements, and therapies)
PubMed	http://www.ncbi.nlm.nih.gov/PubMed	Free	Can limit searches to articles that are identified as having a complementary medicine theme
Quackwatch	http://www.quackwatch.org	Free	Non-profit corporation whose purpose is to 'combat health-related frauds, myths, fads, and fallacies'
Herb quality information ConsumerLab.com	http://www.consumerlab.com	$24	Provides independent test results on many dietary supplements Products that pass testing can display the ConsumerLab seal of approval
Consumer Reports	http://www.consumerreports.org	$24	Occasional articles on herbs and dietary supplements

Continued on page 518

Continued from page 517 Table 23-1 Herb, dietary supplement, and complementary and alternative medicine information on the World Wide Web (selected references)			
Database	URL	Cost per year	Comment(s)
United States Pharmacopeia (USP)	http://www.usp.org	Free	Discusses the Dietary Supplement Verification Program and the meaning of the USP label
Internet information quality			
American Medical Association	http://www.ama-assn.org/ama/pub/category/1905.html	Free	Guidelines for medical and health information sites on the Internet
Health on the Net Foundation	http://www.hon.ch	Free	Promotes guidelines that create a 'code of conduct' for web sites delivering medical information
Regulatory information			
Food and Drug Administration	http://www.cfsan.fda.gov/~dms/supplmnt.html	Free	Nice background on the Dietary Supplement Health and Education Act and current regulatory environment in USA Recent adverse events associated with dietary supplements reported here
Federal Trade Commission	http://www.ftc.gov	Free	Reviews regulations regarding advertising dietary supplements Link to file complaints
Trade or professional information			
American Academy of Medical Acupuncture	http://www.medicalacupuncture.com	Free	The largest national physician acupuncturist organization
National Certification Commission for Acupuncture and Oriental Medicine	http://www.nccaom.org	Free	Accrediting body for acupuncture, eastern medicine, herbology, and Asian body work therapy
National Center for Homeopathy (NCH)	http://www.homeopathic.com	Free	Introduction, links to resources, training, and guide to NCH members
National Ayurvedic Medical Association	http://www.ayurveda-nama.org	Free	National organization Links to annual meeting
Canadian Chiropractic Association	http://www.ccachiro.org	Free	National association with many links, including a searchable association journal index
American Chiropractic Association	http://www.amerchiro.org	Free	Largest chiropractic association in the USA Includes publications and patient information regarding chiropractic

make a concerted effort at discussing integrative medicine approaches as part of the usual physician–patient encounter.

Perhaps one of the most important first steps in discussing integrative medicine with a patient is to simply incorporate questions regarding integrative medicine into the usual routine of the patient interview. In most medical settings, inquiry is made regarding the usage of medications. This simple non-judgmental question can be expanded easily by enquiring regarding the use of herbs, dietary supplements, medicinal teas, megadoses of vitamins, or other supplements. By asking the question simultaneously with enquiries regarding medication use, patients are shown that these other substances are important and are of interest to their medical provider. If asked in a non-judgmental tone, it typically allows patients to be forth-

coming and to share their interests in and/or usage of such therapies openly and freely.

Some physicians find that this is a natural point to also ask about other modalities or therapies that the patient might be employing. This can also be done in a non-judgmental fashion by simply asking, in the context of herbs and other dietary supplements, whether the patient is using any other techniques or therapies to help improve their health or deal with any ongoing issues. The physician can then list a few common examples of things that patients might do, such as taking meditation, seeing a chiropractor, or receiving massage therapy on a periodic basis. By specifying a few concrete examples, the patient can see that this is an important topic and one that the physician is willing to discuss.

The obvious challenge in this setting is for the physician who has not had significant training in integrative medicine or CAM to know how to respond when the patient does reply in the affirmative that they are using or employing integrative medicine approaches. For dietary supplements, there is a wealth of reliable web sites that can be employed. Many institutions now employ physicians or pharmacists who have received extra training in dietary supplements, and their risks and potential benefits, and who can be an excellent resource. To find information regarding specific therapies, again, many online sources are of particular help (Table 23-1).

The goal of discussion regarding integrative medicine with a patient is to allow an opportunity for the education of the patient. This is a critically important goal, as much of the information the patients are otherwise exposed to is commercial in intent and fraught with misinformation. The physician can fulfill a classic role of healers throughout the centuries, that of a teacher, by providing a safe place for the patient to come and seek information about these therapies. By providing the patient with evidence-based, reliable information regarding both the risks and benefits of a possible therapy, and by collaborating with the patient and being a source of evidence-based information, the clinician can be a significant ally to the patient trying to navigate this complex realm of integrative medicine.

REFERENCES

1. Aker PD, Gross AR, Goldsmith CH, et al. Conservative management of mechanical neck pain: systematic overview and meta-analysis. Br Med J 1996; 313:1291–1296.

2. American Dance Therapy Association. About us. Online. Available: http://www.adta.org/about/index.cfm

3. Andrasik F. Behavioral treatment approaches to chronic headache. Neurol Sci 2003; 24(suppl 2):S80–S85.

4. [Anonymous]. About art therapy (American Art Therapy Association). Available: http://www.arttherapy.org/aboutarttherapy/about.htm 28 Jun 2005.

5. [Anonymous]. American Heritage dictionary of the English language. Boston: Houghton Mifflin; 2000.

6. [Anonymous]. NIH consensus conference. Acupuncture. JAMA 1518; 280:1518–1524.

7. [Anonymous]. SAMe for depression. Med Lett 1999; 41:107–108.

8. Assendelft WJ, Morton SC, Yu EI, et al. Spinal manipulative therapy for low back pain. A meta-analysis of effectiveness relative to other therapies. Ann Intern Med 2003; 138:871–881.

9. Assendelft WJJ, Bouter LM, Knipschild PG. Complications of spinal manipulation. J Fam Pract 1996; 42:475–480.

10. Assendelft WJJ, Koes BW, Knipschild PG, et al. The relationship between methodological quality and conclusions in reviews of spinal manipulation. JAMA 1995; 274:1942–1948.

11. Astin J. Mind–body therapies for the management of pain. Clin J Pain 2004; 20:27–32.

12. Astin JA, Harkness E, Ernst E. The efficacy of 'distant healing': a systematic review of randomized trials. Ann Intern Med 2000; 132:903–910.

13. Ball T, Shapiro D, Monheim C, et al. A pilot study of the use of guided imagery for the treatment of recurrent abdominal pain in children. Clin Pediatr 2003; 42:527–532.

14. Balon J, Aker PD, Crowther ER, et al. A comparison of active and simulated chiropractic manipulation as adjunctive treatment for childhood asthma. N Engl J Med 1998; 339:1013–1020.

15. Barrows K, Jacobs B. Mind–body medicine. An introduction and review of the literature. Med Clin North Am 2002; 86:11–31.

16. Barton JW, Margolis MT. Rotational obstruction of the vertebral artery at the atlantoaxial joint. Neuroradiology 1975; 9:117–120.

17. Bedard M, Felteau M, Mazmanian D, et al. Pilot evaluation of a mindfulness-based intervention to improve quality of life among individuals who sustained traumatic brain injuries. Disabil Rehabil 2003; 25:722–731.

18. Belch J, Ansell D, Madhok R, et al. Effects of altering dietary essential fatty acids on requirements for non-steroidal anti-inflammatory drugs in patients with rheumatoid arthritis: a double blind placebo controlled study. Ann Rheum Dis 1988; 47:96–104.

19. Benson H, Beary J, Carol M. The relaxation response. Psychiatry 1974; 37:37–46.

20. Binder A, Parr G, Hazleman B, et al. Pulsed electromagnetic field therapy of persistent rotator cuff tendinitis. A double-blind controlled assessment. Lancet 1984; 1:695–698.

21. Bogduk N, Marsland A. On the concept of the third occipital headache. J Neurol Neurosurg Psychiatry 1986; 49:775–780.

22. Bogduk N. Cervical causes of headache and dizziness. In: Grieve GP, ed. Modern manual therapy of the vertebral column. Edinburgh: Churchill Livingstone; 1986:289–302.

23. Boline PD, Kassak K, Bronfort G, et al. Spinal manipulation vs. amitriptyline for the treatment of chronic tension-type headaches: a randomized clinical trial [see comments]. J Manipulative Physiol Ther 1995; 18: 148–154.

24. Bottiglieri T. S-Adenosyl-L-methionine (SAMe): from the bench to the bedside—molecular basis of a pleiotrophic molecule. Am J Clin Nutr 2002; 76:1151S–1157S.

25. Bove G, Nilsson N. Spinal manipulation in the treatment of episodic tension-type headache: a randomized controlled trial. JAMA 1998; 280:1576–1579.

26. Bovim G, Berg R, Dale LG. Cervicogenic headache: anesthetic blockades of cervical nerves (C2–C5) and facet joints (C2/C3). Pain 1992; 49: 315–320.

27. Browning JE. Pelvic pain and organic dysfunction in a patient with low back pain: response to distractive manipulation: a case presentation. J Manipulative Physiol Ther 1987; 10:116–121.

28. Buckle J. Use of aromatherapy as a complementary treatment for chronic pain. Altern Ther Health Med 1999; 5:42–51.

29. Carlson L, Ursuliak Z, Goodey E, et al. The effects of a mindfulness meditation-based stress reduction program on mood and symptoms of stress in cancer outpatients: 6-month follow-up. Support Care Cancer 2001; 9:112–123.

30. Chally P, Carlson J. Spirituality, rehabilitation, and aging: a literature review. Arch Phys Med Rehabil 2004; 85:S60–S65.

31. Chantre P, Cappelaere A, Leblan D, et al. Efficacy and tolerance of *Harpagophytum procumbens* versus diacerhein in treatment of osteoarthritis. Phytomedicine 2000; 7:177–183.

32. Chapman EH, Weintraub RJ, Milburn MA, et al. Homeopathic treatment of mild traumatic brain injury: a randomized, double-blind, placebo-controlled clinical trial. J Head Trauma Rehabil 1999; 14: 521–542.

33. Cherkin DC, Phillips RB, Mootz R, et al. Chiropractic in the United States: training, practice, and research. Rockville: Agency for Health Care Policy and Research; 1997.

34. Chiu ES, Austin JH. Images in clinical medicine. Acupuncture-needle fragments. N Engl J Med 1995; 332:2.

35. Chrubasik S, Thanner J, Kunzel O, et al. Comparison of outcome measures during treatment with the proprietary *Harpagophytum* extract doloteffin in patients with pain in the lower back, knee or hip. Phytomedicine 2002; 9:181–194.

36. Cohen M, Wolfe R, Mai T, et al. A randomized, double blind, placebo controlled trial of a topical cream containing glucosamine sulfate, chondroitin sulfate, and camphor for osteoarthritis of the knee. J Rheumatol 2003; 30:523–528.

37. Cote P, Kreitz BG, Cassidy JD, et al. The validity of the extension-rotation test as a clinical screening procedure before neck manipulation: a secondary analysis. J Manipulative Physiol Ther 1996; 19:159–164.

38. Davis P, Hulbert JR, Kassak KM, et al. Comparative efficacy of conservative medical and chiropractic treatments for carpal tunnel syndrome: a randomized clinical trial. J Manipulative Physiol Ther 1998; 21: 317–326.

39. Devine E. Meta-analysis of the effect of psychoeducational interventions on pain in adults with cancer. Oncol Nurs Forum 2003; 30:75–89.

40. Dvorak J, Orelli F. How dangerous is manipulation to the cervical spine? Manual Med 1985; 2:1–4.

41. Eisenberg DM, Davis RB, Ettner SL, et al. Trends in alternative medicine use in the United States, 1990–1997: results of a follow-up national survey. JAMA 1998; 280:1569–1575.

42. Eisenberg DM, Kessler RC, Foster C, et al. Unconventional medicine in the United States. Prevalence, costs, and patterns of use. N Engl J Med 1993; 328:246–252.

43. Ernst E, ed. The desktop guide to complementary and alternative medicine. 1st edn. London: Mosby; 2001.

44. Ernst E, White AR. Acupuncture for back pain: a meta-analysis of randomized controlled trials. Arch Intern Med 1998; 158: 2235–2241.

45. Foerster KK, Schmid K, Rovati LC. Efficacy of glucosamine sulfate in osteoarthritis of the lumbar spine: a placebo controlled, randomized, double-blind study. American College of Rheumatology 64th Annual Scientific Meeting, Philadelphia, 2000.

46. Fors E, Sexton H, Gotestam K. The effect of guided imagery and amitriptyline on daily fibromyalgia pain: a prospective, randomized, controlled trial. J Psychiatr Res 2002; 36:179–187.

47. Frumkin LR, Baloh RW. Wallenberg's syndrome following neck manipulation. Neurology 1990; 40:611–615.

48. Garfinkel M, Schumacher H, Husain A, et al. Evaluation of a yoga based regimen for treatment of osteoarthritis of the hands. J Rheumatol 1994; 21:2341–2343.

49. Garfinkel MS, Singhal A, Katz WA, et al. Yoga-based intervention for carpal tunnel syndrome: a randomized trial. JAMA 1998; 280: 1601–1603.

50. Glorioso S, Todesco S, Mazzi A, et al. Double-blind multicentre study of the activity of S-adenosylmethionine in hip and knee osteoarthritis. Int J Clin Pharmacol Res 1985; 5:39–49.

51. Hack GD, Koritzer RT, Robinson WL, et al. Anatomic relation between the rectus capitis posterior minor muscle and the dura mater. Spine 1995; 20:2484–2486.

52. Haldeman S, Chapman-Smith D, Petersen DM, eds. Guidelines for chiropractic quality assurance and practice parameters. Proceedings of the Mercy Center Consensus Conference, Gaithersburg, 1992.

53. Haldeman S, Kohlbeck FJ, McGregor M. Risk factors and precipitating neck movements causing vertebrobasilar artery dissection after cervical trauma and spinal manipulation. Spine 1999; 24:785–794.

54. Haldeman S, Rubinstein SM. Cauda equina syndrome in patients undergoing manipulation of the lumbar spine. Spine 1992; 17: 1469–1473.

55. Han A, Robinson V, Judd M, et al. Tai chi for treating rheumatoid arthritis. Cochrane Database Syst Rev 2004:CD004849.

56. Hanna J. The power of dance: health and healing. J Altern Complement Med 1995; 1:323–331.

57. Hart RG. Vertebral artery dissection. Neurology 1988; 38:987–989.

58. Hurwitz EL, Aker PD, Adams AH, et al. Manipulation and mobilization of the cervical spine. A systematic review of the literature. Spine 1996; 21:1746–1759.

59. Ives JC, Shelley GA. The Feldenkrais method in rehabilitation: a review. Work 1998; 11:75–90.

60. Keefer L, Blanchard E. A one year follow-up of relaxation response meditation as a treatment for irritable bowel syndrome. Behav Res Ther 2002; 40:541–546.

61. Kelly G. The role of glucosamine sulfate and chondroitin sulfates in the treatment of degenerative joint disease. Altern Med Rev 1998; 3:27–39.

62. Kjellman GV, Skargren EI, Oberg BE. A critical analysis of randomised clinical trials on neck pain and treatment efficacy. A review of the literature. Scand J Rehabil Med 1999; 31:139–152.

63. Klein G, Kullich W. Short-term treatment of painful osteoarthritis of the knee with oral enzymes. Clin Drug Invest 2000; 19:15–23.

64. Klougart N, Leboeuf-Yde C, Rasmussen LR. Safety in chiropractic practice. Part II: Treatment to the upper neck and the rate of cerebrovascular incidents. J Manipulative Physiol Ther 1996; 19:563–569.

65. Kokjohn K, Schmid DM, Triano JJ, et al. The effect of spinal manipulation on pain and prostaglandin levels in women with primary dysmenorrhea. J Manipulative Physiol Ther 1992; 15:279–285.

66. Komori T, Fujiwara R, Tanida M, et al. Effects of citrus fragrance on immune function and depressive states. Neuroimmunomodulation 1995; 2:174–180.

67. Konig B. A long-term (two years) clinical trial with S-adenosylmethionine for the treatment of osteoarthritis. Am J Med 1987; 83:89–94.

68. Kreitz BG, Aker PD. Nocturnal enuresis; treatment implications for the chiropractor. J Manipulative Physiol Ther 1994; 17:465–473.

69. Krueger B, Okazaki H. Vertebal-basilar distribution infarction following chiropractic cervical manipulation. Mayo Clin Proc 1980; 55:322–332.

70. Lane D. Music therapy: gaining an edge in oncology management. J Oncol Manage 1993:42–46.

71. Lao L, Hamilton GR, Fu J, et al. Is acupuncture safe? A systematic review of case reports. Altern Ther Health Med 2003; 9:72–83.

72. Leclaire R, Bourgouin J. Electromagnetic treatment of shoulder periarthritis: a randomized controlled trial of the efficiency and tolerance of magnetotherapy. Arch Phys Med Rehabil 1991; 72:284–287.

73. Leeb B, Schweitzer H, Montag K, et al. A metaanalysis of chondroitin sulfate in the treatment of osteoarthritis. J Rheumatol 2000; 27:205–211.

74. Liebl NA, Butler LM. A chiropractic approach to the treatment of dysmenorrhea. J Manipulative Physiol Ther 1990; 13:101–106.

75. Lopes Vaz A. Double-blind clinical evaluation of the relative efficacy of ibuprofen and glucosamine sulphate in the management of osteoarthrosis of the knee in out-patients. Curr Med Res Opin 1982; 8:145–149.

76. Lundblad I, Elert J, Gerdle B. Randomized controlled trial of physiotherapy and Feldenkrais interventions in female workers with neck-shoulder complaints. J Occup Rehabil 1999; 9:179–194.

77. Malmgren-Olsson E, Branholm I. A comparison between three physiotherapy approaches with regard to health-related factors in patients with non-specific musculoskeletal disorders. Disabil Rehabil 2002; 24:308–317.

78. Mannix L, Chandurkar R, Rybicki L, et al. Effect of guided imagery on quality of life for patients with chronic tension-type headache. Headache 1999; 39:326–334.

79. Manocha R, Marks GB, Kenchington P, et al. Sahaja yoga in the management of moderate to severe asthma: a randomised controlled trial. Thorax 2002; 57:110–115.

80. McAlindon TE, LaValley MP, Felson DT. Efficacy of glucosamine and chondroitin for treatment of osteoarthritis. JAMA 2000; 284:1241.

81. Mierau D, Cassidy JD, McGregor M, et al. A comparison of the effectiveness of spinal manipulative therapy for low back pain patients with and without spondylolisthesis. J Manipulative Physiol Ther 1987; 10: 49–55.

82. Morreale P, Manopulo R, Galati M, et al. Comparison of the antiinflammatory efficacy of chondroitin sulfate and diclofenac sodium in patients with knee osteoarthritis. J Rheumatol 1996; 23:1385–1391.

83. Najm W, Reinsch S, Hoehler F, et al. S-adenosyl methionine (SAMe) versus celecoxib for the treatment of osteoarthritis symptoms: a double-blind cross-over trial. BMC Musculoskelet Disord 2004; 5:6.

84. National Center for Complementary and Alternative Medicine. What is complementary and alternative medicine (CAM)? Bethesda: National Institutes of Health–NCCAM; 2002.

85. Nelson CF, Bronfort G, Evans R, et al. The efficacy of spinal manipulation, amitriptyline and the combination of both therapies for the prophylaxis of migraine headache. J Manipulative Physiol Ther 1998; 21:511–519.

86. Nielsen NH, Bronfort G, Bendix T, et al. Chronic asthma and chiropractic spinal manipulation: a randomized clinical trial. Clin Exp Allergy 1995; 25:80–88.

87. Nilsson N, Christensen HW, Hartvigsen J. The effect of spinal manipulation in the treatment of cervicogenic headache. J Manipulative Physiol Ther 1997; 20:326–330.

88. Nykoliation JW, Cassidy JD, Arthur BE, et al. An algorithm for the management of scoliosis. J Manipulative Physiol Ther 1986; 9:1–14.

89. Orme-Johnson D. Medical care utilization and the transcendental meditation program. Psychosom Med 1987; 49:493–507.

90. Parker GB, Tupling H, Pryor DS. A controlled trial of cervical manipulation of migraine. Aust NZ J Med 1978; 8:589–593.

91. Patel C, North W. Randomised controlled trial of yoga and bio-feedback in management of hypertension. Lancet 1975; 2:93–95.

92. Piscoya J, Rodriguez Z, Bustamante S, et al. Efficacy and safety of freeze-dried cat's claw in osteoarthritis of the knee: mechanisms of action of the species *Uncaria guianensis*. Inflamm Res 2001; 50:442–448.

93. Plaugher G, Cremata EE, Phillips RB. A retrospective consecutive case analysis of pretreatment and comparative static radiological parameters following chiropractic adjustments. J Manipulative Physiol Ther 1990; 13:498–506.

94. Powell FC, Hanigan WC, Olivero WC. A risk/benefit analysis of spinal manipulation therapy for relief of lumbar or cervical pain. Neurosurgery 1993; 33:73-78; discussion 8–9.

95. Reginster J, Deroisy R, Rovati L, et al. Long-term effects of glucosamine sulphate on osteoarthritis progression: a randomised, placebo-controlled clinical trial. Lancet 2001; 357:251–256.

96. Reibel D, Greeson J, Brainard G, et al. Mindfulness-based stress reduction and health-related quality of life in a heterogeneous patient population. Gen Hosp Psychiatry 2001; 23:183–192.

97. Rosenstein E. Topical agents in the treatment of rheumatic disorders. Rheum Dis Clin North Am 1999; 25:899–918.

98. Senstad O, Leboeuf-Yde C, Borchgrevink CF. Side-effects of chiropractic spinal manipulation: types, frequency, discomfort and course. Scand J Prim Health Care 1996; 14:50–53.

99. Shekelle PG, Adams AH, Chassin MR, et al. Spinal manipulation for back pain. Ann Intern Med 1992; 117:590–598.

100. Shekelle PG, Coulter I. Cervical spine manipulation: summary report of a systematic review of the literature and a multidisciplinary expert panel. J Spinal Disord 1997; 10:223–228.

101. Shekelle PG. What role for chiropractic in health care? N Engl J Med 1998; 339:1074–1075.

102. Siev-Ner I, Gamus D, Lerner-Geva L, et al. Reflexology treatment relieves symptoms of multiple sclerosis: a randomized controlled study. Mult Scler 2003; 9:356–361.

103. Sloman R. Relaxation and imagery for anxiety and depression control in community patients with advanced cancer. Cancer Nurs 2002; 25:432–435.

104. Smith AL, Kolt GS, McConville JC. The effect of the Feldenkrais method on pain and anxiety in people experiencing chronic low back pain. NZ J Physiother 2001; 29:6–14.

105. Smith M, Neubauer D. Cognitive behavior therapy for chronic insomnia. Clin Cornerstone 2003; 5:28–40.

106. Tarola GA. Manipulation for the control of back pain and curve progression in patients with skeletally mature idiopathic scoliosis: two cases. J Manipulative Physiol Ther 1994; 17:253–257.

107. Tovey P. A single-blind trial of reflexology for irritable bowel syndrome. Br J Gen Pract 2002; 52:19–23.

108. Trice J, Pinals R. Dimethyl sulfoxide: a review of its use in the rheumatic disorders. Semin Arthritis Rheum 1985; 15:45–60.

109. Valente R, Gibson H. Chiropractic manipulation in carpal tunnel syndrome. J Manipulative Physiol Ther 1994; 17:246–249.

110. Wang C, Collet JP, Lau J. The effect of tai chi on health outcomes in patients with chronic conditions: a systematic review. Arch Intern Med 2004; 164:493–501.

111. Watkins G. Music therapy: proposed physiological mechanisms and clinical implications. Clin Nurse Spec 1997; 11:43–50.

112. Williams D. Psychological and behavioural therapies in fibromyalgia and related syndromes. Best Pract Res Clin Rheumatol 2003; 17:649–665.

113. Williams H, Furst D, Dahl S, et al. Double-blind, multicenter controlled trial comparing topical dimethyl sulfoxide and normal saline for treatment of hand ulcers in patients with systemic sclerosis. Arthritis Rheum 1985; 28:308–314.

113a. Winemiller MH, Billow RG, Laskowski ER, et al. Effect of magnetic vs sham-magnetic insoles on plantar heel pain: a randomized controlled trial. JAMA 2003; 290:1474–1478.

113b. Winemiller MH, Billow RG, Laskowski ER, et al. Effect of magnetic vs sham-magnetic insoles on nonspecific foot pain in the workplace: a randomized, double-blind, placebo-controlled trial. Mayo Clin Proc 2005; 80:1138–1345.

114. Wu G. Evaluation of the effectiveness of tai chi for improving balance and preventing falls in the older population—a review. J Am Geriatr Soc 2002; 50:746–754.

115. Zwick D, Rochelle A, Choksi A, et al. Evaluation and treatment of balance in the elderly: a review of the efficacy of the Berg balance test and tai chi quan. NeuroRehabilitation 2000; 15:49–56.

Chapter

24

The Role of Assistive Technology in Rehabilitation
Cathy Bodine and Mary Ellen Buning

CHAPTER OVERVIEW

This chapter provides an overview of assistive technology (AT) devices and services for people with communication disorders, impaired mobility, hearing and visual impairments, and cognitive or learning disabilities. It also describes the selection of appropriate technology and training in its use, suggests ways to avoid the abandonment of AT by clients and caregivers, and discusses the principles of clinical assessment and physician responsibility. Finally, it briefly discusses the future in terms of research and development and the application of emerging technologies to the needs of people with disabilities.

DEFINING ASSISTIVE TECHNOLOGY

The term *assistive technology* is fairly new, although history records the use of tools to enable people with disabilities to walk, eat, and see as far back as the sixth or seventh century BC.[19] Public Law 100-407 currently defines AT as:

> Any item, piece of equipment or product system whether acquired commercially off the shelf, modified, or customized that is used to increase or improve functional capabilities of individuals with disabilities.

This definition also includes a second component defining AT services as 'any service that directly assists an individual with a disability in the selection, acquisition or use of an AT device'. Public Law 100-407 specifies the following.[2]

- Evaluating individuals with disabilities in terms of their goals, needs, and functional abilities in their customary environments.
- Purchasing, leasing, or otherwise providing for the acquisition of AT by persons with disabilities.
- Selecting, designing, fitting, customizing, adapting, applying, retaining, repairing, or replacing AT devices.
- Coordinating and using other therapies, interventions, or services with AT devices, such as those associated with existing education and rehabilitation plans and programs.
- Training or technical assistance for persons with disabilities or, if appropriate, their families.
- Training or technical assistance for professionals (including individuals providing education or rehabilitation services),

employers, or other individuals who provide services to, employ, or are otherwise substantially involved in the major life functions of children with disabilities.

This definition has also been used since 1988 in other federal legislation that authorizes services or supports for persons with disabilities. The Individuals with Disabilities Education Act (IDEA)[3] and Reauthorization of the Rehabilitation Act[1,5] are both examples of legislation that further codify Public Law 100-407.

HISTORY, LEGISLATION, AND UTILIZATION OF ASSISTIVE TECHNOLOGY

Education: the Individuals with Disabilities Education Act (IDEA)

Passed in 1997, IDEA strengthens academic expectations and accountability for the nation's 5.8 million children with disabilities. One important impact of IDEA legislation is that it specifies that AT devices and services are to be provided to children from birth to age 21 to facilitate education in a regular classroom, if such devices and services are required as part of the student's special education, related services, or supplementary aids and services (34CFR 300.308) (Box 24-1). For students with disabilities, AT supports their acquisition of a free and appropriate public education. All individualized education plans developed for children needing special education services must indicate that AT has been considered as a way 'to provide meaningful access to the general curriculum'.[3] AT devices and services included as a component of an individualized education plan must also be provided at no cost to the student or parents. The school can use other public and private sources that are available to fund the AT (34CFR).

Part C of IDEA also includes children before they start school. It covers the needs of children as soon as their developmental differences are noted. It intends that infants and toddlers receive services in natural settings, for example in their home or in other places such as preschool settings, where possible. The services provided for these children are described in individualized family service plans. Individualized family service plans include parents, extended family, early childhood interventionists, and other related services personnel in planning and identifying the goals and necessary services. IDEA also

> **Box 24-1** Summary of the Individuals with Disabilities Education Act assistive technology requirements[3]
>
> - Assistive technology (AT) must be provided by the school district at no cost to the family.
> - Assistive technology must be determined on a case by case basis; if needed to ensure access to free and appropriate public education, AT is required.
> - If the individualized education plan team determines that AT is needed for home use to ensure free and appropriate public education, it must be provided.
> - The student's individualized education plan must reflect the nature of the AT and the amount of supportive AT services required.
> - A parent is accorded an extensive set of procedural safeguards, including the provision of AT to the child.

recognizes that coordination is needed to help families and children with the transition from infant and toddler programs to preschool programs. As a result, students with disabilities are being educated in preschool settings along with typically developing children in an effort to help all children reach the same developmental milestones.

The American with Disabilities Act and the Reauthorization of the Rehabilitation Act

The American with Disabilities Act passed in 1990 clarified the civil rights of persons with disabilities, and specified equal access to public places, employment, transportation, and telecommunications.[39,40] The American with Disabilities Act built on the foundation of the Rehabilitation Act of 1973 (updated in 2003 as the Reauthorization of the Rehabilitation Act) in recognizing the role of employment in enabling individuals with disabilities to become economically self-sufficient and integrated into communities.[4,40]

Vocational rehabilitation services are often key to enabling employment for adults with disabilities. This legislation mandates that AT devices and services are considered and provided as a means to acquire vocational training and to enter into and maintain employment. It also requires that AT be considered during the development and implementation of the individualized worker rehabilitation plan, the document that guides a person's vocational rehabilitation process. For example, if an individual is severely visually impaired and needs to fill out paperwork in order to determine his or her eligibility for vocational rehabilitation services, assistive devices to facilitate reading must be provided at that time. In recent years, Offices of Vocational Rehabilitation have become an important source of funding for AT devices and services to support employment for adults with disabilities.[1,5,18]

Assistive technology and ICIDH-2 (ICF)

The term *disability* is not always precise and quantifiable. The concept of disability is not even agreed by persons who self-identify as having a disability, by professionals who study dis-

ability, or by the general public.[22] This lack of agreement creates an obstacle to the study of disability and to the fair and effective administration of programs and policies intended for people with disabilities.[17,22,23,27] With this issue in mind, the World Health Organization (WHO) developed a global common health language, one that includes physical, mental, and social well-being. The *International Classification of Impairments, Disabilities, and Handicaps* (ICIDH) was first published by WHO in 1980 as a tool for classification of the 'consequences of disease'. The newest version, the *International Classification of Functioning, Disability and Health* (ICF), moves away from a 'consequence of disease' classification (the 1980 version) to a more positive 'components of health' classification. This latest version provides a common framework and language for the description of health and health-related domains, and uses the following language.[42,43]

- *Body functions* are the physiologic functions of body systems (including psychologic functions).
- *Body structures* are anatomic parts of the body such as organs, limbs, and their components.
- *Impairments* are problems in body function or structure, such as a significant deviation or loss.
- *Activity* is the execution of a task or action by an individual.
- *Participation* is involvement in a life situation.
- *Activity limitations* are difficulties an individual may have in executing activities.
- *Participation restrictions* are problems an individual may experience in involvement in life situations.
- *Environmental factors* make up the physical, social, and attitudinal environments in which people live and conduct their lives.

The ICF and the language it uses help professionals define the need for healthcare and related services, such as the provision of AT. It recognizes that physical, mental, social, economic, or environmental interventions can improve lives and levels of functioning for persons with diseases that affect them at the body, person, and social functioning levels.[42] It also characterizes physical, mental, social, economic, or environmental interventions that can improve lives and levels of functioning. Because AT has the potential to improve daily activities and participation in social and physical environments, and improve the quality of life of individuals with disabilities, it clearly fits within the ICF. WHO common health language is used throughout this chapter to discuss the potential impact of appropriate AT.

OVERVIEW OF ASSISTIVE TECHNOLOGY DEVICES

Assistive technology devices are designed to facilitate functional abilities and to meet the needs of humans throughout their varied life stages and roles. It is important to remember that AT device usage and requirements change over time as individuals mature and take on different life roles. Consequently, there is no 'one size fits all' technology available.[12,30,35,36]

Assistive technology devices have the potential to compensate or facilitate immobility; low endurance; difficulty reaching, grasping, or accurately touching keys or switches; problems with seeing or hearing; verbal communication; and the complex skills necessary for reading, writing, and learning. The next sections focus on specific categories of AT devices as they are related to these areas of human function.

The human–technology interface

Considering one's own interaction with technology gives insight into the issues involved in the concept of human–technology interface. Devices await activation or input from the people who use them, and this commonly occurs through dials, switches, keyboards, handlebars, joysticks, or handgrips. This interface typically requires fine motor control, adequate hearing and/or vision, etc. People know they have successfully interacted with devices by the physical, visual, or auditory feedback devices provide (e.g. the sight of brewing coffee, images on a computer monitor, or the sound of a phone ringing).[12,15,24,25,38,41]

Individuals with impairments that affect their interaction with items in their environment need special consideration in the design, function, or placement of the devices they want or need to use.[12,15] For many individuals, it is essential that they are first seated or positioned for optimal use of their residual abilities by means of orthotic or ergonomic seating and positioning interventions (see Ch. 18 for more on this topic).

Direct selection

Once optimal positioning is established, assessment of an individual's reliable, low-effort, high-accuracy hand movements, vision, communication, and hearing helps an evaluator decide whether or not they are able to use a typical 'interface' or need one that is adapted. Using a typical interface (e.g. a computer keyboard, steering wheel, or TV remote control) is called direct selection, because all possible options are presented at once and can be directly selected by the individual. For those without the ability to accurately choose an intended item within the available selection set, a different selection method must be considered.[21]

Scanning or indirect selection

Scanning is the most common indirect selection method used by persons with significant motor impairments. A selection set is presented on a display (e.g. a series of pictures or letters) and is sequentially scanned by a light or cursor on the device. The users choose the desired item by pressing a switch when the indicator reaches the desired location or choice on the display.[12,14,21]

Switches come in many styles and are selected based on the body part that will be activating them (e.g. elbow or chin) and the task or setting for using them (e.g. watching TV in bed or using a communication device while eating). A switch can be as simple as a 'wobble' switch that is activated by a gross motor

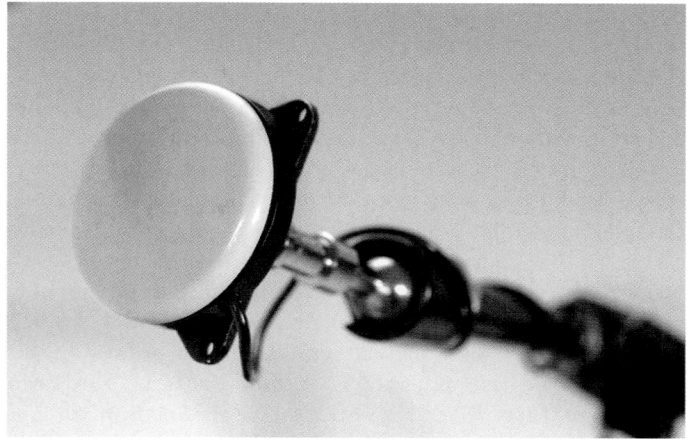

Figure 24-1 A head switch.

movement, such as hitting the switch with the head (Fig. 24-1), hand, arm, leg, or knee. Other switches are activated by tongue touch, by sipping and puffing on a straw, or through very fine movements such as an eye blink or a single muscle twitch. Regardless, switch use and timing accuracy can be very difficult for new users and must be taught. One common method to teach switch activation and use is to interface a switch with battery-operated toys and games, or home or work appliances, to increase motivation and teach the concepts used in indirect selection.

Switches are available in various shapes and sizes. Fairly recent developments in switches include eye gaze switches, which calibrate intentional eye movement patterns and select targets, such as individual keys on an onscreen keyboard. Other new developments include brain wave technology (eye and muscle operated switch, EMOS) that responds to excitation of alpha waves to trigger a selection.

Displays

Human–technology interface also applies to completing the feedback loop from devices back to the user. Examples include software that enlarges images on a computer display for a person with low vision, installing flashing alarms for persons without hearing, and using devices that convert printed text into synthesized speech or Braille for persons with visual impairment or learning disability.

These human–technology interface concepts apply to all forms of AT, whether it is being used for seating, mobility, communication, using a computer, or control of the environment. Good assessment skills, and a focus on clients and their goals and needs, are essential for human–technology interface success and prevention of assistive devices abandonment.

Assistive technology for communication disorders

Vocal communication allows humans to interact, form relationships, and direct the events of their lives. This enables choice and participation. Human communication is based on having both receptive and expressive language abilities, and the physical capacity to reliably produce intelligible speech sounds. Communication impairment can result from congenital conditions such as mental retardation, cerebral palsy, developmental verbal apraxia, and developmental language disorders. Other impairments can be acquired through traumatic brain injury, stroke, multiple sclerosis, amyotrophic lateral sclerosis, tetraplegia, ventilator-dependence, and laryngectomy due to cancer.[6,7,13,16] AT devices that meet the needs of persons with many types of speech and language impairment are commonly called augmentative and alternative communication (AAC) devices, because they can either support or substitute for expressive language impairments. More recently, the term *speech-generating device* has entered into the medical vocabulary to differentiate AAC devices from basic computer devices when seeking third-party funding such as that from Medicaid and Medicare.[6,12]

Some individuals are completely unable to speak, or have such severe expressive difficulties that only those with whom they are very familiar are able to communicate effectively with them. Many devices are available for these individuals, ranging from simple, low-tech picture books to high-end, sophisticated electronic devices (Fig. 24-2). The high-end electronic devices can have digitally recorded or synthetic text to speech output capable of producing complex language interactions.

While AAC devices are extremely useful to non-speaking individuals, they do not replace natural communication. AAC device use should be encouraged along with all other available communication modalities, such as gestures, vocalizations, sign language, and eye gaze.

There are no firm cognitive, physical, or developmental prerequisites for using an AAC device. Instead, comprehensive evaluation techniques are used to match the individual's abilities and communication needs with the appropriate AAC technologies. A qualified team of clinicians perform this evaluation,

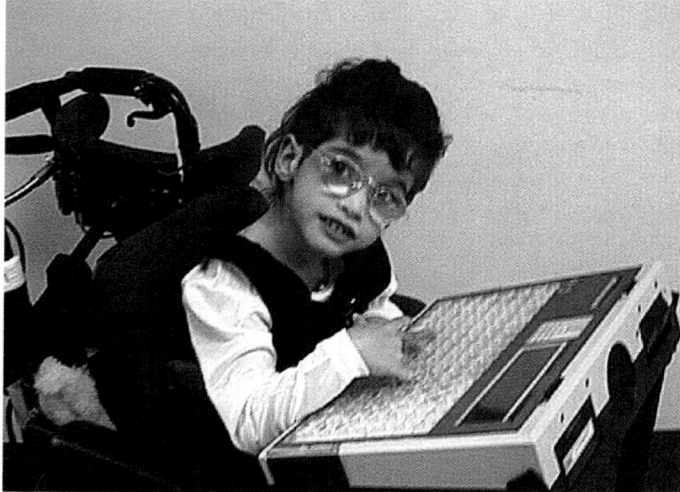

Figure 24-2 Use of the liberator, an augmentative and alternative communication device.

with input from the individual and family members, teachers, employers, and others. Because speaking is considered to be a critical human function, many parents and family members delay seeking out AAC devices, hoping that natural speech will develop. Research shows, however, that using an AAC device can actually support verbal language development. In fact, it can increase the potential for natural speech to develop.[9,29] Children and adults with severe communication impairments can benefit socially, emotionally, academically, and vocationally from using a device that allows them to communicate their thoughts, learn and share ideas, and participate in life activities.

Non-electronic systems

Low-tech, non-electronic AAC systems are often used in addition to an electronic voice output system (or as a backup system in case an electronic device fails or cannot be used during certain activities, such as during a swimming lesson). Low-tech systems can be made by using digital photographs; by using pictures from books or catalogs; or by simply using a marker to draw letters, words, phrases, or pictures. Picture library software is also available commercially. These softwares (e.g. BoardMaker and PCS Symbols) incorporate thousands of line drawings and pictures that can be used to quickly and easily fabricate a low-tech, non-electronic communication system.

Adults with progressive diseases such as amyotrophic lateral sclerosis or multiple sclerosis might also choose to use low-tech picture or alphabet boards as a supplement to verbal communication, due to fatigue during the day or as their ability to verbally communicate decreases. Many of these adults choose to use both low- and high-tech communication systems, depending on the environment they are in and their comfort level with technology.

Electronic voice output systems: digital speech

A variation in low-tech communication systems has developed as a result of the manufacture of low-cost microprocessors capable of storing digitized speech. These low-tech, digital voice output devices work like a tape recorder, allowing recording and storing of simple phrases into memory within the device. When users want to speak, they simply press a button and the device speaks the prerecorded message.

Devices such as One Step, Step by Step, and Big Mac (Fig. 24-3) are simple and relatively inexpensive, and are designed to communicate quick, simple messages such as 'Hi', 'Let's play', or 'Leave me alone'. These technologies are often used with very young children who are beginning communicators, or for those who have significant cognitive impairments. They are not appropriate for individuals needing or wanting to communicate complex thoughts and feelings.

Complex digitized devices store several minutes of recorded voice that is usually associated with representative pictures or icons on a keyboard. These devices are often used by people who are not yet literate, have developmental disabilities, or simply wish to have a simple device to use when going to the

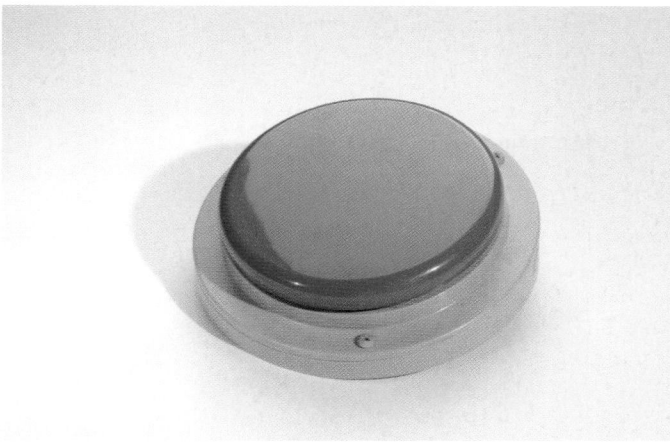

Figure 24-3 The Big Mac electronic voice output system.

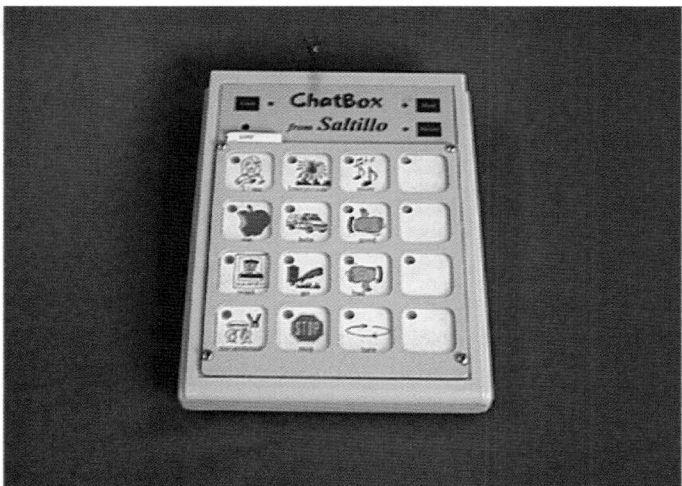

Figure 24-4 The ChatBox electronic voice output system.

store or out to eat. Examples are the Dynamo, the ChatBox (Fig. 24-4), and the Springboard.

Synthesized speech is created by software that uses rules of phonics and pronunciation to translate alphanumeric text into spoken output through speech synthesizer hardware. Voice output systems such as Pathfinder, Dynamyte, and LightWriter are examples of high-tech text to speech devices with built-in speech synthesis. These devices speak words and phrases that have been typed and/or previously stored. The advantage of these systems is that they allow users to speak on any topic and use any words they wish. These systems can encode several thousand words, phrases, and sentences. They are expensive ($6000–9000). They form an essential link to the world, however, for people with severe expressive communication disabilities.

All these voice output systems, whether digital or text to speech, can be activated by direct selection, for example by using a finger or a pointing device such as a mouth stick or head pointer. They can also be activated using indirect selection, for example by using a scanning strategy, or an infrared or wireless switch. In AAC device use, an individual most commonly uses a scanning strategy called row column scanning, in which he or she activates a switch to begin the scan. When the row containing the desired key or icon is highlighted, the user hits the switch again to scan by column. The process is repeated until the desired word or phrase is assembled. While the process can be slow and tedious, indirect selection often provides the only means many people have to communicate with others.

Augmentative and alternative communication devices differ in the mapping and encoding strategies used to represent language, as well as in the storing and retrieving methods used for vocabulary. All systems, however, use either orthographic or pictographic symbols, which vary in ease of learning. When selecting a set of symbols for an individual as part of the user interface, it is important to consider these factors and compare them with the individual's cognitive and perceptual abilities.

Portable amplification systems

For people who speak quietly due to low breath support or who have other difficulties with phonation, portable amplification systems that function like a sound system in a large lecture hall are available. The Speech Enhancer processes speech sounds for people with dysarthria, and enables improved recognition by others. The user typically wears a headset with a microphone attached to a portable device. Their clarified voice is projected via speakers attached to the unit.

ASSISTIVE TECHNOLOGY FOR MOBILITY IMPAIRMENTS

Motor impairments greatly affect the ability of individuals to interact with their environment. Infants are compelled to roll, then crawl and toddle, to explore their surroundings. Any motor impairment can greatly impact overall development. This is often the situation seen in patients with cerebral palsy, spina bifida, arthrogryposis, and other diagnoses that impact motor skills. AT devices can help children achieve developmental milestones when used as an early intervention and with a supportive family.

The loss of acquired motor abilities through trauma or disease is experienced as a severe loss for children and adults, and occurs with spinal cord injury, stroke, multiple sclerosis, amputation, and other conditions. There are many forms of AT that help compensate for impaired motor skills, and they should be introduced as early as possible in rehabilitation to ensure the best outcome possible.

Upper body mobility devices

Given the importance of computer use in education, training, and employment, many AT devices have been developed to provide access to computers to individuals with upper body mobility impairment, such as poor hand control or paralysis. If someone is unable to use a standard mouse and keyboard, there are multiple potential AT options.

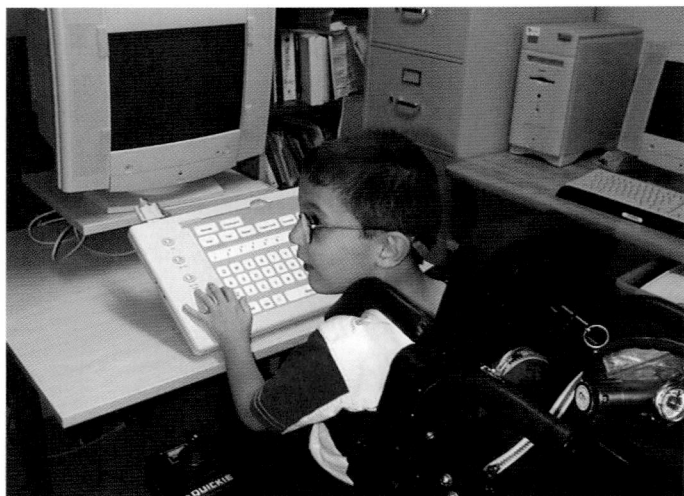

Figure 24-5 The Intellikeys expanded keyboard.

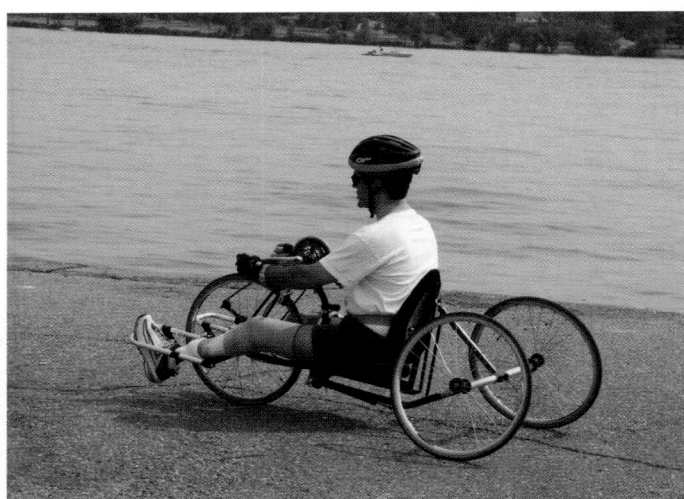

Figure 24-6 The hand bike, an example of a low-tech recreation aid.

Alternative computer keyboards come in many shapes and sizes. There are expanded keyboards, such as the Intellikeys (Fig. 24-5), which provide a larger target or key surrounded by inactive space. Options such as delayed activation response help individuals who have difficulty with pointing accuracy or removing a finger after activating a key. Individuals unfamiliar with a standard QWERTY keyboard layout have the option of an alphabetic layout. This is often helpful for young children who are developing literacy skills, as well as for adults with cognitive or visual impairments.

There are also smaller keyboards (e.g. the Tash Mini Keyboard) designed for persons with limited range of motion and endurance. They are also helpful for individuals who type with one hand, or who use a head pointer or mouth stick to type. These keyboards use a frequency of occurrence layout. The home or middle row in the center of the keyboard holds the space bar and the letters in English words that occur most frequently (e.g. 'a' and 'e'). All other characters, numbers, and functions (including mouse control) fan out from the center of the keyboard based on how frequently they are used in common computer tasks.

Voice recognition (VR) is a mass market technology that has become essential for computer access for many persons with motor impairment. Instead of writing via the keyboard, VR users write or speak words out loud. The computer processor uses information from the user's individual voice file, compares it with digital models of words and phrases, and produces computer text. If the words are accurate, the user proceeds. If not, the user corrects the words to match what was said. As the process continues, the computer updates its voice file, and VR accuracy improves. This software is cognitively demanding but can offer hands-free or greatly reduced keyboarding to many individuals with motor impairment.

Another group of computer input methods include devices that rely on an onscreen keyboard that is visible on the computer monitor, such as the Head Mouse and Tracker 2000. The user wears a head-mounted signaling device or a reflective dot on the forehead to select keys on the onscreen keyboard, choose commands from pull-down menus, or direct mouse movement. Onscreen keyboards are typically paired with rate enhancement options such as word prediction or abbreviation expansion to increase a user's word per minute rate. Because so many tasks can be accomplished through computers, individuals with disabilities—even those with the most severe motor impairments—can fully participate in life. They can perform education- and work-related tasks, and monitor and control an unlimited array of devices or appliances at home, work, and school.

Lower body mobility devices

Individuals with spinal cord injury, spina bifida, or cerebral palsy often have lower body mobility impairments. AT solutions can include crutches, a rolling walker, a powered scooter, or a manual or powered wheelchair. (The prescription of wheelchairs and scooters is covered in Ch. 18.) Simple environmental modifications or adaptations, such as installing a ramp instead of stairs, raising the height of a desk, or widening doorways, can be critical facilitators for these individuals and might be all that is needed. For other activities or to increase participation, it is possible to add automobile hand controls, adapt saddles for horseback riding, or use sit-down forms of downhill skiing (see Fig. 24-6).

There are literally thousands of low-tech assistive devices available for persons with motor impairments. Commonly referred to as aids or adaptive devices for completing activities of daily living, these devices include weighted spoons and scoop plates to facilitate eating, aids for personal hygiene such as bath chairs and long-handled hairbrushes, items for dressing such as sock aids and one-handed buttoners, adapted toys for play, built-up pencil grips for writing and drawing, and many others. Many low-tech mobility aids can be handmade for just a few dollars, while others, such as an adult rolling bath chair, may cost several hundred dollars. All share the common goal of reducing barriers and increasing participation in daily life. (See Ch. 27 for a discussion of aids to daily living devices.)

AT FOR ERGONOMICS AND PREVENTION OF SECONDARY INJURIES

A rapidly growing area of concern for AT practitioners is the development of repetitive strain injuries (RSIs) among both able-bodied and disabled individuals. While specialized keyboards and mouse control have provided computer access for many individuals, the pervasiveness of computer technology has also increased the possibility of RSI. An entire industry of AT has developed over the past few years to deal with repetitive motion disorders.

Computer desks, tables, and chairs used in computer laboratories, classrooms, and offices do not always match the physical needs of users. When people with and without disabilities spend hours repetitively performing the same motor movement, they can and do develop RSI. Potential solutions include properly supporting seated posture, raising or lowering a chair or desk for optimal fit, implementing routine breaks, and using ergonomically designed keyboards and other assistive technologies.

Many of the AT devices described in this chapter (e.g. alternative and specially designed ergonomic keyboards, VR software, and strategies to minimize keystrokes) can also provide useful solutions for individuals with RSI. There are also Internet-based resources that target ergonomic issues, such as those found in Table 24-1.

Electronic aids to daily living (EADLs)

Electronic aids to daily living provide alternative control of electrical devices within the environment, and increase independence in tasks of daily living. This technology is also referred to as environmental control units (ECUs). Within the home, EADLs can control audiovisual equipment (e.g. television, video players and recorders, cable, digital satellite systems, stereo), communication equipment (e.g. telephone, intercom, and call bells), doors, electric beds, security equipment, lights, and appliances (e.g. fan and wave machine). EADLs are controlled directly (by pressing a button with a finger or pointer, or by voice command) or indirectly (by scanning and switch activation). Some AAC devices and some computer systems also provide EADL device control of devices within the environment.

Almost anyone with limited control over her or his environment can benefit from this technology. Children and adults with developmental delays often benefit from low-tech EADLs that increase independence in play through intermittent switch control of battery-operated toys or electrical devices, such as a disco light. For those unable to operate a TV remote control, switches or voice commands to an EADL device allow access to devices they would otherwise be unable to control. Many EADLs also accommodate cognitive and visual deficits. For example, an AAC device can display an icon instead of text for

a client without literacy or who cannot read English. The same device can also use auditory scanning so that choices can be heard if the client has impaired vision.

Electronic aids to daily living are primarily used in the home but can also be used in a work or school setting. An individual can use EADL technology to turn on the lights at a workstation and use the telephone. A child who uses a switch can participate more fully in the classroom by advancing slides for a presentation, or by activating a tape player with a story on cassette for the class.

The term EADL was chosen over ECU for two primary reasons. First, the term more accurately defines this area of AT by emphasizing the task (e.g. communication is a daily living activity) rather than the item being controlled (e.g. the telephone). Second, the term was chosen to improve reimbursement by third-party providers, because the category of ECUs has been poorly funded in the past. In contrast, aids to daily living equipment is traditionally funded very well. Aids to daily living equipment, which is designed to make the client more independent in a specific daily living task, includes bath seats, toileting aids, built-up spoon handles, and zipper pulls. This equipment is defined by the *daily living* task it *aids*.

Environmental control unit devices had the same general goal, but the name failed to reflect the goal, particularly to funding agencies. EADL expands aids to daily living equipment to include equipment that happens to use batteries or plug into the wall, but that still shares the same goal—increasing independence in tasks of daily living.

ASSISTIVE TECHNOLOGY FOR HEARING IMPAIRMENTS

Hearing impairment and deafness affect the feedback loop in the human environment interaction. Because most individuals can hear, it is commonly recognized as a significant barrier in communication, and can compromise safety in situations where sound is used to warn of danger.

Hearing aids

Individuals who have varying degrees of hearing impairment face two major issues: lack of auditory input, and compromised ability to monitor speech output and environmental sound. AT devices such as hearing aids and frequency modulation or radio wave systems can be used to facilitate both auditory input and speech output. Other types of AT device provide a visual representation of the auditory signal. These include flashing lights as an alternative emergency alarm (e.g. for fire or tornado) or the ringing of a phone or doorbell.

Cochlear implants

When the hearing system is impaired at the level of the middle ear or the cochlea, a highly specialized form of AT is used to create an alternative means of stimulating the auditory nerve. This technology is implanted surgically with an electrode array placed within or around the cochlear structure. The external

Table 24-1 Internet-based resources for ergonomics

Organization	Web site address
Government sites	
NASA Ergo Resources	http://ohp.ksc.nasa.gov/topics/ergo/
NIOSH Web	http://www.cdc.gov/niosh/topics/ergonomics/
OSHA Web	http://www.osha.gov/SLTC/ergonomics/index.html
Military sites	
Department of Defense Design Criteria MIL-1472F	http://www.r6.gsa.gov/hac/1472F.htm
Ergonomic Guidelines for Office Furniture Selection	http://www.tobyhanna.army.mil/toby/organize/risk/reg/appen_I.pdf
Educational institution sites	
Cornell University Ergonomics	http://human.cornell.edu/
Ergonomic Design Standard—University of Melbourne	http://www.unimelb.edu.au/ehsm/Ergonomic_design.pdf
Ergonomic Guidelines for Computer Use—Harvard	http://www.hsph.harvard.edu/ccpe/programs/EGCU.shtml
Ergonomic Guidelines for Video Display Terminal	http://www.fiu.edu/~ehs/generalsafety/ergonomics/ergonom.html
Ergonomic Guidelines for Workstation Setup—Radcliffe Institute	http://www.radcliffe.edu/rito/tips/ergonomics.html
Ergonomic Standard and Guidelines—University of Maryland	http://www.otal.umd.edu/guse/standards.html
Ergonomic Workstation Guidelines—NC State University	http://www.ncsu.edu/ehs/www99/right/handsMan/office/ergonomic.html
Loughborough University Ergonomics	http://www.lboro.ac.uk/research/esri/
Louisville University Ergonomics	http://www.louisville.edu/speed/ergonomics/
Office Ergo Guidelines—University of Sydney	http://www.usyd.edu.au/su/ohs/ergonomics/ERGO8a.html
Office Ergonomic Standard—University of Toronto	http://www.utoronto.ca/safety/ergoweb/ErgStd.PDF
Ohio State University Ergonomics	http://osuergo.eng.ohio-state.edu/institute/
University of California, Berkeley Ergonomics	http://www.uhs.berkeley.edu/facstaff/Ergonomics/index.htm
University of California Ergonomics	http://ls.berkeley.edu/lscr/support/faq/ergo/
University of California Los Angeles Ergonomics	http://ergonomics.ucla.edu/
University of California, San Francisco Ergonomics	http://www.me.berkeley.edu/ergo
University of Michigan Ergonomics	http://www.engin.umich.edu/dept/ioe/C4E/research_projects.html
University of Nebraska Ergonomics	http://eeshop.unl.edu/rsi.html
Additional ergonomic resources	
ANSI BHMA Search	http://www.buildershardware.com/20.html
ANSI Document Search	http://www.nssn.org/search.html
Ergo Noise Control—ANSI standard	http://www.quietnoise.com/schools_classrooms/ANSI%20Standard.htm
Ergonomic Center	http://www.ergonomiccenter.com
Ergonomic Edge	http://www.ergonomicedge.com
Ergonomic Product Guidelines	http://www.cccd.edu/ehs/ergo/html/products_guide.html
Ergonomic Resources	http://www.ergonext.com/
Ergonomic Resources	http://www.ergoweb.com/
Ergonomics for Teacher and Student	http://www.ergonomics4schools.com/
Ergoweb	http://www.ergoweb.com/
Next Gen Ergo	http://www.nexgenergo.com/

Continued on page 531

Continued from page 530 Table 24-1	Internet-based resources for ergonomics
Organization	Web site address
Stress Ergonomics	http://www.spineuniverse.com/displayarticle.php/article1484.html
Stress Ergonomics	http://www.spineuniverse.com/displayarticle.php/article1484.html
Taylor and Francis Ergo Group	http://www.ergonomics.tandf.co.uk/ergonomicsarena/homepage.htm
Industry sites 3M Ergo	http://www.3m.com/cws/selfhelp/guidelns.html
American Ergonomics Group	http://www.americanergo.com
Basic Ergo Standard	http://www.iso.ch/iso/en/commcentre/isobulletin/articles/2003/pdf/ergonomic03-06.pdf
Ergonomic for Writers and Editors	http://www.sfwa.org/ergonomics/
Hewlett Packard Ergo Guidelines-Working in Comfort	http://www.hp.com/ergo/ and http://www.hp.com/ergo/pdfs/297660-002.pdf
IBM Ergo Guide-Healthy Computing	http://www.pc.ibm.com/ww/healthycomputing/
Office Ergonomics Training	http://www.office-ergo.com
Office Ergonomics	http://www.healthycomputing.com/office
Repetitive Strain Injury FAQs by CTD Resource Network, Inc.	http://www.tifaq.com/
Work-Related Musculoskeletal Disorders	http://www.nsc.org/ehc/z365/finldrft.htm

portion, a microphone, relays speech and environmental sound to the implanted portion, which is programmed to process, synchronize, and stimulate electrodes appropriately. This system requires a battery pack worn on the body or behind the ear.[12] It also requires an experienced audiologist to teach the individual to use the acoustic cues produced by the cochlear implant as a substitute for natural hearing.

Other hearing technologies
Another recent adaptation for persons with significant hearing impairment is computer-assisted real time translation. This AT solution involves a specially trained typist or stenographer who captures what is being spoken on a computer. The text is then projected on to a display, resulting in close to real time translation. The advantage of this technology is that it can be used by hearing-impaired individuals who are not fluent in sign language, as well as others who might need listening help, such as those who use English as a second language. In addition to use in group environments such as conferences or meetings, a variation of this technology can be used to assist a single student or employee in a small setting.

Environmental adaptations
For individuals who wear hearing aids, there are additional technologies that can facilitate hearing in large rooms or in noisy, crowded environments such as a restaurant. The Conference Mate and Whisper Voice are especially designed for these environments. In the case of the Conference Mate, the person with the hearing loss wears a neck loop, which acts as an antenna and is capable of broadcasting directly to a hearing aid

from a microphone placed near the speaker. It transmits directly to the neck loop, eliminating background sound. This is also an excellent solution for office and school environments. The Whisper Voice is similar, except that it uses a smaller microphone and is more portable. It can be passed from speaker to speaker, with sound transmitted to the neck loop and then on to the hearing aid for amplification.

Environmental adaptations can frequently support individuals who are deaf or hard of hearing. For example, a person speaking to someone who has difficulty hearing can take care not to stand in front of a light source (windows, lamps, etc.) and not to over-exaggerate or hide lip movements. Gestures can be helpful as well.

ASSISTIVE TECHNOLOGY FOR VISUAL IMPAIRMENTS

The term visual impairment technically encompasses all types of permanent vision loss, including total blindness. Low vision refers to a vision loss that is severe enough to impede performing everyday tasks, but that still provides some usable visual information. Low vision *cannot* be corrected to normal by eyeglasses or contact lenses (see http://www.afb.org/section.asp?SectionID=15&DocumentID=1280).

Low-tech visual aids
A variety of AT devices and strategies can help individuals with visual impairments perform daily activities such as reading, writing, personal care, mobility, and recreational activities.

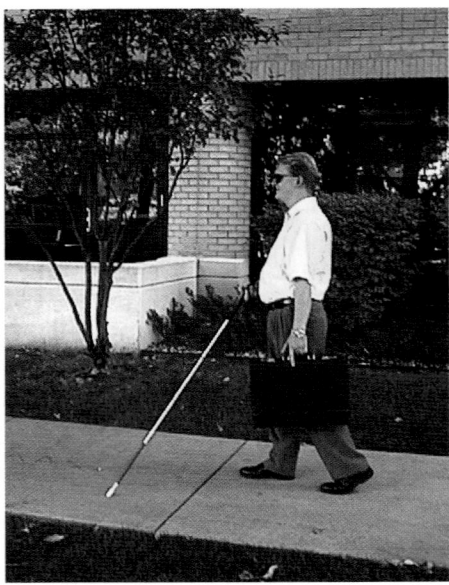

Figure 24-7 Use of a cane by a person with visual impairment.

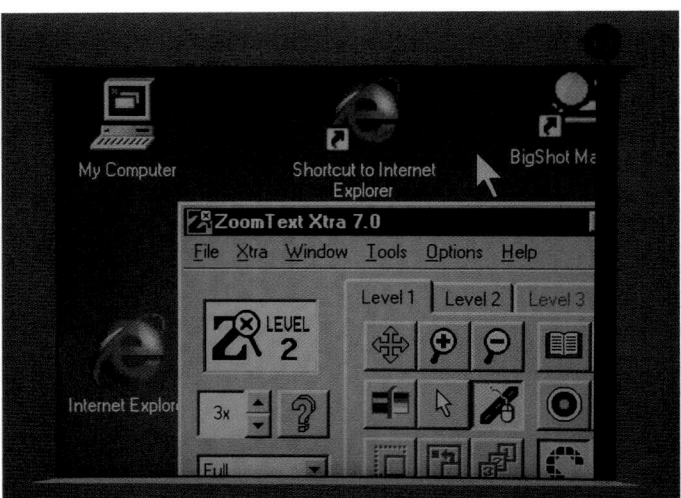

Figure 24-8 Zoomtext screen magnification software for the visually impaired.

Among low-tech solutions are simple handheld magnifiers, the use of large print, or mobility devices (e.g. a white cane, Fig. 24-7) for safe and efficient travel. High-contrast tape or markers can also be used to indicate hazards, what an item is, or where it is located.

Other low-tech solutions include using wind chimes to help with direction finding, using easily legible type fonts such as Verdana (16 point or larger), and using beige paper rather than white to improve the visibility of text. In recreational activities, solutions include beeper balls, three-dimensional puzzles, and outdoor trails with signage (called Braille trails) designed to improve access to the wilderness and other outdoor activities.

Braille text, although less used than in years past due to the advances of computer and other technologies, is still the first choice of many individuals for reading. Many restaurants now provide large-print, Braille, and picture-based menus for customers with a variety of abilities.

Books on tape are another resource for individuals with severe visual impairments. In addition to commercially available tapes for sale and at public libraries, special libraries provide print materials in alternative formats for persons with visual, physical, and learning impairments. Borrowers can arrange to have textbooks and other materials translated into alternate formats. For more information, contact the American Federation for the Blind or the National Library Service for the Blind and Physically Handicapped (http://www.loc.gov/nls/) (see also Box 24-2).

High-tech visual aids

Numerous high-tech solutions exist for persons with visual impairments. Computers outfitted with a speech synthesizer and specialized software, such as Jaws or WindowEyes, allow navigation of the desktop, operating system, applications, and documents, as well as the entire Internet. Any digital text can be heard aloud by the person using this software. For text that is printed, such as menus, memos, and letters, using a technology called optical character recognition allows a page scanner and software to convert print into digital form, where it can then be listened to by way of the computer's speech synthesizer. It can also be converted to Braille or large print.

Another category of high-tech aids are portable note takers with either Braille or speech synthesizer feedback for the user. These devices are specialized personal digital assistants with calendars, contacts, memo, and document capabilities, and can be purchased with either a QWERTY or a Braille keyboard.

For individuals with some degree of visual ability, screen magnification software such as Zoomtext (Fig. 24-8) and MAGic enable the user to choose the amount (2–20 times) and type of magnification preferred for optimal computer access. Many magnification applications combine enlargement with speech synthesis or text to speech.

A recent addition to the list of screen magnification software is called Bigshot. This software is less expensive ($99) and provides fewer features than some other programs. It appears to be an alternative for users who do not need access to the more sophisticated computer functions, however, and it is highly affordable.

Environmental adaptations

Persons with visual impairments usually keep the set-up of their home and work environments constant, because this helps in locating items. They usually need specialized training, however, for mobility in the community. They learn to use environmental cues such as traffic sounds, echoes, or the texture of the sidewalk in combination with mobility aids such as a white cane or a guide dog.

To supplement these less technical aids, some individuals use electronic travel aids that have the capability of detecting obsta-

---

Box 24-2 Resources for persons with low vision or blindness

- American Academy of Ophthalmology
  Public Information Program
  PO Box 7424
  San Francisco, CA 94120
  Tel. 415 561-8555 ext. 214 and 223
  http://www.eyenet.org
- American Council of the Blind in Colorado
  2421 Orchard Avenue
  Grand Junction, CO 81501
  Tel. 888 775-2221
  http://www.acbco.org
- American Council of the Blind
  1155 15th St., NW, #720
  Washington, DC 20005
  Tel. 202 467-5081
  Fax 800 424-8666
  http://www.acb.org
- American Foundation for the Blind
  11 Penn Plaza #300
  New York, NY 10001
  Tel. 800 232-5463
  http://www.afb.org
- American Printing House for the Blind, Inc.
  1839 Frankfort Ave.
  Louisville, KY 40206
  Tel. 502 895-2405
- National Association for Visually Handicapped
  22 W. 21st St., 6th floor
  New York, NY 10010
  Tel. 212 889-3141
- National Braille Association, Inc.
  3 Townline Circle
  Rochester, NY 14623
  Tel. 716 427-8260
- National Braille Press, Inc.
  88 St. Stephen St.
  Boston, MA 02115
  Tel. 617 266-6160
  Fax 617 437-0456
- Recordings for the Blind and Dyslexic
  20 Roszel Road
  Princeton, NJ 08540
  Tel. 609 452-0606

- Rehabilitation Engineering and Assistive Technology Society of
  North America State Technology Projects
  1700 N. Moore St., Suite #1540
  Arlington, VA 22209-1903
  Tel. 703 524-6686
- Aspen Braille Nature Trail
  White River National Forest
  Aspen, CO 81611
  Tel. 970 945-2521
- Assistive Technology Partners
  1245 E. Colfax Ave., Suite 200
  Denver, CO 80218
  Tel. 303 315-1280
  Fax 303 837-1208
  http://www.uchsc.edu/atp
- DVS Home Video (audio captioning)
  125 Western Ave.
  Boston, MA 02134
  Tel. 800 333-1203
- Families of the Blind, Inc.
  3850 Alcott
  Denver, CO 80211-2164
  Tel. 303 433-1500
- Guide Dogs for the Blind, Inc.
  PO Box 151200
  San Rafael, CA 94915-1200
  Tel. 415 499-4000
- Guide Dogs for the Blind, Inc.
  32901 SE Kelso Road
  Boring, OR 97009
  Tel. 503 668-2100
- Helen Keller National Center for Deaf-Blind Youth and Adults
  1880 S. Pierce St., #5
  Lakewood, CO 80232
  Tel. 303 934-9037
- National Federation of the Blind
  1800 Johnson St.
  Baltimore, MD 21230
  Tel. 301 659-9314
- National Library Services for the Blind–Physically Handicapped
  Library of Congress
  1291 Taylor St., NW
  Washington, DC 20542
  Tel. 202 707-5100
  Fax 800 424-8567

---

cles missed by a cane, such as overhanging branches or objects that have fallen. Another technology (Talking Signs) utilizes ultrasound or information embedded in the environment expressly for users who are blind. The demands for independence in community mobility by persons with significant visual impairments are huge, because of the high cognitive demand for remembering routes and because environments constantly change. Many individuals use these types of technologies in order to increase their independent mobility in both familiar areas and in the larger community.

ASSISTIVE TECHNOLOGY FOR COGNITIVE OR LEARNING DISABILITIES

Cognitive disabilities include disorders such as traumatic brain injury, mental retardation, developmental disabilities, autism, Alzheimer disease, learning disability, fragile X syndrome, and other disorders, both developmental and acquired. Most individuals in this group have not had the benefit of using AT devices, because relatively few products have been specifically developed for intellectual impairments. In addition, families, teachers, and others providing support services for individuals with cognitive impairments have generally not been aware of the potential usefulness of AT.

Most have looked to simple solutions for persons with learning and/or cognitive impairments, using strategies such as colored highlighter tape, pencil grips, enlarged text, reminder lists, and calendars. Others try low-tech adaptations such as using a copyholder to hold print materials for easy viewing, and making cardboard windows to help eyes follow text when reading.

In 2004, the US Department of Education, National Institute on Disability Research and Rehabilitation, recognizing the need to increase AT development for persons with cognitive disabilities, funded a Rehabilitation Engineering Research Center for the Advancement of Cognitive Disabilities (RERC-ACT). This RERC-ACT is focusing on developing a wide range of assistive technologies, including vocational and literacy skills, service provision, and enhanced caregiving supports, for persons with significant cognitive impairments. This new field of cognitive technologies promises numerous advances during the next decade (www.rerc-act.org).

Literacy technologies

There are a number of both low- and high-tech solutions available to assist literacy development. Individuals who are unable to read print materials often use books on tape or some of the text to speech software solutions mentioned earlier, such as Jaws. Co:Writer is an example of a specially designed application that predicts the word or phrase an individual is trying to spell as they begin to type a word. Other applications (e.g. Write Outloud and Kurzweil 3000) provide multisensory feedback by both visually highlighting and speaking the text the individual is generating on the computer.

Voice recognition software can be useful for persons with learning disabilities so significant that they are unable to develop writing skills. VR software enables an individual to speak words, phrases, or sentences into a standard computer word-processing program such as Microsoft Word. A review or playback feature in the application allows writers to hear the text they have written repeated back to them. Adding auditory feedback allows them to self-monitor and correct mistakes.

Although VR software is a rapidly developing technology, the user must currently have a fifth grade reading ability in order to read the text used to generate a voice file. This hinders its usability by those with significant learning disabilities. Dragon Naturally Speaking has developed a VR version for children 9 years and older, but its success rate for children with learning and other cognitive disabilities has not yet been published.

Other limitations of VR include reduced accuracy in the presence of ambient noise, such as that found in a typical classroom, and fluctuating vocal abilities related to fatigue for some types of disability. In general, it takes more than 20 hours to train the software to an acceptable level of accuracy (greater than 90%). Although caution is in order when prescribing this type of software, the rapid pace of development bodes well for

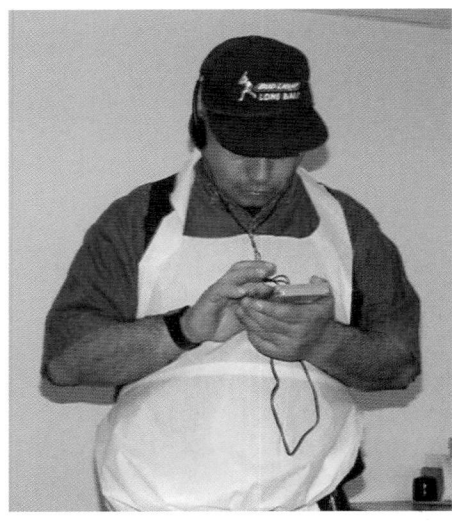

Figure 24-9
Prompting technology: the Pocket Coach.

the future use of this type of software for persons with disabilities.

There are numerous other applications for persons with cognitive impairment that focus on a range of topics, including academics, money management, personal skills development, behavior training, development of cognitive skills, memory improvement, problem solving, time concepts, safety awareness, speech and language therapy, telephone usage, and recreation and games.

Prompting technologies

Recent mainstream technology developments have applications for individuals with cognitive disabilities, and include handheld personal digital assistants. AT software developers (AbleLink Technologies, Inc.) have used this technology and developed software applications (PocketCoach, Fig. 24-9) that provide auditory prompts for individuals with cognitive disabilities. This software can be set up to prompt an individual through each step of a task as simple as mopping a floor, up to the complexity of solving a mathematic problem. The latest version of this software combines voice prompts with visual prompts (Visual Assistant). The individual setting up the system for a user can simply take digital pictures with the accompanying camera, and combine them with digitally recorded voice prompts to further facilitate memory and cognition.

SELECTING APPROPRIATE ASSISTIVE TECHNOLOGIES

Abandonment

Practitioners are sometimes surprised to learn that not everyone with a disability enjoys using technology, however useful it might appear. Depending on the type of technology, non-use or abandonment can be as low as 8% or as high as 75%. On average, one-third of more optional assistive technologies are abandoned, most within the first 3 months.[26,28]

Research has not yet been done to ascertain the number of individuals who are unhappy with their devices, but who must continue to use them because they cannot abandon them without severe consequences.[26,28] For example, an individual who has just received a new wheelchair that does not meet expectations simply cannot stop using the chair, but must wait until third-party funding becomes available again (typically several years). Alternatively, the individual must engage in potentially difficult and unproductive discussions with the vendor, who has more than likely provided the chair as it was prescribed by the assessment team.

Research does tell us that the main reason why individuals with disabilities choose not to use assistive devices is because practitioners fail to consider their opinions and preferences during the process of selecting the device. Typically, it is due to the person with a disability not being included as an active member of the team during the evaluation process.[26,31]

Principles of clinical assessment

The goal of an AT evaluation is to determine if AT devices and services have the potential to help an individual meet activity or participation goals at home, school, work, or play. Other goals of an assessment include the following.

- Providing a safe and supportive environment for the person with a disability, and for his or her family to learn about and review available assistive devices.
- Identifying the need for AT services such as training support staff or integrating an AT device into daily activities.
- Carrying out the modification or customization needed to make the equipment effective.
- Developing a potential list of recommended devices for trial usage before a final selection of technology is made.

The individual and family, as well as the AT team, should specify exactly what they hope to achieve as a result of the evaluation (e.g. equipment ideas, and potential success with vocational or educational objectives).[8,11,12,32,33,34]

When selecting team members to conduct an AT evaluation, professional disciplines should be chosen based on the identified needs of the person with the disability. For example, if the individual presents with both severe motor and communication impairments, team members should include an occupational or physical therapist with expertise in human–technology interface, as well as a speech–language pathologist with a background in working with persons with severe communication impairments and alternative forms of communication. If a cognitive impairment has been identified, someone versed in learning processes, such as a psychologist, neurolinguist, teacher, or special educator, would be an appropriate member of the team. If there is an ergonomic issue (e.g. repetitive stress injury), an evaluator with training in ergonomic assessment or a background in physical or occupational therapy is a necessary component for a successful experience.

It is not appropriate for an AT vendor to be called in to perform an AT evaluation. While vendors can and should be members of the evaluation team, it must be recognized that they have a conflict of interest, because they earn a living by selling products. When working with a manufacturer or vendor, it is important to work with a credentialed provider. When requested by the team, vendors demonstrate their products, discuss pertinent features, and assist in setting up the equipment for evaluation and trial usage. However, other team members, including end users and their families, should perform the evaluation and make the final recommendation(s).

Phase 1 of the assessment process

Knowledge within the field of AT continues to expand and change, sometimes on a daily basis. This directly impacts whether or not the AT device recommended by the assessment team will be used or abandoned by the consumer. As a result of rapidly changing information, the evaluation process continues to be refined. Many researchers are working to develop standardized AT measurement tools,[10,12,20] but the fact remains that there are few available resources to guide practitioners who have not received formalized training in AT assessment.

As mentioned earlier in this chapter, the number one reason AT is abandoned is because the needs and preferences of the consumer are not taken into account during the evaluation process. Other reasons cited for abandonment of devices include the following.[26,27]

- Changes in consumer functional abilities or activities.
- Lack of consumer motivation to use the device or do the task.
- Lack of meaningful training on how to use the device.
- Ineffective device performance or frequent breakdown of the device.
- Environmental obstacles to use, such as narrow doorways.
- Lack of access to and information about repair and maintenance.
- Lack of sufficient need for the device functions.
- Device aesthetics, device's weight, size, and appearance.

Given the relationship that must develop between individuals and AT devices, it is common sense that these factors be considered during the evaluation process. The AT assessment process has evolved from a random process of trying out any number of devices with the individual, to a team process that begins with the technology out of sight.

Phase 1 of the assessment process begins when a referral is received. Standard demographic and impairment-related information is collected, usually over the phone. In the majority of cases, cognitive, motor, vision, and other standard clinical assessments have already been performed, and a release of information is requested from individuals or their caregivers so information can be forwarded to the team. If appropriate assessments have not been conducted, they are scheduled as a component of phase 2 of the assessment process.

Based on the preliminary information, an appropriate team of professionals is assembled and a date is chosen for the evaluation. The team leader takes responsibility for ensuring that the individual with the disability, her or his family, and any other significant individuals are invited to the evaluation.

At the initial meeting, team members spend some time getting to know the individual. Using methods described by Cook and Hussey[12] and Galvin and Scherer,[14] the team identifies the life roles of the consumer (e.g. student, brother, and musician) and the specific activities engaged in by the individual to fulfill those life roles. For example, if a young man is a brother, that means he might play hide and seek with a sibling, squabble over toys, or otherwise engage in brotherly activities. If he is a musician, then he might want or need to have access to musical instruments, sheet music, or simply a radio.

Next, the team identifies any problems that could occur during the individual's daily activities. For example, the musician might not have enough hand control to manage recording equipment, or could experience visual or cognitive difficulties with sheet music. We ask specific questions about where and when these difficulties occur (activity limitations). Perhaps problems occur when the individual is tired or not properly positioned, or when she or he is trying to communicate with others. The individual is also asked to describe instances of success with these activities, and to discuss what made them successful (prior history with and without technology). By now, the team is usually able to recognize patterns of success and failure from the individual's perspective as common limitations across environments emerge.

Finally, the team prioritizes the order in which to address barriers to participation, and a specific plan of action is developed. This specific plan of action contains 'must' statements, such as 'the device must have a visible display in sunlight' or 'the technology chosen must weigh less than 2 lbs'.

It is at this point that the team could be reconfigured. For example, if individuals are not properly seated and positioned, they are referred to the occupational or physical therapist for seating and positioning evaluation before proceeding further. Some members of the team might leave after determining that further assessment from their perspective is not needed. In other situations, as additional needs become apparent, new members are invited to join the team (e.g. a vision specialist). At all times, the assessment team includes the individual and his or her caregivers as the primary members.

Phase 2 of the assistive technology assessment

Once the team has agreed the specific plan of action and those things that 'must' occur, phase 2 of the assessment process begins. The person with the disability and/or his or her caregivers are asked to preview any number of AT devices that could serve to reduce activity limitations and increase participation in chosen environments. These AT devices are tried along with various adaptations, modifications, and placements to ensure an appropriate match of the technology to the individual.

It is at this point that the clinician's AT skills become critical. If trial devices are not properly configured, or if the wrong information is given to the consumer, she or he will be unable to make an appropriate selection. Because many devices require extensive training and follow-up, it is essential that realistic information about training and learning time is provided. It is also important to identify appropriate resources within the local

community. With very few exceptions, the wise course of action involves borrowing or renting the AT device prior to making a final purchase decision. For many individuals, the actual use of technologies on a day to day basis raises new issues that must be resolved. For instance, there might not be the local supports for the technology that is being considered for an individual. In these cases, it is best to first identify local resources or local AT professionals willing to seek additional training before sending the device home with the user. Consumers and their families should always be informed, so that they can make the final decision regarding when and where the equipment will be delivered.

Unexpected benefits of trial use occur as a result of improved functioning, including changes in role and status. In some cases, these unexpected benefits create an entirely new set of problems. These problems can be resolved with time, energy, and patience in the majority of individuals. Other individuals decide that they either prefer the old way of doing things, or that they are interested in adding to or changing the technology once they have had a chance to experiment with it in different settings.

Assistive technology professionals, in consultation with the physician, should also anticipate future needs (e.g. physical and cognitive maturation or degeneration), and final decisions should consider both the expected performance and durability of the device.[14,32]

Writing the report

The evaluation report documents the AT assessment process and must include several components. It is essential to use layperson's terms to help case managers, educators, and others unfamiliar with assistive technologies to understand the process.

In cases where medical insurance is being used to purchase technology, it is essential to document the medical need for the device(s) within the report. This information will be included in the letter of medical necessity required by medical insurers prior to funding approval. For example, the evaluation report might state:

Mr. Jones will use this wheelchair to enable safe and independent mobility in the home and community, and to meet the functional or activities of daily living goals as listed.

In instances where educational or vocational funding is being requested to purchase the technology, the report should focus on the educational or vocational benefit of the assistive devices, and how relevant goals will be met with the recommended equipment.

It is extremely important that all components of the AT device be included in the list of recommended equipment (e.g. cables, ancillary peripherals, warranties, and consumable supplies). In many instances, devices are recommended for purchase as a system. As a result, acquisition can be delayed for months because an item was not included in the initial list. An estimate of the amount of time, cost, and source of training should also be included at this point. Purchasing an AT device without procuring the AT services needed to learn how to use it and how to integrate it into identified activities will result in low use or abandonment.

It is also important to include contact information for the vendors who sell the equipment. Many purchasers are unfamiliar with rehabilitation technology supply companies, and acquisition can be delayed if this information is not included in the report.

PHYSICIAN RESPONSIBILITIES

Prescribing the technologies

The American Medical Association recommends that the following items be considered when prescribing AT and certifying medical necessity: the physician must provide evidence of individual medical necessity for the specific AT being prescribed, and be prepared to talk with insurance company representatives about the medical necessity of complex assistive technologies (e.g. power wheelchairs and AAC devices).[37] Reviewing a comprehensive assessment report from the AT assessment team should supply all the needed information.

Health insurance requires an 'appropriate' prescription that includes mention of the comprehensive assessment process, the individual's motivation, the availability of training, and the potential functional outcome(s) for the patient as compared with the cost of the products. Success with reimbursement also includes using the appropriate medical necessity forms and prior authorization procedures.

Documentation in the medical record

In addition to prescribing and certifying medical necessity on various forms, physicians must maintain complete patient records that include the following.

- Patient diagnosis or diagnoses.
- Duration of the patient's condition.
- Expected clinical course.
- Prognosis.
- Nature and extent of functional limitations.
- Therapeutic interventions and results.
- Past experience with related items.
- Consultations and reports from other physicians, an interdisciplinary team, home health agencies, etc.
- A complete listing of all assistive devices the patient is using, including copies of prescriptions and certification forms or letters.
- A system to track device performance, including follow-up assessment schedules and lists of professionals and vendors to contact if problems occur.

This comprehensive medical record supplies the background information needed to substantiate the need for the AT devices and services, regardless of the funding source.

Letters of medical necessity

Physicians are frequently asked to write letters of medical necessity. Well-written letters of medical necessity help ensure that the AT needs of patients are met. These letters should include the diagnoses (International Center for the Disabled codes) and the functional limitations of the individual (e.g. balance disorder or developmental delay). There should also be a statement about the patient's inability to perform specific tasks, such as activities of daily living, work activities, and ability to walk functionally.

For example, individuals with severe communication disorders typically cannot communicate verbally and/or in writing, and are often unable to communicate independently over the phone. This would also mean they are unable to adequately communicate their healthcare needs to medical personnel, and are therefore unsafe or at risk. These details should be included in a letter of medical necessity.

The letter should also include a paragraph stating why the equipment is necessary. For example, the use of the equipment will allow patients to do the following.

- Function independently or improve their functional ability.
- Perform independent wheelchair mobility in the home and community.
- Return home or move to a less expensive level of care.
- Fulfill the requirement of a lifetime medical need (if for a shorter duration, explain the need).

Next, the letter needs a rationale for choosing this specific equipment. This requires description of the specific equipment features and listing all required components. This might include the following.

- Features that provide safety or safe positioning for an activity.
- Cost-effectiveness of preventing secondary complications (e.g. pressure ulcers).
- Mobility restrictions preventing independent activity.
- Access to areas in the home, such as the bathroom and kitchen.
- Durability of the product over its alternatives.
- Past experience, interventions, and results (failure of less expensive solutions).

Funding assistive technology

The funding sources for AT devices and services fall into several categories. The AT assessment process often helps to identify which source will be used. One source is private or government medical or health insurance. Health insurance defines AT as 'medical equipment necessary for treatment of a specific illness or injury', and a physician's prescription is usually required. When writing a prescription for an AT device, it is important that physicians be made aware of the costs and benefits of the devices, and be prepared to justify their prescriptions to third-party payers. Funding includes not only the initial cost of the device, but also the expense involved in equipment maintenance and patient education or training, as well as the potential economic benefits it provides to the patient (e.g. a return to work).

Assistive technology is usually covered under policy provisions for durable medical equipment, orthoses and prostheses, or aids to daily living and mobility aids. With both private and government health insurance policies, coverage is based on existing law and regulations. In 2002, AAC devices were included for reimbursement by Medicare.[36] AT professionals and other healthcare providers should continually advocate for adequate coverage of AT in all healthcare plans.

Funding for AT is also available from other federal and state government entities, such as the Veterans Administration, State Vocational Rehabilitation Agencies, State Independent Living Rehabilitation Centers, and State Department of Education Services. Local school districts might also fund educational-related AT for children.

Each agency or program sets criteria for the funding of AT devices based on its mission and the purpose of the technology. For example, vocational rehabilitation agencies pay for AT devices and services that facilitate or help maintain paid employment. Education systems fund AT that enables students to perform or participate in school.

Funding is generally available for AT, but persistence and advocacy by the AT provider are required for success.[33,36] The AT provider must keep abreast of the requirements of various funding sources, however, in order to direct the client to the appropriate organizations. Private funding is often available through subsidized loan programs, churches, charitable organizations, and disability-related non-profit groups. Often, funding from several sources is needed to reduce personal out of pocket costs. It is important that the presumed availability of funding not drive the evaluation process and limit the options that are considered for an individual. If the need and the justification for a particular AT solution are clear, then it easier to locate a source of funding and make the case for funding the AT device or service.

Mirenda and Beukelman identify five steps in developing a funding strategy.[7]

1. Survey the funding resources available to the individual.
2. Identify funding sources for the various steps in the AT intervention (e.g. assessment, funding, and training).
3. Prepare a funding plan with the client and family members or advocates.
4. Assign responsibility to specific individuals for the funding of each step of the AT intervention.
5. Prepare the necessary written documentation for the funding source so there is a record in the event that an appeal is needed.

SUMMARY AND FUTURE DIRECTIONS

The world of AT is moving at a very rapid pace, fed in large part by the growth in mainstream technologies and the culture of inclusion that is changing traditional concepts about disability and impairment. Space travel, satellite-supported telecommunications, wireless networks, new materials with advanced performance properties, miniaturization of integrated circuits, and innovation in batteries and power sources are all crossing over into the field of AT. Federal funding supports Rehabilitation and Engineering Research Centers for the development and testing of new AT concepts. Funds also support the transfer of technologies from the federal laboratory system to AT manufacturers. The convergence of these factors is leading to AT products more likely to meet the needs of persons with disabilities.

REFERENCES

1. [Anonymous]. Section 508 of the Rehabilitation Act of 1973, as amended 29 U.S.C. 794 (d). 1998.
2. [Anonymous]. Technology Related Assistance for Individuals with Disabilities Act of 1988. 1988. Federal Register, 19 August 1991:41272.
3. [Anonymous]. The Individuals with Disabilities Education Act Amendments of 1997. 1997.
4. [Anonymous]. The Rehabilitation Act Amendments of 1992 and Assistive Technology. Rehabilitation Engineering and Assistive Technology Society of North America: Assistive Technology Quarterly; 1993.
5. [Anonymous]. The Rehabilitation Act of 1973, as amended. 1973.
6. Ball L, Beukelman D, Patee G. Augmentative and alternative communication: clinical decision making for persons with ALS. 2002:7–12.
7. Beukelman DR, Mirenda P. Augmentative and alternative communication: management of severe communication disorders in children and adults. 2nd edn. Baltimore: Paul H Brookes; 1998:604.
8. Blake DJ, Bodine C. An overview of assistive technology for persons with multiple sclerosis. J Rehabil Res Dev 2002; 39:299–312.
9. Bodine C, Beukelman DR. Prediction of future speech performance among potential users of AAC systems: a survey. Augment Altern Commun 1991; 7:100–111.
10. Bromley BE. Assistive technology assessment: a comparative analysis of five models. In: CSUN 2001. 2001.
11. Chatman A, Hyams S, Neel J, et al. The patient specific functional scale: measurement properties in patients with knee dysfunction. Phys Ther 1997; 77:820–829.
12. Cook AM, Hussey SM. Assistive technologies: principles and practice. 2nd edn. St. Louis: Mosby; 2002.
13. De Ruyter F, Kennedy MR, Doyle M. Augmentative communication and stroke rehabilitation: who is doing what and do the data tell the whole story? In: The National Stroke Rehabilitation Conference, 1990. Boston; 1990.
14. Galvin JC, Scherer M. Evaluating, selecting, and using appropriate assistive technology. Gaithersburg: Aspen Publishers; 1996.
15. Gray DB, Quatrano LA, Lieberman M. Designing and using assistive technology: the human perspective. Baltimore: Paul H Brookes; 1998.
16. Grove N. Augmentative and alternative communication—management of severe communication disorders in children and adults. J Intellect Disabil Res 1994; 38:219–220.
17. Haber PA. High technology in geriatric care. Clin Geriatr Med 1986; 2:491–500.
18. Hager RM. Funding of assistive technology: State Vocational Rehabilitation Agencies and their obligation to maximize employment. Buffalo: Neighborhood Legal Services; 1999.
19. James P, Thorpre N. Ancient inventions. New York: Ballentine Books; 1994.
20. Jutai J. Quality of life impact of assistive technology. Rehabil Eng 1999; 14:2–7.
21. Klund J. A crash course on alternative access. Technol Spec Interest Sect Q 2001:1–3.
22. La Plante MP. The demographics of disability. Milbank Q 1991:55–77.
23. Nagi S. Some conceptual issues in disability and rehabilitation. In: Sussman M, ed. Sociology and rehabilitation. Washington: American Sociological Association; 1965:100–113.
24. Patterson DJ, Liao Lin, Fox D, et al. Inferring high-level behavior from low-level sensors. In: McCarthy AD, et al, eds. UBICOMP 2003: the Fifth International Conference on Ubiquitous Computing. New York: Springer-Verlag; 2003:73–89.
25. Pentland A. Machine understanding of human action. In: 7th International Forum on Frontier of Telecom Technology. 1995.
26. Phillips B, Zhao H. Predictors of assistive technology abandonment. Assist Technol 1993; 5:36–45.

27. Pope AM, Tarlove AR. Disability in America: toward a national agenda for prevention. Washington: National Academy Press; 1991.

28. Riemer-Reiss ML, Wacker Robbyn R. Factors associated with assistive technology discontinuance among individuals with disabilities. J Rehabil 2000:44–49.

29. Romski MA, Sevcik RA. Language learning through augmented means: the process and its products. Baltimore: Paul H Brookes; 1993.

30. Scherer M, Coombs FK. Ethical issues in the evaluation and selection of assistive technology. Online. Available: http://www.gatfl.org/publications/ethical.pdf

31. Scherer M. Assistive technology use, avoidance and abandonment: what we know so far. In: Proceedings of the 6th Annual Technology and Person with Disability Conference, Los Angeles, 1991.

32. Scherer M. Assistive technology: matching device and consumer for successful rehabilitation. Washington: American Psychological Association; 2002.

33. Scherer MJ, Cushman LA. Measuring subjective quality of life following spinal cord injury: a validation study of the assistive technology device predisposition assessment. Disabil Rehabil 2001; 23:387–393.

34. Scherer MJ, McKee BG. Assessing predispositions to technology use in special education: music education majors score with the 'Survey on Technology Use'. In: RESNA '94 Annual Conference. Arlington: Rehabilitation Engineering and Assistive Technology Society of North America; 1994.

35. Scherer MJ. Living in a state of stuck: how technology impacts the lives of people with disabilities. Cambridge: Brookline Books; 1993.

36. Scherer MJ. Living in the state of stuck: how technology impacts the lives of people with disabilities. 3rd edn. Cambridge: Brookline Books; 2000.

37. Schwartzberg JG, Kakavas VK, Malkind S. Guidelines for the use of assistive technology: evaluation, referral, prescription. 2nd edn. Chicago: American Medical Association; 1996.

38. Spruill LC. An individual end-user perspective on converting from manual to power mobility as a result of shoulder pain. In: Thirteenth International Seating Symposium, 1997. Pittsburgh: University of Pittsburgh School of Health and Rehabilitation Sciences; 1997.

39. US Congress. Americans with Disabilities (ADA) accessibility guidelines for buildings and facilities. Washington: US Architectural and Transportation Barriers Compliance Board; 1991:91.

40. US Congress. Americans with Disabilities Act of 1990. 1990.

41. Wehmeyer ML, Kelchner K, Richards S. Individual and environmental factors related to the self-determination of adults with mental retardation. J Vocat Rehabil 1995; 5:291–305.

42. World Health Organization Committee for the International Classification of Functioning. International classification of functioning: ICF checklist. Geneva: WHO: 2002.

43. World Health Organization. International classification of functioning, disability and health: literature review on environmental factors. Geneva: WHO; 2000.

Chapter

25

Peripheral Joint, Soft Tissue and Spinal Injection Techniques

Frank J.E. Falco, C. Obi Onyewu, Franklin Lee Irwin Jr., Daniel W. Kim and Jie Zhu

The use of therapeutic joint injections with corticosteroids for pain relief was first reported by Hollander in 1951 for arthritic joint disease.[42] Hollander demonstrated that hydrocortisone acetate could be effective for the purpose of treating a variety of joint diseases, including osteoarthritis and rheumatoid arthritis. The use of epidural injections was first reported in 1901 by Cathelin, when he injected cocaine through the sacral hiatus for the treatment of lumbar radiculopathy.[14] Robecchi and Capra were the first to report the use of corticosteroids for the treatment of radiculopathy.[77] They performed an S1 nerve root injection with hydrocortisone acetate in a woman suffering from sciatica, with subsequent pain relief. In 1957, Lièvre published the first report on the epidural administration of corticosteroids for the treatment of back and radicular leg pain.[53]

Peripheral joint and axial spine injections are commonly used for both diagnostic and therapeutic purposes. Pain can originate from the peripheral joints and the spine, both of which are frequent causes of disability. Pain sources within articulated joints include the capsule, tendons, ligaments, synovium, and periosteum. Common spine pain generator sites include the facet joint, sacroiliac joint, nerve root (spinal nerve), and intervertebral disk.

Diagnostic injections of an anesthetic with or without a corticosteroid, or the application of provocative injections, can help discern between soft tissue, joint, spine, neurologic, or referred pain. Peripheral joint aspirations can also provide synovial fluid for laboratory analysis. Therapeutic injections can provide pain relief through one of several mechanisms, including aspiration of synovial fluid from an inflammatory joint (arthrocentesis) to reduce pain; and delivering a pharmacologic agent to a painful structure to provide pain relief (whether it be a joint or a neurologic structure), or confirm a painful condition amenable to other interventional means. Many conditions have shown clinical improvement with corticosteroid and/or anesthetic injections, including rheumatoid arthritis, osteoarthritis, seronegative spondyloarthropathies, gout, pseudogout, bursitis, adhesive capsulitis, tendonitis, axial spine pain, sympathetic-mediated disorders, and radiculopathy.

The use of peripheral joint, soft tissue, and spinal injections must always be part of a comprehensive treatment program. This is true whether the injections are used in the setting of acute, subacute, or chronic pain. The decision to perform an injection is determined only after assessing the results of a thorough history and physical examination, laboratory data, electrodiagnostic studies, and imaging studies, as well as the goals of the physician and patient. These injections play an important role in the care of patients, even though they often do not reverse the underlying pathology and typically do not provide permanent pain relief. When these procedures are used in the framework of a well-rounded treatment approach, however, they can deliver long-term pain reduction, increase function, delay or eliminate surgical treatment, and lead to a better overall quality of life.

This chapter presents the injection techniques of the most common joint and soft tissue structures of the upper and lower extremities, as well as spinal procedures that are frequently employed in the treatment of axial, radicular, and limb pain. The different injection solutions, supplies, and equipment to perform the injections are reviewed in this chapter, along with the indications, contraindications, complications, and efficacy.

INJECTION MATERIALS

Local anesthetics are used routinely in a therapeutic and a diagnostic role by confirming or eliminating a specific structure as a pain generator. They are grouped as either esters or amides, depending on the linkage between the lipophilic benzene ring and the amino group at the opposite end of the molecule. The mechanism that allows local anesthetics to provide pain relief is the reversible neural blockade of transmitted neural signals. This is accomplished by blocking sodium channels, which attenuates sodium influx and prevents change in the transmembrane potential.

Local anesthetics can have side effects locally or systemically. Central nervous system effects include seizures, respiratory arrest, convulsions, confusion, and death. Signs of toxicity include tremor, sluggishness, twitches, drowsiness, blurred vision, incoherent speech, and light-headedness. Other systemic reactions include cardiac depression, malignant hypertension, and anaphylaxis.

Corticosteroids have two mechanisms of action. One is as an antiinflammatory agent, and the other is as an immunosuppressive. Their vast array of systemic mechanisms of action involves glucocorticoid, mineralocorticoid, antiinflammatory, and immunosuppressive activities both locally and systemically.

Corticosteroids have been utilized for treatment of musculoskeletal pain because of their antiinflammatory properties. They have also been reported to have a direct membrane-stabilizing effect, which leads to decreased afferent ectopic discharges at the neural membrane. There is also a reversible inhibition of nociceptive C-fiber transmission with local application of corticosteroids. To date, there has been no demonstration of A- or B-fiber transmission interruption.[45] Corticosteroids are also thought to have a modulation effect on spinal cord neural activity.

Several corticosteroids are utilized in joint, soft tissue, and spinal injections, including betamethasone, dexamethasone, hydrocortisone, methylprednisolone, prednisolone, and triamcinolone. Adverse corticosteroid reactions include skin hypopigmentation, subcutaneous fat atrophy, tendon rupture, fluid retention, flushing, hyperglycemia, change in taste, insomnia, malaise, and dyspepsia.[11,32] Systemic suppression of the adrenal glands can happen after a local injection of corticosteroids into any structure, including joint, soft tissues, or the spine. Repeated injections of corticosteroids can lead to a cushingoid appearance.

Non-ionic contrast agents include metrizamide (Amnipaque), iopamidol (Isovue), and iohexol (Omnipaque). These are used in conjunction with fluoroscopy for needle tip localization in performing spinal injection procedures and some peripheral joint injections. The use of contrast significantly reduces the risk of an unintended injection into a vascular area, blood vessel, or subarachnoid space. The adverse effects that can result from the use of contrast agents are due to local tissue toxicity and to anaphylaxis. Greater than 90% of adverse reactions occur within the first 15 min.[36] In addition to anaphylactic reaction, other side effects that have been reported include nausea, headache, and emesis.[55] Pretreatment is recommended with steroids and antihistamines 12 h, and again at 2 h, prior to the procedure in patients with an allergic reaction history.[51] Gadolinium is a viable alternative for patients with contrast material allergies, and provides adequate visualization for spinal injection procedures.[21,22]

Syringes typically utilized in injection procedures are 3 mL, 5 mL, and 10 mL in size. This depends on the required injection volume, needle diameter, and tissue resistance. The needles are available in different diameters (determined by the gauge, which is inversely related to diameter size), lengths, and tips (beveled, pencil point, or blunt) (Fig. 25-1). Beveled tip needles assist in steering needles with flexible shafts (long- or small-diameter needles) through soft tissue structures and/or when the needle tip has to be placed deep within the body. A bend of approximately 10° at the tip of the needle opposite to the bevel increases the steering capability of the needle (Fig. 25-2). Injection tubing can be attached to the needle hub and syringe when performing spinal injection procedures to minimize x-ray exposure. It also reduces needle tip movement by permitting the exchange of syringes at the distal end of the tubing rather than at the needle hub.

Radiation safety when using fluoroscopy for injection procedures requires minimizing exposure to ionizing radiation. This

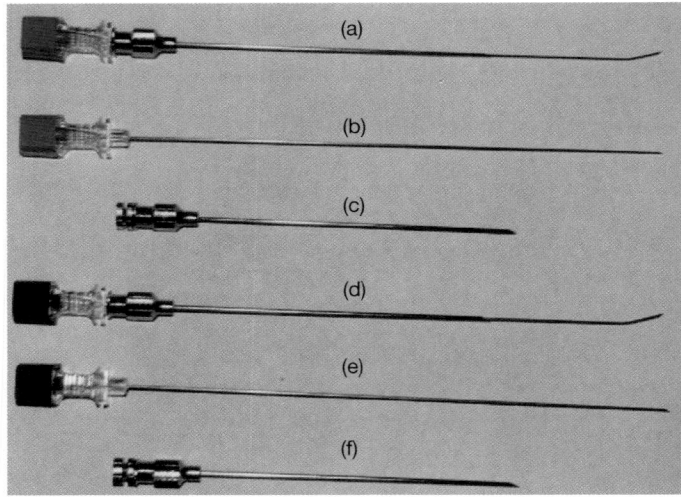

Figure 25-1 Spinal needles. (**a**) Two-needle set: a 6-inch, 25-gauge spinal needle with a distal 10° bend within a 3^1/$_2$-inch, 20-gauge needle; used for lumbar diskography or lumbar transforaminal epidural injections. (**b**) A 6-inch, 25-gauge spinal needle. (**c**) A 3^1/$_2$-inch, 20-gauge spinal needle. (**d**) Two-needle set: a 6-inch, 22-gauge spinal needle with a distal 10° bend within a 3^1/$_2$-inch, 18-gauge needle; used for lumbar diskography or lumbar transforaminal epidural injections. (**e**) A 6-inch, 22-gauge spinal needle. (**f**) A 3^1/$_2$-inch, 22-gauge spinal needle.

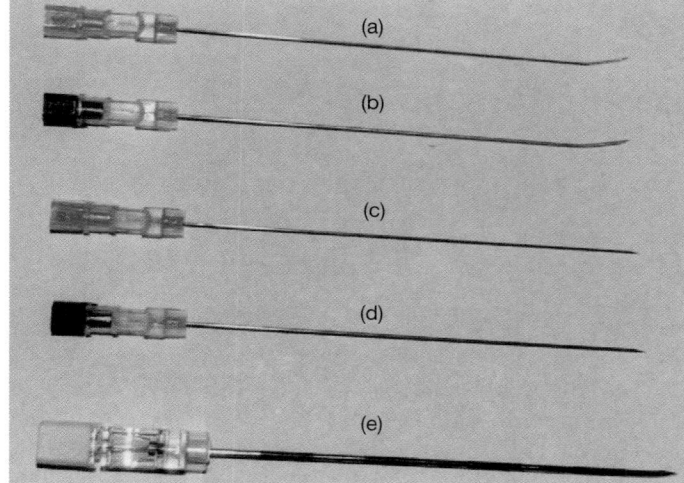

Figure 25-2 Spinal needles. (**a**) A 3^1/$_2$-inch, 20-gauge spinal needle with a distal 10° bend and a radiolucent hub. (**b**) A 3^1/$_2$-inch, 22-gauge spinal needle with a distal 10° bend and a radiolucent hub. (**c**) A 3^1/$_2$-inch, 20-gauge spinal needle with a radiolucent hub. (**d**) A 3^1/$_2$-inch, 22-gauge spinal needle with a radiolucent hub. (**e**) A 3^1/$_2$-inch, 17-gauge Tuohy epidural needle with a radiolucent hub.

exposure can be reduced by decreasing exposure time, by increasing exposure distance, and by maximizing exposure shielding. Appropriate use of image collimation, high- and low-dose modes, image storage capability, and pulsed fluoroscopy can also significantly reduce exposure time. Protective barriers, aprons, and glasses should be used to shield susceptible tissues such as the thyroid, eyes, lungs, colon, and gonads.

GENERAL CONSIDERATIONS

The following are important guidelines that serve as a general protocol in performing joint, soft tissue, and spinal injections. First, always explain the injection to the patient and answer all questions. Obtain informed and documented consent prior to performing the injection, and provide the patient with a clear explanation of the risks and benefits. Instruct patients on how to maintain a pain diary to document their pain activity after the injection procedure. Caution should always be used to avoid the risk of bleeding. Patients using aspirin should discontinue it for at least 7 days. If patients cannot tolerate being off aspirin, a non-selective NSAID can be substituted for at least the 3 days prior to any injection procedure. See the section regarding warfarin (Coumadin) below. Women who are pregnant or suspected to be pregnant should avoid radiation exposure from fluoroscopy.

The patient is properly positioned on the procedure table before beginning the injection. Prepare and drape the injection site in a sterile manner with povidone–iodine (Betadine), chlorhexidine gluconate (Hibiclens), and/or isopropyl alcohol. Sterile gloves are worn during the injection procedure. Gown, cap, and mask are used when performing myelography and diskography. Intravenous or oral antibiotics are used when performing injection procedures in patients with implanted prosthetic devices or with a history of mitral valve prolapse. The injection site can be anesthetized for patient comfort with a local anesthetic, anesthetic cream, or vapocoolant spray prior to the injection. The needle is always aspirated via the syringe before the injection to avoid an intravascular or, in the case of some spinal procedures, an intrathecal injection. Avoid injecting into a ligament, a tendon, or the periosteum. This means repositioning the needle if there is significant resistance. Avoid needle contact with articular cartilage surfaces during joint injections. The injection is given slowly, with steady pressure. A dressing is applied to the injection site after the injection is completed. The patient is encouraged to rest the area after the injection for several days, especially if it is a major weight-bearing joint. All patients should be driven home and should not drive for the next 24 h.

PERIPHERAL JOINT AND SOFT TISSUE INJECTION TECHNIQUES

Indications

Injection of corticosteroid or anesthetic into a joint or soft tissue structure can diagnostically determine if the injected body part is or is not generating local and/or referred pain. Joint aspiration also aids in the diagnosis of the underlying pathologic process through synovial fluid analysis. Therapeutic joint injections provide pain relief and functional improvement in symptomatic pathologic conditions, by either aspiration of fluid from the joint (arthrocentesis) or by delivering a pharmacologic agent to the joint.

Contraindications and complications

Absolute contraindications for performing peripheral joint and soft tissue injections include bacteremia, joint infection, cellulitis, skin ulcerations, osteomyelitis, infectious arthritis, epidural abscess, and joint injections requiring fluoroscopy in the pregnant patient. Relative contraindications include chronic infection distant from the injection site, an allergy to the injection solution, latex allergy, diabetes mellitus, an allergy to contrast agents for fluoroscopically guided joint injections, and altered anatomy from surgical procedures or congenital anomalies. Tendons and ligaments can be ruptured if corticosteroids are injected directly into them (this is estimated to occur in less than 1% of such cases).

Patients requiring anticoagulation medication or with a known bleeding diathesis should be approached with a great deal of caution. Coagulation parameters should be evaluated in these cases, including a prothrombin time, an activated partial thromboplastin time, an international normalized ratio (INR), and a platelet level count. Injections should be avoided with prolonged bleeding times, an INR greater than 1.2, and a platelet count of less than 100 000 per µL.

Efficacy

Most research trials regarding the efficacy of intraarticular steroid injections have been performed on the knee. Rheumatoid arthritis and osteoarthritis are the two most common conditions for which there is an indication for intraarticular joint injections with steroids. Improvement in rheumatoid synovitis has been seen to last for as long as 3 months after injecting glucocorticoids,[37] with improvement in pain and in knee extensor strength.[33] A systematic review by Kirwan found that intraarticular knee injections for osteoarthritis with steroids provided more pain relief than placebo.[50] A randomized controlled trial by Ravaud et al. also demonstrated that intraarticular corticosteroid injections in the knee for osteoarthritis resulted in better pain reduction and function compared with placebo.[74] Jones and Doherty used a double-blind, crossover, placebo-controlled design, and found significant improvement in knee pain at 3 weeks after intraarticular steroid injections, but no significant benefit at 8 weeks.[47] A review of several randomized controlled trials shows that intraarticular injections of hyaluronan (hyaluronic acid, hyaluronate) were more effective than placebo in reducing pain and improving joint function from osteoarthritis of the knee.[74,86]

There are limited data regarding intraarticular injections of joints other than the knee. Although there is evidence of beneficial effects of intraarticular corticosteroid injections for acute exacerbations of osteoarthritis,[23,37,94,98] controlled studies have demonstrated only modest, transient benefits in the case of severe osteoarthritis involving the hip, knee, and ankle.[23,37,72] A small randomized controlled trial found no significant difference between intraarticular injections of methylprednisolone plus lidocaine (lignocaine) versus lidocaine alone for the treatment of shoulder pain, although there was a small improvement in pain and range of motion in both groups at 24 weeks.[76] Plant et al. conducted a prospective open study, injecting a

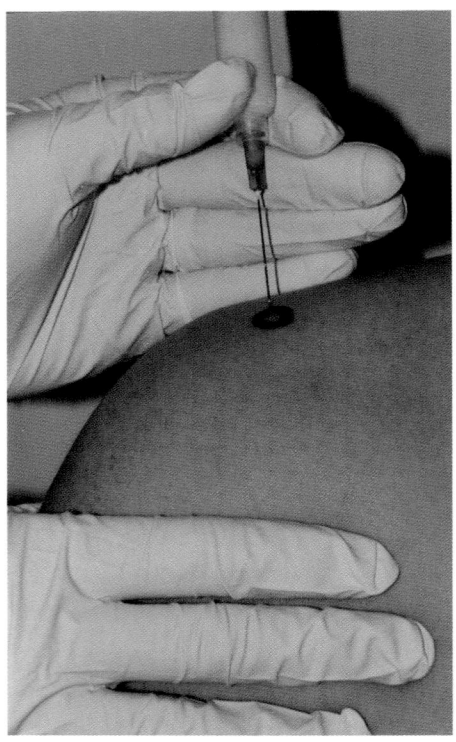

Figure 25-3
Acromioclavicular
joint injection.

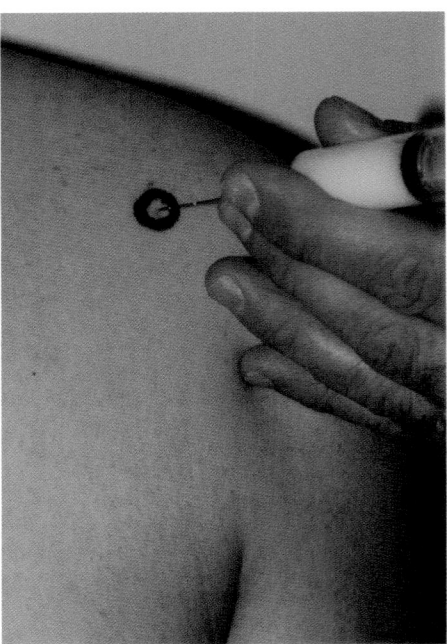

Figure 25-4
Glenohumeral joint
injection, anterior
approach.

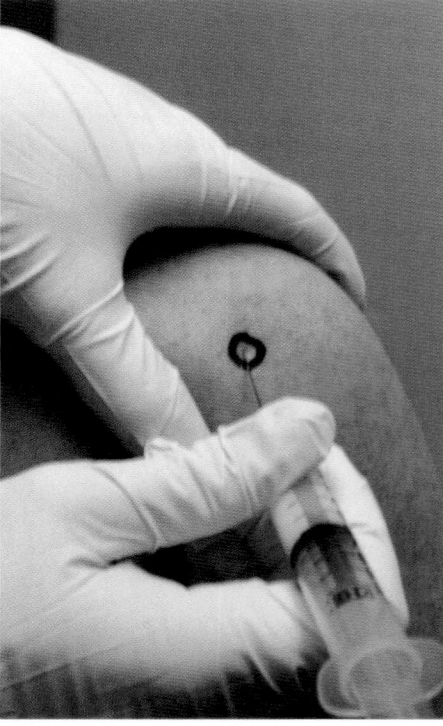

Figure 25-5
Subacromial bursa
injection.

combination of intraarticular steroid and local anesthetic in 45 patients with hip arthritis. This study found significant pain reduction at 2 and 12 weeks, but none at 26 weeks.[71]

Upper limb injection techniques

Acromioclavicular joint
The injection is performed with the patient in the seated position with the upper limb resting comfortably. The acromioclavicular joint is located at a depressed and soft region distal to the end of the clavicle. The injection site is anterior and superior to the acromioclavicular joint (Fig. 25-3). The needle is then advanced inferiorly into the joint.

Glenohumeral joint
The glenohumeral joint is typically injected from either an anterior or a posterior approach. In the anterior approach, a needle is inserted lateral to the coracoid process while avoiding the thoracoacromial artery (Fig. 25-4). The needle is then directed dorsally and medially into the joint space. The posterior approach is set up by placing the patient's hand across the chest on the opposite shoulder. The needle is inserted 2–3 cm below the posterolateral aspect of the acromion. The needle is then advanced toward the coracoid process in an anterior and medial direction into the joint.

Subacromial bursa
The subacromial bursa lies above the supraspinatus tendon and under the acromion. A posterolateral approach is used to place the needle into the subacromial space. The needle is inserted underneath the palpable posterolateral corner of the acromion and advanced toward the coracoid process (Fig. 25-5), which places the needle tip under the acromion.

Ulnohumeral (elbow) joint
The elbow joint consists of three articulations between the humerus, ulna, and radius, with the true elbow joint formed by the humerus and ulna. Injection of the ulnohumeral joint is accomplished from a posterolateral or posterior approach with

the elbow flexed between 50 and 90°. For the posterolateral approach, the needle is inserted in the posterolateral triangle formed by the palpable olecranon, lateral epicondyle, and radial head (Fig. 25-6). The needle is directed medially away from the ulnar nerve and proximally toward the head of the radius. A lack of resistance indicates entry of the needle tip into the joint. The posterior approach to the elbow joint involves inserting the needle in between the posterior olecranon and lateral epicondyle, advancing the needle until there is a loss of tissue resistance (indicating that the needle tip is within the joint).

Medial and lateral epicondyle

Medial epicondylitis, or 'golfer's elbow', results from tendonosis or degenerative changes at the tendon attachment of the wrist flexor and pronator muscle groups. The elbow is positioned in abduction, with the forearm in supination. A needle is inserted at the site of tenderness along the medial epicondyle and advanced until there is contact with the periosteum. The needle is slightly withdrawn before the injection.

Lateral epicondylitis, or 'tennis elbow', is a tendonosis from repetitive wrist extension and forearm supination. The elbow is flexed to 45° and the forearm is placed in pronation. A needle is inserted at the point of tenderness along the lateral epicondyle (Fig. 25-7) and advanced to the periosteum. The injection is delivered after the needle is slightly withdrawn.

Olecranon bursa

Olecranon bursitis, or 'draftsman's elbow', occurs in rheumatoid arthritis, crystal arthropathies, and repetitive trauma. The needle is directed toward the olecranon bursa, which is superficial to the olecranon and external to the elbow joint (Fig. 25-8). Injection of the olecranon bursa should be preceded with

aspiration, and no corticosteroids should be injected if there is a purulent discharge.

Carpal tunnel

Injection of the carpal tunnel can be approached in either an ulnar or a radial orientation, based on positioning relative to the palmaris longus tendon. The ulnar approach is preferred, because it is less likely to injure the median nerve during the injection. The wrist can be flexed to increase the prominence of the palmaris longus tendon. A needle is inserted with the wrist in a neutral position at a 30° angle ulnar to the palmaris longus tendon at the distal wrist crease (Fig. 25-9). The needle is then advanced in a distal and radial direction underneath the transverse carpal ligament. The needle is withdrawn if

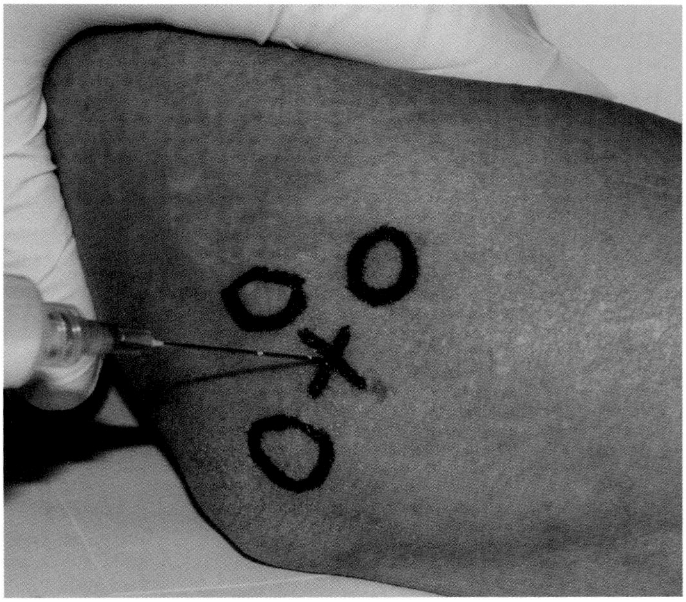

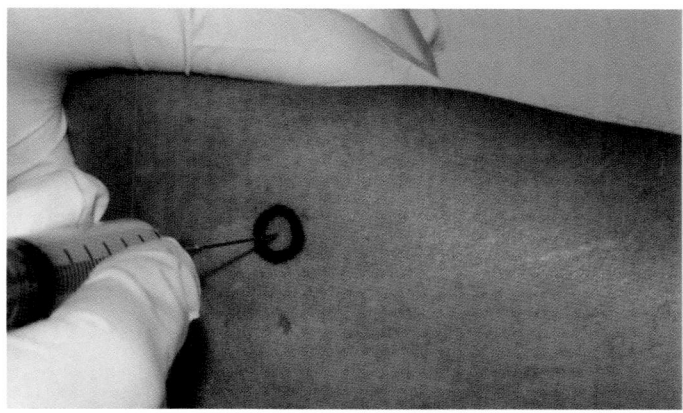

Figure 25-7 Lateral epicondyle injection.

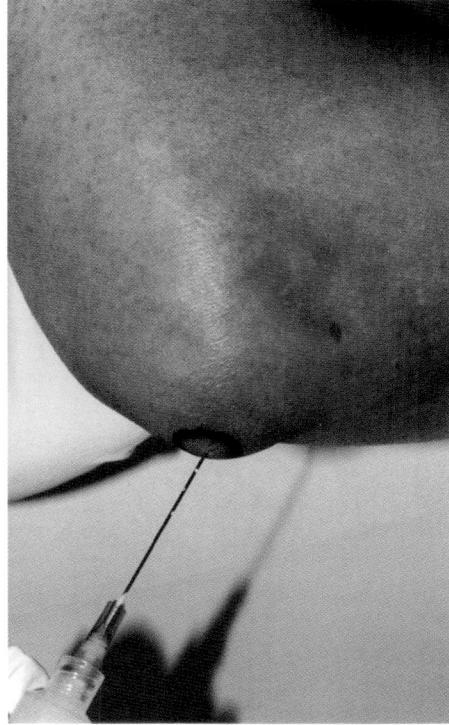

Figure 25-8
Olecranon bursa
injection.

Figure 25-6 Ulnohumeral joint injection, posterolateral approach.

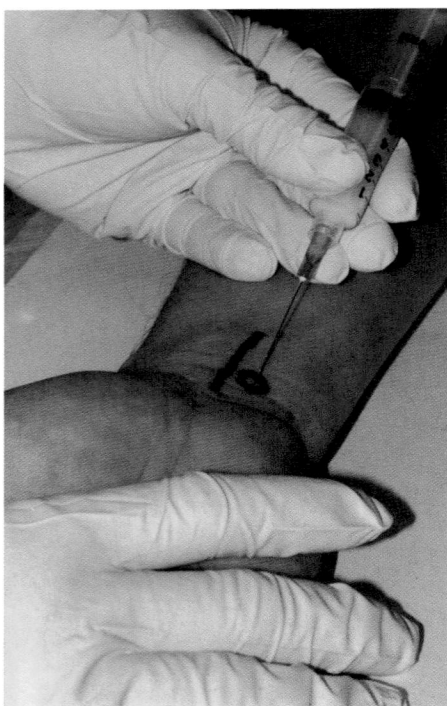

Figure 25-9 Carpal tunnel injection.

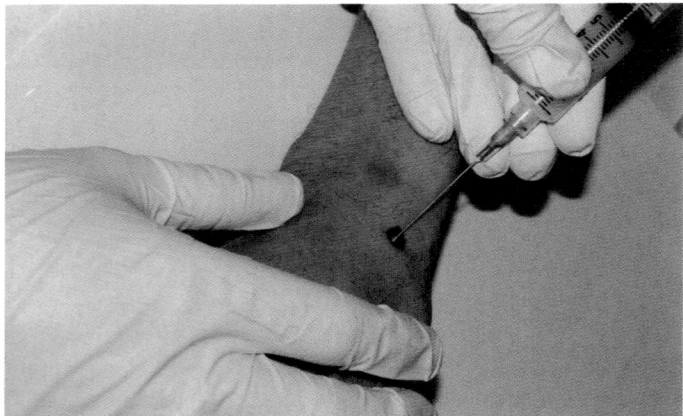

Figure 25-10 De Quervain's tenosynovitis wrist injection.

paresthesias are experienced during the insertion, and redirected within the tunnel.

Abductor and extensor pollicis tendon

De Quervain's tenosynovitis is an inflammatory disorder of the wrist involving the abductor pollicis longus and extensor pollicis brevis tendons. The needle is placed 1 cm proximal to the styloid process at a 45° angle to the forearm alongside either tendon (Fig. 25-10). The needle is repositioned before the injection if there are any paresthesias encountered from the radial nerve during needle insertion.

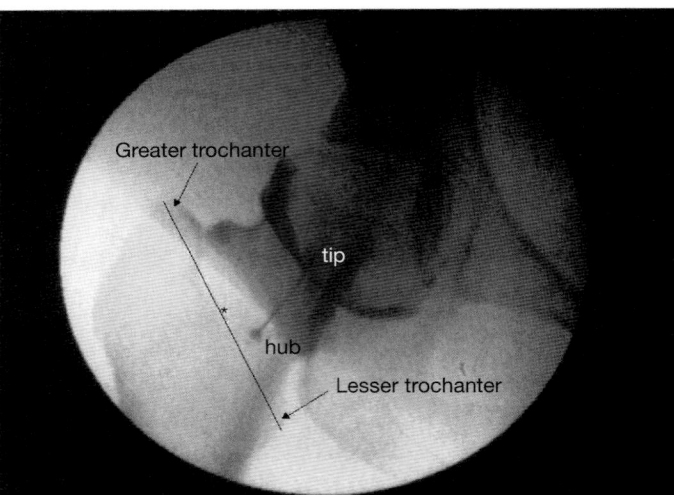

Figure 25-11 Hip joint injection. The spine needle is typically inserted at the midpoint (asterisk) of the intertrochanteric line (black line) between the greater and lesser trochanters. Contrast is visualized extending into the intraarticular hip joint. hub, spine needle hub; tip, spine needle tip.

Lower limb injection techniques
Greater trochanter and ischial bursae

The patient is placed in the lateral decubitus position, with the affected hip upright and the knees flexed to relax the hamstrings. The lateral hip and inferior buttock areas are palpated for the point of greatest tenderness over the greater trochanter and the ischial tuberosity, respectively. For both injection procedures, the needle is inserted through the skin and advanced until contact is made with the periosteum. The needle is then slightly withdrawn so that the tip lies within the bursa.

Hip joint

Intraarticular injections of the hip joint require fluoroscopic guidance and contrast enhancement, whether using a lateral or an anterior approach, in order to identify correct needle tip placement. For the anterior approach, the patient is placed in the supine position with the lower limb in external rotation. The needle is inserted at a site just inferior to the mid trochanteric line. The needle is inserted 45° toward the femoral neck, and advanced under fluoroscopic guidance through the capsule until contact with the periosteum. The needle is slightly withdrawn before aspiration and injection of contrast (Fig. 25-11).

Knee joint

The knee joint is the most common joint site for both injection and aspiration. There are three possible approaches: medial, lateral, and anterior. The patient is positioned supine for aspiration, with the knee fully extended or slightly flexed. The superior medial or superior lateral approaches are generally held to be the best for arthrocentesis. The patella is located by palpation and is the main landmark for localizing the entry site.

For the superior lateral approach, the entry site is about 1 cm superior and lateral to the patella. The skin is penetrated

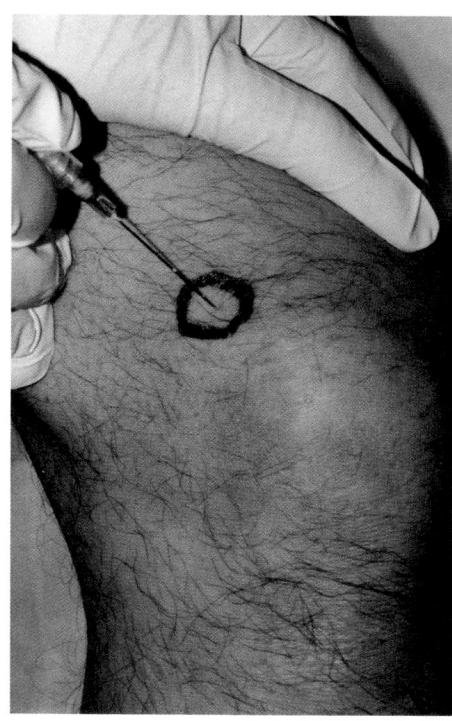

Figure 25-12 Knee joint injection, superior medial approach.

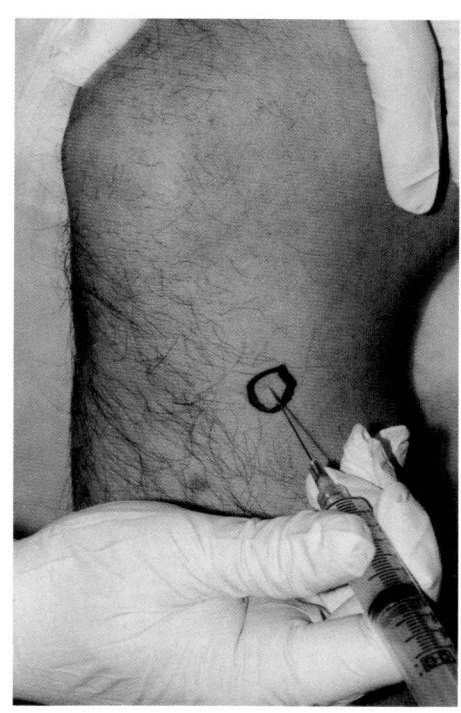

Figure 25-13 Pes anserine bursa injection.

using a large-gauge needle directed at 45° and advanced under the patella toward the medial side of the joint. The needle is advanced into the joint, while applying negative syringe pressure, until synovial fluid starts to enter the syringe. The fluid aspiration can be aided by applying pressure to the medial aspect of the joint to displace the effusion toward the direction of the needle.

For the superior medial approach, needle entry is 1 cm superior and medial to the patella (Fig. 25-12). The needle is directed under the patella and advanced toward the opposite patella midpole, midway between the medial border of the patella and the femur. The advantage of the anterior approach is greater ease of entry into knees with advanced osteoarthritis, as well as for patients who cannot fully extend their knees. The downside to this approach is a greater risk for meniscal and articular cartilage injury.

For injections of corticosteroids without synovial fluid aspiration, the patient is positioned as described or with 90° of knee flexion. The entry site for injection with the knee in the flexed position can be on either the medial or the lateral aspect of the patellar tendon. The joint is entered inferior to the patella, using a needle directed superiorly toward the intercondylar notch. The inferior medial approach is technically easier for injection than the lateral approach if the patient can only slightly flex the knee.

Pes anserine and prepatella bursae

The pes anserine bursa is located between the medial collateral ligament and the confluence of the sartorius, gracilis, and semi-tendinosus tendon insertion at the proximal medial tibia just distal to the joint line. The tendinous border of the medial thigh muscles are identified and traced across the joint line to their insertion at the pes anserine. A needle is inserted at the site of greatest palpable tenderness perpendicular to the tibia, and advanced until contact is made with the periosteum (Fig. 25-13). The needle is slightly withdrawn so that the tip lies in the bursa before the injection. The prepatellar bursa is located between the skin and the anterior surface of the patella. The needle is inserted at the midportion of the superior patellar pole. The bursa can be significant is size from inflammation, which often allows for fluid aspiration that can be aided by direct pressure over the patella before injection.

Ankle joint

The ankle joint is formed by the tibia and talus (tibiotalar mortise), and is not one of the more commonly injected joints. The main indication for injecting the ankle is for pain secondary to osteoarthritis. The two approaches for performing an ankle joint injection are the anterior medial and anterior lateral. The talus is palpated with the foot in the neutral position. A horizontal line can be drawn between the medial and lateral sides of the ankle, just above the malleoli. For the anterior medial approach, a soft spot is identified medial to the anterior tibial tendon and lateral to the medial malleolus. The needle is inserted perpendicular to the tibial joint surface and advanced slightly laterally, superiorly, and posteriorly. The injection is then given slowly after there is a decrease in tissue resistance indicating that the needle has entered the joint. The anterior lateral approach is done with the patient positioned with the foot in plantar flexion. The needle is inserted from the anterior lateral position and directed posteriorly toward the medial malleolus (Fig. 25-14). The needle again is advanced until

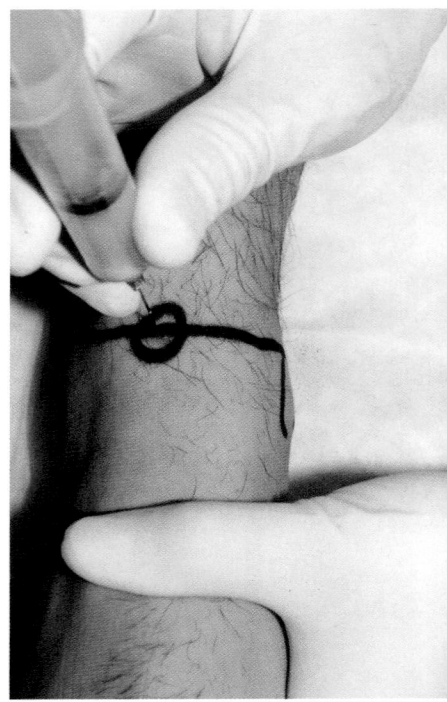

Figure 25-14 Ankle joint injection, anterior lateral approach.

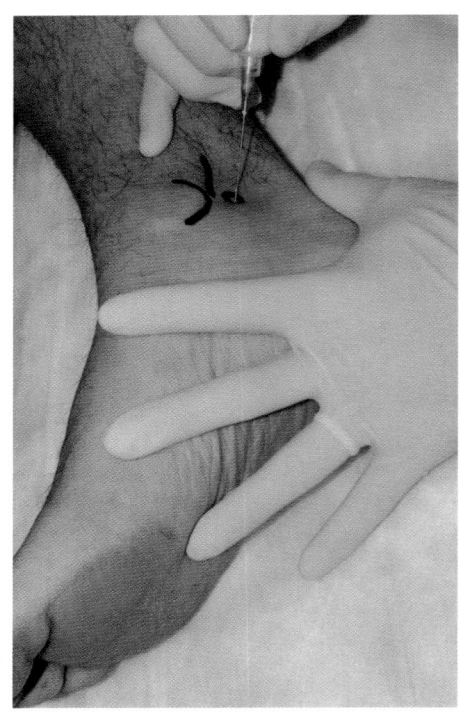

Figure 25-15 Tarsal tunnel injection.

there is a drop in tissue resistance confirming entry into the joint.

Tarsal tunnel

The patient is placed in a lateral decubitus position with the symptomatic foot down. The posterior tibial nerve is posterior to the posterior tibialis tendon, which is identified by resisting foot inversion. The needle is inserted behind the medial malleolus posterior to the tendon (Fig. 25-15) at a 30° angle, and advanced a few centimeters before the injection. The needle is repositioned if there are paresthesias or resistance during the injection.

Plantar fascia

Plantar fasciitis is the most common problem of the hind foot, with inflammation that occurs at its medial attachment to the calcaneus. The site where the medial calcaneus starts to curve superiorly is palpated to confirm the injection site. The needle is inserted at this location perpendicular to the calcaneus, and advanced until it hits periosteum. The needle is then repositioned and advanced distal to the plantar surface of the bone, placing the needle tip superior to the plantar fascia (Fig. 25-16). The injection is then performed in this position, which avoids the superficial fat pad, the subcutaneous tissue, and the fascia that could otherwise lead to fat pad atrophy or tissue necrosis or rupture of the fascia.

Achilles (retrocalcaneal, retro-Achilles) bursae

The retrocalcaneal bursa is located between the calcaneus and the Achilles tendon, whereas the retro-Achilles bursa is located between the Achilles tendon and the skin. Either of these

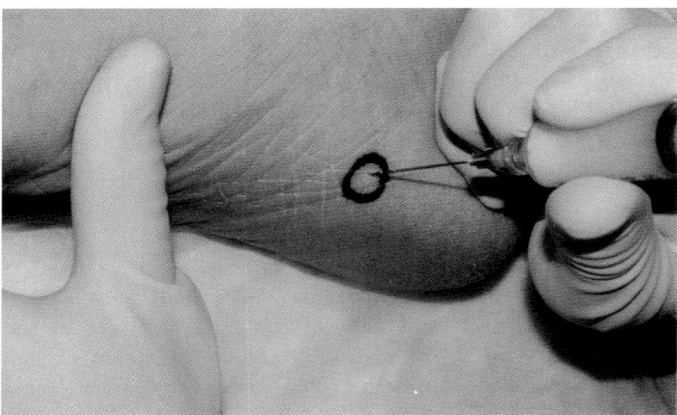

Figure 25-16 Plantar fascia injection.

disorders can be mistaken for Achilles tendonitis or occur in combination with Achilles tendonitis (Haglund syndrome). An injection of the bursa should be considered only in severe, disabling cases after failure of conservative treatment. The patient is forewarned about Achilles tendon rupture as a possible side effect of the corticosteroid injection. To locate the area of maximum tenderness, the Achilles tendon insertion site is palpated deep, superficial, and at the tendon. The retrocalcaneal bursa (Fig. 25-17) is injected deep to the tendon, whereas the retro-Achilles bursa is injected superficial to the tendon. Care must be taken to avoid injecting directly into the Achilles tendon when injecting either bursa.

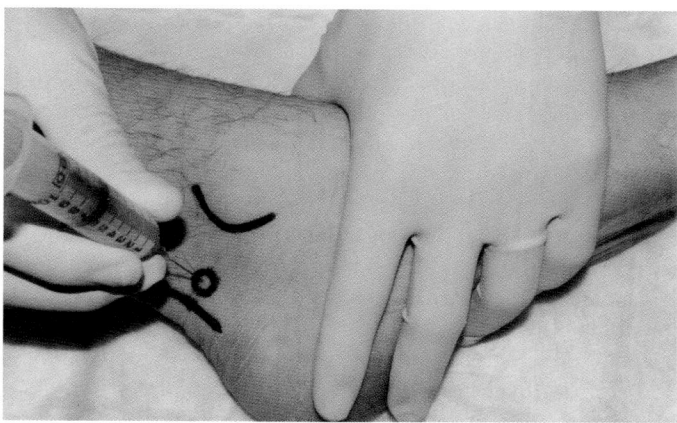

Figure 25-17 Retrocalcaneal bursa injection.

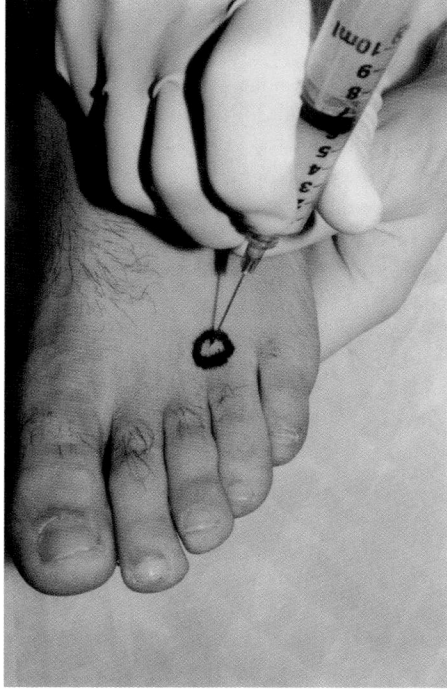

Figure 25-18
Morton's neuroma
injection.

Morton's neuroma

Morton's neuroma is actually a perineural fibrosis of the common digital nerve as it passes between the metatarsal heads. The neuroma most commonly occurs at the distal aspect of the third metatarsal space. A needle is passed through the dorsal surface of the foot (Fig. 25-18), and advanced about 1 cm proximal to the metatarsal web space. The needle is advanced deep enough to place the tip at the level of the neuroma, while at the same time avoiding the plantar fat pad.

SPINAL INJECTION TECHNIQUES

Indications

The history, physical examination, and routine diagnostic studies often fail to provide a diagnosis for spinal disorders. Injection procedures of the spine frequently allow for a definitive diagnosis, which can have an impact on pain control, treatment plan, prognosis, function, and quality of life. Spinal injection procedures with corticosteroids have demonstrated significant pain relief and improved function in the treatment of radiculopathy, as well as with axial low back pain encountered in such conditions as facet joint syndrome and sacroiliac dysfunction. Sympathetic injection procedures with local anesthetics not only help assess the presence or absence of sympathetically mediated pain syndromes, but also provide short- or long-term pain relief. They can also help determine if a patient is a candidate for additional procedures that might provide long-lasting relief.

Other spinal injection procedures, such as epidurography, myelography, and diskography, provide radiologic and diagnostic information for the evaluation and treatment of specific spinal conditions. Epidurography is utilized during epidural procedures to determine proper needle placement and to avoid intravascular or intrathecal injections. Myelography is a diagnostic procedure commonly combined with computed tomography (CT) for the evaluation of spinal pathology, including disk herniations, stenosis, tumors, and infection. Diskography is a procedure used to identify whether or not an intervertebral disk(s) is generating axial spine pain in the cervical, thoracic, or lumbar regions. Diskography is recommended after there has been no response to conservative treatment and traditional diagnostic modalities, such as magnetic resonance imaging (MRI), CT, myelography, and electrodiagnostic studies, are unremarkable or not diagnostic. Diskography is also used for surgical planning when considering an intradiskal procedure, such as intradiskal electrothermal therapy, fusion, or artificial disk replacement.

Contraindications and complications

Complications associated with spinal injection procedures can be general or localized to the procedure site. These include intravascular or subarachnoid injection, allergic or anaphylactic reactions, vasovagal syncope, dural puncture, spinal headache, epidural abscess, and epidural hematoma. Allergic or anaphylactic reactions can occur from either corticosteroids or radiologic contrast material. Typically, contrast allergies occur at the time of the injections, and can quickly progress to an anaphylactic reaction with respiratory compromise. Corticosteroid allergic reactions are often delayed by up to a week, and present as an intense hot, erythematous flushing involving the neck, face, and occasionally the chest area. Corticosteroid anaphylactic reactions often occur within 2–6 h after the injection. While there is concern regarding respiratory compromise, there have been no reported fatalities.

Vasovagal episodes can occur with any type of injection procedure, whether it is a joint injection or a spinal procedure, due to the noxious stimulation effect from the needle. Patients typically become diaphoretic, hypotensive, and bradycardic. Treatment is primarily supportive, including fluids and oxygen, but begins with getting rid of the noxious stimulation by removing the needle.

Dural punctures have a low reported incidence that ranges from 0.5% to 5%.[6,68,73] Headaches resulting from dural puncture[24,25] have been reported to range from 7.5% to 75%.[16] The use of smaller gauge needles with conical non-cutting tips has been associated with fewer episodes of headaches.[35] Dural puncture headaches can occur 1–2 days after a translaminar or transforaminal epidural.

A subarachnoid or intravascular anesthetic injection can lead to periorbital numbness, disorientation, light-headedness, nystagmus, tinnitus, complete sensory or motor block, muscle twitching, respiratory depression, and seizures. The risk of complications from intrathecal and intravascular injections of local anesthetic is proportional to the injected volume.

An epidural abscess is rare from an injection, and is more common with the use of an indwelling catheter. Patients with an abscess present with severe back pain, fever, and chills.

The risk of epidural hematoma increases with anticoagulation but is rare in the presence of normal clotting factors. A hematoma can potentially lead to caudal equina compression in the lumbar spine, or cord compression in the cervical and thoracic spine. The presence of spinal stenosis increases this compression risk. Epidurals should be avoided in patients with a platelet count less than 100 000 per µL and a spinal canal midsagittal diameter less than 12 mm.

Complications of transforaminal epidural steroid injections (TFESIs) include infection, allergic reaction, and bleeding. The negative aspiration of blood appears to be inaccurate in predicting intravascular injection, and contrast injection is recommended to identify vascular uptake.[30,31] Although rare, transforaminal epidurals can lead to cerebral, cerebellar, or spinal cord infarction, leading to cognitive impairment, hemiplegia, quadriplegia, paraplegia, and death.[2,44,67,79,96] Injury to the radicular artery, particularly the artery of Adamkiewicz (lower thoracic and upper lumbar levels), or other collateral arteries within the foramen is believed to occur as a result of spasm, puncture, thrombosis, or embolization by corticosteroid particulate matter.[2,44,67,79,96] This complication might be reduced or eliminated by inserting needles into the posterior portion of the foramen, while avoiding injections in the presence of significant foraminal stenosis, using blunt tip needles,[41] and injecting with non-particulate corticosteroids.

Complications from cervical facet injection include vertebral artery puncture, and motor and sensory block from local anesthetic leaking into the spinal canal. The phrenic and recurrent laryngeal nerve can be temporarily paralyzed during cervical facet joint nerve blocks when using a large volume of local anesthetic. Other complications include spinal cord trauma, spinal anesthesia, dural puncture, intravascular injection, chemical meningitis, hematoma formation, pneumothorax, and infection.

The most common complications of sacroiliac joint injection are due to joint rupture or capsule extravasation. Posterior leakage of contrast into the dorsal sacral foramina, superior recess leakage on to the L5 epidural sheath, and ventral extravasation on to the lumbosacral plexus can affect the nearby neural structures.[26] Further complications include trauma to the sciatic nerve, infection, and adverse drug reactions.

Potential complications from stellate ganglion blocks include pneumothorax, central nervous system toxicity, low blood pressure, phrenic nerve block, brachial plexus block, or blockage of recurrent laryngeal nerve. This procedure is rarely performed bilaterally, because of the risk of blocking the phrenic and recurrent laryngeal nerve. Complications from lumbar sympathetic blocks include lumbar plexus block, renal injection, genitofemoral neuralgia, hypotension, postdural puncture headache, or spinal block.[81,89]

Postdural puncture headache is the most common complication from a myelogram. Minor disturbances in concentration and mentation after myelography are often noted but rarely, if ever, clinically significant. The risk of having a seizure or developing arachnoiditis has essentially been eliminated with the use of water-soluble, non-ionic contrast agents.[46] Epidural hemorrhage is a reported complication of myelography.[91] Spinal cord puncture is another potentially serious complication when cervical myelography is performed with a lateral C1, C2 approach. This risk can be eliminated by using a lumbar puncture to instill contrast for a cervical myelography.

Potential complications from diskography include diskitis, nerve root injury, bleeding, allergic reaction, subarachnoid puncture, soft tissue infection, and chemical meningitis. Although diskitis is a commonly reported complication, the incidence of diskitis is relatively low, with a range of 0.05–4%.[27–29,38,54,69] The incidence of diskitis can be reduced with meticulous aseptic technique, prophylactic antibiotics, styletted needles, and a two-needle technique.[27,29,69]

Efficacy

The largest number of epidural outcome studies has been reported for lumbar epidural steroid injections followed by cervical epidural steroid injections. There are no published randomized studies for thoracic epidural steroid injections. Anecdotal case reports exist describing pain relief after thoracic epidural steroid injections for thoracic radicular pain secondary to disk herniations, idiopathic thoracic neuralgia, herpes zoster, diabetic neuropathy, trauma, and degenerative scoliosis.[24,25,39]

Lumbar epidural steroid injections are effective in the treatment of radiculopathy. The efficacy of lumbar epidural steroid injections is detailed in the Australian National Health and Medical Research Council Advisory Committee report supporting the therapeutic use of caudal injections and TFESIs.[8] Manchikanti reviewed combined randomized, double-blinded, and non-randomized trials for all three approaches to lumbar epidural steroid injections.[64] The evidence for caudal epidurals is strong for short-term relief and moderate for long-term relief. The findings for interlaminar epidurals are moderate for short-term relief and limited for long-term relief of symptoms. The results for TFESIs are strong for both short- and long-term relief.

There are a number of non-randomized studies of cervical epidural steroid injections and a few published randomized trials. Bush and Hillier reported 93% of the patients had good pain relief from TFESI, lasting for 7 months, in a prospective study evaluating cervical epidurals in the treatment of cervical radiculopathy.[10] Cicala[15] and Mangar[66] reported that close to 70% of the patients had positive responses. Randomized studies published by Castagnera[13] and Stav[90] both evaluated interlaminar cervical epidurals, demonstrating positive short- and long-term relief in patients with radiculopathy.

Facet joint dysfunction can result from osteoarthritis or trauma such as a whiplash injury. The prevalence of symptomatic facet joints in chronic axial spine pain has been reported as 25–67% for the neck (cervical),[3,5,7,57] 48% for the mid back (thoracic),[60] and 8–45% for the low back (lumbar).[57,61,85] Fluoroscopically guided facet injections are the only way to identify the facet joint as a pain generator.[1,84] Clinical suspicion by the examiner is the primary indication for diagnostic facet joint injections. Studies demonstrating production of facet joint pain with capsular distention showed that lumbar medial branch blocks were 89% successful at relieving the provoked pain.[48] Other outcome studies of facet joint nerve blocks have demonstrated both short- and long-term relief.[19,63,65] False positive rates have ranged from 27–63% in cervical, to 58% in thoracic, and to 22–47% in lumbar facet joint blocks.[4,5,57–61] The 8% false negative rate in facet joint blocks has most likely been due to inadvertent intravascular uptake.[18]

There is a 10–30% prevalence of sacroiliac joint dysfunction as the cause of low back pain.[70,83] There are no definitive historical, physical examination, or diagnostic findings that are specific for sacroiliac joint pain.[9,56,88] Only 22% of sacroiliac joint injections are successfully performed without fluoroscopic guidance.[78]

Cervical and lumbar sympathetic blockade has been utilized for the diagnosis and treatment of sympathetic-mediated pain such as complex regional pain syndrome type I and II. Cervical and lumbar sympathetic chain neurolysis with either phenol or radiofrequency have demonstrated long-term pain relief.[40,49,95]

Epidurography is an integral part of performing interlaminar and transforaminal steroid injections. Epidurography is used to confirm needle placement in the epidural space prior to instilling therapeutic agents,[20,75,93] and to avoid intravascular[30,31] or intrathecal injection. Epidurography is also used to evaluate the status of the epidural space, such as in the postoperative spine patient.

Myelography is a diagnostic imaging study in which radiopaque contrast material is injected into the intrathecal space under direct fluoroscopic observation. Multiple x-rays are obtained after contrast injection to evaluate specific areas of the spinal canal. Myelography is helpful (particularly when combined with CT) in the evaluation of intrathecal pathology, such as tumors, arachnoiditis, disk pathology, nerve root compression, and spinal stenosis. Myelography with flexion and extension views allows for a dynamic spine evaluation under fluoroscopy that is not possible with MRI or CT. Myelography is also used when MRI or CT are inconclusive.

Although there has been a long and controversial history regarding the value of diskography, it is the opinion of these authors that it has had an impact in the diagnosis of diskogenic pain. This is particularly true in regard to surgical planning and subsequent outcome for surgical fusions.[17,52,87] Diskography has demonstrated a 60% prevalence of diskogenic neck pain in the posttraumatic chronic neck pain population.[7] Diskography has detected a 40% prevalence of diskogenic pain in patients with 6 months of chronic low back pain, who have had an otherwise unremarkable diagnostic work-up including imaging studies.[85] MRI, CT, and/or myelography are commonly inconclusive regarding the presence or absence of diskogenic pain.[34,43,82] Cervical, thoracic, and lumbar diskography performed in asymptomatic volunteers has been demonstrated to be a reliable test.[80,92,97] Psychologic factors have been linked to the results of diskography,[12] whereas others have not found such a link.[62]

Cervical, thoracic, and lumbar epidural injection techniques

Interlaminar approach

Imaging studies (MRI or CT) of the cervical and thoracic spine are recommended to evaluate any possible compromise to the epidural space prior to performing an interlaminar epidural injection at the cervical, thoracic, and upper lumbar levels. The same applies to mid and lower lumbar levels in the postoperative patient. The patient is positioned prone on the fluoroscopy table for the paramedian approach at the cervical, thoracic, or lumbar levels. The entry level for the cervical spine is typically at the C7–T1 level, and at the site of pathology for the thoracic and lumbar spine. Epidural injections are avoided at sites of previous posterior spine surgery, due to the obliteration of the epidural space and the subsequent increased risk of intrathecal penetration.

An epidural needle is advanced through the skin using a paramedian approach under intermittent fluoroscopy until contact is made with the lamina (Fig. 25-19). The needle is 'walked off' the laminar edge on to the ligamentum flavum. The stylet is removed, and a syringe with sterile saline and air is attached to the needle and slowly advanced into the epidural space using a 'loss of resistance' technique. Once the needle is in the epidural space, the syringe is exchanged for one containing non-ionic contrast. A 2- to 3-cc volume of non-ionic contrast is slowly injected under fluoroscopy after negative aspiration to produce an epidurogram to confirm appropriate needle placement. A 1-cc test dose of lidocaine (lignocaine) is injected, after which the anesthetic and corticosteroid solution is slowly injected into the epidural space.

Transforaminal approach

The patient is positioned in the supine position for a cervical TFESI, and the C arm or the patient is positioned obliquely until there is a clear view of the foramen. A spinal needle is inserted and advanced until contact with the superior articular process. The needle is placed within the middorsal, posterior portion of the foramen (Fig. 25-20).

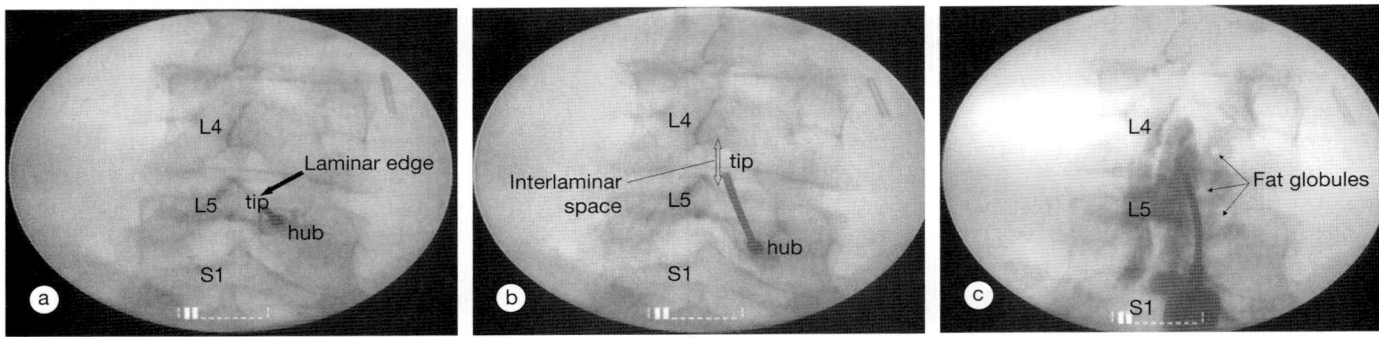

Figure 25-19 Interlaminar lumbar epidural injection. (**a**) Epidural needle in contact with the L5 lamina using a right paramedian approach. (**b**) The epidural needle is 'walked off' the lamina into the L4, L5 interlaminar space. (**c**) Contrast injection produces a lumbar epidurogram demonstrating a fluffy, cloud-like, cobblestone pattern. hub, Epidural needle hub; L4, L4 vertebra; L5, L5 vertebra; S1, S1 vertebra; tip, epidural needle tip.

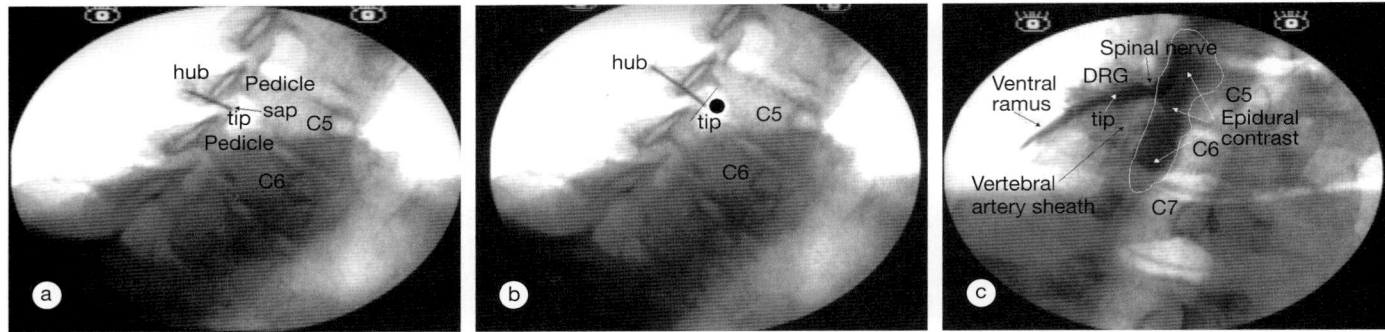

Figure 25-20 Cervical transforaminal epidural steroid injection. (**a**) Spinal needle in contact with the C6 superior articular process. (**b**) Spinal needle advanced into the middorsal (vertical line bisection), posterior portion of the foramen. (**c**) Contrast injection outlining the C6 spinal nerve, dorsal root ganglion (DRG), ventral ramus, and epidural space. •, approximate nerve root position in the foramen; C5, C5 vertebra; C6, C6 vertebra; C7, C7 vertebra; DRG, dorsal root ganglion; hub, spine needle hub; sap, superior articular process; tip, spine needle tip.

The patient is positioned in the prone position for a thoracic or lumbar TFESI, and the C arm or the patient is positioned obliquely until the tip of the ipsilateral subjacent superior articular process divides the pedicle in half. The 'safe triangle' technique commonly described for lumbar TFESI (Fig. 25-21) might not be so safe, in that the needle tip is placed in the anterior foramen (Fig. 25-22), potentially risking an arterial injury and subsequent spinal cord infarction. An alternative method positions the needle tip in the posterior and inferior portion of the foramen (Fig. 25-23). This needle placement is chosen to avoid the radicular or Adamkiewicz artery most commonly located along the superoanterior portion of the nerve.

The patient is placed in a prone position for an S1 TFESI. The S1 foramen is located with fluoroscopy caudad to the S1 pedicle. Repositioning the C arm in a slightly cephalad or lateral position can allow for better visualization of the foramen. A spinal needle is advanced toward the superolateral aspect of the S1 foramen until there is contact with the sacrum, and is then advanced into the foramen (Fig. 25-24).

The needle depth for all transforaminal epidurals is checked with a fluoroscopic anteroposterior and lateral view, to ensure that the needle tip does not extend any further medially than the midpoint of the pedicles. This precaution is taken to avoid penetration of the nerve root dural cuff and the epidural

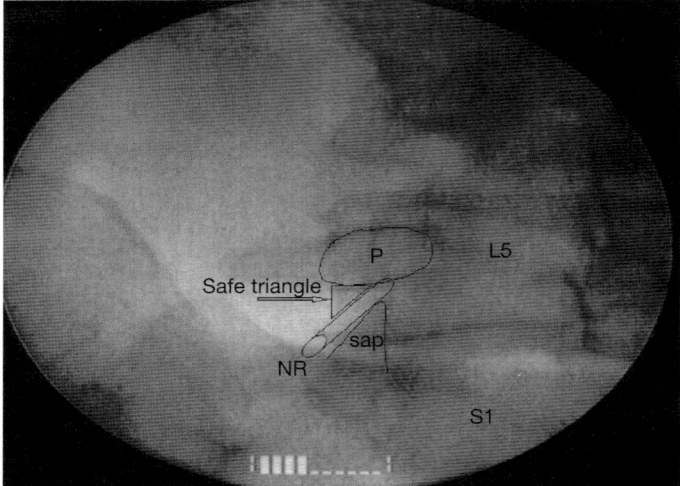

Figure 25-21 'Safe triangle'. This is a triangle created by the lateral edge of the vertebral body (laterally), pedicle (superiorly), and nerve root (medially) that provides a 'safe' area for needle tip placement to avoid contact with the exiting nerve root when performing lumbar transforaminal epidural injections. L5, L5 vertebra; NR, nerve root; P, pedicle; S1, S1 vertebra; sap, superior articular process.

vasculature. Injection tubing is then attached to the needle and to a syringe with contrast. Injection tubing is used mainly to avoid needle tip movement. At least 0.5 cc of non-ionic contrast is injected under fluoroscopy, which outlines the nerve root and spreads into the epidural space. The needle tip is repositioned if there is a venous, arterial, or intrathecal injection. Otherwise, syringes are exchanged for the anesthetic and steroid mixture. The needle tip position is again confirmed by injecting the remaining contrast within the tubing. The solution is slowly injected after a negative 1-cc test dose.

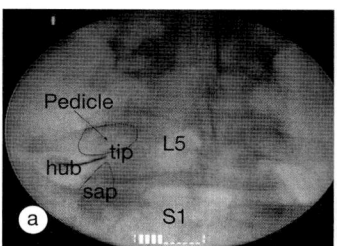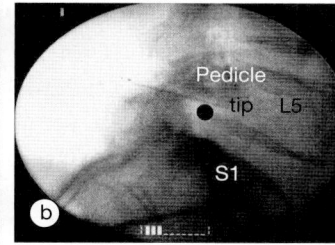

Figure 25-22 Lumbar transforaminal epidural, 'safe triangle' technique. (**a**) Needle placement, oblique view. (**b**) Needle placement, lateral view. •, approximate nerve root position in the foramen; hub, spine needle hub; L5, L5 vertebra; S1, S1 vertebra; sap, superior articular process; tip, spine needle tip.

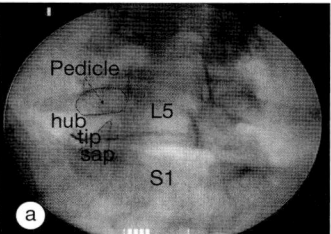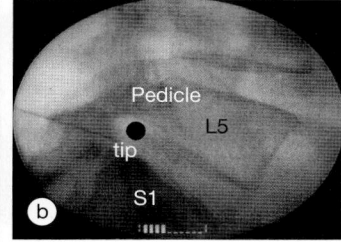

Figure 25-23 Lumbar transforaminal epidural, posterior inferior technique. (**a**) Needle placement, oblique view. (**b**) Needle placement, lateral view. •, approximate nerve root position in the foramen; hub, spine needle hub; L5, L5 vertebra; S1, S1 vertebra; sap, superior articular process; tip, spine needle tip.

Caudal approach

The caudal epidural is a unique third alternative for performing a lumbar epidural injection. The patient is positioned prone, and the sacral hiatus is identified by palpation and with fluoroscopy. A spinal needle penetrates the skin at a 45° angle between the sacral cornu, and is advanced until it contacts the sacrum. The needle is slightly withdrawn and advanced at a shallow 10° angle through the sacrococcygeal ligament into the epidural space. The needle position is confirmed with biplanar fluoroscopy, being careful to keep the needle tip inferior the S2 foramen to avoid thecal sac puncture. After negative aspiration, contrast is injected under fluoroscopy into the epidural space, followed by the injectate solution (Fig. 25-25).

Facet joint and medial branch nerve injection techniques

The cervical nerve roots exit superior to the segmental vertebral pedicle above the C8 nerve root level. For levels below C8, the nerve roots exit below their segmental vertebral pedicle. The thoracic and lumbar medial branch nerve travels across the transverse process below its origin. A specific thoracic or lumbar medial branch nerve is 'blocked' at the transverse process level below its vertebral segment. For example, the right T3 medial branch nerve is injected at the right T4 transverse process.

Cervical spine

The patient is placed in the supine or lateral position for intra-articular cervical facet joint injections. A true lateral cervical spine view is obtained with fluoroscopy regardless of patient position. The articular pillars from each side are superimposed to ensure that the needle tip does not inadvertently pass through the spinal cord. A spinal needle is advanced under fluoroscopy into the ipsilateral symptomatic facet joint. Care is taken to avoid passing the needle beyond the medial aspect of the facet joint into the spinal cord. After negative aspiration, contrast is injected into the joint to confirm needle placement prior to the injection (Fig. 25-26).

The cervical medial branch (facet joint) nerve block is performed by either a posterior or a lateral approach. For the posterior approach, the patient is placed in the prone position

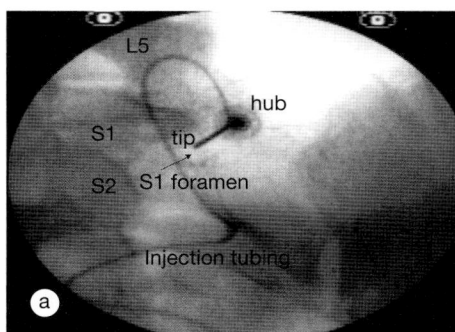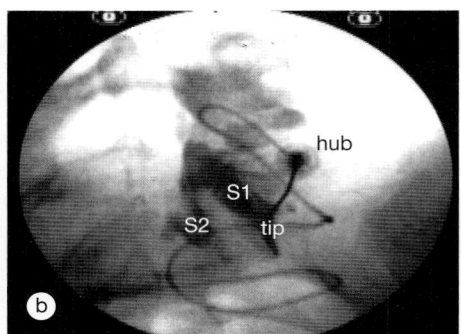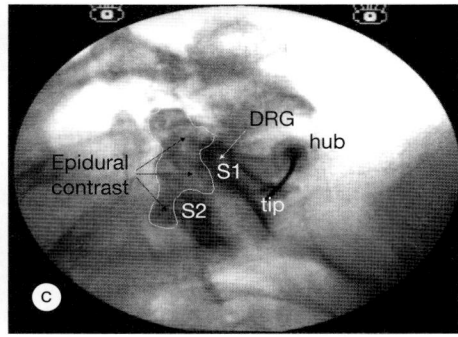

Figure 25-24 Sacral transforaminal epidural. (**a**) Anterior–posterior view of the spinal needle within the S1 foramen, with injection tubing attached to the needle hub. (**b**) Contrast injection. (**c**) Local anesthetic and cortisone injection. DRG, dorsal root ganglion; hub, spine needle hub; L5 (black), L5 vertebra; S1 (white), S1 nerve root; S1 (black), S1 vertebra; S2 (black), S2 vertebra; S2 (white), S2 nerve root; tip, spine needle tip.

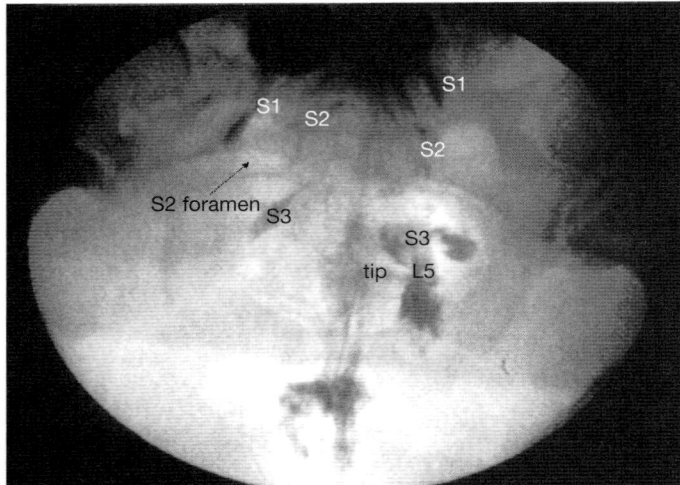

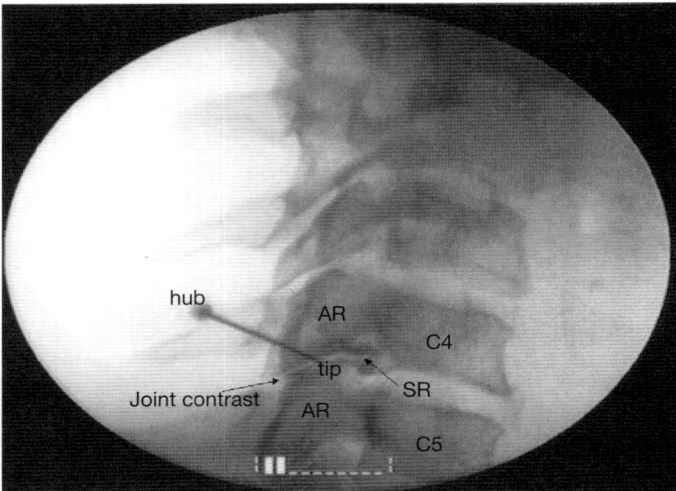

Figure 25-25 Caudal epidural. S1, S1 nerve root; S2, S2 nerve root; S3, S3 nerve root; tip, spine needle tip.

Figure 25-26 Cervical facet joint injection. This is a lateral technique for performing a C4, C5 intraarticular facet joint injection with contrast. AR, articular pillar; C4, C4 vertebra; C5, C5 vertebra; hub, spine needle hub; SR, superior facet joint capsule recess; tip, spine needle tip.

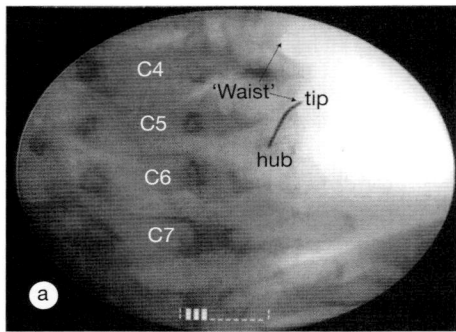
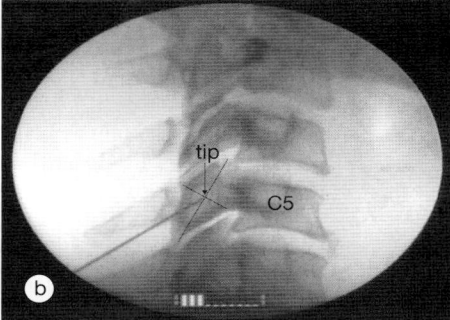
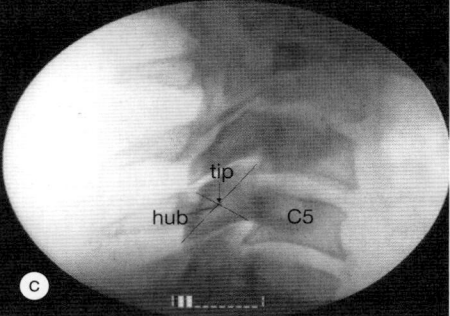

Figure 25-27 Cervical medial branch nerve injection. (**a**) Modified anterior–posterior view of the cervical spine for a right C5 medial branch nerve block using a posterior approach. (**b**) Lateral view of the cervical spine for a C5 medial branch nerve block using a posterior approach. The spine needle tip is at the centroid location of the articular pillar, intersecting lines. (**c**) Lateral view of the cervical spine for a C5 medical branch nerve block. C4, C4 vertebra; C5, C5 vertebra; C6, C6 vertebra; C7, C7 vertebra; hub, spine needle hub; tip, spine needle tip.

with the head turned to the contralateral side. This allows for maximal visualization of the articular pillar concavity or 'waist'. It also positions the vertebral artery anteromedial to the pillar, protecting the vertebral artery from the needle tip, and eliminates superimposition of the mandible over the upper cervical spine injection sites. A spinal needle is inserted just medial to and inferior to the articular waist (the medial branch nerve travels along the waist of the articular pillar), and the needle tip is advanced in a superolateral direction to the articular concavity. A lateral fluoroscopic view assesses needle depth and confirms that the tip is over the centroid, defined as the intersection of the diagonals from the corners of the trapezoid-shaped pillar (Fig. 25-27). The medial branch nerve travels parallel to the articular surfaces along the centroid of the articular pillar, which corresponds to the waist. After negative aspiration, contrast dye can be injected to ensure accurate injectant flow, followed by a 0.3- to 0.5-cc injection of local anesthetic.

Thoracic spine

The patient is placed in a prone position for both thoracic intraarticular facet joint and medial branch nerve injections. For intraarticular injections, the thoracic facet joint is entered at the inferior aspect of the joint, because of its coronal orientation. A spinal needle is inserted one to two segments below the target facet joint, under fluoroscopy in the anteroposterior view. The needle tip is advanced until contact with the subjacent lamina at a point between the 12 o'clock and midpoint of the subjacent superimposed pedicle. The C arm is rotated to provide a lateral view as the needle is inserted into the joint. The tip position is confirmed with another anteroposterior view. After negative aspiration, contrast is injected into the joint to confirm needle placement prior to the anesthetic injection.

The patient is placed in a prone position for T1–4 and T9–10 medial branch nerve blocks. Anteroposterior fluoroscopy is used to visualize each ipsilateral thoracic transverse process. A

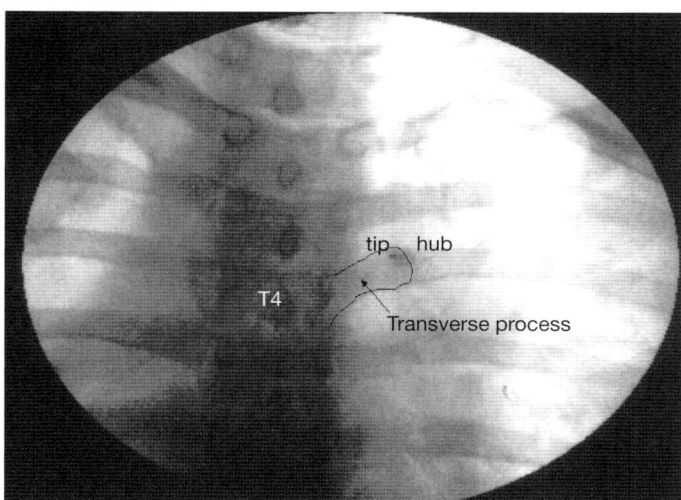

Figure 25-28 Thoracic medial branch nerve injection. Anterior–posterior view of the thoracic spine for a right T3 medial branch nerve block. hub, spine needle hub; T4, T4 vertebra; tip, spine needle tip.

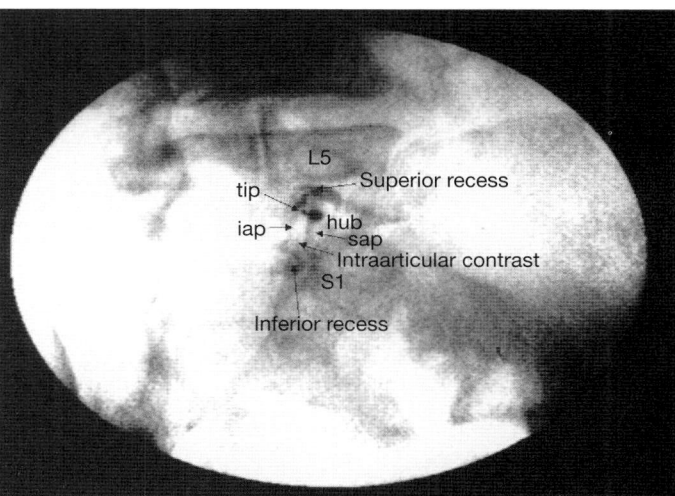

Figure 25-29 Lumbar facet joint injection. An oblique view of an intraarticular contrast injection of the L5–S1 facet joint, with some contrast extravasation beyond the superior recess. hub, spine needle hub; iap, inferior articular process; L5, L5 vertebra; S1, S1 vertebra; sap, superior articular process; tip, spine needle tip.

25° contralateral oblique image can be used if the superolateral transverse process cannot be differentiated from the rib or lamina. A spinal needle is advanced until contact with the superolateral transverse process (Fig. 25-28). The same procedure applies for T5–8 medial branch nerve blocks; however, the needle is advanced in a more cephalad direction to reach the more medial and superior medial branch nerves at these levels. After negative aspiration, 0.3–0.5 cc of local anesthetic is injected, with the bevel oriented in a medial direction. The T11, T12 medial branch nerve blocks are performed in the same manner as lumbar medial branch nerve blocks.

Lumbar spine

The patient or the fluoroscope is placed in a posterior oblique orientation until the joint cavity is first visualized for intra-articular lumbar facet joint injections. A spinal needle is advanced under fluoroscopy toward the midpoint of the facet joint cavity until contact with either articular process. The needle tip is then walked off into the facet joint, taking care not to pass through the joint and into the epidural space. Contrast is injected to confirm needle placement within the joint after negative aspiration (Fig. 25-29).

The procedure for lumbar medial branch block is performed by obtaining oblique views of the specific lumbar vertebra to visualize the 'Scottie dog'. The injection site for L1–4 medial branch is the 'eye' of the Scottie dog over which the nerve travels (Fig. 25-30). Contrast is injected after negative aspiration to assess needle placement. A volume of 0.3–0.5 cc of local anesthetic is injected, with the needle bevel in an inferomedial orientation to prevent flow to the nearby nerve roots (Fig. 25-31). The injection for the L5 dorsal ramus involves placing the C arm in a 10–15° ipsilateral oblique position. The spinal needle is positioned inferior to the superior aspect of the junction of the superior articular process with the sacral ala. The needle bevel should be directed medially to prevent flow into the S1

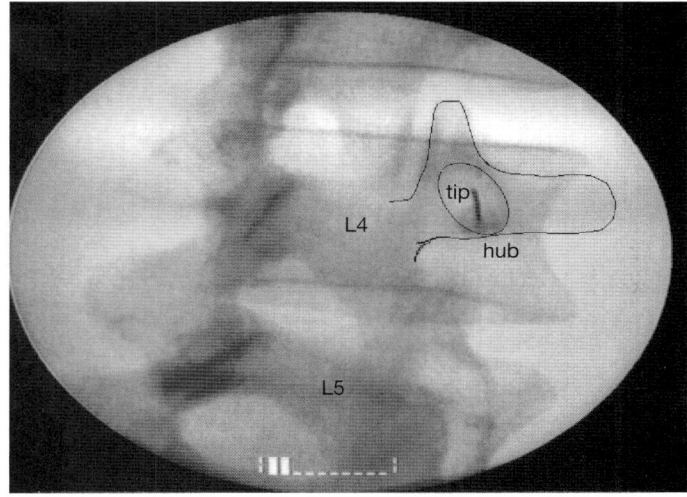

Figure 25-30 Lumbar medial branch nerve injection. An oblique view of spinal needle placement for a right L3 medial branch nerve block. hub, spine needle hub; L4, L4 vertebra; L5, L5 vertebra; tip, spine needle tip.

posterior sacral or the L5 intervertebral foramen. The L5 dorsal ramus is injected with 0.3–0.5 cc of local anesthetic after negative aspiration.

Sacroiliac joint injection technique

The injection is performed with the patient in the prone position. The medial aspect of the joint silhouette corresponds to the posterior limb, and the lateral aspect corresponds to the anterior limb. The C arm is rotated in an attempt to separate the anterior and posterior aspects of the joint, to visualize the most inferior portion of the posterior joint. The C arm rotation continues until direct visualization of the posterior limb is recognized by a very lucent region in the inferior aspect of

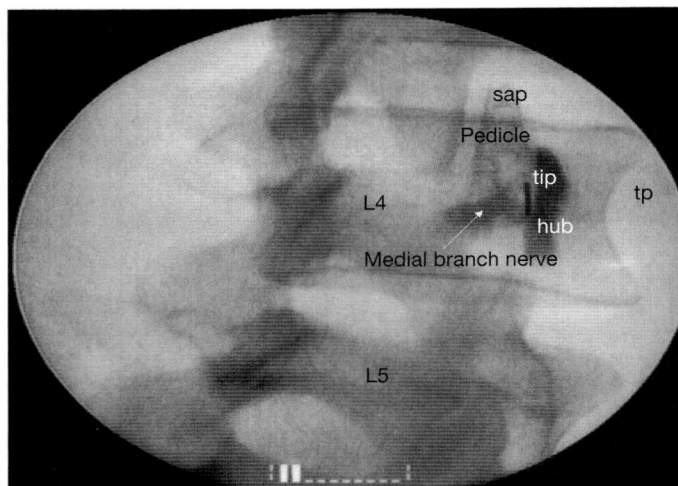

Figure 25-31 Lumbar medial branch nerve injection. An oblique view of a right L3 medial branch nerve block. The first contrast injection demonstrated soft tissue accumulation. A second injection of contrast after repositioning the spinal needle outlined the medial branch nerve. This was followed by an injection of local anesthetic and corticosteroid. hub, spine needle hub; L4, L4 vertebra; L5, L5 vertebra; sap, superior articular process; tip, spine needle tip; tp, transverse process.

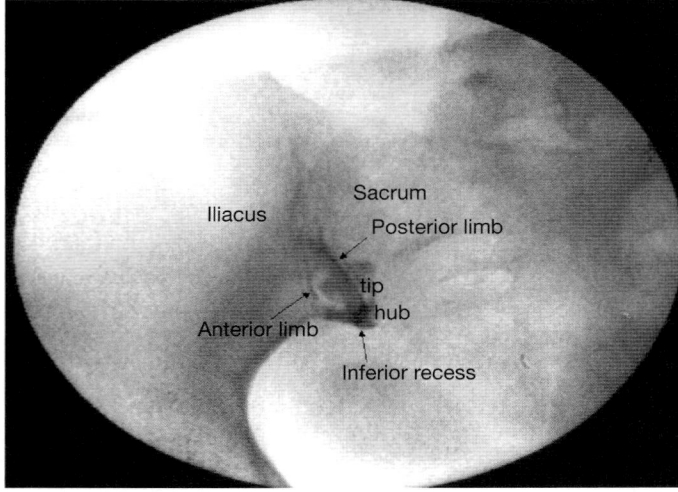

Figure 25-32 Sacroiliac joint injection. Contrast injection outlines the anterior and posterior limbs of the sacroiliac joint as well as the inferior recess. hub, spinal needle hub; tip, spinal needle tip.

the joint, representing overlap with the anterior limb. A spinal needle is inserted 1–3 cm inferior to the joint. The needle pierces the posterior sacroiliac ligament and then enters the joint at the hyperlucent area. Contrast is injected after negative aspiration to produce an arthrogram to confirm needle tip placement (Fig. 25-32).

Sympathetic nerve injection techniques
The technique for sympathetic injection procedures is the same whether performing an anesthetic block or a neurolytic block. Anesthetic blocks are typically performed in a series of four to

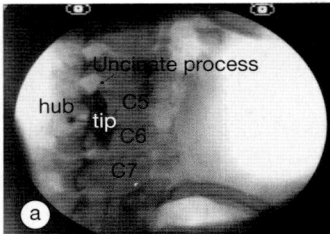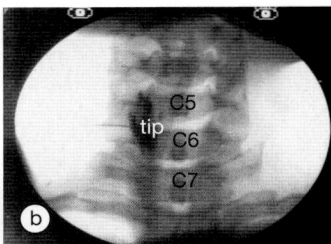

Figure 25-33 Cervical sympathetic injection. (**a**) Oblique view of spinal needle placement and contrast injection. (**b**) Posterior–anterior view of spinal needle placement and contrast injection. C5, C5 vertebra; C6, C6 vertebra; C7, C7 vertebra; hub, spine needle hub; tip, spinal needle tip.

six injections on a weekly basis, unless there is no response after the first injection. A neurolytic block can then be considered in the case of chronic benign pain if there is short-term relief with the injections, without long-term therapeutic relief. Neurolysis should be considered for malignant pain after one anesthetic injection, as long as the patient clearly experiences significant pain relief from the injection.

Cervical sympathetic block
There are two anterior approaches and one posterior approach for a cervical sympathetic block. One anterior technique involves blocking the sympathetic activity at the stellate ganglion by an anterior paratracheal approach at the C6 level, placing the needle at Chassaignac's tubercle. The posterior approach is usually reserved for patients who develop Horner syndrome from an anterior approach without any sympathetic block of the upper extremity. This injection occurs at the T2 or T3 level and provides sympathetic blockade to the upper extremity.

The other anterior technique begins with the patient supine under the fluoroscope. The patient or the fluoroscope is positioned obliquely with the symptomatic side up, to obtain a sharply focused C5, C6 foraminal view. The needle tip is placed along the anterolateral margin of the symptomatic side at the C6 level, by aiming for the superimposed uncinate process. Contrast is injected to outline a fascial plane in the distribution of the cervicothoracic sympathetic chain, observing for any vascular or other unexpected contrast spread (Fig. 25-33). A 10-cc volume of a local anesthetic is injected after a test dose has demonstrated no undesirable effects. The patient is monitored for changes in blood pressure, central nervous system dysfunction, or weakness. The patient should be examined after the block for pain relief, Horner syndrome, and an increase in limb temperature (2–3°C).

Lumbar sympathetic block
The patient is placed in the prone position under the fluoroscope. The C arm or patient is rotated to an oblique position on the symptomatic side, until the tip of the L3 transverse process superimposes with the lateral silhouette of the L3 vertebral body. A spinal needle is inserted over the upper lateral corner of the L3 vertebral body, and advanced until contact with the periosteum (Fig. 25-34). The needle is then advanced

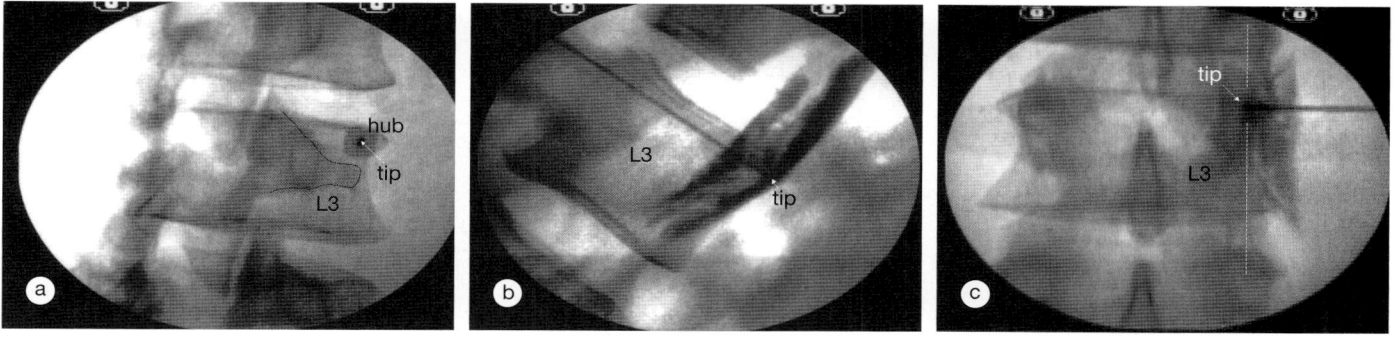

Figure 25-34 Lumbar sympathetic injection. (**a**) Oblique view (with an outline of the transverse process in relationship to the lateral L3 vertebral body border) of spinal needle placement. (**b**) Lateral view of spinal needle placement and contrast injection. (**c**) Anterior–posterior view of spinal needle placement (within the mid pedicular line: dashed white vertical line) and contrast injection. hub, spine needle hub; L3, L3 vertebra; tip, spinal needle tip.

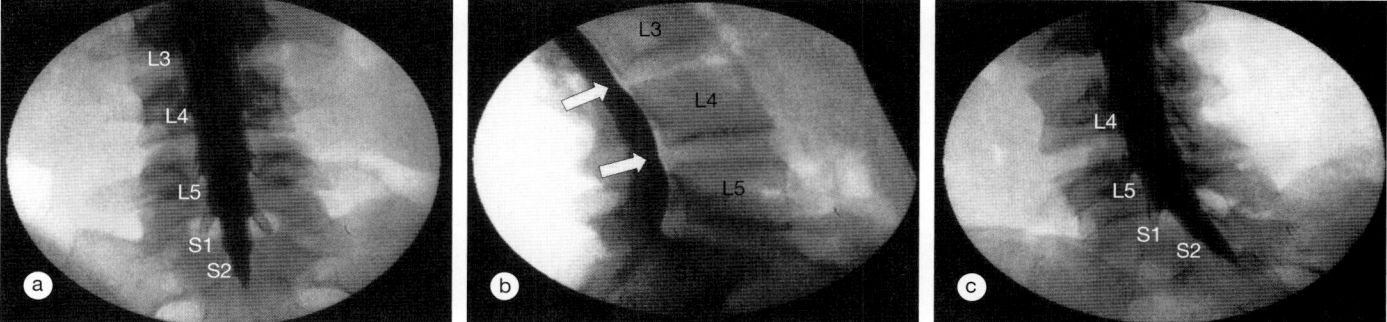

Figure 25-35 Lumbar myelogram. (**a**) Anterior–posterior view of a lumbar myelogram, demonstrating normal nerve root filling. (**b**) Lateral view of a lumbar myelogram, demonstrating ventral deformities (white arrows) of the thecal sac at the L3, L4 and L4, L5 levels. (**c**) Oblique view of the left lumbar spine, showing normal left lumbar nerve root filling. Lumbar nerve roots are labeled in white and lumbar vertebra are labeled in black.

under lateral fluoroscopy along the superior end plate until the tip is just anterior to the vertebral body. The needle tip position is confirmed under anteroposterior fluoroscopy to lie within the mid pedicular line. Before injecting a 10-cc volume of local anesthetic, contrast is injected to confirm spread along the prevertebral fascial plane, as well as to rule out vascular uptake.

Myelography injection technique

The patient is placed prone on the fluoroscopy table, with the head of the table elevated 5–10°. The skin and subcutaneous tissue are anesthetized with 1% lidocaine (lignocaine). A spinal needle is placed midline at the L2, L3 level to ensure the introduction of contrast above the L3 vertebral level. The spinal needle is advanced under fluoroscopy, with the bevel parallel to the long axis of the body. There is resistance as the needle enters the ligamentum flavum, which decreases as it passes through the ligament into the subarachnoid space. The needle tip bevel is turned cephalad, and there is flow of cerebrospinal fluid after removing the stylet. If there is no cerebrospinal fluid flow, a lateral radiographic view is recommended to check the needle depth. If the needle depth is correct, the patient is asked to perform Valsalva's maneuver, which inevitably leads to flow of cerebrospinal fluid through the needle. A catheter is attached

to the needle and to a syringe containing non-ionic contrast. This contrast material is injected into the subarachnoid space under fluoroscopy. Approximately 18–20 cc of contrast is injected to complete the myelogram, after which x-rays are obtained, including anteroposterior, lateral, oblique, flexion, and extension views (Fig. 25-35). A CT scan is performed afterward to complement the myelogram.

For cervical and thoracic myelography, the contrast is injected in the same manner into the lumbar subarachnoid space. The patient is then placed into Trendelenburg's position to allow for flow of contrast into the cervical (Fig. 25-36) and thoracic areas. Care is taken to avoid contrast flow into the foramen magnum. CT and regular x-rays are performed after the myelogram injection. Routine postmyelography instructions include head elevation at 30–45° above the horizontal plane for 12–24 h and oral fluids.

Diskography injection techniques

All diskography procedures are performed under very strict antiseptic technique. Intravenous antibiotics and light intravenous sedation are given to the patient prior to starting the procedure. Intradiskal antibiotics can be given as an alternative or in addition to the intravenous antibiotics for prevention of disk infection.

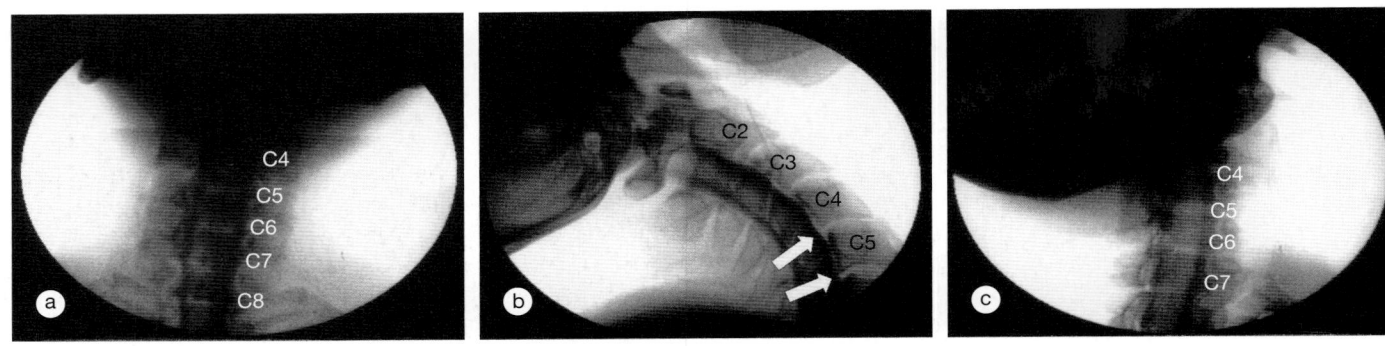

Figure 25-36 Cervical myelogram. (**a**) Anterior–posterior view of a cervical myelogram, demonstrating normal root filling. (**b**) Lateral view of a cervical myelogram, demonstrating ventral deformities (white arrows) of the thecal sac at the C4, C5 and C5, C6 levels. (**c**) Oblique view of the right cervical spine, showing normal right cervical nerve root filling. Cervical nerve roots are labeled in white and cervical vertebra are labeled in black.

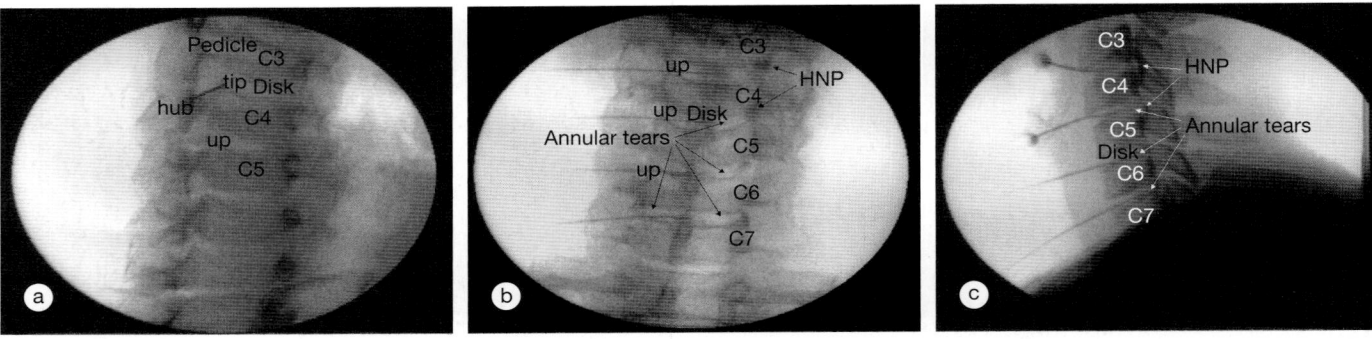

Figure 25-37 Cervical diskogram. (**a**) Foraminal view for initial spinal needle position before entering into the C3, C4 cervical disk. (**b**) Posterior–anterior view of a cervical diskogram, demonstrating left lateral disk herniations at the C3, C4 and C4, C5 levels, with multilevel annular disruption. (**c**) Lateral view of a cervical diskogram, demonstrating disk herniations at the C3, C4 and C4, C5 levels, with multilevel annular disruption. C3, C3 vertebra; C4, C4 vertebra; C5, C5 vertebra; C6, C6 vertebra; C7, C7 vertebra; HNP, herniated nucleus pulposus; hub, spine needle hub; tip, spinal needle tip; up, uncinate process.

The patient is positioned in a modified lateral decubitus position when performing thoracic and lumbar diskography, with the symptomatic side down. The needles are then placed into the disks from the asymptomatic side, in order to avoid any confusion for the patient to distinguish needle-induced annular pain from a provocative pain response. For lumbar diskography, this position also facilitates optimal fluoroscopic imaging and mobilizes the bowel away from the needle path. Although the needle site entry for cervical diskography can be performed with the same methodology, this is not as critical, because the needles are being placed through the anterior portion of the neck. In addition, needle insertion from the left side carries a greater risk of esophageal puncture.

Cervical spine

The anterior and anterolateral approach are the two techniques commonly used today in performing cervical diskography. The patient is placed in the supine position for either approach. A right-sided approach with either technique lessens the risk of puncturing the esophagus at the lower levels of the cervical spine, where it typically is located left of midline. Barium contrast can be swallowed prior to the procedure in order to outline and avoid the esophagus during the study. The needle should enter more laterally at the C2, C3 and C3, C4 disk levels to avoid the hypopharynx, and more medially at the C7–T1 level to avoid the apex of the lung.

The original anterior technique for performing cervical diskography used the non-dominant index finger to compresses the soft tissue structures, while at the same time displacing the great vessels laterally, and the trachea and larynx medially. The dominant hand then places the spinal needles into the disks under continuous fluoroscopy.

The patient or the fluoroscope is oriented in an oblique position for the anterolateral approach, to optimize the view of the foramen at the intended disk level. This allows for advancement of the needle tip at an oblique angle to the disk and posterior to the great vessels, trachea, and esophagus. The spinal needle is advanced from this orientation under intermittent fluoroscopy until contact is made with the uncinate process (Fig. 25-37). The needle tip is then carefully redirected and centered within the disk using biplanar fluoroscopy. The needle tip is only advanced under lateral fluoroscopy in order to prevent spinal cord injury. The advantages of this technique include a significant reduction of x-ray exposure to the physician's hands, greater patient comfort, and potentially a lower risk for disk infection.

Thoracic spine

The patient or the fluoroscope is adjusted to provide a posterior oblique position, with the superior articular process dividing the intervertebral disk space in half. The end plates, the superior articular process, and the rib head form a 'box' (Fig. 25-38) that delineates a safe pathway into the annulus while avoiding the spinal cord and lung. The introducer needle tip is positioned and advanced within the confines of the box to the outer annulus. The procedure needle is then advanced through the introducer needle into the central third of the disk under biplanar fluoroscopic guidance.

Lumbar spine

The patient or the fluoroscope is adjusted to provide a posterior oblique position, with the superior articular process dividing the intervertebral disk space in half (Fig. 25-39). The introducer

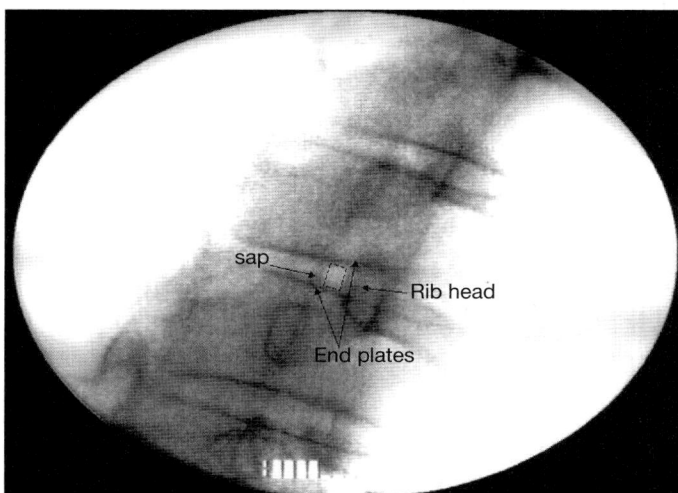

Figure 25-38 Thoracic diskography 'box' view. This oblique starting point allows for safe entry of spinal needles into the thoracic disk.

needle tip is positioned just anterior to the superior articular process and superior to the subjacent end plate. The introducer needle is advanced to the outer annulus, while being aware of any paresthesias from contact with the exiting nerve root at that level. The procedure needle is then advanced through the introducer needle into the central third of the disk under biplanar fluoroscopic guidance.

Once all the needles are positioned in the disks, regardless of the technique, each disk is evaluated by injecting contrast, saline, or a combination of both. The injections are performed under lateral fluoroscopy, after which anteroposterior and lateral x-rays are obtained. The data recorded during the study include injection volume, diskometry (end point), pain level, analgesia, pain quality, and nucleogram. The disk pressure (diskometry) at the onset of pain during lumbar diskography can also be measured and recorded with a pressure gauge in pounds per square inch (p.s.i.). Depending on the measured pressure above the opening pressure, lumbar disks are defined as chemically sensitive (<15 p.s.i.), mechanically sensitive (15–50 p.s.i.), or intermediate (>50 p.s.i.).[17] After the study, the patient undergoes a CT scan of each injected level (Fig. 25-40) for further assessment of disk anatomy.

SUMMARY

Peripheral joint, soft tissue, and spinal injection procedures have become an integral part of the evaluation and treatment of patients suffering from different musculoskeletal disorders. A thorough understanding of the indications, contraindications, and complications of these injections is necessary in order to maximize their effectiveness and safety. Meticulous technique is mandatory to optimize the success of these procedures therapeutically, and to minimize morbidity and in some instances mortality. Although not completely proved by randomized controlled trial studies, these injections are widely held in the field to provide short- and long-term pain relief, improve function,

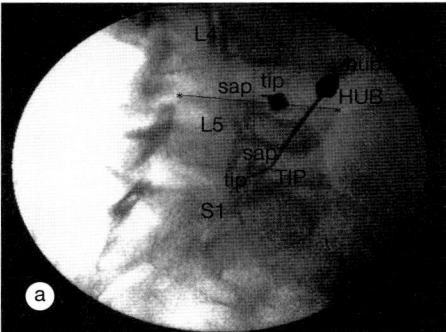 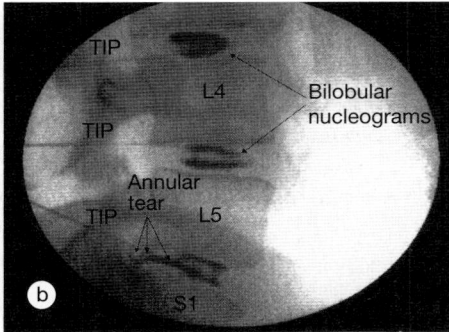 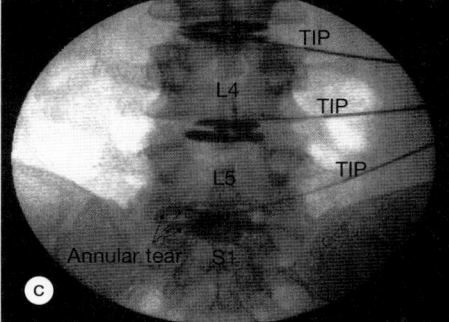

Figure 25-39 Lumbar diskogram. (**a**) Oblique view for initial spinal needle position established by positioning the superior articular process tip (vertical dashed line) until it bisects the intervertebral disk (solid horizontal line between asterisks). (**b**) Lateral view of a lumbar diskogram, demonstrating a L5–S1 posterior full-thickness annular tear with a normal nucleus. The outer annular fibers are intact, otherwise there would be contrast spreading into the epidural space or surrounding soft tissue structures, an important finding when considering percutaneous intradiskal procedures. (**c**) Anterior–posterior view of a lumbar diskogram, showing an L5–S1 left lateral annular tear. The lateral and anterior–posterior views are consistent for a left posterolateral radial annular tear extending from the nucleus to the outer annulus. HUB, introducer spine needle hub; hub, procedure spine needle hub; L4, L4 vertebra; L5, L5 vertebra; S1, S1 vertebra; sap, superior articular process; TIP, introducer spine needle tip; tip, procedure spine needle tip.

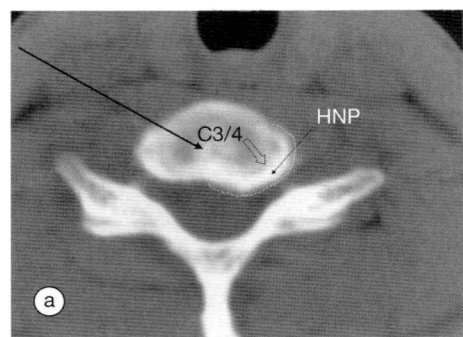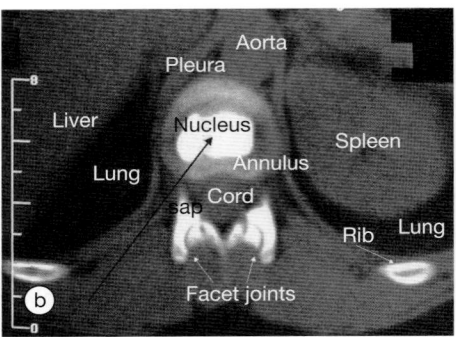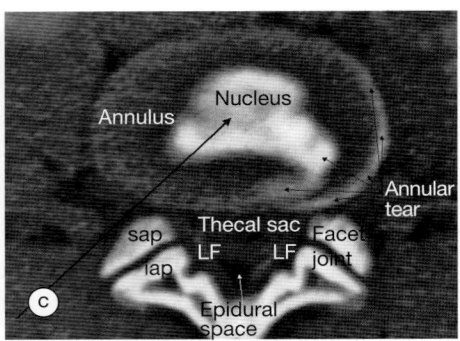

Figure 25-40 Computed tomography (CT) diskogram. (**a**) Cervical CT diskogram demonstrating a left posterolateral disk herniation extending into the left C3, C4 foramen. The open arrow identifies the vertebral edge, and the dashed white line the outer boundary of the disk herniation. The long solid black arrow represents the approximate path of a spinal needle into the disk. (**b**) Thoracic CT diskogram showing a normal disk. The long solid black arrow represents the approximate path of a spinal needle into the disk, avoiding the lung laterally and the spinal cord medially. (**c**) Lumbar CT diskogram revealing a left posterolateral radial annular tear extending into the left lateral outer annulus. The long solid black arrow represents the approximate path of a spinal needle into the disk. HNP, herniated nucleus pulposus; iap, inferior articular process; LF, ligamentum flavum; sap, superior articular process.

and lead to a better quality of life. These techniques should always be used as part of a comprehensive treatment and rehabilitation plan.

REFERENCES

1. Aprill C, Bogduk N. The prevalence of cervical zygapophysial joint pain—first approximation. Spine 1992; 17:744–747.

2. Baker R, Dreyfuss P, Mercer S, et al. Cervical transforaminal injection of corticosteroids into a radicular artery: a possible mechanism for spinal cord injury. Pain 2003; 103:211–215.

3. Barnesley L, Lord S, Bogduk N. Comparative local anaesthetic blocks in the diagnosis of cervical zygapophysial joint pain. Pain 1993; 55:99–106.

4. Barnsley L, Lord S, Wallis B, et al. False positive rates of cervical zygapophysial joint blocks. Clin J Pain 1993; 9:124–130.

5. Barnsley L, Lord S, Wallis BJ, et al. The prevalence of chronic cervical zygapophysial joint pain after whiplash. Spine 1995; 20:20–26.

6. Bodguk N, Cherry D. Epidural corticosteroid agents for sciatica. Med J Aust 1985; 143:402–406.

7. Bogduk N, Aprill C. On the nature of neck pain, discography and cervical zygapophysial joint blocks. Pain 1993; 54:213–217.

8. Bogduk N, Christophidis N, Cherry D, et al. Epidural steroids in the management of back pain and sciatica of spinal origin. Report of the Working Party on Epidural Use of Steroids in the Management of Back Pain. Canberra: National Health and Medical Research Council; 1993.

9. Broadhurst NA, Bond MJ. Pain provocation tests for the assessment of sacroiliac joint dysfunction. J Spine Disord 1998; 11:341–345.

10. Bush K, Hillier S. Outcome of cervical radiculopathy treated with periradicular/epidural corticosteroid injections: a prospective study with independent clinical review. Eur Spine J 1996; 5:319–325.

11. Cardone DA. Joint and soft tissue injection. Am Fam Physician 2002; 66:283–288.

12. Carragee E, Tanner C, Khurana S, et al. The rates of false-positive lumbar discography in select patients without low back symptoms. Spine 2000; 25:1373–1381.

13. Castagnera L, Maurette P, Pointillart V, et al. Long term results of cervical epidural steroid injection with and without morphine in chronic cervical radicular pain. Pain 1994; 58:239–243.

14. Cathelin F. Mode d'action de la cocaine injecte dans l'espace epidural par le procedede de canal sacre. C R Soc Biol 1901; 53:478.

15. Cicala RS, Westbrook L, Angel JJ. Side effects and complications of cervical epidural steroid injections. J Pain Symptom Manage 1989; 4:64–66.

16. Deisenhammer E. Clinical and experimental studies on headaches after myelography. Neuroradiology 1985; 9:99–102.

17. Derby R, Howard M, Grant J, et al. The ability of pressure controlled discography to predict surgical and non-surgical outcome. Spine 1999; 24:364–371.

18. Dreyfuss P, Schwarzer AC, Lau P, et al. Specificity of lumbar medial branch and L5 dorsal ramus blocks. Spine 1997; 22:895–902.

19. Dreyfuss PH, Dreyer SJ, Herring SA. Contemporary concepts in spine care: lumbar zygapophysial (facet) joint injections. Spine 1995; 20:2040–2047.

20. el-Khoury GY, Ehara S, Weinstein JN, et al. Epidural steroid injection: a procedure ideally performed with fluoroscopic control. Radiology 1988; 168:554–557.

21. Falco FJ, Moran JG. Lumbar discography using gadolinium in patients with iodine contrast allergy followed by postdiscography computed tomography scan. Spine 2003; 28:E1–E4.

22. Falco FJ, Rubbani M. Visualization of spinal injection procedures using gadolinium contrast. Spine 2003; 28:E496–E498.

23. Flanagan J, Casale FF, Thomas TL, et al. Intra-articular injection for pain relief in patients awaiting hip replacement. Ann R Coll Surg Engl 1988; 70:156–157.

24. Forrest JB. Management of chronic dorsal root pain with epidural steroid. Can Anesth Soc J 1979; 25:218–220.

25. Forrest JB. The response to epidural steroid injections in chronic dorsal root pain. Can Anesth Soc J 1980; 27:40–46.

26. Fortin JD, Washington WJ, Falco FJE. Three pathways between the sacroiliac joint and neural structures. Am J Neuroradiol 1990; 20:1429–1434.

27. Fraser HF, Osti OL, Vernon-Roberts B. Discitis after discography. J Bone Joint Surg (Br) 1987; 69:26–35.

28. Fraser HF, Osti OL, Vernon-Roberts B. Discitis following chemonucleolysis: an experimental study. Spine 1986; 11:679–687.

29. Fraser HF, Osti OL, Vernon-Roberts B. Iatrogenic discitis: the role of intravenous antibiotics in prevention and treatment. Spine 1989; 14:1025–1032.

30. Furman MB, Giovanniello MT, O'Brien EM. Incidence of intravascular penetration in transforaminal cervical epidural steroid injections. Spine 2003; 28:21–25.

31. Furman MB, O'Brien EM, Zgleszewski TM. Incidence of intravascular penetration in transforaminal lumbosacral epidural steroid injections. Spine 2000; 25:2628–2632.

32. Gallardo MJ. Cutaneous hypopigmentation following a posterior sub-tenon triamcinolone injection. Am J Ophthalmol 2004; 137:779–780.

33. Geborek P, Mansson B, Wollheim FA, et al. Intra-articular corticosteroid injection into rheumatoid arthritis knees improves extensor muscle strength. Rheum Int 1990; 9:265–270.

34. Gibson MJ, Buckley J, Mawhinney R. Magnetic resonance imaging and discography in the diagnosis of disc degeneration. A comparative study of 50 discs. J Bone Joint Surg (Br) 1986; 68:369–373.

35. Grainger RG, Allison D, Adam A, et al. Grainger & Allison's diagnostic radiology: a textbook of medical imaging. 4th edn. New York: Churchill Livingstone; 2001:2422–2423.

36. Grainger RG. Annotation: radiological contrast media. Clin Radiol 1987; 38:3–5.

37. Gray RG, Gottlieb NL. Intra-articular corticosteroids. An update assessment. Clin Orthop 1983; 177:235–263.

38. Guyer RD, Collier R, Stith WJ, et al. Discitis after discography. Spine 1988; 13:1352–1354.

39. Haddox JD. Lumbar and cervical epidural steroid therapy. Anesth Clin N Am 1992; 10:179–201.

40. Haynsworth RF Jr, Noe CE. Percutaneous lumbar sympathectomy: a comparison of radiofrequency denervation versus phenol neurolysis. Anesthesiology 1991; 74:459–463.

41. Heavner JE, Racz GB, Jenigiri B, et al. Sharp versus blunt needle: a comparative study of penetration of internal structures and bleeding in dogs. Pain Practice 2003; 3:226.

42. Hollander JL, Brown EM, Jessar RA, et al. Hydrocortisone and cortisone injection into arthritic joints: comparative effects of and use of hydrocortisone as a local antiarthritic agent. JAMA 1951; 147:1629–1635.

43. Horton WC, Daftari TK. Which disc as visualized by magnetic resonance imaging is actually a source of pain? A correlation between magnetic resonance imaging and discography. Spine 1992; 17:S164–S171.

44. Houten JK, Errico TJ. Paraplegia after lumbosacral nerve root block: report of three cases. Spine J 2002; 2:70–75.

45. Johansson A, Hao J, Sjolund B. Local corticosteroid blocks transmission of normal nociceptive C-fibres. Acta Anaesthesiol Scand 1990; 34:335–338.

46. Johnson AJ, Burrows EH. Thecal deformity after lumbar myelography with iophendylate (Myodil) and meglumine iothalamate (Conray 280). Br J Radiol 1978; 51:196–202.

47. Jones A, Doherty M. Intra-articular corticosteroids are effective in osteoarthritis but there are no clinical predictors of response. Ann Rheum Dis 1996; 55:829–832.

48. Kaplan M. The ability of lumbar medial branch blocks to anesthetize the zygapophysial joint. A physiologic challenge. Spine 1998; 23:1847–1852.

49. Kim JY, Kim KY. Percutaneous radiofrequency thermocoagulation of the stellate ganglion in the treatment of cervical and upper extremity pain: a case report. J Korean Pain Soc 2001; 14:239–244.

50. Kirwan JRR. Intra-articular therapy in osteoarthritis. Baillières Clin Rheumatol 1997;11:769–794.

51. Lasser EC, Berry CC, Talner LB, et al. Pre-treatment with corticosteroids to alleviate reactions to intravenous contrast media. N Engl J Med 1987; 317:845–849.

52. Lee CK, Vessa P, Lee JK. Chronic disabling low back pain syndrome caused by internal disc derangements: the results of disc excision and posterior lumbar interbody fusion. Spine 1995; 20:356–361.

53. Lièvre JA, Block-Michel H, Attali P. L'injection transsscre etude clinique et radiologrique. Bull Soc Med Hosp 1957; 73:1110–1118.

54. Lownie SP, Ferguson GG. Spinal subdural empyema complicating cervical discography. Spine 1989; 14:1415–1417.

55. Maddox TG. Adverse reactions to contrast material: recognition, prevention, and treatment. Am Fam Physician 2002; 66:1229–1234.

56. Maigne JY, Aivakiklis A, Pfefer F. Results of sacroiliac joint double block and value of sacroiliac pain provocation test in 54 patients with low back pain. Spine 1996; 21:1889–1892.

57. Manchikanti L, Pampati V, Fellows B, et al. Prevalence of lumbar facet joint pain in chronic low back pain. Pain Physician 1999; 2:59–64.

58. Manchikanti L, Pampati V, Fellows B, et al. The diagnostic validity and therapeutic value of medial branch blocks with or without adjuvants. Curr Rev Pain 2000; 4:337–344.

59. Manchikanti L, Pampati V, Fellows B, et al. The inability of the clinical picture to characterize pain from facet joints. Pain Physician 2000; 3:158–166.

60. Manchikanti L, Singh V, Pampati S, et al. Evaluation of prevalence of facet joint pain in chronic thoracic pain. Pain Physician 2002; 5:354–359.

61. Manchikanti L, Singh V, Pampati V, et al. Evaluation of the relative contributions of various structures in chronic low back pain. Pain Physician 2001; 4:308–316.

62. Manchikanti L, Singh V, Pampati V, et al. Provocative discography in low back pain patients with or without somatization disorder: a randomized prospective evaluation. Pain Physician 2001; 4:227–239.

63. Manchikanti L, Singh V, Vilms B, et al. Medial branch neurotomy in management of chronic spinal pain: systemic review of the evidence. Pain Physician 2002; 5:405–418.

64. Manchikanti L, Staats PS, Vijay S, et al. Evidence-based practice guidelines for interventional techniques in the management of chronic spinal pain. Pain Physician 2003; 6:3–81.

65. Manchikanti L. Facet joint pain and the role of neural blockade in its management. Curr Rev Pain 1999; 3:348–358.

66. Mangar D, Thomas PB. Epidural steroid injections in the treatment of cervical and lumbar pain syndromes. Reg Anesth 1991; 16:246.

67. Nash TP, Brouwers PJ, Ella JB, et al. A cervical anterior spinal artery syndrome after diagnostic blockade of the right C6-nerve root. Pain 2001; 91:397–399.

68. Okell RW, Sprigge JS. Unintentional dural puncture. A survey of recognition and management. Anaesthesia 1987; 42:1110–1113.

69. Osti OL, Fraser HF, Vernon-Roberts B. Discitis after discography. The role of prophylactic antibiotics. J Bone Joint Surg (Br) 1990; 72:271–274.

70. Pang WW, Mok MS, Lin ML, et al. Application of spinal pain mapping in the diagnosis of low back pain—analysis of 104 cases. Acta Anaesthesiol Sin 1998; 36:71–74.

71. Plant MJ, Borg AA, Dziedzic K, et al. Radiographic patterns and response to corticosteroid hip injection. Ann Rheum Dis 1997; 56:476–480.

72. Postuma P, Stanish WD. The intra-articular and periarticular use of corticosteroids in knee and shoulder. Clin J Sport Med 1994; 4:155–159.

73. Purkis IE. Cervical epidural steroids. Pain Clin 1986; 1:3–7.

74. Ravaud P, Moulinier L, Giraudeau B, et al. Effects of joint lavage and steroid injection in patients with osteoarthritis of the knee: results of a multicenter, randomized controlled trial. Arthritis Rheum 1999; 42:475–482.

75. Renfrew DL, Moore TE, Kathol MH, et al. Correct placement of epidural steroid injections: fluoroscopic guidance and contrast administration. Am J Neuroradiol 1991; 12:1003–1007.

76. Rizk T, Pinals R, Talaiver A. Corticosteroid injections in adhesive capsulitis: investigation of their value and site. Arch Phys Med 1991; 72:20–22.

77. Robecchi A, Capra R. L'idrocortisone (composto F). Prime esperienze cliniche in compo reumatologico. Minerva Med 1952; 98:1259–1263.

78. Rosenburg JM, Quint TJ, de Rosayro AM. Computerized tomographic localization of clinically-guided sacroiliac joint injections. Clin J Pain 2000; 16:18–21.

79. Rozin L, Rozin R, Koehler SA, et al. Death during transforaminal epidural steroid nerve root block (C7) due to perforation of the left vertebral artery. Am J Forensic Med Pathol 2003; 24:351–355.

80. Schellhas KP, Smith MD, Gundry CR, et al. Cervical discogenic pain. Prospective correlation of magnetic resonance imaging and discography in asymptomatic subjects and pain sufferers. Spine 1996; 21:300–312.

81. Schmidt S, Gibbons J. Postdural puncture headache after fluoroscopically guided lumbar paravertebral sympathetic block. Anesthesiology 1993; 78:198–200.

82. Schneiderman G, Flannigan B, Kingston S, et al. MRI in the diagnosis of disc degeneration: correlation with discography. Spine 1987; 12:276–281.

83. Schwarzer AC, April CN, Bogduk M. The sacroiliac joint in chronic low back pain. Spine 1995; 20:31–37.

84. Schwarzer AC, April CN, Derby R, et al. Clinical features of patients with pain stemming from the zygapophysial joints: is the lumbar facet syndrome a clinical entity? Spine 1994; 19:1132–1137.

85. Schwarzer AC, April CN, Derby R, et al. The relative contributions of the disc and zygapophysial joint in chronic low back pain. Spine 1994; 19:801–806.

86. Scott D, Smith C, Lohmander S, et al. Osteoarthritis. Clin Evid 2003; 9:1301–1326.

87. Siebenrock KA, Aebi M. Cervical discography in discogenic pain syndrome and it predictive value for cervical fusion. Arch Orthop Trauma Surg 1994; 113:199–203.

88. Slipman CW, Sterenfeld EB, Chou LH, et al. The predictive value of provocative sacroiliac joint stress maneuvers in the diagnosis of sacroiliac joint syndrome. Arch Phys Med Rehabil 1998; 79:288–292.

89. Sprague R, Rammamurthy S. Identification of the anterior psoas sheath as a landmark for lumbar sympathetic block. Reg Anesth 1990; 15:253–255.

90. Stav A, Ovadra L, Sternbert G, et al. Cervical epidural steroid injection for cervicobrachialgia. Acta Anaesth Scand 1993; 37:562–567.

91. Stevens JM, Kendall BE, Gedroyc W. Acute epidural hematoma complicating myelography. Case report. Br J Radiol 1991; 64:860–864.

92. Walsh TR, Weinstein JN, Spratt KP, et al. Lumbar discography in normal subjects. J Bone Joint Surg (Am) 1990; 72:1081–1088.

93. White AH, Derby R, Wynne G. Epidural injections for the treatment of low back pain. Spine 1980; 5:67–86.

94. Wilke WS, Tuggle CJ. Optimal technique for intra-articular and periarticular joint injections. Mod Med 1988; 56:58–72.

95. Wilkinson HA. Percutaneous radiofrequency upper thoracic sympathectomy. Neurosurgery 1997; 40:216–217.

96. Windsor RE, Falco FJE. Paraplegia following selective nerve root blocks. Int Spinal Injection Soc Newsl 2001: 53–54.

97. Wood KB, Schellas KP, Garvey TA, et al. Thoracic discography in healthy individuals. A controlled prospective study of magnetic resonance imaging and discography in asymptomatic and symptomatic individuals. Spine 1999; 24:1548–1555.

98. Zuckerman JD, Meislin RJ, Rothberg M. Injections for joint and soft tissue disorders: when and how to use them. Geriatrics 1990; 45:45–52.

Chapter

26

Interventional Pain Management Procedures

Frank J.E. Falco, Daniel W. Kim, Jie Zhu, C. Obi Onyewu and Franklin Lee Irwin Jr.

Chronic pain is one of the most common medical problems encountered by physicians (see Ch. 43). Chronic pain has been described as an unpleasant sensation that persists for at least 6 months and often continuing for an indefinite period of time. There are more than 90 million Americans who suffer from a variety of chronic pain syndromes. Chronic pain often disrupts family life, reduces function, and is a financial strain. Chronic pain is more common and causes more disability than cancer and heart disease combined. The drain on the American economy produced by chronic pain is enormous, amounting to more than $100 billion a year in medical expenses, lost work productivity, and insurance costs.

The implementation of interventional pain procedures in the treatment of chronic benign and malignant pain has provided pain relief, improved function, reduced medical costs, and provided a better quality of life and death for those suffering from terminal cancer. This chapter reviews the indications, contraindications, complications, efficacy, and technique of the most common interventional pain management procedures used in the treatment of chronic pain.

The principles regarding patient evaluation, consent, and sterile procedure technique, as discussed in Chapter 25 regarding peripheral and spinal injections, apply to the following interventional pain management procedures as well. Intravenous and/or intradiskal antibiotics are used in most of these procedures, with cap, gown, and sterile gloves. The same precautions are implemented regarding bleeding parameters as well as absolute and relative contraindications. Radiation safety guidelines are followed with these procedures, because they are all performed with fluoroscopic guidance.

RADIOFREQUENCY NEUROLYSIS TECHNIQUES

The basic equipment needed to produce a radiofrequency (RF) tissue lesion from high-frequency waves includes a voltage generator, alternating current, and active and reference electrodes. The patient's tissues serve as a resistor within the circuit and provide impedance. The active electrode is an insulated needle with an exposed tip, while the reference electrode is a large surface adhesive pad. This configuration leads to the greatest current concentration and heat being next to the tip, with diffusion of the current and heat at the large reference electrode.

The current causes vibration of the electrons in the tissues in the vicinity of the RF probe, resulting in an increase in temperature. The greater the voltage and the tissue impedance, the higher the temperature that develops within the tissues.

The advantages of RF include controlled lesion size, accurate temperature monitoring, limited need for anesthesia, precise probe placement, low incidence of morbidity or mortality, and rapid postprocedure recovery. The lesion size is dependent on the probe diameter, the length of the uninsulated tip, the temperature, the time, and the tissue vascularity. In general, the lesion size is greater with a larger probe diameter, longer uninsulated tip, higher temperature, lower tissue vascularity, and longer lesioning time.

Pulsed RF uses 10- to 30-ms bursts of high-frequency alternating current. Lesions created by pulsed RF are low temperature (cold RF) and are non-destructive lesions. When making an RF lesion, the tissue that surrounds the tip of the electrode is exposed to an electromagnetic field (EMF).

Although the mechanism by which pulsed RF treatment works is not known, there are several theories. One theory is that the EMF might have a clinical neuromodulation effect rendering the nerve less likely to transmit painful impulses. Another possibility is that it works in a similar manner to transcutaneous electrical nerve stimulation, activating both spinal and supraspinal mechanisms, which can reduce pain perception.

Radiofrequency neurolysis of the facet joint
Indications
Patients with functionally limited spinal facet joint pain that is resistant to at least 3 months of conservative treatment are candidates for RF neurolysis or ablation (RFA). This condition cannot be definitively diagnosed by history, physical examination, or imaging studies. The current method for diagnosis is through facet joint injections or medial branch (facet joint) nerve blocks. The nerves that supply the facet joints from the cervical to the lumbar spine are the third occipital nerve, the medial branches of the dorsal rami, and the L5 dorsal ramus. Cervical and lumbar medial branch blocks have been shown to be target-specific if anesthetic solutions are injected carefully at specific osseous target points, and contrast is necessary to ensure that inadvertent venous uptake does not occur. A dual injection paradigm of facet joint or medial branch nerve

injections is recommended for a more accurate diagnosis of facet joint pain, because of the false positive rates associated with single lumbar and cervical facet joint or medial branch nerve blocks.

Technique

The patient is positioned prone, with the head turned to the opposite side for cervical facet joint RFA in the same manner as for cervical medial branch nerve injections (see Ch. 25). The C arm is positioned to visualize the segmental articular pillar and its waist. A hypodermic insulated RF probe (needle) is directed just medial to the waist of the articular pillar until contacting bone. The needle is then slowly redirected just off the articular pillar laterally (Fig. 26-1) and repositioned with lateral imaging to the anterior third of the pillar along the centroid plane. Needle placement is confirmed with anterior–posterior (AP) imaging and electrical stimulation that ensures the probe is not close to other nearby neurologic structures.

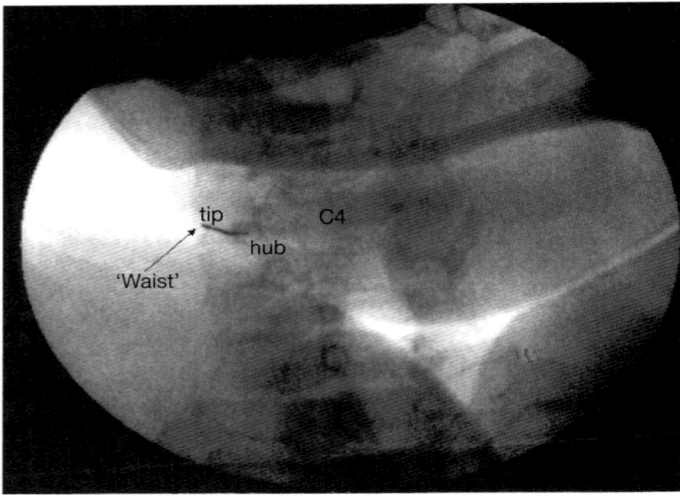

Figure 26-1 Radiofrequency (RF) neurolysis: cervical facet joint. The RF probe in position for left C4 medial branch neurolysis. C4, C4 vertebra; hub, RF probe hub; tip, RF probe tip.

The medial branch nerve is anesthetized before RF lesioning at 80–90°C for 30 s to 2 min per lesion.

The patient is placed prone for RF lesioning of the thoracic facet joints in the same manner as for medial branch nerve injections. The RF needle is inserted over the midline, so that it can be advanced superiorly and laterally to lie parallel to the medial branch nerve as it crosses the target transverse process. The needle is advanced through the skin toward the lateral aspect of the transverse process, and walked off laterally with the tip just over the superolateral edge. The T5 through T8 medial branch nerves are superior to the superolateral transverse process, necessitating a more superior position of the RF needle. Thoracic level RFA lesions are created after electrical stimulation at 80–90°C for 30 s to 2 min.

The patient is placed prone for RF lesioning of the lumbar facet joints. The RF probes are placed parallel to the nerves, as opposed to the perpendicular approach used for medial branch nerve blocks. This allows for optimal denervation of the medial branch nerves. The probe is placed inferior and lateral to the targeted medial branch, and advanced under fluoroscopy until contact at the junction of the superior articular process and the transverse process (Fig. 26-2a). An oblique 'Scottie dog' view (Fig. 26-2b) is then obtained, and the needle should be seen to reside parallel to the target nerve in the osseous groove. The needle is then advanced to the proximal junction of the superior articular process and transverse process for the L1–L4 medial branch nerves (Fig. 26-2b), and the proximal junction of the S1 superior articular process and the sacral ala for the L5 dorsal ramus. A lateral view is then obtained to ensure the needle is placed no further anterior than the posterior aspect of the foramen (Fig. 26-2c). The C arm is then finally repositioned in an AP projection to verify that the needles did not stray laterally while being advanced under oblique imaging. Electrical stimulation is done as a safety precaution, and then the area is anesthetized. This is followed by an RFA lesion at 80–90°C for 30 s to 2 min.

Side effects and complications

Patients can feel increased soreness and local pain, especially in the first 3–5 days, but these symptoms usually disappear within

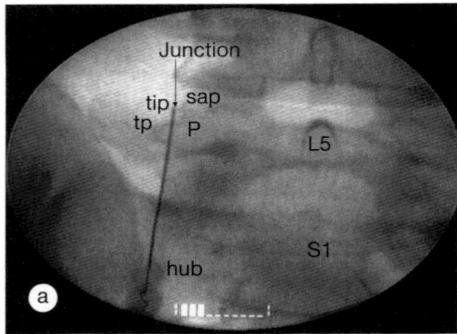
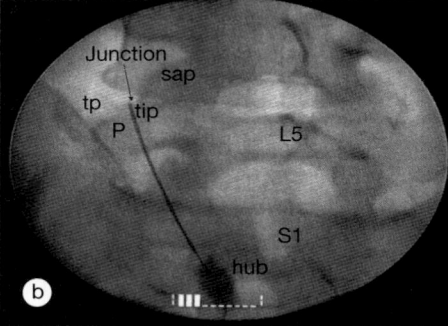
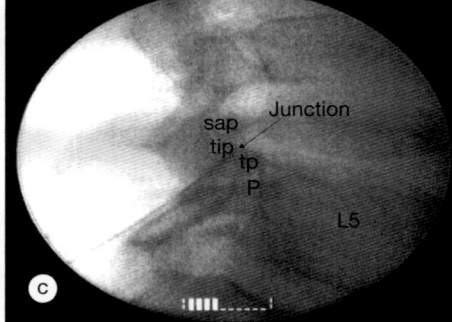

Figure 26-2 Radiofrequency (RF) neurolysis: lumbar facet joint. The RF probe in position for left C4 medial branch neurolysis. (**a**) Anterior–posterior view; (**b**) oblique view; (**c**) lateral view. hub, RF probe hub; Junction, junction of sap and transverse process; L5, L5 vertebra; P, pedicle; S1, S1 vertebra; sap, superior articular process; tip, RF probe tip; tp, transverse process.

2 weeks. Other postoperative symptoms include itching, burning, and hypersensitivity that usually subside in approximately 4–6 weeks. Gabapentin or tricyclic antidepressants can be very helpful for this condition. Improper needle placement can lead to permanent limb weakness, permanent sensory deficit, or persistent neuritis. In the cervical spine, the proximity to the vertebral artery, combined with the vascular nature of this anatomic region, makes intravascular injection or vascular trauma a distinct possibility. The injection of small amounts of local anesthetic into the vertebral arteries can result in seizures. In the thoracic spine, pneumothorax is a potential risk, given the proximity of the pleural space. No long-term complications or serious adverse effects have been described with RF facet ablation procedures when motor stimulation was performed before lesioning to prevent inadvertent ventral ramus or nerve root injury. Needle electromyography (EMG) of the multifidi muscles should be performed if the facet RFA fails to provide pain relief after several weeks. An electromyographic examination should show denervation potentials following this procedure, indicating that there was destruction of the medial branch nerves. If no denervation potentials are seen on EMG and the patient is still symptomatic, the facet RFA can be repeated.

Outcome studies

Lord reported in 1996 the only prospective, double-blind, controlled trial on RFA treatment for chronic cervical facet joint pain. Twenty-four subjects were randomized to an RFA or sham RFA treatment group. RF treatments were conducted at 80°C for 90 s in the RFA group, and at 37°C for the control sham group. The median time that elapsed before pain returned to 50% of the pretreatment level was 263 days for the treatment group versus 8 days for the sham treatment group.[31] Dreyfuss reported the first prospective study to treat only patients with lumbar facet joint pain proved with dual diagnostic medial branch blocks.[15] A 90% denervation rate was confirmed using multifidi EMG 6 weeks after the procedure. At 1-year follow-up, nearly 90% of subjects had at least 60% pain relief, and 60% of subjects had at least 90% pain relief. Overall, one systematic review, two randomized trials, four prospective studies, and three retrospective evaluations of RF medial branch neurotomy have provided the best evidence to date for short-term relief, and moderate evidence for long-term relief, of chronic cervical and lumbar facet joint pain.[35] There have been no reports of long-term adverse side effects secondary to facet joint RF neurolysis, including any risk for creating a Charcot joint.

Radiofrequency neurolysis of the sacroiliac joint
Indications

Candidates for sacroiliac joint (SIJ) RFA are patients who have been diagnosed with chronic SIJ pain resistant to at least 3 months of conservative treatment, and who have experienced significant but transient relief after intraarticular SIJ corticosteroid injections.

Technique

One common technique for SIJ RFA is the bipolar technique, where two RF probes are used to create a bipolar system. Under fluoroscopy, the first RF probe is inserted at the inferior joint margin. The second RF probe is placed more cephalad in the joint, at a distance of less than 1 cm. RF lesions are created at 80°C. Another RF probe is then placed more cephalad in the SIJ, at a distance of less than 1 cm from the second probe, and another lesion is created. Multiple subsequent lesions are then created in a repetitive, alternating, 'leapfrog' manner, going as high in the joint as possible. An alternative approach is to place a single RF probe and advance it cephalad along the posterior capsule, creating overlapping lesions (Fig. 26-3). Another technique is to lesion at the origin of the multiple nerve branches that are believed to innervate the SIJ.

Side effects and complications

The major side effect of SIJ lesioning is postprocedure pain. Care must be taken to avoid placing the RF needle too lateral and traumatizing the sciatic nerve. There is a theoretic risk of dysesthesias if RF lesioning of the L5 dorsal ramus and lateral branches of the S1–S3 dorsal rami is performed, because they provide sensory innervation to the skin of the buttock.

Outcome studies

Formal peer-reviewed outcome studies for SIJ RFA are lacking. An uncontrolled study by Ferrante used a leapfrog technique along the posterior SIJ line. He reported that about 36% of patients experienced a 50% decrease in the visual analog scale (VAS) pain scale for at least 6 months. Ferrante also noted that a significantly higher proportion of non-responders had pain with lateral flexion to the affected side, implying that the presence of facet disease might have prevented these patients from experiencing at least 50% relief of their total back pain.[17]

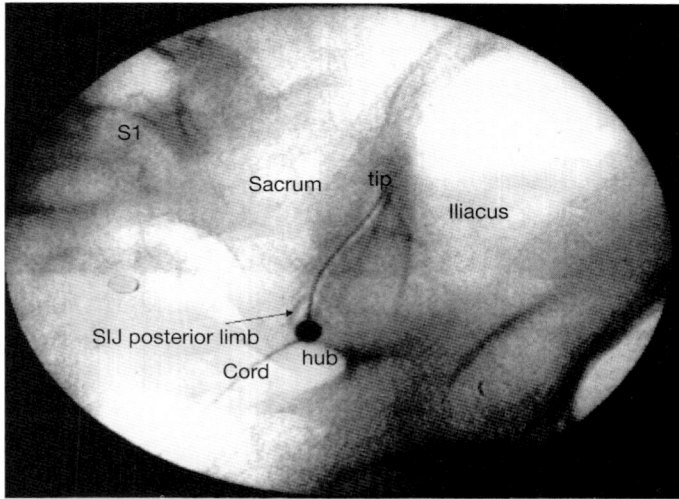

Figure 26-3 Radiofrequency (RF) neurolysis: sacroiliac joint (SIJ). Single RF probe overlapping technique. Note the contrast in the SIJ, confirming probe placement within the posterior limb prior to RF neurolysis. Cord, RF cord to generator; hub, RF probe hub; S1, S1 vertebra; tip, RF probe tip.

Radiofrequency neurolysis of dorsal root ganglia

Indications and contraindications

Selection criteria include radicular pain for more than 6 months with no response to conservative treatment, no indication for surgical intervention, and a positive but short-lived response to a selective nerve root block or transforaminal epidural injection. Contraindications include infection, coagulopathy, platelet dysfunction, neck or back pain alone without any limb pain, deafferentation pain in the involved limb, and severe cardiopulmonary disease for procedures in the cervical and thoracic regions.

Radiofrequency of the dorsal root ganglion (DRG) can be performed with the traditional or pulsed methods. Pulsed RF is being used more frequently to treat dorsal root ganglia than any other application, because the resulting temperature is below the threshold that causes irreversible nerve injury. The use of pulsed RF significantly reduces the risk of developing postprocedure neuritis.

Technique

The technique for probe placement in performing DRG RF neurolysis is the same whether using heat or cold (pulsed) RF. The probe is placed in the dorsal quadrant of the cervical (Fig. 26-4), thoracic, or lumbar foramen. The RF probe is placed anteriorly for DRG RFA of the second DRG (Fig. 26-5). Sensory and motor stimulation is performed as a safety precaution and to improve the success rate of the procedure. The voltage at which the patient first perceives the stimulation in the appropriate dermatome is the sensory threshold. This threshold is usually around 0.4–0.7 V when the tip of the needle is next to the DRG using a frequency of 50 Hz. The frequency is changed to 2 Hz for motor stimulation, and the voltage intensity has to increase to at least twice the sensory threshold before motor activity in the myotomal distribution is typically seen. This is known as the disassociation of stimulation

that occurs at a point over the DRG where the sensory and motor nerves are still separate before crossing over into the ventral and dorsal rami. This is the probe placement site for DRG RFA when using conventional RF. The probe is typically placed next to the DRG for pulsed RF, obtaining a sensory threshold at 0.1–0.2 V. Lesions for traditional RF are created at 80–90°C for 1–2 min, and from 2 to 4 min at 42°C for pulsed RFA.

Side effects and complications

Possible risks include nerve injury, vascular trauma, or entry into the subarachnoid space through the intervertebral foramen.

Outcome studies

A limited case study report showed remarkable effectiveness of pulsed RF in patients with neuropathic pain syndromes whose conditions were poorly controlled with other oral and invasive treatments.[36] One study by Sluijter demonstrated that 56% of patients with radicular pain had a global perceived effect of more than 75% pain relief.[52] Sluijter also showed that 8 of 15 patients were successfully treated at 6 months' follow-up, and 3 of the 7 patients in the unsuccessful group reported that pain had improved on the side that had been treated, but they felt pain on the contralateral side afterward.[52] A more recent pilot study using pulsed RF for chronic cervical pain showed that 72% of patients experienced at least 50% pain relief 8 weeks afterward, and 33% of patients continued to experience good pain relief more than 1 year after treatment.[57] Van Kleef compared conventional RF with a sham group in a prospective double-blind randomized study for cervical DRG RF, and found a significant reduction in pain in the treated compared with the sham group.[56]

Radiofrequency neurolysis cervical sympathectomy

Indications

Cervical sympathectomy RF lesioning is effective in the treatment of sympathetically mediated pain, as well as pain secondary to vascular insufficiency in the face, neck, and upper limbs. This procedure is indicated when the duration of pain relief

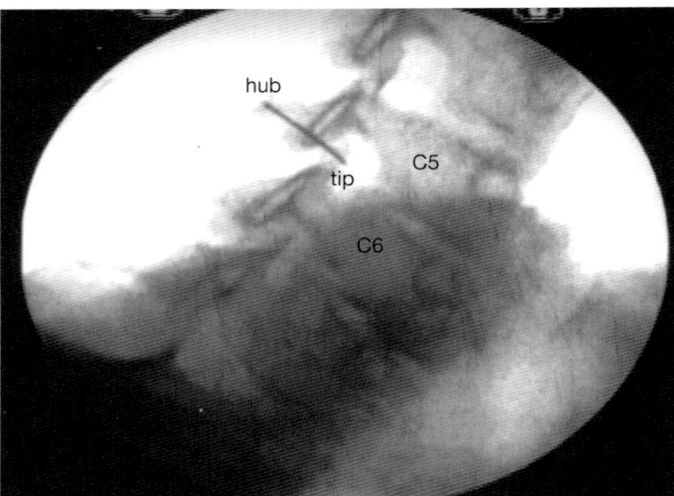

Figure 26-4 Radiofrequency (RF) neurolysis: C6 dorsal root ganglion. C5, C5 vertebra; C6, C6 vertebra; hub, RF probe hub; tip, RF probe tip.

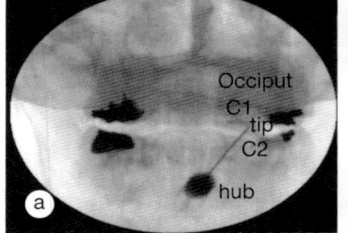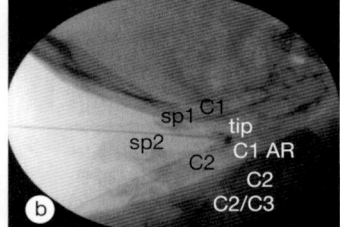

Figure 26-5 Radiofrequency (RF) neurolysis: C2 dorsal root ganglion. (**a**) Anterior–posterior view; (**b**) lateral view. C1 AR, C1 articular pillar; C1, C1 vertebra; C2, C2 vertebra; C2/C3, C2, C3 intervertebral disk; hub, RF probe hub; sp1, C1 spinous process; sp2, C2 spinous process; tip, RF probe tip.

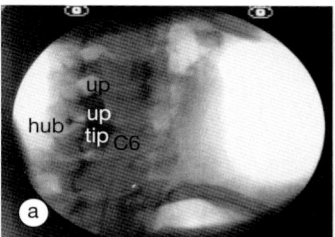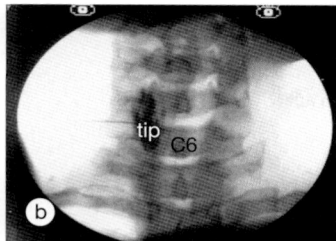

Figure 26-6 Radiofrequency (RF) neurolysis: cervical sympathectomy. (**a**) Oblique (foraminal) view; (**b**) anterior–posterior view. C6, C6 vertebra; hub, RF probe hub; tip, RF probe tip; up, uncinate process.

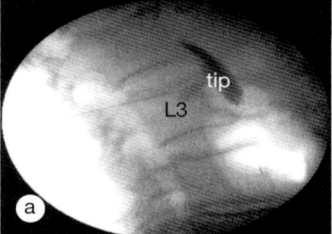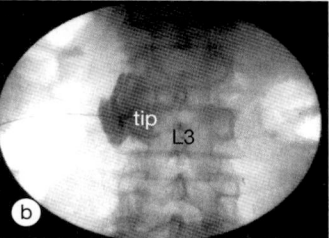

Figure 26-7 Radiofrequency (RF) neurolysis lumbar sympathectomy. (**a**) Lateral view; (**b**) anterior–posterior view. L3, L3 vertebra tip; RF probe tip.

with sympathetic blocks using local anesthetics is not long-lasting.

Technique

The patient is placed supine, with the head rotated to the asymptomatic opposite side. A foraminal view is obtained at the C6, C7 level. An RF needle is advanced through the skin toward the superimposed uncinate process. The needle is then slightly withdrawn after bony contact is made, to bring the needle tip out of the periosteum. Approximately 3–5 mL of contrast is injected after careful aspiration to assure that the RF needle tip is not in a blood vessel (Fig. 26-6). A trial stimulation of both the sensory and the motor nerves is performed prior to RF neurolysis, to assess for any stimulation of nearby neural structures. A small volume of local anesthetic (0.5 mL) should be injected before lesioning. The RF is applied for 60 s at 80°C. The cannula is then redirected for additional lesions at the C6 level. Further lesions can be created at the same session or at another time at the C7 and/or T1 levels.

Side effects and complications

Because of the proximity to the cervical spinal canal, accidental RF lesioning of the neuraxial structures at this level can result in significant neurologic dysfunction, including quadriparesis. Unintentional lesioning of the phrenic nerve can result in diaphragmatic paralysis and respiratory insufficiency. Inadvertent lesioning of the recurrent laryngeal nerve can result in prolonged or permanent hoarseness. A permanent Horner syndrome can occur if the superior cervical sympathetic ganglion is damaged during the procedure. Pneumothorax is a distinct possibility, especially on the right side and with lesioning at the T1 level. The incidence of all the above complications can be decreased with careful use of trial stimulation and fluoroscopic guidance. The anatomic region in this area is highly vascular, increasing the risk for local and systemic anesthetic toxicity as well as hematoma formation.

Outcome studies

A recent retrospective review study demonstrated that 40% of patients who underwent RF lesioning of the stellate ganglion after responding to a diagnostic injection had 50% or more pain relief with a mean follow-up of 52 weeks.[18]

Radiofrequency neurolysis of lumbar sympathectomy

Indications

Radiofrequency lesioning of the lumbar sympathetic chain is indicated for patients who have experienced only short-term pain relief following multiple lumbar sympathetic blocks with local anesthetic. Pain syndromes amenable to treatment include sympathetically mediated pain of the kidneys, ureters, genitalia, and lower limbs such as phantom limb pain, complex regional pain syndrome, and a variety of peripheral neuropathies. Lumbar sympathetic ganglion RF lesioning can also be considered in patients suffering from pain secondary to vascular insufficiency of the lower limb.

Technique

The approach to the lumbar sympathetic chain involves an oblique fluoroscopic technique similar to that used for sympathetic injections. The C arm is positioned obliquely until the L3 transverse process converges with the vertebral body. The RF probe is advanced toward the upper outer quadrant of the L3 vertebral body until contact with the periosteum. The RF is then advanced to the anterior edge of the vertebral body under lateral fluoroscopy. Contrast is injected to confirm probe position and assess for unintentional intravascular placement (Fig. 26-7). Once the needle tip is in the correct position, sensory stimulation at 50 Hz and motor stimulation at 2 Hz are performed to assess for nearby neural structures. During motor stimulation, there should be no movement in the lower limb with intensities up to 3 V. Approximately 1 mL of preservative-free anesthetic is injected before lesioning. An RF lesion is made between the anterior psoas fascia and the anterolateral vertebral body following proper stimulation.

Radiofrequency lesioning at multiple levels is a more effective approach for lumbar sympathectomy. One RF lesion with a 10-mm exposed tip is adequate to produce a 10-mm lesion at the L2 vertebral level along the anterolateral aspect of the vertebral body. The RF probes at the L3 and L4 levels should be positioned initially at a point just posterior to the anterior aspect of the vertebral body for stimulation and lesioning. The RF probes are then moved approximately 5 mm anterior, and a second stimulation followed by lesioning is performed at each of these levels. With this technique, the cannulas are moved further away from the segmental nerves prior to creating the second lesion. This method creates a 15-mm 'strip' lesion at the L3 and L4 levels, and a 10-mm lesion at the L2 level. If the sympathetic disorder involves the foot, another 15-mm lesion might be necessary at the L5 level as well.

Side effects and complications

Damage to the abdominal viscera, puncture of a ureter, or renal trauma during lumbar sympathetic RF lesioning are distinct possibilities. The incidence of this complication is decreased if care is taken to place the needle just beyond the anterolateral margin of the vertebral body. RF lesioning in proximity to the genitofemoral nerve at the L2 vertebral level can result in persistent genitofemoral neuritis that can be difficult to treat. Probe placement that is too medial might result in trauma to the intervertebral disk, spinal cord, and exiting nerve roots.

Outcome studies

Lesioning at multiple lumbar sympathetic levels produced significant lower limb pain relief for 75% of patients over a time period of at least 8 weeks in one prospective case series study.[46]

Nucleoplasty

Nucleoplasty builds on the earlier percutaneous intradiskal treatment concepts of chemonucleolysis, nucleotomy, and RFA. The Food and Drug Administration approved nucleoplasty for treatment of contained herniated disks in June 2001. Nucleoplasty is a non-heat-driven process that uses coblation and bipolar RF technology applied to a conductive medium such as saline to achieve tissue removal with minimal thermal damage to collateral tissues.

Indications

Like other decompressive procedures, nucleoplasty is designed to treat patients with limb pain caused by smaller disk protrusions. Inclusion criteria include chronic diskogenic low back pain with radicular symptoms, contained disk herniation, adequate disk height of at least 50% of normal, and normal psychometric testing. Specific contraindications include severe disk space narrowing, large disk herniation, extruded or sequestered disks, spinal stenosis, spondylolisthesis, spinal fracture, or tumor. The usual general contraindications are the same as for any surgical procedure, and include fever, infection, bleeding diathesis, and anticoagulant therapy.

Technique

The patient is positioned in a modified lateral decubitus position, and the lumbosacral area is prepared in the usual sterile manner. Intravenous antibiotics are given prior to the procedure, with or without intradiskal antibiotics. Using a posterolateral approach under fluoroscopy, a 17-gauge, 6-inch Crawford needle (Fig. 26-8) is inserted through the skin into the center of the nucleus, followed by the injection of non-ionic contrast that produces a nucleogram outlining its borders (Fig. 26-9). A slightly curved wand with a bipolar coil at the distal tip (Fig. 26-8) is then advanced through the Crawford needle until the distal end of the tip touches the inside wall of the anterior

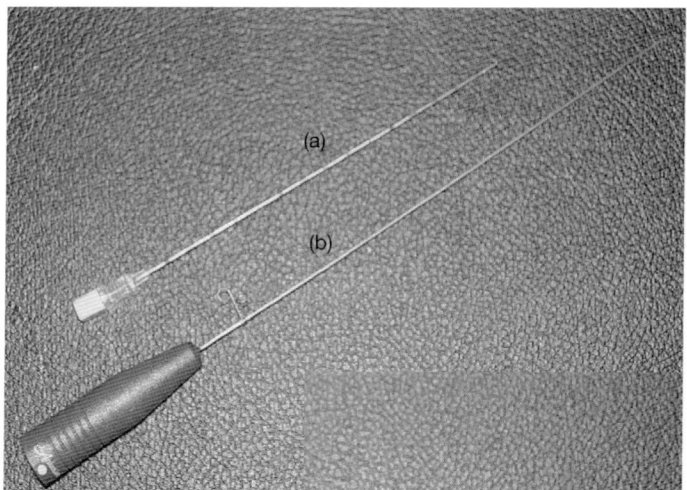

Figure 26-8 Nucleoplasty device: (**a**) Crawford needle; (**b**) bipolar wand.

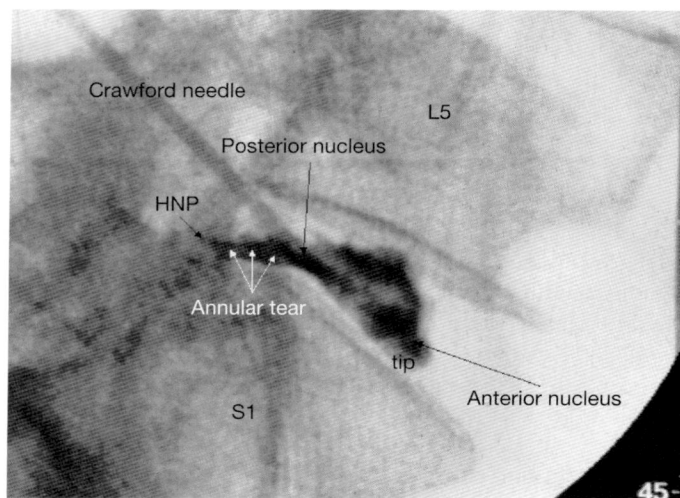

Figure 26-9 Nucleoplasty. Contrast injected through the Crawford needle, outlining the boundaries of the L5–S1 nucleus pulposus as well as revealing a posterior annular tear and disk herniation. HNP, disk herniation; L5, L5 vertebra; S1, S1 vertebra; tip, Crawford needle tip.

annulus (anterior boundary of the nucleus) (Fig. 26-10a). The depth gauge is then advanced down the shaft of the wand to the needle hub (Fig. 26-10b), representing the depth of wand advancement through the Crawford needle for creating channels within the nucleus from coblation. The wand is then withdrawn until the tip is inside the posterior wall of the annulus (Fig. 26-11a), corresponding to the posterior boundary of the nucleus. A reference mark with a surgical pen is made on the wand at the needle hub (Fig. 26-11b). The proximal depth gauge and the distal reference mark on the wand represent the working length of the wand (Fig. 26-11b) for creating channels within that specific nucleus. The dot indicator located on the wand handle (Fig. 26-10b) is oriented to the 12 o'clock position, and the wand is advanced to the depth gauge using the coblation mode. Then the wand is withdrawn to the reference

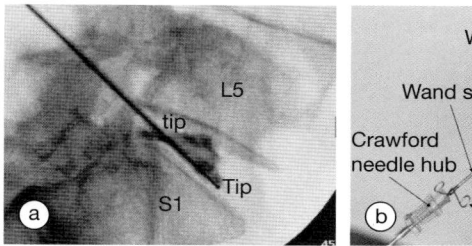
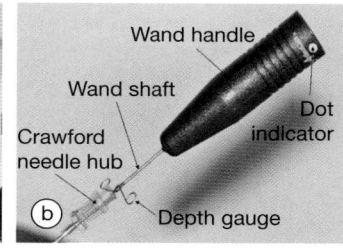

Figure 26-10 Nucleoplasty. (**a**) Nucleoplasty wand tip at the anterior boundary of the nucleus pulposus. (**b**) Depth gauge (clamp-like device) positioned on the wand at the level of the Crawford needle hub, representing the location of the wand tip at the anterior border of the nucleus pulposus. L5, L5 vertebra; S1, S1 vertebra; Tip = nucleoplasty wand tip; tip, Crawford needle tip.

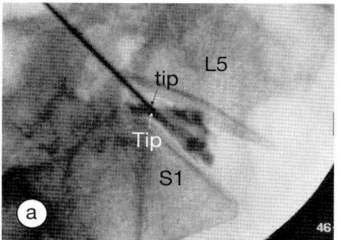
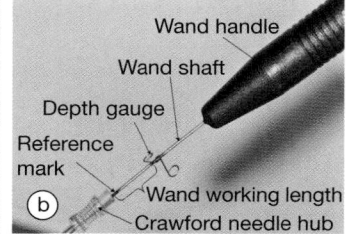

Figure 26-11 Nucleoplasty. (**a**) Nucleoplasty wand tip at the posterior boundary of the nucleus pulposus. (**b**) Reference mark made by surgical pen distal to the depth gauge on the wand, designating the position of the wand tip at the posterior border of the nucleus pulposus. L5, L5 vertebra; S1, S1 vertebra; tip, Crawford needle tip; Tip, nucleoplasty wand tip.

mark using the coagulation mode. The wand is advanced and withdrawn at an approximate rate of 0.5 cm/s to create a single channel. This protocol is repeated to create six different channels by rotating the wand at 2 o'clock increments in either a clockwise or counterclockwise direction.

The result is removal of nuclear material by creating multiple intradiskal channels during coblation with the wand. These channels are then sealed by way of coagulation following withdrawal of the wand. The products of the non-heat-driven process are elementary particles and low molecular weight gases, which are removed quickly from the surgical site through the Crawford needle. The reduction in nuclear tissue volume leads to a decrease in intradiskal pressure that can result in pain reduction. The patient usually does not feel discomfort during the procedure, because the coblation and coagulation take place within the nucleus pulposus that contains little sensory innervation. The practitioner must be aware of any extreme pain or neurologic symptoms in the back or leg that can indicate damage to vital neural structures during the nucleoplasty procedure. If this occurs, the physician should stop and reposition the Crawford needle and/or wand or abort the procedure to avoid potential damage.

Side effects and complications
There have been no reported significant complications after nucleoplasty. However, possible complications include diskitis,

epidural abscess, pneumothorax, trauma to retroperitoneal structures, nerve root or spinal cord trauma, and cauda equina syndrome.

Outcome studies
A recent study demonstrated that, when coblation is performed at the central portion of the disk, there is minimal increased temperature in adjacent neurovascular structures.[8] The effectiveness of nucleoplasty has recently been reported in two prospective trials. Singh et al. observed 41 patients for 12 months and reported that 80% of patients indicated a statistically significant reduction in pain. They also reported improved sitting (62%), standing (59%), and walking (60%) ability.[51] In a prospective cohort study of 48 patients, Sharps reported a 79% decrease in pain scores at 12 months for 13 patients.[50] Derby reported that nucleoplasty gave an overall success rate of 79% and a success rate of 67% in previously operated patients.[14] A cadaveric study demonstrated that nucleoplasty was highly effective at reducing intradiskal pressure in non-degenerated contained disks, but had minimal effect in reducing intradiskal pressure in severely degenerative disks.[7] Nucleoplasty is probably not effective in treating severely degenerated disks because of the nuclear desiccation. Overall, it appears that nucleoplasty seems to be a promising treatment for contained disk herniation with or without radiculopathy, but clinical research in a larger patient population over a longer follow-up period is needed to validate its benefits. Nucleoplasty does not replace microdiskectomy or spinal fusion, but it can fill the gap between conservative treatments and open spinal procedures.[6]

Intradiskal electrothermal annuloplasty
Intradiskal electrothermal annuloplasty (IDET) is a minimally invasive procedure for managing chronic diskogenic low back pain in patients who have failed conservative treatment regimens, and who otherwise are possible candidates for spinal fusion. The IDET procedure might relieve diskogenic pain through numerous potential mechanisms, including thermal nociceptive fiber destruction, biochemical mediation of inflammation, cauterization of vascular ingrowth, induced healing of annular tears, and collagen modification. However, whether collagen modification occurs or not is highly controversial, and the treated disk segment actually exhibits greater instability for a brief period of time after the procedure. Unlike other percutaneous intradiskal procedures, the objective of IDET is not to decrease intradiskal pressure.

Indications
Inclusion criteria include unremitting low back pain for at least 6 months, no significant response to conservative treatment including injections, a negative straight leg-raising test, a magnetic resonance imaging scan unremarkable for a neural compressive lesion, less than 50% decrease in disk height, a small disk protrusion, absence of instability and stenosis, positive low pressure (< 15 p.s.i.) diskography, and no prior surgery. Contraindications include severe radicular symptoms, previous disk surgery at the suspect level, severe loss of disk height

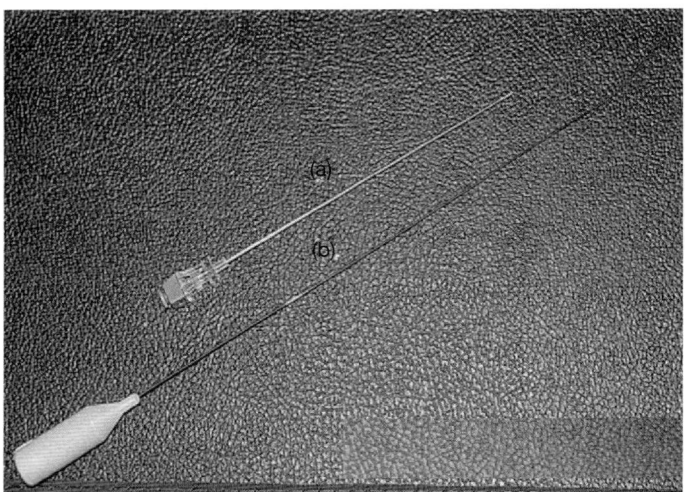

Figure 26-12 Intradiskal electrothermal annuloplasty (IDET) device: (**a**) introducer needle; (**b**) IDET catheter.

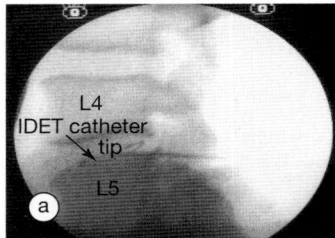
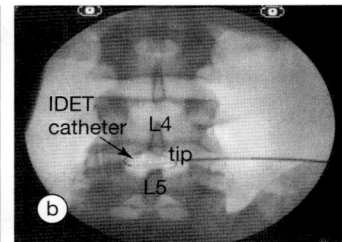

Figure 26-13 Intradiskal electrothermal annuloplasty (IDET), L4, L5: (**a**) lateral view; (**b**) anterior–posterior view. L4, L4 vertebra; L5, L5 vertebra; tip, introducer needle tip.

greater than 50%, imaging studies suggestive of non-diskogenic pathology, segmental instability on flexion and extension radiographs, inflammatory arthritides, extensive solid bone fusion, pregnancy, and psychologic impairment.

Technique

The patient is positioned in a modified lateral decubitus position, and the lumbosacral area is prepared in the usual sterile manner. Intravenous antibiotics are given prior to the procedure, with or without intradiskal antibiotics. A 17-gauge introducer spinal needle (Fig. 26-12) is inserted under fluoroscopic guidance into the center of the disk, using a posterolateral approach. A navigable catheter (Fig. 26-12) with a temperature-controlled thermal resistive coil is then deployed through the needle and positioned intradiskally under two-plane fluoroscopic control. The catheter is navigated as far as possible adjacent to the inner posterior annulus. The catheter temperature is gradually increased according to a uniform protocol to 90°C during a period of 13 min, and maintained at 90°C for an additional 4 min. The catheter should not be heated unless both radiopaque distal markers have exited the needle. The catheter should also be observed in various fluoroscopic views (Fig. 26-13) to make sure that no part of the heating element is in contact with the introducer needle, because heat could be transmitted along the needle. Patients often experience their typical back pain and referred leg pain during the procedure. However, this must be differentiated from true radicular pain, especially if the patient experiences it early in the heating cycle. If this occurs, it is usually indicative of an attenuated posterolateral annulus or extradiskal positioning of the catheter that necessitates repositioning or removal of the catheter. After completing the procedure, the catheter is carefully withdrawn back through the needle to avoid any shearing of the catheter, followed by removal of the introducer needle.

The recommended heating protocol begins at 65°C, and the catheter temperature is increased by 1°C every 30 s until reach-

ing 90°C, which is sustained for a period of 4 min. However, if the patient cannot tolerate the recommended heating protocol, a lower temperature can be used to perform the procedure, based on the belief that the amount of heat delivered over a period of time is more important than the final temperature. Nevertheless, it is strongly suggested that the temperature reach at least 80°C, and should be maintained for 6 min at that particular temperature.

Side effects and complications

Potential complications include bleeding, catheter fracture within the disk, inadvertent puncture of the dura, headache, damage to the thecal sac and its contents, infection including diskitis, and traumatic disk herniation due to the weakened state of the annulus during the first month after the procedure.

Outcome studies

Initial published results for IDET by Derby et al.[13] and Saal et al.[48] showed positive response rates of 73% and 80%, respectively. Subsequent studies showed average decreases in VAS scores of 62–72%, as well as decreases in SF-36 Health Survey body pain of 59–78%. In general, one-third of the patients were significantly better, one-third were slightly better, and one-third were the same or worse. Spinal fusion was subsequently performed in less than 5% of patients treated with IDET, although some patients required spinal surgery 6–18 months after the procedure.[12,29,47] Pauza et al. evaluated the efficacy of IDET for the treatment of chronic diskogenic low back pain after 6 months in a randomized, double-blind, placebo-controlled trial.[40] He reported a statistically significant improvement in bodily pain, VAS scores, overall disability and handicap based on the Oswestry scale, significant improvement in physical functioning on the SF-36, and statistically significant improvement in the Beck Depression Inventory. However, Pauza later reported that, even though mean improvements were statistically significant in the group treated with the IDET procedure, only about 40% of the patients obtained greater than 50% pain relief, while approximately 50% of the patients experienced no appreciable benefit.[41] Kapural showed that IDET was effective in patients with multilevel degenerative disk disease even if all symptomatic disks were not initially treated, but the pain relief and improvement in pain disability index questionnaires were

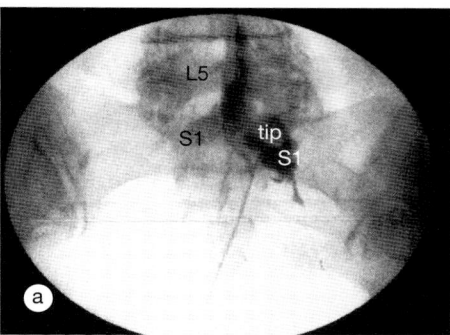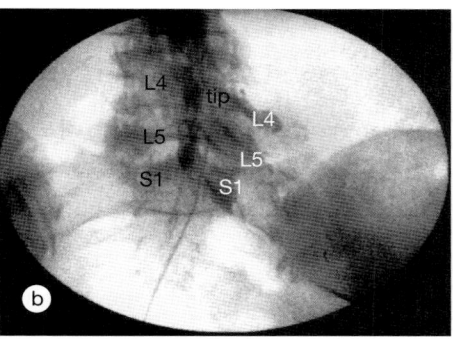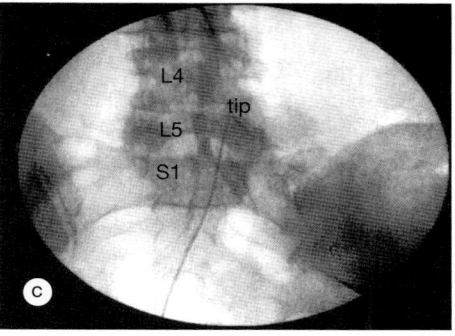

Figure 26-14 Epidural lysis of adhesions. (**a**) Contrast injection revealing right-sided adhesions above the S1 nerve root. (**b**) Contrast injection post epidural lysis, demonstrating elimination of adhesions. (**c**) Injection of local anesthetic and corticosteroid with subsequent washout of contrast. L4 (black), L4 vertebra; L5 (black), L5 vertebra; L5 (white), L5 nerve root; S1 (black), S1 vertebra; L4 (white), L4 nerve root; S1 (white), S1 nerve root; tip, catheter tip.

significantly better in IDET patients with only one or two symptomatic disks.[25]

Epidural lysis of adhesions

Epidural fibrosis with or without adhesive arachnoiditis is a possible complication of spinal surgery. The fibrosis can be caused by manipulation of the supporting structures of the spine, bleeding into the epidural space following surgery, or leakage of disk material. Epidural fibrosis is related to inflammatory reactions that result in the entrapment of nerves within dense scar tissue. Arachnoiditis is most frequently seen in patients who have undergone multiple surgical procedures of the spine. Presumably, inflammation and compression of nerve roots by epidural scar or fibrosis (adhesions) are the mechanism of persistent pain following back surgery, a ruptured or herniated disk, or a vertebral body fracture.

Percutaneous epidural lysis of adhesions (also referred to as epidural neuroplasty or epidural adhesiolysis) has been developed as a conservative procedure to reduce or eliminate adhesions or fibrosis.[23,43–45] A semirigid catheter with a flexible tip is placed into the epidural space to mechanically loosen and/or remove adhesions from the nerve roots. Hypertonic saline can be injected through the catheter at the area of fibrosis to mechanically disrupt adhesions and potentially reduce perineural edema. Hyaluronidase can also be injected to assist with breakdown of scar tissue, and to allow for better infiltration of a local anesthetic and corticosteroid mixture dispensed through the catheter at the site of nerve root involvement.

Indications
The indication for lysis of epidural adhesions includes failed back surgery syndrome, chronic intractable back pain, or chronic radicular leg pain from a disk herniation. Local infection and sepsis are absolute contraindications to this procedure, because of the potential for hematogenous spread via Batson's plexus. Coagulopathy is another absolute contraindication, due to potential compression of the spinal cord or thecal sac from a hematoma.

Technique
The patient is placed in a prone position, and the sacral hiatus is identified by palpation and fluoroscopy. A 16-gauge, $3\frac{1}{2}$-inch styletted needle suitable for catheter placement is inserted and advanced into the sacral hiatus. An AP fluoroscopic view is obtained to ensure that the needle tip is midline and positioned slightly toward the side of pain just below the S3 foramen. The location of the needle in the epidural space is verified with the injection contrast under biplanar fluoroscopy, producing an epidurogram that also identifies the area(s) of adhesions (Fig. 26-14a).

A styletted epidural catheter is used to perform the lysis of adhesions. In order to help steer the catheter in the epidural space, a small bend is made at the distal end of the stylet before it is reinserted into the catheter. The introducer needle stylet is withdrawn, and the epidural catheter is carefully inserted through the needle to the level of the S3 sacral foramina. The catheter is steered gently by alternatively rotating the bent stylet from its proximal end, and advancing or retracting the catheter to lyse the epidural adhesions under a live fluoroscopy. After mechanical lysis of the adhesions with the catheter, an additional 5–10 mL of contrast medium is slowly injected through the catheter to confirm the degree of adhesiolysis (Fig. 26-14b). Hypertonic saline and/or hyaluronidase can be injected at this time through the epidural catheter to assist with removal of scar tissue. Local anesthetic mixed with a corticosteroid is then injected after the lysis of adhesions through the catheter at the location of nerve root involvement, to provide further therapeutic relief (Fig. 26-14c). The catheter is carefully removed after finishing the procedure, so as not to shear any part of the catheter as it is withdrawn through the needle.

Side effects and complications
Possible side effects and complications of this procedure include increasing pain in the injection site or worsening of symptoms, transient increase in back and leg pain, catheter fracture, and ecchymosis or hematoma formation over the sacral hiatus.

More severe complications of epidural lysis of adhesions include local infections, sepsis, bleeding and hematoma formation causing compression of the spinal cord and paralysis, transient nerve compression with temporary paresis, unintended subdural or subarachnoid injection of hypertonic saline, persistent sensory deficit in the lumbar and sacral dermatomes, persistent bowel and/or bladder dysfunction, and sexual dysfunction. Lysis of adhesions in the cervical or thoracic spine must be exercised with caution due to the significant risk for spinal cord trauma.

Outcome studies

Epidural lysis of adhesions can reduce pain in 25% or more of patients who have lumbar radiculopathy plus low back pain refractory to conventional therapies up to 1 year.[23,43,44] Racz reported that 65% of patients had therapeutic pain relief for 1–3 months, but only 13% of patients had the same pain relief for 3–6 months.[45] Manchikanti showed that there were no significant differences in pain relief among 1-day, 2-day, and 3-day procedures.[33] In a prospective randomized controlled study, Manchikanti demonstrated long-term efficacy of pain relief from this procedure, with 97% of patients experiencing significant pain relief at 3 and 6 months, and 47% at 12 months.[34] These patients also showed a significant improvement in mental health and functional status, and a reduction in the use of narcotics. There appears to be no significant difference in treatment efficacy between normal saline and hypertonic saline, or between hyaluronidase and hypertonic saline,[23,33,43,44] although the use of hypertonic saline might reduce the number of patients who require additional treatments.[23]

Vertebroplasty

Traditional treatment of painful compression fractures of spine has been almost exclusively non-operative, including bed rest, non-steroidal antiinflammatory drugs, oral or parenteral analgesics, muscle relaxants, and physical therapy with external back bracing. Surgical treatment for symptomatic vertebral compression fractures has consisted in the past of reduction and internal fixation using an open anterior or posterior approach. In treatment of symptomatic vertebral compression fractures, surgical treatment has traditionally been reserved for actual or impending neurologic compromise. The majority of patients respond favorably to non-operative treatment; however, there are some patients who fail conservative therapy and suffer from prolonged pain and immobility that can persist for life.

Vertebroplasty is a minimally invasive procedure for the treatment of pain and instability caused by a vertebral body compression fracture. The term *vertebroplasty* refers to percutaneous structural reinforcement of the compressed vertebral body using polymethylmethacrylate acrylic cement. The cement hardens on delivery into the vertebral body, providing support and stabilization of the vertebral fracture, or compression by eliminating micromovement of the fracture fragments. Nevertheless, the main goal of vertebroplasty is pain relief from the compression fracture by either stabilizing the fracture or destroying pain fibers from its exothermic reaction. In experienced hands, vertebroplasty is a safe and effective procedure for rapid pain relief due to acute vertebral compression fractures from osteoporosis, hemangiomas, and metastatic tumor.

Kyphoplasty was developed to restore vertebral height and spinal alignment that is not possible with vertebroplasty. Kyphoplasty involves placing a catheter with a balloon tip through a large gauge-size needle into the vertebral body. The balloon is then inflated, which partially restores vertebral height and creates a cavity for cement injection. The balloon is deflated and removed, after which the cement is injected into the vertebral body. In addition to restoring vertebral height and spinal alignment, kyphoplasty allows for the injection of cement under low pressure, potentially reducing the risk for cement extrusion. However, kyphoplasty is performed under general anesthesia in an operating room, and requires considerably more time to complete than vertebroplasty. Nonetheless, the primary goal of both procedures is pain relief, which they both equally provide to patients with compression fractures.

Indications

Vertebroplasty is indicated for patients with osteoporotic compression fractures, from 2 weeks old up to 1 year, causing moderate to severe back pain that is unresponsive to conservative therapy. Vertebroplasty has also been successful for the treatment of spinal compression fracture secondary to metastatic tumor (Fig. 26-15) or benign spinal tumors such as hemangiomas, although the success rate is lower compared with osteoporotic compression fractures. Absolute contraindications for vertebroplasty include infection such as diskitis, osteomyelitis, or sepsis. Relative contraindications include significant compromise of the spinal canal by retropulsed bone fragments or tumor, fracture older than 2 years, greater than 75% collapse of the vertebral body, disruption of the posterior vertebral body wall, fractures above T5, patients who cannot lay prone, and traumatic compression fractures.

Computed tomography (Fig. 26-16) or magnetic resonance imaging is recommended prior to vertebroplasty to access the type of fracture as well as the involvement of the epidural and

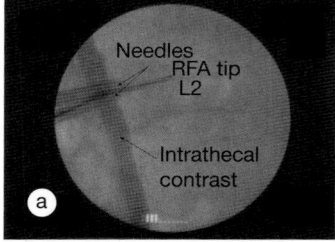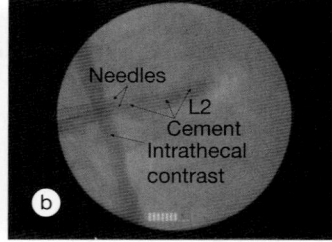

Figure 26-15 Percutaneous vertebroplasty: metastatic tumor. (**a**) Radiofrequency ablation (RFA) with destruction of metastatic tumor within the L2 vertebral body (patient with the computed tomography scan in Fig. 26-13). (**b**) Cement injection into the L2 vertebral body after RFA of metastatic tumor. Note that the L2 posterior vertebral body wall was destroyed by metastatic tumor. Therefore, contrast was injected into the thecal sac at the beginning of the procedure to assess for any retropulsion of radiolucent tumor that could lead to spinal cord compression during the cement injection. L2, L2 vertebra; RFA tip, radiofrequency probe tip.

foraminal space. Compression fractures with a burst fracture of the end plate or a fracture involving the posterior wall of the vertebra might be excluded from vertebroplasty.

A physical examination is performed to localize the level of the pain, and to rule out other causes of back pain such as radiculopathy, disk degeneration, disk herniation, and facet disease. Ideally, the back pain should be at the level of the fracture or within one vertebral body inferior or superior to the fracture, which can be confirmed with an evaluation under fluoroscopy.

Technique

The patient is placed in the prone position, and the C arm is rotated to maximize the oval appearance of the pedicle. The C arm is then tilted to obtain a sharp view of the vertebral end plates. A large-gauge needle is inserted at the center of the pedicle under fluoroscopy, and then advanced through the

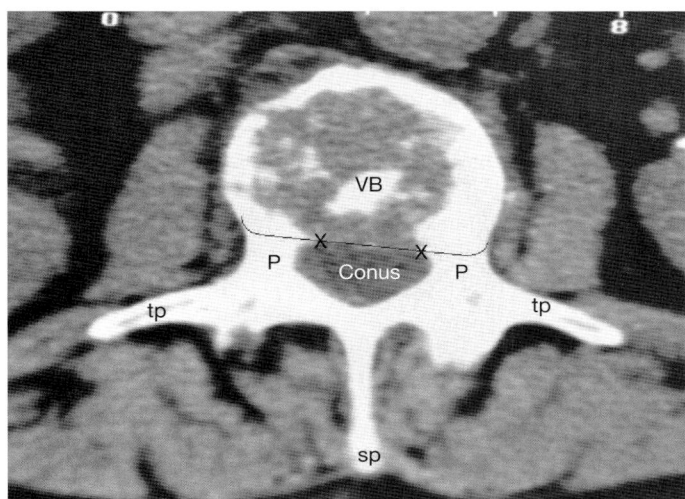

Figure 26-16 Computed tomography scan: L2 vertebra. Soft tissue view demonstrating almost complete replacement of the vertebral body by metastatic tumor (gray material within the vertebral body). The posterior wall (solid line) has been completely destroyed by tumor between the X marks. P, pedicle; sp, spinous process; tp, transverse process; VB, vertebral body.

pedicle (Fig. 26-17a). The needle is kept parallel to the pedicle, and a lateral fluoroscopic view is obtained while the needle is advanced into the anterior third of the vertebral body (Fig. 26-17b) using a twisting motion or gentle tapping of the needle with a sterile hammer. The needle stylet is removed, and 3–5 mL of the cement mixed with contrast is injected into the vertebral body (Fig. 26-17c). The injection is stopped when the cement spreads into the posterior third of the vertebral body. The stylet is placed back into the needle and the needle is removed from the vertebra. Vertebroplasty can be performed using either a single or a bilateral pedicular method depending on the degree of vertebral filling with the cement.

Side effects and complications

The complication rate associated with percutaneous vertebroplasty is 7–10% for treatment of vertebral compression fracture caused by malignant neoplasms, and 1–3% for treatment of osteoporotic vertebral compression fractures.[24,39] The two major complications associated with vertebroplasty are pulmonary compromise and neurologic sequelae. A few cases involving serious complications have been reported, such as pulmonary, fat, and bone marrow embolism.[3,5,27,39] The pulmonary complication rate is higher with vertebroplasty than with kyphoplasty, which appears to be related to the high filling pressure for the bone cement, which can cause extrusion of bone cement into the vertebral venous system.[20,22] Vertebroplasty requires a high-pressure injection using a low-viscosity cement; this can lead to cement leakage in a certain percentage of procedures, because of the vertebral trabeculae structure. However, vertebroplasty in general is a safe procedure to treat those with intractable pain from osteoporotic compression fractures, with fewer than 1% having significant complications.[42] Other complications include fracture of additional vertebral components or the rib, transient fever, increased pain, internal hemorrhage, nerve root irritation, and cord infarction.

Outcome studies

Although no controlled studies have been performed to compare the result of vertebroplasty with that of conservative therapy, positive outcomes have been demonstrated from multiple series of case studies. Vertebroplasty can relieve or completely

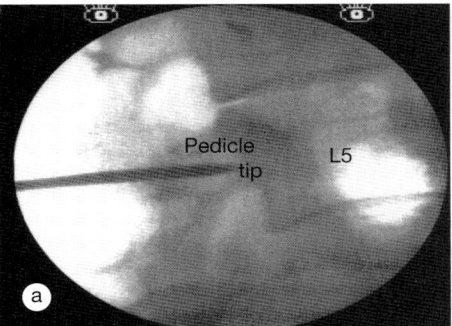
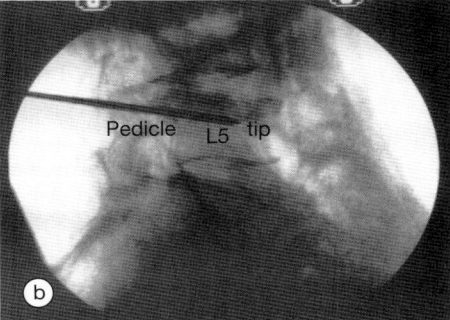
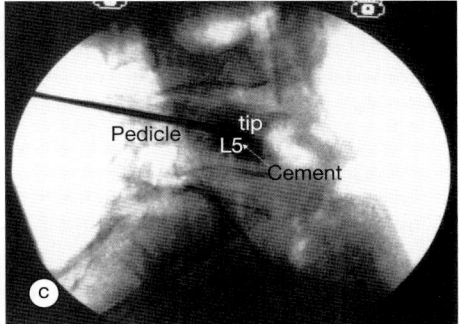

Figure 26-17 Percutaneous vertebroplasty. (**a**) Large-gauge needle within the L5 pedicle. (**b**) Large-gauge needle advanced within the anterior third of the L5 vertebral body. (**c**) Cement injection into the osteoporotic compression fracture of the L5 vertebral body. L5, L5 vertebra; tip, needle tip.

alleviate severe back pain of patients with compression fractures. The study of Jensen et al. on percutaneous vertebroplasty in 231 patients showed a 90% success rate in the treatment of osteoporotic vertebral fractures, and an 80% success rate in painful or unstable neoplastic lesions and vertebral hemangiomas.[24] Cortet conducted an open prospective study, which showed that 90% of patients (29 patients with 47 fractures) with age-related or steroid-induced osteoporosis experienced pain relief and improved mobility at 24 h post vertebroplasty.[11] There were no reports of worsening of pain after the procedure. Another study reported good pain relief in 73% of patients, with at least a 50% reduction in analgesic dose.[49] This study also reported moderate pain relief in 29% of patients (37 patients, 52 vertebrae) with painful malignant vertebral lesions.[49]

Despite a small number of studies published in the literature and the lack of prospective randomized trials, this procedure has gained increasing acceptance as a treatment choice for back pain caused by vertebral fractures. Vertebroplasty is effective in pain control and obtaining spine stability that often improves quality of life.

Spinal cord stimulation

Spinal cord stimulation (SCS) has been used for controlling intractable leg pain for more than 30 years. The SCS system stimulates the dorsal column of the spinal cord by tiny electrical impulses from small electrical wires placed on the spinal cord. This pain modality offers an option to patients with chronic back pain, and can be particularly helpful in patients with chronic leg pain that is unresponsive to other medical treatment. SCS offers the medical community an effective treatment for pain that also reduces the costs associated with the treatment of patients with chronic intractable pain.

Spinal cord stimulation consists of one or two lead wires with a number of electrodes and a pulse generator or battery. The lead wire carries the electrical stimulation from the pulse generator or battery to the posterior column of the spinal cord. The mechanism of spinal cord stimulation is still unknown. Some believe that stimulation of the dorsal columns closes the 'gates' to pain transmission, while others believe that pain relief from SCS results from direct inhibition of pain pathways in the spinothalamic tracts rather than being due to selective large fiber stimulation.[4] The other possible mechanism of SCS might involve producing supraspinal pain inhibition, activation of central inhibitory mechanisms influencing sympathetic efferent neurons, and activation of putative neurotransmitters or neuro-modulators. SCS does not totally eliminate the source of pain, but it interferes with the pain signal, providing relief that varies for each patient.

There are two different types of SCS system, one that is totally implantable and another with an internal SCS lead and an external RF transmitter. An external RF system might be best for the patient who requires a higher voltage or a multilead therapy for pain relief. The power source can be externally worn on a patient's belt to transmit RF energy to the pulse generator that is implanted subcutaneously. The internal battery

system is for a lower voltage or a one- or two-lead therapy, but the battery needs to be surgically replaced every 2–5 years, depending on usage. The SCS leads can be placed into the epidural space either percutaneously or with a small laminotomy. The long-term results from percutaneous epidural SCS implantation are comparable with those obtained from a laminotomy.[55]

Indications

Patients selected for SCS usually have had a disability due to intractable leg pain with or without back pain for more than 12 months. They have also tried all conservative forms of treatment, including medications, physical therapy, manipulations, injections, and other adjuvant treatments, without any significant relief of the pain. Patients who have failed surgical treatment for their back and leg pain are also candidates for this modality. Keeping in mind that this procedure is best for limb rather than for axial pain, the typical candidate should be free of drug dependence, be psychologically suitable and stable, and be a highly motivated individual. The specific types of conditions considered for SCS include radiculopathy, failed neck or back syndrome, epidural fibrosis or arachnoiditis (resulting in radiculopathy), postherpetic neuralgia, peripheral neuropathy, intercostals neuralgia, complex regional pain syndromes types I and II, phantom limb pain, intractable angina, ischemic limb pain, interstitial cystitis, and headaches.

Absolute contraindications for SCS include local or systemic infection, and untreated coagulopathy due to the potential for spinal cord compression from a hematoma. Relative contraindications for SCS are unmotivated and/or psychologically unstable patients, or patients who have exhibited drug-seeking behavior. Patients should try other types of conservative therapy before going on to SCS.

Technique

The patient is placed prone in the procedure, with a bolster under the bottom of the rib cage. A large-gauge epidural needle is advanced under AP fluoroscopy into the T12–L1 interlaminar space using a loss of resistance technique. The needle enters at an angle of approximately 30° from horizontal. The syringe is removed after entering the epidural, and an SCS lead is passed through the needle into the epidural space. The lead is advanced under fluoroscopic guidance, steering it by alternately rotating the needle or lead as well as advancing or retracting the lead, being careful not to shear off the lead into the epidural space. The SCS lead tip should be placed at the top of T8 or T9 (for lumbar coverage) (Fig. 26-18) or the top of C3 (for cervical coverage). The lead should be placed either in the midline for a bilateral stimulation pattern or to the symptomatic side for a unilateral stimulation pattern.

The lead is positioned for the best pain coverage. The patient is then sent home for a trial stimulation for no less than 2 days and typically for 5–7 days. The patient is kept on a prophylactic oral antibiotic during this time period to prevent infection. During the trial, patients keep track of their pain relief, sleeping pattern, stimulation tolerance, pain coverage, use of medica-

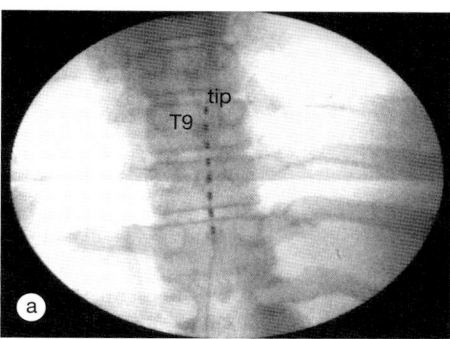
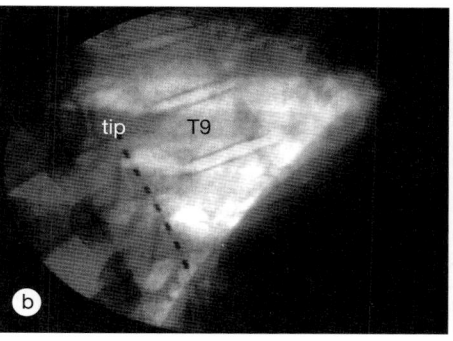
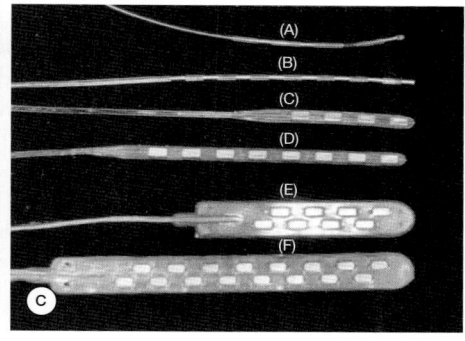

Figure 26-18 Spinal cord stimulator lead placement. Spinal cord stimulator lead positioned in the posterior epidural space at the T9 vertebral level, right of midline, for right lower extremity stimulation. (**a**) Anterior–posterior view; (**b**) lateral view. T9, T9 vertebra; tip, spinal cord stimulator lead tip. (**c**) Spinal cord stimulator leads. Peripheral leads: A, four-electrode lead; B, eight-electrode lead. Laminotomy leads: C, four-electrode lead; D, eight-electrode lead, E, paired four-electrode lead; F, paired eight-electrode lead.

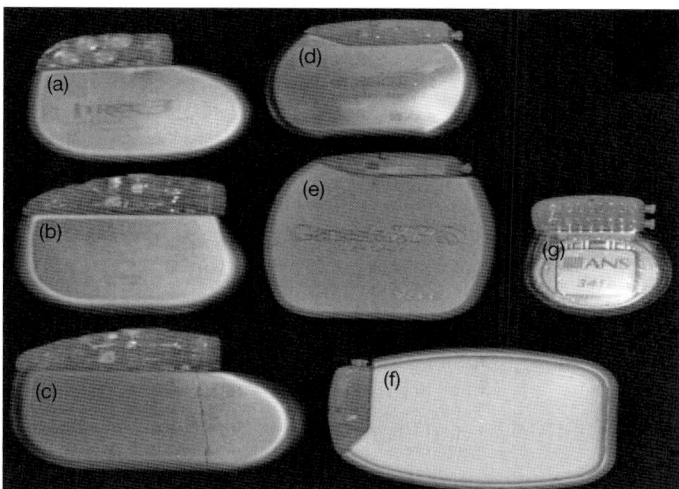

Figure 26-19 Spinal cord stimulator battery or generators. Medtonic: (**a**) Itrel 3 (battery), (**b**) Synergy Versitrel (extended battery), and (**c**) Synergy (extended battery). Advanced Neuromodulation Systems: (**d**) Genesis (battery), (**e**) GenesisXP (extended battery), (**f**) GenesisRC (rechargeable battery), and (**g**) Renew (radiofrequency receiver used with an external battery source).

tions, and functional activities. When the patient returns to the office, these parameters are discussed to determine if the trial was successful or not. If the trial was satisfactory, then the patient is scheduled for a permanent implantation.

The permanent placement procedure is very similar to that used for temporary placement. Once the lead is in place, it is permanently attached to the supraspinous ligament or fascia. The battery or RF receiver (Fig. 26-19) is then implanted into the fatty layer of the lower abdomen, or one of the buttocks, through a small incision. The patient is instructed on how to keep the wound dry and clean for the next 7–10 days to prevent infection. Prophylactic oral antibiotics are prescribed to prevent an infection. Bending or twisting the trunk and/or neck, depending on lead placement, is limited after the procedure, as these movements can dislodge the lead.

Side effects and complications
Complications can occur but are generally minor. The most common complications include scar tissue formation and pain at the pocket or midline incision site. Less common complications include lead migration, lead fracture, and infection. Rare complications include an epidural hematoma, cord compression, paraplegia, and a pulmonary or fat embolism.

Outcome studies
Generally, the more distal the radicular pain, the better the results from SCS. Radicular pain in a unilateral limb responds best to SCS. However, with improved design, dual systems, and multiple electrode leads, it is possible to treat axial pain along with limb pain. Neuropathic pain also tends to respond better to SCS. There does not appear to be any difference in pain relief or complications between cervical and lumbar SCS.[19]

LeDoux demonstrated that 74% of patients with failed back syndrome were receiving 50% or better pain relief with SCS at 2 years.[30] North also found in a prospective randomized study that patients who failed a previous laminectomy did significantly better with SCS compared with a repeat lumbar laminectomy.[37]

In a study by Kelmer and colleagues involving a randomized clinical trial of patients with complex regional pain syndrome, they demonstrated that the SCS group had significant pain reduction and improved quality of life compared with the non-SCS group.[26] In a recent prospective case study by Barolat, patients with chronic low back and leg pain generally did well with SCS for both back and leg pain. At 1 year in this study, 88% of the patients reported fair to excellent relief of leg pain, and 68.8% reported the same for low back pain relief.[1]

Spinal cord stimulation is an option for the improvement of pain and quality of life in a carefully selected subset of patients with chronic intractable pain.[1,16,26,37,38] SCS is generally preferable as a first step when other less invasive treatments have failed to produce acceptable control of the pain, because there are no reported long-term side effects.[37,38] However, because of difficulty in conducting randomized controlled trials, there has been a lack of high-quality studies to test the efficacy and cost-effectiveness of SCS in patients with chronic pain.[4] Despite the positive findings, there is a need for randomized, controlled, long-term studies on the efficacy of SCS involving larger patient populations.[2,21,32,54]

Intrathecal pump therapies

The spinal infusion systems include intrathecal and epidural infusion devices. There are two types of spinal infusion pumps: programmable and non-programmable. The programmable pump is a computerized, battery-operated device (Fig. 26-20) that can dispense medication at different rates throughout the day as well as deliver a bolus. The non-programmable pumps are available in different sizes and different (but fixed) rates. A spinal infusion system consists of a pump and a catheter (Fig. 26-20), both of which are surgically placed under the skin. The catheter is inserted into the intrathecal space and connected to the pump that is implanted into the subcutaneous tissue of the abdomen. The pump releases medication through the catheter into the intrathecal space.

Intrathecal infusion bypasses the blood–brain barrier, allowing for direct access to the brain and spinal cord neuroreceptors. Less medication is required for the desired result, with less chance of side effects from the medications. Currently, morphine, baclofen, and recently ziconotide (an N-type calcium channel blocker) are the only Food and Drug Administration-approved medicines that can be infused into human spinal fluid. However, there are several other medications that have been used off-label in the pump for pain control.

Indications

Intrathecal infusion of preservative-free morphine is designed for patients who suffer from chronic malignant or non-malignant intractable pain. They have failed all types of pain treatment, including physical modalities, manipulations, injections,

surgery, and other adjuvant treatments. Intrathecal infusion of baclofen is designed for patients who have severe spasticity of cerebral or spinal cord origin, and who have failed all forms of treatment without significant improvement. The appropriate candidate for an intrathecal pump has undergone a successful intrathecal trial with either an opioid for pain or baclofen for spasticity. Their body size must be sufficient for implantation of the pump. There should be no issues regarding drug dependence, and the patient must be psychologically suitable and stable. Contraindications for an intrathecal pump include a local or systemic infection as well as a coagulopathy.

Technique

The patient is positioned in a lateral decubitus position to allow for simultaneous access to the spine and abdomen. This avoids the need to prepare the patient twice in the operating room. A relative AP view of the lumbar spine is obtained, and a large epidural needle is advanced through the skin at a cephalad angle into the intrathecal space at the L3, L4 level.

The stylet is removed, allowing free flow of cerebral spinal fluid. A catheter is passed through the needle into the intrathecal space, and is advanced cephalad approximately to the T10 level. An incision is made along the epidural needle, with dissection to the supraspinous ligament or to the fascia. The needle is removed, and an anchor is placed over the catheter and sutured to the ligament or fascia. Next, a subcutaneous pocket is created in the lower abdominal region large enough for the pump. A pump catheter is passed from the abdominal pocket to the midline spine incision through a tunnel in either one or two passes. The pump catheter is attached to the intrathecal catheter as well as to the pump. An extra amount of the pump catheter is placed with the pump in the subcutaneous pocket, and extra intrathecal catheter is placed at the spine incision site, to accommodate for movement by the patient. The spine incision is then sutured closed with layered interrupted sutures follow by skin closure. The pump is sutured into the abdominal pocket typically with silk sutures, and then closed with layered interrupted sutures followed by skin closure.

Side effects and complications

Postsurgical complications can occur, including infection, bleeding, pain, discomfort around the implant site, hematoma, and seroma formation in the pocket. Other potential complications include symptoms of drug overdose and under-dose due to component failure, such as catheter occlusion, catheter fracture or dislodgement, leakage, and catheter migration; arachnoiditis; and toxic spinal cord lesion. Patients can experience the symptoms of urinary retention, nausea, vomiting, itching, weakness, facial flushing, constipation, joint pain, muscle twitching, oversedation, somnolence, respiratory depression, lack of effectiveness, and disorientation.

Intrathecal pump therapies are a safe option for most patients with intractable pain. Most complications are related to the implant procedure, and the incidence of long-term complications is very low. A few cases of spinal cord compression have been reported from an intrathecal catheter tip inflammatory

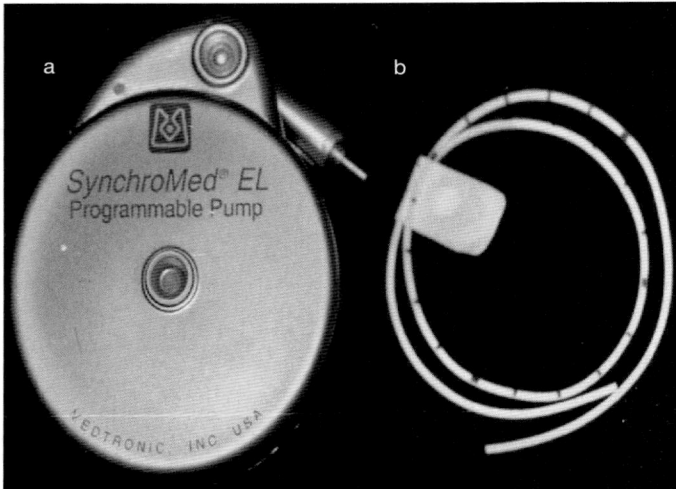

Figure 26-20 Intrathecal pump. (**a**) Medtronic SynchroMed EL programmable pump; (**b**) intrathecal catheter.

mass.[9] To prevent this serious complication, imaging is important in evaluating patients who develop uncontrollable pain and new neurologic findings after intrathecal catheter implantation. Patients who require high-dose intraspinal opioid therapy, and those who receive drugs or mixtures that are not approved for intrathecal use, should be monitored closely for signs of a catheter granulomatous mass or malfunction. Prompt diagnosis and treatment can preserve neurologic function.[9]

Outcome studies

Corrado reported data on a prospective study comparing intrathecal morphine pump patients with those treated with oral medications.[10] He collected data on 40 patients with intractable chronic low back pain who were equally divided into two groups. Those who received the pump did remarkably better, with significantly lower pain and lower disability index scores. Kumar found, in a prospective study of 16 patients with chronic non-malignant pain with a 29-month mean follow-up, that in 12 patients (75%) the therapy was considered a success in terms of improvement in pain and quality of life, whereas it was considered a failure in four patients.[28] Smith et al. demonstrated in a prospective randomized trial that cancer patients with recalcitrant pain had a statistically significant greater clinical response to intrathecal therapy than to medical management.[53] The intrathecal pump patients had a more substantial reduction in VAS scores and drug toxicity, as well as living longer than those who received medical management.

The intrathecal pump is a safe and effective procedure if careful attention is paid to technique. Most patients have a good response to the pump, particularly after a successful trial. The major advantage of an implantable infusion pump is that a very small amount of medication is infused directly into the spine, reducing the risk of systemic side effects observed with equivalent amounts of oral medications. An intrathecal pump might be the only recourse for patients who have severe pain and cannot tolerate the side effects or interactions of oral pain medications.

SUMMARY

Interventional pain management procedures play an important role in the treatment of the nearly 100 million Americans, and an even greater number of patients abroad, who suffer with chronic pain. An understanding of the indications, contraindications, and complications for these procedures is essential to ensure their effectiveness. The use of diagnostic injections and trial applications when possible has a considerable impact on the outcome of these procedures and cannot be overlooked when selecting appropriate candidates. The interventional pain management procedures discussed in this chapter have provided pain relief, increased physical function, reduced medical costs, and a better quality of life for many of these patients with chronic benign and malignant pain. Despite the progress that has been made with interventional pain management, there is still a considerable need for a better understanding of chronic pain, determining the most effective treatment, technology development, technique refinement, and more quality outcome-based research studies.

REFERENCES

1. Barolat G, Oakley J, Law J, et al. Epidural spinal cord stimulation with a multiple electrode paddle lead is effective in treating low back pain. Neuromodulation 2001; 2:59–66.
2. Cameron T. Safety and efficacy of spinal cord stimulation for the treatment of chronic pain: a 20-year literature review. J Neurosurg Spine 2004; 100:254–267.
3. Campbell JN. Examination of possible mechanisms by which stimulation of the spinal cord in man relieves pain. Appl Neurophysiol 1981; 44:181–186.
4. Carter ML. Spinal cord stimulation in chronic pain: a review of the evidence. Anaesth Intensive Care 2004; 32:11–21.
5. Chen HL. A lethal pulmonary embolism during percutaneous vertebroplasty. Anesth Analg 2002; 95:4.
6. Chen YC, Derby R, Lee S. Percutaneous disc decompression in the management of chronic low back pain. Orthop Clin N Am 2004; 35:17–23.
7. Chen YC, Lee SH, Chen D. Intradiscal pressure study of percutaneous disc decompression with nucleoplasty in human cadavers. Spine 2003; 28:661–665.
8. Chen YC, Lee SH, Saenz Y, et al. Histologic findings of disc, endplate and neural elements post coblation of nucleus pulposus: an experimental nucleoplasty study. Spine J 2003; 3:466–470.
9. Coffey RJ, Burchiel K. Inflammatory mass lesions associated with intrathecal drug infusion catheters: report and observations on 41 patients. Neurosurgery 2002; 50:78–86.
10. Corrado P, Gottlieb H, Varga CA, et al. The effect of intrathecal morphine infusion on pain level and disability in pain patients with chronic intractable low back pain. AJPM 2000; 10:160–166.
11. Cortet B, Cotton A, Boutry N, et al. Percutaneous vertebroplasty in the treatment of osteoporotic vertebral compression fractures: an open prospective study. J Rhematol 1999; 26:2222–2228.
12. Derby R, Chen Y, O'Neill C, et al. Intradiscal electrothermal annuloplasty: a novel approach for treating chronic discogenic back pain. Neuromodulation 2000; 3:82–88.
13. Derby R. Intradiscal electrothermal annuloplasty. Paper presented at the North American Spine Society, 13th Annual Meeting. San Francisco, October 28–31, 1998.
14. Derby R. Outcome comparison between IDET, combined IDET nucleoplasty and biochemical injection treatment. Presented at the International Spinal Injection Society, 10th Annual Scientific Meeting. Austin, September 6–8, 2002.
15. Dreyfuss P, Halbrook B, Pauza K, et al. Efficacy and validity of radiofrequency neurotomy for chronic lumbar zygapophyseal joint pain. Spine 2000; 25:1270–1277.
16. Erdek MA, Staats PS. Spinal cord stimulation for angina pectoris and peripheral vascular disease. Anesthesiol Clin N Am 2003; 21:797–804.
17. Ferrante FM, King LF, Roche EA, et al. Radiofrequency sacroiliac joint denervation for sacroiliac syndrome. Reg Anesth Pain Med 2001; 26:137–142.
18. Forouzanfar T, van Kleef M, Weber WE. Radiofrequency lesion of the stellate ganglion in chronic pain syndromes: retrospective analysis of clinical efficacy in 86 patients. Clin J Pain 2000; 16:164–168.
19. Forouzanfar T. Spinal cord stimulation in complex regional pain syndrome: cervical and lumbar devices are comparably effective. Br J Anaesth 2004; 92:348–353.
20. Garfin SR, Yuan HA, Reiley MA. New technologies in spine: kyphoplasty and vertebroplasty for the treatment of painful osteoporotic compression fractures. Spine 2001; 26:1511–1515.
21. Grabow TS. Spinal cord stimulation for complex regional pain syndrome: an evidence-based medicine review of the literature. Clin J Pain 2003; 19:371–383.
22. Groen RJ. Anatomical and pathological considerations in percutaneous vertebroplasty and kyphoplasty: a reappraisal of the vertebral venous system. Spine 2004; 29:1465–1471.

23. Heavner JE. Percutaneous epidural neuroplasty: prospective evaluation of 0.9% NaCl versus 10% NaCl with or without hyaluronidase. Reg Anesth Pain Med 1999; 24:202–207.

24. Jensen ME, Evans AJ, Mathis JM, et al. Percutaneous polymethylmethacrylate vertebroplasty in the treatment of osteoporotic vertebral body compression fractures: technical aspects. Am J Neuroradiol 1997; 18:1897–1904.

25. Kapural L, Mekhail N, Korunda Z, et al. Intradiscal thermal annuloplasty for the treatment of lumbar discogenic pain in patients with multilevel degenerative disc disease. Anesth Analg 2004; 99:472–476.

26. Kelmer MA, Barendse GA, van Kleef M, et al. Spinal cord stimulation in patients with chronic reflex sympathetic dystrophy. N Engl J Med 2000; 343:618–624.

27. Koessler MJ. Fat and bone marrow embolism during percutaneous vertebroplasty. Anesth Analg 2003; 97:293.

28. Kumar K, Kelly M, Pirlot T. Continuous intrathecal morphine treatment for chronic pain of nonmalignant etiology: long-term benefits and efficacy. Surg Neurol 2001; 55:79–88.

29. Lagattuta FB, Brady R, Hudoba P, et al. Incidence of intervertebral fusion in patients treated with intradiscal electrothermotherapy. Paper presented at the American Association of Orthopedic Medicine Annual Meeting. Amelia Island, May 4–6, 2000.

30. LeDoux MS. Spinal cord stimulation for the failed back syndrome. Spine 1993; 18:191–194.

31. Lord S, Barnsley L, Wallis B, et al. Percutaneous radiofrequency neurotomy for chronic cervical zygapophyseal joint pain. N Engl J Med 1996; 335:1721–1726.

32. Mailis-Gagnon A. Spinal cord stimulation for chronic pain. Cochrane Database Syst Rev 2004; 3:CD003783.

33. Manchikanti L, Bakhit CE. Percutaneous lysis of epidural adhesions. Pain Physician 2000; 3:46–64.

34. Manchikanti L, Pampati V, Fellows B, et al. Role of one day epidural adhesiolysis in management of chronic low back pain. Pain Physician 2001; 4:153–166.

35. Manchikanti L, Staats P, Singh V, et al. Evidence-based practice guidelines for interventional techniques in the management of chronic spinal pain. Pain Physician 2003; 6:3–81.

36. Munglani R. The longer term effect of pulsed radiofrequency for neuropathic pain. Pain 1999; 80:437–439.

37. North RG, Kidd DH, Farrokhi F, et al. Spinal cord stimulation versus repeated lumbosacral surgery for chronic pain: a randomized, controlled trial. Neurosurgery 2005; 56:98–106.

38. Oakley JC. Spinal cord stimulation: patient selection, technique, and outcomes. Neurosurg Clin N Am 2003; 14:365–380.

39. Padovani B, Kasriel O, Brunner P, et al. Pulmonary embolism caused by acrylic cement: a rare complication of percutaneous vertebroplasty. Am J Neuroradiol 1999; 20:375–377.

40. Pauza K, Howell S, Dreyfuss P, et al. A randomized, double-blind, placebo-controlled trial evaluating the efficacy of intradiscal electrothermal annuloplasty (IDET) for the treatment of chronic discogenic low back pain: 6-month outcomes. In: Proceedings of the International Spinal Injection Society. Austin, September 7, 2002.

41. Pauza K, Howell S, Dreyfuss P, et al. A randomized, placebo-controlled trial of intradiscal electrothermal therapy for the treatment of discogenic low back pain. Spine J 2004; 4:27–35.

42. Predey TA. Percutaneous vertebroplasty: new treatment for vertebral compression fractures. Am Fam Physician 2002; 66:565.

43. Racz GB, Heavner JE, Raj PP. Epidural neuroplasty. Semin Anesth 1997; 302–312.

44. Racz GB, Heavner JE, Raj PP. Percutaneous epidural neuroplasty. Prospective one-year follow up. Pain Digest 1999; 9:97–102.

45. Racz GB, Holubec JT. Lysis of adhesions in the epidural space. In: Racz GB, ed. Techniques of neurolysis. Boston: Kluwer Academic; 1989:57–72.

46. Rocco AG. Radiofrequency lumbar sympatholysis. The evolution of a technique for managing sympathetically maintained pain. Reg Anesth 1995; 20:3–12.

47. Saal JA, Saal JS. Intradiscal electrothermal treatment for chronic discogenic low back pain: a prospective outcome study with minimum 1-year follow-up. Spine 2000; 25:2622–2627.

48. Saal JS, Saal JA. Management of chronic discogenic low back pain with a thermal intradiscal catheter: a preliminary report. Spine 2000; 25(3):382–388.

49. San Millan Ruiz D, Burkhardt K, Jean B, et al. Pathology findings with acrylic implants. Bone 1999; 25:85S–90S.

50. Sharps LS, Issac Z. Percutaneous disc decompression using nucleoplasty. Pain Physician 2002; 5:121–126.

51. Singh V, Piryani C, Liao K, et al. Percutaneous disc decompression, using coblation (nucleoplasty), in the treatment of discogenic pain. Pain Physician 2002; 5:250–259.

52. Sluijter M, Cosman E, Rittman W III, et al. The effects of pulsed radiofrequency fields applied to the dorsal root ganglion—a preliminary report. Pain Clinic 1998; 11:109–117.

53. Smith TJ, Swainey C, Coyne PJ. Pain management, including intrathecal pumps. Curr Oncol Rep 2004; 6:291–296.

54. Turner JA. Spinal cord stimulation for patients with failed back surgery syndrome or complex regional pain syndrome: a systematic review of effectiveness and complications. Pain 2004; 108:137–147.

55. Urban BJ. Percutaneous epidural stimulation of the spinal cord for relief of pain. Long-term results. J Neurosurg 1978; 48:323–328.

56. Van Kleef M, Liem L, Lousberg R, et al. Radiofrequency lesion adjacent to the dorsal root ganglion for cervicobrachial pain: a prospective double blind randomized study. Neurosurgery 1996; 38:1127–1131.

57. Zundert J. Percutaneous pulsed radiofrequency treatment of the cervical dorsal root ganglion in the treatment of chronic cervical pain syndrome: a clinical audit. Neuromodulation 2003; 6:6–14.

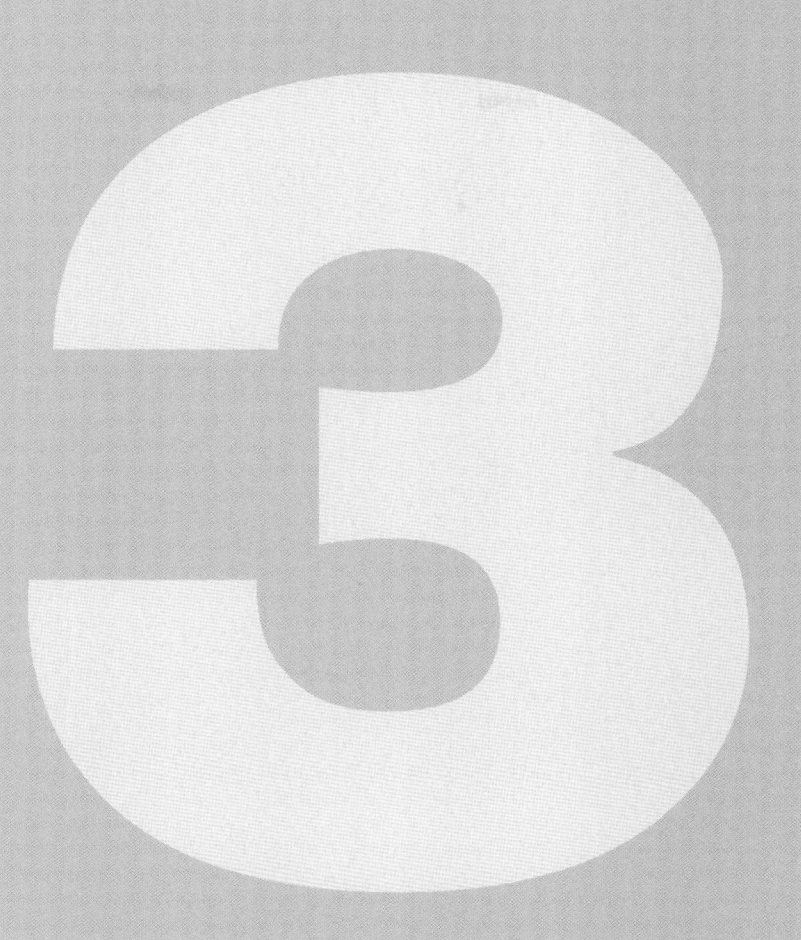

COMMON CLINICAL PROBLEMS

Achieving Functional Independence
Alison E. Lane

Functional independence is the ability to perform daily living tasks without help. The achievement of functional independence ensures that individuals can participate fully in life situations that are meaningful and purposeful. Whether experiencing a physical disability or not, participation in activities of daily living or life occupations is essential to health and well-being.[3] Anthropologists have noted that involvement in the daily routines of self-maintenance, production, and leisure enables humans to express themselves, establish relationships, and build self-identity.[5] The World Health Organization has recognized the importance of participation in life situations to health by reframing the *International Classification of Impairments, Disabilities, and Handicaps*[31] as the *International Classification of Functioning, Disability and Health*.[30] In doing this, understandings of health have shifted significantly, from definitions relating to the absence of disease or impairment to ones that embrace the notion of an individual engaging with and functioning in her or his world. Supporting this shift is emerging evidence of the powerful therapeutic benefit of participation in meaningful daily occupations.[5] Individuals who are able to achieve meaningful participation in life situations are more likely to experience and report increased personal satisfaction and quality of life, increased levels of energy, fewer physical ailments, reduced pain, and improved physical functioning.[17] Ultimately, this impact may decrease the costs of health associated with burden of care, the treatment of physical symptomatology, and poor emotional health.

The goal of medical rehabilitation programs for persons experiencing physical disability as a result of injury, illness, or a developmental condition is to maximize functional independence over time.[7] All members of the rehabilitation team are focused on restoring or enhancing functional capacity such that individuals can engage optimally in daily life tasks that are meaningful and purposeful. Because of the subjective nature of what constitutes 'meaningful' and 'purposeful', it is important to adopt a family- or client-centered frame of reference for care. This frame of reference defines a set of philosophies, attitudes, and approaches to care for persons with special needs and their families.[8] It refers to a relationship between the person, family, and healthcare professional that builds on the person's and family's priorities and that responds to their mutual goals.[4] Some key elements in family- or client-centered care include recognizing family strengths, respecting different methods of coping, facilitating family and professional collaboration at all levels of healthcare, and sharing complete and unbiased information with families on a continuing basis and in a supportive manner. By adopting this frame of reference in practice, the rehabilitation team will be able to plan an evaluation and treatment process that matches the individual's life goals and priorities. Rehabilitation programs that focus their interventions in this way are more likely to achieve the desired outcomes of enhancing productive living, promoting efficient recovery, and reducing the burden of care for individuals with physical disabilities over the long term.[10,16,26]

The aim of this chapter is to overview the current evaluation and treatment principles used by the rehabilitation team to assist an individual experiencing physical disability to achieve functional independence.

EVALUATION

Using a family- or client-centered approach, evaluation of an individual's functional independence necessarily begins with the determination of that person's life goals, premorbid roles and activities, priorities for recovery, and contextual or cultural influences. From here, a more specific evaluation process can be conducted that investigates the individual's actual performance abilities and limitations in key areas of function. It also measures components of functional skill including strength, range of motion, tone, sensation, balance, coordination, visual perception, and cognition. This type of evaluation process is referred to as the top-down approach, and is considered 'the best fit for the emerging system of health-care delivery'.[14] The top-down approach has the advantage of focusing clearly on the roles and activities that are meaningful for patients, consequently increasing motivation for participation in the rehabilitation process and increasing the understanding of the relevance of rehabilitation to daily life. The top-down evaluation approach also allows the definition of outcomes of rehabilitation in terms that are most likely to receive maximum reimbursement. Payers specifically seek outcomes of therapy that allow the patient to function most efficiently and effectively in daily contexts.[14] Top-down evaluation results in rehabilitation goals that are directly related to the individual's performance in life roles.

Determining meaningful life roles and activities

The task of determining a person's life goals, valued functional roles and activities, and priorities for recovery is a complex one. Because of the subjective nature of the content, there are few evaluation tools that provide the rehabilitation team with succinct, quantifiable data relating to this issue. Information about the person's priorities and premorbid activity is usually gained through discussion and interview with the person and/or caregivers. It is important that those team members charged with the responsibility of gathering this information are skilled in techniques of interviewing and counseling, so as to ensure that the individual is able to clearly communicate personal needs and wants.

Within the field of occupational therapy, an evaluation tool has been developed specifically for the purpose of assisting occupational therapists to establish occupational performance (functional performance) goals and priorities with their clients. The Canadian Occupational Performance Measure (COPM)[18] was developed using a client-centered frame of reference, and consists of a semistructured interview approach for gathering patients' perspectives on their needs and wants in areas of self-care, productive living, and leisure. The evaluation process encourages patients to rate their perceptions of their current levels of performance in and satisfaction with participation in key functional tasks. These are then reevaluated and rerated at the end of the rehabilitative process to provide outcome data relating to the patient's perspective on recovery. Evaluation tools such as the COPM provide broad, descriptive information about the person's functional independence needs, which allows the rehabilitation team to target specific areas requiring further evaluation and focus in intervention.

Evaluating specific performance abilities

Once the patient's valued life roles and activities have been identified and goals for rehabilitation determined, more specific evaluation is then completed to establish what performance limitations and abilities exist. A variety of methods can be used to assess functional skill. In many cases, therapists use guided observation and task analysis to determine the level of functional independence demonstrated by the patient. There are a number of more formal measures, however, that have been developed for the purpose of measuring functional capacity. The most commonly used tool in this area is the functional independence measure (FIM).[2] The FIM consists of 18 items examining the functional areas of self-care, sphincter control, transfers, locomotion, communication, and social cognition. Scores on the FIM provide an indicator of level of disability within motor and cognitive domains based on the level of assistance a patient requires to perform key functional tasks.[21] A pediatric version of the FIM, the WeeFIM,[1] has been developed for children aged 6 months to 7 years. It uses a similar structure to the FIM but modifies the items to account for developmental differences in social cognition and communication domains. Data from the FIM and the WeeFIM are being compiled in the Uniform Data System for Medical Rehabilitation to provide a repository of information regarding the functional indepen-

dence of adults and children experiencing physical disability. Other tools used in rehabilitation settings to measure the functional abilities of patients include the following.

- The Barthel Index:[19] a measure of activity of daily living skills, including feeding, transfers, personal hygiene, toileting, bathing, ambulation, stair climbing, dressing, and bowel and bladder control.
- The Assessment of Motor and Process Skills:[9] an observational tool that allows the evaluation of motor and process skills necessary for performance of two or three activities of daily living tasks chosen because of their relevance to the patient. Motor skills observed include stabilization, alignment, positioning, walking, reaching, bending, coordination, manipulation, endurance, and grip. Process skills observed include pacing, attention, choice making, initiation, adjustment, sequencing, organization, navigation, and accommodation.
- The Pediatric Evaluation of Disability Inventory:[13] this measure assesses functional performance in children aged 6 months to 7 years and 6 months in the areas of self-care, mobility, and social function. Scoring includes a rating of functional skill, level of caregiver assistance required, and use of modifications or adaptive equipment.
- The Functional Rehabilitation Evaluation of Sensori-Neurologic Outcomes (FRESNO):[25] this tool assesses functional performance in 0- to 18-year-olds across self-care, motor, communication, cognition, and socialization domains involving 196 items and including a rating of caregiver assistance and adaptive equipment required.

Evaluation tools such as those discussed above provide the rehabilitation team with an overview of the functional skill competence of the patient, and can provide a basis on which to measure the overall effectiveness of the rehabilitation program. These tools do not, however, allow the members of the rehabilitation team to determine the specific components of functional performance that may require remediation.

Evaluation of components of performance

The final step in the top-down evaluation process involves the detailed assessment of the component skills that are necessary for functional independence. Depending on the identified priorities for rehabilitation of the patient and the results of the functional independence measures, all or only some of these component skills might be assessed. Information gathered from this stage of the evaluation will assist the team in determining the most appropriate course for treatment. The following component skills are typically included in an evaluation.

- Joint measurement. Passive and active range of motion is evaluated in joints required for the performance of functional skills (i.e. upper and lower limb joints). The evaluation seeks to determine any limitations in range of motion that might impact on function and require the need for remediation or adaptive equipment.
- Muscle strength. Muscle strength is often affected in disorders of the lower motor neuron system or the muscles

themselves. Muscle weakness can significantly limit functional performance. Muscle strength of good to normal is generally considered necessary for the independent performance of functional tasks.[22]

- Muscle tone, reflexes and reactions, and coordination. Normal muscle tone is essential for the stabilization of joints, movement against gravity, and the ability to shift from stable to dynamic postures. All these movement components are necessary in the independent performance of functional tasks. Evaluation of the degree of hypo- or hypertonicity, the presence or absence of incoordinated movements (such as tremor, ataxia, or athetosis), and the presence or absence of immature reflexes and reactions allows therapists to determine what measures may be necessary to promote independent function.
- Sensation and perception. Intact sensation and perception is essential to the safe and accurate performance of daily living tasks. Elements of sensation commonly assessed include pain, light touch, pressure, thermal sensitivity, discrimination, olfaction, and gustatory sensation.[15,28] Aspects of perception likely to contribute to functional independence include proprioception, stereognosis, body scheme, unilateral neglect, visual form, and space perception and praxis. A combination of both clinical observation and standardized testing can be used to assess these components.
- Cognition. Cognitive skills such as memory, sequencing, problem solving, judgment and decision making, abstract thinking, and calculation underpin the capacity of a person to participate in many productive activities, including home management, paid employment, schooling, and volunteer work. Standardized testing is available to measure cognitive skill level. As well, observations of process skills during the performance of routine tasks can reveal cognitive impairments.
- Oral–motor and swallow function. Intact oral–motor skills and swallowing function is essential for safe and independent eating and drinking. Evaluations in this area are specialized, and generally carried out by trained occupational and speech therapists. Oral muscle tone, coordination, and sensory perception are assessed to determine if food can be effectively managed in the mouth. Further observation of gagging, choking, or coughing while eating can indicate swallowing dysfunction. For diagnosis of swallowing disorders, videofluoroscopic studies should be carried out (see Ch. 28).

Using a top-down approach to evaluation, the rehabilitation team can quickly come to a plan for intervention that involves patients and their families in key decision making that is likely to result in the most effective approach to treatment.

TREATMENT

A number of treatment approaches to achieving functional independence can be used to assist an individual experiencing physical disability. The treatment approach chosen by the therapist and team depends on the nature of the goals set by the individual, the degree of functional limitation experienced, and the type and severity of the component skills impairments noted. Multiple treatment approaches can be used simultaneously with an individual to address different goals. Treatment approaches can generally be understood to fall into two main categories: restorative or compensatory.[14] The goal of restorative or facilitatory treatment approaches is to restore the person's capacity to perform functional skills by restoring the impaired component skills. The aim of this approach is to retrain the individual to perform functional tasks in the same way as was done premorbidly. It is an appropriate treatment strategy when complete or close to complete recovery is expected and few environmental or contextual barriers to functional independence exist. Within this approach, a number of frames of reference for intervention can be adopted depending on the nature of the impairments experienced by the individual. The most common frames of reference used in physical rehabilitation are as follows.

- Developmental. This frame of reference assumes that recovery occurs following a hierarchic, sequential approach where simpler skills form the building blocks for complex ones. Therapy facilitates this progression by assisting in the consolidation of developmentally easier skills before embarking on more complex routines. Examples of treatment techniques that use a developmental frame of reference include sensory integration, neurodevelopmental therapy (Bobath), proprioceptive neuromotor facilitation, Brunnstrom's movement therapy, and Rood's sensorimotor approaches.[11]
- Biomechanical. This frame of reference assumes that remediation of the specific component skills that are impaired will result in a return to functional independence. Treatment techniques using this frame of reference prescribe specific interventions, exercises, and/or graded activities to restore range of motion, strength, endurance, and/or tone. Examples of this approach would include using botulinum toxin type A to weaken hypertonic muscles that impede function, applying a series of casts to increase the length and number of muscle fibers in a hypertonic muscle to reduce tone and increase function, and using a treadmill activity to increase walking endurance.
- Psychosocial. Increasingly in physical medicine and rehabilitation, a psychosocial frame of reference is being used alongside more traditional physical rehabilitative approaches. This is in recognition of the importance of addressing issues surrounding adjustment to illness or injury, social support, and the increased likelihood of chronic emotional disturbance in individuals with significant and life-limiting disabilities. Treatment techniques using this frame of reference can include individual counseling, family therapy, social skills training, and education to patients and significant others about disease or condition

processes. These techniques aim to restore the emotional well-being of the individual and, by doing so, to enhance participation in the rehabilitative plan and prevent secondary illnesses.

The goal of a compensatory or adaptive approach in rehabilitation is to facilitate functional independence through the adaptation or modification of a routine or task, or via the prescription of adaptive equipment that compensates for functional skill limitations. Compensatory or adaptive approaches are useful when full recovery is not expected and significant permanent disability is likely. This approach can involve a variety of solutions for functional difficulties, including the following.

- Changing the method by which a task is completed (e.g. using the tenodesis action to allow gross grasp and release with someone with a spinal cord injury, or teaching a one-handed dressing technique).
- Adapting objects needed for the task or prescribing an assistive device (e.g. building up the handles on eating utensils, or using a long-handled reacher to retrieve objects stored on high shelves).
- Modifying the environment (e.g. redesigning an entire home environment or workplace to allow access for someone in a wheelchair, or removing mats and rugs to prevent falling and allow more independent mobility).[12,14]

With the enormous progress made in recent years in computer and telecommunication technology, individuals with physical disabilities are now able to achieve much higher levels of functional independence than was previously possible through the use of technologic aids. The area of assistive technology is a dedicated field within rehabilitation that specializes in fitting individuals with physical and cognitive disabilities with both low- and high-tech solutions to enhance mobility, communication, community access, and learning. The application of assistive technology in physical disability is discussed in Chapters 18 and 24 of this text.

The remainder of this chapter reviews treatment principles and goals in key areas of functional performance, and outlines commonly used adaptive equipment relevant to each area.

SELF-MAINTENANCE

Feeding

Feeding is a major task of daily living essential for maintaining adequate nutrition and for participation in significant social and cultural routines. Mealtime management is generally identified by patients, families, and the rehabilitation team as a priority for intervention. Within the area of feeding, treatment might focus on developing:

- the underlying oral–motor and oral–pharyngeal coordination necessary for safe oral intake and swallowing;
- the required physical skills for independent self-feeding; and
- the routines and strategies essential to manage the social and behavioral aspects of mealtimes.

Treatment techniques incorporate both restorative and compensatory approaches. Where significant behavioral concerns exist, counseling, parent education and behavior, and group therapy might also be required. Adaptive equipment commonly used to facilitate independence in feeding includes the following.

- Non-slip matting. This is useful to stabilize dishes when bilateral coordination or strength is compromised.
- Scoop dishes or plate guards. These allow food to be stabilized against the raised side, facilitating independence for individuals with functional use of just one hand (Fig. 27-1).
- Weighted utensils and cups, and swivel utensils. These assist in compensating for limited hand control, particularly limited supination.
- Rocker knife. This is useful when bilateral upper limb motor skills are impaired, as with involvement such as hemiplegia. A rocker knife is used by pushing the knife down into food and rocking the knife until the food is cut. This avoids the traditional sliding method, while stabilizing the food with a fork in the opposite hand (Fig. 27-2).
- Adapted and built-up utensils, utensil cuffs, and splints with utensil slots. This equipment assists individuals with weak or absent grasp (Figs 27-2 and 27-3).
- Mobile arm supports or suspension slings. This system supports the forearm while assisting and maximizing such motions as shoulder flexion and extension, horizontal abduction and adduction, external and internal rotation, and elbow flexion and extension. For individuals with limited range of motion for hand to mouth activity, this device may support independence (Fig. 27-3).
- Sippy cups, cutout cups, and spouted cups. A variety of bottles and cups are available to assist children without adequate oral–motor skills such as sucking and lip closure (Fig. 27-4).

Dressing

Achieving functional independence in dressing is also commonly a high priority for patients and the rehabilitation team. Independence in this daily task reduces the physical and time demands of caring for individuals with a disability, and main-

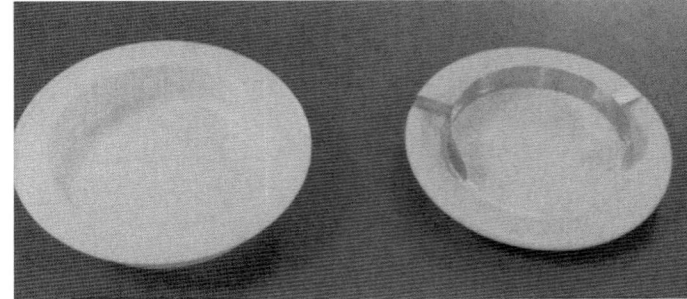

Figure 27-1 A scoop dish and a plate with plate guard are used by pushing food against the rim to scoop; it also helps as a guide.

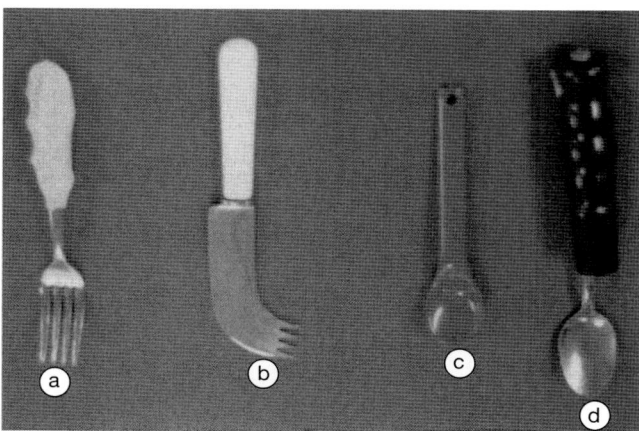

Figure 27-2 Adapted utensils. (**a**) Weighted utensil used by a person with decreased stability. (**b**) Rocker knife used by an individual with functional use of one hand. (**c**) Spoon with plastic shallow bowl. (**d**) Custom-made handle made of putty.

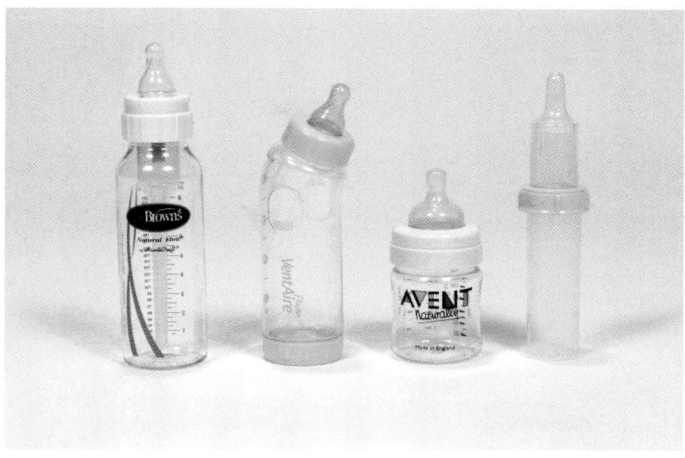

Figure 27-4 Bottles and cups designed to help children without adequate oral–motor skills. (Courtesy of The Children's Hospital, Denver, CO, USA.)

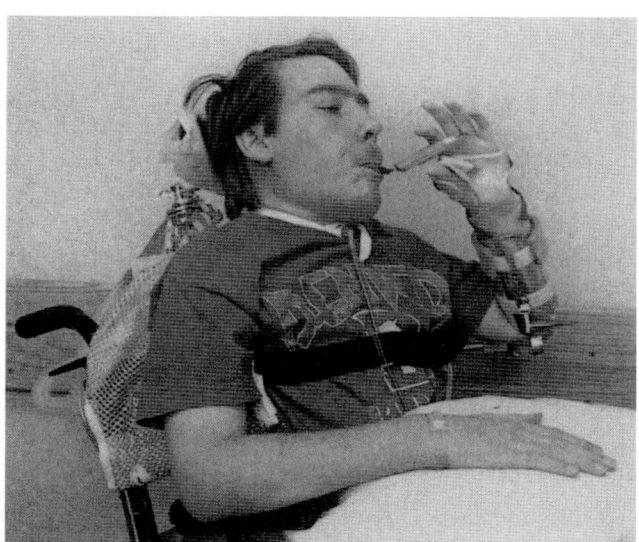

Figure 27-3 The mobile arm supports upper extremity function when shoulder or forearm strength is weak. The subject also has a long opponens splint with a utensil, and a vertical holder for a spoon for feeding.

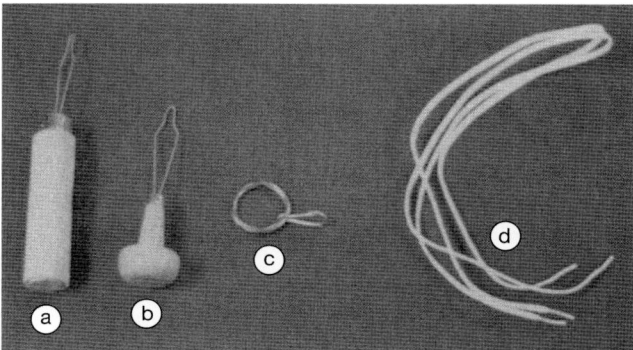

Figure 27-5 Fastener adaptations: (**a**) button aid, (**b**) knob handle button aid, (**c**) zipper pull, and (**d**) elastic laces.

tains the dignity and privacy of those individuals. Within the area of dressing, treatment can focus on developing skills in:

- undressing or removing clothing;
- dressing or donning clothing; and
- managing fasteners (e.g. buttons, zippers, and snaps) and accessories (e.g. belts and shoes).

Treatment techniques incorporate both restorative and compensatory approaches. Substantial gains can be made toward independence, however, through the application of a range of simple compensatory techniques. For example, a range of one-handed dressing techniques can be taught to an individual with a hemiplegia that require neither caregiver assistance nor adaptive equipment. The careful selection of clothing so as to avoid

complex fasteners can also promote increased independence. Modified clothing is now commercially available, but simple, homemade modifications can be effective also. For example, when hand strength is limited, it is useful to put loops on socks to assist in pulling up. Velcro openings on pants can facilitate toileting. In the case of perceptual or cognitive problems, it can help to label clothes so the person can distinguish front from back. Adaptive equipment commonly used to facilitate independence in dressing includes the following.

- Button aids (Fig. 27-5). These devices consist of a wire loop that hooks around the button and is then pulled through the hole. It works especially well for those with reduced manipulation and bilateral motor skills.
- Zipper pulls (Fig. 27-5). These are simple to make and can be chosen or designed by the individual. They can be as simple as a loop tied to the zipper or a wire hook used to pull the zipper up. They are used primarily by those with limited prehension.
- Elastic shoelaces (Fig. 27-5). These are similar to regular cloth laces, except that the elastic laces do not need to be untied or retied each time. They stretch when the foot enters the shoe, adapting to the shoe.

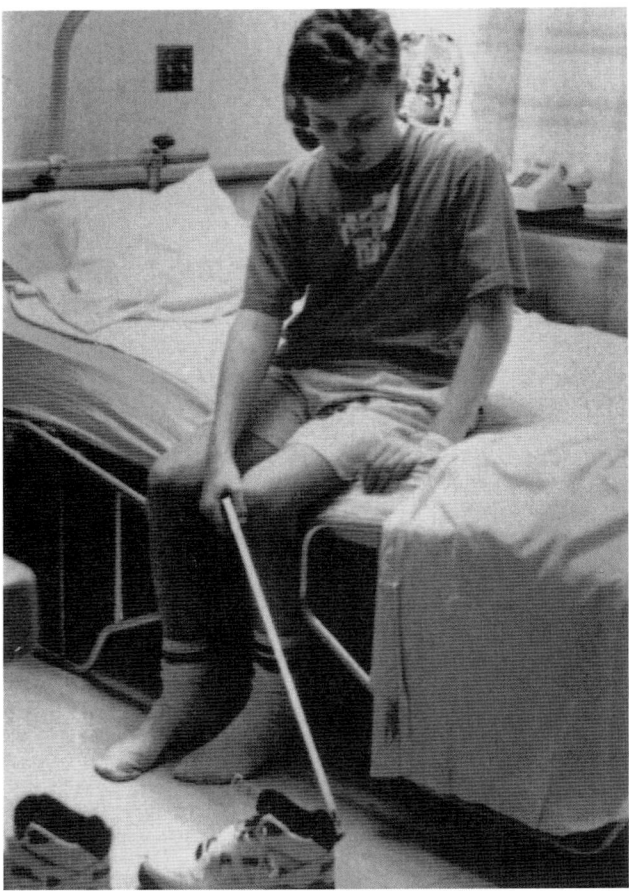

Figure 27-6 A reacher is used to assist in picking up objects from the floor. A reacher helps persons with limited lower extremity and upper extremity mobility. It is operated by squeezing the handle, which opens the tongs. The handle is released to maintain grasp.

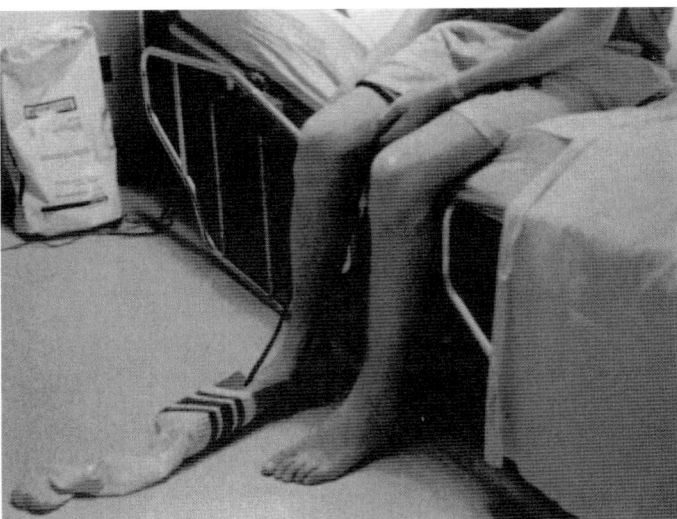

Figure 27-7 A stocking aid is used when a person is limited in reaching down to the feet, or when lower extremity mobility limits bringing the foot near to the hands. A person places the stocking over the sock holder, places the holder in front of the foot, and pulls at the rope to pull it up.

- Reacher (Fig. 27-6). This is useful for retrieving items of clothing when a person has limited reach and mobility. A reacher is an extended stick, usually made of lightweight aluminum, with a grasping unit at the end. It is operated by squeezing the handle, which activates the gripper position to open and close. Reachers come in many lengths and handle types to adapt to a person's ability to grasp.
- Dressing sticks. These are used to aid in pulling up pants and socks.
- Stocking aids (Fig. 27-7). These devices reduce the need to bend at the hips to don socks. They consist of a sock holder and an attached rope. The sock is placed over the sock holder, the foot is slid into the sock holder, and then the rope is used to pull the sock over the person's foot.

Bathing and grooming

In a similar fashion to dressing, achieving independence in bathing and grooming significantly decreases the physical and time burden on caregivers of individuals with disabilities, and can maintain the individual's sense of dignity and privacy. Because bathing and grooming are highly personal activities, independence in this area allows an individual to establish a sense of identity and esteem. The bathroom, where many of these activities take place, however, is a high-risk area for an individual with significant physical and/or cognitive disability. To gain independence in this environment, the individual must be able to safely negotiate slippery floors, small spaces, power outlets, and scalding water temperatures. Within the area of bathing and grooming, treatment focuses on the development of:

- the motor coordination and balance required for performance of various grooming and bathing tasks;
- cognitive and behavioral skills necessary to minimize injury and harm (e.g. from hot water or power outlets); and
- environmental redesign to maximize safety and access in the performance of grooming and bathing tasks.

Restorative treatment approaches would be used to address physical skill competence. Compensatory techniques such as task and environmental modification are most likely to be used to optimize the judgment and decision-making skill required for bathroom safety (e.g. changing the sequence of water mixing so that hot is added after cold to prevent scalds, or turning down the temperature on the home hot water system to minimize scalds). Major bathroom renovation is commonly required to achieve independence in bathing and grooming for an individual using a wheelchair for ambulation (Fig. 27-8). Adaptive equipment commonly used to facilitate independence in dressing includes the following.

- Utensil cuffs and adaptations (e.g. built-up handles and long handles). These tools allow for independent grasp of utensils such as brushes, razors, or toothbrushes where grasp is weak, and enhance reach where range of motion is diminished.

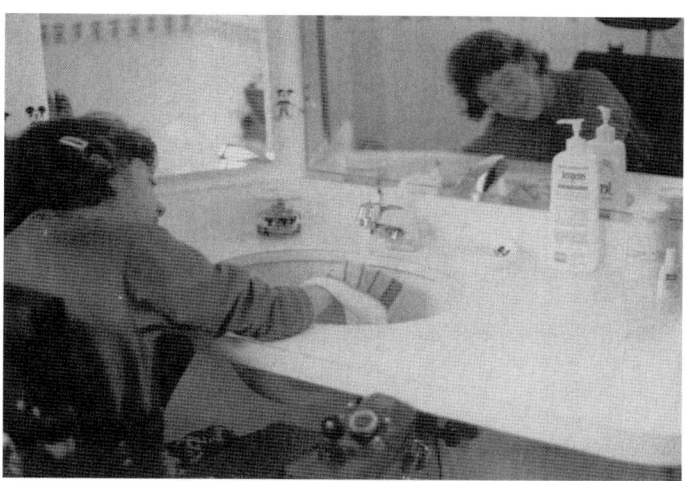

Figure 27-8 Sink with infrared sensor for easily turning water on and off when performing grooming and hygiene activities at the sink.

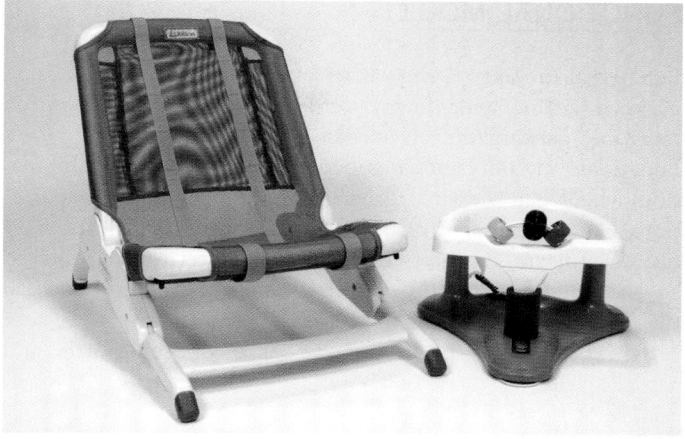

Figure 27-9 A bath chair provides supported positioning for an individual within the bath or shower. (Courtesy of The Children's Hopsital, Denver, CO, USA.)

- Electric shavers and toothbrushes. Without adaptation, these devices can assist those whose strength and endurance are limited.
- Soap on a rope and wash mitts. These allow for the secure grasp of soap to complete face and body washing.
- Suction cups. These can be used to attach utensils such as nail clippers and brushes, and emery boards to facilitate one-handed use or to compensate for reduced bilateral coordination.
- Non-slip matting. This can be used to secure bath mats on a tiled floor or within the bath or shower recess to prevent slipping.
- Grab rails. These can be mounted at various points in the bathroom to facilitate safe transferring into and out of a bath, and to support weaker standing or sitting balance.
- Handheld shower heads. These allow for easier showering in the sitting position and where mobility is limited, facilitating water reaching all parts of the body.
- Bath chairs or rings. These provide supported positioning for the individual within the bath or shower while allowing access to all parts of the body for thorough cleaning (Fig. 27-9).

Hygiene and health routine maintenance

Bowel and bladder management, menstrual care, and the management of health routines and procedures (e.g. skin care and medication regimens) are routine activities of daily living of a highly personal and intimate nature. Achieving functional independence in these areas protects the individual's sense of dignity and privacy, ensures maintenance of social participation and acceptance, and optimizes physical health and well-being. Skills required for dressing, bathing, and grooming are also required to perform basic hygiene and health routine tasks. To enhance independence in these areas, treatment focuses on developing:

- upper limb range of motion, hand function, mobility, and endurance;
- upper and lower body dressing skills;
- modified routines to account for physical or cognitive limitations;
- adapted dispensing equipment or garments; and
- cognitive and behavioral skills to reliably comply with socially accepted hygiene standards.

Restorative treatment approaches would be primarily used to promote improved upper limb dressing, and cognitive and behavioral performance. Compensatory techniques would be used to address the modification of routines, equipment, and garments to enhance independence. Adaptive equipment commonly used to facilitate independence in maintaining hygiene and health includes the following.

- Reaching aids: these devices can assist with dressing components of hygiene tasks, or facilitate the reach for and grasp of items required for hygiene (e.g. toilet tissue).
- Commode chairs, raised toilet seats, and potty chairs: these adapted chairs can assist positioning on the toilet where use of a standard toilet is not possible.
- Dynamic splints: various splints can be manufactured to facilitate self-catheterization or the placement of hygiene products for menstrual care.
- Catheter inserters, clamps, and adapted leg bag emptiers: these facilitate independent management of urinary incontinence in individuals with spinal defects or injuries.
- Adapted suppository inserters and digital stimulators: these devices can be useful for those with weak hand strength or incoordination in managing fecal incontinence.
- Long handled mirror: this allows the personal inspection of skin to check for pressure areas.
- Timers: these can be useful in providing an auditory reminder to perform health routines (e.g. weight shifts to assist in preventing pressure sores, insulin injections, and medication taking).

FUNCTIONAL MOBILITY

Functional mobility is the capacity to move from one position in space (sitting, lying down, standing, etc.) to another position to enable participation in normal daily routines and activities. Functional mobility includes bed mobility, transfers, ambulation, wheelchair mobility, driving, and taking public transportation. The achievement of independence in functional mobility tasks significantly reduces the level of long-term care required by the individual with a disability, and allows the individual to participate in a range of self-care, productive, and leisure activities, thereby promoting a sense of self-worth and actualization.

Bed mobility

Bed mobility includes rolling in bed; scooting up, down, or toward either edge of the bed; and coming to a sitting position at the edge of the bed. Full independence in bed mobility requires being able to get into bed, position or reposition oneself to sleep, and get out of bed without the assistance of another person. Treatment to encourage independence in bed mobility focuses on:

- developing head control, upper limb strength, and motor planning skills;
- improving physical endurance;
- adapting tasks to optimize the use of residual skills; and
- providing modifications to bedroom layout and furniture to assist independent function.

A combination of restorative and adaptive treatment approaches would be used to enhance independent bed mobility. Adaptive equipment commonly used in this area includes the following.

- Loops. Loops attached along the edge of the bed or on to the bed railing can decrease the amount of time needed for bed mobility, and conserve one's energy by providing an anchorage or lever point for the individual. Loops can be useful in both repositioning within the bed and getting into and out of bed.
- Overhead trapeze bar. This fixture can help a person to sit at the edge of the bed or to scoot up or down in bed.
- Step stool. When placed on the floor at the edge of the bed, a step stool can make it easier to get into and out of bed.
- Powered hospital bed. This piece of equipment might be required to improve independence in an individual with significant physical disability. This bed allows for motorized raising or lowering of the head of the bed, bringing the person to a sitting position, and can assist with more comfortable positioning for sleep.

Transfers

The ability to transfer is necessary for anyone who uses a wheelchair for mobility. For a person to be independent in daily living tasks, independent transfers must be performed to wheelchair,

bed, commode, tub, and car (if a van is not adapted for the wheelchair). It is also desirable that all wheelchair users are adept at wheelchair to floor and floor to wheelchair transfers in case of a fall. This is especially helpful for children, who often need to be able to get on the floor to participate in activities with other children. There are many different ways in which a person can perform a transfer. Depending on the functional limitations, certain transfers are faster and more efficient than others, and can change as the person's abilities change. Transfers generally require good upper limb strength and sitting balance. Transfer training would involve:

- development of improved upper limb strength and sitting balance; and
- determination of the most practical and efficient method of transferring within different daily routines and contexts.

Some of the more common methods of performing transfers are described below.

- Stand–pivot transfer. For persons who can attain and maintain standing for short periods of time, the stand–pivot transfer is the most efficient method. Adequate hip and knee extension, and good sitting balance, are required. In this transfer, the person rises from a seated to a standing position and pivots to the adjacent chair to sit down. A modification of the stand–pivot transfer is the sit–pivot transfer, in which good sitting balance and upper limb strength are used to lift the hips up and across to another chair without standing. The feet are usually positioned on the floor. If the legs are too short to reach the floor (frequently the case in children), the feet can remain positioned on the footrests of the wheelchair or on a step stool.
- Sliding board transfer. Sliding boards bridge the gap between transferring surfaces.[20] One end of the sliding board must be positioned securely under the individual's buttocks, and the opposite end placed solidly on the other surface. Once the board is positioned securely between the surfaces, the person scoots his or her hips across the board to the new surface (Fig. 27-10). As with the sit–pivot transfer, the feet can be positioned on the floor or remain on the footrests of the wheelchair. Sliding boards are available in many shapes and sizes, and adaptations can be added according to a person's individual situation.
- Wheelchair to floor transfers. There are various ways to transfer from the wheelchair to the floor. Using the forward method, the footrests are rotated to the side and the feet placed on the floor. Then, flexing far forward in the wheelchair, individuals place their hands on the floor and lower themselves to the floor.

Pivoting to the floor is another method. With the footrests removed or rotated to the side, the person scoots to the edge of the wheelchair and pivots the hips so that she or he is sitting on one buttock. Hands are placed on the seat of the wheelchair. Using strong upper limbs, the body is pivoted out of the wheelchair and the knees are lowered to the floor. From the kneeling

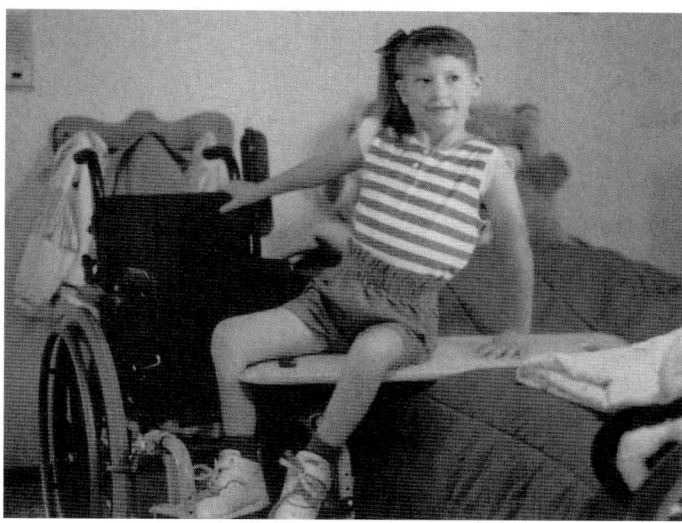

Figure 27-10 Sliding board transfer. The sliding board bridges the gap between the wheelchair and bed. The person uses upper extremities to scoot across the surface from the wheelchair to the bed.

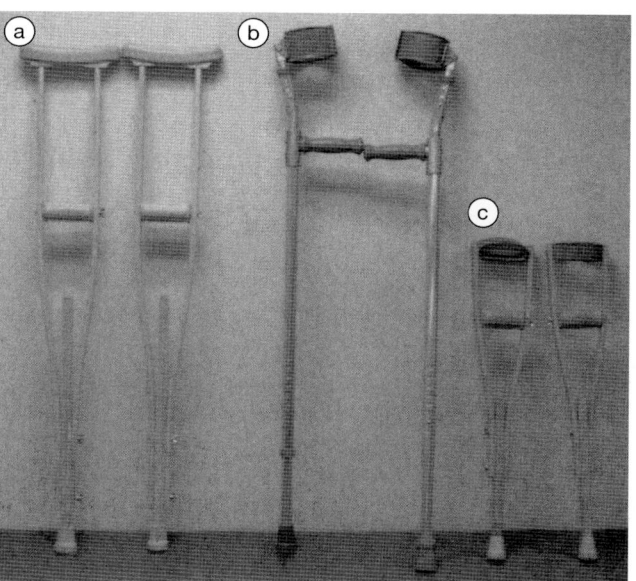

Figure 27-11 (**a**) Axillary crutches are used by individuals with good balance and coordination; the length of time these crutches are required is usually short. (**b**) Forearm crutches have a cuff around the forearm that is open at the front or side, and are used mostly by individuals needing crutches on a long-term basis (e.g. an individual with paraplegia who may require bracing with ambulation). (**c**) Kenny crutches are used mostly by children who need total contact around their forearm.

position facing the wheelchair, the person can then lower the hips to the floor into a side-sitting position.

Yet another method is used when long leg braces are worn. In this case, the footrests must be removed or rotated to the side, hips are moved to the edge of the wheelchair, and the knees are extended with the heels placed on the floor. Then, placing the hands on the forward-most frame of the wheelchair, the person lowers the hips to the floor. This method requires good upper limb strength and long arms for leverage to control the lowering movement for the entire distance to the floor. Children's wheelchairs, with a lower floor to seat height, can help some children perform this type of transfer.

The first two methods can be reversed to transfer from the floor back into the wheelchair. The last method is more difficult, because very good upper limb strength and leverage are important for success.

Ambulation

A person's level of functional independence can be significantly affected by the ability to ambulate. In order to ambulate, one must have sufficient lower limb and trunk strength, as well as balance, coordination, and cognitive skills for safety and timing. Treatment focuses on:

- restoring the underlying physical skills required for independent ambulation;
- gait analysis (see Ch. 5 for a detailed discussion of this process); and
- gait training to promote efficient gait motion.

Independent ambulation is not time- or energy-efficient in some cases, and the use of orthoses and other adaptive equipment might be required. (Lower limb orthoses are discussed in detail in Ch. 16 of this text.) Commonly used walking aids include the following.

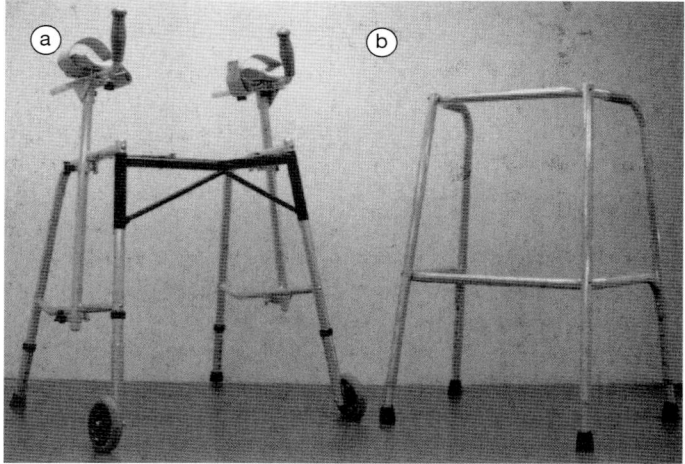

Figure 27-12 (**a**) Rolling walker with platform attachments for a person with limited upper extremity strength and range of motion. The person's forearms rest on the pads and accept the person's weight as the lower extremities take 'steps'. The wheels allow the walker to be pushed forward without having to lift the walker. (**b**) Standard walker. The person must have significant hand strength and range of motion to grip the walker, as well as good standing balance and upper extremity strength to life the walker to advance it forward.

- Walking sticks and crutches (Fig. 27-11). These devices may compensate for an inefficient gait due to reduced muscle power, pain, impaired balance, or joint damage.[29]
- Walking frames or walkers (Figs 27-12 and 27-13). There are a variety of walkers providing differing levels of

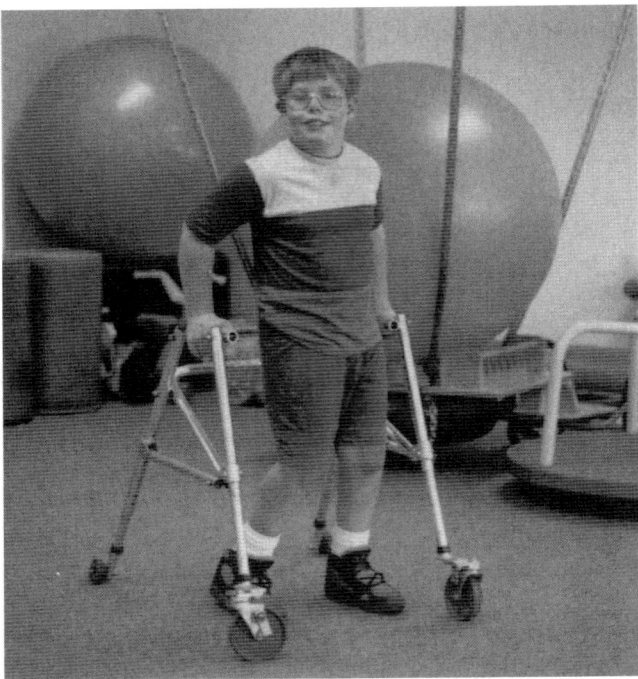

Figure 27-13 A reverse walker is used to facilitate extension posture with a person who tends to maintain a flexed posture while standing.

support for an individual who has unilateral or generalized weakness, has incoordination of the lower limbs, or requires a temporary aid to build confidence.[29]

Wheelchair mobility

For people who are unable to ambulate or are able to ambulate only short distances, use of a wheelchair for mobility can allow increased functional independence in the community. The process for evaluating and prescribing a wheelchair for an individual with a disability is described in detail in Chapter 18 of this text. There are many factors that impact the type of chair prescribed, including many aspects of the individual's skills and abilities, the contexts in which the chair will be used, transportation options, and the availability of maintenance support.[29] After the wheelchair is prescribed, a period of training might be required to fully develop the individual's skills in independent use. With the range of technologies now available in manual and power wheelchairs, it is possible for individuals with high degrees of physical disability to independently mobilize in a wheelchair.

Driving

Being able to drive or be transported in a private car is often an identified priority for individuals with disabilities and their families. Achieving this level of independence in mobility means that individuals have access to a broader range of productive and leisure activities, and can be more easily included in social occasions, vacations, and routine daily errands. A compensatory approach is most commonly used to address issues of independence in driving or traveling in a private car. For self-driving, careful evaluation of residual physical and cognitive skills will determine the level of accommodation needed in car controls and operation. Commonly used car adaptations include the following.[23]

- Hand and finger controls: these allow an individual without lower limb function to perform acceleration and braking functions using the upper limbs.
- Foot controls: in a similar fashion to hand controls, these devices allow for the steering of the car using the lower limbs when upper limb function is insufficient to perform this task.
- Power seats, steering, brakes, and windows: these adaptations may compensate for reduced or weakened motor function.
- Steering wheel knobs and cuffs: these allow for one-handed steering operation or promote better grasp and control of the steering wheel.
- Handles and levers: small handles and levers can be attached to key functions in the car (e.g. windshield wiper stick) to enhance access.

For children or other individuals not able to self-drive, various adaptations can be made to support transportation in a private car. Some examples are as follow.

- Custom car seats: these purpose-built seats allow an older child with a disability to be transported safely in a car.
- Wheelchair tie-down systems: these systems usually require significant modification to be made to the private car or van but allow secure transportation of an individual in a wheelchair inside a car.
- Power lifts and ramps: these devices allow easier access by a person using a wheelchair into and out of the car.

Public transportation

The capacity to use public transport independently can offer older children and adults with disabilities and their families or caregivers additional convenience in the completion of daily routines. Many public transportation systems, including buses, trains, and ferries, make specific accommodations for people with physical and cognitive disabilities. Training in the independent use of these facilities involves:

- determining the availability of suitable public transportation options in the local area;
- understanding the physical and cognitive abilities of the client relative to accessing public transport;
- prescribing appropriate adaptations to wheelchairs to allow for use of tie-down systems; and
- developing organizational, memory, and money management skills to facilitate timetable reading, payment of fares, and negotiation with drivers, etc.

PRODUCTIVE ACTIVITY

Paid or unpaid work

Participation in productive activity via paid or unpaid work can be important to individuals for a number of reasons. It might allow them to be self-sufficient financially; acquire a sense of self-esteem, social status, and group membership; and add structure and routine to their daily lives.[11] Issues surrounding the employment of people with disabilities are discussed in more detail in Chapter 35 of this text. In general, however, to optimize the achievement of functional independence in this area will require consideration of:

- the physical and cognitive requirements of work tasks, and their match with the individual's residual skills;
- the physical access to the work environment and necessary work equipment; and
- the capacity of the individual to participate in necessary work-related behaviors, for example timely and reliable attendance, concentration and application to task, and establishment of appropriate workplace relationships (see Ch. 36).

Household management

Household management is an important aspect of maintaining daily routines and for many adults represents their primary source of productive activity. Assisting an individual to gain functional independence in this area can promote a sense of role identity lost due to illness or injury. Restoring the motor skills required for home maintenance tasks will not be possible or sufficient to ensure full independence in many cases. Integral to successful household management is the combination of motor proficiency (particularly upper limb proficiency) with planning, organization, safety awareness, and money management skills.[6,11] Most commonly, a compensatory approach is required. This generally takes two forms. First, the physical set-up of the home has to be considered in relation to whether it supports access of the individual to all areas of the home to perform cleaning, laundry, yard maintenance, and meal preparation tasks. Second, tasks performed have to be analyzed and modified as necessary to conserve energy and allow independent completion despite physical or cognitive limitations.[6] Clear and open communication with the individual is essential in this process to identify priority household tasks for completion, because home routines are highly individualized and value-based. Commonly used adaptations and modifications that enhance independent household management include the following.

- Home modifications and redesign. Extensive modifications might be required to make a house accessible for a wheelchair user. These can include installing ramps, widening hallways, lowering bench tops, and removing under-sink cabinetry (Fig. 27-14).
- Wheeled carts. These can be used extensively throughout the home to minimize the energy and strength required in

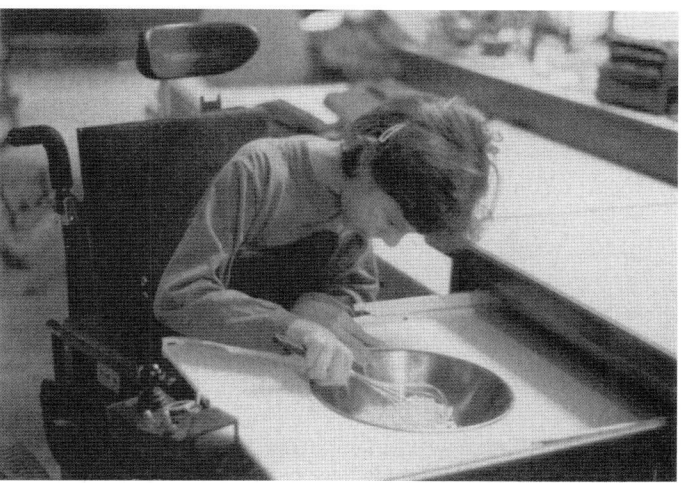

Figure 27-14 A house with a wheelchair-accessible cooking area, so that a child with physical limitations can participate in cooking activities such as mixing ingredients for a cake.

lifting heavy objects (e.g. a basket of laundry, plates and utensils).
- Non-slip matting and suction cups. These can be used to help stabilize pots, jars, or dishes during meal preparation or cleaning.
- Adapted utensils. These can provide for easier completion of tasks requiring cutting, mixing, and reaching.
- Sitting as a preferred position. This position allows for an individual who experiences endurance or mobility difficulties to complete tasks more efficiently.
- Electric appliances. Food processors and electric mixers reduce the labor intensity required for many meal preparation tasks.
- Reorganization of household items. Task efficiency can often be gained through reorganizing the placement and storage of essential equipment, for example by placing hangers near a dryer so that clothes can be hung immediately, reducing the need for ironing; by reducing overall clutter to minimize dusting and the need to search for items; and by removing potential obstacles such as mats and pot plants.

Play and school

For a child, participating in typical play experiences and attending a formal education program constitutes productive activity. Children with disabilities require access to both of these experiences to ensure that there is an opportunity for socialization, learning, and continued development of unaffected skills. Within most public school settings, inclusion of children with disabilities into an individualized educational program is required by public law (in the USA, the Individuals with Disabilities Education Act, Public Law 92-142). The rehabilitation team needs to work with local schools and childcare settings to establish an environment in which children can play and learn in a relatively unrestricted manner. Issues that require consideration when planning for the integration of a child with disabilities into a play or educational setting include the following.

- Can the child physically enter and exit, and mobilize within the school or play environment?
- Are all facilities and equipment (e.g. restrooms, computers, desks, water fountain, and playground equipment) adapted to allow usage by the child?
- Do the play or educational experiences offer the 'just right' challenge to the child, such that learning and development are enhanced?

Treatment approaches used to facilitate independent participation by children in play or educational programs use a combination of restorative and compensatory approaches. Where possible, a child's motor and cognitive abilities will be improved through a therapy program addressing specific skills required for meaningful participation, for example fine motor skills for handwriting and computer access, attention and concentration skills, socialization skills, and self-toileting. Compensatory approaches, however, are often required when disability is significant. Commonly used adaptations and modifications to facilitate typical play and educational experiences include the following.

- Positioning devices. These devices can range from foam wedges to allow a child to participate in an activity on the floor, to custom-made standers or frames to allow for tabletop activities (Fig. 27-15).
- Environmental modifications. Ramps, widened hallways, and boardwalks can enhance a wheelchair user's access to playground and school facilities (Fig. 27-16).
- Equipment modifications. Adapted pencils, computer mice and keyboards, adjustable height tables, and adapted playground equipment can all assist a child with a disability participating in typical play and educational activities (Figs 27-17–27-19).
- Curriculum redesign and accommodations. Depending on the child's skills and abilities, adaptations to the educational curriculum might need to be made to enhance independent performance. This could be as simple as allowing a child more time to complete a writing task when weakness or dexterity is a difficulty, or changing the sequence of activities completed in the day so that more demanding tasks are performed early on to allow for the likelihood of increased fatigue. A child might need an individualized curriculum plan including reduced content and modified expectations in order to enhance the likelihood of educational success.

LEISURE

Time spent in leisure and recreation is considered essential to an individual's psychologic well-being.[5] Leisure activity is activity participated in for its own sake and where enjoyment is the primary goal. The authors believe that leisure is important for self-expression, creativity, relaxation, belongingness, and expe-

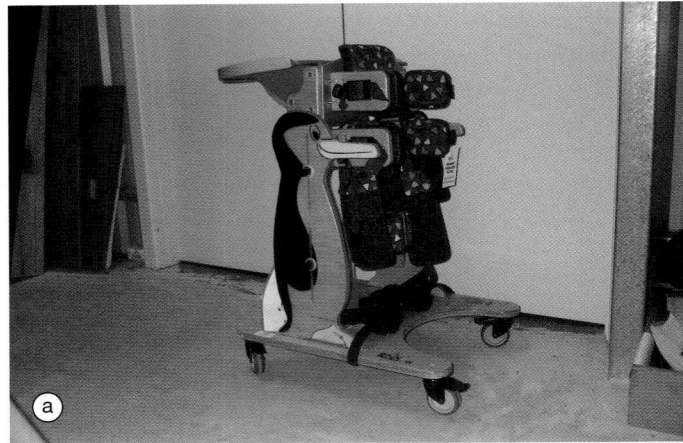

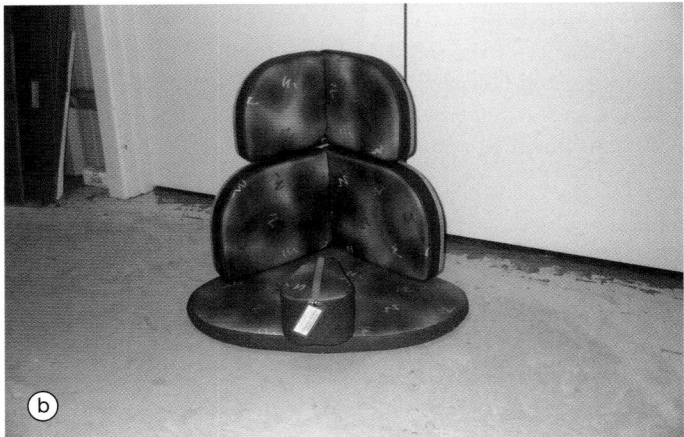

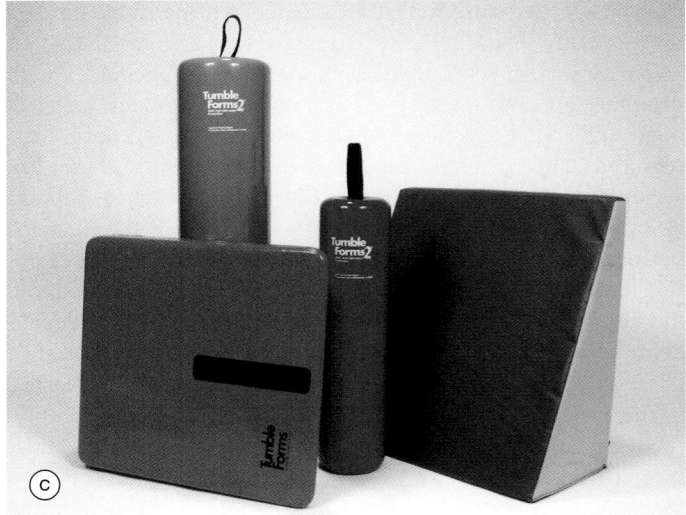

Figure 27-15 Positioning devices range from foam wedges to custom-made standers or frames. ((a) and (b) courtesy of Novita Children's Services, Inc., South Australia, Australia; (c) courtesy of The Children's Hoptial, Denver, CO, USA.)

rience of novelty.[27] Meaningful participation in leisure activities by people with disabilities is highly motivating, and can also facilitate the achievement of independence in other areas such as community integration, self-maintenance, mobility, and organizational and problem-solving skills. The rehabilitation team

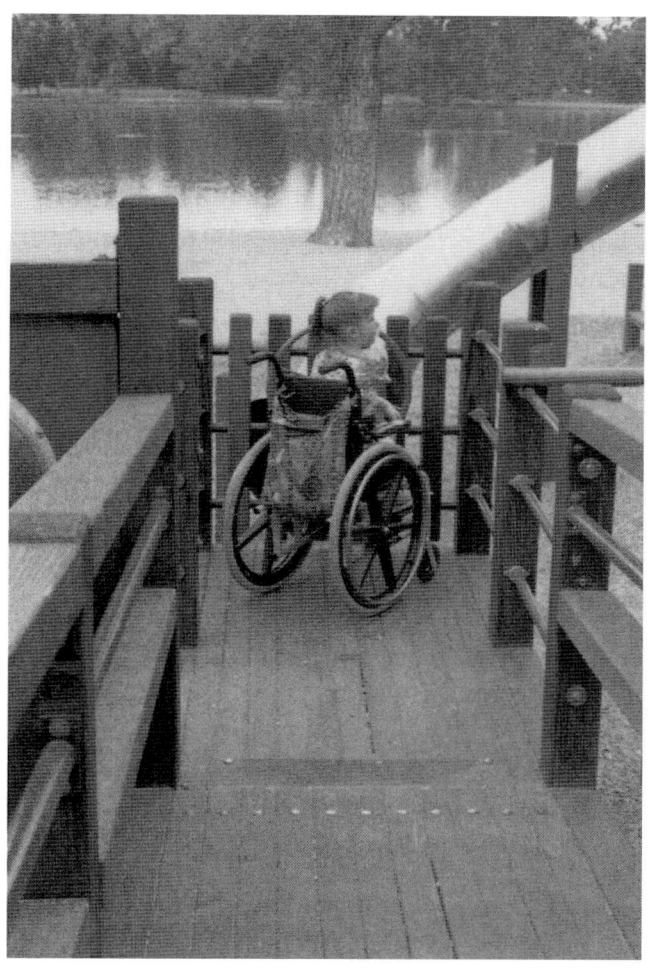

Figure 27-16 Playground equipment accessible by wheelchair, with platforms and ramps.

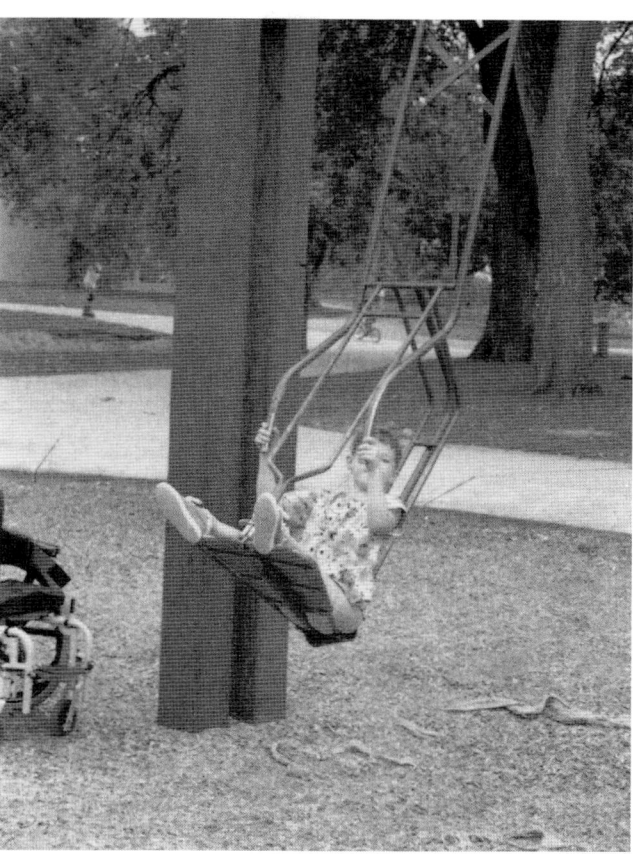

Figure 27-17 An adapted swing. The movement of the swing is achieved by pushing or pulling on the handles, using the arms.

should consider leisure as both a means and an end in terms of the achievement of functional independence.[24] Leisure can take a number of forms, and include quiet recreational activities such as hobbies or crafts, or more active recreation such as sports and travel. Many organizations now exist to facilitate the inclusion of people with disabilities into recreational activities. For example, some city governances have established programs specifically designed for people with physical and cognitive disabilities that are run within community recreation centers. Various advocacy groups and foundations sponsor camping and sports programs for individuals with brain injuries, burns, or chronic conditions. In recent years, more attention has been focused on competitive sports participation by people with disabilities. This is available at local, national, and international levels, culminating in events such as the Paralympics. As in other areas of functional independence, consideration must be given to the interests, priorities, and available resources of individuals and their families; individuals' specific motor and cognitive skills and limitations; and the potential for adaptation of the activity before planning interventions relating to leisure

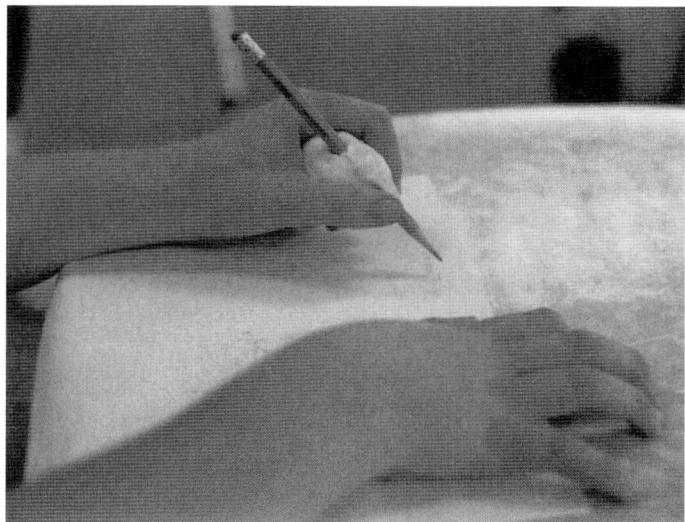

Figure 27-18 A built-up handle made out of setting putty was conformed to a person's grasp to facilitate functional tripod grasp for writing. Modifications can vary from application of foam to commercially available plastic grips.

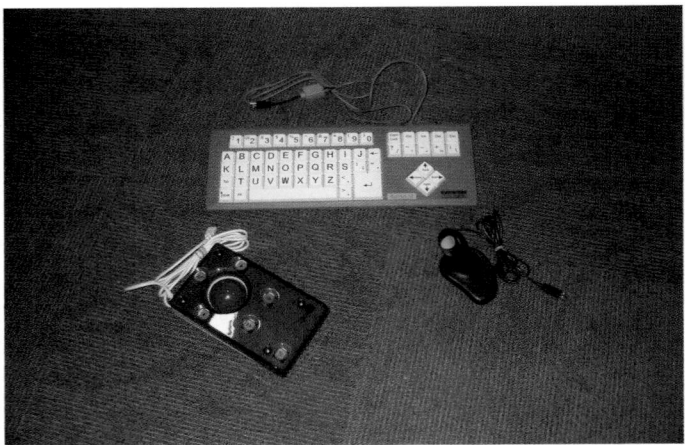

Figure 27-19 Modified equipment can include computer mice and keyboards. (Courtesy of Novita Children's Services, Inc., South Australia, Australia.)

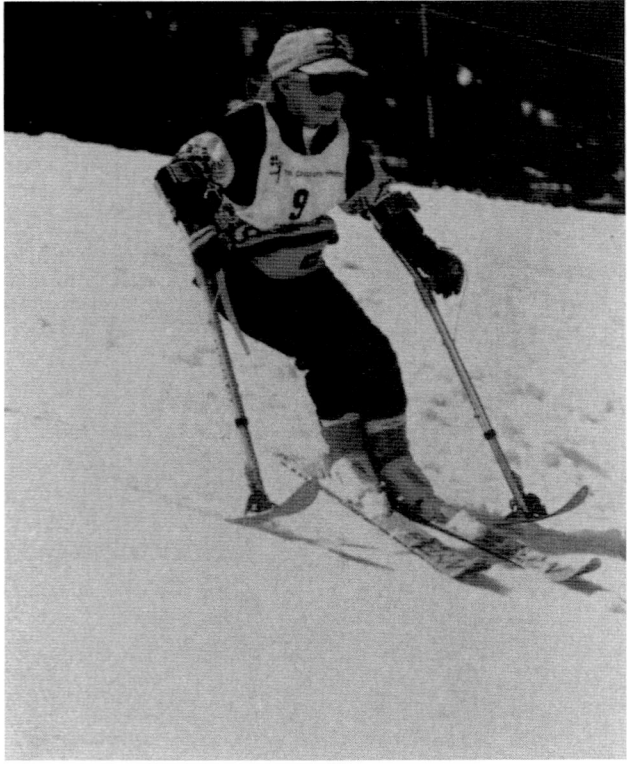

Figure 27-20 Outrigger skis used while skiing by a person who has difficulty shifting weight, maintaining upright stance, and maintaining balance. A person must be able to stand independently but may have difficulty with coordination.

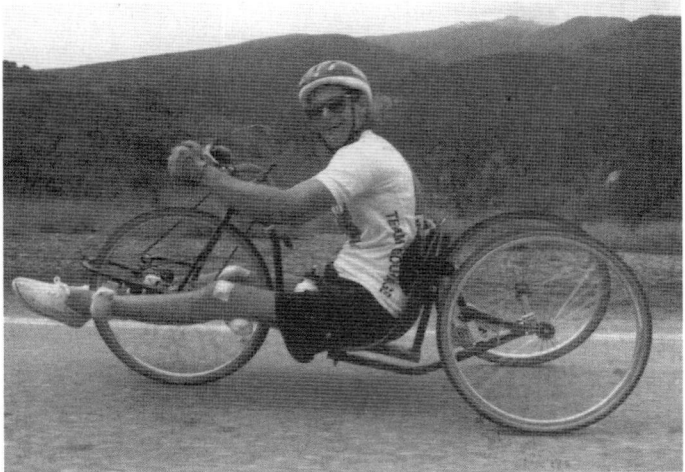

Figure 27-21 A bicycle adapted for a person with spinal cord injury to be propelled with the upper extremities. Bars and straps support the lower extremities while providing adequate seating to maintain sitting balance. (Courtesy of Steve Ackerman, American Wheelsports, Fort Collins.)

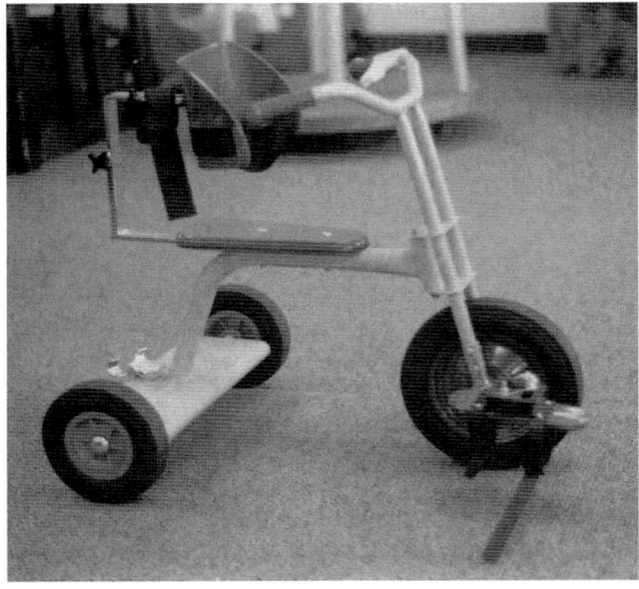

Figure 27-22 A tricycle adapted with footplates and straps, trunk support, and an extended seat for children with limited balance, coordination, and strength.

participation. Figures 27-20–27-24 show examples of adaptations made to common leisure pursuits, enabling people with disabilities to experience enjoyment and achievement.

CONCLUSION

Assisting an individual to achieve optimal functional independence should be the goal of all medical rehabilitation programs.

The benefits to individuals and their families or caregivers are clear. For the individual, an increased sense of personal satisfaction, self-worth, and self-actualization are all coupled with decreased physical ailments and increased vitality. For caregivers, the physical and emotion burden of care associated with physical disability can be reduced or minimized. For rehabilitation programs, a focus on improving outcomes related to functional independence translates into an increased likelihood of reimbursement and enhanced patient satisfaction. There are a number of possible approaches to the facilitation of functional

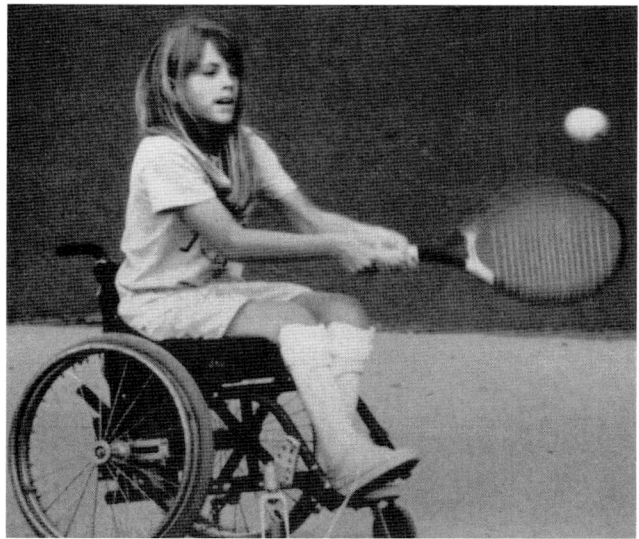

Figure 27-23 Many sports, such as tennis, basketball, and rugby, can be adapted for participation by a person in a wheelchair.

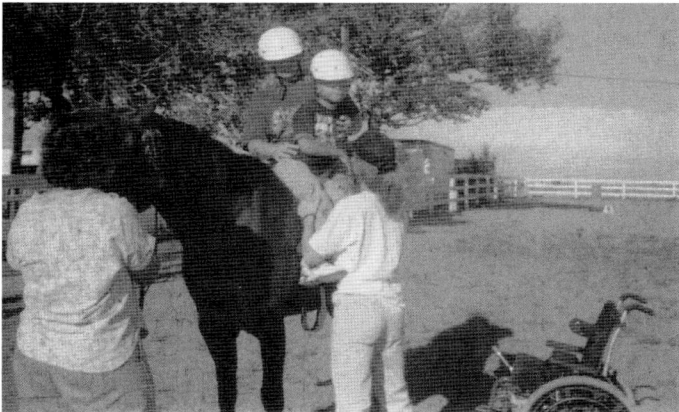

Figure 27-24 Therapeutic horseback riding can be used as an alternative to traditional therapy programs and as a recreational activity. Saddles can be adapted for those with decreased strength in the lower extremities and trunk.

independence in persons with disabilities that are typically either restorative or compensatory in focus. As further advances in technology are made, opportunities for individuals with significant levels of disability to participate independently in life situations will also emerge.

REFERENCES

1. [Anonymous]. Functional independence measure for children (WeeFIM). Outpatient version 1.0. Buffalo: State University of New York at Buffalo; 1994.

2. [Anonymous]. Guide for the uniform data set for medical rehabilitation (adult FIM). Version 4.0. Buffalo: State University of New York at Buffalo; 1993.

3. Baum MC. Participation: its relationship to occupation and health. OTJR: Occup Participation Health 2003; 23(2):46–47.

4. Breske S. When it comes to rehabilitation, family matters. Adv Phys Ther 1992; 23:4.

5. Christiansen C, Baum C. Understanding occupation: definitions and concepts. In: Christiansen C, Baum C, eds. Occupational therapy: enabling function and well-being. 2nd edn. Thorofare: Slack; 1997:2–25.

6. Culler KH. Home management. In: Crepeau EB, Cohn ES, Schell BAB, eds. Willard and Spackman's occupational therapy. Philadelphia: Lippincott Williams & Wilkins; 2003:534–541.

7. Dittmar SS. Overview: a functional approach to measurement of rehabilitation outcomes. In: Dittmar SS, Gresham GE, eds. Functional assessment and outcome measures for the rehabilitation health professional. Gaithersburg: Aspen Publishers; 1997.

8. Edelman L. Getting on board: training activities to promote the practice of family-centered care. Bethesda: Association for the Care of Children's Health; 1991.

9. Fisher A. Assessment of Motor and Process Skills. Report no.: research edition 7.0. Fort Collins: Colorado State University; 1994.

10. Fisher A. The foundation—functional measures, part 2: selecting the right test, minimizing the limitations. Am J Occup Ther 1992; 46(3):278-281.

11. Foster M. Life skills. In: Turner A, Foster M, Johnson SE, eds. Occupational therapy and physical dysfunction. Edinburgh: Churchill Livingstone; 2002:275–314.

12. Foster M. Theoretical frameworks. In: Turner A, Foster M, Johnson SE, eds. Occupational therapy and physical dysfunction. Edinburgh: Churchill Livingstone; 2002:47–81.

13. Hayley SM, Coster WJ, Fass RM. A content validity study of the Pediatric Evaluation of Disability Inventory. Pediatr Phys Ther 1991; 3:177–184.

14. Holm MB, Rogers JC, Stone RG. Person–task–environment interventions: a decision-making guide. In: Crepeau EB, Cohn ES, Schell BAB, eds. Willard and Spackman's occupational therapy. 10th edn. Philadelphia: Lippincott Williams & Wilkins; 2003:460–490.

15. Iyer MB, Pedretti L. Evaluation of sensation and treatment of sensory dysfunction. In: Pedretti L, Early M, eds. Occupational therapy: practice skills for physical dysfunction. 10th edn. St. Louis: Mosby; 2001:422–443.

16. Johnson MV, Maney M, Wilkerson DL. Systematically assuring and improving the quality and outcomes of medical rehabilitation programs. In: DeLisa JA, Gans BM, eds. Rehabilitation medicine: principles and practice. 3rd edn. Philadelphia: Lippincott-Raven Publishers; 1998.

17. Larson E, Wood W, Clark F. Occupational science: building the science and practice of occupation through an academic discipline. In: Crepeau EB, Cohn ES, Schell BAB, eds. Willard and Spackman's occupational therapy. 10th edn. Philadelphia: Lippincott Williams & Wilkins; 2003.

18. Law M, Baptiste S, McColl MA, et al. The Canadian occupational performance measure: an outcome measure for occupational therapy. Can J Occup Ther 1990; 57:82–87.

19. Mahoney F, Barthel DW. Functional evaluation: the Barthel Index. Md State Med J 1965; 14:61–65.

20. Nawoczenski DA, Rinehart ME, Duncanson P, et al. Physical management. In: Buchanan LE, Nawoczenski DA, eds. Spinal cord injury: concepts and management approaches. Baltimore: Williams & Wilkins; 1987:123–184.

21. Ottenbacher KJ, Christiansen C. Occupational performance assessment. In: Christiansen C, Baum C, eds. Occupational therapy: enabling function and well-being. 2nd edn. Thorofare: Slack; 1997.

22. Pedretti L. Muscle strength. In: Pedretti L, Early M, eds. Occupational therapy: practice skills for physical dysfunction. 10th edn. St. Louis: Mosby; 2001:316–359.

23. Pierce S. Restoring competence in mobility. In: Trombly C, Radomski M, eds. Occupational therapy for physical dysfunction. 5th edn. Philadelphia: Lippincott Williams & Wilkins; 2002:665–693.

24. Primeau LA. Play and leisure. In: Crepeau EB, Cohn ES, Schell BAB, eds. Willard and Spackman's occupational therapy. 10th edn. Philadelphia: Lippincott Williams & Wilkins; 2003:567–570.

25. Roberts SD, Wells RD, Brown IS, et al. The FRESNO: a pediatric functional outcome measurement system. J Rehabil Outcomes Meas 1999; 3(1): 11–19.

26. Robertson SC, Colborn AP. Outcomes research for rehabilitation: issues and solutions. J Rehabil Outcomes Meas 1997; 1:15–23.

27. Tinsley HE, Eldredge BD. Psychological benefits of leisure participation. A taxonomy of leisure activities based on their need gratifying properties. J Couns Psychol 1995; 42(2):123–132.

28. Wheatley CJ. Evaluation and treatment of perceptual motor deficits. In: Pedretti L, Early M, eds. Occupational therapy: practice skills for physical dysfunction. 5th edn. St. Louis: Mosby; 2001:444–455.

29. White E. Aids to mobility. In: Turner A, Foster M, Johnson SE, eds. Occupational therapy and physical dysfunction. 5th edn. Edinburgh: Churchill Livingstone; 2002:191–209.

30. World Health Organization. International classification of functioning, disability and health. Geneva: WHO; 2001.

31. World Health Organization. International classification of impairments, disabilities, and handicaps: a manual of classification relating to the consequences of disease. Geneva: WHO; 1980.

Rehabilitation of Patients with Swallowing Disorders

Jeffrey B. Palmer, Denise M. Monahan and Koichiro Matsuo

Swallowing is a complex biologic function essential to human life. Dysphagia, or impaired swallowing, is a common symptom in many disorders. Dysphagia can lead to serious sequelae, such as malnutrition and pneumonia, and can dramatically alter quality of life when it prevents the individual from participating in mealtimes. Dysphagia rehabilitation focuses on the use of therapy and compensatory strategies to improve swallowing and prevent complications. Development of an individualized rehabilitation program requires understanding of the anatomy and physiology of swallowing, the pathophysiology of swallowing dysfunction, and the nature of the underlying disease process, as well as intraindividual and environmental factors.[101] This chapter focuses on oral and pharyngeal swallowing dysfunction, because these are commonly amenable to the rehabilitation approach. We start with the physiology of normal and abnormal swallowing, then discuss the evaluation of swallowing, and finally discuss treatment of dysphagia.

NORMAL SWALLOWING

Physiology

The anatomy of the oral cavity, larynx, and pharynx is shown in Figures 28-1 and 28-2. The swallowing process is traditionally divided into oral, pharyngeal, and esophageal stages (Fig. 28-3). The oral stage is further subdivided into oral preparatory and oral propulsive stages.[78]

When swallowing liquids, food is taken into the mouth and mixed with saliva during the oral preparatory stage. The bolus is collected by the tongue, and positioned between the surface of the tongue and the palate in a 'swallow-ready' position. Premature leakage of food from the oral cavity to the pharynx is prevented by tongue–palate contact behind the bolus.

During the oral propulsive stage, the bolus is propelled from the oral cavity to the pharynx, passing through the faucial isthmus. The tongue surface contacts the palate anteriorly, just behind the upper teeth. The tongue surface moves upward, beginning with the anterior part of the tongue and moving sequentially backward. The area of tongue–palate contact expands posteriorly, squeezing the bolus into the pharynx.

The process is somewhat different when eating solid food (Fig. 28-4).[29,46,105] When the bite of food enters the mouth, it is moved into position for chewing via a mechanism known as stage 1 transport (Fig. 28-4a). During stage 1 transport, the food is first placed on the surface of the tongue. The entire tongue shifts bodily backward in the mouth, carrying the food to the molar region. The tongue then rotates (around the anteroposterior axis) and deposits the bite of food on the occlusal surface of the lower molar teeth.

After stage 1 transport is food processing, in which food particles are reduced in size by mastication and softened with saliva. This is accomplished by rhythmic, linked movements of the jaw, tongue, cheek, and soft palate.[12,45,88,92,102] The jaw opens and closes cyclically. The food is compressed during jaw closing. The tongue and cheek work in conjunction during jaw opening to reposition between the teeth.[12,92]

When a portion of the food reaches a swallow-ready consistency, it is positioned on the surface of the tongue and squeezed back into the pharynx by a mechanism known as stage 2 transport (Fig. 28-4b). The soft palate lifts away from the tongue surface rhythmically during food processing and stage 2 transport to allow bolus transport through the faucial isthmus. The basic mechanism of food propulsion is nearly identical to that described for the oral propulsive phase with a liquid bolus: the tongue compresses the bolus against the palate, and the area of tongue–palate contact expands from anterior to posterior, squeezing the bolus into the oropharynx. Food processing can continue while food accumulates in the oropharynx during multiple stage 2 transport cycles. Bolus aggregation in the oropharynx can last as long as 10 s in normal individuals eating solid food.[46]

In the pharyngeal stage of swallowing, the bolus is propelled from the pharynx into the esophagus (Fig. 28-3). The pharyngeal stage depends on sequential activation of muscles in the oral cavity, tongue, pharynx, and larynx.[19,27,57,108] The soft palate elevates and presses against the lateral and posterior wall of the pharynx, closing off the nasopharynx. The tongue base retracts (pushes backward) to compress the bolus against the pharyngeal wall. The pharyngeal constrictor muscles contract around the bolus sequentially from top to bottom, creating a wave of contraction that squeezes the bolus downward.[56] The pharynx also shortens to reduce pharyngeal volume.[106] The larynx closes to prevent aspiration. The upper esophageal sphincter (UES) opens, permitting the bolus to enter the esophagus.

The hyoid bone and larynx are pulled upward and forward by contraction of the suprahyoid and hypothyroid muscles. These motions are important for protecting the airway and

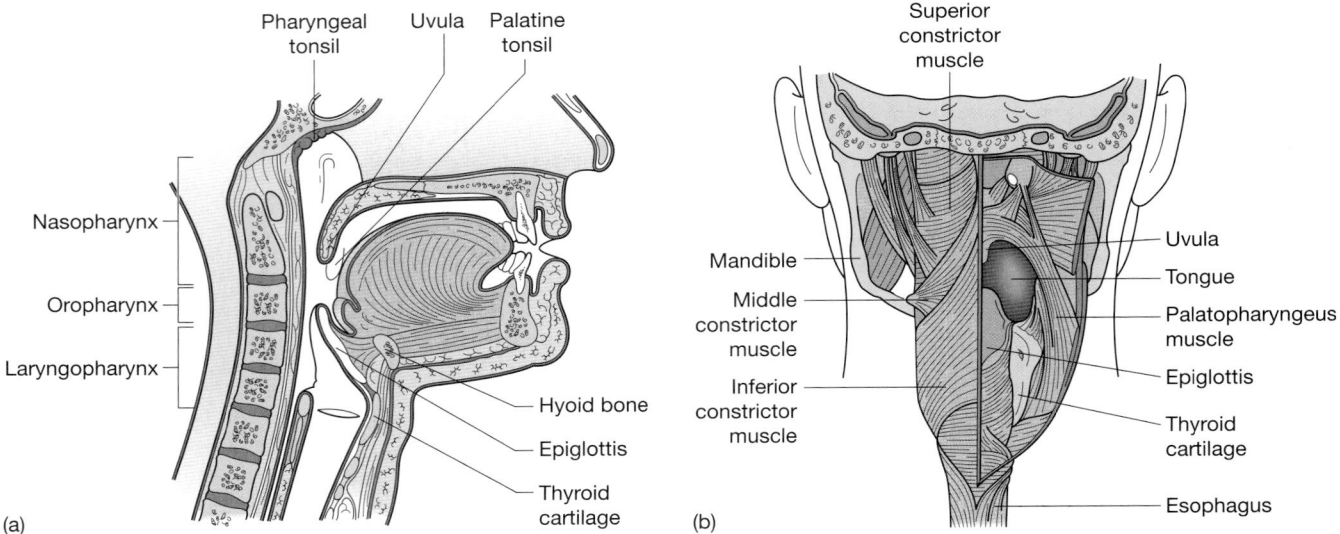

Figure 28-1 Anatomy of the oral cavity and pharynx. (**a**) Divisions of the pharynx. (**b**) Posterior view of the pharynx. (After Banks et al. 2005,[5] with permission.)

opening the UES. Upward movement of the hyoid is highly variable and is influenced by the initial food consistency, while the forward movement is less variable and is related to the opening of the UES.[18,52]

Several protective mechanisms prevent aspiration during swallowing. Breathing pauses briefly during swallowing.[116] The duration of this swallow apnea typically ranges from 0.3 to 1.0 s and increases with bolus volume.[49,111] The hyoid bone and larynx are pulled upward and forward by contraction of the suprahyoid and thyrohyoid muscles. This tucks the larynx under the base of the tongue. The vocal folds close to seal the glottis.[95] The arytenoids tilt forward to contact the base of the epiglottis,[74] and the epiglottis folds backward. This deflects food away from the laryngeal airway.

The UES is held closed between swallows by tonic contraction of the cricopharyngeus muscle, but it opens briefly during each swallow.[32] There are three main factors contributing to UES opening:[18]

1. the cricopharyngeus muscle relaxes, permitting the sphincter to open;
2. contraction of the suprahyoid and thyrohyoid muscles pulls the larynx forward, opening the sphincter; and
3. hydrostatic pressure of the descending bolus pushes outward on the UES, assisting its opening.

The esophagus is quite different from the pharynx; it is primarily composed of striated muscle in its cervical portion, and smooth muscle in its thoracic portion. Because the thoracic esophagus is largely smooth muscle, it has intrinsic contractile activity that can be increased or inhibited by autonomic nerves. Once the bolus has passed through the UES, it is propelled down the esophagus by peristalsis (defined as a wave of inhibition followed by a wave of excitation that propels material down a hollow viscus).[44] In the upright position, gravity assists

peristalsis. The lower esophageal sphincter is held closed by tonic muscle contraction between swallows. It relaxes during a swallow and is pushed open by the pressure of the descending bolus.

Neuroanatomy

Mastication, swallowing, and respiration are controlled by central pattern generators.[11,33,53,84] The neural organization of swallowing requires integration of sensory input, reflexes, and all three of these central pattern generators. The central pattern generator for pharyngeal swallowing is located in the brain stem reticular formation.[53] Sensory information gathered from mechanoreceptors, chemoreceptors, and thermoreceptors in the oral cavity, pharynx, and larynx facilitate swallowing and protect the airway.[91,117] Sensation is carried through the maxillary and mandibular branch of the trigeminal nerve, the glossopharyngeal nerve, and the vagus nerve to a central pattern generator for swallowing. This central pattern generator is located in the nucleus tractus solitarius of the medulla.[53]

When a swallow is initiated, motor neurons in the brain stem produce coordinated contraction of striated muscle fibers in the oropharynx. Swallowing consists of sequential excitation and inhibition of more than 50 muscles. Table 28-1 shows the innervation of major muscles related to swallowing. These lower motor neurons have their cell bodies in the trigeminal (V), facial (VII), and hypoglossal (XII) nuclei, and in the nucleus ambiguus (IX and X).

AGING AND HUMAN DEVELOPMENT

Swallowing in infants

The upper aerodigestive tract of the newborn exhibits anatomic differences from the adult, and these differences support early feeding skills (Fig. 28-5). These differences include a smaller,

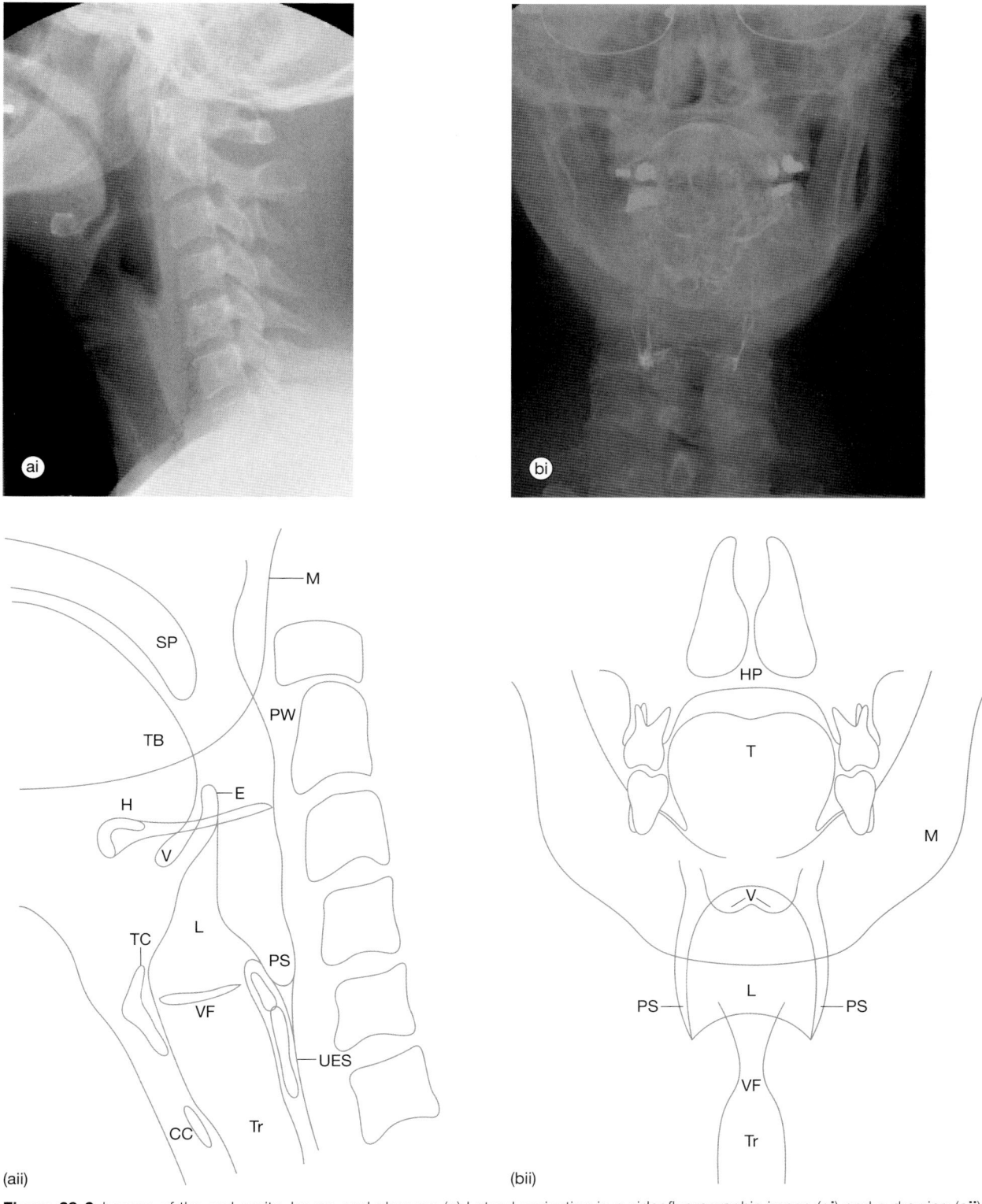

Figure 28-2 Images of the oral cavity, larynx, and pharynx: (**a**) Lateral projection in a videofluorographic image (**ai**) and a drawing (**aii**). (**b**) Posteroanterior projection in a videofluorographic image (**bi**) and a drawing (**bii**). CC, cricoid cartilage; E, epiglotis; H, hyoid bone; HP, hard palate; M, mandible; PW, posterior wall; L, laryngeal vestibule; PS, pyriform sinus; SP, soft palate; T, tongue; TB, tongue base, TC, thyroid cartilage; Tr, trachea; UES, upper esophageal sphincter; V, valleculae; VF, vocal folds.

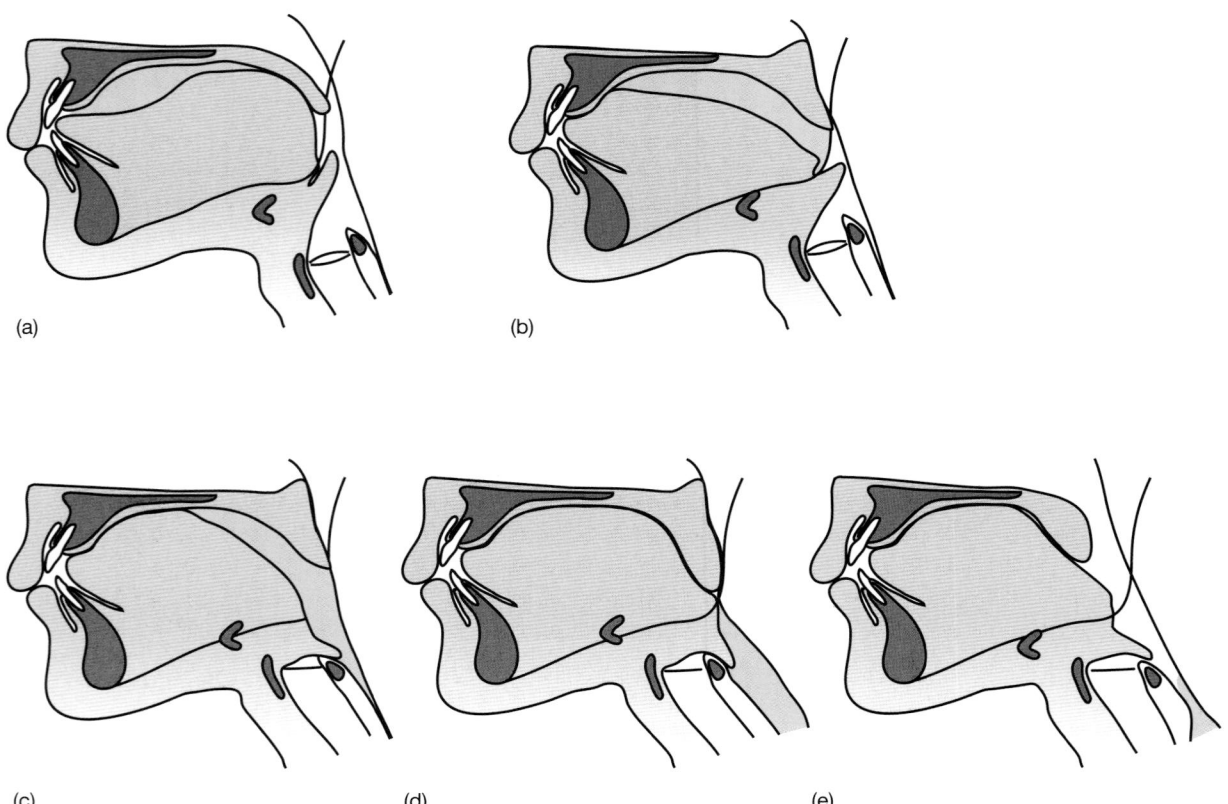

(a)

(b)

(c)   (d)   (e)

Figure 28-3 Normal swallowing of a liquid bolus. These drawings are based on an actual videofluorographic sequence recorded in the lateral projection. (**a**) The bolus is held between the anterior surface of the tongue and hard palate, in a 'swallow-ready' position. The tongue presses against the palate both in front of and behind the bolus to prevent spillage. (**b**) The bolus is propelled from the oral cavity to the pharynx through the fauces. The anterior tongue pushes the bolus against hard palate just behind the upper incisor. The posterior tongue drops away from the palate. (**c**) The soft palate elevates, closing off the nasopharynx. The area of tongue–palate contact spreads posteriorly, squeezing the bolus backward to the pharynx. The larynx elevates and the epiglottis tilts downward. (**d**) The upper esophageal sphincter (UES) opens. The tongue base retracts to contact the pharyngeal wall, which contracts around the bolus, starting superiorly and then progressing downward toward the esophagus. (**e**) The soft palate descends, and the larynx and pharynx reopen. The UES returns to its usual closed state after the bolus passes.

retracted lower jaw; a smaller oral cavity almost completely filled by the tongue; and buccal 'sucking pads' to create stability for early sucking patterns. The larynx rests higher in the neck, and the epiglottis approximates and even slightly overlaps the soft palate. This separates the airway and food way between swallows, allowing the nasopharynx to communicate with the trachea while food can collect in the valleculae, thereby decreasing the risk of aspiration.[63,94] The hyoid bone and larynx descend in the neck during infancy and childhood, and the contact between the epiglottis and the soft palate is lost.[72]

The earliest swallowing pattern is *suckling*, in which the tongue moves in a backward–forward licking motion. As the infant anatomy develops and buccal pads are resorbed, a *sucking* pattern develops. Labial strength is increased and an upward–downward tongue movement emerges. Jaw movement patterns evolve along with developing anatomy. The early phasic up–down jaw motion pattern evolves into a diagonal movement by 6–9 months of age, and to a rotary chewing pattern (in the coronal plane) around 24 months. Oral motor skills continue to mature, and by 24 months infants have established an almost mature oral motor control for swallowing liquids. Maturation for chewing is slower. A mature pattern is reached at 6 or 7 years of age.

Swallowing in the elderly

In the elderly, oral, pharyngeal, and esophageal changes occur related to motor performance and respiratory control during swallowing. Labial and lingual strength and coordination decrease, resulting in slower oral manipulation of food. Dentition is often reduced, resulting in increased mastication time and reduced efficiency.[43] Multiple gestures of the tongue base and hyoid can occur before pharyngeal swallow initiation, along with increased duration of hyoid motion during swallows. An increased latency might be observed from entry of the bolus into the pharynx until onset of laryngeal elevation. Reduction in esophageal function occurs, with decreased amplitude of esophageal peristaltic wave and increased incidence of sliding hiatal hernia. Altered respiratory patterns in the elderly are characterized by an earlier onset and longer duration of swallow apnea, increased incidence of swallow initiation in the inspira-

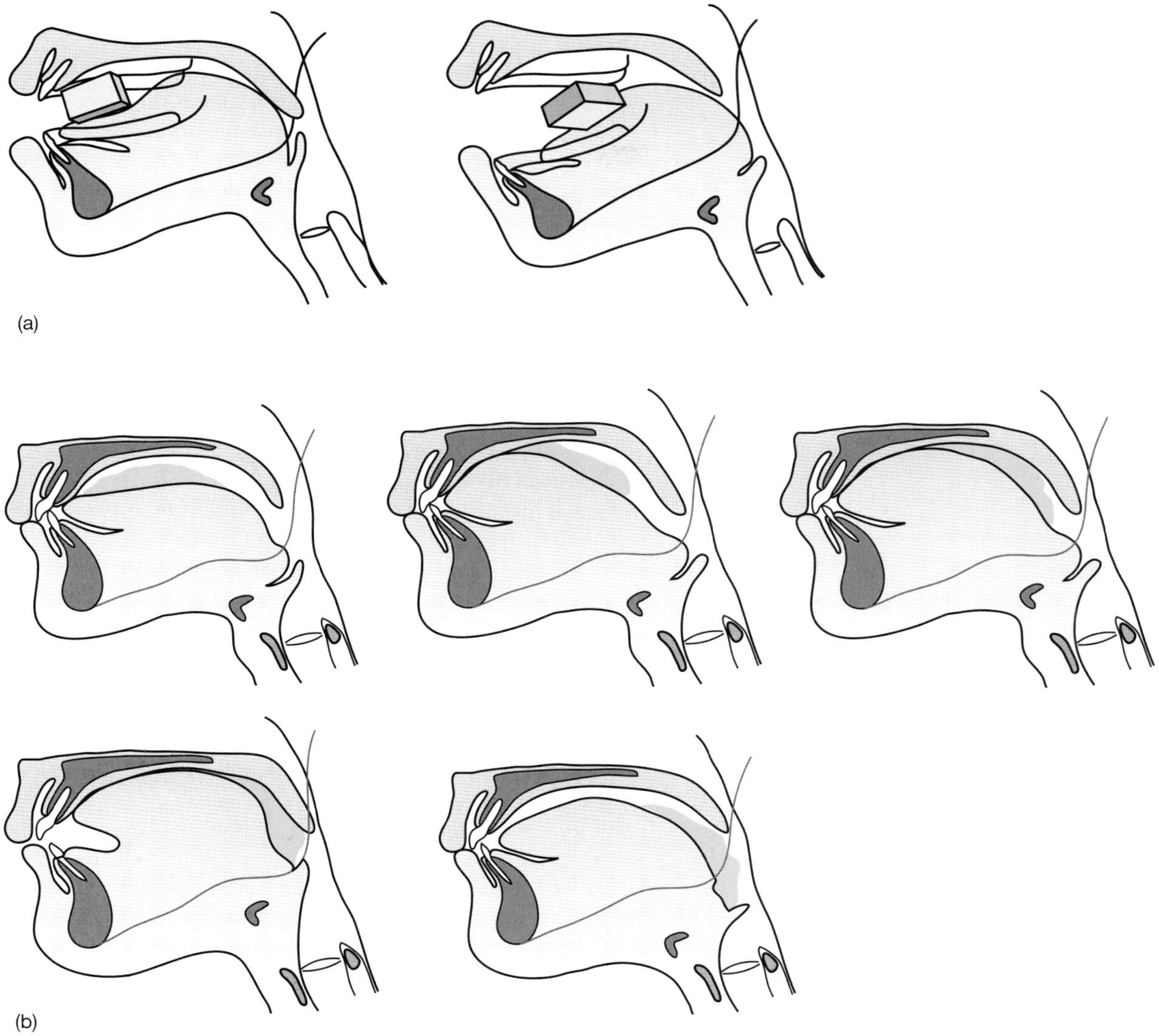

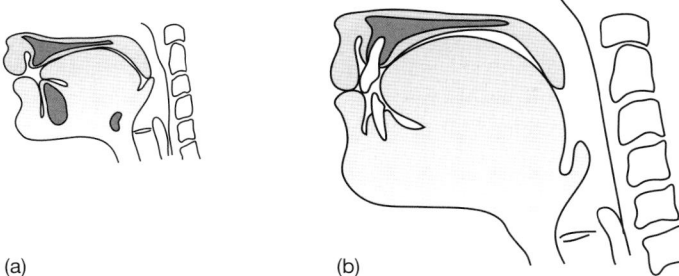

Figure 28-4 Mechanisms of food transport in a normal subject eating solid food. (**a**) Stage 1 transport: the tongue carries the bite of food back to the postcanine region, and then rotates to place it on the occlusal surfaces. (**b**) Stage 2 transport: the tongue squeezes the bolus backward along the palate, through the fauces, and into the pharynx.

(a)   (b)

Figure 28-5 Comparison of infant and adult anatomy: the oral cavity and pharynx in the infant (**a**) and the adult (**b**). In the infant, the epiglottis and soft palate are in contact, and the hyoid bone and larynx are in a relatively higher position. The larynx descends during the first few years of life, so the epiglottis and soft palate lose contact.

tory phase of respiration, and increased respiratory rate immediately after the swallow.[48,49,116] An increased frequency of laryngeal penetration is seen in older adults on consecutive swallows, and might be a normal variation.[20]

PATHOPHYSIOLOGY OF SWALLOWING DYSFUNCTION

Dysphagia can be caused by a wide variety of diseases and disorders affecting the structure and/or function of the oral cavity, larynx, pharynx, or esophagus. Structural deficits can masquerade as functional disorders, so careful diagnostic evaluation is necessary in every case. Dysphagia is commonly classified

Table 28-1 Innervation of major muscles related to swallowing

Cranial nerve	Muscles
Trigeminal nerve (V)	Masticatory muscles Mylohyoid Tensor veli palatini Anterior belly of digastrics
Facial nerve (VII)	Facial muscle Stylohyoid Posterior belly of digastrics
Glossopharyngeal nerve (IX)	Stylopharyngeus
Vagus nerve (X)	Levator veli palatine Palatopharyngeus Salpingopharyngeus Intrinsic laryngeal muscles Cricopharyngeus Pharyngeal constrictors
Hypoglossal nerve (XII)	Intrinsic tongue muscles Hyoglossus Geniohyoid Genioglossus Styloglossus Thyrohyoid

according to the anatomic region affected, i.e. oral, pharyngeal, or esophageal dysphagia. Dysfunction of the oral cavity commonly co-occurs with pharyngeal dysfunction. This is commonly termed *oropharyngeal dysphagia* (although the problem is not limited to the oropharynx). Regardless of site, it is useful to consider whether a given impairment of swallowing affects food transport (preparation and propulsion of the bolus), airway protection (prevention of laryngeal aspiration), or both, because these have implications for treatment. Aspiration of food can occur in structural or functional impairments of the oral cavity, pharynx, or esophagus. It is important to recognize dysphagia, as it can cause dehydration, malnutrition, or respiratory sequelae.

Oral or pharyngeal dysfunction most commonly results from stroke or neurologic disorders. It can also be caused by structural deficits, such as congenital clefts or webs, diverticulae, surgical ablations, cranial nerve injuries, and radiation fibrosis. Impaired oral function can hamper eating, drinking, and swallowing. It might be difficult to maneuver solids or liquids in the mouth; determine whether a bolus is ready for swallowing; contain the bolus in the oral cavity, resulting in leakage from the lips (anteriorly) or into the pharynx (posteriorly); propel the bolus into the pharynx; or initiate swallowing. Deficits in mastication can hamper bolus preparation for swallowing, making the intake of solid food difficult. These are usually manifestations of tongue weakness or incoordination, but sensory impairments can produce similar effects, including excessive retention of food in the oral cavity after swallowing.

Dysfunction of the pharynx can produce impaired swallow initiation, ineffective bolus propulsion, and retention of a portion of the bolus in the pharynx after swallowing. Velopharyngeal incompetence is the inability to close the velopharyngeal isthmus by elevating the soft palate and contracting the pharyngeal walls around it to close off the nasopharynx. In velopharyngeal incompetence, the bolus might be misdirected into the nasal cavity (nasal regurgitation). When tongue base retraction is weak, pharyngeal propulsive force can be inadequate, resulting in retention of all or part of the bolus in the pharyngeal recesses after swallowing. Similar findings can be produced by weakness of the pharyngeal constrictor musculature. If the epiglottis does not invert during swallowing, it might act as a physical barrier, resulting in retention of part of the bolus in the valleculae after swallowing.

Another cause for retention of food in the pharynx after swallowing is impaired opening of the UES. This can be caused by increased stiffness of the UES, as in fibrosis or inflammation, or failure to relax the sphincter's closing muscle (primarily the cricopharyngeus muscle). Because UES opening is an active process, failure of opening can also be caused by weakness of the muscles of sphincter opening, particularly the anterior suprahyoid musculature. This is rarely an isolated finding. Dyscoordination of the swallow can also lead to failure of UES opening. Because the UES is ordinarily closed between swallows, its opening is obligatory for swallowing to occur. This means that failure of UES relaxation and opening can produce obstruction of the food way.

Airway protection is a critical function of swallowing. But airway protection mechanisms are not always effective. The failure of laryngeal protective mechanisms can reflect reduced laryngeal elevation, incomplete closure of the laryngeal vestibule, or inadequate vocal fold closure due to weakness, paralysis, or anatomic fixation. For the purpose of dysphagia rehabilitation, *laryngeal penetration* is defined as passage of material into the larynx, but not through the vocal folds. *Aspiration* is defined as passage of material through the vocal folds (Fig. 28-6). Laryngeal penetration can be observed in normal individuals. Aspiration of microscopic quantities occurs in normal individuals, but aspiration that is visible on fluoroscopy or endoscopy is pathologic, and is associated with increased risk of aspiration pneumonia or airway obstruction.[86] The normal response to aspiration is a strong reflex coughing or throat clearing. However, laryngeal sensation is often abnormal in individuals with severe dysphagia.[38] Silent aspiration, or aspiration in the absence of visible response, has been reported in 25–30% of patients referred for dysphagia evaluations.[38,67,119] The effects of aspiration are highly variable, and some individuals tolerate small amounts of aspiration without apparent ill effects.[37] Several factors determine the effect of aspiration in a given individual, including the quantity of the aspirate, the depth of the aspiration material in the airway, the physical properties of the aspirate (acidic material is most damaging to the lung), and the individual's pulmonary clearance mechanism.[100] Predictors of aspiration pneumonia risk include diagnoses of chronic obstructive pulmonary disease and congestive heart failure,

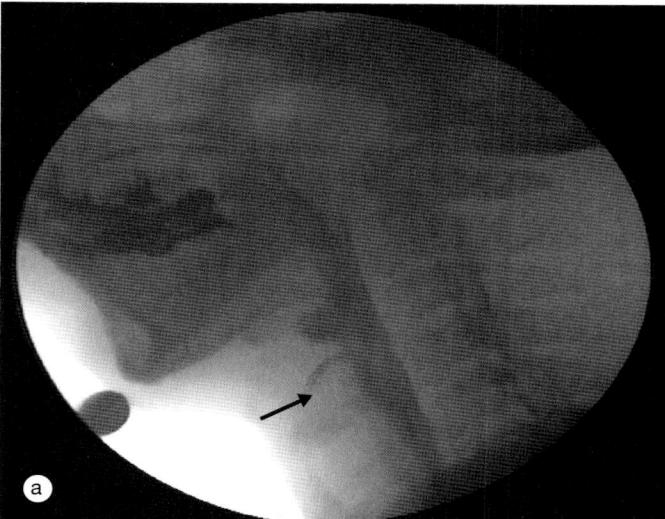
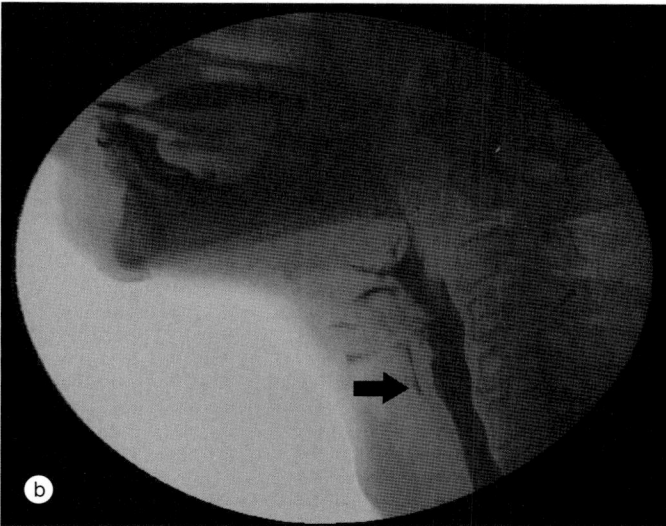

Figure 28-6 Videofluorographic images of laryngeal penetration (**a**, thin arrow) and aspiration (**b**, thick arrow) in dysphagic individuals swallowing liquid barium.

Box 28-1 Selected causes of oral and pharyngeal dysphagia

Neurologic disorder and stroke
- Cerebral infarction
- Brain stem infarction
- Intracranial hemorrhage
- Parkinson disease
- Multiple sclerosis
- Motor neuron disease
- Poliomyelitis
- Myasthenia gravis
- Dementias

Structural lesions
- Thyromegaly
- Cervical hypertosis
- Congenital web
- Zenker diverticulum
- Ingestion of caustic material
- Neoplasm

Psychiatric disorder
- Psychogenic dysphagia

Connective tissue diseases
- Polymyositis
- Muscular dystrophy

Iatrogenic causes
- Surgical resection
- Radiation fibrosis
- Medications

---

presence of a feeding tube, oral–dental status, bedbound status, and presence of dysphagia.[51,64,85]

Dysphagia can result from a wide variety of disorders;[62] see Box 28-1 for a partial list.[13] A major cause of dysphagia is stroke. Dysphagia is found in about half of individuals with a recent stroke.[39,98,109] Most recover within the first 2 weeks, but dysphagia can be severe and persistent. Brain stem lesions can result in particularly severe dysphagia, given their proximity to the major swallow centers.[28,53,127] Reduced laryngeal elevation, insufficient UES opening, vocal fold weakness, and severe weakness of oropharyngeal muscles are common in patients with stroke. Cerebral lesions can result in dyscoordination of the swallow, with impaired oropharyngeal bolus propulsion and airway protection. Swallowing dysfunction is typically more severe in bilateral cerebral lesions, as there is bilateral cortical representation for swallow function. On the other hand, the brain stem motor nuclei innervate only ipsilateral muscles, so lesions of cranial nerves or their nuclei can result in unilateral sensory or lower motor neuron dysfunction.[4]

In neurodegenerative disorders, dysphagia can be the first symptom.[7] Oral-stage dysphagia is common in Parkinson disease, characterized by lingual tremor and tongue-pumping behaviors, which hamper oral food transport.[70] Alzheimer disease can result in agnosia for food within the oral cavity, characterized by oral holding and incoordination of swallowing. In motor neuron disease, progressive degeneration of motor neurons in the brain and spinal cord results in weakness in the muscles of mastication, respiration, and swallowing. Inflammatory muscle diseases, including dermatomyositis and polymyositis, commonly affect striated muscles, resulting in weakness of the pharynx. Progressive systemic sclerosis, on the other hand, affects smooth muscle. It commonly produces esophageal dysfunction, including reduced peristalsis, dilatation of the lower esophagus, and gastroesophageal reflux disease (GERD).

Tumors of the oral cavity, pharynx, and larynx can be treated with surgical excision, deletion of anatomic structures, and chemotherapy or radiation therapy. Dysphagia occurs from tissue loss or dysfunction. Oral cavity cancer often requires partial or complete glossectomy and mandibulectomy, which can limit lingual and mandibular function for bolus formation and propulsion, and significantly increase aspiration risk. Pharyngeal tumor excision can require removal of structures

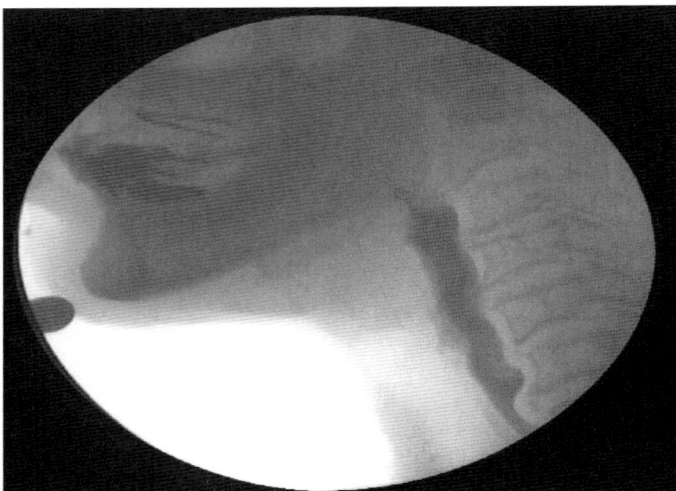

Figure 28-7 Videofluorographic image of a partially obstructive C6–C7 anterior osteophyte. It impinges on the column of barium, narrowing the lumen by more than 50%.

critical for swallowing, including the faucial arches, hyoid bone, epiglottis, and pharyngeal constrictors. Ineffective laryngeal protection and reduced pharyngeal transport are common. Supraglottic laryngectomy, a common cancer surgery, spares the true vocal cords but eliminates the epiglottis, laryngeal vestibule, and false vocal folds. Without these laryngeal protective mechanisms, individuals are at increased aspiration risk. Pharyngeal transport problems are also common. Total laryngectomy separates the airway from the pharynx with a permanent tracheostomy. While there is no risk of aspiration, pharyngeal transport problems due to weakness, tissue fixation, and cricopharyngeal dysfunction are common.

Radiation therapy can cause fibrosis of the oral cavity, pharynx, and larynx immediately following radiation or, in some cases, years later. Xerostomia and edema are common when salivary glands are within the radiation field, hampering bolus formation and timing of oral and pharyngeal transport. The salivary changes are often permanent. Fibrosis can result in delayed swallow initiation, decreased pharyngeal transport, and ineffective laryngeal protection.[60]

Structural abnormalities, whether congenital or acquired, can impair swallow function. Birth defects such as clefts of the lip and palate often produce inadequate labial control for sucking and bolus control, or velopharyngeal insufficiency with nasal regurgitation. The resulting dysphagia can lead to malnutrition, requiring surgical repair of the defect during infancy. Nasogastric tube feedings can be used for short-term alimentation and hydration in severe cases while awaiting surgery.

Structural abnormalities can impair pharyngeal transport and airway protection. Cervical osteophytes are common in the elderly and can impinge on the pharynx (Fig. 28-7).[24] Webs and strictures can obstruct the food pathway. Diverticulae can form along the pharyngeal or esophageal walls. The Zenker diverticulum is a pulsion diverticulum of the hypopharynx. Its mouth is located just above the cricopharyngeus muscle, but the body of

the pouch can extend much lower. Food or liquid collects in the diverticulum and can be regurgitated to the mouth or result in aspiration.

Esophageal dysfunction is common and is often asymptomatic. Webs, rings, or strictures of the esophagus can obstruct the lumen and might require dilatation. Esophageal motor disorders include conditions of either hyperactivity (e.g. esophageal spasm) or hypoactivity (e.g. weakness) of the esophageal musculature. Either of these can lead to ineffective peristalsis with retention of material in the esophagus after swallowing. Retention can result in regurgitation of material from the esophagus back into the pharynx, with aspiration of the regurgitated material.

Gastroesophageal reflux disease can affect swallowing indirectly. In GERD, the lower esophageal sphincter has insufficient tone, rendering it ineffective for preventing gastric contents from passing back through the lower esophageal sphincter into the esophagus. Because the esophageal lining is not resistant to acid (as is the stomach lining), reflux of highly acidic stomach contents can result in inflammation (esophagitis) or scarring (stricture) of the esophagus. This can lead to pain or obstructive symptoms. In severe cases, the refluxate can pass all the way up the esophagus and into the pharynx, passing through the UES. The individual with severe GERD is particularly vulnerable at night, when protective reflexes are less effective. Under these conditions, the refluxate can be aspirated, causing inflammation or scarring of these vital airway structures. Although GERD is not a swallowing disorder per se, it can be an underlying cause of dysphagia or aspiration pneumonia.

Dysphagia is often iatrogenic. Several medications can cause dysphagia through sedation, pharyngeal or esophageal muscle weakness, movement disorders, sensory loss, or impaired salivation (Table 28-2).[118,123] Postsurgical dysphagia is a common complication of anterior cervical fusion, occurring in about one-half of the patients.[121] The mechanism is unclear but may be related to injury of the pharyngeal constrictor muscles or their innervation. Most recover within the first 2 months. Dysphagia can also complicate carotid endarterectomy or surgery for cancer of the esophagus or the head and neck.[8]

Table 28-2 Drug-induced dysphagia	
Medication	Effect on oropharyngeal swallowing
Central nervous system depressants	Depressed brain stem function and control of swallowing
Neuromuscular blockade	Weakness of oropharyngeal musculature and cough
Dopamine antagonists	Extrapyramidal reactions (dystonia, dyskinesia)
Anticholinergic medications	Salivary changes, impaired esophageal peristalsis
Anesthesia	Suppressed laryngeal cough reflex

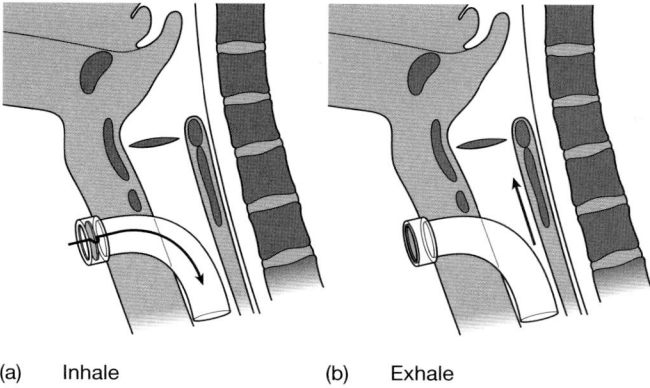

(a)   Inhale   (b)   Exhale

Figure 28-8 Drawing of a tracheostomy tube with speaking valve. The valve permits inspiratory flow (**a**) but prevents expiratory airflow through the tracheostomy tube, providing expiratory flow (**b**) through the larynx and restoring positive subglottic air pressure.

Box 28-2 Symptoms of oropharyngeal dysphagia

Overt
- Coughing
- Choking
- Pain with swallowing
- Throat clearing
- Feeling of food stuck in throat
- Nasal regurgitation
- Difficulty chewing

Subtle
- Shortness of breath
- Changes in vocal quality
- Slowed rate of eating
- Changes in dietary habits
- Difficulty managing saliva

Compromised and altered respiratory function increases the risk of dysphagia. Chronic obstructive pulmonary disease alters the coordination of respiration and deglutition.[93,116] Exacerbations can lead to aspiration. Endotracheal intubation and ventilator dependency can cause decreased laryngeal sensation, pooling of secretions in the pharynx and larynx, impaired swallow initiation, and aspiration.[129] The presence of a tracheostomy tube alters normal pharyngeal aerodynamics, eliminating the positive subglottic pressure normally associated with swallowing and hampering laryngeal protective reflexes. An inflated cuff does not fully eliminate aspiration,[40,61] as secretions can still leak around the cuff into the trachea. A cuffless tracheostomy tube is often better tolerated. A unidirectional tracheostomy speaking valve prevents expiratory airflow through the tracheostomy tube, providing expiratory flow through the larynx and upper airway, and restoring positive subglottic air pressure (Fig. 28-8). Use of a unidirectional valve can improve swallow safety by reducing laryngeal penetration and aspiration.[40]

A number of disorders can mimic dysphagia. GERD with heartburn and retrosternal pain is often accompanied by complaints of dysphagia.[82] Thoracic chest pain due to dysphagia must be differentiated from cardiac disease. Esophageal disorders can occur in up to 50% of individuals who complain of thoracic pain.[81] Globus sensation (the feeling of 'a lump in the throat' in the absence of actual retention of food) can be produced by distal esophageal lesions or hiatal hernia.[41]

Medical history

Dysphagia presents with a variety of symptoms (Box 28-2). A thorough clinical evaluation, including medical history, physical examination, and swallow assessment, is necessary for an accurate diagnosis and rehabilitation plan. Medical history contains information regarding the individual's current swallowing and nutritional status, including a description of complaints related to swallowing. It is especially important to elicit complaints of coughing, choking, or pain with swallowing; change in dietary habits; weight loss; the sensation of food sticking in the neck or chest; or symptoms of GERD (heartburn, and sour or bitter regurgitation). The location of the symptoms (i.e. in the neck versus the chest) is not always a reliable determinant for the location of the pathology or dysfunction. Complaints of thoracic dysphagia are highly suggestive of esophageal dysfunction, but complaints of cervical dysphagia can be caused by either pharyngeal or esophageal disorders. Information on previous swallowing evaluations and results, family history of genetic disorders, the patient's neurologic and surgical history, radiation therapy, and respiratory conditions are important in diagnosis. Current and past medications are noted, as some medications can weaken muscles or exacerbate preexisting conditions. Social history is important in a dysphagia rehabilitation evaluation. The physical and psychologic impact of dysphagia on an individual's family, social, and/or professional life can shape management decisions (e.g. tube feeding versus altered diets).

Physical examination

A general physical examination with examination of all major body systems is essential to a complete dysphagia assessment. Note the general appearance of the patient, including body posturing and respiratory status. As there is a high rate of cognitive dysfunction in patients with feeding and swallowing disorders, cognition and communication function should be evaluated.[87]

Examination of the oral mechanism involves identifying structural abnormalities in the head and neck regions, such as the presence of abnormal spinal curvatures or masses. Palpate the neck, including the hyoid bone and the thyroid and cricoid cartilages, for structural abnormalities. Inspect the oral cavity for structural abnormalities, adequacy of dentition, oral lesions, and secretion management. Respiratory patterns and phonatory function are screened for signs of structural or functional incompetence. A neurologic examination should be conducted, including detailed cranial nerve evaluation. Pupillary constriction, extraocular movement, and visual fields are tested. Hearing should be present bilaterally. Assess facial sensation, palpate muscles of mastication, and observe the muscles of facial expression. Evaluate lingual strength and range of motion in isolated movements and coordinated speech tasks. Evaluate the soft palate and posterior pharyngeal wall for sensation, and for symmetry at rest and with movement, by having the patient phonate and by eliciting a gag reflex. The pharynx and soft palate should contract symmetrically with gagging. The presence or absence of a gag reflex, however, should *not* be considered an indicator of safe swallowing. The reason for this is that normal individuals may have no gag reflex, and individuals with severe dysphagia can have normal gag reflexes.[68]

Bedside swallow evaluation

The BSE is an important step in the clinical evaluation. The BSE includes observation of a dry swallow, as well as trial swallows of food and liquid, and trials of behavioral and dietary modifications. Trials of liquid swallows begin with a small sip of water. If tolerated, larger sips and solid consistencies are observed. The frequently cited 'water test' involves continuously drinking a determined amount of water and monitoring for aspiration or penetration symptoms, including coughing, dyspnea, and throat clearing.[22,128,134] Although this test can be useful in screening for dysphagia, it does not detect silent aspiration or assess swallowing with more advanced consistencies. Most importantly, it does not reveal the mechanism of dysphagia.

During the oral-phase evaluation, note labial seal, rotary mastication, and presence of oral residue, as well as duration of oral phase. Pharyngeal signs of dysphagia include delayed swallow onset, coughing or throat clearing after swallows, wet vocal quality, or dyspnea following trials. Silent aspiration poses a serious problem in clinical assessments, because there are no accurate clinical signs.[73] The clinician's role becomes one of detecting risk factors for aspiration. These include a compromised respiratory system; ineffective protective mechanism, as demonstrated by impaired vocal cord movement and weak cough; and reduced cognitive status (especially related to sedating medications, which can diminish motor control).

Supplemental measures of swallowing contribute to the overall clinical picture. Palpating the hyoid bone and larynx during trial swallows allows the examiner to evaluate swallow timing and presence of laryngeal elevation (although this examination is not reliable for evaluating the amount of laryngeal elevation) (Fig. 28-9). Cervical auscultation allows the clinician to listen to the 'sounds of swallowing'. With a stethoscope placed on the anterior neck, the examiner can listen to characteristics of respiration before and after the swallow, the timing of the swallow in relation to the phase of respiration, and swallow coordination. However, a clear classification of the sounds and their significance is lacking.[71,124] A decrease in oxygen saturation level has been said to indicate aspiration, but this claim has been disputed.[69,120]

The BSE relies on indirect information to make judgments about swallowing safety. Judgments that oral events are abnormal or that pharyngeal swallowing is abnormal are generally

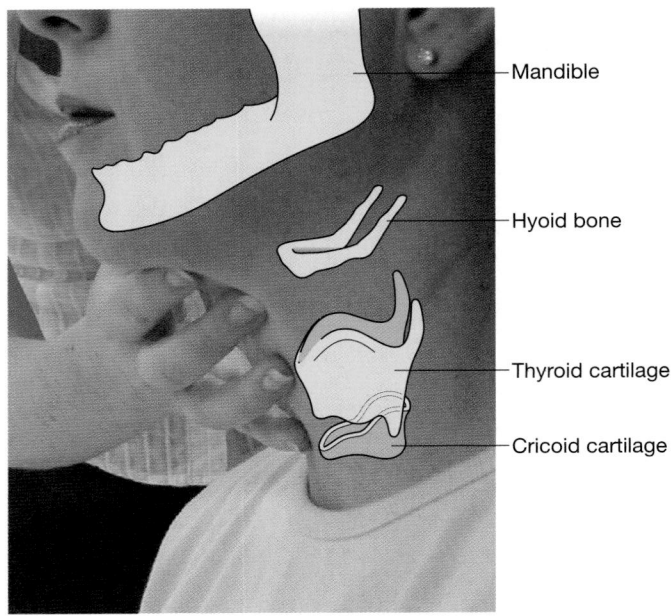

Figure 28-9 Palpating the larynx during swallowing. The middle finger touches the hyoid bone. The fourth finger touches the top of the thyroid cartilage. The fifth finger touches the cricothyroid notch.

reliable, but the presence or absence of aspiration cannot be determined reliably at the bedside.[69,78,128] The best predictors of aspiration appear to be a strong cough response after swallow, and the clinician's overall estimate of the likelihood of aspiration.[77,90] Given the unreliability of BSE alone at identifying aspiration, instrumental examination is essential to the evaluation of individuals with dysphagia.

Videofluorography

The videofluorographic swallow study (VFSS) is the gold standard in dysphagia diagnosis and management. This procedure is typically performed and interpreted jointly by a speech language pathologist and physician (physiatrist or radiologist). During the VFSS, the patient ingests radiopaque foods and liquids, and oral, pharyngeal, and esophageal stages of swallowing physiology are observed and evaluated.

The equipment includes standard fluoroscopy apparatus, a seating system to allow the patient to sit fully upright or be reclined as needed, a videotape recorder (usually S-VHS) with slow motion and freeze-frame capability, a video timer (to insert the actual time on each frame of video), and a microphone (to document activities) (Fig. 28-10).

Using a standardized protocol for the VFSS improves reliability and clinical utility of the examination (Box 28-3). Imaging in both lateral and anteroposterior projections is *essential* to avoid missing major structural or functional abnormalities. Imaging in the lateral projection alone is inadequate, as function and structure on the right and left sides can differ, and they are superimposed in lateral projection.

The VFSS has two key purposes:

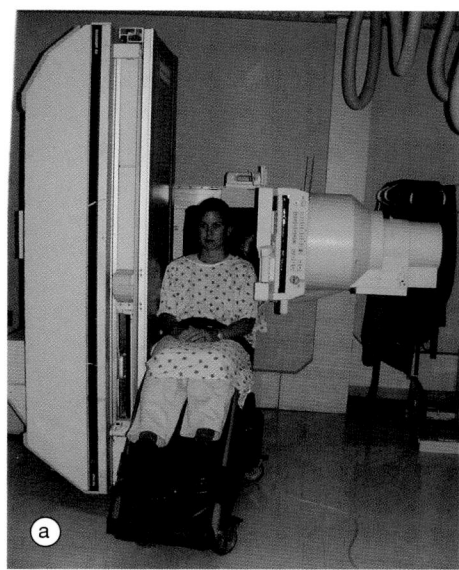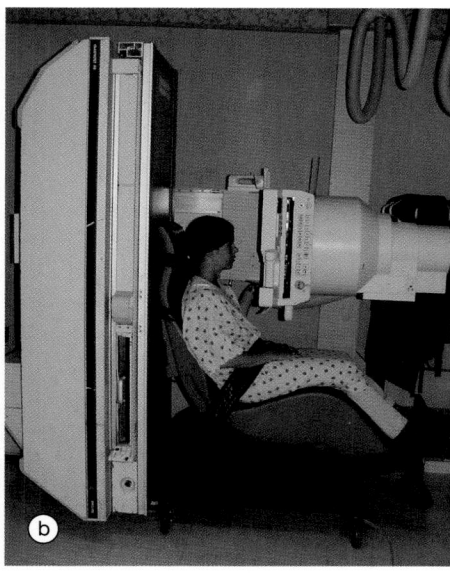

Figure 28-10 Sitting position for a videofluorographic swallowing study in the lateral projection (**a**) and posteroanterior projection (**b**).

Box 28-3 The videofluorographic swallow study protocol[77]

Lateral projection, patient sitting upright in usual position of comfort
- Speech sample ('candy, candy') to visualize velar motion
- Command swallow: 5 mL of thin liquid from a spoon
- Drink thin liquid from a cup (patient controls rate and volume)
- Command swallow: 5 mL of nectar-thick liquid from a spoon
- Drink nectar-thick liquid from a cup (patient controls rate and volume)
- Eat 1 tsp of pudding from a spoon
- Eat 1 tsp of soft food (e.g. chicken salad sandwich spread) from a spoon
- Eat shortbread cookie (e.g. half of a Lorna Doone)
- Compensatory techniques as appropriate
- Other food consistencies as indicated

Anteroposterior projection, sitting upright (neck slightly extended if safe)
- Phonation of 'e' (as in 'he') several times in succession to visualize vocal fold and arytenoids motion
- Command swallow: thin or nectar-thick liquid, 5 or 10 mL
- Compensatory techniques or other foods as appropriate
- Additional swallows as needed for imaging the esophagus

---

1. to identify structural or functional abnormalities related to swallowing; and
2. to identify the circumstances for safe and efficient swallowing.

The VFSS is *not* merely a tool to determine if the patient is aspirating.[99] The VFSS is not a 'pass or fail' examination; it is instead a tool to be used in conjunction with clinical data to develop a rehabilitation program. The examination is not automatically terminated when a patient aspirates. A thorough VFSS include trials of altered consistencies and appropriate compensatory techniques to improve swallow efficiency and

safety (Box 28-3). The results of the study are used to develop a plan for an appropriate diet, therapeutic compensations and exercises, and additional diagnostic studies as needed. In occasional cases, it might be necessary to terminate the study prematurely in the interest of patient safety. Palmer et al. have developed specific criteria for deviating from the standard VFSS protocol in the interest of patient safety.[104] Arvedson and Lefton-Greif have done the same for the VFSS in children.[2]

Videofluoroscopy is the optimal instrumental assessment tool, as it allows for observation of the oral, pharyngeal, and esophageal phases of swallowing. The limitations of VFSS relate to radiation exposure. The radiation dose is quite low, however, and is rarely a limiting factor in adults.[16,133] Pediatric VFSS protocols are designed to further limit radiation exposure.[2]

Fiberoptic endoscopic evaluation of swallowing

The FEES is an instrumental swallowing evaluation tool in which a flexible laryngoscope is passed transnasally to the pharynx to view swallowing events (Fig. 28-11).[40] While VFSS is considered the instrumental tool of choice for oropharyngeal dysphagia assessment, FEES can also provide valuable information. FEES is particularly useful for evaluation of pharyngeal and laryngeal anatomy, and for evaluation of vocal fold function.[58,65] It is also highly sensitive for detecting aspiration.[67] Individuals with physical limitations that prevent fluoroscopy can benefit from FEES. FEES can also be beneficial for more lengthy assessments, because there is no x-ray exposure. The FEES has significant limitations:

- it does not permit visualization of the oral and esophageal stages of swallowing; and
- it does not demonstrate critical events of pharyngeal swallowing, including UES opening, elevation of the larynx, or contraction of the pharynx (Box 28-4).

Standard FEES equipment includes a flexible laryngoscope, a separate light source, and a chip camera for video viewing and

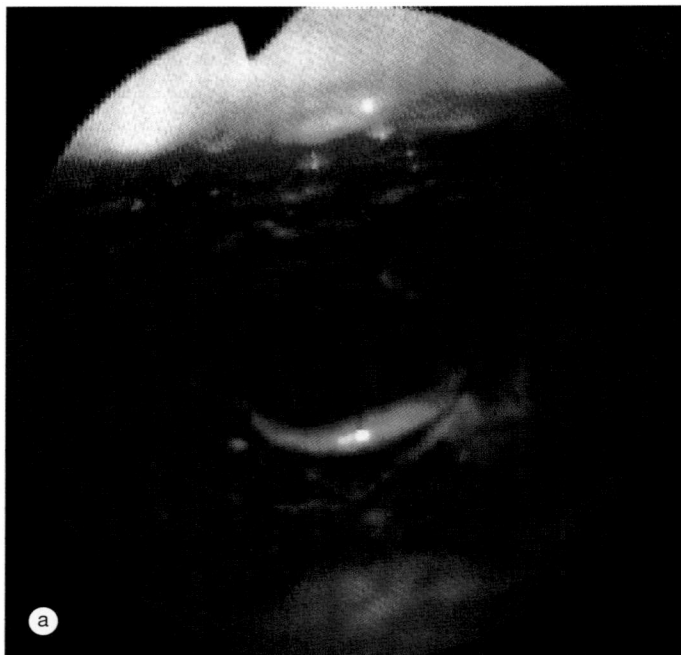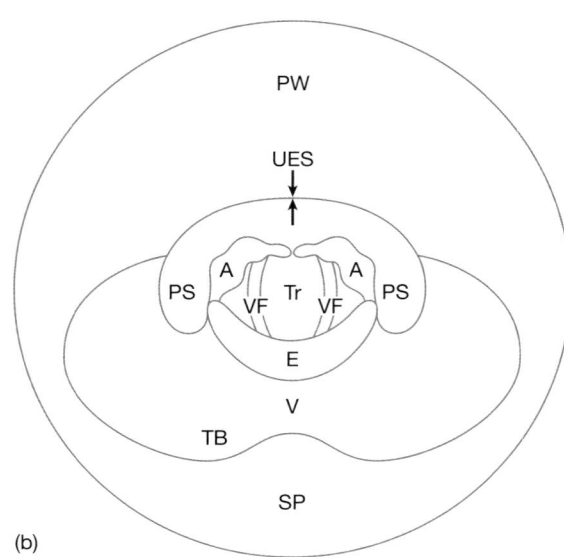

(b)

Figure 28-11 A fibrotic endoscopic image of the pharynx (**a**) and drawing (**b**) of a healthy young subject. A, arytenoid; E, epiglotis; PS, pyriform sinus; PW, posterior pharyngeal wall; SP, soft palate; TB, tongue base; Tr, trachea; UES, upper esophageal sphincter; V, valleculae; VF, vocal folds.

Box 28-4 Advantages and disadvantages of fiberoptic endoscopic evaluation of swallowing

Advantages
- No radiation exposure
- Portability of equipment
- Direct visualization of vocal cord movement
- Direct visualization of anatomy
- Sensitive for showing aspiration
- Sensitive for showing retention in pharynx after swallowing

Disadvantages
- Cannot visualize oral cavity or esophagus
- Cannot visualize the pharyngeal stage of swallowing
- In general, cannot show the mechanism for dysfunction

---

recording. Topical anesthesia or a nasal vasoconstrictor might make the FEES more comfortable. Foods and liquids of various consistencies are colored with blue or green dye to maximize visibility.

Esophagoscopy

Endoscopy is useful for visualizing anatomy but does not directly demonstrate esophageal function. Morphologic changes in the mucosa such as in tumors and esophagitis can be observed and biopsies taken under direct endoscopic guidance. Functional disorders are better assessed with radiologic or manometric studies.

Manometry

Manometry measures pressures in the food way. It is well established as a tool for the evaluation of motor disorders of

the esophagus.[14] Pharyngeal manometry, while it has proved to be extraordinarily useful in research on pharyngeal dynamics, is technically challenging and seldom used in the clinical setting.[79] Concurrent videofluoroscopy assures accurate placement of pressure sensors and accurate interpretation of pressure changes.[97]

Electromyography

Electromyography (EMG) has two main applications related to swallowing:

1. EMG is useful in diagnostic evaluation, because dysphagia can be caused by motor unit disorders;[108] and
2. EMG can be used in biofeedback as an adjunct to dysphagia therapy.

EMG of the muscles of the pharynx and larynx is a reliable method for detecting lower motor neuron dysfunction.[103] EMG is not a sufficient test for demonstration of swallow physiology, however, and should be used only as an adjunct to other instrumental assessments.

TREATMENT OF DYSPHAGIA

Dysphagia treatment rests on five principles:

1. amelioration of the underlying disease process (e.g. with steroids in polymyositis);
2. prevention of complications;
3. improvement of swallowing via therapy;

4. compensations to improve swallowing safety and efficiency; and
5. environmental modifications.

These are not necessarily applied in a temporal sequence, and it is often necessary to proceed with all four approaches at the same time. Early treatment of dysphagia has been shown to reduce the patient's risk of aspiration pneumonia, to reduce medical complications related to malnutrition and dehydration, and to reduce length of hospital stay.[31,110] Treatment of dysphagia, like its evaluation, is best performed by an interdisciplinary team including speech pathology, physiatry, occupational therapy, nursing, nutrition, psychology, and other subspecialties as needed. Rehabilitation of swallowing can involve structured swallowing therapy, surgical management, and pharmacologic management. An important consideration in dysphagia rehabilitation is maintaining adequate alimentation and hydration. Dysphagia can make it quite difficult for an individual to maintain proper alimentation and hydration. This problem can be unintentionally exacerbated by a well-meaning rehabilitation team if the diet is modified so as to make food less appealing.

Structured swallow therapy

Direct swallow therapy uses dietary modifications and postural techniques to improve safety and efficiency while allowing for oral nutrition. Therapy should be based on an understanding of the underlying disease process and the pathophysiology of dysphagia in the individual patient. We will focus on therapy for adults with dysphagia, because treatment of children is quite different.

Individualized therapeutic diets are initiated to maximize safety and efficiency of swallowing, based on the findings of clinical and instrumental assessments. Solid foods can be chopped, soft cooked, or pureed to compensate for oral manipulation and bolus control impairments. Liquid viscosity can be altered to alleviate specific symptoms of dysphagia. In general, thinner (i.e. less viscous) fluids are more easily aspirated, because they are more difficult to control in the oral cavity and pharynx. On the other hand, swallow efficiency (the ability to propel a bolus into the esophagus) is generally higher for thinner liquids, because they are more easily pushed through a small opening (such as a partially obstructed UES). Balancing these considerations requires an individualized approach, and instrumental studies are often necessary. A National Dysphagia Diet has been published by the American Dietetic Association.[89] This diet describes food consistencies that are frequently recommended in dysphagia treatment, but it is by no means comprehensive, nor is it standardized for specific populations (e.g. children). It is important to ensure adequate hydration when patients are placed on thickened liquid diets, because these can make it difficult to get sufficient fluids by mouth. Parenteral fluids might be necessary, especially acutely for the short term. This is especially important in the case of acute stroke, because adequate hydration is critical to recovery.

In addition to diet modifications, dysphagia diets often involve behavioral and postural techniques. Table 28-3 lists common postural techniques and some indications for their use. None of these techniques are effective in all patients. Some are even potentially hazardous, in that they may actually worsen the swallow if applied indiscriminately. Careful clinical and instrumental evaluations are essential in selecting techniques to be utilized in the individual case.[80]

The chin tuck maneuver can reduce laryngeal penetration and aspiration by improving laryngeal vestibule closure and allowing gravity assist oral bolus control (preventing posterior loss of the

Table 28-3 Common postural techniques and some indications for use

Compensatory technique	Indication
Chin tuck	Reduced oral bolus control with aspiration before or during the swallow
Neck extension	Impaired oral bolus propulsion
Head turn (to weak side)	Unilateral pharyngeal weakness with retention after swallowing
Head tilt (to weak side)	Unilateral oral and pharyngeal weakness
Reclining position	Pharyngeal weakness with retention and overflow aspiration after swallowing
Supraglottic swallow	Inadequate or delayed vocal fold closure
Supersupraglottic swallow	Inadequate or delayed closure of laryngeal aditus (entrance)
Effortful swallow	Poor tongue base retraction
Mendelsohn maneuver	Inadequate upper esophageal sphincter opening
Syringe feeding	Impaired oral bolus propulsion
Double swallow	Retention in the pharynx after swallowing
Alternating solids and liquids	Retention in the pharynx after swallowing

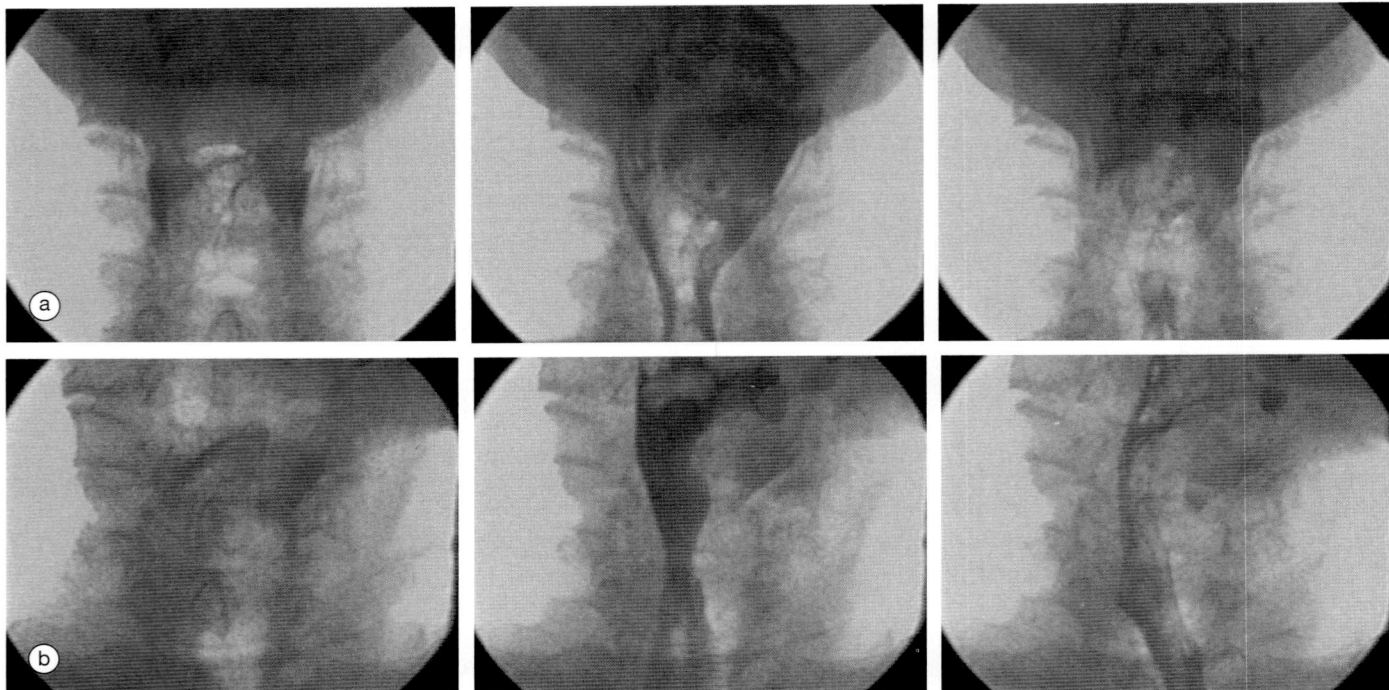

Figure 28-12 Effectiveness of the head rotation maneuver shown with videofluorography image sequences in an individual with lateral medullary infarction. (**a**) Severe left-sided pharyngeal weakness results in retention of barium after swallowing. (**b**) When the same individual turns the head toward the weak left side, the barium is directed preferentially to the stronger right side. This reduces the amount retained after swallowing. The right side of the image is the left side of the patient.

bolus).[131] Neck flexion also reduces pharyngeal peak contraction pressure,[9,10] however, and this can make it ineffective for individuals with weakened pharyngeal constrictor muscles or tongue base retraction.[78] This position can be dangerous in infants.

Rotating the neck to one side diverts the bolus to the contralateral side. In unilateral pharyngeal weakness, head turn to the weak side can divert the bolus to the strong side (Fig. 28-12). This strategy also reduces UES pressure and increases the duration of UES relaxation, facilitating bolus flow into the esophagus.[96] When there is unilateral oral weakness as well, a head tilt toward the stronger side might be helpful. Anteroposterior imaging of the swallow is essential to determine whether there is asymmetric pharyngeal weakness and to assess the utility of this technique.

The neck extension maneuver can assist oral clearance when the tongue is ineffective in oral bolus propulsion. Tilting the head back allows gravity to move the bolus into the hypopharynx. Neck extension should be used cautiously when pharyngeal control is impaired, as it can also cause delayed UES relaxation, incomplete UES relaxation, and premature UES closure.[15]

The reclining posture (anywhere from 30 to 90°) elevates the laryngeal aditus relative to the hypopharynx, which can inhibit aspiration of material retained in the pharynx after swallowing.

Compensatory swallowing techniques are used to reduce aspiration and/or improve pharyngeal clearance. The 'supraglot-tic swallow' involves breath holding prior to swallow onset to close the vocal cords, and an immediate cough after swallow. This technique can be beneficial for individuals with poor bolus control, delayed airway closure, and delayed pharyngeal swallow.[10] The 'supersupraglottic swallow' also protects the airway during the swallow for patients with reduced laryngeal closure through the addition of effortful breath holding.[26] This rotates the arytenoids forward (toward the epiglottis) to promote closure of the laryngeal vestibule. The 'effortful swallow' technique (instruction to 'swallow hard') assists pharyngeal clearance by increasing tongue base movement and lengthening laryngeal vestibule closure.[47] The Mendelsohn maneuver increases the extent and duration of UES opening by voluntarily prolonging contraction of the suprahyoid muscles during swallowing.[25] This can enhance pharyngeal clearance by reducing resistance at the UES. In cases of impaired oral bolus propulsion, syringe feeding can be used to bypass the oral cavity. 'Double swallows' (voluntarily doing a second swallow) can be recommended for patients with pharyngeal constriction resulting in retention after swallow. Alternating solid and liquid consistencies has also been successful in clearing residue from the pharynx. These techniques should be applied with caution, as they can promote aspiration or reduce swallow efficiency. A VFSS can effectively demonstrate when these techniques are indicated, test their effectiveness in the individual case, and demonstrate whether they cause undesirable secondary effects.

Additional pediatric considerations

Positioning is a critical concept in pediatric dysphagia management.[66] Postural modifications are used to compensate for abnormal tone and movement, structural abnormalities, and sensorimotor deficits. Children should be seated upright during meals whenever possible, with neutral neck flexion; elongated neck and trunk; stable shoulder girdle; and neutral positioning of pelvis, hips, and feet. In some children, upright seating maximizes the coordination of respiration and swallowing.[3] Specialty seating and positioning devices maximize stability and control for feeding, including wedges and standers, modified tables, strapping and vesting systems, and head controls. For further information regarding assessment and treatment of infants and children with problems of feeding and swallowing, there are several excellent references.[1,2,113]

The prone position compensates for jaw instability or retraction, tongue retraction, and nasopharyngeal reflux. In children with adequate tone for upright seating, a chin tuck can compensate for tongue retraction and jaw instability. Pharyngeal dysphagia due to inadequate head control and poor trunk stability can be minimized with a reclined position and extended neck.[66] Children with aversive resistance to feeding can benefit from a prone position with head supported in extension. Lethargic resistance to feeding can be minimized by positioning the child upright and away from caregiver's body, but with back and neck support. Swaddling and holding the child close to caregiver's body assists with 'fussy' feeders.[94] Supportive positioning techniques provided by the feeder reduce functional disability with swallowing. Mandibular support, with fingers on jaw, maintains closure and stability. Lingual support for tongue thrust is provided by placing the feeding utensil at midline on the tongue with downward pressure. Labial support during feeding includes finger tapping or vibration to lips and stability maneuvers.

Prosthetic devices

Intraoral prostheses compensate for velopharyngeal insufficiency, loss of lingual or velar tissue due to resection, and velar and lingual paralysis. A palatal obturator can replace a portion of the palate after resection, improving mastication. A palatal augmentation prosthesis effectively lowers the oral surface of the hard palate, maximizing lingual contact with the palate and improving oral food transport.[75] A palatal lift prosthesis elevates the soft palate, reducing velopharyngeal insufficiency. This can potentially improve bolus propulsion and reduce nasal regurgitation during swallow, but the effectiveness of this approach has not been established. In individuals with tracheostomy, use of a one-way speaking valve restores expiratory airflow through the larynx and upper airway, restoring the ability to cough and clear the airway in response to aspiration (Fig. 28-8).[125]

Oral sensory training

Oral sensory awareness therapy can increase the patient's awareness of the bolus and improve swallow coordination. Sour or cold boluses improve oral transit, improve timing of swallow onset, and can secondarily reduce occurrence of aspiration and laryngeal penetration.[54,76,107] Although the efficacy of these techniques has not yet been demonstrated, sensory therapy can also include facial massage, vibration, and tapping of oral musculature.

Electrical stimulation

Surface electrical stimulation is a new modality for treatment of dysphagia. In a typical treatment session, surface electrodes are taped to the skin overlying the submental or anterior cervical strap muscles. Pulsed electrical stimulation is delivered with a commercial device that is marketed specifically for dysphagia therapy. This technique has become quite popular, despite the fact that there is no scientific evidence for its efficacy. The single published report used non-standardized assessment tools of uncertain validity.[34] A physiologic study is currently underway to determine the effects of stimulation on hyolaryngeal motion and swallow safety, but only preliminary data have been presented.[83] This form of therapy cannot be recommended until research shows clearly that it has no deleterious effects on swallowing.

Indirect therapy techniques

Indirect rehabilitation techniques involve the use of oral, pharyngeal, laryngeal, and respiratory exercises to improve flexibility, strength, and coordination (Table 28-4). Oral control exercises include rapid tongue lateralization movements, rotary tongue movements, and movements sweeping the buccal cavities. Bolus formation is improved through simulated manipulation of a bolus within the oral cavity. Simulated chewing exercises with clinician-assisted lateralization and movement of gauze on a string (or sponges) are used to improve bolus manipulation. Suck–swallow exercises are used to improve bolus propulsion.

Exercises for improving flexibility include stretching and range of motion for the soft tissue of the oral cavity, jaws, or neck. Mandibular exercises include jaw rotation, lateralization, and opening–closing. Labial range of motion is improved through labial protrusion and retraction, lateral stretching, and labial opening and closing. Lingual exercises include elevation, depression, lateralization, rotary motion, retraction, protrusion, and stretching posteriorly into each cheek.

Oral muscles are strengthened through resistive movements. Resistance exercises include applying pressure against the jaw during lateral and opening–closing motions; holding a tongue blade between the lips with labial pressure, while pulling the blade anteriorly; squeezing the lips closed against resistance; pushing the tongue against a tongue blade; pushing the tongue into the cheek against manual resistance; and pulling the tongue posteriorly while gripping the tongue tip.

Pharyngeal exercises are designed to increase active range of motion in the larynx, base of tongue, pharynx, and vocal cords. The larynx can be volitionally elevated by sustaining a high pitched 'ee' and by effortful swallows. Tongue protrusion and retraction exercises can increase contact of the tongue base with the posterior pharyngeal wall. Vocal cord adduction exercises (e.g. hard glottal attack, pushing and pulling exercises) can increase vocal cord approximation in cases of laryngeal

Table 28-4 Common indirect therapy techniques

Therapy technique	Description
Oral cavity Oral motor control exercises (jaw, tongue, lip)	Jaw opening and closing Tongue rotation, lateralization, protrusion, retraction Lip protrusion, lateralization, and opening–closing
Relaxation and range of motion (jaw, tongue, lip)	Stretching and increasing range of motion
Resistance exercise (jaw, tongue, lip)	Opening–closing the jaw against resistance Pushing the tongue against resistance
Pharynx Laryngeal elevation exercise	Volitional laryngeal elevation by saying a high-pitched 'ee'
Vocal cord adduction exercise	Pushing wall or table, uttering 'ah' simultaneously
Masako maneuver	Swallowing with the tongue tip held anteriorly outside the mouth
Sensory stimulation	Tactile stimulation of the faucial arches with cold or sour stimuli
Upper esophageal sphincter opening Shaker exercise	Active head raising (neck flexion) in the supine position
Upper esophageal sphincter dilatation	Expansion of a balloon catheter in the upper esophageal sphincter

motion impairment. Sensory stimulation using cold and sour stimuli to the faucial arches can improve pharyngeal swallow timing, when stimuli are applied prior to bolus swallows.[54,112] The Masako maneuver is a technique for increasing tongue base retraction during swallowing.[35] In this maneuver, the tongue tip is gripped anteriorly outside the oral cavity during swallowing.

The Shaker exercise is an isotonic–isometric head raising (neck flexion) exercise performed in the supine position that is designed to strengthen the anterior suprahyoid muscles, and thereby augment UES opening during swallowing (Fig. 28-13). Individuals complete three 1-min head raises with a 1-min break between each one, followed by 30 consecutive head lifts. This exercise can be useful for patients with poor UES opening and retention in the pharynx after swallowing. The effectiveness of the Shaker exercise has been established in a controlled clinical trial.[114,115]

Physiatrists in Japan have pioneered the use of UES dilatation as a technique of rehabilitation for failure of UES relaxation,[50] but this approach has received little attention outside Japan. The patient is taught to perform self-dilatation using a balloon catheter, and performs the technique prior to each meal. It is unclear at this point whether the potential benefits of frequent dilatation outweigh the risks.

Biofeedback involves use of EMG to provide visual feedback during therapy. Surface electrodes are used to record suprahyoid (submental) and infrahyoid muscle activity during exercise, and during direct and indirect swallow therapy. This can improve conscious awareness of the activity in a particular muscle group, fostering the ability to modify that activity. Fiberoptic laryngos-

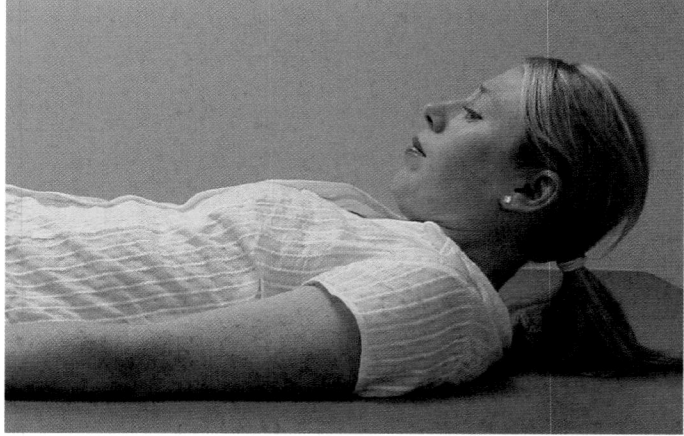

Figure 28-13 The Shaker exercise for augmenting upper esophageal sphincter opening by strengthening the anterior suprahyoid muscles. Starting in the supine position, the neck is flexed without raising the shoulders. The head is raised enough to see the toes without lifting the shoulders.

copy can also be used for biofeedback, especially to demonstrate movements of the larynx involved in swallowing maneuvers (e.g. supraglottic swallow). Biofeedback is not a dysphagia therapy per se, but can be a useful adjunct to therapy.

Surgery for dysphagia

Surgery is rarely indicated for treatment of oropharyngeal dysphagia. Dilatation can be indicated in cases of UES stenosis

Table 28-5 Alternative feeding options

Feeding tube	Insertion	Indication	Possible complications
Nasogastric	Inserted transnasally at bedside; confirmed via stethoscope or x-ray	Short-term feeding	Easily dislodged; can lead to ulceration and stricture
Orogastric	Inserted transorally at bedside	Short-term feeding; patients on ventilator, unable to use nasal passage	—
Gastrostomy	Generally inserted endoscopically	Long-term nutrition and hydration	Infection, bleeding, perforation, clogging, and aspiration
Jejunostomy	Inserted surgically into small intestine	Absence of or inability to use the stomach; severe reflux aspiration	Clogging, diarrhea; questionable benefit for reducing aspiration

when rehabilitation has been unsuccessful. Surgery is often performed for Zenker diverticulum when the diverticulum is large enough to interfere significantly with eating and drinking.[42,132] Cricopharyngeal myotomy is a procedure that disrupts the cricopharyngeus muscle for the purpose of reducing UES pressure, and thereby reducing resistance to flow from the pharynx to the esophagus. However, there is limited evidence of its effectiveness.[17] Botulinum toxin injections are sometimes used to treat dysphagia, especially in cases of oromandibular or lingual dystonia, trismus, or cricopharyngeal dysfunction with failure of UES relaxation.[136] In severe and chronic aspiration, surgery can be necessary to separate the airway from the food way.[122,126] This can be accomplished by combining permanent tracheostomy with laryngectomy or another procedure to close the larynx.[130] Although this definitively prevents aspiration, it has the serious consequence of preventing phonation and can result in significant dysphagia.

Pharyngeal bypass

When adequate and safe oral intake is not possible, pharyngeal bypass procedures eliminate the need for swallowing and provide alternative means for achieving nutrition and hydration (Table 28-5).[59] Short-term feeding options include nasogastric and orogastric tubes, while jejunostomy and gastrostomy tubes are medium- and long-term feeding options. Gastrostomy tube feeding is used safely by thousands of individuals with severe dysphagia.[6] But it should be noted that the use of feeding tubes does not necessarily prevent aspiration, and tube feeding might in fact promote gastroesophageal reflux with secondary aspiration of stomach contents. In one study, up to 44% of acute stroke patients fed with gastrostomy developed pneumonia. Furthermore, 66% of these patients continued to aspirate chronically, with mortality rates greater than 50% after 1 year.[23,30,55] Measures to minimize aspiration include head elevation, good hygiene with bag and line handling, use of slow continuous feeding rather than bolus, and monitoring for gastric residue.[21] Presence of a jejunostomy or gastrostomy permits simultaneous oral feeding. It should be noted that dysphagia

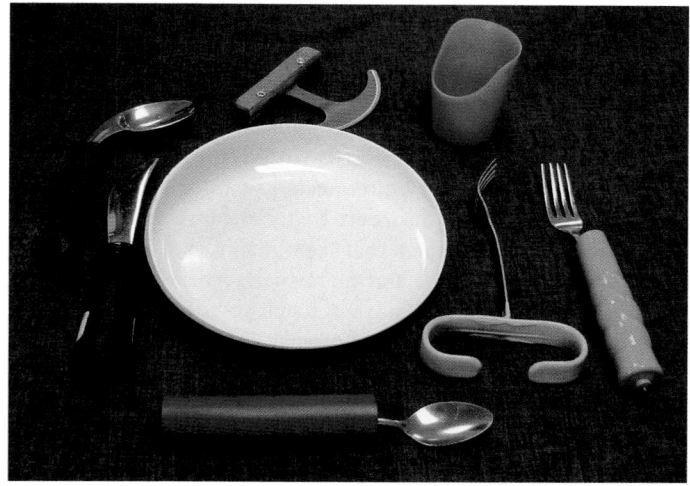

Figure 28-14 Adaptive equipment to support self-feeding.

rehabilitation is often successful in individuals who have been on tube feedings for an extended period of time.

HYGIENIC CONSIDERATIONS

Hygienic considerations have great importance but are often overlooked in dysphagia rehabilitation. These include use of proper oral care, positioning, and adequate nutrition and hydration. Proper oral care reduces potentially pathogenic bacterial colonization, thereby reducing risk of aspiration pneumonia.[85,135]

Upright positioning during and after meals is critical to reduce aspiration risk from food as well as refluxed material, and to maximize the effectiveness of rehabilitation techniques. Special adaptive equipment can be needed to maximize the ability to self-feed (Fig. 28-14). For infants, adaptive nipples control the amount and force needed for an infant to suck liquid. Bottles contain adaptations to improve the ability to hold the bottle, or angled necks to increase natural chin tuck with drinking. Both children and adults with motor incoordination and weakness can benefit from adaptive bowls, plates, cups, and utensils to improve motor stability and efficiency during self-feeding. Nutrition is a concern for individuals with dysphagia, because changes in diet can lead to loss of essential nutrients. Nutritional status should be closely monitored by following body weight and blood chemistries.[36]

PSYCHOLOGIC CONSIDERATIONS

Cognitive and emotional problems occur frequently in individuals with dysphagia, due to the nature of the underlying disease and the social consequences of the symptoms. Cognitive impairment may make it difficult for patients to participate effectively in therapy programs and to use strategies for safe swallowing. The emotional impact of dysphagia can be significant when it prevents the patient from participating in mealtimes. Resulting affective disorders can have a significant impact on participation in therapy and exacerbate social isolation, with negative impact on family and social relationships. Clinicians should be attentive to the mental health of individuals with dysphagia, and psychologic consultation should be requested when appropriate.

Given the variety of disorders that can cause dysphagia, and the serious complications that can result, a comprehensive understanding of normal and abnormal swallow function and prognosis is essential. A team approach to addressing medical, cognitive, physical, and psychosocial aspects of swallowing facilitates as near a return to independence as possible.

REFERENCES

1. Arvedson JC, Brodsky LB. Pediatric swallowing and feeding: assessment and management. 2nd edn. Albany: Singular Publishing Group; 2002.
2. Arvedson JC, Lefton-Greif MA. Pediatric videofluroscopic swallowing studies: a professional manual with caregiver handouts. San Antonio: Communication Skill Builders; 1998.
3. Arvedson JC. Management of pediatric dysphagia. Otolaryngol Clin North Am 1998; 31(3):453–476.
4. Aydogdu I, Ertekin C, Tarlaci S, et al. Dysphagia in lateral medullary infarction (Wallenberg's syndrome): an acute disconnection syndrome in premotor neurons related to swallowing activity? Stroke 2001; 32(9):2081–2087.
5. Banks JC, Nava PB, Petersen D, et al. Atlas of clinical gross anatomy. St. Louis: Mosby; 2005.
6. Britton JE, Lipscomb G, Mohr PD, et al. The use of percutaneous endoscopic gastrostomy (PEG) feeding tubes in patients with neurological disease. J Neurol 1997; 244(7):431–434.
7. Buchholz DW. Neurogenic dysphagia: what is the cause when the cause is not obvious? Dysphagia 1994; 9(4):245–255.
8. Buchholz DW. Oropharyngeal dysphagia due to iatrogenic neurological dysfunction. Dysphagia 1995; 10(4):248–254.
9. Bulow M, Olsson R, Ekberg O. Videomanometric analysis of supraglottic swallow, effortful swallow, and chin tuck in healthy volunteers. Dysphagia 1999; 14(2):67–72.
10. Bulow M, Olsson R, Ekberg O. Videomanometric analysis of supraglottic swallow, effortful swallow, and chin tuck in patients with pharyngeal dysfunction. Dysphagia 2001; 16(3):190–195.
11. Caruana-Montaldo B, Gleeson K, Zwillich CW. The control of breathing in clinical practice. Chest 2000; 117(1):205–225.
12. Casas MJ, Kenny DJ, Macmillan RE. Buccal and lingual activity during mastication and swallowing in typical adults. J Oral Rehabil 2003; 30(1):9–16.
13. Castell DO, Donner MW. Evaluation of dysphagia: a careful history is crucial. Dysphagia 1987; 2(2):65–71.
14. Castell DO. Manometric evaluation of the pharynx. Dysphagia 1993; 8(4):337–338.
15. Castell JA, Castell DO, Schultz AR, et al. Effect of head position on the dynamics of the upper esophageal sphincter and pharynx. Dysphagia 1993; 8(1):1–6.
16. Chan CB, Chan LK, Lam HS. Scattered radiation level during videofluoroscopy for swallowing study. Clin Radiol 2002; 57(7):614–616.
17. Colombo-Benkmann M, Unruh V, Krieglstein C, et al. Cricopharyngeal myotomy in the treatment of Zenker's diverticulum. J Am Coll Surg 2003; 196(3):370–377; discussion 377; author reply 378.
18. Cook IJ, Dodds WJ, Dantas RO, et al. Opening mechanisms of the human upper esophageal sphincter. Am J Physiol 1989; 257(5 part 1):G748–G759.
19. Cook IJ, Dodds WJ, Dantas RO, et al. Timing of videofluoroscopic, manometric events, and bolus transit during the oral and pharyngeal phases of swallowing. Dysphagia 1989; 4(1):8–15.
20. Daniels SK, Corey DM, Hadskey LD, et al. Mechanism of sequential swallowing during straw drinking in healthy young and older adults. J Speech Lang Hear Res 2004; 47(1):33–45.
21. Davis AE, Arrington K, Fields-Ryan S, et al. Preventing feeding-associated aspiration. Medsurg Nurs 1995; 4(2):111–119.
22. DePippo KL, Holas MA, Reding MJ. Validation of the 3-oz water swallow test for aspiration following stroke [see comments]. Arch Neurol 1992; 49(12):1259–1261.
23. Dharmarajan TS, Unnikrishnan D. Tube feeding in the elderly. The technique, complications, and outcome. Postgrad Med 2004; 115(2):51–54, 58–61.
24. Di Vito J Jr. Cervical osteophytic dysphagia: single and combined mechanisms. Dysphagia 1998; 13(1):58–61.
25. Ding R, Larson CR, Logemann JA, et al. Surface electromyographic and electroglottographic studies in normal subjects under two swallow conditions: normal and during the Mendelsohn maneuver. Dysphagia 2002; 17(1):1–12.
26. Donzelli J, Brady S. The effects of breath-holding on vocal fold adduction: implications for safe swallowing. Arch Otolaryngol Head Neck Surg 2004; 130(2):208–210.
27. Doty RW, Bosma JF. An electromyographic analysis of reflex deglutition. J Neurophysiol 1956; 19(1):44–60.
28. Doty RW, Richmond WH, Storey AT. Effect of medullary lesions on coordination of deglutition. Exp Neurol 1967; 17(1):91–106.
29. Dua KS, Ren J, Bardan E, et al. Coordination of deglutitive glottal function and pharyngeal bolus transit during normal eating. Gastroenterology 1997; 112(1):73–83.
30. Dziewas R, Ritter M, Schilling M, et al. Pneumonia in acute stroke patients fed by nasogastric tube. J Neurol Neurosurg Psychiatry 2004; 75(6):852–856.
31. Elmstahl S, Bulow M, Ekberg O, et al. Treatment of dysphagia improves nutritional conditions in stroke patients. Dysphagia 1999; 14(2):61–66.
32. Ertekin C, Aydogdu I. Electromyography of human cricopharyngeal muscle of the upper esophageal sphincter. Muscle Nerve 2002; 26(6):729–739.
33. von Euler C. On the central pattern generator for the basic breathing rhythmicity. J Appl Physiol 1983; 55(6):1647–1659.
34. Freed ML, Freed L, Chatburn RL, et al. Electrical stimulation for swallowing disorders caused by stroke. Respir Care 2001; 46(5):466–474.
35. Fujiu M, Logeman JA. Effect of tongue holding maneuver on posterior pharyngeal wall movement during deglutition. Am J Speech Lang Pathol 1996; 5(1):25–47.
36. Ganger D, Craig RM. Swallowing disorders and nutritional support. Dysphagia 1990; 4(4):213–219.
37. Garon BR, Engle M, Ormiston C. A randomized study to determine the effects of unlimited intake of water in patients with identified aspiration. J Neuro Rehabil 1997; 11(3):139–148.
38. Garon BR, Engle M, Ormiston C. Silent aspiration: results of 1,000 videofluoroscopic swallow evaluations. J Neuro Rehabil 1996; 10(2):121–126.

39. Groher ME, Bukatman R. The prevalence of swallow disorders in two teaching hospitals. Dysphagia 1986; 1(1):3–6.

40. Gross RD, Mahlmann J, Grayhack JP. Physiologic effects of open and closed tracheostomy tubes on the pharyngeal swallow. Ann Otol Rhinol Laryngol 2003; 112(2):143–152.

41. Hajioff D, Lowe D. The diagnostic value of barium swallow in globus syndrome. Int J Clin Pract 2004; 58(1):86–89.

42. Hashiba K, de Paula AL, da Silva JG, et al. Endoscopic treatment of Zenker's diverticulum. Gastrointest Endosc 1999; 49(1):93–97.

43. Hatch JP, Shinkai RS, Sakai S, et al. Determinants of masticatory performance in dentate adults. Arch Oral Biol 2001; 46(7):641–648.

44. Hendrix TR. Coordination of peristalsis in pharynx and esophagus. Dysphagia 1993; 8(2):74–78.

45. Hiiemae KM, Palmer JB, Medicis SW, et al. Hyoid and tongue surface movements in speaking and eating. Arch Oral Biol 2002; 47(1):11–27.

46. Hiiemae KM, Palmer JB. Food transport and bolus formation during complete feeding sequences on foods of different initial consistency [see comments]. Dysphagia 1999; 14(1):31–42.

47. Hind JA, Nicosia MA, Roecker EB, et al. Comparison of effortful and noneffortful swallows in healthy middle-aged and older adults. Arch Phys Med Rehabil 2001; 82(12):1661–1665.

48. Hirst LJ, Ford GA, Gibson GJ, et al. Swallow-induced alterations in breathing in normal older people. Dysphagia 2002; 17(2):152–161.

49. Hiss SG, Treole K, Stuart A. Effects of age, gender, bolus volume, and trial on swallowing apnea duration and swallow/respiratory phase relationships of normal adults. Dysphagia 2001; 16(2):128–135.

50. Hojo K, Fujishima I, Ohkuma R, et al. Balloon catheter treatment methods for cricopharyngeal dysphagia. Jpn J Dysphagia Rehabil 1997; 1(1):45–56 [in Japanese].

51. Holas MA, DePippo KL, Reding MJ. Aspiration and relative risk of medical complications following stroke. Arch Neurol 1994; 51(10):1051–1053.

52. Ishida R, Palmer JB, Hiiemae KM. Hyoid motion during swallowing: factors affecting forward and upward displacement. Dysphagia 2002; 17(4):262–272.

53. Jean A. Brain stem control of swallowing: neuronal network and cellular mechanisms. Physiol Rev 2001; 81(2):929–969.

54. Kaatzke-McDonald MN, Post E, Davis PJ. The effects of cold, touch, and chemical stimulation of the anterior faucial pillar on human swallowing [see comments]. Dysphagia 1996; 11(3):198–206.

55. Kadakia SC, Sullivan HO, Starnes E. Percutaneous endoscopic gastrostomy or jejunostomy and the incidence of aspiration in 79 patients. Am J Surg 1992; 164(2):114–118.

56. Kahrilas PJ, Logemann JA, Lin S, et al. Pharyngeal clearance during swallowing: a combined manometric and videofluoroscopic study. Gastroenterology 1992; 103(1):128–136.

57. Kendall KA, McKenzie S, Leonard RJ, et al. Timing of events in normal swallowing: a videofluoroscopic study. Dysphagia 2000; 15(2):74–83.

58. Kidder TM, Langmore SE, Martin BJ. Indications and techniques of endoscopy in evaluation of cervical dysphagia: comparison with radiographic techniques. Dysphagia 1994; 9(4):256–261.

59. Klose J, Heldwein W, Rafferzeder M, et al. Nutritional status and quality of life in patients with percutaneous endoscopic gastrostomy (PEG) in practice: prospective one-year follow-up. Dig Dis Sci 2003; 48(10):2057–2063.

60. Kotz T, Abraham S, Beitler JJ, et al. Pharyngeal transport dysfunction consequent to an organ-sparing protocol. Arch Otolaryngol Head Neck Surg 1999; 125(4):410–413.

61. Kronenberger MB, Meyers AD. Dysphagia following head and neck cancer surgery. Dysphagia 1994; 9(4):236–244.

62. Kuhlemeier KV. Epidemiology and dysphagia. Dysphagia 1994; 9(4):209–217.

63. Laitman JT, Reidenberg JS. Specializations of the human upper respiratory and upper digestive systems as seen through comparative and developmental anatomy. Dysphagia 1993; 8(4):318–325.

64. Langmore SE, Skarupski KA, Park PS, et al. Predictors of aspiration pneumonia in nursing home residents. Dysphagia 2002; 17(4):298–307.

65. Langmore SE. Endoscopic evaluation and treatment of swallowing disorders. New York: Thieme Medical Publishers; 2001.

66. Larnert G, Ekberg O. Positioning improves the oral and pharyngeal swallowing function in children with cerebral palsy. Acta Paediatr 1995; 84(6):689–692.

67. Leder SB, Sasaki CT, Burrell MI. Fiberoptic endoscopic evaluation of dysphagia to identify silent aspiration. Dysphagia 1998; 13(1):19–21.

68. Leder SB. Gag reflex and dysphagia. Head Neck 1996; 18(2):138–141.

69. Leder SB. Use of arterial oxygen saturation, heart rate, and blood pressure as indirect objective physiologic markers to predict aspiration. Dysphagia 2000; 15(4):201–205.

70. Leopold NA, Kagel MC. Prepharyngeal dysphagia in Parkinson's disease [see comments]. Dysphagia 1996; 11(1):14–22.

71. Leslie P, Drinnan MJ, Finn P, et al. Reliability and validity of cervical auscultation: a controlled comparison using videofluoroscopy. Dysphagia 2004; 19(4):231–240.

72. Lieberman DE, McCarthy RC, Hiiemae KM, et al. Ontogeny of postnatal hyoid and larynx descent in humans. Arch Oral Biol 2001; 46(2):117–128.

73. Linden P, Kuhlemeier KV, Patterson C. The probability of correctly predicting subglottic penetration from clinical observations. Dysphagia 1993; 8(3):170–179.

74. Logemann JA, Kahrilas PJ, Cheng J, et al. Closure mechanisms of laryngeal vestibule during swallow. Am J Physiol 1992; 262(2 part 1):G338–G344.

75. Logemann JA, Kahrilas PJ, Hurst P, et al. Effects of intraoral prosthetics on swallowing in patients with oral cancer. Dysphagia 1989; 4(2):118–120.

76. Logemann JA, Pauloski BR, Colangelo L, et al. Effects of a sour bolus on oropharyngeal swallowing measures in patients with neurogenic dysphagia. J Speech Hear Res 1995; 38(3):556–563.

77. Logemann JA, Veis S, Colangelo L. A screening procedure for oropharyngeal dysphagia. Dysphagia 1999; 14(1):44–51.

78. Logemann JA. Evaluation and treatment of swallowing disorders. 2nd edn. Austin: Pro-Ed; 1998.

79. Logemann JA. Non-imaging techniques for the study of swallowing. Acta Otorhinolaryngol Belg 1994; 48(2):139–142.

80. Logemann JA. Noninvasive approaches to deglutitive aspiration. Dysphagia 1993; 8(4):331–333.

81. Lorenz R, Jorysz G, Classen M. The value of endoscopy and endosonography in the diagnosis of the dysphagic patient. Dysphagia 1993; 8(2):91–97.

82. Lorenz R, Jorysz G, Tornieporth N, et al. The gastroenterologist's approach to dysphagia. Dysphagia 1993; 8(2):79–82.

83. Ludlow C, Ianessa H, Saxon K, et al. Effects of surface electrical stimulation both at rest and during swallowing in chronic pharyngeal dysphagia [abstract]. Dysphagia; in press.

84. Lund JP, Kolta A, Westberg KG, et al. Brainstem mechanisms underlying feeding behaviors. Curr Opin Neurobiol 1998; 8(6):718–724.

85. Marik PE, Kaplan D. Aspiration pneumonia and dysphagia in the elderly. Chest 2003; 124(1):328–336.

86. Marik PE. Aspiration pneumonitis and aspiration pneumonia. N Engl J Med 2001; 344(9):665–671.

87. Martin BJ, Corlew MM. The incidence of communication disorders in dysphagic patients. J Speech Hear Disord 1990; 55(1):28–32.

88. Matsuo K, Hiiemae KM, Palmer JB. Cyclic motion of the soft palate in feeding. J Dent Res 2005; 84(1):39–42.

89. McCallum SL. The National Dysphagia Diet: implementation at a regional rehabilitation center and hospital system. J Am Diet Assoc 2003; 103(3):381–384.

90. McCullough GH, Wertz RT, Rosenbek JC. Sensitivity and specificity of clinical/bedside examination signs for detecting aspiration in adults subsequent to stroke. J Commun Disord 2001; 34(1-2):55–72.

91. Miller AJ. Deglutition. Physiol Rev 1982; 62(1):129–184.

92. Mioche L, Hiiemae KM, Palmer JB. A postero-anterior videofluorographic study of the intra-oral management of food in man. Arch Oral Biol 2002; 47(4):267–280.

93. Mokhlesi B, Logemann JA, Rademaker AW, et al. Oropharyngeal deglutition in stable COPD. Chest 2002; 121(2):361–369.

94. Morris SE, Dunn-Klein M. Pre feeding skills. Tucson: Therapy Skills Builders; 1987.

95. Ohmae Y, Logemann JA, Kaiser P, et al. Timing of glottic closure during normal swallow. Head Neck 1995; 17(5):394–402.

96. Ohmae Y, Ogura M, Kitahara S, et al. Effects of head rotation on pharyngeal function during normal swallow. Ann Otol Rhinol Laryngol 1998; 107(4):344–348.

97. Olsson R, Kjellin O, Ekberg O. Videomanometric aspects of pharyngeal constrictor activity [see comments]. Dysphagia 1996; 11(2):83–86.

98. Paciaroni M, Mazzotta G, Corea F, et al. Dysphagia following stroke. Eur Neurol 2004; 51(3):162–167.

99. Palmer JB, Carden EA. The role of radiology in rehabilitation of swallowing. In: Jones B, ed. Normal and abnormal swallowing: imaging in diagnosis and therapy. 2nd edn. New York: Springer-Verlag; 2003:261–273.

100. Palmer JB, Drennan JC, Baba M. Evaluation and treatment of swallowing impairments. Am Fam Physician 2000; 61(8):2453–2462.

101. Palmer JB, DuChane AS. Rehabilitation of swallowing disorders in the elderly. In: Felsenthal GGS, Steinberg FU, eds. Rehabilitation of the aging and elderly patient. Baltimore: Williams & Wilkins; 1994:275–287.

102. Palmer JB, Hiiemae KM, Liu J. Tongue-jaw linkages in human feeding: a preliminary videofluorographic study. Arch Oral Biol 1997; 42(6):429–441.

103. Palmer JB, Holloway AM, Tanaka E. Detecting lower motor neuron dysfunction of the pharynx and larynx with electromyography. Arch Phys Med Rehabil 1991; 72(3):214–218.

104. Palmer JB, Kuhlemeier KV, Tippett DC, et al. A protocol for the videofluorographic swallowing study. Dysphagia 1993; 8(3):209–214.

105. Palmer JB, Rudin NJ, Lara G, et al. Coordination of mastication and swallowing. Dysphagia 1992; 7(4):187–200.

106. Palmer JB, Tanaka E, Ensrud E. Motions of the posterior pharyngeal wall in human swallowing: a quantitative videofluorographic study. Arch Phys Med Rehabil 2000; 81(11):1520–1526.

107. Pelletier CA, Lawless HT. Effect of citric acid and citric acid-sucrose mixtures on swallowing in neurogenic oropharyngeal dysphagia. Dysphagia 2003; 18(4):231–241.

108. Perlman AL, Palmer PM, McCulloch TM, et al. Electromyographic activity from human laryngeal, pharyngeal, and submental muscles during swallowing. J Appl Physiol 1999; 86(5):1663–1669.

109. Perry L, Love CP. Screening for dysphagia and aspiration in acute stroke: a systematic review. Dysphagia 2001; 16(1):7–18.

110. Poertner LC, Coleman RF. Swallowing therapy in adults. Otolaryngol Clin North Am 1998; 31(3):561–579.

111. Preiksaitis HG, Mayrand S, Robins K, et al. Coordination of respiration and swallowing: effect of bolus volume in normal adults. Am J Physiol 1992; 263(3 part 2):R624–R630.

112. Rosenbek JC, Roecker EB, Wood JL, et al. Thermal application reduces the duration of stage transition in dysphagia after stroke. Dysphagia 1996; 11(4):225–233.

113. Rosenthal SR, Sheppard JJ, Lotze M. Dysphagia and the child with developmental disabilities. San Diego: Singular Publishing Group; 1995.

114. Shaker R, Easterling C, Kern M, et al. Rehabilitation of swallowing by exercise in tube-fed patients with pharyngeal dysphagia secondary to abnormal UES opening. Gastroenterology 2002; 122(5):1314–1321.

115. Shaker R, Kern M, Bardan E, et al. Augmentation of deglutitive upper esophageal sphincter opening in the elderly by exercise. Am J Physiol 1997; 272(6 part 1):G1518–G1522.

116. Shaker R, Li Q, Ren J, et al. Coordination of deglutition and phases of respiration: effect of aging, tachypnea, bolus volume, and chronic obstructive pulmonary disease. Am J Physiol 1992; 263(5 part 1): G750–G755.

117. Shaker R, Ren J, Bardan E, et al. Pharyngoglottal closure reflex: characterization in healthy young, elderly and dysphagic patients with predeglutitive aspiration. Gerontology 2003; 49(1):12–20.

118. Sliwa JA, Lis S. Drug-induced dysphagia. Arch Phys Med Rehabil 1993; 74(4):445–447.

119. Smith CH, Logemann JA, Colangelo LA, et al. Incidence and patient characteristics associated with silent aspiration in the acute care setting [see comments]. Dysphagia 1999; 14(1):1–7.

120. Smith HA, Lee SH, O'Neill PA, et al. The combination of bedside swallowing assessment and oxygen saturation monitoring of swallowing in acute stroke: a safe and humane screening tool. Age Ageing 2000; 29(6): 495–499.

121. Smith-Hammond CA, New KC, Pietrobon R, et al. Prospective analysis of incidence and risk factors of dysphagia in spine surgery patients: comparison of anterior cervical, posterior cervical, and lumbar procedures. Spine 2004; 29(13):1441–1446.

122. Snyderman CH, Johnson JT. Laryngotracheal separation for intractable aspiration. Ann Otol Rhinol Laryngol 1988; 97(5 part 1):466–470.

123. Stoschus B, Allescher HD. Drug-induced dysphagia. Dysphagia 1993; 8(2):154–159.

124. Stroud AE, Lawrie BW, Wiles CM. Inter- and intra-rater reliability of cervical auscultation to detect aspiration in patients with dysphagia. Clin Rehabil 2002; 16(6):640–645.

125. Suiter DM, McCullough GH, Powell PW. Effects of cuff deflation and one-way tracheostomy speaking valve placement on swallow physiology. Dysphagia 2003; 18(4):284–292.

126. Takano Y, Suga M, Sakamoto O, et al. Satisfaction of patients treated surgically for intractable aspiration. Chest 1999; 116(5):1251–1256.

127. Teasell R, Foley N, Doherty T, et al. Clinical characteristics of patients with brainstem strokes admitted to a rehabilitation unit. Arch Phys Med Rehabil 2002; 83(7):1013–1016.

128. Tohara H, Saitoh E, Mays KA, et al. Three tests for predicting aspiration without videofluorography. Dysphagia 2003; 18(2):126–134.

129. Tolep K, Getch CL, Criner GJ. Swallowing dysfunction in patients receiving prolonged mechanical ventilation. Chest 1996; 109(1):167–172.

130. Tomita T, Tanaka K, Shinden S, et al. Tracheoesophageal diversion versus total laryngectomy for intractable aspiration. J Laryngol Otol 2004; 118(1):15–18.

131. Welch MV, Logemann JA, Rademaker AW, et al. Changes in pharyngeal dimensions effected by chin tuck. Arch Phys Med Rehabil 1993; 74(2):178–181.

132. Wisdom G, Blitzer A. Surgical therapy for swallowing disorders. Otolaryngol Clin North Am 1998; 31(3):537–560.

133. Wright RE, Boyd CS, Workman A. Radiation doses to patients during pharyngeal videofluoroscopy. Dysphagia 1998; 13(2):113–115.

134. Wu MC, Chang YC, Wang TG, et al. Evaluating swallowing dysfunction using a 100-ml water swallowing test. Dysphagia 2004; 19(1): 43–47.

135. Yoneyama T, Yoshida M, Ohrui T, et al. Oral care reduces pneumonia in older patients in nursing homes. J Am Geriatr Soc 2002; 50(3): 430–433.

136. Zhao X, Pasricha PJ. Botulinum toxin for spastic GI disorders: a systematic review. Gastrointest Endosc 2003; 57(2):219–235.

Chapter

29

Management of Bladder Dysfunction

Diana D. Cardenas and Michael E. Mayo

The first section of this chapter describes the neuroanatomy and classification of the neurogenic bladder. The discussion then addresses methods of clinical evaluation, management, surgical techniques, and common complications. Bladder dysfunction is commonly found in patients with various neurologic diseases cared for by physiatrists, and basic knowledge of these areas is essential. The diagnosis and treatment of general urologic conditions are beyond the scope of this chapter.

NEUROANATOMY

Structure and function

The detrusor muscle in humans is said to have no gap junctions, which suggests a one on one, nerve to muscle cell innervation. In the striated muscle of the distal sphincter, the majority of fibers are slow twitch, while those in the pelvic floor are a mixture of fast and slow twitch. Contraction of the detrusor muscle is started by phosphorylation of the light myosin chain and relaxed by dephosphorylation. Contraction is initiated by a rise in intracellular calcium concentration from release of calcium from intracellular sources and, more importantly, from an influx of calcium into the cell. This influx is controlled by as many as four calcium channels (three voltage-sensitive and one receptor-sensitive). This probably explains why calcium channel blockers are not effective inhibitors of detrusor activity in the clinical setting. Relaxation of the detrusor is associated with the influx of potassium into the cell. In addition to smooth muscle, collagen forms nearly 50% of the bladder wall in healthy subjects, and this proportion increases considerably in disease states.

Receptors

The receptors active during bladder contraction are cholinergic muscarinic (M_2 and M_3) receptors, and are widely distributed in the body of the bladder, trigone, bladder neck, and urethra. The M_2 receptors predominate structurally in normal bladders, but the M_3 receptors might be more important functionally. Adrenergic receptors are concentrated in the trigone, bladder neck, and urethra, and are predominantly α_1. These have recently been subdivided into α_{1a}, α_{1b}, and α_{1d}. Identification of these α_1 subgroups should allow increased specificity with regard to future therapeutic agents. Noradrenaline (norepinephrine)-containing nerve cells are also found in the paravesical

and intramural ganglia. A few authors describe noradrenaline terminals in the striated muscle of the distal sphincter, although most would dispute this. When these cells are active, they have excitatory effects and maintain continence by contraction of the bladder neck and urethral smooth muscle. β_2 and β_3 adrenergic receptors are found in the bladder neck and also in the body of the bladder. These receptors are inhibitory when activated, and can produce relaxation at the bladder neck on initiation of voiding, and relax the bladder body to enhance storage (Fig. 29-1). In humans, however, the storage role seems to be a minor one. The striated sphincter muscle contains cholinergic nicotinic receptors.

Other lower tract transmitters have been considered, but much of the evidence for their presence and activity is from animal preparations. The role of these other transmitters in normal and disease states in humans is uncertain. Many lower tract transmitters have opposing effects on lower tract function, depending on their site of action. Purine receptors (P_1, stimulated by adenosine, and P_2, stimulated by adenosine triphosphate) have their effects at the pelvic ganglia and the neuroeffector junction, and have inhibitory and facilitative effects, respectively, on the detrusor muscle. Vasointestinal polypeptide, on the other hand, enhances transmission of acetylcholine in pelvic ganglia and inhibits acetylcholine-mediated contraction in the detrusor. Neuropeptide Y has excitatory functions on detrusor muscle and indirect facilitative effects by inhibiting noradrenaline (norepinephrine) release. This transmitter also has inhibitory effects by blocking acetylcholine release and blocks the atropine-resistant bladder contraction. Tachykinins are found mostly in afferent nerves, where their effects are to augment the micturition reflex and also transmit pain sensation. Tachykinins augment the contractile and vascular response in inflammatory states. Prostaglandins cause the slow onset of contractions of the detrusor, while parathyroid hormone-related peptide causes a relaxation.

The main effector transmitter for contraction of the urethra is noradrenaline (norepinephrine), via the α_1 receptors. Smooth muscle relaxation is mediated by the effects of acetylcholine in the pelvic ganglia. This releases nitric oxide in the urethral wall, resulting in relaxation of urethral smooth muscle. Prostaglandins, in contrast to their effects on the detrusor, cause a relaxation of the urethral muscle. Prostaglandins have been tried in various clinical states of urinary retention, but without

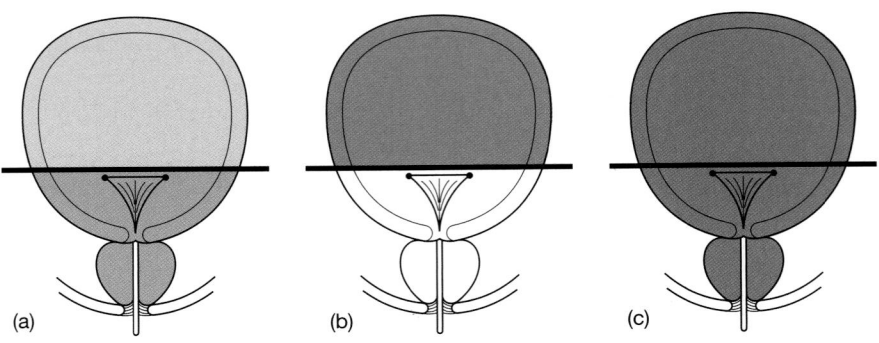

(a)   (b)   (c)

Figure 29-1 (**a**) Distribution of the α-adrenergic receptors, with few in the dome of the bladder and more in the base of the bladder and prostrate. (**b**) Distribution of the β receptors, which are largely in the dome. (**c**) Distribution of the cholinergic receptors, which are widely distributed throughout the dome and the base of the bladder and the urethra.

Table 29-1 Bladder afferent pathways

Receptor	Pelvic (parasympathetic)	Hypogastric (sympathetic)	Pudendal (somatic)
Bladder wall tension	+	−	−
Bladder mucosal nociception (pain, temperature, chemical irritation)	+	+	−
Urethral mucosal sensation (pain, temperature, passage of urine)	−	−	+

consistent results. Serotonin appears to be an antagonist that causes urethral muscle contraction. It might be important in the production of irritable urethral symptoms. The role of estrogens on the lower urinary tract in women is confined to the modification of tissues and receptors. Apparently, estrogens have no direct transmitter effects.

In the brain stem and spinal cord, the various transmitters described above can have a variety of inhibitory and facilitative actions, depending on their site of action. Serotonin might have inhibitory detrusor effects at the midbrain level, and uptake of serotonin might be blocked by tricyclics (which are used in treating nocturnal enuresis). Activation of opiate receptors in the brain stem and sacral spinal cord inhibits voiding. This might partly explain the retention of urine seen with the use of these agents.[36] The pudendal motor neuron bodies are situated in the lateral border of the ventral horn of the sacral cord (Onuf's nucleus). Serotonin and noradrenaline (norepinephrine) reuptake inhibitors prolong the effect of these agents in the synaptic cleft of Onuf's nucleus, and thus increase the activity of the external sphincter. Such a dual agent (duloxetine) is currently under trial for stress incontinence in women and might be useful for some neurologic bladder conditions.[18] A complete discussion of the pharmacology of the lower urinary tract can be found in Steers.[36]

Innervation

The afferent and efferent peripheral pathways include the autonomic by way of the pelvic (parasympathetic) and hypogastric (sympathetic) nerves, and the somatic through the pudendal

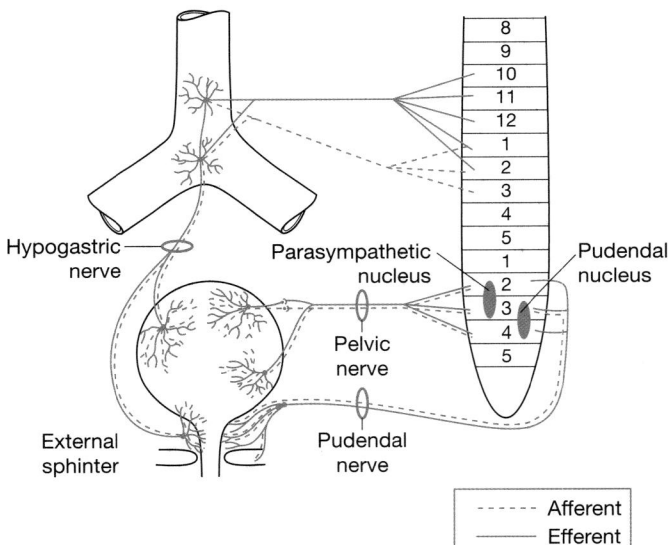

```
----- Afferent
——— Efferent
```

Figure 29-2 The parasympathetic, sympathetic, and somatic nerve supply to the bladder, urethra, and pelvic floor. (From Blaivas 1980,[5] with permission.)

nerves (Table 29-1 and Fig. 29-2). In healthy individuals, the volume of the bladder and the normal voiding reflex is routed via the afferent Aδ fibers. In pathologic states, vanilloid receptor stimulation excites C-afferent fibers, which might mediate the bladder dysfunction due to inflammatory reactions. In suprasacral neurogenic bladder disease, these capsaicin-sensitive

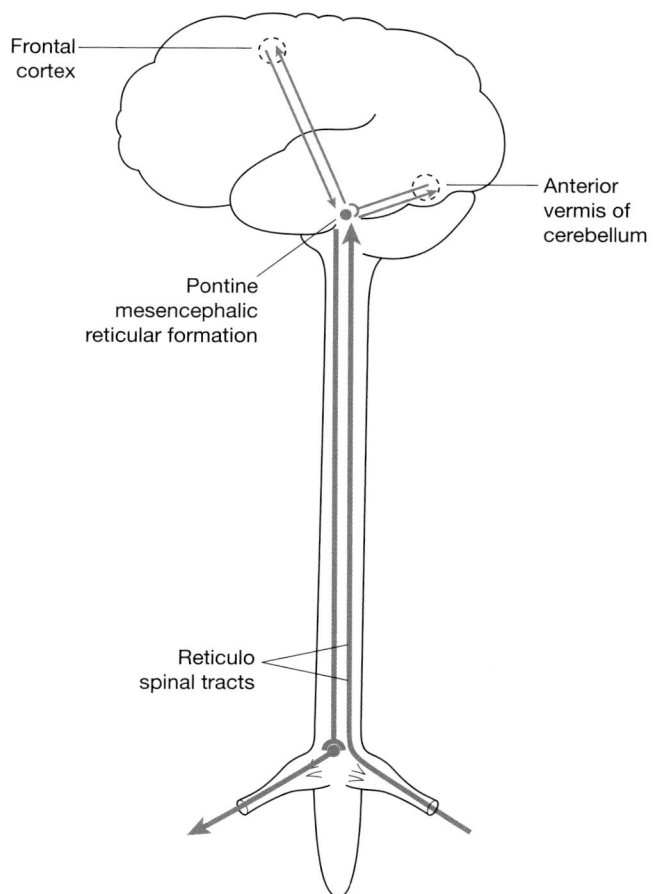

Figure 29-3 The central connections of the bladder reflex are shown, with the afferents ascending possibly in the reticulospinal tracts or the posterior columns to the pontine mesencephalic reticular formation and the efferents running down to the sacral outflow in the reticulospinal tracts. The pontine center is largely influenced by the cortex but also by other areas of the brain, particularly the cerebellum and basal ganglia. (From Bradley and Brantley 1978,[8] with permission.)

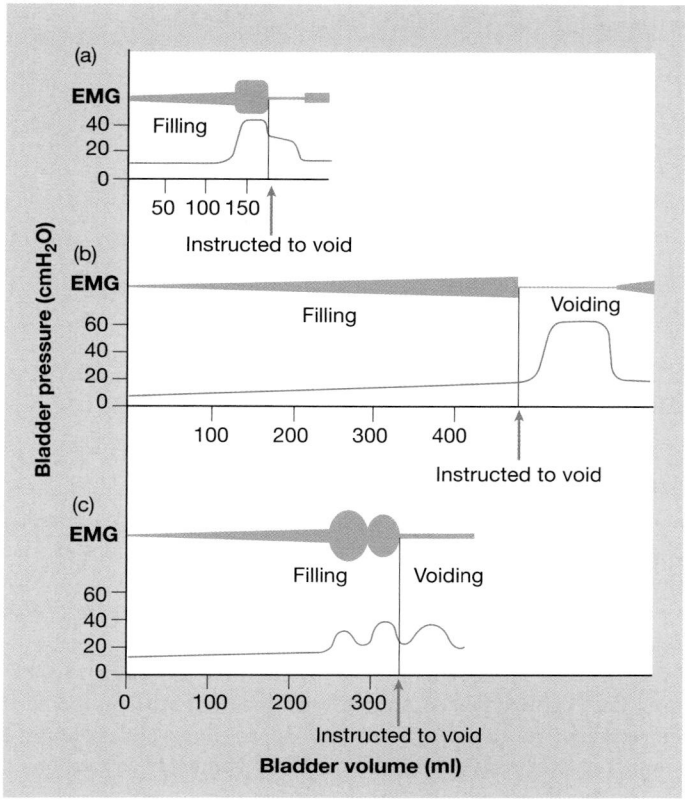

Figure 29-4 Diagram of external sphincter electromyography (EMG) and bladder pressure during filling and voiding in a 2-year-old boy (**a**), a normal male adult (**b**), and an elderly man (**c**). In (**a**), a bladder contraction occurs during filling, which the child attempts to suppress to stay continent by contracting his external sphincter. In (**b**), there are no contractions during filling. Voiding is initiated by a relaxation of the sphincter before the bladder contracts. In (**c**), there are contractions during filling, which the patient tries to suppress. The voiding contraction is low pressure and poorly sustained, leading to incomplete emptying; a condition frequently found in the elderly.

vanilloid receptors and C afferents have a major role in the pathogenesis of hyperactivity. Intravesical capsaicin and resiniferatoxin, which block transmission through C-afferent fibers for several months, have been used experimentally to treat hyperactivity when it does not respond to the usual pharmacologic agents.[22,25]

Central connections and control
The reflex center for the bladder lies in the pons along with the other autonomic centers (Fig. 29-3). Not shown in Figure 29-3 is a reflex with afferent axons originating from the bladder and synapsing on the pudendal nerve nucleus at S2, S3, and S4 (Onuf's nucleus). This allows inhibition of pelvic floor activity during voiding. Another important reflex uses the local segmental innervation of the external sphincter with afferents from the urethra, sphincter, and pelvic floor and efferents in the pudendal nerve. Higher (voluntary) control over the pelvic floor is achieved through afferents that ascend to the sensory cortex.

Descending fibers from the motor cortex synapse with the pudendal motor nucleus.[9]

BLADDER FUNCTION

Urodynamic studies in both intact patients and those with neurologic disease have yielded clinical insights into the normal and abnormal function of the lower urinary tract over the course of life (Fig. 29-4).

Infant and young child
Neonates and infants have truly reflex bladders that empty at approximately 50- to 100-mL volumes. Sometime after the first year of life, the child begins to show some awareness of bladder evacuation and can begin to delay urination for a brief period by contracting the voluntary sphincter. For normal control, the detrusor reflex has to be inhibited by the higher centers at the level of the pontine nucleus. By 5 years of age, approximately 90% of children have normal control. The remaining 10% have

Table 29-2 Functional classification of the neurogenic bladder

Type of failure	Bladder factors	Outlet factors
Failure to store	Hyperactivity Decreased compliance	Denervated pelvic floor Bladder neck descent Intrinsic bladder neck sphincter failure
Failure to empty	Areflexia Hypocontractility	Detrusor–sphincter dyssynergia (striated sphincter and bladder neck) Non-relaxing voluntary sphincter Mechanical obstruction (benign prostatic hypertrophy or stricture)

a more infantile or immature pattern, with detrusor activity between voluntary voidings that produces frequency, urgency, and occasionally urge incontinence and nocturnal enuresis. Most of these children gradually develop inhibition of the detrusor reflex by the onset of puberty.

Adult

With bladder filling, there is only a minimal rise in intravesical pressure (known as accommodation), together with an increase in recruitment of activity in the pelvic floor and voluntary sphincter. Normal voiding is initiated by voluntary relaxation of the pelvic floor, with subsequent release of inhibition of the detrusor reflex at the pontine level. The detrusor contraction is maintained steadily throughout voiding, and the pelvic floor remains quiescent.

Elderly

Frequency, urgency, and incontinence with incomplete emptying are common in the elderly. Urodynamic studies show that many elderly persons have bladder contractions during filling, producing frequency, urgency, and incontinence. These contractions are poorly sustained during voiding and result in incomplete evacuation. Elderly men can have prostatic obstruction, and women can have incontinence related to impaired sphincter activity or stress incontinence. In the absence of these mechanical factors, changes in bladder function in the elderly have been ascribed to loss of cerebral control due to minor strokes, and to changes in the bladder wall due to collagen deposition. Changes in bladder function can also result from polyuria secondary to reduced renal concentrating ability, diuretic use, lack of normal increase in antidiuretic hormone secretion at night, and mobilization of lower extremity edema during sleep.

CLASSIFICATION

The neurogenic bladder has been classified in a variety of ways, beginning with the anatomic classification of Bors and Comarr.[7] The first functional classification was based on cystometric findings, and five basic groups were described: reflex, uninhibited, autonomous, motor paralytic, and sensory neurogenic bladders.[32] This system does not take into account the function of

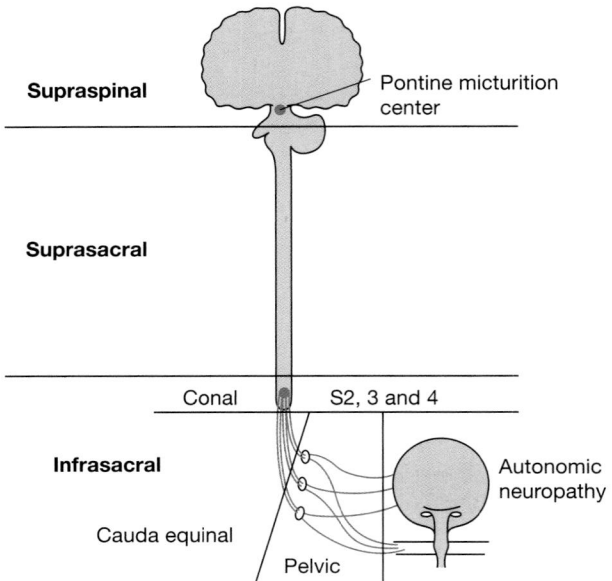

Figure 29-5 Anatomic classification of the neurogenic bladder.

the sphincter mechanisms, however, and there are a few patients in whom the detrusor reflex does not return after spinal cord injury above the sacral outflow. Later, a more anatomic classification system was proposed, in which the neurogenic bladder was subdivided into types such as supraspinal, suprasacral spinal, infrasacral, peripheral autonomic, and muscular lesions (Fig. 29-5). At the same time, others developed functional classifications, all of which were based on conventional urodynamic evaluations. This was an attempt to categorize the lower urinary tract according to the passive storage ability of the bladder, and the activities and coordination of the detrusor and sphincter mechanisms (Table 29-2). In practice it is common to use a combination of both anatomic and functional classifications, with any known neurologic lesion described in anatomic terms (e.g. supraspinal, suprasacral). Clinical management is based on functional changes as demonstrated by conventional urodynamic testing.

HISTORY AND PHYSICAL EXAMINATION

Although the symptoms associated with neuropathologic bladder processes are often misleading and correlate poorly with objective findings, relief of symptoms is one of the patient's main concerns. It is often helpful to have the patient or attendant record fluid intake, output, and incontinence episodes over several 24-h periods. Such record keeping can show whether there is excessive intake or reversed diurnal rhythm of urine production. The history should help determine whether there were voiding symptoms prior to the putative neurologic event, any premorbid conditions (such as diabetes), stroke, and prior urologic or pelvic surgery. The neurologic diagnosis, especially the level of the lesion and its completeness, is important in predicting the type of lower urinary tract dysfunction that might be expected.

The physical examination should assess mental status and confirm the level of the neurologic deficit (if present). The perineal sensation and pelvic floor muscle tone are particularly important in patients with lower spinal cord and peripheral lesions. Reflexes are also important, but the bulbocavernous, cremasteric, and anal reflexes are sometimes difficult to elicit, even in intact subjects. The skin of the perineum and the state of bladder supports should be assessed. The degree of vaginal support and estrogenization should be assessed in women. Evidence of good estrogenization is pink and moist vaginal mucosa with good rugae. Lack of estrogenization is seen as pale, dry, and smooth vaginal mucosa. The prostate in males should be evaluated, but prostate size or consistency alone is not a good indicator of obstruction. It is also important to assess the patient's motivation, lifestyle, body habitus, and other physical impairments.

Table 29-3 Urodynamic definitions

Term	Definition
Bladder	
Hyperactivity	Contractions of the detrusor during filling, due to neurologic disease
Hypocontractility	Unsustained contractions causing failure to empty
Areflexia	Absent contractions with attempt to void
Compliance	Change in volume divided by change in baseline pressure with filling ($<10\,mL/cmH_2O$ abnormal; $10–20\,mL/cmH_2O$ borderline if capacity reduced)
Outlet	
Detrusor–sphincter dyssynergia	
At bladder neck	Usually in high tetraplegic patients with autonomic hyperactivity
At striated sphincter	Uncoordinated pelvic floor and striated sphincter contraction with detrusor contraction during attempts to void
Non-relaxing sphincter	Poor voluntary relaxation of voluntary sphincter in patients with areflexia attempting to void by Valsalva's maneuver
Decreased outlet resistance	Incontinence due to damage to the bladder neck or striated sphincter, pelvic floor descent, or denervation

DIAGNOSTIC TESTS

Indications

The extent of upper and lower urinary tract testing has to be individualized for each patient and each neurologic condition. The upper tracts need evaluation if there are symptoms suggestive of pyelonephritis or prior history of renal disease. Some neurologic conditions—such as strokes, Parkinson disease, and multiple sclerosis—rarely or only occasionally cause upper tract involvement. For these conditions, a simple baseline screening test such as renal ultrasonography (US) is sufficient. Conditions such as those involving a complete spinal cord lesion and myelodysplasia need more extensive and regular upper tract surveillance, with both structural and functional tests. The lower urinary tract evaluation can be quite simple, from urinalysis to urine culture to measurement of postvoid residual (PVR). A full urodynamic evaluation might be necessary, however, especially if incomplete bladder emptying, incontinence, recurrent bacteriuria, or upper tract changes are present.

The bladder findings on urodynamic studies cannot be used alone to determine the level of neurologic lesion. For example, a suprasacral neurogenic bladder from a complete spinal cord injury can remain areflexic, and a conal or cauda equinal bladder

can exhibit high pressures from poor compliance (see Table 29-3). While the anatomic level of the neurologic lesion can suggest to the clinician the most likely pattern of bladder dysfunction, urodynamic testing should be performed to confirm this.

Upper tract tests
Ultrasonography

Ultrasonography is a low-risk and relatively low-cost test for routine evaluation of the upper urinary tract. It is not sensitive enough to evaluate acute ureteral obstruction, and in this clinical setting non-contrast-enhanced computed tomography (CT) should be performed. US is adequate for imaging chronic obstruction and dilatation, scarring, renal masses (both cystic and solid), and renal stones. The ureter is seen on US imaging only if dilated. The bladder, if partially filled, can be evaluated for wall thickness, irregularity, and the presence of bladder stones.

Plain radiography of the urinary tract: kidneys, ureter, and bladder

A plain radiography of the kidneys, ureter, and bladder (KUB) study is often combined with US to identify any possible radio-paque calculi in the ureter or bladder stones not seen on US.

Computed tomography

Computed tomography is often performed without contrast agent enhancement (CT-KUB) and has replaced the regular KUB, US, and excretory urography in the evaluation of the upper tracts when acute obstruction from stones is a possibility. It is also the most sensitive study for detecting small bladder stones in patients with an indwelling catheter, in whom the bladder is collapsed around the catheter.

Excretory urography or CT-IVP

A CT without and then with intravenous contrast, with a delayed plain KUB film (computed tomography–intravenous pyelography, CT-IVP), has largely replaced the excretory urogram. If the serum creatinine concentration is more than 1.5 mg/dL, or if the patient has insulin-dependent diabetes, intravenous contrast agent administration increases the risk of contrast-related nephropathy. In these cases, alternative studies include US, radioisotope renography, and possibly cystoscopy with retrograde pyelography.

Creatinine clearance time

This has been the gold standard for assessing renal function, and is said to approximate the glomerular filtration rate. Its accuracy depends on meticulous urine collection. It can also be misleading in some clinical situations. For example, in tetraplegic patients with low muscle mass and a 24-h creatinine excretion of less than 1000 mg, the calculated creatinine clearance time can be too inaccurate to be clinically useful.

Isotope studies

The technetium-99m dimercaptosuccinic acid (DMSA) scan is still the best study for both differential function and evaluation of the functioning areas of the renal cortex. The renogram obtained with technetium-99m mertiatide (MAG-3) also gives information on urinary tract drainage, as well as a good assessment of differential function. In patients who might have ureteral reflux, these studies should be done only after the bladder has been drained with an indwelling catheter.

Lower tract tests

Urinalysis, culture, and sensitivity testing

These tests are done routinely for all patients with neurogenic bladder disease and should be repeated as often as necessary. Bacteriuria should be treated before any invasive test is performed.

Postvoid residual

By itself, a low PVR of less than 20% of capacity is not indicative of a 'balanced' bladder as it was once defined. High intravesical pressures can be present despite low PVR values. The PVR is simple to determine and clinically useful, especially when compared with prior recordings and taken in conjunction with the bladder pressure, the clinical symptoms, and the appearance of the bladder wall. A catheter insertion has been used for PVR in the past, but there are now simple US machines that non-invasively obtain the PVR.[12]

Cystography

This study is usually performed to test for the presence or absence of ureteral reflux, and it also shows the outline and shape of the bladder. The procedure is usually performed in the radiology department, often with no control over the rate of bladder filling and without any monitoring of intravesical pressure. It is often helpful in planning management to know the level of intravesical pressure at which ureteral reflux occurred. Significant bacteriuria should be treated before the test is performed. Blood pressure should be monitored throughout the test in all patients with spinal cord lesions above T6 who are at risk for autonomic dysreflexia. In many cases, a full videourodynamic study, which includes fluoroscopy of the bladder and monitoring of the intravesical pressure, is more clinically useful. This study is described later.

Cystometrography

Cystometrography (CMG) is a filling study and gives little information about the voiding phase of bladder function. Although carbon dioxide as a filling medium is convenient with the commercially available apparatus, this type of testing has shown considerable variability, poor reproducibility, and the presence of artifacts due to leakage of CO_2 gas around the catheter. Hyperemia of the bladder mucosa has also been noted at cystoscopy immediately after CO_2 use. An advantage of the CO_2 CMG is that any size of catheter can be employed, as there is little resistance to flow and therefore no pressure artifact from the pump.

Water CMGs are best obtained with a two-channel catheter, with one channel used for filling and the other for pressure recording. A rectal pressure trace is also helpful in many patients to help distinguish intravesical pressure variations (due to intraabdominal transmission) from contractions of the detrusor itself. Reported filling rates vary but are usually in the range of 25–60 mL/min. During filling, patients are asked to suppress voiding. Normal values include a capacity of 300–600 mL, with an initial sensation of filling at approximately 50% of capacity. The sensation of normal fullness is said to be appreciated in the lower abdomen, with a sense of urgency in the perineum. The change in volume divided by the rise in baseline pressure during filling (i.e. in the absence of a detrusor contraction) describes the bladder's compliance. This value should be greater than 10 mL/cm H_2O, and 10–20 mL/cm H_2O is borderline if the bladder capacity is reduced. Normal persons are able to suppress detrusor contractions during this test. Any detrusor contraction during the test, usually defined as a phasic pressure change of more than 15 cm H_2O, is abnormal. If the patient is neurologically intact, these contractions were referred to as uninhibited. If the patient has a suprasacral or supraspinal lesion, these contractions are called hyperreflexic.[2] Overactive or hyperactive are terms now used to describe both types of contractions.

Although patients can be instructed to try to void at capacity, many are unable to generate a detrusor contraction. The presence of an easily obtainable involuntary detrusor contraction confirms the presence of hyperactivity in a patient with a suprasacral or supraspinal lesion. The absence of a contraction, however, does not necessarily imply true areflexia in a patient with an infrasacral lesion. The CO_2 CMG is a useful bedside test to monitor the return of a detrusor reflex in the spinal shock phase of spinal cord injury, and to confirm the presence of detrusor hyperactivity in patients with supraspinal or cerebral insult before pharmacotherapy is started.

Sphincter electromyography

Sphincter EMG can be combined with the CMG, or preferably with a full multichannel videourodynamic study.[30] Recordings have been made with a variety of electrodes (monopolar, coaxial needle, and surface electrodes) from the levator, perianal, or periurethral muscles. Because some authors claim there is a functional dissociation between these muscle groups, periurethral recordings are preferred. The integrated EMG is displayed on the same trace as the bladder pressure. EMG activity gradually increases as bladder capacity is reached during bladder filling, and then becomes silent just prior to voiding. Low levels of EMG activity with no recruitment during filling are a common pattern in complete spinal cord injury. When a reflex detrusor contraction occurs in these patients, the EMG activity in the sphincter can increase rather than decrease. With this detrusor–sphincter dyssynergia, voiding often occurs toward the end of the detrusor contraction, as the striated sphincter relaxes more quickly than the smooth muscle of the bladder. This type of sphincter EMG does not display individual motor units, and cannot be used for the evaluation of infrasacral denervation of the pelvic floor musculature (for which standard needle EMG is needed). Diagnostic integrated EMG recordings from the external urethral sphincter are difficult to obtain, and are invasive and painful in patients who are sensate. The fluoroscopic appearance of the urethra is an alternative method of determining sphincter dysfunction, and is preferred after distal sphincterotomy if recurrent distal sphincter dyssynergia is suspected (Fig. 29-6).

Videourodynamics

This study is designed to give the maximum information about the filling and voiding phases of lower urinary tract function, and every effort is made to make it as physiologic as possible.[6] A videourodynamic study is indicated in the following patients:

- those with incomplete spinal cord lesions with incontinence who have some ability to void and inhibit voiding voluntarily but empty incompletely;
- persons with mechanical obstruction (e.g. benign prostatic hyperplasia) with neuropathy;
- candidates for sphincterotomy, to assess detrusor contraction and the presence or absence of bladder neck

obstruction in addition to striated sphincter dyssynergia;
- those who fail to respond to pharmacotherapy;
- those who may be candidates for surgical procedures such as augmentation, continent diversion, or placement of an artificial sphincter or a suprapubic catheter;
- patients who have deterioration of the upper tracts; and
- patients who relapse frequently with symptomatic bacteriuria.

The procedure requires placement of a 7-F two-channel catheter in the bladder and an 8-F balloon catheter in the rectum. EMG of the sphincter can be recorded along with bladder, rectal, and detrusor (bladder minus rectal) pressures. A contrast solution delivered at 50 mL/min is used to fill the bladder, with the patient sitting or lying as appropriate. The blood pressure is recorded in patients with spinal cord lesions above T6 to determine if there is any autonomic dysreflexia. The bladder image is monitored intermittently with fluoroscopy, and the combined radiographic and urodynamic image is mixed on the same screen and can be recorded on videotape (Fig. 29-6). If the patient can sit and void during the study, a flow rate can also be recorded. A videourodynamic study in children with myelodysplasia or spinal cord injury might have to be modified, and adequate clinical information can often be obtained by recording bladder pressure combined with fluoroscopy. Table 29-3 lists urodynamic terms used to categorize bladder and outlet abnormalities.

Cystoscopy

The only routine indication for cystoscopy is the presence of a long-term indwelling suprapubic or urethral catheter, because the presence of the catheter increases the risk of bladder tumor development.[37] Cystoscopy is recommended after 5 years in high-risk patients, such as smokers, or after 10 years in those with no risk factors. Cystoscopy should also be performed after CT-IVP in patients who have gross or microscopic hematuria that cannot be clearly associated with urinary tract infection (UTI), stones, or trauma. Bladder stones can usually be detected on plain radiographs or US, but often CT-KUB is the only study that will pick up small stones, especially if the bladder is collapsed around an indwelling catheter. Repeated lower tract infections can be an indication for cystoscopy and can reveal non-opaque foreign bodies, such as hairs, that have been introduced by catheterization.

Other tests
Urethral pressure profiles

Urethral pressure profiles are obtained by withdrawing a measuring device (microtip transducer or perfused side-hole catheter) gradually down the urethra and measuring the centrally oriented forces. It has limited value except in determining whether a sphincter-active area is still present after a sphincterotomy, which can also be evaluated by videourodynamics.

Bethanechol (Urecholine) stimulation test

The bethanechol stimulation test is based on Cannon's law of denervation, which says that an end organ becomes

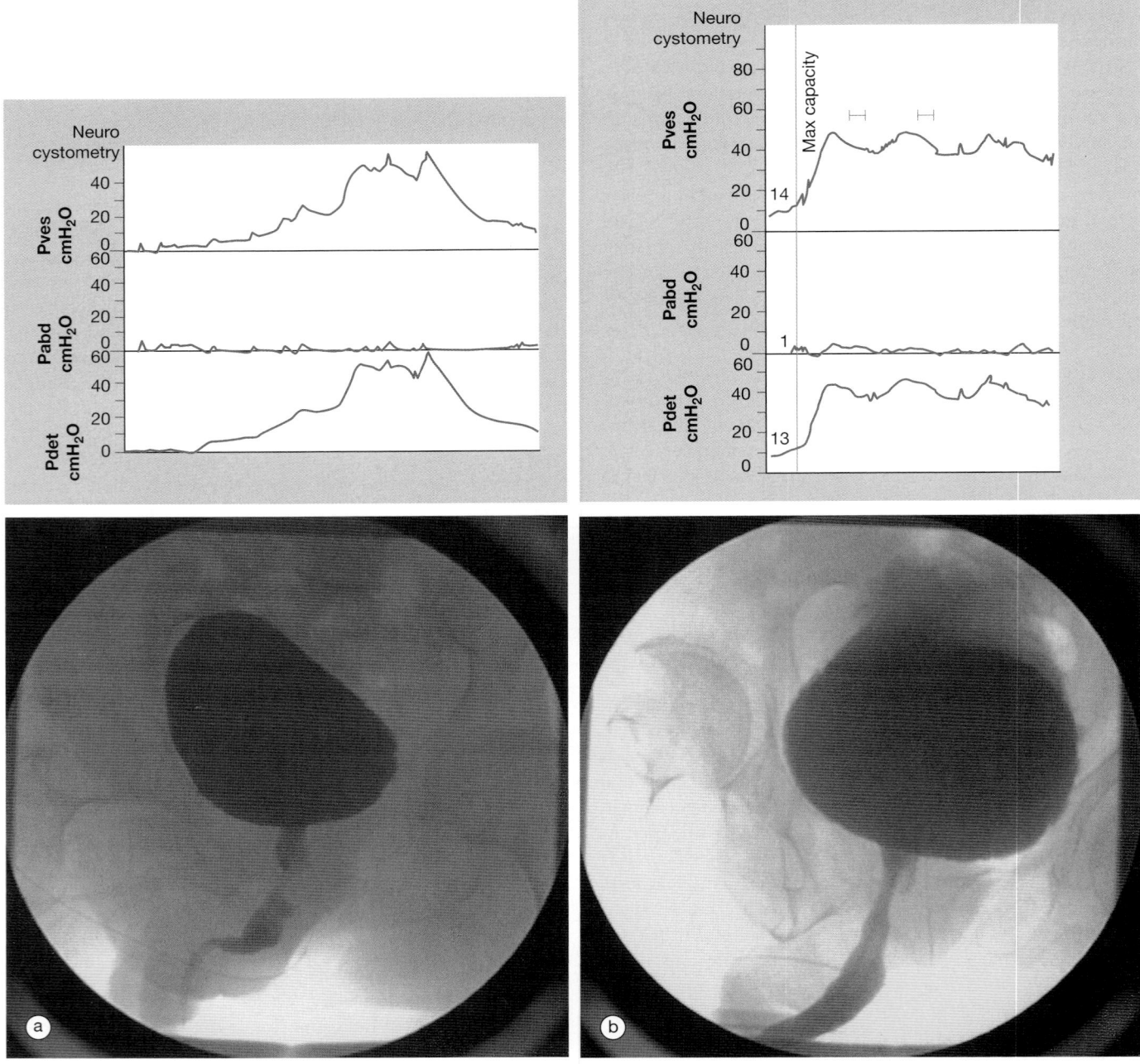

Figure 29-6 (**a**) A videourodynamic study in a male tetraplegic showing recurrent distal sphincter dyssynergia. (**b**) A similar study in a similar patient, showing no evidence of dyssynergia.

supersensitive to its neurotransmitter when denervated. The test is performed in patients with possible infrasacral lesions when the detrusor appears to be areflexic. A rise in baseline pressure of more than 20 cm H_2O on CMG at a volume of 100 mL is considered a positive result. Unfortunately, false positives and false negatives do occur, and the test is positive only in complete decentralization.

MANAGEMENT

General principles

Bladder management should be undertaken in the context of the whole person. Patient goals are to empty the bladder not more than every 3–4 h, remain continent, sleep without interference from the urinary drainage system, and avoid recurrent UTI or other complications. Less than optimal bladder manage-

Table 29-4 Bladder management options

Problem	Options
Failure to store	
Bladder factors	
Behavioral	Timed voids
Collecting devices	Diaper, condom catheter, indwelling catheter
Clean intermittent catheterization	With drugs to lower bladder pressure
Drugs	Anticholinergics, intrathecal baclofen,[a] calcium channel blockers,[a] intravesical vanilloids (resiniferatoxin),[a] botulinum A injection[a]
Surgery	Augmentation, continent diversion, denervation procedures[a]
Outlet factors	
Behavioral	Timed voids, pelvic floor exercises
Collecting devices	Diaper, condom catheter, indwelling catheter
Drugs	α-Agonists, imipramine, estrogens
Surgery	Collagen injection, fascial sling, artificial sphincter, Teflon injection[a]
Failure to empty	
Bladder factors	
Behavioral	Timed voids, bladder stimulation, Valsalva's and Credé's maneuvers
Collecting devices	Indwelling catheter
Clean intermittent catheterization	
Drugs	Bethanechol
Surgery	Neurostimulation[a]
Outlet factors	
Behavioral	Anal stretch void
Collecting devices	Indwelling catheters
Clean intermittent catheterization	
Drugs	α-Blockers, oral striated muscle relaxant, intrathecal baclofen[a]
Surgery	Sphincterotomy incision, stent sphincterotomy, bladder neck incision, prostate resection, pudendal neurectomy[a]
Failure of storage and emptying with non-usable urethra	
Surgery	Suprapubic catheter with or without bladder neck closure, ileal conduit, continent diversion

[a]Experimental or non-standard management.

ment decreases the person's social, vocational, and avocational potential. The following discussion describes specific management approaches (Table 29-4).

Approaches and rationale

Behavioral management

Timed voiding For patients with hyperactivity producing urgency or reflex incontinence, a timed voiding program can help by having the patient urinate before the anticipated detrusor contraction. The limitation to this program is that persons with dementia need continual reminding. It is also useful in patients with sphincter weakness, as the incontinence is worse when the bladder is full, and timed voiding reduces the amount of urine leakage.

Bladder stimulation Various maneuvers have been tried to stimulate the bladder. Stroking or pinching the perineal skin to cause reflex stimulation is only rarely effective. Suprapubic tapping or jabbing over the bladder causes a mechanical stretch of the bladder wall and subsequent contraction. Controlled studies have shown that deeper indentation of the bladder with a jabbing technique is the most effective maneuver.[13] This can be used by spinal cord-injured patients with condom catheters. It is most effective in patients with paraplegia who have good upper limb function.

Valsalva's and Credé's maneuvers   Patients with areflexia and some denervation of the pelvic floor (infrasacral lesions) are able to void by doing a Valsalva maneuver or straining. This is most effective in women, because even the partially paralyzed pelvic floor descends with straining, and the bladder neck opens. Over time, however, the pelvic floor descent increases as the paralyzed muscles atrophy and stretch, and the patient complains of worsening stress incontinence. In men, complete flaccidity of the pelvic floor may allow emptying by straining. Credé's maneuver, usually performed by an attendant, mechanically pushes urine out of the bladder in patients with tetraplegia. The abdominal wall must be relaxed to allow Credé's maneuver to be effective, and there is a theoretic risk of producing ureteral reflux by the long-term use of this method.

Anal stretch voiding   In patients with paraplegia who have a spastic pelvic floor, effective voiding has been achieved by an anal stretch technique. This technique involves relaxing the pelvic floor by first stretching the anal sphincter and then emptying the bladder by Valsalva's maneuver.[26] It requires transfer on to a toilet for bladder emptying, absence of anal sensation, and the ability to generate adequate intraabdominal pressure. For these reasons, it is not widely used, even though the technique was well described more than 20 years ago.

Pelvic floor exercises   Kegel exercises are effective only in female patients with stress incontinence due to pelvic floor descent. Most patients with infrasacral neuropathy need surgery to achieve continence.

Urine collection devices

External condom catheters   External condom catheters are convenient and often the best management for men with tetraplegia who are unable to perform self-catheterization, provided that any outflow obstruction is adequately treated. Although attendants and family members can perform intermittent catheterization, the program often breaks down if the patient is at school or work. Bacteriuria with fever is more common in those who have intermittent catheterization done by an attendant than in those on any other bladder management program, including indwelling catheterization.[14] Problems with skin breakdown and urethral damage can occur if the condom is applied too tightly. There is also an increased risk of UTI because of poor hygiene. The risk is increased in patients who have to do intermittent catheterization because of inadequate emptying and who also need a condom catheter for incontinence.

Indwelling catheters   Indwelling catheters can be either urethral or suprapubic, and are typically used either because other programs have failed or for patient convenience. The combination of sphincterotomy and condom drainage, although ideal for men with tetraplegia, often fails because of inadequate detrusor contractions or penile skin problems. In the past, indwelling catheters had a justifiably bad reputation, but there are recent reports that some patients with indwelling catheters do no worse than those on other methods of management.[17] This change is due to a number of factors, including improved catheter materials. Good catheter care is still very important. Some of the important aspects of care include monthly catheter changes, copious fluid intake, control of hyperactivity with medication, sterilization of the collecting bags with bleach, and avoidance of traction on the catheter. The prevalence of squamous cell carcinoma of the bladder associated with an indwelling catheter might be lower than reported.[37] Most centers continue to recommend yearly cystoscopy, cytology, and biopsy, if indicated, when the patient has had an indwelling catheter in place for 10 years or more, and possibly after only 5 years if there are increased risk factors such as smoking.

Adult diapers and other protective garments   Protective garments have improved considerably over the past few years, and a high-absorbency gel-impregnated material is now used that allows the lining against the patient's perineal skin to stay dry. Protective garments are commonly used in incontinent patients with dementia who have adequate bladder emptying.

Clean intermittent catheterization

Intermittent catheterization using a sterile technique was introduced by Guttmann and Frankel in the 1950s for the treatment of patients with acute spinal cord injury. Lapides et al. in 1972 proposed a non-sterile but 'clean' technique for the management of chronic retention and infection.[27] The technique has since been employed extensively for neurogenic bladder disease. An intermittent catheter program requires a low-pressure bladder of adequate capacity (>300 mL) and enough outflow resistance to maintain continence with normal daily activities. If the bladder is not sufficiently areflexic and compliant, anticholinergics can be used. If these fail, some form of surgery, such as augmentation, can be done to achieve a low-pressure reservoir. Men with lesions at C6 and below, and women with lesions at C7 and below, can usually manage self-catheterization. Patients should restrict fluid intake to maintain an output of not more than 600 mL in the time period chosen. Some patients have enough sensation to be able to catheterize on demand, but most have to do so on a timed schedule. A minimum of three catheterizations per 24 h is recommended, because longer intervals between catheterizations theoretically increase the risk of symptomatic bacteriuria. Most patients wash their catheters with soap and tap water, and reuse the catheters. In those patients with recurrent UTIs, other types of catheters (touchless, enclosed systems, or hydrophilic catheters) or sterilization of catheters can be helpful in reducing infections. It should be noted, however, that evidence for the efficacy of hydrophilic catheters is lacking. A completely sterile technique can also be used but is rarely done in clinical practice.

The most common problems with self-catheterization are symptomatic bacteriuria, urethral trauma, and incontinence. Occasionally, a bladder stone formed on a nidus of hair or lint is found, and patients should be warned to avoid introducing foreign material into the bladder with the catheter. Urethral trauma and catheterization difficulties are usually due to sphincter spasm. This can be managed by using extra lubrication and local anesthetic urethral gel (lidocaine 2%). Sometimes, a curved tip (coudé) catheter is helpful. Repeated urethral bleeding suggests the presence of a break in the urethral mucosa or a false passage, and using an indwelling urethral catheter for a period of time might be necessary for this to resolve. Urethroscopy and unroofing of a false passage is occasionally necessary.

Drugs

Many drugs for lower urinary tract management have been tried, with the rationale for their use often based on animal and organ bath experiments. Bladder management drugs in humans have generally been disappointing. The most effective group is those that inhibit detrusor activity.

Cholinergic agents   The detrusor is innervated by cholinergic muscarinic (M_2 and M_3) receptors. Bethanechol, a cholinergic agonist, can be helpful in detrusor areflexia by increasing detrusor activity. Although a pharmacologic effect can be seen with a parenteral dose when the bladder is partially innervated, oral doses are not effective at levels that can be tolerated by patients. Double-blind, controlled clinical trials have not been performed, and the use of this drug has declined.[20]

Anticholinergic agents   Anticholinergic agents have been used for many years for the suppression of detrusor activity. Propantheline bromide (15–30 mg three times a day) is the prototype, and hyoscyamine (0.125–0.2 mg three or four times a day) has also been used. Oxybutynin hydrochloride, taken at 5–10 mg three times a day has similar actions. Oxybutynin in solution can be administered as an intravesical instillation in patients on intermittent catheterization. It appears to be effective, although somewhat delayed serum levels result that are almost as high as with the oral route. The side effects include mostly dry mouth and constipation, and appear to be less severe than when the drug is given by the oral route.[28] A problem with this technique is that, at present, there is no sterile liquid form, and the 5-mg tablet has to be dissolved in sterile water.

Imipramine is recommended by several authors for its presumed anticholinergic actions. It is said to be additive in its effectiveness when combined with other agents, such as oxybutynin and propantheline. It does not seem to increase side effects. Oxybutynin is now available as a once a day slow-release preparation, which might decrease side effects. A new transdermal preparation is now available that avoids having much of the drug being broken down in the liver (which occurs after oral administration). This is important, because the side effects are due to the breakdown product. Although this is a promising treatment, skin irritation might limit the use of this preparation. Tolterodine, in a dose of 2 mg twice daily, has anticholinergic activity, has fewer troublesome side effects, and is also available as a slow-release oral preparation. Several new, more bladder-specific anticholinergics are on trial and might soon be available (darifenacin, solifenacin, and trospium).

Adrenergic antagonists   The α-adrenergic receptor antagonist phenoxybenzamine (10–30 mg/day) has α_1- and α_2-blocking actions and has been used for inhibiting smooth muscle activity at the bladder neck and in the prostate. Newer agents with more specific α_1-blocking actions are available, such as prazosin, terazosin, and doxazosin.[38] These are typically given in doses of 1–20 mg/day as tolerated. These agents have a number of effects. They appear to reduce the irritative symptoms in men with obstruction due to benign prostatic hyperplasia, and to increase emptying in patients with neurogenic voiding dysfunction. A more specific agent, tamsulosin (0.4–0.8 mg), has been used for the treatment of benign prostatic hyperplasia. This agent has fewer vascular effects and rarely causes hypotension. After suprasacral spinal cord injury, it improved bladder storage and emptying, and decreased the symptoms of autonomic dysreflexia.[1] All these agents are effective in control of the vascular manifestations of autonomic dysreflexia. Phenoxybenzamine, with its α_1- and α_2-blocking action, might be a better choice in this regard than the pure α_1-blocking agents.

Adrenergic agonists   Adrenergic agonists have been used to increase urethral resistance in patients with mild stress incontinence. Anecdotally, ephedrine (25–75 mg/day) has been effective in controlling mild stress incontinence in children with myelodysplasia, but controlled studies are lacking. Adrenergic agonists are rarely used in adults with bladder neuropathy. Prolongation of the α-adrenergic effects on the external urethral sphincter could be possible in future using duloxetine, a serotonin and noradrenaline (norepinephrine) reuptake inhibitor that acts on the pudendal (Onuf's) nucleus in the sacral cord.

Estrogens   Postmenopausal women often have atrophy of the urethral submucosa, which can lead to stress incontinence. Estrogen administration by local application often restores or maintains this tissue and can be helpful in women with a partially denervated pelvic floor and stress incontinence.

Muscle relaxants   Baclofen, tizanidine, and dantrolene sodium are frequently used for skeletal muscle spasticity (see Ch. 31) but have never been shown to be effective in controlled studies in patients with detrusor striated sphincter dyssynergia. Baclofen given intrathecally by infusion pump for severe lower extremity spasticity depresses pelvic floor reflexes but also depresses the detrusor reflex.[35] The net result is a lower pressure bladder that might empty less effectively. Insofar as intrathecal baclofen is indicated in some patients with tetraplegia, this overall decrease in bladder emptying might not be desirable.

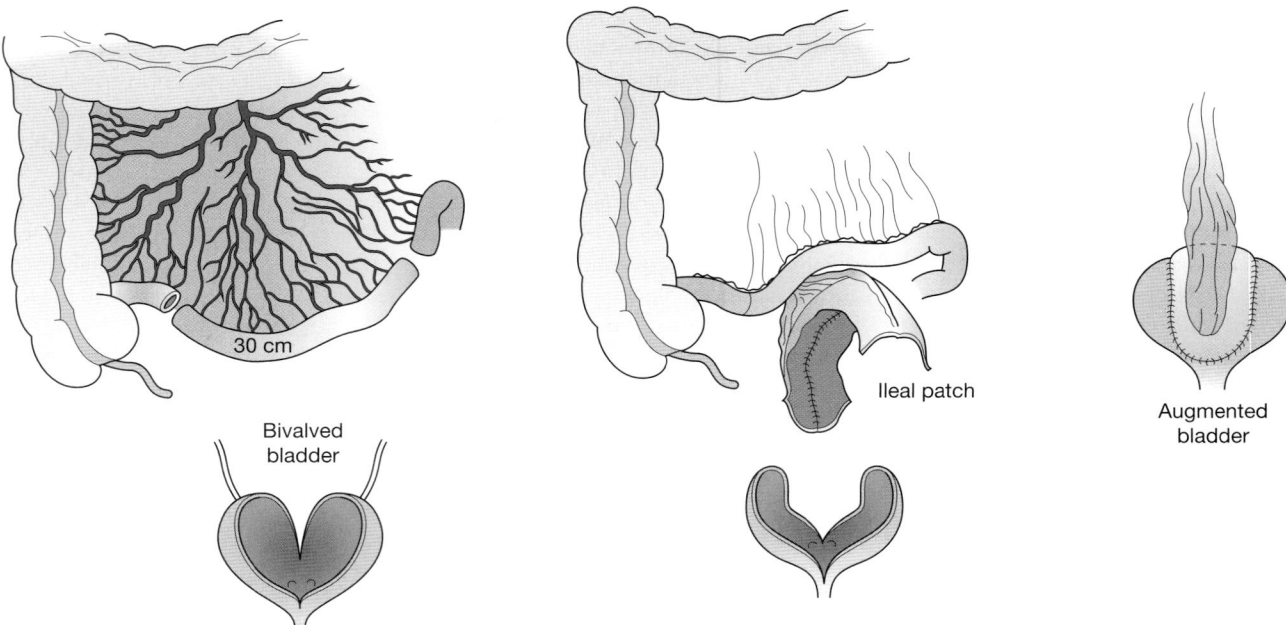

Figure 29-7 Augmentation cystoplasty. A 30-cm segment of small bowel is opened and reconstructed as a U-shaped patch and then sewn into the bivalved bladder.

Intravesical therapy   Two new agents are on trial for intravesical therapy of detrusor hyperactivity. Botulinum A toxin, given by injection at 30–40 sites in the bladder wall to a total dose of 300 units, reduces or abolishes hyperactivity for up to 6 months. Repeated injections have been given with success. Although this is widely available, it is an off-label use for this agent and might not be covered by insurance. Resiniferatoxin instillations are also under trial. These are not as effective as botulinum A toxin but are simpler to administer.[22,25]

Surgery on the bladder or bladder nerves
To increase bladder capacity
Bowel procedures

Augmentation   Bladder augmentation is often recommended for patients who have detrusor hyperactivity or reduced compliance that fails to respond to anticholinergic drugs.[34] The patient must be motivated to continue indefinitely with clean intermittent catheterization and must have adequate outflow resistance. The patient must be fully informed of the immediate surgical risks and the possible long-term sequelae of this procedure. Immediate surgical risks include prolonged intestinal ileus or obstruction, anastomotic leak with peritonitis, wound infection, and pulmonary complications such as pneumonia, and deep venous thrombosis with pulmonary emboli. All the long-term complications are unknown, because bladder augmentation procedures have been performed for only about 20 years. The known long-term complications include chronic bacteriuria, a theoretic risk of neoplastic change, possible diarrhea or malabsorption from a shortened gut or decreased intestinal transit time, and hyperchloremic acidosis due to absorption of urine with secondary mobilization of skeletal calcium (acting as a buffer).

The bladder is opened widely in this procedure, and a detubularized and reconfigured segment of bowel is sewn in. A 20- to 30-cm segment of distal ileum is usually used, but an ileocecal segment, sigmoid, or even a wedge of stomach can be employed (Fig. 29-7). The procedure is intended to result in a 600-mL-capacity, low-pressure reservoir without the use of any drugs. Mucus production is the main day to day problem initially, especially in those with active urinary infection. Mucus production is rarely a problem after the first 3 months if good intermittent catheterization technique and bladder irrigations are used as needed. Because the risk of neoplastic change is unknown with this procedure, yearly cystoscopy should probably begin 10–15 years after the augmentation.

Continent diversion   In this procedure, a section of bowel is used not just to increase effective bladder capacity, but also to form a continent catheterizable channel that opens on to the abdominal wall. It is particularly useful in women for whom intermittent self-catheterization via the urethra is difficult or impossible because of leg spasticity, body habitus, severe urethral incontinence, or the need to transfer from a wheelchair. Men who are unable to perform intermittent catheterization because of strictures, false passages, or fistulas are also potential candidates. It should be noted that severe urethral disease in men is frequently due to poor personal care, and it is inappropriate to perform these procedures on patients who cannot or will not follow through with appropriate techniques. If the patient fails to catheterize after augmentation and continent diversion, the bowel segment can rupture internally before overflow incontinence occurs through the urethra or catheterizable channel.

The procedure involves enlarging the bladder and constructing some form of continent catheterizable channel. The terminal ileum and the ileocecal valve work well, but intussuscepted small bowel, the appendix, and a defunctioned segment of ureter have all been used. The bladder neck might require closure if there is sphincter-related incontinence.

Denervation procedures The denervation technique for bladder hyperactivity is theoretically attractive but is not widely used. Operative approaches include sectioning of the sacral nerve roots or interrupting the peripheral nerve supply near the bladder. Selective sacral rhizotomies have been attempted. The technique involves identifying the nerve root (usually S3 on one side) that carries the detrusor reflex, by doing differential sacral local anesthetic blocks while monitoring the detrusor reflex with CMG. Surgical or chemical destruction of S3 usually results in only temporary areflexia. Over time, the detrusor reflex typically reroutes through the intact sacral nerves. Bilateral S2, S3, and S4 rhizotomies permanently abolish the reflex, but at the expense of loss of reflex erections and worsening of the bowel evacuation problem.[21]

Peripheral denervation of the detrusor has been attempted by transecting the detrusor above the trigone and resuturing it, or by removing the paravesical ganglia via a vaginal approach, or by over-distending the bladder with the intent of damaging the intramural nerves and muscle fibers. In fact, in one clinical study in patients with complete paraplegia, the bladder was intentionally distended in the spinal shock phase with the intent of preventing the return of the bladder reflex. The prevalence of areflexia in the short term following distension was 63%, compared with an expected 15%.[24] None of these peripheral denervation procedures have become commonly accepted, and long-term results of intentional over-distension of the bladder in spinal shock have not yet been reported. Chemical denervation procedures have been discussed under intravesical therapy.

To increase bladder contraction

Electrical stimulation Attempts have been made to stimulate detrusor contraction using electrodes driven by an implanted receiver conveying a stimulus generated by an external transmitter. The electrodes have been implanted on the bladder wall, pelvic nerves, sacral roots, and conus. At present, the only site being used clinically is the sacral roots, and most of the reported series come from Europe.[10] The electrodes are placed on the anterior roots either intradurally or extradurally. To prevent spontaneous hyperactive contractions and antidromic reflex contractions, bilateral S2, S3, and S4 dorsal rhizotomies are usually performed. Pelvic floor contraction with anterior root stimulation will still obstruct voiding, and European centers have elected to stimulate intermittently. This leads to intermittent voiding, as the striated pelvic floor muscle relaxes more quickly than the smooth muscle detrusor. In a center develop-

ing this device in the USA, pudendal neurectomies were performed to decrease outflow resistance.[39] Adequate bladder emptying at acceptable intravesical pressures, with preservation of the bladder wall as well as upper tract morphology and function, has been reported.[10] One important disadvantage of bilateral S2, S3, and S4 rhizotomies is that reflex erections are abolished, and usable erections occurring as a result of sacral root stimulation occur in less than 30% of patients. Bowel evacuation, however, is improved in many patients. Further refinements, such as supraselective rhizotomies with modification of stimulus parameters and electrode design, are future possibilities. This technique has just been approved for routine clinical use in the USA, but there is no company marketing the device at this time.

Surgery on the bladder outlet

To increase outlet resistance Incontinence due to decreased outlet resistance is relatively uncommon in bladder dysfunction secondary to neurologic disease. It is seen in children with myelodysplasia and in women with infrasacral lesions and a denervated pelvic floor. It can occur in active men with complete pelvic floor denervation, but this is rare. Although α-adrenergic agonists might help minor incontinence, more severe leakage typically requires some form of urethral compressive procedure. The options include injection therapy into the bladder neck and urethra to increase the bulk of tissue under and around the bladder neck muscle, a fascial sling, or an artificial sphincter. Electrical stimulation of pelvic floor muscles or nerves, or muscles and nerves, via rectal, vaginal, or implanted electrodes has been tried but has not been effective enough to achieve widespread popularity.

Injection therapy Injections of Teflon have been used for years in the urethra for certain types of stress incontinence, but its use has recently declined because of the danger of particle migration. Autologous fat and bovine collagen have been tried recently, and one to three injections seem to help some proportion of patients. The procedure has few potential side effects and is especially suitable for elderly and poor-risk patients.

External compressive procedures In the fascial sling procedure, a 2-cm strip of fascia is taken from the anterior rectus abdominis fascia or tensor fascia lata. It is wrapped around the bladder neck and fixed anteriorly to the abdominal fascia or pubic tubercle. Patients who are candidates for this procedure must have compliant low-pressure bladders. They will be unable to void by Valsalva's maneuver after a successful sling procedure, and must be willing to perform self-catheterization indefinitely in exchange for being continent.

The artificial urinary sphincter consists of a cuff, a pressure-regulating balloon, and a control pump. The cuff is usually implanted around the bladder neck in both sexes, and less commonly around the bulbar urethra in men. The pump in the labia or scrotum allows the patient to open the cuff for voiding. Reinflation of the cuff is automatic and takes about 3–5 min. Mechanical failure, cuff erosion, and infection can occur with

---

Box 29-1 Preoperative parameters for sphincterotomy

Spontaneous contraction with:

- volume <200 mL
- rise time <20 s
- amplitude >50 cm H_2O
- duration ≥2 min

---

this device. Patients can use Valsalva's maneuver to void and do not usually have to be on self-catheterization. In patients with myelodysplasia, uncontrolled hyperactivity occurs in 10% in the first year after implantation of an artificial sphincter. This is despite the fact that, preoperatively, the detrusor was naturally areflexic or was rendered so by drugs. This probably results from activation of dormant urethrovesical reflexes. Careful follow-up is essential and, if hyperactivity occurs, an augmentation procedure can be done secondarily. It is possible that in the future some intravesical therapy might be helpful in this situation.

To decrease outlet resistance

Sphincterotomy In male spinal cord-injured patients unable or unwilling to do self-catheterization, the use of a condom catheter is a practical alternative. As it is unusual to find a lower urinary tract that has adequate detrusor contraction and a coordinated pelvic floor in these patients, some procedure to decrease outflow resistance is usually indicated. The results are poor in patients without adequate detrusor contractions. Preoperative parameters suggested for a good outcome are presented in Box 29-1. Ablation of the striated sphincter, usually by incision, is the standard procedure. It is now performed anteriorly to avoid the cavernous artery and nerve, which lie lateral to the membranous urethra. Damage of the cavernous artery and nerve can lead to impotence. Some patients also have bladder neck obstruction. This can be due to primary hyperactivity (e.g. in high tetraplegic patients) or to total bladder wall hypertrophy (which follows striated sphincter dyssynergia). These patients need bladder neck ablation either by resection or by incision. In older men, prostatic obstruction from benign disease can also contribute to increased outflow resistance and might require prostatic resection. The immediate morbidity from sphincterotomy—bleeding, clot retention, and infection—is relatively high. The long-term results can be compromised due to recurrent obstruction from stricture or recurrent dyssynergia. An implantable stainless steel stent is now available, and should reduce morbidity and improve long-term results. This stent material is inert, and the epithelium grows through the spaces between the wires of the stent, completely covering it.[31] Unfortunately, the splint is not well tolerated in men with sensory incomplete spinal cord injury.

Other methods of decreasing outflow resistance Intrathecal baclofen given for severe spasticity decreases the pudendal reflexes, but the detrusor reflex and contractions are reduced as well. Consequently, it cannot be used as a chemical sphinc-

terotomy. Botulinum A toxin injected into the striated sphincter has also been used experimentally, but (as in the bladder) its effects last only a few months.[19]

Urinary diversion The use of any urinary diversion procedure should be restricted to patients with severe urethral problems such as stricture, fistula, periurethral abscess, and intractable incontinence with perineal skin breakdown. The simplest method is to insert a suprapubic catheter and close the bladder neck. If the bladder cannot be preserved because of malignant disease, contracture, or ureteral reflux, a standard bowel conduit is recommended, with removal of the bladder in most cases. Usually, a 10- to 15-cm segment of small bowel is used. Because a non-refluxing ureterointestinal anastomosis is desired, the ileocecal segment or sigmoid colon segment is preferred.

MANAGEMENT OF SPECIFIC DISEASES

Diseases of the brain

Stroke

After an initial period of areflexia, stroke patients typically have hyperactivity with frequency and urge incontinence but coordinated voiding and complete emptying (see Ch. 51). Anticholinergics frequently help ameliorate symptoms without adversely affecting emptying. Persistent areflexia and retention can occur with bilateral lesions. Prostatic obstruction can cause retention in elderly men with stroke. Videourodynamic studies are helpful in differentiating these conditions.

Parkinson disease

The prevalence of bladder symptoms in patients with Parkinson disease is high (70%) (see Ch. 52). Most have frequency, urgency, and urge incontinence, and 50% complain of difficulty voiding. Evaluation typically shows bladder hyperactivity, but the contractions are poorly sustained and result in incomplete emptying. Failure to empty can also be due to bradykinesia, be secondary to failure of pelvic floor relaxation, or be due to the adrenergic effects of levodopa, or even the anticholinergic effects of other antiparkinsonian drugs.[4] Treatment is difficult, because there is frequently a combination of incontinence and retention. Detrusor inhibition with drugs makes emptying worse, and α-adrenergic blockers have a marginal effect in decreasing outflow resistance.[38] Intermittent catheterization and detrusor inhibition are often the best choice, but many patients do not have sufficient upper extremity dexterity to catheterize independently.

Dementia, brain tumors, and trauma

Dementia, brain tumors, and trauma can all cause hyperactivity with reflex or urge incontinence with complete emptying. If cognitive impairment is severe, incontinence often persists despite detrusor inhibition. Some type of collecting device is appropriate for many of these patients (see Ch. 50).

Diseases of the brain and spinal cord

Multiple sclerosis is the commonest disease in this category, with 90% of patients developing urinary manifestations in the course of the disease (see Ch. 53). The bladder symptoms usually present because of an incomplete spinal cord lesion with hyperactivity and hypocontractility. Detrusor inhibition with drugs worsens emptying in this case. In the rare, predominantly encephalopathic variety of multiple sclerosis, these agents might be useful. Patients with multiple sclerosis and with a predominantly conal lesion have bladder areflexia. Intermittent catheterization is eventually indicated in most patients with multiple sclerosis, but few are able to undertake it because of poor upper extremity strength and coordination. High-pressure bladders due to hyperactivity and detrusor–sphincter dyssynergia are rare, but sphincterotomy in men is sometimes indicated.[29]

Diseases of the spinal cord

Injury, tumors, and vascular lesions of the spinal cord cause the majority of suprasacral neurogenic bladder problems (see Ch. 56). The detrusor reflex typically returns after a varying period of spinal shock. The center for the detrusor reflex develops in the sacral cord in patients with complete injury. Inhibitory control by the higher center is impaired and, because the long-routed detrusor reflex is interrupted, the detrusor contraction might not be completely sustained. Coordination and control of the pelvic floor are also impaired, leading to lack of voluntary contraction and relaxation. In complete lesions, there is often discoordinated activity during voiding. This discoordination or detrusor–sphincter dyssynergia affects the striated voluntary sphincter, but in high complete tetraplegic patients excessive sympathetic activity can also lead to detrusor–bladder neck dyssynergia. Incomplete spinal cord lesions can produce the supraspinal pattern with urgency and adequate emptying, while patients with complete lesions have reflex incontinence and incomplete emptying due to detrusor–sphincter dyssynergia (in most cases). Some patients have hypocontractility or areflexia and retention. A truly balanced bladder with sustained detrusor contraction and coordinated pelvic floor is uncommon.

The onset and severity of the symptoms vary with the cause of spinal cord dysfunction, but the management discussed here is in relation to spinal cord injury. An indwelling catheter is typically maintained until the patient's medical state is stable and fluid intake can be regulated to achieve a urine output of 1500–2000 mL/day. Intermittent sterile catheterization is then started, preferably by a dedicated catheterization team. The patient should learn self-catheterization when able to do so. A sterile technique is ideal in the hospital, but a clean technique can be used when the patient is discharged home. Maximum allowable bladder volume is 600 mL. In some of these patients, however, retention of interstitial fluid in the lower limbs when the patient is upright, with subsequent mobilization and dumping at night, is frequently a problem. The use of anti-embolism stockings such as TED hose, recumbency early in the evening, and an extra catheterization in the middle of the night might all be necessary to manage this.

In the majority of spinal cord-injured patients, the detrusor reflex returns usually within the first 6 months. Its return is often indicated by episodes of incontinence, but the presence of the detrusor reflex should be confirmed by CMG. Anti-

cholinergics can be given to suppress the reflex and allow intermittent catheterization to continue. Patients with lesions at the level of C7 and below and who can do self-catheterization can continue this in the long term. If the detrusor reflex cannot be suppressed, the patient should consider augmentation, which remains the standard method today for achieving a low-pressure reservoir if medications fail. Intravesical therapy might be an option in the future.

In male patients unable or unwilling to do self-catheterization, and for those who refuse augmentation, sphincterotomy followed by use of an external catheter is probably the best alternative. Other options include intermittent catheterization by an attendant, although this has a greater risk of febrile UTIs.[14] Wearing an external collector alone can be considered, but only 15% of men with spinal cord injury have a suitable, truly 'balanced' bladder with coordinated voiding at low pressure. Some men with tetraplegia end up with an indwelling catheter because of sphincterotomy failure, or inadequate detrusor contractions, or skin breakdown on the penile shaft. Women using intermittent catheterization, but unable to control urinary incontinence with medications, might also choose to use an indwelling catheter. A regular long-term urinary tract surveillance program (Box 29-2) should be set up for spinal cord-injured patients who might, with good care, have a near-normal life expectancy.

Box 29-2 Routine urinary tract surveillance after spinal cord injury

Initial rehabilitation admission
- Urinalysis, initial and as needed
- Urine culture and sensitivity, weekly
- Renal and bladder ultrasound; add KUB in patients with a Foley catheter
- CT-IVP only if ultrasound is abnormal
- Postvoid residuals if voiding
- Cystometrography or urodynamics if clinically indicated
- Creatine clearance, 24-h urine

Routine evaluations (yearly for the first 5 years and, if stable, every other year thereafter)
- Renal ultrasound and KUB for all annual evaluations
- CT-IVP only if indicated by clinical status or ultrasound findings
- Urodynamics determined on an individual basis (often needed annually for the first few years)
- Creatine clearance, 24-h urine, annually
- Postvoid residuals if voiding
- Other tests of renal function as needed

Cystoscopy
Generally performed in patients after 10 years of chronic, continuous indwelling catheterizations (urethral or suprapubic), or earlier (at 5 years) if at high risk (heavy smoker, age >40 years, or history of complicated urinary tract infections) or in any patient with symptoms that warrant such a procedure.

CT-IVP, computed tomography–intravenous pyelography; KUB, kidneys, ureters, and bladder, plain film study.

Diseases of the conus, cauda equina, and peripheral nerves

Trauma, disk disease, lumbar stenosis, arachnoiditis, and tumors are some of the mechanical lesions that can affect this region of the spinal canal. The resulting bladder is typically areflexic or non-contractile and insensate. Pelvic floor innervation is frequently affected in conal lesions, which can lead to incontinence, especially in females. In cauda equinal lesions, the non-myelinated pelvic nerve roots are more easily damaged, and pelvic floor innervation is usually relatively more intact than the detrusor nerve supply. In autonomic neuropathy secondary to diabetes and multiple systems atrophy, the detrusor afferents and efferents are affected and, because of lack of sensation, overstretching contributes to the end result, which is a non-contractile and insensate bladder.

Intermittent catheterization is the initial treatment in all cases if in retention. If the pelvic floor is severely paralyzed, patients might be able to void by straining. Men can be helped by α-adrenergic blocking agents to decrease outflow resistance. Women can often empty by straining but tend to develop severe stress incontinence. Some patients can be candidates for a fascial sling or artificial sphincter. Reduced bladder compliance, usually found in patients after radical pelvic surgery, does not respond well to medications. An augmentation might be indicated in these cases, particularly if the outflow resistance is high and the upper tracts begin to dilate. In the early stages of diabetes, patients can often maintain bladder function and contractility and avoid over-distention by timed voidings.

Diseases of the spinal cord and conus

Myelodysplasia is the most common disease producing a mixed pattern of lower urinary tract dysfunction. Any combination of detrusor and sphincter activity can be found, but it is most common to have a hyperactive or non-compliant bladder with dyssynergia or a non-relaxing sphincter.

Intermittent catheterization is used initially along with medication in infancy and childhood. In many cases, reconstructive surgery is necessary early if more conservative measures fail.

MANAGEMENT OF COMPLICATIONS

Bacteriuria

About one-half of all hospital-acquired infections originate in the urinary tract in association with urinary catheters and other drainage devices. UTIs are a common source of morbidity in patients with neurogenic bladders. Frequent exposure to antibiotics increases the risk of infection with antibiotic-resistant organisms, further complicating the treatment of UTI. The diagnosis of UTI can be delayed or missed in patients with neurologic disorders affecting bladder sensation. In patients with spinal cord disorders, signs and symptoms suggestive of UTI include fever, onset of urinary incontinence, increased spasticity, autonomic dysreflexia, increased sweating, cloudy and odorous urine, malaise, lethargy, or sense of unease.[33] Unexplained signs and symptoms suggestive of UTI in the pres-

ence of pyuria warrant empiric therapy for UTI. The absence of pyuria makes the diagnosis of UTI unlikely but does not exclude it.

Asymptomatic bacteriuria is very common in patients with neurogenic bladder, especially those using intermittent or indwelling catheterization. Most authorities recommend against routine treatment of asymptomatic bacteriuria. However, the presence of significant bacteriuria with urease-producing organisms that are associated with stone formation might warrant treatment.[3]

The spectrum of uropathogens causing catheter-associated UTI is much broader than that causing uncomplicated UTI. *Escherichia coli* causes the majority of uncomplicated UTIs. *E. coli* and organisms such as species of *Proteus, Klebsiella, Pseudomonas, Serratia, Providencia*, enterococci, and staphylococci are relatively more common in patients with catheter-associated UTI.[33] Polymicrobic bacteriuria is the rule in patients with indwelling catheters.

Patients with mild to moderate illness can be treated with an oral fluoroquinolone such as ciprofloxacin, levofloxacin, or gatifloxacin. This group of antibiotics provides coverage for most expected pathogens, including most strains of *Pseudomonas aeruginosa*. Trimethoprim sulfamethoxazole is another commonly used antibiotic for less ill patients, but it does not provide coverage against *P. aeruginosa*. It is less expensive than the fluoroquinolones, and can be used empirically and continued according to the results of susceptibility testing. Amoxicillin, nitrofurantoin, and sulfa drugs are poor choices for empiric therapy because of the high prevalence of resistance to these agents among uropathogens typically involved in complicated UTIs.

In more seriously ill, hospitalized patients, piperacillin plus tazobactam, ampicillin plus gentamicin, or imipenem plus cilastatin provide coverage against most expected pathogens, including *P. aeruginosa* and most enterococci.[11] A number of other parenteral antimicrobial agents can also be used. Patients can be switched to oral treatment after clinical improvement. At least 7–14 days of therapy is generally recommended, depending on the severity of the infection.[3] There is no convincing evidence that regimens longer than this are beneficial. Patients undergoing effective treatment for UTI, with an antibiotic to which the infecting pathogen is susceptible, should have definite improvement within 24–48 h. If not, a repeat urine culture and imaging studies (US or CT) are indicated.

In a patient who has had UTI with high fever or hemodynamic changes suggestive of sepsis, or who is having recurrent symptomatic UTIs, a CT-KUB, cystogram, or urodynamic evaluation might be indicated after successful treatment to look for correctable anatomic or functional abnormalities.

Autonomic dysreflexia

Paroxysmal hypertension, sweating, piloerection, headache, and reflex bradycardia are brought on by increased stimulation into and sympathetic output from the isolated spinal cord below a

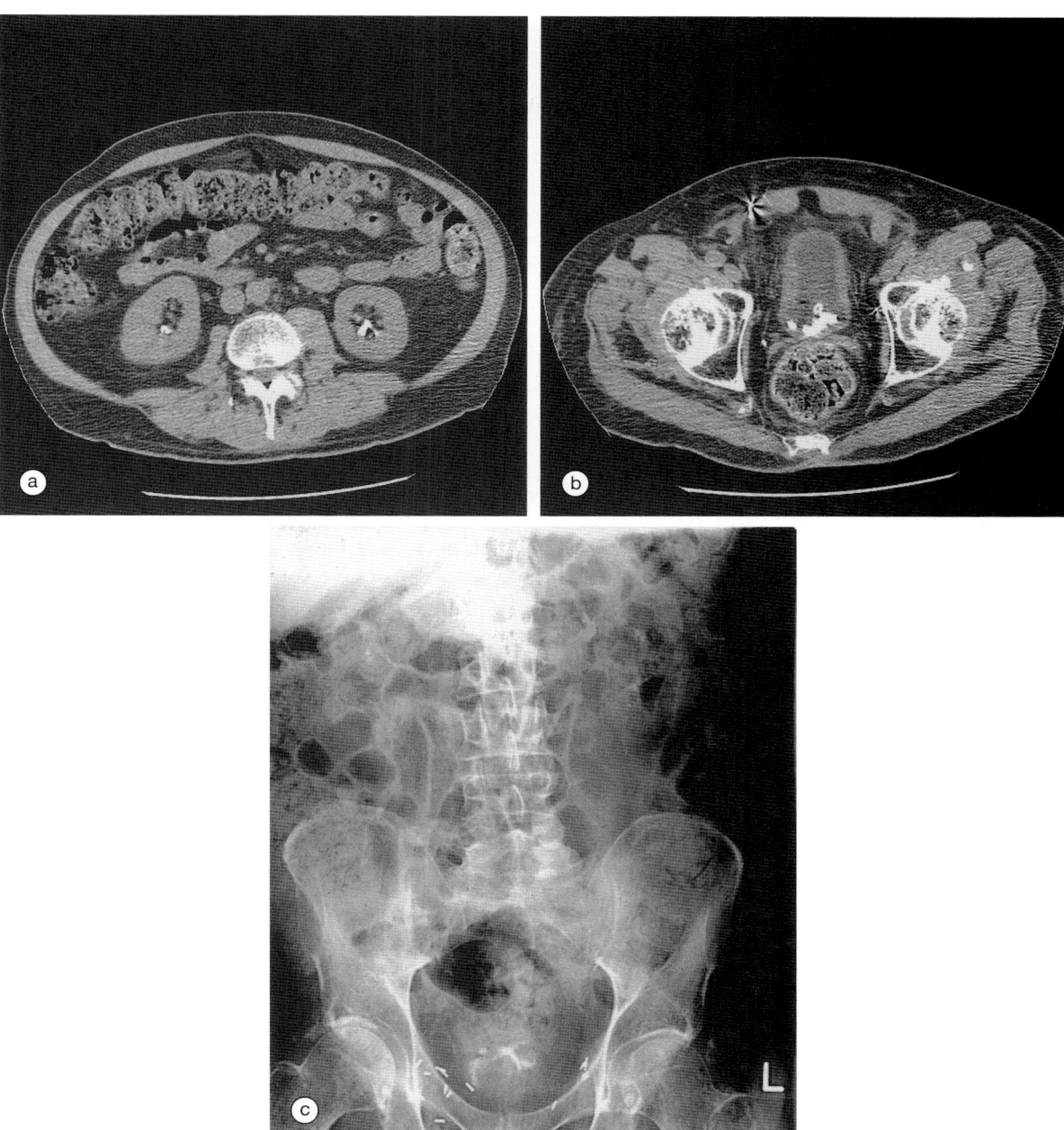

Figure 29-8 A computed tomography of the kidneys, ureter, and bladder (CT-KUB; **a** and **b**) and a standard plain radiograph of the kidneys, ureter, and bladder (KUB; **c**) showing renal and bladder stones in a tetraplegic patient. The stones can be seen on the standard KUB in this patient, but in many patients visualization is difficult due to the size and density of the stones, the size of the patient, and the state of the overlying bowel. CT-KUB is more sensitive.

complete lesion. Spinal cord injuries below T6 are rarely associated with this problem. Stimulation from the bladder from high pressures or over-distention is the most common cause of autonomic dysreflexia. The best treatment is prevention of such stimuli. If symptoms persist when the bladder has been emptied, or if the blood pressure is at a dangerously high level, 10 mg of sublingual nifedipine, a calcium channel-blocking agent, can be given. It is often safer to apply one-half to one inch of Nitropaste on the skin, because this can be wiped off if the blood pressure response is too exaggerated. If a patient has recently ingested sildenafil, prazosin or captopril can be used instead.[15] Long-term management with phenoxybenzamine (10–30 mg/day) has been used to prevent autonomic dysreflexia when all findable causes have been eliminated (see Ch. 55 for further explanation of the treatment of autonomic dysreflexia).

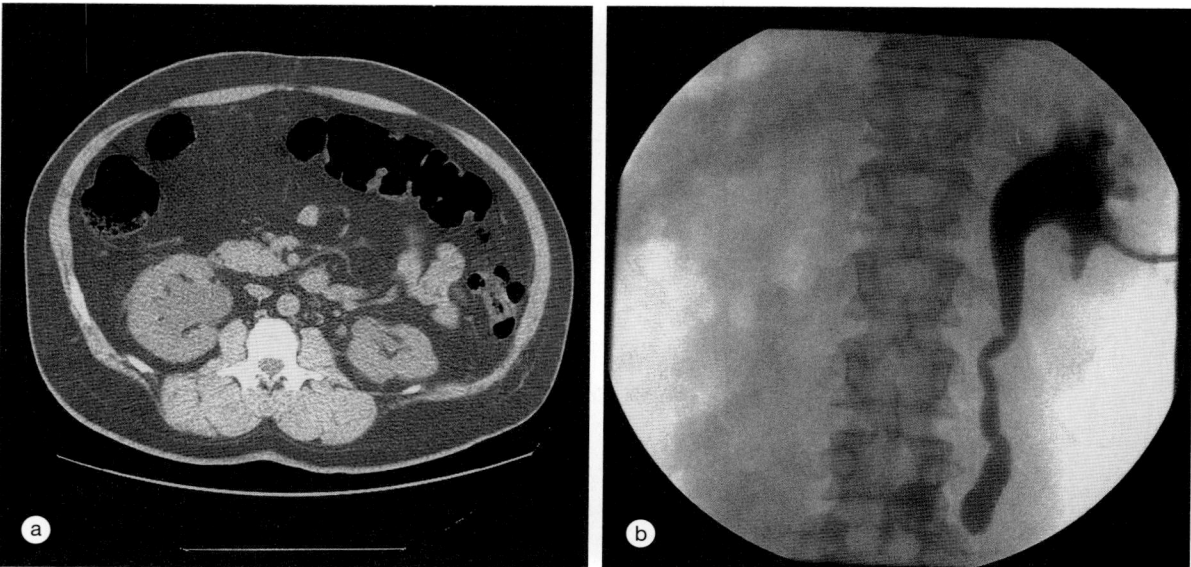

Figure 29-9 A computed tomography of the kidneys, ureter, and bladder (**a**), and a prone antegrade nephrostogram (**b**), demonstrating right hydronephrosis with a dilated ureter down to the ureteroileal junction. The patient is a man with spina bifida whose bladder was augmented and the ureters reimplanted 10 years before. The cause of the obstruction was an inflammatory stricture.

Hypercalciuria and stones

Loss of calcium from the bones occurs in all spinal cord-injured patients and is worse in young males. Increased urinary calcium (>200 mg/24 h) begins about 4 weeks after injury, reaches a maximum at 16 weeks, and can persist for 12–18 months. Renal stone incidence in the first 9 months is approximately 1.0–1.5% and is due mainly to hypercalciuria. Over the next 10 years, upper tract stones are found in 8%, with many of these secondary to infection. The incidence of bladder stones in the first 9 months in patients on intermittent catheterization is 2.3%. In the presence of an indwelling catheter, and despite greater urine output, the prevalence is much higher (8.8%).[16]

Bladder stones are effectively treated with cystoscopy and holmium:yttrium–aluminum–garnet laser lithotripsy. Small stones and particles can be dissolved by daily bladder irrigations with 30 mL of 10% of hemiacidrin (Renacidin) solution, which is left in the bladder for 30 min. Some patients with recurrent stones use this once or twice a week for prophylaxis. In patients who have ureteral reflux, it should be used with caution because of potential nephrotoxicity and absorption of magnesium. Caliceal calculi that are small (<1 cm) and asymptomatic can be followed expectantly, but 50% of these patients become symptomatic over 5 years and half of these will need some sort of invasive procedure.[23] Calculi that are growing or that are located in the renal pelvis should probably be treated before they pass into the ureter and cause obstruction (Fig. 29-8). Extracorporeal shock wave lithotripsy (ESWL) is the standard treatment. For large stones (>3 cm in diameter), a percutaneous approach is preferred, as clearance of fragments is poor if patients are inactive.

Ureteral stones are potentially dangerous in patients with no renal sensation. These can be managed expectantly if they pass down within 2–3 weeks. Patients with reduced sensation might not perceive continuous pain, which would normally suggest severe continuing obstruction. This results in an increased risk of renal damage. When obstruction and infection occur together, they require a drainage procedure as an emergency, with a percutaneous nephrostomy or a retrograde stent. This is typically followed by an endoscopic lithotripsy, stone removal, or ESWL.

Lower urinary tract changes

Trabeculation occurs in the majority of patients after spinal cord injury. In many cases, trabeculation happens despite appropriate management strategies. Sacculation and diverticula can occur when obstruction and high pressure are severe. If a diverticulum occurs at the ureteral hiatus, ureteral reflux is almost inevitable. Chronic infection of dilated prostatic ducts may be an important source for relapsing UTIs in men.

Ureteral reflux and upper tract dilatation

Ureteral reflux or high bladder pressure in the absence of reflux can cause upper tract dilatation (Fig. 29-9). Dilatation without reflux is said to be due to decreased compliance, but data from long-term monitoring suggest that baseline pressure elevations are minimal with natural rates of filling, and that increased phasic activity might be more important.[40] With reflux, or ureteral dilatation without reflux, the bladder pressure should be lowered with intermittent catheterization and anticholinergics. If bladder pressure responds but reflux fails to improve, a surgical procedure to repair the reflux can be considered. If bladder pressures do not improve, the options are to augment the bladder or, in men, to perform a sphincterotomy and rely on free drainage.

SUMMARY

The ultimate goal of bladder management is to prevent renal deterioration and reduce morbidity such as UTIs. The current demands of the healthcare market, however, are to reduce costs and length of hospital stays. These market demands are no doubt affecting daily decisions made by patients and providers regarding bladder management. Time will tell whether these market forces are changing outcomes (morbidity and mortality) related to the neurogenic bladder.

REFERENCES

1. Abrams P, Amarenco G, Bakke A, et al. Tamsulosin: efficacy and safety in patients with neurogenic lower urinary tract dysfunction due to suprasacral spinal cord injury. J Urol 2003; 170(4):1242–1251.

2. Abrams P, Blaivas JG, Stanton SL, et al. Standardization of terminology of lower urinary tract function. In: Krane RJ, Siroky MB, eds. Clinical neurology. 2nd edn. Boston: Little, Brown; 1991:651–669.

3. [Anonymous]. National Institute on Disability and Rehabilitation Research consensus statement. The prevention and management of urinary tract infection among people with spinal cord injuries. J Am Paraplegia Soc 1992; 15:194–204.

4. Berger Y, Blaivas JG, DeLaRocha ER, et al. Urodynamic findings in Parkinson's disease. J Urol 1987; 138(4):836–838.

5. Blaivas JG. Management of bladder dysfunction in multiple sclerosis. Neurology 1980; 30(2):12–18.

6. Blaivas JG. Videourodynamics. In: Krane RJ, Siroky MB, eds. Clinical neurology. 2nd edn. Boston: Little, Brown; 1991:265–274.

7. Bors E, Comarr AE. Neurological urology. Baltimore: University Park Press; 1971.

8. Bradley WE, Brantley SF. Physiology of the urinary bladder. In: Campbell's urology. 4th edn. Philadelphia: Saunders; 1978:106.

9. Bradley WE. Physiology of the urinary bladder. In: Walsh PC, Gittes RF, Perlmutter AD, et al, eds. Campbell's neurology. Philadelphia: Saunders; 1986:129–185.

10. Brindley GS, Rushton DN. Long-term follow-up of patients with sacral anterior root stimulator implants. Paraplegia 1990; 28(8):469–475.

11. Cardenas DD, Hooton TM. Urinary tract infection in persons with spinal cord injury. Arch Phys Med Rehabil 1995; 75(3):272–280.

12. Cardenas DD, Kelly E, Krieger JN, et al. Residual urine volumes in patients with spinal cord injury: measurement with a portable ultrasound instrument. Arch Phys Med Rehabil 1988; 69(7):514–516.

13. Cardenas DD, Kelly E, Mayo ME. Manual stimulation of reflex voiding after spinal cord injury. Arch Phys Med Rehabil 1985; 66(7):459–462.

14. Cardenas DD, Mayo ME. Bacteriuria with fever after spinal cord injury. Arch Phys Med Rehabil 1987; 68:291–293.

15. Consortium for Spinal Cord Medicine. Linsenmeyer TA, Baker ER, et al. Clinical practice guidelines for health-care professionals. Acute management of autonomic dysreflexias: individuals with spinal cord injury presenting to health-care facilities. J Spinal Cord Med 2002; 25(S1):S67–S88.

16. DeVivo MJ, Fine PR, Cutter GR, et al. The risk of renal calculi in spinal cord injury patients. J Urol 1984; 131(5):857–860.

17. Dewire DM, Owens RS, Anderson GA, et al. A comparison of the urological complications associated with long-term management of quadriplegics with and without chronic indwelling urinary catheters. J Urol 1992; 147(4):1069–1071.

18. Dmochowski RR, Miklos JR, Norton PA, et al. Duloxetine versus placebo for the treatment of North American women with stress urinary incontinence. J Urol 2003; 170(4):1259–1263.

19. Dykstra DD, Sidi AA. Treatment of detrusor-sphincter dyssynergia with botulinum A toxin: a double-blind study. Arch Phys Med Rehabil 1990; 71(1):24–26.

20. Finkbeiner AE. Is bethanechol chloride clinically effective in promoting bladder emptying? A literature review. J Urol 1985; 134(3):443–449.

21. Gasparini ME, Schmidt RA, Tanagho EA. Selective sacral rhizotomy in the management of the reflex neuropathic bladder: a report on 17 patients with long-term followup. J Urol 1992; 148(4):1207–1210.

22. Giannantoni A, Di Stasi SM, Stephen RL, et al. Intravesical resiniferatoxin versus botulinum-A toxin injections for neurogenic detrusor overactivity: a prospective randomized study. J Urol 2004; 172(1):240–243.

23. Glowacki LS, Beecroft ML, Cook RJ, et al. The natural history of asymptomatic urolithiasis. J Urol 1992; 147(2):319–321.

24. Iwatsubo E, Komine S, Yamashita H, et al. Over-distension therapy of the bladder in paraplegic patients using self-catheterization: a preliminary study. Paraplegia 1984; 22(4):210–215.

25. Kim JH, Rivas DA, Shenot PJ, et al. Intravesical resiniferatoxin for refractory detrusor hyperreflexia: a multicenter, blinded, randomized, placebo-controlled trial. J Spinal Cord Med 2003; 26(4):358–363.

26. Kiviat MD, Zimmermann TA, Donovan WH. Sphincter stretch: a new technique resulting in continence and complete voiding in paraplegics. J Urol 1975; 114(6):895–897.

27. Lapides J, Diokno AC, Silber SJ, et al. Clean, intermittent self-catheterization in the treatment of urinary tract disease. J Urol 1972; 107(3):458–461.

28. Madersbacher H, Jilg G. Control of detrusor hyperreflexia by the intravesical instillation of oxybutynin hydrochloride. Paraplegia 1991; 29(2):84–90.

29. Mayo ME, Chetner MP. Lower urinary tract dysfunction in multiple sclerosis. Urology 1992; 39(1):67–70.

30. Mayo ME. The value of sphincter electromyography in urodynamics. J Urol 1979; 122(3):357–360.

31. McInerney PD, Vanner TF, Harris SA, et al. Permanent urethral stents for detrusor sphincter dyssynergia. Br J Urol 1991; 67(3):291–294.

32. McLellan FC. The neurogenic bladder. Springfield: Charles C. Thomas; 1939:57–70, 116–185.

33. Montgomerie JZ, Chan E, Gilmore DS, et al. Low mortality among patients with spinal cord injury and bacteremia. Rev Infect Dis 1991; 13(5):867–871.

34. Sidi AA, Becher EF, Reddy PK, et al. Augmentation enterocystoplasty for the management of voiding dysfunction in spinal cord injury patients. J Urol 1990; 143(1):83–85.

35. Steers WD, Meythaler JM, Haworth C, et al. Effects of acute bolus and chronic continuous intrathecal baclofen on genitourinary dysfunction due to spinal cord pathology. J Urol 1992; 148(6):1849–1855.

36. Steers WD. Physiology and pharmacology of the bladder and urethra. In: Walsh PC, Retch AB, et al, eds. Campbell's urology. 7th edn. Philadelphia: Saunders; 1998:870–915.

37. Subramonian K, Cartwright RA, Harnden P, et al. Bladder cancer in patients with spinal cord injuries. BJU Int 2004; 93(6):739–743.

38. Swierzewski SJI, Gormley EA, Belville WD, et al. The effect of terazosin on bladder function in the spinal cord injured patient. J Urol 1994; 151(4):951–954.

39. Tanagho EA, Schmidt RA, Orvis BR. Neural stimulation for control of voiding dysfunction: a preliminary report in 22 patients with serious neuropathic voiding disorders. J Urol 1989; 142(2):340–345.

40. Webb RJ, Styles RA, Griffiths, CJ, et al. Ambulatory monitoring of bladder pressure in low compliance neurogenic bladder dysfunction. J Urol 1992; 48:1477–1488.

Neurogenic Bowel: Dysfunction and Rehabilitation

Steven A. Stiens and John C. King

Neurogenic bowel dysfunction can be a clinically elusive impairment. It is often eclipsed by other, more noticeable associated motor deficits. Neurogenic bowel dysfunction itself can be particularly life-limiting, however, if it is not thoroughly assessed and treated using rehabilitation principles. Interdisciplinary rehabilitative interventions focus on establishing a total management plan for bowel function, termed a *bowel program*, and for assisted defecation, known as *bowel care*.[67] Sensation and mobility might be limited, affecting a person's ability to anticipate the need for and to physically perform independent bowel care and hygiene. Despite many abilities regained during the rehabilitation process, bowel care capabilities at the time of discharge are not always comparable with other skills that would be expected for a given level of function. Bowel continence is one of the greatest predictors of return to home for stroke survivors.[15] In fact, bowel management has been found to be one of the areas of least competence among rehabilitated persons with spinal cord injury (SCI).[6,27] More than one-third of surveyed persons with SCI rated bowel and bladder dysfunction as having the most significant effect on their lives after SCI.[28] In a recent Swedish review of medical problems after SCI, 41% of subjects rated bowel dysfunction as a moderately to severely life-limiting problem.[41]

Bowel programs and techniques for bowel care training should be more effectively pursued during inpatient rehabilitation. Some patients need attendants to help with bowel care, and the attendants must also be well trained.[68,69] The burden of care for persons with neurogenic bowel is much higher if continence is not achieved or if bowel care evacuation times are excessive.[67,76] Careful training of the patient and attendant care is necessary if satisfactory bowel management results are to be achieved.

EPIDEMIOLOGY

Neurogenic bowel dysfunction results from autonomic and somatic denervation, and produces fecal incontinence (FI), constipation, and difficulty with evacuation (DWE). These symptoms are common. The prevalence of FI and fecal impaction ranges from 0.3% to 5.0% in the general population. The prevalence of DWE ranges from 10% to 50% among the hospitalized or institutionalized elderly.[60,76] Although many gastrointestinal disorders can contribute to FI or DWE, disorders that impair the extrinsic (sympathetic, parasympathetic, or somatic)

nervous control of the bowel and anorectal mechanisms are more common among the patient populations seen by physiatrists. Neurogenic bowel difficulties can be a primary disabling and handicapping feature for patients with SCI, stroke, amyotrophic lateral sclerosis, multiple sclerosis, diabetes mellitus, myelomeningocele, and muscular dystrophy.[2,9,15,32,67,79]

IMPACT

Satisfactory functional outcomes depend on an individually designed, patient-centered, and patient-managed bowel program.[68] The three primary objectives of the bowel program that apply to all cases are:

1. to prevent unplanned bowel movements;
2. to promote efficient and effective bowel care; and
3. to prevent complications.

FI decreases the return to home rates for stroke patients.[26] A cross-sectional survey of patients with SCI revealed that the tetrad of constipation, female gender, pressure ulcers, and years post injury were most predictive of an increased need for help in activities of daily living.[42] Almost one-third of persons with SCI report or exhibit worsening of bowel function 5 years beyond their injury, with 33% developing megacolon, suggesting inadequate long-term management.[29,70] Recent evidence has shown some improvement in outcomes for SCI bowel management.[36] Nursing home costs are higher for patients with FI.[76] When restoring normal defecation is not possible, *social continence* becomes the goal. Social continence is defined as predictable, scheduled, adequate defecations without incontinence at other times. It is often achievable by persons with neurogenic bowel dysfunction. Embarrassment and humiliation from FI frequently result in extreme vocational and social disability. Vocational disability and excessive institutionalization add substantial costs to the care related to neurogenic bowel dysfunction. A 1983 report estimated that $8 billion per year is spent in the USA for the care of fecally incontinent institutionalized patients.[60]

BOWEL ANATOMY AND FUNCTION

Anatomy: structure and innervation

The colon is the terminal segment of intestine that has been differentiated for fecal formation, storage, and defecation. The

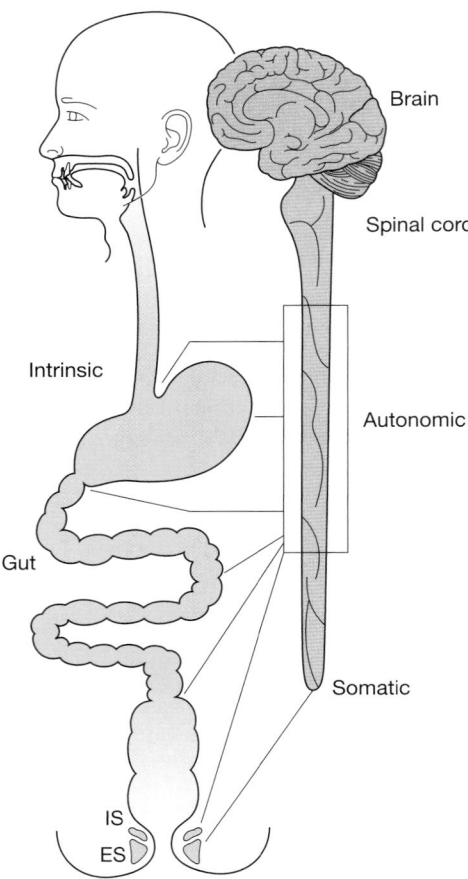

Figure 30-1 The bowel has three nervous systems. IS, internal sphincter; ES, external sphincter.

colon and anorectal mechanisms receive parasympathetic, sympathetic, and somatic innervation (Fig. 30-1). There is also the intrinsic enteric nervous system (ENS) between muscular layers and under the mucosa (Figs 30-2 and 30-3), which traverse from the upper esophagus to the anus. The neurogenic bowel is defined as the loss of direct somatic sensory or motor control functions, with or without impaired sympathetic and parasympathetic innervation.[67] However, the intrinsic ENS remains intact with most presenting injuries and illnesses. The most common exceptions are the developmental disorder of Hirschsprung disease or cases of idiopathic small fiber autonomic neuropathy,[38] most commonly acquired from diabetes mellitus, which can involve the ENS as well. Such diabetic ENS damage, however, does not necessarily correlate with the severity of the peripheral diabetic polyneuropathy. When intact, the intrinsic ENS continues to integrate and modulate bowel function, even without autonomic and somatic nervous system input, and can be the neurologic substrate for bowel habit training.

Physiology: normal function

The colon is a reservoir for food waste until it is convenient for elimination. It also acts as a storage device as long as the colonic pressure is less than that of the anal sphincter mechanism. Fecal

elimination occurs when colonic pressure exceeds that of the anal sphincter mechanism. Other functions of the colon are to reabsorb fluids (up to 30 L/day can be reabsorbed from the large and small bowel walls, with typically only 100 mL of water loss in feces) and gases (90% of the 7–10 L of gases produced by intracolonic fermentation is absorbed rather than expelled). The colon also provides an environment for the growth of bacteria needed to assist in digestion, and serves to absorb certain bacterial breakdown products as well.[25] The layers of the colon wall are depicted in Figure 30-3.

The ENS is the key to proper functioning of the entire gastrointestinal tract. This collection of highly organized neurons is situated in two primary layers: the submucosal (Meissner's) plexus and the intramuscular myenteric (Auerbach's) plexus. These plexuses have an estimated 10–100 million neurons, plus two or three glial cells per neuron. That is more nerve cells than are contained in the spinal cord. The ENS glial cells, which resemble central nervous system astrocytes, are much less abundant than the 20–50 glial cells per neuron in the central nervous system.[24] The coordination of segment to segment function is largely regulated by the ENS, and considered by some as a third part of the autonomic nervous system.[80] The ENS also has its own nerve–blood barrier, similar to that of the central nervous system.[11]

The sympathetic and parasympathetic nervous systems seem to modulate the ENS, rather than directly controlling the smooth muscles of the bowel.[80] The smooth muscles of the bowel also have their own electromechanical automaticity, which is directly modulated by the inhibitory control of the ENS.[11,24] Sympathetic nervous system stimulation tends to promote the storage function by enhancing anal tone and inhibiting colonic contractions, although little clinical deficit occurs from bilateral sympathectomy.[17] Parasympathetic activity enhances colonic motility, and its loss is often associated with DWE, including impactions and functional obstructions, such as Ogilvie pseudoobstructive syndrome.[17]

The normal intact colon wall has a 3- to 6-Hz pattern of slow electrical potential waves, with irregularly occurring bursts of spike activity typically on the apex of these waves every 10–12 s. This spike activity is associated with development of bowel wall tension and with slow peristaltic waves of ring contractions. These ring contractions are several centimeters apart and travel at 1–2 mm/s. These peristaltic waves seem to be paced from the transverse colon, and travel both caudad to the rectum and cephalad to the cecum.[11]

The function of the transverse and ascending colon is largely storage, with propulsion generally retrograde toward the one-way ileocecal valve. This allows the haustral and colonic motility waves to mix and stir contents, and also exposes contents to the colon wall for additional fecal liquid absorption.[11] Occasionally, these proximal-traveling colonic waves reverse, especially during a giant migratory contraction (GMC) of the colon. The GMC is associated with mass movement of feces as far as one-third the length of the colon.[80] In the fasting-emptied colon, GMCs occur approximately four times per day, but twice or less per day in the normal colon.[80] The origin of the GMCs

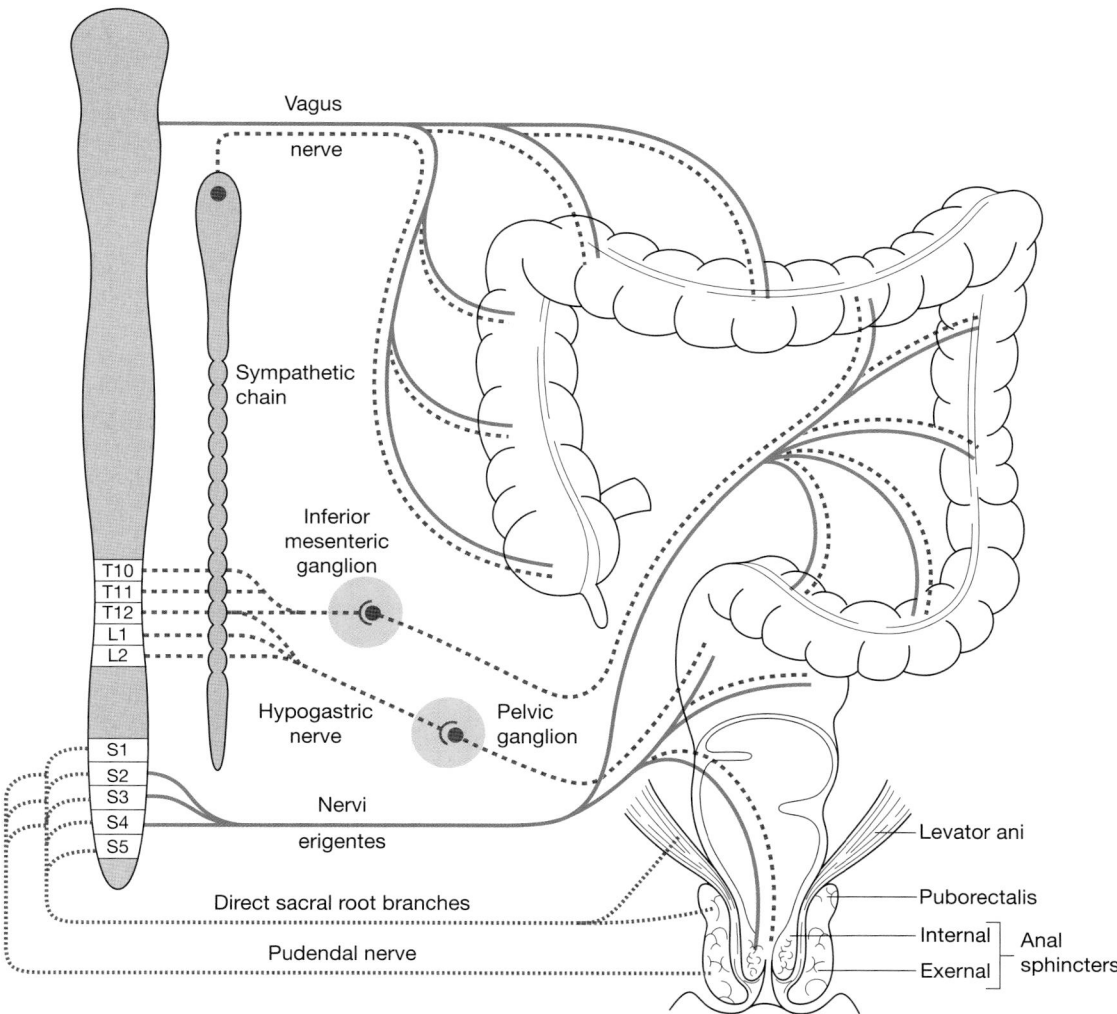

Figure 30-2 Neurologic levels and pathways for the sympathetic, parasympathetic, and somatic nervous system innervation of the colon and anorectum. Not shown is the enteric nervous system, which travels along the bowel wall from esophagus to internal anal sphincter and forms the final common pathway to control the bowel wall smooth muscle.

is poorly understood, but they commonly occur after meals with the gastrocolic response, or due to increased physical activity. The GMC does not seem to be under volitional control.[11]

The rectum is usually empty until just prior to defecation. Perception of rectal contents and pressures[63] is essential for signaling voluntary contraction of the anal sphincter. The resting anal canal pressure is largely determined by the angulation and pressure at the anorectal junction by the puborectalis sling and smooth muscle internal sphincter tone. Continence is maintained by the anal sphincter mechanism,[47,67] which consists of the internal anal sphincter (IAS), the external anal sphincter (EAS), and the puborectalis muscle.[47] Only about 20% of the anal canal pressure is due to the static contraction of the somatically innervated striated EAS.[4] The EAS and puborectalis muscle are the only striated skeletal muscles whose normal resting state is tonic contraction, and these muscles consist mainly of slow-twitch fatigue-resistant type 1 fibers (unlike the situation in non-upright animals such as the cat or dog, in which

it consists of predominately type 2 fibers).[4] Anal pressure can be increased volitionally by contracting the EAS and puborectalis muscles. Maximum volitional squeeze pressures, however, are not as high as can be generated reflexively against Valsalva pressure. The EAS is physically larger than the internal sphincter, and its contraction is under both reflex and volitional control. The volitional control is learned during the course of normal maturation. Normal baseline reflex action of the anorectal mechanism allows spontaneous stool elimination.[61] The EAS is innervated by the S2 through S4 nerve roots via the pudendal nerve, and the puborectalis muscle is innervated by direct branches from the S1 to S5 roots (see Fig. 30-2).[55] The remarkable degree of learned EAS coordination allows the selective discrete passage of gas while juggling a variable mixture of solids, liquids, and gases.

Normal defecation begins with reflexes triggered by rectosigmoid distension of approximately 200 mL of feces (Fig. 30-4).[56] A rectorectal reflex occurs in which the bowel proximal to the distending bolus contracts and the bowel wall distally relaxes, serving to propel the bolus further caudad. Reflex relaxation of the internal sphincter also occurs, which is enhanced by, but does not require, an extrinsic nerve supply. This relaxation, called the rectoanal inhibitory reflex, correlates with the urge

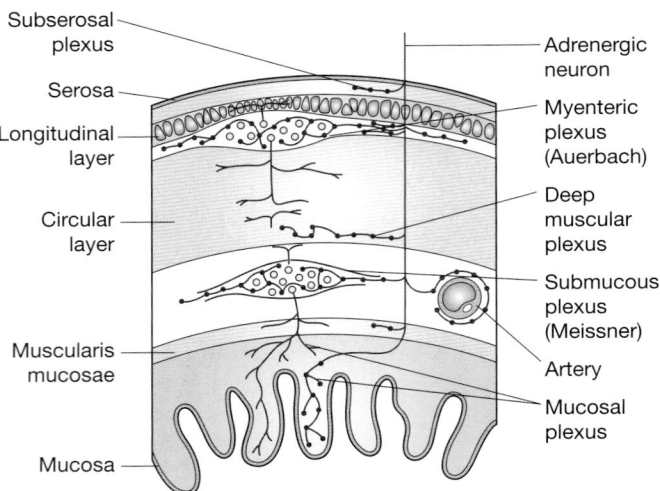

Figure 30-3 A transverse section of the gut, showing the enteric plexus and the distribution of adrenergic neurons. Note the ganglionic plexuses of Auerbach and Meissner. The deep muscular plexus contains a few ganglia, the subserosal contains an occasional ganglion, and the mucosal plexus shows none. The adrenergic fibers are all extrinsic and arise from the prevertebral sympathetic ganglia. The adrenergic fibers are distributed largely to the mesenteric, submucous, and mucosal plexus and to blood vessels. (From Goyal and Crist 1989,[24] with permission.)

labeled 'the call to stool'.[80] One can then volitionally contract the levator ani to open the proximal anal canal and relax the external sphincter and puborectalis muscles. This allows a straighter, shorter, and open anorectal passage (see Fig. 30-4), which permits the bolus to pass. Increasing the intraabdominal pressure by squatting and by Valsalva's maneuver assists bolus elimination. For 90% of normal individuals, only the contents of the rectum are expulsed, whereas 10% will clear the entire contents of the left colon from the splenic flexure distally.[18]

One can elect to defer defecation, however, by volitionally contracting the puborectalis muscle and EAS. The reflexive IAS relaxation subsequently fades, usually within 15 s, and the urge resolves until the IAS relaxation is again triggered. The rectal wall accommodates to the bolus by decreasing its wall tension with time, resulting in less sensory input and less reflex triggering from that particular accommodated bolus. This continence and reflex process is somewhat analogous to the function of the striated external urethral sphincter in volitional control of urinary voiding.

The external sphincter generally tenses in response to small rectal distensions via a spinal reflex, although reflexive relaxation of the external sphincter occurs in the presence of greater distensions.[63] These spinal cord reflexes are centered in the conus medullaris, and are augmented and modulated by higher cortical influences. When cortical control is disrupted, as by SCI, the external sphincter reflexes usually persist and allow spontaneous defecation. During sleep, colonic activity, anal tone, and protective responses to abdominal pressure elevations are all decreased, while rectal tone increases.[11,80]

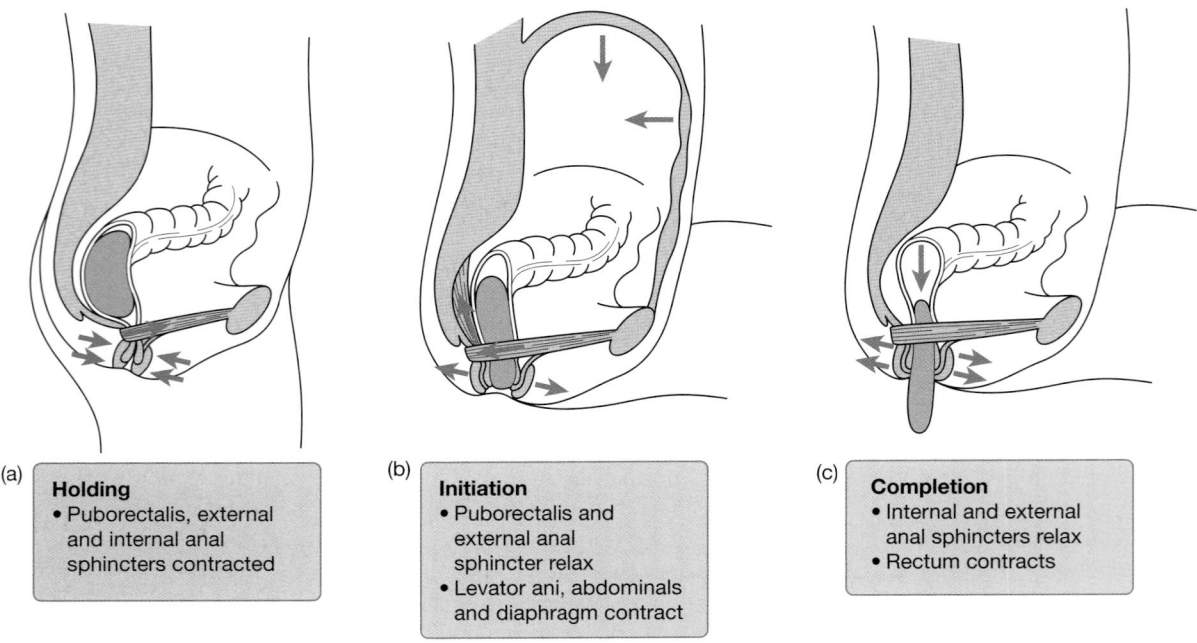

(a) Holding
• Puborectalis, external and internal anal sphincters contracted

(b) Initiation
• Puborectalis and external anal sphincter relax
• Levator ani, abdominals and diaphragm contract

(c) Completion
• Internal and external anal sphincters relax
• Rectum contracts

Figure 30-4 (**a**) Defecation is prevented by a statically increased tone of the internal anal sphincter (IAS) and puborectalis, as well as by the mechanical effects of the acute anorectal angle. Dynamic responses of the external anal sphincter (EAS) and puborectalis to rectal distension reflexes or increased intraabdominal pressures further impede defecation. (**b**) To initiate defecation, the puborectalis muscle and EAS relax while intraabdominal pressure is increased by Valsalva's maneuver, which is facilitated by squatting. The levator ani helps reduce the acute anorectal angle to open the distal anal canal to receive the stool bolus. (**c**) Intrarectal reflexes result in continued IAS relaxation and rectal propulsive contractions, which help expel the bolus through the open canal. (After Schiller 1989,[60] with permission.)

The 'gastrocolonic response' or 'gastrocolic reflex' refers to the increased colonic activity (GMCs and mass movements) that occurs in the first 30–60 min after a meal. This increased colonic activity appears to be modulated both by hormonal effects, from release of peptides from the upper gastrointestinal tract (gastrin, motilin, and cholecystokinin), which increase contractility of colonic smooth musculature, and by a reduction in the threshold for spinal cord-mediated vescicovescical reflexes.[11] Upper gastrointestinal receptor stimulation also results in increased activity in the colon, possibly due to reflexively increased parasympathetic efferent activity to the colon. The possibility of a purely ENS-mediated activation exists, although the small bowel and colon motor activities do not seem to be synchronized. In SCI, the measured increase in colonic activity after a meal is blunted as compared with in normal subjects.[11] The gastrocolonic response is often used therapeutically, even in patients with SCI, to enhance bowel evacuation during this 30- to 60-min postprandial time frame.[1,20] Occasionally, certain foods can serve as trigger foods that are especially likely to induce bowel evacuation shortly after consumption.

PATHOPHYSIOLOGY: NEUROGENIC BOWEL DYSFUNCTION

Upper motor neurogenic bowel

Any destructive central nervous system process above the conus, from SCI to dementia, can lead to the upper motor neurogenic bowel (UMNB) pattern of dysfunction. Spinal cortical sensory pathway deficits lead to decreased ability to sense the urge to defecate. Most persons with SCI, however, sense a vague discomfort when excessive rectal or colonic distension occurs, and 43% have chronic complaints of vague abdominal distension discomfort that eases with bowel evacuation.[46,70] These sensations might be mediated by autonomic nervous system afferent fibers bypassing the zone of SCI via the paraspinal sympathetic chain or by means of vagal parasympathetic afferents.

Colonic compliance and sphincter tone[61] have been experimentally evaluated in subjects with SCI. Studies of colonic compliance in response to a continuous infusion of saline initially suggested rapid pressure rises and a hyperreflexic response.[53,78] More recent studies have demonstrated normal colonic compliances in SCI subjects with UMNB.[45,54] Passive filling of the rectum leads to increases in the resting sphincter tone.[75] These increases are associated with increased external sphincter pressure development due to sacral reflexes that can be abolished by pudendal block.[4] This form of rectal sphincter dyssynergia has unfortunately been labeled decreased colonic compliance, even though intermittent or slow filling in the rectum appears to be associated with normal bolus accommodation and pressure relaxation.[45,60] This contrasts with the true decreased compliance found in ischemic or postinflammatory rectal bowel wall due to fibrosis, which cannot accommodate and relax, regardless of flow rates.

Colonic motility and stool propulsion have been known to be affected by SCI. De Looze et al. use a questionnaire method to study subjects with SCI levels above L2, and found 58% of subjects with chronic SCI had constipation, defined as two or less bowel movements per week or the requirement for digital evacuation.[15] Patients with paraplegia below T10 and above L2, however, were significantly less prone to constipation, at 30% ($P = 0.002$). Actual stool propulsion was studied later by Krogh et al. using swallowed markers and serial radiographs.[40] In subjects with chronic SCI with supraconal lesions, their group found significantly prolonged transit times of the ascending, traverse, and descending colon and rectosigmoid. Total gastrointestinal transit time averaged 3.93 days (1.76 controls) for chronic complete SCI above the conus. In an attempt to demonstrate a difference that may have been conferred by sympathetic innervation, mean total gastrointestinal transit times were compared for patients with lesions above T9 (2.92 ± 2.41) and from T10 down to L2 (2.84 ± 1.93). No significant differences could be found, even with comparison of transit times for individual colonic segments.

Subjects with SCI and complete upper motor neuron bowel lesions were studied during the acute phase (5–21 days) after SCI. These same patients were reevaluated 6–14 months later. Total gastrointestinal transit time was longer during the acute rather than the chronic phase. The upper motor neuron neurogenic colon tended to have slower transit throughout the colon, with less severe rectosigmoid dysfunction.[40] Patients with upper motor neuron neurogenic bowel have spared reflex arc control of the rectosigmoid and pelvic floor. Internal sphincter relaxation on rectal distension occurs in persons with SCI as well as in neurologically intact persons. After sufficient rectal distension, the external sphincter might completely relax, resulting in expulsion of the fecal bolus. Rectal sphincter dyssynergia does not necessarily correlate with bladder sphincter dyssynergia, but it often results in DWE.[55] The protective vesicorectal reflex, whereby the external sphincter pressure increases in response to increased intraabdominal pressure, is usually intact (Table 30-1).[4] Patients with UMNB also have normal or increased anal sphincter tone, intact anocutaneous (or 'anal wink') and bulbocavernosus reflexes,[67] a palpable puborectalis muscle sling, and normal anal verge appearance (Fig. 30-5).

Lower motor neurogenic bowel

Polyneuropathy, conus medullaris or cauda equina lesions, pelvic surgery, vaginal delivery, or even chronic straining during defecation can impair the somatic innervation of the anal sphincter mechanism. Persons with benign joint hypermobility syndrome might be more predisposed to these lesions.[49] These conditions can also produce sympathetic and parasympathetic innervation deficits. If an isolated pudendal insult has occurred, colonic transit times are normal and FI predominates. Distal colonic sluggishness can occur as a result of loss of parasympathetic supply. Segmental stool transit studies demonstrate prolonged transit through the rectosigmoid segments due to the lack of direct innervation from the conus.[40] The addition of constipation and DWE to FI compounds difficulties. This is an especially

Table 30-1 Features of colorectal function in normal subjects and in those with UMNB, UMNB with posterior rhizotomy, and LMNB

	Normal	UMNB	UMNB and posterior rhizotomy	LMNB
Bowel dysfunction	Normal colon activity and defecation	Chronic intractable constipation, fecal impaction, reflex defecation with or without incontinence	Chronic constipation; no reflex defecation	Chronic constipation; fecal impaction maximal in the rectum
Transit time (cecum to anus)	12–48 h	Prolonged >72 h	Very prolonged unless sacral nerve stimulator used	Prolonged >6 days, especially left colon
Colonic motility at rest	GMCs approximately four per 24 h	GMCs may be reduced in frequency	Reduced GMC	Reduced GMC
Colonic motility in response to stimuli	GMCs facilitated by defecation, exercise, and food ingestion	Less GMC facilitation by defecation, exercise, or food ingestion	Less GMC facilitation by defecation, exercise, or food ingestion	Less GMC facilitation by defecation, exercise, or food ingestion
Anal sphincter pressure (mmHg)				
Resting tone	>30	>30	Normal	Reduced
Volitional squeeze	>30 (up to 1800)	Absent	Absent	Absent
Rectal compliance	Normal	Normal but sigmoid compliance decreased	Normal or increased	Rectum dilated; increased distension volume; increased compliance
Rectal balloon distension				
Effect on IAS	Normal rectoanal inhibitory reflex	Normal rectoanal inhibitory reflex	Normal rectoanal inhibitory reflex	Normal rectoanal inhibitory reflex
Effect on EAS	Causes contraction	Causes contraction	No contraction	No contraction
Sensory perception threshold	<20 mL volume	None	None	None
Stimulation of rectal contraction	Induced by balloon distension	Giant rectal contractions stimulated readily	Rectal contraction stimulation	Rectal contraction stimulation
Vesicoanal reflex	Present (>50 mmHg)	Present	Absent	Absent
Valsalva protective reflex				
Reflex defecation	Yes	Yes	Impaired	Impaired
Perianal sensation (cutaneous sensation of touch, pinprick)	Normal	No sensory perception	No sensory perception	Loss of perianal and buttock sensation due to injury to sacral nerves
Anocutaneous reflex ('anal wink')	Present	Present; may be increased	Absent	Absent due to injury to afferent or efferent sacral pathways
Bulbocavernosus reflex	Present	Present; may be increased	Absent	Absent
Anal appearance	Normal	Normal	Normal	Flattened, scalloped, due to loss of EAS bulk

EAS, external anal sphincter; GMCs, giant migratory contractions; IAS, internal anal sphincter; LMNB, lower motor neurogenic bowel; UMNB, upper motor neurogenic bowel.
(After Banwell et al. 1993,[3] and Schiller 1989,[60] with permission.)

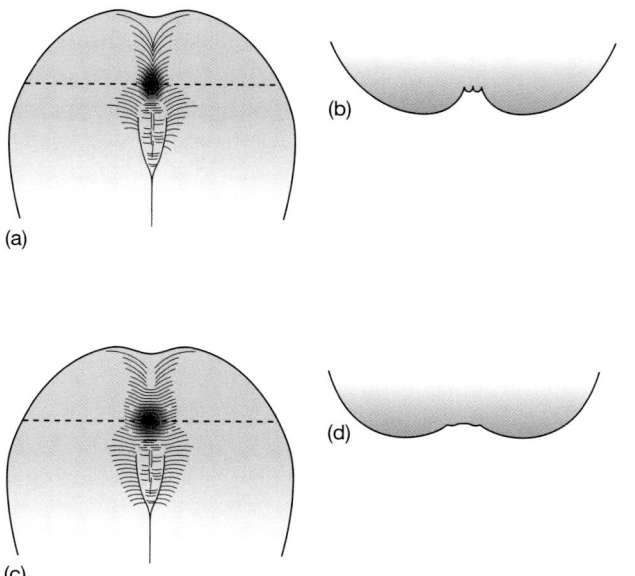

Figure 30-5 Upper motor neurogenic bowel presents an appearance similar to normal (**a**, rear view; **b**, profile from above). Anal contour of the lower motor neurogenic bowel (**c**, rear view; **d**, profile from above), with its atrophic external anal sphincter, shows a flattened, scalloped-appearing anal area.

problematic combination, because the accumulation of a large amount of hard stool that can result from such colonic inertia can overstretch the weakened anal mechanism. This can result in a gaping, patulous, incompetent anal orifice, often with associated rectal prolapse. The denervation, atrophy, and over-stretching of the EAS and IAS lead to loss of the protective IAS tone, which can result in stool soilage from the increased abdominal pressures associated with everyday activities. Rectal distension leads to the expected internal sphincter relaxation, but attenuated or absent external sphincter protective contractions can result in FI or fecal smearing whenever boluses are present at the rectum. The presence of a large bolus in the rectal vault can further compromise the rectoanal angulation at the pelvic floor, and contribute to paradoxical liquid incontinence around a low impaction, called the *ball valve effect*.[4,72,81]

Patients with lower motor neurogenic bowel (LMNB) dysfunction have decreased anal tone due to the smooth muscle that makes up the internal sphincter. If no tone is found initially on inserting the examining finger, the examiner should wait up to 15 s to allow IAS reflex relaxation to recover and restore tone. Chronic overstretching has probably occurred if tone does not return. The anal to buttock contour typically appears flattened and scalloped (see Fig. 30-5), due to atrophy of the pudendal-innervated pelvic floor muscles and EAS.[4] The anocutaneous reflex is absent or decreased (depending on the completeness of the lesion). Likewise, the bulbocavernosus reflex is weak if present (see Table 30-1). The anal canal is shortened (as compared with the normal 2.5- to 4.5-cm length), and the puborectalis muscle ridge may not be palpable. Excessive peri-

neal descent and even rectal prolapse can occur with Valsalva's maneuver.

Evaluation

The gastrointestinal history should not only review cardinal symptoms, but should also address the patient's general neuromuscular and gastrointestinal function. A detailed review of the patient's bowel program includes an assessment of fluids, diet, activity, medications, and aspects of bowel care.[35] A review of the technique and outcome of bowel care should include a description of schedule, initiation method (chemical or mechanical stimulation), facilitative techniques, time requirements, and characteristics of stool results.[67] The history should include premorbid bowel pattern information such as defecation frequency, typical time(s) of the day, associated predefecatory activities, bowel medications and techniques or trigger foods, and stool consistency. It is important to elicit any history of premorbid gastrointestinal disease or dysfunction. The presence of gastrointestinal sensations or pain, warning sensations for defecation, sense of urgency, and ability to prevent stool loss during Valsalva activities such as laughing, sneezing, coughing, or transfers should be noted. Excessively large-caliber hard stool can be ascertained by a history of toilet plugging.[51] The patient's goals and willingness to alter prior bowel patterns or management need to be established.[33]

The physical examination should include the gastrointestinal system and the associated parts of the musculoskeletal and nervous systems required for independent management of the bowel program. The examination should be completed at the onset, and then annually for SCI.[35] The purpose of the examination is to detect functional changes, screen for complications, and identify any new masses or lesions.

The abdomen should be inspected for distension, hernias, and other abnormalities. Percussion and auscultation should precede palpation for masses and tenderness. With the abdomen relaxed, the examiner transabdominally palpates the colon for hard stool. Palpable hard stool should not be present on the right side of the abdomen (ascending colon).

Physical examination continues with inspection of the anus. A patulous gaping orifice suggests a history of over-distension and trauma by a previous regimen. A normal anal–buttock contour (Fig. 30-5) suggests an intact EAS muscle mass, whereas its loss results in a flattened, fanned-out scalloped-appearing anal region. The patient should perform Valsalva's maneuver while the examiner observes the anus and perineum for excessive descent.[73] Perianal cutaneous sharp stimulation normally results in an externally visible anal sphincter reflexive contraction. This is the anocutaneous reflex, mediated by the inferior hemorrhoidal branch of the pudendal nerve (S2–S5). This can be checked by tugging perianal hairs or by the application of the sharp edge of a broken cotton swab stick to the perianal skin. The anocutaneous reflex should be checked in all four quadrants, as selective (especially side to side) deficits can occur. Sensation to pinprick is tested at the same time. A gloved lubricated finger should then be inserted through the anus until no pressure is appreciated at the fingertip. The tone and voluntary squeeze strength of the EAS and tone of the IAS should be assessed. The length of the anus, where pressure is sensed, is normally 2.5–4.5 cm. The point where the pressure decreases marks the anorectal junction. Along the posterior wall, 1.5–2.5 cm from the anal verge, the puborectalis muscular sling can be palpated as a ridge that will push the finger forward as the subject resists defecation. No palpable ridge or push suggests puborectalis atrophy or dysfunction. A shortened length of anal pressure zone suggests EAS muscle atrophy. With the examiner's finger in place, the bulbocavernosus reflex can be elicited by rapidly tapping or squeezing the clitoris or glans penis. Multiple random trials are needed to be certain the vesicorectal Valsalva protective reflexes are not occurring at the same time by random chance. The response can be delayed up to a few seconds in pathologic conditions. A consistent response to the stimulus indicates an intact bulbocavernosus reflex, although the reflex does extinguish when repeatedly elicited. Insertion of the finger in the anal canal occasionally triggers IAS relaxation, but more often triggers a tightening squeeze that is efferently equivalent to the bulbocavernosus reflex. If IAS and EAS relaxation occur, the examiner should wait several seconds for tone to be restored before testing the bulbocavernosus reflex. Ask the patient to volitionally squeeze the anus before removing the finger ('resist defecation') to check for volitional EAS and puborectalis tone and control.

Diagnostic testing

The history and physical examination provide most of the necessary information. The clinical cause of neurogenic bowel dysfunction in most patients who are referred to physiatrists is readily apparent. Additional objective laboratory testing can be helpful when the cause of FI or DWE is obscure, the history appears doubtful, conservative interventions fail, or surgical interventions are contemplated. Table 30-2 lists some of the many tests available.

Basic laboratory tests complement the physical examination. A stool guaiac test is helpful to rule out the presence of blood in the stool. False positives are common after SCI because of hemorrhoids, as well as from anal trauma secondary to bowel care.[67] A flat plate radiograph of the abdomen can be helpful to rule out impaction,[81] megacolon, obstruction, and a perforated viscus.

MANAGEMENT
General principles

A *bowel program* is a comprehensive individualized patient-centered treatment plan focused on preventing incontinence, achieving effective and efficient colonic evacuation, and preventing the complications of neurogenic bowel dysfunction.[67] The subcomponents of a bowel program address diet, fluids, exercise, medications, and scheduled bowel care. *Bowel care* is the individually developed and prescribed procedure for defecation that is carried out by the patient or attendant.[67]

The approach to the problems associated with neurogenic bowel is the same as for all issues that confront the patient in

the rehabilitation process. All aspects of impairment and activity limitation that restrict a person's ability to maintain continence and volitionally defecate must be assessed within the perspective of the entire person. This includes an appraisal of the patient's limit level, bowel pattern, and dietary habits. All aspects of personal performance should be addressed in person-centered rehabilitation, with the overall goal of maximizing independence in bowel management or direction of a bowel program.[64,67]

In children, achieving social continence at the usual developmental age has benefit, especially socially. Riveille, a French psychologist, emphasized the importance of patients with spina bifida becoming continent and independent 'as early as possible' to avoid the irreversible psychologic disturbances that might occur at puberty.[57] Indeed, neurogenic bowel training becomes less effective as children approach puberty, and should begin ideally before public school age.[33]

Neurogenic bowel dysfunction results in problems with fecal storage and elimination. Inability to volitionally inhibit spontaneous defecations leads to incontinence, while the inability to adequately empty leads to constipation and impactions. Paradoxically, impactions can result in diarrhea and incontinence. Providing adequate timely emptying must be combined with the inhibition of spontaneous defecations, except at desired times in order to achieve social continence.

Disablement and rehabilitation models: methods for coordinating efforts of the interdisciplinary team

The method of assessment and intervention for problems caused by neurogenic bowel is the same as for all issues that confront the patient in the rehabilitation process.[67] The rehabilitation evaluation should be interdisciplinary in approach, and include assessment not only of colon and pelvic floor dysfunction but also of impairments of other organs or systems that could affect rehabilitative strategies to make bowel care independent or prevent unplanned bowel movements. The rehabilitation database should specifically note the level and degree of associated comorbid motor and sensory deficits. The examination should assess reflex function to determine the impairment pattern (UMNB or LMNB) of colonic and pelvic floor dysfunction that is present. Next, the problem is succinctly described and included on the rehabilitation problem list as a UMNB or LMNB pattern of impairment.

Activity limitations that limit a person's ability to maintain continence and volitionally defecate must be assessed within the perspective of the entire person. Limitations of functional mobility as well as retained capabilities need to be considered. For example, any residual colonic reflex function can be exploited in bowel care. Task modifications, digital stimulation, or pharmacologic interventions can be utilized to trigger and sustain defecation.[67] The rehabilitation process for development and initiating a bowel program requires knowledge of the individual person and derivation of person-centered goals.[34,66] A single member of the rehabilitation team should coordinate this interdisciplinary intervention effort. Typically, the person

Table 30-2 Laboratory tests of colonic and rectoanal function

Test	Purpose
Colonoscopy, rectosigmoidoscopy, anoscopy	Visualize anatomy to identify lesions Limited benefit to assess function
Anal endosonography	Evaluate structure and continuity of pelvic muscles
Radiography Defecography Barium enema Serial radiographs of tiny radiopaque plastic beads ingested with food	 Visualize kinesiology of defecation Identify structural defects; fluoroscopy time too limited to assess function in any detail Evaluate colonic transit time; useful to confirm constipation history and to identify dysfunctional segments that help plan colostomy level
Manometry	Assess giant migratory contractions and anal pressures; with intrarectal balloon inflation, to evaluate rectoanal inhibitory reflex
Kymography	Measure pressure and volume change by intraluminal balloons
Catheter	Measure pressures by catheter in various compartments of the bowel
Solid sphere retention test	Measure maximal anal resistance force to extraction of spheres of standard sizes
Rectally infused saline continence test	Quantitative reproducible assessment of liquid continence ability
Electromyography Traditional Mucosal electrosensitivity	 Assess motor nerve supply to puborectalis, anococcygeus, levator ani, and external anal sphincter; assess sensory pelvic afferents by nerve conduction studies, bulbocavernosus reflex testing, or somatosensory-evoked potentials Assess degree of mucosal wall sensibility
Intraluminal catheter	Research tool to assess colonic smooth muscle electrical potential activity

(Information compiled from Christensen 1991,[11] Schiller 1989,[60] and Stone et al. 1990.[71])

is the primary nurse, acting in close association with the physiatrist and occupational therapist.

The role performance of the individual that occurs after the acute rehabilitation process is complete determines the timing and content of the new bowel care schedule. The demands of life activities, the duration of bowel care, and the needs of other members of the household should all be considered in scheduling. During inpatient rehabilitation, scheduling can be especially difficult because of the time-consuming nature of bowel care.[4] Evening bowel care often allows for more predictable attendance at daily therapies.

It is crucial to remember that the patient must take a decisive leadership role in designing a bowel program that includes a convenient bowel care schedule. Educating patients about their altered neurogenic bowel physiology and empowering them with options and techniques to construct a bowel care regimen compatible with their life interests are important aspects of the overall rehabilitation process.

Dietary considerations

Food choices are important when colonic transit time is prolonged, as in SCI (96 h versus the 30 h typically found in normal subjects).[4,5,52] Excessive fluid resorption can result in stool hardening and subsequent constipation. Gases and liquids are propelled 30–100 times faster than solids by the colon. Stools that have lost their plasticity might not be kneaded and

folded by the haustra, and instead their transit can be impeded. To maintain a more fluid content, stool softeners, both docusate and food fiber, have been used. No increase in stool bulk, as would be expected with fluid retention, occurs from docusate in normal subjects, which brings its efficacy into question.[4] Fiber does increase stool bulk and plasticity, especially in the more physically coarse forms, which also tend to decrease colonic pressures.[4] Control of excessive stool hardness requires higher fiber foods in preference to lower residual foods.

The American norm has been found to be 100 g (although highly variable, with a range of 35–450 g in males and 5–335 g in females) of solid feces expelled daily or less frequently.[18,60] However, the high pressures involved in moving solid feces probably contribute to the 90% incidence of hemorrhoids in Americans, and to premature diverticula formation and hemorrhoidal complications in more than 70% of patients with SCI.[70] Constant straining at stool can also contribute to peripheral neuropathic deficits in the anal sphincteric musculature.[18] Acceptance of softer stools, from a higher fiber diet, might help reduce these complications and is often recommended for their treatment. A diet that contains at least 15 g of fiber daily is recommended.[35] Increases in the fiber content of the diets of persons with SCI do not decrease colonic transit time[8] but enhance the rectoanal inhibitory reflex.[18] The effects of fiber intake on stool consistency and frequency and the efficacy of evacuation should be evaluated in each individual patient. The longer perineal hygiene time required for softer stools might be a deterrent for some, and should be discussed with patients. Increases in dietary fiber typically result in increased stool bulk, which can require more frequent bowel care.

A wide range of 'normal' bowel patterns exist. Defecation frequencies in non-impaired persons vary dramatically, from several times per day to less than once per week. Ninety-five percent have a frequency of between three times per day and three times per week.[18,58] Stool consistencies vary, from liquid to pudding, pasty, semisolid, soft-formed, medium-formed, and hard-formed. Patients rarely have an adequate vocabulary to describe this socially taboo subject.[69] Fully appreciating an individual's premorbid 'normal' bowel function is important in the planning and goal setting for a new neurogenic bowel program.

Approaches and rationale

Colonic transit time and fecal elimination are enhanced by softer stool. However, if the stool becomes too liquid, the protective angle provided by the puborectalis becomes less effective, and greater EAS pressures are required to maintain continence. Neurogenic bowel resting anal pressures are usually normal to slightly decreased, but are unable to develop the protective increases in EAS tone needed to control more liquid stool.[4] Some degree of stool firmness must be tolerated to prevent incontinence. To avoid incontinence on straining, more firmness (medium-formed) is required for the weaker anal sphincter mechanism of LMNB than for UMNB (semiformed to soft-formed). Docusate is often used to try to increase fluid content and plasticity of the stool, although its clinical efficacy should be individually monitored. Fiber more consistently softens stool but also adds bulk. Bulkier stools can help stimulate the defecatory response more easily in LMNB, although less stimulus is needed in UMNB.[19,44] The presentation of stool to the rectum, triggering defecation, can be associated with GMC and mass movements more than with the slow accumulation of sufficient rectal stool to trigger reflex defecation, and the GMC might be what is actually habituated.[60]

The frequency and specific timing of bowel care to induce adequate colonic emptying can be chosen, based on previous elimination patterns. Regular bowel emptying is recommended as the primary means for enhancing both elimination and decreasing incontinence between stooling. Incontinence is reduced by less stool accumulation, because stool is not presented to the rectum between desired defecation times. Adequate emptying is accomplished by:

- making stools easier to move by means of softening;
- adding bowel stimulant medication if needed; and
- triggering the defecatory reflex at consistent desired times to promote habituation.

Choosing long intervals between elimination allows more fluid reabsorption, resulting in harder stools, which can worsen DWE. Because 95% of unimpaired persons defecate three or more times per week, choosing a frequency of at least as often as every other day would seem more physiologic and less likely to contribute to constipation.[18,35,58] One study of patients with well-managed SCI found frequencies of bowel care to be chosen as daily by 24%, every other day by 46%, and more often than three times a week by 85%.[36] The desire to avoid the unpleasant task of stool elimination leads some to elect longer time intervals between bowel care sessions, but this carries the attendant risk for impaction or sphincter damage caused by rectal distention by larger-caliber, harder stools.

Chronic oral bowel stimulant medication use has been questioned, because of concerns of developing the atonic 'cathartic bowel' syndrome. Certain stimulants, especially in the anthraquinone family (senna, cascara, and aloes), have been shown to damage myenteric neurons with chronic use.[14,65] It has not been established whether late complications from chronic oral bowel stimulant medications occur in those with neurogenic bowel dysfunction. Approaches that appear effective initially need longer term studies to verify their continued benefits, especially because there is a high incidence of late gastrointestinal problems reported in an initially successfully treated SCI population.[70]

Triggering of defecation can be accomplished by digital stimulation, rectal stimulant medications, enemas, or electrical stimulation. All these cause reflex relaxation of the IAS, and if strong enough can reflexly relax the EAS as well. This initiates the rectorectal reflex that helps to eliminate any stool that is present. The GMC and mass movement associated with the 'call to stool' for many intact persons often occurs at consistent times, which can be trainable. If a bowel habit (consistent time or times of day when defecation typically occurs for that individual) existed premorbidly, its consistency should be encouraged by inducing defecation at similar times. Such bowel habits are trainable events that also enhances adequate emptying if consistent training is used. A change from the patient's usual pattern can be habituated, but can take several weeks of inducing defecations at the new desired time before incontinence at the prior time subsides.[33]

There are a variety of rectally administered medications that are utilized to trigger and sustain reflex defecation. The rationale for this prescription is to use the least irritating and most easily inserted and retained medication. Suppositories that are typically utilized include glycerin, vegetable oil-based bisacodyl, and polyethylene glycol-based (PGB) bisacodyl. Options for minienema-triggered bowel care include small-volume phospho soda enema, bisacodyl enema, and Enemeez™. Clinical efficacy studies have been conducted in attempts to measure efficiency and effectiveness of bowel care utilizing various rectally administered triggering medications. In a randomized blinded study, hydrogenated vegetable oil-based (HVB) bisacodyl suppositories were compared with PGB suppositories and the Therevac™ minienema.[30] Subjects with upper motor neuron neurogenic bowel dysfunction were studied, with the events and intervals of bowel care.[30] Bowel care trials with PGB suppositories showed an average time to defecation of approximately 22 min, and a total bowel care time of 50 min. This was much shorter than the average time to defecation of 40 min and total bowel care time of 85 min observed with HVB bisacodyl suppository trials. The use of minienemas had similar efficiency to that of PGB suppositories, and has since been replaced by Enemeez. Results vary in individual patients, and the use of digital stimulation alone is efficient for many SCI persons with upper motor neuron neurogenic bowel.

Theoretically, fewer long-term complications will occur if the following are minimized: anorectal over-distention (as with enemas), anal trauma (as by manual disimpaction), and oral stimulant medication use. An accelerating enema volume required for efficacy should be a warning that chronic rectal over-distention might be leading to less responsiveness.[33] Digital stimulation to induce defecatory reflexes should be favored over manual disimpaction, because the latter can easily result in inadvertent overstretching of the insensate and more delicate anal mechanisms of the neurogenic bowel. Local rectal stimulant suppositories and minienemas with bisacodyl or glycerin do not carry the same risk as that of oral stimulant medications, and do not appear to lead to chronic inflammatory changes of the rectal mucosa.

One approach to initiating neurogenic bowel training is outlined in Box 30-1. Each step is added only after 2 weeks' consistent trial of the previous step has been ineffective. In this approach, obtaining elimination at the desired time is emphasized as the first step, and usually precedes development of complete continence by several weeks. This regimen is designed to enhance responsiveness and emptying at the habituated time, with apparently less responsiveness, or less rectal or stool presentation, during periods between bowel care sessions.

Box 30-1 Protocol for progressive steps in bowel habituation program

1. Perform bowel cleanout if stool is present in the rectal vault or palpable proximal to the descending colon, by multiple enemas or oral cathartic.
2. Titrate to soft stool consistency with diet and bulking agents (fiber) and stool softeners (docusate).
3. Trigger defecation with a glycerin suppository or by digital stimulation 20–30 min after a meal; 10 min later, have the patient attempt defecation on the toilet, limited to less than 40 min, and relieving skin pressure every 10 min.
4. If defecation is not initiated, a trial of a bisacodyl suppository p.r. is initiated.
5. Digital stimulation. Start 20 min after suppository placement and repeat every 5 min.
6. Timed oral medications. Administer casanthranol–docusate sodium (Peri-Colace™), senna (Senokot™), or bisacodyl (Dulcolax™) tablets timed so that bowel movement would otherwise result 30 min to 1 h after anticipated triggered bowel timing.
7. If defecation occurs in less than 10 min after suppository insertion, transition to digital stimulation technique only. Once the patient is well habituated, straining alone may rarely trigger defecations at a desired time.

Note that steps 1–3 are initial interventions and are always followed, with steps 4–6 incorporated only as needed. At least 2 weeks' trial with proper technique is pursued before advancing to the next step.

Bowel function is a very private matter, and patients might be reluctant to seek advice or information despite its major importance to their overall well-being and self-concept.[60,67,68] Information should be freely disseminated in order to enhance the development of healthy habits and minimize bowel complications. Basic education in gastrointestinal function can be presented by lectures, review of SCI care manual chapters,[26] booklets,[68] and videos.[69] Bowel habituation training is more difficult to accept among those with long-established patterns of managing stool hygiene, even if their current methods are ineffective in eliminating incontinence or constipation and are identified by the patient as unsatisfactory.[33] The advantages to a bowel program need to be explicitly communicated and illustrated using the patient's bowel record as evidence for effectiveness.[68]

Intrinsic loss of the ENS, or any segment, including by surgical reanastomosis, can result in loss of the rectoanal inhibitory reflex, causing DWE. Oral laxative abuse can cause dysfunction of the ENS.[14,65] If bowel training is not accomplishing defecation at the desired times, or if repeated involuntary incontinence occurs, further diagnostic evaluation might be indicated (see Table 30-2).

When neurogenic bowel deficits are incomplete and some degree of control and sensation is present, biofeedback might offer a means of enhancing the patient's residual sensory and motor abilities. Improved sensory awareness after biofeedback training is an indicator of success. This typically requires only a few sessions, and most patients improve after just one session.[60] Among more severely impaired non-selected myelomeningocele children, biofeedback and behavioral training are equally effective in restoring continence.[60] For selected individuals with some degree of volitional EAS activation and some degree of anorectal sensation, biofeedback can be a tool to help restore not just social continence, but also normal defecatory control.

Surgical options

Sacral nerve deficits interfere with the action of the puborectalis, levator ani, and EAS (see Fig. 30-2). The resulting pelvic floor descent impairs the protective puborectalis sling angle and decreases the efficacy of protective EAS contractions. Some patients have benefited from transposition of innervated gracilis, adductor longus, gluteus maximus, or free muscle graft palmaris longus to replace puborectalis function and restore the acute anorectal junction angle that this sling provides. Chronic electrical stimulation to enhance development of fatigue resistance is used with these transplants. Sensory deficits are not improved, but continence is somewhat restored, with the ability to inhibit defecation if some degree of sensation remains.[47,60]

Incomplete EAS relaxation during defecation (dyssynergia) results in a functional outlet obstruction and DWE. A prolonged descending colon transit time occurs, which does improve with an IAS and partial EAS myotomy.[17] This procedure relieves constipation in 62% of patients, but results in FI in 16%, and therefore has not become a popular option.[50]

Stimulation of anterior sacral roots S2, S3, and S4 by transrectal electric stimulation or via a stimulator surgically placed for micturition has been performed.[7,10,22,45] Stimulation of S2 tends to promote non-peristaltic, low-pressure colorectal motor activity. Stimulation of S3 causes occasional high-pressure peristaltic waves, especially with repetitive stimulation. Stimulation of S4 increases both rectal and anal tone.[45,77] Electrodefecation has been obtainable by sacral root stimulation in up to 50% of patients, but remains unpredictable.[3,7,10,11] A reliable electroprosthesis for defecation remains an elusive goal.[3,22] Electroprosthesis for both bowel and bladder control has been found to be cost-effective in suprasacral spinal cord-injured persons, although it is unclear how much of this benefit was from improved bowel control.[13] Artificial anal sphincters with a subcutaneous pump reservoir similar to urinary artificial sphincters suffer from high complication rates and poor outcomes, and their use has only been investigative.[47]

In clinical scenarios of prolonged bowel care time, recurrent fecal impactions, or poor or intermittent response to rectal medications to initiate bowel care, the options of the antegrade continence enema should be considered.[12,39,48,74] This is an alternative method of antegrade enema delivery that requires the surgical construction of a catheterizable appendicocecostomy stoma. Through a horizontal right lower quadrant incision, the appendix and right colon are mobilized and brought against the abdominal wall. The tip of the appendix is then amputated and the opening into the appendix lumen is modified into a catheterizable stoma on the abdominal wall. This can now also be performed laparoscopically.[31] This stoma can be catheterized and infused with 200–600 mL of tap water to trigger a propulsive colonic peristalsis and defecation within 10–20 min.[82] Bowel care can then be additionally facilitated with digital stimulation in the usual fashion.

Colostomy has been shown to reduce bowel care time, especially when offered to those with chronic DWE.[59,71] It can be indicated in four general scenarios:

1. when conservative medical measures and training have failed;[35,67]
2. when intrinsic bowel deficits exist, such as in Hirschsprung disease, Chagas disease, and 'cathartic colon';
3. when pressure ulcers or other skin lesions occur that cannot be effectively healed because of frequent soiling; or
4. when recurrent urinary tract seeding by repetitive bowel impactions occurs.[16,59,71]

Although diversion for pressure ulcer healing is usually anticipated to be reversed, those with neurogenic bowel often elect to maintain the colostomy even after the pressure ulcer has healed.[59,71] Colostomy carries a surgical risk, is cosmetically disfiguring, and is seldom necessary to achieve adequate social continence, but it remains a procedure of last resort for the treatment of FI or DWE.[3,16,35,67,70]

Complications
Significant bowel complications requiring medical treatment or lifestyle alterations are reported by 27% of persons with SCI by 5 years or greater beyond their injury, even though bowel management was satisfactory during the first 5 years. Over 80% of persons with SCI had bowel impactions, and 20% had chronic bowel impaction and DWE problems.[70] Impactions have been reported to be complicated by perforation or even death.[81] Impactions have a morbidity ranging between 0% and 6% in the normal population, being higher in the cognitively impaired elderly.[81] Other late gastrointestinal complications reported by patients with SCI include gastroesophageal reflux, premature diverticulosis, and autonomic dysreflexia.[23,37,70] Morbidity from colonic perforation by enema use has also been reported.[43]

Hemorrhoids are more symptomatic when patients have intact sensation, but in one study rectal bleeding due to hemorrhoids was reported by 74% of patients with SCI.[70] Hemorrhoids develop as a result of frequent high pressures in the anorectal marginal veins, and are associated with constipated hard stool passage. Stool softening is the best preventive and chronic treatment measure, but it should be balanced with the requirement to modulate stool consistency to maintain continence.

An overstretched patulous non-competent sphincter associated with rectal prolapse often is the end result of chronic passage of very large hard stools through a weakened anorectal mechanism in LMNB. Over-distention of the weakened neurogenic anal mechanism should be avoided by use of stool softening and gentle care to dilate the sphincter whenever manual disimpaction is required, to minimize trauma to these denervated structures. Although the anus can be significantly dilated to accommodate two fingers for breaking up low impactions, anorectal over-distention has been hypothesized to lead to atonic segments similar to bladder over-distention. The bowel, however, cannot be as easily decompressed and rested to allow recovery as can the bladder. The IAS is smooth muscle that will shorten and remodel to eventually regain competent closure if the overstretching can be eliminated. Unfortunately, this might require months of incontinent, liquid to soft pasty stools, which is seldom tolerated. Should the patient require temporary colostomy for some other disease process, it might be possible, after many months, to then train toward social continence with the decompressed and restored IAS. However, such patients have usually had long courses of constant soiling and often prefer to keep their colostomy and continence rather than pursue surgical reversal and training.

Autonomic dysreflexia occurs in SCI patients with lesions at or above the midthoracic region. FI is a common and potentially dangerous cause of autonomic dysreflexia, because of the substantial time that can be required for its clearance (see Ch. 56). If manual disimpaction is required, lubrication with Lidocaine™ (lignocaine) gel is recommended to decrease additional nociceptive sensory input from the richly innervated anal region.

Bloating and abdominal distention are common complaints of patients with neurogenic bowel dysfunction. These complaints can be reduced in patients with SCI by increasing the frequency of bowel care. This complaint can be especially severe in those with hyperactive EAS protective responses to rectal distention, which can preclude the passing of flatus.

Digital release of flatus might be required, in addition to diet modification to eliminate foods that produce excessive gases. The work-up should also include assessment for any contributing aerophagia (air swallowing).

Treatment outcomes

Bowel habituation training in children with myelomeningocele by means of suppositories, digital stimulation, or both resulted in 83% of compliant patients having less than one incontinent stool per month.[33] The continence catheter enema, which has a distal rectal balloon to avoid immediate enema expulsion, when used daily or every other day, reduced FI to fewer than three episodes per month in children with myelomeningocele.[21,62]

Fecally incontinent nursing home residents with dementia evaluated to have UMNB were treated by medically constipating them (with codeine) and giving biweekly enemas. Those diagnosed to have LMNB had their stools softened with lactulose and received weekly enemas. Fecal continence was restored in 80% of those consistently treated by these protocols.[76]

Although all patients with complete SCI have episodic FI,[46] this is a chronic problem for only 2%.[68] DWE appears to be a progressive problem that develops 5 years or more after SCI. This is rarely reported after training in the first 4 years, but occurs in 20% by a mean of 17 years after injury.[68] Gastrointestinal problems in SCI are not merely nuisances, because they also account for 10% of SCI late mortality.[23]

Patients with multiple sclerosis, parkinsonism, or muscular dystrophy have also been helped by methods to enhance bowel storage or elimination in the setting of deteriorating neuromuscular and anorectal function.[3,9,79] Colostomy can also provide a means of achieving social continence in these patients. Colostomy complications include embarrassing gas problems, appliance loosening and leakage, and cosmetic difficulties.

Patients who develop social bowel continence are enabled to venture into public without fear of malodorous embarrassment and unpredictable social disasters that humiliate as well as require substantial clean-up time. When fear of such adverse events persists, full social and vocational reintegration is impeded. A major hurdle that many patients with neuromuscular compromise can overcome is control of the seemingly automatic neurogenic functions of defecation and bowel elimination. Such patients should not needlessly suffer because inadequate attention has been paid by care providers to this potentially functionally impairing and socially disabling deficit.

Many solutions are yet to come for the large number of persons who cope with neurogenic bowel dysfunction. The colon will continue to be a fertile area for research.[67]

REFERENCES

1. Aaronson MJ, Freed MM, Burakoff R. Colonic myoelectric activity in persons with spinal cord injury. Dig Dis Sci 1985; 30:295–300.

2. Abercrombie JF, Rogers J, Swash M. Faecal incontinence in myotonic dystrophy. J Neurol Neurosurg Psychiatry 1998; 64:128–130.

3. Banwell JG, Creasey GH, Aggarwal AM, et al. Management of the neurogenic bowel in patients with spinal cord injury. Urol Clin North Am 1993; 20:517–526.

4. Bartolo DC, Read NW, Jarratt JA, et al. Differences in anal sphincter function and clinical presentation in patients with pelvic floor descent. Gastroenterology 1983; 85:68–75.

5. Beuret-Blanquart F, Weber J, Gouverneur JP, et al. Colonic transit time and anorectal manometric anomalies in 19 patients with complete transection of the spinal cord. J Auton Nerv Syst 1990; 30:199–207.

6. Boss BJ, Pecanty L, McFarland SM, et al. Self-care competence among persons with spinal cord injury. SCI Nurs 1995; 12:48–53.

7. Brindley GS, Rushton DN. Long-term follow-up of patients with sacral anterior root stimulator implants. Paraplegia 1990; 30:469–475.

8. Cameron K, Nyulasi I, Collier G, et al. Assessment of the effect of increased dietary fibre intake on bowel function in patients with spinal cord injury. Spinal Cord 1996; 34:277–303.

9. Caroscio JT. Amyotrophic lateral sclerosis: a guide to patient care. New York: Thieme; 1986:126.

10. Chia YW, Lee TK, Kour NW, et al. Microchip implants on the anterior sacral roots in patients with spinal trauma: does it improve bowel function? Dis Colon Rectum 1996; 39:690–694.

11. Christensen J. The motor function of the colon. In: Yamada T, ed. Textbook of gastroenterology. Philadelphia: JB Lippincott; 1991:180–196.

12. Christensen P, Kvitzau B, Krogh K, et al. Neurogenic colorectal dysfunction—use of new antegrade and retrograde colonic wash-out methods. Spinal Cord 2000; 38:255–261.

13. Creasey GH, Dahlberg JE. Economic consequences of an implanted neuroprosthesis for bladder and bowel management. Arch Phys Med Rehabil 2001; 82:1520–1525.

14. Cummings JH. Laxative abuse. Gut 1974; 15:758–766.

15. De Looze D, Van Laere M, De Muynck M, et al. Constipation and other chronic gastrointestinal problems in spinal cord injury patients. Spinal Cord 1998; 36:63–66.

16. Deshmukh G, Barkel D, Sevo D, et al. Use or misuse of colostomy to heal pressure ulcers. Dis Colon Rectum 1996; 39:737–738.

17. Devroede G, Lamarche J. Functional importance of extrinsic parasympathetic innervation to the distal colon and rectum in man. Gastroenterology 1974; 66:273–300.

18. Devroede G. Constipation. In: Sleisenger MH, Fordtran JS, eds. Gastrointestinal disease. Philadelphia: Saunders; 1993:837–887.

19. Dikenson VA. Maintenance of anal continence: a review of pelvic floor physiology. Gut 1978; 19:1163–1174.

20. Doughty DB, Jackson DB. Gastrointestinal disorders. St. Louis: Mosby-Year Book; 1993:268.

21. Eire PF, Cives RV, Gago MC. Faecal incontinence in children with spina bifida: the best conservative treatment. Spinal Cord 1998; 36:774–776.

22. Frost F, Hartwig D, Jaeger R, et al. Electrical stimulation of the sacral dermatomes in spinal cord injury: effect on rectal manometry and bowel emptying. Arch Phys Med Rehabil 1993; 74:696–701.

23. Gore RM, Mintzer RA, Calenoff L. Gastrointestinal complications of spinal cord injury. Spine 1981; 6:538–544.

24. Goyal RK, Crist JR. Neurology of the gut. In: Sleisenger MH, Fordtram JS, eds. Gastrointestinal disease. Philadelphia: Saunders; 1989:21–52.

25. Guyton AC. Textbook of medical physiology. 8th edn. Philadelphia: Saunders; 1991:731–735, 742.

26. Hammond MC, Umlauf RL, Matteson B, et al. Yes you can!: a guide to self-care for persons with spinal cord injury. Washington: Paralyzed Veterans Organization of America; 1989:361.

27. Han TR, Kim JH, Kwon BS. Chronic gastrointestinal problems and bowel dysfunction in patients with spinal cord injury. Spinal Cord 1998; 36(7):485–490.

28. Hanson R, Franklin M. Sexual loss in relation to other functional losses for spinal cord injured males. Arch Phys Med Rehabil 1976; 57:291–293.

29. Harari D, Minaker KL. Megacolon in patients with chronic spinal cord injury. Spinal Cord 2000; 38:331–339.

30. House JG, Stiens SA. Pharmacologically initiated defecation for persons with spinal cord injury: effectiveness of three agents. Arch Phys Med Rehabil 1997; 78:1062–1065.

31. Kaname A, Kakizaki H, Machino R, et al. Laparoscopic antegrade continence enema procedure for fecal incontinence in a patient with spina bifida. Int J Urol 2003; 10:401–403.

32. Kerr TP, Robb SA, Clayden GS. Lower gastrointestinal tract disturbance in congenital myotonic dystrophy. Eur J Pediatr 2002; 161:468–469.

33. King JC, Currie DM, Wright E. Bowel training in spina bifida: importance of education, patient compliance, age, and anal reflexes. Arch Phys Med Rehabil 1994; 75:243–247.

34. King JC, Nelson R, Tuturro T, et al. Prescriptions, referrals, and the rehabilitation team. In: DeLisa JA, ed. Rehabilitation medicine principles and practice. 3rd edn. Philadelphia: JB Lippincott; 1998.

35. King R, Biddle A, Braunschweig C, et al. Neurogenic bowel management in adults with spinal cord injury. J Spinal Cord Med 1998; 21:248–293.

36. Kirshblum SC, Gulati M, O'Connor KC, et al. Bowel care practices in chronic spinal cord injury patients. Arch Phys Med Rehabil 1998; 79:20–23.

37. Kirshblum SC, House JG, O'Connor KC. Silent autonomic dysreflexia during a routine bowel program in persons with traumatic spinal cord injury: a preliminary study. Arch Phys Med Rehabil 2002; 83(12):1774–1776.

38. Knowles CH, Scott SM, Wellmer A, et al. Sensory and autonomic neuropathy in patients with idiopathic slow-transit constipation. Br J Surg 1999; 86:54–60.

39. Koyle M, Kaji D, Duque M, et al. The Malone antegrade continence enema for neurogenic and structural fecal incontinence and constipation. J Urol 1995; 154:759–761.

40. Krogh K, Mosdal C, Laurberg S. Gastrointestinal and segmental colonic transit times in patients with acute and chronic spinal cord lesions. Spinal Cord 2000; 38:615–621.

41. Levi R, Hulting C, Nash M, et al. The Stockholm spinal cord injury study: 1. Medical problems in a regional SCI population. Paraplegia 1995; 33:308–315.

42. Liem NR, McColl MA, King W, et al. Aging with a spinal cord injury: factors associated with the need for more help with activities of daily living. Arch Phys Med Rehabil 2004; 85:1567–1577.

43. Liptak GS, Reveli GM. Management of bowel dysfunction in children with spinal cord disease or injury by means of the enema continence catheter. J Pediatr 1992; 120:190–194.

44. Longo WE, Ballantyne GH, Modlin IM. The colon, anorectum, and spinal cord patient. Dis Colon Rectum 1989; 32:261–267.

45. MacDonagh R, Sun W, Smallwood R. Anorectal function in patients with complete supraconal spinal cord lesions. Gut 1992; 33:1532–1538.

46. MacDonagh RP, Sun WM, Smallwood R, et al. Control of defecation in patients with spinal injuries by stimulation of sacral anterior nerve roots. Br Med J 1990; 300:1494–1497.

47. Madoff RD, Williams JG, Caushaj PF. Fecal incontinence. N Engl J Med 1992; 326:1002–1007.

48. Malone P, Ransley P, Kiely E. Preliminary report: the antegrade continence enema. Lancet 1990; 336:1217–1218.

49. Manning J, Korda A, Benness C, et al. The association of obstructive defecation, lower urinary tract dysfunction and the benign joint hypermobility syndrome: a case-control study. Int Urogynecol J 2003; 14:130–132.

50. Martelli H, Devroede G, Arhan P, et al. Mechanisms of idiopathic constipation: outlet obstruction. Gastroenterology 1978; 75:623–631.

51. Martelli H, Devroede G, Arhan P, et al. Some parameters of large bowel motility in normal man. Gastroenterology 1978; 75:612.

52. Menardo G, Baujano G, Corazziari E. Large bowel transit in paraplegic patients. Dis Colon Rectum 1987; 30:924–930.

53. Meshkinpour H, Nowroozi F, Glick M. Colonic compliance in patients with spinal cord injury. Arch Phys Med Rehabil 1983; 64:111–112.

54. Nino-Murcia M, Stone J, Chang P, et al. Colonic transit in spinal cord-injured patients. Invest Radiol 1990; 25:109–112.

55. Pedersen E. Regulation of bladder and colon-rectum in patients with spinal lesions. J Auton Nerv Syst 1983; 7:329–338.

56. Pierce E, Cowan P, Stokes M. Managing faecal retention and incontinence in neurodisability. Br J Nurs 2001; 10:592–601.

57. Ponticelli A, Iacobelli BD, Silveri M, et al. Colorectal dysfunction and faecal incontinence in children with spina bifida. Br J Urol 1998; 81(suppl 3): 117–119.

58. Rendtorff RC, Kashgarian M. Stool patterns of healthy adult males. Dis Colon Rectum 1967; 10:222.

59. Saltzstein R, Romano J. The efficacy of colostomy as a bowel management alternative in selected spinal cord injured patients. J Am Paraplegia Soc 1990; 13:9–13.

60. Schiller LR. Fecal incontinence. In: Sleisenger MH, Fordtran JS, eds. Gastrointestinal disease. Philadelphia: Saunders; 1993:934–953.

61. Shafik A, Shafik AA, Ahmed I. Role of positive anorectal feedback in rectal evacuation: the concept of a second defecation reflex: the anorectal reflex. J Spinal Cord Med 2003; 26:380–383.

62. Shandling B, Gilmour RF. The enema continence catheter in spina bifida: successful bowel management. J Pediatr Surg 1987; 22:271–273.

63. Siproudhis L, Bellissant E, Juguet F, et al. Perception of and adaptation to rectal isobaric distension in patients with faecal incontinence. Gut 1999; 44:687–692.

64. Slater W. Management of faecal incontinence of a patient with spinal cord injury. Br J Nurs 2003; 12:727–734.

65. Smith B. Effect of irritant purgatives on the myenteric plexus in man and mouse. Gut 1968; 9:139–143.

66. Stiens S, Goetz L. Neurogenic bowel dysfunction. In: O'Young B, Young M, Stiens S, eds. Physical medicine and rehabilitation secrets. Philadelphia: Hanley & Belfus; 2002:465–470.

67. Stiens SA, Biener Bergman S, Goetz LL. Neurogenic bowel dysfunction after spinal cord injury: clinical evaluation and rehabilitative management. Arch Phys Med Rehabil 1997; 78:S86–S102.

68. Stiens SA, Braunschweig C, Cowel F, et al. Neurogenic bowel: what you should know. A guide for people with spinal cord injury. Washington: Consortium for Spinal Cord Medicine; 1999:53.

69. Stiens SA, Piddie T, Veland B, et al. Accidents stink. Bowel care 202 video. Washington: Paralyzed Veterans of America Education and Training Foundation. Concepts in Confidence 2002; 1-800-822-4050.

70. Stone J, Nino-Murcia M, Wolf V, et al. Chronic gastrointestinal problems in spinal cord injury patients: a prospective analysis. Am J Gastroenterol 1990; 85:114–119.

71. Stone J, Wolfe V, Nino-Murcia M. Colostomy as treatment for complications of spinal cord injury. Arch Phys Med Rehabil 1990; 71:514–518.

72. Suckling P. The ball-valve rectum due to impacted feces. Lancet 1962; 2:1147.

73. Swash M. New concepts in the prevention of incontinence. Practitioner 1985; 229:895–899.

74. Teichman JMH, Barber DM, Rogenes VJ, et al. Malone antegrade continence enemas for autonomic dysreflexia secondary to neurogenic bowel. J Spinal Cord Med 1998; 160:1278–1301.

75. Tjandra J, Ooi, B, Han W. Anorectal physiologic testing for bowel dysfunction in patients with spinal cord lesions. Dis Colon Rectum 2000; 43:927–931.

76. Tobin GW, Brocklehurst JC. Faecal incontinence in residential homes for the elderly: prevalence, aetiology and management. Age Aging 1986; 15:41–46.

77. Varma J. Autonomic influences on colorectal motility and pelvic surgery. World J Surg 1992; 16:811–819.

78. White J, Verlot M, Ehrentheil O. Neurogenic disturbances of the colon and their investigation by the colon metrogram. Ann Surg 1949; 112: 1042–1057.

79. Wiesel PH, Norton C, Roy AJ, et al. Gut focused behavioural treatment (biofeedback) for constipation and faecal incontinence in multiple sclerosis. J Neurol Neurosurg Psychiatry 2000; 69:240–243.

80. Wingate DL, Ewart WR. The brain–gut axis. In: Yamada T, ed. Textbook of gastroenterology. Philadelphia: JB Lippincott; 1991:50–60.

81. Wrenn K. Fecal impaction. N Engl J Med 1989; 321:658–662.

82. Yang CC, Stiens SA. Antegrade continence enema for the treatment of neurogenic constipation and fecal incontinence after spinal cord injury. Arch Phys Med Rehabil 2000; 81:683–685.

Chapter

31

Spasticity Management

Patricia W. Nance and Jay M. Meythaler

The successful management of spasticity can be a therapeutic challenge. When not excessive, spasticity can assist weakened legs, permit transfer ability, and improve bed mobility. When severe, spastic muscular movements can be violent and uncontrolled, resulting in severe complications such as chronic pain, contractures, long bone fracture, joint dislocations, and chronic skin ulceration. Undesirable complications such as these may be anticipated, prevented, and treated with appropriate management.

The most commonly cited definition is as follows:

Spasticity is a motor disorder that is characterized by a velocity dependent increase in tonic stretch reflexes (muscle tone) with exaggerated tendon jerks, resulting from hyperexcitability of the stretch reflex, as one component of the upper motor neuron syndrome.

American Academy of Neurology (1990)[1]

The specific behavioral features of the upper motor neuron (UMN) syndrome can vary depending on the underlying cause, for example spinal cord injury (SCI) versus cerebral ischemic damage. Spinal interneurons, sensory afferents, and modulatory and motor efferent pathways normally interact to control, coordinate, and modulate spinal motor neuronal activation. The medical literature supports the notion that insufficient descending inhibition results in structural and physiologic reorganization of segmental circuits following injury or dysfunction within the UMN pathways, such as alterations of intrinsic and extrinsic properties of motor neurons and interneurons.

From a clinical standpoint, it is important to distinguish between the positive symptoms related to the UMN syndrome (e.g. spastic dystonia, flexor spasms, exaggerated cutaneous reflexes, autonomic hyperreflexia, and contractures) and the negative symptoms (e.g. paresis, loss of fine dexterity, and fatigability).[198] This difference relates directly to the expectations of outcome following treatment for a positive symptom of spasticity, without necessarily effecting change in the negative symptom of weakness. For example, subjects with spastic hemiparesis with exaggerated flexor patterning and weakness showed greater task-specific functional difficulties in reaching out as compared with reaching up.[199]

This review focuses on a rehabilitative approach to spasticity treatment; that is, first establish the functional problem caused by the spasticity and the related goal of treatment, treat all spasticity-aggravating factors, match the medical therapy to the specific needs of the patient, and finally reevaluate the patient to ensure that the goal of therapy has been met.

CAUSES OF SPASTICITY

Like the UMN syndrome, spasticity can accompany diffuse or localized cerebral or spinal pathology. Anoxic, toxic, or metabolic encephalopathies can cause diffuse cerebral abnormalities, while localized cerebral injury can occur with tumor, abscess, cyst, vascular malformations, infarction, hemorrhage, or trauma. Trauma, inflammation, demyelinating disease, and degenerative and familial disorders, as well as compression by a mass (e.g. neoplasm, infection, or cyst) are examples of spinal cord disorders. An example of a combination of UMN and lower motor neuron pathology is amyotrophic lateral sclerosis, where spasticity can be the dominant feature in some patients. Spasticity is often cited as a significant problem in multiple sclerosis (see Ch. 53), traumatic brain injury (see Ch. 50), cerebral palsy (see Ch. 54), SCI (see Ch. 56), and stroke (see Ch. 51). Problematic spasticity occurs in 40–60% of patients with SCI and multiple sclerosis, which results in a significant influence on social handicap. Almost two-thirds of patients with cerebral palsy present with spastic diplegia.[22,29,123,154,198,199]

Changes in the characteristics of spasticity can help to diagnose problems in parts of the body where the patient no longer has voluntary movement or sensory appreciation. In neurolathyrism, a rare disorder, spasticity can be the main presenting symptom.[132] It is more likely that a healthcare provider will be asked to consider the patient who presents with the sudden worsening of spasticity, possibly due to the onset of a new pathologic process, such as a urinary tract infection, urolithiasis, stool implication, pressure sore, fracture, dislocation, ingrown toe nail or excessively restrictive clothing, irritating condom drainage appliance, or thyrotoxicosis, as reported in a patient with hereditary spastic paraparesis.[168] If there is a remediable cause of spasticity, it must be discovered and treated. If problematic spasticity persists in the absence of a remediable cause, then it is appropriate to pursue treatment until a therapeutic response is obtained. Inevitable complications are the natural history of suboptimal treatment of severe spasticity. These complications include skin abrasion, infection, bone fracture or dislocation, and more frequent inpatient hospitalization.[13,141]

EVALUATION AND MEASUREMENT

Of the many clinical monitoring tools described in the literature to assess the severity of spasticity, most researchers agree that assessment tools should be tailored to meet the individual characteristics of a given patient. The most commonly used assessment method, the Ashworth Scale, has the advantage of ease of use in the clinical setting. This asset has been utilized in a number of pharmaceutical trials of antispasticity medications in which a simple measurement tool can be used easily by the participating clinicians to assess the efficacy of the intervention. There are a number of other spasticity-measuring tools, which range from simple questionnaires and goniometry evaluations to more technologically complicated electromyographic and biomechanical analysis of limb resistance to mechanical displacement, and video monitoring assessment of joint mobility.[26,36,83,151]

As proposed originally, the Ashworth Scale is a simple five-point Likert scale in which the observer's subjective opinion of the subject's resting muscle tone ranges from 'normal' at the lowest grade to 'rigid' at the highest.[7] A recent comprehensive review of engineering and medical literature concluded that the Ashworth Scale is in common use and has significant interrater agreement and good reliability, but it is not a functional outcome measure and can be biased by evaluator subjectivity.[64] A monitoring test should be able not only to assess the change in spasticity during therapy, but also to assess the functional effects of interventions. Such a test should have a well-defined scoring system, be reliable and sensitive to change, and have standard instructions.[151]

The Ashworth Scale,[64,112] Oswestry Scale of Grading,[78] and Degree of Adductor Muscle Tone[181] are some of the tone intensity scales used to assess spasticity in SCI. The original Ashworth Scale is shown in Table 31-1. The original scale was modified by adjusting the lowest number from 0 to 1, and the highest scale from 4 to 5. Another modification from the original scoring scheme was the addition of a point between 1 and 2, where 1 was a 'catch' at the end of joint motion range, and 1+ a catch earlier in the joint motion range nearer to midpoint.[19]

Another method of observing the spasticity phenomenon is to assess the number of episodic spasms. The Penn Spasm Frequency Score[157] is an ordinal ranking of the frequency of leg spasms per day and per hour. One problem with this scale is that patients usually report that the number of spasms occurring per hour is often affected by their activity at the time. For example, they tend to report few spasms if resting comfortably, more if physically active. Also, the duration of each spasm is not taken into consideration.

The casual observation of the free swing of the knee in the 'pendulum test' was formalized and provided objective data by the use of videomotion analysis. The advantages of videomotion analysis of the pendulum test include the ability to do the analysis anywhere a video recorder is available, freedom from the attachment of cumbersome recording devices to the patient, and processing by a non-biased 'blinded' observer (who has had no contact with the patient).[88,140]

Pain can be assessed, whether or not it is associated with spasticity, by a self-administered test such as the Pain Intensity Descriptor Scale[80] or by using a 10-cm visual analog scale.[33,95] Standardized assessments of functional ability or caregiver burden might or might not be sensitive to changes in relative levels of spasticity. These include the Sickness Impact Profile,[17] the 36-Item Short-Form Health Survey,[5] the functional independence measure,[4] and the Caregiver Dependency Scale.[3] Although the Canadian Occupational Performance Measure[161] might have the potential to reveal functional changes should patients state that spasticity was their most functionally limiting problem and of highest importance to them, it has yet to be reported in a clinical trial of an antispasticity treatment.

PHYSIOLOGIC MECHANISMS

There is no single pathophysiologic mechanism to account for all the observable aspects of spasticity. Dysfunction within the central nervous system of descending pathways to and within the spinal cord causes a UMN syndrome that is often associated with exaggerated reflexes and spasticity, which includes velocity-dependent increased muscle tone.[110] While enhanced reflexes are sufficiently common and associated with the spasticity phenomenon to be part of its definition, measurement of the reflex amplitude in some patients (such as patients with stroke or neurologically complete SCI) has shown reductions compared with that in able-bodied subjects.[146,147,167]

Although the spinal alpha motor neuron is considered to be the final common pathway for expression of spasticity, one should consider the more complex motor pathways involved in the disordered movements of spastic brain-injured patients. Spastic hypertonia encompasses a variety of conditions, including dystonia, rigidity, myoclonus, muscle spasm, posturing, and/

Table 31-1	The Ashworth Scale[7]
Score	Definition
0	No increase in muscle tone
1	Slight increase in muscle tone, manifested by a catch and release
2	More marked increase in muscle tone through most of the range of motion, but affected limb is easily moved
3	Considerable increase in muscle tone—passive movement difficult
4	Limb rigid in flexion or extension

or spasticity.[131,138] The following sections briefly review the physiology of segmental reflexes.

The monosynaptic reflex

The physiologic components involved in the spinal stretch reflex response include the muscle spindle stretch receptor, the myelinated sensory neuron, the synapse, the homonymous motor neuron, and the muscle it innervates. As originally described in the decerebrate cat model, the stretch reflex shown a dramatic increase in extensor muscle tone on passive flexion of the extended hind limbs. This stretch reflex has two components: a brisk, short-acting phasic component that responds to the initial dynamic change in length, and a weaker, longer acting tonic component that responds to the steady stretch of the muscle at a new length.[116]

A change in muscle length can evoke a stretch reflex. Modified muscle fibers (intrafusal receptor organs) that detect changes in muscle length are called muscle spindles. Nuclear bag fibers and nuclear chain fibers are two types of specialized spindle fiber. Nuclear bag fibers are further subdivided into dynamic and static nuclear bag fibers. Dynamic nuclear bag fibers are highly sensitive to the rate of change, providing velocity sensitivity to muscle stretch.[122] Static nuclear bag fibers and nuclear chain fibers are more sensitive to the steady-state, static or tonic, muscle length. The structural differences between these fibers are responsible for the physiologic differences in their sensitivities and for the two different components, phasic and tonic, of the stretch reflex. Intracellular muscle fibers are observed to undergo changes as a result of spasticity, as does the extracellular matrix.[117]

Group 1a and group 2 fibers are two types of myelinated sensory afferent fibers that innervate intrafusal fibers. Group 1a, or primary sensory, afferents convey both phasic and tonic stretch information. Group 2 fibers innervate static nuclear bag and nuclear chain fibers, and convey information on the tonic or static change in muscle length. Contained within the muscle spindle unit are contractile elements that stiffen the region of the nuclear bag fibers. These contractile elements maintain spindle sensitivity during skeletal muscle contraction. They are innervated by special motor neurons known as the gamma motor neurons.

The inverse stretch reflex

The Golgi tendon organ is sensitive to intramuscular tension and is innervated by myelinated 1b sensory afferents. The Golgi tendon organ is particularly sensitive to muscle tension created by active muscle contraction, but has a high threshold for detecting passive stretch. Stimulation of 1b afferents leads to inhibition of the homonymous motor neuron and its synergists. The excitation of its antagonistic motor neurons also stimulates 1b afferents. This behavior has been called the inverse myotactic reflex, because its actions oppose those of the stretch (myotactic) reflex. It is also called 1b non-reciprocal inhibition. It should be noted that this reflex is stimulated by muscle tension, whereas the stretch reflex is stimulated by a change in muscle length. The Golgi tendon organ has been hypothesized to function as part of a muscle tension feedback system.[111]

Elevated reflex activity

The stretch reflex can be viewed as a feedback system with muscle length as the regulated variable. Normally, the gain, or input–output relationship, of the stretch reflex to a given change in muscle length is kept low by descending influences when the individual is at rest. The gain is enhanced when physical demand for performance is needed. Hyperreflexia is an example of segmental reflex dysregulation associated with an upper motor lesion. Theoretically, hyperreflexia can result from a number of mechanisms, including decreased spinal inhibitory mechanisms from brain centers, hyperexcitability of alpha motor neurons, peripheral nerve sprouting, and increased gamma fiber activity.

Long-term reductions in inhibition can contribute to hyperreflexia. Examples of inhibition types are as follows: recurrent Renshaw inhibition, reciprocal 1a inhibition, presynaptic inhibition, non-reciprocal 1b inhibition, and inhibition from group 2 afferents. Various lines of research have supported deficient presynaptic and non-reciprocal inhibition as significant contributors to spasticity. The supportive evidence for it being due to deficient group 2 afferent-related and Renshaw inhibition is lacking. Presynaptic inhibition is mediated via a GABAergic mechanism that decreases the efficacy of 1a transmitter release. Interneurons involved in presynaptic inhibition are modulated by descending pathways. Thus the loss or reduction of rostral lesion control can reduce tonic levels of descending facilitation on inhibitory interneurons, leading to increased alpha motor response to normal 1a input.[198]

The 1a inhibitory interneurons are normally controlled by descending excitatory pathways. Reciprocal 1a inhibition decreases the chance for cocontraction of antagonistic and agonistic muscles during the stretch reflex or during voluntary movement. There is evidence for decreased excitability of 1a inhibitory neurons after rostral lesions of the central nervous system. This dysfunction could lead to an increased cocontraction and weakness of voluntary movement.[37] Non-reciprocal 1b inhibition has been found to be decreased or even replaced by facilitation in patients with spastic paresis and spastic dystonia, in this case both stroke and SCI subjects, but not in subjects without spastic dytonia.[48]

Patients with spastic paresis from SCI show increased rather than decreased levels of recurrent Renshaw inhibition. Renshaw cells are inhibitory neurons that are stimulated by collateral axons from alpha motor neurons. When an alpha motor neuron fires, it stimulates a Renshaw cell that, in turn, inhibits the initiating motor neuron and its synergists. The Renshaw cell also inhibits the 1a inhibitory interneuron associated with the initiating motor neuron. Because the Renshaw cell inhibits 1a inhibitory interneurons as well as agonist alpha motor neurons, increased Renshaw cell activity might contribute to spasticity by decreasing reciprocal 1a inhibition.[175] Hyperexcitability of alpha motor neurons might contribute to spasticity. Examples of primary changes in membrane properties that would be expected to produce increased alpha motor neuron discharge include a reduction in the area of dendritic membranes, deafferentation dendritic hyperexcitability, and an increase in the number of excitatory synaptic inputs due to sprouting.[198]

Multisynaptic segmental connections

The majority of spinal segmental connections are polysynaptic. Interposed interneurons connect sensory afferents and antagonistic motor neurons to opposing muscle groups, resulting in a polysynaptic connection. Interneurons also receive excitatory and inhibitory signals from descending pathways. Supraspinal centers can control joint stiffness through the modulation of excitatory and inhibitory input to segmental interneurons and interneuronal networks.[34,90] The interneurons that mediate 1b non-reciprocal inhibition connect inhibitory agonist and excitatory antagonistic motor neurons. At rest, 1b non-reciprocal inhibition opposes the actions of the stretch reflex. Convergent input from 1a spindle afferents is received by 1b interneurons, along with low-threshold cutaneous afferents and joint afferents, excitatory and inhibitory inputs from descending pathways. The afferents for Golgi tendon organs make polysynaptic connections, via interneurons, to homonymous motor neurons, synergist and antagonist motor neurons. Because of Golgi tendon organ sensitivity to active muscle tension and the short-latency convergent input from 1a spindle afferents that 1b interneurons receive, cutaneous afferents, joint afferents, and modulating descending pathways, spinal interneuronal networks are likely to play an important role in exploratory movements of the limbs. A functional example of this network organization would be the reduction of muscle contraction if a limb encountered an unexpected obstacle. The interneuron receiving 1b afferent information would mediate the inhibition of inhibition of the agonist, which would reduce the force against the impediment. Also, 1b inhibition could function to decrease muscle contraction at the extreme range of joint motion. The net effect of 1b inhibition during volitional activity depends on inputs from multiple sources. Recurrent Renshaw inhibition takes place via polysynaptic connections to alpha motor neurons via Renshaw cells and 1a inhibitory interneurons.

The majority of type 2 afferent connections are polysynaptic and involve several classes of interneuron. These interneurons typically arise from muscle spindles, but some afferents originate as free nerve endings or in other types of receptors. Their activation tends to activate flexor synergistic muscles and inhibit physiologic extensors. When unopposed, group 2-mediated activity produces tonic activation of physiologic limb flexors. Group 3 and 4 afferents originate from deep muscle and cutaneous receptors. Group 3 fibers are thinly myelinated. Group 4 fibers are small diameter afferents, often unmyelinated, and originate as free nerve endings serving nociceptive and thermoregulatory functions. Both types of fiber convey impulses generated by extreme pressure, heat, and cold. Similar to type 2 responses, the reflex responses to these stimuli are bilateral flexion predominantly, and are typically proportionate to the stimulus intensity.

The afferent fibers that produce generalized reflexive flexor movements have become known collectively as flexor reflex afferents. Interestingly, the response to cutaneous stimuli is not always one of generalized flexion. The vestibulocollic and cervicocollic reflexes produce patterns of coordinated ipsilateral limb flexion accompanied by contralateral limb extension with activation of group 2 and 3 fibers, to either keep the head level during body tilt or to oppose a fall. Different modalities of stimuli can have differential effects, particularly evident after a neurologic injury. For example, after certain neurologic lesions, pressure applied to the plantar surface of the foot produces a marked extension of the leg, known as extensor thrust. In contrast, a pinprick in the same area leads to flexion withdrawal of the limb. The spinal circuits responsible for ipsilateral flexion and crossed limb extension also receive descending inputs and coordinate voluntary limb movements.

A cutaneous stimulus can modulate the activity of particular motor neurons. Touching an area of skin may cause a reflex contraction of specific muscles, usually those beneath the area of stimulation. This is an example of an exteroceptive response. Cutaneous stimuli might not always produce observable contractions. They may have subthreshold or facilitative effects. Proprioceptive information is transmitted from muscle spindles and Golgi tendon organs via group 1a, 2, and 1b afferents. Finally, there are indications that pathway connectivity and neurotransmitter distribution may account for differential responses comparing the upper limbs to the lower limbs.[126]

GOAL SETTING

Since spasticity results from neurologic dysfunction within several regions in the central nervous system, the associated loss of voluntary motor function can be highly variable among patients with symptomatic spasticity. Consequently, prediction of the functional impact due to the presence of spasticity can be challenging. Compare, for example, an individual with C4 tetraplegia who uses a mouth stick or suck and puff actuator to operate a computer, telephone, and numerous adapted electronic devices, and a head controller to operate an electric wheelchair, to a person with T10 level paraplegia. The presence of mild to moderate spasticity can alter the sitting position so that the control over the adaptive devices is lost for the person with tetraplegia, whereas the paraplegic person does not experience the same functional impact to that level of spasticity intensity. The functional goal for spasticity treatment should be one within the ability of the patient, but the performance of the function is limited mainly by spasticity. Common examples of spasticity-limited functional goals are to improve speed and safety of wheelchair transfers, to improve the performance of activities of daily living such as dressing, and to facilitate perineal hygiene by a caregiver by reducing thigh adductor or pectoral muscle spasticity.

One potential functional goal might be the improvement of gait. While patients with spasticity are reported to have disturbances of gait speed, timing, kinematics, and electromyographic patterns, the relative impact of spasticity on gait remains controversial.[67,69,109,158] While it seems logical that knee extensor muscle torque should correlate with the speed of 'comfortable' walking, by experimental measurement it accounts for only 30% of the variance in gait speed in spastic stroke patients.[18] Young concluded that not all abnormalities underlying 'spastic gait' are caused by spasticity, and consequently are not affected by antispasticity drug treatment.[197]

Pain and fatigue are examples of other factors that can contribute to functional limitations. Spasticity can be caused or exacerbated by pain. The presence of pain is widely acknowledged as a significant negative contributor to the quality of life. Further, the time and energy required to complete a task could change more with the presence of spasticity and its treatment than with the actual ability or inability to complete the task. Increased age, degenerative joint disease, muscle and skin atrophy, and chronic anemia contribute to a generalized decline in health and reduced function that can diminish a patient's ability to cope with spasticity.

NON-PHARMACOLOGIC TREATMENTS

A regular exercise routine that includes daily range of motion exercise[25,86,159] and a high index of suspicion for spasticity-aggravating factors (e.g. urinary tract infection, constipation, skin ulceration, ingrown nails, and fractures) are the mainstays for preventing the change from the simple presence of spasticity to that of spasticity causing loss of function. However, there are a number of other useful physical treatments. For example, spasticity can often be reduced for variable durations by tendon pressure,[113] application of cold, warmth, vibration, splinting, bandaging, massage, low-power laser, and acupuncture.[77,81] Casting a joint with the muscle in a lengthened position can help maintain muscle length. Skin breakdown can occur in the insensate limb, however, and other body damage can occur if the spasticity is severe. In a recent review of the literature pertaining to randomized trials of antispasticity treatments for amyotrophic lateral sclerosis, the recommended treatment included individualized, moderate-intensity, endurance-type exercises for the trunk and limbs.[8] Electrical stimulation of the spinal cord has been reported to result in reduction of spasticity,[12,87] although the measurement of spasticity in these studies has been questioned.[52] Several investigators have shown that electrical stimulation of the peripheral nerves can decrease spasticity in patients with SCI, stroke, or traumatic brain injury.[9,54,114,115,164,165,172,196] Other physical modalities that have been reported to ameliorate spasticity include magnetic stimulation over the thoracic spinal cord[150] and topical application of 20% benzocaine.[166]

PHARMACOLOGIC TREATMENTS

The first treatment that usually springs to mind for spasticity is the pharmacologic. It is hoped that, after reading the preced-

ing paragraphs, what also comes to mind will be excellent medical management, treatment of aggravating factors, and use of physical modalities. Nevertheless, pharmacologic treatment is often required in the management of spasticity, and it is important to have a thorough understanding of the various effects of the medications in this class of therapeutics. The specific pharmacologic effects can be directed toward alteration of transmitters or neuromodulators by suppression of excitation (glutamate), enhancement of inhibition (GABA or glycine), a combination of both (noradrenaline [norepinephrine], serotonin, adenosine, and various neuropeptides), or action on peripheral neuromuscular sites. Although numerous substances have potential antispasticity effects, the US Food and Drug Administration (FDA) has approved only four prescription pharmaceuticals for the treatment of spasticity related to central nervous system disorder. These are baclofen, tizanidine, dantrolene sodium, and diazepam. These four agents will be discussed first, followed by other pharmaceuticals with similar pharmacologic actions but without FDA-approved antispasticity indication.

Enhancement of segmental inhibition via GABA

The main inhibitory neurotransmitters in the central nervous system are GABA and glycine. The physiologic action of GABA on the 1a-mediated spinal reflex is by presynaptic inhibition, as was shown in the 1940s by Sir John Eccles. GABA-containing cells are typically small interneurons. Localized ischemia is a common experimental methodology for eliminating these small GABA-containing interneurons while leaving long tracts intact. A spinal transection, on the other hand, disrupts long tract function but does not diminish the number of GABA interneurons or the concentration of GABA in spinal tissue below the level of transection. Once GABA is released by GABAergic interneurons, free GABA is released to bind to receptors on the postsynaptic membrane. The classic $GABA_A$ receptor has been characterized as having a number of cell membrane protein subunits: alpha, beta, and gamma. GABA-binding activates the receptor, which stimulates the chloride ionophore channel, resulting in membrane hyperpolarization. When an axonal connection exists between a GABAergic interneuron and the terminal of a 1a afferent, then hyperpolarization of that membrane will result in a decrease in excitability, decreased excitatory transmitter release, and subsequently reduced motor neuron firing. For this reason, presynaptic inhibition of the afferent neuronal terminal reduces motor neuron output without direct inhibition of motor neuron excitability. Because GABA does not cross the blood–brain barrier, it would not be useful as an oral antispasticity agent.

Medications with GABA-mimetic and GABA-like actions

Baclofen (Lioresal) Baclofen is β-4-chlorophenyl GABA, which binds to and activates the bicuculline-insensitive $GABA_B$ receptors. Bicuculline is a toxin that antagonizes the inhibitory effects of endogenous GABA at $GABA_A$ receptors, which cause treated animals to convulse. Once a presynaptic GABA$_B$ receptor is activated, potassium conductance is altered, resulting in a net membrane hyperpolarization and a reduction in endogenous transmitter release.[44,93] For example, in a presynaptic sensory neuron, release of GABA by a local inter-neuron and binding at the receptor on the sensory neuron produces inhibition of the primary afferent terminal, and results in a decrease in excitatory neurotransmitter release. Baclofen activation of receptors postsynaptically inhibits calcium conductance and causes inhibition of gamma motor neuron activity, reduced drive to intrafusal muscle fibers, and reduced muscle spindle sensitivity.[189] The overall inhibitory effect of baclofen administration at the spinal cord level reduces sensory and motor neuron activation. It also reduces the activation of monosynaptic spinal reflexes and, to a lesser extent, polysynaptic spinal reflexes. There are numerous clinical reports of the antispasticity effects of oral baclofen for patients with multiple sclerosis or SCI.[57,68,94,95,96,104,155,174] Orally delivered baclofen has recently been studied in patients with cerebral disorders, and was found to have selective efficacy on lower limb spasticity but not on spasticity in the upper limbs.[126]

Baclofen absorption after oral administration occurs mainly in the proximal small intestine. This probably involves two different amino acid transporter systems, due to competitive inhibition of absorption by the neutral and beta amino acids. The kidney normally excretes the baclofen essentially unchanged, but the liver can metabolize as much as 15% of a given dose. This is why periodic liver function testing is advisable during baclofen treatment, and the dosage should be reduced in patients with impaired renal function. The average therapeutic half-life of baclofen is 3.5 h but ranges from 2 to 6 h. Baclofen dosing is usually initiated as 5 mg three times per day and increased gradually to a therapeutic level. The recommended maximum dosage is 80 mg per day in four divided doses. There are reports of improved therapeutic effects with higher dosages,[103] however, and an indication that higher dose prescription is not uncommon.[179] Because baclofen treatment can produce sedation, patients should be cautioned regarding the operation of automobiles or other dangerous machinery and activities made hazardous by decreased alertness. Because baclofen is excreted by the kidneys, patients with renal impairment can require a lower dosage. The effects of chronic baclofen treatment during human pregnancy are largely unknown. In some patients, seizure control has been lost during treatment with baclofen.[107] Abrupt discontinuation of baclofen can produce seizures, confusion, hallucinations, and rebound muscle spasticity with fever.[186]

Oral baclofen is a widely prescribed pharmaceutical in North America, and there are few reports of major toxicity. However, massive overdose with oral baclofen has been reported, including a case report of a 57-year-old woman who ingested 2 g of baclofen, causing coma and hypoventilation. She was given nal-oxone, 50% dextrose, and activated charcoal. Initially, her blood pressure was low, and later systolic hypertension was noted, followed 16 h later by bradycardia and hypotension. Her pupils were small and unresponsive, and muscle stretch reflexes were absent. Plasma baclofen concentrations over time showed first-order elimination kinetics and a half-life of 8 h.[76]

Modulating the monoamines
Tizanidine (Zanaflex)

Tizanidine is an imidazoline derivative and agonist that binds to α_2-receptor sites both spinally and supraspinally,[39,169] similar to the α_2-adrenergic agonist clonidine (see description following). The medical literature supports the notion that the pharmacologic effects include the restoration or enhancement of presynaptic inhibitory modulation of spinal reflexes in patients with spasticity.[49,143,184] Tizanidine has been shown to decrease reflex activity, especially polysynaptic reflex activity, as shown in the spinal transected cat model.[47] This finding has been corroborated by the observation that tizanidine has an antinociceptive effect in animal models.[45,46,98] Several European and American studies have shown that tizanidine is equal in effectiveness to baclofen and diazepam, but with a more favorable tolerability profile. The main advantage appears to be less complaint of treatment-related weakness. Furthermore, two clinical trials demonstrated that patients with spasticity improved muscle strength during tizanidine treatment.[105,129]

Tizanidine has been tested in a number of clinical trials in Europe, and has been found to be safe, well tolerated, and beneficial in treating spasticity of various etiologies.[65] Tizanidine is an α_2 agonist like clonidine, but has a much reduced potency and does not consistently induce a reduction in blood pressure or pulse, as clonidine does.[27] Symptomatic hypotension has been reported when tizanidine is taken with an antihypertensive drug, so the concomitant administration of tizanidine and antihypertensive drugs should be avoided. An important drug interaction between ciprofloxacin, an antibiotic, and tizanidine has prompted the US FDA to approve new safety labeling. Due to ciprofloxacin-induced inhibition of cytochrome P450 1A2, hepatic metabolism of tizanidine is decreased. The resulting increase in tizanidine plasma concentration and clinically significant adverse events is a contraindication to the co-administration of tizanidine, taken orally, and ciprofloxacin, given intravenously.

Tizanidine is well absorbed after an oral dose, with extensive first-pass hepatic metabolism to inactive compounds that are subsequently eliminated in the urine. Therefore tizanidine should be used with caution in patients with known liver abnormality. Because the most common side effects reported during the clinical trials with tizanidine include dizziness and drowsiness, it is recommended that tizanidine therapy begin with a single dose of 2–4 mg at bedtime. The titration of tizanidine should be tailored to the patient. The maintenance dosage is the one at which the therapeutic goals have been met with the least side effects. The scored tizanidine tablets contain 4 mg. Dosage increases of 2–4 mg every 2–4 days are recommended; however, most clinicians experienced with tizanidine recommend a slow and gradual upward titration. This is particularly the case for patients with multiple sclerosis, who tend to experience side effects at lower dosages. The maximum recommended dosage is 36 mg per day. All trials, including those in SCI, multiple sclerosis, or cerebral disorders, have reported somnolence consistently in 42–46% of the patients.[129,140,178]

Alteration of ion channels
Dantrolene sodium (Dantrium)

Dantrolene sodium is a hydantoin derivative whose primary pharmacologic effect is to reduce calcium flux across the sarcoplasmic reticulum of skeletal muscle. This action uncouples motor nerve excitation and skeletal muscle contraction.[62,192] It is indicated for use in chronic disorders characterized by skeletal muscle spasticity, such as SCI, stroke, cerebral palsy, and multiple sclerosis. The oral formulation is prepared as a hydrated sodium salt to enhance absorption (approximately 70%), which occurs primarily in the small intestine. After a dose of 100 mg, the peak blood concentration of the free acid, dantrolene, occurs in 3–6 h. The compound is hydroxylated, and the active metabolite, 5-hydroxydantrolene, peaks in 4–8 h. Dantrolene sodium has been shown to produce a dose-dependent decrease in the stretch reflex[91] and a percentage decrease of grip strength.[70] Dantrolene is lipophilic and crosses cell membranes well, achieving wide distribution and significant placental concentration in the pregnant patient. Liver metabolism by mixed function oxidase and cytochrome P450 produces a 5-hydroxylation of the hydantoin ring and reduction of the nitro group to an amine, which is then acetylated. Urinary elimination of 15–25% of the unmetabolized drug is followed by urinary excretion of the metabolites after oral administration of the drug. The median elimination half-life is 15.5 h after an oral dose, and 12.1 h after an intravenous dose.

The majority of placebo-controlled clinical trials of dantrolene have shown a reduction of muscle tone, stretch reflexes, and increased passive motion. The most consistent finding has been a reduction of clonus in patients with clonus.[160] There have been mixed conclusions regarding the effects of dantrolene sodium on gross motor performance and strength. In comparative trials with spasticity of different etiologies, some have suggested that the best responders to dantrolene sodium are those with stroke and cerebral palsy, and that patients with SCI improve the least, if at all. Most investigators agree, however, that patients with multiple sclerosis do not generally benefit from dantrolene treatment.[119] In four trials of children with cerebral palsy, dantrolene sodium was found to be superior to placebo. The degree of improvement appeared greater in children than in adults. One study found dantrolene to be superior to baclofen, and another suggested equal efficacy to diazepam. In addition to its antispasticity effects, dantrolene has been used in the treatment of malignant hyperthermia and the neuroleptic malignant syndrome.[192] Dantrolene has also been reported to be useful in the treatment of hyperthermia following abrupt baclofen withdrawal.[102,119]

At least 13 clinical reports of overt hepatotoxicity appear in the literature, five of which report hepatonecrosis. The overall incidence of hepatotoxicity in a large group of patients receiving dantrolene sodium for more than 2 months is reported to be 1.8%, with symptomatic hepatitis occurring in 0.6% and fatal hepatitis in 0.3%. The greatest risk was in women older than 30 years who were taking more than 300 mg/day for more than 60 days. Initiation of antispasticity treatment with dantrolene sodium should begin with 25 mg once daily, increasing every 4–7 days, by 25-mg increments, to 100 mg four times per day. The dosage at which the anticipated therapeutic response occurs with least side effects should be the maintenance dose.

Benzodiazepines

Generally, a functionally coupled benzodiazepine–GABA receptor chloride ionophore complex mediates the pharmacologic and antispasticity effects of benzodiazepines.[38,152,171] As described above, the GABA$_A$ receptor supramolecular structure is envisioned as a heteropentameric glycoprotein of about 275 kDa, whose subunits react with GABA, benzodiazepines, steroids, barbiturates, and picrotoxin-like convulsants.[117] More specifically, the duration of action is related to the receptor and pharmacodynamics; certain benzodiazepine subunits are either high-affinity or low-affinity receptors, as well as long-acting and short-acting benzodiazepines. Benzodiazepines enhance GABA$_A$ receptor current, which increases the opening frequency of the chloride ionophore without altering channel conductance or open duration.[185] Also, the relative length of action is related to the duration of activity and rate of metabolism of the pharmacologically active metabolites. Examples of long-acting benzodiazepines are diazepam, chlordiazepoxide, and clonazepam. Oxazepam, alprazolam, and lorazepam are considered to be short acting without significant production of active metabolites. Benzodiazepines cross the placental barrier and are secreted into breast milk. Microsomal enzymes of the liver metabolize the benzodiazepines extensively.

Diazepam (Valium) Diazepam is a benzodiazepine that is sedating, reducing agitation and anxiety. It decreases polysynaptic reflexes and has muscle relaxant, sedation, and antispasticity effects.[50,121,156] Diazepam is usually started with a bedtime dose of 5 mg, increased to 10 mg as needed. Diazepam is well absorbed after an oral dose, with the peak blood level occurring typically in 1 h. Diazepam is metabolized to the active compound N-desmethyldiazepam (nordiazepam), and then to oxazepam. The half-life of diazepam and its active metabolites is 20–80 h, and it is 98–99% protein-bound. In patients with low serum albumin and lower protein-binding capacity, such as is often the case in patients with SCI or stroke, the incidence of undesirable sedation is increased. Daytime therapy is initiated with 2 mg and increased as needed.

Diazepam intoxication causes a range of symptoms from somnolence to coma. While it is generally regarded as having a wide margin of safety, benzodiazepine poisoning has been reported.[173] Near-term infants born with benzodiazepine intoxication are at risk also. There is a case report of a young mother at term, who consumed a diazepam overdose of 250–300 mg and became drowsy but responsive. The fetal heart rate showed decreased variability and absence of accelerations. The benzodiazepine antagonist flumazenil, 0.3 mg, was given to the mother intravenously. Within 5 min, behavioral arousal in the mother and improved fetal heart rate variability were observed.[182]

Typical symptoms of patients in withdrawal from high-dose diazepam (>40 mg per day) are anxiety and agitation; restlessness; irritability; tremor; muscle fasciculation; twitching; nausea; hypersensitivity to touch, taste, smell, light, and sound; insomnia; nightmares; seizures; hyperpyrexia; and psychosis. The intensity of the symptoms and risk of death are related to the prewithdrawal dose. Symptoms of withdrawal from low-dose benzodiazepine (< 40 mg per day) are more likely if the patient has taken the drug consistently for more than 8 months. Long-term usage of diazepam is common. In a study of 23 SCI treatment facilities with the Department of Veterans Affairs, 70% routinely used diazepam as an antispasticity treatment, and 67% of patients had been using it for more than 6 years.[23] Onset of withdrawal symptoms occurs 1–2 days after a short-acting benzodiazepine is stopped, or 2–4 days for a long-acting benzodiazepine. Even when the benzodiazepines are withdrawn slowly over 4–6 weeks, withdrawal symptoms can persist for 6 months.[75]

Clonazepam (Klonopin, Rivotril) Clonazepam is a benzodiazepine that is indicated for the suppression of myoclonic, akinetic, or petit mal seizure activity. It can be used alone or as an adjunct. Well absorbed after an oral dose, the maximum blood concentrations of clonazepam occur in 1–2 h. It is highly protein-bound and is metabolized in the liver. The half-life of clonazepam and its active 7-amino metabolite is 18–28 h. Clonazepam, if used to treat spasticity, can be useful in suppressing spasms at night that disturb sleep. It is most commonly prescribed as 0.5–1 mg at night. If morning sedation is excessive, the tablet can be broken in half and 0.25 mg taken at night.

Gabapentin (Neurontin)

Gabapentin is an approved adjunctive treatment for epileptic seizure disorder. It is a structural derivative of GABA; however, the mechanisms of gabapentin action are not fully elucidated. The off-label use of gabapentin for the treatment of spasticity, spastic hypertonia, and central pain syndromes in patients with SCI and multiple sclerosis has been cited in the literature.[41,74,125,133,149,177] Its plasma level peaks 2–3 h after oral administration, and it has a half-life of 5–7 h. Typically, the required antispasticity dosage is 400 mg t.i.d. or higher to reduce tone in the multiple sclerosis and SCI population.[58,84,133,162] Gabapentin may be associated with mild cognitive or behavioral effects and central nervous system depression, including somnolence, dizziness, ataxia, and fatigue. These adverse effects have been reported regardless of whether the medication is rapidly or slowly titrated. Gabapentin may also cause agitation in cognitively impaired patients.[30] Abrupt cessation must be avoided, as it may cause seizures in patients with brain lesions. Gabapentin awaits a demonstration of efficacy in the pediatric population, but is suggested to be beneficial in treating elderly patients.[11,107,144]

Vigabatrin (Sabril)

Vigabatrin is approved in Canada for the treatment of drug-resistant seizures. It is gamma-vinyl GABA (4-amino-hex-5-enoic acid) that irreversibly inhibits the activity of GABA transaminase. GABA transaminase exists in neurons and glia to regulate the intracellular balance of GABA, glutamate, and intermediate substances in energy metabolism such as α-ketoglutarate. Inhibition of GABA transaminase results in an elevation of GABA levels in the brain.[71,82,85] Vigabatrin is well absorbed after an oral dose, and the peak plasma concentrations occur within 2 h. It is widely distributed in the body and eliminated mainly by the kidney. The plasma half-life is 5–8 h in young adults, and 12–13 h in the elderly. The initial starting dose of vigabatrin is 500 mg twice per day and is often quite sedating. It is well absorbed orally, with peak plasma concentration within 2 h. Like most antiepileptics, somnolence and drowsiness (28%) are unwanted side effects. Other adverse effects associated with vigabatrin are fatigue (28%), dizziness (21%), nystagmus (15%), abnormal vision (11%), agitation (11%), amnesia (10%), depression (10%), aggression psychosis, and paresthesia (9%).[15,191]

Topiramate (Topamax)

Topiramate, another antiepileptic treatment, is a sulfamate-substituted monosaccharide (2,3:4,5-di-O-isopropylidene-B-D-fructopyranose sulfamate). It has been reported to be useful in the treatment of seizures and spasticity in children with Canavan disease, a rare autosomal recessive disease causing early-onset leukoencephalopathy and megalencephaly, as well as the infantile spasms of West syndrome, when combined with vigabatrin.[24,187] It has also been reported to be of therapeutic benefit in an elderly patient with vascular hemichorea–hemiballism.[74] Topiramate is thought to have three possible mechanisms: blockade of state-dependent sodium channels, enhancement of $GABA_A$ receptor activation, and reduction of non-NMDA excitatory amino acid action. It is rapidly absorbed following oral administration, with approximately 80% bioavailability. Peak plasma concentration following a 400-mg dose occurs at approximately 2 h. The half-life is 21 h, and steady state is achieved after approximately 4 days. Topiramate is eliminated unchanged, primarily in the urine. Renal impairment can significantly prolong the elimination half-life of topiramate. Somnolence, dizziness, ataxia, and fatigue were the most frequently reported adverse reactions during clinical trials. The recommended initial dose of topiramate is 50 mg, usually in the evening, with dose increases by 50 mg/day each week to a maximum of 200 mg twice per day. Topiramate is available as 15-mg or 25-mg capsules or as sprinkle capsules.

Lamotrigine (Lamictal)

Lamotrigine is thought to act at voltage-sensitive sodium channels to stabilize neuronal membranes and inhibit the release of excitatory amino acid transmitters; consequently, it has anticonvulsant effects. Lamotrigine has shown analgesic action in animal models of acute and chronic pain.[137] Recent clinical trials with lamotrigine have shown promise in the treatment of chronic pain states, as well as in the treatment of spasticity and concomitant chronic central pain.[20] Skin-related adverse events have been reported during lamotrigine treatment, particularly in patients taking valproic acid.

Riluzole (Rilutec)

Riluzole is approved for symptomatic treatment of amyotrophic lateral sclerosis. It reportedly blocks the action of voltage-sensitive sodium channels, thereby preventing release of excitatory amino acids and producing a reduction in the stiffness associated with amyotrophic lateral sclerosis.[16]

Clonidine (Catapres, Dixarit)

Clonidine is best known as a treatment for hypertension. Because of its effects on the autonomic nervous system, however, clonidine has a number of effects on homeostatic processes. The most commonly described mechanism by which clonidine lowers blood pressure and heart rate appears to be an α_2-mediated inhibition of locus coeruleus neurons and the intermediolateral cell column in the spinal cord. Clonidine has been termed a *partial agonist* because, when injected intravenously, the blood pressure rises as the α receptors on blood vessels cause vasoconstriction and a brief rise in systemic blood pressure. Once the discharge rate of sympathetic preganglionic fibers is decreased via the central mechanism, the blood pressure falls and the heart contraction rate slows.[106,145,183,188]

Clonidine's effect on spinal reflex circuitry is to inhibit short-latency alpha motoneuron response to group 2 muscle afferents, probably by augmenting presynaptic inhibition.[170] It is likely that the antispasticity effect of clonidine is related to its α_2-mediated presynaptic inhibition of sensory afferents.[55,142,143] Clonidine is absorbed well from the gut, as well as through the skin, and has high bioavailability after an oral dose. The half-life is 5–19 h, and 62% is excreted in the urine. Some patients with postural hypotension can develop symptomatic hypotension during clonidine treatment, and some patients can have an improvement of hypotension, so initial dosage should be low to evaluate the patient's blood pressure response. There is a 25-μg formulation available in Canada (Dixarit) that can be taken orally twice per day to begin treatment. Alternatively, a 0.1-mg tablet can be cut into fourths (0.025 mg). The dose can be increased every 3 days by 0.05 mg per day as a three or four times per day dosage regimen. Clonidine is also available as a transdermal patch with two dosage formulations: 0.1 mg or 0.2 mg per day. The clonidine patch has been reported to be a useful treatment for spasticity.[193,195] The patch is designed to deliver the indicated amount of clonidine daily for 7 days. Precaution should be used with individuals who develop an allergic skin reaction to the patch, because they might have become sensitized to clonidine. A cautionary note for insulin-dependent diabetic patients is that clonidine can retard a tachycardia induced by a hypoglycemic reaction to insulin, which can delay the diagnosis. Additional side effects are dry mouth, ankle edema, and depression.

Cyproheptadine (Periactin)

Cyproheptadine has been a prescription pharmaceutical for many years, approved for the treatment of vascular headache, anorexia, and itching associated with hives. It is a non-selective compound with histamine and serotonin antagonist effects. It is deemed safe to use in pregnant women and, in fact, it has been used in the treatment of repetitive spontaneous abortion. Cyproheptadine can decrease the duration of clonus in people with spasticity due to SCI or multiple sclerosis.[10] Cyproheptadine is reported to improve muscle firing patterns and increase walking speed in patients whose gait was limited by clonus.[190] In a comparative clinical trial, cyproheptadine had similar antispasticity efficacy to that of clonidine and baclofen in spinal cord-injured patients.[139] A recent report described a patient who was symptomatic from intrathecal baclofen withdrawal, and who showed significant amelioration of symptoms by the use of cyproheptadine.[130]

Cyproheptadine comes only in a 4-mg size. Treatment should be initiated at 4 mg at bedtime, increasing by a 4-mg dose every 3–4 days. The most commonly effective and tolerable dose is 16 mg in divided doses, such as 4 mg four times per day. The maximum recommended dose is 36 mg per day. The initiation of treatment at full maintenance dosage will produce significant sedation. Patients who take cyproheptadine will also gain weight, typically 10 lbs in the first 2 weeks of treatment.

Chlorpromazine (Thorazine, Largactil)

Chlorpromazine, a phenothiazine derivative developed in 1949, is a well-known sedative–antipsychotic that can depress reflex activity.[21] Chlorpromazine is rarely used as an antispasticity treatment but, in an open clinical trial, resting muscle tone decreased with chlorpromazine and phenytoin (Dilantin) treatment.[35] Adverse effects of chlorpromazine include sedation and the potential risk of tardive dyskinesia.

Inhibition of excitatory amino acids
Orphenadrine citrate (Norflex) and memantine (Namenda)

Orphenadrine citrate is most commonly used as a 'muscle relaxant', but it has shown some efficacy as an antispasticity treatment in patients with SCI when given as an intravenous infusion.[28] A related compound, orphenadrine hydrochloride (Disipal), is a treatment for Parkinson disease. Patch clamp and binding studies have revealed that orphenadrine is an uncompetitive NMDA-type glutamate antagonist. Memantine (1-amino-3,5-dimethyladamantane) has anticonvulsant properties, and has been used to treat Parkinson disease and dementia.[6] Similar to orphenadrine, memantine inhibits binding of the NMDA antagonist MK-801.

Carisoprodol (Soma)

Similar to orphendarine, metaxalone (Skelaxin), and cyclobenzaprine (Flexeril), carisoprodol is a 'centrally acting' muscle relaxant. The antispasticity effects of carisoprodol, an isopropyl derivative of meprobamate, were tested by the then newly described Ashworth Scale in 1964.[7] In that trial of 24 patients with multiple sclerosis, 1 patient was much improved, 16 improved, 2 slightly improved, and 5 showed no change. With an average dose of 350 mg, four times per day, drowsiness is the main side effect.

Cannabinoids

Cannabis (Cesamet, Marinol)   Great controversy exists in the USA concerning the medicinal use of marijuana, despite the long history of the use the leaves of the *Cannabis sativa* plant.[136] The most studied of the various active alkaloids is THC, available as a prescription pharmaceutical dronabinol (Marinol) or as the synthetic cannabinoid nabilone (Cesamet). Several placebo-controlled clinical trials of orally administered compounds cast doubt, however, on the efficacy of THC in objectively reducing spasticity in patients with multiple sclerosis.[180] With the discovery of the endocannabinoid system, and the potential development of selective agonists and endocannabinoid degradation inhibitors, there may be a greater future use of cannabinoids medicinally than that presently.[60] The clinical indication for dronabinol and nabilone is nausea related to chemotherapy treatment. O'Shaughnessy reported the use of hemp extract to treat muscle spasms associated with tetanus in 1842.[153] Reynolds subsequently described the toxic effects and therapeutic use of cannabis in the treatment of epilepsy, chorea, and nocturnal spasms in 1890.[163] Anecdotal reports suggest that smoking marijuana has a muscle-relaxing effect in people with SCI or multiple sclerosis, but users may experience significant rebound spasticity in between doses.[32,59] Further, in an anonymous survey of 131 respondents with amyotrophic lateral sclerosis, 13 reported using cannabis to stimulate the appetite and to alleviate depression, pain, spasticity, and drooling.[2] Dronabinol after an oral dose is 4–12% bioavailable, less than 1% is excreted via the urine, and 95% of the drug is bound to plasma proteins. The half-life is 20–44 h. It is formulated in 2.5-mg, 5-mg, or 10-mg capsules. Nabilone is formulated as a pulvule containing 1 mg, with a recommended dose of 1–2 mg twice per day.

Injectable pharmacologic therapy

The advantage of an injected, locally administered agent is to limit systemic effects while targeting a specific nerve or muscle. There is a good rationale for local therapy in the treatment of spasticity. Local treatment provides the opportunity to target specific muscles and body regions. For example, in a patient with severely spastic distal hand muscles, one can perform intramuscular injections of a given therapeutic agent to achieve a finely graded result. Additional benefits of local therapy include the prevention or amelioration of contracture, and reduction of pain associated with spasticity. Specific targeted alteration of spastic muscle tone can improve sitting posture and reduce the need for splinting or bracing. For example, reducing spastic thigh adductor tone can improve perineal hygiene and ease of nursing care.[181] Finally, local therapies and oral or intrathecal antispasticity treatment may be used in conjunction.

Phenol and alcohol

Prior to the introduction of botulinum toxin and intrathecal baclofen, phenol was the most widely used injectable agent in the treatment of spasticity.[194] Phenol denatures the protein of nerve fibers, and in low concentrations has the property of a reversible local anesthetic. By contrast, alcohol is thought to have a dehydration effect on nerve tissue, resulting in sclerosis of nerve fibers and the myelin sheath. These agents can be injected at motor points identified by electrical stimulation, or directly into or on to nerve. The potential complications of phenol or alcohol injection include pain, dysesthesias that can last from weeks to months, arrhythmias, variable duration of effect, and incomplete irreversibility. Subarachnoid block has been performed with intrathecal phenol or alcohol, although this therapy can result in severe weakness and reduced sphincter function.[148]

Botulinum toxin therapy (Botox, Dysport, Myobloc)

Botulinum toxin is the biologic product of the action of an anaerobic bacterium, *Clostridium botulinum*. The toxin is one of the world's most deadly poisons, and is an extremely potent neuromuscular blocking agent when injected into the area of a motor point. Its primary effects occur at the terminal bouton of a motor nerve. Once actively taken up by the nerve terminal, the toxin permanently prevents the exocytosis of acetylcholine vesicles from the injected cholinergic motor nerve terminals, via interference with a zinc-dependent endopeptidase. This neuromuscular junction blockade results in effective chemical denervation of muscle fibers and failure of contraction. Additionally, intrafusal muscle fibers can be similarly paralyzed, resulting in decreased afferent spindle discharge and decreased reflex activity.

There are seven identified serotypes: A–G. Botulinum toxin serotype A (BTXA) use has been approved by the FDA for the treatment of strabismus, blepharospasm, and related facial dystonia. Botulinum toxin serotype B (BTXB) is approved for the treatment of cervical dystonia. BTXA and BTXB have been demonstrated to be safe and effective in other focal dystonias, such as spasmodic dysphonia (laryngeal dystonia). BTXA and BTXB have been used in the treatment of spasticity.[14,72] The duration of BTXA's clinical effect is variable, but it has been estimated to last approximately 3–4 months in patients with dystonia.[61] Following endocytosis of the toxin, the axons 'recover' by sprouting new nerve terminal boutons.

Generally, there is a dose–effect relationship, such that a greater toxin load per muscle results in a higher degree of weakness. For example, a higher dose of botulinum toxin is typically required to weaken a larger spastic muscle, such as hamstring muscle, than a dystonic finger flexor. Therapy must be individualized for each patient, taking into account the body weight, muscle size, location of muscle, and degree of spasticity. It should also be noted that the serotype, concentration, and volume of the toxin can affect the amount of spread of the toxin and the intensity of the resulting muscle weakening effect.

In 10 non-ambulatory patients with spastic contraction of the thigh adductor muscles due to multiple sclerosis, botulinum toxin improved sitting, positioning, and ease of attaining thigh abduction for urethral catheterization and perineal hygiene.[181] Electromyography-guided botulinum toxin (20–80 U) injections of the urethral rhabdosphincter are reported to reduce detrusor–sphincter dyssynergia in men with SCI.[61] Transient hematuria was noted following the injection. In children with spastic plantar flexors due to cerebral palsy, injection of a total dose of 4 U/kg resulted in significant improvement of ankle position and gait.[31]

A number of open-label studies reported benefits of botulinum toxin injections in the management of spasticity in stroke patients.[42,43,51,124,176] The results indicated that the group receiving high-dose BTXA (300 U total) experienced significant reduction in the elbow and wrist flexor tone, as well as an improvement in physician and patient global assessment scales. However, the functional measures (Fugl-Meyer, Rand 36-Item Health Survey 1.0, functional independence measure, Function Status Index, pain assessment, and caregiver dependency scales) did not improve. Further studies of BTXA in the treatment of spasticity are in progress. To enhance its effectiveness, an additional electrical stimulation protocol seems promising. Most patients tolerate the neurolytic agent well. Two individuals, however, suffered from an intermittent tetraparesis after treatment.[92]

Chronic infusion of medications into the intrathecal space

Intrathecal baclofen (Lioresal)

As noted above, orally administered baclofen is absorbed and has a central site of action, but the intrathecal route of baclofen administration results in a 100-fold increase in potency compared with the oral treatment.[56] Once a reliable implantable drug delivery system was developed, chronic intrathecal baclofen use became possible. Several prospective, randomized studies have demonstrated the effectiveness of intrathecal baclofen for the treatment of spasticity.[13,33,66,89,108,127,128,134,138,141,157,194] Although this form of antispasticity therapy is highly effective, its use is limited by the invasive nature of the treatment and the cost of the implantable devices. However, for patients in whom severe spasticity is the cause for hospitalization, intrathecal baclofen can be cost-effective by reducing the need for inpatient hospitalization or 24-h nursing care.[13,141]

The decision to recommend intrathecal baclofen must involve the determination of the dose at which intrathecal baclofen will be effective. For example, a test dose of 25 μg can be given via lumbar puncture. The muscle tone of the patient should be evaluated hourly for 4–6 h. A decrease in the Ashworth score of a preselected muscle group by one or two grades is often cited as evidence of a threshold dose of intrathecal baclofen.[129,141] If a therapeutic response is not obtained, then trials with 50, 75, or 100 μg could be conducted on following successive days until a therapeutic response is observed. There are two methods

to predict the initial 24-h dose. One way to estimate the 24-h dose is to double the threshold dose. The other is to consider the duration of the antispasticity effect. For example, if the antispasticity effect of the test injection persisted for 8 h, that is one-third of a 24-h period. Consequently, the estimated 24-h dose in this case would be three times the threshold.

Once the implantation and dosage stabilization is complete, the patient is discharged home, and is expected to return for periodic pump refills. When using the electronic, programmable pump, the refill interval is largely based on the programmed daily dosage and flow rate. For patients with very low daily dose requirements, the refill interval can be as long as 4–5 months. The refill procedure must be done with utmost care using strict sterile technique. Following the refill, the pump must be updated and reprogrammed, if needed.

Intrathecal morphine (Infumorph) and midazolam (Versed)

The use of morphine by direct infusion into the epidural or intrathecal space has been reported to be a highly effective antispasticity as well as analgesic treatment.[66] In a series of four patients with the combination of severe pain and spasticity, both conditions were controlled for up to 8 months with daily dosages of 2–4 mg. However, tolerance, pruritis, nausea, hypotension, urinary retention, and respiratory depression can occur with an intrathecal morphine bolus dose as low as 0.4 mg.[40,99] Intrathecal midazolam (Versed) has also been reported to be effective but is limited by sedation.[135]

SURGICAL INTERVENTIONS

Orthopedics and neurosurgery are the two most commonly involved surgical subspecialties involved in the treatment of spasticity. Common goals of surgery are usually to increase mobility, decrease the use of external aids, correct or prevent deformity, and ultimately maximize function.[99] Musculoskeletal compensatory techniques used by the orthopedic surgeons include tendon lengthening, muscle–tendon transfer (e.g. the split anterior tibial transfer), contracture release, capsulotomy, osteotomy, resection arthroplasty, arthrodesis, epiphyseodesis, ankle fusion, and spine fusion.[73,101,120] The neuroablative techniques used by the neurosurgeons involve the interruption of the spinal reflex arc by neurectomy, neurotomy, rhizotomy, selective rhizotomy, dorsal root entry zone lesion, and myelotomy (Bischoff or T-shaped). There is an anecdotal report of two stroke patients with painful spastic hemiparetic leg who experienced improved pain management following unilateral selective posterior rhizotomy.[73] Other procedures include cordotomy, cordectomy, implantation of stimulators, or drug infusion devices. Ideally the procedure would be low in cost, extremely safe, and require a small operation with complete relief of spasticity, and yet produce total preservation of voluntary movement, sensation, and sphincter and sexual function. Unfortunately, a surgical therapy that could achieve this optimal outcome remains a future goal.[100]

CONCLUSION

Spasticity, like the underlying neuropathology it represents, is often in an evolving state of change. Initially, the individual patient should be thoroughly assessed, the goal of treatment determined by agreement between the practitioner and the patient, and a comprehensive treatment plan initiated. This plan should include the avoidance of spasticity-aggravating factors, and frequent range of motion exercise.[101] Patients receiving antispasticity medication should be reviewed periodically to assess response to treatment, as well as side effects and adverse effects; to monitor the optimal use of mobility aids and wheelchair seating (if applicable); and to monitor the accompanying neurologic impairment. Patients who are surgical candidates require a thorough initial investigation. This investigation should establish that skeletal growth and postoperative compliance have been considered, and that the best medical treatment, where appropriate, has failed to benefit the patient. In summary, aggressive diagnosis and management of spasticity, accompanied by the setting of appropriate goals established by dialog between the physician, patient, and caregivers, can lead to substantial improvement in quality of life in affected individuals.

The use of any treatment modality should be tailored to the patient and the diagnosis. A drug that is recommended for a patient with SCI might not be the first-line treatment for a patient with a cerebral cause or spastic hypertonia due to other aspects of the patient's condition (e.g. relative intolerance for sedation as a side effect).[63] Another consideration should be whether these agents, particularly those that have an effect on glutamate (necessary for learning), may slow neurorecovery in the first months following central nervous system injury or illness. For example, one must consider the observation that α-noradrenergic agonists, benzodiazepines, baclofen, and antiepileptic agents might impair neurorecovery in the first weeks and months after injury of illness.[53,79] Considerable research in the different impairment populations, as well as the timing of interventions, remains an ongoing challenge in neurorehabilitation.

REFERENCES

1. American Academy of Neurology. Assessment: the clinical usefulness of botulinum toxin-A in treating neurologic disorders. Report of the Therapeutics and Technology Assessment Subcommittee of the American Academy of Neurology. Neurology 1990; 40:1332–1336.
2. Amtmann D, Weydt P, Johnson KL, et al. Survey of cannabis use in patient with amyotrophic lateral sclerosis. Am J Hosp Palliat Care 2004; 21(2): 95–104.
3. [Anonymous]. Environmental Status Scale, question 4, minimal record of disability for multiple sclerosis. New York: National Multiple Sclerosis Society; 1985:44.
4. [Anonymous]. Guide for the Uniform Data Set for Medical Rehabilitation, version 4.0 (adult FIM). Buffalo: UB Foundation Activities; 1993.
5. [Anonymous]. SF-36 Health Survey. Boston: Medical Outcome Trust; 1992.
6. Areosa SA, Sherriff F, McShane R. Memantine for dementia. Cochrane Database Syst Rev 2005:CD003154.
7. Ashworth B. Preliminary trial of carisoprodol in multiple sclerosis. Practitioner 1964; 192:540–542.
8. Ashworth NL, Satkunam LE, Deforge D. Treatment for spasticity in amyotrophic lateral sclerosis/motor neuron disease. Cochrane Database Syst Rev 2004:CD004156.
9. Bajd T, Gregoric M, Vodovnik L, et al. Electrical stimulation in treating spasticity resulting from spinal cord injury. Arch Phys Med Rehabil 1985; 66:515–517.
10. Barbeau H, Richards CL, Bedard PJ. Action of cyproheptadine in spastic paraparetic patients. J Neurol Neurosurg Psychiatry 1982; 45:923–926.
11. Barnes MP. Spasticity: a rehabilitation challenge in the elderly. Gerontology 2001; 47(6):295–299.
12. Barolat G, Myklebust JB, Wenninger W. Effects of spinal cord stimulation on spasticity and spasms secondary to myelopathy. Appl Neurophysiol 1988; 51:29–44.
13. Becker W, Letts L. Intrathecal baclofen for adults with spinal spasticity. Can J Neurol Sci 1995; 22:122–129.
14. Bell KR, Williams F. Use of botulinum toxin type A and type B for spasticity in upper and lower limbs. Phys Med Rehabil Clin North Am 2003; 14(4):821–835.
15. Ben-Menachem E. Vigabatrin. Epilepsia 1995; 36(suppl 2):S95–S104.
16. Bensimon G, Lacomblez L, Meininger V, et al. A controlled trial of riluzole in amyotrophic lateral sclerosis. N Engl J Med 1994; 330(9): 585–591.
17. Berger M, Bobbitt RA, Carter WB, et al. The Sickness Impact Profile: development and final revision of a health status measure. Med Care 1981; 19:787–805.
18. Bohannon RW, Andrews AW. Correlation of knee extensor muscle torque and spasticity with gait speed in patients with stroke. Arch Phys Med Rehabil 1990; 71:330–333.
19. Bohannon RW, Smith MB. Interrater reliability of a modified Ashworth Scale of muscle spasticity. Phys Ther 1987; 67(2):206–207.
20. Bonicalzi V, Canavero S. Lamotrigine effects on chronic pain: an open-label pilot study [abstract]. In: Proceedings of the 8th World Congress of Pain, 1996.
21. Bradley PB. Tranquilizers: I. Phenothiazine derivatives. In: Root WS, Hofmann FG, eds. Physiological pharmacology. New York: Academic Press; 1963:417–477.
22. Brar SP, Smith MB, Nelson LM, et al. Evaluation of treatment protocols on minimal to moderate spasticity in multiple sclerosis. Arch Phys Med Rehabil 1991; 72:186–189.
23. Broderick CP, Radnitz CL, Bauman WA. Diazepam usage in veterans with spinal cord injury. J Spinal Cord Med 1997; 20:406–409.
24. Buoni S, Zannolli R, Strambi M, et al. Combined treatment with vigabatrin and topiramate in West syndrome. J Child Neurol 2004; 19(5):385–386.
25. Burke D, Andrews C, Ashby P. Autogenic effects of static muscle stretch in spastic man. Arch Neurol 1971; 25:367–372.
26. Burry HC. Objective measurement of spasticity. Dev Med Child Neurol 1972; 14:508–510.
27. Byrd BF, Collins W, Primm RK. Risk factors for severe bradycardia during oral clonidine therapy for hypertension. Arch Intern Med 1988; 148:729–733.
28. Casale R, Glynn C, Buonocore M. Reduction of spastic hypertonia in patients with spinal cord injury: a double-blind comparison of intravenous orphenadrine citrate and placebo. Arch Phys Med Rehabil 1995; 76:660–665.
29. Cervera-Deval J, Morant-Guillen MP, Fenollosa-Vasques P, et al. Social handicaps of multiple sclerosis and their relation to neurological alterations. Arch Phys Med Rehabil 1994; 75:1223–1227.
30. Childers MK, Holland D. Psychomotor agitation following gabapentin use in brain injury. Brain Inj 1997; 11(7):537–540.
31. Chutorian A, Root L. Management of spasticity in children with botulinum-A toxin. Int Pediatr 1994; 9(suppl 1):35–43.
32. Clifford DB. Tetrahydrocannabinol for tremor in multiple sclerosis. Ann Neurol 1983; 13:669–671.
33. Coffey RJ, Cahill D, Steers W, et al. for the Intrathecal Baclofen Multicenter Study Group. Intrathecal baclofen for intractable spasticity of spinal origin: results of a long-term multicenter study. J Neurosurg 1993; 78:226–232.
34. Cohen AH, Rossignol S, Grillner, eds. Neural control of rhythmic movements in vertebrates. New York: Wiley Interscience; 1988.

35. Cohen SL, Raines A, Panagakow J, et al. Phenytoin and chlorpromazine in the treatment of spasticity. Arch Neurol 1980; 37:360–364.

36. Cole B, Finch E, Gowland C, et al, eds. Physical rehabilitation outcome measures. Baltimore: Williams & Wilkins; 1995.

37. Corcos DM, Gottlieb GL, Penn RD, et al. Movement deficits caused by hyperexcitable stretch reflexes in spastic humans. Brain 1986; 109:1043–1058.

38. Costa E, Guidotti A. Molecular mechanisms in the receptor action of the benzodiazepines. Ann Rev Toxicol 1979; 19:531–545.

39. Coward DM, Davies J, Herrling P, et al. Pharmacological properties of tizanidine (DS103-282). Stuttgart: FK Schattattauer Verlag; 1984: 61–71.

40. Craig CL, Zimbler S. Orthopedic procedures. In: Whyte G, ed. The practical management of spasticity in children and adults. Philadelphia: Lea & Febiger; 1990:268–295.

41. Cutter NC, Scott DD, Johnson JC, et al. Gabapentin effect of spasticity in multiple sclerosis: a placebo controlled, randomized trial. Arch Phys Med Rehabil 2000; 81:164–169.

42. Das TK, Park DM. Botulinum toxin in treating spasticity. Br J Clin Pract 1989; 43:401–403.

43. Das TK, Park DM. Effect of treatment with botulinum toxin on spasticity. Postgrad Med J 1989; 65:208–210.

44. Davidoff RA. Antispasticity drugs: mechanisms of action. Ann Neurol 1985; 17:107–116.

45. Davies J, Johnston SE, Hill DR, et al. Tizanidine (DS103-282), a centrally acting muscle relaxant, selectively depresses excitation of feline dorsal horn neurones to noxious peripheral stimuli by an action at alpha adrenoceptors. Neurosci Lett 1984; 48:197–202.

46. Davies J, Johnston SE. Selective antinociceptive effects of tizanidine (DS 103-282), a centrally acting muscle relaxant, on dorsal horn neurones in the feline spinal cord. Br J Pharmacol 1984; 82:409–421.

47. Davies J. Selective depression of synaptic transmission of spinal neurones in the cat by a new centrally acting muscle relaxant, 5-choloro-4-(2-imidazolin-2-yl-amino)-2, 1, 3-benzothiadiazole (DS103 282). Br J Pharmacol 1982; 76:473–481.

48. Delwaide PJ, Gerard P. Reduction of non-reciprocal (Ib) inhibition: a key factor for interpreting spastic muscle stiffness. In: International Congress on Stroke Rehabilitation, Berlin, November 1993.

49. Delwaide PJ. Electrophysiological testing of spastic patients: its potential usefulness and limitations. In: Delwaide PJ, Young RR, eds. Clinical neurophysiology in spasticity. Amsterdam: Elsevier; 1985:185–203.

50. Delwaide PJ. Étude expérimentale de l'hyperréflexie tendineuse en clinique neurologique. Brussels: Arscia; 1971.

51. Dengler R, Neyer U, Wohlfarth K, et al. Local botulinum toxin in the treatment of spastic drop foot. J Neurol 1992; 239:375–378.

52. Dewald JPA, Given JD. Electrical stimulation and spasticity reduction: fact or fiction? In: Katz R, ed. Spasticity. State of the art reviews. Philadelphia: Hanley&Belfus; 1994:507–522.

53. Dikmen SS, Temkin NR, Miller B, et al. Neurobehavioral effects of phenytoin prophylaxis of posttraumatic seizures. JAMA 1991; 265:1271–1277.

54. Dimitrijevic MM. Meshglove 2, modulation of residual upper limb motor control after stroke with whole-hand electrical stimulation. Scand J Rehabil Med 1994; 26:187–190.

55. Donovan WH, Carter RE, Rossi CD, et al. Clonidine effect on spasticity: a clinical trial. Arch Phys Med Rehabil 1988; 69:193–194.

56. Dralle D, Muller H, Zierski J, et al. Intrathecal baclofen for spasticity. Lancet 1985; 2:1003.

57. Duncan GW, Shahani BT, Young RR. An evaluation of baclofen treatment for certain symptoms in patients with spinal cord lesions. Neurology 1976; 26:441–446.

58. Dunevsky A, Perel AB. Gabapentin for relief of spasticity associated with multiple sclerosis. Am J Phys Med Rehabil 1998; 77(5):451–454.

59. Dunn M, Davis R. The perceived effects of marijuana on spinal cord injured males. Paraplegia 1974; 12:175.

60. Duran M, Laporte JR, Capella D. [News about the therapeutic use of cannabis and the endocannabinoid system.] Med Clin (Barc) 2004; 122(10):390–398.

61. Dykstra DD, Sidi AA. Treatment of detrusor-sphincter dyssynergia with botulinum A toxin: a double-blind study. Arch Phys Med Rehabil 1990; 71:24–26.

62. Ellis KO, Carpenter JF. Mechanisms of control of skeletal–muscle contraction by dantrolene sodium. Arch Phys Med Rehabil 1974; 55:362–369.

63. Elovic E. Principles of pharmaceutical management of spastic hypertonia. Phys Med Rehabil Clin North Am 2001; 12:793–816.

64. Elovic EP, Simone LK, Zafonte R. Outcome assessment for spasticity management in the patient with traumatic brain injury: the state of the art. J Head Trauma Rehabil 2004; 19(2):155–177.

65. Emre M. Review of clinical trials with Sirdalud in spasticity. In: Emre M, Benecke R. Spasticity. London: Parthenon Publishing; 1989.

66. Erickson DL, Blacklock JB, Michaelson M, et al. Control of spasticity by implantable continuous flow morphine pump. Neurosurgery 1985; 16: 215–217.

67. Esquenazi A, Hirai BA. Assessment and management of gait dysfunction in patients with spastic stroke or brain injury. In: R Katz, ed. Spasticity. State of the art reviews. Philadelphia: Hanley & Belfus; 1994:523–533.

68. Feldman RG, Kelly-Hayes M, Conomy JP, et al. Baclofen for spasticity in multiple sclerosis: double-blind crossover and three-year study. Neurology 1978; 28:1094–1098.

69. Finch L, Barbeau H. Hemiplegic gait: new treatment strategies. Physiother Can 1986; 38:36–40.

70. Flewellen EH, Nelson TE, Jones WP, et al. Dantrolene dose response in awake man: implications for management of malignant hyperthermia. Anesthesiology 1983; 59:275–280.

71. Francisco GE, Kothari S, Huls C. GABA agonists and gabapentin for spastic hypertonia. Phys Med Rehabil Clin North Am 2001; 12(4): viii, 875–888.

72. Fried GW, Fried KM. Spinal cord injury and use of botulinum toxin in reducing spasticity. Phys Med Rehabil Clin North Am 2003; 14(4): 901–910.

73. Fukuhara T, Kamata I. Selective posterior rhizotomy for painful spasticity in the lower limbs of hemiplegic patients after stroke: report of two cases. Neurosurgery 2004; 54(5):1268–1272.

74. Gatto EM, Uribe Roca C, Raina G, et al. Vascular hemichorea/hemiballism and topiramate. Mov Disord 2004; 19(7):836–838.

75. Geller A. Common additions. Clin Symp 1996; 48:23–24.

76. Gerkin R, Curry SC, Vance MV, et al. First order elimination kinetics following baclofen overdose. Ann Emerg Med 1986; 15(7):115–118.

77. Giebler KB. Physical modalities. In: Glenn MB, Whyte J, eds. The practical management of spasticity in children and adults. Philadelphia: Lea & Febiger; 1990:118–148.

78. Goff B. Grading of spasticity, and its effect on voluntary movement. Physiotherapy 1976; 62:358–361.

79. Goldstein LB. Pharmacologic modulation of recovery after stroke: clinical data. J Neurol Rehabil 1991; 5:129–140.

80. Gracely RH, McGrath P, Dubner R. Rating scales of sensory and affective verbal pain descriptors. Pain 1978; 5:5–18.

81. Gracies JM. Physical modalities other than stretch in spastic hypertonia. Phys Med Rehabil Clin North Am 2001; 12:747–768.

82. Grant SM, Heel RC. Vigabatrin: a review of its pharmacodynamic and pharmacokinetic properties, and therapeutic potential in epilepsy and disorders of motor control. Drugs 1991; 41(6):889–926.

83. Greene WB, Heckman JD, eds. The clinical measurement of joint motion. Rosemont: American Academy of Orthopaedic Surgeons; 1994.

84. Gruenthal M, Mueller M, Olson WL, et al. Gabapentin for the treatment of spasticity in patients with spinal cord injury. Spinal Cord 1997; 35(10):686–689.

85. Guberman A. Vigabatrin. J Neurol Sci 1996; 34:S13–S17.

86. Guissard N, Duchateau J, Hainaut K. Muscle stretching and motoneuron excitability. Eur J Appl Physiol 1988; 58:47–52.

87. Gybels J, van Roost D. Spinal cord stimulation for spasticity. Adv Tech Stand Neurosurg 1987; 15:63–96.

88. Halstead LS, Seager SWJ, Houston JM, et al. Relief of spasticity in SCI men and women using rectal probe electrostimulation. Paraplegia 1993; 31:715–721.

89. Hankey GJ, Stewart-Wynne EG, Perlman D. Intrathecal baclofen for severe spasticity. Med J Aust 1986; 145:465–466.

90. Hepp-Reymond M-C, Marini G. Perspectives on motor behavior and its neural basis. Basel: Karger; 1997.

91. Herman R, Mayer N, Mecomber SA. Clinical pharmaco-physiology of dantrolene sodium. Am J Phys Med 1972; 51:296–311.

92. Hesse S, Mauritz KH. Management of spasticity. Curr Opin Neurol 1997; 10(6):498–501.

93. Hill DR, Bowery NG. ³H-Baclofen and ³H-GABA bind to bicuculline-insensitive GABA_B sites in rat brain. Nature 1981; 290:149–152.

94. Hinderer SR, Lehmann JF, Price R, et al. Spasticity in spinal cord injured persons: quantitative effects of baclofen and placebo treatments. Am J Phys Med Rehabil 1990; 69(6):311–317.

95. Jensen MP, Karoly P, Braver S. The measurement of pain intensity: a comparison of six methods. Pain 1986; 27:117–126.

96. Jerusalem F. A double-blind study on the antispastic action of beta-(4-chlophenyl)-gamma-amino butyric acid (CIBA) in multiple sclerosis. Nervenarzt 1968; 39:515–517.

97. Jones RF, Burke D, Marosszeky JE, et al. A new agent for the control of spasticity. J Neurol Neurosurg Psychol 1970; 33:464–468.

98. Kameyama T, Nabeshima T, Sugimoto A, et al. Antinociceptive action of tizanidine in mice and rats. Naunyn-Schmiedeberg's Arch Pharmacol 1985; 330:93–96.

99. Karol LA. Orthopedic management in myelomeningocele. Neurosurg Clin North Am 1995; 6(2):259–268.

100. Kasdon DL, Abramovitz JN. Neurosurgical approaches. In: Whyte G, ed. The practical management of spasticity in children and adults. Philadelphia: Lea & Febiger; 1990:259–267.

101. Katz RT. Management of spasticity. Am J Phys Med Rehabil 1988; 67:108–116.

102. Khorasani A, Peruzzi WT. Dantrolene treatment for abrupt intrathecal baclofen withdrawal. Anesth Analg 1995; 80:1054–1056.

103. Kirklan LR. Baclofen dosage: a suggestion [letter]. Arch Phys Med Rehabil 1984; 65:214.

104. Knutsson E, Lindblom U, Martensson A. Differences in effects in gamma and alpha spasticity induced by the GABA derivative baclofen (Lioresal). Brain 1973; 96:29–46.

105. Knutsson E, Mårtensson A, Gransberg L. Antiparetic and antispastic effects induced by tizanidine in patients with spastic paresis. J Neurol Sci 1982; 53:187–204.

106. Kobinger W, Walland A. Investigations into the mechanisms of the hypotensive effect of 2,(2,6-dichlorophenylamino)2-imidazoline HCl. Eur J Pharmacol 1967; 2:155–162.

107. Kofler M, Kronenberg MF, Rifici C, et al. Epileptic seizures associated with intrathecal baclofen application. Neurology 1994; 44:25–27.

108. Krach LE. Pharmacotherapy of spasticity: oral medications and intrathecal baclofen. J Child Neurol 2001; 16(1):31–36.

109. Krawetz P, Nance P. Gait analysis of spinal cord injured (SCI) subjects: effects of injury level and spasticity. Arch Phys Med Rehabil 1996; 77:635–638.

110. Lance JW. Symposium synopsis. In: Feldman RG, Young RR, Koella WP, eds. Spasticity: disordered motor control. Chicago: Yearbook Medical; 1980:485–494.

111. Laporte Y, Lloyd DPC. Nature and significance of the reflex connections established by large afferent fibers of muscular origin. Am J Physiol 1952; 169:609–621.

112. Lee KC, Carson L, Kinnin E, et al. The Ashworth Scale: a reliable and reproducible method of measuring spasticity. J Neurol Rehabil 1989; 3:205–209.

113. Leone JA, Kukulka CG. Effects of tendon pressure on alpha motoneuron excitability in patients with stroke. Phys Ther 1988; 68(4):475–480.

114. Levine MF, Hui-Chan CWY. Relief of hemiparetic spasticity by TENS is associated with improvement in reflex and voluntary motor functions. EEG Clin Neurophysiol 1992; 85:131–142.

115. Levine MG, Knott M, Kabat H. Relaxation of spasticity by electrical stimulation of antagonist muscles. Arch Phys Med Rehabil 1952; 33:668–673.

116. Liddell EGT, Sherrington C. Reflexes in response to stretch (myotactic reflexes). Proc R Soc Lond B Biol Sci 1924; 96:212–242.

117. Lieber RL, Steinman S, Barash IA, et al. Structural and functional changes in spastic skeletal muscle. Muscle Nerve 2004; 29(5):615–627.

118. Macdonald RL, Olsen RW. GABA receptor channels. Annu Rev Neurosci 1994; 17:569–602.

119. Mandac BR, Hurvitz EA, Nelson VS. Hyperthermia associated with baclofen withdrawal and increased spasticity. Arch Phys Med Rehabil 1993; 74:96–97.

120. Massagli TL. Spasticity and its management in children. Phys Med Rehabil Clin North Am 1991; 2(4):867–889.

121. Matthew WB. Ratio of maximum H reflex to maximum M response of spasticity. J Neurol Neurosurg Psychiatry 1966; 29:201–204.

122. Matthews PBC. Mammalian muscle receptors and their central actions. Baltimore: Williams & Wilkins; 1972.

123. Maynard FM, Karunas RS, Waring WP. Epidemiology of spasticity following traumatic spinal cord injury. Arch Phys Med Rehabil 1990; 71: 566–569.

124. Memin B, Pollack P, Hommel M, et al. Effects of botulinum toxin on spasticity. Rev Neurol (Paris) 1992; 148(3):212–214.

125. Metz L. Multiple sclerosis: symptomatic therapies. Semin Neurol 1998; 18(3):389–395.

126. Meythaler JM, Clayton W, Davis LK, et al. Orally delivered baclofen to control spastic hypertonia in acquired brain injury. J Head Trauma Rehabil 2004; 19:101–108.

127. Meythaler JM, DeVivo MJ, Hadley M. Prospective study on the use of bolus intrathecal baclofen for spastic hypertonia due to acquired brain injury. Arch Phys Med Rehabil 1996; 77:461–466.

128. Meythaler JM, Guin-Renfroe S, Brunner RC, et al. Intrathecal baclofen for spastic hypertonia from stroke. Stroke 2001; 32:2099–2109.

129. Meythaler JM, Guin-Renfroe S, Johnson A, et al. Prospective assessment of tizanidine for spasticity due to acquired brain injury. Arch Phys Med Rehabil 2001; 82:1155–1163.

130. Meythaler JM, Roper JF, Davis L, et al. Cyproheptadine in intrathecal baclofen withdrawal: a case series. Arch Phys Med Rehabil 2003; 84:638–642.

131. Meythaler JM. Use of intrathecally delivered medications for spasticity and dystonia in acquired brain injury. Yaksh TL, ed. Spinal drug delivery. New York: Elsevier; 1999:513–554.

132. Misra UK, Pandey CM. H reflex studies in neurolathyrism. Electroencephal Clin Neurophysiol 1994; 39:281–285.

133. Mueller ME, Gruenthal M, Olson WL, et al. Gabapentin for relief of upper motor neuron symptoms in multiple sclerosis. Arch Phys Med Rehabil 1997; 78:521–524.

134. Muller H, Zierski J, Dralle D, et al. The effect of intrathecal baclofen in spasticity. In: Muller H, Zierski J, Penn RD, eds. Local spinal therapy of spasticity. Berlin: Springer-Verlag; 1988: 155–214.

135. Müller H, Zierski J. Clinical experience with spinal morphine, midazolam and tizanidine in spasticity. In: Müller H, Zierski J, Penn R, eds. Local-spinal therapy of spasticity. Berlin: Springer; 1988:143–150.

136. Nahas GG, Sutin KM, Harvey DJ, et al, eds. Marijuana and medicine. Totowa: Humana Press; 1999.

137. Nakamura-Craig M, Follenfant RL. Effect of lamotrigine in the acute and chronic hyperalgesia induced by PGE₂ and in the chronic hyperalgia in rats with streptozotocin-induced diabetes. Pain 1995; 63:33–37.

138. Nance P, Meythaler JM. Intrathecal drug therapy. Phys Med Rehabil Clin North Am 1999; 10(2):385–402.

139. Nance P. A comparison of clonidine, cyproheptadine and baclofen in spastic spinal cord injured patients. J Am Paraplegia Soc 1994; 17:151–157.

140. Nance PW, Bugaresti J, Shellenberger K, et al. Efficacy and safety of tizanidine in the treatment of spasticity in patients with spinal cord injury. Neurology 1994; 44(suppl 9):S44–S52.

141. Nance PW, Schryvers OI, Schmidt BJ, et al. Intrathecal baclofen therapy for adults with spinal spasticity: therapeutic efficacy and effect on hospital admissions. Can J Neurol Sci 1995; 22:22–29.

142. Nance PW, Shears AH, Nance DM. Clonidine in spinal cord injury. Can Med Assoc J 1985; 133:41–42.

143. Nance PW, Shears AH, Nance DM. Reflex changes induced by clonidine in spinal cord injured patients. Paraplegia 1989; 27:296–301.

144. Nance PW, Young RR. Antispasticity medications. Phys Med Rehabil Clin North Am 1999; 10:337–355.

145. Nance PW. Alpha adrenergic and serotonergic agents in the treatment of spastic hypertonia. Phys Med Rehabil Clin North Am 2001; 12:889–906.

146. Nance PW. Effects of graded Jendrassik facilitation on type Ia and II mediated reflexes in able-bodied and spinal cord injured humans [abstract]. In: Society for Neuroscience Abstracts; 1990.

147. Nance PW. Reflex characteristics of spinal cord injured humans [abstract]. In: Society for Neuroscience Abstracts; 1989.

148. Nathan PW. Intrathecal phenol to relieve spasticity in paraplegia. Lancet 1959; 2:1099.

149. Nicholson BD. Evaluation and treatment of central pain syndromes. Neurology 2004; 62(5 suppl 2):S30–S36.

150. Nielsen J, Klemar B, Hansen HJ. A new treatment of spasticity with repetitive magnetic stimulation in multiple sclerosis. J Neurol Neurosurg Psychol 1995; 58(2):254–255.

151. Norton BJ, Bomze HA, Chaplin H. Approach to objective measurement of spasticity. Phys Ther 1972; 52:15–23.

152. Olsen RW. GABA–benzodiazepine–barbiturate receptor interactions. J Neurochem 1981; 37:1–13.

153. O'Shaughnessy WB. On the preparation of the Indian hemp or ganja. Trans Med Phys Soc Bombay 1842; 8:421–461.

154. Park TS, Owen JH. Surgical management of spastic diplegia in cerebral palsy. N Engl J Med 1992; 326:745–749.

155. Pedersen E, Arlien-Soborg P, Grynderup V, et al. GABA derivative in spasticity. Acta Neurol Scand 1970; 46:257–266.

156. Pedersen E. Clinical assessment and pharmacologic therapy of spasticity. Arch Phys Med Rehabil 1974; 55:344–354.

157. Penn RD, Savoy SM, Corcos D, et al. Intrathecal baclofen for severe spinal spasticity. N Engl J Med 1989; 320:1517–1554.

158. Perry J. Pathological mechanisms. In: Perry J, ed. Gait analysis: normal and pathological function. Clifton Park: Delmar Learning; 1992:179–181.

159. Petajan JH. Spasticity: effects of physical interventions. J Neurol Rehabil 1990; 4:219–225.

160. Pinder RM, Brogden RN, Speight TM, et al. Dantrolene sodium. A review of its pharmacological properties and therapeutic effects. Drugs 1977; 13:2–23.

161. Pollock N, Baptiste S, Law M, et al. Occupational performance measures: a review based on the guidelines for client-centered practice of occupational therapy. Can J Occup Ther 1990; 57:77–81.

162. Priebe MM, Sherwood AM, Graves DE, et al. Effectiveness of gabapentin in controlling spasticity: a quantitative study. Spinal Cord 1997; 35(3):171–175.

163. Reynolds JR. On the therapeutic uses and toxic effects of *Cannabis indica*. Lancet 1890; 1:637–638.

164. Robinson CJ, Kett NA, Bolam JM. Spasticity in spinal cord injured patients: 1. short-term effects of surface electrical stimulation. Arch Phys Med Rehabil 1988; 69:598–604.

165. Robinson CJ, Kett NA, Bolam JM. Spasticity in spinal cord injured patients: 2. Initial measures and long-term effects of surface electrical stimulation. Arch Phys Med Rehabil 1988; 69:598–604.

166. Sabbahi MA, DeLuca CJ, Powers WR. Topical anesthesia: a possible treatment method for spasticity. Arch Phys Med Rehabil 1981; 62:310–314.

167. Salazar-Torres J, Pandyan AD, Price CI, et al. Does spasticity result from hyperactive stretch reflexes? Preliminary findings from a stretch reflex characterization study. Disabil Rehabil 2004; 26(12):756–760.

168. Sanger TD. Severe resting clonus caused by thyrotoxicosis in a 16-year-old girl with hereditary spastic paraparesis. Mov Disord 2004; 19(6):712–713.

169. Sayers AC, Burki HR, Eichenberger E. The pharmacology of 5-chloro-4-(2-imidazolin-2-yl-amino)-2,1,3-benzothiadiazole (DS 103 282), a novel myotonolytic agent. Arzneimittel-Forsch 1980; 30:793–803.

170. Schomburg ED, Steffens H. The effect of DOPA and clonidine on reflex pathways from group II afferents to alpha-motoneurons in the cat. Exp Brain Res 1988; 71:442–446.

171. Schwarz M, Turski L, Janiszewski W, et al. Is the muscle relaxant effect of diazepam in spastic mutant rats mediated through GABA-independent benzodiazepine receptors? Neurosci Lett 1983; 36:175–180.

172. Seib T, Price R, Reyes MR, et al. The quantitative measurement of spasticity: effect of cutaneous electrical stimulation. Arch Phys Med Rehabil 1994; 75:746–750.

173. Serfaty M, Masterton G. Fatal poisonings attributed to benzodiazepines in Britain during the 1980s. Br J Psych 1993; 163:386–393.

174. Shahani BT, Young RR. Management of flexor spasms with Lioresal. Arch Phys Med Rehabil 1974; 55:465–467.

175. Shefner JM, Berman SA, Young RR. The effect of nicotine on recurrent inhibition in the spinal cord. Neurology 1993; 43:2647–2651.

176. Simpson DM, Alexander DN, O'Brien CF, et al. Botulinum toxin type A in the treatment of upper extremity spasticity: a randomized, double-blind, placebo-controlled trial. Neurology 1996; 46:1306–1310.

177. Sjolund BH. Pain and rehabilitation after spinal cord injury: the case of sensory spasticity? Brain Res Brain Res Rev 2002; 40(1–3):250–256.

178. Smith C, Birnbaum G, Carter JL, et al. Tizanidine treatment of spasticity caused by multiple sclerosis: results of a double-blind, placebo-controlled trial. Neurology 1994; 44(suppl 9):S34–S43.

179. Smith CR, LaRocca N, Giesser BS, et al. High-dose oral baclofen: experience in patients with multiple sclerosis. Neurology 1991; 41:1829–1831.

180. Smith PF. Medicinal cannabis extracts for the treatment of multiple sclerosis. Curr Opin Invest Drugs 2004; 5(7):727–730.

181. Snow BJ, Tsui JK, Bhatt MH, et al. Treatment of spasticity with botulinum toxin: a double-blind study. Ann Neurol 1990; 28:512–515.

182. Stahl MM, Saldeen P, Vinge E. Reversal of fetal benzodiazepine intoxication using flumazenil. Br J Obstet Gynaecol 1993; 100:185–188.

183. Starke K, Borowski E, Endo T. Preferential blockade of presynaptic alpha-adrenoceptors by yohimbine. Eur J Pharmacol 1975; 34:385–388.

184. Stein R, Nordal HJ, Oftedal SI, et al. The treatment of spasticity in multiple sclerosis: a double-blind clinical trial of a new anti-spasticity drug tizanidine compared with baclofen. Acta Neurol Scand 1987; 75:190–194.

185. Study RE, Barker JL. Diazepam and (±) pentobarbital: fluctuation analysis reveals different mechanisms for potentiation of gamma-aminobutyric acid responses in cultured central neurons. Proc Natl Acad Sci USA 1981; 78:7180–7184.

186. Terrence DV, Fromm GH. Complications of baclofen withdrawal. Arch Neurol 1981; 38:588–589.

187. Topcu M, Yalnizoglu D, Saatci I, et al. Effect of topiramate on enlargement of head in Canavan disease: a new option for treatment of megalencephaly. Turk J Pediatr 2004; 46(1):67–71.

188. Unnerstall JR, Kopajtic TA, et al. Distribution of alpha-2 agonist binding sites in the rat and human central nervous system. Brain Res Rev 1984; 7:69–101.

189. Van Hemet JCJ. A double-blind comparison of baclofen and placebo in patients with spasticity of cerebral origin. In: Feldman RG, Young RR, Koella WP, eds. Spasticity: disordered motor control. Chicago: Year Book Medical Publishers; 1980.

190. Wainberg M, Barbeau H. Modulatory action of cyproheptadine on the locomotor pattern of spastic paretic patients [abstract]. In: Society for Neuroscience Abstracts; 1986.

191. Wallace A, Montanez S, Lorio M, et al. Vigabatrin, unlike some anticonvulsants, does not hinder recovery of function. Epilepsia 1996; 37:27.

192. Ward A, Chaffman MO, Sorkin EM. Dantrolene: a review of its pharmacokinetic properties and therapeutic use in malignant hyperthermia, the neuroleptic malignant syndrome and an update of its use in muscle spasticity. Drugs 1986; 32:130–168.

193. Weingarden SI, Belen JG. Clonidine transdermal system for treatment of spasticity in spinal cord injury. Arch Phys Med Rehabil 1992; 73:876–877.

194. Wood KM. The use of phenol as a neurolytic agent. A review. Pain 1978; 5:205–229.

195. Yablon SA, Sipski ML. Effect of transdermal clonidine on spinal spasticity: a case series. Am J Phys Med Rehabil 1993; 72:154–157.

196. Yarkony GM, Roth EJ, Cybulski GR, et al. Neuromuscular stimulation in spinal cord injury II: prevention of secondary complications. Arch Phys Med Rehabil 1992; 73:195–200.

197. Young R. Letters to the editor. J Neurol Neurosurg Psychol 1982; 45:1035–1039.

198. Young RR. Spasticity: a review. Neurology 1994; 44(suppl 9):S12–S20.

199. Zackowski KM, Dromerick AW, Sahrmann SA, et al. How do strength, sensation, spasticity and joint individuation relate to the reaching deficits of people with chronic hemiparesis. Brain 2004; 127(part 5):1035–1046.

Chapter

32

Sexuality Issues in Persons with Disabilities

Fernando Branco, Marca Lee Sipski and Andrew Sherman

Sexuality is one of the most complex areas of human life. It embodies the emotional and physical aspects of human reproductive behavior, with origins in the primal need for procreation. Sexual response is a perhaps unique part of the human body's functioning, because active participation in sexual activity is not necessary for an individual's personal survival. However, it is important for the survival of the human race. When a person becomes disabled, many sexual challenges can arise, including lack of desire for participation, physiologic and mobility changes, and psychologic issues. The goal of this chapter is to review the pertinent issues related to sexuality that a physiatrist should be aware of when caring for a person with a disability.

NORMAL ANATOMY AND PHYSIOLOGY

The penis is a tubular appendage consisting of three distinct cylindric compartments, each one encased by connective tissue. The ventral compartment is the corpus spongiosum, containing the bulbar and penile urethra. The paired dorsal compartments are the corpora cavernosa, or erectile bodies of the penis. The corpora cavernosa are covered by a thick fascial layer called the tunica albuginea. The tunica albuginea in the midline septum is permeable to blood flow, which allows free exchange of nutrients and pharmacologic agents between the corpora cavernosa.[94] The main blood supply is the internal pudendal artery, which is a branch of the internal iliac artery. The common penile artery is the terminal branch of the internal pudendal artery. The penile artery then branches into the bulbourethral, cavernous, and dorsal arteries.[94] The venous drainage of the penis is quite variable. Small venules within the corpora merge to form the subtunical venous plexus and proximally contribute to the emissary veins (Fig. 32-1).

The penis is under both autonomic (parasympathetic–sympathetic) and somatic (sensory–motor) neural regulation. The parasympathetic visceral efferent fibers arise from neurons in the second through the fourth segments of the sacral cord. The pelvic nerves are the preganglionic parasympathetic fibers that synapse on the pelvic plexus, located on the lateral wall of the rectum. Preganglionic sympathetic fibers arise from the 11th thoracic to the third lumbar spinal segments to synapse on sympathetic chain ganglia and subsequently on to the pelvic

plexus via the hypogastric nerve. Parasympathetic stimulation is responsible for erections. Sympathetic stimulation is responsible for seminal emission by inducing the contraction of the prostate and seminal vesicles while simultaneously resulting in closure of the bladder neck. Somatic neural stimulation is important for sensation and contraction of the bulbocavernosus and ischiocavernosus skeletal muscles during the final stages of erection and ejaculation. Somatic neurons originate in the second through fourth sacral spinal cord segments. Somatosensory receptors within the penis converge to form the dorsal nerve of the penis, which converges with other branches more proximally to become the pudendal nerve. With sensory stimulation of the penis, nerve impulses (touch, pain, pressure, and temperature) travel via the pudendal nerve to the spinothalamic tract of the spinal cord and then to the thalamus and cortex.

A summary of male and female neurologic sexual anatomy can be seen in Figures 32-2 and 32-3.

Male anatomy and physiology

Normal ejaculation occurs independent of an erection and has two phases: emission and ejaculation. Emission represents the secretion of fluid from the bulbourethral glands, and its consequent movement through the vas deferens, seminal vesicles, and prostate due to peristalsis of smooth muscle. The thoracolumbar sympathetic outflow from T10 to L2 regulates emission. The sympathetic outflow also closes the bladder neck through the α-adrenergic receptors. The bladder neck is the physiologic sphincter, and prevents the ejaculate from going in a retrograde direction (into the bladder). The external voluntary sphincter is also closed during emission.

Ejaculation occurs when there is projectile movement of the sperm from clonic contractions of the ischiocavernosus and bulbospongiosus muscles. Neurologic impulses are carried by the pudendal nerves (somatic) and sacral parasympathetic nerves (S1–S4). Next, the external voluntary urethral sphincter opens and the bladder neck sphincter remains closed to maintain the anterograde ejaculation. If the bladder sphincter stays open, as it does in some patients with spinal cord injury (SCI), the possibility of retrograde ejaculation is high.

The sympathetic nerve fibers responsible for the detumescence affecting the cavernous smooth muscle are mediated by noradrenaline (norepinephrine), which acts on postsynaptic α receptors. Parasympathetic fibers use acetylcholine (nicotinic

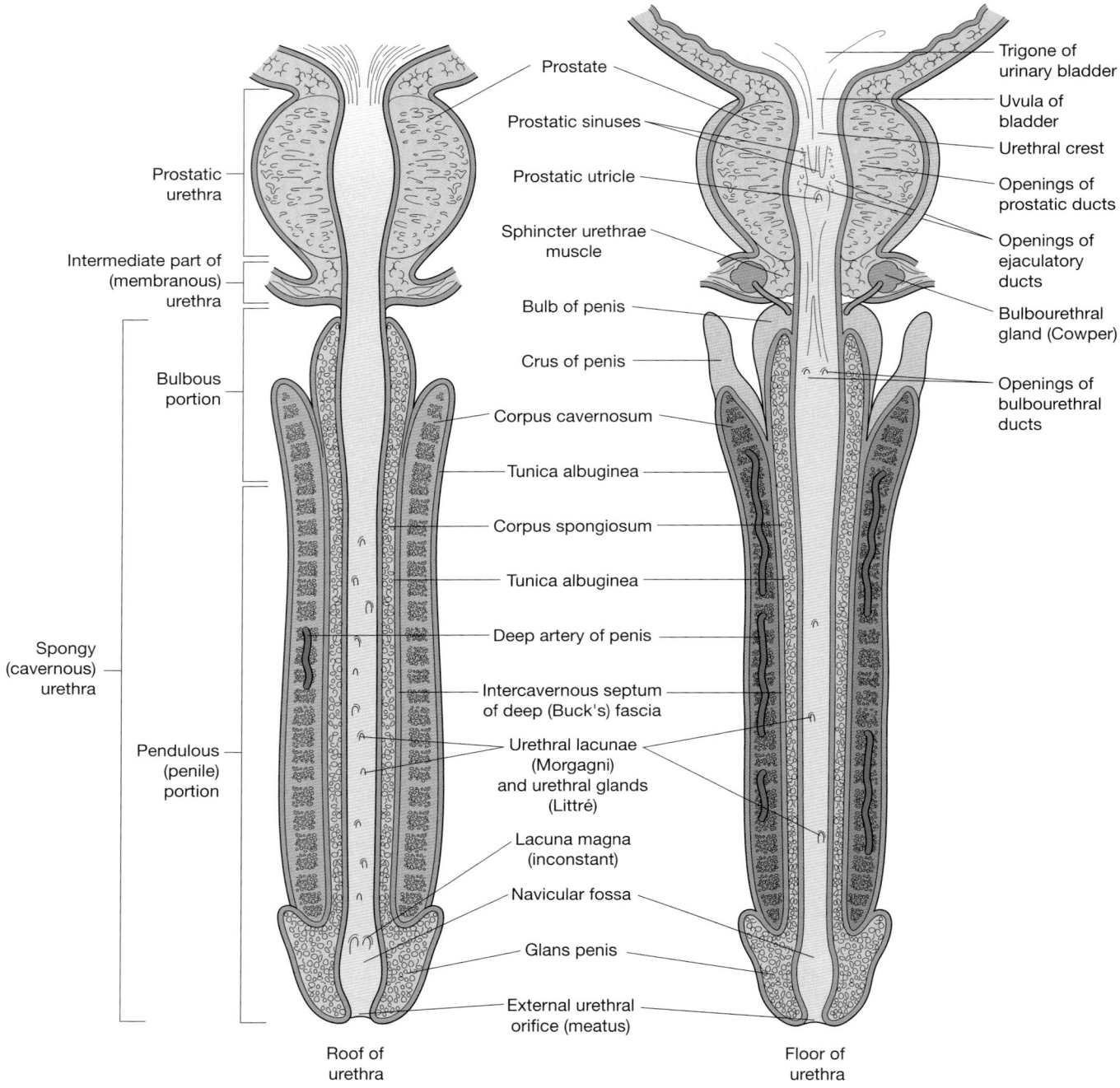

Figure 32-1 Anatomy of the penis. (Courtesy of Novartis Pharmaceutical Corporation.)

receptors for preganglionic and muscarinic receptors for post-ganglionic) as their chemical messenger. Central blockade of catecholamine synthesis has been shown to diminish erectile dysfunction.[86]

Erection can also be achieved through non-adrenergic, non-cholinergic neurons when mediated by nitric oxide. Nitric oxide synthase is an enzyme that produces nitric oxide, a smooth muscle relaxant and vasodilator. Its action is mediated through activation of guanylate cyclase to produce the second messenger

cyclic GMP. The non-adrenergic, non-cholinergic neurons use nitric acid as a neurotransmitter.[22]

Female anatomy and physiology

In the female, the external genitalia consist of the labia majora, the labia minora, and the clitoris. When unstimulated sexually, the major labia normally meet in the midline and provide protection for the subjacent structures: the labia minor, the vaginal outlet, and the urinary meatus. During sexual arousal, the labia

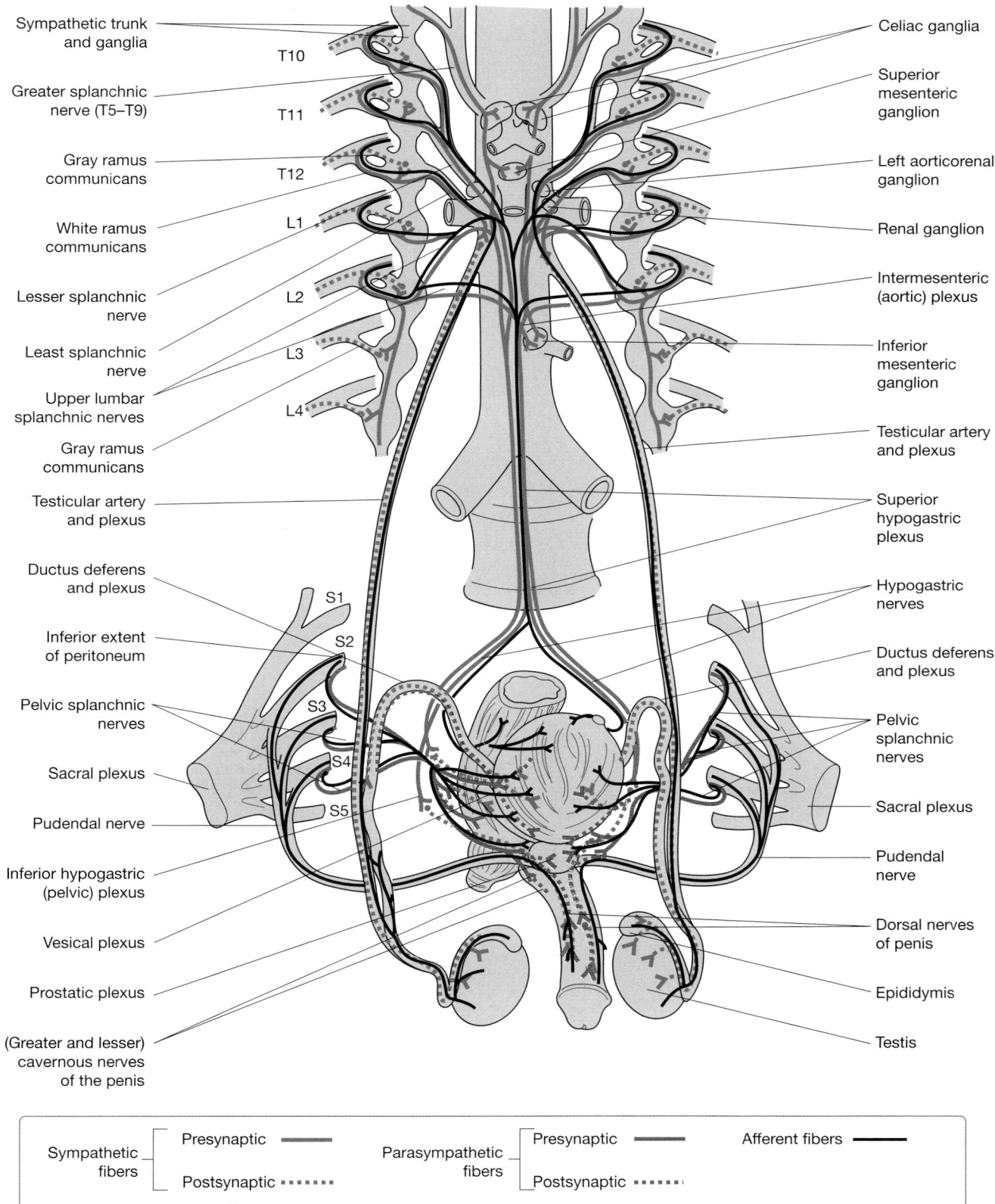

Sympathetic trunk and ganglia

Greater splanchnic nerve (T5–T9)

Gray ramus communicans

White ramus communicans

Lesser splanchnic nerve

Least splanchnic nerve

Upper lumbar splanchnic nerves

Gray ramus communicans

Testicular artery and plexus

Ductus deferens and plexus

Inferior extent of peritoneum

Pelvic splanchnic nerves

Sacral plexus

Pudendal nerve

Inferior hypogastric (pelvic) plexus

Vesical plexus

Prostatic plexus

(Greater and lesser) cavernous nerves of the penis

T10

T11

T12

L1

L2

L3

L4

S1

S2

S3

S4

S5

Celiac ganglia

Superior mesenteric ganglion

Left aorticorenal ganglion

Renal ganglion

Intermesenteric (aortic) plexus

Inferior mesenteric ganglion

Testicular artery and plexus

Superior hypogastric plexus

Hypogastric nerves

Ductus deferens and plexus

Pelvic splanchnic nerves

Sacral plexus

Pudendal nerve

Dorsal nerves of penis

Epididymis

Testis

| Sympathetic fibers | Presynaptic ——— | Parasympathetic fibers | Presynaptic ——— | Afferent fibers ——— |
| | Postsynaptic ······· | | Postsynaptic ······· | |

Figure 32-2 Innervation of the male reproductive organs. (Courtesy of Novartis Pharmaceutical Corporation.)

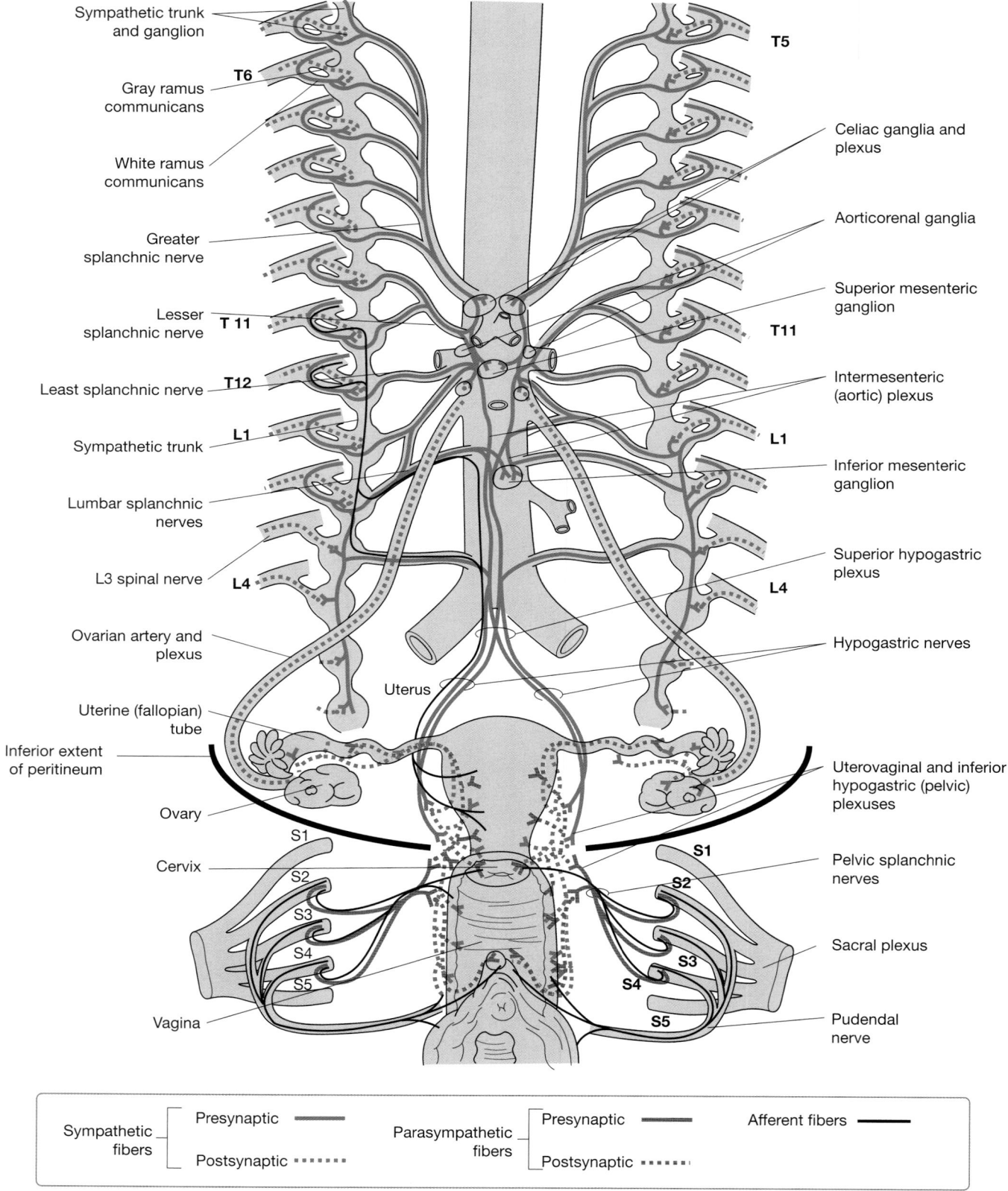

Figure 32-3 Innervation of the female reproductive organs. (Courtesy of Novartis Pharmaceutical Corporation.)

thin out and flatten against the perineum, and there is movement upward and outward away from the vaginal outlet. The labia minora increase in diameter due to vasocongestion and protrude through the labia majora. As the plateau phase approaches, the labia change to a darker color. Bartholin's glands are located in each of the labia minora. They secrete a mucoid material. However, this is not solely responsible for the lubrication necessary for sexual activity. The majority of lubrication occurs during the end of arousal and comes through the vaginal wall.

The clitoris is unique in that it serves as both a receptor and a transformer of sexual stimuli. It consists of two corpora cavernosa enclosed in a dense membrane. A suspensory ligament gives midline support. A dorsal nerve originates from the pudendal nerve and supplies innervation. Ischiocavernosus muscles originating from the ischial rami insert into the crura of the clitoris and provide additional support.[80]

Sexual response

Men and women have similar sexual responses. Masters and Johnson described the four phases of sexual response: arousal (excitement), plateau, orgasm, and resolution. The phases were based on their study of 600 able-bodied subjects. The male pattern has a tendency to be faster and achieve orgasm with a shorter plateau phase. Women have a longer plateau phase, with the possibility of one to several orgasms (climax).

Arousal

Arousal is associated with all four senses (touch, smell, hearing, and vision), as well as memory and fantasy. During the arousal phase, there are increases in heart rate, blood pressure, and respiratory rate, in addition to genital vasocongestion. The limbic system in the brain is associated with sexual arousal, erection, and vaginal lubrication.[48]

Libido (sexual urge or instinct) can be affected by dopamine (increased) and by serotonin (decreased). Depression and its treatment can affect libido. Selective serotonin reuptake inhibitors have a 50–70% chance of delaying orgasm in otherwise normal individuals. The incidence of impotence can be affected in individuals with no other compromising medical conditions.[91]

Plateau

Plateau can be very brief (seconds) or prolonged (minutes), and is described as a pleasurable sense of well-being.[22] During the plateau phase of sexual response, there are further increases in heart rate and respiratory rate, in addition to continued changes in the genitalia. Heart rates from 110 to 180 have been measured near the end of plateau. Hyperventilation occurs as well near the end of the plateau phase, lasting through orgasm and ending in the resolution phase. The female physiologic changes include breast engorgement and clitoral retraction, while the male physiologic changes include testicular elevation and enlargement due to vasocongestion. There is also a slight increase in penile diameter. In women, it is possible to go up to the plateau phase and then go down to resolution without actually achieving orgasm.

Orgasm

Orgasm has been described as a reflex function of the autonomic nervous system that can be facilitated or inhibited by cerebral input.[65] Orgasm is characterized by increases in heart rate, blood pressure, respiratory rate, and involuntary rhythmic contractions of the perineal musculature. There is a significant difference between men and women in relation to orgasm, in that men are known to experience a single orgasm and women are known to have the capability to achieve multiple orgasms.

Resolution

Resolution is the return to the prearousal physiologic state, usually occurring over a period of 5–15 min. It is marked by general perspiration and gradual reversal of blood pressure, heart rate, and respiratory rate to previous levels. The penis loses its filling due to sympathetic tonic discharge that causes contraction of the smooth muscles around the sinusoids and arterioles. However, the penis does not return to its normal size for 30–60 min after an orgasm.

SEXUAL BEHAVIOR AND AGE

The persistent myth that aging and a decline in sexual function are inexorably linked has led healthcare providers to overlook one of the most important quality of life issues in older adults, that of sexuality.[56] Intimacy, love, friendship, and masturbation are all aspects of sexual function that can occur even if coital activity does not. In 1948, Kinsey et al. reported reduced frequency of intercourse to once in every 10 weeks by age 80.[65] Reports of decline in sexual activity, interest, and desire have been reported in numerous studies subsequent to those of Kinsey, and have been reported to be more severe in women than in men.[6,54,63,64,74,96]

Bretschneider and McCoy found that 63% of men and 30% of women aged 80–102 were sexually active; 83% of men and 64% of women reported touching and caressing activity without intercourse, and 72% of men and 40% of women engaged in masturbation.[20] Masturbation decreases in frequency in both men and women with increasing age.[52] Barriers to sexual activity in older individuals include partner availability, health issues, alterations in sex drive, erectile dysfunction in men, dyspareunia in women, impact of medications, and loss of privacy for persons who need assistance with mobility or are nursing home residents.

The physiologic changes in men with aging include a decrease in scrotal vasocongestion and testicular elevation, and a delay in erection. The plateau phase is prolonged, and there is decreased preejaculatory secretion. Orgasm is shorter, with fewer forceful prostatic and urethral secretions, and ejaculation is less forceful.[63] In women, vaginal blood flow, lubrication, and genital engorgement are decreased, as are the changes in breast size that occur in younger women with sexual activity. There is also less uterine and labial elevation. Elderly women retain the ability for multiple orgasms, although these orgasms are usually weaker.[63]

Libido can be decreased, increased, or remain the same in older women and men.[55,102,128] Testosterone plays an important role in libido in both men and women.[97,106,108,113] A great impact of estrogen deficiency has been shown on genital tissue and organs in women, including: shortening of the vagina vault, loss of rugal folds, thinning of vaginal mucosa with concomitant loss of vaginal lubrication, and resulting dyspareunia (painful intercourse).[63] Dyspareunia secondary to estrogen loss and resulting atrophic vaginitis can be corrected with estrogen treatment. These problems occur in one-third of sexually active women over 65 years old.[63] Unlike the loss of testosterone in men and women and its impact on libido, estrogen per se does not appear to be linked to alterations in sex drive.[98]

Psychosocial changes with increasing age include cultural, ethnic, and socioeconomic factors, all of which can impact sexual beliefs, values, attitudes, behaviors, and adaptation to life stresses. Alterations in body image and altered self-perception can be even more important than perceived health in shaping sexual attitude in some individuals.[39] Sexual abuse and early sexual development can affect sexual expression later in life. Marital problems, illness, and deterioration of support networks all have an impact on sexuality.[26] Erectile dysfunction is an increasing problem with aging, occurring in approximately 52% of men aged 40–70[37] to greater than 95% in men over age 70 with diabetes.[52]

Erectile dysfunction is often multifactorial, with common causes including vascular disease, medication use, depression, stress, alcohol and drug abuse, and diabetes. In addition, sensory neuropathy, SCI, cerebrovascular accidents, multiple sclerosis, renal failure, and cirrhosis have also been associated with erectile dysfunction.

Age provides no immunity to sexually transmitted diseases, including AIDS. Ten percent of AIDS cases occur in those over 50 years of age, and only 20% of patients over age 70 have intravenous drug use or homosexuality as risk factors.[137] This indicates that, in the elderly, the great majority of AIDS cases result from heterosexual sex. Because the treatment of HIV with a combination of drugs has begun, survival has increased dramatically. Over the course of time, the demographics of AIDS will reflect even more of an aging population, and the effects on this group have yet to be determined.

PSYCHOSOCIAL ISSUES ASSOCIATED WITH DISABILITY AND SEXUAL ACTIVITY

Sexuality involves an interplay between the psychologic and physical, and their effects are not always discernible or attributable to one factor or another. A myriad of issues, including psychologic, situational, cultural, and couple-related, must be examined when assessing sexuality. This is particularly important for individuals with disabilities, who might have extensive adjustment issues, a decline in self-esteem, and new impair-

ments in mobility. This combination of factors can lead to depression and anxiety, which can exacerbate sexual dysfunction.[117]

An often overlooked issue concerns the age of onset of the disability. For instance, the impact of SCI on a 17-year-old is different from that on a 50-year-old man. The partner of a disabled individual is also deeply affected. Disability and illness lead to stress, and this can exacerbate problems that were preexisting. Couples must be educated about normal sexual response cycles and the impact of their physiologic condition on the sexual response cycle.[131] Changes in partner roles as a result of disability must also be negotiated. These changes can impact sexual desire, activities, and satisfaction. One study reported that 74% of male and 44% of female SCI subjects claimed that their disability significantly and negatively affected the quality of their sexual relationships.[131]

SEXUAL HISTORY

When doing the sexual history taking with disabled individuals, the history should be started by them to describe the chief complaint, allowing them to introduce themselves and the problem. In regard to sexual dysfunction, one should ask the following questions.

- What is the problem?
- Is the problem global and primary, occurring as long as the person has been sexually active, or did the problem start at a specific time? If the problem has only recently started, what are the circumstances that caused the problem to occur? Did the problem occur in relationship to a new disability? Is the problem related to a medical procedure such as surgery or radiation? Or is the problem related to the use of medications?
- Does the person suffer from personal distress as a result of the problem? How does the partner feel about the issue?

Once the problem has been determined to be related to a specific area, issues associated with the problem must be considered. A good history of the problem is important. When did it start? Under what circumstances does it occur, and what medical treatments has the subject undergone?

Many medications, such as antidepressants, antihypertensives, and antispasmodics, can impact sexual functioning, as can treatments such as radiation therapy. Any concomitant medical problems such as diabetes, arthritis, or cardiac disease that can impact sexual functioning should also be noted.

Special issues to consider with regard to the sexual history of a person with disabilities

The history of sexual dysfunction in a person with a disability involves first determining the person's predisability sexual patterns. It is also important to question the preinjury sexual satisfaction and frequency of the person's sexual activity. It is necessary to determine the status of the person's postinjury relationships and ability to participate in sexual activity. It is also important to determine the overall nature of the person's problem, and whether the person has received adequate sexual education. It often becomes apparent that the person with a disability is uncomfortable with sexuality after disability, or that the partner has decided to no longer be sexually active with him or her. It is important to try to identify this subset of people as early as possible, because these individuals and their partners need education, as noted above.

Many questionnaires have been developed to further evaluate sexual function. The Open Ended Sexuality Limited Organizing Worksheet is a semistructured questionnaire that has many open-ended questions and can be used for clinical or training purposes. It is designated for disabled and medically ill populations, and is free of gender bias.[131]

DIAGNOSIS OF SEXUAL DYSFUNCTION

Sexual dysfunction has traditionally been diagnosed using the Diagnostic and Statistical Manual Fourth Edition (DSM-IV) criteria.[4] These criteria base sexual dysfunctions on the sexual response cycle, including desire, excitement, orgasm, and resolution phases. The DSM-IV criteria also direct that sexual dysfunctions should be subtyped into lifelong or acquired disorders, and then into generalized or situational disorders. Subsequent to this, the clinician is asked to indicate whether the etiology is due to psychologic, combined factors, or due to a general medical condition. To qualify as a sexual dysfunction, the disorders must cause marked distress or interpersonal difficulty, and the dysfunction cannot be better accounted for by another psychiatric axis disorder.

The sexual desire disorders include hypoactive sexual desire disorder and sexual aversion disorder. Hypoactive sexual desire disorder is defined as persistently or recurrently deficient or absent sexual fantasies and desire for sexual activity. Sexual aversion disorder is the persistent or recurrent extreme aversion to, and avoidance of, all (or almost all) genital contact with a sexual partner. The arousal disorders include female sexual arousal disorder, the persistent or recurrent inability to attain, or to maintain until completion of the sexual activity, an adequate lubrication–swelling response of sexual excitement. Male erectile disorders include a persistent or recurrent inability to attain, or to maintain until completion of the sexual activity, an adequate erection, and the lack of an adequate erection. Male and female orgasmic disorders are defined as the persistent or recurrent delay or absence of orgasm following a normal excitement phase. Premature ejaculation is defined as persistent or recurrent ejaculation with minimal sexual stimulation before, on, or shortly after penetration and before the person wishes it.

The final category of sexual dysfunctions includes the sexual pain disorders: dyspareunia and vaginismus. Dyspareunia is recurrent or persistent genital pain associated with sexual intercourse in either a man or a woman. Vaginismus is the recurrent or persistent involuntary spasm of the musculature of the outer third of the vagina, which interferes with sexual intercourse.

A recent consensus conference came up with an updated methodology for the diagnosis of sexual dysfunction in women.[7] The guidelines follow the same format at those of the DSM-IV; however, the underlying common thread for all these disorders is that the particular disorder must cause personal distress. A new category, non-coital sexual pain disorder, was also added. It is important to remember that personal distress must be included for a person to have sexual dysfunction. It follows that someone with a neurologic disability might have altered sexual response but not be considered to have sexual dysfunction.[120] For this reason, for women with SCIs, the Female Spinal Sexual Function Classification[122] was recently proposed. It documents whether specific aspects of sexual response, including arousal and orgasm, are anticipated to occur with a particular type of SCI. This can also be used to document the presence or absence of sexual dysfunction in this population.

PHYSICAL EXAMINATION
Physical examination of men
Head, eyes, ears, nose, and throat should be evaluated. Any difficulties with production of saliva and lingual mobility, and swallowing problems should be noted. The neck should be evaluated for pain and range of motion.

Heart and lungs should be monitored for cardiac and breathing rate, arrhythmias, and chest format. An abdominal examination is performed to evaluate bowel sounds, pain, scarring from previous surgeries, and presence of surgical wounds or collection devices.

External genitalia should be examined for presence, shape, and size. Hair distribution, scarring, and collection mechanisms should be noted. Rectal examination should be included.

The neurologic examination should include mental status, and motor and sensory testing, with a sensory examination to focus on T11–L2 and S3–S5 dermatomes, and elicitation of the bulbocavernosus and 'anal wink' reflex, with documentation of whether upper or lower motor neuron dysfunction is present. The limbs should be examined for evidence of peripheral pulses, swelling, and loss of range of motion.

The integrity of the pudendal nerve can be evaluated by compressing the glans penis or the clitoris and checking the anal sphincter or the bulbocavernosus muscle (bulbocavernosus reflex). The pudendal nerve is easily evaluated by the anal sphincter response. It can also be investigated by electrically stimulating the dorsal nerve of the penis or clitoris and recording a response from the bulbocavernosus muscle (Fig. 32-4). This is an important electrical test, as it can be of use in patients with voiding or sexual dysfunction secondary to neurologic causes.[125]

Nocturnal penile tumescence monitoring is helpful to differentiate neurogenic and psychogenic erectile dysfunction.[131] The efferent portion of the circuit (pelvic nerves) can be determined via the nocturnal tumescence monitor (Fig. 32-5). Vascular inflow can be measured non-invasively with Doppler ultrasound, and the venoocclusive mechanism can be assessed with dynamic infusion cavernosometry (Fig. 32-6).

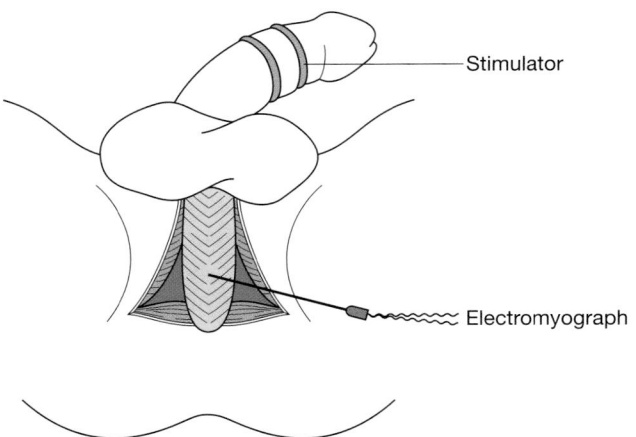

Figure 32-4 Electrical examination of the bulbocavernosus reflex. The dorsal nerve of the penis (or clitoris) is stimulated and the response recorded with a needle electrode located in the bulbocavernosus muscle. (From Smith et al. 1975,[125] with permission.)

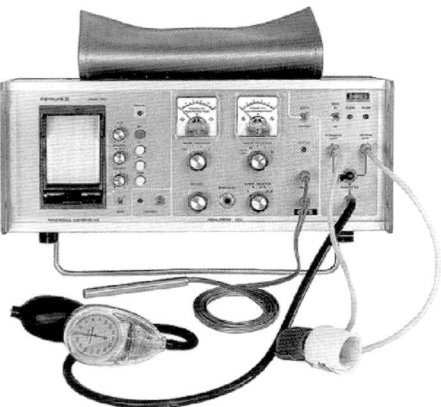

Figure 32-5 A nocturnal tumescence monitor.

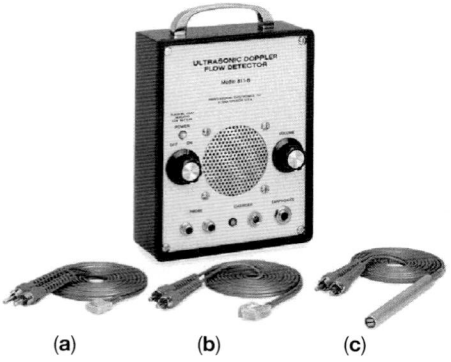

(a)   **(b)**   **(c)**

Figure 32-6 Ultrasound Doppler flow detector. (**a**) Infant flat probe. (**b**) Adult flat probe. (**c**) Standard pencil probe.

Physical examination of women

The physical examination of a woman should include a general medical examination in addition to a gynecologic evaluation. Attention should be paid to the presence of excessive dryness or irritation in the genitals, and to determining a normal appear-

ance in this area. Physiatric examination should include determining the range of motion of the hips and knees, and whether there is hypersensitivity or loss of sensation in the genital area. For those women with SCI, it is useful to perform an American Spinal Injury Association (ASIA) examination and determine the remaining sensation in the T11–L2 and S3–S5 dermatomes (see Ch. 56). It is also useful to determine if the patient has upper motor neuron or lower motor neuron dysfunction in the sacral segments. For persons with diabetes, it should be determined if there are other signs of autonomic dysfunction and neuropathy.

There are no specific testing procedures that have been used clinically to evaluate sexual dysfunction in women. Research studies have used vaginal pulse amplitude through a photoelectric pulse sensor to determine genital vasocongestion,[69] and electromyography of the anal sphincter has been used. Doppler scanning of the clitoris has been advocated by some groups, but this has not achieved general acceptance.

TREATMENT OF FEMALE SEXUAL DYSFUNCTION

Treatment of female sexual dysfunction is a field that has been limited and has traditionally relied on cognitive behavioral therapies. Treatment of sexual dysfunction with medications or other techniques has also recently been explored. Testosterone has been used to treat hypoactive sexual desire, and multiple studies have confirmed its efficacy.[37,84] At the time of this printing, it is anticipated that US Food and Drug Administration (FDA) approval will be received for a testosterone patch to treat female sexual arousal disorder in the near future.

A number of medications have recently been evaluated with regard to improving sexual arousal in women. The use of topical alprostadil has been shown to increase clitoral blood flow.[9] A pilot study in eight patients showed increased subjective and physiologic arousal during visual sexual stimulation.[50] In a laboratory-based study of 41 postmenopausal women, phentolamine was shown to improve vaginal blood flow when women had received estrogenization.[105] The use of sildenafil has also been advocated in small clinical studies to improve female sexual arousal;[14,116] however, its efficacy has not been confirmed in large-scale clinical trials.

For the treatment of anorgasmia, cognitive behavioral therapy has been used for years, and has focused on promoting positive attitudes toward orgasmic ability and satisfaction. Behavioral exercises that have been prescribed include directed masturbation.[72,85] Generally, this involves having the woman view and examine her body with diagrams of female anatomy. This is then followed by instructions for the woman to explore her genitals with an emphasis on finding sensitive pleasurable spots. The woman is encouraged to use lubricants and other sexual aids, and after achieving orgasm independently to include her partner in the process. Sex education has also been used as an adjunctive therapy to treat anorgasmia; however, there has not been any empiric evidence to support its efficacy to treat anorgasmia when used in isolation. Other cognitive behavioral therapies that have been recommended have included the use of Kegel exercises[62] and sensate focus training;[79] however, efficacy has also not been established.

Newer therapies have attempted to use medical means to treat physiologically based sexual dysfunction. The use of ArginMax[51] was compared with placebo in a double-blind, placebo-controlled study in 77 women with unspecified sexual dysfunction. In the ArginMax group, 47% showed an increased frequency of orgasm, as compared with 30% in the placebo group. The use of buproprion-SR[92] was compared with placebo to improve orgasmic function in women with delayed or absent orgasm, with findings of no significant differences between groups. A larger number of studies have addressed the issue of antidepressant-induced anorgasmia;[57,78,89] however, none of these studies have documented efficacy in placebo-controlled trials.

The use of the Eros vacuum clitoral suction device received FDA approval as a means to treat orgasmic dysfunction.[15] Because the device works by stimulating reflex vasocongestion, it might be a particularly useful way to treat orgasmic dysfunction in women with neurologic injuries. Studies are ongoing to test its utility.

The treatment of sexual pain disorders often relies on a multidisciplinary approach. The first step is to treat any organic problems that could be contributing to pain. Psychologic counseling and rehabilitative therapy are then often used to treat these dysfunctions.[13,44]

TREATMENT OF MALE SEXUAL DYSFUNCTION

The occurrence of sexual dysfunction is relatively common among men. More than 10 million men are estimated to have a sexual dysfunction. At least 52% of men older than 40 years have a specific sexual dysfunction according to the Massachusetts Male Aging Study.[122] Ducharme and Gill have suggested that virtually all men with disabilities such as SCI, multiple sclerosis, and brain injury present with sexual dysfunction.[33]

Premature ejaculation

Rosen and Leiblum describe premature ejaculation as one of the most frequent male sexual dysfunctions.[104] Premature ejaculation is defined by the DSM-IV as persistent or recurrent ejaculation with minimal stimulation before, on, or shortly after penetration and before the person wishes it.[4] The clinician must take into account factors that affect duration of the excitement phase, such as age, novelty of the sexual partner or situation, and recent frequency of sexual activity. The disturbance must cause marked distress or interpersonal difficulty, and must not be exclusively linked to the direct effects of a substance. Treatment has historically been based on psychologic interventions that integrate cognitive behavioral systems and dynamic approaches.[141] Manual techniques have included pausing, squeezing the tip or base of the penis, and decreased emphasis on penetration.[33] More recently, clomipramine,[2] sertraline,[87]

fluoxetine[59] and paroxetine[135] have all been shown to be efficacious as oral therapies for the treatment of premature ejaculation.

Inhibited ejaculation

Inhibited ejaculation refers to retarded or delayed ejaculation with or without male anorgasmia, and is common in individuals with disabilities.[53] Most treatment is based on using enhancement of sexual activity with past sexual memories, fantasies, visual or auditory stimulation, and open communication.[53] Unassisted ejaculation rates are very low in men with complete upper motor neuron SCIs and low in men with other patterns of injury. Chemical, vibratory, or electric stimulation can be used to augment ejaculation if the segments between T10 and T12 are intact, but these procedures have primarily been used for fertility purposes (see Ch. 56).

INHIBITED SEXUAL DESIRE

This is very common, affecting possibly 15% of adult males and accounting for up to 50% of cases seen in clinical settings.[10] Inhibited sexual desire is characterized by persistently few or absent sexual fantasies and desire for sexual activity, and does not result from a medical condition, substance abuse, or primary psychiatric disorder.[53] Inhibited sexual desire needs to be distinguished from *sexual aversion*, in which sexual contact is actively avoided because of extreme negative feelings about sex. Sexual abuse or trauma should always be considered.[53] Treatment is through cognitive, behavioral, psychodynamic, and systems approaches.[53] LoPiccolo and Friedman used affective awareness, insight, cognitive restructuring, and behavioral intervention as four components to treat inhibited sexual desire.[73]

PEYRONIE DISEASE

This is characterized by lesion formation in the tunica of the corpora cavernosa, causing curvature and shortening of the penis. According to Jordan, the incidence is 1% in the general male population, increasing in the 45- to 60-year-old population.[53] Trauma to the penis is the main cause. Disabled individuals with diabetes mellitus using injectable treatment for erectile dysfunction are at greater risk. It is uncertain if there is a higher incidence in the population of men with disabilities without other risk factors.[53]

PRIAPISM

This is a persistent erection that does not result from sexual desire, often accompanied with pain and tenderness. It is a rare finding in the general population, and is mostly associated with the use of drugs and with vascular dysfunction.[76] It is a medical emergency, because it can cause permanent erectile dysfunction. In the disabled population, it is commonly associated with penile injections to treat erectile dysfunction.

ERECTILE DYSFUNCTION

Erectile dysfunction is the persistent inability to attain or maintain penile erection sufficient for sexual intercourse. The majority of cases have an organic etiology, most commonly vascular disease that decreases blood flow into the penis.[90] An estimated 10–20 million American men have some degree of erectile dysfunction.[101,122] Specific physical treatments of erectile dysfunction will be discussed in a later section.

SPECIFIC DISABILITIES AND THEIR EFFECTS ON SEXUALITY

Multiple sclerosis

Multiple sclerosis is a demyelinating disease of the central nervous system with the onset generally in the adult years. Approximately 350 000 people in the USA are diagnosed with multiple sclerosis.[5] Although the incidence of sexual dysfunction increases with the severity of disability resulting from multiple sclerosis, sexual dysfunction can also occur early in the course, and sometimes is the presenting symptom.[82] It has been estimated that more than 50% of women and 75% of men with multiple sclerosis experience some form of sexual dysfunction.[81] At baseline, the impact of multiple sclerosis on sexual response is typically related to the location of the neurologic lesions. This issue is compounded by the uncertainty associated with the progression of multiple sclerosis, and the numerous medications that individuals with multiple sclerosis are generally prescribed. Medications used to treat multiple sclerosis that can cause sexual dysfunction include baclofen, antidepressants, antianxiety drugs, and anticholinergics. Sexual complaints can be related to a temporary or long-term disinterest in sex, inability to experience orgasms, difficulty engaging in sexual intercourse due to fatigue, spasticity, muscle weakness, depression, anxiety, bowel and bladder incontinence, decreased sensation and dysesthesia, tremor, and cognitive changes (see Ch. 53).[124]

Stroke

This is the third leading cause of death, and one of the most common diseases leading to major long-term disability. The mean age of stroke patients is higher than that of most other disabled individuals. Although sexual activity is a vital portion of normal life, society tends to deny the sexuality of the elderly and the physically disabled individual. Common problems in the female patient are decline in libido and decreased coital frequency, vaginal lubrication, and orgasm. In the male, decline in libido and poor (or lack of) erection and ejaculation are the most frequent problems.[95] A recent questionnaire study of 192 stroke patients and 94 partners confirmed that a majority of stroke patients reported a marked decline in libido, coital frequency, erectile and orgasmic ability, vaginal lubrication, and general sexual satisfaction. The most important factors associated with these changes included the individuals' general attitude toward sexuality, fear of impotence, inability to discuss sexuality, unwillingness to participate in sexual activity, and

degree of functional disability. Spouses also reported significant decreased libido, sexual activity, and sexual satisfaction as a consequence of their partners' strokes.[66]

Traumatic brain injury

The prevalence of TBI is increasing in the USA due to improved treatment. Young males are at greater risk, and represent a large percentage of the TBI population. Little research has been done on sexual function in patients with TBI, and most of it was done in small populations that were not well characterized. The percentage of subjects who have reported sexual dysfunction after brain injury has varied greatly, probably largely because of the heterogeneity of populations studied.[107] Erectile dysfunction in patients with brain injury occurs in 4–71% across studies.[30,40,67,68,88,136] A well-known possible finding with brain injury is disinhibition, which is associated with orbitofrontal injury. This results in so-called 'hypersexual' or 'inappropriate' behaviors. These behaviors are usually described in the context of interpersonal contacts, but also can be manifested as preservative behaviors, such as excessive masturbation. Hibbard et al. looked at possibly the largest cohort of patients with TBI (322) and their self-reported sexual difficulties, contrasted with persons without TBI (264).[47] Individuals with TBI were found to report more frequent physiologic, physical, and body image difficulties that negatively impacted their sexual function. Associated depression was a predictor for sexual dysfunction in both men and women.

Arthritis

Arthritis patients often present with loss of libido due to pain, joint stiffness, and fatigue. It can also result from the use of steroids and other drugs.[16,27] Osteoarthritis is the most common arthritic condition, with increasing prevalence with age.[41] Treatment is based on patient education highlighting recommended positions, understanding and treating pain, exercise, and psychologic intervention.[100] The Arthritis Foundation offers useful diagrams showing positions for intercourse with various painful joints. Total hip joint replacement has also been shown to be efficacious in the relief of pain associated with sexual intercourse, although care must be taken with positioning after this type of surgery.[29]

Chronic pain and sexual dysfunction

Physicians treating patients with chronic painful conditions have more recently begun to characterize the pain separate from the underlying cause, in terms of a disease itself rather than a symptom. Depression, weight loss or gain, physical deconditioning, and loss of self-image all often accompany chronic pain. The underlying medical conditions causing chronic pain are many, and include lower back or neck injuries, nerve injuries, and terminally malignant cancers.

Each of these conditions that cause chronic pain can limit a person's ability to function mentally and physically, and pain sufferers are left vulnerable to disrupted sexual functioning. There are only a small number of published studies on chronic pain and the effect on sexual function. The complex nature of chronic pain often makes it difficult to tease out the specific effect of pain on sexual interest and function from the other medical and psychologic conditions that can be present. Many patients with pain are maintained on psychotropic drugs, muscle relaxants, or opiate pain medications, many of which cause sexual dysfunction. Finally, in certain types of chronic pain such as pelvic pain, sexual abuse is identified as a contributing cause to their unremitting pain syndrome.

Despite the prevalence of sexual dysfunction in chronic pain syndromes, only a few studies have been published. Ambler et al. surveyed 237 patients with chronic pain.[3] They found that 73% had difficulty with sexual function that the patients self-identified as being related to their pain. These problems included difficulties with arousal, position, low confidence, performance worries, and pain exacerbation. Most responders reported a combination of the above factors. There was no statistically significant difference between men and women. Responders were younger and less depressed than those who did not respond to the survey. No attempt was made to correlate drug use with sexual dysfunction. A smaller study, by Flor et al., found similar percentages.[38]

Ambler et al. also surveyed a subset of 68 patients concerning their preferences for help. In that group, 47% wanted written information only, 26.5% wanted discussion, and 20% wanted both discussion and information. There was no gender difference in these preferences. In a survey by Dunn et al., only one-tenth of the respondents who wanted professional help had previously received such help.[34]

It is evident from these studies that a problem exists on many levels. First, there is a clear disruption of sexual function in patients suffering from chronic pain. Second, the causes of this disruption are many and complex. It appears that comprehensive multidisciplinary medical and psychologic treatment will be required if these patients' needs are to be met and their sexual function improved. Finally, it seems that their needs are not being met by their pain management physicians, despite their wish to have their sexual dysfunction treated along with their pain. It is important for all physicians who treat patients with chronic pain to have an avenue where patients can discuss the sexual problems related to their condition, and then seek treatment in the most appropriate manner.

Diabetes

This is a serious disorder with multisystem effects. Erectile dysfunction can occur in at least 50% of patients with diabetes.[132] The age-adjusted probability of complete loss of erectile function is 28% in treated diabetic patients, compared with 9.6% in the entire sample of the Massachusetts Male Aging Study.[122] The pathogenesis of erectile dysfunction in diabetes is multifactorial, with vascular and neural factors being equally implicated. Hyperglycemia is believed to give rise to biochemical perturbations that lead to microvascular changes resulting in erectile dysfunction.

Women with diabetes have been specifically studied. Eighty-one percent of women, 71% with peripheral neuropathy and 79% without neuropathy, retained libido and sexual activity.[35]

Hulter reported that women growing up with insulin-dependent diabetes reported more frequent sexual problems than control groups did.[49] Studies suggest that the arousal phase was especially affected, which is analogous to the situation with men.

In men with diabetes, the phosphodiesterase inhibitors have revolutionized the management of erectile dysfunction, and oral drug therapy is currently first-line therapy for the condition. These agents act by potentiating the action of intracavernosal nitric oxide, thereby leading to a more sustained erection. The drugs have been shown to improve erectile function domain scores, penetration, maintenance of erection, and more successful intercourse.[8]

Cardiac disease

Cardiac disease, especially coronary artery disease (CAD), is known for its potential to interfere with sexual function.[18] In the Massachusetts Male Aging Study, the probability of any degree of erectile dysfunction in men treated for heart disease was 78.1% in non-smokers and 94.2% in smokers.[122] In both women and men who have undergone a myocardial infarction, little if any information is provided as to when sexual activity can be resumed. Fears of another infarct, angina, fatigue, or decreased libido can alter the pattern of sexual activity. Maximal heart rate and blood pressure occur with exertion and orgasm, regardless of position during sex (see Ch. 34).[74]

Frequency of sexual activity has been examined in both men and women with CAD. Several studies involving large patient populations of men post myocardial infarction showed that 40–70% had both diminished frequency and diminished quality of sexual function.[93] Sexual dysfunction was reported to be related to loss of interest or desire (39%), spouses' reluctance to participate (25%), depression (21%), and anxiety (18%). Anxiety was particularly related to possible recurrence of CAD, coital death, or cardiovascular symptoms in association with sexual activity.[46] Patients generally suffer from three psychologic disturbances after a myocardial infarction: denial, anxiety, and depression.[17] Anxiety develops into a chronic condition in 10–20% of patients. Anxiety tends to be proportionate to the severity of CAD symptoms, and is influenced by the patient's premorbid psychologic makeup. A major source of anxiety is fear of death.[129] Ueno analyzed 5559 cases of sudden death after a myocardial infarction in Japan, and estimated that 0.6% occurred during sexual activity.[134] Silber and Katz studied Americans, and similarly found that 0.5% of postcoronary deaths occurred during sexual activity.[114] In another study, with 1774 patients with myocardial infarction, of whom 858 were sexually active in the prior year, 3% reported sexual activity in the 2 h preceding the onset of their myocardial infarction.[99] Practitioners should educate cardiac patients that the relative risk of myocardial infarction during sexual activity is low, and is similar in people with and without a history of cardiac disease. Data have also revealed that regular exercise can decrease and perhaps eliminate the possibility of myocardial infarction in association with intercourse.[119]

Spinal cord injury

Spinal cord injury affects 250 000 Americans, and 10 000 new cases are added annually. Eighty-two percent of the patients are male, and the majority in their prime reproductive years (mean age 26 years).[93] There are more scientific data about sexual function and sexuality after SCI than for any other disability.[121]

When discussing the impact of an SCI on sexual response, the level and degree of injury must be determined and defined by using the International Standards for Neurological and Functional Classification of SCI (ASIA).[133]

Spinal cord injuries are classified as complete and incomplete, depending on whether there is preservation of voluntary contraction of the external anal sphincter on digital rectal examination, and whether there is preservation of anal sensation. Sexual functioning in SCI depends on both the location and the extent of the injury. In particular, the type of injury affecting the S2–S5 sacral segments is important to determine, as is the degree of sensory function remaining in the T11–L2 dermatomes.

Control of sexual response post SCI

The control of sexual response post SCI can be predicted based on where the injury occurs and the type of lesion affecting the sacral cord. Men with complete tetraplegia and upper motor neuron injury affecting the sacral segments typically have an inability to achieve psychogenic erection but do have reflex erection. Men with complete lower motor neuron injuries affecting their sacral segments typically have inability to achieve reflex erection but can sometimes achieve psychogenic erection. A recent study documented that the loss of psychogenic erection correlates with sympathetic denervation, and loss of somatic and parasympathetic reflex activity correlates with the loss of reflex erection.[109] In women, laboratory-based research has documented that the ability to achieve psychogenic vaginal lubrication is related to the degree of preservation of sensation in the T11–L2 dermatomes, and that reflex lubrication is maintained in women with upper motor neuron injury affecting the sacral segments.[115] The ability to achieve orgasm was also documented in women post SCI, with only 17% of women with complete lower motor neuron injuries affecting their sacral spinal segments reporting the ability to achieve orgasm (as compared with 59% of women with all other levels and degrees of SCI). As compared with able-bodied women, women with SCIs took significantly longer to achieve orgasm. The descriptions of orgasms reported by women with complete or incomplete SCIs or able-bodied subjects could not be distinguished from each other by two blinded psychologists with experience in treating sexual dysfunction.[1] Based on these results, the authors made it clear that treatment of orgasmic dysfunction in women with SCIs should be possible. With exception of the group with lower motor neuron complete injuries affecting their sacral spinal segments, women with SCI appear to maintain the neurologic capability to achieve orgasm.

Treatment of sexual dysfunction in women with SCIs has been studied through the use of sildenafil,[116] through the use of false feedback,[118] and through the use of anxiety-provoking videos.[119] The last technique was designed to increase arousal through stimulation of the sympathetic nervous system, but all these therapies were noted to have some degree of success in a laboratory-based setting. Currently, research is working on improving the ability of women with SCI to achieve orgasm through the use of a clitoral vacuum pump[15] versus via vibratory stimulation (with the mind-set that the control of orgasm is related to a central pattern generator[133]).

Treatment of male sexual dysfunction in SCI requires a holistic approach that not only focuses on creation of an erection and ejaculation, but also on maximizing the pleasurable aspects of sexuality.[36] Most treatments do not center on creating and maintaining a natural erection, but on implementing erection enhancements. Although men with complete upper motor neuron SCI often achieve a reflex erection, the erection might not be sufficient for sexual performance. Ejaculation in men with lower motor neuron or incomplete injuries can occur naturally with sexual contact, but men with complete injuries above T10 typically need to resort to vibrostimulation. Those with injury above T6 should be cautioned about the risk of autonomic dysreflexia. Elliott reports that episodic abdominal and leg contractions, generalized piloerection, scrotal wall retraction, and development of a rigid erection seem to predict a higher likelihood of success with vibrostimulation.

The ability for men with complete SCI to achieve orgasm is more complex. Alexander et al. noted that 38% of men with complete SCI reported the ability to achieve orgasm.[1] This suggests other sexual techniques, not involving stimulation of the genitalia, can create sexual satisfaction in men with SCI.

Fertility in post-SCI men

Men with SCI often ask about fertility. Early studies of semen produced with natural ejaculation in men who were post SCI revealed generally reduced sperm counts and motility. However, multiple studies utilizing vibrostimulation and the technique of electroejaculation have shown mostly normal sperm counts, albeit with lower motility. Several theories for this reduced motility include frequent urinary infections, testicular hyperthermia, sperm stagnation due to anejaculation, and type of urinary management.[127] With careful planning and assistance, pregnancies are possible for the spouses of men with complete SCI.

PENILE PROSTHESIS

In the past, penile prostheses were the only treatment for erectile dysfunction. They are now the treatment of last resort. The first devices used were rigid tubes of synthetic material that provided a permanently erect phallus. Malleable core or hinge types were eventually developed, which permitted manipulation of the penis to conceal it when not in use (Fig. 32-7). Complications are common, and include sensory changes, pressure ulcers from misplacement or displacement of the prosthesis, mechanical failure, infection, or extravasation of fluid

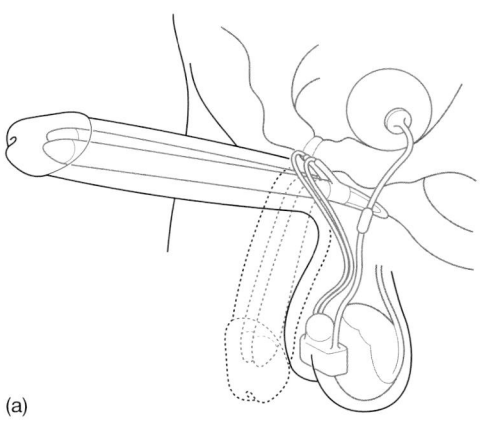
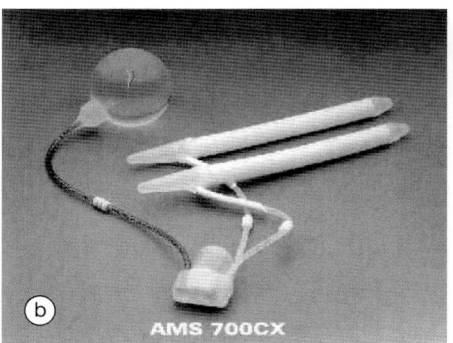
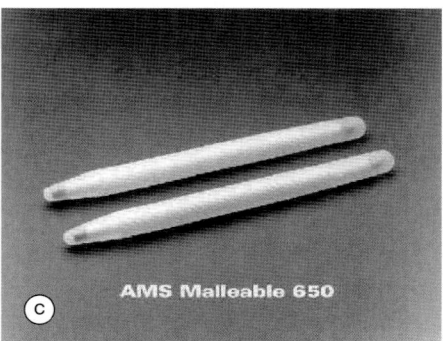

Figure 32-7 Penile prostheses.

from mechanism. The rate of prosthesis infection can be as high as 16.5% in patients with SCI, and infection and extrusion led to a 25% removal rate.[24,25]

VACUUM-ASSISTED DEVICES

Vacuum-assisted devices are used in association with a constriction band, which is a ring placed around the base of the penis to keep it engorged. If a person has enough manual dexterity, a manual pump can be used. Otherwise, battery-operated devices are also available. Complications can occur with excessive vacuum, such as causing a penile hematoma. Patients using any anticoagulant therapy, including warfarin, aspirin, and anti-inflammatories, should not use the pump. A common mistake is the inclusion of the testicles into the constriction band, with dramatic consequences for patients who are insensate. Even when used properly at the base of the penis, the constriction band should not be used longer than 30 min to avoid ischemia (Fig. 32-8).

PENILE INJECTIONS

Intracavernous penile injections are widely accepted as an effective treatment for the restoration of erectile function in men with SCI. They can be highly effective in producing a natural erection in patients with psychogenic or neurogenic erectile dysfunction. Medications are injected into cavernous spaces to induce relaxation of the sinusoidal smooth muscle and enhance corporal filling. The medication spreads to both corporal bodies through intercommunicating channels. The erection noted is remarkably natural in size and rigidity. The duration of the erection is directly proportional to the dose of agent administered.[138] Papaverine alone has had good results. In one study, 98 of 101 patients with SCI had a satisfactory erection sufficient for coital penetration, and only one patient required irrigation of the corpus with saline to achieve detumescence.[58] Several drugs and drug combinations have been used. These include papaverine, with its direct smooth muscle inhibition.

Phentolamine produces smooth muscle relaxation through its α-adrenergic blocking effects, with an increased time and quality of erection. A mixture of papaverine and phentolamine has been effective,[12,112] and the time of erection is longer and the quality of erection better in neurogenic-based impotence.[77] The average frequency of injection is twice a month.[19] Segenreich evaluated 452 patients and used several different protocols, starting with papaverine and phentolamine mesylate (Regitine), and added prostaglandin E_1 or atropine if there was no response. Only 11 patients were referred for a penile prosthesis,[112] as 441 (97.5%) responded to the protocol.

Prostaglandin E_1 by intracavernous injection is generally the drug of choice, because it has a high rate of efficacy and patient satisfaction, and a low risk profile, when compared with other compounds. A study by Beretta demonstrated a positive response with prostaglandin E_1 use alone, with no systemic reactions or priapism noted.[12] A long-term study with prostaglandin E_1 was done by Lundberg, and showed that 57% were still using the intracavernous injection after 47 months, with no major complications noted.[77] Linet and Ogrinc conducted a study with 683 men with erectile dysfunction of varying etiology to study the efficacy and safety of intracavernously injected prostaglandin E_1. The participants reported the ability to engage in sexual intercourse after 94% of the injections. Satisfaction with intercourse was confirmed by 87% of men and 86% of their partners. Penile pain was noted in 50% of subjects during the 6-month study, penile fibrosis in 2%, hematoma or ecchymosis in 8%, and prolonged erections in 5%, but priapism in only 1%. The investigators felt that intracorporal prostaglandin E_1 was effective in the treatment of erectile dysfunction.[71]

Tang, Chu, and Wong studied 15 men with SCI with neurogenic erectile dysfunction using intracavernous injection of prostaglandin E_1. All of them had achieved functional erection adequate for coitus, except one patient who had been proved to have venogenic impotence. No complications were noted, except pain in the injection site in two patients with incomplete lesions.[130]

A combination of papaverine and prostaglandin E_1 was used by Zaslau, with high patient satisfaction and efficacy. From the

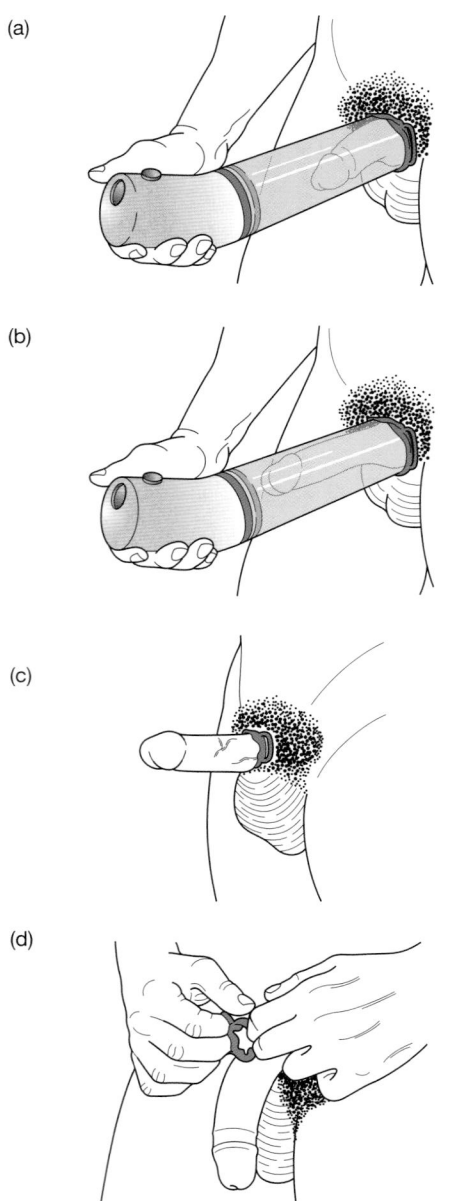

Figure 32-8 Use of a vacuum-assisted device. Patient instructions are as follows. (**a**) You place your penis inside the cylinder and use ErecAid System's specially designed pump to produce the vacuum that pulls blood into the penis. (**b**) The vacuum allows you to create a near-natural erection within a few minutes. (**c**) After you slip the tension ring off the cylinder on to the base of the penis and remove the cylinder, you can safely and easily keep the erection for up to 30 min, using only the tension ring. (**d**) Once you remove the tension ring, your penis returns to its soft state.

37 initial participants, 28 (76%) responded to injection therapy. Five patients dropped out due to lack of current partner or due to pain with injection. The average duration of erection was 43 min. At 3-month follow-up, 85% of patients rated their erections as good or excellent, 43% were using the injection one or more times per week, 77% were moderately or extremely satis-

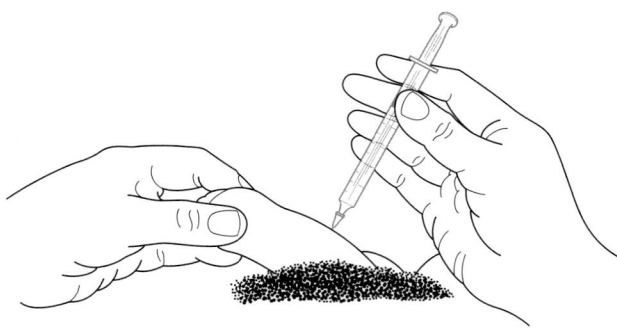

Figure 32-9 Penile injection.

fied with their treatment, and 89% would recommend treatment to a friend.[140]

Complications have been noted with penile injection therapy. The prescribing physician needs to obtain a formal, signed consent to the administration of intracorporal agents before initiating treatment.[138] Chronic administration can cause scarring of the tunica albuginea, which might result in permanent curvature of the erect phallus.[70] Priapism is also a primary risk, with the need for immediate medical attention for aspiration of blood from each corporal body. An α-adrenergic agonist, such as phenylephrine or adrenaline (epinephrine), might be injected to promote contraction of corporal muscle.[75] Patients are advised to limit the frequency of intracorporal injections to every other day to minimize risks (Fig. 32-9).[11]

INTRAURETHRAL THERAPIES

The only medication that has been successfully used transurethrally is alprostadil (prostaglandin E_1). The transurethral delivery system (Muse) was introduced as an alternative to intracavernosal injection. In a study by Wethman and Rajfer of 100 patients, only 7% had well-sustained, rigid erections. Full erections with partial rigidity were obtained by 30%. The remaining 63% of the patients did not achieve erections adequate for penetration. Penile pain occurred in 24% of patients, 3% had a syncopal episode, 3% had urethral bleeding, and one had priapism that required drainage (Fig. 32-10).[139]

ORAL MEDICATIONS
Sildenafil (Viagra)
Several authors have studied sildenafil (Viagra) use for patients with SCI. Schmid studied 41 SCI patients, and demonstrated that sildenafil was a valuable and safe therapeutic management in the erectile dysfunction of patients with SCI. Subject acceptance and satisfaction was high. Penile rigidity sufficient to permit sexual intercourse was achieved by 38 patients (93%). Three patients dropped out because of non-response, despite having increased the doses to 100 mg. Functional erections 1 h after 50 mg were achieved by 22 (58%), whereas 14 (37%)

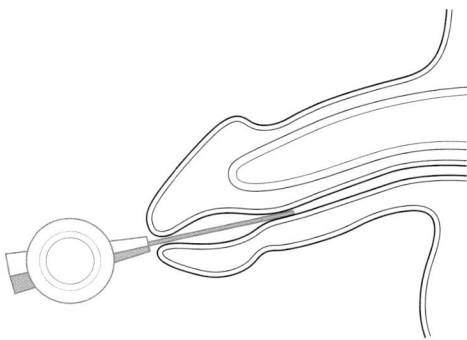

Figure 32-10 Intraurethral therapy.

required higher doses of 75–100 mg. Nearly 10% (4/41) suffered from side effects such as headache or dizziness.[110]

Giuliano showed that sildenafil was an effective and well-tolerated treatment for erectile dysfunction caused by SCI. In his study, there were 178 men with SCI, 143 of whom had residual erectile function at baseline. Some received sildenafil and some placebo, 1 h before sexual activity, for 6 weeks. Improved erections were reported by 127 (76%), and they preferred sildenafil to placebo. In this study, sildenafil improved sexual intercourse in 132 of 166 (80%), compared with 17 of 166 (10%) who experienced improvement with placebo. Sildenafil had a low rate of discontinuation because of treatment-related adverse effects (2% versus 1% for placebo).[42]

A long-term evaluation of patients with SCI and with multiple sclerosis and the use of sildenafil was done by Green. Forty patients were observed for over 2 years, including 33 with SCI. Initially, 36 of 40 (90%) were able to achieve erections sufficient for sexual intercourse. After 2 years, 13 out of 40 were not using sildenafil, but only in six cases was this due to lack of response. Adverse effects were minimal. Green felt that sildenafil was a safe and effective first-line treatment of male neurogenic erectile dysfunction.[45]

A two-part, double-blind, randomized study was done by Maytom with 27 SCI patients. In part 1 of the study, 17 (65%) presented with > 60% rigidity at the penile base after sildenafil use, compared with 2 (8%) with placebo. In part 2, an at-home study, 75% of sildenafil users and 8% of placebo users noted that treatment had improved their erections.[83]

Another double-blind study was done by Derry with 27 patients. Seventy-five percent in the sildenafil group and 7% in the placebo group reported that the treatment helped with their erections. No patient discontinued treatment due to side effects.[32]

A major, multicenter, randomized, double-blind study was done by Hultling in Sweden to evaluate quality of life in 178 men with SCI receiving sildenafil. Significant improvements were seen for overall satisfaction with sex life, sexual relationship with partner, and concerns with erectile problems using the International Index of Erectile Function.

Tadalafil (Cialis)

Tadalafil is one of the new oral agents being used in erectile dysfunction, with most data available related to able-bodied individuals. In a multicenter, randomized, double-blind, crossover study of able-bodied patients comparing tadalafil and sildenafil, it was noted that both medications were well tolerated, with similar adverse reactions. However, most patients preferred to start treatment with sildenafil.[43] Tadalafil was effective up to 36 h after dosing, and was effective regardless of disease severity and causes, and in patients of all ages. The most frequent side effects were headache, dyspepsia, back pain, and myalgia.[23]

Several studies comparing tadalafil and placebo revealed that tadalafil is most effective between 4 and 36 h after ingestion.[103,111,123] At the time of this printing, only one study was completed comparing sildenafil and tadalafil in male SCI patients. In 28 patients, tadalafil allowed the majority of the patients to achieve both erection up to 24 h post dosing, and improved overall sex life satisfaction as well as sexual relations with partner.[31] Tadalafil is a promising treatment option in the treatment of erectile dysfunction in patients with SCI.

Vardenafil hydrochloride (Levitra)

Vardenafil is a potent and highly selective oral phosphodiesterase type 5 inhibitor, and has been studied only in able-bodied individuals. It can be used in mild to severe erectile dysfunction of varying etiologies, as well as in men with erectile dysfunction associated with diabetes mellitus or erectile dysfunction after radical prostatectomy.[60] The most commonly reported adverse events included headache, flushing, rhinitis, dyspepsia, and sinusitis.[61]

Phosphodiesterase-5 inhibitors act by competing with the substrate cyclic GMP for the catalytic site of the enzyme. Even so, sildenafil and vardenafil have minimal differences in molecular structure. Vardenafil has more than 20-fold greater potency than sildenafil for inhibiting purified phosphodiesterase-5.[28] Vardenafil is a very promising treatment of erectile dysfunction in the general and the disabled population, but further studies are needed to determine its efficacy.

Apomorphine sublingual

Apomorphine sublingual is a dopamine D_1 and D_2 receptor agonist, which has been approved for marketing in Europe. It is best selected for treating patients with mild to moderate erectile dysfunction, but it is seldom used in clinical practice due to its limited efficacy and side effects, particularly nausea.[21] The combination of centrally acting agents (apomorphine) with phosphodiesterase-5 inhibitors is an attractive approach, because the two therapies target different mechanisms.[126]

SUMMARY

Sexuality is a complex topic, because it is affected by cultural, social, and personal factors. The physiatrist is faced with a special problem when addressing sexual dysfunction in the individual with disability. The patient's personal sexual experience and outlook need to be addressed. A team approach will be the most appropriate, because different experiences will create a better evaluation and treatment.

New research in the area of sexuality demonstrates that society in general and rehabilitation professionals understand the importance of healthy sexual function in disabled and non-disabled individuals. Female sexual dysfunction, often overlooked in the past, has been discussed and studied as never before. Also, new erectile dysfunction treatments have created the possibility of longer and safer sexual function.

The rehabilitation team must establish that the evaluation and treatment of sexual dysfunction is one of its primary goals. As a group, we have worked for several decades on overcoming the difficulties and prejudice against physical and mental disability.

REFERENCES

1. Alexander CJ, Sipski ML, Findley TW, et al. Sexual activities, desire, and satisfaction in males pre- and post-spinal cord injury. Arch Sex Behav 1993; 22(3):217–228.
2. Althof S, Levine S, Corty E, et al. Clomipramine as a treatment for rapid ejaculation: a double-blind crossover trial of fifteen couples. J Clin Psychiatry 1995; 56(9):402–407.
3. Ambler N, Williams AC, Hill P, et al. Sexual difficulties of chronic pain patients. Clin J Pain 2001; 17:138–145.
4. American Psychiatric Association. Diagnostic and statistical manual of mental disorders. 4th edn. Washington: American Psychiatric Association; 1994.
5. Anderson DW, Ellengerg JH, Levental CA, et al. Revised estimate of prevalence of multiple sclerosis in the United States. Ann Neurol 1992; 31:333–336.
6. Bachman GA. Sexual issues at menopause. Ann NY Acad Sci 1988; 87:87–94.
7. Basson R, Berman J, Burnett A, et al. Report of the International Consensus Development Conference on Female Sexual Dysfunction: definitions and classifications. J Urol 2000; 163:888–893.
8. Basu A, Ryder RE. New treatment options for erectile dysfunction in patients with diabetes mellitus. Drugs 2004; 64:2667–2688.
9. Becher EF, Bechara A, Casabe A. Clitoral hemodynamic changes after a topical application of alprostadil. J Sex Marital Ther 2001; 27: 405–410.
10. Beck JG. Hypoactive sexual desire: an overview. J Consult Clin Psychol 1995; 63(6):919–927.
11. Benard F, Lue TF. The roles of urologist and patient in autoinjection therapy for erectile dysfunction. Contemp Urol 1990; 2:21–26.
12. Beretta G, Zanollo A, Ascani L, et al. Prostaglandin E$_1$ in the therapy of erectile deficiency. Acta Eur Fertil 1989; 20(5):305–308.
13. Bergeron S, Binik Y. The treatment of vulvar vestibulitis syndrome: towards a multimodal approach. Sex Marital Ther 1997; 12:305–311.
14. Berman JR, Berman LA, Lin H, et al. Effect of sildenafil on subjective and physiologic parameters of the female sexual response in women with sexual arousal disorder. J Sex Marital Ther 2001; 27(5):411–420.
15. Billups KL, Berman L, Berman J, et al. A new non-pharmacological vacuum therapy for female sexual dysfunction. J Sex Marital Ther 2001; 27(5):435–442.
16. Blake DJ, Maisiak R, Alarcon GS, et al. Sexual quality of life of patients with arthritis-free controls. J Rheumathol 1987; 14:570–576.
17. Blocker WP. Cardiac rehabilitation. In: Halstead L, Grabois M, eds. Medical rehabilitation. New York: Raven Press; 1985:181–192.
18. Blocker WP. Coronary heart disease and sexuality. Phys Med Rehabil: State Art Rev 1995; 9:387–399.
19. Bodner DR, Leffler B, Frost F. The role of intracavernous injection of vasoactive medications for the restoration of erection in spinal cord injured males: a three year follow up. Paraplegia 1992; 30(2):118–120.
20. Bretschneider JG, McCoy NL. Sexual interest and behavior in healthy 80- to 102-year-olds. Arch Sex Behav 1988; 17(2):109–129.
21. Briganti A, Salonia A, Gallina A, et al. Emerging oral drugs for erectile dysfunction. Expert Opin Emerg Drugs 2004; 9(1):179–189.
22. Burnett AL. Nitric acid control of genitourinary tract functions: a review. Urology 1995; 45:1071–1083.
23. Carson CC, Rajfer J, Eardley I, et al. The efficacy and safety of tadalafil: an update. BJU Int 2004; 93(9):1276–1281.
24. Carson CC, Roberston CN. Late hematogenous infection of penile prosthesis. J Urol 1988; 139(1):50–52.
25. Carson CC. Infections in genitourinary prosthesis. Urol Clin North Am 1998; 16:139–147.
26. Catalan J, Hawton K, Day A. Couples referred to a sexual dysfunction clinic. Psychol Phys Morb. Br J Psychiatry 1990; 156:61–67.
27. Conine TA, Evans JH. Sexual reactivation of chronically ill and disabled adults. J Allied Health 1982; 11:261–270.
28. Corbin JD, Beasley A, Blount MA, et al. Vardenafil: structural basis for higher potency over sildenafil in inhibiting cGMP-specific phosphodiesterase-5 (PDE5). Neurochem Int 2004; 45(6):859–863.
29. Currey HLF. Osteoarthrosis of the hip joint and sexual activity. Ann Rheum Dis 1970; 29:488–493.
30. Dais DL, Schneider LK. Ramifications of traumatic brain injury for sexuality. J Head Trauma Rehabil 1990; 5:31–37.
31. Del Popolo G, Li Marzi V, Mondaini N, et al. Time/duration effectiveness of sildenafil versus tadalafil in the treatment of erectile dysfunction in male spinal cord-injured patients. Spinal Cord 2004; 42(11):643–648.
32. Derry FA, Dinsmore WW, Fraser M, et al. Efficacy and safety of oral sildenafil (Viagra) in men with erectile dysfunction caused by spinal cord injury. Neurology 1998; 51(6):1629–1633.
33. Ducharme SH, Gill KM. Sexuality and disability. In: Diamant L, McAnulty RD, eds. The psychology of sexual orientation, behavior and identity: a handbook. Westport: Greenwood Press; 1995.
34. Dunn KM, Croft PR, Hackett GI. Sexual problems: a study of the prevalence and need for health care in the general population. Fam Pract 1998; 15:519–524.
35. Ellenberg M. Sexual aspects of the female diabetic. Mt Sinai J Med 1977; 44:495–500.
36. Elliott S. Ejaculation and orgasm: sexuality in men with SCI. Top Spinal Cord Inj Rehabil 2002; 8:1–15.
37. Feldman HA, Goldstein I, Hatzchristou G, et al. Impotence and its medical and psychological correlates: results of the Massachusetts Male Aging Study. J Urol 1994; 151:54–61.
38. Flor H, Turk DC, Schloz OB. Impact of chronic pain on the spouse: marital, emotional and physical consequences. J Psychosom Res 1987; 31:63–71.
39. Fooken I. Sexuality in the later years—the impact of health and body image in a sample of older women. Patient Educ Couns 1994; 23:227–233.
40. Garden FH, Bontke CF, Hoffman M. Sexual functioning and marital adjustments after traumatic brain injury. J Head Trauma Rehabil 1990; 5:52–59.
41. Gilliland BC. Degenerative joint disease. In: Braunwald E, Issebacher KJ, Petersdorf RG, et al, eds. Harrison's principles of internal medicine. New York: McGraw-Hill; 1988:1456–1458.
42. Giuliano F, Hultling C, El Masry WS, et al. Randomized trial of sildenafil for the treatment of erectile dysfunction in spinal cord injury. Sildenafil Study Group. Ann Neurol 1999; 46(1):15–21.
43. Govier F, Potempa AJ, Kaufman J, et al. A multicenter, randomized, double-blind, crossover study of patient preference for tadalafil 20 mg or sildenafil citrate 50 mg during initiation of treatment for erectile dysfunction. Clin Ther 2003; 11:2709–2723.
44. Graziottin A. Clinical approach to dyspareunia. J Sex Marital Ther 2001; 27:489–501.
45. Green BG, Martin S. Clinical assessment of sildenafil in the treatment of neurogenic male sexual dysfunction: after the hype. Neurorehabilitation 2000; 15(2):101–105.
46. Hellerstein HK, Friedman EH. Sexual activity and the post coronary patient. Arch Int Med 1970; 125:987–999.
47. Hibbard MR, Gordon WA, et al. Sexual dysfunction after traumatic brain injury. Neurorehabilitation 2000; 15:107–120.

48. Horn LJ, Zasler ND. Neuroanatomy and neurophysiology of sexual function. J Head Trauma Rehabil 1990; 5:1–13.

49. Hulter BM. Sexual problems and life satisfaction in women with insulin controlled dependent mellitus. In: Hulter BM. Sexual function in women with neurological disorders. Uppsala: Acta Universitatis Upsaliensis; 1999:1V1–16.

50. Islam A, Mitachel J, Rosen R, et al. Topical alprostadil in the treatment of female sexual arousal disorder: a pilot study. J Sex Marital Ther 2001; 27:531–540.

51. Ito TY, Trant AS, Polan ML. A double-blind placebo-controlled study of ArginMax, a nutritional supplement for enhancement of female sexual function. J Sex Marital Ther 2001; 27:541–549.

52. Janus SS, Janus CL. The Janus report on sexual behavior. New York: John Wiley; 1993.

53. Jordan GH. Peyronie's disease and its management. In: Krane RJ, Siroky M, Fitzgerald J, eds. Clinical urology. Philadelphia: JB Lippincott; 1994:1282–1297.

54. Kaiser FE, Morley JE. Menopause and beyond. In: Cassel C, ed. Geriatric medicine. 3rd edn. New York: Springer; 1997.

55. Kaiser FE, Viosca SP, Morely JE, et al. Impotence and aging: clinical and hormonal factors. J Am Geriatr Soc 1988; 36:511–519.

56. Kaiser FE. Sexuality in the elderly. Geriatr Urol 1996; 23(1):99–107.

57. Kang B, Lee S, Kim M, et al. A placebo-controlled, double-blind trial of ginkgo biloba for antidepressant-induced sexual dysfunction. Hum Psychopharmacol 2002; 17:279–284.

58. Kappor VK, Chahal AS, Jyoti SP, et al. Intracavernous papaverine for impotence in spinal cord injured patients. Paraplegia 1993; 31(10):675–677.

59. Kara H, Aydin S, Yucel M et al. The efficacy of fluoxetine in the treatment of premature ejaculation: a double-blind placebo controlled study. Am J Psychiatry 1994; 151:1377–1379.

60. Keating GM, Scott LJ. Spotlight on vardenafil in erectile dysfunction. Drugs Aging 2004; 21(2):135–140.

61. Keating GM, Scott LJ. Vardenafil: a review of its use in erectile dysfunction. Drugs 2003; 63(23):2673–2703.

62. Kegel AH. Sexual functions of the pubococcygeus muscle. West J Surg Obstet Gynecol 1952; 60:521–524.

63. Kellett JM. Sexuality in later life. Rev Clin Gerontol 1993; 3:309–314.

64. Kinsey AC, Pomeroy WB, Martin CE. Sexual behavior in the human female. Philadelphia: Saunders; 1953.

65. Kinsey AC, Pomeroy WB, Martin CE. Sexual behavior in the human male. Philadelphia: Saunders; 1948.

66. Korpelainen JT, Nieminen P, Myllyla VV. Sexual functioning among stroke patients and their spouses. Stroke 1999; 30:715–719.

67. Kosteljanetz M, Jensen T, Norgard B, et al. Sexual and hypothalamic dysfunction in the postconcussional syndrome. Acta Neurol Scand 1981; 63:169–180.

68. Kreutzer JS, Zasler ND. Psychosexual consequences of traumatic brain injury: methodology and preliminary findings. Brain Inj 1989; 3:177–186.

69. Laan E, Everaerd W. Physiological measures of vaginal vasocongestion. Int J Impot Res 1998; 10:107–110.

70. Lakin MM, Montague DR, Vanderbrug MS, et al. Intracavernous injection therapy: analysis of results and complications. J Urol 1990; 143:1138–1141.

71. Linet OI, Ogrinc FG. Efficacy and safety of intracavernosal alprostadil in men with erectile dysfunction. N Engl J Med 1996; 334:873–877.

72. LoPiccolo J, Lobitz WC. The role of masturbation in the treatment of orgasmic dysfunction. Arch Sex Behav 1972; 2:163–171.

73. LoPiccolo JL, Friedman MH. Broad spectrum treatment of low sexual desire: integration of cognitive, behavioral and systemic therapy. In: Leiblum SR, Rosen RC, eds. Sexual desire disorders. New York: Guilford Press; 1998:107–144.

74. Ludeman K. The sexuality of the older person: review of literature. Gerontologist 1981; 21:203–208.

75. Lue TF, Tanagho EA. Physiology of erection and pharmacological management of impotence. J Urol 1987; 137:829–836.

76. Lue TF. Physiology of erection and pathophysiology of impotence. In: Walsh PC, Retik AB, Stamey TA, et al. Campbell's urology. Philadelphia: Saunders; 1992:722–725.

77. Lundberg L, Olsson JO, Kihl B. Long-term experience of self-injection therapy with prostaglandin E_1 for erectile dysfunction. Scand J Urol Nephrol 1996; 30(5):395–397.

78. Masand PS, Ashton AK, Gupta S, et al. Sustained-release bupropion for selective serotonin reuptake inhibitor-induced sexual dysfunction: a randomized, double-blind, placebo-controlled, parallel-group study. Am J Psychiatry 2001; 158:805–807.

79. Masters WH, Johnson VE. Human sexual inadequacy. London: Churchill; 1970.

80. Masters WH, Johnson VE. Human sexual response. Boston: Bantam Books; 1980.

81. Mattson DH, Petrie M, Srivasava DK, et al. Multiple sclerosis—sexual dysfunction and its response to medication. Arch Neurol 1995; 52:862–868.

82. Mattson DH. Sexual dysfunction in multiple sclerosis. Mult Scler Clin Issue 1995; 2(3):10–13.

83. Maytom MC, Derry FA, Dinsmore WW, et al. A two-part pilot study of sildenafil (Viagra) in men with erectile dysfunction caused by spinal cord injury. Spinal Cord 1999; 37(2):110–116.

84. Mazer NA. Testosterone deficiency in women: etiologies, diagnosis, and emerging treatments. Int J Fertil 2002; 47(2):77–86.

85. McMullen S, Rosen RC. Self-administered masturbation training in the treatment of primary orgasmic dysfunction. J Consult Clin Psychol 1979; 47:912–918.

86. Melman A, Fersel J, Weinstein P. Further studies on the effect of chronic alpha-methyldopa administration upon the central nervous system and sexual function in male rats. J Urol 1984; 132:804–808.

87. Mendels J. Sertraline for premature ejaculation. J Clin Psychopharmacol 1995; 15(5):341–346.

88. Meyer JE. Die Sexuallen storungen der hirnverletzten. Arch Psychiatrie Z Neurol 1955; 193:449–469.

89. Michelson D, Bancroft J, Targum S, et al. Female sexual dysfunction associated with antidepressant administration: a randomized, placebo-controlled study of pharmacologic intervention. Am J Psychiatry 2000; 157:239–243.

90. Miller TA. Diagnostic evaluation of erectile dysfunction. Am Fam Physician 2000; 61:95–104, 109–110.

91. Modell J, Katholi C. Comparative sexual side effects of buprorion, fluoxetine, paroxetine and sertraline. Clin Pharmocol Ther 1997; 61:476–487.

92. Modell JG, May RS, Katholi CR. Effect of bupropion-SR on orgasmic dysfunction in nondepressed subjects: a pilot study. J Sex Marital Ther 2000; 26:231–240.

93. Mong M, Bernie J, Rajasekaran M. Male infertility and erectile dysfunction in spinal cord injury: a review. Arch Phys Med Rehabil 1999; 80:1331–1339.

94. Monga M, Bernie J, Rajasekaran M. Male infertility and erectile dysfunction in spinal cord injury: a review. Arch Phys Med Rehabil 1999; 80(10):1331–1339.

95. Monga NT, Kerrigan AJ. In: Sipski ML, Alexander CJ, eds. Sexual dysfunction in people with disabilities and chronic illness. Gaithersburg: Aspen Publishers; 1997:189–219.

96. Morley JE, Kaiser FE. Aging and sexuality. In: Albarede JL, Campbell AJ, Grimely-Evans J, et al, eds. Facts and research in gerontology. New York: Springer; 1992.

97. Morley JE, Kaiser FE. Impotence: the internist's approach to diagnosis and treatment. Adv Intern Med 1993; 38:151–168.

98. Morrell MJ, Dixon JM, Carter SM. The influence of age and cycling status on sexual arousability in women. Am J Obstet Gynecol 1984; 148(1):66–71.

99. Muller JE, Mittleman MA, Maclure M, et al. Triggering myocardial infarction by sexual activity: low absolute risk and prevention by regular physical exertion. JAMA 1996; 275:1405–1409.

100. Nadler S. Chapter 14. In: Sipski ML, Alexander CJ, eds. Sexual dysfunction in people with disabilities and chronic illness. Gaithersburg: Aspen Publishers; 1997:261–278.

101. NIH Consensus Development Panel on Impotence. NIH Consensus Conference. Impotence. JAMA 1993; 270(1):83–90.

102. Pfeiffer E, Verwoerdt A, Wang HS. Sexual behavior in aged men and women. Arch Gen Psychiatry 1968; 19:735–758.

103. Porst H, Padma-Nathan H, Giuliano F, et al. Efficacy of tadalafil for the treatment of erectile dysfunction at 24 and 36 hours after dosing: a randomized controlled trial. Urology 2003; 62(1):121–125.

104. Rosen RC, Leiblum SR. Treatment of sexual disorders in the 1990s: an integrated approach. J Consult Clin Psychol 1995; 63(3):877–890.

105. Rubio-Aurioles E, Lopez M, Lipezker M, et al. Phentolamine mesylate in postmenopausal women with female sexual arousal disorder: a psycho-physiological study. J Sex Marital Ther 2002; 28:205–215.

106. Salmon JJ, Geist SH. Effects of androgens on libido in women. J Clin Endocrinol Metab 1943; 3:235–238.

107. Sandel ME. In: Sipski ML, Alexander CJ, eds. Sexual dysfunction in people with disabilities and chronic illness. Gaithersburg: Aspen Publishers; 1997:221–245.

108. Schiavi RC, Schreiner-Engel P, Mandeli J, et al. Healthy aging and male sexual function. Am J Psychiatry 1990; 147:766–771.

109. Schmid DM, Curt A, Hauri D, et al. Clinical value of combined electro-physiological and urodynamic recordings to assess sexual disorders in SCI men. Neurourol Urodyn 2003; 22(4):314–321.

110. Schmid DM, Schurch B, Hauri D. Sildenafil in the treatment of sexual dysfunction in spinal cord-injured male patients. Eur Urol 2000; 38(2):184–193.

111. Seftel AD, Wilso SK, Knapp PM, et al. The efficacy and safety of tadalafil in United States and Puerto Rican men with erectile dysfunction. J Urol 2004; 17(2):652–657.

112. Segenreich E, Israilov S, Shmueli J, et al. Evaluation of 452 patients with erectile dysfunction treated by combinations of vasoactive agents by penile injection. Harefuah 1998; 134(9):673–678.

113. Shifren JL, Braunstein GD, Simon JA, et al. Transdermal testosterone treatment in women with impaired sexual function after oophorectomy. N Engl J Med 2000; 343:682–688.

114. Silber EN, Katz LV. Cardiac activity and sexual response. New York; 1980.

115. Sipski ML, Alexander CJ, Rosen R. Sexual arousal and orgasm in women: effects of spinal cord injury. Ann Neurol 2001; 49:35–44.

116. Sipski ML, Alexander CJ, Rosen RC, et al. Sildenafil effects on sexual and cardiovascular responses in women with spinal cord injury. Urology 2000; 55:812–815.

117. Sipski ML, Alexander CJ. Sexual function in people with disability and chronic illness. Gaithersburg: Aspen Publishers; 1997:7.

118. Sipski ML, Rosen R, Alexander CJ, et al. A controlled trial of positive feedback to increase sexual arousal in women with spinal cord injuries. Neurorehabilitation 2000; 15:145–153.

119. Sipski ML, Rosen RC, Alexander CJ, et al. Sexual responsiveness in women with spinal cord injuries: differential effects of anxiety-eliciting stimulation. Arch Sex Behav 2004; 33(3):295–302.

120. Sipski ML. A physiatrist's view regarding the report of the International Consensus Conference on Female Sexual Dysfunction: potential concerns regarding women with disabilities. J Sex Marital Ther 2001; 27:215–216.

121. Sipski ML. Chapter 9. In: Sipski ML, Alexander CJ, eds. Sexual dysfunction in people with disabilities and chronic illness. Gaithersburg: Aspen Publishers; 1997:149–173.

122. Sipski ML. Documentation of the impact of spinal cord injury on sexual function: the Female Spinal Sexual Function Classification. Top Spinal Cord Inj Rehabil 2002; 8(1):63–73.

123. Skoumal R, Chen J, Kula K, et al. Efficacy and treatment satisfaction with on-demand tadalafil (Cialis) in men with erectile dysfunction. Eur Urol 2004; 46(3):362–369.

124. Smeltzer SC, Kelly CL. Multiple sclerosis. In: Sipski ML, Alexander CJ, eds. Sexual dysfunction in people with disabilities and chronic illness. Gaithersburg: Aspen Publishers; 1997:177–188.

125. Smith DS, Jarlfors U, Cameron BF. Morphological evidence for the participation of microtubules in axonal transport. Ann NY Acad Sci 1975; 253:472–506.

126. Sommer F, Engelmann U. Future options for combination therapy in the management of erectile dysfunction in older men. Drugs Aging 2004; 21(9):555–564.

127. Sonksen J, Ched D. Management of male infertility after spinal cord injury. Top Spinal Cord Inj Rehabil 2002; 8(1):29–41.

128. Starr BD, Weiner MB. The Starr–Weiner report on sex and sexuality in the mature years. New York: Stien & Day; 1981.

129. Stitik TP, Benevento BT. Chapter 16. In: Sipski ML, Alexander CJ, eds. Sexual dysfunction in people with disabilities and chronic illness. Gaithersburg: Aspen Publishers; 1997:303–335.

130. Tang SF, Chu NK, Wong MK. Intracavernous injection of prostaglandin E₁ in spinal cord injured patients with erectile dysfunction. Paraplegia 1995; 33(12):731–733.

131. Tay HP, Juma S, Joseph AC. Psychogenic impotence in SCI patients. Arch Phys Med Rehabil 1996; 77:91–93.

132. Tilton MC. Chapter 15. In: Sipski ML, Alexander CJ, eds. Sexual dysfunction in people with disabilities and chronic illness. Gaithersburg: Aspen Publishers; 1997:279–301.

133. Truitt WA, Coolen LM. Identification of a potential ejaculation generator in the spinal cord. Science 2002; 297(5586):1566–1569.

134. Ueno M. The so-called coital death. Jpn J Legal Med 1963; 17:330–340.

135. Waldinger M, Hengeveld M, Zwinderman A. Paroxetine treatment of premature ejaculation: a double-blind placebo controlled study. J Urol 1996; 156(5):1631–1632.

136. Walker AE, Jablon S. A follow-up study of head wounds in World War II. Veteran's Affairs medical monograph. Washington: Department of Veterans Affairs; 1961.

137. Wallace JI, Paauw DS, Spach DH. HIV in older patients: when to suspect the unexpected. Geriatrics 1993; 48:61–70.

138. Wein AJ, Malloy TR, Hanno PM. Intracavernous injection programs—their place in management of erectile dysfunction. 1987.

139. Wethman P, Rajfer J. MUSE therapy: preliminary clinical observations. Urology 1997; 50(5):809–811.

140. Zaslau S, Nicolis C, Galea G, et al. A simplified pharmacologic erection program for patients with spinal cord injury. J Spinal Cord Med 1999; 22(4):303–307.

141. Zilber B. The new male sexuality. New York: Bantam Books; 1992.

Chapter

33

Prevention and Management of Chronic Wounds

Robert Goldman, Adrian Popescu, Cathy Thomas Hess and Richard Salcido

The financial burden of chronic wound care is immense: in the USA, the chronic wound care bill, including professional expenses, hospital costs, and complications (direct costs only), ranges from $7 billion to $15 billion. The costs for all chronic wound types are increasing at 10% per year, driven by the aging of the 'baby boomers'. Four basic ulcer types present significant economic burden: pressure ulcers ($3–6 billion), ischemic and neuropathic ulcers ($3–5 billion), and venous ulcers (> $2 billion). Because prevention and aggressive treatment of early ulcers reduces costs, there is an economic impetus for growth of outpatient wound centers. In the past 20 years, the number of wound care treatment centers has risen from very few to about 700.[2]

Another trend in wound care derives from the current revolution in molecular biology, gene therapy, biomaterials, and stem cell research. Stem cells are now being applied to animal models of chronic wounds. Chronic wound products derived from recombinant DNA technology have been in place since the late 1990s.[57] Possibly dramatic changes might occur from gene therapy involving growth factors, which are now entering human trials. Human trials involving artificial skin grafts[33] have lead to Food and Drug Administration (FDA) approval for using such grafts with certain ulcer types. Physiatrists can potentially utilize all these interventions.

Physiatrists should be interested and involved in chronic wound care because of the field investment in optimizing the function of patients, managing rehabilitation teams, prescribing orthoses and modalities, and understanding gait biomechanics and protected weight bearing. All these are critical components of conservative or non-surgical chronic wound care. This chapter elaborates the role of the physiatrist as ambulatory wound care consultant, promoting limb salvage and functional preservation.

SCOPE OF THE PROBLEM

Definitions

The National Pressure Ulcer Advisory Panel defines a *pressure ulcer* as an area of unrelieved pressure over a defined area, usually over a bony prominence such as the greater trochanter of the femur, sacrum, or occiput, resulting in ischemia, cell death, and tissue necrosis.[7,47] Pressure ulcers are associated with impaired mental status or sensation, poor hygiene or nutrition,

and multiple comorbidity factors. High standards of nursing and medical management are key to prevention of ulcers in immobilized patients.

Chronic venous or edematous ulcers of the leg typically arise on the gator area of the leg (i.e. the lower third of the leg). They are associated with impaired venous return, incompetence of venous perforators, or loss of fascial integrity of the leg (e.g. from trauma) in patients with normal arterial inflow. The cornerstone of treatment is compression.

Neuropathic ulcers follow repetitive trauma to hyposensate distal extremities (e.g. feet), usually on weight-bearing bony prominences such as metatarsal heads. For uncomplicated neuropathic ulcers, the circulation is usually functionally intact.[61] A cornerstone of treatment is mitigating abnormal axial repetitive pressure and shear.

Ischemic ulcers occur on limbs with impaired arterial inflow due to arteriosclerotic disease, and, in the setting of diabetes, microvascular disease. Often initiated by minor trauma or shoe pressure on the medial or lateral foot margins, they are typically painful and blanched. Ischemic ulcers are frequently associated with neuropathy or edema. Healing of these ulcers primarily depends on reestablishing arterial circulation.

Epidemiology of chronic wounds

Persons with spinal cord injury (SCI) and associated comorbidity are at increased risk for the formation of pressure ulcers. In one community-based sample, the point prevalence of stage 3 or 4 pressure ulcers was 26%.[46] The second population group at risk for pressure ulceration is the elderly. The annual prevalence of pressure ulcers among those 65 years of age and older varies from 0.31% to 0.70%, and such ulcers are most likely to occur in patients 85 years and older.[78]

The prevalence of pressure ulcers of any stage for hospitalized patients ranges from 3.5%[117] to 69%.[1] (The latter prevalence decreased significantly, to 16%, after instituting a multidisciplinary approach to prevention and treatment on the surgical inpatient service at one hospital.) Patients in critical care units can run a higher risk of developing pressure ulcers, as evidenced by a 40% incidence in one study.[9]

Long-term facilities are frequently the disposition for patients with pressure ulcers sustained during acute hospitalization. In one very large study involving 51 nursing homes, 11.3% patients were admitted with stage 2 through stage 4 pressure ulcers.

Long-term care residents are also at risk for the formation of new pressure ulcers. For those residents without pressure ulcers initially, the 1-year incidence was 13.2%, and 2-year incidence 21.6%. Most patients with pressure ulcers had their ulcers healed within 1 year.[13]

Variable implementation of policies and procedures related to incontinence, inspection, turning, positioning, range of motion, and nutrition might partially explain the wide variation in the prevalence of pressure ulcers in long-term care facilities: 2.6–24%.[13] Because of this wide disparity, the prevalence of pressure ulcers is seen or accepted as an important index of care quality, and is monitored by federal and state governments in the Minimum Data Set. It is now becoming recognized, however, that some pressure ulcers could be inevitable, occurring near death in what has been termed *skin failure*.[134]

Diabetes mellitus

Neuropathy, arteriosclerosis, and microvascular disease are all present in diabetes, creating a high risk for chronic wounds developing in the lower limbs, which can result in amputation. There were 54 000 amputations in the USA due to diabetes in 1990, preceded in 85% of cases by foot ulcers. Hospitalization rates for lower extremity amputation are 13 times higher for persons with diabetes than for the general Medicare population.[50] The first major limb amputation for those with diabetes is often followed by a second major amputation, as 28–51% have a contralateral amputation within 5 years.[108]

The cost of a single major amputation is conservatively estimated at $100 000, including the acute hospital stay, surgeries, rehabilitation, and prostheses (unpublished data).[136] Multiplying the cost per amputation and number of amputations among those with diabetes, there is a likely cost burden of $5.4 billion. Because of this cost burden, the US Public Health Service called for a 40% reduction in diabetic-related amputations by the year 2000, and urged prevention and earlier treatment to achieve this goal.[3] Unfortunately, this goal was not met. There was actually a 25% *increase* in dysvascular amputations between 1988 and 1996.[30] These disappointing trends suggest that preventive and early intervention strategies that are elaborated in this chapter need to be more aggressively implemented.

Chronic venous disease

Approximately 1% of the US population and 3% of the population over 65 have venous stasis ulcers, with the incidence rate twice as high for women as for men.[79] An estimated 3.0 million Americans now suffer from venous ulcers. Only 600 000 per year are treated, however, so it is likely that chronic venous disease is under-diagnosed. The cost estimate for healing an uncomplicated venous ulcer is $2500.[102] Intractable venous ulcers are much more expensive, but 20–30% of such ulcers present as intractable. Intractable ulcers are those that are present for more than 1 year, or those whose area exceeds 10 cm^2. The cost can approach $10 000 for each of these intractable cases.[95] At an average cost of $3000 per ulcer, the total direct cost is estimated at $2 billion, which does not factor in the hidden costs of undiagnosed or unreported ulcers.

In addition to the hidden cost of untreated ulcers, there are 2 million lost workdays from this condition.[101]

WOUND PHYSIOLOGY AND PATHOPHYSIOLOGY

Definitions

The Wound Healing Society defines *healing* as complete closing of the integument.[73] Skin wounds that heal by *primary intention* are similar to incisions that are created by a scalpel blade, and then heal rapidly and without complication in 3–14 days. More complicated are the wounds that heal by *secondary intention*. Secondary intention wounds are large tissue defects that fill by granulation followed by epithelialization. Wound closure occurs to some extent because of wound contraction.

Process of normal healing

There are four major phases of wound healing: inflammation, provisional matrix formation, repair, and remodeling.[57] The sequence begins with tissue injury and inflammation. Inflammation is characterized by breakdown of the preexisting tissue scaffolding and clean-up of extracellular and pathogen debris. Matrix breakdown also enables migration of neutrophils, macrophages, epidermal cells, and fibroblasts into the site of injury, enabling its ultimate repair. Repair is analogous to the construction of a new building, with a framework of extracellular matrix components (a provisional matrix of glycosaminoglycans, which are protein–sugar complexes, and fibronectin) attached to 'rivets' (cell attachment sites called integrins). On this framework are laid reinforced 'girders' of type 1 collagen, which are secreted in sections (fibrils) and self-assemble extracellularly. Over this structure (while under construction), a 'roof' of epidermal cells advances over the defect to provide a durable cover, and a 'plumbing' network of neovessels accrete to supply oxygen and nutrients (i.e. neoangiogenesis). After closure, remodeling of dermal matrix occurs, during which collagen fibers are preferentially retained along lines of stress.

Each stage of wound healing is governed by precisely timed signaling between cells and matrix components. These signaling components include cytokines, growth factors, proteases, and protease inhibitors. These components and their interactions, which orchestrate healing, are beyond the scope of this chapter, and are well described elsewhere for the interested reader.[57]

Pathophysiology of chronic wounds

Chronic wounds appear to be in a chronic inflammatory state synonymous with healing arrest. Five commonly identified factors dynamically interact to arrest healing and perpetuate wound status: pathomechanics, reperfusion injury, chronic hypoxia, growth factor abnormalities, and chronic inflammation.

Pathomechanics

Pathomechanics implies noxious application of shear (force tangential to the skin surface) and axial pressure (perpendicular to the skin). Unrelieved static axial pressure is a critical factor in development of pressure ulcers of the buttocks. Prolonged pressure leads to ulcers if tissue capillary pressure of 32 mmHg is exceeded. Known as critical tissue interface pressure, this benchmark is 75 years old and has yet to be substantively amended. It serves as a basis for design of clinical pressure-relieving surfaces.[113]

The critical interface pressure is the pressure above which a tissue cannot be loaded for an indefinite period without resulting ulceration. There is an inverse, hyperbolic relationship between pressure and the duration of pressure application necessary to cause ulcers. Unrelieved axial pressure 4–6 times systolic blood pressure causes necrosis in less than an hour. Pressure below systolic blood pressure, however, might require 12 h to produce a similar lesion. This hyperbolic relationship has been confirmed for several animal models[71] and can serve as the basis for turning patients every 2 h.[109]

Shear forces exacerbate the tendency to ulcerate as a result of axial forces applied to bony prominences or areas of risk, and can lower the ulceration threshold sixfold.[32] The classic example of shear is of a patient sitting semiupright in a hospital bed. This position places the sacrum at increased risk for tissue breakdown. For pressure ulcers, force vectors occur on the time scale of hours. For neuropathic ulcers, force vectors occur over fractions of seconds, consistent with the timing of the gait cycle.[23] Once ulcers form, they are empirically more sensitive to transient or static pressure and shear than is intact skin.

Reperfusion injury

Ischemia from pressure-induced capillary collapse is associated with buildup within the microvasculature of supraoxide free radicals. Supraoxide rises during periods of ischemia. During subsequent reperfusion, an excess of supraoxide causes neutrophils to marginate and traverse the endothelial cell, inducing an inflammatory response that can be important in the pathophysiology of pressure ulcers[114] of the buttocks and heels. Patients with diabetes mellitus are at increased risk of reperfusion injury, because there are decreased levels of microvessel nitric oxide. Nitric oxide is a potent vasodilator that protects endothelium from reperfusion injury.[81]

Chronic hypoxia

Chronic hypoxia results from poor inflow of blood, typically due to arteriosclerotic narrowing proximal to hypoxic skin. Ischemia blunts granulation tissue deposition, mononuclear cell infiltration,[137] and probability of wound closure.[98]

Edema and impaired oxygen and nutrient exchange

Edema is one of the major factors associated with the pathogenesis and maintenance of chronic wounds. Venous ulcers, due to venous congestion and back pressure, extravasate fibrinogen and fluid across the microvasculature endothelium, leading to excess protein-rich interstitial fluid. This fluid is thought to sequester growth factors, which are then unavailable to heal the edematous skin.[37] Venous congestion can also lead to endothelial damage, causing neutrophils to marginate and release free radicals and collagenases. This process further increases membrane permeability to macromolecules, osmotic pressure and fluid shifts, and worsening edema.[39]

Growth factor abnormalities

Growth factor abnormalities can occur in one of four categories:

1. reduced synthesis;
2. increased protein or matrix sequestration;
3. increased breakdown; or
4. insensitivity of target cells (i.e. reduced growth factor receptor concentration).

As wounds heal with optimum conservative treatment, these abnormalities tend to resolve. Growth factor alterations are summarized elsewhere for the interested reader.[57]

Chronic inflammation

Although colonization with bacteria is normal and even helpful, critical colonization and local infection impedes healing. Wounds that have greater than 10^5 organisms per gram of tissue tend not to heal,[63] and are 'stuck' in the inflammatory stage. The process of decreasing bacterial bioburden through 'wound bed preparation' is discussed below.

Comorbidities

The factors that contribute to chronic wound persistence are diverse, interactive, and cumulative, and they affect the whole organism. Predisposing conditions include aging, SCI, and diabetes, among many others (Table 33-1). These comorbidities interact at many levels to contribute to pathomechanics, reperfusion injury, static hypoxia, and local inflammation, and they lead to growth factor abnormalities within wounds.

CLINICAL WOUND ASSESSMENT

Wound area and volume assessment

Assessments are typically performed weekly or biweekly to document the effectiveness of therapy, make changes in treatment if necessary, and support the overall treatment plan.

Wound area

The most straightforward technique is to document the wound's perpendicular linear dimensions (typically in centimeters); the maximum distance is length, and perpendicular distance is width.[17] Although rapidly performed, linear dimensions have limited sensitivity to changes in wound size, have limited information about shape, and overestimate the wound area by up to 25%.[56] To address these concerns, serial wound outlines are now performed. A useful, inexpensive technique is drawing wound outlines on clear plastic (e.g. acetate sheet for transparencies) with an indelible marker; these drawings then become part of the patient's permanent record. Inspection allows immediate appraisal of progress, and if the wound has increased in size, the clinician can modify treatment without delay. Wound area, calculated by computerized planimetry, has excellent inter- and intrarater reliability.[42]

Table 33-1 Comorbidities associated with chronic wounds

Condition	Pathophysiologic effect related to wound healing
Spinal cord injury	Vasomotor instability (>T6 level), insensitivity, denervation atrophy, spasticity, contractures, bowel and bladder alterations[47]
Being elderly	Reduced skin elasticity and altered skin microcirculation,[128] comorbidities, reduced healing rate noted clinically and in animal models[58]
Diabetes	Insensitivity, microangiopathy and altered inflammatory response,[91] foot deformities (intrinsic minus, Charcot), blunted reactive hyperemia, reduced incision breaking strength,[100] and contraction[59] in animal models
Malnutrition	Negative nitrogen balance, cachexia, immunosuppression
Anemia	Local hypoxia
Arteriosclerosis	Local hypoxia
End-stage renal disease	Transient dialysis-related hypoperfusion, arteriosclerosis, microangiopathy
Steroid medications	Reduced healing rate in animal models, immunosuppression
Transplant recipients	Immunosuppression
Smoking	Hypoxia, vasoconstriction, increased blood viscosity
Parkinson disease	Immobility
Osteoporosis	Bony prominences
Upper motor neuron disease	Immobility, contractures, bowel and bladder alterations
Dementia	Immobility, malnutrition, contractures, bowel and bladder alterations
Acutely ill (intensive care unit-related)	Hypotension, immobility, bowel and bladder alteration, malnutrition, increased metabolic demands
Non-compliance, abuse, and neglect	Multifactorial

Wound volume

For a first approximation of volume, area is multiplied by depth to find volume. The volume of a rectangular solid calculated in this manner overestimates the volume of pressure ulcers. Calculating volume of a spheroid is more accurate.[56] By either calculation, using depth is most accurate for deep cavities and least accurate for shallow, irregularly shaped wounds.

Computerized area and volume measurement

Computerized assessment combines digital photography and a technique known as photogrammetry. Photogrammetry calibrates space in the image by means of a target plate to calculate both surface area and volume[72] (many of the illustrations in this chapter include a target plate). One commercially available photogrammetry product is the VeV MD system (Vista Medical Ltd., Winnipeg, Canada).[129]

Wound appearance

To describe wound appearance, the red–yellow–black system is often used (wounds classically transform from black, to yellow, to red as they heal; see Fig. 33-1). One method is to classify a wound as the least advantageous of the three colors that it displays.[76] This method has been criticized as simplistic. The color of the wound surface can be alternatively described as a relative percentage of the three colors. To document appearance, the best method is a digital image, especially when used serially.

Perfusion assessment

It is exceedingly rare that large vessel disease contributes to the formation of pressure ulcers of the trunk, occiput, hips, or buttocks. For more distal wounds of the leg and foot, however, perfusion must be assessed, because:

- in the setting of poor perfusion, therapeutic compression might cause pressure necrosis; and
- perfusion prognosticates wound closure (see also Ch. 57).

Macrocirculation

Macrocirculation refers to blood flow through named anatomic arteries, such as the iliac, femoral, posterior tibial, and plantar.

Ankle brachial index and pulse volume recording Ankle brachial index (ABI) is the ratio of systolic blood pressure of the ankle to that of the arm (brachium).[56] Normal ABI is 0.8–1.3, and can be determined by a portable Doppler instrument and a blood pressure cuff. A series of cuffs determine pulse volume recording, which is continuous monitoring of pressure within cuffs applied to the thigh, calf, and ankle. These segmental pressure traces are checked for bilateral symmetry and

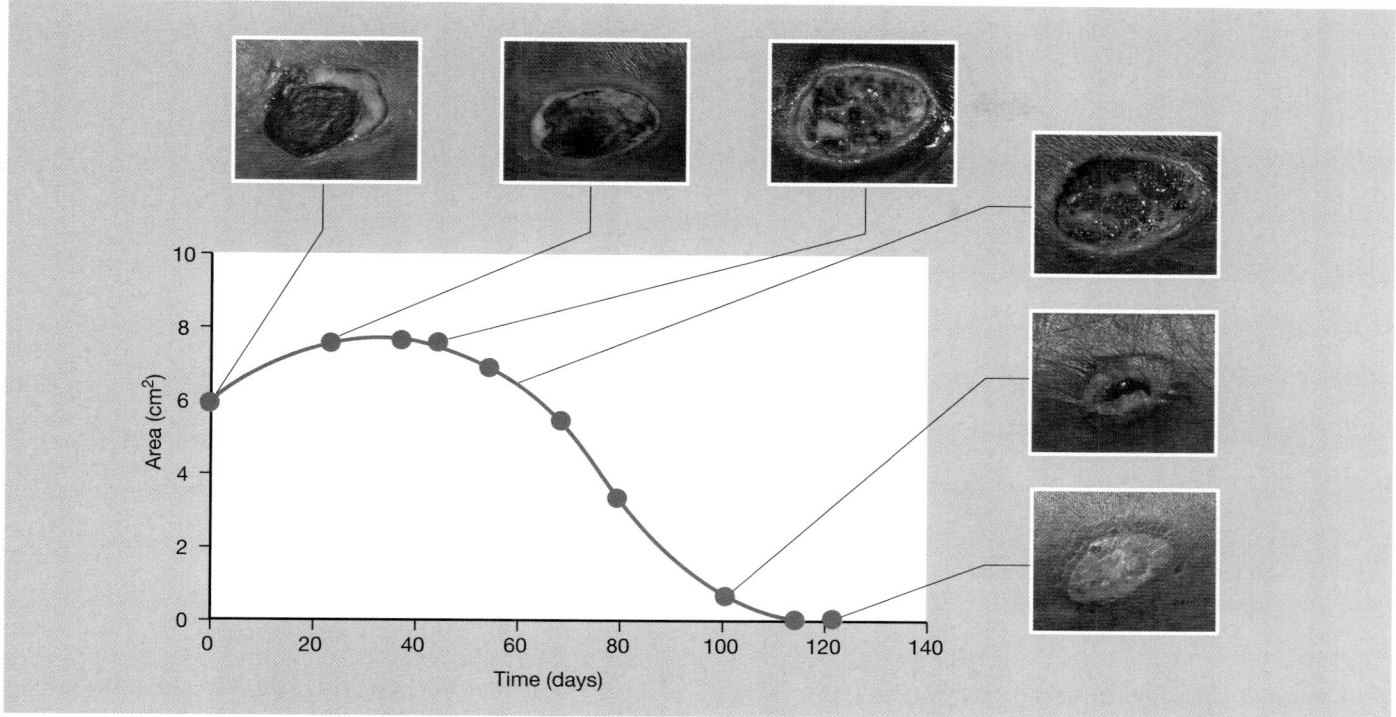

Figure 33-1 Transformation of wound bed from black eschar, to yellow slough, to beefy red granulating base.[56] As the wound bed granulates, area (determined by serial outlines) first increases, then stabilizes, then decreases as epithelialization commences over the granulating wound base. Of the 16 weeks spent in healing this wound, almost half was devoted to wound bed preparation, and half to epithelialization. The patient is a 38-year-old man with type 1 diabetes and 'small vessel disease', which is often associated with black eschar. Pointers connect the wound photographs to corresponding time points. (Used with permission of Lippincott Williams & Wilkins.)

waveform morphology: pulse pressures of normal arteries resemble steep isosceles triangles. Flattened pulse pressure waveforms and/or asymmetric indices suggest proximal flow compromise from arteriosclerosis. For patients with diabetes, calcinosis of the tunica media often falsely elevates ABI. Because calcinosis is less likely to involve foot arteries, it is useful to determine toe pressures. To determine toe pressure, a tiny cuff fits over the hallux and a Doppler probe records systolic pressure. A pressure > 40 mmHg is a good prognostic indicator of healing a foot ulcer. Toe pressure and ABI determination utilize only a portable Doppler instrument and do not require a dedicated vascular laboratory.[10]

Angiography   Angiography typically involves injecting a radiopaque dye into the proximal arterial tree. Conventional dye angiography is the gold standard for imaging macrovessels. It is a good prognosticator of limb salvage based on burden of arteriosclerosis visualized in the lower extremity.[36] A non-invasive alternative to conventional angiography is magnetic resonance angiography, which requires no contrast dye and is superior to conventional angiography in visualizing arteries of the ankle and foot.[84]

Microcirculation

In the skin, blood flows through arterioles, capillaries, and venules in the papillary and reticular dermis.[14] A microcirculation measure that is direct and absolute is transcutaneous oxygen ($TcPO_2$).

$TcPO_2$ is in essence a 'blood gas' of the skin. The normal $TcPO_2$ is greater than 50 mmHg, and the ischemic level is less than 20 mmHg.[98] A typical pattern of electrode placement is the upper leg, foot dorsum, and periwound (see Fig. 33-2).

$TcPO_2$ prognosticates the healing rate of neuropathic and ischemic ulcers. Its predictive value is uniquely strong for diabetic individuals, who have distal arterial calcinosis.[98] For this population, $TcPO_2$ is more accurate than toe pressures to prognosticate healing.[70] The surgical literature reports that $TcPO_2$ also prognosticates success of incisional healing at the transtibial level[110] and foot level.[103] Disadvantages of $TcPO_2$ include the following: the technique is inaccurately low over areas of callus, and it is transiently low in the setting of infection[48] and in the immediate postoperative situation. Measuring instruments are also expensive ($2500–5000 per channel) and time-consuming (20 min to 1 h to obtain a reading).

The most complete picture of lower limb perfusion comes from combining $TcPO_2$ and segmental pressures. For instance, very low distal segmental pressures (i.e. ABI < 0.4) but normal foot $TcPO_2$ could indicate collateralization around an arterial blockage. Under these conditions, normal $TcPO_2$ suggests good healing prognosis and a favorable chance of limb salvage.[56]

Pressure and shear assessment

Sensor arrays and point sensors are commercially available that can help to ensure that insoles and seating cushions minimize

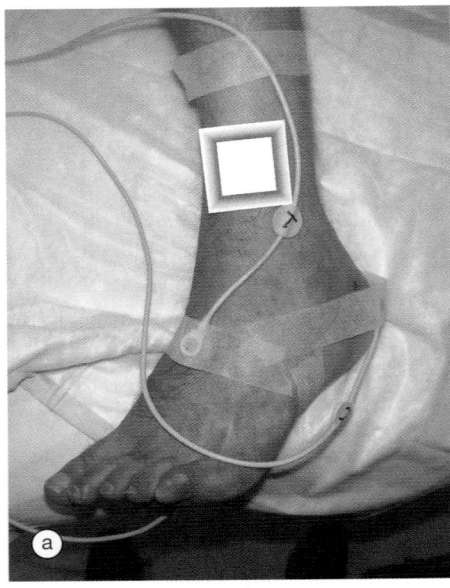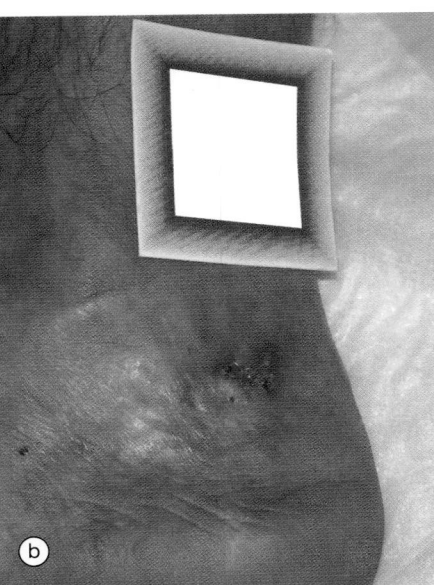

Figure 33-2 Electrode placement for transcutaneous oxygen determination on a 39-year-old man status post iliac artery angioplasty and with a medial ankle wound of 8 months' duration. He also presented with 'blue toe syndrome' (note the violet discoloration over the toes and medial ankle, in a mottled pattern representing livedo). TcPO$_2$ at the medial ankle was 0 mmHg, foot dorsum 40 mmHg, and upper leg (not shown) 50 mmHg. The wound closed after 4 months, coincident with normalization of TcPO$_2$.

axial pressure.[56] Two-dimensional sensor arrays (sensor arrays include resistive, capacitive, piezoresistive types) provide accuracy and good resolution of axial forces highlighting pressure points. Although mechanical axial pressure is well quantified, shear transducers have yet to be perfected for clinical use.

Skin biopsy

Although there are many biopsy types (e.g. excisional, incisional, and shave), the 3-mm punch technique is amenable for physiatric practice (low risk of bleeding and small skin defect). The method for biopsy involves selecting a site over soft tissue that is distant from subcutaneous arteries, fascia, or bone. The site selected should include periwound skin and a small sample of the wound base. Lidocaine (lignocaine) without adrenaline (epinephrine) (1–2 mL) is infused through intact periwound skin toward the wound center. The punch is inserted with a pressing, twisting motion, and a sample is harvested for histologic analysis.[126]

GENERAL PRINCIPLES OF TREATMENT

Wound bed preparation

Chronic wounds (unlike acute wounds) tend to be heavily colonized by bacteria. However, colonization does not equal infection.[85] Wounds exist on a continuum between frank invasion, critical colonization, colonization, and healing. As wounds heal (and bacterial virulence decreases), wound appearance transforms from black, to yellow, to dull red, to bright red (see Fig. 33-1). With beefy granulation tissue formation, there is a substantial decrease of drainage and pain, with management implications. Therapeutic processes for 'coaxing' a chronic wound to granulate have been coined wound bed preparation.[40] Once the wound bed is prepared, the goal is to maintain a moist environment. Epithelium advances and adjoins in a moist environment,

without having to digest eschar (i.e. 'scab'), optimizing healing rate.[133] In addition, wound fluid is well supplied with growth factors that promote closure.

Debridement
Surgical debridement
Surgical debridement is well established as an approach to the care of chronic wounds such as pressure ulcers. Surgical debridement is performed under general or regional anesthesia. It is indicated for abscesses or wounds that traverse tissue planes, and has a moderate to high risk of significant bleeding.

Sharps debridement
Less aggressive outpatient or bedside sharps debridement is performed by many disciplines, including physiatrists, and has been recognized as a distinct debridement method in a recent clinical practice guideline.[47] Usually, a series of sharps debridements are required to have the same effect as one surgical debridement. Sharps debridement is commonly performed in the outpatient setting as part of routine wound care, with minimal blood loss, although pain is always a concern. Pain is managed with topical analgesia. A local anesthetic, lidocaine (lignocaine) 5%, or EMLA cream (lidocaine 2.5% and prilocaine 2.5%)[16] can be applied 5–15 min prior to debridement. Premedication with an opiate analgesic can also be helpful. Debridements should be performed at regular intervals to ward off infection, because devitalized tissue supports the proliferation and growth of pathogens.

Pain is usually not a problem for patients with neuropathic ulcers. These ulcers develop callus that is debrided in an inverted cone pattern using a scalpel and forceps, called 'saucerization'. Debridements should be done periodically, as neuropathic ulcers readily form callus even with very little weight bearing, and a callus paradoxically increases mechanical tension in the wound.[61] Venous ulcers do not develop callus but yellow fibrinous exudate over the wound bed, which can be removed with curettage. If a stasis-like leg ulcer expands after debridement, the diagnosis of pyoderma gangrenosum should be considered.[105]

Note that slough and necrosis can be similarly removed from pressure ulcers. However, because pressure ulcers tend to be deeper than they are wide, knowledge of pelvic anatomy is essential, such as the location of the inferior gluteal artery. Particular concern is raised if the pressure ulcer is 'unstageable', such as when it has a 100% yellow surface. A completely nonviable surface raises concern that the pressure ulcer extends well into deep tissue planes. Such wounds should be sharp debrided with great care (due to the risk of bleeding). Referral to a surgeon is frequently indicated in these cases.

Ischemic wounds also must be sharp debrided with great care, because the blood supply might not be adequate to support a repair response, leading to further necrosis. If eschar appears to be contiguous with bone (e.g. black eschar over the calcaneus), the bone will probably not heal if exposed. In this circumstance, eschar should be left dry unless infection supervenes. Where black eschar overlies soft tissue and reperfusion is possible, the authors advocate topical use of silver sulfadiazine, which has a broad antibacterial spectrum and softens eschar (forming 'pseudoeschar'[90]). This pseudoeschar then self-dislodges or is readily removed by careful periodic sharps debridement.[54,55,85]

Mechanical debridement

Mechanical debridement is accomplished by whirlpool treatments, forceful irrigation, or use of wet to dry dressings. Wet to dry dressings involve placing unraveled, moist gauze into the lesion so that all sections of it are touching the dressing, then allowing the dressing to dry. When the dressing is removed, necrotic tissue is removed with it. Although wet to dry mechanical debridement is a ubiquitous method, it is increasingly criticized as inefficient and unnecessarily painful.[97]

Enzymatic debridement

There are several major types of enzymatic debridement agents currently on the market. These include collagenase (e.g. Santyl) and papain–urea (e.g. Accuzyme and Gladase). Urea denatures protein, which increases the effectiveness of the non-specific protease papain. Because of its specificity, collagenase is said to be better for preparing the wound bed, as it does not digest growth factors or matrix proteins.[40] Enzymatic debriding agents can be the most cost-effective for well-perfused partially necrotic pressure ulcers where sharps debridement is not readily available, such as in the skilled care setting.[85] They are applied with daily change of dressings, until wounds are free of slough or eschar. Note that enzymatic debridement might increase pain and drainage, requiring adjustments to dressing change schedules. The efficiency of enzymatic debriding agents is increased by 'cross-hatching' the eschar with a scalpel.[119]

Autolytic debridement

Autolytic debridement involves the use of natural proteases and collagenases in wound fluid to digest non-viable material. This method can be very effective when utilized under semiocclusive or occlusive dressings. However, autolytic debridement is contraindicated where wounds are infected or critically colonized. If slough or necrotic material is excessive, drainage can also macerate periwound skin, increasing wound size. As a rule of thumb, the amount of viable granulating base ought to be greater than 50% of the entire wound surface.[85]

Dressings[65]

Dressings are typically applied in layers. The primary dressing is contiguous with the wound surface. A secondary dressing is applied external to the primary for absorption, protection, or fixation. For primary or secondary application, the dressing categories shown in Table 33-2, which are organized from most to least absorptive, roughly correspond top down to the order in which they would be used in the process of wound bed preparation. Note the following caveats.

- It would be very unusual to use more than a few categories for a given wound.
- Composites, specialty absorptives, and foams are more likely to be used for a longer period, or until healing.
- Smaller, clean, stage 3 and stage 2 wounds suggest use of hydrocolloids, hydrogels, and films.

DIAGNOSIS AND TREATMENT OF SPECIFIC ULCER TYPES

Pressure ulcers

Presentation

Only a patient who can act to relieve a noxious stimulus can prevent pressure ulcers. Patients who are comatose or severely demented, or who are insensate (e.g. patients with SCI), are at increased risk. Spasticity, contractures, immobility, incontinence, cachexia, diabetes, and advanced age also increase risk. It has been suggested that patients with darkly pigmented skin are at higher risk, because non-blanching erythema of stage 1 pressure ulcers might not be visible on casual inspection.[120]

The most common sites of pressure ulcer formation are the ischium (28%), the sacrum (17–27%), the trochanter (12–19%), and the heel (9–18%). A case history of a sacral pressure ulcer on a geriatric patient is provided in Figure 33-3. Sacral and trochanteric pressure ulcers are also common in patients with SCI. The pressure ulcer staging system is illustrated in Figure 33-4. For the interested reader, there are two excellent guidelines for pressure ulcer assessment and treatment,[7,47] the more recent focusing on pressure ulcers in the setting of SCI.

Treatment

The mainstay of pressure ulcer treatment is good medical and nursing care, including continence care. In the long-term care setting or at home, the debilitated or partially dependent patient with a pressure ulcer should be turned every 2 h.[109] The 90° (lateral decubitus) position should be avoided, however, because

Table 33-2 Advantages, disadvantages, and examples of dressing types[65a]

Product type	Structure	Advantages	Disadvantages	Examples[1]
Composites	Combine physically distinct components into one dressing; include an adhesive border	Well reimbursed Absorbent May be used on infected wounds Easy to apply and remove	Require a border of intact skin for anchoring the dressing	Alldress (Molnlycke Health Care) Telfa Island (Tyco Healthcare/Kendall) 3M Tegaderm Plus Pad Transparent Dressing with Absorbent Pad (3M Health Care)
Antimicrobials	Release ionic silver or polyhexamethylene biguanide to reduce bacterial virulence	Provide a broad range of antibacterial activity Reduce infection	May cause staining, stinging, or sensitization Expensive, not covered by all payers	Acticoat Antimicrobial Dressing (Smith & Nephew Wound Management) Contreet Foam Cavity Dressing with Silver (Coloplast Corp.) Telfa AMD (Tyco Healthcare/Kendall)
Specialty absorptives	Unitized, multilayered fibers of absorbent cellulose, cotton, or rayon; gauze dressings of this type	Very absorbent Can be used as secondary dressings Semi- or non-adherent Easy to apply and remove May have an adhesive border	May not be appropriate as a primary dressing for deep or undermining wounds	Tendersorb Wet-Pruf Abdominal Pads (Tyco Healthcare/Kendall) Primapore Specialty Absorptive Dressing (Smith & Nephew Wound Management) BreakAway Wound Dressing (Winfield Laboratories Inc.)
Alginates	Packaged dry; derived from brown seaweed; absorb up to 20 times their own weight	Very absorbent Fill in dead space Easy to apply and remove	Can dehydrate the wound bed Require a secondary dressing	Aquacel Hydrofiber Wound Dressing (ConvaTec) Sorbsan (Bertex Pharmaceuticals) 3M Tegagen HI Alginate Dressing (3M Health Care)
Foams	Foam of polyurethane, silicone, etc.	Very absorbent May repel contaminants May be used under compression	Not effective for dry wounds May macerate periwound skin if saturated No adhesive; requires secondary dressing for fixation	Allevyn Adhesive Hydrocellular Polyurethane Dressings (Smith & Nephew Wound Management) Mepilex Border Self-adherent Soft Silicone Foam Dressing (Molnlycke Health Care) PolyMem (Ferris Mfg Corp.) 3M Foam Dressing (3M Health Care)
Wound fillers	Beads, pastes, powders, gels, and pads; they absorb several times their weight in exudates	Very absorbent, reduces odor Promote autolytic debridement Easy to apply and remove Fill dead space	Not recommended for use in dry wounds Require secondary dressing	FlexiGel Strands Absorbent Wound Dressing (Smith & Nephew Wound Management) Iodoflex Pad or Iodoflex Gel (Healthpoint) Multidex Maltodextrin Wound Dressing Gel or Powder (DeRoyal)

Continued on page 693

Continued from page 692 Table 33-2   Advantages, disadvantages, and examples of dressing types[a]

Product type	Structure	Advantages	Disadvantages	Examples[1]
Collagens	Sheets, pads, particles, and gels	Promote granulation Absorbent Maintain a moist environment May combine with topical agents	Not recommended for black wounds Require a secondary dressing	BCG Matrix Wound Dressing (Brennen Medical Inc.) Fibracol Plus Collagen Wound Dressing with Alginate (Johnson & Johnson Wound Management) Kollagen-Medifil Pads (Biocore Medical Technologies Inc.) Promogran Matrix (Johnson & Johnson Wound Management)
Contact layers	Thin, porous interface between wound and dressing	Can protect the fragile wound base May be applied beneath topical medications, wound fillers, or gauze dressings for easy removal	Not recommended for stage 1 pressure ulcers or dry wounds Require a secondary dressing	Mepitel Soft Silicone Wound Contact Layer (Molnlycke Health Care) Profore Wound Contact Layer (Smith & Nephew Wound Management) Silon-TSR Temporary Skin Replacement (Bio-Med Sciences Inc.)
Hydrocolloids	Occlusive hydroactive wafers, beads, pastes, or granules; form gel on contact with wound	Provide minimal to moderate absorption Promote autolytic debridement Self-adhesive and protective May be used under compression products	Not for infection, heavy exudates, or high percentage eschar Not for exposed tendon or bone May injure fragile skin on removal Not for most stage 3 or 4 wounds	Comfeel Plus Hydrocolloid Ulcer Dressing (Coloplast Corp.) DuoDerm SignaDress (ConvaTec) Exuderm (Medline Industries Inc.) Replicare Hydrocolloid Dressing (Smith & Nephew Wound Management)
Hydrogels	Glycerin- and water-based products for wound hydration	Provide minimal to moderate absorption Facilitate autolytic debridement Fill in dead space (hydrogel gauzes) Easy to apply and remove	Some require secondary dressing Dehydrate easily if not covered Some may be difficult to secure Some may cause maceration	CarraSmart Gel Wound Dressing with Acemannan Hydrogel (Carrington Laboratories Inc.) ClearSite Hydrogel Wound Dressing (Conmed Corp.) Curagel (Tyco Healthcare/Kendall) Dermagran Hydrophilic Wound Dressing (Derma Sciences Inc.) Vigilon Primary Wound Dressing (Bard Medical Division, CR Bard Inc.)
Transparent films	Semipermeable polyurethane membrane dressings; transparent and waterproof	For wounds with minimal drainage Retain moisture Facilitate autolytic debridement Allow wound observation Do not require secondary dressings	Not indicated for infected wounds, nor on fragile skin Require a border of intact skin May be difficult to apply and handle May dislodge in high-friction areas	Bioclusive Transparent Dressing (Johnson & Johnson Wound Management) Mefilm (Molnlycke Health Care) Opsite (Smith & Nephew Wound Management) 3M Tegaderm Transparent Dressing (3M Healthcare)

[a]*Note that no single product provides optimum coverage for all wounds. Therefore practitioners are urged to understand dressing characteristics and functions. This table is not intended as an exhaustive list, nor does it imply endorsement of any product.*

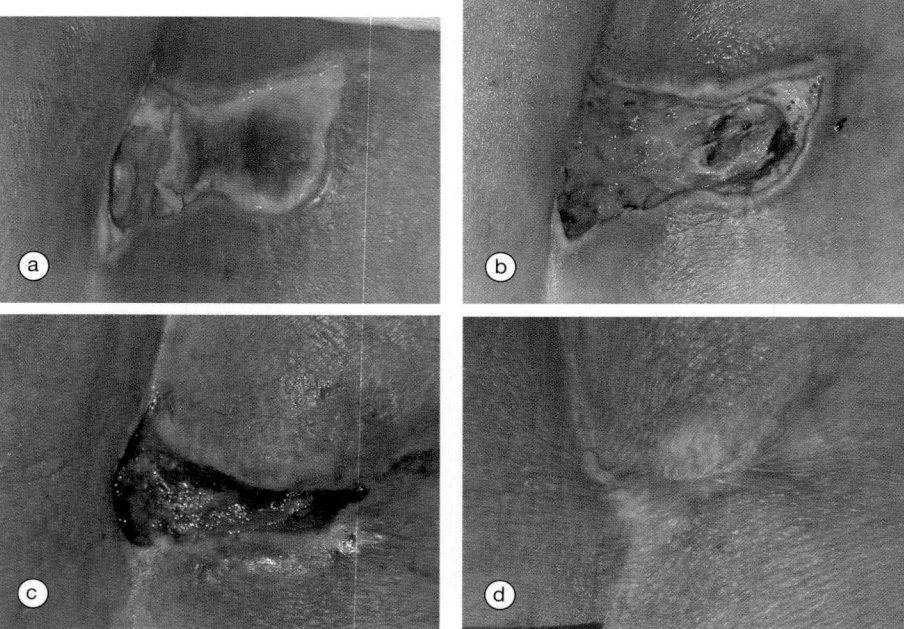

Figure 33-3 The course toward healing for a 66-year-old woman with type 2 diabetes mellitus, who developed a stage 3 sacral pressure ulcer during a prolonged acute hospitalization for bilateral iliofemoral bypass complicated by congestive heart failure. On initial evaluation, 2 months postoperatively, the wound had foul odor and was covered with yellow–green eschar laterally; wound size was 4 by 8 cm and 2.5 cm deep (**a**). The patient received a pressure-relieving surface, nutritional interventions, two sharps debridements, and saline:dilute Betadine (1:100) wet to dry. (**b**) The wound 3 weeks post initial evaluation, after the second sharps debridement. After this, topical treatment included papain–urea–chlorophyllin copper complex (Panafil) with a specialty adsorptive (ABD) and overlying composite (Alldress), changed daily at first. Nine weeks later, the wound is actively contracting (**c**). With contraction, the wound reached 95% closure 28 weeks after initial evaluation, but took an additional 12 weeks to achieve full closure (**d**).

of high pressures against trochanters. Much lower pressures are recorded for the 30° side-lying positions, between which patients should be transferred during position changes.[28] Wound area, depth, undermining, and appearance should be assessed at least weekly, and treatment modified as necessary to maintain healing rate. Nutrition is a critical issue for patients with pressure ulcers (see the *Nutrition* section of this chapter). Total enteral nutrition should be considered if p.o. intake is inadequate and likely to remain so.

Pressure ulcers with necrosis or fibrin must be periodically debrided (e.g. sharps, mechanical, or enzymatic). Deep wounds should be irrigated. For example, irrigation can be done at the bedside with a 50-mL syringe having a 19-gauge Angiocath, and using normal saline. After irrigation, all 'dead space' should be loosely packed. Significant drainage is managed with foams, alginates, or specialty absorptives at an adequate change schedule, so that the dressing can be moist but not soaked. Once drainage is minimal to moderate, and the wound is completely granulating, hydrogels are appropriate. Without an underlying absorptive layer, hydrocolloids (e.g. Duoderm) are appropriate by themselves for stage 2 ulcers or small, clean, stage 3 wounds.

Pressure relief in bed includes placing pillows or other cushioning between trochanteric prominences and the bed for side-lying, keeping the bed as horizontal as possible, and using heel protectors. The maximum efficiency of pressure and shear relief with beds and mattresses correlates with maximum cost (see Table 33-3). The most expensive are called pressure-relieving, because they theoretically maintain tissue interface pressure below the capillary closing pressure of 32 mmHg. Those systems with peak pressures above 32 mmHg, but that are better than hospital mattresses, are called pressure-reducing. Pressure-reducing surfaces work by utilizing air, gel, water,

or foam to passively redistribute pressure, and are referred to as 'static' types of devices. Pressure-relieving devices can also be 'dynamic' (i.e. they require an energy source to redistribute pressure). An example of a dynamic system is a low air loss (e.g. the SAR Low Air Loss Mattress System). Pressure-relieving, dynamic systems are required for high-risk patients (e.g. those with complete SCI) who cannot turn themselves off the ulcerated surface (i.e. they need assistance for bed mobility).

Seating systems for wheelchairs are issued to many patients who lack protective sensation. Examples include air-filled villous cushions (e.g. Roho), contoured foam with a gel insert (e.g. Jay), or contoured foam (e.g. polyurethane) on a solid seat wheelchair. Mechanical weight shift devices (i.e. tilt in space) are appropriate for patients who cannot perform weight shifts. Donut-type devices should be avoided, because they might be more likely to cause pressure ulcers than to prevent them.[27]

In a comprehensive study that included 19 889 elderly residents of 51 nursing homes, and using optimal treatment strategies, 28% of stage 3 and 20% of stage 4 ulcers were healed after 3 months of treatment, and the majority healed within 1 year.[13,111] This report, which might be regarded as a benchmark, illustrates that pressure ulcers are challenging to heal, but that healing is possible. This requires attention to wound bed preparation, pressure relief, moisture balance, and nutrition, all of which are elements of conservative, non-surgical standard care. Recent studies on adjunctive treatments have the goal of improving these outcomes. Those therapies that are commercially available and are supported by prospective randomized controlled clinical trials include electric stimulation[41,49,60] and normal temperature therapy.[131] The use of growth factor therapy platelet-derived growth factor (PDGF)-BB for pressure ulcers,

Stage I

Stage II

Stage III

Stage IV

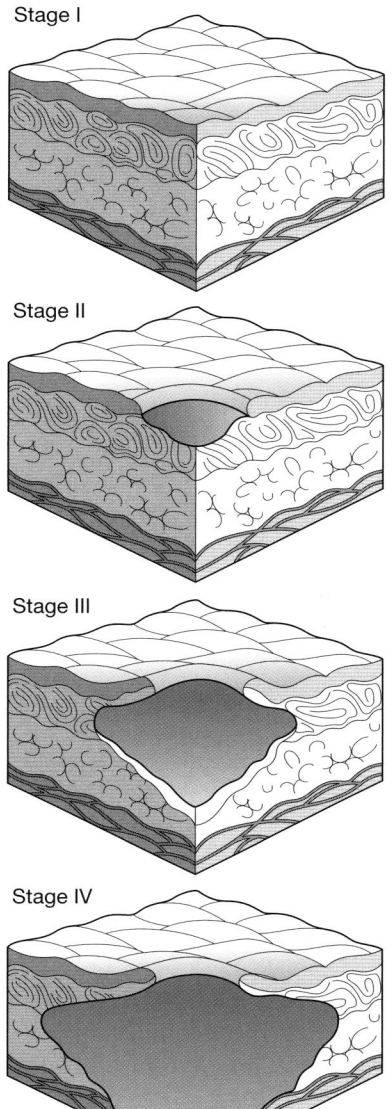

Figure 33-4 Pressure ulcer staging system. Although there is no consensus on generalizing the Shea index to leg ulcer types, for reimbursement purposes, practitioners are frequently asked to describe stasis or neuropathic wounds according to the Shea index. (Used with the permission of the National Pressure Ulcer Advisory Panel.)

Table 33-3 Advantages and disadvantages of support surfaces		
Surface	Advantages	Disadvantages
Static overlays Air	Low maintenance Inexpensive Multipatient use Durable	Can be punctured Requires proper inflation
Gel	Low maintenance Easy to clean Multipatient use Resists puncture	Heavy Expensive Little research
Foam	Lightweight Resists puncture No maintenance	Retains heat Retains moisture Limited life
Water	Readily available in the community Easy to clean	Requires heater Transfers are difficult Can leak Heavy Difficult maintenance Procedures difficult
Dynamic overlays	Easy to clean Moisture control Deflates for transfers Reusable pump	Can be damaged by sharp objects Noisy Assembly required Requires power
Replacement mattresses	Reduced staff time Multipatient use Easy to clean Low maintenance	High initial cost May not control moisture Loses effectiveness

Low air loss	Head and foot of
	  bed can be raised
	Less frequent
	  turning required
	Pressure-relieving
	Reduces shear
	  and friction
	Moisture control
		Noisy
		Difficulty with transfers
		Expensive
		Requires energy
		  source
		Restricts mobility
		Skilled set-up required
		Rental charge

Air-fluidized	Reduces shear
	  and friction
	Lowest interface
	  pressure
	Low moisture
	Less frequent
	  turning required
		Expensive
		Noisy
		Heavy
		Dehydration can
		occur
		Electrolyte imbalances
		can occur
		May cause
		  disorientation
		Difficulty with transfers
		Hot

(After Bryant 1992,[18] with permission.)		

although supported by several randomized clinical trials,[107] remains controversial.[57,96] Negative-pressure therapy (i.e. VAC therapy) is also controversial. Although there are trends in both efficacy[44] and cost-effectiveness,[130] negative-pressure therapy has not, to date, improved healing significantly in randomized prospective trials.

Prevention

There is a good argument that some pressure ulcers cannot be avoided, especially on moribund patients.[134] One large, hospital-based cohort study found that having a 'do not resuscitate' order was a consistent and significant risk factor for pressure ulcer formation.[106] Formation of multiple stage 3 and 4 pressure ulcers near the end of life has been termed skin failure.[134]

For geriatric patients with reasonable chance of long-term survival, education, inspection, and continued pressure and

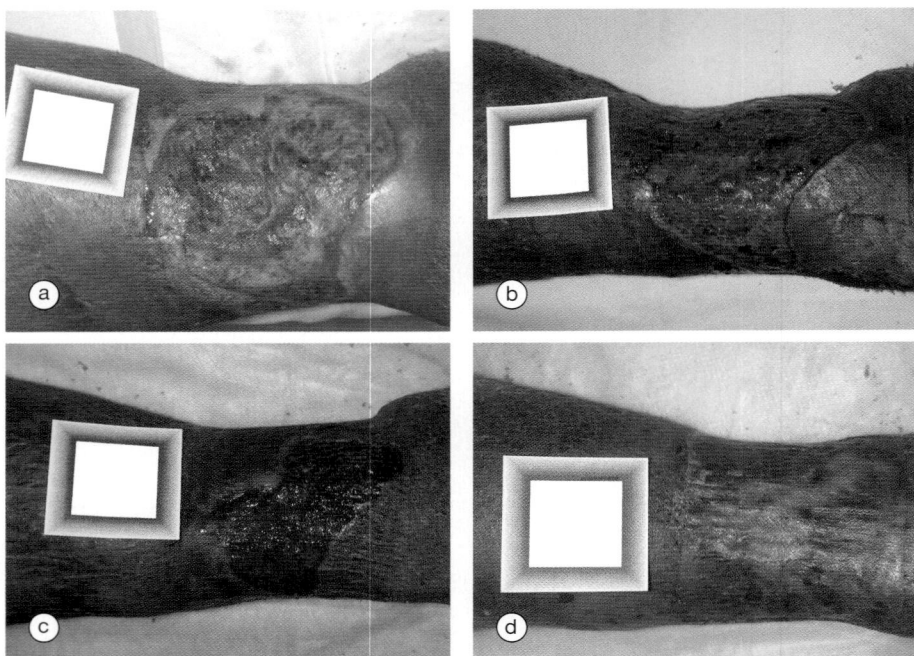

Figure 33-5 The course of healing a venous stasis ulcer of 1-year duration and area greater than 100 cm² on an 81-year-old woman with good blood flow (ankle brachial index = 1.2). On initial presentation, pain was significant (requiring 20 mg of hydrocodone per day), as was edema (+4 pitting). Dramatic edema is also evident in the initial appearance (**a**). Initial care included a course of systemic antibiotics for wound infection without systemic signs (amoxicillin–clavulanate). Topical care included silver sulfadiazine to the wound, with rolled gauze (Kerlex) and loose, long-stretch compression bandaging toe to knee (Coban, 3M), with substantial reduction of edema by week 4 of treatment (**b**). Over the first 4 weeks, to decrease eschar burden, there were twice per week curettage debridements, with daily dressing changes due to significant drainage. Also at 4 weeks and with a moderately red base, silver sulfadiazine was changed to a hydrocolloid with an overlying specialty absorptive dressing. Compression was tapered up to 1.5 rolls of Coban per leg at 4 weeks, and two rolls at 8 weeks of treatment. The wound at week 12 is illustrated (**c**). Opiate intake continued to decrease: at 12 weeks, the patient consumed 5–10 mg of hydrocodone per day, and at 16 weeks, 5 mg per week. With pain decrease, drainage also decreased, resulting in the need for dressing changes twice per week by week 20, and once per week by week 23. The wound closed by week 26 (**d**).

shear optimization are the keys to preventing the first or recurrent ulcerations. In the long-term care setting, assessments by the Norton[94] or Braden[8] scales are reliable and valid. The Braden scale might be more cost-effective,[9] and is widely used in the USA. It comprises six subscales that reflect sensory perception, skin moisture, activity, mobility, friction and shear, and nutritional status. A score of 12 or less indicates high risk, necessitating aggressive inspection, nutritional, and support surface interventions.

Surgery of greater than 4 hours' duration is associated with pressure ulcers that involve the heels and sacrum.[116] A program of risk assessment, pressure ulcer grading, pressure-reducing mattress, and an educational awareness program reduces pressure incidence by about 50% for hip fracture patients who undergo orthopedic surgery and are observed during their inpatient course.[62] Besides surgical patients, a second high-risk group is patients with SCI. An SCI consensus panel advocates education, daily skin inspection, frequent weight shifts, and pressure-reducing or relieving support surfaces for prophylaxis.[47]

Uncomplicated chronic venous ulcers
Presentation
Patients with chronic venous ulcers usually have a history of previous venous ulcer, dependent edema, previous deep venous

thrombosis, pelvic surgery or manipulation, vein stripping, vein harvest for coronary artery bypass graft, or leg graft. Peripheral pulses are typically intact (although it is sometimes difficult to palpate pulses through edematous skin). A well-granulating ulcer with irregular borders positioned about the medial malleolus is typical of saphenous vein dysfunction. Although the gator area (i.e. lower third of the leg) is typical, venous ulcers can be located anywhere on the leg, ankle, or edematous foot dorsum. Frequently associated with the venous ulcer are lower leg hyperpigmentation and a 'knobby' induration of subcutaneous tissue called lipidermosclerosis.[39]

Edema of the leg is a hallmark of venous stasis disease, and stasis ulceration is the end result of longstanding venous congestion (see Fig. 33-5 for a venous leg ulcer case history). In venous congestion, there is breakdown of the ankle pump mechanism. The ankle pump is powered by the contraction of calf muscles during gait within an unyielding leg fascial envelope, creating cyclic pressure peaks, which can reach 100 mmHg.[74] This pressure normally drives venous blood cephalad, with backflow prevented by valves within veins. Veins can become incompetent, however, due to the presence of old clot or proximal vein occlusion (e.g. from organized clot, pelvic mass, or fibrosis). This leads to gravity-induced high static pressure and loss of the ankle pump pressure cycle. Stasis from proximal organized clot is called postphlebitic syndrome.

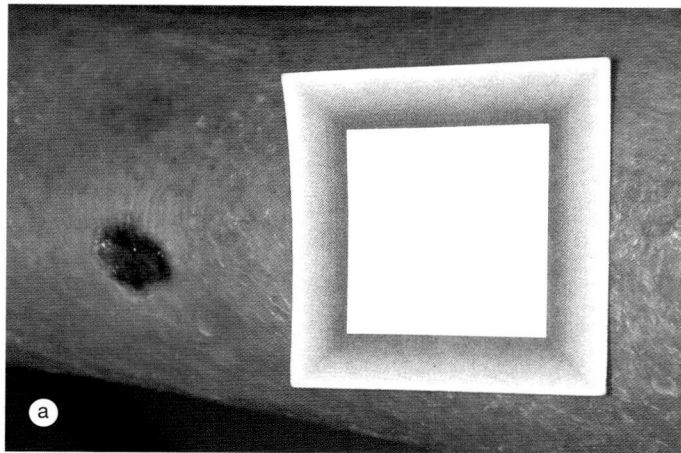

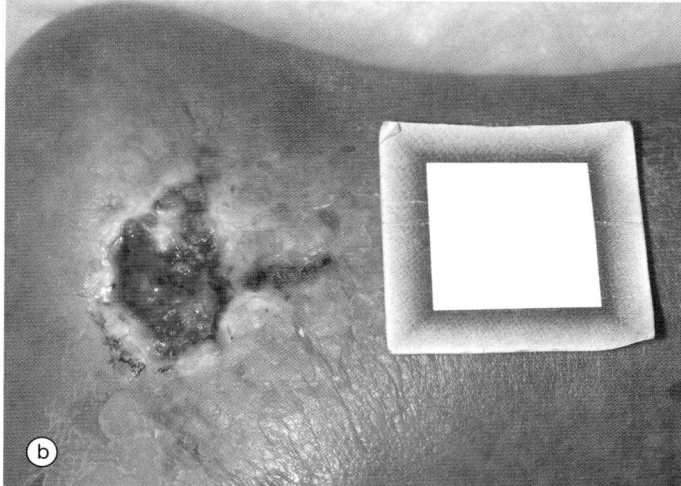

Figure 33-6 Differential diagnosis of venous stasis ulceration. Basal cell carcinoma established by 3-mm punch biopsy for posterior leg stasis-like ulcer on an elderly man with chronic obstructive pulmonary disease (**a**). Kaposi sarcoma (by wedge biopsy) on a 45-year-old man with epidemic AIDS, on his medial ankle (**b**). Both lesions were unresponsive to compression therapy.

The differential diagnosis of venous stasis ulcers includes ulcers related to congestive heart failure, lymphedema, or sickle cell anemia, for which treatment is similar to that for stasis ulceration. Other diagnoses requiring alternative treatment approaches include squamous or basal cell carcinoma, cutaneous T-cell lymphoma, Kaposi sarcoma,[127] cutaneous tuberculosis, vasculitis (i.e. such as in the setting of rheumatoid arthritis), and pyoderma granulosum. If a wound does not respond within 4–6 weeks and/or occurs on an unusual location (i.e. popliteal fossa or foot dorsum), a biopsy is indicated (Fig. 33-6).[102]

Diagnostic tests

A centerpiece of a recent venous leg ulcer guideline is pretreatment determination of ABI.[86] For a normal ABI, standard care including compression (see next paragraph) works well for most stasis ulcers. If arterial disease is suspected, segmental studies (e.g. pulse volume recordings or arterial Doppler studies) are useful to ensure that therapeutic compression is safe. $TcPO_2$ is

considered for ABI < 0.8 or where microcirculation might be impaired (e.g. in diabetes mellitus or end-stage renal disease). If the presentation warrants, venous Doppler is useful to rule out acute venous thrombosis on an urgent basis. On a routine basis, a venous duplex might confirm venous insufficiency or postphlebitic syndrome.

Treatment

Compression therapy has emerged over the centuries as the standard of care for venous stasis ulcers. Edema reduction typically results in pain reduction and wound healing. A common denominator for applying compression is application from toe to knee. There are two major types: elastic and non-elastic (utilizing long-stretch and non-stretch bandaging, respectively). Non-elastic non-stretch compression, classically the Unna paste boot, is effective.[74] Edema is reduced by the inelastic dressing, which serves as a substitute 'fascial envelope', against which calf muscles can increase pressure during ambulation and reestablish a venous ankle pump. Ambulators obtain the best edema reduction.

Elastic compression supplies compression of 30–40 mmHg continuously, depending on the elastic compression brand. Because of the 'high' static pressure, elastic dressings typically have three layers to increase tolerability:

1. a primary dressing over the wound;
2. a secondary layer of padding from toe to knee (e.g. bulky 4-inch Kerlex); and
3. an overlying long-stretch compression layer (e.g. Coban, 3M).

The entire three-layer system can be purchased as a unit (e.g. Profore). Over the counter elastic wraps (e.g. ACE) tend not to supply the adequate compression needed to heal venous ulcers, unless the patient can adhere to most of day leg elevation to waist level.

A common error in the treatment of venous ulcer is inadequate attention to drainage management, such as in the presence of infection. If infection is suspected and is being treated, compression therapy can be used with frequent dressing changes and debridements, or with primary dressings that are more efficient at collecting or 'wicking away' drainage. Frequent dressing changes are also required for draining wounds, to prevent maceration and shear.

Inadequate drainage management is a likely common reason for failure of the weekly applied Unna boot. Another disadvantage is that the Unna boot requires professional expertise to apply. An advantage is that it is durable. Another advantage is that the Unna increases interstitial leg pressure during the toe-off phase of the gait cycle as a substitute for the leg's natural ankle pump, to facilitate flow of venous blood back to the heart.[74] Because it applies transient (rather than constant) pressure, it might be the most appropriate method for mixed venous–arterial ulcers. Elastic compression is, in contrast, relatively easy to apply by lay people in the home setting (with training). Elastic compression is best for non-ambulators.

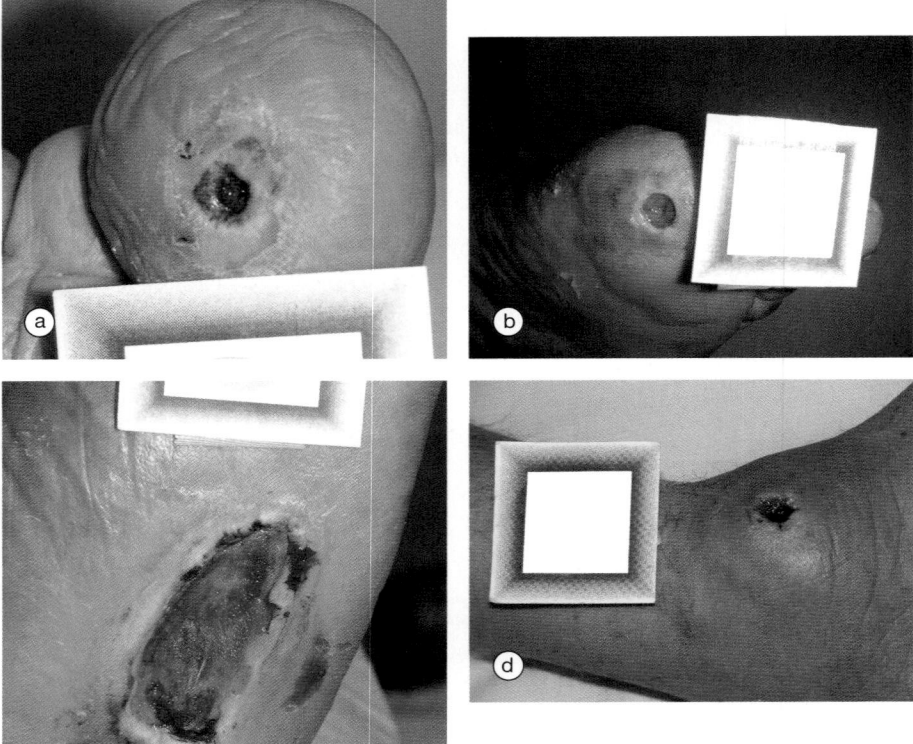

Figure 33-7 Presentations of neuropathic ulceration as circular or ovoid granular wounds surrounded by callus on weight-bearing bony prominences. For each example, weight bearing is excessive due to foot deformity such as claw toe (**a**), subluxation of first metatarsal head (**b**), and Charcot foot with calcaneal bony prominence (**c**). The patients in (a), (b), and (c) have diabetes mellitus with peripheral neuropathy and local insensitivity to the 5.07 monofilament. The patient in (**d**) is a 31-year-old with lumbar meningomyelocele, with a left medial malleolar 'fat pad' as an adaptation to ambulation on pronated feet as a child. As an adult, he no longer ambulates, but a neuropathic ulcer has occurred on this prominence due to repetitive trauma.

McGuckin et al. have incorporated the above set of treatments into a guideline that demonstrates efficacy;[87] if the guideline is not used, healing rates are four times longer and cost six times more than if it is used. With treatment consistent with this guideline, approximately 50% of ulcers heal after 12 weeks of treatment, and another 35% heal after 24 weeks.[75] Wounds that do not close typically have these characteristics in common: ulcer size greater than 10 cm², wound present more than 12 months, and ABI less than 0.8.

For intractable wounds for which the wound bed is optimally prepared,[38] living skin equivalents can be applied beneath compressive dressings with a bolster and without suturing.[33] Because of their high cost, prudence dictates that living skin equivalents should be reserved for venous ulcers that remain open for an extended period despite the best conservative treatment as outlined above.

Prevention: compression stockings
Once venous ulcers heal, the patient remains at risk for recurrence, because the underlying venous or fascial anatomic defect remains. Compression must be a lifelong habit. Compression garments (e.g. Jobst and Juzo) look like stiff stockings, and come in many sizes, colors, and pressures. Most patients do well with 20- to 30-mmHg pressure. If adherent patients ulcerate at the 20- to 30-mmHg level, they are prescribed the 30- to 40-mmHg level. By this stepwise approach, only a few patients require 40- to 50-mmHg compression. Most garments are off the shelf, and only very obese patients or those with unusual-shaped legs (i.e. post trauma) require custom stockings. Several pairs of stockings should be purchased to allow washing, and stockings should be replaced at 6-month intervals. Patient education and 'buy-in' are key to long-term ulcer prevention, and follow-up at 6-month intervals might maximize adherence.

Uncomplicated neuropathic ulcers
Presentation
Neuropathic or 'insensate' foot ulcers can occur as a result of neuropathy of any cause (e.g. diabetes, leprosy[23]) or congenital sensory neuropathy (e.g. hereditary sensory motor neuropathy type 2, lumbar meningomyelocele). The most common type in the USA, however, is neuropathy secondary to diabetes mellitus (see Fig. 33-7). The sensorimotor neuropathy of diabetes is a 'dying back' distal neuropathy leading to preferential denervation atrophy of intrinsic foot muscles. This results in an unbalanced pull of long flexors and extensors, leading to pes cavus, claw toes, and subluxation of the metatarsal heads. This 'intrinsic minus' deformity increases the pressure on bony prominences on already insensate feet. Insensitivity most often affects the plantar forefoot first, so neuropathic ulcers commonly affect plantar toes, hallux, or metatarsal heads. Neurotrophic

osteoarthropathy, or Charcot foot, frequently causes midfoot collapse and plantar-grade subluxation of the navicular or cuboid, leading to especially problematic neuropathic midfoot ulcers.[61]

The physical examination of an uncomplicated ulcer typically shows peripheral pulses to be intact, but sensation is diminished or absent in the vicinity of the ulcer, as measured by the Simmes 5.07 monofilament. Ulcers most frequently are located on bony prominences of the plantar metatarsals, midfoot, or heel. Ulcers can also be associated with digital abnormalities such as claw toes or hallux rigidus. Ulcers usually have regular borders and exuberant surrounding callus (see Fig. 33-7 for examples of neuropathic ulcers). Sensory neuropathy and high plantar pressures (greater than 6 kg/cm^2) are independently associated with ulceration in a diverse diabetic population.[45]

Diagnostic tests

Segmental arterial pressures, including toe pressures, are often used to assess perfusion. If equivocal, TcPO$_2$ can prognosticate healing as long as hyperkeratotic skin is avoided (e.g. plantar foot). If there is clinical suspicion of osteomyelitis, magnetic resonance imaging (MRI) or combined indium–leukocyte bone scan is useful before initiating conservative treatment.

Treatment

Treatment strategies involve 'off-weighting' the ulcer, which reduces mechanical irritation, inflammation, and edema and promotes healing. Neuropathic patients do not feel pain on ambulation, and hence can be challenged to adhere to weight-bearing restrictions. Limited weight bearing must be implemented after a complete physiatric assessment. This assessment should result in prescriptions for appropriate orthoses, assistive devices, weight relief shoes, physical therapy, and limited weight bearing.

Local care of neuropathic ulcers follows general 'good wound care' principles. The moist wound environment can be maintained by antibiotic ointments, such as mupirocin (Bactroban), or a hydrogel. Debridement (i.e. saucerization) is also employed on a weekly or biweekly basis (see under *Debridement*).

Using standard methods, about 24% of wounds are healed at 12 weeks, and 31–47% at 20 weeks.[80] Factors positively associated with healing are area less than 2 cm^2 and duration at time of presentation of less than 2 months.[77] The disappointing results with standard care have prompted many clinicians to seek other alternatives for their patients with neuropathic wounds.

A very effective, time-honored treatment for recalcitrant neuropathic ulcers with good circulation, which many consider the gold standard, is total contact casting.[23,92] The total contact cast has very little padding, usually only around the toes, the malleoli, and the tibial crest. Pressure is distributed axially by virtue of the custom contour of the set plaster. There is no shear, because there is no space inside the cast in which to move. The total contact cast is contraindicated where TcPO$_2$ is less than 35 mmHg or ABI is less than 0.45 in the affected leg.[64]

The effectiveness of the total contact cast has been documented in clinical trials. An open-labeled, controlled trial revealed that in the casting group 90% of neuropathic ulcers healed during 12 weeks of observation. This is in contrast to a conventional treatment group, in which 26% ($P < 0.05$) healed in the same period.[92] Although results using casting are impressive, the cast is a time-consuming, labor-intensive, expensive, and technically challenging process. Even in specialized centers, the technique might be best reserved until other, simpler methods fail to be effective (i.e. the healing rate drops to zero).

Because of the difficulties associated with casting, simpler off-loading techniques are commonly used. These include the healing shoe, the forefoot relief shoe (i.e. 'half shoe'), the removable cast walker, and the DH walker. The DH walker is a well-padded, knee-high 'boot' with a unique insole. The insole comprises hundreds of removable hexagonal pieces, each of which moves freely in multiple directions to reduce shear pressure. For wounds at the toes or metatarsal heads, the DH walker can be just as effective as the total contact cast.

Healing shoe insoles have prominences proximal to, or surrounding, plantar ulcers to relieve high axial pressure. If prepared by trained professionals, healing shoes can be effective in healing digital plantar ulcers. The IPOS forefoot relief shoe (half shoe) reduces axial pressure to forefoot ulcers, as the forefoot is 'hanging in space'. The half shoe, if used as directed, can be effective, but not quite as effective as the total contact cast. In a prospective trial, after 12 weeks of observation, 58.3% and 89.5% of wounds healed, respectively.[5] One problem with healing shoes, half shoes, and walker boots is that they are removable: patients tend to 'cheat', and only a few steps taken without them can defeat healing.[23]

An alternative and very novel strategy is recombinant growth factor technology. Regranex, a formulation of recombinant PDGF, BB isoform (rh-PDGF-BB), has been approved by the FDA for healing of foot ulcers of neuropathic and diabetic etiologies. In a randomized, prospective, double-blind, placebo-controlled trial and after 20 weeks of treatment, 45% of wounds closed in the rh-PDGF-BB group, compared with 25% closure for the standard care group.[121] Application of Regranex is straightforward (topical, once per day, alternated with standard topical care). Disadvantages include the expense ($400 per tube) and storage problems (it must be kept refrigerated). Because of the requirement for daily application, it cannot be used with casting, which is arguably a much more effective technique based on the evidence. However, if a patient with a well-perfused neuropathic ulcer cannot be casted, topical PDGF-BB might be a good choice.

Another method is application of living skin equivalent. Skin equivalents can be used with total contact casting. Where casting is to be done on an immunosuppressed patient with an expected slow healing rate, a living skin equivalent should be considered.

Prevention

The most cost-effective predictor of risk of neuropathic ulceration is testing with the 5.07 Simmes–Weinstein monofilament test. If positive, the subject is at risk of an initial wound or a recurrence. Neuropathic ulcers often recur without periodic follow-up,[21] and by not prescribing orthopedic Oxford shoes. Even if the shoe prescription is filled correctly so that axial pressure and shear are minimized, there is a recurrence rate of up to 30% per year, even with good compliance.[93] Recurrence rates are at least double for patients who refuse to wear prescription shoes.[22,34] Every effort should be made to optimize the shoe prescription.

During the period of skin maturation, a shoe prescription can be filled by a certified pedorthist. A pedorthist has been specifically trained and certified in making specialty shoes, and is well versed in insole and outsole modifications. A typical accommodative shoe prescription is for 'orthopedic Oxford shoes with high toe box, removable PPT–Plastizote insoles and modified rocker bottom'. Each element is important.[68] For example, rocker bottoms reduce pressure at the metatarsal heads.[6] Insoles should be replaced at 3-month intervals (due to tendency to 'bottom out'), and shoes at 1-year intervals. Patient education involves daily inspection of the feet and legs to make sure there are no ecchymoses or excessive callus, which are harbingers of reulceration. Emollients, such as lanolin or Lac-Hydrin, help prevent the drying and cracking of skin, especially between toes, that can be portals for entry of infection.[89] A professional (e.g. podiatrist) should perform nail and callus debridements every 2–3 months on routine follow-up.

Ischemic ulcers

Presentation
Patients with ischemic ulcers usually have peripheral arterial disease, i.e. calcification, stenosis, or blockage of named arteries anywhere from the aortic bifurcation to the plantar and digital arteries. Peripheral arterial disease and cardiovascular disease have similar risk factors:[66] hypertension, diabetes, smoking, family history, and hypercholesterolemia. In addition to arteriosclerosis, patients with ischemic wounds (including those with diabetes and end-stage renal disease) have 'small vessel' or microcirculation abnormality, contributing to local hypoxia. Classic ischemic symptoms such as claudication are very uncommon,[66] partially because patients with ischemic ulcers are very often low-level ambulators, and/or they have peripheral neuropathy.

Ischemic leg and foot ulcers are of multiple subtypes: 'pure', postsurgical, venous, pressure, or neuroischemic. Neuroischemic ulcers (i.e. neuropathy is present) typically occur at areas of trauma or transient repeated pressure. However, neuroischemic ulcers do not occur on the plantar surface, but on the foot margins (e.g. lateral heel, lateral fifth metatarsal head, and medial hallux).[104] Also occurring at the foot margins are pressure-related ischemic wounds. A particularly common scenario seen in the rehabilitation setting is pressure necrosis of the lateral heel margins (which press against the hospital mattress during prolonged immobility and/or on the operating table).

A postsurgical ischemic wound can occur due to dehiscence of an amputation site incision within an ischemic region, such as at a digital or transtibial amputation site. Venous ischemic wounds can occur anywhere on the leg and foot, and are associated with edema or venous insufficiency (see Fig. 33-8 for examples of ischemic ulcers). Pure ischemic ulcers occur in the setting of acute proximal arterial blockage, distal emboli, or macro- or microangiopathy not otherwise classified (see Fig. 33-2).

Ischemic ulcers tend to be exceedingly painful for sensate patients, and are exacerbated by leg elevation and relieved by dependency. Some patients with painful ischemic ulcers are able to sleep only in the sitting position. In addition to wound pain, the skin over the affected area is hairless and appears friable. The ischemic ulcer frequently has a blanched base and 'punched out' appearance, and is painful to probe, and the area surrounding the ulcer might have a bright or dusky red hue that has been termed *ischemic livedo*. The color can be purple or black, signaling the onset of gangrene. The onset of gangrene or cellulitis requires surgical referral.

Diagnostic tests
Vascular studies are critical to establish a prognosis for conservative healing. Pulse volume recordings might show an asymmetric low, and an ABI < 0.4 is not uncommon and tends to carry a poor prognosis. A useful definition of ischemia is periwound $TcPO_2$ < 20mmHg.[54] Healing requires getting more oxygen to the wound.

Treatment
The healing course of ischemic wounds is highly variable, much more than might be expected for other wound types. They might slowly heal, be quasistable for an indefinite period, or aggressively expand. Ischemic wounds that expand eventually can lead to deep soft tissue infection, osteomyelitis, and limb loss.[55] An ischemic wound typically has periwound $TcPO_2$ <20 mmHg,[98] with the most hypoxic wounds (i.e. $TcPO_2$ <10 mmHg) typically demonstrating the most ominous course. A particularly aggressive form of cutaneous gangrene is calciphylaxis, an unusual and grave condition noted in the setting of renal osteodystrophy[83] in a dialysis patient.

If the wound is truly ischemic, a vascular surgical referral is needed to determine if proximal flow can be reestablished by angioplasty or bypass. The outcome in terms of healing and limb salvage is much more favorable with than without revascularization.[125] Whether or not the surgical consultant concludes that bypass or angioplasty is indicated, non-invasive methods contribute immeasurably to reversal of area expansion and even healing. Conservative, non-surgical, standard wound care must be optimized, including liberal use of padding and weight relief strategies. However, the usual guidelines concerning the moist wound environment do not hold for ischemic wounds. Many have advocated keeping ischemic wounds dry in an effort to avoid 'wet gangrene'. Others use dilute Betadine, which is a strong antimicrobial and desiccating agent. There is a good argument to use silver sulfadiazine sparingly (an eschar-softening agent, broad-spectrum antimicrobial, usually well tolerated) on ischemic wounds for which the goal is healing but around which ischemia has not yet resolved.[85,90]

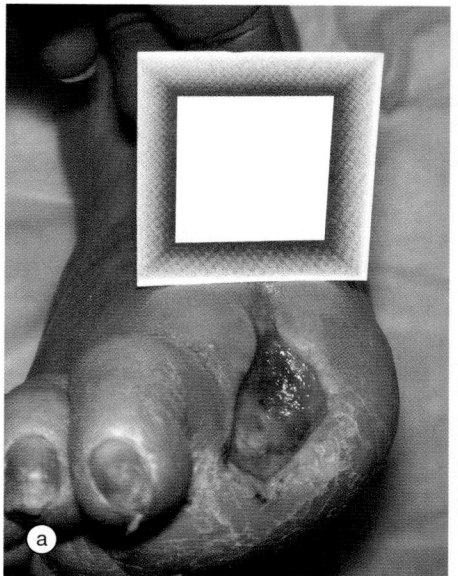 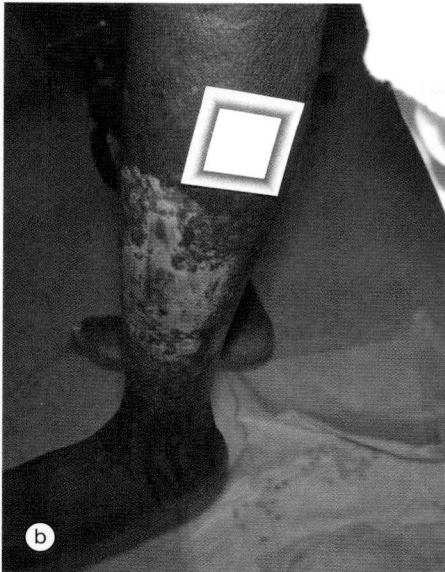 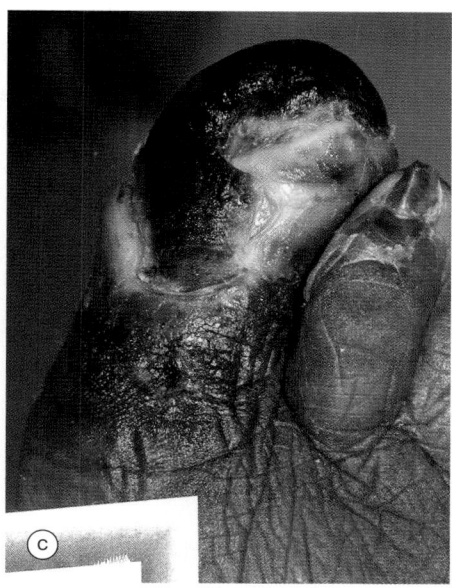

Figure 33-8 Examples of ischemic ulcers. (**a**) An ischemic postsurgical wound on a 70-year-old man with adult-onset diabetes and peripheral neuropathy, who presented with hallux gangrene and an occluded femoral–popliteal bypass. (**b**) A stasis ischemic wound on an elderly nursing home resident, which responded to leg elevation rather than compression. (**c**) An ischemic hallux on an elderly woman with end-stage renal disease. For each case, initial periwound TcPO$_2$ was less than 10 mmHg; each patient had documented peripheral arterial disease, and each ultimately healed, coincident with increase of TcPO$_2$ out of ischemic range. In addition to standard care, the patient in (c) received a 24-week course of daily high volt pulsed current (HVPC) electrotherapy; the patient in (a) received 4 weeks of hyperbaric oxygen, and then 28 weeks of HVPC.

Techniques that address pathomechanics are critical, and involve optimizing gait mechanics, with limited weight bearing to or near the ischemic wound (i.e. limited weight bearing with an assist device). Overly aggressive rehabilitation of a patient with an ischemic wound can be detrimental. For instance, consider the common scenario of a patient with a 'black heel' undergoing preprosthetic inpatient rehabilitation. (A black heel should be considered ischemic until proven otherwise.) Progressive ambulation that involves 'hopping' and repetitive trauma on the ischemic heel wound could worsen inflammation, pain, and ischemia, and cause wound expansion and loss of the second limb. In this case, the short-term goal might best be downgraded to transfers. A useful commandment is 'Thou shalt not walk on a black heel'.

The evidence base is expanding for non-invasive techniques to promote oxygenization and blood flow to ischemic wounds. These treatments are intended for patients for whom revascularization does not lead to healing, who experience graft failure, or who are not revascularization candidates due to multiple high-risk comorbidities. Currently available treatments include hyperbaric oxygen, the circulator boot, and high volt pulsed current (HVPC) electrotherapy. HVPC has been shown in case series,[52,53] a controlled retrospective trial,[55] and a small prospective randomized study[54] to prevent area expansion and promote healing of non-surgical ischemic wounds. Positive outcomes are associated with long-lasting resolution of hypoxia according to serial TcPO$_2$ determination (see Fig. 33-9).

TcPO$_2$ can be helpful in assessing which patients will respond to systemic hyperbaric oxygen treatment.[118] Hyperbaric oxygen treatment typically involves a series of daily 'dives' in 100% oxygen at 2 atmospheres for a 4- to 6-week period. A sea-level air TcPO$_2$ < 15 mmHg combined with an in-chamber TcPO$_2$ < 400 mmHg predicts failure of hyperbaric oxygen therapy with reliability and a positive predictive value of 75%.[43] The circulator boot has been suggested as efficacious on the basis of a large uncontrolled retrospective case series.[31]

Prevention

Prevention of ischemic wounds requires a high index of suspicion. For ischemic wounds with a neuropathic, pressure, or venous component, similar guidelines apply as for uncomplicated wounds of these respective types. For prevention of ischemic pressure wounds, the Braden scale is helpful but might not predict formation of ischemic heel wounds. Frequent skin checks and vigilance are required. Post healing of venous ischemic wounds, careful attention should be paid to compression pressure to avoid necrosis (i.e. use 5- to 10-mmHg anti-embolism stockings, or 10- to 20-mmHg compression hose, rather than 20- to 30-mmHg stockings). Cigarette smoking lowers TcPO$_2$,[123] which complicates healing of chronic wounds

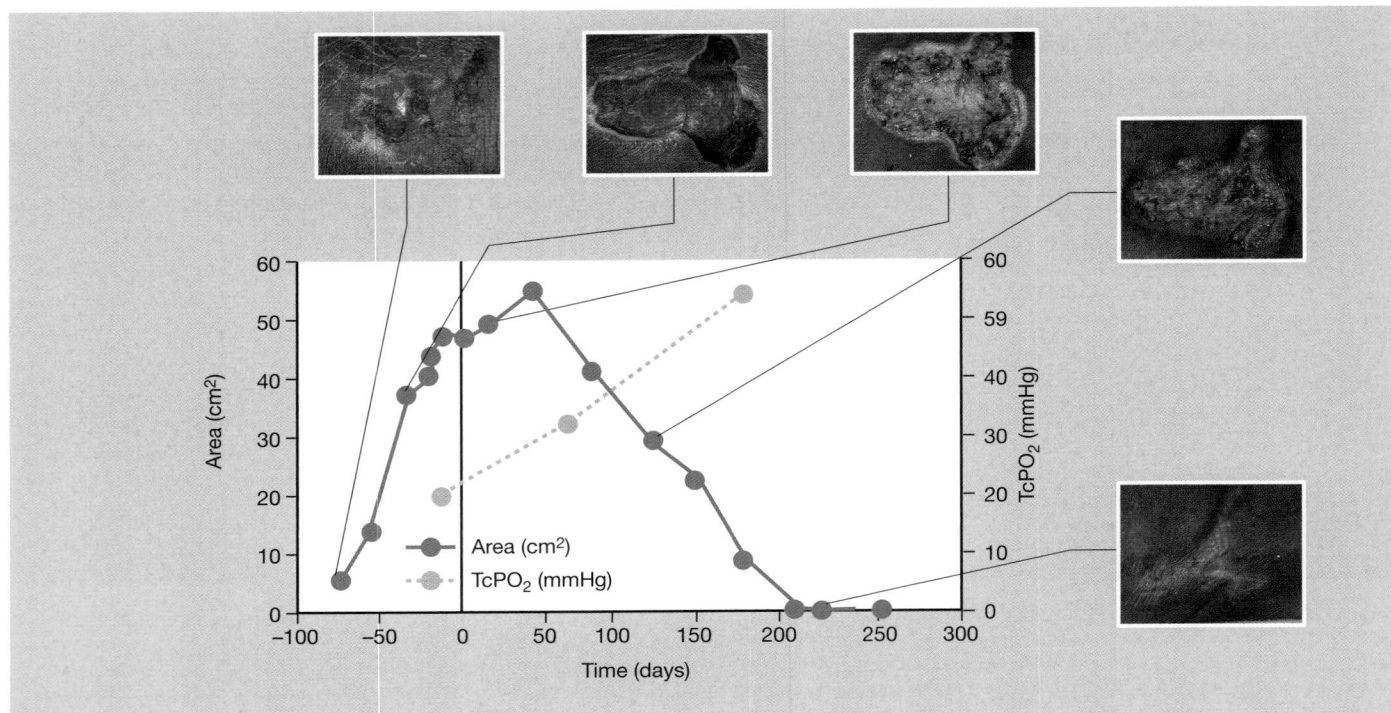

Figure 33-9 A dramatic example of area expansion of ischemic wounds.[52] This wound is on the posterior leg of a 68-year-old woman with end-stage renal disease on hemodialysis (biopsy negative for calciphylaxis). Simultaneously, the patient developed an ipsilateral heel wound that expanded and healed in similar fashion. Two months prior, the patient developed a contralateral ischemic calf ulcer that necessitated transfemoral amputation. Both wounds contralateral to the transfemoral amputation were treated with daily high volt pulsed current (HVPC), beginning at the vertical line of the graph. The graph reveals reversal of area expansion coincident with the start of HVPC (solid line), with subsequent normalization of $TcPO_2$ (dotted line). (Used with permission of Lippincott Williams & Wilkins.)

(especially ischemic wounds) and makes recurrence more likely.

INFECTION, SURGICAL REPAIR, AND THE TRANSITION FROM OUTPATIENT TO ACUTE INPATIENT MANAGEMENT

Presentation

It is critical to make the distinction between wounds that are static (i.e. healing 'arrest') because they are critically colonized or locally infected, and those associated with frank tissue invasion with systemic signs and symptoms of infection. Patients with systemic infection benefit from hospitalization, close monitoring, and intravenous antibiotics. Oral antibiotics, debridement, and topical therapies best manage locally infected wounds. The signs of local infection are increased pain, friable granulation tissue, wound breakdown (i.e. small openings in newly formed epithelial tissue not caused by reinjury or trauma), and foul odor.[48] These 'secondary' signs and symptoms have better sensitivity, specificity, positive predictive, and discriminative value than the classic signs of infection (i.e. rubor, dolor, and tumor).

Systemic signs serve as useful guideposts indicating a need for hospitalization: fever, chills, sweats, nausea, vomiting, or loss of appetite; elevated or depressed temperature; elevated white count; change in mental status; and/or glucose intolerance in

patients with diabetes. For patients with diabetes or of immunosuppressed status (e.g. patients with HIV, organ transplant recipients, and those with end-stage renal disease), there is a lower threshold for hospitalization. For venous leg ulcers, cellulitis is an indication for hospitalization when the erythema extends more than 2 cm from the ulcer margin with systemic signs. Frank purulence or abscess necessitates a surgical referral.

Soft tissue infections: wound culture, microbiology, and antibiotic therapy

Because the surfaces of all ulcers are colonized by bacteria, ulcer cultures should not be routinely performed. Cultures do not have meaning in the absence of suspected 'critical colonization' or infection. To identify the causative organism, there are five major culturing techniques: semiquantitative swab, quantitative swab, needle aspiration, curettage, and quantitative culture. Quantitative cultures are obtained by a punch biopsy. Results are described in terms of colony-forming units per gram of tissue. Many consider quantitative culture to be the gold standard. However, a high false positive rate is observed for quantitative culture of burn wounds.[85] Additionally, not all microbiology laboratories have the capability to perform the technique. Nearly all microbiology laboratories, however, can analyze swabs. Semiquantitative swabs are readily available and straightforward to use; however, they have sensitivity, specificity, and predictive value of less than 50%. Quantitative swabs are more accurate, in that they correlate with quantitative culture if wounds are prewashed before swabbing.[85]

A patient need not be diabetic or immunosuppressed to have mixed bacterial infections. Infection involving deep tissue invasion and hospitalization is almost always polymicrobial, including strict anaerobes and facultative aerobes. Aerobic organisms are usually found in surface swabs, whereas anaerobes are more often isolated from deep tissue or in larger pressure ulcers. Deep tissue isolates can reveal *Proteus mirabilis*, group B or D streptococci, *Escherichia coli*, *Staphylococcus aureus*, *Pseudomonas aeruginosa*, *Peptostreptococcus* species, *Clostridia*, and *Bacteroides fragilis*.[15] *B. fragilis* is often found in blood cultures associated with clinical sepsis. Surgical diabetic foot infections often reveal similar organisms.[19] In recent years, methicillin-resistant *S. aureus* (MRSA) and vancomycin-resistant *Enterococcus* have emerged as important virulent organisms within wounds.[85]

Debridement, antimicrobial dressings, and/or antibiotic topical agents are required for clinically infected wounds. In addition, outpatient infections are treated with broad-spectrum oral antibiotics that cover Gram-positives, Gram-negatives, and anaerobes.[20] Choices for aerobes include cephalexin, sulfamethoxazole–trimethoprim, and quinolone (e.g. ciprofloxacin or levofloxacin). For anaerobes, choices include metronidazole and clindamycin. Clindamycin also covers some Gram-positives, and can be used in simple infections as a single agent.[15] Another choice as a single agent is amoxicillin trihydrate–clavulanate potassium. For MRSA, linezolid is a member of a new antibiotic class, the oxazolidinones, and is broadly active against Gram-positive bacteria, with the advantage of being an oral agent.[122] Intravenous antibiotics for inpatient infections are typically best determined in conjunction with infectious disease or internal medicine consultants.

Osteomyelitis

Subclinical untreated osteomyelitis often leads to non-healing ulcers. Approximately 25% of all non-healing ulcers contain bone infection,[51] and osteomyelitis should be ruled out on the initial presentation if there is a reasonable suspicion. Although bone biopsy is 96% sensitive,[29] surgeons are often reluctant to perform one unless there is some other compelling indication to operate. In the outpatient setting, osteomyelitis is most easily diagnosed by imaging studies.

Imaging studies

Plain films are positive for osteomyelitis if they show reactive bone formation and periosteal elevation. Plain films are the least expensive imaging study, and have a sensitivity of 78% but a specificity of just 50%. Because of the deficiencies of plain films, test combinations have been suggested. A combination of the leukocyte count, erythrocyte sedimentation rate, and plain films provided a sensitivity of 89% and specificity of 88%. If all three test results are positive, the positive predictive value of this combination is 69%. If all are negative, the negative predic-

tive value is 96%.[29] The combination is less helpful if only one or two tests are positive.

Conventional three-phase bone scan is more sensitive for osteomyelitis than plain films, but specificity is still just 50%. Specificity is low because bone scans are poor at differentiating osteomyelitis from soft tissue infection contiguous with bone.[91] Indium leukocyte scanning has been reported to overcome this deficiency, with a sensitivity of 89%. When combined with a three-phase bone scan, the sensitivity of indium white blood cell scanning is 100%, and the specificity is 81%.[15] Radionuclide tests either singly or in combination have the drawback of not revealing anatomic detail.

Magnetic resonance imaging reveals anatomic detail, and is extremely sensitive to the presence of marrow edema on the T2-weighted image. An analysis of 11 studies investigating the diagnosis of osteomyelitis by MRI showed a sensitivity of 95% and a specificity of 88%. One study that used histopathologic findings as the gold standard found excellent predictive value, with a sensitivity of 98% and specificity of 75%.[35] Because the specificity rating of MRI is not 100%, other entities that cause marrow edema, such as resolving fracture or recent surgery, have to be considered.

Adjunctive treatment for osteomyelitis

After a surgical evaluation, with or without surgical debridement and biopsy, management of osteomyelitis includes 6 weeks of antibiotics. Such treatment for up to 12 weeks has been suggested for 'aggressive' treatment of osteomyelitis for diabetic patients.[20] For recurrent osteomyelitis or an initial presentation of osteomyelitis in an immunosuppressed patient (i.e. a transplant recipient), hyperbaric oxygen therapy is considered in parallel with intravenous antibiotics.[124] An oxygen-rich environment in bone enhances leukocytic killing and is synergistic with antibiotics.

Surgical management

The physiatrist on the 'front line' of wound care understands that many, if not most, chronic wounds heal with conservative care. Conservative care is not prudent for scenarios illustrated in the following paragraphs, however, and others as professional judgment dictates.

Surgical management of infection

At no time is the surgeon more appreciated than on presentation of a wound with frank tissue invasion, abscess, frank purulence, fistulae, or acute osteomyelitis, any of which might lead to sepsis (see Fig. 33-10). These infections require operating room debridement and culture (also see under *Debridement* above), because the infection will not resolve with antibiotics alone.

Soft tissue reconstruction

Musculocutaneous flaps are usually the best choice for stage 4 pressure ulcers of the buttocks[4] in spinal cord-injured patients, or when the concomitant loss of muscle function does not contribute to comorbidity. Tissue expanders might optimize

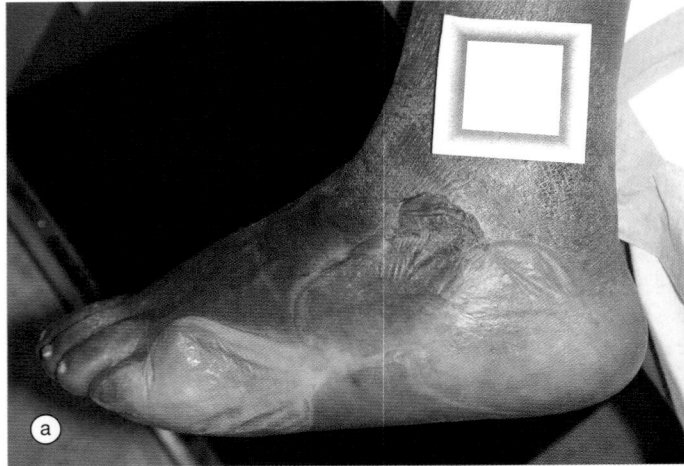

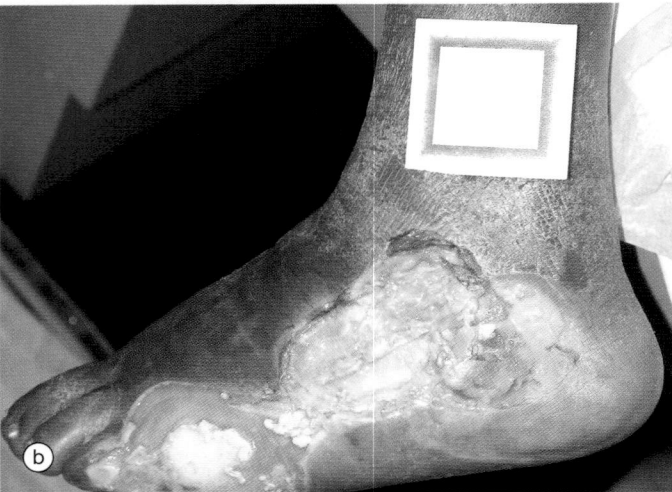

Figure 33-10 An example of a case requiring surgical referral. A 51-year-old man with L3 meningomyelocele complained of a 2-week history of chills and poor appetite. On presentation to the wound clinic, he was afebrile, with a warm, blistered erythematous foot (**a**). Podiatric surgery was immediately called. The surgeon performed a sharps debridement (**b**) and admitted the patient for treatment of abscess–cellulitis with intravenous antibiotics, surgical debridement, and split-thickness skin grafting, which ultimately achieved closure.

coverage.[12] Musculocutaneous flaps are also occasionally employed for well-vascularized pressure ulcers of the heel. Musculocutaneous flaps can help heal osteomyelitis, and limit the damage caused by shearing, friction, and pressure.[82] Split-thickness skin grafts can also be used to repair recalcitrant venous ulcers[115] and neuropathic ulcers.

In geriatric or chronically ill subjects, the benefits of reconstructive surgery might be outweighed by the risks. In addition to the risk of surgery, musculocutaneous flaps have a significant recurrence rate in ulceration, with short-term failure rate (most commonly due to suture line dehiscence) from 5% to 36%. The long-term recurrence rate can be as high as 61%.[112] Recurrence rate can be minimized by attending to mechanical factors. If the pathomechanical defect that led to ulcer in the first place is not corrected (by means of specialty shoes, orthoses, stock-ings, seating systems, or beds), the ulcer is likely to recur postoperatively.

Bone repair and reconstruction

The diabetic foot has deformities that predispose to ulceration. If the ulcer heals and then recurs several times, the orthopedic or podiatric surgeon should evaluate the patient for foot reconstruction, osteotomies, or tendon recessions.

Revascularization

Strides have been made in bypass of infrapopliteal stenoses via femoral–distal bypass.[20] Revascularization is the standard of care for patients with ischemic or gangrenous wounds, understanding that the most appropriate intervention might occasionally be non-surgical, because many high-risk patients are not candidates for arterial bypass. A less invasive option is angioplasty.

Amputation

Dysvascular amputation can be done at the digital, transmetatarsal, Symes, transtibial, or transfemoral level for rapidly expanding gangrene and/or overwhelming infection (see Chs 14 and 57). In these situations, amputation is considered 'curative'.

NUTRITION

Signs of poor nutrition include weight < 90% of ideal body weight. Laboratory markers include albumin < 3.5 g/mL and prealbumin < 15 mg/mL.[25] There is an established link between poor nutrition and pressure ulcer formation.[11]

Nutritional therapy for patients with stage 3 or 4 pressure ulcers includes:

- 30–35 kcal/kg per day;
- 1.2–1.5 g/kg per day protein by means of oral, enteral, or parenteral routes; and
- fluids 1 mL/kcal.[88]

Patients with SCI or AIDS wasting syndrome and pressure ulcers might additionally benefit from oxandrolone to build lean muscle mass. Oxandrolone is an anabolic steroid that is approved by the FDA to promote weight gain after severe physiologic stress (recommended dose of 10–15 mg/day). Oxandrolone is not, however, specifically FDA-approved for the treatment of pressure ulcers.[26]

The evidence basis for vitamin and mineral supplementation is not established for patients without specific vitamin deficits. The relative safety of these compounds, however, suggests that it is reasonable to include these in a complete wound-healing nutritional program. Arginine might enhance collagen concentration and wound breaking strength.[135]

Vitamin C is an essential nutrient in wound healing, due to its role as a cosubstrate in the hydroxylation of proline and lysine, which form collagen cross-links. When specific deficiencies are diagnosed, it is reasonable to recommend up to

750 mg/day for women and 900 mg/day for men).[24] Vitamin A deficiency results in delayed wound healing and increased susceptibility to infection, especially in patients treated with corticosteroids.[67] Zinc is a zymogen for DNA syntheses and metaloproteases. Oral zinc might have a beneficial effect on healing of venous ulcers in people with lower serum zinc level at baseline.[132] Zinc sulfate 220 mg/day is a reasonable dose.

WOUND PAIN

Wound pain bears similarities to both acute and chronic pain: chronic, because the pain is considered long lasting; acute, because the pain (with few exceptions) resolves when the wound heals. As acute pain is of moderate to severe intensity, most patients receive opiate analgesics. They make the patient comfortable, and foster sleep as well as adherence to treatment. In the absence of substance abuse history, nearly all patients easily wean off opiates after the wound heals. (For the elderly or those at fall risk, it is reasonable to prescribe non-opiate analgesics.)

The patient can be dispensed 'as needed' codeine (e.g. 30 mg), oxycodone (e.g. 5 mg), morphine sulfate (e.g. 15 mg), or hydromorphone (e.g. 2 mg), depending on the patient's history of allergies, adverse reactions, or physician preference. If the p.o. morphine-equivalent intake per day exceeds 30 mg, the physician should consider using long-acting opiates, based on opiate equivalence tables. Choices include oxycodone slow release (10 mg q 12) or morphine sulfate slow release (15 mg q 12), or fentanyl transdermal patches (a 25-μg patch applied to the skin q 3 days). Long-acting opioids avoid the high peak–low trough effect associated with on-demand dosing. 'Breakthrough' doses should follow predictable patterns, but total equivalent dose per week should gradually decrease as inflammation subsides and the wound heals. Methadone is often a good choice for a substance abuser with wound pain.

Wound pain requires an assessment scale to judge effectiveness of treatment. The most basic assessment is a numeric rating scale, which is an 11-point scale where 0 is no pain and 10 is the worst possible pain. Patients are asked to quantify their pain levels by choosing a single number from the 11-point scale.[69] The number of 'pain pills' per day consumed by the patient is a concrete and readily understood measure of patient discomfort (see Ch. 43).

WOUND CARE CENTERS

The wound care center concept is probably more than a century old, but it was not until recently that this clinic concept was widely employed. In the USA, there are currently about 700 wound care centers.[2] Wound clinics typically have multidisciplinary staff that can include physicians, podiatrists, physical therapists, nurses, and others. It is said that the ideal wound care clinic 'drives an interdisciplinary stake through institutional silos'. Close periodic follow-up of individual patients is most effective, because patients with wounds that get regular nursing follow-up have an amputation rate 40% lower than expected.[99]

The business aspects of wound care are outside the scope of this chapter. It should be noted, however, that a successful wound clinic must optimize billing practices to mirror the reality that wound care has:

- a medical decision-making component; and
- a supply and personnel (i.e. 'technical') component.

In the USA, the Center for Medicare and Medicaid Services separately reimburses the professional and the hospital. Outpatient hospital-based wound clinics, to be successful in the long term, should utilize both avenues of reimbursement.

CONCLUSION

Prevention and early, aggressive intervention are the cornerstones of chronic wound management. The 'medical' wound care outlined in this chapter can be employed by physiatrists to heal difficult wounds in the outpatient setting, with a minimum of complications, and to proactively save limbs. Chronic wound care offers new practice opportunities for physiatrists in the twenty-first century.

Acknowledgments
Our thanks to the following: Barbara Brewley, RN-C, CRC for photographs; Vista Medical Ltd. (Winnipeg, Canada) Chattanooga Group (Hixson, Tennessee) for equipment; and the National Institutes of Health (NIH 1R41HL61983-01, NIH K08HD01065-01) and University of Pennsylvania Research Foundation for grant funding.

REFERENCES
1. Ameis A, Chiarcossi A, Jimenez J. Management of pressure sores. Comparative study in medical and surgical patients. Postgrad Med 1980; 67:177–184.

2. [Anonymous]. 2005 wound care clinic directory. Malvern: American Association for the Advancement of Wound Care; 2005.

3. [Anonymous]. Healthy people 2000: national health promotion and disease prevention objectives. Washington: Department of Health and Human Services; 1991:73–117.

4. Anthony JP, Huntsman WT, Mathes SJ. Changing trends in the management of pelvic pressure ulcers: A 12-year review. Decubitus 1992; 5(3):50–51.

5. Armstrong DG, Nguyen HC, Lavery LA, et al. Off-loading the diabetic foot wound: a randomized clinical trial. Diabetes Care 2001; 24:1019–1022.

6. Bauman JH, Girling JP, Brand P. Plantar pressures and trophic ulceration: an evaluation of footware. J Bone Joint Surg 1963; 45-B:652–673.

7. Bergstrom N, Bennett MA, Carlson CE. Treatment of pressure ulcers. Rockville: Agency for Health Care Policy and Research; 1994.

8. Bergstrom N, Braden BJ, Laguzza A, et al. The Braden Scale for Predicting Pressure Sore Risk. Nurs Res 1987; 36:205–210.

9. Bergstrom N, Demuth PJ, Braden BJ. A clinical trial of the Braden Scale for Predicting Pressure Sore Risk. Nurs Clin North Am 1987; 22(2):417–428.

10. Bonham PA. Steps for determining the toe brachial pressure index. Adv Skin Wound Care 2004; 17:44–45.

11. Bourdel-Marchasson I, Barateau M, Rondeau V, et al. A multi-center trial of the effects of oral nutritional supplementation in critically ill older

inpatients. GAGE Group. Groupe Aquitain Geriatrique d'Evaluation. Nutrition 2000; 16:1–5.

12. Braddom RL, Leadbetter MG. The use of a tissue expander to enlarge a graft for surgical treatment of a pressure ulcer in a quadraplegic. Am J Phys Med Rehabil 1989; 68:70–72.

13. Brandeis GH, Morris JN, Nash DJ, et al. The epidemiology and natural history of pressure ulcers in elderly nursing home residents [comment]. JAMA 1990; 264:2905–2909.

14. Braverman IM. The cutaneous microcirculation. J Invest Dermatol Symp Proc 2000; 5:3–9.

15. Bridges RM, Deitch EA. Diabetic foot infections: pathophysiology and treatment. Surg Clin North Am 1994; 74:537–555.

16. Briggs M, Nelson EA. Topical agents or dressings for pain in venous leg ulcers. Cochrane Database Syst Rev 2003:CD001177.

17. Brown GS. Reporting outcomes for stage IV pressure ulcer healing: a proposal. Adv Skin Wound Care 2000; 13:277–283.

18. Bryant R. Acute and chronic wounds: nursing management. St. Louis: Mosby Year-book; 1992.

19. Calhoun JH, Overgaard KA, Stevens CM, et al. Diabetic foot ulcers and infections: current concepts. Adv Skin Wound Care 2002; 15:31–42, quiz 44–45.

20. Caputo GM, Cavanagh PR, Ulbrecht JS, et al. Assessment and management of foot disease in patients with diabetes. N Engl J Med 1994; 331:854–860.

21. Chantaleau E, Breuer U, Leisch AC, et al. Outpatient treatment of unilateral diabetic foot ulcers with 'half shoes'. Diabet Med 1993; 10:267–270.

22. Chantelau E, Haage P. An audit of cushioned diabetic footwear: relation to patient compliance. Diabet Med 1994; 11:114–116.

23. Coleman WC, Brand PW, Birke JA. The total contact cast: a therapy for plantar ulceration on insensitive feet. J Am Podiatry Assoc 1984: 74(11):548–552.

24. Collins N. Adding vitamin C to the wound management mix. Adv Skin Wound Care 2004; 17:109–112.

25. Collins N. The difference between albumin and prealbumin. Adv Skin Wound Care 2001; 14:235–236.

26. Collins N. The right mix: using nutritional interventions and an anabolic agent to manage a stage IV ulcer. Adv Skin Wound Care 2004; 17:38–39.

27. Crewe R. Problems of rubber ring nursing cushions and a clinical survey of alternative cushions for ill patients. Care Sci Pract 1987; 5.

28. Defloor T. The effect of position and mattress on interface pressure. Appl Nurs Res 2000; 13:2–11.

29. Deloach ED, Christy RS, Ruf LE. Osteomyelitis underlying severe pressure sores. Contemp Surg 1992; 40:25–32.

30. Dillingham TR, Pezzin LE, Mackenzi EJ. Limb amputation and limb deficiency: epidemiology and recent trends in the United States. South Med J 2002; 95:875–883.

31. Dillon RS. Fifteen years of experience in treating 2177 episodes of foot and leg lesions with the circulator boot. Results of treatments with the circulator boot. Angiology 1997; 48:S17–S34.

32. Dinsdale SM. Decubitus ulcers: role of pressure and friction in causation. Arch Phys Med Rehabil 1974; 55:147–152.

33. Eaglstein WH, Falanga V. Tissue engineering and the development of Apligraf, a human skin equivalent. Adv Wound Care 1998; 11:1–8.

34. Edmonds ME, Blundell MP, Morris ME, et al. Improved survival of the diabetic foot: the role of a specialised foot clinic. Q J Med 1986; 60:763–771.

35. Enderle MD, Coerper S, Schweizer HP, et al. Correlation of imaging techniques to histopathology in patients with diabetic foot syndrome and clinical suspicion of chronic osteomyelitis. The role of high-resolution ultrasound. Diabetes Care 1999; 22:294–299.

36. Faglia E, Favales F, Quarantiello A, et al. Angiographic evaluation of peripheral arterial occlusive disease and its role as a prognostic determinant for major amputation in diabetic subjects with foot ulcers. Diabetes Care 1998; 21:625–630.

37. Falanga V, Eaglstein WH. The 'trap' hypothesis of venous ulceration. Lancet 1993; 341:1006–1008.

38. Falanga V. Classifications for wound bed preparation and stimulation of chronic wounds. Wound Repair Regen 2000; 8:347–352.

39. Falanga V. Venous ulceration. Dermatol Surg Oncol 1993; 19:764–771.

40. Falanga V. Wound bed preparation and the role of enzymes: a case for multiple actions of therapeutic agents. Wounds 2002; 14:47–57.

41. Feedar JA, Kloth LC, Gentzkow GD. Chronic dermal ulcer healing enhanced with monophasic pulsed electrical stimulation. Phys Ther 1991; 71:639–649.

42. Ferrell BA. Assessment of healing. Clin Geriatr Med 1997; 13:575–587.

43. Fife CE, Buyukcakir C, Otto GH, et al. The predictive value of transcutaneous oxygen tension measurement in diabetic lower extremity ulcers treated with hyperbaric oxygen therapy: a retrospective analysis of 1,144 patients. Wound Repair Regen 2002; 10:198–207.

44. Ford CN, Reinhard ER, Yeh D, et al. Interim analysis of a prospective, randomized trial of vacuum-assisted closure versus the healthpoint system in the management of pressure ulcers. Ann Plast Surg 2002; 49:55–61, discussion 61.

45. Frykberg RG, Lavery LA, Pham H, et al. Role of neuropathy and high foot pressures in diabetic foot ulceration. Diabetes Care 1998; 21:1714–1719.

46. Fuhrer M, Garber S, Rintala D. Pressure ulcers in community-resident persons with spinal cord injury: prevalence and risk factors. Arch Phys Med Rehabil 1993; 74(11):1172–1177.

47. Garber SL, Biddle AK, Click CN, et al. Pressure ulcer prevention and treatment following spinal cord injury: a clinical practice guideline for health care professionals. Washington: Paralyzed Veterans of America; 2000.

48. Gardner SE, Frantz RA, Doebbeling BN. The validity of the clinical signs and symptoms used to identify localized chronic wound infection. Wound Repair Regen 2001; 9:178–186.

49. Gardner SE, Frantz RA, Schmidt FL. Effect of electrical stimulation on chronic wound healing: a meta-analysis. Wound Repair Regen 1999; 7:495–503.

50. Gilbertson D, Arneson T, Desai J, et al. Diabetes-related amputations of lower extremities in the Medicare population—Minnesota, 1993–1995. Morb Mortal Wkly Rep 1998; 47:649–652.

51. Goldman R. Pressure ulcers. In: Forciea MA, Lavizzo-Mourey R, Schwab EP, eds. Geriatric secrets. 2nd edn. Philadelphia: Hanley & Belfus; 2000:272–276.

52. Goldman RJ, Brewley BI, Cohen R, et al. Use of electrotherapy to reverse expanding cutaneous gangrene in end-stage renal disease. Adv Skin Wound Care 2003; 16:363–366.

53. Goldman RJ, Brewley BI, Golden M. Electrotherapy re-oxygenates inframalleolar ischemic wounds on diabetic patients—a case series. Adv Skin Wound Care 2002; 15:112–120.

54. Goldman RJ, Brewley BI, Golden M. Home-based electrotherapy improves healing of ischemic wounds: a phase I prospective study. Adv Skin Wound Care 2004.

55. Goldman RJ, Brewley BI, Zhou L, et al. Electrotherapy reverses inframalleolar ischemia: a retrospective, observational study. Adv Skin Wound Care 2003; 16:79–89.

56. Goldman RJ, Salcido R. More than one way to measure a wound: an overview of tools and techniques. Adv Skin Wound Care 2002; 15:236–243.

57. Goldman RJ. Update on growth factors and wound healing: past, present and future. Adv Skin Wound Care 2004; 17:24–35.

58. Goodson WH. Wound healing and aging. J Invest Dermatol 1990; 73:88–91.

59. Greenhalgh DG, Sprugel KH, Murray MH, et al. PDGF and FGF stimulate wound healing in the genetically diabetic mouse. Am J Pathol 1990; 136:1235–1245.

60. Griffin JW, Tooms RE, Mendius RA, et al. Efficacy of high voltage pulsed current for healing of pressure ulcers in patients with spinal cord injury. Phys Ther 1991; 71:433–444.

61. Grunfeld C. Diabetic foot ulcers: etiology, treatment, and prevention. Adv Intern Med 1991; 37:103–132.

62. Gunningberg L, Lindholm C, Carlsson M, et al. Reduced incidence of pressure ulcers in patients with hip fractures: a 2-year follow-up of quality indicators. Int J Qual Health Care 2001; 13:399–407.

63. Heggers JP, Haydon S, Ko F, et al. *Pseudomonas aeruginosa* exotoxin A: its role in retardation of wound healing. J Burn Care Rehabil 1992; 13:512–518.

64. Helm PA, Walker S, Pullium G. Total contact casting in diabetic patients with neuropathic foot ulcerations. Arch Phys Med Rehabil 1984; 65:691–693.

65. Hess CT. Clinical guide to wound care. 5th edn. Philadelphia: Lippincott Williams & Wilkins; 2004.

66. Hirsch AT, Criqui MH, Treat-Jacobson D, et al. Peripheral arterial disease detection, awareness, and treatment in primary care [comment]. JAMA 2001; 286:1317–1324.

67. Hunt TK. Vitamin A and wound healing. J Am Acad Dermatol 1986; 15:817–821.

68. Janisse DJ. Pedorthic care of the diabetic foot. In: Levin ME, O'Neal LW, Bowker JH, eds. The diabetic foot. 5th edn. St. Louis: Mosby Year-book; 1993:549–575.

69. Jensen MP, Turner JA, Romano JM, et al. Comparative reliability and validity of chronic pain intensity measures. Pain 1999; 83:157–162.

70. Kalani M, Brismar K, Fagrell B, et al. Transcutaneous oxygen tension and toe blood pressure as predictors for outcome of diabetic foot ulcers. Diabetes Care 1999; 22:147–151.

71. Kosiak M. Etiology and pathology of ischemic ulcers. Arch Phys Med Rehabil 1959; 40:62–69.

72. Langemo DK, Melland H, Olson B, et al. Comparison of 2 wound volume measurement methods. Adv Skin Wound Care 2001; 14:190–196.

73. Lazarus GS, Cooper DM, Knighton DR, et al. Definitions and guidelines for assessment of wounds and evaluation of healing. Arch Dermatol 1994; 130:489–493.

74. Lippmann HI, Fishman LM, Farrar RH, et al. Edema control in the management of disabling chronic venous insufficiency. Arch Phys Med Rehabil 1994; 75:436–441.

75. Lyon RT, Veith FJ, Bolton L, et al. Clinical benchmark for healing of chronic venous ulcers. Venous Ulcer Study Collaborators. Am J Surg 1998; 176:172–175.

76. Maklebust J. Pressure ulcer assessment. Clin Geriatr Med 1997; 13:455–471.

77. Margolis DJ, Allen-Taylor L, Hoffstad O, et al. Diabetic neuropathic foot ulcers: predicting which ones will not heal. Am J Med 2003; 115:627–631.

78. Margolis DJ, Bilker W, Knauss J, et al. The incidence and prevalence of pressure ulcers among elderly patients in general medical practice. Ann Epidemiol 2002; 12:321–325.

79. Margolis DJ, Bilker W, Santanna J, et al. Venous leg ulcer: incidence and prevalence in the elderly. J Am Acad Dermatol 2002; 46:381–386.

80. Margolis DJ, Kantor J, Berlin JA. Healing of diabetic neuropathic foot ulcers receiving standard treatment. A meta-analysis. Diabetes Care 1999; 22:692–695.

81. van Marum RJ, Meijer JH, Bertelsmann FW, et al. Impaired blood flow response following pressure load in diabetic patients with cardiac autonomic neuropathy. Arch Phys Med Rehabil 1997; 78:1003–1006.

82. Mathes SJ, Feng LJ, Hunt TK. Coverage of the infected wound. Ann Surg 1983; 198:420–429.

83. Mazhar AR, Johnson RJ, Gillen D, et al. Risk factors and mortality associated with calciphylaxis in end-stage renal disease. Kidney Int 2001; 60:324–332.

84. McDermott VG, Meakem JP, Carpenter JP, et al. Magnetic resonance angiography of the distal lower extremity. Clin Radiol 1995; 50:741–746.

85. McGuckin M, Goldman RJ, Bolton L, et al. The clinical relevance of microbiology in acute and chronic wounds. Adv Skin Wound Care 2003; 16:12–23.

86. McGuckin M, Stineman MG, Goin JE, et al. Venous leg ulcer guideline. Philadelphia: Trustees of the University of Pennsylvania; 1997:44.

87. McGuckin M, Waterman R, Brooks J, et al. Validation of venous leg ulcer guidelines in the United States and United Kingdom. Am J Surg 2002; 183:132–137.

88. Mechanick JI. Practical aspects of nutritional support for wound-healing patients. Am J Surg 2004; 188:52–56.

89. Miller OF. Essentials of pressure ulcer treatment: the diabetic experience. J Dermatol Surg Oncol 1993; 19:759–763.

90. Monafo WW, West MA. Current treatment recommendations for topical burn therapy. Drugs 1990; 40:364–373.

91. Morain WD, Colen LB. Wound healing in diabetes mellitus. Clin Plast Surg 1990; 17:493–501.

92. Mueller JJ, Diamond JE, Sinacore DR, et al. Total contact casting in treatment of diabetic plantar ulcers. Diabetes Care 1989; 12:384–388.

93. Myerson M, Papa J, Katulle E, et al. The total contact cast for management of neuropathic plantar ulceration of the foot. J Bone Joint Surg 1992; 74-A:261–269.

94. Norton D. Calculating the risk: reflections on the Norton Scale. Decubitus 1989; 2:24–31.

95. Olin JW, Beusterien K, Childs MB. Medical costs of treating venous stasis ulcers: evidence from a retrospective cohort study. Vasc Med 1999; 4:1–7.

96. Ovington LG. Dressings and adjunctive therapies: AHCPR guidelines revisited. Ostomy Wound Manage 1999; 45:94S–106S, quiz 107S–108S.

97. Ovington LG. Hanging wet-to-dry dressings out to dry. Adv Skin Wound Care 2002; 15:79–84.

98. Padberg FT, Back TLL, Thompson PN, et al. Transcutaneous oxygen (TcPO2) estimates probability of healing in the ischemic extremity. J Surg Res 1996; 60:365–369.

99. Partl M. After-care of patients with diabetic feet by general practitioners or special ambulatory care—effect on rate of amputation. Gesundheitswesen 1994; 56:215–219.

100. Phillips LG, Abdullah KM, Geldner PD, et al. Application of basic fibroblast growth factor may reverse diabetic wound healing impairment. Ann Plast Surg 1993; 31:331–334.

101. Phillips T. A study of the impact of leg ulcers on quality of life: financial, social, and psychologic implications. J Am Acad Dermatol 1994; 31:49–53.

102. Phillips TJ, Dover JS. Leg ulcers. J Am Acad Dermatol 1991; 25:965–985.

103. Pinzur MS, Sage R, Stuck R, et al. Transcutaneous oxygen as a predictor of wound healing in amputations of the foot and ankle. Foot Ankle 1992; 13:271–272.

104. Pitei DL, Lord M, Foster A, et al. Plantar pressures are elevated in the neuroischemic and the neuropathic diabetic foot. Diabetes Care 1999; 22:1966–1970.

105. Powell RJ, Holbrook MR, Stevens A. Pyoderma gangrenosum and its treatment [see comment]. Lancet 1720; 350:1720–1721.

106. Reed RL, Hepburn K, Adelson R, et al. Low serum albumin levels, confusion, and fecal incontinence: are these risk factors for pressure ulcers in mobility-impaired hospitalized adults? Gerontology 2003; 49:255–259.

107. Rees RS, Robson MC, Smiell JM, et al. Becaplermin gel in the treatment of pressure ulcers: a phase II randomized double-blind placebo-controlled study. Wound Repair Regen 1999; 7:141–147.

108. Reiber GE, Boyko EJ, Smith DG, eds. Lower extremity foot ulcers and amputations in diabetes. Washington: US Government Printing Office; 1997:409–428.

109. Reswick JB, Robers JE. Experience at Rancho Los Amigos Hospital with devices and techniques to prevent pressure ulcers. In: Kenedi RM, Cowden JM, Scales JT, eds. Bedsore biomechanics. London: University Park Press; 1976:300.

110. Rhodes GR. Uses of transcutaneous oxygen monitoring in the management of below-knee amputations and skin envelope injuries. Am Surg 1985; 51:701–707.

111. van Rijswijk L. Full-thickness pressure ulcers: patient and wound healing characteristics. Decubitus 1993; 6:16–21.

112. Ruan CM, Escobedo E, Harrison S, et al. Magnetic resonance imaging of nonhealing pressure ulcers and myocutaneous flaps. Arch Phys Med Rehabil 1998; 79:1080–1087.

113. Salcido R, Carney J, Fisher S. A reliable animal model of pressure sore development: the role of free radicals. J Am Paraplegia Soc 1993; 16:61.

114. Salcido R, Donofrio JC, Fisher SB, et al. Histopathology of pressure ulcers as a result of sequential computer-controlled pressure sessions in a fuzzy rat model. Adv Wound Care 1994; 7:23–4, 26, 28 passim.

115. Sanchez S, Eamegdool S, Conway H. Surgical treatment of decubitus ulcers in paraplegics. Plast Reconstr Surg 1969; 43:25–28.

116. Schoonhoven L, Defloor T, Grypdonck MHF. Incidence of pressure ulcers due to surgery. J Clin Nurs 2002; 11:479–487.

117. Shannon ML, Skorga P. Pressure ulcer prevalence in two general hospitals. Decubitus 1989; 2:38–43.

118. Sheffield PJ. Measuring tissue oxygen tension: a review. Undersea Hyperb Med 1998; 25(3):179–187.

119. Silfen R, Amir A, Hauben DJ. Criss-cross scoring of postburn necrotic tissue. Plast Reconstr Surg 2000; 106:510–511.

120. Sprigle S, Linden M, Riordan B. Analysis of localized erythema using clinical indicators and spectroscopy. Ostomy Wound Manage 2003; 49:42–52.

121. Steed DL. Group Diabetic Ulcer Study: clinical evaluation of recombinant human platelet-derived growth factor for the treatment of lower extremity diabetic ulcers. J Vasc Surg 1995; 21:71–81.

122. Stevens DL, Herr D, Lampiris H, et al. Linezolid versus vancomycin for the treatment of methicillin-resistant *Staphylococcus aureus* infections [see comment]. Clin Infect Dis 2002; 34:1481–1490.

123. Strauss MB, Winant DM, Strauss AG, et al. Cigarette smoking and transcutaneous oxygen tensions: a case report. Undersea Hyperb Med 2000; 27:43–46.

124. Strauss MB. Refractory osteomyelitis. J Hyperb Med 1987; 2:147–159.

125. Treiman GS, Oderich GS, Ashrafi A, et al. Management of ischemic heel ulceration and gangrene: an evaluation of factors associated with successful healing. J Vasc Surg 2000; 31:1110–1118.

126. Trent JT, Federman D, Kirsner RS. Skin and wound biopsy: when, why, and how. Adv Skin Wound Care 2003; 16:372–375.

127. Trent JT, Kirsner RS. Cutaneous manifestations of HIV: a primer. Adv Skin Wound Care 2004; 17:116–127.

128. Van den Brande P, von Kemp K, De Coninck A, et al. Laser Doppler flux characteristics at the skin of the dorsum of the foot in young and in elderly healthy human subjects. Microvasc Res 1997; 53:156–162.

129. Verg Inc. Wound measurement system. R3M OA8. Winnipeg: Verg.

130. Wanner MB, Schwarzl F, Strub B, et al. Vacuum-assisted wound closure for cheaper and more comfortable healing of pressure sores: a prospective study. Scand J Plast Reconstr Surg Hand Surg 2003; 37:28–33.

131. Whitney JD, Salvadalena G, Higa L, et al. Treatment of pressure ulcers with noncontact normothermic wound therapy: healing and warming effects. J Wound Ostomy Continence Nurs 2001; 28:244–252.

132. Wilkinson EA, Hawke CI. Oral zinc for arterial and venous leg ulcers. Cochrane Database Syst Rev 2000:CD001273.

133. Winter GD. Epidermal regeneration in the domestic pig. In: Maibach HI, Rovee DT, eds. Epidermal wound healing. Chicago: Year Book Medical Publishers; 1970:71–113.

134. Witkowski JA, Parish LC. The decubitus ulcer: skin failure and destructive behavior. Int J Dermatol 2000; 39:894–896.

135. Witte MB, Barbul A. Arginine physiology and its implication for wound healing. Wound Repair Regen 2003; 11:419–423.

136. Wu F. Relative cost of amputation and total contact casting in rehabilitation medicine. Philadelphia: University of Pennsylvania; 1996:20.

137. Wu L, Brucker M, Gruskin E, et al. Differential effects of platelet-derived growth factor BB in accelerating wound healing in aged versus young animals: the impact of tissue hypoxia. Plast Reconstr Surg 1997; 99:815–822, discussion 823–824.

Cardiac Rehabilitation

Jonathan H. Whiteson

DEFINITION AND GOALS

Cardiac rehabilitation (CR) is an interdisciplinary team approach to patients with functional limitations secondary to heart disease (HD). The focus is on restoring patients to their optimal medical, physical, mental, psychologic, social, emotional, sexual, vocational, and economic status compatible with the severity of their HD. Primary prevention of HD involves screening healthy people to identify and treat risk factors before these illnesses develop. Secondary prevention is initiated during CR to improve HD risk factors and limit further morbidity and mortality.

HISTORICAL DEVELOPMENT

Herrick first described a myocardial infarction (MI) in 1912. Bed rest for 2 months was prescribed, as activity was believed to induce congestive heart failure (CHF), ventricular aneurysm, cardiac rupture, and sudden death. By 1930, pathologic studies revealed stable scar formation by 6 weeks.[136] Bed rest was recommended for 6 weeks, strenuous activity limited for longer, and return to an active lifestyle or work was infrequent. By the 1950s, 'early' ambulation programs at 4 weeks,[161] and then at 14 days,[34] following MI were implemented. These reduced the complications of prolonged bed rest, including deconditioning, venous thrombosis, and pulmonary embolism. During the 1970s, hospital length of stay shortened due to economic pressures. Similar outcomes and safety with early ambulation with no significant difference in occurrence of angina, reinfarction, CHF, or death were noted.[1]

Formalization of post-MI activities into what is now considered phase 1 inpatient CR was initially described by Wenger.[233] Patients progressed from bed rest to independence in activities of daily living (ADL), household ambulation, and stair climbing within 2 weeks. Patients were then discharged home.

Advances in technology and medical management, including catheter-based procedures and minimally invasive and 'off-pump' surgeries, have significantly reduced hospital length of stay. Changes in managed care and Medicare policy, the prospective payment system for inpatient rehabilitation, and the '75% rule' for admission to inpatient rehabilitation units, have also influenced hospital length of stay and inpatient CR. Patients are now discharged within 3–5 days following an uncomplicated MI, and 5–7 days following cardiac surgery. Reductions in hospital length of stay greatly impact the early phases of CR.

EPIDEMIOLOGY OF CARDIOVASCULAR DISEASE

Cardiovascular disease (CVD) is the leading cause of morbidity and mortality in men and women in the USA. Close to 65 million adults have CVD, and the prevalence increases with advancing age: 51% of men and 48% of women between the ages of 55 and 64 years have CVD, and 71% of men and 79% of women over the age of 75 years are affected.[43] In the USA, there is one coronary event every 26 s, and one death every minute from HD. There are 565 000 new MIs each year, as well as 300 000 recurrent MIs. Within 1 year of an MI, 25% of men and 38% of women will die, and 50% will die within 8 years. An average of 11.5 years of life is lost secondary to an MI.

There is also a steady increase in the number of hospital-based interventions for the management of HD. Currently in the USA, there are 1.2 million angiograms, 571 000 angioplasties, 516 000 coronary artery bypass graft (CABG) surgeries, and 2154 heart transplants (HTs) annually. In 2001, 46 000 implantable cardioverter defibrillators (ICDs) and 177 000 pacemakers were placed.

Economic costs are also rising, with estimated costs in the USA in 2004 for all HD of $314 billion. Half is for hospital, physician, and medication costs, and half is due to the lost productivity resulting from morbidity and mortality.

By modifying risk factors for HD, mortality rates have fallen from 228 per 100 000 population in 1970 to 178 per 100 000 in 2001. Life expectancy in the USA is currently 77.2 years (2000 population data). If all CVD was eliminated, estimated life expectancy would increase by 7 years.[7] The impact of CVD is not limited to the USA. Globally, the World Health Organization estimates 16.7 million people die annually from CVD, contributing to nearly 33% of all deaths.

TYPES OF HEART DISEASE

Myocardial infarction remains the primary reason for referral for CR. Increasingly, patients with angina, post-catheter-based

Box 34-1 Risk factors for coronary artery disease

Modifiable
- Physical inactivity
- Hypertension
- Smoking
- Dyslipidemia
- Overweight or obesity
- Diabetes
- Metabolic syndrome
- Emerging factors (see below)

Non-modifiable
- Increasing age
- Gender: male > female
- Prior history: cardiac, peripheral vascular, or cerebrovascular disease
- Family history: genetics
- Cultural or socioeconomic

Box 34-2 Benefits of physical activity on risk factors for coronary artery disease

- Low-density lipoprotein and triglycerides reduced 3–5%[127]
- High-density lipoproteins increased by 4.6%[126]
- Systolic and diastolic resting blood pressures reduced up to 3.4 mmHg (greater reduction seen in hypertensive patients)[60]
- Diabetic control improved: reduction of glycosylated hemoglobin up to 1%[212]
- Weight loss and subsequent weight maintenance enhanced[243]
- Rates of smoking cessation and maintenance of abstinence improved[139]

Table 34-1 Classification of hypertension

	Systolic blood pressure (mmHg)	Diastolic blood pressure (mmHg)
Normal	<120	<80
Prehypertension	120–139	80–89
Stage 1 hypertension	140–159	90–99
Stage 2 hypertension	>160	>100

intervention, CABG, valve surgery, CHF, arrhythmia, and HT are being referred. With an in-depth understanding of the pathophysiology of CVD and the benefits of early mobilization and exercise, there are very few clinical situations where CR is absolutely contraindicated.

RISK FACTORS FOR CORONARY ARTERY DISEASE

Risk factors for CAD are summarized in Box 34-1.

Physical inactivity

Physical inactivity accounts for 250 000 deaths annually. Over 60% of adults in the USA do not participate in regular physical activity. Single women, the elderly, the less educated, the less affluent, African-Americans, and Hispanics are more likely to be inactive.[218] The American College of Sports Medicine recommends at least 30 min of moderate-intensity physical activity on most days of the week, approximating to 600–1200 cal expended per week through exercise. Total energy expenditure, rather than duration or type of activity, has the greatest influence on the development of CAD. Higher levels of energy expenditure significantly predict lower CAD risk.[125]

Physical activity improves other modifiable risk factors for CAD (Box 34-2). Physical activity also reduces the incidence of CAD[24,124] and associated morbidity.[218] The protective effect is maintained only with lifelong exercise.[167] Physical activity and exercise in adults without HD is extremely safe, with the risk of a cardiac event ranging between 1 in 400 000 to 1 in 800 000 h of exercise. The risk of an event is significantly lower among regular exercisers.[64]

Hypertension

Normal blood pressure and hypertension is classified in Table 34-1.

Approximately one billion people worldwide have hypertension, and 7.1 million die annually from its complications. Hypertension is the most significant risk for death worldwide.[247] It affects mostly elderly people,[37] and the incidence increases with age.[225] Nearly 25% of adults in the USA have hypertension that requires treatment.[92] However, despite intensive education campaigns, 30% of people with hypertension do not know they have it, in 25% the condition is suboptimally controlled with medication, and 11% are not medicated. Only one-third of patients with hypertension have their blood pressure controlled with medication,[44] and many elderly patients are not treated to an optimal level.[23] Recent public health programs have improved awareness of and treatment rates for hypertension.

Risk for MI and death increase as blood pressure rises above 115/75.[129] The presence of other CAD risk factors compounds the risk from hypertension.[6] It is significant that a 5-mmHg blood pressure reduction produces a 9% reduction in mortality from CAD.[235]

Management of hypertension requires lifestyle modifications, including increased physical activity and dietary changes[235] for weight management, as well as restriction of sodium and alcohol intake. Lifestyle modification without medication is recommended in stage 1 hypertension for 12 months in those with no other risk factors, or 6 months in people with other risk factors. It can lower systolic blood pressure (SBP) between 3.7 and 4.3 mmHg.[9] Medications are recommended for stage 2 hypertension, or when lifestyle modifications do not normalize blood pressure.

Table 34-2 Classification of dyslipidemia

	Total cholesterol (mg/dL)	Low-density lipoprotein (mg/dL)	Triglycerides (mg/dL)	High-density lipoprotein (mg/dL)
Optimal	<200	<100	<150	>60
Near optimal	–	100–129	–	–
Borderline high	200–239	130–159	150–199	–
High	>240	160–189	200–299	<40
Very high	–	>190	>500	

Smoking

In the USA, over 4000 people start smoking daily.[42] Most people who smoke start before they are 18 years of age. Smoking is more prevalent in those with less education. Despite obvious health consequences, 25% of men and 20% of women continue to smoke. Environmental tobacco smoke is a significant cause of CAD deaths in non-smokers,[41] and many non-smokers report exposure to cigarette smoke at home or work.[169]

Cigarette smoking is the leading preventable cause of illness and premature death in the USA. Over a third of all smoking-related deaths are due to CVD,[41] and up to 30% of all CAD deaths in the USA annually are attributable to smoking.[219] Patients who continue to smoke following CABG have increased morbidity and mortality compared with those who stop smoking.[103] Financial costs are also significant, with over $157 billion annually in medical care and lost productivity.[41]

Prevention of smoking and smoking cessation are essential. With education, fewer youths are starting to smoke, and since 1965 smoking rates have dropped 40% in American adults. Of the 45% of patients who stop smoking spontaneously after a coronary event, 70% relapse within 1 year.[181] A nicotine withdrawal syndrome is responsible for the significant difficulty most people have in quitting smoking.[5] The benefits of smoking cessation are significant. The risk for developing CAD is reduced by 50% within 1 year, and there is a substantial decrease in CAD mortality.[82,187,197] Mortality rates by 3–5 years after MI are reduced by 50%,[241] and sudden cardiac deaths are also reduced.[79]

For smoking cessation, simple brief verbal advice is cost-effective but of limited success. Intensive advice with written instruction is more effective, but more expensive and time-consuming. Individual or group behavioral counseling is most effective, with practical, problem-solving advice and social support from family and healthcare workers. Four nicotine replacement medications are approved for smoking cessation, including gum, inhaler, nasal spray, and patch. They minimize nicotine withdrawal syndrome and are effective and safe.[112] Slow-release bupropion also helps smoking cessation. It acts on central neurochemical pathways, limiting the reduction in dopamine and noradrenaline (norepinephrine) levels that occur with nicotine withdrawal. A combination of behavioral support, nicotine replacement, and bupropion provides the highest success rates for smoking cessation, approaching 20%.[178]

Dyslipidemia

Dyslipidemia is defined according to Table 34-2.[158]

About 105 million adults in the USA have total cholesterol levels of 200 mg/dL or higher, and 50% have a low-density lipoprotein (LDL) level of 130 mg/dL or higher. Up to 40% of caucasian men have a high-density lipoprotein (HDL) level below 40 mg/dL. A raised LDL over 100 mg/dL is an independent risk factor for CAD[242] and predicts risk of recurrent events in preexisting CAD.[246] Reducing LDL is associated with fewer CAD events.[32] Elevated triglycerides are also correlated with CAD.[13] Low HDL is an independent risk factor for CAD, reversed by raising HDL.[242] While genetics is the main factor, 50% of HDL levels are accounted for by overweight, inactivity, smoking, and diabetes.

Achievement of optimal lipid levels is initially done by life-style modification, including dietary changes, increased physical activity, and weight loss. Aerobic exercise, including the use of a bicycle ergometer,[49] and strength training can lower LDL and triglycerides, raise HDL, and reduce the risk for CAD. This benefit is maintained as long as exercise is ongoing.[215]

Reduction of LDL through dietary changes reduces CAD incidence. Plant stanols and sterols, and soluble fibers including oats, barley, and psyllium, can lower LDL.[81] Dietary guidelines for lipid management are summarized in Table 34-3. Medications, including statins,[193] are also effective in reducing total cholesterol, LDL, and triglycerides, and increasing HDL, as well as reducing risk for developing CAD and recurrent events.[189]

Overweight and obesity

Over 60% of American adults are overweight, defined as a body mass index > 25 kg/m². Approximately 30% of all caucasians and African-American men, and 50% of African-American women, are obese (body mass index > 30 kg/m²). Increasing numbers of children are overweight. Currently, 22% of African-American children are overweight.[201] Childhood obesity is linked to greater risk for adult mortality from CVD.

Overweight is associated with 300 000 deaths annually from all causes.[3] Obesity is also related to increased morbidity and

Table 34-3 Dietary guidelines for lipid management

Calorie source	Total daily calories (%)
Total fat	30
Polyunsaturated fat	10
Monounsaturated fat	20
Saturated fat	<7
Carbohydrates	50
Proteins	15
Cholesterol	< 200 mg/day
Fiber	20–30 g/day

Table 34-4 Emerging risk factors for the development of coronary artery disease

Risk factor	Treatment
Lipoprotein a[51]	Nicotinic acid[8]
Homocysteine[236]	Folic acid, vitamins B_6 and B_{12}[135]
Prothrombotic states[148]	Aspirin[102]
High-sensitivity C-reactive protein[118]	Statins[151,164,180]

Box 34-3 Components of the metabolic syndrome[88]

1. Abdominal obesity: waist circumference >102 cm (men), >88 cm (women)
2. Triglycerides >150 mg/dL
3. High-density lipoprotein <40 mg/dL (men), <50 mg/dL (women)
4. Hypertension: >130/85
5. Insulin resistance: fasting blood glucose >110 mg/dL
6. Proinflammatory state
7. Prothrombotic state

poorer quality of life (QOL).[65,67,156] Overweight contributes to hypertension, dyslipidemia, diabetes, and the metabolic syndrome. A 10-lb weight gain increases risk for CVD and mortality.[138] Conversely, weight loss of 10% reduces risk factors for CAD.[159] Direct economic costs of obesity-related CAD, diabetes, and hypertension approach $43 billion. Indirect costs total $31 billion, approximately 9.4% of USA healthcare expenditure.[47]

Diabetes

A fasting blood glucose level over 125 mg/dL defines diabetes. Normal is less than 110 mg/dL. Between 110 and 125 mg/dL is considered an impaired fasting glucose level.[59] About 17 million people in the USA and 5% of all adults have diabetes, and 14.5 million have impaired fasting glucose. There are 800 000 new cases of type 2 diabetes diagnosed annually. One-third of all people with diabetes are undiagnosed and untreated.[97] African-Americans and Hispanic Americans have twice the incidence of diabetes as that of caucasians.[198] The prevalence of diabetes in the USA is currently 7%, and increasing in parallel with increasing rates of obesity and physical inactivity.[96]

Impaired fasting glucose[116] and diabetes increase the incidence of and mortality from CAD.[38] In 65% of patients with diabetes, the mortality is due to CAD.[74] CAD can go undetected, because myocardial ischemia is often silent in people with diabetes, due to autonomic dysfunction.[244] Adequate diabetic control in patients with CAD reduces the incidence of MI, decreases the need for cardiac interventions and surgery, improves QOL, and extends survival.[195] Dietary modification for weight loss and increased physical activity are first-line therapy for hyperglycemia. The addition of oral medications or injectable insulin can be needed to optimize control.

The metabolic syndrome (see below) is a combination of insulin resistance with dyslipidemia, hypertension, and a prothrombotic state.[84] This can precede the development of overt diabetes.

Metabolic syndrome

Key components of the metabolic syndrome are noted in Box 34-3. Three or more of components 1 through 5 must be present for diagnosis.[158]

Approximately 47 million people in the USA have metabolic syndrome. Prevalence increases with age. It is noted in nearly 45% of people over 60 years of age and in one-third of overweight or obese people.[66] Metabolic syndrome is an independent risk factor for CAD[91] and predisposes to diabetes and increased mortality.[120] Treatment focuses on management of underlying risk factors including overweight, physical inactivity, and poor diet. Medications for dyslipidemia, hypertension, hyperglycemia, and thrombosis are considered to optimize control.

Emerging risk factors

Other emerging factors associated with CAD risk are summarized in Table 34-4.

Non-modifiable risk factors

Risk for CAD increases with age, and men have higher rates of CAD at any age than those of women. Women lag about 10–15 years behind men in the incidence of CAD.[242] Previous personal history of CAD, peripheral vascular disease (PVD), and CVD increases the chance of a future cardiac event. Family history also correlates with risk for CAD, although the influence of genetic predisposition is not easily separated from environmental factors and learned behaviors.[192] Men and postmenopausal

Table 34-5 Substrates used in metabolic pathways

	Stored as	Circulating as	Converted to	Metabolic pathways	Net ATP produced
Carbohydrate	Glycogen: liver, muscle	Glucose	Pyruvate, acetyl coenzyme A	Citric acid cycle in mitochondria	36
Fat	Triglycerides: adipose tissue	Three fatty acids, glycerol	Acetyl coenzyme A, glucose	Beta-oxidation, citric acid cycle	460
Protein	Muscle	Amino acids	Pyruvate or acetyl coenzyme A	Deamination	

women are more likely to develop CAD, as are many minorities, partly due to higher rates of hypertension, obesity, and diabetes in these populations.

EXERCISE PHYSIOLOGY

ATP is used to power all organ function, and is produced by one of two metabolic pathways. Unlike anaerobic metabolism, aerobic metabolism is dependent on oxygen to drive the process.

Energy substrates

Energy substrates are the fuels used in metabolic pathways (Table 34-5).

Carbohydrates and fats are the primary sources of metabolic fuel. Protein and amino acids are used as an energy source only with severe caloric deprivation, starvation dieting, or 'overexercising'. Oxygen is required to maximize energy production from carbohydrates and fats. At intense external 'work rates', the body's physiologic mechanisms cannot provide oxygen at the rate it is required by the metabolizing tissues. Aerobic pathways are limited, and anaerobic pathways take over.

Muscles store energy in the form of ATP and phosphocreatine in sufficient quantities to support short burst (10 s) of intense activity. Use of stored ATP and phosphocreatine is considered anaerobic metabolism. Following burst activity, restoration of these stores occurs through aerobic pathways. The production of pyruvate from any substrate does not require oxygen and is also considered anaerobic metabolism. Transport of pyruvate into the mitochondria is oxygen-dependent, and does not occur under anaerobic conditions where pyruvate is converted to lactic acid by lactate dehydrogenase. This pathway has a very limited capacity to produce ATP. The accumulation of lactic acid is associated with impairment of cellular metabolic pathways, muscle soreness, fatigue, significant respiratory stimulation, and a 'forced' decrement or cessation of exercise. Cardiac arrhythmias are more likely to occur under anaerobic conditions. To limit lactic acid accumulation, at least two mechanisms exist to increase its degradation.

First is the Cori cycle, where lactate is transported to the liver, converted back into pyruvate and then into glucose, and released for further muscle metabolism.

Second, buffering systems are important in the energy process. With the production of lactic acid, the pH of the local milieu is lowered, activating buffering mechanisms. Sodium bicarbonate ($NaHCO_3$) is the most abundant and active buffering system for lactic acid, with the production of sodium lactate and carbonic acid (H_2CO_3):

$$\text{lactic acid} + NaHCO_3 \rightarrow \text{sodium lactate} + H_2CO_3.$$

Carbonic acid is rapidly converted to water (H_2O) and carbon dioxide (CO_2):

$$H_2CO_3 \xrightarrow{\text{carbonic acid dehydrogenase}} H_2O + CO_2.$$

Sodium lactate is converted back to lactic acid and then to pyruvate when aerobic conditions are restored.

Detection of a spike in CO_2 production ($\dot{V}CO_2$) with metabolic gas analysis identifies the transition from aerobic to predominantly anaerobic metabolism. During exercise testing, the intensity of exercise when $\dot{V}O_2$ exceeds oxygen consumption ($\dot{V}O_2$) is considered the anaerobic threshold. Anaerobic threshold is one of the key determinants of functional and exercise performance. As patients with HD do not feel well under anaerobic conditions, exercise intensities should be set below anaerobic threshold.

Oxygen consumption

$\dot{V}O_2$ is measured using a metabolic cart, and is the volume of oxygen consumed at any level of activity. Under controlled conditions, at rest, an average 70-kg man consumes 3.5 cc of oxygen per minute for every kilogram of body weight. The unit of oxygen consumption at resting, or 'basal metabolic rate', is referred to as one metabolic equivalent (1 MET). Any increment in activity will produce greater oxygen consumption, or METs. Tables exist of the MET level equivalent for varying intensities of exercise and different activities (Table 34-6).

For any given level of aerobic training, as exercise intensity increases past a critical point, the ability of physiologic systems to provide oxygen is outstripped by the body's oxygen requirements. This represents anaerobic threshold and, using metabolic gas analysis, no further increase in $\dot{V}O_2$ is seen (Fig. 34.1). A rate of maximal $\dot{V}O_2$ has been reached: $\dot{V}O_{2max}$, or aerobic capacity. If further exercise is done after this point, anaerobic mechanisms produce the energy required. Due to lactic acid

Table 34-6 The metabolic equivalent energy expenditure of varying intensity activities

Level	Self-care	Household	Recreational	Vocational
Light (1–3 metabolic) equivalents, METS	Sponge bathing Shaving Dressing or undressing	Preparing light meals Setting table Dusting	Walking 2 mph Writing Reading Playing piano	Typing Light machine work Lifting <10 lbs Using a sewing machine
Light to moderate (3–4 METS)	Showering Climbing stairs Driving	Light gardening Ironing Vacuuming Grocery shopping	Walking 3 mph Slow bicycling Golfing with cart	Light carpentry Working on an assembly line Lifting <20 lbs Bricklaying
Moderate (4–5 METS)	Having sexual intercourse.	Heavy gardening Waxing floors Moving furniture Raking leaves Washing car	Walking 3.5 mph Playing doubles tennis Slow dancing Easy swimming Bicycling 8 mph	Light shoveling Mixing cement Light farming Lifting <50 lbs
Heavy (5–7 METS)		Splitting wood Shoveling snow Climbing ladder	Walking 4–5 mph Playing singles tennis Cross-country skiing at 2.5 mph Doing gymnastics	Heavy farming Heavy industry Lifting 50–100 lbs
Very heavy (>7 METS)		Moving heavy furniture Pushing or pulling hard	Jogging at 5 mph Playing soccer Playing basketball Horseback riding	Heavy construction Lifting 100 lbs

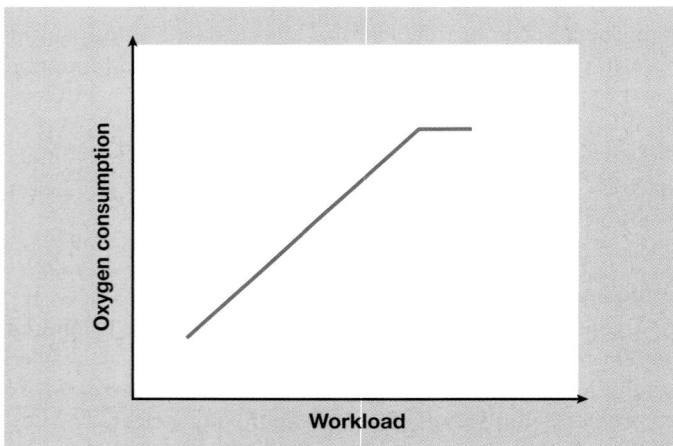

Figure 34-1 Relationship between oxygen consumption and intensity of work being performed.

accumulation, only a short duration of further exercise is possible.

The Fick equation

Complex multicellular organisms utilize organ systems to transport oxygen from the atmosphere to the site of energy production. The efficiency of these systems at any given level of aerobic fitness determines the $\dot{V}O_{2max}$ and the maximal functional capacity. The Fick equation links the significant organ systems involved in the transportation of oxygen—lungs, cardiovascular, and muscle—and is the central theme underlying the enhanced function achieved with aerobic exercise training:

$$\text{oxygen consumption} = \text{cardiac output} \times \text{arteriovenous oxygen difference.}$$

Cardiac output at any degree of aerobic training is a product of the heart rate (HR) and stroke volume (SV) (the volume of blood expelled by the left ventricle during one contraction). The major determinant of SV is the diastolic filling volume. However, diastolic filling volume decreases as HR increases. With slow HR at low exercise intensities, cardiac output initially increases due to increased SV, but at higher intensity levels it increases due to increased HR.[63]

The relationship of exercise intensity to cardiac output is essentially linear (Fig. 34-2). HR also increases in a linear relationship to exercise intensity (Fig. 34-3).

Maximal HR (HR_{max}) is physiologically determined by a person's age, and is estimated by subtracting age from 220. *However, this estimation is never used to determine training HR in CR.*

The arteriovenous oxygen difference reflects the ability of the muscle to extract oxygen from the blood for use with muscle metabolism and energy production. Determinants include the pulmonary, hemopoietic, vascular, and muscular systems (see Box 34-4).

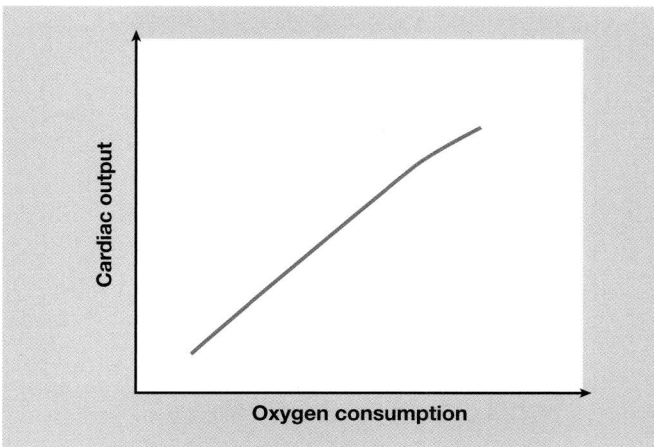

Figure 34-2 Relationship between cardiac output and oxygen consumption.

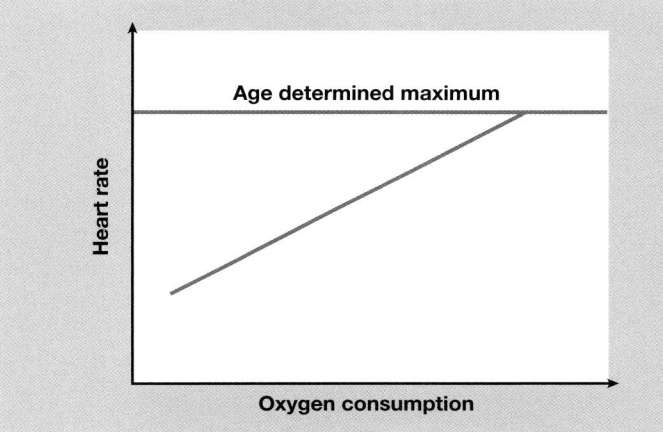

Figure 34-3 Relationship between heart rate and oxygen consumption.

AEROBIC TRAINING

Aerobic training is a habitual dynamic physical activity of sufficient intensity, duration, and frequency to produce physiologic adjustments in the cardiopulmonary response to exercise. For sedentary individuals, aerobic training might constitute increasing levels of general activity and walking. For most active individuals, aerobic training requires progressive exercise. Aerobic training protocols for healthy individuals recommend exercise most days of the week, for 30–60 min, at intensity levels that do not exceed 50–80% of $\dot{V}O_{2max}$.

Training is 'muscle group-specific', and changes in the cardiopulmonary response to exercise will be noted only when the trained muscle groups are tested. For example, a treadmill-training program will not significantly improve the cardiovascular response to bicycling. When designing aerobic training programs, a combination of different aerobic machines using multiple muscle groups is recommended. Significant functional, musculoskeletal, cardiovascular, and psychologic adaptations

---

Box 34-4 Adaptations noted with aerobic training

Functional
- Higher peak work rate
- Reduced disturbance of body function
- Enhanced rate of recovery after exercise

Cardiovascular and pulmonary
- Increased stroke volume and peak CO
- Increased respiratory muscle strength, maximal voluntary ventilation
- Reduced dyspnea

Musculoskeletal
- Increased flexibility
- Increased muscle, tendon, and cartilage strength
- Increased bone density
- Increased lean muscle mass
- Reduced body fat percentage

Biochemical
- Increased aerobic enzyme concentration

Endocrine
- Reduced stress hormone release

Psychologic
- Improved depression and anxiety

---

are noted in 6–10 weeks of starting training, depending on the intensity and frequency (Box 34-4). Biochemical changes are noted within 10 days of starting training. Lack of activity or bed rest can significantly reverse these beneficial effects over the course of 2–3 weeks.

In patients with HD, symptomatic limitation of activity produces a steady decline in aerobic capacity. Following a cardiac event, especially if associated with prolonged bed rest, further significant decline in aerobic capacity occurs. Resting tachycardia is noted, and an exaggerated HR response to lower level activity is common due to reduced vagal tone and enhanced sympathetic drive from circulating catecholamines. Return of HR to normal following completion of exercise is also delayed. Blood pressure responses are variable, but postural hypotension with reduced cardiac output secondary to peripheral blood pooling and loss of vasopostural reflexes is common. Cardiac output can be reduced following MI or with significant fluid overload, as in CHF. Cardiac output is typically improved following valve correction surgery or with resolution of CHF. Myocardial blood flow can be impaired due to progressive coronary narrowing or occlusion, or improved secondary to angioplasty, stent, or CABG. Arteriovenous O_2 difference rapidly decline with bed rest, and accounts for the significant decline in aerobic capacity seen when patients are hospitalized for HD.

Significant muscle changes are noted in CHF, including altered cellular structure, depletion of phosphocreatine and oxidative capacity, and muscle fiber atrophy. Vasomotor changes are common, including increased vasoconstriction and impaired arterial dilatation with increasing exercise intensity.

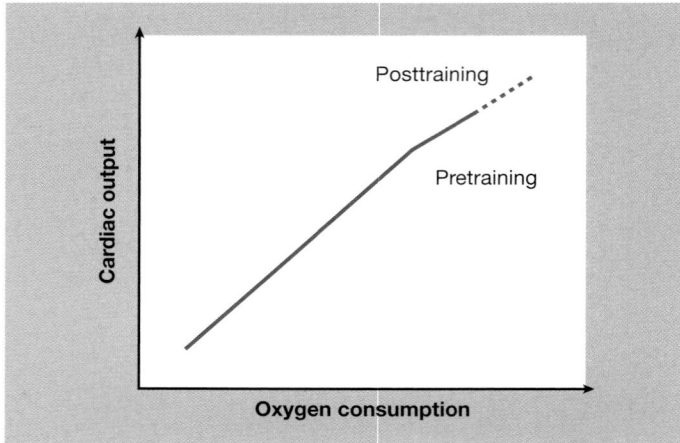

Figure 34-4 Effect of training on the relationship between cardiac output and oxygen consumption.

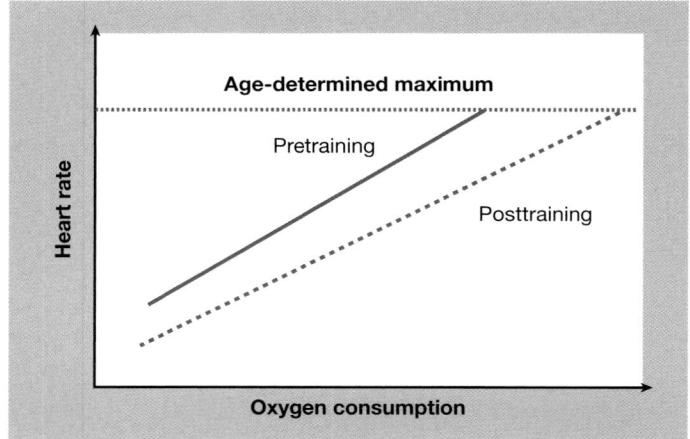

Figure 34-5 Effect of training on the relationship between heart rate and oxygen consumption.

There is a significant change in cardiac physiology and response to exercise following HT. Resting tachycardia is noted, due to loss of vagal tone to the sinoatrial node. The rate of increase in HR and cardiac output with exercise is blunted, as the denervated heart relies on increases in circulating catecholamines to augment these parameters. Peak HR is 25% lower than in age-matched control subjects, and $\dot{V}O_{2max}$ is 33% of predicted. At maximum effort, there is a significantly reduced peak work capacity, cardiac output, HR, and SBP.

Aerobic training influences all determinants of the Fick equation. Following a standard aerobic training program, a small but significant increase is noted in cardiac output at higher work intensities. At rest and submaximal work intensities, however, cardiac output remains the same as that before training (Fig. 34-4).

Heart rate at rest and submaximal work intensities are actually reduced compared with the untrained state, due to enhanced vagal tone producing cardiac slowing. So it is the increased SV noted at rest, submaximal, and maximal work intensities following training that is responsible for the increased cardiac output. The reduced HR allows for longer diastolic filling time (Fig. 34-5).

Arteriovenous O_2 difference is also increased following training. Box 34-5 summarizes the adaptations following training that increase arteriovenous O_2 difference.

The increased peripheral oxygen utilization by aerobically trained muscles accounts for the majority of the increase noted in $\dot{V}O_{2max}$ seen after aerobic training programs. At rest and submaximal levels of exercise intensity, however, there is no difference in $\dot{V}O_2$ from before compared with after the aerobic training program (Fig. 34-6).

Myocardial oxygen consumption

Myocardial oxygen consumption (M $\dot{V}O_2$) increases in a linear fashion with increasing exercise intensity. In a normal heart, the supply of blood and oxygen matches the M $\dot{V}O_2$. The major determinant of myocardial blood flow is the diameter of the

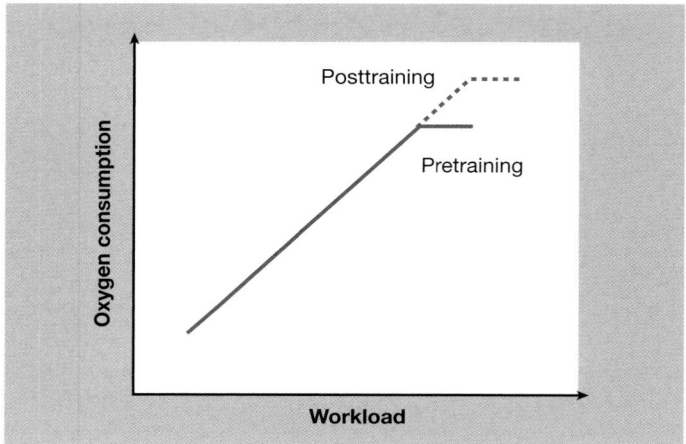

Figure 34-6 Effect of training on the relationship between oxygen consumption and workload.

Box 34-5 Adaptations enhancing arteriovenous O_2 difference following aerobic training

- Increased:
  Hemoglobin oxygen saturation
  Red blood cell hemoglobin concentration
  Size of arteries perfusing type 1 fiber muscles
  Capillary density
  Blood supply to type 1 muscle fiber beds
  Size of the type 1 muscle fibers
  Muscle fiber myoglobin concentration
  Mitochondrial size and concentration
  Aerobic enzymes concentration
- Enhanced minute ventilation

coronary arteries, which normally dilate to increase capacity as myocardial oxygen demand increases. In coronary arteries affected by atherosclerosis, a point is reached where the supply can no longer be increased, and further demand produces a relative lack of myocardial oxygen, or ischemia or angina. The

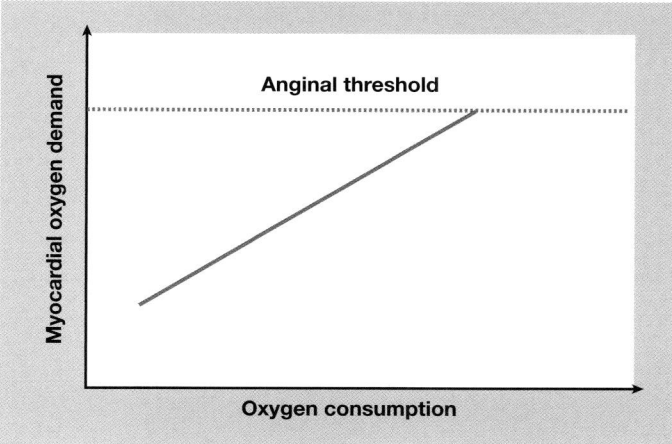

Figure 34-7 Relationship between myocardial oxygen demand and total body oxygen consumption.

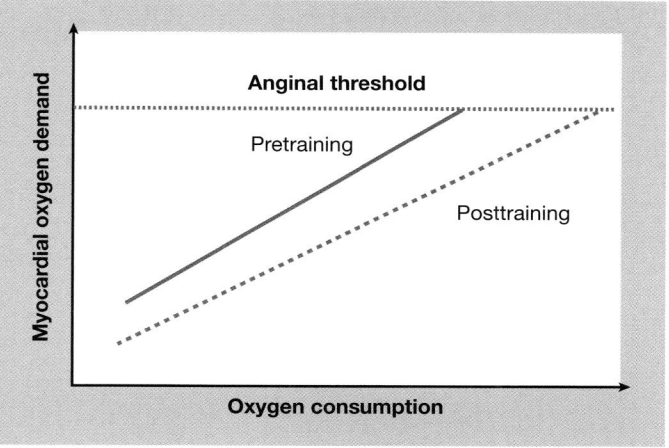

Figure 34-8 Effect of training on the relationship between myocardial oxygen demand and total body oxygen consumption.

exercise intensity when this point is reached is considered the ischemic or anginal threshold (Fig. 34-7).

Ischemia is noted on an electrocardiogram (ECG) as ST segment depression, on echocardiography as wall motion abnormalities, and on nuclear imaging as reversible perfusion deficits. Ischemia can be evident before the symptom of angina is perceived, and is a more sensitive indicator of myocardial hypoperfusion than angina. Without CAD, the ischemic threshold is not reached, and $\dot{V}O_{2max}$ determines maximum M $\dot{V}O_2$. Patients with CAD have narrowed arteries that do not dilate with exercise. Myocardial blood flow is significantly reduced, and at low levels of exercise M $\dot{V}O_2$ overcomes supply. The ischemic threshold is subsequently low.

The muscle group performing the exercise also influences M $\dot{V}O_2$. There is a greater M $\dot{V}O_2$ for the same exercise intensity performed by the upper limbs as compared with by the lower limbs. M $\dot{V}O_2$ is also greater at higher exercise intensities of upright (treadmill) compared with supine (reclining bike) exercise. Exercises with a significant isometric component (rowing machine) generate higher M $\dot{V}O_2$ compared with the same intensity of exercise without the isometric component (step machine).

Measurements of myocardial blood flow and M $\dot{V}O_2$ are only possible with invasive techniques and are not clinically applicable. An estimation of M $\dot{V}O_2$ can be made from the product of HR and SBP, or the double product (DP):

$$M \ \dot{V}O_2 = DP = HR \times SBP.$$

This equation is useful in clinical situations where ischemia is noted or angina is experienced. If the SBP and HR are recorded when ischemia or angina are noted, the DP can be calculated at ischemic threshold. Future exercise should be completed at a HR at least 10 beats below this point.

Exercise training does not affect the ischemic threshold. Only catheter-based coronary interventions or CABG will alter the anatomy of the coronary arteries and enhance blood flow. Combined intensive programs of lifestyle changes, very low-fat vegetarian diets, aerobic exercise, stress management, smoking cessation, and group psychologic support have also produced significant regression of coronary atherosclerosis compared with control subjects, with a significant decline in cardiac events.[166]

M $\dot{V}O_2$ following an aerobic training program is lower at rest and submaximal levels of exercise intensity. This is clinically relevant for patients with CAD, who will be able to perform activities at a greater intensity following an aerobic training program before reaching ischemic threshold as compared with before training. For the same intensity of activity performed after training, a lower M $\dot{V}O_2$ is achieved, providing a wider margin of safety for those with CAD (Fig. 34-8).

CARDIAC EVALUATION

History

The initial evaluation of the patient referred for CR includes a thorough history and physical examination, as well as a review of the available laboratory and physiologic testing data.

The history is the initiation of the physician–patient relationship that nurtures the patient's trust in the physician and promotes adherence with the CR prescription. A patient's trust in the physiatrist's therapeutic recommendations is essential for compliance with a heart-healthy lifestyle. Specific questions identify key areas that influence the CR prescription. Non-solicited information from the patient can provide insight into emotional concerns, as well as disability and handicap. Some patients overlook symptoms that, in hindsight, were cardiac-related. Failure to recognize and report cardiac symptoms is a significant challenge in HD management. A syndrome of overcompensation is typical following a cardiac event, with hypervigilance, anxiety, and overreporting of trivial symptoms. Correlation of these symptoms with physiologic and electrocardiographic data during CR helps allay fears and refocus on potential significant symptoms. Education and counseling are beneficial.

Cardiac causes of *chest pain* must be differentiated from non-cardiac causes (Table 34-7).

Table 34-7 Cardiac versus non-cardiac causes of chest pain

Feature	Cardiac	Musculoskeletal	Gastrointestinal	Pulmonary
Quality	Squeezing, heavy, dull burning	Sharp, stabbing aching	Visceral, burning tightness	Sharp tightness
Nature	Persistent	Intermittent	Variable	Variable
Location	Central chest, diffuse	Discrete pinpoint	Epigastric retrosternal	Discrete pinpoint
Radiation	Neck, back, arms	Dermatomal myotomal	Throat, back	Rare
Duration	Angina <10 min, myocardial infarction >20 min	Minutes to days	Minutes to hours	Minutes to hours
Exacerbating factors	Exercise, emotions (sadness, stress, fear)	Palpation, specific movements and positions	Fasting, spicy foods	Breathing, coughing
Relieving factors	Rest, nitroglycerin	Rest, analgesics, antiinflammatory drugs	Antacids, food	Rest, controlled breathing

Typical ischemic cardiac pain is mediated via the autonomic nervous system, and can be absent in patients with diabetes with autonomic neuropathy. Atypically, and more common in women, dyspnea on exertion is the presenting feature of ischemia. A change in the nature of ischemic pain is important, as it can indicate disease progression or compliance issues with medications. Recurrence of ischemic symptoms following cardiac interventions or CABG can occur due to reocclusion of the vessel or bypass graft.

Palpitations are frequently the presenting feature of an arrhythmia, and are the subjective appreciation of a forceful or irregular heart beat. Palpitations can be due to benign premature atrial or ventricular contractions, or more significant atrial fibrillation and non-sustained ventricular tachycardia (VT). Even malignant arrhythmias, such as sustained VT, might not produce palpitations. Palpitations can be felt only with exertion. A normal resting ECG does not rule out arrhythmia. A 24-h Holter monitor study can be indicated. Exercise stress testing (EST) can provoke arrhythmias that are seen only with exertion.

Dyspnea is the unpleasant sensation of shortness of breath. Dyspnea is often a feature of other diseases: chronic obstructive pulmonary disease (COPD) and restrictive lung disorder, pulmonary embolus, diabetic ketoacidosis, pain syndromes, anxiety, and deconditioning. Shortness of breath at rest, dyspnea on exertion, cough, sputum, edema, and a past smoking history are important in cardiac causes of dyspnea. Shortness of breath can be worse lying flat (referred to as orthopnea), and patients can report waking in the night gasping for breath (referred to as paroxysmal nocturnal dyspnea). HD and COPD often coexist, and differentiation between the two is often difficult. Dyspnea on exertion can be the presenting symptom of ischemia.

Edema is swelling of the extremities and has many potential causes, including CHF, cor pulmonale, deep vein thrombosis (DVT), venous insufficiency, lymphedema, dependent edema, liver disease, hypoalbuminemic states, and cellulitis. In HD, edema implies CHF. Other findings can include weight gain, cough, shortness of breath, engorged jugular veins, pulmonary rales, hepatic congestion, and ascites. The degree of edema, in conjunction with weight fluctuations and features of pulmonary congestion, allows determination of the severity of CHF and its response to therapeutic intervention. Resistant and unilateral lower limb swelling should raise concern for DVT, cellulitis, or lymphedema.

Cough must be differentiated from COPD, pulmonary infections, gastroesophageal reflux disease, postnasal drip, allergy, and a side effect of medications (angiotensin-converting enzyme [ACE] inhibitors). The sputum in HD is typically clear or pink, and frothy as opposed to tenacious. A yellow–green color is typical of a pulmonary infection or COPD exacerbation. A nocturnal cough is frequent with CHF. As pulmonary congestion improves with treatment, the cough should resolve. A persistent cough can indicate mucus plugging or ACE inhibitor-induced cough. Changing to an angiotensin receptor blocker can result in resolution of coughing. Cough developing only on exertion might indicate exercise-induced bronchospasm. Bronchodilators administered before exercise will prevent this.

Dizziness is a sensation that the room is spinning around the patient, and can indicate a failure of cerebral perfusion. Syncope is a loss of consciousness, and can indicate a significant circulatory failure. Seizure disorder and vertebrobasilar insufficiency must be ruled out. HD presenting with dizziness or syncope can be indicative of arrhythmias, aortic stenosis, idiopathic hypertrophic subaortic stenosis with left ventricular (LV) outflow tract obstruction, and LV 'pump' failure. Dizziness soon after rising from bed can be related to orthostatic hypotension, which is a fall in SBP of 10–20 mmHg on standing. Orthostasis can be seen in patients who are on aggressive diuretic regimens combined with vasodilators. It is common in patients with diabetes who have peripheral autonomic neuropathy, and in the Shy–Drager variant of Parkinson disease. Medication adjustment, liberalization of fluid restrictions, and use of lower extremity graduated pressure stockings are helpful. Orthostasis is common in deconditioned individuals following extended bed rest, and improves with mobilization.

Deconditioning, depression, medications including beta-blockers, and poor sleep are common non-cardiac causes of *fatigue*. Deconditioning results from prolonged relative inactivity and improves with increasing activity. Fatigue from depression is common with anergia, poor sleep, and anorexia. Cardioselective beta-blockers have lower incidence of depression. Non-restorative sleep is common in patients with HD due to breathing difficulties, nocturia, anxiety, and depression. Adjustment of diuretic schedules, management of anxiety disorders, and sleep medications are considerations. Cardiac fatigue is related to reduced cardiac output associated with cardiomyopathy. A downward spiral of HD, fatigue, and inactivity leading to further HD is common. Exercise interrupts and reverses this decline. Patient education that cardiac fatigue worsens with further rest and improves with physical exertion is important for compliance with exercise recommendations.

Physical examination

The physiatric examination before CR includes all organ systems that influence the rehabilitation process. Particular attention should be paid to the following.

Pulse rhythm and rate are important. A normal sinus rhythm is a regular pulse between 60 and 100 beats per minute with a P wave preceding every QRS complex on the ECG. Bradycardia is a rate less than 60, can be physiologic in athletes due to increased vagal tone to the heart, and can be pharmacologic due to medications including beta-blockers. It can also be pathologic, as in sick sinus syndrome, heart block, and junctional or ventricular escape rhythms. Tachycardia, a rate above 100, is normal only following exertion. Other causes include pain, dehydration, anemia, CHF, hypotension, and hyperthyroidism. Fear and anxiety can also play a role during CR in a patient who is unfamiliar with the rehabilitation process. Medication (beta-blocker and calcium channel blocker) non-compliance can produce rebound tachycardia.

Sinus arrhythmia is a normal physiologic variant in which the HR increases with inspiration and slows with expiration. An irregularly irregular HR can indicate atrial fibrillation. Atrial flutter, premature atrial contractions, premature ventricular contractions, and second-degree heart block can also produce an irregular pulse.

Arrhythmias are significant if they result in symptoms or signs of ischemia or low SBP. Appropriate treatment must be instituted rapidly to prevent MI or syncope. When there are no hemodynamic consequences, arrhythmias can be considered more benign. A wide complex tachycardia on ECG indicates a more malignant ventricular complex arrhythmia.

Blood pressure normally is *up to* 120/70. Hypertension is over 140/90. In those patients with significant vasculopathy, recording blood pressure from both arms can result in significantly different values due to subclavian artery stenosis. Coarctation of the aorta produces similar findings. A 'low' blood pressure at rest, i.e. 90/60, that is asymptomatic and that increases with walking and exercise is normal and acceptable. Any blood pressure associated with dizziness or fatigue, or that drops on stand-ing or exercise, is abnormal. Deconditioning, dehydration, anemia, and medications are reversible causes of hypotension. Testing for orthostatic hypotension is important. Pulsus paradoxus, a fall in SBP greater than 10 mmHg with inspiration, can indicate pericardial effusion and tamponade requiring urgent surgical evaluation.

A resting blood pressure over 200/110 is a contraindication to exercise. However, many patients present for exercise with elevated blood pressure maintained by anxiety. A patient with asymptomatic elevated blood pressure may be allowed to start CR under close observation, realizing that the pressure most likely will fall toward normal as anxiety dissipates with the onset of exercise.

Heart and lungs are an important part of the physical examination. Auscultation of the heart should correlate with the history of HD. New and unexpected or changed murmurs require further evaluation with echocardiography before the patient can be cleared for exercise. A harsh ejection systolic murmur heard over the aortic region can suggest critical aortic stenosis, a contraindication to CR. Pericardial rubs following heart surgery suggest pericarditis. Treatment includes anti-inflammatory medication. Diminished breath sounds in the lung bases suggest pleural effusions. Wheezes, rales, and rhonchi suggest interstitial edema, pulmonary congestion, and retained secretions or mucus. Oxygen saturation below 90% on pulse oximetry requires supplemental oxygen and treatment of the cardiopulmonary pathology. Coexistent lung disease, asthma, and COPD require appropriate treatment.

Limb examination is also helpful, especially when there is bilateral, symmetric lower limb edema that implies fluid retention. In this case, fluid and sodium restriction and diuretic therapy should be considered. Daily weight gain supports a diagnosis of CHF. Asymmetric lower extremity edema is expected in the limb where vein grafts were removed. Local cellulitis and DVT should be considered, especially when there is unilateral upper limb swelling.

Peripheral pulses should be examined. Carotid bruits and diminished or absent lower extremity pulses indicate widespread vasculopathy. Skin integrity of the feet can be impaired, producing ulceration and gangrene. Lower limb amputation requires special consideration when planning CR.

Musculoskeletal examination is needed to detect generalized or focal muscle atrophy and weakness, significant arthritic conditions, and postoperative myofascial findings (most commonly in the shoulders) and sternal pain (costochondritis). These conditions can require analgesia and modification of the CR program.

Neurologic examination is important because cerebrovascular disease is often associated with CAD. Preexisting or perioperative strokes are not uncommon, especially with atrial fibrillation. Evaluation for focal sensory and motor deficits is essential. Gait and balance disorders also influence planning of the CR program. Peripheral neuropathy is also frequently present in patients with diabetes.

Cognitive examination is helpful, because atherosclerosis underlies CAD, CVD, and some dementias. Post-MI or CABG confusion can be due to preexisting dementia or indicate a new cerebral event. Anesthesia, hypoxia, and medications can result in significant temporary or permanent cognitive deficits, with safety and dependency issues. 'Pump head' is a slang term for an acute confusional state following cardiopulmonary bypass used for cardiac surgeries. Some patients who go through surgery 'off pump' also suffer confusional states. Fluctuating cognitive state following a cardiac event or surgery is consistent with a toxic encephalopathy. This usually resolves over days to weeks. Magnetic resonance imaging (MRI) of the brain can reveal a 'shower' of cerebral emboli, originating from an aortic atheroma or the LV during surgery. Recovery is usually complete. Monitoring for safe use of exercise equipment is necessary during CR in cognitively impaired patients.

CARDIAC TESTING

Rest and exercise tests are required before prescribing CR. Cardiac evaluation during exercise provides a more functional evaluation of cardiovascular responses than at rest.

Resting ECG identifies abnormalities including LV hypertrophy, prior MI, conduction abnormalities, and arrhythmias. Comparison can be made to exercise-induced changes.

Chest roentgenogram identifies cardiomegaly, pulmonary edema, and pleural effusions. Unilateral effusions are common following minimally invasive heart surgery. Other postoperative findings include atelectasis, consolidation, and pneumothorax.

Echocardiogram allows evaluation of the myocardium and valvular apparatus, including ejection fraction (EF), wall motion abnormalities, valve stenosis or regurgitation, and pericardial effusion.

Ambulatory 24-h Holter monitoring identifies intermittent arrhythmias and assists in monitoring results of antiarrhythmic treatments.

Coronary angiography is used to determine the extent of CAD and guide interventions. Standard catheters identify luminal narrowing. Catheters with intravascular ultrasound transducers identify subendothelial lipid-laden plaques. These might not cause luminal narrowing but are at high risk of rupture and subsequent MI. LV and valve function are quantified. Patients with diabetes can have diffuse CAD that is not amenable to intervention, requiring modification of the CR prescription.

Electrophysiologic stimulation allows evaluation of the myocardial conducting system. Arrhythmias and accessory pathways can be ablated. Inducible ventricular arrhythmias warrant an ICD.

Cardiac EST is generally safe, and adverse outcomes are infrequent.[202] Absolute and relative contraindications to EST are summarized in Box 34-6.[78]

Exercise stress testing has been performed safely within 3 days after MI.[190] A low-level **submaximal EST** performed before hospital discharge quantifies functional activity tolerance.[224] Protocols have a predetermined end point, such as a peak HR of 120 beats per minute, 70% of the predicted maximum HR, or a peak MET level of 5.[95] Before commencing

Box 34-6 Contraindications to exercise stress testing

Absolute
- Acute myocardial infarction (within 2 days)
- High-risk unstable angina
- Uncontrolled cardiac arrhythmias causing symptoms of hemodynamic compromise
- Symptomatic severe aortic stenosis
- Uncontrolled symptomatic congestive heart failure
- Acute pulmonary embolus or pulmonary infarction
- Acute myocarditis or pericarditis
- Acute aortic dissection

Relative
- Left main coronary artery disease
- Moderate stenotic valvular heart disease
- Electrolyte abnormalities
- Severe arterial hypertension (> 200 mmHg systolic blood pressure and/or 110 mmHg diastolic blood pressure)
- Tachyarrhythmias or bradyarrhythmias
- Hypertrophic cardiomyopathy and other forms of left ventricular outflow tract obstruction
- Mental or physical impairment leading to inability to exercise adequately
- High-degree atrioventricular block

outpatient CR, a **symptom-limited maximal EST** provides data for exercise risk evaluation and individualization of the CR program. Patients should refrain from eating or drinking caffeinated drinks for 3 h before the EST. Cardiac medications are taken as scheduled. ECG and vital signs are recorded before, during, and after testing. SBP normally rises during an EST by 10–30 mmHg, with a peak > 140 mmHg. Diastolic blood pressure remains stable or decreases.

A normal EST is terminated when 85% of age- and gender-predicted maximum HR is achieved. Other indications for terminating an EST are summarized in Box 34-7.[78]

A poor prognosis is predicted by abnormalities detected on the EST (Table 34-8).

Maximum exercise tolerance is influenced by resting and exercise-induced LV dysfunction. Markers of exercise capacity include exercise duration, MET level, and maximum HR and DP. Translating exercise duration into aerobic capacity, METs, provides a consistent measure of function and performance regardless of exercise modality or protocol. Serial EST allows documentation of physiologic and functional improvements, and modification of the exercise prescription.

Exercise protocols

Exercise stress testing involves cardiac stimulation and cardiac imaging. For a functional evaluation, stimulation is best performed with exercise. Arm ergometry EST is performed when treadmill or bicycle ergometry EST is not possible due to spinal cord injury, amputation, PVD, arthritis, and recent orthopedic surgery. Arm exercise produces an exaggerated HR and SBP response compared with similar workloads performed by the legs. Peak HR, however, is only 70% of that achieved with leg

Table 34-8 Exercise stress test findings associated with poor prognosis

Exercise stress test finding	Associated outcome(s)
Post-myocardial infarction, exercise-induced angina symptoms	Stable angina within 1 year[52,210]
Achieving < 85% of age-predicted maximum heart rate	Increased 2-year mortality[123]
Delayed heart rate recovery after exercise stress test	Increased 6-year mortality[48]
Delayed fall in systolic blood pressure after exercise stress test	Increased mortality[141]
Post-myocardial infarction inadequate increase of systolic blood pressure	Left ventricular dysfunction[57,226]
Post-myocardial infarction rate-pressure product < 21 700	Increased 6-month mortality[227]
A 2-mm ischemic ST segment depression	Increased incidence of myocardial infarction[119,188] 1% annual increased mortality[210,231] Multivessel disease on angiography[146]
Early 1-mm ST segment depression	Increased incidence of myocardial infarction[143] 5% annual mortality[231]
Unable to tolerate exercise stress test	Highest adverse cardiac event rate[133]
Achieve < 5 metabolic equivalents	Increased mortality[162,199]

Box 34-7 Indications for terminating exercise stress testing

Absolute
- Drop in systolic blood pressure (SBP) of > 10 mmHg from baseline, despite an increase in workload, with ischemia
- Moderate to severe angina
- Increasing nervous system symptoms (e.g. ataxia, dizziness, or near-syncope)
- Signs of poor perfusion (cyanosis or pallor)
- Technical difficulties in monitoring electrocardiogram or SBP
- Subject's desire to stop
- Sustained ventricular tachycardia (VT)
- ST elevation > 1.0 mm in leads without diagnostic Q waves (other than V1 or aVR)

Relative
- Drop in SBP of > 10 mmHg from baseline, despite an increase in workload, without ischemia
- ST or QRS changes such as excessive ST depression > 2 mm of horizontal, or down-sloping ST segment depression or marked axis shift
- Arrhythmias other than sustained VT, including multifocal premature ventricular contractions, triplets, or supraventricular tachycardia, heart block, or bradyarrhythmias
- Fatigue, shortness of breath, wheezing, leg cramps, claudication
- Development of bundle branch block or intraventricular conduction delay that cannot be distinguished from VT
- Increasing chest pain
- Hypertensive response: SBP > 250 mmHg and/or diastolic blood pressure > 115 mmHg

testing. The elevated DP is relevant for patients with ischemia. CR protocols will predominantly use arm exercises, and post-CR EST will also be with arm ergometry. This consistency allows accurate evaluation of physiologic changes.

Bicycle ergometry EST can be performed upright or supine. The supine position is most convenient for use with echocardiographic monitoring, and increases the sensitivity of nuclear imaging.[50] The bicycle is either mechanically or electronically braked, and workload is calibrated in watts or kilopond meters per minute. Most protocols begin at a workload of 25 W and increase in 25-W increments every 2 min. Benefits of bicycle ergometry include stability of the thorax, producing less muscle artifact on ECG monitoring, easier blood pressure recording, less influence of a patient's weight on the exercise capacity as compared with treadmill testing, and less anxiety performing exercise seated on a bicycle compared with walking on a mechanically driven treadmill. Cycle ergometers are also smaller, quieter, and less expensive than treadmills. However, patients are less likely to reach $\dot{V}O_{2max}$ or peak predicted target HR on a bicycle as compared with on a treadmill, and early fatigue of the quadriceps muscle on the bicycle is a greater limiting factor than seen with the treadmill.[163] Bicycle ergometry is also associated with a lower $\dot{V}O_{2max}$ and anaerobic threshold than with the treadmill. Treadmill testing applies a more physiologic workload and, in practice, treadmill protocols are used more widely in the evaluation of patients with CAD.

The most frequently used treadmill EST protocol is the Bruce, which starts at 1.7 mph on a 10% grade and increases at 3-min intervals.[33] Limitations of this more aggressive treadmill protocol include the large increases in $\dot{V}O_2$ between stages (5 METs), and the additional energy cost of running as compared with walking that occurs beyond stage 3. The modified

Bruce has two 3-min warm-up stages at 1.7 mph and 0% grade and 1.7 mph and 5% grade. Other protocols, including Naughton,[160] Weber, Balke-Ware,[14] and Cornell,[165] have been developed for patients with CHF, those who are deconditioned, or those who have other causes of limited exercise tolerance.

In patients with an ICD for ventricular arrhythmias, the peak HR must be kept below that which initiates the antitachycardia pacing component of the ICD and eventual discharge. Alternatively, the ICD can be deactivated during the EST to allow the HR to increase while monitoring for the onset of arrhythmias. If VT or ventricular fibrillation (VF) is identified, the device can be reactivated to terminate the arrhythmia.

Other modalities in stress testing

Pharmacologic stress testing is indicated when EST is not possible due to physical limitations, or in patients on beta-blockers who are unable to increase their HR adequately. Intravenous dipyridamole[128] blocks the cellular reuptake of adenosine, a potent vasodilator, increasing local concentrations. Atherosclerotic vessels do not vasodilate with adenosine, whereas normal vessels do, creating relative hypoperfusion in the myocardium supplied by the diseased vessel—a coronary steal syndrome. Adenosine can be infused directly with similar results.[15] Dipyridamole and adenosine are contraindicated in patients with pulmonary disease, as they cause bronchoconstriction. Dobutamine, a cardiac beta agonist that increases $M\dot{V}O_2$, is used instead.[185] In myocardium supplied by diseased vessels, $M\dot{V}O_2$ will exceed supply. Functional information, including duration of exercise, exercise capacity, and symptoms, are not obtained from pharmacologic stimulation. Peak HR is lower without exercise.

Cardiac imaging in stress testing

Cardiac imaging in EST is usually accomplished with ECG, unless it is difficult to interpret (Box 34-8). Echocardiographic imaging of the myocardium overcomes these limitations, and is especially useful in women who are prone to a false positive ECG EST. A baseline echocardiogram is performed before stimulation, noting resting abnormalities. Stimulation is with EST or pharmacologic agents. Exercise protocols for stress echocardiography are available for supine[100] and upright[174] bicycles, and the treadmill.[239] A second echocardiogram is performed immediately following the exercise to identify changes in myocardial contractility compared with in the resting study. The

myocardium should contract normally at rest and be hyperdynamic following exercise. New wall motion abnormalities after exercise indicate ischemia. Echocardiography is more sensitive and specific in identifying ischemia than ECG monitoring is.[186]

Myocardial perfusion can be visualized using radiopharmaceuticals that accumulate in the myocardium in proportion to blood flow. Nuclear imaging is more accurate than stress echocardiography.[182] Examples of radiolabels include thallium-201 and technetium-99m. Imaging is performed with single-photon emission computed tomography (SPECT), where a series of planar images are obtained over a 180° arc around the patient's thorax. Only one injection of thallium-201 is required at peak exercise, with initial imaging performed within 5 min of the injection.[228] Images reflect peak exercise myocardial blood flow. Imaging is repeated 2–4 h later, reflecting myocardial viability. Two separate injections are given with technetium-99m. The first is given during exercise, and imaging within 15 min of this time reflects myocardial perfusion. The second injection is given at rest to evaluate perfusion at this time. Comparison is made between the two images, with regional blood flow abnormalities indicating areas of ischemia.

A normal SPECT image reveals homogeneous uptake of the radiopharmaceutical throughout the myocardium. A relative decrease in uptake signifies a defect. If the defect is present on the initial stress image but reduced or absent from the rest study, reversible ischemia is diagnosed. An unchanged defect, present on both stress and rest images, signifies MI and scar tissue. Detection of LV dilatation on SPECT imaging immediately after exercise is highly indicative of multivessel CAD.[232] Evidence of transient ischemia rather than fixed deficits, and the number of defects and degree of reversibility, are all associated with future cardiac events.[31]

A normal exercise response is defined by an increase in EF by at least 5%. A fall in EF with exercise detected on nuclear imaging from rest to exercise is associated with a poor prognosis.[26] The ventricular response to exercise can have a greater prognostic significance than the extent of CAD.[140]

Computed tomography and magnetic resonance imaging in CAD

Computed tomography[221] and MRI[191] are increasingly useful in the detection of CAD. Catheter-based angiography is invasive, and intravascular ultrasound transducers are required to quantify coronary plaque burden, the strongest determinant of cardiac events.[98] EST is less invasive, but also less sensitive in detecting CAD. Calcium present in coronary plaques can be detected and quantified[2] using a non-invasive electron beam computed tomography (EBCT). A higher total coronary artery calcification score (CACS) correlates well with coronary events.[10] Event rates in asymptomatic patients are significantly higher in those with the highest CACS compared with those with the lowest.[175] Progression of the CACS also identifies greater risk of coronary events compared with stable scores.[176] EBCT allows reliable interpretation of the coronary arteries.[179] However, the absence of calcification does not exclude a vulnerable coronary plaque.[61]

Box 34-8 Cardiac conditions that limit interpretation of the electrocardiogram

- Conduction abnormalities
- Digoxin
- Left bundle branch block
- Left ventricular hypertrophy
- Wolf–Parkinson–White syndrome
- Very low voltage (common following anterior wall infarction)
- Prior bypass surgery

Magnetic resonance imaging is not as accurate in detecting coronary stenosis.[76,136] Technical limitations should improve using ultrafast magnetic resonance scanners. MRI is better at evaluating ventricular function, including EF, SV, and ventricular mass. Wall motion abnormalities can be quantified with cine-MRI.[73] Stress MRI using dobutamine can detect myocardial ischemia[107] and evaluate myocardial viability.[75] MRI is contraindicated in patients with pacemakers and ICDs.

Pulmonary function testing including arterial gas analysis is useful in the differentiation of cardiac and pulmonary diseases, or confirming the presence of both. It completes the evaluation of a dyspneic cardiac patient.

MEDICATIONS IN CARDIAC REHABILITATION

The indications and effects of medications commonly taken by patients involved in CR programs are summarized in Table 34-9.

CARDIAC REHABILITATION AS A CONTINUUM OF CARE

Cardiac rehabilitation was traditionally applied in four distinct phases: acute inpatient care, home-based recuperation, outpatient program, and independent self-care. Programs now represent a flowing continuum of care, individualized according to diagnosis, medical stability, functional ability, and goals, and can be modified based on progress.

Inpatient acute medical setting

Goals are to prevent physiologic deconditioning, achieve safe mobility, and determine disposition (home versus acute rehabilitation). CR is initiated as soon as the patient is medically stable following a cardiac event. Passive range of motion exercises to maintain muscular tone and prevent joint contractures are appropriate for patients in intensive care. Early mobilization to 2–3 METs prevents loss of cardiovascular reflexes associated with prolonged bed rest. Chest physical therapy, including breathing exercises, incentive spirometer and manual techniques, promotes secretion clearance. Nasal cannula oxygen is prescribed to keep oxygen saturations over 90%. Telemetry-monitored seated activities, standing, and ambulation at 3–4 METs follows. Training in ADL to 4–6 METs is initiated, focusing on energy conservation and pacing. Education is initiated regarding nutrition, risk factor modification, potential medical complications, and the ongoing CR process. Length of stay ranges from 3 to 7 days, depending on medical stability, functional ability, and insurance issues. Patients transition home or to inpatient CR.

Inpatient acute rehabilitation setting

Goals include achievement of medical stability, functional independence, and initiation of aerobic conditioning. The ideal setting is a dedicated CR or medically complex unit.

The multidisciplinary team and roles include the following.

- Exercise physiologist: EST, training HR prescription, supervision of aerobic training sessions, and intensity progression.
- Physical therapist: functional independence measure scoring; treatment of physical comorbidities; balance, gait, and stair training; supervision of aerobic training sessions; chest physical therapy; and home equipment recommendations.
- Occupational therapist: functional independence measure scoring, treatment of physical comorbidities, cognitive and safety evaluation, ADL training, energy conservation and pacing education, relaxation and breathing exercises, use of assistive devices, and home equipment recommendations.
- Psychologist: cognitive and psychosocial evaluation and therapy, behavioral modification, and smoking cessation.
- Social worker: psychosocial counseling, patient and family education, discharge planning, and smoking cessation.
- Nutritionist: dietary evaluation, education, and counseling.
- Rehabilitation nurse: wound and skin care, pain management, safety education, and medication education.
- Nurse educator: CVD and risk factor education.
- Physiatrist: prescription of CR program, team supervision and CR program modification, coordination of medical care, and patient education.

Functional and aerobic training is prescribed, based on an admission submaximal EST. Acute CR includes 60 min of telemetry-monitored aerobic exercise, and 60 min each of individual physical and occupational therapy daily. Vital signs are recorded frequently. Patient education and risk factor modification continues. The national average length of stay for CR is 11–13 days. An 'exit' submaximal EST on the day of discharge identifies improvements in aerobic capacity and guides activity during the transitional period.

Transitional period

Goals include reintegration into full community activities and preparation for outpatient CR. The transition period allows for complete wound healing, medical stabilization, and continued functional gains. Patients transition from hospitalization to community independence. Visiting nurse care and home physical therapy are applicable. Unmonitored aerobic exercise is discouraged at this time. The transition time period varies depending on medical and functional recovery.

Outpatient rehabilitation

Goals include progressive aerobic conditioning, education, atherosclerosis risk factor and lifestyle modification, and return to vocational and avocational practices. A symptom-limited EST is performed prior to outpatient CR to complete risk factor stratification.

Risk factor stratification

Risk factor stratification is the extrapolation of medical, functional, and physiologic performance into a safe exercise

Table 34–9 Profile of common medications prescribed in patients involved in cardiac rehabilitation

Class	Example(s)	Physiologic effect(s)	Indication(s)	Side effect(s)	Caution(s)
Beta-blockers	Atenolol Metoprolol Carvedilol	Reduced heart rate, after-load, MV_{O_2}, arrhythmias Improved ejection fraction, left ventricular remodeling	Hypertension Angina Myocardial infarction Congestive heart failure (CHF) Arrhythmia	Fatigue Depression Bradycardia Sexual dysfunction	Diabetic patients: asymptomatic hypoglycemia Peripheral vascular disease: worsens peripheral circulation
Angiotensin-converting enzyme (ACE) inhibitors	Enalapril Lisinopril Ramipril	Inhibits conversion of angiotensin I to angiotensin II, a powerful vasoconstrictor	CHF Coronary artery disease (CAD) Hypertension	Dry cough Angioedema	Worsening renal function in chronic renal insufficiency and renal artery stenosis
Angiotensin receptor blockers	Losartan	Blocks the angiotensin II receptor	Substitute for ACE inhibitor when not tolerated	None greater than placebo	Worsening renal function in chronic renal insufficiency and renal artery stenosis
Calcium channel blockers	Verapamil Diltiazem Nifedipine	Blocks the slow calcium channel, prolonging conduction time through the atrioventricular node	Atrial fibrillation Hypertension	Hypotension Bradycardia Asystole Peripheral edema	Augments effects of beta-blockers
Nitrates	Isosorbide mono- or dinitrate Sublingual nitroglycerin Nitro-paste or patch	Coronary vasodilatation	Acute to chronic stable angina	Headaches Hypotension	Severe hypotension with sildenafil
Statins	Lovastatin Pravastatin Simvastatin Atorvastatin	HMG-CoA reductase inhibitors	Elevated total cholesterol and low-density lipoprotein Reduced high-density lipoprotein	Hepatotoxicity Myopathy Rhabdomyolysis	Muscle soreness
Diuretics	Furosemide Hydrochlorothiazide Spironolactone	Salt and water excretion	Hypertension CHF	Electrolyte abnormalities Worsening renal failure	Dehydration and hypotension, especially with ACE inhibitor
Cardiac glycosides	Digoxin	Increased cardiac inotropy Decreased atrioventricular node conduction velocity	Rate control in atrial fibrillation Symptomatic improvement in CHF	Arrhythmias Nausea Anorexia	Hypokalemia induces toxic effects at lower drug concentration
Antiarrhythmics	Amiodarone	Prolongs action potential duration and refractoriness of all cardiac fibers	Supraventricular tachycardias Ventricular arrhythmias	Pulmonary toxicity Liver failure Thyroid dysfunction Arrhythmias	Potentiates the effects of warfarin (Coumadin) and digoxin Very long half-life Maintenance 200 mg/day

Continued on page 725

Continued from page 724 Table 34-9 Profile of common medications prescribed in patients involved in cardiac rehabilitation

Class	Example(s)	Physiologic effect(s)	Indication(s)	Side effect(s)	Caution(s)
Anticoagulants	Warfarin	Inhibits vitamin K carboxylation Inhibits clotting factors II, VII, IX, and X	Prevention of stroke in atrial fibrillation, clotting on new prosthetic heart valves, and clots in dilated cardiomyopathy Treatment of deep venous thrombosis and pulmonary embolism	Bleeding disorders	Potentiated by other drugs— amiodarone, metronidazole
	Aspirin	Inhibits thromboxane A_2 formation to inhibit platelet aggregation	Secondary prevention of CAD Primary prevention of CAD if uncontrolled risk factors Acute myocardial infarction	Bleeding disorders	Potentiates bleeding disorder if combined with other anticoagulants
	Clopidrogrel	Inhibits ADP-induced platelet aggregation	Prevention of stent thrombosis Acute myocardial infarction	Bleeding disorders	Potentiates bleeding disorder if combined with other anticoagulants
Hypoglycemics	Insulin Metformin Glyburide Glipizide	Reduces blood sugar by increasing circulating insulin or peripheral effects of insulin	Diabetes	Hypoglycemia	Renal insufficiency (metformin), asymptomatic hypoglycemia in patients on beta-blockers
Sildenafil	Sildenafil	Inhibits cyclic GMP-specific phosphodiesterase, resulting in smooth muscle relaxation, vasodilatation, and enhanced penile erection	Male erectile dysfunction	Headache Flushing Mild to severe hypotension	Avoid in those taking nitrates, as combination increases the risk of severe hypotension
Vitamins	Folic acid	Regulates metabolic pathway involved in the metabolism of homocysteine	Treatment of elevated homocysteine as a risk factor for CAD	None	–

prescription, limiting the risk for acute cardiovascular complications during exercise training. Patients are assigned *low, moderate,* or *high* risk for complications, and prescribed an appropriate exercise intensity. Risk of cardiac events during exercise training is greatest in patients with poor LV function, ventricular arrhythmias, or a non-ST elevation MI due to increased risk of later ischemic events.[69] Non-compliance with the exercise prescription[184] and poor compliance with prescribed training HR[106] also increase the risk of mortality. Risk for arrhythmias and ischemia can be highest during recovery following exercise training.[46,240]

Historical data report a range from 1 major complication (cardiac arrest and non-fatal MI) in 26 715 patient exercise hours[99] to 1 in 81 101 h.[222] More recent data indicate a frequency of 1 per 58 451 h.[68] Acute cardiac events might be more likely during the early morning hours.[153] Despite an increased risk of cardiac events during exercise in patients with HD, the overall mortality of patients with HD who exercise regularly is significantly lower than in those who do not.[213]

Risk stratification guidelines are published by the American Association of Cardiovascular and Pulmonary Rehabilitation.[4] Individual CR programs can modify these guidelines. Risk stratification starts with a complete history and physical examination. All test data are reviewed, including ECG, echocardiograms, Holter monitor, coronary angiography, pharmacologic, and EST. Major cardiovascular complications include ongoing ischemia, arrhythmia, and pump failure—failure of the exercising myocardium to maintain adequate cardiac output. These complica-

Table 34-10 Risk assignment for cardiovascular complications that may develop with exercise

	No risk	Low risk	Moderate risk	High risk
Ischemia	No atherosclerosis risk factors No history of coronary artery disease Normal electrocardiogram, echo, angiogram, and exercise stress test (EST)	Atherosclerosis risk factors History of coronary artery disease but no current ischemia or electrocardiogram, echo, or angiographic evidence of atherosclerosis or prior cardiac event Ejection fraction (EF) >50% Normal EST	Ischemia or angina at moderate to high exercise intensity (>7 metabolic equivalents, METs) on EST, controlled at lower intensity exercise levels with medications Stable following an ischemic event, coronary artery bypass graft, or angiographic intervention EF 40–50%	Ischemia or angina at low-intensity exercise levels (<5 METs) on EST despite optimal medications Complex coronary anatomy not amenable to intervention or revascularization EF <40%
Arrhythmia	No history or finding of arrhythmia on testing	Non-sustained, rate-controlled supraventricular arrhythmias with no hemodynamic compromise Unifocal infrequent premature ventricular contractions	Rapid supraventricular arrhythmias with or without symptoms but no hemodynamic compromise Mutifocal premature ventricular contractions, couplets, triplets, or history of non-sustained ventricular tachycardia Paced rhythms	Any arrhythmia with hemodynamic compromise Recent history of ventricular tachycardia, ventricular fibrillation, or asystole, with or without an implantable cardioverter defibrillator
Pump failure	No evidence of congestive heart failure (CHF) Normal rise in systolic blood pressure >20 mmHg with moderate-intensity exercise Normal EF and left ventricular wall motion on imaging	Remote history of CHF controlled with medications Asymptomatic at rest, but mild symptoms at moderate- to high-intensity exercise Mild left ventricular dysfunction, but EF >50% Normal or blunted rise (5–20 mmHg) in systolic blood pressure with moderate-intensity exercise	Active CHF controlled with medications Symptoms with mild- to moderate-intensity exercise Blunted or no rise (0–5 mmHg) in systolic blood pressure with mild-to moderate-intensity exercise Moderate left ventricular dysfunction with EF 40–50%	CHF at rest or with mild-intensity exercise Recent history of a fall in systolic blood pressure with or post exercise Moderate to severe left ventricular dysfunction with EF <40%

tions are often seen in combination. From all available data, a risk is assigned for the development of each complication during exercise (Table 34-10).

Contraindications to exercise

Include unstable angina, resting ST depression > 2 mm, uncontrolled arrhythmias (rate or hemodynamic compromise), critical aortic stenosis, uncompensated CHF, resting SBP > 200 mmHg or diastolic blood pressure > 110 mmHg, fall in SBP > 10 mmHg with exercise, and symptomatic orthostatic SBP drop 10–20 mmHg.

Comorbidities impacting the safety of exercise

Diabetes Blood sugar is tested before and after exercise, and during training if hypoglycemia is suspected. Significant hypoglycemia while exercising is frequent in patients with insulin-dependent diabetes, but is most common several hours after completion of exercise.[131] Guidelines exist to prevent hypogly-

cemia during exercise.[70] A patient having diabetes who has a blood sugar <100 mg/dL before exercise should eat a carbohydrate snack and monitor blood sugar during the exercise session. If blood sugar is > 350 mg/dL, exercise is postponed, as glucose utilization is compromised.

Anticoagulation Unless bruising is progressive, patients on aspirin and clopidogrel can exercise normally. Those with an international normalized ratio > 5.0 are held from exercise until values normalize, to prevent hemarthrosis and muscle hematoma.

Visual and cognitive impairment These are not absolute contraindications to exercise, but close supervision with the use of aerobic machines is required.

Wound and skin integrity Sternal and vein graft wounds should be healing and stable before moderate-intensity exercise is allowed. Sacral pressure sores require pressure relief. With peripheral neuropathy, the skin of the feet must be inspected before and after exercise. Exercise is held if skin integrity is compromised.

Rheumatologic, neurologic, orthopedic, or balance disorders
These also warrant close attention.

Based on the evaluated risk for ischemia, arrhythmia, and pump failure with exercise training, a combined, single risk is assigned. This can be *no, low, moderate,* or *high.* It is prudent to assign a high-risk class even if the patient was high risk for only one parameter. Moderate risk is assigned so long as there were no high-risk parameters, and low risk so long as there were no moderate- or high-risk parameters. There is no indication for monitored CR for those in the no risk class. The assignment of a single risk allows translation of the risk stratification process into a safe exercise training intensity. The HR reserve method described by Karvonen[114] is used to determine the training HR as a measure of exercise intensity:

$$\text{training HR} = \text{RHR} + [(\text{PHR} - \text{RHR}) \times I],$$

where RHR is resting HR from the EST, PHR is peak HR from the EST, and I a coefficient expressed as percentage based on risk stratification class (low risk, 70–85%; moderate risk, 55–70%; and high risk, 40–55%).

The higher the risk for complications, the lower the initial training HR intensity. The training HR can slowly be increased as patients exercise without complication, or reduced if complications develop.

Other methods exist to determine the training intensity. With a benign EST end point, a training HR up to 85% of the maximum HR can be used. More complex end points warrant 60% of maximum HR as an initial training HR. When ischemia limits the EST, a training HR is set 10 beats below the ischemic threshold (the HR when ischemia is first noted). For patients on HR-limiting medications (beta-blockers) with a blunted HR response to exercise, a training HR is set 10–20 beats above resting.

Following HT, abnormal physiologic responses to exercise result in unreliable HR-determined training intensities. EST in HT recipients should include ventilatory gas analysis, and a target training intensity of 50–65% of $\dot{V}O_{2\text{max}}$ should be set. This correlates with a Borg rate of perceived exertion of 12–14, or 'somewhat hard'.[27]

An intense program of education, behavioral and lifestyle modification, smoking cessation, psychologic support, and nutritional counseling continues during the outpatient program. Patients prepare for independent, unsupervised, community-based maintenance exercise. Introduction to local and national peer support groups promotes adherence to a heart-healthy lifestyle.

Maintenance
On completion of outpatient CR, a repeat EST is performed. The new physiologic data enable modification to the training HR and exercise prescription. To maintain achieved gains, exercise must continue at least twice a week. Exercise three to five times a week is needed to continue the training process. Self-monitoring of the training HR using a 'wrist and chest strap' heart monitor is recommended. Maintenance CR is lifelong. Frequent follow-up visits to guide progress are recommended. An annual EST is recommended to update risk stratification and training HR.

Prescription writing for cardiac rehabilitation
Each phase of the CR program requires a physician-directed prescription. All phases require cardiac precautions and telemetry monitoring (except maintenance).

During the inpatient acute medical setting, occupational therapists, physical therapists, and chest therapists each treat the patient for 15–20 min. Goals and an outline of the treatment program have been described above.

The inpatient acute CR program lasts 10–14 days. Both the occupational therapist and the physical therapist provide 60 min each of individual therapy. The physical therapist and exercise physiologist supervise the daily aerobic program, including a 10-min callisthenic warm up, 45–60 min of low-impact aerobic training (three or four modalities up to 15 min each), and a 10-min cooldown including stretching. The warm up prepares the body for more intense aerobic exercise, and might help prevent development of exercise-induced ventricular arrhythmias. The cooldown minimizes postexercise hypotension and subsequent myocardial ischemia. Gentle muscle and joint stretching before and after exercise minimizes postexercise soreness and improves flexibility. Intensity of aerobic exercise training was discussed above. Aerobic modalities typically include stationary bicycle, Schwinn Airdyne, step machine, rowing machine, upper body ergometer, Versaclimber, and treadmill. Training advances initially with duration and then intensity of exercise. Valsalva maneuvers, heavy resistance, and anaerobic exercise are avoided.

The psychologist, social worker, nutritionist, rehabilitation nurse, and nurse educator coordinate further care, depending on the individual needs of the patient.

In the transitional period, regular daily activities are resumed over several weeks. Homecare visiting nurse, physical therapist, and occupational therapist orders are provided if indicated. Patients do not participate in any aerobic exercise during this period.

During outpatient CR, patients attend three exercise sessions per week, supervised by the physical therapist and exercise physiologist, for a total of 36 sessions (depending at times on insurance coverage). The aerobic exercise prescription is as for inpatient acute CR. Light free-weight resistance exercises can be prescribed. Ongoing education is provided by all members of the rehabilitation team.

During maintenance, patients continue with self-directed aerobic training three to five times per week. Training principles and progression mirror previous phases.

CARDIAC REHABILITATION FOR SPECIFIC GROUPS

The principles of evaluation, risk stratification, prescription writing, risk factor modification, patient education, and support discussed previously are central to all programs of CR.

Coronary artery disease

Stable angina

Aerobic training reduces the myocardial oxygen demand for the same activity intensity after training compared with before. More intense activity can be performed before the ischemic threshold is reached (see Fig. 34-8). If anginal symptoms are noted, a brief examination and ECG are indicated before exercise is permitted. Patients who experience exercise-induced angina may take sublingual nitroglycerin prior to exercise. Longer-acting antianginal medications require a 3-h interval before exercising to allow for maximum effect. Exercise intensity is calculated by the Karvonen method, or set 10 beats below the ischemic threshold HR from the EST. CR in patients with CAD is associated with a reduction in morbidity and mortality,[111] in part due to improvement of the autonomic regulation of the heart.[130] Improvement in LV contractile function is also noted.[56] Inpatient CR for severe angina improves physical performance and improves rates of return to work.[203]

Myocardial infarction

In patients with MI, other vessels are also likely to be stenosed, and the exercise prescription is similar to that for stable angina. Following a large MI, exercise training is delayed 4–6 weeks, and a lower intensity level and frequent clinical and echocardiographic monitoring are recommended. Otherwise, exercise training is initiated within 2–4 weeks according to the prescription guidelines previously outlined. Combined resistance and aerobic training improves aerobic fitness and muscle strength more than aerobic training alone without adverse outcomes.[200] Health-related QOL,[108] survival in patients with depression, and rates of non-fatal reinfarction[25] are also improved. Beta-blockers, which are a standard of care following an MI to reduce mortality, do not attenuate the benefits of exercise training.[170]

Following MI, a change in LV dimensions (remodeling) occurs over weeks to months in the infarcted area. It is associated with deteriorating LV function, ventricular arrhythmias, aneurysm formation, and higher mortality. Larger MIs and elevated ventricular pressures increase remodeling. Despite increasing ventricular pressures with moderate-intensity aerobic exercise, training soon after a small MI does not exacerbate remodeling.[40] Exercise frequency also has no effect.[194] ACE inhibitors limit remodeling and improve survival. CR also improves myocardial perfusion[89] and LV electrophysiologic parameters, so reducing risk for malignant ventricular arrhythmias and sudden cardiac death after MI.[113] Overall, following MI, 95% of patients who participate in CR survive 3 years, compared with 64% for non-participants.[245]

Angioplasty and stent

Coronary restenosis following angioplasty, acute stent thrombosis, and later (6–12 month) stenosis due to intimal hyperplasia are common. Clopidogrel with aspirin to prevent thrombosis, and drug-eluting stents to inhibit coronary intimal hyperplasia, reduce rates of acute thrombosis to 0.5% and later stenosis to 2.5%. Close monitoring for symptoms and signs of recurrent ischemia during CR is important. Despite concern that exercise is prothrombotic, there is no increase in the rate of stent restenosis when EST is completed within 1 month of stent placement,[83,183] or with CR participation.[22] Aerobic training programs following angioplasty improve $\dot{V}O_{2max}$ and functional capacity.[121]

Coronary artery bypass surgery

Surgical site integrity and pain initially limit upper body exercise following CABG. Inappropriate transfer techniques or forceful upper body exercises can cause sternal dehiscence. By 6 weeks, postoperative sternal knitting is complete and upper body exercise can be liberalized. Wound breakdown is less of a concern with minimally invasive surgical approaches. Inpatient CR after CABG is well tolerated, and attendance at outpatient sessions is >80%. More intense programs are associated with a more rapid achievement of functional goals and greater patient satisfaction.[171] Improved myocardial perfusion is associated with an increased ischemic threshold.[71] Typical changes in exercise physiologic parameters are noted, with peripheral adaptations accounting for the majority of improvement in $\dot{V}O_{2max}$.[80]

Arrhythmias are noted in one-third of patients during inpatient CR. Predisposing features include hypertension, diabetes, hyperlipidemia, older age, and discontinuation of amiodarone. These comorbidities should be included in risk stratification models for CR, especially if significant arrhythmias were previously noted.[80] Autonomic dysfunction is associated with an increased risk of sudden death following MI and CABG due to ventricular arrhythmias. Aerobic exercise following CABG improves autonomic function[206] and reduces the incidence of arrhythmias.

To overcome strength deficits after CABG, moderate-intensity resistance weight training is safe and effective, but without aerobic exercise does not increase $\dot{V}O_2$.[134] Interval training, such as higher-intensity bursts of exercise interspersed with brief 'rest' at lower-intensity level training, is also beneficial following CABG and gives a more rapid increase in exercise capacity compared with steady-state aerobic training.[144]

Similar sternal wound precautions are also important during CR following heart valve surgery. Prolonged valvular abnormalities and presurgical CHF cause significant deconditioning. Following surgery, with a normal EF, CR proceeds as for CABG. With a reduced EF, CR proceeds as for CHF. With anticoagulation following valve surgery, care must be taken to avoid trauma. High-impact exercises can cause hemarthrosis and bruising.

Cardiomyopathy

Despite EFs < 20%, patients with severe ischemic cardiomyopathy tolerate CR, with increased $\dot{V}O_{2max}$,[16] improved LV systolic and diastolic[17] function, and enhanced QOL.[19] Typically, fewer ventricular arrhythmias[132] and no further myocardial damage[156] are noted. The risk of subsequent cardiac events is inversely related to the degree of functional improvement with CR.[20] Participation also improves survival in a dose–response relationship.[234]

Congestive heart failure

A significant increase in $\dot{V}O_{2max}$ and exercise tolerance is noted with CR for CHF. Most improvement occurs within 3 weeks, but continues for up to 6 months if training continues.[20] This is associated with increased muscle mitochondria,[94] decreased ventilation,[45] reduced catecholamine levels, and improved autonomic function.[93] CR for CHF also improves myocardial perfusion. Fewer cardiac events are noted, with significantly lower rates of hospital readmission for CHF, reduced cardiac mortality,[18,172] and improved QOL.[238] Attenuated LV remodeling underlies these benefits.[77]

Most aerobic programs for CHF utilize a continuous, steady-state training protocol.[45] Interval training, short 60- to 120-s bursts of intense 'work' exercise phases, interspersed with 30- to 60-s 'recovery' exercise phases, also improves $\dot{V}O_{2max}$ and muscle strength.[145] Resistance weight training with weight machines, combined with aerobic training, produces greater improvements in LV function, $\dot{V}O_{2max}$, and strength compared with aerobic training alone.[53] Aerobic training combined with interval and strength training maximizes clinical, physiologic, and functional benefits in CHF.

Over 40% of patients with CHF have conduction abnormalities that exacerbate CHF. Implantation of a biventricular pacemaker with leads placed in both ventricles improves LV–EF significantly. Biventricular pacemakers are often combined with ICDs in one 'box', as both are frequently required. Combination devices significantly improve mortality compared with biventricular pacing alone.[30,248]

Exercise tolerance, $\dot{V}O_{2max}$, anaerobic threshold, and QOL improve with CR in patients with a biventricular pacemaker. Fewer CHF exacerbations requiring hospitalization are noted. These benefits are long-lasting and associated with significant functional improvements. Improved LV function and physiologic chronotropic response to exercise underlie these gains.[90]

Heart transplantation

With improved survival rates following HT, there are increasing numbers of significantly debilitated patients requiring CR. CR is safe for patients on intravenous inotropic support awaiting transplantation.[11] CR is recommended both before and after HT,[220] and protocols include aerobic and resistive exercises[29,117] and respiratory muscle training.[39] The postoperative program is similar to the post-CABG program. Due to the abnormal HR response to exercise and significant limitations in $\dot{V}O_{2max}$, early exercise intensity is set at a Borg score of 11–13, increasing to 13–15 as tolerated.[173] A significant increase in $\dot{V}O_{2max}$ and work capacity with CR is noted.[117] Considering the accelerated rate of atherosclerosis seen after HT, ongoing aerobic exercise needs to be stressed. Long-term continuing care from a multidisci-

plinary HT-specialized CR team is necessary to accommodate the unique needs of these recipients. Needs include the management of complex medication regimens, psychologic adjustment that deals especially with rejection episodes, vocational rehabilitation, and care of significant musculoskeletal and neurologic issues.

Left ventricular assist device

As a bridge to HT, use of the pneumatic LVAD is increasingly popular for end-stage CHF. An LVAD can delay the need for HT, allowing time for medical and functional improvements in patients otherwise too sick for surgery. Ambulation is safely initiated within 7–10 days of insertion of the LVAD, with treadmill training by 3 weeks. Resumption of ADL up to 5 METs is possible within 6 weeks.[150] Patients can survive over 2 years with an LVAD, and exercise during long-term LVAD support is safe.[109] However, functional status is more significantly enhanced following HT compared with LVAD insertion, and transplantation should not be delayed if a suitable organ becomes available.[110]

Arrhythmia

One-third of patients develop atrial tachyarrhythmias immediately following cardiac surgery, most commonly atrial fibrillation. Atrial fibrillation frequently persists during acute inpatient CR. If conversion back to sinus rhythm is not achieved, rate control is essential, as cardiac output is reduced due to impaired LV filling. An HR < 100 is ideal but, in asymptomatic patients with a good blood pressure and a resting HR of 100–120, exercise can be initiated at low intensity levels with close supervision. An HR > 120 at rest or exceeding 140 with light activities is a contraindication to further exercise until the HR response is controlled.

Following MI and CABG, the incidence of ventricular arrhythmias is related to the presence of diabetes, hyperlipidemia, hypertension, and age > 70 years old.[72] Frequent premature ventricular contractions are associated with increased risk of VT and sudden death. VT and VF within 30 days of CABG are rare but account for a significant number of deaths. This is of significance to the CR team, as this coincides with the time period for inpatient CR. Approximately 5% of patients undergoing CR following CABG do not complete the program due to development of an arrhythmia, 25% of which are ventricular.

Aerobic exercise itself may be arrhythmogenic due to a decrease in vagal tone, increased sympathetic neural activity, and circulating catecholamines. Prolonged (10-min) warm up and cooldown before and after exercise training can reduce the frequency of arrhythmias. Patients with ventricular arrhythmias and only minimally reduced EF with good exercise tolerance are far more likely to experience significant complications during CR than patients with very limited exercise capacity. Decreasing exercise intensity and increasing duration and frequency is indicated.[115] Exercise therapy after MI[113] and in patients with EF < 20%[132] can reduce the risk for ventricular arrhythmia.

Nearly 20% of patients with a recent history of ventricular arrhythmia develop VT during inpatient CR. During outpatient CR, nearly 30% develop VT. However, there are very few fatalities noted during EST and CR from ventricular arrhythmias. ICDs are used to manage malignant ventricular arrhythmias. Current indications for an ICD include recurrent or life-threatening VT or VF, and inducible VT or VF on electrophysiologic testing. Mortality rates from VT following MI in patients with reduced EF and treated with an ICD are significantly lower (4%) compared with pharmacologic management (60%).[85] This represents a 27% risk reduction in total mortality with ICD therapy.[85]

Supine exercise is more likely to induce ventricular arrhythmias than upright exercise is. Patients prone to arrhythmias and those with ICDs should exercise with upright activities (walking, biking, and stair climbing) rather than recumbent.[121] CR for patients with an ICD is safe and effective with careful supervision and constant monitoring.[62] Patients with an ICD tolerate an exercise training intensity equal to patients without a device, with a significant increase in $\dot{V}O_{2max}$. About 5% of patients will experience ICD discharge during CR.[223]

Initially after ICD implantation, fear of life-threatening arrhythmias decreases and QOL improves. However, time since implantation and number of ICD discharges predict increasing severity of anxiety, depression, and impairment of QOL. Fear of exercising with an ICD is also common. Social support groups and CR can reverse this fear and improve QOL.[229]

COGNITIVE AND MOOD DISORDERS IN CARDIAC REHABILITATION

Pre-CABG cognitive testing often reveals significant cognitive deficits, especially affecting verbal memory. These deficits are probably related to the presence of coexisting vascular disease.[177] CVD and PVD are risk factors for cognitive decline following CABG.[104] Following CABG, up to 80% of patients experience further cognitive impairments in attention, concentration, short-term memory, and speed of mental responses. Neuropsychologic performance typically declines by day 3 following CABG, with recovery over a week.[155] However, cognitive decline within a week after CABG is a strong indicator of decline at 3 months,[55] and cognitive changes can still be noted 5 years out.[204] A similar pattern is seen after valve surgery.[86] Severe cognitive impairment with encephalopathy is noted in approximately 7% of patients, and is associated with a longer length of stay and a mortality rate five times higher than that of cognitively intact patients.[142] Encephalopathy is associated with a history of previous stroke, hypertension, diabetes, carotid bruit, and longer time on cardiopulmonary bypass.

Metabolic neuronal disturbances indicated by abnormalities on magnetic resonance spectroscopy correlate closely with postoperative cognitive deficits. Anatomic ischemic lesions on MRI, however, do not correlate with impairments.[21]

'Off-pump' surgical techniques and minimally invasive procedures have reduced the incidence of post-CABG cognitive deficits,[249] with equivalent outcomes to on-pump techniques regarding survival and freedom from stroke, MI, and coronary reintervention.

Cognitive dysfunction is also seen with CHF and is associated with a fivefold increase in mortality. In patients with CHF, in-hospital death is significantly increased with cognitive disorder compared to without.[250]

Depression is closely related to HD, including CAD, arrhythmias, MI, CHF, and sudden death.[87] Close to 40% of patients awaiting CABG are depressed. Within 1 week following surgery, 50% are depressed. However, the incidence of depression falls to 23% by 12 months. The presence of preoperative depression is a strong indicator of postoperative depression, and the absence of preoperative depression is a strong indicator of better mood following surgery.[214] Pre-CABG depression also correlates with repeated cardiac hospitalizations, continued surgical pain, failure to resume previous activity levels,[35] and increased 2-year cardiovascular mortality.[36] Depression also predicts greater levels of medical comorbidity following MI,[230] but regular exercise reduces rates of MI and mortality.[25]

A mental health team, including psychiatrist, psychologist, social worker, and occupational therapist, completes a comprehensive neurocognitive and psychosocial evaluation of patients in CR. If cognitive deficits are detected, remediation is provided. Outcome studies evaluating efficacy, however, are lacking. Patient and family education are essential, as cognitive deficits impact functioning and safety at home. Differentiation of anxiety and depression from cognitive dysfunction is important, as they can also present with temporary cognitive changes. Psychiatric treatment of anxiety or depression improves overall outcome. Continuation of cognitive and psychiatric care in outpatient CR is recommended. Behavioral modification for coronary risk factor management should be integrated into the mental health program (see also Ch. 4).

WOMEN AND CARDIAC REHABILITATION

More than 500 000 women die each year from CVD in the USA. More women die from CAD than from all forms of cancer combined, yet most women consider CAD a remote risk. Women have poorer outcomes than men with unstable angina and after MI.[100] Women are also less likely to be referred for CR following MI and CABG, and are less strongly encouraged to participate in CR than men are. Only 7% of the women referred for CR following MI, and only 20% after CABG, actually enroll.[211] Obstacles to participation specific to women include older age, transportation difficulties, a dependent spouse, and lack of spousal support. When enrolled, however, women have adherence rates to CR equivalent to those of men.[216] Following completion of CR, 25% of women stop exercising altogether, and only 48% still exercise after 3 months. Greater social support improves adherence rates.[149]

Education regarding the prevalence and impact of cardiac diseases on women is needed, as well as more aggressive referral styles to encourage women to participate in CR. Programs should be modified to meet the needs of women, and support and education provided to improve lifelong exercise adherence.

DIFFUSE ATHEROSCLEROTIC VASCULAR DISEASE

Atherosclerosis affects all vascular beds, and underlying risk factors were identified above. Endothelial dysfunction in nonobstructive CAD is associated with an increased risk of CVD.[208] Atherosclerotic diseases include CAD, PVD, CVD, renal artery stenosis, and abdominal aortic aneurysm. In patients hospitalized with CAD, 40% have PVD on testing the ankle–brachial index.[54] With more advanced CAD, the greater the likelihood of PVD.[12] In patients admitted for vascular surgery, CAD is noted in 46%, carotid stenosis in 32%, and renal artery stenosis in 5%.[116] In patients with abdominal aortic aneurysm, 71% have CAD, 46% have PVD, and 27% have CVD.[205]

Cardiac rehabilitation programs must take into account the diffuse nature of atherosclerosis. In addition, cardiac precautions should be stipulated during the rehabilitation of patients with thrombotic strokes, PVD, and dysvascular amputation. (see Chs 13, 14, 51 and 57)

RETURN TO WORK

Patients living with CAD are predominantly 35–74 years old and employed when their HD first presents. Lost productivity is a significant part of the $100 billion cost of CAD disease in the USA.[105] Returning a patient with CAD to employment is a major goal of CR, but conventional programs have minimal success in achieving this. Conventional CR improves perception of improved health but has less influence on return to work.[58] CR programs that simulate elements of work, including flexibility and dexterity exercises, return 100% of patients to work compared with 60% for conventional programs. Work simulation CR is also more likely to return patients to the same work they performed prior to the cardiac event. Both programs produce equivalent strength and physiologic improvements.[147]

Psychosocial factors are also closely related to return to work.[217] Additional factors include age, perceived importance of the job, and support from friends and family.[28] The majority of cardiac patients return to work by 6 months. This occurs earlier for those with sedentary jobs, as compared with those with more physically demanding work. More patients return to sedentary (83%) than to heavy (67%) work.[237]

Issues of return to work should be discussed with patients early in the rehabilitation process. Return to sedentary or light work is delayed 2–4 weeks after discharge from inpatient CR. An initial modified schedule is recommended, slowly building to a full schedule over a further 2–4 weeks. For physically demanding jobs, return to work is delayed 4–6 weeks, allowing for surgical wound healing and greater functional recovery. A symptom-limited EST is completed prior to resumption of a physically demanding job to ensure the job MET level requirement is achieved safely. Vocational counseling is indicated if return to prior employment is not feasible. If patients cannot return safely to work, a disability evaluation is indicated (see also Chs 36 and 46).[196]

SEXUAL REHABILITATION IN CARDIAC REHABILITATION

Following CABG, 91% of patients resume sexual activity within 8 weeks, albeit at a decreased frequency.[168] After an MI, 25% of patients report no sexual activity and 50% report a decreased frequency. In those patients with CHF, 40% report they are unable to have sex.[209] A significant concern for patients and partners is whether sexual activity will provoke a further cardiac event. Sexual activity is stated to be as safe as climbing two flights of stairs,[207] but such advice does not reduce the fear of sexual activity. Following CABG, 17% of patients and 35% of partners express concern about resumption of sexual activity.

The majority of patients report no specific sexual activity in the 2 h prior to an MI, and only 1% report sexual activity. It is encouraging to note that the risk of MI during or immediately after sexual activity is reduced or eliminated by regular physical exercise.[152] Despite concerns over sexual activity, up to 90% of 70- to 90-year-old men with CAD report interest in sexual activity. Following an MI, sexual intercourse is not recommended for 2 weeks. An EST guides tolerance for sexual activities. Sexual intercourse between partners who know each other and in a familiar place requires up to 5 METs. Achieving 6 METs on a stress test indicates low risk for a cardiac event during sexual intercourse. Sexual position is not related to safety, but sex in an unfamiliar place or with a different partner produces increased physiologic stress and can trigger a cardiac event.[209]

One member of the CR team should be a resource for questions and concerns regarding resumption of sexual activities. A slow progression from reestablishing a romantic relationship, to foreplay, and then a more intense physically intimate relationship is emphasized. Reassurance that sexual activity in people with CAD is relatively safe, and encouragement to participate in CR, is suggested.[154]

Erectile dysfunction should be discussed. Medications can induce erectile dysfunction (antidepressants and antihypertensives, i.e. beta-blockers), and others treat it. Prescription of sildenafil and other erectile dysfunction medicines should be done only in consultation with the patient's cardiologist.

SUMMARY

Over the past four decades, there have been many advancements in the care of patients with cardiac conditions. Care of these patients has gone from being relatively passive, to emphasizing active and direct interventions that have greatly improved the chances of survival for these patients. The QOL and ultimate longevity of patients with cardiac conditions can be optimized by the use of CR services, especially if administered by an interdisciplinary team.

REFERENCES

1. Abraham A, Sever Y, Weinstein M, et al. Value of early ambulation in patients with and without complications after acute myocardial infarction. N Engl J Med 1975; 292:719–722.

2. Agatston A, Janowitz W, Hildner F, et al. Quantification of coronary artery calcium using ultrafast computed tomography. J Am Coll Cardiol 1990; 15:827–832.

3. Allison D, Fontaine K, Manson J, et al. Annual deaths attributable to obesity in the United States. JAMA 1999; 282:1530–1538.

4. American Association of Cardiovascular and Pulmonary Rehabilitation. Guidelines for cardiac rehabilitation and secondary prevention programs. 4th edn. Champaign: Human Kinetics; 2004.

5. American Psychiatric Association. Substance related disorders. Diagnostic and statistical manual of mental disorders: DSM-IV. 4th edn. Washington: American Psychiatric Association; 1994:242–247.

6. Anderson KM, Wilson PWF, Odell PM, et al. An updated coronary risk profile. A statement for health care professionals. Circulation 1991; 83:356–362.

7. Anderson RN. US decennial life tables for 1989–91, vol 1, no. 4. United States life tables eliminating certain causes of death. Hyattsville: National Center for Health Statistics; 1999.

8. Angelin B. Therapy for lowering lipoprotein(a) levels. Curr Opin Lipidol 1997; 8:337–341.

9. Appel LJ, Champagne CM, Harsha DW, et al. Effects of comprehensive lifestyle modification on blood pressure control. JAMA 2003; 289:2083–2093.

10. Arad Y, Spadaro L, Goodman K, et al. Prediction of coronary events with electron beam computed tomography. J Am Coll Cardiol 2000; 36:1253–1260.

11. Arena R, Humphrey R, Peberdy MA. Safety and efficacy of exercise training in a patient awaiting heart transplantation while on positive intravenous inotropic support. J Cardiopulm Rehabil 2000; 20(4):259–261.

12. Atmer B, Jogestrand T, Laska J, et al. Peripheral artery disease in patients with coronary artery disease. Int Angiol 1995; 14(1):89–93.

13. Austin MA, Hokanson JE, Edwards KL. Hypertriglyceridemia as a cardiovascular risk factor. Am J Cardiol 1998; 81:7B–12B.

14. Balke B, Ware RW. An experimental study of physical fitness of Air Force personnel. US Armed Forces Med J 1959; 10:675.

15. Belardinelli L, Linden J, Berne RM. The cardiac effects of adenosine. Prog Cardiovasc Dis 1989; 32:73–97.

16. Belardinelli R, Georgiou D, Cianci G, et al. Effects of exercise training on left ventricular filling at rest and during exercise in patients with ischemic cardiomyopathy and severe left ventricular systolic dysfunction. Am Heart J 1996; 132(1 part 1):61–70.

17. Belardinelli R, Georgiou D, Cianci G, et al. Exercise training improves left ventricular diastolic filling in patients with dilated cardiomyopathy. Clinical and prognostic implications. Circulation 1995; 91(11):2775–2784.

18. Belardinelli R, Georgiou D, Cianci G, et al. Randomized, controlled trial of long-term moderate exercise training in chronic heart failure: effects on functional capacity, quality of life, and clinical outcome. Circulation 1999; 99:1173–1182.

19. Belardinelli R, Georgiou D, Ginzton L, et al. Effects of moderate exercise training on thallium uptake and contractile response to low-dose dobutamine of dysfunctional myocardium in patients with ischemic cardiomyopathy. Circulation 1998; 97(6):553–561.

20. Belardinelli R, Georgiou D, Purcaro A. Low dose dobutamine echocardiography predicts improvement in functional capacity after exercise training in patients with ischemic cardiomyopathy: prognostic implication. J Am Coll Cardiol 1998; 31(5):1027–1034.

21. Bendszus M, Reents W, Franke D, et al. Brain damage after coronary artery bypass grafting. Arch Neurol 2002; 59:1090–1095.

22. Berlardinelli R, Paolini I, Cianci G, et al. Exercise training intervention after coronary angioplasty: the ETICA trial. J Am Coll Cardiol 2001; 37:1891–1900.

23. Berlowitz DR, Ash AS, Hickey EC, et al. Inadequate management of blood pressure in a hypertensive population. N Engl J Med 1998; 339:1957–1963.

24. Blair SN, Jackson AS. Physical fitness and activity as separate heart disease risk factors: a meta-analysis. Med Sci Sports Exerc 2001; 33:762–764.

25. Blumenthal JA, Babyak MA, Carney RM, et al. Exercise, depression, and mortality after myocardial infarction in the ENRICHD trial. Med Sci Sports Exerc 2004; 36(5):746–755.

26. Bonow RO, Kent KM, Rosing DR, et al. Exercise-induced ischemia in mildly symptomatic patients with coronary artery disease and preserved left ventricular function: identification of subgroup at risk of death during medical therapy. N Engl J Med 1984; 311:1339.

27. Borg G, Linderholm H. Exercise performance and perceived exertion in patients with coronary insufficiency, arterial hypertension and vasoregulatory asthenia. Acta Med Scand 1970; 187(1–2):17–26.

28. Boudrez H, De Backer G, Comhaire B. Return to work after myocardial infarction: results of a longitudinal population based study. Eur Heart J 1994; 15(1):32–36.

29. Braith RW, Limacher MC, Leggett SH, et al. Skeletal muscle strength in heart transplant recipients. J Heart Lung Transplant 1993; 12:1018–1023.

30. Bristow MR, Saxon LA, Boehmer J, et al. Cardiac-resynchronization therapy with or without an implantable defibrillator in advanced chronic heart failure. N Engl J Med 2004; 350(21):2140–2150.

31. Broan KA, Boucher CA, Okada RD, et al. Prognostic value of exercise thallium-201 imaging in patients presenting for evaluation of chest pain. J Am Coll Cardiol 1983; 1:994.

32. Brown BG, Zhao XQ. Lipid therapy to stabilize the vulnerable atherosclerotic plaque: new insights into the prevention of cardiovascular events. In: Grundy SM, ed. Cholesterol lowering therapy: evaluation of clinical trial evidence. New York: Marcel Decker; 2000:249–272.

33. Bruce RA. Exercise testing in adult normal subjects and cardiac patients. Pediatrics 1963; 32(suppl):742.

34. Brummer P, Linko E, Kasanen A. Myocardial infarction treated by early ambulation. Am Heart J 1956; 52:269–272.

35. Burg MM, Benedetto MC, Rosenberg R, et al. Presurgical depression predicts medical morbidity 6 months after coronary artery bypass graft surgery. Psychosom Med 2003; 65(1):111–118.

36. Burg MM, Benedetto MC, Soufer R. Depressive symptoms and mortality two years after coronary artery bypass graft surgery (CABG) in men. Psychosom Med 2003; 65(4):508–510.

37. Burt VL, Whelton P, Roccella EJ, et al. Prevalence of hypertension in the US adult population. Results from the Third National Health and Nutrition Examination Survey, 1998–1991. Hypertension 1995; 25:305–313.

38. Butler WJ, Ostrander LD, Carman WJ, et al. Mortality from coronary heart disease in the Tecumseh Study: long term effect of diabetes mellitus glucose tolerance and other risk factors. Am J Epidemiol 1985; 121:541–547.

39. Cahalin LP, Semigran MJ, Dec GW. Inspiratory muscle training in patients with chronic heart failure awaiting cardiac transplantation: results of a pilot clinical trial. Phys Ther 1997; 77:830–838.

40. Cannistra LB, Davidoff R, Picard MH, et al. Moderate-high intensity exercise training after myocardial infarction: effect on left ventricular remodeling. J Cardiopulm Rehabil 1999; 19(6):373–380.

41. Centers for Disease Control and Prevention. Annual smoking-attributable mortality, years of potential life lost, and economic costs—United States, 1995–1999. Morb Mortal Wkly Rep 2002; 51(14):300–303.

42. Centers for Disease Control and Prevention. Cigarette smoking among high school students—11 states, 1991–1997. Morb Mortal Wkly Rep 1999; 48(31):686–692.

43. Centers for Disease Control and Prevention–National Center for Health Statistics. National Health and Nutrition Examination Survey III (NHANES III, 1998–94). Bethesda: CDC–NCHS.

44. Chabanian AV, Bakris GL, Black HR, et al. Seventh report of the Joint National Committee on the prevention, detection, evaluation and treatment of high blood pressure. Hypertension 2003; 42:1206–1252.

45. Coats AJ, Adamopoulos S, Radaelli A, et al. Controlled trial of physical training in chronic heart failure: exercise performance, hemodynamics, ventilation, and autonomic function. Circulation 1992; 85:2119–2131.

46. Cobb LA, Weaver WD. Exercise: a risk for sudden death in patients with coronary heart disease. J Am Coll Cardiol 1986; 7:215–219.

47. Colditz G. Economic costs of obesity and inactivity. Med Sci Sports Exerc 1999; 31(suppl 11):S663–S667.

48. Cole CR, Blackstone EH, Pashkow FJ, et al. Heart-rate recovery immediately after exercise as a predictor of mortality. N Engl J Med 1999; 341:1351–1357.

49. Crouse SF, O'Brien BC, Grandjean PW, et al. Training intensity, blood lipids, and apolipoproteins in men with high cholesterol. J Appl Physiol 1997; 82:270–277.

50. Currie PJ, Kelly MJ, Pitt A. Comparison of supine and erect bicycle exercise electrocardiography in coronary heart disease: accentuation of exercise induced ischemic ST depression by supine posture. Am J Cardiol 1983; 52:1167–1173.

51. Danesh J, Collins R, Peto R. Lipoprotein(a) and coronary heart disease: meta-analysis of prospective studies. Circulation 2000; 102:1082–1085.

52. Davidson DM, DeBusk RF. Prognostic value of a single exercise test 3 weeks after uncomplicated myocardial infarction. Circulation 1980; 61:236.

53. Delagardelle C, Feiereisen P, Autier P, et al. Strength/endurance training versus endurance training in congestive heart failure. Med Sci Sports Exerc 2002; 34(12):1868–1872.

54. Dieter RS, Tomasson J, Gudjonsson T, et al. Lower extremity peripheral arterial disease in hospitalized patients with coronary artery disease. Vasc Med 2003; 8(4):233–236.

55. van Dijk D, Moons KG, Keizer AM, et al. Octopus Study Group. Association between early and three-month cognitive outcome after off-pump and on-pump coronary bypass surgery. Heart 2004; 90:431–434.

56. Ehsani AA, Biello DR, Schultz J, et al. Improvement of left ventricular contractile function by exercise training in patients with coronary artery disease. Circulation 1986; 74(2):350–358.

57. Ellestad MH. Stress testing, principles and practice. 5th edn. Oxford: Oxford University Press. 2003.

58. Engblom E, Korpilahti K, Hämäläinen H, et al. Quality of life and return to work 5 years after coronary artery bypass surgery: long term results of cardiac rehabilitation. J Cardiopulm Rehabil 1997; 17:29–36.

59. Expert Committee on the Diagnosis and Classification of Diabetes Mellitus. Report of the Expert Committee on the Diagnosis and Classification of Diabetes Mellitus. Diabetes Care 1997; 20:1183–1202.

60. Fagard RH. Exercise characteristics and the blood pressure response to dynamic physical training. Med Sci Sports Exerc 2001; 33(6):S484–S492.

61. de Feyter PJ, Nieman K, van Ooijen P, et al. Non-invasive coronary artery imaging with electron beam computed tomography and magnetic resonance imaging. Heart 2000; 84:442–448.

62. Fitchet A, Doherty PJ, Bundy C, et al. Comprehensive cardiac rehabilitation programme for implantable cardioverter-defibrillator patients: a randomised controlled trial. Heart 2003; 89(2):155–160.

63. Flamm SD, Taki J, Moore R, et al. Redistribution of regional and organ blood volume and effect on cardiac function in relation to upright exercise intensity in healthy human subjects. Circulation 1990; 18:1550.

64. Fletcher GF, Balady GJ, Amsterdam EA, et al. Exercise standards for testing and training: a statement for healthcare professionals from the American Heart Association. Circulation 2001; 104:1694–1740.

65. Fontaine K, Bartlett S. Estimating health-related quality of life in obese individuals. Dis Manage Health Outcomes 1998; 3:61–70.

66. Ford ES, Giles WH, Dietz WH. Prevalence of the metabolic syndrome among US adults: findings from the third National Health and Nutrition Examination Survey. JAMA 2002; 287:356–359.

67. Ford ES, Moriarty DG, Zack MM, et al. Self-reported body mass index and health-related quality of life: findings from the Behavioral Risk Factor Surveillance System. Obes Res 2001; 9:21–31.

68. Franklin BA, Bonzheim K, Gordon S, et al. Safety of medically supervised outpatient cardiac rehabilitation exercise therapy: a 16-year follow-up. Chest 1998; 114:902–906.

69. Franklin BA, ed. ACSM's guidelines for graded exercise testing and participation. 6th edn. Baltimore: Williams & Wilkins; 2000.

70. Franz MJ, Norstrom J. Diabetes: actually staying healthy—your game plan for diabetes and exercise. Wayzata: DCI Publishing; 1990.

71. Froelicher V, Jensen D, Sullivan M. A randomized trial of the effects of exercise training after coronary artery bypass surgery. Arch Intern Med 1985; 145(4):689–692.

72. Galante A, Pietroiusti A, Cavazzini C, et al. Incidence and risk factors associated with cardiac arrhythmias during rehabilitation after coronary artery bypass surgery. Arch Phys Med Rehabil 2000; 81(7):947–952.

73. van der Geest RJ, Reiber JH. Quantification in cardiac MRI. J Magn Reson Imaging 1999; 10:602–608.

74. Geiss LS, Herman WH, Smith PJ. National Diabetes Data Group. Diabetes in America. Bethesda: National Institutes of Health; 1995:233–257.

75. Geskin G, Kramer CM, Rogers WJ, et al. Quantitative assessment of myocardial viability after infarction by dobutamine magnetic resonance tagging. Circulation 1998; 98:217–223.

76. van Geuns RJ, Wielopolski PA, de Bruin HG, et al. Magnetic resonance imaging of the coronary arteries: techniques and results. Prog Cardiovasc Dis 1999; 42:157–166.

77. Giannuzzi P, Temporelli PL, Corra U, et al. ELVD-CHF Study Group. Antiremodeling effect of long-term exercise training in patients with stable chronic heart failure: results of the Exercise in Left Ventricular Dysfunction and Chronic Heart Failure (ELVD-CHF) Trial. Circulation 2003; 108(5):554–559.

78. Gibbons RJ, Balady GJ, Bricker JT, et al. ACC/AHA 2002 guideline update for exercise testing: a report of the American College of Cardiology/American Heart Association Task Force on Practice Guidelines (Committee on Exercise Testing). Online. Available: http://www.acc.org/index.htm

79. Goldenberg I, Jonas M, Tenenbaum A, et al. Current smoking, smoking cessation and the risk of sudden cardiac death in patients with coronary artery disease. Arch Intern Med 2003; 163:2301–2305.

80. Goodman JM, Pallandi DV, Reading JR, et al. Central and peripheral adaptations after 12 weeks of exercise training in post-coronary artery bypass surgery patients. J Cardiopulm Rehabil 1999; 9(3):144–150.

81. Gordon DJ. Cholesterol lowering and total mortality. In: Rifkind BM, ed. Lowering cholesterol in high risk individuals and populations. New York: Marcel Dekker; 1995:333–348.

82. Gordon T, Kannel WB, McGee D, et al. Death and coronary attacks in men after giving up cigarette smoking: a report from the Framingham Study. Lancet 1974; 2:1345–1348.

83. Goto Y, Sumida H, Ueshima K, et al. Safety and implementation of exercise testing and training after coronary stenting in patients with acute myocardial infarction. Circ J 2002; 66:930–936.

84. Gray RS, Fabsitz RR, Cowan LD, et al. Risk factor clustering in the insulin resistance syndrome: the Strong Heart Study. Am J Epidemiol 1998; 148:869–878.

85. Gregoratos G, Abrams J, Epstein AE, et al. ACC/AHA/NASPE 2002 guideline update for implantation of cardiac pacemakers and antiarrhythmia devices: a report of the American College of Cardiology/American Heart Association Task Force on Practice Guidelines 2002. Online. Available: http://www.acc.org/clinical/guidelines/pacemaker/pacemaker.pdf

86. Grimm M, Zimpfer D, Czerny M, et al. Neurocognitive deficit following mitral valve surgery. Eur J Cardio-thorac Surg 2003; 23(3):265–271.

87. Grippo AJ, Johnson AK. Biological mechanisms in the relationship between depression and heart disease. Neurosci Biobehav Rev 2002; 26(8):941–962.

88. Grundy SM, Hansen B, Smith SC, et al. Clinical management of metabolic syndrome. Report of the American Heart Association/National Heart, Lung, and Blood Institute/American Diabetes Association conference on scientific issues related to management. Circulation 2004; 109:551–556.

89. Gunning MG, Walker J, Eastick S, et al. Exercise training following myocardial infarction improves myocardial perfusion assessed by thallium-201 scintigraphy. Int J Cardiol 2002; 84(2–3):233–239.

90. Gururaj AV. Cardiac resynchronization therapy: effects on exercise capacity in the patient with chronic heart failure. J Cardiopulm Rehabil 2004; 24:1–7.

91. Haffner SM, Stern MP, Hazuda HP, et al. Cardiovascular risk factors in confirmed prediabetic individuals: does the clock for coronary heart disease start clicking before the onset of clinical diabetes? JAMA 1990; 263:2893–2898.

92. Hajjar I, Kotchen TA. Trends in prevalence, awareness, treatment, and control of hypertension in the United States, 1998–2000. JAMA 2003; 290:199–206.

93. Hambrecht R, Gielen S, Linke A, et al. Effects of exercise training on left ventricular function and peripheral resistance in patients with chronic heart failure: a randomized trial. JAMA 2000; 283:3095–3101.

94. Hambrecht R, Niebauer J, Fiehn E, et al. Physical training in patients with stable chronic heart failure: effects on cardiorespiratory fitness and ultrastructural abnormalities of leg muscles. J Am Coll Cardiol 1995; 25:1239–1249.

95. Hamm LF, Crow RS, Stull GA, et al. Safety and characteristics of exercise testing early after acute myocardial infarction. Am J Cardiol 1989; 63:1193–1197.

96. Harris MI, Cowie CC, Stern MP, et al, eds. Diabetes in America. 2nd edn. National Institutes of Health publication no. 95-1468. Bethesda: NIH; 1995:631–659.

97. Harris MI, Flegal KM, Cowie CC, et al. Prevalence of diabetes, impaired fasting glucose, and impaired glucose tolerance in US adults: the Third National Health and Nutrition Examination Survey, 1998–94. Diabetes Care 1998; 21:518–524.

98. Hasdai D, Bell MR, Grill DE, et al. Outcome > or = 10 years after successful percutaneous transluminal coronary angioplasty. Am J Cardiol 1997; 79:1005–1011.

99. Haskell WL. Cardiovascular complications during exercise training of cardiac patients. Circulation 1978; 57:920–924.

100. Hayes SN, Long T, Hand MM, et al. Women's ischemic syndrome evaluation: current status and future research directions. Key messages about acute ischemic heart disease in women and recommendations for practice. Circulation 2004; 109:e59–e61.

101. Hecht HS, DeBord L, Sotomayor N, et al. Truly silent ischemia and the relationship of chest pain and ST segment changes to the amount of ischemic myocardium: evaluation of supine bicycle stress echocardiography. J Am Coll Cardiol 1994; 23:369.

102. Hennekens CH, Dyken ML, Fuster V. Aspirin as a therapeutic agent in cardiovascular disease: a statement for healthcare professionals from the American Heart Association. Circulation 1997; 96:2751–2753.

103. Hermanson B, Omenn GS, Kronmal RA. Beneficial six year outcome of smoking cessation in older men and women with coronary artery disease: results from the CASS registry. N Engl J Med 1988; 319:1365–1369.

104. Ho PM, Arciniegas DB, Grigsby J, et al. Predictors of cognitive decline following coronary artery bypass graft surgery. Ann Thorac Surg 2004; 77(2):597–603.

105. Hodgson TA, Cohen AJ. Medical care expenditures for selected circulatory diseases. Med Care 1999; 37:994–1012.

106. Hossack KF, Hartwig R. Cardiac arrest associated with supervised cardiac rehabilitation. J Cardiac Rehabil 1982; 2:402–408.

107. Hundley WG, Hamilton CA, Thomas MS, et al. Utility of fast cine magnetic resonance imaging and display for the detection of myocardial ischemia in patients not well suited for second harmonic stress echocardiography. Circulation 1999; 100:1697–1702.

108. Izawa K, Hirano Y, Yamada S, et al. Improvement in physiological outcomes and health-related quality of life following cardiac rehabilitation in patients with acute myocardial infarction. Circ J 2004; 68(4):315–320.

109. Jaski BE, Kim J, Maly RS, et al. Effects of exercise during long-term support with a left ventricular assist device. Results of the experience with left ventricular assist device with exercise (EVADE) pilot trial. Circulation 1997; 95(10):2401–2406.

110. Jaski BE, Lingle RJ, Kim J, et al. Comparison of functional capacity in patients with end-stage heart failure following implantation of a left ventricular assist device versus heart transplantation: results of the experience with left ventricular assist device with exercise trial. J Heart Lung Transplant 1999; 18(11):1031–1040.

111. Jolliffe JA, Rees K, Taylor RS, et al. Exercise-based rehabilitation for coronary heart disease Cochrane Database Syst Rev 2004;4.

112. Jorenby DE. Smoking cessation strategies for the 21st century. Circulation 2001; 104:E51–E52.

113. Kalapura T, Lavie CJ, Jaffrani W, et al. Effects of cardiac rehabilitation and exercise training on indexes of dispersion of ventricular repolarization in patients after acute myocardial infarction. Am J Cardiol 2003; 92(3):292–294.

114. Karvonen M, Kentala K, Mustala O. The effects of training on heart rate: a longitudinal study. Ann Med Exp Biol Fenn 1957; 35:307–315.

115. Kelly TM. Exercise testing and training of patients with malignant ventricular arrhythmias. Med Sci Sports Exerc 1996; 28:53–61.

116. von Kemp K, van den Brande P, Peterson T, et al. Screening for concomitant diseases in peripheral vascular patients. Results of a systematic approach. Int Angiol 1997; 16(2):114–122.

117. Kobashigawa JA, Leaf DA, Lee N, et al. A controlled trial of exercise rehabilitation after heart transplantation. New Engl J Med 1999; 340:272–277.

118. Koenig W, Sund M, Frohlich M, et al. C-reactive protein, a sensitive marker of inflammation, predicts future risk of coronary heart disease in initially healthy middle-aged men: results from the MONICA (Monitoring Trends and Determinants if Cardiovascular Disease) Augsburg Cohort Study, 1984 to 1982. Circulation 1999; 99:237–242.

119. Krone RJ, Miller JP, Gillespie JA, et al. Usefulness of low level exercise testing early after acute myocardial infarction in patients taking beta-blocking agents. Am J Cardiol 1987; 60:23–27.

120. Lakka HM, Laaksonen DE, Lakka TA, et al. The metabolic syndrome and total and cardiovascular disease mortality in middle-aged men. JAMA 2002; 288(21):2709–2716.

121. Lampman RM, Knight BP. Prescribing exercise training for patients with defibrillators. Am J Phys Med Rehabil 2000; 79:292–297.

122. Lan C, Chen SY, Hsu CJ, et al. Improvement of cardiorespiratory function after percutaneous transluminal coronary angioplasty or coronary artery bypass grafting. Am J Phys Med Rehabil 2002; 81(5):336–341.

123. Lauer MS, Francis GS, Okin PM, et al. Impaired chronotropic response to exercise stress testing as a predictor of mortality. JAMA 1999; 281:524–529.

124. Lee IM, Paffenbarger RS Jr, Hennekens CH. Physical activity, physical fitness and longevity. Aging (Milano) 1997; 9:2–11.

125. Lee IM, Sesso H, Paffenbarger RS Jr. Physical activity and coronary heart disease risk in men: does the duration of exercise episodes predict risk? Circulation 2000; 102:981–986.

126. Leon AS, Sanchez OA. Meta-analysis of the effects of aerobic exercise training on blood lipids [abstract]. Circulation 2001; 104(suppl II):II-414–II-415.

127. Leon AS, Sanchez OA. Response of blood lipids to exercise training alone or combined with dietary intervention. Med Sci Sports Exerc 2001; 33(6):S502–S515.

128. Leppo JA. Dipyridamole thallium-201 imaging: the lazy man's stress test. J Nucl Med 1989; 30:281–287.

129. Lewington S, Clarke R, Qizilbash N, et al. Age-specific relevance of usual blood pressure to vascular mortality: a meta-analysis of individual data for one million adults in 61 prospective studies. Prospective studies collaboration. Lancet 2002; 360:1903–1913.

130. Lucini D, Milani RV, Costantino G, et al. Effects of cardiac rehabilitation and exercise training on autonomic regulation in patients with coronary artery disease. Am Heart J 2002; 143(6):977–983.

131. MacDonald MJ. Postexercise late-onset hypoglycemia in insulin-dependent diabetic patients. Diabetes Care 1987; 10(5):584–588.

132. Mager G, Reinhardt C, Kleine M, et al. Patients with dilated cardiomyopathy and less than 20% ejection fraction increase exercise capacity and have less severe arrhythmia after controlled exercise training. J Cardiopulm Rehabil 2000; 20(3):196–198.

133. Maggioni AP, Turazza FM, Tavazzi L. Risk evaluation using exercise testing in elderly patients after acute myocardial infarction. Cardiol Elderly 1995; 3:88–93.

134. Maiorana AJ, Briffa TG, Goodman C, et al. A controlled trial of circuit weight training on aerobic capacity and myocardial oxygen demand in men after coronary artery bypass surgery. J Cardiopulm Rehabil 1997; 17(4):239–247.

135. Malinow MR, Bostorn AG, Krauss RM. Homocysteine, diet and cardiovascular diseases: a statement for healthcare professionals from the Nutrition Committee, American Heart Association. Circulation 1999; 99:178–182.

136. Mallory G, White P, Sacedo-Salgar J. The speed of healing of myocardial infarction: a study of the pathological anatomy in seventy-two cases. Am Heart J 1939; 18:647–671.

137. Manning WJ, Li W, Edelman RR. A preliminary report comparing magnetic resonance coronary angiography with conventional angiography. N Engl J Med 1993; 328:828–832.

138. Manson JE, Willet WC, Stamfer MJ, et al. Body weight and mortality among women. N Engl J Med 1995; 333:677–685.

139. Marcus BH, Albrecht AE, King TK, et al. The efficacy of exercise as an aid for smoking cessation in women: a randomized controlled trial. Arch Intern Med 1999; 159(11):1229–1234.

140. Mazzotta G, Pace L, Bonow RO. Risk stratification of patients with coronary artery disease and left ventricular dysfunction by exercise radionuclide angiography and exercise electrocardiography. J Nucl Cardiol 1994; 1:529.

141. McHam SA, Marwick TH, Pashkow FJ, et al. Delayed systolic blood pressure recovery after graded exercise: an independent correlate of angiographic coronary disease. J Am Coll Cardiol 1999; 34:754–759.

142. McKhann GM, Grega MA, Borowicz LM, et al. Encephalopathy and stroke after coronary artery bypass grafting. Arch Neurol 2002; 59:1422–1428.

143. McNeer JF, Margolis JR, Lee KL, et al. The role of the exercise test in the evaluation of patients for ischemic heart disease. Circulation 1978; 57:64–70.

144. Meyer K, Lehmann M, Sunder G, et al. Acute cardiovascular and metabolic changes in interval and endurance training in selected patients following aortocoronary bypass operation. Z Kardiol 1990; 79(10):689–696.

145. Meyer K, Samek L, Schwaibold M, et al. Interval training in patients with severe chronic heart failure: analysis and recommendations for exercise procedures. Med Sci Sports Exerc 1997; 29(3):306–312.

146. Miranda CP, Herbert WG, Dubach P, et al. Post-myocardial infarction exercise testing: non-Q-wave versus Q-wave correlation with coronary angiography and long-term prognosis. Circulation 1991; 84:2357–2365.

147. Mital A, Shrey DE, Govindaraju M, et al. Accelerating the return to work (RTW) chances of coronary heart disease (CHD) patients: part 1—development and validation of a training program. Disabil Rehabil 2000; 22(13–14):604–620.

148. Montalescot G, Collet JP, Choussat R, et al. Fibrinogen as a risk factor for coronary heart disease. Eur Heart J 1998; 19(suppl H):H11–H17.

149. Moore SM, Dolansky MA, Ruland CM, et al. Predictors of women's exercise maintenance after cardiac rehabilitation. J Cardiopulm Rehabil 2003; 23:40–49.

150. Morrone TM, Buck LA, Catanese KA, et al. Early progressive mobilization of patients with left ventricular assist devices is safe and optimizes recovery before heart transplantation. J Heart Lung Transplant 1996; 15(4):423–429.

151. Muhlestein JB, Anderson JL, Horne BD, et al. Intermountain Heart Collaborative Study Group. Early effects of statins in patients with coronary artery disease and high C-reactive protein. Am J Cardiol 2004; 94:1107–1112.

152. Muller JE, Mittleman A, Maclure M, et al. Triggering myocardial infarction by sexual activity. Low absolute risk and prevention by regular physical exertion. Determinants of Myocardial Infarction Onset Study Investigators. JAMA 1996; 275:1405–1409.

153. Muller JE. Morning increase of onset of myocardial infarction: implications concerning triggering events. Cardiology 1989; 76:96–104.

154. Muller JE. Sexual activity as a trigger for cardiovascular events: what is the risk? Am J Cardiol 1999; 84:2N–5N.

155. Mullges W, Berg D, Schmidtke A, et al. Early natural course of transient encephalopathy after coronary artery bypass grafting. Crit Care Med 2000; 28:1808–1811.

156. Must A, Spadano J, Coakley E, et al. The disease burden associated with overweight and obesity. JAMA 1999; 282:1523–1529.

157. Myers J, Wagner D, Schertler T, et al. Effects of exercise training on left ventricular volumes and function in patients with nonischemic cardiomyopathy: application of magnetic resonance myocardial tagging. Am Heart J 2002; 144(4):719–725.

158. National Cholesterol Education Program. Third report of the National Cholesterol Education Program (NCEP) Expert Panel on Detection, Evaluation, and Treatment of High Blood Cholesterol in Adults (Adult Treatment Panel III). NIH publication no. 01-3670. Bethesda: National Institutes of Health; 2001.

159. National Institutes of Health. Clinical guidelines on the identification, evaluation and treatment of overweight and obesity in adults: the evidence report. Obes Res 1998; 6:51S–209S.

160. Naughton J, Blake B, Nagle F. Refinements in methods of evaluation and physical conditioning before and after myocardial infarction. Am J Cardiol 1964; 14:837.

161. Newman L, Andrews M, Koblish M. Physical medicine and rehabilitation in acute myocardial infarction. Arch Intern Med 1952; 89:552–561.

162. Nielsen JR, Mickley H, Damsgaard EM, et al. Predischarge maximal exercise test identifies risk for cardiac death in patients with acute myocardial infarction. Am J Cardiol 1990; 65:149–153.

163. Niemeyer MG, van der Wall EE, D'Haene EG, et al. Alternative stress methods for the diagnosis of coronary artery disease. Netherlands J Med 1992; 41:284–294.

164. Nissen SE, Tuzcu EM, Schoenhagen P, et al. Reversal of Atherosclerosis with Aggressive Lipid Lowering (REVERSAL) Investigators. Statin therapy, LDL cholesterol, C-reactive protein, and coronary artery disease. N Engl J Med 2005; 352:29–38.

165. Okin PM, Ameisen O, Kligfield P. A modified treadmill exercise protocol for computer assisted analysis of the ST segment/heart rate slope. J Electrocardiol 1986; 19(4):311–318.

166. Ornish D, Scherwitz LW, Billings JH, et al. Intensive lifestyle changes for reversal of coronary heart disease. JAMA 1998; 280(23):2001–2007.

167. Paffenbarger RS Jr, Hyde RT, Wing AL, et al. A natural history of athleticism and cardiovascular health. JAMA 1984; 252:491–495.

168. Papadopoulos C, Shelley SI, St. Piccolo M, et al. Sexual activity after coronary bypass surgery. Chest 1986; 90:681–685.

169. Pate RR, Pratt M, Blair SN, et al. Physical activity and public health. A recommendation from the Centers for Disease Control and Prevention and the American College of Sports Medicine. JAMA 1995; 273:402–407.

170. Pavia L, Orlando G, Myers J, et al. The effect of beta-blockade therapy on the response to exercise training in postmyocardial infarction patients. Clin Cardiol 1995; 18(12):716–720.

171. van der Peijl ID, Vliet Vlieland TP, Versteegh MI, et al. Exercise therapy after coronary artery bypass graft surgery: a randomized comparison of a high and low frequency exercise therapy program. Ann Thorac Surg 2004; 77(5):1535–1541.

172. Piepoli MF, Davos C, Francis DP, et al. ExTraMATCH Collaborative. Exercise training meta-analysis of trials in patients with chronic heart failure (ExTraMATCH). Br Med J 2004; 328(7433):189.

173. Pina IL, Apstein CS, Balady GJ, et al. American Heart Association Committee on Exercise, Rehabilitation, and Prevention. Exercise and heart failure: a statement from the American Heart Association Committee on Exercise, Rehabilitation, and Prevention. Circulation 2003; 107(8):1210–1225.

174. Presti CF, Armstrong WF, Feigenbaum H. Comparison of echocardiography at peak exercise and after bicycle exercise in evaluation of patients with known or suspected coronary artery disease. J Am Soc Echocardiogr 1988; 1:119.

175. Raggi P, Callister T, Cooil B, et al. Identification of patients at increased risk of first unheralded acute myocardial infarction by electron beam computed tomography. Circulation 2000; 101:850–855.

176. Raggi P, Callister T, Nicholas J, et al. Cardiac events in patients with progression of coronary calcification on electron beam computed tomography [abstract]. Radiology 1999; 213:351.

177. Rankin KP, Kochamba GS, Boone KB, et al. Presurgical cognitive deficits in patients receiving coronary artery bypass graft surgery. J Int Neuropsychol Soc 2003; 9(6):913–924.

178. Raw M, McNeill A, West R. Smoking cessation guidelines for health professionals. A guide to effective smoking cessation interventions for the health care system. Health Education Authority. Thorax 1998; 53(suppl 5 part 1):S1–S19.

179. Rensing BJ, Bongaerts A, van Geuns RJ, et al. Intravenous coronary angiography by electron beam computed tomography: a clinical evaluation. Circulation 1998; 98:2509–2512.

180. Ridker PM, Cannon CP, Morrow D, et al. Pravastatin or Atorvastatin Evaluation and Infection Therapy-Thrombolysis in Myocardial Infarction 22 (PROVE IT-TIMI 22) Investigators. C-reactive protein levels and outcomes after statin therapy. N Engl J Med 2005; 352:20–28.

181. Rigotti NA, Singer DE, Mulley AG, et al. Smoking cessation following admission to a coronary care unit. J Gen Intern Med 1991; 6:305–311.

182. Ritchie L, Trobaugh GB, Hamilton GW, et al. Myocardial imaging with thallium-201 at rest and during exercise: comparison with coronary arteriography and resting and stress electrocardiography. Circulation 1977; 56:66–71.

183. Roffi M, Wenawaser P, Windecker S, et al. Early exercise after coronary stenting in safe. J Am Coll Cardiol 2003; 42:1569–1573.

184. Roitman JL, LaFontaine T, Drimmer AM. A new model for risk stratification and delivery of cardiovascular rehabilitation services in the long-term clinical management of patients with coronary artery disease. J Cardiopulm Rehabil 1998; 18(2):113–123.

185. Ruffolo RR Jr. The pharmacology of dobutamine. Am J Med Sci 1987; 294:244–248.

186. Ryan T, Feigenbaum H. Exercise echocardiography. Am J Cardiol 1992; 69:82H–89H.

187. Salonen JT. Stopping smoking and long-term mortality after acute myocardial infarction. Br Heart J 1980; 43:463–469.

188. Sani M, et al. The prognostic significance of serial exercise testing after myocardial infarction. Circulation 1979; 60:1238.

189. Scandinavian Simvastatin Survival Study Group. Randomized trial of cholesterol lowering in 4444 patients with coronary heart disease: the Scandinavian Simvastatin Survival Study (4S). Lancet 1994; 344: 1383–1389.

190. Senaratne MP, Smith G, Gulamhusein SS. Feasibility and safety of early exercise testing using the Bruce protocol after acute myocardial infarction. J Am Coll Cardiol 2000; 35:1212–1220.

191. Shan K, Constantine G, Sivananthan M, et al. Role of cardiac magnetic resonance imaging in the assessment of myocardial viability. Circulation 2004; 109:1328–1334.

192. Shea S, Ottman R, Gabrielli C, et al. Family history as an independent risk factor for coronary artery disease. J Am Coll Cardiol 1984; 4: 793–801.

193. Shepherd J, Cobbe SM, Ford I, et al for the West of Scotland Coronary Prevention Study Group. Prevention of coronary heart disease with pravastatin in men with hypercholesterolemia. N Engl J Med 1995; 333:1301–1307.

194. Shuichi T, Satoru S, Takeshi B, et al. Predictors of left ventricular remodeling in patients with acute myocardial infarction participating in cardiac rehabilitation. Circ J 2004; 68(3):214–219.

195. Smith SC Jr, Blair SN, Criqui MH, et al. Preventing heart attack and death in patients with coronary disease. Circulation 1995; 92:2–4.

196. Social Security Administration. Disability evaluation under social security. SSA publication no. 64-039, Office of Disability Programs ICN 468600, 2005.

197. Sparrow D, Dawber TR. The influence of cigarette smoking on prognosis after a first myocardial infarction: a report from the Framingham Study. J Chronic Dis 1978; 31:425–432.

198. Stern MP, Mitchell BD. Diabetes in Hispanic Americans. In: Harris MI, Cowie CC, Stern MP, et al, eds. Diabetes in America. 2nd edn. National Institutes of Health publication no. 95-1468. Bethesda: NIH; 1995: 631–659.

199. Stevenson R, Umachandran V, Ranjadayalan K, et al. Reassessment of treadmill stress testing for risk stratification in patients with acute myocardial infarction treated by thrombolysis. Br Heart J 1993; 70: 415–420.

200. Stewart KJ, McFarland LD, Weinhofer JJ, et al. Safety and efficacy of weight training soon after acute myocardial infarction. J Cardiopulm Rehabil 1998; 18(1):37–44.

201. Strauss RS, Pollack HA. Epidemic increase in childhood overweight, 1986–1998. JAMA 2001; 286(22):2845–2848.

202. Stuart RJ Jr, Ellestad MH. National survey of exercise stress testing facilities. Chest 1980; 77:94–97.

203. Stubbe I, Gustafson A, Nilsson-Ehle P, et al. In-hospital exercise therapy in patients with severe angina pectoris. Arch Phys Med Rehabil 1983; 64(9):396–401.

204. Stygall J, Newman SP, Fitzgerald G, et al. Cognitive change 5 years after coronary artery bypass surgery. Health Psychol 2003; 22:579–586.

205. Sukhija R, Aronow WS, Yalamanchili K, et al. Prevalence of coronary artery disease, lower extremity peripheral arterial disease, and cerebrovascular disease in 110 men with an abdominal aortic aneurysm. Am J Cardiol 2004; 94(10):1358–1359.

206. Takeyama J, Itoh H, Kato M, et al. Effects of physical training on the recovery of the autonomic nervous activity during exercise after coronary artery bypass grafting: effects of physical training after CABG. Jpn Circ J 2000; 64(11):809–813.

207. Tardif GS. Sexual activity after a myocardial infarction. Arch Phys Med Rehabil 1989; 70:763–766.

208. Targonski PV, Bonetti PO, Pumper GM, et al. Coronary endothelial dysfunction is associated with an increased risk of cerebrovascular events. Circulation 2003; 107(22):2805–2809.

209. Taylor HA. Sexual activity and the cardiovascular patient: guidelines. Am J Cardiol 1999; 84:6N–10N.

210. Théroux P, Waters DD, Halphen C, et al. Prognostic value of exercise testing soon after myocardial infarction. N Engl J Med 1979; 301: 341–345.

211. Thomas BJ, Miller NH, Lamendola C, et al. National survey on gender differences in cardiac rehabilitation programs. J Cardiopulm Rehabil 1996; 16:402–412.

212. Thompson PD, Crouse SF, Goodpaster B, et al. The acute versus the chronic response to exercise. Med Sci Sports Exerc 2001; 33(6 suppl): S438–S445.

213. Thompson PD. The benefits and risks of exercise training in patients with chronic coronary artery disease. JAMA 1988; 259(10):1537–1540.

214. Timberlake N, Klinger L, Smith P, et al. Incidence and patterns of depression following coronary artery bypass graft surgery. J Psychosom Res 1997; 43(2):197–207.

215. Tokmakidis SP, Volaklis KA. Training and detraining effects of a combined strength and aerobic exercise program on blood lipids in patients with coronary artery disease. J Cardiopulm Rehabil 2003; 23:193–200.

216. Torado JF, Shen BJ, Niaura R, et al. Do men and women achieve similar benefits from cardiac rehabilitation? J Cardiopulm Rehabil 2004; 24:45–51.

217. Trelawny-Ross C, Russell O. Social and psychological responses to myocardial infarction: multiple determinants of outcome at 6 months. J Psychosom Res 1987; 31:125–130.

218. US Department of Health and Human Services. Physical activity and health: a report of the Surgeon General. Atlanta: US Department of Health and Human Services; 1996.

219. US Department of Health and Human Services. Reducing the health consequences of smoking: 25 years of progress. A report of the Surgeon General. Department of Health and Human Services publication (CDC) 89-8411. Washington: DHHS; 1989.

220. US Department of Health and Human Services–Agency for Health Care Policy and Research. Clinical practice guideline no. 17: cardiac rehabilitation. AHCPR publication no. 96-0672. Washington: AHCPR; 1995.

221. Valabhji J, Elkeles RS. Non-invasive measurement of coronary heart disease using electron beam computed tomography. Curr Opin Lipidol 2002; 13:409–414.

222. Van Camp SP, Peterson RA. Cardiovascular complications of outpatient cardiac rehabilitation programs. JAMA 1986; 256:1160–1163.

223. Vanhees L, Kornaat M, Defoor J, et al. Effect of exercise training in patients with an implantable cardioverter defibrillator. Eur Heart J 2004; 25:1120–1126.

224. Vanhees L, Schepers D, Fagard R. Comparison of maximum versus submaximum exercise testing in providing prognostic information after acute myocardial infarction and/or coronary artery bypass grafting. Am J Cardiol 1997; 80:257–262.

225. Vasan RS, Beiser A, Seshardi S, et al. Residual lifetime risk for developing hypertension in middle-aged women and men: the Framingham Heart Study. JAMA 2002; 287:1003–1010.

226. Villella A, Maggioni AP, Villella M, et al for the Gruppo Italiano per lo Studio della Sopravvivenza Nell'Infarto. Prognostic significance of maximal exercise testing after myocardial infarction treated with thrombolytic agents: the GISSI-2 data-base. Lancet 1995; 346:523–529.

227. Villella M, Villella A, Barlera S, et al. Prognostic significance of double product and inadequate double product response to maximal symptom-limited exercise stress testing after myocardial infarction in 6296 patients treated with thrombolytic agents. GISSI-2 Investigators: Grupo Italiano per lo Studio della Sopravvivenza nell'Infarto Miocardico. Am Heart J 1999; 137:443–452.

228. Wackers FJ. The maze of myocardial perfusion imaging protocols anno 1994. J Nucl Cardiol 1994; 1:180.

229. Wallace RL, Sears SF Jr, Lewis TS, et al. Predictors of quality of life in long-term recipients of implantable cardioverter defibrillators. J Cardiopulm Rehabil 2002; 22:278–281.

230. Watkins LL, Schneiderman N, Blumenthal JA, et al. ENRICHD Investigators. Cognitive and somatic symptoms of depression are associated with medical comorbidity in patients after acute myocardial infarction. Am Heart J 2003; 146(1):48–54.

231. Weiner DA, Ryan TJ, McCabe CH, et al. Prognostic importance of a clinical profile and exercise test in medically treated patients with coronary artery disease. J Am Coll Cardiol 1984; 3:772–779.

232. Weiss AT, Berman DS, Law AS, et al. Transient ischemic dilation of the left ventricle on stress thallium-201 scintigraphy: a marker of severe and extensive coronary artery disease. J Am Coll Cardiol 1987; 9:752.

233. Wenger N, Gilbert C, Skoropa M. Cardiac conditioning after myocardial infarction. An early intervention program. J Cardiac Rehabil 1971; 2:17–22.

234. Whellan DJ, Shaw LK, Bart BA, et al. Cardiac rehabilitation and survival in patients with left ventricular systolic dysfunction. Am Heart J 2001; 142(1):160–166.

235. Whelton PK, Appel LJ, Cutler JA, et al. Primary prevention of hypertension: Clinical and public health advisory from the National High Blood Pressure Education Program. JAMA 2002; 288:1882–1888.

236. Whincup PH, Refsum H, Perry IJ, et al. Serum total homocysteine and coronary heart disease: prospective study in middle aged men. Heart 1999; 82:448–454.

237. Wilkund I, Sanne H, Vedin A, et al. Determinants of return to work one year after a first myocardial infarction. J Cardiac Rehabil 1985; 5:62–72.

238. Willenheimer R, Erhardt L, Cline C, et al. Exercise training in heart failure improves quality of life and exercise capacity. Eur Heart J 1998; 19: 774–781.

239. Williams MJ, Marwick TH, O'Gorman D, et al. Comparison of exercise echocardiography with an exercise score to diagnose coronary artery disease in women. Am J Cardiol 1994; 74:435.

240. Willich SN, Lewis M, Lowel H, et al. Physical exertion as a trigger of acute myocardial infarction. N Engl J Med 1993; 329:1684–1690.

241. Wilson K, Gibson N, Willan A, et al. Effect of smoking cessation on mortality after myocardial infarction: meta-analysis of cohort studies. Arch Intern Med 2000; 160:939–944.

242. Wilson PWF, D'Agostino RB, Levy D, et al. Prediction of coronary heart disease using risk factor categories. Circulation 1998; 97:1837–1847.

243. Wing RR, Hill JO. Successful weight loss maintenance. Annu Rev Nutr 2001; 21:323–341.

244. Wingard DL, Barret-Connor EL, Scheidt-Nave C, et al. Prevalence of cardiovascular and renal complications in older adults with normal or impaired glucose tolerance or NIDDM: a population based study. Diabetes Care 1993; 16:1022–1025.

245. Witt BJ, Jacobsen SJ, Weston SA, et al. Cardiac rehabilitation after myocardial infarction in the community. J Am Coll Cardiol 2004; 44:988–996.

246. Wong ND, Wilson PWF, Kannel WB. Serum cholesterol as a prognostic factor after myocardial infarction: the Framingham Study. Ann Intern Med 1991; 115:687–693.

247. World Health Organization. World health report 2002: reducing risks, promoting healthy life. Geneva: WHO; 2002.

248. Young JB, Abraham WT, Smith AL, et al. Combined cardiac resynchronization and implantable cardioversion defibrillation in advanced chronic heart failure (the MIRACLE ICD trial). JAMA 2003; 289:2685–2694.

249. Zamvar V, Williams D, Hall J, et al. Assessment of neurocognitive impairment after off-pump and on-pump techniques for coronary artery bypass graft surgery: prospective randomized controlled trial. Br Med J 2002; 325:1268–1272.

250. Zuccala G, Pedone C, Cesari M, et al. The effects of cognitive impairment on mortality among hospitalized patients with heart failure. Am J Med 2003; 115(2):97–103.

Chapter

35

Pulmonary Rehabilitation

Augusta Alba and Leighton Chan

INTRODUCTION AND PRINCIPLES

The most common form of lung disease in the USA is chronic obstructive pulmonary disease (COPD). Smoking is the main cause of COPD. In 2001, the Centers for Disease Control and Prevention reported that 22.7% of adults 18 years of age or older were current smokers, compared with 41.9% in 1965. Unfortunately, according to the American Cancer Society, 90% of new smokers are children and teenagers. COPD is very rare in non-smokers, and the vast majority of the deaths from this disease can be attributed to cigarette smoking. Statistics regarding COPD are shown in Box 35-1.[51]

Restrictive pulmonary disease is most commonly caused by neuromuscular and orthopedic disorders, such as spinal cord injury (SCI). According to statistics available from the National Spinal Cord Injury Association Resource Center for 1995–8, there are an estimated 250 000–400 000 persons with SCI or spinal cord dysfunction in the USA. Of these patients, 82% are male, 17.5% have complete tetraplegia, and 31.2% have incomplete tetraplegia. Duchenne muscular dystrophy (DMD) is one of the more common neuromuscular diseases that cause restrictive pulmonary dysfunction, with an incidence of 21 per 100 000 births in the USA.

Pulmonary rehabilitation is defined as a multidisciplinary program that provides persons with the ability to adapt to their chronic lung disease.[11] It includes physical conditioning, ongoing medical management, training in coping skills, and psychosocial support. Fear of dyspnea can lead to panic, which increases the work of breathing. Dyspnea also causes progressive inactivity, which further weakens the individual. Pulmonary rehabilitation addresses this fear and uses a greater tolerance of dyspnea to increase strength, endurance, and quality of life.

When there is advanced pulmonary impairment, other treatment options, including mechanical ventilation, may be used. If the impairment is caused by intrinsic lung disease, partial lung resection (lung volume reduction surgery, LVRS) and lung transplant might be helpful.

TREATMENT OPTIONS IN PULMONARY REHABILITATION

There are several modalities used in pulmonary rehabilitation. These include general medical management, oxygen therapy, chest physical therapy, exercise training, and nutritional and psychosocial support.

General medical management

Pharmacologic therapy for COPD can include vaccination against influenza and pneumococcal pneumonia, inhaled quaternary anticholinergic and/or β_2-adrenergic agonist bronchodilators, and inhaled corticosteroids. Oral theophylline can improve respiratory muscle endurance and provide ventilatory stimulation. Leukotriene receptor antagonists, such as montelukast and zafirlukast, reduce the effects of leukotrienes, which include airway edema, smooth muscle constriction, and altered cellular activity associated with the inflammatory process.[23] Environmental and occupational pollution must be prevented and eliminated. For those with emphysema due to α_1-antitrypsin deficiency, α_1-antitrypsin augmentation therapy is efficacious.[47]

Oxygen therapy

Long-term oxygen therapy (LTOT), provided more than 15 h per day, improves survival and quality of life in COPD if hypoxemia is present with arterial oxygen saturation (S_aO_2) of 88%. LTOT is also needed if the patient's S_aO_2 is < 89% and there is evidence of pulmonary hypertension, peripheral edema suggesting congestive cardiac failure, or polycythemia.[17]

Oxygen concentrators have become the most popular method of providing oxygen in the home. DeVilBiss, OxLife, and AirSep are three of the companies offering portable models that can be used with an AC or a DC inverter. The AirSep Lifestyle is the smallest, at 9 lbs, and can be plugged into the 12-V adapter in the car. It has a built-in rechargeable battery that charges in 2 h. It can be carried on a pull cart or on the body with a shoulder strap. It has a pulse-dose feature that conserves oxygen. Generally, 3 L per min (lpm) is the maximum flow recommended from these units. The AirSep Elite provides up to 5 lpm of oxygen and has an oxygen analyzer built into the system. AirSep has produced a model that provides up to 8 lpm of oxygen, and has two flowmeters so that two persons can use oxygen from the same concentrator if the total use is no more than 8 lpm. The Chad Total O_2 System incorporates a refill station as part of the concentrator, so that portable oxygen cylinders can be filled over a period of a couple of hours. An oxygen-conserving regulator allows the oxygen to last four times

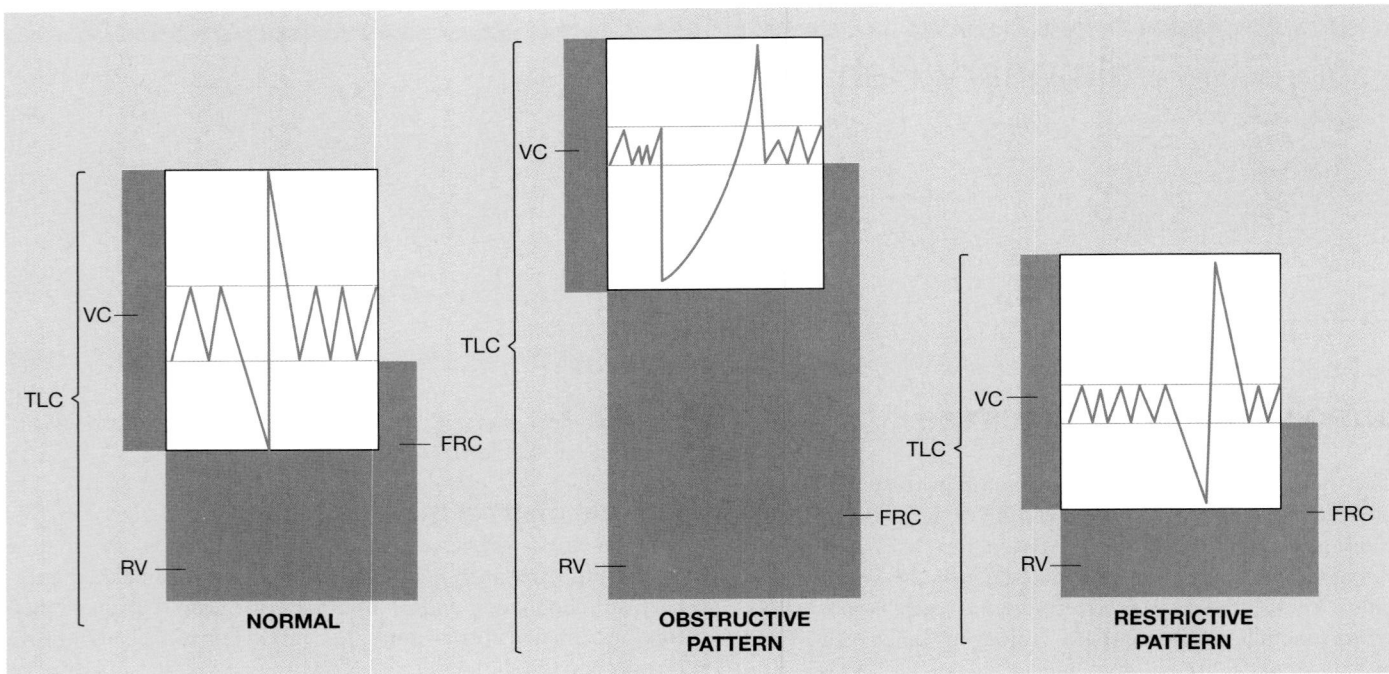

Figure 35-1 Lung volumes in health and disease. FRC, functional residual capacity; RV, residual volume; TLC, total long capacity; VC, vital capacity. The breathing pattern is read from right to left. The obstructive pattern demonstrates prolonged expiration.

Box 35-1 Facts regarding chronic obstructive pulmonary disease

- The majority of patients with chronic obstructive pulmonary disease (COPD) have asthma.
- Asthma is the most common childhood chronic disease.
- Causes of COPD: asthma, chronic bronchitis, emphysema, singly or in combination.
- Between 50 000 and 70 000 cases of COPD in the United States are due to α_1-antitrypsin deficiency; this disorder is under-recognized by physicians.
- COPD is the fifth leading cause of death worldwide.
- Annual worldwide adult deaths from COPD: 2.9 million.
- As of 2000, more women than men die of COPD in the USA.

---

as long. An oxygen cylinder can now be safely mounted on a motorized wheelchair if the motors and batteries are sealed and both are covered by a rigid housing.

Chest physical therapy

A good understanding of pulmonary function tests (Table 35-1 and Fig. 35-1), and the mechanics and work of breathing in normal and diseased states, is essential in planning an effective therapy program for persons with pulmonary disease.[29] Breathing exercises begin with relaxation techniques, which then become the foundation for breathing retraining. Retraining techniques for persons with COPD include pursed lips breathing, head down and bending forward postures, slow deep breathing, and localized expansion exercises or segmental breathing. These

techniques maintain positive airway pressure during exhalation and help reduce over-inflation. Although diaphragmatic breathing is widely taught, it has been shown to increase the work of breathing and dyspnea compared with the natural pattern of breathing in the patient with COPD.[11] The other component occasionally utilized to reduce fatigue is respiratory muscle endurance training, which usually concentrates on inspiratory resistance training. However, training of the expiratory muscles has also been found to be of some value.[59]

Clearance of secretions is mandatory to reduce the work of breathing and to limit infection and atelectasis. In order for chest physical therapy to be effective, mucoactive medications must be given.[48] These include expectorants, mucolytics, bronchodilators, surfactants, and mucoregulatory agents that reduce the volume of mucus secretion. Antitussives must be used for uncontrolled coughing, which can precipitate dynamic airway collapse, bronchospasm, or syncope.

Techniques for clearing secretions include postural drainage, manual or device-induced chest percussion and vibration, device-induced airway oscillation, incentive spirometry, and other devices and measures that improve the ability to cough. In a manually assisted cough, the patient's abdomen is compressed while the patient controls the depth of inspiration and the timing of opening and closing the upper airway. Non-invasive intermittent positive-pressure ventilation (NIPPV) with air stacking or glossopharyngeal breathing (GPB) are used to increase the depth of inspiration when inspiratory muscles are too weak to produce a deep breath. Air stacking is holding a portion of two or more breaths to fully inflate the lungs before exhalation. In GPB, the person uses the tongue to breathe. The

Table 35-1 Typical results of the effect of disease on ventilatory function

Test	Obstructive disease	Restrictive disease
Vital capacity	↔↓	↓↓
Forced expiratory volume	↓↓	↔↓
Midmaximal flow	↓↓	↔↓
Maximal voluntary ventilation	↓↓	↔↓
Residual volume	↑↑	↓↓
Functional residual capacity	↑↑	↓↓
Total lung capacity	↑↑	↓↓

(From Man et al. 2003,[38] with permission.)

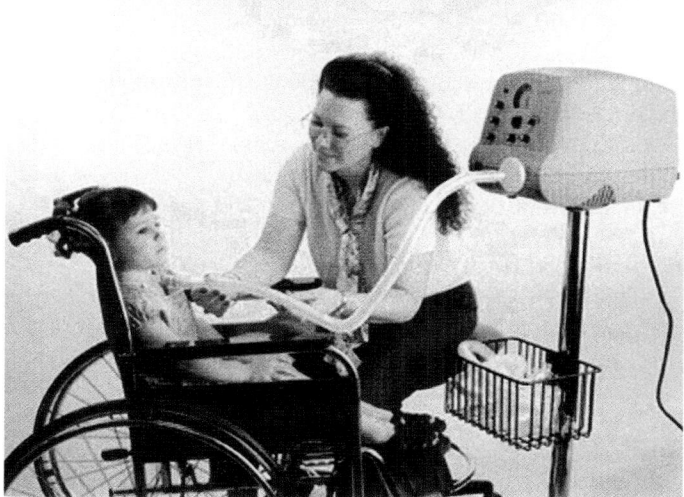

Figure 35-2 CoughAssist Mechanical In-Exsufflator cough machine with mother and child. The mother is using the machine at the child's tracheostomy.

technique is described more fully later in this chapter. When an upper motor neuron lesion above the midthoracic level has paralyzed the abdominal muscles, functional electrical stimulation (FES) of these muscles can produce a cough.[30]

Positive expiratory pressure mask therapy followed by 'huff coughing' is a useful technique when other methods of mobilizing secretions are not tolerated.[37] Autogenic drainage is a secretion clearance technique that combines variable tidal breathing at three distinct lung volume levels, controlled expiratory airflow, and huff coughing. The CoughAssist Mechanical In-Exsufflator cough machine (Fig. 35-2), manufactured by the J.H. Emerson Company (Cambridge, MA), provides a deep inspiration through a face mask or mouthpiece, or with an adapter, to a patient's endotracheal or tracheostomy tube, followed rapidly by controlled suction. It has been shown to provide highly effective secretion removal.[3] The device must be

used with caution and is contraindicated in patients with bullous emphysema, or a history of pneumothorax or pneumomediastinum in the recent past, especially if they are the result of barotrauma.

Exercise conditioning: general considerations

Aerobic exercise is the cornerstone of any pulmonary rehabilitation program. The inclusion criteria for exercise in pulmonary rehabilitation are straightforward. A candidate must demonstrate a decrease in functional exercise capacity due to pulmonary disease. The pulmonary disease should be relatively stable. Medical comorbidities that contraindicate exercise should be absent. Patients should not have orthopedic or cognitive disabilities that prevent exercise. Patients must be motivated to exercise on a consistent basis. Finally, patients should abstain from tobacco products for a number of months.

Cardiopulmonary exercise testing is necessary for the selection and evaluation of individuals in several circumstances prior to exercise conditioning. The American Thoracic Society–American College of Chest Physicians adopted the following indications for cardiopulmonary exercise testing in 2001.[60]

- Evaluation of exercise intolerance.
- Unexplained dyspnea.
- Evaluation of patients with cardiovascular disease.
- Evaluation of patients with respiratory disease:
  COPD;
  interstitial lung disease;
  chronic pulmonary vascular disease;
  cystic fibrosis;
  exercise-induced bronchospasm.
- Preoperative evaluation:
  preoperative evaluation for lung cancer resectional surgery;
  LVRS;
  evaluation for lung or heart–lung transplantation;
  preoperative evaluation of other procedures.
- Exercise prescription for pulmonary rehabilitation.
- Evaluation of impairment or disability.

If the cardiovascular, respiratory, and neuromuscular systems have adequate reserve to undergo a program of progressive exercise, skeletal muscles can develop an increased ability to perform aerobic exercise. After training, a given level of heavy exercise results in lower levels of blood lactate. Lower blood lactate lessens the requirement for oxygen uptake, carbon dioxide production, and ventilation for a given workload. Healthy subjects must train for at least 30 min a day, 3–5 days per week, for 4–8 weeks to achieve this effect. It is well known that gains will be lost if regular exercise at the level achieved is not continued.

The types of exercise usually included in the exercise program are lower limb training on a treadmill, bicycle ergometer, and unsupported or supported arm exercise. Unsupported exercise is carried out with free weights, while supported exercise is performed on the arm ergometer with the arms supported by gripping the ergometer pedals.

Exercise in COPD

All studies of exercise in COPD take into account the severity of the respiratory disability (see Table 35-2).[38] Exercise in a pulmonary rehabilitation program can include only submaximal cycle ergometry and treadmill walking (aerobic or endurance training), and/or weight training (anaerobic or strength training). When both methods are used in patients with severe COPD, pulmonary rehabilitation can produce significant increases in fat-free mass, isokinetic quadriceps strength, and maximal oxygen consumption.[24] One study in elderly patients with severe COPD showed that, although weight training produced significant gains in muscle strength, the measures of endurance and quality of life were not improved beyond that which occurred in the group that received only endurance training.[36]

There have been numerous studies carried out on the effects of exercise on patients with COPD over the past quarter century. These effects are summarized in Box 35-2.[8,9,16,22,25,45,65]

Ambrosino and Strambi described several modalities that are being trialed to reduce the extreme breathlessness and peripheral muscle fatigue that prevent patients with severe COPD from exercising at higher intensities.[2] Continuous positive airway pressure and NIPPV during exercise might reduce the perception of dyspnea. Taking part of the work of breathing away from the respiratory muscles and reducing intrinsic positive end expiratory pressure are considered two of the mechanisms by which these techniques relieve dyspnea. Nocturnal NIPPV in selected patients can improve their ability to exercise during the day. Adding electrical stimulation to strength exercises for peripheral muscles has been shown to further improve muscle strength in patients with COPD. Interval training with rest periods is capable of producing training effects in those who cannot tolerate a sustained period of exercise. Oxygen supplementation even in patients who do not desaturate during exercise allows for higher exercise intensities and produces a superior training effect. High-intensity physical group training in water can produce significant benefits as well.[58]

After an exercise program, patients must not revert to a sedentary lifestyle. To prevent the positive effects of exercise from being lost, continuous outpatient exercise training, home-based or community-based exercise programs, or exercise training in groups of persons with COPD is mandatory.[52]

Exercise in asthma

Asthma severity guidelines published in 1997 and updated in 2002 by the National Heart, Lung, and Blood Institute are based on clinical symptoms during the day and at night, and on the results of pulmonary function testing.[12] The two major categories of asthma patients are those who have it intermittently and those with persistent asthma. Bronchial biopsies in patients with intermittent asthma show evidence of ongoing airway inflammation. Studies have shown that aerobic exercise improves overall fitness and health of asthmatic patients.

Table 35-2 Classification scheme for chronic obstructive pulmonary disease severity: National Heart, Lung, and Blood Institute–World Health Organization Global Initiative for Chronic Obstructive Lung Disease criteria

Stage	Criterion[a]
0	Normal lung function
1 (mild)	FEV_1 ≥80% of predicted
2 (moderate)	50–79% of predicted
3 (severe)	30–49% of predicted
4 (very severe)	FEV_1 <30% of predicted or presence of respiratory failure or clinical signs of right-sided heart failure

[a]In the presence of FEV_1 : FVC ratio of <70%.

BOX 35-2 Improvement seen in exercise reconditioning in moderate chronic obstructive pulmonary disease

Inspiratory muscle training

- Increased maximal inspiratory mouth pressure
- Increased strength of the diaphragm

Pulmonary rehabilitation with or without inspiratory muscle training

- Increased maximal workload
- Improved activities of daily living scores
- Improved anxiety and depression scores
- Increased 6- or 12-min walking distance

Pulmonary rehabilitation (cycle ergometry, 70W)

- Minute volume decrease of 2.5 L/min per blood lactate decrease of 1 mEq/L (normal: minute volume decrease of 7.2 L/min per blood lactate decrease of 1 mEq/L)

A mouse model of atopic asthma has been developed in which the effects of exercise has been studied.[43] Exercise decreased the activation of the transcription factor NF-κB in the lungs of the model. This factor regulates the expression of a variety of genes that encode inflammatory mediators. Moderate-intensity aerobic exercise training of the mice decreased leukocyte infiltration, cytokine production, adhesion molecule expression, and structural remodeling within the lungs. It is suggested that aerobic exercise in patients with asthma might reduce airway inflammation in a similar manner. On the other hand, exercise itself can induce bronchoconstriction in some asthmatic patients.

A study in patients with asthma found that airway vascular hyperpermeability, eosinophilic inflammation, and bronchial hyperactivity are independent factors predicting the severity of exercise-induced bronchoconstriction.[42] Rundell and associates have described a laboratory method, eucapnic voluntary hyperpnea (EVH), that identifies 90% of athletes without known asthma who have exercise-induced bronchoconstriction.[49] The test is done by having athletes breathe 5% carbon dioxide and attempt to breathe for 6 min at a target ventilation equivalent to 30 times baseline FEV_1. If EVH is positive, there is a fall in FEV_1 of 10–19%.

Because exercising in cold air is known to increase bronchial responsiveness as compared with exercising in warm air, a study was done to determine whether facial cooling plays a role in asthmatic children.[64] It was found that facial cooling, combined with either cold or warm air inhalation, caused greater exercise-induced bronchoconstriction than with cold air inhalation. This could indicate that vagal mechanisms play a role in exercise-induced asthma.

Barriero and colleagues have studied the perception of dyspnea in near-fatal asthma patients at both rest and the end point of various forms of exercise as compared with other asthmatic patients.[5] Exercise tolerance was similarly reduced in both groups, but perception of dyspnea both at rest and at peak exercise was significantly lower in the near-fatal asthma group.

Exercise in cystic fibrosis

An estimated 30 000 persons in the USA suffer from cystic fibrosis, which is an autosomal recessive disorder. The basic defect is one of chloride transport, which produces a viscous mucus that inhibits the capability of the lungs to clear infection. The patient ultimately suffers from severe combined obstructive–restrictive pulmonary disease. The abnormal viscosity of the cystic fibrosis secretions is caused to a great extent by degenerating neutrophils that produce extracellular DNA. Dornase alfa (Pulmozyme), or recombinant human deoxyribonuclease, is an enzyme capable of digesting extracellular DNA. It is used by daily long-term nebulization for patients older than 5 years and whose FVC is greater than 40%. Chest physical therapy of all pulmonary segments from one to four times daily is indicated, with increased frequency during exacerbations.

The Vest airway clearance system (Advanced Respiratory, St. Paul, MN) has become a popular method of providing the percussion and vibration necessary to loosen the secretions. An air pulse generator rapidly inflates and deflates an inflatable vest, compressing and releasing the chest wall. This process is called high-frequency chest wall oscillation. It eliminates the need for intensive physical involvement by a caregiver. It also increases airflow velocities, which create repetitive cough-like shear forces and decrease the viscosity of secretions.

Children with cystic fibrosis have reduced anaerobic performance and do not participate in activities requiring short bouts of high-energy expenditure to the same extent as healthy children do. Recently, Klijn and colleagues carried out a study of anaerobic training on children with cystic fibrosis older than 12 years.[31] No child had an FEV_1 below 55% of the predicted level. Subjects were trained 2 days per week for 12 weeks, with sessions lasting 30–45 min. Each anaerobic activity lasted 20–30 s. Three months after the end of training, anaerobic performance and quality of life were significantly higher in the trained group. A measurable improvement in aerobic performance, however, was not sustained.

A multiple regression analysis found that children with cystic fibrosis, whom Klijn studied over a period of 2 years, showed a change in FEV_1 and a change in fat-free mass that explained 47% of the variation of the change in peak oxygen consumption over this period.[32] Children with cystic fibrosis are now surviving into adulthood, with the median survival in 2004 being approximately 32 years.[63] For patients born in the 1990s, the median survival is predicted to be over 40 years. The cornerstones of treatment that have produced this increase in survival are airway clearance, nutritional support, and antibiotic therapy.

The lung function of adults with cystic fibrosis has been studied using FEV_1. Thirty-six percent were found to have normal or mild lung dysfunction (FEV_1 70% predicted), 39% had moderate dysfunction (FEV_1 40–69% predicted), and 25% had severe dysfunction (FEV_1 < 40% predicted). One-third of adults with cystic fibrosis have multiple-resistance Gram-negative organisms. A 3-year study of regular aerobic exercise in adults with cystic fibrosis has found that it reduced the expected decline in pulmonary function throughout that period. Appropriate vigorous aerobic exercise enhances cardiovascular fitness, increases functional capacity, and improves quality of life. However, patients with cystic fibrosis should rarely be exercised in close proximity to one another due to the possibility of transmission of *Burkholderia cepacia*, a highly transmissible bacteria that frequently infects patients with cystic fibrosis.

Survival in cystic fibrosis is correlated with maximal oxygen uptake. Blau and colleagues have found that an intensive 4-week summer camp program for both children and young adults improved exercise tolerance and nutrition in patients with cystic fibrosis.[6]

Exercise in disorders of chest wall function

There are numerous causes of chest wall dysfunction with both mechanical and neuromuscular components. The chest wall can be viewed as encompassing the rib cage, spine, diaphragm, abdomen, shoulder girdles, and neck. Distortions of the trunk are reflected in distortions of the heart, lungs, airway, and abdominal contents as well. There are many conditions that negatively affect the chest wall, including ankylosing spondylitis, pectus excavatum, obesity, the sequelae of thoracoplasty or phrenic nerve crush for the treatment of pulmonary tuberculosis, neuromuscular diseases with weakness of the respiratory bellows mechanism and superimposed spinal curvatures, and Parkinson disease. Ventilatory muscle training in these disorders can reduce respiratory muscle fatigue. Persons with Parkinson disease have shown overall improvement with pulmonary rehabilitation.[10] Patients with developmental disorders are a heterogeneous group in which severe scoliosis is commonly seen. Exercise and other ongoing rehabilitation techniques, such as positioning, and management of spasticity and dysphagia, are of value in their treatment.[56]

Exercise in paradoxical vocal fold dysfunction

Paradoxical vocal fold dysfunction is caused by the vocal folds coming together during inspiration, instead of opening normally. The diagnosis of PVFD is based on patient history and laryngoscopy. The disorder can occur from adolescence to old age. In one study by Patel,[44] 90% of the patients were female, 56% of them had asthma, 12% had laryngeal findings suggestive of gastroesophageal reflux disease, 12% had findings of chronic laryngitis, and 33% had additional findings of laryngomalacia, vocal fold motion impairment, sulcus vocalis, nodules, and subglottic stenosis. These additional findings were mostly seen in the exercise-induced group. If the patient is symptomatic during the examination, a flow-volume loop of the *FVC* shows a flattening of the inspiratory loop, indicative of the low flow associated with partial obstruction in this area during inspiration. Neurologically based dystonias are also a common cause. Throat tightness, dysphonia, and inspiratory difficulty can occur. Speech therapy can provide respiratory retraining. Acute exacerbations can be relieved by administration of helium–oxygen (70% : 30%) with or without NIPPV. Direct vocal cord injection of botulinum toxin A is also used.[57]

Nutritional issues

In moderate to severe COPD, weight loss is common, and is related to decreased exercise capacity and health status, and increased morbidity and mortality. Creutzberg and colleagues studied nutritional treatment of the severely underweight patient in an inpatient program.[13] Nutritional supplementation therapy with two or three oral liquid nutritional supplements daily in these nutritionally depleted patients with COPD produced increases in body weight, fat-free mass, maximal inspiratory mouth pressure, handgrip strength, and peak workload. Symptoms and impact scores on the St. George's Respiratory Questionnaire were improved as well. Maintenance oral glucocorticosteroid treatment blunted the response with respect to maximal inspiratory mouth pressure and peak workload, as well as the symptom score.

Diet counseling and self-management with changes in dietary behavior should start early in the course, when the patient with COPD is still under the care of a primary physician.[7] Practical suggestions for shopping, food preparation, and eating smaller, more frequent meals should be offered. When fatigue, dyspnea, swallowing, or poor appetite interfere with eating, a dietitian can be helpful. Involuntary weight loss is best addressed preventively. Total daily energy expenditure in patients with COPD, whether they were underweight or not, has been shown to be no different than in healthy persons.[54] Insufficient food intake was found to be the cause of the malnutrition. The energy cost of the exercise associated with a pulmonary rehabilitation program was estimated to be 191 kcal/day. Carbohydrate supplementation, however, is necessary where vigorous exercise training results in negative energy balance and weight loss.[53] In selected well-nourished patients, it may actually increase the shuttle walking performance.

Psychosocial support

Biopsychosocial considerations for persons with pulmonary dysfunction include the ongoing education of the patient and family, vocational counseling, and disability evaluation. In addition, occupational therapy may provide patients with severe respiratory disease counseling on energy conservation and techniques for performing the basic activities of daily living.[35] Depression and anxiety are very common comorbidities associated with COPD, due to the often drastic limitations in functional activities, and panic associated with severe dyspnea. Antidepressant and anxiolytic medications are often useful adjuncts to counseling.

MANAGEMENT OPTIONS FOR INDIVIDUALS WITH SEVERE LUNG DISEASE

Mechanical ventilation

The broad array of respiratory assistive devices is shown in Figure 35-3. Within the past 25 years, there has been a dramatic reduction in the use of body ventilators. Their main function is to simulate the function of the inspiratory muscles. The intermittent abdominal pressure ventilator simulates the function of the expiratory muscles. Intermittent positive-pressure ventilation (IPPV) via non-invasive nasal–mouth interfaces or via tracheostomy is now the method of choice, because the equipment is lightweight and portable, and powered by either AC or DC current. There is no contact with the individual other than the nasal–mouth interface or the attachment to the tracheostomy tube (Figs 35-4–35-6). There are more than 30 interfaces commercially available today.

Portable ventilators are volume ventilators designed 25 years ago, high-span bilevel positive airway pressure units and, more recently, laptop volume ventilators (Fig. 35-7). For further information on the wide range of ventilator choices, the reader is referred to a recent publication on the management of neuromuscular disease.[4]

Air stacking, maximal insufflations, assisted coughing, and non-invasive ventilation are described as respiratory muscle aids by Bach.[4] He has also developed an oximetry feedback respiratory aid protocol. In this protocol, the oximeter is used to

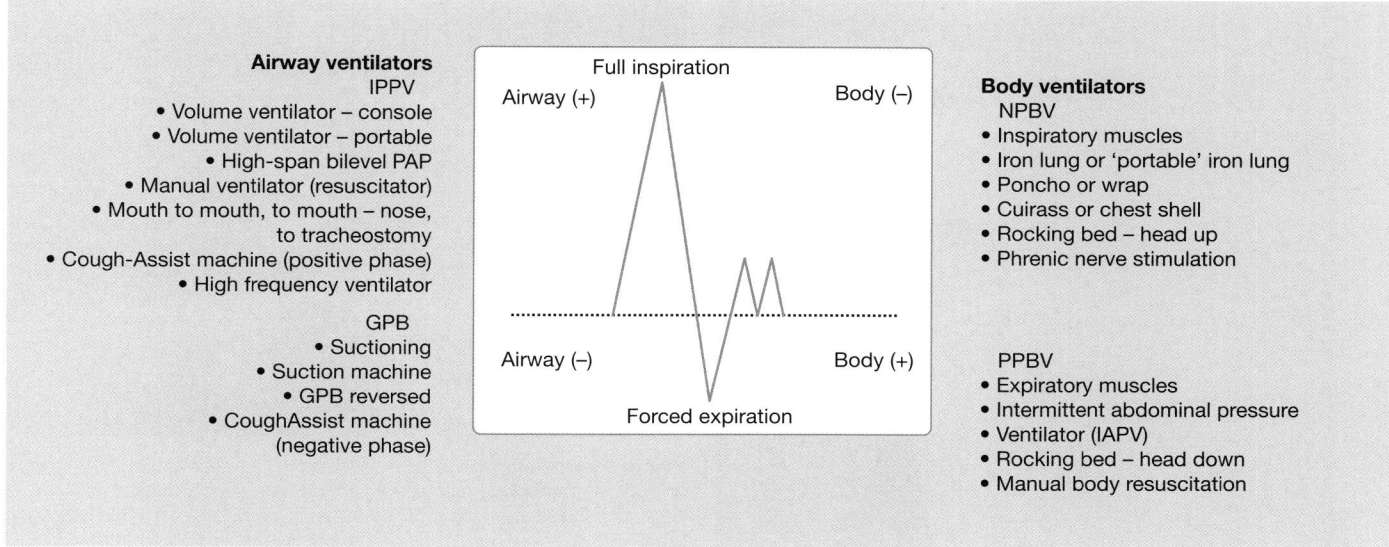

Airway ventilators
IPPV
- Volume ventilator – console
- Volume ventilator – portable
- High-span bilevel PAP
- Manual ventilator (resuscitator)
- Mouth to mouth, to mouth – nose, to tracheostomy
- Cough-Assist machine (positive phase)
- High frequency ventilator

GPB
- Suctioning
- Suction machine
- GPB reversed
- CoughAssist machine (negative phase)

Full inspiration
Airway (+)   Body (–)

Airway (–)   Body (+)

Forced expiration

Body ventilators
NPBV
- Inspiratory muscles
- Iron lung or 'portable' iron lung
- Poncho or wrap
- Cuirass or chest shell
- Rocking bed – head up
- Phrenic nerve stimulation

PPBV
- Expiratory muscles
- Intermittent abdominal pressure
- Ventilator (IAPV)
- Rocking bed – head down
- Manual body resuscitation

Figure 35-3 Respiratory assistive devices superimposed on a graphic representation of the vital capacity, and tidal volume. airway (–), ventilation by negative pressure on airway, producing suctioning; airway (+), ventilation by positive pressure on airway, producing inspiration; body (–), ventilation by negative pressure on body, producing inspiration; body (+), ventilation by positive pressure on body, producing expiration; GPB, glossopharyngeal breathing; IPPV, intermittent positive-pressure ventilation; NPBV, negative-pressure body ventilator; PAP, positive airway pressure; PPBV, positive-pressure body ventilator.

provide patients and their families with feedback to maintain oxyhemoglobin saturation by pulse oximeter (S_pO_2) greater than 94%. This is accomplished by maintaining effective alveolar ventilation and eliminating airway secretion. If the S_pO_2 falls below 95% in the patient with neuromuscular disease, it is due to one or more of three causes: hypoventilation during which there will also be hypercapnia, secretions, or the development of intrinsic lung disease (usually gross atelectasis or pneumonia). Patients and families are taught to pursue airway clearance techniques conscientiously, and to use NIPPV continuously. If these measures fail to bring the S_pO_2 back to normal or to baseline levels, patients must be evaluated by their clinician or in the emergency room. They should be admitted if necessary. Family members or primary care providers need to remain with the patient in the hospital to perform the ongoing routine of secretion removal. The routine itself is typically too time-consuming for hospital personnel to be able to remove secretions with the frequency that is necessary during an acute respiratory infection. When there is inadequate social support, hospital personnel usually find it necessary to intubate the patient for secretion removal and ventilation.

Diaphragmatic pacing (Fig. 35-8) is an alternative method of ventilation that has been available for more than 30 years. The system attained a higher level of reliability and broader application in the early 1990s. Infection and component failure are now rare complications. The need for the patient to retain a tracheostomy because of obstructive sleep apnea remains common. Approximately 1500 phrenic nerve pacers have been implanted worldwide in persons of all ages. Many users have been successfully paced for more than 20 years.[21] Diaphragmatic pacing is indicated in patients with congenital central hypoventilation syndrome (or Ondine's curse), acquired central

hypoventilation syndrome, and high SCI injury. Patients with inadequate social or financial support, poor motivation, or associated medical problems might not be good candidates. Although it is not common, the patient with a diaphragmatic pacer can require a mechanical ventilator as a backup during severe respiratory tract infections.

The pacing system consists of an external transmitter and antenna, and implanted electrodes and receiver. The working life expectancy of the receiver is for the lifetime of the patient, and batteries last for 2–3 weeks. A bipolar electrode is available for use in persons who already have demand cardiac pacers. There is advanced warning of transmitter battery failure, with a gradual decrease in tidal volume over several days. The pacer is thermal-stabilized to allow full outdoor activities with simultaneous pacing. The cervical implant is now recommended in the older child and adult, with 'customized' stimulation parameters that enable pacing with small numbers of residual fibers. Surgery in the supraclavicular region of the neck is relatively simple and hospitalization is typical, although the procedure can be performed in an outpatient setting. Although thoracic phrenic nerve implants for infants and younger children have required thoracotomy in the past, thoracoscopic placement of the electrodes has now been reported in children as young as 5 years.[50] The physician can use transtelephonic monitoring for remote assessment of stimulation effectiveness and diagnosis of problems.

Krieger and associates reported performing 10 nerve transfers in six patients with SCI at the C3 to C5 level, with axonal loss in the phrenic nerves to the extent that pacing was not possible.[33] In their technique, the fourth intercostal nerve was attached to the distal segment of the phrenic nerve 5 cm above the diaphragm. The pacemaker was implanted on the phrenic

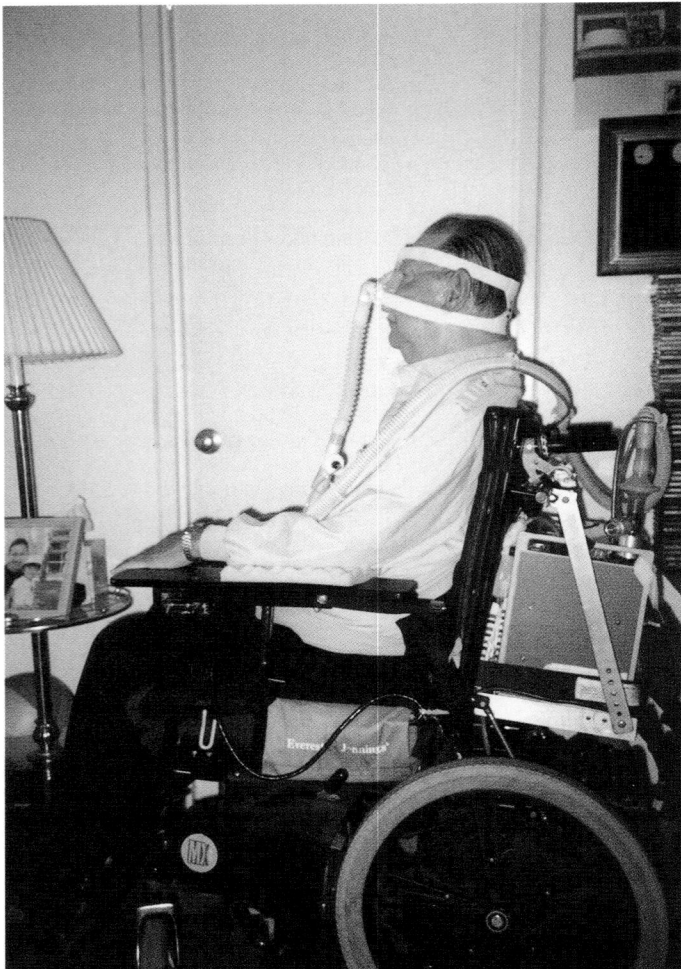

Figure 35-4 Nasal intermittent positive-pressure ventilation in a tetraplegic ventilator user with postpolio syndrome. The ventilator is a typical portable volume ventilator.

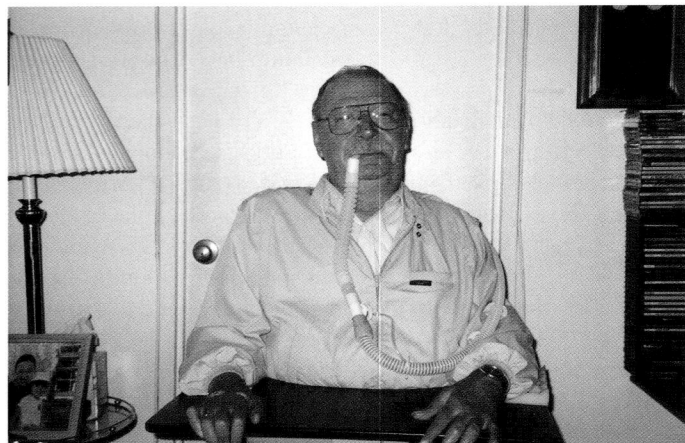

Figure 35-5 Mouth intermittent positive-pressure ventilation with angulated mouthpiece in a tetraplegic ventilator user with postpolio syndrome. The mouthpiece is held with teeth and lips.

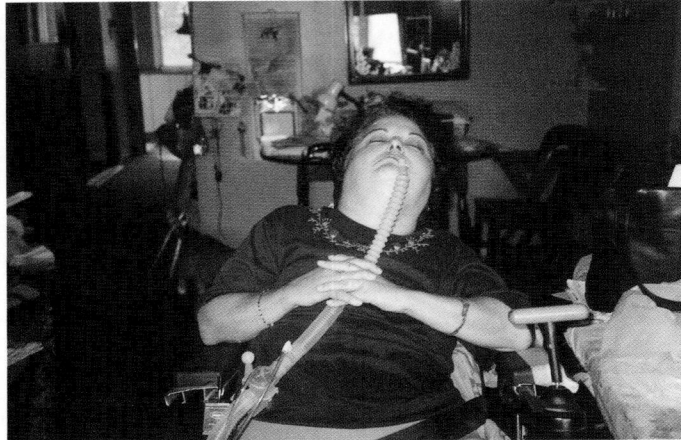

Figure 35-6 Mouth intermittent positive-pressure ventilation (IPPV) with angulated mouthpiece and without lip seal in a ventilator user with postpolio syndrome. She is taking a nap in her wheelchair. She can hold the IPPV hose with her hands on her chest. She has some ability to breathe on her own, and is a good frog breather when she is awake.

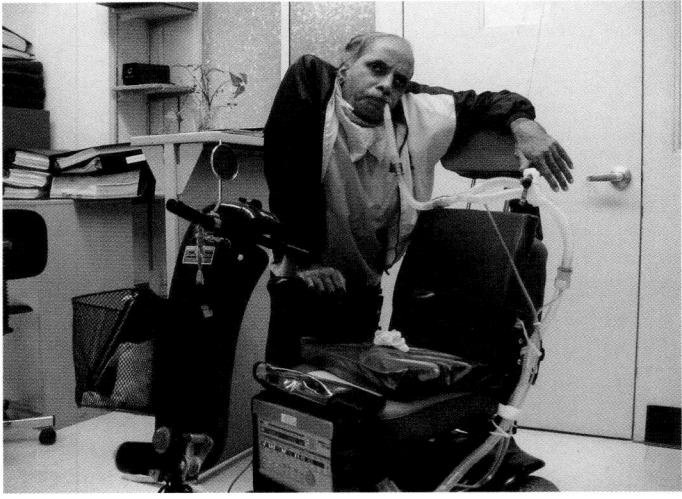

Figure 35-7 Mouth intermittent positive-pressure ventilation (IPVV) in a laptop ventilator user with 'upside-down polio' (upper trunk weaker than lower trunk and legs) and severe kyphoscoliosis. He is breathing continuously, with abdominal muscles when erect. The ventilator allows the muscles to rest. It is mounted in front of the scooter seat. He uses console volume ventilator and tracheostomy IPPV at night. Supine, he has no 'free time' off the ventilator.

nerve distal to the anastomosis. The average interval from surgery to diaphragmatic response to electrical stimulation was 9 months. All patients were able to tolerate diaphragmatic pacing as an alternative to IPPV.

Intramuscular diaphragm electrodes implanted via laparoscopic surgery were reported to successfully stimulate the phrenic nerves in one ventilator-dependent patient with tetraplegia.[18] In patients having only a single phrenic nerve that can be paced, combined intercostal muscle and unilateral phrenic nerve stimulation have also been shown to maintain ventilatory support.[50]

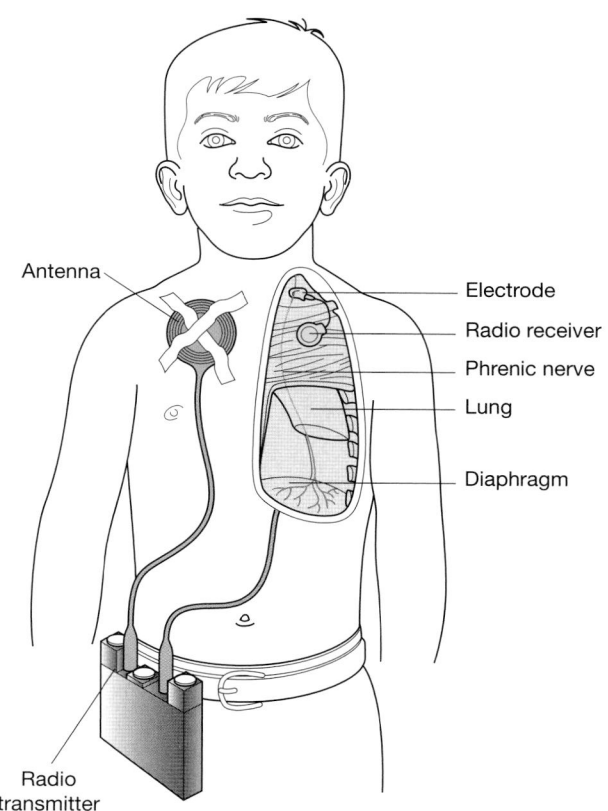

Figure 35-8 Bilateral diaphragmatic pacemaker use in a child with central hypoventilation syndrome.

Labels in figure: Antenna, Electrode, Radio receiver, Phrenic nerve, Lung, Diaphragm, Radio transmitter

Lung volume reduction surgery

Lung volume reduction surgery (LVRS) is utilized in patients with advanced emphysema. In LVRS, 20–30% of one or both lungs (usually at the apices) is removed. Decramer has reported the short-term results of six randomized studies, including the National Emphysema Treatment Trial.[15] These studies have shown reduced hyperinflation (residual volume and total lung capacity decreased), and improved FEV_1 and FVC. The 6-minute walk increased significantly, and quality of life improved. In general, inspiratory muscle function (maximal inspiratory pressure and maximal transdiaphragmatic pressure) also improved. However, this procedure is not for everyone. It has been found that, for patients with an FEV_1 less than 20% predicted and homogeneous disease, or a diffusion capacity less than 20% predicted, mortality increases after LVRS. In addition, the results of the National Emphysema Treatment Trial suggest that all LVRS candidates should first enroll in a pulmonary rehabilitation program, as some patients can improve to the point that they may not qualify for the surgery.[40]

Maxfield has discussed bronchoscopic LVRS as an alternative treatment option.[39] Stapling and plication of the most emphysematous tissue is carried out. Atelectasis can also be induced in these areas by using endobronchial sealants, occluders, or valves. Extraanatomic tracts between the major airways and the emphysematous tissue are created and prevented from collapsing with stents to facilitate expiratory airflow.

Lung transplant

Lung transplants are now performed worldwide. Living donor, lobar, and split-lung procedures are more common in children than in adults. Cystic fibrosis and primary pulmonary hypertension are the two main diseases of children for which lung transplant is performed. COPD is the main reason for lung transplant in adults, although pulmonary hypertension and pulmonary fibrosis are also common presenting diagnoses. Ongoing smoking is an absolute contraindication to lung transplant. Relative contraindications in most programs include prior cancer, psychiatric diagnosis, obesity, and correctable coronary artery disease.[34] Fifty-eight percent of programs in North America that have been queried have a minimum requirement for exercise capacity to be considered for lung transplant. Covering a minimum of 600 ft. on a 6-min walk test is the most common requirement, although some programs require only 250 ft. If an individual can only transfer from bed to chair, 46% of lung transplant centers consider this an absolute contraindication to lung transplant, and 52% consider it a relative contraindication.

SPECIAL CONSIDERATIONS

Obesity-related pulmonary dysfunction

Statistics from the US Department of Health and Human Services in 2004 show that 61% of adults in the USA were overweight or obese (body mass index, BMI, > 25) in 1999. Obesity in children was also common: 13% of adolescents are overweight. The prevalence of obesity in adolescents has tripled in the past 20 years. All racial and ethnic groups, and both genders are affected. Obesity increases the metabolic requirements of breathing, and can lead to pulmonary insufficiency. The respiratory failure of obesity is caused by alveolar hypoventilation from the increased workload of breathing, from obstructive sleep apnea, or both. There is also an increased risk of atelectasis. Daily physical activity is important in preventing and treating overweight and obesity.

Gidding and colleagues have studied the cardiorespiratory morbidity in children and adolescents with a BMI of 40.[26] Four percent had normal fitness, but 80% had peak oxygen consumption < 20 mL of oxygen per min. In 73% of these subjects, asthma treatment, small airway obstruction on pulmonary function testing, or both, were present. Upper airway obstruction was also present in 15% of them. Another study, in adults, found that three of four asthmatic patients who present to the emergency department with acute asthma are either overweight (BMI = 25–29.9; 30%) or obese (BMI ≥ 30; 44%).[55]

Spinal cord injury and pulmonary dysfunction

In SCI, there is diminished cardiopulmonary and circulatory function, as well as lower extremity muscle atrophy and bone mass reduction. Patients with high cervical cord injuries, including children as young as 3 years, can learn neck breathing[27] or GPB as forms of voluntary respiration. This allows some time off the ventilator. In GPB (or frog breathing), air is pumped into the lungs by the patient using the tongue as a piston (Fig.

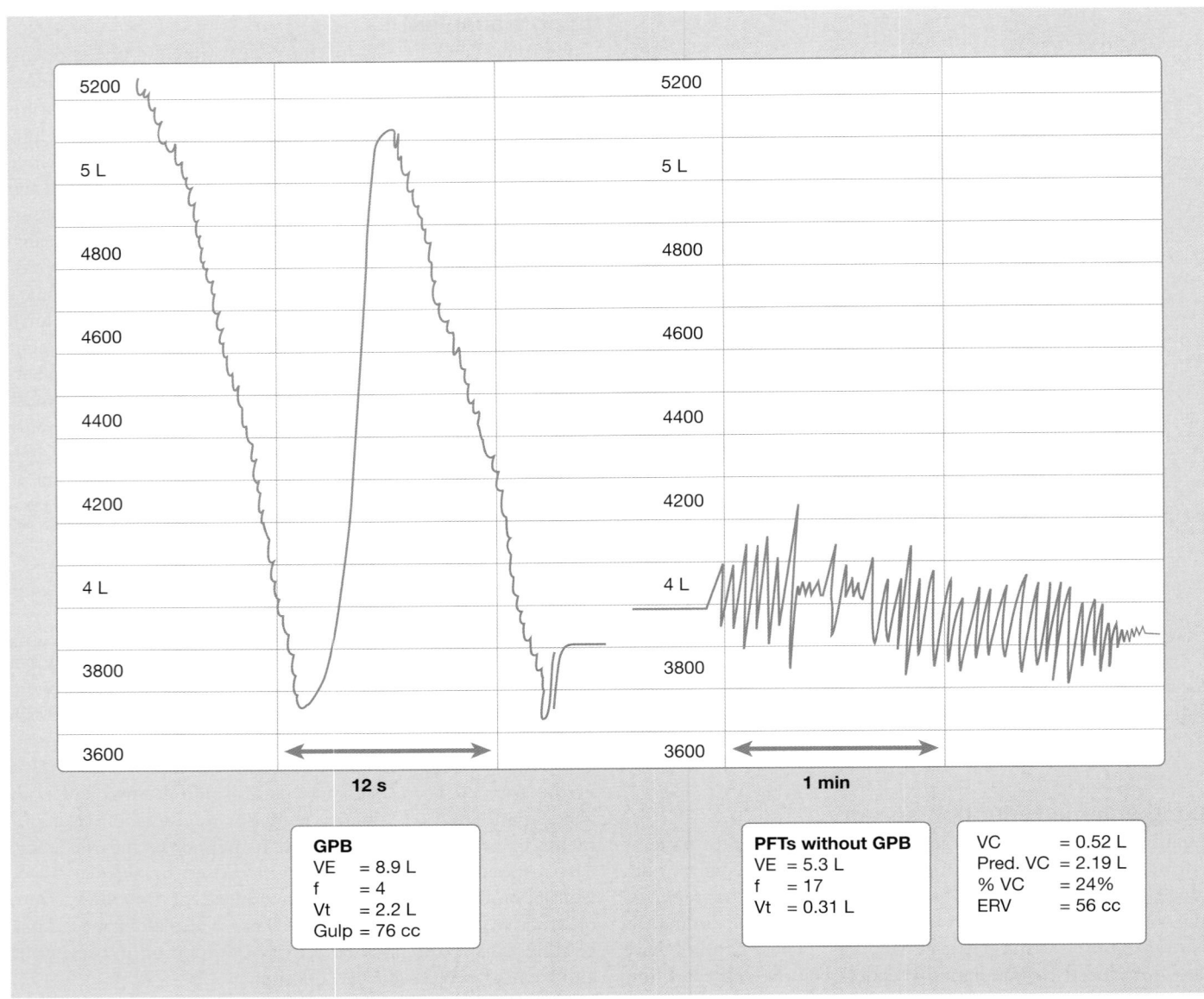

GPB
VE = 8.9 L
f   = 4
Vt = 2.2 L
Gulp = 76 cc

PFTs without GPB
VE = 5.3 L
f   = 17
Vt = 0.31 L

VC   = 0.52 L
Pred. VC = 2.19 L
% VC   = 24%
ERV   = 56 cc

Figure 35-9 Glossopharyngeal breathing (GPB) tracing and results compared with pulmonary function tests without GPB in a tetraplegic ventilator user with postpolio syndrome. ERV, expiratory reserve volume; f, frequency; gulp, volume or single GPB stroke; VE, minute ventilation; VT, tidal volume.

35-9). This technique is known as *glottic press* to speech pathologists. They teach it to patients who have had a laryngectomy, to pump air into the esophagus for esophageal speech. GPB can be used for a number of purposes in addition to being an alternative form of breathing. GPB can improve vocal volume and flow of speech to allow the patient to call for help, and to provide the deep breath needed for an assisted cough.

The person with low cervical or incomplete tetraplegia can perform resistance exercise by pedaling an arm ergometer for 30 min three times a week. FES cycle ergometer training[62] can reverse the detrimental effects of SCI to some degree. A surgically implanted neuroprosthesis that provides FES for exercise, standing, and transfers in individuals with low cervical or thoracic SCI is now available.[1] Body weight-supported treadmill

training[20] with gradually increasing speeds and increasing weight bearing is being studied during early rehabilitation in incomplete SCI (American Spinal Injury Association grades B, C, and D) from C4 to T10.

LONG-TERM RESULTS OF PULMONARY REHABILITATION

Long-term outcomes of mechanical ventilation

Many patients are now surviving significant illness only to become chronically ventilator-dependent. The number of long-term care hospitals in the USA has increased to over 250 in the past 15 years to care for these patients. Acute lung injury survivors weaned from the ventilator have been studied 1 year after hospital discharge.[14] Thirty percent still have generalized cognitive dysfunction, and 78% have decrements in attention, memory, concentration, and/or mental-processing speed. In addition, many have musculoskeletal complications such as weakness and numbness due to critical illness neuropathy and steroid-induced myopathy. Acute respiratory distress syndrome survivors weaned from the ventilator have been studied 1 year after hospital discharge.[14] Emotional dysfunction included the presence of depression, anxiety, and posttraumatic stress disorder.

Long-term outcomes of diaphragm paralysis after acute SCI have been reported.[41] Over a 16-year period, 107 patients required assisted ventilation in the acute phase of injury. Of this group, 31% (33 patients) with a level of injury between C1 and C4 (scale A in the American Spinal Injury Association impairment scale) had diaphragmatic paralysis at the time of respiratory failure. Twenty-one percent of the 33 patients were able to breathe independently after 4–14 months, with a vital capacity > 15 mL/kg. Another 15% (five patients) had some recovery that took more time and for whom the vital capacity remained < 10 mL/kg.

Bach has recently described in detail the long-term outcomes of NIPPV in neuromuscular disease.[4] No patient with DMD has been tracheostomized since 1983 at the Center for Ventilator Management Alternatives and Pulmonary Rehabilitation of the University Hospital in Newark, New Jersey. Some have been using 24-h mechanical ventilation for up to 15–25 years. Cardiomyopathy has become the limiting factor for survival in this population as respiratory deaths are being avoided. Tatara reports similar results in his center in Japan. He had a 5-year cumulative survival rate of 75% for 34 pediatric patients, including 25 with DMD. His patients used full-time mouthpiece–nasal IPPV. Ishikawa reported that, in another center in Japan, he has had a 3-year survival rate of 97.7% and a 10-year survival rate of 93.3% in 44 patients with DMD who started NIPPV in their late teens or early twenties.

Wijkstra and associates reported the long-term outcomes of inpatients with chronic assisted ventilatory care over a period of 15 years.[61] Thirty-six percent of their 50 patients left the hospital to enter a more independent community-based environment. Better outcomes were seen among patients with SCI and neuromuscular disease than in patients with COPD and thoracic restriction.

Gonzalez and coworkers studied long-term NIPPV in kyphoscoliotic ventilatory insufficiency (thoracic restriction) over a period of 3 years.[28] Patients showed improved blood gas levels and respiratory muscle performance, and reduced hypoventilation-based symptoms and number of hospital days.

Long-term results for LVRS

The National Emphysema Treatment Trial began in 1997. By June 2001, slightly over 1000 patients had been randomized to either optimal medical therapy or optimal medical therapy and LVRS. Few patients have been followed for as long as 5 years after surgery, but it appears that the gains from surgery include improvement in dyspnea, reduction or elimination of need for oxygen, and modest gains in FEV_1 and FVC. These improvements might be gradually lost over time.[15]

Long-term results in lung transplant

Three-year survival for the recipients of the 1692 transplants performed during 1997 and 1998 was 59%. Recently, de Perrot and associates reported 15 years of follow-up of 521 lung transplants in 501 patients from 1983 through 2003, with results typical of those found in other centers.[46] The 5-year survival rate was 55.1%, 10-year survival was 35.3%, and 15-year survival was 26.5%. Sepsis and bronchiolitis obliterans were the two most common causes of death.

SUMMARY

To practice pulmonary rehabilitation, physiatrists require a basic knowledge of the anatomy and pathophysiology of the cardiovascular and respiratory systems, as well as of exercise physiology. Patient assessment skills include proficiency in the electromyography of the respiratory muscles, and an understanding of the rapidly expanding field of cardiopulmonary imaging.

The practice of pulmonary rehabilitation can be in a setting limited to this subspecialty but more commonly is practiced as a component of general rehabilitation, where patients have pulmonary dysfunction as a complication of their neurologic or musculoskeletal disabilities or as a medical comorbidity. General rehabilitative therapeutic approaches apply in either setting.

Health policy, legislation, and regulations, including current healthcare delivery systems, must take into account the need for pulmonary rehabilitation at all ages in society. An informed public can facilitate change in this regard. The public is more informed now due to the development of online interest groups, Internet bulletin boards, and almost 350 000 articles pertaining to pulmonary rehabilitation on the Web.

REFERENCES

1. Agarwal S, Triolo RJ, Kobetic R, et al. Long-term user perceptions of an implanted neuroprosthesis for exercise, standing, and transfers after spinal cord injury. J Rehabil Res Dev 2003; 40:241–252.
2. Ambrosino N, Strambi S. New strategies to improve exercise tolerance in chronic obstructive pulmonary disease. Eur Respir J 2004; 24:313–322.
3. Bach JR, Smith WH, Michael J, et al. Airway secretion clearance by mechanical exsufflation in post poliomyelitis ventilator assisted individuals. Arch Phys Med Rehabil 1993; 74:170–177.
4. Bach JR. Management of patients with neuromuscular disease. Philadelphia: Hanley & Belfus; 2004.
5. Barriero E, Gea J, Sanjuas C, et al. Dyspnoea at rest and at the end of different exercises in patients with near-fatal asthma. Eur Respir J 2004; 24:219–225.
6. Blau H, Mussaffi-Georgy H, Fink G, et al. Effects of an intensive 4-week summer camp on cystic fibrosis: pulmonary function, exercise tolerance, and nutrition. Chest 2002; 121(4):1117–1122.
7. Brug J, Schols A, Mesters I. Dietary change, nutrition education and chronic obstructive pulmonary disease. Patient Educ Couns 2004; 52:249–257.
8. California Pulmonary Rehabilitation Collaborative Group. Effects of pulmonary rehabilitation on dyspnea, quality of life, and healthcare costs in California. J Cardiopulm Rehabil 2004; 24:52–62.

9. Casaburi R, Pastesio A, Loli F, et al. Reductions in exercise lactic acidosis and ventilation as a result of exercise training in patients with obstructive lung disease. Am Rev Respir Dis 1991; 143:9–18.

10. Casaburi, R. Principles of exercise training. Chest 1992; 101(suppl 5): 263S–267S.

11. Celli BR. Pulmonary rehabilitation in COPD. UpToDate®. Online. Available: http://www.uptodate.com 2004.

12. Colice GL. The seduction of asthma severity categorization. Chest 2003; 124:2054–2056.

13. Creutzberg EC, Wouters EF, Mostert R, et al. Efficacy of nutritional supplementation therapy in depleted patients with chronic obstructive pulmonary disease. Nutrition 2003; 19:120–127.

14. Curtis JR. The long-term outcomes of mechanical ventilation: what are they and how should they be used? Respir Care 2002; 47:496–505.

15. Decramer M. Treatment of chronic respiratory failure: lung volume reduction surgery versus rehabilitation. Eur Respir J 2003; 22(suppl 47): 47s–56s.

16. Dekhuijzen PN, Beek MM, Folgering HT, et al. Psychological changes during pulmonary rehabilitation and target-flow inspiratory muscle training in COPD patients with ventilatory limitation during exercise. Int J Rehabil Res 1990; 13:109–117.

17. DeWeerdt S, ed. Global initiative for chronic obstructive pulmonary disease: VIII. Component 3: Manage stable COPD. UpToDate®. Online. Available: http://www.uptodate.com 2004:1–25.

18. DiMarco AF, Onders RP, Kowalski KE, et al. Phrenic nerve pacing in a tetraplegic patient via intramuscular diaphragm electrodes. Am J Respir Crit Care Med 2002; 166:1604–1606.

19. DiMarco AF. Neural prostheses in the respiratory system. J Rehabil Res Dev 2001; 38:601–607.

20. Dobkin BH, Apple D, Barbeau H, et al. Methods for a randomized trial of weight-supported treadmill training versus conventional training for walking during inpatient rehabilitation after incomplete traumatic spinal cord injury. Neurorehabil Neural Repair 2003; 17:153–167.

21. Elefteriades JA, Quin JA, Hogan JF, et al. Long-term follow-up of pacing of the conditioned diaphragm in quadriplegia. Pacing Clin Electrophysiol 2002; 25:897–906.

22. Fahy BF. Pulmonary rehabilitation for chronic obstructive pulmonary disease: a scientific and political agenda. Respir Care 2004; 49:28–36.

23. Ferguson GT, Make B. Overview of management of stable chronic obstructive pulmonary disease. UpToDate®. Online. Available: http://www.uptodate.com 2004.

24. Franssen FM, Broekhuizen R, Janssen PP, et al. Effects of whole-body exercise training on body composition and functional capacity in normal-weight patients with COPD. Chest 2004; 125:2021–2028.

25. Garuti G, Cilione D, Dell'Orso D, et al. Impact of comprehensive pulmonary rehabilitation on anxiety and depression in hospitalized COPD patients. Monaldi Arch Chest Dis 2003; 59:56–61.

26. Gidding SS, Nehgme R, Heise C, et al. Severe obesity associated with cardiovascular deconditioning, high prevalence of cardiovascular risk factors, diabetes mellitus/hyperinsulinemia, and respiratory compromise. J Pediatr 2004; 144:766–769.

27. Gilgoff IS, Barras DM, Jones MS, et al. Neck breathing: a form of voluntary respiration for the spine-injured ventilator-dependent quadriplegic child. Pediatrics 1988; 82:741–745.

28. Gonzalez C, Ferris G, Diaz J, et al. Kyphoscoliotic ventilatory insufficiency: effects of long-term intermittent positive-pressure ventilation. Chest 2003; 124: 857–862.

29. Haas F, Axen K, eds. Pulmonary therapy and rehabilitation. Principles and practice. 2nd edn. Baltimore: Williams & Wilkins; 1991:29–42.

30. Jaeger R, Turba RM, Yarkony GM, et al. Cough in spinal cord injured patients: comparison of three methods to produce cough. Arch Phys Med Rehabil 1993; 74:1358–1361.

31. Klijn PHC, Oudshoorn A, van der Ent CK, et al. Effects of anaerobic training in children with cystic fibrosis. Chest 2004; 125:1299–1305.

32. Klijn PHC, van der Net J, Kimpen JL, et al. Longitudinal determinants of peak aerobic performance in children with cystic fibrosis. Chest 2003; 124:2215–2219.

33. Krieger LM, Krieger AJ. The intercostal to phrenic nerve transfer: an effective means of reanimating the diaphragm in patients with high cervical spine injury. Plast Reconstr Surg 2000; 105:1255–1261.

34. Levine SM, on behalf of the Transplant/Immunology Network of the American College of Chest Physicians. A survey of clinical practice of lung transplantation in North America. Chest 2004; 125: 1224–1238.

35. Lorenzi CM, Cilione C, Rizzardi R, et al. Occupational therapy and pulmonary rehabilitation of disabled COPD patients. Respiration 2004; 71:246–251.

36. Mador MJ, Bozkanat E, Agarwal A, et al. Endurance and strength training in patients with COPD. Chest 2004; 125:2036–2045.

37. Mahlmeister MJ, Fink JB, Hoffman GL, et al. Positive-expiratory-pressure mask therapy: theoretical and practical considerations and a review of the literature. Respir Care 1991; 36:1218–1229.

38. Man SFP, McAlister FA, Anthonisen NR, et al. Contemporary management of chronic obstructive pulmonary disease, clinical applications. JAMA 2003; 290:2313–2316.

39. Maxfield RA. New and emerging minimally invasive techniques for lung volume reduction. Chest 2004; 125:777–783.

40. National Emphysema Treatment Trial Research Group. A randomized trial comparing lung-volume-reduction surgery with medical therapy for severe emphysema. N Engl J Med 2003; 348:2059–2073.

41. Oo T, Watt JW, Soni BM, et al. Delayed diaphragm recovery in 12 patients after high cervical spinal cord injury. A retrospective review of the diaphragm status of 107 patients ventilated after acute spinal cord injury. Spinal Cord 1999; 37:117–122.

42. Otani K, Kanazawa H, Fujiwara H, et al. Determinants of the severity of exercise-induced bronchoconstriction in patients with asthma. Asthma 2004; 41:271–278.

43. Pastva A, Estell K, Schoeb TR, et al. Aerobic exercise attenuates airway inflammatory responses in mouse model of atopic asthma. Immunology 2004; 172:4520–4526.

44. Patel NJ, Jorgensen C, Kuhn J, et al. Concurrent laryngeal abnormalities in patients with paradoxical vocal fold dysfunction. Otolarynol Head Neck Surg 2004; 130:686–689.

45. Patessio A, Carone M, Loli F, et al. Ventilatory and metabolic changes as a result of exercise training in COPD patients. Chest 1992; 101:274S–278S.

46. de Perrot M, Chaparro C, McRae K, et al. Twenty-year experience of lung transplantation at a single center: Influence of recipient diagnosis on long-term survival. J Thorac Cardiovasc Surg 2004; 127:1493–1501.

47. Pierson DJ. Translating new understanding into better care for the patient with chronic obstructive pulmonary disease. Respir Care 2004; 40:99–109.

48. Rubin BK, van der Schans CP, Kishioka C, et al. Mucus and mucoactive therapy in chronic bronchitis. Clin Pulm Med 1998; 5(1):l–13.

49. Rundell KW, Anderson AD, Spiering BA, et al. Field exercise vs laboratory eucapnic voluntary hyperventilation to identify airway hyperresponsiveness in elite cold weather athletes. Chest 2004; 125:909–915.

50. Shaul DB, Danielson PD, McComb JG, et al. Thoracoscopic placement of phrenic nerve electrodes for diaphragmatic pacing in children. J Pediatr Surg 2002; 37:974–978.

51. Soriano JB, Kourtney JD, Coleman B, et al. The proportional Venn diagram of obstructive lung disease: two approximations from the United States and the United Kingdom. Chest 2003; 124:474–481.

52. Spruit MA, Troosters T, Trappenburg JC, et al. Exercise training during rehabilitation of patients with COPD: current perspective. Patient Educ Couns 2004; 52:243–248.

53. Steiner MC, Barton RL, Singh SJ, et al. Nutritional enhancement of exercise performance in chronic obstructive pulmonary disease: a randomized controlled trial. Thorax 2003; 58:745–751.

54. Tang NL, Chung ML, Elia M, et al. Total daily energy expenditure in wasted chronic obstructive pulmonary disease patients. Eur J Clin Nutr 2002; 56:282–287.

55. Thomson C, Clark S, Camargo CA. Body mass index and asthma severity among adults presenting to the emergency department. Chest 2003; 124:795–902.

56. Toder DS. Respiratory problems in the adolescent with developmental delay. Adolesc Med 2000; 11:617–631.

57. Vlahakis NE, Patel AM, Maragos NE, et al. Diagnosis of vocal cord dysfunction: the utility of spirometry and plethysmography. Chest 2002; 122:2246–2249.

58. Wadell K, Sundelin G, Henriksson-Larsen K, et al. High intensity physical group training in water—an effective training modality for patients with COPD. Respir Med 2004; 98:428–438.

59. Weiner P, Magadle R, Beckerman M, et al. Specific expiratory muscle training in COPD. Chest 2003; 124:468–473.

60. Weisman IM, Marciniuk D, Martinez FJ, et al. II. Indications for cardiopulmonary exercise testing. ATS/ACCP statement on cardiopulmonary exercise testing. Am J Respir Crit Care Med 2003; 167:211–277.

61. Wijkstra PJ, Avendano MA, Goldstein RS. Inpatient chronic assisted ventilatory care: a 15-year experience. Chest 2003; 124:850–856.

62. Wilder RP, Jones EV, Wind TC, Edlich RF. Functional electrical stimulation cycle ergometer exercise for spinal cord injured patients. Long Term Eff Med Implants 2002; 12:161–174.

63. Yankaskas JR, Marshall BC, Suifan B, et al. Cystic fibrosis adult care—Consensus Conference report. Chest 2004; 125:lS–39S.

64. Zeitoun M, Wilk B, Matsuzaka A, et al. Facial cooling enhances exercise-induced bronchoconstriction in asthmatic children. Med Sci Sports Exerc 2004; 36:767–771.

65. Zu-Wallack RL, Patel K, Reardon JZ, et al. Predictors of improvement in the 12-minute walking distance following a six-week out-patient pulmonary rehabilitation program. Chest 1991; 99:805–808.

Chapter	Employment of Persons with Disabilities
36	*Heidi Klingbeil, Donna Jo Blake and Dan D. Scott*

Disability is a significant public health and social issue in the USA. The number of Americans who experience disability, activity limitations secondary to chronic illnesses, or impairments has risen, while mortality has declined. Approximately 54 million non-institutionalized Americans—almost one person in five—have a mental or physical disability, nearly half of whom can be considered to have a severe disability. Approximately 37.7 million non-institutionalized Americans—almost one person in seven—have limitations severe enough to prevent them from playing, attending school, working, maintaining a household, or caring for themselves. Given these two measures, disability ranks as the nation's largest public health problem.[8,19,21,22,26,29,45]

The growing numbers of Americans with disabilities present new medical, social, and political challenges. The major activity limitations found in those with disabilities include an inability to manage personal care, the inability to work and be financially self-supporting, and the inability to integrate socially and enjoy leisure.[34] These limitations have medical, behavioral, social, and economic implications. In order to help those with disabilities restore functional capacity, prevent further deterioration in functioning, and maintain or improve their quality of life, programs of any type should emphasize rehabilitation and prevention of secondary conditions.[26] These programs must respect disability as multifaceted and foster an interdisciplinary approach to treatment.

Within the medical arena, the specialty of physical medicine and rehabilitation has been concerned with the establishment of physiologic, psychologic, and social equilibrium for persons with disabilities.[17] According to Rusk, 'A rehabilitation program is designed to take a disabled person from his bed back to his job, fitting him for the best life possible commensurate with his disability and more importantly with his ability'.[29] In order to help all persons with disabilities achieve their maximum level of independence, avert further deterioration in functioning, and maintain or improve their quality of life, the physiatrist and the medical rehabilitation team must appreciate the multifaceted character of disability. We must accept the responsibility to initiate appropriate referrals to other collaborating programs that can support these goals beyond the medical arena. One such program is *vocational rehabilitation*.

In this chapter, we examine the subject of employment of people with disabilities. Specifically, we:

- discuss the concept of disability;
- review national data on disability and employment;
- consider the economic impact of disability;
- review policies supporting employment of persons with disabilities;
- discuss economic assistance strategies;
- discuss vocational rehabilitation strategies;
- enumerate the incentives and disincentives for returning to work; and
- postulate that vocational rehabilitation serves as an actual rehabilitation treatment as well as a disability prevention strategy for people with disabilities.

THE CONCEPT OF DISABILITY

Disability itself is not always precise and quantifiable. The concept of disability is not agreed on by persons who consider themselves to have a disability, professionals who study disability, or the general public.[21] This lack of agreement is an obstacle to all studies of disability, and to the equitable and effective administration of programs and policies intended for people with disabilities.[10,11,21,25,26]

The World Health Organization (WHO) has a mandate to develop a global common health language—one that is understood to include physical, mental, and social well-being. The *International Classification of Impairments, Disabilities, and Handicaps* (ICIDH) was first published by WHO in 1980 as a tool for classification of the 'consequences of disease'. A new version, the ICIDH-2 beta-1 draft, was then field-tested. The ICIDH-2 beta-1 draft was designed to provide a common framework for understanding the dimensions of disablement and functioning at three different levels: the body, the person, and society.

The ICIDH-2 reflected the biopsychosocial model of disablement. In this model, disablement and functioning are viewed as outcomes of an interaction between a person's physical or mental condition and the social and physical environment. Human functioning is characterized at three levels: the body or body part, the whole person, and the whole person in social context. Disablements are the dimensions of dysfunctioning that result for an individual at these three levels; these include *impairment*, losses or abnormalities of bodily function and structure; *limitations of activities*; and *restrictions of participation*.

This biopsychosocial model regards functioning and disablement as outcomes of interactions between health conditions (disorders or diseases) and conceptual factors such as social and physical environmental factors and personal factors. The interactions in this paradigm are dynamic, complex, and bidirectional (Fig. 36-1).

Dimensions of dysfunctioning are defined as follows.

- *Impairment* is the loss or abnormality of body structure or of a physiologic or psychologic function.
- *Activity* is the nature and extent of functioning at the level of the person.
- *Participation* is the nature and extent of a person's involvement in life situations in relation to impairment, activities, health conditions, and contextual factors, and may be restricted in nature, duration, and quality.[46]

The concept of disability or disablement continues to be one about which there are many interpretations and opinions. This lack of agreement about the concept of disablement affects epidemiologic studies of disablement and the development of effective treatment and prevention strategies. The biopsychosocial model and the common language of the ICIDH-2 helped to define the need for healthcare and related services; define health outcomes in terms of body, person, and social functioning; provide a common framework for research, clinical work, and social policy; ensure the cost-effective provision and management of healthcare and related services; and characterize physical, mental, social, economic, or environmental interventions that would improve lives and levels of functioning.[46]

The 2001 World Health Assembly subsequently endorsed a revised system, the International Classification of Functioning, Disability and Health (ICF). The ICF provides a common transcultural language across healthcare systems, and is intended to allow comparison of international data and the measurement of health outcomes, quality, and cost, as well as health disparities.

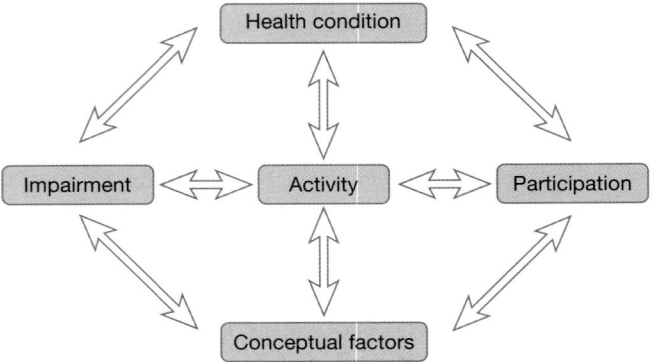

Figure 36-1 Biopsychosocial model of disablement.

DATA: IMPAIRMENT AND DISABILITY

Estimates of impairment and disability come from many sources. In 1990, the National Health Interview Survey found at least 120 million persons with impairments and 33.8 million people with disabilities living in households. Estimates from the 1990 census indicate that 2.3 million residents of institutions can be considered to have a disability. An estimate of the number of people with limitations in life activities, according to the National Health Interview Survey (1992), is 37.7 million, or 15% of the US population.[19]

The Survey of Income and Program Participation (SIPP) from the US Bureau of the Census provides extensive information on the number and characteristics of people with disabilities. SIPP information excludes people living in institutions. Data from the SIPP (1994) indicate that 54 million people, or 20.6% of the US population, have some level of disability.[22] Inability to walk without an assistive device was reported in 1.8 million using a wheelchair, and 5.2 million using another gait aid. Requiring help with one or more activities of daily living was reported in 4.1 million. The International Center for the Disabled (ICD) surveyed 12 500 households in 1986, and found the prevalence of disability to be 15% among Americans aged 16 years and older.[12] While the concept of disability was different for each survey, the results indicate that at least 54 million Americans have disabilities.

Impairments due to chronic disease have become increasingly significant as risk factors of disability.[8,21] Table 36-1 lists the 15 conditions with the highest prevalence of functional compromise or disability.[21] The prevalence of disability with these conditions appears to be due to the prevalence of the condition itself and the chance that the condition will cause a disability. Table 36-2 shows the ranking of persons, by percent of specific conditions, who have functional limitations secondary to that condition.[21] In general, many of the conditions that are significant risk factors for disability are low in prevalence. For example, multiple sclerosis has a low overall prevalence but is a significant risk factor for disability. Examination of this ranking shows seven out of the top 10 disabling conditions to be conditions frequently managed by the physiatrist and the rehabilitation team. These conditions or diseases are typically chronic, requiring a lifetime of rehabilitative management in order to have an effect on the disabling process, prevent secondary conditions, and maintain quality of life.

SOCIOECONOMIC EFFECT OF DISABILITY

Disablement has significant socioeconomic consequences for the individual with disabilities and for society. When a person is unable to participate in her or his social role as a worker or homemaker because of a physical or mental condition, that person is said to have a work disability or a work participation restriction.[6,46] Work participation restriction results in dependency and loss of productivity for that person. Society, in turn, incurs direct and indirect costs.

Table 36-1 Conditions with the highest prevalence of activity limitation

Main cause	Percentage
Orthopedic impairments	16.0
Arthritis	12.3
Heart disease	22.5
Visual impairments	4.4
Intervertebral disk disorders	4.4
Asthma	4.3
Nervous disorders	4.0
Mental disorders	3.9
Hypertension	3.8
Mental retardation	2.9
Diabetes	2.7
Hearing impairments	2.5
Emphysema	2.0
Cerebrovascular disease	1.9
Osteomyelitis or bone disorders	1.1
All causes	
Orthopedic impairments	21.5
Arthritis	18.8
Heart disease	17.1
Hypertension	10.8
Visual impairments	8.9
Diabetes	6.5
Mental disorders	5.6
Asthma	5.5
Intervertebral disk disorders	5.2
Nervous disorders	4.9
Hearing impairments	4.3
Mental retardation	3.2
Emphysema	3.1
Cerebrovascular disease	2.9
Abdominal hernia	1.8

(From La Plante 1991,[21] with permission.)

as Social Security Disability Insurance (SSDI), Supplemental Security Income (SSI), Medicare, and Medicaid. Direct expenditures incurred by our economy in 1986 totaled $169.4 billion.[6]

Disablement is also costly to the individual and society because of the loss of productivity. The indirect monetary costs for the individual are reckoned in terms of losses in job earnings and homemaker services. People with disabilities are less likely to be employed. The employment rate for people 21–64 years of age in 1994 without a disability was 82.1%; for those with a non-severe disability, the employment rate was 76.9%; and for those with a severe disability, the employment rate was 26.1% (Table 36-3).[22]

Disablement is also associated with lower earnings. Thirty percent of persons with a restriction in work participation in 1994 were below the poverty line, while only 8% of non-disabled persons were at the same level.[20] In 1986, the ICD survey found that 50% of all people with disabilities reported household incomes of $15 000 or less, as compared with 25% of non-disabled persons with incomes in that range.[12] In 1994, men 21–64 years of age without a disability had median monthly earnings of $2190. Those with a non-severe disability had $1857 median monthly earnings, and those with a severe disability had $1262 median monthly earnings (Table 36-3).[22] The indirect monetary cost to society is loss from the labor force.[7] For example, in 1988, spinal cord injury alone was estimated to have cost the US economy $2.4 billion in lost productivity.[13]

Disablement imposes indirect non-monetary costs to the individual and to society. Fifty-seven percent of persons with disabilities surveyed by Harris in 1986 believed their disability prevented them from reaching their full potential.[12] Restriction in work participation, in particular, places the individual in a position of dependency on insurance payments or government benefits for income support and medical care. Dependency affects people's feelings about themselves and their overall satisfaction with life.

Pressure from various customers, and especially the third-party payers, for accountability in medical care focuses attention on outcome and cost-effectiveness. Interventions directed at disablement should be assessed with measures of both outcome and cost-effectiveness. Disablement is more than a medical phenomenon: it is a complex socioeconomic process. Assessment of the outcome and cost-effectiveness of an intervention should take into consideration the quality of life and indirect monetary costs, as well as direct expenditures.

Vocational rehabilitation is an intervention that can limit restrictions in work participation. In 1993, the Social Security Administration estimated that, for every dollar spent on vocational rehabilitation services, five dollars in future direct expenditures was saved.[20] While employment is the expected outcome of vocational rehabilitation, the impact of this intervention goes beyond simple employment and saving of direct expenditures. The positive effects of working are demonstrated when the characteristics of working and non-working persons with disabilities are compared. Those who

Direct expenditures include those for medical and personal care, architectural modification, assistive technology, and institutional care, as well as income support for the person with a disability. For the individual, these expenses contribute to impoverishment.[7,42] Society's response to the expenditures related to disablement includes disability-related programs such

Table 36-2 Conditions with the highest risk of disability

Chronic condition	No. of conditions (in thousands)	Causes activity limitation (%)	Rank	Causes major activity limitation (%)	Rank	Causes need for help in basic life activities (%)	Rank
Mental retardation	1202	84.1	1	80.0	1	19.91[a]	9
Absence of leg(s)[a]	289	83.3	2	73.1	2	39.0[a]	2
Lung or bronchial cancer	200	74.8	3	63.5	3	34.5[a]	4
Multiple sclerosis[a]	171	70.6	4	63.3	4	40.7[a]	1
Cerebral palsy[a]	274	69.7	5	62.2	5	22.8[a]	8
Blind in both eyes	396	64.5	6	58.8	6	38.1[a]	3
Partial paralysis in extremity[a]	578	59.6	7	47.2	7	27.5[a]	5
Other orthopedic impairments[a]	316	58.7	8	42.6	8	14.3[b]	12
Complete paralysis in extremity[a]	617	52.7	9	45.5	9	26.1[a]	6
Rheumatoid arthritis[a]	1223	51.0	10	39.4	12	14.9[a]	11
Intervertebral disk disorders[a]	3987	48.7	11	38.2	14	5.3[a]	–
Paralysis in other sites (complete or partial)[a]	247	47.8	12	43.7	10	14.1[b]	13
Other heart disease disorders[c]	4708	46.9	13	35.1	15	13.6[a]	14
Cancer of digestive tract	228	45.3	14	40.3	11	15.9[b]	15
Emphysema	2074	43.6	15	29.8	–	9.6[a]	15
Absence of arm(s) or hand(s)[a]	84	43.1	–	39.0	13	4.1[b]	–
Cerebrovascular disease[a]	2599	38.2	–	33.3	–	22.9[a]	7

[a]Conditions frequently managed by physiatrists.
[b]Figure has low statistical reliability or precision (relative standard error >39%).
[c]Heart failure (9.8%), valve disorders (15.3%), congenital disorders (15.0%), other ill-defined heart conditions (59.9%).
(From La Plante 1991,[21] with permission.)

Table 36-3 Employment and earnings (1994)

	Employment rate of people 21–64 years old (%)	Median monthly earnings of men 21–64 years old ($)	Median monthly earnings of women 21–64 years old ($)
No disability	82.1	2190	1470
Non-severe disability	76.9	1857	1200
Severe disability	26.1	1262	1000

(From McNeil 1994–5,[22] with permission.)

work are better educated, have more money, are less likely to consider themselves disabled and, in general, are more satisfied with life.[12]

Comprehensive rehabilitation of persons with disabilities should include strategies, such as vocational rehabilitation, that reduce work restrictions. The outcomes include increased independence and increased productivity. The cost-effectiveness of comprehensive rehabilitation should be measured in direct and indirect monetary and non-monetary costs over the lifetime of the individual.[3]

DISABILITY-RELATED PROGRAMS AND POLICIES

Programs

There are a plethora of disability-related programs and policies. Each program and policy has its own definition of disablement and/or disability, and differs in the eligibility and application criteria. The programs can be characterized as ameliorative or corrective.[14] *Ameliorative programs* provide payment for income support and medical care. *Corrective programs* facilitate the individual's ability to return to work and to reduce or remove the disablement. Whether ameliorative or corrective, all programs influence the biopsychosocial model of disablement.

Disability-related programs can be categorized into three basic types: cash transfers, medical care programs, and direct service programs. Table 36-4 presents specific programs within these three basic types.[6] Estimates of the expenditures of these disability-related programs provide insight into expenditure trends. In 1970, 61.4% of the disability dollar went for cash transfers, 33% for medical care, and 5.4% for direct services. By 1986, the proportion of the disability dollar for direct services had decreased to 2.1% as the proportion for medical care had increased.[6]

The trend toward ameliorative programs' capturing more resources is a concern. Studies of the socioeconomic conse-

quences of disability support the utility of rehabilitating people with disabilities, allowing them to enter the labor market and thereby decrease their dependency and loss of productivity.

The physiatrist has an important supportive role in initiating referrals to the corrective programs. These programs are in keeping with the philosophy of rehabilitation, which is to maximize individual functioning and lessen disability.

Public disability policies

Public policy in the USA has begun to recognize that many barriers to integration faced by persons with disabilities are the result of discriminatory policy and practices. There is also the view that disability is an interaction between an individual and the environment. This has played a fundamental role in shaping public policy toward disability over the past 20 years. Since the late 1960s, Congress has passed a series of laws aimed at enhancing the quality of life for persons with disabilities. These laws have mandated that housing and transportation be accessible, that education for children with disabilities be appropriate, and that employment practices be nondiscriminatory.[1,9,40]

Three legislative actions deserve to be highlighted. The Rehabilitation Act of 1973 extended civil rights protection to persons with disabilities. This legislation included antidiscrimination and affirmative action in employment. The Rehabilitation Act Amendments of 1978 broadened the responsibility of the Rehabilitation Services Administration to include independent living programs, and created the National Council of the Handicapped (the National Council of the Handicapped became the National Council on Disability in January of 1989). The capstone of this legislative tradition is the Americans with Disabilities Act (ADA) of 1989. This legislation established a clear and comprehensive prohibition of discrimination on the basis of disability.[9,38,40,43]

Table 36-5 reviews the federal disability laws since 1968.[9,38]

VOCATIONAL REHABILITATION

The objective of vocational rehabilitation is to allow persons with physical disabilities to engage in gainful employment. Historically, formal vocational rehabilitation services were instituted to provide returning World War II veterans with disabilities assistance in obtaining suitable occupations.[40]

Before the 1970s, jobs earmarked for persons with disabilities were provided through government-subsidized sheltered workshops. The Comprehensive Employment Training Act of 1973 (CETA) provided public service jobs for persons with disabilities and for the disadvantaged, along with training programs for this population. At its peak in 1980, CETA and sheltered workshops provided more than a million jobs for a broadly defined 'disabled' population. The CETA program lasted from 1973 to 1982, whereon the federal government subsequently returned to state-run vocational rehabilitation agencies for provision of these services to persons with disabilities.

Table 36-4 Disability-related programs	
Type of program	**Specific programs**
Cash transfer	Social insurance: Social Security Disability Insurance Private insurance Indemnity compensation Income support: Supplemental Security Income, veterans' pensions, Aid to Families with Dependent Children
Medical care	Medicare Private disability insurance Veterans' programs Workers' compensation Tort settlements Medicaid
Direct services	Rehabilitation and vocational education veterans' programs Services for persons with specific impairments General funded programs (e.g. food stamps, developmental disabilities, blind, mentally ill) Employment assistance programs, i.e. comprehensive employment training program

(From Berkowitz and Hill 1989,[6] with permission of the ILR Press.)

Table 36-5 Federal disability laws[a]

Year	Public Law No.	Title of law	Key provisions
1968	90-480	Architectural Barriers Act	Requires that buildings built with federal funds or leased by the federal government be made accessible
1970	91-453	Urban Mass Transportation Act	Requires eligible local jurisdictions to plan and design accessible mass transportation facilities and services
1973	98-87	Federal Aid Highway Act	Requires that transportation facilities receiving federal assistance under the act be made accessible; allows highway funds to be used to make pedestrian crosswalks accessible
1973	93-112	Rehabilitation Act	Prohibits discrimination against qualified people with disabilities in programs, or receiving services and benefits, that are federally funded; created Architectural and Transportation Barriers Compliance Board
1975	93-391	Department of Transportation Appropriations Act	Prohibits purchase of mass transit equipment or construction of facilities unless they are accessible to elderly and people with disabilities
1975	94-103	Developmental	Establishes protection and advocacy systems for developmentally disabled people; establishes representative councils in each state for developmentally disabled people
1975	94-142	Education for All Handicapped Children Act	Provides for a free appropriate education for handicapped children in the least restrictive setting possible
1975	94-173	National Housing Act Amendments	Provide for the removal of barriers in federally supported housing; establish Office of Independent Living for disabled people in Department of Housing and Urban Development
1978	95-602	Rehabilitation, Comprehensive Services, and Developmental Disability Amendments	Establish independent living as a priority for state vocational rehabilitation programs; provide federal funding for independent living centers
1980	96-265	Social Security Disability Amendments	Remove certain disincentives to work by allowing people with disabilities to deduct independent living expenses in computing income benefits
1990	101-336	Americans with Disabilities Act	Establishes a clear and comprehensive prohibition of discrimination on the basis of disability

[a]Data from DeJong and Lifchez R 1983[9] and the US Equal Employment Opportunity Commission and the US Department of Justice 1991.[38]

The Rehabilitation Act of 1973 authorized federal funding for state rehabilitation agencies to provide a variety of services to qualified persons with disabilities. Table 36-6 lists the services provided. The federal government supplies 80% of the funding for state vocational rehabilitation agencies, while the states must provide the remaining 20%. State agencies administer the programs under the Rehabilitation Services Administration in the Department of Education. The intent of the Rehabilitation Act was to provide services to persons with disabilities, with emphasis placed on serving those with more severe disabilities (General Accounting Office testimony).[39] State agencies are usually located in the state division or bureau of vocational rehabilitation. The state division provides direct services, and also refers individuals to private rehabilitation agencies and training programs when indicated.

Table 36-6 Services provided by vocational rehabilitation specialists

Diagnosis and evaluation	Adjustment training
Counseling and guidance	Business or vocational training
Restoration[a]	Miscellaneous training
Transportation	Placement
College or university training	Referrals
Income maintenance	On the job training

[a]Includes medical treatment, prosthetic devices, or medically necessary services to correct or modify a physical or mental disorder.

Traditional approaches to vocational rehabilitation

A variety of approaches to vocational rehabilitation have been developed over the years. The traditional approach begins with referral of a person with a disability to a vocational rehabilitation counselor. This referral can be generated by the person with a disability, a physician, a social worker, or a case manager. The initial referral includes medical records, documentation of disabilities and capabilities, and neuropsychologic testing (if available).

The initial interview between the counselor and the client (person with a disability) establishes rapport and provides background information about previous job skills and experiences. The interview also provides information about the individual's educational level, motivation, perceived abilities and disabilities, and areas of interest. If the client was employed prior to the onset of disability, there is often potential for placement with the former employer. This previous employer should be contacted to learn of employment opportunities for the person with a disability. The vocational rehabilitation counselor also assesses the skills the person had premorbidly and the skills needed prior to placement in a suitable position. If no positions are available, vocational testing is performed.

Aptitude matching versus work sample

Vocational testing is performed to assess the client's level of general intelligence, achievement, aptitudes, interests, and work skills. Formal testing consists of administering a battery of paper and pencil standardized tests, examples of which are listed in Table 36-7. This type of approach is known as *aptitude matching*. It determines the client's aptitudes or traits in the areas of general intelligence, visuospatial perception, eye–hand coordination, motor coordination, and dexterity. Performance on the tests is compared against a list of essential aptitudes, grouped by occupation, in the *Dictionary of Occupational Titles* published by the Department of Labor.[23] When a client's apti-

tudes match a particular occupation, a job search is undertaken by the counselor.

A work sample approach is often used in conjunction with aptitude batteries. The work sample approach measures general characteristics such as size discrimination, multilevel sorting, eye–hand–foot coordination, and dexterity. The Valpar Component Work Sample Series (VCWSS) is a good example of the work sample approach. The VCWSS uses complex work apparatus to measure almost exclusively motor responses. There is less focus on general intelligence, aptitude, or academic performance. Work samples can also evaluate the type of 'work group' in which the client is most skilled. This simulated work requires performance of a series of tasks, such as drill press operation or circuit board or bench assembly.[23]

Once the client's skills have been evaluated and interests explored, a vocational goal is developed. The requirements of the potential position must first be determined. This is accomplished by performing a job analysis of the position, then identifying the physical and mental requirements and any necessary job site modifications (e.g. adaptive equipment). If training is proposed, it must be accessible and available to the client. Transportation should be arranged and can be paid for by the vocational rehabilitation agency. Tuition, books, and adaptive equipment to allow performance of the position can also be provided by the agency.

Training programs vary in length depending on the potential vocational goal. They can last from a few weeks to several years. Training can be conducted at a trade school, college, university, or on the job with state vocational rehabilitation agency funding.

On the job training requires job development. The counselor or the client explores community business resources to develop suitable positions. Tax incentives for potential employers can help convince industry to offer training. Sliding scale wages can be arranged to assist in developing positions. For example, the state rehabilitation agency may fund 100% of salary for 3–6 months. The employer gradually assumes that responsibility over the next 3–6 months as the new employee becomes trained. Many employers want to keep the employees they have trained, but some prefer to act in the capacity of trainers for a series of persons with disabilities. In this case, the counselor still has the task of placing the newly trained people.

Once an individual has completed training and has been placed for 60 days, the state vocational rehabilitation agency considers the case a 'success' and closes its file. No follow-up is typically provided.

Sheltered workshops

One of the problems with the traditional approach of the vocational rehabilitation agency has been its poor record of success, especially for persons with severe disabilities. There were 45% fewer people successfully vocationally rehabilitated in 1988 than in 1974, despite increased financial support and larger numbers of persons with disabilities.[40] A 1987 General Accounting Office survey found that, of SSDI recipients receiving vocational rehabilitation, less than 1% left the SSDI rolls.[33]

Table 36-7 Tests administered by vocational rehabilitation counselors or neuropsychologists	
Test	Type
Wechsler Adult Intelligence Scale—Revised	Intelligence
General Aptitude Test Battery	Aptitude
Differential Aptitude Test	Aptitude
Wide Range Achievement Test	Achievement
Strong–Campbell Interest Inventory	Interest
Career Assessment Inventory	Interest
Minnesota Multiphasic Personality Inventory	Personality
Halstead–Reitan	Cognitive evaluation
Luria–Nebraska	Cognitive evaluation

The ICD survey reported that, although 60% of persons with disabilities knew about vocational rehabilitation services, only 10% took advantage of those services. Of those using the services, more than 50% felt they were not useful in securing gainful employment.[12]

As a result of the poor placement record, alternative strategies have been developed for enabling persons with disabilities to obtain gainful employment. These include sheltered workshops, day programs, transitional and supported employment, Projects with Industry, independent living center (ILC)-directed employment, and others. Funding for these programs has come from public, non-profit and private industry, state and federal social service programs, religious entities, corporate and foundation contributions, and individual donations.

A sheltered workshop is a 'public non-profit organization certified by the US Department of Labor to pay "subminimum" wages to persons with diminished earning capacity'.[15] There are more than 5000 of these workshops, including Goodwill, Inc., serving approximately 250 000 persons with disabilities. This form of employment serves persons with severe disabilities, including limited vision, mental illness, mental retardation, and alcoholism. While sheltered workshops provide job experience and income, critics report that sheltered workshops rarely lead to competitive, integrated employment. People with severe disabilities can be competitively employed in the community through the use of some modern strategies, as outlined below.

Day programs

Day programs have existed since before the 1970s, and are meant to provide supervised vocational activity for persons with severe disabilities, usually those with mental retardation or mental illness. These programs are funded by private and corporate sponsors, as well as by state and federal agencies. They are not designed as a transition into competitive employment, nor do they allow community integration. They are geared toward providing supervised day activities while the caretakers of these persons work or perform their own daily routines. Activities are performed in facilities that serve only persons with disabilities.

Home-based programs

Another more traditional method for assisting persons with severe disabilities to obtain employment is the home-based program. Home-based programs can be funded by state vocational rehabilitation, insurance carriers, foundations, and societies, or by other agencies. The person with a disability can perform a variety of jobs, including telephone solicitation, typing, or computer-assisted occupations. Some examples include graphics, accounting, or drafting.

Of these programs—sheltered workshops, day programs, and homebound programs—none emphasizes gainful employment in a non-sheltered integrated setting. It was the failure of these programs to reintegrate their clients into competitive community employment that resulted in the emergence of transitional and supported employment models.

Other programs for employment
Projects with Industry

Projects with Industry is a federally sponsored collaborative program established by the Vocational Rehabilitation Act. Employers design and provide training projects for specific job skills in cooperation with rehabilitation agencies. The goal of Projects with Industry is competitive employment for the participants.

Job fairs have been somewhat successful in matching vacant positions with capable individuals with disabilities. Businesses in a community spend 1 day interviewing applicants with disabilities who have been prescreened by a participating placement agency. The placement agency might provide further services, such as transportation for the potential employee, and make recommendations for work accommodations to the potential employer.

Transitional and supported employment

Transitional and supported employment are two newer strategies for returning disabled persons to competitive, integrated gainful employment. Transitional employment consists of providing the job placement, training, and support services necessary to help persons move into independent or supported employment.[35] Independent employment provides at least a minimum wage to the employee and requires no job subsidy or ongoing support. Transitional employment is a short-term provision of services for a period not to exceed 18 months, and culminates in an independent or supported employment position.

Supported employment has been utilized as a successful strategy for placing or returning the most severely disabled individuals to competitive, integrated community employment. It requires ongoing support after placement, including counseling for the employee and coworkers, and assistance with transportation, housing, and other non-work-related activities.

It began as an alternative to sheltered workshops or day programs and has grown to have modest federal funding and broad community support. This support comes from groups of persons with disabilities, state vocational rehabilitation agencies, and state departments for the developmentally disabled. This concept became a permanent part of the Rehabilitation Act of 1973 with the passage of the 1986 amendments and final regulations published in June 1992.[44]

Box 36-1 Critical criteria for supported employment

- Interventions are provided at the job site.
- Assistance will be long term or permanent.
- Programs will serve only the severely disabled.
- Real pay for real work.
- Work is performed in an integrated setting.

(From Wehman et al 1993,[44] with permission.)

Supported employment is meant to provide ongoing support for persons with severe disabilities. According to Wehman and coworkers, it must meet five critical criteria (Box 36-1).[44] The first is that all interventions, including training, placement, and counseling, be provided at the job site rather than in a therapy room or vocational school. Second, the intervention and services are provided on a permanent or long-term basis as the individual requires them. Third, these programs are intended to serve only those individuals with the most severe disabilities who have been unable to enter the competitive labor market with their disability in the past. Fourth, the work provided is real and meaningful for the employee, and compensation is received equal to that of an able-bodied coworker for the same duties. Fifth, work must occur in an integrated setting allowing interaction with coworkers without disabilities.[44]

The Department of Education's operational definition of supported employment requires that employees be paid for working an average of at least 20 h per week in a position that provides interactions with persons who are not disabled and are not paid caregivers. There must be eight or fewer people with disabilities working together at the job site, and there must be ongoing public funding for providing intervention directly related to sustaining employment. Supportive employment defines the type and level of support needed by an individual to be employable now, not after a non-integrated training program.

Four models of supported employment have been developed. The *enclave* model consists of a small group of persons with disabilities working together at an integrated job site. The *mobile work crew* model uses a small group of workers who travel from job to job and offer contractual services under the direction of a supervisor. The *small business or entrepreneurial* model creates a new small business that produces goods or services using both workers with disabilities and those without them. The most frequently used model is the *job coach with individual placement*.[15]

The job coach, or employment specialist, is an employee of the agency providing supported employment services. The coach works with an individual at the job site to provide interpersonal and coping skills as well as job skills. The coach performs job development prior to placement. Once placement occurs, job training and ongoing job retention services are provided. Job coaches might initially be required to complete the duties not yet mastered by the worker with a disability.

Depending on the disability, behavior modification or cognitive training might be required to enable learning of vital skills. These become the responsibility of the job coach. The job coach should be able to evaluate the ecology of the job site, including attitudes of coworkers, accessibility of the job site, and the necessity for adaptive equipment. The job coach should then be able to educate coworkers and ensure implementation of appropriate accommodations for the person with a disability.

Job coach intervention time can be very significant (almost 8 h/day) initially. Wehman and others conducted a 5-year study of supported employment for persons with traumatic brain injury.[44] They documented an average requirement of 249.1 h per person of job coach time over 6 months. The job coach's intervention time decreased steadily with time on the job to an average of less than 3 h per week per person after 30 weeks of employment.

Some persons require continued significant intervention to assist them in meeting difficulties that arise from changes at the job site; that is, new job duties or changes in personnel or goods produced. Some workers are able to depend on support from employers and coworkers, however, and require little or no further direct job coach support. Supportive employment has been highly successful in allowing persons with severe disabilities to participate competitively in the job market and improve their quality of life and economic situation.

Independent living centers

The ILC movement has traditionally provided a core of non-vocational services such as housing, independent living skills, advocacy, and peer counseling. Just as supported employment has broadened its scope, so has the ILC movement. Both provide a combination of non-vocational and vocational services to persons with severe disabilities. ILCs often employ workers with disabilities as peer counselors and program administrators. The small business approach of supported employment has been successfully implemented by ILCs to place their clients in competitive community employment. As these two philosophies continue to merge and provide similar services to persons with severe disabilities, cooperative ventures between them will allow persons with severe disabilities to fully achieve their maximum level of independence.

Provision of vocational rehabilitation services to persons with disabilities requires a diversity of strategies. The more severe the disability, the more intensive the support and services have to be. Full participation in society is a right of all people. This participation includes being employed in a meaningful job that both gives satisfaction to the worker and contributes to society as a whole. The methods for returning persons with disabilities to work vary, but creative strategies have proved significantly more successful than non-creative strategies.

DISINCENTIVES FOR VOCATIONAL REHABILITATION

Public and political opinion has changed in recent years regarding the ability of persons with disabilities to work. Both persons with disabilities and policy makers have demonstrated a desire to return persons with disabilities to gainful employment. Statements of past presidents of the USA reflect the change of opinion. In 1973, Richard M. Nixon spoke concerning the Rehabilitation Act of 1973, saying it 'would cruelly raise the hopes of the handicapped [for gainful employment] in a way that we could never hope to fulfill'.[15] Advocacy by groups for the rights of persons with disabilities has achieved significant policy changes, as reflected by Ronald Reagan's November 1983 proclamation of the Decade of Disabled Persons, in which the economic independence of all people with disabilities was to become a 'clear national goal'.[35] With the passage of the

Americans with Disabilities Act in July 1990, George H.W. Bush proclaimed the 'end to the unjustified segregation and exclusion of people with disabilities from the mainstream of American life'.[15]

Despite the obvious changes in public and political policies and attitudes, disincentives to entering 'the mainstream' abound for persons with disabilities. In order to become eligible for cash and medical benefits through SSI and SSDI, persons with disabilities must prove that they have total and permanent or long-term disability and must meet strict eligibility criteria. Prior to meeting those criteria, the individual and the family typically must have suffered a series of indignities, including exhausting all personal resources and submitting to significant bureaucratic red tape. 'Red tape' means completing substantial paperwork, obtaining medical reports verifying disability, and enduring long waiting periods for commencement of benefits. This is usually a long and arduous process. Once the person with a disability finally achieves a modest degree of security, an 'opportunity' to give it all up and enter the workforce is made available. Naturally, the person with a disability is suspicious about the assurance that benefits will be preserved and eligibility will not be taken away because of returning to or entering the job market.

Stereotypes about persons with disabilities being unproductive in society are pervasive. Individuals with disabilities often come to view themselves as totally dependent and unable to work. After all, they are placed in a position to prove their dependency and inability to be productive. The government disability entitlement policies state that if you are unable to work, the government will take care of you. In fact, many government policy makers believe that the person with a disability cannot and should not be expected to work. Some even believe that sending a person with a disability a check is much simpler than implementing the provisions of the ADA.

Employers' attitudes serve as another disincentive. Obstacles to qualified applicants with disabilities who want to participate in the workforce include employers' ignorance about the capabilities of a potential employee with a disability, inaccessible work sites, transportation inaccessibility, and discrimination in hiring. The ADA will be instrumental in changing much of this behavior and removing some of these disincentives. As disabled employees take their places, employers and coworkers will become educated and attitudes will change.

The physiatrist and other physicians can also provide disincentives for persons with disabilities by labeling them as 'totally and permanently disabled' or by restricting their activities. Emphasis should be on the capabilities of persons with disabilities and documentation of their functional abilities, both mental and physical.

INCENTIVES FOR VOCATIONAL REHABILITATION

In an effort to overcome disincentives, government policy makers have created incentives for persons with disabilities and for potential employers. These incentives often have a long list of requirements and are very specific in wording in order to prevent abuse.

Incentives for the individual

Since the inception of the SSI program in 1974, only a small number of beneficiaries have been employed. Social Security bulletins note that in 1976 approximately 71 000 beneficiaries were working. By 1997, that number had risen to 305 000. During the same years, the SSI blind and disabled caseload rose from 2 million to 5.1 million. It appears that in 1997 about 6% of those who received an SSI payment were employed. Because these low numbers have been felt to reflect actual disincentives built into the current SSI payment system, a number of incentive programs have been implemented.[18]

Incentive programs are applicable depending on whether the person with a disability receives SSDI or SSI benefits, or both. SSDI work incentives are discussed first. Table 36-8 presents a summary of the terminology and abbreviations for easy reference. Additional references are given here for those wanting more detailed information.[24,27,28,31,33,36,37]

The initial incentive toward a return to work involves a trial work period (TWP). The TWP lets people test their ability to work or run a business without affecting their benefits. This TWP maintains cash benefits for 9 months (not necessarily consecutive) of trial work in a 60-month period. During this period of time, beneficiaries can earn up to $530 per month.[4]

On completion of the TWP and continued employment at or above the substantial gainful activity (SGA) level, benefits continue to be paid for three more months and are then terminated.[24,36,37] Any earnings from work below the monetary limit of the SGA level described in Table 36-8 are excluded when figuring monthly benefit amounts. The SGA dollar amount was increased in 1999 from $500 to $700, and a formula adopted to link this amount in the future to the national average wage index.[4]

The extended period of eligibility (EPE) is a period of 36 consecutive months during which cash benefits can be reinstated if, during that period, the individual's earnings fall below the SGA level. If the individual is unable to maintain earnings at the SGA level, benefits resume automatically and no waiting periods are required. Benefits cease at the end of the EPE, but Medicare continues for three additional months.[24,36,37] The elimination of a second waiting period for both cash benefits and Medicare benefits is also an incentive to perform a trial of work.

Under certain circumstances, the person might be able to participate in a Medicare 'buy-in'. The client must have completed both the TWP and the EPE. In addition, the extended 3 months of Medicare benefits must have passed. Once these conditions are met, Medicare A and B coverage can be purchased. This medical coverage is for those who cannot otherwise obtain health insurance because of preexisting conditions.[24]

Another major incentive program for those receiving SSDI or SSI is for impairment-related work expenses. This allows the cost of certain items and services to be deducted from earnings

Table 36-8 Summary of incentives for the individual receiving benefits to enter work activities

Incentive	Details
Social Security Disability Insurance (SSDI)	Disability benefits program based on medical disability and a worker's earnings covered by social security (Title II—Social Security Act)
Supplemental Security Income (SSI)	Disability benefits program based on medical disability and the amount of income a person receives (Title XVI—Social Security Act)
Trial work period (TWP)	Allows trial return to work to test work ability without affecting benefits (SSDI)
Substantial gainful activity (SGA)	Performance of significant and productive physical or mental work for pay or profit (over $700/month for non-blind [SSDI and SSI]) and $810/month for blind recipients [SSDI only])
Extended period of eligibility	Allows reinstatement of cash benefits without a waiting period if the worker's earnings fall below SGA level within 36 months after TWP (SSDI)
Impairment-related work expenses	Allows costs for certain items to be deducted from earnings when figuring SGA level (SSI and SSDI)
Earned income exclusion	Allows exclusion of a portion of earned income when figuring an individual's monthly benefit (SSI)
Blind work expenses	Allows work-related expenses when figuring benefits (SSI)

when determining the SGA level. Examples include attendant care, medical devices, equipment, and prostheses.[24]

For those persons with disabilities receiving SSI benefits, a different, but often similar, set of incentives applies. These incentives provide SSI recipients with assurances that working will not disadvantage them. Section 1619 of the Social Security Act was made permanent by the Employment Opportunities for Disabled Americans Act passed in November 1986. The incentive of Section 1619 allows receipt of SSI cash benefits, even though earned income exceeds the SGA level. Cash benefits are calculated using the earned income exclusion discussed below. Medicaid benefits continue as an additional incentive even after wages become high enough to cause cessation of SSI cash benefits, provided their continuation is needed to allow the recipient to maintain employment.[24,36,37]

The earned income exclusion allows most of a recipient's earned income to be excluded, including pay received from a sheltered workshop or day activity center, when figuring the SSI monthly amount.[33] 'Blind' work expenses is an incentive that allows a person who has visual impairment to pay for work expenses, such as visual aids, guide dogs, or Braille translations. These allowable expenses are then excluded when calculating benefit amounts.

In an effort to prevent work disincentives, benefit caps have been implemented to decrease excessively generous benefits. These caps utilize various formulas to reduce or limit maximum benefits paid by social security. These formulas take into account other sources of income, such as workers' compensation benefits, but do not exclude veterans' benefits or disability pensions from government jobs.

Another incentive program, Plans for Achieving Self-Support, allows an SSI recipient to set aside income and resources neces-

sary to achieve a work goal. The plan must be approved by the Social Security Administration.[27,36,37]

Incentives for industry

Government policy makers have made various attempts to offer tax incentives to business and industry. These incentives have mainly been directed at making the workplace accessible. Section 190 of the Internal Revenue Code, enacted in 1976 and revised by the Revenue Reconciliation Act of 1990, allows a set amount per year to be deductible for any expenses incurred in barrier removal (making a business or public transportation accessible).[30]

The Revenue Reconciliation Act of 1990 (which was passed 3 months after the ADA) allows an 'access' tax credit with Section 44 of the Internal Revenue Code for small businesses. It allows credit against income taxes for eligible expenditures (auxiliary services for the disabled employee and aids are covered). This access credit is allowed only for expenses incurred for the purpose of enabling a business to comply with the ADA.[30]

Tax credits have also been used as incentives to encourage hiring of target groups, including the 'hard core' unemployed: persons with disabilities and the homeless. The Targeted Jobs Tax Credit (TJTC), originally enacted in 1978, is meant to encourage employers to hire members of these groups. It provides a tax credit for targeted persons, including those persons receiving SSI benefits and vocational rehabilitation referrals (both groups containing large numbers of persons with disabilities). This credit only provides benefits to an employer for 1 year per employee. Many employers use the credit as a windfall; that is, hiring anyone they want and later checking to see if the new employee falls into a targeted group. This practice is called 'retroactive certification'.[30]

The TJTC has, unfortunately, not been particularly useful in increasing the number of disabled people hired. In fact, legislative incentives in general have not been very successful in achieving the goal of vocationally rehabilitating persons with disabilities. There are ongoing efforts in the Congress, however, to improve the incentives for persons with disabilities to return to work. For example, the Work Incentives Improvement Act of 1999 (S.331) provides adequate and affordable health insurance when a person on SSI or SSDI goes to work, by expanding Medicaid options for states and by continuing access to Medicare after returning to work. It encourages SSDI beneficiaries to return to work by assuring that cash benefits remain available if employment proves unsuccessful. An expedited eligibility process is proposed for SSDI beneficiaries who lose benefits due to work and need reinstatement of benefits later. A 'ticket' program would provide a new payment system for SSDI and SSI beneficiaries for employment services. It reimburses vocational rehabilitation, training, and employment service providers a portion of benefit payments saved when the beneficiary earns more than the SGA level, currently $700 per month ($1000 for blind beneficiaries).[4,17] Originally, this program called for sanctions (deductions against social security benefits or suspension of SSI benefits) for refusal of vocational rehabilitation, but this was eliminated as of 1 January 2001.[5]

Approximately 80% of SSI recipients work prior to applying for SSI, and 20% work after they start receiving payments.[31] Scott Muller of the Social Security Administration performed a retrospective analysis of a cohort of over 4000 people who were initially entitled to benefits.[24] Approximately 10% worked during the initial period of entitlement. Of those, 84% were granted a TWP, and of that group, over 70% completed the TWP. More than 50% did not leave the rolls as a result of their efforts. Less than 3% had benefits terminated as a result of return to work.[24]

It is clear from the research conducted by the Social Security Administration that legislating incentives is not the complete answer to rehabilitating persons with work disability. Potential employers and persons with disabilities alike must take the initiative. But the search for feasible means to return the work-disabled to work is well worth it. The General Accounting Office estimates that removing even 1% of disabled beneficiaries from the SSDI and SSI programs each year would result in estimated lifetime savings of $3.0 billion.[32]

DISABILITY PREVENTION

With disability ranking as the nation's largest public health problem, it seems reasonable to interface the public health model of prevention with the ICIDH-2 model of disablement. The public health model defines three categories of prevention: primary, secondary, and tertiary.

Primary prevention is intended for healthy persons, helping them to avoid the onset of a pathologic condition. In persons with disabilities, primary prevention comprises efforts toward preventing a worsening of impairments.

Secondary prevention is aimed at early identification and treatment of a pathologic condition, and reduction of risk factors for disablement. For persons with disabilities, there are many opportunities for preventing impairment from limiting one or more activities. The ameliorative and corrective programs discussed above, including vocational rehabilitation strategies, are aimed at reducing activity limitation. These programs have been effective not only in returning the unemployed to work, but also in preventing job loss in those workers with a disability.[2] Interventions in medical rehabilitation focused on the enhancement of activity, such as provision of assistive technology, can be considered secondary prevention.

The General Accounting Office has studied return to work strategies employed by Germany and Sweden, and recommends that intervention occur as soon as possible after an actual or potentially disabling event to promote and facilitate return to work. Because the current SSI benefit structure in the USA includes a lengthy application process, and then benefits linked to full, permanent disability only, intervention often is only offered long after an applicant has been removed from the workforce—a situation numerous studies have shown to significantly decrease the chance of a successful return to the workforce.[32]

Tertiary prevention focuses on arresting the progression of a pathologic condition and on limiting further disablement. For people with disabilities, tertiary prevention is designed to limit the restriction of a person's participation in some area by the provision of a facilitator or the removal of a barrier.[46] Environmental modifications, provision of services, removal of physical barriers, changes in social attitudes, or reform in legislation and policy are tertiary prevention strategies. Medical rehabilitation is traditionally considered a tertiary prevention strategy. The public disability policies, such as the ADA, are also efforts to reduce environmental and social barriers to participation.[26,41,46]

Considering functioning and disablement as outcomes of interactions between health conditions (disorders or diseases) and conceptual factors (social, environmental, personal), there are many opportunities for the physiatrist and the medical rehabilitation team to intervene. Rehabilitation interventions aimed at prevention of activity limitation or prevention of participation restriction are secondary and tertiary prevention strategies that push the dynamic model of disablement in the direction of function. The physiatrist has a responsibility to be actively involved in therapeutic and public health management of disablement.[16]

CONCLUSION

Comprehensive rehabilitation is an intervention directed at human functioning. The desired outcome is to maximize the physical, mental, social, and economic function of the individual with disabilities. The physiatrist as team leader has the responsibility of encouraging the team to take a holistic approach to the person with disabilities. The holistic approach includes collaboration with professionals outside the traditional medical rehabilitation team, such as those who can facilitate vocational rehabilitation for persons with disabilities.

Vocational rehabilitation is an intervention aimed at preventing an impairment from limiting activities and limiting participation in work. Limitation in work participation has significant socioeconomic consequences for the individual and for society. Employment of persons with disabilities supports a better quality of life and promotes function. Even for people with severe disabilities, vocational rehabilitation strategies have been successful in facilitation of work participation.

Disability is the largest public health problem in the USA. The demands of this public health issue have captured the attention of public policy makers. This has resulted in implementation of significant federal disability laws. The nation's public policies on disability reflect the policy makers' acceptance of disability as a complex process. Disablement is considered to be the result of a dynamic, complex, and bidirectional interaction between health conditions and conceptual factors for each individual.

The physiatrist is positioned to serve a primary role in the functioning and disablement paradigm. As persons with disabilities become a greater segment of our society, the opportunities for physiatrists' involvement are expanded. It is the physiatrist's responsibility to be active in disability prevention, in care and advocacy for persons with disabilities, and in the development of public policy on disablement.

REFERENCES

1. Adams PF, Benson V. Current estimates for the National Health Interview Survey, 1988. Vital Health Stat 10 1989; 173:1–250.
2. Allaire S, Li W, LaValley M. Reduction of job loss in persons with rheumatic diseases receiving vocational rehabilitation: a randomized controlled trial. Arthritis Rheum 2003; 48:3212–3218.
3. Anderson TP. Quality of life of the individual with a disability. Arch Phys Med Rehabil 1982; 63:55.
4. [Anonymous]. Federal Register: rules and regulations 2000; 65(251):82905–82912.
5. [Anonymous]. Federal Register: rules and regulations 68(129):40119–40125.
6. Berkowitz M, Hill MA. Disability and the labor market: an overview. In: Berkowitz M, Hill MA, eds. Disability and the labor market: economic problems, policies, and programs. New York: ILR Press; 1989:1–28.
7. Berkowitz M. The socioeconomic consequences of SCI. Paraplegic News 1994; Jan:18–23.
8. Colvez A, Blanche M. Disability trends in the United States population 1966–76: analysis of reported causes. Am J Public Health 1981; 71:464–471.
9. DeJong G, Lifchez R. Physical disability and public policy. Sci Am 1983; 248:40–50.
10. Haber LD. Identifying the disabled: concepts and methods in the measurement of disability. Soc Secur Bull 1988; 51:11–28.
11. Haber LD. Issues in the definition of disability and the use of disability survey data. In: Daniel LB, Aitter M, Ingram L, eds. Disability statistics, an assessment: report of a workshop. Washington: National Academy Press; 1990:1–71.
12. Harris L. The ICD survey of disabled Americans: bringing disabled Americans into the mainstream. New York: Louis Harris and Associates; 1986.
13. Harvey C. The business of employment: employment after traumatic SCI. Paraplegic News 1993; Oct:10–14.
14. Haveman RH, Halberstandt V, Burkhauser RV, eds. Public policy toward disabled workers: cross-national analyses of economic impacts. New York: Cornell University Press; 1984.
15. Hearne PG. Employment strategies for people with disabilities: a prescription for change. Milbank Q 1991; 69:111–128.
16. Joe TC. Professionalism: a new challenge for rehabilitation. Arch Phys Med Rehabil 1981; 62:245–250.
17. Kennedy EM, et al. The Work Incentives Improvement Act of 1999, Senate Bill 331. Feb 1999.
18. Kenney, L. Earning histories of SSI beneficiaries working in December 1997. Soc Secur Bull 2000; 63(3):34–46.
19. Kraus LE, Stoddard S, Gilmartin D. Chartbook on disability in the United States. Washington: US Department of Education, National Institute on Disability and Rehabilitation Research; 1996.
20. La Plante MP, Kennedy J, Kaye S, et al. Disability and employment, no. 11. Disability statistics abstract series. San Francisco: University of California; 1997.
21. La Plante MP. The demographics of disability. Milbank Q 1991; 69:55–77.
22. McNeil JM. Current population reports, household economic studies, series P70-61. Washington: US Department of Commerce, Bureau of the Census; 1994–5.
23. Menchetti BM, Flynn CC. Vocational evaluation. In: Rusch FR, ed. Supported employment. Sycamore: Sycamore; 1990:111–131.
24. Muller LS. Disability beneficiaries who work and their experience under program work incentives. Soc Secur Bull 1992; 55:2–19.
25. Nagi SZ. Disability concepts revisited: implication to prevention, appendix A. In: Pope AM, Tarlov AR, eds. Disability in America: toward a national agenda for prevention. Washington: National Academy Press; 1991:306–327.
26. Pope AM, Tarlov AR, eds. Disability in America: toward a national agenda for prevention. Washington: National Academy Press; 1991.
27. Rigby DE. SSI work incentive participants. Soc Secur Bull 1991; 54:22–29.
28. Rocklin SG, Mattson DR. The Employment Opportunities for Disabled Americans Act: legislative history and summary of provisions. Soc Secur Bull 1987; 50:25–35.
29. Rusk HA. The growth and development of rehabilitation medicine. Arch Phys Med Rehabil 1969; 50:463–466.
30. Schaffer DC. Tax incentives. Milbank Q 1991; 69:293–312.
31. Scott CG. Disabled SSI recipients who work. Soc Secur Bull 1992; 55:26–36.
32. Sim, J. Improving return-to-work strategies in the United States disability programs, with analysis of program practices in Germany and Sweden. Soc Secur Bull 1999; 59(3):41–50.
33. Social Security Administration. Report of Disability Advisory Council: executive summary. Soc Secur Bull 1988; 51:13–17.
34. Symington DC. The goals of rehabilitation. Arch Phys Med Rehabil 1984; 65:427–430.
35. Thornton C, Maynard R. The economics of transitional employment and supported employment. In: Berkowitz M, Hill MA, eds. Disability and the labor market: economic problems, policies, and programs. New York: ILR Press; 1989:142–170.
36. US Department of Health and Human Services, Social Security Administration. Social security handbook. 13th edn. Washington: Government Printing Office; 1997.
37. US Department of Health and Human Services, Social Security Administration: redbook on work incentives. Washington: Government Printing Office; 1992.
38. US Equal Employment Opportunity Commission, US Department of Justice. Americans with Disabilities Act handbook (EEOC-BK-19). Washington: Government Printing Office; 1991.
39. US General Accounting Office. Testimony before the Subcommittee on Select Education, Committee on Education and Labor, House of Representatives. Vocational Rehabilitation Program: client characteristics, services received, and employment outcomes. Washington: Government Printing Office; 1991.
40. Vachon RA. Employing the disabled. Issues Sci Technol 1989-90; winter:44–50.
41. Vachon RA. Employment assistance and vocational rehabilitation for people with HIV or AIDS: policy, practice, and prospects. In: O'Dell MW, ed.

HIV-related disability: assessment and management. Physical medicine and rehabilitation: state of the art reviews. Philadelphia: Hanley & Belfus; 1993: s203–s224.

42. Vachon RA. Inventing a future for individuals with work disabilities: the challenge of writing national disability policies. In: Woods DE, Vandergoot D, eds. The changing nature of work, society and disability: the impact on rehabilitation policy. New York: World Rehabilitation Fund; 1987:19–45.

43. Verville R. The rehabilitation amendments of 1978: what do they mean for comprehensive rehabilitation? Arch Phys Med Rehabil 1979; 60:141–144.

44. Wehman P, Sherron P, Kregel J, et al. Return to work for persons following severe traumatic brain injury: supported employment outcomes after five years. Am J Phys Med Rehabil 1993; 72:355–363.

45. Wilson RW. Do health indicators indicate health? Am J Public Health 1981; 71:461–463.

46. World Health Organization. Towards a common language for functioning and disablement: ICIDH-2, the international classification of impairments, activities, and participation. Geneva: World Health Organization; 1998.

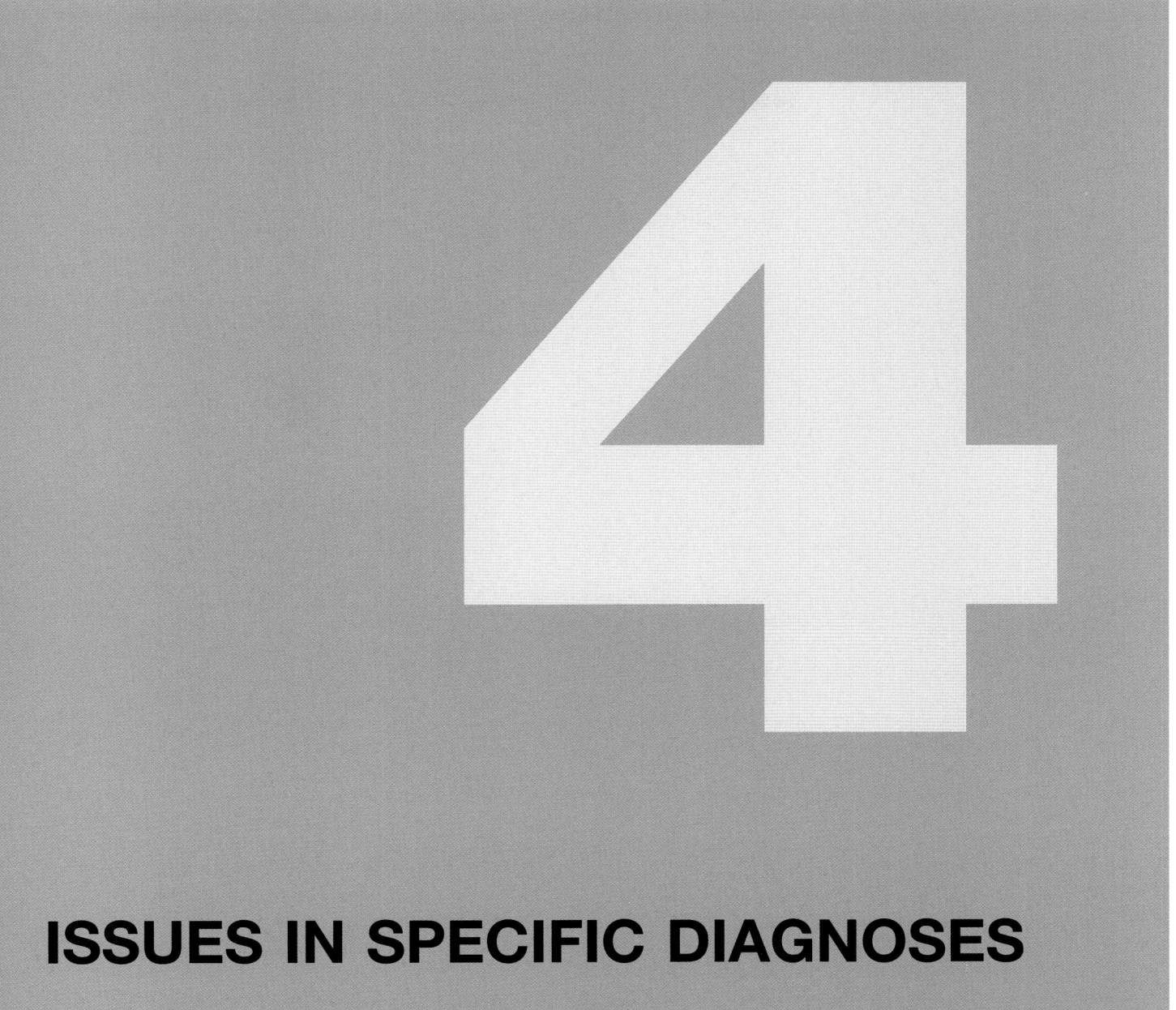

ISSUES IN SPECIFIC DIAGNOSES

Rehabilitation of Patients with Rheumatic Diseases
Jaime Guzman

The rheumatic diseases are more than 100 diverse disorders affecting the musculoskeletal system (Table 37-1).[100] Some of them are common (e.g. osteoarthritis, regional pain syndromes, fibromyalgia, osteoporosis, rheumatoid arthritis, and gout), and many of them are rare (e.g. connective tissue diseases and metabolic disorders of collagen).[100] In many countries, musculoskeletal symptoms and diseases are the most common cause of functional limitations in the adult population.[194] Osteoarthritis and regional pain syndromes (e.g. back pain and neck pain) account for the majority of the disease burden in the population.[16] It has been estimated that osteoarthritis is the eighth leading cause of disability in the world, and accounts for 2.8% of the total years of living with disability.[192] Rheumatoid arthritis affects 0.3–1% of the population in developed countries, and 10% of these patients have severe disability.[192]

This chapter focuses on those rheumatic diseases most likely to be seen by a physiatrist, in particular osteoarthritis and rheumatoid arthritis. Other common disorders, such as fibromyalgia, regional pain syndromes, and osteoporosis, are the subject of separate chapters in this textbook. Osteoarthritis and rheumatoid arthritis are chronic illnesses characterized by variable symptoms, and often take a progressive course.[6,7] There are no known cures, but a number of pharmacologic, surgical, and rehabilitative interventions are known to impact the course of these illnesses and improve the quality of life of people with rheumatic diseases.[121]

Rheumatoid arthritis, the seronegative spondyloarthropathies, and the connective tissue diseases (e.g. vasculitis and systemic lupus) are characterized by aberrant autoimmune responses leading to sustained inflammation and secondary change to tissues in and around the joints.[44] Many of them are actually systemic autoimmune disorders in which joint involvement is only one part of the disease. These disorders are characterized by inflammation, and it is clinically useful to distinguish disease activity from accumulated damage. Disease activity refers to the reversible manifestations of the inflammatory process. Accumulated damage refers to the relatively permanent sequelae of past inflammation and/or treatment side effects. In a patient with rheumatoid arthritis, for example, joint effusions and an elevated sedimentation rate are considered signs of disease activity, while ulnar deviation of the fingers and steroid-associated avascular necrosis of the hip are signs of accumulated damage. This distinction has important implica-

tions for management. Disease activity usually requires adjustment of antiinflammatory and immune-modulating drugs, while accumulated damage calls for surgical and rehabilitation interventions.[6,131]

The goal of this chapter is to describe the condition-specific concepts and principles a physiatrist needs to effectively organize and supervise the rehabilitation of patients with osteoarthritis, rheumatoid arthritis, and related conditions.

PRINCIPLES OF ANATOMY, PATHOPHYSIOLOGY, AND PHARMACOLOGY

Structure and function of the joints

The human body is composed of more than 200 joints with different shapes and functions. Some of these joints (e.g. the glenohumeral joint) allow large displacements in multiple planes, and some serve mostly as bone bridges and in the normal adult allow no movement. According to their anatomy and function, joints can be divided into diarthroses (synovial joints such as the glenohumeral joint), amphiarthroses (cartilaginous joints such as the intervertebral disks) (see Ch. 41), and synarthroses (fibrous, fixed joints such as the parieto-occipital joint).[100]

The typical synovial joint (e.g. the knee joint) consists of two reciprocally shaped bone articular surfaces covered by articular cartilage, a synovial membrane that maintains the joint lubricated by producing synovial fluid, a fibrous joint capsule and ligaments, sometimes periarticular bursa, and the tendons and muscles traversing across the joint (Fig. 37-1). The articular cartilage in synovial joints has a supporting structure of collagen fibers, within which abundant intercellular elastic matrix and some cells (chondrocytes) are contained (Fig. 37-1a).[76] The synovial membrane is composed of two main kinds of cells known as synoviocytes. Type A synovial cells are modified monocytes that produce immune mediators to protect the joint from infectious agents and other insults. Type B synovial cells are modified fibroblasts in charge of producing the intercellular matrix of the synovial membrane and the hyaluronic acid complexes that give the synovial fluid its distinctive viscosity (Fig. 37-1b).[76] The synovial membrane is enclosed by a fibrous capsule attached to the proximal and distal bone. The capsule is reinforced by ligaments, bundles of parallel collagenous fibers with a few embedded fibroblasts (Fig. 37-1c).[76]

Table 37-1 The main types of rheumatic diseases

Disease group and examples	Description
Degenerative and overuse syndromes Osteoarthritis Tendonitis Bursitis	Diseases in which the predominant feature is repetitive trauma and/or 'wear and tear' of cartilage or periarticular tissues, with minor secondary inflammation.
Inflammatory arthropathies Rheumatoid arthritis Psoriatic arthritis Spondylarthropathies	Diseases characterized by chronic or recurrent joint inflammation of unknown cause. Classified according to their pattern of joint involvement and associated features.
Extraarticular rheumatism Fibromyalgia Non-specific neck pain Non-specific back pain	Poorly understood disorders characterized by chronic or recurrent pain with no evidence of inflammation. Primary pathology may be in the perception of pain rather than in the soft tissues.
Connective tissue diseases Systemic lupus erythematosus Polymyositis or dermatomyositis Scleroderma Vasculitis	Autoimmune diseases of unknown etiology characterized by multisystem inflammation and damage.
Inherited disorders of connective tissue Collagenopathies Mucopolysaccharidosis Osteogenesis imperfecta Ehlers–Danlos syndrome	Rare diseases caused by genetic abnormalities affecting the synthesis of structural molecules of the bone and connective tissues.
Crystal-associated arthropathies Gout Calcium pyrophosphate crystals Hydroxyapatite crystals	Diseases characterized by acute or recurrent inflammation due to deposition of crystals in or around the joints.
Infectious arthropathies Viral Bacterial Tuberculosis and fungi	Diseases caused by invasion of joint tissues by microorganisms.
Postinfectious arthropathies Poststreptococcal Postchlamydia Postviral	Diseases triggered by previous exposure to infectious agents.

Periarticular bursae initially develop as herniations of synovial membrane through spaces in the fibrous capsule, and some of them eventually lose their connection with the articular space.[76] They allow for smooth movements of muscles and tendons over bone ridges. Muscles and their tendons are integral parts of the joint functional unit (Fig. 37-1d). They direct and control joint movement, and in some cases provide most of the stability to the joint (e.g. the rotator cuff is the main stabilization structure for the glenohumeral joint). Some tendons slide through extensive tendon sheaths, cuffs of synovial membrane with a few drops of synovial fluid that lubricate and smooth tendon movement (e.g. the extensor tendons of the fingers).[76]

Pathophysiology of inflammation and autoimmunity

Inflammation and autoimmunity play a key role in many rheumatic disorders. Many of the drugs used in rheumatic diseases target immune and inflammatory mediators. Figure 37-2 presents a simplified diagram of the key cells and mediators involved, as well as probable sites of action of commonly prescribed drugs.[44,131]

Lymphocytes are the masterminds behind most immune responses. There are two main types: T lymphocytes and B lymphocytes. T lymphocytes tightly regulate the nature and intensity of immune responses (cellular and humoral). B lymphocytes produce antibodies and other inflammatory mediators, and play an auxiliary role.[44] A subset of T lymphocytes are natural killer cells that eliminate neoplastic or transformed cells. T lymphocytes control the inflammatory response primarily by the production of cytokines. The Th1 cells produce interleukin (IL)-2 and interferon gamma, proinflammatory cytokines that favor a strong cell-mediated response. The Th2 cells produce IL-4, IL-6, and IL-10, which favor humoral or allergic responses and antibody production[38,44]

Monocytes, macrophages, and synovial fibroblasts are the main 'factories' of inflammatory mediators and the 'executors' of cytotoxic responses.[44] Circulating monocytes are directed to inflammatory sites by lymphocytes and humoral factors. In the tissues, the monocytes become resident macrophages and produce large amounts of IL-1, tumor necrosis factor-α, prostaglandins, leukotrienes, and other inflammatory vasoactive mediators.[104] Neutrophils are then recruited into the joint, and release elastase and proteases, which degrade articular cartilage.[44] The complement and coagulation cascade are important additional components of the inflammatory process.[14]

Drug therapy in rheumatic diseases

Many pharmacologic agents are used in the treatment of rheumatic diseases. These include nutraceuticals (food supplements), painkillers, non-steroidal antiinflammatory drugs (NSAIDs), glucocorticoids, disease-modifying antirheumatic drugs (DMARDs), cytotoxics, and biologics (Table 37-2).[131]

Multiple nutraceuticals are promoted for use in rheumatic diseases, but only two groups have been properly tested in humans. These include glucosamine and chondroitin formulations, and polyunsaturated oils. Several randomized trials suggest that glucosamine has an effect on pain in people with osteoarthritis, comparable with the effects of mild antiinflammatories.[113,124,129] Studies in Europe have also shown that glucosamine can retard the loss of articular cartilage in osteoarthritis as judged by x-rays.[138,149] Oils, particularly gamma-linolenic acid, have been shown to have a moderate antiinflammatory effect when consumed in relatively large quantities.[177,197]

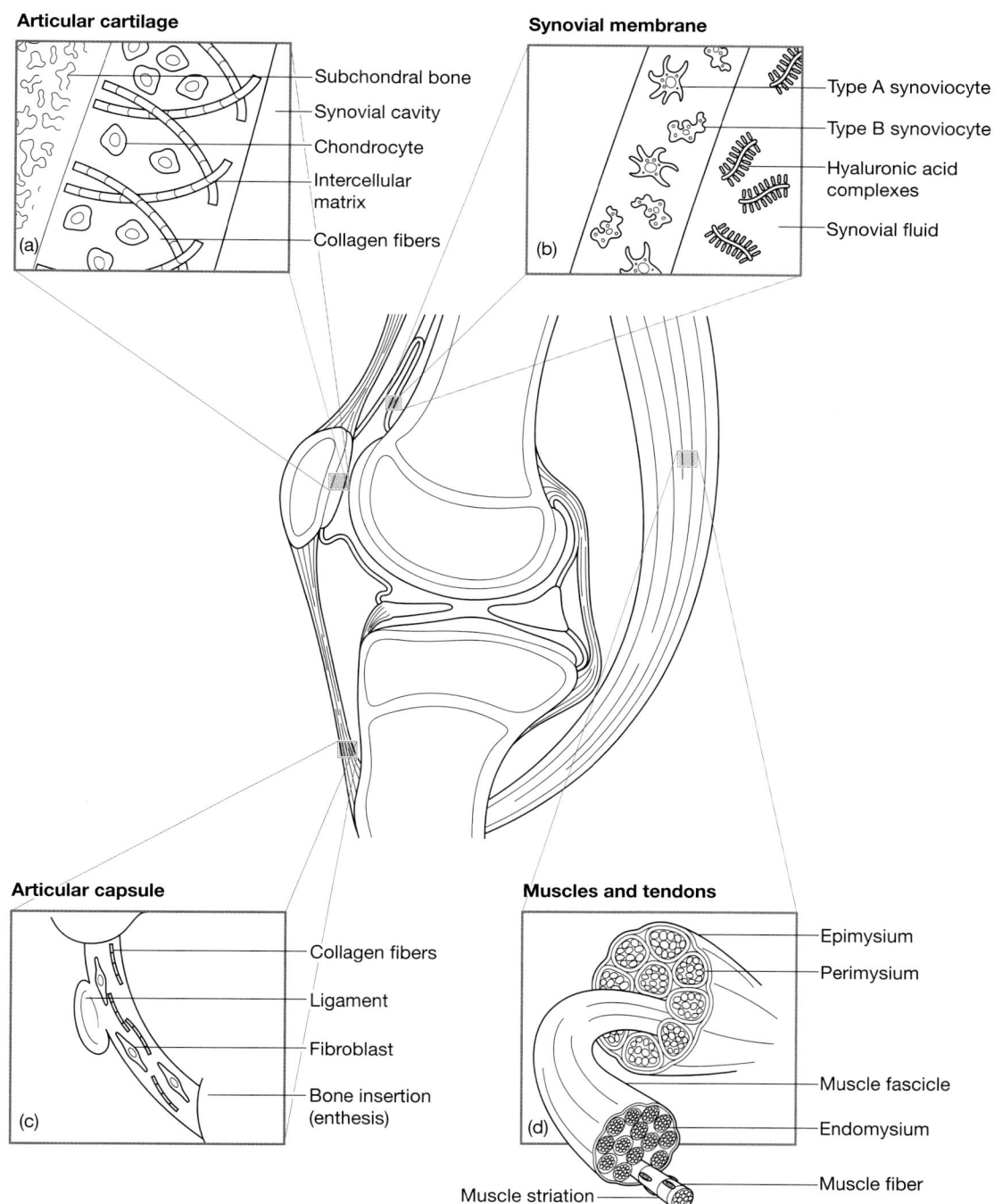

Figure 37-1 Structural components of synovial joints. A synovial joint consists of two reciprocally shaped bone surfaces covered by articular cartilage (**a**), a synovial membrane with type A and B synoviocytes that produce synovial fluid (**b**), a fibrous articular capsule reinforced by ligaments (**c**), and the tendons and muscles traversing across the joint (**d**).

Pain medications, including acetaminophen (paracetamol), tramadol, and opiates, are often used in the treatment of patients with rheumatic diseases.[6] Acetaminophen is the recommended first-line medication in osteoarthritis, and is often used as 'rescue' medication in patients on regular NSAIDs.[7] Codeine and oxycodone alone or in combination with acetaminophen are typically prescribed when NSAIDs and acetaminophen fail to provide adequate pain control.

The NSAIDs are the drugs most commonly prescribed for the management of rheumatic diseases.[131] They can be divided into two large groups: the traditional or non-selective NSAIDs and the selective cyclooxygenase (COX)-2 inhibitors (Table 37-2).[23] The COXs are essential enzymes in the synthesis of prostaglandins, key downstream mediators in the inflammatory cascade (Fig. 37-2).[23] The type 1 COX (COX-1) is expressed in many organs, including the gastric mucosa, platelets, and kidney.

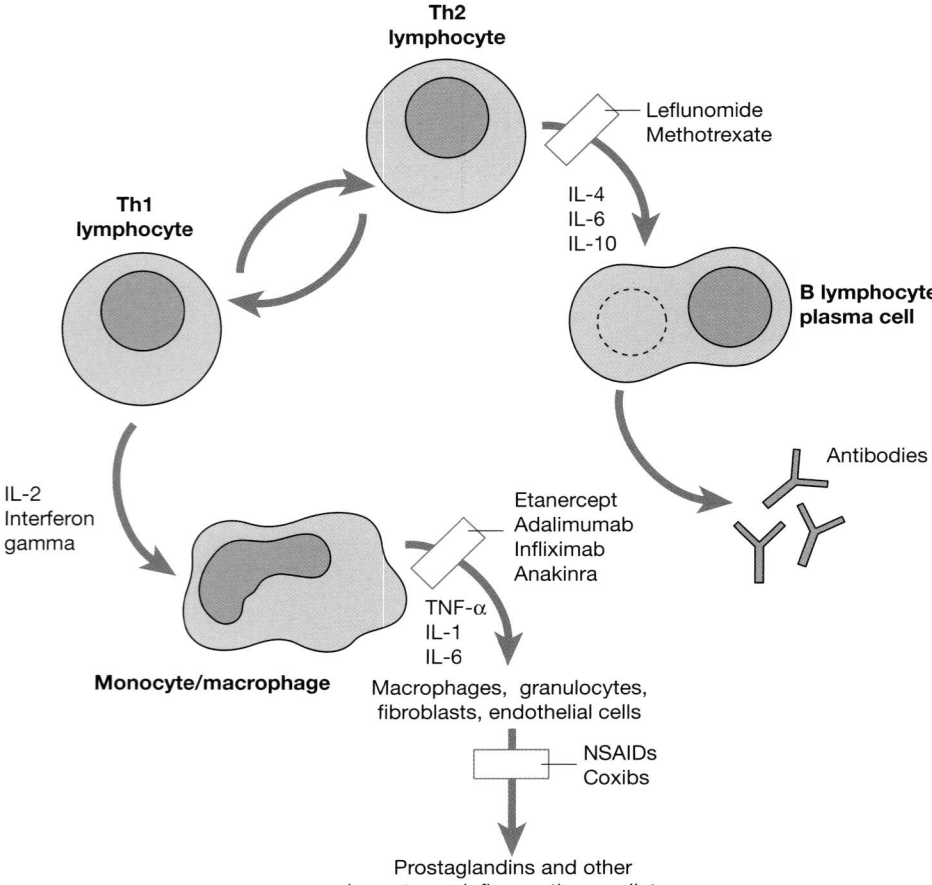

Figure 37-2 The main cells and mediators involved in autoimmune responses. Th1 and Th2 lymphocytes control immune responses by producing cytokines. The Th1 cells produce primarily interleukin (IL)-2 and interferon gamma, which stimulate monocytes and macrophages to produce the potent proinflammatory cytokines IL-1 and tumor necrosis factor-α. The Th2 cells produce primarily IL-4, IL-6 and IL-10, which stimulate B lymphocytes and plasma cells to produce autoantibodies. The proposed site of action of commonly used antirheumatic drugs is marked in the diagram. Coxib, COX-2 inhibitor; NSAID, non-steroidal antiinflammatory drug; TNF-α, tumor necrosis factor-α.

The type 2 COX (COX-2) is primarily induced during the inflammatory process but also plays a role in the kidney and during fetal development.[65]

The main advantage of selective COX-2 inhibitors over traditional NSAIDs is their decreased risk of gastrointestinal ulceration and bleeding.[27,158] They still share the same side effects in the kidney and cognition (fluid retention, increased blood pressure, difficulties with concentration, and occasional confusion).[131] Rofecoxib and valdecoxib, two of the main COX-2 inhibitors, were recalled from the market due to increased risk of myocardial infarction and other cardiovascular events.[31] Other COX-2 inhibitors probably share similar side effects to variable degrees.[130,165] It is possible that some traditional NSAIDS also have an increased risk of cardiovascular events.

Prednisone and other glucocorticoids are often used in the management of rheumatoid arthritis and connective tissue diseases.[131] Intraarticular and periarticular administration of methylprednisolone, triamcinolone, and other depot formulations is common practice in the treatment of osteoarthritis, rheumatoid arthritis, bursitis, and tendonitis. Controlled studies, however, exist only for a few indications.[10,36,117,163] The side effects of oral glucocorticoids are well known.[178] Usual doses in rheumatoid arthritis are between 2.5 and 7.5 mg of prednisone per day. Larger doses are occasionally used for short

time periods. In life-threatening connective tissue diseases, doses of up to 2 mg/kg of prednisone per day are required, and massive doses of intravenous methylprednisolone are occasionally used.[17]

The DMARDs are a heterogenous group of agents grouped together by their presumed effect in slowing permanent damage to the joints in rheumatoid arthritis.[131] Some cytotoxic drugs and newer biologic agents also have a disease-modifying effect. Methotrexate is the most often used DMARD, either alone or in combination.[134] It can be administered once or twice a week by mouth or intramuscularly in doses from 7.5 mg to 30 mg per week.[6,131] Leflunomide is another modern DMARD.[133] Of the older DMARDs, only hydroxychloroquine and sulfasalazine are still in regular use, with intramuscular gold, D-penicillamine, and auranofin used now only sporadically (Table 37-2).[164]

Cytotoxic medications such as azathioprine, cyclophosphamide, mycophenolate, and cyclosporine are primarily used in connective tissue diseases or for refractory cases of rheumatoid arthritis. These medications require close monitoring of blood counts and liver function, and the supervision of a physician experienced in their use (Table 37-2).[6,131]

Biologic agents are relatively new additions to the management of rheumatoid arthritis. They have been synthesized over the past two decades as a result of our advancing knowledge of

Table 37-2 Pharmacologic agents commonly used in the treatment of rheumatic diseases

Drug category	Typical indications and dosages	Precautions and contraindications
Nutraceuticals (Glucosamine, Fish oils, Chondroitin)	For osteoarthritis, glucosamine sulfate 1.5 g/day	Minimal known side effects. Oils can produce bloating and other gastrointestinal symptoms.
Non-steroidal antiinflammatory drugs (NSAIDs)	Ibuprofen 800–3200 mg/day in three or four doses Naproxen 500–1000 mg/day in two doses Diclofenac 50–150 mg/day in two or three doses	Gastrointestinal bleeding, dyspepsia, diarrhea, nausea, and vomiting. Skin reactions. Edema, acute renal insufficiency. Occasional cognitive side effects. Use with caution in patients with conditions that impair renal perfusion or function, and in the elderly. Check complete blood count (CBC), creatinine, and liver function tests at baseline and periodically if high risk.
Selective cyclooxygenase-2 inhibitors (coxibs)	Celecoxib 200–400 mg/day Rofecoxib recalled from the market in 2004 Valdecoxib recalled from the market in 2005	Less risk of gastrointestinal bleeding than with non-selective NSAIDs. Similar effects on kidney and cognition. Increased risk of cardiovascular events. Celecoxib should not be used in patients allergic to sulfonamides.
Glucocorticoids	In rheumatoid arthritis, prednisone or prednisolone 2.5–10 mg/day p.o. In severe lupus and other connective tissue diseases, up to 2 mg/kg per day. Methylprednisolone 10–80 mg for intraarticular or periarticular injection, or triamcinolone hexacetonide 5–20 mg. Methylprednisolone pulses in life-threatening disease 1 g i.v. daily for 1–3 days.	Oral agents: dose-dependent puffing or round face, increase in facial hair, weight gain, osteoporosis, gastrointestinal ulcers and bleeding, depression, insomnia, lowered resistance to infection. Intraarticular injections have a low risk of infection or bleeding. Can produce brief postinjection flare, local skin pigmentation or atrophy. Intratendon injection contraindicated because of risk of tendon rupture.
Synthetic disease-modifying antirheumatic drugs (DMARDs)	Hydroxychloroquine 200–400 mg p.o. q.d. Sulfasalazine 500–2000 mg/day Methotrexate 7.5–30 mg p.o. or i.m. once weekly Leflunomide loading dose of 100 mg p.o. o.d. for 3 days, then 20 mg p.o. o.d.	Risk of macular degeneration. Monitor visual changes, yearly fundoscopy and visual fields. Risk of neutropenia and myelosuppression. Monitor CBC. Consider glucose-6-phosphate dehydrogenase and alanine aminotransferase (ALT) for patients at risk. Risk of mouth ulcers, myelosuppression, hepatic fibrosis, pneumonitis. Monitor CBC, ALT, albumin every 4–8 weeks. Risk of diarrhea, weight loss, myelosuppression, and hepatic fibrosis. Monitor CBC, ALT, albumin every 4–8 weeks
Biologic DMARDs	Etanercept 25 mg s.c. twice weekly or 50 mg s.c. once weekly Infliximab 3 mg/kg i.v. at 0, 2, and 6 weeks, then every 8 weeks Adalimumab 40 mg s.c. every second week Anakinra 100 mg s.c. o.d.	For etanercept, infliximab, and adalimumab, risk of infections. Screen for tuberculosis at baseline. Monitor for symptoms of congestive heart failure or demyelinating disease. Discontinue during active infections. Risk of infections, pneumonia, neutropenia. Screen for asthma. Monitor CBC monthly for months, then every 3 months. Discontinue during active infections.
Cytotoxics	For connective tissue diseases or severe rheumatoid arthritis Azathioprine 1–3 mg/kg p.o. o.d. Cyclosporine 2–4 mg/kg per day p.o. divided b.i.d. Cyclophosphamide 1–3 mg/kg p.o. o.d.	Risk of myelosuppression, infections. Monitor CBC, creatinine, ALT at baseline, then CBC every 2 weeks until dose stable, then every 3 months. Risk of renal insufficiency, anemia, and hypertension. Monitor CBC, creatinine, blood pressure. Risk of hemorrhagic cystitis, infections, myelosuppression, sterility, malignancy. Monitor CBC, urinalysis.

(After American College of Rheumatology 2002,[6] O'Dell 2004,[131] and Olsen and Stein 2004,[133] with permission.)

inflammatory mediators.[133] Many are also used in non-rheumatic autoimmune conditions such as inflammatory bowel disease.[143] The biologic agents currently in use for rheumatoid arthritis target two cytokines: tumor necrosis factor-α and IL-1 (Fig. 37-2). Tumor necrosis factor-α is produced by lymphocytes and macrophages, and induces macrophages, fibroblasts, and endothelial cells to produce a large number of proinflammatory substances.[44] Its action is blocked by etanercept, infliximab, and adalimumab. IL-1 plays a synergistic role to tumor necrosis factor-α and is the target for anakinra.[137]

All these biologic agents are complex proteins and have to be administered subcutaneously (etanercept, adalimumab, and anakinra) or intravenously (infliximab). Their effects are remarkable and fast, often superior to those of methotrexate. Some of them are used primarily in combination with methotrexate, when methotrexate alone fails to achieve a satisfactory response.[133] Some of these biologic agents are also effective in psoriatic arthritis, spondyloarthropathies, and childhood arthritis.[40,109,115] At present, their high cost limits their widespread use.

A large number of other pharmacologic agents are used in the treatment of people with rheumatic diseases. These include tricyclic antidepressants, muscle relaxants, antacids, and gastroprotective agents.[6]

Classification and nosology of rheumatic diseases

Over a 100 rheumatic diseases have been described in the medical literature. As our knowledge of pathophysiology evolves, older syndromes are subdivided into new diseases (Table 37-1). For example, at the end of the nineteenth century, rheumatoid arthritis, gout, and joint manifestations of tuberculosis were grouped together. By the mid twentieth century, they were recognized to be separate disorders. In the second half of the twentieth century, formal ways of separating the rheumatic diseases were established, often in the form of classification or diagnostic criteria.[100] These criteria have been instrumental in facilitating research and clinical practice, because there are seldom pathognomonic findings or laboratory tests that would establish a diagnosis by themselves. Additional criteria have been established for remission, improvement, and outcome measurement in rheumatoid arthritis[29,183] and systemic lupus erythematosus.[27,73]

For many rheumatic diseases, there have historically been two sets of criteria that were supported by the American College of Rheumatology (previously the American Rheumatology Association, http://www.rheumatology.org) or the European League Against Rheumatism. Recent efforts have focused on agreement on unique sets of criteria.[141] This section reviews current classification and response criteria for the most common rheumatic conditions. Outcome measures are reviewed in the following section on evaluation in rheumatic diseases.[98]

Box 37-1 lists criteria for osteoarthritis. Although different sets are applicable to hands, hips, and knees, most require a combination of symptoms (pain and stiffness) and radiologic findings (decreased joint space and osteophytes).[3-5] Table 37-3

Box 37-1 The American College of Rheumatology criteria for the classification of osteoarthritis of the hand, hip and knee

Classification criteria for osteoarthritis of the hand, traditional format[a]

Hand pain, aching, or stiffness, and three or four of the following features.

- Hard tissue enlargement of two or more of 10 selected joints[b]
- Hard tissue enlargement of two or more distal interphalangeal (DIP) joints
- Fewer than three swollen metacarpophalangeal (MCP) joints
- Deformity of at least one of 10 selected joints[b]

Classification criteria for osteoarthritis of the hip, traditional format[c]

Hip pain and at least two of the following three features.

- Erythrocyte sedimentation rate (ESR) (Westergren) < 29 mm/h
- Radiographic femoral or acetabular osteophytes
- Radiographic joint space narrowing (superior, axial, and/or medial)

Criteria for classification of idiopathic osteoarthritis of the knee

Clinical and laboratory

Knee pain plus at least five of the nine following (92% sensitive, 75% specific).

- Age >50 years
- Stiffness <30 min
- Crepitus
- Bony tenderness
- Bony enlargement
- No palpable warmth
- ESR (Westergren) <40 mm/h
- Rheumatoid factor <1:40
- Synovial fluid signs of osteoarthritis (clear, viscous, or white blood cell count <2000/mm[3])

Clinical and radiographic

Knee pain plus at least one of the three following (91% sensitive, 86% specific).

- Age >50 years
- Stiffness <30 min
- Crepitus plus osteophytes

Clinical[d]

Knee pain plus at least three of the six following (95% sensitive, 69% specific).

- Age > 50 years
- Stiffness < 30 min
- Crepitus
- Bony tenderness
- Bony enlargement
- No palpable warmth

[a]This classification method yields a sensitivity of 95% and a specificity of 87%.
[b]The 10 selected joints are the second and third DIP, the second and third proximal interphalangeal, and the first carpometacarpal joints of both hands.
[c]This classification method yields a sensitivity of 89% and a specificity of 91%.
[d]An alternative for the clinical category would be four of six, which is 84% sensitive and 89% specific.
(From Altman et al. 1986,[3] 1990,[4] and 1991,[5] with permission of the American College of Rheumatology.)

Table 37-3 The American College of Rheumatology criteria for the classification of rheumatoid arthritis[a]

Criterion	Definition
1. Morning stiffness	Morning stiffness in and around the joints, lasting at least 1 h before maximal improvement.
2. Arthritis of three or more joint areas	At least three joint areas simultaneously have had soft tissue swelling or fluid (not bony overgrowth alone) observed by a physician. The 14 possible areas are right or left proximal interphalangeal (PIP), metacarpophalangeal (MCP), wrist, elbow, knee, ankle, and metatarsophalangeal (MTP) joints.
3. Arthritis of hand joints	At least one area swollen (as defined above) in a wrist, MCP, or PIP joint.
4. Symmetric arthritis	Simultaneous involvement of the same joint areas (as defined in criterion 2) on both sides of the body (bilateral involvement of PIPs, MCPs, or MTPs is acceptable without absolute symmetry).
5. Rheumatoid nodules	Subcutaneous nodules, over bony prominences, or extensor surfaces, or in juxtaarticular regions, observed by a physician.
6. Serum rheumatoid factor	Demonstration of abnormal amounts of serum rheumatoid factor by any method for which the result has been positive in < 5% of normal control subjects.
7. Radiographic changes	Radiographic changes typical of rheumatoid arthritis on posteroanterior hand and wrist radiographs, which must include erosion or unequivocal bony decalcification localized in or most marked adjacent to the involved joints (osteoarthritis changes alone do not qualify).

[a]For classification purposes, patients shall be said to have rheumatoid arthritis if they have satisfied at least four of these seven criteria. Criteria 1 through 4 must have been present for at least 6 weeks. Patients with two clinical diagnoses are not excluded. Designation as classic, definite, or probable rheumatoid arthritis is not to be made.
(From Arnett et al. 1988,[9] with permission of the American College of Rheumatology.)

presents the 1987 revised criteria for the classification of rheumatic arthritis. The diagnosis requires that four out of seven criteria have to be present for at least 6 weeks.[9] It is clear from this classification that the rheumatoid factor test is not essential for establishing the presence of the disease. The overall picture and constellation of findings are of the most significance.[9] Table 37-4 presents criteria for the classification of systemic lupus erythematosus (last revised in 1997). Four out of 11 criteria have to be present at any time for a patient to be classified as suffering from systemic lupus.[60,140] An antinuclear antibody test, although often positive, is not by itself sufficient, because patients with rheumatoid arthritis and other autoimmune conditions often test positive as well.

The response criteria for rheumatoid arthritis are described in Table 37-5.[61,183] It is now standard practice to report results of clinical trials of new medications using these or similar criteria. Classification or diagnostic criteria exist for many other rheumatic diseases. They can be found in rheumatology textbooks and on the web sites of professional organizations.[100]

PRINCIPLES OF EVALUATION IN RHEUMATIC DISEASE

A successful rehabilitation program for a patient with a rheumatic disease starts with an appropriate evaluation.[121] The general principles of physiatric evaluation are discussed in Chapter 1, and only issues of special application in rheumatic diseases are reviewed here. There are many informal and formal ways to evaluate patients with osteoarthritis and rheumatoid arthritis. A large number of reliable, valid evaluation instruments and techniques have been developed, tested, and translated into several languages.[41,77,152,190]

The International Classification of Functioning, Disability and Health (ICF)[193] provides a good framework to conduct the rehabilitation evaluation of these diseases, and is used here to group commonly used evaluation strategies (Fig. 37-3). Many standard multiitem evaluation instruments were developed before the ICF, and their correspondence to ICF domains is often partial. Each is listed under the domain relevant to most items in the instrument.[172,173]

The initial evaluation seeks to describe the current state (disorder, impairments, activities, and participation), and the environmental and personal factors that can be modified to improve the current state (Table 37-6).[82,113] Subsequent evaluation is used to assess the impact of rehabilitation programs and adjust them accordingly. The detail provided in the evaluation depends on whether the physician is working individually or as part of a rehabilitation team. Working in an interdisciplinary team is ideal, as it facilitates more in-depth formal evaluation and provides different disciplinary perspectives.[184]

Disease and comorbidities

To begin the evaluation, it is important to define the rheumatic disease and associated comorbid conditions. There are significant differences in the pathophysiology and prognosis across the multiple rheumatic diseases (Table 37-1). Current information regarding the diagnosis is important, because inflammatory

Table 37-4 The American College of Rheumatology criteria for the classification of systemic lupus erythematosus[a]

Criterion	Definition
1. Malar rash	Fixed erythema, flat or raised, over the malar eminences, tending to spare the nasolabial folds.
2. Discoid rash	Erythematous raised patches with adherent keratotic scaling and follicular plugging; atrophic scarring may occur in older lesions.
3. Photosensitivity	Skin rash as a result of unusual reaction to sunlight, by patient history or physician observation.
4. Oral ulcers	Oral or nasopharyngeal ulceration, usually painless, observed by a physician.
5. Arthritis	Non-erosive arthritis involving two or more peripheral joints, characterized by tenderness, swelling, or effusion.
6. Serositis	Pleuritis—convincing history of pleuritic pain or rub heard by a physician or evidence of pleural effusion *or* pericarditis—documented by electrocardiogram or rub, or evidence of pericardial effusion.
7. Renal disorder	Persistent proteinuria greater than 0.5 g/day or greater than 3+ if quantitation not performed *or* cellular casts—may be red cell, hemoglobin, granular, tubular, or mixed.
8. Neurologic disorder	Seizures—in the absence of offending drugs or known metabolic derangements (e.g. uremia, ketoacidosis, or electrolyte imbalance) *or* psychosis—in the absence of offending drugs or known metabolic derangements (e.g. uremia, ketoacidosis, or electrolyte imbalance).
9. Hematologic disorder	Hemolytic anemia—with reticulocytosis *or* leukopenia—less than 4000/mm^3 total on two or more occasions *or* lymphopenia—less than 1550/mm^3 on two or more occasions *or* thrombocytopenia—less than 100 000/mm^3 in the absence of offending drugs.
10. Immunologic disorder	Positive lupus erythematosus cell preparation *or* anti-DNA—antibody to native DNA in abnormal titer *or* anti-Sm—presence of antibody to Sm nuclear antigen *or* false positive serologic test for syphilis known to be positive for at least 6 months and confirmed by *Treponema pallidum* immobilization or fluorescent treponemal antibody absorption test.
11. Antinuclear antibody	An abnormal titer of antinuclear antibody by immunofluorescence or an equivalent assay at any point in time and in the absence of drugs known to be associated with 'drug-induced lupus' syndrome.

[a]The *proposed classification* is based on 11 criteria. For the purpose of identifying patients in clinical studies, a person shall be said to have systemic lupus erythematosus if any four or more of the 11 criteria are present, serially or simultaneously, during any interval of observations. (Reprinted from Tan et al. 1982,[176] with permission of the American College of Rheumatology.)

rheumatic diseases evolve over time. A more specific diagnosis can often be established later in the course of the illness. Osteoarthritis and rheumatoid arthritis tend to affect people of middle or advanced age, who often also have comorbidities that require adjustments to the rehabilitation program. It is important to list those comorbidities and the main impairments associated with them (e.g. diabetes with peripheral neuropathy).

Impairments

As noted earlier, it is important to differentiate disease activity from accumulated damage.[6,131] This distinction is needed to tailor the rehabilitation program appropriately, and it also has implications for the overall treatment of the patient. Articular impairments are commonly described by listing and counting the tender, swollen, and deformed joints.[105] This is complemented by measurement of range of joint movement and muscle strength testing (see Ch. 1). The findings are often reported in a listing of joints or on an articular homunculus (Fig. 37-4). Measurement of grip strength by dynamometer or adapted sphygmomanometer is a useful tool in patients with rheumatoid arthritis.[56] X-ray examination usually complements the physical examination. Radiologic changes can be quantified by use of scales, such as Sharp scores, to document severity and assist in long-term follow-up.[84,157]

Activities

Both disease activity and accumulated joint damage can impact the activity level of a person with arthritis. Limitations in reach-

Table 37-5 The American College of Rheumatology preliminary definition of improvement in rheumatoid arthritis

Improvement	Criterion
ACR 20	A 20% improvement in tender and swollen joint counts and 20% improvement in three of the five remaining ACR core set measures: patient and physician global assessments, pain, disability, and an acute-phase reactant.
ACR 50	A 50% improvement in tender and swollen joint counts and 50% improvement in three of the five remaining ACR core set measures: patient and physician global assessments, pain, disability, and an acute-phase reactant.
ACR 70	A 70% improvement in tender and swollen joint counts and 70% improvement in three of the five remaining ACR core set measures: patient and physician global assessments, pain, disability, and an acute-phase reactant.

(From Felson et al. 1993,[61] with permission of the American College of Rheumatology.)

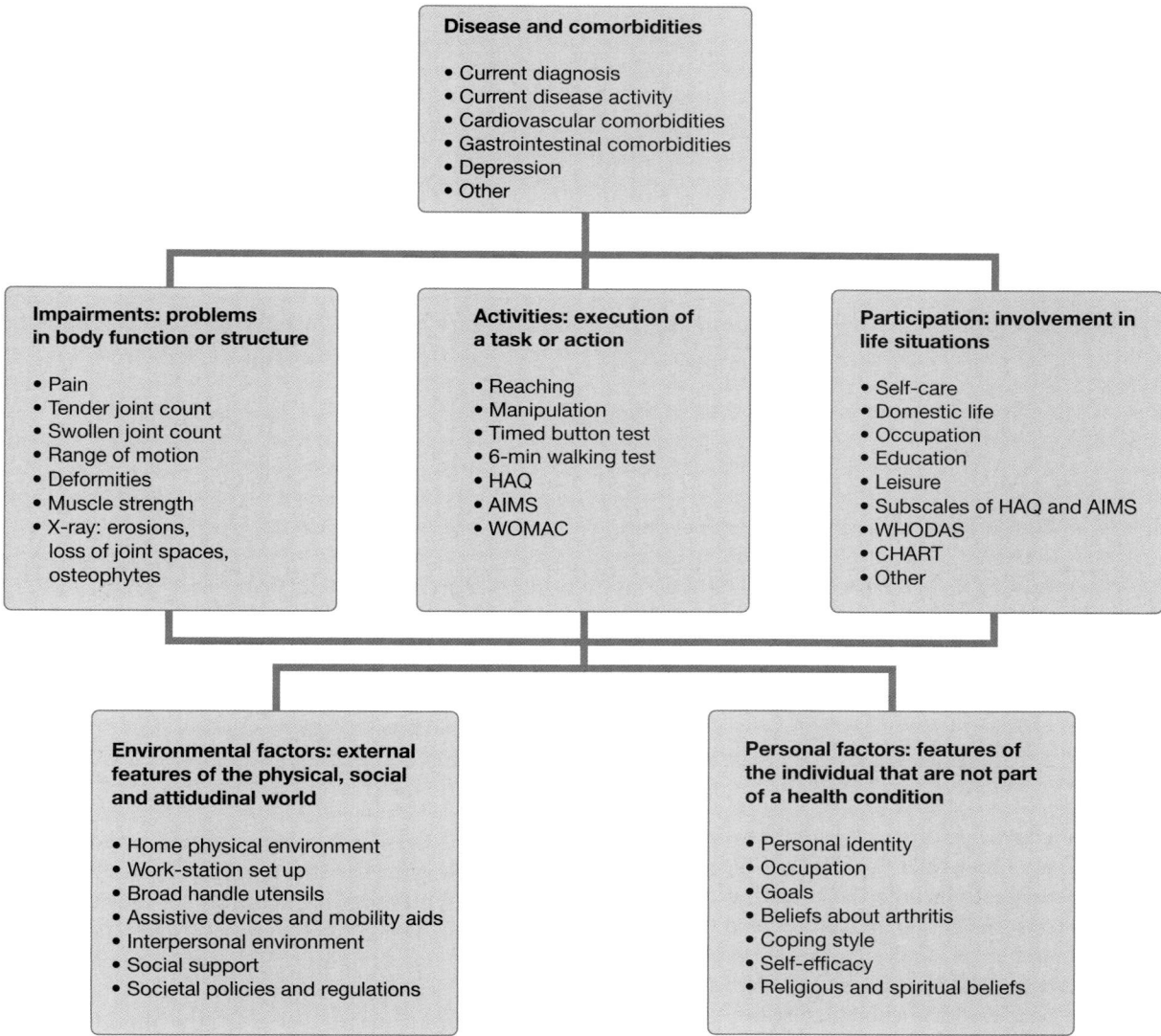

Figure 37-3 Key components of the rehabilitation evaluation of patients with rheumatic diseases. The International Classification of Functioning, Disability and Health provides a good framework to conduct the evaluation by defining six domains of interest: rheumatic disease and comorbidities, impairments, activities, participation, environmental factors, and personal factors. AIMS, Arthritis Impact Measurement Scales; CHART, Craig Handicap Assessment Reporting Technique; HAQ, Health Assessment Questionnaire; WHO DAS, World Health Organization Disability Assessment Schedule; WOMAC, Western Ontario–McMaster Questionnaire.

Table 37-6 Informal and formal methods for the rehabilitation evaluation of patients with rheumatic diseases

Domain	Informal evaluation	Formal evaluation
Impairments	Listing of joints that were tender, swollen, or deformed Manual muscle strength testing	Tender joint count Swollen joint count Deformed joint count Measurement of active and passive range of motion Measurement of grip strength Measurement of muscle strength with dynamometer
Activities	• Do you have any difficulty in reaching, lifting, or handling objects? • Do you have any difficulty in walking? • Do you have any difficulty going up or down stairs?	Health Assessment Questionnaire (HAQ) physical function scale Arthritis Impact Measurement Scales (AIMS) function subscale Western Ontario and McMaster Osteoarthritis Index Timed button test 6-min walking test Get up and go test
Participation	• Please tell me what you do in a normal day, from the time you get up until you go to bed. • Do you have any difficulties at work? • Do you have any difficulty with your house chores? • Do you have any difficulty with leisure or sports?	HAQ subscales AIMS subscales 36-Item Short-Form Health Survey (partially) Craig Handicap Assessment Reporting Technique Canadian Occupational Performance Measure World Health Organization Disability Assessment Schedule Work Limitations Questionnaire
Environmental factors	• Do you have stairs at home? • Is the bathroom easily accessible to you? • Has your home been changed to make it easier for you to go around? • Do you use any aids to grasp objects or move around? • Is your workplace easily accessible? • Who lives with you? • Who do you work with? • Who helps you keep involved at home and at work?	Structured home and workplace visits Physical barriers inventories Social Support Questionnaires
Personal factors	• What would you like to achieve with your rehabilitation? • What do you think caused your arthritis? • What do you think is going to happen with your arthritis? • What do you do to help you cope with your arthritis	Canadian Occupational Performance Measure (elicits patient's goals) Self-efficacy questionnaire Learned helplessness questionnaire Coping strategies questionnaires Beck Depression Inventory Fear avoidance beliefs questionnaire

ing, manipulation, and ambulation are often seen. Activity limitations can be assessed by observation or by self-report. Observer-administered instruments include the timed button test and similar dexterity tests, the get up and go test, and the 6-min walking test.[56] A number of condition-specific instruments have been developed that allow a reliable standardized assessment of activities in people with rheumatic disease.[190]

The Health Assessment Questionnaire (HAQ) was originally developed as a comprehensive tool for assessment of rheumatoid arthritis,[35] but has since been shown to be valuable in the assessment of childhood arthritis[144,159] and other rheumatic conditions. The shortened HAQ physical function scale includes

eight items used in assessing the degree of difficulty in activities, primarily involving the upper extremities. Scores vary from 0 to 3, with higher scores implying more severe activity limitations.[35] The HAQ has been shown to predict subsequent functional status, morbidity, mortality, and healthcare utilization.[35]

The Arthritis Impact Measurement Scales (AIMS) are a comprehensive set of questionnaires that assess the impact of rheumatic disease (primarily rheumatoid arthritis) on patients. It includes subscales for physical function, symptoms, affect, social interaction, and social roles.[118]

The Western Ontario–McMaster Questionnaire (WOMAC) is an instrument designed to assess symptoms and activity limi-

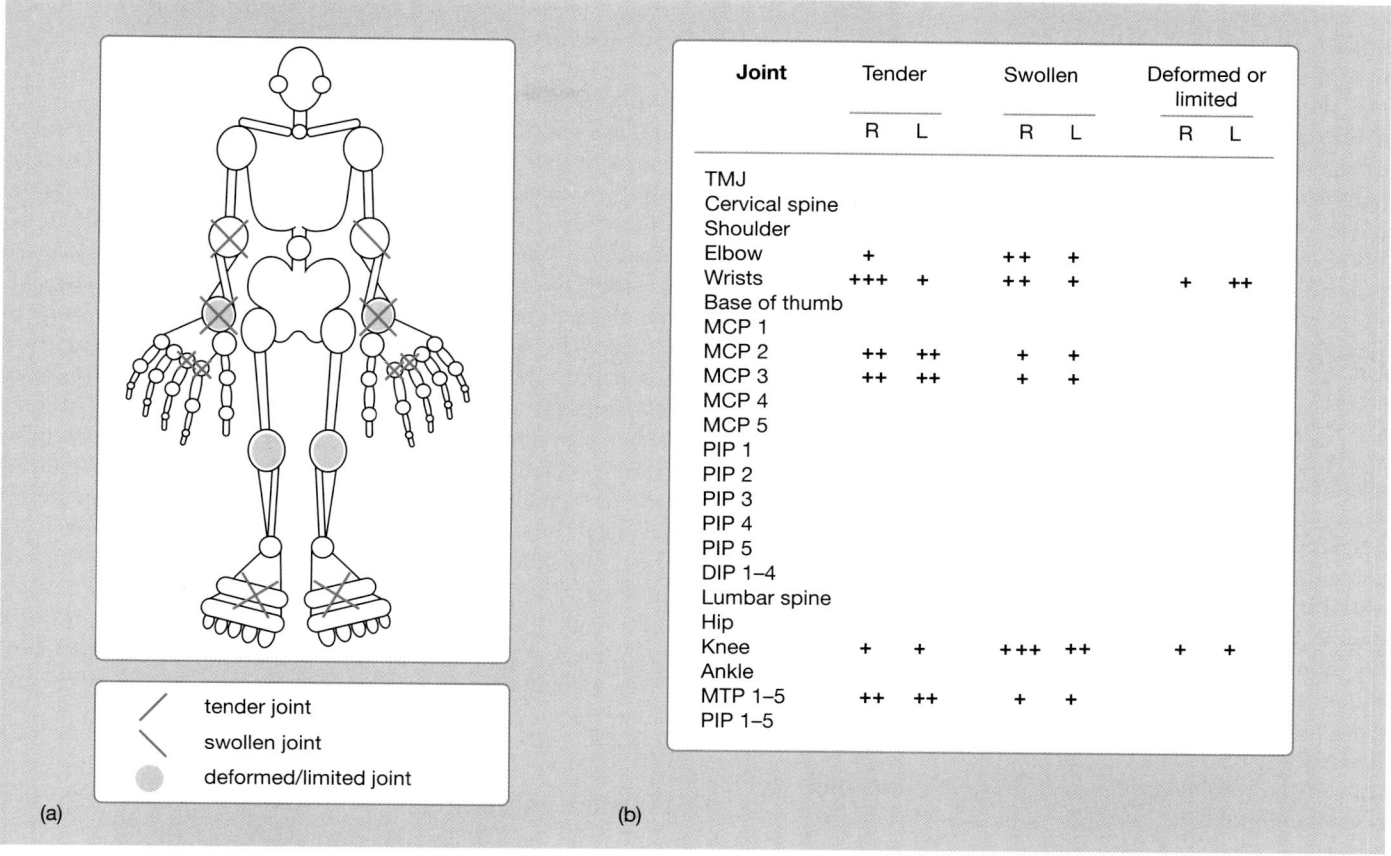

Joint	Tender		Swollen		Deformed or limited	
	R	L	R	L	R	L
TMJ						
Cervical spine						
Shoulder						
Elbow	+		++	+		
Wrists	+++	+	++	+	+	++
Base of thumb						
MCP 1						
MCP 2	++	++	+	+		
MCP 3	++	++	+	+		
MCP 4						
MCP 5						
PIP 1						
PIP 2						
PIP 3						
PIP 4						
PIP 5						
DIP 1–4						
Lumbar spine						
Hip						
Knee	+	+	+++	++	+	+
Ankle						
MTP 1–5	++	++	+	+		
PIP 1–5						

Legend:

/ tender joint

\ swollen joint

● deformed/limited joint

(a)   (b)

Figure 37-4 Documentation of joint impairments. Joint tenderness, swelling, and deformities and limitations of movement are the main impairments in osteoarthritis and rheumatoid arthritis. These can be documented by markings on an articular homunculus (**a**) or in a listing of joints (**b**). DIP, distal interphalangeal; MCP, metacarpophalangeal; MTP, metatarsophalangeal; PIP, proximal interphalangeal; TMJ, temporomandibular.

tations associated with osteoarthritis of the knee and hip.[21,57] It assesses pain, stiffness, and physical limitations, and focuses on ambulation. The WOMAC has proven to be both a reliable and a responsive instrument. It is commonly used in trials of pharmaceutical, surgical, and rehabilitative interventions.

Many more standard questionnaires exist to assist in the evaluation of patients with rheumatic disease, and they have been recently summarized in a monograph.[98]

Participation

The ICF does not provide a single method of separating activities from participation. For the purpose of this chapter, participation includes self-care; domestic life; interpersonal relationships; major life areas (education, work, and economic life); and community, social, and civic life.[193] A simple way of exploring participation during a routine consultation is to enquire about the patient's use of time during a typical day. Both the HAQ and the AIMS questionnaires include subscales that assess participation dimensions in people with arthritis, although they are not as commonly used as the physical function subscales.[35,118]

It should be noted that well-established instruments for assessment of instrumental activities of daily living and assess-

ment of handicap in non-rheumatic conditions, such as the Craig Handicap Assessment Reporting Technique,[185] are easily applicable and helpful in people with rheumatic conditions.[139] More recently, the World Health Organization proposed the Disability Assessment Schedule as a unified, simple way to assess activities and participation across conditions.[180] Rheumatic conditions have a major impact on occupational participation, especially in unemployment and decreased productivity. A number of assessment instruments are being developed to quantify this impact.[15]

Environmental factors

A description of the physical, interpersonal, and societal environment and current environmental adaptations is essential in people with rheumatic conditions, as it is in any person undergoing a rehabilitation assessment.[153] Modifications of the physical environment at home and at work focus on removing obstacles (for reaching and manipulating objects and for ambulation). This can be accomplished by appropriate placement of commonly used objects and use of broad handle utensils and easy to handle doorknobs.

At an interpersonal level, it is important to ask the patient who is aware of their condition and what emotional and material support has been provided.[127] At a societal level, it is important to enquire about the resources and programs the individual has accessed to facilitate activities and participation. Has the person been in contact with patient associations? Has he or she participated in self-help groups? Is the patient aware of the resources of the Arthritis Foundation and its counterparts in other countries?[11,12] A number of standardized instruments exist that assess social support at home and at work.[188] These instruments can be integrated into the rehabilitation assessment.

Personal factors and goals

An assessment of the goals, beliefs, and fears about arthritis is required when designing a rehabilitation program to help improve the function and quality of life of a person living with rheumatic disease.[101,174] Personal characteristics shown to impact prognosis include self-efficacy, coping style, and learned helplessness.[2,148] A number of instruments exist that assess these dimensions and have been extensively validated in people with rheumatic disease.[98] Depressive symptoms are common in people with rheumatic diseases. These symptoms can have a major impact on quality of life, and in the response to rehabilitation interventions.

As in other areas of physiatry, the evaluation of the patient with rheumatic disease concludes with negotiation of the objectives of the rehabilitation program by both the patient and the rehabilitation team.

REHABILITATION INTERVENTIONS OFTEN USED IN RHEUMATIC DISEASES

Many rehabilitation interventions have been recommended for patients with rheumatic disease.[46] This section presents an overview of indications and contraindications of the most common rehabilitation interventions used in patients with rheumatic disease.

Education and self-management

Education and self-management are widely regarded as being fundamental to the comprehensive management of rheumatic diseases, in particular rheumatoid arthritis.[26,28] Patient associations in North America have been instrumental in developing and making available multiple resources.[11,12] Self-management training can be provided by other patients or by healthcare providers. The programs provided by peers have been extensively studied and shown to improve pain, function, self-efficacy, and satisfaction.[86] They can reduce visits to healthcare providers and associated costs. Programs provided by care providers have been less studied but appear to provide similar benefits.[86]

The programs with the best results focus on active learning in peer groups, with an emphasis on problem solving and increasing self-efficacy.[107] They also include information on the nature and prognosis of arthritis; efficacy and side effects of

arthritis medications; and exercise, pacing, and other rehabilitation interventions.[70]

Exercise, rest, and energy conservation

Exercise and exercise-based rehabilitation programs are interventions well supported in controlled trials.[8,79,99] Exercise improves range of motion, strength, and functional activities in osteoarthritis, rheumatoid arthritis, and extraarticular rheumatism.[67,78,79,90,112,169] The exercise program must be individualized according to the disease activity, accumulated joint damage, and the patient's goals and interests.[13,95] The mechanisms of action of therapeutic exercise and its prescription are described in Chapter 19. In general terms, high-impact exercises such as jumping, basketball, etc. should be avoided in patients with significant rheumatic disease.[64] Medium-impact exercises such as walking, jogging, bicycling, and swimming are appropriate, unless there is severe joint inflammation.[96] Severely inflamed joints should only be subjected to gentle mobilization and stretching within the available range of movement.[64]

Strategies for joint protection, energy conservation, and pacing are frequently recommended by occupational therapists. Often, patients develop their own strategies for energy conservation. However, there is limited evidence of efficacy in this regard.[170,171]

Physical modalities

Heat, cold, and other physical modalities have been used to treat rheumatic conditions for centuries.[68,128] Most of these modalities have been accepted by tradition, and only recently have been subjected to controlled trials.[34,66,119,123,150] Local heat can decrease pain, at least temporarily, and can be easily applied by patients or family members if precautions to avoid burns are taken.[120] There is a theoretic possibility that local heat can increase the inflammatory response and possibly increase joint damage, but this has not been supported empirically.[19] The usual contraindications to local heat application apply (see Ch. 21).[19] Local heat can be applied by conduction (heat pads and water bottles), radiation (incandescent lamps and infrared lamps), or immersion (hot water, paraffin baths, and mud baths).[120] There is no solid evidence that one method is preferable to another, and the choice depends on availability and the body part to be treated.[33] For example, paraffin baths are ideally suited to apply heat to the rheumatic hand.[69] Cold and contrast baths (heat alternating with cold) have been described, but there are no adequate studies to support their utility in rheumatic disease.[150] In the absence of conclusive scientific evidence, the patient's comfort and preferences should take precedence.

Ultrasound and diathermy mostly function as conversion methods of applying heat to the deeper tissues, although there might be additional mechanisms at play.[120] Recent studies have reported the use of shock waves to treat tendonitis and fasciitis, but rigorous randomized trials have questioned their efficacy.[36,72] Interferential currents have little application for treating joint disease,[186] but functional electrical stimulation is sometimes used to prevent muscle atrophy during episodes of intense disease activity (see Ch. 22). Transcutaneous electrical nerve stimulation might relieve the pain of rheumatic disease,[33] and animal studies suggest it can also decrease joint swelling.[120,162] Electromagnetic fields have established efficacy in accelerating fracture healing,[1] and available trials suggest some benefit in knee osteoarthritis.[88] Low-power laser has been poorly studied but might provide short-term relief of pain and stiffness.

Manual and mechanical therapies

Manual therapies have been extensively used to treat regional musculoskeletal pain and extraarticular rheumatism.[43,93,181] They are seldom prescribed in rheumatoid arthritis or severe osteoarthritis, because they are typically considered to be alternative or integrative therapies.[69,187] Nevertheless, many patients make use of them outside the medical establishment.[145,146] Traction is sometimes recommended for patients with back or neck pain, but randomized controlled trials have not demonstrated benefit.[22]

Acupuncture could be classified as a mechanical therapy, in that it produces mechanical stimulation by the needle, but diverse theories exist about its mechanism of action.[91,102] Controlled studies are rare, but preliminary evidence suggests benefits in osteoarthritis of the knee (see Ch. 23).[59]

Upper limb orthoses and manipulation aids

Some of the orthoses and utensils often used by patients with rheumatic disease to protect hand joints, prevent or correct deformities, and facilitate function can be seen in Figure 37-5. Details of the biomechanics of and prescription process for upper limb orthoses are provided in Chapter 15. There is some evidence of the usefulness of orthoses in the treatment of patients with rheumatoid arthritis.[171] Resting orthoses can be used for brief periods, particularly during severe inflammatory flares, but their prolonged use should be avoided because it can reduce the joint range of motion and increase muscular atrophy. The orthosis should be removed several times a day for gentle mobilization. Ring orthoses and other variants are frequently used to improve the appearance and function of the fingers (Fig. 37-5). Common indications are swan neck deformities, boutonnière deformities, and ulnar deviation in patients with rheumatoid arthritis.[196]

It is essential that the patient participates in the selection of an orthosis, fully understands its purpose, and complies with the wearing schedule. Rheumatoid arthritis and hand osteoarthritis often decrease grip strength.[56] Broad handle silverware and other utensils can facilitate meal preparation and consumption. Broad handles for covers and doors are often helpful.

Lower limb orthoses and mobility aids

Figure 37-6 shows a number of orthoses and mobility aids often used by patients with rheumatic diseases to protect lower limb joints and facilitate ambulation (see also Ch. 16). There are few controlled studies to establish firm indications and contraindications for lower limb orthotic use in rheumatic diseases. Typically,

it is a matter of trial and error to find out which particular aids help improve function in an individual patient.

Good-quality athletic shoes are often less expensive and better accepted by patients than traditional orthopedic shoes.[94] The shoe should be wide and deep enough to accommodate existing deformities and a fitted orthotic insole.[94] The main goal is not to correct but to accommodate existing deformities to decrease pain and facilitate ambulation. Ankle–foot orthoses can provide mediolateral support to unstable ankles, and prevent tripping if foot drop secondary to rheumatoid vasculitis exists.[106] As shown in Figure 37-6, knee orthoses are often prescribed to unload the medial compartment in patients with osteoarthritis.[137]

Mobility aids are essential for the patient with advanced rheumatic disease to maintain independence at home and in the community. These include canes, axillary and forearm crutches, walkers, and scooters. The occasional patient with advanced rheumatic disease requires a wheelchair for mobility. Wheelchair prescription is discussed in Chapter 18. There are few controlled studies for the use of mobility aids.[20]

SPECIAL REHABILITATION ISSUES IN OSTEOARTHRITIS

Osteoarthritis, also known as degenerative joint disease, is the most common rheumatic disease. Its prevalence increases with age, and is almost universally present in adults 60 years of age and older.[62] The most commonly affected joints are the hips, the knees, the finger joints, and the cervical and lumbar spine (Box 37-1 and Fig. 37-7).[52] The basic pathologic abnormality is fraying, fragmentation, and thinning of the articular cartilage, with associated changes in subchondral bone and mild, secondary inflammation. The vast majority of patients are affected by primary osteoarthritis, possibly caused by a combination of repetitive mechanical stresses and a variable genetic predisposition.[62,63] Secondary osteoarthritis develops in joints previously affected by trauma, sepsis, or inflammatory conditions.[37] Occasional families present with inherited variants of the disease.[108]

When osteoarthritis affects the hip and knee joints, patients most often complain of pain and stiffness on ambulation.[52] The physical examination typically reveals decreased range of motion and bony enlargement at the knee. X-rays show joint space narrowing, subchondral sclerosis, subchondral cysts, and osteophyte formation (Fig. 37-7). Activity limitations often involve difficulty walking on flat surfaces and climbing stairs. In advanced stages, severely curtailed mobility can decrease occupational and non-occupational participation.[192]

When osteoarthritis affects the finger joints, impairments commonly include Heberden and Bouchard nodes (Fig. 37-7) and pain at the base of the thumb,[52] with concomitant joint space narrowing and osteophyte formation. The pain compromises activities that require repetitive use of the thumb and holding loads in the hands, and typing and writing. Participation

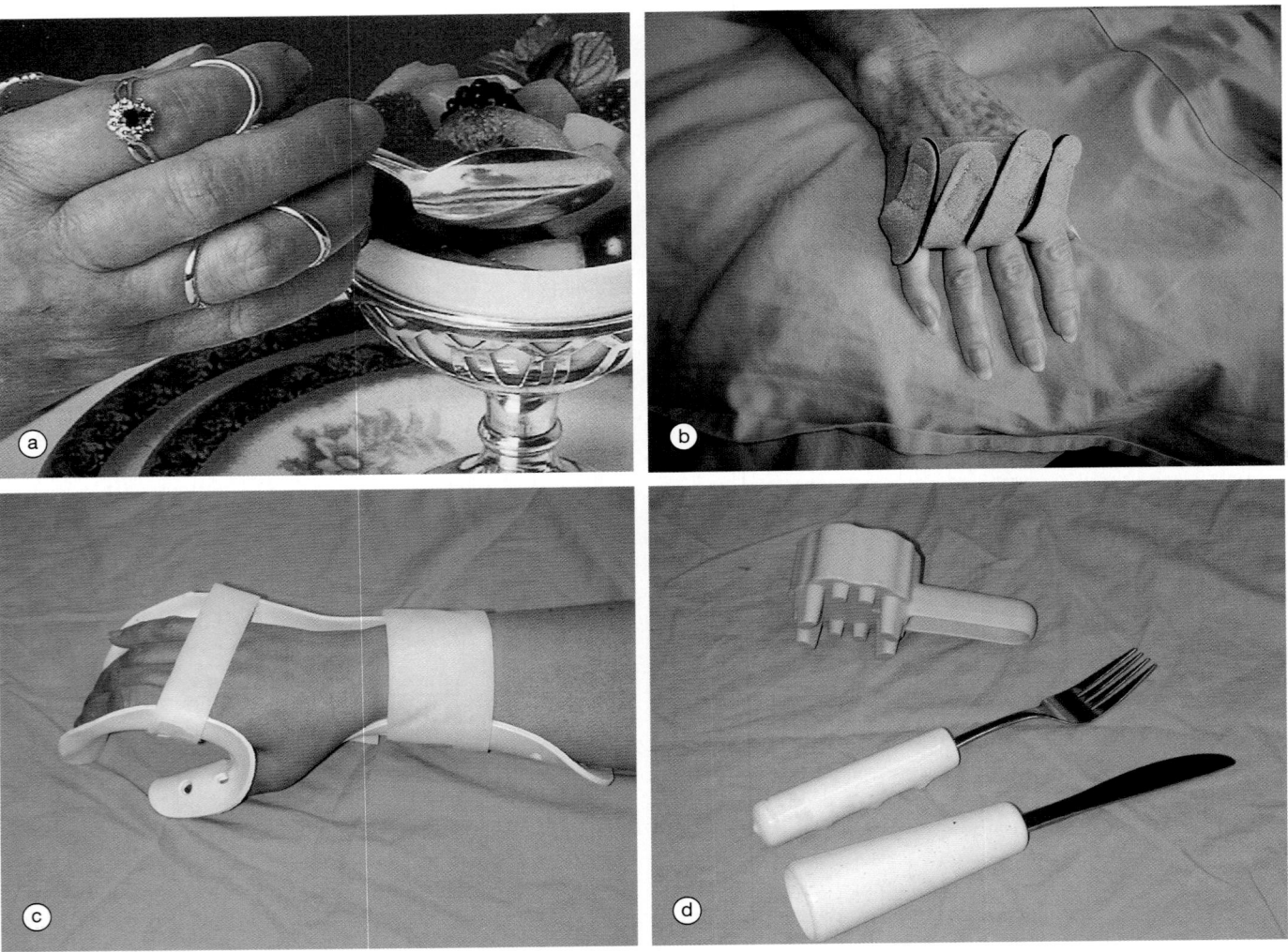

Figure 37-5 Upper limb orthoses and manipulation aids commonly used by patients with rheumatic diseases. (**a**) Ring orthoses to correct swan neck and boutonnière deformities. (**b**) Orthosis to correct ulnar deviation of the fingers. (**c**) Resting orthosis to decrease pain in acutely inflamed joints. (**d**) Broad handle utensils to facilitate meal consumption and opening of faucets.

in jobs that require keyboarding or use of a computer mouse can be restricted.

When osteoarthritis affects the cervical and lumbar spine, pain, stiffness, and decreased range of motion are common. The relationship of pain with the presence of degenerative changes is often complex, because many people with degenerative changes in the spine remain asymptomatic.[51] Advanced osteoarthritis of the facet joints is a common substrate for spinal and foraminal stenosis (Chs 38 and 41).

The comprehensive management of osteoarthritis includes education on self-management, lifestyle modification (weight loss, fitness, and activity pacing), use of medications for pain relief, intraarticular injections of glucocorticoids or hyaluronic acid compounds, surgical interventions with an emphasis on joint replacement, and a plethora of rehabilitation interventions.[16,62,66,97]

Table 37-7 lists known indications and evidence for the rehabilitation interventions most commonly used in osteoarthritis. Figure 37-8 presents a recommended approach for the rehabilitative management of people with osteoarthritis. Rehabilitation post surgical interventions is described later in this chapter.

SPECIAL REHABILITATION ISSUES IN RHEUMATOID ARTHRITIS

Rheumatoid arthritis is an idiopathic inflammatory arthropathy characterized by autoimmune attack to the joints, although it also affects periarticular and extraarticular tissues.[81] It affects approximately 0.3% to 1% of the general population,[192] and is characterized by symmetric waxing and waning inflammation, predominantly affecting the small joints of the hands and feet

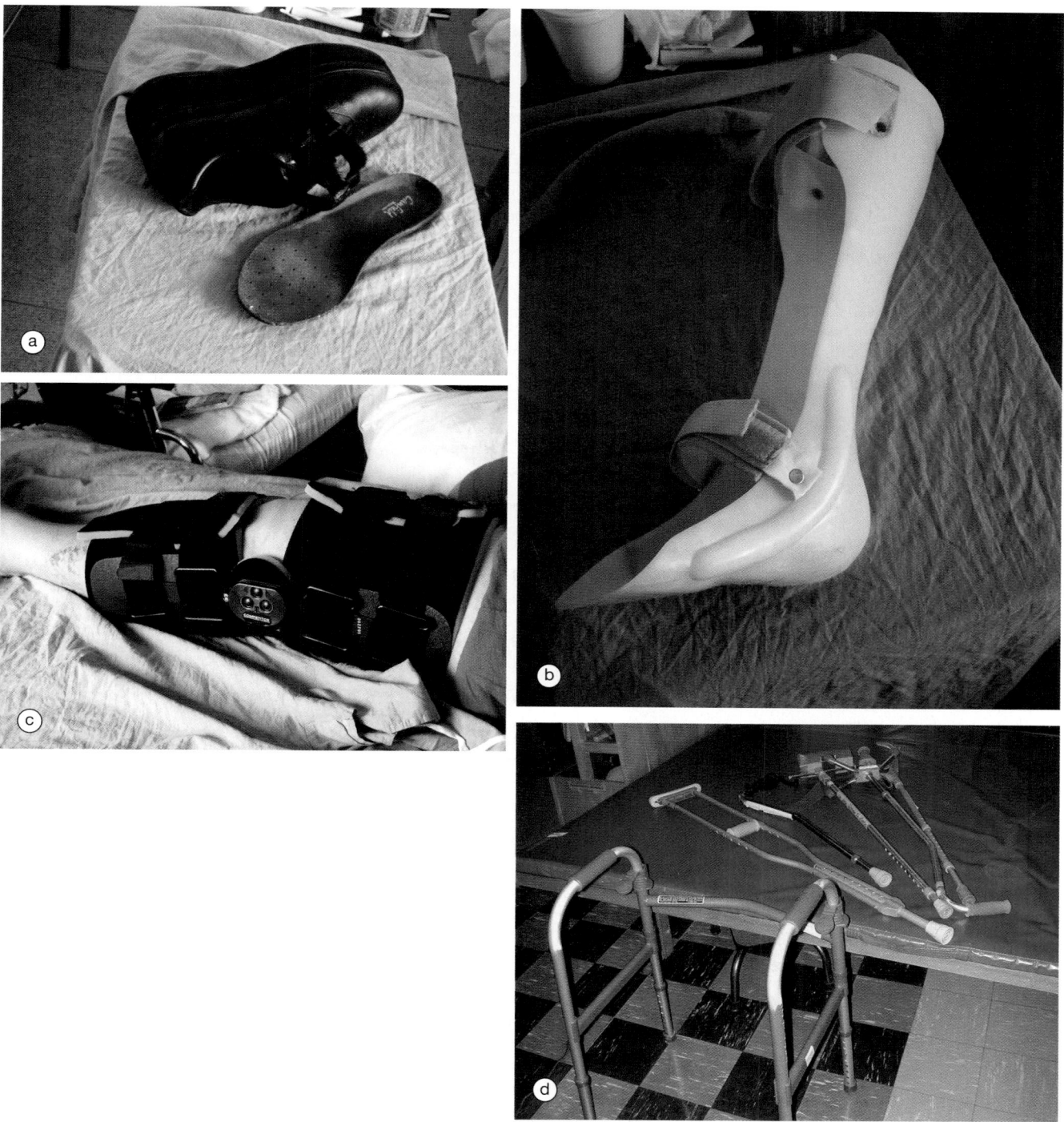

Figure 37-6 Lower limb orthoses and mobility aids. (**a**) Extradepth shoes and molded insoles to accommodate rheumatic foot deformities. (**b**) Ankle–foot orthosis to provide mediolateral ankle support or prevent tripping. (**c**) Knee brace to unload the medial knee compartment. (**d**) Canes and crutches to facilitate ambulation.

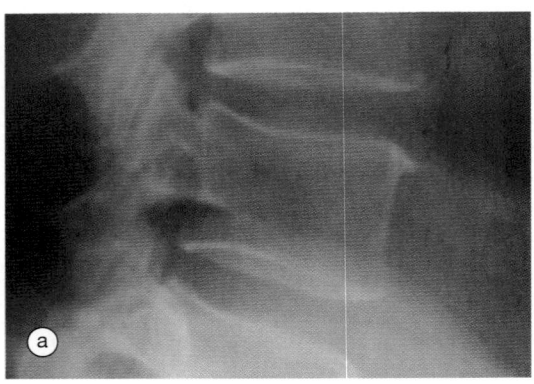

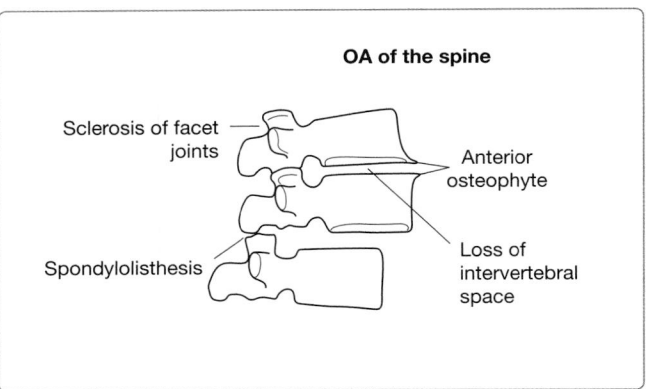

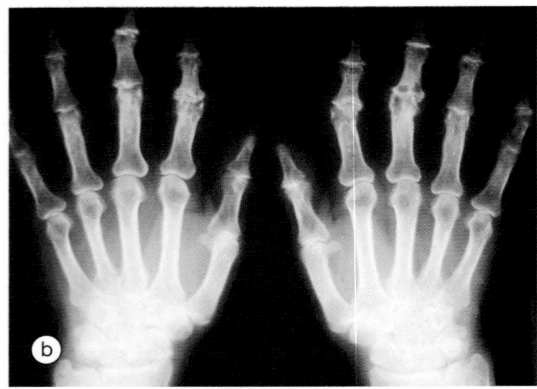

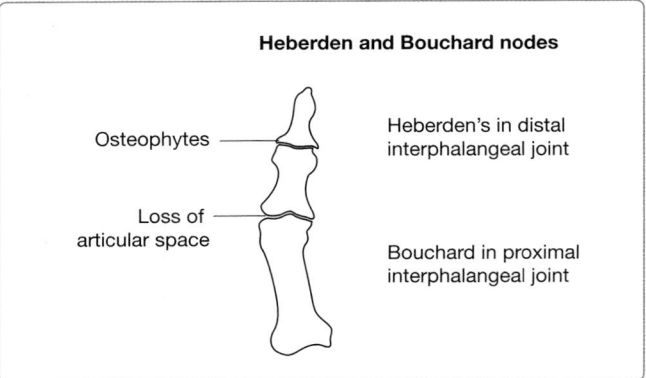

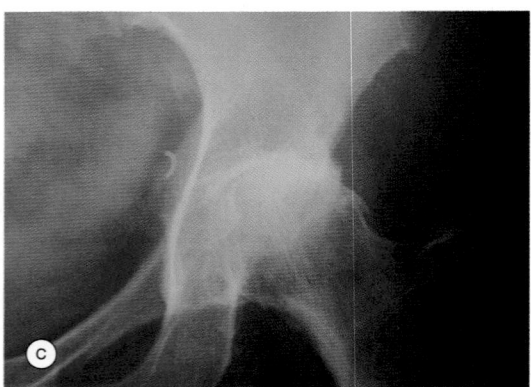

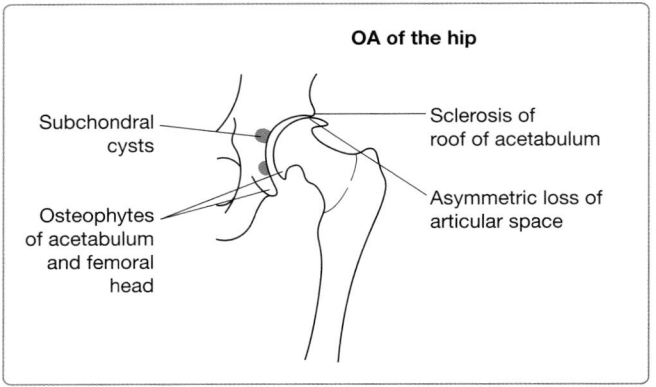

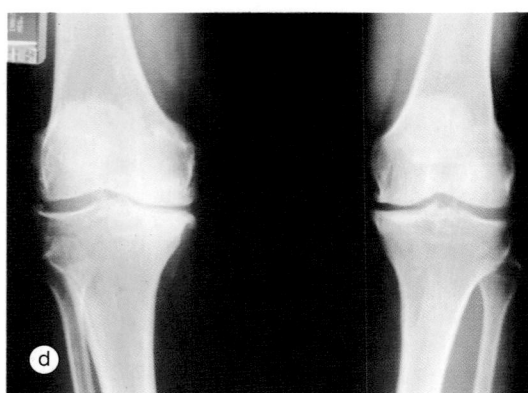

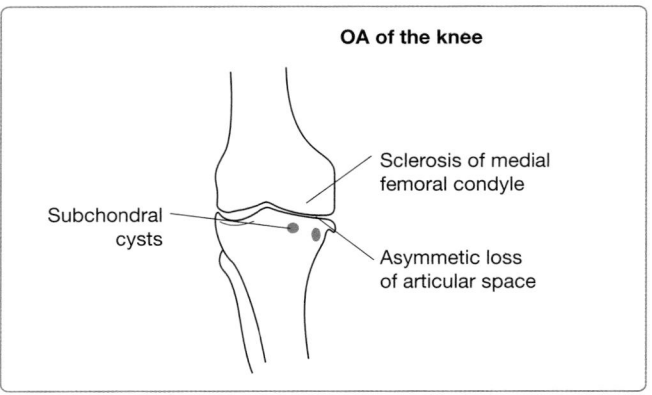

Figure 37-7 Typical deformities and x-ray findings in osteoarthritis of the spine (**a**), hands (**b**), hip (**c**), and knee (**d**).

Table 37-7 Current state of scientific evidence about rehabilitation interventions for osteoarthritis[a]

Intervention	Current evidence
Education and self-management	Widely regarded as beneficial, but some of the trials have mixed patients with osteoarthritis (OA) and rheumatoid arthritis. A recent randomized trial in OA of the knee reported benefits on pain and function for up to 21 months.
Exercise, rest, and energy conservation	Land-based therapeutic exercise has been shown to reduce pain and improve physical function for people with OA of the knee. Both high-intensity and low-intensity aerobic exercise appear to be equally effective in improving functional status, gait, pain, and aerobic capacity.
Physical modalities	Ice massage compared with control had a statistically beneficial effect on range of motion, function, and knee strength. Cold packs decreased swelling. Hot packs had no beneficial effect on edema compared with placebo or cold application. Ultrasound therapy appears to have no benefit over placebo or short-wave diathermy for people with hip or knee OA. Electromagnetic field therapy may provide significant improvements for knee OA, but further studies are required. Transcutaneous electrical nerve stimulation (TENS) and acupuncture-like TENS might be effective in pain control over placebo in OA of the knee, but better studies are required. The results of laser therapy are conflicting in different studies and might depend on the method of application.
Manual and mechanical therapies	No randomized published studies on the use of manual therapies in OA. For pain and function in OA of the knee, there was limited evidence that acupuncture is more effective than being on a waiting list or treatment as usual. For pain, there was strong evidence that real acupuncture is more effective than sham acupuncture.
Upper limb orthoses and manipulation aids	Little evidence specific for OA. The few published trials are in rheumatoid arthritis.
Lower limb orthoses and mobility aids	There is limited evidence that a knee brace is beneficial for OA of the medial compartment of the knee when compared with medical treatment alone or a neoprene sleeve. There is limited evidence that a laterally wedged insole decreases non-steroidal antiinflammatory drug intake compared with a neutral insole.

[a]This table summarizes the author's interpretation of available systematic reviews of randomized trials, primarily Cochrane systematic reviews available in the Cochrane Library.

(Table 37-3 and Fig. 37-9).[81] However, it can affect any synovial joint in the body. Although inflammatory activity waxes and wanes, irreversible damage starts to accumulate early in the disease.[44,131,142]

The approach to the treatment of rheumatoid arthritis has undergone a virtual revolution over the past 20 years. The gradual 'pyramid-like' approaches and original disease-modifying drugs (DMARDs) are no longer used.[131] Instead, aggressive multidrug treatment strategies and biologic agents directed toward cytokines mediating inflammation are used early in the disease to take advantage of a therapeutic window before permanent damage develops.[131]

The most common complaints in rheumatoid arthritis are joint pain, fatigue, and stiffness. Later in the course, decreased range of motion, joint deformities, and muscle atrophy can develop.[81] Impairments shown on x-rays include periarticular osteopenia, erosions, and loss of the joint space (Fig. 37-9).[157] Ultrasound and magnetic resonance imaging (MRI) studies can document earlier signs of joint effusions and subchondral edema.[24,136] Activity limitations often compromise reach, grip,

manipulation of objects, walking, and running.[56,67] Participation restrictions can be experienced in all areas of life, particularly in severe advanced disease, with many patients unable to sustain employment and participate in family activities.[15]

The comprehensive management of rheumatoid arthritis includes education, training in self-management, antiinflammatories, DMARDs, intraarticular steroids, multiple rehabilitation interventions, and surgical intervention including joint replacement.[6,184] The indications and evidence on the rehabilitation interventions most commonly used in rheumatoid arthritis are summarized in Table 37-8. Figure 37-10 presents a recommended rehabilitative approach to patients with rheumatoid arthritis. The timing for use of many rehabilitative interventions depends on the degree of disease activity present. During periods of intense inflammation, rehabilitation interventions focus on providing pain relief with physical modalities, maintaining range of movement, and preventing impairments. During periods of quiescent disease, rehabilitation efforts focus on strengthening, accommodating existing joint damage, and facilitating desired activities and participation.[96]

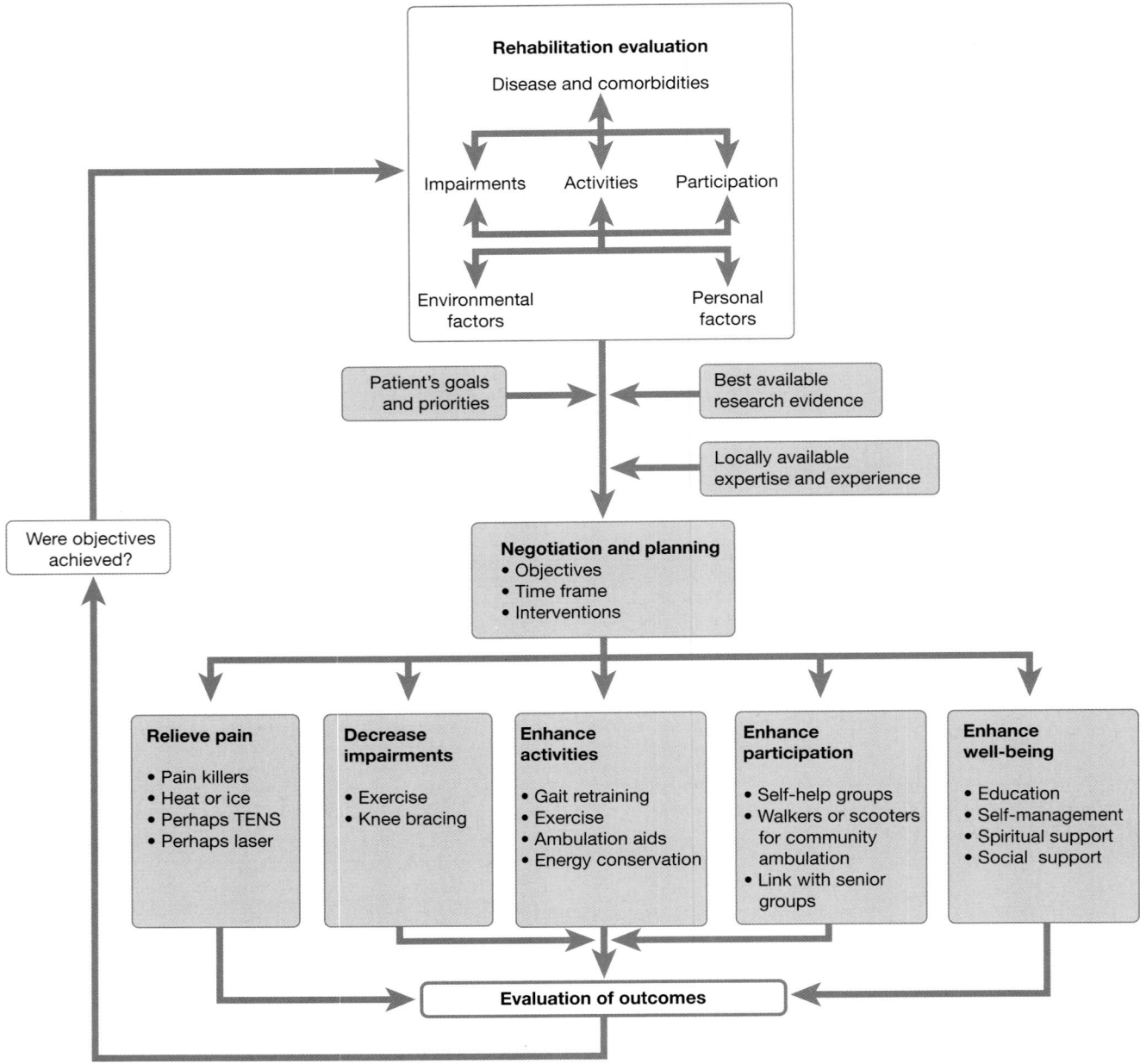

Figure 37-8 A recommended approach to the rehabilitation of patients with osteoarthritis. See Table 37-6 for details on the rehabilitation evaluation. See Table 37-7 for details on best available research evidence on rehabilitation interventions. TENS, transcutaneous electrical nerve stimulation.

REHABILITATION ISSUES IN OTHER RHEUMATIC DISEASES

In addition to osteoarthritis, rheumatoid arthritis, and regional musculoskeletal complaints, physiatrists frequently become involved in the rehabilitation of patients with spondyloarthropathies, inflammatory myopathies, systemic lupus erythematosus, or scleroderma. Patients with these diseases pose special challenges and circumstances.

Spondyloarthropathies

The seronegative spondyloarthropathies are a group of idiopathic inflammatory diseases characterized by spinal inflammation and enthesitis (inflammation at tendon insertion sites). They include ankylosing spondylitis, reactive arthritis, and Reiter syndrome.[182] The arthritis associated with psoriasis and inflammatory bowel disease sometimes manifests as a spondyloarthropathy, with prominent spinal involvement, and sometimes as a peripheral arthritis of small joints.[74]

Typical spondyloarthropathy symptoms include back and neck pain with prolonged morning stiffness, and asymmetric arthralgias involving hip, knee, and feet. Examination can reveal decreased range of movement of the cervical and lumbar spine, tenderness in tendon insertions (patellar and Achilles), and occasional joint effusion.[182] Radiologically, there are initial erosions (better visualized with computed tomography or MRI)

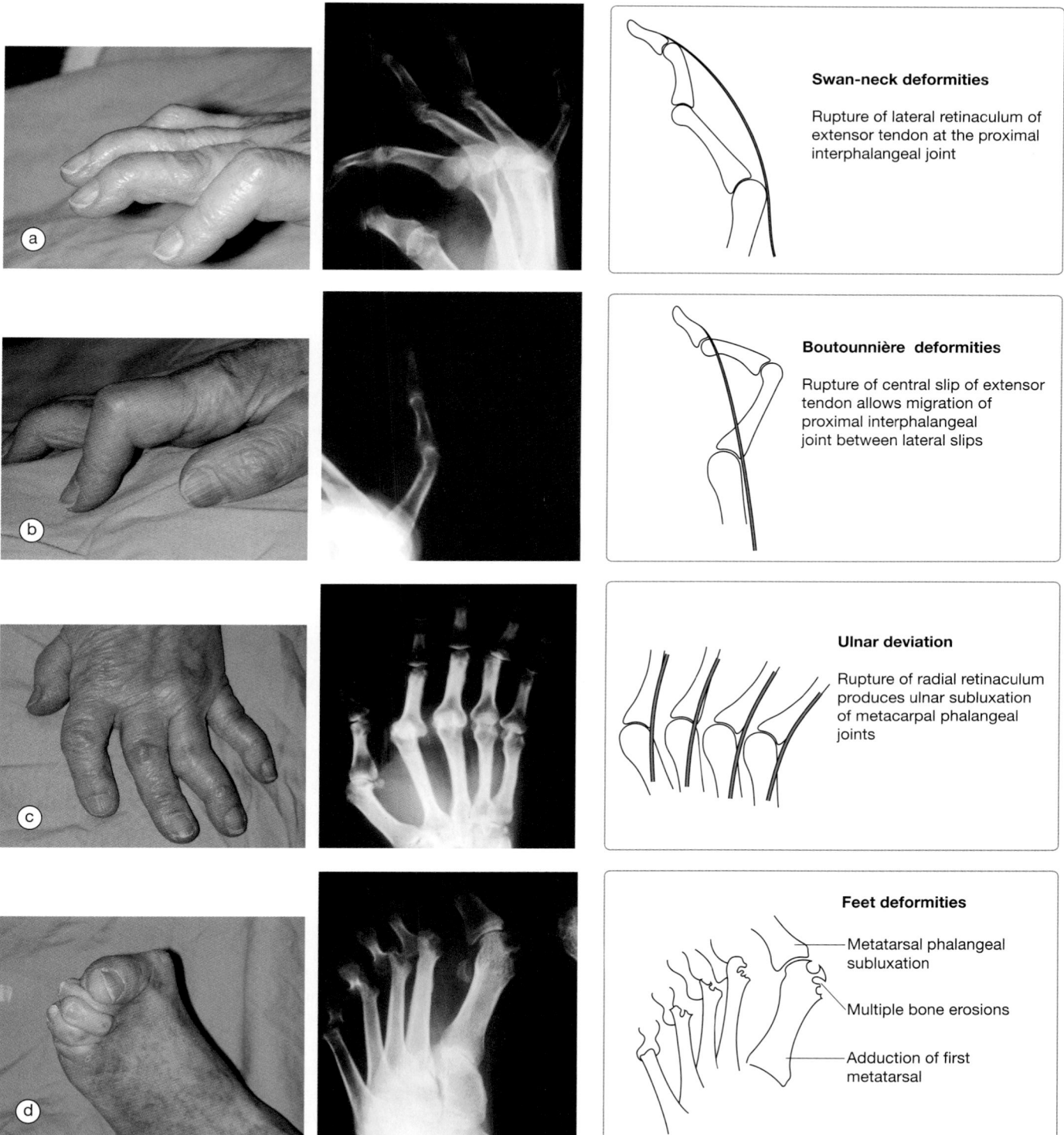

Figure 37-9 Typical deformities and x-ray findings in rheumatoid arthritis of the hands and feet: (**a**) swan neck deformities, (**b**) boutonnière deformities, (**c**) ulnar deviations, and (**d**) feet deformities.

Table 37-8 Current state of scientific evidence about rehabilitation interventions for rheumatoid arthritis[a]

Intervention	Current evidence
Education and self-management	Patient education has shown small short-term effects on disability, joint counts, patient global assessment, psychologic status, and depression.
Exercise, rest, and energy conservation	Several randomized trials suggest that dynamic exercise therapy is effective at increasing aerobic capacity and muscle strength. No detrimental effects on disease activity and pain were observed. There is strong evidence for the efficacy of 'instruction on joint protection' in people with rheumatoid arthritis (RA). T'ai chi does not seem to exacerbate symptoms of RA, and it has significant benefits on lower extremity range of motion.
Physical modalities	A systematic review of thermotherapy for RA found no significant effect of hot and ice pack applications, cryotherapy, and faradic baths on joint swelling, pain, medication intake, range of motion, grip strength, or hand function compared with no treatment or active therapy. No harmful effects of thermotherapy were reported. Two poor-quality trials suggest that hand ultrasound may increase grip strength, and to a lesser extent reduce the number of swollen and painful joints. Several trials of poor quality have reported beneficial effects of balneotherapy in RA. One low-quality trial suggests that electrical stimulation has a beneficial effect on grip strength and fatigue resistance for RA patients with muscle atrophy of the hand. Acupuncture-like TENS seems beneficial for reducing pain intensity and improving muscle power while, conversely, conventional TENS resulted in no clinical benefit on pain intensity compared with placebo. Low-level laser therapy could be considered for short-term relief of pain and morning stiffness for RA patients, particularly because it has few side effects.
Manual and mechanical therapies	One small poor-quality randomized trial suggests that electroacupuncture may be beneficial to reduce knee pain in patients with RA 24 h post treatment.
Upper limb orthoses and manipulation aids	Limited evidence suggests that comprehensive occupational therapy improves functional ability in RA. There is insufficient evidence about the effect of working wrist splints in pain or function for people with RA; some of these splints decrease grip strength and dexterity. Preliminary evidence suggests that resting hand and wrist splints do not seem to affect range of motion or pain, although participants preferred wearing a resting splint to not wearing one.
Lower limb orthoses and mobility aids	There is evidence that extradepth shoes and molded insoles decrease pain during weight-bearing activities such as standing, walking, and stair climbing. Insoles may be effective in preventing progression of hallux abductus angle but do not appear to have significant impact on pain.

[a]This table summarizes the author's interpretation of available systematic reviews of randomized trials, primarily Cochrane systematic reviews available in the Cochrane Library.

that evolve into sclerosis and ankylosis. Typical locations are the sacroiliac joints and the spinal longitudinal ligaments insertion sites.[30,135] The main activity limitations relate to pain and stiffness early in the disease, and to the stooped posture in advanced disease. Involvement of the hips can limit ambulation. Rehabilitative management focuses on exercise to maintain range of movement, and assistive devices for reaching and ambulation in advanced disease.[48]

Inflammatory myopathies

The autoimmune attack in idiopathic inflammatory myopathies can be restricted to striated muscles (polymyositis) or involve the skin as well (dermatomyositis).[82] The myopathy can be a manifestation of other connective tissue diseases such as lupus, or associated with malignant neoplasms.[195] In adults with poly-

myositis in particular, one has to maintain a high degree of suspicion, because malignancy can develop some time after the diagnosis of myopathy.[195] In children, the disease often manifests as dermatomyositis and may occasionally lead to cutaneous vasculitis, subcutaneous calcium deposits, and severe muscle atrophy and mobility restrictions.[49]

The inflammatory myopathies often proceed with episodes of exacerbation and remission. Sometimes they are relatively benign, with one or more flares followed by lifetime remission. Sometimes they have repeated flares, with severe accumulated damage leading to major impairments and restricted mobility.[82] During acute flares, the inflammation can also involve the muscles of the larynx and pharynx, with subsequent difficulties in phonation and swallowing. This might require gastric feedings and assistive devices for communication. Bedridden patients

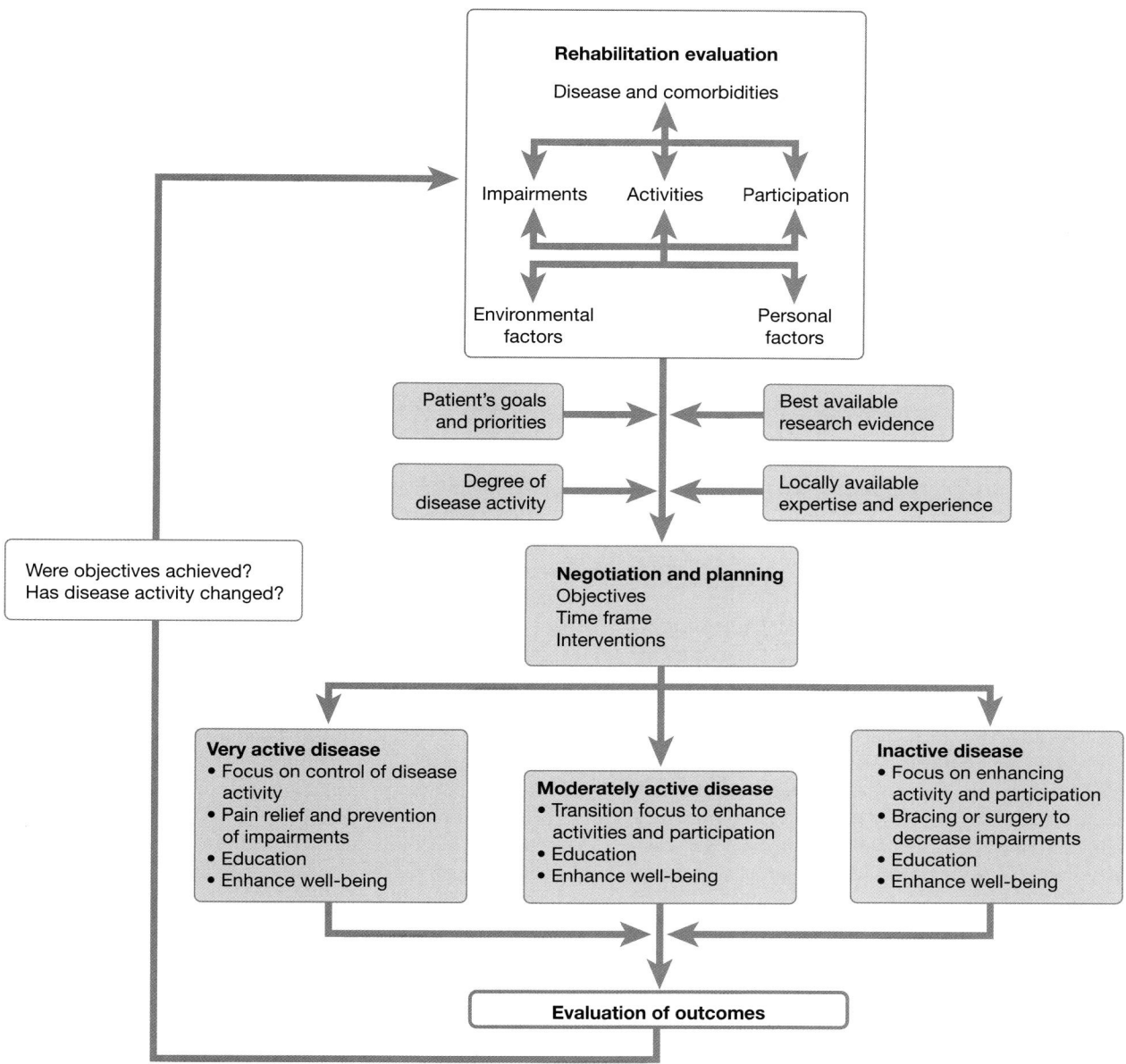

Figure 37-10 A recommended approach to the rehabilitation of patients with rheumatoid arthritis. See Table 37-6 for details on the rehabilitation evaluation. See Table 37-8 for details on best available research evidence on rehabilitation interventions. The specific interventions to decrease impairments, enhance activities and participation, and to enhance wellbeing are similar to those described for osteoarthritis (Fig. 37.8).

are at high risk of pneumonia and pressure ulcers, further complicated by concomitant use of immunosuppressive agents.

During periods of intense muscle inflammation, rehabilitative intervention focuses on passive mobilization to maintain range of movement, and to prevent contractures, pneumonia, and pressure sores.[85] Once the inflammation subsides (usually with normalization of serum levels of muscle enzymes), active-assisted exercises are added and gradually progressed to strengthening exercises.[82] Patients who have been bedridden for prolonged periods typically require gait retraining and assistive devices for ambulation (at least temporarily) (see Ch. 49 for additional details).

Systemic lupus erythematosus

Systemic lupus erythematosus is a heterogeneous disease characterized by autoimmune attack on multiple body systems (Table 37-4).[53] Frequently, the central nervous system involvement, kidney failure, and complications of treatment have greater functional impact than joint involvement. Patients with severe lupus are treated aggressively with glucocorticoids and cytotoxics,[17] and sometimes undergo extended periods of decreased mobility and deconditioning. Both immune suppression and immobility predispose to opportunistic infections, requiring a great degree of suspicion for early recognition and appropriate treatment.

Scleroderma

Progressive systemic sclerosis, most commonly referred to as scleroderma, is a rare disease characterized by accelerated fibrosis of the skin and internal organs.[156] It can involve the kidney, lungs, and gastrointestinal tract. It is a progressive disorder with no known cure, and with variable severity.[156] Some patients develop a 'scleroderma crisis', with sudden progressive kidney failure that requires prompt treatment with angiotensin-converting enzyme inhibitors.[167] In advanced scleroderma, the fibrosis of the periarticular tissues and skin can greatly decrease joint range of movement, mobility, and patient functioning.[116] These predispose patients to pressure ulcers and all the other well-known complications of immobility. Rehabilitation focuses on maintaining functional range of movement or, if this is not possible, on making sure that joints contracture into relatively functional positions.[50] Assistive devices to facilitate activities of daily living and ambulation might be required.

REHABILITATION AFTER SURGERY

Patients with advanced rheumatic disease often undergo surgery to debride, realign, replace, or fuse the joints.[154] Debridement and joint lavage are often performed in osteoarthritis and septic arthritis.[91,111] A recent randomized trial suggests that in absence of mechanical blocking by intraarticular debris, however, debridement for knee osteoarthritis is only as useful as sham surgery.[123] There is agreement for the need to remove fluid and debris in septic arthritis. Synovectomy to remove the inflamed synovial membrane (pannus) in rheumatoid arthritis is decreasing in frequency, but still occasionally used in joints refractory to systemic agents.[39]

Surgery to realign the joints often takes the form of osteotomies (e.g. lateral tibial proximal osteotomy to correct genu varus and modify loads at the knee),[122] or tendon and ligament transposition to realign deformed finger joints. Other examples include bunionectomy and resection of metatarsal heads to realign the toes.

Joint replacement surgery is a well-established procedure at the hip and the knee that greatly improves the quality of life of people with advanced osteoarthritis and rheumatoid arthritis.[58,125] The prostheses and surgical techniques for shoulder and elbow replacement are improving, but results still lag behind those seen in hip and knee replacement.[42,47] Replacement of finger joints with flexible implants is sometimes performed, but the cosmetic results are often better than the functional results.[179]

Arthrodesis or surgical fusion of the joints is sometimes performed to decrease pain in joints with advanced destruction not suitable for prosthetic implants. For example, arthrodesis of ankle and foot joints often improves function by decreasing pain on ambulation in patients with severe rheumatoid involvement.

The rehabilitation of younger patients with hip and knee replacement has changed in the past decades from prolonged inpatient rehabilitation, to rapid discharge after early weight bearing and mobilization followed by home or outpatient rehabilitation.[71] Older patients and those with a number of comorbidities still need inpatient rehabilitation. These patients with increased rehabilitation needs are often older women with severe preoperative activity limitations and use of ambulation devices, and who have nobody to assist them at home after surgery.[132] The rehabilitation issues after hip replacement for rheumatic disease are similar to those in hip replacement after femoral neck fractures.

Rehabilitation after hip replacement

In hip replacement surgery, the femoral head and the acetabulum are replaced by a metal stem and head, and a plastic acetabular component.[89] Variations of this basic design include alternative joint surfaces made of ceramics and other materials.[80] The femoral stem can be cemented or 'press fit' in place.[54] Hip replacement is highly effective in relieving pain and improving function. The mean implant life is from 10 to 20 years.[126] The surgery is indicated in any person with advanced hip disease that is refractory to conservative management, and who has low to moderate surgical risks.[126]

Those with uncomplicated surgery and cemented components can start full weight bearing the day after surgery, and progress rapidly to independent ambulation and discharge.[83] Non-cemented components traditionally require delayed weight bearing, although recent studies challenge this notion.[25] Revision surgery (to replace the old implant) and surgery involving femoral osteotomies or intraoperative complications require more prolonged rehabilitation.

The overall rehabilitation approach to uncomplicated hip replacement surgery is depicted in Figure 37-11. Most hospitals now have established standard protocols for the rehabilitation of patients with an uncomplicated hip replacement.[151] Typical programs start with a preoperative visit to assess the patient's situation, clarify expectations, and instruct patients on a home exercise program (with emphasis on hip muscles and the quadriceps) and necessary environmental modifications to allow discharge as soon as possible.[55,74,114] In the postoperative period, activity training progresses rapidly from bed to chair transfers to standing, and then to ambulation with aids and stair climbing.[83] Rehabilitation continues at home with the assistance of relatives or community care providers.[102] The rehabilitation approach to those who require more prolonged rehabilitation in an inpatient facility is the same, but the progression from one stage to the next is slower.

The complications of hip replacement surgery are well known, and the rehabilitation program includes measures to prevent falls, deep vein thromboses, hip dislocation, wound infection, and dehiscence. Nerve palsies of the sciatic or common peroneal nerves sometimes complicate hip replacement surgery and can require use of an ankle–foot orthosis.[18] Delayed complications include septic arthritis, aseptic loosening of the implant, heterotopic ossification, and premature implant failure. The usual posterolateral surgical approach requires postoperative 'hip precautions' to avoid hip dislocation. They include avoiding

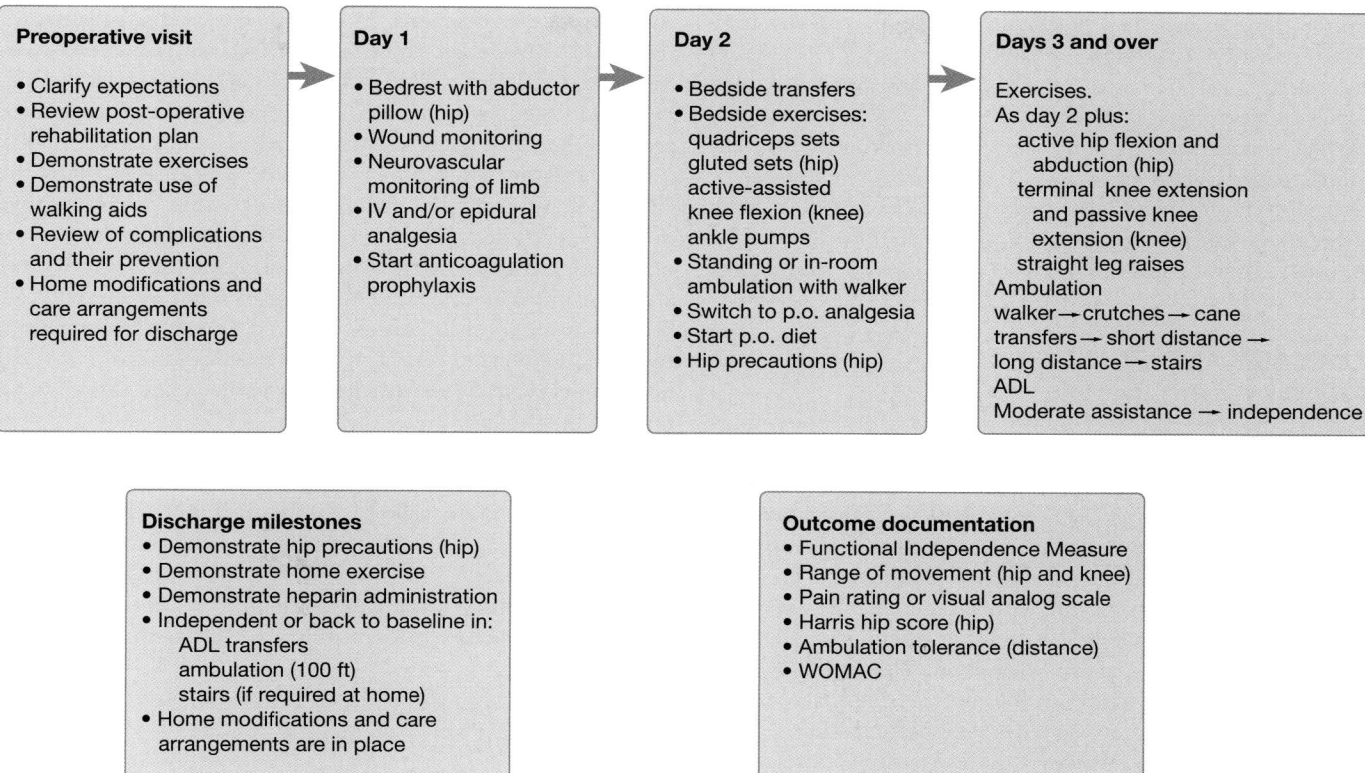

Preoperative visit	Day 1	Day 2	Days 3 and over

• Clarify expectations
• Review post-operative rehabilitation plan
• Demonstrate exercises
• Demonstrate use of walking aids
• Review of complications and their prevention
• Home modifications and care arrangements required for discharge
	• Bedrest with abductor pillow (hip)
	• Wound monitoring
	• Neurovascular monitoring of limb
	• IV and/or epidural analgesia
	• Start anticoagulation prophylaxis
		• Bedside transfers
		• Bedside exercises: quadriceps sets gluted sets (hip) active-assisted knee flexion (knee) ankle pumps
		• Standing or in-room ambulation with walker
		• Switch to p.o. analgesia
		• Start p.o. diet
		• Hip precautions (hip)
			Exercises.
			As day 2 plus:
			  active hip flexion and abduction (hip)
			  terminal knee extension and passive knee extension (knee)
			  straight leg raises
			Ambulation
			walker → crutches → cane
			transfers → short distance → long distance → stairs
			ADL
			Moderate assistance → independence

Discharge milestones
• Demonstrate hip precautions (hip)
• Demonstrate home exercise
• Demonstrate heparin administration
• Independent or back to baseline in:
   ADL transfers
   ambulation (100 ft)
   stairs (if required at home)
• Home modifications and care arrangements are in place

Outcome documentation
• Functional Independence Measure
• Range of movement (hip and knee)
• Pain rating or visual analog scale
• Harris hip score (hip)
• Ambulation tolerance (distance)
• WOMAC

Figure 37-11 A recommended approach to rehabilitation after joint replacement of the hip and knee. ADL, activities of daily living; WOMAC, Western Ontario–McMaster Questionnaire.

hip flexion beyond 90°, and adduction and internal rotation.[166] Twisting of the trunk when getting up from the toilet or a car seat, or tying the shoes, are typical risk activities.[110] A postoperative abduction pillow or hip abduction brace is used in some centers.[29]

Rehabilitation after knee replacement

In knee replacement surgery, the femoral condyles and the tibial plateaux are replaced by a metal femoral stem and condyles, and a plastic tibial component. Resurfacing of the patella with a plastic component is optional.[37,160,161] The implants are usually cemented in place, although press fit components are also occasionally used. Design options exist to preserve the posterior cruciate ligament or to substitute for its function.[155] Overall results and implant life are approaching those for hip replacement.

The rehabilitation program after knee replacement proceeds much the same way as that after hip replacement, with the use of care pathways in most hospitals (Fig. 37-11).[147] The usefulness of continuous passive motion machines to flex and extend the knee after surgery has been debated, and it is unclear if its benefits are worth the cost.[32] Complications after knee replacement include falls, deep vein thromboses (less common than in hip surgery), common peroneal nerve palsy, infection, and wound dehiscence.

Rehabilitation after hand surgery

Hand surgery in a patient with rheumatic disease can include joint replacement, osteotomies, and tendon repairs or transfers.[160,161,175,179] The rehabilitation program includes a period of initial immobilization, followed by gentle range of movement exercises, then progressing to strengthening and retraining of hand activities.[191] Controlled studies do not exist, and the speed and particularities of each program are usually dictated by the experience and preference of the surgeon and the rehabilitation professionals.

Hand orthoses are commonly used in the rehabilitation post surgery to control and to assist the range of movement of operated joints, as well as to gradually increase the stress applied to repaired tendons.[45] Tendon rupture, infections, and wound dehiscence are the common complications.[160,161]

Other upper limb surgery, such as shoulder and elbow replacements, is being increasingly performed. The functional outcomes have greatly improved over the past 10 years.[42,47]

Rehabilitation after foot surgery

Foot surgery can include joint debridement, tendon repair, osteotomies, and arthodesis.[160,161] The results of ankle arthroplasty are at present much less impressive than for hip or knee arthroplasty.[168] 'Triple arthrodesis' or pantalar arthrodesis is sometimes performed to reduce pain in patients with advanced joint destruction. It produces a 'solid ankle' that often requires shoe adaptations, such as a cushioned heel and/or rocker soles, to allow a more functional ambulation.[189]

When extensive foot surgery is performed, patients can require extended periods of non-weight bearing.[87] These can be particularly problematic in patients with concomitant arthritis of the upper limbs, which interferes with the use of crutches and other mobility aids.

SUMMARY AND CONCLUSIONS

Many of the over 100 recognized rheumatic diseases require physiatrist involvement. This chapter has described the main concepts and principles a physiatrist uses to effectively organize and supervise the rehabilitation of patients with common rheumatic conditions, with a focus on osteoarthritis, rheumatoid arthritis, and rehabilitation after joint replacement.

The rehabilitation of a person with a rheumatic disease starts, as in other areas of rehabilitation, with a careful assessment of impairments, activities, and participation. This is followed by consideration of the environmental and personal factors that can be modified to improve activities and participation. A complete assessment often involves a professional interdisciplinary team.[123] The evaluation concludes with a negotiation between the patient and team members to agree on common goals and the essential elements of the individualized rehabilitation program.

In the evaluation of a patient with inflammatory rheumatic disease, it is important to differentiate those changes related to active inflammation (disease activity) from permanent impairments (accumulated damage). During episodes of intense disease activity, the rehabilitative emphasis is on providing pain relief with physical modalities, and maintaining range of movement and preventing contractures, while the disease is brought under better control with pharmacologic agents. Once the disease activity decreases, emphasis shifts to active exercise, strengthening, and retraining of functions and ambulation. In advanced disease, orthoses and assistive devices can be tried to enhance activities and allow participation. Modifications of the environment can also help facilitate such participation.

Outpatient-based physiatrists can also have direct input in osteoarthritis management by providing intraarticular administration of glucocorticoids or hyaluronic acid polymers, and prescribing orthoses and assistive devices. The injection techniques are reviewed in Chapter 25. The role of the physiatrist in diagnosis and management of regional pain syndromes is reviewed in detail in Chapters 38–41.

Figures 37-8 and 37-10 present summaries of the general rehabilitation approach to patients with osteoarthritis and rheumatoid arthritis. Patient education and self-management are essential components of the rehabilitation of most patients with rheumatic disease. In North America, these are often championed or provided outside traditional medical settings by patient and advocacy associations.[11,12] Controlled studies have shown significant impacts of these efforts on pain, function, well-being, and satisfaction.[86] Exercise is another essential component supported by controlled trials,[99] while the evidence for physical modalities and assistive devices is still sparse.[68,171]

Rehabilitation after surgery requires coordination with the orthopedic surgeon, and involves gradual transition from range of movement exercises to muscle strengthening and retraining of activities of daily living. This transition can be relatively fast after uncomplicated hip and knee replacement, often requiring brief in-hospital rehabilitation followed by home or outpatient rehabilitation (Fig. 37-11).[55,83] More prolonged inpatient rehabilitation is typically needed in older patients and those with a number of comorbidities.

Rehabilitation interventions and strategies are a core component of the management of people with rheumatic diseases. Physiatrists are often called to assist in the development and coordination of appropriate individual rehabilitation programs for these patients. Until a cure for these diseases is found, rehabilitative intervention will continue to be an essential part of good healthcare for patients with rheumatic diseases.

REFERENCES

1. Aaron RK, Ciombor DM, Simon BJ. Treatment of nonunions with electric and electromagnetic fields. Clin Orthop 2004; Feb(419):21–29.
2. Abraido-Lanza AF, Vasquez E, Echeverria SE. Religious and other forms of coping among Latinos with arthritis. J Consult Clin Psychol 2004; 72(1):91–102.
3. Altman R, Alarcon G, Appelrouth D, et al. The American College of Rheumatology criteria for the classification and reporting of osteoarthritis of the hand. Arthritis Rheum 1990; 33(11):1601–1610.
4. Altman R, Alarcon G, Appelrouth D, et al. The American College of Rheumatology criteria for the classification and reporting of osteoarthritis of the hip. Arthritis Rheum 1991; 34(5):505–514.
5. Altman R, Asch E, Bloch G, et al. Development of criteria for the classification and reporting of osteoarthritis: classification of osteoarthritis of the knee. Arthritis Rheum 1986; 29(8):1039–1049.
6. American College of Rheumatology. Guidelines for the management of rheumatoid arthritis. Arthritis Rheum 2002; 46(2):328–346.
7. American College of Rheumatology. Recommendations for the medical management of osteoarthritis of the hip and knee. Arthritis Rheum 2000; 43(9):1905–1915.
8. American Geriatrics Society Panel on Exercise and Osteoarthritis. Exercise prescription for older adults with osteoarthritis pain: consensus practice recommendations. J Am Geriatr Soc 2001; 49(6):808–823.
9. Arnett FC, Edworthy SM, Bloch DA, et al. The American Rheumatism Association 1987 revised criteria for the classification of rheumatoid arthritis. Arthritis Rheum 1988; 31(3):315–324.
10. Arroll B, Goodyear-Smith F. Corticosteroid injections for osteoarthritis of the knee: meta-analysis. Br Med J 2004; 328(7444):869.
11. Arthritis Foundation. Online. Available: http://www.arthritis.org/ Nov 2004.
12. Arthritis Society. Online. Available: http://www.arthritis.ca Nov 2004.
13. Ashe MC, Khan KM. Exercise prescription. J Am Acad Orthop Surg 2004; 12(1):21–27.
14. Atkinson JP. Complement system. In: Harris D, Budd C, Genovese MC, et al, eds. Kelley's textbook of rheumatology. 7th edn. Philadelphia: Elsevier; 2005:342–355.
15. Backman CL. Employment and work disability in rheumatoid arthritis. Curr Opin Rheumatol 2004; 16(2):148–152.
16. Badley EM, DesMeules M. Scientific editors: arthritis in Canada. An ongoing challenge. Ottawa: Health Canada; 2003.

17. Badsha H, Edwards CJ. Intravenous pulses of methylprednisolone for systemic lupus erythematosus. Semin Arthritis Rheum 2003; 32(6): 370–377.

18. Barrack RL. Neurovascular injury: avoiding catastrophe. J Arthroplasty 2004; 19(4 suppl 1):104–107.

19. Batavia M. Contraindications for superficial heat and therapeutic ultrasound: do sources agree? Arch Phys Med Rehabil 2004; 85(6): 1006–1012.

20. Bateni H, Maki BE. Assistive devices for balance and mobility: benefits, demands, and adverse consequences. Arch Phys Med Rehabil 2005; 86(1):134–145.

21. Bellamy N. WOMAC: a 20-year experiential review of a patient-centered self-reported health status questionnaire. J Rheumatol 2002; 29(12): 2473–2476.

22. Beurskens AJ, de Vet HC, Henrica C, et al. Efficacy of traction for nonspecific low back pain: 12-week and 6-month results of a randomized clinical trial. Spine 1997; 22(23):2756–2762.

23. Bingham CO. Development and clinical application of Cox-2-selective inhibitors for the treatment of osteoarthritis and rheumatoid arthritis. Cleve Clin J Med 2002; 69(suppl 1):S5–S12.

24. Bird P, Conaghan P, Ejbjerg B, et al. The development of the EULAR-OMERACT rheumatoid arthritis MRI reference image atlas. Ann Rheum Dis 2004; 64(suppl 1):i8–i10.

25. Boden H, Adolphson P. No adverse effects of early weight bearing after uncemented total hip arthroplasty: a randomized study of 20 patients. Acta Orthop Scand 2004; 75(1):21–29.

26. Bodenheimer T, Lorig K, Holman H, et al. Patient self-management of chronic disease in primary care. JAMA 2002; 288(19):2469–2475.

27. Bombardier C, Gladman DD, Urowitz MB, et al. Derivation of the SLEDAI. A disease activity index for lupus patients. Arthritis Rheum 1992; 35(6):630–640.

28. Brady TJ, Kruger J, Helmick CG, et al. Intervention programs for arthritis and other rheumatic diseases. Health Educ Behav 2003; 30(1): 44–63.

29. Branson JJ, Goldstein WM. Primary total hip arthroplasty. AORN J 2003; 788(6):947–953, 956–969; quiz 971–974.

30. Braun J, Golder W, Bollow M, et al. Imaging and scoring in ankylosing spondylitis. Clin Exp Rheumatol 2002; 6(28):s178–s187.

31. Bresalier RS, Sandler R, Quan H, et al. Cardiovascular events associated with rofecoxib in a colorectal adenoma chemoprevention trial. N Engl J Med 2005; 352:1092–1102.

32. Brosseau L, Milne S, Wells G, et al. Efficacy of continuous passive motion following total knee arthroplasty: a metaanalysis. J Rheumatol 2004; 31(11):2251–2264.

33. Brosseau L, Welch V, Wells G, et al. Low level laser therapy (classes I, II and III) for treating osteoarthritis. Cochrane Database Syst Rev 2004: CD002046.

34. Brosseau L, Yonge KA, Robinson V, et al. Thermotherapy for treatment of osteoarthritis. Cochrane Database Syst Rev 2003; 4:CD004522.

35. Bruce B, Fries JF. The Stanford Health Assessment Questionnaire: a review of its history, issues, progress, and documentation. J Rheumatol 2003; 30(1):167–178.

36. Buchbinder R. Clinical practice: plantar fasciitis. N Engl J Med 2004; 350(21):2159–2166.

37. Buckwalter JA, Saltzman C, Brown T. The impact of osteoarthritis. Clin Orthop 2004; 247S:s6–s15.

38. Budd RC, Fortner KA. T lymphocytes. In: Harris D, Budd C, Genovese MC, et al, eds. Kelley's textbook of rheumatology. 7th edn. Philadelphia: Elsevier; 2005:133–152.

39. Bynum CK, Tasto J. Arthroscopic treatment of synovial disorders in the shoulder, elbow and ankle. J Knee Surg 2002; 15(1):57–59.

40. Calin A, Dijkmans BAC, Emery P, et al. Outcomes of a multicentre randomized clinical trial of etanercept to treat ankylosing spondylitis. Ann Rheum Dis 2004; 63:1514–1600.

41. Cardiel MH, Abello-Banfi M, Ruiz-Mercado R, et al. How to measure health status in rheumatoid arthritis in non-English speaking patients: validation of a Spanish version of the Health Assessment Questionnaire Disability Index (Spanish HAQ-DI). Clin Exp Rheumatol 1993; 11(2): 117–121.

42. Chafik D, Lee TQ, Gupta R. Total elbow arthroplasty: current indications, factors affecting outcomes and follow-up results. Am J Orthop 2004; 33(10):496–503.

43. Cherkin DC, Sherman KJ, Deyo RA, et al. A review of the evidence for the effectiveness, safety, and cost of acupuncture, massage therapy, and spinal manipulation for back pain. Ann Intern Med 2003; 138(11): 898–906.

44. Choy EHS, Panayi GS. Cytokine pathways and joint inflammation in rheumatoid arthritis. N Engl J Med 2001; 344(12):907–916.

45. Chu MM. Splinting programmes for tendon injuries. Hand Surg 2002; 7(2):243–249.

46. Clark BM. Rheumatology: 9. Physical and occupational therapy in the management of arthritis. CMAJ 2000; 163(8):999–1005.

47. Collins DN, Harryman DT, Wirth MA. Shoulder arthroplasty for the treatment of inflammatory arthritis. J Bone Joint Surg Am 2004; 86-A(11): 2489–2496.

48. Dagfinrud H, Kvien TK, Hagen KB. Physiotherapy interventions for ankylosing spondylitis. Cochrane Database Syst Rev 2004; 18(4):CD002822.

49. Dalakas MC, Hohlfeld R. Polymyositis and dermatomyositis. Lancet 2003; 362(9338):971–982.

50. Denton CP, Black CM. Scleroderma—clinical and pathological advances. Best Pract Res Clin Rheumatol 2004; 18(3):271–290.

51. Deyo RA, Weinstein JN. Low back pain. N Engl J Med 2001; 344(5): 363–370.

52. Dougados M. Clinical features of osteoarthritis. In: Harris D, Budd C, Genovese MC, et al, eds. Kelley's textbook of rheumatology. 7th edn. Philadelphia: Elsevier; 2005:1514–1527.

53. Edworthy SM. Clinical manifestations of systemic lupus erthematosus. In: Harris D, Budd C, Genovese MC, et al, eds. Kelley's textbook of rheumatology. 7th edn. Philadelphia: Elsevier; 2005:1201–1224.

54. Emerson RH. Proximal ingrowth components. Clin Orthop Relat Res 2004; Mar(420):130–134.

55. Enloe LJ, Shields RK, Smith K, et al. Total hip and knee replacement treatment programs: a report-using consensus. J Orthop Sports Phys Ther 1996; 23(1):3–11.

56. Escalante A, Haas RW, Rincon I, et al. Measurement of global functional performance in patients with rheumatoid arthritis using rheumatology function tests. Arthritis Res Ther 2004; 6(4):R315–R325.

57. Escobar A, Quintana JM, Bilbao A, et al. Validation of the Spanish version of the WOMAC questionnaire for patients with hip or knee osteoarthritis. Western Ontario and McMaster Universities Osteoarthritis Index. Clin Rheumatol 2002; 21(6):466–471.

58. Ethgen O, Bruyere O, Richy F, et al. Health-related quality of life in total hip and total knee arthroplasty. A qualitative and systematic review of the literature. J Bone Joint Surg Am 2004; 86-A(5):963–974.

59. Ezzo J, Hadhazy V, Birch S, et al. Acupuncture for osteoarthritis of the knee: a systematic review. Arthritis Rheum 2001; 44(4):819–825.

60. Feletar M, Ibanez D, Urowitz MB, et al. The impact of the 1997 update of the American College of Rheumatology revised criteria for the classification of systemic lupus erythematosus: what has been changed? Arthritis Rheum 2003; 48(7):2067–2069.

61. Felson DT, Anderson JJ, Boers M, et al. The American College of Rheumatology preliminary core set of disease activity measures for rheumatoid arthritis clinical trials. The Committee on Outcome Measures in Rheumatoid Arthritis Clinical Trials. Arthritis Rheum 1993; 36(6): 729–740.

62. Felson DT, Lawrence RC, Hochberg MC, et al. Osteoarthritis: new insights. Part 2: treatment approaches. Ann Intern Med 2000; 133(9):726–737.

63. Felson DT. Risk factors for osteoarthritis. Clin Orthop 2004; 427S: S16–S21.

64. Finckh A, Iversen M, Liang MH. The exercise prescription in rheumatoid arthritis: primum non nocere. Arthritis Rheum 2003; 48(9):2393–2395.

65. FitzGerald GA, Patrono C. The coxibs, selective inhibitors of cyclooxygenase-2. N Engl J Med 2001; 345(6):433–442.

66. Fitzgerald GK, Oatis C. Role of physical therapy in management of knee osteoarthritis. Curr Opin Rheumatol 2004; 16 (2):143–147.

67. Fransen M, McConnell S, Bell M. Therapeutic exercise for people with osteoarthritis of the hip or knee. A systematic review. J Rheumatol 2002; 29(8):1737–1745.

68. Fransen M. Dietary weight loss and exercise for obese adults with knee osteoarthritis: modest weight loss targets, mild exercise, modest effects. Arthritis Rheum 2004; 5(5):1366–1369.

69. Fransen M. When is physiotherapy appropriate? Best Pract Res Clin Rheumatol 2004; 18(4):477–489.

70. Fries JF, Lorig K, Holman HR. Patient self-management in arthritis? Yes! J Rheumatol 2002; 29(2):362–368.

71. Ganz SB, Wilson PD, Cioppa-Mosca J, et al. The day of discharge after total hip arthroplasty and the achievement of rehabilitation functional milestones: 11-year trends. J Arthroplasty 2003; 18(4):453–457.

72. Gerdesmeyer L, Wagenpfeil S, Haake M, et al. Extracorporeal shock wave therapy for the treatment of chronic calcifying tendonitis of the rotator cuff: a randomized controlled trial. JAMA 2003; 290(19):2573–2580.

73. Gladman DD, Goldsmith CH, Urowitz MB, et al. The Systemic Lupus International Collaborating Clinics/American College of Rheumatology (SLICC/ACR) damage index for systemic lupus erythematosus international comparison. J Rheumatol 2000; 27(2):373–376.

74. Gladman DD. Psoriatic arthritis. In: Harris D, Budd C, Genovese MC, et al, eds. Kelley's textbook of rheumatology. 7th edn. Philadelphia: Elsevier; 2005:1155–1164.

75. Gocen Z, Sen A, Unver B, et al. The effect of preoperative physiotherapy and education on the outcome of total hip replacement: a prospective randomized controlled trial. Clin Rehabil 2004; 18(4):353–358.

76. Goldring SR, Goldring MB. Biology of the normal joint. In: Harris D, Budd C, Genovese MC, et al, eds. Kelley's textbook of rheumatology. 7th edn. Philadelphia: Elsevier; 2005:1–34.

77. Gonzalez VM, Stewart A, Ritter PL, et al. Translation and validation of arthritis outcome measures into Spanish. Arthritis Rheum 1995; 38(10): 1429–1446.

78. Gowans SE, deHueck A. Effectiveness of exercise in management of fibromyalgia. Curr Opin Rheumatol 2004; 16(2):138–142.

79. Hakkinen A. Effectiveness and safety of strength training in rheumatoid arthritis. Curr Opin Rheumatol 2004; 16(2):132–137.

80. Hannouche D, Hamadouche M, Nizard R, et al. Ceramics in total hip replacement. Clin Orthop Relat Res 2005; Jan(430):62–71.

81. Harris ED. Clinical features of rheumatoid arthritis. In: Harris D, Budd C, Genovese MC, et al, eds. Kelley's textbook of rheumatology. 7th edn, Philadelphia: Elsevier; 2005:1043–1100.

82. Harris-Love MO. Physical activity and disablement in the idiopathic inflammatory myopathies. Curr Opin Rheumatol 2003; 15:679–690.

83. Healy WL, Ayers ME, Iorio R, et al. Impact of a clinical pathway and implant standardization on total hip arthroplasty: a clinical and economic study of short-term patient outcome. J Arthroplasty 1998; 13(3): 266–276.

84. van der Heijde D, Landewe R, Klareskog L, et al. Prevention and analysis of data on radiographic outcome in clinical trials. Arthritis Rheum 2005; 52(1):49–60.

85. Hicks JE. Role of rehabilitation in the management of myopathies. Curr Opin Rheumatol 1998; 10(6):548–555.

86. Holman H, Lorig K. Patient self-management: a key to effectiveness and efficiency in care of chronic disease. Public Health Rep 2004; 119(3): 239–243.

87. Horst F, Nunley JA. Ankle arthodesis. J Surg Orthop Adv 2004; 13(2): 80–91.

88. Hulme J, Robinson V, DeBie R, et al. Electromagnetic fields for the treatment of osteoarthritis. Cochrane Database Syst Rev 2002; 1:CD003523.

89. Huo MH, Mullers MS. What's new in hip arthroplasty? J Bone Joint Surg Am 2004; 86-A(10):2341–2353.

90. Hurley MV. Muscle dysfunction and effective rehabilitation of knee osteoarthritis: what we know and what we need to find out. Arthritis Rheum 2003; 49(3):444–452.

91. Ilan DI, Rettig ME. Rheumatoid arthritis of the wrist. Bull Hosp Jt Dis 2003; 61(3-4):179–185.

92. Irnich D, Behrens N, Gleditsch JM, et al. Immediate effects of dry needling and acupuncture at distant points in chronic neck pain: results of a randomized, double-blind, sham-controlled crossover trial. Pain 2002; 99(1-2):83–89.

93. Irnich D, Behrens N, Molzen H, et al. Randomized trial of acupuncture compared with conventional massage and 'sham' laser acupuncture for treatment of chronic neck pain. Br Med J 2001:3221–3226.

94. Janisse DJ. Prescription footwear for arthritis of the foot and ankle. Clin Orthop 1998; Apr(349):100–107.

95. Jones KD, Clark SR. Individualizing the exercise prescription for persons with fibromyalgia. Rheum Dis Clin North Am 2002; 28(2):419–436.

96. de Jong Z, Munneke M, Zwinderman AH, et al. Is a long-term high-intensity exercise program effective and safe in patients with rheumatoid arthritis? Results of a randomized controlled trial. Arthritis Rheum 2003; 48(9):2415–2424.

97. Jordan KD, Arden NK, Doherty M, et al. EULAR recommendations 2003: an evidence based approach to the management of knee osteoarthritis: report of a task force of the standing committee for international clinical studies including therapeutic trials (ESCISIT). Ann Rheum Dis 2003; 62:1145–1155.

98. Katz PP. Introduction to special patient outcomes in rheumatology issue of arthritis care and research. Arthritis Rheum 2003; 49(5):S1–S4.

99. Kettunen JA, Kujala UM. Exercise therapy for people with rheumatoid arthritis and osteoarthritis. Scand J Med Sci Sports 2004; 14(3): 138–142.

100. Klippel JH. Primer on the rheumatic diseases. 11th edn. Atlanta: Arthritis Foundation; 1997.

101. Kramer BJ, Harker JO, Wong AL. Arthritis beliefs and self-care in an urban American Indian population. Arthritis Rheum 2002; 47(6):588–594.

102. Kuisma R. A randomized, controlled comparison of home versus institutional rehabilitation of patients with hip fracture. Clin Rehabil 2002; 16(5):553–561.

103. Langevin HM, Churchill DL, Wu J, et al. Evidence of connective tissue involvement in acupuncture. FASEB J 2002; 16(8):872–874.

104. Lee DM, Kiener HP, Brenner MB. Synoviocytes. In: Harris D, Budd C, Genovese MC, et al, eds. Kelley's textbook of rheumatology. 7th edn. Philadelphia: Elsevier; 2005:175–188.

105. Leeb BF, Andel I, Sautner J, et al. Disease activity measurement of rheumatoid arthritis: comparison of the simplified disease activity index (SDAI) and the disease activity score including 28 joints (DAS28) in daily routine. Arthritis Rheum 2005; 53(1):56–60.

106. Lin SS, Sabharwal S, Bibbo C. Orthotic and bracing principles in neuromuscular foot and ankle problems. Foot Ankle Clin 2000; 5(2):235–264.

107. Lorig KR, Holman H. Self-management education: history, definition, outcomes, and mechanisms. Ann Behav Med 2003; 26(1):1–7.

108. Loughlin J. Familial inheritance of osteoarthritis. Clin Orthop 2004; 427S: S22–S25.

109. Lovell D. Biologic agents for the treatment of juvenile rheumatoid arthritis: current status. Paediatr Drugs 2004; 6(3):137–146.

110. Mahoney CR, Pellicci PM. Complications in primary total hip arthroplasty: avoidance and management of dislocations. Instr Course Lect 2003; 52:247–255.

111. Manadin AM, Block JA. Daily needle aspiration versus surgical lavage for treatment of bacterial septic arthritis in adults. Am J Ther 2004; 11(5):412–415.

112. Mannerkorpi K, Iversen MD. Physical exercise in fibromyalgia and related syndromes. Best Pract Res Clin Rheumatol 2003; 17(4):629–647.

113. Masi AT, White KP, Pilcher JJ. Person-centered approach to care, teaching, and research in fibromyalgia syndrome: justification from biopsychosocial perspectives in populations. Semin Arthritis Rheum 2002; 32(2):71–93.

114. McGregor AH, Rylands H, Owen A, et al. Does preoperative hip rehabilitation advice improve recovery and patient satisfaction? J Arthroplasty 2004; 19(4):464–468.

115. Mease PJ, Kivitz AJ, Burch FX, et al. Etanercept treatment of psoriatic arthritis. Arthritis Rheum 2004; 50(7):2264–2272.

116. Medsger TA. Natural history of systemic sclerosis and the assessment of disease activity, severity, functional status, and psychologic well-being. Rheum Dis Clin North Am 2003; 29(2):255–273.

117. Meenagh GK, Patton J, Kynes C, et al. A randomized controlled trial of intra-articular corticosteroid injection of the carpometacarpal joint of the thumb in osteoarthritis. Ann Rheum Dis 2004; 63:1260–1263.

118. Meenan RF, Mason JH, Anderson JJ, et al. AIMS2. The content and properties of a revised and expanded Arthritis Impact Measurement Scales health status questionnaire. Arthritis Rheum 1992; 35(1):1–10.

119. Michener LA, Walsworth MK, Burnet EN. Effectiveness of rehabilitation for patients with subacromial impingement syndrome: a systematic review. J Hand Ther 2004; 17(2):152–164.

120. Minor MA, Sanford MK. The role of physical therapy and physical modalities in pain management. Rheum Dis Clin North Am 1999; 25(1): 233–248.

121. Minor MA. Editorial overview: meeting the challenges of evidence-based rheumatology rehabilitation. Curr Opin Rheumatol 2004; 16(2):130–131.

122. Mont MA, Stuchin SA, Paley D, et al. Different surgical options for monocompartmental osteoarthritis of the knee: high tibial osteotomy versus unicompartmental knee arthroplasty versus total knee arthroplasty: indications, techniques, results and controversies. Instr Course Lect 2004; 53:265–283.

123. Moseley JB, O'Malley K, Petersen NJ, et al. A controlled trial of arthroscopic surgery for osteoarthritis of the knee. N Engl J Med 2002; 347(2): 81–88.

124. Muller-Fassbender H, Bach GL, Hasse W, et al. Glucosamine sulfate compared to ibuprofen in osteoarthritis of the knee. Osteoarthritis Cartilage 1994; 2(1):61–69.

125. Murray DG, Crown RS, Dickersin K, et al. Total hip replacement. JAMA 1995; 273(24):1950–1956.

126. National Institutes of Health Consensus Development Panel on Total Hip Replacement. NIH consensus conference: total hip replacement. JAMA 1995; 273(24):1950–1956.

127. Neugebauer A, Katz PP. Impact of social support on valued activity disability and depressive symptoms in patients with rheumatoid arthritis. Arthritis Rheum 2004; 51(4):586–592.

128. Nicholas JJ. Physical modalities in rheumatological rehabilitation. Arch Phys Med Rehabil 1994; 75(9):994–1001.

129. Noack W, Fischer M, Forster KK, et al. Glucosamine sulfate in osteoarthritis of the knee. Osteoarthritis Cartilage 1994; 2(1):51–59.

130. Nussmeire NA, Whelton AA, Brown MT, et al. Complications of the COX-2 inhibitors parecoxib and valdecoxib after cardiac surgery. N Engl J Med 2005; 352(11):1081–1091.

131. O'Dell JR. Therapeutic strategies for rheumatoid arthritis. N Engl J Med 2004; 350:2591–2602.

132. Oldmeadow LB, McBurney H, Robertson VJ. Predicting risk of extended inpatient rehabilitation after hip or knee arthroplasty. J Arthoplasty 2003; 18(6):775–779.

133. Olsen NJ, Stein CM. New drugs for rheumatoid arthritis. N Engl J Med 2004; 350:2167–2179.

134. Ortendahl M, Holmes T, Schettler JD, et al. The methotrexate therapeutic response in rheumatoid arthritis. J Rheumatol 2002; 29(10):2084–2091.

135. Ory PA, Gladman DD, Mease PJ. Psoriatic arthritis and imaging. Ann Rheum Dis 2005; 64(2):1155–1157.

136. Ostergaard M, Ejbjerg B, Szkudlarek M. Imaging in early rheumatoid arthritis: roles of magnetic resonance imaging, ultrasonography, conventional radiography and computed tomography. Best Pract Res Clin Rheum 2005; 19(1):91–116.

137. Paluska SA, McKeag DB. Knee braces: current evidence and clinical recommendations for their use. Am Fam Physician 2000; 61(2):411-418, 423–424.

138. Pavelka K, Gatterova J, Olejarova M, et al. Glucosamine sulfate use and delay of progression of knee osteoarthritis. Arch Intern Med 2002; 162:2113–2123.

139. Perenboom RJ, Chorus AM. Measuring participation according to the International Classification of Functioning, Disability and Health (ICF). Disabil Rehabil 2003; 25(11-12):577–587.

140. Petri M, Magder L. Classification criteria for systemic lupus erythematosus: a review. Lupus 2004; 13(11):829–837.

141. Petty RE, Southwood TR, Manners P, et al. International League of Association for Rheumatology classification for juvenile idiopathic arthritis. J Rheumatol 2004; 31(2):390–392.

142. Pincus T, Sokka T, Wolfe F. Premature mortality in patients with rheumatoid arthritis: evolving concepts. Arthritis Rheum 2001; 44(6):1234–1236.

143. Podolsky DK. Inflammatory bowel disease. N Engl J Med 2002; 347(6): 417–429.

144. Pouchot J, Ecosse E, Coste J, et al. Validity of the childhood health assessment questionnaire is independent of age in juvenile idiopathic arthritis. Arthritis Rheum 2004; 51(4):519–526.

145. Ramos-Remus C, Gamez-Nava JI, Gonzalez-Lopez L, et al. Use of alternative therapies by patients with rheumatic disease in Guadalajara, Mexico: prevalence, beliefs, and expectations. Arthritis Care Res 1998; 11(5): 411–418.

146. Ramos-Remus C, Watters CA, Dyke L, et al. Assessment of health locus of control in the use of nonconventional remedies by patients with rheumatic diseases. J Rheumatol 1999; 26(11):2468–2474.

147. Ranawat CS, Ranawat AS, Mehta A. Total knee arthroplasty rehabilitation protocol. J Arthroplasty 2003; 18(3):27–30.

148. Rapp SR, Rejeski WJ, Miller ME. Physical function among older adults with knee pain: the role of pain coping skills. Arthritis Care Res 2000; 13(5):270–279.

149. Reginster JY, Deroisy R, Rovat LC, et al. Long-term effects of glucosamine on osteoarthritis progression: a randomized, placebo-controlled clinical trial. Lancet 2001; 357:251–256.

150. Robinson V, Brosseau L, Casimiro L, et al. Thermotherapy for treating rheumatoid arthritis. Cochrane Database Syst Rev 2004; 2: CD002826.

151. Roos EM. Effectiveness and practice variation of rehabilitation after joint replacement. Curr Opin Rheumatol 2003; 15(2):160–162.

152. Russak SM, Croft JD, Furst DE, et al. The use of rheumatoid arthritis health-related quality of life patient questionnaires in clinical practice: lessons learned. Arthritis Rheum 2003; 49(4):575–584.

153. Schneidert M, Hurst R, Miller J, et al. The role of environment in the International Classification of Functioning, Disability and Health (ICF). Disabil Rehabil 2003; 25(11-12):588–595.

154. Schurman DJ, Smith RL. Osteoarthritis. Current treatment and future prospects for surgical, medical, and biologic intervention. Clin Orthop Relat Res 2004; 427S:S183–S189.

155. Scuderi GR, Clarke HD. Cemented posterior stabilized total knee arthroplasty. J Arthroplasty 2004; 19(4 suppl 1):17–21.

156. Seibold JR. Scleroderma. In: Harris D, Budd C, Genovese MC, et al. Kelley's textbook of rheumatology. 7th edn. Philadelphia: Elsevier; 2005: 1279–1308.

157. Sharp JJ, Young DY, Bluhm GB, et al. How many joints in the hands and wrists should be included in a score of radiologic abnormalities used to assess rheumatoid arthritis? Arthritis Rheum 1985; 28(12):1326–1335.

158. Silverstein RE, Faich G, Goldstein JL, et al. Gastrointestinal toxicity with celecoxib vs nonsteroidal anti-inflammatory drugs for osteoarthritis and rheumatoid arthritis. JAMA 2000; 284(10):1247–1255.

159. Singh G, Athreya BH, Fries JF, et al. Measurement of health status in children with juvenile rheumatoid arthritis. Arthritis Rheum 1994; 37(12): 1761–1769.

160. Sledge CB. Introduction to surgical management of patients with arthritis. In: Harris D, Budd C, Genovese MC, et al, eds. Kelley's textbook of rheumatology. 7th edn. Philadelphia: Elsevier; 2005:1829–1835.

161. Sledge CB. Principles of reconstructive surgery for arthritis. In: Harris D, Budd C, Genovese MC, et al, eds. Kelley's textbook of rheumatology. 7th edn. Philadelphia: Elsevier; 2005:1836–1916.

162. Sluka KA, Walsh D. Transcutaneous electrical nerve stimulation: basic science mechanisms and clinical effectiveness. J Pain 2003; 4(3):109–121.

163. Smidt N, van der Windt DA, Assendelft WJ, et al. Corticosteroid injections, physiotherapy, or a wait-and-see policy for lateral epicondylitis: a randomized controlled trial. Lancet 2002; 359(9307):657–662.

164. Sokka T, Pincus T. Contemporary disease modifying antirheumatic drugs (DMARD) in patients with recent onset rheumatoid arthritis in a US private practice: methotrexate as the anchor drug in 90% and new DMARD in 30% of patients. J Rheum 2002; 29(12):2521–2524.

165. Solomon SD, McMurray JJV, Pfeffer MA, et al. Cardiovascular risk associated with celecoxib in a clinical trial for colorectal adenoma prevention. N Engl J Med 2005; 352(11):1071–1080.

166. Soong M, Rubash HE, Macauly W. Dislocation after total hip arthroplasty. J Am Acad Orthop Surg 2004; 12(15):314–321.

167. Steen VD. Scleroderma renal crisis. Rheum Dis Clin North Am 2003; 29(2):315–333.

168. Stengel D, Bauwens K, Ekkernkamp A, et al. Efficacy of total ankle replacement with meniscal-bearing devices: a systematic review and meta-analysis. Arch Orthop Trauma Surg 2005; 125(2):109–119.

169. Stenstrom CH, Minor MA. Evidence for the benefit of aerobic and strengthening exercise in rheumatoid arthritis. Arthritis Rheum 2003; 49(3):428–434.

170. Steultjens EMJ, Dekker J, Bouter LM, et al. Occupational therapy for community dwelling elderly people: a systematic review. Age Ageing 2004; 33(5):453–460.

171. Steultjens EMJ, Dekker J, Bouter LM, et al. Occupational therapy for rheumatoid arthritis: a systematic review. Arthritis Rheum 2002; 47(6): 672–685.

172. Stucki G, Cieza A, Geyh S, et al. ICF core sets for rheumatoid arthritis. J Rehabil Med 2004; Suppl 44:87–93.

173. Stucki G, Cieza A. The International Classification of Functioning, Disability and Health (ICF) core sets for rheumatoid arthritis: a way to specify functioning. Ann Rheum Dis 2004; 63(suppl II):ii40–ii45.

174. Suarez-Almazor ME. Patient–physician communication. Curr Opin Rheumatol 2004; 16:91–95.

175. Takigawa S, Meletiou S, Sauerbier M, et al. Long-term assessment of Swanson implant arthroplasty in the proximal interphalangeal joint of the hand. J Hand Surg Am 2004; 29(5):785–795.

176. Tan EM, Cohen AS, Fries JF, et al. The 1982 revised criteria for the classification of systematic lupus erythematosus (SLE). Arthritis Rheum 1982; 25:1271–1277.

177. Tidow-Kebritchi S, Mobarhan S. Effects of diets containing fish oil and vitamin E on rheumatoid arthritis. Nutr Rev 2001; 59(10):335–341.

178. Townsend HB, Saag KG. Glucocorticoid use in rheumatoid arthritis: benefits, mechanism, and risks. Clin Exp Rheumatol 2004; 22(5 suppl 35): S77–S82.

179. Trail IA, Martín JA, Nuttall D, et al. Seventeen-year survivorship analysis of silastic metacarpophalangeal joint replacement. J Bone Joint Surg Br 2004; 87(7):1002–1006.

180. van Tubergen A, Landewe R, Heuft-Dorenbosch L, et al. Assessment of disability with the World Health Organization Disability Assessment Schedule II in patients with ankylosing spondylitis. Ann Rheum Dis 2003; 62(2):140–145.

181. van Tulder M, Koes B, Bombardier C. Low back pain. Best Pract Res Clin Rheumatol 2002; 16(5):761–775.

182. van der Linden S, van der Hiejde D, Braun J. Ankylosing spondylitis. In: Harris D, Budd C, Genovese MC, et al, eds. Kelley's textbook of rheumatology. 7th edn. Philadelphia: Elsevier; 2005:1125–1141.

183. Van Gestel AM, Prevoo ML, Van't Hof MA, et al. Development and validation of the European league against rheumatism response criteria for rheumatoid arthritis. Arthritis Rheum 1996; 39(1):34–40.

184. Vliet Vlieland TP. Multidisciplinary team care and outcomes in rheumatoid arthritis. Curr Opin Rheumatol 2004; 16(2):153–156.

185. Walker N, Mellick D, Brooks CA, et al. Measuring participation across impairment groups using the Craig Handicap Assessment Reporting Technique. Am J Phys Med Rehabil 2003; 82(12):936–941.

186. Watson T. The role of electrotherapy in contemporary physiotherapy practice. Man Ther 2000; 5(3):132–141.

187. Weiner DK, Ernst E. Complementary and alternative approaches to the treatment of persistent musculoskeletal pain. Clin J Pain 2004; 20(4): 244–255.

188. Williams P, Barclay L, Schmied V. Defining social support in context: a necessary step in improving research, intervention and practice. Qual Health Res 2004; 14(7):942–960.

189. Winson IG, Robinson DE, Allen PE. Arthroscopic ankle arthrodesis. J Bone Joint Surg Br 2005; 87(3):343–347.

190. Wolfe F, Pincus T, Thompson AK, et al. The assessment of rheumatoid arthritis and the acceptability of self-report questionnaires in clinical practice. Arthritis Rheum 2003; 49(1):59–63.

191. Wong JM. Management of stiff hand: an occupational therapy perspective. Hand Surg 2002; 7(2):261–269.

192. Woolf AD, Pfleger B. Burden of major musculoskeletal conditions. Bull World Health Organ 2003; 81(9):646–656.

193. World Health Organization. International Classification of Functioning, Disability and Health. Online. Available: http://www.who.org Feb 2002.

194. World Health Organization. The burden of musculoskeletal conditions at the start of the new millennium. World Health Organ Tech Rep Ser 2003; 919.

195. Wortmann RL. Inflammatory diseases of muscle and other myopathies. In: Harris D, Budd C, Genovese MC, et al, eds. Kelley's textbook of rheumatology. 7th edn. Philadelphia: Elsevier; 2005:1309–1335.

196. Zijlstra TR, Heijnsdijk-Rouwenhorst L, Rasker JJ. Silver ring splints improve dexterity in patients with rheumatoid arthritis. Arthritis Rheum 2004; 51(6):947–951.

197. Zurier RB, Rossetti RG, Jacobson EW, et al. Gamma-linolenic acid treatment of rheumatoid arthritis. A randomized, placebo-controlled trial. Arthritis Rheum 1996; 39(11):1808–1817.

Chapter

38

Treatment of Common Neck Problems

Michael J. DePalma and Curtis W. Slipman

INTRODUCTION AND EPIDEMIOLOGY

Successful treatment of cervical spinal disorders requires an accurate assessment of the underlying spinal condition, which can involve a broad range of biomechanical and biochemical disorders. The clinician needs to conceptualize a process of diagnosis and treatment that incorporates an understanding of the pathophysiology of cervical spine injury and the associated potential symptom manifestations, an awareness of the advantages and disadvantages of the myriad of diagnostic tools, and knowledge of the potential therapeutic alternatives. The initial step in this process is the history taking. It is important that one distinguish between axial cervical pain (neck pain) and upper limb pain. As eloquently stated by Bogduk,[26] the neck is not the upper limb, and the upper limb is not the neck. Pain in the upper limb is not pain in the neck, and vice versa.

Axial cervical pain must not be mistaken for cervical radicular pain. Cervical axial pain is defined as pain occurring in all or part of a corridor extending from the inferior occiput inferiorly to the superior interscapular region, localizing to the midline or just paramidline. The patient perceives it as stemming from the neck. Cervical radicular pain, defined as pain involving the shoulder girdle and distally, manifests as pain in the upper limb. The etiologies of these two different sets of symptoms vary, as does the diagnosis and management of each. Equating cervical axial and cervical radicular pain can result in misdiagnosis, inappropriate investigation, and institution of suboptimal treatment.[26] Such confusion can easily occur, because both disorders result from injury to the cervical spine. Each of these injuries or conditions differs in occurrence, mechanism, pathophysiology, treatment, and rehabilitation.

Epidemiologic reports have sometimes clustered neck and limb pain, but neck complaints are ubiquitous. The prevalence of neck pain with or without upper limb pain ranges from 9 to 18% of the general population,[121,135,223,234] and one out of three individuals can recall at least one incidence of neck pain in their lifetime.[121] Cervical pain is more frequently encountered in clinical practice than low back pain is,[242] and traumatic neck pain becomes chronic in up to 40% of patients, with 8–10% experiencing severe pain.[49] The occurrence increases in the workplace, with a prevalence of 35–71% among Swedish forest and industrial workers.[91,93] The frequency of occupational cervical complaints increases with age. Approximately 25–30% of workers less than 30 years of age report neck stiffness, and 50% of workers over 45 years old report similar complaints.[92,223,234]

Cervical radiculopathy occurs less commonly, with an annual incidence of 83.2 per 100 000, and peaks at 50–54 years of age.[175] Five to ten percent of workers less than 30 years old complain of pain referring into the upper limb, while 25–40% of those over 45 years experience pain in the upper limb.[92] Overall, 23% of working men have experienced at least one episode of upper limb pain.[92] Neck pain and/or cervical radicular pain are common complaints across different patient profiles.

Evaluating and treating common cervical spine conditions calls for a probability analysis of what injured structure is most likely causing the patient's complaints. An astute spine clinician recognizes individual symptom composites to accurately diagnose and treat these injuries. This chapter is intended to be a foundation for approaching common cervical spine disorders, and provides a view of a tiered treatment algorithm that incorporates both conservative and invasive interventions.

PATHOPHYSIOLOGY OF CERVICAL PAIN AND THE SIGNIFICANCE OF REFERRAL PATTERNS

A working knowledge of the anatomic interrelationships within the cervical spine (Fig. 38-1) is important in order to comprehend the pathomechanisms of cervical spine disorders. The cervical spine is a discrete segment of the axial skeleton (Fig. 38-2), and functions to support and stabilize the head; allow the head to move in all planes of motion; and protect the spinal cord, nerve roots, spinal nerves, and vertebral arteries.[163] There are seven cervical vertebrae and eight cervical nerve roots. The atlantooccipital (C0–1) articulation permits 10° of flexion and 25° of extension. The C1–2 level or the atlantoaxial joint forms the upper cervical segment, and is responsible for 40–50% of all cervical axial rotation, demonstrated clinically by 45° of rotation in either direction.[54,55,63,236] Below the C2–3 level, lateral flexion of the cervical spine is coupled with rotation in the same direction. This spinal segment marks a transition where permitted motion changes from rotation to flexion, extension, and lateral bending.[63,228] This motion is accomplished by the 45° sagittal inclination of the cervical zygapophyseal joints.[137] The zygapophyseal joints allow motion within the

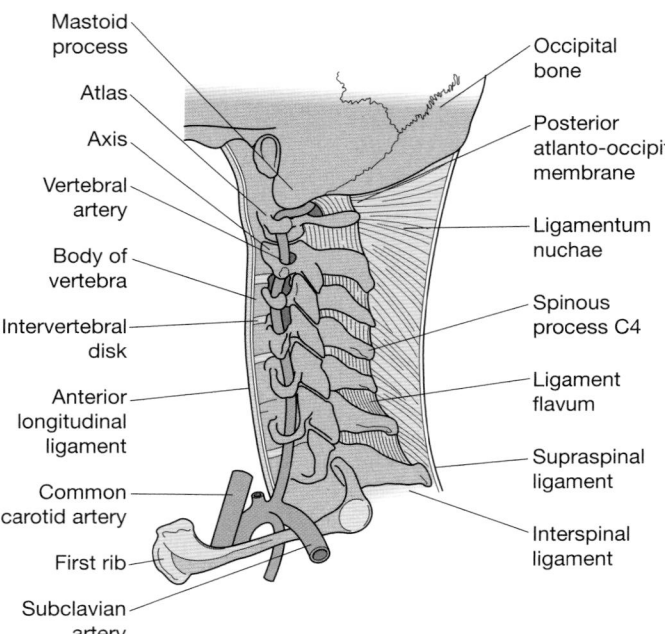

Figure 38-1 Anatomic relationship of cervical spine ligaments to other structures in the neck. (From Crafts 1979,[44] with permission of John Wiley.)

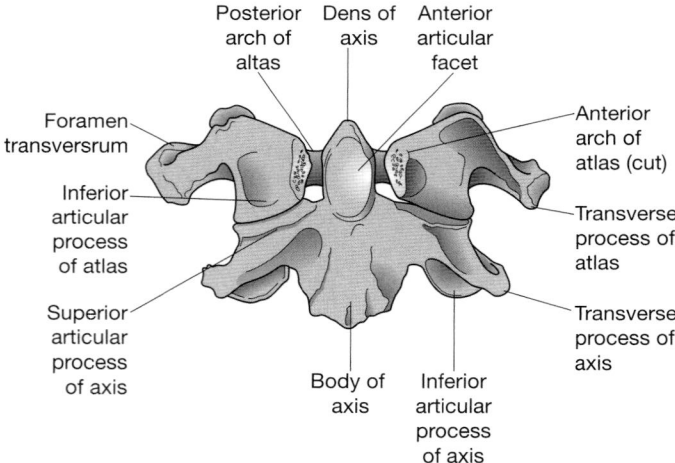

Figure 38-2 Anterior view of the atlas and axis. The anterior tubercle of the atlas has been removed to reveal the odontoid process of the axis. (From Crafts 1979,[44] with permission of John Wiley.)

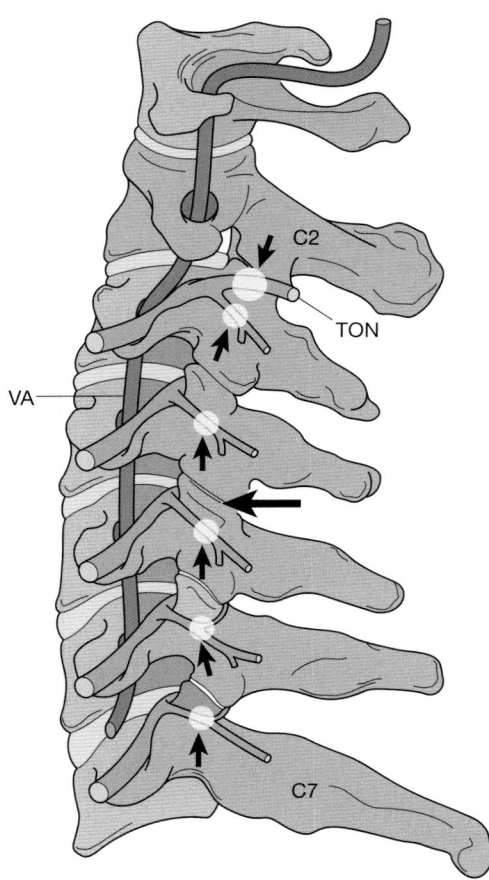

Figure 38-3 Target zones for cervical medial branch block. Lateral illustration of the cervical spine, showing target zones (arrows pointing to circles) located at the midportion of the C2 through C7 articular pillars. The third occipital nerve is a relatively large nerve branch that may require three separate blocks at the level of the C2 inferior facet–C3 superior facet and where it courses lateral to the C2–3 facet joint.

cervical spine, connect each vertebral segment,[202] and are innervated by medial branches from the cervical dorsal rami (Fig. 38-3).[27] In addition, the C0–1 joint is innervated by the C1 ventral ramus,[122] and the C1–2 joint by the C2 ventral ramus laterally[122] and the sinuvertebral nerves of C1, C2, and C3 medially.[112] The greatest amount of flexion occurs at C4–5 and C5–6, while lateral bending occurs primarily at C3–4 and C4–5.[63,228] The lower cervical vertebrae (C3–7) have unique synovial joint-like articulations, uncovertebral joints or joints of Luschka, located between the uncinate processes (Fig. 38-4).[153] These joints commonly develop osteoarthritic changes, which can narrow the diameter of the intervertebral foramina (Fig. 38-5).[74,90,219] These intervertebral foramina are widest at C2–3 and progressively decrease in size to the C6–7 level. The radicular complex of dorsal root ganglia, nerve roots, spinal nerve, and surrounding sheath accounts for 20–35% of the cross-sectional area of the intervertebral foramina.[74,90,219] The remaining intervertebral foramina volume is filled by loose areolar or adipose tissue, Hoffman's ligaments, radicular artery, and numerous venous conduits that usually encircle the nerve roots.[202] The neuroforamina are bordered anteromedially by the uncovertebral joint, superiorly and inferiorly by successive pedicles, and medially by the edge of the vertebral end plate and intervertebral disk (Fig. 38-5).[202]

The intervertebral disks are located between the vertebral bodies of C2 through C7. Each is composed of an outer annulus fibrosis innervated posterolaterally by the sinuvertebral nerve, comprising branches from the vertebral nerve and ventral ramus, and innervated anteriorly by the vertebral nerve (Fig. 38-6).[22] The inner portions of the disks comprise the gelatinous nucleus pulposus, providing transmission of axial loads to dissipate forces throughout various ranges of motion.[202] Each

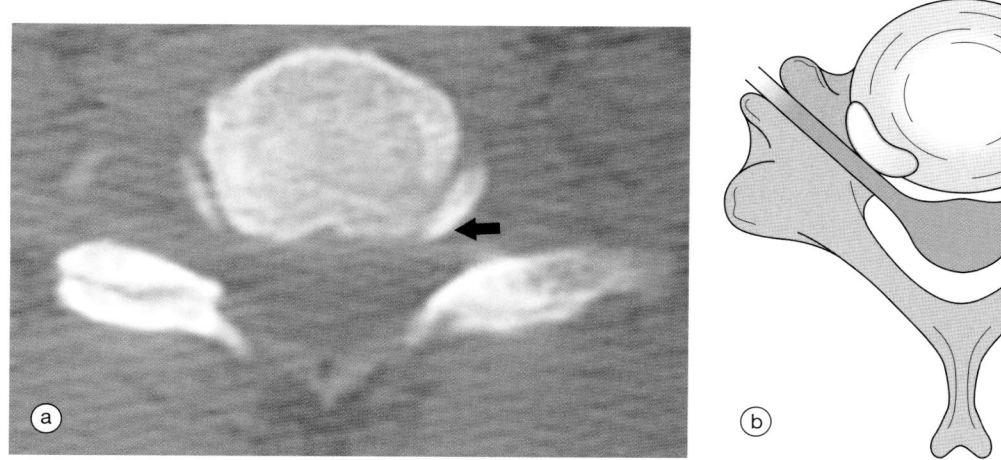

Figure 38-4 Luschka's (uncovertebral) joints. (**a**) The cervical spine, displaying Luschka's joint (arrow). (**b**) Proximity of uncovertebral joints (UV) to cervical nerve roots (NR). (Panel b from Macnab and McCulloch 1994,[134] with permission of Williams & Wilkins.)

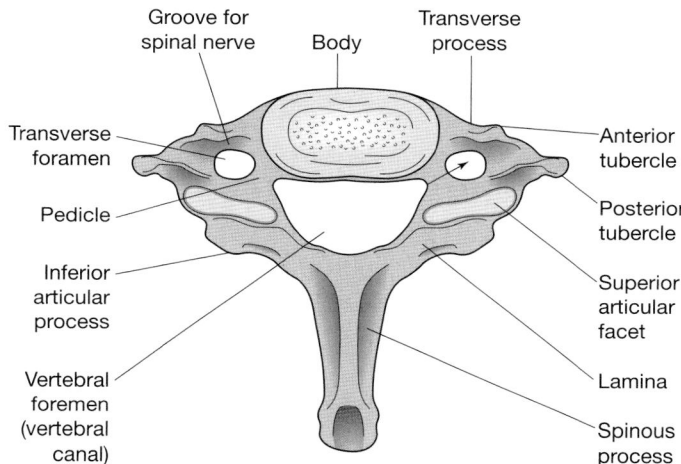

Figure 38-5 Axial view of the seventh cervical vertebrae, illustrating the intervertebral foramen (black arrow).

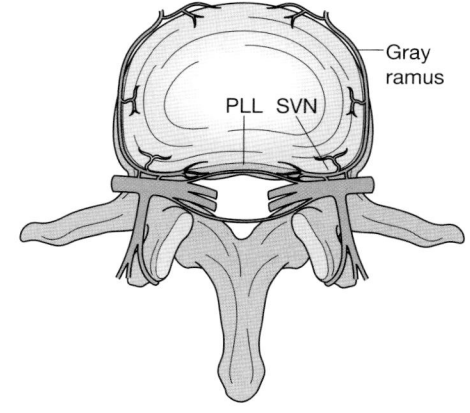

Figure 38-6 Nerve supply of the cervical intervertebral disk. ALL, anterior longitudinal ligament; PLL, posterior longitudinal ligament; SVN, sinovertebral nerve. (From Bogduk and Twomey 1991,[21] with permission.)

intervertebral disk is thicker anteriorly than posteriorly, which contributes to the natural cervical lordotic curvature.[202] Normal cervical spine anatomy can undergo degenerative or traumatic changes, leading to various cervical spine disorders.

Three essential requirements are needed for a structure to serve as a source of pain. It must be innervated, capable of producing pain similar to that seen clinically, and susceptible to disease or injury known to be painful.[25] Non-neural structures of the neck, such as the intervertebral disk, zygapophyseal joint, posterior longitudinal ligament, and muscles, can serve as a nidus for pain and produce somatic referral of pain into the upper limb.[34,62,108–110,119] Classic experiments have demonstrated that stimulation of these posterior midline structures produces local neck pain as well as somatically referred pain into the upper limb.[34,62,108–110,119] Kellegren was first to investigate the pain referral patterns of non-neural spinal structures by stimulating periosteum, fascia, tendon, and muscle with hypertonic saline.[109,110] He hypothesized that a central nervous system phe-

nomenon mediated the pain referral, because anesthetizing the corresponding peripheral nerve distal to the site of stimulation did not diminish the distally referred pain. These experiments were the first to demonstrate this phenomenon of somatically referred pain, and that cervical spinal disorders could produce pain in the upper limb as well as headache.[34,62,108–110,119] These symptoms were produced without irritation of neural tissue. Such pain referral has been termed *somatic*, previously labeled as sclerotomal, and occurs when a mesodermal structure such as a ligament, joint capsule, intervertebral disk annulus, or periosteum is stimulated, leading to symptoms referred into another mesodermal tissue structure of similar embryonic origin.[202] This mechanism of somatically referred symptoms involves convergence.[26] Afferents from both the cervical spine and the distal upper limb converge on second-order neurons within the spinal cord, allowing spinal pain to be misperceived as arising from those distal limb sites.[26] It is via this mechanism that cervical intervertebral disks and zygapophyseal joints create upper limb symptoms.[202]

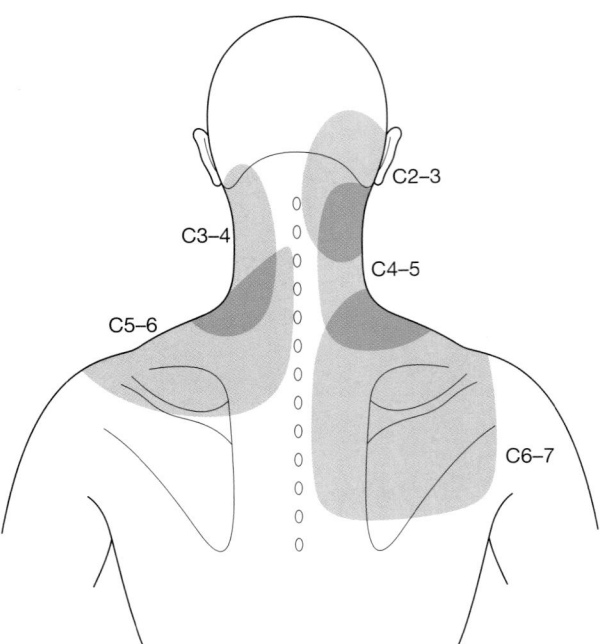

Figure 38-7 Pain referral from C2 to C3 through C6–C7 facet joints. (From Dwyer et al. 1990,[56] with permission.)

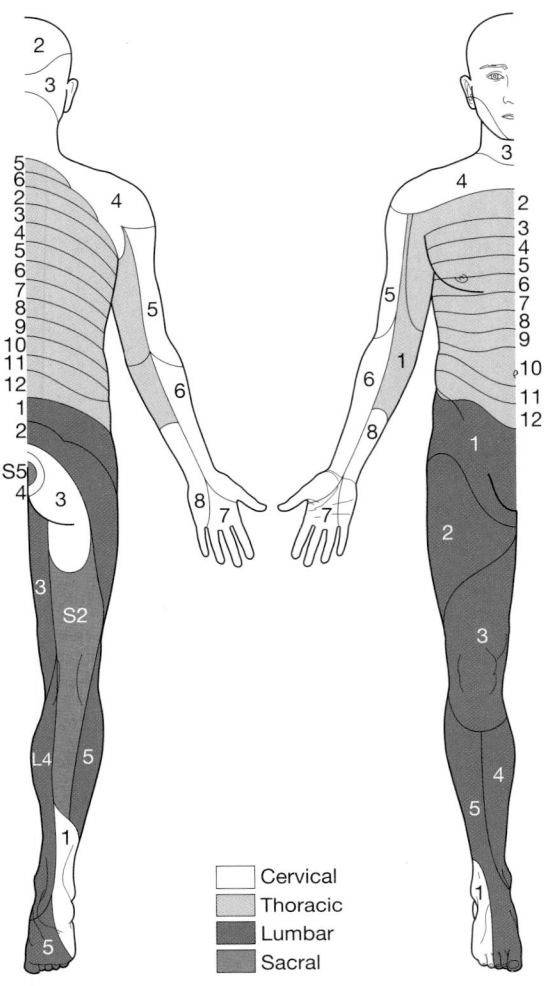

Figure 38-8 Dermatomal distribution of the cervical nerve roots. (From Ellis 1976,[58] with permission of Blackwell.)

It is believed that biomechanical and/or biochemical insults to non-neural structures can trigger nociceptive nerve fibers, via compression or inflammation, causing pain referral.[202] Mechanical stimulation of the cervical zygapophyseal joints or their innervating nerves has been shown to produce head and neck pain with upper limb referral patterns (Fig. 38-7).[9,53,56,66] Anesthetizing symptomatic joints has revealed similar patterns of symptomatic referral from the cervical joints.[20,205]

Pain emanating from the cervical zygapophyseal joints tends to follow relatively constant and recognizable referral patterns. The C1–2 and C2–3 levels refer rostrally to the occiput. The C3–4 and C4–5 joints produce symptoms over the posterior neck. Pain from the C5–6 joint spreads over the supraspinatus fossa of the scapula, whereas pain from the C6–7 joint spreads further caudally over the scapula.[9,20,26,53,56,66] Additionally, C1–2, C2–3, C3–4, and C4–5 zygapophyseal joints can refer pain to the face, and C3–4, C4–5, and C5–6 can refer symptoms to the head.[20] Each joint can produce unilateral or bilateral symptomatology. It is not intuitive that a unilateral joint could trigger only contralateral pain, and this manifestation has never been formally investigated.[204]

Very similar pain patterns have been produced by mechanical stimulation of the cervical intervertebral disks (Fig. 38-8).[40,72,188] In our experience, bilateral paramidline upper neck pain without associated headaches is commonly due to cervical intervertebral disk disruption (CIDD) rather than zygapophyseal joint-mediated pain. Our observations are supported by Grubb's recent study that found that 34–50% of cervical disks produced bilateral pain at each cervical disk level.[72] Furthermore, a more detailed study from the Penn Spine Center revealed that 30–62% of cervical disks produced bilateral pain during cervical diskography.[210] When taken together, these findings support the notion that the pattern of pain stemming from a particular structure is a consequence of that structure's innervation rather than the structure itself.[26] In line with this logic is the finding that stimulation of the upper cervical musculature can produce pain in the head.[46] Discriminating CIDD-mediated pain from zygapophyseal joint pain or pain emanating from the cervical spine soft tissues requires systematic and meticulous interpretation of history and physical examination findings.

Cervical radicular pain is a fundamentally different clinical picture, because the presenting chief complaint is typically upper limb pain. The etiology of upper limb symptoms can be confusing when a non-radicular disorder creates symptoms in a radicular distribution, or when a usually radicular disorder causes pain in an uncharacteristic dermatomal pattern (dynatomal pattern—pattern of referred symptoms).[211] Regardless, radicular pain is most consistent with arm symptoms that are more intense than axial complaints.[202] Upper limb pain due to cervical radiculopathy can refer symptoms into the arm, forearm, and/or hand (Fig. 38-9).[57] However, periscapular or trapezial pain greater than neck pain can be due to upper cervi-

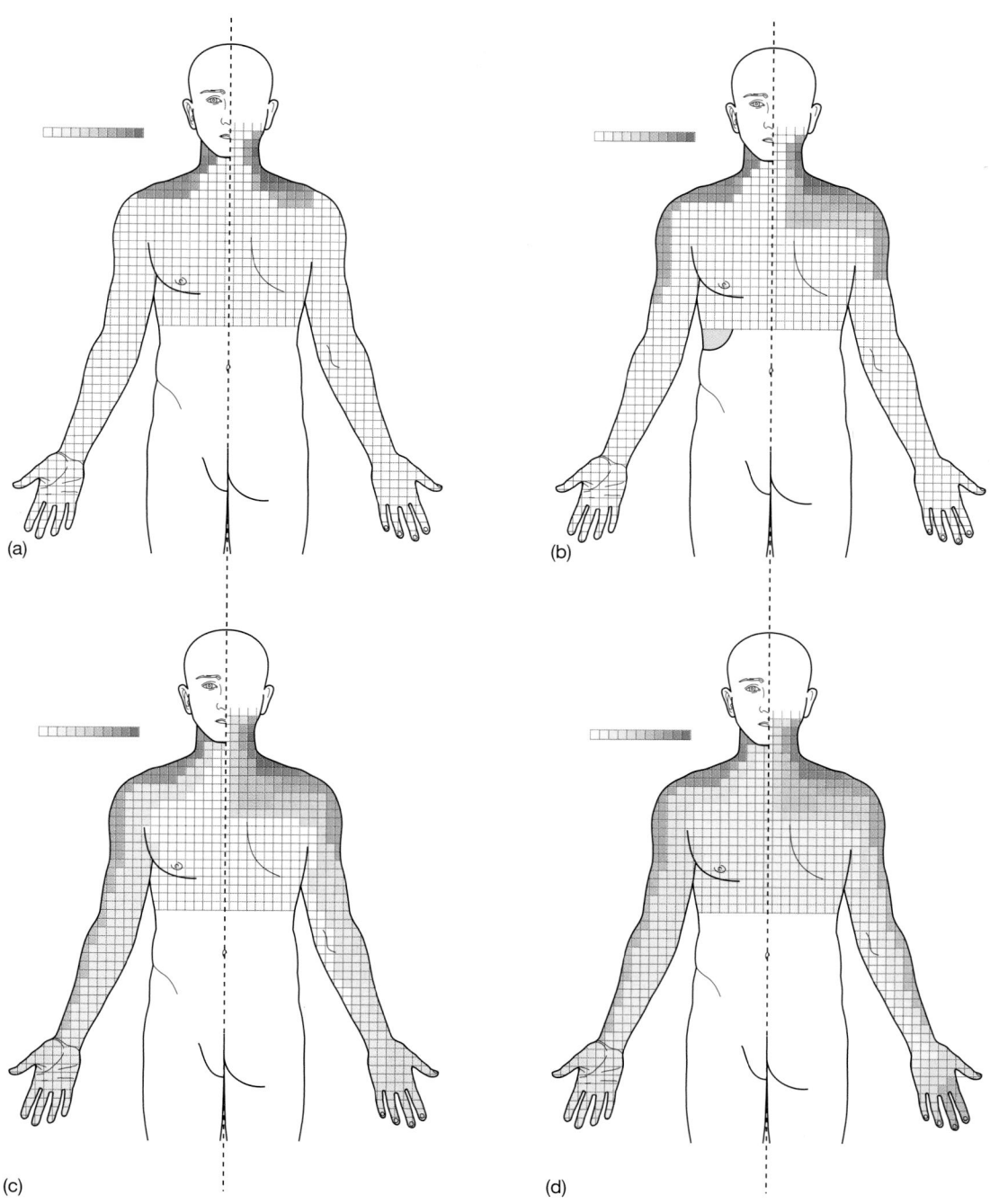

Figure 38-9 Dynatomal mapping of cervical radicular pain from mechanical stimulation of cervical nerve roots C4 (**a**), C5 (**b**), C6 (**c**), and C7 (**d**). (Courtesy of CW Slipman, M.D.)

cal nerve root involvement such as C4 or C5.[211] Radicular pain from C5 tends to remain in the arm, but pain from C6, C7, and C8 extends into the forearm and hand. Nevertheless, pain that is primarily in the upper back with or without arm symptoms can emanate from the C4 through C6 roots. When experienced in the middle to lower aspect of the ipsilateral scapula, C7 or C8 roots could be the culprit.

Nerve vulnerability within the intervertebral foramina arises consequent to changes in one or more of three separate structures: the zygapophyseal joints, the uncovertebral joints, and the intervertebral disk. The most common cause of cervical radiculopathy is a herniated cervical intervertebral disk,[94] followed by cervical spondylosis[245] with or without cervical myelopathy (Box 38-1). The precise mechanism by which disk herniation or spondylosis causes radicular pain is still unclear. Direct neurocompression of the nerve root does not necessarily cause pain,[89] and pure myotomal weakness can occur.[127] Proposed mechanisms for pain in cervical radiculopathy include nerve root inflammation,[26] increased discharge of the dorsal root ganglion, mechano- or chemosensitivity of the nerve root

---

Box 38-1 Disorders affecting the neck

Mechanical
- Cervical sprain
- Cervical strain
- Herniated nucleus pulposus
- Osteoarthritis
- Cervical spondylosis
- Cervical stenosis

Rheumatologic
- Ankylosing spondylitis
- Reiter syndrome
- Psoriatic arthritis
- Enteropathic arthritis
- Rheumatoid arthritis
- Diffuse idiopathic skeletal hyperostosis
- Polymyalgia rheumatica
- Fibrositis (fibromyalgia)

Infectious
- Vertebral osteomyelitis
- Diskitis
- Herpes zoster
- Infective endocarditis
- Granulomatous process
- Epidural, intradural, and subdural abscesses
- Retropharyngeal abscess
- AIDS

Endocrinologic and metabolic
- Osteoporosis
- Osteomalacia
- Parathyroid disease
- Paget disease
- Pituitary disease

Tumors
Benign tumors
- Osteochondroma
- Osteoid osteoma

- Osteoblastoma
- Giant cell tumor
- Aneurysmal bone cyst
- Hermangioma
- Eosinophilic granuloma
- Gaucher disease

Malignant tumors
- Multiple myeloma
- Solitary plasmacytoma
- Chondrosarcoma
- Ewing sarcoma
- Chordoma
- Lymphoma
- Metastases

Extradural tumors
- Epidural hemangioma
- Epidural lipoma
- Meningioma
- Neurofibroma
- Lymphoma

Intradural tumors
- Extramedullary, intradural
  Neurofibroma
  Meningioma
  Ependymoma
  Sarcoma
- Intramedullary
  Ependymoma
  Astrocytoma

Others
- Arteriovenous malformations
- Syringomyelia

---

itself, or direct pressure on chronically injured axons or on a normal dorsal root ganglion.[89,177] Other potential causes of cervical radiculopathy include tumor,[231] trauma,[170] sarcoidosis,[10] arteritis,[186] and athetoid or dystonic cerebral palsy.[65]

Cervical intervertebral disk injury can be categorized into two broad categories: internal disruption and herniation. *Disk herniation* is a generalized term, which is further divided into protrusion, extrusion, and sequestration (Fig. 38-10). A more thorough discussion of disk herniation occurs below. Internal disk disruption is a descriptive phrase used to detail pathologic changes within the nucleus pulposus and/or annular fibers with little or no external deformation.[45] The process of disk degeneration occurs over a spectrum of disk abnormalities (Fig. 38-11). Initially, circumferential outer annular tears secondary to repetitive microtrauma are associated with interruption in blood and nutritional supply to the disk. These tears eventually coalesce to form radial tears occurring concurrently with a decrement in the water-imbibing ability of the nucleus pulposus. The mechanical integrity of the intervertebral disk suffers

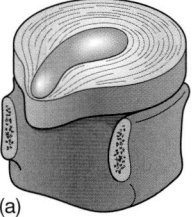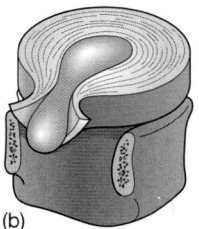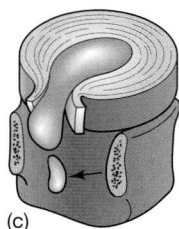

(a)   (b)   (c)

Figure 38-10 Cervical intervertebral disk herniations: (**a**) small subligamentous herniation or protrusion, (**b**) extrusion, and (**c**) sequestered fragment (arrow).

as disk space narrows, more tears develop, and type 2 proteoglycans continue to be destroyed.[113] Biochemical insults have been purported to occur prior to these biomechanical alterations.[185] The end result is a cervical disk that is biomechanically incompetent and prone to biochemical insult.

Cervical zygapophyseal joint injury can occur due to osteoarthritis or trauma resulting from both macrotraumatic and

Sagittal view

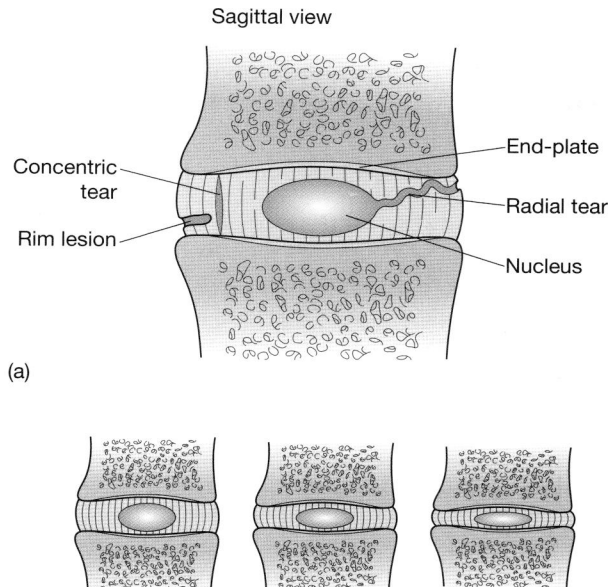

(a)

(b)

Figure 38-11 Intervertebral disk degeneration. (**a**) Sagittal view. Concentric tears eventually coalesce to form radial tears. (**b**) This leads to disk space collapse.

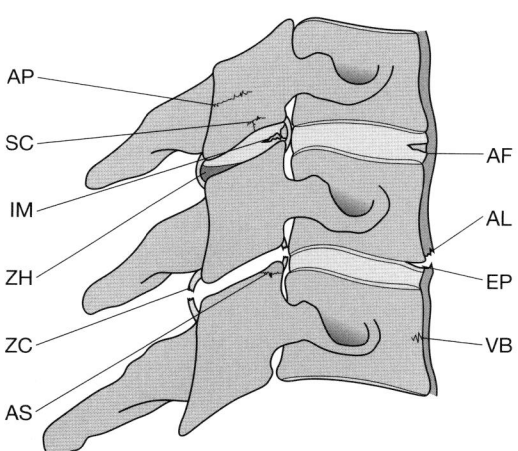

Figure 38-12 The more common lesions affecting the cervical spine following whiplash: AF, tear of the annulus fibrosus of the intervertebral disc; AL, tear of the anterior longitudinal ligament; AP, articular pillar fracture; AS, fracture involving the articular surface; EP, endplate avulsion/fracture; IM, contusion of the intra-articular meniscus of the zygapophyseal joint; SC, fracture of the subchondral plate; VB, vertebral body fracture; ZC, rupture or tear of the zygapophyseal joint capsule; ZH, hemarthrosis of the zygapophyseal joint.

microtraumatic events. Acceleration–deceleration zygapophyseal joint injuries can result in osseous injury to the articular pillars, articular surface, or subchondral bone; intraarticular hemarthrosis; contusion of the intraarticular meniscus; or tears of the zygapophyseal joint capsule (Fig. 38-12).[1,2,17,38,98,120] We have successfully treated patients suffering from cervical zygapophyseal joint synovitis, who had experienced the onset of

symptoms on awakening after sleeping in an awkward position. Painful cervical zygapophyseal joint arthropathy can result as a consequence of cervical intervertebral disk degeneration as well. Biochemical and biomechanical effects can both cause cervical zygapophyseal joint symptom manifestation.

COMMON CLINICAL DISORDERS

Cervical strain and sprains

Epidemiology

A cervical strain is a musculotendinous injury produced by an overload injury due to excessive forces imposed on the cervical spine.[43] In contrast, cervical sprains are overstretching or tearing injuries of spinal ligaments. Muscular strains are seen most frequently because many cervical muscles do not terminate in tendons, but rather attach directly to bone via myofascial tissue that blends seamlessly with periosteum.[171] Cervical sprain and strain injuries account for approximately 85% of neck pain resultant from acute, repetitive, or chronic neck injuries.[97] These injuries are the most common type of injury to motor vehicle occupants in the USA,[173] and are one of the most common causes of pain after non-catastrophic sports injuries.[43] Approximately one-third of motor vehicle accident victims develop neck pain within 24 h of the injury.[193] Automobile-related cervical strain and sprain injuries are more common in western societies and in metropolitan areas having higher densities of motor vehicles.[218] The incidence is higher in women and individuals 30–50 years old.[218]

Pathophysiology

Differing pathomechanisms are causal in cervical strain and sprain injuries, depending on the nature of the abnormal stress applied to the cervical spine. Acceleration–deceleration injuries result in excursions of the cervical spine that result in an S-shaped curvature approximately 100 ms after a rear-end impact.[105] By 200–250 ms after impact, the head initiates forward flexion of the neck after maximally extending to approximately 45°.[142] Posterior neck muscle activation occurs by 90–120 ms[222] and coincides with the deceleration of the head moving forward.[142] As the head continues to move forward, the neck extensors eccentrically contract to decelerate the head, placing them at increased risk of injury (Fig. 38-13).[156] These experimental findings lend support for a simple muscle or ligamentous strain injury during motor vehicle accidents. Partial and complete muscle tears and hemorrhage have been visualized by ultrasound[139] and magnetic resonance imaging (MRI),[168] and observed in postmortem examinations.[102] Tears of the anterior longitudinal ligament have been reported in surgical explorations[30] and identified at postmortem.[29] Anatomic studies have demonstrated that the anterior longitudinal ligament merges imperceptibly with the intervertebral disks and can be injured with injury to the cervical disk.[178]

Physiologic forces acting on a relatively normal cervical spine result in typical soft tissue strain seen in non-athletes. In individuals with thoracic kyphosis and consequential cervical lordosis and extension, strain occurs in the levator scapulae, superior

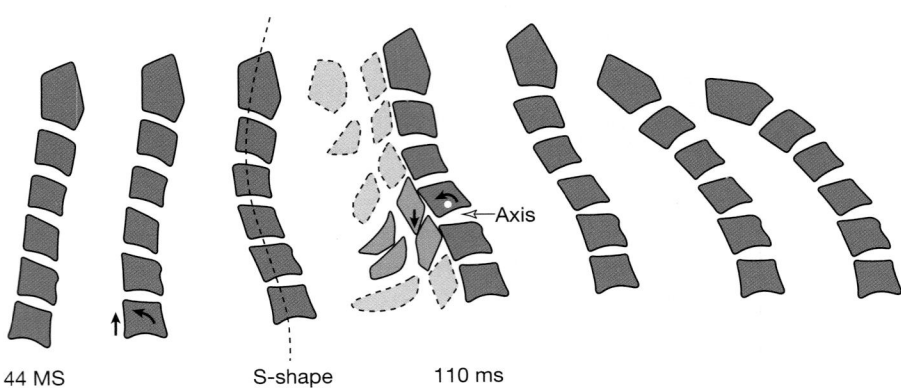

44 MS   S-shape   110 ms

←Axis

Figure 38-13 The appearance of sequential radiographs of the cervical spine during the extension phase of whiplash. At 110 ms, the C5 vertebra rotates about an abnormally high axis of rotation, causing the vertebral body to separate anteriorly from C6 (white arrow), and the inferior articular process of C5 to chisel into the superior articular process of C6 (black arrow). (After Kaneoka et al. 1997,[105] with permission).

trapezius, sternocleidomastoid, scalene, and suboccipital muscles.[43] Traumatic blows often incurred in sporting injuries can result in a more acute cervical strain or sprain.[43] Repetitive motions, as occur in recreational activities, can tax shortened and deconditioned cervical rotators, extensors, and lateral flexors that are frequently present in those with cervical spondylosis.[43]

Diagnosis

The history and physical examination findings guide the treating clinician in diagnosing cervical soft tissue injury. A thorough history of the mechanism of injury should be elicited from the patient. An acute event such as a motor vehicle accident, sports injury, fall, or industrial accident can create forces significant enough to injury cervical soft tissues. Details that should be sought are the exact onset of pain relative to a traumatic event, location of the symptoms, any referral pattern, or other associated symptoms. Cervical strain and sprain injuries can be associated with headaches. These headaches are typically sharp or dull and localize to the cervical or shoulder girdle musculature. The patient can also report neck fatigue or stiffness that lessens with gradual activity. Aggravating factors include passive or active motion.

Decreased cervical range of motion can be detected on gross examination. This is due to muscle guarding and splinting to avoid pain. Palpation of the involved region is usually uncomfortable or moderately painful. The most commonly involved areas are the upper trapezius and sternocleidomastoid muscles. Neurologic signs are typically absent, and neuroforaminal closure techniques should not elicit referral pain into the distal upper limb. Motor examination can reveal give-way weakness due to pain, but this pattern can be differentiated from true neuromuscular weakness.

Further diagnostic testing such as imaging or electrodiagnostic evaluations are not indicated unless neurologic or motor abnormalities are detected, or significant pain into the limbs is reported. Plain radiography would be ordered first to evaluate for bony malalignment or fractures. It is reasonable to examine cervical flexion and extension x-rays to evaluate for instability prior to prescribing functional restoration. In most instances, these images are normal or reveal non-specific loss of cervical lordosis due to muscle splinting (Fig. 38-14).

Treatment

Initial care includes controlling pain and inflammation to curb the injury response, mitigate deconditioning, and facilitate active participation in a functional restoration program. Nonsteroidal antiinflammatory drugs (NSAIDs) and acetaminophen (paracetamol) aid in controlling pain and nurturing restorative sleep patterns. We do not typically prescribe muscle relaxants, but some clinicians utilize these medications to improve sleep. If patients complain of substantial 'spasm' not ameliorated by analgesics and proper positioning, tizanidine or tricyclic antidepressants might be successful.

Physical modalities such as massage, superficial and deep heat, electrical stimulation, and a soft cervical collar can be employed in the treatment program. Light massage causes sedation, reduction of adhesions, muscular relaxation, and vascular changes (see Ch. 20).[241] Superficial heat[123] and deep heat with ultrasound[60] produce analgesia and muscle relaxation, help resolve inflammation, and increase connective tissue elasticity (see Ch. 21). Transcutaneous electrical nerve stimulation (TENS) can also be effective in modulating musculoskeletal pain (see Ch. 22).[136] A soft cervical collar can be prescribed to ease painful sleep disturbances and reduce further neck strain. The collar can be worn while awake, but should be restricted to the first 72 h after the injury to minimize interference with healing and prevent development of soft tissue tightening.[144] A gradual return to activities should be initiated by 2–4 weeks after injury, and should include a functional restoration program to address postural reeducation and functional biomechanical deficits.[43]

Once the acute pain has improved, proper spinal biomechanics must be restored with the establishment of proper movement patterns. Healthy cervical segmental motion requires efficient stabilization throughout the cervical and thoracic spines. Proprioceptive retraining, balance, and postural conditioning should be incorporated into the exercise regimen. Flexibility and range of motion are improved by mobilization and stretching exercises. Proprioception is improved by utilizing visual feedback during exercises and functional tasks. These should be performed with simultaneous dynamic demands on the patient's base of support.[43,116] Such a program (Table 38-1) enhances the healthy dissipation of forces across the cervical spine with efficient myofascial efforts.

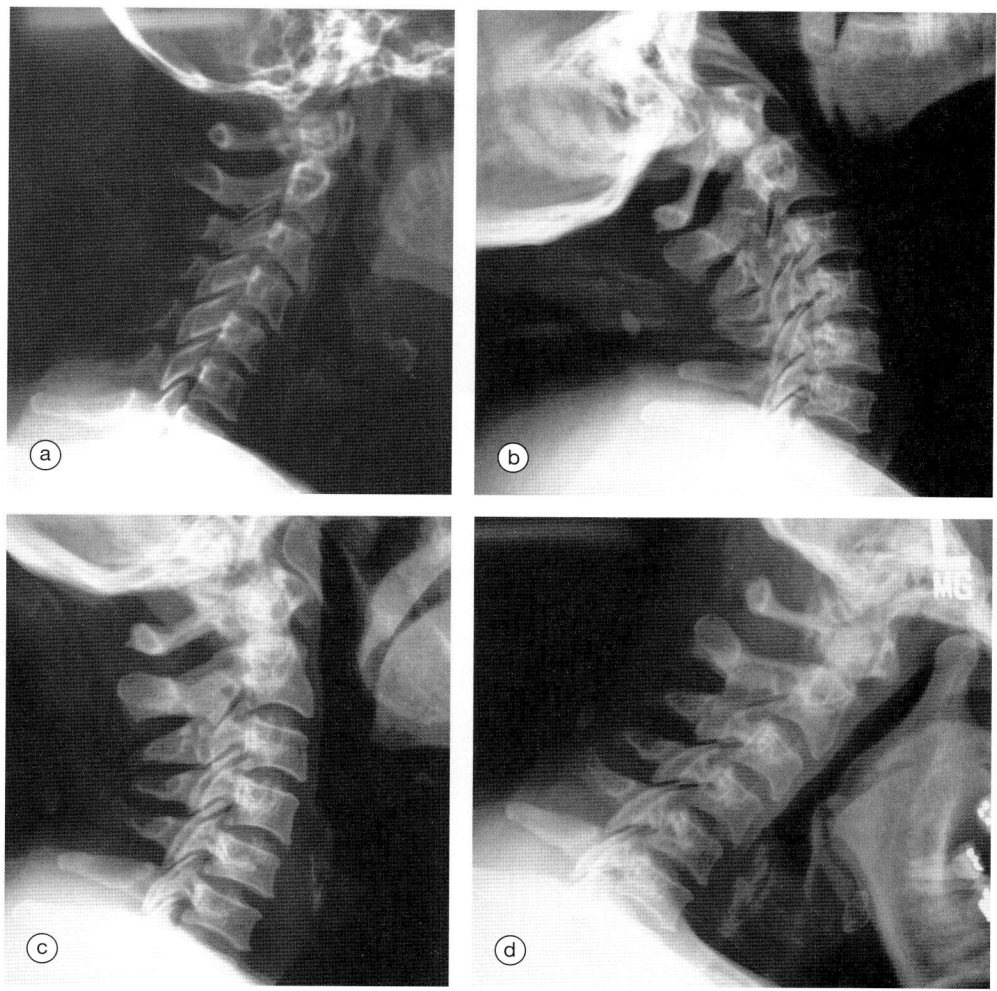

Figure 38-14 Lateral plain radiographs of the cervical spine, showing decreased lordosis (**a**), extension (**b**), neutral (**c**), and flexion (**d**).

Cervical radiculopathy and radicular pain

Epidemiology

Cervical radiculopathy is a pathologic process involving neurophysiologic dysfunction of the nerve root.[57] Signs and symptoms of cervical radiculopathy include myotomal weakness, paresthesias, sensory disturbances, and muscle stretch reflex changes.[57] Cervical radicular pain is not necessarily caused by a loss of nerve root function. Cervical radiculopathy, on the other hand, involves reflex and strength changes due to pathologic changes in nerve root function.[26] Separating cervical radicular pain from cervical radiculopathy is important, because it can change the treatment strategies.

A large epidemiologic study of 561 patients in Rochester, Minnesota, found an average annual age-adjusted incidence of cervical radiculopathy of 83.2 per 100 000 for cervical radiculopathy.[175] The peak incidence occurred between the ages of 50 and 54 years in the study cohort.[175] A history of trauma or physical exertion preceding the onset of symptoms occurred in just under 15% of patients.[175] The order of decreasing frequency of involved levels was C7, C6, C8, and C5.[175]

Pathophysiology

Cervical nerve root injury is most commonly due to cervical intervertebral disk herniation (CIDH)[94] and secondly to spondylitic spinal changes (Fig. 38-15).[245] The causal role of neural compression in CIDH-induced radiculopathy was first introduced by Semmes and Murphey in 1943.[194] Subsequent radiologic studies have demonstrated the existence of asymptomatic cervical disk abnormalities.[18,140,145,225] A growing body of evidence has emerged attesting to the etiologic role of an inflammatory response to a CIDH in some way triggering painful radicular signs and symptoms.[67,106,107] Animal studies have shown disrupted nerve root physiology due to gradient pressure[183] and inflammation in the absence of compression.[160] Nerve roots are anatomically less resilient than peripheral nerves to both biomechanical and biochemical insults, and respond to each with the same pathologic sequence of events.[154]

Cervical spondylosis (or degenerative osteoarthritic changes) is manifested by ligamentous hypertrophy, hyperostosis (bony overgrowth), disk degeneration, and zygapophyseal joint arthropathy.[245] Hypertrophy of the zygapophyseal joints and

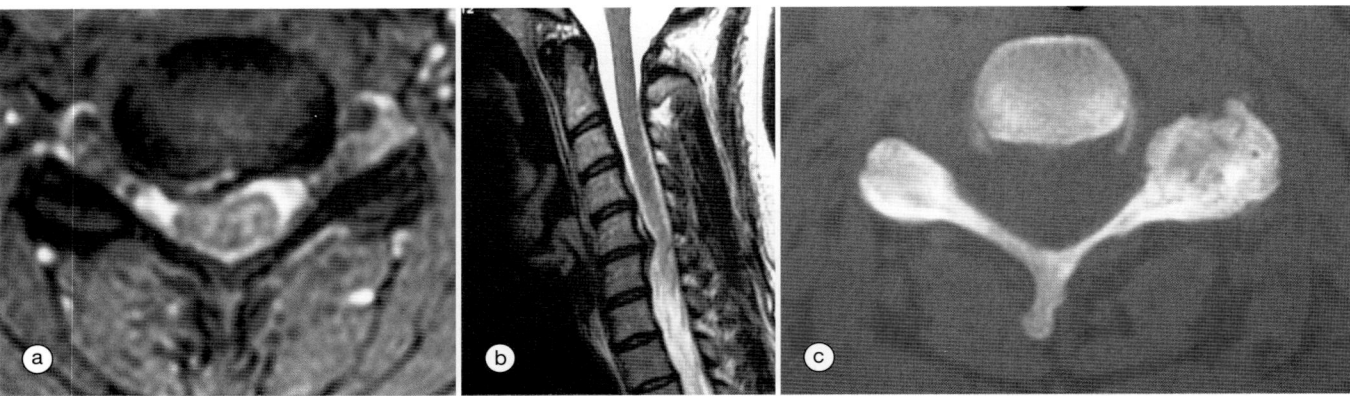

Figure 38-15 Axial (**a**) and sagittal (**b**) magnetic resonance imaging views revealing a central and rightward C5–6 intervertebral disk extrusion. (**c**) Axial computed tomography view of the C3–4 segmental level, revealing moderate to severe left C4 foraminal stenosis due to zygapophyseal joint arthrosis and uncovertebral joint hypertrophy.

Table 38-1 Cervicothoracic stabilization exercises

Type of exercise	Cervicothoracic stabilization level		
	Level 2 (basic)	Level 2 (intermediate)	Level 3 (advanced)
Direct cervical stabilization	Cervical active range of motion	Cervical gravity	Cervical active
	Cervical isometrics	Resisted isometrics	Range gravity-resisted
Indirect cervical stabilization exercises			
Supine, head supported	Theraband chest press	Unsupported dying bug	Chest flies
	Bilateral arm raise		Bench press
	Supported dying bug		Incline dumbbell press
Sit	Reciprocal arm raise	Swiss ball reciprocal	Swiss ball bilateral
	Unilateral arm raise	Arm raises	Shoulder shrugs
	Bilateral arm raise	Chest press	Supraspinatus raises
	Seated row		
	Latissimus pull-down		
Stand	Theraband reciprocal	Standing rowing	Upright row
	Chest press	Biceps pull-down	Shoulder shrugs
	Theraband straight arm latissimus pull-down		Supraspinatus raises
	Theraband chest press		
	Theraband latissimus pull-down		
	Standing rowing		
	Crossovers		
	Triceps press		
Flexed hip-hinge position	0–30°	30–60°	60–90°
	Reciprocal arm raise	Incline prone flies	Bilateral anterior
	Unilateral arm raise	Reciprocal deltoid raise	Deltoid raises
	Bilateral arm raise	Cable crossovers	Interscapular flies
	Interscapular flies		
Prone	Reciprocal arm raise	Quadruped	Head supported
	Unilateral arm raise	Head unsupported	Prone flies
	Bilateral arm raise	Swiss ball bilateral	Latissimus flies
		Anterior deltoid raises	
		Swiss ball prone	
		Rowing	
		Swiss ball prone flies	
Supine, head unsupported	Not advised for level 1	Partial sit-ups	Swiss ball chest flies
		Arm raises	Swiss ball reciprocal

(From Sweeney et al. 1990,[220] with permission of Hanley & Belfus.)

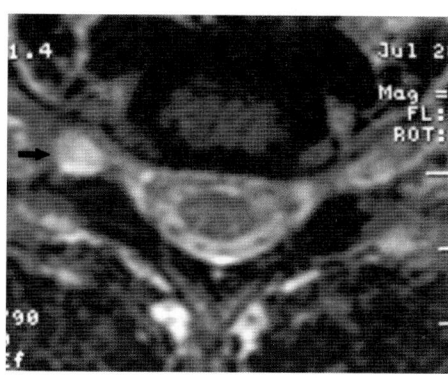

Figure 38-16 Axial view of the C7–T1 intervertebral disk, revealing an apparent zygapophyseal joint cyst (black arrow) emanating from the right C7–T1 joint.

Table 38-2	Nerve root levels, peripheral nerves, and muscles of the upper limb commonly evaluated in the patient with neck pain	
Nerve root level	Nerve	Muscle
C5, C6	Axillary	Deltoid
C5, C6	Musculocutaneous	Biceps brachii
C5, C6	Suprascapular Suprascapular	Supraspinatus Infraspinatus
C7	Radial Median	Triceps Pronator teres
C8, T1	Median Ulnar	Abductor pollicis brevis First dorsal interossei

uncovertebral joints results in intervertebral foramina stenosis and nerve root impingement.[202,245] Vertebral body osteophytes and disk material can form a 'hard disk' that can also compress the adjacent nerve root.[175,245] Although cervical zygapophyseal joint cysts are rare,[132] patients with cervical zygapophyseal joint-induced radiculopathy have been treated at the Penn Spine Center (Fig. 38-16). In these cases, it is not clear to what extent biochemical versus biomechanical influences affect the neural elements.

Diagnosis

History and physical examination   Patients suffering from acute CIDH-related radiculopathy typically report a history of axial cervical pain that is typically followed by an explosive onset of upper limb pain. In contrast, spondylitic radicular pain presents more gradually. Cervical radicular pain can masquerade as a deep dull ache or sharp lacinating pain. It can occur in a number of locations, including the medial scapular edge (C5–7), superior trapezius (C5–6), precordium (C5–6), deltoid and lateral arm (C5–6), posteromedial arm (C7–T1), anterolateral forearm (C6–7), posterior forearm (C7–8), and any of the upper extremity digits (C6–T1).[57,211]

Exacerbating factors include activities that raise subarachnoid pressure, such as coughing, sneezing, or Valsalva maneuvers. If a significant component of stenosis is present, cervical extension can amplify the symptoms. Alleviation of the radicular pain by elevating the ipsilateral humerus is known as the shoulder abduction relief sign.[48,61]

The physical examination begins with the clinical observation of neck position, as patients characteristically tilt toward the side of the disk herniation. Atrophy can be detected with more severe or longstanding lesions. Muscle wasting in the supra- or infrascapular fossae or deltoid suggests C5 or C6 involvement; triceps in C7 injury; thenar eminence in C8; and first dorsal interossei in T1.[175] Manual muscle testing has greater specificity than reflex or sensory abnormalities (Table 38-2),[243] and might need to be performed repetitively or with the muscle at a mechanical disadvantage to elicit subtle weakness. Severe weakness (<3/5 MRC) is less consistent with a single root lesion, and should alert the clinician to the presence of a possible multilevel radiculopathy, alpha motor neuron disease, plexopathy, or focal peripheral neuropathy. Sensation to light touch, pinprick, and

vibration can be altered. The patient should be assessed for the presence of long tract signs such as Hoffman's sign and Babinski's response to ensure that there is no spinal cord involvement.

Provocative maneuvers such as neuroforaminal closure and root tension signs help localize the lesion to the cervical spine. Spurling's maneuver,[216] cervical extension, lateral flexion, and ipsilateral axial rotation reproducing radicular symptoms is highly specific but not sensitive for cervical radiculopathy.[232] L'hermitte's sign,[126] which is rapid passive cervical flexion while the patient is seated, can produce an electric shock sensation down the spine and occasionally into the limbs in patients with cervical cord involvement due to tumor, spondylosis, or multiple sclerosis.[164]

Imaging studies   Although plain cervical radiography is not very sensitive in detecting disk pathology, it remains the initial radiographic examination in almost every assessment of musculoskeletal injury.[151] Plain films of anteroposterior, lateral, open mouth, and flexion and extension views are indicated to evaluate spinal stability in cases of rheumatoid arthritis or ankylosing spondylitis,[57] spondylolisthesis, post fusion, or after traumatic injury.[151] Computed tomographic myelography is regarded as the gold standard against which other imaging modalities ought to be judged in evaluating degenerative cervical spine conditions.[182] However, most clinicians reserve unenhanced computed tomography (CT) for the evaluation of osseous details such as foraminal stenosis,[151] bone tumors, and fractures.[104]

Magnetic resonance imaging is the imaging modality of choice in investigating cervical radiculopathy,[104,138] because it details diskal, ligamentous, osseous, and neural tissue very well (see Ch. 7).[152] The MRI is non-invasive and does not expose the patient to radiation. Although it has become a widely prescribed imaging test, it is expensive, requires patient cooperation to minimize artifact, and is often not tolerated by claustrophobic patients. Patients with embedded metallic objects such as pacemakers or prosthetic heart valves cannot undergo MRI. Contrast-enhanced CT can accurately evaluate disk pathology[151] in these cases. Because cervical intervertebral disk abnormalities occur in asymptomatic patients,[18,86,140,145,225] the clinical findings have to be correlated with the imaging findings to accurately diagnose the lesion responsible for the patient's signs and symptoms.

Electrodiagnostic evaluation   Nerve conduction studies and electromyography can be used to assess the neurophysiologic function of the nerve roots, plexus, and peripheral nerves. Electrodiagnostic examinations, if performed by an appropriately trained physician, can clarify or confirm the suspected diagnosis. Electrodiagnostic examination is also helpful in determining the prognosis of nerve injury. The American Association of Neuromuscular and Electrodiagnostic Medicine guidelines for the electrodiagnostic examination for a radiculopathy include abnormalities in two or more muscles innervated by the same root but different peripheral nerves, provided that normal findings are observed in muscles innervated by adjacent nerve roots.[238] At least one corresponding motor and sensory nerve conduction study should be performed in the involved limb to ensure the absence of a concomitant plexus or peripheral process. If abnormalities are found, the correlating contralateral muscle and nerves should be examined to exclude a generalized process such as peripheral neuropathy or motor neuron disease. A screening examination of six upper limb muscles in addition to the cervical paraspinals can identify 94–99% of cervical radiculopathies.[51] These studies can effectively exclude other problems such as brachial plexus lesions (such as Pancoast tumor or Parsonage–Turner syndrome) and focal peripheral entrapments (such as carpal tunnel syndrome and ulnar entrapment at the elbow or wrist). If the amplitude of the affected muscle's compound muscle action potential is reduced by less than 50% of that of the contralateral limb (Fig. 38-17), functional motor recovery will probably return with conservative

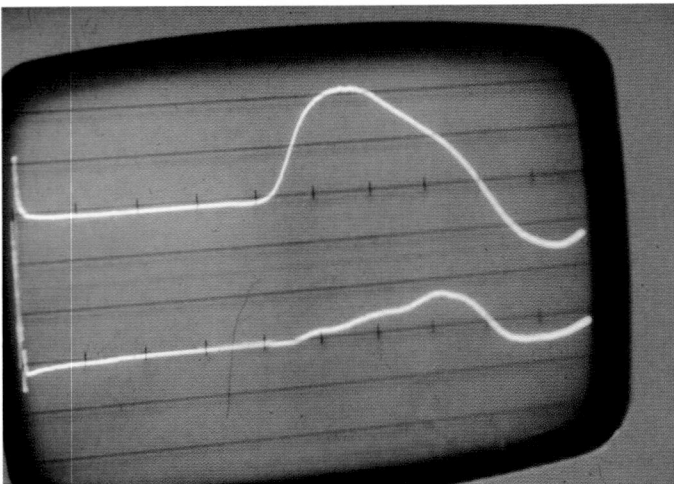

Figure 38-17 Oscilloscope screen waveform of bilateral abductor pollicis brevis compound muscle action potential (CMAP) amplitudes. The top trace demonstrates a healthy waveform with normal amplitude and duration. The bottom trace illustrates a 65% reduction of the CMAP amplitude of the contralateral muscle, with slightly increased duration.

care, and repeat studies can be performed to document neurophysiologic healing (see Chs 10–12).[100]

Treatment

Physical medicine and rehabilitation   The primary objectives of treatment of cervical radiculopathy include the resolution of pain, improvement in myotomal weakness, avoidance of spinal cord complications,[57,240] and prevention of recurrence.[240] Despite few outcome studies comparing surgical to medical rehabilitation and interventional (conservative) care, accumulated evidence supports the natural resolution of cervical radicular symptoms with conservative care.[47,80,184,203] The treatment approach must be molded to the individual patient. A definitive indication for a surgical approach is a progressive neurologic deficit. Otherwise, the patient's necessary level of posttreatment function can help dictate how aggressively to intervene. For example, a relatively sedentary patient might decide to tolerate a low level of discomfort after conservative care. An athlete, on the other hand, might not want to settle for symptoms that are exacerbated by extreme physical activity. The design of the treatment plan has to take into account the individual and how he or she functions at home, at work, and in the community.

Modalities   Patient education, activity modification, and relief of pain are the initial treatment steps. The treating physician should explain to the patient the mechanism of how the injury occurred, and the most likely treatment outcomes. This explanation should emphasize the importance of proper posture, biomechanics, and the utility of an ergonomic evaluation.[240]

Repetitive and heavy lifting must be avoided, as well as positioning the cervical spine in extension, axial rotation, and ipsilateral flexion. Severe pain can prohibit continued work or athletic activity, and restrict activities of daily living. Mild to moderate symptoms can usually be tolerated by the patient, allowing continued but restricted activities.

Thermotherapy is often used to modulate pain and to increase muscle relaxation.[125,149] No definitive guideline has been published to date regarding the role of thermal modalities in cervical radiculopathy.[179] Cold can be applied for 15–30 min one to four times a day, and superficial heat can be applied up to 30 min two to three times a day. The decision regarding which thermal agent to use is driven by the patient's perception of which provides the best pain relief.[124] Deep heating modalities such as ultrasound should be avoided in the treatment of cervical radiculopathy, because an increased metabolic response and subsequent inflammation can aggravate the nerve root injury.[125,179]

Transcutaneous electrical nerve stimulation is helpful in the management of various musculoskeletal and neurogenic disorders (see Chs 21 and 22). It can be utilized early in the treatment course of cervical radiculopathy to help modulate pain and enable the patient to engage in other therapeutic modalities. TENS is believed to act via the gate theory. Stimulating large myelinated fibers presumably blocks nociceptive transmission in smaller fibers at the level of the spinothalamic

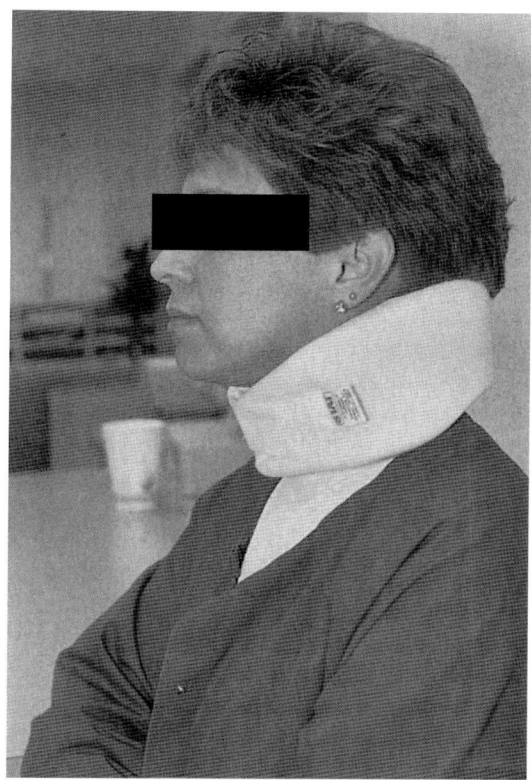

Figure 38-18 Cervical orthosis. A cervical soft collar with the widest side posteriorly and the narrowest side anteriorly.

tract neurons.[147] Although TENS theory has been shown to provide some relief of low back pain,[214] no studies have been published demonstrating conclusive evidence of its efficacy in cervical radicular pain.

Cervical orthoses function to limit painful range of motion and facilitate patient comfort during the acute injury phase (see Ch. 17).[179] Soft cervical collars limit flexion and extension by approximately 26%,[101] and are prescribed as kinesthetic reminders of proper cervical positioning.[240] The narrower segment should be positioned anteriorly to maintain the neck in the neutral or slightly flexed position (Fig. 38-18).[57,184,240] The exceptions to this include patients with a positive L'hermitte's sign, and those with rheumatoid arthritis, or atlantoaxial subluxation. The use of a soft collar should be limited to the first week or two of symptoms[48,118] to minimize adverse outcomes related to further soft tissue deconditioning.

Cervical traction applies a distractive force across the cervical intervertebral disk space. It is commonly used by patients with cervical radiculopathy, despite a lack of proven efficacy.[57,240] It is presumed to work via the decompression of cervical soft tissues and intervertebral disks.[42,221] Superficial heat, massage, and/or TENS therapy can be performed prior to and during traction to relieve pain and to help relax the muscles.[41,42] Twenty-five pounds of force are required to distract the mid-cervical segments when applied for 25 min at an angle of pull of 24°.[41] Cervical traction can be executed with an intermittent heavy-weight or a continuous light-weight regimen in the

therapy gym or home setting.[42] Traction is contraindicated in patients with myelopathy, positive L'hermitte's sign, rheumatoid arthritis, or atlantoaxial subluxation (see Ch. 20).[42]

Medications A role for antiinflammatory medications is logical in light of the evidence of an inflammatory component to CIDH-related radiculopathy.[67,106,107] NSAIDs are the first line of pharmacologic intervention prescribed to treat cervical radiculopathy. At low doses, they provide an analgesic effect, and at high doses an antiinflammatory effect. Side effects associated with the use of NSAIDs relate to their irritation of the gastrointestinal mucosa, platelet inhibition, and renal function. Antiinflammatory agents that target the cyclooxygenase-2 pathway provide similar analgesia and antiinflammatory properties to those of their non-selective counterparts, but with better gastrointestinal tolerability and less antiplatelet effect.[78] For these reasons, these newer agents may be preferable to traditional NSAIDs for cervical radiculopathy patients, and because diagnostic and therapeutic spinal injections can be performed without interrupting these therapeutic medications. However, recent findings have emerged suggesting that caution should be exercised when prescribing valdecoxib or celecoxib at high doses for an extended length of time, due to a supposed increase in cardiovascular risk (National Cancer Institute Adenoma Prevention with Celecoxib trial).

Adjunct medications are often utilized in conjunction with antiinflammatory medications and include muscle relaxants, tricyclic antidepressants, and antiepileptics. Muscle relaxers are sedating and secondarily relax skeletal muscle. They may be used to aid sleep if disrupted by painful muscular guarding. Low-dose tricyclic antidepressant medications such as amitriptyline or nortriptyline, prescribed at 10–25 mg at bedtime, can be beneficial in decreasing radicular pain and aiding sleep.[57] Associated side effects are largely anticholinergic, such as dry mouth, urinary retention, drowsiness, and constipation. Antiepileptic medication such as gabapentin can be effective in modulating neuropathic pain. The therapeutic dose varies from 300 to 900 mg/day up to 3600 mg/day. The most common side effects are lethargy, fatigue, ataxia, and dry mouth. Hence it is recommended to start at a low dose, 300 mg at bedtime, and titrate upward until either symptoms are controlled or side effects curtail the dosage curve. Other options include tiagabine (Gabitril), zonisamide (Zonegran), and oxcarbazepine (Trileptal). We typically reserve antiepileptic medications for patients suffering with persistent radicular pain postoperatively or who are not appropriate surgical candidates after failure of other therapeutic interventions.

Opiate analgesics can be necessary at times when radicular pain is severe and disrupts sleep. Short-acting opioid–analgesic combination medications can be prescribed to facilitate restorative sleep patterns by controlling the radicular pain (sometimes in conjunction with the use of a soft cervical collar). Opiate medications typically should not be prescribed after the acute phase, and other interventions should be maximized before resorting to long-term use of opioids (see Ch. 43)

Stabilization and functional restoration Rehabilitation requires approaching the patient as a whole, addressing both the psychologic and behavioral consequences of injury, in addition to the physical impairments (E.W. Johnson, personal communication, Columbus, 2002). Functional restoration includes biomechanical concerns, physical conditioning, and strength training. All these are needed to facilitate injury healing and prevent recurrence of injury.

Cervicothoracic stabilization is the functional restoration of spinal biomechanics, and is used to limit pain, maximize function, and prevent injury progression or recurrence.[43,220] Integral parts of this stabilization include restoration of spinal flexibility, postural reeducation, and conditioning. Normal range of motion and good posture are essential to prevent repetitive microtrauma to cervical structures due to poor movement patterns.[32] The patient must be taught how to control activity throughout the kinetic chain. The stabilization program is initiated by establishing the pain-free interval of cervical range of motion, and then progressively adding motion outside this range as the symptoms subside. Any restriction of range of motion in the spine or soft tissues is aggressively treated to achieve full or functional range of motion. Proper cervical biomechanics are restored using passive range of motion, spine and soft tissue mobilization techniques, self-stretching, and correct posture. Improved neuromuscular control is developed first for static positions, and then advanced to dynamic and functional activities.[43]

Cervical strengthening begins with isometric exercises of the flexor, extensor, rotator, and lateral flexor muscles. The exercises are performed first in the supine position and then progressed to the seated and standing positions.[43] The patient is carefully progressed to concentric isotonic exercises, avoiding combined movements unless pain-free. Muscles that are stretched or weakened as a result of poor posture are targeted during this phase.[43] One of the main goals of the exercise program is improved muscular balance and flexibility of the cervicothoracic and capital muscle groups.[43]

Attention is also paid to the shoulder girdles and upper limb conditioning. Mid to upper cervical radiculopathies with myotomal weakness can disrupt scapulothoracic and glenohumeral stabilization. The trapezius, serratus anterior, rhomboids, and rotator cuff muscles must be strengthened.[43] Proper scapulothoracic kinetics and glenohumeral coupling allow mechanically efficient spinal posture, as well as efficient dissipation of energy by the upper limbs in functional activities.

Interventional spine physiatry Interventional spine physiatry is a relatively young and developing subspecialty within the field of physiatry. The scope of this subspecialty involves the judicious use of precision, image-guided spinal procedures to both diagnose and treat painful spinal disorders. Interventional spine physiatrists rely on a knowledge-based algorithmic approach, which is a combination of evidence-based medicine and extensive clinical experience.

Diagnostic selective nerve root block If imaging reveals a structural lesion at the nerve root level that corroborates the

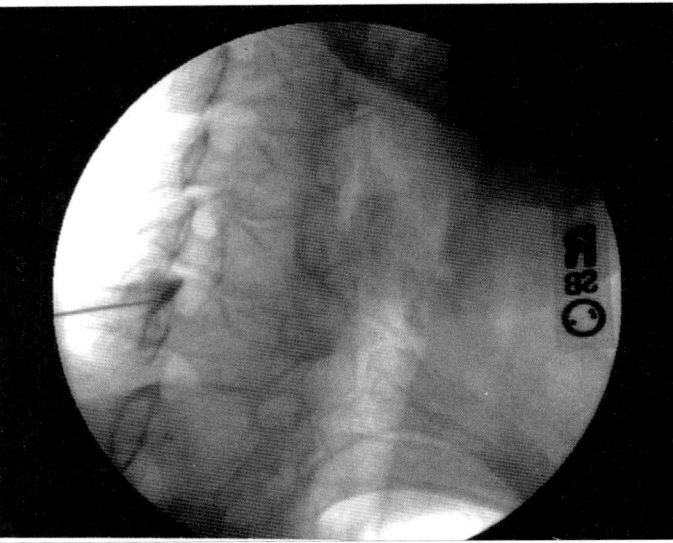

Figure 38-19 Fluoroscopic image of a diagnostic C6 selective nerve root block.

physical examination findings, and an electrodiagnostic evaluation confirms the clinical suspicion, therapeutic interventions can be indicated. However, if the physical examination and electrodiagnostic studies are equivocal in the setting of an abnormal MRI, the diagnosis can often be clarified with a fluoroscopically guided diagnostic selective nerve root block (SNRB) at the suspected segmental level (Fig. 38-19). If the diagnostic block is negative, the next step in the diagnostic algorithm is pursued.[202] The specificity of cervical diagnostic SNRBs has been suggested to range from 87 to 100%,[6,111] and the sensitivity has been shown to be 100%.[6] The utility of diagnostic lumbar SNRBs has been explored in the literature,[52,77,118,191,217,230] and the observed specificity and sensitivity values for lumbar diagnostic SNRBs closely mirror these values for their cervical counterparts. A diagnostic SNRB is a functional diagnostic test, because the patient's cooperation and understanding is imperative in gaining accurate and valid diagnostic information.[202] Because of a relative lack of methodological investigations configuring the sensitivity and specificity of cervical diagnostic SNRBs, we must extrapolate from the lumbar data (see also Chs 25–26).

Therapeutic selective nerve root injection The natural history of radiculopathy due to CIDH or spondylosis is a gradual resolution of symptoms with conservative care in 65–83% of patients.[80,175,184,207] Two of these studies,[184,207] however, incorporated fluoroscopically guided cervical epidural or selective nerve root injections (SNRIs) of corticosteroids. Heckman et al. retrospectively observed 65% of 60 cervical radiculopathy (90% due to CIDH, 10% due to spondylosis) patients improve significantly with conservative care that did not involve spinal injections.[80] Several studies have examined the utility of cervical therapeutic SNRIs to treat cervical radiculopathy after failure of more conservative care.[15,31,47,184,208,229] Good to excellent results have ranged from 50 to 83%, with follow-up intervals from 6 to 21 months.[15,31,47,184,208,229] More successful results have been obtained in the presence of CIDH[31,47,184] than with spondylotic changes.[15,47,208,229] Not surprisingly, traumatically induced cervical radiculopathy portends a poorer prognosis.[206,207] 'Whiplash'-induced cervical radicular pain in the absence of concomitant foraminal stenosis, and traumatic spondylotic cervical radicular pain are successfully treated with conservative care including up to 2–4 SNRIs in 14%[207] and 20%[206] of cases, respectively. In this patient profile, if an initial SNRI achieves no improvement in radicular pain, then further injections should be aborted, as probably less than 20% of patients will respond to further injections.[206,207]

Despite a growing concern regarding the safety of cervical SNRIs, they have been demonstrated to be safe[96] and offer a valid minimally invasive treatment intervention to treat painful, non-traumatic cervical radicular symptoms. The goal of SNRI is to modulate the inflammatory response to the CIDH by injecting steroids close to the disk–nerve root interface. This is intended to control pain and to start the process of nerve root healing, while the intervertebral disk herniation naturally resorbs and/or becomes inert tissue. A proportion of cases will eventually require decompression due to persistent intervertebral disk herniation volume and/or continuation of the inflammatory response.

Percutaneous disk decompression   Percutaneous diskectomy has been investigated as a non-surgical alternative for treating persistent cervical radiculopathy.[36,76,82,88,115,197] Various technologies have been employed to achieve cervical intervertebral disk decompression, including laser,[36,76,88,115,197] enzymatic,[82] and mechanical[36,88] decompression. The follow-up intervals have been relatively short[76,82,197] or unspecified.[88] The two studies with the longest outcome data demonstrated disparate results[36,115] and included a heterogeneous study cohort.[115]

Nucleoplasty is a technology that uses coblation energy to vaporize nuclear tissue into gaseous elementary molecules. It has recently been developed and applied to the spine.[196] In a recent study conducted at the Penn Spine Center,[203] nucleoplasty was combined with SNRI to treat both the biomechanical and biochemical causes of CIDH-related cervical radicular pain that had been unresponsive to conservative care. These patients demonstrated a contained CIDH without stenosis and persistent radicular pain, and had been deemed appropriate surgical candidates. At 6 months, 91–95% of these 21 patients experienced an average 83% reduction in their pain level, with the greatest rate of reduction occurring within the first 2 weeks.[203] At 12 months, 17 of 21 had a good or excellent result. It should be noted that each of the 21 patients in this consecutive cohort had been considered candidates for surgery by a fellowship-trained spine surgeon, yet only two ultimately required surgery. No major complications were encountered, and the procedure was performed with light intravenous sedation on an outpatient basis. On the basis of this study at least, it appears that percutaneous diskectomy with coblation technology combined with SNRI can be safe and effective in reliev-

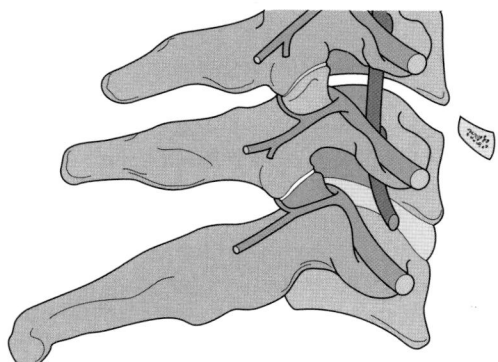

Figure 38-20 Anterior cervical diskectomy and fusion using the Smith–Robinson technique. The offending disk has been removed, and the block of bone graft is placed into the intervertebral level. The graft increases the disk height, thereby opening the foramen, and allows fusion. (From An and Simpson 1994,[5] with permission.)

ing cervical radicular pain. It can be offered as a non-operative alternative to surgery if more conservative measures fail.

Surgery   Indications for surgical treatment of CIDH or spondylotic-related cervical radiculopathy include intractable pain, severe myotomal deficit (progressive or stable), or progression to myelopathy. Surgical outcome studies have demonstrated good or excellent results in 80–96% of patients.[4,71,83,114] At 3 months postoperatively, surgical intervention such as anterior cervical diskectomy and fusion (Fig. 38-20) or posterior foraminotomy has achieved quicker improvement in radicular pain, strength, and sensation than has conservative care.[167] These differences between conservative and surgical approaches equalize at 1 year.[167] Our goal is to effectively modulate and enhance the body's natural response to a CIDH, beginning with conservative antiinflammatory measures, then moving to minimally invasive interventions, and culminating in open surgical decompression if necessary.

Cervical joint pain
Epidemiology
The cervical zygapophyseal joints are a common source of chronic posttraumatic neck pain.[8] Chronic traumatic cervical zygapophyseal joint-mediated neck pain has an estimated prevalence of 54–64%.[14,19,130] Painful cervical zygapophyseal joints most commonly occur in association with a symptomatic intervertebral disk at the same level.[19] In patients with chronic zygapophyseal joint pain, 58–88% complain of associated headaches.[14,130,131] The prevalence of C2–3 zygapophyseal joint pain has been estimated to be 50–53% in patients whose chief complaint is posterior headaches after whiplash injury.[130,131] Traumatically induced lower cervical pain attributable to a zygapophyseal joint most commonly involves the C5–6 level.[14,19,130] More than one structure can be injured in traumatically induced cervical zygapophyseal joint pain.[202] Spontaneous (non-traumatic) cervical zygapophyseal joint pain affects usually one joint and can be due to spondylosis or improper biomechanics.

Diagnosis

History and physical examination   A detailed examination should be completed on any patient who sustains a whiplash injury to understand the mechanism of injury and to exclude spinal cord injury, plexopathy, or traumatic brain injury. Details of the accident, including the neck position at the time of impact, can help predict which structures are the most likely to be injured. However, the clinical history cannot provide pathognomonic findings to distinguish zygapophyseal joint-mediated pain from other sources of axial neck pain.[20] In our experience, traumatic upper zygapophyseal joint involvement such as at the C2–3 joint is more likely to cause unilateral occipital headaches rather than neck pain. Unilateral paramidline neck pain, with or without periscapular symptoms, that is more painful than any associated headaches, suggests zygapophyseal joint pain rather than disk or root injury.

The physical examination must assess neurologic function and cervical range of motion. The clinician should suspect zygapophyseal joint injury when the patient can pinpoint a localized spot of maximal pain, or define an area of pain typical for the referral distribution of a particular zygapophyseal joint. Focal tenderness to palpation posterolaterally over a joint lends further support for an underlying painful zygapophyseal joint.[103] Increased focal suboccipital pain that occurs or is exacerbated with 45° of cervical flexion and sequential axial rotation suggests a painful C1–2 joint.[53] Despite these suggestions, to date there have been no well-designed investigations of clinical examination findings that are diagnostic of cervical zygapophyseal joint pain.

Imaging studies   Cervical zygapophyseal joint subluxation can be detected by plain radiography, and CT can better delineate joint fracture. Soft tissue injury, however, is largely undetected by advanced imaging. This means that imaging has a limited role in determining the pain generator.[28,224] Nuclear imaging might demonstrate increased radiotracer uptake if there is an abnormality within the zygapophyseal joint, but it cannot discriminate between symptomatic and asymptomatic abnormalities.

Treatment

Physical medicine and rehabilitation   During the acute phase of injury, the treatment focuses on analgesia and antiinflammatory modalities. NSAIDs are indicated to provide pharmacologic control of pain and inflammation. If the pain is not controlled with these medications, opiates can be prescribed to facilitate restorative sleep patterns and participation in functional restoration. Physical modalities should be used in the acute phase of injury to modulate pain and inflammation, and can be used to reduce or eliminate the need for opiates.

Superficial cryotherapy such as with ice application is preferred to superficial heat, due to its analgesic and antiinflammatory qualities. Although superficial heat has analgesic effects and relaxes muscles, its metabolic effects preclude its use in treating acute cervical zygapophyseal joint injuries. Cryotherapy should initially be applied for 20 min three or four times a day

to cause vasoconstriction and decrease the release of pain and inflammatory mediators.[123] Soft tissue mobilization and massage can help break muscular guarding or splinting, but should not be the mainstay of treatment. Soft cervical collars can be worn for a short period of time, up to 72 h after the initial injury. These are used for comfort, especially when sleeping. Patient education regarding proper positioning to avoid aggravating factors should occur concurrently with analgesic and antiinflammatory medications.

The restorative phase encompasses stabilization and functional restoration by normalizing the range of motion, soft tissue length, and biomechanical deficits, and strengthening the spinal musculature. Transition to this phase begins after there is a reduction in pain caused by the acute injury. Restoration of cervical spine motion helps achieve a balanced posture that decreases strain of the injured joints and also allows optimal strengthening to occur. Cervicothoracic stabilization addresses flexibility, posture reeducation, and strengthening, all of which reduce pain, improve function, and prevent recurrent injury.[220] Proprioceptive skills are implemented during strengthening exercises to achieve these goals.[43] The patient is discharged to a home exercise maintenance program to maintain mobility and strength.

Interventional spine physiatry   The natural history of whiplash-induced neck pain is of gradual recovery in a majority of patients. It is imperative, however, that an accurate diagnosis is formulated to maximize treatment if a patient's pain is moderate or severe, or persists beyond this natural historical time frame. Determining which exact joint(s) is the source of symptoms requires the meticulous use of fluoroscopically guided intraarticular injections.

Diagnostic zygapophyseal joint blocks   The close anatomic relationship and overlapping referral patterns of spinal structures necessitate the use of fluoroscopically guided diagnostic zygapophyseal joint blocks (Fig. 38-21) to confirm a clinically suspected painful joint. Diagnostic blocks offer a definitive means by which to target symptomatic joints. Local anesthetic can be injected into the joint or on the innervating nerves to the joint to anesthetize a joint. The diagnosis is based on the concept that if the symptomatic structure is blocked, the patient's pain will be relieved. If the pain is unrelieved, the tested joint is excluded as the source of the symptoms. Approximately one-third of responders can represent false positives.[12] Consequently, comparative blocks[129] using anesthetics of varying duration of effect might need to be performed before considering more invasive treatment options. Our approach to cervical zygapophyseal joint pain entails instituting therapeutic injections after a positive single intraarticular diagnostic block. If intraarticular injections of corticosteroid are ineffective, comparative blocks incorporating a placebo injection are performed prior to performing a medial branch neurotomy.

Therapeutic zygapophyseal joint injections   Therapeutic intraarticular cervical zygapophyseal joint injections can be appropriate in individuals who have not improved from phar-

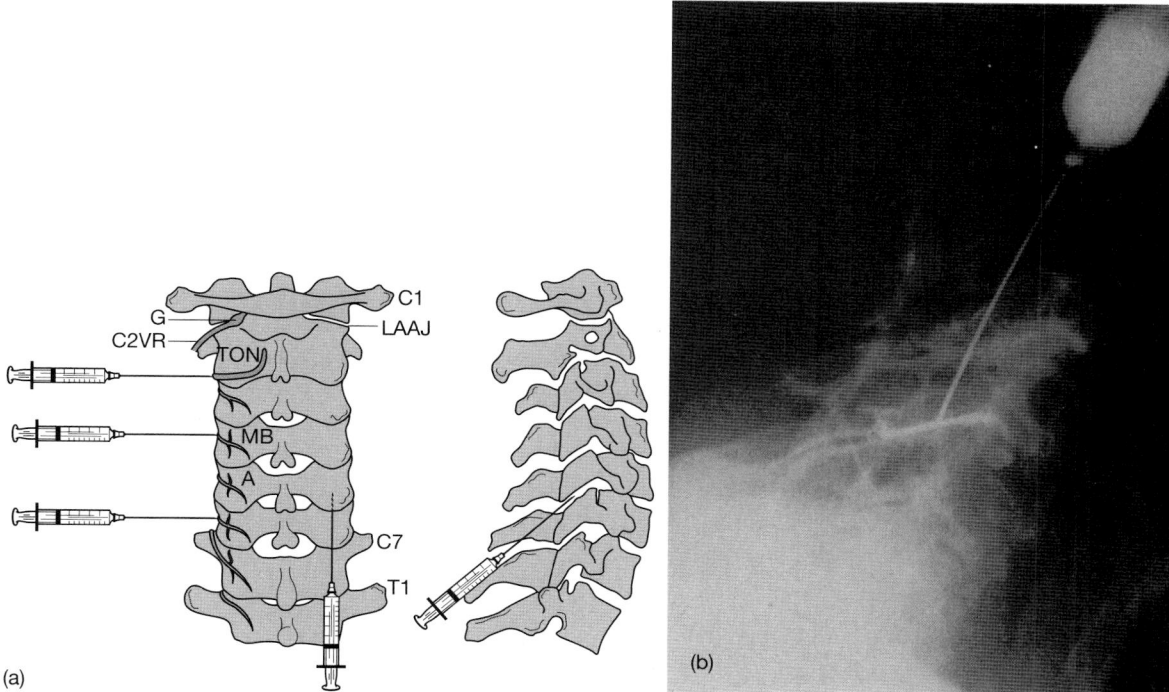

Figure 38-21 Cervical facet injections. (**a**) Needle placement for medial branch nerve and intraarticular zygapophyseal injections. Left: posterior view of the cervical spine, showing the location of the C2 ganglion (G) behind the lateral atlantoaxial joint (LAAJ), the C2 ventral ramus (C2VR), and the location of the medial branches of the cervical dorsal rami (MB), their articular branches (A), and the third occipital nerve (TON). Needles are positioned for injection of the C4 and C6 medial branches and the third occipital nerve. The articular pillar of C7 may be obscured by the shadow of the large C7 transverse process, in which case the C7 medial branch can be located midway between the lateral convexities of the C6–7 and C7–T1 zygapophyseal joints. Right: lateral view of the cervical spine, showing the course of the needle in the facet joint cavity of the C5–6 facet joint, using a posterior approach. (**b**) Lateral cervical radiograph showing precise needle placement into the zygapophyseal joint, producing a characteristic arthrogram. The joint was entered using a lateral approach to the cervical spine. (From Bogduk 1988,[23] with permission of JB Lippincott.)

macologic and physical modalities. Barnsley et al. reported that single intraarticular steroid injections were not effective for the treatment of chronic whiplash-related cervical zygapophyseal joint pain.[13] However, in this study the authors treated patients with only one therapeutic injection, utilized one outcome measure, and did not restrict physical therapy exercises.[13] In our experience, fluoroscopically guided therapeutic intraarticular steroid injections have been efficacious in treating cervical zygapophyseal joint pain. Slipman et al. demonstrated good to excellent results in 61% of patients suffering from daily whiplash-related occipital headaches originating from the C2–3 joints.[209] Patients who benefited from these injections underwent an average of two therapeutic injections.

Percutaneous radiofrequency neurotomy If patients fail to obtain satisfactory relief from steroid injections, then radiofrequency ablation of the joint's innervating medial branches can be offered. Lord et al. established the efficacy of radiofrequency neurotomy in patients with chronic cervical zygapophyseal joint pain through a randomized, double-blind, placebo-controlled trial.[128] The median time that elapsed before return of pain to preneurotomy level in the treatment group was 9 months, compared with 1 week in the sham control group. A subsequent study by McDonald et al. observed that repeat neurotomy can provide the same pain relief if the

patient's symptoms returned after an initially successful procedure.[143] Radiofrequency neurotomies of the atlantooccipital, atlantoaxial, and C2–3 joints have not been investigated. There is currently no technique for denervating the atlantooccipital and atlantoaxial joints, and denervation of the C2–3 joint has not been studied, due to the adverse effect of suboccipital hypoesthesia from neurotomy of the third occipital nerve. We have successfully employed radiofrequency neurotomy of the C2–3 zygapophyseal joint, and most patients are not distressed by the suboccipital hypoesthesia.

Cervical internal disk disruption
Epidemiology
Internal disk disruption was first described by Crock over 30 years ago, and indicates that an intervertebral disk has lost its normal internal architecture but maintains a preserved external contour in the absence of nerve root compression.[45] In traumatically induced chronic neck pain, 20% of patients may be suffering from CIDD, and another 41% may be suffering from CIDD and a concomitant zygapophyseal joint injury.[19] Litigation might adversely affect treatment outcomes for CIDD,[50] but this potential litigation effect has not been substantiated in other investigations.[158,174,187] In non-litigation cases, non-operative and operative outcomes are similar to those for CIDD.[50]

Diagnosis

History and physical examination   The symptom complex of CIDD includes posterior neck pain, occipital and suboccipital pain, upper trapezial pain, inter- and periscapular pain, non-radicular arm pain, vertigo, tinnitus, ocular dysfunction, dysphagia, facial pain, and anterior chest wall pain.[68,190] Patients often report a history of preceding trauma such as a motor vehicle accident with acute onset. In the absence of a precipitating event, CIDD symptoms can start spontaneously and gradually, or explosively. If referral symptoms are present, the patient's chief complaint is primarily axial pain associated with nondescript upper limb symptoms. Exacerbating factors usually include prolonged sitting, and coughing, sneezing, or lifting. Lying supine or recumbent with head support typically alleviates the patient's symptoms.

The physical examination can show only subtle cervical range of motion restrictions, unless there has been prior cervical surgery. A thorough neuromusculoskeletal examination should be performed to exclude myelopathy or radiculopathy. If spondylosis is present, cervical extension and lateral bending are more restricted than flexion and axial rotation are. Palpation over the cervical spinous processes of the involved level can elicit pain in that region or a portion of the patient's axial pain. Separating these patients from those with non-organic neck pain can be achieved by eliciting non-organic signs, such as superficial or non-anatomic tenderness, pain with rotation of head and pelvis together, non-anatomic sensory loss, give-way weakness, and overreaction.[213]

Imaging studies   Distinguishing painful from non-painful cervical disks solely on imaging characteristics can be difficult. Disk abnormalities have been noted in asymptomatic patients,[18,140,225] and CIDD by definition displays an age-appropriate appearance on MRI.[45] Plain films can reveal hyperostosis and disk space collapse but frequently do not correlate with pain symptoms. Disk desiccation, loss of disk height, annular fissure, osteophytosis, and reactive end-plate changes are markers of disk degeneration (Fig. 38-22).[151] Decreased intradiskal signal on T_2-weighted images correlates well with histologic degeneration of the disk.[151] MRI features are not useful, however, in detecting symptomatic cervical disks.[189] Consequently, functional diagnostic testing such as provocative diskography is relied on to diagnose the painful disk level. Our understanding of pain distribution from CIDD or degenerative disks has been expanded by studies of these functional diagnostic tests.[40,72,188]

Treatment
Physical medicine and rehabilitation

Treating cervical intervertebral disk injury without radiculopathy is similar to treating radicular symptoms. The initial step is to control pain and inflammation. NSAIDs can be used on a short-term basis unless contraindicated due to renal disease or gastrointestinal intolerance to NSAIDs. The American College of Rheumatology guidelines state that renal function in healthy patients should be checked at 6 weeks after initiating NSAIDs. If renal function is normal at 6 weeks, it should be checked again at 12 months. Adjunct medications such as tricyclic antidepressants can help modulate pain and aid in sleep regulation. Opiate analgesics are typically used sparingly and only for short periods of time.

Physical modalities should be prescribed to modulate pain and transition the patient from passive treatment to active functional restoration. Superficial modalities and TENS therapy can be used for pain. Heat modalities can also be used to increase soft tissue elasticity prior to and during cervical traction. In uncontrolled studies, electrical stimulation (TENS) has been found to be helpful in cervical pain. Traction might be beneficial by distracting painful intervertebral disks. Cervical collars can help maintain comfortable positioning but should not be worn by the patient for more than 72 h. These passive modalities should be utilized early in the treatment process and later on an as-needed basis, and should not replace activity-based therapies.

As with all other mechanical cervical pain disorders, CIDD requires a thorough evaluation of spinal biomechanics. As the acute pain starts to subside, the patient is enrolled in an active stretching and flexibility program with transition to conditioning and stabilization. The independent effects of exercise and stabilization, specifically in the treatment of cervical disk injury, have not been scientifically validated.[215] The effects can be inferred from a lumbar stabilization research report that demonstrated a statistically significant reduction in pain and disability in a group of patients with spondylosis and spondylolisthesis.[161] The only methodologically correct way to study outcomes in patients with true cervical diskogenic pain would be to enroll and treat a cohort of patients after diskography-proven concordant axial neck pain. No such studies exist.

Interventional spine physiatry

Provocative diskography   Provocative diskography is a functional diagnostic test in which the accuracy of the investigation relies heavily on patient input. Smith and Nichols first described cervical diskography in the early 1950s,[212] and its utility has been contested ever since.[19] Provocative diskography is the only test that can address the symptomatic status of the disk, and

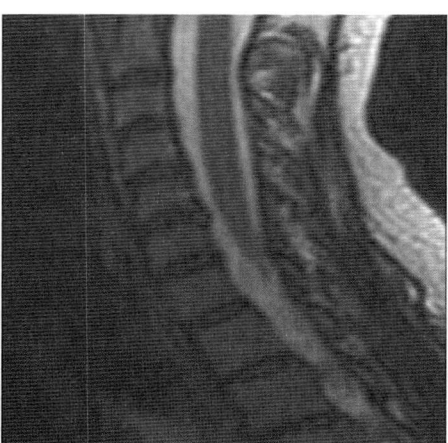

Figure 38-22
Magnetic resonance imaging scan depicting degenerative intervertebral disk space changes such as desiccation and mild loss of disk height.

is typically used when CIDD is in question. It is also used as a presurgical evaluation. A positive response requires evidence of structural internal derangement that corroborates production of the patient's usual pain (a concordant response).

Proponents of diskography suggest that healthy disks accept a finite volume of contrast and do not produce symptoms with mechanical stimulation.[192,237] Diskography should be considered valid only when an asymptomatic control disk injection accompanies a concordantly painful disk. Although false positives have been demonstrated in asymptomatic volunteers,[87] these findings can be dismissed due to technical insufficiencies. Cervical provocative diskography has not produced false positive pain responses in asymptomatic volunteers.[189] On occasion, a provocative diskogram can produce a false positive in the presence of a painful cervical zygapophyseal joint.[19] Bogduk warns that concluding that a positive cervical diskogram in traumatic chronic cervical pain is conclusive might be misleading, and recommends completing diagnostic zygapophyseal joint blocks at the level of the painful disk before pursuing treatment interventions.[19] Cervical intervertebral disks have been shown to refer pain into the head and face both unilaterally and bilaterally,[210] and overlap pain referral patterns produced by painful zygapophyseal joints.

Transforaminal epidural steroid injections Instillation of steroids into the anterior epidural space to bathe the posterior surface of the intervertebral disks and posterior longitudinal ligament can address biochemically stimulated nociception.[202] A C7 transforaminal epidural steroid injection (TFESI) is performed if the symptoms behave like diskogenic pain and are primarily located at the base, or refer outward from the base, of the cervical spine. The identical procedure is performed at the C5 or C6 level to treat upper neck pain with or without headaches, facial, or upper limb symptoms.[202] If a steroid effect, defined as a 50% reduction in preinjection pain level lasting for 2 days within 7 days after the procedure, is not experienced by the patient, cervical diskography or diagnostic zygapophyseal joint blocks are typically pursued.

The efficacy of TFESIs has not been systematically studied. Interlaminar epidural steroid injections have been investigated in a heterogeneous group of patients with axial and radicular pain.[37,172,181,196] Most of the patients in these studies had ill-defined symptoms of axial pain and/or radicular pain. The injections were completed posteriorly via the interlaminar approach without fluoroscopic guidance, using the loss of resistance technique. Outcomes were successful in approximately 40–84% of treated patients.[37,172,181,196] Medication injected posteriorly between the laminae might not diffuse anteriorly[117] to reach the potential pain generator. Despite the paucity of literature regarding the utility of TFESIs in treating diskogenic cervical pain, the authors typically perform two injections initially before assessing the clinical response. In our experience, approximately 50% of patients experience significant and lasting relief. The more acute or subacute the symptom duration, the better the results, presumably due to a relatively acute inflammatory disk injury.

Surgery

Patients suffering from severe and recalcitrant axial cervical pain felt to be diskogenic in origin may be candidates for surgery. Our approach to patients with CIDD is to consider cervical diskography if the patient does not realize a pain-relieving steroid effect after two TFESIs. If the diskogram reveals one or two contiguous levels producing concordant pain, then the patient might be a surgical candidate. If three or more levels are concordant, two levels are non-contiguous, or any concordantly painful disks are lobular, then the patient requires a comprehensive chronic pain-modulation program.

The only surgical treatment for CIDD or symptomatic cervical degenerative disks is fusion,[70,95,235] which can be accomplished by anterior cervical diskectomy and fusion or by posterior fusion. The rationale is that, by fusing the bony vertebral elements, motion is eliminated, thereby reducing diskogenic pain. The utility of provocative diskography to determine the level(s) to fuse is controversial. Some authors have reported 'good or excellent' results in 70–96% of patients after cervical fusion of levels determined by diskography.[71,192,198,237] Seibenrock observed a pain reduction of greater than 75% in 96% of 27 patients who underwent cervical fusion of a total of 39 levels.[192] The review was retrospective, and the authors might have included some patients who had primarily radicular complaints. Garvey et al. found that 82% of 87 patients reported their self-perceived outcome as good, very good, or excellent at a mean of 4.4 years after fusion.[69] Ninety-three percent of these patients reported greater than 50% reduction in their pain rating postsurgically. Interestingly, a statistically significant difference was obtained for patients who were treated based on a truly positive diskogram.

Cervical myelopathy and myeloradiculopathy
Epidemiology

Cervical spondylitic myelopathy is the most common cervical cord lesion after middle age,[239] but not as common as spondylitic cervical radiculopathy.[3] The average age at onset is after 50 years, and men predominate.[39] Other causes of myelopathy have to be ruled out, including multiple sclerosis, motor neuron disease, vasculitis, neurosyphilis, subacute combined degeneration, syringomyelia, and spinal tumors.[245] One of these other conditions can be present in up to 17% of patients having spondylitic myelopathy.[33]

Diagnosis

History and physical examination Symptom onset is typically insidious, although a minority of patients can experience acute onset with or without a preceding traumatic event. Myelopathic patients often complain of numbness and paresthesias in the distal limbs and extremities, weakness more often in the lower than upper limbs, and intrinsic hand muscle wasting.[245] Cervical axial pain can be the primary complaint in up to 70% of patients at one point in the disease course.[245] The natural history typically involves an initial deterioration, followed by a static period that can last several years.[159] Bladder function disturbances occur in approximately one-third of cases and suggest more severe spinal cord injury.[245] Patients can concurrently complain of unilateral or bilateral radicular pain due to nerve root involvement at the stenotic level. The combination of cord and radicular involvement is referred to as cervical spondylitic myeloradiculopathy.

A common examination finding is myelopathic weakness in the lower limbs and, to a lesser extent, in the upper limbs. The upper extremities will demonstrate intrinsic hand muscle weakness and wasting due to anterior horn cell damage.[245] Pain and temperature disturbances representing injury to the spinothalamic tracts appear as a level of sensory disruption in the thoracic or lumbar region, or glove and stocking distribution. Proprioception and vibratory deficits indicating posterior column malfunction are more common in the lower limbs than in the upper.[245] Upper motor neuron signs such as Hoffman's sign, brisk reflexes, and Babinski's signs are often present. The signs and symptoms might or might not be symmetric, and complete sparing of the upper limbs is rare. The clinical level of spinal involvement might not correlate with the radiologic level of maximum compression, and there can be a difference of one to two segments.[245] Asymmetric reflexes in the upper limbs, or myotomal weakness, can indicate concomitant radiculopathy.

Imaging studies   Radiographic evaluations typically demonstrate the cervical cord compression. Most are spondylitic in nature. Other causes include a superimposed CIDH impinging on the thecal sac, or ossification of the posterior longitudinal ligament (the etiology in 27% of middle-aged patients[227]). Plain radiography provides information regarding the osseous diameter of the central canal and decreased height of the intervertebral disk spaces, and the presence of posterior hyperostosis, foraminal encroachment, and subluxation. A central canal diameter less than 10 mm in a symptomatic patient supports the existence of myelopathy.[245] Asymptomatic central cervical spinal stenosis has been observed in 16% of individuals under age 64.[226] A 30% reduction in the cross-sectional area of the cervical spine is the minimum decrement in symptomatic patients.[166] In order to accurately diagnose cervical spondylitic myelopathy, approximately one-third of the central canal must be compromised, and objective central canal changes ought to be evident. These include a complete lack of cerebrospinal fluid flow, cord deformation, or intracord signal abnormalities. MRI allows detection of myelomalacia, which reflects progressive cord compression, signal alteration, atrophy,[176] and the amount of cerebrospinal fluid volume surrounding the cord (Fig. 38-23). The preoperative transverse area of the spinal cord at the site of maximal compression tends to correlate with the eventual clinical outcome, while the postoperative dimension of the cord strongly correlates with clinical recovery.[154]

Electrodiagnostic evaluation   Electromyography and nerve conduction studies can be performed to diagnose nerve root injury, as discussed under cervical radiculopathy. In cases of cervical myelopathy, the needle electrode examination can reveal rate-coding abnormalities in muscles below the injured

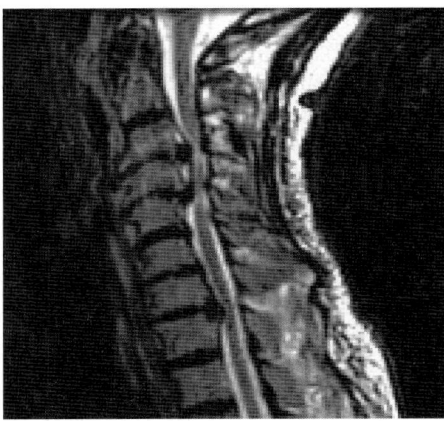

Figure 38-23
Sagittal magnetic resonance imaging scan of central spinal stenosis and myelomalacia. Notice the lack of cerebrospinal fluid anterior and posterior to the cord at C3–4 and C4–5.

segment, in which the patient recruits normal-appearing motor unit potentials but in a less than full interference pattern at maximal effort, indicative of upper motor neuron injury.

The utility of somatosensory evoked potentials to evaluate cervical myelopathy has been investigated.[35,244] Somatosensory evoked potentials with the median, ulnar, and posterior tibial nerve stimulation are more sensitive in detecting posterior column dysfunction than clinical testing is. Somatosensory evoked potentials can be used to detect subclinical cord involvement, when the chief complaint is cervical axial or radicular pain. Cervical myelopathy can be distinguished from multiple sclerosis by the pattern of abnormalities obtained by somatosensory evoked potentials. Changes in peripheral nerve conduction studies, when combined with central slowing, are indicative of myeloradiculopathy.[35,244]

Treatment

Non-operative care   Conservative care can include physical therapy and cervical orthoses in patients with mild or static symptoms without hard evidence of gait disturbances or pathologic reflexes.[59,169] Improvement of sensory and motor deficits occurs in 33–50% of patients.[33,39,169]

Surgery   Surgery is indicated for patients with severe or progressive symptoms, or those for whom conservative measures failed.[99] If a CIDH alone is causing cord compression, then anterior cervical diskectomy and fusion at the appropriate level(s) is indicated.[84] In the case of impingement from degenerative spondylosis or ossification of the posterior longitudinal ligament, surgical intervention aims to remove either the offending anterior structures (such as osteophytes) or the calcified posterior longitudinal ligament (to decompress posteriorly). Both these interventions allow more space for the cord. Anterior decompression is frequently accomplished by corpectomy, in which a vertebral body is removed in addition to the adjacent intervertebral disks, and the segment is then fused with a fibula autograft or allograft of a bone cage.[16] Posterior decompression involves laminectomy with or without fusion,[73] or laminoplasty (Fig. 38-24).[85] Extensive laminectomy without fusion can lead to postoperative deformity and kyphosis.[150] This has led to the

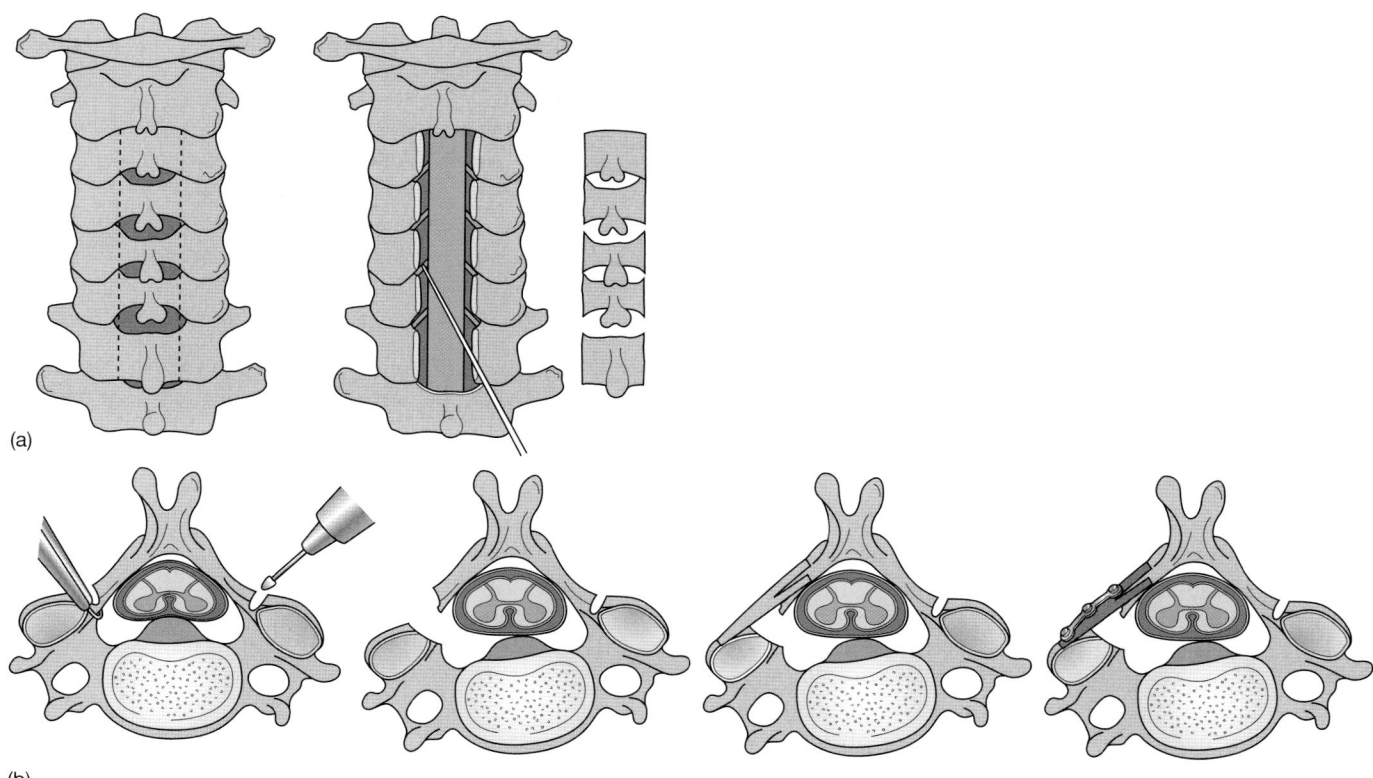

Figure 38-24 Laminectomy and laminoplasty. (**a**) Laminectomy involves excision of the posterior elements laterally to the level of the pedicles. (**b**) Laminoplasty is achieved by completely cutting the laminae on one side while burring the contralateral laminae, allowing this side to act as a hinge. The posterior elements will eventually heal with a widened canal as a graft is placed in the opening.

frequent use of the technique of laminoplasty, in which deformity and kyphosis are much less common and motion is preserved due to absence of a fusion.[150]

The decision to decompress anteriorly or posteriorly is predicated on the number of stenotic levels and the contour of the cervical spine. If three or fewer levels are stenotic, anterior corpectomy and fusion is preferred.[84] In cases of three or more stenotic levels with lordosis preserved, laminoplasty is preferred.[5,84] If, however, three or more levels are involved, with loss of normal cervical lordosis, laminectomy and posterior fusion is performed to maintain cervical spinal stability.[219]

Effective treatment is afforded by anterior decompression, with symptomatic improvement in 85–99% of patients.[133,141] Performing corpectomy at more than two levels can result in a less stable construct, and is generally avoided due to complications arising from dislodgement of the graft[84] or non-union.[81] Laminoplasty has been found to be more effective than laminectomy, with fewer complications in treating cervical myelopathy.[81]

Cervicogenic headaches

Cervicogenic headaches are a constellation of symptoms that represent the common referral patterns of cervical spinal structures. The term *cervicogenic headache* was first coined in 1983.[199] Its definition has been augmented or adjusted several times since.[79,146,148,200] This underscores the myriad of pain generators and manifestations that comprise cervicogenic headaches, and also points out the lack of consensus regarding the definition.

Epidemiology and pathophysiology

The prevalence of cervicogenic headache has been reported to range from 0.4 to 2.5% in the general population,[201] to as high as 36.2% in patients with a complaint of headaches.[7,157] Women are more commonly affected (79.1%) than men (20.9%),[233] with a mean age of 42.9 years and an average symptom duration of 6.8 years.[75]

Various spinal structures have been implicated in cervicogenic headache, including nerve roots and spinal nerves, dorsal root ganglia, uncovertebral joints, intervertebral disks, facet joints, ligaments, and muscles.[199] Circumstantial evidence supports the convergence theory to explain why cranial symptoms can occur due to cervical spine pain generators. Convergence of two separate primary afferents derived from two different body regions on the same second-order intraspinal neurons allows the nociceptive activity of one afferent nerve to be perceived as pain in the distribution of the other afferent nerve.[24] The cervicogenic headache can be due to degenerative changes, a direct result of trauma, or occur without any underlying biomechanical insult to the various cervical spinal structures subserved by cervical afferent fibers. The C2–3 zygapophyseal joint,[130,131] and the C2–3, C3–4, C4–5, and C5–6 intervertebral disks,[210]

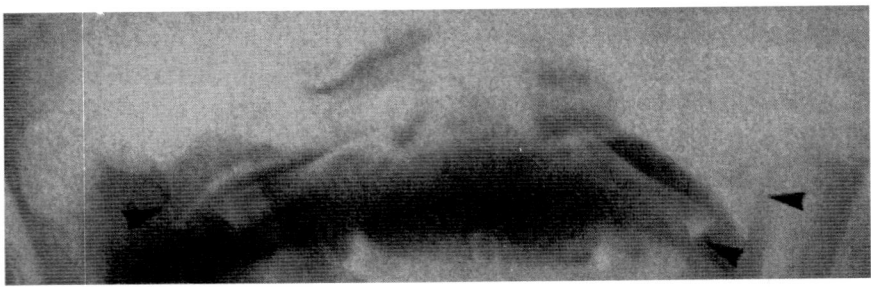

Figure 38-25 Open mouth view of the cervical spine, showing a burst fracture of the atlas (Jefferson fracture). Offsetting of the lateral masses of the atlas with those of the axis (arrowheads) confirms the burst fracture. (From Pavlov and Torg 1987,[165] with permission.)

have been primarily implicated as sources of cervicogenic headache.

Diagnosis

History and physical examination Support for a structural source within the cervical spine as the etiology of the patient's headaches is obtained by eliciting any history of prior head or neck trauma such as a whiplash event.[200] Whiplash events such as motor vehicle accidents have been associated with injury to the cervical zygapophyseal joints, intervertebral disks, or nerve roots, either in isolation or in combination.[14,130,224] Cervicogenic headaches have been conceptualized as being primarily unilateral and stemming from the posterior occipital region. The referral of pain is toward the vertex of the scalp, ipsilateral anterolateral temple, forehead, midface, or ipsilateral shoulder girdle.[200,204,205,210] Symptoms can spread to involve the contralateral side,[204] but typically the side of the initial referral source remains most intense.[200] The character of the pain can vary from a deep ache to sharp and stabbing. The duration of the painful symptoms fluctuates from initial episodic bouts of pain, progressing to more chronic and constant pain. Patients often describe the pain as initiating in the cervical region, and traveling to the head and the neck as the pain becomes severe. The cervicogenic headache can then become the primary complaint, overshadowing the original cervical axial pain.

The duration of the symptoms ranges from a few hours to a few weeks, but characteristically lasts longer than that associated with migraine headaches. The pain intensity in cervicogenic headache is less excruciating than for cluster headaches, and is usually non-throbbing in character.[200] Autonomic complaints such as photophobia, phonophobia, and nausea are less apparent than in a migraine attack but can still occur.[64,200] Accompanying complaints of dizziness or vertigo sometimes associated with near-syncopal episodes have also been described but are not common.[64]

Physical examination of the patient with complaints of cervicogenic headache typically reveals reduced active range of motion due to muscle guarding, arthritic changes, or soft tissue inflexibility. If the cervicogenic headache is being produced by a cervical zygapophyseal joint, the patient can usually pinpoint with one finger or with the palm of the hand a unilateral area of maximal pain. Cervical intervertebral disk-induced cervicogenic headache typically begins as midline pain that spreads across the spine and into the head or face. However, unilateral occipital headache symptoms that are greater than the neck pain following a traumatic event are more suggestive of zygapophyseal joint pain than diskogenic symptoms.[14,130] Certain head and neck movements can precipitate painful symptoms, such as axial rotation or cervical extension. We have commonly seen patients report an onset after sleeping in an awkward position. Spurling's maneuver does not reproduce upper limb radicular symptoms but usually aggravates the axial pain, and patients report reproduction of their paramidline zygapophyseal joint-mediated pain. This pain can also often be reproduced with deep palpation over the involved joint.

Imaging studies A history of trauma requires cervical flexion and extension lateral radiographs to detect abnormal segmental motion. It also requires anteroposterior views, including an open mouth view of the odontoid process, to rule out fractures (Fig. 38-25).[151] Any suspicion for fracture mandates a subsequent cervical CT scan performed with multiplanar reformatted images to better delineate the osseous injury.[151] MRI is better than CT at evaluating the intervertebral disks for desiccation, decreased disk height, and frank herniation. However, MRI has a false positive rate of 51% and a false negative rate of 27% in detecting painful disks identified by diskography.[246] Abnormalities seen on imaging studies should be clinically correlated, as such findings can occur in lifelong asymptomatic individuals.[18,140,225]

Functional diagnostic tests and treatment Once the etiology of cervicogenic headache has been identified, the offending structure is treated in a similar fashion as that outlined above. Cervicogenic headaches due to upper cervical zygapophyseal joint pain can be studied with confirmatory diagnostic blockade. The traditional algorithm includes intraarticular diagnostic injections performed sequentially in the C2–3, C3–4, and C1–2 joints.[14] Following a zygapophyseal joint mapping study, we now also incorporate blockade of C4–5 zygapophyseal joints if the headaches include anterior head or facial symptoms. Once the painful joint is identified, therapeutic injections are performed as outlined under treatment of cervical zygapophyseal joint pain. If patients experience short-term relief from a minimum of two and a maximum of four therapeutic intraarticular injections, a double-block paradigm is exercised to minimize the false positive rate of single diagnostic injections.[12] Radiofrequency ablation of the medial branches to the painful joint can be successful in alleviating cervicogenic headaches due to cervical zygapophyseal joint injury that fails to respond to other measures.[128] Radiofrequency ablation of the third occipital nerve to treat C2–3 zygapophyseal joint-mediated headaches has been successfully performed at the Penn Spine Center, but this has not been studied in a large cohort.[128]

Whiplash syndrome

Whiplash (hyperflexion–hyperextension) should be conceptualized as having three components. The *whiplash event* is the biomechanical effect incurred by the occupants of one vehicle when struck by another vehicle. The *whiplash injury* is the impairment, or injured structure, resulting from the whiplash event. The *whiplash syndrome* is the set of symptoms arising from the whiplash injury.[11] During a whiplash event, the head and neck do not suffer a direct blow, but each undergoes an excursion due to the inertial response of the body to forces imparted on it.[11] Rear-end collisions represent the most common pattern of whiplash-related injury, but injury due to head-on and side collisions can also occur.[11]

Regardless of the direction of impact, whiplash is defined by the passive movement of the neck. Muscular control to stabilize the cervical spine does not react quickly enough to prevent injurious forces from occurring across the cervical functional spinal units. Both the lack of muscular pillaring and the generation of abnormal forces resulting in movements around abnormal axes of rotation subject the passive restraining structures to abnormal strain.[11,105] For example, at 110 ms after rear-end impact, the C5–6 disk space widens anteriorly, causing abutment of the articular processes of the C5–6 zygapophyseal joint[105] and posterior shear within the disk.[162] The anterior disk, anterior longitudinal ligament, posterior disk or annulus, and cervical zygapophyseal joints are all at risk of injury during a whiplash event.[11,105,162] Injury also occurs to the cervical soft tissues, resulting in strain and sprain injuries.[156] These injuries typically heal over a relatively short time period, as would be expected for soft tissue injury. The most commonly reported symptoms of whiplash injury include neck pain and headaches, followed by shoulder girdle pain, upper limb paresthesias, and weakness. Less common symptoms include dizziness, visual disturbances, and tinnitus.[11]

Most patients suffering from whiplash syndrome are destined to recover within the first 2–3 months after the injury, and after 2 years 82% are symptom-free.[174] Severely afflicted patients account for only 6% of all whiplash patients at 3 months, and this percentage decreases minimally to 4% at 2 years.[174] Studies have demonstrated that chronicity of whiplash symptoms develops independent of litigation,[158] and litigation does not alter response to treatment.[187] The clinician should pursue evaluation and treatment of whiplash-related symptoms, rather than just assume that the pain is due to mitigating circumstances such as secondary gain considerations.

CONCLUSION

Neck pain is one of the most common complaints of patients seeking medical attention. Knowledge of spinal biomechanics and pathophysiology helps determine the most likely pain generators in each case. A variety of spinal structures can produce overlapping or obscure symptomatology. An accurate diagnosis provides the best opportunity for effective treatment. The building blocks for successful therapeutic interventions include controlling pain and inflammation while at the same time educating the patient about the injury, the treatment objectives, and the prognosis. As technology advances and our knowledge of cervical spine disorders grows, our clinical pathways for treatment of cervical problems will continue to evolve and improve. It is important to view the patient as a whole, and institute physical, pharmacologic, behavioral, and interventional treatments in the broad context of achieving what is best for the patient's physiologic and psychologic well-being.

REFERENCES

1. Abel MS. Occult traumatic lesions of the cervical vertebrae. Crit Rev Clin Radiol Nucl Med 1975; 6:469–553.
2. Abel MS. The radiology of chronic neck pain: sequelae of occult traumatic lesions. Crit Rev Diagn Imaging 1982; 20:27–78.
3. Adams C. Cervical spondylitic radiculopathy and myelopathy. In: Vinken PJ, Bruyn GW, ed. Handbook of clinical neurology, 26. Amsterdam: North-Holland Publishing; 1977:97–112.
4. Aldrich F. Posterolateral microdiscectomy for cervical monoradiculopathy caused by posterolateral soft cervical disc sequestration. J Neurosurg 1990; 72:370–377.
5. An HS, Simpson JM. Surgery of the cervical spine. London: Martin-Dunitz; 1994.
6. Anderberg L, Annertz M, Brandt L, et al. Selective diagnostic cervical nerve root block—correlation with clinical symptoms and MRI-pathology. Acta Neurochir 2004; 146(6):559–565.
7. Anthony M. Cervicogenic headache: prevalence and response to local steroid therapy. Clin Exp Rheumatol 2000; 18(2 suppl 19): S59–S64.
8. Aprill C, Bogduk N. The prevalence of cervical zygapophyseal joint pain: a first approximation. Spine 1992; 17:744–747.
9. Aprill C, Dwyer A, Bogduk N. Cervical zygapophyseal joint pain patterns. II: A clinical evaluation. Spine 1990; 15:458–461.
10. Atkinson R, Ghelman B, Tsairis P, et al. Sarcoidosis presenting as cervical radiculopathy. A case report and literature review. Spine 1987; 7:412–416.
11. Barnsely L, Lord S, Bogduk N. The pathophysiology of whiplash. Spine State Art Rev 1998; 12(2):209–242.
12. Barnsley L, Lord SM, Wallis BJ, et al. False-positive rates of cervical zygapophysial joint blocks. Clin J Pain 1993; 9:124–130.
13. Barnsley L, Lord SM, Wallis BJ, et al. Lack of effect of intraarticular corticosteroids for chronic pain in the cervical zygapophyseal joints. N Engl J Med 1994; 330(15):1047–1050.
14. Barnsley L, Lord SM, Wallis BJ, et al. The prevalence of chronic cervical zygapophyseal joint pain after whiplash. Spine 1995; 20:20–26.
15. Berger O, Dousset V, Delmer O, et al. Evaluation of CT-guided periganglionic foraminal steroid injections for treatment of radicular pain in patients with foraminal stenosis. J Radiol 1999; 80:917–925.
16. Bernard TN Jr, Whitecloud TS III. Cervical spondylotic myelopathy and myeloradiculopathy: anterior decompression and stabilization with autogenous fibula strut graft. Clin Orthop 1987; 221:149–160.
17. Binet EF, Moro JJ, Marangola JP, et al. Cervical spine tomography in trauma. Spine 1977; 2:163–172.
18. Boden SD, McCowin PR, Davis DO, et al. Abnormal magnetic resonance scans of the cervical spine in asymptomatic subjects: a prospective investigation. J Bone Joint Surg 1990; 72(8):1178–1184.
19. Bogduk N, Aprill C. On the nature of neck pain, discography and cervical zygapophysial joint blocks. Pain 1993; 54:213–217.
20. Bogduk N, Marsland A. The cervical zygapophysial joints as a source of neck pain. Spine 1988; 13:610–617.

21. Bogduk N, Twomey LT. Clinical anatomy of the lumbar spine. New York: Churchill Livingstone; 1991:117.

22. Bogduk N, Windsor M, Inglis A. The innervation of the cervical intervertebral discs. Spine 1988; 13:2–8.

23. Bogduk N. Back pain: zygapophyseal joint blocks and epidural steroids. In: Cousins MJ, Bridenbaugh PO, eds. Neural blockade in clinical anesthesia and pain management. 2nd edn. Philadelphia: JB Lippincott; 1988:939.

24. Bogduk N. Cervicogenic headache: anatomic basis and pathophysiologic mechanisms. Curr Pain Headache Rep 2001; 5(4):382–386.

25. Bogduk N. Low back pain. In: Bogduk N, ed. Clinical anatomy of the lumbar spine and sacrum. 3rd edn. New York: Churchill Livingstone; 1997:199–200.

26. Bogduk N. The anatomy and pathophysiology of neck pain. Phys Med Rehabil Clin North Am 2003; 14:455–472.

27. Bogduk N. The clinical anatomy of the cervical dorsal rami. Spine 1982; 7:319–330.

28. Borchgrevink GE, Smevik O, Nordby A, et al. MR imaging and radiography of patients with cervical hyperextension–flexion injuries after car accidents. Acta Radiologica 1995; 36:425–428.

29. Bucholz RW, Burkhead WZ, Graham W, et al. Occult cervical spine injuries in fatal traffic accidents. J Trauma 1979; 119:768–771.

30. Buonocore E, Hartman JT, Nelson CL. Cineradiograms of cervical spine in diagnosis of soft tissue injuries. JAMA 1966; 198:143–147.

31. Bush K, Hillier S. Outcome of cervical radiculopathy treated with periradicular/epidural corticosteroid injections: a prospective study with independent clinical review. Eur Spine J 1996; 5:319–325.

32. Cailliet R. Neck and arm pain. 3rd edn. Philadelphia: FA Davis; 1991.

33. Campbell AMG, Phillips DG. Cervical disk lesions with neurologic disorder. Differential diagnosis, treatment and prognosis. Br Med J 1960; 2:481–485.

34. Campbell DG, Parsons CM. Referred head pain and its concomitants. J Nerv Ment Dis 1944; 99:544–551.

35. Chan KM, Nasathurai S, Chavin JM, et al. The usefulness of central motor conduction studies in the localization of cord involvement in cervical spondylitic myelopathy. Muscle Nerve 1998; 21:1220–1223.

36. Chiu JC, Clifford TJ, Greenspan M, et al. Percutaneous microdecompressive endoscopic cervical discectomy with laser thermodiskoplasty. Mt Sinai J Med 2000; 67(4):278–282.

37. Cicala RS, Thoni K, Angel JJ. Long term results of cervical epidural steroid injections. Clin J Pain 1989; 5(2):143–145.

38. Clark CR, Igram CM, el Khoury GY, et al. Radiographic evaluation of cervical spine injuries. Spine 1988; 13:742–747.

39. Clarke E, Robinson PK. Cervical myelopathy: a complication of cervical spondylosis. Brain 1956; 75:187–225.

40. Cloward RB. Cervical diskography. A contribution to the aetiology and mechanism of neck, shoulder and arm pain. Ann Surg 1959; 130:1052–1064.

41. Colachis S, Strohm B. A study of tractive forces angle of pull on vertebral interspaces in the cervical spine. Arch Phys Med Rehabil 1965; 46:820.

42. Colachis SC Jr, Strohm BR. Effect of duration of intermittent cervical traction on vertebral separation. Arch Phys Med Rehabil 1966; 47:353–359.

43. Cole AJ, Farrell JP, Stratton SA. Functional rehabilitation of cervical spine athletic injuries. In: Kibler WB, Herring SA, Press JM, et al, eds. Functional rehabilitation of sports and musculoskeletal injuries. New York: Aspen; 1998

44. Crafts RC. Textbook of human anatomy. 2nd edn. New York: John Wiley; 1979.

45. Crock HV. A reappraisal of intervertebral disc lesions. Med J Aust 1970; 1:983–989.

46. Cyriax J. Rheumatic headache. Br Med J 1938; 2:1367–1368.

47. Cyteval C, Thomas E, Decoux E, et al. Cervical radiculopathy: open study on percutaneous periradicular foraminal steroid infiltration performed under CT control in 30 patients. Am J Neuroradiol 2004; 25:441–445.

48. Davidson RI, Dunn EJ, Metzmaker JN. Shoulder abduction test in diagnosis of radicular pain in cervical extradural compressive monoradiculopathies. Spine 1981; 6:441–446.

49. Deans G, Magalliard J, Kerr M, et al. Neck pain: a major cause of disability following car accidents. Injury 1987; 18:10–21.

50. DePalma AF, Rothman RH, Levitt RL, et al. The natural history of severe cervical disc degeneration. Acta Orthop Scand 1972; 43:392–396.

51. Dillingham TR, Lauder TD, Andary M, et al. Identification of cervical radiculopathies. Optimizing the electromyographic screen. Am J Phys Med Rehabil 2001; 80(2):84–91.

52. Dooley JF, McBroom RJ, Taguchi T, et al. Nerve root infiltration in the diagnosis of radicular pain. Spine 1988; 13(1):79–83.

53. Dreyfuss P, Michaelsen M, Fletcher D. Atlanto-occipital and lateral atlanto-axial joint pain patterns. Spine 1994; 19:1125–1131.

54. Dvorak J, Panjabi MM, Grob D, et al. Validation of flexion extension radiographs of cervical spine. Spine 1987; 18:120–127.

55. Dvorak J, Panjabi MM, Novotny J, et al. In vivo flexion/extension of the normal cervical spine. J Orthop Res 1991; 9:828–834.

56. Dwyer A, Aprill C, Bogduk N. Cervical zygapophyseal joint pain patterns. I: A study in normal volunteers. Spine 1990; 15:453–457.

57. Ellenberg MR, Honet JC, Treanor WJ. Cervical radiculopathy. Arch Phys Med Rehabil 1994; 75:342–352.

58. Ellis H. Clinical anatomy: a revision and applied anatomy for clinical students. 6th edn. London: Blackwell; 1976:205.

59. Emery SE. Cervical spondylitic myelopathy: diagnosis and treatment. J Am Acad Orthop Surg 2001; 9(6):376–388.

60. Falconer J, Hayes KW, Chang RW. Therapeutic ultrasound in the treatment of musculoskeletal conditions. Arthritis Care Res 1990; 3:85–91.

61. Fast A, Parikh S, Marin E. The shoulder abduction relief sign in cervical radiculopathy. Arch Phys Med Rehabil 1989; 70(5):402–403.

62. Feinstein B, Langton JBK, Jameson RM, et al. Experiments on referred pain from deep somatic tissues. J Bone Joint Surg (Am) 1954; 36A:981–997.

63. Fielding J. Cineroentgenography of the normal cervical spine. J Bone Joint Surg (Am) 1957; 39:1280–1284.

64. Fredriksen T, Sjaastad O. Cervicogenic headache (CEH): notes on some burning issues. Funct Neurol 2000; 15(4):199–203.

65. Fuji T, Yonenobu K, Fujiwara K, et al. Cervical radiculopathy or myelopathy secondary to athetoid cerebral palsy. J Bone Joint Surg 1987; 69A: 815–821.

66. Fukui S, Ohseto K, Shiotani M, et al. Referred pain distribution of the cervical zygapophyseal joints and cervical dorsal rami. Pain 1996; 68:79–83.

67. Furusawa N, Baba H, Miyoshi N, et al. Herniation of cervical intervertebral disk. Immunohistochemical examination and measurement of nitric oxide production. Spine 2001; 26:1110–1116.

68. Garvey TA, Transfeldt E, Malcolm JR, et al. Outcome of anterior cervical discectomy and fusion as perceived by patients treated for dominant axial–mechanical cervical spine pain. Spine 2002; 27(1): 1887–1894.

69. Garvey TA, Transfeldt EE, Malcolm JR, et al. Outcome of anterior cervical discectomy and fusion as perceived by patients treated for dominant axial–mechanical cervical spine pain. Spine 2002; 27(17):1887–1894.

70. Gore DR, Sepic SB, Gardner GM, et al. Neck pain: a long term follow up of 205 patients. Spine 1987; 12:1–5.

71. Gore DR, Sepic SB. Anterior cervical fusion for degenerated or protruded discs. A review of one hundred forty-six patients. Spine 1984; 9:667–671.

72. Grubb SA, Kelly CK. Cervical discography: clinical implications from 12 years of experience. Spine 2000; 25:1382–1389.

73. Guigui P, Benoist M, Deburge A. Spinal deformity and instability after multilevel cervical laminectomy for spondylotic myelopathy. Spine 1998; 15:440–447.

74. Hadley LA. Anatomicroradiographic studies of the spine: changes responsible for certain painful back conditions. NY J Med 1939:969–974.

75. Haldeman S, Dagenais D. Cervicogenic headaches: a critical review. Spine J 2002; 2(2):162.

76. Harada J, Dohi M, Fukuda K, et al. CT-guided percutaneous laser disk decompression (PLDD) for cervical disk hernia. Rad Med 2001; 19(5):263–266.

77. Haueisen DC, Smith BS, Myers SR, et al. The diagnostic accuracy of spinal nerve injections studies: their role in the evaluation of recurrent sciatica. Clin Orthop Relat Res 1985; 198:179–183.

78. Hawkey DJ. Cox-2 inhibitors. Lancet 1999; 353:307–314.

79. Headache Classification Committee of the International Headache Society. Classification and diagnostic criteria for headache disorders, cranial neuralgias, and facial pain. Cephalgia 1988; 8(suppl 7):1–96.

80. Heckmann JC, Lang CJ, Zobelein I, et al. Herniated cervical intervertebral discs with radiculopathy: an outcome study of conservatively or surgically treated patients. J Spinal Disord 1999; 12:396–401.

81. Heller JG, Edwards CC II, Murakami H, et al. Laminoplasty versus laminectomy and fusion for multilevel cervical myelopathy: an independent matched cohort analysis. Spine 2001; 26(12):1330–1336.

82. Hellinger J, Linke R, Heller H. A biophysical explanation for Nd:YAG percutaneous laser disc decompression success. J Clin Laser Med Surg 2001; 19(5):235–238.

83. Herkowitz H, Kurz LT, Overhohlt DP. Surgical management of cervical soft disc herniation: a comparison between the anterior and posterior approach. Spine 1990; 15:1026–1030.

84. Herkowitz HN. The surgical management of cervical spondylitic radiculopathy and myelopathy. Clin Orthop 1989; 239:94–108.

85. Hirabayashi K, Watanabe K, Wakano K, et al. Expansive open-door laminoplasty for cervical spine stenotic myelopathy. Spine 1983; 8:693–699.

86. Hitselberger WE, Witten RM. Abnormal myelograms in asymptomatic patients. J Neurosurg 1968; 28:204–206.

87. Holt EP. Fallacy of cervical discography: report of 50 cases in normal subjects. JAMA 1964; 188:799–801.

88. Hoogland T, Scheckenbach C. Low-dose chemonucleolysis combined with percutaneous nucleotomy in herniated cervical disks. J Spinal Disord 1995; 8(3):228–232.

89. Howe JF, Loeser JD, Calvin WH. Mechanosensitivity of dorsal root ganglia and chronically injured axons: a physiological basis for the radicular pain of nerve root compression. Pain 1977; 3:25–41.

90. Hoyland JA, Freemont AJ, Jayson MI. Intervertebral foramen venous obstruction. A cause of periradicular fibrosis? Spine 1989; 14(6):558–568.

91. Hult L. Cervical, dorsal, and lumbar spinal syndromes. Acta Orthop Scand (Suppl) 1954; 17:39–102.

92. Hult L. Frequency of symptoms for different age groups and professions. In: Hirsch C, Zotterman Y, eds. Cervical pain. New York: Pergamon Press; 1971:17–20.

93. Hult L. The Munkfors investigation. Acta Orthop Scand (Suppl) 1954; 17:1–38.

94. Hunt WE, Miller CA. Management of cervical radiculopathy. Clin Neurosurg 1986; 33(29):485–502.

95. Hunt WE. Cervical spondylosis: natural history and rare indications for surgical decompression. Clin Neurosurg 1980; 27:466–480.

96. Huston CW, Slipman CW, Garvin C. Complications and side effects of cervical and lumbosacral nerve root injections. Arch Phys Med Rehabil 2005; 86(2):277–283.

97. Jackson R. Cervical trauma: not just another pain in the neck. Geriatrics 1982; 37:123.

98. Jeffreys E. Disorders of the cervical spine. 2nd edn. Oxford: Butterworth-Heinemann; 1993:105–112.

99. Jeffreys RV. The surgical treatment of cervical myelopathy due to spondylosis and disc degeneration. J Neurol Neurosurg Psychiatry 1986; 49:353–361.

100. Johnson EW, Melvin JL. Value of electromyography in lumbar radiculopathy. Arch Phys Med Rehabil 1971; June:239–243.

101. Johnson RM, Hart DL, Simmons EF, et al. Cervical orthoses: a study comparing their effectiveness in restricting cervical motion in normal subjects. J Bone Joint Surg (Am) 1977; 59:332.

102. Jonsson H Jr, Brin G, Rauschning W, et al. Hidden cervical spine injuries in traffic accident victims with skull fractures. J Spinal Disord 1991; 4:251–263.

103. Jull G, Bogduk NK, Marsland A. The accuracy of manual diagnosis for cervical zygapophysial joint pain syndromes. Med J Aust 1988; 148:233–236.

104. Kaiser JA, Holland BA. Imaging of the cervical spine. Spine 1998; 23:2701–2712.

105. Kaneoka K, Ono L, Inami S, et al. Abnormal segmental motion of the cervical spine during whiplash loading. J Jpn Orthop Assoc 1997; 71: S1680.

106. Kang JD, Georgescu HI, Larkin L, et al. Herniated cervical intervertebral discs spontaneously produce matrix metalloproteinases, nitric oxide, interleukin-6, and PGE_2. Spine 1995; 20:2373–2378.

107. Kang JD, Stefanovic-Racic M, McIntyre L, et al. Toward a biochemical understanding of human intervertebral disc degeneration and herniation: contributions of nitric oxide, interleukins, prostaglandins, and matrix metalloproteinases. Spine 1997; 22:1065–1073.

108. Keegan JJ, Garrett GD. The segmental distribution of the cutaneous nerves in the limbs of man. Anat Rec 1948; 102:409–437.

109. Kellgren JH. Observations on referred pain arising from muscle. Clin Sci 1938; 3:175–190.

110. Kellgren JH. On the distribution of pain arising from deep somatic structures with charts of segmental pain. Clin Sci 1939; 3:35–46.

111. Kikuchi S, Macnab I, Moreau P. Localisation of the level of symptomatic cervical disc degeneration. J Bone Joint Surg Br 1981; 63B(2):272–277.

112. Kimmel DL. Innervation of the spinal dura mater of the posterior cranial fossa. Neurology 1960; 10:800–809.

113. Kirkaldy-Willis WH. The pathology and pathogenesis of low back pain. In: Kirkaldy-Willis WH, ed. Managing low back pain. New York: Churchill Livingstone; 1988:49.

114. Klein BR, Vaccaro AR, Albert TJ. Health outcome assessment before and after anterior cervical discectomy and fusion for radiculopathy: a prospective analysis. Spine 2000; 25:801–803.

115. Knight MTN, Goswami A, Patko JT. Cervical percutaneous laser disc decompression: preliminary results of an ongoing prospective outcome study. J Clin Laser Med Surg 2001; 19(1):3–8.

116. Knott M, Voss D. Proprioceptive neuromuscular facilitation: patterns and techniques. New York: McGraw-Hill; 1956.

117. Kraemer J, Ludwig J, Bickert U, et al. Lumbar epidural perineural injection: a new technique. Eur Spine J 1997; 6:357–361.

118. Krempen JF, Smith BS. Nerve root injection: a method for evaluating the etiology of sciatica. J Bone Joint Surg 1974; 56A:1435–1444.

119. Kuslich SD, Ahern JW, Garner MND. An in vivo, prospective analysis of tissue sensitivity of lumbar spinal tissues. Presented at the 12th Annual Meeting of the North American Spine Society, New York, 1997.

120. LaRocca H. Acceleration injuries of the neck. Clin Neurosurg 1978; 25:209–217.

121. Lawrence JS. Disc degeneration. Its frequency and relationship to symptoms. Ann Rheum Dis 1969; 28:121.

122. Lazorthes G, Gaubert J. L'innervation des articulations interapophysaire vertebrales. C R Assoc Anat 1956; 43:488–494.

123. Lehman JF. Therapeutic heat and cold. 4th edn. Baltimore: Williams & Wilkins; 1990.

124. Lehmann JD, Brunner GD, Stow RW. Pain threshold measurements after therapeutic application of ultrasound, microwaves and infrared. Arch Phys Med Rehabil 1958; 39:560–565.

125. Lehmann JF, DeLateur BJ. Therapeutic heat. In: Lehmann JF, ed. Therapeutic heat and cold. 3rd edn. Baltimore: William & Wilkins; 1982:413–414.

126. L'Hermitte J. Etude de la commation de la moele. Rev Neurol 1932; 1:210–239.

127. Liversedge LA, Hutchinson EC, Lyons JB. Cervical spondylosis simulating motor neuron disease. Lancet 1953; 2:652–659.

128. Lord SM, Barnsley L, Bogduk N. Percutaneous radiofrequency neurotomy in the treatment of cervical zygapophysial joint pain: a caution. Neurosurgery 1995; 36:732–739.

129. Lord SM, Barnsley L, Bogduk N. The utility of comparative local anaesthetic blocks versus placebo-controlled blocks for the diagnosis of cervical zygapophysial joint pain. Clin J Pain 1995; 11:208–213.

130. Lord SM, Barnsley L, Wallis BJ, et al. Chronic cervical zygapophyseal joint pain after whiplash. A placebo-controlled prevalence study. Spine 1996; 21:1737–1745.

131. Lord SM, Barnsley L, Wallis BJ, et al. Third occipital nerve headache: a prevalence study. J Neurol Neurosurg Psychiatry 1994; 57:1187–1190.

132. Lunardi P, Acqui M, Ricci G, et al. Cervical synovial cysts: case report and review of the literature. Eur Spine J 1999; 8:232–237.

133. Macdonald RL, Fehlings MG, Tator CH, et al. Multilevel anterior cervical corpectomy and fibular allograft fusion for cervical myelopathy. J Neurosurg 1997; 26:990–997.

134. Macnab I, McCulloch J. Neck ache and shoulder pain. Baltimore: Williams & Wilkins; 1994.

135. Makela M, Heliovara M, Sievers D, et al. Prevalence, determinants, and consequences of chronic neck pain in Finland. Am J Epidemiol 1991; 134:1356–1367.

136. Malacca R, Jeans ME, Stratford JG, et al. Ice massage and transcutaneous electrical stimulation: comparison of treatment for low back pain. Pain 1980; 9:209–217.

137. Malanga G. The diagnosis and treatment of cervical radiculopathy. Med Sci Sports Exerc 1997; 29(suppl):S236–S245.

138. Manelfe C. Imaging of the spine and spinal cord. Radiology 1991; 3:5–15.

139. Martino F, Ettore GC, Cafaro E, et al. L'ecographia musculo-tendinea nei traumi distorvi acuti del collo. Radiol Med Torino 1992; 83:211–215.

140. Matsumoto M, Fujimura Y, Suzuki N, et al. MRI of cervical intervertebral discs in asymptomatic subjects. J Bone Joint Surg 1998; 80B:19–24.

141. Mayr MT, Subach BR, Comey CH. Cervical spinal stenosis: outcome after anterior corpectomy, allograft reconstruction, and instrumentation. J Neurosurg 2002; 96(1S):10–16.

142. McConnell WE, Howard RP, Guzman HM, et al. Analysis of human test subject kinematic responses to low velocity rear end impacts. Proceedings of the 37th STAPP Car Crash Conference. Warrendale: Society for Automotive Engineers; 1993:2130.

143. McDonald GJ, Lord SM, Bogduk N. Long-term follow up of patients treated with cervical radiofrequency neurotomy for chronic neck pain. Neurosurgery 1999; 45:61–67.

144. McKinney LA. Early mobilization of acute sprain of the neck. Br Med J 1989; 299:1006–1008.

145. McRae DL. Asymptomatic intervertebral disc protrusions. Acta Radiol 1956; 46:9–27.

146. Meloche J, et al. Painful intervertebral dysfunction: Robert Maigne's original contribution to headache of cervical origin. The Quebec Headache Study Group. Headache 1995; 33(6):328–334.

147. Melzack R, Wall PD. Pain mechanisms: a new theory. Science 1965; 150:971–979.

148. Merskey H, Bogduk N. Classification of chronic pain. Descriptions of chronic pain syndromes and definitions of pain terms. In: Merskey H, Bogduk N, eds. Cervicogenic headache. Seattle: International Association for the Study of Pain; 1994.

149. Michlovitz S. Cryotherapy: the use of cold as a therapeutic agent. In: Michlovitz S, ed. Thermal agents in rehabilitation. 2nd edn. Philadelphia: Davis; 1990:88–108.

150. Mikawa Y, Shikata J, Yamamuro T. Spinal deformity and instability after multilevel cervical laminectomy. Spine 1987; 12:6–11.

151. Mink JH, Gordon RE, Deutsch AL. The cervical spine: radiologist's perspective. Phys Med Rehabil Clin North Am 2003; 14:493–548.

152. Modic M, Masaryk T, Mulopulos G, et al. Cervical radiculopathy: prospective evaluation with surface coil MR imaging, CT with metrizamide, and metrizamide myelography. Radiology 1986; 161:753–759.

153. Moore KL, Agur AM. Essential clinical anatomy. Baltimore: Williams & Wilkins; 1995.

154. Morio Y, Teshima R, Nagashima H, et al. Correlation between operative outcomes of cervical compression myelopathy and MRI of the spinal cord. Spine 2001; 26:1238–1245.

155. Murphy RW. Nerve roots and spinal nerves in degenerative disk disease. Clin Orthop Relat Res 1977; 129:46–60.

156. Newham DJ. The consequences of eccentric contractions and their relationship to delayed-onset muscle pain. Eur J Appl Physiol 1988; 57:353–359.

157. Nilsson N. The prevalence of cervicogenic headache in a random population sample of 20–59 year olds. Spine 1995; 20(17):1884–1888.

158. Norris H, Watt I. The prognosis of neck injuries resulting from rear-end vehicle collisions. J Bone Joint Surg 1983; 65B:608–611.

159. Nurick S. The natural history and the results of surgical treatment of the spinal cord disorder associated with cervical spondylosis. Brain 1972; 95:101–108.

160. Olmarker K, Rydevik B, Nordborg C. Autologous nucleus pulposus induces neurophysiologic and histologic changes in porcine cauda equina nerve roots. Spine 1993; 18:1425–1432.

161. O'Sullivan PB, Phyty GD, Twomey LT, et al. Evaluation of specific stabilizing exercise in the treatment of chronic low back pain with radiologic diagnosis of spondylosis or spondylolisthesis. Spine 1997; 22:2959–2967.

162. Panjabi M, Ito S, Pearson A, et al. Injury mechanisms of the cervical intervertebral disc during simulated whiplash. Spine 2004; 29(11):1217–1225.

163. Parke WW. Applied anatomy of the spine. In: Rothman RH, Simeone FA, eds. The spine. 3rd edn. Philadelphia: Saunders; 1992.

164. Parminder SP. Management of cervical pain. In: DeLisa JA, ed. Rehabilitation medicine: principles and practice. Philadelphia: Lippincott; 1988: 753.

165. Pavlov H, Torg JS. Roentgen examination of cervical spine injuries in the athlete. Clin Sports Med 1987; 6:761.

166. Penning L, Wilmink JT, Van Woerden HH, et al. CT myelographic findings in degenerative disorders of the cervical spine: clinical significance. AJR Am J Roentgenol 1986; 7:119–127.

167. Persson LC, Moritz U, Brandt L. Cervical radiculopathy: pain, muscle weakness and sensory loss in patients with cervical radiculopathy treated with surgery, physiotherapy or cervical collar. A prospective, controlled study. Eur Spine J 1997; 6:256–266.

168. Pettersson K, Hildingsson C, Toolanen G, et al. MRI and neurology in acute whiplash trauma: no correlation in prospective examination of 39 cases. Acta Orthop Scand 1994; 65:525–528.

169. Phillips DG. Surgical treatment of myelopathy with cervical spondylosis. J Neurol Neurosurg Psychiatry 1973; 36:879–884.

170. Poindexter DP, Johnson EW. Football shoulder and neck injury: a study of the 'stinger'. Arch Phys Med Rehabil 1984; 65:601–602.

171. Press JM, Herring SA, Kibler WB. Rehabilitation of musculoskeletal disorders. In: The textbook of military medicine. Borden Institute: Office of the Surgeon General; 1996.

172. Purkis IE. Cervical epidural steroids. Pain Clinic 1986; 1:3–7.

173. Quinlan KP, Annest JL, Myers B, et al. Neck strains and sprains among motor vehicle occupants—United States, 2000. Accid Anal Prev 2004; 36:21–27.

174. Radanov BP, Sturzenegger M, Di Stefano G. Long-term outcome after whiplash injury: a 2-year follow-up considering features of injury mechanism and somatic, radiologic, and psychosocial findings. Medicine 1995; 74:281–297.

175. Radharkrishnan K, Litchy WJ, O'Fallon WM, et al. Epidemiology of cervical radiculopathy. A population-based study from Rochester, Minnesota, 1976–1990. Brain 1994; 117(part 2):325–335.

176. Ramanauskas W, Wilner H, Metes J. MR imaging of compressive myelomalacia. J Comput Assist Tomogr 1989; 13:399–404.

177. Rappaport ZH, Dever M. Experimental pathophysiological correlates of clinical symptomatology in peripheral neuropathic pain syndrome. Stereotact Funct Neurosurg 1990; 54–55:90–95.

178. Rauschning W. Anatomy of the normal and traumatized spine. In: Sances A, Tomas DL, Ewing CL, et al, eds. Mechanisms of head and spine trauma. Deer Park: Aloray; 1986:531–563.

179. Redford JB, Patel A. Orthotic devices in the management of spinal disorders. Spine State Art Rev 1995; 9:673–688.

180. Reitman C, Esses S. Modalities, manual therapy, and education: a review of conservative measures. Spine State Art Rev 1995; 9:661–672.

181. Rowlingson JC, Kirschenbaum LP. Epidural analgesic techniques in the management of cervical pain. Anesth Analg 1986; 65:938–942.

182. Russell EJ. Computed tomography and myelography in the evaluation of cervical degenerative disease. Neuroimaging Clin North Am 1995; 5(3):329–348.

183. Rydevik B, Brown M, Lundborg G. Pathoanatomy and pathophysiology of nerve root compression. Spine 1984; 9:7–15.

184. Saal J, Saal J, Yurth E. Nonoperative management of herniated cervical intervertebral disc with radiculopathy. Spine 1996; 21(16):1877–1883.

185. Saal J. The role of inflammation in lumbar pain. Spine 1995; 20:1821–1827.

186. Sanchez MC, Arenillas JIC, Gutierrez DA, et al. Cervical radiculopathy: a rare symptom of giant cell arteritis. Arthritis Rheum 1983; 26:207–209.

187. Sapir D, Gorup J. Radiofrequency medial branch neurotomy in litigant and non litigant patients with cervical whiplash. Spine 2001; 26(12):E268–E273.

188. Schellhas KP, Smith MD, Gundry CR, et al. Cervical discogenic pain: prospective correlation of magnetic resonance imaging and discography in asymptomatic subjects and pain sufferers. Spine 1996; 21:300–312.

189. Schellhas KP, Smith MD, Gundry CR, et al. Cervical discogenic pain: prospective correlation of magnetic resonance imaging and discography in asymptomatic subjects and pain sufferers. Spine 1996; 21(3): 300–312.

190. Schofferman J, Garges K, Goldthwaite N, et al. Upper cervical anterior diskectomy and fusion improves discogenic cervical headaches. Spine 2002; 27(20):2240–2244.

191. Schutz H, Lougheed WM, Wortzman G, et al. Intervertebral nerve-root in the investigation of chronic lumbar disc disease. Can J Surg 1973; 16:217–221.

192. Seibenrock KA, Aebi M. Cervical discography in discogenic pain syndrome and its predictive value for cervical fusion. Arch Orthop Trauma Surg 1994; 113:199–203.

193. Selecki BR. Whiplash. Aust Fam Phys 1984; 13:243–247.

194. Semmes RE, Murphey MD. The syndrome of unilateral rupture of the sixth cervical intervertebral disk with compression of the seventh cervical nerve root. A report of four cases with symptoms simulating coronary disease. JAMA 1943; 121:1209–1214.

195. Sharps LS, Isaac Z. Percutaneous disc decompression using nucleoplasty. Pain Physician 2002; 5(2):121–126.

196. Shulman M. Treatment of neck pain with cervical epidural injection. Reg Anesth 1986; 11:92–94.

197. Siebert W. Percutaneous laser discectomy of cervical discs: preliminary clinical results. J Clin Laser Med Surg 1995; 13(3):205–207.

198. Simmons EH, Segil CM. An evaluation of discography in the localization of symptomatic levels in discogenic disease of the spine. Clin Orthop 1975; 108:57–69.

199. Sjaastad O, et al. 'Cervicogenic' headache. A hypothesis. Cephalgia 1983; 3:249–256.

200. Sjaastad O, Fredriksen T, Pfaffenrath V. Cervicogenic headache: diagnostic criteria. The Cervicogenic Headache International Study Group. Headache 1998; 38(6):442–445.

201. Sjaastad O, Fredriksen T. Cervicogenic headache: criteria, classification and epidemiology. Clin Exp Rheumatol 2000; 18(2 suppl 19):S3–S6.

202. Slipman CW, Chow DW, Isaac Z, et al. An evidence-based algorithmic approach to cervical spinal disorders. Crit Rev Phys Med Rehabil Med 2001; 13(4):283–299.

203. Slipman CW, DePalma MJ, Bhargava A, et al. Treatment of cervical radiculopathy with combined percutaneous plasma field discectomy and nerve root glucocorticoid injection: a pilot study.

204. Slipman CW, Isaac Z, Oleski C, et al. Does the cervical zygapophyseal joint refer symptoms to the neck bilaterally?: preliminary data from 100 patients. Arch Phys Med Rehabil 2002; 83(11):1665.

205. Slipman CW, Isaac Z, Thomas J, et al. Cervical zygapophyseal joint syndrome and referral to the head and face: preliminary data from 100 patients. Arch Phys Med Rehabil 2002; 83(11):1665.

206. Slipman CW, Lipetz JS, DePalma MJ, et al. Therapeutic selective nerve root block in the nonsurgical treatment of traumatically induced cervical spondylitic radicular pain. Am J Phys Med Rehabil 2004; 83(6):446–454.

207. Slipman CW, Lipetz JS, Jackson HB, et al. Outcomes of therapeutic selective nerve root blocks for whiplash induced cervical radicular pain. Pain Physician 2001; 4(2):167–174.

208. Slipman CW, Lipetz JS, Jackson HB, et al. Therapeutic selective nerve root block in the nonsurgical treatment of atraumatic cervical spondylitic radicular pain: a retrospective analysis with independent clinical review. Arch Phys Med Rehabil 2000; 81:741–746.

209. Slipman CW, Lipetz JS, Plastaras CT, et al. Therapeutic zygapophyseal joint injections for headaches emanating from the C2–3 joint. Am J Phys Med Rehabil 2001; 80(3):182–188.

210. Slipman CW, Plastaras C, Patel R, et al. Provocative cervical discography symptom mapping. Spine J 2005; 5(4):381–388.

211. Slipman CW, Plastaras CT, Palmitier RS, et al. Symptom provocation of fluoroscopically guided cervical nerve root stimulation: are dynatomal maps identical to dermatomal maps? Spine 1998; 23:2235–2242.

212. Smith GW, Nichols PJ. The technique of cervical discography. Radiology 1957; 68:718–720.

213. Sobel JB, Sollenberger P, Robinson R, et al. Cervical nonorganic signs: a new clinical tool to assess abnormal illness behavior in neck pain patients: a pilot study. Arch Phys Med Rehabil 2000; 81:170–175.

214. Spitzer W, Leblanc F, Dupuis M, et al. Scientific approach to the assessment and management of activity-related spinal disorder: a monograph for clinicians. Report of the Quebec Task Force on Spinal Disorders. Spine 1987; 12(suppl):S1–S57.

215. Spitzer WO, Skovron ML, Salmi LR, et al. Scientific monograph of the Quebec Task Force on Whiplash-associated Disorders: redefining 'whiplash' and its management. Spine 1995; 20(suppl 8):3S–73S.

216. Spurling RG, Scoville WB. Lateral rupture of the cervical intervertebral discs. A common cause of shoulder and arm pain. Surg Gynecol Obstet 1944; 78:350–358.

217. Stanley D, McLaren MI, Euinton HA, et al. A prospective study of nerve root infiltration in the diagnosis of sciatica: a comparison with radiculography, computed tomography, and operative findings. Spine 1990; 15(6): 540–543.

218. Su HC, Su RK. Treatment of whiplash injuries with acupuncture. Clin J Pain 1988; 4:233.

219. Swanberg H. The intervertebral foramina in man. Chicago: Scientific Publishing; 1995.

220. Sweeney T, Prentice C, Saal JA, et al. Cervicothoracic muscular stabilizing technique. Phys Med Rehabil State Art Rev 1990; 4:335–360.

221. Swezey RL, Swezey AM. Efficacy of home cervical traction therapy. Am J Phys Med Rehabil 1999; 78:30–32.

222. Szabo T, Welch J. Human subject electromyographic activity during low speed rear impacts. Presented at the 40th STAPP Car Crash Conference. Warrendale: Society for Automotive Engineers; 1996.

223. Takala J, Sievers K, Klaukka T. Rheumatic symptoms in the middle-aged population in southwestern Finland. Scand J Rheumatol (Suppl) 1982; 47:15–29.

224. Taylor JR, Twomey LT. Acute injuries to cervical joints. An autopsy study of neck sprain. Spine 1993; 9:1115–1122.

225. Teresi LM, Lufkin RB, Reicher MA, et al. Asymptomatic degenerative disk disease and spondylosis of the cervical spine: MR imaging. Radiology 1987; 164:83–88.

226. Teresi LM, Lufkin RB, Reicher MA, et al. Asymptomatic degenerative disk disease and spondylosis of the cervical spine: MR imaging. Radiology 1987; 164:83–88.

227. Tomita K, Nomura S, Umaeda S, et al. Cervical laminoplasty to enlarge the spinal canal in multilevel ossification of the posterior longitudinal ligament with myelopathy. Arch Orthop Trauma Surg 1988; 107:148–153.

228. Und B, Schlbom H, Nordwall A, et al. Normal range of motion in cervical spine. Arch Phys Med Rehabil 1989; 70:692–695.

229. Vallee JN, Feydy A, Carlier RY, et al. Chronic cervical radiculopathy: lateral approach periradicular corticosteroid injection. Radiology 2001; 218:886–892.

230. VanAkkerveeken PF. The diagnostic value of nerve root sheath infiltration. Acta Orthop Scand 1993; 251 (suppl):61–63.

231. Vargo MM, Flood KM. Pancoast tumor presenting as cervical radiculopathy. Arch Phys Med Rehabil 1990; 71:606–609.

232. Viikari-Juntura E, Porras M, Laasonen EM. Validity of clinical tests in the diagnosis of root compression in cervical disc disease. Spine 1989; 14:253–257.

233. Vincent M. Cervicogenic headache: a comparison with migraine and tension-type headache. Cephalgia 1999; 1(suppl 25):11–16.

234. Westerling D, Jonsson BG. Pain from the neck–shoulder region and sick leave. Scand J Soc Med 1980; 8:131–136.

235. White AA III, Southwick WO, Deponte RJ, et al. Relief of pain by anterior cervical spine fusion for spondylosis. A report of sixty-five patients. J Bone Joint Surg (Am) 1973; 55A:525–534.

236. White AA, Panjabi MM. The problem of clinical instability in the human spine: a systematic approach. In: Clinical biomechanics of the spine. 2nd edn. Philadelphia: Lippincott; 1990.

237. Whitecloud TS, Seago RA. Cervical discogenic syndrome: results of operative intervention in patients with positive discography. Spine 1987; 12:313–316.

238. Wilbourn AJ, Aminoff MJ. AAEM minimonograph 32: the electrodiagnostic examination in patients with radiculopathies. Muscle Nerve 1998; 21:1612–1631.

239. Wilkinson M. The morbid anatomy of cervical spondylosis and myelopathy. Brain 1960; 83:589–616.

240. Wolff MW, Levine LA. Cervical radiculopathies: conservative approaches to management. Phys Med Rehabil Clin North Am 2002; 13:589–608.

241. Wood EC. Beard's massage: principles and techniques. Philadelphia: Saunders; 1974.

242. Ylinen J, Ruuska J. Clinical use of isometric neck strength measurement in rehabilitation. Arch Phys Med Rehabil 1994; 75:465–469.

243. Yoss RE, Corbin KB, McCarthy CS, et al. Significance of symptoms and signs in localization of involved root in cervical disc protrusion. Neurology 1957; 7:673–683.

244. Yu YL, Jones SJ. Somatosensory evoked potentials in cervical spondylosis: correlation of median, ulnar, and posterior tibial nerve responses with clinical and radiological findings. Brain 1985; 108:273–300.

245. Yu YL, Woo E, Huang CY. Cervical spondylitic myelopathy and radiculopathy. Acta Neurol Scand 1987; 75:367–373.

246. Zheng Y, Liew S, Simmons E. Value of magnetic resonance imaging and discography in determining the level of cervical discectomy and fusion. Spine 2004; 29(19):2140–2145.

Chapter

39

Musculoskeletal Problems of the Upper Limb

Jonathan T. Finnoff

'The whole is greater than the sum of its parts'. This statement is surely reflected in the upper limb. Through the complex interplay of neuromusculoskeletal elements in the upper limb, activities as dichotomous as playing a piano and throwing a shot put can be achieved. The diversity of functional roles played by the upper limb is reflected by the multitude of injuries that can occur in this anatomic region. This chapter addresses musculo-skeletal problems that occur in the upper limb.

UPPER LIMB PHYSICAL EXAMINATION

There are multiple special tests for the upper limbs. This section describes several important tests for each region of the upper limb.

Shoulder tests

Anterior apprehension (crank) and relocation tests

These are tests for anterior glenohumeral joint instability. The patient is placed in the supine position. The examiner abducts the patient's shoulder 90°, and flexes the elbow 90°. The examiner uses one hand to slowly externally rotate the patient's humerus, using the patient's forearm as the lever. At the same time, the examiner's other hand is placed posterior to the patient's proximal humerus, and exerts an anteriorly directed force on the humeral head. The test is considered positive if the patient indicates a feeling of impending anterior dislocation. If the examiner then removes their hand from behind the proximal humerus, places it over the anterior proximal humerus, and exerts a posteriorly directed force, and the patient reports a reduction in their apprehension, then a positive relocation test has occurred.[95]

Posterior apprehension test

This test evaluates posterior glenohumeral joint stability. The patient's affected shoulder is forward flexed to 90°, then maximally internally rotated. A posteriorly directed force is then placed on the patient's elbow by the examiner. A positive test causes a 50% or greater posterior translation of the humeral head, or a feeling of apprehension in the patient.[95]

Sulcus sign

The sulcus sign is used to evaluate inferior glenohumeral joint instability. The patient is seated or standing with the arm relaxed in shoulder adduction. The patient's forearm is grasped by the examiner, and a distal traction force is placed through the patient's arm. In the presence of inferior instability, a sulcus will develop between the humeral head and the acromion.[95]

O'Brien's test

This test evaluates for acromioclavicular joint and/or labral abnormalities. The patient's shoulder is flexed to 90° with the elbow fully extended. The arm is then adducted 15°, and the shoulder is internally rotated so that the patient's thumb is pointing down. The examiner applies a downward force against the arm, which the patient is instructed to resist. The shoulder is then externally rotated so that the patient's palm is facing up, and the examiner applies a downward force on the patient's arm, which the patient is instructed to resist. A positive test is indicated by pain during the first part of the maneuver with the patient's thumb pointing down, which is then lessened or eliminated when the patient resists a downward force with the palm facing up. Pain in the region of the acromioclavicular joint is indicative of acromioclavicular pathology, while pain or painful clicking deep inside the shoulder suggests labral pathology.[120]

Speed's test

This test is for biceps tendonitis. The patient's shoulder is forward flexed to 90°, the elbow is fully extended, and the palm is facing up. The examiner applies a downward force against the patient's active resistance. Pain in the region of the bicipital groove suggests bicipital tendonitis.[95]

Neer–Walsh impingement test

The patient's shoulder is internally rotated while at the side. The examiner passively forward flexes the patient's shoulder to 180° while maintaining the internal rotation. Pain in the sub-acromial area suggests rotator cuff pathology.[95]

Hawkins–Kennedy impingement test

The patient's shoulder and elbow are each passively flexed to 90°. The examiner then grasps the patient's forearm, stabilizes the patient's scapulothoracic joint, and uses the forearm as a lever arm to internally rotate the glenohumeral joint. A positive test is indicated by pain in the subacromial region with internal rotation.[95]

Drop arm test

The examiner passively abducts the patient's shoulder 90°. The patient is then asked to slowly lower the arm back to the side. A positive test is indicated by pain and an inability to slowly lower the arm to the side. This suggests a rotator cuff tear.[95]

Elbow tests

Cozen's test

The patient is asked to fully extend the elbow, pronate the forearm, and make a fist. The examiner then resists the patient's attempt to extend and radially deviate the wrist. Pain over the lateral epicondyle represents a positive test and suggests the presence of lateral epicondylitis.[93]

Ligamentous instability test

The examiner flexes the patient's elbow 20–30°, and stabilizes the patient's arm by placing a hand at the elbow and a hand on the distal forearm. A varus and valgus force is placed across the elbow by the examiner to test the stability of the radial and ulnar collateral ligaments, respectively.[93]

Wrist and hand tests

Finkelstein's test

This test is used to detect tenosynovitis of the extensor pollicis brevis and abductor pollicis longus tendons (de Quervain tenosynovitis). The patient makes a fist with the thumb inside the fingers, and the examiner passively deviates the wrist in an ulnar direction. A positive test causes pain in the affected tendons.[94]

Watson's test

This test assesses scapholunate stability. The patient's wrist begins in an ulnarly deviated position. The examiner places a dorsally directed force against the proximal volar pole of the scaphoid. The examiner then radially deviates the wrist while continuing to place the same force against the scaphoid. A 'pop' or subluxation of the scaphoid indicates a positive test.[94]

Tinel's sign

The examiner taps over the carpal tunnel. A positive sign is indicated by paresthesias into the thumb, index, and middle fingers. A positive sign is suggestive of carpal tunnel syndrome.[94] Tinel's sign can be elicited over any superficial sensory or mixed nerve.

Phalen's test

The examiner maximally flexes the patient's wrists and holds them in this position for 1 min. Production of paresthesias in the median sensory distribution of the hand suggests carpal tunnel syndrome.[94]

REHABILITATION PRINCIPLES OF UPPER LIMB INJURY

The importance of making the correct diagnoses in planning an appropriate treatment program cannot be overemphasized. A complete diagnosis includes whether the injury is acute, chronic, or an acute exacerbation of a chronic injury. Understanding the mechanism of injury is very important. Tissues that are overloaded by the injury, as well as those directly injured, must be identified. Functional biomechanical deficits such as strength and flexibility imbalances are frequently present. The patient often tries to compensate for the injury by altering movement patterns and using muscle substitutions, which leads to reduction in functional performance and secondary injuries at distant sites in the kinetic chain.

Once an accurate diagnosis has been made with a thorough history, physical examination, and appropriate diagnostic testing, an effective treatment program can be developed. Kibler has proposed three broad stages of rehabilitation: the acute stage, the recovery stage, and the functional stage.[78] The acute stage of rehabilitation focuses on reducing the patient's symptoms and facilitating tissue healing. In specific circumstances, immobilization through splinting or casting might be utilized during the acute stage of rehabilitation.

The acronym RICE, which stands for rest, ice, compression, and elevation, is frequently used in this phase of rehabilitation. Rest should not be absolute. It is important for the patient to maintain cardiovascular fitness, strength, and flexibility during this phase. The patient should be instructed on appropriate activities that can be performed during the acute stage of rehabilitation that will not aggravate symptoms nor be detrimental to tissue healing. For example, if a volleyball player has rotator cuff tendonitis, she or he might be allowed to perform passive glenohumeral joint range of motion exercises to maintain flexibility and glenohumeral joint health, ride a stationary bicycle for cardiovascular fitness, and perform scapular stabilizing exercises in preparation for more advanced rehabilitative exercises of the shoulder.

During the acute phase of rehabilitation, cryotherapy can be used for acute injuries to decrease pain, inflammation, muscle guarding, edema, and local blood flow.[65,77] Heat increases blood flow, reduces muscle spasm, and reduces pain, and can be utilized in the acute phase of rehabilitation for chronic injuries.[77] High-frequency electrical stimulation is often used during the acute phase of rehabilitation to reduce muscle guarding and increase local circulation.[174]

Opioid and non-opioid analgesics might be required for pain control during the acute phase of rehabilitation. Non-steroidal antiinflammatory drugs (NSAIDs) are often utilized for their analgesic and antiinflammatory properties. Randomized, placebo-controlled trials have demonstrated reduced pain, reduced edema and tenderness, and a faster return to activity in NSAID-treated athletes than in those treated with placebo.[5,171] It is important to remember, however, that NSAIDs are not entirely benign and can result in gastropathy, peripheral edema, renal toxicity, and other conditions.[31,56] There is recent evidence that at least the cyclooxygenase-2 NSAIDs might have cardiac side effects if used chronically. Due to these concerns, NSAIDs should be used only if local physical modalities and less toxic medications such as acetaminophen (paracetamol) are not effective.

Oral and injected corticosteroids have also been used for pain control and reduction of inflammation during the acute phase of rehabilitation. Due to the possibility of significant systemic and localized consequences of corticosteroid use, however, their use should be limited to very select cases.[49,145] These side effects include suppression of the hypothalamic–pituitary–adrenal axis, osteoporosis, avascular necrosis, infection, and tendon or ligament rupture.

The patient can advance to the recovery phase of rehabilitation when the pain has been adequately controlled and tissue healing has occurred.[78] This is indicated by full pain-free range of motion and the ability to participate in strengthening exercises for the injured limb. The emphasis of the recovery phase of rehabilitation involves the restoration of flexibility, strength, and proprioception in the injured limb. Strength and flexibility imbalances, and maladaptive movement patterns and muscle substitutions, should be corrected in this phase of rehabilitation. Open kinetic chain exercises can be beneficial when correcting strength imbalances, while closed kinetic chain exercises are frequently used to provide joint stabilization through muscle cocontraction. The patient's cardiovascular and general fitness should continue to be maintained. Progression to functional activities is initiated toward the end of this phase.

The patient can begin the functional stage of rehabilitation when the injured limb has regained 75–80% of normal strength as compared with the uninjured limb, and when there are no strength and flexibility imbalances.[78] The patient's rehabilitation needs to continue to address maladaptive movement patterns and muscle substitutions, and full strength needs to be obtained. Functional activities should be incorporated into the rehabilitation program, with a vocational or an avocational specific progression eventually leading to return to normal activities.

MUSCULOSKELETAL PROBLEMS OF THE UPPER LIMB

Conditions of the shoulder

Sternoclavicular joint sprains

Sternoclavicular joint sprains can be graded on a scale of 1 to 3 (Table 39-1). Grade 1 injuries are mild sprains without instability or significant ligament disruption. Grade 2 injuries are moderately severe ligamentous sprains with associated subluxation of the sternoclavicular joint. A grade 3 injury results in complete disruption of the sternoclavicular ligaments, with anterior or posterior dislocation.[37]

Sternoclavicular joint dislocations account for less than 1% of all joint dislocations. Two-thirds of sternoclavicular joint dislocations occur anteriorly, while a third of dislocations occur posteriorly. The etiology is usually traumatic.[37]

The diagnosis of sternoclavicular joint injuries is made with an accurate history, physical examination, and radiologic evaluation. Anterior sternoclavicular joint injuries can cause the medial end of the clavicle to become more prominent, while posterior joint injuries typically have more pain with a less prominent medial clavicular end. Posterior dislocations can also

Table 39-1 Ligamentous injury grading scale	
Grade	Sign
1	Tenderness to palpation without joint laxity
2	Tenderness to palpation with joint laxity but a good end point
3	Tenderness to palpation with significant joint laxity and no end point

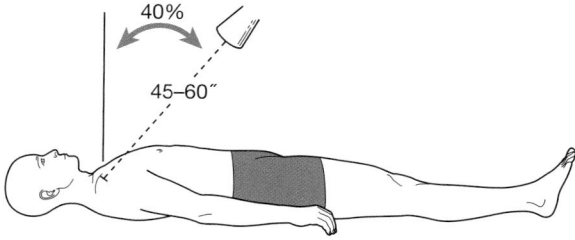

Figure 39-1 The serendipity view of the sternoclavicular joints.

be associated with vascular compromise to the ipsilateral upper limb, neck and/or upper limb venous congestion, difficulty breathing, or difficulty swallowing. The presence of tenderness at the sternoclavicular joint without subluxation or dislocation indicates a grade 1 injury, tenderness with subluxation indicates a grade 2 injury, and tenderness with associated dislocation indicates a grade 3 injury.[175]

The radiologic evaluation of sternoclavicular joint injuries should include not only an anteroposterior radiograph of the chest or sternoclavicular joint, but also the serendipity view, which involves a 40° cephalic tilt view of the sternoclavicular joints (Fig. 39-1).[146] Often, standard radiographs leave the diagnosis in question, and computed tomography (CT) scan is frequently used for definitive evaluation of sternoclavicular joint injuries.

The treatment of grade 1 and 2 injuries involves ice for the first 24–48 h and sling immobilization for comfort and protection. NSAIDs and other analgesics might be required for adequate pain control. Activity can progress as tolerated, with an anticipated return to activity after 1–2 weeks for a grade 1 injury and 4–6 weeks for a grade 2 injury.

Controversy exists in the treatment of grade 3 sternoclavicular joint sprains. De Jong and Sukui reported that a majority of patients treated non-operatively with analgesics and sling immobilization for anterior grade 3 dislocations had good or excellent outcomes at 5-year follow-up.[73] Most acute anterior dislocations remain unstable post reduction, however, and surgical intervention is usually done.[175]

Because complications frequently arise with grade 3 posterior dislocations, a thorough evaluation to rule out pulmonary or vascular damage should be undertaken. After serious associated injuries have been ruled out, closed reduction of posterior grade

3 dislocations can be performed. If mediastinal compression is present, posterior grade 3 dislocations require immediate surgical intervention.[175] The practitioner should never attempt to reduce a posterior sternoclavicular joint dislocation 'on the field', because there is a great risk of significant vascular complications. In this situation, the closed reduction should take place in the hospital setting in the presence of a vascular surgeon.

Clavicle fractures

A majority of clavicular fractures occur in childhood and in adults under 25 years of age. Eighty percent of clavicular fractures occur in the middle third of the clavicle, while approximately 15% occur in the lateral one-third and 5% in the medial one-third. Most clavicular fractures occur due to a direct blow to the point of the shoulder, but a small percentage occur due to a fall on to an outstretched arm.[17]

Clavicular fractures can be classified as group 1 (middle third), group 2 (distal third), or group 3 (proximal third) fractures.[4] Neer proposed three additional classifications for group 2 fractures.[113] Type 1 fractures were interligamentous with minimal displacement. Type 2 fractures occurred medial to the coracoclavicular ligaments and were displaced. Type 3 fractures were intraarticular fractures of the distal clavicle in the acromioclavicular joint.

Most patients know when they have fractured their clavicle. It is important to rule out associated injuries to neurovascular and pulmonary structures during the physical examination and radiologic evaluation. Routine anteroposterior radiographs of the clavicle are usually adequate for visualization of clavicular middle third fractures. For proximal third fractures, the addition of a serendipity view is often employed. When a lateral third fracture is suspected, a 15° cephalic tilt anteroposterior view centered on the acromioclavicular joint using a soft tissue technique (Zanca view) and an axillary lateral view are usually diagnostic when combined with anteroposterior radiographs. Occasionally, CT scanning is required for more definitive evaluation.[17]

If the fracture has good alignment, partial immobilization is the treatment of choice using an immobilization device such as a sling or figure of eight bandage. For group 1 fractures with more than 100% displacement, a reduction maneuver should be performed. If crepitus is felt between the bone ends during the procedure, this suggests that there is no tissue interposition to prevent healing. However, if no crepitus is felt, tissue is frequently interposed between the fracture ends. This has been suggested as a cause of non-union and is an indication for surgical intervention. Other common indications for surgical intervention include open fractures, neurovascular compromise, comminuted and/or shortened fractures in the dominant arm of a throwing athlete, tenting of the skin over the fracture site that might lead to tissue necrosis, and group 2 type 2 fractures.[17]

Acromioclavicular joint sprains

Acromioclavicular joint sprains account for only 9% of all shoulder injuries, are most frequent in men in their third decade of

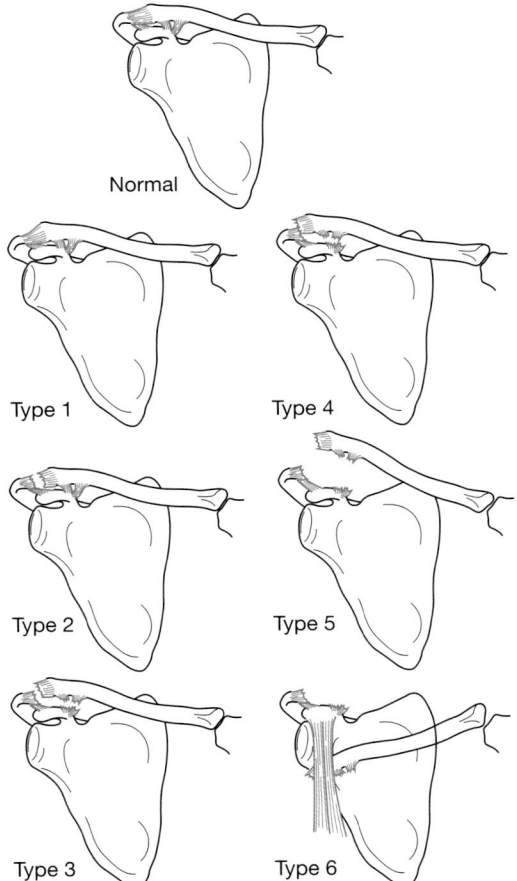

Figure 39-2 The Rockwood classification of acromioclavicular joint sprains.

life, and are usually partial rather than complete sprains.[99] Most injuries occur due to direct trauma from a fall or blow to the acromion. Physical examination shows point tenderness, a positive horizontal adduction test, and a positive O'Brien's test.

Rockwood classified acromioclavicular joint sprains into six types (Fig. 39-2).[147] Type 1 sprains are mild injuries in which the coracoclavicular and acromioclavicular ligaments are intact and radiologic evaluation is normal. Type 2 injuries involve the complete disruption of the acromioclavicular ligaments, but with intact coracoclavicular ligaments. Radiographs might demonstrate clavicular elevation relative to the acromion, but less than 25% displacement. Type 3 sprains result in the complete disruption of the acromioclavicular and coracoclavicular ligaments, but the deltotrapezial fascia remains intact. Radiographs reveal a 25–100% increase in the coracoclavicular interspace relative to the normal shoulder. Type 4 sprains involve complete disruption of the coracoclavicular and acromioclavicular ligaments, with posterior displacement of the distal clavicle into the trapezius muscle. In type 5 sprains, the coracoclavicular and acromioclavicular ligaments are fully disrupted, along with a rupture of the deltotrapezial fascia. This results in an increase in the coracoclavicular interspace to greater than 100% of the normal shoulder. Type 6 sprains involve complete disruption of the coracoclavicular and acromioclavicular ligaments, and the deltotrapezial muscular attachments, with displacement of the distal clavicle below the acromion or the coracoid process.

Radiographic evaluation of the acromioclavicular joint should include anteroposterior and lateral views of the acromioclavicular joint, and a Zanca view. While stress views might help the clinician differentiate between type 2 and type 3 injuries, this has not been shown to outweigh the additional cost, time, and patient discomfort associated with stress views.[99]

Type 1, 2, and 3 acromioclavicular joint sprains are usually treated non-operatively with a brief period of sling immobilization, ice, and analgesics. The patient's activities are allowed to progress as the pain subsides. During the acute phase of rehabilitation, a program to regain full upper limb range of motion and restore shoulder girdle strength and function is employed. Indications for surgical intervention for type 3 sprains include persistent pain or unsatisfactory cosmetic results. Sprains that fall into the type 4, 5, or 6 categories require surgical treatment.[99]

Intraarticular acromioclavicular joint fractures are treated similarly to type 1 through 3 acromioclavicular joint sprains, unless the injury is open or involves neurovascular compromise. Posttraumatic arthrosis in the acromioclavicular joint can occur. Persistent pain, despite an appropriate non-operative treatment program, necessitates surgical resection of the distal clavicle.[99]

Osteolysis of the distal clavicle

Repetitive overload of the distal clavicle can result in osteolysis. Young weightlifters who perform a significant amount of bench press and military press lifts, especially with suboptimal technique, are the most susceptible to this condition.[26] The athlete usually presents with gradual onset of acromioclavicular joint pain that is increased with bench press, particularly when the bar is lowered all the way to the chest, because this results in a significant sheer stress to the acromioclavicular joint. The condition frequently occurs bilaterally.[156]

Radiographic evaluation is the same as for acromioclavicular joint injuries. The pathologic changes found on radiographs include distal clavicular subchondral bone loss and cystic changes. Widening of the acromioclavicular joint can occur in late stages. Bone scans are positive during active disease and can be used to confirm the diagnosis.[99]

Non-operative treatment of distal clavicular osteolysis involves avoidance of the aggravating activities. Ice, NSAIDs, and occasional acromioclavicular joint intraarticular corticosteroid injections can assist in pain control. For many athletes, however, activity modification is not practical and/or does not result in significant pain relief. In those athletes who fail non-operative measures, or are unable to adequately modify their activities, distal clavicular resection is the surgical procedure of choice.[156]

Scapulothoracic crepitus

Multiple authors have reported the occurrence of pathologic sounds at the scapulothoracic joint, often referred to as a snapping scapula or scapular crepitus.[109,132,134] The three primary types of sound that can occur at this joint include a gentle friction sound, a louder grating sound, and a loud snapping. While the gentle friction sound is probably physiologic, a loud grating sound is suggestive of soft tissue disease such as bursitis, fibrotic muscle, muscular atrophy, or anomalous muscular insertions.[109] Occasionally, an excessive thoracic kyphosis or thoracic scoliosis can cause pathologic crepitus at the scapulothoracic articulation. Scapulothoracic dyskinesis or scapular winging can also cause painful friction between the scapula and the thorax.[79] A loud snapping sound is frequently caused by bony pathology such as an osteophyte, a rib or scapular osteochondroma, a hooked superomedial angle of the scapula, or a malunion of rib fractures.[108,132,143]

The physical examination of individuals with symptomatic scapulothoracic crepitus or snapping should include localization of pain and crepitus or snapping through palpation, evaluation of scapulothoracic mechanics for quality and quantity of scapulothoracic motion, and a neurologic examination of the upper limb. Electrodiagnostic studies should be employed when a peripheral neurologic injury is suspected. Tangential and anteroposterior radiographic evaluation of the scapula can be helpful when evaluating for osseous causes of the scapular crepitus or snapping. The radiologic work-up might require further evaluation by CT or magnetic resonance imaging (MRI) for selected cases.

Treatment is warranted when the scapular snapping or crepitus is symptomatic. Non-operative treatment involves correction of biomechanical deficits such as scapulothoracic dyskinesis, strength and flexibility imbalances, and poor posture. Soft tissue mobilization of the scapulothoracic articulation in individuals with restricted motion is frequently helpful. Anti-inflammatory medications and local modalities can assist in pain control. An injection of corticosteroids into the painful area has been advocated by some authors,[32,100] but caution must be exercised because complications such as pneumothorax can occur. For those who fail non-operative measures, several surgical procedures have been described for treatment of this condition.[100]

Rotator cuff tendonitis/tendinopathy and impingement

Injuries to the rotator cuff are a common malady. While macrotrauma can cause rotator cuff injuries, traditionally the cause of rotator cuff tendonitis was thought to be repetitive microtrauma to the musculature and outlet impingement between the acromion and greater tuberosity of the humerus.[107] Neer categorized this type of rotator cuff injury into three stages.[114] Stage 1 injuries involved inflammation and edema in the rotator cuff. Stage 2 rotator cuff injuries had progressed to fibrosis and tendonitis. When a partial or complete rotator cuff tear occurred, this was considered a stage 3 injury. In the overhead athlete, underlying instability patterns of the glenohumeral joint with associated excessive translation of the humeral head frequently lead to outlet impingement and rotator cuff disease.[7]

On cadaveric examination, Bigliani found a relationship between the acromial shape and the presence of rotator cuff

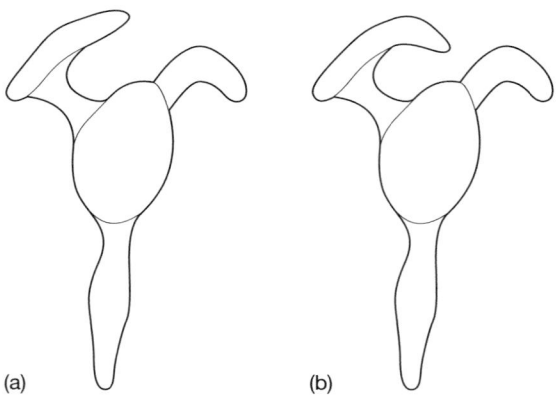

Figure 39-3 (**a**) Type 1 acromion; (**b**) type 3 acromion.

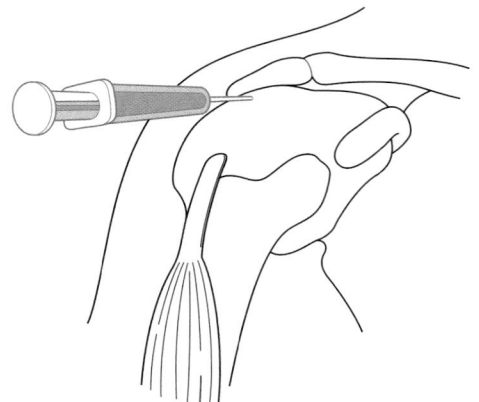

Figure 39-4
Subacromial injection of 1% lidocaine (lignocaine) can assist in the diagnosis of subacromial impingement.

tears.[21] He classified the acromions into three types (Fig. 39-3). Type 1 acromions were relatively flat, while type 2 acromions demonstrated a curve. Type 3 acromions were hooked. The incidence of rotator cuff tears increased as the acromion progressed from a type 1 to a type 3 shape. This was presumably related to the greater outlet impingement of the rotator cuff caused by an increasing acromial curve.

A phenomenon referred to as internal impingement has recently been reported in young overhead athletes.[39,169] When the arm is abducted 90° and then maximally externally rotated, there is contact between the undersurface of the rotator cuff and the posterosuperior glenoid rim. This is augmented by anterior glenohumeral joint instability. This can result in an internal impingement and leads to pathologic changes to the undersurface of the rotator cuff, which are exacerbated by overhead activities.

Impingement can be primary or secondary. Examples of causative factors leading to primary impingement include a hooked acromion or a thick coracoacromial ligament. Secondary impingement has many causes. Instability patterns of the glenohumeral joint can lead to narrowing of the scapular outlet or an increase in the acuity of the angle between the glenoid rim and humerus during overhead activities.[62] Lack of adequate scapular control or weakness in the scapular stabilizers can lead to poor positioning of the scapula during arm elevation. In this situation, the acromion might not be retracted during overhead activities and secondary impingement can occur.[61] During the follow-through phase of the throwing motion, eccentric contraction of the rotator cuff occurs. Musculotendinous fiber microfailure can occur over time due to the 'eccentric overload' of the rotator cuff, leading to secondary outlet impingement. Regardless of whether the impingement is primary or secondary, the underlying cause must be determined in order to formulate an appropriate treatment program.

Rathbun and Macnab performed vascular studies of the rotator cuff.[138] They found a relatively hypovascular zone in the leading edge of the supraspinatus tendon when the arm was in an adducted position as compared with an abducted position. Further studies by Lohr and Unthoff found that the articular surface of the supraspinatus tendon was hypovascular compared

with the bursal surface.[91] These hypovascular areas of the blood supply to the rotator cuff have been implicated as a cause of rotator cuff degeneration, and correlate well with the higher incidence of articular-sided partial-thickness tears of the rotator cuff.

Patients with rotator cuff injuries frequently note anterior shoulder pain that occurs with overhead activity, and also at night while trying to sleep. Symptoms such as stiffness, weakness, and catching might also be present. It is important to try to elicit any symptoms of underlying glenohumeral joint instability, such as numbness, tingling, feelings of subluxation, or previous 'dead arm' episodes.

The physical examination of patients with suspected rotator cuff pathology should include an evaluation of the cervical spine, because problems originating in the cervical spine frequently refer symptoms to the shoulder. During inspection, the examiner should be sure to assess for proper scapulothoracic mechanics. Strength testing of the rotator cuff muscles can detect weakness as a result of a rotator cuff tear, or pain inhibition due to tendonitis or tendinosis. The Neer and Hawkins impingement tests should be performed. If the Neer and/or Hawkins impingement tests elicit pain, injection of 10 mL of 1% lidocaine (lignocaine) into the subacromial space will eliminate the pain of repeat testing if subacromial impingement is truly the cause of the patient's pain (Fig. 39-4).

The examination of individuals with suspected rotator cuff pathology should also include maneuvers to detect underlying glenohumeral joint instability. The anterior apprehension test can be used to detect both anterior instability of the glenohumeral joint and also internal impingement. If the patient has a sensation of anterior apprehension during the test that is relieved with the relocation test, then there is probably anterior instability. However, if there is pain in the posterior aspect of the shoulder during the anterior apprehension test that is relieved with the relocation test, then internal impingement is occurring.

Radiographic evaluation of patients with suspected rotator cuff pathology should include anteroposterior, supraspinatus outlet, and axillary radiographs. Anteroposterior radiographs should be performed in the neutral, external, and internal rotation positions to adequately visualize the glenohumeral joint, and the greater and lesser tuberosities. Large rotator cuff tears can be indicated by an acromiohumeral distance of less than 5 mm and sclerosis on the undersurface of the acromion. The supraspinatus outlet view allows for categorization of the acromion type, and will reveal any osteophytes of the acromioclavicular joint that might be encroaching on the subacromial space.

Double-contrast arthrograms can be used to detect full-thickness rotator cuff tears, and also for the visualization of the intraarticular portion of the long head of the biceps tendon. Bursal-sided partial-thickness rotator cuff tears are poorly evaluated with this technique. MRI appears to be the best imaging technique for rotator cuff pathology, with reported sensitivity of 100% and specificity of 95% for full-thickness rotator cuff tears.[68]

Non-operative treatment should begin with measures to reduce pain, including activity modification, local modalities, and antiinflammatory medications. If this is not effective, some patients can benefit from a subacromial corticosteroid injection, although studies of corticosteroid injections have shown mixed results.[63,105,112] Patients who continue to be resistant to the above pain control measures, or have underlying calcific tendonitis, might respond to extracorporeal shock wave therapy. Success rates for treating rotator cuff tendinosis and calcific tendonitis with extracorporeal shock wave therapy have been reported to be between 47% and 70%.[122]

As pain resolves, full passive and active range of motion should be reestablished. This should be followed by neuromuscular reeducation for normalization of the scapulothoracic rhythm. A structured strengthening program of the scapular stabilizing and rotator cuff musculature should be instituted. Underlying kinetic chain deficits need to be identified and corrected. A planned progression of return to functional activity completes the rehabilitation program. If the patient fails to respond to the above measures, there might be a need for a surgical evaluation.

Patients who have sustained an acute full-thickness rotator cuff tear should receive early surgical intervention to maximize their postoperative recovery potential. If the rotator cuff tear is chronic, an initial trial of non-operative rehabilitation measures can be employed with the goal of restoring the patient to a functional level. However, in the young or active subgroups, non-operative measures frequently fail to restore the patient to an adequate level of function and surgical intervention is required.

Long head of the biceps tendon strains

Rupture of the long head of the biceps brachii tendon usually occurs in patients over 40 years of age with a prolonged history of outlet impingement and rotator cuff disease. The patient frequently experiences a pop at the time of the injury, which often occurs during lifting or pulling activities. However, some patients just present with a painless retraction of the biceps distally, resulting in an exaggeration of the biceps muscle contour. Pain can occur with an acute rupture but is not usually a factor in chronic cases. Because rupture of the long head of

the biceps brachii tendon results in a loss of approximately 8% of elbow flexion strength and 21% of supination strength,[97] function is not significantly affected in most individuals.

This injury is best evaluated radiographically with MRI, which demonstrates the ruptured biceps tendon retracted from the bicipital groove.

Treatment in patients over 40 years of age who are relatively sedentary includes sling immobilization for comfort if needed, NSAIDs, and local cryotherapy. Range of motion exercises should begin with gentle passive range of motion, and progress to more aggressive active range of motion as the patient's symptoms improve. Strengthening exercises of the rotator cuff, shoulder girdle, and arm musculature should be undertaken when the patient is able to tolerate it. This allows for maximal restoration of function.

In younger or physically active patients, early surgical intervention can be warranted. Mariani et al. reported that 93% of the surgically treated patients and 63% of the nonsurgically treated patients were able to return to full work capacity.[97]

Pectoralis major strain

Pectoralis major muscle strains are most commonly seen in athletes who perform forceful shoulder adduction and/or internal rotation against resistance, such as weightlifters and football players.[104] Pectoralis muscular strains can be categorized into three grades, with grade 1 being minimal muscle disruption, and grade 3 a complete rupture of the muscle (which can occur in the muscle belly or at the musculotendinous junction). Rupture of the pectoralis major tendon can also occur.

The onset of a pectoralis major muscle strain is usually characterized by sudden pain in the pectoral region during a forceful activity employing shoulder adduction or internal rotation. Edema and ecchymosis on the chest wall and/or proximal anterior arm region can develop, and the anterior axillary fold often demonstrates a visible defect when the shoulder is abducted 90°. The defect in the muscle can also be palpable on examination. Weakness and pain with shoulder adduction and internal rotation is usually present.

Standard plain film radiographic evaluation is normal. However, ultrasound or MRI examinations can demonstrate the injury.

Treatment is conservative for grade 1 or grade 2 strains, intramuscular grade 3 strain, or rupture from the sternal or clavicular origins. Conservative treatment should include ice, NSAIDs or mild analgesics, and sling immobilization for comfort if needed. Early gentle passive range of motion should progress to active range of motion as able, and a progressive strengthening program should be employed.

If the patient sustains a complete rupture of the pectoralis major tendon at the humeral insertion, non-athletes can undergo a conservative treatment program if they are willing to accept that they will not regain their full preinjury strength. However, in athletes and those who wish to improve their postinjury strength potential, surgical intervention is needed.

Glenohumeral joint instability

The glenohumeral joint is an endarthroidial joint with a rather large humeral head in relation to the small glenoid fossa. This anatomic relationship allows for the significant mobility seen in the glenohumeral joint, but comes at the price of poor bony stability. Glenohumeral joint stability is provided by a combination of static and dynamic stabilizers.

The static stabilizers of the glenohumeral joint include the bony congruence between the humeral head and the glenoid fossa, the glenoid labrum, the negative intraarticular pressure, the glenohumeral joint capsule, and the glenohumeral ligaments.[1]

The dynamic stabilizers of the glenohumeral joint include the scapular stabilizing muscles, the rotator cuff muscles, and the long head of the biceps.[84] The importance of optimal scapular function for glenohumeral joint stability cannot be overemphasized. The scapular stabilizing muscles orient the scapula properly in relation to the humerus for optimal static and dynamic stability of the glenohumeral joint, and stabilize the scapula during glenohumeral joint movements.[47] The scapular stabilizing muscles include the serratus anterior, trapezius, pectoralis minor, rhomboideus minor and major, latissimus dorsi, and levator scapulae.[47]

The rotator cuff muscles include the supraspinatus, infraspinatus, subscapularis, and teres minor. These muscles contribute to dynamic glenohumeral joint stability through a number of mechanisms. Concavity compression, first described by Lippitt et al.,[89] refers to the compressive forces placed on the glenohumeral joint during rotator cuff muscle cocontractions. These forces press the humeral head into the glenoid fossa, center the humeral head within the glenoid fossa, and help resist glenohumeral translation. Because the glenohumeral ligaments are lax in the midranges of glenohumeral joint motion, coordinated rotator cuff muscle contraction and concavity compression are particularly important mechanisms for glenohumeral joint stability in these ranges.[84]

At the distal insertion of the rotator cuff muscles on the humerus, there is an intertwining of the joint capsule with the rotator cuff tendons. With rotator cuff muscle contraction, it is possible that the glenohumeral joint capsule develops tension and increases in stiffness, consequently acting as a dynamic musculoligamentous stabilizing system.[84]

The rotator cuff muscles also provide glenohumeral joint stability through passive muscle tension, and act as barriers to glenohumeral joint translation during active motion.[25,30] The subscapularis appears to be an especially important stabilizer of both anterior and posterior glenohumeral joint stability.[22,40]

Proprioception and neuromuscular control refer to the mechanism by which the position and movements of the shoulder girdle are sensed (proprioception), processed, and result in an appropriate motor response (neuromuscular control).[111] Glenohumeral joint instability is often associated with a concomitant decrement in proprioception.[87] The abnormal proprioception is restored following surgical correction of the joint instability, suggesting that one of the mechanisms causing proprioceptive

Table 39-2 Classification of the degree of glenohumeral joint instability	
Grade	Signs
Subluxation	Humeral head extends to the edge of the glenoid fossa without dislocation, followed by spontaneous reduction
Dislocation	Humeral head becomes fully dislodged from the glenoid fossa; this usually requires manual relocation
Microinstability	Repetitive microtraumatic or congenital laxity of the glenohumeral ligaments

deficits in unstable glenohumeral joints is a lack of appropriate capsuloligamentous tension.[88]

The classification of glenohumeral joint instability includes the degree, frequency, etiology, and direction of instability.[14] The degree includes dislocation, subluxation, or microinstability (Table 39-2). A dislocation implies that the humeral head is disassociated from the glenoid fossa, and often requires manual reduction. A subluxation occurs when the humeral head translates to the edge of the glenoid, beyond normal physiologic limits, followed by self reduction. Microinstability is due to excessive capsular laxity, is multidirectional, and is frequently associated with internal impingement of the rotator cuff.[14]

The frequency of instability can be either acute or chronic.[14] Acute instability involves a new injury resulting in subluxation or dislocation of the glenohumeral joint. Chronic instability refers to repetitive instability episodes.

The etiology of glenohumeral joint instability can be traumatic or atraumatic.[14] Unidirectional instability is frequently caused by a traumatic event resulting in disruption of the glenohumeral joint. Atraumatic instability refers to glenohumeral joint instability due to congenital capsular laxity or repetitive microtrauma. Atraumatic instability can be subclassified into voluntary and involuntary categories. Voluntary instability refers to an individual who can volitionally sublux or dislocate the glenohumeral joint, while those with involuntary instability cannot. Some patients with voluntary instability have associated psychologic pathology, which often portends a poor outcome if surgical stabilization is performed.[150]

Glenohumeral joint instability can be unidirectional or multidirectional. Unidirectional instability refers to instability only in one direction. The most frequent type of unidirectional instability is traumatic anterior instability.[14] Multidirectional instability is instability in two or more directions, and is usually due to congenital capsular laxity or chronic repetitive microtrauma.[14]

Anterior instability is most frequently caused by a tear in the anterior–inferior glenohumeral joint capsule (involving the middle glenohumeral ligament and/or anterior band of the inferior glenohumeral ligament), or detachment of the anterior–inferior glenoid labrum from the glenoid rim.[84] The latter of these two entities is frequently referred to as a Bankart lesion.[16] Bankart lesions can also involve a fracture of the anterior–inferior glenoid rim, commonly referred to as a 'bony Bankart lesion'.[153] Variations of the Bankart lesion include the Perthes lesion and the anterior labroligamentous periosteal sleeve avulsion lesion.[153] Other anatomic lesions that contribute to anterior glenohumeral joint instability include humeral avulsion of the glenohumeral ligament, superior labral anterior to posterior (SLAP) lesions, injury to the rotator interval, or rotator cuff tears (particularly to the subscapularis muscle).[84] Acute anterior glenohumeral joint dislocations are also frequently associated with a compression fracture of the posterolateral aspect of the humeral head, referred to as a Hill–Sachs defect.[153]

Inferior glenohumeral joint instability typically does not occur in isolation. However, causes of inferior glenohumeral joint instability include capsuloligamentous laxity, absence of the glenoid fossa upward tilt, and lesions to the rotator interval, the inferior glenohumeral ligament, the superior glenohumeral ligament, the coracohumeral ligament, and the inferior glenoid labrum.

Congenital glenoid hypoplasia, or excessive glenoid or humeral retroversion, has been reported to contribute to posterior glenohumeral joint instability. However, the more common lesions that lead to posterior glenohumeral joint instability include excessive capsuloligamentous laxity, or an injury to the rotator interval, superior glenohumeral ligament, posterior band of the inferior glenohumeral ligament, coracohumeral ligament, or subscapularis muscle.[10] A tear of the posterior inferior glenoid labrum causing separation from the glenoid fossa rim, often referred to as a 'reverse Bankart lesion', or a fracture of the posterior inferior glenoid fossa rim, can also cause posterior glenohumeral joint instability.[10,136] A 'reverse Hill–Sachs defect' can also be present, representing an impaction fracture of the anterior humeral head.[10,136]

Multidirectional instability can be due to primary or secondary capsuloligamentous laxity. It is frequently seen bilaterally, and can be accompanied by generalized joint laxity.[14] Recurrent unilateral joint instability occasionally stretches the glenohumeral capsuloligamentous structures to the point that multidirectional instability develops secondarily.[14] Another possible cause for secondary multidirectional instability is the presence of an underlying connective tissue disorder such as Marfan or Ehlers–Danlos sydrome.[14]

While many patients with glenohumeral joint instability have vague symptoms, common complaints of patients with shoulder instability include pain, popping, catching, locking, an unstable sensation, stiffness, and swelling.[18] A history of acute trauma or chronic, repetitive microtrauma should be obtained. Some patients might have a history of glenohumeral joint dislocation, and the examiner should find out the direction of dislocation, the duration of the dislocation, whether it has reoccurred, and whether it required manual reduction or spontaneously reduced. Subluxation episodes are commonly associated with a burning or aching dead feeling in the arm. Repetitive overhead activities such as baseball pitching can cause enough microtrauma to lead to symptomatic laxity.[18] Patients should be asked whether they or their family has a history of generalized ligamentous laxity or connective tissue disorders.

The physical examination should include inspection, palpation, glenohumeral joint range of motion, analysis of scapulothoracic kinesis, upper limb strength, sensation (including proprioception), and reflex evaluations, as well as special tests for glenohumeral joint instability.

The most common initial radiographic views for the evaluation of glenohumeral joint instability include the anteroposterior shoulder view, axillary lateral view, and scapular Y view.[14] The anteroposterior view allows visualization of the osseous structures of the shoulder, including the scapula, clavicle, upper ribs, humeral head, and glenoid rim.[153] With internal rotation, the anteroposterior view can also allow visualization of a Hill–Sachs defect.[153] The scapular Y view can help in the assessment of glenohumeral joint alignment following acute dislocations.[153] The axillary lateral view can assess anterior or posterior subluxation or dislocation, as well as fractures of the anterior or posterior glenoid rim.[153] Other specialized views include the Garth view and the West Point view, both of which are useful in the detection of Bankart fractures. The Stryker Notch view can be used for evaluation of Hill–Sachs defects, and stress views for the documentation of the degree of glenohumeral joint instability.[153]

Computed tomography was previously the gold standard for glenoid labral evaluation. However, with the advent of MRI and magnetic resonance arthrography, CT scan now has a limited role. MRI and magnetic resonance arthrography provide superior visualization of the labrum, cartilage, and joint capsule without the ionizing radiation of CT. Visualization of nondisplaced injuries to the inferior glenohumeral ligament and/or anteroinferior glenoid labrum is improved by placing the arm in an abducted and externally rotated position.

The treatment options for glenohumeral joint instability and dislocation include non-operative and operative approaches. Following glenohumeral joint subluxation episodes and in patients with multidirectional instability or unidirectional posterior or inferior instability, a comprehensive rehabilitation program that addresses kinetic chain deficits, scapulothoracic mechanics, and shoulder girdle strength, flexibility, and neuromuscular control is appropriate. Only in those patients who have failed a comprehensive non-operative treatment program should operative intervention be considered.

For patients with glenohumeral joint instability, the strengthening program should begin with closed kinetic chain exercises, which promote cocontraction of the glenohumeral joint stabilizing musculature. The initial closed kinetic chain exercises can be performed with the patient weight bearing through the shoulder, such as weight bearing in a quadruped position. As the patient's pain is reduced, and the stability improves, closed kinetic chain exercises that allow the shoulder to pass through more functional ranges of motion can begin. An example of this type of exercise would involve having the patient forward flex the shoulder to approximately 90°, placing the hand against a wall with a small hand towel between the hand and the wall, and performing circular or diagonal patterned shoulder movements while weight bearing through the shoulder by leaning against the wall. The patient can eventually progress to functional open kinetic chain exercises as stability is achieved.

Proprioceptive closed and open kinetic chain exercises are also important to recoordinate the stabilizing shoulder girdle musculature and attain engrams that respond appropriately to a dynamically changing environment. Initial proprioceptive exercises can include closed kinetic chain shoulder exercises by weight bearing through the shoulders in a quadruped position with the hands on wobble boards, or with the legs on an exercise ball. An example of an open kinetic chain proprioceptive exercise is using a body blade in functional shoulder ranges of motion.

For patients who have suffered a first-time traumatic anterior glenohumeral joint dislocation, the decision between a trial of non-operative treatment versus immediate surgical stabilization is more controversial. In the older, less active patient, non-operative management frequently is successful.[3] In the younger, more active patient involved in contact sports, studies have shown a very high redislocation rate in those treated non-operatively, when compared with those receiving early operative intervention.[12,13,80,161]

Regardless of whether a patient opts for early surgical intervention, closed reduction confirmed by radiologic examination should be performed on all patients who sustain an acute glenohumeral joint dislocation that does not spontaneously reduce. Radiologic studies should be performed in two planes, such as anteroposterior with the humerus in internal rotation and axillary lateral views, to confirm relocation and exclude an associated fracture.[153] Sensory testing over the deltoid muscle is important, because the axillary nerve is the most common associated nerve injury following shoulder dislocation.[14] Medications such as NSAIDs and mild opioid analgesics can be considered for initial pain control.

Previous research suggested that immobilization of the glenohumeral joint following relocation did not appear to affect the rate of glenohumeral joint redislocation, and was therefore only recommended as a comfort measure.[66,67,155] However, MRI studies have demonstrated an improved anatomic approximation of Bankart lesions when the shoulder immobilization occurs with the humerus externally rotated 30°.[71,72] Preliminary data also suggest that, in patients who have sustained an anterior glenohumeral joint dislocation, 3 weeks of sling immobilization with the shoulder in 30° of external rotation results in a significant reduction in redislocation rates following non-operative treatment of acute anterior glenohumeral joint dislocations.[70] Therefore, if non-operative treatment is employed following traumatic anterior glenohumeral joint dislocation, it appears that 3 weeks of immobilization with the shoulder in 30° of external rotation is appropriate. This period of immobilization should be followed by a comprehensive rehabilitation program that restores full glenohumeral and scapulothoracic motion; corrects scapulothoracic dyskinesis; and restores the normal strength, endurance, and neuromuscular control to the rotator cuff and shoulder girdle musculature.

Adhesive capsulitis

Codman first described 'frozen shoulder' as a painful restriction in shoulder range of motion in a patient with normal radiographs.[57] Neviaser introduced the more descriptive term *adhesive capsulitis* for this syndrome.[115] Adhesive capsulitis occurs in approximately 2–5% of the general population, is two to four times more common in women than in men, and is most frequently seen in individuals between 40 and 60 years of age.[27,34]

Adhesive capsulitis is usually an idiopathic condition, but it can be associated with diabetes mellitus or inflammatory arthritis. Pathologic evaluation can reveal some perivascular inflammation, but the predominant abnormality seen on pathologic examination includes fibroblastic proliferation with increased collagen and nodular band formation.[27]

Adhesive capsulitis has been divided into four stages (Table 39-3).[59] Stage 1 occurs for the first 1–3 months, and involves pain with shoulder movements but no significant glenohumeral joint range of motion restriction when examined under anesthesia. Stage 2, or the 'freezing stage', lasts for approximately 3–9 months, and is characterized by pain with shoulder motion and progressive glenohumeral joint range of motion restriction in forward flexion, abduction, and internal and external rotation. During stage 3, or the 'frozen stage', symptoms last for 9–15 months and include a significant reduction in pain but maintenance of the restricted glenohumeral joint range of motion. Stage 4, frequently referred to as the 'thawing stage', lasts for approximately 15–24 months and involves a progressive restoration of range of motion.

Routine radiographic evaluation is usually normal. However, glenohumeral joint arthrography will reveal a significant reduction in the capsular volume.

Hannafin et al. advocate the early use of intraarticular corticosteroid injections during stages 1 and 2 in order to decrease the initial inflammatory stage in an attempt to reduce the development of fibrosis.[59] With the judicious use of oral anti-

Table 39-3 Stages of adhesive capsulitis		
Stage	Duration (months)	Signs and symptoms
1	1–3	Painful shoulder movement, minimal restriction in motion
2	3–9	Painful shoulder movement, progressive loss of glenohumeral joint motion
3	9–15	Reduced pain with shoulder movement, severely restricted glenohumeral joint motion
4	15–24	Minimal pain, progressive normalization of glenohumeral joint motion

inflammatory medications and a closely monitored home exercise program involving shoulder range of motion and shoulder girdle strengthening, most patients will attain complete restoration of normal function over a 14-month period.[110]

Despite the favorable results seen with non-operative treatment, due to the prolonged course of recovery, several authors have advocated such treatments as manipulation of the shoulder under anesthesia, hydrodilatation of the glenohumeral joint, arthroscopic capsular release, open surgical release, and postoperative rehabilitation facilitated by an interscalene block for pain control.[20,34,58,123,133] The response to these treatments has been mixed, and non-surgical intervention appears to be the initial treatment of choice for this condition.

Superior labral anterior to posterior lesions

Andrews and colleagues were the first to report the importance of the superior labrum and biceps tendon complex as a source of pain and shoulder dysfunction.[8] The term *SLAP lesion*, which stands for superior labral anterior to posterior injury, has been used to name injuries to the superior labrum and biceps tendon complex.[158] The glenoid labrum, which serves to deepen the glenoid socket, increases the contact area of the humeral head by approximately 70%.[135] In addition to increasing the static stability of the glenohumeral joint, the superior aspect of the glenoid labrum serves as an attachment point for the long head of the biceps tendon. Research has demonstrated the importance of the long head of the biceps in providing dynamic stability to both anterior–posterior and superior–inferior humeral head translation.[127,148]

Snyder and colleagues proposed a classification system for SLAP lesions (Fig. 39-5).[158] Type 1 lesions involve a fraying injury to the superior labrum without detachment of the biceps tendon. In type 2 lesions, the biceps tendon is detached from the supraglenoid tubercle. Type 3 lesions are characterized by bucket handle tearing of the superior labrum without detachment of the biceps tendon. Type 4 lesions involve a tear of the superior labrum that extends into the biceps tendon.

Several mechanisms of injury have been proposed for SLAP lesions. A fall on an outstretched arm, which causes superior translation of the humeral head and compression of the superior glenoid labrum, was reported by Snyder and colleagues.[158] During the deceleration phase of the overhead throw, the biceps fires at its greatest rate according to electromyographic studies. Andrews and coworkers suggested that this significant traction force by the biceps on the superior labrum could result in a SLAP lesion.[8] The late cocking phase of an overhead throw also creates a torsional peeling-back stress to the superior glenoid labrum that can result in a SLAP lesion.[28] Traction injuries to the shoulder, such as when workers fall from a scaffold and catch themselves, can also cause a SLAP injury.[92]

The most common complaints of individuals with a SLAP lesion are pain with overhead throwing, and mechanical symptoms such as clicking, catching, or grinding. SLAP lesions can, however, mimic the symptoms of many different diagnoses, such as impingement, acromioclavicular joint pain, bicipital tendonitis, or glenohumeral joint instability. Consequently, a

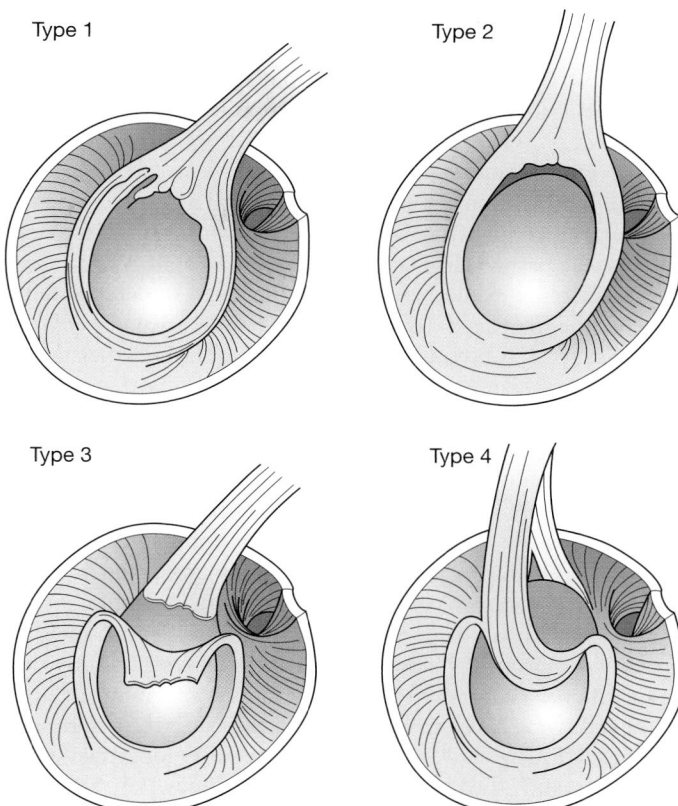

Figure 39-5 Classification of superior labral anterior to posterior lesions.

high degree of suspicion is important in order to make this diagnosis. Physical examination often reveals underlying glenohumeral joint instability. A positive O'Brien's test is also suggestive of a SLAP lesion.

Standard radiographic imaging of the shoulder is usually normal. Gadolinium-enhanced magnetic resonance arthrograms scans of the shoulder have improved the ability to detect SLAP lesions. However, the gold standard for diagnosing SLAP lesions remains arthroscopy.

There currently are no studies of non-operative SLAP lesion treatment, and surgery is the standard treatment. However, correction of strength and flexibility deficits and normalization of scapulothoracic mechanics should help with the postsurgical recovery. Patients who have been diagnosed with SLAP lesions should be referred for surgical consultation in order to receive definitive treatment.

Conditions of the elbow
Lateral epicondylitis

Lateral epicondylitis is a common tendinopathy about the elbow, and is frequently referred to as tennis elbow. The history of this malady dates back to 1883, when it was described as an injury resulting from lawn tennis.[38] Modern tennis players continue to be afflicted with this condition, which is reported to occur in up to 50% of tennis players.[117] Any activity that places excessive repetitive stress on the lateral forearm musculature, however, can cause this condition.

Lateral epicondylitis is more common in patients over 35 years of age and peaks in those between 40 and 50 years old.[76,118] It is more common in male than in female tennis players, but does not display a gender predilection in the general population.[36] When lateral epicondylitis results from a work-related injury, conservative measures are less successful and surgical intervention occurs more frequently.[54]

Lateral epicondylitis is actually a misnomer for this condition, because the pathologic changes are not inflammatory but rather degenerative. Nirschl reported the presence of vascular granulation in the damaged tissue and termed it *angiofibroblastic hyperplasia*.[118] Subsequent studies have confirmed that this is the lesion present in tennis elbow.[140] It appears that a more appropriate term for this condition is *lateral epicondylosis* rather than epicondylitis.

The degenerative tendinosis of lateral epicondylosis occurs most commonly in the extensor carpi radialis brevis origin, but also involves the extensor digitorum communis origin in 30% of cases.[118] Only in rare instances are the origins of the extensor carpi radialis longus or extensor carpi ulnaris involved.

Patients with lateral epicondylosis frequently report a gradual onset of symptoms, which usually occur after specific activities. Traumatic or sudden onset of symptoms can also occur. The backhand swing in tennis frequently exacerbates the symptoms, as does gripping and activities that require repetitive wrist extension and forearm pronation and supination. Physical examination can reveal point tenderness over the lateral epicondyle and a positive Cozen's test. Entrapment of the posterior interosseous branch of the radial nerve can mimic lateral epicondylosis, but the tenderness associated with this condition is 3–4 cm distal to the lateral epicondyle rather than directly over it.[172]

While standard anteroposterior and lateral radiographs are usually normal, an oblique view of the lateral epicondyle might reveal punctuate calcifications in the extensor tendon origin.[36]

The initial treatment for lateral epicondylosis involves discontinuation of provocative activities, and antiinflammatory medications. Localized cryotherapy is frequently helpful, and galvanic electrical stimulation can assist in pain control. Iontophoresis can also be utilized for pain control, but one double-blind placebo-controlled study did not show any efficacy of this treatment in patients with lateral epicondylosis.[152] If the patient continues to be symptomatic, corticosteroid injection can be helpful, but it is important to be aware that these injections can lead to further tendon degeneration and can predispose to tendon rupture. Studies also have not shown consistent improvement with corticosteroid injections, and one study revealed no difference between patients who received rehabilitation combined with a corticosteroid injection when compared with patients who received rehabilitation combined with a sham injection.[6,116] Using a 'peppering' needling technique in the area of tendinosis by repetitively inserting and withdrawing the needle can improve the efficacy of injections.[6] Extracorporeal shock wave therapy for lateral epicondylosis has been reported to be successful in 48–73% of cases recalcitrant to other non-

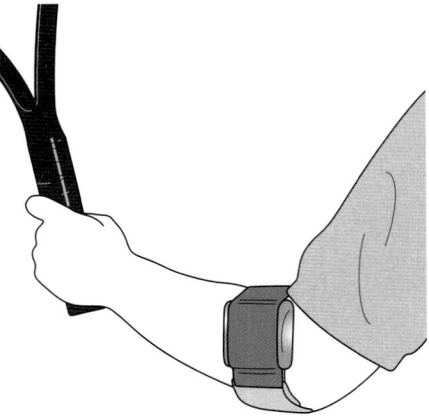

Figure 39-6 Lateral counterforce strap for lateral epicondylosis.

operative measures.[122] In a prospective study by Edwards and Calandruccio,[44] injection of 2 mL of autologous blood under the extensor carpi radialis brevis tendon showed a 79% success rate in patients for whom other non-operative measures had failed. Correction of kinetic chain deficits distal or proximal to the symptomatic site can be performed early in the treatment program.

Following adequate pain control, an exercise program to address strength, endurance, and flexibility deficits should be instituted. Eccentric strengthening exercises of the wrist extensor musculature have been advocated as a form of treatment for lateral epicondylosis.[163] Lateral counterforce straps, commonly referred to as tennis elbow straps, can be used during activity (Fig. 39-6). Aggravating activities should be analyzed to ensure that the patient is using the appropriate equipment and proper technique. Correct grip size of tennis rackets is very important. Training errors should also be addressed.

Those who do not respond to non-operative treatment can be referred for surgical evaluation. Nirschl reported complete pain relief and return to full activities in 85% of his surgically treated patients, and significant pain relief but mild activity limitations in another 12% of surgically treated patients.[117] Only 3% of patients in this series reported a lack of improvement postoperatively.

Medial epicondylitis

Medial epicondylitis, frequently referred to as golfer's elbow, has the same degenerative pathologic changes as those described in lateral epicondylitis, and is therefore more correctly termed *medial epicondylosis*.[124] Risk factors for medial epicondylosis include training errors; faulty equipment; repetitive activities requiring wrist flexion and forearm pronation; and biomechanical abnormalities such as poor strength, flexibility imbalances, and joint instability. This condition occurs three to seven times less frequently than lateral epicondylosis, and the degenerative changes are most frequently found in the pronator teres and flexor carpi radialis origins.[124]

Patients often report a gradual onset of pain over the medial epicondyle that is exacerbated by activities that require repetitive gripping, wrist flexion, and forearm pronation and supination. The patient might report a feeling of grip strength weakness. This condition occasionally occurs traumatically as a result of an acute rupture of the ulnar collateral ligament of the elbow. Symptoms of a concomitant ulnar neuropathy can be present. Physical examination demonstrates tenderness to palpation over the medial epicondyle, weakness in grip strength, pain when a tight fist is made, and pain with resisted wrist flexion and forearm pronation.

Oblique radiographs of the medial epicondyle can reveal punctuate calcifications in the region of the flexor tendon origins.[36] It is also important to rule out degenerative changes in the posterior medial aspect of the olecranon, because this condition can cause symptoms similar to those seen with medial epicondylosis.

Non-operative treatment should include discontinuation of aggravating activities, antiinflammatory medications, and local cryotherapy. Other physical modalities, such as galvanic electrical stimulation or iontophoresis, can be used if initial treatment is unsuccessful. Corticosteroid injections have been employed to treat this condition but can lead to further tendon degeneration and predispose to tendon rupture. Medial epicondylosis can also be responsive to extracorporeal shock wave therapy.[122] Correction of kinetic chain abnormalities should be undertaken early in the treatment program.

After pain control has been obtained, a program should be initiated that addresses strength, endurance, and flexibility imbalances and deficits. A medial counterforce strap can be employed to facilitate an appropriate exercise program. Training errors should be corrected. The patient's aggravating activities should be analyzed to establish whether equipment or technique modifications need to be implemented. For those who fail conservative measures, operative treatment can be warranted.

Distal biceps tendonitis and rupture

Distal biceps brachii tendonitis is not a common clinical entity. Throwing athletes can develop an eccentric overload of the distal biceps brachii during the deceleration or follow-through phase of throwing. Patients report pain in the antecubital fossa with activities that require repetitive elbow bending or during the follow-through phase of throwing. Physical examination will reveal tenderness to palpation over the distal biceps tendon and pain with resisted elbow flexion. Radiologic evaluation is usually normal.

Treatment of distal biceps brachii tendonitis begins with activity modification, ice, and antiinflammatory medications. Kinetic chain abnormalities should be addressed early in the rehabilitation process. When the patient is able to participate in an active strengthening program, eccentric exercises should be employed. The patient should resume functional activities in a planned, gradually escalating manner, and should not return to full unrestricted activity until full strength and range of motion has been restored.

Rupture of the distal biceps brachii tendon is also an uncommon injury. This usually occurs in patients between 30 and 50 years of age, with a significant predilection for men and the dominant limb.[11,15,41] The injury usually occurs during a heavy lifting activity while the elbow is at 90° of flexion.[52] The rupture usually involves the distal biceps brachii tendon proper at the radial tuberosity insertion site, with variable involvement of the lacertus fibrosus.[41] Although prodromal symptoms are usually absent, pathologic examination of the avulsed tendon frequently reveals degenerative changes in the distal biceps brachii tendon.[137]

Patients with distal biceps brachii tendon ruptures present with a history of acute pain and a popping or tearing sensation in the antecubital fossa during a heavy lifting activity. They might or might not report a reduction in elbow flexion or forearm supination strength. Clinical findings include ecchymosis, edema, and erythema in the antecubital fossa, and a palpable absence of the distal biceps brachii tendon. The biceps brachii muscle belly might have a deformity during contraction due to balling up of the muscle, but elbow flexion and forearm supination should still be intact due to the presence of the brachialis and supinator muscles, respectively.

Radiologic evaluation should be performed to rule out avulsion fracture from the radial tuberosity. MRI or ultrasound can be helpful in cases where the diagnosis is not clear.

Treatment of biceps brachii tendon ruptures is surgical, and early intervention is recommended.

Distal triceps tendonitis and rupture

The triceps brachii muscle inserts distally on to the olecranon process. Its primary function at the elbow is elbow extension. Activities that require repetitive elbow extension, such as throwing, weightlifting, or using a hammer, can result in an overuse injury to the distal triceps brachii, causing tendonitis. This condition can be found in conjunction with loose bodies in the posterior compartment of the elbow or with lateral epicondylitis.[159]

Symptoms of triceps brachii tendonitis include aching and burning pain in the distal triceps. The pain frequently occurs following specific aggravating activities in the early manifestations of this condition, but eventually the symptoms are experienced during activity. Physical examination reveals tenderness over the distal triceps tendon and pain with resisted elbow extension. Radiologic evaluation is usually normal.

Treatment for triceps tendonitis includes activity modification, ice, and antiinflammatory medications for pain control. Early range of motion exercises should be employed. As pain resolves, a more aggressive strengthening program should begin. Eccentric strengthening exercises of the triceps brachii should be considered in those who have experienced chronic symptoms. Surgical intervention is rarely required.

Triceps tendon rupture can occur in individuals who fall on to an outstretched hand or receive a direct blow to the distal triceps brachii tendon. Minimal trauma might be required for tendon disruption in those who have received previous steroid injections around the distal triceps tendon, or in people who have been treated with chronic oral steroids for other system conditions.[159,168] The most common site of disruption is at the distal insertion site on the olecranon, and a small avulsion fracture from the olecranon might be present.

Patients with this condition typically report a fall on an outstretched hand or direct blow to the triceps tendon. An audible pop might have occurred at the time of the injury. Elbow extension weakness, and erythema, ecchymosis, and edema at the area of the tendon rupture usually develop. Physical examination demonstrates these findings, along with a palpable defect. The ability to actively extend the elbow can be present due to an intact anconeus muscle, but the strength will be significantly reduced when compared with that of the opposite limb.

Standard radiographs of the elbow might reveal a small avulsion fracture on the lateral view.[48] Ultrasonography or MRI readily demonstrates the pathology.[164]

Surgical repair of the triceps tendon disruption is recommended.

Snapping triceps tendon

Occasionally, a pathologic band over the medial side of the distal triceps can cause a snapping sensation over the medial epicondyle during elbow flexion and extension.[43] The astute clinician should try to differentiate this condition from ulnar nerve subluxation, but certainly both conditions can occur at the same time. The patient might report a history of medial elbow popping or snapping during elbow flexion and extension activities. The snapping of the band over the medial epicondyle is frequently palpable on examination. Conservative treatment for this condition includes deep tissue massage, stretching of the triceps muscle, and occasionally local corticosteroid injection. Patients who do not respond to this regimen might require surgical intervention.

Olecranon bursitis

The olecranon bursa lies subcutaneously over the olecranon process. Olecranon bursitis can be septic or aseptic. Aseptic bursitis is either acute hemorrhagic bursitis due to a macrotraumatic insult to the bursa, or chronic bursitis due to repetitive microtrauma. Septic bursitis can occur due to a localized or systemic infection. Aseptic bursitis is frequently seen in athletes who participate in football or hockey.[82]

The history of aseptic bursitis can begin with a direct blow to the area, but some patients report an insidious onset of symptoms following a small abrasion or laceration to the area. If the injury is chronic and recurrent, the patient can experience an initial period of swelling that feels like a small liquid pouch that eventually organizes into a permanently thickened bursa with intrabursal bands. Septic bursitis is associated with significant edema, erythema, and hyperthermia in the area of the infected bursa, and frequently is accompanied by systemic symptoms of infection. Physical examination reveals an edematous area over the olecranon that is usually tender to palpation. Elbow range of motion can be limited due to tissue tightness and pain. If the bursa is infected, the area can feel warm, and the patient might have an increased white blood cell count.

Radiographic evaluation should be performed to determine if the patient has an osteophyte over the tip of the olecranon, or calcification within the bursal sac.

The initial treatment of an acute traumatic aseptic bursitis includes sterile aspiration of the bursa followed by application of a compressive dressing. The patient should begin an antiinflammatory medication and frequently apply ice to the area. The olecranon should be protected from further insult by using an elbow pad.

For those with chronic bursitis, treatment should include ice, intermittent antiinflammatory medications, and protection of the area from further insult. If edema is present, a compressive dressing should be applied. An intrabursal injection of corticosteroid medications can be helpful in patients who have aseptic bursitis. For aseptic bursitis that is recalcitrant to standard treatment, sclerotherapy using a tetracycline injection into the bursa has been advocated.[60] Surgical excision is also an option for patients who do not obtain relief with the above measures.

For patients with septic bursitis, the bursa should be aspirated for symptomatic relief and to obtain a fluid sample for laboratory analysis including Gram stain, culture, and sensitivity, and crystal analysis. The area should then be wrapped in a compressive dressing, and the patient should be instructed to elevate the arm. Intravenous antibiotics are warranted in patients with systemic symptoms, but oral antibiotics might be adequate for those experiencing only localized symptoms. If the patient does not improve with the above measures, referral for incision and drainage should be made.

Ulnar collateral ligament sprain

Injuries to the ulnar collateral ligament of the elbow are a result of valgus stress to the elbow. This can be due to a single traumatic episode, but is frequently seen with the repetitive microtrauma associated with throwing. The late cocking phase of overhead throwing is characterized by a valgus torque of approximately 64 N-m across the elbow.[50] During the acceleration phase of overhead throwing, the valgus forces across the elbow are increased, leading to further stress on the ulnar collateral ligament (Fig. 39-7).

The ulnar collateral ligament comprises an anterior, posterior, and transverse bundle. It is primarily stabilized by the anterior bundle.[165] The anterior bundle has a thin superficial and thick deep layer, and the superficial or deep layer can be torn individually or as a unit.[166]

Patients with ulnar collateral ligament injuries complain of medial elbow pain, which is exacerbated by the late cocking and acceleration phases of throwing. If the injury was acute, an audible pop might have been heard, but more frequently the symptoms have an insidious onset. Throwing athletes can report a decrement in throwing velocity and accuracy. Ulnar nerve traction can occur due to the increased laxity of the elbow, and resulting symptoms of ulnar neuritis can be present. Physical examination often reveals a 5° elbow flexion contracture,

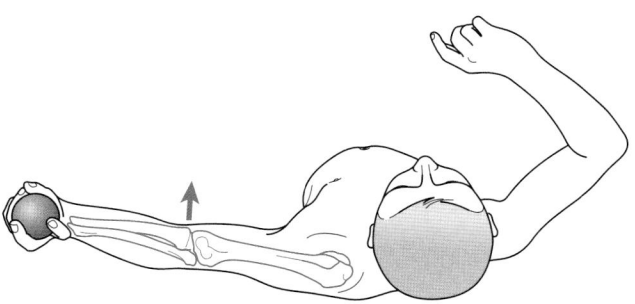

Figure 39-7 Valgus stress at the elbow during the acceleration phase of the throwing cycle.

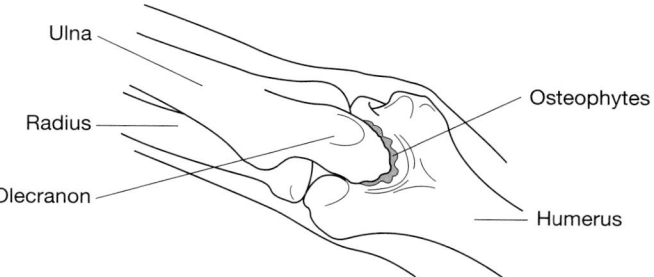

Figure 39-8 Posteromedial osteophytes of the olecranon due to valgus extension overload.

tenderness over the ulnar collateral ligament, and pain with valgus stress to a slightly flexed elbow.

Anteroposterior, lateral, and oblique radiographs of the elbow should be obtained. Calcification of the ulnar collateral ligament can occur, and avulsions from the humeral or ulnar attachments should be ruled out.[154] CT or MRI arthrograms can help further define the injury, particularly if the injury is a partial tear of the ulnar collateral ligament that involves only the deep fibers.[154] MRI has the advantage of excellent soft tissue visualization.

Partial ulnar collateral ligament injuries should be initially treated with non-operative measures. Conservative treatment should include discontinuation of throwing activities for 3–6 weeks, and initiation of gentle elbow range of motion, localized modalities, and antiinflammatory medications. A progressive strengthening program of the medial forearm musculature should be done, because these muscles are dynamic stabilizers of the medial elbow against valgus stress. Occasionally, a hinged elbow brace is used for initial support and comfort. Taping the medial elbow to resist valgus stress can be helpful. When the patient has full pain-free range of motion and symmetric strength, an interval throwing program can be initiated with the overhead throwing athlete (Box 39-1). Proper throwing mechanics should be ensured. Patients who fail conservative management can be candidates for ulnar collateral ligament reconstruction.

Patients with full-thickness ulnar collateral ligament injuries are less likely to respond favorably to non-operative measures, and ligament reconstruction is often required for definitive treatment.

Valgus extension overload of the elbow

Valgus extension overload is a common disorder in overhead throwing athletes, accounting for approximately 65% of surgeries for medial elbow pain in professional baseball players.[9] This disorder is characterized by impingement of the posteromedial olecranon against the medial wall of the olecranon fossa from the valgus elbow stress during overhead throwing. Over time, repetitive impingement at this site can result in olecranon osteophyte formation, intraarticular loose bodies, and deposition of fibrous tissue in the olecranon fossa (Fig. 39-8).[173]

The patient often presents with posteromedial elbow pain during the acceleration phase or follow-through phase of throw-

---

Box 39-1 Interval throwing program

Athletes are allowed to progress from one phase to the next as soon as they are able to complete the phase pain-free.

45-ft phase
- Step 1: warm up, 25 45-ft throws × 2 with 15-min rest between sets
- Step 2: warm up, 25 45-ft throws × 3 with 15-min rest between sets

60-ft phase
- Step 1: warm up, 25 60-ft throws × 2 with 15-min rest between sets
- Step 2: warm up, 25 60-ft throws × 3 with 15-min rest between sets

90-ft phase
- Step 1: warm up, 25 90-ft throws × 2 with 15-min rest between sets
- Step 2: warm up, 25 90-ft throws × 3 with 15-min rest between sets

120-ft phase
- Step 1: warm up, 25 120-ft throws × 2 with 15-min rest between sets
- Step 2: warm up, 25 120-ft throws × 3 with 15-min rest between sets

150-ft phase
- Step 1: warm up, 25 150-ft throws × 2 with 15-min rest between sets
- Step 2: warm up, 25 150-ft throws × 3 with 15-min rest between sets

180-ft phase
- Step 1: warm up, 25 180-ft throws × 2 with 15-min rest between sets
- Step 2: warm-up, 25 180-ft throws × 3 with 15-min rest between sets
- Step 3: begin throwing off of the mound or return to their respective positions

---

ing. The pain associated with valgus extension overload can be differentiated from the pain seen with an ulnar collateral ligament injury, because the pain with valgus extension overload is localized over the posterior medial tip of the olecranon. Physical examination shows tenderness to palpation over the posterior medial tip of the olecranon, and pain with repetitive passive elbow hyperextension with a valgus force across the elbow.

Radiographic evaluation should include anteroposterior, lateral, and axial radiographs. These can demonstrate an olecranon osteophyte or intraarticular loose bodies. The osteophyte is best viewed on lateral views. MRI can provide further delineation of the pathologic lesions, but normal radiographs and MRI do not exclude this condition.

The initial treatment of valgus extension overload is conservative. The patient should discontinue aggravating activities, particularly throwing, and localized modalities and range of motion exercises should be initiated. Antiinflammatory medications can help reduce the pain and facilitate the rehabilitation program. It is important to address kinetic chain deficits, ensure proper throwing mechanics, and strengthen the medial forearm musculature to reduce the valgus stress across the elbow during throwing activities. Once all the above factors have been addressed and the patient has full pain-free elbow range of motion and full strength, an interval throwing program can be initiated (see Box 39-1). Symptoms frequently return when the athlete returns to throwing activities, and surgical intervention might be required.

Medial epicondylar traction apophysitis and stress fracture

Injuries to the medial elbow in young throwing athletes have been referred to as 'Little Leaguer's elbow', and include medial epicondylitis, traction apophysitis, stress fractures through the medial epicondylar epiphyses, and avulsion fractures of the medial epicondyle.[24] These injuries classically occur in the dominant arm of throwing athletes between the ages of 9 and 12 years.[23] Excessive throwing causes chronic repetitive valgus stress to the medial elbow, resulting in a traction injury to the immature medial epicondyle. The medial epicondylar apophysis does not close until 14 years of age in girls and 17 years of age in boys, and is the last elbow physis to close (Fig. 39-9).[23]

The patient frequently presents with medial elbow pain exacerbated by throwing. Physical examination reveals tenderness over the medial epicondyle, and there can also be mild edema in the painful region and a slight flexion contracture of the elbow.

Radiologic evaluation should include anteroposterior, lateral, axial, and comparison views of the elbow. Common radiologic abnormalities associated with medial elbow traction injuries in young throwing athletes include medial epicondylar enlargement, fragmentation, beaking, and avulsion of the medial epicondyle (Fig. 39-10).[24] In the past, the studies done included a three-phase bone scan followed by tomograms or CT scan through the areas of increased activity. MRI currently has the advantage of evaluating for both osseous and soft tissue injuries that might not be identified with other techniques.

Treatment should begin with a 4- to 8-week period of rest from throwing activities. Ice, antiinflammatory medications, and elbow range of motion exercises should be instituted early. As symptoms resolve, progressive strengthening of the medial forearm musculature should be performed. An interval throw-

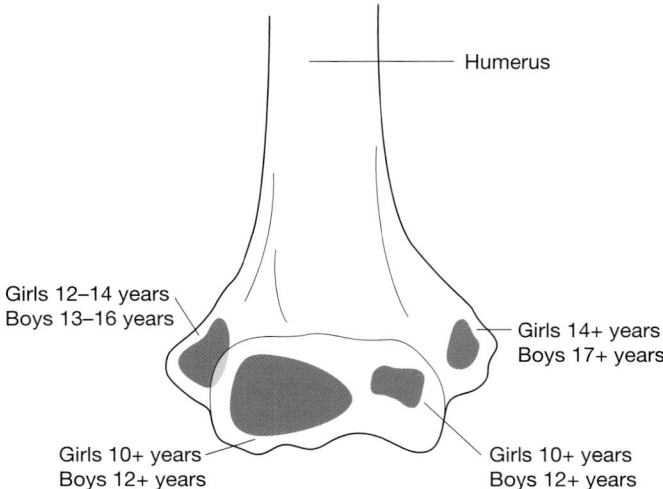

Figure 39-9 The average age for distal humeral ossification centers to fuse.

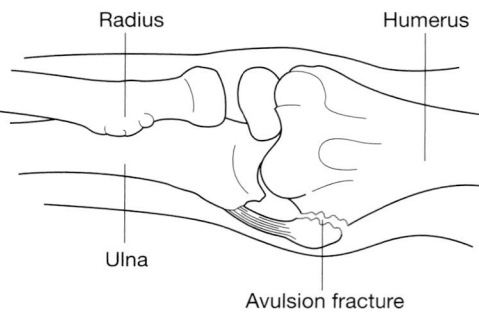

Figure 39-10 Valgus stress to the immature elbow can result in an avulsion fracture of the medial epicondylar ossification center.

ing program can begin when full pain-free range of motion has been restored and there are no strength asymmetries (see Box 39-1). If pain resumes with throwing activities, a more prolonged period of rest extending for several months should be initiated. This should be followed by the same gradually progressive resumption of throwing activities. If after 6 months of treatment the patient is still symptomatic, surgical consultation is warranted.

If a displaced avulsion fracture occurs, surgical treatment for appropriate anatomic reduction is required.

Osteochondrosis and osteochondritis dissecans of the capitellum

Panner disease is an osteochondrosis of the capitellum that occurs in children between the ages of 7 and 10 years, and begins with degeneration or necrosis of the capitellum, with eventual regeneration and calcification of this area.[131] The etiology of Panner disease is unknown, but it appears to be related to disordered endochondral ossification in association with trauma or vascular impairment.

Clinically, patients with Panner disease present with dull, aching lateral elbow pain aggravated by throwing activities.

Effusion of the elbow is frequently present, but range of motion is usually not restricted.

Treatment of Panner disease is non-operative and initially involves discontinuation of throwing activities. Occasionally, a posterior long arm splint is used for pain control. Repeat radiographs should be performed to ensure adequate healing, because late articular collapse of the capitellum, although uncommon, can occur.

Osteochondritis dissecans can also occur to the capitellum. This entity has several unique characteristics that enable clinicians to differentiate it from osteochondrosis of the capitellum. Osteochondritis dissecans occurs in throwing athletes between 9 and 15 years of age, whereas osteochondrosis occurs in 7- to 10-year olds.[23] Osteochondritis dissecans involves focal lesions to the capitellum, while osteochondrosis involves the entire capitellum.[23] Osteochondritis dissecans frequently leads to loose body formation, and osteochondrosis is usually self-limited, resolving with rest and time.[23]

Patients with osteochondritis dissecans present with the insidious onset of lateral elbow pain, accompanied by an elbow flexion contracture of 15° or more. Catching and/or locking can also be present. The elbow might also have an effusion.

Radiographic evaluation should include anteroposterior, lateral, and oblique views of the elbow. While CT arthrogram and tomograms were previously used to define the lesion, MRI is quickly becoming the study of choice for osteochondritis dissecans.

Treatment should begin with rest, ice, and antiinflammatory medications. Elbow immobilization with a posterior long arm splint might provide symptomatic relief. Gentle progressive range of motion and strengthening exercises should begin once pain has resolved, and protection from forceful activities should continue for a minimum of 6 weeks to allow healing. Once full strength and range of motion have been restored, the patient can begin a gradual return to functional activities. Serial radiographic evaluation should be performed to ensure adequate healing of the lesion, although in some cases symptomatic improvement can occur despite persistent radiologic abnormalities. In patients with large loose bodies, persistent mechanical symptoms, or pain recalcitrant to non-operative measures, surgical intervention might be required.

Elbow dislocations

Elbow dislocations involving the proximal ulna and distal humerus most frequently occur in a posterolateral direction, and are a result of a fall on an outstretched arm with the elbow in hyperextension (Fig. 39-11).[121] Anterior, lateral, and posteromedial dislocations also occur but are much less frequent. When a posterolateral elbow dislocation occurs, associated injuries include disruption of the ulnar and radial collateral ligaments of the elbow, and occasionally disruption of the flexor pronator forearm musculature, or periarticular and intraarticular fractures.[75,119,167] Injuries to the brachial artery, or the median, ulnar, or radial nerves, should be identified and treated. Acute anterior forearm compartment syndrome can also occur with elbow dislocations.

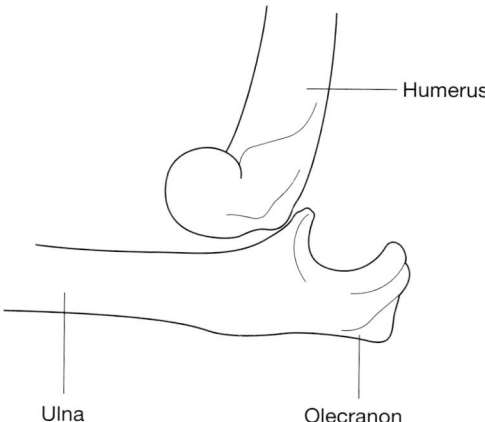

Figure 39-11 Posterior dislocation of the elbow.

Clinical evaluation should include a complete neurovascular examination of the injured limb and standard anterior–posterior, lateral, and oblique radiographs to correctly classify the direction of the dislocation and identify any associated fractures.

Treatment should begin with reduction of the dislocation. Pre- and postreduction films should be obtained to ensure proper reduction. If the elbow cannot be reduced in a closed manner, then open reduction should be performed. Postreduction neurovascular examination is very important to rule out new or continued neurovascular compromise. If the flexor–pronator musculature has been disrupted along with the ulnar collateral ligaments, early surgical intervention is warranted.[119] Gross medial elbow instability without flexor–pronator musculature rupture can be treated non-operatively if the patient does not participate in overhead throwing sports. However, overhead throwing athletes with complete disruption of the ulnar collateral ligament frequently require surgical intervention to reduce their postinjury morbidity.

Conservative treatment of elbow dislocations includes a sling or posterior long arm splint for 2–3 days, followed by progressive range of motion exercises. Prolonged immobilization is important to avoid, because flexion contractures are a frequent complication of this injury. A hinged elbow brace that allows flexion and extension of the elbow can assist in early range of motion activities. Ice and antiinflammatory medications can assist in patient comfort. Progressive strengthening activities should begin as the patient pain allows, and full return to activities should be expected in approximately 8 weeks. A majority of patients have had a 90% restoration of function by 3 months post injury.[74,144] In addition to the surgical indications previously mentioned, surgical intervention can be warranted in patients who experience chronic recurrent elbow instability.

Disorders of the forearm and wrist
Flexor carpi ulnaris tendonitis
Flexor carpi ulnaris tendonitis occurs due to repetitive microtrauma from activities requiring wrist flexion and ulnar deviation, such as racket sports or golf.[64] Because the pisiform bone

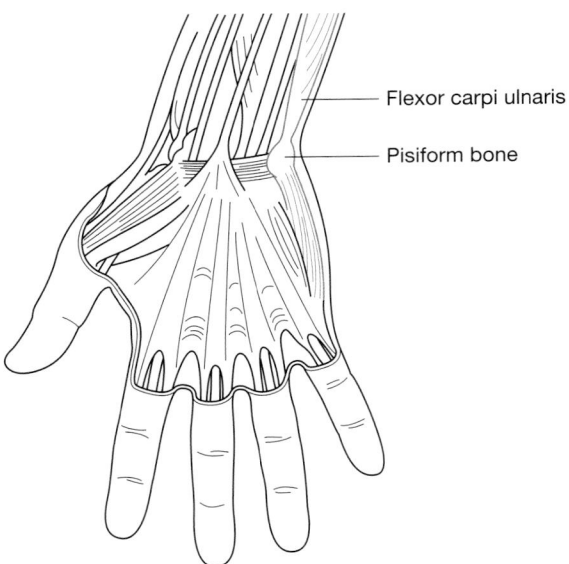

Figure 39-12 Pisiform bone embedded in the flexor carpi ulnaris tendon.

is embedded in the flexor carpi ulnaris tendon, a condition frequently associated with flexor carpi ulnaris tendonitis is pisotriquetral compression syndrome with eventual pisotriquetral osteoarthritis (Fig. 39-12).[142]

Patients with flexor carpi ulnaris tendonitis report pain in the volar ulnar aspect of the wrist that developed insidiously. Activities requiring repetitive wrist flexion and ulnar deviation frequently aggravate this condition. The patient might also experience crepitus in the region of the pisotriquetral joint during wrist movement. Physical examination can reveal localized edema and tenderness to palpation over the distal flexor carpi ulnaris tendon. Compression of the pisiform against the triquetrum can cause pain if osteoarthritis is present in this joint. Lateral wrist radiographs with slight supination and extension can also demonstrate the pisotriquetral joint osteoarthritis.[142]

Treatment includes activity modification, ice, and antiinflammatory medications. Wrist–hand orthoses with the wrist in 25° of volar flexion can assist in symptom control.[142] The splint should be removed at least twice daily to allow for wrist range of motion, to prevent the complications associated with immobilization. Galvanic electrical stimulation and iontophoresis can be beneficial adjuncts to treatment. Recalcitrant cases can respond to a localized corticosteroid injection. When symptoms have been reduced, a gradually progressive rehabilitation program addressing forearm strength, flexibility, and endurance deficits should begin. A functional progression to return patients to their previous activities should be employed. Training and technique errors should be corrected.

Patients who do not respond to a comprehensive non-operative treatment program can respond to surgical resection of the pisiform bone with or without Z plasty lengthening of the flexor carpi ulnaris tendon.[130]

Flexor carpi radialis tendonitis

The flexor carpi radialis tendon passes through a tunnel formed by the transverse carpal ligament, trapezial ridge, and scaphoid tuberosity prior to inserting on the second metacarpal base.[142] While tendonitis in the flexor carpi radialis is relatively uncommon, activities that require repetitive gripping with wrist flexion and radial deviation predispose to this condition.[42]

Symptoms usually develop slowly and include radial wrist pain with gripping, and forceful wrist flexion with radial deviation. Physical examination reveals tenderness to palpation over the distal flexor carpi radialis tendon, and pain with passive wrist extension or with resisted wrist flexion combined with radial deviation.

Treatment includes discontinuation of aggravating activities, ice, and antiinflammatory medications. If splinting is required, a wrist–hand orthosis with 25° of wrist flexion is appropriate.[142] The patient should be instructed to remove the splint at least twice daily for wrist range of motion exercises in order to prevent the complications associated with prolonged immobilization. Galvanic electrical stimulation or iontophoresis can be used as adjunct treatments. A peritendinous injection with corticosteroid medication might be beneficial in recalcitrant cases. It should be kept in mind, however, that complications associated with corticosteroid injection can occur, such as tendon rupture.

Following adequate pain control, a rehabilitation program to correct strength, endurance, and flexibility deficits of the forearm musculature should be employed. Kinetic chain deficits should be identified and corrected. Ensure that the athlete is using correct technique in their sport, and that they are not training inappropriately. A gradually progressive return to functional activity should occur as the patient's symptoms resolve.

De Quervain's syndrome

The first dorsal compartment of the wrist contains the abductor pollicis longus and extensor pollicis brevis tendons. These tendons run beneath a sheath over the dorsal aspect of the radial styloid process. Shear and repetitive microtrauma in this area can result in a stenosing tenosynovitis referred to as de Quervain's syndrome.[142] De Quervain's syndrome is the most common tendonitis of the wrist, and is most frequently seen in patients who perform activities requiring forceful gripping with radial deviation of the wrist, or repetitive use of the thumb.[33,90]

Patients with this condition present with insidious onset of pain over the dorsal radial aspect of the wrist, aggravated by activities such as racket sports, golf, or fly fishing. Patients can also report a sensation of crepitation in the wrist. Physical examination frequently demonstrates some mild edema localized to the dorsal radial wrist, and tenderness to palpation over the first dorsal compartment. Finkelstein's test is pathognomonic for the diagnosis.[142]

Treatment for de Quervain's syndrome includes rest, ice, antiinflammatory medications, and a thumb spica splint. The patient should remove the splint several times a day to perform gentle range of motion exercises in order to prevent the complications of prolonged immobilization. Galvanic electrical stimulation or iontophoresis can help with inflammation and pain control. Corticosteroid injection into the peritendinous region of the first dorsal compartment results in successful treatment in 62–100% of cases.[81,176] However, the wary clinician should always consider the possible detrimental effects of corticosteroid injection, such as tendon rupture.

Following adequate pain control, a rehabilitation program should be instituted that includes addressing flexibility, strength, and endurance deficits of the forearm musculature. Training and technique errors frequently lead to this condition and should be addressed as part of the treatment program. Kinetic chain deficits should be identified and corrected. If the patient does not respond to the above treatment program, surgical intervention might be warranted.

Intersection syndrome

The abductor pollicis longus and extensor pollicis brevis tendons cross the extensor carpi radialis longus and brevis tendons 4–6 cm proximal to Lister's tubercle. An inflammatory condition can develop at this crossing due to the friction from the tendons repetitively rubbing against each other. This condition is called intersection syndrome, and is most frequently seen in oarsmen, weightlifters, and racket sport athletes.[35,126,142]

Intersection syndrome presents with the insidious onset of dorsoradial distal forearm pain that is aggravated by activities requiring repetitive wrist extension.[142] Physical examination reveals mild edema and acute tenderness 4–6 cm proximal to Lister's tubercle, frequently associated with crepitation during wrist flexion and extension.

Treatment for this condition includes rest, ice, antiinflammatory medications, and splinting with a neutral wrist–hand orthosis. The orthosis should be removed approximately twice daily for wrist range of motion and hand range of motion in order to prevent immobilization complications. Deep tissue massage, galvanic electrical stimulation, or iontophoresis can be used as adjuncts to treatment. Strength, endurance, flexibility, and kinetic chain deficits should be addressed as a part of the comprehensive rehabilitation program. Corticosteroid injection into the point of maximal tenderness is used if the patient does not respond to initial treatment. The potential for tendon rupture post corticosteroid injection should be discussed with the patient prior to their use. This condition requires surgical treatment only rarely.

Extensor carpi ulnaris tendonitis and subluxation

The second most frequent tendonitis of the wrist is extensor carpi ulnaris tendonitis. Repetitive wrist extension with ulnar deviation, such as occurs in the non-dominant hand of the two-handed backhand, predisposes to this condition.[142] Rupture or attenuation of the overlying tendon sheath can result in subluxation of the extensor carpi ulnaris tendon.[151]

Extensor carpi ulnaris tendonitis usually presents with insidious onset of dorsoulnar wrist pain that occurs during activities requiring forceful or repetitive wrist extension and ulnar deviation. Patients with tendon subluxation often report a history of a pop following a forceful wrist volar flexion and ulnar deviation, with subsequent pain.[151] Physical examination of patients with tendonitis reveals tenderness to palpation over the extensor carpi ulnaris tendon, and pain with resisted wrist extension with ulnar deviation. Subluxation can be induced by having the patient actively ulnarly deviate the wrist while the forearm is in full supination. The extensor carpi ulnaris tendon might palpably and/or visually sublux ulnarly over the ulnar styloid process.[142]

Treatment of extensor carpi ulnaris tendonitis involves rest, ice, antiinflammatory medications, and a neutral wrist–hand orthosis. The orthosis should be removed twice daily for wrist range of motion exercises to prevent complications from immobilization. Galvanic electrical stimulation or iontophoresis can be added in cases not responding to initial treatment. Local peritendinous corticosteroid injection can assist in the treatment of this condition, but the complications of corticosteroid injections need to be kept in mind.

Following adequate pain control, a rehabilitation program that focuses on correcting strength, flexibility, and endurance deficits of the forearm musculature should be employed. Kinetic chain deficits should be identified and addressed. Training and technique errors should be identified and corrected. If the patient does not respond to the above treatment program, a search for other diagnoses that mimic extensor carpi ulnaris tendonitis, such as triangular fibrocartilage complex (TFCC) injury, should be undertaken.

Acute extensor carpi ulnaris tendon subluxations can be treated with cast immobilization of the wrist in a pronated and dorsiflexed position for 6 weeks.[29] However, early surgical repair for acute injuries has also been advocated to improve predictability of outcome.[151] In injuries characterized by chronic recurrent subluxation, surgical reconstruction of the subsheath should be performed.

Scapholunate instability

Scapholunate instability due to ligamentous injury is the most common type of ligament injury in the wrist.[98] This can occur when a person falls on the pronated outstretched hand with the wrist in extension and ulnar deviation. Following scapholunate ligament disruption, the scaphoid moves into a flexed position, while the lunate and triquetrum become extended. This pattern is referred to as a dorsal intercalated segmental instability (DISI) pattern (Fig. 39-13).[86] If this injury is not diagnosed early and treated properly, joint stress will ultimately lead to progressive wrist arthrosis and scapholunate advanced collapse.[141]

Patients who sustain a scapholunate injury report falling on their outstretched hand with subsequent wrist edema, ecchymosis, and restricted range of motion. Physical examination will reveal tenderness over the scapholunate joint, particularly on the dorsum of the wrist. The patient typically has a positive Watson's test, which is indicated by a pop and reproduction of the pain.[94]

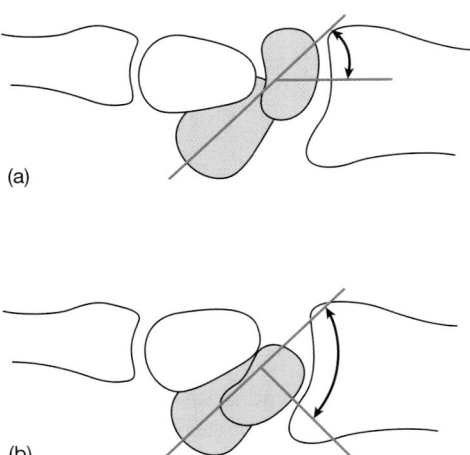

(a)

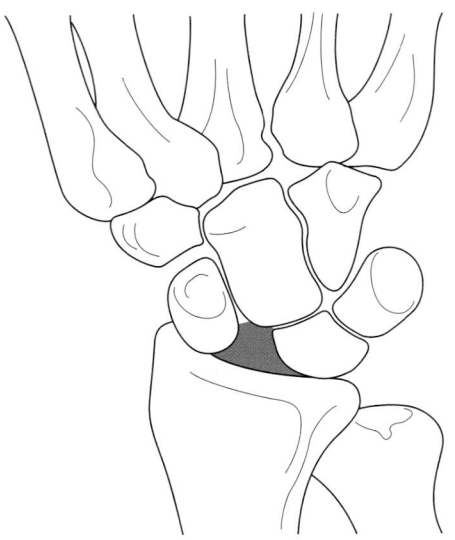

(b)

Figure 39-13 (a) Normal scapholunate angle between 30 and 60°. (b) Scapholunate angle greater than 60°, indicating a dorsal intercalated segmental instability pattern suggestive of scapholunate dissociation.

Figure 39-14 A gap between the scaphoid and lunate on anteroposterior radiographs indicates scapholunate dissociation.

Radiographic evaluation should include anteroposterior, anteroposterior with a clenched fist, lateral, and oblique radiographs.[141] The presence of associated fractures should be determined. The lateral radiograph can reveal the presence of a DISI pattern injury (see Fig. 39-13). This is characterized by a dorsally directed angle of more than 60° between the scaphoid and the lunate.[141] A gap of more than 3 mm between the scaphoid and lunate on anteroposterior radiographs is also diagnostic for scapholunate instability (Fig. 39-14).[141] The clenched fist view exaggerates this finding. Radiographic evaluation should include comparison studies with the opposite wrist.

If standard radiographs are not diagnostic, further studies including arthrography or MRI can be obtained. However, the sensitivity and specificity of these studies are variable.[141] Wrist arthroscopy has become the gold standard for diagnosing this entity.

Acute scapholunate ligament injuries should be treated surgically. Chronic scapholunate injuries are more difficult to treat

but continue to require surgical intervention. Partial wrist arthrodesis can be required for chronic scapholunate instability, and a proximal row carpectomy is frequently utilized to treat scapholunate advanced collapse.[141]

Scaphoid fracture

Approximately 6% of all fractures involve the carpal bones, and 70% of carpal fractures involve the scaphoid.[45] The scaphoid is positioned distal to the radius and is part of the proximal row of carpals. The scaphoid is the primary restraint to excessive wrist extension, and is therefore prone to injury. The scaphoid fractures in the middle third 80% of the time, the proximal third 15% of the time, and the distal third 4% of the time. Only 1% of scaphoid fractures occur through the distal tubercle.[45]

The scaphoid receives its blood supply from a branch of the radial artery. The blood supply enters the scaphoid through its distal pole, and the proximal scaphoid is dependent on the distal blood supply. It is for this reason that proximal or middle third fractures of the scaphoid are prone to avascular necrosis and non-union.[45]

Patients who sustain scaphoid fractures usually fall on an extended wrist. They usually complain of pain in the radial aspect of the wrist, particularly dorsally, along with slight edema and ecchymosis in the area of the anatomic snuffbox. On physical examination, the anatomic snuffbox will be tender to palpation. Neurovascular function should be assessed.

Radiologic evaluation of the wrist should include anteroposterior, lateral, right and left oblique, and anteroposterior clenched fist views.[45] Scaphoid fractures can be very subtle and not readily apparent on radiographs. Associated carpal instability patterns should be assessed radiographically, with particular attention paid to scapholunate dissociation. Scapholunate dissociation is suggested by a 3 mm or larger gap between the scaphoid and lunate during clenched fist anteroposterior views, or with a DISI pattern on lateral radiographs.[45]

Because minimal edema occurs with this fracture, early cast immobilization can be utilized. For non-displaced middle or proximal third fractures, the first 6 weeks of immobilization should use a long arm thumb spica cast with the elbow in 90° of flexion and the wrist in neutral flexion–extension and neutral deviation incorporating the first metacarpophalangeal joint with the thumb in slight extension and abduction.[45]

If the fracture occurs in the distal third of the scaphoid, or if there is a high index of suspicion for a fracture of the scaphoid that was not seen on radiographs, a short arm thumb spica cast with the wrist and thumb positioned the same as described for the long arm cast can be used.[45]

Patients with non-displaced middle or proximal third fractures can be switched from the long arm thumb spica cast to a short arm thumb spica cast after 6 weeks, with the total duration of immobilization being for 12–20 weeks depending on when radiographic union occurs.[45] Patients with non-displaced distal third fractures typically require between 10 and 12 weeks of immobilization in a short arm thumb spica cast.[45] The fracture should be re-x-rayed every 2–3 weeks until radiographic union is documented.[45]

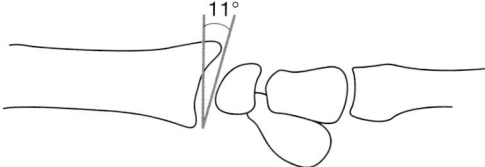

Figure 39-15 Normal scaphoid volar tilt is approximately 11°, radial inclination is 23°, and the distance between the distal ulnar articular surface and the tip of the radial styloid process is 12 mm.

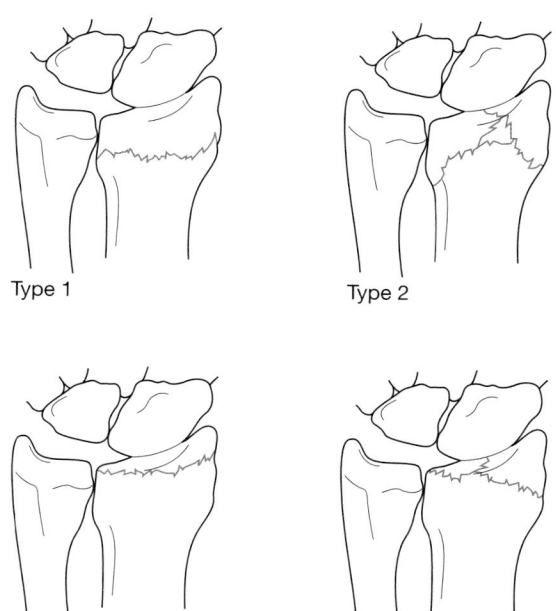

Type 1   Type 2

Type 3   Type 4

Figure 39-16 Frykman's classification of distal radius fractures.

If a scaphoid fracture is suspected, and following 2 weeks of short arm thumb spica cast immobilization the patient continues to have anatomic snuffbox tenderness and repeat radiographs are still negative, then a bone scan or MRI can be performed to confirm or exclude this diagnosis. If the bone scan or MRI reveals a non-displaced fracture, then standard treatment as outlined above should be performed.

During cast immobilization, the patient should be encouraged to perform range of motion and strengthening exercises with the upper limb regions that are not immobilized. Following completion of the immobilization period, the patient should begin an exercise program to restore full pain-free range of motion in the immobilized joints, and strengthening of the immobilized musculature.

Patients with displaced fractures, those who sustain scapholunate dissociation, or those who develop avascular necrosis or a non-union should be referred to an orthopedist for treatment.

Distal radial fractures

The distal radius is one of the most frequently fractured areas of the body. Postmenopausal women and children appear to be particularly susceptible to this fracture.[46] The distal radius has three articulations: the distal radioulnar joint, the radioscaphoid joint, and the radiolunate joint. The distal radius normally displays a volar tilt of approximately 11°, a radial inclination along the articular surface as viewed on the anterior–posterior radiograph that is 23°, and a 12-mm distance between the tip of the radial styloid process to a line drawn perpendicular to the distal ulnar articular surface (this can be measured on a standard anteroposterior radiographic image) (Fig. 39-15).[46]

Frykman proposed a classification system for distal radial fractures.[46] Type 1 and 2 fractures are extraarticular fractures, and types 3 and 4 are intraarticular fractures involving the radiocarpal joint. Type 5 and 6 fractures are intraarticular fractures involving the radioulnar joint, while types 7 and 8 are intraarticular fractures that involve both the radioulnar and the radiocarpal joints (Fig. 39-16). The even-numbered fractures indicate the presence of an associated ulnar styloid fracture. The potential for adverse outcome increased as the Frykman classification number increased.

A majority of patients who sustain a distal radius fracture report falling on an extended wrist. Physical examination often reveals localized edema and ecchymosis along with deformity at the fracture site. There will be tenderness to palpation over

the fracture site. It is important to document normal neurovascular function during the examination.

Distal radial fractures can be assessed using anteroposterior, lateral, and oblique radiographs.[46] The anteroposterior view allows measurements of the radial inclination and length, while the lateral view allows evaluation of the volar tilt.

The most common distal radius fracture is a Frykman type 1 fracture called the Colles fracture.[46] This fracture is characterized by a fracture line 2 cm proximal to the distal radius, with dorsal angulation of the distal fragment and radial shortening. Minimally displaced Frykman type 1 or 2 fractures can be managed with closed reduction, and immobilization with a double sugar tong splint with the wrist in slight flexion and ulnar deviation.[46] The forearm should be in a neutral position, and the elbow should be flexed 90°.[46] Satisfactory reduction requires that there is less than 5 mm of radial shortening, no dorsal tilt of the distal radius, and less than 2 mm of displacement of fracture fragments. The patient should be followed-up in 3 days for repeat radiographs.[46]

By approximately 3 days post injury, patients with a non-displaced fracture can be placed in a short arm cast with the wrist in a neutral position for approximately 6 weeks, with repeat radiographs every 2 weeks for the first 6 weeks.[46] Patients with a minimally displaced fracture who are status post reduction should receive repeat radiographs at the 3-day follow-up to ensure maintenance of the reduction, and should be placed in a long arm cast with the wrist in slight flexion and ulnar deviation, the forearm in a neutral position, and the elbow flexed to 90° for 3–4 weeks.[46] This can then be switched to a short arm cast with the wrist in a neutral position for 3–4 more weeks until healing has occurred.[46] Patients with minimally displaced fractures status post reduction should receive repeat

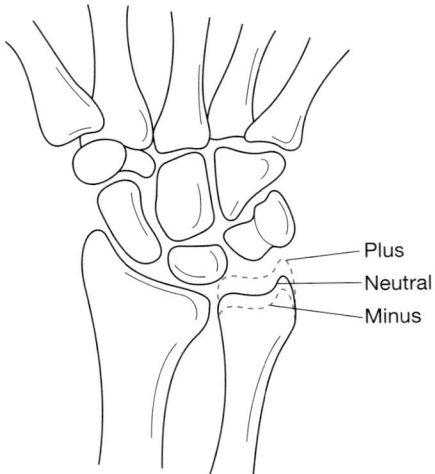

Figure 39-17 Ulnar variance.

radiographs weekly for the first 3 weeks, then every 2 weeks until healing is complete.[46]

The patient should be instructed on range of motion exercises for the joints that are not immobilized and, following discontinuation of the cast, a rehabilitation program should be instituted to ensure restoration of full joint range of motion and upper limb strength.

Patients with Frykman type 3 fractures or higher, comminuted fractures, fractures with significant displacement or that are unstable should be referred to an orthopedist for management.

Kienbock disease

Kienbock first described a condition characterized by progressive collapse of the lunate in 1910.[101] This entity, now commonly referred to as Kienbock disease, is hypothesized to result from repetitive compressive forces to the wrist causing microfractures in the lunate, leading to vascular compromise, avascular necrosis, and eventual collapse of the lunate.[53,101] This condition occurs more frequently in patients who have ulnar minus variant wrists (Fig. 39-17).[53]

Kienbock disease presents with pain and stiffness in the wrist. Physical examination can reveal limited wrist range of motion, and tenderness to palpation over the lunate on the dorsum of the wrist.

Radiographic evaluation typically reveals an ulnar minus variant in the wrist.[53] The lunate can appear normal in early cases, but frequently becomes sclerotic with cystic changes, followed by fragmentation and collapse.[101] Bone scans might demonstrate increased uptake, while radiographs are still negative.[101] MRI can also be helpful in diagnosing Kienbock disease.

In early cases of Kienbock disease, the wrist should also be immobilized in an attempt to allow revascularization.[160] If the patient has an ulnar minus wrist variant, an attempt at relieving lunate trauma through an ulnar lengthening procedure or radial shortening procedure can be performed.[101] For more advanced cases of Kienbock disease, partial wrist arthrodesis, or lunate

excision with soft tissue or silicone replacement, might be required.[101]

Triangular fibrocartilage complex injuries

The TFCC is composed of an avascular central articular disk and vascular dorsal and palmar radioulnar ligaments.[141] The TFCC is the primary stabilizer of the distal radioulnar joint, and can be injured in an acute traumatic event such as falling on an outstretched hand, or through repetitive microtrauma such as in gymnastics. Axially loading of the wrist results in 18% of the load being born through the TFCC and the remaining 82% through the radiocarpal joint.[129] A positive ulnar variance results in an increase in the load-bearing function of the TFCC, which results in a higher incidence of TFCC injuries (see Fig. 39-17).[129]

When individuals sustain a TFCC injury, they can report either a single traumatic event resulting in the injury, or an insidious onset. Traumatic tears occur more frequently in young athletes, while degenerative tears are more common in older patients. Patients with acute injuries often report an axial load to the wrist associated with rotational stress.[141] The patient can also report wrist catching and locking. The physical examination can reveal tenderness to palpation in the hollow between the flexor carpi ulnaris tendon and the extensor carpi ulnaris tendon, just distal to the ulnar styloid process.[141]

Radiographic evaluation of the wrist can reveal an ulnar plus variant on the anteroposterior view. Tricompartment wrist arthrogram, MRI, and MRI arthrogram can provide more specific information regarding TFCC pathology.[141]

When the central articular disk of the TFCC has been acutely injured, surgical debridement is the treatment of choice. A 90% good to excellent result with this treatment was reported by Bednar and Osterman.[19] Peripheral tears of the TFCC also respond well to surgical intervention, but the postoperative recovery process is slower than that for central articular disk injuries.[141] Patients with degenerative tears of the TFCC should be evaluated for an ulnar plus variant and, if this is present, an ulnar shortening procedure should be considered along with surgical debridement of the TFCC.[141]

Extensor tendon central slip disruption

A rupture of the central slip of the extensor tendon at the base of the middle phalanx results in a boutonnière injury (Fig. 39-18). A boutonnière injury is characterized by the inability to actively extend the proximal interphalangeal joint, but patients with this injury are able to maintain full proximal interphalangeal joint extension if they are passively placed in this position.[55] The reason the proximal interphalangeal joint is held in flexion is due to the migration of the lateral bands of the extensor mechanism volarly below the axis of rotation in the proximal interphalangeal joint, resulting in a flexion force at this joint.[55] However, the lateral bands continue to exert an extension force on the distal interphalangeal joint.

The central slip injury can be due to a rupture of the central slip or an avulsion fracture at the distal insertion point of the central slip on the dorsal proximal aspect of the middle phalanx.

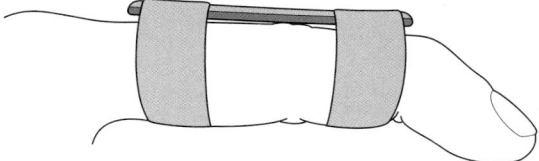

Figure 39-19 Dorsal extension splint of the proximal interphalangeal joint.

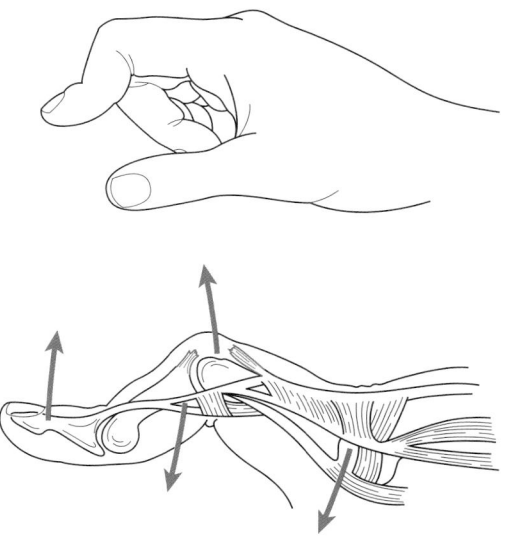

Figure 39-18 A boutonnière deformity due to rupture of the central slip and volar migration of the lateral bands.

This injury can be a result of direct trauma to the area, forced flexion of the interphalangeal joints, or after a lateral volar dislocation of the proximal interphalangeal joint.[142]

The patient usually reports a specific injury to the digit, resulting in an inability to extend the flexed proximal interphalangeal joint. Physical examination will reveal a boutonnière's deformity of the affected digit, and can reveal tenderness to palpation over the dorsum of the proximal interphalangeal joint. In acute cases, when the proximal interphalangeal joint is fully extended, the patient will be able to actively maintain the extension.

Standard radiographic evaluation of the proximal interphalangeal joint should be performed to evaluate for an associated avulsion fracture of the dorsal proximal aspect of the middle phalanx. If the injury is evaluated within approximately 6 weeks, and the patient has full passive extension of the proximal interphalangeal joint, then treatment should involve continuous extension splinting of the proximal interphalangeal joint for 5–6 weeks (Fig. 39-19).[55] The distal interphalangeal joint can be left unsplinted, and flexion exercises of the distal interphalangeal joint should be initiated early in the treatment program. It is important to educate the patient that even a single episode of proximal interphalangeal joint flexion over this time period can prevent successful treatment of this condition, so compliance is critical.

In patients who have a chronic boutonnière deformity, or if the proximal interphalangeal joint is not able to be passively extended, an aggressive rehabilitation program involving serial casting or splinting to restore full passive range of motion should be implemented.[142] If adequate passive joint range of motion is obtained, and symptoms are minimal, no further treatment can be required. However, if the patient is not able to regain significant proximal interphalangeal joint extension range of

motion, then surgical intervention to repair the extensor mechanism can be warranted. However, surgical results are variable, and therefore a trial of non-operative treatment should be utilized in all patients prior to considering surgical intervention.[55]

If a large displaced avulsion fracture from the dorsal proximal aspect of the middle phalanx accompanies the boutonnière deformity, early surgical intervention is the treatment of choice.[142]

Terminal extensor tendon disruption

Disruption of the distal extensor tendon at its insertion on the dorsal proximal aspect of the distal phalanx results in an injury called a mallet finger (Fig. 39-20).[55] This can be due to a tendon rupture, or an avulsion fracture of the dorsal proximal distal phalanx. This injury usually occurs due to a hyperflexion force to an extended distal interphalangeal joint. A zone of hypovascularity within the distal extensor tendon can predispose to this injury.[170]

The patient frequently reports an injury resulting in distal interphalangeal joint pain and the inability to extend the distal interphalangeal joint. Physical examination reveals a distal interphalangeal joint in a flexed position that the patient is unable to extend actively. The patient can experience tenderness to palpation over the dorsal aspect of the distal interphalangeal joint and, if the injury was recent, there can be accompanying erythema, ecchymosis, and edema.

Radiologic studies of the distal interphalangeal joint should be performed to evaluate for an avulsion fracture of the dorsal proximal aspect of the distal phalanx.

The treatment for this injury is usually non-operative, unless a large avulsion fracture is present, in which case surgical intervention can be required.[55] Non-operative treatment involves splinting the distal interphalangeal joint in extension 24 h per day for 6–8 weeks (Fig. 39-21).[55] Patients should be educated on the importance of never allowing their distal interphalangeal joint to flex during this period, because any flexion in this area can prevent adequate healing and predispose to a permanent extension lag. Following an adequate period of

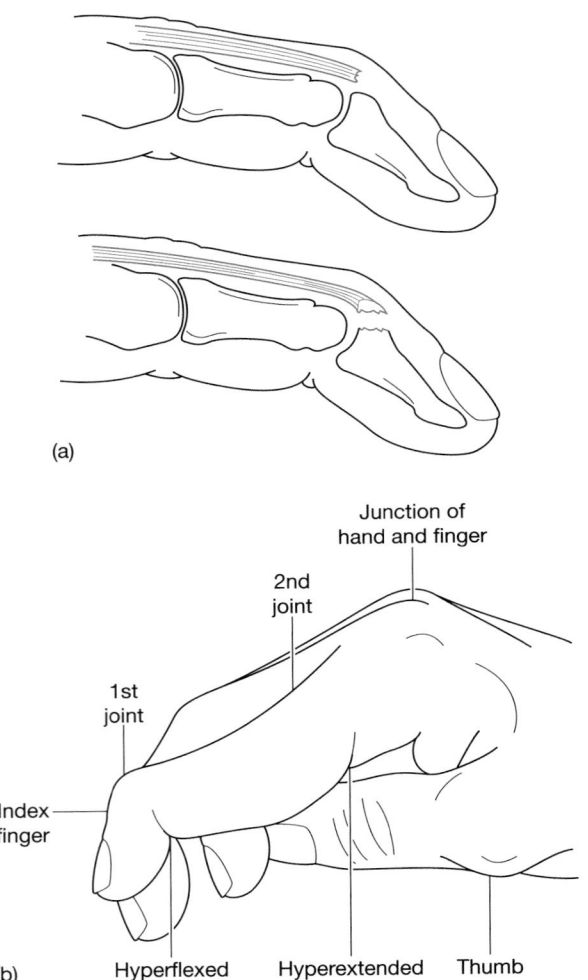

(a)

(b)

Figure 39-20 (**a**) An extensor tendon rupture (top) or avulsion fracture (bottom) resulting in a mallet finger deformity (**b**).

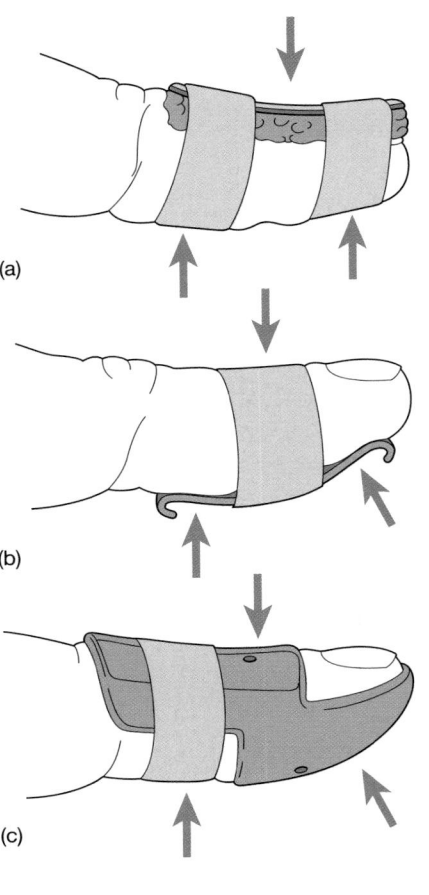

(a)

(b)

(c)

Figure 39-21 The distal interphalangeal joint can be splinted in extension with a dorsal padded aluminum splint (**a**), a volar aluminum splint without a pad (**b**), or a stack splint (**c**).

splinting, the patient should be placed in a rehabilitation program to restore full joint range of motion, and to ensure adequate strength, flexibility, and endurance in the forearm and hand musculature.

Flexor digitorum profundus rupture

Distal disruption of the flexor digitorum profundus tendon can occur with vigorous gripping activities, such as when a football player is making a tackle by gripping the opponent's jersey. Due to this mechanism of injury, distal flexor digitorum profundus tendon disruptions are frequently referred to as a jersey finger.[83] Biomechanical studies have revealed that the flexor digitorum tendon to the ring finger has a lower breaking strength than the other flexor digitorum profundus tendons, which might explain the increased incidence of disruption in the tendon to this digit when compared with other digits.[96]

The history of patients with a jersey finger usually includes a vigorous gripping activity resulting in a sudden severe pain, frequently associated with a pop. The patient will subsequently be unable to actively flex the affected distal interphalangeal

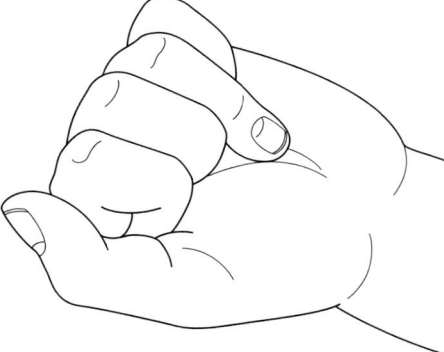

Figure 39-22 When asked to make a fist, patients with a ruptured flexor digitorum profundus tendon will be unable to flex the affected digit (in this case, the ring finger).

joint. Physical examination reveals the inability to actively flex the distal interphalangeal joint, which becomes apparent when the patient is asked to make a fist (Fig. 39-22). The retracted tendon mass can be palpable in the palm of the hand.

Radiographic evaluation of the distal interphalangeal joint should be performed to rule out associated avulsion fracture of the proximal volar aspect of the distal phalanx.

The treatment for this injury is surgical repair. If the tendon has retracted to the palm, then the repair should be performed within 7–10 days of the injury to prevent adhesion formation.[83]

However, if the tendon does not retract below the proximal interphalangeal joint, then delayed repair can be performed within 6–8 weeks of the injury.[83] Associated fractures should be addressed at the time of surgery.

Proximal interphalangeal joint dislocations

The proximal interphalangeal joint is the most frequently dislocated joint in the hand.[55] Dislocations can occur in dorsal, volar, and lateral directions, with dorsal dislocations being the most frequent.[142] Dorsal dislocations occur due to an axial load to the joint combined with hyperextension.[142] Dorsal dislocations result in various levels of injuries to the volar plate of the proximal interphalangeal joint, and radial and ulnar collateral ligaments, and can also be accompanied by a fracture.

Volar proximal interphalangeal joint dislocations are usually due to a varus or valgus force across the joint combined with a volar force to the middle phalynx.[142] Associated injuries with volar proximal interphalangeal joint dislocations include radial and ulnar collateral ligament sprains, central slip injuries, partial volar plate injuries, and fractures.

Dislocations usually present with deformity, pain, ecchymosis, and edema. The patient can report falling on the affected joint. Physical examination reveals tenderness to palpation over the injured structures. Following reduction, radial and ulnar collateral ligament injuries can be assessed by performing varus and valgus stress to the proximal interphalangeal joint. Disruption of the central slip can be assessed by determining if the patient is able to passively extend a flexed proximal interphalangeal joint. Dorsal and volar instability can be determined by first performing a digital block for anesthesia, followed by stabilizing the proximal phalanx and exerting a translational volar and dorsal force to the middle phalanx.

Radiologic evaluation should include standard radiographs of the proximal interphalangeal joint to assess for associated fractures. Avulsion fractures from the volar proximal aspect of the middle phalanx are commonly seen with dorsal dislocations. Postreduction films should also be performed to ensure that adequate reduction has been achieved. Following a digital block for local anesthesia, the joint's stability can be assessed by having the patient actively flex and extend the proximal interphalangeal joint under fluoroscopy.[55]

Following relocation, treatment for dorsal dislocations of the proximal interphalangeal joint includes an extension block splint of the proximal interphalangeal joint to allow for healing of the volar plate injury and associated collateral ligament injuries (Fig. 39-23).[55] The dorsal extension block splint should begin at approximately 45° of flexion for the first week. This can be reduced by 10° each week, with a return to full extension in the fifth week. When the splinting is discontinued, buddy taping the injured finger to the adjacent finger for a few weeks can provide some stability for the joint as tissue healing continues and range of motion exercises are instituted.

If stable closed reduction of a volar proximal interphalangeal joint dislocation can be attained, then non-operative treatment can proceed with splinting of the proximal interphalangeal joint in full extension for 4–5 weeks (see Fig. 39-19).[55] This can be

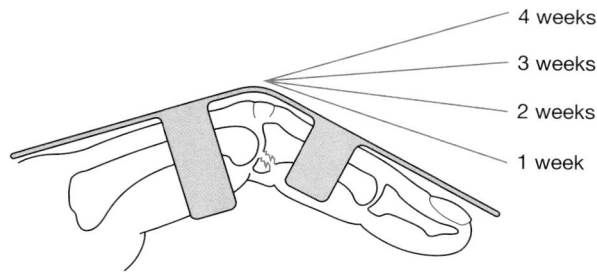

Figure 39-23 A dorsal extension splint with a reduction in extension block by 10° each week for 4 weeks.

followed by buddy taping the injured finger to an adjacent digit for approximately 2 weeks and resumption of normal activities as tolerated.

Surgical indications for proximal interphalangeal joint injuries include radiologic or gross instability following reduction, fractures involving greater than 50% of the articular surface, inability to reduce the dislocation, pilon fractures, or recurrent instability.[55]

First metacarpophalangeal joint ulnar collateral ligament sprain

Radially directed forces across the first metacarpophalangeal joint can result in an ulnar collateral ligament injury. This injury, often referred to as gamekeeper's thumb, is frequently seen in skiers and athletes who participate in sports such as basketball and football.[142] Ulnar collateral ligament injuries to the first metacarpophalangeal joint can be categorized into the standard three-grade severity scale of ligament sprains (see Table 39-1).

When a grade 3 sprain to the ulnar collateral ligament of the first metacarpophalangeal joint occurs due to avulsion of the distal end of the ligament from the base of the first proximal phalanx, there is the possibility of interposition of the adductor pollicis aponeurosis between the base of the first proximal phalanx and the ruptured end of the ulnar collateral ligament.[162] This is called a Stener lesion and can prevent adequate healing of this injury, leading to chronic joint pain and instability.

Patients who sustain this injury report a radially directed force across the first metacarpophalangeal joint. They might report an associated pop and a feeling of instability in the joint. Physical examination reveals tenderness to palpation over the ulnar collateral ligament. If a Stener lesion is present, a palpable mass on the ulnar side of the first metacarpophalangeal joint might be present, representing the avulsed ulnar collateral ligament.[2]

Ulnar collateral ligament stress examination should be performed following local anesthesia via a wrist block, although an initial examination without local anesthesia can be attempted. The stress examination should be performed with the joint in both full extension and 30° of flexion. A complete tear is indicated by an angular difference between the injured and uninjured first metacarpophalangeal joint during stress examination of greater than 15–30°.[69,128] A lack of an end point during stress examination also suggests complete ulnar collateral ligament disruption.

Radiologic evaluation should include anteroposterior, lateral, and oblique radiographs to detect the presence of fractures or joint subluxation. MRI allows better visualization of the soft tissue injuries, but its sensitivity and specificity for this condition is still being examined.

Treatment of partial tears involves ice, antiinflammatory medications, and immobilization in a thumb spica cast for 10–14 days, followed by a wrist–hand–thumb spica orthosis for 2 weeks, and a hand-based thumb spica orthosis for 2–4 more weeks.[55] Patients who participate in contact sports should continue to wear a thumb spica splint during competition for the remainder of the season. Local taping for stability during activity can be used after the period of splinting has been completed. Gentle progressive range of motion exercises should begin following cast immobilization by removing the splint twice daily, and activity should be progressed as tolerated.

Early surgical repair has been advocated for complete ruptures of the ulnar collateral ligament.[51,85,102,125,157] Surgery is also indicated for individuals with an avulsion fracture of the base of the proximal phalanx with angulation and displacement greater than 3 mm, or with chronic recurrent instability.[106]

Collateral ligament injuries of the second to fifth proximal and distal interphalangeal joints

Radial and ulnar collateral ligament injuries to the proximal and distal interphalangeal joints can be associated with multiple ligament injuries and/or dislocation, but they can also occur in isolation. Collateral ligament injuries of the interphalangeal joints can be classified according to the standard three-grade ligamentous sprain scale (see Table 39-1).

The mechanism of injury for the ulnar or radial collateral ligaments of the proximal or distal interphalangeal joints is a radial or ulnar stress to the joint, respectively. Physical examination reveals associated tenderness over the injured ligament, and ligament stability can be assessed with radial or ulnar stress to the joint following a digital block for local anesthesia.

Radiologic evaluation of radial or ulnar collateral ligament injuries involves standard anteroposterior, lateral, and oblique radiographs to assess for a fracture. If the dynamic stability of the joint is in question, active flexion and extension of the joint can be performed under fluoroscopy while the joint is anesthetized with a digital block.

Partial tears of the radial or ulnar collateral ligaments of the proximal or distal phalangeal joints can be treated with ice, antiinflammatory medications, and buddy taping the digit to an adjacent digit for 3–6 weeks. Activities can be allowed as tolerated. If there is a complete disruption of the ligament with significant instability, an attempt at non-operative treatment can be performed, but some authors advocate early open repair of this injury.[103,139,149]

CONCLUSION

There are many common injuries and syndromes that affect the upper limbs. Most of them are well described in the literature, and most can be treated non-surgically. After the acute treatment has achieved pain control and stabilization, rehabilitation should be undertaken to restore the strength, range of motion, and proprioception of the limb. The patient also typically needs an evaluation of the kinetic chain to prevent recurrent injuries.

REFERENCES

1. Abboud J, Soslowsky LJ. Interplay of the static and dynamic restrains in glenohumeral instability. Clin Orthop 2002; 400:48–57.
2. Abrahamsson S, Sollerman C, Lundborg G, et al. Diagnosis of displaced ulnar collateral ligament of the metacarpophalangeal joint of the thumb. J Hand Surg Am 1990; 15:457–460.
3. Abrams J, Savoie FH III, Tauro JC, et al. Recent advances in the evaluation and treatment of shoulder instability: anterior, posterior, and multidirectional. Arthroscopy 2002; 18:1–13.
4. Allman F. Fractures and ligamentous injuries of the clavicle and its articulation. J Bone Joint Surg Am 1967; 18:433–438.
5. Almekinders L. The efficacy of nonsteroidal anti-inflammatory drugs in the treatment of ligament injuries. Sports Med Arthrosc Rev 1990; 9:137–142.
6. Altay T, Gunal I, Ozturk H. Local injection treatment for lateral epicondylitis. Clin Orthop 2002; 398:127–130.
7. Altchek D, Dines DM. Shoulder injuries in the throwing athlete. J Am Acad Orthop Surg 1995; 3:159–165.
8. Andrews J, Carson WG, McLeod WD. Glenoid labrum tears related to the long head of the biceps. Am J Sports Med 1985; 13:337–341.
9. Andrews J, Timmerman LA. Outcome of elbow surgery in professional baseball players. Am J Sports Med 1995; 23:404–413.
10. Antoniou J, Harryman DT. Posterior instability. Orthop Clin North Am 2001; 32:463–473.
11. Anzel S, Covey KW, Weiner AD, et al. Disruption of muscles and tendons: an analysis of 1,014 cases. Surgery 1959; 45:406.
12. Arciero R, Wheeler JH, Ryan JB, et al. Arthroscopic Bankart repair versus nonoperative treatment for acute, initial anterior shoulder dislocations. Am J Sports Med 1994; 22:589–594.
13. Aronen J, Regan K. Decreasing the incidence of recurrence of first time anterior shoulder dislocations with rehabilitation. Am J Sports Med 1984; 12:283–291.
14. Backer M, Warren RF. Glenohumeral instabilities. In: DeLee J, Drez D, Miller MD, eds. DeLee and Drez's orthopaedic sports medicine principles and practice. Philadelphia: Saunders; 2003:1020–1034.
15. Baker B, Bierwagen D. Rupture of the distal tendon of the biceps brachii: operative versus non-operative treatment. J Bone Joint Surg Am 1985; 67:414–417.
16. Bankart A. The pathology and treatment of recurrent dislocation of the shoulder joint. Br J Surg 1938; 26:23–29.
17. Basamania C. Clavicle fractures in adult athletes. In: Jesse DDJ, DeLee C, eds. Orthopaedic sports medicine principles and practice. Philadelphia: Saunders; 2003:958–969.
18. Beasley L, Faryniarsz DA, Hannafin JA. Multidirectional instability of the shoulder in female athletes. Clin Sports Med 2000; 19:331–349.
19. Bednam J, Osterman AL. The role of arthroscopy in the treatment of traumatic triangular fibrocartilage injuries. Hand Clin 1994; 10:605–614.
20. Bell S, Coghlan J, Richardson M. Hydrodilatation in the management of shoulder capsulitis. Australas Radiol 2003; 47:247–251.
21. Bigliani L, Morrison DS, April EW. The morphology of the acromion and its relationship to rotator cuff tears. Orthop Trans 1986; 10:228.
22. Blasier R, Soslowsky L, Malicky D, et al. Posterior glenohumeral subluxation: active and passive stabilization in a biomechanical model. J Bone Joint Surg 1997; 79A:433–440.
23. Bradley J, Petrie RS. Elbow injuries in children and adolescents. In: DeLee J, Drez D, Miller MD, eds. Orthopaedic sports medicine principles and practice. Philadelphia: Saunders; 2003:1249–1264.
24. Brogdon B, Crowe NE. Little Leaguer's elbow. Am J Roentgenol 1960; 83:671–675.

25. Browne A, Hoffmeyer P, Tanaka S, et al. Glenohumeral elevation studies in three dimensions. J Bone Joint Surg 1990; 72B:843.

26. Brunet M, Reynolds M, Cook S. Atraumatic osteolysis of the distal clavicle: histological evidence of synovial pathogenesis. Orthopedics 1986; 9:557–559.

27. Bunker R, Anthony PP. The pathology of frozen shoulder: a Dupuytren-like disease. J Bone Joint Surg Br 1995; 77:677–683.

28. Burkhart S, Morgan CD. The peel-back mechanism: its role in producing and extending posterior type II SLAP lesions and its effect on SLAP repair rehabilitation. Arthroscopy 1998; 14:637–640.

29. Burkhart S, Wood M, Linscheid RL. Post-traumatic recurrent subluxation of the extensor carpi ulnaris tendon. J Hand Surg 1982; 7:1.

30. Cleland A. Notes on raising the arm. J Anat Physiol 1884; 18:275.

31. Clive D, Stoff JS. Renal syndromes associated with nonsteroidal anti-inflammatory drug-induced gastroduodenal ulceration. N Engl J Med 1984; 327:1575–1580.

32. Cobey M. The rolling scapula. Clin Orthop Relat Res 1968; 60:193–194.

33. Conklin J, White W. Stenosing tenosynovitis and its possible relation to the carpal tunnel syndrome. Surg Clin North Am 1960; 40:531–540.

34. Connolly J. Unfreezing the frozen shoulder. J Musculoskel Med 1998; Nov:47–58.

35. Cooney W. Sports injuries to the upper extremity. Postgrad Med 1984; 76:45–50.

36. Coonrad R, Hooper WR. Tennis elbow: its course, natural history, conservative and surgical management. J Bone Joint Surg Am 1973; 55:1177–1182.

37. Cope R, Riddervold HO, Shore JL, et al. Dislocations of the sternoclavicular joint: anatomic basis, etiologies, and radiologic diagnosis. J Orthop Trauma 1991; 5:379–384.

38. Cyriax H. The pathology and treatment of tennis elbow. J Bone Joint Surg Am 1936; 18:921–940.

39. Davidson P, ElAttrache NS, Jobe CM, et al. Rotator cuff and postero-superior glenoid labrum injury associated with increased glenohumeral motion: a new site of impingement. J Shoulder Elbow Surg 1995; 4:384–390.

40. DePalma A, Coker AJ, Probhaker M. The role of the subscapularis in recurrent anterior dislocation of the shoulder. Clin Orthop 1969; 54:35.

41. Dobbie R. Avulsion of the lower biceps brachii tendon: analysis of 51 previously reported cases. Am J Surg 1941; 51:661.

42. Dobyns J, Sim FH, Linscheid RL. Sports stress syndromes of the hand and wrist. Am J Sports Med 1978; 6:236.

43. Dugas J, Andrews JR. Throwing injuries in the adult. In: DeLee J, Drez D, Miller MD, eds. Orthopedic sports medicine principles and practice. Philadelphia: Saunders; 2003:1236–1249.

44. Edwards S, Calandruccio JH. Autologous blood injections for refractory lateral epicondylitis. J Hand Surg 2003; 28:272–278.

45. Eiff M, Hatch RL, Calmbach WL. Carpal fractures. In: Eiff M, Hatch RL, Calmbach WL, eds. Fracture management for primary care. Philadelphia: Saunders; 1998:65–77.

46. Eiff M, Hatch RL, Calmbach WL. Radius and ulna fractures. In: Eiff M, Hatch RL, Calmbach WL, eds. Fracture management for primary care. Philadelphia: Saunders; 1998:79–95.

47. Ellen M, Gilhool JJ, Rogers D. Scapular instability: the scapulothoracic joint. Phys Med Rehabil Clin North Am 2000; 11:755–770.

48. Farrar E, Lippert FG. Avulsion of the triceps tendon. Clin Orthop 1981; 161:242–246.

49. Fitzgerald R. Intrasynovial injection of steroids. Mayo Clin Proc 1976; 51(10):655–659.

50. Fleisig G, Andrews JR, Dillman CJ, et al. Kinetics of baseball pitching with implications about injury mechanisms. Am J Sports Med 1995; 23:233–239.

51. Frank W, Dobyns J. Surgical pathology of collateral ligamentous injuries of the thumb. Clin Orthop 1972; 83:102–114.

52. Friedmann E. Rupture of the distal biceps brachii tendon. JAMA 1963; 184:60–63.

53. Gelberman R, Salamon PB, Jurist JM, et al. Ulnar variance in Kienbock's disease. J Bone Joint Surg Am 1975; 57:674–676.

54. Gellman H. Tennis elbow (lateral epicondylitis). Orthop Clin North Am 1992; 23:75–82.

55. Graham T, Mullen DJ. Athletic injuries of the adult hand. In: DeLee J, Drez D, Miller MD, et al. Orthopaedic sports medicine principles and practices. Philadelphia: Saunders; 2003:1381–1431.

56. Greene J, Winickoff RN. Cost-conscious prescribing of nonsteroidal anti-inflammatory drugs for adults with arthritis. Arch Intern Med 1992; 152:1995–2002.

57. Griffin L. The female athlete. In: DeLee J, Drez D, Miller MD, et al. Orthopaedic sports medicine principles and practices. Philadelphia: Saunders; 2003:505–520.

58. Hamdan T, Al-Essa KA. Manipulation under anaesthesia for the treatment of frozen shoulder. Int Orthop 2003; 27:107–109.

59. Hannafin J, Chiaia TA. Adhesive capsulitis. Clin Orthop 2000; 372:95–109.

60. Hassell A, Fowler PD, Dawes PT. Intra-bursal tetracycline in the treatment of olecranon bursitis in patients with rheumatoid arthritis. Br J Rheumatol 1994; 33:859–860.

61. Hawkins R, Abrams JS. Impingement syndrome in the absence of rotator cuff tear (stages 1 and 2). Orthop Clin North Am 1987; 18:373–382.

62. Hawkins R, Kennedy JC. Impingement syndrome in athletes. Am J Sports Med 1980; 8:151–158.

63. Hay E, Thomas E, Paterson SM, et al. A pragmatic randomised controlled trial of local corticosteroid injection and physiotherapy for the treatment of new episodes of unilateral shoulder pain in primary care. Ann Rheum Dis 2003; 62:394–399.

64. Helal B. Racquet player's pisiform. Hand Clin 1978; 10:87–90.

65. Herring S. Rehabilitation of muscle injuries. Med Sci Sports Exerc 1990; 22:453.

66. Hovelius L, Eriksson K, Fredin H, et al. Recurrences after initial dislocation of the shoulder. Results of a prospective study of treatment. J Bone Joint Surg 1983; 65:343.

67. Hovelius L. Anterior dislocation of the shoulder in teenagers and young adults: five year prognosis. J Bone Joint Surg 1987; 69A:393–399.

68. Iannotti J, Zlatkin MB, Esterhai JL, et al. Magnetic resonance imaging of the shoulder: sensitivity, specificity and predictive value. J Bone Joint Surg Am 1991; 73:17.

69. Isani A, Melone CP. Ligamentous injuries of the hand in athletes. Clin Sports Med 1986; 5:757–772.

70. Itoi E, Hatakeyama Y, Kido T, et al. A new method of immobilization after traumatic anterior dislocation of the shoulder: a preliminary study. J Shoulder Elbow Surg 2003; 12:413–415.

71. Itoi E, Hatakeyama Y, Urayama M, et al. Position of immobilization after dislocation of the shoulder. J Bone Joint Surg Am 1999; 81:385–390.

72. Itoi E, Sashi R, Minagawa H, et al. Position of immobilization after dislocation of the glenohumeral joint. J Bone Joint Surg Am 2001; 83:661–667.

73. de Jong K, Sukui DM. Anterior sternoclavicular dislocation: a long-term follow-up study. J Orthop Trauma 1990; 4:420–423.

74. Josefsson P, Johnell O, Gentz CF. Long-term sequelae of simple dislocation of the elbow. J Bone Joint Surg Am 1984; 66:927–930.

75. Jossefsson P, Johnell O, Wendeberg B. Ligamentous injuries in dislocations of the elbow joint. Clin Orthop 1987; 21:221–225.

76. Kamien M. A rational management of tennis elbow. J Sports Med 1990; 9:173–191.

77. Kaul M, Herring SA. Superficial heat and cold. Phys Sports Med 1994; 22:65.

78. Kibler W. A framework for sports medicine. Phys Med Rehabil Clin North Am 1994; 5:1.

79. Kibler W. Role of the scapula in the overhead throwing motion. Contemp Orthop 1991; 22:525–532.

80. Kirkley A, Griffin S, Richards C, et al. Prospective randomized clinical trial comparing the effectiveness of immediate arthroscopic stabilization versus immobilization and rehabilitation in first traumatic anterior dislocations of the shoulder. Arthroscopy 1999; 15:507–514.

81. Lapidus P, Guidotti FP. Stenosing tenovaginitis of the wrist and fingers. Clin Orthop 1972; 83:87–90.

82. Larson R, Osternig LR. Traumatic bursitis and artificial turf. J Sports Med 1974; 2:183–188.

83. Leddy J, Packer JW. Avulsion of the profundus tendon insertion in athletes. J Hand Surg 1977; 2:66.

84. Levine W, Flatow EL. The pathophysiology of shoulder instability. Am J Sports Med 2000; 28:910–917.

85. Linscheid R, Grainger RW, Johnson EW. The thumb metacarpophalangeal joint injuries. Minn Med 1972; 55:1037–1040.

86. Linscheid RL, Beabout JW, Bryan RS. Traumatic instability of the wrist. Diagnosis, classification, and pathomechanics. J Bone Joint Surg Am 1972; 54:1612–1632.

87. Liphart S, Henry TJ. The physiological basis for open and closed kinetic chain rehabilitation for the upper extremity. J Sport Rehabil 1996; 5:71–87.

88. Liphart S, Warner JP, Borsa PA, et al. Proprioception of the shoulder joint in healthy, unstable, and surgically repaired shoulders. J Shoulder Elbow Surg 1994; 3:371–380.

89. Lippitt S, Vanderhooft E, Harris SL, et al. Glenohumeral stability from concavity–compression: a quantitative analysis. J Shoulder Elbow Surg 1993; 2:27–35.

90. Lipscomb P. Stenosing tenosynovitis at the radial styloid process (de Quervain's disease). Am J Surg 1951; 134:110–115.

91. Lohr J, Uhthoff HK. The microvascular pattern of the supraspinatus tendon. Clin Orthop 1990; 254:35.

92. Maffet M, Gartsman GM, Moseley B. Superior labrum–biceps tendon complex lesions of the shoulder. Am J Sports Med 1995; 23:93–98.

93. Magee D. Elbow. In: Magee D, ed. Orthopedic physical assessment. Philadelphia: Saunders; 2006.

94. Magee D. Forearm, wrist, and hand. In: Magee D, ed. Orthopedic physical assessment. Philadelphia: Saunders; 2006.

95. Magee D. Shoulder. In: Magee D, ed. Orthopedic physical assessment. Philadelphia: Saunders; 2006.

96. Manske P, Lesker PA. Avulsion of the ring finger flexor digitorum profundus tendon: an experimental study. Hand Clin 1978; 10:52–55.

97. Mariani E, Cofield RH, Askew LJ, et al. Rupture of the tendon of the long head of the biceps brachii. A surgical versus nonsurgical treatment. Clin Orthop Relat Res 1988; 228:233–239.

98. Mayfield J, Johnson RP, Kilcoyne RK. Carpal dislocations: pathomechanics and progressive perilunar instability. J Hand Surg Am 1980; 5:226–241.

99. Mazzocca A, Sellards R, Garretson R, et al. Injuries to the acromioclavicular joint in adults and children. In: DeLee J, Drez D, Miller MD, eds. Orthopedic sports medicine practices and principles. Philadelphia: Saunders; 2003:912–934.

100. McCluskey GI, Bigliani LU. Surgical management of refractory scapulothoracic bursitis. Orthop Trans 1991; 15:801.

101. McCue F, Bruce JF, Koman JD. Wrist and hand. In: DeLee J, Drez D, Miller MD, eds. Orthopaedic sports medicine principles and practice. Philadelphia: Saunders; 2003:1337–1431.

102. McCue F, Hakala MW, Andrews JR, et al. Ulnar collateral ligament injuries of the thumb in athletes. J Sports Med 1975; 2:70–80.

103. McCue F, Honner R, Johnson ME, et al. Athletic injuries of the proximal interphalangeal joint requiring surgical treatment. J Bone Joint Surg Am 1970; 52:937–956.

104. McEntire J, Hess WE, Coleman S. Rupture of the pectoralis major muscle. J Bone Joint Surg Am 1972; 54:1040–1046.

105. McInerney J, Dias J, Durham S, et al. Randomised controlled trial of single, subacromial injection of methylprednisolone in patients with persistent, post-traumatic impingement of the shoulder. Emerg Med J 2003; 20:218–221.

106. Melone C, Beldner S, Basuk RS. Thumb collateral ligament injuries: an anatomic basis for treatment. Hand Clin 2000; 16:345–357.

107. Meyer A. Chronic functional lesions of the shoulder. Arch Surg 1937; 35:646–674.

108. Milch H, Burman MS. Snapping scapula and humerus varus: report of six cases. Arch Surg 1933; 26:570–588.

109. Milch H. Snapping scapula. Clin Orthop Relat Res 1961; 20:139–150.

110. Miller M, Wirth MA, Rockwood CA Jr. Thawing the frozen shoulder, the 'patient' patient. Orthopedics 1996; 19:849–853.

111. Myers J, Lephart SM. Sensorimotor deficits contributing to glenohumeral instability. Clin Orthop 2002; 400:98–104.

112. Naredo E, Cabero F, Beneyto P, et al. A randomized comparative study of short term response to blind injection versus sonographic-guided injection of local corticosteroids in patients with painful shoulder. J Rheumatol 2004; 31:308–314.

113. Neer C, Foster CR. Fractures of the distal third of the clavicle. Clin Orthop 1968; 58:43–50.

114. Neer CI. Impingement lesions. Clin Orthop 1983; 173:70–77.

115. Neviaser J. Adhesive capsulitis of the shoulder. J Bone Joint Surg Am 1945; 27:211–222.

116. Newcomer K, Laskowski ER, Idank DM, et al. Corticosteroid injection in early treatment of lateral epicondylitis. Clin J Sport Med 2001; 11:214–222.

117. Nirschl R, Petrone FA. Tennis elbow: the surgical treatment of lateral epicondylitis. J Bone Joint Surg Am 1979; 61:832–839.

118. Nirschl R. The etiology and treatment of tennis elbow. Am J Sports Med 1974:2.

119. Norwood L, Shook JA, Andrews JR. Acute medial elbow ruptures. Am J Sports Med 1981; 9:16–19.

120. O'Brien S, Pagnani MJ, Fealy S, et al. The active compression test: a new and effective test for diagnosing labral tears and acromioclavicular joint abnormality. Am J Sports Med 1998; 26:610–613.

121. O'Driscoll S, Morrey BF, An KN. Elbow dislocation and subluxation: a spectrum of instability. Clin Orthop 1992; 280:186–197.

122. Ogden J, Alvarez RG, Levitt R, et al. Shock wave therapy (orthotripsy) in musculoskeletal disorders. Clin Orthop 2001; 387:22–40.

123. Ogilvie-Harris D, Biggs DJ, Fitsialos DP, et al. The resistant frozen shoulder: manipulation vs. arthroscopic release. Clin Orthop 1995; 319:238–248.

124. Olliviere C, Nirschl RP, Pettrone FA. Resection and repair for medial tennis elbow. Am J Sports Med 1995; 23:214–221.

125. Osterman A, Hayken GD, Bora FW. A quantitative evaluation of thumb function after ulnar collateral repair and reconstruction. J Trauma 1981; 21:854–861.

126. Osterman A, Moskow L, Low DW. Soft tissue injuries of the hand and wrist in racquet sports. Clin Sports Med 1988; 7:329–348.

127. Pagnani M, Speer KP, Altchek DW, et al. Arthroscopic fixation of superior labral lesions using a biodegradable implant: a preliminary report. Arthroscopy 1995; 11:194–198.

128. Palmer A, Louis DS. Assessing ulnar instability of the metacarpophalangeal joint of the thumb. J Hand Surg Am 1978; 3:542–546.

129. Palmer A, Werner FW. Biomechanics of the distal radioulnar joint. Clin Orthop 1984; 187:26–35.

130. Palmieri T. Pisiform area pain treatment by pisiform excision. J Hand Surg 1982; 7A:477–480.

131. Panner H. A peculiar affectation of the capitellum humeri resembling Calve–Perthes' disease of the hip. Acta Radiol 1929; 10:234.

132. Parsons T. The snapping scapula and subscapular exostoses. J Bone Joint Surg Br 1973; 55:345–349.

133. Pearsall A, Speer KP. Frozen shoulder syndrome: diagnostic and treatment strategies in the primary care setting. Med Sci Sports Exerc 1998; 30(suppl 4):S33–S39.

134. Percy E, Birbrager D, Pitt MJ. A review of the literature and presentation of 14 patients. Can J Surg 1988; 31:248–250.

135. Perry J. Anatomy and biomechanics of the shoulder in throwing, swimming, gymnastics, and tennis. Clin Sports Med 1983; 2:247–251.

136. Petersen S. Posterior shoulder instability. Orthop Clin North Am 2000; 31:263–283.

137. Postacchini F, Pudda G. Subcutaneous rupture of the distal biceps brachii tendon. J Sports Med Phys Fitness 1975; 15:84–90.

138. Rathbun J, Macnab I. The microvascular pattern of the rotator cuff. J Bone Joint Surg Br 1970; 52:540.

139. Redler I, Williams JT. Rupture of a collateral ligament of the proximal interphalangeal joint of the finger: analysis of 18 cases. J Bone Joint Surg Am 1967; 49:332.

140. Regan W, Wold L, Coonrad R, et al. Microscopic pathology of lateral epicondylitis. Am J Sports Med 1992; 20:746.

141. Rettig A. Athletic injuries of the wrist and hand. Part I: traumatic injuries of the wrist. Am J Sports Med 2003; 31:1038–1048.

142. Rettig A. Athletic injuries of the wrist and hand. Part II: overuse injuries of the wrist and traumatic injuries to the hand. Am J Sports Med 2004; 32:262–273.

143. Richards R, McKee MD. Treatment of painful scapulothoracic crepitus by resection of the superomedial angle of the scapula. Clin Orthop Relat Res 1989; 247:111–116.

144. Roberts P. Dislocations of the elbow. Br J Surg 1969; 56:806–815.

145. Robinson J, Brown PB. Medications in low back pain. Phys Med Rehabil Clin North Am 1991; 2:97–126.

146. Rockwood CJ. Disorders of the sternoclavicular joint. In: Rockwood CJ, Matsen FA, eds. The shoulder. Philadelphia: Saunders; 1990:477–525.

147. Rockwood CJ. Injuries to the acromioclavicular joint. In: Rockwood CJ, ed. Fractures in adults. Philadelphia: Lippincott; 1984:860–910.

148. Rodosky M, Harner CD, Fu FH. The role of the long head of the biceps muscle and superior glenoid labrum in anterior stability of the shoulder. Am J Sports Med 1994; 22:121–130.

149. Rodriguez A. Injuries to the collateral ligaments of the proximal interphalangeal joints. Hand Clin 1973; 55:55.

150. Rowe C, Pierce DS, Clark JG. Voluntary dislocation of the shoulder: a preliminary report on a clinical, electromyographic and psychiatric study of twenty-six patients. J Bone Joint Surg 1973; 62A:897–908.

151. Rowland S. Acute traumatic subluxation of the extensor carpi ulnaris tendon at the wrist. J Hand Surg 1986; 11A:809.

152. Runeson L, Haker E. Iontophoresis with cortisone in the treatment of lateral epicondylalgia (tennis elbow)—a double blind study. Scand J Med Sci Sports 2002; 12:136–142.

153. Sanders T, Morrison WB, Miller MD. Imaging techniques for the evaluation of glenohumeral instability. Am J Sports Med 2000; 28:414–433.

154. Schwartz M, Al-Zahrani SA. Diagnostic imaging of elbow injuries in the throwing athlete. Oper Tech Sports Med 1996; 4:84–90.

155. Simonet W, Cofield R. Prognosis in anterior shoulder dislocation. Am J Sports Med 1984; 12:19.

156. Slawski D, Cahill B. Atraumatic osteolysis of the distal clavicle: results of open surgical excision. Am J Sports Med 1994; 22:267–271.

157. Smith R. Post-traumatic instability of the metacarpophalangeal joint of the thumb. J Bone Joint Surg Am 1977; 59:14–21.

158. Snyder S, Karzel RP, Del Pizzo W, et al. SLAP lesions of the shoulder. Arthroscopy 1990; 6:274–279.

159. Sollender J, Rayan GM, Barden GA. Triceps tendon rupture in weight lifters. J Shoulder Elbow Surg 1998; 7:151–153.

160. Stahl F. On lunatomalacia (Kienbock's disease), a clinical and roentgenological study, especially on its pathogenesis and the late results of immobilization treatment. Acta Chir Scand (Suppl) 1947; 126:1–133.

161. Stein D, Jazrawi L, Bartolozzi AR. Arthroscopic stabilization of anterior shoulder instability: a review of the literature. Arthroscopy 2002; 18:912–924.

162. Stener B. Displacement of the ruptured ulnar collateral ligament of the metacarpophalangeal joint of the thumb. J Bone Joint Surg Br 1962; 44:869–879.

163. Svernlov B, Adolfsson L. Non-operative treatment regime including eccentric training for lateral humeral epicondylalgia. Scand J Med Sci Sports 2001; 11:328–334.

164. Tiger E, Mayer DP, Glazer R. Complete avulsion of the triceps tendon: MRI diagnosis. Comput Med Imaging Graph 1993; 17:51–54.

165. Timmerman L, Andrews JR. The histologic and arthroscopic anatomy of the ulnar collateral ligament of the elbow. Am J Sports Med 1994; 22:667–673.

166. Timmerman L, Andrews JR. Undersurface tear of the ulnar collateral ligament in baseball players: a newly described lesion. Am J Sports Med 1994; 22:33–36.

167. Timmerman L, McBride DG. Elbow dislocations in sports. Sports Med Arthrosc Rev 1995; 3:210–218.

168. Twinning R, Marcus WY, Garey JL. Tendon ruptures in systemic lupus erythematosus. J Am Med Assoc 1964; 187:123–124.

169. Walch G, Liotard JP, Boileau P, et al. Postero-superior glenoid impingement. Another impingement of the shoulder. J Radiol 1993; 74:47–50.

170. Warren R, Kay NR, Norris SH. The microvascular anatomy of the distal digital extensor tendon. J Hand Surg Br 1988; 13:161–163.

171. Weiler J. Medical modifiers of sports injury. The use of nonsteroidal anti-inflammatory drugs (NSAIDs) in sports soft-tissue injury. Clin Sports Med 1992; 11:625–644.

172. Werner C. Lateral elbow pain and posterior interosseous nerve entrapment. Acta Orthop Scand Suppl 1979; 174:1–62.

173. Wilson F, Andrews JR, Blackburn TA, et al. Valgus extension overload in the pitching elbow. Am J Sports Med 1983; 11:83–88.

174. Windsor R, Lester JP, Herring SA. Electrical stimulation in clinical practice. Phys Sports Med 1993; 21:85.

175. Wirth M, Rockwood CA Jr. Injuries to the sternoclavicular joint in the adult and child. In: DeLee J, Drez D, Miller MD, eds. Orthopedic sports medicine. Philadelphia: Saunders; 2003:934–958.

176. Wood M, Dobyns J. Sports-related extra-articular wrist syndromes. Clin Orthop 1986; 202:93–102.

Chapter

40

Musculoskeletal Disorders of the Lower Limb

Pamela A. Hansen and Stuart E. Willick

This chapter reviews musculoskeletal disorders of the lower limb, including soft tissue, bone, and joint pathology. The chapter is organized by anatomic region within diagnostic categories. Although the authors acknowledge that this organizational scheme is arbitrary, it was chosen to decrease redundancy in describing certain conditions that can occur in multiple anatomic locations, such as osteoarthritis or stress fractures. The authors also acknowledge that space does not permit a comprehensive discussion of all musculoskeletal disorders of the lower limbs. The conditions of primary interest to the practitioner of musculoskeletal and sports medicine are covered in greater detail.

The first section of this chapter discusses disorders of muscle and tendon groups in the lower limb, with a special focus on kinetic chain considerations. The second section of the chapter reviews disorders of the joints of the lower limbs. The final section discusses the spectrum of bone overload conditions.

Over the past decade, a new lexicon has evolved among practitioners of musculoskeletal rehabilitation. There are several terms that are used throughout the chapter that might not be familiar to all readers. For the sake of clarity, we would like to first define some of these terms.

First and foremost, the term *kinetic chain* refers to the model of human motion that analyzes and treats dysfunction along connected anatomic regions, rather than focusing only on the location of pain. This model recognizes that dysfunction in one anatomic region can cause dysfunction in other anatomic regions that are linked to the first region during motion. Treatment plans that address only the painful site, and ignore underlying pathology at other sites along the motion chain, have less chance of success than a treatment plan that restores proper function along the entire chain. Kinetic chain considerations are most relevant when discussing muscle and tendon pathology, but should not be ignored when addressing bone and joint pathology.

The term *biomechanical deficits* refers to any deficiencies in range of motion, flexibility, strength, endurance, or motor control. The term *muscle imbalance* refers to the divergence from normal function of different muscle groups that work as agonists or antagonists to stabilize a body part or create motion. Muscle imbalances often occur between muscles on the anterior versus posterior side of a joint, such as the hip flexors versus the hip extensors, or the medial versus lateral side of a joint,

such as hip adductors versus hip abductors. Recent literature has suggested that these types of muscle imbalances predispose to injury.[31,68,137]

The term *functional exercise* refers to exercise movements that stimulate muscle groups to work in a way that they normally work during functional or athletic activities. Functional exercise is distinguished from more conventional types of exercise that tend to isolate muscle groups, rather than have various muscle groups within a kinetic chain working together. For example, a previously accepted method to strengthen the peroneal muscles after a lateral ankle sprain was to have the patient evert the foot against the resistance of a Theraband. While this method is effective in strengthening the peroneal muscles, it is not a motion that people normally perform during everyday activities or athletic activities. A more sophisticated and functional ankle rehabilitation exercise program might have the patient standing on the affected leg while performing movements with the other leg, or standing on the affected leg while performing movements with the upper limbs and torso in patterns that the body uses during real life activities. 'Sport-specific' exercises are functional exercises that use motion patterns that athletes must perform in their athletic events. Finally, the terms *tendonitis* and *tendinosis*, while sometimes used interchangeably, more correctly refer to acute and chronic overload conditions of tendons, respectively.[76,104]

DISORDERS OF MUSCLE–TENDON GROUPS OF THE LOWER LIMB

Disorders of the iliotibial band, including trochanteric bursitis

The iliotibial band (ITB) is a strong fascial band that runs along the lateral aspect of the thigh from the level of the greater trochanter to the proximal, anterolateral tibia (Fig. 40-1). ITB motion is controlled proximally primarily by the gluteus maximus and tensor fascia lata, the two muscles that insert into it. The ITB inserts distally on to a bony prominence at the proximal, anterolateral tibia called Gerdy's tubercle. The ITB can therefore exert forces at the hip and at the knee. Conversely, alterations in various lower limb mechanics, such as genu valgum, pes planus, and tibial internal or external rotation, can affect ITB function. There are three clinically important bursae related to the ITB.[108] The proximal bursa is positioned

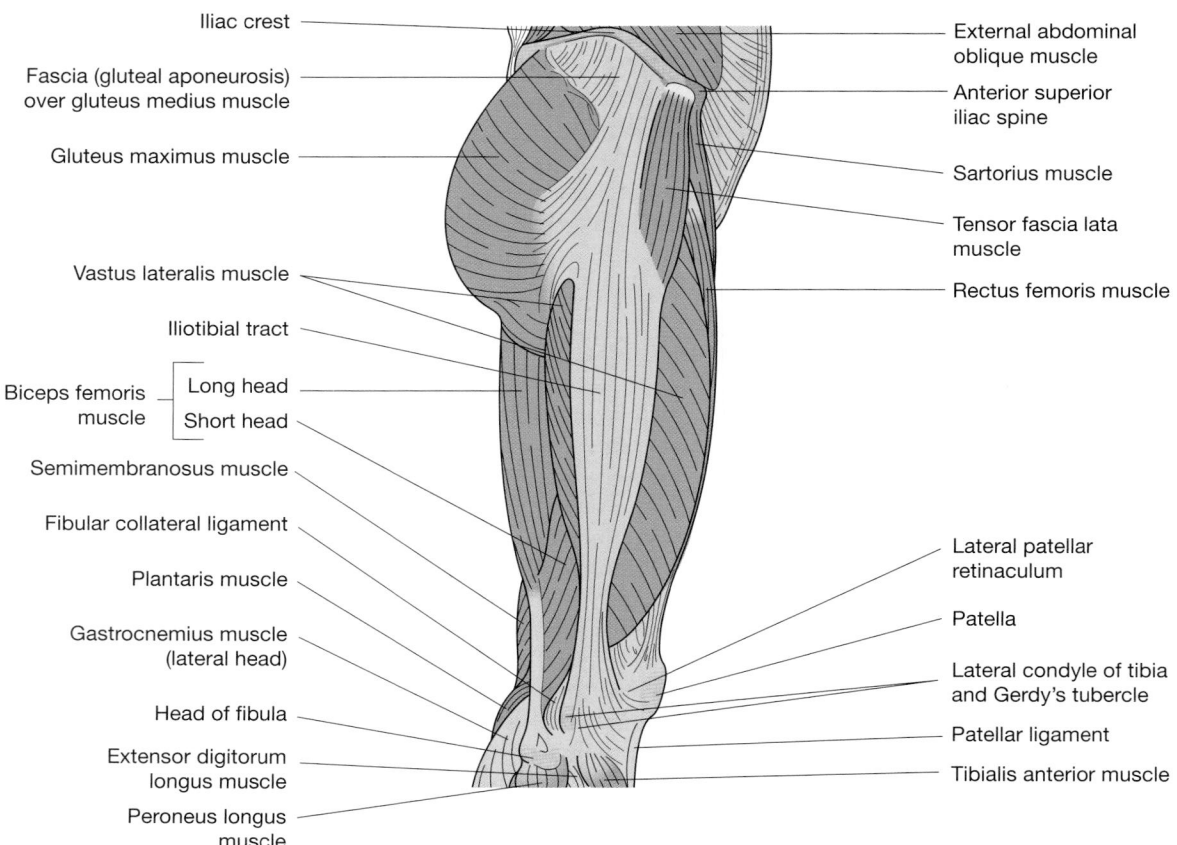

Iliac crest

Fascia (gluteal aponeurosis) over gluteus medius muscle

Gluteus maximus muscle

Vastus lateralis muscle

Iliotibial tract

Biceps femoris muscle — Long head / Short head

Semimembranosus muscle

Fibular collateral ligament

Plantaris muscle

Gastrocnemius muscle (lateral head)

Head of fibula

Extensor digitorum longus muscle

Peroneus longus muscle

External abdominal oblique muscle

Anterior superior iliac spine

Sartorius muscle

Tensor fascia lata muscle

Rectus femoris muscle

Lateral patellar retinaculum

Patella

Lateral condyle of tibia and Gerdy's tubercle

Patellar ligament

Tibialis anterior muscle

Figure 40-1 The iliotibial band is a strong fascial band that runs from the lateral hip to the lateral knee.

to decrease friction between the ITB and the greater trochanter of the femur. Another site of potential friction is where the ITB runs over the lateral epicondyle of the femur.[18] The third lies at the ITB's distal attachment on the tibia.

While a bursa can become inflamed from direct trauma, it is far more common for a bursa to become gradually inflamed due to improper training techniques or abnormal biomechanics. In these cases, the bursal inflammation is not a primary process, but rather secondary to muscle imbalance around the hip girdle or other abnormalities along the kinetic chain. The purpose of a bursa is to allow for low-friction gliding of soft tissues over a bony prominence. Any imbalance or dysfunction of the hip muscles can result in abnormal ITB motion and trochanteric bursitis. Patients with trochanteric bursitis can usually localize pain to the lateral hip. The pain is sometimes felt along the path of the ITB in the lateral thigh. On examination, there is tenderness to palpation directly over the greater trochanter or immediately posterior to it. There is often weakness of the gluteus medius[41] and the hip external rotators, which can be detected with manual resistance testing. A typical hip girdle muscle imbalance seen in the setting of trochanteric bursitis includes tensor fascia lata tightness and gluteus maximus inhibition or weakness. The modified Thomas test is an excellent physical examination maneuver to assess for inflexibility around the hip girdle. One should always check the function of the deep hip

external rotators as well as muscle function along the entire kinetic chain, from the core region to the ankle. The function of the hip external rotators can be tested statically and dynamically. In runners and cyclists with ITB symptoms, it is important to perform a biomechanical assessment while the patient is running or riding. Occasionally, an audible snap can be heard as the ITB rubs over the greater trochanter. This is sometimes referred to as lateral snapping hip syndrome. This condition is contrasted with the so-called internal snapping hip syndrome, in which a deeper, more medial snap is appreciated by the patient.[52] Internal snapping hip is felt to be due to the iliopsoas tendon rubbing over the iliopectineal eminence or the femoral head. The same kinetic chain abnormalities that can cause ITB pain at the lateral hip can also cause pain and tenderness where the ITB passes over the lateral epicondyle of the femur, or at its insertion on to Gerdy's tubercle. Symptoms are exacerbated by repetitive activities such as running or cycling.

Regardless of the location of symptoms related to ITB dysfunction, the treatment principles remain the same. The patient should reduce or eliminate the exacerbating activities. Ice is helpful for reducing pain and inflammation, and for facilitating a stretching program. The exercise prescription should be based on the patient's relevant biomechanical deficits, which are determined by the office examination and a functional examination of the patient while she or he is participating in activities.

Providing standardized exercise handouts or prescribing non-specific rehabilitation protocols can result in non-specific patient outcomes. One common example of prescribing non-specific exercises for an ITB problem is to prescribe ITB stretches, when the primary deficit is hip abductor weakness. Another common mistake is to focus on hip abductor strengthening if the most relevant biomechanical deficit is impaired eccentric control of the hip external rotators. Because all the hip girdle muscles originate on the pelvis, the core musculature must be able to adequately stabilize the pelvis in order for the hip girdle muscles to perform their functions during dynamic activities. Other interventions, such as ITB massage and myofascial release, ultrasound, and local injection of corticosteroid may facilitate the patient's rehabilitation program. Off the shelf and custom-made foot orthoses can be helpful in reducing impact and improving subtalar positioning and tibial rotation. If errors in training technique are felt to have contributed to the onset of symptoms, then appropriate training regimens should be discussed with the patient.

Disorders of the hamstring muscle group

Strains of the thigh muscles are common in individuals participating in ballistic activities. The most commonly strained muscle group in the thigh is the hamstring group. The hamstring group includes semimembranosus, semitendinosus, and short and long heads of the biceps femoris. Hamstring strains most commonly occur with forceful eccentric contraction of the hamstring muscles, especially when the muscle is at a mechanical disadvantage near full flexion or full extension (Fig. 40-2). The patient will usually be able to describe an appropriate, acute overload mechanism. On examination, hamstring pain can

be reproduced by passive stretch of the muscle, by resistance testing of the muscle, and by direct palpation of the injured area. The strain can occur near the hamstring origin at the ischial tuberosity, in the belly of the muscle, or in the region of the distal musculotendinous junction. Severe hamstring strains will produce visible ecchymosis at and distal to the site of injury. A large muscle tear might produce a palpable defect. Imaging is usually not necessary to establish the diagnosis. If needed, magnetic resonance imaging (MRI) is the imaging modality of choice.[75,131,144] Acute treatment consists of relative rest, ice, early gentle range of motion exercises, and gently progressive strengthening exercises as tolerated. Exercises should be progressed to higher weight and include more ballistic and sport-specific movements when tolerated. It is not uncommon for an acute hamstring strain to keep an individual from their usual athletic activities for 6 weeks or more.

With proximal hamstring injuries, occasionally the bone fails before the muscle or tendon fails, resulting in an ischial avulsion injury. The most common age group for ischial avulsion fractures is 15–25 years of age.[22,145] The most common activities that cause ischial avulsion fractures include gymnastics, hurdling, and dance. The patient can usually describe sudden onset of pain at the ischial tuberosity after a forceful movement involving hamstring contraction, while the muscle was at maximum length with full hip flexion and knee extension. On physical examination, there is typically point tenderness at the ischial tuberosity, pain with passive hamstring stretch, and pain with knee flexion or hip extension against resistance. Plain films are usually adequate to visualize the avulsion (Fig. 40-3). These fractures usually do not need surgery and can be treated similar to other hamstring injuries, although the period of relative rest

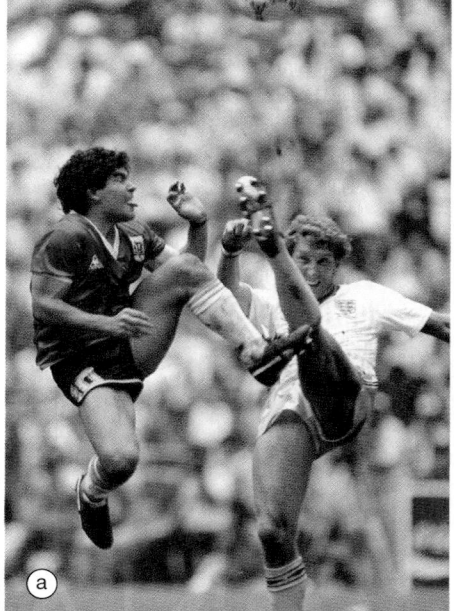
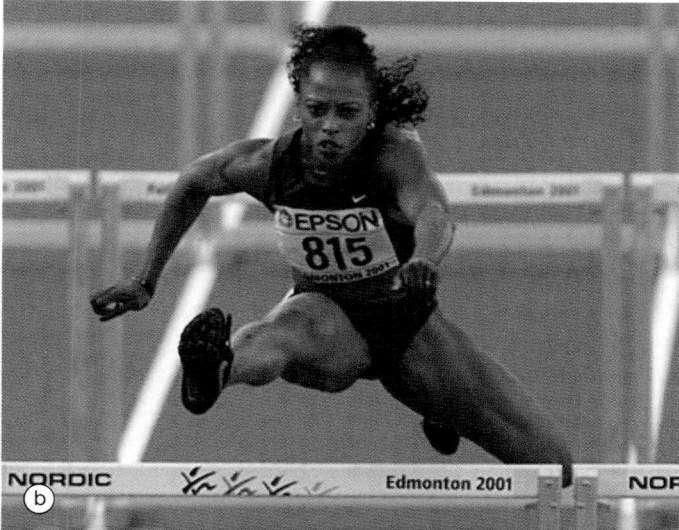

Figure 40-2 The primary function of the hamstring muscle group is to slow down knee extension during open kinetic chain movements. This muscle group is at risk for acute overload during ballistic activities.

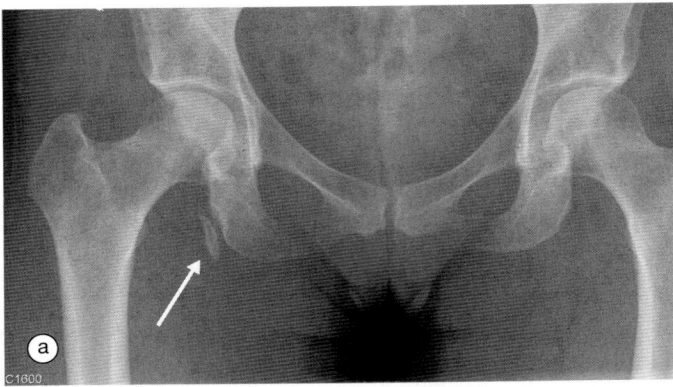

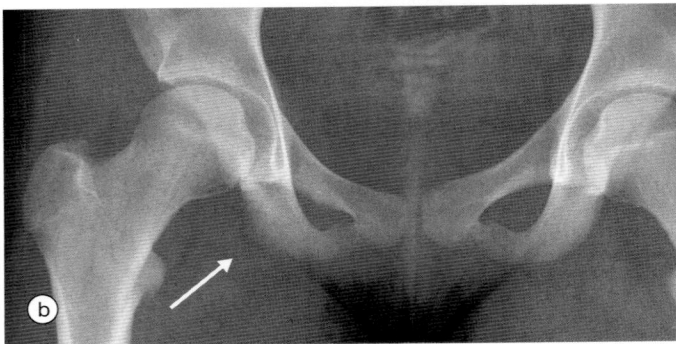

Figure 40-3 Examples of ischial avulsion fractures. (**a**) Anteroposterior x-ray of the pelvis, showing an old ischial avulsion fracture. The patient was a 17-year-old female cheerleader who had sudden onset of buttock pain with a high-kicking maneuver 9 months prior to presentation. (**b**) Anteroposterior x-ray of the pelvis, showing irregularity of the right ischial tuberosity. The patient was a 14-year-old cheerleader with acute onset of right buttock pain after a high-kicking maneuver. In both cases, symptoms resolved completely after a period of relative rest followed by progressive rehabilitation.

might be longer to allow for bone healing. If initial symptoms are severe enough to prevent comfortable ambulation, crutches can be used for a few days. Ice should be applied frequently over the first few days to decrease pain and swelling. Anti-inflammatory medication can be taken for the same reasons. Although surgical intervention is rarely needed, orthopedic consultation should be obtained if the avulsion fragment is displaced greater than 2 cm, or if resolution of symptoms does not occur in the expected time period. As pain decreases over the first 1–2 weeks, slowly progressive hamstring stretching and strengthening should be started. The rehabilitation program must be undertaken very cautiously during first several weeks to avoid further displacement of the avulsion. There is no predetermined amount of time, however, that one should wait prior to starting a stretching and strengthening program for the hamstring muscle group after this injury.[15,27,139] A general guideline is that the patient should experience no discomfort or only mild discomfort with the rehabilitation program.

In older (skeletally mature) individuals, the proximal hamstring tendon might avulse, because in these individuals the weakest link is the tendon rather than the bone. The mechanism of injury is the same as described above. In high-demand athletes, surgical reattachment is usually indicated, and although

late repair is feasible, early identification and surgical intervention usually produce the best outcomes.[139]

Hamstring muscle disorders can also have an insidious onset. Hamstring tendonopathy can occur at the ischial tuberosity or distally in the medial or lateral hamstring tendons. In addition to pain with activities, a careful history often reveals a change in the patient's activity level, such as a recent rapid increase in running. The physical examination findings are similar to, but usually less dramatic than, those seen with an acute hamstring strain. In addition to the usual rehabilitation protocols such as relative rest, ice, non-steroidal antiinflammatory drugs (NSAIDs), and hamstring stretching and strengthening, one should try to identify and correct errors in training technique, running gait, cycling or jumping mechanics, and relevant biomechanical deficits. Eccentric training of the hamstring group helps the muscle to absorb more loading force, and restoring as much balance as possible to the quadriceps–hamstring force couple is also important. A local injection of steroid in the region of the ischial bursa might help facilitate the active exercise program during rehabilitation, but potential side effects need to be kept in mind.

Disorders of the adductor muscle group

The adductor muscle group consists of adductor magnus, adductor longus, adductor brevis, sartorius, gracilis, and pectineus. As with other muscle or tendon injuries, strains of the hip adductor muscles usually occur with forceful activation of the muscles, especially when in a lengthened position. Adductor strains can be due to acute or repetitive overload. These injuries can occur in anyone, but are particular common in those involved in soccer, hockey, and skiing.[33,142] Strains of the adductor group most commonly occur at or near their origin off the inferior pubic ramus. Intramuscular strains also occur. The adductor longus is the most commonly involved.[91,103] Isolated sartorius muscle strains can also occur. A sudden, forceful contraction of sartorius can result in an avulsion fracture at the muscle's proximal attachment at the anterior superior iliac spine (ASIS). This injury is treated similarly to other acute tendon strains, although a longer period of relative rest might be required prior to progressing the patient to stretching and strengthening exercises.

The physical examination is most notable for reproduction of the patient's pain with passive stretch and active resistance testing of the adductor group. Radiographs are not needed to establish a diagnosis of adductor strain, but are useful when looking for bone injuries such as avulsion factures. If needed, MRI can frequently show signal change in the area of injury (Fig. 40-4). Treatment includes early, gradually progressive range of motion exercises and careful strengthening exercises, with return to sport-specific exercises when tolerated. If the rehabilitation program is performed too aggressively in the early stages, there is a risk of further injury. While the rehabilitation program focuses on the adductor muscle group, one needs to address the entire kinetic chain and the hip adductor–abductor force couple in order to decrease the chance of recurrent injury. Because the adductors arise from the pelvis, the pelvis must be stabilized with a core exercise program. The rehabilitation

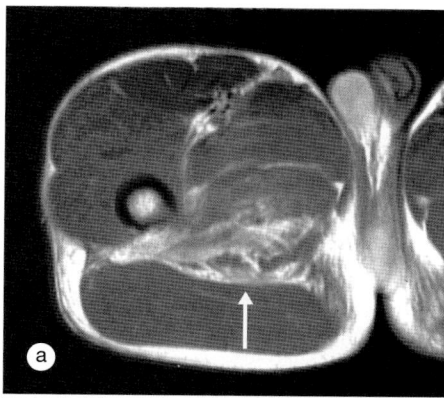

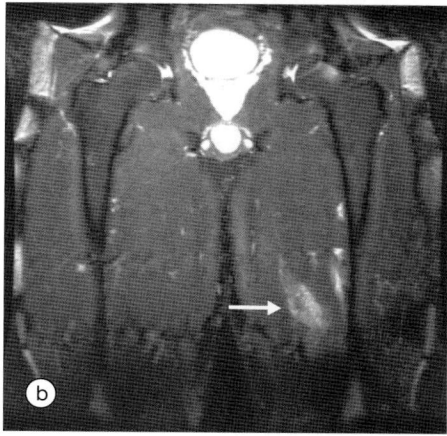

Figure 40-4 Examples of adductor strains. (**a**) T2-weighted axial magnetic resonance imaging (MRI) of the proximal thigh, showing a hemorrhagic tear in the proximal adductor muscle group. The patient was an Olympic hockey player who got checked from the right side while the right leg was in an abducted position. (**b**) T2-weighted coronal MRI of the thighs, showing a more distal, less severe strain of the left adductor muscle group than that seen in (a). This patient was also a hockey player.

program should also seek to maximize flexibility, strength, motor control, and endurance of the hip flexors, hamstrings, hip abductors, and hip extensors. One should check for and correct tightness of the ITB, which if present can inhibit strengthening of the adductors.

Combined muscle group injuries
Pes anserine tendonitis or bursitis
One hamstring muscle (semitendinosus) and two adductor muscles (sartorius and gracilis) course together along the medial aspect of the knee to insert on the proximal, anteromedial tibia (Fig. 40-5). The anatomist who coined the name *pes anserinus* thought that the insertion of these three tendons looked like a goose's foot. Acute inflammation of one or more of these three tendons near their insertion is called pes anserine tendonitis. Subacute or chronic irritation of one or more of these tendons near their tibial attachment is called pes anserine tendinosis. Inflammation of the bursa that lies just under the tendons near their insertion is termed pes anserine bursitis. Clinical differentiation between these conditions is difficult or impossible.

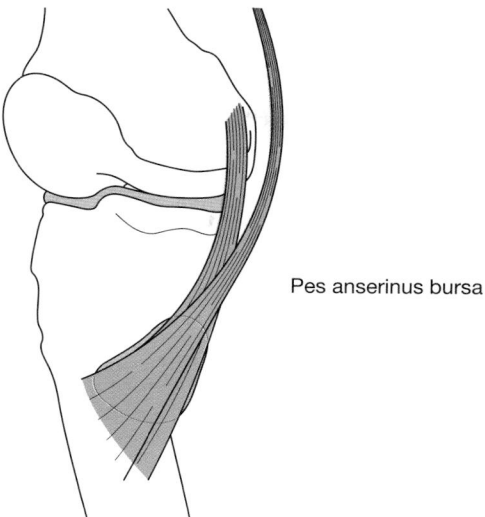

Pes anserinus bursa

Figure 40-5 The semitendinosus, sartorius, and gracilis tendons form a conjoined tendon on the anteromedial aspect of the proximal tibia referred to as the pes anserinus.

Bursal pathology is usually secondary to dysfunction of the overlying tendons. The patient typically complains of pain in the region of the pes anserine insertion. The patient might sometimes provide a history of a sudden increase in activity level. On palpation, there is usually local tenderness at the pes anserine insertion. Common biomechanical deficits that are associated with this condition include a weak core, weak medial hamstrings, and weak hip adductors. Initial treatment includes ice and NSAIDS to decrease pain and swelling. While the rehabilitation program focuses on maximizing flexibility, strength, endurance, and motor control of the pes anserine muscles, the entire kinetic chain must be addressed. Core control should be maximized to allow for proper hamstring and hip adductor function. Anterior to posterior and medial to lateral muscle imbalances should be identified and rehabilitated. Impaired subtalar motion and abnormal tibial rotation should also be addressed. In runners and cyclists, running gait and cycling mechanics need to be observed, and modified if necessary. Running shoes and inserts need to be appropriate for each individual's biomechanical characteristics. Imaging is usually not indicated unless there is suspicion for stress fracture or intraarticular pathology, such as an injury to the meniscus. Underlying bone and joint injuries can sometimes cause secondary dysfunction of the pes anserine tendons. A local steroid injection can help facilitate the active exercise program at times.

Athletic pubalgia and sportsman's hernia
Athletic pubalgia and sportsman's hernia refer to a spectrum of disorders that cause pain in the lower abdomen and groin. Pain generators can include overload of one or more of the lower abdominal muscles near the superior pubic ramus, a strain of the hip flexors and/or hip adductors, stress response or stress fracture of the pubic rami, and pubic symphysitis

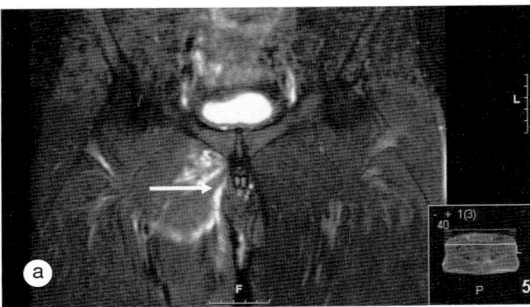
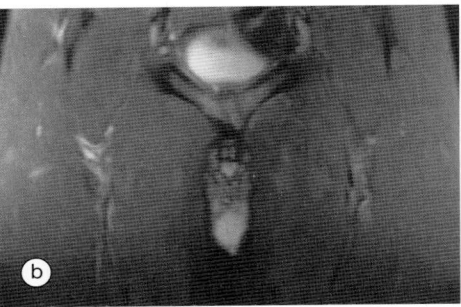
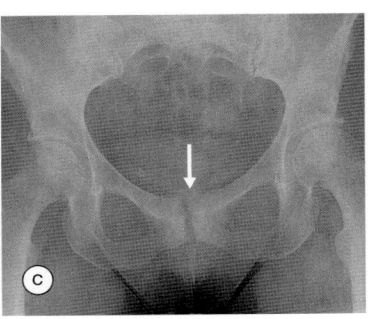

Figure 40-6 Examples of the spectrum of conditions seen in athletic pubalgia. (**a**) T2-weighted, short tau, inversion recovery, coronal magnetic resonance imaging (MRI) of a college football place kicker, showing a hemorrhagic tear of the right hip adductor muscles off the pubic ramus. (**b**) T2-weighted, fat suppression, coronal MRI of the pelvis of a collegiate pole vaulter, showing increased signal intensity of both pubic rami and the pubic symphysis, consistent with stress responses of the superior pubic rami and pubic symphysitis. (**c**) Anteroposterior x-ray of the pelvis, showing irregularity, subchondral cyst formation, and subchondral sclerosis of the symphysis pubis, consistent with symphysitis. The patient was a 22-year-old soccer player with chronic, bilateral groin pain.

(Fig. 40-6).[8,42,43,65,84] A defect in the fascia of the lower, anterior abdominal wall has also been described. Overload injury in this region is most commonly seen in football, soccer, and hockey.[7,32,42,50,77,92] There can be a delay in accurate diagnosis, and rehabilitation is often incomplete. Because symptoms of athletic pubalgia can easily become chronic, it is imperative to establish an accurate and complete diagnosis and to institute comprehensive rehabilitation as early as possible. Maximizing core stability and restoring full range of motion, strength, endurance, and motor control of the core muscles, hip flexors, and adductors are keys to successful rehabilitation. Functional exercises to work these muscle groups should be started as soon as the patient is able to tolerate them. Surgical consultation should be considered if there is a suspicion for a fascial defect of the anterior abdominal wall or a true inguinal hernia.[130] Impact or repetitive loading activities should be avoided in the setting of bone overload, such as pelvic stress response or stress fracture.

Injuries to the quadriceps muscle group
Patellar tendonopathy

A common term for patella tendinopathy is jumper's knee. Symptoms of patella tendon overload most commonly start insidiously. When the patient is able to localize a point of maximal pain, it is usually at the inferior pole of the patella. The pain, however, can occur anywhere along the course of the tendon. Individuals at risk for patella tendon overload include those who participate in repetitive knee flexion and extension activities, such as basketball players, volleyball players, bicyclists, rowers, and mogul skiers.[59] The diagnosis is usually made primarily by history. Patients might or might not have tenderness along the course of the tendon. The examiner should look for biomechanical deficits that can lead to unequal distribution of forces along the links in the kinetic chain that are most involved with jumping. For example, the knee extensor mechanism can become overloaded during repetitive flexion and extension if more proximal muscle groups, such as the lumbar and hip extensors, are not adequately activating. Distally, the

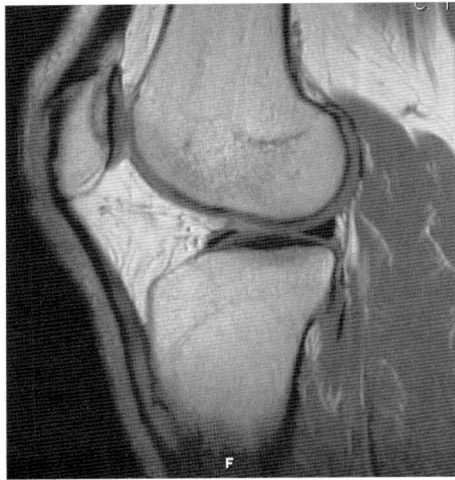

Figure 40-7 T1-weighted sagittal magnetic resonance imaging of the knee, showing extensive signal change within the distal patellar tendon, consistent with patellar tendonosis. The patient was a 37-year-old ultramarathoner whose symptoms failed to improve with cessation of running, appropriate physical therapy, various non-steroidal antiinflammatory drugs, and modalities including extracorporeal shock wave treatment. He ultimately underwent surgical debridement of the tendon and was able to return to running 6 months later.

knee extensor mechanism can be placed at a biomechanical disadvantage if the individual lacks adequate ankle dorsiflexion, which is a necessary motion for squatting. Ankle dorsiflexion is also necessary for maximal activation of the calf muscles, which assist the quadriceps in jumping and eccentrically controlling the landing motion. The muscle groups involved in the jumping motion should be evaluated for their eccentric as well as concentric function, because both types of muscle action are involved in jumping and landing. Imaging is usually not necessary to make the diagnosis. For refractory cases, or when the clinical diagnosis is in question, MRI and ultrasound both provide adequate visualization of the tendon (Fig. 40-7).

Treatments include ice, NSAIDs, cross-friction massage, modalities, quadriceps stretching, and strengthening exercises, and addressing relevant biomechanical deficits. Some patients gain symptomatic relief from a patellar tendon or 'Chopat' strap. Identifying and correcting errors in training technique can prevent recurrence. For longstanding, refractory cases that will not respond to an appropriate rehabilitation program, surgical debridement of the tendon might be of benefit.

Osgood–Schlatter disease and Sinding–Larsen–Johansson disease

When a young adolescent presents with pain at the tibial tuberosity that is exacerbated with activities and direct contact, Osgood–Schlatter disease should be considered. The underlying cause of this relatively common condition is not clear, but repetitive overload at the patella tendon insertion can cause inflammation, irregularity, and/or partial avulsions of the secondary ossification center of the tibial tuberosity. Clinically, the diagnosis is made when there is significant pain and tenderness at the tibial tubercle. The radiographic hallmark of Osgood–Schlatter disease is irregularity and fragmentation of the tibial tuberosity (Fig. 40-8). Although far less common then Osgood–Schlatter disease, similar findings can be seen at the origin of the patella tendon at the inferior pole of the patella, in which case the condition is called Sinding–Larsen–Johansson disease. For both conditions, the mainstays of treatment include ice, NSAIDs, gently progressive quadriceps stretching, careful pain-free quadriceps strengthening, and activity modification. Activity modification is sometimes the most difficult part of the treatment regimen, because the individuals who suffer from these conditions are usually very active adolescents. Realistically, activity modification can mean encouraging the patient to participate in one sport per season rather than two or three. Symptoms might be intermittent or persistent until the growth plates close, at which point symptoms usually resolve spontaneously.

Quadriceps strains, and quadriceps and patella tendon rupture

Forceful quadriceps contraction with the foot planted can cause injury to the quadriceps muscle itself or failure of either the quadriceps or patella tendon (Fig. 40-9).[59] The patient can usually describe an appropriate mechanism of injury, and might describe a sense of having an unstable knee. On examination, there is anterior knee swelling and a palpable defect just proximal or just distal to the patella. The patient will be unable to extend the knee. When asked to do so, the patella will not move if there is a quadriceps tendon rupture, but will elevate without causing knee extension with a patella tendon rupture. A careful musculoskeletal and neurovascular examination should be performed to assess for associated injuries such as anterior cruciate ligament (ACL) tear and femoral neuropathy. A patient with an acute quadriceps or patella tendon rupture should be placed in a knee immobilizer and made non–weight bearing with crutches. Rupture of the quadriceps or patella tendons requires surgical repair within a few days for optimal results.

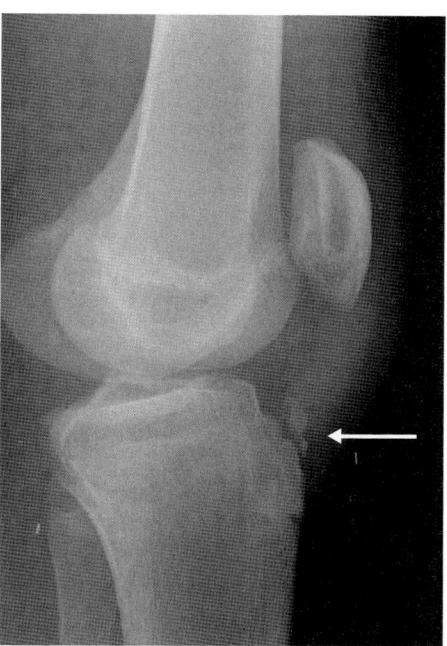

Figure 40-8 Lateral x-ray of the knee, showing the typical appearance of Osgood–Schlatter disease. There is irregularity and fragmentation of the tibial tuberosity. The patient was a 16-year-old wrestler with a 3-month history of increasing anterior knee pain. His other knee and his brother's knees all had a similar radiographic appearance.

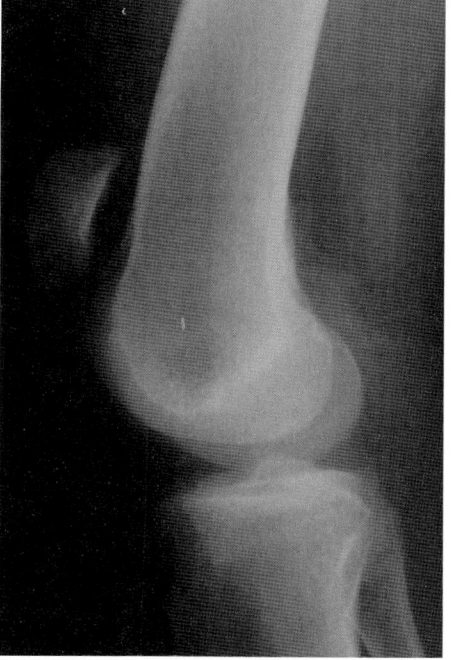

Figure 40-9 Lateral x-ray of the knee, showing an abnormally high-riding patella after an acute patella tendon rupture. The patient was a 40-year-old airline pilot who described 'landing a little aft of center' while alpine skiing. A sudden forceful quadriceps contraction while attempting to regain balance resulted in this injury.

Rectus femoris avulsion from the AIIS

A forceful contraction of rectus femoris can result in an avulsion fracture of the anterior inferior iliac spine. This diagnosis is distinguished from a simple muscle strain by radiographs, but treatment follows the same rehabilitation guidelines, with ice, relative rest, and gently progressive stretching and strengthening exercises when tolerated. Surgery is indicated only for dramatically displaced avulsion fragments, which are uncommon.[96,97]

Quadriceps contusions and myositis ossificans

Contusions of the quadriceps muscle group due to a direct and forceful blow to the area are fairly common (Fig. 40-10). The patient can usually provide a history of direct trauma to the front of the thigh. The patient typically reports pain at the site of the injury, and might report stiffness and difficulty with weight bearing. An antalgic gait is usually noted, along with tenderness, ecchymosis, and swelling in the anterior thigh. Knee flexion can be severely restricted. Extension is often preserved. Radiographs should be obtained to look for an underlying femur fracture. Ice should be applied aggressively to decrease swelling and pain. Early range of motion should be started as soon as it is tolerated in order to decrease muscle stiffness, which invariably ensues. Some practitioners advocate immobilizing the knee in flexion for a few days to decrease contracture of the quadriceps muscle.[58]

Following a severe quadriceps contusion, the intramuscular hematoma can undergo calcific transformation, resulting in myositis ossificans.[11,12,28] Myositis ossificans occurs in up to 10–20% of all thigh contusions, and the quadriceps is the most common location for myositis ossificans to occur.[70] Aspirin and standard antiinflammatory medications should be avoided in the first few days, because of the theoretically increased risk of promoting additional bleeding into the injury site. Cyclooxygenase-2 inhibitors, which do not interfere with platelet function, can be used. If pain and stiffness persist or worsen after several weeks of appropriate care, consideration should be given to repeating radiographs and obtaining advanced imaging with a bone scan or MRI to look for calcification in the muscle. Bone scan and MRI are more sensitive in the early stages of myositis ossificans than plain films. If myositis ossificans develops, first-line treatment includes progressive range of motion and medication. Radiation therapy can be tried for recalcitrant symptoms. Surgical resection of the calcified tissue is indicated for unresponsive cases, but should not be undertaken prior to maturation of the mass because of the high risk of recurrence. A cold bone scan provides evidence that osteoblastic activity has ceased.

Patellofemoral arthralgia

As its name implies, the term *patellofemoral arthralgia* refers to pain in the joint between the patella and the femur. Other terms that have been used to refer to this condition include *patellofemoral pain syndrome* and *chondromalacia*. The latter term is discouraged, because it lacks specificity. Patellofemoral arthralgia is the most common cause of knee pain seen in the

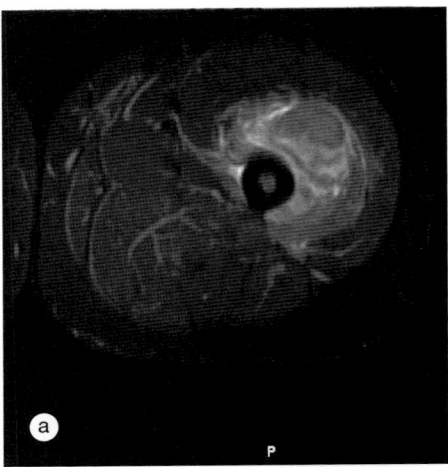

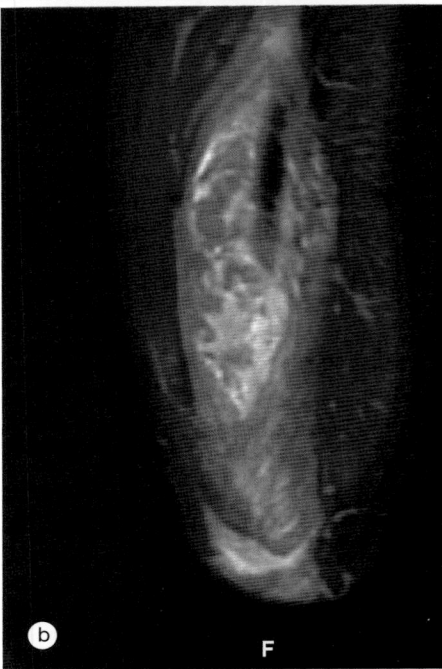

Figure 40-10 Quadriceps contusion. (**a**) T2-weighted axial and (**b**) sagittal magnetic resonance images of the thigh, showing a massive contusion of the vastus intermedius muscle. The patient was a female Olympic hockey player who was struck by the knee of a male player during a scrimmage. The forces were efficiently transferred through the superficial quadriceps muscles, which were spared injury, to the deep quadriceps muscle. With aggressive rehabilitation, the athlete was able to compete during the Olympics and led her team in scoring. She did not develop myositis ossificans, demonstrating the capricious nature of the condition.

younger population. Although patellofemoral pain can arise from an acute traumatic event, such as a fall on to the knee with injury to the bone or subchondral cartilage, it is more commonly gradual in onset. As the knee goes through flexion and extension, the patella normally tracks proximally and distally within the trochlear groove.

Abnormal mechanics along the kinetic chain can cause improper tracking of the patella. There are several typical biomechanical abnormalities that one should look for during a comprehensive assessment. A tight quadriceps muscle can cause the patella to ride high within the trochlear groove, and therefore create abnormal forces on the retropatellar cartilage. A tight ITB, via fibers that attach to the lateral retinaculum of the patella, can cause the patella to track laterally. An ineffective oblique portion of the vastus medialis will not be able to oppose the lateral pulling of a tight ITB. Pes planus is associated with tibial internal rotation, which may position the patella medially within the trochlear groove through the pull of the patella tendon. On the proximal side of the kinetic chain, ineffective eccentric function of the hip external rotators might fail to adequately control femoral internal rotation during running, which can also cause abnormal patellofemoral tracking, and weak hip abductors can place increased load on the ITB.

The patient with patellofemoral arthralgia can usually localize the pain to the anterior knee, or even say that the pain is 'under the kneecap'. At times, one can elicit a history of a recent increase in activity, such as putting in a new floor without using knee pads, or a rapid increase in running. A mainstay of clinical diagnosis is tenderness to palpation under the medial and lateral aspects of the patella. Pain or apprehension with medial–lateral glide and tilt maneuvers of the patella also supports the diagnosis. The functional examination should look for all the biomechanical deficits listed in the previous paragraph. Conditions such as patellar tendonitis that share predisposing biomechanical risk factors can coexist with patellofemoral arthralgia. The differential diagnosis includes infra- or suprapatellar bursitis, synovial plica, quadriceps tendonitis, patellar tendonitis, Sinding–Larson–Johansson disease, and intraarticular pathology such as a meniscus tear.

Initial treatment protocols employ the usual principles of musculoskeletal rehabilitation, including ice, NSAIDs, strengthening weak or imbalanced muscle groups in the core and lower limbs, and stretching tight structures such as the ITB. Activity modification, such as temporarily substituting swimming for running, is important. Many advocate the use of patellofemoral taping techniques to improve patellofemoral tracking and decrease pain. Specific patellofemoral control braces can also decrease pain and improve muscle activation in up to 50% of patients.[118] Two prospective studies have shown that improving quadriceps strength strongly correlates with symptomatic improvement.[63,100] Patellofemoral forces can be minimized during quadriceps strengthening by performing closed kinetic chain strengthening exercises between 0 and 30° of flexion.[135]

Despite the best efforts of the patient and the treatment team, patellofemoral symptoms can become refractory. Although there is not sufficient literature to support their use, consideration should be given for trials of steroid injection, hyaluronate injections, acupuncture, and arthroscopy if a patient fails to respond non-interventional measures. In very carefully selected patients, surgical release of the lateral retinaculum and tightening or reconstruction of the medial patellofemoral ligament can improve patellar positioning within the groove and improve symptoms.

Injuries to the anterior leg muscle group

Tibialis anterior, extensor hallucis longus, and extensor digitorum longus

Overload injuries to these muscles are less common than overload injuries to other muscle–tendon groups of the lower limbs. A common history for overload of tibialis anterior is onset of anterior leg pain following an increase in downhill running. During downhill running, the ankle dorsiflexors can become overloaded as they work eccentrically during and just after heel strike to slow down ankle plantar flexion. Pain can be experienced in the belly of the muscle, at the musculotendinous junction, or at the insertion of tibialis anterior on the anteromedial midfoot. On examination, symptoms are usually reproduced with resisted ankle dorsiflexion. If symptoms are mild, the sensitivity of the examination may be increased if performed after the patient has run to fatigue. Treatment consists of ice, NSAIDs, strengthening the ankle dorsiflexors, stretching the heel cord, and a period of relative rest without running downhill followed by a slower progression of hill running and other activities. The differential diagnosis includes stress fracture and anterior compartment syndrome.

Injuries to the posterior leg muscle group and associated soft tissue structures

Gastrocnemius, soleus, tibialis posterior, flexor hallucis longus, and flexor digitorum longus

Any of the muscles of the deep or superficial compartments of the posterior leg can become acutely or insidiously overloaded.[5] As with other overload injuries, these muscles are more prone to sudden or repetitive eccentric overload. Achilles tendon overload is common, and can be either chronic or acute. In the chronic setting, typical changes of tendinosis can be seen clinically by way of a swollen, nodular, tender Achilles tendon.[62] Although not usually necessary for diagnosis, ultrasound and MRI show typical changes that correspond to microscopic features of breakdown in the normal collagen orientation, vacuole formation, and microscopic tearing (Fig. 40-11). Treatment consists of ice, NSAIDs, activity modification, stretching, and strengthening exercises. Muscle groups along the kinetic chain that work synergistically with the ankle plantar flexors must also be tested and rehabilitated, if indicated. For example, in the running, jumping, and cycling motions, the ankle plantar flexors work synergistically with the knee and hip extensors. Additionally, one must address errors in training technique, such as increasing the volume of running or jumping too rapidly, and technique issues, such as toe running. Toe running can place excessive eccentric demands on the ankle plantar flexors. Eccentric strength training has been shown to be especially effective in the rehabilitation of chronic Achilles tendinopathy.[1]

A sudden, powerful eccentric force can cause an acute rupture of the Achilles tendon. Patients can almost always describe such a mechanism, usually during ballistic sporting activities such as basketball. The event is sometimes accompanied by an audible pop, with inability to continue the activity. Patients commonly relate that they feel as if they were 'kicked

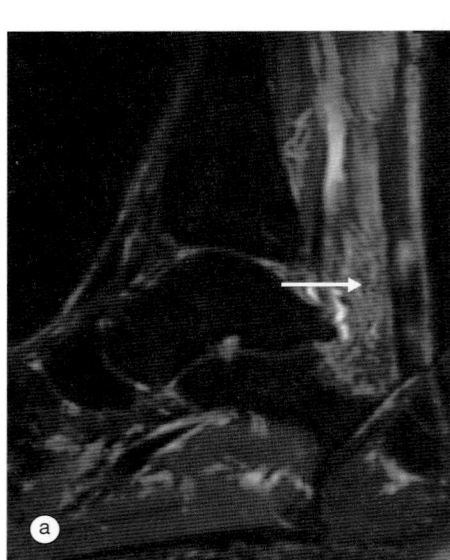 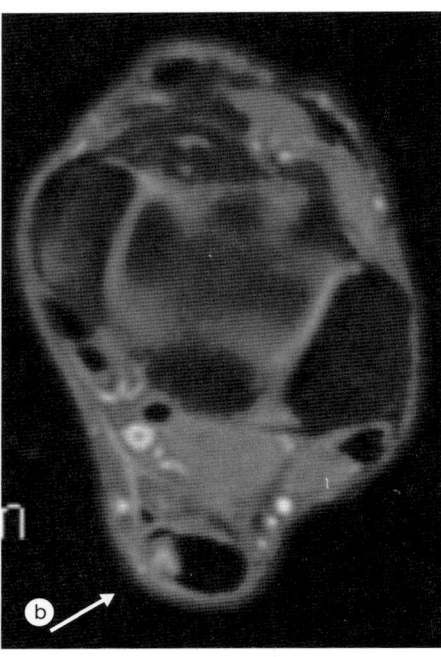

Figure 40-11 Achilles tendonopathy. T2-weighted, fat suppression, sagittal (**a**) and axial (**b**) magnetic resonance imaging of the ankle, showing diffuse thickening and increased signal in the Achilles tendon consistent with Achilles tendonosis. The patient was a 42-year-old ultradistance runner who presented with acute on chronic posterior heel pain.

in the calf'. On examination, there will be swelling in the region of the Achilles tendon, and often the examiner can appreciate a palpable defect in the tendon. The patient typically has difficulty with plantar flexion, although some plantar flexion activity might be provided by the other posterior leg muscles. This compensation limits the sensitivity of Thompson's test, in which the examiner squeezes the calf muscles of the prone patient and looks for passive plantar flexion in response. The treatment of acute Achilles tendon rupture includes surgical reconstruction followed by immobilization and then aggressive rehabilitation, versus immobilization followed by aggressive rehabilitation.[112] The period of immobilization can be as long as 3 months. Which treatment to pursue depends on multiple factors, including the age, health, and activity level of the patient; the presence of a partial versus complete tear; the amount of retraction of the torn ends; and the preference of the patient and practitioner. Although good outcomes have been reported with and without surgery, the incidence of a repeat Achilles tendon rupture is lower following surgical reconstruction.[8,74,102,105,147]

Sever's disease

Sever's disease is a traction apophysitis of the Achilles tendon insertion on the posterior calcaneus. Like Osgood–Schlatter disease, it is most commonly seen in active adolescents at a time of rapid growth, during which muscles and tendons become tighter as bones become longer. The primary symptom is pain at the Achilles insertion that is exacerbated with activities and improved with rest. The primary physical examination finding is tenderness at the Achilles insertion. The gastrocnemius–soleus complex can be tight. X-rays are usually not necessary to make the diagnosis but can reveal irregularity of the posterior calcaneus apophysis. Treatment includes ice, NSAIDs, relative rest,

gently progressive heel cord stretching, and gently progressive pain-free calf-strengthening exercises. A heel lift can be used for a short period to unload the area. Symptoms resolve with skeletal maturity.

Flexor hallucis longus overload

Overload of the flexor hallucis longus tendon is seen in dancers, gymnasts, and other active individuals who perform repetitive and forceful toe flexion.[119] The patient can present with pain anywhere along the course of the flexor hallucis longus muscle–tendon unit. Symptoms are reproduced with flexion of the great toe against resistance and direct palpation of the tendon. Passive stretch of the muscle–tendon does not reproduce symptoms as reliably as with some other injuries, such as hamstring strains. Imaging studies are not initially indicated, but when necessary, MRI is the study of choice (Fig. 40-12). As with other muscle and tendon overload conditions, treatment consists of ice, NSAIDs, activity modification, and strengthening exercises. Local injection of anesthetic and corticosteroid around the tendon can decrease pain and inflammation, and facilitate progress with the exercise program.

Tibialis posterior overload or medial tibial stress syndrome

Dysfunction of the tibialis posterior muscle is common. The muscle serves many roles. It functions concentrically as an ankle inverter and weak plantar flexor. It creates a force couple with tibialis anterior to support the medial longitudinal arch. It can easily be placed at a biomechanical disadvantage in the setting of anatomic abnormalities such as pes planus and calcaneal eversion. Certain conditions, most notably rheumatoid arthritis, are associated with dysfunction and pathologic rupture of the tibialis posterior tendon. One can assess for tibialis posterior

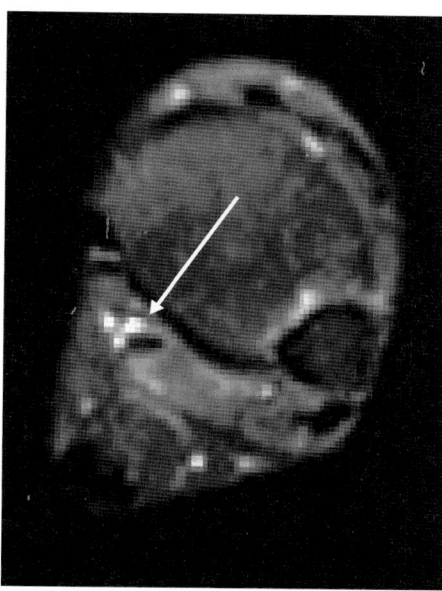

Figure 40-12 T2 axial magnetic resonance imaging of the ankle, showing increased signal around the flexor hallucis longus tendon. The patient was a professional dancer.

function by performing a resistance test of ankle inversion combined with plantar flexion, and by viewing calcaneal motion from behind as the patient performs slow heel raises. A normally functioning tibialis posterior tendon will permit the calcaneus to rise in line with the leg or in slight calcaneal varus. A dysfunctional tibialis posterior allows the calcaneus to rise in valgus.

There is a spectrum of overload pathology in the medial leg that is collectively referred to as medial tibial stress syndrome. The common term is *shin splints*. There are several tissues that can be involved when a patient presents with medial or posteromedial leg pain. As mentioned above, tibialis posterior can hurt along its origin at the posteromedial border of the tibia. Overload of medial gastrocnemius or medial soleus can also cause pain in this region. Persistent stress can cause progression of pathology to involve the periosteum of the tibia, a condition called periostitis. When further stress is placed on the bone, frank breakdown of the osseous microarchitecture ensues, resulting in stress reaction in the bone and finally stress fracture.

Patients with medial tibial stress syndrome present with pain and tenderness along the medial and/or posteromedial border of the tibia. One can often elicit a history of a rapid increase in running or other athletic activities. Walking and running gait evaluations can show that the patient is a toe walker or a toe runner, which can cause excessive eccentric overload to the ankle plantar flexors. One should look for static and dynamic pes planus, which can place the tibialis posterior at a biomechanical disadvantage. Conversely, if tibialis anterior is weak or inhibited, it may be unable to perform its function as a supporter of the medial longitudinal arch of the foot. A kinetic chain evaluation should focus on other muscle groups that work synergistically with tibialis posterior during functional activities.

It can be difficult or impossible to clinically distinguish exactly which of the above-mentioned tissues are involved in the overload process when a patient presents with medial leg pain. Clinically, one often proceeds with a course of rehabilitation at the time of the initial evaluation. Usual rehabilitation principles apply, including ice, NSAIDs, activity modification, tibialis posterior strengthening, and kinetic chain functional exercises, if needed. Off the shelf or custom-made foot orthoses can be helpful to provide shock absorption and accommodate for a pes planus. A gradual return to higher level activities is prescribed. If the patient fails to adequately improve with an appropriate rehabilitation program, consideration should be made for imaging to look for periostitis, stress reaction, or stress fracture. These bone overload conditions are rarely appreciated with plain films. MRI has replaced bone scan in most centers as the study of choice to look for stress reaction and stress fracture. If the patient initially presents with point tenderness or risk factors for stress fracture, such as the female athlete triad, one should proceed with imaging at the time of the initial visit. The differential diagnosis also includes chronic exertional compartment syndrome (CECS). Further discussion of compartment syndromes and bone overload conditions in the lower limbs is presented later in the chapter.

Injuries to the lateral leg muscle group
Fibularis longus and brevis

The correct anatomic name for the peroneus muscle has been changed to fibularis. However, for the purpose of this discussion we will refer to this muscle group in terms of its widespread usage, which is peroneus. The peroneal muscles can be injured either from a sudden, forceful contraction or from repetitive overload. Acute injuries sometimes occur at the time of a lateral ankle sprain, when the peroneal muscles will activate eccentrically to counteract the inversion moment.[114,115] On physical examination, there is tenderness over the lateral leg, usually approximately 12 cm proximal to the medial malleolus at the level of the musculotendinous junction. On MRI, a longitudinal tear of peroneus longus, peroneus brevis, or both can be seen (Fig. 40-13). While many of these injuries respond well to ankle rehabilitation, persistent cases can require surgical intervention.

Two other conditions of the peroneal muscles should be familiar to the musculoskeletal physician. The peroneal muscles are held in place behind the lateral malleolus of the ankle by the superior peroneal retinaculum. An incompetent retinaculum allows for subluxation of a peroneal tendon around the lateral malleolus. Damage to the retinaculum that causes peroneal tendon subluxation can occur with a severe ankle sprain. If subluxation is recurrent, symptoms are often best addressed with a surgical procedure entailing peroneal tendon groove deepening and retinacular repair. Rarely, the peroneus longus muscle herniates through a fascial defect on the lateral aspect of the leg, usually near the junction of the middle and distal thirds. This is usually a benign condition and infrequently requires surgical consultation.

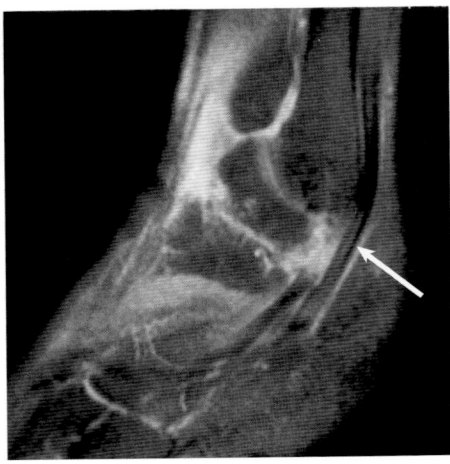

Figure 40-13
T2-weighted sagittal short inversion time–inversion recovery magnetic resonance imaging of the ankle, showing a longitudinal split tear of the peroneus brevis tendon.[116]

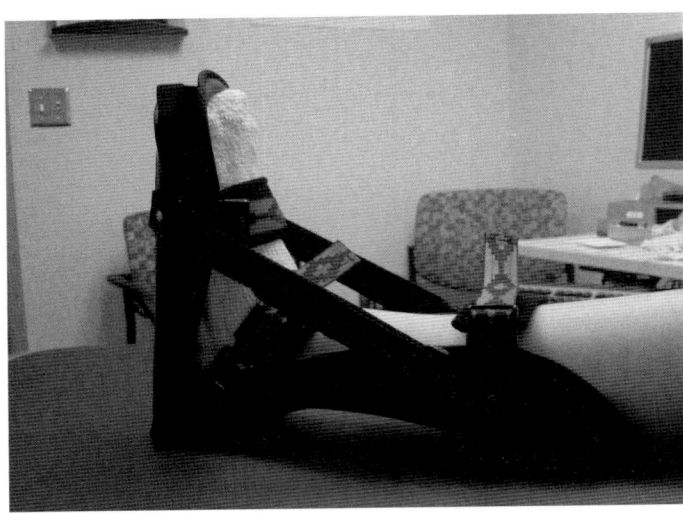

Figure 40-14 Resting night splint.

Compartment syndrome

The term *compartment syndrome* refers to a condition in which the pressure within a given muscle compartment is abnormally elevated. There are two types of compartment syndrome: acute and chronic. Acute compartment syndrome is usually due to significant trauma, such as a fracture or crush injury, and is a surgical emergency. CECS of the lower extremity is seen most commonly in high-volume runners.[116] Symptoms can mimic those of tendonopathy or stress fracture. Patients with CECS complain of recurrent leg cramping or pain with activities. Symptoms usually come on at a predictable time point in their exercise routine. Occasionally, the patient can localize the cramping to a particular compartment of the leg (anterior, lateral, superficial posterior, and deep posterior). More often, however, the cramping is difficult to localize. Neurologic symptoms, such as temporary foot drop during activities, can occur when high compartment pressures cause ischemia to the tibial or peroneal nerves. Definitive diagnosis is by intramuscular compartment pressure testing. In addition to a history and physical examination that are consistent with CECS, one or more of the following criteria must be met to formally establish the diagnosis:

- preexercise pressure $\geq$ 15 mmHg;
- 1-min postexercise pressure $\geq$ 30 mmHg; or
- 5-min postexercise pressure $\geq$ 20 mmHg.[116]

Newer MRI imaging techniques that measure increased T2 signal in a specific compartment after exercise might provide a non-invasive way of documenting selective compartment pressure increase.[3,35,78,110] Treatment can be challenging. The primary non-surgical treatment is avoiding the inciting activities. Massage therapy can sometimes be helpful. If prolonged activity modification and rehabilitation are unsuccessful, fasciotomy or fasciectomy should be considered, and in the carefully selected patient can be very effective.[136]

Injury to the plantar foot muscles and plantar fascia; plantar fasciitis

Four plantar foot muscles take their origin from the volar calcaneus: adductor hallucis, quadratus plantae, flexor digitorum brevis, and abductor digiti minimi quinti. Overload of these muscles can result in an enthesopathy at the calcaneus, causing volar heel pain. The same process can cause inflammation and pain in the plantar fascia. This condition is referred to as plantar fasciitis. Patients with plantar fasciitis present with volar heel pain that is often, but not always, worse with their first few steps in the morning. Tenderness to palpation is present at the volar aspect of the heel, usually slightly medial to midline. Imaging studies are usually not indicated, unless there is a history of acute trauma or symptoms become recalcitrant. The presence or absence of a calcaneal traction spur correlates poorly with symptoms of plantar fasciitis.[69]

As with other musculotendinous injuries, a similar biomechanical approach should be taken when treating plantar fasciitis. The rehabilitation plan should focus on restoring range or motion, strength, endurance, and motor control of the heel cord and foot intrinsic muscles. If pain with the first few steps in the morning is a prominent symptom, then a resting night splint can be very helpful in preventing overnight tightening of the heel cord and plantar structures (Fig. 40-14). A kinetic chain evaluation might reveal predisposing biomechanical deficits. If the patient is a toe runner, then the foot intrinsic muscles can become eccentrically overloaded. Similarly, a tight heel cord or a tight hamstring can prevent proper heel strike and result in excessive forces being placed on the plantar foot muscles. If tibialis posterior and/or tibialis anterior are not doing their assigned job of supporting the medial longitudinal arch, the plantar foot muscles can become overloaded as they try to compensate for their more proximal agonists. More proximally still, the dynamic function of the hip external rotators should be assessed. The hip external rotators eccentrically control femoral internal rotation during the weight-bearing phase of running, and therefore have an indirect effect on tibial rotation and subtalar pronation. Local injection of corticosteroid can assist in decreasing local inflammation and pain, but the patient must be cautioned that corticosteroid can increase the risk of rupture of the plantar fascia (Fig. 40-15).

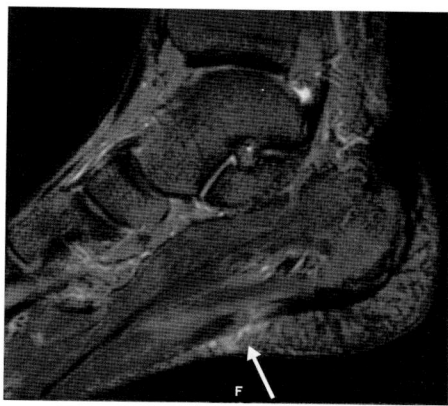

Figure 40-15 T2-weighted fat suppression magnetic resonance imaging of the foot, showing increased signal in the midportion of the plantar fascia, indicating an acute rupture of that structure. The patient was an Olympic bobsledder who was unable to compete with this injury.

DISORDERS OF THE JOINTS OF THE LOWER LIMB

Osteoarthritis

Osteoarthritis in the weight-bearing joints is very common. Osteoarthritis affecting the hip, knee, ankle, and foot are discussed together, because the principles of diagnosis and treatment are similar. Patients with lower limb osteoarthritis typically complain of joint pain that is worse with weight bearing and improved with rest. Pain and stiffness are common first thing in the morning but typically last less than an hour. This is in contrast to inflammatory arthropathies, in which morning pain often lasts longer than 1 h. Joint effusions can be noted with overuse of an arthritic joint. Joint trauma and obesity both predispose an individual to developing osteoarthritis in the weight-bearing joints. There is a clear genetic predisposition to early and diffuse osteoarthritis in some families.

Pain from hip osteoarthritis is often felt in the groin region, and is less commonly described as being posterior or lateral. The pain can be referred into the anterior thigh. The differential diagnosis of hip osteoarthritis includes referred pain from the lumbar spine. The physical examination is most notable for an antalgic gait on the affected side, and reproduction of groin pain with passive hip internal rotation.

Knee osteoarthritis can affect the medial tibiofemoral compartment, the lateral tibiofemoral compartment, the patellofemoral joint, or all three compartments. The medial compartment is often involved first, with varus alignment noted on inspection. Other findings can include joint line tenderness, crepitus, and palpable osteophytosis. Ankle and foot arthritis often occurs years after trauma to these joints or with malalignment that loads joints abnormally. Frequent locations of osteoarthritis include the first metatarsophalangeal joint of the great toe, the subtalar joint, and the ankle joint. Osteoarthritis of the first metatarsophalangeal joint (hallux rigidus) results in loss of dorsiflexion, joint swelling, and pain. Pain from subtalar arthritis is appreciated when walking on uneven surfaces and is often

especially painful. Ankle arthritis is characterized by pain, swelling, and stiffness in the anterior ankle.

Plain films are the study of choice to assess for osteoarthritis. The radiologic hallmarks of osteoarthritis include decreased joint space, marginal osteophytosis, subchondral cyst formation, and subchondral sclerosis (Fig. 40-16).[85]

There are many treatment options for lower limb osteoarthritis. A patient can sometimes modify symptoms simply by modifying activities. Switching from higher impact activities such as basketball to lower impact activities such as bicycling or swimming can decrease or eliminate joint pain.[80,143] Ice, acetaminophen (paracetamol), and NSAIDs can all reduce joint pain. Glucosamine and chondroitin sulfate have been shown in some studies to reduce pain in knee osteoarthritis.[79,90,121,122,140] Strength training and aerobic exercise can improve joint control and decrease pain.[109] Strategies aimed at reducing loads on joints include weight loss, cushioned shoes, and walking aids such as a cane.[146] Intraarticular injection of anesthetic and steroid can be helpful both diagnostically and therapeutically.[111,134] Injections of the foot, ankle, and hip joints are best performed under fluoroscopic guidance with contrast confirmation. Research into the efficacy of hyaluronate injections is ongoing. Several investigations looking at knee osteoarthritis have concluded that intraarticular injections relieve pain and improve function in patients with mild and moderate knee osteoarthritis.[2,60,71,83] For patients with recalcitrant pain or severe functional limitations, arthroplasty can provide substantial improvement in pain and function.

Disorders of the hip joint

Avascular necrosis

Avascular necrosis, also called osteonecrosis, is the death of bone due to a lack of blood supply. This can lead to microfractures and eventually collapse of the bone. The femoral head is the most commonly affected location. Disruption of the normal blood supply to the femoral head can be caused by various conditions, including trauma; high doses of corticosteroids; alcohol abuse; and systemic illness such as diabetes, lupus, and sickle cell anemia.[81] The severity of symptoms with avascular necrosis is usually related to the degree of articular surface disruption. Symptoms are similar to those experienced with hip osteoarthritis, including groin pain that increases with weight bearing. Often, there is limited motion and pain with internal rotation, flexion, and abduction of the hip. X-rays can reveal sclerosis of the femoral head, or in severe cases collapse of the femoral head (Fig. 40-17). In mild cases, the plain films can be normal. MRI and computed tomography (CT) can detect the condition in its earlier stages. Conservative treatment might include keeping weight off the affected joint and use of pain medications. Once collapse occurs, joint replacement surgery is indicated to improve pain and function.

Legg–Calve–Perthes disease

Legg–Calve–Perthes disease is idiopathic osteonecrosis of the femoral head in children. It occurs most frequently in boys

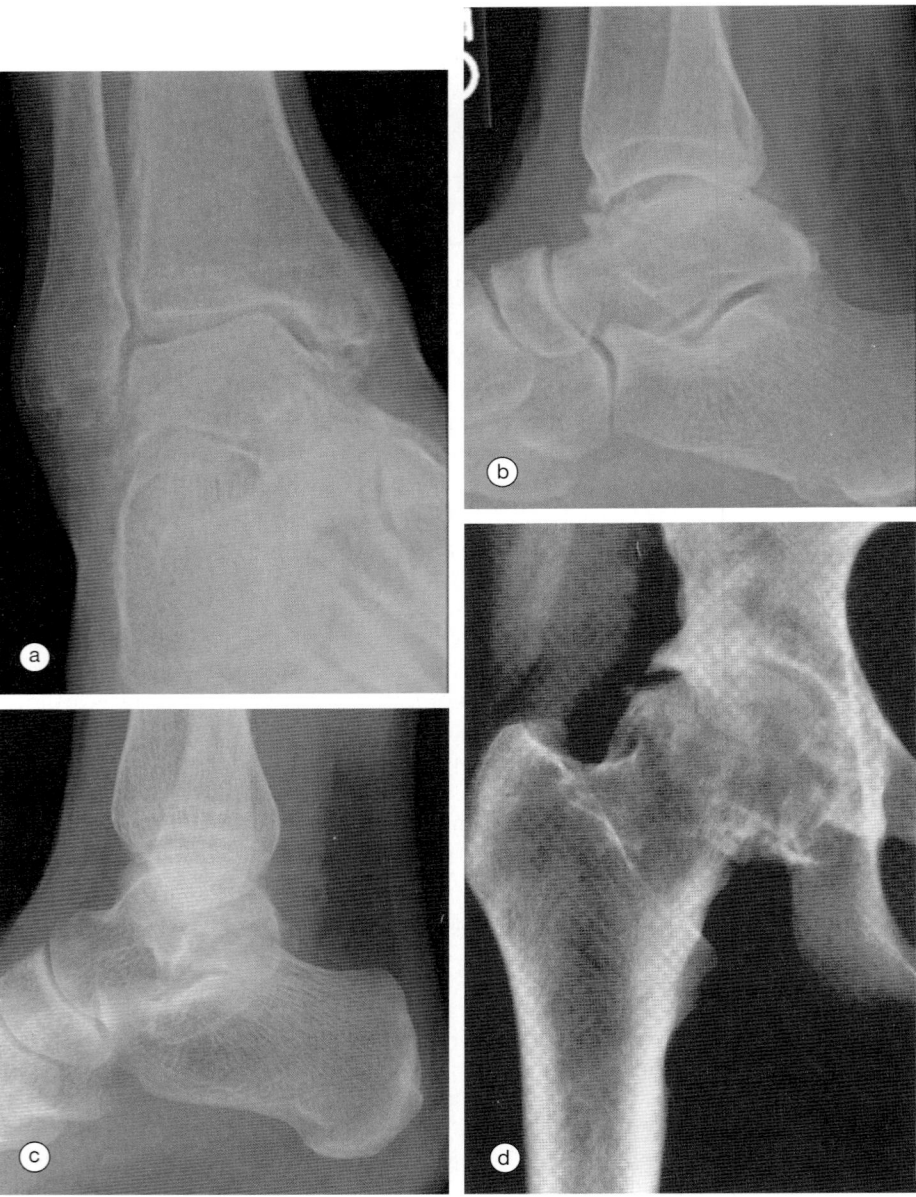

Figure 40-16 Examples of osteoarthritis. Anteroposterior (**a**) and lateral (**b**) x-rays of the ankle, showing advanced osteoarthritis in the ankle joint. There are large dorsal spurs, small intraarticular calcific bodies, and varus alignment is present at the joint, with widening of the joint space laterally, consistent with chronic ligamentous laxity. (**c**) Lateral x-ray of the ankle, showing advanced osteoarthritis of the posterior subtalar joint. There is significant irregularity of the joint margins, with subchondral sclerosis and cyst formation. (**d**) Anteroposterior x-ray of the hip, showing very severe osteoarthritis, with near-complete obliteration of the joint space and extensive remodeling of the femoral head.

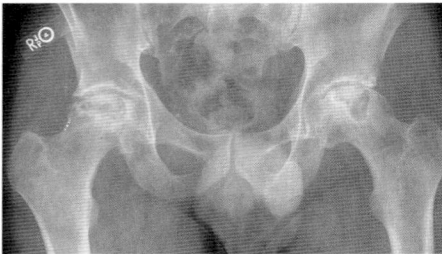

Figure 40-17 Anteroposterior x-ray of the pelvis, showing advanced avascular necrosis of both femoral heads.

tion of the femoral head and remodeling of the bone. The prognosis is better in younger children and with mild involvement. In children under the age of 6, observation and use of an abduction brace to maintain the femoral head in a spherical state is reasonable. Osteotomy is often performed in older children.[82]

Slipped capital femoral epiphysis

The most common hip disorder in adolescents is slipped capital femoral epiphysis. Injury to the physeal plate of the proximal femur with medial displacement of the femoral head relative to the femoral shaft can be due to acute trauma or repetitive microtrauma. Slipped capital femoral epiphysis is rare in boys under age 11 and girls under age 9, and is more common in overweight boys.[82] There can be an association with hypothyroidism and renal osteodystrophy.[45] Slipped capital femoral

between the ages of 4 and 8. Because bone repair is relatively rapid in children, the prognosis is significantly better compared with for adults with avascular necrosis. Signs of Legg–Calve–Perthes disease in a child include limping and restriction in hip motion, especially abduction. The child may complain of groin or thigh pain. Healing can occur in children with revasculariza-

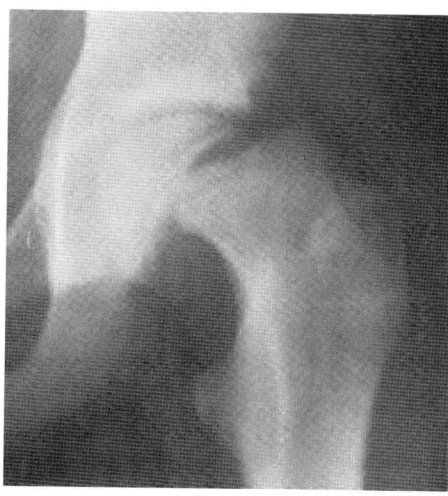

Figure 40-18
Anteroposterior x-ray of a severe, acute slipped capital femoral epiphysis.

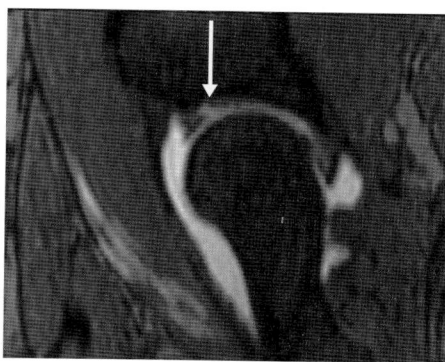

Figure 40-19
Gadolinium-enhanced sagittal magnetic resonance imaging of the hip, showing an anterior labrum tear.

epiphysis is bilateral about 50% of the time.[82] An adolescent with an acute slip presents with severe hip pain that is exacerbated with any motion. The individual tends to hold the hip flexed and externally rotated. Anteroposterior and lateral radiographs confirm the diagnosis (Fig. 40-18). A mild slip can be treated conservatively.[123] Otherwise, one attempt at closed reduction can be attempted. If this is unsuccessful, then open reduction should be pursued. After reduction, gentle range of motion can be started within a few days, but weight bearing is restricted for 4–6 weeks.[123] After this time period, gradually progressive strengthening and functional exercises are advanced. Complications include non-union, avascular necrosis of the femoral head, rotational deformity, and osteoarthritis.[82,132]

Hip dislocation

Because of the depth of the acetabulum, dislocation of the femoral–acetabular joint requires significant trauma. In children, hip dislocation is more common than hip fractures. In adults, fractures of the acetabulum often accompany hip dislocations. Most commonly, the head of the femur dislocates posteriorly relative to the acetabulum.[98] The patient with an acute posterior hip dislocation presents with severe hip pain and tends to hold the hip in flexion, internal rotation, and adduction. With the less common anterior dislocations, the hip is held in an extended, abducted, and externally rotated position. On physical examination, there will be an obvious deformity. The patient will not tolerate range of motion or resistance testing due to pain. A complete neurologic examination should be performed to assess for lumbosacral plexopathy, sciatic neuropathy, and femoral neuropathy.[89] One should always assess for associated injuries, in particular spine and ipsilateral knee trauma, which can be masked by hip pain. Radiographs are indicated to confirm the clinical diagnosis and look for associated injuries. Hip dislocations are an orthopedic emergency, and closed reduction under anesthesia should be performed as soon as possible. Postreduction x-rays are obtained to confirm anatomic alignment. At times, CT or MRI is obtained if further characterization of associated injuries is needed. Surgery is indicated if attempts at closed reduction are unsuccessful, and to repair displaced or comminuted fractures and remove intra-articular loose bodies.[34] Most clinicians recommend non-weight bearing for 3–4 weeks, followed by protected weight bearing for an additional 3 weeks.[123] Gradually progressive rehabilitation can start a few days to a couple of weeks after reduction, depending on the patient's comfort level and whether or not surgery was performed. The most concerning complications of hip dislocation include posttraumatic osteoarthritis and avascular necrosis, which occurs in up to 10% of patients.[132] The risk of avascular necrosis increases with age greater than 5, reduction delayed greater than 6 h, and more severe trauma to the hip joint.

Labral injuries

Acetabular labral tears are analogous to glenoid labral tears, with some notable exceptions. Patients with acetabular labral tears often present with painful catching of the hip, especially when the hip is at a particular angle.[87] There might or might not be a clear history of acute or repetitive trauma. Femoral–acetabular grind maneuvers might reproduce symptoms. Historical features and physical examination maneuvers are even less specific for acetabular labral tears than they are for glenoid labral tears. This may be because the hip is a larger, deeper joint with less sensitive innervation than the shoulder joint. Magnetic resonance arthrography with gadolinium contrast is the imaging study of choice to assess for these injuries (Fig. 40-19). Definitive diagnosis is by arthroscopy or open surgery.

Treatments include NSAIDs, relative rest, intraarticular steroid injections, and surgical debridement or repair. The arthroscopic and open surgical approaches to labral injuries of the hip continue to evolve.[19,20,37,66]

Impingement syndromes

In recent years, there has been greater attention given to the concept of hip impingement. This condition is somewhat analogous to the subacromial impingement syndrome of the shoulder. Certain anatomic variants, such as acetabular retroversion and decreased femoral head–neck offset, can increase the likelihood of the femur impinging on the superior acetabular lip during hip flexion activities. In our anatomy laboratory, we have seen the hip flexor and adductor muscles impinge under the inguinal ligament during full passive hip flexion, which might be another source of anterior hip pain.

Disorders of the knee joint

Knee ligament injuries

Four ligaments provide static stability to the knee. The most commonly injured knee ligaments are the medial collateral ligament (MCL) and ACL. The MCL courses from the medial femoral condyle to the proximal, medial tibia, and provides restraint against valgus force. Patients presenting with an MCL sprain will often be able to describe sustaining a sudden valgus force with the foot planted. They will often be able to localize the pain to the medial side of the knee. The physical examination will be most notable for tenderness along the course of the MCL and a positive valgus stress test. If the patient is apprehensive with valgus stress testing but a firm end feel is appreciated, then the injury is most likely a grade 1 sprain with no gross tearing of the ligament (Fig. 40-20). If the medial joint line opens up without apparent restraint, the injury is a grade 3 sprain, representing complete disruption of the ligament. Depending on the degree of ligament injury, medial knee swelling may be present, but an intraarticular effusion is usually absent in isolated MCL sprains, because the MCL is extra-articular. Although plain films are usually unremarkable in an isolated MCL injury, anteroposterior and lateral x-rays are useful to rule out an associated bony injury. MRI is the imaging study of choice to evaluate the MCL, but is usually obtained only if other injuries are suspected or if the patient is an elite athlete. Initial treatment most commonly consists of aggressive use of ice and elevation to decrease swelling and pain. A knee immobilizer may be used for 1–2 weeks to provide joint stability and allow reparative scar tissue to begin forming. Early,

gentle knee flexion and extension exercises are initiated in the first 1–2 weeks, and gradual return to full activities as tolerated is progressed over 1–4 weeks, depending on the severity of the injury. Isolated MCL tears, even grade 3, rarely if ever require surgery.[53]

Tears of the ACL are the most functionally devastating, because of the ACL's crucial role in the dynamic stability of the knee, especially during activities involving side to side or cutting maneuvers. The ACL courses from the medial wall of the lateral femoral condyle anteromedially to the anterior spine of the tibial plateau. The ACL restrains anterior displacement of the tibia relative to the femur, and internal rotation of the tibia relative to the femur.[106] ACL tears can occur as the result of contact or non-contact injuries. Although different mechanisms can place the ACL at risk, the individual is often rotated on a planted foot with the knee in flexion and the quadriceps activating strongly.[25] The patient will often report hearing or feeling a 'pop'. The patient will also describe a sense of knee instability, especially with twisting activities such as changing direction when walking. Return to sports participation is usually impossible or associated with repeated episodes of instability. In the acute setting, pain might not be a prominent symptom. When significant pain is present acutely, it can suggest the presence of an associated injury, such as a bone contusion or meniscus tear. On physical examination, an effusion is usually present, and the anterior drawer and Lachman's test may reveal increased anterior displacement of the tibia relative to the femur. Lachman's test is reported to have greater sensitivity for detecting ACL insufficiency compared with the anterior drawer test.[141] Plain films can show an effusion. The presence of a small capsular avulsion fracture off the lateral tibial plateau is termed a *Segond fracture*, and is considered pathognomic of the presence of an ACL tear (Fig. 40-21).[25] An MRI is often obtained to confirm the clinical diagnosis and look for associated injuries, such as meniscal tears, capsular injuries, other ligament injuries, bone bruises, and popliteus injuries (Fig. 40-22).

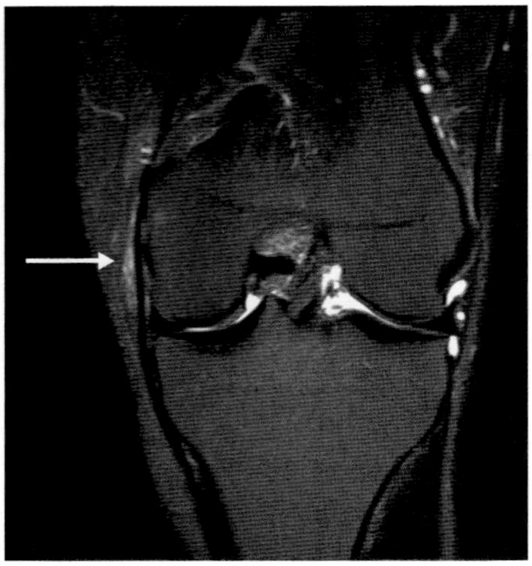

Figure 40-20 T2-weighted, fat suppression, coronal magnetic resonance imaging of the knee, showing increased signal surrounding the medial collateral ligament with intact fibers of the ligament, consistent with grade 1 strain. The patient was a football player who sustained a valgus injury to the knee with his foot planted on the ground.

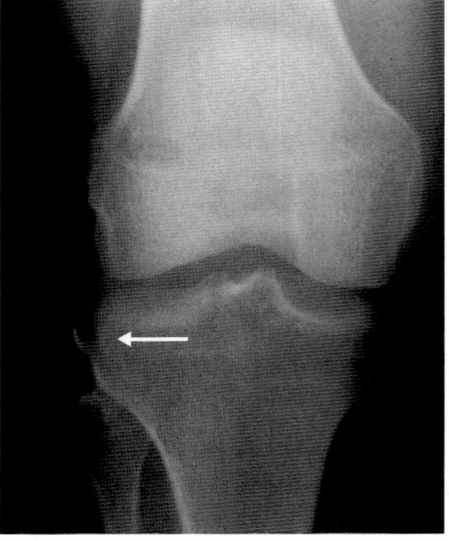

Figure 40-21
Anteroposterior x-ray of the knee, showing a large Segond fracture, indicating the likely presence of an anterior cruciate ligament tear.

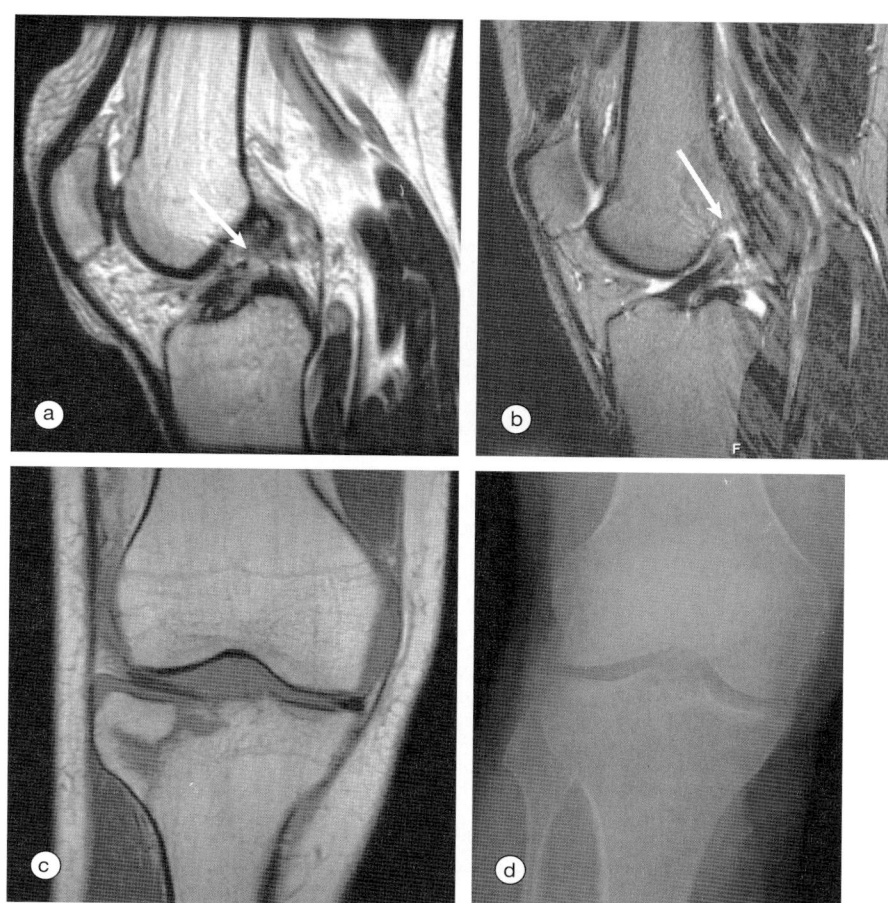

Figure 40-22 Examples of anterior cruciate ligament (ACL) tears and associated injuries. (**a**) T1 sagittal magnetic resonance imaging (MRI) showing a mid-substance tear of the ACL. (**b**) T1 sagittal MRI showing an ACL tear from the proximal attachment site on the femur. (**c**) Coronal T1-weighted MRI showing a non-displaced tibial plateau fracture that was associated with an ACL injury. (**d**) The fracture was not appreciated on initial x-rays, which were normal.

The management of acute ACL tears includes aggressive use of ice, elevation, and compression. A knee immobilizer or hinged knee brace can be used initially to provide stability. Crutches can also be used if needed. Early, gentle knee flexion and extension exercises can minimize the development of stiffness. Quadriceps inhibition is almost ubiquitous after ACL tears, and atrophy in this muscle group can be fairly dramatic even within a few weeks of injury. Straight leg raises performed in the knee immobilizer promote safe quadriceps activation and decrease atrophy. The longer term treatment of ACL tears depends primarily on the patient's desired activity level. Young healthy individuals who participate in cutting sports should strongly consider ligament reconstruction to increase knee stability and decrease the chance of developing posttraumatic osteoarthritis from a chronically unstable knee.[4,23] Sedentary individuals or individuals participating primarily in straight ahead activities such as walking and cycling might opt for aggressive rehabilitation to maximize muscular control of the joint. It is also reasonable for patients to pursue aggressive rehabilitation and defer surgical reconstruction if they are not experiencing episodes of instability and are willing to avoid impact and aggrevise cut/pivot activities. Most knee surgeons recommend waiting at least 1–2 weeks prior to reconstruction, in order to allow time for swelling and stiffness to decrease. The use of functional knee braces in ACL-deficient patients seems to provide some benefit in moderate activities

and appears to limit subluxation events, although the mechanism for this is unclear. There is no evidence to show that these braces prevent ACL injury.[24]

Injuries of the posterior cruciate ligament (PCL) are less common than injuries of the ACL. PCL deficiency generally results in less significant functional limitations compared with the ACL-deficient knee. The PCL courses posteriorly and inferiorly from the femoral intercondylar notch to the posterior tibial spine. It serves to restrain posterior displacement of the tibia relative to the femur. A common mechanism for PCL disruption is a forceful blow to the proximal, anterior leg. This can drive the tibia posterior relative to the femur. PCL disruptions have occurred in soccer goalkeepers who get kicked in the shin when sliding to make a save, in individuals who fall on to their shins, and in motor vehicle accidents when a front seat passenger has the shin driven into the dashboard (the so-called 'dashboard injury'). The clinical diagnosis of a PCL tear is primarily based on a positive posterior drawer test. Plain films are usually negative in isolated PCL injuries. MRI can be obtained to confirm the diagnosis and look for associated injuries. Acute management includes ice, elevation, pain control if needed, and early gentle range of motion exercises. If the individual is having difficulty with walking, a knee immobilizer and crutches can be used for 1–2 weeks. Most individuals with isolated PCL injuries can return to full activities, including athletics, with functional rehabilitation.[113] On rare occasions, surgical reconstruction of the PCL is undertaken if the individual continues to experience instability symptoms or functional limitations.

The lateral collateral ligament, also called the fibular collateral ligament, courses from the lateral femoral condyle to the fibular head, and resists varus forces at the knee.[64] The lateral collateral ligament is rarely injured in isolation but can be torn in multiligament injuries and knee dislocations.

Posterolateral corner injuries

The posterolateral corner of the knee has received increasing attention over the past decade. This is a complicated anatomic region that includes the lateral collateral ligament, popliteus tendon, posterolateral joint capsule, biceps femoris tendon, peroneal nerve, lateral head of gastrocnemius, lateral meniscus, and posterior meniscofemoral ligament. Injury to any or all of these structures can accompany a severe knee sprain such as an ACL tear or a knee dislocation. Accurate diagnosis of injuries to the posterolateral corner of the knee can be difficult, but is important to ensure complete management of these types of injuries. MRI is helpful to determine the extent of structural involvement, and early surgical evaluation is important to optimize outcome.

Meniscal injuries

Injuries to the menisci are common. They can be the result of acute trauma or gradual degeneration. A sudden or forceful twisting motion on a planted foot is the most common mechanism of injury for acute meniscus tears. The patient typically reports a slow onset of swelling after the injury (often the day after injury), pain with weight bearing and twisting maneuvers, and sometimes clicking within the knee. Locking of the knee suggests the presence of a bucket handle meniscus tear that has flipped up into the intercondylar notch (Fig. 40-23). The hallmarks of the physical examination include medial or lateral joint line tenderness, effusion, and a positive McMurray's test. MRI is the study of choice to look for meniscus tears. Initial treatments include ice, elevation, NSAIDs, and bracing. Additional treatments depend on healing potential and the patient's goals. Simple tears have a greater chance of healing than complex tears. Tears in the outer portion of the meniscus, referred to as the vascularized 'red zone', have greater healing potential than tears located centrally in the avascular 'white zone'. Vascular zone tears in younger individuals can be amenable to arthroscopic meniscal repair procedures. In older athletes, if there are no mechanical symptoms present, it is reasonable to allow 3–6 weeks of relative rest and rehabilitation to see if symptoms improve. Referral for consideration of arthroscopic intervention is indicated if the patient remains limited in function, has persistent mechanical symptoms, or has recurrent episodes of pain and swelling. Patients who need to return to full activities quickly, such as elite athletes, can proceed with arthroscopy sooner. Arthroscopic treatment options include repair of the meniscus tear versus debridement of the meniscus with partial meniscectomy.

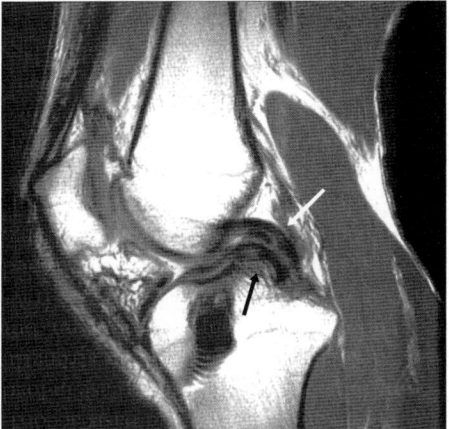

Figure 40-23 T1 sagittal magnetic resonance imaging of a knee, showing a bucket handle meniscus tear that flipped up into the notch, creating the so-called double posterior cruciate ligament (PCL) sign. The patient was an Olympic alpine ski racer who had a prior anterior cruciate ligament (ACL) reconstruction and who sustained this meniscus injury during competition. The tibial tunnel and screw were not placed anterior enough in the tibia, essentially creating a non-functional ACL graft and leaving the knee unstable. The superior black line, denoted by the white arrow, is the real PCL. The inferior black line, denoted by the black arrow, is the bucket handle meniscus tear that displaced into the notch.

Osteochondral lesions (osteochondritis dissecans)

Osteochondritis dissecans is a lesion of subchondral bone with or without involvement of the overlying articular cartilage. These lesions are classified into four categories. Grade 1 involves compression of subchondral trabeculae with preservation of the cartilage. Grade 2 involves incomplete detachment of an osteochondral fragment. Grade 3 involves complete avulsion of an osteochondral fragment without dislocation. Grade 4 involves complete avulsion of an osteochondral fragment with dislocation (loose body).[16] The most common site for osteochondritis dissecans is the inferior portion of the medial femoral condyle, but they can also occur in the lateral femoral condyle or retropatellar cartilage. Symptoms include recurrent swelling and pain with activity that is lessened with rest. Wilson's test, which involves extending the knee the last 30° with the foot internally rotated, can be positive. Because these symptoms might be caused by other injuries, such as meniscus tears and articular cartilage defects, formal diagnosis usually awaits imaging studies or direct arthroscopic visualization. Treatment depends on the grading of the lesion and the severity of symptoms, and can include anything from relative rest to surgery.[40]

Prepatellar bursitis

Prepatellar bursitis, also known as housemaid's knee, is a common cause of swelling and pain anterior to the patella. The term housemaid's knee comes from its association with individuals whose work necessitates kneeling for extended periods of time. Prepatellar bursitis is common in professions such as carpet laying and gardening, and is also seen in wrestlers secondary to irritation or friction from the wrestling mat. Knee range of motion can be mildly limited. The swelling is within the bursa, not within the knee joint itself. Treatment of prepatellar bursitis begins with avoiding the aggravating activities. Ice, compression, and NSAIDs are useful to decrease swelling and pain. Aspiration followed by instillation of corticosteroid can be helpful, but a septic bursitis needs to be ruled out first. In some individuals, drainage or excision of the bursa might be indicated.

Disorders of the ankle and subtalar joints
Sprains

Ankle sprains are the most common musculoskeletal injury in the lower limb. They account for 25% of all sports injuries. The strongest predictor of ankle sprains is a history of prior sprain. The most commonly injured ligament is the anterior talofibular ligament, which has the weakest tensile strength of the lateral ankle ligament complex. The most common mechanism for ankle sprains is inversion, usually combined with plantar flexion. Syndesmotic injuries involving the thick ligaments connecting the tibia and fibula are often referred to as 'high' ankle sprains; they require more time to heal and are more likely to require surgical stabilization. Sprains of the deltoid ligament on the medial aspect of the ankle are far less common than lateral ankle sprains. These occur during forceful and sudden ankle eversion.

Ankle injuries are graded from simple distortion or partial tear in the ligament with no instability (grade 1) to partial or complete tear of the ligament with instability (grades 2 and 3, respectively). Accurate diagnosis can be difficult immediately after an injury, due to the presence of diffuse pain and swelling. Grading the degree of ligament damage with the physical examination is sometimes more reliable a few days after the injury. The combination of pain over the anterior talofibular ligament, hematoma discoloration, and a positive anterior drawer test has a sensitivity of 96% and specificity of 84% for diagnosing a grade 2 or 3 sprain.[29] A positive squeeze test (compressing the tibia and fibula at midcalf) and external rotation test (externally rotating the dorsiflexed foot) is suggestive of a syndesmotic injury. When tenderness is present over the distal fibula, ankle joint, syndesmosis, base of the fifth metatarsal, or other bony structures, radiographs should be obtained to rule out fracture. Avulsion fractures of the base of the fifth metatarsal can occur from the pull of peroneus brevis (Fig. 40-24). If non-displaced or mildly displaced, these fractures can usually be treated non-operatively with use of an orthopedic shoe for 1–2 weeks or until pain subsides. Greater displacement of the avulsion fragment might require screw or pin fixation.

Acute treatment includes icing and compressive wrapping of the ankle. Icing and elevation can help minimize swelling, and early mobilization and use of a brace for support can be helpful initially. Crutches are used only when pain precludes full weight bearing. Sensorimotor control is reduced in persons with persistent instability complaints after injury. Balance and proprioceptive training improves sensorimotor control and can reduce the risk of future injury. As a patient progresses in therapy, dynamic strengthening and sport-specific functional drills

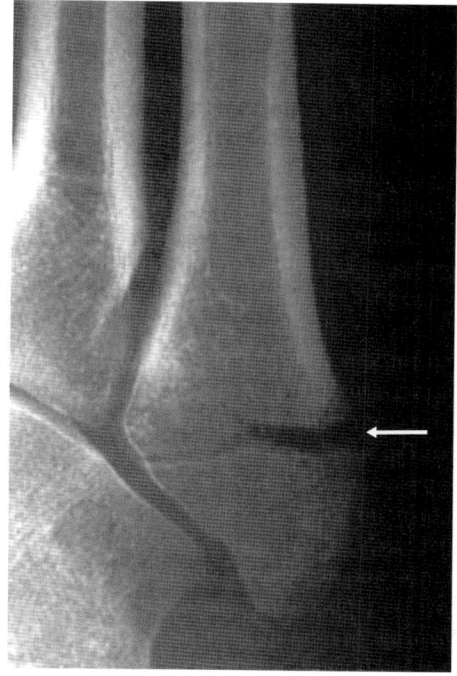

Figure 40-24
Anteroposterior x-ray of the foot, showing a minimally displaced avulsion fracture of the base of the fifth metatarsal. The patient was a division 1 cross-country runner who sustained an inversion ankle sprain during a race. This injury is usually treated non-operatively with short-term immobilization and progressive ankle rehabilitation.

should be incorporated into the exercise program.[86] Functional tests to determine readiness to return to activity include 'shuttle runs' and single-leg hopping. In returning to sport, taping or bracing have been shown in some studies to be helpful in reducing the risk of recurrent ankle sprains. These effects are probably due to mechanical restriction as well as neuromuscular and sensory mechanisms. Bracing is often favored over taping, as it better restricts ankle motion without affecting performance, it retains its restrictive property longer, and it is more cost-effective in the long term.[13,21,38,95] Medial ankle sprains and syndesmotic injuries require longer healing times than lateral sprains. A walking boot can be used for the first 2–4 weeks with these injuries. About one-third of patients have mild to moderate residual pain with activity.

In cases of a complete syndesmotic injury, screw fixation is indicated. Most other ankle injuries heal without complication. With a functional rehabilitation program, the patient can return to full activity within a few days to weeks, depending on the severity of the sprain. Residual symptoms are more likely if the rehabilitation is incomplete. It has been reported that up to 40% of ankle sprains lead to persistent problems with pain and instability.[46] Occult injuries must be suspected in these individuals. The most commonly overlooked injuries include fractures, osteochondral lesions, injuries to the subtalar joint or syndesmosis, peroneal tendonopathy or rupture, proprioceptive deficit, and impingement syndrome. Pain is the most common cause of subjective or 'functional' instability. In these patients, physiologic range is not exceeded on examination. A few of the common causes include peroneal muscle weakness, proprioceptive deficit, and subtalar instability. If pain is not present between episodes of instability, there might be true mechanical instability. These patients have ankle mobility beyond the

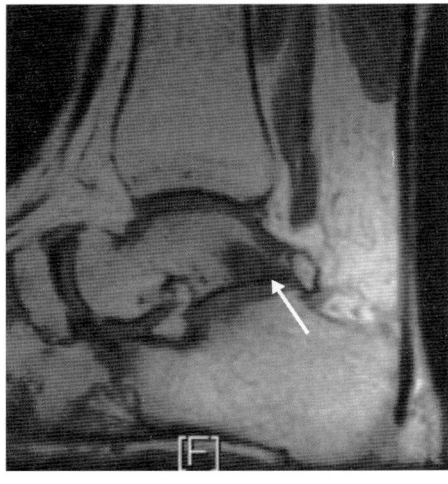

Figure 40-25
Sagittal T1-weighted magnetic resonance imaging of the ankle, showing a large osteochondral lesion in the inferior posterior talus.

physiologic range of motion, with abnormal laxity on examination. Studies have shown that balance exercises and peroneal strengthening can restore functional stability to even the mechanically unstable ankle. Surgery can be indicated after failure of an extended period of appropriate aggressive ankle strength and stability treatment in patients with symptomatic mechanical instability.

Osteochondral lesions of the ankle

The talus ranks third in location after the knee and elbow for osteochondral lesions. Osteochondral lesions occur in about 6.5% of all ankle sprains. There is a history of trauma in about 80% of cases.[138] Patients present with deep ankle pain that is worse with weight bearing and improved with rest. Tenderness can sometimes be elicited with palpation in the region of the subtalar joint and with subtalar joint play maneuvers. MRI is more sensitive than plain films for visualizing the lesion and assessing soft tissue structures (Fig. 40-25). Osteochondral lesions can affect the medial or lateral talus. Medial lesions usually occur following a compressive force with an inversion–flexion movement. Medial lesions are less commonly related to acute trauma, tend to be less severe, and are more likely to undergo spontaneous healing. Lateral talus osteochondral lesions often occur following forced eversion and dorsiflexion. Symptoms are more pronounced, and self-healing occurs less frequently. Osteoarthritic changes may develop earlier in these patients. Non-operative treatment of symptomatic osteochondral lesions of the talus fails in 30–40% of patients. Generally, stage 1 disease is treated non-operatively. Stage 4 is treated operatively. Stages 2 and 3 are treated conservatively on the medial side and surgically on the lateral side.[138]

Miscellaneous disorders of the foot

Several miscellaneous disorders of the foot deserve mention.

Morton's interdigital neuroma, metatarsalgia, and sesamoiditis

Although distinct clinical entities, these conditions are reviewed jointly because they have similar presentations. Morton's neuroma is due to irritation of one of the interdigital nerves of the foot as it passes below the transverse ligament of the metatarsal heads. The most common location for an interdigital neuroma is between the third and fourth metatarsal heads, but it can also occur between the other metatarsal heads.[39] Symptoms usually start insidiously. The patient typically presents with pain in the region of the metatarsal heads. There can be referral of pain or paresthesias into the two toes innervated by the interdigital nerve in question. Patients sometimes describe a sensation of having a pebble in their shoe or a wrinkle in their sock. Pain is exacerbated with forefoot weight bearing, narrow toe boxes, and high heels, all of which can load the region of the metatarsal heads and interdigital nerves. If there are no neurologic symptoms referred to the toes, the challenge of the physical examination is to distinguish between pain coming from between two metatarsal heads versus pain coming from the metatarsal heads themselves, which would be more consistent with metatarsalgia. Occasionally, the examiner appreciates a click when palpating a larger or firmer neuroma, especially when palpation is combined with squeezing the metatarsal heads together from the medial and lateral sides. Metatarsalgia, as its name implies, is pain coming from the metatarsal heads. Jumping, toe running, and high heels can all cause overload of the metatarsal heads, just as they can cause entrapment or irritation of the interdigital nerve beneath the transverse metatarsal ligament. The second metatarsal head is the most commonly involved.

When the pain is in the region of the first metatarsal head, the differential diagnosis includes injury to the sesamoid bones in the flexor hallucis tendon, such as stress response or stress fracture. Pain coming from an injured sesamoid bone is sometimes referred to as *sesamoiditis*. Distinguishing between metatarsalgia, sesamoid stress response, and sesamoid fracture can be clinically challenging. A bipartite sesamoid seen on plain films can be a normal variant, and advanced imaging with MRI or bone scan might be required to diagnose a fracture of the sesamoid.

For interdigital neuromas, metatarsalgia, and sesamoiditis, first-line interventions aim to unload the forefoot. Avoiding high heels is recommended. Shoes that have larger toe boxes can also be helpful. Gel inserts are effective at distributing forces more evenly. Custom-made foot orthoses with premetatarsal pads, or simply using premetatarsal pads alone, can transfer forces from the region of the metatarsal heads to slightly more proximal and therefore unload the painful area. Local injection with anesthetic and steroid is often useful both diagnostically and therapeutically for interdigital neuroma. There is no role for injections for metatarsalgia. For recalcitrant neuroma symptoms that are unresponsive to these measures, surgical excision can be considered, with the understanding that recurrence can occur.

Iselin's disease

Apophysitis of the fifth metatarsal base, or Iselin disease, is an overuse osteochondrosis seen in growing children. Although amenable to treatment, it is a self-limiting disorder, disappearing spontaneously with completion of growth.

Turf toe

Sudden and forceful hyperextension (or less commonly hyper-flexion) of the first metatarsophalangeal joint can cause a sprain of the joint capsule and ligaments, with subsequent swelling and pain. The incidence of this injury has increased since the advent of artificial turf. Radiographs should be obtained to exclude fracture. Initial treatment consists of ice and stiff-soled shoes to protect the joint. Although many of these injuries resolve within 3–4 weeks, some can result in functional limitations for a much greater period of time.

BONE INJURIES OF THE LOWER LIMB

A comprehensive discussion of acute fractures of the lower limbs is beyond the scope of this chapter. Many acute fractures of the lower limb can be successfully treated without surgical intervention. Examples include non-displaced pubic rami fractures, pelvic avulsion fractures, many non-displaced or minimally fibular fractures, and non-displaced or minimally displaced foot fractures. The most important take home point for the non-surgeon who is treating fractures is to consult with your orthopedic colleagues frequently to make sure that a surgical injury is not being under-treated. The final section of this chapter focuses on the spectrum of repetitive overload injuries of the bones of the lower limb.

Stress reactions and stress fractures

Injuries to bone can be due to acute trauma, chronic repetitive overload, metabolic disorders, and neoplasm. Although a musculoskeletal physician must be able to recognize and appropriately treat or triage any of these conditions, space does not allow for a full discussion of all disorders of bone. This section focuses on repetitive overload injuries to the bones of the lower limb.

These types of injury are common in physically active individuals, especially those who participate in endurance activities such as distance running. In cases of repetitive stress, or in the setting of impaired bone metabolism, bone strain occurs on a continuum from 'stress response' or 'stress reaction' to overt stress fracture. Bone overload can occur in any location in the lower limb (Fig. 40-26). The ability of bone to withstand repetitive forces without breaking down depends on several factors. The stronger the bone is prior to being subjected to repetitive loading, the better it is able to withstand the loads applied to it. Both intrinsic and extrinsic factors are important to consider in determining the risk for stress reactions or stress fractures. Intrinsic risk factors include poor dietary habits, altered menstrual status, and biomechanical abnormalities that do not allow for proper distribution of forces along the kinetic chain. Extrinsic factors can include training surface type, training errors, footwear, and insoles.

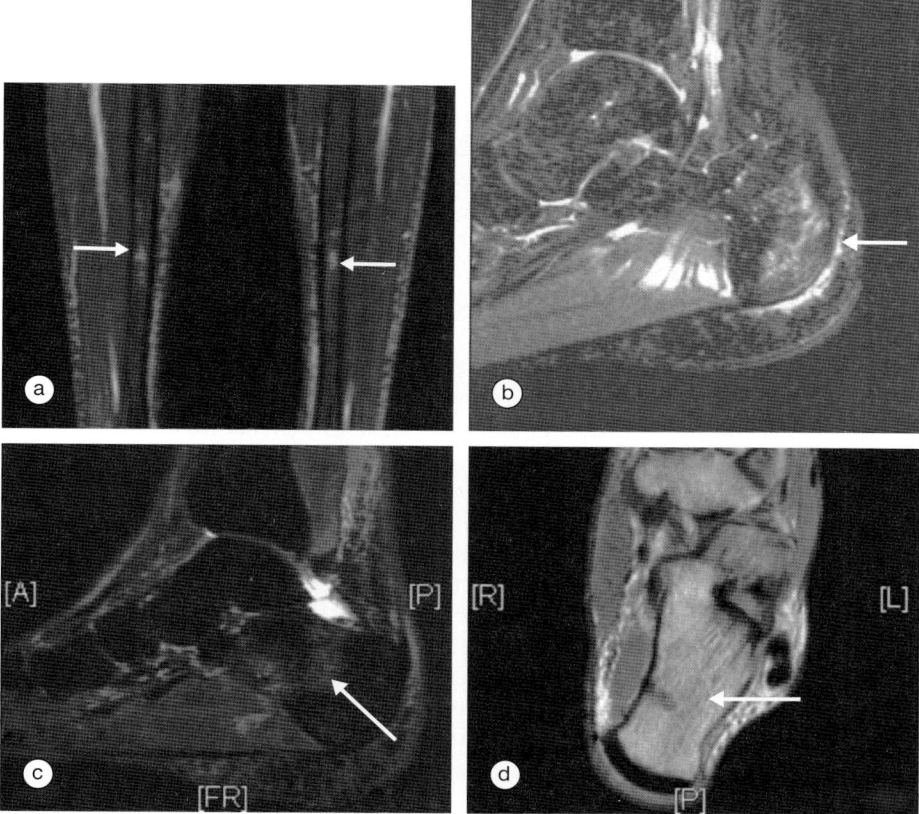

Figure 40-26 Examples of stress responses and stress fractures. (**a**) T2-weighted, fat suppression, coronal magnetic resonance imaging (MRI) of the legs shows increased signal in the medullary cavity of both tibiae, consistent with stress response or stress reaction. There is no discrete line indicative of a stress fracture. The patient was a division 1 cross-country runner with oligomenorrhea and disordered eating. (**b**) T2-weighted, fat suppression MRI of the foot, showing increased signal in the calcaneus, consistent with a stress response. The patient was an Olympic freestyle skiing aerialist who had bilateral heel pain. The contralateral heel MRI had a similar appearance. T2-weighted, fat suppression, sagittal (**c**) and T1-weighted, axial (**d**) magnetic resonance images showing a calcaneal stress fracture. The patient was a 29-year-old ultramarathoner.

Athletes report a greater frequency of disordered eating patterns than the general population, especially in sports emphasizing leanness.[117] Individuals with disordered eating can have insufficient dietary intake of calories, protein, calcium, and other nutrients to achieve optimal bone quality. The triad of disordered eating, amenorrhea, and osteopenia that occurs in athletic females is referred to as the female athlete triad. Restrictive eating behaviors increase the likelihood of stress fractures in women.[14,15,44,101] Low caloric intake with negative protein balance has been hypothesized as one of the mechanisms for menstrual disturbances in female athletes.[150] There is evidence that menstrual and hormonal disturbances increase the risk of stress fracture and lead to premature bone loss, particularly at trabecular sites.[61,99]

Flexibility, although difficult to study, can play a role in fracture risk. Some studies have suggested that increased hip external rotation and decreased ankle dorsiflexion might increase the risk for stress fractures in certain populations.[47,48,57]

Skeletal alignment affects the amount of force absorbed by the foot, and how much force is transferred to proximal structures during ground contact. A rigid pes cavus foot is less able to absorb shock during and just after heel strike, and can therefore transmit greater forces to proximal bones than a foot that is able to undergo normal pronation. Similarly, a pes planus foot does not allow the normal pronation mechanism to properly absorb forces. Either foot alignment can increase the risk of a stress fracture, the location of which can vary depending on the foot type and activity.[88,129] Other studies looking at alignment have suggested that leg length discrepancy and increased Q angle can increase the risk of stress fracture.[26]

While it is clear that training errors contribute to stress fractures, there is limited research identifying the contribution of various training components. Furthermore, appropriate training regimens vary greatly among individuals. Athletes should be encouraged to keep training logs documenting type of training, volume, intensity, and rest periods. A rapid increase in training volume and intensity often precedes a stress fracture, just as it might precede a muscle–tendon overload injury. Articles about training in the military situation have shown that elimination of running and marching on concrete, preentry physical conditioning, and inclusion of rest periods were felt to reduce stress fracture risk.[51,126,127]

Shoes and insoles can be an important component in minimizing stress fracture risk. Proper shoe fit that matches an individual's foot type, as well as adequate support and shock absorption, are essential. Studies looking at the effect of insoles or other footwear modifications on the prevention of stress fractures have shown a reduction in the number of stress fractures by over 50%.[49,93,94]

The patient presenting with a suspected stress fracture usually provides a history of a recent acceleration in the intensity or duration of training prior to the onset of symptoms. The patient most frequently complains of insidious onset of focal pain that is exacerbated with weight-bearing activities. In cases of certain stress fractures, such as femoral neck and navicular fractures, symptoms can be vague, thus increasing the time to diagnosis. The differential diagnosis usually includes tendonopathy, enthesopathy, and CECS.

Imaging studies are not always necessary. A 6-week period of relative rest with non-impact rehabilitation and alternative training methods such as pool running can be instituted. Imaging can be reserved for individuals who remain symptomatic and are unable to return to full activities. In these cases, or when complete diagnosis is required sooner, the initial imaging study of choice is radiographs. It should be kept in mind, however, that plain films are relatively insensitive and detect less than 50% of stress fractures.[72,73] When radiographs are normal but the suspicion for stress fracture remains high, advanced imaging studies are appropriate. Bone scans are sensitive for detecting stress fractures but lack anatomic definition. They can also remain positive long after symptoms have resolved. This limits the ability of bone scans to aid in return to sport decisions.[133] MRI provides excellent anatomic information, and can be more useful in grading lesions and assessing soft tissue structures.[6] At our institution, MRI is the study of choice to look for stress fractures. CT provides optimal definition of bony architecture.

Multiple factors influence the length of time required to safely return to full activities following a stress fracture. These include duration of symptoms, stage of stress reaction, site of stress fracture, and level of activity or competition. Most stress fractures heal without complication with activity modification, and allow return to sport in 4–8 weeks. There are a few high-risk stress fractures, however, that require more aggressive treatment (these are discussed below).

Initial treatment includes pain management, activity modification, strengthening, fitness maintenance, and risk factor modification. Once healing is well underway and pain is minimal, the gradual resumption of the impact-loading phase of rehabilitation begins.

Pain can be a problem mainly during weight bearing with lower extremity stress fractures. It might be appropriate to use crutches to minimize weight bearing for the first 7–10 days. Modalities such as ice can also be helpful. Analgesics such as acetaminophen (paracetamol) are appropriate. There is some debate about the use of NSAID medications after a stress fracture. On a theoretic basis at least, the mode of action of these medications might prevent optimal repair of the stress fracture, with reduction in the bone-remodeling process.

Activity modification includes eliminating impact activities for a period of time until daily ambulation is pain-free. During this time, it is important to continue muscle strengthening and cross-training to keep the cardiopulmonary system fit.

Reduced muscle size and strength have been shown to predispose to stress fractures.[56] In endurance events, muscle fatigue can increase the strain on bone.[149] Muscle mass is important to build and maintain, because the load placed on bone can be reduced at sites when muscles are better able to absorb repetitive impact.[125] A strengthening program should therefore begin immediately after a diagnosis of stress fracture is made. The exercises prescribed should not cause pain at the fracture site.

Inactivity has negative impacts on the cardiovascular system, metabolism, and skeletal muscle after even brief periods of rest. It is important that the physician and the patient understand that fitness should be maintained in ways that avoid overloading the bone. The most common cross-training activities include cycling, swimming, water running, rowing, and Stairmaster. The more sport-specific the cross-training is, the better the carryover effect of the training. It is for this reason that deep water running has become so popular among runners with stress fractures. Studies have shown no significant differences in maximal oxygen uptake, anaerobic threshold, running economy, stride length, and 2-mile performance after 4–8 weeks of land versus deep water running training.[36,55,148] In sports requiring specific skills, the neuromuscular adaptations are not easily duplicated with cross-training, and it is important to find appropriate ways to resume these isolated sport-specific skills as soon as possible.

When walking is pain-free, the graduated impact phase of rehabilitation should progress on an individualized basis according to fracture site and symptoms. A progressive increase in load is necessary to allow bone to adapt with increases in strength. Resumption of activity should not be accompanied by pain, but it is not uncommon to have some mild discomfort at the fracture site. If bony pain occurs, then activity should be stopped for 1–2 days. When the individual is pain-free while walking, the activity is resumed at a level prior to where symptoms occurred. When training resumes, it is important to allow adequate recovery time after hard sessions or hard weeks of training. Progress should be monitored clinically by the presence or absence of symptoms and local signs. It is not necessary to monitor progress by imaging studies. Radiologic healing lags behind clinical healing.

Although most stress fractures heal without incident using the above treatment strategies, there are particular stress fractures that tend to develop complications and therefore require specific treatment. These include femoral neck, anterior cortex of the middle third of the tibia, navicular, and proximal fifth metatarsal fractures.

In femoral neck stress fractures, symptoms are often vague, and one should have a high index of suspicion to catch this diagnosis early and avoid complications such as displacement or avascular necrosis. If suspicion is present, an MRI should be obtained (Fig. 40-27). Fractures on the tension side (lateral) are less common and require immediate surgical referral. Fractures on the compression side (medial) are more common. If the fracture line extends over 50% of the width of the femoral neck, percutaneous fixation should be considered, as the likelihood of displacement is higher.[6,30,128] When the fracture line is < 50% of the width of the femoral neck, strict non-weight-bearing status is necessary for about 4 to 6 weeks until the patient is pain-free. This should be followed by functional rehabilitation with progressive weight bearing over the next 4–8 weeks according to symptoms. If the athlete is not progressing as expected, additional radiologic evaluation should be considered.

Navicular fractures have a higher likelihood of delayed union, non-union, or avascular necrosis. There is evidence that contin-

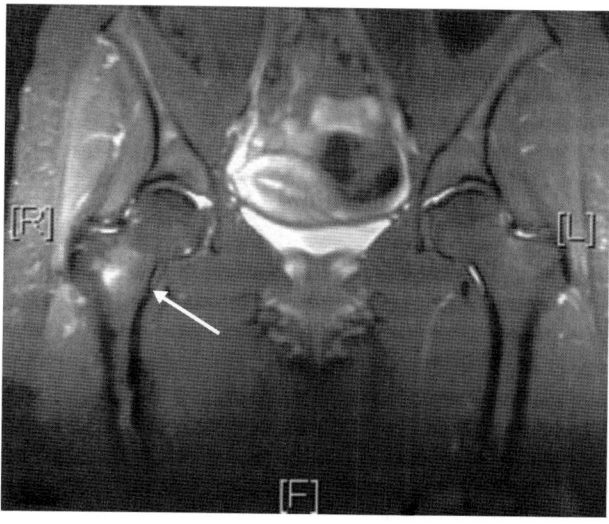

Figure 40-27 T2-weighted, fat suppression, coronal magnetic resonance imaging of the pelvis, showing increased signal in the right femoral neck consistent with stress fracture. The patient was an elite cross-country ski racer who had onset of symptoms after 'bounding' exercises, which involve running uphill on one leg.

ued weight bearing on a tarsal navicular fracture is associated with a 74% failure rate of healing.[67] Therefore early diagnosis and treatment are important. Radiographs are often normal, and an MRI or bone scan can confirm the diagnosis. If positive, a CT scan is often the most appropriate study to optimally visualize the bone. Navicular fractures involving a cortical break at the dorsal aspect of the navicular alone have the best prognosis, typically healing by 3 months. With propagation of the fracture into the navicular body, healing time is slightly longer. Initial management of these fractures consists of non-weight bearing, with boot immobilization for 6–8 weeks. If symptoms persist, one should consider use of a bone stimulator or surgical fixation.[54] Navicular fractures that propagate across the body and involve another cortex have a significantly higher risk of complication, and early surgical intervention should be considered.[120,124]

The 'dreaded black line' is a tension-type stress fracture of the anterior cortex of the middle third of the tibia. These fractures are well known for their progression to non-union or complete fracture. With continued activity, the risk of complete fracture is 60%.[10] Even with appropriate activity modification for 9–12 months, non-surgical treatment fails in 25–60% of cases.[9] Initial treatment may consist of activity modification and pneumatic leg splints. Intramedullary fixation, however, can also be considered as an appropriate initial treatment.[17]

Stress fractures of the fifth metatarsal are prone to non-union and refracture (Fig. 40-28). Early stress fractures (bony edema only) are typically treated with non-weight-bearing immobilization for 6 weeks, followed by 6 weeks of protected weight bearing. If healing still has not occurred, surgical fixation is appropriate. Surgery is usually considered as first-line treatment in cases where a clear fracture line is present or in elite athletes.[17,107]

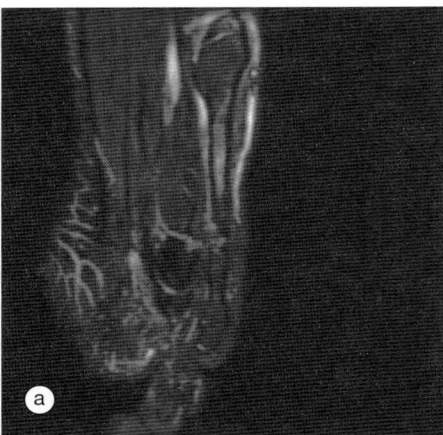

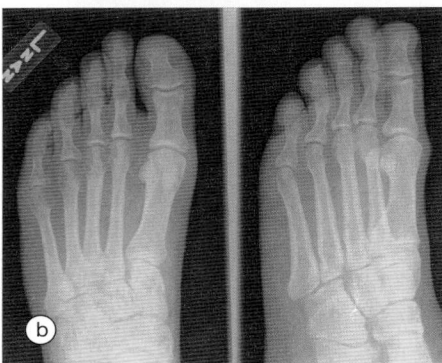

Figure 40-28
(**a**) T2-weighted, short inversion time–inversion recovery, fat suppression, axial magnetic resonance imaging of the foot, showing increased signal in the fifth metatarsal consistent with stress fracture. (**b**) No lesion in the bone was appreciated on the initial x-rays.

Stress fractures of the lower limbs are common, and should be recognized and treated early to maximize successful outcome. Although most individuals go on to heal with an appropriate functional rehabilitation program, there is a subset of fractures that are at high risk of complications and need to be identified early and managed appropriately.

SUMMARY

Having a sound understanding of anatomy and kinetic chain biomechanics, in conjunction with fundamental history and physical examination skills, permits a practitioner to establish appropriate diagnoses for patients presenting with soft tissue, bone, and joint disorders of the lower limbs. Ancillary testing, such as imaging studies, can help confirm or disprove clinical diagnoses and establish the severity of injury. The majority of lower limb injuries can be successfully treated with non-operative measures that include medications, activity modification, and intelligent exercise strategies. The practitioner should be able to recognize injuries that require surgical consultation.

REFERENCES

1. Alfredson H, Pietila T, Jonsson P, et al. Heavy-load eccentric calf muscle training for the treatment of chronic Achilles tendinosis. Am J Sports Med 1998; 26(3):360–366.

2. Altman RD, Moskowitz R. Intra-articular sodium hyaluronate (Hyalgan) in the treatment of patients with osteoarthritis of the knee: a randomized clinical trial. Hyalgan Study Group. J Rheum 1998; 25:2203–2212. (Correction in: J Rheum 1999; 26:1216)

3. Amendola A, Rorabeck CH, Vellett D, et al. The use of magnetic resonance imaging in exertional compartment syndromes. Am J Sports Med 1990; 18(1):29–34.

4. Andersson C, Odensten M, et al. Knee function after surgical or nonsurgical treatment of the acute rupture of the anterior cruciate ligament: a randomized study with a long-term follow-up period. Orthopaedics 1991; 264:255–263.

5. Andrews JR. Overuse syndromes of the lower extremity. Clin Sports Med 1983; 2:137.

6. Arendt EA, Griffiths HJ. The use of MR imaging in the assessment and clinical management of stress reactions of bone in high-performance athletes. Clin Sport Med 1997; 16:291–306.

7. Ashby EC. Chronic obscure groin pain is commonly caused by enthesopathy: 'tennis elbow' of the groin. Br J Surg 1994; 81:1632–1634.

8. Bahndari M, Guyatt GH, Siddiqui F, et al. Treatment of acute Achilles tendon ruptures a systematic overview and metaanalysis. Clin Orthop 2002; 400:190–200.

9. Batt ME, Kemp S, Kerslake R. Delayed union stress fractures of the anterior tibia: conservative management. Br J Sports Med 2001; 35:74–77.

10. Beals RK, Cook RD. Stress fractures of the anterior tibial diaphysis. Orthopedics 1991; 14:869–875.

11. Beiner JM, Jokl P. Muscle contusion injuries: current treatment options. J Am Acad Orthop Surg 2001; 9(4):227–237.

12. Beiner JM, Jokl P. Muscle contusion injury and myositis ossificans traumatica. Clin Orthop 2002; 403S:S110–S119.

13. Bennell K, McCrory P. The role of ankle support in the prevention of ankle injury. Sport Health 1992; 10:13–16.

14. Bennell KL, Malcolm SA, Thomas SA, et al. Risk factors for stress fractures in track and field athletes: a 12-month prospective study. Am J Sports Med 1996; 24:810–818.

15. Bennell KL, Malcolm SA, Thomas SA, et al. Risk factors for stress fractures in female track-and-field athletes: a retrospective analysis. Clin J Sports Med 1995; 5:229–235.

16. Berndt AL, Harty M. Transchondral fractures (osteochondritis dissecans) of the talus. J Bone Joint Surg 1959; 41A:988–1020.

17. Boden BP, Osbahr DC. High-risk stress fractures: evaluation and treatment. J Am Acad Orthop Surg 2000; 8:344–353.

18. Brukner P, Khan K. Clinical sports medicine. Sydney: McGraw-Hill; 1993:310.

19. Byrd JW, Jones KS. Hip arthroscopy in athletes. Clin Sports Med 2001; 20(4):749–761.

20. Byrd JW, Jones KS. Prospective analysis of hip arthroscopy with 2-year follow-up. Arthroscopy 2000; 16(6):578–587.

21. Callaghan MJ. Role of ankle taping and bracing in the athlete. Br J Sports Med 1997; 31:102–108.

22. Canale ST, Beaty JH. Pelvic and hip fractures. In: Rockwood CA Jr, Wilkins KE, Beaty JH, eds. Fractures in children. 4th edn. Philadelphia: JB Lippincott; 1996.

23. Casteleyn P, Handeberg F. Non-operative treatment of anterior cruciate ligament injuries in the general population. J Bone Joint Surg 1996; 78(3):446–451.

24. Cawley PW, France E, Paulos LE. The current state of functional knee bracing research. A review of the literature. Am J Sports Med 1991; 19:226–233.

25. Clancy W, Ray J. Acute tears of the anterior cruciate ligament. J Bone Joint Surg 1988; 70A:1843–1848.

26. Cowan DN, Jones BH, Frykman PN, et al. Lower limb morphology and risk of overuse injury among male infantry trainees. Med Sci Sports Exerc 1996; 28:945–952.

27. Croisier J, Forthomme B, et al. Hamstring muscle strain recurrence and strength performance disorders. Am J Sports Med 2002; 30(2):199–203.

28. Diaz JA, Fischer DA, Rettig AC, et al. Severe quadriceps muscle contusions in athletes—a report of three cases. Am J Sports Med 2003; 31:289–293.

29. Dijk van CN, Lin LSL, Bossuyt PMM, et al. Diagnosis of sprained ankles. J Bone Joint Surg 1997; 79:1039–1040.

30. Egol KA, Koval KJ, Kummer F, et al. Stress fractures of the femoral neck. Clin Orthop 1998; 348:72–78.

31. Ekstrand J, Gillquist J. The frequencies of muscle tightness and injuries in soccer players. Am J Sports Med 1982; 10:75–78.

32. Emery CA, Meeuwisse WH, Powell JW. Groin and abdominal strain injuries in the National Hockey League. Clin J Sports Med 1999; 9(3):151–156.

33. Emery CA, Meeuwisse WH. Risk factors for groin injuries in hockey. Med Sci Sports Exerc 2000; 33(9):1423–1433.

34. Epstein HC. Traumatic dislocations of the hip. Clin Orthop 1973; 92: 116.

35. Eskelin MK, Lotjonen JM, Mantysaari MJ. Chronic exertional compartment syndrome: MR imaging at 0.1 T compared with tissue pressure measurement. Radiology 1998; 206(2):333–337.

36. Eyestone ED, Fellingham F, George J, et al. Effect of water running and cycling on maximum oxygen consumption and 2-mile run performance. Am J Sports Med 1993; 21:41–44.

37. Farjo LA, Glick JM, Sampson TG. Hip arthroscopy for acetabular labral tears. Arthroscopy 1999; 15(2):132–137.

38. Firer P. Effectiveness of taping for the prevention of ankle ligament sprains. Br J Sports Med 1990; 24:47–50.

39. Fitzgibbons T, Keown B, Sampson C, et al. Foot problems in athletes. In: Mellion M, ed. Office sports medicine. 2nd edn. Philadelphia: Hanley and Belfus; 1996:318–336.

40. Flynn JM, Kocher MS, Ganley TJ. Osteochondritis dissecans of the knee. J Pediatr Orthop 2004; 22(4):434–443.

41. Frederickson M, Cookingham CL, Chaudhari AM, et al. Hip abductor weakness in distance runners with iliotibial band syndrome. Clin J Sport Med 2000; 10(3):169–175.

42. Fricker PA, Taunton JE, Ammann W. Osteitis pubis in athletes: infection, inflammation or injury? Sports Med 1991; 12(4):266–279.

43. Fricker PA. Management of groin pain in athletes. Br J Sports Med 1997; 31(2):97–101.

44. Frusztajer NT, Dhuper S, Warren MP, et al. Nutrition and the incidence of stress fractures in ballet dancers Am J Clin Nutr 1990; 51: 779–783.

45. Garrick J, Webb DR. Pelvis, hip, thigh injuries. In: Sports injuries: diagnosis and management. Philadelphia: Saunders; 1990:175–196.

46. Gerber JP, Williams GN, Scoville CR, et al. Persistent disability associated with ankle sprains: a prospective examination of an athletic population. Foot Ankle Int 1998; 19(10):653–660.

47. Giladi M, Milgrom C, Simkin A, et al. Stress fractures: identifiable risk factors. Am J Sports Med 1991; 19:647–652.

48. Giladi M, Milgrom C, Stein M, et al. External rotation of the hip. A predictor of risk for stress fractures. Clin Orthop Relat Res 1987; 216:131–134.

49. Gillespie WJ, Grant I. Interventions for preventing and treating stress fractures and stress reactions of bone of the lower limbs in young adults. Cochrane Database Syst Rev 2000; 2:CD000450.

50. Gilmore J. Groin pain in the soccer athlete: fact, fiction and treatment. Clin Sports Med 1998; 17(4):787–793.

51. Greaney RB, Gerber RH, Laughlin RL, et al. Distribution and natural history of stress fractures in US marine recruits. Radiology 1983; 146:339–346.

52. Gruen GS, Scioscia TN, Lowenstein JE. The surgical treatment of internal snapping hip. Am J Sports Med 2002; 30(4):607–613.

53. Haimes J, Wroble R, Grood E, et al. The role of the medial structures in the intact and ACL-deficient knee. Am J Sports Med 1994; 22(4):401–410.

54. Harmon KG. Lower extremity stress fractures. Clin J Sports Med 2003; 13(6):358–364.

55. Hertler L, Provost-Craig M, Sestili D. Water running and the maintenance of maximum oxygen consumption and leg strength in runners [abstract]. Med Sci Sports Exerc 1992; 24:S23.

56. Hoffman JR, Chapnik L, Shamis A, et al. The effect of leg strength on the incidence of lower extremity overuse injuries during military training. Mil Med 1999; 164:153–156.

57. Hughes LY. Biomechanical analysis of the foot and ankle for predisposition to developing stress fractures. J Orthop Sports Phys Ther 1985; 7:96–101.

58. Jackson DW, Feagin J. Quadriceps contusions in young athletes: relation of severity of injury to treatment and prognosis. J Bone Joint Surg Am 1973; 55:95–105.

59. Jaivin JS, Fox JM. Thigh injuries. In: Nickolas JA, Hershman EB, eds. The lower extremity. St. Louis: Mosby; 1995:999–1023.

60. Jones AC, Pattrick M, Doherty S, et al. Intra-articular hyaluronic acid compared to intra-articular triamcinolone hexacetonide in inflammatory knee osteoarthritis. Osteoarthr Cartil 1995; 3:269–273.

61. Jonnavithula S, Warren MP, Fox RP, et al. Bone density is compromised in amenorrheic women despite return of menses: a 2-year study. Obstet Gynecol 1993; 81:669–674.

62. Kader D, Saxena A, Movin T, et al. Achilles tendonopathy: some aspects of basic science and clinical management. Br J Sports Med 2002; 36: 239–249.

63. Kannus P, Nittymaki S. Which factors predict outcome in the nonoperative treatment of patellofemoral pain syndrome? A prospective follow-up study. Med Sci Sports Exerc 1994; 26:289.

64. Kannus P. Nonoperative treatment of grade II and III sprains of the lateral ligament compartment of the knee. Am J Sports Med 1989; 17(1): 83–88.

65. Karlsson J, Sward L, Kalebo P, et al. Chronic groin injuries in athletes: recommendations for treatment and rehabilitation. Sports Med 1994; 17(2):141–148.

66. Kelly BT, Williams RJ, Phillippon MJ. Hip arthroscopy: current indications, treatment options, and management issues. Am J Sports Med 2003; 31:1020–1037.

67. Khan KM, Fuller PJ, Bruckner PD, et al. Outcome of conservative and surgical management of navicular stress fracture in athletes: eighty-six cases proven with computerized tomography. Am J Sports Med 1992; 20:657–666.

68. Kibler WB, Chandler TJ, Uhl TL. A musculoskeletal approach to the preparticipation physical examination preventing injury and improving performance. Am J Sports Med 1989; 17:525.

69. Kibler WB, Goldberg C, Chandler TJ. Functional biomechanical deficits in running athletes with plantar fasciitis. Am J Sports Med 1991; 19:66–71.

70. King JB. Post-traumatic ectopic calcification in the muscles of athletes: a review. Br J Sports Med 1998; 32(2):287–290.

71. Kirwan JR, Rankin E. Intra-articular therapy in osteoarthritis. Baillières Clin Rheumatol 1997; 11:769–794.

72. Kiuru MJ, Pihlajamaki HK, Hietanen HJ, et al. MR imaging, bone scintigraphy, and radiography in bone stress injuries of the pelvis and the lower extremity. Acta Radiol 2002; 43:207–212.

73. Knapp TP, Garrett WE. Stress fractures: general concepts. Clin Sports Med 1997; 16:339–355.

74. Kocher MS, Bishop J, Marshall R, et al. Operative versus nonoperative management of acute Achilles tendon rupture. Am J Sports Med 2002; 30(6):783–790.

75. Koulouris G, Connell D. Evaluation of the hamstring muscle complex following acute injury. Skeletal Radiol 2003; 32:582–589.

76. Kraushaar BS, Nirschl RP. Tendinosis of the elbow. Clinical features and findings of histological, immunohistochemical, and electron microscopy studies. J Bone Joint Surg Am 1999; 81:259–278.

77. Lacroiz UJ. A complete approach to groin pain. Phys Sports Med 2000; 28(1):66–86.

78. Lauder TD, Stuart MJ, Amrami KK, et al. Exertional compartment syndrome and the role of magnetic resonance imaging. Am J Phys Med Rehabil 2002; 81(4):315–319.

79. Leeb BF, Schweitzer H, Montag K, et al. A meta-analysis of chondroitin sulfate in the treatment of osteoarthritis. Arthritis Rheum 1998; 41(suppl): S198.

80. Lequesne MG, Dang N, Lane NE. Sport practice and osteoarthritis of the limbs. Osteoarthr Cartil 1997; 5(2):75–86.

81. Lloyd-Smith R, Clement DB, Mckenzie DC, et al. A survey of overuse and traumatic hip and pelvis injuries in athletes. Phys Sports Med 1995; 13:131–141.

82. MacEwen GD, Bunnell WP, Ramsey PL. The hip. In: Lovell WW, Winter RB, eds. Pediatric orthopaedics. Philadelphia: Lippincott; 1986.

83. Marshall KW, Manolopoulos V, Mancer K, et al. Amelioration of disease severity by intraarticular hylan therapy in bilateral canine osteoarthritis. J Orthop Res 2000; 18(3):416–425.

84. Martens MA, Hansen L, Mulier JC. Adductor tendinitis and musculus rectus abdominis tendopathy. Am J Sports Med 1987; 15: 353–356.

85. Martin JA, Buckwalter JA. Articular cartilage aging and degeneration. Sports Med Arthrosc Rev 1996; 4:263–275.

86. Mascaro TB, Swanson LE. Rehabilitation of the foot and ankle. Orthop Clin North Am 1994; 25:147–160.

87. Mason JB. Acetabular labral tears in the athlete. Clin Sports Med 2001; 20(4):779–790.

88. Matheson GO, Clement DB, McKenzie DC, et al. Stress fractures in athletes. A study of 320 cases. Am J Sports Med 1987; 15:46–58.

89. Matsumoto K, Sumi HS, Sumi Y, et al. An analysis of hip dislocations among snowboarders and skiers: a 10-year prospective study from 1992 to 2002. J Trauma Inj Infect Crit Care 2003; 55:946–948.

90. McAlindon TE, LaValley MP, Gulin JP, et al. Glucosamine and chondroitin sulfate for treatment of osteoarthritis: a systematic quality assessment and meta-analysis. JAMA 2000; 283(11):1469–1475.

91. Merrifield HH, Cowan RFJ. Groin strain injuries in ice hockey. J Sports Med 1973; 1(2):41–42.

92. Meyers WC, Foley DP, Garrett WE, et al. Management of severe lower abdominal or inguinal pain in the high-performance athletes. Am J Sports Med 2000; 28(1):2–8.

93. Milgrom C, Finestone A, Shlamkovitch N, et al. Prevention of overuse injuries of the foot by improved shoe shock attenuation. A randomized, prospective study. Clin Orthop 1992; 281:189–192.

94. Milgrom C, Giladi M, Kashtan H, et al. A prospective study of the effect of a shock-absorbing orthotic device on the incidence of stress fractures in military recruits. Foot Ankle 1985; 6:101–104.

95. Miller EA, Hergenroeder AC. Prophylactic ankle bracing. Pediatr Clin North Am 1990; 37:1175–1185.

96. Miller ML. Avulsion fractures of the anterior superior iliac spine in high school track athletic training. Athl Train 1982; 17:57.

97. Miller ML. Avulsion fractures of the pelvis. Am J Sports Med 1985; 13:349–358.

98. Moorman CT, Warren RF, Hershman EB, et al. Traumatic posterior hip subluxation in American football. J Bone Joint Sirg 2003; 85A: 1190–1196.

99. Myburgh KH, Bachrach LK, Lewis B, et al. Low bone mineral density at axial and appendicular sites in amenorrheic athletes. Med Sci Sports Exerc 1993; 25:1197–1202.

100. Natri A, Kannus P, Jarvinen M. Which factors predict the long term outcome in chronic patellofemoral pain syndrome? A 7-yr prospective follow-up study. Med Sci Sports Exerc 1998; 30:1572.

101. Nattiv A, Puffer JC, Green GA. Lifestyles and health risks of collegiate athletes: a multi-center study. Clin J Sport Med 1997; 7:262–272.

102. Nelson G, Martens M, Burssens A. Surgical treatment of chronic Achilles tendonitis. Am J Sports Med 1989; 17:754.

103. Nicholas SJ, Tyler TF. Adductor muscle strains in sport. Sports Med 2002; 32(5):339–344.

104. Nirschl RP. Elbow tendinosis/tennis elbow. Clin Sports Med 1992; 11:851–870.

105. Nistor L. Surgical and non-surgical treatment of Achilles tendon ruptures. J Bone Joint Surg 1981; 63A:394.

106. Noyes F, Butler D, Grood E. Biomechanical analysis of human ligament grafts used in knee ligament repairs and reconstructions. J Bone Joint Surg 1984; 66A:344–352.

107. Nunley JA. Fractures of the base of the fifth metatarsal. Orthop Clin North Am 2001; 32:171–180.

108. Orchard JW, Fricker PA, Abud AT, et al. Biomechanics of iliotibial band friction syndrome in runners. Am J Sports Med 1996; 24(3):375–379.

109. O'Reilly SC, Muir KR, Doherty M. Effectiveness of home exercise on pain and disability from osteoarthritis of the knee: a randomized controlled trial. Ann Rheum Dis 1999; 58:15–19.

110. Ota Y, Senda M, Hashizume H, et al. Chronic compartment syndrome of the lower leg: a new diagnostic method using near-infrared spectroscopy and a new technique of endoscopic fasciotomy. Arthroscopy 1999; 15(4):439–443.

111. Owen DS, Weiss JJ, Wilke WS. When to aspirate and inject joints. Patient Care 1990; 24(14):128–145.

112. Paavola M, Kannus P, Jarvinen T, et al. Achilles tendinopathy. J Bone Joint Surg 2002; 84A(11):2062–2076.

113. Parolie JM, Bergfeld JA. Long-term results of non-operative treatment of isolated PCL injuries in the athlete. Am J Sports Med 1986; 14:35–38.

114. Patterson JO. Ankle injuries. In: Lillegard WA, Rucker KS, eds. Handbook of sports medicine. Boston: Andover; 1993:172–183.

115. Patterson MJ, Cox WK. Peroneus longus tendon rupture as a cause of chronic lateral ankle pain. Clin Orthop Relat Res 1999; 365:163–166.

116. Pedowitz RA, Hargens AR, Murbarak SJ, et al. Modified criteria for the objective diagnosis of chronic compartment syndrome of the leg. Am J Sports Med 1990; 18:35.

117. Picard CL. The level of competition as a factor for the development of eating disorders in female collegiate athletes. J Youth Adolesc 1999; 28:583–594.

118. Powers CM. The effects of patellar bracing on clinical changes and gait characteristics in subjects with patellofemoral pain [abstract]. Phys Ther 1998; 30:S48.

119. Quirk R. Common foot and ankle injuries in dance. Orthop Clin North Am 1994; 25:123–133.

120. Quirk R. Stress fractures of the navicular. Foot Ankle Int 1998; 19:494–496.

121. Reginster J-Y, Deroisy R, Paul I, et al. Glucosamine sulfate significantly reduces progression of knee osteoarthritis over 3 years: a large randomized, placebo-controlled, double-blind, prospective trial [abstract]. Arthritis Rheum 1999; 42(suppl 9):S400.

122. Reginster JY, Deroisy R, Rovati LC, et al. Long-term effects of glucosamine sulphate on osteoarthritis progression: a randomized, placebo-controlled clinical trial. Lancet 2001; 357(9252):251–256.

123. Reid DC. Problems of the hip, pelvis, and sacroiliac joint. In: Sports injury assessment and rehabilitation. New York: Churchill Livingstone; 1992: 626–661.

124. Saxena A, Fullem B, Hannaford D. Results of treatment of 22 navicular stress fractures and a new proposed radiographic classification system. J Foot Ankle Surg 2000; 39:96–103.

125. Scott SH, Winter DA. Internal forces at chronic running injury sites. Med Sci Sports Exerc 1990; 22:357–369.

126. Scully TJ, Besterman F. Stress fracture: a preventable training injury. Mil Med 1982; 147:285–287.

127. Shaffer RA, Brodine SK, Almeida SA, et al. Use of simple measures of physical activity to predict stress fractures in young men undergoing a rigorous physical training program. Am J Epidemiol 1999; 149:236–242.

128. Shin AY, Gillingham BL. Fatigue fractures of the femoral neck in athletes. J Am Acad Orthop Surg 1997; 5:293–302.

129. Simkin A, Leichter I, Giladi M, et al. Combined effect of foot arch structure and an orthotic device on stress fractures. Foot Ankle 1989; 10:25–29.

130. Simonet WT, Saylor HL III, Sim L. Abdominal wall muscle tears in hockey players. Int J Sports Med 1995; 20:31–37.

131. Slavotinek JP, Verrall GM, Fon GT. Hamstring injury in athletes: using MR imaging measurements to compare extent of muscle injury with amount of time lost from competition. AJR Am J Roentgenol 2002; 179: 1621–1628.

132. Spector T, Harris PA, Hart DJ. Risk of osteoarthritis associated with long-term weight bearing sports. Arthritis Rheum 1996; 39:995–998.

133. Spitz DJ, Newberg AH. Imaging of stress fractures in the athlete. Radiol Clin North Am 2002; 40:313–331.

134. Stefanich RJ. Intra-articular corticosteroids in treatment of osteoarthritis. Orthop Rev 1986; 19:65–71.

135. Steinkamp LA, Dillingham MF, Markel MD. Biomechanical considerations in patellofemoral joint rehabilitation. Am J Sports Med 1993; 21: 438–444.

136. Styf JR, Korner LM. Chronic anterior-compartment syndrome of the leg: results of treatment by fasciotomy. J Bone Joint Surg 1986; 68A:1338.

137. Taimela S, Kujalu U, Osterman K. Intrinsic risk factors and athletic injuries. Sports Med 1990; 9:205.

138. Tol JL, Struijis PA, Bossuyt PM, et al. Treatment strategies in osteochondral defects of the talar dome: a systematic review. Foot Ankle 2000; 21: 11–126.

139. Tornese D, Bandi M, Melegati G, et al. Principles of hamstring strain rehabilitation. J Sports Traumatol 2000; 22(2):70–85.

140. Towheed TE. Glucosamine sulfate in osteoarthritis: a systematic review. Arthritis Rheum 1998; 41(suppl):S198.

141. Tria AJ, ed. Ligaments of the knee. New York: Churchill Livingstone; 1995.

142. Tyler TF, Nicholas SJ, et al. The association of hip strength and flexibility with the incidence of adductor muscle strains in professional ice hockey players. Am J Sports Med 2001; 29(2):124–128.

143. Vad V, Hong H, Zazzali M, et al. Exercise recommendations in athletes with early osteoarthritis of the knee. Sports Med 2002; 11:729–773.

144. Verrall GM, Slavotinek JP, Barnes PG, et al. Diagnostic and prognostic value of clinical findings in 83 athletes with posterior thigh injury—comparison of clinical findings with magnetic resonance imaging documentation of hamstring muscle strain. Am J Sports Med 2003; 31:969–973.

145. Waters PM, Millis MB. Hip and pelvic injuries in the young athlete. Clin Sports Med 1988; 7(3):513–526.

146. Watterson JR, Esdaile JM. Therapeutic mechanisms and clinical potential in osteoarthritis of the knee. J Am Acad Orthop Surg 2000; 8(5): 277–284.

147. Weber M, Niemann M, Lanz R, et al. Nonoperative treatment of acute rupture of the Achilles tendon: results of a new protocol and comparison with operative treatment. Am J Sports Med 2003; 31:685–691.

148. Wilber RL, Moffatt RJ, Scott BE, et al. Influence of water-run training on running performance [abstract]. Med Sci Sports Exerc 1994; 26:S4.

149. Yoshikawa T, Mori S, Santiesteban AJ, et al. The effects of muscle fatigue on bone strain. J Exp Biol 1994; 188:17–33.

150. Zanker CL, Swaine IL. Relation between bone turnover, estradiol, and energy balance in women distance runners. Br J Sports Med 1998; 32: 167–171.

Chapter

41

Low Back Pain

Karen P. Barr and Mark A. Harrast

Low back pain has become a costly burden to society and a leading cause of disability and loss of productivity. This chapter outlines the anatomy and biomechanics of the lumbar spine, and our current understanding of the physiology of low back pain. We discuss the clinical evaluation and treatment of various etiologies of low back pain and leg pain caused by lumbar spine disease.

EPIDEMIOLOGY

Low back pain is a symptom, not a disease, and has many causes. It is generally described as pain between the costal margin and the gluteal folds. It is extremely common. About 40% of people say that they have had low back pain within the last 6 months.[213] Studies have shown a lifetime prevalence as high as 84%.[220] Onset usually begins in the teens to early forties. Most patients have short attacks of pain that are mild or moderate and do not limit activities, but these tend to recur over many years. Most episodes resolve with or without treatment. The median time off work for a back injury is 7 days, and many people with low back pain never alter their activity. However, a small percentage of low back pain becomes chronic and causes significant disability. In most studies, about half the amount of sick days used for back pain are accounted for by the 15% of people who are home from work for more than a month. Between 80 and 90% of the healthcare and social costs of back pain are for the 10% who develop chronic low back pain and disability. Just over 1% of adults in the USA are permanently disabled by back pain, and another 1% are temporarily disabled.[140]

The percentage of patients disabled by back pain, as well as the cost of low back pain, has steadily increased over the past 25 years. This appears, however, to be more from social causes than from a change in the conditions that cause low back pain. The two most commonly cited factors are the increasing societal acceptance of back pain as a reason to become disabled, and changes in the social system that pay benefits to patients with back pain.

ANATOMY AND BIOMECHANICS OF THE LUMBAR SPINE

General concepts

The lumbar spine has a dichotomous role in terms of function, which is strength coupled with flexibility. The spine performs a major role in support and protection (*strength*) of the spinal canal contents (spinal cord, conus, and cauda equina) but also give us inherent *flexibility*, allowing us to place our limbs in appropriate positions for everyday functions.

The strength of the spine results from the size and arrangements of the bones, as well as from the arrangement of the ligaments and muscles. The inherent flexibility results from the large number of joints placed so closely together in series. Each vertebral segment can be thought of as a three-joint complex (one intervertebral disk with vertebral end plates, and two zygapophyseal joints). The typical lordotic framework of the lumbar spine assists with this flexibility but also increases the ability of the lumbar spine to absorb shock, which is an important role due to the amount of forces that travel through the spine on a regular basis.

The vertebrae

The bony anatomy of the lumbar spine consists of five lumbar vertebrae. A smaller percentage of the population has four (the fifth vertebrae is sacralized) or six (the first sacral segment is lumbarized). There are also anatomic variants consisting of a partially lumbarized S1, where there can be a pseudoarthrosis between the transverse process of the lowest lumbar vertebrae and the sacral alae, or the articulation might be entirely united through bony fusion. It is important to recognize this articulation, when it exists, as it has been hypothesized to be a potential source of pain.

The lumbar vertebrae have distinct components, which include the vertebral body, the neural arch, and the posterior elements (Fig. 41-1). The vertebral bodies increase in size as you travel caudally in the spine. The lower three are typically more wedge-shaped (taller anteriorly), which helps create the normal lumbar lordosis. The structure of these large vertebral bodies serves its weight-bearing function well to support axially directed loads; however, they would fracture more routinely were it not for the shock-absorbing intervertebral disks placed strategically between the vertebral bodies.

The sides of the bony neural arch are the pedicles, which are thick pillars that connect the posterior elements to the vertebral bodies. They are designed to resist bending, and to transmit forces back and forth from the vertebral bodies to the posterior elements. The posterior elements consist of the laminae, the articular processes, and the spinous processes. The superior and inferior articular processes of adjacent vertebrae create the zygapophyseal joints. Finally, the pars interarticularis is a part

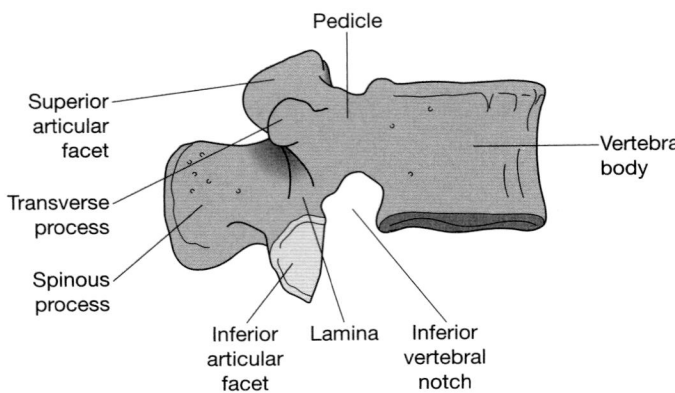

Figure 41-1 Lateral view of the lumbar vertebrae. (From Parke 1999,[154] with permission.)

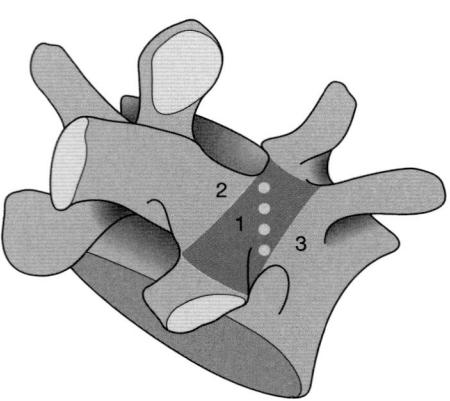

Figure 41-2 An oblique dorsal view of an L5 vertebra, showing the parts of the vertebral arch: 1, pars interarticularis (crosshatched area); 2, pars laminaris; and 3, pars pedicularis. The dotted line indicates the most frequent site of mechanical failure of the pars interarticularis. (From Parke 1999,[154] with permission.)

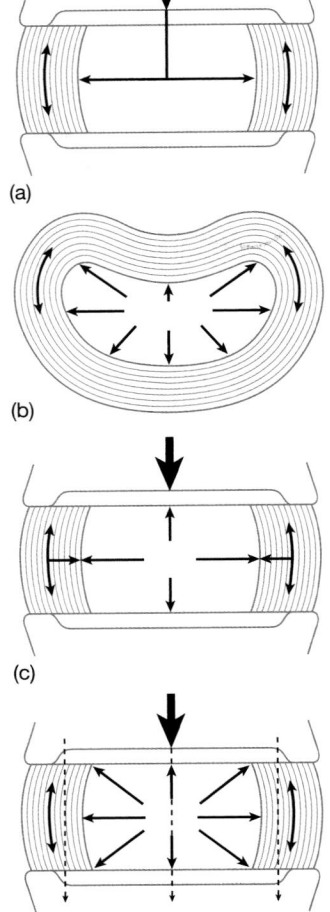

Figure 41-3 The mechanism of weight transmission in an intervertebral disk. (**a**) Compression raises the pressure in the nucleus pulposus. This is exerted radially on to the annulus fibrosus, and the tension in the annulus rises. (**b**) The tension in the annulus is exerted on the nucleus, preventing it from expanding radially. Nuclear pressure is then exerted on the vertebral end plates. (**c**) Weight is borne, in part, by the annulus fibrosus and by the nucleus pulposus. (**d**) The radial pressure in the nucleus braces the annulus, and the pressure on the end plates transmits the load from one vertebra to the next. (From Bogduk 1977,[26] with permission.)

of the lamina between the superior and inferior articular processes (Fig. 41-2). The pars is the site of stress fractures (spondylolysis), because it is subjected to large bending forces as the forces transmitted by the vertically oriented lamina undergo a change in direction into the horizontally oriented pedicle.[23]

The joints

The intervertebral disk

The intervertebral disk and its attachment to the vertebral end plate are considered a secondary cartilaginous joint, or symphysis. The disk consists of the internal nucleus pulposus and the outer annulus fibrosus. The nucleus pulposus is the gelatinous inner section of the disk. It consists of water, proteoglycans, and collagen. At birth, the nucleus pulposus is 90% water. Disks desiccate and degenerate as we age, and lose some of their height, which is one reason we are slightly shorter in our geriatric years.

The annulus fibrosus consists of concentric layers of fibers at oblique angles to each other, which help to withstand strains in any direction. The outer fibers of the annulus comprise more collagen, and less proteoglycans and water, than the inner fibers.[19] The varying composition supports the outer fibers' functional role in acting more as a ligament to resist flexion, extension, rotation, and distraction forces.

The main function of the intervertebral disk is shock absorption (Fig. 41-3). However, it is primarily the annulus that acts as the shock absorber, and not the nucleus, which is primarily a liquid (and incompressible). When an axial load occurs, the increase in force in the incompressible nucleus pushes on the annulus and stretches its fibers. If the fibers break, then a herniated nucleus pulposus results.

The zygapophyseal joints

The zygapophyseal joints (or Z joints) are paired synovial joints, i.e. they have a synovium and a capsule (Fig. 41-4). Their alignment or direction of joint articulation determines the direction of motion of the adjacent vertebrae. The lumbar zygapophyseal joints lie in the sagittal plane, and thus primarily allow flexion and extension, although some lateral bending and very little rotation are allowed, which limit torsional stress on the lumbar disks. Rotation is more a component of thoracic spine motion. The majority of flexion and extension (90%) occurs at the L4–5

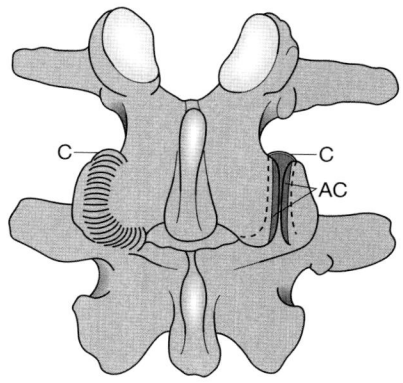

Figure 41-4 A posterior view of the L3–4 zygapophysial joints. On the left, the capsule of the joint (C) is intact. On the right, the posterior capsule has been resected to reveal the joint cavity, the articular cartilages (AC), and the line of attachment of the joint capsule (dashed line). The upper joint capsule (C) attaches further from the articular margin than the posterior capsule does. (From Bogduk 1977,[27] with permission.)

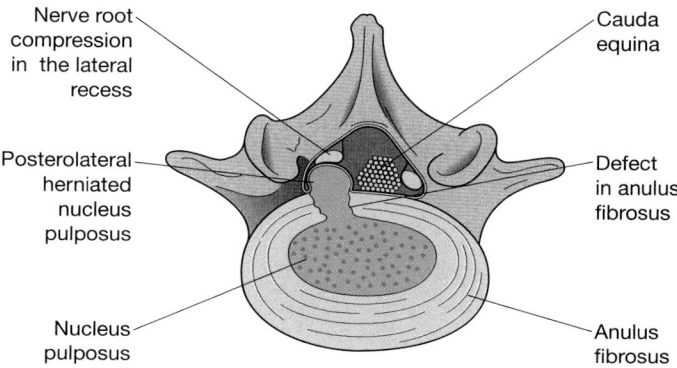

Figure 41-5 Posterolateral intervertebral disk herniation.

to S1 levels, thus contributing to the high prevalence of disk problems at these levels.

Biomechanics

Because flexion loads the anterior disk, the nucleus is displaced posteriorly.[102] If the forces are great enough, the nucleus can herniate through the posterior annular fibers. The lateral fibers of the posterior longitudinal ligaments are thinnest, however, making posterolateral disk herniations the most common (Fig. 41-5). The posterolateral portion of the disk is most at risk, with forward flexion accompanied by lateral bending (i.e. bending and twisting). Finally, when in flexion the zygapophyseal joints can no longer resist rotation. This increases torsional shear forces in the lumbar spine, making rotary movements in a forward-flexed posture probably the most risky for lumbar disks.

The ligaments

There are two main sets of ligaments of the lumbar spine: longitudinal ligaments and segmental ligaments. The two longitudinal ligaments are the anterior and posterior longitudinal ligaments. They are named according to their position on the vertebral body. The anterior longitudinal ligament acts to resist extension, translation, and rotation, whereas the posterior longitudinal ligament acts to resist flexion. Disruption of either ligament primarily occurs with rotation rather than with flexion or extension. The anterior longitudinal ligament is twice as strong as the posterior longitudinal ligament.

The main segmental ligament is the ligamentum flavum, which is a paired structure joining adjacent laminae and is the ligament that is pierced when performing lumbar punctures. It is a very strong ligament but also elastic enough to allow flexion. Flexing the lumbar spine puts this ligament on stretch, decreasing its redundancy and making it easier to pierce during a lumbar puncture.

The other segmental ligaments are the supraspinous, interspinous, and intertransverse. The supraspinous ligaments deserve mention, as they are the strong ligaments that join the tips of adjacent spinous processes and act to resist flexion. These ligaments, along with the ligamentum flavum, act to restrain the spine and prevent excessive shear forces in forward bending. This is supported by electromyographic studies that have shown that there is no active contraction of the erector spinae and hip extensor muscles when resting in lumbar flexion.

The muscles

Muscles with origins on the lumbar spine

These muscles can be divided anatomically into posterior and anterior muscles. The posterior muscles include the latissimus dorsi and the paraspinals. The lumbar paraspinals consist of the erector spinae (iliocostalis, longissimus, and spinalis), which act as the chief extensors of the spine, and the deep layer (rotators and multifidi) (Figs 41-6 and 41-7). The multifidi are tiny segmental stabilizers that act to control lumbar flexion, because they cannot produce enough force to truly extend the spine. Their more important function has been hypothesized as more of a sensory organ to provide proprioception for the spine, given the predominance of muscle spindles seen histologically in these muscles.

The anterior muscles of the lumbar spine include the psoas and quadratus lumborum. Because of the direct attachment of the psoas on the lumbar spine, tightening this muscle accentuates the normal lumbar lordosis. This can increase forces on the posterior elements and can contribute to zygapophyseal joint pain. The quadratus lumborum acts in side bending and can assist in lumbar flexion.

Abdominal musculature

The superficial abdominals include the rectus abdominis and external obliques (Fig. 41-8a). The deep layer consists of internal obliques and the transversus abdominis (Fig. 41-8b). The transversus abdominis has received significant attention over the recent past as an important muscle to train in treating low back pain. Its connection to the thoracolumbar fascia (and consequently its ability to act on the lumbar spine) has

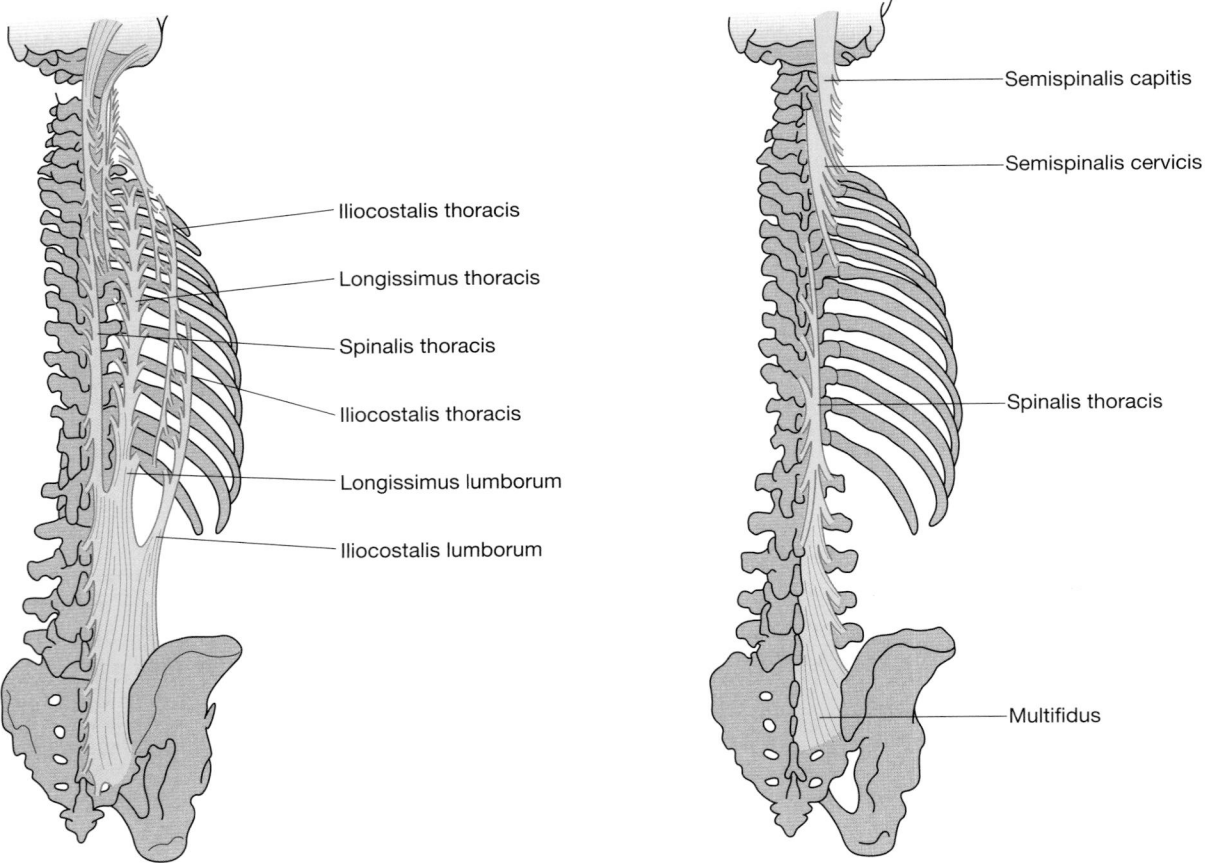

Figure 41-6 The intermediate layer of back muscles: the erector spinae.

Figure 41-7 The deep back muscles: the multifidi.

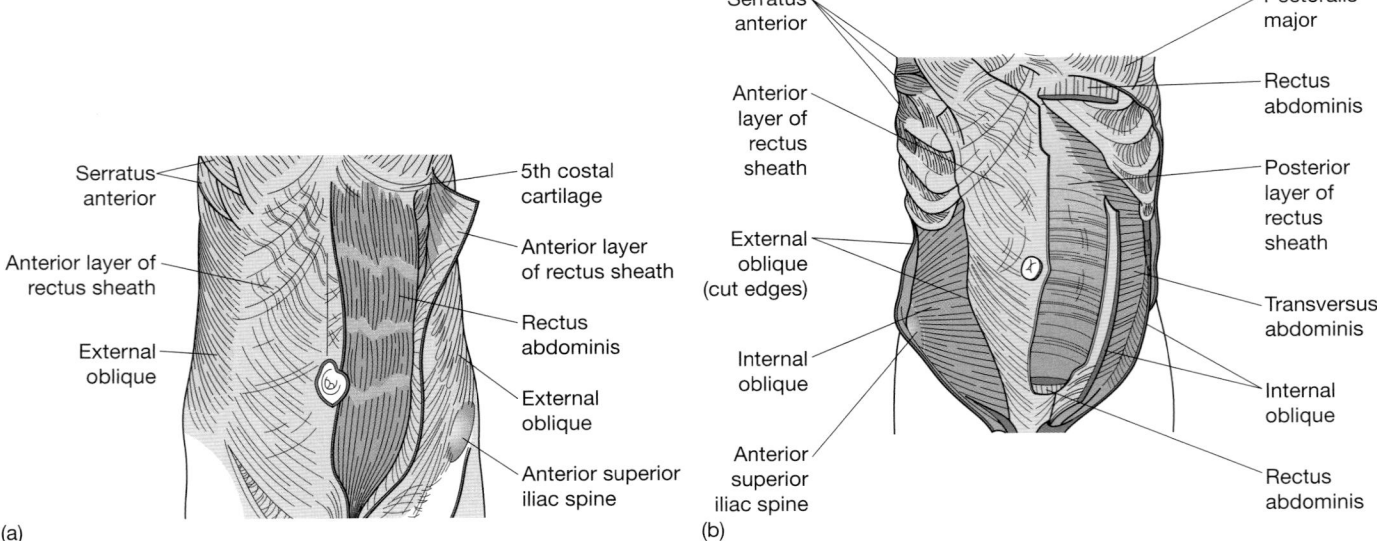

Figure 41-8 (**a**) The superficial abdominal muscles. (**b**) The deep abdominal muscles.

probably been the major reason it has received such attention of late.

Thoracolumbar fascia

The thoracolumbar fascia, with its attachments to the transversus abdominis and internal obliques, acts as an abdominal and lumbar 'brace'. It decreases some of the shear forces that other muscles and lumbar motions create. This abdominal bracing mechanism results from contraction of these deep abdominal muscles, which creates tension in the thoracolumbar fascia, which then creates an extension force on the lumbar spine without increasing shear forces.[71]

Pelvic stabilizers

The pelvic stabilizers are considered 'core' muscles due to their indirect effect on the lumbar spine, even though they do not have a direct attachment to the spine. The gluteus medius stabilizes the pelvis during gait. Weakness or inhibition of this muscle results in pelvic 'instability', which introduces lumbar side bending and rotation, creating increased shear or torsional forces on the lumbar disks.

The piriformis, as a hip and sacral rotator, can cause excessive external rotation of the hip and sacrum when it is tight. This can result in increased shear forces at the lumbosacral junction (i.e. the L5–S1 disk).

Biomechanical lifting in relation to muscular activity and disk loads

The activity of the lumbar muscles correlates well with intra-diskal pressures (i.e. when back muscles contract, there is an associated rise in disk pressure). These pressures change depending on spine posture and the activity undertaken. Figure 41-9 demonstrates these changes in L3 disk pressure under various positions and exercises.[141,142] Adding rotation to the already flexed posture increases the disk pressure substantially. Comparing lifting maneuvers, it has been shown that there is not a significant difference in disk pressure when lifting with the legs (i.e. with the back straight and knees bent) versus lifting with the back (i.e. with a forward-flexed back and straight legs).[6,7] What decreases the forces on the lumbar spine is lifting the load close to your body, as the farther the load is from the chest, the greater the stress on the lumbar spine.[7]

The nerves

The conus medullaris ends at about bony level L2, and below this level is the cauda equina. The cauda equina consists of the dorsal and ventral rootlets, which join together in the intervertebral neuroforamen to become the spinal nerves (Fig. 41-10). The spinal nerve gives off the ventral primary ramus, which, together from the other levels, forms the lumbar and lumbosacral plexus to innervate the limbs. The dorsal primary ramus, with its three branches (medial, intermediate, and lateral), innervates the posterior half of the vertebral body, the paraspinal muscles, and the zygapophyseal joints, and provides sensation to the back. The medial branch is the most important to remember, as it innervates the zygapophyseal joints and lumbar multifidi and is the target during radiofrequency neurotomy for presumed zygapophyseal joint pain (Fig. 41-11).[25]

BIOCHEMISTRY AND PATHOPHYSIOLOGY

Radiculitis and radiculopathy

Many patients with radicular pain have no neural impingement noted on magnetic resonance imaging (MRI). Studies have shown that disk herniations can cause an inflammatory response.[121,124,174] The mechanism stems from the fact that the

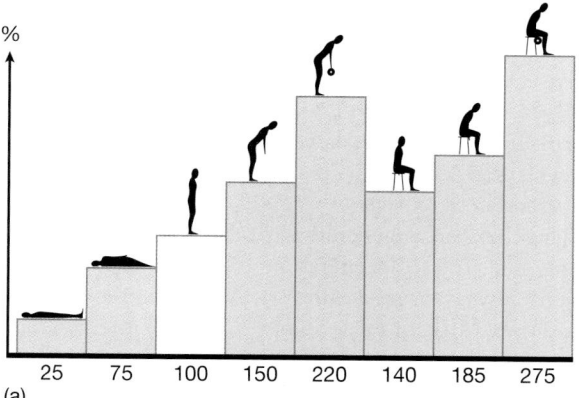

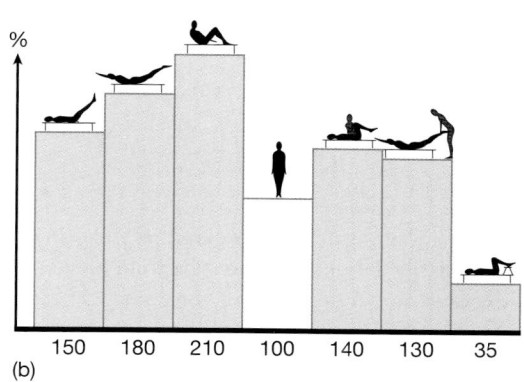

%

25 75 100 150 220 140 185 275

(a)

%

150 180 210 100 140 130 35

(b)

Figure 41-9 (a) Relative change in pressure (or load) in the third lumbar disk in various positions in living subjects. (b) Relative change in pressure (or load) in the third lumbar disk during various muscle-strengthening exercises in living subjects. Neutral erect posture is considered 100% in these figures; other positions and activities are calculated in relationship to this. (From Nachemson with permission of Lippincott Williams & Wilkins.)

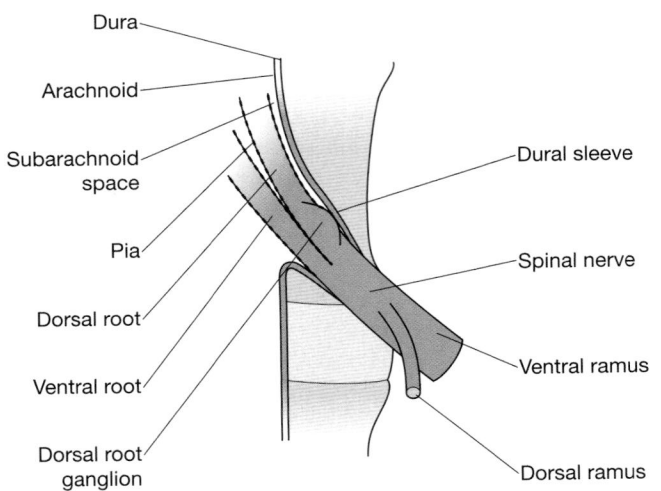

Figure 41-10 A lumbar spinal nerve, its roots and meningeal coverings. The nerve roots are invested by pia mater, and covered by arachnoid and dura as far as the spinal nerve. The dura of the dural sac is prolonged around the roots as their dural sleeve, which blends with the epineurium of the spinal nerve. (From Bogduk 1977,[24] with permission.)

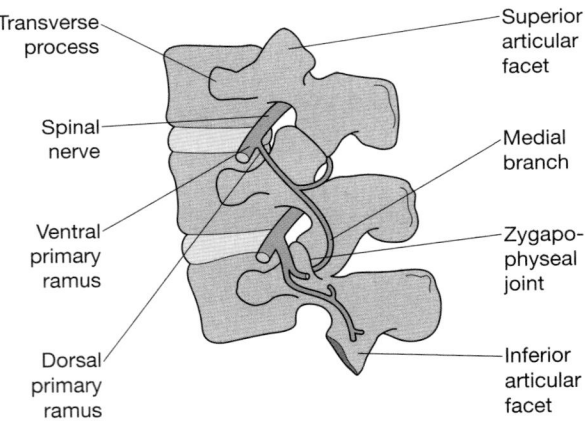

Figure 41-11 Observe that the innervation of the zygapophyseal joints derives from the medial branch off the dorsal primary ramus.

nucleus pulposus, being in an immunoprotected setting in non-pathologic states, is highly antigenic. When the fluid of the nucleus pulposus is exposed to neural tissue of the spinal canal and neuroforamen through a defect in the annular fibers, an autoimmune-mediated inflammatory cascade begins. The inflammatory mediators generated can cause swelling of the nerves. This can alter their electrophysiologic function, sensitizing these neurons and enhancing pain generation without specific mechanical compression.

Multiple inflammatory mediators have been identified at the site of disk injury, indicating their role in the pathogenesis of chemical radiculitis. These mediators include phospholipase A_2, cyclooxygenase-2, prostaglandin E_2, nitric oxide, cytokines, interleukins, and immunoglobulins.[62,70,136,174] Although these inflammatory mediators have all been implicated in the biochemical pathogenesis of radicular symptoms, the role of the inflammatory cells, including macrophages and neutrophils, has not yet been elucidated.[74,97]

The mechanism of mechanical compression of the nerve roots has been studied as well.[13,171,172] Compression of nerve roots can induce structural and vascular changes as well as inflammation.[142] Neural compression can result in impairment of intraneural blood flow, subsequently decreased nutrient supply to the neural tissue, local ischemia, and formation of intraneural edema. This can set off an inflammatory cascade similar to that described above. Mechanical stimulation of lumbar nerve roots has also been shown to stimulate production of substance P, the neuropeptide known to modulate sensory nociceptive feedback.[13] With these biochemical reactions, the local structural effects of mechanical compression (demyelination and axonal transport block) just compound the symptomatic response.

The degenerative spine cascade

Kirkaldy-Willis et al. have supplied us with the most accepted theory describing the cascade of events in degenerative lumbar spine disease that results in spondylotic changes, disk herniations, and eventually multilevel spinal stenosis (Fig. 41-12).[100] At the heart of this theory is the fact that, although the posterior zygapophyseal joints and the anterior intervertebral disks are separated anatomically, forces and lesions affecting one certainly alter and affect the other. For example, axial compressing injuries can damage the vertebral end plates, which can lead to degenerative disk disease, which eventually stresses the posterior joints, leading to the common degenerative changes seen in them over the course of time. Torsional stress can injure the posterior joints and/or the disks, which in turn leads to increased stress on both these elements, resulting in further degenerative changes over time. When these degenerative changes affect one level, say L4–5, a chain reaction occurs, placing stress on the levels above and below the currently affected level, and eventually resulting in more generalized multilevel spondylotic changes.

In studying lumbar degenerative disease, the question of which came first (disk degeneration or zygapophyseal joint degeneration) always arises. Fujiwara has answered this by studying multiple MRIs of aging spines.[63] He hypothesizes that disk degeneration precedes zygapophyseal joint osteoarthritis, and that it might take 20 years for zygapophyseal joint disease to occur after the onset of disk degeneration.

To describe the degenerative cascade in more detail, we will separate our discussion of the changes that occur in the posterior joints from those in the disk, but fully realizing that they

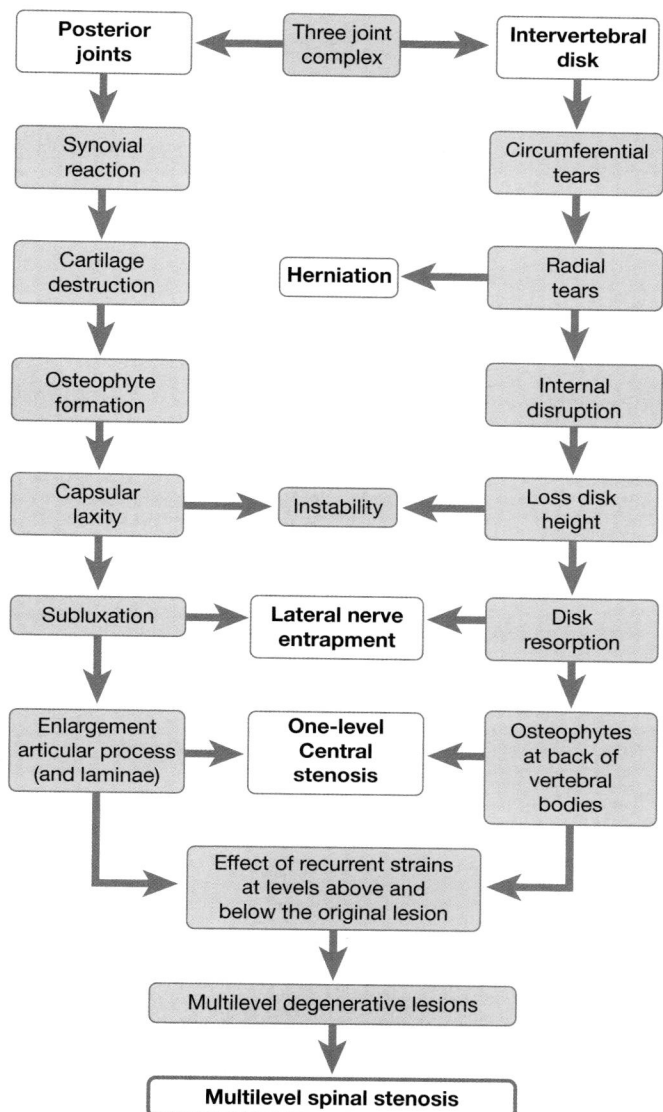

Figure 41-12 The spectrum of degenerative change that leads from minor strains to marked spondylosis and stenosis. (From Kirkaldy-Willis et al. 1978,[100] with permission of Lippincott Williams & Wilkins.)

A similar process is occurring anteriorly at the disk level from repetitive microtrauma of primarily shearing forces. Tears in the annulus are thought to be the first anatomic sign of degenerative wear. When the annulus is weakened enough, typically posterolaterally, the internal nucleus pulposus can herniate. However, internal disk disruption can occur without herniation as age and repeated stresses acting on the spine cause the gelatinous nucleus to become more fibrous over time. Tears in the annulus can progress to tears in the fibrous disk material, resulting in 'internal disk disruption' without frank herniation. All this results in a loss of disk height, which causes instability (as the end-plate connection to the disk is degenerated), as well as lateral recess and foraminal narrowing, and potential nerve root impingement. The loss of disk height also places new stresses on the posterior elements, resulting in further instability of the zygapophyseal joints and further degeneration and nerve root impingement.

The above description is a well-accepted theory of how mechanical compression of lumbar nerve roots and the cauda equina occurs to result in the neurogenic claudication symptoms of lumbar stenosis. More recently, there are newer theories that support a spinal vascular role in stenosis symptoms. Because there are many people with anatomic stenosis on imaging studies without symptoms, the following vascular theories have credence.

If mechanical compression were the sole problem in spinal stenosis, decompressive surgeries would be the only needed cure. We know that this is untrue, and consequently alternative theories on the pathogenesis of symptomatic spinal stenosis have been studied. Two theories supporting a vascular component to symptoms of spinal stenosis are the venous engorgement and arterial insufficiency theories.[1]

In the venous engorgement theory, the spinal veins of patients with stenosis dilate, causing venous congestion and stagnating blood flow.[42] This pooling of blood in the spinal veins increases epidural and intrathecal pressures, leading to a microcirculatory, neuroischemic insult (i.e. an ischemic neuritis), which in turn leads to the typical neurogenic claudication symptoms of stenosis.

The arterial insufficiency theory of spinal stenosis is based on the arterial dilatation of the lumbar radicular vessels during lower limb exercise to provide increased blood flow and nourishment to the nerve roots. In patients with spinal stenosis, this reflex dilatation might be defective.[14] As patients with spinal stenosis are typically elderly, they are also at higher risk for atherosclerosis, which in turn just amplifies the arterial insufficiency.

Pain generators of the lumbar spine

The low back is an anatomically diverse set of structures, and there are many potential sources of pain. This makes low back pain often complex and confusing for those inexperienced in spine medicine. One particularly useful strategy to clarify these potential sources of pain is learning what low back structures

both can occur simultaneously and affect each other (Fig. 41-12). The degenerative changes that occur in the zygapophyseal joints from aging and repetitive microtrauma are similar to those that occur in the appendicular skeletal joints. Initially, the synovium hypertrophies, which eventually results in cartilage degeneration and destruction. With lessened and weakened cartilage and capsular laxity, the joint can become unstable. With the repetitive abnormal joint motion that results from this instability, the bony joint hypertrophies. This narrows the central canal and lateral recesses, potentially impinging nerve roots.

Box 41-1 Potential pain generators of the back

A useful classification system to understand the potential sources of low back pain depends on knowing what structures are innervated (and can transmit pain) and what structures have no innervation.

Innervated structures
- Bone: vertebrae
- Joints: zygapophyseal
- Disk: only the external annulus and potentially diseased disk
- Ligaments: anterior longitudinal ligament, posterior longitudinal ligament, interspinous
- Muscles and fascia
- Nerve root

Non-innervated structures
- Ligamentum flavum
- Internal annulus
- Disk: nucleus pulposus

Box 41-2 Most common indications from history and examination for pathologic findings needing special attention and sometimes immediate action (including imaging)

- Back pain in children <18 years old with considerable pain, or onset in those > 55 years old
- History of violent trauma
- Constant progressive pain at night
- History of cancer
- Systemic steroids
- Drug abuse, HIV infection
- Weight loss
- Systemic illness
- Persisting severe restriction of motion
- Intense pain with minimal motion
- Structural deformity
- Difficulty with micturition
- Loss of anal sphincter tone or fecal incontinence, saddle anesthesia
- Widespread progressive motor weakness or gait disturbance
- Inflammatory disorders (ankylosing spondylitis) suspected
- Gradual onset <40 years
- Marked morning stiffness
- Persisting limitation of motion
- Peripheral joint involvement
- Iritis, skin rashes, colitis, urethral discharge
- Family history

(From Nachemson and Vingard 2001,[138] with permission of Lippincott Williams & Wilkins.)

---

are innervated (and thus can transmit pain through neural pain fibers) and what structures have no innervation (Box 41-1).

The sinuvertebral nerve innervates the anterior vertebral body, the external annulus, and the posterior longitudinal ligament. The posterior longitudinal ligament is a highly innervated structure, and can play a significant role in low back pain perception with lumbar disk herniations. The medial branch of the dorsal primary ramus innervates the zygapophyseal joints and interspinous ligaments, as well as the lumbar multifidi. The other small branches of the dorsal primary ramus innervate the posterior vertebral body and other lumbar paraspinal musculature and fascia. The anterior longitudinal ligament is innervated by the gray rami communicans, which branch off the lumbar sympathetic chain. The internal annulus fibrosus and nucleus pulposus do not have innervation and in non-disease states cannot transmit pain.

THE HISTORY AND PHYSICAL EXAMINATION OF THE LOW BACK

A complete history and physical examination is important in the evaluation of low back pain to determine the cause of the symptoms, rule out serious medical pathology, and determine if further diagnostic evaluation is needed.

The history

The causes of back pain are often very difficult to determine. For as many as 85% of patients, no specific cause for back pain is found.[46] A common rule of thumb quoted in medicine is that 85% of a diagnosis is made using the history alone. There is no reason to think that back pain should be significantly different. Therefore a thorough history is very important for the patient with back pain.

As with any pain history, features of back pain that should be explored include location; character; severity; timing, including onset, duration, and frequency; alleviating and aggravating factors; and associated signs and symptoms. Each of these features can assist the clinician in obtaining a diagnosis and prognosis, and determining the appropriate treatment.

A careful pain history such as this can identify serious medical pathology that can cause back pain, such as metastatic cancer, infection, and rheumatologic disease. Elements of historical information that suggest a serious underlying condition as the cause of the pain are called red flags (Box 41-2). When these are present, further work-up is necessary. Specific questions should be asked to clarify if any red flags are present. The sensitivity and specificity of the history in identifying red flags has been perhaps the best studied aspect of the low back pain history (Tables 41-1 to 41-3).

Besides determining specific facts about the pain, a purpose of the history is to explore the patient's perspective and illness experience. Certain psychosocial factors are valuable in determining prognosis (Box 41-3). Factors such as poor job satisfaction, catastrophic thinking patterns about pain, the presence of depression, and excessive rest or downtime are much more common in patients in whom back pain becomes disabling. These are called yellow flags, because the clinician should proceed with caution, and further psychologic evaluation or

Table 41-1 Sensitivities and specificities of different elements of the history and examination for some specific causes of low back pain

Disease or group of diseases	Symptom or sign	Sensitivity	Specificity
Spinal malignancy	Age > 50 years	0.77	0.71
	Previous history of cancer	0.31	0.98
	Unexplained weight loss	0.15	0.94
	Pain unrelieved by bed rest	0.90	0.46
	Pain lasting > 1 month	0.50	0.81
	Failure to improve with1 months' conservative therapy	0.31	0.90
	Erythrocyte sedimentation rate > 20 mm	0.78	0.67
Spinal infection	Intravenous drug abuse, urinary tract infection, skin infection	0.4	—
	Fever	0.27–0.83[a]	0.98
	Vertebral tenderness	'Reasonable'	'Low'
	Age > 50 years	0.84	0.61
Compression fracture	Age > 70 years	0.22	0.96
	Corticosteroid use	0.66	0.99
Herniated intervertebral disk	Sciatica	0.95	0.88

[a]The sensitivity of 'fever'.
(From Nachemson and Vingard 2001,[138] with permission.)

Table 41-2 Patterns of back pain

	Pattern	Where pain is worst	Aggravating movement	Relieving movement	Onset	Duration	Probable cause
Back-dominant pain or mechanical cause	1	Back or buttocks (<90% back pain); myotomes seldom affected; dermatomes not affected	Flexion; stiff in morning	Extension	Hours to days	Days to months (sudden or slow)	Disk involvement (minor herniation, spondylosis), sprain, strain
	2	Back or buttocks; myotomes seldom affected; dermatomes not affected	Extension or rotation	Flexion	Minutes to hours	Days to weeks (sudden)	Facet joint involvement, strain
Leg pain dominant or non-mechanical cause	3	Leg (usually below knee); myotomes commonly affected (especially in chronic cases); pain in dermatomes	Flexion	Extension	Hours to days	Weeks to months	Nerve root irritation (most likely cause is disk herniation)
	4	Leg (usually below knee); (may be bilateral); myotomes commonly affected (especially in chronic cases); pain in dermatomes	Walking (extension)	Rest (sitting) and/or postural change	With walking	—	Neurogenic intermittent claudication (stenosis)

(From Magee 2002,[115] with permission.)

Table 41-3 Some implications of painful reactions

Activity	Reaction of pain	Possible structural and pathologic implications
Lying sleeping	↓ ↑	Decreased compressive forces: low intradiskal pressures Absence of forces produced by muscle activity Change of position: noxious mechanical stress Decreased mechanoreceptor input Motor segment 'relaxed' into a position compromising affected structure Poor external support (bed) Non-musculoskeletal cause
First rising (stiffness)	↑	Nocturnal imbibition of fluid, disk volume greatest Mechanical inflammatory component (apophyseal joints) Prolonged stiffness, active inflammatory disease (e.g. ankylosing spondylitis)
Sitting	↑	Compressive forces High intradiskal pressure
With extension	↓ ↑	Intradiskal pressure reduced Decreased paraspinal muscle activity Greater compromise of structures of lateral and central canals Compressive forces on lower apophyseal joints
With flexion	↓ ↑	Little compressive load on lower apophyseal joints Greater volume, lateral and central canals Reduced disk bulge posteriorly Very high intradiskal pressures Increased compressive loads, upper and midapophyseal joints Mechanical deformation of spine
Prolonged sitting	↑	Gradual creep of tissues
Sitting to standing	↑	Creep, time for reversal, difficulty in straightening up Extension of spine, increase disk bulge posteriorly
Walking	↑	Shock loads greater than body weight Compressive loads (vertical creep) Leg pain Neurologic claudication Vascular claudication
Driving	↑	Sitting: compressive forces Vibration: vibro creep repetitive loading, decreased hysteresis loading, decreased hysteresis Increased dural tension sitting with legs extended Short hamstrings: pull lumbar spine into greater flexion
Coughing, sneezing, straining	↑	Increased pressure in subarachnoid space (increased blood flow, Batson's plexus, compromises space in lateral and central canal) Increased intradiskal pressure Mechanical 'jarring' of sudden uncontrolled movement

(From Magee 2002,[115] with permission.)

treatment should be considered if they are present. Some of these psychosocial factors are addressed by specific questions, and some become evident through statements that patients make during the history as they describe their illness experience. Questions about, for example, what patients believe is causing the pain, their fear and feelings surrounding this belief, their expectations about the pain and its treatment, and how back pain is affecting their lives (including work and home life) can yield valuable information. Many of these yellow flags are better prognostic indicators than the more traditional medical diagnoses.[214]

The physical examination
Table 41-4 outlines a thorough examination of the lumbar spine.

Observation
Observation should include a survey of the skin, muscle mass, and bony structures, as well as observation of overall posture (Fig. 41-13), and the position of the lumbar spine in particular (Fig. 41-14). Gait should also be observed for clues regarding etiology and contributing factors.

Table 41-4 Physical examination for low back pain

Examination component	Specific activity	Reason for this part of the examination
Observation	Observation of overall posture	Determine if structural abnormality or muscle imbalances are present
	Observation of lumbar spine	Further define muscle imbalance and habitual posture
	Observation of the skin	Search for diagnoses such as psoriasis, shingles, or vascular disease as cause of the pain
	Observation of gait	Screen the kinetic chain and determine if muscular, neurologic, or joint problems are contributing to symptoms
Palpation	Bones	Search for bony problems such as infection or fracture
	Facet joints	Identify if specific levels are tender
	Ligaments and intradiskal spaces	Determine if these are tender
	Muscles	Search for trigger points, muscle spasms, muscle atrophy
Active range of motion	Forward flexion	Amount, quality if painful
	Extension	—
	Side bending	Same, also side to side differences
	Rotation	—
Neurologic examination	Manual muscle testing of L1–S1 myotomes	Determine weakness
	Pinprick and light touch sensation, L1–S1 dermatomes	Determine sensory loss
	Reflexes: patellar, hamstring, Achilles	Test injury to L4, L5, or S1 roots if diminished, upper motor neuron disease if brisk
	Balance and coordination testing	Signs of upper motor neuron disease
	Plantar responses	Same
	Straight leg raise	Neural tension at L5 or S1
	Femoral nerve arch	Neural tension at L3 or L4
Orthopedic special tests	Abdominal muscle strength	Determines weakness and deconditioning
	Pelvis stabilizer strength, i.e. gluteus medius, maximus, etc.	Determines weakness and deconditioning
	Tightness or stiffness of hamstrings	Determines areas of poor flexibility
	Tightness or stiffness of hip flexors	—
	Tightness or stiffness of hip rotators	—
	Prone instability test	Signs of instability

Box 41-3 Some common 'yellow flags'

- The presence of catastrophic thinking: there is no way the patient can control the pain, that disaster will occur if the pain continues, etc.
- Expectations that the pain will only worsen with work or activity
- Behaviors such as avoidance of normal activity, and extended rest
- Poor sleep
- Compensation issues
- Emotions such as stress and anxiety
- Work issues, such as poor job satisfaction and poor relationship with supervisors
- Extended time off work

Palpation

Palpation should begin superficially and progress to deeper tissues. It can be done with the patient standing, or to ensure that the back muscles (Fig. 41-15) are fully relaxed, this is often done with the patient lying prone, perhaps with a pillow under the abdomen to slightly flex the spine into a position of comfort. It should proceed systematically to determine what structures are tender to palpation. Sometimes pressure over isolated vertebrae is applied to look for the painful level; this is known as prone instability testing.

Range of motion

Quantity of range of motion There are several ways to measure spinal range of motion (ROM). These include using a

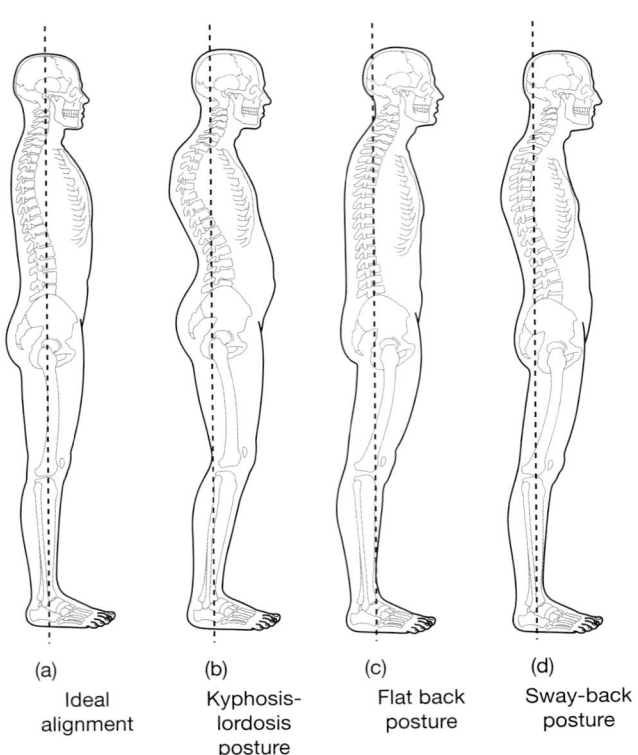

(a)
Ideal
alignment

(b)
Kyphosis-
lordosis
posture

(c)
Flat back
posture

(d)
Sway-back
posture

Figure 41-13 The four types of postural alignment: (**a**) ideal alignment, (**b**) kyphosis–lordosis posture, (**c**) flat back posture, (**d**) sway-back posture. (From Kendall and McCreary 1983,[97a] with permission.)

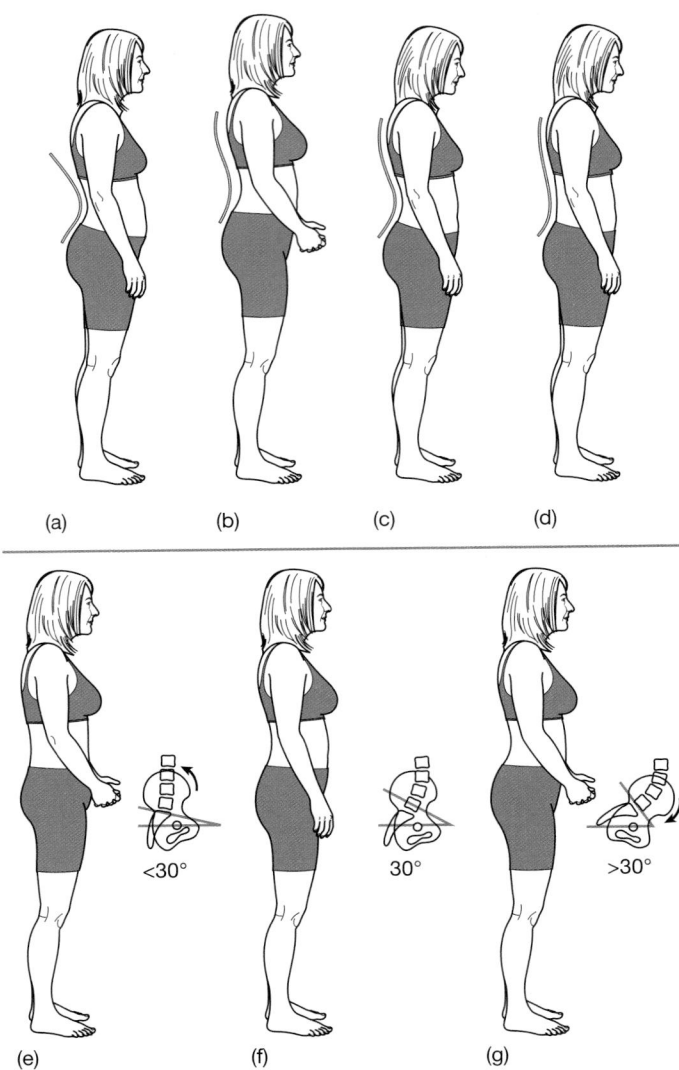

(a)   (b)   (c)   (d)

(e)   (f)   (g)

<30°   30°   >30°

Figure 41-14 Faulty pelvic alignment as a result of weak and long abdominal muscles (**a**), short and stiff hip flexors (**b**), apparent anterior tilt (**c**), and posterior tilt (**d**). The effect of pelvic tilting on the inclination of the base of the sacrum to the transverse plane (sacral angle) during upright standing is shown. (**e**) Tilting the pelvis backward reduces the sacral angle and flattens the lumbar spine. (**f**) During relaxed standing, the sacral angle is about 30°. (**g**) Tilting the pelvis forward increases the sacral angle and accentuates the lumbar spine. (From Sahrmann 2002,[176] with permission.)

single or double inclinometer; measuring the distance of finger-tips to floor; and, for forward flexion, the Schober test (measuring distraction between two marks on the skin during forward flexion). Of these methods, the double inclinometer has been shown to correlate the closest to measurements on radiographs.[73,192] The literature varies on inter- and intrarater reliability and the use of inclinometers. Fingertip to floor has good inter- and intrarater reliability, but this takes into account the movement of the pelvis, and is affected by structures outside the spine such as tight hamstrings.[158] The Schober test is commonly used to assess a decrease in forward flexion in ankylosing spondylitis. It is sensitive for this condition but is not specific. General figures for normal ROM are forward flexion, 40–60°; extension, 20–35°; lateral flexion, 15–20°; and rotation, 3–18°. Studies to determine normal ROM in asymptomatic adults have found large variations within the normal range.[155] The normal ROM of people without back pain, and the ROM in patients with back pain, overlap. It is unclear what the significance of decreased ROM is in patients with back pain, because many people without back pain also have limited range. ROM can also change depending on the time of day, the effort the patient expends, and many other factors.[230]

Quality of range of motion The examiner should record if there are abnormalities in the patient's movement pattern during ROM, such as a 'catch' in the range or whether it causes pain. This can give clues to the diagnosis. For example, pain with forward flexion can signify disk disease, and pain with

extension can signify spondylolisthesis, zygapophyseal joint disease, or spinal stenosis.

The neurologic examination

The neurologic examination of the lower extremities can rule out clinically significant nerve root impingement and other neurologic causes of leg pain (Tables 41-5 and 41-6). The physical examination should logically proceed to discover if a particular root level is affected by combining the findings of weakness, sensory loss, diminished or absent reflexes, and special tests such as straight leg raise. In addition, an upper motor neuron condition should be ruled out. The accuracy of the neurologic

Table 41-5 Factors that affect posture

Reason for abnormality	Clinical example
Bone structure	Compression fractures Scheuermann disease
Ligamentous laxity	Hyperextension of the knees, elbows
Muscle and fascial length	Tight hamstrings that cause a posterior pelvic tilt Weak and long abdominal muscles that allow an anterior pelvic tilt
Body habitus	Obesity or pregnancy causes changes in force and increased lumbar lordosis
Neurologic disease	Spasticity causes an extension pattern of the lower limb
Mood	Depression causes forward slumped shoulders
Habit	Long-distance cyclists have increased thoracic kyphosis and flat spine from prolonged positioning while riding

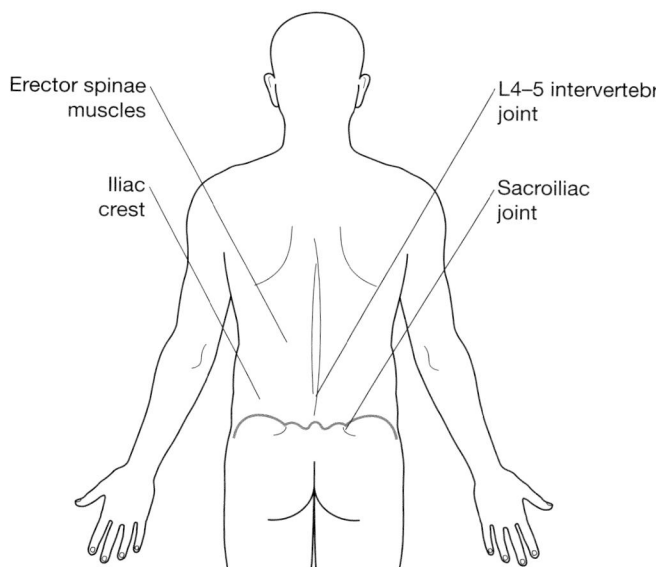

Erector spinae muscles

Iliac crest

L4–5 intervertebral joint

Sacroiliac joint

Figure 41-15 Anatomy of the low back surface anatomy.

examination in diagnosing herniated disk is moderate. However, combinations of findings increase the accuracy considerably.[46] The sensitivity and specificity of different findings for lumbar radiculopathy have been well studied (Table 41-7).

Orthopedic special tests to assess for relative strength and flexibility

Back pain can be caused by deconditioning, poor endurance, and muscle imbalances. Therefore, any inefficient or abnormal movement patterns of muscles that control the movement of the spine and the position of the pelvis should be identified. Because of their stabilizing effect on the spine, abdominal muscle strength and endurance is important. There are several different ways to measure abdominal muscle strength and

control. Kendall recommends two tests to grade abdominal muscles: the curl trunk sit up (Fig. 41-16), and holding the low back flat during leg lowering (Fig. 41-17).

Because of the great amount of strength needed for both these tests, and the inability of many patients with back pain even to perform the lowest grades, other tests have been developed to test abdominal strength. One grading system assesses whether the patient is able to maintain a neutral spine position while adding increasingly more challenging leg movements (Fig. 41-18).

Besides determining the strength of the abdominals, strength testing of the hip abductors and the ability to activate the gluteus maximus are often assessed to examine pelvic stability. Assessing for areas of relative inflexibility is also important. Commonly performed tests are hip flexor flexibility, hamstring flexibility, other hip extensors' length, and gastrocnemius/soleus length. Balance challenges, such as the ability to maintain single-footed stance, are also helpful to determine a patient's baseline status.

Orthopedic special tests for lumbar segmental instability

Many clinicians and researchers believe that one cause of mechanical low back pain is segmental instability that responds to specific stabilization treatments. Therefore accurately identifying this group from other forms of mechanical low back pain is important. These special tests include passive intervertebral motion testing and the prone instability test.

Passive intervertebral motion testing The patient lies prone. The examiner applies a firm steady pressure over the spinous process anteriorly, and assesses the amount of vertebral motion and whether pain is provoked.[85]

Prone instability test The patient lies prone, with the torso on the examining table and the legs over the edge of the table with the feet resting on the floor. The examiner performs passive intervertebral motion testing at each level and notes

Table 41-6 Lumbar root syndromes

Root	Dermatome	Muscle weakness	Reflexes or special tests affected	Paresthesias
L1	Back, over trochanter, groin	None	None	Groin, after holding posture, which causes pain
L2	Back, front of thigh to knee	Psoas, hip abductor	None	Occasionally front of thigh
L3	Back, upper buttock, front of thigh and knee, medial lower leg	Psoas, quadriceps–thigh wasting	Knee jerks sluggish, protein kinase B-positive, pain on full straight leg raise	Inner knee, anterior lower leg
L4	Inner buttock, outer thigh, inside of leg, dorsum of foot, big toe	Tibialis anterior, extensor hallucis	Straight leg raise limited, neck flexion pain, weak knee jerk; side flexion limited	Medial aspect of calf and ankle
L5	Buttock; back and side of thigh; lateral aspect of leg; dorsum of foot; inner half of sole and first, second, and third toes	Extensor hallucis, peroneals, gluteus medius, ankle dorsiflexors, hamstrings–calf wasting	Straight leg raise limited to one side, neck flexion pain, ankle jerk decreased, crossed leg raising pain	Lateral aspect of leg, medial three toes
S1	Buttock, back of thigh, and lower leg	Calf and hamstrings; wasting of gluteals, peroneals; plantar flexor	Straight leg raise limited	Lateral two toes, lateral foot, lateral leg to knee, plantar aspect of foot
S2	Same as S1	Same as S1, except peroneals	Same as S1	Lateral leg, knee, heel
S3	Groin, inner thigh to knee	None	None	None
S4	Perineum: genitals, lower sacrum	Bladder, rectum	None	Saddle area, genitals, anus, impotence

(From Magee 2002,[115] with permission.)

Table 41-7 Lumbosacral radiculopathy in patients with sciatica[a]

Finding[b]	Sensitivity (%)	Specificity (%)	Positive lumbosacral radiculopathy	Negative lumbosacral radiculopathy
Motor examination				
Weak ankle dorsiflexion	54	89	4.9	0.5
Ipsilateral calf wasting	29	94	5.2	0.8
Sensory examination				
Leg sensation abnormal	16	86	NS	NS
Reflex examination				
Abnormal ankle jerk	48	89	4.3	0.6
Other tests				
Straight leg-raising maneuver	73–98	11–61	NS	0.2
Crossed straight leg–raising maneuver	23–43	88–98	4.3	0.8

NS, Not significant.
[a]Diagnostic standard: for lumbosacral radiculopathy, surgical finding of disk herniation compressing the nerve root.
[b]Definition of findings: for ipsilateral calf wasting, maximum calf circumference at least 1 cm smaller than on contralateral side; for straight leg raising maneuvers, flexion at hip of supine patient's leg, extended at the knee, causes radiating pain in affected leg (pain confined to back or hip is a negative response); for crossed straight leg raising maneuver, raising contralateral leg provokes pain in the affected leg.
(From McGee 2001,[125] with permission.)

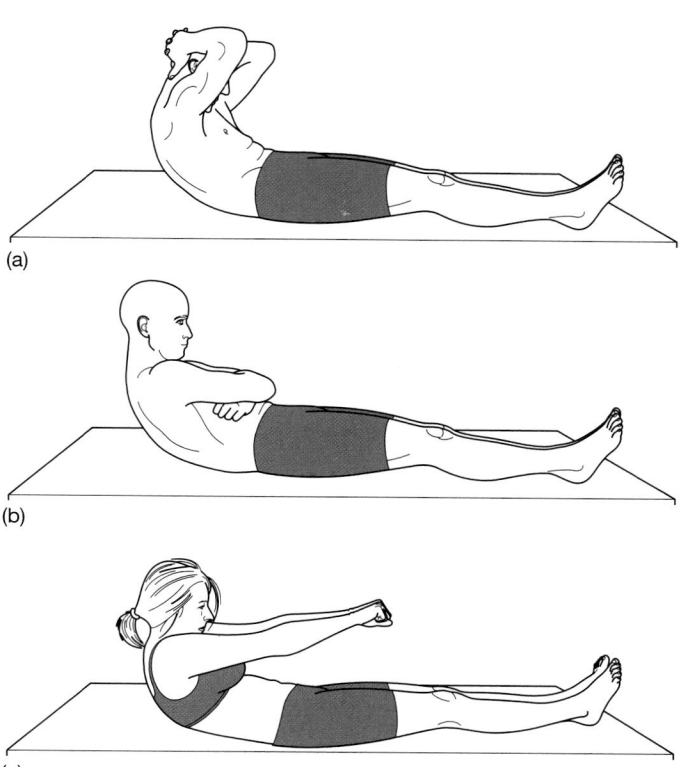

(a)

(b)

(c)

Figure 41-16 Trunk raising forward: grading. The curl trunk sit up is performed with the patient lying supine and with the leg extended. The patient posteriorly tilts the pelvis and flexes the spine, and slowly completes a curled trunk sit up. Kendall states that the 'crucial point in the test for the abdominal muscle strength is at the moment the hip flexors come into strong action. The abdominal muscle at this point must be able to oppose the force of the hip flexors in addition to maintain the trunk curl'. At the point where the hip flexors strongly contract, patients with weak abdominal muscles will tilt the pelvis anteriorly and extend the low back. (**a**) A 100% or normal grade is the ability to maintain spinal flexion and come into the sitting position with the hands clasped behind the head. (**b**) An 80% or good grade is the ability to do this with the forearms folded across the chest. (**c**) A 60% or fair grade is the ability to do this with the forearms extended forward. A 50% or fair grade is the ability to begin flexion but not maintain spinal flexion with the forearms extended forward. (From Kendall and McCreary 1983,[97a] with permission.)

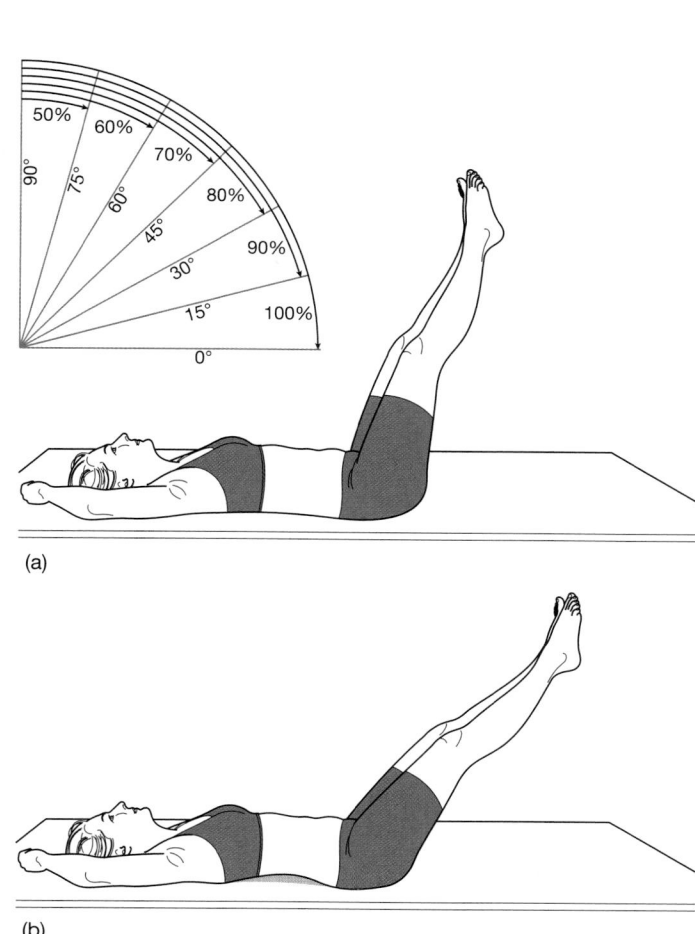

(a)

(b)

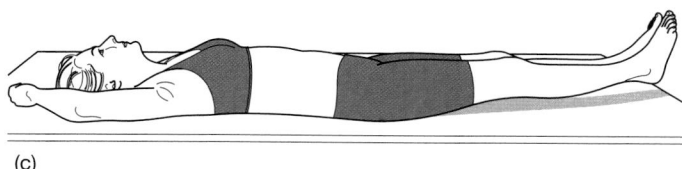

(c)

Figure 41-17 Leg lowering: grading. In the second test, the patient raises the legs one at a time to a right angle, and then flattens them back on the table. The patient slowly lowers the legs while holding the back flat. A 100% or normal grade is the ability to hold the low back flat on the table as the legs are lowered to the fully extended position. An 80% or good grade is the ability to hold the low back flat and lower the legs to a 30° angle. (**a**) A 60% or fair plus grade is the ability to lower the legs to 60° with the low back flat. (**b**) The pelvis tilted anteriorly and the low back arched as the legs were lowered. (**c**) The final position. Kendall notes that this second test is more important than the first (Fig. 41-16) in grading muscles essential to proper posture, and that often patients who do well on the first test do poorly on the second. (From Kendall and McCreary 1983,[97a] with permission.)

provocation of pain. Then the patient lifts the legs off the floor, and the painful levels are repeated. A positive test is when the pain disappears when the legs are lifted off the table. This is because the extensors are able to stabilize the spine in this position.[85,126]

Examining the area above and below the lumbar spine

Generally, in musculoskeletal medicine, the joint above and the joint below the painful area should be assessed to make sure nothing is missed. This is a good idea for the examination of the lumbar spine as well. ROM of the hip joints should be assessed, and a quick screen of the knee and ankle joint can determine if pathology in these areas is contributing to the back problem. The thoracic spine can be quickly screened as well during ROM and palpation.

Illness behavior and non-organic signs seen on physical examination

There are multiple reasons why patients with back pain might display symptoms out of proportion to injury. Illness behaviors are learned behaviors, and are responses that some patients use to convey their distress. Several studies have found that patients with chronic low back pain and chronic pain syndrome experience significant anxiety during the physical examination, even

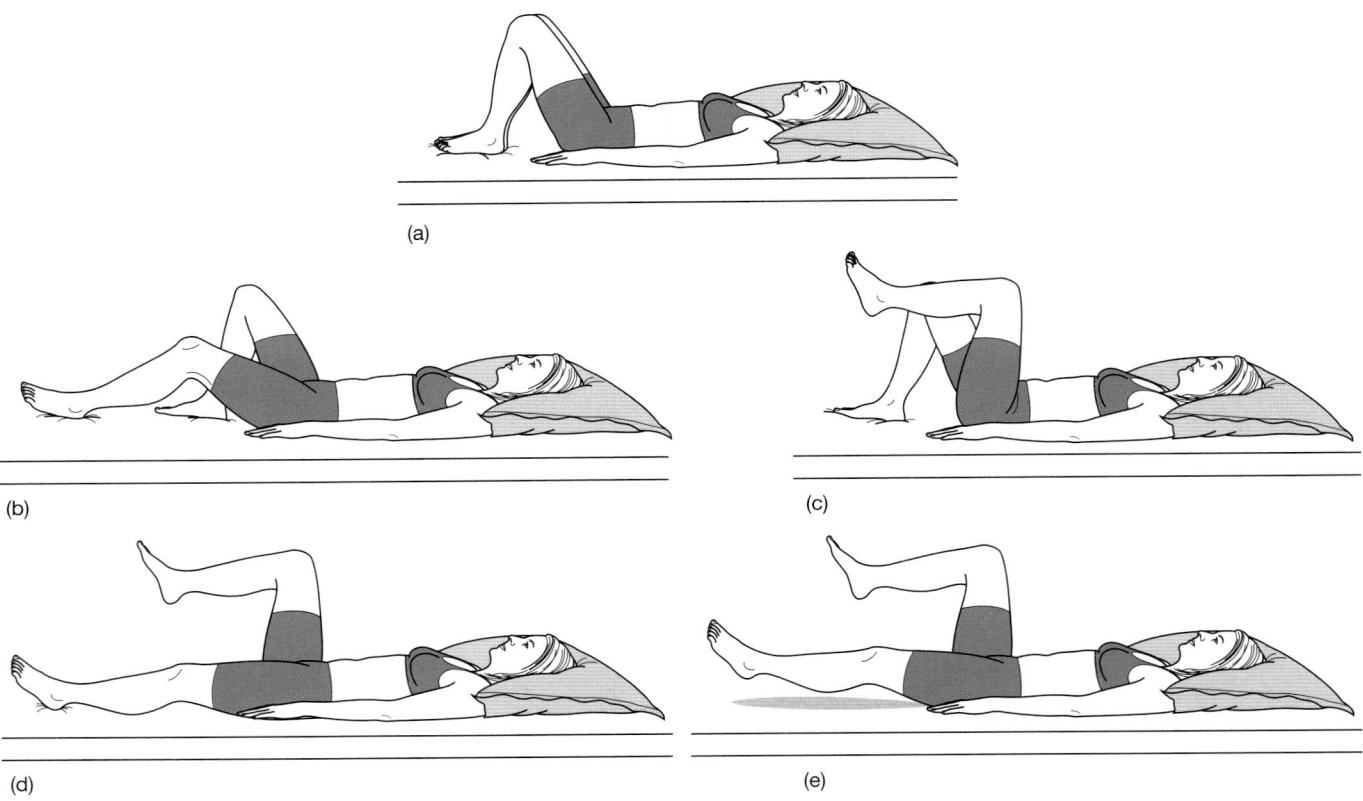

Figure 41-18 Abdominal strength grading. (**a**) The patient lies supine with the knees bent (supine crook lying). The physician cues the patient to activate the transversus abdominis ('Pull your belly button toward your backbone'), and a very slight lumbar lordosis is maintained in a neutral position in which the spine is neither flexed nor extended. The ability to maintain the neutral spine is progressively challenged by loading the spine via lower extremity movements. Grading is as follows. (**b**) Grade 1: the patient is able to maintain a neutral spine while extending one leg by dragging the heel along the table; the other leg remains in the starting position. (**c**) Grade 2: the patient is able to maintain a neutral spine while holding both legs flexed 90° at the hip and 90° at the knee, and touching one foot to the mat and then the other. (**d**) Grade 3: the patient is able to maintain a neutral spine while extending one leg by dragging the heel along the table. The other leg is off the mat and flexed 90° at the hip and 90° at the knee. (**e**) Grade 4: the patient is able to maintain a neutral spine while extending one leg hovered an inch or two above the table, while the other leg is off the mat and flexed 90° at the hip and 90° at the knee. Grade 5: the patient is able to extend both legs a few inches off the mat and back again while maintaining the spine in neutral.

to the level experienced during panic attacks. This complicates the assessment by altering the clinical presentation of the condition. This anxiety is generally manifest as avoidance behavior, such as decreased ROM or poor effort with muscle testing.[77] Other reasons for illness behavior include a desire to prove to physicians how disabling the pain is and malingering. One way to assess for illness behavior on physical examination is to perform parts of the examination to search for Waddell's signs. Waddell's signs are forms of illness behavior.[219] They are non-organic findings on physical examination that correlate with psychologic distress. They are as follow.

- Inappropriate tenderness that is widespread or superficial.
- Pain on testing that only simulates loading the spine, such as light pressure applied to the top of the head, which reproduces back pain, or rotating the hips and shoulders together to simulate twisting without actually moving the spine, which reproduces back pain.
- Inconsistent performance when testing the same thing in different positions, such as a difference in outcome of the straight leg-raising test with the patient supine versus sitting.

- Regional deficits in strength or sensation that do not have an anatomic basis.
- Overreaction during the physical examination.

Findings in three out of these five categories are suggestive of psychologic distress.

CLINICAL EVALUATION: DIAGNOSTICS

Imaging studies

Imaging of the lumbar spine should be used in the evaluation of low back pain if specific pathology needs to be confirmed after a thorough history and physical examination.

Plain radiography

Conventional radiographs are indicated in trauma to evaluate for fracture, and to look for bony lesions such as tumor when red flags are present in the history. As an initial screening tool for lumbar spine pathology, however, they have very low sensitivity and specificity.[68] Anterior–posterior and lateral views are the two commonly obtained views. Oblique views can be obtained to examine for a spondylolysis by visualizing the pars interarticularis and the 'Scottie dog' appearance of the lumbar spine (Fig. 41-19). Lateral flexion–extension views are obtained to check for dynamic instability, although the literature does not support their usefulness.[51] They are potentially most helpful from a surgical screening perspective when evaluating a spondylolisthesis. They are commonly obtained in posttrauma and postsurgical patients.

Magnetic resonance imaging

Magnetic resonance imaging is the preeminent imaging method for evaluating degenerative disk disease, disk herniations, and radiculopathy (Fig. 41-20) (see also Ch. 7). On T_2-weighted imaging, the annulus can be differentiated from the internal nucleus, and annular tears can be seen as high-intensity zones. These zones are of unclear clinical significance but are thought to be potential pain generators.

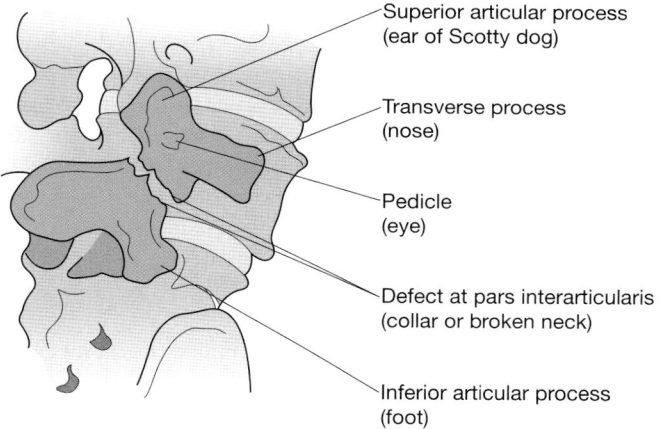

Figure 41-19 Oblique drawing of the lumbosacral junction, outlining the 'Scottie dog' and the area of spondylolysis.

Superior articular process
(ear of Scotty dog)

Transverse process
(nose)

Pedicle
(eye)

Defect at pars interarticularis
(collar or broken neck)

Inferior articular process
(foot)

Adding gadolinium contrast enhancement helps to identify structures with increased vascularity. Contrast is always indicated in evaluating for tumor or infection, or to determine scar tissue (vascular) versus recurrent disk herniation (avascular) in postsurgical patients with recurrent radicular symptoms.

The downside of MRI is that, although it is a very sensitive test, it is not very specific in determining a definite source of pain. It is well established that many people without back pain have degenerative changes, disk bulges, and protrusions on MRI. Boden demonstrated that one-third of 67 asymptomatic subjects were found to have a 'substantial abnormality' on MRI of the lumbar spine.[21] Of the subjects younger than 60, 20% had a disk herniation, and 36% of those older than 60 had a disk herniation and 21% had spinal stenosis. Bulging and degenerative disks were even more commonly found. In another study of lumbar MRI findings in people without back pain, Jensen demonstrated that only 36% of 98 patients had normal disks.[91] They found that bulges and protrusions were very common in asymptomatic subjects, but that extrusions were not. In a more recent study in 2001, Jarvik confirmed these findings.[90] In studying 148 asymptomatic subjects, he concluded that the less common findings on MRI of moderate or severe central stenosis, root compressions, and disk extrusions are likely to be clinically relevant. MRI is rarely appropriate in an initial work-up unless there has been a major acute injury or there are symptoms of infection, tumor, or progressive neurologic loss.[84]

Computed tomography

Because of the resolution of anatomic structures in MRI, it has essentially replaced computed tomography (CT) scanning as the imaging study of choice for low back pain and/or radiculopathy. However, CT scanning is still more useful than MRI in evaluating bony lesions. CT scans are also useful in the postsurgical patient with excessive hardware that can obscure magnetic resonance images, and in patients with implants (aneurysm clips or pacemakers) that preclude MRI.

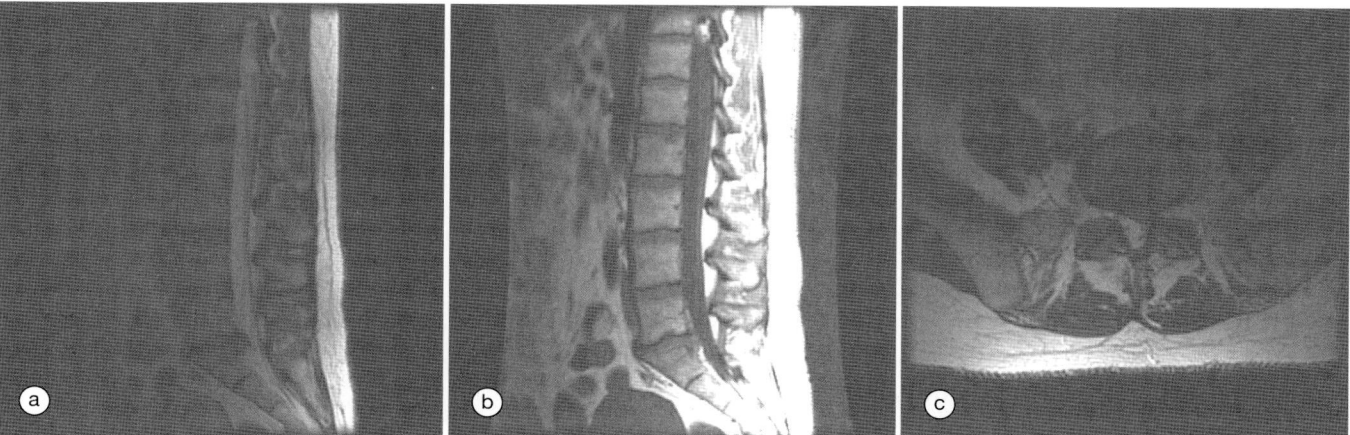

Figure 41-20 Disk extrusion in a 48 year old woman with back and left leg pain. (**a** and **b**) Sagittal T_2 and T_1-weighted MRI showing L5–S1 disk extrusion with caudal extension. (**c**) Axial T_2-weighted MRI showing the extrusion is left paracentral in the lateral recess, occupying the space where the S1 root resides.

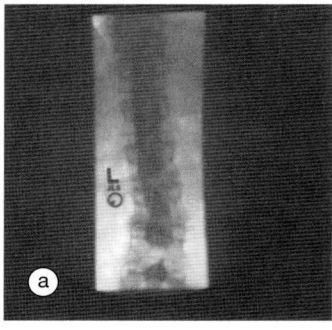
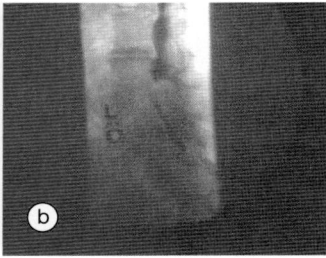

Figure 41-21 Anteroposterior (**a**) and lateral (**b**) myelograms of a 59-year-old woman with severe L4–5 central stenosis due to a large left L4–5 zygapophyseal joint synovial cyst. Note the obvious filling defect at the L4–5 level. She had symptoms of cauda equina syndrome and regained full neurologic function after decompression surgery.

Myelography

In myelography, contrast dye is injected into the dural sac and plain radiographs are performed to produce images of the borders and contents of the dural sac (Fig. 41-21). CT images can also be obtained after contrast injection to produce axial cross-sectional images of the spine that enhance the distinction between the dural sac and its surrounding structures. This is typically reserved as a potential presurgical screening tool but has been utilized less with the advancement of MRI.

Scintigraphy

Radionuclear bone scanning is a fairly sensitive but not specific imaging modality that can be used to detect occult fractures, bony metastases, and infections. To increase anatomic specificity, single-photon emission computed tomography (SPECT) bone scanning is used to obtain bone scans with axial slices. This allows the diagnostician to differentiate uptake in the posterior elements from more anterior structures of the spine. The diagnostic utility of this study with regard to altering clinical decision making is controversial and has not been well studied.

Electromyography

Electromyography is useful in evaluating radiculopathy, as it provides a physiologic measure for detecting neurogenic changes and denervation with good sensitivity and high specificity. It can help to provide information as to which anatomic lesions found in imaging studies are truly physiologically significant.[169] See Chapters 10, 11, and 12 for further details.

Laboratory studies

Bloodwork is rarely used in isolation as a diagnostic strategy for low back pain. It is helpful as an adjunct in diagnosing inflammatory disease of the spine (with such markers of inflammation as sedimentation rates and C-reactive proteins) and some neoplastic disorders, such as multiple myeloma with a serum protein electrophoresis and urine protein electrophoresis.

DIFFERENTIAL DIAGNOSIS AND TREATMENT: THE PROTOTYPE OF BACK PAIN GREATER THAN LEG PAIN

Mechanical low back pain

Nearly 85% of those who seek medical care for low back pain do not receive a specific diagnosis.[46] The majority of these patients most probably have a multifactorial cause for back pain, which includes functional instability; deconditioning; abnormal posture; poor muscle recruitment; emotional stress; and changes associated with aging and injury such as disk degeneration, arthritis, and ligamentous hypertrophy. This type of back pain can be given many names; simple backache, nonspecific low back pain, lumbar strain, and spinal degeneration are a few of the common names for this condition. The name given to a condition sends certain messages to the patient who receives the diagnosis. For example, the term *simple backache* may cause a patient to think that the physician misunderstands because, from the patient's perspective, the pain is not simple if it has not resolved in a few days. The label *non-specific low back pain* can cause the patient to continue to seek care from multiple providers in order to receive a specific diagnosis. *Lumbar strain* suggests that the condition was caused by overactivity, which is often not the case, and that further physical activity would cause it to recur, which is not true. *Spinal degeneration* sends the message that the changes are permanent and will probably worsen.[214] The term *mechanical low back pain* is perhaps the best term for this multifactorial axial backache. It suggests the mechanism of injury better than terms such as *strain* or *sprain*. It does not imply permanence. It is precise, and it suggests that, by changing biomechanics, improvement can occur.

The biomechanics of the spine are not unlike the biomechanics of other systems, in that longevity of the components and efficiency of the system depend on precise movements of each segment. In the spine, this means both an alignment in sustained postures and movement patterns that reduce tissue strain and allow for efficient muscle action without trauma to the joints or soft tissue.[176] The biomechanical model for the treatment of mechanical low back pain is that movement patterns which are altered because of faulty strength and flexibility, fatigue from poor endurance, or abnormal neural control can eventually cause tissue damage. Tissue damage can also lead to abnormal movement patterns and further damage, which is the basis for the Kirkaldy-Willis degenerative cascade.[115] One of the goals of rehabilitation is to categorize faulty alignment and abnormal movement patterns so that specific treatment can be given. Clinicians and researchers alike theorize that, when alignment and movement patterns deviate from the ideal, degeneration and tissue overload is more likely, just like abnormal tire wear occurs on a car out of alignment. Unlike machinery, the body can adapt with time to stress on the segments. This adaptation can be the healthy response of tissue to loading (as is seen with exercise), such as muscle hypertrophy or increased bone density, or it can begin a cycle of microtrauma that can lead to macrotrauma.[115,128,176] The theoretic model for this approach is strong, and research is beginning to validate many of these concepts, although this is not easy given the complex nature of the system.

Physical factors associated with mechanical low back pain

Segmental instability   The biomechanical model is particularly complex in the spine, because of the presence of global movement patterns and segmental movement patterns. Two interrelated muscular tasks must be carried out at the same time: maintaining overall posture and position of the spine, and control of individual intersegmental relationships. Sufficient joint stiffness is required at the segmental level to prevent injury and allow for efficient movement. This stiffness is achieved with specific patterns of muscle activity, which differ depending on the position of the joint and the load on the spine. The inability to achieve this stiffness, and the resulting segmental instability, is thought to be a common factor in mechanical low back pain.[166]

Instability can be a result of tissue damage, poor muscular endurance, or poor muscular control, and is usually a combination of all three factors. Structural changes from tissue damage, such as strained or failed ligaments that cause joint laxity, vertebral end-plate fractures, and loss of disk height, can lead to segmental instability because of the altered anatomy. However, muscles provide the most critical component of spinal stability. A cadaver spine in which the bones and ligaments are intact but the muscles have been removed will buckle under only 20 lbs of compressive load. The human spine with muscles functioning properly, however, can handle many times that load.[127]

In normal situations, only a small amount of muscular coactivation, about 10% of maximal contraction, is needed to provide segmental stability. In a segment damaged by ligamentous laxity or disk disease, slightly more might be needed. Because of the gentle force required to perform activities of daily living, muscular endurance is more important than absolute muscle strength for most patients, although some strength reserve is needed for unpredictable activities such as a fall, a sudden load to the spine, or quick movements. In sports and heavy physical work, both strength and endurance needs increase. For example, in rapid breathing caused by exertion, there is rhythmic contraction and relaxation of the abdominal wall. A fit person can simultaneously provide spine support with abdominal wall muscles, and meet breathing demands, but a less fit person might not be able to and therefore could more easily become injured or have pain.[127]

Muscular imbalances and neural processing problems   It has been known for many years that disk disease, ligamentous injury, and arthritis can cause low back pain. More recently, a significant amount of research is emerging with the following aims.

- To determine what muscular abnormalities exist in patients with back pain.

- To ascertain if exercise training can lead patients with low back pain to develop more normal firing patterns, endurance, and strength ratios.
- To see whether this in turn will improve pain.

If these three things can be shown, then the next step will be determining if patients at risk for back pain can be identified and treated before they develop problems.

There appear to be consistent muscular problems in patients with persistent low back pain. Some of these factors might exist preinjury and make the spine more susceptible to injury, and some are adaptations to injury. Just as is seen in other areas of the body such as the knee, muscle function and strength around the spine is altered after injury. Studies of patients with back pain have found significant muscle recruitment abnormalities. For example, a group working at the University of Queensland in Australia studied patients with no history of low back pain, and found that contraction of the transversus abdominis preceded contraction of muscles that move the arms and legs when subjects were instructed to move their limbs in a certain direction in response to a stimulus. These contractions happened without conscious effort by the pain-free subjects to stabilize the spine before limb contractions began, so that unwanted trunk movements would not occur with limb movement. However, in patients with low back pain, firing of the transversus abdominis is delayed, often occurring after the limb movement is completed.[165] Other studies have also uncovered abnormal firing patterns in the deep stabilizers of the spine with activities such as accepting a heavy load and responding to balance challenges. Other researchers have found strength ratio abnormalities and endurance deficits in patients with low back pain, such as abnormal flexion to extension strength ratios and lack of endurance of torso muscles.[128]

Lumbar paraspinal abnormalities   Studies of lumbar paraspinals have found several abnormalities in patients with low back pain. Multiple imaging studies have demonstrated paraspinal muscle atrophy, particularly multifidi atrophy, in patients with chronic low back pain. In a study using ultrasound to measure the multifidi in patients with unilateral acute and subacute low back pain compared to subjects without low back pain, the side to side difference in multifidi size was $3 \pm 4\%$ in the normal subjects and $31 \pm 8\%$ in the patients with low back pain. The atrophy was found on the same side as the symptoms, and was usually confined to one vertebral level. One subject was measured within 24 h of developing pain and displayed asymmetry, and the researchers interpreted this as the result of segmental inhibition of the multifidus.[166]

Recovery of the multifidi does not appear to occur spontaneously with the resolution of back pain. The same researchers performed a randomized trial of 39 subjects with acute first-episode unilateral low back pain with multifidus atrophy. Subjects were randomized to a control group and a treatment group. The treatment group received specific exercises for multifidus activation and strengthening; the control group received education and usual care. Both groups had near resolution of back pain and return to baseline function at 4 weeks. However, in the control group, the multifidi remained almost unchanged at 4 and 10 weeks, while in the treatment group the multifidus cross-sectional area was restored to normal within 4 weeks of treatment. Long-term follow-up revealed that 30% in the treatment group suffered a recurrence of back pain within a year, and 80% of the control group suffered a recurrence. After 3 years, people in the control group were 12.4 times more likely to have further episodes of pain than those in the exercise group.[86]

Biopsies of multifidi in patients with low back pain also show abnormalities. Atrophy of type 2 muscle fibers is found, and internal structural changes of type 1 fibers that give them moth-eaten appearance are seen. In a study of patients undergoing surgery for lumbar disk herniations with duration of symptoms from 3 weeks to 1 year, multifidi biopsies collected at the time of surgery revealed type 2 muscle atrophy and type 1 fiber structural changes. Biopsies were repeated 5 years postoperatively. Type 2 fiber atrophy was still found in all patients, both those who had improved with surgery and those who had not. However, in the positive outcome group, the percentage of type 1 fibers with abnormal structures had decreased, and in the negative outcome group there was a marked increase in abnormal type 1 fibers.[161]

There is increasingly strong scientific support for the multifactorial nature of low back pain, which includes both structural and dynamic factors. This gives a theoretic basis for treatment aimed at improving spine biomechanics as a means of treating mechanical low back pain, along with other treatments aimed at pain management. The research in this area is intriguing but not yet conclusive. As is further discussed in the *Prevention of back pain* section, it is unclear whether these muscular abnormalities are the result of back pathology that leads to pain, or the cause of back pain. Study results conflict regarding consistent deficits in patients with back pain. This again reflects the heterogeneous nature of the group of patients classified as having mechanical low back pain, and that different factors predominate for different patients.

Psychosocial factors and low back pain

Pain is an individual experience, and biomechanical factors alone do not explain much of the variance seen clinically in patients with back pain. Multiple psychosocial factors have been found to play a role in low back pain. This is briefly discussed here, and more thoroughly discussed in the chapter on chronic pain, as these issues are shared by multiple painful conditions and not just low back pain.

Depression and anxiety　It appears that between 30 and 40% of those with chronic back pain also have depression.[107] This rate is so high because depressed patients are more likely to develop back pain and to become more disabled by pain, and because some patients with persistent pain become depressed. Patients who are depressed are at increased risk of developing back and neck pain. In a recent analysis of factors leading to the onset of back and neck pain, those in the highest quartile for depression scores had a fourfold increased risk of developing low back pain than those in the lowest quartile for depression

scores.[37] There is also strong evidence that psychosocial factors are closely linked to the transition from acute pain to chronic pain and disability. In a study of 1628 patients with back pain seen at a pain clinic, those with a comorbid diagnosis of depression were over three times more likely to be in the worst quartiles of physical and emotional functioning on the 36-Item Short-Form Health Survey than those who were not depressed.[65] Multiple other studies have found that depression, anxiety, and distress are strongly related to pain intensity, duration, and disability.[110]

Patient beliefs about pain and pain cognition　Beliefs about back pain can be highly individual and are often not based on facts. Some patients with back pain, especially those with chronic low back pain that keeps them from working, have a great deal of fear about back pain. These include fears that their pain will be permanent, that it is related to activity, and that exercise will damage their back. This set of beliefs is labeled fear-avoidance. For example, studies have found that patients with chronic low back pain who perform poorly on treadmill exercise tests,[178] walk slower on treadmill tests,[3] and perform more poorly on spinal isometric exercise testing[4] were the ones with more anticipation of pain than those who did well on these tests. Fear-avoidance beliefs rather than actual pain during testing predicted their performance. Fear-avoidance levels explain self-reported disability and time off work more accurately than actual pain levels or medical diagnosis do.[117] This has led Waddell and other experts to state that 'the fear of pain may be more disabling than pain itself'.[219]

A large, population-based study found that subjects with high levels of pain catastrophizing, characterized by excessively negative thoughts about pain, and high fear of movement and injury or reinjury (kinesophobia), who had back pain at baseline were much more likely to have especially severe or disabling pain at follow-up compared to those who did not catastrophize. For those without back pain at the initial questionnaire, catastrophizers were more likely to have developed low back pain with disability at follow-up than non-catastrophizers.[159] Thought processes, such as the presence of catastrophizing, are not limited to back pain and are often part of a larger pattern of relationships and thought processes.

Patients' beliefs about pain and their approach to dealing with pain have been consistently found to affect outcomes. Fortunately, changes in these beliefs and cognitive patterns are possible. Multidisciplinary pain programs have proven effective in decreasing fear-avoidant beliefs and catastrophizing (see Ch. 43).[188]

These changes in beliefs can also improve function. For example, a study in which a group of patients with chronic low back pain underwent a cognitive behavioral treatment program found that, although there were not significant changes in pain intensity, those with reductions of fear-avoidance beliefs had significant reductions in disability. Changes in fear-avoidant beliefs accounted for 71% of the variance in reduction in disability in this study.[229]

History, physical examination, and diagnostic tests in mechanical low back pain

The history and physical examination in mechanical low back pain is variable. There are no specific diagnostic tests for mechanical low back pain. Tests and imaging are used to exclude other diagnoses.

Treatment of mechanical low back pain

Reassurance and patient education   Education should include providing as much of an explanation as patients need in terms they can understand. In addition, the physician should provide empathy and support, and impart a positive message. Reassurance that there is no serious underlying pathology, that the prognosis is good, and that the patient can stay active and get on with life despite the pain can help counter negative thoughts and misinformation that the patient might have about back pain.[214]

There is strong evidence from systematic reviews that the advice to continue ordinary activity as normally as possible fosters faster recovery and can lead to less disability than the advice to rest and 'let pain be your guide'.[215] It is controversial whether patients with low back pain fare better with a specific diagnosis or not. Education and explanations, however, should be adequate. As Waddell states in his book *The Back Pain Revolution*, 'Simply saying that "I can't find anything wrong" may imply that you are not sure and make patients worry more!'[214] On the other hand, some diagnoses carry negative messages to patients that suggest permanent damage and the need to 'get fixed', such as degenerative disk disease or arthritis.[214] Mechanical low back pain is a useful diagnostic term, because it implies the mechanism of the pain and the way it is best treated without suggesting permanence.

Beyond a diagnosis, there is other information that patients want about low back pain. In a study of patients who presented with low back pain to their primary care doctors in a health maintenance organization setting, the information that patients wanted from their doctor included the likely course of their back pain, how to manage their pain, how to return to usual activity quickly, and how to minimize the frequency and severity of recurrences. They ranked each of these areas of education a higher priority than finding a cause or receiving a diagnosis for their pain.[214] Providing this information in an amount and in a way that patients can understand helps build a therapeutic doctor–patient relationship and, it is hoped, help reduce anxiety and speed recovery.

Back schools   The term *back school* is generally used for group classes that provide education about back pain. The content and length of these classes varies a great deal, but generally they include information about the anatomy and function of the spine, common sources of low back pain, proper lifting technique and ergonomic training, and sometimes advice about exercise and remaining active. In general, studies have found back school to be effective in reducing disability and pain for chronic low back pain.[203]

Exercise   There are no well-controlled studies that show that exercise is effective for the treatment of *acute* low back pain. Many practitioners believe that exercise for patients with acute low back pain is appropriate to prevent deconditioning, to reduce the chance of recurrence of symptoms, and to reduce the risk of the development of chronic pain and disability. This is consistent with rehabilitation principles for other acute injuries, such as sports-related injuries or rehabilitation after joint replacement surgery.[218] Perhaps because of problems with long-term exercise compliance, however, the overall favorable prognosis for each episode of acute back pain, or the outcome measures used, this principle is not yet supported by scientific research.

In contrast, multiple high-quality studies have found that exercise results in positive outcomes in the treatment of *chronic* low back pain.[205] This includes a wide variety of exercises used, although the most common type studied is a combination of strengthening and flexibility exercises.[86] This is not surprising, because it is generally believed that the purpose of exercises for the treatment of low back pain is to strengthen and increase endurance of muscles that support the spine and improve flexibility in areas where this is lacking. This is combined with motor retraining to establish normal patterns of muscle activity, and treatment of deficits of the kinetic chain that interfere with biomechanical efficiency.

Adverse effects of exercise for low back pain are rarely reported, so it is generally a very safe treatment. One reason that studies have not been able to determine what exercises are best could be that multiple forms of exercise can achieve the goal of restoring full function and regaining physical fitness.[108,204,218] Because endurance is a big problem with many patients with persistent back pain, activity levels should be increased by planned, fixed increments based on realistic goals rather than symptoms, because it is the normal course of low back pain that there will be temporary exacerbations of pain along the way. Beyond the physiologic benefits of exercise, increasing activity has positive effects on beliefs and behaviors about pain. Small doses of exercise that are not sufficient to cause physiologic change have been found to increase function and decrease pain. When specifically studied, this appeared to be from decreased fear-avoidance beliefs and reduced anxiety. By exposing fearful patients to physical activity through gradually increasing activity levels despite pain, they receive positive reinforcement by meeting goals, and personal experience can reduce fear of movement, reinjury, and catastrophizing.[22]

Specific exercise treatment for low back pain   *Postural retraining*   Exercise prescriptions for mechanical low back pain generally begin with the goal of improving alignment and posture. Although researchers have not been able to consistently identify which specific postural faults are associated with chronic low back pain,[52] the correction of posture is important for at least two reasons. One is that exercises are more effective if they are done from a position of proper alignment that promotes optimal joint function and movement patterns. The second is that, for virtually all patients, much more time will be spent in habitual postures such as sitting and standing than will ever be spent exercising. If these habitual postures can reduce abnormal tissue strains, there is a better chance of reducing pain and promoting healing.[175]

Posture should be evaluated in both sitting and standing, and faulty positions corrected. Common faulty postures in standing include either excessive lumbar lordosis or a flat back. In sitting, common faults include patients who tend to lean to one side, often leaning on an armrest that is too low. This causes prolonged lateral flexion of the trunk that can lead to pain, especially if the lateral flexion is abnormally occurring at only a few segments. Short patients whose feet do not reach the floor when they sit can overuse hip flexors to hold the legs in position, which can increase forces on the spine. Tall patients might sit with the knees higher than the hips, causing increased lumbar flexion.[176] Some of these postural faults are habitual and can be improved with education, cuing, and practice. Some postural faults are structural problems that do not change with exercise, such as the kyphosis of Scheuermann disease or idiopathic scoliosis, and should be addressed with aids such as higher armrests or a chair with increased lumbar support. Many postural faults begin as habitual, and then become structural as tight muscles and tendons do not allow immediate correction with cuing, and weak muscles cannot maintain the proper position even if it can be reached. This is what is seen with typical postural faults such as long standing lordosis, in which hip flexors and lumbar paraspinals become tight from prolonged positioning in lordosis, and abdominal muscles become long and weak from disuse and their prolonged lengthened position.

These types of faults can be addressed with the proper exercises to stretch tight areas and strengthen weak areas. However, this is harder to achieve in patients with persistent back pain. Multiple studies have shown that subjects with chronic low back pain have deficits in spinal proprioception and make repositioning errors. For example, in a study in which asymptomatic patients were compared with patients with chronic low back pain in an activity in which participants were assisted into neutral spine posture and then asked to reproduce this position after periods of relaxed full lumbar flexion, the group with back pain had significantly more repositioning errors.[152] This has important implications for treatment, as those with back pain may need extensive training by a physical therapist to change their posture, rather than just education regarding posture or a few simple demonstrations.

Lumbar stabilization   Either after or at the same time as postural therapy and retraining, exercise training is added that addresses the issues of decreased muscular endurance, abnormal strength ratios, and poor motor control in patients with low back pain. Generally, this includes lumbar stabilization exercises. This is also called core strengthening. It includes training in the proper use of muscles to increase stiffness and support in areas that are weak and deconditioned, and improving flexibility in areas of excessive stiffness. One of the principles of physics is that movement occurs along the path of least resistance. In the case of the body, the greatest degree of motion

occurs at the most flexible segment. In the spine, pathology is often seen at the most flexible segments. Increasing muscular strength, endurance, and neural firing patterns around these segments can stiffen them and decrease abnormal flexibility. Proper treatment also addresses the issue, however, that sometimes segments or areas with reduced flexibility can be the problem. The reduced flexibility of some segments contributes to compensatory motion at the most flexible segments and leads to injury.

Many exercises can be stabilizing exercises. The key is practicing these exercises so that optimal or at least improved motor patterns can be learned that ensure a stable spine. Achieving stability is not just a matter of activating a few targeted muscles. It is the ability to continually change motor strategies as needed to support posture, to endure unexpected loads, to prepare for moving quickly, and to provide sufficient stiffness in any degree of freedom of the joint so that it is not subjected to further injury. This end result is achieved by approaching the problems in stages. The usual stages of a lumbar stabilization exercise program are outlined below. For patients currently experiencing back pain, exercises should be chosen that impose low loads on the spine so that pain is not increased.

Awareness of spine position and muscle contraction in various positions and with different activities   This begins with the postural training as discussed above, and progresses to include movement patterns and activities of daily living. This is key for further training. Patients need to be able to appreciate the position of their bodies while bending, reaching, moving the arms and legs, and doing activities such as washing dishes or working on the computer. They also need to be able to determine motor patterns of movement. For example, patients should be able to distinguish lumbar flexion from hip flexion when bending forward, and need to assess whether the spine is moving excessively or abnormally during exercises. This type of training can be accomplished with a combination of simple exercises and education.

Obtaining and maintaining mild abdominal contraction and multifidi activation   Some patients with low back pain learn this step easily and can contract the proper muscles for stabilization, such as the transversus abdominis, very easily. For them, simple cuing such as 'Bring your belly button toward your backbone' will activate the proper muscles. For other patients, this can be a long process of training that can take significant effort by the physical therapist and might even need further techniques such as biofeedback. This step is essential, however, before moving to the next step, which demands further strength and endurance of the muscles and more sophisticated motor strategies.[165]

Stabilization exercises to establish motor patterns and build endurance   Many exercises can be stabilization exercises. A balanced program addresses the need for sufficient anterior abdominal strength with exercises such as curl-ups, leg lifts, oblique strengthening, bridging, and other exercises chosen based on baseline strength, ability to maintain the appropriate position while doing the exercises, and reducing spinal forces in those with back pain. The quadratus lumborum is an important lateral stabilizer of the spine, and can be strengthened with exercises such as side bridging. Extensor strengthening can be accomplished by various extension patterns in quadruped as well as other exercises. Pelvic floor exercises and appropriate breathing patterns are also addressed.

Modifications for those in whom exercises aggravate pain McGill and colleagues have done extensive research evaluating spinal forces generated during exercise. For example, sit ups cause over 3000 N of compressive loads on the spine because of psoas activity, about the same as moderately heavy lifting. Leg raises also cause relatively high compressive forces. Curl-ups cause lower forces on the spine, so are a better choice for anterior abdominal strengthening in the early stages of rehabilitation, or in those who have increased pain and cannot tolerate exercises with increased spinal loading. Lying prone and extending the spine while extending the arms and legs causes over 6000 N of compression to the spine, and might be much too intense for those with back injuries. The quadruped position with the leg extended, however, also activates spinal extensors but causes less than half the amount of spinal compression if done properly with the abdominal muscles engaged and the spine in neutral.[126] These examples show how modification of exercises can reduce spinal forces and increase exercise tolerance.

Some patients, especially those with persistent pain, can have high fear-avoidant behavior and develop kinesophobia, a fear of movement and a belief that movement will increase pain or cause them to be injured. This fear of pain, rather than forces on the spine or spinal pathology, leads to poor exercise tolerance. If this is the reason for poor exercise tolerance, it can be addressed by graded reactivation and gradual increases in activity. A positive experience with this might decrease fears. For more severe cases, a multidisciplinary approach that includes psychologic counseling to explore these dysfunctional thought processes can be needed. The physician should emphasize to patients that exercise needs to become a daily habit. Lack of compliance is one of the main reasons why exercise treatments fail. The health benefits of the stabilization program should be discussed, and patients should be reminded that exercising needs to continue even after symptoms decrease.

Flexion exercises for low back pain Once popular for the treatment of acute low back pain, using a series of flexion exercises has not been found to be more helpful for acute low back pain than other interventions, such as spinal manipulation, in several studies. No research has been done on the effectiveness of flexion exercises for chronic low back pain.[202]

Extension exercises for low back pain Still commonly used by therapists in the treatment of low back pain, and in particular back pain accompanied by radicular leg pain, extension-based exercises are often done using the principles of the McKenzie method of physical therapy. This therapy approach divides the diagnosis for back pain into three categories: derangement, dysfunction, and postural syndrome. The most common

of these are derangements, and exercises are chosen that centralize the pain, i.e. move the pain from the leg or buttock into the low back. Although early studies were very promising, later studies have found this type of physical therapy to be helpful for low back pain but no more effective than other types of exercise.[38,202]

Aerobic activity Increasing aerobic activity is a cornerstone of most exercise programs for low back pain. Studies in this area are often difficult to interpret because, both in the clinical setting and in research studies, aerobic activity is usually combined with strengthening and flexibility exercise. Studies have found that group classes that combine low-impact aerobics with strengthening and stretching floor exercises can be as effective in reducing pain and decreasing disability as individualized physical therapy and strengthening with weight machines.[118] Many clinicians have found that patients with chronic low back pain tend to have very low fitness levels, but research in this area has had conflicting results. For example, one study, in which prediction equations to estimated VO_{2max} (a measure of aerobic fitness) in patients with chronic low back pain were compared with normal values, found that values for chronic low back pain patients did not differ from age-matched normal values for sedentary men and women.[227,228] This could be because those who agreed to participate in the study were not representative of all patients with chronic low back pain, or it might simply demonstrate the poor aerobic fitness of sedentary people in general. Perhaps this poor fitness level is related more to lifestyle than to back pain.

No particular type of aerobic activity has been found to be more effective for gaining fitness or decreasing pain than another for patients with back pain. A willingness to regularly participate in the activity at an intensity level to improve fitness is a more important factor than the specific type of exercise. One small study that compared symptom-limited exercise tests performed on the treadmill, stationary bicycle, or upper extremity ergometer by patients with low back pain found that pain scores were higher at the end of the treadmill test than the test on the other two pieces of equipment. However, this appeared to be because patients prematurely stopped the bicycle and arm ergometer tests because of muscular fatigue, and patients were able to reach significantly higher heart rates and peak VO_2 on the treadmill test despite pain complaints.[228] If increasing aerobic fitness in a commonly used activity is the goal, then walking might be the best way to achieve this, despite pain complaints in patients with back pain. Patients with chronic low back pain tend to walk slower during gait analysis than those without pain. This is linked more with fear of pain and high scores on fear-avoidance and catastrophic thinking scales than with pain ratings.[4] Interestingly, a slow stroll reduces spine motion and causes almost static loading of tissues, overall higher spine loading, and therefore more pain than faster walking with arm swings. Faster walking causes cyclic loading of tissues and results in lower spine torques, muscle activity, and loading. Swinging the arms facilitates efficient storage and use of elastic energy, which reduces the need for concentric muscle contractions with each step.[128] Fast walking has been shown to be therapeutic for low back pain, as has other aerobic activity.[128,181]

Aquatic exercises for mechanical low back pain Patients who have not tolerated land-based exercises are often able to participate in pool exercises. There are several benefits to exercising in the water. One is buoyancy and reduction of gravitational stress. The greater the amount of the body that is submerged, the greater the effect. For example, there is a 90% reduction in gravitational stresses when exercising in the vertical position when the patient is immersed to the neck.[101] Water can also decrease pain via the gate theory, in which the sensory input from the water temperature, hydrostatic pressure, and turbulence cause the patient to feel less pain. Muscle guarding and muscle overactivity might also be decreased in warm water. For those patients fearful of movement and reinjury, moving in the pool can increase their confidence as they see that they can progress without pain. The same principles for progressing therapy apply to aquatic exercise as to land-based exercise. Patients can learn neutral position, stabilizing, and other strengthening exercise, and by walking, jogging (these can be done in deep water using a buoyancy belt or vest), or swimming can add an aerobic component.[101] There has not been a great deal of research in this area, but small case series have found it an effective exercise form for patients with low back pain.[11,101]

Exercise after spine surgery Most of the research in this area has been done on patients who have undergone lumbar disk surgery. One systematic review of this subject found no evidence that exercising after disk surgery increases injury rate or need to reoperate.[148] Overall, exercise appears effective to decrease pain and increase return to work rates. Those who used high-intensity exercise compared with low-intensity exercise found significantly better short-term pain relief, functional status, and faster return to work with the high-intensity program. However, there was no difference between the high- and low-intensity groups at 1-year follow-up, perhaps because of long-term compliance issues with the high-intensity exercises. Another study found home exercise programs equally effective to a supervised exercise program when all patients are given the same exercises.[148]

Overall, exercise has been found to be one of the most effective treatments for decreasing pain and increasing function in chronic low back pain. The many other health benefits of exercise, along with the low risk of causing harm, make it a first-line treatment for mechanical low back pain.

Medication

Non-steroidal antiinflammatory drugs Multiple studies provide strong evidence that NSAIDS prescribed at regular intervals provide pain relief for both acute and chronic low back pain. Studies comparing the effectiveness of NSAIDs have not found any particular NSAID to be superior to others.[204,208]

NSAIDS are associated with some risk, especially gastrointestinal bleeding. Other side effects include decreased hemostasis and renal dysfunction or failure in patients with abnormal renal function or hypovolemia.[16] The deleterious cardiovascular effects of the cyclooxygenase-2 inhibitors have received much attention as of late.

Muscle relaxants The use of muscle relaxants remains controversial. One reason is that it is unclear what role muscle 'spasms' play in mechanical low back pain. Some object to the term *muscle spasm* for skeletal muscle, because only smooth muscles have the syncytial innervation pattern needed to actually spasm. They prefer the term *muscle guarding*. Other experts do not believe that pain in the low back is generally caused by muscle spasms. Others think that, if muscle spasms are present, they can contribute to the healing process by immobilizing the back and are therefore efficacious in acute low back pain. Despite this controversy, 35% of patients who visit a primary care physician for low back pain are prescribed muscle relaxants.[207] These medications fall into three classes of drug: the benzodiazepines, the non-benzodiazepines that are antispasmodics, and antispasticity medication.

The mechanism of action for benzodiazepines is the enhancement of GABA inhibitory activity. The limited research done on this class of medication has found them to be effective for both acute and chronic low back pain for short-term pain relief and decrease of muscle spasm. However, they have significant adverse effects, such as sedation, dizziness, and mood disturbances. Rapid withdrawal can cause seizures. These medications have serious abuse and addiction potential, and they are not recommended for mechanical low back pain except in unusual cases for a short time.[41,207]

Non-benzodiazapine antispasmodics include medications with multiple mechanisms of action. Cyclobenzaprine has a structure similar to that of tricyclic antidepressants and is believed to act in the brain stem. Carisoprodol blocks interneuronal activity in the spinal cord and descending reticular formation. The mechanism of action of methocarbamol is not known but may be due to central nervous system depression.[8] There are multiple high-quality studies showing that these medications are effective for patients with acute low back pain for short-term pain relief. The most common side effects are drowsiness and dizziness. There is not currently any evidence that one is more efficacious than another. Carisoprodol is metabolized to meprobamate, an antianxiety agent. It has significant potential for abuse and can result in psychologic and physical dependence.[207] Because of this risk, and the fact that it is not more efficacious than other muscle relaxants, it should not be used except in rare cases. There is not much literature on the use of muscle relaxants for chronic pain, and the drug manufacturers in this class state that they are not for long-term use.[8,41]

Antispasticity medication has also been used to treat low back pain. Baclofen is a GABA derivative that inhibits transmission at the spinal level and brain. One study has shown this medication to be effective for short-term pain relief in acute low back pain. Dantrolene works on the muscle, blockading the sarcoplasmic reticulum calcium channels. A small study of 20 patients found it to be effective for acute low back pain. It does not have the drowsiness side effect of the other muscle relaxants, but there is a risk of severe hepatotoxicity.[207]

Antidepressants Tricyclic antidepressants are an effective treatment for many painful conditions, such as diabetic neuropathy, postherpetic neuralgia, fibromyalgia, and headaches. There are no adequate studies to show if they are effective for the treatment of acute low back pain. Multiple studies and reviews have shown their effectiveness, however, for chronic low back pain. Staiger and colleagues did a best evidence synthesis of randomized, placebo-controlled trials on this topic, which included 440 patients.[189] They found that the tricyclics and tetracyclics had significant effects in reducing pain. These reductions were seen in studies in which depressed patients were excluded, so the mechanism is independent of any treatment of underlying depression. The doses used in almost all these studies were within the Agency for Health Care Policy and Research guidelines for treatment of depression. The most common side effects seen with the use of tricyclic antidepressants are dry mouth, blurry vision, constipation, dizziness, tremors, and urinary disturbances.

The selective serotonin reuptake inhibitors and trazodone are not effective in treating chronic low back pain, which is consistent with the findings in studies for other painful conditions, such as diabetic neuropathy.[189]

Opioids Many providers use short-acting opioids to treat acute low back pain. The use of opioids for chronic nonmalignant pain is much more controversial. Randomized controlled trials in this area are lacking. Most studies on opioid use and pain include pain in many sites of the body, although back pain generally makes up a large percentage of the pain complaints. These studies also tend to suffer from high dropout rates, because of either medication side effects or lack of efficacy. Studies with long-term follow-up are lacking.

In one randomized controlled trial of pain relief with oral sustained-release morphine versus placebo, in which 44% of the patients had low back pain, the morphine group had less pain but no psychologic or functional improvement.[17] In a randomized open-label trial of 36 patients with chronic low back pain, one-third of the subjects were treated with naproxen, one-third with set doses of oxycodone, and one-third with as-needed doses of oxycodone plus sustained-relief morphine titrated for pain intensity. Both opioid groups had significantly less pain but no improvement in sleep or activity levels. In a larger, non-randomized, open-label trial, about half of patients treated with opioids had 50% or more pain relief, about 25% had less than 50%, and about 25% did not respond. It is not clear what percent had changes in function.[17]

Side effects are substantial, and in many studies occur in well over half the participants. These effects include nausea, constipation, somnolence, dizziness, and pruritis.[17]

In studies that have compared long-acting with short-acting opioids, the long-acting medications appear to generally give better pain relief, are better tolerated, and are thought to have less abuse potential.

Generally, because of side effects, abuse potential, tolerance, and unknown long-term effects on pain and neuronal functioning, opioid medications are avoided, and a more global approach to mechanical low back pain is used. As with other treatments, long-term opioid treatment should be used only after careful analysis of the positive and negative impacts on function and quality of life. Outcomes beyond simple pain reduction should be used, and a rational end point of treatment and criteria for tapering and discontinuing the medications should be determined. Opioid medications should not be used without regular follow-up (see Ch. 43).[16,17]

Anticonvulsants The anticonvulsants, particularly gabapentin, are widely used for neuropathic pain. Large, randomized, controlled trials have not yet been conducted with these medications for the treatment of mechanical low back pain. Some pain experts believe that chronic back pain is maintained long after the acute noxious stimuli have ceased by processes similar to neuropathic pain, such as central sensitization in the spinal cord and a disinhibition of inhibitory neurotransmitters. If this is the case, then it is a type of neuropathic pain and should respond to treatment by anticonvulsants. This has not yet been proved or disproved in the medical literature.

Topical treatments Lidocaine (lignocaine) patches have been found effective by some patients for the treatment of back pain. No large studies have proved or disproved its efficacy. A variety of creams and lotions are used by patients, including irritants and antiinflammatory creams. Some people find them effective, but they have not been subjected to extensive research. These treatments carry little risk and have low incidence of side effects.

Injections and needle therapy for mechanical low back pain

Myofascial pain and trigger point injections The theory that irritable foci in skeletal muscle can cause both local and referred pain is generally accepted, although some physicians doubt the diagnosis of myofascial pain because, in general, the research supporting the biochemical and mechanical basis of trigger points is inconclusive (see Ch. 44). In regard to mechanical low back pain, it is thought that acute trauma or overload, chronic overwork and fatigue, or altered neurologic input causes trigger points to develop. They are treated by a combination of techniques, which include reducing biomechanical stress in the area by avoiding tissue overload and making postural changes, ischemic compression, stretching, and injections.[198,199] Of this treatment approach, the injection component has been most studied. A Cochrane review of injection therapy for low back pain pooled the results of multiple studies that have found injections of trigger points to be effective in the treatment of low back pain. These included studies that evaluated dry needling, lidocaine (lignocaine) alone, and lidocaine with steroid injections. The reviewers concluded that trigger point injections are better than placebo injections for long-term pain relief based on these studies.[143]

Acupuncture Acupuncture has been used for the treatment of pain conditions for thousands of years (see Ch. 23). From a western medicine perspective, it appears to have multiple mechanisms of action, including effects on the endogenous opioid peptide system, an effect on the sympathetic nervous system, and alterations in pain processing in the spinal cord and brain.[83] The efficacy of acupuncture in the treatment of low back pain is difficult to determine. Like other physical treatments, it is difficult to perform blinded studies. When comparing acupuncture with other standard treatments for low back pain, such as exercise, the results are difficult to interpret, because the placebo effect is thought to increase with more invasive procedures. There are great variations in the diagnosis and treatment of low back pain by acupuncturists. Much like other treatments for low back pain, such as physical therapy and medication regimens, treatments are patient- and provider-specific, and acupuncture treatments vary from one another by the points chosen, what type of needle stimulation is done, and the duration of the treatment.[87,93]

Despite these difficulties, the effectiveness of acupuncture to treat low back pain is increasingly being studied. It has also been the subject of multiple systematic reviews and metaanalyses (more than 45 from the late 1980s to 2004). Most of these reviews comment primarily on the quality of studies done, and most studies are considered to be of poor quality, so only limited conclusions on the efficacy of acupuncture can be made. There seems to be general consensus in multiple reviews, however, that the evidence for acupuncture in relieving low back pain is either positive or inconclusive. For example, the British Medical Association's rigorous analysis in 2002 of acupuncture found it to be effective for low back pain, whereas the Canadian/Alberta Health Authorities report's rigorous analysis done the same year found the results inconclusive for low back pain.[20]

More high-quality definitive studies and clinical experience is obviously needed to reach a final conclusion in this area. Acupuncture is safe for the treatment of low back pain, with very low complication rates and side effects. The most common side effects are bruising and pain at the site of needle insertion.[20]

Experimental injection procedures Botulinum toxin injections are increasingly being used to treat low back pain. The mechanism of action could be through changes in sympathetic tone, reduction of muscle spasms, or another unknown mechanism. Studies in this area are currently small, and the results are inconclusive as to whether this will be an effective treatment for back pain.

Prolotherapy is another controversial procedure gaining popularity in certain parts of the country. It consists of a series of injections into spinal ligaments to cause inflammation and thickening of the ligaments. Based on the scientific literature, the ability of this procedure to treat low back pain has not yet been validated.

Steroid injections and other spinal procedures See Chapter 25 for other specific spinal procedures used in the treatment of low back pain.

Manual mobilization or manipulation Historical references to manual medicine go back over 4000 years. In the nineteenth century, an increased interest in manual medicine began in Great Britain and the USA. There are multiple theories as to how manual medicine works. One theory is that it restores normal motion to restricted segments. Another is that it changes neurologic control via reflex mechanisms, especially the interaction between the autonomic nervous system and the spinal cord.[72]

Multiple randomized controlled trials and systematic reviews have been done to assess the efficacy of manual therapy. In most countries with national guidelines for the treatment of low back pain, spinal manipulation is recommended for acute low back pain,[216] although this is not universal. The recommendations for chronic back pain are much more varied. Assendelft and colleagues performed a metaanalysis of the effectiveness of this treatment for low back pain and found many high-quality studies.[12] This metaanalysis had weaknesses common to all metaanalyses, including the variety in quality of the studies, the possibility of publication bias, and statistical issues. Its strengths were the size of the patient pool, thoroughness, and inclusion of the most recent available data up to 2002. The metaanalysis included a total of 5486 patients. For both acute and chronic low back pain, the authors found spinal manipulation more effective than placebo (which was either sham manipulation or treatments judged to be ineffective) for short-term pain relief. There was an improvement in function noted, but this did not reach statistical significance. When spinal manipulation was compared with other treatments known to be effective, such as analgesics, exercise, and physical therapy, the authors could find no statistically significant benefits as compared with other therapies. Results did not change when they looked at studies in which only manipulation and not mobilization was used. They also could not identify any particular subgroup of patients for whom manipulation was particularly effective, although they theorized that, if such a group existed, it would be small.

Of note, the authors also did not find other commonly used treatments, such as physical therapy and medication, to be statistically more effective than spinal manipulation, so their conclusion was that spinal manipulation is more effective than placebo, and is one of several options of modest effectiveness for patients with low back pain.

Traction The literature in this area has been criticized because of disagreement as to whether studies done have used the appropriate weight of traction, frequency of treatment, and length of treatment session. For example, many studies have been of traction used once per week, while some practitioners believe traction should be done daily and that outcomes of studies with frequency less than this are invalid.[81] Multiple randomized controlled trials using different doses of traction have been done, however, and most have not found traction to be effective for the treatment of back pain. No well-done study has shown that a specific weight or frequency of traction is effective over sham treatment.[204,208]

Heel lifts and correction of leg length discrepancy   There is no consensus in the literature as to whether small differences in leg length lead to increased back pain. Part of the controversy stems from the multiple reasons that legs can appear to be of different length. Limb length discrepancy can be secondary to either anatomic limb length inequality (in which there is a true difference in length between the head of the femur and the ankle), or to functional or apparent limb length inequality, which may be from many diverse causes. The apparent limb length inequality sources range from foot biomechanics (e.g. increased pronation and decreased arch height causing a functionally shorter limb) to imbalances of soft tissue around the pelvis (e.g. quadratus lumborum shortening causes hiking of the pelvis so that the legs appear a different length). There is little consensus on what level of leg length discrepancy is clinically significant, or how prevalent leg length discrepancies are. Studies range from a 4% to 95% prevalence based on different populations, measurement techniques, and cutoffs for clinical significance from 5 mm to 11 mm. Small, unblinded studies have found that correction of leg length discrepancy decreases low back pain, but this has not yet been evaluated in large, controlled trials.[29]

Lumbar supports   Lumbar supports are used to both treat and prevent low back pain. There are multiple types of lumbar support. They vary from a simple elastic wrap to custom-molded plastic braces. High-quality studies comparing the effectiveness of different braces are generally lacking, although one study showed that patients who wore a lumbar support plus a rigid insert in the back had more subjective improvement than those who wore a brace without a rigid support.[134]

Several mechanisms of action have been proposed as to why lumbar supports would be effective. One hypothesis is that they prevent excessive spinal motion, either by physically blocking extremes of motion or by providing sensory feedback to remind the patient not to bend excessively. Another theory is that they increase intraabdominal pressure without increasing abdominal muscle activity, and therefore could reduce muscle force, fatigue, and compressive loading on the spine.[160] A review of the literature regarding the mechanisms of action of lumbar supports showed that neither of these theories has been proven. In general, lumbar supports decrease ROM, but the results are not consistent. Decreases in ROM vary between subjects, with some subjects even showing increased range while wearing a brace, and the plane of motion that is reduced varies between subjects and the types of braces tested. For example, some types of brace reduce rotation, while others reduce flexion and extension. There is no evidence that lumbar supports actually increase intraabdominal pressure or decrease muscle forces and fatigue.[160] Regarding the efficacy of lumbar supports, there is limited evidence that lumbar supports provide some pain relief for low back pain when compared with no treatment, but when compared with other treatments they are no more effective.

Studies also show that overall there is poor compliance for subjects to consistently wear lumbar supports. There is no consistent evidence that lumbar supports prevent the occurrence of back pain.[205]

Transcutaneous electrical nerve stimulation   The development of TENS was based on the gate theory of pain of Melzack and Wall. In this theory, the stimulation of large afferent fibers inhibits small nociceptive fibers, and so the patient feels less pain. There are multiple types of TENS applications, such as high frequency moderate intensity, low frequency high intensity, and burst frequency (see Ch. 22). Clinically, many patients find TENS helpful for temporary relief of low back pain. Evaluating the research in this area is difficult because of the difficulty of an equivalent placebo and the different types of TENS applications used between studies, and because most studies use patients' memory of their pain, which is frequently inaccurate, as an outcome measure.[30] Metaanalyses of TENS outcomes show trends toward better pain reduction, better function, and satisfaction with treatment as compared with placebo, but these trends do not reach statistical significance and, given the small changes, are of unclear clinical significance. Larger, methodologically sound studies are still needed to evaluate the efficacy of this treatment.[135]

Massage   Massage is one of the most commonly used complementary therapies for low back pain. The mechanism of action is thought to include relaxation and stress reduction, the therapeutic benefits of touch, and beneficial effects on the structure or function of tissues and pain sensation.[64] Research that included massage has generally fallen into two categories: studies that measure the effect of massage, and studies that assess the effectiveness of other interventions and use massage as a control with hands-on effects. Interestingly, in studies in which massage was used as the control, massage was not generally found to be more beneficial. This could be because of the effectiveness of both interventions, explaining why no differences were found, or it could have been due to publication bias. In studies in which massage was one of the main interventions, massage has been found to be effective for pain relief and in restoring function. For example, Cherkin and colleagues performed an interesting study that compared massage, acupuncture, and self-care education for chronic low back pain.[39] After 10 weeks in which up to 10 treatments were allowed, the massage group showed improvements on disability scales, had decreased medication use, and had less time with restricted activity than the control group. After 1 year, many of these gains were maintained.[39] Other high-quality studies have also found massage to be effective for improving symptoms and functions in subacute and chronic low back pain. High-quality studies on the effects of massage on acute low back pain have not yet been done (see also Ch. 20).

Complementary movement therapies   There are many movement therapies being used in the treatment of low back pain. A few of the most commonly used therapies are listed below. These therapies have been found helpful in case series but have not been subjected to stringent randomized controlled trials (see also Ch. 23).

- Yoga: both an exercise system and philosophy that promotes relaxation, acceptance, and breathing techniques while various stretching and strengthening exercises are done.
- Pilates: a form of core-strengthening exercises that stress alignment and proper form.
- Alexander technique: an educational approach to posture and normalizing movement patterns.
- Feldenkrais: a combination of classes and hands-on work with therapeutic exercise to promote natural and comfortable movement patterns and improve body awareness.

Multidisciplinary pain treatment programs　There is strong evidence that a multidisciplinary program with a goal of functional restoration is helpful for severe chronic pain.[204] This is discussed further in Chapter 42 on chronic pain.

Treatment of comorbidities　Multiple comorbidities are often seen with back pain. Issues commonly associated with low back pain include depression, anxiety, and sleep disturbances. Treating these conditions often diminishes pain and increases function. Those who suffer from low back pain often also have other illnesses associated with an unhealthy and sedentary lifestyle, such as obesity, non-insulin-dependent diabetes, and cardiovascular disease. This must be taken into account when formulating a rehabilitation plan.

Other causes of back pain greater than leg pain
Lumbar spondylosis

The degenerative cascade of Kirkaldy-Willis has already been described above. Because degenerative disease of the zygapophyseal joints generally coexists with degenerative disk disease, it is difficult to separate the two entities. Both can cause axial back pain. Both can also cause referred pain into the buttocks and legs. Mooney and McCall have studied the sclerotomal distribution of zygapophyseal joint pain in detail.[123,137] Zygapophyseal joint pain has even been described to refer below the knee in some cases.

Delineating a degenerative zygapophyseal joint as the primary pain generator in axial low back pain, however, is difficult. Imaging studies are not particularly useful, because many asymptomatic people have spondylotic changes in their spines. This diagnosis is also made more commonly in older patients. Those in the older population have multiple findings in their history, in their physical examination, and on imaging studies that complicate arriving at specific diagnoses or specific pain generators as the cause of their complaints. Spondylotic zygapophyseal joints are seen quite commonly with other potential sources of low back pain such as degenerative disks and lumbar stenosis. On physical examination, patients with these imaging findings commonly have postural abnormalities, poor pelvic girdle mechanics, and potentially multiple myofascial sources

for pain. They typically have an accentuated lumbar lordosis, in part due to tight hip flexors, which exacerbates the problem by increasing stress on the posterior elements.

From biomechanical studies and knowledge of anatomy, we know that lumbar extension and rotation increase forces placed on the posterior zygapophyseal joints. This specific maneuver, however, has not been shown to be diagnostic for zygapophyseal joint pain in clinical settings (by either history or examination). There actually are no unique identifying features in the history, physical examination, or radiologic imaging that are diagnostic for zygapophyseal joint pain. The only diagnostic maneuvers for zygapophyseal joint pain are fluoroscopically guided zygapophyseal joint injections with local anesthetic, and medial branch blocks (i.e. local anesthetic blocks of the medial branches of the dorsal primary rami that innervate the zygapophyseal joints).[48,120] Using these injection techniques, the prevalence of facet-mediated pain has been estimated to be 15% in the younger population and 40% in older age groups.[179,180] Schwarzer's 1994 study demonstrated that the vast majority of lumbar zygapophyseal joint pain originates from the L4–5 and L5–S1 zygapophyseal joints. Consequently, if injections are used as treatment, most can be directed to those two lumbar levels.

There are more conservative management options for the spondylotic spine and facet-mediated pain that should be trialed before resorting to invasive procedures such as intraarticular zygapophyseal joint corticosteroid injections or medial branch neurotomies. The conservative treatments are similar to treatments for osteoarthritic joints, and can be categorized as lifestyle and activity modification, medications, and exercise.

Lifestyle and activity modifications include weight control, relative rest, and initially limiting activities that result in increased pain (e.g. sleeping prone generally is to be avoided). Medications used include analgesics such as acetaminophen (paracetamol) and NSAIDs. There might be a role for glucosamine, because it has demonstrated a good response for pain relief with knee osteoarthritis. Exercise programs are generally designed to decrease the forces acting on the zygapophyseal joints. This can include improving postural control by reducing any exaggerated lumbar lordosis through hip flexor stretching and pelvic tilts, but also developing the spine's supportive musculature, including the deep abdominals, quadratus lumborum, and gluteal muscles, to stabilize the pelvis and lessen potential shearing forces in the lumbar spine. There is no single proven exercise program, however, for standardized treatment with an exercise protocol for zygapophyseal joint-mediated pain. If land-based exercise is initially too aggravating, aquatic therapy can be the best starting place. Finally, lumbar braces or corsets have not proven useful in the long term, but for an overweight patient with a protuberant abdomen or large pannus (which can certainly increase zygapophyseal joint stress by increasing the lordotic posture) it could be the best alternative.

Interventional treatments for zygapophyseal joint pain have been briefly mentioned above. A more detailed discussion can be found in Chapter 26.

Lumbar disk disease

Diskogenic causes of low back pain generally fall into three categories: degenerative disk disease, internal disk disruption, and disk herniation. Diskogenic pain is classically described as bandlike and exacerbated by lumbar flexion, but this is not always the case. It can be unilateral, can radiate to the buttock, and can even be worsened by extension or side bending (depending on the site of disk pathology).

Internal disk disruption

Bogduk defines internal disk disruption as a condition in which the internal architecture of the disk is disrupted, but its external surface remains essentially normal (i.e. there is no bulge or herniation).[23] It is characterized by degradation of the nucleus pulposus and radial fissures that extend to the outer third of the annulus (high-intensity zone areas on MRI).[9] It can be diagnosed only by postdiskography CT, which shows the degradation of the nucleus and the presence and extent of the annular fissures. Although the use of diskography is controversial, most believe that annular tears (especially those that reach the outer third of the annulus, i.e. the innervated fibers) can be a source of low back pain. It must be remembered, however, that, like most abnormalities on lumbar spine imaging, annular tears or high-intensity zone areas are seen commonly in asymptomatic subjects.

The proposed mechanisms for pain generation from internal disk disruption are similar to those previously described for disk herniation and radiculopathy; that is, chemical nociception from inflammatory mediators and mechanical stimulation. Similar to other general causes of low back pain, treatment generally encompasses NSAIDs and non-opiate analgesics, relative rest, and exercise programs designed to strengthen the lumbar supportive musculature. Epidural steroids might have a potential role in treatment as well. Recently, Butterman supplied us with some potential criteria for the role of epidural steroid injections in degenerative disk disease.[36] There are many novel, interventional treatment approaches that are discussed in detail in Chapters 25 and 26, including intradiskal steroids and intradiskal electrothermal annuloplasty. However, it should be kept in mind that these interventional treatments are still awaiting rigorous scientific studies. Fusion surgery is another controversial treatment for degenerative disk disease. Because of the variable and controversial results of fusion surgery, much hype is being generated about disk replacement surgery, which has gained popularity in Europe and was, in October 2004, approved in the USA.

Disk herniation

The terminology used to describe disk material that extends beyond the intervertebral disk space is confusing. *Herniated disk*, *herniated nucleus pulposus*, *disk protrusion*, *disk bulge*, *ruptured disk*, and *prolapsed disk* are all commonly used terms, and sometimes are used (incorrectly) synonymously. Displaced disk material can be initially classified as a bulge (disk material is displaced >50% of its circumference) or as a herniation

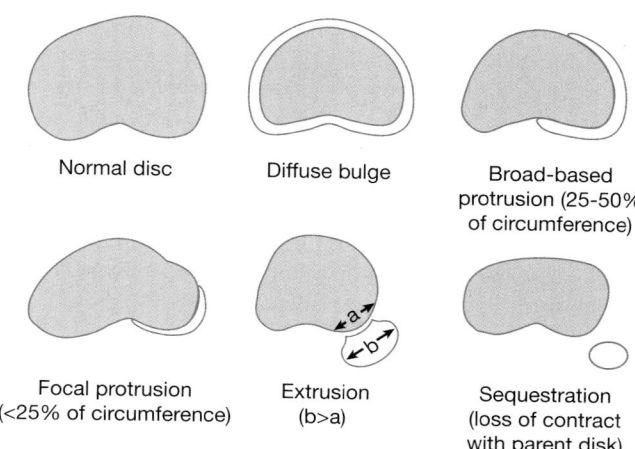

Figure 41-22 Disk herniation, protrusion, and extrusion. (From Maus 2002,[122] with permission.)

(<50% of its circumference) (see Fig. 41-22).[53] Disk herniations can then be subclassified into protrusions or extrusions. A disk protrusion is defined as a herniation with the distance of the edges of the herniated material less than the distance of the edges at its base. A disk extrusion occurs when the distance of the edges of the herniated material is greater than the distance of the edges at its base. A disk extrusion can be further subclassified as a sequestered or sequestrated disk if the extruded disk material has no continuity with the disk of origin. Finally, disk herniations can be described as contained or uncontained depending on the integrity of the outer annular fibers. If the outer annular fibers are still intact, it is described as a contained disk herniation. This classification has no relevance to the integrity of the posterior longitudinal ligament.

Over 95% of lumbar disk herniations occur at the L4–5 and L5–S1 levels.[45,187] Next most common is L3–4, followed by L2–3. The most common lumbosacral radiculopathies are consequently L5 and S1. Posterolateral disk herniations are most common because the annulus fibrosus is weakest posterolaterally. Posterolateral disks can affect the nerve root as it descends in the lateral recess or just before it enters the neural foramen. Far lateral or extraforaminal herniations can affect the nerve root as it exits the neural foramen, and central disk herniations may affect any part of the cauda equina depending on the level.

As noted above, disk herniations can cause an inflammatory response that can affect the nerve root, or there can be mechanical compression, both of which can cause radicular symptoms. However, disk herniations can cause solely axial pain. Diagnosing diskogenic low back pain is a challenge, because we know asymptomatic subjects can have disk herniations present on MRI.[21,90,91] Diskography is a controversial diagnostic tool for diskogenic pain (see Ch. 26). It is typically used as a presurgical screening tool.

The mainstay of treatment for diskogenic back pain is conservative. The literature is rather poor for discerning effective conservative management for diskogenic low back pain or, for that matter, axial low back pain in general. The primary reason is that most studies do not have a well-defined patient population, because it is quite difficult to discern the exact etiology of low back pain (e.g. diskogenic, facet, ligamentous, or muscular). Studies evaluating conservative measures (such as rehabilitation programs and exercise) might have different patients who would respond to different forms of exercise and not all be suitable for the one standardized exercise program used in the study. Many other studies do not even define the exercise program well enough to truly make any appropriate conclusions about one form of exercise over another.

Even when it is agreed that the etiology of low back pain is diskogenic, patients still respond differently to various exercise regimens, primarily because the location of the disk herniation typically dictates which lumbar spine movements can enhance pain and which do not (i.e. posterolateral disks cause more pain with flexion, central disks are usually more painful in extension, and for lateral disks there is more pain with ipsilateral side bending). It is appropriate to individualize rehabilitation programs according to which movements patients can do with little pain, and slowly progress their exercise program or movement patterns to include more planes of motion (that might initially have been painful) to improve the patients' functioning with less pain.

Prior to exercise treatment, some patients need a limited period of convalescence. During this initial period, these patients have relative rest with avoidance of activities that enhance pain (e.g. lifting, repetitive bending and twisting, and prolonged sitting). It might also be helpful to use pain medications (acetaminophen [paracetamol], NSAIDs, or a limited prescription of an opiate analgesic) and modalities such as lumbar traction to decrease pain prior to initiating a rehabilitation program. Prolonged bed rest greater than 3 days is not indicated, as it has not been shown to reduce disability from low back pain.[44] Getting the patient moving and educated on proper body mechanics for sitting and standing postures, as well as for lifting, is important early on in the course of treatment.

Most patients with diskogenic pain do well with conservative management alone. There are still some patients who do not respond to these conservative measures. Over the past few years, there has been an insurgence of interventional procedures to tackle the problem of diskogenic back pain, in order to prevent the need for surgical management. There is growing literature to support epidural steroid injections as a pain management strategy for disk herniations with radiculitis. Because it is well accepted that a disk herniation can cause an inflammatory response, epidural steroid injections for diskogenic pain (i.e. without radicular symptoms) have been used and probably are indicated, although there is no proven literature to support this. There are many other procedures that are gaining in popularity, including intradiskal steroid injections, annuloplasty, and nucleoplasty (see Ch. 26).

The literature on surgical management for diskogenic pain is similar to that regarding epidural steroid injections, i.e. surgery is most effective in improving radicular leg symptoms and is less impressive for axial back complaints. The most common surgical procedure is diskectomy. However, if there is concern for instability (say, in patients with significant multilevel degenerative disease), spinal fusion is sometimes considered. Only recently have prosthetic disk replacements been given considerable thought to replace spinal fusion as a motion-sparing procedure.

Spondylolysis

Spondylolysis is a defect of the pars interarticularis, and is a common cause of back pain in children and adolescents. The most common hypothesized mechanism of injury is repetitive hyperextension loading in the immature spine, and is commonly reported in adolescent gymnasts and football linemen.[56,89] Acute fracture from a severe hyperextension injury is also possible but less commonly reported.[55] Pars defects have been reported in non-athletic individuals as well. In growing children, the defect is rarely seen before walking begins and most commonly occurs at age 7–8 years.[144] An increase in incidence occurs during the adolescent growth spurt between ages 11 and 15 years. The pars defect appears to result from a combination of hereditary dysplasia of the pars and repetitive stressing of the spine by walking and extension loading.[47] Unilateral or bilateral defects can occur; however, bilateral involvement may result in spondylolisthesis. Ninety percent of these lesions occur at the L5–S1 level.

Patients typically present with low back pain that is exacerbated by extension and alleviated by rest or activity limitation. Physical examination can demonstrate focal tenderness, pain with lumbar extension, and hamstring tightness (Fig. 41-23). The neurologic examination is usually normal. If a spondylolisthesis is present, a palpable step-off with examination of the spinous processes might be evident.

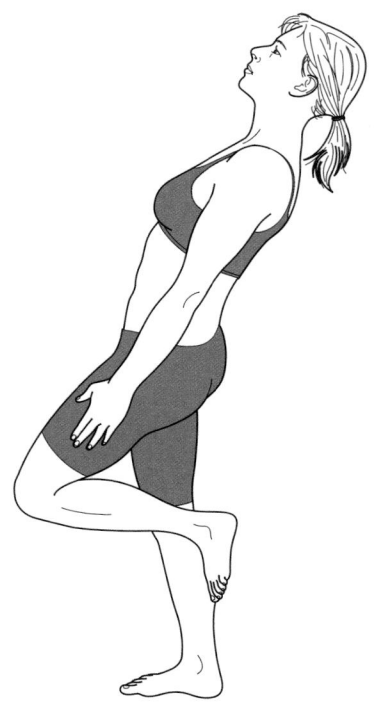

Figure 41-23 The standing one leg hyperextension test.

Radiologic assessment of a suspected pars injury begins with plain films to include oblique views of the lumbar spine. Oblique views demonstrate the typical Scottie dog appearance of the lumbar vertebrae, and a pars defect will show up as a break in the dog's collar or neck (Fig. 41-19).[163] Bone scanning is a more sensitive test for a pars injury, and is indicated if the plain films are normal or if the plain films show a fracture that could be old. The bone scan demonstrates increased bony turnover at the site of a recent fracture, healing fracture, or bony stress injury. SPECT is even more sensitive and specific for an active spondylolysis than planar bone scans are.[164] Thin-cut CT scanning through the level of the pars injury can be useful to determine if a fracture is old (sclerotic borders at the fracture edges) or acute. MRI can sometimes miss a spondylolysis but is very sensitive for other etiologies of a young athlete's back pain, such as disk herniation.

A spectrum of successful management strategies for spondylolysis have been employed. Conservative management is most common, typically beginning with relative rest and avoidance of activities that increase pain (repetitive extension). Bracing is quite common for symptomatic spondylolysis. Micheli advocates use of a modified Boston overlap brace constructed with 0° of lumbar flexion 23 h a day for at least 6 months.[131] He demonstrated that 32% of young athletes healed their fracture, and 88% were able to resume pain-free activity even if fracture union did not occur.[133] From these data, it is obvious that fracture union should be considered a hope, but it is not a necessary goal to be asymptomatic and fully functional in sports and everyday life. Bracing is not an absolute necessity, however, and some consider it only for those patients who cannot or will not comply with their activity restrictions, or for those who need a stigma of disability to show an overzealous coach or intrusive parent.

In any event, braced or not, the young athlete is at risk for deconditioning. When pain allows, the patient should be encouraged to begin aerobic conditioning and eventually enter a spinal rehabilitation program before return to a sport. Once the athlete has mastered a basic core stabilization program, functional progression back to the specific sport is appropriate, with a focus on neuromuscular proprioceptive control and sport-specific drills before full return to play. For the patient with chronic low back pain and spondylolysis, O'Sullivan et al. demonstrated that a specific exercise program focused on training the lumbar multifidi and deep abdominals can be very effective.[153] Surgical treatment is rarely indicated for the patient with spondylolysis alone, but is more common when spondylolysis is in the setting of spondylolisthesis and/or radiculopathy.

The natural history of spondylolysis and low-grade (<2) spondylolisthesis is benign, i.e. it is rare to have progressive slippage. Saraste demonstrated this in a study of 225 patients with a 20-year follow-up period.[177] Most cases of progressive slippage occur during the adolescent growth spurt, however, so for very young athletes monitoring with lateral flexion–extension plain films during this time is appropriate. Besides the adolescent growth spurt, a listhesis >50% is considered a risk factor for progressive slip.

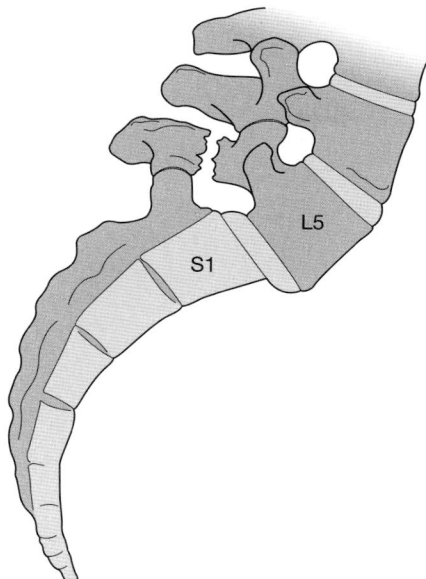

Figure 41-24 Grade 1 isthmic spondylolisthesis.

Spondylolisthesis

There are many causes of lumbar spondylolisthesis or anterior slippage of one vertebra on another. Spondylolisthesis can be grouped into six different categories by etiology. The most common is the isthmic spondylolisthesis (Fig. 41-24). The isthmic slip occurs due to a spondylolysis or 'stress fracture' of the pars interarticularis (as described above). The dysplastic spondylolisthesis is a congenital slip, and is caused by dysplasia of the facet joints of the upper sacrum, leading to an inability to resist shear stresses; consequently forward slippage results. Degenerative spondylolisthesis is seen in the older spine, and is related to longstanding intersegmental instability from degenerative facet or disk disease. The most common level affected in a degenerative slip is the L4–5 level. Traumatic spondylolisthesis is rare, and is caused by acute fracture secondary to trauma. Pathologic spondylolisthesis is due to medical causes of generalized or local bone disease that can cause decreased bony strength. This form can present as an isthmic defect or an elongated, intact pars. The final category is postsurgical and is due to resulting instability from an extensive decompression, which is quite uncommon now due to the amount of hardware used for fusions after extensive decompression.

The patient with spondylolisthesis typically presents with low back pain. Sometimes, there is a complaint of intermittent radicular symptoms related to a dynamic radiculitis, i.e. nerve root irritation caused by subtle instability at the listhetic segment. Physical examination is not different from that seen in spondylolysis. When imaging a patient with suspected spondylolisthesis, lateral flexion–extension views are helpful for presurgical screening. With lateral plain films, the degree of slip is graded 1–5 (Table 41-8).

The natural history of spondylolisthesis is spontaneous stabilization. It is generally accepted that significant slip progression

Table 41-8 Meyerding's grading system for spondylolisthesis[a]

Grade	Percentage slip
1	<25
2	25–49
3	50–74
4	75–99
5	≥100 (spondyloptosis)

[a]Meyerding divided the anterior–posterior diameter of the superior surface of the first sacral vertebral into quarters and assigned the grade accordingly.[226]

rarely occurs in adults.[177,182] There is some controversy regarding slip progression in adolescents. Harris studied youths with grade 3 or 4 slips in a long-term follow-up study, and noted that there was a higher incidence of progression of the slip until skeletal maturity was reached.[80] Saraste and Seitsalo had similarly large long-term observational studies that demonstrated that slip progression in youths and adults was quite small overall.[177,182] Possible factors positively correlating with slip progression include degree of slip, degenerative disk disease at the level of slip, adolescent age, and ligamentous laxity that manifests as hypermobility on imaging (i.e. motion on flexion–extension views).

Treatment for an isthmic spondylolisthesis in a young patient is similar to that for the athlete with spondylolysis, as described in the prior section. Fusion surgery is generally considered in adolescents if the slip is grade 3 or greater. For the degenerative spondylolisthesis, non-operative management with a rehabilitation program similar to that described in the section on degenerative zygapophyseal joint and disk disease is appropriate, because both are typical findings with a degenerative slip. Operative intervention with fusion is generally considered only for recalcitrant pain after an appropriate rehabilitation program, persistent radiculopathy, or progressive instability.

Other spinal fractures

There are many other types of spinal fracture, the most common of which are briefly discussed below. Many are secondary to trauma. Evidence-based guidelines have not yet been developed for the treatment of traumatic spine fractures. Current literature in this area is mainly of retrospective case series. Outcomes appear to be most dependent on the amount of neurologic injury at the time of injury, and on the time elapsed between injury and surgery if a neurologic injury exists.[210]

The three-column structural concept of Denis is the most common way to classify spinal fractures. This concept divides the spine into anterior, middle, and posterior columns. The anterior column is made up of the anterior longitudinal ligament and the anterior half of the vertebral body and disk. The middle column is made up of the posterior longitudinal ligament and the posterior half of the vertebral body and disk. The posterior column is made up of the rest of the bony and soft tissues of the spine. If two of the three columns are intact, the spine is stable and treatment with pain management and rehabilitation is generally indicated.

Posterior column fractures   This includes transverse process and spinous process fractures. These are stable injuries. They are treated by pain management techniques and avoiding contact sports until the fractures have healed.

Anterior column fractures   These are compression fractures and generally are caused by flexion injuries. These fractures usually do not cause neurologic deficits and do not require surgery. If greater than 50% of the height of the vertebral body is lost, there is an increased chance that the fracture can be unstable, because posterior injury might also be involved, and further investigation can be warranted. The treatment of traumatic compression fractures remains controversial.

Anterior and middle column fractures   These are burst fractures and are usually the result of compression and flexion injuries. Instability and cord compression should be ruled out with plain films, a CT scan, and a thorough neurologic assessment. If patients are neurologically intact and there is no evidence of posterior instability, they can often be treated with a brace, usually a thoracic–lumbar–sacral orthosis for 12 weeks. If there is injury to the posterior longitudinal ligament, then surgery is usually required. Burst fractures in which there is loss of 50% or more of the height of the vertebral body, greater than 50% impingement into the spinal canal, or greater than 20° of kyphosis require surgery to achieve stability.

Anterior and posterior column fractures   These are caused by flexion and distraction injuries, and are called chance fractures. They are usually caused by seat belt injuries in high-impact motor vehicle accidents. They are unstable fractures. They are sometimes treated with bracing but often require surgery.[156]

Osteoporotic compression fractures   Osteoporotic compression fractures are important to diagnose, both because they are a significant source of morbidity and because they also can herald the risk for subsequent fractures, particularly hip fractures, which have a high morbidity and mortality. Patients who have had a previous vertebral fracture have 3.8 times the risk of suffering a hip fracture compared with those who have not. The risk of compression fractures increases as bone density decreases. Genetic factors account for much of the risk, as well as exercise, calcium intake, smoking, alcohol use, and age at puberty (see Ch. 42).

Compression fractures can be a significant cause of pain, and are generally the reason that there is a higher incidence of back pain in elderly women as compared with in men. Pain is especially prevalent if three or more fractures are present. These subjects have twice as much back pain as those without compression fractures.[61] Fractures can be asymptomatic or can present with sudden onset of severe pain. Pain can radiate anteriorly, and usually gradually improves over several weeks.

Diagnostic evaluation for vertebral fractures   Up to 30% of those with osteoporotic compression fractures have an underlining cause, which is called secondary osteoporosis. Common causes of secondary osteoporosis are use of oral steroids, hyperthyroidism, metastases, and multiple myeloma. An underlying cause should always be ruled out. This can be done with a complete blood count, sedimentation rate, reactive protein, thyroid function tests, bone profile, and biochemical profile (such as liver function test, electrolytes, and albumin).[147] Bone mineral density measurements are useful to confirm the diagnosis of osteoporosis and to assess the efficacy of treatment.

Treatment   A balance should be found between alleviating pain and the pain medication side effects. Calcitonin, either subcutaneous or intranasal, has been found in multiple studies to decrease pain without significant side effects. Adjunct treatment and modalities such as TENS might be helpful. Intercostal nerve blocks are sometimes used to treat the pain.

Vertebroplasty is a procedure in which bone cement is injected into the bone for pain relief and to strengthen the bone. Studies so far have mainly been case series or uncontrolled prospective studies, but it appears that up to 80% of patients treated obtain significant pain relief, and complications are rare. The complications can include compression of the spinal nerve roots and spinal cord, and pulmonary embolism.[61]

Osteoporosis requires treatment with a combination of medication, lifestyle modification, and exercise (see Ch. 42).

Cancer and low back pain

Cancer is the second leading cause of death in the USA, and two-thirds of patients with cancer develop metastases. The third most common site of metastases is to bone. The spine is the most common site for bony metastases, and vertebral body metastases are found in over one-third of cancer patients. The most common cancers that involve the spine are lung, breast, prostate, and renal cell.[157]

Back pain is by far the most common symptom of metastatic disease. It is caused by stretching of the periosteum and tumor mass effect. Most commonly, the thoracic region of the spine is involved, although the lumbar spine is a more common site for colorectal cancer.[162] The pain can start gradually and increase as the bone is destroyed. It is a constant ache not exacerbated by movement. Sometimes, the pain has a more sudden onset because of a pathologic fracture, and this type of pain can be worse with movement, especially if the spine is unstable. Deyo found that the most specific historical feature for malignancy is a previous history of cancer (98% specific), and the authors considered it prudent to consider new-onset back pain in a patient with a history of cancer to be malignant disease until proven otherwise. This historical feature has a sensitivity of only

0.31, however, so only about one-third of patients with spinal malignant neoplasm have a history of cancer. Consequently, other features suggestive of malignancy must be explored in the history. Back pain unrelieved by bed rest is greater than 90% sensitive so, if the pain is relieved by bed rest, malignancy is unlikely. This is not specific, so many patients without malignancy will complain that their pain is not relieved by bed rest. Other historical features related to cancer include unexplained weight loss and failure to improve with conservative care. New onset of back pain after age 50 is suspicious for malignancy, because many other common causes of back pain begin at an earlier age. These features can be combined to give the clinician confidence in determining if cancer should be included in the differential diagnosis. For example, in Deyo's study of nearly 2000 patients with back pain, no patient under 50 had cancer involving the spine without a history of cancer, unexplained weight loss, and failure to improve with conservative care, giving a combined sensitivity of 100%.[46]

Neurologic deficits occur much less commonly than back pain, but 5–20% of patients with spinal metastases will develop neurologic deficits either from mechanical pressure of the tumor or from bone extruded from a collapsed vertebral body.[201] Deficits often occur several months after the back pain began.[67]

Imaging for suspected spinal metastasis

Because significant vertebral body destruction must occur before changes are seen on plain films, the sensitivity of plain films is low, especially early in the course of the disease. In the thoracic and lumbar spine, the most common finding on plain films is pedicle erosion. Compression fractures can also be seen. Technetium-99 bone scintigraphy is more sensitive for most types of metastases than plain films are, but the specificity is low. Trauma or degenerative disease can cause false positives. Certain highly vascular metastases, such as renal cell and thyroid, can be missed on bone scans.[67,162] CT is the best imaging modality to examine bone anatomy, but it does not give nearly as much information about neural compression as MRI does. It is useful for surgical planning. MRI is the imaging modality of choice for a full evaluation of spinal metastases. It is very sensitive and can show early changes in the bone marrow. It also shows both bony destruction and neural compression.[67,162]

Spinal infections

Spinal infections include osteomyelitis, diskitis, pyogenic facet arthropathy, and epidural infections. These structures are often all infected at the same time. The incidence of spinal infections is increasing. Some of the causes of this include the growing numbers of immunocompromised patients who are at high risk, drug resistance of some infections, and the recent increases in tuberculosis.[194] It is important to diagnose and treat spinal infections quickly to prevent increased morbidity and mortality, and to prevent complications such as epidural abscesses that can cause paralysis. However, this is not always easy. In Tali's review article of spinal infection, he describes the 'rule of 50' to assist in the diagnosis of spinal infections: 50% of the patients are older than 50, 50% will have a fever, and 50% will have a normal white blood count. The urinary tract is the source in 50%, *Staphylococcus aureus* is the organism in 50%, the lumbar spine is affected in 50%, and symptoms are present for greater than 3 months in 50%.[194]

Vertebral osteomyelitis can occur from hematogenous spread or secondary to a contiguous focus of infection. Hematogenous spread occurs via spinal arteries, and infection can quickly spread from the end plate of one vertebral body into the disk and then into the adjacent vertebral body. The most common source is urinary tract infections, often caused by *Escherichia coli* and other enteric bacilli. Hematogenous spread is also seen from other sources, such as infected intravenous lines or endocarditis. Patients with diabetes, those on hemodialysis, intravenous drug users, and other immunocompromised patients are at increased risk.[116,194] The most common location is the lumbar spine, and the most common symptom is back pain, although 15% of patients also have radicular pain. Symptoms can begin slowly and progress over months. Many patients do not have a fever or elevated white blood count. The erythrocyte sedimentation rate, however, is usually elevated. The infection can spread to surrounding tissues, and epidural, paraspinal, and psoas abscesses can also be present. Epidural abscesses are particularly serious because of the risk of spinal cord injury. Early diagnosis is important to prevent bone necrosis and other complications of a spreading infection.[98]

Plain films are usually normal the first 2 weeks, and then the first sign is a periosteal reaction. As the infection progresses, plain films show irregular erosions in the end plates of adjacent vertebral bodies and narrowing of the disk space. This appearance is nearly pathognomonic for infection, as tumors and other causes of irregular erosions rarely cross the disk space. Bone scan shows changes as soon as 24 h after symptoms begin but is not specific. MRI is as sensitive as bone scan and can give important anatomic information, so is generally the imaging technique that should be used.[98,100]

Treatment for spinal infections is usually a 4- to 6-week course of intravenous antibiotics. Sensitivity can often be determined by blood cultures but, if these are negative, samples from a bone biopsy might be necessary. Following the erythrocyte sedimentation rate is helpful to determine the effectiveness of treatment. Surgery is generally necessary only if the spine has become unstable, there are progressive neurologic deficits, or medical treatment fails. Spontaneous fusion of the infected segments often occurs after treatment.[98]

Osteomyelitis secondary to a contiguous focus of infection is seen after surgical procedures and with extension of infection from adjacent soft tissue. The most common organism is *S. aureus*.[116,194] Risk factors for development of postoperative osteomyelitis include history of smoking, obesity, poor nutrition, uncontrolled diabetes, administration of steroids, history of malignancy, and radiation treatment in the area of surgery.[98] These infections usually present about 14–30 days after surgery.[98] Diagnosis is sometimes difficult, as symptoms such as

pain or fever can be attributed to soft tissue infection or the surgical procedure. Imaging studies can also be less conclusive because of surgical or soft tissue changes. Erythocyte sedimentation rate is usually elevated after surgery, so is not as useful in making the diagnosis in the first weeks after surgery.[98] Treatment for these types of infection usually requires surgical debridement and then a course of antibiotics.[116,194]

Diskitis can occur from contiguous spread of infection, or iatrogenically from procedures such as diskectomy and diskography. The incidence of these types of infection is low, as studies report a 0–3% incidence with procedures, but morbidity if infection occurs is significant. One study found that 55–87% of patients were unable to return to their normal work after diskitis. One reason for this poor outcome is the difficulty of using antibiotics to treat the infection because of the relative avascularity of disks.[31]

Spondyloarthropathies

Spondyloarthropathies are a group of diseases associated with the HLA-B27 allele. They include ankylosing spondylitis, Reiter syndrome, reactive arthritis, psoriatic arthritis, enteropathic arthritis, and undifferentiated spondyloarthropathy. It is hypothesized that, in genetically susceptible individuals, an interplay of environmental and immunologic factors leads to clinical manifestations. Although the diseases are grouped together, each has unique features on clinical presentation.[95]

Ankylosing spondylitis

Ankylosing spondylitis is the prototype for the spondyloarthropathies. It is three times more common in men than in women. Symptoms usually begin in the late teens or twenties. It generally first presents with morning stiffness and a dull ache in the low back or buttocks. On physical examination, there is decreased spinal mobility, decreased chest expansion, and tenderness of the sacroiliac joints with direct pressure and with maneuvers that stress the joints.[95]

Findings outside the spine are also common. Hip or shoulder arthritis is seen in about 30% of patients, and asymmetric peripheral joint arthritis is also seen in about 30% of patients. Bony tenderness and enthesitis at multiple sites, such as the heels, greater trochanters, iliac crests, and tibial tuberosities, is common. Systemic disease manifestations include anterior uveitis, heart disease, and inflammatory bowel disease.[195]

The modified New York criteria are widely used for diagnosis. These are the presence of sacroiliitis on x-ray and one of the following: history of inflammatory back pain (insidious onset of back pain before age 40 that lasts longer than 3 months, is accompanied by morning stiffness, and improves with activity), decreased ROM of the spine, and limited chest expansion. Blood work can also be helpful in establishing the diagnosis. The HLA-B27 gene is present in 90% of patients with ankylosing spondylitis. Most patients also have an elevated sedimentation rate. Beyond the changes to the sacroiliac joints of erosions and sclerosis, as the disease progresses there are typical changes in the lumbar spine, including reactive sclerosis and erosions. This can lead to squaring of the vertebral body, and eventually to bony bridging between vertebrae.[195]

The initial treatment includes exercises that promote spinal extension. There is evidence that exercise promotes mobility, improves function, and prevents severe deformity in many cases.[195] NSAIDs are helpful to relieve pain and inflammation, so that the exercises can be done and function maintained. Indomethacin is particularly effective for this condition. Sulfasalazine and methotrexate are sometimes used, especially if there is peripheral arthritis. Disease-modifying agents such as the tumor necrosis factor inhibitors are also being used to treat ankylosing spondylitis, and large studies to determine their effectiveness are needed.[95] Sacroiliac injections under fluoroscopy can reduce symptoms acutely but do not cause long-term benefit.[195]

Other spondyloarthropathies

Reiter syndrome and reactive arthritis can affect the spine. Asymmetric sacroiliitis and discontinuous spondylitis are seen. These usually begin after a genitourinary or gastrointestinal infection. Systemic symptoms are common, and conjunctivitis is seen in up to 50% of patients. Psoriatic arthritis can affect the spine, but an oligoarticular pattern of distal joints is much more common. Enteropathic spondyloarthropathies occur in about 20% of patients with inflammatory bowel disease and can be indistinguishable from ankylosing spondylitis. The term *undifferentiated spondyloarthropathies* is used if a patient has some features of, but does not fully meet, the diagnostic criteria for a well-defined spondyloarthropathy. Treatment of these conditions from a rehabilitation standpoint is similar to the treatment of ankylosing spondylitis.[95]

DIFFERENTIAL DIAGNOSIS AND TREATMENT: LEG PAIN GREATER THAN BACK PAIN

The differential diagnosis for those with leg pain greater than back pain is shorter than that for whom back pain predominates. Common causes of this are discussed below, as are common mimickers of radicular pain that are not to be missed.

Lumbosacral radiculopathy

Radicular symptoms can be the result of overt mechanical compression of a nerve root, or a chemically mediated inflammatory process. The most common compressing lesion by far is a disk protrusion. Less than 1% of patients who present with radicular symptoms have other causes, including infection, malignancy, or fracture.[43] Rare presentations of radiculopathy, i.e. those with fever, weight loss, night pain, cancer history, or osteoporosis risk factors, certainly warrant special attention to evaluate for the less common but potentially more catastrophic causes of radiculopathy.

The most common levels of disk herniation are L4–5 and L5–S1, with L5 and S1 being the most common nerve roots involved in radiculopathy. Multiple nerve roots can be affected by a single disk herniation, given the organization of the cauda equina. Central disk herniations can affect nerve rootlets that are descending in the cauda equina. The affected nerve root level might not correlate with the level of the disk herniation. For example, a central L3–4 disk herniation could impact the L5 or S1 rootlets as they descend through the thecal sac before exiting out of their expected neural foramen. True cauda equina syndrome occurs when the lowest sacral rootlets are affected, resulting in bowel, bladder, and sexual dysfunction. Up to 1% of all disk herniations present as cauda equina syndrome.[184] In the appropriate clinical setting, a large postvoid residual of urine is a good predictor of cauda equina syndrome.[43] Cauda equina syndrome is a surgical emergency. Recovery of neurologic deficits, including bowel and bladder dysfunction, is greatest if decompressive surgery is performed within 48 h.[220]

The natural history of lumbosacral radiculopathy resulting from disk herniation tends to favor spontaneous resolution of symptoms over time.[35] There have been multiple reports that disk protrusions and extrusions can regress without surgical treatment.[196] Conservative treatment is best used to decrease pain and improve the patient's level of functioning during acute management of radiculopathy. Even with some neurologic injury, conservative management should be considered, as various studies have documented the same neurologic recovery in groups treated surgically and non-surgically.[223]

The specifics of conservative management of lumbosacral radiculopathies, however, are still debatable. Given that radicular pain is thought to have some inflammatory component, antiinflammatory medications are commonly implemented in the initial management. NSAIDs are useful medications for the short-term symptomatic relief of acute low back pain; however, they have been found to be less effective in patients with radiculopathy.[206] There is also no definite support for oral steroids in the treatment of acute radiculopathy.[40] The neuropathic pain agents (anticonvulsants and tricyclic antidepressants) are often used for radicular pain, although no studies have proven their efficacy.[40] They are sometimes more useful for their known side effect of sedation in those patients with an associated sleep disturbance.

Although exercise therapy has not specifically been demonstrated to alter the course of acute radiculopathy, there is probably a role for exercise.[202] Relative rest is initially indicated for the first 1–3 days. After that, increasing activity level is important. Whether to do this in a structured, supervised setting (i.e. in physical therapy) or alone is debatable, as the studies that evaluate exercise programs are not specific to an anatomic diagnosis. This is due to the fact that most studies lump together patients with variable causes of back pain and radiculopathy (far lateral disk herniation versus central disk herniation versus stenosis) when analyzing an exercise approach. Saal reported very favorable outcomes using aggressive non-operative care (an active exercise program potentially with epidural steroid injections) in the treatment of lumbar disk herniation with radiculopathy.[173] Their protocol is the basis for many exercise programs used in the treatment of lumbar disk herniations with radiculopathy today.

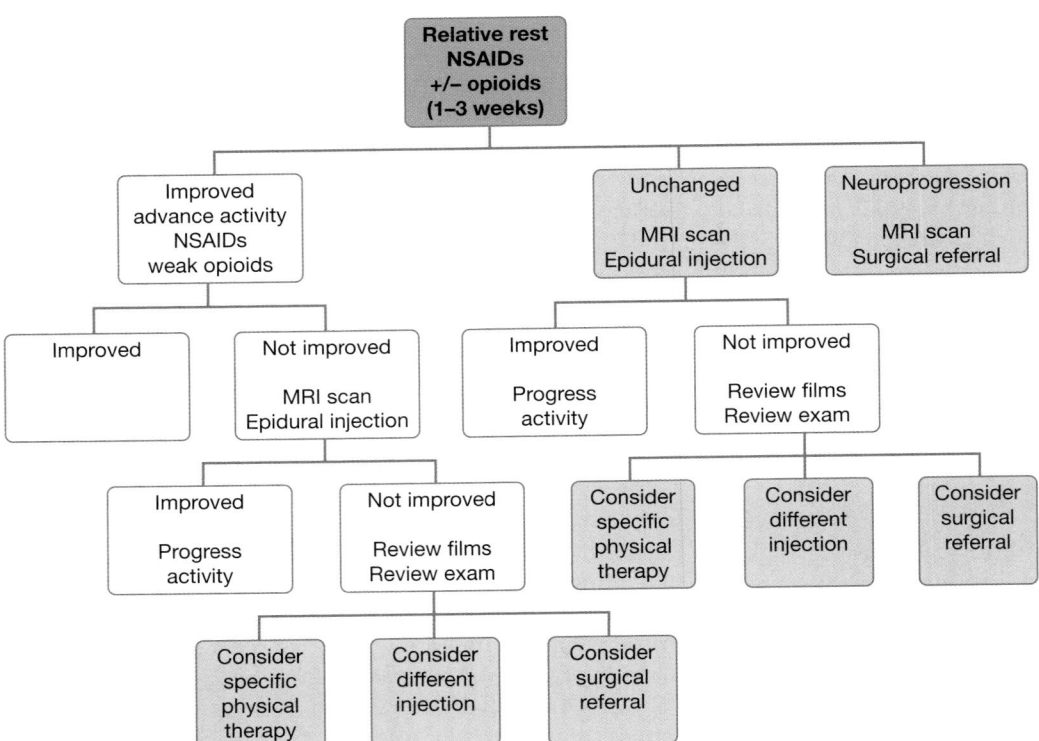

Figure 41-25 Algorithmic approach to acute lumbosacral radiculopathy (without cauda equina). (From Chiodo and Haig 2002,[40] with permission.)

Lumbar epidural steroid injections have become a common adjuvant for the treatment of lumbosacral radiculopathy. The more recent literature supports the use of fluoroscopically guided transforaminal epidural injections for early pain relief, and potentially a more rapid recovery and reduced need for surgical intervention.[94,111,167,209] They are best used in combination with an active rehabilitation program, and are commonly used to facilitate active therapy by decreasing pain and inflammation.

Surgical management of lumbosacral radiculopathy is best reserved for those patients who have significant persistent radicular symptoms despite 6–8 weeks of maximized conservative management, neurologic progression, or cauda equina syndrome. Common decompressive procedures with favorable outcomes include lumbar hemilaminotomy with diskectomy, and lumbar hemilaminectomy.[190] Patients need to be counseled regarding appropriate expectations following surgery for lumbar disk herniation with radiculopathy. Surgery might slightly accelerate the resolution of neurologic deficits for the typical radiculopathy; however, the major benefit of surgical intervention is pain relief.[45] Relief of leg pain should be expected; however, back pain relief is more difficult to predict. Patients should be counseled that they are likely to have recurrent back difficulties even after a successful decompressive surgery. Figure 41-25 shows a useful algorithmic approach to the management of acute lumbosacral radiculopathy.

Lumbar spinal stenosis

The symptoms of spinal stenosis result from a complex series of changes within the lumbar spine.[66] Generally, these changes are related to aging. The narrowing of the spinal canal that occurs in stenosis results from the degenerative changes described by Kirkaldly-Willis.[100] Not all patients with significant narrowing, however, have symptoms. There are probably vascular and biochemical factors involved that add to the mechanical compression (resulting from narrowing of the canal), which ultimately leads to symptomatic spinal stenosis. These have been described earlier in this chapter. Box 41-4 gives a classification schema for spinal stenosis, and Table 41-9 outlines a radiologic grading scale.

The variable symptoms of spinal stenosis are due to the fact that a single nerve or multiple nerve roots can be affected at one or multiple locations within the lumbar spine. Mechanical compression of the nerves can occur due to central canal narrowing, lateral recess narrowing, and intervertebral foraminal narrowing. This results in variable symptoms, from a monoradiculopathy to polyradiculopathy to the hallmark symptoms of neurogenic claudication.

Neurologic claudication is the most common presenting symptom of lumbar stenosis, and results from central canal narrowing. It is classically described as bilateral leg pain initiated by walking, prolonged standing, and walking downhill (relative lumbar extension). Typically, it is relieved by sitting or

Table 41-9 Grading lumbar stenosis on magnetic resonance imaging

Grade	Percentage of the anteroposterior canal dimensions at a normal level
Mild	75–99
Moderate	50–74
Severe	<50

Box 41-4 Classification of spinal stenosis

- Congenital
  Achondroplasia or dwarfism
  Idiopathic or congenital
- Acquired
  Degenerative
  Iatrogenic or postsurgical
- Traumatic
- Combined

bending forward. If foraminal or lateral recess stenosis is the primary pathologic issue, then patients can present with more standard radicular pain in the typical dermatomal distribution. Most patients default to a forward-flexed posture to widen the central canal, subsequently decreasing mechanical compression of the nerve roots. This can lead to significant hip flexion contractures.

The natural history of lumbar spinal stenosis is fairly favorable overall. Johnsson followed patients with lumbar stenosis over a 4-year period with conservative treatment.[92] Based on subjective patient reports, 70% remained unchanged, 15% improved, and 15% worsened. Walking capacity improved in 42% of patients, remained unchanged in 32%, and decreased in 26%. Amundson reported on a 10-year study of patients randomly assigned to surgical or non-surgical treatment.[5] Non-surgical treatment consisted of bracing for 1 month followed by physical therapy. He demonstrated that neurologic deterioration was rare, that delaying surgery (with conservative management) had no effect on postoperative outcomes and that, at 4 years, half the conservative treatment group and four-fifths of the surgical group had favorable outcomes. During the final 6 years of study, clinical deterioration of symptoms was rare. In general, most patients with symptomatic stenosis remain unchanged, while some improved and others worsened. It is impossible to predict which patients will fall into each of these categories. It is useful information that a diagnosis of lumbar stenosis does not mean rapid neurologic deterioration, and that conservative management for those with mild to moderate symptoms is warranted.

The primary goals of conservative management are pain control, and reducing the functional limitations that result from the lessened activity and pain of stenosis. There are multiple facets to this management program, including oral medications, epidural steroids, and a comprehensive functional rehabilitation program. The oral medications are no different than what have been described previously for treatment of radiculopathy. Even more attention needs to be placed on side effects, however, as most patients with lumbar stenosis are elderly and potentially have multiple medical problems that already require multiple medications.

Botwin has demonstrated that there probably is a role for epidural steroid injections in the non-operative treatment of symptomatic lumbar stenosis.[28] He performed transforaminal epidural steroid injections in stenosis patients who were deemed surgical candidates. They also received oral medications and physical therapy. Even at 1-year follow-up, 64% of his patients felt subjectively better. Only 17% of patients went on to surgery within the 1-year follow-up period.

Although there is a paucity of studies examining specific rehabilitation protocols, there is certainly a role for a therapeutic exercise program in the management of lumbar spinal stenosis. The basis of any protocol should be flexion-based lumbar stabilization exercises. This includes strengthening the abdominals and pelvic girdle stabilizers, including the gluteals. Improving hip mobility through stretching, especially of the anterior muscles (iliopsoas and rectus femoris), is also key. Aerobic conditioning is the final component of a comprehensive rehabilitation program for stenosis. Bracing with an abdominal corset might be beneficial for overweight patients with a protuberant abdomen, to lessen the forces creating an exaggerated lordotic posture. However, there is a lack of clear data supporting the role of lumbosacral orthoses in spinal stenosis.

Surgical consideration for lumbar stenosis should be given to patients with intractable pain recalcitrant to non-operative management, profound or progressive neurologic deficit, or lifestyle impairment.[170] Age is not a contraindication to surgery, although the patient's general health status must be considered.[10,82] Laminectomies are the most common decompressive procedures.[170] When spinal stenosis is associated with instability, degenerative spondylolisthesis, deformity, or recurrent stenosis, fusion is often performed. Instrumentation often improves the fusion rate but does not influence the clinical outcome.[183] If selectively chosen, most patients with neurogenic claudication do quite well with surgical management. However, if the chief symptomatic complaint is axial low back pain, the surgical outcome is generally poorer.[96]

Non-lumbar spine causes of 'radicular' leg symptoms

There are a number of non-spinal disorders that mimic lumbar radiculopathy, because they generate pain referral patterns similar to lumbosacral dermatomes. Their etiology is diverse and includes joint, soft tissue, vascular, and peripheral nerve sources. A thorough history and physical examination can typically help differentiate these disorders from lumbosacral radiculopathy; however, other diagnostic studies might be necessary.

Joint disorders

The sacroiliac joint is now generally accepted as a potential pain generator that can refer into the lower limb. Other than true sacroiliitis (associated with the spondyloarthropathies), the exact pathologic structure or source of pain from the sacroiliac joint is still uncertain. In 2002, Vilensky reported that substance P may be found in the posterior sacroiliac ligament.[211] However, it is still not known whether it is the synovium, the articular cartilage, the capsule, the ligamentous structures, the muscular support of the sacroiliac joint, or a combination that is the primary source of pain referred to as sacroiliac joint pain.

Although there are multiple physical examination maneuvers created to stress the sacroiliac joint and reproduce pain, rigorous studies have demonstrated that no one physical examination maneuver (nor combination) correlates well to diagnose sacroiliac joint pain confirmed from diagnostic local anesthetic injections into the joint.[49] The gold standard for diagnosing sacroiliac joint pain is a fluoroscopically guided injection of local anesthetic into the sacroiliac joint.

Guided injections have helped to delineate the sclerotomal referral pattern of pain emanating from the sacroiliac joint.[59,60] Sacroiliac joint pain generally does not radiate above the lumbosacral junction. It can radiate into the groin, thigh, and even below the knee, with significant overlap of lumbosacral radicular pain patterns.

Disorders involving the hip joint generally refer pain into the groin and sometimes the anterior thigh. The prototypical disorder is osteoarthritis of the hip. This pain pattern is easily confused with L1–2 to 3 nerve root involvement. Plain films of the hip as well as hip ROM on physical examination are generally most helpful in differentiating an intraarticular hip source of pain from spinal referred pain.

Soft tissue disorders

Piriformis syndrome is thought to cause sciatica via the piriformis muscle putting local pressure on the sciatic nerve in the pelvis. Pain generally emanates into the posterior thigh but can refer below the knee in an L5 or S1 dermatomal pattern. The patient also describes buttock pain and typically has tenderness over the sciatic notch. There are multiple examination maneuvers used to reproduce sciatica resulting from piriformis syndrome.[18] Pace's maneuver is described as resisted abduction and external rotation of the thigh. Freiberg's maneuver is forceful internal rotation of the extended thigh. Beatty described his maneuver as deep buttock pain produced by the side-lying patient holding a flexed knee several inches off the table. Fishman described an electrophysiologic approach to diagnose piriformis syndrome using H waves.[58]

Greater trochanteric pain syndrome is a descriptive term for a regional pain syndrome focused about the greater trochanter, buttock, and lateral thigh.[185] It is often initially diagnosed as trochanteric bursitis but, given its recalcitrant nature and not always responding to well-placed greater trochanter bursa injections, is probably multifactorial in etiology. There is probably an association with gluteal muscle (medius and minimus) pathology, potentially tendonopathy, tears, or myofascial pain. On physical examination, besides the generalized tenderness in the region, typically there is significant gluteal muscle inhibition and deconditioning that can manifest as hip abductor weakness. Generally, a comprehensive rehabilitation program focusing initially on pain control and neuromuscular reeducation of the gluteal muscles is important prior to progressing to strength-building exercises for the gluteals.

Iliotibial band syndrome can be confused with an L4 or L5 radiculopathy. The iliotibial band is an extension of the tensor fascia lata that traverses the lateral aspect of the thigh, attaching at Gerdy's tubercle on the proximal lateral tibia. Iliotibial band syndrome typically presents as lateral knee pain, but it can also present with more proximal (lateral thigh) pain or radiate distally into the calf. When the iliotibial band is tight, it can also exacerbate trochanteric bursitis and be associated with lateral hip and buttock pain. Iliotibial band tightness is evaluated with Ober's maneuver.[114]

Myofascial pain syndromes are quite common, and are thought to arise from active trigger points within a muscle or its fascia.[186] Activation of trigger points in various muscles have typical pain referral patterns that can mimic lumbosacral dermatomes (see Ch. 42).

Vascular disorders

Vascular claudication from peripheral vascular disease can be difficult to differentiate from neurogenic claudication secondary to lumbar spinal stenosis, especially because both are common in elderly patients. Symptoms from both are exacerbated by walking; however, flexing forward or sitting is necessary to alleviate the symptoms of neurogenic claudication. On the contrary, just stopping ambulation typically improves the vascular symptoms. Leaning forward on a grocery cart or walker while ambulating can also reduce neurogenic claudication but does not help with vascular claudication. The bicycle test can be used to differentiate between the two, because any lower extremity exercise should exacerbate vascular claudication; however, stationary cycling (while sitting with lumbar flexion) should not exacerbate neurogenic claudication. Finally, a patient with neurogenic claudication typically has more pain with downhill walking, due to the relative lumbar extension and resultant narrowing of the spinal canal, whereas uphill walking is more strenuous and thus brings on symptoms of vascular disease.

Peripheral nerve disorders

Peripheral polyneuropathy is a common cause of paresthesias in the distal lower extremities and feet that can mimic symptoms of lumbar stenosis. They are often seen together in elderly patients with diabetes. Electrodiagnostic studies are used to diagnose a superimposed peripheral polyneuropathy in patients who have MRI findings of lumbar stenosis. Epidural steroid injections can sometimes be helpful in this situation to help determine how much of the patient's leg and foot symptoms are related to spinal stenosis over peripheral polyneuropathy.

PREVENTION OF BACK PAIN

Because back pain is so common, and because it results in enormous expense to society, the question of whether or not back pain is an inevitable consequence of life or is preventable is often asked. The answer is still not completely known, but certain factors appear to reduce the risk of developing first episodes of back pain and the risk of a particular episode becoming chronic.

Psychosocial factors

It is unclear how much of a role psychosocial factors play in the new onset of low back pain, but probably the strongest preventions against the development of chronic back pain are psychologic and social factors. Strong work and family relationships, a sense of being connected to a community, good mental health, proactive beliefs about pain that do not include catastrophizing and fear-avoidance, the management of any depression and anxiety that exists, and high job satisfaction all appear to be protective against the development of chronic pain.[217]

Physical factors

Studies have found conflicting results of whether physical fitness is protective in the development of low back pain. In Linton and van Tulder's review of prevention of back pain, they identified six randomized controlled trials. Four of the six trials found a benefit of exercise in reducing the occurrence of back pain and work-related absenteeism. One trial was inconclusive, and one found no difference between advice to exercise and a health club membership, although it is unclear how much exercise was being done. Overall, it appears that exercise is beneficial in reducing the incidence of back pain.[109]

Smoking and low back pain

Smoking is a risk factor for the development of back pain, most probably because degenerative changes of the lumbar spine are increased and the blood flow and nutrition to disks are decreased in smokers.[139]

Education

Studies are conflicting as to whether back schools (educational courses to teach about ergonomics, good lifting techniques, and other back-related issues) prevent back pain and disability or make no difference.[109]

Lumbar supports

Although the results of some non-randomized controlled trials looked promising for back pain prevention, the majority of randomized controlled trials do not show that lumbar supports prevent back pain.

PROGNOSIS OF LOW BACK PAIN

Prognosis is difficult to fully ascertain for several reasons. One is that low back pain is a symptom caused by a vast spectrum of pathology with a variety of prognostic outcomes. Another is that the pain experience is individual, and treatment expectations vary. There is a huge body of medical literature that highlights the complex cultural, psychologic, social support, and economic factors that influence pain and rehabilitation outcome.[110]

That being taken into account, the prognosis for low back pain is being better defined. The much quoted view that 90% of cases of acute low back pain will recover within 6 weeks does not include the entire story of low back pain, either in clinical practice or in reviews of the scientific literature. Most studies are performed with subjects who seek medical care for their low back pain, and this might be a select population not generalizable to all those who develop back pain. A recent meta-analysis of patients who sought medical care for back pain of less than 3 weeks' duration was done. They included both those in treatment arms of studies and in the placebo arms, so that both the natural course and the clinical course of back pain could be evaluated. The study found that most patients rapidly improved within 1 month, and that most continued to have pain decrease, although more slowly, until about 3 months. From 3 months to a year, little change in pain was seen. The risk of a recurrence within 3 months varied between 19 and 34%, and the risk of a recurrence within a year was between 66 and 84%. This was a heterogeneous diagnostic population, although the vast majority of patients fell under the diagnosis of mechanical low back pain.

LOW BACK PAIN IN SPECIAL POPULATIONS
Low back pain in pregnancy

Low back pain is a common problem in pregnancy. Multiple studies have estimated the prevalence at 49–76%.[54,103,150,151,221] Risk factors for the development of low back pain during pregnancy include a history of prior back pain, previous pregnancy-related back pain, and low back pain during menses.[32,221] Low back pain is also correlated with the pregnant woman's age.[221] The risk of development of back pain during pregnancy decreases with age. Studies differ on the timing of low back pain during a pregnancy. Earlier studies demonstrated that back pain was generally present in the first 5–7 months of pregnancy, and that pain then decreased subsequently thereafter.[54] More recent studies demonstrate occurrences at any time during the pregnancy, generally reaching a peak at 36 weeks.[103,151,221] Pain decreases after this point and is substantially improved by 3 months postpartum.[151]

The specific etiology of low back pain in pregnancy is unclear. The potential pain generators in pregnant women are probably multiple, and probably similar in etiology to those in the non-pregnant patient with mechanical low back pain. However, there is a very different reason that the tissue is stressed and generating pain in the pregnant patient. Pain drawings have shown that the pain location is variable. In some, it is localized to the sacroiliac areas, and in others more to the lumbar spine.[150]

Lumbar disk herniation is uncommon as a cause of pain, as the prevalence is only 1 in 10 000 pregnant women.[105] The prevalence of disk abnormalities on MRI is the same for pregnant and non-pregnant women.[225]

The etiology of low back pain in the pregnant woman is hypothesized to be increased biomechanical strain or an altered hormonal influence. The biomechanical alterations are due to changes in spine posture related to the anterior movement of the pregnant woman's center of gravity. However, an argument against purely biomechanical factors as the primary cause is that the back pain often starts prior to significant weight gain by the mother, and the incidence does not parallel the weight gain.[33]

There probably is a hormonal influence in the etiology of low back pain in pregnancy. The hypothesis is that the hormonal changes during pregnancy alter the lumbopelvic ligaments, influencing the stability of the lumbosacral spine and making it more vulnerable to loading.[103] However, a direct correlation between circulating levels of the hormone relaxin and pelvic and back pain is controversial.[2,78,104,113]

There are only a few high-quality studies evaluating therapeutic interventions in pregnancy-related low back pain, and there is not much evidence on which to base recommendations for management.[191] To decrease pain, individualized physical therapy, water aerobics, acupuncture, and massage therapy can be recommended.[57,99,146,224] Instruction on a home exercise program, use of a sacroiliac belt, and back school have not been shown to significantly diminish pain intensity.[50,119,130,145] There are no good data to offer an opinion on the use of lumbar–abdominal orthoses that are designed to support the pregnant woman's abdomen.

Pediatric low back pain

Back pain in the pediatric population has traditionally been considered to be relatively rare and, if present, a concern for serious pathology was generally raised. This belief is now known to be untrue. In a subset of studies involving greater than 300 children each, the prevalence of back pain was cited between 30 and 51%.[15,69] Severe back pain, which is either relapsing or permanent, was reported in 3–15%.[15] There is a noted increase in back pain prevalence as the child ages. In a Finnish cohort study, back pain prevalence was reported as 1% in children 7 years old, 6% when 10 years old, and 18% when 14 years old.[193] Another reported the prevalence at 12% for 11-year olds and 50% for 15- to 18-year olds, which approaches the adult prevalence.[34] The same study reported that the pain is often recurrent, but that the experience of back pain is frequently forgotten. Other studies demonstrate that the prevalence of low back pain has the greatest increase during puberty and the time of the maximum growth spurt.[106,212] Risk factors for non-specific low

back pain in the pediatric population include increase in age, female gender, parents with low back pain, hyperlordotic posture, history of spinal trauma, participation in competitive sports or a high level of physical activity, and depression.[15] The literature does not support the following as risk factors for pediatric back pain: being overweight, hamstring tightness, a low level of physical activity, and poor school performance.[15] In the pediatric population, sitting appears to be the main exacerbating factor of low back pain.[15] There also appears to be a positive correlation between low back pain in adolescence and the presence of pain as an adult.[79]

There has been more recent attention focused on the role of backpack use in the development of pediatric low back pain; however, there is still not a proven correlation. Carrying a backpack greater than 7.5–15% of the wearer's body weight increases the metabolic demands over what is required to move a person's body weight alone.[112,168] The general recommendation for a child's backpack weight is limited to 10% of body weight.[112] This limit is based on concerns of increasing metabolic costs, and not on the risk of back pain development (there are conflicting reports in the literature regarding backpack weight and back pain).[76,112,200,222] There are many new backpack designs to improve ergonomic fit; however, there are no studies demonstrating their effectiveness in reducing back pain.[112]

Some of the specific causes of low back pain in the pediatric population are listed in Box 41-5. Spondylolysis and isthmic spondylolisthesis often present in young athletes with back pain, and have been reported as the most common underlying cause of persistent low back pain among children and adolescents.[132] Most believe the etiology is from overuse, particularly during the growth spurt. The presence of isthmic defects in children in the western world is between 2 and 7%, and as high as 30% in elite athletes.[149]

Scheuermann disease typically presents in the adolescent as painless exaggerated thoracic kyphosis. From a postural standpoint, the teenager typically presents with excessive thoracic kyphosis (which is demonstrated to be fixed in attempted hyperextension), with a compensatory lumbar hyperlordosis. Radiographic criteria for the diagnosis of Scheuermann disease include anterior wedging of at least three adjacent vertebrae, end-plate irregularities, Schmorl's nodes, and disk space

---

Box 41-5 Etiology of pediatric low back pain

- Non-specific
- Spondylolysis with or without spondylolisthesis
- Lumbar disk herniation
- Slipped vertebral apophysis
- Scheuermann disease
- Diskitis
- Vertebral osteomyelitis
- Neoplasm
- Rheumatic disease
- Somatization

narrowing.[75] These findings are present equally in the adolescent population without back pain, but there is a higher prevalence of concomitant degenerative disk changes in those with pain.[197]

The etiology of Scheuermann disease is uncertain. Some believe that it is due to repetitive loading of the immature spine that might have some preexisting abnormality of the cartilaginous end plate.[88] There does appear to be a familial link.[129] Scheuermann disease can have a benign course, although some untreated patients develop progressive structural kyphosis. Brace wearing is recommended until skeletal maturity is reached to help prevent the progressive kyphosis.

Idiopathic scoliosis is not generally painful. If associated with pain, often there is more serious underlying pathology such as tumor, infection, or spondylolisthesis. The curve direction in idiopathic scoliosis is typically right thoracic and left lumbar. If an atypical curve is encountered, further evaluation beyond plain films is generally warranted.

Neoplastic disease of the pediatric spine is fortunately rare. Most pediatric spinal tumors are primary (not metastatic), benign bone tumors arising from the vertebrae.[88] The most common tumors of the pediatric spine include osteoid osteoma, osteoblastoma, and aneurysmal bone cysts. The classic pain of osteoid osteoma is nocturnal pain that responds to aspirin. The most frequent malignant lesion affecting the pediatric spine is Ewing's sarcoma.

Acknowledgments

The authors would like to thank Nilda Gatchalian for her assistance in preparing this manuscript.

REFERENCES

1. Akuthota V, Lento P, Sowa G. Pathogenesis of lumbar spinal stenosis pain: why does an asymptomatic stenotic patient flare? Phys Med Rehabil Clin North Am 2003; 14(1):17–28.
2. Albert H, Godskesen M, Westergaard JG, et al. Circulating levels of relaxin are normal in pregnant women with pelvic pain. Eur J Obstet Gynecol Reprod Biol 1997; 74(1):19–22.
3. Al-Obaidi SM, Al-Zoabi B, Al-Shuwaie N, et al. The influence of pain and pain-related fear and disability beliefs on walking velocity in chronic low back pain. Int J Rehabil Res 2003; 26(2):101–108.
4. Al-Obaidi SM, Nelson RM, Al-Awadhi S, et al. The role of anticipation and fear of pain in the persistence of avoidance behavior in patients with chronic low back pain. Spine 2000; 25(9):1126–1131.
5. Amundsen T, Weber H, Nordal HJ, et al. Lumbar spinal stenosis: conservative or surgical management? A prospective 10-year study. Spine 2000; 25(11):1424–1435.
6. Andersson GBJ, Johnsson B, Nachemson AL. Intradiscal pressure, intraabdominal pressure and myoelectric back muscle activity related to posture and loading. Clin Orthop 1977; 129:156–164.
7. Andersson GBJ, Johnsson B, Nachemson AL. Quantitative studies of back load lifting. Spine 1976; 1:178–164.
8. [Anonymous]. Physicians' desk reference. Montvale: Thomson Healthcare; 2004:3296.
9. Aprill C, Bogduk N. High-intensity zone: a diagnostic sign of painful lumbar disc on magnetic resonance imaging. Br J Radiol 1992; 65(773):361–369.
10. Arinzon ZH, Fredman B, Zohar E, et al. Surgical management of spinal stenosis: a comparison of immediate and long term outcome in two geriatric patient populations. Arch Gerontol Geriatr 2003; 36(3):273–279.
11. Ariyoshi M, Sonoda K, Nagata K, et al. Efficacy of aquatic exercises for patients with low-back pain. Kurume Med J 1999; 46(2):91–96.
12. Assendelft WJ, Morton SC, Yu EI, et al. Spinal manipulative therapy for low back pain. A meta-analysis of effectiveness relative to other therapies. Ann Intern Med 2003; 138(11):871–881.
13. Badalamente MA, Dee R, Ghillani R, et al. Mechanical stimulation of dorsal root ganglia induces increased production of substance P: a mechanism for pain following nerve root compromise? Spine 1987; 12(6):552–555.
14. Baker AR, Collins TA, Porter RW, et al. Laser Doppler study of porcine cauda equina blood flow. The effect of electrical stimulation of the rootlets during single and double site, low pressure compression of the cauda equina. Spine 1995; 20(6):660–664.
15. Balague F, Troussier B, Salminen JJ. Non-specific low back pain in children and adolescents: risk factors. Eur Spine J 1999; 8(6):429–438.
16. Ballantyne J. Nonsteroidal anti-inflammatory drugs. In: Ballantyne J, Fishman SM, Abdi S, eds. The Massachusetts General Hospital handbook of pain management. 2nd edn. Philadelphia: Lippincott Williams & Wilkins; 2002:87–102.
17. Bartleson JD. Evidence for and against the use of opioid analgesics for chronic nonmalignant low back pain: a review. Pain Med 2002; 3(3) 260–271.
18. Beatty RA. The piriformis muscle syndrome: a simple diagnostic maneuver. Neurosurgery 1994; 34(3):512–514.
19. Best BA, Guilak F, Setton LA, et al. Compressive mechanical properties of the human annulus fibrosus and their relationship to biomechanical composition. Spine 1994; 19:212–221.
20. Birch S, Hesselink JK, Jonkman FA, et al. Clinical research on acupuncture: part 1. What have reviews of the efficacy and safety of acupuncture told us so far? J Altern Complement Med 2004; 10(3):468–480.
21. Boden SD, Davis DO, Dina TS, et al. Abnormal magnetic-resonance scans of the lumbar spine in asymptomatic subjects. A prospective investigation. J Bone Joint Surg Am 1990; 72(3):403–408.
22. Boersma K, Linton S, Overmeer T, et al. Lowering fear-avoidance and enhancing function through exposure in vivo. A multiple baseline study across six patients with back pain. Pain 2004; 108(1–2):8–16.
23. Bogduk N. Clinical anatomy of the lumbar spine and sacrum. Edinburgh: Churchill Livingstone; 1997.
24. Bogduk N. Nerves of the lumbar spine. In: Bogduk N. Clinical anatomy of the lumbar spine and sacrum. 3rd edn. Edinburgh: Churchill Livingstone; 1977.
25. Bogduk N. The innervation of the lumbar spine. Spine 1983; 8(3):286–293.
26. Bogduk N. The inter-body joint and the intervertebral discs. In: Bogduk N. Clinical anatomy of the lumbar spine and sacrum. 3rd edn. Edinburgh: Churchill Livingstone; 1977.
27. Bogduk N. The zygapophysial joints. In: Bogduk N. Clinical anatomy of the lumbar spine and sacrum. 3rd edn. Edinburgh: Churchill Livingstone; 1977.
28. Botwin KP, Gruber RD, Bouchlas CG, et al. Fluoroscopically guided lumbar transformational epidural steroid injections in degenerative lumbar stenosis: an outcome study. Am J Phys Med Rehabil 2002; 81(12):898–905.
29. Brady RJ, Dean JB, Skinner TM, et al. Limb length inequality: clinical implications for assessment and intervention. J Orthop Sports Phys Ther 2003; 33(5):221–234.
30. Brosseau L, Milne S, Robinson V, et al. Efficacy of the transcutaneous electrical nerve stimulation for the treatment of chronic low back pain: a meta-analysis. Spine 2002; 27(6):596–603.
31. Brown EM, Pople I, de Louvois J, et al. Spine update: prevention of postoperative infection in patients undergoing spinal surgery. Spine 2004; 29(8):938–945.
32. Brynhildsen J, Hansson A, Persson A, et al. Follow-up of patients with low back pain during pregnancy. Obstet Gynecol 1998; 91(2):182–186.
33. Bullock JE, Gwendolen AJ, Bullock MI. The relationship of low back pain to postural changes during pregnancy. Aust J Physiother 1987; 33:10–17.
34. Burton AK, Clarke RD, McClune T, et al. The natural history of low back pain in adolescents. Spine 1996; 21(20):2323–2328.
35. Bush K, Cowan N, Katz DE, et al. The natural history of sciatica associated with disc pathology. A prospective study with clinical and independent radiologic follow-up. Spine 1992; 17(10):1205–1212.
36. Buttemann GR. The effect of spinal steroid injections for degenerative disc disease. Spine J 2004; 4:495–505.

37. Carroll LJ, Cassidy JD, Cote P. Depression as a risk factor for onset of an episode of troublesome neck and low back pain. Pain 2004; 107(1-2): 134–139.

38. Cherkin DC, Deyo RA, Battie M, et al. A comparison of physical therapy, chiropractic manipulation, and provision of an educational booklet for the treatment of patients with low back pain. N Engl J Med 1998; 339(15): 1021–1029.

39. Cherkin DC, Eisenberg D, Sherman KJ, et al. Randomized trial comparing traditional Chinese medical acupuncture, therapeutic massage, and self-care education for chronic low back pain. Arch Intern Med 2001; 161(8): 1081–1088.

40. Chiodo A, Haig AJ. Lumbosacral radiculopathies: conservative approaches to management. Phys Med Rehabil Clin North Am 2002; 13(3):vii, 609–621.

41. Cluff RS. Adjuvant treatments. In: Ballantyne J, ed. The Massachusetts General Hospital handbook of pain management. Philadelphia: Lippincott Williams & Wilkins; 2002:125–137.

42. Crock HV. The applied anatomy of spinal circulation in spinal stenosis. In: McNeill TW, ed. Lumbar spinal stenosis. St. Louis: Mosby; 1992: 91–101.

43. Della-Giustina DA. Emergency department evaluation and treatment of back pain. Emerg Med Clin North Am 1999; 17(4):vi-vii, 877–893.

44. Deyo RA, Diehl AK, Rosenthal M. How many days of bed rest for acute low back pain? A randomized clinical trial. N Engl J Med 1986; 315(17): 1064–1070.

45. Deyo RA, Loeser JD, Bigos SJ. Herniated lumbar intervertebral disk. Ann Intern Med 1990; 112(8):598–603.

46. Deyo RAR, Kent D. What can the history and physical examination tell us about back pain? JAMA 1992; 268(6):760–765.

47. Dietrich M, Kurowski P. The importance of mechanical factors in the etiology of spondylolysis. A model analysis of loads and stresses in human lumbar spine. Spine 1985; 10(6):532–542.

48. Dreyer SJ, Dreyfuss PH. Low back pain and the zygapophyseal (facet) joints. Arch Phys Med Rehabil 1996; 77:290–300.

49. Dreyfuss P, Michaelsen M, Pauza K, et al. The value of medical history and physical examination in diagnosing sacroiliac joint pain. Spine 1996; 21(22):2594–2602.

50. Dumas GA, Reid JG, Wolfe LA, et al. Exercise, posture, and back pain during pregnancy. Part 2. Exercise and back pain. Clin Biomech 1995; 10:104–109.

51. Dvorak J, Panjabi MM, Novotny JE, et al. Clinical validation of functional flexion–extension roentgenograms of the lumbar spine. Spine 1991; 16(8):943–950.

52. Fann AV. The prevalence of postural asymmetry in people with and without chronic low back pain. Arch Phys Med Rehabil 2002; 83(12): 1736–1738.

53. Fardon DF, Milette PC. Nomenclature and classification of lumbar disc pathology. Recommendations of the Combined Task Forces of the North American Spine Society, American Society of Spine Radiology, and American Society of Neuroradiology. Spine 2001; 26(5):E93–E113.

54. Fast A, Shapiro D, Ducommun EJ, et al. Low-back pain in pregnancy. Spine 1987; 12(4):368–371.

55. Ferguson RL, Allen BLJ. A mechanistic classification of thoracolumbar spine fractures. Clin Orthop 1984; Oct(189):77–88.

56. Ferguson RL, McMasters MC, Stanitski CL. Low back pain in college football. J Bone Joint Surg 1974; 56:1300.

57. Field T, Hernandez-Reif M, Hart S, et al. Pregnant women benefit from massage therapy. J Psychosom Obstet Gynaecol 1999; 20(1):31–38.

58. Fishman LM, Zybert PA. Electrophysiologic evidence of piriformis syndrome. Arch Phys Med Rehabil 1992; 73(4):359–364.

59. Fortin JD, Aprill CN, Ponthieux B, et al. Sacroiliac joint: pain referral maps upon applying a new injection/arthrography technique. Part II: clinical evaluation. Spine 1994; 19(13):1483–1489.

60. Fortin JD, Dwyer AP, West S, et al. Sacroiliac joint: pain referral maps upon applying a new injection/arthrography technique. Part I: Asymptomatic volunteers. Spine 1994; 19(13):1475–1482.

61. Francis RM, Baillie SP, Chuck AJ, et al. Acute and long-term management of patients with vertebral fractures. Q J Med 2004; 97(2):63–74.

62. Franson RC, Saal JS, Saal JA. Human disc phospholipase A_2 is inflammatory. Spine 1992; 17(6):S129–S132.

63. Fujiwara A, Tamai K, Yamato M, et al. The relationship between facet joint osteoarthritis and disc degeneration of the lumbar spine: an MRI study. Eur Spine J 1999; 8(5):396–401.

64. Furlan AD, Brosseau L, Imamura M, et al. Massage for low back pain. Cochrane Database Syst Rev 2002; 2:CD001929.

65. Gallagher RM, Mossey JM. Impact of co-morbid depression on self-reported pain and physical and emotional functioning in low back pain patients. Pain Med 2001; 2(3):242.

66. Garfin SR, Rydevik BL, Lipson SJ, et al. Spinal stenosis: pathophysiology. In: Rothman RH, Simeone FA, eds. The spine. 4th edn. Philadelphia: Saunders; 1999:779–796.

67. Gerrard GE, Franks KN. Overview of the diagnosis and management of brain, spine, and meningeal metastases. J Neurol Neurosurg Psychiatry 2004; 75(2):ii37–ii42.

68. Gibson ES. The value of preplacement screening radiograph of low back pain. Spine State Art Rev 1987; 2:91–107.

69. Goodman JE, McGrath PJ. The epidemiology of pain in children and adolescents: a review. Pain 1991; 46(3):247–264.

70. Goupille P, Jayson MI, Valat JP, et al. The role of inflammation in disk herniation-associated radiculopathy. Semin Arthritis Rheum 1998; 28(1): 60–67.

71. Gracovetsky S, Farfan H, Helleur C. The abdominal mechanism. Spine 1985; 10(4):317–324.

72. Greenman PE. Pelvic girdle dysfunction. In: Butler JP, ed. Principles of manual medicine. 2nd edn. Baltimore: Williams & Wilkins; 1996: 305–367.

73. Gronblad M, Hurr H, Kouri JP. Relationships between spinal mobility, physical performance tests, pain intensity and disability assessments in chronic low back pain patients. Scand J Rehabil Med 1997; 29(1):17–24.

74. Gronblad M, Virri J, Seitsalo S, et al. Inflammatory cells, motor weakness, and straight leg raising in transligamentous disc herniations. Spine 2000; 25(21):2803–2807.

75. Guanciale AF, Dillin WH, Watkins RG. Back pain in children and adolescents. In: Rothman RH, Simeone FA, eds. The spine. 4th edn. Philadelphia: Saunders; 1999:187–220.

76. Guyer L. Backpack = back pain. Am J Public Health 2001; 91:16–19.

77. Hadjistavropoulos HD, LaChapelle DL. Extent and nature of anxiety experienced during physical examination of chronic low back pain. Behav Res Ther 2000; 38(1):13–29.

78. Hansen A, Jensen DV, Larsen E, et al. Relaxin is not related to symptom-giving pelvic girdle relaxation in pregnant women. Acta Obstet Gynecol Scand 1996; 75(3):245–249.

79. Harreby M, Neergaard K, Hesselsoe G, et al. Are radiologic changes in the thoracic and lumbar spine of adolescents risk factors for low back pain in adults? A 25-year prospective cohort study of 640 school children. Spine 1995; 20(21):2298–2302.

80. Harris IE, Weinstein SL. Long-term follow-up of patients with grade-III and IV spondylolisthesis. Treatment with and without posterior fusion. J Bone Joint Surg Am 1987; 69(7):960–969.

81. Harte AA, Baxter GD, Gracey JH. The efficacy of traction for back pain: a systematic review of randomized controlled trials. Arch Phys Med Rehabil 2003; 84(10):1542–1553.

82. Hee HT, Wong HK. The long-term results of surgical treatment for spinal stenosis in the elderly. Singapore Med J 2003; 44(4):1750–1780.

83. Helms JM. The basic, clinical, and speculative science of acupuncture. In: Acupuncture energetics—a clinical approach for physicians. Berkeley: Medical Acupuncture Publishers; 1995:19–70.

84. Herzog RJ, Ghanayem AJ, Guyer RD, et al. Magnetic resonance imaging: use in patients with low back pain or radicular pain. Spine J 2003; 3(3 suppl):6S–10S.

85. Hicks GE, Fritz JM, Delitto A, et al. Interrater reliability of clinical examination measures for identification of lumbar segmental instability. Arch Phys Med Rehabil 2003; 84(12):1858–1864.

86. Hodges PW. Core stability exercise in chronic low back pain. Orthop Clin North Am 2003; 34(2):245–254.

87. Hogeboom CJ, Sherman KJ, Cherkin DC. Variation in diagnosis and treatment of chronic low back pain by traditional Chinese medicine acupuncturists. Complement Ther Med 2001; 9(3):154–166.

88. Hollingworth P. Back pain in children. Br J Rheumatol 1996; 35(10): 1022–1028.

89. Jackson DW, Wiltse LL, Cirincoine RJ. Spondylolysis in the female gymnast. Clin Orthop 1976; Jun(117):68–73.

90. Jarvik JJ, Hollingworth W, Heagerty P, et al. The Longitudinal Assessment of Imaging and Disability of the Back (LAIDBack) Study: baseline data. Spine 2001; 26(10):1158–1166.

91. Jensen MC, Brant-Zawadzki MN, Obuchowski N, et al. Magnetic resonance imaging of the lumbar spine in people without back pain. N Engl J Med 1994; 331(2):69–73.

92. Johnsson KE, Rosen I, Uden A. The natural course of lumbar spinal stenosis. Clin Orthop 1992; Jun(279):82–86.

93. Kalauokalani D, Sherman KJ, Cherkin DC. Acupuncture for chronic low back pain: diagnosis and treatment patterns among acupuncturists evaluating the same patient. South Med J 2001; 94(5):486–492.

94. Karppinen J, Ohinmaa A, Malmivaara A, et al. Cost effectiveness of periradicular infiltration for sciatica: subgroup analysis of a randomized controlled trial. Spine 2001; 26(23):2587–2595.

95. Kataria RK, Brent LH. Spondyloarthropathies. Am Fam Physician 2004; 69(12):2853–2860.

96. Katz JN, Lipson SJ, Chang LC, et al. Seven- to 10-year outcome of decompressive surgery for degenerative lumbar spinal stenosis. Spine 1996; 21(1):92–98.

97. Kawakami M, Tamaki T, Matsumoto T, et al. Role of leukocytes in radicular pain secondary to herniated nucleus pulposus. Clin Orthop 2000; 376:268–277.

97a. Kendall FP, McCreary EK. Trunk Muscles in Muscle Testing and Function. Philadelphia: Williams and Wilkens 1983, p 194.

98. Khan IA, Vaccaro AR, Zlotolow DA. Management of vertebral diskitis and osteomyelitis. Orthopedics 1999; 22(8):758–765.

99. Kihlstrand M, Stenman B, Nilsson S, et al. Water-gymnastics reduced the intensity of back/low back pain in pregnant women. Acta Obstet Gynecol Scand 1999; 78(3):180–185.

100. Kirkaldy-Willis WH, Wedge JH, Yong-Hing K, et al. Pathology and pathogenesis of lumbar spondylosis and stenosis. Spine 1978; 3(4):319–328.

101. Konlian C. Aquatic therapy: making a wave in the treatment of low back pain. Orthop Nurs 1999; 18(1):11–20.

102. Krag MH, Seroussi RE, et al. Internal displacement distribution from in vitro loading of human thoracic and lumbar spinal motion segments: experimental results and theoretical predictions. Spine 1987; 12:1001–1007.

103. Kristiansson P, Svardsudd K, von Schoultz B. Back pain during pregnancy: a prospective study. Spine 1996; 21(6):702–709.

104. Kristiansson P, Svardsudd K, von Schoultz B. Serum relaxin, symphyseal pain, and back pain during pregnancy. Am J Obstet Gynecol 1996; 175(5):1342–1347.

105. LaBan MM, Perrin JC, Latimer FR. Pregnancy and the herniated lumbar disc. Arch Phys Med Rehabil 1983; 64(7):319–321.

106. Leboeuf-Yde C, Kyvik KO, Bruun NH. Low back pain and lifestyle. Part II—obesity. Information from a population-based sample of 29,424 twin subjects. Spine 1999; 24(8):779–783, discussion 783–784.

107. Levy HI, Hanscom B, Boden SD. Three-question depression screener used for lumbar disc herniations and spinal stenosis. Spine 2002; 27(11):1232–1237.

108. Liddle SD, Baxter GD, Gracey JH. Exercise and chronic low back pain: what works? Pain 2004; 107(1–2):176–190.

109. Linton SJ, van Tulder MW. Preventive interventions for back and neck pain. In: Nachemson AL, Johnsson B, eds. Neck and back pain: the scientific evidence of causes, diagnosis, and treatment. Philadelphia: Lippincott Williams & Wilkins; 2000:127–147.

110. Linton SJ. Psychological risk factors for neck and back pain. In: Nachemson AL, Jonsson E, eds. Neck and back pain: the scientific evidence of causes, diagnosis, and treatment. Philadelphia: Lippincott Williams & Wilkins; 2000:57–78.

111. Lutz GE, Vad VB, Wisneski RJ. Fluoroscopic transforaminal lumbar epidural steroids: an outcome study. Arch Phys Med Rehabil 1998; 79(11):1362–1366.

112. Mackenzie WG, Sampath JS, Kruse RW, et al. Backpacks in children. Clin Orthop 2003; 409:78–84.

113. MacLennan AH, Nicolson R, Green RC, et al. Serum relaxin and pelvic pain of pregnancy. Lancet 1986; 2(8501):243–245.

114. Magee DJ. Hip. In: Magee DJ, ed. Orthopedic physical assessment. Philadelphia: Saunders; 1992:333–371.

115. Magee DJ. Lumbar spine. In: Magee DJ, ed. Orthopedic physical assessment. 4th edn. Philadelphia: Elsevier; 2002:467–566.

116. Maguire JH. Osteomyelitis. In: Braunwald E, Fauci AS, Kasper DL, et al, eds. Harrison's principles of internal medicine. 15th edn. New York: McGraw-Hill; 2001:825–829.

117. Main CJ, Waddell G. Beliefs about back pain. In: The back pain revolution. Edinburgh: Churchill Livingstone; 2004:323–342.

118. Mannion AF, Muntener M, Taimela S, et al. Comparison of three active therapies for chronic low back pain: results of a randomized clinical trial with one-year follow-up. Rheumatology (Oxford) 2001; 40(7):772–778.

119. Mantle MJ, Holmes J, Currey HL. Backache in pregnancy II: prophylactic influence of back care classes. Rheumatol Rehabil 1981; 20(4):227–232.

120. Marks RC, Houston T, Thulbourne T. Facet joint injection and facet nerve block: a randomized comparison in 86 patients with chronic low back pain. Pain 1992; 49(3):325–328.

121. Marshall LL, Trethewie ER, Curtain CS. Chemical radiculitis. A clinical, physiological, and immunological study. Clin Orthop 1979; 129:61–67.

122. Maus TP. Imaging of the spine and nerve roots. In: Kraft GH, ed. Physical medicine and rehabilitation clinics of North America. Philadelphia: Saunders; 2002:13.

123. McCall IW, Park WM, O'Brien JP. Induced pain referral from posterior lumbar elements in normal subjects. Spine 1979; 4(5):441–446.

124. McCarron RF, Wimpee MW, Hudkins PG, et al. The inflammatory effect of nucleus pulposus. A possible element in the pathogenesis of low-back pain. Spine 1987; 12(8):760–764.

125. McGee SR. Evidence-based physical diagnosis. Philadelphia: Saunders; 2001.

126. McGill S. Developing the exercise program. In: Low back disorders: evidence-based prevention and rehabilitation. Champaign: Human Kinetics; 2002:239–257.

127. McGill S. Lumbar spine stability: myths and realities. In: Low back disorders: evidence-based prevention and rehabilitation. Champaign: Human Kinetics; 2002:137–146.

128. McGill S. Normal and injury mechanics of the lumbar spine. In: Low back disorders: evidence-based prevention and rehabilitation. Champaign: Human Kinetics; 2002:87–136.

129. McKenzie L, Sillence D. Familial Scheuermann disease: a genetic and linkage study. J Med Genet 1992; 29(1):41–45.

130. Mens JM, Snijders CJ, Stam HJ. Diagonal trunk muscle exercises in peripartum pelvic pain: a randomized clinical trial. Phys Ther 2000; 80(12):1164–1173.

131. Micheli LJ, Hall JE, Miller ME. Use of modified Boston brace for back injuries in athletes. Am J Sports Med 1980; 8(5):351–356.

132. Micheli LJ, Wood R. Back pain in young athletes. Significant differences from adults in causes and patterns. Arch Pediatr Adolesc Med 1995; 149(1):15–18.

133. Micheli LJ. Back injuries in gymnastics. Clin Sports Med 1985; 4(1):85–93.

134. Million R, Nilsen KH, Jayson MI, et al. Evaluation of low back pain and assessment of lumbar corsets with and without back supports. Ann Rheum Dis 1981; 40(5):449–454.

135. Milne S, Welch V, Brosseau L, et al. Transcutaneous electrical nerve stimulation (TENS) for chronic low back pain. Cochrane Database Syst Rev 2001; 2:CD003008.

136. Miyamoto H, Saura R, Harada T, et al. The role of cyclooxygenase-2 and inflammatory cytokines in pain induction of herniated lumbar intervertebral disc. Kobe J Med Sci 2000; 46(1–2):13–28.

137. Mooney V, Robertson J. The facet syndrome. Clin Orthop 1976; Mar-Apr(115):149–156.

138. Nachemson A, Vingard E. Assessment of patients with neck and back pain: a best-evidence synthesis. In: Nachemson AL, Jonsson E, eds. Neck and back pain: the scientific evidence of causes, diagnosis, and treatment. Philadelphia: Lippincott Williams & Wilkins; 2001.

139. Nachemson AL, Vingard E. Influences of individual factors and smoking on neck and low back pain. In: Nachemson AL, Jonsson E, eds. Neck and back pain: the scientific evidence of causes, diagnosis, and treatment. Philadelphia: Lippincott Williams & Wilkins; 2000:79–95.

140. Nachemson AL, Waddell G, Norlund AI. Epedemiology of neck and low back pain. In: Nachemson AL, Johnsson B, eds. Neck and back pain: the scientific evidence of causes, diagnosis, and treatment. Philadelphia: Lippincott Williams & Wilkins; 2000:165–187.

141. Nachemson AL. Disc pressure measurements. Spine 1981; 6(1):93–97.

142. Nachemson AL. The lumbar spine: an orthopaedic challenge. Spine 1976; 1:59.

143. Nelemans PJ, de Bie RA, de Vet HCW, et al. Injection therapy for subacute and chronic benign low-back pain (Cochrane review). Cochrane Database Syst Rev 2000; 2:CD001824.

144. Newman PH. The etiology of spondylolisthesis. J Bone Joint Surg 1963; 45B:39–59.

145. Nilsson-Wikmar L, Holm K, Oijerstedt R, et al. In: Tilscher H, Dorman T, Snijders CH, eds. Third Interdisciplinary World Congress on Low Back and Pelvic Pain, Vienna, 1998:330–331.

146. Noren L, Ostgaard S, Nielsen TF, et al. Reduction of sick leave for lumbar back and posterior pelvic pain in pregnancy. Spine 1997; 22(18):2157–2160.

147. Old JI, Calvert M. Vertebral compression fractures in the elderly. Am Fam Physician 2004; 69(1):111–116.

148. Ostelo RW, de Vet HC, Waddell G, et al. Rehabilitation following first-time lumbar disc surgery: a systematic review within the framework of the Cochrane Collaboration. Spine 2003; 28(3):209–218.

149. Osterman K, Schlenzka D, Poussa M, et al. Isthmic spondylolisthesis in symptomatic and asymptomatic subjects, epidemiology, and natural history with special reference to disk abnormality and mode of treatment. Clin Orthop 1993; 297:65–70.

150. Ostgaard HC, Andersson GB, Karlsson K. Prevalence of back pain in pregnancy. Spine 1991; 16(5):549–552.

151. Ostgaard HC, Zetherstrom G, Roos-Hansson E. Back pain in relation to pregnancy: a 6-year follow-up. Spine 1997; 22(24):2945–2950.

152. O'Sullivan PB, Burnett A, Floyd AN, et al. Lumbar repositioning deficit in a specific low back pain population. Spine 2003; 28(10):1074–1079.

153. O'Sullivan PB, Phyty GD, Twomey LT, et al. Evaluation of specific stabilizing exercise in the treatment of chronic low back pain with radiologic diagnosis of spondylolysis or spondylolisthesis. Spine 1997; 22(24):2959–2967.

154. Parke WW. Applied anatomy of the spine. In: Rothman RH, Simeone FA, eds. The spine. 4th edn. Philadelphia: Saunders; 1999.

155. Parks KA, Crichton KS, Goldford RJ, et al. A comparison of lumbar range of motion and functional ability scores in patients with low back pain: assessment for range of motion validity. Spine 2003; 28(4):380–384.

156. Patel RV, DeLong W Jr, Vresilovic EJ. Evaluation and treatment of spinal injuries in the patient with polytrauma. Clin Orthop 2004; May(422):43–54.

157. Patel SR, Benjamin RS. Soft tissue and bone sarcomas and bone metastases. In: Braunwald E, Fauci AS, Kasper DL, et al, eds. Harrison's principles of internal medicine. 15th edn. New York: McGraw-Hill; 2001:625–628.

158. Perret C, Poiraudeau S, Fermanian J, et al. Validity, reliability, and responsiveness of the fingertip-to-floor test. Arch Phys Med Rehabil 2001; 82(11):1566–1570.

159. Picavet HS, Vlaeyen JW, Schouten JS. Pain catastrophizing and kinesophobia: predictors of chronic low back pain. Am J Epidemiol 2002; 156(11):1028–1034.

160. van Poppel MN, de Looze MP, Koes BW, et al. Mechanisms of action of lumbar supports: a systematic review. Spine 2000; 25(16):2103–2113.

161. Rantanen J, Hurme M, Falck B, et al. The lumbar multifidus muscle five years after surgery for a lumbar intervertebral disc herniation. Spine 1993; 18(5):568–574.

162. Ratliff JK, Cooper PR. Metastatic spine tumors. South Med J 2004; 97(3):246–253.

163. Ravichandran G. A radiologic sign in spondylolisthesis. AJR Am J Roentgenol 1980; 134(1):113–117.

164. Read MT. Single photon emission computed tomography (SPECT) scanning for adolescent back pain. A sine qua non? Br J Sports Med 1994; 28(1):56–57.

165. Richardson C, Jull G, Hodges P, et al. General considerations in motor control and joint stabilization: the basis of assessment and exercise techniques. In: Therapeutic exercise for spinal segmental stabilization in low back pain: scientific basis and clinical approach. Edinburgh: Churchill Livingstone; 1999:79–91.

166. Richardson C, Jull G, Hodges P, et al. Traditional views of the function of the muscles of the local stabilizing system of the spine. In: Therapeutic exercise for spinal segmental stabilization in low back pain: scientific basis and clinical approach. Edinburgh: Churchill Livingstone; 1999:21–40.

167. Riew KD, Yin Y, Gilula L, et al. The effect of nerve-root injections on the need for operative treatment of lumbar radicular pain. A prospective, randomized, controlled, double-blind study. J Bone Joint Surg Am 2000; 82-A(11):1589–1593.

168. Robertson RJ, Caspersen CJ, Allison TG, et al. Differentiated perceptions of exertion and energy cost of young women while carrying loads. Eur J Appl Physiol Occup Physiol 1982; 49(1):69–78.

169. Robinson LR. Electromyography, magnetic resonance imaging, and radiculopathy: it's time to focus on specificity. Muscle Nerve 1999; 22(2):149–150.

170. Russell MD, Hanley EN. Surgical management of lumbar spinal stenosis. In: Rothman RH, Simeone FA, eds. The spine. 4th edn. Philadelphia: Saunders; 1999:806F–806M.

171. Rydevik B, Brown MD, Lundborg G. Pathoanatomy and pathophysiology of nerve root compression. Spine 1984; 9(1):7–15.

172. Rydevik B, Holm S. Pathophysiology of the intervertebral disc and adjacent neural structures. In: Rothman RH, Simeone FA, eds. The spine. Philadelphia: Saunders; 1990:208–227.

173. Saal JA, Saal JS, Herzog RJ. The natural history of lumbar intervertebral disc extrusions treated nonoperatively. Spine 1990; 15(7):683–686.

174. Saal JS, Franson RC, Dobrow R, et al. High levels of inflammatory phospholipase A_2 activity in lumbar disc herniations. Spine 1990; 15(7):674–678.

175. Sahrmann SA. Concepts and principles of movement. In: Diagnosis and treatment of movement impairment syndromes. St. Louis: Mosby; 2002:9–50.

176. Sahrmann SA. Movement impairment syndromes of the lumbar spine. In: Diagnosis and treatment of movement impairment syndromes. St. Louis: Mosby; 2002:51–119.

177. Saraste H. Long-term clinical and radiological follow-up of spondylolysis and spondylolisthesis. J Pediatr Orthop 1987; 7(6):631–638.

178. Schmidt AJ. Cognitive factors in the performance level of chronic low back pain patients. J Psychosom Res 1985; 29(2):183–189.

179. Schwarzer AC, April CN, Derby R, et al. Clinical features of patients with pain stemming from the lumbar zygapophysial joints. Is the lumbar facet syndrome a clinical entity? Spine 1994; 19(10):1132–1137.

180. Schwarzer AC, Wang SC, Bogduk N, et al. Prevalence and clinical features of lumbar zygapophysial joint pain: a study in an Australian population with chronic low back pain. Ann Rheum Dis 1995; 54(2):100–106.

181. Sculco AD, Paup DC, Fernhall B, et al. Effects of aerobic exercise on low back pain patients in treatment. Spine J 2001; 1(2):25–101.

182. Seitsalo S. Operative and conservative treatment of moderate spondylolisthesis in young patients. J Bone Joint Surg Br 1990; 72(5):908–913.

183. Sengupta DK, Herkowitz HN. Lumbar spinal stenosis. Treatment strategies and indications for surgery. Orthop Clin North Am 2003; 34(2):281–295.

184. Shapiro S. Medical realities of cauda equina syndrome secondary to lumbar disc herniation. Spine 2000; 25(3):348–351.

185. Shbeeb MI, Matteson EL. Trochanteric bursitis (greater trochanter pain syndrome). Mayo Clin Proc 1996; 71(6):565–569.

186. Simons DG, Travell JG. Myofascial pain syndromes. In: Melzack R, ed. Textbook of pain. New York: Churchill Livingstone; 1989:368–385.

187. Spangfort EV. The lumbar disc herniation. A computer-aided analysis of 2,504 operations. Acta Orthop Scand Suppl 1972; 142:1–95.

188. Spinhoven P, Ter Kuile M, Kole-Snijders AM, et al. Catastrophizing and internal pain control as mediators of outcome in the multidisciplinary treatment of chronic low back pain. Eur J Pain 2004; 8(3):211–219.

189. Staiger TO, Gaster B, Sullivan MD, et al. Systematic review of antidepressants in the treatment of chronic low back pain. Spine 2003; 28(22):2540–2545.

190. Storm PB, Chou D, Tamargo RJ. Surgical management of cervical and lumbosacral radiculopathies: indications and outcomes. Phys Med Rehabil Clin North Am 2002; 13(3):735–759.

191. Stuge B, Hilde G, Vollestad N. Physical therapy for pregnancy-related low back and pelvic pain: a systematic review. Acta Obstet Gynecol Scand 2003; 82(11):983–990.

192. Sullivan MS, Shoaf LD, Riddle DL. The relationship of lumbar flexion to disability in patients with low back pain. Phys Ther 2000; 80(3): 240–250.

193. Taimela S, Kujala UM, Salminen JJ, et al. The prevalence of low back pain among children and adolescents. A nationwide, cohort-based questionnaire survey in Finland. Spine 1997; 22(10):1132–1136.

194. Tali ET. Spinal infections. Eur J Radiol 2004; 50(2):120–133.

195. Taurog JD, Lipsky PE. Ankylosing spondylitis, reactive arthritis, and undifferentiated spondyloarthropathy. In: Braunwald E, Fauci AS, Kasper DL, et al, eds. Harrison's principles of internal medicine. 15th edn. New York: McGraw-Hill; 2001:1949–1955.

196. Teplick JG, Haskin ME. Spontaneous regression of herniated nucleus pulposus. Am J Roentgenol 1985; 145(2):371–375.

197. Tertti MO, Salminen JJ, Paajanen HE, et al. Low-back pain and disk degeneration in children: a case–control MR imaging study. Radiology 1991; 180(2):503–507.

198. Travell JG, Simons DG. Apropos of all muscles. In: Myofascial pain and dysfunction—the trigger point manual—the upper extremities, vol 1. Baltimore: Williams & Wilkins; 1983:45–102.

199. Travell JG, Simons DG. Background and principles. In: Myofascial pain and dysfunction—the trigger point manual—the upper extremities, vol 1. Baltimore: Williams & Wilkins; 1983:5–44.

200. Troussier B, Marchou-Lopez S, Pironneau S, et al. Back pain and spinal alignment abnormalities in schoolchildren. Rev Rheum Engl Ed 1999; 66(7–9):370–830.

201. Tschirhart CE, Nagpurkar A, Whyne CM. Effects of tumor location, shape and surface serration on burst fracture risk in the metastatic spine. J Biomech 2004; 37(5):653–660.

202. van Tulder M, Malmivaara A, Esmail R, et al. Exercise therapy for low back pain: a systematic review within the framework of the Cochrane collaboration back review group. Spine 2000; 25(21):2784–2796.

203. van Tulder MW, Esmail R, Bombardier C, et al. Back schools for nonspecific low back pain. Cochrane Database Syst Rev 2000; 2:CD000261.

204. van Tulder MW, Goossens M, Waddell G, et al. Conservative treatment of chronic low back pain. In: Nachemson AL, Jonsson E, eds. Neck and back pain: the scientific evidence of causes, diagnosis, and treatment. Philadelphia: Lippincott Williams & Wilkins; 2000:271–304.

205. van Tulder MW, Jellema P, van Poppel MN, et al. Lumbar supports for prevention and treatment of low back pain (Cochrane review). Cochrane Database Syst Rev 2000; 3:CD001823.

206. van Tulder MW, Scholten RJ, Koes BW, et al. Nonsteroidal anti-inflammatory drugs for low back pain: a systematic review within the framework of the Cochrane Collaboration Back Review Group. Spine 2000; 25(19):2501–2513.

207. van Tulder MW, Touray T, Furlan AD, et al. Muscle relaxants for nonspecific low back pain: a systematic review within the framework of the Cochrane Collaboration. Spine 2003; 28(17):1978–1992.

208. van Tulder MW, Waddell G. Conservative treatment of acute and subacute low back pain. In: Nachemson AL, Jonsson E, eds. Neck and back pain: the scientific evidence of causes, diagnosis, and treatment. Philadelphia: Lippincott Williams & Wilkins; 2000:241–269.

209. Vad VB, Bhat AL, Lutz GE, et al. Transforaminal epidural steroid injections in lumbosacral radiculopathy: a prospective randomized study. Spine 2002; 27(1):11–16.

210. Verlaan JJ, Diekerhof CH, Buskens E, et al. Surgical treatment of traumatic fractures of the thoracic and lumbar spine: a systematic review of the literature on techniques, complications, and outcome. Spine 2004; 29(7):803–814.

211. Vilensky JA, O'Connor BL, Fortin JD, et al. Histologic analysis of neural elements in the human sacroiliac joint. Spine 2002; 27(11):1202–1207.

212. Viry P, Creveuil C, Marcelli C. Nonspecific back pain in children. A search for associated factors in 14-year-old schoolchildren. Rev Rheum Engl Ed 1999; 66(7-9):381–388.

213. Von Korff M, Dworkin SF, Le Resche L, et al. An epidemiologic comparison of pain complaints. Pain 1988; 32(2):173–183.

214. Waddell G, Burton K. Information and advice for patients. In: The back pain revolution. Edinburgh: Churchill Livingstone; 2004:323–342.

215. Waddell G, Feder G, Lewis M. Systematic reviews of bed rest and advice to stay active for acute low back pain. Br J Gen Pract 1997; 47(423): 647–652.

216. Waddell G, van Tulder M. Clinical guidelines. In: The back pain revolution. Edinburgh: Elsevier Science; 2000:283-322.

217. Waddell G, Waddell H. A review of social influences on neck and back pain and disability. In: Nachemson AL, Jonsson E, eds. Neck and back pain: the scientific evidence of causes, diagnosis, and treatment. Philadelphia: Lippincott Williams & Wilkins; 2000:13–55.

218. Waddell G, Watson PJ. Rehabilitation. In: The back pain revolution. Edinburgh: Churchill Livingstone; 2004:371–399.

219. Waddell G. Illness behavior. In: The back pain revolution. Edinburgh: Churchill Livingstone; 2000:72–89.

220. Walker BF. The prevalence of low back pain: a systematic review of the literature from 1966 to 1998. J Spinal Disord 2000; 13(3):205–217.

221. Wang SM, Dezinno P, Maranets I, et al. Low back pain during pregnancy: prevalence, risk factors, and outcomes. Obstet Gynecol 2004; 104(1): 65–70.

222. Watson KD, Papageorgiou AC, Jones GT, et al. Low back pain in schoolchildren: the role of mechanical and psychosocial factors. Arch Dis Child 2003; 88(1):12–17.

223. Weber H. Lumbar disc herniation. A controlled, prospective study with ten years of observation. Spine 1983; 8(2):131–140.

224. Wedenberg K, Moen B, Norling A. A prospective randomized study comparing acupuncture with physiotherapy for low-back and pelvic pain in pregnancy. Acta Obstet Gynecol Scand 2000; 79(5):331–335.

225. Weinreb JC, Wolbarsht LB, Cohen JM, et al. Prevalence of lumbosacral intervertebral disk abnormalities on MR images in pregnant and asymptomatic nonpregnant women. Radiology 1989; 170(1 part 1):125–128.

226. Wiltse LL, Winter RB. Terminology and measurement of spondylolisthesis. J Bone Joint Surg Am 1983; 65(6):768–772.

227. Wittink H, Hoskins MT, Wagner A, et al. Deconditioning in patients with chronic low back pain: fact or fiction? Spine 2000; 25(17): 2221–2228.

228. Wittink H, Michel TH, Kulich R, et al. Aerobic fitness testing in patients with chronic low back pain: which test is best? Spine 2000; 25(13): 1704–1710.

229. Woby SR, Watson PJ, Roach NK, et al. Are changes in fear-avoidance beliefs, catastrophizing, and appraisals of control, predictive of changes in chronic low back pain and disability? Eur J Pain 2004; 8(3):201–210.

230. Zuberbier OA, Hunt DG, Kozlowski AJ, et al. Commentary on the American Medical Association guides' lumbar impairment validity checks. Spine 2001; 26(24):2735–2737.

Chapter

42

Prevention and Treatment of Osteoporosis

Mehrsheed Sinaki

> Bone, to be maintained, needs to be mechanically strained—within its biomechanical limits.
>
> Mehrsheed Sinaki, M.D.

Through an interdisciplinary approach, we can add quality to the years of life of patients with osteoporosis. Osteoporosis is the most prevalent metabolic bone disease in the USA and is a major public health problem. The direct and indirect cost of osteoporosis in the USA alone is estimated to be more than $14 billion annually.[42] Much of this expense relates to hip fractures. In 15–20% of hip fracture cases, the outcome is fatal.[45,50]

Osteoporosis consists of a heterogeneous group of syndromes in which there is reduced bone mass per unit volume in otherwise normal bone, resulting in fragile bone. The increment in bone porosity results in architectural instability of bone and increases the likelihood of fracture. The ratio of mineral to matrix is normal in osteoporosis, but in osteomalacia the mineral content is significantly reduced.

The World Health Organization has defined osteoporosis as bone mineral density 2.5 standard deviations below the peak mean bone mass of young normal adults.[91] Z score is the number of standard deviations from the mean bone density for age-matched, sex-matched, and ethnic-matched individuals. For instance, a 75-year-old woman with a Z score of −1.0 is one standard deviation below the bone mineral density of an average 65-year-old woman, but her T score may be −3.0 because she is three standard deviations below the bone mineral density of an average 30-year-old woman. Normal bone mineral density is T score ≥ −1; osteopenia is T between −1 and −2.5, osteoporosis T ≤ −2.5, and severe osteoporosis T ≤ −2.5 with fracture. In the asymptomatic stage of osteoporosis, it is characterized simply by a low bone mass without fractures. Osteoporosis becomes clinically problematic only when the bone fractures.

BONE FUNCTION AND STRUCTURE

Bone serves as a mechanical support for musculoskeletal structures; as protection for vital organs; and as a metabolic source of ions, especially calcium and phosphate. Despite its appearance, bone is a very active tissue. To maintain its biomechanical competence, bone tissue undergoes continuous change and renewal so that older bone tissue is replaced by newly formed bone tissue. Approximately 20% of bone tissue is replaced annually by this cyclic process. There are two types of bone cells: osteoclasts, which resorb the calcified matrix, and osteoblasts, which synthesize new bone matrix.[53]

Osteoclasts are localized on the endosteal bone surfaces; their origin is hematopoietic, and they share a common precursor with the monocyte macrophage. Osteoclasts are large multinucleated cells with an average of 10 to 20 nuclei. Osteoclasts have a special cell membrane with folds that invaginate at the interface with bone surface, called the 'ruffled border'. To induce resorption of bone and the mineralized bone matrix, osteoclasts produce proteolytic enzymes in this ruffled border.

Osteoblasts are derived from mesenchymal cells. The role of osteoblasts is mineralization of the matrix through budding of vesicles from their cytoplasmic membrane. These vesicles are rich in alkaline phosphatase. Osteoblasts secrete all the growth factors that are trapped in the matrix.

BONE REMODELING

Bone is continuously being turned over by the two processes of modeling and remodeling. This process allows maintenance of the biomechanical integrity of the skeleton, and it supports the role of bone in provision of an ionic bank for the body and mechanical support. Bone remodeling is a process that allows removal of old bone and replacement with new bone tissue.

Bone remodeling has five phases.

1. Activation: osteoclastic activity is recruited.
2. Resorption: osteoclasts erode bone and form a cavity.
3. Reversal: osteoblasts are recruited.
4. Formation: osteoblasts replace the cavity with new bone.
5. Quiescence: bone tissue remains dormant until the next cycle starts.

This process is cyclic, starting with bone resorption and finishing with bone formation. In adult human bone, each cycle of remodeling lasts 3–12 months. The signal that stops osteoclastic activity is not yet completely defined. After bone resorption, the reversal phase starts, which involves osteoblastic activity. Then the osteoblasts start to fill the resorption cavity. During the process of osteoclastic activity, the growth factors, stored in the bone matrix, are released and subsequently can stimulate osteoblastic proliferation.

This process of bone resorption and formation is called *coupling*. The ideal situation in the coupling process is equilibrated bone formation and resorption. In osteoporosis, however, there is a disequilibrium between resorption and formation, favoring resorption that results in bone loss.

The number of active remodeling units in trabecular bone is about three times higher than that in cortical bone. The physical endurance of any bone is affected by the percentage of cortical bone involved in its structure. Trabecular bone is more active metabolically than cortical bone because of the significant surface exposure areas. Consequently, more bone loss occurs at the trabecular areas when resorption is greater than formation. The vertebrae consist of 50% trabecular bone and 50% cortical bone, whereas the femoral neck consists of 30% trabecular bone and 70% cortical bone. When bone turnover increases, bone loss and osteoporosis occur in the vertebrae before the femoral neck.

PATHOGENESIS

Peak adult bone mass is achieved between ages 30 and 35 years. Bone mass at any point thereafter in life is the difference between the peak adult bone mass and the amount that has been lost since the peak was reached. Age-related bone loss is a universal phenomenon in humans. Any circumstances that limit bone formation or increase bone loss increase the likelihood that osteoporosis will develop later in life. Measures that can maximize peak adult bone mass are clearly desirable.

Trabecular (or cancellous) bone represents about 20% of skeletal bone mass and makes up 80% of the turnover media. The cortex makes up only 20% of the turnover media, and is made of compact bone. The cortex represents 80% of skeletal bone mass. In both cortical and trabecular bone, bone remodeling is initiated with activation of osteoclasts, which erode the bone, resulting in bone resorption. The resorption sites are then refilled by osteoblastic activities, a process called bone formation. If the amount of bone resorbed equals the amount formed, the bone loss is zero. The remodeling process does not result in zero balance after age 30 to 35 years. After this age, the normal process of remodeling results in bone loss.[51]

Certain conditions, such as hyperparathyroidism or thyrotoxicosis, can increase the rate of bone remodeling. These conditions increase the rate of bone loss, which results in high-turnover osteoporosis. The secondary causes of osteoporosis are associated with an increased rate of activation of the remodeling cycle. Although environmental factors such as calcium intake, smoking, alcohol, physical exercise, and menopause are important factors in determining bone mineral density, genetic factors are the major determinant and contribute to 80% of the variance in peak bone mineral density.[11] Fracture incidence related to osteoporosis is lower in men than in women, because the diameter of vertebral bodies and long bones is greater in men at maturity and bone loss is less (about half that of women) throughout life in men.[56]

CLASSIFICATION OF OSTEOPOROSIS

Osteoporosis can be primary or secondary to other disorders that result in bone loss. The most common osteoporosis is either postmenopausal or age-related.[44] Primary osteoporosis is the rare disorder of idiopathic juvenile osteoporosis, the cause of which is unknown. This typically occurs before puberty (between ages 8 and 14 years), and patients present with osteoporosis that is progressive over 2–4 years in association with the occurrence of multiple fractures, axial or axioappendicular.[27] Remission usually occurs by the end of the 2- to 4-year course. In this type of osteoporosis, the process of bone formation is normal but there is an increase in osteoclastic activity, resulting in increased bone resorption. This type of osteoporosis is most evident in the thoracic and lumbar spine, and needs to be distinguished from juvenile epiphysitis or Scheuermann disease. This disorder is usually self-limiting, but the radiographic appearance might not return to normal. The laboratory values are typically normal, and the diagnosis is made by exclusion. The most common causes of osteoporosis are listed in Box 42-1.

Box 42-1 Common causes of osteoporosis

Hereditary, congenital
- Osteogenesis imperfecta, neurologic disturbances (myotonia congenita, Werdnig–Hoffmann disease), gonadal dysgenesis

Acquired (primary and secondary)
Generalized
- Idiopathic (in premenopausal women and middle-aged or young men; juvenile osteoporosis)
- Postmenopausal
- Age-related

Secondary
- Nutrition: malnutrition, anorexia or bulimia, vitamin deficiency (C or D), vitamin overuse (A or D), calcium deficiency, high sodium intake, high caffeine intake, high protein intake, high phosphate intake, alcohol abuse
- Sedentary lifestyle, immobility, smoking
- Gastrointestinal diseases (liver disease, malabsorption syndromes, alactasia, subtotal gastrectomy) or small bowel resection
- Nephropathies
- Chronic obstructive pulmonary disease
- Malignancy (multiple myeloma, disseminated carcinoma)
- Drugs: phenytoin, barbiturates, cholestyramine, heparin
- Endocrine disorders: acromegaly, hyperthyroidism, Cushing syndrome (iatrogenic or endogenous), hyperparathyroidism, diabetes mellitus(?), hypogonadism

Localized
- Inflammatory arthritis, fractures and immobilization in cast, limb dystrophies, muscular paralysis

(From Sinaki 1993,[83] with permission of the Mayo Foundation.)

HORMONES AND PHYSIOLOGY OF BONE

The rate of bone remodeling can be increased by parathyroid hormone (PTH), thyroxine, growth hormone, and vitamin D [1,25(OH)$_2$D$_3$]; it can be decreased by calcitonin, estrogen, and glucocorticoids.[33]

The major hormone for calcium homeostasis is *parathyroid hormone*. PTH is secreted by the parathyroid glands, which are located behind the thyroid glands. The level of plasma calcium is the major moderator of the secretion of PTH. PTH regulates the plasma calcium ion (Ca^{2+}) concentration in three ways.

1. In the presence of active vitamin D, it stimulates bone resorption and the release of calcium and phosphate.
2. Through production of calcitriol in the kidneys, it indirectly increases intestinal absorption of calcium and phosphate.
3. It increases active reabsorption of calcium ions in the renal distal tubal area.

PTH also reduces proximal tubular reabsorption of phosphate. In general, PTH increases serum calcium and mostly tends to lower serum phosphate.

Calcitonin is a hormone secreted by the parafollicular cells of the thyroid gland. The major stimulus of calcitonin is the serum level of calcium. Through inhibition of osteoclastic activity, calcitonin directly prohibits calcium and phosphate resorption, lowering the serum calcium level.

The main regulators of vitamin D synthesis are the serum concentrations of 1,25(OH)$_2$D$_3$ itself, calcium, phosphate, and PTH. Vitamin D also can be synthesized through exposure to the sun and conversion in the liver. PTH is the major inducer of the active form of vitamin D formation in the kidney. This function is accomplished through the effect of the enzyme 1α-hydroxylase, which transforms the inactive form of vitamin D to the potent form. The active form of vitamin D increases intestinal absorption of calcium and phosphate. Vitamin D also is required for appropriate bone mineralization. The effect of the active form of vitamin D is both a direct stimulation of osteoblastic activity and an indirect effect through increasing the intestinal absorption of calcium and phosphorus.

ROLE OF SEX STEROIDS

The main endocrine function that occurs at menopause is loss of secretion of estrogen and progesterone from the ovaries.[25,34,56] The premenopausal ovary produces primarily estradiol. Progesterone secretion, which occurs cyclically after ovulation in the premenopausal state, also declines to very low levels at the postmenopausal stage. These changes in circulating sex steroids are gradual in a woman's sexual reproductive life. The premenopausal ovary also produces androgens, especially testosterone. The circulating testosterone levels decrease after menopause. The major source of estrogen in postmenopausal women is conversion from dihydroepiandrostenedione. This is converted into androstenedione, which changes into estrone in fat cells. Estrone is the major source of estrogen in postmenopausal women. Men do not have the equivalent of menopause but, in some elderly men, bone mass decreases along with a decline in gonadal function. The testosterone level in men decreases with age as a result of a decreased number of Leydig cells in the testes. Male hypogonadism is typically associated with bone loss.[30]

OTHER FACTORS AFFECTING BONE MASS

Several other factors can contribute to the reduction of sex-related steroids. In hyperprolactinemia, which is due to a prolactin-secreting pituitary tumor, failure of the gonadal axis results in a significant loss of bone. Amenorrheic athletes who exercise excessively (such as high-mileage runners) and have lower than normal body weight have lower circulating estradiol, progesterone, and prolactin levels. Their amenorrhea is associated with hypothalamic hypogonadism, which leads to excessive bone loss. This bone loss can be partly reversible when training distances are decreased.[10,35]

Reduction of sex steroids is not the only cause of bone loss. Other factors, such as race, genetics, nutrition, physical exercise, and lifestyle, can also contribute to the rate of bone loss after ovariectomy or natural menopause.[74] It is well known that bone must be physically stressed to be maintained. A significant body of data shows that the rate of strain change also influences bone growth and remodeling.[41]

EFFECT OF AGING ON BONE MASS

In the normal aging process, there is a deficit between resorption and formation, because osteoblastic activity is not equal to osteoclastic activity. The result of the remodeling process is bone loss during each cycle of remodeling. Bone loss occurs even when the remodeling process is not increased. In fact, activation of skeletal remodeling is decreased as a result of the process of aging. This gives rise to the concept of low-turnover osteoporosis, which occurs concomitantly with the aging process.

Age plays a significant role in the rate of bone turnover. It has been clearly determined that bone turnover increases in women at menopause, but bone turnover does not increase significantly in men with aging. Most studies have shown that plasma levels of 1,25(OH)$_2$D$_3$ decrease with age by about 50% in both men and women.

Growth hormone stimulates renal production of the active form of vitamin D [1,25(OH)$_2$D$_3$]. Growth hormone decreases with age. Growth hormone secretion is reduced in osteoporosis. Growth hormone and insulin-like growth factor-I have several positive effects on calcium homeostasis, including synthesis of 1,25(OH)$_2$D$_3$, osteoblast proliferation, osteoclast differentiation, and bone resorption.

It appears that special forms of vitamin K therapy in the elderly can be associated with a reduction in the rate of bone resorption, demonstrated by decreased excretion of urinary

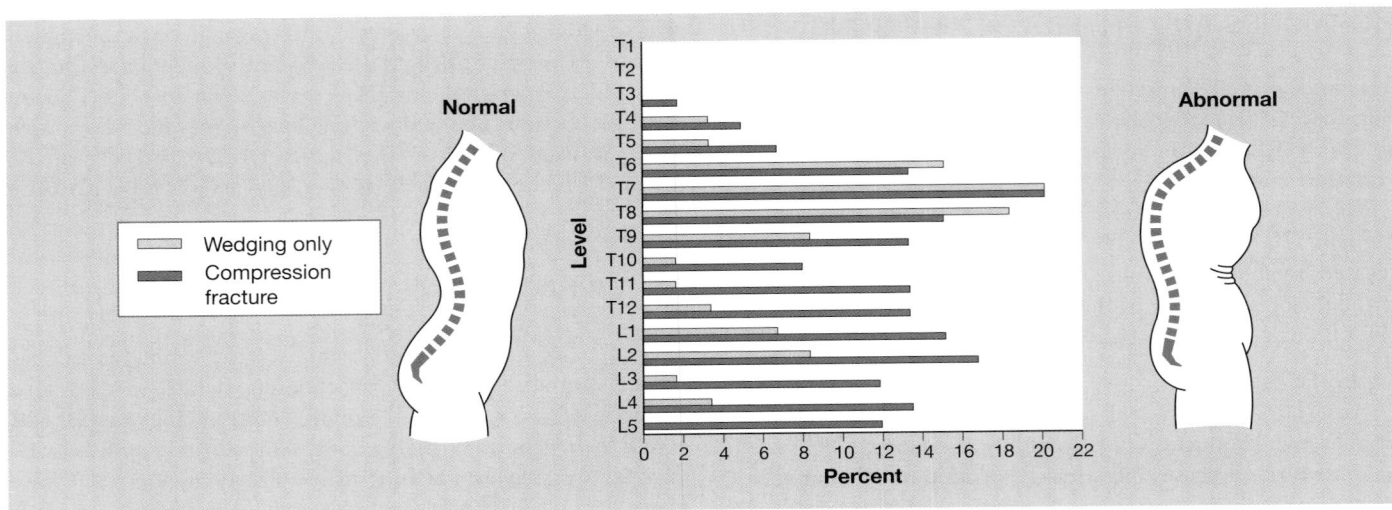

Figure 42-1 Incidence of wedging and compression fractures at various levels of the spine. (From Sinaki and Mikkelsen 1984,[66] with permission of the American Congress of Rehabilitation Medicine and the American Academy of Physical Medicine and Rehabilitation.)

hydroxyproline. Further studies are needed to support this. Studies have shown that calcium absorption is less efficient in the elderly.[23] Bone loss also has been related to deficiencies in trace metal elements such as copper, zinc, and magnesium, but this issue is not fully resolved.

Plasma calcitonin levels are higher in men than in women. Calcitonin levels do not change with age. Studies have shown that estrogens stimulate calcitonin secretion.[87,88] Thyroid hormone levels typically show no change or are slightly decreased with age. PTH level increases with age, perhaps due to mild hypocalcemia and decreased $1,25(OH)_2D_3$. This reduction in the active form of vitamin D can be due to lower consumption of dietary vitamin D, lower exposure to sunlight, lower skin capacity for vitamin D conversion, reduced intestinal absorption, and reduced 1α-hydroxylase activity.

Several studies have demonstrated that the level of physical activity decreases with aging.[74] Physical strain and mechanical load also affect bone mass.[16] Exercise is known to stimulate the release of growth hormone or other trophic factors that can stimulate osteoblastic activity.[14] Optimal nutrition and physical activity are necessary to achieve the genetic potential for bone mass. The peak bone mass attained by young adulthood is a major determinant of bone mass in later life. Female gymnasts, both children and college-aged athletes, reportedly have higher bone mineral density than swimmers.[4,13] Nutrition also can affect both bone matrix formation and bone mineralization. The recommended adequate calcium intake for ages 9–18 years is 1300 mg/day (Table 42-1).[38]

CLINICAL MANIFESTATIONS OF OSTEOPOROSIS

Osteoporosis is typically a 'silent disease' until fractures occur. Osteoporotic vertebral fractures can go unnoticed until incidentally seen on a chest radiograph. Appendicular fractures, however, require immediate attention. The fact that the frac-

Table 42-1 Optimal calcium intake: National Institutes of Health recommendations

Group	Calcium (mg/day)
Infants, children, and young adults	
Birth to 6 months	400
6 months to 1 year	600
1–10 years	800–1200
11–24 years	1200–1500
Adult women	
>24 years, pregnant and lactating	1200–1500
<24 years, pregnant and lactating	1200
25–49 years (premenopausal)	1000
50–64 years (postmenopausal), taking estrogen	1000
50–64 years (postmenopausal), no estrogen	1500
>65 years	1500
Adult men	
25–64 years	1000
>65 years	1500
(From Anonymous 1994,[2] with permission.)	

ture results from osteoporosis should not affect the orthopedic method of management. The most common areas for osteoporotic fractures are the midthoracic and upper lumbar spine (Fig. 42-1),[66] hip (proximal femur), and distal forearm (Colles fracture). The highest incidence of fractures is in white females. The female : male ratio is about 7 : 1 for vertebral fractures, 2 : 1 for hip fractures, and 5 : 1 for Colles fractures. It has been estimated that, after menopause, a woman's lifetime risk of sustaining an osteoporotic fracture is 1 in 2 or 3.[40]

The most concern is for hip fracture, because the risk of death with osteoporotic hip fracture is 15–20%, despite all the developments in surgical and non-surgical intervention. The management of an osteoporotic spine fracture requires immobilization of the involved vertebral bodies and analgesia. Fortunately, these fractures heal through becoming more condensed, and typically do not require any specific treatment process, as is usually needed for the appendicular fractures. If there is non-union of the appendicular fracture, one needs to look for conditions other than osteoporosis, such as osteomalacia or hyperparathyroidism. The duration of immobilization should be for only a limited time, sufficient to ensure the primary fracture-healing process. Prolonged immobilization is discouraged, because it can contribute to additional osteoporosis.

The orthopedic management for most osteoporotic fractures is generally non-controversial, except for the management of hip fracture. The management of femoral neck fracture creates a great deal of controversy because of the high complication rate. There is an ongoing effort to try to solve these controversies through prospective studies. Despite these efforts, the treatment of hip fracture remains a challenge, and each case creates an emergency situation. Shoulder fracture, especially the surgical neck of the proximal humerus, is not uncommon in elderly women. This type of fracture usually occurs from an impact force directly on to the shoulder during a fall. This fracture is typically such that a conservative treatment regimen suffices.

FRACTURES AND MANAGEMENT

The relationship between bone mass and spinal fractures has been studied extensively, and it is known that, as bone mass decreases, fracture risk increases. For every standard deviation of decrease in bone mineral density, the risk of osteoporotic fracture of the spine increases 1.5- to 2-fold, and the risk of hip fracture increases 2.6-fold.[22] Another predictor of fracture risk is age itself. The risk of fracture due to osteoporosis doubles every 5–7 years.[22] It is not clear whether age-related changes in bone density and bone quality are factors that increase the risk of fractures due to falls.

Vertebral fracture

The incidence of vertebral fractures is poorly understood, because 50% of these fractures can be subclinical and the patient might not seek medical attention. Vertebral fractures can create both acute and chronic pain.

Acute pain that occurs in the absence of a previous fracture is usually due to compression fractures in the vertebrae. Sometimes a minor fall or even an affectionate hug can lead to a compression fracture. The compressed vertebrae might not be apparent on radiographs for up to 4 weeks after the injury.[44] Compression fracture usually results in acute pain that later

---

Box 42-2 Management of acute pain in patients with osteoporosis

- Bed rest (2 days): significant bone loss is not likely to occur with 2 days of bed rest
- Analgesics: avoid constipating medicines such as codeine derivatives
- Avoidance of constipation
- Physical therapy: initially cold packs, then mild heat and stroking massage
- Avoidance of exertional exercises
- Teaching of lifting and standing principles to avoid excessive spinal strain
- Back supports, if needed, to decrease pain and expedite ambulation
- Gait aids if needed

(From Sinaki 1993,[83] with permission of the Mayo Foundation.)

---

resolves (Box 42-2).[83] The spinal deformity as a result of these fractures can produce chronic pain.[79]

Kyphotic postural change is the most physically disfiguring and psychologically damaging effect of osteoporosis.[61] The incidence of osteoporosis can be substantially decreased only by early detection and subsequent intervention in the high-risk patient population.

Disproportionate weakness in back extensor musculature relative to body weight or flexor strength considerably increases the possibility of compressing vertebrae in the fragile osteoporotic spine. Recognition and improvement of decreased back extensor strength enhance the ability to maintain proper vertical alignment.[72] The geriatric population has an increased risk for debilitating postural changes because of several factors, the two most apparent being a greater prevalence of osteoporosis and involutional loss of functional muscle motor units.[20,39] Development of kyphotic posture not only can predispose to postural back pain but also can increase the risk of falls.[37] Several other factors also can contribute to the risk of falls (Box 42-3).[81]

Chronic pain can be due to the development of deformity caused by vertebral wedging, compression, and secondary ligamentous strain. This is often difficult to distinguish from associated disk deterioration. The intervertebral disks undergo the most dramatic age-related changes of all connective tissues.[1] With aging, the number and diameter of the collagen fibril portion of the disk increase. This change is accompanied by a progressive decrease in disk compliance. Loss of distinction between the nucleus pulposus and the annulus fibrosus occurs eventually.

Chronic back pain secondary to osteoporosis is related to postural changes due to vertebral fractures.[61] Strong back muscles contribute to good posture and skeletal support (Fig. 42-2).[24,70,71] One controlled study showed the long-term effects of back extensor resistance training 8 years after cessation of the exercise.[62,63] The women in the study were not receiving hormone replacement therapy. Compared with the exercise

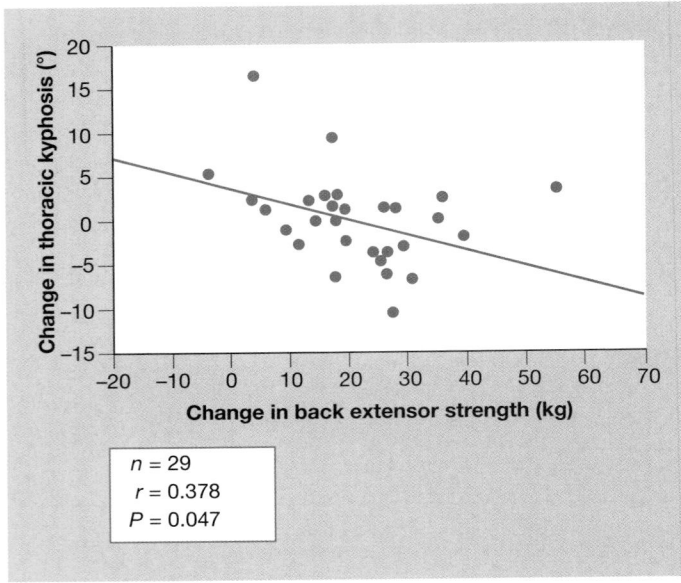

Figure 42-2 Correlation between change in back extensor strength and change in thoracic kyphosis in 29 healthy estrogen-deficient women with hyperkyphosis (34.1° or more). A significant negative correlation was found. (From Itoi and Sinaki 1994,[24] with permission of the Mayo Foundation for Medical Education and Research.)

Box 42-3 Risk of falls: contributing factors

Extrinsic

- Environmental: obstacles, slippery floors, uneven surfaces, poor illumination, stairs not well defined, pets, icy sidewalks
- Extraskeletal: inappropriate footwear, obstructive clothing

Intrinsic

- Intraskeletal: lower extremity weakness (neurogenic or myopathic), balance disorder (vestibular, peripheral neuropathy, hyperkyphosis), visual impairment, bifocals, vestibular changes, cognitive decline, decreased coordination (cerebellar degeneration), postural changes, imbalance, gait unsteadiness, gait apraxia, reduced muscle strength, reduced flexibility, respiratory (orthopnea), postural hypotension, cardiovascular deconditioning, iatrogenically reduced alertness

(From Sinaki 2004,[77] with permission of Current Science.)

Box 42-4 Management of chronic pain in patients with osteoporosis

- Improve faulty posture; may need Posture Training Support.
- Manage pain (ultrasound, massage, or transcutaneous electrical nerve stimulation).
- If beyond correction, apply back support to decrease painful stretch of ligaments.
- Avoid physical activities that exert extreme vertical compression forces on vertebrae.
- Prescribe a patient-specific therapeutic exercise program.
- Start appropriate pharmacologic intervention.

(From Sinaki 1993,[88] with permission of the Mayo Foundation.)

---

as codeine sulfate or its derivatives, because they can cause constipation.[76]

Vertebroplasty (kyphoplasty)

Vertebroplasty (kyphoplasty) has recently been used for the management of vertebral fractures. This procedure involves the injection of acrylic cement (such as polymethylmethacrylate) into a partially collapsed vertebral body. Jensen et al. found that 63% of osteoporotic patients who underwent vertebroplasty decreased their use of opiates and analgesics for pain control, 7% increased their use, and 30% remained the same.[26] However, vertebroplasty does not substitute for rehabilitative measures that are needed after fracture.[47]

Hip fracture

Hip fracture is an emergency situation. In typical cases, the extremity is rotated outward (externally rotated) and shortened. It is difficult to tell from the clinical evaluation whether the fracture is intracapsular (femoral neck fracture) or extracapsular (trochanteric fracture). Radiographs are necessary to make this distinction, because the operative treatment and the outcome of intracapsular versus extracapsular hip fractures differ considerably. The consensus is that surgery is the treatment of choice for femoral neck fracture and trochanteric hip fracture. In some unusual cases of impacted fracture, conservative treatment might be advisable, however, particularly in a patient who is severely debilitated and has impaired general health. Femoral neck fracture requires fixation, and the type of fixation varies among surgeons. Because of the high incidence of operative failures after internal fixation of these fractures, most orthopedists prefer performing arthroplasties. Some orthopedists prefer total joint replacement, whereas some prefer hemiarthroplasty only for the femoral neck and head. The rationale is that total hip arthroplasties are considered to stay intact longer than hemiarthroplasties. The only concern is that the hemiarthroplasty is a considerably smaller surgical trauma for the patient, and hence is advocated in the very old or frail patient with a prognosis of limited mobility.

The trochanteric hip fracture creates lesser problems, despite the fact that the fracture engages more bone than does the femoral neck fracture. The operative treatment of choice is internal fixation (Fig. 42-4). The postoperative course for all

group, those in the control group had a 2.7 times greater number of vertebral fractures at 10-year follow-up.[63] The pain and skeletal deformity associated with osteoporosis might secondarily reduce muscle strength. The reduction in muscle strength can further exacerbate the postural abnormalities associated with this condition (Fig. 42-3).

Chronic pain can also be due to microfractures that are visible only on bone scanning and that occur continuously. Management of chronic osteoporosis-related pain is outlined in Box 42-4. One should be hesitant about using opiate analgesics such

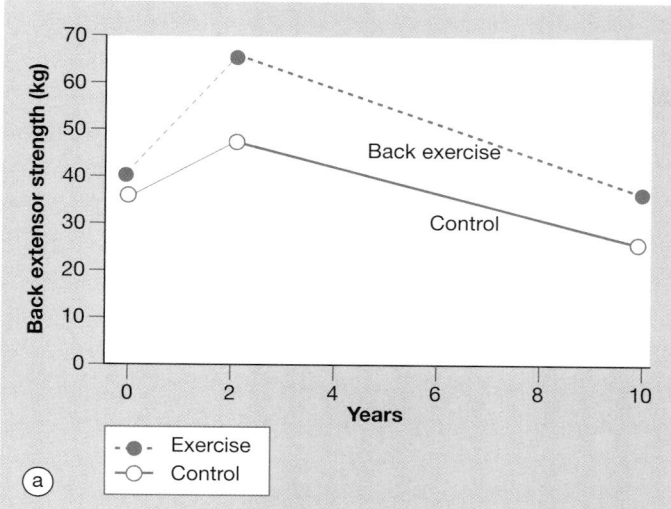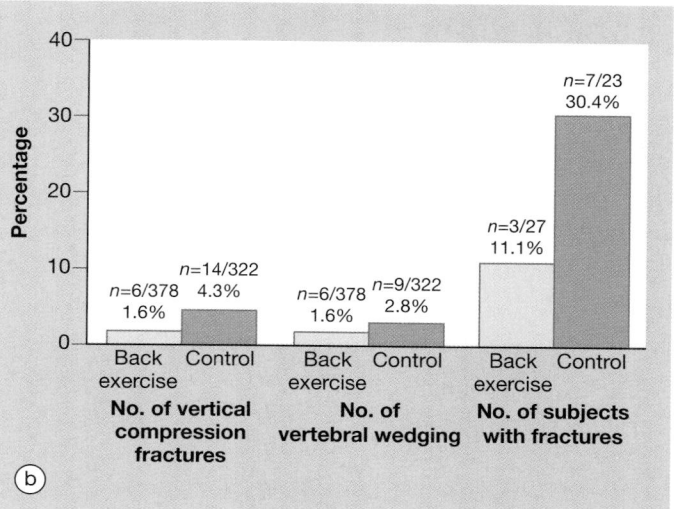

Figure 42-3 (**a**) Back extensor strength in two study groups: back exercise (n = 27) and control (n = 23). Subjects participated in self-selected physical activities during years 3 through 10. In both groups, back extensor strength increased at 2 years (P = 0.0001) and decreased at 10 years (P = 0.0001). The back extensor strength of the back exercise group was significantly greater than that of the control group at both 2 years (P = 0.0005) and 10 years (P = 0.0357). The values are mean ± SD. (**b**) At 10-year follow-up, the number of vertebral compression fractures was 14 out of 322 vertebral bodies examined (4.3%) in the control group and 6 fractures out of 378 vertebral bodies examined (1.6%) in the back exercise group (chi-square test, P = 0.029). The number of control subjects with vertebral fractures was three times greater than in the back exercise group. (a, from Sinaki et al. 2002,[63] with permission of Elsevier Science; b, from Sinaki 2003,[73] with permission of Springer-Verlag.)

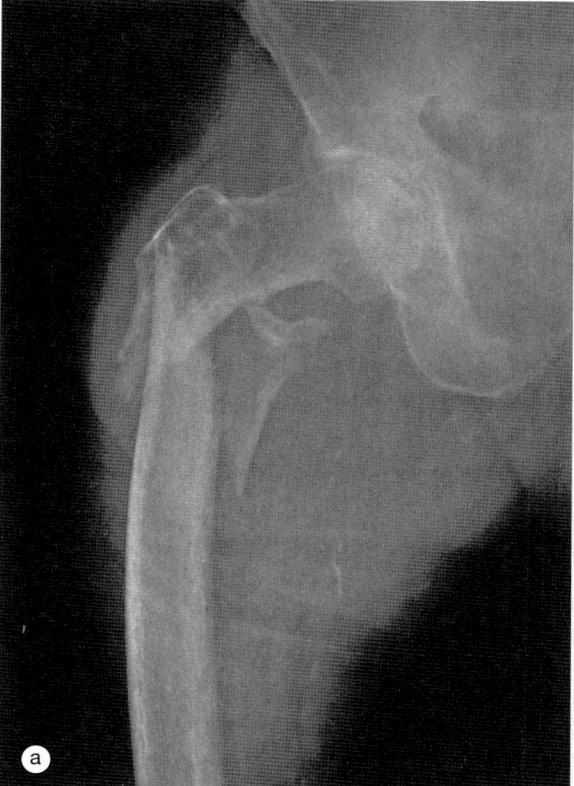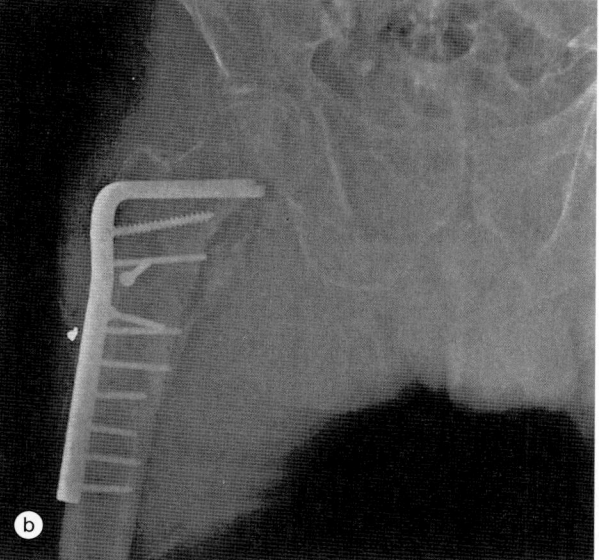

Figure 42-4 (**a**) The right femur with medial displacement of a large fragment containing lesser trochanter and lateral angulation across the fracture. (**b**) Internal nail, plate, and screw fixation in the same patient.

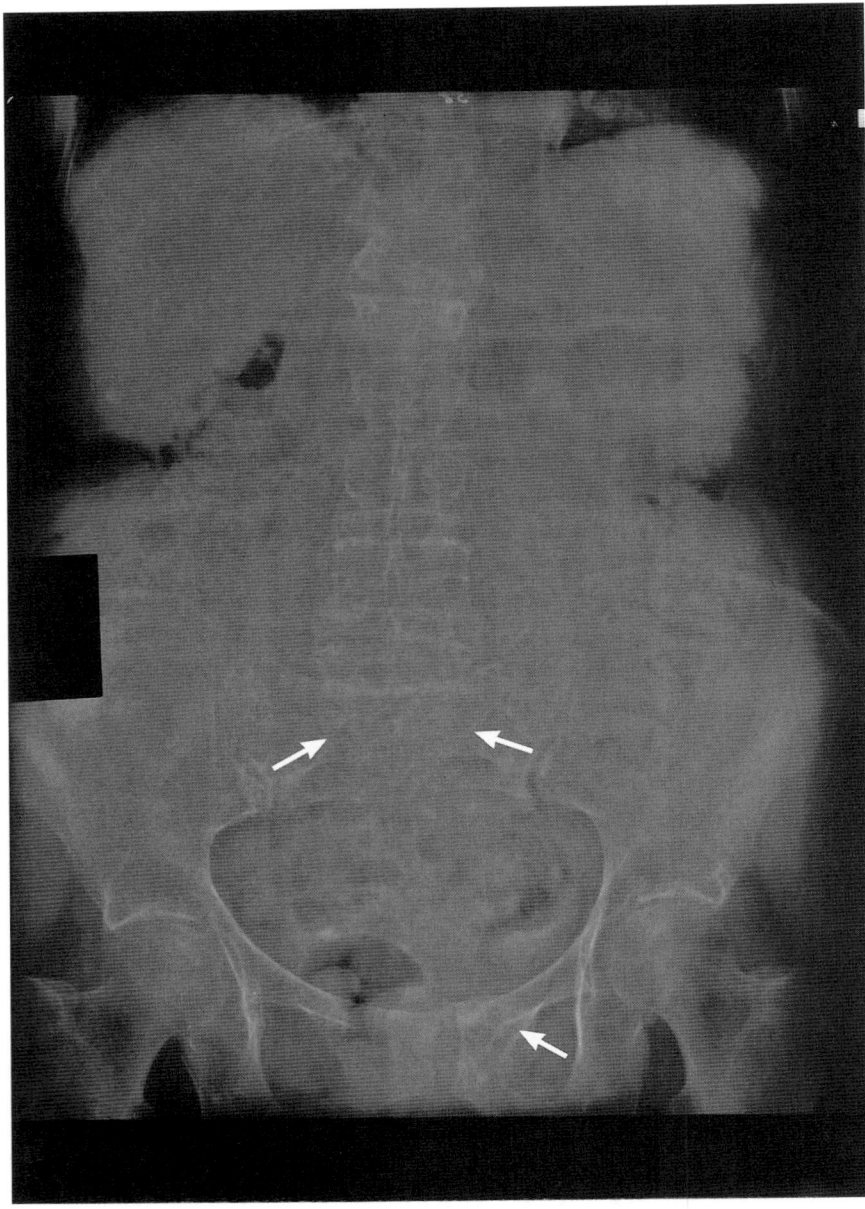

Figure 42-5 A 75-year-old woman with osteoporosis who had insufficiency fractures of left pubic bone and in both sacral alae. (From Sinaki 1998,[78] with permission of Editrice Kurtis.)

hip fractures, regardless of whether internal fixation or joint arthroplasty is done, is less eventful if physical therapeutic measures are used postoperatively, such as use of gait aids with partial weight bearing on the operative side. Only in severely comminuted fractures, or fractures in which the operative result has been unsatisfactory, is the restriction of weight bearing to no weight bearing needed.

Hip pads for fracture prophylaxis

There is conflicting evidence as to whether hip protectors can reduce the incidence of hip fractures in the elderly, high-risk population. One randomized controlled trial showed that hip protector pads can protect against hip fractures in an elderly nursing home population (average age 81 years), but compliance with use of the hip protectors has been a concern.[28]

Another study showed no significant difference in the incidence of hip fractures, even in the participants who were compliant with use of the hip protectors.[55] It appears that at-risk elderly individuals, especially those with a history of falls, impaired balance, and decreased cognition, would benefit from the use of hip pads, in addition to use of gait aids.[77]

Sacral insufficiency fracture

Other axial skeletal fractures, such as fractures of the sacral alae and pubic rami, can also occur (Fig. 42-5). Pelvic fractures are particularly common in patients with osteoporosis. Fractures of the pubic rami can occur with minimal strain, and most patients can hardly recall having an incident of severe strain. Healing typically occurs without invasive procedures. Ambulatory activities are reduced temporarily, and a wheeled

Table 42-2 Some of the diagnostic evaluations for osteoporosis

Evaluation	Details
History and physical examination	Family history of osteoporosis, type and location of pain, general dietary calcium intake, level of physical activity, height and weight
Radiography of chest and spine	To rule out lymphomas, rib fractures, compression fractures, etc.
Bone mineral density (spine and hip)	At menopause and every 2 years for high-risk patients and every 5 years for low-risk patients
Complete blood cell count	To rule out anemias associated with malignancy, etc.
Chemistry group (serum calcium, phosphorus, vitamin D, parathyroid hormone, alkaline phosphatase, osteocalcin)	To assess the level of alkaline phosphatase, which can be increased in osteomalacia, Paget disease, bony metastasis and fracture, intestinal malabsorption, vitamin D deficiency, chronic liver disease, alcohol abuse, phenytoin (Dilantin) therapy, hypercalcemia of hyperparathyroidism, hypophosphatemia of hyperparathyroidism and osteomalacia, malabsorption, malnutrition (these tests will also demonstrate an increase in calcium in hyperparathyroidism)
Erythrocyte sedimentation rate and serum protein electrophoresis	To determine changes indicative of multiple myeloma or other gammopathies
Total thyroxine	Increased total thyroxine may be a cause of osteoporosis because of increased bone turnover
Immunoreactive parathyroid hormone	Hyperparathyroidism (accompanied by hypercalcemia)
25-Hydroxyvitamin D and 1,25-dihydroxyvitamin D	Gastrointestinal disease, osteomalacia
Urinalysis and 24-h urine	To check for proteinuria due to nephrotic syndrome and for low pH due to renal tubular acidosis. A 24-hour urine test can exclude hypercalciuria (normal calcium value in men is 25–300 mg/specimen; in women, 20–275 mg/specimen[75])
Optional: bone scan, iliac crest biopsy	After tetracycline double-labeling for bone histomorphometry, bone marrow biopsy may be indicated to exclude multiple myeloma and metastatic malignancy
Biochemical markers of bone turnover	Formation: serum osteocalcin, alkaline phosphatase (bone), procollagen peptides Resorption: serum acid phosphatase, pyridinoline, deoxypyridinoline, urinary calcium or creatinine

walker is initially recommended for decreasing pain. Later in the treatment, crutches and a cane can be used. Weight bearing is limited, as dictated by the level of pain in the pelvic area. Fracture of the sacrum with minimal trauma also can occur, and the goal of management is to decrease weight-bearing pain with the use of proper assistive devices for ambulation.[89] For management of pelvic pain, sedative physical therapeutic measures are recommended.

DIAGNOSTIC STUDIES IN OSTEOPOROSIS

The diagnosis of osteoporosis requires a thorough history and physical examination, including family history of osteoporosis, type and location of musculoskeletal pain, general dietary calcium intake, level of physical activity, and height and weight measurements (Table 42-2).

Several biochemical indices also are used in the differential diagnosis of metabolic bone disease or, in some instances, for therapeutic follow-up.[8] For example, biochemical markers for bone formation are calcium, phosphorus, PTH, bone-specific alkaline phosphatase, and serum osteocalcin. Resorption markers include 24-h urinary calcium excretion corrected by creatinine excretion, hydroxyproline, and pyridinium cross-links (in urine).[17] The interpretation of these tests is unfortunately clouded in patients with osteoporosis, because of the high intra- and inter-individual variations of these parameters. Indices of bone turnover show seasonal and circadian variations (Table 42-2).

Radiographic findings consist of increased lucency of the vertebral bodies with loss of horizontal trabeculae and increased prominence of the cortical end plates and vertically oriented trabeculae, reduction in cortex thickness, and anterior wedging of vertebral bodies.[9,18] The degree of wedging that indicates a true fracture varies from a 15% to 25% reduction in anterior height relative to the posterior height of the same vertebra. There are other morphologic changes, such as biconcavity of vertebral bodies and complete compression fractures (reduction in both the anterior and the posterior height by at

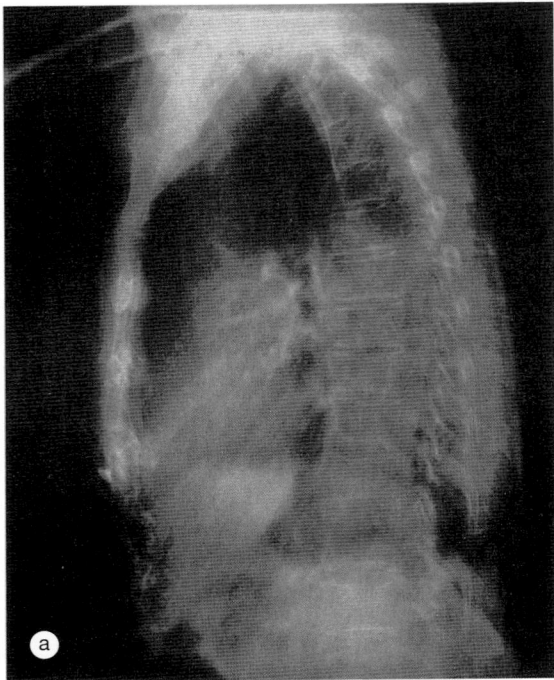
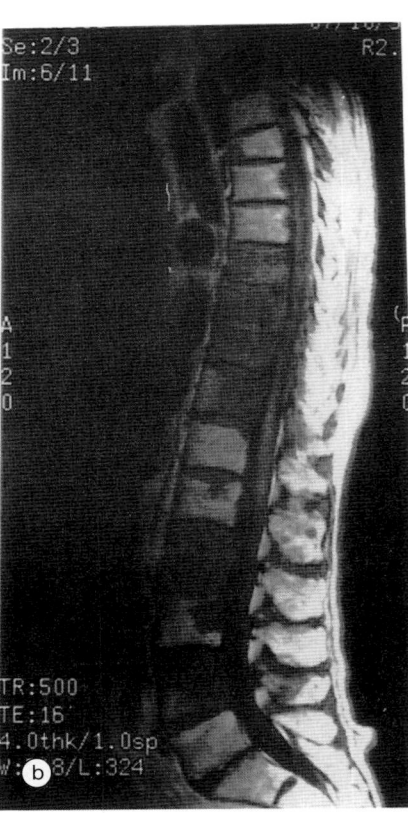

Figure 42-6 (a) Lateral radiograph of the spine in a 77-year-old man with persistent back pain. No evidence of metastatic lesion was identified. **(b)** Magnetic resonance imaging demonstrates extensive skeletal metastases from T3 through lower lumbar spine, with involvement of nearly every vertebral body. The most extensive involvement is at T3, T8 through T11, T12, and L4.

least 25% compared with the adjacent normal vertebrae).[18,54] Bone scan and magnetic resonance imaging can further define the cause of bone loss (Fig. 42-6), if needed.

Osteoporosis is typically not visible on conventional radiographs until at least 25–30% of bone mineral has been lost. Consequently, evaluation of bone mineral density through absorptiometry techniques is recommended.[90] These are also helpful in treatment, because calculated bone loss or gain is required in therapeutic trials of agents affecting bone mass. The different methods for evaluation of bone mass have different levels of precision.[89] Available methods include photon absorptiometry (single or dual), finger x-ray spectrometry, ultrasound densitometry, qualitative computed tomography, and dual x-ray absorptiometry. The most commonly used technique is dual-energy absorptiometry. Dual-energy x-ray absorptiometry has high precision and is commonly used for research and clinical evaluations to measure the bone mineral density of the spine and hips (Fig. 42-7). More commonly measured is the bone mineral density of the femoral neck, because spinal bone density can be erroneously high as a result of osteoarthritis of the spine. It also can be used to measure total-body bone mass. It is x-ray-based and has a precision of about 1%. The amount of radiation used is less than 3 mrad.[90]

TREATMENT

Osteoporosis is a multifactorial condition and its treatment has several facets, so it requires a team approach.[3] Endocrine con-

sultation is needed, along with interventions from specialists in physical medicine and rehabilitation, pharmacology, psychology, and nutrition.[3] The World Health Organization has defined osteoporosis as bone mineral density T score ≤ -2.5. Detailed definitions for normal bone mineral density, osteopenia, and osteoporosis are provided earlier in the text of this chapter. These definitions facilitate decision making for therapeutic trials. They are also helpful for prescription of a proper exercise program.

Because fractures generally occur with falls, the prevention of falls decreases the risk of fracture.[80] A recent study showed that patients with osteoporosis who had kyphosis were significantly more at risk of falls than control subjects without osteoporosis–kyphosis.[58] A recent controlled trial demonstrated significant improvement in risk of fall, balance, and unsteadiness of gait after a 4-week spinal proprioceptive extension exercise dynamic (SPEED) program.[59] Through utilization of a weighted kypho-orthosis and SPEED program, back pain decreased and level of physical activity increased. The SPEED program opens a new area of investigation for reducing risk of falls in kyphotic, osteoporotic individuals with balance disorder.[57]

Exercise

The efficacy of exercise for improving bone mass is supported by hormonal and nutritional factors (Box 42-5). To meet the challenge of mechanical load, skeletal tissue must have enough bone mass and proper architecture to withstand the physical

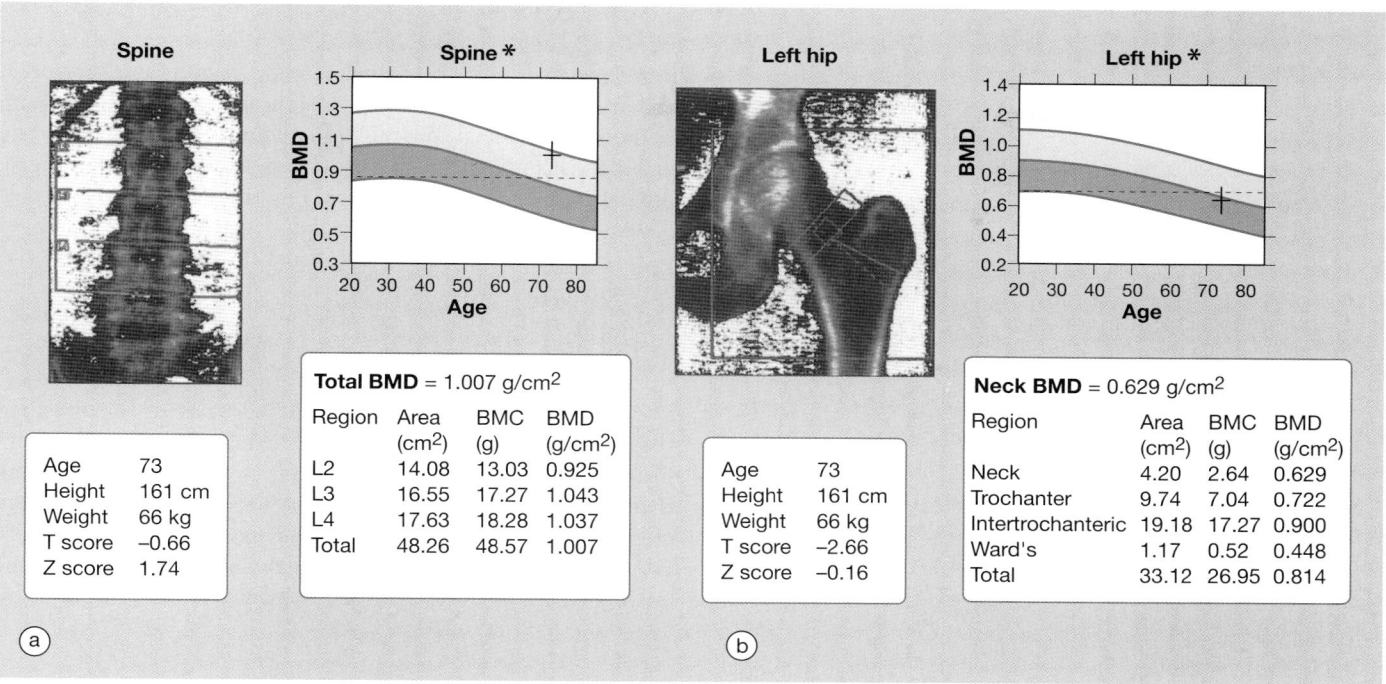

Figure 42-7 Reports of bone mineral density (BMD) studies with dual-energy x-ray absorptiometry of spine and hip in a patient with osteoporosis. (**a**) Lumbar spine BMD. (**b**) Femoral neck BMD. BMD of the spine can be erroneously high due to osteoarthritis of the spine. *, Age- and sex-matched; BMC, bone mineral content; T, peak bone mass; Z, age-matched.

strain that is imposed on it. It is fortunate that normal musculoskeletal structure is highly adaptable and can meet the challenge of usual mechanical loads. The challenge in osteopenia and osteoporosis from mechanical load and strain might not be tolerated without damage to the architecture of bone. A supervised, non-strenuous, progressive, resistive exercise program can improve bone mass in inactive individuals.[69] By understanding both the benefits and the shortcomings of nutritional and exercise approaches for musculoskeletal management of osteoporosis, we can create a better prophylactic program for osteoporosis.

High rates and magnitude of bone strain are produced during high-impact sports activities such as gymnastics, badminton, tennis, volleyball, and basketball. The high-impact bone loading results in site-specific increases in bone mineral density. One study showed a significant difference in bone mineral density between gymnasts and volleyball players. The lower extremities are loaded differently in these two athletic activities.[13] Gymnasts had higher bone mineral density than that of volleyball players, except for the pelvic bone.

According to Frost's theory, a minimum threshold of mechanical loading is needed to evoke an increased level of bone mineral density.[15] This theory is referred to as that of the minimum effective strain stimulus. Lanyon suggested that the greatest osteogenic effect from mechanical loading is promoted when the strain is vigorous enough to produce high strain, repeated daily, short in duration, and applied to a specific bone site.[29] Mechanical loading, when applied properly, can stimulate

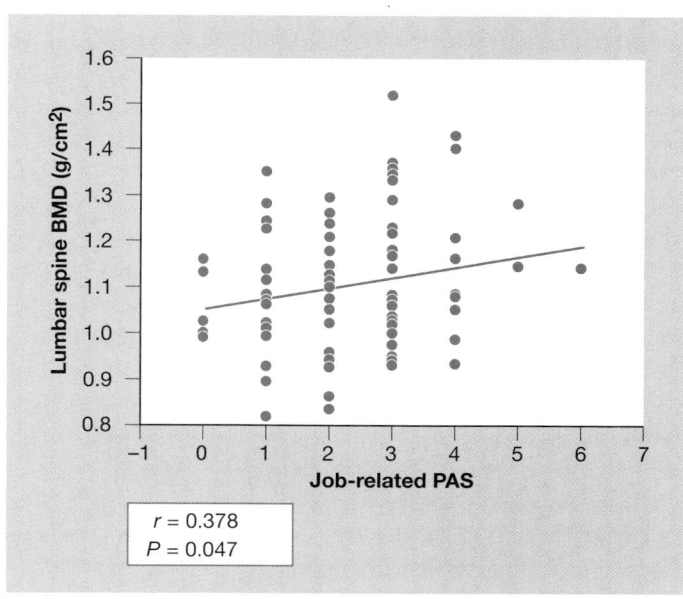

Figure 42-8 Job-related physical activity score (PAS) significantly correlated with spinal bone mineral density (BMD). (From Sinaki et al. 1998,[60] with permission of Williams &Wilkins.)

osteogenic activity. Axial loading of the skeleton during lifting activities at one's job or in the care of children can be as osteogenic as working out in a gym (Fig. 42-8).[60] Individuals with normal bone mineral density can perform high-impact exercises such as aerobics, jogging, and skiing. For persons with osteo-

Box 42-5 Suggested rehabilitation guidelines on the basis of bone mineral density T scores[a]

Reduction to −1 SD (normal)
- No treatment
- Patient education, preventive measures
- Lifting techniques
- Proper diet (calcium and vitamin D)
- Jogging (short distances)
- Weight training
- Aerobics
- Abdominal and back-strengthening exercises[b]
- Postural exercises?

−1 to −2.5 SD (osteopenia)[c]
- Consultation for treatment
- Patient education, preventive interventions
- Pain management
- Back-strengthening exercises
- Limit load lifting (10–20 lbs)
- Aerobic exercises, walking 40 min/day
- Exercises: weight training three times a week
- Postural exercises: Posture Training Support combined with pelvic tilt and back extension
- Frenkel exercises, prevention of falls
- T'ai chi, if desired
- Antiresorptive agents

−2.5 SD or more (osteoporosis)[c]
- Pharmacologic intervention
- Pain management
- Range of motion, strengthening, coordination
- Midday rest, heat or cold, stroking massage if needed
- Back extensor strengthening
- Walking 40 min/day, as tolerated; Frenkel exercises
- Aquatic exercises once or twice a week
- Fall prevention program (see Box 42-3)
- Postural exercises: Posture Training Support combined with pelvic tilt and back extension
- Prevention of vertebral compression fractures (orthoses, as needed)
- Prevention of spinal strain (lifting 5–10 lbs)
- Evaluation of balance, gait aid
- Safety and facilitation of self-care through modification of bathroom (grab bars), kitchen (counter adjustment), occupational therapy consultation
- Start strengthening program with 1–2 lbs and increase as tolerated to 5 lbs in each hand
- Hip protective measures

[a]T score: standard deviation below peak normal young adult bone mass.
[b]See Figures 42-9 and 42-10 for proper exercise program and posture.
[c]Osteopenia or osteoporosis as defined by the World Health Organization.[91]

Spinal extension exercises should be used along with exercises to reduce lumbar lordosis.[62,73] Weakness in abdominal muscles adds to the problems of poor posture and protruded abdomen. To complement a posture training exercise program, isometric abdominal muscle-strengthening exercises should be included (Figs 42-9 and 42-10). Our osteoporosis back exercise program has been studied extensively through controlled trials and has been proven to be safe and effective.[24,63,66]

Strenuous spinal flexion and spinal flexion exercises should be avoided in patients with osteoporosis (Fig. 42-11).[66] In our study comparing the effect of flexion and extension exercises on the spine, we found that, even without pharmacotherapy, patients with osteoporosis who performed back extension exercises (Fig. 42-9k) had a significantly lower rate of fracture than those who performed spinal flexion exercises or no exercise.[66] Osteoporotic women generally have weaker back extensors than normal women of comparable age (Fig. 42-12). The choice of physical activity is important and has to be individualized. Fitness programs, such as swimming or short periods of stationary biking, are not significantly osteogenic[12,46] but can fulfill the

Figure 42-9 Non-strenuous exercises for patients with severe osteoporosis. (**a–c**) Upper back and shoulder extension exercise performed with spine supported. (**d** and **e**) Flexibility of the shoulder joint may contribute to improvement of upper back posture. To avoid upper back and neck strain in a fragile skeleton, shoulder rotation exercises can be performed in the supine position. (**f**) Pectoral stretching exercise performed in the sitting position. This is used to reduce kyphotic posturing. (**g**) Back extension exercise in the sitting position. This position avoids or minimizes pain in patients with severe osteoporosis. (**h**) Deep-breathing exercise combined with pectoral stretching and back extension exercise. The patient sits on a chair, places hands at the level of the head, and inhales deeply while gently extending the elbows backward. While exhaling, the patient returns the arms to the starting position. This is repeated 10–15 times. (**i**) Exercise to decrease lumbar lordosis with isometric contraction of lumbar flexors. (**j**) Isometric exercise to strengthen abdominal muscles. (**k**) Extension exercises in the prone position with a pillow under the abdomen (to avoid hyperextension). (**k3**) To increase the effect of back extension strengthening, weight is added. (**l**) Exercise for improving strength in lumbar extensors and gluteus maximus muscles. (**m**) Specificity of exercises: muscle-strengthening and weight-loading exercises that may decrease bone loss. (These exercises were developed for the osteopenic spine by M. Sinaki through a grant from the Retirement Research Foundation. These techniques are designed to decrease strain on the spine despite weight lifting.) (**m1**) Shoulder extensors contribute to reduction of kyphotic posturing. Shoulder extensors can be strengthened with a proper combination of weight-lifting and weight-bearing exercises while balance is maintained. One knee is bent to avoid lumbar strain. To avoid straining the spine and to maintain balance, leaning or holding on to a steady object for support is recommended. Note: the amount of weight lifted is about 1–2 lbs in each hand, not to exceed 5 lbs in each hand. The amount of weight needs to be prescribed according to the patient's bone mineral density (status of osteoporosis) and the condition of the upper extremities. (**m2**) Bilateral or unilateral spine and hip weight-loading exercise. When weight is lifted above the head, the knees should be bent slightly to avoid straining the lumbar spine. Note: the amount of weight lifted is about 1–2 lbs in each hand, not to exceed 5 lbs in each hand. The amount of weight needs to be prescribed according to the patient's bone mineral density (status of osteoporosis) and the condition of the upper extremities. (a–h2, l, and m, from Sinaki 1993,[83] with permission of the Mayo Foundation; i, j, k1, and k2, from Sinaki 1988,[76] with permission of the Mayo Foundation; k3, from Sinaki 1993,[82] with permission of the Mayo Foundation.)

porosis, non-straining exercises such as walking for 45 min three times a week or daily walking for 30 min are recommended. In-water exercises are recommended for patients who are unable to perform antigravity exercises because of pain or weakness. The non-strenuous, low-resistance exercises can be advanced to antigravity and strengthening exercises as permitted by a patient's musculoskeletal status.

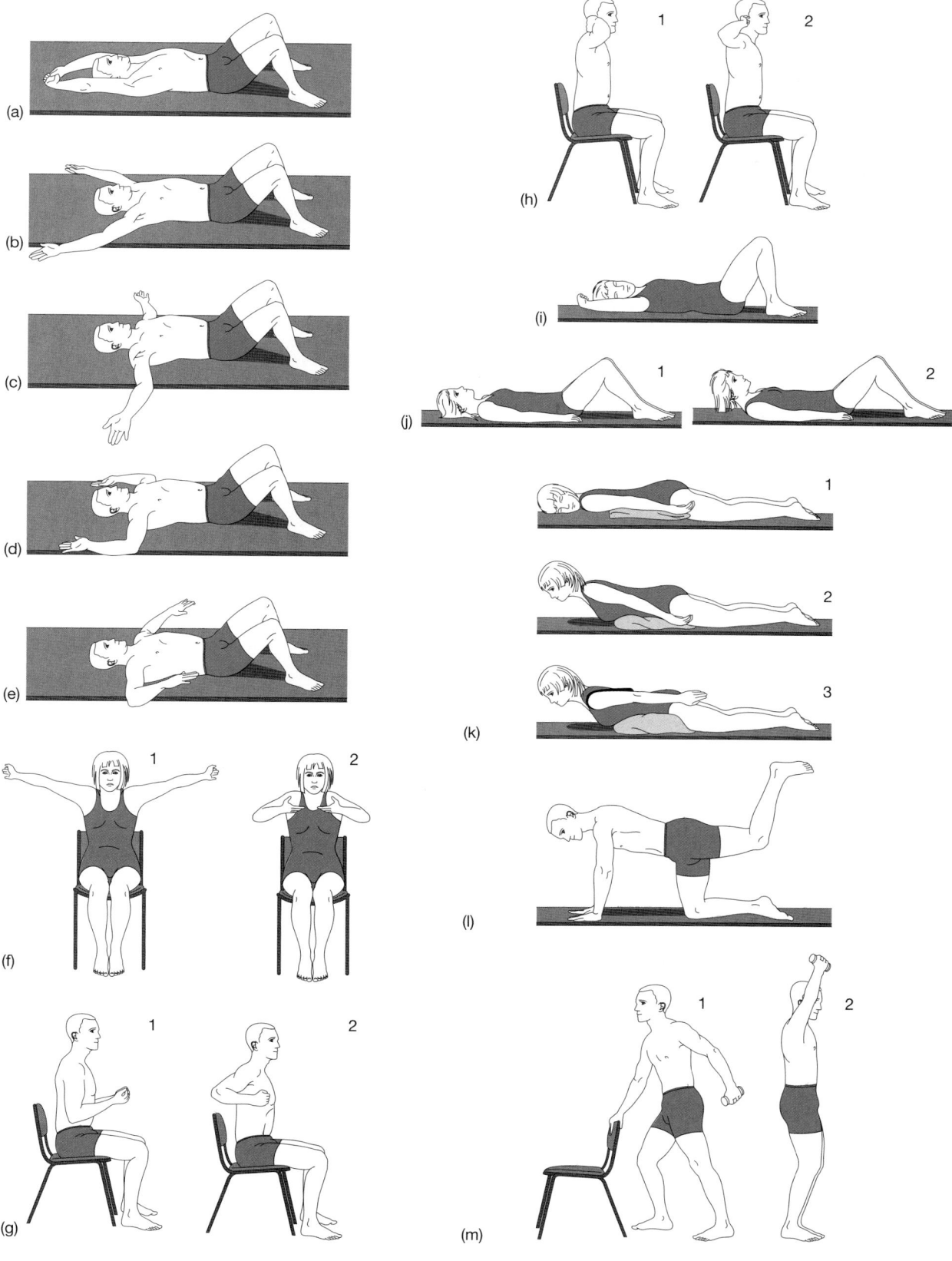

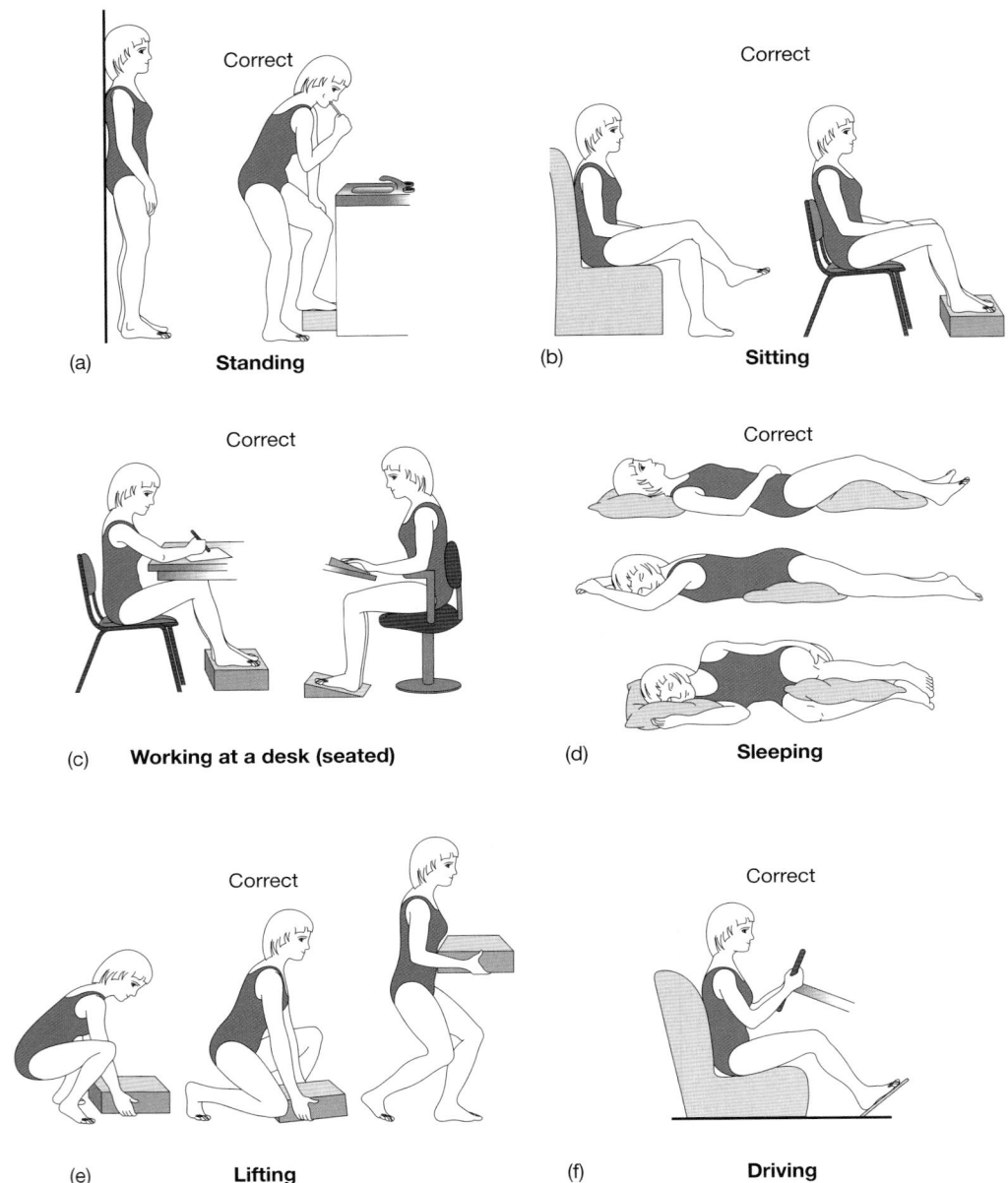

(a) **Standing**

(b) **Sitting**

(c) **Working at a desk (seated)**

(d) **Sleeping**

(e) **Lifting**

(f) **Driving**

Figure 42-10 Static and dynamic correct postures. (From Sinaki and Mokri 1996,[64] with permission of Saunders.)

need for cardiovascular fitness without straining the osteoporotic frame. Walking for 40 min at least three times a week is effective for maintaining lower extremity bone density. Knowledge of the bone mineral density is helpful before recommending a weight-training program.

Posture training program and the osteoporotic skeletal frame

Any support that can improve posture and decrease pain-related paraspinal muscle cocontraction is desirable. The number and diameter of collagen fibrils of the intervertebral disks decrease with aging. This results in loss of resiliency of the disks. In addition, reduced paraspinal muscle strength[68] and forward tendency of head and trunk related to the effect of gravity can cause iliocostal friction syndrome and flank pain. This pain does

not respond to the use of conventional orthoses. Indeed, orthoses such as corsets can make the pain worse through pressure over the lower rib cage (Fig. 42-13). Posture training programs that are intended to decrease kyphosis can also subsequently reduce iliocostal friction syndrome.[29,78] Posture training programs such as the application of a weighted kyphoorthosis for half an hour twice a day or for 1 h twice a day while trying to contract back extensors can provide reeducation for improvement of kyphotic posturing and reduction of the risk of falls (Fig. 42-14).[65]

Orthoses and the osteoporotic spine

Acute compression fracture usually results in severe pain and, if not managed well, can lead to prolonged immobility. The final outcome is creation of chronic pain behavior and subsequent

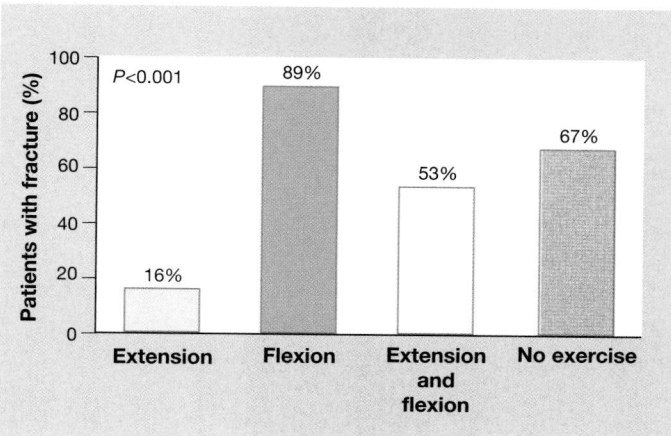

Figure 42-11 Percentage of patients with spinal fracture after spinal extension exercise, spinal flexion exercise, extension and flexion exercise, and no exercise. (Data from Sinaki and Mikkelsen 1984.[66])

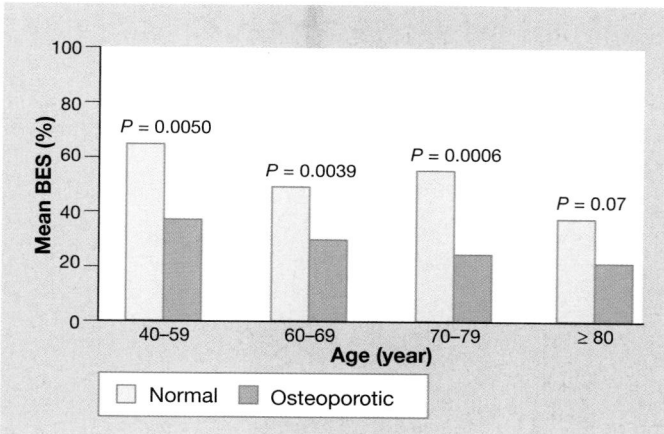

Figure 42-12 Back strength in normal women vs women with osteoporosis. BES, back extensor strength. (Data from Sinaki et al. 1993.[64])

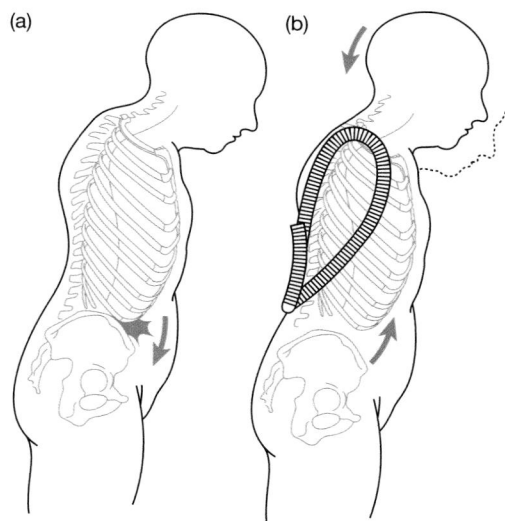

Figure 42-13 Severe kyphosis can result in iliocostal contact or iliocostal friction syndrome (**a**). Application of a weighted kypho-orthosis provides counteracting forces, which enable users to contract their erector spinae muscles better and decrease kyphotic posturing (**b**). (From Sinaki 1995,[86] with permission of Edizioni Medico-Scientifiche.)

be taught in the rehabilitative program for patients with osteoporosis.

Pharmacologic interventions

Several pharmacologic agents can be used for treatment of osteoporosis. Estrogen, calcium, and vitamin D are the most commonly advocated pharmacologic treatments for involutional osteoporosis. Antiresorptive agents include estrogens, androgens, calcitonin, and bisphosphonates. Osteoblast stimulator agents include fluoride and PTH. Fluoride is not approved by the Food and Drug Administration at this time for the treatment of osteoporosis, because of an increased risk of appendicular fractures. Studies on the effect of PTH 1–34 (Teriparatide) on fractures and bone mineral density have been very promising. PTH 1–34 decreases the risk of vertebral fractures and increases vertebral, femoral, and total body bone mineral density. The preferred dosage is 20 μg daily, self-administered subcutaneous injections, which result in fewer side effects than the 40-μg dosage.[43] There can reportedly be a 9–13% increase in bone mineral density of the spine and 65–69% reduction of risk of new vertebral fractures compared with in a placebo-treated group. PTH is contraindicated in subjects who have a history of cancer. Side effects include nausea, dizziness, leg cramps, headache, and hypercalcemia. Studies are currently in progress evaluating new agents that can improve bone mass.

It is obvious that cessation of tobacco and alcohol abuse are necessary. An adequate calcium intake is required (Table 42-1) to permit normal bone development and potentially to decrease bone loss. Adequate calcium and vitamin D intakes appear to have only a modest effect on bone loss after menopause. Inadequate intakes of calcium and vitamin D are common, especially in elderly nursing home residents. One study showed the

psychologic consequences. Acute pain needs to be actively managed with proper physical measures. Sedative physical therapy, including application of cold and later heat, and isometric muscle contractions of the paraspinal muscles can be helpful. Rigid thoracolumbar orthoses to promote extension of the spine are helpful (Fig. 42-15) (also see Ch. 17). If thoracolumbar orthoses are not tolerated because of postural changes, a thoracic weighted kypho-orthosis (Fig. 42-16) or a combination of a kypho-orthosis and lower back support (elastic abdominal support) might suffice. In some cases, long-distance ambulatory activities can require use of a cane or a wheeled walker. Temporary use of a wheelchair with a supportive back cushion is indicated in some cases. Every effort needs to be taken to prevent the patient's confinement to one room or prolonged bed rest. Every effort should be made to limit immobility and its resulting reactive depression. Safety during ambulation is paramount, and prevention of falls and fracture should

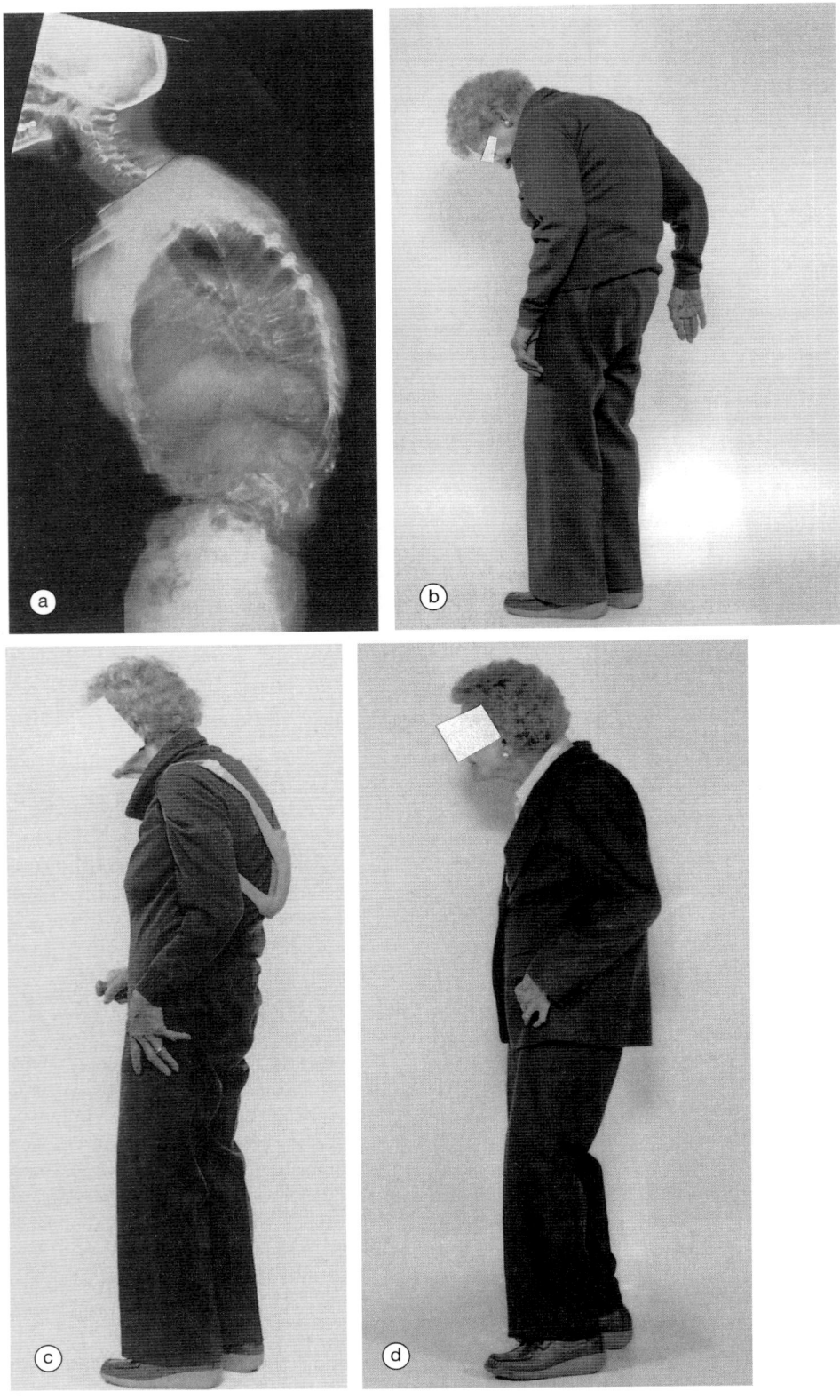

Figure 42-14 An 86-year-old woman with osteoporosis. (**a**) Radiograph of the spine depicts osteoporotic and postural changes. (**b**) Severe kyphotic posturing, which made ambulation difficult. (**c**) The same patient wearing a weighted kypho-orthosis. (**d**) The same woman's postural correction at age 92 after a 6-year trial with weighted kypho-orthosis and posture training program; the patient is not wearing the kypho-orthosis. (a and d: from Sinaki 1998,[78] with permission of Editrice Kurtis; b and c, from Sinaki 1995,[84] with permission of Hanley and Belfus.)

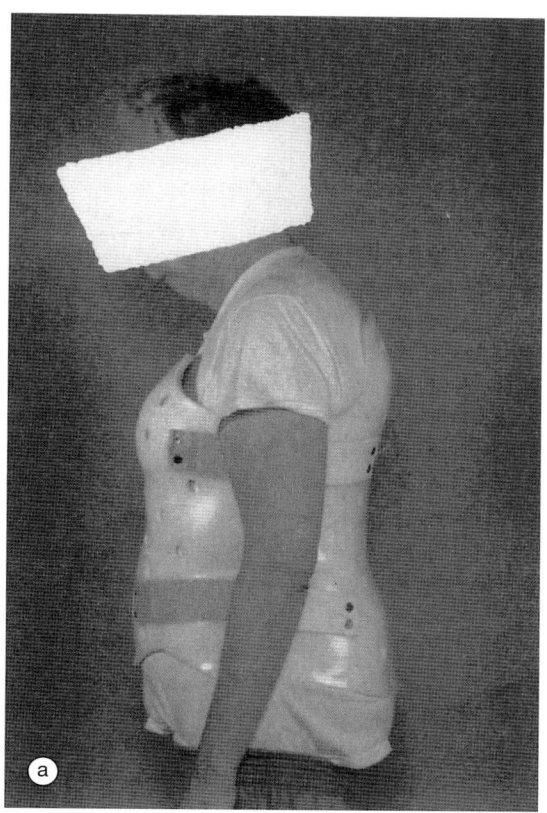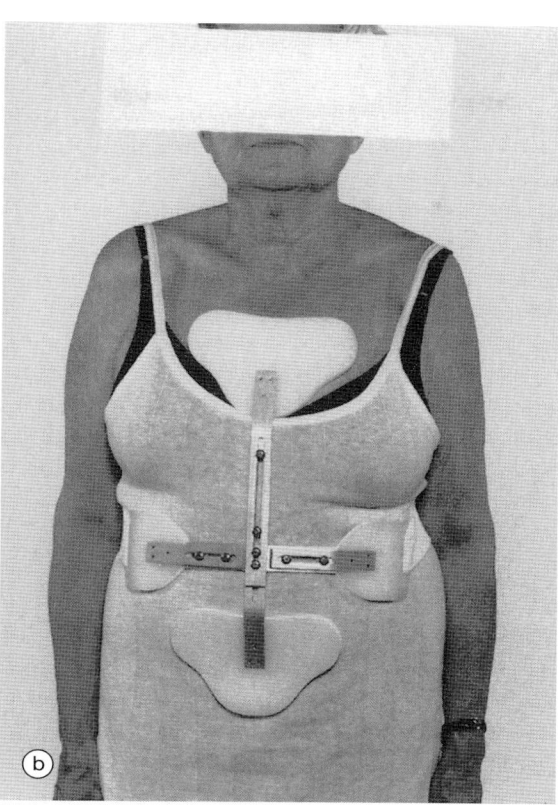

Figure 42-15 (**a**) Rigid back support: bivalved body jacket. The brace is made of polypropylene and is custom-fitted. (**b**) Cruciform anterior spinal hyperextension (CASH) brace. A patient with osteoporosis of the spine and compression fractures was unable to tolerate increased intraabdominal pressure with the use of abdominal back support because of hiatal hernia. The patient was fitted with a CASH brace satisfactorily. (a, from Sinaki 1996,[81] with permission of Georg Thieme Verlag; b, from Sinaki 1988,[76] with permission of the Mayo Foundation.)

efficacy of supplementation of calcium and vitamin D for reduction of the risk of hip fracture in elderly subjects.[5] Typical recommendations are 1500 mg of elemental calcium daily in divided doses (Table 42-1). The recommended vitamin D dosage is between 600 and 800 IU/day. The dose of vitamin D varies, and depends on the patient's exposure to the sun and dietary intake of vitamin D. It is necessary to determine the serum level of $1,25(OH)_2D_3$ in some cases (the normal levels are at least 20 ng/mL and preferably 30 ng/mL). These values can differ in different laboratories and locations. In the upper Midwestern region of the USA, they are 15–80 ng/mL in the summer and 14–42 ng/mL in the winter.

Estrogen acts directly on bone cells, and is an antiresorptive agent that has been shown to decrease the rate of bone loss and fractures in postmenopausal women, whether the menopause is natural or surgical. Estrogen is not as commonly used now because of the alarming results of the Women's Health Initiative studies.[19] When a patient with an intact uterus is treated with estrogen, progesterone also should be used under a proper regimen to prevent the development of endometrial hyperplasia and possibly endometrial carcinoma. There are several regimens for estrogen and progesterone use. They can be used concur-

rently (combination pills) or cycled. The proper regimen needs to be individualized.

Minimal effective doses of some forms of oral estrogen are usually used (conjugated equine estrogens, 0.3 mg; estradiol, 50 μg/day). Parenteral estrogens can be administered in the form of patches, implants, or gels. The implants are inserted subcutaneously, where they slowly release estradiol. Estrogen patches can deliver estradiol through the skin. Patches are changed once or twice weekly, and implants are usually inserted every 6 months. Implants are not popular in the USA. The advantage of parenteral estrogen is that metabolism in the liver is bypassed, making smaller doses sufficient. The commonly used transdermal estradiol 17 (patch) strength can vary from 0.05 mg (usual dose) to 0.1 mg (high dose). In some instances, a low dose of 0.025 mg is used.

Contraindications to estrogen replacement therapy include liver or gallbladder disease, recent history of thromboembolism or thrombophlebitis, and suspected breast or endometrial carcinoma. Estrogens also can have an adverse effect on existing hypertension, hyperlipidemia, migraine headaches, chronic thrombophlebitis, and endometriosis. Administration of progestins can result in uncomfortable side effects such as fatigue,

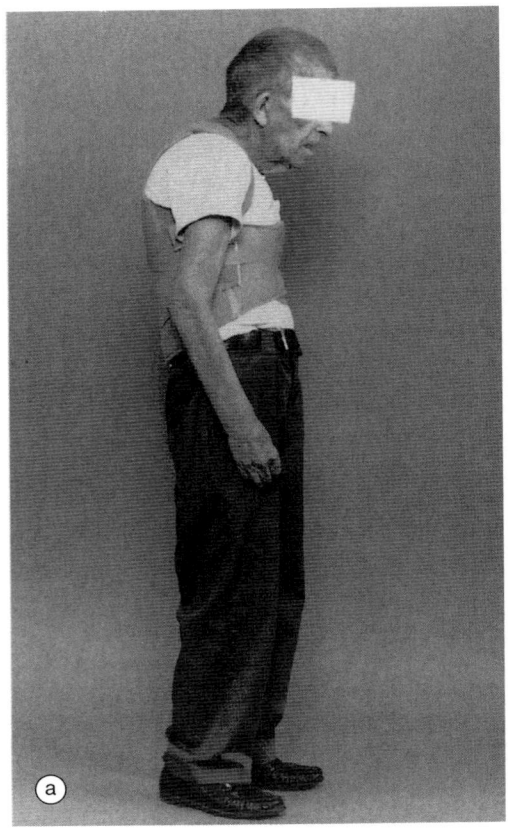
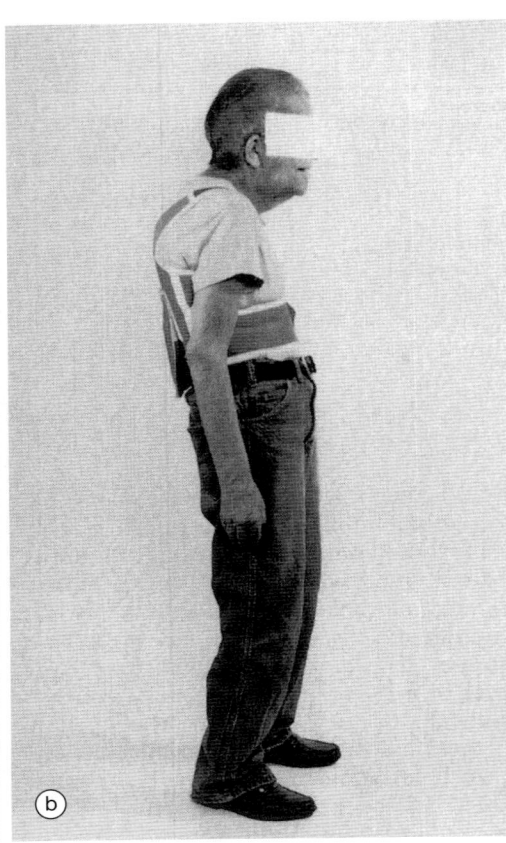

Figure 42-16 (**a**) Thoracolumbar support (rigid stays). A problem with fitting due to spinal deformities. (**b**) Posture Training Support vest sometimes is tolerated better than conventional thoracolumbar support. Weight in the pouch can range from 1 to 2½ lbs, as required.

depression, breast tenderness, bloating, menstrual cramps, and headaches.[48] Progesterone in the form of medroxyprogesterone acetate (Provera) at a dosage of 2.5–5 mg/day is often used for the first 10 days at the beginning of the cycle. Estrogen protects against both osteoporosis and cardiovascular disease. However, many postmenopausal women discontinued their use of hormone replacement therapy after the results of the Women's Health Initiative studies became available.[32] Of all breast cancer cases, 78% occur in women after age 50 years. There are reports that hormone replacement therapy increases the risk of breast cancer by 2.3% per year, and this risk increases to 3.5% per year after 5 years. Women who have cardiovascular disease should not use hormone replacement therapy for prevention. Estrogen therapy should also be discontinued if a woman has an acute cardiovascular event. In general, decision making for use of the therapy is better based on non-coronary benefit. The patient's preference is important for management of menopausal symptoms, usually hot flashes and bone health.

Calcitonin, an antiresorptive agent, acts directly on the osteoclasts. Calcitonin has a few disadvantages that limit its use.[52] It is most effective in patients whose rate of bone turnover is high. Calcitonin is approved for therapy of established osteoporosis, but the long-term fracture-reducing efficacy of calcitonin has not been clearly demonstrated. The subcutaneous or intramuscular injection of 50–100 units of salmon calcitonin or 0.5 mg of human calcitonin, given every other day, is commonly used.

The use of nasal calcitonin might improve the patient's compliance. Side effects of parenteral use, such as flushing or nausea, and development of antibodies can limit its use. The nasal spray can cause nasal irritation, crusting, and ulcerations, which usually require discontinuation of its use.

Bisphosphonates affect trabecular bone, especially in the lumbar spine, where bone mineral density increases of 5–10% occur during the first 2 years of treatment. Alendronate sodium, an amino-bisphosphonate, has been shown to normalize the rate of bone turnover and increase bone mass.[6] Alendronate must be taken with a full glass of water on awakening. The patient should not eat or recline for 30–45 min after taking the medication. Patient education and compliance are very important for the use of alendronate. One potential adverse effect of alendronate is esophageal irritation, particularly in patients with reflux or other esophageal dysfunction. Risedronate is another bisphosphonate that has been recently introduced for the treatment of osteoporosis. Treatment with risedronate, 5 mg per day, was shown to significantly decrease the incidence of vertebral and non-vertebral fractures in postmenopausal osteoporosis.[21] Table 42-3 reflects the weekly doses of bisphosphonates that are commonly recommended.

Anabolic steroids have an osteoblastic effect. They are used only under the most extreme circumstances, however, because they can have significant androgenic effects and induce liver function abnormalities. Thiazide diuretics inhibit urinary

Table 42-3 Commonly used agents in osteoporosis

Agent	Common dosage	Potential side effects
Progesterone (Provera), oral	2.5–5 mg (days 1–10 of cycle)	–
Alendronate sodium (Fosamax)	10 mg/day (70 mg once a week dose)	Esophageal irritation
Risedronate (Actonel)	5 mg/day (35 mg once a week dose)	Esophageal irritation
Calcitonin	200 units nasal spray (Miacalcin) or 50–100 mg every other day injections	Nasal irritation or ulceration
Raloxifene (Evista)	60 mg/day (oral)	Leg cramps, hot flashes, deep vein thrombosis
Calcium	1000–1500 mg/day (Table 42-1)	–
Vitamin D (multivitamin)	600–800 IU/day	–
Estrogen		–
Conjugated equine (Premarin)	0.3 mg (oral) per day	Headache, weight gain, change of mood or depression, increased blood pressure, gallbladder or liver disease, thrombophlebitis and increased blood clotting, increased serum triglyceride and blood glucose levels, abnormal vaginal bleeding, overgrowth of the uterine lining, breast and endometrial cancer
Transdermal estradiol 17 (patch)	0.05–0.1 mg	

excretion of calcium, and can retard bone loss and reduce the rate of fractures in patients with osteoporosis.

Sodium fluoride stimulates osteoblastic activity. It can increase bone density up to 8% per year in the lumbar spine and 4% in the proximal femur. However, it decreases cortical bone density in the radius by approximately 2% per year. There also have been reports of an increased rate of non-vertebral fractures in patients treated with fluoride. Sodium fluoride, although it is being used as a therapeutic measure in European countries, remains an investigational agent in the USA and should not be used as a routine form of treatment in patients with osteoporosis.[49]

The estrogen receptor mixed agonist–antagonists tamoxifen and raloxifene protect against bone loss in ovariectomized rats. They have an antiestrogenic effect on breast tissue. These agents also are known as selective estrogen receptor modulators.[7] However, the mechanism by which these compounds affect bone is not completely defined. Recent studies in humans have been promising,[36] but the percentage increment in bone mineral density has not been as much as that with alendronate sodium. One of the side effects related to tamoxifen is uterine hyperplasia, but this is not a concern in treatment with raloxifene. Raloxifene decreases total cholesterol and serum low-density lipoprotein levels. Raloxifene is currently used only in the postmenopausal stage of osteoporosis (Table 42-3 and Box 42-6).

Treatment of osteoporosis in men includes the usual supplementation with calcium and vitamin D, limitation of alcohol use, and cessation of smoking. In cases of hypogonadism in men, endocrine consultation is necessary, and testosterone replacement therapy is a possibility. Bisphosphonates have also been

Box 42-6 Pharmacologic options in osteoporosis

Antiresorption
Act on osteoclasts and stabilize bone

- Calcium
- Estrogen
- Calcitonin
- Bisphosphonates
- Selective estrogen receptor modulators
- Thiazide diuretics
- Ipriflavone (investigational)

Formation
Act on osteoblasts and increase bone formation

- Vitamin D
- Anabolic steroids
- Parathyroid hormone
- Growth factors (investigational)
- Fluoride (investigational)

helpful as antiresorptive agents for management of osteoporosis in men.

Management of steroid-induced osteoporosis requires calcium and vitamin D supplementation, use of oral antiresorptive agents such as alendronate sodium (70 mg once a week dose or risedronate 35 mg once a week dose), and implementation of a proper exercise program. In advanced stages of bone loss and muscle weakness, the use of assistive devices or a wheelchair might be necessary.[76] If hyperparathyoidism or thyrotoxicosis is present, proper management should be implemented. In the case of hyperparathyroidism, surgical removal of the parathyroid adenoma is recommended.

A balanced diet is needed for maintenance of musculoskeletal health. Excessive dietary intake of sodium and phosphorus should be avoided. Studies of young women with malnutrition due to anorexia nervosa have demonstrated poor muscle strength, significant loss of bone mass, irregularity of menstrual periods, and estrogen deficiency.

In regard to osteoporosis, the distinct effects of nutrition, exercise, hormones, and lifestyle on osteoporosis cannot be separated.[85] The patient's quality of life can certainly be affected by musculoskeletal changes related to osteoporosis. Practical treatment of patients with osteoporosis requires pharmacologic interventions, physical and rehabilitative measures, and good nutrition. It also requires consideration of the psychologic consequences and reactions experienced by the patients. Public education can contribute to prevention, better understanding, and management of the consequences of osteoporosis.

REFERENCES

1. Adams P, Eyre DR, Muir H. Biochemical aspects of development and ageing of human lumbar intervertebral discs. Rheumatol Rehabil 1977; 16:22.

2. [Anonymous]. Optimal calcium intake. NIH Consensus Statement June 6–8. 1994; 12:1.

3. Bonner FJ Jr, Sinaki M, Grabois M, et al. Health professional's guide to rehabilitation of the patient with osteoporosis. Osteoporos Int 2003; 14(suppl 2):S1–S22.

4. Cassell C, Benedict M, Specker B. Bone mineral density in elite 7- to 9-yr-old female gymnasts and swimmers. Med Sci Sports Exerc 1996; 28:1243.

5. Chapuy MC, Arlot ME, Duboeuf F, et al. Vitamin D_3 and calcium to prevent hip fractures in the elderly woman. N Engl J Med 1992; 327:1637.

6. Chesnut CH III, McClung MR, Ensrud KE, et al. Alendronate treatment of the postmenopausal osteoporotic woman: effect of multiple dosages on bone mass and bone remodeling. Am J Med 1995; 99:144.

7. Delmas PD. Clinical use of selective estrogen receptor modulators. Bone 1999; 25:115.

8. Delmas PD, Hardy P, Garnero P, Dain M. Monitoring individual response to hormone replacement therapy with bone markers. Bone 2000; 26(6):553–560.

9. Doyle FH, Gutteridge DH, Joplin GF, et al. An assessment of radiological criteria used in the study of spinal osteoporosis. Br J Radiol 1967; 40:241.

10. Drinkwater BL, Nilson K, Ott S, et al. Bone mineral density after resumption of menses in amenorrheic athletes. JAMA 1986; 256:380.

11. Econs MJ, Speer MC. Genetic studies of complex diseases: let the reader beware [editorial]. J Bone Miner Res 1996; 11:1835.

12. Emslander HC, Sinaki M, Muhs JM, et al. Bone mass and muscle strength in female college athletes (runners and swimmers). Mayo Clin Proc 1998; 73:1151.

13. Fehling PC, Alekel L, Clasey J, et al. A comparison of bone mineral densities among female athletes in impact loading and active loading sports. Bone 1995; 17:205.

14. Felsing NE, Brasel JA, Cooper DM. Effect of low and high intensity exercise on circulating growth hormone in men. J Clin Endocrinol Metab 1992; 75:157.

15. Frost HM. A determinant of bone architecture: the minimum effective strain. Clin Orthop 1983; 175:286.

16. Frost HM. Why do marathon runners have less bone than weight lifters? A vital-biomechanical view and explanation. Bone 1997; 20:183.

17. Garnero P, Darte C, Delmas PD. A model to monitor the efficacy of alendronate treatment in women with osteoporosis using a biochemical marker of bone turnover. Bone 1999; 24:603.

18. Genant HK, Vogler JB, Block JE. Radiology of osteoporosis. In: Riggs BL Jr, Melton LJ III, eds. Osteoporosis: etiology, diagnosis, and management. New York: Raven Press; 1988:181–220.

19. Grady D, Herrington D, Bittner V, et al. Cardiovascular disease outcomes during 6.8 years of hormone therapy: Heart and Estrogen/progestin Replacement Study follow-up (HERS II). JAMA 2002; 288:49. Erratum in: JAMA 2002; 288:1064.

20. Gutmann E. Age changes in the neuromuscular system and aspects of rehabilitation medicine. In: Buerger AA, Tobis JS, eds. Neurophysiologic aspects of rehabilitation medicine. Springfield: Charles C Thomas; 1976:42–61.

21. Harris ST, Watts NB, Gerant HK, et al. Effects of risedronate treatment on vertebral and nonvertebral fractures in women with postmenopausal osteoporosis: a randomized controlled trial. JAMA 1999; 282:1344.

22. Hiu SL, Slemenda CW, Johnston CC Jr. Age and bone mass as predictors of fracture in a prospective study. J Clin Invest 1988; 81:1804.

23. Ireland P, Fordtran JS. Effect of dietary calcium and age on jejunal calcium absorption in humans studied by intestinal perfusion. J Clin Invest 1973; 52:2672.

24. Itoi E, Sinaki M. Effect of back-strengthening exercise on posture in healthy women 49 to 65 years of age. Mayo Clin Proc 1994; 69:1054.

25. Jackson JA, Kleerekoper M. Osteoporosis in men: diagnosis, pathophysiology, and prevention. Medicine (Baltimore) 1990; 69:137.

26. Jensen ME, Evans AJ, Mathias JM, et al. Percutaneous polymethylmethacrylate vertebroplasty in the treatment of osteoporotic vertebral body compression fractures: technical aspects. AJNR Am J Neuroradiol 1997; 18:1897.

27. Jones ET, Hensinger RN. Spinal deformity in idiopathic juvenile osteoporosis. Spine 1981; 6:1.

28. Kannus P, Parkkari J, Niemi S, et al. Prevention of hip fracture in elderly people with use of a hip protector. N Engl J Med 2000; 343:1506.

29. Kaplan RS, Sinaki M, Hameister MD. Effect of back supports on back strength in patients with osteoporosis: a pilot study. Mayo Clin Proc 1996; 71:235.

30. Khosla S. Role of hormonal changes in the pathogenesis of osteoporosis in men. Calcif Tissue Int 2004: Aug; 75(2):110–113.

31. Lanyon LE. Using functional loading to influence bone mass and architecture: objectives, mechanisms, and relationship with estrogen of the mechanically adaptive process in bone. Bone 1996; 18(suppl 1):37S.

32. de Lignieres B. Hormone replacement therapy: clinical benefits and side-effects. Maturitas 1996; 23(suppl):S31.

33. Lindsay R, Cosman F, Herrington BS, et al. Bone mass and body composition in normal women. J Bone Miner Res 1992; 7:55.

34. Lindsay R, Hart DM, Sweeney A, et al. Endogenous oestrogen and bone loss following oophorectomy. Calcif Tissue Res 1977; 22(suppl): 213.

35. Lindsay R. Estrogen deficiency. In: Riggs BL Jr, Melton LJ III, eds. Osteoporosis: etiology, diagnosis, and management. 2nd edn. Philadelphia: Lippincott-Raven; 1995:133–160.

36. Lufkin EG, Whitaker MD, Nickelsen T, et al. Treatment of established postmenopausal osteoporosis with raloxifene: a randomized trial. J Bone Miner Res 1998; 13:1747.

37. Lynn SG, Sinaki M, Westerlind KC. Balance characteristics of persons with osteoporosis. Arch Phys Med Rehabil 1997; 78:273.

38. Matkovic V, Heaney RP. Calcium balance during human growth: evidence for threshold behavior. Am J Clin Nutr 1992; 55:992.

39. McComas AJ, Fawcett PR, Campbell MJ, et al. Electrophysiological estimation of the number of motor units within a human muscle. J Neurol Neurosurg Psychiatry 1971; 34:121.

40. Melton LJ III, Kan SH, Frye MA, et al. Epidemiology of vertebral fractures in women. Am J Epidemiol 1989; 129:1000.

41. Mosley JR, Lanyon LE. Strain rate as a controlling influence on adaptive modeling in response to dynamic loading of the ulna in growing male rats. Bone 1998; 23:313.

42. National Osteoporosis Foundation. Capitol Hill rallies Americans to take a walk! America walks for strong women. Washington: National Osteoporosis Foundation; 5 Aug 1998.

43. Neer RM, Arnaud CD, Zanchetta JR, et al. Effect of parathyroid hormone (1-34) on fractures and bone mineral density in postmenopausal women with osteoporosis. N Engl J Med 2001; 344:1434.

44. Nordin BE, Horsman A, Crilly RG, et al. Treatment of spinal osteoporosis in postmenopausal women. Br Med J 1980; 280:451.

45. Peck WA, Riggs BL, Bell NH, et al. Research directions in osteoporosis. Am J Med 1988; 84:275.

46. Petrie RS, Sinaki M, Squires RW, et al. Physical activity, but not aerobic capacity, correlates with back strength in healthy premenopausal women from 29 to 40 years of age. Mayo Clin Proc 1993; 68:738.

47. Pfeifer M, Sinaki M, Geusens P, et al. Musculoskeletal rehabilitation in osteoporosis: a review. J Bone Miner Res 2004; 19(8):1208–1214.

48. Prelevic GM, Bartram C, Wood J, et al. Comparative effects on bone mineral density of tibolone, transdermal estrogen and oral estrogen/progestogen therapy in postmenopausal women. Gynecol Endocrinol 1996; 10:413.

49. Riggs BL, Melton LJ III, eds. Osteoporosis: etiology, diagnosis, and management. New York: Raven Press; 1988.

50. Riggs BL, Melton LJ III. Involutional osteoporosis. N Engl J Med 1986; 314:1676.

51. Riggs BL, Wahner HW, Melton LJ III, et al. Rates of bone loss in the appendicular and axial skeletons of women. Evidence of substantial vertebral bone loss before menopause. J Clin Invest 1986; 77:1487.

52. Riggs BL. Overview of osteoporosis. West J Med 1991; 154:63.

53. Rodan GA, Rodan SB. The cells of bone. In: Riggs BL Jr, Melton LJ III, eds. Osteoporosis: etiology, diagnosis, and management. 2nd edn. Philadelphia: Lippincott-Raven; 1995:1–39.

54. Sartoris DJ, Clopton P, Nemcek A, et al. Vertebral-body collapse in focal and diffuse disease: patterns of pathologic processes. Radiology 1986; 160:479.

55. van Schoor NM, Smit JH, Twisk JW, et al. Prevention of hip fractures by external hip protectors: a randomized controlled trial. JAMA 2003; 289:1957.

56. Seeman E. The dilemma of osteoporosis in men. Am J Med 1995; 98:76S.

57. Sinaki M, Brey R, Hughes C, et al. Significant reduction of risk of fall in osteoporotic women: a four-week proprioceptive dynamic program [abstract]. J Bone Miner Res 2004; 19(suppl 1):S174.

58. Sinaki M, Brey RH, Hughes CA, et al. Balance disorder and increased risk of falls in osteoporosis and kyphosis: significance of kyphotic posture and muscle strength. Osteoporos Int 2005; 16(8):1004–1010.

59. Sinaki M, Brey R, Hughes C, Larson D, Kaufman K, Sinaki M, Brey RH, Hughes CA, Larson DR, Kaufman KR. Significant reduction in risk of falls and black pain in osteoporotic-kyphotic women through a proprioceptive dynamic program. Mayo Clinic Proc 2005; 80(7):849–855.

60. Sinaki M, Fitzpatrick LA, Ritchie CK, et al. Site-specificity of bone mineral density and muscle strength in women: job-related physical activity. Am J Phys Med Rehabil 1998; 77:470.

61. Sinaki M, Grubbs NC. Back strengthening exercises: quantitative evaluation of their efficacy for women aged 40 to 65 years. Arch Phys Med Rehabil 1989; 70:16.

62. Sinaki M, Itoi E, Rogers JW, et al. Correlation of back extensor strength with thoracic kyphosis and lumbar lordosis in estrogen-deficient women. Am J Phys Med Rehabil 1996; 75:370.

63. Sinaki M, Itoi E, Wahner HW, et al. Stronger back muscles reduce the incidence of vertebral fractures: a prospective 10 year follow-up of postmenopausal women. Bone 2002; 30:836.

64. Sinaki M, Khosla S, Limburg PJ, et al. Muscle strength in osteoporotic versus normal women. Osteoporosis Int 1993; 3:8.

65. Sinaki M, Lynn S. Reducing the risk of falls through proprioceptive dynamic posture training in osteoporotic women with kyphotic posturing: a randomized pilot study. Am J Phys Med Rehabil 2002; 81(4):241–246.

66. Sinaki M, Mikkelsen BA. Postmenopausal spinal osteoporosis: flexion versus extension exercises. Arch Phys Med Rehabil 1984; 65:593.

67. Sinaki M, Mokri B. Low back pain and disorders of the lumbar spine. In: Braddom RL, ed. Physical medicine and rehabilitation. Philadelphia: Saunders; 1996.

68. Sinaki M, Nwaogwugwu NC, Phillips B, et al. Effect of gender, age, and anthropometry on axial and appendicular muscle strength. Am J Phys Med Rehabil 2001; 80:330.

69. Sinaki M, Wahner HW, Bergstralh EJ, et al. Three-year controlled, randomized trial of the effect of dose-specified loading and strengthening exercises on bone mineral density of spine and femur in nonathletic, physically active women. Bone 1996; 19:233.

70. Sinaki M, Wahner HW, Offord KP, et al. Efficacy of nonloading exercises in prevention of vertebral bone loss in postmenopausal women: a controlled trial. Mayo Clin Proc 1989; 64:762.

71. Sinaki M, Wollan PC, Scott RW, et al. Can strong back extensors prevent vertebral fractures in women with osteoporosis? Mayo Clin Proc 1996; 71:951.

72. Sinaki M. Beneficial musculoskeletal effects of physical activity in the older woman. Geriatr Med Today 1989; 8:53.

73. Sinaki M. Critical appraisal of physical rehabilitation measures after osteoporotic vertebral fracture. Osteoporos Int 2003; 14(9):773–779.

74. Sinaki M. Effect of physical activity on bone mass. Curr Opin Rheumatol 1996; 8:376.

75. Sinaki M. Exercise and osteoporosis. Arch Phys Med Rehabil 1989; 70:220.

76. Sinaki M. Exercise and physical therapy. In: Riggs BL Jr, Melton LJ III, eds. Osteoporosis: etiology, diagnosis, and management. New York: Raven Press; 1988:457–479.

77. Sinaki M. Falls, fractures, and hip pads. Curr Osteoporos Rep 2004;2:131–137.

78. Sinaki M. Musculoskeletal challenges of osteoporosis. Aging Clin Exp Res (Milano) 1998; 10:249.

79. Sinaki M. Musculoskeletal rehabilitation. In: Riggs BL Jr, Melton LJ III, eds. Osteoporosis: etiology, diagnosis, and management. 2nd edn. Philadelphia: Lippincott-Raven; 1995:435–473.

80. Sinaki M. Nonpharmacologic interventions: exercise, fall prevention, and role of physical medicine. Clin Geriatr Med 2003; 19:337.

81. Sinaki M. Prevention of hip fracture: physical activity. In: Ringe JD, Meunier JP, eds. Osteoporotic fractures in the elderly: clinical management and prevention. Stuttgart: Georg Thieme Verlag; 1996:99–115.

82. Sinaki M. PTS: Posture Training Support brochure Y32255. Jackson: Camp International; 1993.

83. Sinaki M. Rehabilitation in metabolic bone disease. In: Sinaki M, ed. Basic clinical rehabilitation medicine. 2nd edn. St Louis: Mosby; 1993:209–236.

84. Sinaki M. Rehabilitation of osteoporotic fractures of the spine. In: Physical medicine and rehabilitation: state of the art reviews, vol 9. Philadelphia: Hanley and Belfus; 1995:105–123.

85. Sinaki M. Spectrum and management of musculoskeletal changes in osteoporosis. In: The official program, IX Congresso Nazionale Societa Italiana dell'Osteoporosi e delle Malattie Metaboliche dell'Osso. Parma, Italy, October 1–4, 1997.

86. Sinaki M. The influence of exercise on bone and the rehabilitation of osteoporotic patients. In: Passeri M, ed. The opinion of the orthopedist and physiatrist. Pavia: EDIMES Publishing; 1995.

87. Stevenson JC, Abeyasekera G, Hillyard CJ, et al. Calcitonin and the calcium-regulating hormones in postmenopausal women: effect of oestrogens. Lancet 1981; 1:693.

88. Stevenson JC. Regulation of calcitonin and parathyroid hormone secretion by oestrogens. Maturitas 1982; 4:1.

89. Wahner HW, Dunn WL, Brown ML, et al. Comparison of dual-energy x-ray absorptiometry and dual photon absorptiometry for bone mineral measurements of the lumbar spine. Mayo Clin Proc 1988; 63:1075.

90. Wahner HW. The evaluation of osteoporosis: dual energy x-ray absorptiometry in clinical practice. London: M Dunitz; 1994.

91. World Health Organization Study Group. Assessment of fracture risk and its application to screening for postmenopausal osteoporosis. Technical report series/WHO 843. Geneva: WHO; 1994.

Chapter

43

Management of Chronic Pain

Steven P. Stanos, Mark D. Tyburski and R. Norman Harden

There are among us those who haply please
to think our business is to treat disease.
And all unknowingly lack this lesson still
'tis not the body, but the man is ill.
              S. Weir Mitchell (cited by Schofield 1902)

HISTORICAL OVERVIEW

Pain defined

Pain is a subjective and entirely individually personal experience influenced by learning, context, and multiple psychosocial variables.[189] Pain is not merely the end product of peripheral receptor stimulation and afferent signaling, but a complicated dynamic process of neural interplay with the noxious environment along ascending and descending peripheral, spinal cord, and brain networks. The International Association for the Study of Pain (IASP) defines pain as 'an unpleasant sensory and emotional experience associated with actual or potential tissue damage, or described in terms of such damage'.[193] Pain serves an adaptive function, a warning system designed to protect the organism from harm. With chronicity and/or neuraxial pathology, however, the nociceptive system can become maladaptive and reflect endogenous pathology instead of exogenous state.[256] Acute pain is usually a response to a 'noxious' event (i.e. a mechanical, thermal, or chemical insult) causing depolarization of the non-specialized transducers (the nociceptors). It is time-limited, and treatment should be aimed at removing the underlying pathologic process. Concurrent behaviors will be designed to avoid or remove the offending noxious stimulus. In contrast, chronic pain is designated 3–6 months following the initiating event, and in many cases may not be associated with any obvious ongoing noxious event or pathologic process.[208] Behavior can become pathologic as attempts to avoid the noxious element fail, fight or flight responses escalate to no purpose, etc. Chronic pain can differ from acute pain conditions in that underlying tissue pathology or injury begins to less directly correlate with levels of pain report. Whereas acute pain can be considered a physiologic response to tissue trauma or damage, chronic pain involves a more dynamic interplay of additional psychologic and behavioral mechanisms (Table 43-1).[48] Chronic pain often is associated with disrupted sleep and declining function, and eventually can cease to serve any protective role, becoming a source of dysfunctional behaviors, suffering, and disability,

often completely perplexing to the patient and the unprepared physician.

Environmental and affective factors can contribute to the persistence of pain and subsequent illness behaviors. The individual's subjective response to chronic pain is shaped by the cognitive repertoire involved in attending to and anticipating noxious sensory signals, and in appraising events associated with those signals (Fig. 43-1). Chronic painful conditions, when left untreated, can result in multiple problems, including unnecessary personal suffering for the patient, increased medical care utilization, overuse or misuse of psychoactive medications, iatrogenic complications secondary to inappropriate surgeries, excess disability, comorbid emotional problems (including increased risk of suicide), and increased economic and social costs. A multidisciplinary approach that addresses psychosocial as well as biologic factors and focuses on functional restoration in all areas of life is sine qua non.

The prepared physiatrist can offer a unique perspective and skill set to the assessment and management of chronic pain and the psychosocial sequelae. The rehabilitative interdisciplinary team approach, a model for the treatment of other chronic disability conditions (e.g. spinal cord injury, stroke-related disorders, and amputee-related conditions), is focused on maximizing independent physical function, improving psychosocial state, and returning patients to work and previous leisure pursuits, as well as maximizing patients' reintegration into the community and subsequent improvement of general quality of life. To achieve these ambitious goals, as well as adding the goal of decreasing the pain to tolerable levels, the physiatrist must thoroughly understand and appreciate the biologic, psychologic, and socioeconomic implications of pain and pain-related disability. A list of cogent pain terminology and definitions is included for review (Table 43-2).

This chapter offers the foundation for comprehensive pain management skills; a review of historical aspects that shaped the field of pain management and research; a review of our current understanding of both physiologic and pathophysiologic mechanisms of pain, the impact of psychosocial factors on the experience of pain, and their role in pain assessment and treatment; and a review of multidisciplinary treatment options that pertain to various chronic pain conditions. A multidisciplinary approach will be proposed as unequivocally the best model for successful and comprehensive chronic pain management.

Table 43-1 Basic differentiation of major temporal pain classifications

Character	Acute	Subchronic	Chronic
Duration	Seconds	Hours to days	Months to years
Temporal features	Instantaneous and simultaneous to cause	Resolves on recovery	Persistent, long-term disease; may exceed resolution of tissue damage
Major characteristics	Proportional to cause	Primary and secondary hyperalgesia, allodynia, spontaneous pain	Subchronic characteristics plus paresthesias, dysesthesias, pronounced affective component
Class	Nociceptive	Principally nociceptive; neuropathic	Principally neuropathic; nociceptive
Source of pain	Transient nociceptive activation	Peripheral and central mechanisms	Peripheral and central mechanisms
Adaptive value	High; preventive	Protective: recovery	None: maladaptive
Adaptive response	Withdrawal, escape	Quiescence, avoidance of contact with injured tissue	Cognitive-behavioral, catastrophizing, pain-related anxiety and fear, helplessness
Examples	Contact with hot surface	Inflamed wound	Chronic low back pain, muscle pain syndromes

(After Millan 1999,[194] with permission.)

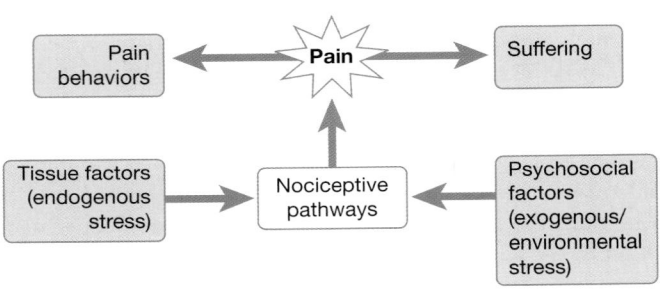

Figure 43-1 Processes of chronic pain. (From Kidd and Urban 2001,[144] with permission.)

Prevalence

Chronic pain and related suffering and disability represent an accelerating public health concern and a fiscal 'black hole' in the US economy. Prevalence rates of chronic pain vary widely, from 2% to 55% in general population studies,[42,69,115,295] and probably realistically represent 30–40%.[5,29] Prosaic diagnoses (i.e. chronic arthritic and musculoskeletal conditions and spine-related disorders) account for a large portion of reported pain and correlate with a high concurrent risk for disability.[44,311] By 2030, physician-diagnosed arthritis and related disability is predicted to affect 71 million Americans.[44] Projected expansion of the elderly population, as well as increased survival rates of the disabled population and individuals with life-shortening or (previously) terminal conditions, will lead to further increases in prevalence.

Reviews of chronic pain as a secondary problem in patients with a primary disability, such as spinal cord injury, amputation, cerebral palsy, and multiple sclerosis, have demonstrated even higher prevalence rates of intolerable pain (>70%), which can substantially add to disability. For instance, a longitudinal study of chronic pain in adult cerebral palsy patients found that pain remained steady over a 2-year period, and that pain was unlikely to decrease spontaneously without treatment.[126] Pain associated with rehabilitation diagnoses is often reported in multiple sites, not just the focal site of the primary injury,[68,292] and can contribute to a more generalized loss of function and related disability.

The cost of chronic pain

The progression from 'acute' to 'chronic' pain inevitably includes a greater impact in related psychologic and social functioning. Chronic pain-related impairment and disability has significant socioeconomic consequences due to high healthcare costs, lost wages and productivity, and the growing costs of disability benefits and other compensation.[286] Conservative estimates of cost related to healthcare expenditure and lost productivity range from $70 to $120 billion annually.[89,211] Chronic pain is responsible for 90 million physician visits, 14% of all prescriptions, and 50 million lost workdays per year.[24,52] One-third of the population suffers from chronic pain-related conditions, at a cost of $100 billion in related compensation, healthcare, and litigation costs.[158] Stewart et al. found that 75% of pain-related productivity loss was on the job, not due to absence from work.[274]

HISTORY

The concept of 'pain' has been part of the human experience closely woven into the cultural fabric of philosophy, politics, and religion since early times, including the documented periods in ancient China, India, and Egypt. In a quest for analgesia and

Table 43-2 Terminology utilized in the discussion of pain

Term	Definition
Addiction	A chronic biopsychosocial disease characterized by impaired control over drug use, compulsive use, continued use despite harm, and craving
Allodynia	Pain due to a stimulus that does not normally provoke pain
Analgesia	Absence of pain in response to stimulation that would normally be painful
Central pain	Pain initiated or caused by a primary lesion or dysfunction in the central nervous system
Dependence	A maladaptive pattern of drug use marked by tolerance and a drug class-specific withdrawal syndrome that can be produced by abrupt cessation, rapid dose reduction, decreasing blood levels of drug, or administration of an antagonist
Dysesthesia	An unpleasant abnormal sensation, whether spontaneous or evoked
Hyperalgesia	An increased response to a stimulus that is normally painful
Hyperesthesia	Increased sensitivity to stimulation, excluding the special senses
Neurogenic pain	Pain initiated or caused by a primary lesion, dysfunction, or transitory perturbation in the peripheral or central nervous system
Neuropathic pain	Pain initiated or caused by a primary lesion or dysfunction in the nervous system[a]
Nociception	A receptor preferentially sensitive to a noxious stimulus or to a stimulus that would become noxious if prolonged
Noxious stimulus	A noxious stimulus is one that is damaging to normal tissues
Pain	An unpleasant sensory and emotional experience associated with actual or potential tissue damage
Paresthesia	An abnormal sensation, whether spontaneous or evoked, that is not unpleasant
Peripheral neurogenic pain	Pain initiated or caused by a primary lesion, dysfunction, or transitory perturbation in the peripheral nervous system
Peripheral neuropathic pain	Pain initiated or caused by a primary lesion or dysfunction in the peripheral nervous system
Psychogenic pain	Pain not due to an identifiable, somatic origin and that may reflect psychologic factors
Tolerance	A state of adaptation in which exposure to a drug induces changes that result in diminution of one or more of the drug's effects over time

[a]See also neurogenic pain and central pain. Peripheral neuropathic pain occurs when the lesion or dysfunction affects the peripheral nervous system. Central pain may be retained as the term when the lesion or dysfunction affects the central nervous system.
(After Merskey and Bogduk 1994,[193] with permission of IASP Press.)

decreased suffering, individuals have tolerated rather barbaric and ineffective treatments, including purging, cupping, blistering, bleeding, leeching, heating, and freezing.[259] In ancient Greece, Hippocrates (460–370 BC) hypothesized that four bodily fluids ('humors') were responsible for the state of one's personality, and with any physical and psychologic illness an imbalance of these humors could lead to pain. Early medical practitioners continued this quest for relief from pain and suffering with the use of various concoctions including the use of mandrake, one of the earliest known medicinal plants, as a means of inducing analgesia and anesthesia. Crude forms of opium have also been used. The 'somniferant' sponge, a sponge saturated with a mixture of opium juices, mandrake root, and other plant extracts, was used for pain relief and in everyday medical treatments, and as a crude anesthetic for the inevitable and almost always painful surgical procedures.[23]

The history of our understanding of pain physiology and treatments evolved in parallel (to some extent) with general advancements in the field of medicine. During the European Dark Ages (400–1300 AD), a time of little progress in any field of science, Middle Eastern medicine and the treatment of pain flourished. For instance, the writings of Turkish surgeon Subancuoglu eloquently described procedures involving 'cauterization' for the treatment of migraine headaches, dental pain, low back pain, and 'sciatica'.[97]

The seventeenth century Renaissance offered a more biomedical reductionism approach, separating mind from body, spearheaded by advancements in modern science (anatomy, physiology, and physics). Physicians slowly began to break away from the Galvanic tradition of bodily humors. Still, by the eighteenth century, pain management was primarily relegated to the practice of quackery. Charlatans used various concoctions and tonics, with many including opium. Opium continued to be used widely for a number of pain and non-pain-related ailments, including diarrhea and dysentery. Animal studies led to significant advancement in the understanding of neurophysiology, including work by Charles Bell describing sensory responses of posterior spinal nerves, and motor responses associated with anterior spinal nerves.

The nineteenth and twentieth centuries included important advances in pharmacologic treatment for pain. Before this, crude forms of analgesia included the use of laudanum, a mixture of opium, alcohol, and other ingredients given with whiskey or other types of alcohol, for analgesia and also prior to surgical procedures. Serturner isolated morphine from opium in 1806, leading to advancement in isolation techniques and the subsequent production of morphine (in the 1820s), codeine (in 1832), and synthetic opioids such as methadone and fentanyl (in the 1940s). The chemist Felix Hoffman developed acetylsalicylic acid (aspirin) from extracts of willow tree bark, as the first reliable analgesic for the relief of moderate pain.[54] Alexander Wood's development of the syringe made parenteral administration practical and convenient, but also led to increased abuse and misuse of the opioids. Diacetylated morphine (heroin) was later introduced by the Bayer Company in 1898 as a cough suppressant.[117] Abusers soon learned that the compound could be crushed into a powder and snorted, injected, or smoked with significant euphoric effects. The Harrison Narcotic Control Act was passed in 1914, limiting the use of morphine and other opiates to the care of a physician. Controversies related to the use of opioid medications for ongoing treatment of chronic non-malignant and cancer-related pain has been a primary focus of federal regulatory and legislative scrutiny. Fear of iatrogenic addiction in the use of chronic opioid management, and variability between federal, state, and community-based laws, has led to ongoing physician fears for aggressive management of pain-related conditions. It remains an important evolving contemporary issue related to the treatment of chronic pain.

Many of the advancements in anesthesiology pain management developed from experiences in treating injured soldiers. Twentieth century surgical advancements included the works of Rene Leriche and his experience with treating wounded World War I soldiers. He eloquently described chronic pain states including phantom limb pain. His work also included descriptions of 'sympathetic pain' arising from smooth muscle in peripheral blood vessels. Leriche championed surgical procedures directed at relieving sympathetic-mediated pain, with aggressive surgical procedures involving sympathetic ganglia and surgical 'periarterial' sympathectomies. Another surgeon, William K. Beecher, helped to put forward the importance of psychologic factors in the experience of pain. As a young army physician in World War II, he observed significantly less pain reported and fewer requests for pain medication by soldiers severely wounded in battle, as compared with civilian patients in his practice with similar injuries.[20] He went on to describe the 'power of placebo', underscoring the importance of meaning and distraction as important factors in the experience of pain.

The success of the gate control theory in the 1960s helped initiate pain management as a formal field of study. John Bonica formalized the idea of pain management as a multidisciplinary collaboration in the late 1940s. In 1974, Bonica organized a scientific meeting of leaders in the field of pain medicine, which established the IASP. The publication of the IASP's journal, *Pain*, occurred 1 year later. The IASP created the first Taxonomy of Pain in 1979, and continues to publish clinical updates and guidelines regarding a number of pain-related conditions (i.e. headache, cancer pain, chronic non-malignant pain, and complex regional pain syndrome). It also cultivates research related to further understanding of pain mechanisms, and treatment developments. A number of agencies and professional societies remain active in the field of pain science and treatment, including the American Pain Society, American Academy of Pain Medicine, and multispecialty spine intervention-based societies such as the North American Spine Society and International Spinal Injection Society. In the past two decades, there has been an explosive growth of modern neuroscience that has led to advancement in understanding pain mechanisms and treatment. This is due in part to the financial impetus from the analgesic area, and the development of new tools such as functional imaging studies (positron emission tomography and functional magnetic resonance imaging), which have helped to demonstrate evidence of complex cortical networks related to pain perception.[224,227]

Recently, the number of physiatrists becoming interested in pain medicine as a subspecialty has exponentially increased, with many pursuing formal fellowship training. Subspecialty certification in pain medicine is now offered by the American Board of Physical Medicine and Rehabilitation in cooperation with the American Board of Psychiatry and Neurology and the American Board of Anesthesiology. With the growing availability of pain fellowships and the increasing number of physiatrists specializing solely in pain medicine, advanced interventional pain management procedures (including fluoroscopically guided spinal interventions and placement of implantable pain devices) are increasingly being performed by physiatrists as part of a comprehensive treatment plan for chronic pain disorders.

Early history of pain theory: a peripheral perspective

The development of pain medicine as a more formal science has been closely related to advancements in pain theory. Understanding historical factors related to the works of scientists and physicians can help the clinician better understand the complexities of the multidimensional experience of pain and suffering. Below is an overview of key factors related to pain theory, beginning with specificity theory up through and including contemporary theories.

The dualistic or mind–body controversy started with Rene Descartes' (1596–1650) biomedical theories, and can be seen as a precursor to specificity theory. He likened the pain system to a bell-ringing mechanism. The individual on the ground pulls the rope, ringing the bell in the tower. Similarly, placing the foot next to a burning flame would set particles in the foot in motion, traveling up the leg, back, and to the head, causing activation of pain. This theory, traditionally ascribed to Descartes, actually has earlier antecedents of Galen, based on the central position of the pineal gland, the center of the soul, and the sensory motor system.[191]

The specificity theory remained somewhat unchallenged until the nineteenth century, with the emergence of physiology as a more formal scientific field of study. Magendie (1783–1855) and his student, Claude Bernard (1813–1878), revolutionized the field of physiology by codifying the principles of observation, data recording, and analysis (considered heretic at the time!). Bernard was the first to publish observations about the relationship of the autonomic nervous system to pain, and one of his students, the American Civil War surgeon Silas Weir Mitchell, would go on to elucidate what he called 'causalgia' (now complex regional pain syndrome type 2). The qualities of pain experience were thought to be associated with properties of sensory nerves. Johannes Müller was the first to elaborate on more specific neural pathways for pain in his theory of 'specific nerve energies' (1842). Müller's concept included the distinction of four major cutaneous modalities (i.e. touch, warmth, cold, and pain), each with its own projection system to the brain.[191]

Max von Frey expanded Müller's idea of specific nerve energies to include a theory based on specific receptors. Von Frey proposed the presence of cutaneous sensitivity maps on the skin 'mapped out' by anatomists of the day with a brand new experimental device, the microscope. First, a spotlike distribution of warmth and cold cutaneous sensitivity was mapped out with two devices: a pin on a string, to gauge pressure thresholds for pain, and snippets of horsetail hairs attached to a piece of wood, to map out distributions of 'touch spots'. More formal standardized versions of these instruments continue to be used in contemporary sensory testing (i.e. von Frey filaments and von Frey hairs, respectively). Second, von Frey included his theory, later disproved, that there were specific pain receptors (free nerve endings) that varied in their distribution on the body to complement other specialized receptors identified around the same time (Meissner corpuscles, touch; Krause end bulbs, cold; and Ruffini end organs, warmth). Sherrington later postulated the existence of specialized cells or 'nociceptors', which could detect noxious sensations in terms of the lowest 'lumen' or threshold.[260]

An alternative to these specificity theories, the intensive (summation) theory, was formulated by Erb in 1874. Intensive theory proposed that each sensory transducer was capable of producing pain only if the stimulus reached a sufficient intensity.[27] Later, Goldscheider (1894) refined the stimulus intensity and summation theories and proposed the pattern theory. In pattern theory, pain results after total output at the cellular level reaches a critical level, either by stimulation by non-noxious stimuli or by pathologic conditions that enhance summation. The theory centered on the contention that all nerve fibers are alike, and that pain is produced by spatiotemporal patterns of neuronal impulses versus activity on 'specific' nerve fibers.

Central theories of pain

Until the late 1800s, pain theory was based primarily on peripheral mechanisms, and failed to explain persistent pain states.

William Livingston's work with injured soldiers in World War II, and later in chronic work-related injuries, suggested that some portion of chronic pain mechanisms might be related to more specific central nervous system dysfunction.[157] Livingston's summation theory stated that pathologic stimulation of sensory nerves after nerve injury could lead to reverberating circuits in neuron pools of the spinal cord, which could later be triggered by peripheral non-noxious inputs. This volley of nerve impulses could lead to a 'vicious cycle' between central and peripheral processes.[151]

Although debate continued among three basic pain theories, specificity ultimately prevailed and was universally accepted and practiced. An appreciation for cognitive and psychologic aspects of pain processing, although secondary, slowly emerged within the fourth theory of pain, proposed by Hardy, Wolff, and Goodell. Pain was separated into two components: the perception of pain (afferent) and the reaction to pain (efferent). Pain perception was thought as a more hardwired physiologic process, whereas reaction to pain was under the influence of complex psychologic and physiologic processes influenced by past experiences, the environment, and emotional state.[113]

The Dutch surgeon Willem Noordenbos suggested that pain transmission was not a one to one synaptic transmission system, but involved a multisynaptic modification process with complex interactions (such as convergence) between synapses. The sensory interaction theory of Noordenbos (1959) proposed two systems involving transmission of pain and other sensory information: a slow system (unmyelinated and thinly myelinated fibers) and a fast-acting system (large myelinated fibers). Large fibers could inhibit transmission of impulses from small fibers. This set the stage for Melzack and Wall's seminal work on the gate control theory of pain modulation in 1965 (discussed in more detail below). Although controversial then and now, it brought an emphasis to a more convergent view of central pain processing at the spinal cord and cerebral levels.

Melzack and Wall's gate control theory championed a more convergent view of pain processing. The spinal cord is not just a passive conduit for pain transmission, but an active modulator of pain signals. Activity in large myelinated afferent fibers theoretically activates dorsal horn encephalogenic interneurons that inhibit cephalad transmission in small unmyelinated primary afferent nociceptive fibers and the secondary transmission cells in the lateral spinothalamic tracts.[190] Somatic afferents activate convergent wide dynamic range cells deep in the dorsal horn (lamina V), which project in the spinothalamic tract to higher somatosensory processing in the thalamus and cortex. In theory, inhibiting pain by rubbing the skin activates large-diameter afferents inhibiting small-diameter fiber activation of wide dynamic range cells, 'closing' the 'gate'.

Additional work by Melzack and Casey 3 years later emphasized motivational, affective, and cognitive aspects of the pain experience. Neural pathways could activate both sensory discriminative information about the location and intensity of pain, and more emotional and motivational effects of pain experience. Descending inhibition from cortical structures could also influence pain. Descending modulation of the gate theoretically could block nociceptive signals at the dorsal horn and provide the basis for behavioral-induced reduction of pain. In turn, psychologic processes such as depression could potentially increase pain by 'opening' gating mechanisms at the dorsal horn. This modulation, carried down to the dorsal horn in the dorsolateral funiculus, and ramifying throughout the entire neuraxis, provides a way for the central nervous system to actively modulate the afferent input at multiple levels of the central nervous system. This impacts all aspects of the pain experience, including affective, subjective, and evaluative components. The gate control theory offered a new model for the successful integration of experimental and clinical observations related to the study of pain. The gate control theory, although challenged as somewhat incomplete, has remained the core of contemporary pain science. It has spurred the development of new clinical treatments, including neurophysiologically based procedures (transcutaneous electrical nerve stimulation, spinal cord stimulation), pharmacologic, cognitive, and behavioral treatments.

Melzack has extended his work with the gate control theory to include the more central 'neuromatrix' theory based on concepts from cognitive neuroscience network theory.[242] Dimensions of the pain experience are considered as output of the neuromatrix, which proposes a 'neurosignature' of pain experience that is unique to each individual and is influenced by sensory, psychosocial, and genetic factors. This pattern is modulated by various sensory inputs from the environment, and by cognitive events such as psychologic stress. In turn, these multiple parallel processing inputs contribute to the sensory, affective, and cognitive dimensions of the pain experience and subsequent behavior.

Recent advances in neuroimaging and the exploding field of neuroscience networking have offered greater insight into higher level cerebral plasticity related to acute and chronic pain. Apkarian et al. studied brain morphologic changes with the use of high-resolution magnetic resonance imaging in a group of patients with chronic low back pain.[6] Significant evidence of discrete central nervous system degeneration (gray matter atrophy) in the chronic pain patient group was demonstrated. Discrete thalamic and prefrontal cortex atrophy was reported at a rate approximately 5–10 times greater that of normal age-related atrophy. This underscores the importance of appropriate and aggressive treatment of pain as a means of preventing possible long-term or permanent central nervous system changes. In addition, these findings add to the ongoing developments in neural plasticity of pain, as these changes are not plastic but are perhaps permanent (Fig. 43-2). The use of positron emission tomography and functional magnetic resonance imaging has offered accelerating insight into the main cerebral components of human nociceptive processing and networking at the brain and spinal cord levels.[131]

History of contemporary advancements in psychologic aspects of pain

The twentieth century also provided significant growth in the fields of psychiatry and psychosomatic medicine. Sigmund Freud emphasized the potential link between psychologic and

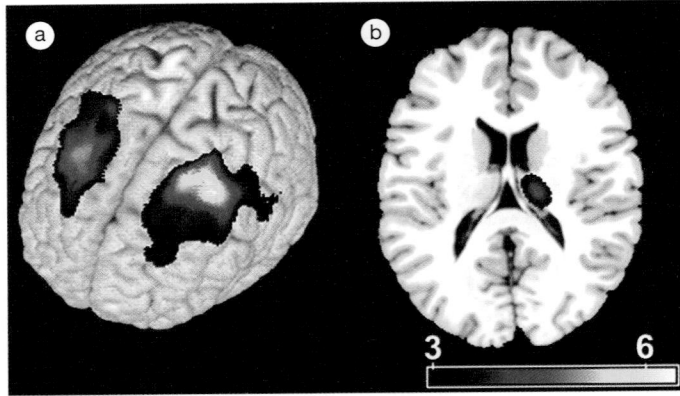

Figure 43-2 Regional gray matter density decreases in subjects with chronic low back pain. (From Apkarian et al. 2004,[6] with permission.)

physical factors in a number of medical conditions. Later, disenchantment with Freud's psychoanalytic principles led to the development of the field of psychosomatic medicine, and the subsequent rapid development of the fields of health psychology and behavioral medicine in the 1970s.[100] Physicians such as George Engel (1959) challenged the biomedical model of disease as inadequate, in that it failed to include the social, psychologic, and behavioral dimensions of illness. Engel's classic article *'Psychogenic' pain and the pain-prone patient* discussed various contextual meanings of persistent pain and the importance of an individual's interpretation of his or her pain. Sternbach argued that physiologic and affective perceptions of pain should be understood as learned responses under the control of environmental forces, and addressed psychophysiologic pain syndromes including 'stress-induced pain disorders'.[273] Wilbert Fordyce later proposed an operant conditioning model of chronic pain, based on an ends approach of identifying and treating pain behaviors. More contemporaneously, higher cognitive functioning in pain states (such as memory and emotive components) were embraced in the cognitive behavioral approach, led by health psychologists such as Dennis Turk and Frances Keefe, emphasizing the role of attributions, efficacy, personal control, and problem solving. Thoughts and beliefs could influence, and be influenced by, emotional and physiologic responses.[290] This has contributed to the evolution of a more clinically pragmatic school of pain assessment and treatment, the biopsychosocial model. This model incorporates the physical, cognitive, affective, and behavioral components related to ongoing pain experience. In this context, biologic factors can initiate a physical disturbance, but psychosocial factors often influence pain perception, pain behavior, and the ongoing pain experience.[81,289]

PHYSIOLOGY AND PATHOPHYSIOLOGY OF PAIN

In a normal homeostatic state, cutaneous, visceral, and musculoskeletal pain serve as an alarm system to the body

Table 43-3 Signal processing

Stage	Description
Transduction (receptor activation)	One form of energy (thermal, mechanical, or chemical stimulus) is converted electrochemically into nerve impulses (action potentials) in primary afferents
Transmission	Coded information is transferred from primary afferent fibers to spinal cord dorsal horn and on to brain stem, thalamus, and higher cortical structures
Modulation	Involves activity- and signal-induced dorsal horn neural plasticity, which includes altered receptor and channel function (i.e. wind-up and central sensitization), gene expression,[312] and changes in brain-mediated descending inhibition and facilitation
Perception	Begins with activation of sensory cortex. The cortex is in intimate communication with motor and prefrontal cortices, which initiate efferent responses as well as more primitive structures involved in the emotive aspects of pain

that indicates damage or potential damage in the environment. The purpose of nociception is to alert the organism to this potential damage so that avoidance behavior can be initiated. In contrast, chronic pain states may represent an alteration involving damage or injury to the central nervous system that serves no real protective role, reflecting a 'pathologic' as opposed to 'physiologic' state. The complex interaction between the initial stimulus of tissue injury and the subjective experience of nociception and acute and/or chronic pain can be described by four general processes known as transduction, transmission, modulation, and perception (Table 43-3).

Normal pain, or *nociception*, is characterized primarily by the processes of transduction and transmission, with minimal emphasis on modulation and a 'normal' perception process. With chronic or persistent pain states, there is a shift of focus to the processes of modulation and perception. These four general processes are reviewed below, and serve as an important foundation for a more clear understanding of complex pain mechanisms and possible rational pharmacotherapeutic, interventional, and cognitive behavioral treatment approaches.

Transduction

The principle receptor for pain is the branched endings of C and Aδ fibers (Table 43-4) in the skin, muscles, and joints. Damaging (or potentially damaging) energy in the cellular environment impacts the free nerve endings, and the complicated cellular processes of nociceptive transduction occur. Inflammatory cascades are concurrently activated (prostaglandin, leuko-

triene, etc.) and immediately become principle players in the transduction process. Recent histochemical studies have revealed two broad categories of C fibers: peptidergic and isolectin B4-binding. Peptidergic fibers contain a variety of peptide neurotransmitters, including substance P and calcitonin gene-related peptide (CGRP), and expresses tyrosine receptor kinase A receptors, which show high affinity for nerve growth factors. Peptidergic neurons appear to be key players in neurogenic inflammation (where the transduction cells themselves become active participants in the local inflammatory process) and other chronic inflammatory states.[38,60,313] The other class, isolectin B4-binding, contains few neuropeptides but expresses a surface carbohydrate group selectivity binding to the plant lectin isolectin B4, and is supported by glial-derived neurotropic factor.[277] Isolectin B4 expresses P2X3 receptors, a subtype of ATP-gated ion channels.[136] Differences in supporting tropic factors might be responsible for differing functional responses to painful stimuli between these distinct C-fiber types. Neurotropins have emerged as potential factors for activity-dependent changes at the synapse and possibly subsequent central nervous system plasticity.[161]

There are probably multiple arachidonic acid residue receptors involved (prostaglandin, leukotriene, etc.), and the 'chaos' level of complexity is further complicated by the very active presence of the support cells (glia and myelin) and the efferent input by the central nervous system itself, primarily via the sympathetic nervous system. There are noradrenergic receptors on the transduction cell, and these can be 'uncovered' or activated in inflamed tissue.

Aδ nociceptors (also responders to noxious, thermal, and chemical stimuli) are most easily classified on functional grounds. Type 2 exhibit short response latencies to heat and are activated at relatively higher thresholds (43°C). Type 2 Aδ are responsible for the initial sensation of a burn stimulus. Type 1 Aδ exhibit longer response latencies and are activated at much higher temperatures (>50°C). Type 1 Aδ and nociceptive C fibers are more commonly associated with persistent painful sensations.[43]

Transmission

Cutaneous peripheral afferent neurons can be classified into three types based on diameter, structure, and conduction velocity of action potentials. In general, C fibers (thin, unmyelinated, slowly conducting; $0.5-2.0$ m s^{-1}) and Aδ fibers (medium, thinly myelinated, rapidly conducting; $12-30$ m s^{-1}) carry noxious stimuli, and Aβ fibers (large, myelinated, and fast; $30-100$ m s^{-1}) carry innocuous stimuli (touch, vibration, and pressure), except in situations of peripheral or central sensitization (Table 43-4). The percentage of distribution of nociceptors in the skin is roughly proportioned 70%, 10%, and 20%, respectively. With peripheral and central neuroplastic changes in Aβ fibers, innocuous stimuli might be perceived as painful, resulting in allodynia. Aδ nociceptors respond to intense mechanical and temperature stimuli, and with sensitization contribute to the process called hyperpathia, in which noxious stimuli become frankly more painful and the pain perception may last longer,

Table 43-4 Nerve fiber classification

Sensory and motor fibers	Sensory fibers	Diameter (μm)	Myelinated	Velocity (m/s)	Motor function	Sensory function
Aα	1a 1b	10–20 10–20	Yes Yes	0–120 50–120	Alpha motor neurons —	Muscle spindle afferents Golgi tendon organs, touch, pressure
Aβ	2	4–12	Yes	25–100	Motor neurons to intrafusal and extrafusal muscle fibers	Secondary muscle spindle afferents, touch, pressure, vibration
Aγ		2–8	Yes	10–50	Motor neurons to intrafusal muscle fibers	—
Aδ (types 1 and 2)	3	1–5	Lightly	3–30	—	Touch, pain, and temperature
B		1–3	No	3–15	Preganglionic autonomic fibers	—
C	4	<1	No	0.5–2	Postganglionic autonomic fibers	Pain and temperature

even after the initial stimulus is removed. Most C fibers are polymodal transducers. Aβ fibers demonstrate encapsulated nerve endings involved in non-nociceptive function. Aδ fibers mediate the fast, prickling quality of pain, whereas C fibers mediate the slow, burning quality of pain. An additional class of nociceptors, the so-called silent or sleeping nociceptors, make up approximately 10–20% of C fibers in the skin, joints, and viscera, and are normally unresponsive to acute noxious stimuli. With inflammation and tissue injury, these 'silent' nociceptors are sensitized via activation of second-messenger systems and the release of a number of local chemical mediators (i.e. bradykinin, prostaglandins, serotonin, and histamine), and may contribute to temporal and spatial summation, increasing afferent input at the dorsal horn.[46,101,253]

Peripheral sensitization

C fibers and Aδ receptors undergo changes in response to tissue injury such as inflammation, ischemia, and compression. These changes are marked at the peripheral terminals by the release of chemical mediators from damaged and inflammatory cells. The so-called inflammatory soup, rich in algesic substances, causes a lowering of threshold for activation and subsequent evoked pain. Algogenic substances also activate second-messenger systems, which induce gene expression in the cell. Excitatory amino acids and neuropeptides (substance P, CGRP, and neurokinins) are released by peripheral and central nociceptive C fibers, inducing neurogenic inflammation. Neurogenic inflammation involves retrograde release of algogenic substances, which in turn excites other nearby nociceptors, creating local feed forward loops of sensitization and activation.

Modulation

Primary afferents subserving distinct input from cutaneous, muscle, and visceral tissues converge at the dorsal horn. Several

ascending pathways are involved in transferring and modulating this nociceptive input. At the cellular level, the influx of sodium is fundamental to electrical signaling and subsequent generation of action potentials and excitatory postsynaptic potentials. This is followed by calcium channel opening, contributing to more prolonged depolarization, as well as second-messenger molecular changes involved in more permanent neuroplastic central nervous system changes. At the synaptic terminal of the axon, action potentials lead to the release of neurotransmitters. Neurotransmitter release is dependent on specific ion channels, which are either ligand-gated, opening in response to binding of ligands to receptors, or voltage-gated, opening in response to changes in membrane potentials.[246] Other targeted receptor and ion channels include vanilloid (capsaicin) receptor, heat-activated, ATP-gated purinergic receptor (P2X), proton-gated or acid-sensing ion channels, and voltage-gated sodium channels. The vanilloid receptor is a non-selective cation channel (vanilloid receptor 1) activated by elevated temperature (>43°C) and acidification.

Aδ and C fibers convey nociceptive information primarily to superficial laminae (I and II) and deep laminae (V and VI) of the dorsal horn. Lamina I plays an important role in relaying information on the current state of tissues, including damaging mechanical stress, heat and cold, local metabolism (acid pH, hypoxia), cell breakdown (ATP, glutamate), mast cell activation (serotonin, bradykinin), and immune activity (cytokines).[55] Aβ fibers transmit innocuous, mechanical stimuli to deeper laminae (III–VI). Lamina I cells are activated by nociceptive-specific neurons, whereas lamina V cells respond to wide dynamic range neurons of 'wide' stimulus intensities. Wide dynamic range neurons receive input from mechanoreceptive Aβ fibers and nociceptive (Aδ and C) fibers (Fig. 43-3). Normal synaptic transmission conduction of action potentials at the dorsal horn

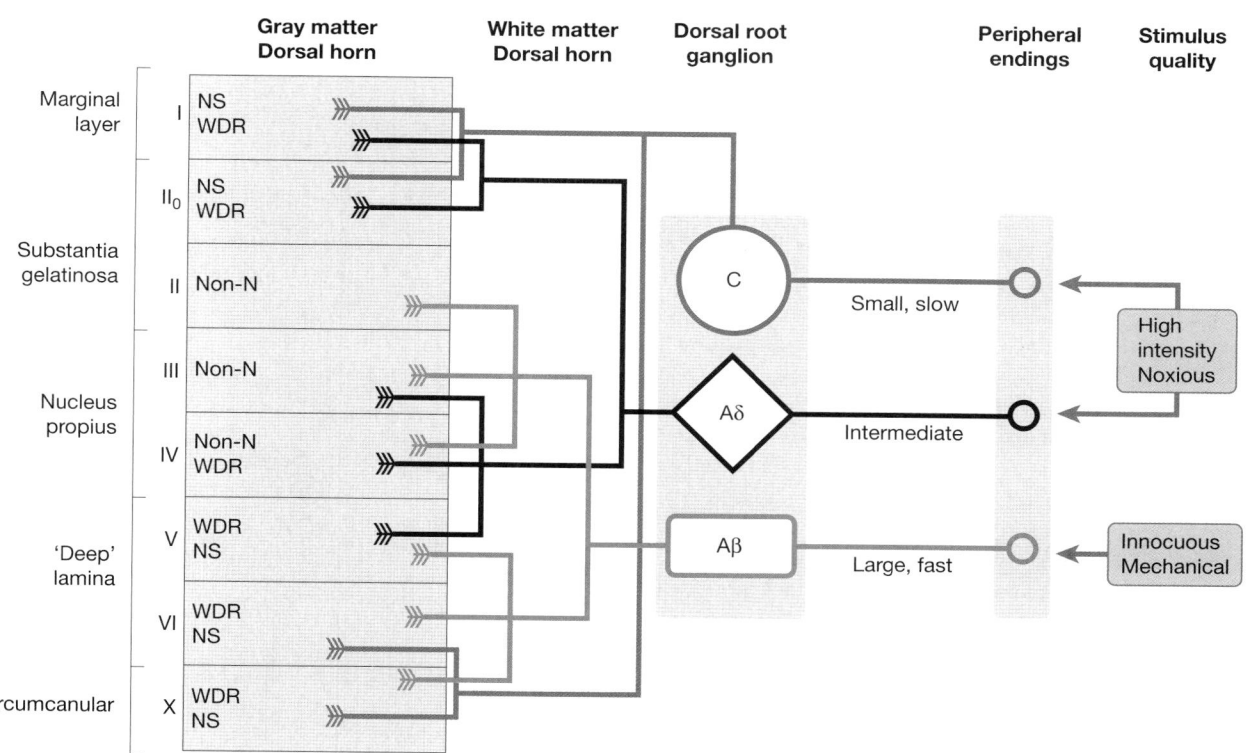

Figure 43-3 Organization of cutaneous, primary afferent input to the dorsal horn of the spinal cord. (From Millan 1999,[194] with permission.)

initiates neurotransmitter release. Low-intensity stimulations (i.e. brush, touch, or vibration) activate Aβ fibers only, releasing fast, glutamate-mediated postsynaptic currents. Fast excitatory transmission glutamate is coreleased presynaptically with neuropeptides such as substance P, CGRP, cholecystokinin, proteins (brain-derived neurotropic factor), and glial-derived factors.[170] Glutamate acts on a range of transmission cell receptors, such as NMDA (slow current), AMPA (fast current), metabotropic glutamate receptors, and kainate ligand-gated ion channels. With normal transmission, sodium flows only through the AMPA receptor, while the NMDA receptor is blocked by magnesium. Prolonged depolarization of the postsynaptic cell causes voltage-dependent magnesium removal, opening the channel and allowing additional sodium and calcium to enter the cell. This amplified evoked response to subsequent input describes the process of 'wind-up'.[170]

Central sensitization

The term *central sensitization* describes a complex set of activation-dependent posttranslational changes occurring at the dorsal horn, brain stem, and higher cerebral sites. For instance, at the dorsal horn, nociceptors release neurotransmitters (glutamate, substance P, and brain-derived neurotropic factor) on to the transmission cells, which results in changes in activation of related receptors and channels (as described above). This results in an increase in calcium influx (and efflux from cytoplasmic organelles), contributing to potentiation of the cell by activation of calcium-dependent enzyme protein kinases (protein kinase

C, cyclic AMP, and tyrosine receptor kinase).[166] Posttranslational changes also include phosphorylation of NMDA and AMPA receptors, activation of second messengers such as nitric oxide, and central prostaglandin production.[312]

Ascending and descending modulation

Melzack and Casey's classic descriptions of neuroanatomic pathways make a distinction between the lateral and medial pain systems corresponding to their relationship with the thalamus.[189] The two systems are highly interdependent, the lateral (neospinothalamic) system generally representing sensory-discriminative dimensions, versus the medial (paleospinothalamic) system involving more motivational-affective and cognitive-evaluative dimensions of the pain experience. Additional ascending pathways, including the spinothalamic, spinomesencephalic, spinoreticular, spinolimbic, spinocervical, and dorsal column pathways, are described elsewhere.[308]

The lateral system projects to the ventral posterolateral and ventral posteromedial thalamic nuclei prior to projecting to the somatosensory and premotor cortices. The motor input is nearly as large as the sensory input, and this theoretically prepares the recipient of the painful input for the appropriate efferent (behavioral) response. The more medial pathway projects to the medial thalamic nuclei and limbic cortices, which include the anterior cingulated cortex, orbitofrontal cortex, and amygdala. The medial system involves important connections with periaqueductal gray, a key area involved in modulating nociceptive inhibition and behavioral responses to potentially threatening stimuli.[208] Animal and human studies have identified the anterior cingulated cortex in regulating avoidance behaviors and the perception of pain unpleasantness.[148] Only a small portion of these action potentials normally reach the thalamus and higher brain centers, due to significant modulating or filtering effects at the spinal cord and brain stem. Of course, with prolonged pathology and inflammation these filters 'break down', contributing to central sensitization.

In addition to descending inhibition, the endogenous inhibitory system also includes local endogenous opioids (from periaqueductal gray), biogenic amines (serotonin and noradrenaline [norepinephrine]), and GABA, which generally act to inhibit pain signals. Important excitatory transmitters in this system include glutamate and substance P.[144,315] Besides descending inhibition from cortical areas, recent studies have suggested that descending facilitatory pathways may link brain stem and spinal cord areas via pronociceptive serotonergic[281] and opioid mechanisms.[74] These pronociceptive pathways may help explain the possible mechanism of persistent pain signs and symptoms, such as allodynia and hyperalgesia, that are common to chronic pain conditions.[223]

Pathways originating from the spinal cord dorsal horn activate brain structures involved in rudimentary aspects of the autonomic system response (i.e. escape, arousal, and fear), including the medulla and midbrain reticular formation, amygdala, hypothalamus, and thalamic nuclei.[227] Activation of somatosensory cortices (S1–S2) provides information regarding the quality and intensity of pain.[118] Affective aspects of the pain experience, such as pain unpleasantness, reflect more of the aversive qualities of the pain experience, such as the 'suffering' component. Higher processing involves parietal and insular regions, contributing to an overall sense of intrusion and unpleasantness.[231] Finally, convergence of these pathways with more frontal regions, such as the anterior cingulate cortex, is responsible for attention and 'emotional valence' of the overall pain experience.

Although cutaneous and visceral pain share common cortical and subcortical networks, differences in response pattern, frequency, and processing might underlie differences in quality, affect, and resultant behavioral responses.[276] Visceral pain has a more indistinct quality, poor localization, and in general is associated with autonomic markers such as bradycardia and hypotension. Cutaneous nociceptive reactions more classically involve protective reflexes such as tachycardia and hypertension.

PSYCHOLOGIC ISSUES RELATED TO CHRONIC PAIN

The physiatric approach to chronic pain conditions must include an understanding of the wide array of important psychologic (affective and cognitive) factors that impact the multidimensional experience of pain. Psychologic factors can serve to decrease or increase the subjective perception of pain and adjustment to ongoing pain-related disability. Affective factors

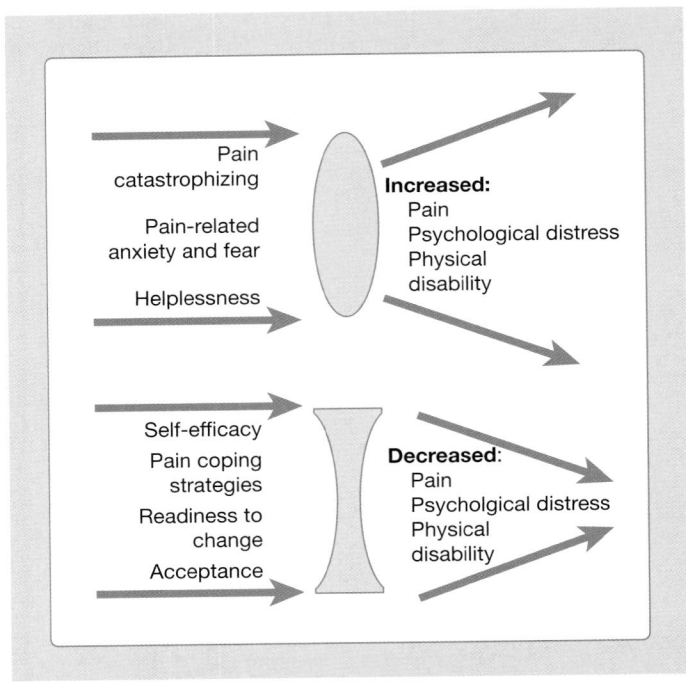

Figure 43-4 Factors associated with adjustment to pain. (From Keefe et al. 2004,[140] with permission.)

usually include more negative emotions, such as depression, pain-related anxiety, and anger. Cognitive factors include catastrophizing, fear, helplessness, decreased self-efficacy, pain coping, readiness to change, and acceptance (Fig. 43-4).

Affective factors
Depression
A strong association between chronic pain and depression has been suggested.[96,237,278] The prevalence estimates of major depression in patients with chronic pain conditions vary from 5% to 87%, and this variation may be due to a number of analytic factors, including the diagnostic criteria used, type of pain studied, and selection bias.[9,78,93] Somatic symptoms of major depressive disorder can also be common in patients with chronic pain (i.e. change in appetite, change in weight, loss of energy, and sleep disturbance). The incidence of depression among chronic pain patients can be higher than with other chronic medical conditions.[14] The presence of chronic pain may be related to longer durations of depressive symptoms.[70,209] In general, most systematic reviews on the relationship between pain and depression suggest that chronic pain precedes depression.[77] Predictors of depression in chronic pain include pain intensity, number of painful areas reported, frequency the severe pain is experienced, and a number of related psychosocial factors. Depressed patients can report higher levels of pain, be less active, report greater disability and life interference related to pain, and are more likely to display overt pain behaviors.[141,149] Brown et al. examined the mediating factors of the relationship between chronic pain in patients with rheumatoid arthritis and decreased cognitive functioning, which included

measures of inductive reasoning and working memory. Elevated depression mediated the relationship between higher levels of pain and reduced cognitive functioning,[31] underscoring the importance of the complex relationship between depression, chronic pain, and functional impairment.

Anxiety

Anxiety related to pain is an important factor involved in maladaptive responses, behavioral interference, and affective distress. Heightened pain-related anxiety has been described as one of the most disabling aspects of ongoing chronic pain. It is closely related to avoidance activities (discussed below), which serve to promote ongoing pain, physical deconditioning, and social isolation.[111] Anxiety as a psychologic construct in chronic pain has been developed by McCracken and colleagues as *pain-related anxiety*. Pain-related anxiety encompasses fear reactions across the cognitive, behavioral, and physiologic dimensions of pain. In chronic pain, it has been found to be a significant predictor of pain severity, disability, and pain behaviors.[179]

Anger

Ongoing failure to achieve pain relief and repeated unsuccessful attempts to escape pain have been shown to be associated with increased levels of anger and physiologic responses to pain, independent of pain intensity.[3,125] In a study of patients presenting for chronic pain management, Okifuji et al. reported 70% of participants with angry feelings, most commonly with themselves (74%) and healthcare professionals (62%). In this study, anger toward oneself was associated with pain and depression, whereas 'only anger' was related to perceived disability.[210]

Conceptualizations of anger in chronic pain vary. A more classic definition of anger has been described as a 'feeling involving a belief that a person one cares for has, intentionally or through neglect, been treated without respect, and a want to have that respect reestablished'.[264] Anger as a construct has also been considered to be related to personality dispositions associated with unconscious conflicts,[88] or as a reaction to the presence of ongoing unrelieved pain.[73] Others have suggested that chronic pain might develop as a conversion-like symptom in order to 'suppress' feelings of anger, and suppressed anger could be related negatively to adjustment to ongoing chronic pain.[142] In contrast, 'anger out' has also been linked to poor adjustment.[34] These styles of anger management—suppression (anger in) and expression (anger out)—are distinguished from overt hostility. *Hostility* has been defined as 'an attitude of cynical mistrustfulness, resentment, and interpersonal antagonism'.[267] Burns has demonstrated how anger management style and hostility can affect maintenance and exacerbation of chronic low back pain via symptom-specific physiologic responses (i.e. increased muscle stress reactivity in lumbar paraspinals in patients with low back pain).[34] This work was based on the studies of Flor and colleagues, which showed that patients with chronic low back pain exhibited greater stress-induced increases in electromyogram readings in lower paraspinal muscles as compared with normal subjects.[80,82] Anger and related physiologic responses are additional targets for pharmacologic and behavioral treatments, including relaxation training and other mind–body treatments.

Cognitive factors

Many patients with chronic pain demonstrate a reduction in goal-directed activities and assume a more passive sedentary lifestyle. This further contributes to a downward spiral of inactivity, deconditioning, and increased somatic focus. Individual responses to pain are recognized as important variables of the pain experience and can be associated with a greater risk of maintaining pain-related disability. Patients who frequently have excessively negative thoughts about themselves, others, and the future are more likely to experience high levels of depression, low levels of activity, and increased tension.[102,280] Pain beliefs (pain-related fear and self-efficacy), anger, and passive coping are important affective factors, which can significantly affect pain response, behavior, and function. Other neurocognitive factors, unique to each patient, including attention, expectation or anticipation, and appraisals, can contribute to maladaptive behaviors and can represent important targets for cognitive and behavioral interventions.[47]

Learning factors
Operant learning

Fordyce's operant conditioning approach to pain serves as one of the earliest psychologic models for chronic pain.[83] The model focuses primarily on observable behavioral manifestations of pain, which are subject to both reinforcement and avoidance learning. When an individual is exposed to a stimulus that causes tissue damage, an immediate response occurs that involves withdrawal and/or attempts to escape the stimulus. By successfully avoiding pain (i.e. 'punishment'), the individual achieves a reduction in pain, thus rewarding the avoidance behavior. The acquisition of pain behaviors may be determined initially by the history of learned avoidance behaviors. In these cases, pain becomes a discriminating stimulus signaling behaviors that are pain-reducing, such as rest and analgesic medication consumption. With time, pain-eliciting situations such as movement and activity cause anticipatory fear and are avoided. Over time, pain avoidance behaviors can generalize to other potentially painful stimuli, contributing to more inactivity and passivity.[156,300] In a similar way, verbal expression of pain (e.g. complaining) and non-verbal pain behaviors (e.g. limping and grimacing) may be maintained by external reinforcement contingencies such as subtle rewards by significant others or family members who respond to these behaviors.

Waddell has identified a set of 'non-organic' signs that can be used as a simple clinical screening tool to help identify signs and symptoms of pain behavior (tenderness, simulation, distraction, and regional sensory and motor impairments). Although controversial, a study of non-organic signs in a group of patients with low back pain found that demonstration of at least three of the five signs correlated with psychologic distress.[301]

Respondent learning

The development of chronic pain can also be initiated and maintained by classical or respondent learning. In this case, an aversive stimulus is paired with a neutral stimulus and, with repeated exposures over time, the neutral stimulus will come to elicit an aversive response (i.e. fear). For example, a work-related lifting injury elicits an automatic response such as increased muscle tension and sympathetic arousal (fear and anxiety). Over time, fear and anxiety become associated with the once neutral stimuli of simple work-related activities, and lead to increased avoidance of the behavior.[299] With chronic pain, the patient learns to anticipate negative consequences of activity, even in the absence of the noxious stimulus.

Fear of movement

Kinesophobia, a term that describes an irrational and excessive fear of movement, physical activity, and reinjury, is exhibited by many patients with chronic pain.[147] Fear of movement may be initially induced by classical conditioning but reinforced through operant learning; by avoiding the conditioned anxiety and fear associated with movement, the patient never extinguishes the fear. It has been shown in studies to strongly correlate with other responses, such as catastrophic thinking and subsequent increased fear and avoidance behaviors in chronic low back pain patients. In this way, increased levels of fear and disability can occur independently of the experienced pain intensity.[298] McCracken found that increased fear and anxiety in low back pain subjects correlated with decreased range of motion and increased expectation of pain.[181] Other studies in chronic low back pain have found pain-related fear and fear-avoidance beliefs as predictors of disability, decreased activities of daily living, and lost work time.[184] In a Dutch study of patients presenting to a primary care clinic with chronic low back pain, approximately 70% of participants agreed to the statement 'Simply being careful not to make unnecessary movements is the safest thing I can do to prevent back pain', and approximately 50% endorsed the statement 'Back pain always means that the body is injured'. In addition, patients who reported pain-related fear had increased risk for disability at 6 months (odds ratio = 4.6, 95% confidence interval).[218]

A cognitive behavioral model emphasizes two opposing behavioral responses: confrontation and avoidance. Waddell and colleagues' conclusion that 'fear of pain and what we do about pain can be more disabling than pain itself'[302] underscores the importance of identifying and treating such maladaptive thinking and behavior in a physiatric approach to effectively managing chronic pain.

BEHAVIORAL TREATMENT APPROACHES

Operant behavioral techniques

Operant behavioral therapy refers to interventions focused on the observed behavior of the patient. As proposed by Fordyce, operant models of pain are based on both positive and negative reinforcement contingencies.[83] Environment and social factors serve to maintain pain behaviors. For example, the verbal expression of pain and non-verbal pain behaviors (e.g. grimacing and guarding) can be maintained by both positive (attention

from others, potential monetary gain) and negative reinforcement (non-occurrence of aversive stimuli, avoidance of activity).[139] Once identified, these behaviors serve as targets for treatment. Many times, these behaviors need to be reinforced only intermittently. Operant behavioral therapy can be most useful and practical with patients demonstrating excessive pain behaviors despite limited tissue pathology, poor insight into the relationship of their own behavior and subjective experiences of pain, and operant-related issues (secondary gain).

Goals of operant behavioral therapy include encouraging the development and acquisition of more adaptive pain management strategies, which include establishing 'wellness' behaviors and discouraging or reducing reinforcement of pain behaviors.[53] The theory suggests that both wellness and pain behaviors can be shaped. Management techniques target unlearning these behaviors, and serve as the basis of most functional restoration-based programs developed by Mayer and Gatchel.[176] Operant behavioral therapy approaches can be delivered in individual sessions and in group settings. Operant behavioral therapy techniques that patients can master and apply include pacing and graded exercise, scheduling and/or limiting pain medications and passive treatments, and social reinforcement via spouse and family training.

Cognitive behavioral techniques

Cognitive therapy techniques are based on the notion that one's cognitions can have an impact on mood, behavior, and physiologic function.[17] Techniques used in pain management are designed to help patients notice and modify the negative thought patterns that contribute to ongoing pain and affective distress. These include cognitive restructuring, problem solving, distraction, and relapse prevention.[304] Five primary assumptions underlie all cognitive behavioral therapy interventions (Box 43-1).[28] Cognitive behavioral therapy is a flexible, viable, and empirically validated approach for effectively treating patients with persistent pain.[53,201]

Box 43-1 Five primary assumptions that underlie all cognitive behavioral therapy interventions

1. Individuals actively process information regarding internal stimuli and environmental events.
2. Cognitions interact with emotional and physiologic reactions as well as with behavior.
3. There are reciprocal interactions between an individual's behavior and environmental responses.
4. Effective treatment interventions must address the cognitive, emotional, and behavioral dimensions of the presenting problem.
5. It is necessary to help individuals become active participants in learning adaptive methods of responding to their problems.

(After Bradley et al. 2003,[28] with permission.)

SLEEP AND CHRONIC PAIN

Sleep is a dynamic, complex physiologic process that is required for survival. During sleep, there is decreased sensitivity to the external environment and increased activity of the parasympathetic nervous system. Sympathetic nervous system activity is similar to that in wakefulness, except for during periods of rapid eye movement (REM). Breathing is irregular, and control of body temperature is altered. Sleep comprises alternating REM and non-REM (NREM) states that cycle at an ultradian rhythm of approximately 90 min.[240]

Sleep of 8–8.5 h is considered restorative in adults. Sleep is entered through NREM, and the NREM–REM cycle occurs three to six times during a normal 8-h sleep period. The stages of sleep are stage 1 (light sleep), stage 2, stage 3, stage 4 (deep or delta-wave sleep), and REM sleep. Stage 1 is a transitional stage between wakefulness and sleep. It comprises 2–5% of total sleep time, and occurs when initially falling asleep and during brief arousal periods within sleep. Stage 2 is marked by sleep spindles and K complexes, and occurs throughout the sleep period, accounting for 45–55% of total sleep time. NREM stages 3 and 4 occur primarily during the first third of sleep, and are commonly referred to as delta-wave, slow-wave, or deep sleep. They account for approximately 20% of total sleep time. REM sleep is characterized by fast electroencephalograph activity, skeletal muscle atonia, REM, and bursts of autonomic activity. The last third of sleep is primarily spent in REM.[240]

The determinants of sleep are numerous, and include homeostasis, the circadian rhythm, control via the ventrolateral preoptic nucleus, age, drugs, external temperature, medical and psychiatric disease, and other environmental factors.[240,244] The ventrolateral preoptic nucleus has been shown to contain GABAergic and galaninergic neurons that are necessary for normal sleep.[251] Lesions to this region have been shown to decrease both REM and NREM sleep by 55%, verifying their function in inhibiting the firing of cells involved in wakefulness.[162] These inhibited neurons contain the neurotransmitters histamine, norepinephrine, serotonin, hypocretin, and glutamate. Age represents a strong determinant of sleep, as time spent in stages 3 and 4 decreases by 10–15%, latency to fall asleep increases, and the number and duration of overnight arousal periods increases in the elderly when compared with in young adults.[244]

The interrelationship between disturbed sleep and chronic pain conditions is well documented.[198,199,219,266] Prevalence estimates of disturbed sleep range from approximately 50% to 90% depending on the clinical study population under evaluation.[37,198,199] While the nature of the relationship between pain and disturbed sleep is not well understood, a reciprocal association is suggested.[2,266] Patients with chronic pain can display frequent sleep fragmentation, longer sleep latency, and decreased overall quality of sleep.[37] Sleep fragmentation is characterized by repetitive short interruptions in sleep, and is a recognized factor in the cause of excessive daytime sleepiness.[271] This inability to maintain sleep can be the most important factor in the treatment of disturbed sleep in individuals with chronic pain.

ASSESSMENT

The assessment of chronic pain involves a thorough physical examination as well as a comprehensive evaluation of pain intensity and psychosocial factors related to ongoing pain experience, interference with sleep, daily activities, family life, and employment. Subjective reports of pain intensity are an important part of the initial assessment and subsequent visits, and can include pain intensity numeric rating scales, visual and verbal analog scales, and pain drawings. Self-monitored pain intensity ratings are both reliable and valid.[128] Patient variability remains, however, when interpreting self-report measurement scales. Recent work has examined the level of change that best represents a clinically important improvement with the use of the numeric rating scale in monitoring pain response with drug treatment trials. Farrar et al. found that a reduction of approximately 30% represented a clinically important difference.[71] A commonly used comprehensive measure of pain intensity, the McGill Pain Questionnaire Short Form, measures three dimensions of pain: sensory, affective, and evaluative. It utilizes 20 subclasses or groupings of pain adjectives, including sensory (e.g. 'sharp', 'dull', and 'heavy') and affective (e.g. 'annoying', 'tiring', and 'exhausting'); it also includes pain drawings and the visual analog scale.[192]

Additional psychometric measures can also be included in the initial assessment focusing on psychosocial factors such as mood (depression, anxiety, and anger), attitudes, beliefs, functional capacity, activity interference, and personality traits (Table 43-5). The use and combination of these different methods depend largely on the goal of the assessment. A semistructured interview by an experienced psychologist is the most comprehensive means of evaluating the psychologic state of the patient.[28] A packet of self-reported questionnaires completed by the patient prior to the evaluation, measuring a wide spectrum of the multidimensional factors related to pain, can be used in isolation or as an adjunct to the psychologic and medical interview.

The comprehensive evaluation should include a complete medical history and physical examination identifying related impairments, pain behaviors, and postural and soft tissue abnormalities (i.e. regional myofascial pain). The psychologic interview, administered by a psychiatrist or pain psychologist (structured or semistructured), can lead to the diagnosis according to the *Diagnostic and Statistical Manual Fourth Edition* criteria. The pain disorder criteria include the following.

- Pain is in one or more anatomic sites.
- Pain causes clinically significant distress or impairment.
- Psychologic factors are judged to play an important role.
- Symptoms(s) are not intentionally produced.
- Pain is not better accounted for by another condition.

Pain disorder can be associated with a psychologic and/or a general medical condition.[4]

Table 43-5 Psychometric assessment tools

Psychometric measure	Psychometric assessment tool	Description	Reference
Pain intensity	Numeric rating scale Visual analog scale Verbal rating scale	0–10, 0–100, 'no pain' to 'worst pain' Straight line, 0–10 cm List of adjectives or descriptors	—
Pain affect	McGill Pain Questionnaire—Short Form (MPQ-SF)	20 descriptors (sensory, affective, evaluative), pain drawing, visual analog scale; four-point Likert scale from 0 (none) to 3 (severe)	Melzack (1975)[192]
	Brief Pain Inventory (BPI) and Brief Pain Inventory—Short Form (BPI-SF)	Measures the impact of pain on everyday activities and mood	Cleeland and Ryan (1994)[51]
Anxiety and coping	Pain Anxiety Symptoms Scale (PASS)	40 items; anxiety related to pain on six-point scale, subscales: cognitive anxiety symptoms, escape and avoidance, fearful appraisals, physiologic symptoms	McCracken et al. (1992)[184]
	Spielberger State–Trait Anxiety Inventory (STAI)	40 items; differentiates between the temporary condition of 'state anxiety' and the more general and longstanding quality of 'trait anxiety'	Spielberger et al. (1970)[269]
	Survey of Pain Attitudes (SOPA)	57-item, five-point scale assessing control, disability, medical cures, solicitude, medication, emotion, and harm	Jensen et al. (1987)[127]
Depression	Beck Depression Inventory (BDI)	21-item, four-point scale assessing mood and neurovegetative dimensions of depression	Beck and Steer (1987)[18]
	Center for Epidemiologic Studies Depression Scale (CES-D)	Less compromised validity by somatic symptoms as compared with the BDI, more sensitive to changes in severity of depression	Radloff (1977)[230]
	Zung Self-Rating Depression Scale	20-item, rapid assessment tool for severity of depression	Zung (1965)[319]
Mood and personality	Minnesota Multiphasic Personality Inventory (MMPI)	567 true-false items, 60–90 min to administer	Butcher et al. (1989)[35]
	Symptom Checklist 90 (SCL-90-R)	90-item, five-point scale, global index score, and nine subscales of general emotional distress	Derogatis (1983)[63]
	Millon Behavioral Health Inventory	150 true–false items, assesses styles of relating to providers, psychosocial stressors, and response to illness	Millon et al. (1979)[196]
Functional capacity and activity interference	Sickness Impact Profile (SIP)	136 items, 12 dimensions of function	Bergener et al. (1981)[22]
	36-Item Short-Form Health Survey (SF-36)	Eight scales to measure limitations in physical and social activities due to physical and emotional problems, bodily pain, vitality, and general health perceptions	Ware and Sherbourne (1992)[303]
	West Haven-Yale Multidimensional Pain Inventory (WHYMPI or MPI)	52-item, seven-point scale, 12 dimensions (pain experience, perceptions of others, common daily activities), classifies patients primarily into three classes (dysfunctional, interpersonally distressed, and adaptive copers)	Kerns et al. (1985)[143]

Continued on page 965

Continued from page 964 Table 43-5	Psychometric assessment tools		
Psychometric measure	Psychometric assessment tool	Description	Reference
	Pain Disability Index (PDI)	Seven questions: degree of interference with functioning, home, recreation, social activities, occupations, sexual behavior, self-care, life support	Trait et al. (1987)[285]
	Oswestry Disability Questionnaire	10 sections, assesses the effect of back and leg pain on activities of daily living and patient's everyday life	Leclaire et al. (1997)[154]
Coping and beliefs	Coping Strategies Questionnaire (CSQ)	50 items, cognitive and behavioral coping strategies assessed	Rosenstiel and Keefe (1983)[238]
	Survey of Pain Attitudes (SOPA)	57 items, subscales (control, disability, medical cures, solicitude, medication, emotion, and harm)	Jensen et al. (1987)[127]

TREATMENT

The ultimate goal of a rehabilitation-based approach to chronic pain is the reduction of pain and the restoration of function. The physiatrist plays a critical role in the assessment and management of chronic pain conditions, and leads the team of healthcare professionals in achieving this goal of maximal functional recovery. The treatment of chronic pain conditions has been practiced according to a number of different patient care models. Regardless of the setting, recent data suggest that chronic pain management is best addressed utilizing a biopsychosocial assessment and approach to treatment.[110,183,291] The traditional biomedical model fails, as it focuses on the identification and treatment of a specific anatomic pain generator without accounting for the psychologic determinants involved in the pain experience. The treatment goals of chronic pain management encompass the acceptance and reduction of pain, maximal restoration of functional mobility, restoration of sleep, improvement in mood, return to leisure activity, and return to work (Box 43-2).

Pain treatment programs

The IASP classifies four types of pain treatment program (Table 43-6).[159] In general, multidisciplinary treatment centers or clinics may or may not include a formal interdisciplinary collaboration model. Although the terms *multidisciplinary* and *interdisciplinary* are many times used interchangeably, *multidisciplinary* more formally refers to a collaboration with members of different disciplines (including various medical specialists and therapists) managed by a leader who directs a range of ancillary services. Team members assess and treat patients independently and then share information. *Interdisciplinary* describes a deeper level of a consensus-based collaboration where the entire process (i.e. evaluation, goal setting, and

Box 43-2 Chronic pain management: goals of treatment

- Maximize and maintain physical activity and function.
- Reduce the misuse or abuse of dependency-producing medications, invasive procedures, and passive modalities, fostered by a change toward active patient self-management.
- Return to previous levels of activity at home, in the workplace, and in leisure pursuits.
- Reduce subjective reported pain intensity and maladaptive pain behaviors.
- Assist patients in obtaining resolution and/or closure of contentious work-related or litigation aspects of the pain condition.

treatment delivery) is orchestrated by the team, facilitated by regular face to face meetings, and primarily delivered within a single facility.[177] Multi- and interdisciplinary program facilities may be accredited by the Commission on Accreditation of Rehabilitation Facilities, with established treatment standards and ongoing outcome measurement. The interdisciplinary team is commonly led by a physiatrist or other pain specialist, and includes physical and occupational therapists, pain psychologists, relaxation training experts, vocational rehabilitation and therapeutic recreational specialists, social workers, and nurse educators (Box 43-3). A key process in multidisciplinary treatment is the comprehensive evaluation. This usually incorporates a thorough musculoskeletal evaluation, psychologic assessment and, in patients with work-related injuries, a vocational rehabilitation interview. The evaluation enables the team to assess patient motivation and realistic goals for return to function and/or work. Those patients accepted for treatment are placed in a structured outpatient environment with one on one and group-based treatments.

Table 43-6 Classification of pain treatment centers

	Multidisciplinary pain center	Multidisciplinary pain clinic	Pain clinic	Modality-oriented clinic
Comprehensive assessment and management	Yes	Yes	Yes	No
Physicians	Multispecialty	Multispecialty	Single specialty	Single specialty
Psychologists	Yes	Yes	Variable	No
Other healthcare professionals	Physical, occupational, recreation therapists; nurses; biofeedback, relaxation specialists; movement-based therapy practitioners; vocational counselors; other specialists	Physical, occupational, recreation therapists; nurses; biofeedback, relaxation specialists; movement-based therapy practitioners; vocational counselors; other specialists	Variable	No
Therapeutic modalities	Multiple	Multiple	Variable	Focused
Affiliation	Major health science institutions	Variable	Variable	Variable
Research and educational activity	Yes	Variable, not typical	Variable, not typical	Variable, not typical
General or specific focus of care	Comprehensive, acute and chronic pain	Comprehensive, chronic pain	Specific, chronic pain (i.e. regional focus such as headaches)	Specific, acute and chronic pain (i.e. nerve block clinics)

Box 43-3 Interdisciplinary pain team members

- Physiatrist
- Physical therapist
- Occupational therapist
- Pain psychologist
- Social worker
- Recreational therapist
- Biofeedback specialist
- Nursing educator
- Vocational counselor

Multidisciplinary and interdisciplinary approaches

Interdisciplinary treatment

Interdisciplinary biopsychosocial rehabilitation-based programs have been increasingly and successfully utilized in the treatment of patients with chronic pain and related psychosocial dysfunction.[8,94,110,134,235] Comprehensive reviews of the clinical and cost-effectiveness of interdisciplinary programs have demonstrated significant improvements in return to work, function, reduced healthcare utilization, and closure of disability claims.[19,291] Positive functional results have been shown in patients classified as having both short-term and long-term disability at the onset of care.[134] These comprehensive programs have also shown clear benefits over conventional management in regard to decreasing pain behavior and improving mood.

Scope and intensity varies, with most outpatient-based centers offering part-time (2 days per week) or full-time (5 days per week, 6–8 h per day) programs lasting 4–6 weeks in total duration. The interdisciplinary model provides ongoing communication for all members of the treatment team, helping to facilitate patient progress while they progress the behavioral, cognitive, and active therapy treatments. Patients are discussed individually, in a team conference format, on a weekly basis, enabling ongoing communication of progress and adjustment of treatment goals. Physician follow-up visits two or three times per week are ideal for ongoing pharmacologic trials (targeted for improving mood, disturbed sleep, and analgesia) and encouraging progress across the multiple therapy domains.

At completion of treatment, patients are encouraged to continue with their own individually structured home exercise, aerobic, and stretching program. They should also be independent in their own use of various relaxation and pacing techniques. The identification of a chronic pain condition as a chronic *disease* imparts an important facet into the continued care of these patients. As with a chronic disease such as diabetes or hypertension, self-control and self-management of symptoms are critical for successful treatment. It logically follows that chronic pain should be treated as any other chronic disease or illness, in that regular follow-up and reassessment of psychosocial and physical function be performed.[21,152,291]

Table 43-7 Modalities utilized in the treatment of chronic pain

Modality	Superficial or deep	Mechanism of action	Example	Indication	Precautions and contraindications
Heat	Superficial	Conduction Conduction Convection Convection	Hydrocollator packs Paraffin baths Whirlpool baths Fluidotherapy	Pain, contracture, hematoma, chronic inflammation, muscle spasm, arthritis, prior to stretching program to increase collagen extensibility	Acute trauma, hemorrhage, bleeding diathesis, impaired sensation, altered thermal regulation, malignancy, ischemia, cognitive deficits or inability to report pain
	Deep	Conversion Conversion Conversion	Ultrasound Shortwave diathermy Microwave		
Cold	Superficial	Conduction Conduction Conduction	Ice Cold packs Cryotherapy-compression units	Pain, acute trauma, acute inflammation, joint effusion, hemorrhage, muscle spasm, spasticity	Cold hypersensitivity, ischemia, impaired sensation, cognitive deficits, areas over superficial peripheral nerves, Raynaud phenomenon or disease, cryoglobulinemia, arterial vascular disease
		Convection Evaporative	Whirlpool baths Vapocoolant spray		
Electrical stimulation	Superficial	Gate control, endogenous opioid release, direct peripheral effects Direct stimulation of muscle fibers	Transcutaneous electrical nerve stimulation Interferential current therapy	Rheumatoid arthritis, osteoarthritis, deafferentation pain syndromes, visceral pain, sympathetically mediated pain, tension headache, acute postoperative pain, Raynaud disease, ischemic pain, urogenital dysfunction	Demand-type cardiac pacemaker; carotid sinus, laryngeal or pharyngeal muscles, eyes, and mucosal membranes; cognitive deficits; abdominal, lumbosacral, or pelvic areas of pregnant women; edema; open wounds or skin irritation

Multidisciplinary team

Physical therapy and occupational therapy Physical and occupational therapists utilize active and passive therapeutic exercises, manual techniques, and passive physical modalities (Table 43-7) to address deficits in flexibility, strength, balance, neuromuscular control, posture, functional mobility, locomotion, and endurance. Both types of therapists help patients to overcome fear of movement. While there is some crossover between the skill sets of physical and occupational therapists, they possess established core competencies that are fairly universal. Physical therapists specialize in gait training and locomotion, core stability, lower extremity biomechanics, and functional mobility, as well as activities of daily living such as bed mobility and transfers. They are also experts in the development of aerobic conditioning programs aimed at improving cardiopulmonary health and endurance. Occupational therapists typically concentrate on educating patients regarding proper posture and ergonomics related to upper limb functional activities such as lifting and computer usage. They address upper extremity-related activities of daily living including feeding, hygiene, grooming, bathing, and dressing. Physical and occupational therapists also play a primary role in the education of patients, family members, and other caregivers.

Physical and occupational therapists involved in interdisciplinary chronic pain treatment programs must be adept in their ability to assess initial levels of functional ability, and then monitor and progressively increase the level and complexity of therapeutic exercises. The majority of chronic pain patients have secondary impairments in addition to their primary pain-related diagnoses (i.e. general inflexibility, deconditioning, myofascial pain, and other postural abnormalities), which are important focuses of treatment. A functional cognitive behaviorally mediated therapeutic approach may be necessary in order to maximize outcomes. This approach may help foster patient optimism, decrease fear of reinjury, and maximize patient compliance.

Psychology Pain psychology assessment and therapeutic interventions focus on both cognitive and behavioral factors related to pain. As noted earlier, key psychologic factors involved in the development of and adaptation to chronic pain include anxiety and fear-avoidance behavior,[140,180,299] pain catastrophizing,[140,258,279,293] and helplessness.[140] Factors identified with improvement in adjustment to chronic pain include self-efficacy, pain coping strategies, readiness to change, and acceptance.[140] Psychologic intervention focuses on unlearning maladaptive responses and reactions to pain, while fostering self-efficacy, wellness, improved coping, perceived control, decreased catastrophizing, and acceptance (see Fig. 43-4).[140] Phases of individual and group-based treatment include education, skills training, application, and relapse prevention.

Relaxation training can be provided by a number of team disciplines, including psychology, physical therapy, nursing, or certified biofeedback specialists. Formal techniques include guided relaxation response training (guided imagery, visual or auditory guided biofeedback), meditation, and hypnosis. These techniques help to encourage the patient's role as an active participant in ongoing self-management (see *Mind–body medicine* section).

Vocational rehabilitation   The Centers for Medicare and Medicaid Service define vocational rehabilitation as 'the process of facilitating an individual in the choice of or return to a suitable vocation'.[45] Title I of the Rehabilitation Act of 1973 describes the goods or services provided in order to render a handicapped individual employable. Vocational rehabilitation counselors should be involved with patient care early in the process of chronic pain management to ensure identification of employment as a long-term goal for the patient.

Vocational counselors participate in the analysis of current or prior job descriptions, provide suggestions for work accommodation or modification, and if necessary facilitate vocational testing and targeted retraining. At the end of the rehabilitation process, vocational rehabilitation can help coordinate functional capacity evaluation testing and finalize return to work issues (i.e. restrictions and level of work). Vocational rehabilitation counselors acquire information from the physical therapists, occupational therapists, and physician to address instructions as to limitation of duty (full or limited) and the functional restrictions or modifications that might be required. These restrictions or modifications include sitting or standing tolerance, walking, pushing, pulling, stair usage, bending at the waist, sustained postures, hot or cold tolerance, data entry or other repetitive tasks, grip, tool usage, and vibration factors.

Nurse facilitator   The program nurse or nursing staff member plays an essential role in coordinating patient progress and care during evaluation, treatment, and ongoing follow-up. Nursing plays a critical role in educational aspects of treatment, including basic instruction on pain pathways, pharmacology, nutrition, and sleep hygiene. The nurse facilitator can also serve as a patient advocate in ongoing communication with all team members.

Therapeutic recreation   Therapeutic recreation specialists evaluate and plan leisure activities for the promotion of mental and physical health. They help patients establish and incorporate the functional and cognitive behavioral pain management strategies learned from other disciplines of treatment into social and community situations. Techniques incorporated from other disciplines include biomechanical and postural correction, pacing, and relaxation strategies. An individualized recreational assessment with short- and long-term goal setting is typically followed by individual and group projects, as well as supervised outings.

Medications

Pharmacotherapy is a critical component in the treatment of chronic pain conditions. The importance of specific treatment targets can vary considerably from those addressed in acute pain treatment paradigms. While acute pain treatment primarily focuses on analgesia and control of inflammation, drug therapy in chronic pain states requires a more comprehensive focus including mood and sleep disturbances. A mechanistic approach to rational pharmacology is an important component of the practitioner's armamentarium for managing the diverse nature of chronic pain. This approach incorporates the use of oral and topical medications including traditional and newer generation antidepressants, anticonvulsants, sleep agents, non-opioid analgesics, antiinflammatories and, in selected cases, chronic opioid therapy.

This section reviews current updates in pharmacotherapy as it applies to a broad range of chronic pain conditions, including neuropathic pain and manifestations of chronic pain conditions (pain, affective distress, and sleep disturbance). The section includes an overview related to controversies in the use of cyclooxygenase (COX)-2 inhibitors, pharmacologic use of opioids, tricyclic antidepressants (TCAs) and novel antidepressants, anticonvulsant medications, sleep-related drugs, and topical analgesics.

NSAIDs and COX-2 inhibitors

Conventional (i.e. non-specific) non-steroidal antiinflammatory drugs (NSAIDs) have been first-line treatment for analgesia and the treatment of inflammatory conditions including osteoarthritis, rheumatoid arthritis, and various musculoskeletal-related conditions.[275,287] COX-1 and COX-2 isoforms catalyze the conversion of arachidonic acid to prostaglandins. More recent classification of NSAIDs is as follows.

- Conventional or non-selective NSAIDs, those that inhibit both the COX-1 isoenzyme and the COX-2 isoenzyme.
- NSAIDs that are more selective for the COX-2 isoenzyme (COX-2 inhibitors).

Conventional non-selective NSAIDs were found to offer effective analgesic responses but are limited by potential upper gastrointestinal bleeding and ulceration, renal toxicity, and platelet dysfunction.[49]

The isolation of the COX-2 protein in the early 1990s led to the development and release of a new class of NSAIDs, the COX-2 inhibitors. The new oral COX-2 inhibitors include celecoxib (Celebrex), rofecoxib (Vioxx), and valdecoxib (Bextra). Meloxicam (Mobic) is an NSAID with preferential COX-2 selectivity that spares COX-1 at approved doses. It can be considered as a special agent in the COX-2 class (Table 43-8).[214] COX-1 is constitutively expressed in most tissues, being responsible for homeostatic functions such as platelet aggregation and the maintenance of upper gastrointestinal mucosa integrity by producing protective prostaglandins. COX-2, a largely cytokine 'inducible' constitutive isoenzyme, is primarily responsible for producing inflammation and pain. Animal neuropathic pain models have demonstrated up-regulation of COX-2 by early inflammatory changes in various types of peripheral nerve injury,[165] as well as COX-2 induction in dorsal horn neurons and other regions of the central nervous system.[249]

Table 43-8 Commonly prescribed non-steroidal antiinflammatory medications

Class	Generic name (trade name)	Dose (elderly/adult)	Half-life (onset)	Mechanism of action	Other
Cyclooxygenase-2 inhibitors	Rofecoxib (Vioxx)[a]	12.5/25 mg daily Acute pain: 50 mg daily × 5 days maximum	17 h (45 min)	Suppress prostaglandin synthesis; selective cyclooxygenase (COX)-2 inhibition; analgesic, antipyretic, and antiinflammatory actions	Selective COX-2 inhibitors do not inhibit platelet aggregation; sulfonyl moiety
	Celecoxib (Celebrex)	100/100–200 mg b.i.d., or 200 mg daily	9–10 h (<60 min)	Suppresses prostaglandin synthesis; selective COX-2 inhibition; analgesic, antipyretic, and antiinflammatory actions	Does not inhibit platelet aggregation; crosses placenta; sulfonamide moiety
	Valdecoxib (Bextra)[b]	10/10–20 mg daily. Acute pain: 20 mg b.i.d. for short periods of time (i.e. primary dysmenorrhea)	8–11 h (<60 min)	Suppresses prostaglandin synthesis; selective COX-2 inhibition; analgesic, antipyretic, and antiinflammatory actions	No effect on platelet aggregation; sulfonamide moiety
Oxicam derivatives	Meloxicam (Mobic)	7.5/7.5–15 mg daily	15–20 h	Prostaglandin synthetase inhibition; some selectivity for COX-2; analgesic, antipyretic, and antiinflammatory actions	Does not generally affect platelet counts, prothrombin time, or partial thromboplastin time; patients with coagulation disorders or patients receiving anticoagulants should be carefully monitored
Propionic acid derivatives	Ibuprofen (Motrin, Advil, Ibuprin, Nuprin, Rufen, Saleto)	200/200–800 mg q.i.d.	2–4 h (30 min)	Reversible non-selective COX inhibitor—inhibits formation of prostaglandin and thromboxane A_2; various effects on leukotriene production; inhibition of platelet aggregation	Analgesic action at dosages <1600 mg/day; doses >1600 mg/day needed for antiinflammatory action; available in over the counter preparations
	Naproxen (Anaprox, Naprelan, Naprosyn, Aleve)	250/250–500 mg b.i.d.; acute pain 1.5 g/day in divided doses	12–15 h (60 min)	Reversible non-selective COX inhibitor—inhibits formation of prostaglandin and thromboxane A_2; various effects on leukotriene production; inhibition of platelet aggregation	Available in over the counter preparations

Continued on page 970

Continued from page 969 Table 43-8   Commonly prescribed non-steroidal antiinflammatory medications

Class	Generic name (trade name)	Dose (elderly/adult)	Half-life (onset)	Mechanism of action	Other
Acetic acid derivatives	Etodolac (Lodine)	400/400–600 mg b.i.d.	7.3 h (30 min)	Reversible non-selective COX inhibitor—inhibits formation of prostaglandin and thromboxane A_2; various effects on leukotriene production; inhibition of platelet aggregation	Relative COX-2 selectivity
	Ketorolac (Toradol; Acular [ophthalmic])	i.m. single dose 30/60 mg; i.m. multidose (maximum 5 days) 15/30 mg q. 6 h (maximum 120 mg/day)	2.4–8.6 h (10 min i.m.)	Reversible non-selective COX inhibitor—inhibits formation of prostaglandin and thromboxane A_2; various effects on leukotriene production; inhibition of platelet aggregation	Also available in i.v., ophthalmic, and p.o. formulations; p.o. indicated only for continuation of parenteral therapy; not for chronic use—total treatment should not exceed 5 days
	Diclofenac (Cataflam, Voltaren, Solaraze; with misoprostol, Arthrotec)	50 mg b.i.d./50 mg b.i.d.–q.i.d.; or 75 mg b.i.d.	2 h (30 min)	Reversible non-selective COX inhibitor—inhibits formation of prostaglandin and thromboxane A_2; various effects on leukotriene production; inhibition of platelet aggregation	Alternate formulation: diclofenac with misoprostol (Arthrotec)
Salicylate derivatives	Aspirin (Aspirin CR, Easprin, Ascriptin, Bayer, Ecotrin, Empirin, Bufferin)	325/325–650 mg/day (maximum 4 g/day)	3–6 h (15–30 min)	Inhibition of prostaglandin synthesis and release, formation of thromboxane A_2; inhibition of platelet aggregation	Therapeutic response may take 2 weeks for arthritis treatment
	Salsalate (Amigesic, Disalcid, Argesic-SA, Salflex, Mono-Gesic, Salsitab)	500/500–750 mg b.i.d.–t.i.d. (max 3 g/day)	7–8 h	Inhibition of prostaglandin synthesis	Does not inhibit platelet aggregation; onset of antiinflammatory action in 3–4 days
Para-aminophenol derivatives	Acetaminophen (Tylenol, Panadol, Neopap, Apacet, Acephen)	325–1000 mg q. 4–6 h (4 g daily maximum)	3–4 h (10–30 min)	COX inhibitor in central nervous system; analgesic and antipyretic; no antiinflammatory properties	Severe adverse effects include hepatic and renal failure; available in alternate forms (rectal, drops, elixir)

Continued on page 971

Class	Generic name (trade name)	Dose (elderly/adult)	Half-life (onset)	Mechanism of action	Other
	Continued from page 970 Table 43-8 Commonly prescribed non-steroidal antiinflammatory medications				
Barbituric acid derivatives	Butalbital compounds (butalbital plus acetaminophen or aspirin plus caffeine); with acetaminophen and caffeine (Fioricet, Medigesic, Endolor, Americet); with codeine (Fioricet with codeine); with acetaminophen (Phrenilin, Triaprin); with acetylsalicylic acid and caffeine (Fiorinal, Farbital); with codeine (Fiorinal with codeine)	One or two tablets q. 4 h (maximum six tablets/day)	3–4 h	Analgesic properties of acetaminophen, aspirin, caffeine; anxiolytic and muscle relaxant properties of butalbital	Risk of psychologic or physical dependence

[a]Voluntarily withdrawn from the US market in September 2004.
[b]Voluntarily withdrawn from the US market in April 2005.

This suggests COX-2 involvement with peripheral and central sensitization processes, and involvement in key mechanisms underlying neuroplastic changes in chronic pain states.

Major studies, including the Vioxx Gastrointestinal Outcomes Research (VIGOR) trial, the Celecoxib Long-term Arthritis Safety Study (CLASS), and the Safety and Efficacy Large Scale Evaluation of COX Inhibition Therapies (SELECT) trial, demonstrated significant safety benefits of COX-2 inhibitors as compared with non-selective NSAIDs with regard to reduced incidence of symptomatic gastric ulcers and renal toxicity.[26,62,216,261] The VIGOR trial reported a 2.38-fold increase in relative risk of cardiovascular events among study patients with rheumatoid arthritis randomly assigned to rofecoxib treatment.[26] Reevaluation of the VIGOR study suggested that the higher rate of cardiovascular events in the treatment group (rofecoxib) as compared with in the naproxen group could be due to additional cardioprotective effects of naproxen,[57] although ongoing questions remain.

Despite billions of dollars in sales and the widespread use of COX-2 inhibitors, questions and concerns reemerged regarding the potential increased risk of cardiac events, including myocardial infarction and sudden cardiac death.[145,203] Some have proposed that selective COX-2 inhibitors can decrease vascular prostacyclin (PGI_2) production, interfering with the balance between prothrombotic and antithrombotic eicosanoids (thromboxane A_2), and increasing the likelihood of a prothrombotic state manifested by possible cardiac events.[112] Merck voluntarily withdrew rofecoxib from the market in 2004, after a trial involving the use of high-dose rofecoxib in adenomatous polyp disease found an increased risk for serious cardiovascular events in patients taking the drug, as compared with those patients on a traditional NSAID. Other studies have found conflicting results when looking at other agents and possible 'class effects' with increased incidence of myocardial and renal events. Other studies subsequently demonstrated similar cardiac effects with naproxen, causing many practitioners to reassess the chronic use of non-selective NSAIDs and COX-2 inhibitors for management of chronic spine and osteoarthritic conditions.

Based on a 2004 review of available data from long-term placebo- and active-controlled clinical trials of NSAIDs, the US Food and Drug Administration (FDA) concluded that an increased risk of serious adverse cardiovascular events may be a class effect for NSAIDs (excluding aspirin), and requested that the package insert for all NSAIDs be revised to include a boxed warning to highlight the potential increased risk of cardiovascular events and the risk of serious and potentially life-threatening gastrointestinal bleeding.[281] Physicians need to assess relative risks versus potential benefits (analgesia, decreased stiffness, and improved function) on an individual case by case basis. Ongoing monitoring of blood pressure, cardiac, and renal status is recommended with acute and chronic use of both non-selective NSAIDs and selective COX-2 inhibitors.[10,222]

Opioid analgesics

Opioid and opioid-like medications are potent analgesics (Table 43-9). Opioids work by binding to three receptor types (μ, δ,

Table 43-9 Commonly prescribed opioid analgesics

Class	Name (trade names)	Dose (elderly/adult)	Half-life (onset)	Mechanism of action	Other
Natural opium alkaloids	Morphine (Astramorph, Avinza, Duramorph, Infumorph, Kadian, MS Contin, MSIR, Oramorph SR, RMS, Roxanol)	p.o.: 5–30 mg q. 4 h s.c./i.m.: 4–15 mg q. 4 h i.v.: 4–15 mg in 4–5 mL of H_2O for injection over 5 min p.r.: 10–20 mg q. 4 h p.o. sustained release: 15–60 mg q. 8–12 h (based on 24-h requirements of immediate-release p.o. MSO_4)	2.5–3 h (s.c./i.m., 10–30 min; i.v., p.r., p.o. suspension)	Opioid agonist activity at multiple receptors: μ (supraspinal analgesia and euphoria), κ (spinal analgesia and sedation), and δ (dysphoria, psychotomimetic effects)	Sustained release oral form available; epidural or intrathecal injectable solution available; treat overdose with naloxone 0.2–0.8 mg i.v.
	Codeine (with acetaminophen or acetylsalicylic acid) (Tylenol #2, #3, #4; Empirin #3, #4; Robitussin AC; Capital, Aceta, Phenaphen, Fioricet with codeine, Fiorinal with codeine)	p.o.: 15–60 mg q. 4 h (maximum daily acetaminophen/ acetylsalicylic acid dose 4 g)	2.5–3.5 h (p.o.: 30–60 min)	Opioid agonist activity at multiple receptors: μ (supraspinal analgesia and euphoria), κ (spinal analgesia and sedation), and δ (dysphoria, psychotomimetic effects)	Compared with MSO_4: decreased analgesia, constipation, respiratory distress, sedation, emesis, and physical dependence; increased antitussive effects
Phenanthrene derivatives	Hydrocodone (with acetylsalicylic acid or acetaminophen) (Lortab, Lortab ASA, Vicodin, Norco, Vicoprofin, Entuss-D, Ztuss, S-T Forte, P-V-Tussin, Tussanil, Tussafed HC)	p.o.: 5–10 mg q. 4–6 h (maximum daily acetaminophen/ acetylsalicylic acid dose 4 g)	3.8 h (10–30 min)	Opioid agonist activity at multiple receptors: μ (supraspinal analgesia and euphoria), κ (spinal analgesia and sedation), and δ (dysphoria, psychotomimetic effects)	Compared with MSO_4: decreased analgesia, respiratory depression, and physical dependency; equivalent antitussive effects
	Oxycodone (± acetaminophen or acetylsalicylic acid) (Oxycontin, Oxy IR, Percolone Oxyfast, Roxicodone); with acetylsalicylic acid (Percodan, Endodan, Roxiprin); with acetaminophen (Percocet, Endocet, Tylox, Rixicet, Roxilox)	p.o.: 5 mg q. 6 h (4 g maximum dose of acetylsalicylic acid or acetaminophen) Sustained release: 10/10–160 mg q. 12	2–5 h (10–15 min)	Opioid agonist activity at multiple receptors: μ (supraspinal analgesia and euphoria), κ (spinal analgesia and sedation), and δ (dysphoria, psychotomimetic effects)	Compared with MSO_4: equivalent analgesia, constipation, antitussive effects, respiratory depression, sedation, emesis, and physical dependence

Continued on page 973

Continued from page 972 *Table 43-9* Commonly prescribed opioid analgesics					
Class	Name (trade names)	Dose (elderly/adult)	Half-life (onset)	Mechanism of action	Other
	Hydromorphone (Dilaudid)	p.o.: 1–4 mg q. 4–6 h ER: 12–32 mg q. 24 h p.r.: 3 mg q. 6–8 h	2.6 h (<15 min)	Opioid agonist activity at multiple receptors: μ (supraspinal analgesia and euphoria), κ (spinal analgesia and sedation), and δ (dysphoria, psychotomimetic effects)	Compared with MSO_4: equivalent analgesia, constipation, sedation, respiratory depression; decreased emesis; available in i.v., i.m., s.c. formulations; sustained release preparation recently FDA-approved with 24-h dosing schedule
Diphenylheptane derivative	Methadone (Dolophine)	p.o.: 2.5–10 mg q. 6 h s.c./i.m.: 2.5–10 mg q. 3-4 h Maintenance of dependency p.o.: 20–120 mg/day	13–47 h (p.o., 30–60 min; s.c./i.m., 10–20 min)	Opioid agonist activity at multiple receptors: μ (supraspinal analgesia and euphoria), κ (spinal analgesia and sedation), and δ (dysphoria, psychotomimetic effects); NMDA receptor antagonist	Compared with MSO_4: equivalent analgesia, antitussive effects, respiratory distress, and constipation; less sedation, emesis, physical dependence; commonly utilized for the detoxification and maintenance of opiate dependence; possible NMDA antagonist effects of reduced central sensitization and reduced opioid tolerance
	Propoxyphene (±acetaminophen) (Darvon, Dolene; Darvon-N); with acetaminophen (Darvocet, Propacet, Wygesic)	p.o.: 65 mg q. 4 h (maximum 390 mg/day) Napsylate 100 mg q. 4 h (maximum 600 mg/day)	6–12 h (15–60 min)	Opioid agonist activity at multiple receptors: μ (supraspinal analgesia and euphoria), κ (spinal analgesia and sedation), and δ (dysphoria, psychotomimetic effects)	Compared with MSO_4: less analgesia, sedation, emesis, respiratory depression, and physical dependence
Phenylpiperidine derivative	Fentanyl (Sublimaze); transdermal (Duragesic); transmucosal) (Actiq, Oralet)	Transdermal: 25/25–100 μg/h q. 72 h Transmucosal: 200, 400, 600, 800, 1200, 1400, 1600 μg	2.5–4 h (p.o., 5–15 min; i.m., 7–15 min; i.v., 1–2 min) Transdermal: half-life 17 h after patch removal, steady state at 24 h	Opioid agonist activity at multiple receptors: μ (supraspinal analgesia and euphoria), κ (spinal analgesia and sedation), and δ (dysphoria, psychotomimetic effects)	Compared with MSO_4: equivalent analgesia; less respiratory depression and emesis; transdermal delivery for use in chronic pain—other forms utilized for perioperative anesthesia

and κ) belonging to a G-protein receptor family. Presynaptic effects of opioids decrease calcium into the cell, inhibiting subsequent release of excitatory neurotransmitters (serotonin, norepinephrine, substance P, and glutamate). Postsynaptic effects include increasing potassium efflux, resulting in hyperpolarization of the neuron, decreasing synaptic transmission.[284] At the brain stem level, opioids inhibit GABAergic transmission, leading to excitation of descending inhibition.[120]

The use of chronic opioid analgesic therapy (COAT) in chronic pain management should incorporate the use of longer acting medications and the judicious use of short-acting medications for breakthrough pain episodes. Maintaining steady serum levels with long-acting agents can help to maintain consistent opioid serum levels. This offers numerous advantages, including convenient dosing schedules, more sustained analgesia, and uninterrupted sleep. It also limits frequent episodes of breakthrough pain and over-reliance on the use of excessive daily consumption of short-acting opioids.

Longer acting oral opioid medications are available, and include extended release morphine (MS Contin, Avinza, and Kadian) and oxycodone (OxyContin) formulations. Recent advancements in opioid management include novel fentanyl oral and transdermal delivery systems, transmucosal (Actiq), and transdermal (Duragesic). The highly lipophilic character of fentanyl allows for rapid absorption across the buccal mucosa, with transmucosal delivery providing peak serum levels at approximately 22 min after initiating dosing. Transdermal fentanyl systems deliver the medication across the skin into a drug reservoir or depot beneath the dermis, enabling steady release directly into the bloodstream over a 72-h period, again bypassing first-pass metabolism.

It is important to understand basic pharmacologic principles related to these agents, including absorption, bioavailability, plasma half-life, peak onset, and duration of analgesia, when selecting appropriate agents (Table 43-9). For example, sustained release oxycodone (OxyContin) provides a bimodal release system with bimodal peak serum release at 0.6 and 6.8 h dosed on a b.i.d. schedule. Variability of pharmacokinetics between patients can necessitate adjustment from standard dosing regimens. A recent survey of a large university-based chronic pain clinic found that a significant number of patients on chronic sustained release oxycodone management required dosing more frequently than twice daily (every 8 h dosing) (67%). Many patients in this clinic required greater than half the amount of rescue medication as compared with the every 12 h dosing group.[172]

Methadone   The use of methadone has experienced a rebirth in its use as a 'novel' opioid analgesic. Long used in addiction medicine and opioid maintenance programs, this synthetic opioid has a number of potentially unique advantages compared with other opioids. Methadone hydrochloride is a relatively potent NMDA receptor antagonist. NMDA activation has been implicated as a key player in behavioral and neural plasticity (i.e. central sensitization)[185] and as a mediator of opioid tolerance.[109] Methadone offers other potential advantages, including

low price and no active metabolites. Clinicians prescribing methadone need to use caution,[306] because methadone accumulates in tissues with repeated dosing, creating an extensive reservoir, and is highly protein-bound. Half-life varies from 7 h to 5 days. Dosing changes must be done at least every 5–6 days. Morley and Makin describe standardized conversion regimens for converting oral morphine equivalents to methadone. For example, with 24-h doses less than 300 mg, a fixed dose one-tenth the actual morphine dose every 3 h as required (p.r.n.) for 5 days. On day 6, the amount taken over the previous 2 days is averaged to a daily dose, which is then taken on a regular fixed twice a day schedule.[200]

Outcomes of opioid management for chronic pain   Controversy continues regarding the use of chronic opioid therapy for chronic non-malignant pain, and relates primarily to fears of possible development of iatrogenic addiction and abuse.[133,288] Studies have demonstrated modest to moderate levels of analgesia in chronic pain, but varied results when examining improvement in functional status.[124,225,255] Moulin et al. examined the effects of morphine SR with active placebo in a double-blind randomized controlled trial in soft tissue or musculoskeletal pain, and failed to demonstrate any functional or psychologic improvements despite significant pain reduction.[202] In a study of patients on long-term opioid therapy, stable long-term pain control was achieved in those patients who finished a 12-month trial (56%) with sustained transdermal fentanyl at doses of approximately 90 μg/h.[195] Others have demonstrated that chronic opioid therapy can lead to a so-called pain opioid downhill spiral characterized by loss of functional capacity and corresponding increase in depressed mood.[255] Studies attempting to corroborate these findings found support for the downhill spiral, but that opioid use independently failed to explain a comparable amount of variance in illness behavior. On the contrary, associated benzodiazepine use was found to be associated with functional impairment, increased healthcare utilization, depression, and pain.[50] Assessing patients' individual psychosocial factors and analgesic response to COAT should incorporate ongoing monitoring of functional improvements and assessment for signs or symptoms of possible addictive or aberrant use (see Table 43-2 for definitions).[305] The physician should be aware of local, state, and federal laws and regulations guiding controlled substance use. Careful individual patient assessment and monitoring, which can include urine and serum toxicology testing, is recommended.[138]

Legislative and federal scrutiny   The more liberal prescribing practices of the late 1990s have been slowed after the realization of increased incidence of abuse and diversion. Increased focus on more comprehensive patient pain and psychologic assessment, as well as standardized office screening and monitoring practices (formal patient–physician contracts or treatment agreements), have become basic standards of practice for physicians choosing to prescribe opioids and other controlled substances. Patient–physician treatment agreements have been published by a number of national pain organizations, including the American Pain Society and the American Academy of Pain

Medicine. Potential complications of agreements include per-petuating stigmas on the patient due to the patient believing opioid prescribing to be a problem, the binding nature of con-tracts remaining unclear, and the existence of significant varia-bility among the content of agreements. This variability includes many contracts with statements limiting driving, although such limitations are not clearly supported in the literature.[79] The use of a 'trilateral' opioid contract has been proposed, which includes the collaboration of primary care physicians, as well as the pain physician and the patient, as a means of effectively transferring care and responsibility for long-term opioid man-agement back to the primary care physician once the individual opioid regimen is stabilized.[79]

Controversies related to COAT   Physicians continue to disa-gree about COAT and the level of symptom relief and physical and psychologic functioning. Questions remain regarding impaired cognitive functioning, endocrine effects, and the pos-sible iatrogenic contribution of opioid-induced hypersensitivity with long-term high-dose opioid management.

Cognitive functioning with opioid therapy   Controversy remains regarding the effects of COAT on psychomotor func-tioning.[316] Haythornthwaite et al. studied the effects of chronic opioid therapy on cognition and mood in a group of chronic pain patients before and after achieving stable opioid doses. Besides reducing pain, long-acting opioid medication reduced anxiety and hostility without declines in cognition, while dem-onstrating improvements on measures of psychomotor speed and sustained attention.[116] Fishbain and colleagues' recent com-prehensive review of studies found that there was moderate, generally consistent evidence for no impairment of psycho-motor abilities, inconclusive evidence for no impairment on cognitive functioning, and strong consistent findings of no evidence of greater incidence of motor vehicle accidents or violations.[76] Others have argued that transient cognitive and psychomotor impairment can be more evident during dose escalation and in opioid-naive patients.[32]

Endocrine effects of long-term high-dose opioid manage-ment   Animal models and some case study reviews in humans have suggested that chronic high-dose opioid therapy can cause abnormalities in hypothalamic–pituitary–adrenal axis and hypothalamic–pituitary–gonadal secretion.[58,236] Endocrine effects can include deceased testosterone, progesterone, and estradiol (resulting in decreased libido in men and women); amenorrhea; and reduced cortisol response to stress. These effects can be more common with administration of intraspinal opioids.[1,213] The syndrome of opioid-induced androgen defi-ciency has been described in case series, and can require addi-tional screening and treatment (testosterone supplementation) by the prescribing physician.

Opioid hyperalgesia and pronociceptive effects   Progress in understanding cellular and neuromodulatory mechanisms involved in addiction and pain treatment point to possible pro-nociceptive effects of chronic opioid therapy, independent of more widely accepted and understood neural mechanisms

involved with the 'desensitization' process of tolerance (a phar-macologic phenomena characterized by the need to increase the dose over the course of time in order to maintain the same opioid analgesic effect). Several mechanisms contribute to these cellular adaptive processes, including receptor desensitization most probably mediated by the NMDA receptor cascade.[171] Repeated administration of opioids might not only contribute to tolerance, but might also lead to a pronociceptive cascade of events (opioid-induced abnormal pain sensitivity) representing a 'sensitization' process supported by evidence of increased spinal dynorphin, descending central facilitation, and activation of pronociceptive glutamate. Some clinicians have suggested maintaining opioid doses at the lowest level required to achieve analgesia as a means of limiting these cellular processes. Periodic opioid rotation and the use of NMDA receptor antagonists and other non-opioid medications within a rational polypharmacy approach have been suggested to limit escalating doses of opioids and possible pronociceptive and tolerance effects.[13] Opioid NMDA antagonists include methadone and propoxyphene. Non-opioid NMDA antagonists include dextromethorphan, ketamine, and memantine. Formal randomized placebo-controlled studies are lacking on the use of these medications.

Anticonvulsant medications as a treatment for neuropathic pain conditions

Neuropathic pain has been defined as pain 'initiated or caused by a primary lesion or dysfunction in the nervous system'.[193] Neuropathic pain manifests as spontaneous pain (stimulus-independent, i.e. paresthesia and dysesthesia) or pain hyper-sensitivity caused by a stimulus after damage or changes in the sensory neurons (stimulus-evoked pain: allodynia and hyperal-gesia).[66] Peripheral mechanisms include sensitization of noci-ceptors by local chemical inflammatory changes (substance P, serotonin, bradykinin, histamine, and COX and lipoxygenase pathways); ectopic activity from damaged, demyelinated, or regenerating nerve sprouts; noradrenergic sensitivity; lowering of neuronal threshold for firing at ectopic areas by accumulation of sodium and calcium channels; and changes at the more proximal dorsal root ganglion (i.e. spontaneous activity).[15] Peripheral changes can also lead to loss of central GABAergic inhibition, opioid receptor down-regulation, and interneuron cell death.[307] Central nervous system changes are primarily due to phenotypic changes of Aβ and C fibers, sprouting of nerve fibers in deeper layers of dorsal horn laminae,[314] and effects of central sensitization. Central sensitization is primarily mediated by the release of neurotransmitters (e.g. substance P, glutamate, CGRP, neurokinin A, and GABA), increased calcium flux, and activation of NMDA receptors.[270]

Understanding basic physiologic neurotransmitter changes can help target the use of a single or a number of anticonvul-sants in the management of chronic neuropathic pain states, including postherpetic neuralgia, diabetic peripheral neuropa-thy, spinal radiculopathy, trigeminal neuralgia, HIV-related neuropathic pain states, and small-fiber neuropathy. Recent treatment recommendations highlight the importance of a mechanistic approach to diagnosis and treatment, and to proposed 'first-line' medications (i.e. gabapentin, 5% lidocaine [lignocaine] patch, opioid analgesics, tramadol, and TCAs) based on positive results from multiple randomized trials, as well as to 'second-line' agents based on positive results from a single randomized controlled trial or inconsistent finding. Second-line agents in some cases have shown greater efficacy but are awaiting future randomized controlled trials.[66]

First-generation anticonvulsants include phenytoin and carbamazepine, which exert membrane-stabilizing effects by blocking sodium channels and reducing neuronal excitability, presumably in sensitized C nociceptors.[64] The use of newer generation anticonvulsants has made their incorporation into outpatient management more practical, given their more favorable metabolic and interaction profiles as compared with traditional anticonvulsants. Older generation antiepileptic drugs (i.e. phenytoin, phenobarbital, carbamazepine, and valproic acid) are effective agents for a number of seizure-related disorders, but they may be less practical options in outpatient chronic pain management due to much less favorable metabolic and interaction profiles when compared with newer generation agents, which may necessitate serum blood level and organ monitoring during titration.[217] To follow is a brief update on newer generation anticonvulsant and neuropathic agents, including key individual pharmacokinetic profiles and suggested therapeutic doses for chronic pain conditions. Most of the anticonvulsant agents have been used off-label, except those with FDA approval, including the 5% lidocaine patch (Lidoderm) and gabapentin (Neurontin) for postherpetic neuralgia and carbamazepine (Tegretol) for trigeminal neuralgia.

Gabapentin has also found wide off-label use for a number of chronic neuropathic pain conditions. Randomized, double-blind, placebo-controlled studies have demonstrated efficacy with analgesia in diabetic peripheral neuropathy (titrated from 900 to 3600 mg/day)[11] and postherpetic neuralgia.[241] These studies showed significant improvement in pain (average daily pain 4.2 versus 6.0 with placebo), sleep, and physical function at similar maximum doses of 3600 mg/day and heterogeneous groups of neuropathic pain.[257] Gabapentin, although structurally related to GABA, is an $\alpha_2\delta$ ligand. The $\alpha_2\delta$ receptor is a protein associated with neuronal voltage-gated calcium channels. Binding to this channel reduces presynaptic calcium influx into the cell at the dorsal horn, reducing the release of several neurotransmitters (glutamate, substance P, norepinephrine, and CGRP). A number of indirect GABAergic mechanisms have also been proposed. Multiple studies have demonstrated significantly reduced pain, and improved sleep, mood, and quality of life, at dosages between 1800 mg/day and 3600 mg/day. Side effects include somnolence and dizziness. Gabapentin's unique pharmacokinetics lend to the necessity of using higher doses as compared with other newer generation anticonvulsants. With escalating dose titration, the intestinal active transport absorption system becomes saturated, decreasing the percentage of bioavailability, resulting in a non-linear relationship between serum concentration and dosage. When this occurs, a significant increase in dosage is needed to see a relative increase in therapeutic response.

Pregabalin is also an $\alpha_2\delta$ ligand and is structurally related to gabapentin, with no intrinsic GABA activity. Studies have demonstrated efficacy in the management of postherpetic neuralgia,[67,84,245] diabetic peripheral neuropathy,[85,234,239] general peripheral neuropathy,[87,122] and generalized anxiety disorder[72,215] with doses between 150 mg/day and 600 mg/day. Pregabalin demonstrates linear pharmacokinetics, and has a rapid onset of actions (within 1 h), stable bioavailability independent of dose (approximately 90%), and an affinity for the $\alpha_2\delta$ subunit that is six times greater than that of gabapentin. Pregabalin appears to work by modulating voltage-gated calcium channels, decreasing calcium influx into the cell, and limiting release of excitatory neurotransmitters (substance P, glutamate, aspartate, and norepinephrine).[75] Pregabalin (Lyrica) is FDA-approved for postherpetic neuralgia and diabetic peripheral neuropathy in the USA, and approved for neuropathic pain in Europe. Pregabalin's relatively increased potency, linear pharmacokinetics, and stable bioavailability, as compared with gabapentin, may diminish the need for prolonged dose titration.

Lamotrigine blocks voltage-dependent sodium channels and N-type calcium channels, and inhibits glutamate release.[108,187] Dosages range from 50 to 400 mg/day. Efficacy has been demonstrated in studies of patients resistant to other therapies with trigeminal neuralgia[317] and central poststroke pain.[296] Oxcarbazepine is an analog of carbamazepine, without the epoxide metabolite. It is felt that the epoxide metabolite is a possible contributor to drug interactions and adverse events associated with carbamazepine use.[186] Oxcarbazepine has shown efficacy in postherpetic neuralgia, trigeminal neuralgia, and diabetic peripheral neuropathy at doses averaging between 600 and 1200 mg/day.[41]

Tiagabine is a novel selective GABA reuptake inhibitor, indicated for partial seizures, that has also been used off-label for chronic neuropathic pain, anxiety, and insomnia. Theoretically, increasing GABA levels at the synaptic cleft (dorsal horn and brain) might help to increase GABA's inhibitory effects on neuronal excitability. Increased GABA levels have been associated with improved sleep, characterized by increasing time in NREM stage 3 and stage 4 sleep.[173]

Topiramate and zonisamide are broad-spectrum anticonvulsants with a number of proposed mechanisms, including inhibition of voltage-gated sodium channels, potentiation of GABAergic inhibition, and blocking excitatory glutamate activity and voltage-gated calcium channels. Inhibition of carbonic anhydrase and antiglutamate effects have been considered as mechanisms responsible for the clinically significant weight loss associated with these medications.[30,90] The mechanism of levetiracetam, an agent with a chemical structure unrelated to that of other anticonvulsants, remains unclear but might include calcium channel effects.[163] It is similar to gabapentin, having minimal drug–drug interactions, and is easily renally excreted.

Antidepressants

Antidepressants have demonstrated mixed efficacy in a number of chronic pain-related conditions (i.e. nociceptive, neuropathic, inflammatory, poststroke pain conditions, central pain states, and headache) and chronic pain-related disorders (i.e. depression, anxiety, and insomnia).[40,247] Antidepressants can be divided into general classes: TCAs, selective serotonin reuptake inhibitors (SSRIs), selective serotonin–norepinephrine reuptake inhibitors, and triazolopyridines (i.e. trazodone and nefazodone). Analgesic effects of antidepressants have primarily been associated with peripheral and central norepinephrine and serotonin effects, but may also involve binding to opioid and NMDA receptor complexes, reducing intracellular Ca^{2+} accumulation, and binding to α adrenoceptors and a number of ion channels (i.e. Na^+, Ca^{2+}, and K^+).[252] Emotional and painful symptoms of depression may be regulated by overlapping pathways for serotonin and norepinephrine at the brain and spinal cord, affecting mood, sleep, coping, and painful symptoms. A more divergent view of transmitter effects has also suggested that the noradrenergic system is involved with motivational activities including energy, interest, and concentration, as compared with serotonergic systems influencing behavioral activity (i.e. sexual function, appetite, and impulsiveness).[61]

Tricyclic antidepressants and SSRIs Tricyclic antidepressants have been found to be effective in controlled trials for a variety of chronic pain conditions.[164] Their use as both potent antidepressants and sedating medications can fit into a number of therapeutic targets related to symptom management of chronic pain syndrome (pain, depression, and disturbed sleep) (Table 43-10). Dosing these medications initially at night can be of benefit for the relatively potent serotonergic, noradrenergic, and antihistaminergic effects. Noradrenergic side effects can be associated with autonomic (i.e. orthostatic hypotension, dizziness, and urinary retention), cardiac (i.e. tachycardia), and ocular (i.e. blurred vision) disturbances. Serotonergic effects can include increased gastric distress, agitation, and headaches.[220] Antihistamine-mediated effects can include decreased gastric acid secretion and sedation. The so-called serotonin syndrome[272] is a rare, reversible clinical syndrome and medical emergency associated with toxic serum and cerebrospinal fluid levels of serotonin. The syndrome is characterized by mental state dysfunction as well as autonomic and neurologic

Table 43-10 Commonly used medications for the treatment of disturbed sleep

Class	Drug	Typical dose (elderly/adult)	Half-life	Mechanism of action	Comments
Non-benzodiazepine hypnotics	Zaleplon (Sonata)	5/10 mg	1 h	Interacts with GABA–benzodiazepine complex to facilitate GABA transmission	Especially useful for sleep initiation disorders
	Zolpidem (Ambien)	5/10 mg	2–4 h	Interacts with GABA–benzodiazepine complex to facilitate GABA transmission	Useful for initiation of sleep; few residual effects with dosages up to 30 mg
	Eszopiclone (Lunesta)	2/3 mg	4–6 h	Exact mechanism unknown; interacts with GABA–benzodiazepine complex to facilitate GABA transmission	Binds BZD-1 receptor with greater affinity than benzodiazepines; FDA-approved for long-term management of insomnia
Benzodiazepines	Triazolam (Halcion)	0.125/0.25 mg	1.5–5.5 h	Enhances inhibitory action of GABA	Useful for initiation of sleep; anterograde amnesia with higher dosages; no active metabolites
	Temazepam (Restoril)	7.5–15/15–30 mg	8–15 h	Enhances inhibitory action of GABA	Useful for initiation of sleep; intermediate duration; no active metabolites
	Lorazepam (Ativan)	0.5–1/1–2 mg	12–15 h	Enhances inhibitory action of GABA	No active metabolites; not marketed as a hypnotic

Continued on page 978

Class	Drug	Typical dose (elderly/adult)	Half-life	Mechanism of action	Comments
	Flurazepam (Dalmane)	7.5–15/15–30 mg	30–100 h	Enhances inhibitory action of GABA	Risk of significant accumulation, especially in the elderly
Tricyclic antidepressants: tertiary amines	Doxepin (Sinequan, Adapin)	25/50–100 mg	8–24 h	Serotonin > noradrenaline (norepinephrine) reuptake inhibition, strong anticholinergic effect, antagonize α_2 and H_1 receptors, Na^+ channel blockade	Sedative effect at lower doses than antidepressant effect
	Amitriptyline (Elavil); with chlordiazepoxide (Limbitrol); with perphenazine (Triavil)	25/50–100 mg	10–28 h (nortriptyline metabolite 18–60 h)	Serotonin > noradrenaline (norepinephrine) reuptake inhibition, strong anticholinergic effect, antagonize α_2 and H_1 receptors, Na^+ channel blockade	Beneficial for patients with depression and early morning awakening; neuropathic pain; strong anticholinergic action; sedative effect at lower doses than antidepressant effect
	Imipramine (Tofranil, Tofranil PM)	10/25–75 mg	6–20 h	Serotonin > noradrenaline (norepinephrine) reuptake inhibition, strong anticholinergic effect, antagonize α_2 and H_1 receptors, Na^+ channel blockade	Sedative effect at lower doses than antidepressant effect
Tricyclic antidepressants: secondary amines	Nortriptyline (Aventyl, Pamelor)	10/25 mg	28–31 h	Serotonin > noradrenaline (norepinephrine) reuptake inhibition, anticholinergic effects, antagonize α_2 and H_1 receptors, Na^+ channel blockade	Less sedation and fewer anticholinergic effects
	Desipramine (Norpramin)	10/25 mg	14–62 h	Noradrenaline (norepinephrine) > serotonin reuptake inhibition, anticholinergic effects, antagonize α_2 and H_1 receptors, Na^+ channel blockade	Less sedation and fewer anticholinergic effects
Triazolopyridine derivatives	Trazodone (Desyrel)	25/50–100 mg	Biphasic (3–6 h, 5–9 h)	Serotonin receptor antagonist, serotonin reuptake inhibition	Shorter half-life than tricyclic antidepressants; lower anticholinergic profile
Non-prescription antihistamines	Diphenhydramine (Benadryl, Banaril, Dytuss, Hyrexin), with acetaminophen (Excedrin PM, Tylenol PM, Sominex Pain Relief)	12.5/25–50 mg	3.5–17.5 h	Antihistamine, H_1 receptor	Mild sedation; effect may be lost after 3–4 days of use; strong anticholinergic effects

Continued from page 977 Table 43-10 Commonly used medications for the treatment of disturbed sleep symptoms, and can occur with concomitant use of TCAs and other medications, including SSRIs[197] and tramadol (a synthetic codeine analog with noradrenergic and serotonergic effects).[104,233]

Analgesic effects of TCAs can be evident within 1 week of dose initiation, and followed later by antidepressant effects with escalating dose titration.[164,221] Although SSRI use has surpassed the use of traditional antidepressants due to a more tolerable side effect profile, analgesic effects of these compounds have been mixed in a number of controlled studies including diabetic peripheral neuropathy[174,175,262,263,265] and fibromyalgia.[106,310] Studies involving the use of triazolopyridines, which are compounds with similar chemical properties to those of TCAs (including trazodone and nefazodone), have demonstrated little to no analgesic effects, although they can be beneficial in restoring sleep.[59,86] A more rational polypharmacy approach can include the use of SSRIs dosed in the morning, in conjunction with a more sedating TCA or TCA-like medication at night for pain-related insomnia.

Serotonin–norepinephrine reuptake inhibitors The newest class of antidepressants, dual monoamine reuptake inhibitors, was developed for the treatment of depression with a goal of providing shorter onset of antidepressant effects and less side effects due to their relative serotonin and norepinephrine selectivity. Mirtazapine is a potent antagonist of central α_2-adrenergic receptors, an antagonist of 5-HT$_2$ and 5-HT$_3$ receptors, and an enhancer of norepinephrine and serotonin neurotransmission. Mirtazapine is indicated for the treatment of depression, and can be used to enhance the efficacy of SSRIs. Its relatively sedating effects can have additional benefits for improving sleep in patients with chronic pain. Venlafaxine is a potent dual reuptake inhibitor of serotonin (at lower doses), and of norepinephrine and possibly dopamine (at higher doses), without binding to cholinergic, histaminic, or α_1-adrenergic receptor sites. Analgesic effects have been found in animal models,[153] and in human studies including a number of case reports and case series of heterogeneous chronic pain conditions,[268,283] neuropathic pain states,[282] and fibromyalgia.[65] The newest selective serotonin–norepinephrine reuptake inhibitor, duloxetine, is a potent balanced reuptake inhibitor of both serotonin and norepinephrine, and demonstrates a higher affinity for monoamine transporters as compared with venlafaxine.[36] Duloxetine is indicated for major depressive disorder, diabetic peripheral neuropathy, and postherpetic neuralgia. Additional benefit has been reported in a randomized, double-blind, placebo-controlled study of patients with primary fibromyalgia. Duloxetine (titrated to 60 mg twice daily) improved fibromyalgia-related symptoms and pain severity independent of baseline depression in women greater than in men.[7]

Medication for insomnia

Pain is an important factor related to sleep problems in community-based studies,[105] and may reflect a bidirectional relationship where pain may interrupt onset and quality of sleep while pain intensity may be exacerbated by insufficient or non-restorative sleep patterns.[2] Pain clinic studies report greater than 70% of patients reporting disturbed sleep.[199,219] In one study of patients with chronic pain, McCracken and Iverson reported at least 90% of patients reporting at least one sleep disturbance.[182] Severity of sleep disturbance has also been correlated with greater pain, depression, and disability.[182,199,309] Multiple classes of medications with a number of differing mechanisms are available for pain-related insomnia and may be incorporated into a rational polypharmacy approach (Table 43-10).

From a historical perspective, treatment for pain-related insomnia has primarily relied on pharmacotherapy. Barbiturates, barbiturate-like compounds, and antihistamines were commonly used until the introduction of the benzodiazepines, which had fewer safety concerns and less potential for the development of tolerance. However, over the past decade, the use of benzodiazepines has declined with the introduction of the non-benzodiazepine hypnotics, also commonly referred to as the Z drugs (zolpidem and zaleplon).[254] Like the benzodiazepines, the Z drugs facilitate GABA$_A$ transmission by preferential binding at the 1a receptor subunits (corresponding to benzodiazepine receptor subtype 1), and therefore are devoid of the significant muscle relaxant, anxiolytic, and anticonvulsant activity of traditional full agonist benzodiazepines.[250] A third non-benzodiazepine hypnotic, eszopiclone, is FDA-approved for the long-term management of insomnia, and retains a greater half-life (5–5.8 h) with evidence of greater sleep maintenance efficacy as compared with the current relatively shorter half-life Z drugs.[318]

In addition to medications that affect the benzodiazepine receptor complex, there are a number of other drugs that have profound effects on sleep and wakefulness. Medications such as the TCAs and trazodone are especially useful in patients with disturbed sleep that is present with concurrent chronic conditions such as elevated anxiety levels, depression, and myofascial or neuropathic pain. These drugs increase total sleep time as well as NREM stage 2 sleep. They act by inhibition of norepinephrine and serotonin uptake, and block histamine and acetylcholine. When choosing a medication to address disturbed sleep, the half-life of the medication should be considered to ensure that the medication is appropriate for the particular sleep disturbance. Patients with trouble initiating sleep may require shorter acting medications, while those with fragmented sleep and frequent awakenings may more ideally benefit from medications with an intermediate to long half-life.

There is little evidence to support the long-term use of benzodiazepines for the management of insomnia and anxiety in chronic pain.[107] Some have suggested that chronic use might simply prevent rebound insomnia rather than promote restorative sleep.[226,248] Chronic benzodiazepine use can lead to associated cognitive impairment, and it can increase risk for falls, produce rebound insomnia with prolonged use, disrupt normal sleep architecture, and promote misuse and abuse in patients with histories of substance-related disorders.[107,135,150,243] Medications with other secondary sedating qualities may also be considered as part of this approach (i.e. muscle relaxers, TCAs and tricyclic-like antidepressants, and novel antidepressants). Older and newer generation anticonvulsants have been shown to decrease sleep latency and to increase total sleep time and slow-wave sleep.[229] In general, opiates tend to produce sedation, and have the effect of increasing sleep fragmentation and decreasing REM and stage 2 sleep. Antidepressants in the SSRI class are associated with both insomnia and somnolence, depending on the specific medication. Overall, they tend to decrease total sleep time and are less sedating than the TCAs. SSRIs can reduce REM sleep. A complete sleep history can help determine behavioral issues impacting insomnia, as well as the excessive use of nicotine and alcohol prior to bedtime. Nicotine use may lead to delayed sleep onset. Alcohol's relatively sedating qualities may facilitate sleep by increasing slow-wave and reducing REM sleep, but it also may cause a rebound increase in sleep fragmentation later in the sleep cycle.

Topical analgesics

The use of over the counter and prescription topical analgesics continues to grow. An increased understanding of nociceptor physiology, including a greater understanding of thermosensation, has been spurred by identification of proteins called vanilloid receptors, detectors of noxious heat, and subsequent identification of a new family of thermosensation receptors, the transient receptor protein vanilloid channel (TRPV) family.[137] The vanilloid receptor (TRPV1) is a non-selective cation receptor activated by capsaicin, the pungent agent found in chili peppers. Another TRPV receptor, the cold- and menthol-sensitive receptor, has been identified and might contribute to a better understanding of cold thermosensation and the possible development of targeted cold-producing analgesics. Pharmacologic studies of menthol have suggested a possible κ-opioid receptor effect, providing additional analgesic properties to the substance.[92] A number of prescription and over the counter topical therapies are available for the treatment of musculoskeletal and neuropathic pain states, including the lidocaine (lignocaine) patch, topical TCAs, capsaicin creams, and topical NSAIDs.

Prescription medications include lidocaine 5% patches that are indicated for postherpetic neuralgia. Lidocaine acts peripherally by blocking sodium channels. Randomized placebo-controlled studies have demonstrated analgesic efficacy in postherpetic neuralgia[241] and focal peripheral neuropathic pain syndromes.[188] Safety and decreased risk for systemic effects with multiple patches worn up to 24 h at a time has more recently been reported.[95]

More widely used in Europe, topical TCAs such as doxepin and amitriptyline have demonstrated efficacy in a number of neuropathic pain states.[103,178] Topical capsaicin, which depletes substance P and CGRP, leading to a pharmacologic desensitization of nociceptors, has demonstrated efficacy in a number of trials, including diabetic peripheral neuropathy, HIV-associated neuropathic pain, and painful distal polyneuropathy.[39,160,212] More widespread use in chronic pain is limited by poor patient tolerability of the necessary 'desensitization' application process.

Over the counter topical analgesics include NSAIDs, capsaicin, and menthol-based products. Compounding pharmacies can serve a unique service in providing customized compounding of various creams and gels for topical use, including ketamine, gabapentin, cyclobenzaprine, and various NSAIDs.[132]

Mind–body medicine

Mind–body medicine describes a subset of medical care that attempts to tie together methods of ancient traditional eastern healing techniques with the modern biopsychosocial model of healthcare. Therapies that fall under the guise of mind–body medicine include but are not limited to relaxation therapy, biofeedback, meditation, hypnosis, guided imagery, yoga, and t'ai chi. Many of these methods, such as meditation and relaxation therapy, display significant overlap in basic theory and mechanism, while other methods, such as t'ai chi and yoga, can be further subclassified as movement-based therapies. Two of the more commonly used mind–body medicine techniques, relaxation training and biofeedback, are described below.

Relaxation training

Relaxation techniques are incorporated to some extent as an element of almost all mind–body medicine therapies, most notably in meditation, guided imagery, hypnosis, and biofeedback. The technique of progressive muscle relaxation as developed by Jacobson in 1938[123] is perhaps the most popular form of relaxation training, although it has been modified and abbreviated by various practitioners. Progressive muscle relaxation teaches the patient to sequentially voluntarily contract and then relax various muscle groups. Through this voluntary cycle, the patient gains insight into the sensation of muscle tension, which can then facilitate subsequent muscular relaxation.

Progressive muscle relaxation has been studied in various chronic conditions, with strong support for its use in the treatment of anxiety, depression, headache, and insomnia, as well as chronic pain.[12,16,25,119,205] Treatments are commonly combined with guided imagery or meditation, and a brief form of progressive muscle relaxation known as self-control relaxation can be taught to patients to practice during periods of acute flare-ups. Relaxation therapies are ideal behavioral techniques for patients with chronic pain conditions, because they are easy to learn, utilize minimal healthcare resources, and are without side effects.

Biofeedback

Biofeedback is a therapeutic technique that utilizes various forms of auditory and visual physiologic monitoring to teach patients to modify physiologic functions that are not normally under conscious control. Common target responses include heart rate, blood pressure, skin temperature, and muscle tension. Clinical approaches utilized during biofeedback training are similar to those utilized in relaxation therapy, and include diaphragmatic breathing, imagery, progressive muscle relaxation, and autogenic training.

The positive effects of biofeedback have been documented in numerous chronic pain conditions, including low back pain, headache, temporomandibular disorders, and fibromyalgia.[16,33,56,297] It is an important form of therapeutic training for chronic pain conditions, because it allows and encourages the patient to achieve an improved sense of self-control and self-efficacy.

Movement-based therapies
Aquatic rehabilitation
The physical properties of water make it an ideal setting for the rehabilitation of selected chronic pain patients, such as those with significant fear and anxiety related to movement. The pool-based environment affords numerous advantages to land-based therapy, due to the buoyancy and viscosity provided by water. The buoyant force reduces the effective weight of the patient in proportion to the depth of water. Weight-bearing loads are reduced to 40% of total body weight when standing in chest-deep water.[114] With the patient in a floating state, the effects of gravity are eliminated. Aquatic-based therapy programs allow for graduated loads to tissue by progressively decreasing the depth at which therapy is performed. The viscosity of water provides resistance to movement equal to that of the force exerted by the patient. This resistance also varies with the speed of movement performed.[228]

Reduced self-reported levels of pain, anxiety, and depression have been shown in patients with fibromyalgia who participated in a pool-based physical therapy program.[129] Other studies have reported improvements in pain, fatigue, social and physical function, and quality of life.[168,169] Effects can last up to 24 months after participation in a pool-based exercise program.[168] Other benefits include muscle relaxation, improved body awareness, cardiorespiratory fitness, balance, and coordination.[228]

Pilates
The Pilates method was developed by Joseph Pilates in the early 1920s as a training process that utilizes specially designed resistance training equipment to perform ordered exercise sequences that focus on core strengthening, power, concentration, breathing, and kinesthetic awareness. While the method has traditionally been practiced by ballet dancers, it has now progressed to the mainstream world of fitness.

There is a scant body of literature supporting its role in the treatment of chronic pain syndromes, and its use is experiential. There are reports of improvements in strength and flexibility, as well as static and dynamic posture in selected populations.[121]

Yoga
With its name derived from the Sanskrit *yug*, which means 'to join', yoga dates back to the third century BC. The *Yoga Sutra*, a philosophic guidebook for the practice of yoga, was initially compiled by the Indian sage Patanjali, who is considered to be the father of classic yoga. He described eight limbs of the philosophy to be followed for achieving a moral, meaningful life: *yama* (moral behavior), *niyama* (healthy habit), *asana* (physical postures), *pranayama* (breathing exercises), *pratyahara* (sense withdrawal), *dharana* (concentration), *dhyana* (contemplation), and *samadhi* (higher consciousness). There are six branches of yoga that each offers a particular approach to life. *Raja* yoga calls for strict adherence to the eight limbs described in the *Yoga Sutra*, while *hatha* yoga techniques focus more on physical postures (*asanas*).

While there are a number of different yoga styles, the most popular forms of yoga focus on the performance of various postures (asanas), stretches, and controlled breathing (pranayamas). Yoga programs have been reported to improve balance and flexibility;[91,232] decrease disability and depression;[91] reduce blood pressure, heart rate, and anxiety;[232] and improve range of motion, muscular endurance, and lung capacity.[232] The beneficial effects on pain might be derived from the control of stress and depression, and the relaxation, stretching, and strengthening of targeted muscles.[91,98,99,206] Yoga can also be practiced in a group setting or with individual instruction.

Feldenkrais
The Feldenkrais method is a system of body retraining created by Moshe Feldenkrais, a Russian-born Israeli physicist. The method incorporates gentle stretching, reaching, and postural change sequences with a goal of improved kinesthetic awareness and psychologic well-being. The two complementary components of the Feldenkrais method—'awareness through movement', which consists of verbal cues to movement, and 'functional integration', which involves touch to facilitate movement—can be practiced together or independently of each other. Movement sequences can replicate activities of daily living or can be abstract in nature.

Feldenkrais therapy has been reported to improve health-related quality of life and self-efficacy of pain in patients with persistent non-specific musculoskeletal complaints.[167] Other effects of the Feldenkrais method include decreased perceived stress, lowered anxiety,[130] and improvement in mood.[207] The slow, fluid movements can be performed by patients at any functional level. In addition, the technique can be taught in gravity-eliminated positions such as lying down.

T'ai chi
T'ai chi chuan, commonly referred to as t'ai chi, translates as 'supreme ultimate boxing'. However, the method itself incorporates both a health regimen and a Chinese martial art with a common set of principles and movements. T'ai chi is known for the integration of sharp mental focus with slow, rhythmic, dancelike movement sequences and postures that unite the mind and body by facilitating the flow of *qi* throughout the body. The gentle nature of the technique allows for the practice by patients of various functional levels and chronic disease processes.

In a sample of women diagnosed and treated for breast cancer, those involved in a program of t'ai chi demonstrated improvements in health-related quality of life and self-esteem compared with those who solely received psychosocial support.[204] Other reported beneficial effects of t'ai chi include improved functional balance,[146,155] quality of life, activity tolerance, cardiovascular function, pain management, flexibility, strength, and kinesthetic sense.[146]

CONCLUSION

The quest to relieve pain and suffering has challenged human-kind for centuries. Treatment and a better understanding of the complex multidimensional experience of pain have historically evolved with the growth in understanding of anatomy and physiology, psychology, and behavioral and cognitive aspects of human behavior. A crude understanding of basic pain pathways as a peripheral 'specific' mechanism has evolved into a more 'central' comprehensive understanding of the nature of complicated pain pathways, cellular mechanisms of pain transmission (peripheral and central sensitization), complex interactions of cerebral inputs into pain processing, and effects of previous experiences in shaping the experience of pain and pain-related suffering.

A biopsychosocial physiatric approach to understanding and treating pain (acute or chronic) can be the most pragmatic one. Psychologic factors, including levels of affective distress, maladaptive beliefs, operant issues, fears, and level of social support, can be important contributors to the subjective experience of pain and are therefore appropriate targets for treatment. A thorough pain assessment and likelihood of a more accurate clinical diagnosis can be achieved with the incorporation of related psychometric measures and diagnostic tests in conjunction with a comprehensive history and physical examination.

A rational approach to treatment incorporates goals for achieving realistic levels of analgesia, improvement of mood and sleep, and restoration of function with the use of one or a number of medications with complementary pharmacologic activity at different sites along the pain pathway. Successful use of a rational polypharmacy approach (i.e. TCAs, NSAIDs, novel antidepressants, and opioids) is based on appropriate patient selection, understanding of medication mechanisms of action, pharmacokinetics, pharmacodynamics, side effect profiles, and risks for potential aberrant use. Appropriate goal-oriented treatment can include active and passive therapies, cognitive behavioral therapy, relaxation training, and other mind–body therapies. Formal multidisciplinary and/or inter-disciplinary functional restoration treatment programs may be necessary for those patients who have failed more unimodal approaches. The physiatrist is encouraged to approach all patients with persistent pain from a diagnostic and therapeutic perspective in a multidisciplinary biopsychosocial manner as a means of improving psychosocial function, decreasing pain, and improving quality of life.

REFERENCES

1. Abs R, Verhelst J, Maeyaert J, et al. Endocrine consequences of long-term intrathecal administration of opioids. J Clin Endocrinol Metab 2000; 85:2215–2222.

2. Affleck G, Urrows S, Tennen H, et al. Sequential daily relations of sleep, pain intensity, and attention to pain among women with fibromyalgia. Pain 1996; 68:363–368.

3. Aldrich S, Eccleston C, Crombez G. Worrying about chronic pain: vigilance to threat and misdirected problem solving. Behav Res Ther 2000; 38:457–470.

4. American Psychiatric Association. Diagnostic and statistical manual of mental disorders. 4th edn. Washington: APA; 1994.

5. Andersson HI. The epidemiology of chronic pain in a Swedish rural area. Qual Life Res 1994; 3:S19–S26.

6. Apkarian AV, Sosa Y, Sonty S, et al. Chronic back pain is associated with decreased prefrontal and thalamic gray matter density. J Neurosci 2004; 24:10410–10415.

7. Arnold LM, Crofford LY, Wohlreich M. A double-blind, multicenter trial comparing duloxetine with placebo in the treatment of fibromyalgia patients with or without major depressive disorder. Arthritis Rheum 2004; 50:2974–2984.

8. Ashburn MA, Staats PS. Management of chronic pain. Lancet 1999; 353:1865–1869.

9. Atkinson JH, Slater MA, Grant I, et al. Depressed mood in chronic low back pain: relationship with stressful life event. Pain 1988; 35: 47–55.

10. Aw TJ, Haas SJ, Liew D, et al. Meta-analysis of cyclooxygenase-2 inhibitors and their effects on blood pressure. Arch Intern Med 2005; 165:1–7.

11. Backonja M, Beydoun A, Edwards KR, et al. Gabapentin for the symptomatic treatment of painful neuropathy in patients with diabetes mellitus: a randomized controlled trial. JAMA 1998; 280:1831–1836.

12. Baird CL, Sands L. A pilot study of the effectiveness of guided imagery with progressive muscle relaxation to reduce chronic pain and mobility difficulties of osteoarthritis. Pain Manage Nurs 2004; 5:97–104.

13. Ballantyne JC, Mao J. Opioid therapy for chronic pain. N Engl J Med 2003; 349:1943–1953.

14. Banks SM, Kerns RD. Explaining high rates of depression in chronic pain: a diathesis–stress framework. Psychol Bull 1996; 119:95–110.

15. Baron R. Peripheral neuropathic pain: from mechanisms to symptoms. Clin J Pain 2000; 16(2 suppl):S12–S20.

16. Barrows KA, Jacobs BP. Mind–body medicine. An introduction and review of the literature. Med Clin North Am 2002; 86:11–31.

17. Beck AT, Rush AJ, Shaw BF, et al. Cognitive therapy of depression. New York: Guilford Press; 1979.

18. Beck AT, Steer RA. Beck Depression Inventory manual. New York: Psychological Corp.; 1987.

19. Becker E, Horn S, Hussla B, et al. Guidelines for the sociomedical assessment of performance in patients suffering from discopathy or associated diseases. Gesundheitswesen 2003; 65(1):19–39 (in German).

20. Beecher HK. Measurement of subjective responses: quantitative effects of drugs. New York: Oxford University Press; 1959.

21. Bendix AF, Bendix T, Lund C, et al. A prospective, randomized, 5-year follow-up study of functional restoration in chronic low back pain patients. Eur Spine J 1998; 7:111–119.

22. Bergener M, Bobbit RA, Carter WB. The Sickness Impact Profile: development and final revision of a health status measure. Med Care 1981; 19:787–805.

23. Bergman NA. The genesis of surgical anesthesia. Park Ridge: Wood Library–Museum of Anesthesiology; 1998:18.

24. Berry PH, Chapman CR, Covington EC, et al. Pain: current understanding of assessment, management, and treatments. Oakbrook Terrace: Joint Commission on Accreditation of Healthcare Organizations; 2001.

25. Blanchard EB, Nicholson NL, Taylor AE, et al. The role of regular home practice in the relaxation treatment of tension headache. J Consult Clin Psychol 1991; 59:467–470.

26. Bombardier C, Lain L, Reicin A, et al. Comparison of upper gastrointestinal toxicity of rofecoxib and naproxen in patients with rheumatoid arthritis. VIGOR Study Group. N Engl J Med 2000; 343:1520–1528.

27. Bonica JJ, Loeser JD. History of pain concepts and therapies. In: Loeser JD, Butler SH, Chapman CR, et al, eds. Bonica's management of pain. Philadelphia: Lippincott Williams & Wilkins; 2001:3–16.

28. Bradley LA, McKendree-Smith NL, Cianfrini LR. Cognitive-behavioral therapy interventions for pain associated with chronic illness. Semin Pain Med 2003; 1:44–54.

29. Brattberg G, Thorslund M, Wikman A. The prevalence of pain in a general population. The results of a postal survey in a county of Sweden. Pain 1989; 37:215–222.

30. Bray GA, Hollander P, Klein S, et al. A 6-month randomized, placebo-controlled, dose-ranging trial of topiramate for weight loss in obesity. Obes Res 2003; 11(6):722–733.

31. Brown SC, Glass JM, Park DC. The relationship of pain and depression to cognitive function in rheumatoid arthritis patients. Pain 2002; 96:279–284.

32. Bruera E, Macmillan K, Hanson K, et al. The cognitive effects of the administration of narcotic analgesics in patients with cancer pain. Pain 1989; 39:13–16.

33. Buckelew SP, Conway R, Parker J, et al. Biofeedback/relaxation training and exercise interventions for fibromyalgia: a prospective trial. Arthritis Care Res 1998; 11:196–209.

34. Burns JW. Anger management style and hostility: predicting symptom-specific physiological reactivity among chronic low back pain patients. J Behav Med 1997; 20:505–522.

35. Butcher JN, Dahlstrom WG, Graham JR. MMPI-2: manual for administration and scoring. Minneapolis: University of Minnesota Press; 1989.

36. Bymaster FP, Dreshfield-Ahmad LJ, Threlkeld PG, et al. Comparative affinity of duloxetine and venlafaxine for serotonin and norepinephrine transporters in vitro and in vivo, human serotonin receptor subtypes and other neuronal receptors. Neuropsychopharmacology 2001; 25:871–880.

37. Call-Schmidt TA, Richardson SJ. Prevalence of sleep disturbance and its relationship to pain in adults with chronic pain. Pain Manage Nurs 2003; 4:124–133.

38. Cao YQ, Mantyh PW, Carlson EJ, et al. Primary afferent tachykinins are required to experience moderate to intense pain. Nature 1998; 392:390–394.

39. Capsaicin Study Group. Treatment of painful diabetic peripheral neuropathy with topical capsaicin. A multicenter, double-blind, vehicle-controlled study. Arch Intern Med 1991; 151:2225–2229.

40. Cardenas DD, Warms CA, Turner JA, et al. Efficacy of amitriptyline for relief of pain in spinal cord injury: results of a randomized controlled trial. Pain 2002; 96:365–373.

41. Carrazana E, Mikoshiba I. Rationale and evidence for the use of oxcarbazepine in neuropathic pain. J Pain Symptom Manage 2003; 25(5 suppl): S31–S35.

42. Catala E, Reig E, Artes M, et al. Prevalence of pain in the Spanish population: telephone survey in 5000 homes. Eur J Pain 2002; 6:133–140.

43. Caterina MJ, Julius D. Sense and specificity: a molecular identity for nociceptors. Curr Opin Neurobiol 1999; 9:525–530.

44. Centers for Disease Control and Prevention. 2001.

45. Centers for Medicare and Medicaid Services. Glossary. Online. Available: http://www.cms.hhs.gov/glossary 20 June 2005.

46. Cervero F. Sensory innervation of the viscera: peripheral basis of visceral pain. Physiol Rev 1994; 74:95–138.

47. Chapman CR, Okifuji A. Pain: basic mechanisms and conscious experience. In: Breitbart D, ed. Psychosocial aspects of pain: a handbook for healthcare providers, progress in pain research and management, vol 27. Seattle: IASP Press; 2004.

48. Chapman CR, Stillman M. Pathological pain. In: Kruger L, ed. Pain and thought. 2nd edn. New York: Academic Press; 1996.

49. Cheng JF, Harris RC. Cyclooxygenases, the kidney, and hypertension. Hypertension 2004; 43:525–530.

50. Ciccone DS, Just N, Bandilla EB, et al. Psychological correlates of opioid use in patients with chronic nonmalignant pain: a preliminary test of the downhill spiral hypothesis. J Pain Symptom Manage 2000; 20:180–192.

51. Cleeland CS, Ryan KM. Pain assessment: global use of the Brief Pain Inventory. Ann Acad Med 1994; 23:129–138.

52. Coda BA, Bonica JJ. General considerations of acute pain. In: Lowese JD, Bonica JJ, eds. Bonica's management of pain. 3rd edn. Philadelphia: Lippincott Williams & Wilkins; 2001: 222–240.

53. Compas BE, Keefe FJ, Haaga DA, et al. Sampling of empirically supported psychological treatments from health psychology: smoking, chronic pain, cancer, and bulimia nervosa. J Consult Clin Psychol 1998; 66:89–112.

54. Costiglione A. The renaissance of medicine in Italy. Baltimore: Johns Hopkins Press; 1934.

55. Craig AD. Pain mechanisms: labeled lines versus convergence in central processing. Annu Rev Neurosci 2003; 26:1–30.

56. Crider AB, Glaros AG. A meta-analysis of EMG biofeedback treatment of temporomandibular disorders. J Orofac Pain 1999; 13:29–37.

57. Dalen JE. Selective COX-2 inhibitors, NSAIDs, aspirin, and myocardial infarction. Arch Intern Med 2002; 162:1091–1092.

58. Daniell HW. Hypogonadism in men consuming sustained-action oral opioids. J Pain 2002; 3(5):377–384.

59. Davidoff G, Guarracini M, Roth E, et al. Trazodone hydrochloride in the treatment of dysesthetic pain in traumatic myelopathy: a randomized, double-blind, placebo-controlled study. Pain 1987; 29:151–161.

60. De Felipe C, Herrero JF, O'Brien JA, et al. Altered nociception, analgesia and aggression in mice lacing the receptor for substance P. Nature 1998; 392:394–397.

61. Delgado PL. Common pathways of depression and pain. J Clin Psychiatry 2004; 65(suppl 12):16–19.

62. Dequeker J, Hawkey C, Kahan A, et al. Improvement in gastrointestinal tolerability of the selective cyclooxygenase COX-2 inhibitor, meloxicam, compared with piroxicam: results of the Safety and Efficacy Large Scale Evaluation of COX Inhibition Therapies (SELECT) trial in osteoarthritis. Br J Rheumatol 1998; 37:946–951.

63. Derogatis LR. The SCL-90-R manual II: administration, scoring, and procedures. Towson: Clinical Psychometric Press; 1983.

64. Dray A. Kinins and their receptors in hyperalgesia. Can J Physiol Pharmacol 1997; 75:704–712.

65. Dwight MM, Arnold LM, O'Brien H, et al. An open clinical trial of venlafaxine treatment of fibromyalgia. Psychosomatics 1998; 39:14–17.

66. Dworkin RH, Backonja M, Rowbotham MC, et al. Advances in neuropathic pain: diagnosis, mechanisms, and treatment recommendations. Arch Neurol 2003; 60:1524–1534.

67. Dworkin RH, Corbin AE, Young JP, et al. Pregabalin for the treatment of postherpetic neuralgia: a randomized, placebo-controlled trial. Neurology 2003; 60:1274–1283.

68. Ehde DM, Jensen MP, Engel JM, et al. Chronic pain secondary to disability: a review. Clin J Pain 2003; 19:3–17.

69. Elliott AM, Smith BH, Penny KI, et al. The epidemiology of chronic pain in the community. Lancet 1999; 354(9186):1248–1252.

70. Estlander AM, Takala EP, Verkasalo M. Assessment of depression in chronic musculoskeletal pain patients. Clin J Pain 1995; 11:194–200.

71. Farrar JT, Young JP Jr, LaMoreaux L, et al. Clinical importance of changes in chronic pain intensity measured on an 11-point numerical pain rating scale. Pain 2001; 94:149–158.

72. Feltner DE, Crockatt JG, Dubovsky SJ, et al. A randomized, double-blind, placebo-controlled, fixed-dose, multicenter study of pregabalin in patients with generalized anxiety disorder. J Clin Psychopharm 2003; 23:240–249.

73. Fernandez E, Turk DC. The scope and significance of anger in the experience of chronic pain. Pain 1995; 61:165–175.

74. Fields H. State-dependent opioid control of pain. Nat Rev Neurosci 2004; 5(7):565–575.

75. Fink K, Dooley DJ, Meder WP, et al. Inhibition of neuronal Ca^{2+} influx by gabapentin and pregabalin in the human neocortex. Neuropharmacology 2002; 42(2):229–236.

76. Fishbain DA, Cutler RB, Rosomoff HL, et al. Are opioid-dependent/tolerant patients impaired in driving-related skills? A structured evidence-based review. J Pain Symptom Manage 2003; 25(6):559–577.

77. Fishbain DA, Cutler RB, Rosomoff HL, et al. Chronic pain associated depression: antecedent or consequence of chronic pain? A review. Clin J Pain 1997; 13:116–137.

78. Fishbain DA, Goldeberg M, Meagher BR, et al. Male and female chronic pain patients categorized by DSM-III psychiatric diagnostic criteria. Pain 1986; 26:181–197.

79. Fishman SM, Kreis PG. The opioid contract. Clin J Pain 2002; 18: S70–S75.

80. Flor H, Birbaumer N, Schugens MM, et al. Symptom-specific psychophysiological responses in chronic pain patients. Psychophysiology 1992; 29:452–460.

81. Flor H, Birbaumer N, Turk DC. The psychobiology of chronic pain. Adv Behav Res Ther 1990; 12:47–84.

82. Flor H, Turk DC, Burbaumer N. Assessment of stress-related psychophysiological reactions in chronic back pain patients. J Consult Clin Psychol 1985; 53:354–364.

83. Fordyce WE. Behavioral methods of chronic pain and illness. St. Louis: Mosby; 1976.

84. Frampton JE, Foster RH. Pregabalin: in the treatment of postherpetic neuralgia. Drugs 2005; 65:1111–1118.

85. Frampton JE, Scott LJ. Pregabalin: in the treatment of painful diabetic peripheral neuropathy. Drugs 2004; 64:2813–2820.

86. Frank RG, Beck NC, Parker JC, et al. Depression in rheumatoid arthritis. J Rheumatol 1988; 15:920-925.

87. Freynhagen R, Strojek K, Griesing T, et al. Efficacy of pregabalin in neuropathic pain evaluated in a 12-week, randomized, double-blind, multicentre, placebo-controlled trial of flexible- and fixed-dose regimens. Pain 2005; 115:254–263.

88. Fromm-Reichmann F. Principles of intensive psychotherapy. Chicago: University of Chicago Press; 1950.

89. Frymoyer JW, Durett CL. The economics of spinal disorders. In: Frymoyer JW, ed. The adult spine. Philadelphia: Lippincott-Raven; 1997.

90. Gadde KM, Franciscy DM, Wagner HR II, et al. Zonisamide for weight loss in obese adults: a randomized controlled trial. JAMA 2003; 289(14):1820–1825.

91. Galantino ML, Bzdewka TM, Eissler-Russo J, et al. The impact of modified Hatha yoga on chronic low back pain: a pilot study. Altern Ther Health Med 2004; 10:56–58.

92. Galeotti N, Mannelli LD, Mazzanti G, et al. Menthol: a natural analgesic compound. Neurosci Lett 2002; 322:145–148.

93. Gallagher RM, Moore P, Chernoff I. The reliability of depression diagnosis in chronic low back pain. Gen Hosp Psychiatry 1995; 17:399–413.

94. Gallagher RM. Treatment planning in pain medicine. Integrating medical, physical, and behavioral therapies. Med Clin North Am 1999; 83:823–849.

95. Gammaitoni AR, Davis MW. Pharmacokinetics and safety of continuously applied lidocaine patches 5%. Am J Health-Syst Pharm 2002; 59:2215–2220.

96. Gamsa A. The role of psychological factors in chronic pain: II. A critical appraisal. Pain 1994; 57(1):17–29.

97. Ganidagli S, Cengiz M, Aksoy S, et al. Approach to painful disorders by Serefeddin Sabuncuoglu in the fifteenth century Ottoman period. Anesthesiology 2004; 100:165–169.

98. Garfinkel MS, Schumacher HR, Husain A, et al. Evaluation of a yoga based regimen for treatment of osteoarthritis of the hands. J Rheumatol 1994; 21:2341–2343.

99. Garfinkel MS, Singhal A, Katz WA, et al. Yoga-based intervention for carpal tunnel syndrome. JAMA 1998; 280:1601–1603.

100. Gatchel RJ. Perspectives on pain: a historical overview. In: Gatchel RJ, Turk DC, eds. Psychosocial factors in pain. New York: Guilford Press; 1999.

101. Gebhart GF. Visceral pain. Seattle: IASP Press; 1995:516.

102. Geisser ME, Roth RS, Theisen ME, et al. Negative effect, self-report of depressive symptoms, and clinical depression: relation to experience of chronic pain. Clin J Pain 2000; 16:110–120.

103. Gerner P, Kao G, Srinivasa V, et al. Topical amitriptyline in healthy volunteers. Reg Anesth Pain Med 2003; 28:289–293.

104. Gilliam PK. Serotonin syndrome: history and risk. Fundam Clin Pharmacol 1998; 12:482–491.

105. Giron MS, Forsell Y, Bernsten C, et al. Sleep problems in a very old population: drug use and clinical correlates. J Gerontol A Biol Sci Med Sci 2002; 57:M236–M240.

106. Goldenberg DL, Simms RW, Geiger A, et al. High frequency of fibromyalgia in patients with chronic fatigue seen in a primary care practice. Arthritis Rheum 1990; 33:381–387.

107. Griffiths RR, Weerts EM. Benzodiazepine self-administration in humans and laboratory animals—implications for problems of long-term use and abuse. Psychopharmacology 1997; 134:1–37.

108. Grunze H, von Wegerer J, Greene RW, et al. Modulation of calcium and potassium currents by lamotrigine. Neuropsychobiology 1998; 38(3):131–138.

109. Gudehithlu KP, Reddy PL, Bhargava HN. Effect of morphine tolerance and abstinence on the binding of MK-801 to brain regions and spinal cord of the rat. Brain Res 1994; 639:269–274.

110. Guzman J, Esmail R, Karjalainen K, et al. Multidisciplinary rehabilitation for chronic low back pain: systematic review. Br Med J 2001; 322:1511–1516.

111. Hadjistavropoulos HD, LaChapelle DL. Extent and nature of anxiety experienced during physical examination of chronic low back pain. Behav Res Ther 2000; 38:13–29.

112. Hankey GJ, Eikelboom JW. Cyclooxygenase-2 inhibitors. Are they really atherothrombotic, and if not, why not? Stroke 2003; 34:2736–2740.

113. Hardy JD, Wolff HG, Goodell H. Pain sensations and reactors. New York: Williams & Wilkins; 1952.

114. Harrison RA, Hillman M, Bulstrode S. Loading of the lower limb when walking partially immersed: implications for clinical practice. Physiotherapy 1992; 78:164.

115. Hasselström J, Liu-Palmgren J, Rasjo-Wraak G. Prevalence of pain in general practice. Eur J Pain 2002; 6:375–385.

116. Haythornthwaite JA, Menefee LA, Quatrano-Piacentini AL, et al. Outcome of chronic opioid therapy for non-cancer pain. J Pain Symptom Manage 1998; 15:185–194.

117. Higby GJ. Heroin and medical reasoning: the power of analogy. NY State J Med 1986; 86:137–142.

118. Hofbauer RK, Rainville P, Duncan GH, et al. Cortical representation of the sensory dimension of pain. J Neurophysiol 2001; 86:402–411.

119. Holland JC, Morrow GR, Schmale A, et al. A randomized clinical trial of alprazolam versus progressive muscle relaxation in cancer patients with anxiety and depressive symptoms. J Clin Oncol 1991; 9:1004–1011.

120. Inturrisi CE. Clinical pharmacology of opioids for pain. Clin J Pain 2002; 18:S3–S13.

121. Ives JC, Sosnoff J. Beyond the mind–body exercise hype. Phys Sports Med 2000; 28:67–81.

122. Jaaskelainen SK. Pregabalin for painful peripheral neuropathy. Lancet Neurol 2005; 4:207–208.

123. Jacobson E. Progress relaxation. Chicago: University of Chicago Press; 1938.

124. Jamison RN, Raymond SA, Slawsky EA, et al. Opoid therapy for chronic noncancer back pain. Spine 1996; 23:2591–2600.

125. Janssen SA, Philip S, Arntz A. The effect of failing to control pain: an experimental investigation. Pain 2004; 107:227–233.

126. Jensen MP, Engel JM, Hoffman AJ, et al. Natural history of chronic pain and pain treatment in adults with cerebral palsy. Am J Phys Med Rehabil 2004; 83:439–445.

127. Jensen MP, et al. The development and preliminary validation of an instrument to assess patients' attitudes toward pain. J Psychosom Res 1987; 31:393–400.

128. Jensen MP, Karoly P. Self-report scales and procedures for assessing pain in adults. In: Turk DC, Melzack R, eds. Handbook of pain assessment. New York: Guilford Press; 2001:15–34.

129. Jentoft ES, Kvalvik AG, Mengshoel AM. Effects of pool-based and land-based aerobic exercise on women with fibromyalgia/chronic widespread muscle pain. Arthritis Care Res 2001; 45:42–47.

130. Johnson SK, Frederick J, Kaufman M, et al. A controlled investigation of bodywork in multiple sclerosis. J Altern Complement Med 1999; 5:237–243.

131. Jones AK, Kulkarni B, Derbyshire SW. Pain mechanisms and their disorders. Br Med Bull 2003; 65:83–93.

132. Jones M. Chronic neuropathic pain: pharmacological interventions in the new millennium. Int J Pharm Compound 2000:4.

133. Joranson DE, Ryan KM, Gilson AM, et al. Trends in medical use and abuse of opioid analgesics. JAMA 2000; 283:1710–1714.

134. Jordan KD, Mayer TG, Gatchel RJ. Should extended disability be an exclusion criteria for tertiary rehabilitation? Socioeconomic outcomes of early versus late functional restoration in compensation spinal disorders. Spine 1998; 23:2110–2116.

135. Judd LL, Ellinwood E, McAdams LA. Cognitive performance and mood in patients with chronic insomnia during 14-day use of flurazepam and midazolam. J Clin Psychopharmacol 1990; 10:56S–67S.

136. Julius D, Basbaum AI. Molecular mechanisms of nociception. Nature 2001; 413:203–210.

137. Julius D. The molecular biology of thermosensation. In: Dostrovsky JO, Carr DB, Koltzenburg M, eds. Proceedings of the 10th World Congress on Pain, Progress in Pain Research and Management, vol 24. Seattle: IASP Press; 2003.

138. Katz N, Fanciullo G. Role of urine toxicology testing in the management of chronic opioid therapy. Clin J Pain 2002; 18:S76–S82.

139. Keefe FJ, Lefebvre JC. Behavior therapy. In: Melzack R, Wall P, eds. Textbook of pain. London: Churchill Livingstone; 1999:1445–1462.

140. Keefe FJ, Rumble ME, Scipio CD, et al. Psychological aspects of persistent pain: current state of the science. J Pain 2004; 5:195–211.

141. Keefe FJ, Wilkins RH, Cook WA, et al. Depression, pain and pain behavior. J Consult Clin Psychol 1986; 54:665–669.

142. Kerns RD, Rosenberg R, Jacob MC. Anger expression and chronic pain. J Behav Med 1994; 17:57–67.

143. Kerns RD, Turk DC, Rudy TE. The West Haven-Yale Multidimensional Pain Inventory (WHYMPI). Pain 1985; 23:345–356.

144. Kidd BL, Urban LA. Mechanisms of inflammatory pain. Br J Anaesth 2001; 87:3–11.

145. Kimmel SE, Berlin JA, Reily M, et al. Patients exposed to rofecoxib and Celebrex have different odds of nonfatal myocardial infarction. Ann Intern Med 2005; 142(3):157–164.

146. Klein PJ, Adams WD. Comprehensive therapeutic benefits of Taiji: a critical review. Am J Phys Med Rehabil 2004; 83:735–745.

147. Kori SH, Miller RP, Todd DD. Kinesophobia: a new view of chronic pain behavior. Pain Manage 1990; 3:35–43.

148. Koyana T, Kato K, Mikami A. During pain-avoidance neurons activated in the macaque anterior cingulated and caudate. Neurosci Lett 2000; 283:17–20.

149. Krause SJ, Weiner RL, Tait RC. Depression and pain behavior in patients with chronic pain. Clin J Pain 1994; 10:122–127.

150. Kripke DF, Hauri P, Ancoli-Israel S, et al. Sleep evaluation in chronic insomniacs during 14-day use of flurazepam and midazolam. J Clin Psychopharmacol 1990; 10:32S–43S.

151. Kucharski A, Todd E. Pain: historical perspectives. In: Warfield CA, Bajwa Z, eds. Principles and practice of pain medicine. 2nd edn. New York: McGraw-Hill; 2004.

152. Lanes TC, Gauron EF, Spratt KF, et al. Long-term follow-up of patients with chronic back pain treated in a multidisciplinary rehabilitation program. Spine 1995; 20:801–806.

153. Lang E, Hord AH, Denson D. Venlafaxine hydrochoride relieves thermal hyperalgesia in rats with an experimental mononeuropathy. Pain 1996; 68:151–155.

154. Leclaire R, Blier F, Fortin L, et al. A cross-sectional study comparing the Oswestry and Roland-Morris Functional Disability Scales in two populations of patients with low back pain of different levels of severity. Spine 1997; 22:68–71.

155. Li F, Harmer P, Fisher KJ, et al. Tai chi: improving functional balance and predicting subsequent falls in older persons. Med Sci Sports Exerc 2004; 36:2046–2052.

156. Linton SJ, Melin L. Behavioral analysis of chronic pain and its management. In: Hersen ABM, Iesler M, eds. Progress in behavior modification. New York: Academic Press; 1985:1–42.

157. Livingston WK. Pain and suffering. Seattle: IASP Press; 1998.

158. Loeser JD, Butler SH, Chapman CR, et al, eds. Bonica's management of pain. Philadelphia: Lippincott; 2001.

159. Loeser JD. Desirable characteristics for pain treatment facilities. Seattle: IASP Press; 1992.

160. Low PA, Opfer-Gehrking T, Dyck PJ, et al. Double-blind, placebo-controlled study of the application of capsaicin cream in chronic distal painful polyneuropathy. Pain 1995; 62:163–168.

161. Lu B. BDNF and activity-dependent synaptic modulation. Learn Mem 2003; 10:86–98.

162. Lu J, Greco MA, Shiromani P, et al. Effect of lesions of the ventrolateral preoptic nucleus on NREM and REM sleep. J Neurosci 2000; 20:3830–3842.

163. Lukyanetz EA, Shkryl VM, Kostyuk PG. Selective blockade of N-type calcium channels by levetiracetam. Epilepsia 2002; 43(1):9–18.

164. Lynch ME. Antidepressants as analgesics: a review of randomized controlled studies. J Psychiatry Neurosci 2001; 261:30–36.

165. Ma W, Eisenach JC. Cyclooxygenase-2 in infiltrating inflammatory cells in injured nerve is universally up-regulated following various types of peripheral nerve injury. Neuroscience 2003; 121:691–704.

166. Malenka RC, Nicoll RA. Long-term potentiation—a decade of progress. Science 1999; 285(5435):1870–1874.

167. Malmgren-Olsson EB, Branholm IB. A comparison between three physiotherapy approaches with regard to health-related factors in patients with non-specific musculoskeletal disorders. Disabil Rehabil 2002; 24: 308–317.

168. Mannerkorpi K, Ahlmén M, Ekdahl C. Six- and 24-month follow-up of pool exercise therapy and education for patients with fibromyalgia. Scand J Rheum 2002; 31:306–310.

169. Mannerkorpi K, Nyberg B, Ahlmen M, et al. Pool exercise combined with an education program for patients with fibromyalgia syndrome: a prospective, randomized study. J Rheumatol 2000; 27:2473–2481.

170. Mannion RJ, Woolf CJ. Pain mechanisms and management: a central perspective. Clin J Pain 2000; 16:S144–S156.

171. Mao J, Price DD, Mayer DJ. Experimental mononeuropathy reduces the antinociceptive effects of morphine: implications for common intracellular mechanisms involved in morphine tolerance and neuropathic pain. Pain 1995; 61:353–364.

172. Marcus DA, Click RM. Sustained-release oxycodone dosing survey of chronic pain patients. Clin J Pain 2004; 20:363–366.

173. Mathias S, Wetter TC, Steiger A, et al. The GABA uptake inhibitor tiagabine promotes slow wave sleep in normal elderly subjects. Neurobiol Aging 2001; 22(2):247–253.

174. Max MB, Culnane M, Schafer SC, et al. Amitriptyline relieves diabetic neuropathy pain in patients with normal or depressed mood. Neurology 1987; 37:589–596.

175. Max MB, Lynch SA, Muir J, et al. Effects of desipramine, amitripyline, and fluoxetine on pain in diabetic neuropathy. N Engl J Med 1992; 326:1250–1256.

176. Mayer TG, Gatchel RJ. Functional restoration for spinal disorders: the sports medicine approach. Philadelphia: Lea & Febiger; 1988.

177. McCallin A. Interdisciplinary practice—a matter of teamwork: an integrated literature review. J Clin Nurs 2001; 10:419–428.

178. McCleane G. Topical application of doxepin hydrochloride, capsaicin and a combination of both produces analgesia in chronic human neuropathic pain: a randomized, double-blind, placebo-controlled study. Br J Clin Pharmacol 2000; 49:574–579.

179. McCracken LM, Gross RT, Aikens J, et al. The assessment of anxiety and fear in persons with chronic pain: a comparison of instruments. Behav Res Ther 1996; 34:927–933.

180. McCracken LM, Gross RT, Eccleston C. Multimethod assessment of treatment process in chronic low back pain: comparison of reported pain-related anxiety with directly measured physical capacity. Behav Res Ther 2002; 40:585–594.

181. McCracken LM, Gross RT, Sorg PJ, et al. Prediction of pain in patients with chronic low back pain: effects of inaccurate prediction and pain-related anxiety. Behav Res Ther 1993; 31:647–652.

182. McCracken LM, Iverson GL. Disrupted sleep patterns and daily functioning in patients with chronic pain. Pain Res Manage 2002; 7(2): 75–79.

183. McCracken LM, Turk DC. Behavioral and cognitive-behavioral treatment for chronic pain. Outcome, predictors of outcome, and treatment process. Spine 2002; 27:2564–2573.

184. McCracken LM, Zayfert C, Gross RT. The Pain Anxiety Symptom Scale: development and validation of a scale to measure fear of pain. Pain 1992; 50:67–73.

185. McDonald JW, Johnson MV. Physiological and pathophysiological roles of excitatory amino acids during central nervous system development. Brain Res Rev 1990; 15:41–70.

186. McLean MJ, Schmutz M, Wamil AW, et al. Oxcarbazepine: mechanisms of action. Epilepsia 1994; 35(suppl 3):S5–S9.

187. McNamara JO, Patel M, He XP, et al. Glutamate receptor autoimmunity in Rasmussen's encephalitis. Cold Spring Harb Symp Quant Biol 1996; 61:327–332.

188. Meier T, Wasner G, Faust M, et al. Efficacy of lidocaine patch 5% in the treatment of focal peripheral neuropathic pain syndromes: a randomized, double-blind, placebo-controlled study. Pain 2003; 106:151–158.

189. Melzack R, Casey KL. Sensory, motivational and central control determinants of pain: a new conceptual model. In: Kenshalo D, ed. The skin senses. Springfield: Thomas; 1966: 423–443.

190. Melzack R, Wall PD. Pain mechanisms: a new theory. Science 1965; 150:971–976.

191. Melzack R. The puzzle of pain. New York: Basic Books; 1973.

192. Melzack R. The Short Form McGill Pain Questionnaire: major properties and scoring methods. Pain 1975; 1:277–299.

193. Merskey H, Bogduk N. IASP Task Force on Taxonomy classification of chronic pain: description of chronic pain syndromes and definition of pain terms. Seattle: IASP Press; 1994.

194. Millan MJ. The induction of pain: an integrative review. Prog Neurobiol 1999; 57:1–164.

195. Milligan K, Lanteri-Minet M, Borchert K, et al. Evaluation of long-term efficacy and safety of transdermal fentanyl in the treatment of chronic noncancer pain. J Pain 2001; 2(4):197–204.

196. Millon T, Breen JC, Meagher RB. Professional Psychol 1979; 10:529–539.

197. Mittino D, Mula M, Monaco F. Serotonin syndrome associated with tramadol–sertraline coadministration. Clin Neuropharmacol 2004; 27:150–151.

198. Moldofsky H. Management of sleep disorders in fibromyalgia. Rheum Dis Clin North Am 2002; 28:353–365.

199. Morin CM, Gibson D, Wade J. Self-reported sleep and mood disturbance in chronic pain patients. Clin J Pain 1998; 14:311–314.

200. Morley JS, Makin MK. The use of methadone in cancer pain poorly responsive to other opioids. Pain Rev 1998; 5:51–58.

201. Morley S, Eccleston C, Williams A. Systematic review and meta-analysis of randomized controlled trials of cognitive behavior therapy and behavior therapy for chronic pain in adults, excluding headache. Pain 1999; 80:1–13.

202. Moulin DE, Iezzi A, Amireh R, et al. Randomised trial of oral morphine for chronic non-cancer pain. Lancet 1996; 347(8995):143–147.

203. Mukherjee D, Nissen SE, Topol EJ. Risk of cardiovascular events associated with selective COX-2 inhibitors. JAMA 2001; 286(8):954–959.

204. Mustian KM, Katula JA, Gill DL, et al. Tai chi chuan, health-related quality of life and self-esteem: a randomized trial with breast cancer survivors. Support Care Cancer 2004; 12:871–876.

205. National Institutes of Health Technology Assessment Panel on Integration of Behavioral and Relaxation Approaches into the Treatment of Chronic Pain and Insomnia. Integration of behavioral and relaxation approaches into the treatment of chronic pain and insomnia. JAMA 1996; 276(4):313–318.

206. Nayak NN, Shankar K. Yoga: a therapeutic approach. Phys Med Rehabil Clin North Am 2004; 15:783–798.

207. Netz Y, Lidor R. Mood alterations in mindful versus aerobic exercise modes. J Psychol 2003; 137:405–419.

208. Nicholson K, Martelli MF. The problem of pain. J Head Trauma Rehabil 2004; 19:2–9.

209. Ohayon MM, Schatzberg AF. Using chronic pain to predict depressive morbidity in the general population. Arch Gen Psychiatry 2003; 60:39–47.

210. Okifuji A, Turk DC, Curran SL. Anger in chronic pain: investigations of anger targets and intensity. J Psychosom Res 1999; 47:1–12.

211. Okifuji A, Turk DC, Kalauokalani D. Clinical outcome and economic evaluation of multidisciplinary pain centers. In: Block AR, Kremer EF, Fernandez E, eds. Handbook of pain syndromes. Mahwah: Erlbaum; 1999:77–97.

212. Paice JA, Ferrans CE, Lashley FR, et al. Topical capsaicin in the management of HIV-associated peripheral neuropathy. J Pain Symptom Manage 2000; 19:45–52.

213. Paice JA, Penn RD, Ryan WG. Altered sexual function and decreased testosterone in patients receiving intraspinal opioids. J Pain Symptom Manage 1994; 9:126–131.

214. Pairet M, van Ryn J, Schierok H, et al. Differential inhibition of cyclooxygenase-1 and -2 by meloxicam and its 4′-isomer. Inflamm Res 1998; 47:270–276.

215. Pande AC, Crockatt JG, Feltner DE, et al. Pregabalin in generalized anxiety disorder: a placebo-controlled trial. Am J Psychiatry 2003; 160:533–540.

216. Pavelka K, Recker DP, Verburg KM. Valdecoxib is as effective as diclofenac in the management of rheumatoid arthritis with a lower incidence of gastroduodenal ulcers: results of a 26-week trial. Rheumatology (Oxford) 2003; 42:1207–1215.

217. Perucca E. Established antiepileptic drugs. In: Brodie MJ, Treiman DM, eds. Modern management of epilepsy. Baillière's clinical neurology, vol 5. London: Baillière-Tindall; 1996:693–722.

218. Picavet SJ, Vlaeyen JWS, Schouten J. Pain catastrophizing and kinesophobia: predictors of chronic low back pain. Am J Epidemiol 2002; 156:1028–1034.

219. Pillowsky I, Crettenden I, Townley M. Sleep disturbance in pain clinic patients. Pain 1985; 23:27–33.

220. Polatin PB, Dersh J. Psychotropic medication in chronic spinal disorders. Spine J 2004; 4:436–450.

221. Polatin PB, Mayer TG. Occupational disorders and the management of chronic pain. Orthop Clin North Am 1996; 27:881–890.

222. Pope JE, Anderson JJ, Felson DT. A meta-analysis of the effects of nonsteroidal anti-inflammatory drugs on blood pressure. Arch Intern Med 1993; 153:477–484.

223. Porreca F, Ossipov MH, Gebhart GF. Chronic pain and medullary descending facilitation. Trends Neurosci 2002; 25(6):319–325.

224. Porro CA, Baraldi P, Pagoni G, et al. Does anticipation of pain affect cortical nociceptive systems? J Neurosci 2002; 22(8):3206–3214.

225. Portenoy RK. Opioid therapy for chronic nonmalignant pain: a review of the critical issues. J Pain Symptom Manage 1996; 11:203–217.

226. Poyares D, Guilleminault C, Ohayon MM, et al. Chronic benzodiazepine usage and withdrawal in insomnia patients. J Psychiatr Res 2004; 38:327–334.

227. Price DD. Psychological and neural mechanisms of the affective dimension of pain. Science 2000; 288:1769–1772.

228. Prins J, Cutner D. Aquatic therapy in the rehabilitation of athletic injuries. Clin Sports Med 1999; 18:447–461.

229. Qureshi A, Lee-Chiong T. Medications and their effects on sleep. Med Clin North Am 2004; 88:751–766.

230. Radloff L. J Appl Psychol Measurement 1977; 1:385–401.

231. Rainville P, Duncan GH, Price DD, et al. Pain affect encoded in human anterior cingulated but not somatosensory cortex. Science 1997; 277:968–971.

232. Raub JA. Psychophysiologic effects of Hatha yoga on musculoskeletal and cardiopulmonary function: a literature review. J Altern Complement Med 2002; 8:797–812.

233. Reus VI, Rawitscher L. Possible interaction of tramadol and antidepressants. Am J Psychiatry 2000; 157:839.

234. Richter RW, Portenoy R, Sharma U, et al. Relief of painful diabetic peripheral neuropathy with pregabalin: a randomized placebo-controlled trial. J Pain 2005; 6:253–260.

235. Robbins H, Gatchel RJ, Noe C, et al. A prospective one-year outcome study of interdisciplinary chronic pain management: compromising its efficacy by managed care policies. Anesth Analg 2003; 97:156–162.

236. Roberts LJ, Finch PM, Pullan PT, et al. Sex hormone suppression by intrathecal opioids: a prospective study. Clin J Pain 2002; 18:144–148.

237. Romano JM, Turner JA. Chronic pain and depression: does the evidence support a relationship? Psychol Bull 1985; 97:18–34.

238. Rosenstiel AK, Keefe FJ. The use of coping strategies in chronic low back pain patients: relationship to patient characteristics and current adjustment. Pain 1983; 17:33–44.

239. Rosenstock J, Tuchman M, LaMoreaux L, et al. Pregabalin for the treatment of painful diabetic peripheral neuropathy: a double-blind, placebo-controlled trial. Pain 2004; 110:628–638.

240. Roth T. Characteristics and determinants of normal sleep. J Clin Psychiatry 2004; 65(suppl 16):8–11.

241. Rowbotham MC, Davies PS, Verkempinck C, et al. Lidocaine patch: double-blind controlled study of a new treatment method for post-herpetic neuralgia. Pain 1996; 65:39–44.

242. Rumelhart DE, McClelland JL, PDP Research Group. Parallel distributed processing: explorations in the microstructure of cognition. Cambridge: MIT Press; 1986.

243. Rush CR, Griffiths RR. Zolpidem, triazolam, and temazepam: behavioral and subject-rated effects in normal volunteers. J Clin Psychopharmacol 1996; 16:146–157.

244. Russo MB. Normal sleep, sleep physiology, and sleep deprivation: general principles. eMedicine 2004. Online. Available: http://www.emedicine.com/neuro/topic444.htm 13 Feb 2005.

245. Sabatowski R, Galvez R, Cherry DA, et al. Pregabalin reduces pain and improves sleep and mood disturbances in patients with post-herpetic neuralgia: results of a randomized placebo-controlled clinical trial. Pain 2004; 109:26–35.

246. Sadock BJ, Sadock VA. The brain and behavior. In: Kaplan & Sadock's synopsis of psychiatry. 9th edn. Philadelphia: Lippincott Williams & Wilkins; 2003.

247. Salerno SM, Browning R, Jackson JL. The effects of antidepressant treatment on chronic back pain: a meta-analysis. Arch Intern Med 2002; 162:19–24.

248. Salzman C, Watsky E. Rational prescribing of benzodiazepines. In: Hallstrom C, ed. Benzodiazepine dependence. Oxford: Oxford University Press; 1993:13–33.

249. Samad TA, Moore KA, Sapirstein A, et al. Interleukin-1β-mediated induction of Cox-2 in the CNS contributes to inflammatory pain hypersensitivity. Nature 2001; 410:471–475.

250. Sanger DJ, Depoortere H. The pharmacology and mechanism of action of zolpidem. CNS Drug Rev 1998; 4:323–340.

251. Saper CB, Chou TC, Scammell TE. The sleep switch: hypothalamic control of sleep and wakefulness. Trends Neurosci 2001; 24:726–731.

252. Sawynok J, Esser MJ, Reid AR. Antidepressants as analgesics: an overview of central and peripheral mechanisms of action. J Psychiatry Neurosci 2001; 26:21–29.

253. Schaible HG, Schmidt RF. Time course of mechanosensitivity changes in articular afferents during a developing experimental arthritis. J Neurophysiol 1988; 60:2190–2195.

254. Scharf MB, Roth T, Vogel GW, et al. A multicenter, placebo-controlled study evaluating zolpidem in the treatment of chronic insomnia. J Clin Psychiatry 1994; 55:192–199.

255. Schofferman J. Long-term use of opioid analgesics for the treatment of chronic pain of non-malignant origin. J Pain Symptom Manage 1993;8: 279–288.

256. Scholz J, Woolf CJ. Can we conquer pain? Nat Neurosci 2002; 5(suppl):1062–1067.

257. Serpell MG, Neuropathic Pain Study Group. Gabapentin in neuropathic pain syndromes: a randomised, double-blind, placebo-controlled trial. Pain 2002; 99:557–566.

258. Severijns R, van den Hout M, Vlaeyen J, et al. Pain catastrophising and general health status in a large Dutch community sample. Pain 2002; 99:367–376.

259. Shapiro AK. Psychological aspects of medication. In: Lief HI, Lief VF, Lief RN, eds. The psychological bases of medical practice. New York: Hoeber; 1963.

260. Sherrington CS. Integrative action of the nervous system. New York: Scribner's Sons; 1906.

261. Silverstein FE, Faich G, Goldstein JL, et al. Gastrointestinal toxicity with celecoxib vs. nonsteroidal anti-inflammatory drugs for osteoarthritis and rheumatoid arthritis: the CLASS study: a randomized controlled trial. JAMA 2000; 284:1247–1255.

262. Sindrup SH, Bjerre U, Dejgaard A, et al. The selective serotonin reuptake inhibitor citalopram relieves the symptoms of diabetic neuropathy. Clin Pharmacol Ther 1992; 52:547–552.

263. Sindrup SH, Gram LF, Brosen K, et al. The selective serotonin reuptake inhibitor paroxetine is effective in the treatment of diabetic neuropathy symptoms. Pain 1990; 42:135–144.

264. Smedslund J. How shall the concept of anger be defined? Theory Psychol 1992; 3:5–34.

265. Smith AJ. The analgesic effects of selective serotonin reuptake inhibitors. J Psychopharmacol 1998; 12:407–413.

266. Smith MT, Haythornthwaite JA. How do sleep disturbance and chronic pain inter-relate? Insights from the longitudinal and cognitive-behavioral clinical trials literature. Sleep Med Rev 2004; 8:119–132.

267. Smith TW, Frohm KD. What's so unhealthy about hostility? Construct validity and psychosocial correlates of the Cook and Medley Ho scale. Health Psychol 1985; 4:503–520.

268. Songer DA, Schulte H. Venlafaxine for the treatment of chronic pain. Am J Psychiatry 1996; 153:737.

269. Spielberger CD, et al. Manual of the STAI. Palo Alto: Consulting Psychologists Press; 1970.

270. Stacey BR. Management of peripheral neuropathic pain. Am J Phys Med Rehabil 2005; 84(3 suppl):S4–S16.

271. Stepanski E, Lamphere J, Badia P, et al. Sleep fragmentation and daytime sleepiness. Sleep 1984; 7:18–26.

272. Sternbach H. The serotonin syndrome. Am J Psychiatry 1991; 148: 705–713.

273. Sternbach RA. Principles of psychophysiology. New York: Academic Press; 1966.

274. Stewart WF, Ricci JA, Chee E, et al. Lost productive time and cost due to common pain conditions in the US workforce. JAMA 2003; 290:2443–2454.

275. Stovitz SD, Johnson RJ. NSAID and musculoskeletal treatment. Phys Sports Med 2003; 31(1).

276. Strigo IA, Duncan GH, Boivin M, et al. Differentiation of visceral and cutaneous pain in the human brain. J Neurophysiol 2003; 89:3294–3303.

277. Stucky CL, Gold MS, Zhang X. Mechanisms of pain. Proc Natl Acad Sci USA 2001; 98(21):11845–11846.

278. Sullivan MJ, Reesor K, Mikail S, et al. The treatment of depression in chronic low back pain: review and recommendations. Pain 1992; 50:5–13.

279. Sullivan MJ, Stanish W, Waite H, et al. Catastrophizing, pain, and disability in patients with soft tissue injuries. Pain 1998; 77:253–260.

280. Sullivan MJ, Thorn B, Haythornthwaite JA, et al. Theoretical perspectives on the relation between catastrophizing and pain. Clin J Pain 2001; 17:52–64.

281. Suzuki R, Rygh LJ, Dickenson AH. Bad news from the brain: descending 5-HT pathways that control spinal pain processing. Trends Pharmacol Sci 2004; 25(12):613–617.

282. Tasmuth T, Hartel B, Kalso E. Venlafaxine in neuropathic pain following treatment of breast cancer. Eur J Pain 2002; 6:17–24.

283. Taylor K, Rowbotham MC. Venlafaxine hydrochloride and chronic pain. West J Med 1996; 165:147–148.

284. Terman G, Bonica JJ. Spinal mechanisms and their modulation. In: Loeser JD, Butler SD, Chapman CR, et al, eds. Bonica's management of pain. 3rd edn. Philadelphia: Lippincott Williams & Wilkins; 2001:73–152.

285. Trait RC, Pollard CA, Margolis RB, et al. The Pain Disability Index: psychometric and validity data. Arch Phys Med Rehabil 1987; 68:438–441.

286. van Tulder MW, Koes BW, Bouter LM. A cost-of-illness study of back pain in the Netherlands. Pain 1995; 62:233–240.

287. van Tulder MW, Scholten RJ, Koes BW, et al. Nonsteroidal anti-inflammatory drugs for low back pain: a systematic review within the framework of the Cochrane Collaboration Back Review Group. Spine 2000; 25:2501–2513.

288. Turk DC, Brody MC, Okifuji EA. Physicians' attitudes and practices regarding the long-term prescribing of opioids for non-cancer pain. Pain 1994; 59:201–208.

289. Turk DC, Flor H. Chronic pain: a biobehavioral perspective. In: Gatchel RJ, Turk DC, eds. Psychosocial factors in pain: critical perspectives. New York: Guilford Press; 1999: 18–34.

290. Turk DC, Meichenbaum D, Genest M. Pain and behavioral medicine. A cognitive-behavioral perspective. New York: Guilford Press; 1983.

291. Turk DC. Clinical effectiveness and cost effectiveness of treatment for patients with chronic pain. Clin J Pain 2002; 18:355–365.

292. Turner JA, Cardenas DD, Warms CA, et al. Chronic pain associated with spinal cord injuries: a community survey. Arch Phys Med Rehabil 2001; 82:501–509.

293. Turner JA, Jensen M, Warms C, et al. Catastrophizing is associated with pain intensity, psychological distress, and pain-related disability among individuals with chronic pain after spinal cord injury. Pain 2002; 98:127–134.

294. US Food and Drug Administration. Alert for healthcare professionals: prescription non-steroidal anti-inflammatory drugs (NSAIDs). April 7, 2005. Online. Available: http://www.fda.gov/cder/drug/InfoSheets/HCP/NS_NSAIDsHCP.pdf 16 June 2005.

295. Verhaak PF, Kerssens JJ, Dekker J, et al. Prevalence of chronic benign pain disorder among adults: a review of the literature. Pain 1998; 77: 231–239.

296. Vestergaard K, Andersen G, Gottrup H, et al. Lamotrigine for central poststroke pain: a randomized controlled trial. Neurology 2001; 56(2): 184–190.

297. Vlaeyen JW, Haazen IW, Schuerman JA, et al. Behavioral rehabilitation of chronic low back pain: comparison of an operant treatment, an operant-cognitive treatment and an operant-respondent treatment. Br J Clin Psychol 1995; 34:95–118.

298. Vlaeyen JW, Kole-Snijders AM, Boeren RG, et al. Fear of movement/(re)injury in chronic low back pain and its relation to behavioral performance. Pain 1995; 62:363–372.

299. Vlaeyen JW, Linton SJ. Fear-avoidance and its consequences in chronic musculoskeletal pain: a state of the art. Pain 2000; 85:317–332.

300. Vlaeyen JW, Seelen HA, Peters M, et al. Fear of movement/(re)injury and muscular reactivity in chronic low back pain patients: an experimental investigation. Pain 1999; 82:297–304.

301. Waddell G, McCulloch JA, Kummel E, et al. Nonorganic physical signs in low-back pain. Spine 1980; 5:117–125.

302. Waddell G, Newton M, Henderson I, et al. A Fear-Avoidance Beliefs Questionnaire (FABQ) and the role of fear-avoidance beliefs in chronic low back pain and disability. Pain 1993; 52:157–168.

303. Ware JE, Sherbourne CD. The MOS 36-Item Short Form Health Survey (SF-36). Med Care 1992; 30:473–483.

304. Waters SJ, Campbell LC, Keefe FJ, et al. The essence of cognitive-behavioral pain management. In: Dworkin RH, Breitbart WS, eds. Psychosocial aspects of pain: a handbook for health care providers. Progress in pain research and management, vol 27. Seattle: IASP Press; 2004:261–283.

305. Weaver M, Schnoll S. Abuse liability in opioid therapy for pain treatment in patients with an addiction history. Clin J Pain 2002; 18:S61–S69.

306. Wheeler WL, Dickerson ED. Clinical application of methadone. Am J Hosp Palliat Care 2000; 17(3):196–203.

307. Willis WD, Coggeshall RE. Sensory mechanisms of the spinal cord. New York: Plenum Press; 1991.

308. Willis WD, Westlund KN. Neuroanatomy of the pain system and of the pathways that modulate pain. J Clin Neurophysiol 1997; 14:2–31.

309. Wilson KG, Eriksson MY, D'Eon JL, et al. Major depression and insomnia in chronic pain. Clin J Pain 2002; 18:77–83.

310. Wolfe F, Cathey MA, Hawley DJ. A double-blind placebo-controlled trial of fluoxetine in fibromyalgia. Scand J Rheumatol 1994; 23:255–259.

311. Woolf AD, Pfeger B. Burden of major musculoskeletal conditions. Bull World Health Organ 2003; 81:646–656.

312. Woolf CJ, Costigan M. Transcriptional and posttranslational plasticity and the generation of inflammatory pain. Proc Natl Acad Sci USA 1999; 96:7723–7730.

313. Woolf CJ, Mannion RJ, Neumann S. Null mutations lacking substance: elucidating pain mechanisms by genetic pharmacology. Neuron 1998; 20:1063–1066.

314. Woolf CJ, Shortland P, Coggeshall RE. Peripheral nerve injury triggers central sprouting of myelinated afferents. Nature 1992; 355:75–78.

315. Woolf CJ. Pain: moving from symptom control toward mechanism-specific pharmacologic management. Ann Intern Med 2004; 140:441–451.

316. Zacny JP. A review of the effects of opioids on psychomotor and cognitive functioning in humans. Exp Clin Psychopharmacol 1995; 3:432–466.

317. Zakrzewska JM, Chaudhry Z, Nurmikko TJ, et al. Lamotrigine (Lamictal) in refractory trigeminal neuralgia: results from a double-blind placebo controlled crossover trial. Pain 1997; 73(2):223–230.

318. Zammit GK, McNabb LJ, Caron J, et al. Efficacy and safety of eszopiclone across 6-weeks of treatment for primary insomnia. Curr Med Res Opin 2004; 20:1979–1991.

319. Zung WWK. A self-rating scale depression scale. Arch Gen Psychol 1965; 12:63–70.

Chapter

44

Muscle Pain Syndromes

James P. Robinson and Lars Arendt-Nielsen

We all have experienced pain and tenderness in our muscles. These routinely and predictably occur after unaccustomed exercise, producing a syndrome labeled delayed-onset muscular soreness (DOMS).[43] Fortunately, DOMS predictably resolves within a few days and is not a cause of chronic musculoskeletal pain.

Muscle pain also appears to be common among patients with clinically significant musculoskeletal pain. There are a large number of patients who have these complaints:

- diffuse pain;
- pain with an aching quality, and described as muscular soreness;
- tenderness in muscles where aching pain is reported.

We will use these three simple criteria in this chapter as descriptive criteria for muscle pain.

Most physicians who treat musculoskeletal disorders would probably agree that many of their patients meet the above criteria for muscle pain. There are marked differences in the opinions of physicians regarding the pathophysiology underlying the complaints of muscle pain, however, as well as the importance physicians should place on such complaints. Even the terminology to describe muscle pain is a potential battleground. As a first approximation, we can say that muscle pain has a great deal of overlap with the term *myofascial pain* that some physicians use. As discussed below, a major difference between the two terms is that *muscle pain* is a descriptive term, whereas the term *myofascial pain* is embedded in an elaborate theory.

Proponents of myofascial pain theory assert that myofascial pain exists, and that it plays a major role in chronic musculoskeletal pain. At the opposite extreme, many physicians ignore myofascial pain entirely. For example, the term *myofascial pain* does not appear in the index of *Essentials of Musculoskeletal Medicine*[96a] or *Campbell's Operative Orthopaedics*.[37] Still others criticize the concept of myofascial pain, suggesting that patients diagnosed with myofascial pain actually have chronic pain syndromes with somatoform features.[33]

This chapter has three distinct purposes. First, we will discuss some of the controversies about the existence and significance of muscular (myofascial) pain. Second, we will discuss recent experimental research on muscular pain. Finally, we will describe strategies for evaluating and treating patients with suspected muscular pain.

MUSCLE PAIN: BASIC CONCEPTS AND CONTROVERSIES

Terminology: muscle pain versus myofascial pain

As noted above, we use *muscle pain* in a descriptive sense—to denote widespread, aching pain that appears to emanate from muscles, together with tenderness over the muscles. *Myofascial pain* is a more complex term, however, that has meaning only in relation to a complex theory. Simons, a leading proponent of myofascial pain, states:

> The myofascial pain syndrome, in its strict sense, is a regional pain syndrome characterized by the presence of myofascial trigger points (TrPs) . . . The most distinctive clinical characteristics of TrPs include circumscribed spot tenderness in a nodule that is part of a palpably tense band of muscle fibers, patient recognition of the pain that is evoked by pressure on the tender spot as being familiar, pain referred in the pattern characteristic of TrPs in that muscle, a local twitch response, painful limitation of stretch range of motion, and some weakness of that muscle.
>
> (Mense and Simons 2001,[166] p. 205.)

You might surmise from the above that myofascial pain is essentially equivalent to muscle pain, and that trigger points are more or less equivalent to tender areas in muscle. In fact, many authors have used the term *myofascial pain syndrome* (MPS) in a loose sense to describe a syndrome in which a patient presents with muscle tenderness and complaints of muscular pain. Simons describes this situation as follows:

> [The term *MPS*] has acquired both a general and a specific meaning, which need to be distinguished . . . The general meaning includes a regional muscle pain syndrome of any soft tissue origin that is associated with muscle tenderness . . . and it is commonly used in this sense by dentists . . . The other meaning is specifically a MPS caused by TrPs.
>
> (Mense and Simons 2001,[166] p. 211.)

However, there are several considerations that challenge the equation of myofascial pain with muscle pain, and trigger points with tender areas in muscle.

One is that the descriptive criteria given above for designating pain as muscle pain are fairly simple. In contrast, the clinical phenomena used to identify trigger points are more complex and difficult for clinicians to master. Although these criteria are nominally objective, research has demonstrated that the actual situation is more complex. A necessary condition for a clinical finding to be considered objective is that different observers are able to agree about when it is present, i.e. that there be acceptable interrater reliability. As discussed below, interrater reliability for many of the indicators of trigger points appears to be obtainable only under unusual circumstances.

Another issue that bears on the objectivity of trigger points is that different clinicians appear to have markedly different thresholds for deciding that a trigger point exists and/or that a patient has significant myofascial pain. We are not aware of published literature on this issue, but informal observation supports the view that some clinicians diagnose myofascial pain in a very high proportion of patients with musculoskeletal pain, whereas others use the diagnosis much less frequently (and still others essentially do not consider myofascial pain to be a legitimate medical diagnosis).

While muscle pain can in principle be discussed without any hypotheses about its pathophysiology, *trigger points* and *myofascial pain* are embedded in a complex theory about muscle dysfunction and related muscular pain. A recent formulation of this theory has been named the integrated trigger point hypothesis.[166] A key element is the 'energy crisis' hypothesis regarding the pathophysiology underlying trigger points. It states that, under a variety of circumstances in which muscles become overloaded, excessive and prolonged release of calcium from the sarcoplasmic reticulum of muscle cells occurs. The influx of calcium stimulates prolonged contractile activity within the cells, increasing metabolic activity within them to such an extent that localized ischemia develops. The ischemia then stimulates the release of vasoactive substances. These have two major effects. First, they sensitize nociceptors in muscles, producing the pain that patients with myofascial pain report. Second, they precipitate a train of events that aggravate ischemia of the muscle, thereby creating a vicious circle (Fig. 44-1).

The integrated hypothesis contains multiple postulates, and allows for multifactorial causation of the pain that patients with myofascial pain report. For example, it allows for the possibility that nociceptive input from muscles can produce central nervous system sensitization. Consequently, the pain in a patient with chronic myofascial pain might be a product of a combination of ongoing nociceptive input from the affected muscle and central nervous system sensitization. However, the integrated hypothesis proposes that myofascial pain is initiated by events that occur in a muscle (muscle overload), and that the primary pathophysiologic process in myofascial pain is a metabolic abnormality within muscles that activates nociceptors in the muscles. The integrated hypothesis embodies the broader hypothesis that individuals who experience muscle pain are accurately registering abnormalities in the structure and function of their muscles. To put the matter differently, the energy crisis hypothesis assumes that myofascial pain stems in a fairly

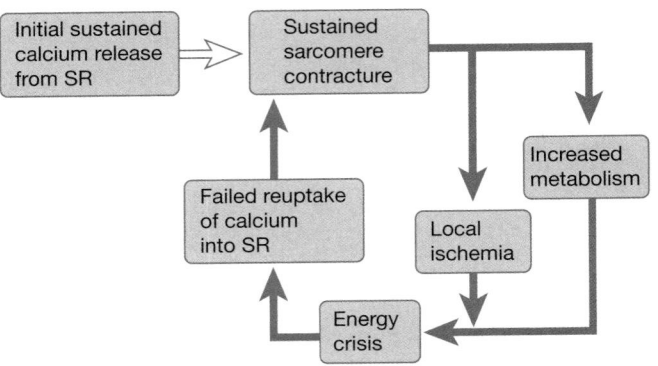

Figure 44-1 The energy crisis hypothesis, which postulates a vicious cycle of events that appear to contribute significantly to trigger points. The function of the sarcoplasmic reticulum is to store and release unused calcium that induces activity of the contractable elements, which causes sarcomere shortening. An initiating event, such as trauma or a marked increase in the end-plate release of acetylcholine, can result in excessive release of calcium from the sarcoplastic reticulum. This calcium produces minimal contracture of a segment of muscle, which creates a minimal energy demand and chokes off local circulation. The ischemia interrupts energy supply, which causes failure of the calcium pump of the sarcoplastic reticulum, completing the cycle. (From Simons et al. 1999,[207] with permission of Williams & Wilkins.)

straightforward way from nociceptive input from an injured or dysfunctional muscle. This perspective might seem self-evident but, as discussed below, several lines of evidence challenge its validity.

A key assumption of myofascial theory is that trigger points represent 'upstream' biologic abnormalities that put an individual at risk for pain, but are not synonymous with pain. In effect, Travell and Simons view a trigger point as an indicator of deranged function in a muscle that predisposes an individual to muscular pain. The relation between trigger points and muscular pain could be seen as analogous to the relation between coronary artery stenosis and angina. The distinction that Travell and Simons make between trigger points and muscular pain permits them to introduce the concept of latent trigger points.[244,245] These are points that meet the criteria for trigger points when they are examined, but are not associated with clinically significant pain.

One might conceptualize relations between trigger points and muscle pain in a Venn diagram (Fig. 44-2). As this diagram suggests, a substantial overlap between trigger points and muscle pain can be postulated. It is possible for individuals to have trigger points, however, but not clinically significant muscle pain (i.e. latent trigger points). Another logical possibility shown in the diagram is that there might be individuals who have clinically significant muscle pain but not trigger points. Although Simons mentions this possibility, we are not aware of any detailed discussions of non-myofascial muscular pain by myofascial pain proponents.[166]

Confusion between *muscle pain* as a descriptive term and *myofascial pain* as a theory-laden term is aggravated by the fact that many researchers use the term *myofascial pain* even though they have not followed the evaluation procedures necessary to

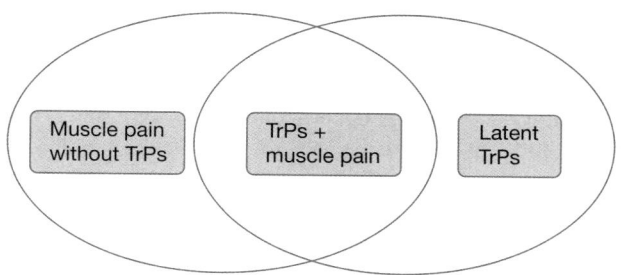

Figure 44-2 Venn diagram showing the overlap between muscle pain and trigger points.

determine whether subjects had trigger points. Consequently, at the present time, it is difficult if not impossible to determine whether studies on 'myofascial pain' address the construct defined by Travell and Simons. In this chapter, we will use the terminology used by authors of studies without attempting to determine whether their terminology is accurate.

Divergent perspectives on myofascial pain

Informal observation suggests that only a minority of physicians who specialize in the management of musculoskeletal disorders subscribe to the principles outlined by Simons and other proponents of myofascial theory. If this observation is valid, it raises an obvious question: why do so many specialists in musculoskeletal medicine not follow the tenets proposed by Simons? The question is difficult to answer, because many physicians simply ignore myofascial theory without elaborating their reasons for doing so.

We assume that physicians who do not subscribe to the tenets of myofascial theory notice that muscular pain is present in some of their patients, i.e. notice that some patients report pain in muscles and demonstrate tenderness to palpation of muscles. We believe that they reject the myofascial model for one of two reasons. Some follow what has been called the structural lesion model of musculoskeletal pain.[192] This model, which dominates in orthopedics, holds that musculoskeletal pain typically follows injury or dysfunction in joints, periarticular tissues, or nerves. From the standpoint of the structural lesion model, muscular pain would be construed as a secondary phenomenon that is not an appropriate target for treatment. Just as an infectious disease specialist addresses the pathogen causing an infection rather than directly treating the fever that occurs during an infection, so an orthopedist is likely to direct attention to joints, periarticular tissues, or nerves rather than to the muscle pain that might result from dysfunction in these tissues. Other physicians argue that patients who present with muscular pain are actually demonstrating abnormal pain behavior[187] that reflects psychiatric dysfunction (e.g. a somatoform disorder) rather than a genuine musculoskeletal disorder.

Fibromyalgia

Physicians dating back to the nineteenth century have pondered the significance and etiology of aching, muscular pain and muscular tenderness. They used a number of terms to describe

muscular pain, and developed a variety of theories to explain it.[166,191] In 1904, Gowers introduced the term *fibrositis*. This term was used sporadically during the early part of the twentieth century, but during the 1960s and 1970s came to be used with increasing frequency by rheumatologists.

In the 1960s, rheumatology was a relatively new specialty. Patients with widespread pain were often referred for rheumatologic evaluation to determine whether their symptoms were the result of a systemic inflammatory process, such as rheumatoid arthritis. Some rheumatologists became interested in patients who presented with widespread, seemingly muscular pain but who did not have evidence of a well-defined rheumatologic disorder. During the 1960s and 1970s, articles describing these patients began to be published in the rheumatologic literature.[213,214] Rheumatologists typically used the label *fibrositis* to describe a syndrome characterized by widespread, seemingly muscular pain; tenderness to palpation of certain muscles; and the absence of markers of a well-defined rheumatologic syndrome. The first attempt to provide specific clinical criteria for the diagnosis of fibrositis was made by Smythe and Moldofsky.[215] In 1981, Yunus et al. recommended the term *fibromyalgia* as preferable to fibrositis, because the inflammatory process suggested by the term *fibrositis* was not found.[271]

During the 1980s, research on fibrositis/fibromyalgia increased sharply. Rheumatologists gradually adopted the term *fibromyalgia* as the preferable one. A key advance came in 1990, when a multicenter study was undertaken by rheumatologists to identify optimal criteria for identifying fibromyalgia, at least for the purposes of research.[267] After considering several different diagnostic criteria, the researchers concluded that only two were needed to create maximal sensitivity and specificity: a history of widespread musculoskeletal pain of at least 3 months' duration, and a report of pain in at least 11 of 18 designated sites during deep palpation of the sites.

At a descriptive level, fibromyalgia has similarities to and differences from MPS. The two are similar, in that patients with both kinds of problems report aching pain that, to an evaluating physician, appears to be muscular in origin. But the tender points that define fibromyalgia do not necessarily have all the characteristics (such as taut bands and referred pain) of myofascial trigger points.[266] Fibromyalgia is also by definition a widespread pain syndrome, whereas MPS is usually thought of as a regional pain syndrome. At this time, there is consensus that fibromyalgia is distinctly different from MPS.[166] It is worth noting, however, that during the 1980s, when little was known about fibromyalgia, careful consideration was given to the hypothesis that the widespread muscular tenderness reported by fibromyalgia patients actually reflected the fact that they had multiple myofascial trigger points.[208]

It is beyond the scope of this chapter to review the voluminous research that has been done on fibromyalgia, or to consider the multiple pathophysiologic hypotheses that have been advanced to explain it. It is interesting to note, however, that much of the research on fibromyalgia during the 1980s addressed the possibility that the disorder was fundamentally a disorder of muscle.[30] This seemed like a plausible hypothesis, because fibromyalgia patients reported significant pain during deep palpation of muscles.

During the past 15 years, researchers on fibromyalgia have shifted away from explaining the disorder on the basis of peripheral pathology (i.e. abnormalities in muscles), and have instead reached the conclusion that the fundamental problem in the disorder is a disturbance in central nervous system processing of sensory information. Recent formulations of the pathophysiology of fibromyalgia have relied heavily on basic neurobiologic findings regarding central nervous system sensitization.[220,222] In a similar vein, a recently published review of treatments for fibromyalgia highlights the fact that the best-supported treatments address fibromyalgia as a systemic problem rather than as a local or multifocal disorder of muscles.[83]

Because there is now significant doubt that fibromyalgia is a muscle pain syndrome, it will not be considered further in this chapter. It is worth noting, however, that the history of concepts regarding fibromyalgia over the past 25 years forms a cautionary tale. Early researchers took the seemingly obvious perspective that, because fibromyalgia patients reported muscular tenderness, they must have some abnormality in their muscles.[30] In contrast, current thinking emphasizes that the muscular tenderness of fibromyalgia patients is essentially an epiphenomenon of a disturbance in central nervous system function. As discussed at several points in this chapter, the same type of analysis might turn out to be appropriate for myofascial trigger points.

RESEARCH ON CLINICAL AND EXPERIMENTAL MUSCLE PAIN

Preliminaries and basic distinctions

Key portions of the theory of myofascial pain date back to the 1940s.[243] The theory was based largely on the observations of astute clinicians, particularly Janet Travell and later David Simons. Their viewpoint was well enough developed to permit them to publish a comprehensive book on myofascial pain in 1983.[244] Empiric research of myofascial pain in particular or muscle pain in general, however, was virtually non-existent during the time period when Travell and Simons were developing concepts related to myofascial pain. In the preface to their seminal book *Muscle Pain*, Mense and Simons described the situation as follows:

The history of this book reaches back to the year 1978, when the authors met for the first time in Montreal on the occasion of the Second World Congress on Pain, organized by the . . . IASP. Contact between the authors was maintained and intensified in ensuing years. The contacts were used for long and vivid discussions of all aspects of muscle pain. In 1978, the mechanisms of muscle pain were largely unknown.

Very often, [our] discussions started with an effort to account for a clinical observation and ended with the frustrating conclusion that it could not be solved because too little was known about the neurobiology and pathophysiology of muscle pain. In the late 1970s, pain research in general was a relatively new discipline, and the bulk of the available knowledge was obtained in experiments on cutaneous pain. Although many mechanisms controlling cutaneous pain could be assumed to be functioning also in muscle pain, it became increasingly clear that muscle pain differed from cutaneous pain in many aspects.

(Mense and Simons 2001,[166] p. vii, 30.)

Fortunately, research on clinical phenomena associated with muscle pain has mushroomed during the past 30 years. It is now possible at least to identify points of convergence and divergence between myofascial theory and experimental findings, and to clarify problems for which further research is needed. A summary of relevant experimental findings is given below (see Mense and Simons 2001[166] for a more extended discussion). However, the research that bears on muscle pain is diffuse, and you need to keep several distinctions and limitations in mind when you review it.

Proponents of myofascial pain have used the term *myofascial pain* essentially only in the context of patients with clinically significant pain. It is not clear how the term applies to experimentally induced muscle pain. To determine whether experimental muscle pain is relevant to an understanding of myofascial pain, one would have to address three issues.

1. To what extent is myofascial pain defined on the basis of distinctive clinical findings (taut band, exquisitely tender site within a band, local twitch response, etc.) as opposed to historical information that suggests that the pain was initiated by overload of the symptomatic muscle? If a history of muscle overload is viewed as a necessary condition for myofascial pain, then most research on experimental muscle pain would, by definition, be irrelevant to an understanding of myofascial pain.

2. What percentage of patients with experimentally induced muscle pain have the clinical findings associated with myofascial pain, such as taut bands or local twitch responses? We are not aware of data that address this issue, because we are not aware of research in which examination criteria for the identification of myofascial pain have been used on normal subjects in whom muscle pain has been experimentally induced.

3. What is the time course for the development of myofascial pain following muscle overload? In experimental research, subjects report onset of muscle pain almost immediately after a noxious stimulus (such as a hypertonic saline injection) is administered. Consequently, the time course between the inciting event (injection) and pain onset might be too brief for experimentally induced muscle pain to faithfully simulate myofascial pain.

Some data and theory related to muscle pain come from animal research. This research is very important, because experimenters studying pain in animals can use very tight experimental controls, and can perform invasive procedures that would be ethically unacceptable in human research. There is a problem, however, of generalizing from animal research to human muscle pain. A key example of this issue is central nervous system sensitization.[186] This phenomenon has been identified in animals on the basis of electrophysiologic events typically recorded in the dorsal horn of the spinal cord. Correlates of central nervous system sensitization have been identified in such research, for example animals with central nervous system sensitization show more rapid temporal summation of responses to repeated noxious stimuli than do animals with no evidence of such sensitization.[270] Researchers on human muscle pain have proposed by analogy that rapid temporal summation can be used as an indicator of central nervous system sensitization.[219] You should be aware, however, that references to central nervous system sensitization in humans are not based on the electrophysiologic activity that is used to identify this phenomenon in animals.

Tenderness is studied in muscle pain research by applying pressure to subjects at various anatomic sites. Typically, such an application elicits an awareness of pressure at first. As the pressure is increased, the subject reports a change, such that the stimulation becomes painful. The pressure at which this conversion from painless pressure to painful pressure occurs is called the pressure pain threshold.[66]

Hyperalgesia refers to abnormally intense pain in response to relatively mild sensory input to an area. In research on muscle pain, hyperalgesia can be operationally defined as a reduction in the pressure pain threshold. However, hyperalgesia can occur in response to sensory input other than mechanical stimulation. It is possible, for example, to study hyperalgesia in response to electrical stimulation or thermal stimulation.[56]

In most research on muscle pain, pain is assessed when a subject is at rest, consequently spontaneous pain is assessed, rather than pain associated with physical activity.

In experimental research on muscle pain, pain in a muscle is typically induced by noxious stimulation, such as with electrical stimulation or injection of hypertonic saline into a muscle. This methodology permits an experimenter to distinguish clearly between the primary site of pain and sites of referred pain. For example, research demonstrates that, following a hypertonic saline injection into the tibialis anterior muscle, subjects reliably report pain not only immediately around the injection site (the primary source) but also in the dorsum of the foot (referred pain). In clinical practice and in clinical research on patients with muscular pain, the patients are usually asked about their typical pain, or about the pain they are having at the time of the experiment. With this methodology, there is inevitable ambiguity about whether the pain described by patients represents a primary site or a referred site.

In addition to spontaneous pain in a referral site, individuals can report paresthesias. They also can demonstrate hyperalgesia in these sites (e.g. reduced pressure pain threshold).

Investigators frequently focus on a single site when they study patients who appear to have muscle pain. However, if a patient has pain and/or hyperalgesia in a specific muscle, an obvious question arises: is the pain limited to the identified muscle, or is the identified pain or hyperalgesia simply a single manifestation of sensitivity that is much more diffuse? For example, fibromyalgia patients might report pain and demonstrate hyperalgesia in the right upper trapezius muscle, but further evaluation is almost certain to reveal that the patients also have pain and hyperalgesia in several other parts of their bodies. Moreover, there is evidence in fibromyalgia that the pain or hyperalgesia is not limited to muscles, because they also demonstrate hyperalgesia to palpation of various bony prominences.[173]

A paradigm for experimental muscle pain: technique and typical findings

During the past 10 years, extensive research has been done on experimentally induced muscle pain in normal human volunteers. In a typical study, subjects receive an injection of hypertonic saline (5%) into the tibialis anterior muscle of one leg. They are then asked to indicate the location of their resultant pain on human figure drawings, and to indicate the severity of their pain at various sites on a 10-cm visual analog scale. The pain ratings are provided repeatedly (e.g. every 5 s).[88]

When a single bolus of hypertonic saline is injected over a 20-s period, subjects typically report pain that lasts for approximately 3 min and is rated at approximately 5 over 10 in severity (see Fig. 44-3). When hypertonic saline is injected over a period of 15 min rather than in a single bolus, subjects report pain lasting up to 25 min (see Fig. 44-4).[89]

Subjects typically indicate pain both immediately around the injection site (primary pain) and over the ventral aspect of the ankle (referred pain). Pain at the primary site is typically rated as more severe than pain at the referred site. When pressure is applied to the injected leg, subjects typically demonstrate hyperalgesia (reduced pressure pain threshold) in sites where they report spontaneous pain.

Within this general paradigm, the effects of a host of modifications can be examined. Muscles other than the tibialis anterior can be studied. In particular, extensive research has been done on the effects of injections to the masseter muscle.[261] Pain can be provoked by intramuscular electric stimulation, and by a variety of chemicals other than hypertonic saline. These include capsaicin, bradykinin, serotonin, and substance P.[10,16] Following injections, pain threshold and pain tolerance can be studied in response to several different sensory modalities, including pressure, thermal stimuli, and electric stimulation.[56] Experiments can be carried out on both normal subjects and patients with significant musculoskeletal pain, for example ones with fibromyalgia or persistent neck pain following whiplash injuries.[22]

When combined with clinical studies of patients with muscle pain, experimental research on muscle pain has made it possible to investigate empirically several hypotheses about muscle pain. The discussion below addresses three areas: referred pain, hyperalgesia, and motor responses in individuals with muscle pain.

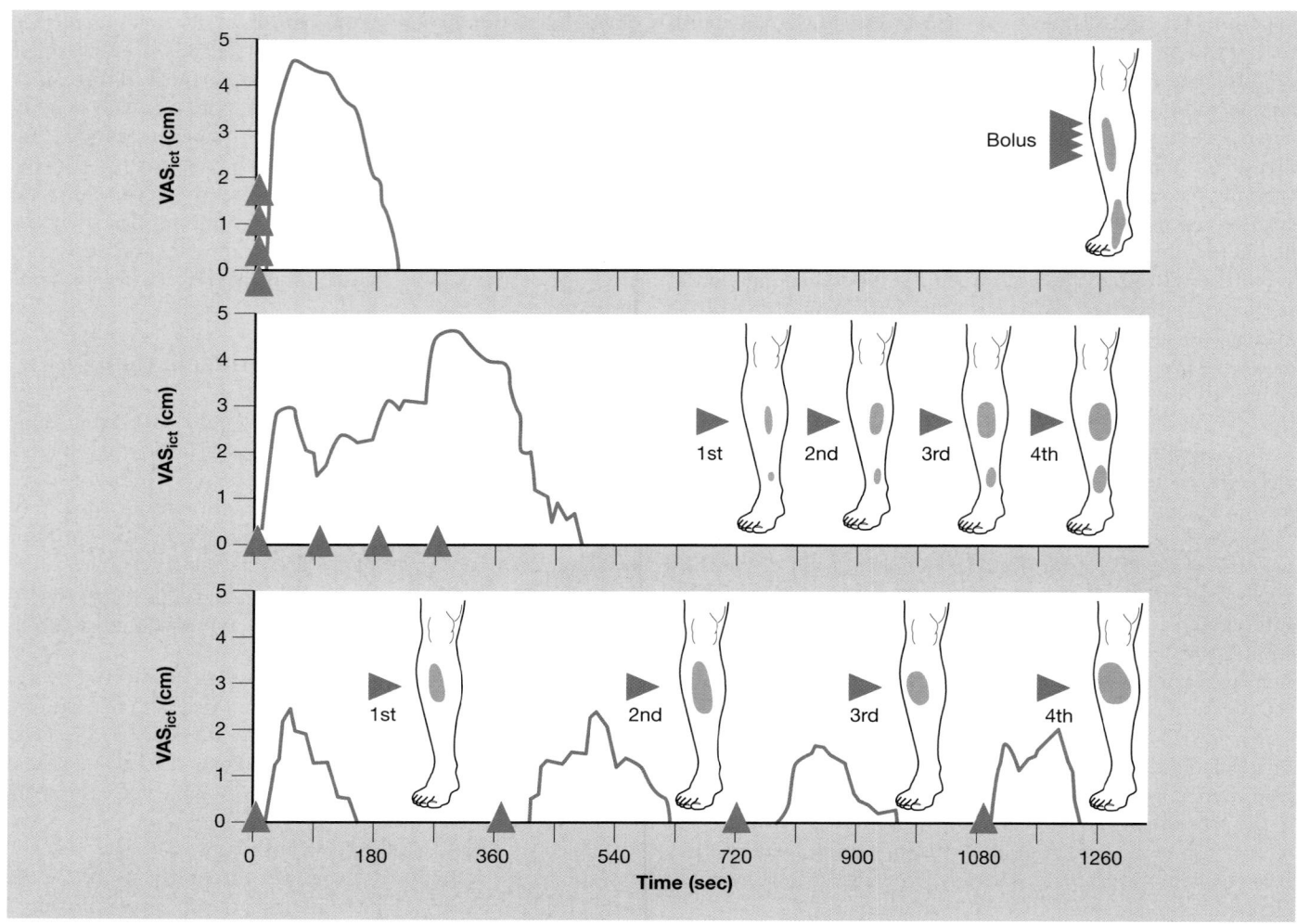

Figure 44-3 The plots show the mean (± SE) development (n = 11) in visual analog scale scores (VAS$_{tot\ peak}$, VAS$_{loc}$, and VAS$_{ref}$), the size of local and referred pain areas after bolus, and the four sequential infusions given at 90 s and 360 s ISI. The mean values are shown against the cumulative infusion volume. There is significant correlation between the raw measures and the cumulative infusion volume (significant differences: Friedman, $P < 0.05$; SNK, $P < 0.05$) compared with the other series of infusions (bolus and after four sequential infusions), where 0.4 mL of saline has been infused. (From Graven-Nielsen et al. 1997,[88] with permission.)

Referred pain

Referred pain has been known and described for more than a century, and has been used extensively as a diagnostic tool in the clinic. Originally, the term *referred tenderness and pain* was used. Pain from deep structures such as muscle, joints, ligaments, tendons, and viscera is typically described as diffuse and difficult to locate precisely, in contrast to superficial types of pain (e.g. skin and mucosal pains).[34,142,170] Consequently, the perceived localization of deep pain might be different from the original source of pain. Pain located at the source of pain is termed *local pain* or *primary pain*, whereas pain felt in a different region away from the source of pain is termed *referred pain* or *heterotopic pain*.[34] A clear distinction between spread of pain and referred pain is not possible at the moment, and these phenomena may also share common pathophysiologic mechanisms.

Pain drawings can be used as valuable tools to illustrate the localization and extent of myofascial pain areas,[64,155] although the perceived size of body areas is labile and can be influenced by pain-induced changes in central somatosensory maps.[75] Furthermore, patients might have difficulties transferring their perception of pain areas to a two-dimensional standardized anatomic map. Photographs of their own involved pain areas could eventually be an improvement on this simple technique.

Pain drawings have so far not been used on a regular basis in clinical research on MPS. Only a few studies have applied systematic pain maps to patients with myofascial pain in the trigeminal region.[96,99,250] One study showed that only about 19% of patients referred to a facial pain clinic have pain confined to the trigeminal regions, whereas 66% have widespread pain outside the trigeminal and cervical regions.[250] Information on these concomitant sites of pain seems to have been largely neglected, even though their presence draws attention toward the involvement of more widespread pathophysiologic mechanisms in some patients with myofascial pain.[251]

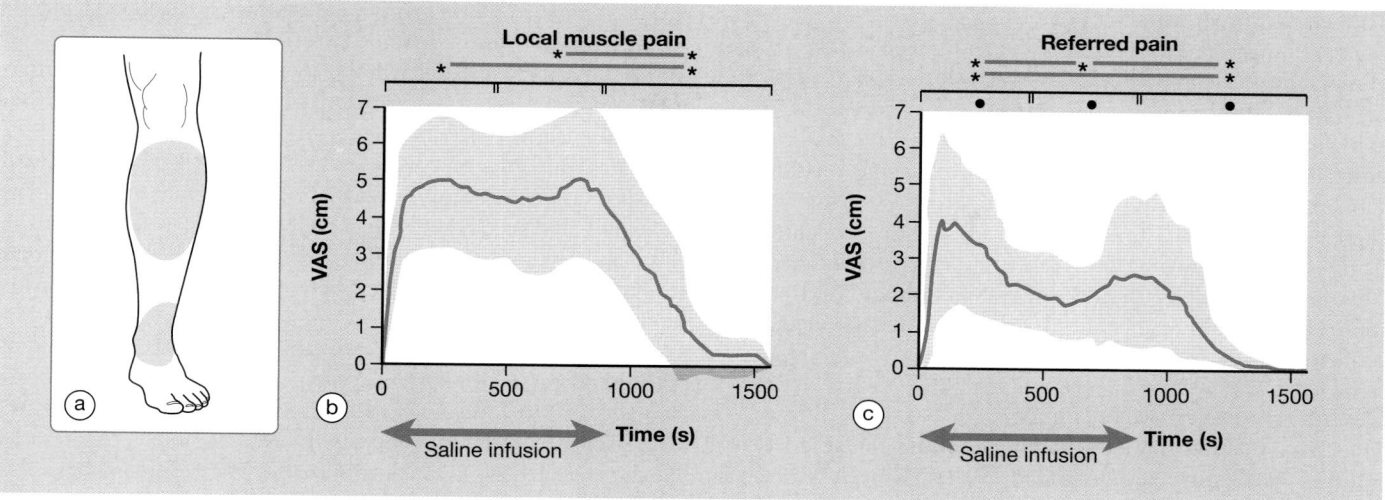

Figure 44-4 The distribution of local muscle and referred pain (**a**) and their main visual analog scale (VAS) scores (± SD, shaded area) for the local muscle (**b**) and referred (**c**) pain after infusion of hypertonic saline into muscle. TA (n = 11). Significantly (Friedman, $P < 0.0001$; SNK, $P > 0.05$) lower, referred mean VAS score compared with mean VAS score of local muscle pain (•), and different mean VAS scores within local muscle or referred pain (*) are indicated for the three intervals (20–460 s, 460–900 s, and 900–1600 s). (From Graven-Nielsen et al. 1997,[89] with permission.)

Neurophysiologic models for referred pain

Inman and Saunders systematically investigated the distribution of referred pain in relation to the activated muscle groups.[109] Based on their observations, it was suggested that referred pain followed more frequently the distribution of sclerotomes (muscle, fascia, and bone) than the classic dermatomes.[70]

Experimentally referred pain can be induced by stimulation of a given muscle by hypertonic saline or electrical stimulation (Fig. 44-3). The hypertonic saline model has been widely used for experimental and clinical studies (Fig. 44-4).

Several neuroanatomic and neurophysiologic theories regarding the appearance of referred pain have been suggested, and basically they state that nociceptive dorsal horn or brain stem neurons receive convergent inputs from various tissues. Consequently, higher centers cannot identify correctly the actual input source.[7,8] Most recently, the models have included newer theories in which sensitization of dorsal horn and brain stem neurons play a central role.

Several theories for referred pain have been suggested and will briefly be summarized.

Convergent projection theory

Based on the ideas of Sturge[229] and Ross,[194] Ruch[196] proposed that afferent fibers from different tissues converge on to common spinal neurons. The core of this suggestion is that the nociceptive activity from the spinal cord is misinterpreted as originating from other structures. This could explain the segmental nature of referred muscle pain and the increased referred pain intensity recorded when local muscle pain was intensified.[9,54,94,134] It does not adequately explain, however, the apparent delay in the development of referred pain following onset of local pain.[88,89,109,134] Referred pain has also not been demonstrated to be a stereotyped bidirectional phenomenon (e.g. muscle pain in the anterior tibial muscle produces pain in the

ventral part of the ankle, but the opposite condition has not been demonstrated). However, jaw muscle pain can be referred to the teeth, and tooth pain can be referred to the jaw muscles. Finally, the threshold for eliciting local and referred muscle pain is different.[105,109,134,211,241]

Convergence facilitation theory

MacKenzie[149] was also inspired by the ideas of Sturge[229] and Ross.[194] He believed that viscera were totally insensitive, and that non-nociceptive afferent input to the spinal cord created an irritable focus in the spinal cord. This focus would make other somatic inputs appear in an abnormal fashion, and in some cases even be perceived as referred pain. The theory was not recognized, mainly because it did not accept true visceral pain. But, in recent years, MacKenzie's simple idea of an irritable focus has reclaimed awareness under another term: *central sensitization*. The somatosensory sensitivity changes reported in referred pain areas could in part be explained by similar mechanisms in the dorsal horn and brain stem neurons, and the delay in appearance of referred pain demonstrated in various studies[94,134] could also be explained because the creation of central sensitization may take time.

Axon reflex theory

Bifurcation of afferents from two different tissues has been suggested as an explanation of referred pain.[211] Although bifurcation of nociceptive afferents from different tissues (muscle and skin,[164] and intervertebral disks and skin[238]) exists, it is generally agreed that these types of neurons are rare.[159] Moreover, this theory cannot explain the time delay in the appearance of referred pain, the different thresholds required for eliciting local and referred muscle pain, and the somatosensory sensitivity changes associated with referred pain.

Thalamic convergence theory

Theobald suggested that referred pain appeared as a summation of input from the injured area and the referred pain area within neurons in the brain, and not in the spinal cord.[239] A study, applying computer simulations, of referred pain in monkeys has demonstrated several pathways, which converge on different subcortical and cortical neurons.[4] Numerous experimental and clinical studies (e.g. Laursen et al., 1999[133]) have documented pain reduction following anesthetization of a referred pain area. This finding suggests that peripheral processes contribute to referred pain, although central processes are assumed to be predominant.

Central hyperexcitability theory

The above theories do not account for all the characteristics of referred pain previously described in this chapter. Mense has suggested an interesting theory, especially from a referred muscle pain point of view, which is known as the central hyperexcitability theory.[170]

Recordings from dorsal horn neurons in animals have revealed that, within minutes after noxious stimuli were applied to a receptive field in a muscle, new receptive fields at a distance from the original receptive field emerged.[8,103] That is, following nociceptive input, dorsal horn neurons that were previously responsive to only one area within a muscle began to respond to nociception from areas that previously had not provoked a response. The appearance of new receptive fields could indicate that latent convergent afferents on the dorsal horn neuron might be opened by noxious stimuli arising from muscle tissue,[170] and that this facilitation of latent convergence connections could appear as referred pain. Observations from the same group have demonstrated that substance P released from the terminal ends of primary afferents plays a role in the connectivity in the dorsal horn.[53] Furthermore, an expansion of the receptive fields proximal to the normal receptive field was found in a study where experimental myositis was induced, and afterward application of antagonists to three different neurokinin receptors was effective in preventing the induced hyperexcitability.[106]

The central hyperexcitability theory is consistent with several of the characteristics of referred muscle pain (dependency on stimulus and a delay in appearance of referred pain compared with local pain). However, if the emergence of new receptive fields is construed as the neurophysiologic basis for referred pain, the fact that such fields are sometimes *proximal* to a site of nociceptive input conflicts with the majority of studies on experimentally induced referred pain in healthy subjects.[6,88,89,94,109,127,133–136] These studies demonstrate the development of referred pain distal to a site of induced pain, but not proximal to it. Clinical studies looking at the spread of experimentally induced referred pain in patients suffering from whiplash syndrome and fibromyalgia have demonstrated proximal as well as distal referral of pain.[90,122] We have seen proximal spread of referred muscle pain in a few healthy volunteers following intramuscular injection of capsaicin in only one study. A possible explanation of the divergence between findings in healthy humans versus ones in people with clinically significant pain is that the preexisting pain in the latter people might have induced a state of hyperexcitability in the spinal cord, resulting in proximal and distal referral compared with the predominant distal referral in healthy subjects (Fig. 44-5).

The hyperexcitability theory[103,169,170,209] is based on animal studies in which receptive fields appeared within minutes. This does not fit exactly with the development of referred pain in humans that occurs within seconds. We think, however, that the idea of latent connections between dorsal horn neurons is convincing.

In summary, referred pain probably reflects a combination of central processing and peripheral input. As far as central processing is concerned, research conducted in relation to the central hypersensitivity theory supports the role of altered functioning in the dorsal horn as a contributor to referred pain. It is also likely that supraspinal mechanisms contribute to referred pain, although they have not been extensively studied. Also, there are multiple questions about referred pain that have not yet been resolved fully by research, and have not been incorporated into theories of referred pain.

Kellgren found evidence of hyperalgesia, i.e. increased tenderness to pressure, in areas of referred pain following experimentally induced muscle pain.[127] This finding parallels observations for cutaneous secondary hyperalgesia, where the hyperalgesic area is related to the capsaicin-induced pain intensity. However, not all later studies have been able to reproduce Kellgren's findings. Similarly, skin sensitivity in the referred pain area has been reported to depend on the stimulus modality tested.[87,134,252] Increased visual analog scale response to electrical cutaneous stimulation and decreased sensitivity to radiant heat or pinprick stimulation have been reported in referred pain areas.[87,138] This modality-specific somatosensory change found in the referred muscle area is similar to findings in secondary hyperalgesic areas of the skin after injury.

The neuropharmacology of central sensitization has been described in detail. In particular, the NMDA and neurokinin-1 receptors and nitric oxide synthesis may play a crucial role for hyperexcitability and spontaneous hyperactivity.[104] It has been shown that chronic musculoskeletal pain responds better to NMDA receptor antagonist (ketamine) treatment than to conventional morphine management,[218] indicating a role of central sensitization in these patients. The reason is that NMDA antagonists in many animal, experimental, and clinical studies are found to inhibit wind-up and hyperalgesia. Therefore it is plausible to propose that muscle pain conditions[170] may evoke central sensitization, which may play an important role in chronic musculoskeletal pain syndromes (see later section).

Central sensitization of dorsal horn or brain stem neurons initiated by nociceptive activity from muscles may explain the expansion of pain with referral to other areas, and probably also hyperalgesia in these areas. However, facilitated neurons cannot account for research indicating *decreased sensation* to certain sensory stimuli in the referred area. For example, it was found that saline-induced muscle pain resulted in deep tissue hypoalgesia in extrasegmental areas distant from the pain focus.[91,233]

Referred Muscle Pain

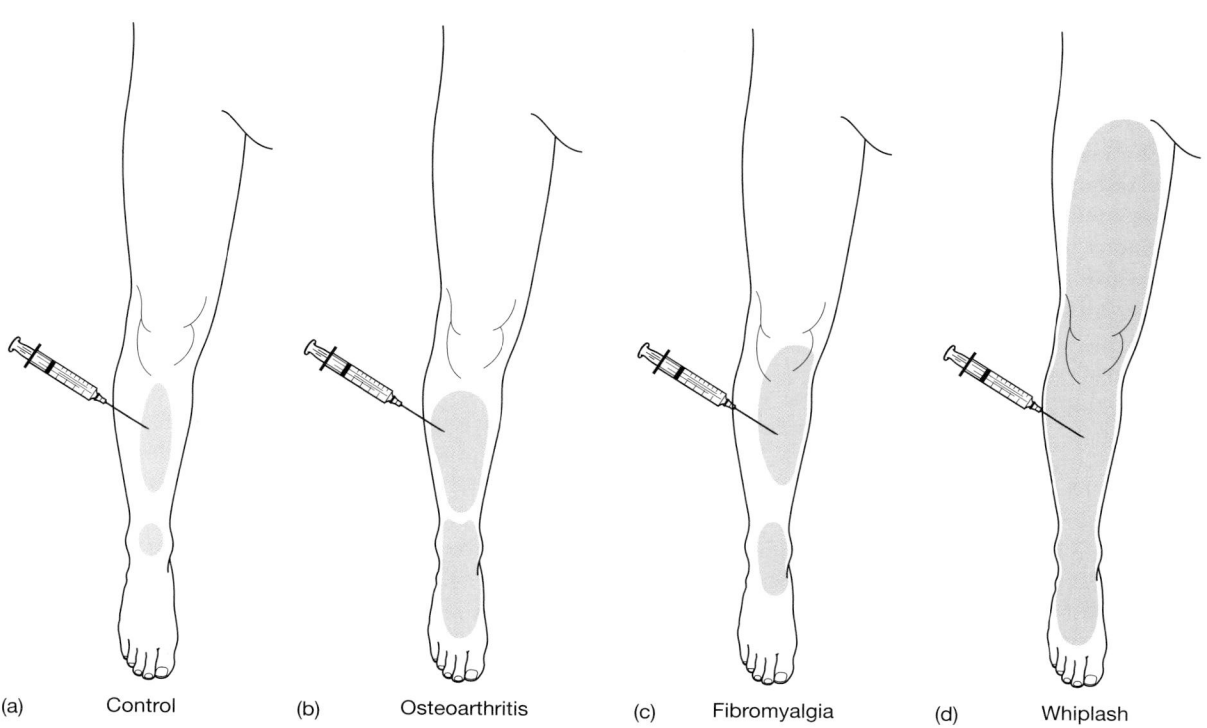

Hypertonic (6%, 0.5ml) in tibialis anterior

Figure 44-5 Patterns of referred pain following injection of hypertonic saline (6%, 0.5 mL, into the tibialis anterior). (**a**) Control subjects demonstrate local spread of pain around the injection site plus an area of referred pain over the dorsum of the foot. (**b**) Patients with lower extremity osteoarthritis demonstrate a pattern of local spread plus referred pain similar to that of control subjects, although encompassing a somewhat larger area. Patients with fibromyalgia (**c**) and (**d**) whiplash demonstrate referred pain both proximally and distally from the injection site. (Courtesy of Lars Arendt-Nielsen.)

Similar findings have been reported for cutaneous touch perception.[225] Descending inhibitory control of dorsal horn neurons may explain the decreased response to additional noxious stimuli in the referred pain area. Segmental inhibition at the spinal cord or brain stem level might also contribute to the decreased sensitivity. In animals, intramuscular capsaicin injections have been shown to produce inhibition of C-fiber activity from the contralateral leg. This inhibition was blocked by cooling the spinal cord,[79] and by spinal cord application of naloxone and phentolamine.[80] One practical implication of research demonstrating hypoalgesia in areas distant from a pain focus is that descending inhibitory mechanisms and/or segmental inhibition at the spinal cord level might mask increases in somatosensory sensitivity caused by muscle pain.

The involvement of peripheral input from the referred pain area is not clear. Anesthetizing this area has produced reductions in referred pain intensity in some studies, but no effects in others. For example, Laursen et al. found that it is possible to induce referred pain to limbs with complete sensory loss due to an anesthetic block.[133] Conversely, Vecchiet et al. demonstrated that infiltration of muscle tissue with anesthetics 30 min after injection of hypertonic saline (i.e. no ongoing pain) completely reversed cutaneous and muscular hyperalgesia.[254] This

effect of a peripheral block on muscle hyperalgesia could suggest peripheral sensitization. Alternatively, deep and especially cutaneous hyperalgesia after muscle pain might be caused by a central mechanism in which peripheral input is needed, which is also a necessary condition for referred pain.[87] Recently, we found hyperalgesia to pressure distal to the referred pain area produced by experimental pain induced in the tibialis anterior muscle.[92] The referred hyperalgesic area was innervated by the deep peroneal nerve, which also innervates the tibialis anterior muscle. This suggests involvement of summation between muscle afferents and the somatosensory afferents from the hyperalgesic area, with facilitation by central sensitization.

Central sensitization and referred pain in musculoskeletal conditions

Recent studies have provided good evidence of central sensitization in chronic musculoskeletal pain (Fig. 44-5). In the first study, it was found that fibromyalgia patients experienced stronger pain and larger referred areas after intramuscular injection of hypertonic saline.[218] The most interesting aspect was the fact that these manifestations were present in lower limb muscles, in which the patients normally do not experience ongoing pain. One could argue that the subjective pain ratings could be a result of, for example, hypervigilance, but the patients had no clues of the normal referred pain area to injection of hypertonic saline in the tibialis anterior muscle. Normally, pain from the tibialis anterior is projected distally to the ankle and only rarely proximally. In these patients, substantial proximal spread of the referred areas was found. This corresponds to basic neurophysiologic experiments in rats, in which dorsal horn neuron recordings from various spinal segments were investigated before and after muscle nociception.[103] In these experiments, the muscle nociception caused a proximal spread of sensitization, which possibly could explain the clinical findings. Moreover, intramuscular electrical stimulation was used to assess the efficacy of temporal summation of painful muscle stimuli in fibromyalgia patients, and temporal summation was found to be more pronounced in the patients compared with in control subjects.[218] The increased efficacy of temporal summation in fibromyalgia patients has recently been reproduced with cutaneous heat stimulation.[221] Temporal summation of pain stimuli applied to skin, joint, and muscle was most pronounced for muscle tissue,[268] illustrating the importance of testing the temporal summation from deep tissue, as this might specifically be affected by central sensitization in musculoskeletal pain conditions. Increased referred pain areas and facilitated temporal summation in pain patients suggest that the efficacy of central processing is increased (central sensitization) in these patients. Moreover, in fibromyalgia patients, the expanded referred pain areas and exaggerated temporal summation were partly inhibited by ketamine (an NMDA antagonist) targeting central sensitization.[93]

Similar findings of enlarged referred pain areas from the tibialis anterior muscle have been shown in patients suffering from chronic whiplash pain.[122] The increased areas of referred pain were found both in the neck–shoulder region (painful region) and in distant areas in which the patient does not normally experience pain (i.e. lower leg). Central sensitization in whiplash patients is also suggested to be based on increased sensitivity to intramuscular electrical stimulation of the tibialis anterior muscle compared with healthy subjects.[51] These findings could only partly be a manifestation of central sensitization of second-order neurons, but suggests that more generalized pathologic mechanisms also are involved in the whiplash syndrome. One possibility to explain the widespread changes could be a decreased efficacy of endogenous pain inhibitory systems, or even increased action of descending facilitatory pathways. In patients suffering from chronic osteoarthritic knee pain,[19] extended areas of saline-induced referred pain have been found. This indicates that noxious joint input to the central nervous system may facilitate the referred pain mechanisms possibly due to central sensitization. Similarly, in patients with myofascial temporomandibular disorder (TMD) pain, enlarged pain areas were found with painful injections of hypertonic saline into the masseter muscle.[236] There is also preliminary evidence that the perceived areas of experimentally induced pain are larger in patients with chronic tension-type headache, another condition with a distinct role of pathophysiologic changes in musculoskeletal tissues. Similarly, enlarged referred pain areas are also found after visceral stimulation in patients with chronic visceral pain.

The significance of referred pain for models of clinical muscle pain

When a patient complains of pain, an examining physician who is aware of the subtleties surrounding referred pain would probably consider whether the site that the patient identifies as painful represents the primary site of injury or irritation, or an area of referral. Unfortunately, there are no definite markers to facilitate this distinction. A related problem is that, if there is clinical evidence that a site designated by a patient as painful is in reality a site of referred pain, there are no definite indicators of where the primary site might be. The history of medical concepts regarding sciatica highlights the difficulties involved in distinguishing between referred pain and 'primary pain', and in identifying the primary site underlying referred pain. The symptom complex of sciatica was recognized by Hippocrates, but over the subsequent 2300 years physicians looked for local pathology in the lower extremity to explain the symptoms, and failed to appreciate that sciatica usually reflects pathology in the lumbar spine.[2]

Travell and Simons have indicated that one of the hallmarks of a trigger point is that pressure exerted on it by an examiner produces both localized pain and pain in a characteristic referral pattern.[244] Their theory of myofascial pain highlights the fact that irritation or injury in one muscle can cause referred pain in another muscle. But they do not systematically explore the possibility that irritation of structures other than muscles can yield referred pain to muscles. This possibility has been explored by other investigators. They have found that irritation of a variety of non-muscular structures—including intervertebral disks,[183] facet joints,[60,73,74] and spinal ligaments[98,126]—can produce referred pain that can mimic myofascial pain. This can be seen by comparing the pain pattern described by Travell and Simons for a myofascial syndrome affecting the levator scapulae muscle (Fig. 44-6) with a composite picture of pain indicated

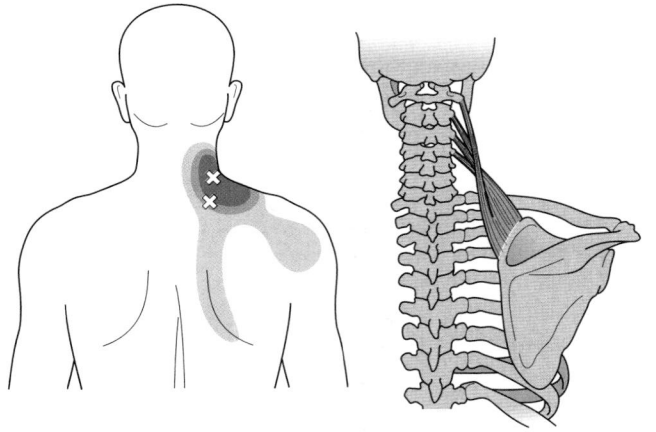

Figure 44-6 Consolidated referred pain pattern of the two trigger point locations (indicated by crosses) for the right levator scapulae muscle. The essential pain pattern is solid, and the spillover pattern is stippled.

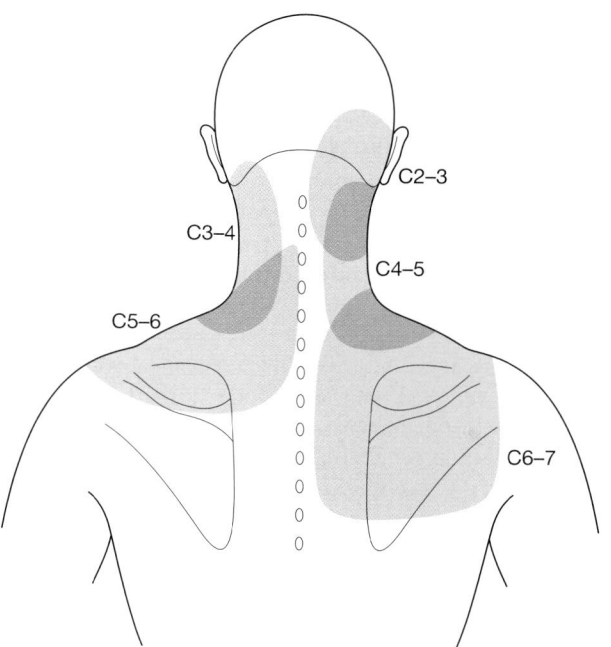

Figure 44-7 A composite map of the results in all volunteers, depicting the putative characteristic distribution of pain from zygapophyseal joints at segments C2–3 to C6–7. (From Dwyer et al. 1990,[60] with permission.)

by normal volunteers following cervical facet joint injections with hypertonic saline (Fig. 44-7). Other research has shown that referred muscular pain can result from irritation of visceral structures associated with conditions such as gallbladder disease, endometriosis, and colonic distention.[18,55,223]

The idea that muscular pain might reflect referred pain secondary to irritation of non-muscular structures invites a conceptualization of muscular pain that is fundamentally different from the one proposed by Travell and Simons. Travell and Simons emphasized that, although myofascial pain is influenced by a wide range of factors (such as postural abnormalities or hypothyroidism), it is fundamentally a reflection of an abnormality in muscles. Research on referred pain raises the possibility that myofascial pain might in fact be a secondary phenomenon in which a combination of irritation of non-muscular structures plus altered central nervous system processing of sensory input causes referred pain to muscles. Some writers have specifically argued that phenomena meeting the descriptive criteria for muscle pain can be caused by neuropathies[12,97] or spinal disorders.[129] Orthopedic texts have largely ignored the topics of myofascial pain and referred pain, but the structural lesion model of musculoskeletal disorders emphasized in orthopedics[192] implies that muscular pain is a secondary phenomenon.

The idea that muscle pain reflects referred pain rather than a primary abnormality in muscles undercuts the rationale for the attention that myofascial pain proponents devote to diagnosing myofascial pain and treating it directly. If myofascial pain is an epiphenomenon of some other kind of disorder, clinicians might be wasting their time when they attempt to dissect its nuances or make it a target for therapy.

Hyperalgesia in musculoskeletal pain conditions

Mechanical stimuli have been used extensively to assess the sensitization of myofascial tissues in humans. The most widely used technique is pressure algometry.[65,85,117] Pressure algometry is actually recommended as one of the diagnostic procedures for evaluation of patients with tension-type headache,[101] but so far not for examination of MPS or other musculoskeletal pain conditions. Methodological concerns such as short-term and long-term reproducibility,[67,84,111,116,143,181,188] influence of pressure rates and muscle contraction levels,[137,144,161] and examiner expectancy[180] have all been addressed carefully. Provided that proper standardization is applied, pressure pain thresholds are generally considered an improvement on the manual palpation technique of muscles. However, a palpometer device has been developed[24,25] and tested in patients with tension-type headache and fibromyalgia.[27,28] This device might also provide useful information in patients with MPS.

A large number of studies have consistently reported lower pressure pain thresholds in the jaw-closing muscles of patients with myofascial TMD pain compared with in normal subjects.[39,143,152,160,182,189,198,232] Patients with episodic or chronic tension-type headache have been reported to have lower pressure pain thresholds in craniofacial muscles,[132,199] but other studies have failed to show this difference between tension-type headache patients and control subjects.[82,118,120] The degree of chronicity and probably the daily levels of pain might influence the pressure pain thresholds.[121,197] Furthermore, there might be differences related to measurement on tender points or trigger points versus on fixed anatomic locations.[121,182]

The pathophysiologic mechanism responsible for lower pain thresholds in deep tissues could be a sensitization of peripheral nociceptors. Animal studies have shown that a deep noxious input causes sensitization of the peripheral receptors.[31] Endogenous substances released by tissue trauma, such as bradykinin, serotonin, prostaglandin E_2, adrenaline (epinephrine), and hypoxia, lower the mechanical threshold of nociceptors into the innocuous range, making weak stimuli able to excite nociceptors and elicit pain.[95,165,168,169,171] It is also the case that experimental myositis in animals is associated with an increased density of substance P- and nerve growth factor-immunoreactive nerve fibers, which could contribute to the peripheral sensitization process.[190] It is also an intriguing finding that myofascial TMD pain seems to be associated with local changes in serotonin levels as revealed by microdialysis techniques.[63] These authors suggested that peripheral serotonin could be involved in the hyperalgesia to pressure stimuli in patients with myofascial TMD pain, in accordance with a direct hyperalgesic action of intradermally applied serotonin in rats.[237] Furthermore, there is some evidence that histidine decarboxylase and formation of histamine could be linked to muscle fatigue and pain.[262] Although peripheral sensitization might cause deep tissue hyperalgesia, there is substantial evidence that sensitization of second-order neurons in the spinal cord or brain stem also are involved in the pathophysiologic process.[46,57,108,169,204]

The obvious question is: how site-specific and localized are these changes in deep hyperalgesia? So far, much research has focused on local changes in the pain sensitivity in the areas of the trigger points and those to which pain referral occurs. However, the studies of Scudds et al.[203] and Vecchiet et al.[255] address the question of whether there is also a generalized change in pain perception in patients with MPS. In the study of Scudds et al., the MPS patients were unfortunately not compared with pain-free control persons, but with other patients suffering from chronic pain. The patients with MPS clearly proved to be less sensitive to painful pressure than the patients suffering from fibromyalgia. This was valid not only for the typical tender point areas of the fibromyalgia but also for loci, which according to their definition are not hyperalgesic in either syndrome. In this connection, an especially elucidating study was carried out by Vecchiet and his colleagues[255] on 22 patients with MPS, 13 fibromyalgia patients, and 30 persons who were pain-free. They measured the electrical pain threshold at a myofascial trigger point, demonstrated hyperalgesia at a fibromyalgic tender point (both located in the trapezius muscle), and at a control point. Both groups of patients presented hyperalgesic when their problematic area was stimulated, whether it was the trigger point or the tender point. It is of interest to note that this was equally valid for the stimulation of a cutaneous, a subcutaneous, or a muscle tissue. This indicates that the hyperalgesia found in trigger points or tender points involves multiple tissues, rather than just muscle tissue. In contrast to the fibromyalgia patients, the patients suffering from MPS displayed completely normal pain sensitivity outside these areas. Consequently, as of yet there is no evidence for the existence of a generalized hyperalgesia in MPS.

Malow et al. reported that the pressure pain sensitivity in the finger was increased in patients with myofascial TMD pain.[154] Maixner et al. have presented good evidence that patients with myofascial TMD pain are hyperalgesic to stimulation of deep tissues outside the craniofacial region.[151,152] These results are in contrast, however, to the findings from Carlson et al.[39] and Svensson et al.[232] They found no significant differences in pressure pain thresholds in the finger between patients with myofascial TMD pain and control subjects. It is difficult to explain the observed differences, because strict inclusion criteria for the diagnosis of TMD pain were followed[58] and comparable pressure algometers were used in these studies[39,152,232] The levels and duration of pain also seem to be similar in the studies. Discrete differences are, however, apparent in the pressure stimulation technique, such as the number of repetitions, diameter of stimulation tip, and response criteria (push button, raise hand, or verbal sign). It is still unclear, nevertheless, how comparable results can be obtained from the jaw-closing muscles but opposing results from a remote site. It should be noted that the pressure pain thresholds were relatively more reduced (22–30%) in the jaw-closing muscles than in the wrist (12%) in patients with myofascial TMD pain.[152] This could imply a graded effect of changes in deep hyperalgesia. In contrast, more pronounced changes in deep pressure sensitivity were observed in the finger than in the temporalis muscles in patients with chronic tension-type headache compared with in healthy controls.[26] It remains an open question whether the deep sensitivity

to painful stimuli is generally or specifically altered in patients with myofascial TMD pain, and if graded responses exist eventually corresponding to transitions from localized pain complaints to more widespread pain complaints.

Only a few clinical studies exist on referred hyperalgesia. Leffler et al. assessed somatosensory function in referred pain in long-term trapezius myalgic patients.[140] Hyperalgesia to pressure and hypoalgesia to light mechanical stimulation were found in the referred pain area, suggesting a modality or tissue-specific change of the somatosensory function similar to previous experimental findings.[87] However, in patients with lateral epicondylalgia, only hypoalgesia to light mechanical stimulation was found in the referred pain area produced by muscle contractions.[139] A factor that might influence the somatosensory changes is the duration of habitual pain. The patients in whom referred hyperalgesia was found on average had experienced pain for 6 years,[140] whereas the patients on average had pain for 6 months in the study where hyperalgesia was not detected.[139] Increased sensitivity to pressure in a non-painful area was found in rheumatoid arthritis patients suffering more than 5 years, in contrast to patients with pain for less than 1 year.[140] This fits well with the concept of central sensitization, as a certain period of nociceptive input is needed to induce central sensitization. Interestingly, widespread pain in musculoskeletal pain disorders is frequently initiated by localized deep pain, indicating the development of central sensitization over time.

Another manifestation of central sensitization may be the number of palpable trigger points; recently, we found a significantly higher number of these points in lower limb muscles in patients suffering from knee osteoarthritis compared with in control subjects.[20] The presence of central sensitization may facilitate low-intensity input and hence result in the experience of pain when a possible latent trigger point is activated. This may also be one of the reasons why a localized painful condition can spread and become generalized.

A dysfunction of the descending inhibitory control systems might have similar effects to those of central sensitization. In healthy subjects, generalized hypoalgesia to pressure is found during strong experimentally induced pain. In contrast, fibromyalgia patients do not show such modulation, indicating a dysfunction of the descending inhibitory control.[130] The mechanism of descending inhibition is intact in short- and long-term rheumatoid arthritis patients compared with control subjects.[140] Before surgery (e.g. hip replacement), osteoarthritis patients lacked the generalized hypoalgesic effect to pressure during a strong experimental pain, in contrast to the normalized descending inhibition after hip surgery.[131] This might reflect the fact that the descending system is maximally involved in the condition with continuous pain (before surgery), and that after surgery the dynamic of the system is reestablished and effectively modulates the sensitivity to pressure. Thus a dysfunction of the descending inhibitory control system might be involved in chronic muscle pain conditions, although it has not been a systematic finding in different groups of patients.

Motor responses

The completely resting muscle is characterized by the absence of any electromyography (EMG) activity. However, with the jaws at rest there is weak EMG activity present in the human jaw-closing muscles.[265] This might serve to counteract the effects of gravity on the lower jaw, i.e. postural activity. There is a general consensus that healthy, non-painful jaw muscles exhibit only very low levels of EMG activity in the range of 3–5 μV, but no scientific evidence for any exact threshold values is present.[148]

We recorded the resting muscle activity by intramuscular wire and surface electrodes during saline-induced muscle pain.[234] In this study, there was a transient increase in the EMG activity during infusion of hypertonic saline compared with infusion of isotonic saline. After the infusion and during ongoing muscle pain, there was no significant difference in the resting EMG level. Ongoing muscle pain did not produce sustained increased EMG activity. Moreover, experimental muscle pain does not cause any changes in resting EMG activity between repeated maximal voluntary contractions (MVCs).[87] Elert et al. reported an increase in the resting EMG activity between contractions in fibromyalgia patients.[61] Others report no increase in the resting muscle EMG activity in fibromyalgia,[272] TMD,[38] and low back pain patients.[1,48] Observation of muscle spasms in the referred pain area from trigger point activation is also reported.[242] In addition, saline-induced muscle pain produced increased resting muscle activity in muscles away from the painful muscle,[24,210] but this finding was inconstant and based on limited material.

There is no consensus on the surface EMG activity of jaw-closing muscles in conditions with myofascial TMD pain. A number of studies have indicated no significant difference in postural activity,[38,153] while other studies have found a small increase,[81,145] and some studies have shown a small decrease.[110] The same controversy is present for tension-type headache, because studies have reported significant increases in pericranial surface EMG activity[119,253] or no significant increases or relationships to pain.[45,156] This confusing picture also applies to several other myofascial pain conditions, for example low back pain and fibromyalgia (for a review see Lund et al.[147]). Many of the published studies have been criticized for the lack of proper matching between the MPS patients and control groups with regard to age and gender.[146,148] Two well-controlled studies, however, have shown a small, significant increase in surface EMG activity in patients with persistent myofascial pain in the masticatory muscles[81] and chronic tension-type headache.[118] The specificity of a slightly increased surface EMG activity in these muscles has, however, also been questioned because it could easily be contaminated with the cross-talk of EMG activity from mimic muscle (e.g. eye muscles or platysma).[228] Cross-talk between deep and superficial layers of, for example, the neck and shoulder muscles could also be a potential problem for the interpretation of surface EMG recordings in MPS. Pain is reflected in the facial expressions and mimic responses,[141] which seems to support a potential contribution from mimic muscles to the surface EMG recordings of jaw-closing muscles.

Finally, the pathophysiologic importance of such small increases in postural EMG activity, if they exist, has been discussed.[228] The described EMG increases are calculated to represent less than 1% of the mascimal voluntary contraction (MVC) level, and there is no evidence that this can lead to the development of muscle pain.[228]

Increased postural EMG activity has for a long time been believed to play a very important role in the pathophysiologic mechanisms in many muscle pain disorders. Increased EMG activity in painful muscles would also intuitively explain the clinical impression of increased tension or hardness in the same muscles. Evidence has been presented for increased hardness of pericranial muscles in patients with tension-type headache.[13] Travell et al. are usually given credit for the description of the vicious cycle that proposed a mutually reinforcing relationship between chronic pain and muscle hyperactivity.[243] In this respect, confusion on the terminology has existed for a long time, because the terms *muscle tension*, *muscle spasms*, *muscle contractures*, and *muscle hyperactivity* have been used interchangeably but can represent entirely different conditions.[166] DeVries suggested that muscle pain and soreness were caused by tonic local spasm of motor units, and that the pain reflex sustained the tonic muscle contraction, setting up a vicious cycle.[53] Later, Johansson and Sojka presented a model to explain muscle tension and pain, which integrated the gamma-motor neuron system in the pathophysiologic mechanism.[123] Mense discussed a modified vicious cycle concept in which the central component was local ischemia.[169] It was pointed out, however, that at present there is no evidence for the suggested chain of events. Finally, Mense and Simons have proposed that tension in painful muscles is electrically silent, and that muscle contracture and not contraction could cause tension.[166] The minute loci of trigger points could be associated with localized EMG activity,[166] but the question of increased EMG activity in trigger points of jaw-closing muscles has not been unambiguously answered yet.[71,121,147,269]

The MVC during saline-induced muscle pain is significantly lower than the control condition.[87,235] A clinical demonstration of the observed decrease in muscle strength during voluntary isometric contractions of a painful muscle has also been made in fibromyalgia,[17,112,113] TMD,[176] and low back pain patients.[3,240] In fibromyalgia patients, the reduction in strength is suggested to be due to a deficit in central activation of motor units, because supramaximal stimulation of the ulnar nerve shows no difference in the strength of the adductor pollicis muscle between patients and a control group.[17] The nociceptive activity most likely modulates the motor neuron firing, as a correlation between pain intensity and EMG changes is found.[5,84]

During a static contraction (80% of the MVC before pain), muscle pain causes a significant reduction in endurance time.[87] Contractions at 10% of MVC after injection of hypertonic saline were previously found to cause no changes in EMG activity.[15] Submaximal, static contraction of the trapezius muscle in unilateral shoulder pain patients produces progressively increased EMG amplitude until endurance is reached, but the recordings from the painful and non-painful side are similar.[100]

The different findings between submaximal and maximal contractions[87] might be explained by changes in the descending neural drive to motor neurons. The descending neural drive cannot be voluntarily increased during MVC, and an inhibitory mechanism controlling the motor neurons might therefore explain decreases in MVC. When submaximal contractions are performed, it might be possible to increase the voluntary neural drive and consequently compensate for the potential inhibitory mechanism.

In accordance with experimental findings,[87] the endurance time is decreased in muscle pain patients.[29,44,62,77] The decline of motor neuron firing in fatigued muscles is proposed to be reflex-mediated by group III and IV excitation.[32,76] Thus a similar mechanism may be involved in muscle pain, as a decreased endurance time is demonstrated during saline-induced muscle pain.[87] If submaximal contractions during muscle pain are obtained by increased voluntary neural drive, the decreased endurance time could alternatively be due to a more pronounced central fatigue.[115] In clinical studies, various physiologic factors within the muscle (e.g. microcirculation) could influence endurance time,[102] but this is not likely to occur in healthy volunteers.

The lumbar muscle EMG activity during a flexion–extension exercise is higher in low back pain patients in full flexion than in control subjects, in whom it is normally silent.[1,206,246] Moreover, the muscle activity is lower during the extension phase in low back pain patients compared with controls.[206] This indicates that the pain modulation of muscle activity is dependent on the specific muscle function (agonist or antagonist phases). This has been found in several previous clinical studies (for review, see Lund et al.[147]). The lumbar muscle EMG activity in low back pain patients and during saline-induced lumbar muscle pain is increased in phases where the EMG activities is normally silent, and not affected or decreased in the phases with strong EMG activity in controls.[5] During dynamic contractions, muscle pain causes decreased EMG activity in the agonistic phase[30,146,230,231,235] and increased EMG in the antagonistic phase[87,146,224,227,235] of the muscle activity in painful muscles.

Reduced movement amplitudes have been reported in low back pain patients,[1,5,69,125] in TMD patients,[59] and during saline-induced muscle pain.[5,87,150,179,231] The increased EMG activity of the muscle (antagonistic phase) opposite to the painful muscle[87] and the decreased EMG activity of the painful muscle (agonistic phase)[231] are probably a functional adaptation of muscle coordination to limit movements.[226] This adaptation can protect the painful muscle by reducing the muscle activity and contraction force.

The relationship between work-related muscle pain and muscle activity has been studied extensively in an attempt to find a valid predictor for the development of myalgia. The question is why some people develop myalgia when performing work at a low level of force. A decreased frequency of unconscious gaps in the low-level EMG activity was found to predict the patients who developed myalgia.[257] Experimental models of muscle pain have also been used in occupational settings (low load, repetitive work), in which it was found that saline-induced

neck muscle pain caused a decreased working rhythm and a muscle coordination change that could be interpreted as protective.[150]

The adaptation to muscle pain can change from the acute pain phase to the chronic pain condition. Nevertheless, the initial adaptation from experimental acute muscle pain is similar to the adaptation seen in chronic muscle pain patients.[147] This suggests that the protective adaptation is maintained in the transition from acute to chronic muscle pain.

In interpreting the above data, it is important to remember that all voluntary muscle activity is controlled by complex motor programs in the central nervous system.[23,125] We believe that the above-described anomalies in motor function among individuals with muscle pain usually reflect changes in these programs. We further postulate that the patterns of motor behavior associated with pain-induced alterations in motor programs are often dyskinetic. These dyskinetic motor patterns can lead to persistent strains in the musculoskeletal system. As an example, an individual with a painful knee might develop movement patterns characterized by simultaneous activation of flexors and extensors of the knee. This cocontraction would produce strains on the muscles around the knee, because, for example, extension of the knee would be associated with excessive eccentric contractions of the hamstrings. The strains caused by the dyskinetic motion patterns might in turn set the stage for persistent pain in the affected muscles.

A model depicting our hypotheses is shown schematically in Figure 44-8. The model must be considered speculative, because we are not aware of systematic research that validates the various steps postulated. In our opinion, the model represents an alternative conceptual model of the way in which chronic muscular pain may develop.

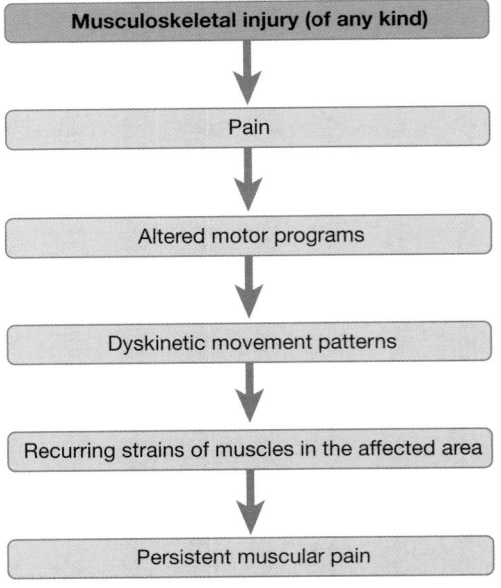

Figure 44-8 A postulated pathway linking musculoskeletal injury with chronic muscle pain.

RESEARCH ON MYOFASCIAL PAIN

Epidemiology and general features of myofascial pain

As discussed earlier, opinions diverge dramatically regarding virtually all aspects of myofascial pain. The epidemiology of myofascial pain is one example of this. Some research indicates a high prevalence of myofascial pain among various patient populations, with rates ranging from 30% among patients in a general medical clinic[212] to 85% among patients treated at a pain center.[68] As is the case with other forms of chronic muscle pains, women seem to be more often afflicted than men. The differences in gender, however, are not very large when it concerns MPS.[72] Even among young adults with no clinical muscle pain, the prevalence of latent trigger points (manifested by physical examination findings indicative of trigger points) has been reported to be approximately 50%.[217] These data suggest that myofascial pain is a major cause of musculoskeletal pain. Obviously, physicians who are not proponents of myofascial pain have a different perspective, because the term *myofascial pain* is not even listed in the indexes of standard orthopedic texts.

The pain present in MPS is often very persistent and of the same dull quality as other kinds of deep pain.[256] Systematic studies of the intensity of pain, for example by measurement using visual analog scales or other validated ratio interval scales, have hardly been done. It is, however, probable that both the sensory-discriminative and affective-motivational dimension of pain in MPS, as well as the extent of functional impairment, are only marginally less pronounced compared with the levels in fibromyalgia or chronic back pain.[163,247,266]

Further symptoms of MPS include impaired mobility accompanied by partial parafunctional habits of movement, general fatigue, and sleep disorders.[216] It is scarcely known whether MPS patients suffer from psychologic problems, because the disorder has traditionally been treated purely somatically as being due to a protracted muscular trauma, muscular injuries, or overstraining of the muscles. In a study of 283 patients in a pain clinic, of which 85% had been diagnosed as suffering from MPS, point prevalence between 40 and 50% for anxiety disorder, somatoform disorder, and depression was found.[68] The opinion that psychologic disorders in MPS play only a minor role can be called into question because of such data.

As a general rule, an acute pain due to muscular injury, an overstraining of a muscle, or muscle fatigue is thought to precede chronic MPS. This massive nociceptive input to the central nervous system in these acute conditions is presumably able to generate an hyperalgesic area in the form of trigger points, which may continue to exist even after the muscular pain has subsided.[157,167] A trigger point pool can gradually develop, which, under further strain, can suddenly lead to the surprisingly persistent and intense pain in chronic MPS.[216] It should be emphasized that this transition from acute pain in muscle tissues to a chronic pain disorder is a working hypothesis that not has been validated, but which seems likely from a clinical perspective. Longitudinal studies with clear case definitions and operationalized measures of pain and somatosensory function will be needed to test this hypothesis. It is also noteworthy that an extensive literature demonstrates that unaccustomed, strenuous muscle activity produces a characteristic syndrome of muscle pain (called DOMS), but that individuals with DOMS almost always recover uneventfully within a few days.[42] The literature on DOMS is difficult to reconcile with the assertion of myofascial pain proponents that muscle overload can have severe and long lasting effects.

Trigger points in myofascial pain syndrome

Trigger points are often believed to be the initiator of myofascial pain, but frequently are not located in its direct vicinity, sometimes not even in the same muscle.[216] Another important aspect of MPS is that manipulation of these trigger points can cause pain or paresthesia experienced by the patients in other and sometimes remote regions.[72] Interestingly, this spread or referral of pain is not limited to dermatomes or myotomes.[169] Nevertheless, the experience of the diffuse pain appears to be a rather consistent phenomenon that has allowed one to determine where the trigger points are located.[244,245] How precisely the trigger points can be determined from the mere description and location of pain has not been investigated, i.e. the sensitivity, specificity, and predictive value of this clinical procedure have never been established.

The trigger points, which are believed to have a diameter of between 2 and 5 mm, are embedded in a band of hardened muscle fibers, which is responsible for the tenseness and restriction of the mobility of the befallen muscle. Squeezing or pressing this band results in local muscle spasms and a burst activity in the EMG.[72,209] The muscles in which the trigger point is located are marked by an increased EMG activity and tendency to become fatigued, which is probably due to the decrease in the phosphates that deliver the energy.[30] It should, however, be noted that serious methodological problems may arise when assessing the intramuscular EMG activity from such a small volume as constituted by the trigger point.

Trigger points are identified on the basis of physical examination findings, although ancillary tests such as EMG may substantiate their presence.[166] As noted earlier, Simons identifies multiple clinical findings that are characteristic of trigger points, including:

- a circumscribed spot of tenderness in a nodule that is part of a palpably taut band of muscle fibers;
- patient recognition of the pain provoked by pressure on the tender spot as being familiar;
- referral of pain in a characteristic pattern;
- a local twitch response;
- painful limitation of range of motion; and
- some weakness of the involved muscle.[166]

At another point, Simons indicates that the minimal acceptable criteria for identifying a trigger point are 'spot tenderness in a palpable band and subject recognition of the pain' (Mense and Simons 2001,[169] p. 225).

Several studies have been performed to determine whether different phenomena thought to be associated with trigger points can be reliably identified by examiners. Research during the early 1990s suggested that interrater reliability for at least some of the key features of trigger points was poor.[178,266] Subsequently, Gerwin et al. demonstrated that, under ideal conditions, experts in myofascial pain could achieve acceptable interrater reliability for several phenomena associated with trigger points, including tenderness, presence of taut bands, referred pain, and patient recognition of typical pain.[78] Agreement for local twitch responses was less impressive. Sciotti et al. subsequently demonstrated that, under ideal conditions, experts in myofascial pain could agree on the presence of trigger points in the upper trapezius muscles of subjects, and could agree within a few millimeters regarding the precise location of the trigger points.[200] It is noteworthy that these positive results were obtained only when clinicians who were already experienced in the diagnosis and treatment of myofascial pain trained together in order to improve the consistency of their examinations and interpretation of findings. When experts did not undergo joint training to improve consistency, interrater reliability was poor.[78] Moreover, even with training, clinicians who did not previously have extensive experience in the management of myofascial pain failed to achieve acceptable agreement with a myofascial expert regarding trigger point phenomena.[107]

These studies do not permit a simple conclusion to be reached about the reliability with which trigger points can be identified. There is substantial evidence that clinicians can agree regarding the presence of muscular tenderness.[177,247] But it appears that adequate interrater reliability for other phenomena associated with myofascial pain can be achieved only under extraordinary conditions that are not at all reflective of the settings in which clinicians and most researchers make decisions about whether or not individuals have trigger points. Problems associated with achieving interrater reliability are greatly magnified by the tendencies of researchers to use the term *myofascial pain* loosely, and to fail to describe the operational definition for myofascial pain used in studies. Gerwin et al. state the issue as follows:

> One implication of this study is that researchers studying MPS or the MTrP need to define the TrP for the purposes of their study. The criteria by which a TrP is identified, or the diagnosis of MPS made, needs to be clearly stated in order to properly interpret the reliability of the study.
>
> (Gerwin et al. 1997,[78] p. 72.)

The neurophysiologic mechanisms assumed to be responsible for the spread and referral of pain from trigger points are convergences of nociceptive afferent fibers from the trigger points and from the area to which the pain is transferred to the same second-order neuron in the spinal cord or brain stem, or even at higher levels in the somatosensory system. The area of the zone to which pain is referred depends on the sensitivity of the trigger point: highly sensitive trigger points can induce pain in large areas. In principle, trigger points can develop in every muscle and often correlate, in their localization, with acupuncture points.[157] Empirical research has demonstrated, however, that trigger points are not distributed uniformly through the body, but, rather, are most likely to be found in the regions of the head and neck, the shoulder ligaments, and in the lower back.[59]

An important question in MPS is whether the pain sensitivity at the trigger points is indeed as markedly increased as would be expected according to its definition. Reeves and his colleagues examined nine patients suffering from myofascial pain in the head and neck areas using a pressure dolorimeter, and compared the pain thresholds from five typical trigger point areas in the head and neck areas with thresholds from control areas throughout the same muscles.[188] All the thresholds measured in the trigger point areas were significantly lower. Reeves et al. unfortunately did not make any statements as to whether there were any trigger points in these areas.[188] The study of Schiffman et al., in which 45 patients with myofascial pain were examined, also displays this weakness.[198] The 15 areas examined were indeed typical loci of myofascial trigger points; however, the trigger points were not confirmed diagnostically. The thresholds for painful pressure of the patients were significantly lower in every locus examined than the thresholds of the control persons who were free of pain.

The importance of a diagnostic verification of the trigger points is demonstrated in a further study by Reeves and his colleagues with 20 patients suffering from unilateral and bilateral myofascial neck and head pain.[114] Using palpation, Jaeger and Reeves first identified the trigger points in the muscles of the neck and shoulders. The thresholds for painful pressure at these verified trigger points were markedly lower than the thresholds of their earlier study,[188] in which no trigger point localization had taken place. In patients with a unilateral pain syndrome, the thresholds at the trigger point on the symptomatic side were significantly lower than those measured contralaterally at the same muscle area.

Jaeger and Reeves[114] also examined the influence of the classic therapy for myofascial pain, which involved a prespraying of the muscles that contained the trigger points with cold and then passively stretching them.[244,245] This treatment carried out by Jaeger and Reeves led not only to a decrease in ongoing pain, but also to a reduction of the local hyperalgesia at the trigger point. One cannot, however, conclude from this that the intensity of the myofascial pain is solely dependent on the pain sensitivity of the trigger point. The correlation between both variables was too low for such a conclusion.[114] Furthermore, improvements in the clinical symptomatology, for example by using transcutaneous electrical stimulation,[86] were possible without eliminating the trigger point hyperalgesia.

Vecchiet and his colleagues examined the pain thresholds for electrical stimuli at the myofascial trigger points and in the zones to which pain referral occurred of 10 patients suffering pain in the head and neck.[256] In both areas, the pain thresholds of the patients were significantly lower than those of pain-free control persons. Treating the trigger points with a local anesthesia led not only to an increase in pain thresholds here, but also in the zones to which pain referral occurred. This points to a close correlation between the pain sensitivity at both places. The findings of Jaeger and Reeves,[114] as well as those of Graff-Radford et al.,[86] showed, however, that a similar close relationship does not necessarily exist between the pain sensitivity at the trigger point and the intensity of the clinical pain.

Summary of experimental muscle pain research

This section has briefly reviewed the rapidly growing area of experimental human muscle pain research. This research has provided important insights into issues that are fundamental to an understanding of muscle pain, including hyperalgesia, referred pain, and the roles of central and peripheral nervous system sensitization in persistent pain.

As is often the case in a new area of investigation, research on muscle pain has frequently generated controversies and questions rather than definitive answers. But, like any scientific endeavor, muscle pain research offers the promise of incremental knowledge that, in the long run, will provide insights greater than those gleaned by even the most gifted clinician. We have summarized this research because we are convinced that the time is rapidly approaching when physicians who treat muscular pain will need to be conversant with experimental muscle pain research, just as cardiologists need to be conversant with research on the physiology of the heart.

The focus of the majority of human muscle pain research has been on the basic neurobiology of muscle pain, rather than on issues of central importance to clinicians. One practical consequence of this focus is that there has been only a modest amount of research on linkages between phenomena demonstrated in laboratory research and phenomena observed in patients with clinically significant muscular pain. For example, we are not aware of any studies in which the clinical indicators of myofascial trigger points have been assessed in normal subjects who have been exposed to experimentally induced muscle pain. Also, experimental research to date has not identified any dramatically new therapies for muscle pain. Thus results of experimental muscle pain studies are not used to support recommendations in the discussion below on clinical management of muscle pain.

MANAGEMENT OF MUSCLE PAIN

Initial issues

Breadth of the field

Muscle pain or muscle dysfunction has been proposed as an explanation for a wide range of medical syndromes. To consider a short list, muscle pain has been proposed to play an important role in tension headaches, temporomandibular joint dysfunction, spinal pain, and pelvic pain. Correspondingly, it has been studied by neurologists, dentists, orthopedists, and gynecologists. One consequence of this diversity is that there are pockets of information about muscle pain that are available to specialists in a single organ system, but are difficult to interpret by other health practitioners. A good example of this problem is the literature of myofascial pain in relation to temporomandibular joint dysfunction. A strong case could be made for the thesis that research on the role of myofascial pain in temporo-

mandibular joint dysfunction has advanced farther than research on myofascial pain in any other clinical setting, but very few non-dentists have enough skill in dentistry or orofacial pain to interpret the research findings. As a practical matter, this chapter will focus on muscle pain in relation to spinal disorders.

Differences of opinion

The discussion above indicates that physicians have fundamental differences in perspective regarding muscle pain. These differences, together with the lack of definitive empiric evidence regarding the best ways to manage muscle pain, make it impossible to describe management strategies that are evidence-based or uniformly accepted.

Although clinical aspects of muscle pain have been discussed in detail only by proponents of myofascial theory, it is possible to discern three different general perspectives that physicians bring to bear on muscle pain.

1. Muscle pain reflects dysfunction and hypersensitivity in muscles. This is the perspective of Simons. It is consistent with treatments that focus on muscle pain and dysfunction.
2. Muscle pain is a secondary phenomenon. Irritation of other structures (e.g. spinal joints) causes referred pain to muscles. From this perspective, the most appropriate way to treatment muscle pain is to rectify the 'upstream' pathology that is viewed as the cause of the muscle pain.
3. Muscle pain is essentially a somatoform disorder. This position, articulated most forcefully by Bohr,[33] suggests that physicians should avoid reifying muscle pain with labels suggesting a known pathophysiologic mechanism, and should focus on modifying patients' perceptions of their bodies.

The discussion below reflects the following assumptions on the part of the authors.

- Muscle pain syndromes are heterogeneous with respect to pathophysiology.
- In many instances, they reflect a combination of altered central nervous system functioning, guarding, and deconditioning, rather than a primary abnormality within muscles.
- Muscle pain usually coexists with other sources of pain (e.g. a patient may have spinal pain based on a combination of facet joint irritation plus surrounding muscular hypersensitivity).
- Clinically significant muscular pain usually occurs in the context of chronic pain, so that treatment of muscular pain should be based on insights that have come from the management of chronic muscle pain in general.

Patient evaluation: history

Symptoms and history of present injury or illness

The most important historical information to elicit involves the duration of pain, the location of pain, and the issue of whether pain has spread since its onset. The issue of chronicity is

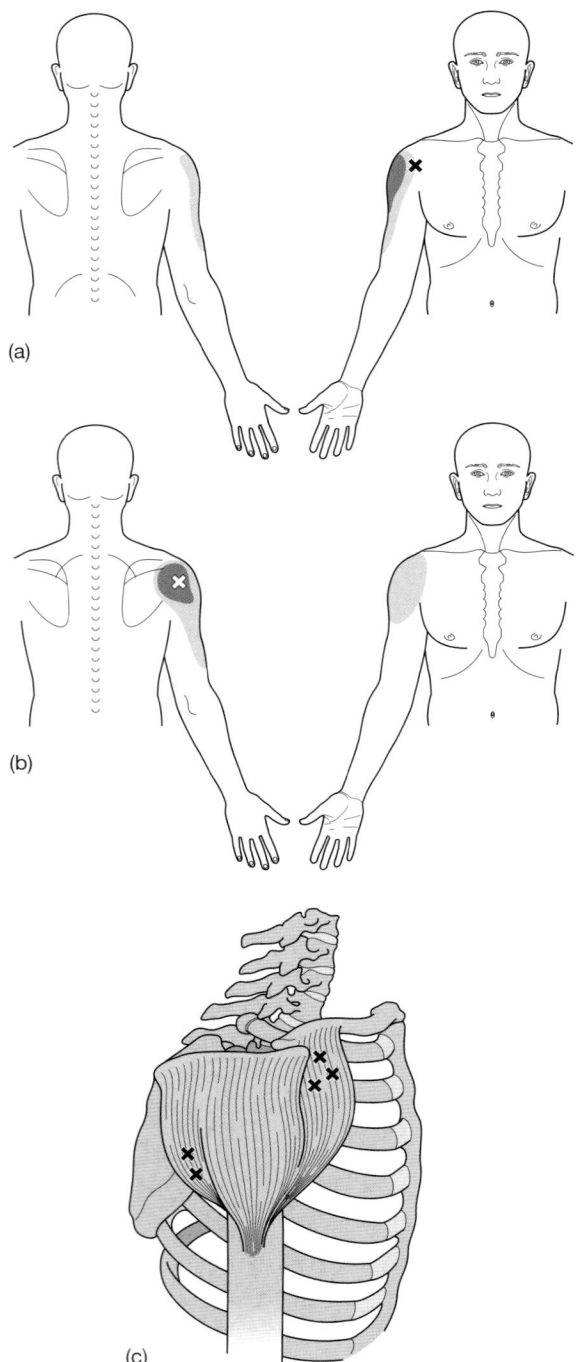

Figure 44-9 Referred pain patterns from trigger points (indicated by crosses) in the right deltoid muscle. (**a**) Pain pattern from trigger points in the anterior part of the muscle. (**b**) Pain patterns from the posterior part. (**c**) Usual location of trigger points in the muscle, lateral view.

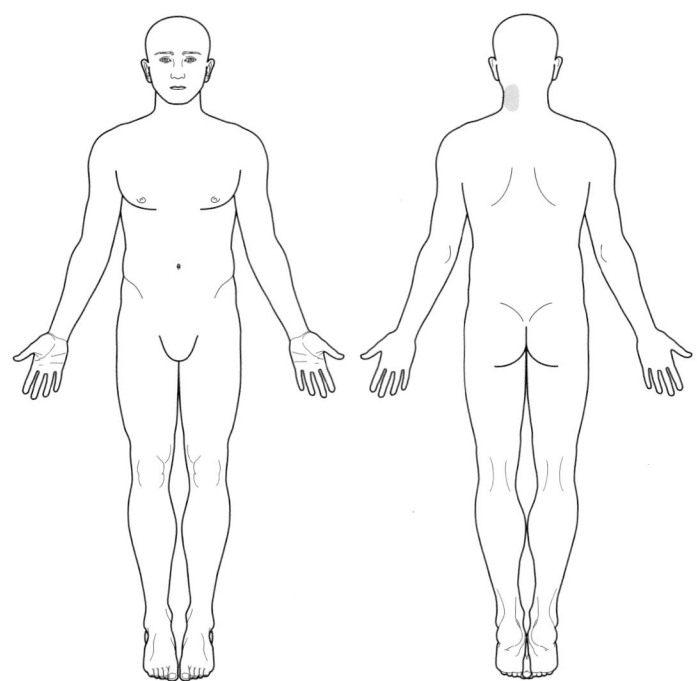

Figure 44-10 Localized axial spinal pain that suggests irritation of a cervical facet joint.

addressed below. The location of pain can give important clues about whether or not a patient is likely to have myofascial pain. A pain diagram is extremely helpful as a first step in determining where a patient is symptomatic.

In the simplest case, a patient will describe an area of pain that is classic for myofascial pain—one that closely matches one of the patterns described in *Myofascial Pain and Dysfunction*

(Fig. 44-9).[244,245] This type of pain diagram would greatly increase the probability that the patient actually has myofascial pain. But you can see at least four other patterns of pain on the musculoskeletal pain diagram. Some patients describe very localized pain, for example slightly off center in the lower cervical region (Fig. 44-10). This type of drawing is suggestive of joint pain (such as a C5–6 facet arthropathy) rather than myofascial pain. Other patients indicate pain in a pattern that is classic for a radiculopathy (Fig. 44-11). The presence of a radiculopathy does not rule out concurrent myofascial pain. Indeed, some experts in muscular pain argue that myofascial pain is common in radiculopathies, and at least one[97] argues that myofascial pain is essentially always a by-product of a radiculopathy or neuropathy. A pain diagram in a classic radicular pattern, however, should alert you to the strong possibility that your patient has something going on other than straightforward myofascial pain. It implies that, even if you find evidence of myofascial pain in your examination, you should consider directing your treatment toward the radiculopathy rather than toward the myofascial pain. A third pattern that you will commonly see is very widespread pain (Fig. 44-12). This should increase your level of suspicion that your patient's problem could best be described as fibromyalgia rather than regional myofascial pain. Finally, you will encounter many patients whose drawings indicate that their pain is limited to one body region, but is diffuse within that region and does not correspond in any obvious way to a classic MPS (Fig. 44-13). It is possible that the pain of such patients reflects myofascial pain, but is complex because it is a product of multiple trigger points. However, it is equally likely that these

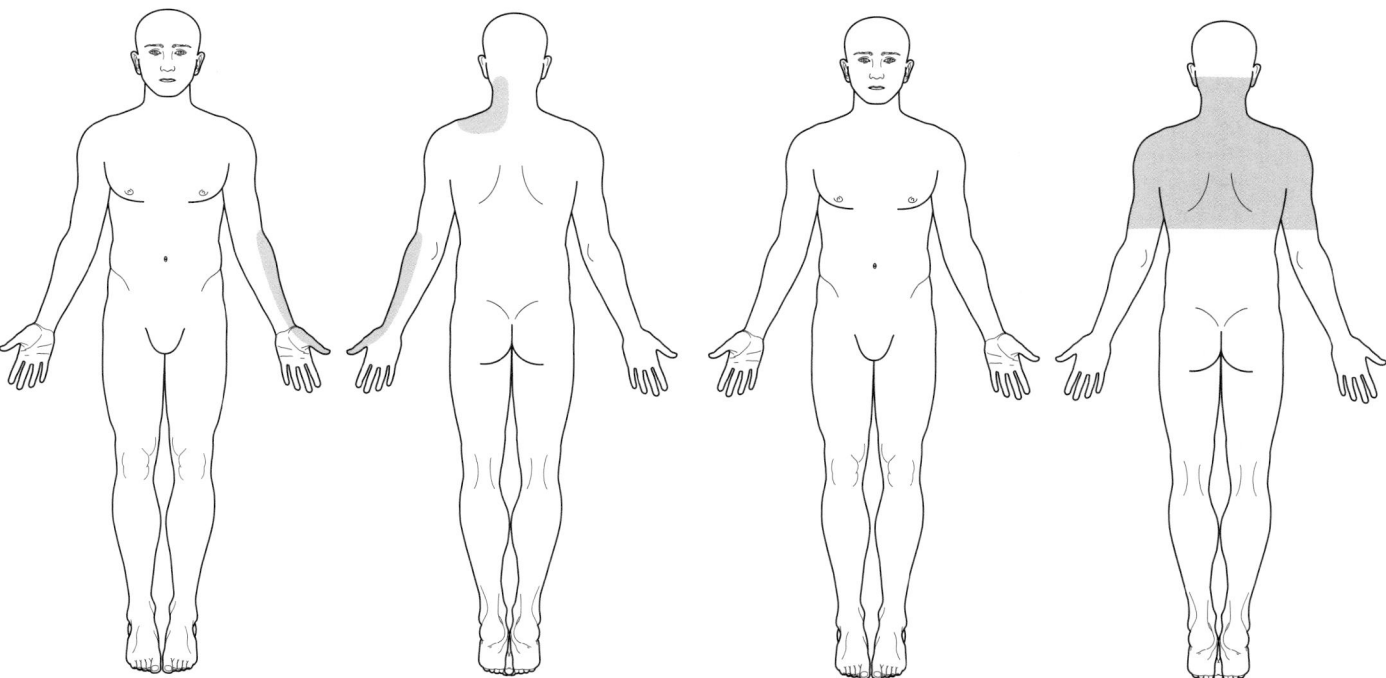

Figure 44-11 Neck and upper extremity pain in a pattern suggesting a cervical radiculopathy involving the C6 nerve root.

Figure 44-13 Widespread regional pain that does not conform to a well-accepted pattern of myofascial pain and whose etiology is uncertain.

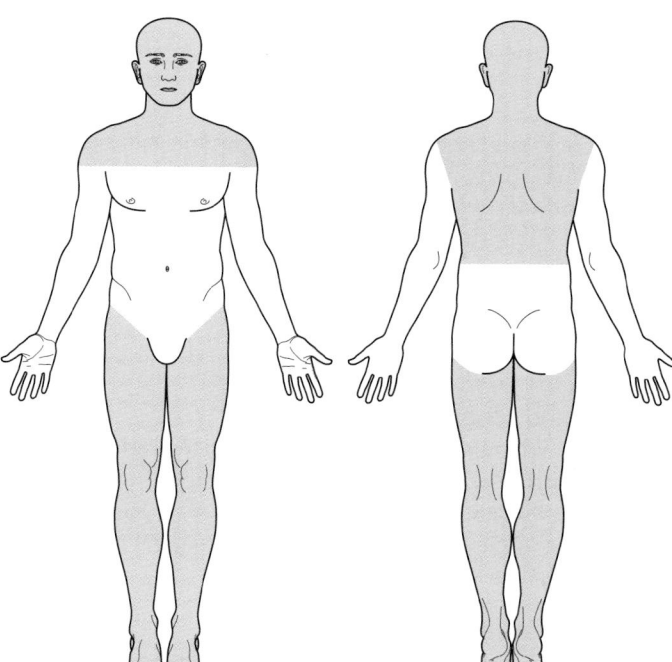

Figure 44-12 Widespread musculoskeletal pain suggestive of fibromyalgia.

patients have muscle pain that is not readily construed as myofascial pain.

Obviously, you should use a pain diagram only as a starting point in determining your patient's musculoskeletal symptoms. You need to supplement the drawing with detailed questioning

of the patient. This permits you to better determine the distribution of the patient's pain, as well as its quality and associated symptoms, including numbness, paresthesias, and focal weakness. If your patient reports multiple areas of pain, it is important for treatment planning to ask her or him about the area that is most symptomatic.

You also need information about the diagnostic evaluations and prior treatments patients have received for their pain problem. If these have been extensive, they should allow you to determine how likely it is that your patient has pain secondary to a radiculopathy or to an irritation or injury to one of the joints of the spine (e.g. a symptomatic disk or a facet arthropathy). The presence of these sources of pain does not negate the possibility that your patient also has myofascial pain, but your ultimate treatment plan should take into account all the factors that may be contributing to the pain.

Chronicity

If patients are referred to you for consultation regarding the presence of myofascial pain, they are likely to have muscle pain disorders that are chronic or at least subacute. You should explore at least three issues related to chronicity:

1. the patient's level of function prior to the injury that you are evaluating;
2. the chronicity (time since symptom onset) of the current injury; and
3. whether or not the patient has signs of a chronic pain syndrome.

As far as the first issue is concerned, it is important for you to know whether you are dealing with a previously healthy individual who has developed persistent pain following a distinct injury or, at the opposite extreme, an individual with virtually lifelong pain. If you obtain information indicating the latter, you should anticipate that your chances of helping the patient are likely to be only modest.

You should be very attentive to the issue of chronicity of the presenting pain problem. It is helpful to divide patients into three groups on the basis of the duration of their problem: acute (0–4 weeks), subacute (4–12 weeks), and chronic (>12 weeks). These categories are only approximate, but most experts in pain believe that an individual who remains symptomatic for more than 3–6 months should be designated as a chronic pain patient.[248] The significance of chronicity is that patients who have had protracted muscle pain are less likely to respond to a new treatment program than are patients who are relatively acute. It is worth nothing that many proponents of myofascial theory argue that chronicity among patients with myofascial pain is a by-product of the failure of other physicians to properly diagnose them, and that even delayed treatment of myofascial pain can be highly effective. This optimistic appraisal must be balanced, however, against the overwhelming body of evidence indicating that people with chronic pain are difficult to treat (see Ch. 43).[42,193]

There are probably multiple reasons why patients with chronic muscle pain are relatively refractory to treatment. However, there is abundant evidence that, as pain persists, some patients demonstrate worsening pain and activity limitations over time, somatic preoccupation, excessive fear of activity, dramatic functional limitations on examination, and psychologic dysfunction. The term *chronic pain syndrome* has been used to describe such individuals.[249] Although this term is controversial,[172,184] it (or some congener such as *abnormal illness behavior*) is useful because it refers to a constellation of attitudes and behaviors that is frequently seen in patients with chronic pain, presumably because, over time, some patients gradually develop a dysfunctional set of methods for coping with their pain. Chronicity is not associated, however, with chronic pain syndrome in a one to one fashion. Some individuals with very persistent pain do not show evidence of a chronic pain syndrome. Conversely, some individuals demonstrate abnormalities suggesting chronic pain syndrome almost immediately after they are injured. In fact, pain researchers have proposed a set of 'yellow flags'[128] to identify individuals who, shortly after injury, demonstrate behavioral abnormalities suggestive of an incipient chronic pain syndrome.

There is not a single, definitive set of criteria for identifying a patient as having a chronic pain syndrome. The criteria set out in Box 44-1 have been developed by the workers' compensation system in Washington State. They include indicators of a chronic pain syndrome, as well as other factors thought to increase the risk that an injured worker will demonstrate long-term disability.

Pain experts have different views about how to construe chronic pain syndrome. Some view chronic pain syndrome as a behavioral or psychologic syndrome that fits into the broad grouping of somatoform disorders in the American Psychiatric Association's *Diagnostic and Statistical Manual of Mental Disorders*.[11] Others point to recent research on altered central nervous system processing in response to nociceptive input (see above), and construe chronic pain syndrome as a disorder of central nervous system functioning that is a more or less predictable consequence of nociceptive barrages.[192,259] It is beyond the scope of this chapter to address the complex issues underlying these two perspectives, but regardless of which one is more valid, the implication of chronic pain syndrome for treatment is clear. A patient who has evidence of a chronic pain syndrome is likely to be refractory to treatment. You need to determine whether your patient has evidence of a chronic pain syndrome for at least two reasons:

1. patients with chronic pain syndromes have a relatively poor prognosis with any kind of treatment; and
2. patients with chronic pain syndromes are probably better served by rehabilitative treatments than by highly interventional ones.

Severity of disability

Some patients with muscle disorders continue to function in all major areas of their lives, including work and family activities. Others might have similar medical findings but report overwhelming disability associated with their disorders. For example, they might report that they have been out of work for years, or that they are virtually bedbound most of the time. To some extent, you can capture the issue of severity of disability when you inquire about factors that indicate a chronic pain syndrome. However, disability is such a crucial issue that you should strongly consider reporting about it separately. There are two simple rules about severity of disability. First, among patients with musculoskeletal disorders, it correlates only modestly with medical findings.[260] Second, independent of medical factors, patients who report severe disability have a relatively poor prognosis for response to treatment.

General medical history

Some general medical problems are thought to predispose individuals to myofascial pain. For example, people with hypothyroidism are thought to be susceptible.[244,245] Factors that act as predisposing or perpetuating factors for myofascial pain are not discussed further in this chapter.

Patient evaluation: examination

You should always perform a thorough overall musculoskeletal examination on a patient with suspected myofascial pain. The reason for this is simple: many patients with evidence of myofascial pain also have evidence of other sources of pain, such as painful spinal joints or radiculopathy.

As far as an examination for muscle pain, myofascial pain, or trigger points is concerned, several points are important. First, the text by Travell and Simons[244,245] gives detailed information about techniques for identifying trigger points in specific muscles. You should review this material to get hints about

Box 44-1 Proposed list of risk factors for prolonged disability

Medical factors
- Presence of secondary medical condition
- Injury to dominant hand
- Hospitalization within 28 days of injury for reasons unrelated to industrial injury
- Preexisting psychiatric conditions

Injury descriptions
- Non-overt injury: injury occurring in course of usual work activities
- No objective findings on examinations
- Diagnosis not consistent with injury description
- Time gap in report of injury
- Unwitnessed accident

Provider and patient factors
- No identifiable treatment plan or goals
- Overutilization of healthcare delivery systems and services by either patient or provider, or over-referral by physician; may include frequent changes of attending physician
- Misuse of scheduled medications by patient
- Physician fostering illness beliefs
- Number of surgeries both related and unrelated to work-related problem; may include a number of unsuccessful surgeries in the same area
- Spread of diagnosis over time; newly contended diagnosis
- No documented medical progress

Psychosocial factors
- Exaggerated illness behavior: presence of non-organic signs (Waddell signs), no objective findings
- Evidence of abuse of alcohol, illicit drug, or prescription medication
- Presence of depression or avoidance anxiety, posttraumatic disorder, or other dysphoric affects (e.g. anger at employer, supervisor, or Labor and Industries)
- History of childhood abuse, physical or sexual abuse, substance abuse in caretaker, or family instability
- Presence of personality traits or disorders (e.g. presence of specific somatization traits or problematic interpersonal relationships); arrests

Demographic factors
- Low educational level, including illiteracy
- English not primary language
- Age greater than 50 and employed in heavy industry
- Back or lower extremity injury with medium or heavy labor employment
- Nearing retirement age

Job factors
- Anger at employer
- Employer anger at worker
- Miscellaneous employer factors: seasonal work, strike, plant closure, job becoming obsolete, etc.
- Loss of job in which the injury occurred
- Singular work history in heavy industry
- Complaints of inability to function
- History of poor job performance, frequent job change, short duration of employment, job dissatisfaction, or job termination prior to claims filing
- Employer or worker not active in return to work efforts
- Worker is not clearly headed back to work
- Perception of the worker that he or she will be retrained 'for a better job' or other misperceptions of Labor and Industries vocational entitlement

Administrative factors
- Third-party involvement
- Recent claim closures; application for reopening
- Employer protest
- Current income, including time loss, compares favorably with net income prior to injury
- Multiple Labor and Industries claims (may include a number of previous claims)
- Loss of driver's license or other credentials
- Loss of medical insurance
- Originally non-time loss claim that has become time loss
- Non-compliance with medical or vocational treatment
- Worker or physician perception that Labor and Industries is unresponsive or adversarial

(From Department of Labor and Industries 1999,[52] with permission.)

patient positioning and specific examination techniques. Second, you should be prepared for situations in which you obtain only some of the findings associated with trigger points. For example, you will frequently encounter patients with tenderness over muscles but without local twitch responses, taut bands, or other findings thought to be markers of trigger points. These patients can probably benefit from treatment for myofascial pain, even though they do not have all the classic findings for trigger points. Third, you need to be careful about the amount of force you exert when you examine muscles for trigger points or tenderness. As the abundant literature on pressure pain threshold demonstrates, any person will complain of pain when an examiner pushes very forcefully on his or her muscles. It is probably best to use the criterion proposed by the American College of Rheumatology for the diagnosis of fibromyalgia. In their landmark paper on research criteria for the diagnosis of fibromyalgia,

several rheumatologists with expertise in fibromyalgia recommended that an examiner push on a muscle with a force of up to 4 kg.[267] If a patient does not report localized or referred pain by then, the site should be considered negative for muscle tenderness or trigger point. Finally, you should strongly consider doing a screening examination for fibromyalgia in any patient whom you are evaluating for myofascial pain. Regardless of the precise relations between pain in fibromyalgia and pain in MPS,[35] the presence of widespread tenderness should warn you that your patient has something more complex than an MPS affecting one or a few muscles.

Patient evaluation: assessment
Musculoskeletal diagnoses

When you have completed your history and physical examination, you should address the issue of whether your patient has myofascial pain. It is possible that you will find that the patient has a local or regional pain syndrome that meets all the classic criteria for myofascial pain. However, you should be prepared for several variants. Some patients have a muscle pain syndrome but do not have all the classic findings of MPS. Others might or might not have clear-cut myofascial pain in a single region, but will have evidence of a fibromyalgia-like syndrome. You should comment on these variations in your assessment.

You should also comment on whether there are other musculoskeletal problems in addition to myofascial pain that contribute to your patient's pain. You should be prepared for the common co-occurrence of myofascial pain with painful spinal joints or irritation of spinal nerve roots (radiculopathy).

Other factors contributing to pain

If your patient has subacute or chronic pain, you should comment on factors other than strictly musculoskeletal ones that might be contributing to the persistence of his or her musculoskeletal symptoms. As described above, you should assess the patient for factors associated with chronic pain syndrome, and render some opinion about whether there is strong evidence for this entity. In particular, you should comment on exaggerated pain behavior or dramatic functional limitations on examination, reports of severe disability with respect to work and/or activities of daily living, and evidence of psychologic dysfunction.

Treatment

Initial treatment decisions

Once you have made a diagnosis of myofascial pain, your initial treatment plan depends on multiple factors related to characteristics of your patient and the manner in which the patient was referred to you. One important determinant of your initial treatment plan is your assessment of whether or not the patient's pain derives from factors other than just myofascial pain. For example, if you believe that your patient has radicular pain, you may opt for epidural injections or other therapies directed toward radiculopathy prior to instituting treatment for myofascial pain. It is worth noting in this regard that many specialists in musculoskeletal medicine observe muscle pain when they evaluate patients, but essentially ignore it for purposes of treatment planning. They seem to assume that muscle pain is a secondary phenomenon that will resolve on its own if an underlying structural abnormality in the spine is addressed.

If you receive a referral from an orthopedist with the specific request of performing myofascial treatment on the patient, you can move immediately to some form of trigger point injections (see below). Conversely, if a patient with very chronic muscle pain comes to your office with the expectation that you will assume care of her or his pain, you might want to move more slowly and follow the preliminary steps described below.

Comprehensive treatment: preliminary steps

Assume that you will become the primary pain management physician for a 40-year-old woman who is 1 year status post a neck injury from a rear-end motor vehicle accident, has evidence of myofascial pain involving several neck and shoulder girdle muscles, and does not have definite evidence of a cervical radiculopathy or a disk or facet syndrome as contributors to her pain. This is the type of patient for whom you should seriously consider a comprehensive treatment plan that is based on the premise that she has a chronic pain problem.

The first step in this plan should be communication with the patient about the way you approach muscle pain, the responsibilities you expect her to take on, and the probable duration of your treatment. You should avoid the temptation to promise a cure for her, because she has a chronic pain problem. A more realistic goal is for her to get enough pain relief, and to develop good enough pain coping strategies, so that she can return to important roles and activities despite some residual pain.

Comprehensive treatment: treatment modalities

Once ground rules have been established, you should have your patient start a multimodal treatment program, usually including the following.

Patient education At a minimum, you should require that your patient learn something about the complexities of chronic pain, and the need for her to develop strategies to manage it. She should be advised to buy one of the many user-friendly books for patients with chronic muscle pain. At our clinic, we rely on *Managing Pain Before It Manages You*.[40]

In addition to reading about chronic pain, your patient ideally would have an opportunity to interact with a nurse in your office who has skills in patient education, or (for particularly complex patients) with a psychologist who specializes in chronic pain.

Physical therapy A well-designed physical therapy program carried out by a therapist with whom you interact regularly can help your treatment plan in a variety of ways. First, an active program in physical therapy gives a clear message to your patient: that she has to do a lot of the work required to get better. You should support this message by emphasizing to patients that, although physical therapists have skills in several areas, their main role is to act as training coaches who teach patients how to perform therapeutic exercises. Second, serial assessments by a physical therapist can help determine your patient's baseline level of physical performance, and help interpret her responses to various treatment interventions. Third, some interventions thought to be relatively specific to myofascial pain can be carried out by physical therapists. The most obvious example is spray and stretch techniques,[244,245] but a variety of myofascial release treatments can also be performed. Fourth, the physical therapist establishes an exercise program for your patient, and helps her move toward a self-directed exercise program. For a patient with myofascial pain involving several neck or shoulder girdle muscles, this program should include a well-constructed stretching program for the affected muscles (as described, for example, by Travell and Simons[244,245]). It should also include strengthening exercises for neck, shoulder girdle, and upper extremity muscles, and a progressive aerobics program.

Medications Most of the medication options for a patient with chronic myofascial pain following a whiplash injury are not at all specific to myofascial pain, but have been found to be useful in chronic muscle pain in general. The information below briefly reviews several classes of medications that might be helpful for your patient. You need to know at the outset that a wide range of medication regimens need to be considered for your patient precisely because there is no single regimen that reliably produces dramatic benefit. The problem of unreliability in the effects of various pharmacologic regimens is aggravated by the enormous heterogeneity of the medical conditions in which myofascial pain is thought to play a role. Cohen et al. state the problem as follows:

> Myofascial pain comprises a heterogeneous group of disorders. Therefore, it is not surprising to find conflicting outcomes as to the pharmacologic efficacy of different drugs.
>
> (Cohen et al. 2004,[47] p. 519.)

Two reviews of pharmacologic management of myofascial pain have recently been published.[47,264] You should consult them for additional details regarding different classes of drugs that have been used in myofascial pain, and for the research supporting their use. You also need to consult standard pharmacology texts to consider the full spectrum of therapeutic and adverse effects associated with various medication regimens.

Non-steroidal antiinflammatory drugs There is no evidence that myofascial pain is an inflammatory disorder, therefore you would not expect NSAIDs to be particularly helpful for your patient. However, it is possible that the patient's pain is a result of both myofascial pain and a spinal joint disorder such as degenerative disease of a cervical facet joint. Because this kind of multifactorial pain is common in myofascial pain patients, a trial on NSAIDs might be warranted.

Tricyclic antidepressants Tricyclic antidepressants have been supplanted by newer antidepressant medications for the management of depression, but they have demonstrated significant efficacy in the treatment of a variety of chronic pain disorders. Their efficacy has been demonstrated most clearly in the treatment of pain from neuropathic disorders such as diabetic neuropathies,[158] but there is also evidence for their efficacy in the treatment of fibromyalgia[83] and tension headaches.[14] Of note is the fact that the effects of tricyclic antidepressants on pain appear to be independent of their antidepressant effects, because they occur at much lower doses than those required to treat depression. In addition to their potential for reducing pain, tricyclic antidepressants might help patients with myofascial pain by improving their sleep.

Other antidepressants A recent comprehensive review of treatments for fibromyalgia concluded that fluoxetine has some efficacy.[83] Other selective serotonin reuptake inhibitors have not been studied systematically in fibromyalgia, and research on other painful conditions suggests that they are relatively ineffective in the treatment of chronic pain.[36,174] In contrast, dual reuptake inhibitors such as duloxetine and to some extent venlafaxine have demonstrated efficacy in the treatment of fibromyalgia and other chronic pain conditions.[83] They would be reasonable choices for patients with myofascial pain who did not benefit from tricyclic antidepressants.

Muscle relaxers Medications used as muscle relaxers or spasmolytics in myofascial pain include drugs with a variety of pharmacologic actions, including ones that presumably exert a muscle-relaxing effect as a consequence of their sedative action on the central nervous system (e.g. benzodiazepines and carisoprodol), medications that affect the neuromuscular system peripherally (dantrolene and quinine), an α_2-adrenergic agonist (tizanidine), and an agent that is structurally related to the tricyclic antidepressants (cyclobenzaprine). Tizanidine and cyclobenzaprine have the best-documented efficacy in reducing myofascial pain.[101] Although patients often report short-term symptom relief from sedatives such as benzodiazepines, pain specialists have expressed concern over long-term use of these agents because of the risk of drug dependence.

Anticonvulsants Anticonvulsants increase the response threshold of neurons by affecting voltage-activated sodium channels, and by enhancing GABA-mediated synaptic inhibition.[162] Some of them, particularly carbamazepine and gabapentin, have documented efficacy in the treatment of neuropathic pain states including diabetic neuropathy, postherpetic neuralgia, and trigeminal neuralgia. Although clinicians have used anticonvulsants for myofascial pain and a wide range of other chronic pain conditions, there are no well-controlled studies demonstrating their efficacy in myofascial pain. It is of interest, however, that pregabalin, a gabapentin analog that has recently been released, has demonstrated efficacy in the treatment of pain among fibromyalgia patients.[49]

Opiates Physicians and basic scientists have been unable to define the parameters for appropriate use of long-term opiate therapy for non-malignant pain in general. The situation is no better for myofascial pain, and perhaps somewhat more ambiguous because of the uncertain nature of myofascial pain. Several randomized controlled trials lasting from one to a few weeks have been conducted on opiates for the treatment of several different chronic pain disorders.[185,195] These have generally demonstrated modest benefit for opiates, but the relevance of these findings to long-term treatment (perhaps lasting years) is uncertain. Pain specialists are also appropriately concerned about the risk of drug abuse or progressive tolerance when opiates are used over months or years.[41] Many of the issues surrounding long-term opiate therapy are addressed in a recent review article.[21] Based on the unequivocal short-term analgesic properties of opiates, you can be confident that, if you start your patients on an opiate, they will initially report pain relief. The problem is that the patient is at significant risk to report a loss of efficacy from the opiate after a period of a few weeks, and might well request dose increases to cover this. You then face the difficult challenge of deciding whether to continue the opiates or, if not, how to taper the patient off them. One middle ground strategy is to use opiates only for targeted purposes that are inherently time-limited. For example, you might prescribe an opiate for your patient as she gets started in her functionally oriented physical therapy program.

It is worth noting that, while the above discussion focuses on the effects of different categories of medication on pain in myofascial syndrome, drugs can be used for problems other than pain. For example, some investigators have proposed a vicious circle between myofascial pain and disturbed sleep.[175] It might be appropriate to describe a sedating antidepressant (e.g. trazodone and amitriptyline) for the specific purpose of helping your patient sleep better. Also, like many patients with chronic pain, your patient may have associated depression. If so, she should be considered for treatment with a tricyclic antidepressant at a full antidepressant dose, or for treatment with one of the newer antidepressants.

Comprehensive treatment: injections

Most of the interventions described above are relevant to any patient with chronic musculoskeletal pain, regardless of whether or not there is evidence of myofascial pain. In contrast, injection therapies (often called trigger point injections) represent a group of treatments that are fairly specific for myofascial pain. In fact, it is typical for proponents of myofascial theory to at least implicitly convey the sense that injections represent a definitive form of treatment for myofascial pain.

In our opinion, injections play a much more modest, albeit important, role. They can be extremely valuable in demonstrating both to you and to your patient that the pain is myofascial in nature. In fact, a 'diagnostic' trigger point injection done at the outset of treatment might help your patient commit to a strenuous program designed to improve the myofascial pain. At a later point, your patient's treatment might get 'stuck' (e.g the patient might reach a performance plateau in physical therapy, or report that the pain continues at an unacceptable level despite an appropriate pharmacologic regimen and an apparently sincere effort on the patient's part to develop coping strategies to manage the pain). Judicious use of injection therapy in such a situation might act as a catalyst that stimulates a sustained improvement in your patient's functional ability and pain level.

But neither of these reasons for performing injections embodies the notion that the injections represent a cure for your patient. In fact, there is no convincing evidence that myofascial pain patients are cured by trigger point injections.[48] Injections also represent a passive form of therapy that has the potential to create dependency on the part of patients because of short-term pain relief. This is true even if the injections are not producing sustained functional and symptomatic improvement.

Regardless of whether injections are construed as cures for myofascial pain (as proponents generally imply) or as adjuncts to an overall rehabilitation program (as we advocate), it is important to consider how often they should be performed, and how many represent an optimal course of treatment. The latter issue has been largely neglected in the literature on injection therapy for myofascial pain. There is no known cumulative

toxicity from the substances that are typically injected (local anesthetic, saline, water, or nothing, as in dry needling). If injection therapy is construed as an adjunct to an active rehabilitation program for myofascial pain patients, however, it seems prudent to limit the number of injections that are offered to patients. In our myofascial pain clinic, we typically recommend a maximum of three to six injections during an initial treatment program designed to improve a patient's myofascial disorder, with the possibility of additional injections on a sporadic basis during maintenance treatment.

It is beyond the scope of this chapter to describe specific techniques for performing injections on patients with myofascial pain. Excellent pictures and descriptions of several technical issues related to at least certain kinds of injections are given in the Travel and Simons text.[244,245] A few issues in addition to those raised by Travel and Simons are worth discussing, however.

What should be injected? In their classic descriptions of trigger point injections, Travel and Simons[244,245] indicated that the injectate should be the local anesthetic procaine. Other physicians have injected different local anesthetics, such as lidocaine (lignocaine) or bupivacaine. Still others have injected either saline or water (Garvey and Fine[63,73]). Finally, the technique of intramuscular stimulation (also called dry needling) popularized by Dr. Chan Gunn[97] involves stimulating trigger points with acupuncture needles, but not injecting any fluid. In this ambiguous situation, a comprehensive review by Cummings and White[50] is extremely informative. After an extensive literature search, they identified 23 randomized controlled trials involving comparisons between different injectates during injection therapy for myofascial trigger points. They stated:

> No trials were of sufficient quality or design to test the efficacy of any needling technique beyond placebo in the treatment of myofascial pain. Eight of the 10 trials comparing injection of different substances and all 7 higher quality trials found that the effect was independent of the injected substance. All 3 trials that compared dry needling with injection found no difference in effect.
>
> (Cummings and White 2001,[50] p. 986.)

Based on the Cummings and White review, it is reasonable to conclude that the results of trigger point injections are likely to be comparable when a variety of different local anesthetics are used, or when saline or water are used. Also, trigger point injections and dry needling appear to be roughly equal in efficacy. A more difficult issue is that of the appropriateness of botulinum toxin in myofascial pain. Botulinum toxin injections are relatively new to medicine. The earliest Medline citation regarding them is from 1973, when the use of botulinum injections was described in the treatment of strabismus.[201,202] During the past 20 years, botulinum toxin injections have been tried in a wide range of conditions, including torticollis, cerebral palsy, hyperhidrosis, various urologic conditions, and cosmetic surgery. Published reports on their role in myofascial pain are relatively recent; a Medline search on 26 September 2004 using the key words *botulinum* and *myofascial* yielded 17 citations, with the earliest one from 2001.

It is plausible to assume that botulinum toxin would be helpful in disorders in which pain is related to abnormal muscle tone. It is not at all clear, however, that abnormal muscle tone is a problem in patients with myofascial pain. Moreover, two comparisons between botulinum toxin injections and other types of injections for patients with myofascial pain have failed to demonstrate any superiority for botulinum.[124,263]

Another possible agent to inject in trigger points is a corticosteroid. However, because myofascial pain is not considered to be an inflammatory condition, and because corticosteroids have the potential to cause significant adverse effects, we would not recommend them in injection therapy for myofascial pain.

What if you cannot identify definite trigger points on your preinjection examination? Proponents of myofascial theory give the impression that they can always find trigger points to inject. In our experience, however, it is not uncommon to find patients who appear to have muscular pain, but in whom it is difficult to identify discrete trigger points. The reasons for this are multiple. For example, some patients tolerate a trigger point examination poorly and report pain everywhere you palpate. As a result, it is difficult to identify especially sensitive areas in their muscles. Palpatory findings can also be difficult to interpret in obese patients, or in ones who have trigger points in relatively inaccessible muscles. In such situations, it is reasonable to inject at the site that seems to be most sensitive, even if it does not meet all the criteria for a trigger point. If you have got pretty close to a trigger point, you can usually find it by probing with your needle after it is in the affected muscle, and noting sites that cause your patient to wince and report severe pain.

How many sites should you inject? This is a concern in a patient with multiple trigger points or widespread muscular tenderness. In addressing this issue, it is important to remember that trigger point injections frequently cause short-term pain. This fact can challenge the coping resources of a chronic pain patient who is emotionally very reactive to pain. As a practical indicator of the difficulty that many patients with myofascial pain have tolerating the pain of trigger point injections, one of us (JPR) has had to abort several trigger point injections over the years because of vasovagal reactions on the part of patients. Also, during that time several patients have called to complain of a major flare-up of their pain after trigger point injections. The likelihood of either of these problems can probably be reduced if you are very cautious when you first do trigger point injections. For example, even in a patient with multiple potential targets for injection, it is wise to inject only a very limited number of sites during the first session of trigger point injections. If the patient tolerates the procedure well, you can be more aggressive in following injection sessions.

What can you do to minimize emotional distress in patients as they undergo trigger point injections? This question is important because many patients with myofascial pain are emotionally reactive when confronted with situations that might aggravate their pain. Their emotional distress, in turn, can aggravate their pain by causing increased muscular tension or hyper-

vigilance.[258] As a practical matter, you need to conduct trigger point injections in an environment that is as non-threatening as possible. If possible, you should use a procedure room in which the lighting and sounds foster relaxation rather than stress. You should be careful about your demeanor as you prepare and carry out injections. It is often helpful to allow your patient to stay in the procedure room for about 10 min after trigger point injections. During this time, the room should be quiet. It can also help patients relax if they can apply a heating pad to the area you have injected.

Monitoring progress

As your patients progress in your myofascial pain treatment program, you need some way to monitor their progress. Given the complexity of chronic myofascial pain, the parameters you should ideally monitor are likely to be multiple. They include the following.

- The patient's knowledge of myofascial pain and chronic pain generally: their belief systems regarding the nature of the problem, and the treatment that the patient perceives as being necessary.
- The patient's depression and anxiety level, including the fear of activity or reinjury.
- The patient's participation and progress in physical therapy.
- The patient's sleep pattern.
- The patient's functional status (e.g. ability to work).
- The patient's involvement in the treatment program, in particular the willingness to play an active role in rehabilitation.
- The patient's pain level.

Ideally, your patient will demonstrate progressive improvement in most of the above domains. It is possible, however, that treatments will provide only temporary benefit. For example, trigger point injections that you perform might yield pain relief and improved function that last a few days or weeks but are followed by a return to baseline. This pattern is often seen in patients with very chronic pain. If the short-term benefits of treatment are very definite, you might reconceptualize the goals of your treatment program, and define success on the basis of short-term benefit rather than progressive and sustained improvement. This reconceptualization of goals is particularly appropriate for a chronic patient who functions well much of the time but has recurring flare-ups of myofascial pain that are quite debilitating. For such a patient, trigger point injections (or other interventions) could be viewed as targeted therapy for pain flare-ups, rather than as definitive therapy.

If you determine that your patient is not improving, you should consider alternatives to your treatment program. One possibility is to revisit the issue of treatment directed toward a joint or neurologic injury rather than toward myofascial pain. This embodies the idea that myofascial pain typically co-occurs with radiculopathy or with spinal joint injury or dysfunction. Another possibility would be to consider psychophysiologic or psychologic treatments, such as biofeedback, relaxation training, and cognitive behavioral therapy. Finally, it might be appropriate to consider the large group of alternative or complementary treatments that have been used on patients with myofascial pain. Based on published literature, these include chiropractic, neuroreflexology, acupuncture, and several other approaches (see Chs 20 and 23).

Terminating care

A multimodal treatment program for a patient with myofascial pain should produce maximal benefit within about 3 months. The main exception to this generalization is that your treatment program is likely to take longer if it includes multiple medication trials. In the ideal situation, your treatment would lead to significant improvements in your patient's functional level, understanding of myofascial pain or chronic pain, and pain level. You should anticipate, however, that the patient will not be completely symptom-free and might need long-term treatment.

One option when your patient reaches maximal benefit is to refer the patient back to the primary care provider. Alternatively, you might continue to treat the patient, but with the understanding that you are providing maintenance care. Whichever model you choose, you should be prepared to see the patient for reevaluation if, in the future, there is a significant recurrence of myofascial pain.

SUMMARY

Muscle pain has interested and confounded physicians for at least 100 years. For at least the past 30 years, the dominant paradigm for understanding clinically significant muscle pain has been the theory of myofascial pain initially articulated by Travell[242-245] and currently described by Simons[166] and others. During the past 20 years, research in several areas has provided insights that in some instances challenge postulates of myofascial pain theory. At least five lines of research are relevant.

1. Simons and many other proponents of myofascial theory have been active in researching various issues related to trigger points and the diagnosis and treatment of myofascial pain. For example, recent studies have addressed the electrophysiology of trigger points and the biochemical environment at trigger points.[205]
2. Research on experimental muscle pain in normal humans has proliferated, and systematic comparisons have been made between the responses of normal subjects and those of patients with clinically significant muscle pain to experimentally induced muscle pain.
3. Several studies have expanded our understanding of referred pain in response to irritation of a variety of musculoskeletal structures, such as intervertebral disks and facet joints. Although these studies have generally not directly addressed muscle pain, they have provided insights about interactions between muscle pain and pain emanating from other musculoskeletal structures.
4. Research on chronic pain in humans has expanded greatly during the past 20 years. Studies have demonstrated that myofascial pain is common among patients with chronic muscle pain, and have identified strategies for chronic pain management that are relevant to the treatment of patients with myofascial pain.
5. Animal research on the neurobiology of pain has provided insights that need to be considered in the clinical management of chronic pain. In particular, this research has elaborated the contribution of central nervous system sensitization in persistent pain.

At the present time, these insights have not been brought together to provide a coherent perspective on the pathophysiology of muscular pain, or on the appropriate management of it. A major goal of this chapter has been to identify different perspectives on muscle pain, and to look for parallels and points of divergence among these perspectives. Much more work is needed on this type of integration. At this point, the discrepancies among different perspectives are so large that it is even difficult to formulate questions about muscle pain in a way that is acceptable to the general community of physicians and researchers. In particular, this chapter has pointed out differences between the theory-laden term *myofascial pain* and the more neutral term *muscle pain*.

In the absence of conclusive evidence about optimal ways to diagnose and treat clinically significant muscle pain, management strategies are of necessity empiric. The perspective taken in this chapter is that clinically significant muscle pain occurs primarily in patients with chronic musculoskeletal pain. Consequently, the treatment of muscle pain should be based on principles that have been developed for the treatment of chronic pain in general. Proponents of myofascial pain theory would almost certainly disagree with this perspective.

One of our goals in this chapter has been to acquaint readers not only with controversies related to muscle pain, but also with the advances that are occurring in our understanding of muscle pain as a result of research in several areas. Our hope is that further research in the areas outlined above will lead to some convergence among the currently disparate views regarding muscle pain. Currently, we can only dimly view the shape of such a convergence. At one extreme, it is possible that further research will firmly establish trigger points as clinically important entities that can be reliably diagnosed and effectively treated. At the opposite extreme, further research might show that most clinically significant muscle pain is in actuality an epiphenomenon driven by a combination of injury or degeneration in other musculoskeletal structures and central nervous system sensitization.

The good news is that, as a result of multiple vigorous research programs around the world, there is room for optimism that, within the next several years, we will be able to answer basic questions about muscle pain that until now have been answered strictly by clinical intuition.

REFERENCES

1. Ahern DK, Follick MJ, Council JR, et al. Comparison of lumbar paravertebral EMG patterns in chronic low back pain patients and non-patient controls. Pain 1988; 34:153–160.

2. Allan DB, Waddell G. An historical perspective on low back pain and disability. Acta Orthop Scand Suppl 1989; 234:1–23.

3. Alston W, Carlson KE, Feldman DJ, et al. A quantitative study of muscle factors in the chronic low back syndrome. J Am Geriatr Soc 1966; 14(10):1041–1047.

4. Apkarian AV, Brüggemann J, Shi T, et al. A thalamic model for true and referred visceral pain. In: Gebhart GF, ed. Visceral pain, progress in pain research and management. Seattle: IASP Press; 1995:217–259.

5. Arendt-Nielsen L, Graven-Nielsen T, Svarrer H, et al. The influence of low back pain on muscle activity and coordination during gait: a clinical and experimental study. Pain 1996; 64:231–240.

6. Arendt-Nielsen L, Graven-Nielsen T, Svensson P, et al. Temporal summation in muscles and referred pain areas: an experimental human study. Muscle Nerve 1997; 20:1311–1313.

7. Arendt-Nielsen L, Laursen RJ, Drewes AM. Referred pain as an indicator for neural plasticity. Prog Brain Res 2000; 129:343–356.

8. Arendt-Nielsen L, Svensson P. Referred muscle pain: basic and clinical findings. Clin J Pain 2001; 17:11–19.

9. Arendt-Nielsen L. Induction and assessment of experimental pain from human skin, muscle and viscera. In: Jensen TS, Turner JA, Wiesenfeld-Hallin Z, eds. Proceedings of the 8th World Congress on Pain. Seattle: IASP Press; 1997:393–425.

10. Arima T, Svensson P, Arendt-Nielsen L. Capsaicin-induced muscle hyperalgesia in exercises and non-exercised human masseter. J Orofacial Pain 2000; 14:213.

11. Aronoff GM, Livengood JM. Pain: psychiatric aspects of impairment and disability. Curr Pain Headache Rep 2003; 7(2):105–115.

12. Asbury AK, Fields HL. Pain due to peripheral nerve damage: an hypothesis. Neurology 1984; 34(12):1587–1590.

13. Ashina M, Bendtsen L, Jensen R, et al. Muscle hardness in patients with chronic tension-type headache: relation to actual headache state. Pain 1999; 79:201–205.

14. Ashina S, Ashina M. Current and potential future drug therapies for tension-type headache. Curr Pain Headache Rep 2003; 7(6):466–474.

15. Ashton-Miller JA, McGlashen KM, Herzenberg JE, et al. Cervical muscle myoelectric response to acute experimental sternocleidomastoid pain. Spine 1990; 15(10):1006–1012.

16. Babenko UV, Graven-Nielsen T, Svensson P, et al. Experimental human muscle pain induced by intramuscular injections of bradykinin, serotonin, and substance P. Eur J Pain 1999; 3:93.

17. Bäckman E, Bengtsson A, Bengtsson M, et al. Skeletal muscle function in primary fibromyalgia. Effect of regional sympathetic blockade with guanethidine. Acta Neurol Scand 1988; 77:187–191.

18. Bajaj P, Bajaj P, Madsen H, et al. Endometriosis is associated with central sensitization: a psychophysical controlled study. J Pain 2003; 4(7):372–380.

19. Bajaj P, Graven-Nielsen T, Arendt-Nielsen L. Osteoarthritis and its association with muscle hyperalgesia: an experimental controlled study. Pain 2001; 93:107–114.

20. Bajaj P, Graven-Nielsen T, Arendt-Nielsen L. Trigger points in patients with lower limb osteoarthritis. J Musculoskelet Pain 2001; 9:17–33.

21. Ballantyne JC, Mao J. Opioid therapy for chronic pain. N Engl J Med 2003; 349(20):1943–1953.

22. Banic B, Petersen-Felix S, Andersen OK, et al. Evidence for spinal cord hypersensitivity in chronic pain after whiplash injury and in fibromyalgia. Pain 2004; 107(1–2):7–15.

23. Basmajian JV, DeLuca CJ. Muscles alive: their functions revealed by electromyography. 5th edn. Baltimore: Williams & Wilkins; 1985.

24. Bendtsen L, Jensen R, Jensen NK, et al. Muscle palpation with controlled finger pressure: new equipment for the study of tender myofascial tissues. Pain 1994; 59:235–239.

25. Bendtsen L, Jensen R, Jensen NK, et al. Pressure-controlled palpation: a new technique which increases the reliability of manual palpation. Cephalalgia 1995; 15(3):205–210.

26. Bendtsen L, Jensen R, Olesen J. Decreased pain detection and tolerance thresholds in chronic tension-type headache. Arch Neurol 1996; 53:373–376.

27. Bendtsen L, Jensen R, Olesen J. Qualitatively altered nociception in chronic myofascial pain. Pain 1996; 65:259–264.

28. Bendtsen L, Nørregaard J, Jensen R, et al. Evidence of qualitatively altered nociception in patients with fibromyalgia. Arthritis Rheum 1997; 40:98–102.

29. Bengtsson A, Bäckman E, Lindblom B, et al. Long term follow-up of fibromyalgia patients: clinical symptoms, muscular function, laboratory test—an eight year comparison study. J Musculoskelet Pain 1994; 2(2):67–80.

30. Bennett RM. Beyond fibromyalgia: ideas on etiology and treatment. J Rheumatol 1989; 16 (suppl 19):185–191.

31. Berberich P, Hoheisel U, Mense S. Effects of carrageenan-induced myositis on the discharge properties of group III and IV muscle receptors in the cat. J Neurophysiol 1988; 59:1395–1409.

32. Bigland-Ritchie B, Dawson NJ, Johansson RS, et al. Reflex origin for the slowing of motoneurone firing rates in fatigue of human voluntary contractions. J Physiol 1986; 379:451–459.

33. Bohr TW. Fibromyalgia syndrome and myofascial pain syndrome. Do they exist? Neurol Clin 1995; 13(2):365–384.

34. Bonica JJ. General considerations of acute pain. In: Bonica JJ, ed. The management of pain. 2nd edn. Philadelphia: Lea & Febiger; 1990:159–179.

35. Borg-Stein J, Stein J. Trigger points and tender points: one and the same? Does injection treatment help? Rheum Dis Clin North Am 1996; 22(2):305–322.

36. Briley M. Clinical experience with dual action antidepressants in different chronic pain syndromes. Hum Psychopharmacol 2004; 19(suppl 1): S21–S25.

37. Canale ST, ed. Campbell's operative orthopaedics. 10th edn. St. Louis: Mosby; 2003.

38. Carlson CR, Okeson JP, Falace DA, et al. Comparison of psychologic and physiologic functioning between patients with masticatory muscle pain and matched controls. J Orofacial Pain 1993; 7(1):15–22.

39. Carlson CR, Reid KI, Curran SL, et al. Psychological and physiological parameters of masticatory muscle pain. Pain 1998; 76:297–307.

40. Caudill MA. Managing pain before it manages you. New York: Guilford Press; 2002.

41. Chabal C, Erjavec MK, Jacobson L, et al. Prescription opiate abuse in chronic pain patients: clinical criteria, incidence, and predictors. Clin J Pain 1997; 13(2):150–155.

42. Cheadle A, Franklin G, Wolfhagen C, et al. Factors influencing the duration of work-related disability: a population-based study of Washington state workers' compensation. Am J Public Health 1994; 84:190–196.

43. Cheung K, Hume PA, Maxwell L. Delayed onset muscle soreness. Sports Med 2003; 33(2):145–164.

44. Clark GT, Beemsterboer PL, Jacobson R. The effect of sustained submaximal clenching on maximum bite force in myofascial pain dysfunction patients. J Oral Rehabil 1984; 11(4):387–391.

45. Clark GT, Sakai S, Merrill R, et al. Cross-correlation between stress, pain, physical activity, and temporalis muscle EMG in tension-type headache. Cephalalgia 1995; 15:511–518.

46. Coderre TJ, Katz J, Vaccarino AL, et al. Contribution of central neuroplasticity to pathological pain: review of clinical and experimental evidence. Pain 1993; 52:259–285.

47. Cohen SP, Mullings R, Abdi S. The pharmacologic treatment of muscle pain. Anesthesiology 2004; 101(2):495–526.

48. Collins GA, Cohen MJ, Nailboff BD, et al. Comparative analysis of paraspinal and frontalis EMG, heart rate and skin conductance in chronic low back pain patients and normals to various postures and stress. Scand J Rehabil Med 1982; 14:39–46.

49. Crofford L, Russell IJ, Mease P, et al. Pregabalin improves pain associated with fibromyalgia syndrome in a multicenter, randomized, placebo-controlled monotherapy trial. Arthritis Rheum 2002; 46:S613.

50. Cummings TM, White AR. Needling therapies in the management of myofascial trigger point pain: a systematic review. Arch Phys Med Rehabil 2001; 82:986–992.

51. Curatolo M, Petersen-Felix S, Arendt-Nielsen L, et al. Central hypersensitivity in chronic pain after whiplash injury. Clin J Pain 2001; 17:306–315.

52. Department of Labor and Industries. Attending doctor's handbook. Olympia: Department of Labor and Industries; 1999.

53. DeVries HA. Quantitative electromyographic investigation of the spasm theory of muscle pain. Am J Phys Med 1966; 45(3):119–134.

54. Drewes AM, Arendt-Nielsen L, Jensen JH, et al. Experimental pain in the stomach: a model based on electrical stimulation guided by gastroscopy. Gut 1997; 41:753–757.

55. Drewes AM, Petersen P, Rossel P, et al. Sensitivity and distensibility of the rectum and sigmoid colon in patients with irritable bowel syndrome. Scand J Gastroenterol 2001; 36(8):827–832.

56. Drewes AM, Schipper KP, Dimcevski G, et al. Multi-modal induction and assessment of allodynia and hyperalgesia in the human oesophagus. Eur J Pain 2003; 7(6):539–549.

57. Dubner R. Hyperalgesia in response to injury to cutaneous and deep tissues. In: Fricton JR, Dubner R, eds. Orofacial pain and temporomandibular disorders. Advances in pain research and therapy, vol 21. New York: Raven Press; 1995:61–71.

58. Dworkin SF, LeResche L, eds. Research diagnostic criteria for temporomandibular disorders: review, criteria, examinations and specifications, critique. J Craniomandib Disord Facial Oral Pain 1992; 6:301–355.

59. Dworkin SF, LeResche L, Truelove E. Epidemiology of signs and symptoms in temporomandibular disorders: clinical signs in cases and controls. J Am Dent Assoc 1990; 120:273–281.

60. Dwyer A, Aprill C, Bogduk N. Cervical zygapophyseal joint pain patterns. I: A study in normal volunteers. Spine 1990; 15(6):453–457.

61. Elert JE, Dahlqvist SBR, Henriksson-Larsén K, et al. Increased EMG activity during short pauses in patients with primary fibromyalgia. Scand J Rheumatol 1989; 18:321–323.

62. Elert JE, Dahlqvist SR, Almay B, et al. Muscle endurance, muscle tension and personality traits in patients with muscle or joint pain—a pilot study. J Rheumatol 1993; 20(9):1550–1556.

63. Ernberg M, Hedenberg-Magnusson B, Alstergren P, et al. Effect of local glucocorticoid injection on masseter muscle level of serotonin in patients with chronic myalgia. Acta Odontol Scand 1998; 56:129–134.

64. Escalante A, Lichtenstein MJ, Lawrence VA, et al. Where does it hurt? Stability of recordings of pain location using the McGill Pain Map. J Rheumatol 1996; 23(10):1788–1793.

65. Fischer AA, ed. Muscle pain syndromes and fibromyalgia. Pressure algometry for quantification of diagnosis and treatment outcome. New York: Haworth Medical Press; 1998:1–158.

66. Fischer AA. Algometry in diagnosis of musculoskeletal pain and evaluation of treatment outcome: an update. J Musculoskelet Pain 1998; 6(1):5–32.

67. Fischer AA. Pressure algometry over normal muscles. Standard values, validity and reproducibility of pressure threshold. Pain 1987: 30(1):115–126.

68. Fishbain DA, Goldberg M, Meagher BR, et al. Male and female chronic pain patients categorized by DSM-III psychiatric diagnostic criteria. Pain 1986; 26(2):181–197.

69. Floyd WF, Silver PHS. The function of the erectores spinae muscles in certain movements and postures in man. J Physiol 1955; 129:184–203.

70. Foerster O. The dermatomes in man. Brain 1933; 56:1–39.

71. Fricton JR, Auvinen MD, Dykstra D, et al. Myofascial pain syndrome: electromyographic changes associated with local twitch response. Arch Phys Med Rehabil 1985; 66:314–317.

72. Fricton JR. Musculoskeletal measures of orofacial pain. Anesth Prog 1990; 37(2–3):136–143.

73. Fukui S, Ohseto K, Shiotani M, et al. Distribution of referred pain from the lumbar zygapophyseal joints and dorsal rami. Clin J Pain 1997; 13(4):303–307.

74. Fukui S, Ohseto K, Shiotani M, et al. Referred pain distribution of the cervical zygapophyseal joints and cervical dorsal rami. Pain 1996; 68(1):79–83.

75. Gandevia SC, Phegan CM. Perceptual distortions of the human body image produced by local anaesthesia, pain and cutaneous stimulation. J Physiol 1999; 514(part 2):609–616.

76. Garland SJ. Role of small diameter afferents in reflex inhibition during human muscle fatigue. J Physiol 1991; 435:547–558.

77. Gay T, Maton B, Rendell J, et al. Characteristics of muscle fatigue in patients with myofascial pain-dysfunction syndrome. Arch Oral Biol 1994; 39:847–852.

78. Gerwin RD, Shannon S, Hong C, et al. Interrater reliability in myofascial trigger point examination. Pain 1997; 69:65–73.

79. Gjerstad J, Tjolsen A, Svendsen F, et al. Inhibition of evoked C-fibre responses in the dorsal horn after contralateral intramuscular injection of capsaicin involves activation of descending pathways. Pain 1999; 80:413–418.

80. Gjerstad J, Tjolsen A, Svendsen F, et al. Inhibition of spinal nociceptive responses after intramuscular injection of capsaicin involves activation of noradrenergic and opioid systems. Brain Res 2000; 859:132–136.

81. Glaros AG, Glass EG, Brockman D. Electromyographic data from TMD patients with myofascial pain and from matched control subjects: evidence for statistical, not clinical, significance. J Orofacial Pain 1997; 11:125–129.

82. Göbel H, Weigle L, Kropp P, et al. Pain sensitivity and pain reactivity of pericranial muscles in migraine and tension-type headache. Cephalalgia 1992; 12:142–151.

83. Goldenberg DL, Burckhardt C, Crofford L. Management of fibromyalgia syndrome. JAMA 2004; 292(19):2388–2395.

84. Goulet J-P, Clark GT, Flack VF, et al. The reproducibility of muscle and joint tenderness detection methods and maximum mandibular movement measurement for the temporomandibular system. J Orofacial Pain 1998; 12:17–26.

85. Gracely RH, Reid KI. Orofacial pain measurement. In: Fricton JR, Dubner R, eds. Orofacial pain and temporomandibular disorders. Advances in pain research and therapy, vol 21. New York: Raven Press; 1995:117–143.

86. Graff-Radford SB, Reeves JL, Baker RL, et al. Effects of transcutaneous electrical nerve stimulation on myofascial pain and trigger point sensitivity. Pain 1989; 37(1):1–5.

87. Graven-Nielsen T, Arendt-Nielsen L, Svensson P, et al. Effects of experimental muscle pain on muscle activity and co-ordination during static and dynamic motor function. Electroencephalogr Clin Neurophysiol 1997; 105:156–164.

88. Graven-Nielsen T, Arendt-Nielsen L, Svensson P, et al. Quantification of local and referred muscle pain in humans after sequential i.m. injections of hypertonic saline. Pain 1997; 69:111–117.

89. Graven-Nielsen T, Arendt-Nielsen L, Svensson P, et al. Stimulus–response functions in areas with experimentally induced referred muscle pain—a psychophysical study. Brain Res 1997; 744:121–128.

90. Graven-Nielsen T, Aspegren-Kendall S, Henriksson KG, et al. Ketamine attenuates experimental referred muscle pain and temporal summation in fibromyalgia patients. Vienna; 1999:516.

91. Graven-Nielsen T, Babenko V, Svensson P, et al. Experimentally induced muscle pain induces hypoalgesia in heterotopic deep tissues, but not in homotopic deep tissues. Brain Res 1998; 787:203–210.

92. Graven-Nielsen T, Gibson SJ, Laursen RJ, et al. Opioid insensitive hypoalgesia to mechanical stimuli at sites ipsilateral and contralateral to experimental muscle pain in human volunteers. Exp Brain Res 2002 (in press).

93. Graven-Nielsen T, Kendall SA, Henriksson KG, et al. Ketamine reduces muscle pain, temporal summation, and referred pain in fibromyalgia patients. Pain 2000; 85:483–491.

94. Graven-Nielsen T, McArdle A, Phoenix J, et al. In vivo model of muscle pain: quantification of intramuscular chemical, electrical, and pressure changes associated with saline-induced muscle pain in humans. Pain 1997; 69:137–143.

95. Graven-Nielsen T, Mense S. The peripheral apparatus of muscle pain: evidence from animal and human studies. Clin J Pain 2001; 17:2–10.

96. Gray RJ. How reliable is your patient? A comparison of subjective complaints and clinical findings in a group of temporomandibular joint patients. J Dent 1986; 14(5):223–225.

96a. Greene WB (ed). Essentids of musculoskeletal medicine. Second edition. Rosemount, IL: American Academy of Orthopedic Surgeons; 2001.

97. Gunn CC. Gunn approach to the treatment of chronic pain: intramuscular stimulation for myofascial pain of radiculopathic origin. 3rd edn. Philadelphia: Churchill Livingstone; 1996.

98. Hackett G. Ligament and tendon relaxation (skeletal disability) treated by prolotherapy (fibro-osseous proliferation). 3rd edn. Springfield: Charles C. Thomas; 1958.

99. Hagberg C. General musculoskeletal complaints in a group of patients with craniomandibular disorders (CMD). A case control study. Swed Dent J 1991; 15(4):179–185.

100. Hagberg M, Kvarnström S. Muscular endurance and electromyographic fatigue in myofascial shoulder pain. Arch Phys Med Rehabil 1984; 65:522–525.

101. Headache Classification Committee of the International Headache Society. Classification and diagnostic criteria for headache disorders, cranial neuralgias and facial pain. Cephalalgia 1988; 8(suppl 7):1–96.

102. Henriksson KG, Mense S. Pain and nociception in fibromyalgia: clinical and neurobiological considerations on aetiology and pathogenesis. Pain Rev 1994; 1:245–260.

103. Hoheisel U, Mense S, Simons DG, et al. Appearance of new receptive fields in rat dorsal horn neurons following noxious stimulation of skeletal muscle: a model for referral of muscle pain? Neurosci Lett 1993; 153:9–12.

104. Hoheisel U, Sander B, Mense S. Myositis-induced functional reorganisation of the rat dorsal horn: effects of spinal superfusion with antagonists to neurokinin and glutamate receptors. Pain 1997; 69(3):219–230.

105. Hong CZ, Chen YN, Twehous D, et al. Pressure threshold for referred pain on the trigger point and adjacent areas. J Musculoskelet Pain 1996; 4:61–79.

106. Howell JN, Chilla AG, Ford G, et al. An electromyographic study of elbow motion during postexercise muscle soreness. J Appl Physiol 1985; 58(5):1713–1718.

107. Hsieh C, Hong C, Adams AH, et al. Interexaminer reliability of the palpation of trigger points in the trunk and lower limb muscles. Arch Phys Med Rehabil 2000; 81:258–264.

108. Hu JW, Sessle BJ, Raboisson P, et al. Stimulation of craniofacial muscle afferents induces prolonged facilitatory effects in trigeminal nociceptive brain-stem neurones. Pain 1992; 48:53–60.

109. Inman VT, Saunders JBCM. Referred pain from skeletal structures. J Nerv Ment Dis 1944; 99:660–667.

110. Intrieri RC, Jones GE, Alcorn JD. Masseter muscle hyperactivity and myofascial pain dysfunction syndrome: a relationship under stress. J Behav Med 1994; 17:479–500.

111. Isselee H, De Laat A, Bogaerts K, et al. Short-term reproducibility of pressure pain thresholds in masticatory muscles measured with a new algometer. J Orofacial Pain 1998; 12:203–209.

112. Jacobsen S, Danneskiold-Samsoe B. Isometric and isokinetic muscle strength in patients with fibrositis syndrome. New characteristics for a difficult definable category of patients. Scand J Rheumatol 1987; 16(1):61–65.

113. Jacobsen S, Wildschiødtz G, Danneskiold-Samsøe B. Isokinetic and isometric muscle strength combined with transcutaneous electrical muscle stimulation in primary fibromyalgia syndrome. J Rheumatol 1991; 18:1390–1393.

114. Jaeger B, Reeves JL. Quantification of changes in myofascial trigger point sensitivity with the pressure algometer following passive stretch. Pain 1986; 27(2):203–210.

115. James C, Sacco P, Jones DA. Loss of power during fatigue of human leg muscles. J Physiol 1995; 484(1):237–246.

116. Jensen K, Andersen HØ, Olesen J, et al. Pressure-pain threshold in human temporal region: evaluation of a new pressure algometer. Pain 1986; 25:313–323.

117. Jensen K, Tuxen C, Pedersen-Bjergaard U, et al. Pain and tenderness in human temporal muscle induced by bradykinin and 5-hydroxytryptamine. Peptides 1990; 11:1127–1132.

118. Jensen R, Bendtsen L, Olesen J. Muscular factors are of importance in tension-type headache. Headache 1998; 38:10–17.

119. Jensen R, Fuglsang-Frederiksen A, Olesen J. Quantitative surface EMG of pericranial muscles in headache. A population study. Electroencephalogr Clin Neurophysiol 1994; 93:335–344.

120. Jensen R, Rasmussen BK, Pedersen B, et al. Muscle tenderness and pressure pain thresholds in headache. A population study. Pain 1993; 52:193–199.

121. Jensen R. Pathophysiological mechanisms of tension-type headache. A review of epidemiological and experimental studies. Doctoral thesis, University of Copenhagen, 1999.

122. Johansen MK, Graven-Nielsen T, Olesen AS, et al. Generalised muscular hyperalgesia in chronic whiplash syndrome. Pain 1999; 83:229–234.

123. Johansson H, Sojka P. Pathophysiological mechanisms involved in genesis and spread of muscular tension in occupational muscle pain and in chronic musculoskeletal pain syndromes: a hypothesis. Med Hypotheses 1991; 35:196–203.

124. Kamanli A, Kaya A, Ardicoglu O, et al. Comparison of lidocaine injection, botulinum toxin injection, and dry needling to trigger points in myofascial pain syndrome. Rheumatol Int 2005; 25(8):604–611.

125. Kandell ER, Schwartz JH, Jessell TM, ed. Principles of neural science. 4th edn. New York: McGraw-Hill; 2000.

126. Kellgren J. On the distribution of pain arising from deep somatic structures with charts of segmental pain areas. Clin Sci 1939; 4:35–46.

127. Kellgren JH. Observation on referred pain arising from muscle. Clin Sci 1938; 3:175–190.

128. Kendall NA. Psychosocial approaches to the prevention of chronic pain: the low back paradigm. 1: Baillières Best Pract Res Clin Rheumatol 1999; 13(3):545–554.

129. Korr IM. The facilitated segment: a factor in injury to the body framework. In: Peterson B, ed. The collected papers of Irvin M. Korr. Newark: American Academy of Osteopathy; 1979.

130. Kosek E, Hansson P. Modulatory influence on somatosensory perception from vibration and heterotopic noxious conditioning stimulation (HNCS) in fibromyalgia patients and healthy subjects. Pain 1997; 70:41–51.

131. Kosek E, Ordeberg G. Lack of pressure pain modulation by heterotopic noxious conditioning stimulation in patients with painful osteoarthritis before, but not following, surgical pain relief. Pain 2000; 88:69–78.

132. Langemark M, Jensen K, Jensen TS, et al. Pressure pain thresholds and thermal nociceptive thresholds in chronic tension-type headache. Pain 1989; 38:203–210.

133. Laursen R, Graven-Nielsen T, Jensen TS, et al. The effect of compression and regional anaesthetic block on referred pain intensity in humans. Pain 1999; 80(1–2):257–263.

134. Laursen RJ, Graven-Nielsen T, Jensen TS, et al. Quantification of local and referred pain in humans induced by intramuscular electrical stimulation. Eur J Pain 1997; 1:105–113.

135. Laursen RJ, Graven-Nielsen T, Jensen TS, et al. Referred pain is dependent on sensory input from the periphery: a psychophysical study. Eur J Pain 1998; 1:261–269.

136. Laursen RJ, Graven-Nielsen T, Jensen TS, et al. The effect of differential and complete nerve block on experimental muscle pain in humans. Muscle Nerve 1999; 22:1564–1570.

137. Lavigne GJ, Thon MT, Rompré P, et al. Sensory descriptors from touch to pressure-pain and experimental variables: a psychophysiological study in human on pressure-pain threshold. In: Gebhart GF, Hammond DL, Jensen TS, eds. Proceedings of the 7th World Congress on Pain. Progress in pain research and management, vol 2. Seattle: IASP Press; 1994:831–842.

138. Leffler AS, Kosek E, Hansson P. Injection of hypertonic saline into musculus infraspinatus resulted in referred pain and sensory disturbances in the ipsilateral upper arm. Eur J Pain 2000; 4:73–82.

139. Leffler AS, Kosek E, Hansson P. The influence of pain intensity on somatosensory perception in patients suffering from subacute/chronic lateral epicondylalgia. Eur J Pain 2000; 4:57–71.

140. Leffler AS, Kosek E, Lerndal T, et al. Somatosensory perception and function of diffuse noxious inhibitory controls (DNIC) in patients suffering from rheumatoid arthritis. Eur J Pain 2002; 6(2):161–176.

141. LeResche L, Dworkin SF. Facial expressions of pain and emotions in chronic TMD patients. Pain 1988; 35(1):71–78.

142. Lewis T. Suggestions relating to the study of somatic pain. Br Med J 1938; 1:321–325.

143. List T, Helkimo M, Falk G. Reliability and validity of a pressure threshold meter in recording tenderness in the masseter muscle and the anterior temporalis muscle. J Craniomandibular Pract 1989; 7:223–229.

144. List T, Helkimo M, Karlsson R. Influence of pressure rates on the reliability of a pressure threshold meter. J Craniomandibular Disord Facial Oral Pain 1991; 5:173–178.

145. Lous I, Sheikoleslam A, Møller E. Postural activity in subjects with functional disorders of the chewing apparatus. Scand J Dent Res 1970; 78:404–410.

146. Lund JP, Donga R, Widmer CG, et al. The pain-adaptation model: a discussion of the relationship between chronic musculoskeletal pain and motor activity. Can J Physiol Pharmacol 1991; 69:683–694.

147. Lund JP, Stohler CS, Widmer CG. The relationship between pain and muscle activity in fibromyalgia and similar conditions. Lund JP, Stohler CS, Widmer CG, eds. Progress in fibromyalgia and myofascial pain. Amsterdam: Elsevier Science; 1993:311–327.

148. Lund JP, Widmer CG, Schwartz G. What is the link between myofascial pain and dysfunction? In: Lund JP, Widmer CG, Schwartz G, eds. EMG of jaw reflexes in man. Leuven: Leuven University Press; 1989:427–444.

149. MacKenzie J. Some points bearing on the association of sensory disorders and visceral disease. Brain 1983; 16:321–353.

150. Madeleine P, Lundager B, Voigt M, et al. Shoulder muscle co-ordination during chronic and acute experimental neck-shoulder pain. An occupational pain study. Eur J Appl Physiol 1999; 79(2):127–140.

151. Maixner W, Fillingim R, Booker D, et al. Sensitivity of patients with painful temporomandibular disorders to experimentally evoked pain. Pain 1995; 63:341–351.

152. Maixner W, Fillingim R, Sigurdsson A, et al. Sensitivity of patients with painful temporomandibular disorders to experimentally evoked pain: evidence for altered temporal summation of pain. Pain 1998; 76:71–81.

153. Majewski RF, Gale EN. Electromyographic activity of anterior temporal area pain patients and non-pain subjects. J Dent Res 1984; 63:1228–1231.

154. Malow RM, Grimm L, Olson RE. Differences in pain perception between myofascial pain dysfunction patients and normal subjects: a signal detection analysis. J Psychosom Res 1980; 24:303–309.

155. Margolis RB, Chibnall JT, Tait RC. Test-retest reliability of the pain drawing instrument. Pain 1988; 33(1):49–51.

156. Martin PR, Mathews AM. Tension headaches: psychophysiological investigation and treatment. J Psychosom Res 1978; 22:389–399.

157. McCain GA, Scudds RA. The concept of primary fibromyalgia (fibrositis): clinical value, relation and significance to other chronic musculoskeletal pain syndromes. Pain 1988; 33(3):273–287.

158. McCleane G. Pharmacological strategies in relieving neuropathic pain. Expert Opin Pharmacother 2004; 5(6):1299–1312.

159. McMahon SB. Mechanisms of cutaneous, deep and visceral pain. In: Wall PD, Melzack R, eds. Textbook of pain. Edinburgh: Churchill Livingstone; 1994:129–151.

160. McMillan AS, Blasberg B. Pain-pressure threshold in painful jaw muscles following trigger point injection. J Orofacial Pain 1994; 8:384–390.

161. McMillan AS, Lawson ET. Effect of tooth clenching and jaw opening on pain-pressure thresholds in the human jaw muscles. J Orofacial Pain 1994; 8:250–257.

162. McNamera JO. Drugs effective in the therapy of the epilepsies. In: Hardman JG, Limbird LE, eds. Goodman and Gilman's the pharmacologic basis of therapeutics. 9th edn. New York: McGraw-Hill; 1996.

163. Melzack R, Katz J, Jeans ME. The role of compensation in chronic pain: analysis using a new method of scoring the McGill Pain Questionnaire. Pain 1985; 23(2):101–112.

164. Mense S, Light AR, Perl ER. Spinal terminations of subcutaneous high-threshold mechanoreceptors. In: Brown AG, Réthelyi M, eds. Spinal cord sensations. Edinburgh: Scottish Academic Press; 1981:79–84.

165. Mense S, Meyer H. Bradykinin-induced modulation of the response behaviour of different types of feline group III and IV muscle receptors. J Physiol (Lond) 1988; 398:49–63.

166. Mense S, Simons DG. Muscle pain. Understanding its nature, diagnosis, and treatment, Philadelphia: Lippincott Williams & Wilkins; 2001.

167. Mense S. Considerations concerning the neurobiological basis of muscle pain. Can J Physiol Pharmacol 1991; 69(5):610–616.

168. Mense S. Muscular nociceptors. J Physiol (Paris) 1977; 73(3):233–240.

169. Mense S. Nociception from skeletal muscle in relation to clinical muscle pain. Pain 1993; 54(3):241–289.

170. Mense S. Referral of muscle pain. APS J 1994; 3:1–9.

171. Mense S. Sensitization of group IV muscle receptors to bradykinin by 5-hydroxytryptamine and prostaglandin E_2. Brain Res 1981; 225(1):95–105.

172. Merskey H, Bogduk N, ed. Classification of chronic pain. 2nd edn. Seattle: IASP Press; 1994.

173. Mikkelsson M, Latikka P, Kautiainen H, et al. Muscle and bone pressure pain threshold and pain tolerance in fibromyalgia patients and controls. Arch Phys Med Rehabil 1992; 73(9):814–818.

174. Mochizucki D. Serotonin and noradrenaline reuptake inhibitors in animal models of pain. Hum Psychopharmacol 2004; 19(suppl 1):S15–S19.

175. Moldofsky HK. Disordered sleep in fibromyalgia and related myofascial facial pain conditions. Dent Clin North Am 2001; 45(4):701–713.

176. Molin C. Vertical isometric muscle forces of the mandible. Acta Odont Scand 1972; 30:485–499.

177. Nilsson N. Measuring cervical muscle tenderness: a study of reliability. J Manipulative Physiol Ther 1995; 18(2):88–90.

178. Njoo KH, Van der Does E. The occurrence and inter-rater reliability of myofascial trigger points in the quadratus lumborum and gluteus medius: a prospective study in non-specific low back pain patients and controls in general practice. Pain 1994; 58(3):317–323.

179. Obrez A, Stohler CS. Jaw muscle pain and the effect on gothic arch tracings. J Prosthet Dent 1996; 75:393–398.

180. Ohrbach R, Crow H, Kamer A. Examiner expectancy effects in the measurement of pressure pain thresholds. Pain 1998; 74:163–170.

181. Ohrbach R, Gale EN. Pressure pain thresholds in normal muscles: reliability, measurement effects and topographic differences. Pain 1989; 37:257–263.

182. Ohrbach R, Gale EN. Pressure pain thresholds, clinical assessment, and differential diagnosis: reliability and validity in patients with myogenic pain. Pain 1989; 39:157–169.

183. O'Neill CW, Kurgansky ME, Derby R, et al. Disc stimulation and patterns of referred pain. Spine 2002; 27(24):2776–2781.

184. Pearce JM. Chronic regional pain and chronic pain syndromes. Spinal Cord 2005; 43(5):263–268.

185. Peloso PM, Bellamy N, Bensen W, et al. Double blind randomized placebo control trial of controlled release codeine in the treatment of osteoarthritis of the hip or knee. J Rheumatol 2000; 27(3):764–771.

186. Petrenko AB, Yamakura T, Baba H, et al. The role of N-methyl-D-aspartate (NMDA) receptors in pain: a review. Anesth Analg 2003; 97(4):1108–1116.

187. Pilowsky I. Low back pain and illness behavior (inappropriate, maladaptive, or abnormal). Spine 1995; 20(13):1522–1524.

188. Reeves JL, Jaeger B, Graff-Radford SB. Reliability of the pressure algometer as a measure of myofascial trigger point sensitivity. Pain 1986; 24(3):313–321.

189. Reid KI, Gracely RH, Dubner RA. The influence of time, facial side, and location on pain-pressure thresholds in chronic myogenous temporomandibular disorder. J Orofacial Pain 1994; 8:258–265.

190. Reinert A, Kaske A, Mense S. Inflammation-induced increase in the density of neuropeptide-immunoreactive nerve endings in rat skeletal muscle. Exp Brain Res 1998; 121:174–180.

191. Reynolds MD. The development of the concept of fibrositis. J Hist Med Allied Sci 1983; 38:5–35.

192. Robinson JP, Ricketts D, Hanscom DA. Musculoskeletal pain. In: Merskey H, Loeser JD, Dubner R, eds. The paths of pain 1975–2005. Seattle: IASP Press, 2005.

193. Robinson JP, Turk DC. Introductory essay. In: Schmidt RF, Willis WD, eds. Encyclopedic reference of pain. Heidelberg: Springer, 2005.

194. Ross J. On the segmental distribution of sensory disorder. Brain 1988; 10:333–361.

195. Roth SH, Fleischmann RM, Burch FX, et al. Around-the-clock, controlled-release oxycodone therapy for osteoarthritis-related pain: placebo-controlled trial and long-term evaluation. Arch Intern Med 2000; 160(6):853–860.

196. Ruch TC. Pathophysiology of pain. In: Ruch TC, Patton HD, Woodbury JW, et al, eds. Neurophysiology. Philadelphia: Saunders; 1961:350–368.

197. Sand T, Zwart JA, Helde G, et al. The reproducibility of cephalic pain pressure thresholds in control subjects and headache patients. Cephalalgia 1997; 17:748–755.

198. Schiffman E, Fricton JR, Haley D, et al. A pressure algometer for myofascial pain syndrome: reliability and validity testing. In: Dubner R, Gebhart GF, Bond MR, eds. Proceedings of the 5th World Congress on Pain. Pain research and clinical management, vol 3. Amsterdam: Elsevier; 1988:407–413.

199. Schoenen J, Bottin D, Hardy F, et al. Cephalic and extracephalic pressure pain thresholds in chronic tension-type headache. Pain 1991; 47:145–149.

200. Sciotti VM, Mittak VL, DiMarco L, et al. Clinical precision of myofascial trigger point location in the trapezius muscle. Pain 2001; 93:259–266.

201. Scott AB, Rosenbaum A, Collins CC. Pharmacologic weakening of extra-ocular muscles. Invest Ophthalmol 1973; 12(12):924–927.

202. Scott AB. Botulinum toxin injection into extraocular muscles as an alternative to strabismus surgery. J Pediatr Ophthalmol Strabismus 1980; 17(1):21–25.

203. Scudds RA, Trachsel LC, Luckhurst BJ, et al. A comparative study of pain, sleep quality and pain responsiveness in fibrositis and myofascial pain syndrome. J Rheumatol 1989; 16(suppl 19):120–126.

204. Sessle BJ. Masticatory muscle disorders: basic science perspectives. In: Sessle BJ, Bryant PS, Dionne RA, eds. Temporomandibular disorders and related pain conditions. Progress in pain research and management, vol 4. Seattle: IASP Press; 1995:47–61.

205. Shah J. The dynamic role of sensitization in chronic muscle pain: a novel approach for assaying local tissue abnormalities. Presentation at the 65th Annual Assembly of the American Academy of Physical Medicine and Rehabilitation, October 2004.

206. Sihvonen T, Partanen J, Hänninen O, et al. Electric behavior of low back muscles during lumbar pelvic rhythm in low back pain patients and healthy controls. Arch Phys Med Rehabil 1991; 72:1080–1087.

207. Simons DG, Travell J, Simons LS. Travell and Simons' myofascial pain dysfunction: the trigger point manual, vol 1. 2nd edn. Baltimore: Williams & Wilkins; 1999.

208. Simons DG. Fibrositis/fibromyalgia: a form of myofascial trigger points? Am J Med 1986; 81(suppl 3A):93–98.

209. Simons DG. Muscular pain syndromes. In: Fricton JR, Awad EA, eds. Myofascial pain and fibromyalgia. Advances in pain research and therapy, vol 17. New York: Raven Press; 1990:1–41.

210. Simons DJ, Day E, Goodell H, et al. Experimental studies on headache: muscle of the scalp and neck as sources of pain. Assoc Res Nerv Ment Dis 1943; 23:228–244.

211. Sinclair DC, Weddell G, Feindel WH. Referred pain and associated phenomena. Brain 1948; 71:184–211.

212. Skootsky SA, Jaeger B, Oye RK. Prevalence of myofascial pain in general internal medicine practice. West J Med 1989; 151:157–160.

213. Smythe H. Fibrositis syndrome: a historical perspective. J Rheumatol 1989; 16(suppl 19):2–6.

214. Smythe H. Tender points: evolution of concepts of the fibrositis/fibromyalgia syndrome. Am J Med 1986; 81(suppl 3A):2–6.

215. Smythe HA, Moldofsky H. Two contributions to understanding of the 'fibrositis' syndrome. Bull Rheum Dis 1977; 28:928–931.

216. Sola AE, Bonica JJ. Myofascial pain syndromes. In: Bonica JJ, Loeser JD, Chapman CR, et al, eds. The management of pain. 2nd edn. Philadelphia: Lea & Fibiger; 1990:352–367.

217. Sola AE, Rodenberger ML, Gettys BB. Incidence of hypersensitive areas in posterior shoulder muscles. Am J Phys Med 1955; 34:585–590.

218. Sörensen J, Graven-Nielsen T, Henriksson KG, et al. Hyperexcitability in fibromyalgia. J Rheumatol 1998; 25:152–155.

219. Staud R, Cannon RC, Mauderli AP, et al. Temporal summation of pain from mechanical stimulation of muscle tissue in normal controls and subjects with fibromyalgia syndrome. Pain 2003; 102(1–2):87–95.

220. Staud R, Price DD, Robinson ME, et al. Maintenance of windup of second pain requires less frequent stimulation in fibromyalgia patients compared to normal controls. Pain 2004; 110(3):689–696.

221. Staud R, Vierck CJ, Cannon RL, et al. Abnormal sensitization and temporal summation of second pain (wind-up) in patients with fibromyalgia syndrome. Pain 2001; 91:165–175.

222. Staud R. New evidence for central sensitization in patients with fibromyalgia. Curr Rheumatol Rep 2004; 6(4):259.

223. Stawowy M, Bluhme C, Arendt-Nielsen L, et al. Somatosensory changes in the referred pain area in patients with acute cholecystitis before and after treatment with laparoscopic or open cholecystectomy. Scand J Gastroenterol 2004; 39(10):988–993.

224. Stohler CS, Ashton-Miller JA, Carlson DS. The effects of pain from the mandibular joint and muscles on masticatory motor behaviour in man. Arch Oral Biol 1988; 33(3):175–182.

225. Stohler CS, Kowalski CJ, Lund JP. Muscle pain inhibits cutaneous touch perception. Pain 2001; 92:327–333.

226. Stohler CS, Lund JP, Morimoto T. Psychophysical and orofacial motor response to muscle pain—validation and utility of an experimental model. In: Stohler CS, Lund JP, Morimoto T, eds. Brain and oral functions. Amsterdam: Elsevier Science; 1995:227–237.

227. Stohler CS, Yamada Y, Ash MM Jr. Antagonistic muscle stiffness and associated reflex behaviour in the pain-dysfunctional state. Helv Odont Acta 1985; 29(2):13–20.

228. Stohler CS, Zhang X, Lund JP. The effect of experimental jaw muscle pain on postural muscle activity. Pain 1996; 66:215–221.

229. Sturge WA. The phenomena of angina pectoris and their bearing upon the theory of counter-irritation. Brain 1983; 5:492–510.

230. Svensson P, Arendt-Nielsen L, Houe L. Muscle pain modulates mastication: an experimental study in humans. J Orofacial Pain 1998; 12:7–16.

231. Svensson P, Arendt-Nielsen L, Houe L. Sensory-motor interactions of human experimental unilateral jaw muscle pain: a quantitative analysis. Pain 1996; 64:241–249.

232. Svensson P, Arendt-Nielsen L, Nielsen H, et al. Effect of chronic and experimental jaw muscle pain on pain-pressure thresholds and stimulus–response curves. J Orofacial Pain 1995; 9:347–356.

233. Svensson P, Graven-Nielsen T, Arendt-Nielsen L. Mechanical hyperesthesia of human facial skin induced by tonic painful stimulation of jaw muscles. Pain 1998; 74(1):93–100.

234. Svensson P, Graven-Nielsen T, Matre DA, et al. Experimental muscle pain does not cause long-lasting increases in resting EMG activity. Muscle Nerve 1998; 21:1382–1389.

235. Svensson P, Houe L, Arendt-Nielsen L. Bilateral experimental muscle pain changes electromyographic activity of human jaw-closing muscles during mastication. Exp Brain Res 1997; 116(1):182–185.

236. Svensson P, List T, Hector G. Analysis of stimulus-evoked pain in patients with myofascial temporomandibular pain disorders. Pain 2001; 92:399–409.

237. Taiwo YO, Levine JD. Serotonin is a directly-acting hyperalgesic agent in the rat. Neuroscience 1992; 48:485–490.

238. Takahashi Y, Sato A, Nakamura SI, et al. Regional correspondence between the ventral portion of the lumbar intervertebral disc and the groin mediated by a spinal reflex. A possible basis of discogenic referred pain. Spine 1998; 23:1853–1859.

239. Theobald GW. The role of the cerebral cortex in the apperception of pain. Lancet 1949; 257:41–47.

240. Thorstensson A, Arvidson Å. Trunk muscle strength and low back pain. Scand J Rehabil Med 1982; 14:69–75.

241. Torebjörk HE, Ochoa JL, Schady W. Referred pain from intraneural stimulation of muscle fascicles in the median nerve. Pain 1984; 18:145–156.

242. Travell J, Berry C, Bigelow N. Effects of referred somatic pain on structures in the reference zone [abstract]. APS 1944; 3:49.

243. Travell JG, Rinzler S, Herman M. Pain and disability of the shoulder and arm. JAMA 1942; 120(6):417–422.

244. Travell JG, Simons DG. Myofascial pain and dysfunction, vol 1. Baltimore: Williams & Wilkins; 1983.

245. Travell JG, Simons DG. Myofascial pain and dysfunction, vol 2. Baltimore: Williams & Wilkins; 1992.

246. Triano JJ, Schultz AB. Correlation of objective measure of trunk motion and muscle function with low-back disability ratings. Spine 1987; 12(6):561–565.

247. Tunks E, McCain GA, Hart LE, et al. The reliability of examination for tenderness in patients with myofascial pain, chronic fibromyalgia and controls. J Rheumatol 1995; 22(5):944–952.

248. Turk DC, Okifuji A. Pain terms and taxonomies of pain. In: Loeser JD, ed. Bonica's management of pain. 3rd edn. Philadelphia: Lippincott Williams & Wilkins; 2001.

249. Turk DC, Robinson JP, Loeser JD, et al. Pain. In: Cocchiarella L, Andersson GBJ, eds. Guides to the evaluation of permanent impairment. 5th edn. Chicago: AMA Press; 2001.

250. Turp JC, Kowalski CJ, O'Leary N, et al. Pain maps from facial pain patients indicate a broad pain geography. J Dent Res 1998; 77(6):1465–1472.

251. Turp JC, Kowalski CJ, Stohler CS. Pain descriptors characteristic of persistent facial pain. J Orofacial Pain 1997; 11(4):285–290.

252. Tuveson B, Lindblom B, Fruhstorfer H. Experimental muscle pain and sensory changes at the site of referred pain [abstract]. SASP, 22th Annual Meeting, Reykjavik, 1999:77.

253. Vaughn R, Pall ML, Haynes SN. Frontalis EMG response to stress in subjects with frequent muscle-contraction headaches. Headache 1977; 16:313–317.

254. Vecchiet L, Galletti R, Giamberardino MA, et al. Modifications of cutaneous, subcutaneous and muscular sensory and pain thresholds after the induction of an experimental algogenic focus in the skeletal muscle. Clin J Pain 1988; 4:55–59.

255. Vecchiet L, Giamberardino MA, de Bigontina P, et al. Comparative sensory evaluation of parietal tissues in painful and nonpainful areas in fibromyalgia and myofascial pain syndrome. In: Gebhart GF, Hammond DL, Jensen TS, eds. Proceedings of the 7th World Congress on Pain. Progress in pain research and management, vol 2. Seattle: IASP Press; 1994:177–185.

256. Vecchiet L, Giamberardino MA, Saggini R. Myofascial pain syndromes: clinical and pathophysiological aspects. Clin J Pain 1991; 7(suppl 1): S16–S22.

257. Veiersted KB, Westgaard RH, Andersen P. Electromyographic evaluation of muscular work pattern as a predictor of trapezius myalgia. Scand J Environ Health 1993; 19:284–290.

258. Vlaeyen JWS, Linton SJ. Fear-avoidance and its consequences in chronic musculoskeletal pain: a state of the art. Pain 2000; 85:317–332.

259. Waddell G. Compensation for chronic pain. London: Stationery Office; 2004.

260. Waddell G. The back pain revolution. Philadelphia: Churchill Livingstone; 1998.

261. Wang K, Sessle BJ, Svensson P, et al. Glutamate evoked neck and jaw muscle pain facilitate the human jaw stretch reflex. Clin Neurophysiol 2004; 115(6):1288–1295.

262. Watanabe M, Tabata T, Huh JI, et al. Possible involvement of histamine in muscular fatigue in temporomandibular disorders: animal and human studies. J Dent Res 1999; 78(3):769–775.

263. Wheeler AH, Goolkasian P, Gretz SS. A randomized, double-blind, prospective pilot study of botulinum toxin injection for refractory, unilateral, cervicothoracic, paraspinal, myofascial pain syndrome. Spine 1998; 23:1662–1666.

264. Wheeler AH. Myofascial pain disorders. Drugs 2004; 64(1):45–62.

265. Woda A, Piochon P, Palla S. Regulation of mandibular postures: mechanisms and clinical implications. Crit Rev Oral Biol Med 2001; 12(2):166–178.

266. Wolfe F, Simons DG, Fricton J, et al. The fibromyalgia and myofascial pain syndromes: a preliminary study of tender points and trigger points in persons with fibromyalgia, myofascial pain syndrome and no disease. J Rheumatol 1992; 19(6):944–951.

267. Wolfe F, Smythe HA, Yunus MB, et al. The American College of Rheumatology 1990 Criteria for the Classification of Fibromyalgia. Report of the Multicenter Criteria Committee. Arthritis Rheum 1990; 33(2):160–172.

268. Wright A, Graven-Nielsen T, Davies I, et al. Temporal summation of pain from skin, muscle and joint following nociceptive ultrasonic stimulation in humans. Exp Brain Res 2002; 144:475–482.

269. Yemm R. A neurophysiological approach to the pathology and aetiology of temporomandibular dysfunction. J Oral Rehabil 1985; 12(4):343–353.

270. You HJ, Morch CD, Arendt-Nielsen L. Electrophysiological characterization of facilitated spinal withdrawal reflex to repetitive electrical stimuli and its modulation by central glutamate receptor in spinal anesthetized rats. Brain Res 2004; 1009(1–2):110–119.

271. Yunus M, Masi AT, Calabro JJ, et al. Primary fibromyalgia (fibrositis): clinical study of 50 patients with matched normal controls. Semin Arthritis Rheum 1981; 11:151–171.

272. Zidar J, Bäckman E, Bengtsson A, et al. Quantitative EMG and muscle tension in painful muscles in fibromyalgia. Pain 1990; 40:249–254.

Chapter

45

Concepts in Sports Medicine
William F. Micheo

Sports medicine is an important area of practice for many physical medicine and rehabilitation specialists. Because of their training in anatomy, biomechanics, pathophysiology of musculoskeletal injury, and functional rehabilitation, physiatrists are well prepared to care for individuals who exercise to achieve health-related benefits and those who participate in recreational and competitive sports. The rehabilitation medicine model applies well to the field of sports medicine, because the majority of injuries related to sports and exercise participation do not require surgical management and should be treated by aggressive conservative care. Sports medicine care should be delivered in an interdisciplinary team approach, which is one of the strengths of the specialty of physical medicine and rehabilitation. This interdisciplinary team includes the athlete and many professionals, including physicians, dentists, physical therapists, athletic trainers, psychologists, nutritionists, and coaches.

The goal of rehabilitation is to return the individual to normal form and function. The injured athlete should achieve normal flexibility, strength, and muscle balance, as well as neuromuscular coordination, before returning to participation in sports.

The process of rehabilitation should start as early as possible after the injury, and minimize functional losses associated with acute or chronic recurrent injury. Evaluation, management, and rehabilitation of sports injury require an accurate diagnosis, and specific treatment addressing not only the area of injury but the complete kinetic chain.

EPIDEMIOLOGY OF INJURY

Understanding the incidence and prevalence of injuries based on variables such as type and nature of the injury, age group, type of sports, gender, and time since the onset of symptoms, among others, has contributed to the development of programs aimed at prevention, treatment, and rehabilitation of sports injuries.[44] Athletic injuries occur from an overload on the muscles, nerves, tendons, bones, or joints. The knee, foot, and ankle are common sites of injury in athletes, and frequent diagnoses include tendinopathies, ligament sprains, and patellofemoral pain.[43]

The location and type of injuries seen in athletes is influenced by the particular sport involved. Overhead sports such as baseball, tennis, or volleyball often lead to injuries in the shoulder

and elbow. Sports that require trunk rotation, flexion, and extension, such as gymnastics and diving, lead to trunk and spine injuries (Fig. 45-1). Running and jumping sports result in injuries to the knee and ankle.

The specific diagnoses seen by the clinician also vary depending on the sport. Running and jumping sports lead to ankle sprains, patellofemoral pain, and anterior cruciate ligament (ACL) tears of the knee. Overhead sports athletes can present with rotator cuff tendinopathy, shoulder instability, and suprascapular neuropathy. Athletes who participate in sports that require twisting and flexion, such as judo and wrestling, present with spondylolysis, disk disease, and facet joint syndrome (Fig. 45-2).

The age and gender of the individual also influences the type of athletic injury.[43,44] Young and female athletes can present with injuries as a result of overuse and ligamentous laxity, while older individuals can present with degenerative conditions exacerbated by athletic activity.

Physiatrists working as team physicians or traveling with sports teams to different competitions should be prepared to deal with medical problems in addition to musculoskeletal injuries. Frontera reported on the utilization of health services during international sports competitions and showed that, although the most common reason for evaluation was musculoskeletal injury (39.1%), a significant number of individuals presented with medical problems, including respiratory (17.2%), gastrointestinal (12.2%), and skin (5.8%) complaints.[42]

ETIOLOGY OF INJURY

Athletic injury can be caused by extrinsic factors such as training errors, inappropriate equipment, and irregular running surfaces. Training errors account for 60% of running injuries. These include increasing running to more than 40–45 miles per week, running hills excessively, and doing interval training, which significantly increases the rate of injury.[40] Continued exposure to repetitive activity such as throwing is associated with increased risk of injury.

Individual or intrinsic factors such as ligamentous laxity, poor flexibility, and malalignment can also predispose to injury. Young athletes can present with back pain due to a lack of flexibility and trunk weakness associated with growth.[60] Female athletes

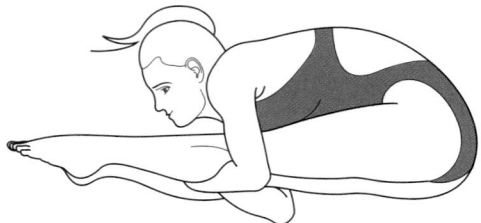

Figure 45-1 Trunk flexion. Platform diving.

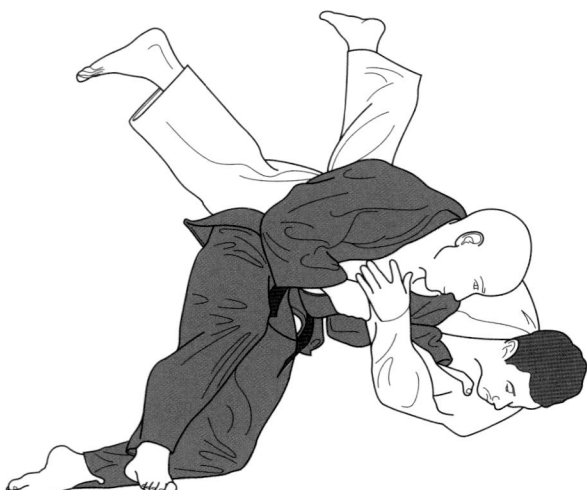

Figure 45-2 Back flexion and rotation. Judo.

Box 45-1 Patient evaluation

History

- Type of sports
- Mechanisms of injury
- Severity of injuries
- Previous history of injury
- Previous treatment strategies
- Growth and development
- Menstrual history
- Associated medical problems
- Associated psychologic issues

Physical examination
- Limitation of motion
- Loss of flexibility
- Muscle weakness
- Muscle imbalance
- Neurologic deficits
- Proprioceptive deficits
- Core muscle strength
- Dynamic flexibility
- Sports-specific techniques

---

with patellar laxity and lower limb malalignment can present with knee extensor mechanism disorders.[6] Older athletes with muscle weakness or imbalance often present with Achilles tendonitis associated with sports participation.[78]

CLASSIFICATION OF INJURY

For practical purposes, an injury can be defined as a pathologic process that interrupts training or competition and leads the athlete to seek medical treatment. Sports injuries are usually divided into two basic types: those that result from macrotrauma, and those associated with overuse and repetitive microtrauma. In traumatic injuries, there is a clear inciting event that results in damage to previously normal tissue. Microtraumatic overuse injury occurs when repetitive exposure to sports activity results in a failure of normal homeostasis and an inability of tissue to recover from athletic-related trauma.[67]

Athletic injury can be classified as acute, chronic, or an acute exacerbation of a chronic injury. The athlete can present with an acute injury such as an ankle sprain, a chronic injury such as rotator cuff tendinopathy associated with a gradual increase in symptoms, or acute presentation of a chronic injury such as lateral epicondylitis that was not appropriately treated and led to reduced performance.

PATIENT EVALUATION

The history and physical examination are very important in evaluating an injured athlete. Pertinent information that should be obtained in the history includes the type of sport, the mechanism of injury, the severity of the injury, and the previous treatment strategies (if any). In addition, information regarding growth and development, menstrual history, previous history of similar or related injuries, and associated medical problems should be obtained. Psychologic issues that should be investigated include anxiety associated with competition, parental involvement in sports, and abnormal attitude toward eating.

The physical examination should identify limitation of motion, lack of flexibility, muscle weakness and imbalance, neurologic as well as proprioceptive deficits, and ligamentous laxity. It is also important to evaluate core trunk and pelvic muscle strength, dynamic flexibility, and sports specific techniques (Box 45-1).

The treating physician also has the responsibility of ordering and interpreting the diagnostic studies needed to make an accurate diagnosis. Some important studies include ulnar deviation wrist x-rays for suspected scaphoid fracture, bone scan to rule out tibial stress fracture, computed tomography of the lumbar spine with fine cuts at the level of the pars interarticularis to confirm spondylolysis, and magnetic resonance imaging (MRI) of the shoulder for rotator cuff tears. Complete diagnosis of athletic injury can be established using a modification of the musculoskeletal injury complex model described by Kibler.[67] This model identifies the anatomic site of injuries, the clinical symptoms, and the functional deficits (Box 45-2).

The clinical symptoms complex addresses the main complaints of the injured athlete. Symptoms such as pain, swelling,

Box 45-2 Framework for musculoskeletal injuries

Clinical alterations
- Symptoms

Anatomic alterations
- Tissue injuries
- Tissue overload

Functional alterations
- Biomechanical deficits
- Subclinical adaptations

Box 45-3 Rehabilitation of musculoskeletal injuries: goals

Acute phase
- Treat symptom complex.
- Protect anatomic injury site.

Recovery phase
- Correct biomechanical deficits.
- Improve muscle control and balance.
- Retrain proprioception.
- Start sports-specific activity.

Functional phase
- Increase power and endurance.
- Improve neuromuscular control.
- Work on entire kinematic chain.
- Return to competition.

Box 45-4 Rehabilitation of athletic injury: therapeutic interventions

Acute phase
- Active rest
- Cryotherapy
- Electrical stimulation
- Protected motion
- Static and closed chain exercises
- General conditioning
- Non-steroidal antiinflammatory drugs

Recovery phase
- Modalities: superficial heat, ultrasound, electrical stimulation
- Range of motion exercises, static and dynamic flexibility exercises
- Closed chain exercises, proprioceptive neuromuscular facilitation patterns
- Dynamic strengthening exercise
- Sports-specific exercises, surgical tubing, multiplanar joint exercises, for trunk and extremities

Functional phase
- Plyometric exercises, diagonal and multiplanar motions with tubing-light weights, medicine balls
- Increase multiple-plane neuromuscular control
- Maintenance in general flexibility strengthening, power and endurance exercise, sports-specific progression, return to sports

a feeling of instability, numbness, weakness, or change in performance should be identified in order to be appropriately treated. A typical clinical symptom complex associated with an acute ankle sprain would be pain secondary to inversion injury, swelling over the lateral ankle, and inability to participate in a basketball game.

The anatomic alterations complex identifies the site of the primary injury causing the patient's symptoms and the associated areas of tissue overload. An example of this could be the young baseball pitcher who presents with injury to the rotator cuff and overload of the scapular stabilizer muscles.

The functional alterations complex addresses the biomechanical deficits that result from an athletic injury, and the adaptations used by the athletes in order to try to continue to participate in sports. A clinical scenario in which this could be seen is the soccer athlete with lumbar disk disease, a previous history of back pain, tight hamstrings, and weak hip muscles who changes kicking techniques because of loss of hip mobility and presents with an adductor strain.

PRINCIPLES OF SPORTS REHABILITATION

Rehabilitation of the injured athlete can be divided into acute, recovery, and functional phases. Each phase has specific goals (Box 45-3). These phases can be correlated with the inflammatory, repair, and remodeling stages of tissue injury.[31] Athletic rehabilitation combines therapeutic modalities, exercise, and functional sports-specific training to return the competitor to unrestricted sports participation as soon as possible (Box 45-4). Rehabilitation should start early in the postinjury period to reduce the deleterious effects of inactivity and immobilization, and to reduce the overall level of physical impairment.

The acute phase addresses the clinical symptoms complex and should focus on treating tissue injury. This phase correlates with the inflammatory stage of injury, in that primary tissue damage is followed by secondary injury resulting from hypoxia and inflammatory enzymatic activity. The goal at this stage should be to reduce pain and inflammation and allow tissue healing. Reestablishment of non-painful range of motion, prevention of muscle atrophy, and maintenance of general fitness should be addressed.

Therapeutic strategies used in this phase include ice, electrical stimulation, static exercise, and protected range of motion exercise. Cryotherapy, transcutaneous nerve or high-voltage galvanic electrical stimulation, and analgesic or non-steroidal antiinflammatory drugs (NSAIDs) should be used early in the rehabilitation process to reduce pain and inflammation. In addition, use of orthotic equipment can be required to protect the injured part.

Static or isometric muscle contractions can be used to maintain muscle strength and mass if isotonic exercise is not possible or inadvisable. Isometric contractions are well tolerated in the early stages of injury rehabilitation and should be performed at multiple joint angles, using a maximal voluntary effort, with repetitions lasting 5–10 s. If pain or swelling inhibits voluntary muscle contraction, low-voltage electrical stimulation can be used in combination with static exercise to facilitate muscle recruitment.[45] Active exercise should be started as soon as the patient can tolerate a minimal external load through a pain-free range of motion. Pain and swelling control is essential and should be accomplished prior to progressing to the next rehabilitation phase.

The recovery phase is the longest rehabilitation phase and correlates with the fibroblastic repair stage, in that inflammatory changes are replaced by granulation tissue. This phase should focus on obtaining normal passive and active range of motion, improving muscle control, achieving normal muscle balance, and working on proprioception. Loading of injured tissues should be done in a gradual progressive manner, because the tensile strength of affected tissue is reduced. Biomechanical and functional deficits, including lack of flexibility and inability to run or jump, should be addressed in this phase.

Therapeutic strategies used in this stage include superficial heat, ultrasound, electrical stimulation, and stretching and strengthening exercises. In addition, proprioceptive retraining for the upper and lower extremities should be undertaken. Dynamic exercise for strengthening is the most important component of this stage. Combinations of open and closed kinetic chain techniques can be used in this phase. Open chain exercises are ones in which the distal portion of the limb is free to move in space. Closed chain exercises are ones in which the distal portion of the limb is fixed.

Flexibility training includes both static and dynamic techniques. Muscles that cross two or more joints are prone to become tight as a result of injury and require static stretching. The hamstrings are a classic example of a two-joint muscle. Schwellmus reported that improvement in static flexibility could result from hamstring stretching, and recommends stretching for 30 s, at least three times a day, for a total of three repetitions. Changes in muscle length can be expected after 7 days, and the benefits of daily stretching can last to up to 21 days.[111]

Proprioceptive neuromuscular facilitation techniques that include contract–relax and contract–relax–antagonist-contract methods can be used in combination with static stretching. These techniques require a knowledgeable therapist in order to be performed appropriately, but the duration of the stretches is usually shorter, with each repetition lasting only 10 s.[74]

Dynamic flexibility, in which training is performed in the sagittal, frontal, and transverse planes of motion, has become popular recently in the rehabilitation of the injured athlete. Progressive motion in all three planes that combines eccentric, isometric, and concentric muscle actions in a functional manner can be incorporated in this stage of rehabilitation.

Dynamic strengthening exercises are very important during the recovery phase of rehabilitation. Open kinetic chain exercises allow joint isolation, and train both the concentric and eccentric phases of muscle contraction. Dynamic strengthening can also be used to address specific muscles that are weak. Eccentric muscle contractions generate the greatest muscle force (see Ch. 19) and can cause injury due to muscle and tendon overload. Consequently, strengthening with the use of eccentric exercises is important in the rehabilitation of tendinopathy.[78] Eccentric muscle contractions for gaining strength have to be used judiciously and carefully, because this type of exercise can result in muscle damage. Loading the muscle gradually allows recovery of tissue tensile strength, and reduces the pain and swelling associated with delayed-onset muscle soreness. Multiplanar resistive exercise that attempts to reproduce sports-specific actions should be added to the rehabilitation program when isolated single-joint exercises can be performed through a full range of motion. An example of this is resistive training for the shoulder abductors and external rotators with exercise tubing or light weight that reproduces the pitching motion.

Closed kinetic chain exercises that involve multiple joints and muscle cocontraction are also used in this stage of rehabilitation. These exercises emphasize the sequential movement of functionally related joints, control joint centers of motion, and transfer of applied loads.[68] In addition, these exercises can reduce strain, translation loads, and shear in injured or operated knee ligaments, and allow the transition to functional activities of the lower limb following injury (Fig. 45-3).[34,85] In patients with shoulder instability and rotator cuff tendinopathy, closed chain exercises that result in scapular and rotator cuff muscle coactivation are beneficial, particularly in the early stages of rehabilitation that emphasizes proximal stability.[69]

Core muscle strengthening has also been incorporated into functional rehabilitation programs. Strengthening of the abdominal, gluteal, hip girdle, paraspinal, and pelvic floor muscles is important, because these core muscles stabilize the spine and allow a stable platform for sports activity. The core muscles can act as force generators, transfer links in the kinetic chain, and force attenuators or decelerators. The dynamic stabilization program used for the rehabilitation of lumbar disk disease has been used as a base for the development of progressive functional core exercise.[2] McGill has described the abdominal curl-up with one knee bent, the side bridge, and the bird-dog (or quadruped) exercises as basic stabilization exercises (Fig. 45-4).[81]

Proprioceptive training and rehabilitation is also an important component of this phase. Proprioception can be defined in the clinical context as a complex neuromuscular process that involves afferent input and efferent responses. It also allows the body to maintain stability during static and dynamic activities. Deficits in proprioception can occur after athletic injury to the ankle, knee, shoulder, and spine. Proprioception has been found to be trainable, and improvement in function can be expected despite changes in joint laxity following injury.[75] Exercises to retrain proprioception and balance typically progress from standing on both legs on a stable supported surface to single-limb exercises with eyes open and closed.

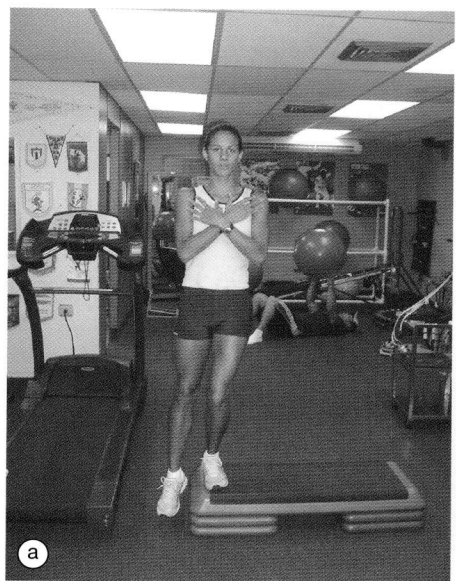
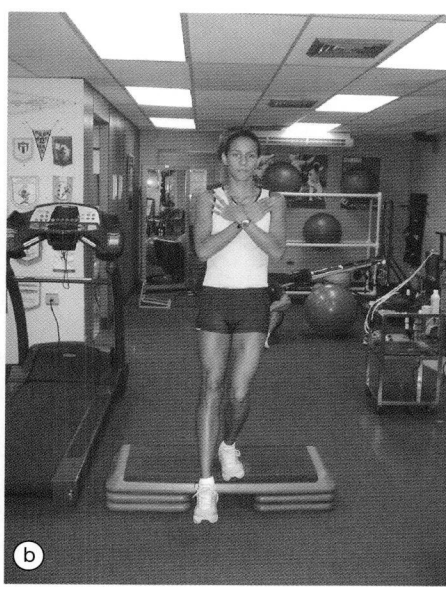

Figure 45-3 Closed kinetic chain exercises: (**a**) side step-down exercise; (**b**) front step-down exercise.

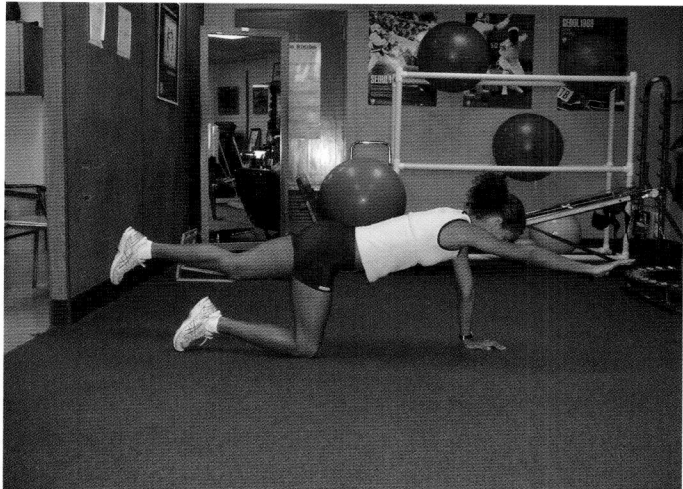

Figure 45-4 Quadriped stabilization exercise.

Sports-specific training should be initiated in this stage. Progression of the training without recurrence of symptoms is necessary prior to advancing to the functional phase of rehabilitation.

The functional phase correlates well with the maturation and remodeling stage of tissue healing, in which the tensile strength of the granulation tissue increases and the collagen fibers are realigned. This phase should focus on increasing power and endurance while improving neuromuscular control. Rehabilitation at this stage should work on the entire kinematic chain, addressing specific functional deficits. This program should be continuous, with the ultimate goal of prevention of recurrent injury.

Therapeutic strategies used in this stage typically include plyometric exercises. These combine eccentric muscle activity prior to a concentric contraction. An example of a plyometric exercise that can be used for training is the counter-movement jump in which the athlete starts from a standing position, squats, jumps, and lands on two legs. Plyometrics are used to gain power, used in sports-specific training to improve technique, for maintenance strengthening, and in flexibility programs.[45]

Once the athlete returns to practice and competition, prevention of recurrent injury is very important. For this reason, the concept of *prehabilitation* has been developed. Prehabilitation is defined as conditioning strategies in formerly injured athletes to prepare them for the stresses and demands of their sport. Prehabilitation focuses on sport-specific musculoskeletal areas in the athlete that have been shown to be weak or susceptible to injury, or have already been injured in a specific sport.[65]

Components of a prehabilitation program include stretching, strengthening, proprioception, and plyometric exercises. Thacker reported that, while stretching has been found to improve flexibility (especially static flexibility), it has not been conclusively shown to reduce the risk of injury.[117] In the immediate poststretching period, loss of strength has been reported to occur, as well as adverse effects on jumping performance and in some instances even reduced running economy.[134] Conditioning strategies and appropriate warm-up using sports-specific dynamic movements can be better alternatives to reduce injury risk.

Strengthening exercises are known to reduce the risk of injury. Eccentric exercise, in particular, has been found to reduce the risk of hamstring strains in elite athletes, and should be included as part of the training and prehabilitation program for the running athlete.[14] Balance training, learning how to fall from a jump, modifying cutting techniques, and plyometric exercises that activate the hamstrings have been found to reduce the risk of ACL injuries in females, and should be integrated into injury prevention programs (Fig. 45-5).[58,91]

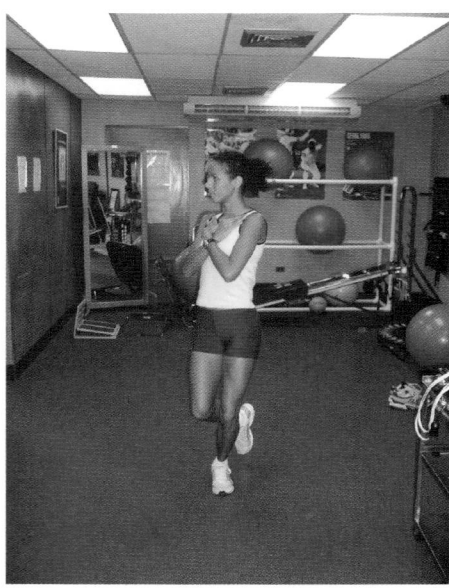

Figure 45-5 Single-leg balance training.

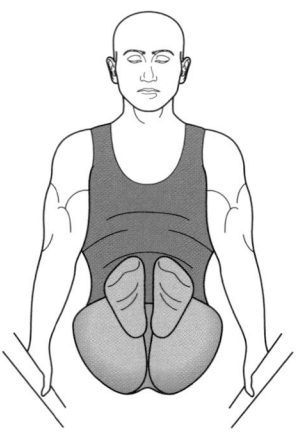

Figure 45-6 Rotator cuff overload. High-bar exercise in men's gymnastics.

MANAGEMENT OF UPPER LIMB INJURIES

Shoulder injury

The glenohumeral joint has a high degree of mobility at the expense of stability. Static and dynamic restraints maintain the shoulder in place with overhead activity. Muscle action, particularly of the rotator cuff and scapular stabilizers, is important in maintaining joint congruity in midranges of motion. Static stabilizers such as the glenohumeral ligaments, joint capsule, and glenoid labrum are important for stability in the extremes of motion.[115] Injury can occur secondary to trauma or to overuse from repeated activity, such as in gymnastics, throwing sports, and swimming (Fig. 45-6).

Traumatic injuries

Glenohumeral dislocation   In the case of traumatic instability of the glenohumeral joint, the individual usually falls on the outstretched, externally rotated, and abducted arm, with a resulting anterior dislocation. A blow to the posterior aspect of

the externally rotated and abducted arm can also result in anterior dislocation. Posterior dislocation usually results from a fall on the forward-flexed and adducted arm, or by direct blow in the posterior direction when the arm is above the shoulder. An acutely dislocated shoulder can usually be recognized by the position of the arm. In anterior dislocation, the arm is held in external rotation while the humeral head can be palpated anterior to the glenoid. Posterior dislocations present with internal rotation and posterior fullness of the shoulder.[8]

In the case of acute anterior dislocation, the injured individual presents with pain, decreased active motion, and deformity. If the injury was observed or the mechanism of injury is clear, and no evidence of neurologic or vascular damage is evident on the clinical examination, reduction can be attempted with traction in forward flexion and slight abduction, and followed by gentle internal rotation.[8] If this fails, the patient should be transported away from the playing area and reduction can be attempted by placing the patient prone, sedating the individual, and allowing the injured arm to hang from the bed with a 5- to 10-lb weight attached to the wrist.

If there is a suspicion of fracture or posterior dislocation, the patient should undergo radiologic evaluation prior to attempting a reduction. The x-rays should be repeated after the reduction. There is some controversy regarding the treatment of first-time anterior dislocations. Although some clinicians have recommended immobilization for as long as 6 weeks, it is not clear that this improves the long-term outcome. Many authors advocate functional rehabilitation following a period of immobilization until the patient is pain-free and able to progress in the treatment program.

Age is a very important factor in management, because younger patients have a higher rate of recurrence. The young athlete returning to competition after the shoulder dislocation should be advised about the possibility of recurrence and the future need for surgical intervention. In the case of the overhead athlete with a dislocation of the throwing arm, early surgical intervention might be recommended.[93]

Acromioclavicular dislocation   Dislocations of the acromioclavicular joint are caused by a direct blow on the posterior aspect of the acromion and spine of the scapula, such as when a player falls on the tip of his or her shoulder. These dislocations are classified from Type 1 to Type 6 based on the anatomic relationship between the acromion and the clavicle following the injury. Type 1 acromioclavicular dislocations represent complete tears of the joint capsule, with no major break in continuity between the acromion and clavicle. Type 2 dislocations involve a complete tear of the joint capsule, but the coracoclavicular ligaments are intact. Point tenderness is associated with this ligamentous disruption, and on visual examination the distal end of the clavicle is very prominent. Type 3 lesions involve a complete disruption of both the joint capsule and the coracoclavicular ligaments. Type 4 injury results in posterior dislocation of the clavicle relative to the acromion, Type 5 shows superior displacement of the clavicle through the trapezius, tenting the skin to more than 100% of clavicle displacement, and Type 6 shows inferior displacement of the clavicle.[131]

Physical examination reveals an obvious depression of the scapula with what appears to be an elevation of the clavicle, localized tenderness to palpation, and limited active shoulder motion. Radiographic examination should be performed with the patient upright, and a study holding weights can be used in the diagnosis of Type 1 or Type 2 injuries.

Non-operative treatment is used for Type 1 and Type 2 injuries. A sling is used to support the arm, and the upper limb should be kept at rest. Heavy lifting or contact sports should be avoided until full range of motion is restored, with no pain on joint palpation. In Type 1 injuries, this process usually takes 2 weeks, but it can take up to 6 weeks in Type 2 injuries. Normal motion should be accompanied by normal scapular muscle control and rotator cuff strength prior to allowing the patient to return to competition.

The treatment of a Type 3 acromioclavicular dislocation is somewhat controversial. Some recommend surgical intervention, while others prefer conservative treatment and rehabilitation after a period of immobilization. Type 4 to Type 6 injuries require surgical treatment.[13]

Overuse injuries

Rotator cuff injury   Overload of the rotator cuff can occur with recurrent overhead activity such as pitching a baseball, serving a tennis ball, or swimming freestyle. The resulting symptoms of reduced motion, muscle weakness, and pain can interfere with activity. In the young patient, this rotator cuff overload is often associated with shoulder instability.[22] The repeated stresses of overhead activity place great demands on the dynamic and static stabilizers of the glenohumeral joint, including the rotator cuff, ligaments, capsule, and glenoid labrum.[17] These biomechanical stresses lead to increased translation of the humeral head, and to pain associated with external subacromial or secondary impingement of the rotator cuff. The individual might report that the shoulder slips out of the joint, or that the arm goes 'dead'. Weakness with overhead activity is also a frequent complaint. Less commonly, the patient presents with symptoms associated with internal impingement. In these cases, the rotator cuff tendon is compressed against the superoposterior aspect of the glenoid labrum with repeated abduction and external rotation.[1]

Older athletes can present with primary impingement associated with a curved or hooked acromion, osteophytes of the acromioclavicular joint, or thickened coracoacromial ligament. These can cause rotator cuff symptoms with abduction of the arm.[1,17] Symptoms of pain at rest, particularly at night in the older athlete, can be due to a rotator cuff tear.

The physical examination should start with inspection for the presence of deformity, atrophy of muscle, asymmetry, and scapular winging. The individual should be observed from the anterior, lateral, and posterior positions. Palpation of soft tissue and bone should be systematic, and includes the rotator cuff, biceps tendon, subacromial and acromioclavicular regions, and glenohumeral joints.

Passive and active range of shoulder motion should be evaluated. Differences between passive and active motion can be secondary to pain, weakness, or neurologic damage. Repeated overhead activity in baseball can lead to an increase in measured external rotation accompanied by a reduction in internal rotation. Participation in tennis can result in an internal rotation deficit with less of an increase in external rotation. Strength testing should be performed to identify weakness of specific muscles of the rotator cuff and the scapular stabilizers. The supraspinatus muscle can be tested in the scapular plane with internal rotation or the so-called empty can position. The external rotators can be tested with the arm at the side of the body, and the subscapularis muscle can be tested by using the 'liftoff test', in that the palm of the hand is lifted away from the lower back. The scapular stabilizers, such as the serratus anterior and the rhomboid muscles, can be tested in isolation or by doing standing push-ups against a wall. Sensory and motor examination of the shoulder girdle should always be performed to rule out nerve injuries.[23]

Rotator cuff external impingement can be assessed by testing the shoulder in 90° of forward flexion with internal rotation, or extreme forward flexion with the forearm supinated. It should be noted whether symptoms are reproduced by these maneuvers. Glenohumeral translation testing looking for laxity or instability should be documented. Apprehension testing can be performed with the patient sitting, standing, or in the supine position. The shoulder joint is stressed in abduction and external rotation, looking for reproduction of the feeling of instability in the patient. A relocation maneuver that reduces the symptoms also aids in the diagnosis.[82] The individual with internal impingement presents with posterior shoulder pain rather than apprehension in this position of shoulder abduction and external rotation.

Other tests include the load and shift maneuver to document humeral head translation in anterior or posterior directions, the sulcus sign to document inferior humeral head laxity, and the active compression test. This test, as described by O'Brien, involves a downward force being applied to the forward-flexed, adducted, and internally rotated shoulder, trying to reproduce pain associated with labral tears or acromioclavicular joint pathology.[94] The across chest adduction maneuver can also be used to reproduce acromioclavicular symptomatology.

Management of rotator cuff injury should begin as soon after the injury as possible. The goals of non-surgical management include reducing pain, restoring full motion, correction of muscle strength deficits, achieving muscle balance, and returning to full activity free of symptoms.[73] The treatment can be divided into acute, recovery, and functional phases, with key points of the rehabilitation presented in Box 45-5.

The acute phase of treatment should focus on treating tissue injury, treating clinical symptoms of pain, and protecting the rotator cuff as well as the shoulder-stabilizing structures. The goal in this stage should be to allow tissue healing while reducing pain and inflammation. Non-painful range of motion, prevention of muscle atrophy, and maintenance of general fitness should be addressed. Treatment strategies in the acute stage

---

Box 45-5 Rehabilitation of rotator cuff injury: key points

Acute phase
- Reduce shoulder pain.
- Maintain range of motion.
- Promote scapular control.

Recovery phase
- Correct shoulder internal rotation deficit.
- Strengthen scapular stabilizer muscles.
- Strengthen rotator cuff in functional range of motion.
- Work on trunk and lower limb strength and balance.

Functional phase
- Increase power of the trunk and limb muscles.
- Correct inappropriate technique.

---

include the use of cryotherapy and high-voltage galvanic stimulation to the shoulder, combined with static and closed chain exercises to the rotator cuff and scapular muscles. Pain-free range of motion of the shoulder as well as strengthening of the trunk and lower extremities should be started.[66,73]

The recovery phase should focus on obtaining normal passive and active glenohumeral range of motion, improving scapular muscle control, and regaining normal muscle strength and balance. Biomechanical and functional deficits such as glenohumeral internal rotation deficits and throwing motion abnormalities should be addressed.

Treatment strategies include superficial heat, ultrasound, shoulder girdle mobilization, posterior capsule stretching, and strengthening exercises. The strengthening program should include closed kinetic chain exercises for the rotator cuff and scapular stabilizers, including push-ups against a wall. Pain-free strengthening of the rotator cuff muscles and scapular stabilizers could be undertaken with the use of light weights or surgical tubing in an open kinetic chain mode of exercise. Functional activities should be started, including squats, lunges, and rotational exercises to improve core trunk, pelvis, and lower extremities muscle strength. Sports-specific training should also be incorporated into the treatment program. A supervised return to a sport program in which the patient progresses without symptoms is required before starting the next rehabilitation phase.[1]

The functional phase of treatment should focus on increasing the power and endurance of the upper extremities while improving neuromuscular control. Rehabilitation at this stage should work on the entire kinematic chain and address specific functional deficits in muscle balance, dynamic flexibility, and throwing technique. This program should be continuous with prehabilitation and has the ultimate goal of preventing a recurrent injury.

Recurrent shoulder instability   The spectrum of shoulder instability ranges from acute traumatic dislocation (which is usually unidirectional) to recurrent subluxation that is usually not related to trauma. Patients with recurrent instability can have a history of recurrent dislocations, but more commonly

that of subluxation or pain associated with repeated overhead activity.[89] The patient can also complain of weakness, locking, transient giving way of the shoulder, or having a 'dead arm'. Some patients present with impingement symptoms of the rotator cuff secondary to failure of the capsuloligamentous structures that stabilize the shoulder at the extremes of range of motion.[83]

The key to diagnosing recurrent shoulder instability is the demonstration of asymmetry of glenohumeral translation from side to side. This is particularly important in the patient with evidence of generalized ligamentous laxity, who might also exhibit laxity of other joints as demonstrated by hyperextension of the elbow and knee. Apprehension testing can be performed with the patient sitting, standing, or in the supine position. The shoulder joint is stressed in abduction and external rotation, trying to reproduce the patient's feeling of instability. A relocation maneuver that reduces the symptoms also aids in the diagnosis. Other tests include the load and shift maneuver, to document humeral head translation in anterior or posterior directions; the sulcus sign, to document inferior humeral head laxity; and the active compression test, looking for labral pathology.

The initial treatment of patients with multidirectional or microtraumatic shoulder instability is non-operative. Symptom reduction is the first goal. This is followed by rehabilitation addressing weakness of the scapular stabilizers and rotator cuff muscles. The appropriate sports-specific mechanics should be undertaken before surgery is considered. Emphasis should be placed on working the scapular and rotator cuff muscles in a 'closed chain' cocontraction method. This method emphasizes joint stabilization, which requires synergism of the static stabilizers and the muscles.

If the patient continues to have recurrent episodes of instability, surgical reconstructive surgery should be considered. Open versus arthroscopic repair techniques can be considered, depending on such factors as age and the cause of the instability (such as previous shoulder dislocations or generalized ligamentous laxity).[41,93,118]

Elbow injuries

Elbow injuries resulting from repetitive overuse can be seen in overhead sports such as baseball and tennis. In other sports, such as gymnastics, judo, and basketball, elbow injuries are less common, but they can occur if there is either repeated upper limb activity or trauma such as falling on an outstretched arm. Forces that can damage the elbow include valgus stress on the medial structures, compression of the lateral structures, and extension overload of the posterior structures. Because of a stable joint structure, single traumatic events require substantial forces to result in fracture or dislocation.

Traumatic injuries
Dislocation: fracture   Single-event injuries are most often a result of collision of an outstretched hand with the ground. If the elbow is somewhat flexed, posterolateral dislocation can

occur. If the elbow is fully extended, transmission of force up the radius can result in a fracture of the radial head or capitellum. Varus or valgus shear forces at the time of impact can result in fracture of the condylar and supracondylar structures. Direct impact on the elbow is another mechanism of injury that can result in fractures about the elbow, usually to the olecranon.[99]

The basics of treatment of fractures of the elbow region include early reduction, management of associated fractures, ongoing assessment of the neurovascular status, and early protected range of motion to minimize the risk of flexion ankylosis. In most cases, complete immobilization should not exceed 2 weeks, because prolonged lack of movement has a higher risk of flexion contractures with associated pain. A removable splint that permits active elbow range of motion, including flexion–extension and supination–pronation, can be used early in the rehabilitation process. By 10–14 days, if the fracture or dislocation is stable, the splint should be discontinued and full elbow flexibility and strengthening begun.[128] On return to play, the elbow can be braced or taped to limit elbow hyperextension and for protection from valgus forces.

Overuse injuries

Soft tissue injuries Injuries to the soft tissue include lateral epicondylitis, medial epicondylitis, ulnar collateral ligament injury, and ulnar neuropathy. Although these are more common in throwing and racquet sports, they can occur in other sports such as gymnastics and basketball.

The patient having lateral epicondylitis presents with pain anterior and distal to the lateral elbow associated with excessive use of the wrist extensor musculature, usually the extensor carpi radialis brevis, and less commonly the extensor digitorum communis, extensor carpi radialis longus, and extensor carpi ulnaris.[37] The pain is commonly increased on resisted wrist extension with the elbow extended and the forearm pronated. The athlete might also complain of pain with gripping activities. The examination typically shows localized tenderness anterior to the lateral epicondyle over the forearm extensors origin. There can also be weakness of wrist extension that is due to pain inhibition of function, as well as loss of passive wrist flexion in chronic cases.

Management includes control of acute symptoms with relative rest, icing, and therapeutic modalities, as well as NSAIDs. Stretching of the wrist extensors is initially done with the elbow bent, and progresses to stretching with extended elbow and pronated forearm. This should be combined with eccentric strengthening in different wrist positions. Generalized conditioning and specific strengthening of the shoulder and trunk muscles should be included. A local corticosteroid injection allows a more rapid progression in the rehabilitation program in some cases. The use of a counterforce brace to reduce the force load on the extensor muscles has been advocated when athletes return to practice or competition.[102] Evaluation of appropriate sports-specific technique is important prior to allowing return to sports. An example of this would be a tennis player who leads to the elbow when hitting the backhand, uses little contribution of the lower extremities and trunk muscles when generating power for the stroke, and gets recurrent symptoms on returning to play.

Athletes with medial epicondylitis typically have injury to the forearm flexor and pronator muscle groups associated with tensile overload. Pain occurs distal to the medial epicondyle, at the origin of the flexor–pronator group, and increases with resisted forearm pronation or wrist flexion.[37] Weakness of shoulder girdle and trunk muscles is also present in many individuals who present with this condition.

Management includes symptomatic treatment combined with stretching and strengthening of the flexor–pronator muscle group. The program should also include strengthening of the shoulder girdle, trunk, and lower limb muscles, as well as a program of generalized conditioning. In severe cases, local injection and counterforce bracing can be used as previously described for lateral epicondylitis. Improving the technique of hitting the tennis forehand or pitching the curve in baseball might be required to reduce recurrence.

Some patients with chronic medial elbow region symptoms have injury to the capsule and ligamentous structures, or to the ulnar nerve. The symptoms are related to repeated activity in which valgus and extension forces are applied to the elbow. The athlete typically complains of medial elbow pain during the late cocking and acceleration phases of throwing. As a result, there is some loss of both throwing velocity and control. Physical examination shows tenderness over the medial side of the elbow joint. Stability testing with the elbow in 20–30° of flexion can reproduce pain symptoms in ulnar collateral ligament injury.[96] Patients with ulnar neuropathy can present with pain or paresthesias in the distribution of the nerve. In many instances, sensory symptoms might not be present at rest and are only reproduced following activity.

Management of medial injury to the ulnar collateral ligament includes avoiding activities with valgus stress, strengthening of the whole upper limb kinetic chain, and improvement of sports-specific technique such as leading with the elbow when pitching. Surgical repair is needed in some cases, but only after failure of an appropriate rehabilitation program of 3–6 months' duration.

Ulnar neuropathy in the elbow region typically occurs in the cubital tunnel, and can be treated with an elbow pad to avoid direct pressure over the nerve. In severe cases, it might be necessary to use an elbow orthosis made of a rigid thermoplastic material that holds the elbow in 45° of flexion. In the early stages of recovery, the orthosis should be worn during most of the day. As the patient's symptoms improve, it should be used only at night. Appropriate stretching, strengthening of the whole kinetic chain, and sports biomechanics should also be addressed.

Wrist and hand injuries

Hand and upper limb injuries are among the most common injuries sustained by athletes. Unfortunately, there is a tendency to minimize their severity, as the hand does not bear weight and the injuries rarely render the athlete unable to compete. Wrist and hand injuries are fairly common, comprising 3–9% of all athletic injuries.[103] Although soft tissue injuries are more common, fractures are also seen quite frequently. Hand and wrist injuries are more common in adolescents than in adults, due to epiphyseal trauma. The most common hand and wrist injuries in sports that engage the hand with a ball include metacarpal, phalangeal and scaphoid fractures, proximal interphalangeal (PIP) joint dislocations, and mallet finger.[106]

Hand and wrist injuries can occur secondary to throwing, repeated overhead activity, or weight bearing, or be due to direct impact.[100] Throwing typically causes injuries mainly by overuse and repetition, including de Quervain's tendonitis, and subluxation and tendonitis of the extensor carpi ulnaris. Weight bearing on the dorsiflexed wrist and hand causes dorsal scaphoid and lunate impaction against the radius (carpal impingement), distal radial physis stress fractures, and triangular fibrocartilage injuries. Impact stresses on the hand and wrist can cause scaphoid fracture of the wrist, scapholunate dissociation, metacarpal fractures, and PIP dorsal dislocation and mallet finger.[127]

Traumatic injuries

Fractures   The scaphoid navicular is the most commonly fractured carpal bone, and the injury occurs in sports in which the participants are subjected to violent forces. The mechanism of injury is usually a fall on the outstretched hand, causing hyperextension of the wrist.

The patient presents with complaints of wrist pain localized to the anatomic snuffbox area, and x-rays including ulnar deviation views should be obtained. If the x-rays are negative but there is a strong clinical suspicion of fracture, a thumb spica splint could be applied for 2 weeks. This is followed by a reexamination to confirm that the pain has disappeared. If the patient is still symptomatic, repeat x-rays and a bone scan or MRI should be performed to rule out a fracture. This is very important to avoid postfracture aseptic necrosis of the scaphoid bone.[104]

The treatment of a non-displaced scaphoid fracture consists of a thumb spica cast for approximately 6–8 weeks until the fracture is clinically and radiographically healed. The more proximal the fracture of the scaphoid, the longer it will take to heal, due to compromise of its blood supply. Early open reduction and internal fixation are recommended as the treatment of choice if the scaphoid fracture is proximal or displaced. An open reduction and internal fixation is frequently used in the elite competitive athlete to shorten the recovery time. The athlete usually returns to sports within 3–4 months of an open reduction of a scaphoid fracture.[104]

Fractures due to athletic trauma are typically stable because of the low energy involved as a cause of the injury. Phalangeal fractures are common and usually associated with crush injury or a direct blow to the hand. These fractures constitute more than half of all hand fractures. In basketball, the most common fracture is in distal phalanx of the middle finger. These fractures are usually stabilized by the nail plate dorsally and the pulp

septa volarly. The treatment for proximal phalanx fractures that are non-displaced is with a distal interphalangeal (DIP) extension splint for 3 weeks. Displaced distal phalanx fracture requires referral for possible surgical treatment.

Middle and proximal phalanx fractures usually occur as a result of a direct blow to the finger. It is important to determine and assure the stability of the fracture. Fractures having no malrotation, minimal angulation, or motion can be treated with splinting or 'buddy taping' to the next finger. The athletes can return to competition as soon as there is no tenderness over the fracture site. Closed reduction and percutaneous pin fixation might be required if the alignment is unacceptable or the fracture is displaced. Special attention is required when dealing with adolescents, because the physeal plate at the base of the phalanx can be involved.[105]

Metacarpal fractures are very common and represent up to 36% of all hand injuries. Metacarpal fractures that involve the middle and ring fingers are usually more stable than those of the index and small finger. This is due to the support provided by the transverse metacarpal ligament. The treatment of metacarpal fractures is closed reduction and splinting for 3–4 weeks followed by active range of motion. Fractures through the diaphysis of the metacarpals tend to shorten or rotate as well as angulate, and surgery is necessary in some cases.[86]

The thumb is frequently traumatized because of its unprotected position. Thumb fractures are usually caused by impact to the radial side of the thumb, and typically occur at the proximal one-third of the thumb metacarpal. Fracture angulation is usually in adduction and volar flexion. Closed treatment can be used if there is only minimal angulation. Fractures to moderate degrees of angulation or malrotation usually require open reduction and internal fixation.

Dislocations   Dorsal dislocation of the PIP joint is probably the most common dislocation in sports. For a dorsal dislocation to occur, the volar plate must be torn, leading to a dorsal displacement of the middle phalanx of the finger.

The treatment of this dislocation is immediate reduction on the field, followed by buddy taping for 3–6 weeks. The player can return to competition immediately after a reduction using the buddy-taping technique but, when not playing, the athlete should have the affected joint immobilized with a dorsal splint in 30° of flexion to promote the healing of the volar plate.[51] Inadequately treated dorsal dislocations can develop a pseudoboutonnière deformity.

Closed tendon injuries   These injuries result from trauma to either the flexor or the extensor tendons of the hand, and are commonly seen in basketball players. These injuries are often believed to be minor and go untreated. If these injuries are not diagnosed and treated early in the course, however, permanent deformity can result.

The most common of the closed tendon injuries of the hand is the mallet finger, also referred to as baseball finger or dropped finger. It is caused by direct impact against an extended DIP joint of any finger. The patient presents with pain, swelling on the dorsum of the DIP joint, and an inability to extend the joint. This injury usually results from trauma directly to the terminal extensor tendon, but it can also be associated with an avulsion fracture of the dorsal aspect of the distal phalanx at the DIP joint. The treatment of the mallet finger when it occurs in the substance of the extensor tendon consists of applying a dorsal splint in extension of the DIP joint. The splint is used continuously for 6 weeks, followed by an additional 4 weeks of dorsal night splinting to prevent the occurrence of the deformity. It is important that the athlete wears a protective splint maintaining the DIP joint in extension for approximately 2 months, to protect the joint from reinjury during competition. It should be noted that good results can be obtained with late treatment.[105] This is true even if treatment is delayed by as much as 3–4 months after the injury.

If an avulsion fracture at the dorsal aspect of the DIP joint does not involve the articular surface, it can still be treated with dorsal splinting. Surgery might be required if the fracture involves more than a third of the articular surface.

A traumatically induced boutonnière (French word meaning buttonhole) deformity occurs as a result of an injury to the central slip of the extensor tendon at or near its insertion into the base of the middle phalanx. The cause is usually a blow to the dorsal aspect of the middle phalanx that forces the digit into flexion while the athlete is actively extending the PIP joint. It can also be caused by unrecognized palmar dislocation of the PIP joint that spontaneously reduced or was reduced on the field by the athlete.

The clinical presentation of the boutonnière deformity is that of weakness of PIP extension or an extensor lag at the PIP joint, accompanied by swelling, pain, and tenderness at the dorsal aspect of the joint. The classic deformity consisting of flexion of the PIP joint and hyperextension of the DIP joint is rarely seen acutely. If the injury goes untreated, the central slip retracts, the triangular ligament becomes stretched, and the lateral bands fall palmar to the axis of rotation. In this case, the lateral bands actually become flexors of the PIP joint and retract proximally, hyperextending the DIP joint.

The treatment of choice of an acute boutonnière deformity is the use of a volar or palmar splint as early as possible after the injury. This palmar splint holds the metacarpophalangeal and PIP joint in extension, while allowing active and passive flexion of the DIP joint. This DIP flexion is important, because it helps the lateral bands assume and maintain the anatomic position at the PIP joint. The splint should be worn continuously for 5–6 weeks, with an additional 2 weeks as a night splint. After 5 weeks of splinting, gentle active and passive range of motion exercises are begun at the PIP joint. In the event that the injury has been overlooked and the classic boutonnière deformity has developed, surgical release with reconstruction might be necessary.

Avulsion of the flexor digitorum profundus tendon, also known as the 'Jersey finger', is a relatively common injury seen in many sports. It is most common in American football. It usually occurs in the ring finger, with the mechanism of injury being forceful extension of the finger during maximum contraction of the profundus. The athlete presents acutely with swelling and pain of the palmar aspect of the hand, and inability to actively flex the DIP joint of the involved finger.

This injury is classified into three types. In Type 1, the profundus tendon retracts into the palm of the hand, and the patient presents with pain and swelling at the level of the lumbrical muscles. In Type 2, the profundus tendon retracts back to the level of the PIP joint, and is held there by the intact long vinculum. The patient presents with pain and swelling as well as loss of active flexion at the level of the DIP joint. In Type 3, the avulsion of the profundus tendon is associated with a large bony fragment that is held in place by the A-4 pulley. Type 3 presents with pain and swelling over the distal aspect of the middle phalanx. Radiographs of the hand usually show a bony fragment just proximal to the DIP joint. The treatment for this injury is usually surgical, but Type 1 can require early intervention because the tendon retracted to the palm has compromised blood supply.[86]

Ligament injuries   Gamekeeper's thumb is the most common soft tissue injury of the thumb, and is due to rupture of the ulnar collateral ligaments. This injury can occur from a fall on the hand or from trauma associated with excessive thumb abduction and hyperextension. The ligaments can be partially or completely torn. Failure to diagnose this injury can lead to chronic instability. First- and second-degree tears can be treated with immobilization with a short-arm thumb spica cast for 4 weeks. After 2 weeks, the cast can be changed, and if the patient is pain-free a removable splint can be used and range of motion exercises started.

Stress radiographs can help make the diagnosis when the ulnar collateral ligament is completely torn. The radiographs are also helpful in detecting an avulsion fracture. A non-displaced avulsion fracture can be treated with a cast for 4–6 weeks. Operative treatment should be considered if the avulsion fracture is greater than 10–15% of the articular surface, displacement is more than 2–3 mm, or angulation is present.[51]

The most common wrist ligament injury is scapholunate dissociation, which usually results from a fall on the outstretched hand with excessive wrist extension and ulnar deviation. The patient presents with pain and swelling in the dorsal aspect of the wrist. The scaphoid shift maneuver (also known as Watson's test) can be performed by applying dorsal stress to the scaphoid as the wrist is moved from ulnar to radial deviation. Reproduction of the pain and/or hearing a pop constitutes a positive test.[104]

In a severe injury, a separation of 2–3 mm between the scaphoid and the lunate can be seen on posteroanterior radiographs. Less severe injuries with dynamic partial scapholunate dissociations can sometimes be demonstrated on clenched fist or radial–ulnar deviation views.[77]

Treatment of acute static scapholunate ligament dissociation is surgical, with closed reduction and pinning, or with open reduction and repair of the ligament. Acute partial ligament injuries without any of the collapse deformities are best treated in a short-arm thumb spica cast for at least 6 weeks.[130]

Overuse injuries

Dorsal wrist impingement syndromes are common in all sports where repetitive dorsiflexion of the wrist occurs during axial loading. Gymnasts have a high incidence of wrist pain that can be associated with dorsal wrist capsulitis, dorsiflexion impaction syndrome, and distal radius stress reaction or fractures. In addition, ulnar impaction syndrome and triangular fibrocartilage complex damage can occur with repeated pronation and ulnar deviation on the weight-bearing forearm.[100] The patient presents with swelling and tenderness of the distal wrist, and has limited wrist extension and pain with motion. Management includes splinting, rest from weight-bearing activities, NSAIDs, and in some instances local injection.

De Quervain's syndrome results from an overuse of the hand and the wrist. It is a tenosynovitis of the abductor policies longus and the extensor policies brevis that occurs in activities requiring forceful grasp, coupled with radial and ulnar deviation, as well as repetitive use of the thumb. Pain over the radial aspect of the wrist is the most common presenting symptom. The physical examination shows tenderness of the first dorsal compartment of the wrist and reproduction of symptoms with Finkelstein's test. This test is done by having the patient place the thumb inside a fist with the wrist radially deviated. The wrist is then radially deviated, with reproduction of the patient's pain. The treatment for this condition is initially rest, immobilization, and NSAIDs. Physical therapy modalities such as ultrasound and electrical stimulation can also be helpful. If the patient does not improve, a steroid injection in the first dorsal compartment of the wrist can be done. In the rare case in which conservative measures fail, a surgical release of the first dorsal compartment is indicated.

The extensor carpi ulnaris is the second most common site for tenosynovitis in the upper limb. It presents as pain and swelling along the dorsal ulnar aspect of the wrist. It commonly occurs in tennis players due to repetitive twisting and ulnar deviation of the wrist. The initial treatment is NSAIDs and splinting. If this fails, an injection into the area of the tendon sheath usually takes care of the problem. In rare recalcitrant cases, surgical release of the tendon sheath along with repair might have to be performed. Technical factors such as extreme ulnar deviation with the forehand stroke in tennis players needs to be addressed.

Trigger finger is an overuse syndrome of the hand that can be associated with racquet sports because of repeated grasping. Repetitive impact at the level of the metacarpophalangeal joint can cause thickening of the A-1 pulley, resulting in swelling and pressure over the flexor tendon sheath. Initial treatment includes relative rest and NSAIDs. It usually responds to a steroid injection of the flexor tendon sheath under the A-1 pulley. Surgical release of the A-1 pulley is needed in some cases.

Rehabilitation concepts that are important in the management of overuse injuries of the wrist and hand include reduction of swelling, protection and splinting of the injured part in the acute phase, maintenance of range of motion of the uninvolved joints, and recovery of strength prior to returning to activity. Strengthening should be performed in a pain-free manner, isolating the specific joint involved in the initial phases of rehabilitation. Conditioning of the unaffected limb should be maintained throughout the recovery process.

MANAGEMENT OF LOWER LIMB INJURY

Knee injury

Athletes participating in sports activities involving running, jumping, or changing directions often present with traumatic or overuse injuries to the knee. Acute knee injury can result from a contact that induces a valgus stress, such as a tackle in football, non-contact deceleration and change of direction resulting from a cut in basketball, and forced flexion associated with a squat. Overuse injuries can result from repeated activity such as running downhill, jumping, or lifting weights. In our sports medicine clinic, the knee is the most commonly injured anatomic area evaluated.[43]

Traumatic injuries

Anterior cruciate ligament tears   Anterior cruciate ligament injury is very common in sports.[121] It is commonly injured in female athletes participating in high-demand sports such as soccer and basketball.[5] The ACL is a collagenous structure approximately 38 mm in length and 10 mm in width. It arises from a wide base in the tibia anterolateral to the anterior tibial spine. It then traverses the knee in a posterolateral direction, attaching in a broad fan-like fashion at the posterolateral corner of the intercondylar notch of the femur. The ACL is a static stabilizer of the knee, with a primary function of resisting hyperextension and anterior tibial translation in flexion and providing rotatory control. It is also a secondary restraint to valgus and varus forces. Biomechanical studies of the ACL have shown that forces in the ligament are the highest in the last 30° of extension and in hyperextension. ACL forces are also high during anterior tibial translation, internal rotation, and varus.[132]

Anterior cruciate ligament injury usually presents with pain, immediate swelling, and limited range of motion associated with a non-contact injury. The injury usually results from a sudden deceleration during a high-velocity movement, and requires a forceful contraction of the quadriceps muscle. ACL injury has also been described as a result of a valgus stress, hyperextension, and external rotation, such as when landing from a jump. Injury can also occur with severe internal rotation of the knee, or hyperextension with internal rotation. Traumatic injury to the ligament can occur with valgus stress to the knee in combination with injury to the medial collateral ligament and the medial meniscus.[20]

Some patients present with a history of recurrent episodes of knee instability, associated with swelling and limited motion. These patients often give a history of a remote injury to the knee, which was rested and immobilized but not rehabilitated.[88]

The physical examination is usually very sensitive and specific in the diagnosis of ACL tears and other pathologic processes of the knee.[95] The examiner should observe the knee for asymmetry, palpate for areas of tenderness, measure active and passive range of motion, and document muscle atrophy. Special maneuvers such as the apprehension test to rule out patellar subluxation, collateral ligament testing, and flexion–rotation tests such as McMurray's test to rule out meniscal injury should be done. Testing for the integrity of the ACL in the patient with an acute injury should include a Lachman's test. This is done by applying an anterior force to the tibia, with the knee in 30° of flexion, while the examiner tries to reproduce anterior migration of the tibia on the femur. Another important test in the acute setting is the lateral pivot shift maneuver, in which the examiner attempts to reproduce anterolateral rotatory instability by internally rotating the leg and applying a valgus stress to the knee as it is flexed. In the patient with chronic ACL insufficiency, the anterior drawer test, in which an anterior force is applied to the tibia with the knee flexed to 90°, can also be used.

The patient with the non-operated ACL-deficient knee can present with an acute or a recurrent injury. Complaints vary from a swollen, painful knee to a recurrently unstable joint with associated muscle weakness and atrophy.

Protection of secondary structures is of paramount importance in the acutely injured knee. The rate of progression of rehabilitation depends on the extent of damage to other knee structures. Special care should be taken not to stress the knee in terminal extension, because the ACL is stressed in full extension and hyperextension. Early use of closed kinetic chain exercises, in which the distal segment of the limb is fixed and the proximal segments are free to move, allows progression of strengthening to the presumption of reduced shear forces to the knee.[34] These exercises allow quadriceps strengthening with hamstring muscle cocontraction, which theoretically reduces ACL strain and minimizes patellofemoral joint reaction forces.

The individual with a recurrently unstable knee frequently benefits from a trial of rehabilitation. This involves correction of muscle weakness and proprioceptive deficits, and functional retraining in combination with activity modification. This can often reduce the episodes of instability.[88]

Recurrent anterolateral instability is a functionally unacceptable outcome in the athlete who wants to continue in high-level sports that require change of direction and jumping. Athletes with chronic ACL deficiency typically have an increased incidence of meniscal injuries that can lead to early osteoarthritis. Reconstruction of the ligament using the central portion of the patellar ligament or semitendinosus–gracilis tendon grafts has become the treatment of choice for this athletic population.[46,47] The choice of graft depends on several factors, including a history of patellofemoral pain and the preference of the surgeon.

Rehabilitation should begin after reconstructive surgery on the first postoperative day. See Box 45-6 for the key features of the rehabilitation program for the patient with a reconstructed ACL. The early use of cryotherapy, compression, and elevation has been shown to reduce swelling postoperatively. It

Box 45-6 Anterior cruciate ligament injury: key points

Acute phase
- Reduce postoperative swelling.
- Achieve full extension.
- Mobilize patella to reduce scarring.
- Avoid loading the anterior cruciate graft in the last 30° of extension.

Recovery phase
- Obtain full knee range of motion.
- Achieve quadriceps muscle control.
- Strengthen gluteal and core muscles.
- Work on proprioception and balance.
- Integrate functional activities in three planes of motion.

Functional phase
- Strengthen the whole kinetic chain.
- Work on power activities.
- Return to sports-specific training and activity.
- Transition to prehabilitation with proprioception and balance training.

is very important to achieve full passive extension and to initiate early active flexion in the first few days post surgery. Partial weight bearing with crutches is usually started immediately after the operation.[50]

Rapid progression of the rehabilitation program has reduced complications usually associated with ACL surgery, such as stiffness, muscle weakness and atrophy, and patellofemoral pain.[7] Early in the rehabilitation, it is important to avoid excessive strain of the reconstructed ligament with terminal (0–30°) extension open kinetic chain resisted quadriceps exercises. Open kinetic chain exercises can be safely used in the 90–45° range at this stage. Use of closed kinetic chain exercises such as minisquats, steps, and lunges causes quadriceps strengthening with tolerable shear forces to the graft. Aquatic exercises that allow progressive weight bearing while benefiting from the effects of buoyancy can be started as soon as the sutures are removed.

Individuals vary in the rate they can achieve full range of motion, normal strength, normal proprioception, and adequate sports-specific skills. Achievement of these goals should be accomplished prior to allowing the individual to return to sports activity. Although some programs have reported very early return to activity following reconstruction, the majority of accelerated rehabilitation programs lead to return to competitive sports 6 months after surgery.[21]

Prevention of ACL injury has become very important for athletes participating in basketball, handball, and soccer. Neuromuscular training has been shown to reduce the incidence of ACL injury in female athletes, and has been incorporated as a prehabilitation strategy in this population.[58,61,91]

Meniscal tears The menisci serve as shock absorbers, decrease load concentrations, and help guide normal knee kinematics. As much as 50% of the compressive load across the knee is transmitted through the menisci, and this increases during flexion. Any injury to the menisci reduces the weight contact area of the knee, placing the articular cartilage at risk for failure or degenerative changes.[97] Common causes of injury include acute macrotrauma following hyperflexion or twisting, and chronic microtrauma due to running or jumping. Meniscus cartilage is subject to the aging process, and can tear by shear failure in the older runner without acute trauma.

Symptoms of meniscal tears include pain with activity or mechanical symptoms of catching, grinding, locking, and slight swelling. Clinical signs include joint line tenderness, and pain on hyperflexion or hyperextension.

Many patients with a small meniscal tear improve with a trial of rehabilitation for 4–6 weeks that includes ice, NSAIDs, reductions of weight-bearing activity, and strengthening. Surgical consultation is recommended in refractory cases, if the patient continues to have mechanical symptoms and swelling with sports activity. The surgical options include meniscal repair of a peripheral tear, or partial meniscectomy. In the young athlete, repair of the meniscus is the preferred option if clinically possible. Meniscectomy and debridement are often the only alternatives in the older athlete.[28]

Rehabilitation after meniscal surgery has progressed in recent years. Accelerated rehabilitation programs that allow early weight bearing and progressive range of motion have replaced more conservative protocols in which the patient was maintained on non-weight bearing and limited in range of motion post surgery.[112] Special precautions, however, should be taken with extreme flexion and rotation, and axial loading in the postoperative period. The patient with meniscal repair and an ACL-deficient knee needs to be counseled about the possibility of recurrent instability and failure of the meniscal repair.

Overuse injuries

Patellofemoral pain syndrome Overuse injuries of the extensor mechanism of the knee are very common in sports. The athlete with patellofemoral pain syndrome usually presents with pain associated with activity such as running down hills, climbing stairs, or jumping. Female or young athletes can present with painful patellar instability.

Anterior knee pain is very common in runners and jumpers, and can be secondary to more than one pathologic process. The pain generators in extensor mechanism disorders include the subchondral bone of the patella, synovial capsular and retinacular soft tissues, and tendon insertions on the patella. The resulting pain can be associated with stimulation of free nerve endings, secretion of inflammatory mediators, and abnormal transmission of forces through the cartilage to the subchondral bone.[10]

Biomechanical abnormalities associated with anterior knee pain can include increased femoral internal rotation; tight structures including the hip flexors, hamstrings, iliotibial band, and Achilles tendon; and increased foot pronation. Quadriceps muscle weakness can also be associated with patellar pain.[39]

Symptoms include dull, aching retropatellar or peripatellar pain of insidious onset. It typically worsens with activities in knee flexion, such as squatting, sitting for prolonged periods (theater sign), descending stairs, or running hills. The physical examination usually shows patellar crepitus, pain with patellar compression or quadriceps contraction, and quadriceps muscle atrophy. Tightness of the hip flexors and hamstrings is also frequently found. In the patients with coexisting patellar instability, apprehension can be identified in addition to pain over the superior lateral facet. Proximal muscle weakness can also be present, as evidenced by the patient having difficulty with single-leg stance and eccentric muscle control.

Acute treatment of the patellofemoral pain syndrome includes modified rest, ice, and NSAIDs. Stretching the iliotibial band and strengthening the quadriceps with both open and closed chain exercises should be instituted early, in combination with cross-training strategies. In some patients, closed chain exercises are the preferred mode of strength training because of reduced patellofemoral joint stress. Other important considerations include gluteal strengthening to reduce femoral internal rotation with weight-bearing activities, and strengthening the ankle muscles in combination with heel cord stretching to manage hyperpronation. These help control patellofemoral forces across the knee.[39]

Patellar taping such as that described by McConnel can be used in the early stages of training with good clinical results.[80] Taping is typically done in a manner that forces the patella to track more medially. Other interventions include neoprene knee sleeves or other patellofemoral orthoses that attempt to control patellar laxity to promote proper patellar tracking. Shoe orthoses to control hyperpronation can also be helpful.

Arthroscopic surgery is rarely indicated in the patient with patellofemoral pain, and should be used judiciously when approaching this problem. In patients with lateral pressure syndrome, an arthroscopic lateral release can relieve patellar tilt.[98]

Leg and foot injuries Leg and foot injuries are common occurrences, especially in athletes who participate in sports that emphasize repetitive lower limb activity, such as track and field, jogging, and soccer. Athletes who compete in martial arts, such as karate and tae kwon do, can present with traumatic injuries to the leg and foot as well. In our practice, leg, ankle, and foot injuries represent close to 20% of the cases evaluated in our sports medicine clinics.[43]

Ankle sprains Acute ankle sprains are a very common cause of lost playing time and disability among athletes. Although they are considered by many to be benign injuries, many athletes present with recurrent sprains, functional instability, and inability to return to their sport at the previous level of performance.[4]

Stability of the ankle depends on its bony architecture, static effects of the ligaments, and dynamic effects of muscles. The lateral ligamentous complex consists of the anterior talofibular (ATFL), calcaneofibular (CFL), posterior talofibular, and lateral talocalcaneal ligaments. The ATFL is the weakest of the lateral ankle ligaments and the one most commonly injured. The CFL is the second weakest ligament and crosses both the tibiotalar and the subtalar joints, both of which can be involved in an acute ankle sprain.[29]

The most common mechanism of injury to the lateral ankle ligaments occurs from a forced plantar flexion and inversion of the ankle, with the body's center of gravity rolling over the ankle. The sequence of ligament tears in an inversion injury is first the ATFL, followed by the anterolateral capsule, and finally the distal tibiofibular ligament. Progressive inversion strains also result in a CFL tear.[108]

The patient complains of acute lateral ankle pain that is usually accompanied by swelling, difficulty with weight bearing, and ecchymosis. The physical examination shows diffuse swelling, tenderness over the lateral ligament complex, pain with inversion, and in many instances peroneal muscle weakness. Palpation of bony structures such as the posterior malleoli, the fifth metatarsal, and the navicular should be performed to rule out associated fractures. The anterior drawer test stresses the ATFL and should be performed to document ligamentous laxity. The talar tilt test evaluates the CFL in inversion but can be somewhat limited in the acute stage by pain.

Management of the acute stage emphasizes reduction of ankle effusion and pain, as well as protection of the lateral ligament complex. Ice, NSAIDs, elevation, taping, or wrapping with lateral felt pads can be useful in the early stages of recovery. Physical therapy emphasizing movement in a pain-free range of motion can be combined with the use of functional stirrup braces and early weight bearing.

In the recovery phase, static and dynamic exercises for strengthening are started, but inversion stress to the ankle should be avoided. Gentle stretching of the Achilles tendon is done to avoid a plantar flexion contracture. Electrical stimulation combined with ultrasound can aid in reduction of pain and inflammation. Proprioceptive training instituted early in the rehabilitation process reduces the risk of functional instability following the injury. Ankle board training and gradual closed chain exercises can be instituted in this stage of rehabilitation.[109]

The functional rehabilitation phase emphasizes dynamic strengthening of the ankle muscles. Balance and proprioception training is done that includes exercises on stable surfaces that gradually progress to unstable surfaces. The goal at this stage is to normalize the strength of the whole lower limb, transition to sports activity, and prevent dynamic instability. The use of ankle bracing during athletic activity should be considered for up to 6 months following an injury to the ankle.[54]

The timing of allowing the athlete to return to activity varies depending on the severity of the sprain. Athletes with grade 1 sprains usually return to play in 1–2 weeks, but those with grade 2 sprains can be out of competition for up to 6 weeks. Athletes with grade 3 sprains can take several months to return to their sports.

The role of proprioceptive balance board training for the prevention of ankle sprains has been studied by Verhagen.[123] He demonstrated that significantly fewer ankle sprains developed in volleyball players who followed a prescribed balance board training program, when compared with control subjects who followed the normal team training routine. This type of proprioceptive training should be integrated into the prehabilitation program, and is recommended for all athletes who participate in running or jumping sports.

Medial tibial stress syndrome Medial tibial stress syndrome (MTSS), also known as shin splints, is a common example of an overuse injury seen in running sports. Although runners are most commonly afflicted, individuals involved in jumping activities such as basketball, volleyball, or track and field can also develop MTSS. Although the exact anatomic changes that cause MTSS have been debated, most experts agree that there is an inflammatory process at the periosteum of the tibia, caused by overuse and by biomechanical abnormalities. Recent information has pointed to the fascial insertion of the medial soleus muscles into the tibia as the possible cause of the pain symptoms. Biomechanical factors that can be associated with the syndrome include excessive foot pronation, loss of leg flexibility, and limited ankle range of motion.[72]

The clinical presentation is pain associated with activity, which initially improves with warm up but recurs at the end of the workout. Commonly, symptoms arise when athletes are beginning a training program or when abruptly increasing the intensity of their training. The physical examination shows diffuse tenderness over the posteromedial aspect of the distal third of the tibia, with occasional localized edema in the region. Initial x-rays are usually negative, and the diagnosis can be confirmed with the aid of a three-phase bone scan that reveals patchy areas of increased uptake along the medial border of the tibia.[15] In chronic cases, there can be periosteal thickening on plain radiographs, and a bone scan can be helpful to rule out a tibial stress fracture.

The initial treatment of this condition includes relative rest with cross-training, ice, NSAIDs, and gentle stretching of the gastrocnemius and soleus. Other therapeutic modalities, such as iontophoresis and ultrasound, can be useful adjuncts in the rehabilitation of MTSS.[129] As symptoms begin to subside, a gradual return to activities is recommended, but with a decrease in training intensity, and running on soft, flat surfaces. Additional measures include flexibility exercises for the entire lower limb, strengthening of the whole kinetic chain, and cross-training activities to maintain cardiovascular conditioning. Management of foot pronation might include the use of motion control shoes with a straight last, and/or the prescription of shoe orthoses.

Stress fractures Stress fractures are very common injuries, and the site of the stress fractures varies from sport to sport. In a series of 196 stress fractures, Iwamoto found that basketball players predominantly sustained stress fractures of the tibial shaft, medial malleolus, and metatarsal bones.[63] Tennis and volleyball players predominantly had fractures of the tibial shaft.[63] Stress fractures are overuse injuries to bone, which is a dynamic tissue that is constantly remodeling when exposed to repetitive stress. Stress injury occurs when bone breakdown exceeds bone remodeling. Stress to bone can range from a simple stress reaction to edema, to a stress fracture that can progress to a complete fracture. The diagnosis and treatment of these fractures depends on their location and potential for spontaneous healing. Fractures that are low risk with good potential for healing include those of the posteromedial tibial cortex, fibula, and metatarsal shaft. Higher risk fractures with a lower potential for healing include those of the anterior cortex of the tibia, the base of the fifth metatarsal, and the tarsal navicular.[59]

Clinically, this injury presents with a gradual increase in activity-related pain that is aggravated by repetitive loading of the lower limb and improved by rest. Physical examination shows localized discrete tenderness that reproduces the symptoms of pain. Minimal soft tissue swelling is often present as well. Maneuvers that reproduce the pain symptoms, such as hopping on one leg or jumping, can also aid in making the diagnoses.

X-rays are usually negative for the first 2–4 weeks following the stress fracture. If the clinical picture is highly suspicious for stress fracture, then a bone scan or an MRI should be considered. Bone scan and MRI are both sensitive and specific examinations for the diagnosis of stress fractures. MRI provides anatomic information about the surrounding structures, and can be superior to bone scan for following up the healing fracture.[59] Bone scan usually reveals a focal increase in uptake at the site of the fracture, but can remain positive for 1–2 years following the fracture. MRI is more expensive but can reveal the fracture line and the degrees of subsequent healing.

Treatment during the acute phases consists of relative rest, ice, and NSAIDs. High-risk stress fractures such as those of the fifth metatarsal or navicular can require non-weight bearing, casting, and in some instances surgery. Low-risk stress fractures such as the tibial shaft and metatarsals can be treated with functional activity progression. To maintain cardiovascular fitness, cross-training with the bicycle or in the pool is recommended. When the patient is asymptomatic at rest, a program of progressive return to running should be instituted. Initially, runs are allowed on even, soft surfaces and progression is allowed weekly provided that no symptoms recur.

Achilles tendonitis   The Achilles tendon is the largest and strongest tendon in the body, and during sports activities is under large tensile loads that can result in injury. Achilles tendon disorders are very common in sports, particularly in running sports. There is a 7–9% annual incidence of Achilles tendon disorders reported in elite runners.[129] Constant repetitive exercise eventually leads to progressive degenerative changes at the tissue level.

The terminology describing tendon injury has been modified in recent years. Although the term *tendonitis* is often used in clinical practice to depict tendon injury, inflammatory cells are infrequently seen in biopsy specimens of injured tendons. The term *tendonosis* should be used in the majority of individuals to describe the Achilles tendon injury, because the most common pathologic finding is intratendonous degeneration without inflammation. In the athlete with acute symptoms, the Achilles tendon develops acute edema and inflammation in the paratenon. Chronic Achilles tendon symptomatology usually includes thickening of the tendon, and localized tenderness with palpation. There is limited sports-specific performance that results from these degenerative changes that are referred to as tendinopathy.[114]

Achilles tendon injuries frequently affect mature male athletes who are active in running and jumping activities. The typical history is one of gradual onset of pain that worsens with activity, associated with changes in intensity of the exercise, running surfaces, or footwear. Physical examination shows tenderness to palpation of the Achilles tendon 2–6 cm from its insertion, inflexibility of the ankle dorsiflexors, and weakness of the ankle plantar flexors.

Conservative treatment for Achilles tendonitis includes relative rest, as well as physical modalities and exercises that address the biomechanical deficits. Exercise prescription for tendinopathy has a bias toward eccentric exercises,[25] and eccentric programs for stretching and strengthening the gastrocnemius muscle have been developed. One exercise that is very important in the rehabilitation of these disorders is the heel drop. This exercise is performed standing on a bench, and the individual allows the heel to drop eccentrically with the knee extended, and subsequently returns the foot to a neutral position.[114] As symptoms improve, the rehabilitation program should progress to include fast eccentric exercises, adding concentric gastrocnemius strengthening, and functional dynamic exercises such as lunges and squats. A gradual running and jumping program can be started when the patient is asymptomatic at rest. A heel lift used in the initial stages can relieve pain by reducing tensile loading, but long-term use can perpetuate the inflexibility.

Achilles rupture   Degenerative changes in the Achilles tendon associated with poor tendon vascularity can lead to an Achilles tendon rupture. The mechanisms of rupture include forefoot push-off with the knee in extension, sudden unexpected dorsiflexion of the ankle resulting from a fall in a hole, and arising following violent dorsiflexion of the plantar-flexed foot when falling from a jump.[79] Clinically, the patient presents with pain and a history of hearing an audible snap when falling from a jump or starting to sprint. In many instances, the patients are unable to walk or bear weight. A high level of suspicion is required not to miss the diagnosis, because some patients are able to plantar flex the foot using other muscles.

On physical examination, there is a palpable defect proximal to the tendon insertion. Significant swelling can be present, making the examination difficult. The patient can plantar flex the foot but cannot perform a toe raise. Thompson's test, which evaluates the integrity of the tendon, can be performed by squeezing the posterior calf in the prone position and observing passive plantar flexion. This test can be falsely negative, because the intact plantaris muscle can plantar flex the ankle when the calf is squeezed.

In the case of a complete tear, non-surgical management with casting and functional bracing can be used. This treatment, however, carries a higher risk of rerupture and should be reserved for patients who are not interested in high levels of activity. Open surgical repair of the Achilles tendon can restore the anatomy and allow transition to early rehabilitation. Recently, shorter immobilization periods and the use of functional bracing has gained popularity, with an earlier recovery of range of motion.[79]

Plantar fasciitis   Plantar fasciitis is the most common cause of heel pain and affects 15–20% of runners.[40] The plantar fascia is a tough, fibrous, aponeurotic structure arising from the medial calcaneal tubercle and inserting into the plantar plates of the metatarsophalangeal joints, the bases of the proximal phalanges of the toes, and the flexor tendon sheaths. It provides shape and support to the longitudinal arch and acts as a shock absorber on foot impact.

Plantar fasciitis is an overload injury usually associated with biomechanical abnormalities. Tight plantar flexors and short foot flexor muscles, as well as weakness of posterior calf muscles, can be associated with increased pronation, and these factors can cause an increased load in the plantar fascia insertion. Other biomechanical abnormalities of the lower limb, such as hip abductor weakness, external rotation of the leg, and supinated high arch feet, can also be factors.[113]

Patients usually complain of heel pain on first arising in the morning that decreases during the day and then worsens with increased activity. Commonly, this is not associated with trauma and presents insidiously. It can be diffuse initially, but over time it localizes to the medial calcaneus. Patients often relate the onset of symptoms to a rapid increase in distance, speed, intensity, or frequency of running. Other factors can include changing to a flexible shoe having minimal rear foot control.

The diagnosis is based mainly on the history and physical examination. The patient presents with tenderness with palpation over the medial calcaneal tubercle and, in more advanced cases, over the proximal medial longitudinal arch. Slight swelling in the area and Achilles tendon tightness are present in most patients. Other findings on the examination can include pronated and everted foot, supinated foot, tightness of the hamstrings, and weakness of the leg and intrinsic foot muscles.

Treatment is initially directed to relieve pain, and includes NSAIDs and icing to the affected area. Heel pads and arch supports to maintain the longitudinal arch during ambulation can aid in symptom management.

Rehabilitation includes an exercise program to correct the biomechanical deficits. Stretching of plantar flexors, hamstrings, and plantar fascia should be combined with strengthening of short foot flexors and plantar flexors.

Localized steroid and anesthetic injection can provide initial pain relief, but superficial injections that cause fat pad atrophy should be avoided. The use of night splints, or in severe cases casting, can reduce pain. Surgery should be considered only if the pain has not responded to appropriate conservative treatment for 6–12 months. The athlete can return to activity when pain is absent and the biomechanical deficits have been corrected.

BACK INJURY

The patterns of back injury (also see Chs 17, 41, and 42) differ in child and adolescent athletes and adults.[3] Young athletes involved in sports that require trunk rotation and hyperextension usually present with posterior elements injury. Repeated stresses associated with gymnastics, diving, and wrestling places the athlete at increased risk of pars interarticularis injury such as spondylolysis.[60] These athletes can present with acute or gradual onset of pain and limited motion that restricts activity.

Older athletes can present with injuries to the anterior elements of the spine, including the vertebral end plate and the intervertebral disks.[133] These individuals usually present with symptoms associated with trunk flexion and rotation. They can present with episodes of axial back pain and limited motion followed by episodes of sciatica.

Repeated exposure to rotational activities can lead to progressive degenerative disk and facet joint disease associated with spinal stenosis. These athletes can present with leg pain, weakness, or numbness associated with activity that improves with sitting or trunk flexion.

The physical examination shows limited back motion, with a lateral trunk list that can be associated with an annulus fibrosus tear or with muscle–ligament injury. Flexibility testing of the hip rotators, flexors, and hamstring muscles should be performed. Neurologic examination should address areas of sensory loss, abnormal muscle stretch reflexes, and focal muscle weakness. Special tests to identify abnormal neural tension and reproduce leg symptoms, such as the straight leg-raising maneuver; the slump test, in which the sitting patient's knee is extended after flexion of the cervical spine; or the femoral stress test, in which the hip is extended while flexing the knee, should be performed.

The direction of motion that worsens the patient's pain should be identified. Increased pain with flexion and rotation is usually associated with diskogenic injury, while pain with extension and rotation is usually associated with posterior element injury. A useful test in the patient with suspected spondylosis is the one-legged hyperextension maneuver, on which the patient extends the lumbar spine while standing in one leg, reproducing the patient's ipsilateral symptoms.[48] The other factors that should be identified include inflexibility of the hip and hamstring muscles, and weakness of the core muscles, as well as abnormalities in balance. Rehabilitation of the athlete with a back injury should start as soon as the injury occurs. Key points in the rehabilitation of back injury are shown in Box 45-7. During the acute phase, the focus is on reducing pain and protecting injured or inflamed tissue. Bed rest should be kept to less than 3 days for non-radicular low back pain. It is not clear what the optimal bed rest period is for patients with radicular pain, but patients should be mobilized as soon as they tolerate it.[56]

In the initial phase of treatment, modalities such as ice and electrical stimulation can be used in combination with isometric exercises. Identification of the neutral spine position of comfort,

---

Box 45-7 Rehabilitation of back injury: key points

Acute phase
- Limit bed rest to 2–3 days.
- Identify direction of pain exacerbation.
- Identify neutral spine position.
- Initiate recruitment of core muscles.

Recovery phase
- Exercise in the direction that reduces or centralizes pain.
- Work on trunk stabilization.
- Strengthen the core muscles in three planes of motion.
- Integrate sports-specific training.

Functional phase
- Advance dynamic flexibility program.
- Continue advanced core strengthening.
- Return to activity to correct sports-specific technique.
- Emphasize correct spine mechanics in sport activity.

---

and education about proper spine biomechanics, should be done at this stage. Isometric and static exercises should be initiated to retrain proper muscle firing patterns in patients with muscle inhibition and abnormal firing patterns. Light aerobic exercise that does not exacerbate the pain can also be included in the treatment program. Analgesics and NSAIDS that facilitate participation in the rehabilitation program should also be used.

In the recovery phase of treatment, flexion- or extension-biased exercise should be used, depending on the direction that exacerbates the symptoms. Patients with sciatica secondary to diskogenic disease can benefit from extension exercises, while patients with facet syndrome or spondylolysis benefit from flexion exercises.[30] Superficial heat, electrical stimulation, and in some cases ultrasound can be used as part of the treatment program. Back stabilization exercises in the neutral spine position are used to strengthen the back and pelvic core musculature. The muscles that are targeted for exercise training include the multifidi, quadratus lumborum, abdominals, and hip girdle muscles.[2,81] Dynamic flexibility training in sagittal, frontal, and transverse planes of motion should be started gradually as the core strength improves. As the patient's pain improves, specific inflexibilities of the hip flexors, rotators, and hamstrings, as well as muscle imbalances, are addressed. An aerobic and conditioning program is progressed as tolerated during this phase.

In the maintenance treatment phase, the progression of trunk strengthening is emphasized. Exercises with gym balls, rotational patterns, and eccentric loading of the spine are done. Normal spine mechanics for sports activities and progression of sports-specific training are required prior to allowing the athlete to return to competition.

Consideration should be given to the use of spinal bracing in patients with spondylolysis who do not respond to treatment. The use of epidural steroids and other injection techniques can be considered in patients who have a radiculopathy severe enough to inhibit them from participation in the rehabilitation program.

Surgery can be required in the rare case of failure of conservative treatment for diskogenic pain. Return to play after surgical treatment is variable, but aggressive rehabilitation frequently allows a rapid return to competition. Patients with percutaneous diskectomy or microdiskectomy can return to sports activities several months after their injury; however, patients having a surgical spinal fusion typically take up to a year to return to non-contact sports.[32]

Prevention of low back pain is very important for the athlete, because a history of previous symptoms statistically predisposes to recurrent injury.[52] Hip muscle imbalance has been considered as one of the predisposing factors for back pain, and core strengthening programs for the correction of these imbalances show promise as a prehabilitation strategy.[92]

MANAGEMENT OF HEAD AND CERVICAL SPINE INJURIES

The physician covering athletic events, particularly contact sports, needs to be prepared to deal with the athlete who presents with head or neck injuries. These injuries can result in significant morbidity, and rarely even in mortality. Proper management requires planning ahead by the sports medicine team prior to the event.

Head injuries occur more commonly than spine injuries in athletes. Head injuries occur at a rate of 132–367 cases per 100 000 people per year, with sports activities accounting for approximately 14% of these injuries.[49] It has been estimated that 5–10% of the 10 000 cervical injuries occurring in the USA every year result from sports activity. The sports having the highest risk of cervical injuries include American football, wrestling, gymnastics, and diving.[70] A recent review of the causes of fatalities in American football from 1945 to 1999 showed that 69% of the deaths were associated with brain injury and 16% with cervical spine injuries.[18]

Head injuries (also see Ch. 50)
Recognition of a severe head injury is relatively easy, especially if the athlete has had a complete loss of consciousness. However, mild head injuries are much more frequent in contact collision sports. In mild head injuries, there is no loss of consciousness, but rather a transient loss of alertness or a brief period of post-traumatic amnesia that can be difficult to recognize. More than 90% of all cerebral concussions fall into this mild category.[19]

The majority of these mild traumatic brain injuries result in a transient neurologic syndrome without structural damage to the brain. Concussion is defined as a clinical syndrome having the immediate and transient posttraumatic impairment of neural function, such as alteration of consciousness, disturbance of vision, or disturbance of equilibrium due to brain stem involvement.[64]

Signs and symptoms of concussion include amnesia, loss of consciousness, headache, dizziness, blurred vision, attention deficit, and nausea. There is also a wide variety of other complaints that can be encountered in concussed athletes. These include descriptions of vacant stare, irritability, emotional liability, impaired coordination, sleep disturbance, noise or light intolerance, lethargy, behavioral disturbance, and altered sense of taste or smell.[120] The time required for resolution of these signs and symptoms is extremely variable.

In assessing an athlete with a head injury who is conscious, the level of consciousness or alertness is the most sensitive criteria for both establishing the nature of the head injury and subsequently treating the athlete. Orientation to person, place, and time should be ascertained, as well as the presence or absence of posttraumatic amnesia. The physician should gauge the athlete's ability to retain new information, such as the ability to repeat words immediately or after 15 min, as well as the ability to repeat one's assignments on certain plays in the contest (see Box 45-8).[53] It is also important to do a complete neurologic examination and to establish the presence and severity of neurologic symptoms such as headache, lightheadedness, difficulty with balance, incoordination, and deficits in sensory or motor function.

The severity of the injury can be classified based on the presence or absence of loss of consciousness and posttraumatic amnesia. Multiple classification scales exist that attempt to establish the severity of concussion. Examples of scales of severity classifying the injuries into mild, moderate, and severe categories are shown in Table 45-1.[18]

Sequelae to mild traumatic brain injury include irreversible cognitive deficits, and death due to second impact syndrome. Return to play before the brain recovers from an injury can lead to either of these serious complications, although prolonged cognitive deficits can be seen after a single initial insult. Postconcussion syndrome is a less serious, yet potentially debilitating result of a concussion. Postconcussion syndrome involves prolonged, disabling, and sometimes permanent symptoms such as headache, dizziness, nausea, tinnitus, depression, irritability, slowed mental processing, impaired attention, and deficits in memory.

After a diagnosis of concussion has been made, there are many factors that can influence the return to play decision. These include injury severity, past history of the athlete, demands of the chosen sport, the presence of postconcussive symptoms, and the speed of resolution of the acute symptoms. While scientifically validated return to play guidelines do not yet exist, the consensus of experts in this field suggests that complete resolution of concussion symptoms (both at rest and during exercise) is mandatory prior to the resumption of training or playing. The use of neuropsychologic testing can also be considered in the return to play decision making, particularly in the case where baseline test values were established prior to the injury. An example of guidelines to return to competition after concussion endorsed by the American College Sports of Medicine is seen in Table 45-2.[19]

It is important to keep in mind that the risk of recurrent concussions is greater for individuals who have a history of previous concussion.[55,135] Younger athletes also appear to be at risk for a more protracted recovery from concussion.[38]

Box 45-8 Sideline tests of memory

- Immediate recall of three words
- Recall of three words after 15 min
- Recent memory items (game score, period or quarter, who scored last or who won, describe last play, field location)
- Months in reverse order
- Orientation (name, date of birth, age, year)

(After Grindel et al. 2001,[53] with permission.)

Table 45-1 Severity of concussion

Grade	Cantu (1986)	Colorado (1991)	American Medical Society for Sports Medicine
Mild	No LOC PTA <30 min Confusion	No LOC No PTA	No LOC Symptoms <5 min
Moderate	LOC <5 min PTA >30 min Symptoms 5 min to 24 h Confusion	No LOC PTA	LOC <1 min
Severe	LOC >5 min PTA >24 h Symptoms >24 h	LOC	LOC >1 min

LOC, loss of consciousness; PTA, posttraumatic amnesia.
(After Johnston et al. 2001,[64] with permission.)

Table 45-2 Guidelines for return to play after concussion

Grade	First concussion	Second concussion	Third concussion
1 (mild)	Return if symptom-free for 1 week	Return in 2 weeks if symptom-free for 1 week	Terminate season; return next season if symptom-free
2 (moderate)	Return if symptom-free for 1 week	Return in 1 month if symptom-free for 1 week; consider terminating season	Terminate season; return next season if symptom-free
3 (severe)	After 1 month, return if symptom-free for 1 week	Terminate season; return next season if symptom-free	–

(From Cantu 1996,[19] with permission of Williams & Wilkins.)

Rare but severe brain injury associated with sports includes second-impact syndrome or malignant brain edema, hematomas, and intracranial hemorrhages. The second-impact syndrome occurs when an athlete is still symptomatic from an initial head injury and sustains a second head injury. Usually within seconds to minutes of the second impact, the initially conscious but stunned athlete precipitously collapses, with rapidly dilating pupils, loss of eye movement, and evidence of respiratory failure. The management of severe brain injury in an athlete who has collapsed includes protection of the cervical spine, cardiopulmonary resuscitation, and prompt transportation to a medical facility having the capability of performing computed tomography or MRI of the brain.[49]

Cervical spine injuries

Cervical spine injuries (see also Ch. 56) usually result when the accelerating head and neck strike a stationary object. This is typically associated with axial loading of the flexed cervical spine, seen with tackling in football or hitting the ground with the vertex of the head in contact sports. The cervical injury can range in severity from sprain or strain to cervical spinal cord injury with resultant tetraplegia. Management of the injury depends on the severity of the trauma and the findings on the physical examination.

The sports medicine team should be prepared to deal with a cervical spine emergency during practice or competition. This includes practice on how to treat a football player who receives trauma to the cervical spine while wearing a helmet. In this situation, special precautions need to be taken to protect the cervical spine. Physicians and emergency personnel should only remove the helmet if it does not hold the head securely during immobilization or transportation, or the helmet does not allow appropriate ventilation, or the face mask cannot be removed. If helmet removal is indicated, both the helmet and the shoulder pads should be removed simultaneously, while protecting the cervical spine.[49,125]

Sports-related tetraplegia is the most dreaded complication that can result from spinal cord injury. Incorrect tackling techniques in which the head is used as a spear to make initial contact with the opponent can lead to this injury. A reduction of spinal cord injury in American football has resulted from a prohibition of this tackling method, and educating coaches and athletes on the consequences of tackling the opponent with a flexed cervical spine. Management of tetraplegia includes assessment of the airway, breathing, and circulation as well as protection from further damage to the spinal cord. The athlete should be transported to the hospital for radiologic evaluation and emergency management. Methylprednisolone can be used for the management of acute tetraplegia and administered intravenously at a dose of 30 mg/kg, followed by an infusion of 5.4 mg/kg per h for 24–48 h.[70]

Athletes with cervical cord neurapraxia and temporary loss of strength or sensation merit special attention. The decision regarding returning to play following a reversible spinal injury is a challenging and controversial one.[90] Athletes with a history of transient cervical cord neurapraxia, who have a normal neurologic examination and normal imaging studies, as well as normal cervical strength and range of motion, are permitted by some clinicians to return to sports.[120] Others counsel the athletes against returning to sports following this injury.[19,35] The athlete with spinal stenosis documented by MRI (or spear tackler's spine), in which there is loss of cervical lordosis documented by x-rays, should be advised about the possibility of irreversible neurologic injury when returning to contact sports and should be excluded from participation.[35]

A burner or stinger is a transient neurologic event characterized by pain and paresthesias in a single upper limb following a blow to the neck or shoulder. The players present with tingling or burning sensations, and numbness of the involved limb. One mechanism of injury seen in young American football players is depression of the shoulder accompanied by lateral flexion of the neck in the opposite direction. This causes traction to the upper branches of the brachial plexus. The other mechanism is rotation and extension of the neck toward the ipsilateral shoulder, affecting the cervical roots by compression in the neural foramina. Stinger is usually reversible, but some athletes have recurrent symptoms that require protective equipment, and improvement in technique and cervical muscle strength. Return to play should only be permitted when the athlete has a normal examination, including range of motion and strength of the upper limb and cervical spine.

The athlete with a soft tissue injury to the cervical region should be evaluated to rule out neurologic injury. Once a neurologic injury has been ruled out, the management includes NSAIDs, therapeutic modalities, and a stretching and strengthening program. Postural abnormalities that need to be corrected typically include forward head with tight pectoral muscles, increased thoracic kyphosis, scapular protraction, and hypermobility of the cervical spine.[126] Strengthening of the scapular stabilizers, shoulder girdle, and cervical muscles is very important, because weakness of these can predispose the athlete to recurrent injury.

SPECIAL ISSUES IN SPORTS MEDICINE

Older athletes (see also Ch. 60)

With improvement in medical care, there has been a significant increase in the aging population that is participating in exercise and competitive sports. This trend is accelerating, and by 2030 approximately 20% of Americans will be elderly. The elderly can be divided into three categories: the young old, that correspond to ages 65–74; the old, that correspond to ages 75–85; and the old old, that correspond to those older than 85. Between 1960 and 1980, the population of the old increased by 140%. It is anticipated that the number of old old in the US will grow from 4 million to 13 million by 2040.[101]

Structured physical activity in the form of regular exercise appears to have a significant role in preventing and reversing some of the changes typically associated with age (Table 45-3). Regular exercise benefits older adults through improved overall health and physical fitness, increased opportunities for social contacts, gains in cerebral function, lower rates of mortality, and fewer years of disability in later life (see Chs 19 and 34). Walking and to some extent running are forms of regular exercise that can be performed throughout life and result in physiologic as well as functional benefits, that in turn improve the quality of life of the elderly.[26]

The older athlete, however, can be at a higher risk of injury. This is due to a number of factors, including prior joint injuries, loss of flexibility, and strength deficits associated with the aging process.[119] It is important for the practitioner treating older athletes to consider the demands of the sport in which they participate, the physiologic changes seen in the elderly, their response to a sports-specific training program, and the treatment of specific injuries in this patient population.

An important issue in the older athlete is the relationship of exercise and osteoarthritis. Available information about the effects of sports on the synovial joint and the development of osteoarthritis are not conclusive and sometimes contradictory. A systematic review of randomized clinical trials, published by Van Baar et al. in 1999, found exercise therapy benefits in pain control, self-reported disability, walking performance, and patient's global assessment.[122] Controlled studies of running in dogs have shown an increase in cartilage thickness, proteoglycan content, and indentation stiffness with moderate running after

Table 45-3 Physiologic changes associated with typical aging and exercise

Physiologic variable	Aging	Exercise
Cardiovascular		
$\dot{V}O_2$ maximum	↓	↑
Maximum heart rate	↓	No changes
Maximum stroke volume	↓	↑
A–V O_2 difference	↓	↑
Neuromuscular changes		
Muscle strength	↓	↑
Type 1 fibers	↑	↑
Type 2 fibers	↓	↑
No. of fibers	↓	No changes
Fiber size	↓	↑
Muscle fiber area	↓	↑
Muscle oxidative capacity	↓	↑
Motor unit function	↓	↑
Bone and connective tissue changes		
Tensile strength	↓	↑
Bone resorption	↑	↓
Bone mass	↓	↑
Stiffness	↑	↓

(After Pu and Nelson 1999,[101] with permission of Human Kinetics.)

40 weeks. With more strenuous running, the cartilage and proteoglycan content decreased, but the animals did not develop joint degeneration.[71] Buckwalter reviewed some of the clinical studies in humans, and concluded that lifelong jogging or moderate low-impact running does not appear to increase the risk for development of osteoarthritis in people with normal strength and joints, but appears to lead to an increased risk of developing marginal osteophytes not associated with articular cartilage degeneration.[16] On the other hand, there appears to be an increased risk of lower limb osteoarthritis in participants of repetitive, high-impact sports, and this is strongly associated with a history of joint injury.[24]

Many of the patients with osteoarthritis eventually benefit from arthroplasty to improve function, decrease pain symptoms, and allow the return to sports after joint replacements. Visuri et al. found that recreational exercises increase after total hip replacement, with walking increasing from 2% to 55% and cycling from 7% to 29%.[124] Bradbury et al. found that 65% of patients who participated in sports previously returned to doing exercise after total knee replacement.[12] The majority of patients return to low-impact sports such as golf and bowling. Patients who did not participate in sports preoperatively are less likely to begin sports after surgery.

There is still debate about the long-term effect of sports activity on prosthesis wear, loosening, and revision rates. It appears that light exercise has no deleterious effect on replaced hips, and some authors have found the risk of loosening to be lower in patients who returned to sports.[107] Patients should be advised against high-impact activity but allowed to participate in low-impact sports. Potential complications of returning to sports should be balanced by the beneficial effects of exercise on the cardiovascular and musculoskeletal systems.

Female athletes

Female athletes participating in competitive sports, particularly the ones involving weight categories and scoring systems that can be affected by physical appearance, are under intense pressure to have a low percentage of body fat because of perceived benefits on performance. This can lead to abnormal eating behavior and the development of the female athlete triad. The triad involves disordered eating, amenorrhea, and osteoporosis.[110]

Physicians treating female athletes should have a high index of suspicion for this condition, particularly in the athlete who presents with a stress fracture. Management of the female athlete triad involves adequate nutrition to achieve a positive energy balance, supplementation with calcium and vitamin D, weight-bearing exercise that is not excessive, and in some instances medications that can include oral contraceptives. Education of athletes aimed at preventing this condition is key in the young female athlete, because bone health and reduced risk of osteoporosis in later life depends on achieving normal peak bone mass in early adulthood.

Approximately 25 million Americans currently have osteoporosis, with nearly 1.5 million fractures reported every year in older individuals.[26] Risk factors for developing osteoporosis, in addition to excessive exercise and menstrual dysfunction, include sedentary lifestyle as one of its modifiable factors. Weight-bearing exercise is an important part of the prevention and treatment of the disease. Exercisers who report lifelong, strenuous or moderate exercise have a higher bone mass density of the hip than those who report using mild exercises. Postmenopausal women who receive exercise plus calcium supplementation have less bone loss than those who receive calcium supplementation alone (see Ch. 42).

High-intensity strength training is effective in maintaining femoral neck bone mass density as well as improving muscle mass, strength, and balance in postmenopausal women when compared with unexercised control subjects. Resistance training should take place at least two non-consecutive days per week, and include two or three sets of 8–12 repetitions for each muscle, with short rests between sets to allow for an intensity that can approach muscular fatigue. The amount of weight that is lifted should increase as strength builds, keeping resistance to approximately 60–80% of one repetition maximum. Sessions of exercise lasting 20–30 min are recommended, because sessions lasting 60 min or more lead to reduced compliance.

Another issue in the female athlete is the susceptibility to specific musculoskeletal injuries, such as ACL tears, patellofemoral pain, and stress factures. Multiple factors have been identified as possible causes of these injuries in women, including ligamentous laxity, hormonal influences, anatomic variants, muscle strength, and muscle recruitment deficits. Factors that appear to play a significant role in ACL injury include weakness of proximal muscles, and dynamic movement patterns such as landing on a single limb with an extended knee that falls into a valgus position.[57,62]

Young athletes

Sports injuries in children and adolescents are the most common cause of musculoskeletal injury that requires emergency treatment. Damore reported that 41% of pediatric patients with musculoskeletal injuries presenting for evaluation at the emergency department of a university hospital had sports injuries, and the most common diagnoses were sprains, contusions, and fractures. Head injuries were associated with biking, hand injuries with American football and basketball, knee injuries with soccer, and ankle and foot injuries with basketball.[27]

The risk of developing sports injuries in the young athlete is associated with modifiable factors such as lack of preseason conditioning and poor endurance. Other factors include non-modifiable factors such as sex, age, and history of previous injury.[33] Biomechanical considerations related to overuse injuries include timing of the adolescent growth spurt, quality of movement control, and imbalances between flexibility and muscle strength. It is our clinical experience that the injuries in the young athlete that are related to these biomechanical factors include tibial tubercle and calcaneal apophysitis, patellofemoral pain, and rotator cuff impingement associated with shoulder instability.

Identification of these injury risk factors is very important for planning the medical care of the pediatric athlete. The structured preparticipation examination (PPE) is a valuable tool for the physician practicing sports medicine, and possibly the only encounter that the young athlete has with a physician. It has the objectives of identifying medical and orthopedic conditions that would make sports participation unsafe, screening for underlying medical illness, and facilitating the development of preventive conditioning programs.[84] Components of the PPE include a brief medical and family history, a general medical examination, and a clinical evaluation of the major joints. The scheduling of the PPE should be one that allows sufficient time to address the treatment and the rehabilitation issues identified prior to the competitive season. Usually, performing the PPE 6–8 weeks prior to the beginning of the season allows the medical team time to address the rehabilitation needs of the athlete and establish prehabilitation programs when needed.

The benefits of strength training for the pediatric athlete have been debated over the past several years. It appears that strength training in this population can have health-related benefits that include an increase in bone mass and a loss of body fat. Fitness-related benefits with strength training include an increase in power and strength. Strength training can also lead to a reduction in sports injuries. Strength-training programs also appear to be safe when they are structured appropriately and emphasize light weights lifted with correct technique for 10–15 repetitions. The program should combine single-joint, open chain exercises with multijoint, closed chain exercises.[36]

Physically challenged athletes

The opportunity to participate in sports competition has increased for physically challenged athletes in recent years. It has been estimated that over 2 million disabled athletes participate in sports competition in the USA.[11] In addition, many athletes have had the opportunity to represent their country in international competitions and participate at an elite level.

The type of physical impairment of the athlete and the sports in which they participate typically determine the type of injury that the competitor is most likely to suffer. Wheelchair athletes who compete in track and field or basketball usually present with soft tissue injuries of the upper limb, particularly the shoulder. Abrasions and lacerations of the hands are also common. Disabled skiers usually have injuries affecting the lower extremities if they ski upright, and injuries to the upper extremities if they ski in a sitting position.[76]

Medical issues that need to be addressed in physically challenged athletes include skin integrity, risk of thermal injury, and coexisting illnesses that can affect the use of medication such as NSAIDs. The proper fit of adaptive equipment, wheelchairs, prostheses, and orthoses should be carefully assessed. Other factors that can affect exercise performance include venous pooling of the lower extremities in the sitting athlete, poor trunk muscle control that affects upper limb function, and muscle imbalances secondary to neurologic injury. Bernard described the isokinetic torque of the shoulder rotator muscles in athletes with disabilities, and found that the relationship of these depended on the neurologic level of injury, and that the external rotators had a significantly higher peak torque than the internal rotators.[9]

Rehabilitation of the disabled athlete should follow the same principles as for the rehabilitation of the able-bodied athlete. Management of the clinical symptoms and protecting the injured tissue should be followed by a flexibility, strengthening, and proprioceptive training program that addresses the kinetic chain used for the sports activity. For example, a wheelchair tennis player with a rotator cuff tendinopathy typically would require training of the rotator cuff and scapular stabilizers, as well as the available trunk muscles, in a functional, sports-specific manner prior to returning to play.

Medical concerns

The team physician should be prepared to deal with medical issues that arise in the care of their athletes. These issues can include management of respiratory problems such as exercise-induced asthma, gastrointestinal problems such as gastroenteritis, and fluid and electrolytes balance. Other issues that also need to be addressed include inappropriate weight loss behavior, the use of ergogenic aids, and doping rules in sports competition.

The use of anabolic steroids, stimulants, and other ergogenic substances has become widespread in sports as athletes look to develop an advantage on their competitors. Anabolic agents have been shown to contribute to an increase in body weight, lean body mass, and muscle strength in the athlete who uses them in combination with high-intensity exercise and adequate nutrition. The side effects of these agents are multiple, particularly when used in very high doses, and include decreased testicular size, infertility, increased cholesterol, elevated blood pressure, and aggressive behavior (also known as 'roid rage').[116]

The sports medicine physician and the members of the healthcare team need to be aware of the risks associated with the use of these agents, counsel the athletes about them, and instill in the athlete the importance of fair play and competition.

REFERENCES

1. Akuthota V, Chou LH, Drake DF, et al. Sports and performing arts medicine: shoulder and elbow overuse injuries in sports. Arch Phys Med Rehabil 2004; 85(3 suppl 1):52–58.

2. Akuthota V, Nadler SF. Core strengthening. Arch Phys Med Rehabil 2004; 85(3 suppl 1):86–92.

3. Anderson GB. Diagnostic considerations in patients with back pain. Phys Med Rehabil Clin N Am 1998; 9:309–322.

4. Anderson SJ. Acute ankle sprains. Phys Sports Med 2002; 30(12):29–35.

5. Arendt E, Dick R. Knee injury patterns among men and women in collegiate basketball and soccer: NCAA data and review of literature. Am J Sports Med 1995; 23:694–701.

6. Arendt EA. Orthopaedic issues for active and athletic women. Clin Sports Med 1994; 13(2):483–503.

7. Arnold T, Shelbourne KD. A perioperative rehabilitation program for anterior cruciate ligament surgery. Phys Sports Med 2000; 28:31–49.

8. Bahr R, Craig E, Engerbretsen L. The clinical presentation of shoulder instability including on-field management. Clin Sports Med 1995; 14:761–776.

9. Bernard PL, Codine P, Minier J. Isokinetic shoulder rotator muscles in wheelchair athletes. Spinal Cord 2004; 42(4):222–229.

10. Biedert RM, Sanchis-Alfonso V. Sources of anterior knee pain. Clin Sports Med 2002; 21:335–347.

11. Birrer RB. The Special Olympics: an injury overview. Phys Sports Med 1984; 12:95–97.

12. Bradbury N, Borton D, Spoo T, et al. Participation in sports after total knee replacement. Am J Sports Med 1998; 26(4):530–535.

13. Bradley JP, Elkousy H. Decision making: operative versus nonoperative treatment of acromioclavicular joint injuries. Clin Sports Med 2003; 22:277–290.

14. Brockett CL, Mongan DL, Proske V. Predicting hamstrings strain injury in elite athletes. Med Sci Sports Exerc 2004; 36(3):379–387.

15. Brukner P. Exercise related lower leg pain: bone. Med Sci Sports Med 1999; 32(3 suppl):15–26.

16. Buckwalter JA, Lane NE. Athletics and osteoporosis. Am J Sports Med 1997; 25(6):873–881.

17. Burkhart SS, Morgan CD, Kibler WB. Shoulder injuries in overhead athletes: the 'dead arm' revisited. Clin Sports Med 2000; 19:125–158.

18. Cantu RC, Mueller FO. Brain injury related fatalities in American football, 1945–1999. Neurosurgery 2003; 54(4):846–852.

19. Cantu RC. Head and neck injuries. In: Kibler WB, ed. ACSM's handbook for the team physician. Baltimore: William & Wilkins; 1996:188–204.

20. Carborn DNM, Johnson BM. The natural history of the anterior cruciate ligament deficient knee: a review. Clin Sports Med 1993; 12:625–636.

21. Cascio BM, Culp L, Cosgarea AJ. Return to play after anterior cruciate ligament reconstruction. Clin Sports Med 2004; 23:395–408.

22. Cavallo RJ, Speer KP. Shoulder: instability and impingement in throwing athletes. Med Sci Sports Exerc 1998; 30(S):18–25.

23. Clarnette RC, Miniaci A. Clinical exam of the shoulder. Med Sci Sports Exerc 1998; 30(S):1–6.

24. Conaghan PG. Update on osteoarthritis. Part I: current concepts and the relation to exercise. Br J Sports Med 2002; 36(5):330–333.

25. Cook JL, Purdam CR. Rehabilitation of lower limb tendinopathies. Clin Sports Med 2003; 22(4):777–789.

26. Crespo CJ. Exercise and the prevention of chronic disabling illness. In: Frontera WR, ed. Exercise in rehabilitation medicine. Champaign: Human Kinetics; 1999:151–172.

27. Damore DT, Metzl JD, Ramundo M, et al. Patterns in childhood sports injury. Pediatr Emerg Care 2003; 19(2):65–67.

28. DeHaven KE, Bronstein RD. Arthroscopic medial meniscal repair in the athlete. Clin Sports Med 1997; 16(1):69–86.

29. DiGiovanni BF, Partal G, Baumhauver JF. Acute ankle injury and chronic lateral instability in the athlete. Clin Sports Med 2004; 23:1–19.

30. Donelson R. The McKenzie approach to evaluating and treating low back pain. Orthop Rev 1990; 19(8):681–686.

31. Dugan SA, Frontera WR. Rehabilitation in sports medicine. In: Micheli L, Smith A, Bachl N, et al, eds. Team physician manual. Hong Kong: Lippincott Williams & Wilkins, Asia; 2001:162–186.

32. Eck JC, Riley LH. Return to play after lumbar spine conditions and surgeries. Clin Sports Med 2004; 23:367–379.

33. Emery CA. Risk factors for injury in child and adolescent sport: a systematic review of the literature. Clin J Sport Med 2003; 13(4):256–268.

34. Escamilla RF, Fleisig GS, Zheng N, et al. Biomechanics of the knee during closed kinetic chain and open kinetic chain and open kinetic chain exercises. Med Sci Sports Exerc 1998; 30:556–569.

35. Fagan K. Transient quadriplegia and return to play criteria. Clin Sports Med 2004; 23:409–419.

36. Faigenbaum AD. Strength training for children and adolescents. Clin Sports Med 2000; 19(4):593–619.

37. Field LD, Altchek DW. Elbow injuries. Clin Sports Med 1995; 14(1):59–78.

38. Field M, Collins MW, Lovell MR, et al. Does age play a role in recovery from sports related concussion?: a comparison of high school and collegiate athletes. J Pediatr 2003; 142(5):546–553.

39. Fredericson M, Powers CM. Practical management of patellofemoral pain. Clin J Sports Med 2002; 12:36–38.

40. Fredericson M. Common injuries in runners. Sports Med 1996; 21(1):49–72.

41. Freedman KB, Smith AP, Romeo AA, et al. Open Bankart repair versus arthroscopic repair to transglenoid sutures or bioabsorbable tracks for recurrent anterior instability of the shoulder: a meta-analysis. Am J Sports Med 2004; 32(6):1520–1527.

42. Frontera WR, Micheo WF, Aguirre G, et al. Patterns of disease and utilization of health services during international sports competitions. Arch Med Deporte 1997; 14:479–484.

43. Frontera WR, Micheo WF, Amy E, et al. Patterns of injuries evaluated in an interdisciplinary clinic. P R Health Sci J 1994; 3:65–170.

44. Frontera WR. Epidemiology of sports injuries: implications for rehabilitation. In: Frontera WR, ed. Rehabilitation of sports injuries: scientific basis. Massachusetts: Blackwell; 2003:3–9.

45. Frontera WR. Exercise and musculoskeletal rehabilitation: restoring optimal form and function. Phys Sports Med 2003; 31(12):39–45.

46. Fu FH, Bennett CH, Latterman C, et al. Current trends in anterior cruciate ligament reconstruction: part I: biology and biomechanics of reconstruction. Am J Sports Med 1999; 27(6):821–890.

47. Fu FH, Bennett CH, Ma B, et al. Current trends in anterior cruciate ligament reconstruction: part II: operative procedures and clinical correlations. Am J Sports Med 2000; 28(1):124–130.

48. Gerbino PG, Micheli LJ. Low back injuries in the young athlete. Sports Med Arthrosc Rev 1996; 4:122–131.

49. Ghiselli G, Schaadt G, McAllister DR. On the field evaluation of an athlete with a head or neck injury. Clin Sports Med 2003; 22:445–465.

50. Gotlin RS, Huie R. Anterior cruciate ligament injuries: operative and rehabilitative options. Phys Med Rehabil Clin N Am 2000; 11:895–924.

51. Graham TJ, Mullen DJ. Athletic injuries of the adult hand. In: DeLee J, Drez D, Miller M, eds. DeLee & Drez's orthopedic sports medicine principles and practice. Philadelphia: Saunders; 2003:1381–1431.

52. Greene HS, Cholewicki J, Galloway MT, et al. A history of low back injury is a risk factor for recurrent back injuries in varsity athletes. Am J Sports Med 2001; 29(6):795–800.

53. Grindel SH, Lovell MR, Collins MW. The assessment of sport-related concussion: the evidence behind neuropsychological testing and management. Clin J Sport Med 2001; 11:134–143.

54. Gross MT, Liu HY. The role of ankle bracing for prevention of ankle sprain injuries. J Orthop Sports Phys Ther 2003; 33(10):572–577.

55. Guskiewicz KM, McCrea M, Marshall SW, et al. Cumulative effects associated with recurrent concussion in collegiate football players: the NCAA Concussion Study. JAMA 2003; 19(19):2549–2555.

56. Hagen KB, Hilde G, Jamtvedt G, et al. Bed rest for acute low-back pain and sciatica. Cochrane Rev 2004; 2.

57. Harmon KG, Ireland ML. Gender differences in noncontact anterior cruciate ligament injuries. Clin Sports Med 2000; 19(2):287–302.

58. Harmon KG, Ireland ML. Gender differences in non-contact anterior cruciate ligament injuries. Clin Sports Med 2000; 19(2):287–302.

59. Harmon KG. Lower limb stress fractures. Clin J Sports Med 2003; 13:358–364.

60. d'Hemecourt PA, Gerbino PG II, Micheli LJ. Back injuries in the young athlete. Clin Sports Med 2000; 19(4):663–679.

61. Hewett TE, Lindenfeld TN, Riccobene JV, et al. The effect of neuromuscular training on the incidence of knee injury in female athletes. Am J Sports Med 1999; 27(6):699–706.

62. Ireland ML. The female ACL: why is it more prone to injury? Orthop Clin N Am 2002; 33(4):637–651.

63. Iwamoto J, Takeda T. Stress fractures in athletes: review of 196 cases. J Orthop Sci 2003; 8(3):273–278.

64. Johnston KM, McCrory P, Mohtadi NG, et al. Evidence-based review of sport-related concussion: clinical science. Clin J Sport Med 2001; 11:150–159.

65. Kibler WB, Chandler TJ. Functional rehabilitation and return to training and competition. In: Frontera WR, ed. Rehabilitation of sports injuries: scientific basis. Massachusetts: Blackwell; 2003:288–300.

66. Kibler WB, Livingston B, Bruce R. Current concepts in shoulder rehabilitation. Adv Oper Orthop 1995; 3:249–300.

67. Kibler WB. A framework for sports medicine. Phys Med Rehabil Clin N Am 1994; 5:1–8.

68. Kibler WB. Closed kinetic chain rehabilitation for sports injuries. Phys Med Rehabil Clin N Am 2000; 11:369–384.

69. Kibler WB. Rehabilitation of rotator cuff tendinopathy. Clin Sports Med 2003; 22:837–847.

70. Kim DH, Vaccaro AR, Berta SC. Acute sports related spinal cord injury: contemporary management principles. Clin Sports Med 2003; 22:501–512.

71. Kiviranta I. Articulate cartilage thickness and glycosminoglycan distribution in the canine knee joint after strenuous exercises. Clin Orthop 1992; 283:302–308.

72. Kortebein PM, Kaufman KR, Basford JR, et al. Medial tibial stress syndrome. Med Sci Sports Med 1999; 32(3 suppl):27–33.

73. Krabak BJ, Sugar R, McFarland EG. Practical nonoperative management of rotator cuff injuries. Clin J Sports Med 2003; 13(2):102–105.

74. Krivickas L. Training flexibility. In: Frontera WR, Dawson DM, Slovik DM, eds. Exercise in rehabilitation medicine. Champaign: Human Kinetics; 1999:83–102.

75. Laskowski ER, Newcomer-Aney K, Smith J. Proprioception. Phys Med Rehabil Clin N Am 2000; 11:323–340.

76. Laskowski ER. Rehabilitation of the physically challenged athlete. Clin Sports Med 1994; 5(1):215–233.

77. Lewis DM, Osterman AL. Scapholunate instability in athletes. Clin Sports Med 2001; 20:131–140.

78. Maffulli N, Wong J, Almekinders LC. Types and epidemiology of tendinopathy. Clin Sports Med 2003; 22:675–692.

79. Maffulli N, Wong J. Rupture of the Achilles and patellar tendons. Clin Sports Med 2003; 22:761–776.

80. McConnel J. The physical therapist's approach to patellofemoral disorders. Clin Sports Med 2002; 21:3663–387.

81. McGill S. Low back disorder: evidence-based prevention and rehabilitation. Champaign: Human Kinetics; 2002.

82. Meister K. Current concepts. Injuries to the throwing athlete. Part two: evaluation/treatment. Am J Sports Med 2000; 28:587–601.

83. Meister K. Current concepts. Injuries to the throwing athlete. Part one: biomechanics/pathophysiology/classification of injury. Am J Sports Med 2000; 28:265–275.

84. Metzl JD. The adolescent preparticipation physical examination: is it helpful? Clin Sports Med 2000; 19(4):577–592.

85. Micheo W, Amy E. Anterior cruciate ligament sprain. In: Frontera WR, Silver JK, eds. Philadelphia: Hanley & Belfus; 2002:301–307.

86. Micheo W, Amy E. Basketball injuries: upper limb considerations. In: McKeag DB, ed. Handbook of sports medicine and science. Massachusetts: Blackwell; 2003:177–190.

87. Micheo W, Esquenazi A. Orthoses in the prevention and rehabilitation of injuries. In: Frontera WR, ed. Rehabilitation of sports injuries: scientific basis. Massachusetts: Blackwell; 2003:301–315.

88. Micheo W, Frontera WR, Amy E, et al. Rehabilitation of the patient with an anterior cruciate ligament injury: a brief review. Bol Assoc Med P R 1995; 87:29–36.

89. Micheo WF, Ramos E. Glenohumeral instability. In: Frontera WR, Silver JK, eds. Essentials of physical medicine and rehabilitation. Philadelphia: Hanley & Belfus; 2001:76–89.

90. Morganti C. Recommendations for return to sports following cervical spine injuries. Sports Med 2003; 33(8):563–573.

91. Myklebust G, Engebretsen L, Hoff Braekken I, et al. Prevention of anterior cruciate ligament injuries in female team handball players: a prospective intervention study over three seasons. Clin J Sports Med 2003; 13:71–78.

92. Nadler SF, Malanga GA, Bartoli LA, et al. Hip muscle imbalance and low back pain in athletes: influence core strengthening. Med Sci Sports Exerc 2002; 34(1):9–16.

93. Nelson BJ, Arciero RA. Arthroscopic management of glenohumeral instability. Am J Sports Med 2000; 28:602–614.

94. O'Brien SJ, Pagnani MJ, Fealy S, et al. The active compression test: a new and effective test for diagnosing labral tear and acromioclavicular joint abnormality. Am J Sports Med 1998; 26:610–613.

95. O'Shea KJ, Murphy KP, Heekin D, et al. The diagnostic accuracy of history, physical examination, and radiographs in the evaluation of traumatic knee disorders. Am J Sports Med 1996; 24:164–167.

96. Pandya RD, Gillogly SD, Andrews JR. Throwing injuries to the elbow. In: Andrews JR, Zarins B, Wilk, KE, eds. Injuries in baseball. Philadelphia: Lippincott-Raven; 1998:223–228.

97. Petrosini AV, Sherman OH. A historical perspective on meniscal repair. Clin Sports Med 1996; 15(3):445–453.

98. Pidoriano AJ, Fulkerson JP. Arthroscopy of the patellofemoral joint. Clin Sports Med 1997; 16(1):17–28.

99. Plancher KD, Lucas TS. Fracture dislocations of the elbow in athletes. Clin Sports Med 2001; 20:59–76.

100. Plancher KD, Minnich JM. Sports specific injuries. Clin Sports Med 1996; 15(2):201–218.

101. Pu CT, Nelson ME. Aging, function and exercise. In: Frontera WR, ed. Exercise in rehabilitation medicine. Champaign: Human Kinetics; 1999:391–424.

102. Renstrom PA. Elbow injuries in tennis. In: Renstrom PA, ed. Handbook of sports medicine and science tennis. Oxford: Blackwell Science; 2002:233–247.

103. Rettig AC, Patel DV. Epidemiology of elbow, forearm, and wrist injuries in the athlete. Clin Sports Med 1995; 14(2):289–298.

104. Rettig AC. Athletic injuries of the wrist and hand: part I: traumatic injuries of the wrist. Am J Sports Med 2003; 31(6):1038–1048.

105. Rettig AC. Athletic injuries of the wrist and hand: part II: overuse injuries of the wrist and traumatic injuries to the hand. Am J Sports Med 2004; 32(1):262–273.

106. Rettig AC. Epidemiology of hand and wrist injuries in sports. Clin Sports Med 1998; 17(3):401–406.

107. Ritter MA, Meding JB. Total hip replacement: can the patient play sports again? Orthopedics 1987; 10:1447–1452.

108. Safran MR, Benetetti RS, Bartolozzi AR, et al. Lateral ankle sprains: a comprehensive review. Part 1: etiology, pathoanatomy, histopathogenesis, and diagnosis. Med Sci Sports Exerc 1999; 31(7 suppl):429–437.

109. Safran MR, Zachazewski JE, Benedetti RS, et al. Lateral ankle sprains: a comprehensive review. Part 2: treatment and rehabilitation with an emphasis on the athlete. Med Sci Sports Exerc 1999; 31(7 suppl):438–447.

110. Sanborn CF, Horea M, Siemers BJ, et al. Disordered eating and the female athlete triad. Clin Sports Med 2000; 19(2):199–213.

111. Schwellnus M. Flexibility and joint range of motion. In: Frontera WR, ed. Rehabilitation of sports injuries: scientific basis. Massachusetts: Blackwell; 2003:232–257.

112. Shelbourne KD, Patel DV, Adsit WS, et al. Rehabilitation after meniscal repair. Clin Sports Med 1996; 15(3):595–612.

113. Simons SM. Foot injuries in the runner. In: O'Connor FG, Wilder RP, eds. Textbook of running medicine. New York: McGraw-Hill; 2001:213–226.

114. Sorosky B, Press J, Plastaras C, et al. The practical management of Achilles tendinopathy. Clin J Sports Med 2004; 14:40–44.

115. Speer KP. Anatomy and pathomechanics of shoulder instability. Clin Sports Med 1995; 14:751–760.

116. Sturmi JE, Diorio DJ. Anabolic agents. Clin Sports Med 1998; 17(2):261–282.

117. Thacker SB, Gilchrist J, Stroup DF, et al. The impact of stretching on sports injury risk: a systematic review of the literature. Med Sci Sports Exerc 2004; 36(3):371–378.

118. Ticker JB, Warner JJ. Selective capsular shift technique for anterior and anterior–inferior glenohumeral instability. Clin Sports Med 2000; 19(1):1–17.

119. Ting AJ. Running and the older athlete. Clin Sports Med 1991; 10:319–325.

120. Torg JS, Gennarelli TM. Head and cervical spine injuries. In: DeLee JC, Drez D, eds. Orthopaedic sports medicine. Philadelphia: Saunders; 1994:417–462.

121. Uhorchak JM, Scoville CR, Williams GN, et al. Risk factors associated with noncontact injury of the anterior cruciate ligament: a prospective four-year evaluation of 859 West Point cadets. Am J Sports Med 2003; 31(6):831–842.

122. Van Baar MA, Assendelft WJ, Dekker J, et al. Effectiveness of exercise therapy in the patients with osteoarthritis of the hip and knee. Arthritis Rheum 1999; 42(7):1361–1369.

123. Verhagen E, van der Beek A, Twik J. The effect of a proprioceptive balance board training program for the prevention of ankle sprains. Am J Sports Med 2004; 32(6):1385–1393.

124. Visuri T, Honkanen R. Total hip replacement: its influence on spontaneous recreation exercise habits. Arch Phys Med Rehabil 1980; 61:325–328.

125. Warninger KN. Management of the helmeted athlete with suspected cervical spine injury. Am J Sports Med 2004; 32(5):1331–1350.

126. Weinstein SM. Assessment and rehabilitation of the athlete with a stinger. Clin Sports Med 1998; 17:127–135.

127. Werner SL, Plancher KD. Biomechanics of wrist injuries in sports. Clin Sports Med 1998; 17(3):407–420.

128. Wiesner ST. Rehabilitation of elbow injuries in sports. Phys Med Rehabil Clin N Am 1994; 5:81–113.

129. Wilder RP, Sethi S. Overuse injuries: tendinopathies, stress fractures, compartment syndrome, and shin splints. Clin Sports Med 2004; 23:55–81.

130. Wilson RL, McGinty LD. Common hand and wrist injuries in basketball players. Clin Sports Med 1993; 12:265–291.

131. Wolin PM. Shoulders injuries. In: Kibler WB, ed. ACSM's handbook for the team physician. Baltimore: Williams & Wilkins; 1996:253–271.

132. Woo Sly, Debski RF, Wtithrow JD, et al. Biomechanics of knee ligaments. Am J Sports Med 1999; 27:533–543.

133. Young JL, Press JM, Herring SA. The disc at risk in athletes: perspectives on operative and nonoperative care. Med Sci Sports Exerc 1997; 29(S):222–232.

134. Young WB, Behm DG. Should static stretching be used during a warm-up for strength and power activities? Streng Cond J 2002; 24(6):33–37.

135. Zemper ED. Two year prospective study of relative risk of a second cerebral concussion. Am J Phys Med Rehabil 2003; 82(9):653–659.

Chapter

46

Occupational Rehabilitation

Brian S. Foley and Ralph M. Buschbacher

Appropriate handling of an injured worker requires a thorough understanding of medical principles, detailed history taking, and a musculoskeletal evaluation with emphasis on the neuromuscular system. Teamwork with an interdisciplinary approach to the treatment of the patient is more effective than the standard medical model.

Occupational musculoskeletal injuries are much the same as other injuries, except that they occur at work. In the USA, the federal government oversees workers' compensation only for small specific groups such as railroad workers. Other employer workers' compensation systems are generally governed by state law. Each state can decide for itself how to define a work injury, how cases will be managed, and what benefits are provided.

EPIDEMIOLOGY

Occupational injuries are both common and expensive. Occupational low back pain occurs in 2% of workers per year. Low back pain is the most common cause of disability in those under age 45. *Direct costs* include medical expenses; *indirect costs* include lost worker productivity. The total annual direct costs are in excess of $65 billion, with indirect costs over $106 billion. Occupational injuries and illnesses are insufficiently appreciated contributors to the total burden of healthcare costs in the USA.[18]

Work-related musculoskeletal disorders account for the largest and most expensive source of injuries. A National Academy of Sciences study found that musculoskeletal disorders of the back and arm cause over one million workers to miss time from their job each year, at an annual cost of over $50 billion.[26] When one takes into account such indirect costs as reduced productivity, loss of customers due to errors made by replacement workers, and regulatory compliance, the total yearly cost of all workplace injuries is estimated to be well over $1 trillion, or 10% of the US gross domestic product.[21,22,25] A small percentage of injured workers account for a large percentage of costs. For example, 7.4% of cases of absence from work for 6 months in a cohort of occupational back pain claimants accounted for about 70% of lost days, medical costs, and wage replacement costs.[1]

HISTORY

Occupational health and safety is not a new concept. Many of our common treatments—such as splints, surgery, dressings, and ointments—were referred to in the Edwin Smith papyrus, dating to about 3000 BC. The Code of Hammurabi in Babylon, *c*.2000 BC, contained clauses dealing with proper handling of injuries, physician fees, and monetary damages for those who harm others.

The Egyptians established the first fully staffed 'occupational health clinic' under the guidance of Ramses II in about 1500 BC. In order to maintain a healthy workforce to build temples and canals, the pharaoh had physician civil servants regularly examine the workers, enforce hygiene, and isolate the sick. Treatments were further advanced by the Greek physicians Hippocrates and Galen, who documented more environmental hazards. The Romans' concern over work site dangers prompted them to make many improvements in ventilation, waste disposal, and construction methods.

The basic principles of compensation for injury began in the Middle Ages. The code of King Rothari in 643 clarified a sliding scale of payments for various injuries and disabilities, part of which went to the victim. King Canute specified payments for specific injuries that gave rise to our current impairment guides. For example, the compensation for the loss of a thumb was twice that for the loss of the second digit, and two and a half times that given for the loss of the third digit. The first monograph dealing with the diseases of a specific occupational group, *On the Miners' Sickness and Other Miners' Diseases* by Paracelsus, was published in 1567.

Many observers in the seventeenth century commented on the diseases of certain workers, but it was not until the eighteenth century that the first comprehensive treatise on the diseases of workers was published. Bernardino Ramazzini noted in his *Discourse on the Diseases of Workers* that workers can be harmed by either 'the harmful character of the materials that they handle' or 'certain violent and irregular motions and unnatural postures of the body, by reason of which the natural structure of the vital machine is so impaired that serious diseases gradually develop therefrom'. Ramazzini consistently emphasized the link between occupation and health, earning him the title 'father of occupational medicine'.

Workers' compensation acts were passed near the end of the nineteenth century in Germany (1884), Austria (1887), Great Britain (1897), and France (1898). In the USA, the Bureau of Labor Statistics was established in 1869 to study industrial accidents. The Employer's Liability Law (1877) established the potential for employer liability in workplace accidents. Workers' compensation legislation was finally passed into law in the USA in 1911, after a long study of the German insurance plan. Further concerns over workers' safety led to the formation of the Occupational Safety and Health Act of 1970.[10,12]

Prior to the current workers' compensation system, an injured worker's only recourse was to sue the employer. Eighty percent of these lawsuits were lost by the plaintiff. In those cases, the injured worker often had no source of income for long periods, as well as no medical benefits. After the unsuccessful lawsuit, they might have been fired as well. On the employer's side, there was tremendous unlimited liability in the event that the injury suit was successful. The injured worker had to prove that the employer was in some way at fault for the injury.

The current system in the USA is a *no fault* system. This means that the injured worker does not need to prove that the employer is at fault, and vice versa. Under the current system, if the injury occurred at work, medical costs and partial payment of lost income are covered. The amount of income covered varies with each state, but generally does not replace 100% of the workers' entire salary or wage. Workers who are required to be off work typically receive medical treatment for the injury and a portion of their normal wage while recovering.

Because workers' compensation is run differently in each state, there is considerable variability in the rules of coverage. The international approach to injured workers varies even more markedly. In economies with a strong social benefit system, such as that of France, the injured workers do not return to work as quickly as in the USA. Throughout much of the world, low back pain is not considered a severely disabling injury, but rather a normal part of life. This approach to low back pain is probably healthier and more cost-effective. Individuals in the USA are more disabled given the same level of back injury compared with those in other countries.[30]

Once injured workers agree to receive workers' compensation benefits, they forgo their right to sue their employer. The employee still has the right to sue third parties. For example, a truck driver injured in a motor vehicle accident due to a tire exploding can accept workers' compensation benefits for lost earnings and medical expenses. The worker would not be able to sue the employer (the trucking company), but would still have the option of suing the tire manufacturer for product liability.

PRINCIPLES

An *injury* occurs after a specific event that can be pinpointed at a particular place and time. This generally refers to minor trauma or a specific lifting injury. A typical example of an occupational injury would be a lumbosacral sprain or strain after lifting a patient in a hospital. An *occupational illness*, on the other hand, comes on gradually. This can occur after repetitive microtrauma and result in a *cumulative trauma disorder* such as carpal tunnel syndrome. Cumulative trauma disorder, repetitive motion disorder, and repetitive strain injury are among the terms used to refer to the work-related musculoskeletal disorders associated with occupational illness. Cumulative trauma disorder causation is multifactorial, and generally is thought to include diagnoses such as carpal tunnel syndrome and lateral epicondylitis. A cumulative trauma disorder is not a medical diagnosis, but is actually only a label. A pathoanatomic diagnosis is not always possible in these cases. Cumulative trauma disorders account for 56% of all occupational injuries. Occupational injuries currently affect 15–20% of all Americans. The mean cost per case of upper extremity cumulative trauma disorders is nearly 10 times that of other workers' compensation cases. Sixty percent of new occupational illnesses in 1992 were associated with repetitive motion.[23]

Although occupational risk factors have been identified, the recent literature is showing less of a direct causation of overuse syndromes than was previously thought. For example, studies have shown that computer use does not pose a severe occupational hazard for developing symptoms of carpal tunnel syndrome.[2] Although there are psychologic risk factors for developing symptoms, there appears to be little scientific evidence for the effectiveness of biopsychosocial rehabilitation on repetitive strain injuries.[16]

There are few high-quality studies of effective injury prevention. One such large-scale, randomized, controlled trial of an educational program to prevent work-associated low back injury found no long-term benefits associated with training.[3] Many employers include education regarding lifting techniques in new employee orientation. Nurses with mechanical lifting devices and lifting teams in their workplace are significantly less likely to have a musculoskeletal injury or disorder.[8,13,14,32]

There are multiple known risk factors for occupational injury claims. These include smoking, low educational status, job dissatisfaction, lower socioeconomic status, deconditioning, and previous history of injuries or disabilities. Other physical risk factors include repetitive motion, improper positioning, forceful movement, contact stresses, whole body vibration, cold temperatures, and unaccustomed work. It is less well known how altering these risk factors will affect injury rates.[26] Workers with the greatest physical work requirements and those with the shortest duration of employment are at the highest risk of back injuries.[11]

Improving one's flexibility, strength, and aerobic fitness reduces pain, improves sleep, and improves workplace functioning. A review of controlled trials looking at education, lumbar supports, exercises, ergonomics, and risk factor modification found that only exercise demonstrated sufficient evidence of back or neck pain prevention.[19,33] A cohort study suggested that correct dynamic trunk extension performance can protect against back-related permanent work disability.[29]

The value of musculoskeletal fitness as a vital component of the overall health-related fitness equation has not been appreciated fully. Achieving an adequate level of muscle strength and flexibility enhances dynamic joint stabilization. This helps prevent excessive load transmission to joint structures, and reduces the abnormal movement patterns that can predispose one to injury.[15] There is a relationship between subjective well-being and work ability in the general population. Life dissatisfaction predicts subsequent work disability, especially among the physically healthy.[17]

Personal modifiable factors are major influences in the recovery from work-related disorders. Factors associated with better recovery include exercise or physical activity outside work and lower stress levels. Factors associated with higher disability levels over time are cigarette smoking and bed rest.[28] Although risk factors for developing occupational disability have been identified, the overall predictive power of such regression models is low.[27]

Risk factors for delayed recovery have been identified and have been called *yellow flags*. Identifying those individuals and using more aggressive case management with them can be helpful in reducing workers' compensation costs, because they typically account for the largest costs. Focusing on reducing the perception of disability at the time of injury is critical to preventing time loss.[31] Non-return to work is associated with higher psychosocial morbidity.[20] The doctor's proactive communication regarding return to work can improve outcomes. A positive return to work recommendation was associated with about a 60% higher return to work rate during the subacute or chronic phase (> 30 days of disability), according to a prospective study on doctor–patient communication.[4]

One conceptual model to improve functional outcomes in occupational injuries (and reduce costs) is called BICEPS. This stands for brevity, immediacy, centrality, expectancy, proximity, and simplicity. Brevity: the initial and subsequent visits should be brief and problem-focused. Immediacy: early intervention correlates with early resolution. Centrality: evaluations and treatments should ideally occur in one convenient location. Expectancy: the physician must be clear in communicating an expectation of recovery. The physician's statement that a full and speedy recovery is expected helps the injured worker toward that goal. Proximity: the worker should remain at work as much as possible. This allows the worker to maintain the ability to produce, continue appropriate work habits, maintain a feeling of self-worth, and continue relationships with fellow workers. Simplicity: a return to healthy functioning can be facilitated by clear explanations and reassurance.

EVALUATIONS

Job descriptions are generally available for each injured worker and should be reviewed to help identify whether that person can return to the regular job. *Job site analyses* done by ergonomists or occupational therapists can help to evaluate whether a worker can perform the particular job safely. They can also help

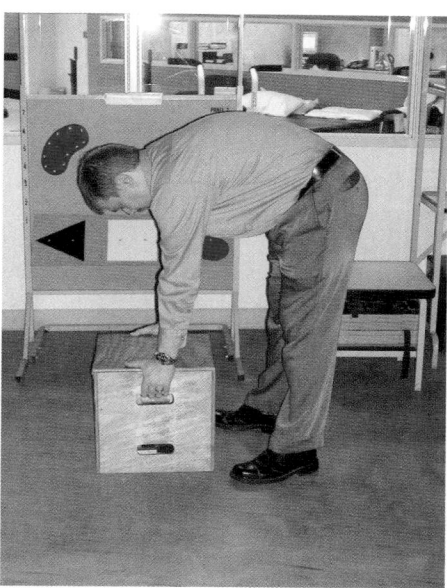

Figure 46-1
Demonstration of improper lifting technique. Note the man's lumbar flexion.

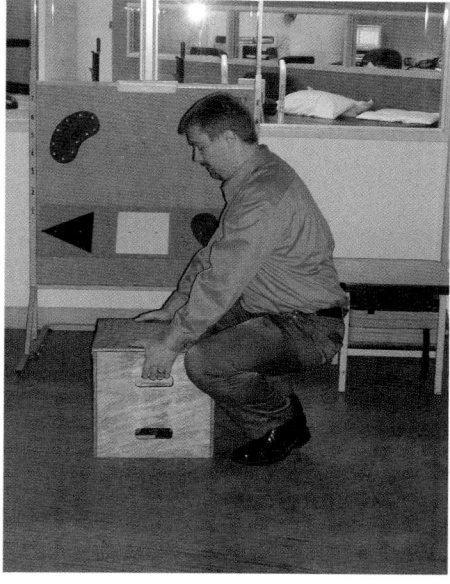

Figure 46-2
Demonstration of proper lifting technique. Note the man's knee flexion.

determine if job modifications are needed to permit the worker to perform the job safely. *Ergonomics* refers to the study of how the human body interacts with the environment. There are certain physical arrangements that increase work-related musculoskeletal disorders. Ergonomists are experts in making modifications and suggestions to reduce the risks of injury (see Figs 46-1 and 46-2).

Preplacement evaluations can be helpful in finding work for an individual who has a higher than average risk for injury. Such persons should not be placed in a job that is known to have a high injury rate. Many employers, such as automotive manufacturers, perform median nerve conduction studies on new hires. These tests are considered a baseline and can be used for comparison purposes later on if the employees develop carpal tunnel symptoms.

Functional baseline testing, which is also called human performance evaluations, can be done to clarify the individual's physical ability and to help guide safe job placement. The testing is less extensive than a functional capacity evaluation (FCE; see explanation below) and does not include consistency and validity testing.

Restricted duty allows the injured worker to maintain current function and employment without risking further injury. This is often a better option than being off work. The Department of Labor has published a book called the *Dictionary of Occupational Titles*[34] that clarifies categories of work. They are as follow: sedentary, light, medium, heavy, and very heavy. The occasional maximal lifting that corresponds to each of these is 10 lbs, 20 lbs, 50 lbs, 100 lbs, and greater than 100 lbs, respectively (Tables 46-1 and 46-2).

INDEPENDENT MEDICAL EXAMINATIONS

Independent medical examinations are sometimes required in workers' compensation cases. Often, controversies regarding causation, maximal medical improvement (MMI), work restrictions, impairments, and disability prompt a request for an IME. The intent is to have an independent review of a complex medical case. It combines a thorough review of all available medical records and tests, with an extensive history and physical examination. There is no doctor–patient relationship established during this IME, and a true IME cannot be done by any physician with a treatment role with the patient. The diagnosis and recommendations sections of the report are often detailed, but treatment is not ordered by the examining physician. The reader of these reports is typically an insurance adjuster or an attorney, so the concluding remarks should be stated in layman's language with as little medical jargon as possible. The most useful IMEs are thorough, unbiased, clear, and legally defensible.

TREATMENT

Acute injury

An acute injury is defined as one that has persisted for 6 months or less. For musculoskeletal or work-related injuries, the acute phase can actually be considered much shorter. A condition becomes chronic when it persists beyond the expected normal healing time. Musculoskeletal injuries generally resolve within 12 weeks and should be considered chronic beyond 3 months. Many consider the subacute phase to be between 6 and 12 weeks.

Longer durations of the initial episode of care or work disability are among the most powerful predictors of recurrence. This implies that shorter episodes of care and early

Table 46-1 Material handling limits		
	Percentage of day	Handling repetitions
Infrequent	1–2	1–4
Occasional	3–33	5–32
Frequent	34–66	33–250
Constant	67–100	251–2000

(After US Department of Labor 1986,[34] with permission of the US Government Printing Office.)

Table 46-2 Material handling limits for different demands of work			
Physical demand	Occasionally	Frequently	Constantly
Sedentary duty	Lift or carry up to 10 lbs Sit 6–8 h Stand or walk 0–2 h	Negligible – –	Negligible – –
Light duty	Lift or carry up to 20 lbs Stand 4–8 h Walk 0–4 h	Up to 10 lbs – –	Negligible – –
Medium duty	Lift or carry up to 50 lbs Stand or walk 8 h	Up to 20 lbs –	Up to 10 lbs –
Heavy duty	Lift or carry up to 100 lbs Stand or walk 8 h	Up to 50 lbs –	Up to 20 lbs –
Very heavy duty	Lift or carry over 100 lbs Stand or walk 8 h	Over 50 lbs –	Over 20 lbs –

(After US Department of Labor 1986,[34] with permission of the US Government Printing Office.)

return to work contribute to better outcomes.[35] There is a direct correlation between the number of days to first recheck and the days to final release of patients with back pain injuries. On average, reducing time between initial visit and first recheck by 1 day shortens the number of days to final release by 3.1 days.[6] One study of occupational medicine physicians found that those with the best patient outcomes placed only 35% of their patients with low back pain on restrictions and kept < 1% off work.[7]

Subacute phase of care

Increasing evidence points to the subacute stage of care as a critical period in preventing disability. Interventions in this stage that address maladaptive cognitions and behavior, and focus on return to work, have demonstrated reductions in lost work time and disability.[9] Imaging is often indicated at the start of the subacute phase to rule out more serious pathology. Injections can be helpful for both diagnostic and therapeutic purposes at this point. Injections can be performed with an anesthetic agent and/or a steroid medication, depending on the intended purposes. Physical therapy is often indicated in this phase to maximize functional recovery. The goal is to reduce pain as well as restore function and prevent reinjury.

Chronic phase of care

Illness behaviors are often seen in the patient with *chronic pain syndrome*. In chronic pain syndrome, the symptoms become the central focus of the patient's life. They may include grimacing, loud sighing, inconsistency on examination, slow movements, doting family members, etc. Pain management can be the only indicated treatment for ongoing pain, and might be appropriate even after a worker's injury case is 'closed'. Even after MMI has been reached, ongoing symptomatic pain management is sometimes required. Chronic pain is typically associated with depression and anxiety. Screening for borderline personality disorders, somatoform disorders, antisocial personality disorder, and histrionic personality is often appropriate.

CASE CLOSURE

Case closure is considered by employers to be the ultimate goal for any workers' compensation case, but there are other goals as well. The physician would like injured workers to be either fully recovered or independent in their functioning. The employer would like the individual to return to her or his job or to another job within the company. The case manager and insurer have an incentive to return the injured worker as soon as is safely possible to their maximal level of functioning. Injured workers need to put the injury behind them as quickly as possible and move on.

Workers' compensation cases ultimately end at the point after which minimal change over the course of the following year is expected. This used to be quantified as less than 3% change over the course of 1 year. The number is less critical and should not be emphasized, but it can be used as a guide to indicate how much change is appropriate in the time before a case is closed.

Maximal medical improvement is attained once the medical condition has resolved or has become fixed and stable. At this point, further diagnostic testing or intervention is not recommended. At MMI, the injured worker is not expected to significantly change in pain level or functional ability in the near future.

A *permanent partial impairment* (PPI) rating might be appropriate once the point of MMI has been attained. The PPI rating is designed to compensate the individual for any future lost earnings due to their residual dysfunction following the work-related injury. If there was a preexisting condition, an adjustment or apportionment can be needed (Table 46-3).

The most widely accepted methodology for evaluating impairment is the *AMA Guides to the Evaluation of Permanent Impairment*, published by the American Medical Association. It is periodically updated and is currently in its fifth edition. Several states require its use in PPI determinations; while other states allow or require the use of other editions or their own state guide.

There are a number of tools that can be used for measuring impairments. *Goniometry* measures joint angle and documents restricted range of motion. *Dynamometry* measures such voluntary forces as grip strength. Validity tests can be used to measure the consistency of grip strength testing with a dynamometer (most commonly the Jamar dynamometer). *Inclinometry* can be used to measure the range of motion in the cervical, thoracic, or lumbar spine. Specific techniques as well as normal values are illustrated in the *AMA Guides*.

Work conditioning refers to the process of increasing the injured worker's strength and cardiovascular fitness after a prolonged period of decreased activity. This process is in preparation for return to full employment but might not be specifically tailored toward a particular job.

Although there is some overlap with work conditioning, *work hardening* generally refers to the process of preparing a particular worker for a specific job by improving strength, conditioning, flexibility, and overall functional ability.

Table 46-3 Terminology of apportionment	
Term	Definition
Precipitation	Injury causes a 'latent' disease process to appear
Acceleration	Injury hastens appearance of an underlying disease process
Aggravation	*Permanent* worsening of a prior condition by a particular event
Exacerbation	*Temporary* worsening of a prior condition by an injury
Recurrence	Signs or symptoms of a prior illness or injury occur in the absence of a new provocative event
(After Demeter et al. 2003,[5] with permission.)	

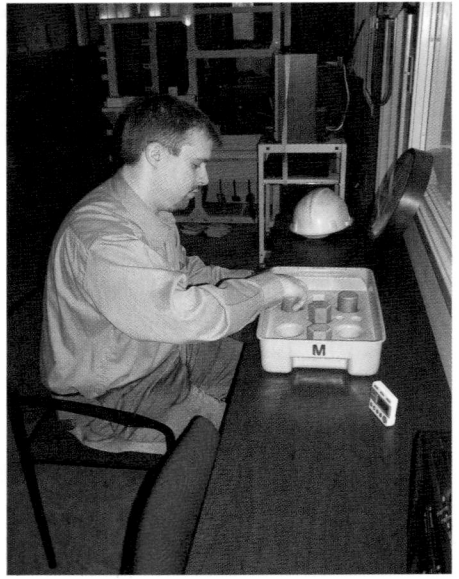

Figure 46-3
Evaluation of fine
motor skills.

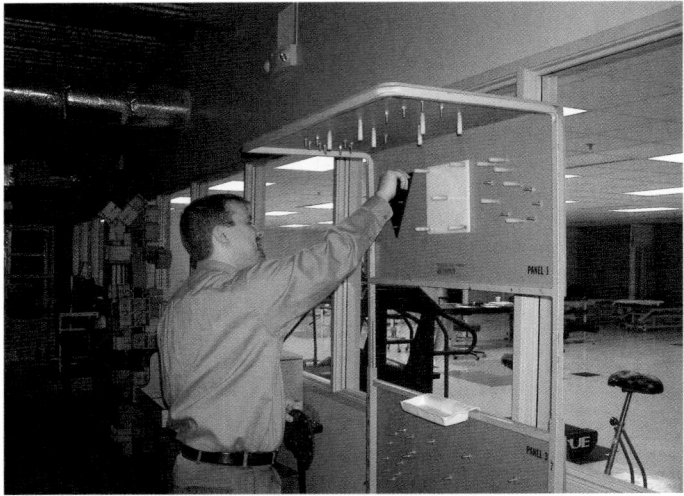

Figure 46-5 Simulation of work that is above the shoulder level.

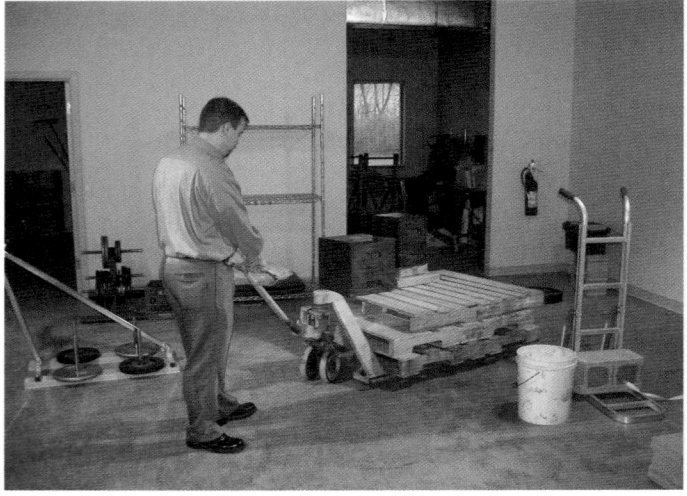

Figure 46-4 Simulated pulling of a loaded pallet.

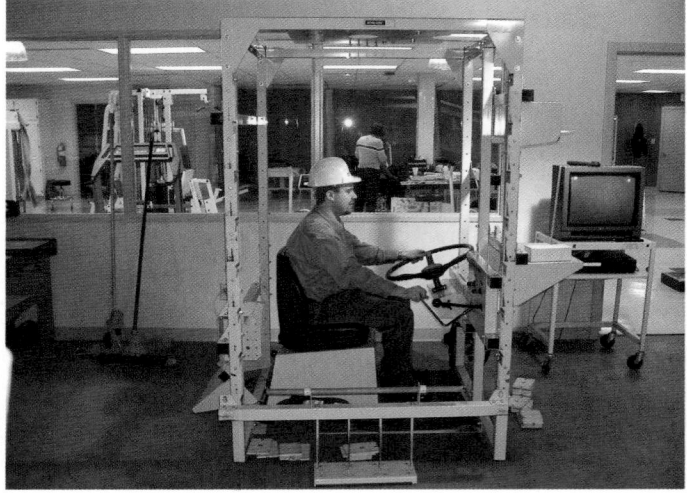

Figure 46-6 Commercial vehicle-driving simulation.

Job matching can be appropriate when selecting specific jobs for particular workers of specified abilities.

Functional capacity evaluations

Functional capacity evaluations are extensive and formalized physical and occupational testing. FCEs are done typically by specially trained physical and occupational therapists. These evaluations last 1 or 2 days. They assess many aspects of the person's functioning. FCEs emphasize validity and consistency, overall functional ability, and the ability to perform a particular type of employment. Often, the FCE can guide or clarify what *Dictionary of Occupational Titles* category job the injured worker can perform. Occasionally, FCE testing is helpful in documenting inconsistencies, decreased effort, and lack of validity on repeat testing (see Figs 46-3–46-6).

Disability

Disability can result from impairment. Disability is defined as a patient's deficits in functional activities. It takes into account other aspects of a person's function, such as education, age, occupational history, and skills. An application for social security disability income can be appropriate in severely disabled individuals.

Vocational rehabilitation

Vocational rehabilitation varies regionally in its availability and quality. Vocational rehabilitation is often recommended, after case closure has been reached, if an individual has persistent impairment and disability limiting their potential employment. This is particularly the case if workers are unable to return to their previous employment.

MEDICOLEGAL ASPECTS OF OCCUPATIONAL REHABILITATION

Workers' compensation involves an interaction between the medical and legal systems. Physiatrists are often thrown into this environment, and it is helpful to learn some basics of the legal system to practice more effectively. A few of these critical legal concepts are as follow.

The Americans with Disabilities Act

The ADA is a federal law designed to help protect the rights of disabled citizens. Employers cannot avoid hiring impaired persons solely because of their impairment and disability, as long as they are able to perform the key components of the job. *Preemployment* physicals are not allowed under the ADA. After an individual has been hired, however, a preplacement physical can be used to help find the most appropriate job for that individual. Employers are also responsible for making *reasonable accommodations* to allow disabled individuals to perform their job functions. There is an approved list of diagnoses that are considered disabilities. The list also includes some diagnoses that can be perceived as disabilities (e.g. an able-bodied HIV-positive worker). This federal legislation is broad-sweeping and has not yet been fully tested in the courts, although case law continues to accumulate.

Depositions and testimony

Workers' compensation cases are sometimes contested and might require the physician to perform a deposition, video deposition, or courtroom testimony. Before providing testimony, it is important to thoroughly review all medical records of the case and be comfortable with the legal protocols. Remember the five Ps: 'proper preparation prevents poor performance'.

While the treating physician often needs to provide testimony or deposition, an actual appearance in court is rarely needed. Issues in question typically involve the mechanism of injury, preexisting conditions, contributing factors, and whether the resulting impairment or disability is consistent with the injury. Although expert witnesses are not usually involved in this process, physiatrists often have the opportunity to perform in the role of medical expert. Recent controversies over the reliability of expert testimony in lawsuits have resulted in efforts to encourage evidence-based testimony.

Daubert refers to a federal Supreme Court case decision that has had a major impact on giving expert testimony. Expert witnesses will now be held to the Daubert standard and can be subject to a Daubert hearing. This process is designed to eliminate testimony that is based on only the expert's opinion. It is felt that juries can be too easily persuaded to accept 'junk science', so it should never be allowed into the courtroom. Information given by expert testimony must be generally well accepted in the medical community, published in peer-reviewed literature, have a scientific basis, and have a known error rate. If these four criteria are not met, the expert witness can be barred from testifying.

Fraud

Malingering is the intentional misrepresentation of signs or symptoms with the intent to receive secondary gain. Malingering is a fraudulent activity and is uncommon. The term should not be used to describe subtle exaggeration of symptoms, functional overlay, or even symptom magnification. The term should be used rarely and only when proper documentation supports such a serious accusation.

Surveillance can be used to document malingering. Occasionally, insurance companies or other interested parties will hire a private investigator to observe an injured worker for 1 or 2 days. If the video records activities that are inconsistent with that injured worker's reported abilities, it might document inconsistency. The footage can provide useful and sometimes startling evidence of functional ability, but it needs to be used with great caution due to the severity of the implication of fraud.

Causation

When doctors state an opinion on a medicolegal issue, they need to state it within 'a reasonable degree of medical certainty'. This means that, based on the available evidence, the truth of the statement is more likely than not corresponding to the civil law standard 'preponderance of the evidence'. Our scientific training prepares us to meet a higher standard of certainty (normally 95%), corresponding to the criminal law standard of 'beyond a reasonable doubt'. We are not expected to be that certain of our opinions in medicolegal cases.[24]

FUTURE ROLE OF THE PHYSICAL MEDICINE AND REHABILITATION PHYSICIAN

The future of physiatrists in occupational rehabilitation is quite bright. The quality, availability, and variety of educational and training programs in occupational rehabilitation are expanding, as is the level of interest in occupational rehabilitation among a growing number of 'outpatient' physiatrists. Due to extensive training in teamwork and musculoskeletal evaluations, physiatrists are well positioned to be the future leaders of occupational rehabilitation. The growing emphasis on evidence-based medicine provides opportunities for basic and clinical research in improving rehabilitation of the injured worker.

REFERENCES

1. Abenhaim L, Suissa S. Importance and economic burden of occupational back pain: a study of 2,500 cases representative of Quebec. J Occup Med 1987; 29:670–674.

2. Andersen JH, Thomsen JF, Overgaard E, et al. Computer use and carpal tunnel syndrome: a 1-year follow-up study. JAMA 2003; 289(22): 2963–2969

3. Daltroy LH, Iversen MD, Larson MG, et al. A controlled trial of an educational program to prevent low back injuries. N Engl J Med 1997; 337:322–328

4. Dasinger LK. Doctor proactive communication, return-to-work recommendation, and duration of disability after a workers' compensation low back injury. J Occup Environ Med 2001; 43:515–525.

5. Demeter SL, Andersson GBJ, eds. Disability evaluation. 2nd edn. St. Louis: Mosby; 2003

6. Derebery J, Anderson JR. From Concentra Health Services analysis based on year-to-date [November 1999] data. Low back pain: an evidence-based, biopsychosocial model for clinical management. Beverly Farms: OEM Press; 2002.

7. Derebery J, Anderson JR. Low back pain: an evidence-based, biopsychosocial model for clinical management. Beverly Farms: OEM Press; 2002.

8. Engkvist IL, Hjelm EW, Hagberg M, et al. Risk indicators for reported overexertion back injuries among female nursing personnel. Epidemiology 2000; 11:519–522.

9. Feldman JB. The prevention of occupational low back pain disability: evidence-based reviews point in a new direction. J Surg Orthop Adv 2004; 13(1):1–14.

10. Felton JS. History of occupational health and safety. Introduction to occupational health and safety. National Safety Council; 1986.

11. Gardner L, Landsittel DP, Nelson NA, et al. Risk factors for back injury in 31,076 retail merchandise store workers. Am J Epidemiol 1999; 150(8):825–833.

12. Goetsch DL. Occupational safety and health. 2nd edn. Prentice-Hall; 1996.

13. Guthrie PF, Westphal L, Dahlman B, et al. A patient lifting intervention for preventing the work-related injuries of nurses. Work 2004; 22:79–88.

14. Hignett S, Crumpton E, Ruszala S, et al. Evidence-based patient handling: systematic review. Nurs Stand 2003; 17(33):33–36.

15. Hunt A. Musculoskeletal fitness: the keystone in overall well-being and injury prevention. Clin Orthop Relat Res 2003; 1(409): 96–105.

16. Karjalainen K, Malmivaara A, van Tulder M, et al. Biopsychosocial rehabilitation for upper limb repetitive strain injuries in working age adults. Cochrane Database Syst Rev 2003; 1.

17. Koivumaa-Honkanen H, Koskenvuo M, Honkanen RJ, et al. Life dissatisfaction and subsequent work disability in an 11-year follow-up. Psychol Med 2004; 34(2):221–228.

18. Leigh JP, Markowitz SB, Fahs M, et al. Occupational injury and illness in the United States. Estimates of costs, morbidity, and mortality. Arch Intern Med 1997; 157(14):1557–1568.

19. Linton SJ, van Tulder MW. Preventive interventions for back and neck pain problems: what is the evidence? Spine 2001; 26:778–787.

20. Mason S. Outcomes after injury: a comparison of workplace and nonworkplace injury. J Trauma 2002; 53:98–103.

21. Melhorn JM, Gardner P. How we prevent prevention of musculoskeletal disorders in the workplace. Clin Orthop 2004; 419:285–296.

22. Melhorn JM, Wilkinson LD, O'Malley MD. Successful management of musculoskeletal disorders. Human and ecological risk assessment 2001; 7(7):1801–1810.

23. Melhorn JM. Cumulative trauma disorders and repetitive strain injuries. Clin Orthop Relat Res 1998; 351:107–126.

24. Melhorn, JM. Impairment and disability evaluations: understanding the process. J Bone Joint Surg 2001; 83-A(12):1905–1911.

25. National Academy of Sciences, National Research Council, Institute of Medicine. Work related musculoskeletal disorders: report, workshop summary, and workshop papers. Washington: National Academy of Sciences, National Research Council, Institute of Medicine; 1999:1–240.

26. National Academy of Sciences. Musculoskeletal disorders and the workplace: low back and upper extremities. National Academy of Sciences; 2001.

27. Okurowski L, Pransky G, Webster B, et al. Prediction of prolonged work disability in occupational low-back pain based on nurse case management data. J Occup Environ Med 2003; 45:763–770.

28. Oleske DM, Neelakantan J, Andersson GB, et al. Factors affecting recovery from work-related, low back disorders in autoworkers. Arch Phys Med Rehabil 2004;85(8):1362–1364.

29. Rissanen A, Heliovaara M, Alaranta H, et al. Does good trunk extensor performance protect against back-related work disability? J Rehabil Med 2002; 34:62–66.

30. Sanders SH, Brena SF, Spier CJ, et al. Chronic low back pain patients around the world: cross-cultural similarities and differences. Clin J Pain 1992; 8:317–320.

31. Tate RB, Yassi A, Cooper J. Predictors of time loss after back injury in nurses. Spine 1999; 24(18):1930–1936.

32. Trinkoff AM, Brady B, Nielsen K. Workplace prevention and musculoskeletal injuries in nurses. J Nurs Adm 2003; 33(3):153–158.

33. Tveito TH, Hysing M, Eriksen HR. Low back pain interventions at the workplace: a systematic literature review. Occup Med 2004; 54:3–13.

34. US Department of Labor. Dictionary of Occupational Titles. US Government Printing Office; 1986.

35. Wasiak R. Risk factors for recurrent episodes of care and work disability: case of low back pain. J Occup Environ Med 2004; 46:68–76.

Useful web sites

In addition to the listed references, there are many excellent web sites and organizations that can provide additional information in the field of rehabilitation of the injured worker. Some of them are as follow.

American Academy of Disability Evaluating Physicians (http://www.AADEP.org)

American Academy of Physical Medicine and Rehabilitation (http://www.AAPMR.net)

American Board of Independent Medical Examiners (http://www.ABIME.org)

American College of Occupational and Environmental Medicine (http://www.ACOEM.org)

The Cochrane Collaboration (http://www.cochrane.org)

SEAK, Inc. (http://www.SEAK.com)

Chapter

47

Motor Neuron Diseases

Priti Khanna, Sharon P. Nations and Jaya R. Trivedi

When Lou Gehrig gave his famous speech at Yankee Stadium on July 4, 1939, many people had never heard of amyotrophic lateral sclerosis (ALS). Now, ALS, frequently referred to as Lou Gehrig disease, is the most common adult motor neuron disease. It is a progressive neuromuscular condition that causes degeneration of motor neurons in the cortex, brain stem, and spinal cord, usually resulting in paralysis, and ultimately death. Motor neuron diseases are classified according to the types of motor neurons that are affected. ALS affects both upper and lower motor neurons. Primary lateral sclerosis (PLS) and hereditary spastic paraplegia (HSP) affect upper motor neurons. Lower motor neurons can be affected in several diseases, including the many forms of spinal muscular atrophy (SMA), cancer, and viruses such as polio and West Nile.

Regardless of the type of motor neuron disease, the patient is best treated by an interdisciplinary team. This team can include physicians; dieticians; psychologists; social workers; orthotists; physical, occupational, and respiratory therapists; and speech pathologists. The benefits of a team approach include improved communication among the various healthcare professionals, better access for patients, and efficient and comprehensive management of the various issues that typically arise during the course of the disease.

CLASSIFICATION OF MOTOR NEURON DISEASES

Motor neuron diseases can be sorted into three categories based on the target of the disease process. Box 47.1 gives an outline of these disorders.

Combined upper and lower motor neuron disorders

Amyotrophic lateral sclerosis
Amyotrophic lateral sclerosis is one of the most devastating of the motor neuron diseases in its effects on the patient. It is a progressive degenerative disorder, which typically involves both upper and lower motor neurons. Initially, ALS can present as predominantly either upper or lower motor neuron in type, making diagnosis more difficult. The worldwide prevalence is 5–7 per 100 000,[68,80] with men affected more commonly than women (ratio of about 1.5:1.0).[15,66] ALS usually begins in middle age (mean onset 58 years), but it can present in any

decade of adult life. Rare cases appear in the adolescent years.

Skeletal muscles become weak and atrophic, but ocular muscles are typically spared. It is not yet known why the ocular muscles are spared. The patient eventually loses the ability to move independently, speak, or swallow. Death is usually due to respiratory failure. The prognosis varies, partly depending on patient decisions regarding interventions such as gastrostomy and mechanical ventilation. Genetic factors might also play a role. Patients with a homozygous deletion in the survival motor neuron (SMN) 2 gene have a shorter life expectancy.[101] The overall 5-year survival rate in ALS is 28%.[68,80] Patients in whom the disease begins with bulbar symptoms tend to have a poorer prognosis, as only 50% of these patients are alive 1 year after symptom onset.[11]

Familial amyotrophic lateral sclerosis
The majority of cases of ALS are sporadic, but approximately 10% are familial. The inheritance pattern is usually autosomal dominant. About 15% of patients with familial ALS have a mutation in the gene encoding copper zinc superoxide dismutase (SOD1).[11] Over 60 different SOD1 mutations have been identified.[88] The SOD1 mutation results in a 'toxic gain of function', whereby the conformational change in the enzyme results in a new interaction that is detrimental to the cell.[30] The discovery of the relationship of some familial ALS cases to SOD1 mutations in 1993[83] led to the development of transgenic animal models of the disease. This allowed an experimental system to test hypotheses regarding pathogenic mechanisms and potential therapies.

Juvenile amyotrophic lateral sclerosis
Juvenile ALS is a form of familial ALS characterized by combined upper and lower motor neuron symptoms and signs with onset prior to age 25 years.[77] Autosomal dominant and recessive forms of juvenile ALS have been described. Mutations of the alsin gene on chromosome 2q33 are seen in a recessive form.[103] Patients with the recessive type present in their first decade with spasticity, weakness, pseudobulbar affect, and mild distal amyotrophy. Another recessive form that localizes to chromosome 15q12–21[35] presents with predominantly lower motor neuron symptoms, with onset in the second decade. Senataxin gene mutations on chromosome 9q34 cause an autosomal

---

Box 47-1 Classification of motor neuron diseases

Combined upper and lower motor neuron diseases
- Amyotrophic lateral sclerosis (ALS), sporadic
- ALS, hereditary
  Autosomal dominant
  Autosomal recessive
  Juvenile ALS
- ALS variants
  ALS with frontotemporal dementia
  Western Pacific ALS parkinsonism–dementia complex
  Progressive muscular atrophy
  Brachial amyotrophic diplegia

Upper motor neuron diseases
- Primary lateral sclerosis
- Hereditary spastic paraparesis
- Viral (HIV, human T-cell leukemia virus types 1 and 2)

Lower motor neuron diseases
- Spinal muscular atrophy
- Fazio–Londe disease
- Bulbospinal muscular atrophy (Kennedy syndrome)
- Poliomyelitis and postpolio syndrome
- West Nile virus infection
- Paraneoplastic

Box 47-2 Revised clinical criteria for diagnosis of amyotrophic lateral sclerosis[9]

The presence of:
- evidence of lower motor neuron degeneration by clinical, electrophysiologic, or neuropathologic examination;
- evidence of upper motor neuron degeneration by clinical examination; and
- progressive spread of symptoms or signs within a region or to other regions, as determined by history or examination.

Together with the absence of:
- electrophysiologic or pathologic evidence of other disease processes that might explain the signs of lower and/or upper motor neuron degeneration; and
- neuroimaging evidence of other disease processes that might explain the observed clinical and electrophysiologic signs.

---

dominant form.[17] The onset is also in the second decade with spasticity, hyperreflexia, extensor plantar responses, distal weakness, and atrophy. Juvenile ALS typically progresses very slowly and over decades, with the need for wheelchair use in the fifth or sixth decade.

Sporadic amyotrophic lateral sclerosis

The etiology of sporadic ALS is unknown. Potential factors that have been investigated that might lead to apoptosis and cell death include oxidative stress, glutamate excitotoxicity to which motor neurons are more susceptible than other central nervous system neurons, damage to axonal transport, and abnormal proteosome function.[20]

Clinical features

Clinical features of ALS include asymmetric weakness and atrophy of muscles, usually beginning in distal limbs or in bulbar muscles. At time of presentation, the patient usually has a history of progression for a number of months and up to 2 years. Patients might have vague sensory complaints, such as 'heaviness' or 'numbness' in weakened limbs, but sensory loss is usually not demonstrated on physical examination. Muscle stretch reflexes are typically brisk or preserved in the presence of weakened muscles. Tone can be increased. Fasciculations are usually seen in limb, trunk, and/or tongue muscles. Speech can be slurred or have a strained, spastic quality. As the disease progresses, patients develop dysphagia, initially for thin liquids, then for all foods. Dyspnea and orthopnea can present late in the course, or earlier if the onset is in bulbar or cervicothoracic muscles. Respiratory insufficiency can occasionally be the presenting symptom.

Currently, there are no biologic markers for the disease that can be reliably identified in the serum or cerebrospinal fluid to diagnose ALS. Confirmation of the diagnosis is based on clinical presentation and elimination of potentially confounding diagnoses, such as spinal cord compression or tumor, syringomyelia, multiple sclerosis, lymphoma, multifocal motor neuropathy, myasthenia gravis, or HIV infection. An electrodiagnostic study is almost always mandatory, and in a typical case demonstrates widespread muscle membrane irritability, including positive waves and fibrillations in muscles of different nerve and myotome distributions. Fasciculations are usually present as well. Electromyography (EMG) changes are subtle in the earliest stages of the disease or when upper motor neuron signs predominate. A repeat study may be required. An EMG showing fibrillations in the tongue is very helpful in the diagnosis, because it documents disease above the foramen magnum.

Muscle biopsy is not routinely performed, but can be indicated in atypical cases to rule out an inflammatory process or inclusion body myositis. The World Federation of Neurology Research Committee on Motor Neuron Diseases published revised criteria for the diagnosis of ALS in 1998 (see Box 47-2).[9]

Pathology

Autopsy findings include atrophy of the frontal cortex, particularly the precentral gyrus. Brain stem and spinal cord motor neurons are replaced by gliosis. Corticospinal tract degeneration is common, particularly in sporadic ALS. Neurons of the nucleus of Onuf in the sacral cord are spared. Within the remaining motor neurons can be seen eosinophilic intracytoplasmic granular inclusions called Bunina bodies, or rod-shaped filamentous inclusions called Hirano bodies. There is degeneration of Clarke's nucleus, but dorsal spinal columns show degeneration only rarely in sporadic ALS. Neurofibrillary tangles and plaques are rare in the cortex.[97]

Amyotrophic lateral sclerosis variants

ALS with frontotemporal dementia   Many investigators have reported an association between ALS and dementia.[65] Patients and their families have noted changes in personality, planning, organization, language, and other frontal lobe functions.[12,13,74,78] These symptoms are characteristic of frontotemporal dementia (FTD), a syndrome resulting from degeneration of frontal and anterior temporal lobe neurons. Ubiquitin-positive inclusions in motor neurons as well as in frontal and temporal lobes have been demonstrated in patients with both ALS and dementia.[47,62] The incidence of dementia in patients with ALS had been considered uncommon until recently. But the work of Lomen-Hoerth and colleagues has shown diminished word generation (which is a test of frontal lobe function) in 31 of 100 consecutive ALS patients without a prior diagnosis of dementia. Of the 44 patients who agreed to formal neuropsychologic testing, 23 demonstrated possible, probable, or definite FTD. The bulbar-onset patients in this study were more likely to have evidence of FTD.[52]

Western Pacific ALS–parkinsonism–dementia complex An unusual clustering of cases of ALS with parkinsonism–dementia complex (PDC) has been reported among the Chamorro people of Guam, on other islands of the Mariana group in the Western Pacific, and on the Kii peninsula of Japan. Patients develop dementia, as well as such extrapyramidal features as rigidity of trunk and limbs, and postural instability. Tremor is uncommon. Some patients also develop a striking amyotrophy with upper motor neuron signs similar to those of ALS.

The etiology of this disorder is still puzzling, but environmental exposures have been investigated. Chronic consumption of a neurotoxin found in a member of the cycad plant family, one of the staples of the Chamorro diet, has been considered as a possible although unproven inciting factor.[61] Intracytoplasmic filamentous inclusions composed of aberrant tau protein are hallmarks of the disease, as they are in Alzheimer's disease, progressive supranuclear palsy, corticobasal degeneration, and other neurodegenerative diseases known as 'tauopathies'. A distinct genetic basis for the disease has not yet been proven, despite efforts to identify tau gene mutations in this population.[100] The incidence of both Guamanian ALS and PDC has declined in recent decades. The incidence of PDC seems to have stabilized somewhat compared with that of ALS, which has continued to decline.[61] The reasons for this are unknown, but changing environmental factors could be responsible.

Progressive muscular atrophy

Progressive muscular atrophy is a term that has been used to refer to cases of sporadic motor neuron disease in which upper motor neuron signs are not found on examination. Even in cases of apparent pure lower motor neuron dysfunction, high signal intensities in corticospinal tracts can sometimes be demonstrated on magnetic resonance imaging (MRI).[5,40] While not specific for ALS, such changes might provide evidence of upper motor neuron abnormality. Progression is frequently cited as being slower in progressive muscular atrophy. Many of these patients eventually develop upper motor neuron signs characteristic of typical ALS.

Brachial amyotrophic diplegia

Brachial amyotrophic diplegia is a sporadic motor neuron disorder that remains largely restricted to the upper limbs for years. Patients present with progressive proximal and distal upper limb weakness along with decreased reflexes. The arms hang flaccidly by the patients' sides. This is similar to the 'man in the barrel syndrome' described in patients with infarction in the watershed zones between the anterior and middle cerebral artery distributions. It typically spares the lower limbs, respiratory, and bulbar musculature, and there are usually no pyramidal signs. Over a period of many years, these patients can also develop lower extremity weakness. This disease is considered to be a very slowly progressive variant of ALS. It is important to recognize this entity, as it aids in predicting the prognosis.[46]

Upper motor neuron disorders
Primary lateral sclerosis

Primary lateral sclerosis is a rare, non-familial upper motor neuron degenerative disorder of unknown etiology. It involves dysfunction of the corticospinal tracts, with sparing of the lower motor neurons of the brain and spinal cord.[85] The mean age of onset was 53.4 years in one series.[21]

Clinical features Clinical presentation can be heterogeneous. The disease onset is insidious, with very slow progression. In contrast with ALS, patients with PLS can live for many years. There are long periods of stabilization in PLS. In Forestier's series of patients, the presentation typically began with spasticity in lower limbs, followed by hyperactive muscle stretch reflexes, and Babinski's and Hoffman's signs.[21] These patients often have severe spasticity, leading to the use of a walker or wheelchair. Muscle weakness in the limbs can be relatively mild in comparison with the spasticity. Pseudobulbar weakness and emotional lability can also occur, but less so than in ALS. Urinary urgency is not uncommon, and is related to detrusor hyperreflexia and a spastic internal sphincter. Cognitive involvement can rarely be seen, due to frontal lobe dysfunction. The lack of lower motor neuron involvement in PLS is a key feature in distinguishing it from ALS. However, EMG in rare cases shows sparse distal fibrillations and positive sharp waves suggestive of active denervation, implying lower motor neuron involvement.[21]

Pathology Autopsy findings in a patient with PLS showed atrophy of the precentral gyrus with loss of Betz cells in layer 5, and decreased numbers of pyramidal neurons in layers 3 and 5. Other findings included pallor and degeneration in the dorsolateral quadrant of the white matter at all levels of the spinal cord. Onuf's nucleus and the number of anterior horn cells were normal.[75]

Hereditary spastic paraplegia

Hereditary spastic paraplegia is a clinically and genetically heterogeneous group of degenerative disorders in which patients present with spastic paraparesis. Inheritance patterns can be autosomal dominant, autosomal recessive, or X-linked recessive.[33] Ten different loci have been identified in the autosomal dominant forms, and five genes have been described so far.[69]

Clinical features   Hereditary spastic paraplegia can be divided into two groups, depending on whether the syndrome is 'pure' or not. Pure HSP implies the presence of spastic paraparesis in isolation. The complicated forms of HSP can be associated with distal amyotrophy, sensory polyneuropathy, mental retardation and macular degeneration, optic atrophy, dystonia, or cerebellar involvement.[33] The age of onset varies and can be before age 20. In the early-onset cases, developmental delay and spasticity of the lower limbs are commonly seen. Patients have a tendency to stumble and have leg stiffness, and also have poor athletic performance. Over the course of time, the upper extremities also become involved. The jaw jerk and upper limb reflexes tend to be brisk, while those in the lower limbs are markedly increased, with clonus and extensor plantar responses. Vibratory and proprioceptive loss occurs in only 10% of cases, and usually in the later stages. Sphincter dysfunction with urinary urgency is seen in about half of the patients.[34] Pes cavus is seen in more than 50% of patients.[58] The clinical characteristics of the early- and late-onset forms are similar, except that urinary symptoms and sensory loss are more frequent in the early form.

Pathology   The abnormalities are mostly confined to the spinal cord. There have been reports of corticospinal tract degeneration from the medullary pyramids downward that increases caudally. Posterior column degeneration that increases caudally can also occur, without loss of posterior root fibers.[6]

Viral infectious disorders of upper motor neurons

HIV-related myelopathy   Neurologic disorders associated with HIV-type infection include central nervous system infections, neoplasms, vascular complications, peripheral neuropathies, and myopathies. One of the major neurologic manifestations of the infection includes vacuolar myelopathy. In these patients, CD4 counts are usually less than 200 cells/mm^3.[89] Presenting symptoms include gait difficulty, lower extremity weakness, and bladder dysfunction. Physical examination typically demonstrates spastic paraparesis, Babinski's signs, and sensory abnormalities. Radiologic studies of the brain and spine, as well as cerebrospinal fluid studies, are usually normal or reveal only minor, non-specific abnormalities. These studies, however, must always be performed to exclude other treatable infections or neoplasms.[89] The pathologic findings of vacuolar myelopathy include vacuolization of myelin sheaths due to the accumulation of foamy macrophages and microglia, with relative preservation of axons.[89]

Human T-cell leukemia virus type 1-associated myelopathy   Human T-cell leukemia virus type 1-associated myelopathy is also referred to as tropical spastic paraparesis. It is endemic in the Caribbean area, southern Japan, equatorial Africa, South Africa, and parts of Central and South America. It produces a slowly progressive chronic myelopathy that typically starts after age 30. Some patients also develop optic atrophy, cerebellar ataxia, or polyneuropathy. Definitive diagnosis requires a positive serology in blood or cerebrospinal fluid.[58]

Lower motor neuron disorders
Spinal muscular atrophy

Spinal muscular atrophy is a hereditary disorder causing degeneration of motor neurons and leading to weakness and atrophy of skeletal muscles. Most pedigrees show an autosomal recessive pattern of inheritance, and more than 90% of these are due to a homozygous deletion in the SMN 1 gene on chromosome 5q11.2–13.3.[39] Another type of autosomal recessive SMA, SMA with respiratory distress, is not associated with the SMN deletion. Autosomal dominant forms of SMA occur, and a severe form associated with arthrogryposis and bone fractures has been shown to be X-linked.[48] The International SMA Consortium on Childhood SMA devised a classification system in 1991 that was based on age at onset and achievement of milestones (Table 47-1).[60]

Clinical features   Typical clinical features include proximal more than distal weakness, hypo- or areflexia, fasciculations of the tongue and other muscles, and hand tremor. If SMN gene deletion testing is negative, then electrodiagnostic and muscle biopsy can be used to help confirm the diagnosis. The electrodiagnostic studies typically show normal sensory nerve conduction studies and neurogenic changes on EMG. Muscle biopsy usually shows neurogenic atrophy.[39] Infants with type 1 SMA (also known as Werdnig–Hoffman disease) have profound weakness and hypotonia, often with voluntary movement only in the hands and feet. Malnutrition results from poor ability to suck and fatigue with feeding. Respiratory insufficiency leads to death unless the child is placed on mechanical ventilation. These children rarely survive to the second decade.[39] Patients with type 2 SMA are hypotonic but achieve motor milestones up to about age 6 months. They usually can sit without support if placed in a sitting position. Age at death ranges from 7 months to 7 years.[10] SMA type 3 (Kugelburg–Welander disease) usually presents in late childhood or adolescence, and may be mistaken for muscular dystrophy due to the presence of proximal weakness and elevated creatine kinase levels. There is little progression of weakness over the years. Muscle stretch reflexes are normal or depressed but never hyperactive. Patients have a thin body habitus, with atrophy of muscles in the arms and legs. Complications of SMA include restrictive lung disease, with respiratory insufficiency sometimes occurring during sleep before it is otherwise clinically apparent.[39] Clubfoot, scoliosis, kyphosis, and flexion contractures are also seen.[39] These patients are typically very intelligent and can suffer from lack of intellectual challenge.[39]

Adult-onset SMA (onset after age 20), sometimes referred to as type 4, comprises less than 10% of SMA cases. The history is one of slowly progressive proximal weakness due to neurogenic atrophy, and prognosis for normal life expectancy is good. Most cases are autosomal recessive, but autosomal dominant inheritance has been described.[70,71,79] SMA with predominantly distal weakness is rare and also has a relatively benign course.[32]

Table 47-1 Spinal (bulbospinal) muscular atrophies of infancy and childhood

Disease	Age at onset	Weakness distribution	Sit	Stand	Walk	Course
Werdnig–Hoffmann disease						
Type 1	<2 months	Proximal legs abducted; face, fingers, toes normal	–	–	–	Usually die by age 2–3 years
Type 2	2–12 months	Proximal thigh and hip muscles	+	+	–	Most die during first decade, some live through second decade
Kugelberg–Welander disease	2–17 years (mean 9 years)	Normal early development; shoulder and hip girdle atrophy (Gower's sign frequently present)	+	+	May walk for 20–40 years after onset	—

+, Ability present; –, ability not present.
(After Swaiman 1989,[96] with permission.)

Pathology Autopsy reveals thinned ventral spinal roots, and loss of motor neurons in spinal cord and brain stem. Dorsal columns and lateral corticospinal tracts are spared.[97]

Spinal and bulbar muscular atrophy (Kennedy syndrome)

Kennedy syndrome is an uncommon X-linked recessive disorder due to excessive numbers of cytosine-adenine-guanine (CAG) triplets in the androgen receptor gene.[50] The number of trinucleotide repeats in normal subjects is 17–26, while the number in patients with Kennedy disease is between 40 and 65.

Clinical features Patients have progressive weakness and atrophy of bulbar musculature as well as proximal more than distal limb muscles. Peripheral neuropathy, decreased muscle stretch reflexes, and tremor are also seen in a majority of the patients. Gynecomastia is very common, and diabetes mellitus occurs in a higher incidence than in the general population. Age of onset ranges from 20 to 40 years.[97] Female carriers are asymptomatic, but there is a report of mild subclinical abnormalities on electrodiagnostic testing and muscle biopsy.[92] Diagnosis can be suspected in adult men with typical clinical features and neurogenic changes on EMG. Genetic testing for confirmation of the diagnosis is commercially available.

Pathology The CAG expansion in the gene does not result in complete absence of androgen receptor function. Decreased function of the receptor also does not appear to be the cause of the neurologic symptoms in Kennedy disease, because patients with complete androgen insensitivity syndrome do not develop neurologic symptoms.[57] Instead, the presence of nuclear inclusions containing mutant androgen receptor protein in motor neurons of the brain stem and spinal cord (a pathologic hallmark of the disease[51]) appears to play an as yet undetermined role in the pathogenesis.[45,84,98]

Fazio–Londe disease

This disorder was first described by Fazio and Londe in families with progressive bulbar paralysis. It is a degenerative disorder of the motor neurons affecting the motor cranial nerve nuclei throughout the brain stem, with onset in childhood. There are at least three distinct subtypes: a very rare autosomal dominant form, and two variants with probable autosomal recessive inheritance in which onset may be early or late. In the early-onset type, respiratory failure and rapid progression to death occur. The clinical course is protracted, with less respiratory involvement[54] in the late-onset type.

Poliomyelitis and postpolio syndrome

Poliomyelitis is a viral infection involving the anterior horn cells (lower motor neurons), producing weakness in affected bulbar and/or spinal myotomes. Prior to the advent of the polio vaccine, polio was the most common viral infection of the central nervous system.[59] Only about 1% of patients developed paralysis. Initial symptoms were fever, malaise, headache, and gastrointestinal or upper respiratory tract symptoms. In rare cases, the symptoms would progress to worsening headache and neck stiffness, followed in 2–5 days by myalgias and paralysis.[59] Spinal fluid protein and cell count could be normal initially, but within a few days would be mild to moderately elevated. Weakness was typically asymmetric, and more common in the lower extremities. Careful neurologic examination or EMG testing could often demonstrate more widespread weakness than the patient had noticed. Maximal recovery could take years, and could be complete or partial. Initial medically approved therapy consisted of splinting or casting affected limbs. An Australian nurse named Sister Kenny began advocating in 1944 a program of early mobilization and application of moist heat packs. Although her ideas were initially rejected by established medicine, many were later adopted.[59] After development of the

---

Box 47.3 Postpolio syndrome: criteria for establishing a diagnosis[31]

- Confirmed history of paralytic polio
- Partial to fairly complete neurologic and functional recovery
- Period of neurologic and functional stability for at least 15 years
- Onset of two or more of the following symptoms since achieving stability:
  Unaccustomed fatigue
  New weakness in muscles previously affected and/or unaffected
  Muscle and/or joint pain
  Functional loss
  Cold intolerance
  New atrophy
- No other medical explanation for the new health problems

---

polio vaccine, acute poliomyelitis became rare in the USA, primarily occurring only in immunocompromised patients exposed to live-virus vaccine. It is, unfortunately, still a public health problem in some developing countries.

Patients with a history of polio infection may develop fatigue and worsening muscle weakness several years or even decades after the initial infection. This phenomenon was first recognized in the nineteenth century by Raymond, Charcot, and others,[67] and has been termed the *postpolio syndrome* (PPS). PPS has been reported to affect 28.5–64% of polio survivors.[44,102] The diagnosis of PPS is usually one of exclusion. It might be helpful to use the criteria established by Halstead and Rossi when evaluating a patient's complaints (see Box 47-3).

Many symptoms appear to be related to overuse of weak muscles: abnormal muscle fatigue with delayed recovery after heavy use; myalgias; and pain from chronic stress on joints, ligaments, and tendons in paretic limbs.[43] Progressive scoliosis, uneven limb size, and poor posture can also contribute to the development of pain. Pain then leads to limitation of physical activity, which results in disuse weakness and atrophy.[43] The cause of PPS is unknown, but the most accepted hypothesis is that excess metabolic demand on residual motor neurons leads to their eventual deterioration.[43,53]

Studies to determine the presence of other potential causes for the patient's symptoms should be performed. These should include electrodiagnostic studies to investigate possible neuropathy, radiculopathy, or myopathy. Neuroimaging (MRI or computed tomography [CT] scan) should be considered to exclude such disorders as spinal foraminal or canal stenosis. A sleep study can demonstrate sleep apnea or another sleep disorder that could cause fatigue and daytime somnolence.

West Nile virus

West Nile virus infection has recently been associated with a poliomyelitis-like syndrome. It is a mosquito-borne illness that was first identified in 1937 in the West Nile district of Uganda. It was eventually found to be widespread in the Eastern hemisphere.[73] In August 1999, a cluster of 59 cases of meningo-

encephalitis associated with muscle weakness occurred in New York City. This was soon discovered to have paralleled an illness causing deaths of large numbers of birds in the area. The epidemics in both humans and in birds were eventually shown to be due to the West Nile virus.[63] Since then, there has been spread of illness to other regions of the USA. Most human infections are not clinically apparent. According to surveys conducted in New York City in 1999 and 2000, only 1 in 150 infections results in meningitis or encephalitis. Risk factors for severe neurologic symptoms include advanced age and immunosuppression. Typical early symptoms include malaise, nausea, vomiting, eye pain, headache, myalgias, and rash. About half of hospitalized patients in the USA during 1999 and 2000 had severe muscle weakness, and about 10% of patients in the New York outbreak had complete flaccid paralysis.[63] The usually asymmetric paralysis has been associated with significant active denervation changes on EMG, and abnormal signal in anterior spinal cord or spinal roots on MRI. Autopsies have shown inflammation and loss of anterior horn cells in the spinal cord.[42] Neurologic symptoms can be attributed to West Nile virus only if antiviral IgM antibody is detected in cerebrospinal fluid by enzyme-linked immunosorbent assay, West Nile virus nucleic acid is detected in cerebrospinal fluid, there is a fourfold increase in neutralizing IgG antibodies between acute and convalescent sera, or virus is isolated from brain or spinal cord.[82] Management is primarily supportive, although possible treatment with intravenous gamma globulin prepared from Israeli donors (where the disease is endemic) is being tested.[82]

Paraneoplastic motor neuron disease

Rarely, motor neuron disorders have been reported in association with an underlying cancer. These can be pure lower motor neuron, pure upper motor neuron, or a combination compatible with a diagnosis of ALS. Underlying cancer types include lymphoma (both Hodgkin and non-Hodgkin), breast cancer, renal cell carcinoma, small cell lung carcinoma, and ovarian carcinoma.[22,104] Some patients have been reported to have positive paraneoplastic antibodies, such as anti-Hu[22] and anti-Purkinje cell (anti-Yo) antibodies.[49] Improvement occurs following treatment of the underlying malignancy in some cases.

CLINICAL EVALUATION IN MOTOR NEURON DISEASES

History

The first step in the diagnosis of any motor neuron disorder is obtaining the history from the patient and/or the patient's family. The location of symptoms at onset and their rate of progression should be noted. The pattern of weakness, whether more proximal or distal, can provide clues to the diagnosis. With proximal weakness, patients can complain of difficulty rising from a chair, climbing stairs, reaching into cabinets, or washing their hair. With distal weakness, patients might complain of tripping, or difficulty writing or grasping objects. Leg stiffness, leg 'dragging', or difficulty walking can be symptoms of spasticity. Difficulty swallowing, malnourishment as evidenced by weight loss, or changes in speech quality suggest bulbar muscle weakness. Respiratory muscle involvement is suggested by shortness of breath when supine or with minimal exertion, or early morning headaches. Muscle twitches (fasciculations) might be noted by the patient or family. Although cramps are frequent complaints in patients with ALS, myalgias, sharp or shooting pain, tingling, or burning are not typical and should raise a question of an alternative or possibly superimposed disorder. Details of the family history (including ascertainment of any members affected with any gait disorder, progressive weakness, or need for a wheelchair) are important, because many motor neuron diseases are inherited. Finally, assessing the patient's ability for self-care and level of support from family or community is important in planning long-term care or determining the need for assistive devices.

Physical examination

Muscles should be inspected for the presence of atrophy or fasciculations. Passive movement of the limbs allows detection of contractures or of changes in tone. Manual muscle testing in adults or children able to cooperate demonstrates the level of muscle function and reveals the pattern of weakness. Patients with SMA typically have symmetric proximal weakness, while ALS patients typically have asymmetric weakness that, at least initially, is worse distally. In upper motor neuron disorders, muscle stretch reflexes should be increased or relatively preserved in weak limbs. Reflexes will be decreased or absent in lower motor neuron disorders. Gait often demonstrates the waddling and lumbar lordosis associated with proximal weakness, the foot drop associated with distal weakness, or the slow 'scissoring' gait associated with spasticity. The sensory examination should be normal.

Laboratory investigations

Electrodiagnostic testing is important in the evaluation of any patient suspected of having a motor neuron disease. The presence of sensory nerve conduction abnormalities argues for an alternative diagnosis in lieu of or in addition to motor neuron disease (except in Kennedy disease, see above). Motor nerve conduction studies can be normal or show low-amplitude responses, if there has been significant loss of motor neurons to the muscle that is being used to record a response. Conduction velocities should be normal or near normal, and there should be no evidence of conduction block. EMG typically demonstrates fibrillations or positive waves in muscles affected by lower motor neuron degeneration. Chronic neuropathic changes, such as high-amplitude and long-duration polyphasic potentials and reduced recruitment of motor units, are seen, particularly in the more slowly progressing diseases such as SMA. In pure upper motor neuron disorders, the EMG, with rare exceptions (see above), should not show signs of active or chronic denervation.

Muscle biopsy is often necessary in the evaluation of patients with suspected childhood SMA, or in any case in which the differential diagnosis includes myopathy. If the ALS patient presents with typical upper and lower motor neuron signs and with electrodiagnostic evidence of widespread active denervation, muscle biopsy is not usually necessary. The biopsy of an affected muscle shows denervation atrophy. In infants and young children, this is seen as areas with numerous small rounded muscle fibers. In older children and adults, small angular fibers that are typical of acute denervation, and fiber-type grouping that is evidence of chronic denervation with reinnervation, are seen. Significant inflammation or vasculitis suggests an inflammatory condition rather than a motor neuron disorder.

Neuroimaging studies are important to search for evidence of a structural cause for muscle atrophy or hyperreflexia. It should be directed by the localization of the symptoms and signs found during the patient interview and examination. MRI is the method of choice for evaluating brain, spinal cord, and nerve roots or plexuses. If an MRI is contraindicated (i.e. in a patient with a cardiac pacemaker or other contraindication), CT scan with contrast of the brain or CT myelography of the spine might be necessary. Table 47.2 lists other laboratory tests that might be indicated to rule out other causes of the patient's symptoms. Spinal fluid protein levels can be mildly elevated in ALS, but not usually over 100 mg/dL, and cell count and immunoglobulin index and synthetic rate should be normal. Serum creatine kinase levels are usually normal in SMA types 1 and 2, but often mildly elevated in SMA type 3, adult-onset SMA, ALS, and Kennedy disease. They can also be elevated rarely in PPS. The elevation does not usually exceed 10 times the upper limit of normal.

Pharmacologic treatment

Because the etiology and pathogenesis of most motor neuron diseases is still uncertain, treatment remains mostly symptomatic. There are various potential treatments that are being studied worldwide, however, that might one day prove beneficial in curing or halting the progression of some of these disorders.

Pharmacologic treatment of amyotrophic lateral sclerosis

Riluzole is a Food and Drug Administration (FDA)-approved agent used in the treatment of ALS. It is a neuroprotective drug that modulates glutamatergic transmission. Prospective, double-blind, placebo-controlled studies have shown that riluzole slows the progression of ALS, and it may improve the survival in patients with bulbar-onset ALS.[7] The dosage used in the study was 100 mg/day in two divided doses given orally. Subsequently, studies showed a significant difference in the speed of progression between the riluzole and placebo groups in less severely affected ALS patients, suggesting that riluzole maintained patients in milder health states longer.[81] Adverse effects include asthenia, spasticity, and usually mild elevations in

Table 47-2 Laboratory evaluation of amyotrophic lateral sclerosis

Test	Condition mimicking amyotrophic lateral sclerosis
Serum protein electrophoresis with immunofixation	Lymphoma with paraneoplastic myelopathy
Vitamin B_{12} level	Vitamin B_{12} deficiency myeloneuropathy
Methylmalonic acid level	
Homocysteine	
Human T-cell leukemia virus types 1 and 2	Infectious myelopathy
HIV types 1 and 2	
Rapid plasma reagin treponemal antibodies	
Lyme antibodies	
Angiotensin-converting enzyme	Sarcoid myelopathy
Parathyroid hormone	Weakness, muscle pain, fasciculations
Thyroid hormone	
Hexosaminidase A and B levels	Hereditary lower motor neuronopathy
Spinal fluid analysis for IgG synthetic rate and index, protein, cells; IgG index, synthetic rate normal	Inflammatory myelopathy
Creatine kinase	Myopathy

aminotransferase levels. It is a very expensive drug and does not improve survival beyond an average of 3 months.

Other agents have been or are being studied in the treatment of ALS. Minocycline holds promise, as it has been shown to delay disease onset and improve survival in rodent models of ALS. Phase 3 trials are currently underway to study its effects in individuals with ALS.[28] Creatine monohydrate, celecoxib, antiretroviral drugs, and antioxidants are other agents that have been and are being studied. Various growth factors, including brain-derived neurotrophic factor, insulin-like growth factor-1,[8] and ciliary neurotrophic factor,[55] have failed to show any beneficial effect. With the lack of a cure for ALS, stem cell transplantation is an attractive option for future research.

Pharmacologic treatment of other motor neuron diseases

Sodium butyrate[16] and valproic acid[95] have been found to increase the amount of SMN protein, and are being studied extensively as treatment options in SMA. In patients with spinal and bulbar muscular atrophy, leuprorelin, a luteinizing hormone-releasing hormone agonist that reduces testosterone release from the testes, might be a potential treatment option. It has been reported to rescue motor dysfunction and nuclear accumulation of mutant androgen receptors in male transgenic mice.[45] Highly active antiretroviral therapy, composed of multiple anti-HIV drugs, is recommended in patients with HIV-related myelopathy. In cases of tropical spastic paraparesis, no antiviral agents effectively treat the condition. However, reports have suggested a favorable immunomodulatory effect of high doses of vitamin C in such patients.[44]

Symptomatic treatment

Sialorrhea causes significant stress to the patient, and can be controlled with pharmacologic intervention. Options include glycopyrrolate, amitriptyline, benztropine, trihexyphenidyl hydrochloride, and transdermal hyoscine.[55] Suction machines and mechanical insufflation–exsufflation are effective in extracting mucus from the airway (see Ch. 35).[55] Additional treatments include botulinum toxin A injections,[25] surgery,[27] and radiotherapy of the salivary glands.[93]

Pseudobulbar affect or emotional lability, in which there is pathologic crying or laughing, is encountered in about 50% of patients with ALS. Agents used to control this include amitryptiline,[55] fluvoxamine,[55] fluoxetine, and sertraline. Many patients may also have sleep, appetite, and other mood symptoms such as depression. These factors must be kept in mind while choosing the appropriate drug for pseudobulbar affect.

Spasticity can occasionally cause pain and limit ambulation. It can also affect speech and swallowing, leading to increased bulbar difficulties. Various agents can be tried to treat spasticity, with baclofen being the most commonly used. Baclofen dosage varies from 10 mg to 80 mg given orally in divided doses. The baclofen intrathecal pump has been used to treat severe spasticity when other agents have failed. Adverse effects of baclofen include fatigue, weakness, and drowsiness. Other agents that can be tried include tizanidine, diazepam, and dantrolene sodium. Botulinum toxin A can also be used as an antispasticity agent,[91] although it is not FDA-approved for this indication. It is not recommended in ALS, because it can increase weakness. Further details of spasticity management are discussed in Chapter 31.

Other pharmacologic agents

Quinine sulfate has been used to treat cramps, as have baclofen and gabapentin. Barring a single case report of modafinil in ALS,[94] there have been no published reports of treatment of fatigue in ALS. Amantadine and modafinil, however, have been reported to be useful in patients with fatigue from other neurologic diseases, including multiple sclerosis. It can be considered for use in patients with ALS as well. Pain is a common complaint of patients with longstanding weakness and limitation of ability to change position. Some authors suggest the use of non-steroidal antiinflammatory drugs for initial treatment of pain in patients with ALS.[41] Opiate medications can be used for intractable pain, but have the potential to exacerbate respiratory insufficiency and constipation in these patients.[41] Other symptoms often encountered in treating patients with motor neuron diseases include insomnia and anxiety. Zolpidem tartrate, lorazepam, or opioids may be used to treat insomnia, while buspirone hydrochloride, alprazolam, and opioids can be used for anxiety.

GENERAL PRINCIPLES OF REHABILITATION

Supportive care is just as important as medications in treating patients with motor neuron disease and in managing the multitude of issues that arise as the disease progresses. An interdisciplinary team that includes neurologists, physiatrists, physical and occupational therapists, speech pathologists, orthotists, dieticians, social workers, psychologists, and others can work effectively to provide the needed care for patients and their families. One of the most important goals of treatment in physical medicine and rehabilitation is to maximize functional independence. This goal holds true for patients with motor neuron disease as well. It is critical to educate patients and caregivers on the expected disease progression, so that they can prepare themselves for the future.

The role of exercise

The use of exercise in patients with a neuromuscular disease is often controversial. The possible deleterious effects of exercise on muscle fibers are sometimes conveyed to patients, but the scientific data to support this are not clear. It appears that some form of exercise is both physically and psychologically beneficial throughout the disease process. Physical and occupational therapists should be consulted to instruct patients on an appropriate exercise routine, and to provide education in various other areas important to functional independence.

Therapies at each stage of motor neuron disease

Although each motor neuron disease has a different presentation and clinical progression, it can be helpful to use Sinaki and Mulder's description of the six stages of ALS as a guide in formulating therapies and treatment.[18,90] During stage 1, the patient is independent in mobility and activities of daily living. Therapy for this stage focuses on patient and caregiver education, psychologic support, home safety evaluation, and energy conservation techniques. Normal physical activities should be continued, and active range of motion exercises, submaximal aerobic strengthening, and general conditioning exercises should be prescribed. Patients should be advised to avoid overuse and fatigue, and to pace themselves appropriately.

During stage 2, the patient with ALS will have moderate generalized weakness, resulting in slightly decreased independence in mobility and activities of daily living. The patient might benefit from bracing, especially with ankle–foot orthoses, mobile arm supports, and wrist supports. Occupational therapists can be particularly helpful in fabricating upper limb orthoses, which can help facilitate fine motor coordination of the upper limbs (see Chs 15 and 16). Adaptive equipment needs for activities of daily living can be assessed and provided (see Ch. 27). Passive range of motion of upper and lower extremities should be taught to patients and caregivers, and incorporated into a daily routine. Depending on the level of disability, it might still be possible for some patients to perform muscle strengthening and endurance exercises with appropriate instruction. A stationary bicycle is often a safe mode of aerobic exercise for patients during this stage.

Patients in stage 3 of ALS are still ambulatory, but typically have marked weakness of certain muscle groups. They usually require assistance for transfers and activities of daily living. Patients often need further bracing in this stage, and should also be assessed for a wheelchair. A lightweight manual wheelchair might be useful initially, but patients with ALS almost always require a power wheelchair to maintain their independence (see Ch. 18). Many funding agencies in the USA limit the number of wheelchairs a patient can receive in a specific time period. For example, a typical rule is one wheelchair for 5 years. If the patient has such a funding agency rule, then it is important that the patient be prescribed the expensive power chair. The less expensive manual wheelchair can often be obtained as a loan from charitable organizations.

Neck extensor weakness often starts to occur in this stage, and patients report fatigue and difficulty holding their head up. A cervical collar should be considered for this situation.

Passive range of motion exercises should continue, with a particular focus on the shoulder joints to prevent loss of shoulder range of motion and painful adhesive capsulitis as the disease progresses. Spasticity can develop due to the upper motor neuron involvement. Drory et al. reviewed the effect of exercise on patients with ALS and found that, at 3 months, patients performing 15 min of exercise twice daily had significantly less spasticity than control patients.[19] If patients are safe doing so, they should continue using aerobic exercises such as riding a stationary bicycle or walking in a pool with supervision. Home modifications, including bathroom revisions, ramp installations, and grab bars, should be well underway or completed by this time if it is clinically apparent that the patient will need them.

Stage 4 is characterized by severe lower extremity and mild upper extremity weakness. Patients will be exclusively wheelchair users during this time. Some can perform activities of daily living at a wheelchair level. A power wheelchair with features including, but not limited to, a reclining back, tilt in space, custom seating, and a modifiable control system should strongly be considered (see Ch. 18). A hospital bed with a pressure-relieving mattress can help with bed mobility and reduce skin breakdown. Lifting aids such as a Hoyer lift or a pivot lift can be very helpful for patients and caregivers. Proper instruction on the use of these devices is critical to avoid injury. Active and passive range of motion exercises should be continued during this stage of ALS.

Patients in stage 5 have sufficient weakness that they will require assistance with transfers, activities of daily living, and all types of mobility. Pain arising from spasticity or musculoskeletal conditions might need to be the focus of the therapies. Family training on safe transfers, lifting, and positioning should be completed at this point. The caregiver should continue to administer passive range of motion exercises.

Stage 6 is the final stage of ALS, at which time the patients are usually in bed on a full-time basis and dependent for all activities. Cardiopulmonary physical therapy techniques can be important in optimizing ventilatory perfusion matching, to mobilize secretions, and to provide cough assistance (see Ch. 35).[18] The administration of passive range of motion continues, and hospice care is often instituted at this time to help meet the other needs of the patient and caregiver.

Although the stages described above are specific to ALS, physicians treating patients with other motor neuron diseases can follow a similar protocol depending on the specific disease and resulting level of disability. It is important to explain the disease process and expected progression to patients and caregivers. An exercise program involving physical and occupational therapists should include instructing patients on proper techniques and guidelines for their individual exercise routine. It is prudent to have patients avoid overuse and fatigue when exercising, and to restrict their activities to those where safety will not be compromised.

Speech and swallowing therapy

Speech and swallowing problems during the course of motor neuron disease can be a major cause of frustration, anxiety, and depression for both patients and caregivers. Patients should be monitored closely by family members and healthcare professionals for progressive dysphagia (see Ch. 28). A speech–language pathologist can perform a bedside swallowing evaluation or a more involved imaging study to evaluate the degree of dysphagia. The information obtained can then be used to guide treatment and recommendations on diet. Mild dysphagia can

often be managed with adjustments of head position and/or by diet modifications, such as adding thickening agents to liquids. As dysphagia progresses, supplemental tube feedings might be needed. Neuromuscular electrical stimulation is a fairly new form of therapy that can be tried for patients with dysphagia as well. It is a non-invasive treatment that consists of transcutaneous electrical stimulation applied through electrodes placed on the neck to stimulate inactive swallowing muscles.[24]

A registered dietician can be a valuable adjunct to the dysphagia evaluation and treatment described above. Close monitoring of body weight and options for supplemental calories or complete meals are some of the issues about which a dietician can educate the patient and family. Both the dietician and speech–language pathologist can provide insight into when tube feedings should be implemented. Sometimes tube feedings are indicated for patients who can still safely swallow, but are unable to fulfill their nutritional needs because of excessive fatigue of the swallowing muscles. In many cases, patients choose to continue to eat what they enjoy and can still manage orally, while the feeding tube reduces the burden of eating for calories.[23] In other cases, patients might need to rely completely on tube feedings if they are at severe risk of aspirating with any oral nutrition. Poor nutritional status is associated with severe respiratory muscle weakness and diminished pulmonary function,[3] further stressing the importance of ensuring adequate nutritional support.

There are various types of tubes available for nutritional supplementation. Nasogastric tubes are an option, but in most cases a more permanent option is indicated due to the nature of the disease. A percutaneous endoscopic gastrostomy can be safely and conveniently placed under local anesthesia, and can avoid the gastrointestinal symptoms often associated with a jejunostomy.[23] Patients and caregivers should be educated on the proper care of the feeding tube to maintain its functionality. Education should also be provided on body positioning to decrease the risk of aspiration.

Bulbar involvement can lead to dysarthria. In motor neuron disease, dysarthria will usually be one of three types: flaccid, spastic, or mixed (see Ch. 3).[57] Speech–language pathologists can assist in evaluating the type of dysarthria, and advising on the appropriate treatment and compensatory strategies. In the initial stages of treatment, the focus is usually to maximize intelligibility strategies and introduce energy conservation techniques. With worsening dysarthria and/or anarthria, the incorporation of augmentative communication devices plays an important role.[57] Augmentative communication devices should be customized to meet the needs of the patient. For example, if the upper extremities are too weak to point to letters on a communication board or to type words on a keyboard, a device that utilizes a visual scanning mechanism can be helpful.

Respiratory management

Most patients with motor neuron disease develop respiratory compromise. Patients with ALS have at least 84% of the mortality from pulmonary complications and respiratory failure.[4] Pulmonary complications can result from bulbar or respiratory muscle weakness, or a combination of these. Symptoms can include dyspnea on exertion or when lying supine, difficulty with coughing and talking, difficulty falling asleep, morning headaches, nightmares, tremor, nervousness, hyperhidrosis, tachycardia, and anorexia.[87] Healthcare professionals should be aware of and constantly monitor patients' pulmonary function. Early intervention includes a frank discussion of possible progression of symptoms, to allow time for patients and their families to think about their options and the desired level of aggressiveness in treatment. One of the best ways to accomplish this is through referral to a pulmonologist who is familiar with motor neuron diseases.

Management can initially include chest physiotherapy and postural drainage, especially if the patient has difficulty clearing secretions from the chest.[87] Preventing pulmonary infections is a primary goal in respiratory management, and pneumococcal and influenza vaccines should be administered as well. Respiratory muscle exercise can be instituted. In many cases, a training program can delay the onset of ventilatory failure in ALS.[86] A suction machine is a very helpful device for patients who are unable to clear their secretions.

As respiratory compromise worsens, various non-invasive devices can be considered. One of the most practical options to consider is non-invasive intermittent positive-pressure ventilation. Using it at night can alleviate many of the symptoms that patients experience secondary to respiratory compromise.[87] Non-invasive ventilation can postpone initiation of tracheostomy with mechanical ventilation by several months, prolong life, and improve comfort in the patient who refuses total mechanical ventilation. It can also be used to give the patient a limited form of mechanical ventilation, while still considering the option of full invasive mechanical ventilation.[86]

Psychologic management

Traditionally, motor neuron disease is thought of as a disease process that affects the body but spares the mind. Dementia due to involvement of the frontotemporal area of the brain can occur, and can occasionally even be the presenting feature of the disease.[38] Patients with this variant of motor neuron disease usually exhibit changes in personality and cognitive dysfunction; however, verbal and non-verbal memory are often well preserved.[64,72] Neuropsychologic cognitive evaluations can be especially helpful in determining the type of dementia and recommending strategies for coping with it.

Patients with motor neuron disease commonly experience a wide range of emotions, including anxiety, denial, anger, and depression. Studies have shown the prevalence of depression ranging from 5 to 75%.[23] A study by Hogg et al. examined correlations between the level of impairment and psychologic symptoms.[36] This study found that 44% of the sample had depression, and noted that patients who were more physically impaired were more depressed. It also found that more severe impairments of speech correlated with increased anxiety.

In addition to the psychologic impact of motor neuron disease on patients, caregivers may also be affected. A study by Goldstein et al. found that anxiety and depression were reported by caregivers, with the levels of depression correlating to some extent with the degree of patients' functional limitations.[26] They also noted that the greater the caregiver's level of current strain in caring for their partner, the greater was the caregiver's perception of a loss of intimacy between them.[26]

Addressing the psychologic issues that arise should be an important focus of treatment. Psychologists and social workers can be helpful in providing individual and family therapy, and can serve as a resource for patients and families. Emotional support is also provided by established organizations, such as the Muscular Dystrophy Association, the ALS Association, and other community groups. Patients and their families should be strongly encouraged to utilize the available resources, because coping with the illness can be very difficult and can have a strong emotional impact on a family.

In addition to psychologic supportive therapy, medications such as antidepressants and anxiolytics should be used as needed. Many patients are resistant to taking these types of medications. However, if they are indicated, their use should be discussed with patients and their families. Side effect profiles should be considered before prescribing these medications. In some instances, the side effects of certain medications can be beneficial for the patient. For example, the anticholinergic side effects of tricyclic antidepressants can be helpful for patients experiencing sialorrhea.

Bracing and equipment

Equipment needs vary depending on the disease process and the patient's level of disability. Orthoses can be simple in design, but can offer patients an opportunity to improve their comfort and/or functional independence. Cervical collars can provide much needed support for patients with neck extensor weakness. If the neck extensor weakness is mild, a soft foam collar may be adequate. Sometimes these are not well tolerated due to skin irritation and excessive sweating. A wire frame cervical collar can provide support even as weakness progresses, and might be better tolerated than the foam collar.

An ankle–foot orthosis can allow safer ambulation for patients with lower limb weakness. Assessment of the degree of support the ankle–foot orthosis needs to provide the patient requires a careful evaluation. An analysis of gait and specific muscle testing of muscles providing inversion, eversion, dorsiflexion, plantar flexion, and knee extension provides the most valuable input on the type of brace to be fabricated.[37] Consideration should also be given to the progression of the disease, and the prescribed brace should be designed to permit later modifications.

In addition to aiding ambulation, an ankle–foot orthosis can also function to passively stretch the ankle plantar flexors. Tightness and contractures that limit ankle dorsiflexion can occur rapidly. Patients and caregivers should be educated on the importance of monitoring the skin for increased pressure areas or breakdown, and adjustments should be made as needed. Lightweight material should be used to fabricate the orthosis when possible, because a heavy brace can prove too difficult to use.

Occupational therapists can provide valuable assistance in fabricating or recommending orthoses that help maximize positioning and upper extremity function. Some of these include wrist splints, dynamic finger extension splints, or thumb shell splints.[14] A mobile arm support or a balanced forearm orthosis can be beneficial for patients who have proximal upper extremity weakness. It supports the weight of the arm and forearm against gravity. This type of orthosis can allow for self-feeding by enabling the user to flex the elbow and bring the hand to the mouth. Utensils with a lightweight built-up grip or an angled shape, plate guards, rocker knives, and lightweight mugs can also be useful for feeding. Occupational therapists can also provide excellent advice on dressing techniques and adaptive equipment, such as button hooks, Velcro straps instead of laces, and long-handled shoehorns that can make the task of dressing easier and less energy-consuming (see Ch. 27).

An assistive device for ambulation can be helpful in some patients. These are usually prescribed progressively, beginning with straight or quad canes, then a walker. Rolling walkers can be beneficial to those with upper limb weakness who are unable to lift a standard walker. Other features that are sometimes helpful include a handheld braking mechanism, basket attachment, or an attached seat (see Ch. 16).

A wheelchair should be considered for patients who can ambulate for only a short distance or who are non-ambulatory. A wheelchair that is both lightweight and portable is initially the most appropriate.[37] Appropriate seating in any wheelchair is necessary to provide adequate support. A solid back improves trunk alignment and helps prevent shoulder and back dysfunction more than a sling type back.[99] Children are frequently placed in larger wheelchairs to allow room for growth. Unfortunately, in many cases these wheelchairs do not provide the support the child needs, and increase the risk of developing contractures and subsequent joint deformities. When a patient can no longer propel a wheelchair, a powered wheelchair might be needed. Before prescribing a power wheelchair, however, a brief cognitive assessment of the patient's ability to manage such a wheelchair should be performed. If the patient is deemed cognitively able to safely use a power wheelchair, an appropriate seating evaluation should be performed to ensure adequate support. It is important to note that a scooter type of wheelchair will not provide the support that a patient with motor neuron disease needs.

The progressive nature of motor neuron diseases should be taken into consideration when developing the features of the wheelchair. The power wheelchair should incorporate mechanisms for pressure relief, facilitation of transfers, reduction of dependent edema, and specialty drive controls that can be adjusted as needed (see Ch. 18) (Fig. 47-1).

It is helpful to review with the patient and family all the potential features of a power wheelchair before prescribing it. Motorized wheelchairs offer patients a slightly greater opportunity for increased activity, comfort, and maneuverability, but are more difficult to load and transport than manual wheelchairs.[99] Because wheelchairs in general and power chairs in particular are expensive, it is important to have a social worker

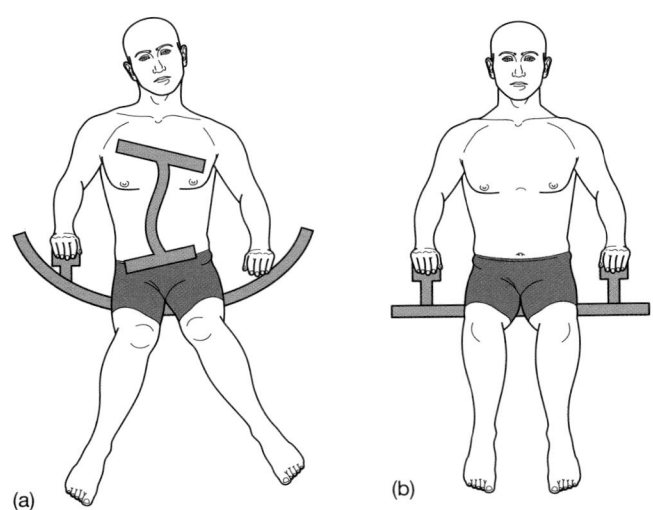

(a)   (b)

Figure 47-1 (**a**) A wide hammock seat promotes deformity. (**b**) Proper positioning includes a firm seat and correct arm height.

involved who can assist in obtaining all available funding resources.

Lifts are often essential for lifting and transferring patients with motor neuron disease. Fully electric hospital beds can help make position changes easier and provide pressure relief. These beds also allow the patient to be positioned high enough for caregivers to assist them with less chance of back injury. Patients and caregivers should be instructed on the importance of turning every 2 h to decrease the risk of skin breakdown. A mattress overlay might also be indicated to alleviate pressure on susceptible areas and prevent pressure ulcers (see Ch. 33).

Toileting is an area that often becomes very difficult for patients with motor neuron diseases, despite the fact that bowel and bladder function are often preserved. A variety of equipment is available to assist in toileting, but should only be prescribed after obtaining an understanding of the patient's level of function, available assistance, and home environment. Equipment such as a raised toilet seat with armrests, bedside commode, or urinal for men can help the patient be as independent as possible with toileting activities. In the later stages of motor neuron disease, protective undergarments and/or indwelling or condom catheters might need to be utilized. Toileting can sometimes be a very stressful activity for patients with impaired mobility, because the entire process involves many skills and is energy-consuming. It is not unusual to discover that some patients limit their oral intake in the hope of requiring fewer trips to the commode. These patients should be monitored for signs of dehydration and nutritional deficits.

Bathing is also quite challenging in many patients, especially in the later stages of the disease. Bathroom modifications, specialized equipment, or a combination of these can be helpful. A tub bench and/or handheld shower can be useful if the patient is still able to safely bathe in the bathroom. As mobility declines, sponge baths by a caregiver are often the safest option, minimizing risk of injury to either the patient or the caregiver.

Rehabilitation management of postpolio syndrome

Many patients who have had a history of poliomyelitis can develop new musculoskeletal and neuromuscular symptoms several years after their initial illness. Although symptoms of PPS can vary, it has been reported that the most common complaint of patients is that of decreased endurance, limiting their ability to perform their activities of daily living.[29] Because the diagnosis of PPS is usually one of exclusion, physicians should evaluate for other possible causes of symptoms before diagnosing PPS.

The treatment of PPS can include medications, assistive devices, adaptive equipment, and exercise. Physicians or physical therapists should provide education on the types of exercise that the patient can use. Studies have shown that non-fatiguing exercise programs can improve mild to moderate weakness without laboratory evidence of muscle damage[1,19,44] or overwork weakness. A key point to stress in an exercise regimen is to avoid fatigue and overuse, and to pace oneself appropriately. Muscle fatigue is a common complaint of patients with PPS, and can usually be improved with bouts of activity interspersed with frequent rest breaks.[2] Swimming might be a beneficial option, as the buoyancy of water reduces strain on joints. Flexibility and cardiorespiratory fitness have also been shown to improve in patients with PPS who have participated in aquatic exercise programs.[76]

Musculoskeletal pain is often a major issue in patients with PPS. Residual weakness from the initial bout of polio can result in long-term overuse and stressing of joints.[43] The pain can limit physical activity, which if not recognized and treated early on, can contribute to further deterioration of function due to deconditioning, as well as other complications of immobility.

SUMMARY

Motor neuron diseases can affect any age, with ALS being the most common type in adults. The various motor neuron diseases differ in their clinical presentation and course. Optimal patient care and treatment require a clear understanding of the individual disease process and clinical progression. An interdisciplinary team of healthcare professionals can combine their efforts to maximize comprehensive care to the patient, with the main goal of improving the quality of life.

DEDICATION

This chapter is dedicated to Mr. Tilak Raj Khanna, whose battle with ALS ended on November 4, 2003. His goal of educating his family continued even throughout his illness as he gracefully demonstrated important lessons about life and death. He will always be remembered. May he rest in peace.

REFERENCES

1. Agre JC, Rodriquez AA, Franke TM. Strength, endurance, and work capacity after muscle strengthening exercise in postpolio subjects. Arch Phys Med Rehabil 1997; 78:681–686.
2. Agre JC, Rodriquez AA. Intermittent isometric activity. Arch Phys Med Rehabil 1991; 72:971–977.
3. Arora NS, Rochester DF. Respiratory muscle strength and maximal voluntary ventilation in undernourished patients. Am Rev Respir Dis 1982; 126:5–8.
4. Bach JR. Amyotrophic lateral sclerosis communication status and survival with ventilatory support. Am J Phys Med Rehabil 1993; 72(6):343–349.
5. Basak M, Erturk M, Oflazoglu B, et al. Magnetic resonance imaging in amyotrophic lateral sclerosis. Acta Neurol Scand 2002; 105:395–399.
6. Behan WMH, Maia M. Strumpell's familial spastic paraplegia: genetics and neuropathology. J Neurol Neurosurg Psychiatry 1974; 37:8–20.
7. Bensimon G, Lacomblez L, Meininger V, for the ALS/Riluzole Study Group. A controlled trial of riluzole in amyotrophic lateral sclerosis. N Engl J Med 1994; 330:585–591.
8. Borasio GD, Robberecht W, Leigh PN, et al. A placebo-controlled trial of insulin-like growth factor-I in amyotrophic lateral sclerosis. European ALS/IGF-I Study Group. Neurology 1198; 51:583–586.
9. Brooks BR, Miller RG, Swash M, et al. El Escorial revisited: revised criteria for the diagnosis of amyotrophic lateral sclerosis. ALS and other motor neuron disorders 2000; 1:293–299.
10. Byers RK, Banker BQ. Infantile muscular atrophy. Arch Neurol 1961; 5:140–164.
11. Carter GT, Krivickas LS, Weydt P, et al. Drug therapy for amyotrophic lateral sclerosis: where are we now? J Invest Drugs 2003; 6:147–153.
12. Caselli RJ, Windebank AJ, Petersen RC, et al. Rapidly progressive aphasic dementia and motor neuron disease. Ann Neurol 1993; 33:200–207.
13. Cavalleri F, De Renzi E. Amyotrophic lateral sclerosis with dementia. Acta Neurol Scand 1994; 89:391–394.
14. Chan CW, Sinaki M. Rehabilitation management of the ALS patient. In: Belsh JM, Schiffman PL, eds. Amyotrophic lateral sclerosis: diagnosis and management for the clinician. Armonk: Futura; 1996:315–331.
15. Chancellor AM, Warlow CP. Adult onset motor neuron disease: worldwide mortality, incidence, and distribution since 1950. J Neurol Neurosurg Psychiatry 1992; 55:1106–1115.
16. Chang JG, Hsieh-Li HM, Jong YJ, et al. Treatment of spinal muscular atrophy by sodium butyrate. Proc Natl Acad Sci USA 2001; 98: 9808–9813.
17. Chen YZ, Bennett CL, Huynh HM, et al. DNA/RNA helicase gene mutations in a form of juvenile amyotrophic lateral sclerosis (ALS4). Am J Hum Genet 2004; 74:1128–1135.
18. Dal-Bello-Haas V, Kloos AD, Mitsumoto H. Physical therapy for a patient through six stages of amyotrophic lateral sclerosis. Phys Ther 1998; 78:1312–1323.
19. Drory VE, Goltsman E, Reznik JG, et al. The value of muscle exercise in patients with amyotrophic lateral sclerosis. J Neurol Sci 2001; 191(1-2): 133–137.
20. Festoff BW, Suo A, Citron BA. Prospects for the pharmacotherapy of amyotrophic lateral sclerosis: old strategies and new paradigms for the third millennium. CNS Drugs 2003; 17:699–717.
21. Forestier NL, Maisonobe T, Piquard A, et al. Does primary lateral sclerosis exist? A study of 20 patients and a review of the literature. Brain 2001; 124:1989–1999.
22. Forsyth PA, Dalmau J, Graus F, et al. Motor neuron syndromes in cancer patients. Ann Neurol 1997; 41:703–705.
23. Francis K, Bach JR, DeLisa JA. Evaluation and rehabilitation of patients with adult motor neuron disease. Arch Phys Med Rehabil 1999; 80: 951–963.
24. Freed ML, Freed L, Chatburn RL, et al. Electrical stimulation for swallowing disorders caused by a stroke. Respiratory Care 2001; 46(5):466–474.
25. Giess R, Naumann M, Werner E, et al. Injections of botulinum toxin A into the salivary glands improve sialorrhoea in amyotrophic lateral sclerosis. J Neurol Neurosurg Psychiatry 2000; 69:121–123.
26. Goldstein LH, Adamson M, Jeffrey L, et al. The psychological impact of MND on patients and carers. J Neurol Sci 1998; 160(suppl 1):S114–S121.
27. Good RL, Smith RA. Surgical management of sialorrhea. Laryngoscope 1970; 80:1078–1089.
28. Gordon PH, Moore DH, Gelinas DF, et al. Placebo-controlled phase I/II studies of minocycline in amyotrophic lateral sclerosis. Neurology 2004; 62:1845–1847.

29. Grimby G, Jonsson AL. Disability in poliomyelitis sequelae. Phys Ther 1994; 75(5):415–424.

30. Gurney MR, Pu H, Chiu AY, et al. Motor neuron degeneration in mice that express a human Cu, Zn superoxide dismutase mutation. Science 1994; 264:1772–1775.

31. Halstead LS, Rossi CD. Post-polio syndrome: clinical experience with 132 consecutive outpatients. In: Halstead LS, Wiechers DO, eds. Research and clinical aspects of the late effects of poliomyelitis. White Plains: March of Dimes Birth Defects Foundation; 1987:3–26.

32. Harding AE, Thomas PK. Hereditary distal spinal muscular atrophy: a report on 34 cases and a review of the literature. J Neurol Sci 1980; 45:337–348.

33. Harding AE. Classification of the hereditary ataxias and paraplegias. Lancet 1983; 1:1151–1155.

34. Harding AE. Hereditary spastic paraplegias. Semin Neurol 1993; 13:333–336.

35. Hentati A, Ouahchi K, Pericak-Vance MA, et al. Linkage of a commoner form of recessive amyotrophic lateral sclerosis to chromosome 15q15-q22 markers. Neurogenetics 1998; 2:55–60.

36. Hogg KE, Goldstein LH, Leigh PN. The psychological impact of motor neurone disease. Psychol Med 1994; 24:625–632.

37. Howell C. Physical therapy interventions in the management of amyotrophic lateral sclerosis. In: Mitsumoto H, Norris FH, eds. Amyotrophic lateral sclerosis: a comprehensive guide to management. New York: Demos Publications; 1994:93–117.

38. Hudson AJ. Amyotrophic lateral sclerosis and its association with dementia, parkinsonism and other neurological disorders: a review. Brain 1981; 104:217–247.

39. Iannaccone S. Spinal muscular atrophy. Semin Neurol 1998; 18:19–25.

40. Iwasaki Y, Ikeda K, Ichikawa Y, et al. MRI in ALS patients. Acta Neurol Scand 2003; 107:426.

41. Jackson CA, Bryan WW. Amyotrophic lateral sclerosis. Semin Neurol 1998; 18:27–39.

42. Jeha LE, Sila CA, Lederman RJ, et al. West Nile virus infection: a new paralytic illness. Neurology 2003; 61:55–59.

43. Jubelt B, Agre JC. Characteristics and management of postpolio syndrome. JAMA 2000; 284:412–414.

44. Kataoka A, Imai H, Inayoshi S, et al. Intermittent high-dose vitamin C therapy in patients with HTLV-1 associated myelopathy. J Neurol Neurosurgery Psychiatry 1993; 56:1213–1216.

45. Katsuno M, Adachi H, Doyu M, et al. Leuprorelin rescues polyglutamine-dependent phenotypes in a transgenic model of spinal and bulbar muscular atrophy. Nat Med 2003; 9:768–773.

46. Katz JS, Wolfe GI, Anderson PB, et al. Brachial amyotrophic diplegia. A slowly progressive motor neuron disorder. Neurology 1999; 53:1071–1076.

47. Kawashima T, Dohura K, Kikuchi H, et al. Cognitive dysfunction in patients with amyotrophic lateral sclerosis is associated with spherical or crescent-shaped ubiquitinated intraneuronal inclusions in the parahippocampal gyrus and amygdala, but not in the neostriatum. Acta Neuropathol 2001; 102:467–472.

48. Kobayashi H, Baumbach L, Matise T, et al. A gene for a severe lethal form of X-linked arthrogryposis (X-linked infantile spinal muscular atrophy) maps to human chromosome Xp11.3-q11.2. Hum Mol Genet 1995; 4:1213–1216.

49. Kwaja S, Sripathi N, Ahmad BK, et al. Paraneoplastic motor neuron disease with type 1 Purkinje cell antibodies. Muscle Nerve 1998; 21:943–945.

50. La Spada AR, Wilson EM, Lubahn DB, et al. Androgen receptor gene mutations in X-linked spinal and bulbar muscular atrophy. Nature 1991; 4:77–79.

51. Li M, et al. Nuclear inclusions of the androgen receptor protein in spinal and bulbar muscular atrophy. Ann Neurol 1998; 44:249–254.

52. Lomen-Hoerth C, Murphy J, Langmore S, et al. Are amyotrophic lateral sclerosis patients cognitively normal? Neurology 2003; 60:1094–1097.

53. McComas AJ, Quartly C, Griggs RC. Early and late losses of motor units after poliomyelitis. Brain 1997; 120:1415–1421.

54. McShane MA, Boyd S, Harding B, et al. Progressive bulbar paralysis of childhood. A reappraisal of Fazio–Londe disease. Brain 1992; 115:1889–1900.

55. Miller RG, Rosenberg JA, Gelinas DF, et al. Practice parameter: the care of the patient with amyotrophic lateral sclerosis (an evidence based review). Report of the quality standards subcommittee of the American Academy of Neurology. Neurology 1999; 52:1311–1323.

56. Mitsumoto H, Chad DA, Pioro EP. Speech and communication management. In: Reinhardt RW, Wissler BM, Zuckerman DW, et al, eds. Amyotrophic lateral sclerosis. Philadelphia: FA Davis; 1998:405–418.

57. Mitsumoto H, Cwik VA, Neville H, et al. Motor neuron diseases, part A. Continuum 1997; 3:41–46.

58. Mitsumoto H. Disorders of upper and lower motor neurons. In: Bradley WG, Daroff RB, Fenichel GM, et al, eds. Neurology in clinical practice: the neurological disorders. Boston: Butterworth-Heinemann; 2000:1985–2018.

59. Mulder DW. Clinical observations on acute poliomyelitis. Ann NY Acad Sci 1995; 753:1–10.

60. Munsat TL. Workshop report: International SMA collaboration. Neuromuscul Disord 1991; 1:81.

61. Murakami N. Parkinsonism–dementia complex on Guam—overview of clinical aspects. J Neurol 1999; 246(suppl 2):16–18.

62. Nakano I. Frontotemporal dementia with motor neuron disease (amyotrophic lateral sclerosis with dementia). Neuropathology 2000; 20:68–75.

63. Nash D, Mostashari F, Fine A, et al. The outbreak of West Nile virus infection in the New York City area in 1999. N Engl J Med 2001; 344:1807–1814.

64. Neary D, Snowden JS, Mann DM, et al. Frontal lobe dementia and motor neuron disease. J Neurol Neurosurg Psychiatry 1990; 53:23–32.

65. Neary D, Snowden JS, Mann DMA. Cognitive change in motor neurone disease/amyotrophic lateral sclerosis (MND/ALS). J Neurol Sci 2000; 180:15–20.

66. Nelson LM, Matkin C, Longstreth WT Jr, et al. Population-based case-control study of amyotrophic lateral sclerosis in western Washington State. II. Diet. Am J Epidemiol 2000; 151:164–173.

67. Nollet F, de Visser M. Postpolio syndrome. Arch Neurol 2004; 61:1142–1144.

68. Norris F, Sheperd R, Denys E, et al. Onset, natural history and outcome in idiopathic adult motor neuron disease. J Neurol Sci 1993; 118:48–55.

69. Orlacchio A, Kawarai T, Totaro A, et al. Hereditary spastic paraplegia. Clinical genetic study of 15 families. Arch Neurol 2004; 61:849–855.

70. Pearn J. Autosomal dominant spinal muscular atrophy: a clinical and genetic study. J Neurol Sci 1978; 38:263–275.

71. Pearn JH, Hudgson P, Walton JN. A clinical and genetic study of spinal muscular atrophy of adult onset: the autosomal recessive form as a discrete disease entity. Brain 1978; 101:591–606.

72. Peavy GM, Herzog AG, Rubin NP, et al. Neuropsychological aspects of the dementia of motor neurone disease: a report of two cases. Neurology 1992; 42:1004–1008.

73. Petersen LR, Marfin AA. West Nile virus: a primer for the clinician. Ann Intern Med 2002; 137:173–179.

74. Portet F, Cadihac C, Touchon J, et al. Cognitive impairment in motor neuron disease with bulbar onset. Amyotroph Lateral Scler Other Motor Neuron Disord 2001; 2:23–29.

75. Pringle CE, Hudson AJ, Munoz DG, et al. Primary lateral sclerosis. Clinical features, neuropathology diagnostic criteria. Brain 1992; 115:495–520.

76. Prins JH, Hartung H, Merritt DJ, et al. Effect of aquatic exercise training in persons with poliomyelitis disability. Sports Med Train Rehabil 1994; 5:29–39.

77. Rabin BA, Griffin JW, Crain BJ, et al. Autosomal dominant juvenile amyotrophic lateral sclerosis. Brain 1999; 122:1539–1550.

78. Rakowicz WP, Hodges JR. Dementia and aphasia in motor neuron disease: an underrecognised association? J Neurol Neurosurg Psychiatry 1998; 65:881–889.

79. Rietschel M, Rudnik-Schoneborn S, Zerres K. Clinical variability of autosomal dominant spinal muscular atrophy. J Neurol Sci 1992; 107:65–73.

80. Ringel SP, Murphy JR, Alerson MK, et al. The natural history of amyotrophic lateral sclerosis. Neurology 1993; 43:1316–1322.

81. Riviere M, Meningier V, Zeisser P, et al. An analysis of extended survival in patients with amyotrophic lateral sclerosis treated with riluzole. Arch Neurol 1998; 55:526–528.

82. Roos KL. West Nile encephalitis and myelitis. Curr Opin Neurol 2004; 17:343–346.

83. Rosen DR, Siddique T, Patterson D, et al. Mutations in Cu/Zn superoxide dismutase gene are associated with familial amyotrophic lateral sclerosis. Nature 1993; 362:59–62.

84. Ross CA. Polyglutamine pathogenesis: emergence of unifying mechanisms for Huntington's disease and related disorders. Neuron 2002; 35: 819–822.

85. Rowland LP. Primary lateral sclerosis: disease, syndrome, both or neither? J Neurol Sci 1999; 170:1–4.

86. Schiffman PL. Pulmonary function and respiratory management of the ALS patient. In: Belsh JM, Schiffman PL, eds. Amyotrophic lateral sclerosis: diagnosis and management for the clinician. Armonk: Futura; 1996:333–355.

87. Shaw P. Motor neurone disease. In: Greenwood RJ, Barnes MP, McMillan TM, et al, eds. Handbook of neurological rehabilitation. 2nd edn. New York: Psychology Press; 2003:641–661.

88. Shaw PJ. Genetic inroads in familial ALS. Nat Genet 2001; 29: 103–104.

89. Simpson DM, Tagliati M. Neurologic manifestations of HIV infection. Ann Intern Med 1994; 121:769–785.

90. Sinaki M, Mulder DW. Rehabilitation techniques for patients with amyotrophic lateral sclerosis. Mayo Clinic Proc 1978; 53:173–178.

91. Snow BJ, Tsui JK, Bhatt MH, et al. Treatment of spasticity with botulinum toxin: a double-blind study. Ann Neurol 1990; 28:512–515.

92. Sobue G, Hashizume Y, Mukae E, et al. Subclinical phenotypic expressions in heterozygous females of X-linked recessive bulbospinal neuronopathy. J Neurol Sci 1993; 117:74–78.

93. Stalpers LJA, Moser EC. Results of radiotherapy for drooling in amyotrophic lateral sclerosis. Neurology 2002; 58:1308.

94. Sternbach H. Adjunctive modafinil in ALS. J Neuropsychiatry Clin Neurosci 2002; 14:239.

95. Sumner CJ, Huynh TN, Markowitz JA, et al. Valproic acid increases SMN levels in spinal muscular atrophy patient cells. Ann Neurol 2003; 54:647–654.

96. Swaiman KF. Anterior horn cell and cranial motor neuron disease. In: Swaiman KF, ed. Pediatric neurology: principles and practice, vol 2. St. Louis: Mosby Year-Book; 1989:1083–1103.

97. Tandan R. Disorders of the upper and lower motor neurons. In: Bradley WG, Daroff RB, Fenichel GM, et al, eds. Neurology in clinical practice. Boston: Butterworth Heinemann; 1996:1823–1852.

98. Taylor JP, Fischbeck KH. Altered acetylation in polyglutamine disease: an opportunity for therapeutic intervention? Trends Mol Med 2002; 8:195–197.

99. Trail M, Nelson N, Van JN, et al. Wheelchair use by patients with amyotrophic lateral sclerosis: a survey of user characteristics and selection preference. Arch Phys Med Rehabil 2001; 82:98–102.

100. Trojanowski JQ, Ishihara T, Higuchi M, et al. Amyotrophic lateral sclerosis/parkinsonism dementia complex: transgenic mice provide insights into mechanisms underlying a common tauopathy in an ethnic minority on Guam. Exp Neurol 2002; 176:1–11.

101. Veldink JH, van den Berg LH, Cobben JM, et al. Homozygous deletion of the survival motor neuron 2 gene is a prognostic factor in sporadic ALS. Neurology 2001; 56:749–752.

102. Windebank AJ, Litchy WF, Daube JR, et al. Late effects of the paralytic poliomyelitis in Olmsted County, Minnesota. Neurology 1991; 41: 501–507.

103. Yang Y, Hentati A, Deng HX, et al. The gene encoding alsin, a protein with three guanine-nucleotide exchange factor domains, is mutated in a form of recessive amyotrophic lateral sclerosis. Nat Genet 2001; 29:160–165.

104. Younger DS, Rowland LP, Latov N, et al. Lymphoma, motor neuron disease, and amyotrophic lateral sclerosis. Ann Neurol 1991; 30: 431–433.

Rehabilitation of Patients with Neuropathies

Andrea Peterson and John C. Kincaid

Neuropathies can be generalized or localized, proximal or distal. They can be due to compression, metabolic derangements, toxic exposure, autoimmune inflammation, hereditary causes, infection, and neoplasm. Because many of these produce similar manifestations, determining a specific etiology requires a thorough history of the mode of onset and symptoms produced. Determining if other family members have been similarly affected is also very important. The results of the physical examination help to better define the scope of the problem. The electrodiagnostic evaluation and the results of the laboratory studies of blood, urine, and at times spinal fluid help to further refine the diagnosis. In selected cases, a nerve biopsy might be needed to make the diagnosis.

NERVE ANATOMY AND PHYSIOLOGY

Most peripheral nerves contain both afferent and efferent neurons. There are 12 cranial nerves and 31 spinal nerves, which together form the peripheral nervous system. In the cervical and lumbosacral regions, axons intermingle to form plexuses.

Each spinal nerve innervates a characteristic sensory area (dermatome) (Fig. 48-1) and group of muscles (myotome) (Table 48-1). Individual peripheral nerves also have their own distinctive sensory and motor territories (Fig. 48-2). Knowledge of the usual patterns of sensory and motor innervation is essential in determining the specific nerve or nerve root level of involvement in disease states.

Each peripheral nerve is surrounded by an outer connective tissue sheath called the epineurium. Inside the epineurium, the axons are arranged in fascicles, which are surrounded by a perineurium. Axons can intermingle and cross from one fascicle to another along the course of the nerve. Each individual nerve fiber is surrounded by a membrane called the endoneurium (Fig. 48-3).[133]

Each axon is enclosed by a Schwann cell (see Ch. 10). Unmyelinated axons have only a single layer of the cell membrane and can share the Schwann cell with several other axons. Myelinated fibers are wrapped by multiple layers of Schwann cell membrane and are thereby more effectively insulated. Nodes of Ranvier are longitudinal gaps located between individual Schwann cells. Depolarization occurs in myelinated axons only at these nodes, allowing the nerve impulse to 'jump'

from one node to the next in what is called saltatory conduction or propagation. This process allows for faster impulse transmission with minimal expenditure of energy. Within peripheral nerves, there are an array of axon diameters and degrees of myelination. Tables 48-2 and 48-3 show the common classification systems of nerve fiber types.

CLASSIFICATION OF NEUROPATHIES

Neuropathies are generally divided into two major categories, demyelinating and axonal, depending on whether the primary lesion is in the myelin sheath or the axon.[39] *Demyelination* can be localized, as in a focal neuropathy such as carpal tunnel syndrome (CTS). It can be generalized, as in Guillain–Barré syndrome (GBS). *Axonal* lesions also can be focal or generalized. These can be traumatic in origin, arising secondary to compression, traction, or transaction. They can also occur in generalized polyneuropathies caused by toxic or metabolic derangements. Peripheral neuropathies can also have a mixture of demyelinating and axonal pathology. Localized nerve injuries can be further classified by the amount of myelin versus axonal involvement and the degree of severity. There are two main classification schemes: the Seddon system[125] and the Sunderland system[133] (Table 48-4). The Sunderland system is an expansion of Seddon's divisions. Both are in common usage.

ETIOLOGIES OF NEUROPATHY

There is a wide array of neuropathic disorders, which are usually categorized by etiology. These include hereditary disorders (Box 48-1), toxic disorders (Box 48-2), those associated with systemic diseases and inflammatory processes (Box 48-3), idiopathic disorders (Box 48-4), entrapment disorders (Table 48-5), nutritional disorders (Box 48-5), and those secondary to infectious processes (Box 48-6; Figs. 48-4 and 48-5).

The inherited neuropathies, such as hereditary motor and sensory neuropathy (HMSN) or Charcot–Marie–Tooth (CMT) disease, have been increasingly linked to specific chromosomal abnormalities.[94,98,104,106,116,143,149,156] The predominant cause of neuropathy worldwide is still leprosy. However, the most common causes of diffuse peripheral neuropathies seen in the developed world are diabetes and alcoholism. A specific cause

Text continued on p. 1076

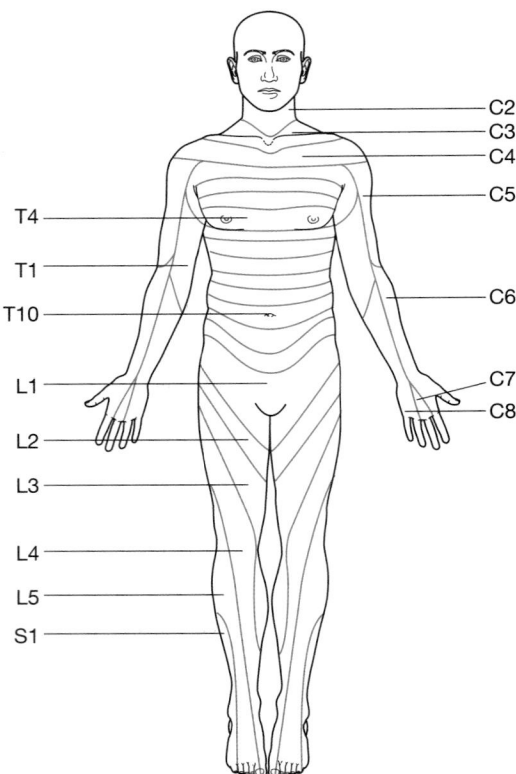

Figure 48-1 Dermatomal innervation pattern of the spinal nerves. Each spinal nerve goes on to provide sensation to a band of skin. This is done through a variety of peripheral nerves and is remarkably constant. (From Buschbacher 2002,[28] with permission of Butterworth-Heinemann.)

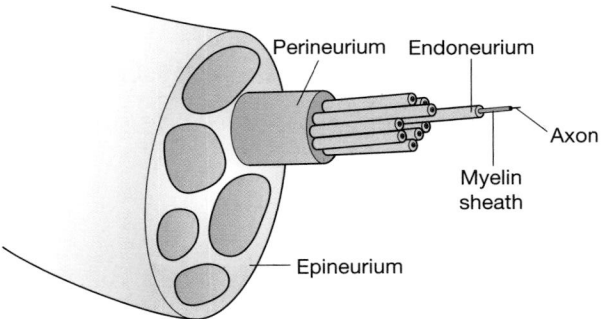

Figure 48-3 The internal anatomy of a nerve. The surrounding structure is called the epineurium. Internally, the nerve fibers are arranged in bundles, or fasciculi, surrounded by a perineurium. Each individual nerve fiber is enveloped by a sheath of myelin and an endoneurium. (From Buschbacher 1994,[26] with permission of Butterworth-Heinemann.)

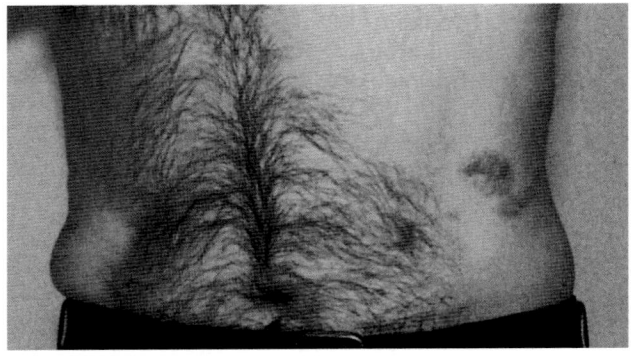

Figure 48-4 Patient with acute shingles (herpes zoster).

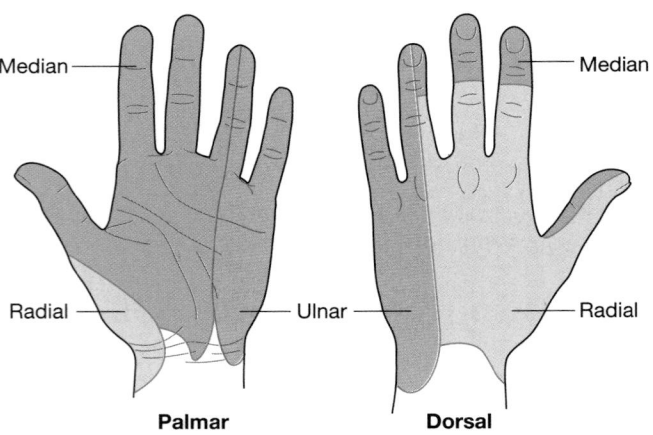

Figure 48-2 A sample of peripheral nerve patterns of innervation from the hand. Although overlap can occur with the dermatomal pattern, knowledge of both systems helps the examiner to distinguish spinal from peripheral nerve pathologic features. (From McNeil and Buschbacher 2002,[96] with permission of Butterworth-Heinemann.)

Box 48-1 Hereditary peripheral neuropathies

- Charcot–Marie–Tooth disease (hereditary motor and sensory neuropathy [HMSN] types 1 and 2)
- Dejerine–Sottas disease (HMSN type 3)
- Refsum disease (HMSN type 4)
- Neuropathies associated with:
  Spinocerebellar degeneration (HMSN type 5)
  Optic atrophy (HMSN type 6)
  Retinitis pigmentosa (HMSN type 7)
- Friedreich ataxia
- Pressure-sensitive hereditary neuropathy
- Acute intermittent porphyria
- Familial amyloid neuropathy
- Fabry disease
- Hereditary sensory neuropathy
- Giant axonal neuropathies
- Lipoprotein neuropathies
- Roussy–Lévy syndrome
- Riley–Day syndrome
- Pelizaeus–Merzbacher disease
- Metachromatic leukodystrophy
- Krabbe leukodystrophy
- Tangier disease

Table 48-1 Common spinal nerve level and peripheral nerve innervation patterns of common muscle groups

Muscle group	Major cranial nerve or spinal nerve level	Peripheral nerve
Upper extremity		
Shoulder muscles		
Elevators	Cranial nerve XI, C4, C5	Spinal accessory nerve, posterior branches of spinal nerves
Protractors	C5–C7	Long thoracic nerve, pectoral nerves
Retractors	C5–C8	Dorsal scapular nerve, spinal accessory nerve, thoracodorsal nerve
Upward rotators	Cranial nerve XI, C5, C6	Long thoracic nerve, spinal accessory nerve
Downward rotators	C6–C8	Thoracodorsal nerve, pectoral nerves
Abductors	C5, C6	Axillary and suprascapular nerves
Extensors	C6–C8	Thoracodorsal, axillary, and pectoral nerves
Flexors	C5, C6	Axillary, musculocutaneous, and pectoral nerves
Internal rotators	C5, C6	Pectoral nerves, thoracodorsal and subscapular nerves
External rotators	C5, C6	Axillary and suprascapular nerves
Elbow flexors	C5, C6	Musculocutaneous nerve
Elbow extensors	C7	Radial nerve
Wrist extensors	C6, C7	Radial nerve
Wrist flexors	C7, C8	Median and ulnar nerves
Finger extensors	C7	Radial nerve
Finger flexors	C7, C8	Median and ulnar nerves
Intrinsic hand muscles	T1	Ulnar and median (thumb) nerves
Trunk and back		
Abdominal muscles	T7–T12	Segmental innervation
Back muscles	C2–C5	Segmental innervation
Lower extremity		
Hip flexors	T12, L1, L2	Lumbosacral plexus
Hip extensors	L5, S1, S2	Inferior gluteal nerve
Hip abductors	L4, L5, S1	Superior gluteal nerve
Hip adductors	L2–L4	Obturator nerve
Knee flexors	L5, S1	Sciatic nerve
Knee extensors	L2–L4	Femoral nerve
Foot dorsiflexors	L4, L5	Deep peroneal nerves
Foot plantar flexors	S1	Tibial nerve
Foot inverters	L4	Deep peroneal and tibial nerves
Foot everters	L5, S1	Superficial peroneal nerve

(After Buschbacher 2002,[27] with permission of Butterworth-Heinemann.)

Table 48-2 Nerve fiber types in mammalian nerve

Fiber type	Function(s)	Fiber diameter (μm)	Conduction velocity (m/s)	Spike duration (ms)	Absolute refractory period (ms)
A					
α	Proprioception, somatic motor	12–20	70–120		
β	Touch, pressure	5–12	30–70	0.4–0.5	0.4–1.4
γ	Motor to muscle spindles	3–6	15–30		
δ	Pain, temperature, touch	2–5	12–30		
B	Preganglionic autonomic	<3	3–15	1.2	1.2
C					
Dorsal root	Pain, reflex responses	0.4–1.2	0.5–2.5	2	2
Sympathetic	Postganglionic sympathetics	0.3–1.3	0.7–2.3	2	2

(From Ganong 1987,[56] with permission of Appleton & Lange.)

Box 48-2 Toxic peripheral neuropathies

Drugs
- Amiodarone
- Chloramphenicol
- Corticosteroids
- Dapsone
- Diphenylhydantoin
- Disulfiram
- Halogenated hydroxyquinolones
- Heroin
- Hydralazine
- Isoniazid
- Lysergide (LSD)
- Misonidazole
- Nitrofurantoin
- Pyridoxine
- Sodium cyanate
- Tetanus toxoid
- Thalidomide

Heavy metals
- Antimony
- Arsenic
- Gold
- Lead
- Mercury
- Thallium

Organic compounds
- Acrylamide
- Carbon disulfide
- Dichlorophenoxyacetic acid
- Ethyl alcohol
- Ethylene oxide
- Methyl butyl ketone
- Triorthocresyl phosphate

Box 48-3 Diseases associated with peripheral neuropathy

- Alcoholism
- Amyloidosis
- Benign monoclonal gammopathy (IgG, IgA, IgM)
- Chronic liver disease
- Chronic obstructive pulmonary disease
- Cryoglobulinemia
- Diabetes mellitus
  Distal symmetric neuropathy
  Autonomic neuropathy
  Proximal asymmetric painful motor neuropathy
  Cranial mononeuropathies
- Giant cell arteries
- Gout
- Hypothyroidism
- Necrotizing angiopathy
- Neuropathies in malignant diseases
  Lymphomas: focal and systemic
  Multiple myeloma
  Bronchogenic carcinoma
  Tumors of the ovary, testes, penis, stomach, or oral cavity
  Meningeal carcinomatosis
  Oat cell carcinoma
  Osteosclerotic myeloma
  Vasculitis or connective tissue disease

Box 48-4 Idiopathic neuropathies

- Brachial neuritis (Parsonage–Turner syndrome)
- Chronic inflammatory polyradiculopathy
- Chronic relapsing polyneuropathy
- Fisher syndrome
- Acute inflammatory demyelinating polyradiculoneuropathy (Guillain–Barré syndrome)
- Steroid-responsive polyneuropathy
- Multifocal motor neuropathy

Table 48-3 Numeric classification sometimes used for sensory neurons

No.	Origin	Fiber type
1a	Muscle spindle, annulospiral ending	Aα
1b	Golgi tendon organ	Aα
2	Muscle spindle, flower spray ending; touch, pressure	Aβ
3	Pain and temperature receptors; some touch receptors	Aδ
4	Pain and other receptors	Dorsal root C

(From Ganong 1987,[56] with permission of Appleton & Lange.)

Box 48-5 Nutritional neuropathies

- Beriberi or pellagra: thiamine (vitamin B_1) deficiency
- Riboflavin (vitamin B_2) deficiency
- Pyridoxine (vitamin B_6) deficiency
- Pernicious anemia (vitamin B_{12} deficiency)
- Protein or calorie deficiency in children

Box 48-6 Infectious causes of peripheral neuropathy

- Cytomegalovirus in HIV infection
- Diphtheria
- Herpes zoster
- Leprosy
- Rabies

Table 48-4 The Seddon and Sunderland classification systems

Seddon[125]	Sunderland[133]	Description
Neurapraxia	First-degree injury	Focal conduction block; axons remain intact
Axonotmesis	Second-degree injury	Axonal damage and Wallerian degeneration; intact supporting structures
Neurotmesis	Third-degree injury Fourth-degree injury Fifth-degree injury	Interruption of axon and endoneurium Interruption of perineurium and endoneurium All supporting structures and axon damaged

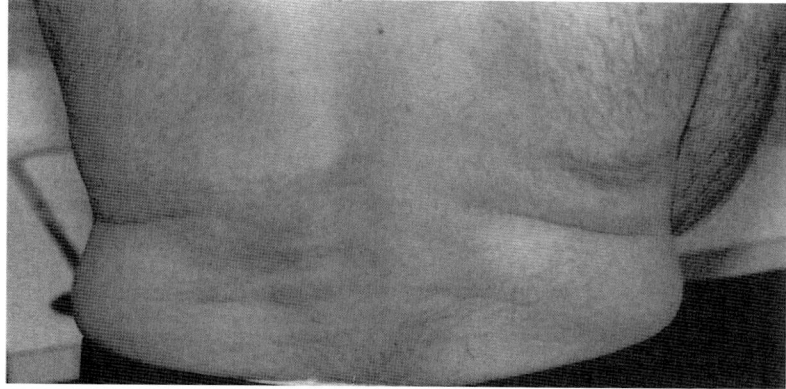

Figure 48-5 Patient with acute shingles (herpes zoster).

Table 48-5 Common peripheral nerve injury and entrapment syndromes	
Nerve	Entrapment
Radial nerve	At the radial groove of the humerus ('Saturday night palsy') Posterior interosseous nerve syndrome
Ulnar nerve	At the olecranon groove Tardy ulnar palsy Cubital tunnel syndrome Injury at the wrist (can be at the canal of Guyon)
Median nerve	At the supracondylar ligament of Struthers (at elbow) Pronator teres syndrome Carpal tunnel syndrome Anterior interosseous syndrome
Sciatic nerve	Injection palsy—injury to lateral division Injury to medial division
Femoral nerve	Above or below the inguinal ligament
Peroneal nerve	At head of fibula
Tibial nerve	Tarsal tunnel syndrome

for peripheral neuropathy cannot be identified in up to one-third of the cases.[154]

While classification systems allow for a labeling framework, they are not always helpful for the diagnosis and treatment of the individual patient. A diagnostic algorithm is presented in Figure 48-6. What follows is a more practical clinical approach.

Evaluation of the patient with neuropathy

History

The diagnostic process begins with the physician obtaining a careful history. Some key questions are as follows.

- Is the onset sudden or gradual?
- Is the progression rapid or slow?
- Is the predominant manifestation sensory, motor, or both?
- Is the distribution focal or generalized, distal or proximal, symmetric or asymmetric?
- Is there autonomic involvement?
- Does the patient have any associated diseases?

The family, social, and occupational histories are important for identifying familial occurrences or toxic exposures.

Physical examination

Sensory examination Sensory modalities including light touch, pinprick, proprioception, vibration, and cold temperature should be tested. If these are preserved, it is unlikely that a significant sensory deficit is present. If sensory deficits are detected, carefully documenting the extent and pattern of the

loss is important, because this information helps track the progress of the disease. The information is also important for identifying patients who need to be counseled about protecting hypoesthetic skin.

Motor examination Muscle strength should be graded by functional tests of multiple muscles and muscle groups (see Ch. 1). Patterns of atrophy should also be recorded. Normal patients vary widely in their strength, due to differences both in muscle bulk and in level of motivation, understanding, and cooperation. Pain can also prevent a patient from exerting full muscle force (pain inhibition of function).

Reflex testing In generalized peripheral neuropathy, the muscle stretch reflexes (MSRs) are often decreased or absent distally. In some of the polyneuropathies, MSRs can be absent throughout. Focal depression of reflexes indicates a local lesion such as radiculopathy or plexopathy. Abnormally brisk reflexes suggest that a central nervous system process is present, rather than a peripheral nerve problem.

Electrodiagnostic examination in neuropathy

Nerve conduction studies Nerve conduction studies are usually the most helpful part of the electrodiagnostic examination for the evaluation of peripheral nerve disorders (see Chs 10–12). These studies determine the conduction velocity of the nerve as well as the amplitude of the resulting action potential. The distal latency provides information about function in the terminal segments of the nerve where terminal axonal branching prohibits calculating a uniform conduction velocity.[88] The large diameter myelinated axons of both motor and sensory populations are evaluated by these tests.

In disease of the myelin sheath, the conduction velocity is typically slowed to <70% of the lower limit of normal. The distal latency is typically prolonged to >130% of the normal values. When more severe demyelination is present, the action potential can fail to conduct at all. This situation is termed conduction block. If conduction block is present, the amplitude of the evoked response drops by a greater than normal amount between distal and proximal stimulation sites (see Chs 10, 11, and 12). The amount of drop reflects the number of axons affected.

In diseases where axonal degeneration predominates (see Box 48-7), the conduction velocity remains relatively normal or is only decreased by amounts of <30% below the low limit of normal. More typical of axonopathy, however, is a reduction in amplitude of the responses evoked from distal stimulus sites. This is especially true when recording directly from nerves, as is done in sensory conduction studies. Sensory responses tend to become abnormal earlier and more severely than motor responses. This is thought to occur because sensory axons lack the redundancy inherent in the motor axon's innervation of multiple muscle fibers. Hence changes in sensory axon number are more clearly reflected in the action potential amplitude. Temporal dispersion between distal and proximal sites is usually minimal.

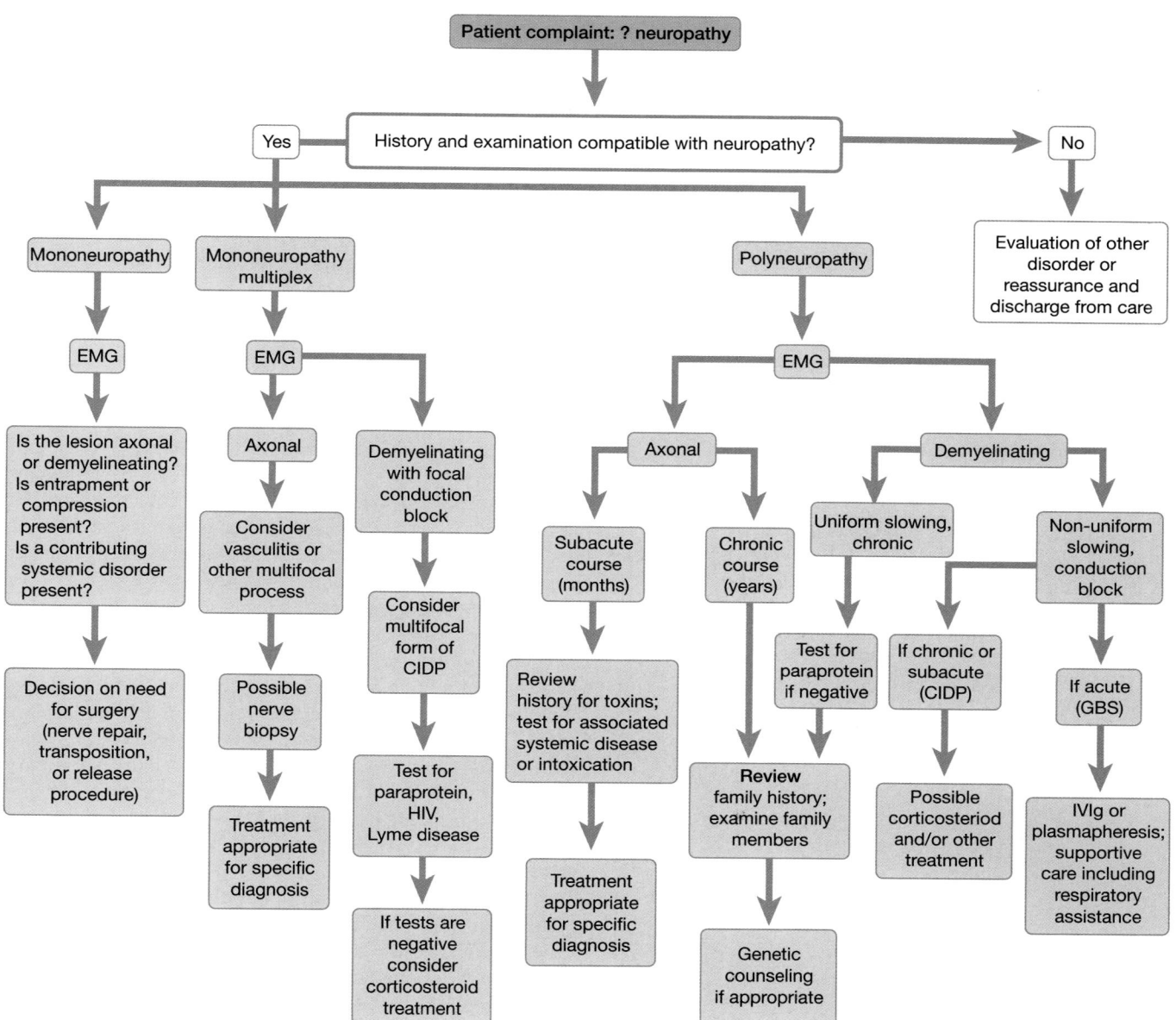

Figure 48-6 Diagnostic algorithm for neuropathies.

Many peripheral neuropathies involve a mixed component of both axonal degeneration and demyelination (see Box 48-7). This combination of pathologies may result in a pattern of findings, with slowing below 70% of the lower limit of normal or prolongation of distal latency beyond 130%, and abnormal temporal dispersion, as well as decreased amplitude of the responses recorded from distal stimulus sites (see Chs 10, 11, and 12).

Electromyography The electromyography (EMG) needle records the summated activity of the muscle fibers controlled by individual anterior horn cells. The activities recorded are motor unit potentials. In pathologic states producing breakdown of the axon or motor neuron, spontaneous action

potentials of single muscle fibers resulting from electrical instability of the muscle membrane may be recordable in the form of fibrillations or positive waves. The distribution of these findings is useful in localizing lesions. The pattern of EMG findings can also aid in determining the time course of the lesion, and helps in analyzing the progress of reinnervation (see Ch. 11).

In mild generalized peripheral neuropathy, the EMG findings are usually minimal and will be limited to the distal muscles. In mildly affected muscles, the changes in chronic cases include changes in motor unit action potential architecture, such as mild enlargement in size and increased polyphasicity. In more severe axonal-type neuropathies, there is muscle membrane instability manifesting as fibrillations and positive waves. As

---

> **Box 48-7** Peripheral neuropathies: electrodiagnostic classification
>
> **Sensorimotor, uniform demyelinating**
> - Hereditary motor and sensory neuropathy (HMSN) types 1, 3, and 4
> - Metachromatic leukodystrophy
>
> **Motor > sensory axonal**
> - Porphyria
> - HMSN types 2 and 5
> - Lead neuropathy
> - Vincristine neuropathy
> - Axonal Guillain–Barré syndrome
>
> **Sensorimotor axonal and demyelinating**
> - Diabetes
> - Uremia
>
> **Sensorimotor axonal**
> - Amyloidosis
> - Folate deficiency
> - Thiamine deficiency
> - Alcoholic neuropathy
> - Mercury toxicity
> - Gold toxicity
> - Rheumatoid arthritis
> - AIDS neuropathy
>
> **Motor > sensory segmental demyelinating**
> - Guillain–Barré syndrome
> - Chronic inflammatory demyelinating polyneuropathy
> - Leprosy
> - Amiodarone neuropathy
> - AIDS neuropathy
> - Ulcerative colitis neuropathy
> - Hypothyroidism
> - Diphtheria
> - Acute arsenic polyneuropathy
>
> **Sensory axonal**
> - Hereditary sensory neuropathy
> - Friedreich ataxia
> - Cisplatin toxicity
> - Vincristine toxicity
> - Isoniazid toxicity
> - Pyridoxine toxicity
> - Sjögren syndrome
> - AIDS neuropathy
> - Vitamin B_{12} deficiency

reinnervation progresses, membrane instability lessens and polyphasic motor units of prolonged duration and high amplitude are seen. When reinnervation is completed, the motor unit action potentials have the characteristic neuropathic appearance of being long in duration and high in amplitude. Demyelination typically causes little abnormal muscle membrane irritability, and fibrillation potentials and positive sharp waves are only occasionally seen.[39] The major finding in demyelinating lesions is a reduced number of motor unit potentials firing, which results from conduction block in individual axons.

COMMON COMPLICATIONS OF NEUROPATHY

Muscle weakness, sensory loss, neuropathic pain, and autonomic problems occur commonly in patients with neuropathies.

Muscle weakness

Joint contractures and muscle shortening are associated with muscle weakness. These complications can be prevented with daily range of motion and muscle-stretching exercises. Depending on the degree of weakness, this exercise can be passive, active-assistive, or active. A program of gentle strengthening, which can include isometric, isotonic, isokinetic, manual-resistive, and progressive-resistive exercise, should be carefully tailored to the patient. While improvement of strength is desirable, the muscles should not be overworked, as this can result in paradoxical weakening (overwork weakness).[11,69] Patients with strength levels of $^3/_5$ or less are most at risk of developing overwork weakness. These patients should not be denied the opportunity to exercise. However, they need close monitoring to make certain that the exercise is making them stronger rather than weaker.

When the patient's ability to change position voluntarily is impaired, proper passive positioning is essential. Splinting might be required to help prevent contractures in patients with prolonged, severe muscle weakness (see Chs 15 and 16). Orthoses should be appropriately prescribed for the patient to increase function and aid in positioning. Peripheral nerves can be compressed between bony prominences and the bed or chair. Injury to the ulnar nerve at the elbow or the common peroneal nerve at the fibular head is the most common lesion of this type.

Sensory loss

When protective sensation is compromised, the hypoesthetic or anesthetic areas should be examined daily by the caregivers or the patient. Because they are the most distal body part, the feet are most commonly and most severely affected by loss of sensation in peripheral neuropathy. The patient can traumatize the skin unknowingly, causing breakdown and ulceration. Repetitive joint trauma can lead to the development of neuro-arthropathic (Charcot) joints. In either case, the prescription of custom-molded shoe inserts or even custom-molded shoes is frequently indicated. Plastizote or other materials that more evenly distribute pressure forces can be used to make shoe inserts that prevent calluses and ulcers over the metatarsal heads. Other orthotic modifications, such as metatarsal pads, can be built into the inserts. Rocker bottom soles also help redistribute pressure to help prevent foot trauma and ulcers.[22,32]

In addition to careful daily skin examination, the patient should be instructed in thorough, gentle cleaning and soaking techniques. Patients with peripheral neuropathy frequently have autonomic neuropathy as well, putting them at risk for dry and scaly skin over the distal legs and feet due to a lack of normal sweating. This can be treated by applying a moisturizing cream to the entire foot surface, except between the toes. This helps prevent fissuring and scaling of the skin that can lead to ulcers and infections. Patients should test the temperature of bath water with a thermometer to prevent scalding. The feet should be inspected daily for callus formation, erythema, abrasions, and bruising. The toenails should be cut square to help prevent ingrown toenails. Waiting too long to treat can lead to irreversible sequelae, which can ultimately result in amputation.

Autonomic dysfunction

Autonomic problems are seen in a variety of neuropathies but are perhaps most commonly associated with diabetes mellitus and GBS. Cardiovascular symptoms can include orthostatic intolerance or cardiac arrhythmias. Genitourinary symptoms include a flaccid bladder and male impotence. Gastrointestinal symptoms can include vomiting, dysphagia, diarrhea, and constipation.[155] Sweating abnormalities are seen with autonomic involvement as well.

The autonomic dysfunction in GBS can be life-threatening. These patients should have cardiac monitoring with close observation for dysrhythmias and blood pressure instability during the early stages of their disease.

Pain

Neuropathic pain is a common problem in peripheral neuropathy, and it can be difficult to treat effectively. Reduction of pain rather than elimination should be the goal in most cases. The current first line of treatment for neuropathic pain is typically one of the antiepileptic medications, such as gabapentin. Carbamazepine is an alternative medication. Anticonvulsant drugs such as gabapentin and carbamazepine should be dosed no more aggressively than the manufacturer's recommendations. Both these medications probably work best for the prickling and tingling sensations, and also to some degree for the burning discomfort. If these medications are going to work, some relief is typically noted by the patient in a day or two. If carbamazepine is used long term, the white blood cell count should be monitored periodically.

The second line of treatment for pain due to autonomic dysfunction is the tricyclic antidepressants, such as amitriptyline. These should be started at a low dose and increased slowly over time in accordance with the manufacturer's recommendation. The side effects of these drugs include sedation, orthostatic hypotension, and worsening of urinary retention. This type of medication works best for aching or burning type of pain, and can also reduce allodynia, such as the discomfort some patients experience from bed sheets touching bare toes. (Allodynia is pain due to a stimulus that is not normally painful.) Nortriptyline can be tried if the cholinergic side effects from amitriptyline are too great. Trazodone can be tried in patients who do not tolerate the tricyclics.

Analgesics also have a role in treatment. Non-opioid medications such as acetaminophen (paracetamol) or non-steroidal antiinflammatory drugs (NSAIDs) should be tried first. Propoxyphene or hydrocodone is required at times. Rarely, opioids such as oral morphine, methadone, or transdermal fentanyl are required in patients who experience extremely severe pain. A multiple drug regimen might be needed to treat neuropathic pain in some patients. In such instances, care should be taken to avoid problematic drug interactions.[146] Topical capsaicin and transdermal lidocaine (lignocaine) patches[38] can be beneficial in some patients. Transcutaneous electrical nerve stimulation can be tried as well.[10]

MONONEUROPATHIES

Mononeuropathies, often caused by nerve entrapment, can potentially occur in most nerves in the body. Certain nerves are more vulnerable, however, and some of the most common mononeuropathies will be discussed below.

Median nerve

Carpal tunnel syndrome

The median nerve is most commonly entrapped at the wrist, as it passes through the carpal tunnel. The volar surface of the carpal tunnel is formed by the flexor retinaculum, and the dorsal side by the carpal bones. The contents of the carpal tunnel include the median nerve, the flexor pollicis longus tendon, and four tendons each from the flexor digitorum superficialis and profundus muscles. Swelling or increased pressure inside the carpal tunnel can lead to compression of the median nerve, producing symptoms of CTS.

The presentation of CTS most commonly includes paresthesias (numbness, tingling, and burning) involving the median nerve distribution (first $3\frac{1}{2}$ digits), along with a deep aching pain in the hand and wrist. At times, the pain will radiate into the forearm, and even rarely to the shoulder. The patient might report subjective swelling of the hand but, on inspection, no swelling is usually apparent. Nocturnal worsening of symptoms is common. The patient often reports awakening with hand paresthesias, which are then relieved by shaking the involved hand ('flick' sign). In advanced cases of CTS, sensory symptoms last longer or become persistent, and thenar weakness develops. The patient might also report dropping objects frequently.

Carpal tunnel syndrome is more common in women, and occurs bilaterally in about 50% of the cases. It is often associated with repetitive hand and wrist movements or the use of vibrating machines. The great majority of the cases are idiopathic in origin. Certain systemic conditions, such as diabetes mellitus, amyloidosis, hypothyroidism, and rheumatoid arthritis, can predispose to CTS. Obesity[10] and pregnancy are also risk factors for CTS. Increased susceptibility to CTS has been thought to occur in patients with a ratio of anteroposterior diameter to mediolateral diameter at the wrist crease ≥ 0.7 (more square wrist).[61] More recent studies have challenged this observation.[130,153]

Physical examination findings in CTS vary according to the severity. The physical examination can be normal in mild cases. Abnormalities in median sensory testing can be found as the syndrome progresses. Motor testing in more advanced cases shows weakness and atrophy of the abductor pollicis brevis and

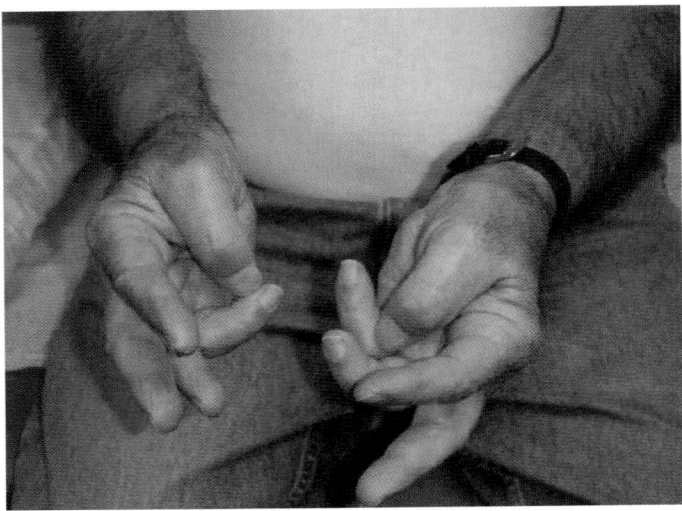

Figure 48-7 Patient with severe carpal tunnel syndrome and weakness with thumb opposition.

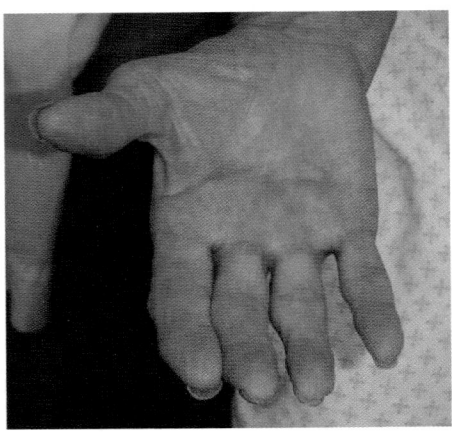

Figure 48-8 Patient with severe carpal tunnel syndrome with atrophy of the opponens pollicis and abductor pollicis brevis muscles.

opponens pollicis muscles (Figs. 48-7 and 48-8). Provocative tests include Tinel's sign, Phalen's sign, and the median nerve compression test. Kuhlman and Hennessey found that the sensitivities for Phalen's, Tinel's, and median nerve compression were all low (51%, 23%, and 28%, respectively). Specificities ranged from 66% to 87%.[86] Another diagnostic help is the flick sign, where a patient gives a history of flicking their wrists to alleviate pain and numbness. The flick sign was found to have a sensitivity of 37% and a false positive rate of 26%.[68]

Electrodiagnostic studies are an important electrophysiologic extension of the history and physical in diagnosing CTS (see Chs 10–12). Nerve conduction studies and EMG can determine the presence and the severity of median neuropathy at the wrist. They are also useful in ruling out other potential diagnoses, such as C6 radiculopathy, brachial plexopathy, or a more proximal median neuropathy.

Treatment of CTS begins conservatively with measures of rest, removal of aggravating factors, antiinflammatory medications, and treatment of associated medical conditions.

It has been hypothesized that idiopathic CTS is a manifestation of vitamin B_6 deficiency. Although this is controversial, treatment with vitamin B_6 in doses of 50–300 mg daily can be tried.[7] Using custom or prefabricated nocturnal wrist splints, which hold the wrist in 0–30° of extension, often provide good relief of symptoms, at least while being worn. Range of motion exercises of the wrist and upper extremity are important in maintaining function. Corticosteroid injection into the carpal tunnel can decrease inflammation and may be of benefit, especially in patients with mild symptoms of less than 1 year in duration.[57] Kaplan et al. found the risks for poor outcome in non-operative treatment to include age greater than 50, symptoms for more than 10 months, constant paresthesias, stenosing flexor tenosynovitis, and a positive Phalen's test in less than 30 s.[80] A failure rate of 93% was found in those patients with three risk factors, and those with four or more had a 100% failure rate. In severe cases of CTS, or those refractory to conservative treatment, surgery is performed. Surgery can be performed openly or by endoscopic release, with the goal being decompression of the median nerve in the carpal tunnel. Both surgeries are equally effective at improving symptoms, and evidence is conflicting as to whether endoscopic release results in earlier return to work or improved level of function.[58] Predictors of poor outcome after surgery include older age, heavy vibration exposure, severe symptoms during activities of daily living, or duration longer than 3 years.[6,37]

Ulnar nerve

Ulnar neuropathy at the elbow

Ulnar neuropathy at the elbow (UNE), also known as cubital tunnel syndrome, is the second most common entrapment neuropathy. The ulnar nerve enters the cubital tunnel between the medial epicondyle and the olecranon, and beneath the humeroulnar aponeurotic arcade. Potential sites of nerve entrapment include the ulnar groove just proximal to the epicondyle, the humeroulnar aponeurotic arcade, and the exit site from the deep flexor pronator aponeurosis.

Symptoms of UNE include paresthesias of the fourth and fifth digits, and the ulnar aspect of the dorsum of the hand. Weakness and muscle atrophy occur later and, when present, most commonly affect the intrinsic hand muscles (Fig. 48-9). Side to side confrontational strength testing is a useful test in detecting weakness of the intrinsic muscles of the hand (Fig. 48-10).[25] The flexor carpi ulnaris and flexor digitorum profundus to digits 4 and 5 are significantly involved in more severe cases.

A Tinel's sign can be present at the elbow. Reproduction of symptoms occurs in some patients with elbow flexion or ulnar groove compression. Loss of elbow range of motion or elbow valgus deformity can also be seen with UNE.

There are many potential causes for development of UNE. Chronic external compression of the ulnar nerve at the elbow can occur with certain arm positions, such as routinely resting the elbow on a hard surface. Acute lesions can develop secondary to prolonged periods of having the arm in unfavorable posi-

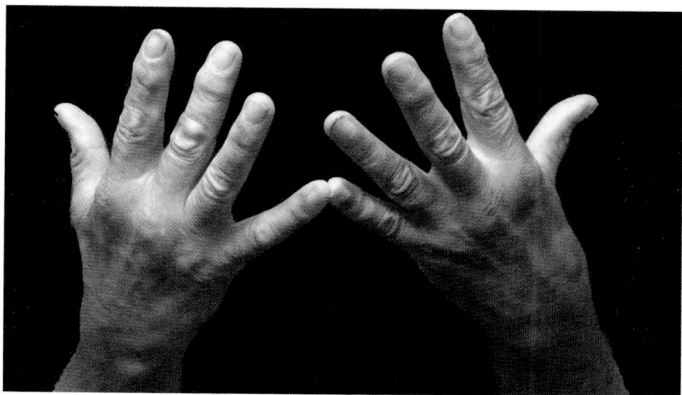

Figure 48-9 Left-sided intrinsic hand muscle weakness in ulnar neuropathy at the elbow. The left hand is unable to hold a piece of paper without using the flexor pollicis longus (Froment's sign). Ulnar sensory deficits are present.

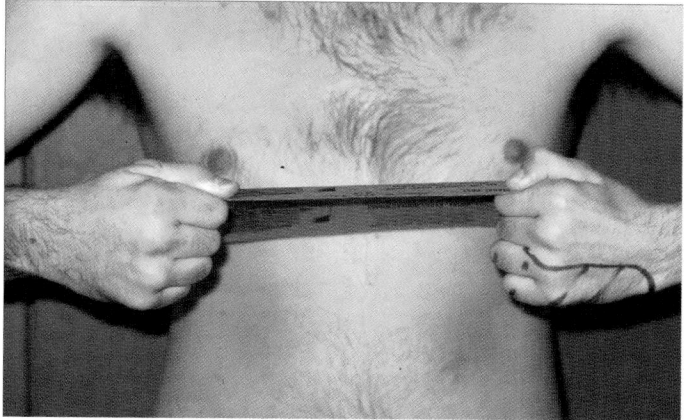

Figure 48-10 Side to side confrontational strength testing in a patient with left ulnar neuropathy at the elbow, demonstrating the giving way of the left abductor digiti minimi (Buschbacher's sign).

tions, like pronation or flexion, such as during surgery when a patient is under general anesthesia, or in a coma. If the cubital tunnel is congenitally small, repeated elbow flexion and extension can produce a lesion at the elbow when combined with the effect of normal constriction that occurs during elbow flexion. Other potential etiologies include elbow joint derangement secondary to trauma or arthritis, intraarticular loose bodies, ligamentous thickening, soft tissue calcifications, and ganglion cysts. When UNE occurs years after elbow trauma, it is referred to as 'tardy ulnar palsy'. Although debate exists, some feel that repeated subluxation of the ulnar nerve at the ulnar groove can contribute to the development of UNE.

Electrodiagnostic studies are used to confirm the diagnosis of UNE and help define the probable pathology. Ulnar motor nerve conduction studies should be performed with the elbow in 70–90° of flexion.[29] This position helps lessen variation in nerve conduction velocities between different segments of the nerve encountered with elbow in extension. When demyelination is present, ulnar motor nerve conduction velocities across

the elbow will be decreased, and will be slow relative to the forearm segment. However, if there are primarily axonal changes, the ulnar motor nerve conduction studies can be mildly slowed in both the elbow and the forearm segments. 'Inching' studies are often useful to help localize the lesion.[30] Sensory nerve conduction studies of the ulnar nerve at the wrist and dorsal ulnar cutaneous nerve can show reduction of amplitude if the lesion is axonal. At times, both demyelination and axonal loss are present, giving a mixed presentation on electrodiagnostic studies. A demyelinating lesion will eventually produce a reduced number of motor units firing and changes in recruitment. This is also seen in the axonal type, with the addition of signs of abnormal muscle membrane irritability, such as positive waves and fibrillations. The pattern of EMG abnormalities is helpful in making certain that the lesion is UNE rather than C8 radiculopathy or brachial plexopathy such as a lower trunk injury. It is of interest that the flexor carpi ulnaris muscle is resistant to showing EMG changes in UNE, at least as compared with other ulnar innervated muscles (see Ch. 11–12).

Imaging studies can assist in the diagnosis of UNE. Plain x-rays can help evaluate the bony architecture of the elbow, but they are not directly informative about the nerves or soft tissue. Ultrasonography has been shown to detect morphologic changes and the extent of the ulnar lesion at the elbow, and shows promise as a screening and follow-up imaging modality in patients with UNE.[108] Magnetic resonance imaging (MRI) or computed tomography (CT) may be required to evaluate deeper structural lesions in the elbow (see Ch. 7).

Conservative treatment of UNE consists of eliminating any underlying aggravating factors. For example, prolonged extreme elbow flexion at night can be prevented by use of a splint that holds the elbow in mild flexion. External pressure on the nerve can be remedied by the use of an elbow pad. Select patients benefit from education in avoiding repetitive elbow flexion and extension. Antiinflammatory medications are helpful in some patients. If 3–6 months of conservative treatment fail or severe weakness exists, surgical evaluation is recommended. The surgical options include decompression of the nerve under the humeroulnar aponeurotic arcade, transposition of the nerve anterior to the medial epicondyle, or medial epicondylectomy. A clear consensus about the most optimal procedure has not yet emerged.

Radial nerve

The radial nerve is the largest nerve in the upper limb. It is involved in entrapment syndromes less frequently than the median and ulnar nerves, but is more commonly injured from trauma, such as a humeral shaft fracture affecting the radial nerve near the radial groove. The radial nerve supplies motion to the primary agonists for elbow extension, wrist extension, and finger extension, as well as contributing to elbow flexion, forearm supination, and thumb extension. It supplies sensation to the skin overlying the posterior arm, forearm, and hand.

Radial neuropathy at the spiral groove

The most common radial neuropathy occurs at the spiral groove.[113] This neuropathy is often referred to as 'Saturday night palsy', due to the nerve being compressed when the arm is draped over a chair or hard surface while the patient is sedated by alcohol or drugs. During the normal sleep cycle, enough body movement occurs that such nerve entrapments do not occur. But during stupor and/or coma produced by alcohol and other drugs, the protective movement during the sleep cycle is suppressed. This can also occur when an inebriated couple sleep with the head of one on the midarm of the other for a protracted period. In this case, it is known as 'honeymooner's paralysis'. Other potential etiologies include humeral fracture,[111] strenuous triceps contraction,[93] and vasculitis.

Patients with radial nerve injury usually present with a wrist drop. Strength testing reveals weakness of wrist and finger extensors. Patients also report weakness with elbow flexion, apparently due to weakness of the brachioradialis. They also complain at times of weakness of thumb abduction and forearm supination secondary to involvement of the brachioradialis, abductor pollicis longus, and supinator muscles. Elbow extension (triceps) is spared in most cases, as the majority of the triceps muscle is innervated above the site of radial injury. Patients can also complain of sensory disturbance over the posterolateral hand, which corresponds to the distribution of the superficial radial sensory nerve (Fig. 48-11).

Examination typically shows some degree of sensory deficit in the territory of the superficial radial sensory nerve. Sensation over the posterior arm and forearm should be normal. MSRs show a reduced or absent brachioradialis reflex, with normal triceps, biceps, and finger flexor responses. Motor and sensory

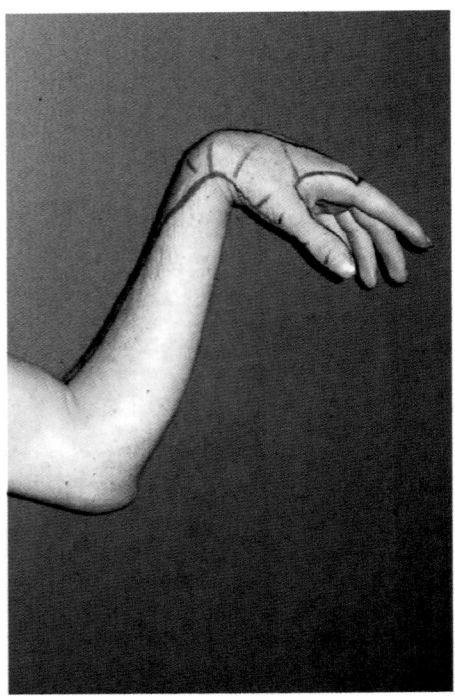

Figure 48-11
Sensory loss involving the superficial radial nerve distribution.

examination involving the median and ulnar distribution should be normal, but the weakness of the wrist extensors can produce an apparent weakness of the ulnar innervated interosseous muscles. This is due to the fact that the fingers normally cannot be abducted as well when the metacarpophalangeal joints are in flexion, due to the shape of the metacarpal heads. This pseudoweakness of the interosseous muscles can be eliminated by supporting the fingers in extension, such as by placing the hand on a bedside table or other supportive surface.

Electrodiagnostic studies can be useful in identifying and localizing the lesion. Motor nerve conduction study of the radial nerve should be performed, with stimulation at the elbow, over the spiral groove of the humerus, and even more proximally if technically possible. The recording electrode should be placed on a radial innervated forearm muscle, such as the extensor digitorum or extensor indicis. This technique is useful in localizing the lesion and in quantitating the degree of conduction block versus axon loss at the spiral groove.[150] Conduction block can be diagnosed when stimulation above the site of the lesion results in at least a 50% drop in the amplitude of the evoked response, as compared with stimulating below the lesion. If axonal loss is present, the amplitude of the compound muscle action potential will be reduced with stimulation above and below the site of the nerve lesion. Fibrillation potentials and positive sharp waves are present in the radial innervated muscles distal to the spiral groove when the lesion is of the axon loss type. Sensory involvement is evaluated by testing the superficial radial sensory nerve action potentials.[3]

In addition to electrodiagnostic studies, imaging studies such as plain films and MRI can be helpful in evaluating potential underlying causes of nerve involvement and in helping to eliminate other possible diagnoses, such as C7 or C8 radiculopathy. Sonographic studies have also been useful in detecting radial nerve entrapment within a humeral fracture.[18]

Spontaneous recovery usually occurs over a time frame of several weeks to a few months in compressive radial nerve lesions, as long as the underlying source of injury is eliminated or does not recur. Neurapraxic lesions that are due to demyelination can recover in days, whereas axonal lesions require axonal regrowth that can take months. Radial nerve transection is uncommon and is usually associated with an open fracture.[51]

During the recovery phase, wrist splints can be used to help assist with wrist and finger extension. Upper extremity range of motion exercises should be instituted to avoid contractures. Serial electrodiagnostic studies can follow nerve recovery and, if signs of reinnervation are absent after 4 months, surgical exploration might be required.[46,123] In cases where nerve injury is irreparable or nerve repair has failed, tendon transfer should be considered to help compensate for the weakness in radial nerve innervated muscles.[128]

Posterior interosseous neuropathy

The posterior interosseous nerve (PIN) is a deep branch of the radial nerve, which pierces the interosseous membrane between the radius and the ulna, and supplies the extensor carpi ulnaris, finger and thumb extensors, and abductor pollicis longus. It does not contain any cutaneous sensory fibers, as the superficial radial sensory nerve comes off the radial nerve proximal to the PIN. Posterior interosseous neuropathy is most often caused by entrapment in the radial tunnel or at the arcade of Frohse (supinator syndrome).[40] Other reported causes of PIN lesions include Monteggia fractures (proximal ulna and radial head posterior dislocation),[101] elbow joint fractures,[40] rheumatoid elbow synovitis,[100] lipomas,[13] hematomas,[36] ganglion cysts,[84] and fibromas.[40] The use of an aluminum forearm orthosis (Canadian crutch) has been associated with PIN syndrome.[126]

Patients present with weakness of finger and thumb extension at the metacarpophalangeal joint. Thumb abduction can also be weak. The wrist typically deviates radially during extension due to the weakness of the extensor carpi ulnaris (Fig. 48-12). Lateral elbow and proximal forearm pain can be present due to involvement of deep sensory fibers of the PIN that supply the interosseous membrane and joint capsules.[113]

Needle EMG is the most useful electrodiagnostic test in localizing PIN. The findings depend on whether the lesion is demyelinating or axonal. Both types of lesions result in a reduction in the number of motor units firing and changes in recruitment. Axonal lesions also produce abnormal muscle membrane irritability, such as positive waves and fibrillation potentials. The findings are limited to those muscles innervated by the PIN, which helps separates the lesion from a more proximal radial nerve lesion. The supinator muscle has variable involvement. Nerve conduction studies show a normal superficial radial sensory study, while radial motor studies to the extensor digitorum or extensor indicis can show reduced muscle action potential amplitude.

Imaging studies such as plain films, CT, and MRI can also be useful to evaluate for underlying fracture or space-occupying lesion. Conservative treatment includes NSAIDs, splinting, and upper limb range of motion exercises. Repetitive pronation and supination of the forearm should be avoided in radial tunnel or supinator syndrome. Kaplan found that 80% of patients with electrophysiologically confirmed PIN lesions treated conservatively had resolution of symptoms at 5 years.[78] In cases with progressive weakness or failed conservative treatment after 3–6 months,[84] surgery should be considered. In PIN lesions due to underlying mass, surgical exploration and resection is usually required. Tendon transfers can help restore function in those with persistent hand weakness. In complete lesions, an extensor tenodesis splint can aid in developing pinch force (see Ch. 15).

Long thoracic nerve

The long thoracic nerve originates from the ventral rami of the fifth through seventh cervical roots. It travels beneath the brachial plexus and clavicle, and passes over the first rib. It then descends superficially along the lateral chest wall to the eighth or ninth rib, where it innervates the serratus anterior muscle.[151] The serratus anterior functions to protract and upwardly rotate the scapula, pulling the scapula forward to fix it against the rib cage.

With injury to the long thoracic nerve, scapular winging results (Fig. 48-13). The inferior angle of the scapula is rotated upward, and there is medial displacement of the medial scapular border. Most long thoracic palsies are a result of brachial plexitis or neuralgic amyotrophy. Injury to the long thoracic nerve can occur iatrogenically, such as during surgical procedures like radical mastectomy, first rib resection, and transaxillary sympathectomy.[82] The nerve can also be injured by blunt trauma to the shoulder or arm that stretches the nerve.

Patients frequently report periscapular pain and a general weakness of shoulder and upper arm function. Shoulder abduction is usually limited to 90°. Medial winging of the scapula is present at rest. When the patient extends the arms out in front

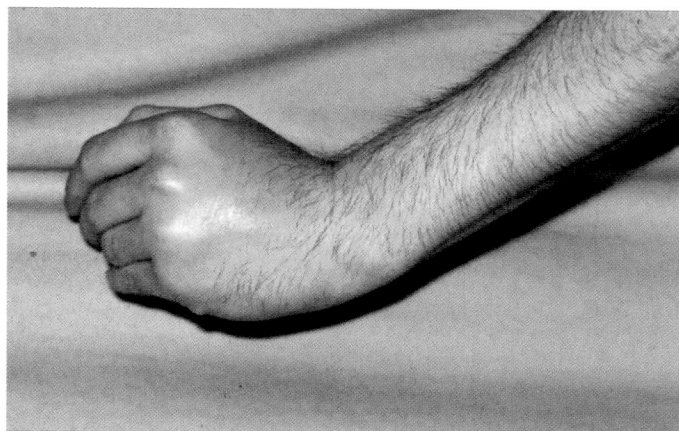

Figure 48-12 Patient with a posterior interosseous nerve injury and radial deviation of the wrist during extension, due to weakness of the extensor carpi ulnaris.

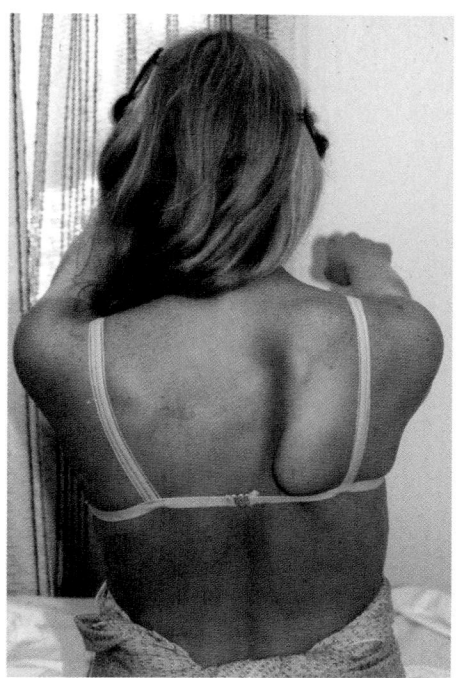

Figure 48-13 Long thoracic nerve injury with medial scapular winging, due to weakness of the serratus anterior.

of the body, three signs are present. The scapular wings medially, the scapula moves away from the chest wall, and forward flexion of the shoulder is weak and limited to 90°. Sensation should be normal. A careful neurologic examination is necessary to rule out cervical radiculopathy or brachial plexopathy.

Imaging studies of the cervical spine, shoulder, and chest should be considered. Electrodiagnostic studies are useful in confirming a long thoracic neuropathy. Motor and sensory nerve conduction studies of the contralateral upper limb will generally be normal, but they should be performed to rule out other diagnoses, such as brachial plexopathy. The EMG abnormalities are limited to the serratus anterior muscle.

Nerve recovery can be followed with serial EMG examinations. However, unlike other focal neuropathies, electrodiagnostic findings in long thoracic neuropathies have not been found to correlate with functional outcome.[54]

Most long thoracic neuropathies recover spontaneously within 1 year.[107] While recovery is taking place, range of motion exercises are important to avoid development of adhesive capsulitis of the shoulder. Scapulothoracic bracing is available but is usually poorly tolerated.[148] If clinically indicated, penetrating injuries should be treated with surgical exploration and early repair.[87] In patients who remain symptomatic after 1 year and have EMG evidence of total denervation, surgery can be performed in an attempt to alleviate pain and improve function. Options for surgery include scapulothoracic fusion, fascial sling suspension, and muscle transfer.[87] Currently, the most used method is muscle transfer. Transfer of the tendon of the pectoralis major's sternocostal head to the scapula is the most common surgical treatment used to treat serratus anterior paralysis. This technique has a 70–91% success rate in decreasing pain and scapular winging, as well as restoring shoulder motion.[62,72,90,112]

Spinal accessory nerve

The spinal accessory, or 11th cranial nerve, is a pure motor nerve. It supplies the sternocleidomastoid and trapezius muscles. The trapezius muscle functions to elevate, retract, and rotate the scapula. Injury to the spinal accessory nerve can occur with surgery in the posterior cervical triangle, such as cervical lymph node biopsy,[41] radical neck dissection,[120] and carotid endarterectomy.[134] The nerve can also be damaged by blunt trauma or traction injuries.

Patients complain of pain and weakness around the shoulder and periscapular regions. The affected shoulder is depressed, and atrophy of the trapezius muscle can be evident on inspection. Weakness of shoulder shrug, shoulder flexion, and shoulder abduction is found on examination. Lateral winging of the scapula is magnified during shoulder abduction. This has the effect of deepening the axilla. Secondary problems, such as adhesive capsulitis of the shoulder, subacromial impingement, and radicular type pain from traction on the brachial plexus, can be present due to impaired scapulothoracic function.[87]

Routine upper extremity motor and sensory nerve conduction studies will be normal. The compound motor action potential amplitude of the spinal accessory nerve will be low or absent on the involved side, and should be compared with the unaffected side. Needle EMG of the trapezius muscle shows signs of denervation and/or reinnervation. The sternocleidomastoid muscle is usually normal, unless the lesion is more proximal, in which case both the trapezius and the sternocleidomastoid will have EMG abnormalities. Other shoulder girdle and paraspinal muscles should be studied to rule out underlying cervical radiculopathy, plexopathy, or other proximal neuropathy.

Treatment options for spinal accessory neuropathy are similar to those for long thoracic neuropathy. For patients who fail conservative treatment after 1 year, surgery can be considered. As with long thoracic neuropathy, muscle transfer surgery is preferred over scapulothoracic fusion and fascial-sling suspensions.[87] Muscle transfer surgery for trapezius winging commonly consists of lateral transfers of the levator scapula, rhomboideus minor, and rhomboideus major muscles. In one study, 91% of patients had significant pain improvement and 87% had improved function after undergoing the above muscle transfer surgery for trapezius winging.[14]

Common peroneal nerve

Peroneal entrapment neuropathy occurs most frequently at the fibular head, and is the most common lower limb compressive neuropathy. The common peroneal nerve arises from the sciatic nerve at the popliteal fossa. It divides near the fibular head into the deep and superficial peroneal nerves. The deep peroneal nerve passes around the neck of the fibula. It innervates the tibialis anterior, peroneus tertius, extensor digitorum longus and brevis, and extensor hallucis brevis, and provides sensation to the first web space. The superficial peroneal nerve innervates the peroneus longus and brevis, and provides sensation to the dorsum of the foot and lateral lower leg.

Symptoms of common peroneal neuropathy at the fibular head (CPNFH) can vary, but typically include partial or complete foot drop and sensory loss involving the dorsum of the foot and lower lateral leg. The patient can report frequent tripping or falls, secondary to foot drop. Pain is rare. If there are complaints of low back pain or radicular leg pain, L5 radiculopathy should be ruled out.

The peroneal nerve is most commonly injured secondary to external compression as it courses around the fibular head. At this level, the nerve is more susceptible to compression injury, because it is only covered by subcutaneous tissue and is directly apposed to bone. Predisposing factors to CPNFH include prolonged immobilization and altered consciousness (such as in coma, prolonged bed rest, or anesthesia). Other sources of external pressure include plaster casts, knee braces, frequent crossing of legs (especially when weight loss has occurred), and prolonged squatting or kneeling.[103] Peroneal nerve palsy has been reported after use of intermittent sequential pneumatic compression[110] and ankle–foot orthoses.[122] Rarer causes of CPNFH include an underlying nerve tumor, cyst, ganglion, or lipoma. Direct nerve trauma from fibular fracture, knee dislocation, knee surgery, lacerations, and blunt injuries can result in CPNFH.

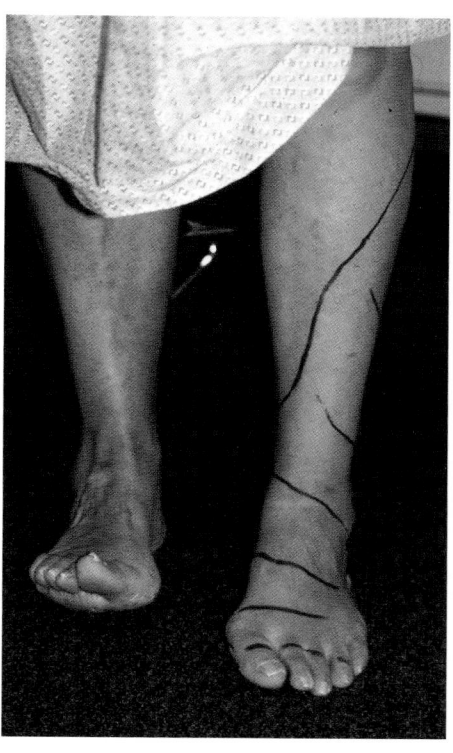

Figure 48-14 A patient with a peroneal nerve injury at the fibular head, with involvement of both the superficial and the deep branches. The patient's sensory loss pattern is marked. The patient is unable to fully dorsiflex the foot due to weakness of the tibialis anterior muscle.

When patients present with a foot drop, it is always important to carefully differentiate between L5 radiculopathy, CPNFH, injury to the lateral division of the sciatic nerve, or even a more central cause such as stroke. Physical examination in CPNFH shows non-spastic weakness of ankle and toe dorsiflexion, and ankle eversion. Sensory changes on the dorsum of the foot and lower lateral leg are present (Fig. 48-14). Posterior tibial muscle weakness, a depressed medial hamstring reflex, and a positive straight leg-raising test are more suggestive for L5 radiculopathy. A Tinel's sign over the peroneal nerve at the fibular neck can be present. In some instances, only the deep peroneal nerve is involved. This gives the same sensory loss as CPNFH, except that sensation will be normal in the first web space and ankle eversion strength will be normal.

Electrodiagnostic studies are important in ruling out other diagnoses, the most common being L5 radiculopathy. EMG and nerve conduction studies also provide information on the nature of the lesion (demyelinating and/or axonal) and site of lesion, and allow predictions about the expected course of recovery. A motor nerve conduction study of the common peroneal nerve should be performed above and below the fibular head, with recording at the extensor digitorum brevis or anterior tibialis. In CPNFH, the pattern of findings can include focal slowing, conduction block, and/or temporal dispersion across the fibular head. Sensory nerve conduction study of the superficial peroneal nerve can be normal in mild cases but, if abnormal, it is very helpful in excluding an L5 radiculopathy. Needle EMG should cover the peroneally innervated muscles, including the short head of the biceps femoris as well as other non-peroneal L5 innervated muscles, such as the posterior tibial and the gluteus medius. The short head of the biceps femoris typically has normal needle EMG findings, because this peroneal innervated muscle lies proximal to the fibular head.

Conservative treatment consists of patient education in decreasing aggravating activities, such as prolonged squatting (often seen in gardeners, carpet layers, and roofers). Any external compressive source, such as a cast, needs to be adjusted or replaced. Thin patients who frequently cross their legs might respond to the use of kneepads placed at the fibular head and neck. In patients with foot drop, ankle–foot orthoses can help with ankle support and fall prevention. Ankle range of motion exercise should be encouraged to avoid joint contracture. Spontaneous improvement should occur over 2–3 months in lesions with conduction block, as long as further compression is eliminated. Repeat EMG can aid in monitoring the recovery process. Surgery is reserved for severe cases with axonal loss, which after 4–6 months have not responded to conservative care,[81] or when a mass lesion such as a tumor, cyst, or ganglion is present. Surgical intervention is also required in cases of complete nerve laceration, and should be done early in the course.

Lateral femoral cutaneous nerve

The lateral femoral cutaneous nerve of the thigh supplies sensation to the anterolateral aspect of the thigh. The nerve arises from the second and third lumbar roots, and is a pure sensory nerve. It courses through the lumbar plexus and then around the pelvic brim to exit beneath the inguinal ligament adjacent to the anterior superior iliac spine.[29]

Meralgia paresthetica is an entrapment syndrome of the lateral femoral cutaneous nerve at the anterior superior iliac spine. Patients present with pain, paresthesias, and sensory loss in the anterolateral thigh. Prolonged compression of the nerve secondary to lower abdominal or upper thigh obesity is the most frequent cause. Diabetes and thyroid disease can be predisposing factors. Other sources of compression include pregnancy and the wearing of excessively tight clothing or belts. Mass effect on the nerve is a much less common etiology. Reported cases include uterine leiomyoma,[132] psoas muscle tumor,[2] and metastases in the lumbar spine.[117] The nerve can be directly traumatized by pelvic fractures and during abdominal or pelvic surgeries.

Diagnosis is made primarily by the history and physical examination. Examination shows sensory changes in the anterolateral thigh (Fig. 48-15). Symptoms are often exacerbated by hip extension. Relief of symptoms following a nerve block with local anesthetic can confirm the diagnosis.[77] Nerve conduction studies of the lateral femoral cutaneous nerve are often challenging even in non-obese patients. However, if a reliable response can be elicited, it can be compared with the unaffected side. Electrodiagnostic studies are important to rule out other diagnoses, such as lumbar radiculopathy, plexopathy, and other neuropathy. Imaging studies are needed if underlying mass or trauma is suspected.

Treatment for meralgia paresthetica is dependent on the underlying disorder, and can include weight loss, avoidance of constrictive clothing, relative rest, application of ice, NSAIDs,

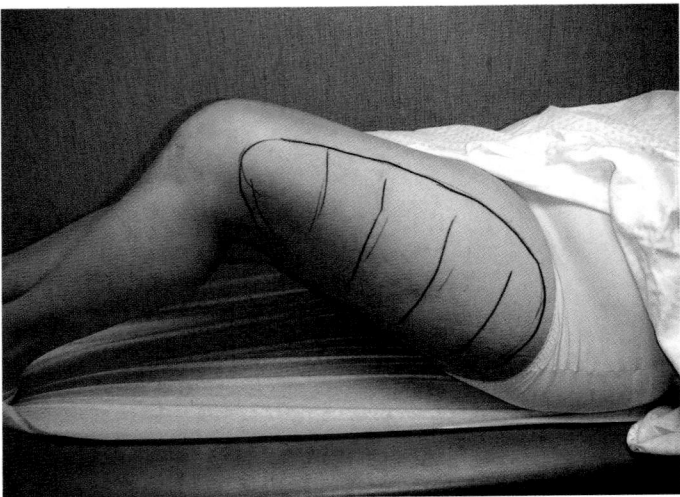

Figure 48-15 Sensory involvement of the lateral femoral cutaneous nerve in meralgia paresthetica.

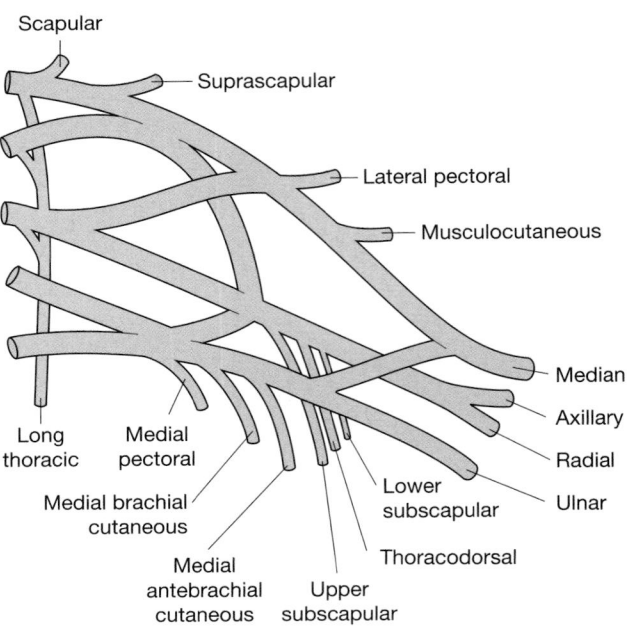

Figure 48-16 The brachial plexus. Ventral branches of the spinal nerves from C5 through T1 intermingle to form the peripheral nerves of the upper limb. (From Buschbacher 1994,[26] with permission of Butterworth-Heinemann.)

injection of local anesthetic, and decompressive surgery. Treatment of neuropathic pain can include tricyclic antidepressants, antiseizure medications, topical capsaicin, or lidocaine–prilocaine cream. Most patients improve with conservative therapy over a few months.[152]

Tibial nerve

Tarsal tunnel syndrome is an entrapment of the tibial nerve under the flexor retinaculum at the level of the medial malleolus. The contents of the tarsal tunnel include the tibial nerve, flexor hallucis longus tendon, flexor digitorum longus tendon, and posterior tibial artery.

The exact etiology of tarsal tunnel syndrome is often unknown. It can be associated with ankle trauma, excessive pronation or supination of the foot, edema, pes planus, or an underlying ganglion cyst. Symptoms include tingling and burning along the medial ankle and sole of foot. The medial, lateral, or both aspects of the sole can be affected, depending on whether the medial or lateral plantar branches or the main trunk of the tibial nerve are affected. The pain commonly occurs at rest and is often intensified after walking.

On examination, tenderness is present over the tarsal tunnel, which is just posterior to the medial malleolus. A Tinel's sign can be present at this location, and the test often reproduces some of the symptoms. Sensation can be altered along the distribution of the lateral and medial plantar branches of the tibial nerve on the plantar aspect of the foot. Weakness of the intrinsic foot musculature can be present but is frequently difficult to assess clinically.

Imaging studies, such as radiographs or MRI of the foot and ankle, can identify underlying bony pathology or ganglion. Electrodiagnostic testing can help confirm the diagnosis by demonstrating prolonged distal latencies in the medial and/or lateral plantar nerves. Needle examination may show signs of membrane instability and neurogenic-type motor unit potentials in the abductor hallucis and/or abductor digiti quinti.

Treatment options include orthoses to correct foot pronation or supination, NSAIDs, and corticosteroid–local anesthetic injection. Surgical release for tarsal tunnel syndrome does not have as high a rate of success as that of carpal tunnel release. However, when the patient has significant symptoms that do not respond to conservative management, surgery should be considered. In one surgical series, patients who had space-occupying lesions as the etiology of tarsal tunnel syndrome had better surgical outcomes than those in which the etiology was idiopathic, posttraumatic, or due to foot deformities.[142]

Brachial plexus

The brachial plexus is a complex structure originating from the C5–T1 nerve roots (Fig. 48-16). The plexus is divided into roots, trunks, divisions, cords, and terminal branches. Lesions are typically described as involving the upper, middle, and lower trunks, or lateral, posterior, and medial cords. At times, a complete lesion can occur with involvement of the entire plexus.

Trauma is the most common cause of brachial plexopathy. Open injuries can occur from stab wounds or gunshot wounds. Closed injuries typically produce injury due to traction on the plexus, such as after a fall. Intraoperative brachial plexus injuries can occur during median sternotomies or thoracotomies. Injuries that cause the head and shoulder to be stretched apart, such as in newborn deliveries or falls on the shoulder, typically result in upper trunk plexopathies with involvement of C5 and C6 fibers and/or the upper trunk, typically referred to as Erb paralysis (Fig. 48-17). The resulting weakness in shoulder abduction, elbow flexion, and forearm supination causes the

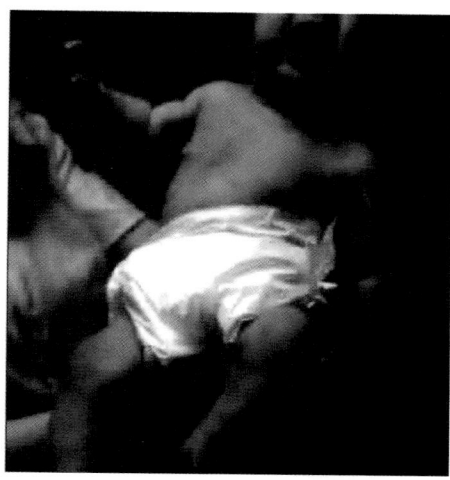

Figure 48-17
Newborn baby with Erb palsy of the left limb.

upper limb to be held in shoulder adduction and internal rotation, and wrist flexion, the so-called 'waiter's tip' deformity. Lower trunk plexopathies affect the C8–T1 fibers, resulting in severe hand weakness, known as Klumpke palsy. This can occur after an injury in which there is forceful upward traction on the arm.

Brachial plexopathy can also occur with an underlying mass, such as a Pancoast tumor of the lung, lymphoma, or breast cancer. At times, the presentation must be differentiated from a radiation plexitis (see Ch. 58). Neuralgic amyotrophy or Parsonage–Turner syndrome can affect the brachial plexus, and is described in more detail later in this chapter.

The diagnosis of a brachial plexopathy can be supported by electrodiagnostic studies. Sensory nerve conduction studies are abnormal in the affected territory, unless the lesion is preganglionic, as in a root avulsion. Motor nerve conduction studies also can be abnormal, depending on the portion of the plexus involved and on the amount of axonal loss. Needle examination shows evidence of denervation and/or reinnervation in affected muscles of more than a single root or peripheral nerve distribution. Lack of abnormalities on needle examination of the cervical paraspinal muscles further supports a diagnosis of brachial plexopathy rather than cervical radiculopathy. With underlying tumor, the extent of cord or rootlet disruption can be assessed with MRI of the cervical spine or axilla.

Treatment for brachial plexopathy has several components. Positioning is important to prevent edema and to provide support. Range of motion exercises are needed to prevent contracture. Orthoses might be necessary to improve upper extremity function and provide stabilization. Pain medications such as anticonvulsants, tricyclic antidepressants, NSAIDs, cyclooxygenase-2 inhibitors, and opioids can be of benefit. Muscle reeducation should be started once pain is controlled and patients are able to tolerate strengthening exercises. Surgery is typically considered if there is no recovery by 3 months, or if recovery has plateaued before 6 months following injury.[79] Options for surgical treatment include neurolysis, primary nerve repair, grafting, and nerve transfers.[79]

Idiopathic brachial neuritis (Parsonage–Turner syndrome)

Idiopathic brachial neuropathy, or brachial neuritis, is a peripheral neuropathy that most commonly affects the radial, long thoracic, phrenic, suprascapular, or spinal accessory nerves.[85,147] Men are affected twice as frequently as women.[83] In approximately one-third of the cases, the shoulders are affected bilaterally, although one side can be more severely involved.[39] This condition classically begins with spontaneous onset of a deep aching pain in one shoulder. The pain often is excruciating. One to two weeks later, the patient notes weakness in the affected muscles. Atrophy typically develops several weeks later.[39,85] The motor nerves are usually more affected than the sensory nerves. If sensory nerves are affected, the most likely deficits are the axillary, radial, or cutaneous nerves of the upper extremity.[39]

Electrodiagnostic studies show that motor conduction velocities are normal in the nerve fibers to the unaffected muscles. Latencies from Erb's point to the affected muscles can be slightly prolonged, with decreased amplitude and temporal dispersion.[85] Needle examination reveals signs of acute denervation in the affected muscles.[19,85] The most affected muscles should also be sampled contralaterally, as abnormality can be present that has not been detected clinically.

Prognosis is generally good,[39] but recovery can take several years in severe cases.[85,141] Rehabilitation management includes maintaining shoulder range of motion and preventing contractures, so that the limb is functional when recovery eventually occurs. Orthotic prescription is also often appropriate. For example, a wrist–hand orthosis can be useful if wrist drop is present.

Lumbosacral plexus

The lumbosacral plexus is formed by the lumbar and sacral plexuses (Fig. 48-18). Injuries of the lumbosacral plexus can be associated with underlying trauma, such as with pelvic fractures. Colorectal and gynecologic tumors can cause lumbosacral plexopathies, as can radiation treatment (see Ch. 58). Damage to the lumbosacral plexus can occur intraoperatively during hip surgery, and intrapartum from labor and delivery. Other underlying causes include inflammation, ischemia, or hemorrhage. Diabetic amyotrophy commonly affects the femoral and obturator nerves, and is discussed later in the chapter.

The symptoms of a lumbosacral plexopathy vary depending on the area of involvement. Plexopathies involving the lumbar plexus cause weakness in hip flexion, knee extension, and hip adduction. Sensory loss involves the anterolateral thigh and medial lower leg. Pain occurs with retroperitoneal hemorrhage or tumor. It tends to be felt in the groin and radiates to the thigh when the hip is extended. With involvement of the lower lumbar and sacral roots, there is weakness in hip extension, abduction, and knee flexion. Weakness in dorsiflexion, plantar flexion, eversion, and inversion of the ankle can be present also. Sensory changes typically involve the lower leg, foot, or posterior thigh.

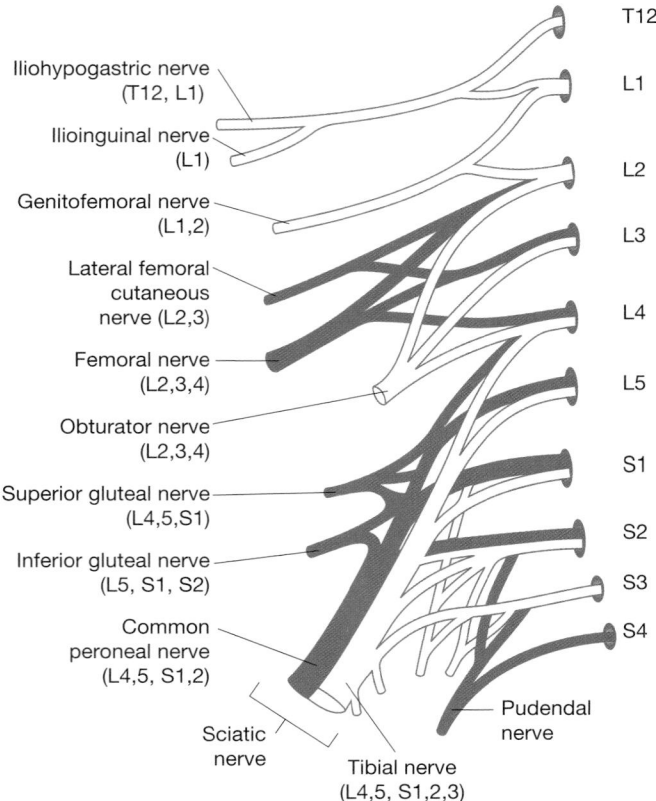

Figure 48-18 Diagram of the lumbosacral plexus. Posterior nerves are shaded. (From Tan 1998,[136] with permission.)

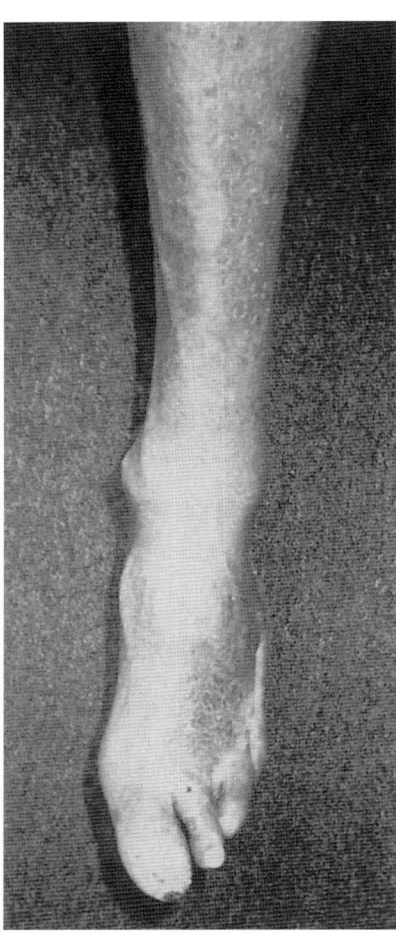

Figure 48-19 Typical appearance of a foot with changes of diabetic peripheral neuropathy and peripheral vascular disease.

Electrodiagnostic studies are important for localizing the lesion and aiding in prognosis. Distinguishing a lumbosacral plexopathy from a radiculopathy is important (sensory nerve conduction studies can be abnormal in plexopathy). The lumbar paraspinal EMG is normal in lumbar plexopathy, but shows signs of denervation and/or reinnervation in affected muscles of more than a single root or peripheral nerve distribution. When axonal loss is present, motor and sensory nerve action potentials can show decreased amplitudes in the affected nerves. Other tests that can help make a specific diagnosis include vascular studies (if ischemia is suspected) and imaging studies (for identifying tumors or hemorrhage).

Treatment for lumbosacral plexopathy is similar to that for brachial plexopathy, except that gait training is also often needed. Assistive devices, such as a walker or cane, can be helpful in stabilizing gait. Acute surgical intervention might be indicated, depending on the underlying etiology.

POLYNEUROPATHIES

The following is a discussion of the rehabilitation management of several representative polyneuropathies. This list is not all-inclusive, but the principles described can readily be adapted to other, similar disorders.

Diabetic neuropathies

Both insulin-dependent and non-insulin-dependent diabetes mellitus can cause neuropathies. These are classified by whether the manifestations are symmetric or asymmetric (Figs. 48-19 to 48-21). In the symmetric group are polyneuropathies, including:

- a primarily sensory peripheral neuropathy, the most common of the diabetic neuropathies (acroneuropathy);
- autonomic peripheral neuropathy, which is often seen in conjunction with the sensory form;
- acute painful neuropathy; and
- subclinical neuropathy.

The asymmetric neuropathies include:

- mononeuropathies and radiculopathies;
- proximal lower extremity motor neuropathy, also known as diabetic amyotrophy; and
- entrapment neuropathies (see above).

It should be kept in mind that these neuropathies can also be caused by other diseases, and every neuropathy in a patient having diabetes should not automatically be diagnosed as a diabetic neuropathy. Hyperglycemia in a newly diagnosed diabetic patient or one whose diabetes is poorly controlled can also cause

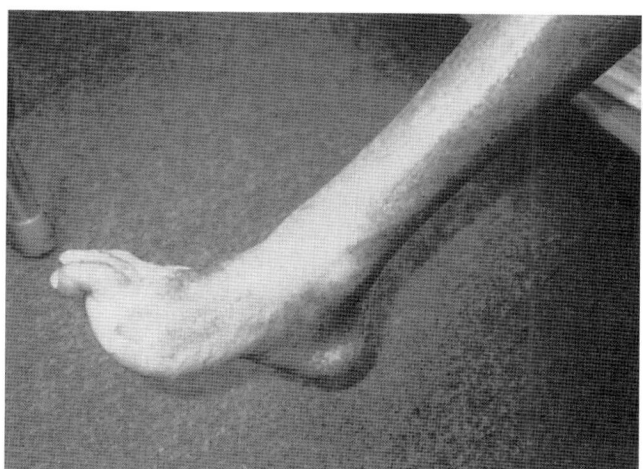

Figure 48-20 Foot with changes of diabetic peripheral neuropathy and peripheral vascular disease.

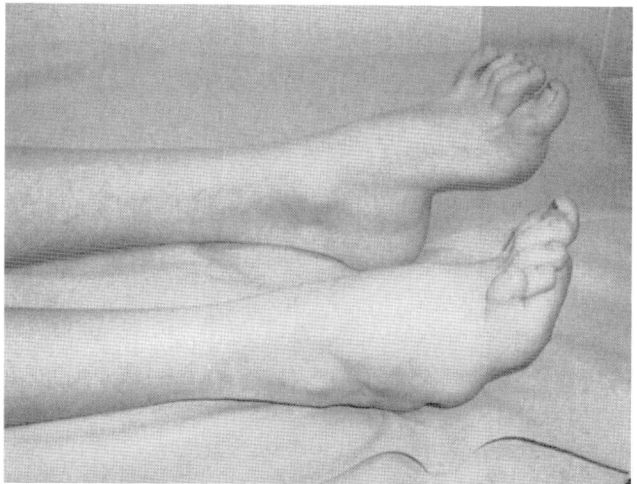

Figure 48-21 'Intrinsic minus' foot deformity in a patient with diabetic peripheral neuropathy.

a reduction in nerve conduction velocity, which can be asymptomatic. This slowing might be reversible.[139] Diabetes predisposes the patient to the development of focal neuropathies such as CTS.

Descriptions

Symmetric peripheral neuropathy in diabetes   The initial symptoms of diabetic symmetric polyneuropathy are usually sensory and located distally. They include burning, itching, and a 'pins and needles' sensation. Patients can also complain of muscle cramping or tightness, especially at night. On physical examination, the greatest abnormalities are in light touch and vibration, with preservation of proprioception until late in the course. The symptoms begin in the toes and progress proximally over the course of months to years. The longest nerves are

affected first. The fingers and hands can become involved later, giving the typical stocking and glove distribution.[119] If the diabetic patient with severe peripheral sensory impairment does not care for the affected areas meticulously, repeated undetected trauma can result in skin ulceration, Charcot joint, and ultimately even amputation.

Weakness is generally seen later in the course of diabetic neuropathy. It starts distally and progresses proximally. A 'foot slap' due to foot dorsiflexor weakness is often the first sign of weakness. Patients with diabetic polyneuropathy can also have an ataxic gait. This can be due to weakness of ankle musculature or, in later stages of the illness, abnormal proprioception.

An acute painful diabetic neuropathy occurs rarely but can be very troublesome. It is characterized by severe symmetric pain in the distal lower extremities, described as a burning dysesthesia. It is often associated with depression, insomnia, and weight loss.[139] Examination reveals only mild, if any, sensory loss.[4] Allodynia might be found on sensory examination. This type of neuropathy has been referred to inappropriately as diabetic 'neuritis'.

Lower extremity proximal motor neuropathy   Lower extremity proximal motor neuropathy was earlier called 'diabetic amyotrophy'. It was initially described as being a unilateral proximal leg weakness, but is now known to at times occur bilaterally as well.[138]

It was once thought that the cause of this disorder was a spinal cord lesion, but electrodiagnostic studies have shown that the lesion is located in the nerve roots and plexus.[138]

The onset of this neuropathy can be acute or subacute. Pain is often the initial complaint and is worse at night.[138] It can be located in the low back, hip, or proximal leg. The pain is described as a deep ache and can be severe in degree. Weakness appears several weeks after the onset of the pain, and is located in the quadriceps, iliopsoas, or thigh adductors, individually or more often in combination.[138] The gluteal muscles, hamstrings, and gastrocnemius can also be weak. Sensation tends to become abnormal about the same time the motor dysfunction appears, and is most often located in the femoral nerve territory, including the region of the saphenous nerve. Recovery occurs over a 12- to 24-month period, and the prognosis for significant improvement is generally good.[138]

Mononeuropathy and entrapment neuropathy   Individual cranial or peripheral nerves can be affected as a manifestation of diabetic neuropathy. The oculomotor cranial nerve is most commonly affected, although the abducens, trochlear, and facial nerves can be involved as well.[138] The pupil is usually spared in oculomotor palsy.[60] Individual peripheral nerves such as the median at the wrist, ulnar at the elbow, and peroneal at the knee can be affected in isolation.

Multiple nerves can also be affected in an asymmetric fashion. This is referred to as mononeuropathy multiplex. In this condition, the onset tends to be subacute or insidious. This is in contrast to mononeuritis multiplex, as seen in polyarteritis nodosa or other systemic vasculitides, where the onset tends to be acute and then progress in a stepwise fashion over days to weeks.

Persons with diabetes have long been thought to be at increased risk for entrapment neuropathies. Fraser et al. found no clear-cut relationship between the mononeuropathies and duration of diabetes, diabetic control, or the presence of other diabetic complications.[52] The preponderance of evidence, however, seems to support the common belief that diabetes does indeed predispose to the development of focal pressure neuropathies.[74,139]

Truncal radiculopathy   Thoracoabdominal or truncal neuropathy or radiculopathy occurs most often in diabetic patients older than age 50.[119] Onset is usually acute, but in some cases can be gradual. The distribution is usually unilateral, involving primarily T3 through T12.[131] The condition is often painful and includes a differential diagnosis of myocardial infarction, an intraspinal pathologic process, abdominal disease, or malignancy.[119] Sensory loss and allodynia can be found in the painful area. This type of neuropathy can occur in isolation or with the proximal asymmetric type of neuropathy described above. Symptoms tend to gradually improve over several months.

Management of diabetic peripheral neuropathy

Medical management   The exact pathophysiology of diabetic neuropathy remains undetermined, so there is consequently no definitive treatment. Two current hypotheses are that the nerve injury is due to metabolic or ischemic processes.[23,140] These processes are not mutually exclusive. Pathologic studies provide evidence for ischemic microvascular disease,[55] while metabolic abnormalities include an accumulation of sorbitol and a reduction of myoinositol.[55,63] Because glucose is converted to sorbitol by aldose reductase, it was once thought that aldose reductase inhibitors could improve the course of disease. They have not, however, been shown to be significantly helpful in the treatment of peripheral neuropathy, or have produced potentially significant side effects.[75] Because there is a reduced myoinositol content in diabetic peripheral nerves, it was hypothesized that supplementation with this substance could be a useful treatment. In animal studies, myoinositol has improved nerve conduction velocities,[63] but clinical trials in humans have not shown any significant benefit.[64] The most important preventive measure for diabetic neuropathy is generally believed to be good glucose control.

Sensory changes   Sensory loss is the most common symptom of diabetic peripheral neuropathy. Because decreased protective sensation is frequently compounded by vascular insufficiency and dry skin (due to autonomic impairment), skin breakdown can occur. Careful daily inspection of the affected areas is necessary, with daily soaks followed by the use of a moisturizing cream or lotion. Toenails must be cut carefully straight across to prevent ingrown nails. Proper footwear, with appropriate in-shoe orthoses, is imperative. The patient should avoid use of heat on the affected limbs, and avoid foot trauma. When there is concern for skin breakdown, a podiatrist should be involved in the patient's care. If such preventive measures are not undertaken, ulceration and neuroarthropathy are common. Poor healing of ulcers can lead to gangrene, and ultimately to amputation.

Pain   Neuropathic pain in patients with diabetes is often difficult to manage. The treatment approach is generally the same as that described above. The pain of diabetic neuropathy typically decreases spontaneously over time, and patients should be encouraged to remain active to avoid the complications of inactivity.

Autonomic dysfunction   Autonomic dysfunction is often seen together with sensory loss. This can involve various body functions, including the cardiovascular, genitourinary, gastrointestinal, and thermoregulatory systems.

The primary cardiovascular abnormalities are orthostatic hypotension, cardiac arrhythmias, and impaired heart rate control.[70] Orthostatic hypotension might be the only one of these to actually produce symptoms. The cause of orthostatic hypotension is most likely an impaired vasoconstriction reflex.[70] Heart abnormalities include a resting tachycardia, fixed heart rate, and loss of sleep bradycardia.[47] Postural hypotension should be managed with the least invasive measures. The initial treatment is to teach the patient to change position slowly and to consider sleeping with the head of the bed elevated.[138] Compression stockings and an abdominal binder can improve venous return and decrease symptoms. When these fail, use of a mineralocorticoid such as fludrocortisone or the α agonist midodrine might benefit the patient.[138]

Gastrointestinal dysautonomia can manifest as esophageal dysmotility,[129] gastroparesis,[95] bowel incontinence,[124] and constipation or diarrhea.[121,124] Patients with diabetic gastroparesis often complain of abdominal bloating, nausea, vomiting, early satiety with eating, and heartburn. Gastroparesis diabeticorum is typically treated with metoclopramide.[95] Diarrhea or constipation can be treated with a proper diet. A course of tetracycline or another broad spectrum antibiotic can also be used to help alleviate diarrhea.[145]

Common genitourinary abnormalities include erectile dysfunction[121] and neurogenic bladder.[76] Diabetic impotence is common in the male and is usually irreversible.[49] Treatment choices include counseling, medication, suction erection devices, and penile implants (see Ch. 32). The early signs of neurogenic bladder include decreased urinary frequency, followed by difficulties with initiating micturition. The bladder eventually becomes flaccid, and urinary retention with overflow voiding occurs as the neuropathy worsens.[24,48] The management of neurogenic bladder depends on the severity of the condition (see Ch. 29). Postvoiding residual measurement often helps in determining the severity. In cases of mild to moderate impairment of bladder function, the patient should be encouraged to empty the bladder every 2–3 h while awake. As severity increases, an intermittent catheterization program might be necessary to assure adequate drainage. Use of a parasympathomimetic agent can also be helpful (see Ch. 29).

When the thermoregulatory system is also affected, there can be impaired distal sweating. It can leave the skin dry and subject to cracking and fissuring. Regular skin care and lubrication are necessary (see Chs 33 and 57).

Acute inflammatory demyelinating polyradiculopathy

Acute inflammatory demyelinating polyradiculopathy, also known as Guillain–Barré syndrome, was first described by Landry in the 1860s, but derived its eponym from a description in 1916 by Georges Guillain and Jean Alexander Barré. Guillain and Barré recognized that this was a paralyzing condition associated with an increased concentration of protein, but not cells, in the cerebrospinal fluid. This laboratory finding was termed cytoalbuminologic disassociation, and distinguished the condition from other causes of acquired acute paralysis such as poliomyelitis. Since their original description, other related disorders have been identified. These include a relapsing–remitting form, the Miller–Fisher variant, in which there is ataxia, ophthalmoplegia, and depressed MSRs but preserved strength,[50] and a slowly progressive (chronic) steroid-responsive form.

Guillain–Barré syndrome is an acquired symmetric polyneuropathy that usually affects the lower extremities initially. It often begins with paresthesias in the toes or fingertips, followed shortly by weakness, which begins distally and then ascends proximally. Pain is a less common symptom but can be present in the form of a deep backache, or less commonly as painful limb paresthesias. The weakness progresses over days to about 4 weeks and can, in severe cases, produce total body paresis, including of the muscles of respiration. GBS can involve somatic, cranial, and autonomic nerves. The extraocular muscles and sphincters are generally spared.

The etiology of GBS is not fully established, but the condition often begins several weeks following a viral or bacterial infection, immunization, or surgery.[9] Diagnostic criteria[118] for typical GBS include the required features of areflexia and acquired, progressive weakness in all extremities. Features that strongly support the diagnosis include progression over a period of up to 4 weeks, relative symmetry, mild sensory symptoms, cranial nerve involvement, recovery beginning 2–4 weeks after progression ceases, autonomic dysfunction, elevated concentration of protein in the cerebrospinal fluid with <10 cells per mm³, and typical electrodiagnostic features.

On physical examination, GBS shows symmetric limb weakness. Bilateral facial weakness is also present in one-third of the patients. The MSRs are absent. Sensory deficits are usually mild. If respiratory muscles are involved, the vital capacity is usually one-half the predicted value. The vital capacity should be carefully monitored, because weakness can progress rapidly and the patient might require ventilatory support. Autonomic function is often affected (71%)[59] and can produce abnormalities in heart rate, heart rhythm, and blood pressure. A period of observation in an intensive care unit is necessary. Patients who require ventilatory support generally have a longer period of recovery that can extend over months.[99]

The damage to the nerve in GBS appears to be primarily of a demyelinating type, but in more severe cases there can also be prominent axonal loss.[39] Histologic examination of the nerves reveals lymphocytes and macrophages surrounding the endoneurial vessels.[5] The neuropathy is thought to be produced by a cell-mediated attack on the myelin sheath, although in some cases the axons appear to be the target instead. In general, antibodies have not been shown to be causative of the nerve dysfunction. The role of other humoral mediators, such as cytokines, has also not been established thus far.

The nerves are affected earliest at the root level.[9] Shortly thereafter, the most distal part of the nerve becomes involved, with the intervening segments being affected last.

Electrodiagnostic findings in Guillain–Barré syndrome

Because the earliest involvement of GBS is at the nerve root level, the earliest electrodiagnostic abnormalities are prolongation or absence of the late responses (F wave and H reflex). A few days later, there can be a prolongation of distal latency, and then slowing of motor nerve conduction velocity. Temporal dispersion of the evoked responses and partial conduction block between distal and proximal stimulus sites can also be seen. The EMG in patients with weakness tends to show a reduction in the number of motor units firing on maximal effort.

If serial studies are performed, the electrodiagnostic findings frequently lag behind the clinical course, both during worsening and recovery phases.[8] EMG signs of denervation indicate that the patient has a component of axonopathy rather than just demyelination. A poorer short-term outcome is suggested when axonal change is seen with the amplitude of the distal compound muscle action potential < 10% of normal.

Management of Guillain–Barré syndrome

Patients with acute GBS should be hospitalized for observation and monitoring of the progression of the disease. It is particularly important to serially monitor the pulmonary and cardiovascular systems. If the vital capacity is rapidly declining, especially if it is <18 mL/kg of body weight,[118] or if there is cardiovascular dysautonomia, the patient should be monitored in an intensive care unit. Mechanical ventilation might become necessary.

Due to their immobility, these patients are at risk for developing deep venous thrombosis, pressure ulcers, and other complications of immobility. Appropriate preventive and treatment measures should be undertaken. Treatment with plasmapheresis or high-dose intravenous immunoglobulin (IVIg) is effective in shortening the course of an attack of GBS.[97] Plasmapheresis is done in a series of three to five plasma exchanges, performed on an approximately every other day schedule.[65] Intravenous gamma globulin is usually administered daily at 0.4 g/kg of body weight for five consecutive days.[105]

Intravenous immunoglobulin has some advantages over plasmapheresis. It is easier to administer, has fewer complications, and is more comfortable for the patient.[105] IVIg can cause self-limited flu-like symptoms such as fever, myalgia, headache, nausea, and vomiting.[92] It should be used cautiously in patients with congestive heart failure and renal failure, due to the resulting increased plasma volume.[105]

Contraindications to plasma exchange include recent myocardial infarction, angina, sepsis, or cardiovascular dysautonomia.[118] A rare complication of plasmapheresis is sepsis, thought to be secondary to immunoglobulin depletion.[53] There is a risk of acquiring viral infections, such as hepatitis or HIV, if fresh frozen plasma is used. GBS does not respond to corticosteroids.[71]

Rehabilitation methods   In the early stages of GBS, the patient can be bedridden due to weakness and even tetraplegia. During this time, it is important to prevent contractures with range of motion exercise, positioning, and the use of static splints. Careful positioning and turning are necessary to prevent peripheral nerve compression and pressure ulcer formation. Meticulous pulmonary care is indicated to prevent atelectasis and pneumonia.

The rehabilitation program is gradually advanced in intensity as the patient improves. Because the patient with GBS is susceptible to overwork weakness, the strengthening program should initially be non-fatiguing. When muscles regain greater than antigravity strength, they can generally be stressed with more aggressive strengthening exercises. If the exercises are advanced too quickly, however, there can be a regression of strength (the so-called overwork weakness).[10] This occurrence should alert the clinician and therapist to reduce the activity level.

During recovery, patients with GBS often benefit from the use of orthoses and assistive devices. Rocker feeders are helpful, as are clothing adaptations and other assistive devices (see Ch. 27). Ankle–foot and wrist orthoses can be useful in preventing contractures and enhancing function. It is more common for GBS patients to develop tightness of two-joint muscles than joint contractures. Stretching of these muscles alleviates this problem, and should include the hamstrings, tensor fascia lata, and gastrocnemius muscles.

Gait retraining typically begins with the use of the tilt table. The tilt table is actually valuable well before gait training is possible, as it helps prevent orthostatic intolerance. Tilt table training can be instituted as soon as the patient is medically stable. This can also be started by elevating the head of the bed and having the patient sit upright for extended periods as tolerated. Cardiovascular and autonomic adaptation occur as the patient is gradually elevated to the upright position. Patients are eventually allowed to stand in a standing table, which improves their muscular endurance and permits them to work on other tasks. When muscle strength improves sufficiently, the patient is advanced to the parallel bars. This is done with the close assistance of a therapist to assist in movement and to prevent falls. As gait skills improve, the patient can be advanced to an assistive device for ambulation, such as a walker, and then to crutches or canes. The patient is ultimately advanced to ambulation without assistance or with assistive devices. Lower extremity orthoses are used as indicated throughout the course of treatment (see Ch. 16).

In addition to progressive ambulation training, patients develop upper limb strength and endurance through a combination of functional and weight-training exercises. The goal is to achieve independent self-care using assistive devices as needed (only temporarily, it is hoped). Most patients tolerate such a rehabilitation program and go on to an essentially complete recovery. Approximately 85% of patients with GBS achieve a full and functional recovery within 6–12 months.[105] The 7–15% or so who do not recover completely from GBS[118] benefit from the long-term use of assistive devices and rehabilitation strategies. Relapse of GBS can occur, but only at a rate of 3–5%.[67]

HIV neuropathy

There are several types of peripheral neuropathy associated with HIV infection (Box 48-8). The most common is distal symmetric sensory polyneuropathy (DSPN). DSPN presents with distal pain, paresthesias, hyporeflexia, and relatively normal strength. Symptoms tend to manifest later in the course of the illness, develop over weeks to months, and persist once present. Risk factors for DSPN include increased age, depressed CD4 cell count, and elevated plasma HIV viral load.[33] This type of neuropathy occurs in approximately 30% of patients with a CD4 cell count at or below 200 per μL.[135] DSPN is treated similarly to other painful neuropathies. Incomplete control of symptoms is a common problem.

Another painful axonal neuropathy is due to necrotizing vasculitis, which affects the vasa nervorum of the peripheral nerve trunks. This condition occurs relatively early in infection, has a more rapid onset, and has asymmetric clinical features that are typical of mononeuritis multiplex. With vasculitic neuropathy,

---

Box 48-8 Classification of peripheral nerve complications in HIV disease

Early HIV disease
- Seroconversion-related neuropathies
- Guillain–Barré syndrome
- Mononeuropathies

Moderately advanced HIV disease
- Chronic inflammatory demyelinating polyneuropathy
- Mononeuritis multiplex
- Diffuse infiltrative lymphocytosis syndrome
- Syphilitic polyradiculopathy
- Hepatitis C infection-related neuropathy
- Human T-lymphotropic virus infection type 1-related neuropathy
- Motor neuron disease syndrome

Advanced HIV disease
- Distal symmetric sensory polyneuropathy
- Autonomic neuropathy
- HIV-related lumbosacral polyradiculopathy
- Cytomegalovirus infection-related polyradiculopathy
- Cytomegalovirus infection mononeuritis multiplex

Medication-related neuropathy
- Antiretroviral drugs: didanosine, stavudine, and zalcitabine
- Other drugs: ethambutol, HMG-CoA reductase inhibitors, isoniazid, paclitaxel (Taxol), thalidomide, vinblastine, and vincristine

(From Brew 2003,[21] with permission.)

IVIg and corticosteroid treatments can lead to rapid relief, followed by arrest of the neuropathic process.[20,21]

Medication-induced (iatrogenic) neuropathies in HIV infection present in a similar manner to DSPN, but over a shorter time. The most likely sources are the antiretroviral treatments ddI, d4T, and ddC.[34,115] In the case of ddC treatment, peripheral neuropathy is the most common dose-limiting adverse effect and is generally reversible on discontinuation.[1] Symptoms may continue, however, for up to 6–8 weeks after withdrawal of the offending drug.[21] Other medications used in HIV disease and the treatment of its complications that can be associated with a neuropathy include vincristine, vinblastine, paclitaxel (Taxol), isoniazid, ethambutol, dapsone, thalidomide, and the HMG-CoA reductase inhibitors.[21]

Progressive polyradiculomyelopathy is a rare, severe infection of nerve roots and the cauda equina. This infection is commonly caused by cytomegalovirus and less often by *Mycobacterium tuberculosis*.[35,89,127] Symptoms and signs include extreme lower extremity pain, weakness, and sphincter dysfunction. Rapid diagnosis is important, because treatment can arrest or partly reverse this otherwise fatal infection.[114] Treatment involves anticytomegalovirus therapy, antituberculous drugs, and highly active antiretroviral therapy.[21,35]

Charcot–Marie–Tooth disease (HMSN types 1 and 2)

Charcot–Marie–Tooth disease includes a group of hereditary symmetric distal polyneuropathies.[17] It is one of the most frequently inherited neurologic diseases, with an estimated prevalence of 125 000 persons in the USA.[31] The inherited CMT defects have been mapped to chromosome 17 (CMT1A), chromosome 1 (CMT1B), the X chromosome (CMTX), and others.[12,16,31,66,73,102,144] The most common type is CMT type 1 (HMSN 1). It is usually inherited in an autosomal dominant fashion.[116] CMT type 2 (HMSN 2) is one-third as common.[31]

Charcot–Marie–Tooth disease is usually detected in the first or second decade of life, although foot deformities can be noted even during infancy.[31] The initial symptoms include progressive distal lower limb weakness and then atrophy. Pes cavus deformity is common, and is exaggerated (if not caused) by the distal motor dysfunction. The most severely affected muscles are the intrinsic foot muscles and peroneal muscles.[31] Distal sensory deficits are often present.

Physical examination typically reveals peripheral weakness. The ankle MSRs are often absent, and other reflexes can be hypoactive.[98] Gait abnormalities are common, and include drop foot, foot slap, and steppage gait. As the disease progresses, the distal upper limbs can become involved, resulting in weakness and atrophy of intrinsic hand muscles and producing impaired dexterity (Fig. 48-22). Nerves can be palpably enlarged.[31]

In HMSN 1, there is segmental demyelination with secondary Schwann cell proliferation. The Schwann cells form 'onion bulbs'—concentric arrays around the axon—which account for the peripheral nerve enlargement.[45] HMSN 2 is sometimes known as the 'axonal' form of CMT disease. Histologically, it

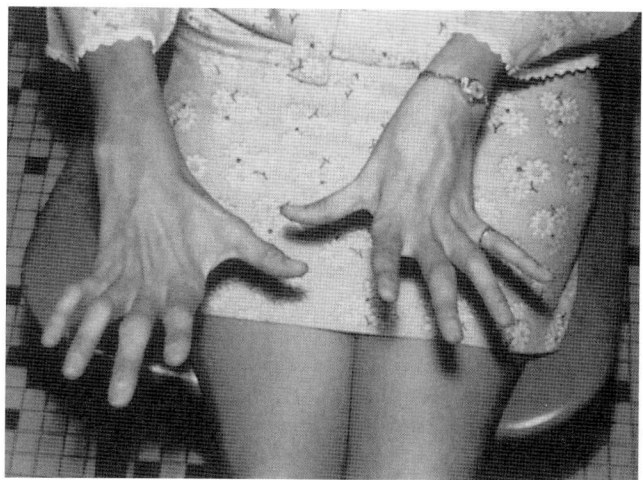

Figure 48-22 Hands of a patient with advanced Charcot–Marie–Tooth disease.

is characterized by axonal loss with subsequent Wallerian degeneration.[43]

Charcot–Marie–Tooth disease has variable penetrance.[15] A carrier might have only mild asymptomatic foot deformities, while other members of the same family exhibit significant difficulties with ambulation and hand dexterity. The symptoms of HMSN 1 and HMSN 2 are similar, although they tend to be milder in type 2.[43] In both conditions, the abnormalities progress very slowly over years to decades, with only gradual deterioration in function. Despite distal weakness, these patients typically remain ambulatory throughout their lives[43] and their lifespan is normal.[44]

Electrophysiologic studies are helpful in diagnosing CMT disease and in distinguishing type 1 from type 2. In HMSN 1, the motor nerve conduction velocities are severely reduced (to about one-half of normal) and the distal latencies prolonged.[43] As the disease progresses, the compound muscle action potential amplitudes decrease.[31] Sensory nerve action potential amplitudes are significantly decreased.[31] Needle EMG examination can show signs of denervation in the affected muscles as the axons are eventually involved also.[39] In HMSN 2, the conduction velocity is normal to near normal, while both the motor and sensory action potential amplitudes are diminished. On needle EMG, signs indicative of denervation are present.[39]

Management of Charcot–Marie–Tooth disease

Treatment of CMT disease is aimed primarily at maintenance of function, because currently there is no known direct treatment. Ankle–foot orthoses might be indicated if there is significant leg weakness or ankle instability. Careful selection of shoes is important. Custom-molded can be necessary in some cases.

The patient with CMT disease is at risk for decreased joint range of motion and contractures, especially loss of ankle dorsiflexion. The patient should be taught appropriate range of motion and stretching exercises. Careful daily inspection of hypoesthetic areas should be encouraged.

Mononeuritis multiplex

Mononeuritis multiplex is characterized by onset of sensory and motor dysfunction[42,137] that occurs asymmetrically, asynchronously, and abruptly. Pain is usually a prominent feature. It is most commonly due to multiple nerve infarctions, and is commonly seen in association with the systemic vasculitides. These include polyarteritis nodosa, rheumatoid vasculitis, Wegener granulomatosis, systemic lupus erythematosus, Lyme disease, Sjögren syndrome, cryoglobulinemia, temporal arteritis, scleroderma, sarcoidosis, leprosy, acute viral hepatitis, and AIDS.[42,109] Prompt diagnosis is critical if mononeuropathy multiplex is due to a vasculitis, because treatment with steroids, and at times additional immunosuppressive medications, can arrest or limit the condition. The neuropathy can be the initial manifestation of the systemic condition. Failure to recognize and then treat vasculitis can have serious and even fatal consequences.

Electrodiagnostic studies show an axonal-type involvement of multiple individual nerves. One nerve of an adjacent pair, such as the median or ulnar, might be abnormal while the other is spared. Over time, the condition can evolve into more of a generalized symmetric pattern as additional nerves are affected. Biopsy of affected nerves shows inflammatory infiltration of white cells around the intraneural blood vessels.

The rehabilitation management depends on the sites involved, and generally includes positioning, bracing (static and functional), and a strengthening program, as tolerated. The precautions for insensate areas as described above should be instituted if appropriate.

Ischemic monomelic neuropathy

Ischemic monomelic neuropathy results from infarction of all nerves of a distal extremity. It can be caused by spontaneous or iatrogenic arterial occlusion or embolization, such as during surgical procedures. The patient complains of deep burning pain that persists even after arterial flow has been restored. Symptoms are predominantly due to a distal sensory loss in all nerve distributions. In more severe cases, there is weakness as well, although the motor involvement is not usually as severe.[91] Sensory symptoms can persist for months and are treated with antidepressants or anticonvulsants.

Electrodiagnostic evaluation reveals sensory and motor axonal loss distally. Treatment is supportive, with gait aids and orthoses as indicated. Sensory loss guidelines are to be followed as well.

CONCLUSION

Neuropathy is a common diagnosis with many causes and varied prognoses. It is of utmost importance to accurately diagnose the disease in order to be able to treat the patient with neuropathy appropriately, and to give a reasonable prognosis. Much of the symptomatic treatment discussed in this chapter is similar for the different diseases, and can be used for other forms of peripheral neuropathy that have not been discussed in detail.

Rehabilitation treatment in patients with neuropathy can significantly improve their quality of life.

REFERENCES

1. Adkins JC, Peters DH, Faulds D. Zalcitabine. An update of its pharmacodynamic and pharmacokinetic properties and clinical efficacy in the management of HIV infection. Drugs 1997; 53(6):1054–1080.
2. Amoiridis G, Wohrle J, Grunwald I, et al. Malignant tumour of the psoas: another cause of meralgia paraesthetica. Electromyogr Clin Neurophysiol 1993; 33(2):109–112.
3. de Araujo MP. Electrodiagnosis in compression neuropathies of the upper extremities. Orthop Clin N Am 1996; 27(2):237–244.
4. Archer AG, Watkins PJ, Thomas PK, et al. The natural history of acute painful neuropathy in diabetes mellitus. J Neurol Neurosurg Psychiatry 1983; 46(6):491–499.
5. Asbury AK, Arnason BG, Adams RD. The inflammatory lesion in idiopathic polyneuritis. Its role in pathogenesis. Medicine (Baltimore) 1969; 48(3):173–215.
6. Atroshi I, Johnsson R, Ornstein E. Patient satisfaction and return to work after endoscopic carpal tunnel surgery. J Hand Surg 1988; 23(1):58–65.
7. Aufiero E, Stitik TP, Foye PM, et al. Pyridoxine hydrochloride treatment of carpal tunnel syndrome: a review. Nutr Rev 2004; 62(3):96–104.
8. Bannister RG, Sears TA. The changes in nerve conduction in acute idiopathic polyneuritis. J Neurol Neurosurg Psychiatry 1962; 25:321–328.
9. Barohn RJ, Saperstein DS. Guillain–Barré syndrome and chronic inflammatory demyelinating polyneuropathy. Semin Neurol 1998; 18(1):49–61.
10. Becker J, Nora DB, Gomes I, et al. An evaluation of gender, obesity, age, and diabetes mellitus as risk factors for carpal tunnel syndrome. Clin Neurophysiol 2002; 113(9):1429–1434.
11. Bensman A. Strenuous exercise may impair muscle function in Guillain–Barré patients. JAMA 1970; 214:468–469.
12. Bergoffen J, Trofatter J, Pericak-Vance MA, et al. Linkage localization of X-linked Charcot–Marie–Tooth disease. Am J Hum Genet 1993; 52(2):312–318.
13. Bieber EJ, Moore JR, Weiland AJ. Lipomas compressing the radial nerve at the elbow. J Hand Surg 1986; 11(4):533–535.
14. Bigliani LU, Compito CA, Duralde XA, et al. Transfer of the levator scapulae, rhomboid major, and rhomboid minor for paralysis of the trapezius. J Bone Joint Surg Am 1996; 78(10):1534–1540.
15. Bird TD, Kraft GH. Charcot–Marie–Tooth disease: data for genetic counseling relating age to risk. Clin Genet 1978; 14(1):43–49.
16. Bird TD, Ott J, Giblett ER. Evidence for linkage of Charcot–Marie–Tooth neuropathy to the Duffy locus on chromosome 1. Am J Hum Genet 1982; 34(3):388–394.
17. Bird TD. Hereditary motor-sensory neuropathies. Charcot–Marie–Tooth syndrome. Neurol Clin 1989; 7(1):9–23.
18. Bodner G, Huber B, Schwabegger A, et al. Sonographic detection of radial nerve entrapment within a humerus fracture. J Ultrasound Med 1999; 18(10):703–706.
19. Bradley WG, Madrid R, Thrush DC, et al. Recurrent brachial plexus neuropathy. Brain 1975; 98(3):381–398.
20. Bradley WG, Verma A. Painful vasculitic neuropathy in HIV-1 infection: Relief of pain with prednisone therapy. Neurology 1996; 47(6):1446–1451.
21. Brew BJ. The peripheral nerve complications of human immunodeficiency virus (HIV) infection. Muscle Nerve 2003; 28(5):542–552.
22. Brown D, Wertsch JJ, Harris GF, et al. Effect of rocker soles on plantar pressures. Arch Phys Med Rehabil 2004; 85(1):81–86.
23. Brown MJ, Asbury AK. Diabetic neuropathy. Ann Neurol 1984; 15(1):2–12.
24. Buck AC, Reed PI, Siddiq YK, et al. Bladder dysfunction and neuropathy in diabetes. Diabetologia 1976; 12(3):251–258.
25. Buschbacher R. Side-to-side confrontational strength-testing for weakness of the intrinsic muscles of the hand. J Bone Joint Surg Am 1997; 79(3):401–405.
26. Buschbacher RM. Basic tissue organization and function. In: Buschbacher RM, ed. Musculoskeletal disorders: a practical guide for diagnosis and rehabilitation. Stoneham: Butterworth-Heinemann; 1994:17–18.

27. Buschbacher RM. Musculoskeletal disorders: a practical guide for diagnosis and rehabilitation. 2nd edn. Stoneham: Butterworth-Heinemann; 2002: 57.

28. Buschbacher RM. The musculoskeletal examination. In: Buschbacher RM, ed. Musculoskeletal disorders: a practical guide for diagnosis and rehabilitation. 2nd edn. Stoneham: Butterworth-Heinemann; 2002:59.

29. Campbell WW. Essentials of electrodiagnostic medicine. Baltimore: Williams & Wilkins; 1999.

30. Campbell WW. The value of inching techniques in the diagnosis of focal nerve lesions. Muscle Nerve 1998; 21(11):1554–1556.

31. Chance PF, Pleasure D. Charcot–Marie–Tooth syndrome. Arch Neurol 1993; 50(11):1180–1184.

32. Chen WP, Ju CW, Tang FT. Effects of total contact insoles on the plantar stress redistribution: a finite element analysis. Clin Biomech 2003; 18(6): S17–S24.

33. Childs EA, Lyles RH, Selnes OA, et al. Plasma viral load and CD4 lymphocytes predict HIV-associated dementia and sensory neuropathy. Neurology 1999; 52(3):607–613.

34. Connolly KJ, Allan JD, Fitch H, et al. Phase I study of 2′-3′-dideoxyinosine administered orally twice daily to patients with AIDS or AIDS-related complex and hematologic intolerance to zidovudine. Am J Med 1991; 91(5):471–478.

35. Corral I, Quereda C, Casado JL, et al. Acute polyradiculopathies in HIV-infected patients. J Neurol 1997; 244(8):499–504.

36. Davison BL, Kosmatka PK, Ferlic RJ. Acute radial nerve compression following routine venipuncture in an anticoagulated patient. Am J Orthop 1996; 25(10):712–713.

37. DeStefano F, Nordstrom DL, Vierkant RA. Long-term symptom outcomes of carpal tunnel syndrome and its treatment. J Hand Surg 1997; 22(2): 200–210.

38. Devers A, Galer BS. Topical lidocaine patch relieves a variety of neuropathic pain conditions: an open-label study. Clin J Pain 2000; 16(3): 205–208.

39. Dumitru D, Zwarts M, Amato A. Peripheral nervous system's reaction to injury. In: Dumitru D, Amato A, Zwarts M, eds. Electrodiagnostic medicine. 2nd edn. Philadelphia: Hanley & Belfus; 2002:115–156.

40. Dumitru D, Zwarts M. Focal peripheral neuropathies. In: Dumitru D, Amato A, Zwarts M, eds. Electrodiagnostic medicine. 2nd edn. Philadelphia: Hanley & Belfus; 2002:1043–1126.

41. Dunn AW. Trapezius paralysis after minor surgical procedures in the posterior cervical triangle. South Med J 1974; 67(3):312–315.

42. Dyck PJ, Benstead TJ, Conn DL, et al. Nonsystemic vasculitic neuropathy. Brain 1987; 110(part 4):843–853.

43. Dyck PJ, Chance PJ, Lebo RV, et al. Hereditary motor and sensory neuropathies. In: Dyck PJ, Thomas PJ, Griffin JW, et al, eds. Peripheral neuropathy, vol 2. Philadelphia: Saunders; 1993:1094–1136.

44. Dyck PJ, Lambert EH. Lower motor and primary sensory neuron diseases with peroneal muscular atrophy. I. Neurologic, genetic and electrophysiologic findings in hereditary polyneuropathies. Arch Neurol 1968; 18(6): 603–618.

45. Dyck PJ. Histologic measurements and fine structure of biopsied sural nerve: normal, and in peroneal muscular atrophy, hypertrophic neuropathy, and congenital sensory neuropathy. Mayo Clin Proc 1966; 41(11): 742–774.

46. Eaton CJ, Lister GD. Radial nerve compression. Hand Clin 1992; 8(2): 345–357.

47. Ewing DJ, Borsey DQ, Travis P, et al. Abnormalities of ambulatory 24-hour heart rate in diabetes mellitus. Diabetes 1983; 32(2):101–105.

48. Fagerberg SE, Kock NG, Petersen I, et al. Urinary bladder disturbances in diabetics. A comparative study of male diabetics and controls aged between twenty and fifty years. Scand J Urol Nephrol 1967; 1:19–27.

49. Fairburn CG, Wu FC, McCulloch DK, et al. The clinical features of diabetic impotence: a preliminary study. Br J Psychiatry 1982; 140:4 47–452.

50. Fisher M. An unusual variant of acute idiopathic polyneuritis (syndrome of ophthalmoplegia, ataxia and areflexia). N Engl J Med 1956; 255(2): 57–65.

51. Foster RJ, Swiontkowski MF, Bach AW, et al. Radial nerve palsy caused by open humeral shaft fractures. J Hand Surg 1993; 18(1):121–124.

52. Fraser DM, Campbell IW, Ewing DJ, et al. Mononeuropathy in diabetes mellitus. Diabetes 1979; 28(2):96–101.

53. French Cooperative Group on Plasma Exchange in Guillain–Barré syndrome. Efficiency of plasma exchange in Guillain–Barré syndrome: role of replacement fluids. Ann Neurol 1987; 22(6):753–761.

54. Friedenberg SM, Zimprich T, Harper CM. The natural history of long thoracic and spinal accessory neuropathies. Muscle Nerve 2002; 25(4): 535–539.

55. Gabbay KH, Merola LO, Field RA. Sorbitol pathway: presence in nerve and cord with substrate accumulation in diabetes. Science 1966; 151(707): 209–210.

56. Ganong WF. Review of medical physiology. 13th edn. East Norwalk: Appleton & Lange; 1987.

57. Gelberman RH, Aronson D, Weisman MH. Carpal-tunnel syndrome. Results of a prospective trial of steroid injection and splinting. J Bone Joint Surg Am 1980; 62(7):1181–1184.

58. Gerritsen AA, Uitdehaag BM, van Geldere D, et al. Systematic review of randomized clinical trials of surgical treatment of carpal tunnel syndrome. Br J Surg 2001; 88(10):1285–1295.

59. Gibbels E, Giebisch U. Natural course of acute and chronic monophasic inflammatory demyelinating polyneuropathies (IDP). A retrospective analysis of 266 cases. Acta Neurol Scand 1992; 85(4):282–291.

60. Goldstein JE, Cogan DG. Diabetic ophthalmoplegia with special reference to the pupil. Arch Ophthalmol 1960; 64:592–600.

61. Gordon C, Johnson EW, Gatens PF, et al. Wrist ratio correlation with carpal tunnel syndrome in industry. Am J Phys Med Rehabil 1988; 67(6): 270–272.

62. Gozna ER, Harris WR. Traumatic winging of the scapula. J Bone Joint Surg Am 1979; 61(8):1230–1233.

63. Greene DA, Lattimer SA, Sima AA. Sorbitol, phosphoinositides, and sodium-potassium-ATPase in the pathogenesis of diabetic complications. N Engl J Med 1987; 316(10):599–606.

64. Gregersen G, Borsting H, Theil P, et al. Myoinositol and function of peripheral nerves in human diabetics. A controlled clinical trial. Acta Neurol Scand 1978; 58(4):241–248.

65. Guillain–Barré Syndrome Study Group. Plasmapheresis and acute Guillain–Barré syndrome. Neurology 1985; 35(8):1096–1104.

66. Guiloff RJ, Thomas PK, Contreras M, et al. Linkage of autosomal dominant type 1 hereditary motor and sensory neuropathy to the Duffy locus on chromosome 1. J Neurol Neurosurg Psychiatry 1982; 45(8):669–674.

67. Hadden RD, Karch H, Hartung HP, et al. Preceding infection, immune factors, and outcome in Guillain–Barré syndrome. Neurology 2001; 56(6): 758–765.

68. Hansen PA, Micklesen P, Robinson LR. Clinical utility of the flick maneuver in diagnosing carpal tunnel syndrome. Am J Phys Med Rehabil 2004; 83(5):363–367.

69. Herbison GJ, Jaweed MM, Ditunno JF Jr. Exercise therapies in peripheral neuropathies. Arch Phys Med Rehabil 1983; 64(5):201–205.

70. Hilsted J, Parving HH, Christensen NJ, et al. Hemodynamics in diabetic orthostatic hypotension. J Clin Invest 1981; 68(6):1427–1434.

71. Hughes RA, Wijdicks EF, Barohn R, et al. Practice parameter: immunotherapy for Guillain–Barré syndrome: report of the Quality Standards Subcommittee of the American Academy of Neurology. Neurology 2003; 61(6):736–740.

72. Iceton J, Harris WR. Treatment winged scapula by pectoralis major transfer. J Bone Joint Surg Br 1987; 69(1):108–110.

73. Ionasescu VV, Trofatter J, Haines JL, et al. Mapping of the gene for X-linked dominant Charcot–Marie–Tooth neuropathy. Neurology 1992; 42(4):903–908.

74. Johnson EW. Sixteenth annual AAEM Edward H. Lambert lecture. Electrodiagnostic aspects of diabetic neuropathies: entrapments. American Association of Electrodiagnostic Medicine. Muscle Nerve 1993; 16(2): 127–134.

75. Judzewitsch RG, Jaspan JB, Polonsky KS, et al. Aldose reductase inhibition improves nerve conduction velocity in diabetic patients. N Engl J Med 1983; 308(3):119–125.

76. Kahan M, Goldberg PD, Mandel EE. Neurogenic vesical dysfunction and diabetes mellitus. NY State J Med 1970; 70(19):2448–2455.

77. Kallgren MA, Tingle LJ. Meralgia paresthetica mimicking lumbar radiculopathy. Anesth Analg 1993; 76(6):1367–1368.

78. Kaplan PE. Posterior interosseous neuropathies: natural history. Arch Phys Med Rehabil 1984; 65(7):399–400.

79. Kaplan RJ. Physical medicine and rehabilitation pearls of wisdom. Lincoln: Boston Medical Publishing; 2003.

80. Kaplan SJ, Glickel SZ, Eaton RG. Predictive factors in the non-surgical treatment of carpal tunnel syndrome. J Hand Surg 1990; 15(1): 106–108.

81. Katirji MB, Wilbourn AJ. Common peroneal mononeuropathy: a clinical and electrophysiologic study of 116 lesions. Neurology 1988; 38(11): 1723–1728.

82. Kauppila LI, Vastamaki M. Iatrogenic serratus anterior paralysis: long-term outcome in 26 patients. Chest 1996; 109(1):31–34.

83. Kimura J. Polyneuropathies. In: Kimura J, ed. Electrodiagnosis in diseases of nerve and muscle: principles and practice. 2nd edn. Philadelphia: Davis Publications; 1989.

84. Kleinert JM, Mehta S. Radial nerve entrapment. Orthop Clin N Am 1996; 27(2):305–315.

85. Kraft GH. Axillary, musculocutaneous and suprascapular nerve latency studies. Arch Phys Med Rehabil 1972; 53(8):383–387.

86. Kuhlman KA, Hennessey WJ. Sensitivity and specificity of carpal tunnel syndrome signs. Am J Phys Med Rehabil 1997; 76(6):451–457.

87. Kuhn JE, Plancher KD, Hawkins RJ. Scapular winging. J Am Acad Orthop Surg 1995; 3(6):319–325.

88. Lange D, Tolunsky E. Infections and peripheral neuropathy. In: Brown W, Bolton C, Aminoff M, eds. Neuromuscular function and disease. Philadelphia: Saunders; 2002:1251–1262.

89. Lange DJ. AAEM minimonograph #41: neuromuscular diseases associated with HIV-1 infection. Muscle Nerve 1994; 17(1):16–30.

90. Leffert RD. Pectoralis major transfer for serratus anterior paralysis. Orthop Tran 1992–3; 16:761.

91. Levin KH. AAEE case report #19: ischemic monomelic neuropathy. Muscle Nerve 1989; 12(10):791–795.

92. Lindenbaum Y, Kissel JT, Mendell JR. Treatment approaches for Guillain–Barré syndrome and chronic inflammatory demyelinating polyradiculoneuropathy. Neurol Clin 2001; 19(1):187–204.

93. Manske PR. Compression of the radial nerve by the triceps muscle: a case report. J Bone Joint Surg Am 1977; 59(6):835–836.

94. Martini R, Zielasek J, Toyka KV. Inherited demyelinating neuropathies: from gene to disease. Curr Opin Neurol 1998; 11(5):545–556.

95. McCallum RW, Ricci DA, Rakatansky H, et al. A multicenter placebo-controlled clinical trial of oral metoclopramide in diabetic gastroparesis. Diabetes Care 1983; 6(5):463–467.

96. McNeil BE, Buschbacher RM. Wrist and hand. In: Buschbacher RM, ed. Musculoskeletal disorders: a practical guide for diagnosis and rehabilitation. 2nd edn. Stoneham: Butterworth-Heinemann; 2002:167.

97. van der Meche FG, Schmitz PI. A randomized trial comparing intravenous immune globulin and plasma exchange in Guillain–Barré syndrome. Dutch Guillain–Barré Study Group. N Engl J Med 1992; 326(17): 1123–1129.

98. Mendell JR. Charcot–Marie–Tooth neuropathies and related disorders. Semin Neurol 1998; 18(1):41–47.

99. Meythaler JM, DeVivo MJ, Braswell WC. Rehabilitation outcomes of patients who have developed Guillain–Barré syndrome. Am J Phys Med Rehabil 1997; 76(5):411–419.

100. Millender LH, Nalebuff EA, Holdsworth DE. Posterior interosseous-nerve syndrome secondary to rheumatoid synovitis. J Bone Joint Surg Am 1973; 55(4):753–757.

101. Morris AH. Irreducible Monteggia lesion with radial-nerve entrapment. A case report. J Bone Joint Surg Am 1974; 56(8):1744–1746.

102. Mostacciuolo ML, Muller E, Fardin P, et al. X-linked Charcot–Marie–Tooth disease. A linkage study in a large family by using 12 probes of the pericentromeric region. Hum Genet 1991; 87(1):23–27.

103. Nagler SH, Rangell L. Peroneal palsy caused by crossing the legs. JAMA 1947; 133:755–761.

104. Nelis E, Haites N, Van Broeckhoven C. Mutations in the peripheral myelin genes and associated genes in inherited peripheral neuropathies. Hum Mutat 1999; 13(1):11–28.

105. Newswanger DL, Warren CR. Guillain–Barré syndrome. Am Fam Physician 2004; 69(10):2405–2410.

106. Ouvrier R. Correlation between the histopathologic, genotypic, and phenotypic features of hereditary peripheral neuropathies in childhood. J Child Neurol 1996; 11(2):133–146.

107. Overpeck DO, Ghormley RK. Paralysis of the serratus magnus muscle caused by lesions of the long thoracic nerve. JAMA 1940; 114: 1194–1196.

108. Park GY, Kim JM, Lee SM. The ultrasonographic and electrodiagnostic findings of ulnar neuropathy at the elbow. Arch Phys Med Rehabil 2004; 85(6):1000–1005.

109. Parry GJ. Mononeuropathy multiplex (AAEE case report #11). Muscle Nerve 1985; 8:493–498.

110. Pittman GR. Peroneal nerve palsy following sequential pneumatic compression. JAMA 1989; 261(15):2201–2202.

111. Pollock FH, Drake D, Bovill EG, et al. Treatment of radial neuropathy associated with fractures of the humerus. J Bone Joint Surg Am 1981; 63(2):239–243.

112. Post M. Pectoralis major transfer for winging of the scapula. J Shoulder Elbow Surg 1995; 4(1 part 1):1–9.

113. Preston DC, Shapiro BE. Electromyography and neuromuscular disorders. Boston: Butterworth-Heinemann; 1998.

114. Price RW. Neurological complications of HIV infection. Lancet 1996; 348(9025):445–452.

115. Rana KZ, Dudley MN. Clinical pharmacokinetics of stavudine. Clin Pharmacokinet 1997; 33(4):276–284.

116. Reilly MM. Genetically determined neuropathies. J Neurol 1998; 245(1):6–13.

117. Rinkel GJ, Wokke JH. Meralgia paraesthetica as the first symptom of a metastatic tumor in the lumbar spine. Clin Neurol Neurosurg 1990; 92(4):365–367.

118. Ropper AH. The Guillain–Barre syndrome. N Engl J Med 1992; 326(17):1130–1136.

119. Ross MA. Neuropathies associated with diabetes. Med Clin N Am 1993; 77(1):111–124.

120. Roy PH, Beahrs OH. Spinal accessory nerve in radical neck dissections. Am J Surg 1969; 118(5):800–804.

121. Rundles RW. Diabetic neuropathy: general review with report of 125 cases. Medicine 1945; 24:111–160.

122. Ryan MM, Darras BT, Soul JS. Peroneal neuropathy from ankle-foot orthoses. Pediatr Neurol 2003; 29(1):72–74.

123. Samardzic M, Grujicic D, Milinkovic ZB. Radial nerve lesions associated with fractures of the humeral shaft. Injury 1990; 21(4): 220–222.

124. Schiller LR, Santa Ana CA, Schmulen AC, et al. Pathogenesis of fecal incontinence in diabetes mellitus: evidence for internal-anal-sphincter dysfunction. N Engl J Med 1982; 307(27):1666–1671.

125. Seddon HJ. Three types of nerve injury. Brain 1943; 66(4):237–288.

126. Siegel IM. Dorsal interosseous nerve compression syndrome from the use of a Canadian crutch. Muscle Nerve 1988; 11(12):1273–1274.

127. Simpson DM, Wolfe DE. Neuromuscular complication of HIV infection and its treatment. AIDS 1991; 5(8):917–926.

128. Skoll PJ, Hudson DA, de Jager W, et al. Long-term results of tendon transfers for radial nerve palsy in patients with limited rehabilitation. Ann Plast Surg 2000; 45(2):122–126.

129. Smith B. Neuropathology of the oesophagus in diabetes mellitus. J Neurol Neurosurg Psychiatry 1974; 37(10):1151–1154.

130. Sposato RC, Riley MW, Ballard JL, et al. Wrist squareness and median nerve impairment. J Occup Environ Med 1995; 37(9):1122–1126.

131. Stewart JD. Diabetic truncal neuropathy: topography of the sensory deficit. Ann Neurol 1989; 25(3):233–238.

132. Suber DA, Massey EW. Pelvic mass presenting as meralgia paresthetica. Obstet Gynecol 1979; 53(2):257–258.

133. Sunderland S. A classification of peripheral nerve injuries producing loss of function. Brain 1951; 74(4):491–516.

134. Swann KW, Heros RC. Accessory nerve palsy following carotid endarterectomy. J Neurosurg 1985; 63(4):630–632.

135. Tagliati M, Grinnell J, Godbold J, et al. Peripheral nerve function in HIV infection: clinical, electrophysiologic, and laboratory findings. Arch Neurol 1999; 56(1):84–89.

136. Tan CJ. Practical manual of physical medicine and rehabilitation. Diagnostics, therapeutics, and basic problems. St. Louis: Mosby; 1998:743.

137. Taylor RA. Heredofamilial mononeuritis multiplex with brachial predilection. Brain 1960; 83:113–137.

138. Thomas PK, Thomlinson DR. Diabetic and hypoglycemic neuropathy. In: Dyck PF, Thomas PK, Griffin JW, eds. Peripheral neuropathy, vol 2. Philadelphia: Saunders; 1993:1219–1250.

139. Thomas PK. Classification, differential diagnosis, and staging of diabetic peripheral neuropathy. Diabetes 1997; 46(suppl 2):S54–S57.

140. Thomas PK. Diabetic neuropathy: models, mechanisms and mayhem. Can J Neurol Sci 1992; 19(1):1–7.

141. Tsairis P, Dyck PJ, Mulder DW. Natural history of brachial plexus neuropathy. Report on 99 patients. Arch Neurol 1972; 27(2):109–117.

142. Urguden M, Bilbasar H, Ozdemir H, et al. Tarsal tunnel syndrome—the effect of the associated features on outcome of surgery. Int Orthop 2002; 26(4):253–256.

143. Valentijn LJ, Baas F. Genetic basis of peripheral neuropathies. Prog Brain Res 1998; 117:249–264.

144. Vance JM, Barker D, Yamaoka LH, et al. Localization of Charcot–Marie–Tooth disease type 1a (CMT1A) to chromosome 17p11.2. Genomics 1991; 9(4):623–628.

145. Virally-Monod M, Tielmans D, Kevorkian JP, et al. Chronic diarrhea and diabetes mellitus: prevalence of small intestinal bacterial overgrowth. Diabetes Metab 1998; 24(6):530–536.

146. Virani A, Mailis A, Shapiro LE, et al. Drug interactions in human neuropathic pain pharmacotherapy. Pain 1997; 73(1):3–13.

147. Walsh NE, Dumitru D, Kalantri A, et al. Brachial neuritis involving the bilateral phrenic nerves. Arch Phys Med Rehabil 1987; 68(1):46–48.

148. Warner JJ, Navarro RA. Serratus anterior dysfunction. Recognition and treatment. Clin Orthop 1998; 349:139–148.

149. Warner LE, Garcia CA, Lupski JR. Hereditary peripheral neuropathies: clinical forms, genetics, and molecular mechanisms. Annu Rev Med 1999; 50:263–275.

150. Watson BV, Brown WF. Quantitation of axon loss and conduction block in acute radial nerve palsies. Muscle Nerve 1992; 15(7):768–773.

151. Wiater JM, Bigliani LU. Long thoracic nerve injury. Clin Orthop 1999; 368:17–27.

152. Wilton TD. Tegretol in the treatment of diabetic neuropathy. S Afr Med J 1974; 48(20):869–872.

153. Winn FJ Jr, Habes DJ. Carpal tunnel area as a risk factor for carpal tunnel syndrome. Muscle Nerve 1990; 13(3):254–258.

154. Wolfe GI, Barohn RJ. Cryptogenic sensory and sensorimotor polyneuropathies. Semin Neurol 1998; 18(1):105–111.

155. Younger DS, Rosoklija G, Hays AP. Diabetic peripheral neuropathy. Semin Neurol 1998; 18(1):95–104.

156. Zlotogora J. Dominance and homozygosity. Am J Med Genet 1997; 68(4):412–416.

Chapter

49

Myopathic Disorders

Craig M. McDonald, Jay J. Han, Richard T. Abresch and Gregory T. Carter

CLINICAL AND DIAGNOSTIC APPROACH TO THE PATIENT WITH A SUSPECTED MYOPATHY

Disease history

The common presenting chief complaints from parents or children with suspected myopathic disorders include infantile floppiness or hypotonia, delay in motor milestones, feeding and respiratory difficulties, abnormal gait characteristics, frequent falls, difficulty ascending stairs or arising from the floor, and muscle cramps or stiffness.[53,122,123] Teenagers with later onset disorders typically present with chief complaints of strength loss or decreasing endurance, falls, difficulty ascending stairs, exercise intolerance, episodic weakness, muscle cramps, focal wasting of muscle groups, and breathing difficulties.

Information should be obtained about whether the process is getting worse, staying the same, or getting better. If strength is deteriorating, it is important to ascertain the rate of progression (i.e. is weakness increasing over days, weeks, months, or years?). Is the distribution of the weakness predominantly proximal, distal, or generalized? It is also important to identify factors that worsen or help primary symptoms.

A comprehensive past medical history and surgical history should be obtained (Box 49-1). A history of recent illnesses should be carefully elucidated, including respiratory difficulties, aspiration pneumonias, or recurrent pulmonary infections. In addition, such cardiac symptoms as dizziness, syncope, chest pain, orthopnea, or exertional complaints may indicate superimposed involvement of the myocardium. A review of pulmonary symptoms should be obtained. A history of weight loss may be due to recurrent illnesses, nutritional compromise, swallowing difficulty, or progressive lean tissue atrophy.

A detailed history regarding pregnancy (e.g. quality of fetal movement or pregnancy complications) and perinatal problems (evidence of fetal distress, respiratory difficulties in the recovery room, need for resuscitation or ventilation problems in early infancy, ongoing respiratory difficulties, swallowing or feeding difficulties, and persistent hypotonia) should be obtained. Perinatal respiratory distress in the delivery room may be seen in some of these disorders.

History regarding the child's acquisition of developmental milestones should be ascertained relating to head control, independent sitting, crawling, standing with and without support, walking with and without support, fine motor prehension, bimanual skill acquisition (bringing objects to midline and trans-

fer of objects), and language acquisition. Information regarding gait characteristics (toe walking, excessive lordosis, etc.), running ability, transitions from floor to standing, stair climbing, falls, recreational or athletic performance, pain or muscle cramps, and easy fatigue or lack of endurance may be important clues to the presence of a myopathic disorder. History regarding mental development, type of school, and school performance may be important indicators of superimposed cognitive involvement, which is common in Duchenne and myotonic muscular dystrophy (MMD). For the older child, a detailed history regarding the age of onset of symptoms, progression, distribution of weakness, presence of muscle cramps, fatigue, episodic weakness, presence of atrophy, performance in physical education, current and past ambulatory distances, ability to move from floor to standing, problems climbing stairs, and problems reaching overhead or dressing can all be important functional information.

A thorough anesthetic history should be obtained. A history of muscle cramps at rest or with exertion can be associated with a muscular dystrophy, metabolic myopathy, toxic myoglobinuria, or inflammatory myositis. Malignant hyperthermia is associated with primary familial malignant hyperthermia, central core congenital myopathy, Duchenne muscular dystrophy (DMD), and Becker muscular dystrophy (BMD).[15] Other myopathic conditions occasionally associated with malignant hyperthermia include Fukuyama congenital muscular dystrophy, limb girdle muscular dystrophy (LGMD), facioscapulohumeral muscular dystrophy (FSHMD), periodic paralysis, myotonia congenita, mitochondrial myopathy, and the Schwartz–Jampel syndrome.[15,23,65,76,125]

Family history

If a neuromuscular disease is suspected, it is important to get a detailed family history and pedigree chart. Autosomal dominant conditions have pedigrees with multiple generations affected, with equal predilection for males and females. Typically, one-half of offspring within a pedigree are affected.[13,14,41]

In autosomal recessive conditions, typically only one generation is affected, with equal incidence in males and females. One-fourth of offspring are usually clinically affected. Parents in earlier generations may be normal, and the parents of affected children are presumptive heterozygote carriers of the

Box 49-1 Clinical history

- History of weakness, fatigue, or lack of endurance
  Anatomic distribution and pattern of weakness and focal
    wasting of muscle groups: arms versus legs, proximal versus
    distal, symmetric versus asymmetric. Myopathies have
    weakness that is usually proximal greater than distal.
    Neuropathies typically have sensory loss and weakness usually
    distal greater than proximal.
  Information regarding gait characteristics (toe walking, excessive
    lordosis, etc.): running ability, transitions from floor to standing,
    stair climbing, falls, and recreational or athletic performance.
  Fatigue or lack of endurance
  Muscle cramps or stiffness
  Identify factors that worsen or help primary symptoms
  Course of weakness (acute, days to weeks; chronic, months to
    years; episodic): is the weakness getting worse, staying the
    same, or getting better? Ascertain the rate of progression
    (days, weeks, months, or years).
  Onset age (neonatal, childhood, teen, adult [20–60 years], or
    geriatric)
- History of recent illnesses (e.g. respiratory difficulties, pneumo-
  nia, pulmonary infection)
- Pain
- Feeding difficulties, nutritional status, and body composition
- Cardiac symptoms (dizziness, syncope, chest pain, orthopnea,
  cardiac complaints with exertion)
- Pulmonary symptoms (breathing difficulties, sleep disturbance,
  morning headaches)
- Anesthetic history
- History regarding the child's acquisition of developmental
  milestones
  Ascertain when the child was able to control her or his head, sit
    independently, crawl, stand with and without support, walk
    with and without support, gain fine motor prehension, and
    acquire bimanual skills (bringing objects to midline, transfer of
    objects).
  For the older child, obtain a detailed history of current and past
    ambulatory distances, ability to move from floor to standing,
    problems climbing stairs, problems reaching overhead,
    problems dressing, and performance in physical education.
- History regarding language acquisition, mental development,
  and school performance
- History regarding pregnancy
  Quality of fetal movement
  Pregnancy complications
  Perinatal problems
  Fetal distress
  Evidence of fetal distress
  Respiratory difficulties in the recovery room
  Need for resuscitation or ventilation problems in early infancy
  Persistent hypotonia

condition.[41] In many instances of autosomal recessive inherit-ance, no other members of the nuclear family unit are affected, making the confirmation of inheritance pattern difficult unless a molecular genetic marker is present or a protein abnormality is confirmed by immunohistochemistry techniques.[7,10] In X-linked recessive conditions, males on the maternal side of the family are affected in approximately 50% of instances, and females are carriers in 50% of instances. Males can have the condition but cannot otherwise be carriers.[41,64]

Examination of the affected relatives is important. The medical records and diagnostic evaluations of affected family members should be reviewed and the diagnosis confirmed if possible. Did other members have disease onset at the same time and similar progression? In some instances, the examina-tion of a parent can help establish the diagnosis in an affected infant or child, as is frequently the case in MMD. In this dis-order, genetic anticipation with abnormal CTG trinucleotide expansion of unstable DNA results in progressively earlier onset of the disease in successive generations, with increasing severity.[7,95]

In the case of the dystrophic myopathies, a definitive molecu-lar genetic or pathologic diagnosis can often be found in a sibling or close relative. The clinician can establish the diagnosis in a child or adult based on clinical examination, easily obtained laboratory data, creatine kinase, or molecular genetic testing, thus avoiding further invasive testing such as muscle biopsy.

Physical examination

Physical examination findings typically help focus the remain-der of the diagnostic evaluation, such as electrodiagnosis, molecular genetic testing, and histopathologic analysis of biopsy specimens. All diagnostic information must be interpreted within the context of relevant clinical information. In many instances, a precise molecular genetic diagnosis is not medically possible. However, the diagnostic work-up should determine the most likely clinical syndrome, and allow the clinician to provide the patient and family with accurate prognostic infor-mation and guidance. Table 49-1 shows the typical time of onset of the physical findings observed in the most common myo-pathic diseases.

Specific aspects of the physical examination include simple inspection for the presence of focal or diffuse muscle wasting. Focal enlargement of muscles or 'pseudohypertrophy' is seen in such dystrophic myopathies as DMD and BMD. The increase in calf circumference in DMD is caused by an increase in fatty connective tissue rather than true muscle fiber hypertrophy.[18,19] Other neuromuscular disorders can show calf pseudohyper-trophy, such as childhood-type acid maltase deficiency. Focal atrophy of particular muscle groups may provide diagnostic clues to specific myopathic disorders such as Emery–Dreifuss muscular dystrophy (EDMD), FSHMD, and LGMD.[61–63,102]

A thorough general physical examination of cardiac, pulmo-nary, and gastrointestinal systems should be performed on all patients suspected of having a neuromuscular disease. Hepatomegaly can be seen in such metabolic myopathies as acid maltase deficiency (type 2 glycogenosis) and type 3 and 4 gly-cogenosis.[41,108] The skin should be evaluated for characteristic skin rashes and nail bed capillary changes if an inflammatory myopathy such as dermatomyositis is suspected. Craniofacial changes and dental malocclusion are common in congenital MMD, congenital myopathies, and congenital muscular dystro-phy. A neurologic examination should include a thorough evalu-ation of cranial nerve function, muscle tone, muscle strength, sensory and cerebellar function, deep tendon reflexes, and assessment for the presence of percussion and/or grip myotonia

Table 49-1 Onset of common clinical findings

Clinical sign	Muscular dystrophy or dystrophies							
	Duchenne	Becker	Myotonic	Congenital myotonic	Facioscapulohumeral	Limb girdle	Oculopharyngeal	Emery–Dreifuss
Onset of symptoms	Child	Child to adult	Child to adult	Child	Child to adult	Child to adult	Adult	Child
Skeletal muscle weakness	Child	Child to adult	Child to adult	Child	Child to adult	Child to adult	Adult	Child
Facial weakness	—	—	Child to adult	—	Child to adult	—	Adult	—
Difficulty standing up	Child	Child to adult	Adult	Child to adult	Teen to adult	Child to adult	Adult	Child to teen
Difficulty running and climbing stairs	Child	Child to adult	Adult	Child to adult	Child to adult	Child to adult	Adult	Child to teen
Focal atrophy	Teen	Ault	Adult	Child to adult	Child to adult	Child to adult	Adult	Child
Focal enlargement of calf muscles	Child	Child	—	—	—	Child to adult	Adult	—
Gower's sign	Child	Child to adult	—	—	Teen to adult	Child to adult	Adult	Child to teen
Weakness of shoulder and upper arm muscles	Child	Child to adult	Child to adult	Child to adult	Child to adult	Child to adult	Adult	Child
Contractures	Child	Child to adult	Adult	Child	Teen to adult	Child to adult	—	Child
Scoliosis	Teen	Adult (rare)	—	Teen	Teen to adult	Teen to adult	—	—
Ptosis	—	—	Adult	Child to adult	Child to adult	—	Adult	—
Hypothyroidism	—	—	Child to adult	Child to adult	—	—	—	—
Insulin resistance	—	—	Teen to adult	Teen to adult	—	—	—	—
Myotonia	—	—	Child to adult	Child	—	—	—	—
Cataracts	With steroids	—	Adult	Teen to adult	—	—	—	—
Respiratory distress	Teen to adult	Adult	Adult	Child to adult	Teen to adult	Teen to adult	Adult	Adult
Cardiac conduction defects	Teen to adult	Adult	Adult	Teen to adult	Adult	Teen to adult (variable)	Adult (sporadic)	Child
Cardiac ventricular dysfunction	Teen to adult	Teen to adult	Adult	Teen to adult	—	Teen to adult (variable)	Adult (sporadic)	Teen to adult
Dysphagia	Teen to adult	Adult	Adult	Child to adult	Adult	Teen to adult	Adult	Adult
Gastrointestinal motility or constipation	Teen to adult	Adult	Adult	Child to adult	Adult	Teen to adult	Adult	Adult

in situations where a myotonic syndrome is suspected. Musculo-skeletal examination will reveal the presence of limb contractures and spinal deformity. Flexion contractures are particularly common in the hips, knees, and ankles, and are most easily assessed with the patient lying supine on the examination table.

Significant intellectual impairment can occur in some myopathic disorders, such as congenital MMD, Fukuyama congenital muscular dystrophy, selected cases with mitochondrial encephalomyopathies, and a small proportion of DMD cases.[51,76,100,118,174,189]

A thorough functional examination is essential in the diagnostic evaluation of a patient with suspected neuromuscular disease. This includes assessment of head control, bed or mat mobility, transitions from supine to sit and from sit to stand, sitting ability without hand support, standing balance, gait, stair climbing, and overhead reach.

Careful assessment of scapular winging, scapular stabilization, and scapular rotation is very helpful in the assessment of patients with FSHMD and limb girdle syndrome (Fig. 49-1). The scapula is stabilized for overhead abduction by the trapezius, rhomboids, and serratus anterior. Shoulder abduction to 180° requires strong supraspinatus and deltoid, in addition to strong scapular stabilizers.

Patients with proximal weakness involving the pelvic girdle muscles often rise from the floor using the classic Gower's sign. The patient usually assumes a four-point stance on knees and hands, brings the knees into extension while leaning forward the upper extremities, substitutes for hip extension weakness by pushing off the knees with the upper extremities, and sequentially moves the upper extremities up the thigh until an upright stance with full hip extension is achieved. A Gower's sign is not specific to any myopathic condition but can be seen in DMD and many forms of LGMD, including severe childhood autosomal recessive muscular dystrophy (SCARMD), congenital muscular dystrophy, and congenital myopathy.[2,21,22,24,44]

Patients with proximal lower extremity weakness often exhibit a classic myopathic gait pattern (Fig. 49-2). Initially, weakness of the hip extensors produces anterior pelvic tilt and a tendency for the trunk to be positioned anterior to the hip joints.[45] Patients compensate for this by maintaining lumbar lordosis to position their center of gravity or weight line posterior to the hip joints. This stabilizes the hip in extension on the anterior capsule of the hip joints. Patients subsequently develop weakness of the knee extensors, producing a tendency for knee instability and knee buckling with falls. Patients compensate for this by decreasing stance-phase knee flexion and posturing the ankle increasingly over time into plantar flexion. This produces a knee extension moment at foot contact and the plantar flexion of the ankle during the mid to late stance phase of gait. This helps position the weight line or center of gravity anterior to the knee joint, producing a stabilizing knee extension moment. Patients with DMD progressively demonstrate toe walking with initial floor contact with the foot increasingly forward on to the midfoot, and finally the forefoot, as they reach the transitional phase of ambulation before wheelchair reliance. Weakness of

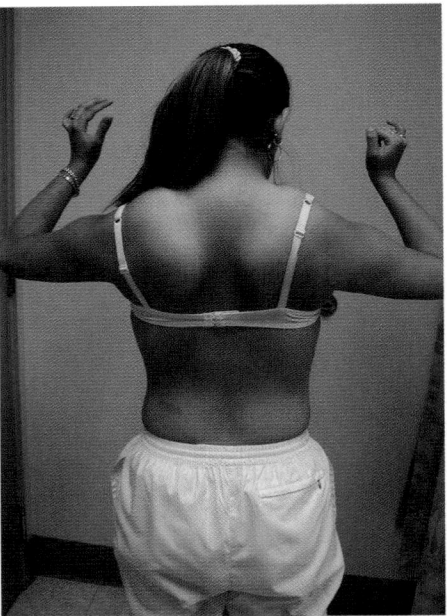

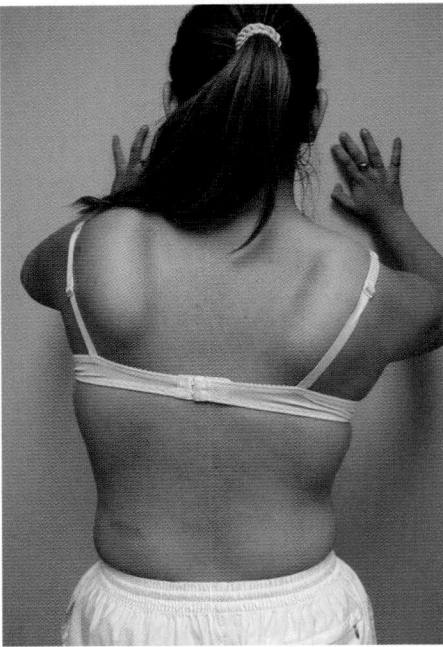

Figure 49-1
Scapular winging in a patient with facioscapulohumeral muscular dystrophy.

the hip abductors produces a tendency toward lateral pelvic tilt and pelvic drop of the swing-phase side. Patients with proximal weakness compensate for this by bending or lurching the trunk laterally over the stance-phase hip joint.[150] This produces the so-called 'gluteus medius lurch' or compensated Trendelenburg gait pattern.

Patients with distal weakness affecting the ankle dorsiflexors and ankle everters in less severe proximal weakness (e.g. EDMD, MMD, and FSHMD) often exhibit a foot slap at floor contact, with a steppage gait pattern to facilitate swing-phase clearance of the plantar-flexed ankle. Alternatively, these patients may clear the plantar-flexed ankle using some degree of circumduction at the hip, or by vaulting on the stance-phase side. Milder

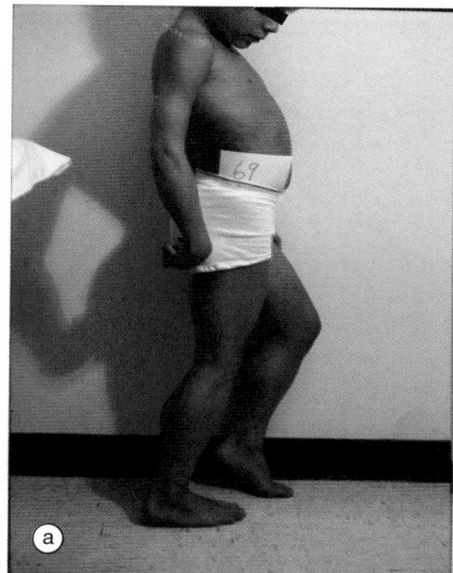

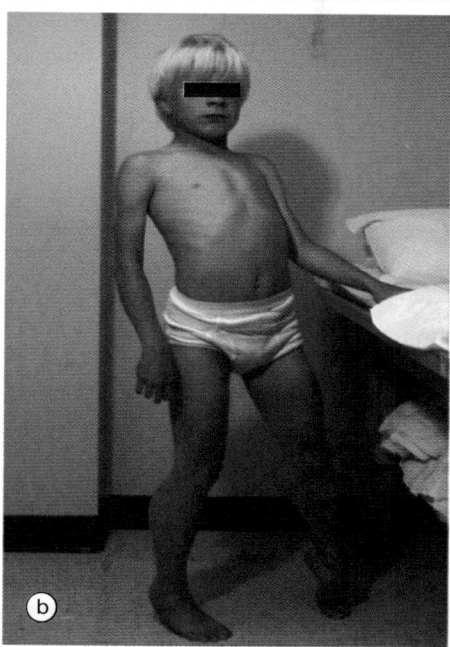

Figure 49-2
Myopathic gait pattern due to pelvic girdle and knee extension weakness. (**a**) Lumbar lordosis to keep the center of mass posterior to the hip joint, anterior pelvic tilt due to hip extensor weakness, weight line or center of mass maintained anterior to an extended knee, and forefoot ground contact with stance-phase plantar flexion (toe walking) to maintain a knee extension movement and knee stability. (**b**) Trendelenburg or 'gluteus medius' gait with lateral lean over the stance side due to hip abductor weakness; ankle dorsiflexion weakness necessitates swing-phase circumduction for clearance.

50–100 times normal.[30] A normal creatine kinase value helps exclude the diagnosis of DMD and BMD. Overlap in creatine kinase values occurs between DMD and BMD. Other forms of muscular dystrophy, such as EDMD, LGMD, FSHMD, and congenital muscular dystrophy, can show moderate elevations in creatine kinase. However, in congenital muscular dystrophy, the creatine kinase value is extremely variable, ranging from normal to a fairly marked elevation. Neuromuscular disease severity is not closely associated with creatine kinase values. In all dystrophic myopathies, the creatine kinase values tend to decrease over time as the patient has progressive loss of muscle fiber due to irreversible cell death. A 3-year-old with DMD might have a creatine kinase value of 25 000, while a 10-year-old with DMD could show a creatine kinase value of only 2000. This is due to the fact that, as muscle cells die, there are fewer of them left to leak creatine kinase into the serum.[28,29,47]

Other conditions with significant elevations in creatine kinase include polymyositis, dermatomyositis, acute rhabdomyolysis, and malignant hyperthermia.[41] In many of the congenital structural myopathies, such as central core disease, nemaline rod myopathy, and fiber-type disproportion syndrome, a serum creatine kinase is likely to be normal or only mildly elevated. In a child with muscle weakness, a normal creatine kinase does not exclude a myopathy.[111,126,141] However, a severely elevated creatine kinase is highly suggestive of a dystrophic myopathy or inflammatory myopathy.[73]

Serial creatine kinase measurement in the morning after several days of sedentary activity is still useful in the evaluation of potential female DMD carriers who do not have a detectable gene deletion on molecular genetic studies. Three normal creatine kinase values in these female subjects give approximately 90% specificity for ruling out carrier status.[41,73] Even one elevated creatine kinase makes carrier status a possibility.

Lactate and pyruvate levels are useful in the evaluation of possible metabolic myopathy. The presence of a lactic acidosis can be seen in such mitochondrial encephalomyopathies as Kearns–Sayre syndrome, myoclonic epilepsy and ragged red fibers (MERRF), and mitochondrial encephalomyopathy with lactic acidosis and stroke-like episodes (MELAS). Whenever clinical evidence suggests a disorder of oxidative metabolism, blood lactate and pyruvate levels should be obtained.[137,171] Arterial lactate values are a more reliable guide. Lactate elevations under ischemic or exercise stress suggest mitochondrial dysfunction. When lactic acidemia is present, the lactate:pyruvate ratio can aid in the differential diagnosis. Children with suspected encephalomyopathy should be evaluated with cerebrospinal fluid lactate levels, because these values are less subject to flux than are either venous or arterial values. The ischemic forearm test, initially utilized by McArdle, is the most widely used means of assessing muscle in aerobic metabolism in older, more cooperative patients.[43,171]

distal lower extremity weakness can be found by testing heel walking and toe walking.

Serum laboratory studies

Most myopathic conditions show significant elevations in transaminases, aldolase, and creatine kinase.[33,52,57,58] In the setting of a muscle disease, serum gamma-glutamyl transferase is the only reliable indication of true hepatocellular disease. The creatine kinase enzyme catalyzes the release of high-energy phosphates from creatine phosphate. It is present mainly in muscle, and leaks into the serum in large amounts in any disorder involving muscle fiber injury.[30,31,34] The MM fraction is specific to skeletal muscle. The creatine kinase value is significantly elevated in the early stages of DMD and BMD, with values up to

Electrodiagnostic studies

Nerve conduction and electromyography (EMG) are an extension of the clinician's physical examination, and a powerful tool for the localization of lesions within the motor unit. EMG and nerve conduction studies can help guide further studies, such as muscle biopsies, by providing information about the most appropriate muscle site for the biopsy. Needle EMG can initially narrow the differential diagnosis by excluding primarily neurogenic processes such as spinal muscular atrophy, which may sometimes be clinically difficult to distinguish from a myopathy.[35,49,107] Typically in myopathies, the proximal muscles of the lower limbs exhibit more prominent EMG findings.[73] It is critical to sample a sufficient number of muscles to establish a diffuse myopathic process as opposed to a focal injury. Muscles that are severely weak, i.e. less than 2 on manual muscle testing, are not good to sample, as the muscle tissue can be too deteriorated to provide a good signal.[49] The more revealing findings will be obtained in muscles of intermediate involvement with respect to weakness.

The motor unit action potentials (MUAPs) in patients with myopathic disorders have variable (normal to reduced) amplitudes and are typically polyphasic.[107] This results from the variability in muscle fiber diameters. There may be a population of short-duration, non-polyphasic MUAPS as well. Early MUAP recruitment is a hallmark of myopathy, with the interference pattern rapidly filling up. However, if muscle fiber loss is severe, then there may be some motor unit dropout, with the appearance of fast-firing individual 'spikes'. This can be distinguished from neurogenic processes by the low amplitudes.

Myopathic disorders will generally display abnormal rest activity on EMG, including fibrillation potentials and positive sharp waves.[49] However, it is important to note that, in many metabolic, mitochondrial, and congenital myopathies, abnormal rest activity may not be present. In the setting of myopathy, fibrillation potentials and positive sharp waves represent spontaneously depolarizing muscle fibers that have been effectively denervated due to muscle necrosis destroying the motor end plate or separating it from other portions of the muscle fiber. In longstanding myopathies, there may be little residual rest activity, due to the loss of muscle fiber. Further, these waveforms may be of smaller amplitude than those seen from a neurogenic etiology. Therefore the clinician might need to use a higher sensitivity setting on the EMG recording unit.

Other forms of rest activity are critical to note. Increased insertional activity is common in most myopathies. Myotonic discharges, with waxing and waning of the amplitude and frequency of the motor units, along with a characteristic dive-bomber sound, are prominent in the myotonic disorders, including MMD. Complex repetitive discharges, sometimes referred to as 'pseudomyotonic' discharges, are a non-specific finding that may be seen in longstanding myopathic or neuropathic conditions.[35,36]

A more thorough discussion is provided in the chapters on electrodiagnosis.

Molecular genetic studies

The application of molecular genetic techniques has resulted in enormous gains in our understanding of the molecular and pathophysiologic basis of many myopathic diseases. In addition, molecular genetic studies now aid in the diagnostic evaluation of the dystrophin-deficient muscular dystrophies (DMD and BMD), MMD, FSHMD, and some forms of LGMD.[41] The clinical application of molecular genetic studies is described in the following sections on specific neuromuscular disease conditions.

Muscle biopsy evaluation
Muscle biopsy technique

The two techniques for obtaining a muscle biopsy specimen are the traditional open biopsy and the needle biopsy.[126,135] Either technique can be performed under local anesthesia, although most clinicians in the USA use general anesthesia for open biopsies and local anesthesia for needle biopsies. There can be some disruption in the architecture of the tissue with the needle biopsy technique. This can affect the histologic examination and electron microscopy. Most electromyographers limit their needle EMG study to one side of the body, so that the contralateral side can be biopsied with any potential interference from the needle tracks or minor hemorrhage. Immunocytochemistry analyses, such as western blot and metabolic studies, do not require strict maintenance of the muscle cellular architecture.

Muscle biopsy site selection

Selection of the muscle is based on the distribution of muscle weakness found clinically, in addition to the electrodiagnostic findings. In a dystrophic myopathy, the muscle biopsy should be clinically affected, but not so severely affected that it is largely replaced by fat and connective tissue with minimal residual muscle fiber present for evaluation. The insertional activity on EMG or muscle imaging studies can be helpful in this respect. Severely reduced insertional activity suggests that muscle tissue has been replaced by fat or fibrotic tissue.[107] Sufficient normative information about proportional fiber type and fiber diameter should be available with age-appropriate norms. A diagnosis of congenital myopathy with fiber type disproportion cannot be made without careful consideration of the normal fiber type predominance in a given muscle. For example, the vastus lateralis is two-thirds type 2 fibers (with equal proportions of type 2a and type 2b fibers) and one-third type 1 fibers. The anterior tibialis, however, has predominantly type 1 fibers, and the anconeus is mostly type 1 fibers.[38] Some muscles, such as the quadriceps and biceps, have longitudinally running fibers that facilitate orientation of the specimen for preparation of cross-sectional slices. The gastrocnemius muscle, on the other hand, can be difficult to orient because fibers run in different plains.

For routine diagnostic studies, the vastus lateralis muscle in the lower extremity and the triceps or biceps in the upper extremity are often preferred. When proximal muscles are severely affected or only distal muscles are involved, the extensor carpi radialis or anterior tibialis muscles are often biopsied.[73,126]

Histology and histochemistry

The histopathologic study is likely to provide information about whether the basic disease process is primarily a myopathy or a neurogenic process. In some instances, a specific diagnosis can be made (such as dystrophic myopathy or inflammatory myopathy). When analyzing paraffin sections, basic pathologic reactions of muscle can include fiber necrosis, central nuclei indicative of regeneration, abnormalities of muscle fiber diameter (atrophy, hypertrophy, abnormal variation, and fiber size), fiber splitting, vacuolar change, inflammatory infiltrates, and proliferation of connective tissue or fibrosis.[126] A dystrophic myopathy frequently is characterized by the presence of normal fibers, hypertrophied fibers, degenerating fibers, atrophic fibers, regenerating fibers, and connective tissue and fatty infiltration (Fig. 49-3). Neurogenic changes can be characterized by small or large groups of atrophic fibers with or without target fibers, and frequently by hypertrophy of the non-atrophic fibers.

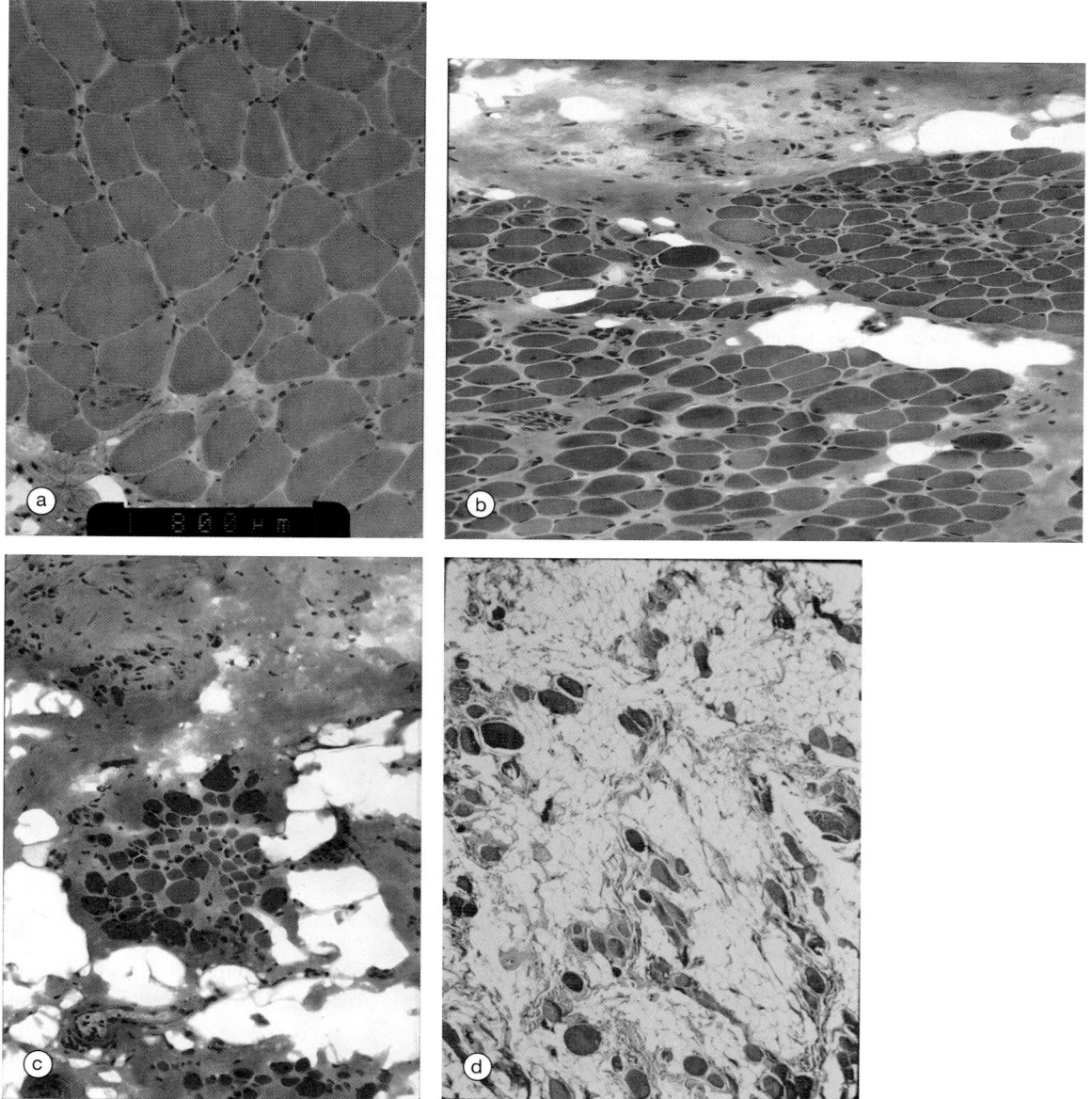

Figure 49-3 Muscle biopsy specimens of the vastus lateralis from (**a**) an able-bodied control subject, (**b**) a 3-year-old patient with Duchenne muscular dystrophy (DMD), (**c**) a 9-year-old DMD patient, and (**d**) a 19-year-old DMD patient, stained with hematoxylin and eosin. Whereas the biopsy from the control subject (a) consists of angulated fibers with peripheral nuclei, the muscle tissue from the 3-year-old with DMD (b) are characterized by both dystrophic and hypertrophied fibers, regenerating fibers with central nuclei, inflammatory cells, and fibrosis with fat infiltration. The biopsy from the 9-year-old with DMD (c) exhibits more extensive loss of muscle fiber, with dystrophic fibers, hypertrophied fibers, and central nucleated regenerating fibers. Note the extensive fibrosis and fat infiltration. The postmortem muscle biopsy specimen in a 19-year-old with end-stage DMD (d) has very few remaining muscle fibers, and tremendous replacement of muscle fibers by fat and connective tissue.

A variety of histochemical stains can be used to differentiate between fiber types (types 1, 2a, 2b, and 2c). Based on the histochemical analyses, information is obtained about the following.

- Pattern of fiber types (e.g. normal predominance, fiber-type predominance, selective fiber-type involvement, or reinnervation evidenced by fiber-type grouping).
- Analysis of muscle fiber diameters (e.g. fiber hypertrophy or atrophy, increased variability in fiber diameter, or denervation atrophy with a narrow range of diameters among atrophic and non-atrophic fibers).
- Alterations in the muscle fiber (e.g. central nuclei, necrosis, splitting or branching, regeneration, or the presence of a variety of other accumulations and fiber alterations, both specific to certain conditions and non-specific).

Congenital myopathies are a group of structural myopathies whose diagnosis is based on classic histologic characteristics seen on muscle biopsy (e.g. centronuclear or myotubular, central core, nemaline rod, and fiber-type disproportion myopathies).

Immunoblotting and immunostaining

Immunoblotting of a muscle sample provides information about amounts of specific muscle protein, such as dystrophin or other structural proteins important in maintaining the structural integrity of the muscle membrane.[48,54,55] Immunoblotting can be performed with as little as 10 mg of frozen tissue. Quantitative dystrophin analysis using western blot technique can differentiate DMD from BMD, and thus help determine the prognosis in a young symptomatic patient, which is not determined by standard molecular genetic analysis of the dystrophin gene.[66,87-89] Dystrophin quantity ≤ 3% is consistent with DMD. Dystrophin levels of 3–20% of normal are seen in some with less severe 'outlier' DMD or severe BMD, and either 20–80% dystrophin or normal quantity with reduced or increased molecular weight dystrophin is consistent with BMD. A normal dystrophin level in a patient with histologic evidence of a dystrophic myopathy is suggestive of an LGMD (Table 49-2). Immunofluorescent staining of muscle biopsy sections for dystrophin helps identify symptomatic female DMD carriers and some female BMD carriers.[126]

Table 49-2 Dystrophin western blot analysis	
Finding(s)	Phenotype
<3% dystrophin quantity	Duchenne
3–20% dystrophin quantity	'Outlier'
20–80% dystrophin quantity, or 90–100% dystrophin quantity and abnormal structure	Becker
100% dystrophin quantity and abnormal dystrophic fibers	Limb girdle

The progressive loss of muscle fibers evident in muscular dystrophy is now thought to be caused by primary muscle sarcolemmal membrane abnormalities due to inherited structural abnormalities (abnormal molecular weight, deficiency, or absence) of dystrophin or dystrophin-associated transmembrane glycoproteins. Membrane instability leads to membrane injury from mechanical stresses, transient breaches of the membrane, and membrane leakage. Ultimately, after multiple cycles of degeneration and regeneration, irreversible muscle cell death occurs.[71,74,75,86] The muscle fiber is then replaced by connective tissue and fat, and this fibrotic replacement of the muscle can be exceedingly aggressive. This has given rise to the concept of diseases of the dystrophin–glycoprotein complex. Primary genetic abnormalities lead to abnormalities of intracellular dystrophin, transmembrane sarcoglycans, or transmembrane dystroglycans. Specific muscle cytoskeletal protein abnormalities lead to specific dystrophic disease phenotypes.[17,82,83,90] An abnormality in the muscle protein merosin, located in the extracellular matrix, gives rise to one of the forms of congenital muscular dystrophy. Immunoblotting and/or immunofluorescent staining of the proteins of the dystrophin–glycoprotein complex now allows many patients with LGMD to be subtyped.[28,212]

Electron microscopy

Electron microscopy is used to evaluate ultrastructural changes of muscle fiber organelles or internal components, as well as changes in the muscle fiber.[141] At times, this provides additional complementary information to the histologic and histochemical assessment of muscle fibers that can be diagnostically relevant. For example, ultrastructural alterations of the mitochondria can provide important information and direct additional metabolic studies in the work-up of mitochondrial myopathy.

Metabolic studies

Depending on clinical suspicion and on histologic and ultrastructural changes on muscle biopsy, additional metabolic studies may be obtained to evaluate for the presence of metabolic myopathies, including glycogenoses, lipid disorders, or mitochondrial myopathies.

SPECIFIC MYOPATHIES

Dystrophinopathies

Duchenne muscular dystrophy

Duchenne muscular dystrophy is an X-linked disorder caused by an abnormality at the Xp21 gene loci.[106,142] The gene for DMD and BMD occupies 2.5 million base pairs of DNA on the X chromosome, and is about 10 times larger than the next largest gene identified to date.[6] The gene contains 79 exons of coding sequence.[106,160] Its primary protein product is called dystrophin, which is found in the plasma membrane of all myogenic cells, in certain types of neurons, and in small amounts in other cell types.[79,132,136,166] Dystrophin deficiency at the plasma membrane of muscle fibers disrupts the membrane cytoskeleton, and leads to the secondary loss of other components of the muscle cytoskeleton.[31,34,184] The primary consequence of the cytoskeleton abnormalities is membrane instability, leading to membrane injury from mechanical stresses, transient breaches of the membrane, and membrane leakage. Chronic dystrophic myopathy is characterized by aggressive fibrotic replacement of the muscle, and eventual failure of regeneration with muscle fiber death and fiber loss. The common characteristics of dystrophinopathies are shown in Table 49-3.

The incidence of DMD has been estimated to be around 1 in 3500 male births.[64] Approximately one-third of isolated cases are due to new mutations, which is considerably higher than observed in other X-linked conditions. This high mutation rate might be due to the large size of the gene.

While a history of hypotonia and delayed motor milestones are often reported in retrospect, the parents are often unaware of any abnormality until the child starts walking. There has been variability reported in the age of onset of DMD. In 74–80% of instances, onset is noted before the age of 4 years.[129] The vast majority of cases are identified by 5–6 years of age. The most frequent presenting symptoms are abnormal gait, frequent falls, and difficulty climbing stairs. Difficulty negotiating stairs is an early feature, as is a tendency to fall due to the child tripping or stumbling on a plantar-flexed ankle, or the knee buckling or giving way due to knee extensor weakness. There is progressive difficulty getting up from the floor, with presence of a Gower's sign (Fig. 49-4). Parents frequently note the toe walking, which is a compensatory adaptation to knee extensor weakness. They also note a lordotic posture of the lumbar spine, which is a compensatory change due to hip extensor weakness.

Duchenne muscular dystrophy is occasionally identified presymptomatically in situations where a creatine kinase value is obtained with a markedly elevated value, or when malignant hyperthermia occurs during general anesthesia for an unrelated surgical indication. Early identification also occurs when the

Table 49-3 Characteristics of dystrophinopathies

Character	Duchenne muscular dystrophy	Becker muscular dystrophy
Inheritance	X-linked recessive	X-linked recessive
Gene location	Xp21.2	Xp21.2
Protein	Dystrophin	Dystrophin
Onset	3–5 years	>7 years
Severity and course	Relentlessly progressive Reduced motor function by 2–3 years Steady decline in strength Loss of ambulation: 9–13 years Death between 15 and 25 years	Slowly progressive Severity and onset correlate with muscle dystrophin levels Loss of ambulation: 16–18 years
Weakness	Proximal > distal Symmetric Legs and arms	Proximal > distal Symmetric Calf pain with exercise
Muscle size	Calf hypertrophy	Calf hypertrophy
Musculoskeletal	Contractures: ankles, hip, and knees Scoliosis: onset after loss of ambulation	Contractures: ankles and others
Cardiac	Dilated, especially >18 years	Cardiomyopathy may occur before weakness
Respiratory	Failure in second decade	—
Intelligence	Mean IQ about 88	Slightly reduced, especially with deletion of Dp140 transcription unit
Sensory	Night blindness	—
Muscle pathology	Endomysial fibrosis Variable fiber size Myopathic grouping Fiber degeneration Fiber regeneration Dystrophin: absent Sarcoglycans: reduced	Variable fiber size Endomysial connective tissue Fiber degeneration Fiber regeneration Dystrophin: reduced
Blood chemistry and hematology	Creatine kinase: very high High aspartate aminotransferase and alanine aminotransferase Elevated troponin I	Creatine kinase: 5000–20 000 Lower levels with increasing age

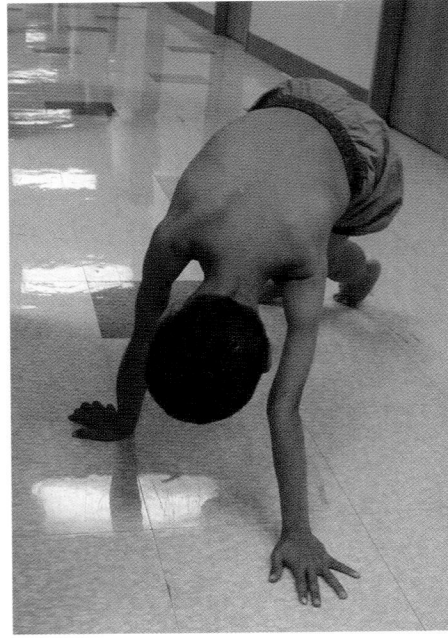
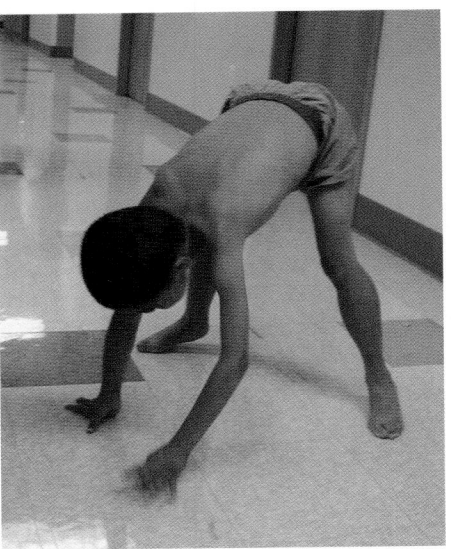
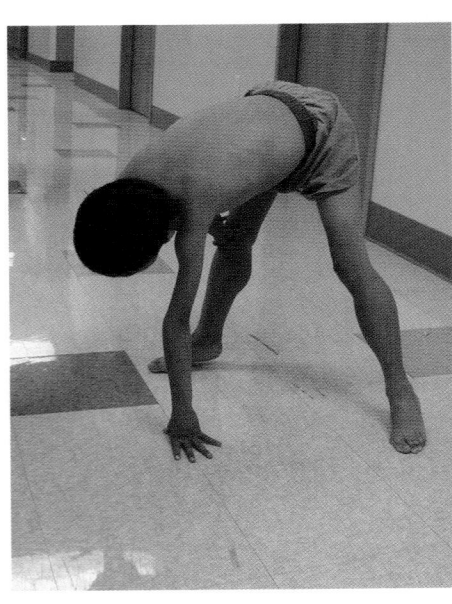
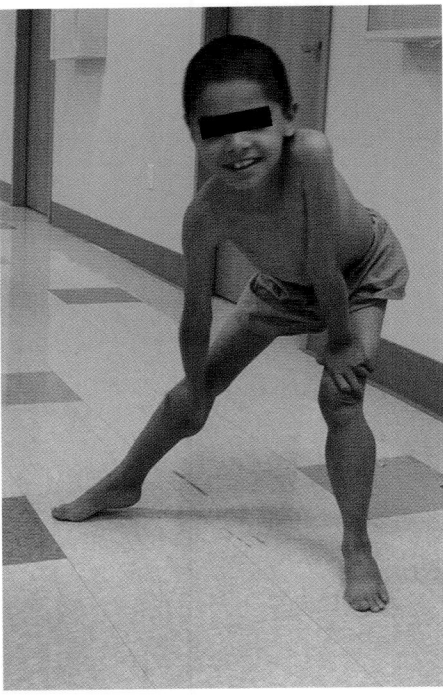

Figure 49-4 Gower's sign in a 9-year-old boy with Duchenne muscular dystrophy.

diagnosis is pursued in a male subject with an affected older sibling.

Pain in the muscles, especially the calves, is a common symptom. Enlargement of muscles, particularly the calves, is commonly seen (Fig. 49-5). Recently, children aged 8–11 years with DMD have been noted to exhibit an unusual clinical examination sign that results from selective hypertrophy and wasting in different muscles in the same region.[150] When viewing these patients from behind with their arms abducted to 90° and elbows flexed to 90°, DMD patients demonstrate a linear or oval depression (due to wasting) of the posterior axillary fold,

with hypertrophied or preserved muscles on its two borders (i.e. infraspinatus inferomedially and deltoid superolaterally), as if there were a valley between the two mounts (Fig. 49-6).

The tongue is also frequently enlarged. An associated wide arch to the mandible and maxilla with separation of the teeth is frequently seen, presumably secondary to the macroglossia. The earliest weakness is seen in the neck flexors during the preschool years. Early in the disease course, weakness is generalized but predominantly proximal. Pelvic girdle weakness pre-dates shoulder girdle weakness by several years. Ankle dorsiflexors are weaker than ankle plantar flexors, ankle everters

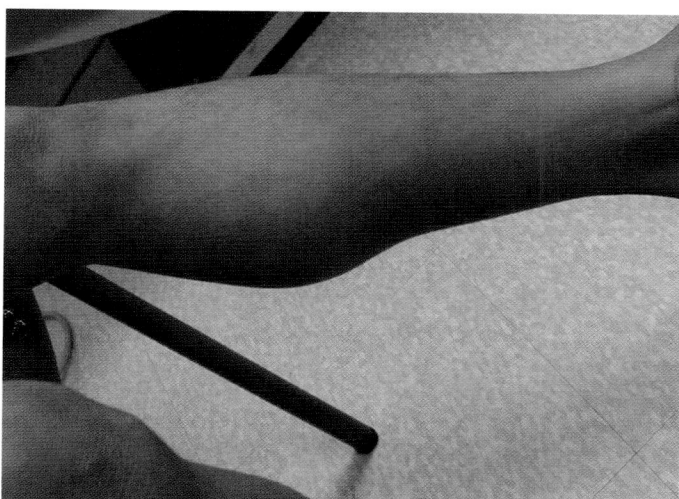

Figure 49-5 Calf pseudohypertrophy in a boy with Duchenne muscular dystrophy.

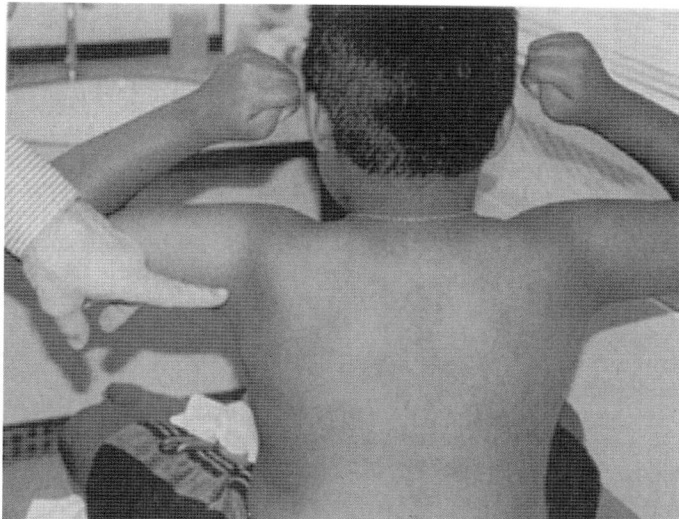

Figure 49-6 Posterior axillary depression sign in Duchenne muscular dystrophy. Note the prominent deltoid superolaterally and infraspinatus inferomedially.

are weaker than ankle inverters, knee extensors are weaker than knee flexors, hip extensors are weaker than hip flexors, and hip abductors are weaker than hip adductors.[9,11]

The weakness progresses steadily, but the rate can be variable during the disease course. Quantitative strength testing shows greater than 40–50% loss of strength by 6 years of age.[101,123,169,173] With manual muscle testing, DMD subjects exhibit loss of strength in a fairly linear fashion from ages 5–13, and measurements obtained several years apart will show fairly steady disease progression. However, a variable course is often noted when analyzing individuals over a shorter period of time.[169,190] Investigators have shown a flattening in the rate of the strength loss curve at approximately ages 14–15.[123,169] Therefore investigators doing studies involving the natural history of DMD

should be cautious about including subjects transitioning to the teenage years, because of the flattening of the manual muscle testing strength curve with increasing age.[123] This caution is particularly important in studies of potential therapeutic agents. Quantitative strength measures have been shown to be more sensitive for demonstrating strength loss than manual muscle testing when strength is graded 4–5.[123]

The average age of wheelchair use in an untreated DMD population is 10 years, with a range of 7–13 years.[26,27,123] Timed motor performance is a useful predictor of time when ambulation will be lost without provision of long leg braces. One large natural history study showed that all DMD subjects who took 9 s or longer to ambulate 30 ft. lost ambulation within 2 years.[123] All DMD subjects who took 12 s or longer to ambulate 30 ft. lost ambulation within 1 year.[123] Ambulation past the age of 14 should raise the suspicion of a milder form of muscular dystrophy, such as BMD or LGMD. Ambulation beyond 16 years was previously used as an exclusionary criterion for DMD.[25] Immobilization for any reason can lead to a marked and often precipitous decline in muscle power and ambulatory ability. A fall with resultant fracture leading to immobilization and loss of ambulatory ability is not an uncommon occurrence.

Significant joint contractures have been found in nearly all DMD children older than age 13.[123,196,197] The most common contractures include ankle plantar flexion and inversion, knee flexion, hip flexion, iliotibial band, elbow flexion, and wrist flexion contractures.[123] Shortening of two joint muscles occurs particularly in the iliotibial band and gastrocnemius.[67] Significant contractures have been shown to be rare in DMD before age 9 for all joints. There is no association between muscle imbalance around a specific joint (defined as grade 1 or greater difference in flexor and extensor strength) and the frequency or severity of contractures involving the hip, knee, ankle, wrist, and elbow in DMD.[123]

The presence of lower extremity contractures in DMD has been shown to be strongly related to the onset of wheelchair reliance.[123,170] Lower extremity contractures were rare while DMD subjects were still upright, but developed soon after they began using a wheelchair for most of the day. The occurrence of elbow flexion contractures also appears to be directly related to prolonged static positioning of the limb, and these contractures develop soon after wheelchair reliance as well. There is a relationship between wheelchair reliance and hip and knee flexion contractures.[123,168] Mild contractures of the iliotibial bands, hip flexor muscles, and heel cords occur in most DMD patients by 6 years of age.[96] Limitations of knee, elbow, and wrist extension occur about 2 years later; however, these early observed contractures were relatively mild.[96] Given the tremendous replacement of muscle by fibrotic tissue in subjects with DMD, it is not surprising that a muscle of less than antigravity extension strength, statically positioned in flexion in a wheelchair, would develop a flexion contracture. The lack of lower extremity weight bearing probably contributes to the rapid acceleration in the severity of these contractures after transition to wheelchair. Ankle plantar flexion contractures are not likely a significant cause of wheelchair reliance, as few subjects exhibit plantar flexion contractures of ≥15° before their transition to a wheelchair.[123] Natural history data suggest that weakness is the major cause of loss of ambulation in DMD, rather than contracture formation.

The reported prevalence of scoliosis in DMD varies from 33% to 100%.[116,117,123,156] This marked variability is primarily because of retrospective selection for scoliosis, the inclusion or exclusion of functional curves, and dissimilar age groups. The prevalence of scoliosis is strongly related to age. Fifty percent of DMD patients acquire scoliosis between ages 12 and 15, corresponding to the adolescent growth spurt. At least 90% of older DMD subjects with no specific treatment for scoliosis have clinical spinal deformity. This is consistent with Oda's report that 15% of older DMD patients show mild non-progressive curves (usually 10–30°).[143] The rate of progression of the primary or single untreated lateral curve is reported to range from 11° to 42° per year, depending on the age span studied. Johnson and Yarnell reported an association between side of curvature, convexity, and hand dominance.[98] McDonald's study, on the other hand, showed no correlation between side of primary convexity and handedness.[123] Oda and colleagues reported that the likelihood of severe progressive spinal deformity could be predicted by type of curve and early pulmonary function measurements.[143] Those without significant kyphosis or hyperlordosis and a peak absolute forced vital capacity (FVC) greater than 2000 mL tend not to show severe progressive scoliosis.

No cause and effect relationship has been established between the onset of wheelchair reliance and the occurrence of scoliosis.[84,123] Wheelchair reliance and scoliosis are both an age-related phenomenon. The causal relationship between loss of ambulatory status and scoliosis is doubtful, given the substantial time interval between the two variables in most subjects (scoliosis usually develops after 3–4 years in a wheelchair). Both wheelchair reliance and spinal deformity can be significantly related to other factors (e.g. age, adolescent growth spurt, increase in weakness of trunk musculature, and other unidentified factors) and appear to represent coincidental signs of disease progression.

Absolute FVC volumes increase in patients with DMD during the first decade, and plateau during the early part of the second decade.[81,123] A linear decline in percent predicted FVC is apparent between 10 and 20 years of age in DMD.[123] Rideau reported that the FVC was predictive of the risk of rapid scoliosis progression.[157] In the most severe DMD cases, maximal FVC reached a plateau of less than 1200 mL. This was associated with loss of ability to walk before age 10 and severe progressive scoliosis. Maximum FVCs plateau between 1200 mL and 1700 mL. Spinal deformity was present consistently in these cases but varied in intensity. The least severe DMD cases reached plateaus in FVC of greater than 1700 mL. Similarly, McDonald and colleagues also found that those patients with higher peak FVC (>2500 mL) had a milder disease progression, losing 4% of predicted FVC per year.[123] Those with peak predicted FVC less than 1700 mL lost 9.6% of predicted FVC per

year.[123] The peak obtained absolute values of FVC that usually occur early in the second decade are an important prognostic indicator for severity of spinal deformity, as well as of the severity of restrictive pulmonary compromise due to muscular weakness.

Reduced maximal static airway pressures (both maximal inspiratory pressure and maximal expiratory pressure) are the earliest indicators of restrictive pulmonary compromise in DMD.[10,20] Impaired values are usually noted between 5 and 10 years of age. Vital capacity typically increases concomitant with growth between 5 and 10 years of age, with the percent of predicted FVC remaining relatively stable and close to 100% of predicted. Patients with DMD typically show a linear decline in percent predicted FVC between 10 and 20 years of age. An FVC falling below 40% of predicted can contraindicate surgical spinal arthrodesis, irrespective of scoliotic severity, because of increased perioperative morbidity.[91,156] Patients who need surgical intervention for scoliosis or other deformities should have surgery before the vital capacity drops below 40% of predicted.[156]

Respiratory failure in DMD is insidious in its onset, and results from a number of factors, including respiratory muscle weakness and fatigue, alteration in respiratory system mechanics, and impairment of the central control of respiration. Noninvasive forms of both positive- and negative-pressure ventilatory support are increasingly being offered to patients with DMD. This will be discussed in more detail later in the chapter, under management of restrictive lung disease.

The dystrophin protein is present in both the myocardium and the cardiac Purkinje fibers.[4,140] Abnormalities of the heart can be detected by clinical examination, electrocardiogram (ECG), echocardiography, and Holter monitoring. Cardiac examination is notable for the point of maximal impulse palpable at the left sternal border due to the marked reduction in anteroposterior chest dimension common in DMD. A loud pulmonic component of the second heart sound suggests pulmonary hypertension in patients with restrictive pulmonary compromise. Nearly all patients over the age of 13 demonstrate abnormalities of the ECG.[42,77,123] Q waves in the lateral leads are the first abnormalities to appear, followed by elevated ST segments and poor R wave progression, increased R/S ratio, and resting tachycardia and conduction defects. ECG abnormalities have been demonstrated to be predictive for death from the cardiomyopathy, with the major determinants including R wave in lead V1 less than 0.6 mV; R wave in lead V5 less than 1.1 mV; R wave in lead V6 less than 1.0 mV; abnormal T waves in leads II, III, AVF, V5, and V6; cardiac conduction disturbances; premature ventricular contraction; and sinus tachycardia.[112,113,148] Sinus tachycardia can be due to low stroke volume from the progressive cardiomyopathy, or in some cases can be sudden in onset and labile, suggesting autonomic disturbance or direct involvement of the sinus node by the dystrophic process.[131]

Autopsy studies and thallium-201 single-photon emission computed tomography (CT) imaging show left ventricular lateral and posterior wall defects that might explain the lateral Q waves and the increased R/S ratio in V1 seen on ECG.[134,138,209]

Localized posterior wall fibrosis is peculiar to DMD and is not seen in other types of muscular dystrophy. Pulmonary hypertension leading to right ventricular enlargement is also known to cause prominent R waves in V1, and has been demonstrated in patients with DMD.[213]

Ventricular ectopy is a known complication of the cardiomyopathy in DMD that probably explains the observed cases of sudden death.[181] Yanagisawa and colleagues reported an age-related increase in the prevalence of cardiac arrhythmias detected by ambulatory 24-h ECG recordings.[210] They also noted an association between ventricular arrhythmias and sudden death in DMD. Clinically evident cardiomyopathy is usually first noted after age 10, and is apparent in nearly all patients over age 18.[140] Development of cardiomyopathy is a predictor of poor prognosis.[123] Echocardiography has been used extensively to follow the development of cardiomyopathy and predict prognosis in patients with DMD. The onset of systolic dysfunction noted by echocardiography is associated with a poor prognosis.[123] The myocardial impairment remains clinically silent until late in the course of the disease, possibly caused by the absence of exertional dyspnea, secondary to lack of physical activity. Death has been attributed to congestive heart failure in as many as 40–50% of patients with DMD by some investigators.[123,140] Regular cardiac evaluations with ECG, echocardiography, and Holter monitor should be employed in teenagers with preclinical cardiomyopathy.

The dystrophin isoform is present in the brain.[142,145,174] Previous studies on intellectual function in children with DMD have generally revealed decreased IQ scores when these children are compared with both control and normative groups.[123,174] A mean score for the DMD population of 1.0–1.5 standard deviations below population norms has been reported. There has generally been a considerable consistency in the degree of impairment across measures, reflecting a rather mild global deficit. Some studies have demonstrated relative deficits in verbal IQ.[174] In a longitudinal assessment of cognitive function, McDonald and colleagues found the IQ measure in DMD to be stable over time.[123] On neuropsychologic testing, a large proportion of DMD subjects fell within the 'mildly impaired' or 'impaired' range according to normative data.[123] These findings probably reflect a mild global deficit rather than focal nervous system impairment.

Substantial anthropometric alterations have been described in DMD. Short stature and slow linear growth with onset shortly after birth have been reported.[60,128,153] Accurate measurement of linear height is extremely difficult in this population. Arm span measurements can be used as an alternative measure of linear growth, but this measurement can also be difficult, as elbow flexion contractures of greater than 30° are frequently present in patients older than 13. Forearm segment length has been proposed as an alternative linear measurement in DMD patients with proximal upper extremity contractures, and radius length can be followed for those with wrist and finger contractures.[153]

Obesity is a substantial problem in DMD, subsequent to the loss of independent ambulation.[39,59,172] Weight control during early adolescence facilitates ease of care, in particular ease of transfers during later adolescence.

Longitudinal weight measurements in DMD confirm significant rates of weight loss in subjects aged 17–21.[59,121] This is probably caused by relative nutritional compromise during the later stages, when boys with DMD have higher protein and energy intake requirements because of hypercatabolic protein metabolism.[78] Protein and calorie requirements can often be 160% of that predicted for able-bodied populations during the later stages of DMD.[180] Restrictive lung disease becomes more problematic during this time, and this can also influence caloric intake and requirements. Self-feeding often becomes impossible during this period, because of biceps weakness. Some subjects with DMD also develop signs and symptoms of upper gastrointestinal dysfunction.[16,92]

The overall care of DMD can be a challenging task, and will encompass most of the rehabilitation modalities discussed later in this chapter. Ultimately, the clinician will also be faced with helping the patient and family deal with end of life issues.

Becker muscular dystrophy

Becker muscular dystrophy is a form of muscular dystrophy with a similar pattern of muscle weakness to that seen in DMD. It also has X-linked inheritance, but with later onset and a much slower rate of progression than in DMD. It was first described by Becker and Kiener in 1955.[13] The disorder has the same gene location as the DMD gene (Xp21) and is allelic. On immunoblotting or immunostaining of muscle biopsy specimens, the presence of altered molecular weight dystrophin or decreased abundance of dystrophin suggests a BMD phenotype.[6] Some subjects have 20–80% of the normal level of dystrophin, while other subjects may have reduced or increased molecular weight dystrophin.[6] BMD has a lower incidence than DMD, with prevalence rates for BMD ranging from 12 to 27 per million and a recent estimated overall prevalence of 24 per million.[62,63,122]

The demonstration of a deletion in the Xp21 gene with cDNA probes is useful in the diagnostic evaluation of dystrophin-deficient myopathies.[41] In the gene deletion test, small blood samples are used as a source of patient DNA, and the dystrophin (DMD, BMD) gene is tested to determine whether it is intact or not. This is done by polymerase chain reaction or Southern blotting, and the methods determine whether all segments of the gene are present. If any segment is missing, the findings indicate the presence of a deletion mutation. Not all DMD and BMD patients have deletion mutations. Many have point mutations that cannot be detected by these methods. Because the gene is so large and complex, it is currently not feasible to routinely test for the other types of smaller mutation. About 55% of DMD patients and 70% of BMD patients show deletion mutations of the gene on currently available tests.[41] A positive DNA test result (presence of a deletion) is diagnostic of a dystrophinopathy (Duchenne or Becker dystrophy). There are no false positives if the test is done appropriately.[41]

Differential diagnosis between DMD and BMD is best done by family history of clinical phenotype. If the patient is still ambulating at 16–20 years of age and has a deletion mutation, then the correct diagnosis is BMD. Some laboratories will report the reading frame. This information can differentiate between a DMD and a BMD diagnosis in approximately 90% of deletion-positive cases.[122,126] Mutations at the Xp21 locus, which maintain the translational reading frame (in-frame mutations), result in an abnormal but partially dysfunctional dystrophin, whereas in DMD the mutations shift the reading frame (out of frame mutations), so that virtually no dystrophin is produced.[41] The reading frame interpretation is most accurate for deletions in the center of the gene (exons 40–60), and is least accurate for deletions at the beginning of the gene (exons 1–20).

Absent dystrophin or levels less than 3% of normal generally are considered diagnostic of DMD; however, 5% of such patients have BMD phenotypes. The dystrophin in BMD typically has an abnormally small molecular weight (< 427 kDa). A minority of patients have dystrophin of larger than normal molecular weight (> 427 kDa) or normal molecular weight. Most BMD patients with larger or smaller molecular weight dystrophin also have decreased quantities of the protein.[122,126] All BMD patients with normal molecular weight dystrophin have decreased quantities, usually less than 30% of normal. Smaller size dystrophin typically is caused by deletion mutations, and larger size dystrophin by duplication mutations. A further refinement is the use of antibodies specific to the carboxy terminal region of dystrophin. Using such antibodies, immunohistochemistry reveals that the carboxy terminal region is almost always absent in DMD but invariably present in BMD.[6]

Studies have shown significant overlap in the observed age of onset between DMD and BMD.[122] Determination of the quantity and molecular weight of dystrophin has substantially improved the early differentiation of BMD, outlier DMD, and the more common and rapidly progressive DMD phenotype. However, Bushby and colleagues found no clear correlation between abundance of dystrophin and clinical course within the BMD group.[25]

The series of Bushby and Gardner-Medwin included 67 BMD subjects, and supported the presence of two major patterns of progression in BMD: a 'typical' slowly progressive course, and a more 'severe' and rapidly progressive course.[24] All the severe BMD patients showed difficulty climbing stairs by age 20, whereas none of the typical BMD patients had difficulty climbing stairs before age 20. Abnormal ECGs were seen in 27% of typical BMD subjects and 88% of subjects with the more severe phenotype. Bushby and Gardner-Medwin found BMD subjects to have a mean age of onset of 12 years in the typical group and 7.7 years in the severe group.[24] Some patients with BMD present with major muscle cramps as an isolated symptom.[19]

The most useful clinical criterion to distinguish BMD from DMD is the continued ability of the patient to walk into the late teenage years. Those with BMD will typically remain ambulatory beyond 16 years. Some patients become wheelchair users in their late teens or twenties, whereas others continue walking into their forties, fifties, or later. Outlier DMD patients generally stop ambulating between 13 and 16 years of age.[122,123]

As in DMD, preclinical cases are often identified by the finding of a grossly elevated creatine kinase value. There is also considerable overlap in creatine kinase values between DMD and BMD cases at the time of presentation, and creatine kinase values cannot be used to differentiate DMD from BMD.

Patients with BMD have a distribution of weakness that is similar to that in those with DMD.[122] Proximal lower limb muscles are involved earlier in the disease course. Gradual involvement of the pectoral girdle and upper limb musculature occurs 10–20 years from onset of disease. Extensors have been noted to be weaker than flexors.[122] The muscle groups that are most severely involved early in the course of disease include the hip extensors, knee extensors, and neck flexors.[122]

Calf enlargement is a non-specific finding in BMD, as is the presence of a Gower's sign. Over the course of time, the gait becomes similar to that in other neuromuscular disease conditions with proximal weakness. Patients often ambulate with a lumbar lordosis, forefoot–floor contact, decreased stance-phase knee flexion, and a modified Trendelenburg or gluteus medius lurch, often described as a waddle.

Early development of contractures does not appear to be a feature of BMD.[96,122] As with DMD, non-ambulatory BMD subjects can develop equinus contractures, knee flexion contractures, and hip flexion contractures. Subjects with BMD are more likely to develop flexion contractures subsequent to wheelchair reliance.

Spinal deformity is not nearly as common or severe in BMD as it is in DMD. Spinal instrumentation is rarely required by patients with BMD.[122]

Compromised pulmonary function is also much less problematic in BMD.[15,122] The percent predicted FVC does not appear substantially reduced until the third or fourth decade.[122] The percent predicted maximal expiratory pressure appears relatively more reduced at younger ages than the percent predicted maximal inspiratory pressure, a finding seen in DMD and other neuromuscular diseases.[15] This might be due to more relative involvement of the intercostals and abdominal musculature, with relative sparing of contractile function in the diaphragm with BMD. Predicted maximal expiratory pressure can be a useful quantitative measure of impairment and perhaps disease progression early in the course of BMD.

The pattern of occasional life-threatening cardiac involvement in otherwise mild and slowly progressive BMD has been reported.[139,162,211] A significant percentage of BMD patients develop cardiac abnormalities. The rate of progression of cardiac failure can be more rapid than the progression of skeletal myopathy.[177,211] In fact, successful cardiac transplantation has been increasingly reported in BMD subjects with cardiac failure.[40,50] Approximately 75% of BMD patients have been found to exhibit ECG abnormalities.[122] The abnormal findings most commonly reported include abnormal Q waves, right ventricular hypertrophy, left ventricular hypertrophy, right bundle branch block, and non-specific T-wave abnormalities. Unlike in DMD, resting sinus tachycardia has not been a frequent finding. Echocardiography has shown left ventricular dilatation in 37%, whereas 63% have subnormal systolic function because of global hypokinesis.[99,198] The cardiac compromise can be disproportionately severe, relative to the degree of restrictive lung disease, in some BMD subjects. The evidence for significant myocardial involvement in BMD is sufficient to warrant screening of all these patients at regular intervals using ECG and echocardiography. The slowly progressive nature of this dystrophic myopathy, which is compatible with many years of functional mobility and longevity, makes these patients suitable candidates for cardiac transplantation if end-stage cardiac failure occurs.[151]

Some patients with BMD present with an isolated cardiomyopathy with no clinical manifestation of skeletal muscle involvement.[109] The diagnosis can be established by demonstration of a deletion in the Xp21 gene or by muscle biopsy. Isolated cases of cardiomyopathy in children, particularly those with family histories indicative of X-linked inheritance, should be screened for BMD with an initial serum creatine kinase estimation and molecular genetic studies of the Xp21 gene.

Cognitive testing in BMD subjects has shown large variability in IQ scores and neuropsychologic test measures. Mildly reduced intellectual performance has been noted in a subset of BMD patients; however, the degree of impairment is not as severe as noted in DMD.[125]

Other atypical clinical presentations include a complaint of cramps on exercise in individuals with no muscle weakness.[62] Patients with focal wasting of the quadriceps who have previously been diagnosed with quadriceps myopathy have recently been diagnosed with BMD. This is based on molecular genetic testing and/or dystrophin analysis on muscle biopsy.[122]

Limb girdle muscular dystrophy

Advances in molecular biology have shown that LGMD is a very heterogeneous group of dystrophic myopathies, usually with childhood or adolescent onset (although there are late-onset forms), no sex linkage, and a distribution and pattern of weakness similar to those in DMD but with a much slower rate of progression.[125] There are at least 15 different subtypes of LGMD, most of which have been linked to abnormalities of the dystrophin-associated glycoproteins (DAGs), especially α-sarcoglycan (adhalin), a 50-kDa DAG, and γ-sarcoglycan.[120] The 50-kDa DAG protein has been linked to the 17q12–q21.33 locus, and more recently the children with this have been referred to as having severe, childhood-onset, autosomal recessive muscular dystrophy (SCARMD), which is also classified as LGMD 2D.[120,147] Cases in other families with SCARMD have been linked to chromosome 13q12; these individuals with LGMD 2C may show a primary deficiency of γ-sarcoglycan and a secondary deficiency of α-sarcoglycan.[117] LGMD 2E patients (chromosome 4q12) show a primary deficiency in β-sarcoglycan, and LGMD 2F patients (chromosome 5q33–q34) show a primary deficiency of δ-sarcoglycan.[66,117] Most of the primary sarcoglycan abnormalities lead to secondary deficiencies of α-sarcoglycan. All the DAGs are reduced in DMD patients,

because the carboxy terminal portion of dystrophin binds to the dystrophin-associated proteins and maintains their integrity.[6,159] A less severe autosomal recessive dystrophic myopathy (LGMD 2A) has been linked to chromosome 15q1–q21.1, the gene for the protein calpain-3.[41,117] Diagnosis of SCARMD or LGMD subtypes is confirmed by muscle biopsy.[158] Table 49-4 lists the characteristics of the most common autosomal recessive limb girdle muscular dystrophies, and Table 49-5 lists the characteristics of the most common autosomal dominant limb girdle muscular dystrophies.

Dystrophin analysis is generally normal in subjects with LGMD.[41] Of the seven recessive loci identified to date, four are sarcoglycan genes.[41,126] Their four proteins make up the sarcoglycan complex, which is felt to interact directly with the 43-kDa DAG and with dystrophin.[41,145] DAGs probably provide connections between the extracellular matrix (the protein merosin) and the intracellular membrane cytoskeleton (attached to dystrophin).[41,117,126,145] An abnormality of the dystrophin–glycoprotein complex, resulting from primary deficiencies of one or more of the DAGs, results in a disruption in the linkage between the intracellular sarcolemmal cytoskeleton and the extracellular matrix. Disruption of the membrane cytoskeleton is common to the pathophysiology of most muscular dystrophies, the dystrophinopathies.

Patients with SCARMD can exhibit calf hypertrophy and a Gower's sign. Loss of ambulation generally occurs between 10 and 20 years but occasionally after 20 years of age. In one series, several differences between DMD and SCARMD were noted.[125] In contrast to in DMD, the limb extensors were not weaker than the limb flexors. In particular, ankle dorsiflexors were similar in strength to ankle plantar flexors, knee extensors showed similar strength compared with knee flexors, and hip extensors and hip flexors showed similar strength values. The severity and rate of progression often varies between and within the families of SCARMD patients. Contractures appear to be much less prevalent and severe in SCARMD compared with in DMD. The prevalence of joint contractures in SCARMD subjects was found to be similar to that observed in BMD subjects in one series.[96]

Spinal deformity appears to be much less problematic in SCARMD than in DMD. Less than 50% of SCARMD subjects were found to have curves of mild to moderate severity, ranging from 5° to 30°.[125] The prevalence and severity of spinal deformity in SCARMD appears to be similar to that observed in BMD.

Restrictive pulmonary insufficiency occurs in SCARMD but is not as severe as that seen in DMD. The prevalence of severe restrictive lung disease in SCARMD is similar to that observed in BMD.[15,125]

Few studies have systematically evaluated the cardiac manifestations of SCARMD and other limb girdle dystrophies. In one series, the prevalence of abnormal ECG findings in SCARMD was 62%.[125] ECG abnormalities include evidence of infranodal conduction defects, evidence of left ventricular hypertrophy, increased R/S ratio in V1, and abnormal Q waves.

Table 49-4 Characteristics of autosomal recessive limb girdle muscular dystrophies

Character	Type of limb girdle muscular dystrophy			
	2A	2B	2C	2D
Inheritance	Autosomal recessive	Autosomal recessive	X-linked recessive	X-linked recessive
Gene location	4p21	2p13	13q12	17q21
Protein	Calpain-3	Dysferlin	γ-Sarcoglycan	α-Sarcoglycan (adhalin)
Onset	Early onset: <12 years Leyden–Mobius type: 13–29 years Late onset: >30 years	Mean 19 ± 3 years Range 12–39 years	Mean 5–6 years C283Y mutation: <2 years	2–15 years

Severity and course	Variable progression
	Mild phenotype in
	  majority
	Early onset has more
	  homogeneous and severe
	  progression
	Loss of ambulation:
	  10–30 years after onset
		Slow progression
		Loss of ambulation:
		  10–30 years after
		  onset
		Mild weakness
			Variable progression
			  (some like Duchenne,
			  others like Becker)
			Loss of ambulation: 10–
			  37 years (mean 16 years)
			No relation between
			  death and age of onset
				Variable progression
				Absent adhalin: rapidly
				  progressive (Duchenne-
				  like phenotype)—earlier
				  onset
				Reduced adhalin: later
				  onset, milder weakness,
				  ambulation may be
				  preserved—later onset

Weakness	Proximal legs, rectus
	  abdominis, arms, and
	  periscapular
	Quadriceps: may be
	  spared
		Weakness in
		  gastrocnemius,
		  quadriceps, and psoas
		Weakness in biceps
		  occurs approximately
		  9 years after in legs
			Proximal > distal
			Quadriceps: spared
				Proximal > distal
				Symmetric
				Quadriceps weakness

Muscle size	Limbs, pelvic, and
	  shoulder: atrophy of
	  posterior compartments
		Hypertrophy: uncommon	Hypertrophy of calf and
			  tongue in some patients
				Calf hypertrophy in some
				  patients

Musculoskeletal	Contractures: calf
	  (toe-walking may be
	  presenting sign)
		Contractures: calf
		  (toe-walking may be
		  presenting sign)
			Lumbar hyperlordosis,
			  scapular winging
				Scapular winging

Cardiac	No involvement	No involvement	Occasional, especially late in disease course	Dilated cardiomyopathy
Intelligence	Normal or mild mental retardation	Normal	Normal	—

Muscle pathology	Myopathic
	Necrosis and
	  regeneration
	Large size variability
	Endomysial fibrosis
	Type 1 predominance
	  with increasing
	  weakness
	Normal dystrophin and
	  sarcoglycan
		Myopathic
		Necrosis and
		  degeneration
		Variable fiber size
		Increased endomysial
		  connective tissue
		Absent or reduced
		  dysferlin staining
		Normal dystrophin and
		  sarcoglycan
			Myopathic
			Inflammation: occasional
			Severe disease: absent
			  γ-sarcoglycan
			Slowly progressive:
			  reduced γ-sarcoglycan
			Dystrophin: normal or
			  reduced
				Myopathic
				Degeneration and
				  regeneration
				Variable fiber size
				Increased endomysial
				  connective tissue
				Myopathic grouping of
				  fibers
				Absent or reduced adhalin
				  (α-sarcoglycan)
				Other sarcoglycans:
				  reduced or absent

Creatine kinase	7–80 times normal	10–72 times normal	Very high	Very high (often >5000)

Continued on page 1115

Continued from page 1114 Table 49-4	Characteristics of autosomal recessive limb girdle muscular dystrophies				
Character	Type of limb girdle muscular dystrophy				
	2E	2F	2G	2I	2J
Inheritance	Autosomal recessive	Autosomal recessive	Autosomal recessive	X-linked recessive	Autosomal recessive
Gene location	4q12	5q33	17q12	19q13.3	2q31
Protein	β-Sarcoglycan	δ-Sarcoglycan	Telethonin	Fukutin-related protein	Titin
Onset	3 years to teens Intrafamilial variability	2–10 years	Mean 12.5 years Range 9–15 years	0.5–27 years 61% less than 5 years	Usually childhood Range: less than 10 years to third decade
Severity and course	Moderate progression and severity Often in wheelchair by 10–15 years, usually by 25 years	Rapid progression Loss of ambulation: 9–16 years Death in second decade	Slow progression, 40% non-ambulatory in third or fourth decade	Variable progression and severity Early onset: non-ambulant by teens Later onset: slowly progressive, 30% non-ambulatory by fourth to sixth decade	Slowly progressive, but variable Loss of ambulation typically occurs before 30 years Some patients ambulatory at 60 years
Weakness	Proximal	Proximal Symmetric	Arms: proximal Legs: proximal and distal (foot drop)	Proximal > distal Legs: thigh adductors, psoas, quadriceps Arms: periscapular, deltoid, biceps, triceps Face: mild weakness in older patients	Proximal > distal
Muscle size	Prominent muscle hypertrophy Tongue is occasionally hypertrophic	Calf hypertrophy Cramps	Calf hypertrophy: 50% Calf atrophy: 50%	Calf, tongue, and thigh hypertrophy Wasting in regions of weakness	Anterior tibialis wasting
Musculoskeletal	Shoulders: scapular winging and muscle wasting	—	—	Contractures in ankles (especially in non-ambulant) Scoliosis	—
Cardiac	Occasional cardiomyopathy	Dilated cardiomyopathy described that may occur without muscle myopathy	Cardiac involvement in 55% of patients	Dilated cardiomyopathy in 30–50%	None
Intelligence	–	Normal	—	Normal	—
Muscle pathology	Myopathic Sarcoglycans: usually absent Dystrophin: often reduced, but not absent	Myopathic Fiber degeneration Fiber regeneration δ-Sarcoglycan absent Other sarcoglycans absent or reduced	Myopathic Fiber degeneration Fiber regeneration Rimmed vacuoles Telethonin absent from muscle	Myopathic Necrosis and degeneration Variable fiber size Increased connective tissue Type 1 fiber predominance Reduced staining for adhalin (α-sarcoglycan)	Myopathic No vacuoles Loss of calpain-3
Creatine kinase	Very high (often >5000)	10–50 times normal	3–30 times normal	Very high: 1000–8000	High

Table 49-5 Characteristics of autosomal dominant limb girdle muscular dystrophies

Character	Type of limb girdle muscular dystrophy		
	1A	1B	1C
Inheritance	Autosomal dominant	Autosomal dominant	Autosomal dominant
Gene location	5q31	1q11–q21	3p25
Protein	Myotilin	Lamin A/C	Caveolin-3
Onset	Variable Third to seventh decade Anticipation: age of onset decreases in succeeding generations	<20 years	5 years
Severity and course	Slow progression	Slow progression Upper limbs involved by third or fourth decade	Moderately severity and progression Adults with Gower's maneuver
Weakness	Legs and arms Symmetric Proximal at onset Distal with disease progression	Lower limb Symmetric Proximal	Proximal
Muscle size	—	—	Calf hypertrophy
Musculoskeletal	Contractures: ankles	No contractures	Cramps after exercise
Cardiac	Cardiomyopathy: 50%	Cardiomyopathy: 62% Arteriovenous conduction block	—

Muscle pathology	Myopathic
	Variable fiber size
	Fiber degeneration and regeneration
	Rimmed vacuoles
	Normal levels of myotilin
	Normal sarcoglycans
	Reduced laminin-γ1
		Mild myopathy
		Laminin A subcellular localization
			Myopathic
			Reduced caveolin-3 staining
			Reduced dysferlin on muscle fiber
			  sarcolemma but normal by
			  western blot

Creatine kinase	0–15 times normal, commonly twice normal	Normal to mildly elevated	4–25 times normal

Intellectual functioning in SCARMD has generally been found to be normal.[125]

Facioscapulohumeral muscular dystrophy

Facioscapulohumeral muscular dystrophy is a slowly progressive dystrophic myopathy with predominant involvement of facial and shoulder girdle musculature. The condition is autosomal dominant with linkage to the chromosome 4q35 locus.[41,192,193,203] Prevalence has been difficult to ascertain because of undiagnosed mild cases, but has been estimated at 10–20 per million.[64,102]

Facial weakness is an important clinical feature of FSHMD (Fig. 49-7). The initial weakness affects the facial muscles, especially the orbicularis oculi, zygomaticus, and orbicularis oris. These patients often have difficulty with eye closure but not ptosis. Subjects with FSHMD often have an expressionless appearance and exhibit difficulty whistling, pursing the lips, drinking through a straw, or smiling. Even in the very early stages, forced closure of the eyelids can be easily overcome by the examiner. Masseter, temporalis, extraocular, and pharyngeal muscles characteristically are spared in FSHMD.

Patients with FSHMD show characteristic patterns of muscle atrophy and scapular displacement. Involvement of the latissimus dorsi, trapezius, rhomboids, and serratus anterior results in a characteristic appearance of the shoulders, with the scapula positioned more laterally and superiorly, giving the shoulders a forward-sloped appearance (Fig. 49-1). The upper border of the scapula rises into the trapezius, falsely giving it a hypertrophied appearance. From the posterior view, the medial border of the scapula may exhibit profound posterior and lateral winging. The involvement of shoulder girdle musculature in FSHMD can be quite asymmetric.

The typical onset is in adolescence or early adult life. Initially, patients show predominant involvement of facial and shoulder girdle musculature. Scapular stabilizers, shoulder abductors, and shoulder external rotators may be significantly affected, but at times the deltoids are surprisingly spared if tested with the scapulae stabilized. Both the biceps and triceps may be more affected than the deltoids. Over time, ankle dorsiflexion weakness often becomes significant in addition to pelvic girdle weakness. Late in the disease course, patients can show marked wrist extension weakness. Some authors

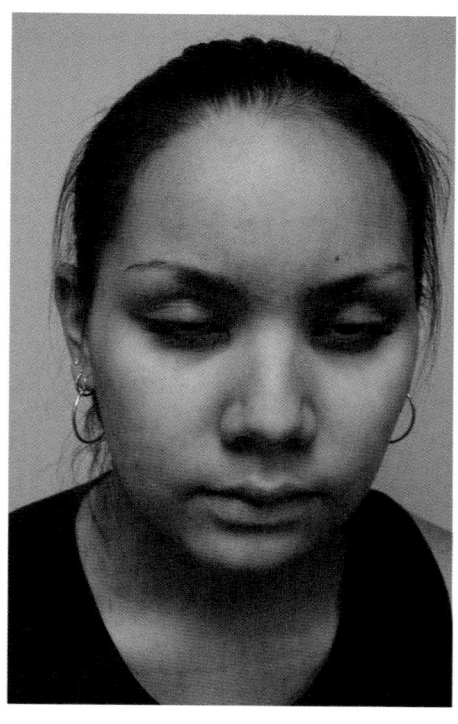

Figure 49-7 Facial involvement in facioscapulohumeral muscular dystrophy. Eye closure is weak, and weakness in orbicularis oris produces difficulty smiling, puffing out the cheeks, and pursing the lips.

have found asymmetric weakness in the dominant upper limb.[97,102]

A sensory neural hearing deficit was originally observed in Coates syndrome (early-onset FSHMD). These individuals have a myopathy that presents in infancy. The disease progression is fairly rapid, with most individuals becoming wheelchair users by the late second or third decade.[146] These individuals also have a progressive exudative telangiectasia of the retina. Early recognition and photocoagulation of the abnormal retinal vessels can often prevent loss of vision. Several audiometry studies have demonstrated hearing deficits in many later onset FSHMD patients in addition to those with Coates syndrome, suggesting that impaired hearing function is more common than expected in FSHMD.[130,193] All patients with FSHMD should have screening audiometry and ophthalmologic evaluation.

Contractures are relatively uncommon in FSHMD. In the most comprehensive study to date, 22 subjects had range of motion (ROM) testing of major upper and lower extremity joints.[102] Clinically significant loss of ROM (defined as a reduction in ROM greater than 20°) was present in two subjects (9%) at the wrist and in one subject (5%) at the hip, knee, and ankle. This subject had been wheelchair-reliant for 15 years at the time of ROM testing. Although active motion is severely restricted, subjects with FSHMD typically maintain full passive ROM.

Spinal deformity is common, with 80% of FSHMD subjects exhibiting hyperlordosis, alone or in combination with scoliosis. Rarely, severe and progressive hyperlordosis is associated with FSHMD. Patients with severe hyperlordosis might utilize their lordotic posturing to compensate for hip extensor weakness. Scoliosis alone accounts for only 20% of spinal deformity in

FSHMD.[84] FSHMD patients with scoliosis typically have mild and non-progressive curves.

Mild restrictive lung disease has been reported in nearly one-half of patients with FSHMD.[15,32,102] Expiratory musculature appears to be more affected than inspiratory muscles in FSHMD.[32] A recent Dutch study identified 10 FSHMD patients on nocturnal ventilatory support at home, representing approximately 1% of the Dutch FSHMD population.[207] Severe muscle disease, wheelchair dependency, and kyphoscoliosis appeared to be risk factors for respiratory failure.[207]

The presence of cardiac abnormalities in FSHMD is still debated. While diverse ECG abnormalities have been noted, one study showed no abnormalities on ECG, chest radiography, Holter monitoring, and echocardiography.[198] Nuclear scanning with thallium-201 has demonstrated diffuse defects consistent with diffuse fibrosis.[198] Abnormalities in systolic time intervals on echocardiography and elevations in atrial natriuretic peptide are consistent with subclinical cardiomyopathy.[102,198] Cardiac complications in FSHMD are rare, and patients in general have normal longevity. There is usually no associated intellectual involvement in this dystrophic myopathy.

Changes on muscle biopsy are relatively slight, with the most consistent finding being the presence of isolated small atrophic fibers. Other fibers may be hypertrophied. Serum creatine kinase levels are normal in the majority of patients. Molecular genetic testing for the FSH gene is now available for diagnostic confirmation.

Myotonic muscular dystrophy

Myotonic muscular dystrophy is an autosomal dominant multi-system muscular dystrophy with an incidence of 1 per 8000.[64,95] The disorder affects skeletal muscle, smooth muscle, myocardium, brain, and ocular structures. Associated findings include frontal pattern baldness and gonadal atrophy (in male patients), cataracts, and cardiac dysrhythmias. Insulin insensitivity can be present. The gene has been localized to the region of the DM protein kinase (DMPK) gene at 19q13.3.[90,154] Patients demonstrate expansion of an unstable CTG trinucleotide repeat within the region. Normal individuals generally have < 37 repeats that are transmitted from generation to generation. Patients with MMD may have 50 to several thousand CTG repeats with remarkable instability. The age of onset is inversely correlated with the repeat links.[90] Mild, late-onset MMD usually is associated with 50–150 repeats; classic adolescent or young adult-onset MMD shows 100–1000 repeats; and congenital MMD patients show greater than 1000 repeats.[41,90,154] The expanded CTG repeat further expands as it is transmitted to successive generations, providing a molecular basis for 'genetic anticipation'. Both maternal to child and paternal to child transmission occurs. However, it can be more severe if transmitted from the mother, with repeat size in offspring exceeding 1000 CTG repeats or more frequently occurring in maternal transmission. Affected fathers seldom transmit alleles larger than 1000 copies to offspring, due to a lack of sperm containing such alleles, presumably due to the poor motility of sperm containing alleles of that size, although this has not been proven.

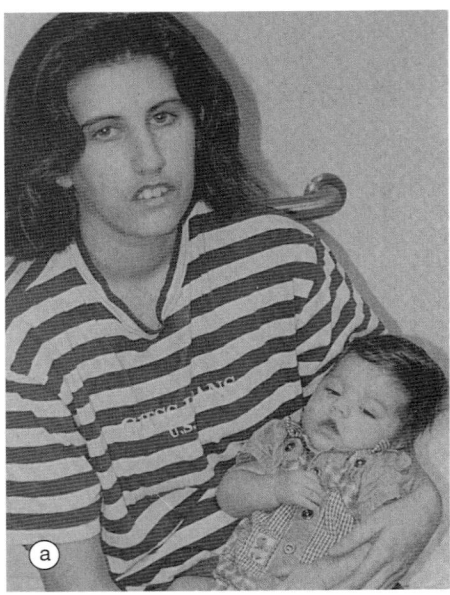

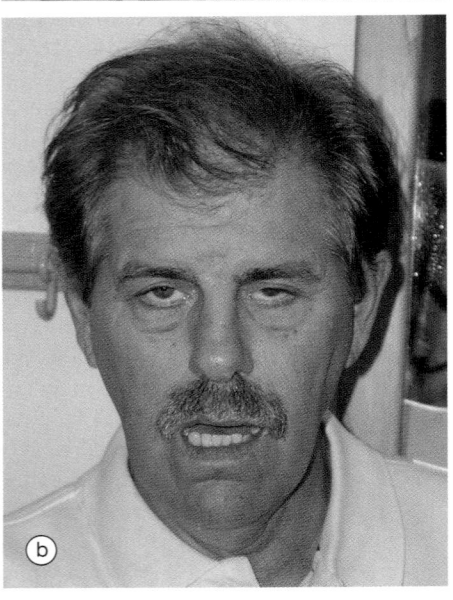

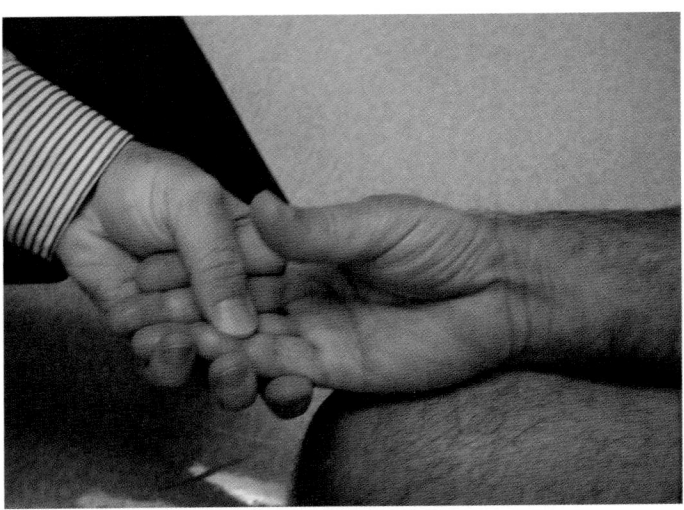

Figure 49-9 Percussion myotonia of the thenar eminence in a patient with myotonic muscular dystrophy.

Figure 49-8 Typical facial characteristics in myotonic muscular dystrophy (MMD). (a) A mother with MMD and an infant with congenital MMD; the symptomatic mother has 560 trinucleotide CTG repeats at the DM protein kinase (DMPK) gene loci in chromosome 19q13.3, while the infant has 1330 repeats. (b) An adult man with MMD and temporal wasting, receding hairline, long drawn face, and myopathic tenting of the mouth.

Several characteristic facial features of MMD may be seen on inspection (Fig. 49-8). The adult with longstanding MMD often has characteristic facial features. The long, thin face with temporal and masseter wasting is drawn and has been described by some as lugubrious or 'hatchet' face. Adults of both sexes often exhibit frontal balding.

Myotonia is a state of delayed relaxation or sustained contraction of skeletal muscle that is easily identified in children with MMD. Grip myotonia can be demonstrated by delayed opening of the hand, with difficulty extending the fingers following tight grip. Percussion myotonia can be elicited by striking the thenar eminence with a reflex hammer, producing adduction and flexion of the thumb, with slow return (Fig. 49-9). Needle EMG shows myotonic discharges, which are spontaneous waxing and waning spikes that produce a characteristic dive-bomber sound.[107]

Myotonic muscular dystrophy is one of the few dystrophic myopathies with greater distal weakness than proximal weakness.[119] Although neck flexors, shoulder girdle musculature, and pelvic girdle musculature can become significantly involved over decades, the weakness is initially most predominant in the ankle dorsiflexors, ankle everters and inverters, and hand muscles.[95] Significant muscle wasting can occur over time. In MMD patients with infantile onset, a congenital clubfoot or talipes equinovarus frequently occurs. In adult-onset MMD, contractures at the wrist, ankle, and elbows are relatively uncommon and mild.[95,96] Patients with congenital-onset MMD may develop spinal deformity requiring surgical spinal arthrodesis.[84]

Abnormalities on ECG and echocardiography are demonstrated in approximately 70–75% of patients with MMD.[95,113,133] Prolongation of the PR interval, abnormal axis, and infranodal conduction abnormalities are all suggestive of conduction system disease, which might explain the occurrence of sudden death in less than 5% of MMD patients.[113] Ventricular tachycardia can also contribute to the syncope and sudden death associated with MMD. Some patients have required implantation of cardiac pacemakers. Q waves have been reported on screening ECGs in MMD patients, and this abnormality might reflect myocardial fibrosis.[95,113] Any MMD patient with dyspnea, chest pain, syncope, or other cardiac symptoms should receive thorough cardiac evaluation.

Subjects with MMD have a very high incidence of restrictive lung disease.[95,191] Involvement of respiratory muscles is a major cause of respiratory distress and mortality in affected infants with MMD. Swallowing difficulties that produce aspiration of material into the trachea and bronchial tree, along with weakened respiratory muscles and a weak cough have been reported as factors that may result in pulmonary complications in MMD patients. Care should be taken during general anesthesia in MMD, due to the risk of cardiac arrhythmias and malignant hyperthermia.

Constipation is a fairly common complaint in congenital MMD, due to smooth muscle involvement. Patients with MMD should also be screened for diabetes mellitus, as there is an increased incidence of insulin insensitivity.

Those with congenital MMD usually show significantly reduced IQ, often in the mentally retarded range.[95] In adult-onset MMD, there is evidence for a generally lower intelligence of a mild degree (full-scale IQs have been reported to be in the 86–92 range).[95] However, there is a wide range of IQ values found in this population, with many subjects scoring in the above-average range. Cognitive functioning also appears to be directly related to the size of the CTG expansion at the MMD gene locus.

There is a newly discovered form of MMD known as type 2 MMD (MMD2 or DM2). It has also been referred to as proximal myotonic myopathy.[41,90] MMD2 is now known to be caused by a mutation on chromosome 3, and is thought to be clinically less severe than either typical MMD or congenital MMD. MMD2 may be associated with insulin insensitivity, diabetes, and low testosterone levels in males.

Other myotonic disorders
Myotonia congenita

Myotonia congenita (Thomsen disease) is inherited as an autosomal dominant condition. It is a condition in which the patient has myotonia but not weakness. Symptoms can be present from birth but usually develop later. The myotonia can manifest as difficulty in releasing objects or as difficulty walking or climbing stairs. The myotonia is exacerbated by prolonged rest or inactivity. Myotonia may be aggravated by cold. Patients can demonstrate grip myotonia or lid lag following upward gaze or squint, and diplopia following sustained conjugate movement of the eyes in one direction. The other common feature of myotonia congenita is muscle hypertrophy. Patients can have a 'Herculean' appearance.[73,126]

A recessive form of myotonia congenita (Becker form) also exists with later onset, more marked myotonia, more striking hypertrophy of muscles, and associated weakness of muscles. The dominant form seems more prone to aggravation of the myotonia by cold.[126]

The diagnosis is essentially made clinically with confirmation of classic myotonic discharges on EMG. Muscle biopsy is essentially normal apart from the presence of hypertrophy of fibers and an absence of type 2B fibers.[126,135]

Paramyotonia congenita

Paramyotonia congenita is an autosomal dominant myotonic condition characterized by generalized hypertrophy, mild involvement of proximal muscles, and more severe involvement of hands and muscles of the face. Myotonic episodes usually subside within a matter of hours but are significantly aggravated by cold temperatures. This is usually not a severe disease, and these patients have a good overall prognosis and normal life expectancy.[41,126]

Schwartz–Jampel syndrome

Schwartz–Jampel syndrome is an autosomal recessive disorder with myotonia, dwarfism, diffuse bone disease, narrow palpebral fissures, blepharospasm, micrognathia, and flattened facies.[110,175] Limitation of joint movement can be present, along with skeletal abnormalities, including short neck and kyphosis. Muscles are typically hypertrophic and clinically stiff. The symptoms are not progressive, and the overall prognosis is good.

Electrodiagnostic studies show continuous electrical activity, with electrical silence being difficult to obtain. There is relatively little waxing and waning in either amplitude or frequency of complex repetitive discharges. Abnormal sodium channel kinetics in the sarcolemma of muscle has been demonstrated.[110] Some therapeutic benefit has been reported with procainamide and carbamazepine.[175]

Emery–Dreifuss muscular dystrophy

Emery–Dreifuss muscular dystrophy is an X-linked recessive progressive dystrophic myopathy with a gene locus identified at Xq28.[41,61,63,199] The muscle protein that is deficient in EDMD has been termed *emerin*. The condition usually presents in adolescence or early adult life, and many clinical features can be seen in early childhood. Patients can present with a selective scapulohumeral peroneal distribution weakness with striking wasting of the biceps, accentuated by sparing of the deltoids and forearm muscles. However, this is clinically differentiated from FSHMD by the lack of facial involvement. Ankle dorsiflexors often are weaker than ankle plantar flexors. Significant atrophy usually is present in the upper arms and legs, due to focal wasting of the calf muscles and biceps.

An associated cardiomyopathy usually presents with arrhythmia and can lead to sudden death in early adult life.[63,200] The cardiomyopathy can progress to four-chamber dilated cardiomyopathy with complete heart block and ventricular arrhythmias.[200] Atrial arrhythmia usually appears prior to complete heart block. Reported features include first-degree heart block, followed by Wenckebach phenomenon, and then complete atrial ventricular dissociation and atrial fibrillation or flutter with progressive slowing of the rate.[200] Syncope or near syncope commonly occurs later in the second decade or early in the third decade.[200] Evidence of cardiac arrhythmia, sometimes present only at night, might be detected on 24-h Holter monitoring. The provision of a cardiac pacemaker to the patient with arrhythmia may be life-saving and considerably improve life expectancy.

Some patients with EDMD may show evidence of nocturnal hypoventilation as a result of restrictive expansion of the chest in association with the rigid spine, and partly due to involvement of the diaphragm.[63,199]

Creatine kinase can be moderately elevated, with a value between two and five times the upper limit of normal. EMG usually shows a myopathic pattern. Muscle biopsy shows a myopathic process, with variation in fiber size, clusters of atrophic fibers, mild proliferation of connective tissue, and some focal necrosis of fibers.

A hallmark of EDMD clinically is the early presence of contractures of the elbow flexors with limitation of full elbow extension. Heel cord tightness might be present early in the disorder, concomitant with ankle dorsiflexion and toe walking. Unlike in DMD, the toe walking in EDMD usually is secondary to ankle dorsiflexion weakness and not a compensatory strategy to stabilize the knee due to proximal limb weakness. Tightness of the cervical and lumbar spinal extensor muscles, resulting in limitation of neck and trunk flexion, with inability to flex the chin to the sternum and to touch the toes, also has been reported in EDMD.

A dominantly inherited disorder with a similar phenotype has been reported, but the gene locus is unknown. Some reported cases of 'rigid spine syndrome', a form of congenital muscular dystrophy, may be EDMD cases in view of the marked predominance of male patients in this disorder and the associated contractures reported at the elbows and ankles.[199]

Congenital muscular dystrophy

The term *congenital muscular dystrophy* has been widely used for a group of infants presenting with hypotonia, muscle weakness at birth or within the first few months of life, congenital contractures, and a dystrophic pattern on muscle biopsy. The dystrophic changes noted on biopsy separate this group of disorders from the congenital myopathies. The condition tends to remain relatively static. However, some subjects show slow progression, whereas others gain developmental milestones and achieve the ability to walk.

There are several syndromes of congenital muscular dystrophy with central nervous system abnormality. Fukuyama congenital muscular dystrophy is associated with mental retardation, structural brain malformations evident on magnetic resonance imaging (MRI), and a dystrophic myopathy. The gene locus has recently been identified to be at 9q31–33.[76,185]

Muscle–eye–brain disease describes a syndrome comprising congenital muscular dystrophy, mental retardation, and ocular abnormality. Infants present with congenital hypotonia, muscle weakness, elevated creatine kinase, myopathic EMG, and dystrophic changes on muscle biopsy.[163–165] Ophthalmologic findings include severe visual impairment, with uncontrolled eye movements associated with severe myopia. Patients often deteriorate around 5 years of age, with progressive occurrence of spasticity. CT scans have shown ventricular dilatation in low density of the white matter.

Cases with more pure congenital muscular dystrophy without central nervous system involvement have been identified. The main clinical features are muscle weakness and hypotonia; congenital contractures; histologic changes of a dystrophic nature, often with extensive connective tissue or adipose proliferation but no substantial evidence of necrosis or regeneration; normal to moderately elevated creatine kinase; normal intellect; and brain imaging that may be either normal or show changes in the white matter on CT or MRI. One form results from deficiency of merosin, an extracellular protein important for maintenance of sarcolemmal membrane stability in the muscle fiber.[186] The loci for merosin-deficient congenital muscular dystrophy have

been linked to chromosome 6q.[41] A further subtype of congenital muscular dystrophy without central nervous system involvement and normal merosin has been reported, but the genetic locus has not been established.

Patients with congenital muscular dystrophy often exhibit early contractures, including equinovarus deformities, knee flexion contractures, hip flexion contractures, and tightness of the wrist flexors and long finger flexors. The contractures can become more severe over time with prolonged static positioning and lack of adequate ROM and splinting or positioning.

Congenital myopathies

The term *congenital myopathy* is used to describe a group of heterogenous disorders, usually presenting with infantile hypotonia, due to genetic defects causing primary myopathies with the absence of any structural abnormality of the central nervous system or peripheral nerves. The specific diagnosis of each entity is made on the basis of specific histologic and electron microscopic changes found on muscle biopsy. While patients can be hypotonic during early infancy, they later develop muscle weakness that is generally non-progressive and static. The weakness is predominantly proximal, symmetric, and in a limb girdle distribution.

The serum creatine kinase values are frequently normal, and the EMG can be normal or show mild, non-specific changes, usually of a myopathic nature (small-amplitude polyphasic potentials). The only congenital myopathy consistently associated with EMG abnormalities is myotubular (centronuclear) myopathy.[49,107] In this disorder, the EMG shows myopathic MUAPs with frequent complex repetitive discharges and diffuse fibrillation potentials. These myopathies can be considered primarily structural in nature. Patients do not actively lose muscle fibers.

Central core myopathy

This is an autosomal dominant disorder with the autosomal dominant gene locus at 19q13.1, the same gene locus as for the malignant hyperthermia gene.[100] Indeed, these patients have a high incidence of malignant hyperthermia with inhalational anesthetic agents. Muscle fiber histology shows amorphous-looking central areas within the muscle that may be devoid of enzyme activity. Electron microscopy shows the virtual absence of mitochondria and sarcoplasmic reticulum in the core region, and a marked reduction in the interfibrillary space and an irregular zigzag pattern (streaming) of the Z lines.[145] There is a predominance of high oxidative, low glycolytic type 1 fibers, and a relative paucity of type 2 fibers, resulting in a relative deficiency of glycolytic enzymes.

Patients generally demonstrate mild and relatively non-progressive muscle weakness, either proximal or generalized, presenting in either early infancy or later. Mild facial weakness can be seen. Patients often achieve gross motor milestones such as walking rather late, and they continue having difficulty going upstairs. They may show a Gower's sign. The disorder typically remains fairly static over the years. A frequent occurrence of congenital dislocation of the hip is observed.

Central core myopathy and familial malignant hyperthermia appear to be allelic, as the ryanodine receptor chain implicated in malignant hyperthermia has the same locus.[41,145]

Nemaline myopathy

Nemaline myopathy, also referred to as rod body myopathy, represents a varied group of disorders with different modes of inheritance, but the most typical form is autosomal recessive. While the rods can be easily overlooked on routine hematoxylin and eosin staining, they can be readily demonstrated with the Gomori trichrome stain. The rods are readily demonstrated on electron microscopy. They are thought to be abnormal depositions of Z-band material of a protein nature, and possibly alpha actinin.[108]

A severe form of the disease can present in the neonatal period with very severe weakness, respiratory insufficiency, and often a fatal outcome. Most cases present with a mild, non-progressive myopathy with hypotonia and proximal weakness. In more severe cases, swallowing difficulty can be present in the neonatal period. Skeletal abnormalities such as kyphoscoliosis, pigeon chest, pes cavus feet, high-arched palate, and an unusually long face have been noted. Cardiomyopathy has been described in both severe neonatal and milder forms of the disease.

Autosomal dominant inheritance has been described in a few instances, with the gene localized to chromosome 1, q21–q23.[108] The locus of the more common autosomal recessive forms has not yet been located.

Myotubular myopathy (centronuclear myopathy)

Patients with non-X-linked myotubular myopathy have muscle biopsies showing a striking resemblance to the myotubes of fetal muscle. Patients typically present with early hypotonia, delay in motor milestones, generalized weakness of both proximal and distal musculature, and ptosis with weakness of the external ocular muscles as well as weakness of the axial musculature. Nocturnal hypoventilation has been described.[111] The gene locus has not been identified to date, but most known non-X-linked forms appear to show autosomal dominant inheritance.

Severe X-linked (congenital) myotubular myopathy

Cases with neonatal onset and severe respiratory insufficiency have been identified with an X-linked recessive mode of inheritance. The gene for this disorder has been located to Xq28.[41] Muscle biopsy shows characteristic fetal-appearing myotubes.

Patients present with severe generalized hypotonia, associated muscle weakness, swallowing difficulty, and respiratory insufficiency. They often become ventilator-dependent at birth. If they are able to be weaned from the ventilator, subsequent death due to pulmonary complications is not uncommon. Aspiration pneumonias are common. Additional clinical features include congenital contractures, facial weakness, and weakness of the external ocular muscles. EMG shows many fibrillations and positive sharp waves.[107]

Mini core disease (multicore disease)

This is a relatively rare congenital myopathy, with muscle biopsies showing multiple small randomly distributed areas in the muscle with focal decrease in mitochondrial oxidative enzyme activity and focal myofibrillar degenerative change. Characteristic changes are present on electron microscopy. There is a predominance of type 1 fiber involvement.[23]

Clinically, patients present with hypotonia, delays in gross motor development, and non-progressive symmetric weakness of the trunk and proximal limb musculature. There may be mild facial weakness, and there is also associated diaphragmatic weakness, placing patients at risk for nocturnal hypoventilation. Subtle ultrastructural changes allow this condition to be distinguished from central core disease. Inheritance is autosomal recessive, but the gene location is not yet known.

Congenital fiber-type disproportion

Congenital fiber-type disproportion represents a heterogenous group of conditions most probably with varied genetic defects. The condition was initially delineated by Brooke on the basis of the muscle biopsy picture, demonstrating type 1 fibers that are smaller than type 2 fibers by a margin of more than 12% of the diameter of the type 2 fibers.[53] Congenital muscular dystrophy, MMD, and severe spinal muscular atrophy all may show small type 1 fibers and should be excluded. The diagnosis of congenital fiber-type disproportion should be made only in the presence of normal-sized or enlarged type 2 fibers, and not in cases where both type 1 and type 2 fibers are small.

Patients typically present with infantile hypotonia and delay in gross motor milestones. The severity has been noted to be quite variable, but it is generally non-progressive. There is generally short stature and low weight. Patients may exhibit a long narrow face, high-arched palate, and deformities of the feet including either flatfeet or occasionally high-arched feet. Kyphoscoliosis has been reported. Lenard and Goebel documented a case with fairly severe weakness and associated respiratory deficit, necessitating tracheostomy.[111] The mode of inheritance for congenital fiber-type disproportion is varied, with both autosomal recessive and autosomal dominant patterns of inheritance reported. Genetic loci have not been identified to date.

REHABILIATION OF MYOPATHIC DISORDERS

Clinical evaluation

A multidisciplinary approach is the best way to deliver effective care for these patients. The Muscular Dystrophy Association sponsors clinics designed specifically to care for patients with muscular dystrophy and other neuromuscular disorders. Once the diagnosis is confirmed, the rehabilitation physician and team can manage clinical problems, and the patient can be enrolled in any ongoing research trials. Enrollment in a clinical trial, if available, should be encouraged and facilitated. It not only furthers science but also provides some hope for the family and ensures frequent follow-up. The clinic team needs staff members in neurology, physiatry, pulmonology, genetics, and therapies, including physical and occupational. Because of the learning disabilities experienced by some of the patients, a neurodevelopmental speech–language pathologist can also be a valuable member of the team.

At initial evaluation, the parents should be thoroughly educated about the expected outcome and what problems might be encountered. The physician should assess the patient or parental goals, and orchestrate a rehabilitative program that matches those goals. The family should be informed of the expected clinical problems that are likely to be encountered over the course of time, including progressive weakness, decreased endurance, limb contractures, spinal deformity, body composition changes, decreased mobility, decreased pulmonary function, and cardiac impairment if the myocardium is affected. Rehabilitation approaches directed at improving impairment and/or resultant disability can substantially improve the quality of life and community integration of these patients.

In childhood muscular dystrophies, parents will often report early walking problems, hypotonia, and delayed developmental milestones. The most frequent presenting symptoms are abnormal gait, frequent falls, and difficulty climbing stairs. Pain in the muscles, especially the calves, is a common symptom. Parents frequently note the toe walking, which is a compensatory adaptation to knee extensor weakness. Difficulty negotiating stairs is an early feature, as is a tendency to fall due to tripping or stumbling on a plantar-flexed ankle. Knee buckling or giving way due to knee extensor weakness also contributes to falling or stumbling. Progressive difficulty in getting up from the floor or a deep-seated position is also noted.

In many muscle diseases, the earliest weakness is seen in the neck flexors, which can be a subtle clinical finding. The weakness ultimately is generalized but typically, early in a myopathic disease course, strength loss is most predominant proximally. Pelvic girdle weakness often pre-dates shoulder girdle weakness by several years. Ankle dorsiflexors are weaker than ankle plantar flexors, ankle everters are weaker than ankle inverters, knee extensors are weaker than knee flexors, hip extensors are weaker than hip flexors, and hip abductors are weaker than hip adductors.

Because of proximal weakness involving the pelvic girdle muscles, patients will exhibit a 'myopathic' gait pattern. The early weakness of the hip extensors produces anterior pelvic tilt and a tendency for the trunk to be positioned anterior to the hip joint. Lumbar lordosis is maintained, which positions the center of gravity or weight line posterior to the hip joints. This stabilizes the hip in extension on the anterior capsule and the ligamentous support of the hip joint. Later, as the weakness of the knee extensors increases, this produces knee instability and knee buckling with falls. To gain more stability during the stance phase, patients compensate by positioning the ankle increasingly into more plantar flexion. This produces a knee extension moment at foot contact and the plantar flexion of the ankle during the mid to late stance phase of gait, and helps position the weight line or center of gravity anterior to the knee joint. This produces a stabilizing knee extension moment. Ultimately, weakness of the hip abductors produces a tendency toward lateral pelvic tilt and pelvic drop of the swing-phase side. Bending or lurching the trunk laterally over the stance-phase hip joint compensates for proximal hip abduction weakness. This produces a waddle or modified Trendelenburg gait. The process can occur over 5 years in DMD, but may take decades in slowly progressive adult myopathies, which show a similar pattern of weakness and changes in physical functioning to those in DMD, yet the loss of function takes place over a much longer time period.

A thorough functional examination is essential in the diagnostic evaluation of any patient with suspected muscular disease. This includes the evaluation of head control, bed or mat mobility, transitions from supine to sit, sit to stand, sitting ability without hand support, standing balance, gait, stair climbing, and overhead reach.

Rehabilitation management

Limb contractures and scoliosis: the role of stretching, bracing, and surgery

Although there is some variability in reported incidence, significant joint contractures and scoliosis develop in a large percentage of patients with DMD.[96,127] Joint contracture and scoliosis can occur but are not usually major clinical problems in the slowly progressive myopathies.[96] However, all patients with muscle disease should have an examination of their spine and major joints at each clinic visit.

The occurrence of contractures appears to be directly related to prolonged static positioning of the limb, and these contractures often develop soon after wheelchair reliance.[127] Several studies have shown that wheelchair use and lack of lower extremity weight bearing contribute to the rapid acceleration of contractures.[127] Upper limb contractures can occur in ambulatory patients with focal, proximal atrophy, particularly at the shoulder girdle. This can be worsened by glenohumeral subluxation. Slings might be helpful in supporting the joint but cannot prevent contracture formation or subluxation. Gentle static stretching and splinting might slow the progression of contractures, but this has not been well studied. Although orthopedic contracture release allows a patient to be braced and might prolong ambulation, it appears that weakness is the major factor that limits ambulation, and not joint contracture per se. In a randomized trial, Manzur and colleagues showed no benefit to early surgical treatment of contractures in DMD.[117] This is discussed further in the next section.

Wheelchair reliance and scoliosis were both found to be age-related phenomena but not necessarily causally linked. Several investigators note no relationship between the age of wheelchair reliance and subsequent progression of scoliosis.[116,123] Lord et al. reported a 3.5-year difference between wheelchair dependency and scoliosis in DMD.[116] The causal relationship between loss of ambulatory status and scoliosis is doubtful, given the substantial time interval between the two variables in most subjects. Further, a significant percentage of DMD patients develop scoliosis before they become wheelchair-dependent.[143] It is more likely that both wheelchair reliance and scoliosis are related to other factors (e.g. age, adolescent growth spurt, increasing weakness of trunk musculature, or other unidentified factors) and are coincidental signs of disease progression.

Upper limb contractures typically do not have a major impact on function if they are mild. Patients with EDMD typically get elbow flexion contractures, but they rarely cause a physical impairment. Joint ROM should be objectively monitored on a regular basis. Severe elbow flexion contractures of >60° are associated with decreased distal upper extremity function and can produce difficulty when dressing.

Passive stretching of the elbow flexors can be combined with passive stretching toward forearm supination to help prevent contractures. Prophylactic occupational therapy management of the wrist and hand is recommended in DMD to slow the development of contractures and to maintain fine motor skills. Daily passive stretching of the wrist flexors and the intrinsic and extrinsic muscles of the hand and wrist are recommended, as are active ROM exercises for the wrist and long finger flexors. Nighttime resting splints that promote wrist extension, metacarpophalangeal extension, and proximal interphalangeal flexion are recommended. Daytime positioning should emphasize wrist and finger extension, but splints should not compromise sensation or function.

Shoulder contractures are less problematic in patients with profound proximal muscle weakness. Combined shoulder internal rotation, adduction contracture, and elbow flexion deformity can interfere with self-feeding. Severe shoulder internal rotation deformities can complicate dressing, produce pain on passive ROM, and cause pain during sleep.

Patients with DMD develop scoliosis most commonly between the ages of 13 and 15 years, corresponding closely with the adolescent growth spurt.[123] While there is evidence on CT for asymmetric involvement of the erector spinae in DMD, it is extremely difficult to clinically detect asymmetric paraspinous muscle strength.[101] Studies on trunk flexor or extensor strength in neuromuscular disease patients with or without scoliosis showed no significant difference in manual muscle testing, although this method is not capable of measuring asymmetric strength.[101] Several studies confirm that primary or single thoracolumbar curves are more common than lumbar curves. Spinal bracing has not been shown to be effective in preventing progression of scoliosis in this population.[84] Any muscle disease patient with scoliosis should be observed closely with serial radiographs. Appropriate and timely spinal instrumentation and fusion should be done before the primary curve becomes greater than 25°. It is also critical that the vital capacity has not gone below 40% of its predicted value, as that can lead to increased surgical complications.[84] Although progressive neuromuscular scoliosis creates significant positioning and musculoskeletal problems, it has not been shown to directly affect pulmonary function.[172] However, complications will increase substantially if the patient already has compromised breathing. If the surgery is done in curves that have progressed much beyond 40°, the likelihood of successful correction and fusion are diminished.[172] Before and after surgery, wheelchairs should always have custom-fitted, fully supportive seating systems that help promote correct spinal positioning.

Bracing to prolong or maintain ambulation

The purpose of bracing at any level is to improve function and stability. The use of long leg bracing prolongs ambulation time and has been advocated in DMD partly on the presumption that this will delay scoliosis.[179,194] Several studies, however, have suggested that the ability to continue ambulation with long leg braces for several years could also be indicative of a slower disease progression rate, with relatively less weakness of trunk musculature present at a given age.[85,195,201,202] Although this is debated, and there is no consensus of expert opinion, any perceived association between prolonged ambulation with long leg bracing and delayed or decreased scoliosis in DMD might not be directly causal. Because of weakness in both proximal (hip and knee extension) and distal (ankle plantar and dorsiflexion) muscle groups in DMD, a long leg brace or knee–ankle–foot orthosis is generally needed if bracing is used.[9,11]

Patients with other muscle diseases might also benefit from bracing, depending on the distribution of weakness, gait problems, and joint instability created by the weakness. The clinician should consider the weight of the brace, and whether or not the patient is actually willing to use a brace. An off the shelf brace, combined with careful assessment by the clinician, can often help determine whether braces are truly indicated. Most patients will require a short course of physical therapy after the braces are made to help them use it effectively. Because of the predominance of distal weakness, some MMD patients with dorsiflexion weakness may benefit from short leg braces or ankle–foot orthoses. These should be custom-made of a lightweight polymer such as polypropylene or carbon fiber resin.[176] They should fit intimately to provide good stability and prevent pressure ulcers. The older, traditional, double-metal upright ankle–foot orthoses built into the shoe can be too heavy and actually hinder ambulation. If there is severe distal muscle weakness and ankle instability, the braces should be high profile, coming around the ankle in front of the malleoli.

Weakness and the role of exercise

Skeletal muscle weakness is the ultimate cause of the majority of clinical problems in this patient population. There have been several well-controlled studies looking at the effect of exercise as a means to gain strength in neuromuscular disorders.[3,103–105,114,167,187,208] Most of this literature unfortunately mixes myopathic and neuropathic subjects together. In slowly progressive neuromuscular disorders, a 12-week moderate resistance (30% of maximum isometric force) exercise program resulted in strength gains ranging from 4% to 20% without any notable deleterious effects.[3] A 12-week home aerobic program also improved endurance.[208] However, in the same population, a 12-week high-resistance exercise program (training at the maximum weight a subject could lift 12 times) showed no further added beneficial effect compared with the moderate-resistance program, and there was evidence of overwork weakness in some of the subjects.[103] In a comparative study, patients having Charcot–Marie–Tooth disease, a hereditary motor and sensory neuropathy, appeared to benefit significantly from a strengthening program, whereas MMD patients showed neither beneficial nor detrimental effects.[114] It is likely that the most effective exercise regimens for neuropathies and myopathies are different, but further studies are needed to confirm this. Because of the active muscle degeneration in the rapidly progressive myopathic disorders such as DMD, the risk for overwork weakness is great, and exercise should be prescribed cautiously, using a common sense approach.

Dystrophin-deficient muscle is very susceptible to exercise-induced muscle injury.[149,152,155,178,182,206] We studied the effects of exercise on skeletal muscle from both normal and mdx mice, a genetically homologous murine model of DMD, using voluntary running protocols.[188,206] In contrast to normal mice, the mdx mice show considerable avoidance behavior for exercise, which might be an innate survival strategy. After exercise on a mouse wheel ad libitum, the extensor digitorum longus and soleus muscles of adult mdx mice became significantly weaker and showed histochemical signs of further damage when compared with control mdx muscles.[206]

All patients with muscle disease should be advised not to exercise to exhaustion, due to the risk of muscle damage and dysfunction. Patients participating in an exercise program should be cautioned of the warning signs of overwork weakness, which include feeling weaker rather than stronger within 30 min post exercise, or excessive muscle soreness 24–48 h following exercise. Other warning signs include severe muscle cramping, heaviness in the extremities, and prolonged shortness of breath.

Early intervention with gentle, low-impact aerobic exercise such as walking, swimming, and stationary bicycling improves cardiovascular performance and increases muscle efficiency, and lessens fatigue. Fatigue in this population is multifactorial, and is due in part to impaired muscular activation, generalized deconditioning, and diminished cardiopulmonary performance caused by immobility.[208] Aerobic exercise not only improves physical functioning, but is beneficial in fighting depression, maintaining ideal body weight, and improving pain tolerance.[208] Based on the available investigations, we believe that there is adequate evidence to generally advocate a submaximal strengthening program for persons with slowly progressive neuromuscular disorders. There seems to be no additional benefit to high-resistance, low-repetition training sets, and the risk of actually increasing weakness becomes greater. It is hoped that improvement in strength translates to more functional issues such as improved endurance and mobility.

Exercise can induce muscle cramping, presumably due to sarcolemmal instability.[73] Membrane-stabilizing agents such as mexiletine or phenytoin might be helpful, particularly in the myotonic disorders, although this is off-label use, and these drugs are not approved by the US Food and Drug Administration (FDA) for this indication. Slow (30 s sustained), static muscle stretching is also helpful. The benzodiazepines and other centrally acting muscle relaxants can be used for cramping but induce somnolence and respiratory suppression. Dantrolene, by impairing excitation–contraction coupling, is effective at reducing muscle cramps, but will induce more weakness and should not be used in the muscle disease population.

Restrictive lung disease

Restrictive lung disease is actually a misnomer in this patient population, because the lung tissue itself is normal. The problems stems from weakness of the diaphragm, chest wall, and abdominal musculature. Restrictive lung disease can become quite severe in DMD, MMD, and some of the congenital myopathies. Patients should be educated early in the disease process so that informed decisions can be made further down the line. Pulmonary function tests should be done routinely, at least once a year in slowly progressive diseases and as clinically indicated in more severe myopathies. The FVC is the most useful single laboratory value to follow, although the peak cough flow and the maximal inspiratory and expiratory pressures may also be helpful. The peak cough flow and maximal expiratory pressure reflect chest wall and abdominal muscle strength and the ability to cough and clear secretions. The maximal inspiratory pressure reflects diaphragmatic strength and the ability to ventilate.

Most patients with severe restrictive lung disease eventually develop hypoventilation, which leads to elevated CO_2 levels.[15,56] Measuring only O_2 saturation levels with pulse oximetry can be inadequate. End tidal CO_2 levels or arterial blood gases should be measured periodically, depending on the clinical condition of the patient. A thorough review of systems can help define any problems. Hypoventilating patients will often become hypercapnic at night and complain of a morning headache, restlessness or nightmares, and poor-quality sleep. This is because hypoventilation is prominent first in the supine position. This can cause daytime somnolence. Insufficient respiration with hypoxia may occur later, especially if the lung is damaged by chronic aspiration.

Options for non-invasive interventions include a chest cuirass or portalung, which mechanically inflates the lung by creating negative chest wall pressure, similar to the iron lungs used commonly during the polio outbreaks. Although effective, these devices are cumbersome and are often poorly tolerated.[46] Tracheostomies can be associated with significant morbidity, and should be avoided if at all possible.[10,12] Intermittent positive pressure ventilation by mouth avoids the need for tracheostomy and maintains reasonable quality of life.[1,8] Bimodal positive airway pressure is the best initial form. This can be done in the home, and should be considered the preferred modality of assisted ventilation in this population.[8,15] It generally takes some work with a respiratory therapist to get a good face or lip seal on the mask or nasal–oral orthotic interface. Patients may benefit initially from using assisted ventilation mainly at night. This is covered in more detail in Chapter 35.

Cardiac complications

As noted earlier, significant cardiac involvement occurs in DMD, BMD, MMD, EDMD, and some cases of the SCARMD subtype of LGMD. The evidence for significant myocardial involvement in these diseases is sufficient to warrant screening of all these patients at regular intervals using ECG and echocardiography. The myocardial impairment can remain clinically silent until late in the course of the disease, possibly due to the absence of exertional dyspnea secondary to lack of physical activity. It is important to note that manifesting DMD carriers (carriers who exhibit some signs of muscle disease) can manifest cardiac disease as well.[123]

Close follow-up will be needed for all patients with myocardial involvement. The slowly progressive nature of this dystrophic myopathy, which is compatible with many years of functional mobility and longevity, makes some of these patients suitable candidates for cardiac transplantation if end-stage cardiac failure occurs. Successful cardiac transplantation has been increasingly reported in BMD subjects with cardiac failure who are otherwise still quite physically functional.[152]

Medical management of cardiomyopathy in this setting includes after-load reduction with angiotensin-converting enzyme inhibitors, along with positive ionotropic agents such as digoxin. If significant tachyarrhythmia is present, then beta-blockers may be indicated.[113] All muscle disease patients with significant cardiac involvement should be referred to a cardiologist skilled in this area for treatment.

Nutritional management

As mobility decreases, there is an increasing tendency toward obesity, especially in the more severe myopathies. This typically occurs shortly after losing independent ambulation. An obesity prevalence of 54% has been reported in DMD.[121,144] However, in prior studies, obesity was unrelated to strength decline, age of wheelchair reliance, functional grade status, timed motor performance, pulmonary function, likelihood of ECG abnormalities, or age at death.[123] Weight control has its primary rationale in facilitating ease of care, especially ease of transfers and skin care. A recent case series shows some potential use of topiramate as a weight reduction agent in DMD.[39]

Malnutrition can be a significant problem in the advanced stages of a severe myopathy such as DMD. Nutritional compromise is particularly problematic if there is severe respiratory compromise with increased work of breathing, which can also influence caloric intake.[144,204] Self-feeding often becomes impossible during this period. Patients with DMD can develop signs and symptoms of upper gastrointestinal dysfunction, making feeding more difficult.[92,205] Nutritional counseling with energy intake and energy allowance estimations should be done for all patients with severe (FVC < 50% of predicted) restrictive lung disease. Placement of a percutaneous endoscopic gastrostomy tube can facilitate nutrition even if the patient can swallow, because it allows for rapid and easy delivery of large amounts of calories and fluids. Patients should be reassured that they will still be able to eat food orally for enjoyment.

Chronic pain: psychosocial and vocational considerations

Chronic pain appears to substantially impair function in this population.[93,94] It would appear that pain, depression, and other indicators of altered personality profiles can substantially impact social integration and employment rates, and might be as important as physical abilities with respect to this. A large percentage of these patients exhibited elevated scores for bodily pain and depression on standardized testing, including the 36-Item Short-Form Health Survey, Brief Pain Inventory, and Minnesota Multiphasic Personality Inventory test.[93,95,122,123] Thus these factors should be assessed and treated.

Except for DMD, MMD, and some of the congenital and mitochondrial myopathies, the majority of people with muscle disease show intellectual levels within the normal range.[95,122,123] However, employment rates for this population are substantially lower than for the able-bodied.[95,122,123] Indicators of emotional pathology appeared to be associated with unemployment, whereas loss of ambulation and arm function was not.[95] Higher levels of education correlated with higher employment rates and improved self-esteem in this group.[95] Level of education appears to be very important with respect to employability and self-esteem, and should be emphasized.

Reactive clinical depression can occur in advanced disease. Family, social, and religious support systems are helpful in the prevention and treatment of depression. Antidepressant medicine can provide assistance with mood elevation, appetite stimulation, and sleep. Referral to a psychiatrist or clinical psychologist is required in some cases. Depression in the spouse or significant other, family, or friends should not be overlooked, and group or family counseling can be helpful. Patients should be referred to a support group. Support groups are often a great resource, not only for psychologic support but also for problem solving and recycling of durable medical equipment.

Equipment

There are a number of additional useful equipment items that can substantially improve quality of life, including handheld showers, bath tub benches, grab bars, raised toilet seat, hospital beds, commode chairs, activities of daily living aids (sock aid, grabbers, etc.), and wheelchair ramps (see Ch. 27). At some time point as the disease progresses, the extent of muscle weakness or the energy requirements for ambulation will necessitate that a patient use a wheelchair for mobility. In the milder cases of myopathy, a manual wheelchair, preferably lightweight or ultralightweight, can be used for traveling long distances to conserve energy. As the disease progresses, a power wheelchair system tailored to the patient's current and potential future needs should be prescribed. If the patient has too much upper extremity weakness to propel a manual wheelchair, a small, removable electric motor ('power pack') can be attached directly to the rear wheels. The advantage of this system is that a specialized transportation system is not required. This can be disassembled and the wheelchair folded to fit inside the trunk of a car or the back of a van. Power wheelchairs are much less portable, having large powered rear wheels and front casters. In a power wheelchair, the motor or drive train section is independent of the seating system and its attendant components. A power wheelchair can be rear-wheel drive, midwheel drive, and even four-wheel drive in some of the newer models.

Power scooters are an alternative to a power wheelchair, and might be suitable for the myopathy patient who has adequate upper extremity and trunk strength. However, scooters cannot be fitted with more extensive and supportive seating systems.

Therefore, if the patient requires significant trunk support, then a power wheelchair would be more appropriate. Scooters are also much longer and have a greater turning radius than a power wheelchair, and this can be limiting in terms of use in tight spaces. It is important to note that most insurance companies will not pay for a power wheelchair if the patient has already been reimbursed for a scooter or manual wheelchair, because these are all considered locomotion mobility devices. Power wheelchairs can cost upward of $20 000, while scooters typically cost under $5000 and manual wheelchairs even less. Therefore, the patient may be best purchasing the manual wheelchair and scooter, and saving their insurance benefit for the power wheelchair if it is anticipated that they will need one in the near future. The Muscular Dystrophy Association does cover part of the cost of any wheelchair, and that can be a good financial resource for the myopathy patient.

A power wheelchair should have a high back and adequate head and neck support to support weakened trunk muscles, as well as a reclining (tilt in space) seat that allows the patient the capability of doing independent postural changes for comfort and pressure relief.[115] In addition to adequate trunk and spine support, the wheelchair should also have a good cushion to avoid pressure ulcers.[26,27] Because of the remarkable expense, along with potential reimbursement restrictions, the patient should be carefully evaluated by the entire rehabilitation team, preferably in a specialized mobility and seating clinic, in order to determine the exact type of power wheelchair system that is going to be recommended. This is covered in further detail in Chapter 18. A pressure-relieving mattress (air or dense foam) should be used on the bed at home, along with foam wedges to facilitate proper positioning. This helps prevent pressure ulcers and contractures. Wheeled walkers, quad (four-point) canes, and Lofstrand crutches can also help by providing a broader base of support. However, patients must have the upper extremity strength to appropriately use a cane or walker. These devices should be used on a trial basis first, under supervision, before they are prescribed. Frequently, severe weakness in the neck flexors and extensors results in a 'floppy head', associated with severe neck pain and tightness. This might be helped by a hard cervical (Philadelphia-type) or Freeman collar.

Future areas of research

Major advances in the understanding of the molecular basis of many myopathies have greatly enhanced diagnostic accuracy, and can provide the basis for therapeutic intervention. There has been significant improvement in the functional imaging of muscle, particularly in the field of MRI. This may someday help facilitate earlier and more physiologically accurate diagnosis of myopathy.[124] There are various myotrophic growth factors currently in development that might enhance muscle repair and growth.

Major pharmacologic advances have occurred over the past decade. Although a comprehensive discussion of clinical trials is beyond the scope of this chapter, some of the major advances

will be noted. Because DMD is the most common severe myopathy, it has received a fair degree of study. Although not FDA-approved for this use, prednisone, at 1 mg/kg per day, given to boys with DMD aged 4–8 years, has been shown to prolong the time of ambulation and at least should be considered for use in this disease.[5,37,68–71,80] Major side effects of prednisone include weight gain, osteoporosis, and mood lability. Deflazacort has similar beneficial effects and may have slightly less side effects than prednisone has; however, it is not currently available in the USA. There have also been several recent randomized, crossover, double-blind, placebo-controlled pilot studies of extended-release albuterol in patients with dystrophinopathies (DMD and BMD) and FSHMD.[72,161] Outcomes were isometric knee extensor and flexor strength, and manual muscle testing. There was some small evidence of benefit in the dystrophinopathies but not in FSHMD. Therefore, 12-week treatment with extended-release albuterol may increase strength in patients with dystrophinopathies, but clearly larger, double-blind, randomized studies are necessary to confirm these results. There is also some literature showing a modest positive benefit of the protein creatine monohydrate in DMD for transient improvement of strength.[183] Further study is warranted before conclusive recommendations can be made.

Stem cell therapy holds some promise for replacing diseased muscle. However, it is important for the clinician and patient to realize that these diseases would not be cured by stem cell treatment, as this would not correct the underlying genetic defect. Despite this, it may be possible to significantly improve function by growing new muscle tissue through stem cell therapy. Further, it may be possible to treat these diseases with genetically modified (corrected) stem cells, which would not only improve function but partially correct the genetic abnormality.

Increased understanding of the molecular basis of many muscle diseases has greatly enhanced diagnostic accuracy and the ability to do prenatal diagnostic screening. This has also provided the groundwork for therapeutic intervention. Techniques are being developed for gene insertion and DNA repair using a number of vectors, including gutted viruses. This could ultimately lead to a true cure.

Important advances in the use of reliable functional assessment tools have made it easier to judge the effectiveness of experimental interventions. The Timed Motor Performance assessment developed by Brooke et al. is a good example of a simple measurement scale that can be used at routine clinic visits.[21,22]

Major advances have been made in the fields of biomedical engineering and computer science, providing patients with myopathy with refined, more functional equipment and allowing better strategies for improvement of quality of life.[1,73] As progress continues to change our management, it also changes patients' expectations. For example, now many patients with DMD are living well into adulthood, going to college, and starting careers. A comprehensive approach to the treatment of these patients can help them enjoy an enhanced quality of life.

REFERENCES

1. Abresch RT, Carter GT, Jensen MP, et al. Assessment of pain and health-related quality of life in slowly progressive neuromuscular disease. Am J Hosp Palliat Care 2002; 19(1):39–48.

2. Aitkens S, Lord J, Bernauer E, et al. Relationship of manual muscle testing to objective strength measurements. Muscle Nerve 1989; 12(3):173–177.

3. Aitkens SG, McCrory MA, Kilmer DD, et al. Moderate resistance exercise program: its effect in slowly progressive neuromuscular disease. Arch Phys Med Rehabil 1993; 74(7):711–715.

4. Akita H, Matsuoka S, Juroda Y. Predictive electrocardiographic score for evaluating prognosis in patients with Duchenne muscular dystrophy. Tokushima J Exp Med 1995; 40:55–67.

5. Alman BA, Raza SN, Biggar WD. Steroid treatment and the development of scoliosis in males with Duchenne muscular dystrophy. J Bone Joint Surg Am 2004; 86(3):519–524.

6. Arahata K, Beggs AH, Honda H, et al. Preservation of the c-terminus of dystrophin molecule in the skeletal muscle from Becker muscular dystrophy. J Neurol Sci 1992; 101:1488–1494.

7. Ashizawa T, Dubel JR, Dunne PW, et al. Anticipation in myotonic dystrophy: II. Complex relationships between clinical findings and structure of the GCT repeat. Neurology 1992; 42:1877–1881.

8. Bach JR, Campagnolo DI, Hoeman S. Life satisfaction of individuals with Duchenne muscular dystrophy using long-term mechanical ventilatory support. Am J Phys Med Rehabil 1991; 70:129–135.

9. Bach JR, McKeon J. Orthopedic surgery and rehabilitation for the prolongation of brace-free ambulation of patients with Duchenne muscular dystrophy. Am J Phys Med Rehabil 1991; 70(6):323–331.

10. Bach JR. Pulmonary rehabilitation: the obstructive and paralytic conditions. Philadelphia: Hanley & Belfus; 1995:303–310.

11. Bakker JP, De Groot IJ, Beelen A, et al. Predictive factors of cessation of ambulation in patients with Duchenne muscular dystrophy. Am J Phys Med Rehabil 2002; 81(12):906–912.

12. Baydur A, Kanel G. Tracheobronchomalacia and tracheal hemorrhage in patients with Duchenne muscular dystrophy receiving long-term ventilation with uncuffed tracheostomies. Chest 2003; 123(4):1307–1311.

13. Becker PE, Kiener G. Eine Neue X-Chromosomale Muskeldystrophie. Arch Psychiatr Z Neurol 1955; 193:427–430.

14. Becker PE. Two new families of benign sex-linked recessive muscular dystrophy. Rev Can Biol 1962; 21:551–555.

15. Benditt JO. Management of pulmonary complications in neuromuscular disease. Phys Med Rehabil Clin North Am 1998; 9(1):167–185.

16. Benson ES, Jaffe ES, Tarr PI. Acute gastric dilatation in Duchenne muscular dystrophy: a case report and review of the literature. Arch Phys Med Rehabil 1996; 77:512–519.

17. Bione S, Maestrini, E, Rivella S, et al. Identification of a novel x-linked gene responsible for Emery–Dreifuss muscular dystrophy. Nat Genet 1994; 8:323–331.

18. Bonsett CA. Pseudohypertrophic muscular dystrophy: distribution of degenerative features as revealed by anatomical study. Neurology 1963; 13:728–737.

19. Bradley WG, Jones MZ, Mussini JM, et al. Becker-type muscular dystrophy. Muscle Nerve 1978; 1:111–116.

20. Braun NMT, Aurora NS, Rochester DF. Respiratory muscle and pulmonary function in poliomyositis and other proximal myopathies. Thorax 1983; 38:316–321.

21. Brooke MH, Fenichel GM, Griggs RC, et al. Clinical investigation in Duchenne dystrophy. II. Determination of the 'power' of therapeutic trials based on the natural history. Muscle Nerve 1983; 6:91–98.

22. Brooke MH, Fenichel GM, Griggs RC, et al. Duchenne muscular dystrophy: patterns of clinical progression and effects of supportive therapy. Neurology 1989; 39:745–758.

23. Brooke MH. A neuromuscular disease characterized by fibre type disproportion. In: Kakulas BA, ed. Clinical studies in myology. Proceedings of the Second International Congress on Muscle Diseases, Perth, Australia, 1971. Part II. Amsterdam: Excerpta Medica; 1973:295–315.

24. Bushby KMD, Gardner-Medwin D, Nicholson LVB, et al. The clinical, genetic and dystrophin characteristics of Becker muscular dystrophy: II. Correlation of phenotype with genetic and protein abnormalities. J Neurol 1993; 240:105–112.

25. Bushby KMD, Thambyayah M, Gardner-Medwin D. Prevalence and incidence of Becker muscular dystrophy. Lancet 1991; 337:1022–1029.

26. Butler C, Okamoto G, McKay T. Motorized wheelchair driving by disabled children. Arch Phys Med Rehabil 1984; 65:95–103.

27. Butler C, Okamoto G, McKay T. Powered mobility for very young disabled children. Dev Med Child Neurol 1983; 25:472–480.

28. Campbell KP, Kahl SD. Association of dystrophin and an integral membrane glycoprotein. Nature 1989; 338:259–262.

29. Campbell KP. Three muscular dystrophies: loss of cytoskeleton–extracellular matrix linkage. Cell 1995; 80:675–677.

30. Carter GT, Abresch RT, Fowler WM. Adaptations to exercise training and contraction-induced muscle injury in animal models of neuromuscular disease. Am J Phys Med Rehabil 2002; 81(suppl):151–161.

31. Carter GT, Abresch RT, Walsh SA, et al. The mdx mouse diaphragm: exercise-induced injury. Muscle Nerve 1997; 20:393–394.

32. Carter GT, Bird TD. Facioscapulohumeral muscular dystrophy presenting as respiratory failure. Neurology 2005; 64(2):401–402.

33. Carter GT, Kikuchi N, Abresch RT, et al. Effects of exhaustive concentric and eccentric exercise on murine skeletal muscle. Arch Phys Med Rehabil 1994; 75(5):555–559.

34. Carter GT, Kikuchi N, Horasek S, et al. The use of fluorescent dextrans as a marker of sarcolemmal injury. Histol Histopathol 1994; 9(3):443–447.

35. Carter GT, Longley KJ, Entrikin RK. Electromyographic and nerve conduction studies in the mdx mouse. Am J Phys Med Rehabil 1992; 71(1):2–5.

36. Carter GT, Longley KJ, Walsh SA, et al. Lack of effect of amitriptyline in murine myotonia. Am J Phys Med Rehabil 1992; 71(5):279–282.

37. Carter GT, McDonald CM. Preservation of function in Duchenne dystrophy with long-term pulse prednisone therapy. Am J Phys Med Rehabil 2000; 79(5):455–458.

38. Carter GT, Wineinger MA, Walsh SA, et al. Effect of voluntary wheel-running exercise on muscles of the mdx mouse. Neuromuscul Disord 1995; 5(4):323–331.

39. Carter GT, Yudkowsky MP, Han JJ, et al. Topiramate for weight reduction in Duchenne muscular dystrophy. Muscle Nerve 2004; 31(6):788–789.

40. Casazzo F, Banbilla SG, Salvato A, et al. Cardiac transplantation in Becker muscular dystrophy. J Neurol 1988; 235:496–499.

41. Chance P, Ashizawa T, Hoffman E, et al. Molecular basis of neuromuscular disease. Phys Med Rehabil Clin North Am 1998; 9:49–82.

42. Chenard AA, Becane HM, Tertrain F, et al. Systolic time intervals in Duchenne muscular dystrophy: evaluation of left ventricular performance. Clin Cardiol 1998; 11:407–412.

43. Coleman RA, Stajich JM, Pact VW, et al. The ischemic exercise test in normal adults and in patients with weakness and cramps. Muscle Nerve 1986; 9:216–221.

44. Comi GP, Prelle A, Bresolin N, et al. Clinical variability in Becker muscular dystrophy. Genetic, biochemical and immunohistochemical correlates. Brain 1994; 117:1–10.

45. Cross D, Harnden P, Pellsier JF, et al. Muscle hypertrophy in Duchenne muscular dystrophy. A pathological and morphometric study. J Neurol 1989; 236:43–49.

46. Curran FJ. Night ventilation by body respirators for patients in chronic respiratory failure due to late stage Duchenne muscular dystrophy. Arch Phys Med Rehabil 1981; 62:270–276.

47. De Lateur BJ, Giaconi RM. Effect on maximal strength of submaximal exercise in Duchenne muscular dystrophy. Am J Phys Med 1979; 58:26–35.

48. Di Mario JX, Uzman A, Strohman RC. Fiber regeneration is not persistent in dystrophic (mdx) mouse skeletal muscle. Dev Biol 1991; 148:314–321.

49. Dillingham TR. Electrodiagnostic approach to patients with suspected generalized neuromuscular disorders. Phys Med Rehabil Clin North Am 2001; 12(2):253–277.

50. Donofrio D, Challa V, Hackshaw B, et al. Cardiac transplantation in a patient with Becker muscular dystrophy and cardiomyopathy. Arch Neurol 1980; 46:705–712.

51. Dorman C, Hurley AD, D'Avignon J. Language and learning disorders of older boys with Duchenne muscular dystrophy. Dev Med Child Neurol 1988; 30:316–321.

52. Dorsher PT, Sinaki M, Muller DW, et al. Wohlfart–Kugelberg–Welander syndrome: serum creatine kinase and functional outcome. Arch Phys Med Rehabil 1991; 72:587–595.

53. Dubowitz V. Muscle disorders in childhood. 2nd edn. London: Saunders; 1995:14–62.

54. Duggan DJ, Fanin M, Pegoraro E, et al. Alpha-sarcoglycan (adhalin) deficiency: complete deficiency patients are 5% of childhood-onset dystrophin-normal muscular dystrophy and most partial deficiency patients do not have gene mutations. J Neurol Sci 1996; 140:30–41.

55. Duggan DJ, Hoffman EP. Autosomal recessive muscular dystrophy and mutations of the sarcoglycan complex. Neuromuscul Disord 1996; 6:475–481.

56. Eagle M, Badouin SV, Chandler C, et al. Survival in Duchenne muscular dystrophy: improvement in life expectancy since 1967 and the impact of home nocturnal ventilation. Neuromuscul Disord 2002; 12(10): 26–929.

57. Eagle M. Report on the Muscular Dystrophy Campaign Workshop: Exercise in Neuromuscular Diseases, Newcastle, January 2002. Neuromuscul Disord 2002; 12(10):975–983.

58. Edwards RT, Jones DA, Newham DJ, et al. Role of mechanical damage in pathogenesis of proximal myopathy in man. Lancet 1984; 8376:548–556.

59. Edwards RT, Round JM, Jackson MJ, et al. Weight reduction in boys with muscular dystrophy. Dev Med Child Neurol 1984; 26:384–392.

60. Eiholzer U, Boltshauser E, Frey D, et al. Short stature: a common feature in Duchenne muscular dystrophy. Eur J Pediatr 1988; 147:602–609.

61. Emery AH, Dreifuss FE. Unusual type of benign x-linked muscular dystrophy. J Neurol Neurosurg Psychol 1966; 29:338–345.

62. Emery AH, Skinner R. Clinical studies in benign (Becker type) x-linked muscular dystrophy. Clin Genet 1976; 10:189–195.

63. Emery AH. Emery–Dreifuss muscular dystrophy and other related disorders. Br Med Bull 1989; 45:772–780.

64. Emery AH. Population frequencies of inherited neuromuscular diseases. A world survey. Neuromuscul Disord 1991; 1:19–25.

65. Engel WK, Foster JM, Hughes BP, et al. Central core disease—an investigation of a rare muscle cell abnormality. Brain 1961; 84:167–175.

66. Ervasti JM, Ohlendieck K, Kahl SD, et al. Deficiency of a glycoprotein component of the dystrophin complex in dystrophic muscle. Nature 1990; 345:315–321.

67. Eyring EJ, Johnson EW, Burnett C. Surgery in muscular dystrophy. JAMA 1972; 222:1067–1075.

68. Fenichel G, Pestronk A, Florence J, et al. A beneficial effect of oxandrolone in the treatment of Duchenne muscular dystrophy: a pilot study. Neurology 1997; 48(5):1225–1234.

69. Fenichel GM, Florence JM, Pestronk A, et al. Long-term benefit from prednisone therapy in Duchenne muscular dystrophy. Neurology 1991; 41:1874–1881.

70. Fenichel GM, Mendell JR, Moxley RT, et al. A comparison of daily and alternate-day prednisone therapy in the treatment of Duchenne muscular dystrophy. Arch Neurol 1991; 48:575–582.

71. Fong P, Turner PR, Denetclaw WF, et al. Increased activity of calcium leak channels in myotubes of Duchenne human and mdx mouse origin. Science 1990; 250:673–676.

72. Fowler EG, Graves MC, Wetzel GT, et al. Pilot trial of albuterol in Duchenne and Becker muscular dystrophy. Neurology 2004; 62(6):1006–1008.

73. Fowler WM, Carter GT, Kraft GH. Role of physiatry in the management of neuromuscular disease. Phys Med Rehabil Clin North Am 1998; 9(1):1–8.

74. Franco A, Lansman JB. Mechanosensitive ion channels in skeletal muscle from normal and dystrophic mice. J Physiol 1994; 481:299–309.

75. Friedrich O, Both M, Gillis JM, et al. Mini-dystrophin restores L-type calcium currents in skeletal muscle of transgenic mdx mice. J Physiol 2004; 15(555):251–265.

76. Fukuyama Y, Kawazura M, Haruna H. A peculiar form of congenital progressive muscular dystrophy. Report of 15 cases. Pediatria Universitatis Tokyo 1960; 4:5–12.

77. Gilroy J, Cahalan J, Berman R, et al. Cardiac and pulmonary complications in Duchenne progressive muscular dystrophy. Circulation 1963; 27:484–491.

78. Goldstein M, Meyer S, Freund HR. Effects of overfeeding children with muscular dystrophies. J Parenter Enteral Nutr 1989; 13:603–609.

79. Gospe SM, Lozaro RP, Lava NS, et al. Familial x-linked myalgia and cramps: a non-progressive myopathy associated with a deletion in the dystrophin gene. Neurology 1989; 39:1277–1281.

80. Griggs RC, Moxley RT, Mendell JR, et al. Duchenne dystrophy: randomized, controlled trial of prednisone (18 months) and azathioprine (12 months). Neurology 1993; 43:520–534.

81. Hahn A, Bach JR, Delaubier A, et al. Clinical implications of maximal respiratory pressure determinations for individuals with Duchenne muscular dystrophy. Arch Phys Med Rehabil 1997; 78:1–12.

82. Harley H, Rundle SA, MacMillan JC, et al. Size of the unstable CTG repeat sequence in relation to phenotype and parental transmission in myotonic dystrophy. Am J Hum Genet 1993; 52:1164–1171.

83. Harley HG, Brook JD, Rundle SA, et al. Expansion of an unstable DNA region and phenotypic variation in myotonic dystrophy. Nature 1992; 355:545–551.

84. Hart DA, McDonald CM. Spinal deformity in progressive neuromuscular disease: natural history and management. Phys Med Rehabil Clin North Am 1998; 9:213–225.

85. Heckmatt JZ, Dubowitz V, Hyde SA, et al. Prolongation of walking in Duchenne muscular dystrophy with lightweight orthoses: review of 57 cases. Dev Med Child Neurol 1985; 27:149–157.

86. Hocherman SD, Bezanilla F. A patch-clamp study of delayed rectifier currents in skeletal muscle of control and mdx mice. J Physiol 1996; 493:113–128.

87. Hoffman EP, Brown RH Jr, Kunkel LM. Dystrophin: the protein product of the Duchenne muscular dystrophy locus. Cell 1987; 51:919–928.

88. Hoffman EP, Fischbeck KH, Brown RH, et al. Dystrophin characterization in muscle biopsies from Duchenne and Becker muscular dystrophy patients. N Engl J Med 1988; 318:1363–1376.

89. Houzelstein D, Lyons GE, Chamberlain J, et al. Localization of dystrophin gene transcripts during mouse embryogenesis. J Cell Biol 1992; 119:811–826.

90. Hunter A, Tsilfidis C, Mettler G, et al. The correlation of age of onset with CTG trinucleotide repeat amplification in myotonic dystrophy. J Med Genet 1992; 29:774–781.

91. Iannaccone ST, Owens H, Scott J, et al. Postoperative malnutrition in Duchenne muscular dystrophy. J Child Neurol 2003; 18(1):17–20.

92. Jaffe KM, McDonald CM, Ingman E, et al. Symptoms of upper gastrointestinal dysfunction: case-control study. Arch Phys Med Rehabil 1990; 71:742–744.

93. Jensen MP, Abresch RT, Carter GT, et al. Chronic pain in persons with neuromuscular disease. Arch Phys Med Rehabil 2005; 86(6):1155–1163.

94. Jensen MP, Abresch RT, Carter GT. The reliability and validity of a self-reported version of the functional independence measure in persons with neuromuscular disease and chronic pain. Arch Phys Med Rehabil 2005; 86(1):116–122.

95. Johnson ER, Abresch RT, Carter GT, et al. Profiles of neuromuscular diseases: myotonic dystrophy. Am J Phys Med Rehabil 1995; 74: S104–S117.

96. Johnson ER, Fowler WM Jr, Lieberman JS. Contractures in neuromuscular disease. Arch Phys Med Rehabil 1992; 73:807–815.

97. Johnson EW, Braddom R. Overwork weakness in facioscapulohumeral muscular dystrophy. Arch Phys Med Rehabil 1971; 52:333–339.

98. Johnson EW, Yarnell S. Hand dominance and scoliosis in Duchenne muscular dystrophy. Arch Phys Med Rehabil 1976; 57:462–471.

99. Katlyer BC, Misra S, Somani PN, et al. Congestive cardiomyopathy in a family of Becker x-linked muscular dystrophy. Postgrad Med J 1977; 53:12–18.

100. Kausch K, Lehmann-Horn F, Janka M, et al. Evidence for linkage of the central core disease locus to the proximal long arm of human chromosome 19. Genomics 1991; 10:765–777.

101. Kilmer DD, Abresch RT, Fowler WM Jr. Serial manual muscle testing in Duchenne muscular dystrophy. Arch Phys Med Rehabil 1993; 74:1168–1175.

102. Kilmer DD, Abresch RT, McCrory MA, et al. Profiles of neuromuscular diseases: facioscapulohumeral muscular dystrophy. Am J Phys Med Rehabil 1995; 74:S131–S145.

103. Kilmer DD, McCrory MA, Wright NC, et al. The effect of a high resistance exercise program in slowly progressive neuromuscular disease. Arch Phys Med Rehabil 1994; 75(5):560-563.

104. Kilmer DD. Response to aerobic exercise training in humans with neuromuscular disease. Am J Phys Med Rehabil 2002; 81:S148–S150.

105. Kilmer DD. Response to resistive strengthening exercise training in humans with neuromuscular disease. Am J Phys Med Rehabil 2002; 81: S121–S126.

106. Koenig M, Hoffmann EP, Bertelson CK, et al. Complete cloning of the Duchenne muscular dystrophy (DMD) cDNA and preliminary genomic organization of the DMD gene in mouse and affected individuals. Cell 1987; 50:509–516.

107. Krivickas LS. Electrodiagnosis in neuromuscular disease. Phys Med Rehabil Clin North Am 1998; 9(1):83–115.

108. Laing N, Majda B, Akkari P, et al. Assignment of a gene (NEM1) for autosomal dominant nemaline myopathy to chromosome 1. Am J Hum Genet 1992; 50:576–581.

109. Lazzeroni E, Favaro L, Botti G. Dilated cardiomyopathy with regional myocardial hypoperfusion in Becker muscular dystrophy. Int J Cardiol 1989; 22:126–131.

110. Lehmann-Horn F, Iaizzo P, Franke C, et al. Schwartz–Jampel syndrome: II. Na^+ channel defect causes myotonia. Muscle Nerve 1990; 13:528–537.

111. Lenard HG, Goebel HH. Congenital fibre type disproportion. Neuropaediatrie 1975; 6:220–225.

112. Leth A, Wulff K. Myocardiopathy in Duchenne progressive muscular dystrophy. Acta Paediatr Scand 1976; 65:28–33.

113. Lewis W, Sanjay Y. Management of cardiac complications in neuromuscular disease. Phys Med Rehabil Clin North Am 1998; 9:145–157.

114. Lindeman E, Leffers P, Spaans F, et al. Strength training in patients with myotonic dystrophy and hereditary motor and sensory neuropathy: a randomized clinical trial. Arch Phys Med Rehabil 1995; 76(7):612–620.

115. Liu M, Mineo K, Hanayama K, et al. Practical problems and management of seating through the clinical stages of Duchenne muscular dystrophy. Arch Phys Med Rehabil 2003; 84(6):818–824.

116. Lord J, Behrman B, Varzos N, et al. Scoliosis associated with Duchenne muscular dystrophy. Arch Phys Med Rehabil 1990; 71:13–27.

117. Manzur AY, Hyde SA, Rodillo E, et al. A randomized controlled trial of early surgery in Duchenne muscular dystrophy. Neuromuscul Disord 1992; 2:379–387.

118. Marsh GG, Munsat TL. Evidence of early impairment of verbal intelligence in Duchenne muscular dystrophy. Arch Dis Child 1974; 49:118–139.

119. Mathieu J, Boivin H, Richards CL. Quantitative motor assessment in myotonic dystrophy. Can J Neurol Sci 2003; 30(2):129–136.

120. Matsumura K, Tome FMS, Collin H, et al. Deficiency of the 50K dystrophin-associated glycoprotein in severe childhood autosomal recessive muscular dystrophy. Nature 1992; 359:320–327.

121. McCrory M, Wright N, Kilmer D. Nutritional aspects of neuromuscular diseases. Phys Med Rehabil Clin North Am 1998; 9:127–144.

122. McDonald CM, Abresch RT, Carter GT, et al. Profiles of neuromuscular diseases: Becker muscular dystrophy. Am J Phys Med Rehabil 1995; 74: S93–S110.

123. McDonald CM, Abresch RT, Carter GT, et al. Profiles of neuromuscular diseases: Duchenne muscular dystrophy. Am J Phys Med Rehabil 1995; 74:S70–S82.

124. McDonald CM, Carter GT, Fritz RC, et al. Magnetic resonance imaging of denervated muscle: comparison to electromyography. Muscle Nerve 2000; 23(9):1431–1434.

125. McDonald CM, Johnson ER, Abresch RT, et al. Profiles of neuromuscular diseases: limb-girdle syndromes. Am J Phys Med Rehabil 1995; 74: S117–S130.

126. McDonald CM. Clinical approach to the diagnostic evaluation of progressive neuromuscular disorders. Phys Med Clin North Am 1998; 9(1):9–48.

127. McDonald CM. Limb contractures in progressive neuromuscular disease and the role of stretching, orthotics and surgery. Phys Med Rehabil Clin North Am 1998; 9(1):187–212.

128. McDonald DG, Kinali M, Gallagher AC, et al. Fracture prevalence in Duchenne muscular dystrophy. Dev Med Child Neurol 2002; 44(10):695–698.

129. Mendell JR, Province MA, Moxley RT, et al. Clinical investigation of Duchenne muscular dystrophy: a methodology for therapeutic trials based on natural history controls. Arch Neurol 1987; 44:808–815.

130. Meyerson MD, Lewis E, Ill K. Facioscapulohumeral muscular dystrophy and accompanying hearing loss. Arch Otolaryngol 1984; 110(4): 261–268.

131. Miller G, D'Orsogna L, O'Shea JP. Autonomic function and the sinus tachycardia of Duchenne muscular dystrophy. Brain Dev 1989; 22:247–256.

132. Monaco AP, Bertelson CJ, Liechti-Gallati S, et al. An explanation for the phenotypic differences between patients bearing partial deletions of the DMD locus. Genomics 1988; 2:90–96.

133. Moorman JR, Coleman RE, Packer D, et al. Cardiac involvement in myotonic muscular dystrophy. Medicine 1985; 64(6):371–378.

134. Mori H, Utsunomiya T, Ishijima M, et al. The relationship between 24-hour total heart beats or ventricular arrhythmias and cardiopulmonary function in patients with Duchenne muscular dystrophy. Jpn Heart J 1990; 31(5):599–612.

135. Mubarak SJ, Chambers HG, Wenger DR. Percutaneous muscle biopsy in the diagnosis of neuromuscular disease. J Pediatr Orthop 1992; 12:191–198.

136. Mulley JC, Kozman HM, Phillips HA, et al. Refined genetic localization for central core disease. Am J Hum Genet 1993; 52:398–404.

137. Munsat TL. Standardized forearm ischemic exercise test. Neurology 1970; 20:1171–1174.

138. Nagai T. Prognostic evaluation of congestive heart failure in patients with Duchenne muscular dystrophy. Retrospective study using non-invasive cardiac function tests. Jpn Circ J 1989; 53(5):406–410.

139. Nigro G, Comi LI, Politano L, et al. Evaluation of the cardiomyopathy in Becker muscular dystrophy. Muscle Nerve 1995; 18(3):283–291.

140. Nigro G, Comi LI, Politano L, et al. The incidence and evolution of cardiomyopathy in Duchenne muscular dystrophy. Int J Cardiol 1990; 26(3):277–289.

141. Nonaka I, Miyoshino S, Miike T, et al. An electron microscopical study of the muscle in congenital muscular dystrophy. Kumamoto Med J 1972; 25:68–75.

142. Nudel L, Zuk D, Zeelan E, et al. DMD gene product is not identical in muscle and brain. Nature 1989; 337:76–81.

143. Oda T, Shimizu N, Yonenobu K, et al. Longitudinal study of spinal deformity in Duchenne muscular dystrophy. J Pediatr Orthop 1993; 13:478–491.

144. Okada K, Manabe S, Sakamoto S, et al. Predictions of energy intake and energy allowance of patients with Duchenne muscular dystrophy and their validity. J Nutr Sci Vitaminol 1992; 38:155–161.

145. Ozawa E, Yoshida M, Suzaki A, et al. Dystrophin-associated proteins in muscular dystrophy. Hum Mol Genet 1995; 4:1711–1714.

146. Padberg GW, Brouwer OF, de Keizer RJ, et al. On the significance of retinal vascular disease and hearing loss in facioscapulohumeral muscular dystrophy. Muscle Nerve 1995; 2:S73–S81.

147. Passos-Bueno MR, Oliveira JR, Bakker E, et al. Genetic heterogeneity for Duchenne-like muscular dystrophy (DLMD) based on linkage and 50 DAG analysis. Hum Mol Genet 1993; 2:1945–1951.

148. Perloff JK. Cardiac rhythm and conduction in Duchenne muscular dystrophy. J Am Coll Cardiol 1984; 3:1263–1281.

149. Petrof BJ, Shrager JB, Stedman HH, et al. Dystrophin protects the sarcolemma from stresses developed during muscle contraction. Proc Natl Acad Sci USA 1993; 90:3710–3714.

150. Pradhan S. New clinical sign in Duchenne muscular dystrophy. Pediatr Neurol 1994; 11:298–301.

151. Quinlivan RM, Dubowitz V. Cardiac transplantation in Becker muscular dystrophy. Neuromuscul Disord 1992; 2:165–171.

152. Rafael JA, Cox GA, Corrado K, et al. Forced expression of dystrophin deletion constructs reveals structure–function correlations. J Cell Biol 1996; 134:93–102.

153. Rappaport D, Colleto GM, Vainzof M, et al. Short stature in Duchenne muscular dystrophy. Growth Regul 1991; 1:11–21.

154. Redman JB, Fenwick RG, Fu Y, et al. Relationship between parental trinucleotide GCT repeat length and severity of myotonic dystrophy in offspring. JAMA 1993; 269:1960–1972.

155. Reimann J, Irintchev A, Wernig A. Regenerative capacity and the number of satellite cells in soleus muscles of normal and mdx mice. Neuromuscul Disord 2000; 10:276–282.

156. Rideau Y, Glorion B, Delaubier A, et al. The treatment of scoliosis in Duchenne muscular dystrophy. Muscle Nerve 1984; 7:281–290.

157. Rideau Y, Jankowski L, Grellet J. Respiratory function in the muscular dystrophies. Muscle Nerve 1981; 4:155–167.

158. Ringel SP, Carroll JE, Schold C. The spectrum of mild x-linked recessive muscular dystrophy. Arch Neurol 1977; 34:408–412.

159. Roberds SL, Leturcq F, Allamand V, et al. Missense mutations in the adhalin gene linked to autosomal recessive muscular dystrophy. Cell 1994; 78:625–631.

160. Roberts RG, Coffey AJ, Bobrow M, et al. Exon structure of the human dystrophin gene. Genomics 1993; 16:536–542.

161. Rose MR, Tawil R. Drug treatment for facioscapulohumeral muscular dystrophy. Cochrane Database Syst Rev 2004; 2:CD002276-2283.

162. Sakata C, Sunohara N, Nonaka I, et al. A case of Becker muscular dystrophy presenting with cardiac failure as an initial symptom. Rinsho Shinkeigaku 1990; 30:210–215.

163. Santavuori P, Leisti J, Kruus S. Muscle, eye and brain disease: a new syndrome. Neuropaediatrie 1977; 8(suppl):553–561.

164. Santavuori P, Pihko H, Sainio K, et al. Muscle–eye–brain disease and Walker–Warburg syndrome. Am J Med Genet 1990; 36:371–380.

165. Santavuori P, Somer H, Sainio K, et al. Muscle–eye–brain disease (MEB). Brain Dev 1989; 11:147.

166. Sanyal SK, Johnson WW, Thapar MK, et al. An ultrastructural basis for the electrocardiographic alteration associated with Duchenne progressive muscular dystrophy. Circulation 1978; 57:1122–1133.

167. Scott OM, Hyde SA, Goddard C, et al. Effect of exercise in Duchenne muscular dystrophy: controlled six-month feasibility study of effects of two different regimes of exercises in children with Duchenne dystrophy. Physiotherapy 1981; 67:174–182.

168. Scott OM, Hyde SA, Goddard C, et al. Prevention of deformity in Duchenne muscular dystrophy. A prospective study of passive stretching and splintage. Physiotherapy 1981; 67:177–185.

169. Scott OM, Hyde SA, Goddard C, et al. Quantitation of muscle function in children: a prospective study in Duchenne muscular dystrophy. Muscle Nerve 1982; 5:291–297.

170. Siegel IM, Miller JE, Ray RD. Subcutaneous lower limb tenotomy in the treatment of pseudohypertrophic muscular dystrophy. J Bone Joint Surg 1986; 50:1437–1444.

171. Sinkeler SPT, Daanen HAM, Wevers RA, et al. The relation between blood lactate and ammonia in ischemic handgrip exercise. Muscle Nerve 1985; 8:523–531.

172. Smith PFM, Calverley PMA, Edwards RHT, et al. Practical problems in the respiratory care of patients with muscular dystrophy. N Engl J Med 1987; 316:1197–2004.

173. Sockolov R, Irwin B, Dressendorfer RH, et al. Exercise performance in 6 to 11 year old boys with Duchenne muscular dystrophy. Arch Phys Med Rehabil 1977; 58:195.

174. Sollee ND, Latham EE, Kinndlon DJ, et al. Neuropsychological impairment in Duchenne muscular dystrophy. J Clin Exp Neuropsychol 1985; 7:486–494.

175. Spaans F, Wagenmakers A, Saris W, et al. Procainamide therapy, physical performance and energy expenditure in the Schwartz–Jampel syndrome. Neuromuscul Disord 1991; 1:371–382.

176. Spencer GE, Vignos PJ Jr. Bracing for ambulation in childhood progressive muscular dystrophy. J Bone Joint Surg 1962; 44:234–340.

177. Steare SE, Benatar A, Dubowitz V. Subclinical cardiomyopathy in Becker muscular dystrophy. Br Heart J 1992; 68:304–308.

178. Stedman HH, Sweeney HL, Shrager JB, et al. The mdx mouse diaphragm reproduces the degenerative changes of Duchenne muscular dystrophy. Nature 1991; 352:536–539.

179. Steffensen BF, Lyager S, Werge B, et al. Physical capacity in non-ambulatory people with Duchenne muscular dystrophy or spinal muscular atrophy: a longitudinal study. Dev Med Child Neurol 2002; 44(9):623–632.

180. Stewart PM, Walser M, Drachman DB. Branched-chain ketoacids reduce muscle protein degradation in Duchenne muscular dystrophy. Muscle Nerve 1982; 5:197–205.

181. Takenaka A, Yokota M, Iwase M, et al. Discrepancy between systolic and diastolic dysfunction of the left ventricle in patients with Duchenne muscular dystrophy. Eur Heart J 1993; 14(5):669–678.

182. Tanabe Y, Esaki K, Nomura T. Skeletal muscle pathology in X chromosome-linked muscular dystrophy (mdx) mouse. Acta Neuropathol (Berl) 1986; 69:91–95.

183. Tarnopolsky MA, Mahoney DJ, Vajsar J, et al. Creatine monohydrate enhances strength and body composition in Duchenne muscular dystrophy. Neurology 2004; 62(10):1771–1777.

184. Tinsley JM, Blake DJ, Zuelling RA, et al. Increasing complexity of the dystrophin-associated protein complex. Proc Natl Acad Sci USA 1994; 91:8307–8311.

185. Toda T, Segawa M, Nomura Y, et al. Localization of a gene for Fukuyama type congenital muscular dystrophy to chromosome 9q31–33. Nat Genet 1993; 5:283–291.

186. Tome FS, Evangelista T, Leclerc A, et al. Congenital muscular dystrophy with merosin deficiency. Life Sci 1994; 317:351–357.

187. Topin N, Matecki S, Le Bris S, et al. Dose-dependent effect of individualized respiratory muscle training in children with Duchenne muscular dystrophy. Neuromuscul Disord 2002; 12(6):576–583.

188. Torres LFB, Duchen LW. The mutant mdx inherited myopathy in the mouse. Brain 1987; 110:269–299.

189. Tuikka RA, Laaksonen RK, Somer HVK. Cognitive function in myotonic dystrophy: a followup study. Eur Neurol 1993; 33:436–442.

190. Uchikawa K, Liu M, Hanayama K, et al. Functional status and muscle strength in people with Duchenne muscular dystrophy living in the community. J Rehabil Med 2004; 36(3):124–129.

191. Ugalde VO, Breslin EH, Walsh SA, et al. Pursed lip breathing improves ventilation in myotonic muscular dystrophy. Arch Phys Med Rehabil 2000; 81:472–478.

192. Upadhyaya M, Lunt PW, Sarfarazi M, et al. DNA marker applicable to presymptomatic and prenatal diagnosis of facioscapulohumeral disease. Lancet 1990; 336:1320–1327.

193. Verhagen WI, Huygen PL, Padberg GW. The auditory, vestibular and oculomotor system in facioscapulohumeral dystrophy. Acta Otolaryngol 1995; 1:140–152.

194. Vignos PJ Jr, Archibald KC. Maintenance of ambulation in childhood muscular dystrophy. J Chronic Dis 1960; 12:273–281.

195. Vignos PJ Jr, Watkins MP. Effect of exercise in muscular dystrophy. JAMA 1966; 197:843–849.

196. Vignos PJ Jr. Management of musculoskeletal complications in neuromuscular disease: limb contractures and the role of stretching, braces and surgery. Phys Med Rehabil State Art Rev 1988; 2:509–521.

197. Vignos PJ Jr. Physical models of rehabilitation in neuromuscular disease. Muscle Nerve 1983; 6:323–327.

198. de Visser M, de Voogt WG, la Riviere GV. The heart in Becker muscular dystrophy, facioscapulohumeral dystrophy, and Bethlem myopathy. Muscle Nerve 1992; 15:591-603.

199. Voit T, Krogmann O, Lennard HG, et al. Emery–Dreifuss muscular dystrophy: disease spectrum and differential diagnosis: Neuropediatrics 1988; 19:62–69.

200. Waters DD, Nutter DO, Hopkins LD, et al. Cardiac features of an unusual x-linked humeroperoneal neuromuscular disease. N Engl J Med 1975; 293:1017–1023.

201. Wenneberg S, Gunnarsson LG, Ahlstrom G. Using a novel exercise programme for patients with muscular dystrophy. Part I: a qualitative study. Disabil Rehabil 2004; 26(10):586–594.

202. Wenneberg S, Gunnarsson LG, Ahlstrom G. Using a novel exercise programme for patients with muscular dystrophy. Part II: a quantitative study. Disabil Rehabil 2004; 26(10):595–602.

203. Wijmenga C, Frants RR, Brouwer OF, et al. The facioscapulohumeral muscular dystrophy gene maps to chromosome 4. Lancet 1990; 2:651-58.

204. Willig TN, Carlier L, Legrand M, et al. Nutritional assessment in Duchenne muscular dystrophy. Dev Med Child Neurol 1993; 35:1074–1089.

205. Willig TN, Paulus J, Lacau Saint Guily J, et al. Swallowing problems in neuromuscular disorders. Arch Phys Med Rehabil 1994; 75:1175–1183.

206. Wineinger MA, Abresch RT, Walsh SA, et al. Effects of aging and voluntary exercise on the function of dystrophic muscle from mdx mice. Am J Phys Med Rehabil 1998; 77(1):20–27.

207. Wohlgemuth M, van der Kooi EL, van Kesteren RG, et al. Ventilatory support in facioscapulohumeral muscular dystrophy. Neurology 2004; 63(1):176–178.

208. Wright NC, Kilmer DD, McCrory MA, et al. Aerobic walking in slowly progressive neuromuscular disease: effect of a 12-week program. Arch Phys Med Rehabil 1996; 77:64–72.

209. Yamamoto S, Matsushima H, Suzuki A, et al. A comparative study of thallium-201 single photon emission computed tomography and electrocardiography in Duchenne and other types of muscular dystrophy. Am J Cardiol 1988; 61:836–847.

210. Yanagisawa A, Miyagawa M, Yotsukura M, et al. The prevalence and prognostic significance of arrhythmias in Duchenne type muscular dystrophy. Am Heart J 1992; 124:1244–1249.

211. Yazawa M, Ikeda S, Owa M, et al. A family of Becker progressive muscular dystrophy with severe cardiomyopathy. Eur Neurol 1987; 26:13–19.

212. Yoshida K, Ikeda S, Nakamura A, et al. Molecular analysis of the Duchenne muscular dystrophy gene in patients with Becker muscular dystrophy presenting with dilated cardiomyopathy. Muscle Nerve 1993; 16:1161–1172.

213. Yotsukura M, Miyagawa M, Tsuya T, et al. Pulmonary hypertension in progressive muscular dystrophy of the Duchenne type. Jpn Circ J 1988; 52:321–325.

Chapter

50

Rehabilitation after Traumatic Brain Injury

David X. Cifu, Jeffrey S. Kreutzer, Daniel N. Slater and Laura Taylor

TERMINOLOGY

Traumatic brain injury (TBI), as opposed to *brain injury*, should be used to describe all injuries to the brain caused by an external force.[165] *Concussion* is a term to describe any closed (i.e. no dural disruption) TBI; however, it is most commonly applied to mild injuries. *Open* or *penetrating* TBI identifies an injury where the dura has been disrupted by a missile, stab wound, or other injury. *Non-traumatic* brain injuries are best identified by the etiology and pathology associated with them, such as hypoxic or anoxic encephalopathy, stroke or ischemic brain injury, brain tumor, and toxic metabolic brain injury or encephalopathy. Severity of TBI is typically determined by the initial scores on the Glasgow Coma Scale (GCS), a 15-point scale assessing eye opening, verbalization, and command following (see Table 50-1).[258] An individual who has sustained a mild TBI has had an immediate period of altered or lost consciousness, with a GCS score by 30 min post injury of 13–15. Moderate TBI signifies an immediate period of altered or loss of consciousness for more than 30 min, and a 6-h GCS score of 9–12. Severe TBI signifies an immediate loss of consciousness without regaining consciousness for more than 6 h (GCS score 3–8).[37]

EPIDEMIOLOGY

Incidence

The annual incidence of TBI requiring hospitalization and overall is estimated to be 200 and 500 cases, respectively, per 100 000 population in the USA, with approximately 1.4 million receiving documentable urgent care.[11,35,79,80,140–143,163,246] TBI results in 1.11 million emergency department visits, 235 000 hospitalizations, and 50 000 deaths annually.[163] The vast majority (~80%) of hospitalized and virtually all the non-hospitalized injuries can be classified as mild TBI. The remaining 20% of the hospitalized new injuries can be evenly divided between moderate and severe injuries.[49,248] Approximately 20 per 100 000 people per year survive TBI with moderate to severe physical or neurobehavioral deficits.[139]

Demographics

Males are 1.5 times as likely to sustain and 3–4 times more likely to die from a TBI.[80,91,140,163,246] The higher risk in males is true of all age groups, although the increase diminishes in the geriatric population.[163,254] The peak risk of TBI occurs between the ages of 18 and 25 (200–225/100 000).[246] Smaller peaks also occur in older adults (>70 years) and children (<5 years). The leading cause of death among children aged 1–14 is trauma, with brain injury accounting for 40% of this total.[7] Older adults have the highest mortality rate.[6] Minorities have a slightly higher incidence of TBI.[35,89,105]

Etiology

Alcohol abuse is the largest indirect cause of TBI.[50,54] Falls are the most common cause of TBI necessitating evaluation in an emergency department.[163] Nearly half of all TBIs requiring admission to the hospital are transportation-related, most commonly due to motor vehicle crashes, followed by auto–pedestrian and bicycle crashes. Assaults are another common cause of TBI. Auto–pedestrian and bicycle crashes are most common among children, while falls are most common among both children and older adults.[35,80,142,143,163]

Prevention

The economic and social impact of TBI has not been extensively studied, but given its high incidence and specific demographics, both are likely to be significant. The single most preventable risk factor in TBI is alcohol usage.[19,50,54,166] Seat belt usage and air bags, when used in conjunction with seat belts, have been shown to decrease injury severity and concomitant injuries.[56,61,255,293] Helmet use by both motorcyclists and bicyclists has also been demonstrated to reduce the severity of TBIs. Bicycle helmets potentially reduce the risk of TBI by 85%.[230,247,275] Child safety seats for automobiles, when correctly installed, reduce the risk of death by 70% for infants and 54% for toddlers.[255] Specific interventions, such as improving environmental factors to reduce the incidence of falls (e.g. lighting, room obstacles, and throw rugs), has been shown to be effective in reducing the risk of TBI in older adults.[240,262,263] Prevention of falls in young children can be improved with education programs.[4] It is unfortunate that many of the specific 'preventable' risk factors for TBI are also increasingly challenging problems in our society (e.g. substance abuse, crime, poor workplace conditions, and child and elder abuse). These might be difficult to significantly improve.

Table 50-1 Glasgow Coma Scale[a]

Patient's response	Score
Eye opening	
Eyes open spontaneously	4
Eyes open when spoken to	3
Eyes open to painful stimulation	2
Eyes do not open	1
Motor	
Follows commands	6
Makes localizing movement to pain	5
Makes withdrawal movements to pain	4
Flexor (decorticate) posturing to pain	3
Extensor (decerebrate) posturing to pain	2
No motor response to pain	1
Verbal	
Oriented to place and date	5
Converses but is not oriented	4
Utters inappropriate words, not conversing	3
Makes incomprehensible non-verbal sounds	2
Not vocalizing	1

[a]Instructions: rate best response in the verbal and motor categories and the stimulus needed to elicit eye opening. Sum the three ratings to obtain the score.

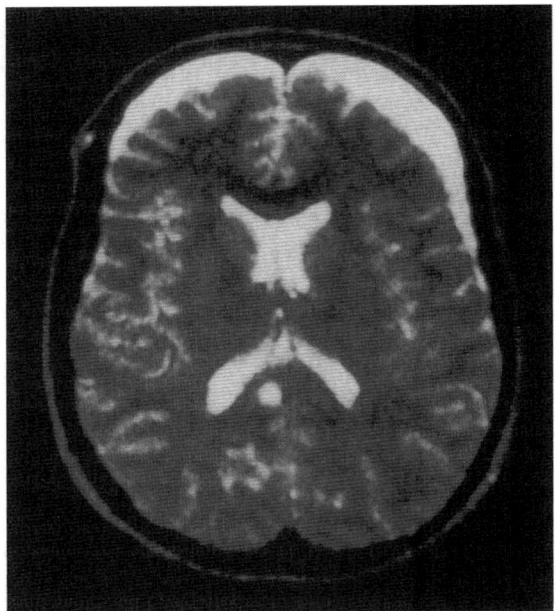

Figure 50-1 T2-weighted magnetic resonance imaging (MRI) scan of severe traumatic brain injury. T2-weighted MRI scan of a 32-year-old woman who was injured in an automobile–pedestrian accident 1 month earlier. Initial computed tomography (CT) scan revealed a right frontal subdural hematoma. This image shows bifrontal subdural fluid collections and a shear injury in the splenium of the corpus callosum. The corpus callosum lesion, which is a classic sign of diffuse axonal injury, was not visualized on CT scans. In general, MRI can visualize a larger number of traumatic lesions than can CT, especially lesions that are non-hemorrhagic or are located near bony areas. The patient, who had an initial Glasgow Coma Scale score of 7, underwent inpatient and postacute rehabilitation. She returned to work as a secretary and lives independently.

PATHOPHYSIOLOGY

Primary injury

Primary injury occurs at the moment of impact, and in TBI is predominantly the result of acceleration–deceleration and rotational forces. These forces result in diffuse axonal injury (DAI), petechial hemorrhages, parenchymal contusions, and cranial nerve injury. DAI is the term used to describe the often widespread stretching of axons caused by the rapid rotation of the brain around its axis, and is a distinguishing feature of TBI, as compared with other types of brain injury.[85,190] The actual cause of DAI is not well defined, but is related to impairments in axoplasmic transport and eventually axonal disconnection.[190,210] DAI can occur with TBI, but in mild TBI it is often microscopic and therefore is not visible on neuroimaging studies. It is more likely to be macroscopic and appear on neuroimaging studies in more severe injuries (Fig. 50-1). Lesions tend to be found where the injury forces on the axons are greatest (i.e. nearest to the surface of the brain), and are most often seen at the gray–white matter interface. More severe injuries are more likely to produce deeper lesions. Visible lesions, or petechial hemorrhages, are most common in the midbrain, pons, corpus callosum, and white matter of the cerebellum.[1,17,93,170,200,224]

DAI is the mechanism of initial loss of consciousness after TBI,[1] and results in more generalized deficits (e.g. confusion and incoordination). Recovery from DAI is usually gradual.[127]

Parenchymal contusions or cortical bruising occur at the crests of gyri, primarily on the undersurface of the frontal lobes and at the temporal tips. This is where both the proximity of the brain to the skull and the irregularities of the skull surface increase the risk of injury. These lesions can result from even low-velocity injuries, such as ground level falls or local blunt trauma. More severe injuries are likely to produce larger and/or deeper contusions. Cortical contusions elevate the risk for seizures and are more likely to produce focal deficits (e.g. aphasias and motor weakness).[93] A less common cause of parenchymal injury is direct laceration of brain tissue caused by metallic or bony fragments. This can occur with a gunshot (Fig. 50-2) or other missile injury; a depressed skull fracture, most often due to significant blunt trauma; or due to a penetrating injury (e.g. knife or other foreign object). The mechanism of injury associated with these parenchymal lacerations is unfortunately likely to also cause subdural and epidural hemorrhage. Conversely, these injuries are most often not associated with other bodily injury. If survivable, they are associated with more focal deficits.

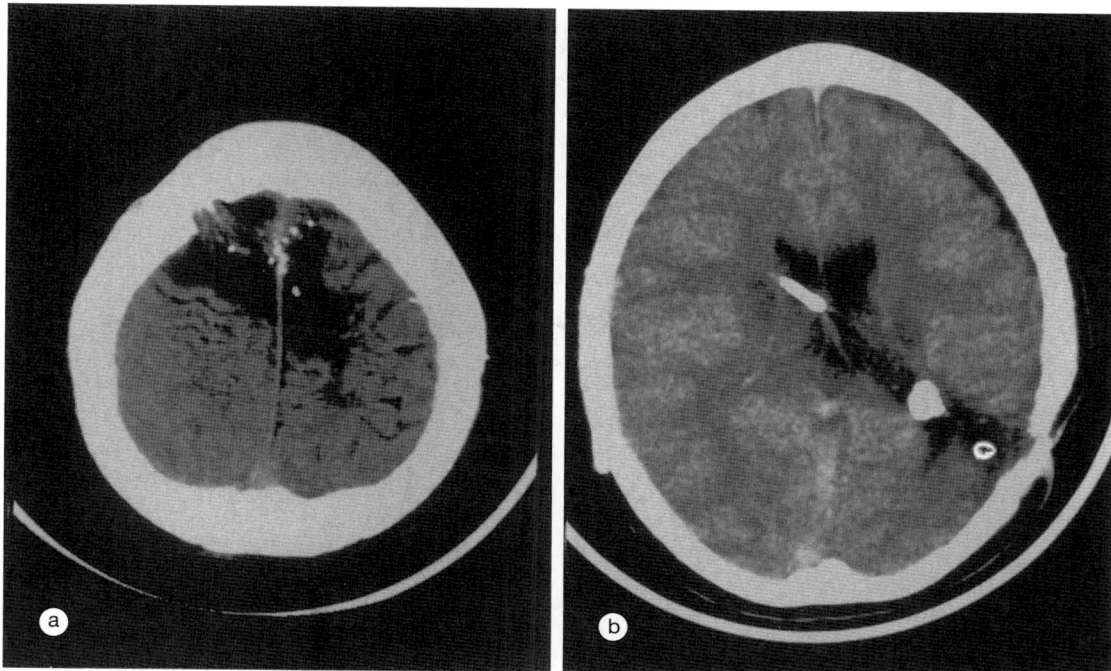

Figure 50-2 Penetrating traumatic brain injury caused by gunshot. Initial computed tomography scan images of the brain of a 14-year-old boy shot at close range during an assault involving a playground altercation with another teenager. (**a**) Entry wound in the superior right frontal area with bullet track crossing the midline. In-driven bone fragments underlie the entry wound. (**b**) Exit wound in the left temporal-parietal area. Destruction of brain tissue is seen along the bullet path. Focal injuries to the bilateral superior frontal area and to the left parietal-temporal area correlate with chronic bilateral lower extremity paresis and written language deficits. After extended physical and occupational therapy, the patient gained independence in feeding with set-up and mobility using a motorized wheelchair.

Secondary injury

Secondary injury mechanisms are physiologic and pathologic processes, triggered by the initial injury, that can cause additional brain insult and injury. These secondary injury cascades include intracranial hemorrhage (e.g. epidural, subdural, and intracerebral hematomas), vasogenic or cytogenic brain edema, excitotoxicity, oxidant injury, and hypoxia (Fig. 50-3). Elevations in intracranial pressure (ICP), which can be caused by both primary and secondary mechanisms (e.g. enlarging hematoma and edema), can cause decreases in cerebral perfusion pressures and subsequent ischemic damage.[93,97,178] The mass effect from focal (e.g. hematoma) or generalized (e.g. hydrocephalus) increases in pressure can cause further secondary injury from brain shift or herniation. Each of these factors can affect both the rate and the extent of recovery from TBI.

ACUTE MANAGEMENT (see Figs 50-4 and 50-5)

Initial assessment

In order to provide standardized and coordinated systems of care, the American College of Surgeons, in partnership with state and local organizations, has adopted a system of trauma triaging to prioritize the high-intensity services available at comprehensive medical centers for trauma victims with corresponding needs.[71,268] All individuals who sustain a TBI significant enough to cause persistent alteration or loss of consciousness should be urgently transported to a level 1 (highest level of services) trauma center for assessment. Individuals who sustain only transient (< 1 min) alterations in consciousness, and who have returned to their normal baseline without any evidence or elevated risk for other organ injury, can be transported to a level 2 (medium level of services) trauma center for evaluation. The ABCs (airway, breathing, and circulation) of basic life support must be instituted concomitantly with the multiorgan assessment and stabilization of trauma management. The homeostasis of the brain must be reestablished in parallel with the remainder of the body. To this end, a multidisciplinary approach is recommended by the American College of Surgeons, headed by trauma surgeons who are able to coordinate their acute efforts with the neurosurgical consultants.[25]

Acute neurosurgical management focuses on urgent assessment of primary brain injury and prevention of secondary brain injury. Initial assessment is accomplished by neurologic examination, computed tomography (CT) scanning of the brain, and evaluation of ICP (if indicated by neurologic and imaging testing). Neurologic assessment must address neuromuscular, sensory (including special senses), cognitive, communication, and behavioral impairments. Pupillary inspection is a vital component of acute evaluation. When compared with baseline documentation, it can be accurately used to assess for potentially life-threatening problems (such as brain stem herniation). Serial follow-up evaluations performed by members of both the neurosurgical and the rehabilitation teams are extremely important in monitoring for recurrent and new problems.

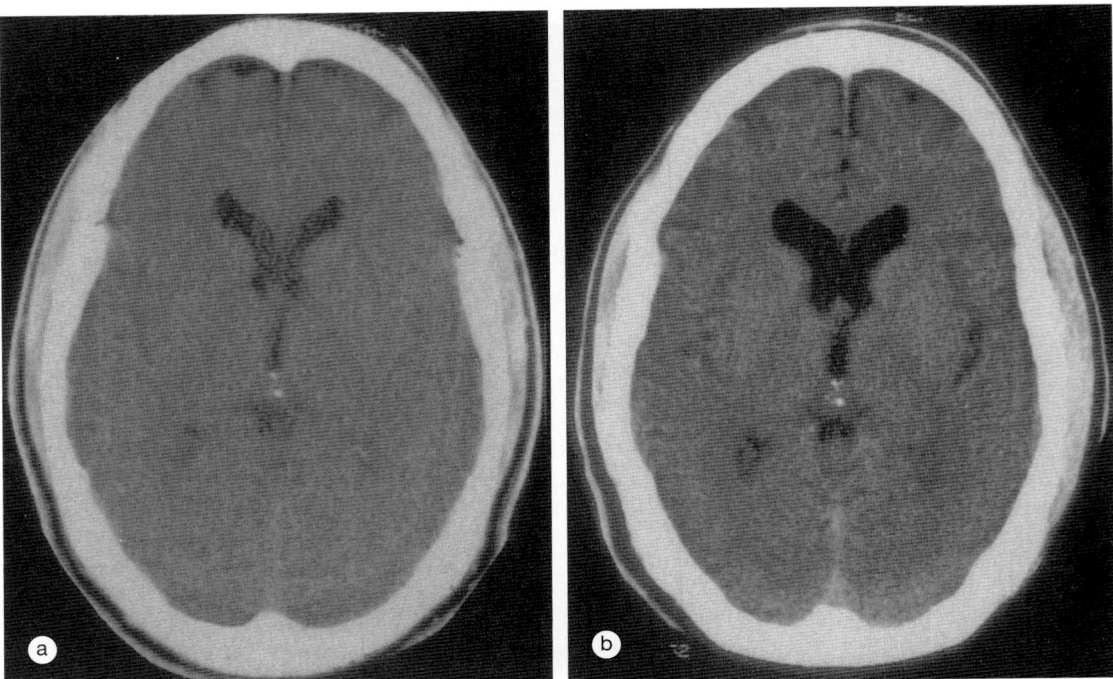

Figure 50-3 Anoxic brain injury. Computed tomography images showing anoxic brain injury in a 32-year-old man who sustained a mild traumatic brain injury and facial injury (zygomatic arch fracture) in a fall from a ladder, and then suffered a 10-min cardiac arrest during facial surgery. Images are in the horizontal plane through the level of the lateral ventricles, performed before and after the brain injury. (**a**) Day of injury scan, performed to clear him for surgery, revealed no intracranial abnormality. (**b**) Follow-up scan, performed 20 days later, revealed atrophic changes predominantly in the frontal and temporal lobes. During the first month post injury, he was agitated and confused, but he gradually recovered independence in ambulation and self-care. Follow-up at 4 months post injury indicated severe amnesia, for which he received full-time supervision. By 1 year post injury, his level of functioning had improved to allow part-time supervision. The patient has never resumed working, driving, or going unsupervised for a 24-h period.

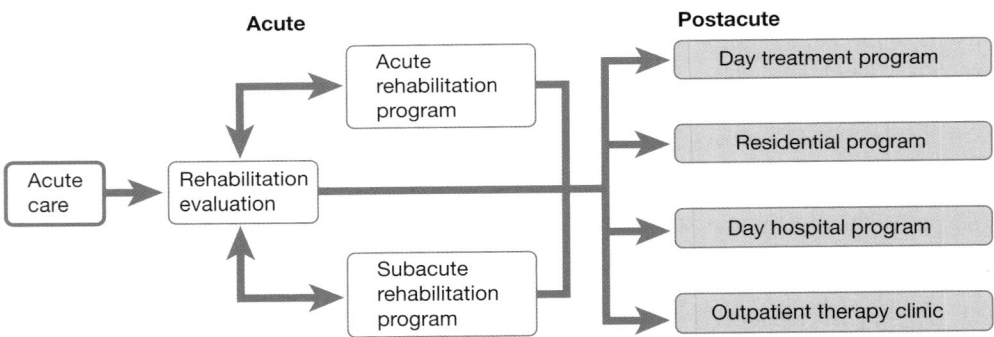

Figure 50-4 Rehabilitation pathway following brain injury. Flowchart showing typical pathways followed by patients from injury through the acute and postacute phases of rehabilitation. Evaluation by a rehabilitation physician is the initial, necessary step before patients are transferred from acute care to rehabilitation programs. Patients may be transferred between acute and subacute rehabilitation programs, depending on individual needs. The choice of postacute program may depend on local availability.

Early prognosis

There are a number of early and late factors that have been demonstrated to have a significant association with outcome after TBI (Box 50-1) but, even when used in combination, these factors account for a small amount of the total outcome variance observed. Initial brain injury severity (Table 50-2) is an important 'predictor' of morbidity and mortality. The GCS is the 'gold standard' measurement of initial TBI severity (see Table 50-1).[258] The GCS is a 15-point scale that allows rating

of an individual's best motor (rated 1–6) response, best verbal (rated 1–5) response, and the weakest stimulus needed to elicit eye opening (rated 1–4). The three ratings are summed to yield a score from 3 (lowest) to 15 (highest). A score of 8 or less is defined as comatose (not following commands, not uttering understandable words, not opening eyes), and persistence at or below a GCS score of 8 for more than 6 h indicates a severe TBI.[37] The depth of initial alteration in consciousness is an important measure of severity, and as measured by the GCS

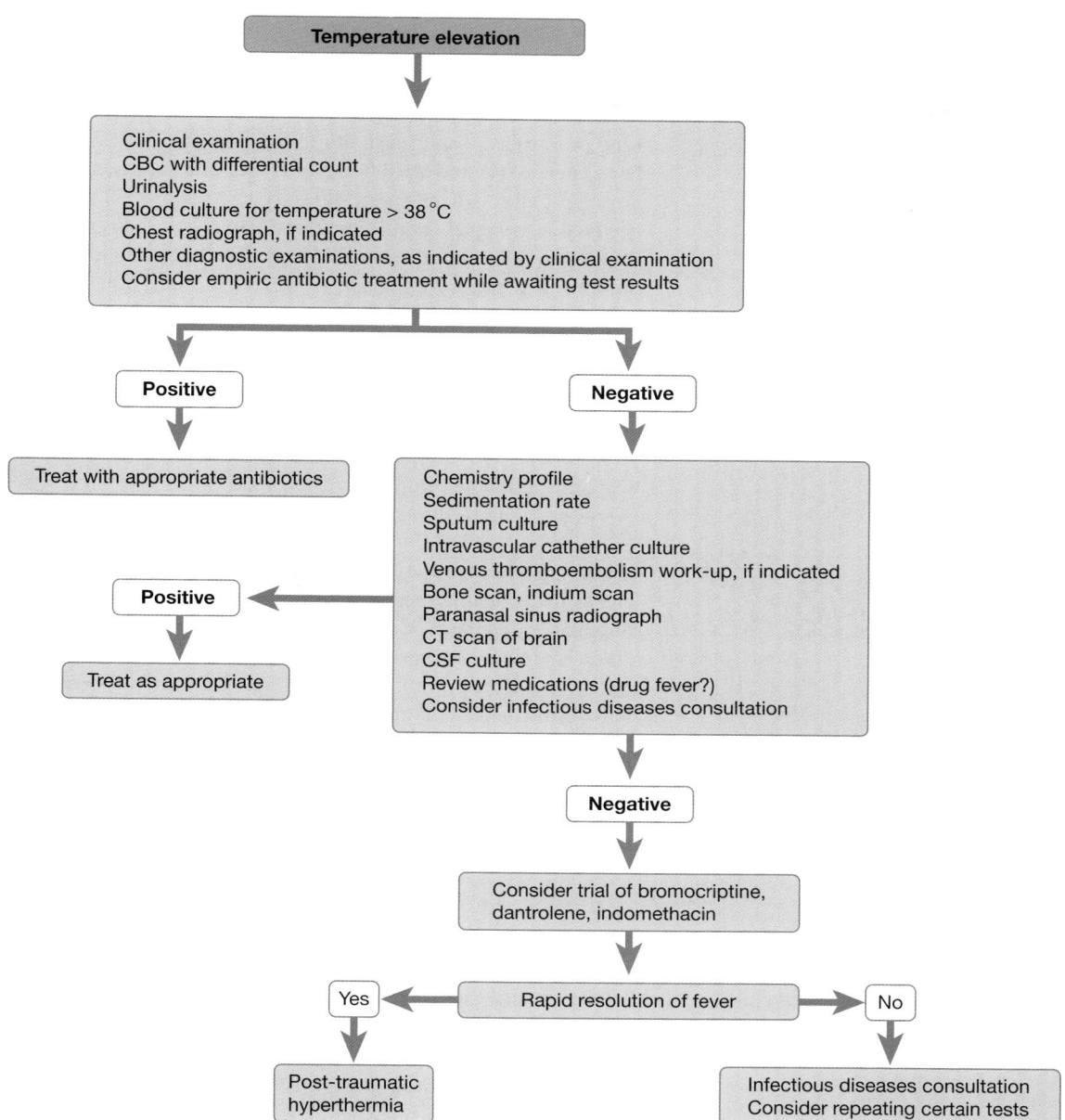

Figure 50-5 Suggested fever work-up algorithm for the patient with brain injury. CBC, complete blood count; CSF, cerebrospinal fluid; CT, computed tomography.

Box 50-1 Factors useful in determining prognosis acutely after traumatic brain injury

- Glasgow Coma Scale score (initial 7 days post traumatic brain injury)
- Duration of coma
- Duration of posttraumatic amnesia
- Sustained intracranial pressure > 20 mmHg
- Brain stem reflexes (Glasgow–Liège Scale)
- Multimodal evoked potentials (limited utility)
- Neuroimaging (limited utility)
- Age (> 55 years)

has been strongly associated with both acute and chronic neuro-behavioral outcomes after TBI. This strong association persists for at least the first week post TBI.[24,37,269] An individual in coma is defined as having no meaningful interaction with the environment and no definable sleep–wake cycling. Individuals who progress to clear sleep–wake cycles, but who continue to have an inability to react to or interact with the environment, are termed 'vegetative'.[87] While the transition period between being comatose and interacting with the environment is often hard to distinguish, the progression from a motor GCS score of 5 (inconsistently follows commands) to 6 (consistently follows commands) has been suggested as a reliable technique.[280]

Table 50-2 Classifying severity of traumatic brain injury	
Severity	Classification
Mild	Definite alteration or loss of consciousness. Glasgow Coma Scale (GCS) score of 13–15 at worst after resuscitation. Non-focal neurologic examination.
Uncomplicated	Normal head computed tomography (CT) scan.
Complicated	Brain abnormality on head CT scan.
Grade 1	No loss of consciousness. Alteration in consciousness lasts less than 15 min.
Grade 2	No loss of consciousness. Alteration in consciousness lasts more than 15 min, but resolves by 30 min.
Grade 3	Any loss of consciousness lasting up to 30 min.
Moderate	Alteration or loss of consciousness. Any loss of consciousness lasting >30 min but <6 h. GCS score of 9–12 at worst after resuscitation.
Severe	Loss of consciousness lasting >6 h. GCS score of 6–8 at worst after resuscitation.
Very severe	Loss of consciousness lasting >6 h. GCS score of 3–5 at worst after resuscitation

The leading causes of coma in descending frequency are trauma, drug overdose, and cardiac arrest. Traumatic coma has a better prognosis than non-traumatic coma. Clinical parameters indicating an unfavorable prognosis in individuals with coma (in particular brain injury associated with anoxia) include persistent absence of pupillary light reaction by day 3, persistent absence of motor response to pain by day 3, and persistent GCS score <5 by day 3.[13]

Moderate TBI is defined as an initial alteration or loss of consciousness, with a GCS score < 12 for more than 30 min and a GCS score of between 9 and 12 (non-comatose) by 6 h post injury. A mild TBI (commonly called a concussion) requires an initial alteration or loss of consciousness with a GCS score of 13–15 by 30 min post injury. An individual with an initial GCS score of 15 can only be described as having sustained a mild TBI if there has been a demonstrable alteration in consciousness at the time of the initial injury. Reports of altered or lost consciousness 'recalled' weeks or months after the initial injury have questionable validity. Mild TBI has been further subdivided into complicated mild (presence of TBI-related CT scan abnormalities) and uncomplicated mild (normal CT scan). An individual's lowest postresuscitation GCS score is the best measure of injury-related severity.[58,59,64] The utility of the GCS to measure injury severity might be limited in the presence of secondary injuries (e.g. eye trauma, tracheal injury, and spinal cord injury), necessary treatment (e.g. intubation, sedation, and chemical paralysis), or premorbid conditions (e.g. aphasia and dementia). A modified version of the GCS for children is available.[273]

Measures of brain injury severity are most useful as 'predictors' of morbidity and mortality in the first 48 h. These factors have been associated with both short- and long-term outcomes after TBI, although, as noted, they account for a small percentage of the variances seen in outcome. Duration of altered consciousness is an important measure of severity, particularly the duration of coma (GCS score < 8) and the duration of post-traumatic amnesia (PTA).[16,24,28,37,225,269] During PTA, individuals are no longer comatose (i.e. they have a GCS score > 8) but are disoriented and amnesic for day to day events. The Galveston Orientation and Amnesia Test (GOAT) provides a reliable and validated measure of emergence from PTA. A GOAT score of >70 indicates emergence from PTA.[169] A modified pediatric version is available. Duration of PTA has been associated with short- and long-term outcome after TBI.[16,28,37,58,59,127,225]

Neuroprotective agents

The acute release of excitotoxic neurotransmitters, such as glutamate, has been demonstrated in the post-TBI period. These neurotransmitters activate cell receptors that, in turn, increase neuronal influx of sodium and calcium. As this electrolyte imbalance is corrected by these neurons, energy stores must be utilized. Additionally, free radicals, lipases, and proteases are released, which can further increase glutamate release. This cycle of activity results in further cell injury.[190,294] Neuroprotective drugs and hypothermia have been demonstrated, in animals, to decrease the adverse effects and secondary injury caused by the release of these excitatory neurotransmitters after TBI. This protective effect has, unfortunately, not been clearly demonstrated in humans.[46,135,267,294]

Intracranial pressure management

Intracranial pressure monitoring is recommended in individuals with severe TBI (GCS score 3–8) and an abnormal CT scan (demonstrating hematomas, contusions, or evidence of edema), or a normal CT scan but two of three risk factors (age > 40, unilateral or bilateral posturing, or systolic blood pressure < 90 mmHg).[25] Elevated ICP is a common cause of secondary brain injury, because it contributes to a decrease in cerebral perfusion pressure, which comprises the difference between mean arterial blood pressure and ICP. While sustained elevations of ICP > 20 mmHg have been associated with poorer outcome, it now appears that a decline in cerebral perfusion pressure to < 70 mmHg is a more specific cause of cerebral ischemia. Acute management includes maintenance of mean arterial blood pressure (via fluid replacement and vasopressors), reduction of ICP, and limiting environmental stimuli, as well as chemical sedation. More aggressive management of elevated ICP is indicated only for acute neurologic deterioration and refractory elevations. This management includes hyperventilation, barbiturate-induced coma, bolus dosing of mannitol, and craniectomy. The use of glucocorticoids has no proven value after TBI.[25,221]

Hydrocephalus

Cerebrospinal fluid (CSF) protects and provides nutrients and oxygen to the brain. It is produced at a rate of approximately 150 cc/h in the lateral ventricle by the choroid plexus, and is reabsorbed at an equal rate in the sagittal sinus by the arachnoid granulations. The entire 500-cc volume of CSF found in adults is completely recycled every 4–5 h. An increase in total CSF volume or a non-physiologic distribution of CSF is known as hydrocephalus, a condition that often results in the classic findings of altered mentation, ataxia, and urinary incontinence. These findings can be difficult, however, to clearly differentiate from TBI-related deficits. Serial CT scans of the brain are recommended in patients who are recovering slowly, or who have atypical recovery patterns or symptoms (e.g. new-onset hypertension, late seizures, and late agitation) (Fig. 50-6). The main mechanisms leading to hydrocephalus include an increase in production of CSF (e.g. from a chordoma), an obstruction of the ventricular system (e.g. from a blood clot or mass effect), or an obstruction in reabsorption (e.g. 'clogging' of the arachnoid granulations with blood clots, bone spicules, or by infectious material). Hydrocephalus might develop slowly after TBI, especially if there is underlying (i.e. atrophy) or TBI-related excess space within the cranial vault. Treatment with temporary or permanent ventricular shunting is warranted in symptomatic patients.[25,175]

Surgical intervention

Common interventions to reduce secondary injury include focal evacuation of hematomas that are causing mass effect, and debridement of parenchymal contusions that are causing edema or could be at risk for infection. Focal skull flaps are sometimes used temporarily (usually for 6 weeks) to relieve focal swelling. Bifrontal craniectomies, while extreme, can also be used for intractable elevations in ICP.[12]

Neuroimaging

During the acute stage of TBI, CT scanning is the preferred neuroimaging modality. This is because of the ease of obtaining adequate images quickly, and the lack of contraindications of its use in the presence of various life-saving situations. CT scanning is also preferred, most importantly, because of its sensitivity to show the presence of blood, facial and skull fractures, and the variety of intracranial injuries that would require emergent neurosurgical intervention. While serial brain-imaging studies are commonplace in patients with recent TBI, special attention should be paid to the presence of late or delayed bleeding and hydrocephalus. A second imaging study (typically a CT scan) performed between 2 and 4 weeks post injury can rule out these abnormalities, particularly if there has not been the expected clinical improvement. Indications for a magnetic resonance imaging (MRI) (or dynamic imaging studies) in the acute period after TBI include unexplained clinical findings, such as brain stem pathology or a concomitant ischemic event. After the acute management period, CT scanning is useful in detecting or monitoring hydrocephalus.

The greater resolution of MRI makes it a more sensitive tool to assess injuries after TBI, particularly small petechial hemorrhages, non-hemorrhagic white matter injury (DAI), and contusions of the frontal and brain stem regions.[134,259] Recent advances in MRI technology (magnetic transfer and fluid-attenuated inversion recovery) have improved its sensitivity to white matter injury, although the MRI can still be normal in the presence of a documented mild TBI.[121,184,196,249]

Single-photon emission computed tomography scanning (SPECT) is a functional imaging modality that is used to determine blood flow based on the distribution of a radiopharmaceutical agent in the brain. It provides an even more sensitive assessment of brain functioning, and can be useful in better defining abnormalities in individuals who remain unconscious or who have mild TBI. Newer 'triple-head' cameras provide a resolution of approximately 1 cm, and also assist in more precise anatomic localization. Literature linking SPECT findings with neuropsychologic or functional sequelae are lacking.[10,21,38,88,180,199] Positron emission tomography (PET), which utilizes labeled metabolic substrates or blood components to measure metabolic activity, can have a role in identifying focal areas of abnormal cortical activity.[78,133] Newer PET scanners have a resolution of approximately 4 mm, but the imaging cost (approximately $2000) is more than double that of a comparable SPECT scan. PET scans have been demonstrated to provide reproducible data with anatomic-structural studies, and with studies involving cognitive activation of the brain.[171,265] Studies correlating specific brain injury with behavioral–functional deficits are limited.[77]

Functional magnetic resonance imaging (fMRI) assesses activity-related changes in cerebral blood flow without the use of ionizing radiation. In addition to the lack of radiation exposure, fMRI also offers the advantages of being available using many existing MRI scanners and anatomic resolution down to 1 mm. fMRI appears to be similar to PET scanning for cognitive activation tasks, but presently it has no defined clinical role after TBI.[288] Magnetic resonance spectroscopy (MRS) uses the basic principles of MRI (measurement of the protons in water and lipids) to quantify the neurochemicals within the brain as markers of neural integrity or pathology. Values are typically expressed as a ratio relative to the levels of creatine (considered relatively stable in the brain). Similar to fMRI, MRS can be performed on many existing MRI scanners, and does not expose the individual to ionizing radiation. The ability of MRS to assess cellular level abnormalities, while still experimental, might make it a highly sensitive and specific diagnostic tool in even mild TBI.[9,82] The role of these newer dynamic imaging studies in the standard assessment or management of individuals with acute or chronic TBI is unclear at present.

Electrophysiologic evaluation

Electrophysiologic evaluations after TBI generally have limited clinical value, especially when a detailed physical examination can be performed. Multimodal-evoked potentials (MEPs) can be done, including somatosensory-evoked potentials, visual-evoked potentials, and auditory brain stem-evoked potentials.

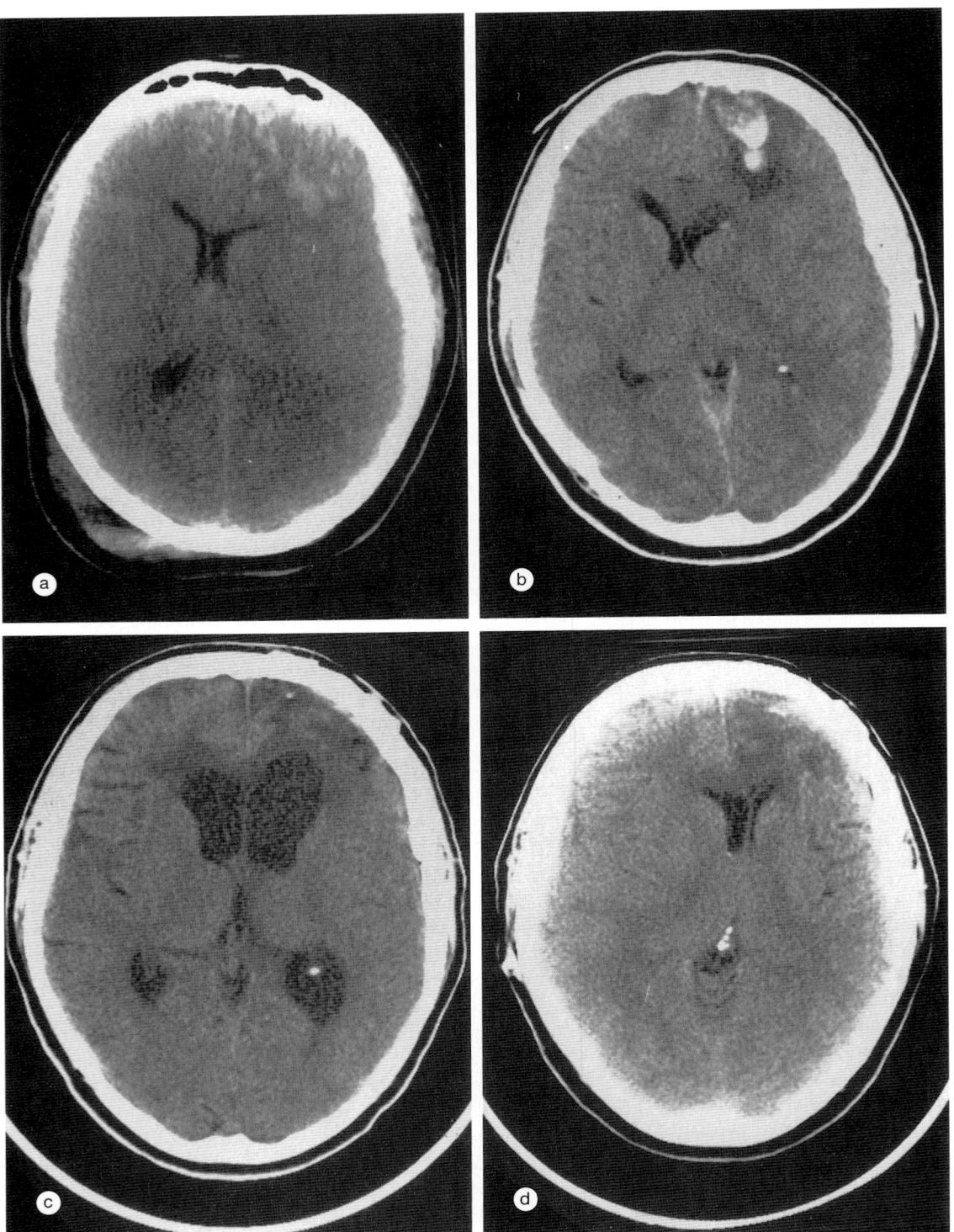

Figure 50-6 Severe traumatic brain injury complicated by hydrocephalus. Computed tomography scan images of the brain of a 47-year-old woman who suffered a severe traumatic brain injury in a fall from a horse. Glasgow Coma Scale score was 14 at the scene but later decreased to 8. (**a**) Initial day of injury scan reveals hemorrhagic contusions in the left frontal lobe and swelling of the left cerebral hemisphere, with less extensive contusions in the right frontal and anterior left temporal lobes. (**b**) Follow-up scan at 4 days post injury reveals increased swelling of the left cerebral hemisphere, causing early herniation and mass effect. Partial lobectomy of the left frontal lobe was then performed. The patient regained independence in ambulation and self-care but remained in posttraumatic amnesia (PTA). (**c**) Follow-up scan at 2 months post injury, obtained because of an early plateau in functional recovery, reveals generalized enlargement in the ventricular system consistent with communicating hydrocephalus. After placement of a ventriculoperitoneal shunt, she promptly cleared from PTA. (**d**) Follow-up scan at 7 months post injury, obtained because of worsening cognitive and behavioral problems, reveals a chronic right frontal-parietal subdural hematoma. After drainage of the hematoma, functional recovery progressed for several more months. By 15 months post injury, she had passed a driving evaluation and was independent in shopping and cooking, but had not returned to work. Neuropsychologic evaluation revealed moderate, selective deficits in recent memory and right-hand coordination.

MEPs might have some utility in determining the locations of specific lesions, demonstrating the presence of injury in mild TBI, or demonstrating the presence of specific deficits (e.g. vision and hearing) in comatose or uncooperative individuals.

Electroencephalographs (EEGs) can provide general information about the severity and location of injury, although many changes (e.g. generalized slowing) might persist despite functional improvements.[55,95,222] EEGs have a low sensitivity in predicting seizure risk.[118,229,239] Quantitative EEG has not been demonstrated to have a role in the clinical management of TBI.[63,219]

Deep venous thrombosis prophylaxis

Immobility, fractures, soft tissue trauma, and venous catheterizations for blood drawing and monitoring are common after TBI, and create significant risk for development of deep venous thrombosis (DVT) of both the upper and lower limbs. DVT occurs in 16–54% of all TBI cases, including nearly 20% of all individuals with TBI admitted to inpatient rehabilitation units.[43,188] Studies have demonstrated that screening of all patients for DVT before admission to the rehabilitation unit is cost-effective.[43,188] Morbidity and possible fatality from pulmonary embolism warrant aggressive preventive measures. The postphlebitic syndrome is also a potential problem. It is a chronic condition characterized by intermittent limb swelling with associated pain; varicosities; skin changes; and elevated risk for skin breakdown, infection, and recurrent DVT. It occurs in as many as 30% of untreated patients with DVT. It is important to note that the incidence of upper limb DVTs, with the associated risk of pulmonary embolus, might be as high in these patients as lower limb DVT's.[253]

Swelling, pain, and provocative maneuvers such as Homan's sign are not consistently present in patients with a DVT. Therefore, standardized screening tests are indicated in all patients at risk (i.e. all patients with a TBI necessitating inpatient or skilled nursing facility–level rehabilitation stay, as well as those with limited mobility). Doppler ultrasound is a non-invasive, relatively easy, and sensitive diagnostic tool in detecting DVT. Impedance plethysmography is of similar sensitivity but is less often used. D-dimer assay is highly sensitive for DVT, but is of poor specificity because it is often positive due to the initial trauma. While venography remains the gold standard in detecting DVT, it is also invasive, carries a risk for DVT and bleeding, and is rarely clinically necessary.

Prophylaxis for DVT (Box 50-2) should be carefully considered for all individuals with TBI on acute admission to the hospital. Graded compression stockings are of low utility.[84] The presence of intracranial bleeds and the postsurgical state often delay the decision to start chemical prophylaxis. A clinical standard is unfortunately still not available to predict which patients with TBI specifically require chemical prophylaxis with anticoagulants, which prophylaxis is maximally effective, and when to begin such therapy. For example, prepubescent children have minimal risk and are rarely prophylaxed. Generally, a minimum of 5000 units of unfractionated heparin sodium subcutaneously administered every 12 h is recommended for

---

Box 50-2 Managing deep venous thrombosis risk after traumatic brain injury

- Encourage early ambulation and mobility in all patients, as soon as injury allows.
- TED hose and aspirin do not reduce deep venous thrombosis (DVT) risk.
- Thigh-high intermittent compression devices help reduce DVT risk but are not appropriate primary prophylaxis.
- Duplex Doppler ultrasonography has been shown to have clinical utility and is cost-effective in all patients admitted for inpatient rehabilitation.
- Utilize 5000 units of subcutaneous unfractionated heparin sodium in all patients who are not fully ambulatory in 24 h (may be utilized 12 h after surgery for control of major bleeding).
- Utilize prophylactic dosing of low molecular weight heparin sodium in all patients with long bone fractures, prior DVT, or > 4 total risk factors for DVT (may be utilized 36–72 h after major trauma or 12 h postoperatively).
- Vena cava filters alone are not appropriate DVT prophylaxis. Appropriate chemical prophylaxis should be initiated as soon as is feasible.
- All upper extremity and lower extremity DVTs must be treated with adjusted dose warfarin or low molecular weight heparin for at least 3 months.

---

all individuals with a TBI who are unable to resume full mobility within 24 h. If surgery is required or active bleeding prevents such anticoagulation, thigh-high intermittent compression devices should be used temporarily. The subcutaneous heparin should be reinstituted as early as 12 h after surgery has been completed or bleeding has been controlled. Patients with long bone or pelvic fractures, prior DVT or other coagulopathies, or other identified elevated risk for DVT should be considered for more intensive anticoagulation with low molecular weight heparin (LMWH) until fully mobilized.[84,114] The earliest proven safe time period for initiating this prophylaxis is a minimum of 36 h post TBI.[83]

Seizure prophylaxis

Symptomatic seizures are an important complication following TBI, with potentially consequent functional limitation and social isolation. The incidence of such seizures varies depending on time after injury and several risk factors. *Late seizures*, defined as occurring 7 days or more post TBI, affect 14–53% of moderate to severe TBI survivors.[68] They also account for 5% of all epilepsy and 20% of symptomatic epilepsy.[106,270] *Immediate seizures* occur within 24 h, whereas *early seizures* occur after 1 day but before 7 days post injury. The work of Temkin and colleagues demonstrated a significant reduction in the incidence of early, but not late, seizures using prophylaxis with phenytoin for the first 7 days post TBI.[260] The American Academy of Physical Medicine and Rehabilitation and the American Association of Neurological Surgeons now recommend such prophylaxis as a treatment standard (see Box 50-3).

Box 50-3 Managing posttraumatic seizure risk

- All patients with a postresuscitation Glasgow Coma Scale score < 12 require 7 days of post-traumatic brain injury therapeutic phenytoin sodium. Longer prophylaxis has not been shown to be beneficial.
- Immediate (< 24 h post injury) posttraumatic seizures do not require any additional prophylaxis after 7 days.
- Early (24 h to 7 days post injury) seizures should be treated with at least 12 months of an antiepileptic medication, unless a time-limited intracranial abnormality was causal (e.g. hydrocephalus, infection, and active hemorrhage).
- Late (> 7 days post injury) seizures should be treated with an antiepileptic medication for at least 12 months.
- Any seizure that lasts > 2 min (i.e. status epilepticus) warrants treatment with an antiepileptic medication for at least 12 months.

Box 50-4 Rehabilitation assessment after traumatic brain injury

- Serial neurologic, medical, and functional (including swallowing) examinations.
- Monitoring participation and progress in formal therapy and nursing care.
- Ensure appropriate prophylactic treatments (e.g. deep venous thrombosis, seizure, and removal of Foley catheters) are being performed.
- Assessment of patient's preinjury status and current social support systems.
- Assessment of patient's resources for rehabilitation needs. Facilitating procurement of necessary additional resources.
- Partnering with acute care team to optimize care, communicate with patient and family, and plan and institute rehabilitation program.

REHABILITATION MANAGEMENT (see Fig. 50-4)

Inpatient consultation

Rehabilitation services after TBI should begin as soon as the individual is admitted to the hospital. These services include appropriate preventive care, active medical management, family education, and supportive therapies (e.g. positioning, range of motion, establishing communication and cognition status, and self-care activities). Individuals who are assessed in the emergency department only, but not admitted to the hospital, should be reassessed by a skilled brain injury specialist (preferably a physiatrist) in the first several weeks after injury. For inpatients, early rehabilitative interventions can prepare the patient for more formal services as medical stability and brain recovery allow. Specific activity retraining (e.g. muscle strengthening) might need to wait until discharge from the intensive care unit (ICU) or at least 3–4 days post injury. All individuals with acute physical, cognitive, behavioral, and/or functional deficits as a result of a TBI should receive the most intensive rehabilitation appropriate in the least restrictive environment possible in order to maximize outcome. A return to the most familiar, preinjury living environment is the first choice for discharge. When this is not feasible, another community setting (family member's home, adult group home, or assisted living) is a good second option.

When an individual with TBI is admitted to the hospital, the physiatrist should perform serial evaluations of progress to optimize acute care and help to establish an aftercare program. Follow-up rehabilitation consultations entail both an assessment of the ongoing medical and functional needs, as well as an assessment of the individual's response to rehabilitation interventions (e.g. medication and therapy). When an individual no longer requires inpatient medical or surgical care, a definitive recommendation should be made for ongoing rehabilitation care. This recommendation can range from transfer to an inpatient brain injury rehabilitation unit, to a non-inpatient setting for ongoing focused therapies, to outpatient physician clinic follow-up. A variety of alternatives to traditional inpatient rehabilitation for individuals with brain injury have developed in the past 10 years in the USA. While financial factors have been a major driving force, the need for either a less intensive or a less restrictive treatment setting for many individuals has also played an important role. The advent of automobile air bags and improved resuscitation and neurosurgical techniques has allowed for increased survival from even severe TBI, often with less physical and cognitive impairment than in the past.[8,24,56,71,255,268,293] These individuals might move through the acute and inpatient rehabilitation settings more rapidly, but still require some degree of services. A second group of individuals, who might not have previously survived the initial injury, are left with devastating impairments that do not allow them to participate fully in traditional rehabilitation services. While efficacy data supporting the utility of alternative rehabilitation programs for specific diagnostic groups are limited and variable, they do offer therapeutic options for those patients who do not meet traditional admission criteria. Fitting the needs and resources of an individual who has survived a TBI into these therapeutic options, as part of continuum of available rehabilitation services in a community, is a key role of the physiatrist and is vital to successfully reintegrate these individuals back into society.

Physiatric assessment

Physiatric assessment after TBI (Box 50-4) should occur as soon after the injury as is logistically feasible, optimally in the first 24 h. Clearly, individuals who are medically or surgically unstable will be able to undergo only limited examinations; however, substantial information may still be obtained regarding injury characteristics, premorbid issues, social supports available, and understanding family goals. As soon as possible, a comprehensive assessment of the acute medical and neurologic status of the individual should be performed. In individuals with moderate to severe TBI, particular attention should be paid to the following areas: DVT prophylaxis, posttraumatic seizure prophylaxis, feeding and nutritional status, neuroendocrine disturbances, bowel functioning, bladder management, pain control, skin care, sleep hygiene, fluctuation in cognition, and behavioral issues.[32] Serial neurologic examinations should be done, focusing on level of alertness and attention, awareness of environment, command following, extremity movement and coordination, and balance. Information gleaned from these examinations can provide the acute therapy treatment team with useful information on ways to optimally interact with the patient. In older adults in particular, an assessment of the clinical manifestations of cerebrovascular, cardiovascular, metabolic, pulmonary, bone, and joint disease allows one to best structure the rehabilitation interventions. All appropriate rehabilitation therapies, including physical therapy, occupational therapy, and speech and language pathology, should be initiated as soon as the injured individual can be assessed and determined to be able to tolerate this activity. Appropriate positioning and joint range of motion can be initiated immediately, while more functional tasks might need to wait until ICPs are normal and intensive neurosurgical procedures (e.g. ventriculostomies and other cerebrospinal drains) are completed.

In individuals with mild TBI, there will typically be less of a focus on physical abilities and medical issues, and more of a focus on an assessment of cognitive and behavioral functioning. Occasionally, emergency room physicians, traumatologists, intensivists, and even neurosurgeons can miss the presence of some of the more subtle sequelae of a mild TBI. Consequently, a heightened awareness for mild TBI must accompany all assessments of trauma victims. New cognitive findings in individuals with preexisting deficits can also be overlooked, such as in a nursing home resident after a fall. The rehabilitation consultant should evaluate these individuals closely. Focused and often rapidly delivered education must be provided to the patient, family, and caretakers on common difficulties. Appropriate outpatient referrals should be made for follow-up care (e.g. return to school or work, return to driving, increase in level of nursing home care, and postconcussive syndrome care). Formal neuropsychologic evaluations have little role in this acute period but can prove to be invaluable in the postacute phase of rehabilitation. Individuals with mild TBI who have had only an alteration, but no loss, of consciousness will not typically undergo extensive diagnostic testing (e.g. a head CT scan) or be counseled regarding their potential short- and long-term deficits. The persistence of neurologic deficits, particularly in the areas of balance, cognition, behavior, headache, and auditory and visual processing, for more than 2 weeks after a defined mild TBI is often labeled 'postconcussive syndrome'. While full recovery is common, rapid, structured, and skilled assessment and care is vital to optimize long-term outcome.

The rehabilitation approach to an individual who has sustained a TBI is similar to the general rehabilitation approach, with additional attention paid to the neurologic system and areas of secondary injury. An understanding of preinjury activity levels (including school or work level, as appropriate), cognitive limitations, behavioral issues, and chronic medical conditions is vital. This information assists in the assessment of the potential physiologic reserve present prior to acute injury. This can assist in the acute determination of an individual's readiness and

appropriateness for specific rehabilitation interventions (i.e. specificity, intensity, and goal setting for therapies). A thorough review of the patient's preinjury and current medication routine is important in optimizing treatments. For example, premorbid medications might not have been restarted, and numerous medications that are especially cognitive-impairing might no longer be necessary. This review can also define therapy parameters (e.g. anticoagulant use and antihypertensive use) and prevent secondary conditions (e.g. antithrombotics are often underutilized in the frail older adult patient).

A complete rehabilitation assessment must include a comprehensive review of the social support network relevant to the individual with TBI, which involves an understanding of both the formal and the informal support systems available. Formal support systems in the USA include federal (Medicare and Social Security), state (Medicaid, Department of Rehabilitation Services, welfare, and area agencies on aging), and local (adult day health programs, school systems, transportation, and Meals on Wheels) resources. Informal support systems include family, friends, and religious affiliations. Early involvement of family and friends in planning and implementing the rehabilitation program is vital. Many older adults tend to have significant others who are older, disabled, or deceased. This makes it more likely that they will need to have increased involvement of extended families in their systems of support. Daughters and female caregivers are more likely to play a major support role, particularly a physical or hands-on one, than male caregivers. It is essential to clearly understand the individual's premorbid and/or present role in the social structure to which you are attempting to return them. It is also important to assess the role of organized religion in the individual's life, and the goals of the patient and the caregiver (e.g. are they the same?), and determine if there are any applicable advance directives. Sensitivity to cultural factors is needed in working successfully within existing support systems.

A working knowledge of the most common funding mechanisms available for post-TBI care is extremely important. In the USA, 98% of older adults are primarily funded by Medicare. The majority of the chronically disabled also have Medicare funding. Recent changes to Medicare reimbursement for inpatient care have resulted in a reduction in funding for TBI care (in older adults) that might have an impact on future referral and resource utilization patterns.[109] Medicare is a federally sponsored program with uniform coverage across the USA. Increasingly, however, managed-care Medicare plans are becoming available that have variable benefits. Medicaid is a state-sponsored program (e.g. MediCal in California). It funds health insurance for the medically indigent, pregnant women, and children. Medicaid inpatient, outpatient, home health, nursing home, durable medical equipment, and physician benefits vary from state to state. Numerous managed-care Medicaid programs have recently become available, which has further increased the diversity of covered services. In Canada, Australia, New Zealand, and most European countries, the government funds the overwhelming majority of rehabilitation care. Other sources of coverage for individuals with TBI can include commercial insurance, workers' compensation (for work and workplace-related injuries), and auto insurance coverage (for those involved in auto accidents) for their rehabilitation services. An understanding of the resources these different payment sources make available and an open communication with the insurer or designated case manager is important in optimizing care.

Prognosis (Box 50-5)

The initial severity of TBI is one of the major factors that 'predict' the short-term (up to 3 months) and long-term outcomes after TBI.[24] Greater severity of TBI, as measured by GCS score in the first 7 days post injury, coma duration, and pupillary dilatation, has been associated with poorer outcomes on measures of global functioning such as the Glasgow Outcome Scale (GOS).[117] The addition of brain stem reflex measurement to the GCS score, measuring the so-called Glasgow–Liège Scale score, adds even greater predictive value.[22] MEPs appear to have similar sensitivity in augmenting the gross predictive value of the GCS and other acute severity measures.[96,122,216] Additional prognostic factors include increased ICP (> 20 mmHg for more than 24 h),[24] decreased cerebral blood flow (< 18 mL/100 g per min),[23] and hypoxic injuries.[273] These measures unfortunately have only limited value in prognosticating the specific outcomes of individual patients, and consequently have more of a research than a clinical utility.[193,194] Duration of PTA might have a better clinical utility in correlating with lengths of rehabilitation needs and outcomes, especially in patients with DAI.[127,225] Additional factors that might have clinical utility in outcome 'prediction',

include age,[45] Disability Rating Scale (DRS) score at rehabilitation admission,[208] early assessment of balance,[96] and presence of acute medical complications.[69] Overall, however, the actual predictive value of these factors is small.

The assumption is often made that brain injury in children has a better prognosis for functional and cognitive recovery due to brain *plasticity*. This term describes structural and functional adaptations of the brain after injury. It is also assumed that the younger the child, the more plasticity the injured brain possesses. Unfortunately, research has not supported this assumption.[231] The brain injury might greatly impair development of a child's full potential, or even result in a specific motor or cognitive dysfunction. Worsening of impairments and appearance of new impairments have also been observed in children maturing after TBI.[2]

Outcome measures

The GOS and the Glasgow Outcome Scale—Extended (GOS-E) are the most widely used outcome measures in TBI research, in particular in acute-care clinical trials.[74,116] Their clinical utility is limited by the global nature of their measurement. The GOS is a five-point scale (death and vegetative state plus three levels of independent functioning) that can be completed in less than 30 s. While it is extremely easy to complete, the lack of specific, objective criteria that separate the three functional levels limit its accuracy (see Table 50-3). The eight-level GOS-E is more sensitive to changes in functioning, and the increased divisions of functioning allow for more accurate assessment. However, the need for a structured interview increases the time to complete this scale (see Table 50-4). The DRS is a measure of neurologic status and the cognitive ability to perform functional tasks, and provides a somewhat more patient-specific measure that has utility in both research and clinical realms (see Table 50-5).[215] The utility of the DRS is greatly limited by the need for input from multiple treatment team members over the course of several days to accurately portray an individual's level of functioning. Inter- and intrarater reliability is often poor. The Rancho Los Amigos Levels of Cognitive Functioning Scale is a useful descriptive tool for both clinicians and family members to identify and follow an individual patient's cognitive and behavioral functioning on an eight-point scale (see Table

---

Box 50-5 Factors useful in determining prognosis postacutely after traumatic brain injury

- Duration of coma
- Duration of posttraumatic amnesia (especially with diffuse axonal injury)
- Age (> 55 years)
- Disability Rating Scale score (at rehabilitation admission)
- Sitting and standing balance
- Presence of medical complications

Table 50-3 Glasgow Outcome Scale

Patient's abilities	Definition	Score
Death	–	1
Persistent vegetative state	No cerebral cortical function as judged behaviorally; unable to interact with environment; unresponsive	2
Severe disability	Conscious and able to follow commands but dependent on 24-h care and unable to live independently	3
Moderate disability	Disabled but capable of independent care; unable to return to work or school	4
Good recovery	Mild impairment with persistent sequelae but able to participate in a normal social life, including able to return to work or school	5

Table 50-4 Glasgow Outcome Scale—extended[a]

Patient's abilities	Score
Death	1
Persistent vegetative state	2
Lower severe disability	3
Upper severe disability	4
Lower moderate disability	5
Upper moderate disability	6
Lower good recovery	7
Upper good recovery	8

[a]Directed interview required to complete.

Table 50-5 Disability Rating Scale

	Score[a]
Patient's response	
Eye opening	0–3
Verbal	0–4
Motor	0–4
Cognitive ability for feeding	0–3
Cognitive ability for toileting	0–3
Cognitive ability for grooming	0–3
Dependence on others	0–5
Employability	0–3
Summed total	0–30
Disability	
No disability	0
Mild disability	1
Partial disability	2–3
Moderate disability	4–6
Moderately severe disability	7–11
Severe disability	12–16
Extremely severe disability	17–21
Vegetative state	22–24
Extreme vegetative state	25–29
Death	30

[a]0, No disability.

50-6).[101] It has limited research utility but is a practical clinical measure for categorizing patients. The Functional Independence Measure (FIM)[94] and associated pediatric version (WeeFIM)[201] are widely used in brain injury rehabilitation centers. The limited cognitive and behavioral focus of these measures, however, restricts their practical utility in individuals with TBI. A modified version of the FIM, with expanded cognitive and behavioral measures, called the Functional Assessment Measure (FAM),[102] was used for a brief period of time in clinical and research arena but has limited current use.

Rehabilitation settings (Table 50-7)

Inpatient, interdisciplinary rehabilitation units have been the standard post-TBI care setting for more than 30 years in the USA. Distinct units (often separate, secured sections or floors of more generalized rehabilitation units) specialized for the rehabilitation of individuals with TBI have been the preferred settings. These units provide on average 3 h/day of structured therapy, 24 h/day nursing services, daily physician services, and an interdisciplinary model of care.[44] Limited research supports the advantages of this model over non-specialized settings.[234] A greater intensity of inpatient services, particularly cognitively focused therapies, has been associated with improved outcomes.[44] Individuals who are most appropriate for maximally intensive (≥15 h per week of formal therapy services) interdisciplinary rehabilitation programs are those demonstrating the following characteristics:

- an acute or new brain injury-related disability that is significantly below premorbid baseline abilities;
- a support system that permits return to the community (i.e. a residential setting);
- the ability to tolerate, participate in, and improve with therapies; and
- appropriate funding to pay for services and aftercare needs.

Individuals who are particularly frail due to advanced age, premorbid medical conditions, or the severity and/or complexity of the new TBI might have difficulty tolerating the intensity of 3 h per day therapy services. These individuals might not be able to benefit maximally from inpatient rehabilitation. If they can be safely treated in the community, then a progressively more intensive home or outpatient therapy program might be beneficial. If they cannot be safely treated in the community, an institutionally based program of subacute rehabilitation services might be optimal. Individuals who can benefit from 3 or more hours of structured therapy a day, but who do not require inpatient management, are best treated in a day rehabilitation program. The admission and discharge criteria for these specialty programs vary considerably from site to site.

Subacute programs offer lower intensity, interdisciplinary rehabilitation settings designed to meet the needs of individuals with acute and often devastating disabilities who are not yet able to return home, and who cannot tolerate the level of intensity of services provided in a traditional rehabilitation unit (and thus comply with the so-called 'three-hour rule').[42,252,272] These individuals would otherwise remain in the acute units (or

Table 50-6 Rancho Los Amigos Levels of Cognitive Functioning Scale[a]

Patient's abilities	Level
No response The individual appears to be in deep sleep and is completely unresponsive to any stimuli.	1
Generalized response The individual reacts inconsistently and non-purposefully to stimuli. Responses are limited in nature and often the same regardless of the stimuli presented. Responses may include gross motor movements, vocalization, and physiologic changes. Response time is likely to be delayed. Deep pain evokes the earliest response.	2
Localized response The individual responds specifically but inconsistently to stimulus. Responses are directly related to the type of stimuli presented. For example, an individual's head will turn toward a sound or his or her eyes will focus on an object when presented. The individual may follow simple commands and may respond better to some people (i.e. family and friends) than to others.	3
Confused: agitated The individual is in a heightened state of activity, with severely decreased ability to process information. Behavior is non-purposeful relative to the immediate environment. Attempts to climb out of bed, remove restraints, and hostility are common. The individual requires maximum assistance to perform self-care activities. An individual may sit, reach, or walk, but will not necessarily perform these activities on request.	4
Confused: inappropriate The individual appears alert and responds to simple commands fairly consistently. Agitation, which is out of proportion (but directly related) to stimuli, may be evident. Lack of external structure results in random or non-purposeful responses. Inappropriate verbalizations and high distractibility are common. Memory is severely impaired, but the individual may self-feed with supervision and requires only assistance for self-care activities.	5
Confused: appropriate The individual shows goal-oriented behavior but is dependent on external input for direction. Response to discomfort is appropriate. Responses are incorrect due to memory problems, but are appropriate to the situation. Simple commands are followed consistently, and carryover for relearned activities is evident. Orientation is inconsistent, but awareness of self, family, and basic needs is increased.	6
Automatic: appropriate The individual appears appropriate within hospital and home settings, goes through daily routine automatically, but is robotlike, with shallow recall of activities performed. Has absent to minimal confusion and lacks insight. The individual frequently demonstrates poor judgment and problem solving, and expresses unrealistic future plans. With structure, the individual is able to initiate tasks or social and recreational activities.	7
Purposeful: appropriate The individual is alert and oriented, able to recall and integrate past and recent events, and is aware of and responsive to the environment. Independence in the home and community has returned. Carryover for new learning is present, and the need for supervision is absent once activities have been learned. Social, emotional, and cognitive abilities may still be decreased.	8

[a]The Rancho Los Amigos Levels of Cognitive Functioning (RLA) were designed to measure and track an individual's progress early in the recovery period. They have been used as a means to develop 'level-specific' treatment interventions and strategies designed to facilitate movement from one level to another. An RLA level is determined based on behavioral observations.

even ICUs) of hospitals for extended periods of time, due to the complexity of their medical issues and their tendency to develop significant complications. If transferred to custodial nursing homes or returned home, they are likely to worsen medically and lose functional skills, frequently requiring hospital readmission.

On transfer to a subacute rehabilitation program, individuals must demonstrate the ability to functionally benefit from this ongoing lower intensity therapy (specifically physical therapy and occupational therapy, as speech and language pathology services are utilized only intermittently). Subacute programs are particularly well suited for individuals with severe TBI or non-traumatic brain injury who have persistent altered consciousness (coma or near-coma), prolonged ICU or acute-care stays with resultant severe deconditioning, or previously deconditioning (e.g. frail elder) or preexisting disabilities (e.g. prior stroke). These patients often require significant amounts of nursing and medical care, including wound care, tracheostomy and feeding tube management, and infection treatment interventions. Programs typically provide from 1 to 2 h of individual therapy time a day, with the remainder of the day spent with nursing staff focusing on improved physical tolerance and

Table 50-7 Rehabilitation settings after traumatic brain injury

Setting	Service intensity	Common deficits
Acute care (hospital)	30–90 min of physical therapy (PT), occupational therapy (OT), and speech and language pathology (SLP) 5–7 times/week. 1–3 times/week physiatry assessment. Intense nursing care.	Full range of motoric, cognitive, behavioral, and communication deficits.
Subacute (skilled nursing facility or specialty unit)	30–120 min of PT and OT 5–6 times/week. Intermittent SLP evaluation. 1–3 times/week physiatry evaluation. Intense nursing care. Intermittent social work.	Significant generalized motoric, cognitive, and communication deficits. Also for significant non-weight-bearing limitations. Significant spasticity with high contracture and skin breakdown risk. Usually Rancho Los Amigos Scale (RLAS) of 1–3, but occasional agitation. Hypoarousal common.
Inpatient rehabilitation	2–4 h of PT, OT, SLP, and psychology 5–7 times/week. 5–7 times/week physiatry evaluation. Moderate nursing care. Intensive social work.	Moderate focal to generalized motoric, cognitive, behavioral, and communication deficits. RLAS 4–6. Decreased attention and agitation common.
Day	2–4 h of PT, OT, SLP, and psychology 5 times/week. Minimal to moderate nursing care and social work. 1–2 times/week physiatry evaluation. Increasing therapeutic recreation and vocational involvement. Transportation usually available.	Moderate focal to mild generalized motoric (usually imbalance), cognitive, and communication deficits. Occasional behavioral dysfunction. RLAS 5–7.
Outpatient	30–90 min of PT, OT, SLP, and psychology 3 times/week. Physiatry evaluation every 1–3 months. Increasing therapeutic recreation and vocational involvement.	Mild to moderate focal motoric, cognitive, and communication deficits. Intermittent behavioral dysfunction may be amenable. RLAS 5–8.
Home	30–60 min of PT and OT 2–3 times/week. Physiatry evaluation every 1–3 months. Rare SLP available.	Significant generalized motoric deficits or weight-bearing limitations. May be used to train family or slowly improve endurance. Rarely effective.

medical stability. Physical and occupational therapy provide the mainstay of therapy services, with speech and language pathology services used more for assessment purposes. Neuropsychology services are rarely available. These programs are traditionally located in specialized areas of nursing homes (so-called skilled nursing facilities or SNFs), rehabilitation units, or acute hospitals. Therapy services are typically offered 5–6 days per week.

Physical therapy in a subacute setting tends to focus on maintaining and increasing range of motion, modulating extremity tone, improving tolerance to sitting or standing, and basic mobility tasks (e.g. transfers and early ambulation skills). Similarly, occupational therapy addresses maintaining and increasing range of motion, modulating extremity tone, facilitating functional tasks in sitting, and basic activities of daily living skills training. Cotreatment between the physical therapies and occupational therapies is common, to allow for advancing functional activities during standing activities. Intermittent speech and language pathology services (i.e. one or two times weekly) are predominantly utilized in this setting for monitoring and upgrading swallowing abilities (e.g. upgrading diets) and to improve basic communication skills. Nursing care focuses on monitoring health status, replicating activities performed in physical or occupational therapy sessions, promoting maximal time out of bed, and patient and family education. Physician involvement

is often once or twice weekly and is focused on facilitating interdisciplinary activities of the team, ongoing medical monitoring, medication adjustments, patient and family education, and liaising with other medical professionals. Physician management can include both a physiatrist and an internist, based on the acuity of medical involvement. Case management and social work services are also an integral aspect of a subacute rehabilitation program, but often these services are integrated into other team member's roles.

The admission criteria of subacute rehabilitation programs are similar to those of inpatient rehabilitation units. Functional progress, however, might be anticipated in different areas (e.g. time out of bed, sitting tolerance, and participating in therapy) and at a different pace (e.g. objective gains every 2–3 weeks). Regularly scheduled interdisciplinary team meetings and monthly educational sessions, as well as regular unscheduled interactions as needed, are keys to success. These interdisciplinary activities are the differentiating features that allow subacute rehabilitation programs to succeed with highly challenging patients, when seemingly similar physical therapy and occupational therapy services in an acute or a custodial nursing home more frequently do not.

Lengths of stay are dictated by the needs and progress of the patients, and can range from 4 to 16 weeks. A patient must require at least two therapy disciplines and daily nursing or physician care to remain in the program. Costs range (depending on therapy needs and intensity) from $300 to $1500 per day, which is comparable with the cost of inpatient care. Insurance coverage is often available, usually as a specialized benefit.

Day programs are intense, interdisciplinary rehabilitation settings designed to meet the needs of individuals with acute disabilities (or exacerbations of underlying chronic conditions) who are no longer hospitalized but require ongoing therapy (at least two disciplines), nursing, and medical care.[176,284] Patients are more likely to have cognitive and behavioral impairments limiting their function than individuals who qualify for inpatient rehabilitation stays (the inpatients are typically physically, medically, cognitively, and behaviorally impaired). Programs typically provide up to 3 h of individual therapy time, in addition to structured group activities. While the traditional physical therapy, occupational therapy, and speech and language pathology are a mainstay of treatment, increasing emphasis is placed on neuropsychologic and therapeutic recreation services. Day rehabilitation programs are usually offered 5 days per week, and can be full-day or half-day treatments. Lower intensity options (e.g. 3 days per week) are often used to initiate disabled individuals who have significant concomitant deconditioning into a gradual reconditioning program, or to offer older individuals a 'trial' period to assess their ability to tolerate the program. Treatment sites are usually located in the community (as opposed to at a major medical center) to facilitate access and allow greater availability of 'real life' settings for disabled individuals to be trained. Van transportation to the location(s) is commonly provided.

Physical therapy, occupational therapy, and speech and language pathology specialists address traditional skills training in day rehabilitation programs, although usually for patients with a higher level of physical functioning than those admitted to an inpatient unit. Neuropsychologic services focus on cognitive and behavioral deficits that might prevent successful maintenance in the home environment and successful return to productivity (work, school, chores, hobbies, driving, etc.). Neuropsychologists are often team leaders of these programs, particularly when TBI is the primary focus. Therapeutic recreation specialists focus on both leisure skills retraining and community reintegration. Community outings address advanced activities of daily living training (shopping and errands), driving, prevocational skills, and leisure. Daily nursing care is a vital component of an interdisciplinary day rehabilitation program, because it often is necessary to allow the disabled individual to remain out of the hospital setting. These services often include medication management, wound care, laboratory and vital signs monitoring, tube feeding, and liaising with medical providers. Other interventions include patient and family education and teaching, bowel and bladder care training, and assessing day to day health status. Physician involvement is often once or twice weekly, and focused on facilitating interdisciplinary activities of the team, ongoing medical monitoring (e.g. anticoagulation levels), medication adjustments, patient and family education, and liaising with other medical professionals. Case management and social work services are also an integral aspect of a day rehabilitation program; however, often these tasks are integrated into other team member's roles.

Day rehabilitation programs admission criteria are similar to those of inpatient rehabilitation units. However, functional progress might be anticipated in different areas (e.g. balance skills, high-level cognitively based activities of daily living tasks, and community reintegration) and at a different pace (e.g. objective gains every 2 weeks). The keys to success include regularly scheduled interdisciplinary team meetings and monthly educational sessions, as well as regular unscheduled interactions as needed. These interdisciplinary activities are the differentiating features that allow day rehabilitation programs to succeed with highly challenging patients, where seemingly similar outpatient or home health therapy programs do not. Lengths of stay are dictated by the needs and progress of the patients, and range from 2 to 8 weeks, based on ongoing needs and demonstrated functional progress. A patient must require at least two therapy disciplines and weekly nursing and physician care to remain in the program. Costs range (depending on therapy needs and intensity) from $200 to $500 per day, which is comparable with home or outpatient therapy services and approximately one-third the cost of inpatient care. Insurance coverage is often available, either as a specialized benefit or as a combination of individualized therapy billings.

Deep venous thrombosis management

Treatment of DVT and pulmonary embolus requires anticoagulation generally for at least 3 and 6 months, respectively.[114] Some debate exists as to whether a DVT distal to the popliteal fossa should be treated, due to much lower risk of embolization.[114] Proponents cite the possibility of developing postphlebitic syndrome, as well as the elevated risk of extension or propagation of the thrombus without treatment. All upper limb thromboses above the wrist warrant similar treatment as that for lower extremity DVT.[114] Mobilization of the patient should be restricted to bed rest for the first 24 h after detection of a thrombus, but can be liberalized once full anticoagulation is achieved. LMWH is particularly practical in the acute rehabilitation phase, as the patient is not encumbered with an intravenous line and frequent laboratory work is not necessary. While full anticoagulation with LMWH can be used as the sole long-term treatment, patients are typically transitioned to oral anticoagulation with warfarin. Warfarin is usually given in combination with LMWH until the international normalized ratio (INR) reaches a level of 2. Thereafter, the INR should be maintained at a level between 2 and 3 by adjusting the warfarin dosage. Changes in INR typically require at least 3 days of dosing, so too-frequent laboratory assessment or dose changes are not recommended. There is also no role for initial bolus dosing with warfarin. Anticoagulation of the agitated, impulsive, medically frail, elderly, or mobility-impaired individual warrants careful consideration and diligent monitoring due to elevated fall, bleeding, and non-compliance risks. Vena cava (or Greenfield) filters are generally reserved for patients who develop pulmonary emboli despite full anticoagulation, or for patients with DVT in whom the anticoagulation is contraindicated.[114] These filters are of questionable long-term efficacy, and pulmonary embolus can occur despite their placement.[220]

Seizure management

Posttraumatic seizures occurring after the first week following TBI affect 14–53% of moderate to severe TBI survivors,[68] and account for 5% of all epilepsy and 20% of symptomatic epilepsy.[106,270] In patients who will develop posttraumatic seizures, the initial onset of late seizures occurs in more than half of patients within 1 year post injury and in about 76% within 2 years.[106,270] The identification of high-risk patients and targeting prophylaxis accordingly has not been shown to be effective,[260] but risk factors for the development of late seizures have been identified. A recent multicenter study identified imaging abnormalities and corresponding risk for posttraumatic epilepsy.[68] Seizures most often followed biparietal contusion, followed by dural penetration with metal fragments, multiple intracranial surgeries, subdural hematoma with evacuation, midline shift greater than 5 mm, and multiple or bilateral cortical contusions. Surprisingly, the study found severity of TBI measured with initial GCS score not to be predictive of subsequent late seizure. Other studies have shown that injury severity is predictive of early and late seizures. These studies have also identified such factors as chronic alcoholism, age, intracranial hemorrhage, length of PTA, depressed skull fracture, lesion location, and early glucocorticoid administration.[5,68,70,92,276] Prophylaxis for late seizures longer than the universally recognized standard of 7 days post injury in response to a perceived elevated risk, such as the above-mentioned factors, warrants further investigation and is not at present recommended.

Regardless of etiology, the development of late seizures warrants treatment (see Fig. 50-7). Complex partial seizures are the most common presentation, followed by simple partial and then generalized or tonic–clonic seizures. Absence seizures are rare following TBI. The use of carbamazepine for the management of partial seizures and valproate for generalized posttraumatic epilepsy has been advocated.[289] Phenytoin, carbamazepine, valproate, and phenobarbital are all sedating and probably somewhat detrimental to cognition and long-term neurologic recovery.[60] Newer agents, while often less sedating and easier to use, are less studied specifically for TBI-related late seizures.[60] Lamotrigine might improve post-TBI mood and behavior, and be less sedating than older medications. Gabapentin is more often used as second-line adjuvant seizure medication or first-line neuropathic pain treatment, but it can be sedating. Topiramate (Topamax) can precipitate psychosis and depression, but this is less likely if the medication is started at a low dose.

Several theories explaining the etiology of late seizures have been postulated and could lead to new treatment and prevention. Seizure threshold is probably lowered through 'disinhibition' of excitatory neural cells. The recovery of such inhibition has been seen to occur in animal models within 1 week. Such temporary loss of inhibition might lead to cellular reorganization and raise the likelihood of later epilepsy. Recent animal

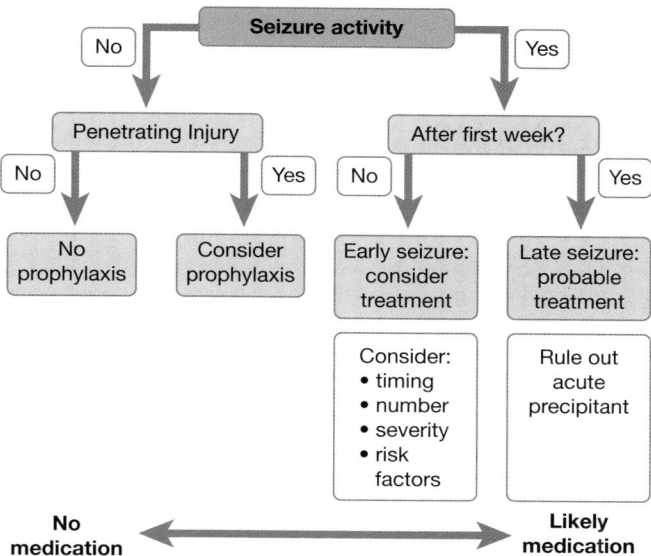

Figure 50-7 Guidelines for the initiation of antiepileptic medications.

studies in which delayed seizure was induced revealed anatomic changes described as 'mossy fiber sprouting' in coronal brain sections. These findings were reproduced in studies in which seizure was induced by a different method.[290] The immediate administration of antiepileptic medication after TBI has been shown to reduce delayed seizure in similar models.[291] Human studies are needed in this regard.

Swallowing and feeding

Providing sufficient nutrition in a safe and tolerable manner is vital after TBI. The hypermetabolic state described after brain injury is more difficult to alleviate due to commonly occurring post-TBI sequelae, including dysphagia, gastroparesis, gastric ulcer, abnormal tone, cognitive impairment, and nausea. Adequate enteral nutrition that is initiated within 24 h of injury and meets caloric requirements has been demonstrated to result in fewer postinjury complications.[257]

Total parenteral nutrition has been previously avoided due to fear of increasing serum osmolality and exacerbating ICP.[292] Several studies have demonstrated no such result from total parenteral nutrition. The initiation of total parenteral nutrition is advocated if caloric demands with enteral feeding are not met by 72 h after injury.

Dysphagia, or impaired swallowing, affects 25–60% of TBI inpatients admitted for rehabilitation (see Ch. 28).[292] Aspiration, the penetration of oral contents beyond the vocal folds, occurs in as many as 42% of TBI patients. The development of aspiration pneumonia is a serious sequela, with a 10% mortality rate. Cranial nerve involvement, oral and pharyngeal trauma, cognitive impairment, and impaired airway function all can contribute to dysphagia.[73] Field and Weiss identified the following most common problems of swallowing in descending frequency: prolonged oral transit, delayed swallowing reflex, valleculae pooling, and pyriform sinus pooling. Delayed or absent swallow reflex has been demonstrated in 81% of patients with moderate to severe TBI, followed by reduced tongue control (50%) and reduced esophageal peristalsis (33%).[73]

Bedside evaluation of swallow has poor sensitivity, as nearly 40% of aspiration is 'silent' or without symptoms.[164,285] Evaluation using dynamic radiographic or endoscopic techniques is consequently the standard of care. Any doubt of a patient's ability to swallow warrants study by these methods, which have been demonstrated to have acceptable sensitivity.[73,98,191] Videofluoroscopy or modified barium swallow has been the study of choice to evaluate for dysphagia. The swallow of a barium contrast bolus is observed for delayed transit, pooling, and penetration with varying consistencies. The efficacy of compensatory strategies for dysphagia can also be observed during fluoroscopy. Another, more recent technique, fiberoptic endoscopic evaluation of swallowing, provides real time images similar to those of videofluoroscopy, with additional advantages. The procedure can be performed at the bedside, utilizes food rather than contrast, can be repeated without radiation exposure, and is tolerable for longer periods of time.[98]

After aspiration risk is determined, recommendations for limiting or modifying oral feeding should be implemented. Thin liquids are generally the most difficult to handle without aspiration, due to the effects of gravity. Differing thickness of liquids and consistency of foods are recommended, based on observations of swallowing studies. Unfortunately, there are no controlled studies documenting the efficacy or guiding the use of these dietary modifications. If the patient is at risk for aspiration of all food consistencies and is not allowed any food by mouth (n.p.o.), enteral nutrition can be achieved with nasogastric or endogastric means. Nasogastric feeding provides little protection against aspiration, however, with one study reporting a 50% aspiration rate in TBI patients.[227] Nasogastric feeding can also hinder effective swallowing, cause nasal and esophageal irritation and erosion, and worsen agitation. It is therefore recommended that, if more than 3 weeks of non-oral feeding are required after TBI, a percutaneous endoscopic gastrostomy, gastrojejunostomy, or jejunostomy tube be placed.[227]

Nausea is a commonly encountered problem on initiating enteral feeding after TBI. Possible etiologies are gastroesophageal reflux, gastroparesis, vestibular dysfunction, gastric ulcer, and constipation. Gastroparesis is another commonly encountered problem after TBI. Gastric emptying time in TBI patients has been observed to be twice that of healthy individuals.[277] The coexistent relaxation of the lower esophageal sphincter after brain injury creates a risk for reflux, nausea, and aspiration. Close monitoring of gastric residual volumes, elevation of the head of the bed, and coloring of enteral fluids are helpful preventive measures. Low-dose oral erythromycin is an often utilized prokinetic agent for gastroparesis. Metoclopramide is another agent, but it has significant side effects, including sedation, an elevated risk to develop tardive dyskinesia, and potential worsening of motor recovery (due to dopamine-blocking properties). Metoclopramide has also been found not to have a significant impact on gastric emptying in one study of acutely brain-injured patients.[177] Postpyloric feeding via gastrojejunostomy or jejunostomy tube is a sometimes necessary and effective way to circumvent gastroparesis.[206] Such feeding does not impart a decreased risk for aspiration, and can impair absorption of medications generally absorbed in the stomach.

Gastric ulcers are common acutely after TBI, as a result of concomitant medical stressors, excessive secretion of adrenocorticoids, frequent medication adjustments, alterations in swallowing and oral intake, and endogastric instrumentation. Prophylaxis with a proton pump inhibitor medication is prudent and can also alleviate symptoms of reflux. These medications are available both orally and intravenously. Use of histamine (H_2) blockers is discouraged due to their potential sedation effects.

Nutrition

Following TBI, patients experience a significant increase in metabolism and catabolism that peaks 48–72 h after injury.[57] The simultaneous release of glucagon, adrenaline (epinephrine), noradrenaline (norepinephrine), cortisol, and insulin stimulates this response. The increased energy demand results in compensatory breakdown of carbohydrates, amino acids, and fat. This creates a catabolic state and a negative nitrogen balance. The additional energy demand for a patient with TBI has been estimated to be between 40 and 69% above normal.[57] Meeting nutritional demands is further complicated by the significant variability that exists in the metabolism of individual TBI patients. Formulas for calculating resting metabolic expenditure that factor in GCS score, heart rate, and days after injury are available and should be utilized. However, portable 'metabolic carts', which measure V_{O_2}, give a more accurate measurement of caloric demand and are becoming more widely available.[25]

Assessment and proper ongoing management of nutrition and dysphagia (Box 50-6) are essential to prevent malnutrition, aspiration pneumonia, and poor rehabilitative outcomes.[164,285] Initiating proper nutrition as soon as possible after TBI has been shown to improve outcome.[257] A positive nitrogen balance, in which nitrogen intake exceeds loss, indicates adequate protein

---

Box 50-6 Managing nutritional status after traumatic brain injury

- Additional energy demand after traumatic brain injury (TBI) is 40–69% above that of the normal uninjured individual. Appropriate nutrition should be initiated within 24 h of injury.
- The recommended diet after significant TBI is 2–2.5 g protein/kg per day and 25–35 non-protein kcal/kg per day.
- Dysphagia can occur in more than 60% and aspiration in more than 40% of individuals with severe TBI.
- Bedside evaluations have poor reliability.
- Modified barium swallows are recommended for all patients with significant injury. Flexible endoscopic evaluation of swallowing is an acceptable alternative.
- Nasogastric feeding does not prevent aspiration risk, increases ulcer risk, and may alter sleep hygiene and behaviors.
- Percutaneous endoscopic gastrojejunostomy tubes are recommended if non-oral nutrition and hydration cannot be achieved by 2–3 weeks post TBI.

intake. Achieving such a positive balance might be impossible during the early catabolic state after injury. A 24-h urine urea nitrogen level is often utilized for such an assessment, and should range between 12 and 20 g per day.[25] A general target proposed for intake is 2–2.5 g protein/kg per day and 25–35 non-protein kcal/kg per day.[257]

Bowel and bladder management

Incontinence is common after brain injury and is often due in large part to frontal lobe damage. Such injury leads to an uninhibited neurogenic bladder and bowel (see Chs 29 and 30). Similar to the voiding patterns of an infant or an adult with dementia, the bladder contracts at a certain volume and the individual is unable to consciously prevent an incontinent episode by maintaining the integrity of the external sphincter. Bladder incontinence typically presents as multiple small voids without urinary retention, and is due to detrusor hyperreflexia. Impairments in speech, mobility, and cognition are also important contributory factors. Retention of urine with overflow incontinence due to dyssynergia can also have iatrogenic causes, such as overuse of opiates, use of medications with anticholinergic side effects, and clogged catheters. Urinary tract injury and urinary tract infection should be ruled out first. Retention can be measured by monitoring the postvoid residual volumes. Detrusor hyperreflexia can be managed in the acute stage with external collection such as condom catheters and pads. These methods are temporary, and carry a risk of infection and skin breakdown. As early as is feasible, a bladder retraining program, consisting of scheduled voiding and careful fluid management, should be initiated. The timing and frequency of micturition can be adjusted to the needs of the patient, and decreased as continence is gained. Once patients have few or no episodes of incontinence, they should be encouraged to initiate voiding without prompts.

Anticholinergic medications can decrease hyperreflexia but should be reserved for patients who fail a trial of timed micturition. Use of these medications carries the risk of sedation, memory impairment, constipation, and urinary retention, and is not often necessary.

Brain stem (especially pontine) injury can lead to detrusor–sphincter dyssynergia, similar to the upper motor neuron bladder abnormalities seen from a cervical or high thoracic spinal cord injury, requiring an intermittent catheterization program or chronic indwelling catheter. An intermittent catheterization program carries a lower risk of urinary tract infection and other complications, but can be challenging to teach to patients with cognitive impairment.

Incontinence of bowel can also be addressed with a scheduled daily bowel program. High-fiber nutrition assists in preventing constipation, as well as controlling diarrhea that is not due to infectious etiology. The use of glycerin suppositories, if needed, should be scheduled after a meal to take advantage of the gastrocolic reflex. Diarrhea is a common problem after brain injury, most commonly due to an infectious etiology, due to impaction with secondary leakage around the site, and as a result of tube feeding. Use of antibiotics in the acute care of brain-injured patients is common, and the presence of diarrhea should alert the clinician to test for *Clostridium difficile* colitis. Treatment with metronidazole is generally successful, but oral vancomycin might be a better alternative, as there is no systemic absorption. Converting to lower osmotic feeding solutions and refraining from oral magnesium supplementation can correct osmotic diarrhea.

Secondary injuries

Delayed diagnosis of limb and axial fracture is common after brain injury.[217] Multiple and complex acute issues, along with altered consciousness, communication skills, and cognitive impairment all can hinder detection. A thorough reexamination of the musculoskeletal system is warranted as soon as patient is able to more fully cooperate. Additionally, each time the TBI patient's rehabilitation treatment setting changes (e.g. from inpatient to outpatient), a focused reexamination for occult injuries should be undertaken. Swelling, pain, deformity, or something less obvious (such as increased agitation) can all be indicative of an underlying fracture. It is unclear whether pain and delayed mobility from fractures can hinder long-term recovery, but the presence of a fracture is a significant risk factor for DVT, functionally limiting heterotopic ossification (HO), and a worsening of short-term outcomes.[69,84,130] Prompt fixation of the fracture can often expedite mobilization. When indicated, open reduction and fixation of fractures can allow patients to undergo therapy unencumbered by weight-bearing precautions or pain, while simultaneously hospital stay and healthcare costs are reduced.[209]

The common etiologies of spinal cord injury, such as motor vehicle accidents, falls, and violence, parallel those of TBI. Coexistence of TBI and spinal cord injury is common, as documented by studies that show that 20–50% of patients with cervical spinal cord injury also have sustained a TBI.[48] Unfortunately, a paucity of literature and guidelines exists for treating such patients. The complex education necessary for independent self-care after spinal cord injury is adversely impacted by cognitive impairment due to TBI. Effective rehabilitation will ultimately require not only expertise in each pathology, but also innovation to adapt to the very unique needs of each patient.

Peripheral nerve entrapment can occur after TBI, due to a number of factors, including direct trauma with swelling, HO, prolonged positioning during periods of therapeutic sedation, fracture repair and other corrective surgery, the use of restraints or specialized safety devices, and the need for frequent vascular access acutely. Prompt diagnosis is often limited by cognitive impairment, language deficits, and coexistent pathology. A high index of suspicion is always warranted, as early treatment of causative factors can prevent permanent nerve palsy. As with occult fractures, thorough reexamination is warranted as soon as patient cooperation improves. Each time the rehabilitation treatment setting of an individual with TBI changes, a focused approach to detect occult injuries should be undertaken. Electromyography is useful to clarify the diagnosis and localize the lesion (see Chs 10–12). Compression neuropathies are most

Table 50-8	Common problems observed by medical professionals during the acute stages post injury, and the symptoms and associated problems characterizing these problems	
Problematic behavior	Symptoms and commonly associated problems
Agitation	Combativeness and verbal or physical aggression Irritability Confusion and disorientation Motor restlessness Limited self-awareness and insight Impulsivity Drooling or spitting Difficulties with verbal expression Sleep problems
Hypoarousal	Problems awakening or remaining awake Decreased alertness Sleep problems Attention and concentration problems
Depression	Depressed or labile mood Flat affect Crying spells Expressions suggesting feelings of hopelessness, pessimism, or worthlessness Anhedonia Psychomotor retardation Sleep problems Poor appetite or weight loss Hypoarousal Limited energy, persistence, or motivation

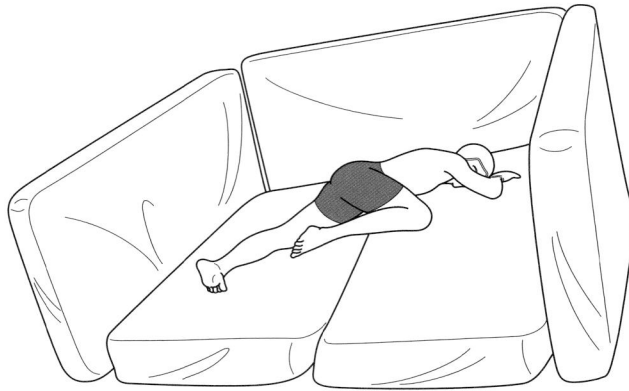

Figure 50-8 The Craig bed. Agitated non-ambulatory patients often benefit from the use of a floor (Craig) bed. Mattresses can be laid on the floor and 3- to 4-ft padded walls on four sides allow the patient to roll around. The use of a floor bed with close supervision, together with the use of mittens and a helmet (if necessary), often eliminates the need for restraints.

common in the ulnar and peroneal nerves, due to their subcutaneous location. Pressure relief with fitted pads and positioning often results in significant pain relief.

Behavioral dysfunction

In the early stages following TBI, patients might demonstrate a variety of problematic behaviors. The most common include agitation, hypoarousal, and depression. Table 50-8 illustrates symptoms medical professionals might notice acutely with each of these problematic behaviors.

Agitation

Agitation and restlessness are among the most commonly reported acute behavioral symptoms.[26,169] Agitation can be problematic during hospitalization secondary to physical and verbal aggression, which often accompanies agitation. Behavioral observation is the most common method for identifying agitation.[182]

Two questionnaires can also be used to assess and track agitation: the Agitated Behavior Scale (ABS)[53] and the Neurobehavioral Rating Scale.[168] The ABS is particularly useful clinically, because it can be rapidly (5 min) and reliably used by different caregivers. The scores generated can also be used to both determine treatment interventions (e.g. an ABS score > 28 implies moderate agitation and warrants scheduled medication) and

monitor the success of these interventions (e.g. graphing of scores every 8 h). The environment might need to be altered when agitation is problematic. For example, the patient's comfort level can be monitored, and physical irritants can be reduced (e.g. placing the patient in a private room, reducing outside noise or number of visitors, ensuring diapers are clean, and removing potentially hazardous items).[182] Physical activity can also be increased to divert energy to safer and more useful behaviors.[182] Medications can be prescribed to manage agitation. Common medications include atypical antipsychotics, psychostimulants, beta-blockers, and anticonvulsants. The reader is referred to the section on *Maladaptive behavior and agitation* presented in the *Inpatient rehabilitation* section of this chapter for a comprehensive discussion of medication alternatives. Physical restraints are the most restrictive mode of intervention, and are generally discouraged but can be necessary when agitation leads to self-harm or harm of others (see Fig. 50-8).[182] Review of state laws and facility guidelines are strongly encouraged prior to pursuing use of physical restraints.

Hypoarousal

Hypoarousal is particularly problematic during hospitalization, because the patient's ability to remain awake and alert during treatment is compromised. Frequently, patients with impaired arousal difficulties are able to tolerate only a few minutes of therapy prior to falling asleep or experiencing a decline in alertness.[182] Indicators of hypoarousal include patients complaining of fatigue or asking to return to their rooms, patients falling asleep frequently and in unusual locations, staff complaining about the patient's inability to remain alert or awake during therapies, and patients having difficulty completing tasks. Environmental management is important for addressing hypoarousal problems. Schedules should be established that include frequent breaks and efforts for building stamina over time. The patient might benefit most if challenging tasks are scheduled during peak periods of alertness, and if there is a balance, with alteration between challenging and less intense tasks. Staff can also monitor the patient for signs of decreased alertness, and reduce task demands prior to severe deterioration. Several medications have been shown to improve arousal, particularly psychostimulants such as methylphenidate and amantadine sulfate.[184]

Depression

Evaluation and treatment of depression is critical. Depression often hinders patients' ability to participate in and benefit from rehabilitation.[182] Depression can be assessed via observation and clinical interview. Many questionnaires have been developed for the purpose of identifying depression (e.g. the Beck Depression Inventory, Hamilton Depression Inventory, and Zung Depression Inventory). The Neurobehavioral Functioning Inventory,[149] designed to assess common neurobehavioral symptoms following TBI, includes a scale focusing on symptoms of depression (see Ch. 4).

There are many alternative treatment options for depression. First, environmental management is important during hospitalization. The physical setting should be positive (e.g. cheerful decor and pictures of family and friends).[182] Second, staff behavior plays an important role in managing patients' depression.[182] Staff should encourage patients and be positive about the benefits of treatment. Normalization of reactions to disability is critical. Humor and focus on accomplishments are also helpful. Third, group, family, and individual therapy are common components of inpatient rehabilitation programs, which are often recommended during inpatient consultation. Group therapy provides an avenue for normalization of problems and social support. Individual and family psychotherapy are often utilized for support of patients and their family members, education about recovery and treatment options, and normalization of problems. Antidepressant medication is also a useful adjunct to psychotherapy. Careful consideration of side effects is encouraged, and the side effect profiles should be reviewed with the patient and family whenever possible.

INPATIENT REHABILITATION

Spasticity

Spasticity, a velocity-dependent increase in muscular resistance to passive range of motion, is common after TBI. This is due to the loss of supraspinal inhibition of the muscle stretch reflex. The disorder can have direct positive and negative functional implications. Resultant complications can include pain, skin breakdown, and muscle contracture. The increased tone can occasionally be useful, however, as in compensating for weakness of the legs during a stand–pivot–transfer. For this reason, functional assessment is imperative to individualize treatment. Intervention should be pursued only to assist in reaching tangible functional goals, such as improving gait, motor control, positioning, hygiene, preventing deformity, and reduction of pain. Consideration of exacerbating factors, such as pain and its underlying etiology, infection, skin breakdown, positioning, and stage of recovery is also imperative prior to intervention. Rarely

Table 50-9 Modified Ashworth scale

Physical examination	Score
No increase in muscle tone	0
Slight increase in muscle tone, manifested by a catch and release or by minimal resistance at the end of the range of motion when the affected part(s) is moved in flexion or extension	1
Slight increase in muscle tone, manifested by a catch, followed by minimal resistance throughout the reminder (less than half) of the range of movement	2
More marked increase in muscle tone through most of the range of movement, but affected part(s) easily moved	3
Considerable increase in muscle tone passive, movement difficult	4
Affected part(s) rigid in flexion or extension	5

can moderate to severe spasticity be addressed with a single modality. A complement of interventions tailored to the specific patient needs is generally the most effective. Objective evaluation of the severity of spasticity using scales such as the Modified Ashworth Scale (see Table 50-9) is helpful in initial examination as well as to monitor the efficacy of subsequent therapeutic intervention.[189] Measurement of range of motion using goniometry, and observation for hyper- or hypokinesis, gait, coordination, and synergy patterns is also warranted (see Ch. 31).

Attention to spasticity acutely after TBI (see Table 50-10) is prudent to prevent long-term impairment resulting from its complications, such as contracture (see Fig. 50-9). Acutely, bedside range of motion exercises and appropriate positioning both in and out of bed can generally be performed, without compromising management of airway and elevated ICP. Modalities such as heat, cold, vibration, or tapping can be used to directly treat mild spasticity. They can also be used to assist in stretching techniques, and as a method of analgesia for pain. Close attention to the skin to prevent damage from spasticity and the abnormal and prolonged postures that can be assumed is imperative. This is especially true because many persons with TBI and spasticity have impaired communication and cognition, and because peripheral nerve palsies are common among brain-injured patients. During acute and postacute rehabilitation, proper positioning remains an important consideration, with goals of improving function, symmetry, and alignment. Specific splints and orthoses that place joints in positions that promote the reduction of tone, while simultaneously stretching relevant soft tissues, are frequently valuable. Serial casting can be used for relieving contractures. This involves the intermittent removal and reapplication of a cast to a limb that places the involved joint in a state of constant passive stretch. The anticipated goal is a stepwise increase in range of motion. While unproven, serial casting seems to be useful in many challenging patients.

Table 50-10 Management of spasticity after traumatic brain injury

Agent	Indications and limitation
Eliminating irritants	Vital first-line step in management. Difficult to always assess relationship to tone. Rarely completely eliminates spasticity. Low cost.
Range of motion and positioning	Vital first-line step in management. Often difficult for nursing staff to perform and maintain consistently. When performed appropriately, can reduce need for secondary measures. Must be performed frequently. Low cost but moderately labor-intensive.
Modalities	Second-line agent with limited utility when used in isolation. May assist in range of motion or positioning. Often labor-intensive. Risk of thermal burns in cognitively and tactile-impaired patients.
Splinting and casting	Important second-line agent. Limited long-term effectiveness due to inconsistent use, difficulty in repositioning devices, and elevated risk for skin breakdown. Need to be used with regular range of motion. Low cost but high labor intensity. Limited efficacy data.
Systemic medications	Third-line agent with fair efficacy. Side effects limit utility in focal (single-limb) spasticity. Sedation, hepatotoxicity, and hypotension are not uncommon. Dantrolene sodium is recommended as first line.
Neurolytics	Good third-line agent for focal (one- or two-limb) spasticity. Neuromuscular blockade (botulinum toxin or phenol) most common. A 3- to 6-month duration with limited side effects. High cost for botulinum toxin. Electrodiagnostic or ultrasound-guided placement is recommended. Good efficacy data.
Intrathecal baclofen pump	Good fourth-line agent, particularly for lower extremity involvement. Extensive postplacement therapy required. High short- and long-term costs. Good efficacy data.
Surgery	Poor to fair fifth-line intervention. Irreversible. Very surgeon-dependent. Limited efficacy data.

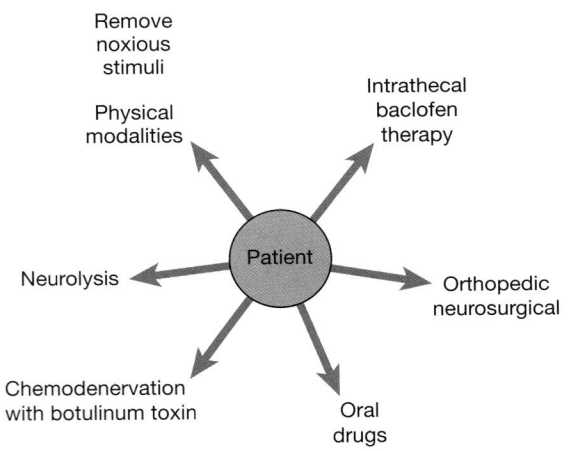

Figure 50-9 The complementary approach to the management of spasticity of cerebral origin.

Vigilance in ensuring adequate padding of the splints and monitoring skin for pressure ulcers is necessary.

Systemic spasticity due to TBI can require additional measures, including system antispasticity medications such as dantrolene sodium, baclofen, tizanidine, and diazepam. Each has potential adverse side effects, particularly sedation, that must be weighed against other potential benefits of their administration. Dantrolene is usually recommended as a first-line agent, due to its lower potential to cause cognitive impairment. Despite the peripheral mechanism of dantrolene (inhibition of release of calcium from the sarcoplasmic reticulum), it can cause transient and dose-dependent cognitive side effects.[32] The reported, but rare, hepatotoxicity caused by the drug warrants initial and ongoing monitoring of liver enzyme levels during administration. Baclofen, a GABA analog, and diazepam, a GABA-potentiating substrate, have considerable potential to cause sedation. Tizanidine acts centrally by an α_2-receptor agonist mechanism (similar to that of clonidine), and appears to indirectly decrease the release of excitatory amino acids and increases presynaptic inhibition. Tizanidine can be quite sedating, and rarely can cause hypotension and also exacerbate orthostatic symptoms. Baclofen, dantrolene sodium, and diazepam can be used in children, but close monitoring is required for untoward effects.

Intrathecal delivery of antispasticity agents is ideal for treating severe and generalized spasticity resistant to oral drugs, and can often be done without sedative effects. Baclofen is frequently administered continuously via a surgically implanted and programmable pump into the spinal CSF. The dosage is much lower compared with enteral baclofen, while drug delivery to the site of action in the central nervous system is substantially increased. Intrathecal administration minimizes potential systemic side effects, while simultaneously achieving improved spasticity control. As in cerebral palsy, the medication is most efficacious in brain-injured patients with predominantly lower limb spasticity.[189] The intervention is usually not considered until at least 1 year post injury to allow for spontaneous recovery, but earlier usage can be indicated in severely affected individuals. While the modality has proven efficacy, several factors must be considered prior to pump implantation. These include the surgical risks, cost, potential for malfunction, ability to comply with frequent pump refills, and acceptance of cosmesis. Equally important is the ability of the patient and/or caregiver to understand, assess, and address potential complications. Symptoms of withdrawal, such as increased tone and mental status changes, warrant emergent attention. Problems such as pump failure, catheter obstruction, and failure to refill the medication are not uncommon. More severe symptoms of withdrawal, such as seizure, rhabdomyolysis, and hyperthermia, can lead to fatality without expedient readministration of oral or intrathecal baclofen. Baclofen overdose, although less common, is most often seen during initial administration. This can be counteracted by administration of physostigmine, which should be readily available for this complication.

Neurolytic techniques, such as intramuscular injection of phenol and botulinum toxin, are commonly utilized for individuals with more focal spasticity. Similarly, functional deterioration and the weakness resulting from the procedure must be considered. Phenol works through neurolysis, and is most often administered with the aid of electromyography or ultrasound guidance to help to localize the muscles' motor points or the nerve to the hypertonic muscle. Complications include bleeding, swelling, pain, DVT, and weakness. The procedure can be quite painful and can warrant sedation in children or cognitively impaired adults, especially when multiple sites are to be injected. After injection, acute swelling and pain should be appropriately addressed using limb elevation, antiinflammatory analgesics, and cold compresses. Dysesthesia can be addressed by repeat injection of phenol to complete neurolysis of the sensory component of the targeted nerve, or by administration of oral agents commonly used for neuropathic pain.

Botulinum toxin is also injected intramuscularly but works by adhering to the presynaptic membrane, with blockage of the release of acetylcholine. This prevents synapse conduction past the neuromuscular junction. Administration of the drug is usually less painful than that of phenol, but it is far more expensive and can have a shorter period of efficacy, lasting typically no longer than 3 months. Electromyography or ultrasound guidance for administration of botulinum toxin is not generally required, but should be used to help localize small (e.g. forearm, hand, or foot) or deep (e.g. tibialis posterior) muscles. Common potential complications include infection, bleeding, and weakness. Immunotolerance leading to decreased drug efficacy is rarely observed. This can be addressed by switching the serotype of toxin utilized, and by limiting repeat administration to no more frequently than every 4 months.[66] The therapeutic benefit of the drug is not generally seen for 5–10 days. Dosage exceeding 8 U of serotype A or 200 U of serotype B per kg body weight at one time is not recommended. Better efficacy research defining dosing limitations, specific indications, and injection site specifics is needed.

Orthopedic and neurosurgical management of spasticity due to TBI is occasionally indicated, in concert with bracing, medication, and appropriate therapy. Rhizotomy is the lysis of either the dorsal or anterior root of spinal nerves involved in the reflex arc of hypertonic musculature. This procedure has permanent consequences and is rarely conducted on adults. The surgery is generally reserved for children thought to have significant postintervention rehabilitative potential. Orthopedic tendon lengthening procedures can be utilized for contractures resulting from spasticity. The two most common procedures include Achilles tendon lengthening and the split lateral anterior tibialis tendon transfer (SPLATT) procedure. Achilles tendon lengthening is used to treat ankle plantar flexion contractures. Ankle inversion contractures are surgically treated by the SPLATT procedure. The long-term efficacy of these procedures, as well as that of multimodal interventions aimed at individuals with severe or end stage contractures, has not been well studied.

Heterotopic ossification

Neurogenic HO, i.e. the formation of mature lamellar bone in periarticular areas, has been reported in the wide range of 11–76% of patients with TBI.[32,76,81] Functionally limiting neurogenic HO that warrants intervention occurs much less frequently, with an incidence between 10 and 20%.[76,81] The pathophysiology of HO remains elusive. Recent theory postulates that central nervous system damage can alter signals to nerves identified in bone, with subsequent alteration in neuroendocrine signals controlling bone formation.[120,130] The disease in neurotrauma process should not be mistaken with another subset of HO, myositis ossificans, which is bone formation within soft tissue following focal trauma. In neurogenic HO, bone formation occurs between layers of fascia, a key difference in differentiating pathology.

The symptoms of HO include pain; decreased range of motion; and periarticular warmth, redness, and swelling. Unfortunately, these are also the symptoms commonly seen in other TBI problems, such as DVT, fracture, and infection. These symptoms justify expedient diagnosis and appropriate treatment. Initial evaluation for HO with plain film is relatively inexpensive but is often negative early (i.e. in the first 3–4 weeks) in the process of HO, prior to calcification. Strong clinical suspicion in a symptomatic patient with a negative x-ray warrants a triple-phase bone scan. The first or flow phase is most diagnostic of the increased periarticular activity seen with HO. Laboratory measurement of serum alkaline phosphatase has no role in the initial diagnosis, but can be useful to monitor efficacy of therapy and maturity of bone formed in HO. Initial testing is performed to attain baseline values, and is likely to be elevated from multifactorial sources resultant from trauma.

Heterotopic ossification is associated with poorer functional outcome and longer hospitalization in inpatient rehabilitation facilities.[119] Functionally limiting consequences of HO include pain, limited joint range of motion, and nerve and vascular compression. It most commonly affects the neurologically involved side and major joints, including the shoulder, hip, knee, and elbow. Risk factors include spasticity, prolonged coma, immobilization, and fractures. Prophylaxis with anti-

Table 50-11 Neuroendocrine abnormalities seen after traumatic brain injury

Abnormality	Comment
Hyponatremia	The syndrome of inappropriate antidiuretic hormone secretion is treated with fluid restriction, whereas salt repletion is treatment for cerebral salt wasting.
Hypernatremia	Nasally administered desmopressin is the treatment for diabetes insipidus, and should be titrated to serum sodium, beginning with one 'squirt'.
Anterior pituitary–hypothalamic dysfunction Adrenocorticotropic hormone deficiency (Addison disease)	Fatigue and weakness common.
Hypothyroidism	Cold intolerance and fatigue are common.
Gonadotropin deficiency	Impotence, amenorrhea, poor libido, and fatigue are common.
Growth hormone deficiency	Results in decreased energy, depression, fatigue and, most importantly, increased mortality.

inflammatory medications or joint irradiation, while occasionally prescribed in high-risk patients undergoing hip arthroplasty, has not been specifically demonstrated to be either clinically or cost-effective in brain-injured patients.

Early detection of neurogenic HO and treatment with range of motion exercises and bisphosphonates might halt or slow down the progress of the disorder. Such efforts might specifically prevent further functional loss, limit joint ankylosis, alleviate pain, and obviate the need for subsequent surgical excision, which is rarely effective. Treatment of HO by surgical removal should be reserved for patients for whom significant functional gain is expected. The maturity of the ectopic bone formation must be assured so as to decrease the likelihood of recurrence. This can be achieved by delaying surgery for at least 18 months after injury, awaiting decline in serum alkaline phosphatase levels, and demonstrating no evidence of increased activity on all phases of a triple-phase bone scan. Typically, the third phase of such a test will be the last to 'cool'.

Neuroendocrine dysfunction

Hormonal abnormalities (see Table 50-11) affect as many as 30–50% of patients after severe TBI.[251] The resulting symptoms, such as fatigue and cognitive impairment, can also appear similar to the typical post-TBI sequelae. The benefits of vigilant and routine screening abnormalities after brain injury are unfortunately not well studied. During the acute stage of moderate and especially severe TBI, hormonal abnormalities can be associated with the effects of acute hospitalization and secondary conditions. Treatment of apparent hormonal disturbances in the TBI patient, even without specific clinical correlates, is generally warranted.

Alteration in serum sodium is a common electrolyte abnormality after TBI. Damage to the posterior pituitary gland or its neuroendocrine axis can result in hyper- or hyponatremia. In either case, close monitoring of sodium levels with gradual correction is prudent. Hyponatremia can be due to the syndrome of inappropriate antidiuretic hormone secretion (SIADH), cerebral salt-wasting syndrome, thyroid dysfunction, the use of hypotonic enteral feeding formulas, or diuretic use. Distinguishing the two etiologies can be achieved through analysis of urine and serum osmolality and sodium. SIADH is a blood volume-expanded condition with hypotonic serum and urine that is associated with either normal or elevated urine osmolality and sodium.[146] Cerebral salt-wasting syndrome is a blood volume-contracted condition with hypertonic serum and urine with low osmolality and high sodium. Making the distinction is important, as each diagnosis is treated differently.[203] Fluid restriction is the first step in the treatment of SIADH. Salt repletion is the treatment for cerebral salt-wasting syndrome. Correction of sodium should be a gradual process in both conditions, because too rapid a correction can result in neuronal death with central pontine myelinosis. Nasally administered desmopressin is the treatment of choice for hypernatremia caused by diabetes insipidus.

Dysfunction of the anterior pituitary gland in patients with TBI has been a focus of more recent study.[129] Effective screening and treatment can have significant implications on quality of life and function of patients after TBI.[129] Fatigue is a well-known and common problem after brain injury and can be addressed, at least partially, by detecting and treating hormone deficiencies. Damage to the fragile hypothalamic–pituitary axis can result in low levels of growth hormone, prolactin, thyroid hormone, adrenocorticotropic hormone (ACTH), follicle-stimulating hormone (FSH), and luteinizing hormone (LH). Continual deficiency of ACTH can result in Addison disease, with weakness and fatigue. Hypothyroidism typically results in cold intolerance and fatigue. FSH and LH deficiencies can result in impotency and fatigue. Growth hormone deficiency can result in decreased energy, depression, and fatigue. Most importantly, growth hormone deficiency can result in increased mortality. Whether growth hormone deficiency is a factor in the shorter life expectancy seen after TBI is unknown.

Providing growth hormone can result in improved lipid profile, increased exercise tolerance, increased sense of well-being, and improved bone density.[129]

Little or no guidelines exist for appropriate timing of screening for neuroendocrine dysfunction. A recent consortium agreed that, aside from the typical sodium abnormalities described, other pituitary dysfunction can also be common, but resolves quickly and is too difficult to treat acutely after acute TBI. The recommendations were made for a battery of serum hormone levels to be drawn prospectively, at 3 months and 12 months, for the following patients:

- patients after moderate to severe TBI;
- patients with mild TBI who have delayed recovery; and
- patients with remote injuries and symptoms consistent with a pituitary dysfunction.

The hormone levels recommended for assessment include a morning (9 a.m.) cortisol, free thyroxine and triiodothyronine, thyroid-stimulating hormone, insulin-like growth factor-1, prolactin, FSH, LH, testosterone (in men), and estrogen (in women).

Amenorrhea in female patients is common after TBI, and usually resolves in the first 5–12 months. Pregnancy testing should be done in the acutely injured patient of childbearing age who is unable to reliable relate her sexual history. Pregnancy has an obvious impact on imaging studies, as well as on the choice of anticoagulation and antiepileptic medications employed. The physiatrist should emphasize the value of safe and effective pregnancy prevention measures (with consideration of cultural and religious values), at least for the time of the acute and rehabilitative phases of treatment.

While sexual dysfunction after TBI can have an endocrine component, it is more likely to be due to complex psychosocial factors. This topic is further reviewed in later sections (see also Ch. 32).

Motor and balance recovery

Prognosis of functional recovery of coordination and motor function is generally favorable, even in severe TBI. However, subtle persistent deficits can be detected remotely even after mild TBI. One retrospective study demonstrated that around 85% of patients ambulated independently after severe TBI. The same study reported that the most rapid recovery takes place within the first 2–3 months after injury. Around 95% of patients who will ambulate do so within this time frame. If independence is not achieved in this period, the prognosis is much worse, with approximately 14% achieving subsequent independence.[129] The timing of recovery is similar for upper limb function, but prognosis is slightly better if function is not achieved by 2 months.[126] Motor processes requiring speed, such as finger tapping, have been found to be impaired as late as 1 year post injury. The functional significance of such findings is unclear.[100] Studies of pediatric populations reveal that gait, hand, and gross motor function deficits persist in comparison with age-matched controls after 8 months, despite significant rehabilitation

gains.[161] The long-term consequence of such differences and impact on further motor development is less studied.

Balance and coordination can be impacted by a variety of peripheral and central neurologic lesions. A careful assessment of movement and function, along with a consideration of findings on neuroimaging, can allow the physiatrist to target appropriate therapy. Damage to the visual and vestibular pathways can lead to an array of deficits that impair balance. Cerebellar insult can lead to ataxia of gait as well as upper limb impairment. Basal ganglia damage can lead to tremor and bradykinesia.[195]

Vestibular dysfunction and dizziness are common sequelae after mild TBI. Commonly prescribed 'sedating' medications, such as meclizine, can theoretically slow recovery due to their mechanism of decreasing the sensation of causative stimuli. Focused vestibular rehabilitation programs with purposeful exposure to and habituation and coping strategies for exacerbating movements have proven efficacy.[47] Benign paroxysmal positional vertigo is a condition that is caused by movement of otolithic debris or granules within the semicircular canals. Trauma can lead to the release of such debris. Specific therapy like the Dix–Hallpike maneuver and the Liberatory technique can be utilized for both diagnosis and therapy. Anxiolytic agents, such as buspirone and trazodone, can also have some positive effects on symptoms.

Improving function with upper limb ataxia, myoclonus, or tremor is often difficult. Use of weighted instruments for activities of daily living can sometimes be helpful. Strength must obviously be preserved for these aids to have utility. Splinting can also be utilized to stabilize proximal joints and improve fine motor function. Beta-blocking and dopaminergic agonist medications can also be of help but should be utilized with functional goals in mind.

Slowness of movement and response is often a persistent complication after brain injury that has clear functional and vocational implications. This problem can be more due to delayed processing than to actual alterations in signal speed from the motor cortex, and is difficult to address therapeutically.[296] If natural recovery, repetitive tasking, or cognitively enhancing medications do not have the desired impact, then educating the patient and potential employer regarding the persistence of these deficits is imperative to ensure successful community reintegration.

Cognitive interventions
Therapy

Early after injury, problems with disorientation, confusion, and limited self-awareness are common and challenging. Patients who are disoriented to person, place, time, and situation often have difficulty making sense of their environment and circumstances of their injury, and become very confused. Often, confusion and disorientation are accompanied by bizarre or disinhibited behavior, severe amnesia and cognitive impairments, wandering, agitation, aggression, and anxiety, as well as perseverative speech, thoughts, and/or behaviors.[182]

Assessment of orientation is a common practice that is often carried out via the GOAT. Maintaining a rigid structure and quiet environment can help ameliorate disorientation and confusion. Repeatedly reminding patients where they are and why they are there (e.g. 'You're in the hospital to recover from an injury to your brain') is also beneficial. Calendars and clocks should be mounted in locations where patients can easily see them, and staff should direct patients to check these devices on a regular basis until problems with disorientation subside. Decorating the patient's room with pictures of family and close friends, and familiar objects can increase their comfort level. Family and friends can also be encouraged to discuss familiar topics and review current events and photographs of familiar people and places.[182]

Self-awareness deficits can reflect the inability to appreciate or difficulty acknowledging injury-related changes.[238] Limited self-awareness contributes to safety concerns, as patients can overestimate their abilities and engage in potentially dangerous tasks.[182] Given the potential dangers associated with poor awareness, evaluation and early identification is critical. Awareness can be assessed by comparing patients' reports of difficulties with those of rehabilitation team members, family members, and caregivers.[182]

Awareness problems can also be indicated by frequent requests to engage in behaviors that staff members deem beyond the patient's capabilities. Another indication is the insistence by the patient that they can independently complete activities deemed unsafe. Additional indicators of awareness difficulties include blaming others for problems, complaints about the irrelevance of rehabilitation therapies, failures despite initial confidence about performance, and comments about the difference between the patient and others on the unit.[182]

Group therapy provides a useful technique for addressing self-awareness problems, because patients might receive feedback from their peers. Matthies and colleagues outlined several other strategies rehabilitation team members can use to facilitate improved self awareness, including the following.[182]

- Compare the patient's performance to a standard.
- Mutually review and evaluate task performances as compared with standards.
- Mutually review results of neuropsychologic, cognitive, and functional assessments with patients, identifying areas of strengths and weakness and making comparisons with average functioning.
- Allow patients to 'practice' in real world settings to provide opportunities for realizing the difference between the protected hospital setting and the outside world.
- Provide constructive feedback about strengths, weakness, and effort.
- Encourage the patient to self-monitor their performance and behavior.

Medications

Pharmacologic intervention to enhance cognitive recovery (see Table 50-12) after TBI remains an understudied and controversial topic. New psychoactive medications are becoming available, further complicating the selection of appropriate pharmacotherapy. Randomized, placebo-controlled studies that evaluate the efficacy of even the oldest agents utilized for attention and arousal are nearly non-existent. Medications should be used to target specific components of cognitive impairment elucidated with careful and well-documented examinations. The conservative use of such agents is also warranted, as brain-injured patients are often more vulnerable to medication side effects. If a patient is recovering at a quick pace, the need for medication is questionable. Using single agents is recommended, rather than the polypharmacy that is often seen. If the target

Table 50-12 Medications to enhance cognition after traumatic brain injury	
Medication(s)	Comments
Amantadine sulfate	Best available data on improving arousal and cognition in lower functioning patients (i.e. Rancho Los Amigos Scale 3). Recommend 50–150 mg b.i.d. Probable increased seizure risk above 300 mg/day. Limited side effects. Inexpensive.
Methylphenidate	Best available data on improving arousal and attention. Recommend 5–20 mg b.i.d. Long-acting available. Limited side effects. Inexpensive. Abuse potential.
Neurostimulants (e.g. dextroamphetamine, modafinil)	Little to no objective data available. Theoretically would expect similar results as those of methylphenidate. Expensive. Abuse potential.
Atomoxetine	Newer agent for attention deficit–hyperactivity disorder is a selective noradrenaline (norepinephrine) inhibitor. Little to no objective data available. Anticipate an effect similar to that of methylphenidate. May cause initial sedation. Recommend 40–80 mg b.i.d. Expensive. No known abuse potential.
Physostigmine inhibitors (e.g. donepezil, rivastigmine, memantine)	Anti-Alzheimer disease agents with anecdotal data supporting efficacy in memory deficits after traumatic brain injury. Significant gastrointestinal side effects. Expensive. Limited clinical efficacy.

impairment is not clearly improving and a therapeutic dosing of the medication has been reached, the medication should be appropriately discontinued.

Patients at a Rancho 3 level of cognition only respond and localize to noxious stimulation, due to impairment in arousal. Dopaminergic medications, such as amantadine sulfate, are often selected to help patients improve beyond this level. Studies of amantadine sulfate reveal conflicting results with no definitive evidence of efficacy, only 'positive trends'.[187,232] Another less well-studied dopaminergic drug is bromocriptine. The drug is contraindicated in patients with ischemic heart disease and uncontrolled hypertension. One study also showed modest efficacy of bromocriptine in the treatment of non-fluent aphasia.[99] Levodopa is another agent less utilized for arousal, but it has also not been studied in a clinically usable way.

Patients at Rancho 4 and 5 levels of cognition respond but have difficulty maintaining attention to stimuli. Agitation can partially be due to an inability to interpret and focus on one stimulus. It is somewhat intuitive that medications used for attention deficit might be of benefit for this state. Methylphenidate has been shown in several small studies to improve sustained attention, phasic arousal, speed of processing, and distractibility.[125,281,282] Dextroamphetamine works by a similar mechanism and is thought to have similar efficacy. Little evidence exists to support the common concern that such medications lower seizure threshold. However, both medications have addiction and abuse potential. Modafinil is a stimulant that increases activity in more discrete areas of the brain. It is designed to treat narcolepsy, and can be an ideal drug in the brain-injured patient with notable and impairing sleepiness. Atomoxetine, a newer agent for attention deficit–hyperactivity disorder, is a selective noradrenaline (norepinephrine) inhibitor. While initially sedating, this drug can be an option in patients with substance abuse history, or who suffer anxiety or agitation with more classic stimulants. None of these newer agents have been clearly documented to be effective in patients with TBI. If targeted impairments are seen to improve with these stimulant medications, then efforts at weaning down to the lowest effective dose should be initiated periodically (e.g. every 2–3 months at first, and then every 6 months for chronic usage). A goal of eliminating all non-essential medications must remain paramount in the physiatrist's mind when treating individuals with TBI.

Pharmacologic treatment of memory impairment after TBI is a relatively new field, given great attention due to increased awareness of treatments for Alzheimer disease. The use and study of donepezil, rivastigmine, and memantine is increasing rapidly.[214,271] A recent randomized, placebo-controlled, double-blind crossover trial of donepezil in patients with postacute TBI revealed positive treatment results.[295] A significant increase in short-term memory and sustained attention was observed. Memantine is an NMDA agonist, and is thought to enhance memory and also to be a neuroprotective agent, but research remains to be done to demonstrate any clinical efficacy in TBI. Patients with TBI and the ApoE4 gene have been demonstrated to be more likely to develop Alzheimer disease, although whether memantine can delay or prevent onset of Alzheimer disease after TBI has not been studied.[75]

Behavioral interventions
Maladaptive behavior and agitation
Common behaviors after TBI, such as thrashing, yelling, cursing, punching, and public masturbation, are often quite distressing to family members and clinicians unfamiliar with TBI. While the emergence of such behavior can be a sign of neurologic recovery and improved arousal, a thorough investigation to rule out other etiologies should first be pursued. Agitation has been defined as a special subtype of delirium specific to TBI, and includes PTA and behaviors such as disinhibition, emotional lability, aggression, and akathisia.[226] As with other presentations of delirium, a number of causes, including iatrogenic and physiologic, other than the actual brain injury are possible. Some of the most common etiologies include hydrocephalus, intracranial bleeding, seizure, pulmonary embolism, electrolyte disturbance, infection, cognitively impairing medication, under-treated pain, and disturbed sleep.

Therapy interventions
Disruptive and dangerous behaviors can hinder a patient's ability to benefit from rehabilitation services, and interrupt the patient's social functioning at work, at home, or in treatment facilities. Behavior management is an important tool for addressing problems with disruptive or dangerous behavior, and refers to a planned and coordinated process of managing patients' behavior. Behavior management often involves the use of rewards and punishments to increase the frequency of positive behaviors and decrease the frequency of negative behaviors. Behavior management plans are typically developed by the staff psychologist, but can be implemented by other rehabilitation providers (e.g. nursing staff and rehabilitation therapists), family members, and other individuals involved in patients' care. For example, redirection and time-out can be used by staff to divert agitated patients' attention from sources of irritation. Reinforcement can be offered in circumstances where patients engage in more appropriate behaviors.[182] The reader is also referred to the section on *Behavioral dysfunction* presented in the *Inpatient consultation* section of this chapter for information about environmental alterations and medication alternatives to address problems with agitation. Experienced staff members typically have the knowledge and skills necessary to positively influence patients' behavior. Box 50-7 illustrates strategies and guidelines that can be utilized to sensitize staff and help them understand their power to influence patients' behavior.[182]

Medications
Medications (see Table 50-13) should be utilized only when environmental modification and behavioral strategies fail, or when the safety of the patient or others is immediately threatened. Medication usage should be consistent and target specific behavior. The ABS is an objective method to rate severity of agitation, monitor improvement or exacerbation, and ensure

Table 50-13 Medications to improve agitated behavior after traumatic brain injury

Medication(s)	Comments
Methylphenidate	Most commonly used in children. Improvements in attention may help reduce agitated behavior. Inexpensive. Well tolerated.
Antipsychotics (e.g. haloperidol)	Effective in similarly agitated psychiatric patients. Unclear long-term effects on recovery. Sedating, but often used only at night. Low cost. Rarely used with new antipsychotics secondary to risk of neuroleptic malignant syndrome and tardive dyskinesias.
Atypical antipsychotics (e.g. olanzapine)	Effective in similarly agitated psychiatric patients. Unclear long-term effects on recovery. Sedating, but often used only at night. Moderate cost. Well tolerated.
Beta-blockers (e.g. propranolol)	Limited research supports use, particularly in 'aggressive or violent' patients. Low cost. Should be dosed up rapidly and then gradually removed once effective. Recommend 10–240 mg t.i.d. Close monitoring of blood pressure.
Antiepileptics (e.g. valproate, carbamazepine)	Limited research supports use, particularly in 'irritated' and hyperkinetic patients. Should be dosed to a therapeutic level. Low cost. May be sedating.
Trazodone	Effective sleep medication, but unclear role as an as needed medication for agitation. Low cost. Recommend 50–200 mg q.h.s.
Physostigmine inhibitors (e.g. donepezil, rivastigmine, memantine)	Anti-Alzheimer disease agents with anecdotal data supporting efficacy in memory deficits after traumatic brain injury. Significant gastrointestinal side effects. Expensive. Limited clinical efficacy.

Box 50-7 Guidelines to help sensitize staff to their power to influence patients' behavior

- Plan patient interactions in advance to increase intervention effectiveness. Anticipating the diversity of patients' reactions and your responses, and role-playing or visualizing difficult or frightening encounters, is potentially valuable.
- Behavior that can be influenced in a negative manner can probably be influenced in a positive manner as well. Be reasonable. Try to change the balance gradually by increasing positive behaviors and reducing or avoiding the negative ones.
- Be aware of your feelings toward the patient and your competence in handling the patient's problems. If you are uncertain about your effectiveness, consult with other staff, enlist their assistance, or seek another assignment.
- Good intentions don't guarantee positive behavioral influence. Be sensitive to the possibility that you may inadvertently contribute to negative behavioral patterns.
- Decide on the limits of acceptable behavior in advance, explain the contingencies for unacceptable behavior, provide warnings when behavior approaches limits, and follow through consistently on the application of contingencies.
- Carefully consider the level of experience and training, especially of new staff, before assigning patients.
- Keep in mind that aggression is a common occurrence following brain injury. Staff should always be prepared to deal with a wide variety of aggressive behavior.
- Enlist the open support of family members, friends of the patient, and other staff to help increase the patient's responsiveness to your interventions.
- Your level of confidence influences the patient's reactions to you. Patients are often very competent at judging your level of confidence. Remember, you have been empowered by your experience, your employer, your colleagues, and the patient's family to help.

(From Matthies et al. 2004,[182] with permission of the National Resource Center for Traumatic Brain Injury.)

that medication is utilized only when needed. Medications often employed for other delirious patients, such as benzodiazepines and older neuroleptics, can cause paradoxical delusion and worsen agitation in TBI. Rancho 4 patients are beginning to be receptive to and probably have difficulty in distinguishing and interpreting stimuli. These and other medications can further impair such abilities. The sometimes unpredictable results of medication use justify conservative and symptom-specific employment of medication.

Newer, atypical antipsychotic medications are increasingly being utilized to manage agitation and other maladaptive behavior after brain injury. These drugs target more specific dopamine receptors and might be expected to produce differing results. This has been found to be true in retrospectively performed human and laboratory animal studies.[67,285] The clinician should be aware of the risk of neuroleptic malignant syndrome in using any neuroleptic. While rare, the disorder can appear similar to agitation and cause delays in expedient treatment. Neuroleptic malignant syndrome differs from agitation in that patients have hyperthermia, autonomic instability, and rigidity. Rapid treatment with dantrolene is needed to reverse the potentially life-threatening condition.[124]

The use of stimulating agents, such as methylphenidate, early in the presentation of agitation can be efficacious. This is thought to be due to a positive impact on sustained arousal and focused attention.[283] In the pediatric TBI population in particular, the use of methylphenidate for agitation is most common and well accepted. Centrally acting beta-blocking medication has been shown effective for agitation. Propranolol has specifically been shown to decrease the intensity but not the number of outbursts in episodic agitation.[27] Anticonvulsant medications have also been utilized for agitation. Valproic acid, carbamazepine, and lamotrigine have all been utilized, but with few studies addressing their efficacy.[131,202] Trazodone is an often used sleep medication that is also prescribed for as needed use in mild to moderate agitation. Regardless of the medication utilized, ongoing assessment of efficacy and periodic reevaluation of necessity is prudent. Once a patient progresses and is more able to interpret environmental stimuli, the need for medication is probably eliminated.

Pain management

The high-speed accidents that often lead to TBI are also often accompanied by bony fractures, nerve impingement, and muscular injuries. Pain-related behaviors can develop in an attempt to avoid or delay pain-producing activities, and often impede rehabilitation efforts. These behaviors include requests to discontinue the activity, lack of cooperation with treatment, complaints of illness, pulling or moving away, inappropriate behavior, distraction attempts, topic changes, or requests for breaks to go to the bathroom or to get something to eat or drink.[182]

The diagnosis and treatment of resultant pain is important, not only to relieve the patient, but also to enhance effective rehabilitation. Patients often volunteer information about the nature and extent of pain. Reports of pain may be impacted, however, by the patient's perception of the meaning of pain and by their cultural beliefs about pain. In addition, because communication and cognition are often impaired with TBI, it is often helpful to rely on other signs and symptoms when assessing pain, such as agitation, tachycardia, deformity, and swelling. Observation of the patient's behavior and interview of staff members can provide valuable information about pain and pain-related behaviors. Direct questioning and patient and/or family interview can also yield helpful information about pain levels. Patients can be asked to rate their level of pain on a visual analog scale (e.g. 1–5 or 1–10), with higher numbers reflecting more intense pain. Pain questionnaires, such as the McGill Pain Inventory and the Robert Jones and Agnes Hunt Pain Inventory, can also provide an opportunity to gather additional information about intensity, duration, reactions, and precipitants in a systematic manner.[182]

Treatment of pain in persons with TBI poses a challenge, because opiate and neuropathic medications can often cause sedation. If poorly controlled, pain can undoubtedly be distracting and cognitively impairing. During treatments and therapies,

staff might be able to redirect the patient's thinking to more positive activities through distraction.[182] Reminding the patient of the benefits of painful therapies can lead to more effortful performance during treatment. Rehabilitation team members can also teach patients to engage in more appropriate behaviors (e.g. counting, clenching fist, squeezing inanimate objects, and deep abdominal breathing) rather than disruptive reactions to pain.[182] Conservative measures including modalities (heat, cold, transcutaneous electrical nerve stimulation, and ultrasound) should be tried first. Early treatment with acetaminophen (paracetamol) should be initiated, using a scheduled administration rather than on an 'as needed' basis, particularly in cognitive or communication-impaired individuals. Non-steroidal antiinflammatory drugs (NSAIDs) are also ideal, because they are generally non-sedating. Recent evidence, however, indicates such drugs might impair bone healing and could be relatively contraindicated in the face of acute fractures. Whether the effect of NSAIDs on bone healing is clinically significant in the often young population that suffers TBI remains to be researched. Tramadol is a less sedating alternative to opiate medications that has a significant effect on pain. Stomach upset and dizziness can often be avoided if the drug is started at a low dose. Tramadol can lower seizure threshold. Antiepileptic agents are often used for neuropathic pain and, when possible, should be scheduled at night to prevent sedation and normalize sleep–wake cycles.

OUTPATIENT CONSULTATION

Neurobehavioral consequences of brain injury
Acute neurobehavioral changes
Acutely following injury, persons with TBI exhibit numerous neurobehavioral changes. European and American researchers have investigated the acute neurobehavioral consequences of TBI for the past 20 years, and have identified a high incidence of disorientation, memory impairment (Fig. 50-10), conceptual disorganization, irritability, disinhibition, agitation, aggression, restlessness, decreased insight and awareness, decreased energy, fatigue, slowness, mood swings, decreased initiation and motivation, and poor planning early following brain injury.[18,26,166–168,185,238] Keyser and colleagues conducted a multicenter study involving survivors of mild to severe TBI 2–260

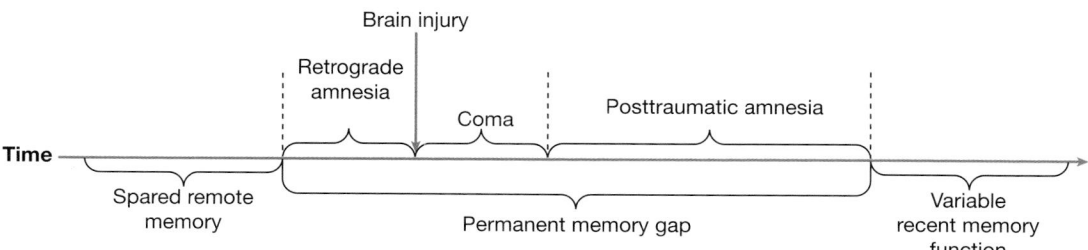

Figure 50-10 Recovery of memory after brain injury. Time line showing the stages of cognitive recovery that apply to most survivors of severe brain injury. Mild and moderate traumatic brain injury will demonstrate the same stages as depicted, except for coma. Some survivors do not recover from unconsciousness or from posttraumatic amnesia (PTA). The majority of patients emerge from PTA and have a permanent memory gap for experiences that occurred during unconsciousness, PTA, and a shorter preinjury period (retrograde amnesia).

days post injury.[132] The most significant symptoms that were endorsed by experienced clinicians on the Neurobehavioral Rating Scale included memory deficits, impaired insight, attentional problems, fatigue, and blunted affect.

Long-term neurobehavioral consequences

Neurobehavioral consequences of TBI have been found to continue for years and decades post injury. Thomsen investigated relatives' perceptions of survivors' difficulties up to 5 years post injury and found that emotional and behavioral difficulties were commonly reported, including irritability, temper problems, restlessness, and problems with initiation.[261] Thomsen interviewed the same sample 10–15 years post injury and found that neurobehavioral problems persisted, particularly slowness, memory deficits (Fig. 50-10), social withdrawal, and irritability. In a study of patients 7 years post injury, Oddy and colleagues found that patients reported difficulties following instructions, visual disturbance, getting lost, anger management problems, and clumsiness.[197] Their relatives described the patients as having problems with limited insight, childishness, impatience, fatigue, and speaking difficulties. Both patients and their relatives reported memory problems, concentration difficulties, alcohol sensitivity, and lack of interest. Brooks and colleagues interviewed relatives of patients with severe TBI who were 5 years post injury.[29] The five most commonly reported symptoms were memory problems, personality changes, slowness, irritability, and bad temper.

Witol and colleagues examined the long-term neurobehavioral consequences of TBI among survivors who were 5–34 years post injury.[286] The symptoms most frequently endorsed by patients 5–9 years post injury included boredom; moving, thinking, reading, and writing slowly; frustration; difficulty lifting heavy objects; poor concentration; trouble making decisions; tiredness; losing train of thought; being easily distracted; impatience; balance problems; and feeling misunderstood by others. Many of these problems were also reported by those 10–34 years post injury, including the following: frustration; impatience; feeling misunderstood by others; boredom; losing train of thought; moving, thinking, reading, and writing slowly; tiredness; and trouble making decisions. Additional problems related to memory deficits, slowed learning, word-finding problems, restlessness, and difficulty following instructions.

Psychologic consequences

Psychiatric disorders are common post TBI, particularly depression, anxiety disorders, and substance abuse disorders. Hibbard and colleagues evaluated the pre- and postinjury prevalence rates of psychiatric disorders in a sample of 100 adult patients with TBI using the Structured Clinical Interview for *Diagnostic and Statistical Manual Fourth Edition* (DSM-IV) Diagnoses.[108] Fifty-one percent of the sample met criteria for DSM-IV axis 1 disorders before injury, most commonly depression and substance abuse. Post injury, 80% of the sample met criteria for one or more axis 1 disorders at some point following the TBI. The most common diagnoses included major depression (61%

of the sample), substance abuse (28% of the sample), post-traumatic stress disorder (19% of the sample), obsessive-compulsive disorder (15% of the sample), and panic disorder (14% of the sample). Twenty-five percent of the sample met criteria for comorbid major depression and an anxiety disorder.

Substance abuse

Substance abuse is a significant problem for many individuals who sustain TBI.[54,256] Among patients with TBI, research suggests that preinjury alcohol abuse rates range from 44% to 79%.[19,51,54,137,158,159,223] In addition, 21–37% report a history of illicit drug use.[136,156,158,159,223] Alcohol and illicit drug use appears to decline at first after injury, but increases again as time post injury elapses.[52,54,150,154,156,158,228]

Psychotherapeutic approaches to intervention

Long-term psychiatric difficulties often are obstacles to successful community reintegration, and negatively impact patients' rehabilitation outcomes, interpersonal relationships, and vocational potential.[20,28,30,72,108] Given the negative outcomes associated with psychiatric disturbance post TBI, treatment of psychiatric disturbances is imperative. Many rehabilitation professionals identify psychotherapy as a critical component of holistic treatment for patients with TBI.[34,220–213] Individual therapy provides an arena for psychoeducation, coping skills training, and support. Family members are often invited to sessions to provide input about the patient's functioning, or for psychoeducation related to TBI, strategies for improved coping, and ways they can support the patient. Substance abuse often hinders progress in rehabilitation. Substance abuse assessment, prevention, and treatment are critical following TBI. Special attention should be paid to those who were intoxicated at injury, as research suggests they are more likely to be heavier drinkers pre- and postinjury.[159] Education is a principal component of prevention and treatment programs. Patients and their families are provided with information about the dangers of alcohol and drug use, risk factors, warning signs of relapse, and treatment alternatives.[156,162] Patients and family members can also be encouraged to plan for high-risk situations and educated about relapse prevention strategies.[162] Referral is often needed to specialized substance abuse treatment programs and to support groups for patients and families, such as Alcoholics Anonymous, Narcotics Anonymous, Al-Anon, and Alateen.[162,233,256] The effectiveness of these interventions in patients with persistent cognitive and behavioral difficulties may be limited.

Neuropsychologic assessment

Comprehensive neuropsychologic evaluation is an important step in the development of individualized treatment plans for patients following TBI. Holistic assessment typically focuses on cognitive, academic, neurobehavioral, and emotional functioning, with an emphasis on identifying areas of strength and limitations. Impaired judgment and safety issues, pain, substance abuse, vocational potential, motivation, and effort are also areas

---

Box 50-8 Common referral questions for neuropsychologic assessment after traumatic brain injury

- How has the neurologic injury impacted the patient's cognitive, emotional, or neurobehavioral functioning? Describe levels of functioning in each area relative to preinjury.
- Within each area of cognitive, intellectual, and psychomotor functioning, compare the patient's performance to that of the normal population. Which areas would you consider to be relative strengths and which areas would you consider to be weaknesses?
- Is there evidence of posttraumatic stress disorder, depression, anxiety, or other psychologic disorders? Is there evidence that emotional or psychologic difficulties contribute to cognitive deficits?
- Is there any evidence of preexisting cognitive, emotional, or neurobehavioral difficulties? If so, are current symptoms consistent with preexisting difficulties, traumatic brain injury, or a combination of factors?
- Please provide information about the patient's judgment and safety (e.g. driving, independent living, financial and/or medication management).
- How has the injury impacted the patient's academic and vocational potential?
- What is the prognosis for the future, with and without intervention, with respect to vocational or academic functioning, independent living, driving, financial management, and improvements or declines?
- What types of intervention have the potential to benefit the patient? What kinds of training, accommodations, and interventions are most likely to increase his or her potential for academic or vocational success?
- Is the patient eligible for special services or benefits?
- Compare the patient's functioning in each area to the patient's last evaluation. Which skills have improved, declined, and remained stable?

---

of emphasis in neuropsychologic assessment. In addition, neuropsychologists are often called on to assess the impact of injury on family functioning. Test findings are utilized for diagnosis, treatment planning, and prognostication about the future impact of injury and future rehabilitation needs.

Common referral questions

Patients are referred for neuropsychologic assessment by a variety of sources, including physicians, psychologists, rehabilitation therapists, and family. Clarifying the referral question(s) is critical for appropriate test selection, writing beneficial reports, and developing appropriate recommendations. Referrals might be made for a number of reasons. Referral sources often request information pertaining to the following: neuropsychologic, neurobehavioral, and emotional functioning diagnosis; functional abilities; judgment and safety; prognosis; and treatment and rehabilitation needs. Box 50-8 depicts the most common referral questions observed by neuropsychologists.

Behavioral observation

During the course of the neuropsychologic evaluation, the neuropsychologist has the opportunity to observe the patient's behavior in a variety of situations, including clinical interview, standardized testing process, and interactions with family members and staff. Observation can also be conducted in the rehabilitation unit, at home, and at work or school. Behavioral observation provides the neuropsychologist with the opportunity to assess behaviors, which are not readily evaluated by quantitative testing instruments. If observation is not feasible, family members, caregivers, employers, teachers, and rehabilitation staff may be able to provide additional information about behavior observed in the home. Behavioral observation often serves as the foundation for development of behavioral management plans and rehabilitation treatment plans.

Quantitative assessment

Quantitative assessment of cognitive and behavioral deficits begins with the clinical interview, which allows for identification of presenting complaints, clarification of information from the records, and history gathering. Standardized tests are subsequently administered to evaluate cognitive, academic, neurobehavioral, and emotional functioning. Tests are selected to address problem areas endorsed by the patient and her or his family, and questions posed by the referral source. Administration of standardized assessment tests allows the neuropsychologist to compare individuals' functioning with normative data and to compare their functioning over repeated testing sessions.[173] Readers interested in a comprehensive review of this subject are referred to Lezak's seminal text *Neuropsychological Assessment* (see also Ch. 4).[172,173]

Developing practical recommendations and reports

Developing practical recommendations and communicating assessment results to referral sources, clinicians, patients, and their families are critical tasks for neuropsychologists. Comprehensive neuropsychologic assessment culminates in the development of practical, feasible, and meaningful recommendations that can enhance patients' and families' well-being and optimize functioning. Recommendations often include development of compensatory strategies and referral for services in the community (e.g. medical follow-up, psychologic services, psychiatric intervention, support groups, and vocational or academic assistance). Repeated neuropsychologic testing is often also suggested to monitor progress or deterioration and to modify the existing treatment plan.

Test results and recommendations must be communicated in a clear and concise manner in order for the reader to understand the necessary information to meaningfully improve the patient's life. Otherwise, the utility of the assessment process comes into question. Reports should include a thorough injury description and review of the patient's pre- and postinjury history. The impact of preexisting conditions, psychologic and emotional issues, motivation, effort, self-awareness, and pain should also be considered. Reports are most effective when they are written in a language lay people can understand, are disseminated in a timely fashion, address the referral source's questions, highlight strengths as well as deficits, and are tailored to the specific patient.

Cognitive interventions

Cognitive rehabilitation and therapy

Impaired cognition is typically distressing for persons with TBI. Many neurocognitive symptoms, such as attention and concentration, memory, learning, planning, and academic skills, have been found to be amenable to cognitive remediation and retraining efforts.[39–41,128,205,242–245] Through cognitive rehabilitation, patients are taught to use compensatory strategies that enhance functioning compromised by neurologic damage. Typical compensatory strategies include use of memory logs, checklists, mnemonic devices, and self-monitoring. Strengths are often exploited to overcome areas of relative weakness. Table 50-14 depicts neurocognitive problems that are often problematic post injury, and intervention strategies that can be employed by rehabilitation professionals.[182]

Family functioning

Effects of TBI on the family

With decreases in third-party payments for treatment, and decreases in the length of hospital and rehabilitation stays,[104] family members often take the role of principal caregiver soon after injury.[110,152] Caregiving places significant burden on the family members, and is associated with increased risk of emotional difficulties.[86,103,145,146,174,179,198,204,207] Research has shown that over one-third of family caregivers report clinically significant levels of depression and anxiety.[179]

Family needs

Many empiric investigations have examined the needs of families following TBI.[34,123,138,144,155,160,181,183,191,235,236,241,250,287] The Family Needs Questionnaire[144] has been a prevalent assessment tool in many of these studies. Research reveals that family members commonly cite health information, reassurance, and clear and honest portrayal of complete information as their most important needs.[143,155] Personal needs are typically rated as less important by families (i.e. spending time with friends, and discussing his or her feelings).[144,155] Research has shown that high levels of unmet needs are associated with significantly higher levels of psychiatric morbidity and lower perceived quality of life.[192]

The impact on the parents of a child with TBI must be recognized and addressed, given the vital role of their participation and support during recovery.[3] Parents can be invaluable in offering insight into the individual needs and changes in a child after brain injury. However, the significant emotional and financial impact of such injury can promote feelings of isolation and lack of support among parents. Posttraumatic stress disorder is a constellation of symptoms, such as recurrent thoughts and experience of the incident leading to the injury. It is common both in the patient and in the parent.[241] Substantial stress results from the expense, complex planning for recovery, reintegration into the home and school, and other continuing needs of the child. Proactive efforts to promote education about the care system and transitions in rehabilitation milieux, along with development of peer support systems, can help alleviate these feelings. Such efforts can allow the parents to be more effective in offering appropriate support and ultimately help improve functional outcome for their child.

Approaches to intervention

Research reveals that many families do not receive professional emotional support after TBI.[138] Given the critical role family members play in caring for survivors of TBI, intervention should focus on ensuring family members are coping well and have supports needed to perform their caregiver role effectively.

Holistic interventions to help family members often reflect a core set of goals.

- To educate family members about the normal effects of injury.
- To educate the family about the survivor's cognitive and personality changes consequent to the injury.
- To help family members appreciate the effects of injury on themselves.
- To help family members develop effective coping and communication skills.
- To help family members identify resources in their home community.
- To provide emotional support and help family members adjust to injury-related life changes.

Helping family members problem solve and manage stress effectively is a key component of many family support programs. Clinicians also often help identify long-term needs and provide life care planning.

The Brain Injury Family Intervention (BIFI) is one example of a holistic approach to family intervention. The BIFI was developed over the past decade, and is based on considerable clinical experience and research review.[147] It is a structured approach to helping families address their most common and salient issues, concerns, and challenges. Bibliotherapy is a component of the BIFI, and is a common method chosen by rehabilitation professionals to facilitate communication of vital medical knowledge. For example, in the BIFI, information about the consequences of TBI and the recovery process that are presented in the book *Getting Better and Better After Brain Injury: a Guide for Families, Friends, and Caregivers* is reviewed and discussed during sessions.[148] Family members are reminded that they will be unable to optimally support the survivor if they do not take care of themselves. The BIFI also focuses on teaching compensatory strategies to cope with common injury-related sequelae and life changes, and on providing information about area resources. Community-based support groups for survivors and their families are recommended as valuable sources of emotional support, social networking, and information.

Sexuality

Sexual dysfunction is commonly reported following TBI, and many sexual issues include inappropriate behavior, impulsivity, decreased libido, and inadequate sexual performance.[65,107] Hibbard and colleagues compared individuals with TBI to

Table 50-14 Common neurocognitive impairments observed by rehabilitation professionals following traumatic brain injury, and intervention techniques

Neurocognitive deficits	Intervention strategies
Attention and concentration problems	• Reduce distractions in the environment (e.g. wear ear plugs, sit facing wall, clear desk before beginning work). • Avoid interruptions (e.g. use 'do not disturb' sign). • Use self-coaching (or talking self through a task) to stay on track. • Schedule regular breaks throughout the day to reduce fatigue. • Alternate between cognitively challenging and less demanding tasks. • Set goals to sustain attention for longer periods of time, using timers to signify when time has elapsed. • Be sure you have the patient's full attention before beginning to present information (e.g. say the patient's name, make eye contact with the patient) and redirect the patient to the task if attention wanes. • Avoid multitasking when possible; if not possible, record information about stopping point before changing tasks. • Consider medication alternatives (e.g. psychostimulants).
Learning and memory deficits	• Use assistive devices such as memory books, calendars, 'to do' lists, cameras, alarms, and tape recorders. • Establish routines and maintain structure. • Present information in many forms (e.g. auditory, visual, kinetic) and demonstrate tasks. • Repeat information. • Have clients tape record and replay information in order to listen to material several times. • Use pillboxes and alarms to aid in recall of medication. • Teach patients mnemonic strategies, imagery techniques, and rhymes to facilitate recall of important information. • Break tasks down into small steps and introduce new steps as earlier steps are accomplished.
Planning and problem-solving deficits	• Ask patients how they plan to approach task prior to beginning, and help them evaluate potential for success with their plan. • Encourage patients to stop and think before acting. • Teach patients to use structured problem-solving techniques (i.e. define the problem, brainstorm alternatives, evaluate options, select best option, assess success of solution). • Encourage patients to develop and maintain mentor relationship with a trusted family member or friend who can provide constructive feedback.
Language problems	• Use short, simple sentences and enunciate clearly when presenting information to the patient. • Provide instructions in multiple formats (e.g. oral and written). • Teach the patient to repeat and paraphrase information to ensure they heard the information correctly. • Encourage the patient to ask others to repeat information and speak slowly and clearly. • Be patient and allow patients time to find words and complete sentences. • Provide contextual and phonemic cues. • Encourage patients to use gestures, drawings, and descriptions when speaking. • Support efforts to speak and be alert for social withdrawal. • Educate family members and caregivers about the nature of deficits and techniques to ensure successful communication.
Academic impairments	• Teach patients to use a calculator for all but the most basic mathematic operations and check work carefully. • Rely on family for financial management. • Encourage patients to take notes and highlight or underline key words while they are reading. • Teach the PQRST method for reading comprehension (preview, question, read, study, test). • To aid in spelling difficulties, encourage use of electronic spelling aid, word processing spell checker, or speller's dictionary. • Encourage patients to make flash cards to review words frequently missed, play Scrabble, and work crossword and other puzzles. • Focus on quality versus quantity, and allow ample time for task completion.

persons with other types of disabilities with respect to sexuality, and found that individuals with TBIs have more frequent physiologic problems and body image difficulties.[107] Sexual dysfunction often has a profound negative effect on the maintenance and development of romantic relationships. Psychotherapeutic approaches are designed to help TBI survivors and their family members cope with difficulties such as impaired sexual performance or disinhibition.[61]

Traditional sex therapists often assert that poor-quality relationships often underlie complaints about intimate relations. Professionals should not neglect to appreciate how brain injury has affected survivors' physical functioning. However, improving the quality of the marital relationship, especially positive communication and mutual support, can greatly benefit physical aspects of the couple's relationship. Some researchers have asserted that a majority of spouses and patients suffer from major depressive disorder. Depression affects sexuality, and treatment of depression can have a myriad of important benefits (see also Ch. 32).

Return to school and work
Return to school or return to work assessments
Research suggests that the majority of patients who sustained moderate or severe TBI are unable to sustain employment post injury or return to their preinjury school environment.[30,90,115,153] Given that TBI most often affects young men who are in the most productive years of their working lives, return to work is typically an important goal for patients and their families.[62,286] School and vocational issues are also primary concerns of referral sources. Commonly, the referral questions focus on vocational disability, readiness to return to school or work, ability to maintain current employment status, workplace safety issues, and needs for vocational rehabilitation services and school or workplace accommodations. Neuropsychologists are often called on to conduct comprehensive neuropsychologic evaluations to reveal strengths and limitations, identify potential obstacles to successful return to work, and make recommendations for intervention.

Evaluation and subsequent rehabilitation for cognitive and linguistic difficulties is a long-term endeavor, and is especially challenging in the pediatric population. Cognitive and communication deficits are difficult to measure and address, due to a relative paucity of assessment tools.[113] Examination and treatment must be further tailored to the age and expected cognition of the child. Although many children regain lower level language ability within 3 months, they remain at risk for later academic failure and difficulty with higher order cognition.[36] Deficits in attention and information processing can significantly impair future learning in both daily and academic environments, and may lead to global cognitive dysfunction. Rehabilitative efforts must be flexible and ongoing through maturation to maximize potential cognitive ability.

Intervention models
Following comprehensive evaluation, neuropsychologists offer recommendations and provide treatment to address potential obstacles to employment. For example, patients can be taught strategies to compensate for cognitive difficulties. Social, coping, and relaxation skills training are often provided. Psychotherapy can be offered to facilitate adjustment to postinjury life changes and to psychologic and neurobehavioral difficulties. Treatment also focuses on the development of reasonable vocational and life goals, and effective problem solving. In addition, neuropsychologists advocate for services required for successful return to work.

Following TBI, patients often need additional support, such as supported employment, to supplement traditional vocational rehabilitation. With supported employment, individuals are placed in paid positions and work with individuals with and without disabilities.[237] Vocational specialists, or job coaches, assist with job placement, skills training, and on the job supports. In contrast to center-based rehabilitation models, most of the vocational rehabilitation professional's time is spent helping patients after they find a job, rather than before. Vocational specialists reduce their time on the job site as the patient exhibits proficiency with the job requirements, but continue to provide ongoing support services to aid in job retention.[237,278,279] Wehman and colleagues evaluated the effectiveness of a supportive employment program for patients following severe TBI.[278] Preliminary assessments were conducted to match participants to job openings. Participants received assistance to address common obstacles to employment, such as transportation or housing issues and interpersonal difficulties. Interventions included vocational training, social skills training, employment accommodations and modifications, and counseling. On and off site work supports were also provided. Results revealed that all participants were able to return to work with supported employment services. Wehman and colleagues conducted a long-term follow-up study evaluating the costs and efficiency of supported employment.[279] The findings supported the assertion that supported employment is cost-effective for persons with disabilities.

Driving assessment and intervention
Driving evaluation
Given the inherent danger associated with driving, driving safety is a common area of concern for families of persons with TBI and referral sources following TBI. Evaluation of driving abilities is a complex matter. Patients typically are eager to regain their independence through driving. Awareness issues can hamper their ability to recognize driving safety. Alternatively, patients who have been involved in motor vehicle crashes might be fearful of driving. Family members can have a variety of reactions as well. Some might be impatient about having their loved one return to driving, due to the inconvenience of transporting the individual to appointments, while others might be very protective of the patient and fear return to driving.

Hopewell and van Zomeren recommend a multistage model of decision making with respect to driving.[111] Predriving assessments are typically encouraged prior to in vivo driving evaluations[111,186] Predriving assessments usually involve assessment of the basic skills necessary for driving. Neuropsychologic evaluation provides information about areas of neuropsychologic functioning that are important for safe driving, including attention and concentration, speed of information processing, learning, memory, executive functioning, visuoperception, visuomotor functioning, motor functioning, and personality.[31,112,186] During the predriving assessment, patients and their family members might also be asked about their concerns, and about recent accidents or traffic violations.

The Judgment and Safety Screening Inventory (JASSI)[157] can be utilized to gain both patient and informant perspectives, allowing for cross-informant comparisons. The JASSI was designed to assess patient and informant concern levels (none, little, much, or very) about patients' judgment and safety concerns in the following areas: travel; financial management; interpersonal functioning; food and kitchen; use of appliances, tools, and utensils; household issues; medications and alcohol; fire safety; and firearm safety. Within the travel domain, respondents are asked to provide information about driving safety (e.g. having accidents, distractibility, and failing to yield right of way) and other travel-related issues (e.g. traveling in dangerous neighborhoods, failing to look both ways when crossing the street, and not using a helmet). Medical evaluation is also necessary to rule out the presence of seizures and other physical problems that might hinder the ability to drive safely.

After passing predriving assessments, patients can progress to evaluation via driving simulator or in vivo driving.[111,186] Simulators yield information about the patient's ability to maintain control of the vehicle and operate the vehicle. Behind the wheel driving assessments can be conducted in specified courses (e.g. parking lot maneuvering) or on the road.

Driver's training

After identifying areas of weakness, driver's training can be offered to remediate problems. Classes can be provided to teach defensive driving techniques and compensatory strategies to address cognitive deficits. In addition, simulated and in vivo driver's training offers opportunities to practice strategies taught in the classroom setting, and allows for practice to improve response time.[186] Many hospitals and rehabilitation facilities offer driver's training, and community organizations such as the American Association of Retired Persons offer classes in defensive driving. Following driver's training, reevaluation might be valuable to determine whether or not the patient is capable of driving safely.

Disability determination

Disability determination involves ascertaining whether or not the patient has the capacity to engage in gainful employment. Clinicians are asked to determine if patients are disabled secondary to physical or mental impairments associated with TBI. When conducting disability evaluations, physicians must determine the nature and extent of the medical impairment, and the impact of the medical condition on the patients' ability to work long term. Neuropsychologists are typically involved in identifying the nature and extent of cognitive and psychologic impairments that can preclude working. Results from compre-

hensive neuropsychologic evaluation yield valuable information about the impact of TBI on neurobehavioral, emotional, cognitive, and academic functioning. Assessment of vocational issues is also valuable. The reader is referred to the section entitled *Return to school or return to work assessments* for additional information. The neuropsychologist uses the findings to determine whether or not the patient can successfully return to their prior job or perform other jobs (see also Chs 6 and 36).

Questions also arise surrounding the ability to drive, to live independently, and to manage finances and medications. Evaluation of patients' judgment is critical to disability determination. To do so, the clinician can ask patients and their family members about daily functioning. The JASSI[157] was developed to assess judgment and safety in daily functioning. With the JASSI, medication issues are assessed (such as forgetting medications, using alcohol while taking medications, and not taking medications as prescribed). With respect to financial management, the JASSI includes questions about forgetting to pay bills, losing money, giving others personal financial information, and misplacing credit cards and checkbooks. Concerns are also evaluated in the areas of driving, kitchen safety, household management, interpersonal issues, fire safety, and firearm safety. When assessing the extent of disability, the clinician is also called on to determine if the patient's ability to live independently is negatively impacted by factors such as mobility issues and impaired smell.

Medicolegal involvement

Motor vehicle crashes are the primary reasons for hospitalization for persons with TBI. Following injury, many patients seek legal counsel for assistance in obtaining treatment or compensation for their injuries and healthcare costs. Medical professionals and neuropsychologists are often asked to serve as experts in legal cases. Common questions posed by attorneys during the litigation process include the following.[157]

- Did the patient sustain a TBI?
- How severe was the TBI?
- Describe pre- and postinjury levels of functioning and indicate if the injury exacerbated prior problems.
- What are the long-term physical, neuropsychologic, cognitive, neurobehavioral, and emotional sequelae of the injury?
- Are the sequelae consistent with those expected following similar injuries?
- Are there other factors that better account for presenting complaints and observed deficits (e.g. preexisting problems, psychologic issues, level of motivation or effort, and secondary gain issues)?
- What is the potential long-term impact of the injury in terms of vocational, academic, interpersonal, and daily functioning?
- What is the prognosis for improvement with and without treatment?

- Are current treatments reasonable, necessary, and likely to be beneficial?
- What type of treatments and services will be necessary to optimize functioning?

Comprehensive review of records is typically the first step in medicolegal evaluations. Records review is critical for understanding the potential impact of preexisting problems, and for gaining information about mechanism of injury, injury severity, and treatment history. Records can also provide information about history of litigation or benefit seeking. Following the record review, comprehensive evaluation is typically warranted to evaluate the nature and extent of the injury and resulting impairments. Evaluation of motivation and effort is a standard component of comprehensive neuropsychologic evaluation. To assess level of effort, standardized tests are administered, such as the Portland Digit Recognition Test,[14,15] Recognition Memory Test,[274] Rey 15-Item Test,[218] and Test of Memory Malingering.[264] Consistency in performance on various tests, consistency of deficits with the level of injury, and consistency between test results and observed behaviors and presenting complaints are considered. Information is also gathered about potential secondary gain issues (e.g. revenge, financial gain, and disability) and history of litigation and benefit seeking.

Medicolegal evaluation culminates in production of a report that presents conclusions derived from records review and evaluation. Successful reports address questions posed by referral sources in a thorough manner. Factors that are often addressed in the context of a thorough report include educational, vocational, legal, and interpersonal history; family medical and mental health history; history of premorbid and postinjury medical and mental health problems and treatment; injury information and injury-related treatment history; presenting complaints; patients' attributions for problems; behavioral observations; motivation and effort during testing; level of self-awareness; test results; consistency of test data; conclusions about the nature and extent of injury and injury-related effects; treatment needs; and prognosis.[151]

SUMMARY

Traumatic brain injuries occur to 1.4 million Americans annually, cutting across all age and ethnic categories. The rehabilitation of individuals with TBI requires a wide range of expertise, and entails a variety of treatment teams and settings. Primary prevention and early management of injuries to prevent secondary damage are vital to successful outcomes. Impairment and disability can include a combination of medical, physical, cognitive, behavioral, and functional difficulties that are best managed by specialized clinicians working in dedicated TBI teams. Short- and long-term outcomes after TBI are typically good, and can be monitored using well-accepted measurement tools. Ongoing research is focused on prevention of secondary brain injury following initial trauma, and improving pharmacologic and rehabilitative treatments for neuromedical, cognitive, and behavioral sequelae.

REFERENCES

1. Adams JH, Doyle D, Ford I, et al. Diffuse axonal injury in head injury: definition, diagnosis and grading. Histopathology 1989; 15:49–59.
2. Agency for Health Care Policy and Research. Rehabilitation for traumatic brain injury in children and adolescents. Evidence report/technology assessment. No. 2, supplement. September 1999.
3. Aitken ME, Mele N, Barrett KW. Recovery of injured children: parent perspectives on family needs. Arch Phys Med Rehabil 2004; 85(4): 567–572.
4. American Academy of Pediatrics. Falls from heights: windows, roofs, and balconies. Pediatrics 2001; 107:1188–1191.
5. Annegers JF, Grabow JD, Broover RV, et al. Seizures after head trauma: a population study. Neurology 1980; 30:683–689.
6. Annegers JF, Grabow JD, Kurland LT. The incidence, causes and secular trends of head injury in Olmstead County, Minnesota. Neurology 1980; 30:912–919.
7. Annegers JF. The epidemiology of head trauma in children. In: Shapiro K, ed. Pediatric head trauma. Mt. Kisco: Futura; 1983.
8. [Anonymous]. Fatality reduction by safety belts for front-seat occupants of cars and light trucks. Ann Emerg Med 2001; 37:728–729.
9. Ariza M, Junque C, Mataro M, et al. Neuropsychological correlates of basal ganglia and medial temporal lobe NAA/Cho reductions in traumatic brain injury. Arch Neurol 2004; 61:541–544.
10. Audenaert K, Jansen HM, Otte A, et al. Imaging of mild traumatic brain injury using ^{57}Co and ^{99m}Tc HNPAO SPECT as compared to other diagnostic procedures. Med Sci Monit 2003; 9:MT112–MT117.
11. Barth JT, Macciocchi SN, Diamond PT. Mild head injury: current research and clinical issues. In: Rosenthal M, Griffin ER, Kreutzer JS, et al, eds. Rehabilitation of the adult and child with traumatic brain injury. 3rd edn. Philadelphia: FA Davis; 1999:471–478.
12. Beaumont A, Marmarou A. Treatment of raised intracranial pressure following traumatic brain injury. Crit Rev Neurosurg 1999; 9(4):207–216.
13. Berek K, Jeschow M, Aichner F. The prognostication of cerebral hypoxia after out-of-hospital cardiac arrest in adults. Eur Neurol 1999; 37:135–145.
14. Binder LM, Willis SC. Assessment of motivation after financially compensable minor head trauma. Psychol Assess J Consult Clin Psychol 1991; 3:175–181.
15. Binder LM. Assessment of malingering after mild head trauma with the Portland Digit Recognition Test. J Clin Exp Neuropsychol 1993; 15:170–182.
16. Bishara SN, Partridge FM, Godfrey HPD, et al. Posttraumatic amnesia and Glasgow Coma Scale related to outcome in survivors in a consecutive series of patients with severe closed-head injury. Brain Inj 1992; 6: 373–380.
17. Blumbergs PC, Scott G, Manavis J, et al. Topography of axonal injury as defined by amyloid precursor protein and the sector scoring method in mild and severe closed head injury. J Neurotrauma 1995; 12:565–572.
18. Boake C, Freeland JC, Ringholz GM, et al. Awareness of memory loss after severe closed-head injury. Brain Inj 1995; 9(3):273–283.
19. Bogner JA, Corrigan JD, Mysiw WJ, et al. A comparison of substance abuse and violence in the prediction of long-term rehabilitation outcomes after brain injury. Arch Phys Med Rehabil 2001; 82:571–577.
20. Bond MR. The psychiatry of closed head injury. In: Brooks N, ed. Closed head injury: psychological, social and family consequences. New York: Oxford Press; 1984.
21. Bonne O, Gilboa A, Louzoun Y, et al. Cerebral blood flow in chronic symptomatic milt traumatic brain injury. Psychiatry Res 2003; 124: 141–152.
22. Born JD, Albert A, Hans P, et al. Relative predictive value of best motor response and brain stem reflexes in patients with severe head injury. Head Inj 1985; 71:54–58.
23. Bouma GJ, Muizelaar JP, Stringer WA, et al. Ultra-early evaluation of regional cerebral blood flow in severe head injured patients using xenon-enhanced computerized tomography. J Neurosurg 1992; 77:360–368.
24. Brain Trauma Foundation–American Association of Neurological Surgeons–Joint Section on Neurotrauma and Critical Care. Early indicators of prognosis in severe traumatic brain injury. J Neurotrauma 2000; 17:449–554.
25. Brain Trauma Foundation–American Association of Neurological Surgeons–Joint Section on Neurotrauma and Critical Care. Guidelines for the

management of severe traumatic brain injury. J Neurotrauma 2000; 17:454–560.

26. Brooke M, Questad K, Patterson D, et al. Agitation and restlessness after closed head injury: a prospective study of 100 consecutive admissions. Arch Phys Med Rehabil 1992; 73:320–323.

27. Brooke MM, Patterson DR, Questad KA. The treatment of agitation during initial hospitalization after traumatic brain injury. Arch Phys Med Rehabil 1992; 73:917–921.

28. Brooks N, Campsie L, Symington C, et al. The effects of severe head injury on patient and relative within seven years post injury. J Head Trauma Rehabil 1987; 2:1–13.

29. Brooks N, Campsie L, Symington C, et al. The five year outcome of severe blunt head injury: a relative's view. J Neurol 1986; 49:764–770.

30. Brooks N, McKinlay W, Symington C, et al. Return to work within the first seven years of severe head injury. Brain Inj 1987; 1:5–19.

31. Brouwer WH, Withaar FK, Tant ML, et al. Attention and driving in traumatic brain injury: a question of coping with time-pressure. J Head Trauma Rehabil 2002; 17(1):1–15.

32. Burnett DM, Watanabe TK, Greenwald BD. Congenital and acquired brain injury. 2. Brain injury rehabilitation: medical management. Arch Phys Med Rehabil 2003; 84(suppl 1):S8–S11.

33. Butler R, Satz P. Individual psychotherapy with head injured adults: clinical notes for the practitioner. Prof Psychol Res Pract 1988; 19(5): 536–541.

34. Campbell CH. Needs of relatives and helpfulness of support groups in severe head injury. Rehabil Nurs 1988; 13(6):320–325.

35. Centers for Disease Control and Prevention. Traumatic brain injury in the United States: a report to Congress. Atlanta: CDC; 1999. Online. Available: http://www.cdc.gov/ncipc/pub-res/tbicongress.htm

36. Chapman SB, McKinnon L, Levin HS, et al. Longitudinal outcome of verbal discourse in children with traumatic brain injury: three-year follow-up. J Head Trauma Rehabil 2001; 16(5):441–455.

37. Choi SC. Predicting outcome in the head-injured patient. In: Narayan RK, Wilberger JE, Povlishock JT, eds. Neurotrauma. New York: McGraw-Hill; 1996:593–611.

38. Choskey MS, Costa DC, Iannotti F, et al. [99]TcMHMPAO SPECT studies in traumatic intracerebral haematoma. J Neurol Neurosurg Psychiatry 1991; 54:6–11.

39. Cicerone K, Dahlberg C, Kalmar K, et al. Evidence based cognitive rehabilitation: recommendations for clinical practice. Arch Phys Med Rehabil 2000; 81:1596–1615.

40. Cicerone KD, Wood JC. Planning disorder after closed head injury: a case study. Arch Phys Med Rehabil 1987; 68:111–115.

41. Cicerone KD. Remediation of 'working attention' in mild traumatic brain injury. Brain Inj 2002; 16:185–195.

42. Cifu DX, Johns J. Subacute rehabilitation programs. Do they really produce good outcomes? Adv Med Directors Rehabil 1998; 7:35–39.

43. Cifu DX, Kaelin DL, Wall BE. Deep venous thrombosis: incidence on admission to a brain injury rehabilitation program. Arch Phys Med Rehabil 1996; 77(11):1182–1185.

44. Cifu DX, Kreutzer JS, Kolakowsky-Hayner MA, et al. The relationship between therapy intensity and rehabilitative outcomes after traumatic brain injury: a multicenter analysis. Arch Phys Med Rehabil 2003; 84:1441–1448.

45. Cifu DX, Kreutzer JS, Marwitz JH, et al. Functional outcomes of older adults with traumatic brain injury: a prospective, multicenter analysis. Arch Phys Med Rehabil 1996; 77(9):883–888.

46. Clifton GL, Miller ER, Choi SC, et al. Lack of effect of induction of hypothermia after acute brain injury. N Engl J Med 2001; 344:556–563.

47. Cohadon F, Richer E, Reglade C, et al. Psychological consequences of vertigo and the effectiveness of vestibular rehabilitation for brain injury patients. Brain Injury 2001; 15(5):387–400.

48. Cook N. Respiratory care in spinal cord injury with associated traumatic brain injury: bridging the gap in critical care nursing interventions. Intensive Crit Care Nurs 2003; 19(3):143–153.

49. Coonley-Hoganson R, Sachs N, Desai BT, et al. Sequelae associated with head injuries in patients who were not hospitalized: a follow-up survey. Neurosurgery 1984; 14:315–317.

50. Corrigan JD, Bogner JA, Lamb-Hart GL. Substance abuse and brain injury. In: Rosenthal M, Griffin ER, Kreutzer JS, et al, eds. Rehabilitation of the adult and child with traumatic brain injury. 3rd edn. Philadelphia: FA Davis; 1999:556–571.

51. Corrigan JD, Bogner JA, Mysiw WJ, et al. Life satisfaction after traumatic brain injury. J Head Trauma Rehabil 2001; 16(6):543–555.

52. Corrigan JD, Smith-Knapp K, Granger CV. Outcomes in the first 5 years after traumatic brain injury. Arch Phys Med Rehabil 1998; 79(3): 298–305.

53. Corrigan JD. Development of a scale for assessment of agitation following traumatic brain injury. J Clin Exp Neuropsychol 1989; 11(2):261–277.

54. Corrigan JD. Substance abuse as a mediating factor in outcome from traumatic brain injury. Arch Phys Med Rehabil 1995; 76:302–309.

55. Courjon J. A longitudinal electro-clinical study of 80 cases of posttraumatic epilepsy observed from the time of original trauma. Epilepsia 1970; 11:29–36.

56. Crandall CS, Olson LM, Sklar DP. Mortality reduction with air bag and seat belt use in head-on passenger car collisions. Am J Epidemiol 2001; 153:219–224.

57. Cuthbertson DP. Alterations in metabolism following injury: part 1. Injury 1980; 11:175.

58. Dikmen S, Machamer JE. Neurobehavioral outcomes and their determinants. J Head Trauma Rehabil 1995; 10:74–86.

59. Dikmen SS, Ross BL, Machamer JE, et al. One year psychosocial outcome in head injury. J Int Neuropsychiatr Soc 1995; 1:67–77.

60. Dodrill CB, Troupin AS. Neuropsychological effects of carbamazepine and phenytoin: a reanalysis. Neurology 1991; 41:141–143.

61. Dombrowski LK, Petrick JD, Strauss D. Rehabilitation treatment of sexuality issues due to acquired brain injury. Rehabil Psychol 2000; 45(3):299–309.

62. Doninger N, Heinemann A, Bode R, et al. Predicting community integration following traumatic brain injury with health and cognitive status measures. Rehabil Psychol 2003; 48(2):67–76.

63. Duffy FH, Hughes JR, Miranda F, et al. Status of quantitative EEG (QEEG) in clinical practice, 1994. Clin Electroencephalogr 1994; 25(4):6–22.

64. Eisenberg HM. Outcome and head injury: general considerations and neurobehavioral recovery—part 1, general considerations. In: Becker DP, Povlishock JT, eds. Central nervous system status report. Bethesda: National Institute of Neurological and Communicative Diseases and Stroke; 1985:271–280.

65. Elliott ML, Biever LS. Head injury and sexual dysfunction. Brain Inj 1996; 10(10):703–717.

66. Elovic E, Zafonte RD. Spasticity management in traumatic brain injury. Phys Med Rehabil State Art Rev 2001; 15:327–348.

67. Elovic EP, Lansang R, Li Y, et al. The use of atypical antipsychotics in traumatic brain injury. J Head Trauma Rehabil 2003; 18(2):177–195.

68. Englander J, Bushnik T, Duong T, et al. Analyzing risk factors for late posttraumatic seizures: a prospective, multicenter investigation. Arch Phys Med Rehabil 2003; 84:365–373.

69. Englander J, Cifu DX, Zafonte R, et al. Impact of medical complications on outcome after traumatic brain injury. J Head Trauma Rehabil 1996; 11:15–26.

70. Evans JH. Post-traumatic epilepsy. Neurology (Minneap) 1962; 12:6665–6674.

71. Fakhry SM, Trask AL, Waller MA, et al. Management of brain-injured patients by an evidence based medicine protocol improves outcomes and decreases hospital charges. J Trauma 2004; 56:292–499.

72. Fann JR, Katon WJ, Uomoto JM, et al. Psychiatric disorders and functional disability in outpatients with traumatic brain injuries. Am J Psychiatry 1995; 152:1493–1499.

73. Field LH, Weiss CJ. Dysphagia with head injury. Brain Inj 1989; 3:19–26.

74. Flannery J. Using the levels of cognitive functioning assessment scale with patients with traumatic brain injury in an acute care setting. Rehabil Nurs 1998; 23(2):88–94.

75. Fleminger S, Oliver DL, Lovestone S, et al. Head injury as a risk factor for Alzheimer's disease: the evidence 10 years on; a partial replication. J Neurol Neurosurg Psychiatry 2003; 74:857–862.

76. Flin C, Curalucci H, Duvocelle A, et al. Heterotopic ossification and brain injury. Ann Readapt Med Phys 2002; 45(9):517–520.

77. Fontaine A, Azouvi P, Remy P, et al. Functional anatomy of neuropsychological deficits after severe traumatic brain injury. Neurology 1999; 53:1963–1968.

78. Foster NL, Chase TN, Fedio P, et al. Alzheimer's disease: focal cortical changes shown by positron emission tomography. Neurology 1983; 33:961–965.

79. Frankowski RF, Annegers JF, Whitman S. The descriptive epidemiology of head injury in the United States. In: Becker DP, Povlishock JT, eds. Central nervous system status report. Bethesda: NINCDS; 1985:33–43.

80. Frankowski RF. The demography of head injury in the United States. In: Miner M, Wagner KA, eds. Neurotrauma, vol 1. Boston: Butterworths; 1986:1–17.

81. Garland DE, Blum CE, Waters RL. Periarticular heterotopic ossification in head-injured adults. Incidence and location. J Bone Joint Surg 1980; 62:1143–1146.

82. Garnett MR, Corkill RG, Blamire AM, et al. Altered cellular metabolism following traumatic brain injury: a magnetic resonance imaging study. J Neurotrauma 2001; 18:231–240.

83. Geerts WH, Code KI, Jay RM, et al. A prospective study of venous thromboembolism after major trauma. N Engl J Med 1994; 331(24): 1601–1606.

84. Geerts WH, Heit JA, Clagett GP, et al. Prevention of venous thromboembolism. Chest 2001; 119(suppl):132S–175S.

85. Genarelli TA. Cerebral concussion and diffuse brain injuries. In: Cooper PA, ed. Head injury. 3rd edn. Baltimore: Williams & Wilkins; 1993: 137–158.

86. Gervasio A, Kreutzer J. Kinship and family member's psychological distress after traumatic brain injury: a large sample study. J Head Trauma Rehabil 1997; 12(3):14–26.

87. Giancino JT, Ashwal S, Childs N, et al. The minimally conscious state: definition and diagnostic criteria. Neurology 2002; 58:349–353.

88. Goldenberg G, Oder W, Spatt J, et al. Cerebral correlates of disturbed executive function and memory in survivors of severe closed head injury: a SPECT study. J Neurol Neurosurg Psychiatry 1992; 55:362–368.

89. Goldstein FC, Levin HS. Neurobehavioral outcome of traumatic brain injury in older adults: initial findings. J Head Trauma Rehabil 1995; 10(1):57–73.

90. Gollaher K, High W, Sherer M, et al. Prediction of employment outcome one to three years following traumatic brain injury. Brain Inj 1998; 12:255–263.

91. Gordon WA, Mann N, Willer B. Demographic and social characteristics of the Traumatic Brain Injury Model System Database. J Head Trauma Rehabil 1993; 8:12–25.

92. Grafman J, Jonas B, Salazar A. Epilepsy following penetrating head injury to the frontal lobes. Adv Neurol 1992; 57:369–378.

93. Graham DI. Neuropathology of head injury. In: Narayan RK, Wilberger JE, Povlishock JT, eds. Neurotrauma. New York: McGraw-Hill; 1996:43–59.

94. Granger CV, Hamilton BB, Sherwin FS. Guide for use of the uniform data set for medical rehabilitation. Buffalo: State University of New York; 1986.

95. Greenberg RP, Becker DP, Miller JD, et al. Evaluation of brain function in severe head trauma with multimodality evoked potentials: part 2. Localization of brain dysfunction and correlation with posttraumatic neurologic conditions. J Neurosurg 1977; 47:163–177.

96. Greenberg RP, Stablein DM, Becker DP. Noninvasive localization of brainstem lesions in the cat with multimodality evoked potentials: correlation with human head injury data. J Neurosurg 1981; 54:740–750.

97. Greenwald BD, Burnett DM, Miller MA. Congenital and acquired brain injury: 1. Brain injury: epidemiology and pathophysiology. Arch Phys Med Rehabil 2003; 84(suppl 1):S3–S7.

98. Groher ME, Picon-Nieto L. Evaluation of communication and swallowing disorders. In: Rosenthal M, Griffith ER, Kreutzer JS, et al, eds. Rehabilitation of the adult and child with traumatic brain injury. 3rd edn. Philadelphia: FA Davis; 1999:183–198.

99. Gupata SR, Mlcoh AG. Bromocriptine treatment of nonfluent aphasia. Arch Phys Med Rehabil 1992; 73:373–376.

100. Haaland KY, Temkin N, Randahl G, et al. Recovery of simple motor skills after head injury. J Clin Exp Neuropsychol 1994; 16(3):448–456.

101. Hagen C, Malkmus D, Durham P. Levels of cognitive functioning. Downey: Rancho Los Amigos Hospital; 1972.

102. Hall KM, Hamilton BB, Gordon WA, et al. Characteristics and comparisons of functional assessment indices: Disability Rating Scale, Functional Independence Measure and Functional Assessment Measure. J Head Trauma Rehabil 1993; 8(2):60–74.

103. Harris J, Godfrey H, Partridge F, et al. Caregiver depression following traumatic brain injury (TBI): a consequence of adverse effects on family members? Brain Inj 2001; 15(3):223–238.

104. Harrison-Felix C, Newton CN, Hall K, et al. Descriptive findings from the Traumatic Brain Injury Model Systems national database. J Head Trauma Rehabil 1996; 11(5):1–14.

105. Harrison-Felix C, Zafonte R, Mann N, et al. Brain injury as a result of violence: preliminary findings from the traumatic brain injury model systems. Arch Phys Med Rehabil 1998; 79:730–737.

106. Hauser WA, Annegers JF, Kurland LT. Prevalence of epilepsy in Rochester, Minnesota: 1940–1980. Epilepsia 1991; 32:429–445.

107. Hibbard MR, Gordon WA, Flanagan S, et al. Sexual dysfunction after traumatic brain injury. Neurorehabilitation 2000; 15(2):107–120.

108. Hibbard MR, Uysal S, Kepler K, et al. Axis I psychopathology in individuals with traumatic brain injury. J Head Trauma Rehabil 1998; 13(4):24–39.

109. Hoffman JM, Doctor JN, Chan L, et al. Potential impact of the new Medicare prospective payment system on reimbursement for traumatic brain injury inpatient reimbursement. Arch Phys Med Rehabil 2003; 84(8):1165–1172.

110. Holland D, Shigaki CL. Educating families and caretakers of traumatically brain injured patients in the new health care environment: a three-phase model and bibliography. Brain Inj 1998; 12(12):993–1009.

111. Hopewell CA, van Zomeren AH. Neuropsychological aspects of motor vehicle operation. In: Tupper DE, Cicerone KD, eds. The neuropsychology of everyday life: assessment and basic competencies. Boston: Kluwer; 1990.

112. Hopewell CA. Driving assessment issues for practicing clinicians. J Head Trauma Rehabil 2002; 17(1):48–61.

113. Hotz G, Helm-Estabrooks N, Nelson NW. Development of the Pediatric Test of Brain Injury. J Head Trauma Rehabil 2001; 16(5): 426–440.

114. Hyers TM, Agnelli G, Hull RD, et al. Antithrombotic therapy for venous thromboembolic disease. Chest 2001; 119(suppl 1):176S–193S.

115. Jacobs HE. The Los Angeles head injury survey: procedures and findings. Arch Phys Med Rehabil 1988; 69:425–431.

116. Jennett B, Bond M. Assessment of outcome after severe brain damage. Lancet 1975; i:480–487.

117. Jennett B, Teasdale G. Management of head injuries. Philadelphia: FA Davis; 1981.

118. Jennett B. EEG prediction of post-traumatic epilepsy. Epilepsia 1975; 16:251–256.

119. Johns JS, Cifu DX, Keyser-Marcus L, et al. Impact of clinically significant heterotopic ossification on functional outcome after traumatic brain injury. J Head Trauma Rehabil 1999; 14(3):269–276.

120. Jones KB, Mollano AV, Morcuende JA, et al. Bone and brain: a review of neural, hormonal, and musculoskeletal connections. Iowa Orthop J 2004; 24:123–132.

121. Jordan BD, Zimmerman RD. Magnetic resonance imaging in amateur boxers. Arch Neurol 1988; 45:1207–1208.

122. Judson JA, Cant BR, Shaw NA. Early prediction of outcome from cerebral trauma by somatosensory evoked potentials. Crit Care Med 1990; 18:363–368.

123. Junque C, Bruna O, Mataro M. Information needs of the traumatic brain injury patient's family members regarding the consequences of injury and associated perception of physical, cognitive, emotional and quality of life changes. Brain Inj 1997; 11(4):251–258.

124. Kadyan V, Colachis SC, Depalma MJ, et al. Early recognition of neuroleptic malignant syndrome during traumatic brain injury rehabilitation. Brain Inj 2003; 17(7):631–637.

125. Kaelin DL, Cifu DX, Matthies B. Methylphenidate effect on attention deficit in the acutely brain-injured adult. Arch Phys Med Rehabil 1996; 77:6–9.

126. Katz DI, Alexander MP, Klein RB. Recovery of arm function in patients with paresis after traumatic brain injury. Arch Phys Med Rehabil 1998; 79(5):488–493.

127. Katz DI, Alexander MP. Traumatic brain injury: predicting course of recovery and outcome for patients admitted to rehabilitation. Arch Neurol 1994; 51:661–670.

128. Katz DI, Mills V. Traumatic brain injury: natural history and efficacy of cognitive rehabilitation. In: Stuss D, Winocur G, Robertson IH, eds. Cognitive rehabilitation. Cambridge: Cambridge University Press; 1999: 279–301.

129. Katz DI, White DK, Alexander MP, et al. Recovery of ambulation after traumatic brain injury. Arch Phys Med Rehabil 2004; 85(6): 865–869.

130. Keenan MA, Haider T. The formation of heterotopic ossification after traumatic brain injury: a biopsy study with ultra-structural analysis. J Head Trauma Rehabil 1996; 11(4):8–22.

131. Kennedy R, Burnett DM, Greenwald BD. Use of antiepileptics in traumatic brain injury: a review for psychiatrists. Ann Clin Psychiatry 2001; 13:163–171.

132. Keyser L, Witol AD, Kreutzer JS, et al. Multi-center investigation of neurobehavioral outcome after traumatic brain injury. Neurorehabilitation 1995; 5:255–267.

133. Kirby BS, Van Horn JE, Ostrem JL, et al. Cognitive activation during PET: a case study of monozygotic twins discordant for closed head injury. Neuropsychologia 1996; 34:689–697.

134. Kishore PR, Lipper MH, Girevendulis AK, et al. Posttraumatic hydrocephalus in patients with severe head injury. Neuroradiology 1978; 16:261–265.

135. Knoller N, Levi L, Shoshan I, et al. Dexanabinol (HU-211) in the treatment of severe closed head injury: a randomized, placebo controlled, phase II clinical trial. Crit Care Med 2002; 30:548–554.

136. Kolakowsky-Hayner SA, Gourley EV, Kreutzer JS, et al. Pre-injury substance abuse among persons with brain injury and persons with spinal cord injury. Brain Inj 1999; 13(8):571–581.

137. Kolakowsky-Hayner SA, Kreutzer JS. Pre-injury crime, substance abuse, and neurobehavioural functioning after traumatic brain injury. Brain Inj 2001; 15(1):53–63.

138. Kolakowsky-Hayner SA, Miner KD, Kreutzer JS. Long-term life quality and family needs after traumatic brain injury. J Head Trauma Rehabil 2001; 16(4):374–385.

139. Kraus JF, Black MA, Hessol N, et al. The incidence of acute brain injury and serious impairment in a defined population. Am J Epidemiol 1984; 119:186–201.

140. Kraus JF, McArthur DI, Silverman TA, et al. Epidemiology of brain injury. In: Narayan RK, Wilberger JE Jr, Povlishock JT, eds. Neurotrauma. New York: McGraw-Hill; 1996:13–30.

141. Kraus JF, McArthur DI. Epidemiologic aspects of brain injury. Neurol Clin 1996; 14:435–450.

142. Kraus JF, McArthur DI. Incidence and prevalence of, and costs associated with traumatic brain injury. In: Rosenthal M, Griffin ER, Kreutzer JS, et al, eds. Rehabilitation of the adult and child with traumatic brain injury. 3rd edn. Philadelphia: FA Davis; 1999:3–18.

143. Kraus JF, Sorenson SB. Epidemiology. In: Silver JM, Yudofsky SC, Hales RE, eds. Neuropsychiatry of traumatic brain injury. Washington: American Psychiatry Press; 1994:3–41.

144. Kreutzer J, Devany C, Keck S. Family needs following brain injury: a quantitative analysis. J Head Trauma Rehabil 1994; 9(3):104–115.

145. Kreutzer J, Gervasio A, Camplair P. Patient correlates of caregiver's distress and family functioning after traumatic brain injury. Brain Inj 1994; 8(3):211–230.

146. Kreutzer J, Gervasio A, Camplair P. Primary caregiver's psychological status and family functioning after traumatic brain injury. Brain Inj 1994; 8(3):197–210.

147. Kreutzer J, Kolakowsky-Hayner S, Demm S, et al. A structured approach to family intervention after brain injury. J Head Trauma Rehabil 2002; 17(4):349–367.

148. Kreutzer J, Kolakowsky-Hayner S. Getting better (and better) after brain injury: a guide for family, friends, and caregivers. Richmond: National Resource Center for Traumatic Brain Injury; 1999.

149. Kreutzer J, Seel RT, Marwitz JH. The Neurobehavioral Functioning Inventory. San Antonio: Psychological Corporation; 1999.

150. Kreutzer JS, Doherty KR, Harris JA, et al. Alcohol use among persons with traumatic brain injury. J Head Trauma Rehabil 1990; 5(3):9–20.

151. Kreutzer JS, Harris-Marwitz J, Myers SL. Neuropsychological issues in litigation following traumatic brain injury. Neuropsychology 1990; 4:249–259.

152. Kreutzer JS, Kolakowsky-Hayner SA, Ripley D, et al. Charges and lengths of stay for acute and inpatient rehabilitation treatment of traumatic brain injury 1990–1996. Brain Inj 2001; 15(9):763–774.

153. Kreutzer JS, Marwitz JH, Walker W, et al. Moderating factors in return to work and job stability after traumatic brain injury. J Head Trauma Rehabil 2003; 18(2):128–138.

154. Kreutzer JS, Marwitz JH, Witol AD. Interrelationships between crime, substance abuse, and aggressive behaviours among persons with traumatic brain injury. Brain Inj 1995; 9(8):757–768.

155. Kreutzer JS, Serio CD, Berquist S. Family needs after brain injury: a quantitative analysis. J Head Trauma Rehabil 1994; 9(3):104–115.

156. Kreutzer JS, Wehman PH, Harris JA, et al. Substance abuse and crime patterns among persons with traumatic brain injury referred for supported employment. Brain Inj 1991; 5(2):177–187.

157. Kreutzer JS, West DD, Marwitz JH. Judgment and Safety Screening Inventory: administration manual. Richmond: National Resource Center for Traumatic Brain Injury; 2001.

158. Kreutzer JS, Witol AD, Marwitz JH. Alcohol and drug use among young persons with traumatic brain injury. J Learn Disabil 1996; 29(6): 643–651.

159. Kreutzer JS, Witol AD, Sander AM, et al. A prospective longitudinal multicenter analysis of alcohol use patterns among persons with traumatic brain injury. J Head Trauma Rehabil 1996; 11(5):58–69.

160. Kreutzer JS. Family Needs Questionnaire. Richmond: Rehabilitation Research and Training Center on Severe Traumatic Brain Injury; 1988.

161. Kuhtz-Buschbeck JP, Hoppe B, Golge M, et al. Sensorimotor recovery in children after traumatic brain injury: analyses of gait, gross motor, and fine motor skills. Dev Med Child Neurol 2003; 45(12):821–828.

162. Langley MJ, Lindsay WP, Lam CS, et al. A comprehensive alcohol abuse treatment programme for persons with traumatic brain injury. Brain Inj 1990; 4(1):77–86.

163. Langlois JA, Rutland-Brown W, Thomas KE. Traumatic brain injury in the United States. Emergency department visits, hospitalizations, and deaths. Atlanta: Centers for Disease Control and Prevention; 2004.

164. Leder S. Fiberoptic endoscopic evaluation of swallowing in patients with acute traumatic brain injury. J Head Trauma Rehabil 1999; 14(5): 448–453.

165. Lehmkuhl LD. Brain injury glossary. Houston: HDI Press; 1993.

166. Levin HS, Benton AL, Grossman RG. Neurobehavioral consequences of closed head injury. New York: Oxford University Press; 1982.

167. Levin HS, Grossman RG. Behavioral sequelae of closed head injury. Arch Neurol 1978; 35:720–727.

168. Levin HS, High WM, Goethe KE, et al. The Neurobehavioral Rating Scale: assessment of the behavioural sequelae of head injury by the clinician. J Neurol Neurosurg Psychiatry 1987; 50(2):183–193.

169. Levin HS, O'Donnell VM, Grossman RG. The Galveston orientation and amnesia test: a practical scale to assess cognition after head injury. J Nerv Ment Dis 1979; 167:675–684.

170. Levin HS, Williams D, Crofford MJ, et al. Relationship of depth of brain lesions to consciousness and outcome after closed head injury. J Neurosurg 1988; 69:861–866.

171. Levine B, Cabeza R, McIntosh AR, et al. Functional reorganization of memory after traumatic brain injury: a study with $H_2^{15}O$ positron emission tomography. J Neurol Neurosurg Psychiatry 2002; 73:173–181.

172. Lezak MD, Howieson DB, Loring DW. Neuropsychological assessment. 4th edn. New York: Oxford University Press; 2004.

173. Lezak MD. Neuropsychological assessment. 3rd edn. New York: Oxford University Press; 1995.

174. Livingston MG, Brooks DN, Bond MR. Three months after severe head injury: psychiatric and social impact on relatives. J Neurol Neurosurg Psychiatry 1985; 48:870–875.

175. Luerssen TG. Intracranial pressure: current status in monitoring and management. Semin Pediatr Neurol 1997; 4:146–155.

176. Malec JF, Basford JS. Postacute brain injury rehabilitation. Arch Phys Med Rehabil 1996; 77:198–207.

177. Marino LV, Kiratu EM, French S, et al. To determine the effect of meto-clopramide on gastric emptying in severe head injuries: a prospective, randomized, controlled clinical trial. Br J Neurosurg 2003; 17(1):24–28.

178. Marmarou A. Pathophysiology of intracranial pressure. In: Narayan RK, Wilberger JE, Povlishock JT, eds. Neurotrauma. New York: McGraw-Hill; 1996:413–429.

179. Marsh NV, Kersel DA, Havill JH, et al. Caregiver burden at 1 year following severe traumatic brain injury. Brain Inj 1988; 12(12):1045–1059.

180. Masdeu JC, Abdel-Dayem H, Van Heertum RL. Head trauma: use of SPECT. J Neuroimag 1995; 5(suppl 1):S53–S57.

181. Mathis M. Personal needs of families of critically ill patients with and without brain injury. J Neurosurg Nurs 1984; 16:36–44.

182. Matthies BK, Kreutzer JS, West DD. The behavior management handbook: a practical approach to patients with neurological disorders. Richmond: National Resource Center for Traumatic Brain Injury; 2004.

183. Mauss-Clum N, Ryan M. Brain injury and the family. J Neurosurg Nurs 1981; 13:165–169.

184. McElligott JM, Greenwald BD, Watanabe TK. Congenital and acquired brain injury. 4. New frontiers: neuroprotective agents, cognitive-enhancing agents, new technology, and complementary medicine. Arch Phys Med Rehabil 2003; 84(suppl 1):S18–S22.

185. McKinlay W, Watkins A. Cognitive and behavioral effects of brain injury. In: Rosenthal M, Griffith E, Kreutzer J, et al, eds. Rehabilitation of the adult and child with traumatic brain injury. 3rd edn. Philadelphia: FA Davis; 1999:167–182.

186. McNeny R. Activities of daily living. In: Rosenthal M, Griffith E, Kreutzer J, et al, eds. Rehabilitation of the adult and child with traumatic brain injury. 3rd edn. Philadelphia: FA Davis; 1999:242–253.

187. Meythaler JM, Brunner RC, Johnson A, et al. Amantadine to improve neurorecovery in traumatic brain injury-associated diffuse axonal injury: a pilot double-blind randomized trial. J Head Trauma Rehabil 2002; 17:300–313.

188. Meythaler JM, DeVivo MJ, Hayne JB. Cost-effectiveness of routine screening for proximal deep venous thrombosis in acquired brain injury patients admitted to rehabilitation. Arch Phys Med Rehabil 1996; 77(1):1–5.

189. Meythaler JM, Guin-Renfore S, Grabb P, et al. Long-term continuously infused intrathecal baclofen for spastic dystonic hypertonia in traumatic brain injury: 1-year experience. Arch Phys Med Rehabil 1999; 80:13–19.

190. Meythaler JM, Peduzzi JD, Eleftheriou E, et al. Current concepts: diffuse axonal injury-associated traumatic brain injury. Arch Phys Med Rehabil 2001; 82:1461–1471.

191. Morgan AS. Causes and complications associated with swallowing disorders in traumatic brain injury. J Head Trauma Rehabil 1999; 14(5):454–461.

192. Moules S, Chandler BJ. A study of the health and social needs of carers of traumatically brain injured individuals served by one community rehabilitation team. Brain Inj 1999; 13(12):983–993.

193. Multi-society Task Force on PVS. Medical aspects of the persistent vegetative state. Part I. New Engl J Med 1994; 330:1499–1508.

194. Multi-society Task Force on PVS. Medical aspects of the persistent vegetative state. Part II. New Engl J Med 1994; 330:1572–1579.

195. Nayernouri T. Posttraumatic parkinsonism. Surg Neurol 1985; 24:263–264.

196. Noguchi K, Ogawa T, Inugami A. Acute subarachnoid hemorrhage: fluid-attenuated inversion recovery pulse sequences. Radiology 1995; 196:773–777.

197. Oddy M, Coughlan T, Tyerman A, et al. Social adjustment after closed head injury: a further follow-up seven years after injury. J Neurol Neurosurg Psychiatry 1985; 49:564–568.

198. Oddy M, Humphrey M, Uttley D. Subjective impairment and social recovery after closed head injury. J Neurol Neurosurg Psychiatry 1978; 41:611–616.

199. Oder W, Podrecka I, Spatt J, et al. Cerebral function following catastrophic brain injury: relevance of single photon emission computed tomography and positron emission tomography. In: Levin HS, Benton AL, Muizelaar JP, et al, eds. Catastrophic brain injury. New York: Oxford University Press; 1996:51–76.

200. Ommaya AK, Gennarelli TA. Cerebral concussion and traumatic unconsciousness: correlation of experimental and clinic observation on blunt head injuries. Brain 1974; 97:633–654.

201. Ottenbacher KJ, Msall ME, Lyon N, et al. Measuring developmental and functional status in children with disabilities. Dev Med Child Neurol 1999; 41:186–194.

202. Pachet A, Friesen S, Winkelaar D, et al. Beneficial behavioural effects of lamotrigine in traumatic brain injury. Brain Inj 2003; 17(8):715–722.

203. Palmer BF. Hyponatremia in patients with central nervous system disease: SIADH versus CSW. Trends Endocrinol Metab 2003; 14(4):182–187.

204. Panting A, Merry PH. The long term rehabilitation of severe head injuries with particular reference to the need for social and medical support for the patient's family. Rehabilitation 1972; 38:33–37.

205. Park N, Ingles JL. Effectiveness of attention rehabilitation after acquired brain injury: a meta-analysis. Neuropsychology 2001; 15(2):199–210.

206. Pepe J, Barba CA. The metabolic response to acute traumatic brain injury and implications for nutritional support. J Head Trauma Rehabil 1999; 14(5):462–474.

207. Perlesz A, Kinsella G, Crowe S. Psychological distress and family satisfaction following traumatic brain injury: injured individuals and their primary, secondary, and tertiary carers. J Head Trauma Rehabil 2000; 15(3):909–929.

208. Ponsford JL, Olver JH, Curran C. Prediction of employment status 2 years after traumatic brain injury. Brain Inj 1995; 9:11–20.

209. Poole GV, Miller JD, Agnew SG, et al. Lower extremity fracture fixation in head-injured patients. J Trauma 1992; 32(5):654–659.

210. Povlishock JT, Christman CW. The pathobiology of traumatically-induced axonal injury in animals and humans: a review of current thoughts. J Neurotrauma 1995; 12(4):55–64.

211. Prigatano G, Ben-Yishay Y. Psychotherapy and psychotherapeutic interventions in brain injury rehabilitation. In: Rosenthal M, Kreutzer J, Griffith E, et al, eds. Rehabilitation of the adult and child with traumatic brain injury. Philadelphia: FA Davis; 1999: 271–282.

212. Prigatano G. Disordered mind, wounded soul: the emerging role of psychotherapy in rehabilitation after brain injury. J Head Trauma Rehabil 1991; 6(4):1–10.

213. Prigatano G. Psychotherapy after brain injury. In: Prigatano G. Neuropsychological rehabilitation after brain injury. Baltimore: Johns Hopkins University Press; 1986.

214. Rao VL, Dogan A, Todd KG, et al. Neuroprotection by memantine, a noncompetitive NMDA receptor antagonist after traumatic brain injury in rats. Brain Res 2001; 911(1):96–100.

215. Rappaport M, Hall KM, Hopkins K. Disability Rating Scale for severe head trauma: coma to community. Arch Phys Med Rehabil 1982; 63:118–123.

216. Rappaport M. Evoked potential and head injury in a rehabilitation setting. In: Miner M, Wagner K, eds. Neurotrauma: treatment, rehabilitation, and related issues. Boston: Butterworths; 1986.

217. Reed MJ. A case of multiple missed fractures. Eur J Emerg Med 2004; 11(6):343–345.

218. Rey A. L'examen clinique en psychologie. Paris: Presses Universitaires de France; 1964.

219. Rodin EA. Some problems in the clinical use of topographic EEG analysis. Clin Electroencephalogr 1991; 22:23–29.

220. Rodriguez JL, Lopez JM, Proctor MC, et al. Early placement of prophylactic vena caval filters in injured patients at high risk for pulmonary embolism. J Trauma 1996; 40:797–804.

221. Rosner MJ, Daughton S. Cerebral perfusion pressure management in head injury. J Trauma 1990; 30:933-940, discussion 940–941.

222. Rowe MJ III, Carlson C. Brainstem auditory evoked potentials in postconcussion dizziness. Arch Neurol 1980; 37:679–683.

223. Ruff RM, Marshall LF, Klauber MR, et al. Alcohol abuse and neurological outcome of the severely head injured. J Head Trauma Rehabil 1990; 5(3):21–31.

224. Sahuquillo J, Vilalta J, Lamarca J, et al. Diffuse axonal injury after severe head trauma. Acta Neurochir 1989; 101:149–158.

225. Sandel ME, Bell KR, Michaud LJ. Brain injury rehabilitation. 1. Traumatic brain injury: prevention, pathophysiology, and outcome prediction. Arch Phys Med Rehabil 1998; 79(suppl 1):S3–S9.

226. Sandel ME, Mysiw WJ. The agitated brain injured patient. Part 1: definitions, differential diagnosis, and assessment. Arch Phys Med Rehabil 1996; 77:617–623.

227. Saxe JM, Ledgerwood AM, Lucas CF, et al. Lower esophageal sphincter dysfunction precludes safe gastric feeding after head injury. J Trauma 1994; 37:581–584.

228. Sbordone RJ, Liter JC, Pettler-Jennings P. Recovery of function following severe traumatic brain injury: a retrospective 10-year follow-up. Brain Inj 1995; 9(3):285–299.

229. Scherzer E, Wessely P. EEG in posttraumatic epilepsy. Eur Neurol 1978; 17:38–42.

230. Schieber RA, Sacks JJ. Measuring community bicycle helmet use among children. Public Health Rep 2001; 116:113–121.

231. Schneider GE. Is it really better to have your brain lesion early?: a revision of the Kennard principle. Neuropsychologia 1979; 17:557–583.

232. Schneider WN, Drew-Catest J, Wong TM, et al. Cognitive and behavioral efficacy of amantadine in acute brain injury: an initial double-blind placebo-controlled study. Brain Inj 1999; 13:863–872.

233. Seaton JD, David CO. Family role in substance abuse and traumatic brain injury rehabilitation. J Head Trauma Rehabil 1990; 5(3):41–46.

234. Semlyen J, Summers S, Barnes M. Traumatic brain injury: efficacy of multidisciplinary rehabilitation. Arch Phys Med Rehabil 1998; 79(6): 678–683.

235. Serio CD, Kreutzer JS, Gervasio AH. Predicting family needs after brain injury: implications for intervention. J Head Trauma Rehabil 1995; 10(2): 32–45.

236. Serio CD, Kreutzer JS, Witol AD. Family needs after traumatic brain injury: a factor analytic study of the Family Needs Questionnaire. Brain Inj 1997; 11(1):1–9.

237. Shafer MS, Wehman P, Kregel J, et al. National supported employment initiative: a preliminary analysis. Am J Ment Retard 1990; 95:316–327.

238. Sherer M, Boake C, Levin E, et al. Characteristics of impaired awareness after traumatic brain injury. J Int Neuropsychol Soc 1998; 4(4):380–387.

239. da Silva AM, Nunes B, Vaz AR, et al. Posttraumatic epilepsy in civilians: clinical and electroencephalographic studies. Acta Neurochir Suppl 1992; 55:56–63.

240. Sinaki M, Lynn SG. Reducing the risk of falling through proprioceptive dynamic posture training in osteoporotic women with kyphotic posturing: a randomized pilot study. Am J Phys Med Rehabil 2002; 81:241–246.

241. Sinnakaruppan I, Williams DM. Family carers and the adult head-injured: a critical review of carers' needs. Brain Inj 2001; 15(8):653–672.

242. Sohlberg M, Mateer C. Effectiveness of an attention training program. J Clin Exp Neuropsychol 1987; 19:117–130.

243. Sohlberg M, Mateer C. Introduction to cognitive rehabilitation. New York: Guilford Press; 1989.

244. Sohlberg M, Mateer C. Training use of compensatory memory books: a three stage behavioral approach. J Clin Exp Neuropsychol 1987; 11: 871–891.

245. Sohlberg M, White O, Evans E, et al. Background and an initial investigation of the effects of prospective memory training. Brain Inj 1992; 5:139–154.

246. Sorenson SB, Kraus JF. Occurrence, severity, and outcomes of brain injury. J Head Trauma Rehabil 1991; 6(2):1–10.

247. Sosin DM, Sacks JJ, Holmgreen P. Head injury-associated deaths from motorcycle crashes. Relationship to helmet use laws. JAMA 1990; 264: 2395–2399.

248. Sosin DM, Sniezek JE, Thurman DJ. Incidence of mild and moderate brain injury in the United States: 1991. Brain Inj 1996; 10:47–54.

249. de Souza NM, Hajinal JV, Baudouin CJ. Potential for increasing conspicuity of short-T1 lesions in the brain using magnetization transfer imaging. Neuroradiology 1995; 37(4):278–283.

250. Stebbins P, Leung P. Changing family needs after brain injury. J Rehabil 1998; 64(4):15–22.

251. Stewart DG, Cifu DX. Neuroendocrinologic management after TBI. Phys Med Rehabil Clin North Am 1997; 8(4):827–842.

252. Stewart DG, Miller M, Cifu DX. Subacute rehabilitation after TBI. Neurorehabilitation 1998; 10:13–23.

253. Stone LR, Keenan MA. Deep venous thrombosis of the upper extremity after traumatic brain injury. Arch Phys Med Rehabil 1992; 73(5): 486–489.

254. Susman M, DiRusso SM, Sullivan T, et al. Traumatic brain injury in the elderly: increased mortality and worse functional outcome at discharge despite lower injury severity. J Trauma 2002; 53(2):219–223.

255. Task Force on Community Preventive Services. Recommendations to reduce injuries to motor vehicle occupants: increasing child safety seat use, increasing safety belt use, and reducing alcohol-impaired driving. Am J Prev Med 2001; 21(4 suppl):16–22.

256. Taylor LA, Kreutzer JS, Demm SR, et al. Traumatic brain injury and substance abuse: a review and analysis of the literature. Neuropsychol Rehabil 2003; 13:165–168.

257. Taylor SJ, Fettes SB, Jewkes C, et al. Prospective, randomized, controlled trial to determine the effect of early enhanced enteral nutrition on clinical outcome in mechanically ventilated patients suffering head injury. Crit Care Med 1999; 27:2525–2529.

258. Teasdale G, Jennett B. Assessment of coma and impaired consciousness. Lancet 1974; 2:81–84.

259. Teasdale G, Mendelow D. Pathophysiology of head injuries. In: Brooks N, ed. Closed head injury: psychological, social, and family consequences. Oxford: Oxford University Press; 1984:4–36.

260. Temkin NR, Dikmen SS, Wilensky AJ, et al. A randomized double-blind study of phenytoin for the prevention of post-traumatic seizures. N Engl J Med 1990; 323:497–502.

261. Thomsen IV. Late outcome of very severe blunt head trauma: a 10–15 year second follow-up. J Neurol Neurosurg Psychiatry 1984; 48:260–268.

262. Tinetti ME, Baker DI, McAvay G, et al. A multifactorial intervention to reduce the risk of falling among elderly people living in the community. N Engl J Med 1994; 331:821–827.

263. Tinetti ME, Speechley M. Prevention of falls in the elderly. N Engl J Med 1989; 321(23):1055–1059.

264. Tombaugh TN. Test of Memory Malingering (TOMM). New York: Multi Health Systems; 1996.

265. Umile EM, Sandel ME, Alavi A, et al. Dynamic imaging in mild traumatic brain injury: support for the theory of medial temporal vulnerability. Arch Phys Med Rehabil 2002; 83:1506–1513.

266. Vandiver V, Johnson J, Christofero-Snider C. Supporting employment for adults with acquired brain injury: a conceptual model. J Head Trauma Rehabil 2003; 18(5):457–463.

267. Verma A. Opportunities for neuroprotection in traumatic brain injury. J Head Trauma Rehabil 2000; 15:1149–1161.

268. Vitaz T, McIlov L, Rague G, et al. Development and implementation of a clinical pathway for severe traumatic brain injury. J Trauma 2001; 51:369–375.

269. Vollmer DG. Prognosis and outcome of severe head injury. In: Cooper PR, ed. Head injury. 3rd edn. Baltimore: Williams & Wilkins; 1993: 553–581.

270. Walker AE, Jablon S. A follow-up of head injured men of World War II. J Neurosurg 1959; 16:600–610.

271. Walker W, Seel R, Gibellato M, et al. The effects of donepezil on traumatic brain injury acute rehabilitation outcomes. Brain Inj 2004; 18(8): 739–750.

272. Walker WC, Kreutzer JS, Witol AD. Level of care options for the low-functioning brain injury survivor. Brain Inj 1996; 10:65–75.

273. Ward JD. Pediatric head injury. In: Narayan RK, Wilberger JE, Povlishock JT, eds. Neurotrauma. New York: McGraw-Hill; 1996:859–868.

274. Warrington EK. Recognition Memory Test: manual. Berkshire: NFER-Nelson; 1984.

275. Wasserman RC, Buccini RV. Helmet protection from head injuries among recreational bicyclists. Am J Sports Med 1990; 18:96–97.

276. Watson NF, Barber JK, Doherty MJ, et al. Does glucocorticoid administration prevent late seizures after head injury? Epilepsia 2004; 45(6): 690–694.

277. Weekes E, Elia M. Observations on the patterns of 24-hour energy expenditure changes in body composition and gastric emptying in head-injured patients receiving nasogastric tube feedings. J Parenter Nutr 1996; 20:31–37.

278. Wehman P, Kregel J, Keyser-Marcus L, et al. Supported employment for persons with traumatic brain injury: a preliminary investigation of long-term follow-up costs and program efficiency. Arch Phys Med Rehabil 2003; 84:192–196.

279. Wehman P, West M, Kregel J, et al. Return to work for persons with severe traumatic brain injury: a data-based approach to program development. J Head Trauma Rehabil 1995; 10(1):27–39.

280. Whyte J, Cifu DX, Dikmen S, et al. Prediction of functional outcomes after traumatic brain injury: a comparison of two measures of duration of unconsciousness. Arch Phys Med Rehabil 2001; 82:1355–1359.

281. Whyte J, Hart T, Schuster K, et al. Effects of methylphenidate on attentional function after traumatic brain injury. Am J Phys Med Rehabil 1997; 76:440–450.

282. Whyte J, Vaccaro M, Grieb-Neff P, et al. Psychostimulant use in the rehabilitation of individuals with traumatic brain injury. J Head Trauma Rehabil 2002; 17:284–299.

283. Whyte J. Clinical drug evaluation. J Head Trauma Rehabil 1988; 3(4):95–99.

284. Willer B, Corrigan JD. Whatever it takes: a model for community-based services. Brain Inj 1994; 8:647–659.

285. Wilson MS, Gibson CJ, Hamm RJ. Haloperidol, but not olanzapine, impairs cognitive performance after traumatic brain injury in rats. Am J Phys Med Rehabil 2003; 82(11):871–879.

286. Witol AD, Sander AM, Kreutzer JS. A longitudinal analysis of family needs following traumatic brain injury. Neurorehabilitation 1996; 7:175–187.

287. Witol AD, Sander AM, Seel RT, et al. Long term neurobehavioral characteristics after brain injury: implications for vocational rehabilitation. J Vocat Rehabil 1996; 7:159–167.

288. Xiong J, Rao S, Gao JH, et al. Evaluation of hemispheric dominance for language using functional MRI: a comparison with positron emission tomography. Hum Brain Mapp 1998; 37:42–58.

289. Yablon SA. Posttraumatic seizures. Arch Phys Med Rehabil 1993; 74(9):983–1001.

290. Yang L, Benardo LS. Epileptogenesis following neocortical trauma from two sources of disinhibition. J Neurophysiol 1997; 78:2804–2810.

291. Yang L, Benardo LS. Valproate prevents posttraumatic seizure activity in an in vitro model in neocortical slices. Epilepsia 2000; 41:1507–1513.

292. Young B, Ott L, Twyman D, et al. The effect of nutritional support on outcome from severe head injury. J Neurosurg 1987; 67:76–80.

293. Zador PL, Ciccone ME. Automobile driver fatalities in frontal impact: airbags compared with manual belts. Am J Public Health 1993; 83(5):661–666.

294. Zafonte RD, Lansand R, Giap B. Pathophysiology of traumatic brain injury: an overview of the neuroprotective strategies. Phys Med Rehabil State Art Rev 2001; 15:229–244.

295. Zhang L, Plotkin RC, Wang G, et al. Cholinergic augmentation with donepezil enhances recovery in short-term memory and sustained attention after traumatic brain injury. Arch Phys Med Rehabil. 2004; 85(7): 1050–1055.

296. van Zommeren AH, Brower WH, Deelman BG. Attention deficits: the riddles of selectivity, speed, and alertness. In: Brooks N, ed. Closed head injury: psychological, social, and family consequences. Oxford: Oxford University Press; 1984:74–107.

Chapter

51

Rehabilitation in Stroke Syndromes

Richard L. Harvey, Elliot J. Roth and David Yu

Providing rehabilitation care for patients with stroke is at once a compelling and complicated endeavor. Stroke is a common syndrome, and care of the stroke patient is often thought of as a prototype rehabilitation effort, because of its high frequency and its reliance on virtually all members of the typical rehabilitation team. However, the fact that no two strokes are alike and no two patients react similarly to their situations means that caring for patients with stroke is also a distinct experience requiring individual attention. Most patients who experience stroke can and do have improvement in functional ability, but the amount, rate, timing, pattern, type, and ultimate outcome of the improvements differ across patients and across situations. The approach that is required for appropriate assessment and treatment of stroke patients therefore demands specialized knowledge, skills, and creativity.

The past 10 years has witnessed a transformation in the therapeutic approach to the rehabilitation of stroke, spurred by a growing literature on motor recovery after focal brain injury.[127] It is now evident both clinically and scientifically that improvement in motor control after stroke is *use-dependent*, responding best to repetitive training mixed with continuous modification of the program in order to keep training tasks challenging to the patient.[167] Newer research is now leading beyond just therapeutic exercise, adding novel interventions such as pharmacology, new modalities, and robotics as potentially enhancing the results of motor retraining.

The emergence of use-dependent recovery has pushed rehabilitation clinicians to carefully assess the balance between restoration of neurologic control and training in functional independence with compensatory techniques. This is particularly challenging in the acute inpatient rehabilitation setting, where the desire to facilitate neurologic recovery is most desirable but the need to discharge the patient home safely is most imminent. Fortunately, our tradition of the interdisciplinary rehabilitation team is well suited to addressing these modern challenges.

While formal therapeutic interventions, exercise, and neurologic retraining comprise the most prominent components of the rehabilitation process, other aspects of the program are important as well. Many rehabilitation activities extend beyond the specific therapy treatment sessions. For example, integrating functional activities learned in formal therapy into self-care under the supervision of inpatient nursing staff or later in the home environment can significantly reinforce newly gained skills. Recreational programs often serve as major therapeutic interventions. Dealing with psychologic and social issues can be a more significant clinical activity than the more obvious motor control enhancement strategies. Interactions among patients can provide both emotional support and practical suggestions regarding skill performance. Most critically, the amount and nature of the interactions between patients and professionals can be highly motivating and instructive for patients and their families. A positive and encouraging rehabilitation milieu typically provides the opportunity for these 'less formal' therapeutic interactions.

The major underlying theme of all rehabilitation interventions is to maximize quality of life for patients with stroke. It is quality of life, and not simply improved motor control, functional independence, or community placement, that is the real goal of the rehabilitation program. Indeed, for some stroke survivors, complete independence in daily living skills might be undesirable or impractical for physical, psychologic, or social reasons. The goal of enhancing quality of life is paramount, and affects both the choices of specific interventions and the manner in which clinical activities are performed. The comprehensive rehabilitation management program is characterized by a holistic approach, in which patients as a whole and their overall situation are considered, rather than focusing on isolated aspects of existence. This goal usually, but not always, includes helping the patient to achieve as much functional independence as possible.

Understanding stroke and the rehabilitation of patients who sustain stroke is important, not only because stroke is a common diagnosis among patients in rehabilitation programs, but also because it provides an opportunity to learn about the functioning of the central nervous system, and the application of rehabilitation principles in general. This chapter reviews the mechanisms and clinical features of stroke; the preventive, diagnostic, and acute management techniques; and the principles and practices of stroke rehabilitation assessment and intervention that enable rehabilitation providers to assist the patient in achieving the ultimate goal of maximizing quality of life. Special emphasis is placed on new and recent developments in stroke rehabilitation. In light of the many challenges to both providing and investigating stroke rehabilitation, the recent developments in stroke care and research are striking. An important recurring theme during both acute management and rehabilitation care, which has been consistent over time, is the centrality of an attitude that replaces therapeutic nihilism with optimism and aggressiveness.[19]

DEFINITIONS

Stroke or cerebrovascular accident?

Ancient writers of history, science, and poetry used the word *apoplexy*, meaning a sudden strike of paralysis, dumbness, or fainting from which the victim frequently failed to recover. Such a stroke of illness, whether delivered by the gods or disease, was a spontaneous event of the same character as a 'stroke of genius', a 'stroke of luck', or a 'stroke of misfortune'. The word *stroke* then connotes the presence of strong external forces causing the disease that would render treatment useless. The more modern term *cerebrovascular accident* or *CVA* merely perpetuates this nihilistic view of stroke care.[19] Clinicians today have retained the name *stroke* because of the sudden and surprising nature of symptomatic cerebrovascular disease, and yet we recognize that stroke is associated with known risk factors and that both acute medical care and rehabilitation can reduce mortality and disability.

We define stroke as a non-traumatic brain injury, caused by occlusion or rupture of cerebral blood vessels, that results in sudden neurologic deficit characterized by loss of motor control, altered sensation, cognitive or language impairment, disequilibrium, or coma. This definition includes an array of etiologic sources, but excludes non-vascular conditions that can present with stroke-like symptoms, such as seizure, syncope, hypoxemia, traumatic brain injury, or brain tumor.

STROKE PATHOPHYSIOLOGY

Stroke is a neurologic syndrome caused by a heterogeneous group of vascular etiologies requiring different management.[44] The causes can be grossly categorized as hemorrhagic or ischemic. Intracranial hemorrhage accounts for 15% of all strokes, and can be further divided into intracerebral (10%) and subarachnoid (5%) hemorrhage. Subarachnoid hemorrhages (SAHs) typically result from aneurysmal rupture of a cerebral artery with blood loss into the space surrounding the brain. Rupture of weakened vessels within brain parenchyma as a result of hypertension, arteriovenous malformation (AVM), or tumor causes intracerebral hemorrhage (ICH).

The remaining 85% of strokes are caused by ischemic brain injury resulting from large vessel (40%) or small vessel (20%) thrombosis, cerebral embolism (20%), and other less common causes (5%) such as cerebral vasculitis or cerebral hypoperfusion. Vessel occlusion from thrombosis in both large and small arteries is most commonly caused by atherosclerotic cerebrovascular disease. Vascular changes or lipohyalinosis found in small, deep, perforating arteries as associated with chronic hypertension can lead to small vessel thrombosis. Cerebral emboli are usually of cardiac origin, and are frequently a result of valvular disease or atrial fibrillation. In addition, they can arise from chronic ischemic cardiovascular disease with secondary ventricular wall hypokinesis, which can also increase the risk for intracardiac thrombus formation.

Ischemic stroke

The unifying pathophysiology of thrombotic, embolic, and lacunar stroke is cerebral ischemia from compromise of cerebral blood flow (CBF). The location and temporal development of cerebral injury vary with the etiology.

Thrombosis

The entire pathophysiology of infarction from cerebral thrombosis remains controversial, but it is strongly associated with atherosclerotic cerebrovascular disease. Atherosclerotic plaque formation occurs frequently at major vascular branching sites, including the common carotid and vertebrobasilar arteries. Atherosclerosis is an inflammatory disease that often develops in the presence of chronic hypertension, beginning with increased permeability of vascular intima followed by leukocyte adhesion and infiltration. Monocyte and T-cell accumulation produce lipid-laden foam cells within the vessel wall, and fatty streaks appear on the endothelial surface. Eventually, smooth muscle cell migration, continued inflammatory activity, and the formation of a fibrous cap compromise blood flow, leading to turbulence. Rupture of the fibrous cap can rapidly promote initial thrombus formation by stimulating platelet aggregation and activation of the extrinsic pathway of the coagulation system. The loosely attached thrombus, or 'white clot', that forms is composed of platelet cells and fresh fibrin.[252]

It is unclear whether symptoms of transient ischemic attack (TIA) are caused by transient thrombotic occlusion of major cerebral arteries or by microemboli that break away from a thrombus, but both phenomena might be important. Symptoms of transient monocular blindness, or amaurosis fugax, are probably due to microemboli from the internal carotid artery that cause a branch occlusion of the ipsilateral ophthalmic artery.[227] Other intracranial branch occlusions can similarly result from microemboli arising in the extracranial vessels, leading to injury or infarction in focal regions.[339]

In contrast, a large arterial thrombus can occlude a major extracranial artery, producing a low-flow state that causes ischemic injury to neural tissue supplied by the most distal arterial branches.[23] The volume of damage that results from such hemodynamic compromise can be quite large, but it is dependent on the length of time the vessel is occluded, the rate of flow through the occluded site, and the effectiveness of the collateral circulation. Fibrinolytic enzymes are released that control acute thrombus formation, potentially dissolving the clot within minutes to hours. However, recanalization might fail or be delayed, permitting the arterial thrombus to completely or partially occlude blood flow. Collateral circulation can support the compromised cortical zone, but it can be less effective in elderly persons or in those with diffuse atherosclerotic disease or diabetes.

Ischemic injury from a cerebrovascular thrombus probably results in simultaneous distal branch occlusions from microemboli and compromise of blood flow proximally. The neurologic outcome of cerebral thrombi varies widely and can include brief TIAs, minor strokes without functional compromise, or major strokes resulting in significant impairment and functional disability.

Embolism

Beyond the microemboli produced by cerebrovascular thrombi, the majority of embolic strokes have a cardiac origin. Thrombus formation within the cardiac chambers is generally caused by structural or mechanical changes within the heart. Atrial fibrillation is a significant risk factor for embolic stroke as a result of poor atrial motility and outflow, with stasis of blood and atrial thrombus formation. Atrial fibrillation is often caused by rheumatic valvular disease or coronary artery disease, but it can be idiopathic. Mural thrombus within the left ventricle after myocardial infarction, in the presence of cardiomyopathy or after cardiac surgery, is the other major cause of embolic stroke.[43,48] Mechanical heart valves universally cause cerebral emboli if anticoagulation is insufficient. Infectious endocarditis can lead to septic emboli.

Cerebral emboli lodge within arterial branches of the major arteries, causing single or multiple branch occlusions resulting in sudden, focal neurologic impairment. These branch occlusions significantly compromise flow distally, inducing ischemic injury to neural tissue, glia, and vascular endothelium. Reperfusion of the occluded vessel can occur in response to endogenous fibrinolysis, but because ischemic damage to the vascular bed is often significant, the capillaries become incompetent and secondary cerebral hemorrhage ensues.

In contrast to thrombotic stroke, microemboli probably do not precede cardioembolic strokes, as TIAs are uncommon. Frequently, no cardiac thrombus can be found after the event, and the only clue to an embolic cause is the sudden neurologic deficit without previous or progressive symptoms.

Lacunes

Lacunar infarcts are small, circumscribed lesions that measure less than 1.5 cm in diameter and are located in subcortical regions of the basal ganglia, internal capsule, pons, and cerebellum.[203] The area of a lacune (meaning 'little lake') roughly corresponds to the vascular territory supplied by one of the deep perforating branches from the circle of Willis or major cerebral arteries. Lacunar strokes are strongly associated with hypertension, and pathologically associated with microvascular changes that often develop in the presence of chronic hypertension. Histologic changes such as arteriolar thickening and evenly distributed deposition of eosinophilic material, called *lipohyalinosis* and *fibrinoid necrosis*, are commonly seen in the subcortical perforating arteries of hypertensive persons who have had lacunar strokes. Microatheromas within deep perforating arteries are also important causes of lacunar infarction. In addition to hypertension, diabetes mellitus is associated with lacunar stroke as a result of chronic microvascular changes.

Hemorrhagic stroke
Intracerebral hemorrhage

The deep perforating cerebral arteries are also the site of rupture preceding ICH. However, unlike lacunar strokes, ICH does not obey the anatomic distribution of a vessel but dissects through tissue planes. Such damage can be significant, resulting in increased intracranial pressure, disruption of multiple neural tracts, ventricular compression, and cerebral herniation. Acute mortality is high, but those who survive ICH often experience rapid neurologic recovery during the first 2 or 3 months after the hemorrhage.

Nearly one-half of all ICHs occur within the putamen and the cerebral white matter.[101] Sudden hemorrhage into brain parenchyma is related to both acute elevations in blood pressure and chronic hypertension. Microvascular changes associated with hypertensive hemorrhages include lipohyalinosis and Charcot–Bouchard aneurysms.[92] The latter are not true aneurysms of the vessel wall but are pockets of extravasated blood or 'pseudoaneurysms', a sign of previous microscopic ruptures within the vascular wall. The bleeding typically lasts no more than 1–2 h, corresponding to the usual time course of acute symptom development. Late neurologic decline is related to posthemorrhagic edema or rebleeding.

Cerebral amyloid angiopathy is unusual but is gaining recognition as an important cause of ICH in the elderly.[88] Lobar hemorrhages located near the cortex that occur in patients older than 55 years who have some premorbid history of mild dementia are characteristic of this disease, but in the absence of tissue staining for Congo red amyloid deposits within the adventitia of cerebral vessels, diagnostic uncertainty remains. Other notable causes of ICH include the use of anticoagulants, intracranial tumor, and vasculitis.

Subarachnoid hemorrhage

Subarachnoid hemorrhage, or bleeding that occurs within the dural space around the brain and fills the basal cisterns, is most commonly caused by rupture of a saccular aneurysm or an AVM. Saccular aneurysms develop from a congenital defect in an arterial wall followed by progressive degeneration of the adventitia, which causes ballooning or out-pouching of the vessel. The risk of bleeding from unruptured aneurysms is speculative but appears greatest for aneurysms greater than 10 mm in diameter.[299]

Saccular aneurysms often rupture during the fifth or sixth decade of life. When a rupture occurs, the extravasation of blood into the subarachnoid space is irritating to the dura and results in a severe headache often described as 'the worst in my life'. Because of a sudden drop in cerebral perfusion pressure, acute loss of consciousness is frequent. Focal neurologic changes or coma can ensue. As many as one-third of patients with aneurysmal hemorrhage die immediately. Patients who present with coma, stupor, or severe hemiplegia have the worst prognosis for proximate survival. The risk of rebleeding from an unoperated aneurysm is as high as 30% within the first month after hemorrhage, and declines thereafter. The risk for long-term rebleeding remains 3% per year.[328]

Saccular aneurysms are most often found in the anterior region of the circle of Willis, particularly near branches of the anterior communicating, internal carotid, and middle cerebral arteries, but they can also be found at the junction of almost any branch site within the cerebral circulation. Early surgical and endovascular management using modern neurosurgical clipping techniques and cooling are as safe as late surgery, and it significantly reduces risk of rebleeding.

Arteriovenous malformations present with hemorrhage earlier in life than do aneurysms, often in the second or third decade. Although they cause nearly 9% of all SAHs, vascular malformations are also important causes of ICH and intraventricular hemorrhage.[224] An AVM is a congenital structure consisting of a tangled web of vascular tissue that contains multiple arteriovenous fistulas, which permit arterial to venous shunting of blood. They can be located anywhere in the central nervous system and can grow quite large, displacing normal neural structures, usually without disruption of function. Seizure, migraine, and hemorrhage are typical presenting symptoms.

The incidence of lifetime hemorrhage with AVM is 40–50%,[201] with a rebleeding rate of 4% per year and a mortality rate of 1% per year.[217] Treatment options include endovascular embolization, surgical resection, and radiotherapy (gamma knife).

Hydrocephalus

Acute and chronic hydrocephalus can complicate both SAH and intraventricular hemorrhage by obstructing cerebrospinal fluid (CSF) outflow. Blood coagulum within the ventricular system can block the foramen of Sylvius or the fourth ventricle, causing acute obstructive hydrocephalus over minutes to hours after hemorrhage, leading to lethargy, coma, or death if not treated. Placement of an external ventriculostomy device can be lifesaving, but if the obstruction does not resolve, a ventriculoperitoneal shunt is placed for long-term decompression.

Normal pressure hydrocephalus is very common after SAH and often develops during rehabilitation care. The pathophysiologic cause is a functional disruption of CSF resorption due to fibrosis of the arachnoid granulations from subarachnoid blood.[142] The classic symptoms of subcortical dementia, incontinence, and gait disorder are clues to the presence of hydrocephalus, but the physiatrist should also have a high level of suspicion when a patient with recent hemorrhage is not making expected functional gains in a rehabilitation program. That suspicion is often confirmed when the patient makes a remarkable recovery after shunting.

THE ANATOMIC BASIS OF STROKE SYNDROMES

Disability in stroke is a result of central nervous system injury by which physical, cognitive, and psychologic functioning become impaired. Specific impairments appear when focal regions and neural systems within the brain are damaged by

vascular compromise. Neurologic brain mapping has been an active area of research dating back to 1800, when Franz Joseph Gall developed phrenology. He interpreted personality and mental capacity by studying the bumps on the human skull. Although phrenology has been discredited, the study of brain topography has proved quite useful for predicting neurologic impairment after focal brain injury.

Motor control and strength
Anatomy
The primary motor area is located along the cortex of the precentral gyrus anterior to the central sulcus of both hemispheres, and extends from the paracentral lobule within the longitudinal fissure to the frontal operculum within the Sylvian fissure. The classic 'motor homunculus' is useful for visualizing the topography of motor control along the precentral gyrus. Axons from these cortical cells descend via the internal capsule to the pyramidal tract in the brain stem and the corticospinal tract in the spinal cord.

Recovery
With hemiplegia, weakness and poor control of voluntary movement are present initially, associated with reduced resting muscle tone. As voluntary movement returns, non-functional mass flexion and extension of the limbs are first noted (Table 51-1). Synergy patterns, or mass contraction of multiple muscle groups, are seen.[309] Later, movement patterns can be independent of synergy.[270]

Motor coordination and balance
Trunk control and stability, coordination of movement patterns, and balance all involve complex extrapyramidal systems that are frequently disrupted by stroke. Extrapyramidal disorders can be a major impediment to functional recovery but are often amenable to therapeutic exercise.

Table 51-1 Synergy patterns in motor recovery

	Upper limb	Lower limb
Flexor synergy	Shoulder retraction Shoulder abduction Shoulder external rotation Elbow flexion Forearm supination Wrist flexion Finger flexion	Hip flexion Hip abduction Hip external rotation Knee flexion Ankle eversion Dorsiflexion Toe extension
Extensor synergy	Shoulder protraction Shoulder adduction Elbow extension Forearm pronation Wrist extension Finger flexion	Hip extension Hip adduction Knee extension Ankle inversion Plantar flexion Toe flexion

Anatomy

Anterior to the precentral gyrus within the frontal lobe is the premotor area, which is important in motor planning. Multiple fiber tracts from this region descend via the anterior limb of the internal capsule to the basal ganglia and the cerebellum, with input from the vestibular, visual, and somatosensory systems. Injury to either the efferent or the afferent systems (or both) can cause poor static and dynamic balance as well as movement disorders such as ataxia, chorea, hemiballismus, and tremors.

Spasticity

Spasticity is a velocity-dependent increase in resistance to muscle stretch that develops after an upper motor neuron injury within the central nervous system.[177] When severe, spasticity can cause reduced flexibility, posture, and functional mobility, as well as joint pain, contracture, and difficulty with positioning for comfort and hygiene. In stroke, an increase occurs in both tonic and phasic reflexes. Loss of upper motor neuron control causes disinhibited alpha and gamma motor neuron activity and heightened sensitivity to class 1a and 2 muscle spindle afferents.[117] Consequently, monosynaptic and multisynaptic spinal reflexes become hyperactive.

Spasticity develops shortly after completed stroke, and is initially manifested as an increased phasic response to tendon tap and a slight catch with passive ranging. Later, ranging can become difficult, and the patient might show tonic positioning in flexion or extension. Often, as voluntary motor activity returns, a reduction in tone and reflex response is noted, but if recovery is incomplete, spasticity usually remains (see Ch. 31).

Sensation

Loss of sensation after stroke can have a significant effect on joint and skin protection, balance, coordination, and motor control.

Anatomy

Pain and temperature sensation are relayed centrally by fibers that enter the spinothalamic tract from the contralateral dorsal root ganglion and ascend to the ventral posterior lateral nucleus of the thalamus. Some spinothalamic fibers enter the superior colliculus and ascending reticular formation.

Sensory fibers for joint proprioception and stereognosis ascend ipsilaterally from the dorsal root ganglion within the dorsal column, and cross to the contralateral side within the lower medulla after synapsing with the nucleus gracilis and cuneatus. The fibers then ascend in the medial lemniscus to the ventral posterior lateral thalamus. The ventral posterior lateral thalamus relays sensory information to the primary sensory cortex, located posterior to the central sulcus in the postcentral gyrus.

Although injury to the sensory pathways typically causes hypoesthesia or reduced sensation, patients with lesions in the thalamus or spinothalamic tract occasionally experience severe pain that can interfere with functional recovery and rehabilitative care.

Language and communication

Aphasia is an impairment of language, but typical lesions that cause aphasia affect comprehension and the use of symbolic material for the purpose of communication and meaning (see also Ch. 3). Testing of language should include an examination of oral expression, verbal comprehension, naming, reading, writing, and repeating. The classic aphasia syndromes are listed in Table 51-2. Although this anatomic classification of aphasia is useful for functionally describing communication problems after stroke, it is not very useful for guiding therapy. There is a newer trend to describe aphasia, using a psycholinguistic approach that is presently being worked out in the aphasiology literature.[42]

Although language is considered a function of the left or dominant hemisphere, some elements of communication such

Table 51-2 Clinical characteristics of the aphasia syndromes

Syndrome	Fluency	Expression	Comprehension	Repetition	Naming
Broca	Impaired	Impaired	Mildly impaired	Impaired	Impaired
Wernicke	Normal	Impaired	Impaired	Impaired	Impaired
Global	Impaired	Impaired	Impaired	Impaired	Impaired
Transcortical motor	Impaired	Mildly impaired	Normal	Normal	Mildly impaired
Transcortical sensory	Normal	Mildly impaired	Mildly impaired	Normal	Mildly impaired
Conduction	Normal	Mildly impaired	Normal	Impaired	Mildly impaired
Anomic	Normal	Normal	Normal	Normal	Impaired
Isolation of language zone	Impaired	Impaired	Impaired	Normal	Impaired
Pure motor speech disorder	Impaired	Impaired	Normal	Impaired	Impaired
Pure word deafness	Normal	Normal	Impaired	Impaired	Normal

as *prosody* have non-dominant hemisphere control. Prosody is the rhythmic pattern and vocal intonation of speech that adds emphasis and emotional content to language. There is some clinical and pathologic evidence that prosody might have similar anatomic topography as verbal language in the non-dominant hemisphere.[251]

Anatomy

Patients with Broca-type aphasia have lesions near the frontal operculum, anterior to the precentral gyrus. This location has been aptly named *Broca's area* and is considered a motor association area, as it is adjacent to the oral motor area of the primary motor cortex. However, the Broca-type aphasia is a primary language deficit with mildly compromised comprehension as well as impaired oral expression. It cannot be considered a purely motor impairment. The topographic location for the Wernicke type of aphasia is *Wernicke's area*, which is found in the posterior superior portion of the first temporal gyrus near the primary auditory cortex, and is considered an auditory association area. Lesions near but not involving Broca's or Wernicke's area are associated with transcortical motor and sensory aphasias, respectively.[5]

Ross has described aprosodia that is associated with lesions of the frontal operculum of the right or non-dominant hemisphere.[251] Patients who have aprosody speak at an even tempo with flat intonation when asked to express a sentence with an emotional tone. However, they are able to hear and comprehend the emotional content of language. In contrast, patients with a lesion in the temporoparietal region have an affective agnosia, in that they are unable to recognize the emotional prosody of spoken language. Despite the agnosia, these patients express prosody without difficulty.

Conduction aphasia, with severely impaired repetition of language, is associated with a lesion of the arcuate fasciculus, which is a bundle of fibers that pass from the temporal to the frontal lobe.[108] Disorders of reading (alexia) and writing (agraphia) are associated with disconnection of the primary language area from the primary visual cortices, which correlates to lesions in the angular gyrus at the junction of the occipital and temporoparietal lobes.[98]

Apraxia

Disorders of skilled movement in the absence of motor, sensory, or cognitive impairment are called *apraxia*. Patients with apraxia often have difficulty performing simple functional activities such as using a spoon or a comb, or they will perform them in a clumsy manner. It is often difficult to test for apraxia in the presence of a language deficit, because the examiner must be assured that the patient understands the command. However, patients with apraxia can have difficulty waving goodbye or using a gesture for hitchhiking when asked to demonstrate these maneuvers. Apraxia is most commonly seen in left hemisphere strokes and affects the left non-hemiplegic limb. Geshwind attributes apraxia in this situation to a disconnection of the right cortical motor association area from the left hemisphere due to an injury of the anterior callosal fibers.[109] Under these circum-stances, the right brain cannot know what the left brain wants to do!

Patients with right parietal strokes often have significant difficulty in dressing, despite adequate strength and flexibility. This has been called 'dressing apraxia', but it is not a true apraxia, because it is not a disorder of skilled motor function. It is actually a disorder of spatial perception that impairs the patient's ability to find the sleeves and neck of a shirt. Similarly, patients with 'constructional apraxia' have difficulty copying a figure due to visuospatial deficits consistent with right parietal stroke.

Neglect syndrome

Heilman et al. define hemispatial neglect as a failure to report, respond, or orient to novel or meaningful stimuli presented to the side opposite a brain lesion.[129] It is important to exclude visual, somatosensory, or motor impairments that would explain the lack of response before attributing it to neglect. Hemispatial neglect significantly contributes to disability after stroke, because it has a negative impact on sitting balance, visual perception, wheelchair mobility, safety awareness, skin and joint protection, and fall risk. Patients with neglect have difficulty completing hygiene and self-care on the affected side, fail to eat food items in the neglected visual space, and frequently run into objects and walls. Neglect is a disorder of visual and spatial attention, and is associated with temporoparietal strokes and lesions of the frontal eye fields, cingulate gyrus, thalamus, and reticular formation.[197]

Dysphagia

Dysphagia is common after stroke, occurring in 30–65% of patients with unilateral or bilateral hemispheric and brain stem infarctions.[7,14,61,116,137–139,182] Risk for aspiration pneumonia is strongly associated with a delayed initiation of pharyngeal swallow and reduced pharyngeal transit times frequently seen on videofluoroscopic swallow evaluation.[148,149] Other neurologic factors that influence risk for aspiration after stroke include reduced labial and lingual mobility and sensation, unilateral neglect, pooling of pharyngeal residue within the vallecula and pyriform sinuses, and cricopharyngeal dysmotility. Laryngeal elevation during swallow normally declines with age, and can have a negative influence on aspiration risk after stroke (see also Ch. 28).

Uninhibited bladder and bowel

Bladder and bowel incontinence are frequent consequences of stroke. Because the pontine micturition center is typically preserved, reflex voiding usually shows normal synchronous internal sphincter relaxation with detrusor contraction. Post-void residual volumes are generally low in the absence of prostatic hypertrophy or other forms of bladder outlet obstruction. Incontinence is caused by a lack of voluntary inhibition to void from upper motor neuron injury, and results in urgency of urination. In alert individuals, awareness of the need to void is unaffected, but immobility, unilateral neglect, and communication deficits often impair a patient's ability to use equipment or call for assistance when the need arises. Although most stroke survivors with diabetes have uninhibited voiding, some might have a hypotonic bladder from a parasympathetic autonomic neuropathy to the detrusor muscle. Special care should be taken to check post-void residual volumes in these patients. Bowel incontinence results from uninhibited reflex rectal emptying by the same mechanism as the uninhibited bladder.

CLINICAL STROKE SYNDROMES

Anatomic localization of lesions within the central nervous system predicts physical or cognitive impairment and disability. Understanding the clinical syndromes associated with defined cerebrovascular lesions in ischemic stroke can be a valuable tool to the physiatrist leading the rehabilitation team.

Middle cerebral artery syndromes

Strokes within the middle cerebral artery (MCA) distribution are very commonly seen within the inpatient rehabilitation setting. The anatomic distribution of the MCA includes a large proportion of cerebral cortex, and ischemia within the MCA imparts significant impairment and disability, often requiring intensive rehabilitation care. The MCA is particularly vulnerable to both cardioembolic and thrombotic disease, which can result in a variety of stroke syndromes.

Anatomy

The anterior circulation of the brain consists of both internal carotid arteries derived from the right and left common carotid arteries. The right carotid is usually a branch of the right subclavian; the left is a direct branch of the aorta. After the internal carotid artery passes intracranially through the carotid siphon, it provides the ophthalmic branch to the orbit and then bifurcates at the circle of Willis into the anterior cerebral artery (ACA) and MCA. The MCA stem or M1 segment turns laterally, passing along the base of the brain to the Sylvian fissure overlying the insular cortex, where it typically bifurcates into an upper and a lower division. Along the path of the M1 segment, small, deep, perforating branches called *lenticulostriate arteries* are supplied to the putamen, globus pallidus, caudate, and internal capsule. The M2 segment comprises the upper and lower divisions of the MCA as they travel posteriorly and superiorly along the insular cortex. Branches of the divisions pass laterally along the frontal, parietal, and temporal opercula constituting the M3 segment. The M4 segment includes the branches supplying the frontal, parietal, and temporal convexities.

Middle cerebral artery stroke

Main stem The impairments following occlusion of the MCA main stem (M1 segment) are listed in Box 51-1. The hemiplegia in a main stem stroke is complete, affecting the upper and lower limbs and lower portions of the face equally. This results primarily from ischemia from within the deep lenticulostriate circulation to the posterior limb of the internal capsule through

---

Box 51-1 Middle cerebral artery stroke: main stem

- Contralateral hemiplegia
- Contralateral hemianesthesia
- Contralateral hemianopia
- Head or eye turning toward lesion
- Dysphagia
- Uninhibited neurogenic bladder

Dominant hemisphere
- Global aphasia
- Apraxia

Non-dominant hemisphere
- Aprosody and affective agnosia
- Visuospatial deficit
- Neglect syndrome

Box 51-2 Middle cerebral artery stroke: upper division

- Contralateral hemiplegia[a]
- Contralateral hemianesthesia
- Contralateral hemianopia
- Head or eye turning toward lesion
- Dysphagia
- Uninhibited neurogenic bladder

Dominant hemisphere
- Broca aphasia
- Apraxia

Non-dominant hemisphere
- Aprosody
- Visuospatial deficit
- Neglect syndrome

[a]Leg relatively more spared than hand and face.

---

which the descending fibers of the primary motor cortex pass. In contrast, the hemisensory deficit is not as severe, because the ascending sensory fibers are not affected, and only the inferior portion of the primary sensory cortex is supplied by the MCA. Although the MCA perforators supply only the upper half of the visual radiations, complete hemianopias are frequently described. Dysphagia and uninhibited voiding are commonly found, even in unilateral strokes.

Upper division Middle cerebral artery upper division strokes are listed in Box 51-2. The clinical presentation is very similar to that of a main stem infarction, but hemiplegia and language comprehension deficits are usually not as severe. Because the M1 segment of the MCA is spared, the vascular supply to the internal capsule is preserved, and ischemia is limited to the inferolateral portion of the primary motor cortex. As a result, motor strength and control are better in the lower limb than in

> **Box 51-3** Middle cerebral artery stroke: lower division
>
> - Contralateral homonymous hemianopia
> **Dominant hemisphere**
> - Wernicke aphasia
> **Non-dominant hemisphere**
> - Affective agnosia

> **Box 51-4** Anterior cerebral artery stroke
>
> - Contralateral hemiplegia[a]
> - Contralateral hemianesthesia
> - Head or eye turning toward lesion
> - Grasp reflex—groping
> - Paratonia (or Gegenhalten)
> - Disconnection apraxia
> - Akinetic mutism (abulia)
>
> [a]Hand relatively more spared than arm and leg.

the hand and face. A classic Broca-type aphasia is typical in a dominant hemisphere stroke, and aprosodia without affective agnosia is found in non-dominant hemisphere stroke.

Lower division   Branch obstruction of the MCA lower division is much less common than upper division stroke, and is usually caused by an embolic event. Motor and sensory function is generally intact. Despite this, patients with stroke of the MCA lower division can have significant functional disability from impaired language and vision, and poor awareness of deficits. Box 51-3 lists the impairments associated with lower division strokes.

Anterior cerebral artery syndromes
Anatomy
The ACA supplies the interhemispheric cortical surface of the frontal and parietal lobes. The A1 segment branches medially from the internal carotid bifurcation to the anterior communicating artery. Turning superiorly, the artery passes over the optic nerve, along the rostrum of the corpus callosum (A2), and around the genu (A3); it passes posteriorly to the coronal suture (A4) and terminates at the parietal lobe (A5). The ACA divides during its course into two major branches, the pericallosal and callomarginal branches, which provide smaller branches to the cortical surface. The recurrent artery of Heubner is a branch from the A1 or proximal A2 segment that deeply perforates to supply important structures such as the head of the caudate, the anterior limb of the internal capsule, the anterior putamen and globus pallidus, and the hypothalamus.

Anterior cerebral artery stroke
The disorders resulting from an ACA infarction are listed in Box 51-4. The hemiplegia in ACA strokes shows weakness of the shoulder and foot with relative sparing of the forearm, hand, and face, because the focus of ischemia is over the paracentral lobule of the interhemispheric cortex. Unilateral foot drop can be a long-term impairment requiring orthotic management. A left upper limb apraxia to verbal commands can also result from an infarction of the anterior corpus callosum, which disconnects the right hemisphere prefrontal area from the left hemisphere language area.

Occlusion involving the anterior communicating artery and the recurrent artery of Heubner can extend the infarction through the anterior limb of the internal capsule, causing complete hemiplegia. The proximity of such a stroke to Broca's area

> **Box 51-5** Posterior cerebral artery stroke
>
> - Hemisensory deficit
> - Visual impairment
> - Visual agnosia
> - Prosopagnosia
> - Dyschromatopsia
> - Alexia without agraphia
> - Memory deficits

can also result in a transcortical motor aphasia. Frontal lobe injury can result in ipsilateral or bilateral rigidity characterized by a force-dependent resistance in passive limb movement called paratonia or Gegenhalten. This is also often associated with a grasp reflex.

Posterior cerebral artery syndromes
Anatomy
The vertebral arteries typically branch from the right and left subclavian arteries, passing rostrally through the transverse foramina of the cervical vertebra and intracranially via the foramen magnum. At the junction of the medulla and pons, the vertebral arteries unite to form the basilar artery, which again divides into the two posterior cerebral arteries (PCAs) near the top of the midbrain. The P1 segment extends from the basilar to the posterior communicating artery, and the P2 segment extends beyond. Supplying the thalamus are the deep perforating arteries from the P1 and the stem of the P2 segments, called the *thalamoperforants* and *thalamogeniculates*. The branches of the P2 segment include the anterior and posterior inferior temporal, occipital temporal, calcarine, and occipitoparietal arteries.

Posterior cerebral artery stroke
The syndrome of PCA infarction is listed in Box 51-5. The blood supply of the thalamus is provided by the perforating arteries of the PCA. Infarcts in the region can cause hemisensory deficits, including hypoesthesia, dysesthesia, and occasionally hyperesthesia or pain. Thalamic pain syndrome was first described by Dejerine and Roussy in 1906,[68] but nearly any disruption of sensory afferent fibers within the central nervous

system can cause a central poststroke pain syndrome. Visual disturbances result from injury to the lateral geniculate, temporal, and occipital visual radiations and the calcarine cortex of the occipital lobe. In addition, damage to visual association areas can cause dyschromatopsia, or altered color discrimination. A disorder of reading without impaired writing (alexia without agraphia) associated with a right visual field deficit results from an infarction of the left occipital cortex and posterior corpus callosum, disconnecting the intact right visual cortex from the primary language area of the left hemisphere. Impaired memory can result from infarction of the temporal lobe and the hippocampal gyri.

Vertebrobasilar syndromes
Anatomy
The major arterial branches supplying the brain stem and cerebellum are the posterior inferior cerebellar artery (PICA), the anterior inferior cerebellar artery (AICA), and the superior cerebellar artery (SCA). The PICA originates from the distal vertebral artery and wraps dorsally around the medulla, whereas the AICA is a branch of the basilar artery circling around the pons. Both supply the inferior lobe of the cerebellum. The superior lobe of the cerebellum receives its blood supply from the SCA branching from the basilar artery at the level of the midbrain. Throughout the course of the basilar artery and its major tributaries, small, deep, perforating arteries branch to supply the brain stem. These branches include paramedian penetrators supplying the medial and basal portions of the brain stem, and the short and long circumferential arteries supporting the lateral brain stem.

Brain stem stroke syndromes
The brain stem is a complex structure containing cranial nerves, bulbar nuclei, and tracts. The bulbar nuclei form afferent and efferent cranial nerves that innervate the ipsilateral side of the body, whereas the ascending and descending bulbar and spinal tracts innervate contralaterally. Consequently, unilateral brain stem strokes often cause loss of cranial nerve function ipsilaterally and sensorimotor dysfunction contralaterally.[110] Cerebellar strokes result in ipsilateral ataxia, whereas brain stem strokes can cause ipsilateral, contralateral, or bilateral limb ataxia. The common brain stem syndromes are listed in Table 51-3, along with their anatomic correlates.

The *Wallenberg* or lateral medullary syndrome is a commonly occurring stroke that frequently requires inpatient rehabilitation. It is characterized by ipsilateral limb ataxia, loss of pain and temperature sensation on the ipsilateral face and contralateral body, ipsilateral Horner syndrome (myosis, ptosis, and anhydrosis), dysphagia, dysphonia, and nystagmus. Vertebral artery thrombosis near the PICA branch is the usual cause. The prognosis for functional improvement is excellent.

Most of the remaining brain stem syndromes occur with basilar artery thrombosis. The *locked-in* syndrome is a severe pontine stroke causing quadriplegia, oral motor and laryngeal weakness, and disruption of conjugate eye movements. Oral communication is impaired, but because upward gaze is controlled at the midbrain level within the tectum, patients usually have voluntary vertical eye movements that they can use for communication.

Cerebellar strokes are common, and can cause life-threatening obstruction of the fourth ventricle and

Table 51-3 Brain stem syndromes and their anatomic correlates

Syndrome	Location	Structural injury	Characteristics
Weber	Medial basal midbrain	Third cranial nerve Corticospinal tract	Ipsilateral third nerve palsy Contralateral hemiplegia
Benedikt	Tegmentum of midbrain	Third cranial nerve Spinothalamic tract Medial lemniscus Superior cerebellar peduncle Red nucleus	Ipsilateral third nerve palsy Contralateral loss of pain and temperature sensation Contralateral loss of joint position Contralateral ataxia Contralateral chorea
Locked in	Bilateral basal pons	Corticospinal tract Corticobulbar tract	Bilateral hemiplegia Bilateral cranial nerve palsy (upward gaze spared)
Millard–Gubler	Lateral pons	Sixth cranial nerve Seventh cranial nerve Corticospinal tract	Ipsilateral sixth nerve palsy Ipsilateral facial weakness Contralateral hemiplegia
Wallenberg	Lateral medulla	Spinocerebellar tract Fifth cranial nerve Spinothalamic tract Vestibular nuclei Sympathetic tract Nucleus ambiguus	Ipsilateral hemiataxia Ipsilateral loss of facial pain and temperature sensation Contralateral loss of body pain and temperature sensation Nystagmus Ipsilateral Horner syndrome Dysphagia and dysphonia

Table 51-4 Lacunar syndromes and their anatomic correlates

Syndrome	Anatomic sites
Pure motor stroke	Posterior limb internal capsule Basis pontis Pyramids
Pure sensory stroke	Thalamus Thalamocortical projections
Sensory–motor stroke	Junction of internal capsule and thalamus
Dysarthria—clumsy hand	Anterior limb internal capsule Pons
Ataxic hemiparesis	Corona radiata Internal capsule Pons Cerebellum
Hemiballismus	Head of caudate Thalamus Subthalamic nucleus

hydrocephalus if cerebellar edema develops. Such strokes occur with PICA, AICA, or SCA occlusion. PICA and AICA strokes are generally caused by arterial thrombosis of the vertebrobasilar system, but SCA strokes are more commonly cardioembolic.[108]

Lacunar strokes

Lacunar strokes are located within the deep cerebral white matter, basal ganglia, thalamus, and pons, and result from occlusion of single, small, perforating arteries.[203] Strokes are common and present with a wide variety of neurologic and functional deficits. The most common syndromes are listed in Table 51-4.

ACUTE STROKE MANAGEMENT

Epidemiology
Stroke incidence, mortality, prevalence, and survival
Data from several population-based study cohorts estimate that the yearly incidence of stroke in the USA is 700 000, which comprise 500 000 new strokes and 200 000 recurrent strokes.[8] Stroke continues to result in significant morbidity, mortality, and disability, particularly among people older than 65 years.

Stroke is primarily a disease of older individuals, but 28% of strokes occur in persons younger than 65 years. Children have an annual incidence of 2.7 strokes per 100 000. In adults, the primary cause of ischemic stroke is atherosclerosis, whereas in children the causes include cerebrovascular anomalies, congenital heart disease, carotid dissection, sickle cell disease, inherited disorders of coagulation, and previous infection with varicella zoster.[186] Hemorrhagic strokes can occur as a result of moya-moya disease and hemophilia.

The incidence of stroke is 19% higher among adult men than in women of all races. Among black men less than 65 years old, stroke incidence is two- to threefold higher than among whites. The relative incidence of stroke among black women compared with white women is even higher. Many important risk factors for stroke are found in higher frequency among black people, including hypertension, diabetes mellitus, heart disease, smoking, excessive alcohol use, and sickle cell disease. The rate of stroke in Asian countries is higher than in the USA, with a greater proportion of strokes caused by intracranial hemorrhage.

Stroke was the primary cause of death in 163 538 persons in 2001, and it remains the third leading cause of death in the USA; it is exceeded only by cardiovascular disease and cancer.[8] However, a well-documented reduction in annual stroke mortality has taken place within the USA in the past century.[141] In particular, there was a sharp decline in the annual stroke deaths for both men and women that began in the 1970s and continued well into the 1980s before the slope flattened in the early 1990s.[165,194] Approximately 200 000 fewer fatal strokes occurred in this period than would have been predicted from data of the previous decade.[165] It can be argued that the improved detection and treatment of hypertension that began in the 1960s, and escalated in 1973 with introduction of the National High Blood Pressure Education and Control Program, is directly responsible for the steep decline in stroke mortality.[165,194]

Stroke survivors, many of whom require rehabilitation services, presently number nearly 5 million in the US population. Although the mortality from stroke has declined in the USA, hospitalizations for stroke increased by 18.6% between 1988 and 1997.[86] As our population ages, the incidence and prevalence of stroke will continue to rise. Stroke rehabilitation will have an important role in reducing the burden of long-term stroke care on society.

Stroke risk factors
Hypertension remains the most important public health concern today, because it is the leading risk factor for two of the top three causes of death in the USA: coronary heart disease and stroke. Hypertension is treatable, and its control has the potential for widespread reduction in death and disability in the USA. The combination of stroke and heart disease is not unusual, and can have a significant impact on medical care and rehabilitation.[259] When faced with a patient with a recent stroke, TIA, or asymptomatic carotid bruit, the clinician must be concerned about the presence of coronary heart disease. Similarly, any patient who presents with known heart disease and chronic atrial fibrillation should be considered a candidate for stroke prophylaxis. A major but often neglected part of physiatric care for stroke survivors and their families is stroke and coronary heart disease prevention and risk factor reduction.

Modifiable risk factors
Hypertension There is a 35% prevalence of hypertension within the US adult population. Defined as a systolic pressure greater than 165 mmHg, or a diastolic pressure greater than

95 mmHg, hypertension increases the relative risk of stroke by a factor of six. Among stroke survivors, 67% have chronic hypertension.[121] Several meta-analyses of randomized trials of antihypertensive medications have demonstrated that a 10- to 12-mmHg reduction of systolic and a 5- to 6-mmHg reduction of diastolic pressure is associated with a 35% reduction in stroke risk in both hypertensive and normotensive subjects.[55,188] Interestingly, no threshold diastolic value was found below which further pressure reduction lacked an additional effect on stroke risk. Consequently, reductions in diastolic blood pressure below traditionally normotensive values contributed to further risk reduction in these studies.

The Hypertension Detection and Follow-up Program was the first major study to demonstrate a reduction in stroke incidence with antihypertensive treatment. This was a population-based randomized clinical trial with a 5-year follow-up involving 11 000 hypertensive persons who were either provided with a stepped care antihypertensive program or referred for traditional care. There was a 1.9% incidence of stroke among patients on stepped care treatment, compared with 2.9% on a referred care program, equaling a 35% reduction in stroke incidence and a 44% reduction in fatal strokes.[145] Isolated systolic hypertension is more common among individuals older than 60 years, and is an independent risk factor for stroke and cardiovascular disease.[159] The Systolic Hypertension in the Elderly Program[276] randomized more than 4700 subjects aged 60 years and older with systolic pressures greater than 160 mmHg and diastolic pressure less than 90 mmHg to antihypertensive treatment or placebo. Over the 5-year study period, subjects treated with antihypertensive medication had an average reduction in systolic blood pressure of 17 mmHg and a 36% reduction in the incidence of stroke when compared with control subjects.

More recently, the role of angiotensin-converting enzyme inhibitors in the prevention of stroke has been appreciated. The Heart Outcomes Prevention study demonstrated that ramipril provides a 32% relative reduction in stroke occurrence in patients with a history of myocardial infarction, stroke, peripheral vascular disease, or other risk factors.[136] The Perindopril Protection Against Recurrent Stroke Study randomized patients with stroke or TIA with or without hypertension to perindopril versus placebo, finding a 28% relative risk reduction with antihypertensive treatment. The combination of a diuretic with the angiotensin-converting enzyme inhibitor improved blood pressure reduction and provided better risk reduction.[236]

Ample evidence supports public health efforts aimed at reducing the prevalence of poorly controlled blood pressure, thereby reducing the risk of stroke and heart disease. Improved public education, detection, and treatment of hypertension will have a positive impact on the further decline of stroke incidence and mortality.

Smoking   It has been known for many years that cigarette smoking is an important risk factor for cardiovascular disease, but its negative influence on stroke was questioned. More recently, community-based data from the Framingham Study have confirmed that smoking is independently associated with an increased risk of atherothrombotic stroke in both men and women. The relative risk of stroke for heavy smokers (>40 cigarettes per day) is twice that of light smokers (<10 cigarettes per day). Cessation of smoking reverses risk to that of non-smokers within 5 years after quitting.[329] Smoking is also a significant risk factor for SAH and ICH in both men and women.[174,175,263]

Hypercholesterolemia   The role of elevated serum cholesterol has not been epidemiologically linked to increased stroke incidence per se, but its strong influence on the development of coronary artery disease and atherosclerosis[253] indicates that hypercholesterolemia is at least an indirect risk factor for stroke. Indeed, an association between carotid artery atherosclerosis and increased serum cholesterol levels has been noted.[216,265] The use of HMG-CoA reductase inhibitors or statins can reduce the risk of stroke,[40] but their role in prevention can have as much to do with their ability to stabilize atherosclerotic plaques and reduce inflammation as their ability to reduce serum cholesterol.[191,286] Still, there is a role for dietary reduction of cholesterol and saturated fatty acids in the prevention of stroke. Current targets for patients with coronary heart disease and stroke are a low-density lipoprotein <100 mg/dL and a total cholesterol <200 mg/dL. High-density lipoprotein levels >60 mg/dL are desirable.[3]

Diabetes mellitus and other risk factors   Diabetes mellitus increases the relative risk of ischemic stroke to three to six times that of the general population. This risk can be partly attributed to the higher prevalence of hypertension and heart disease among persons with diabetes, but even after controlling for these factors, diabetes independently doubles stroke risk.[1,16,158] The prevalence of diabetes among stroke survivors is 20%.[1,121,200]

Whether obesity is a risk factor for stroke has been challenged. Hypertension and diabetes mellitus are more common in the obese and are strong influences for stroke risk. Weight loss has a positive influence on blood pressure and diabetic control, and probably has a risk-reducing effect on stroke and cardiovascular disease. Although obesity can indirectly increase stroke risk, its independence as a risk factor remains questionable.

Heart disease, including electrocardiographic evidence of left ventricular hypertrophy, cardiac failure, and non-valvular atrial fibrillation, increases stroke risk by two to six times normal. Control of hypertension, cessation of smoking, and reduction of serum cholesterol can reduce the development of heart disease as well as prevent stroke. However, in the presence of established conditions such as atrial fibrillation or left ventricular failure, the use of medical means to reduce stroke risk can become important. Prevention of heart disease through lifestyle changes has a positive influence on stroke prevention.

Elevated plasma levels of homocysteine have been associated with increased risk of stroke and carotid artery disease.[274] Hyperhomocysteinemia can result from inherited enzyme deficiencies or acquired deficiencies of required enzyme cofactors such as folate, vitamin B_{12}, or vitamin B_6. The hyperviscosity that can occur with hyperhomocysteinemia can lead to hyper-coagulability or enhanced atherogenesis by microvascular damage from traumatic shearing forces against vessel walls. Patients with acute stroke who have elevated plasma homocysteine are at risk for recurrent stroke, and supplementation with folate, vitamin B_{12}, and vitamin B_6 is advised.[28]

Non-modifiable risk factors

Certain important risk factors for stroke that are not modifiable include age, sex, race, and previous stroke. The epidemiology of age, sex, and race as they relate to stroke were reviewed earlier in the chapter. Once an individual has a stroke, the risk of recurrent stroke is significant. Although the presence of a stroke is not in itself modifiable as a risk factor, a careful work-up to determine the cause of the stroke can provide valuable information for clinical decisions regarding secondary stroke prevention.

The first 6 hours

A basic pathophysiologic understanding of cerebral ischemia clarifies the actions necessary to protect the brain during acute stroke. Cerebral tissue necrosis occurs when CBF, normally under tight autoregulation, is compromised from either arterial thrombosis or embolism. Normal cerebral autoregulation maintains a cerebral perfusion rate of 50 mL/100 g of cerebral tissue per min, which remains constant regardless of acute changes in systemic mean arterial pressure. During cerebrovascular compromise, normal neural activity can be sustained with a CBF as low as 20 mL/100 g per min, but a rate below 10 mL/100 g per min results in cellular death. Within the CBF range between 10 and 20 mL/100 g per min, basic cellular functions are supported but the sodium–potassium pump fails, rendering the neural cells 'electrically silent'.[280] In an acute stroke, these surviving but inactive neural cells are located at the rim of the ischemic injury, where collateral circulation provides the minimal tissue perfusion needed. This rim has been called the *ischemic penumbra*, after the partial shadow surrounding a solar eclipse. Improved blood flow to the ischemic penumbra can theoretically restore normal neurologic function. However, the longer the ischemic period before reperfusion, the less likely is the ischemic penumbra to survive. Recent acute stroke management protocols have focused on vascular reperfusion in order to maximally save the ischemic penumbra. From the standpoint of public education regarding stroke, the National Stroke Association has emphasized that, to reduce neural impairment, acute stroke management should be implemented within the first 6 h of the event.

There are a number of treatments that are available and are being employed more frequently for acute ischemic stroke. The most commonly used treatment is intravenous recombinant tissue plasminogen activator (rt-PA), a thrombolytic agent that was approved for use in the USA in 1996. Because rt-PA can be only safely given within 3 h of stroke onset, considerable effort has been taken to educate the public about the signs and symptoms of stroke and the need to seek immediate treatment. Similarly, more and more hospitals are developing clinical programs to manage acute ischemic stroke. Currently, the Joint Commission on Accreditation of Healthcare Organizations is in the process of certifying acute stroke centers throughout the USA that meet basic criteria for the rapid identification and treatment of acute stroke.[6]

The efficacy of intravenous rt-PA is well supported when given early after onset of stroke symptoms, reducing the absolute risk of being dead or dependent by 16%.[321] Better outcomes are achieved in patients with mild to moderate neurologic impairment, in persons younger than 75 years, and when the drug is administered within 90 min of onset.[2] In the definitive US trial, there was a 12% absolute increase in patients with little or no disability 3 months after treatment. The major risk of giving intravenous rt-PA is intracranial bleeding, which can be fatal. Symptomatic brain hemorrhage occurred in 6.4% of patients treated with rt-PA and only 0.6% in the placebo group. Yet 3 months after treatment, mortality was similar in both groups.[211] Strict adherence to the Food and Drug Administration-approved intravenous rt-PA protocol can maximally reduce serious hemorrhagic complications.

In addition to intravenous rt-PA, many experienced centers are now providing intraarterial rt-PA to patients with large vessel occlusions of the MCA or basilar artery who present within 6 h of onset. Although there are no intraarterial thrombolytics approved for treatment of acute stroke, there are data to support the use of this technique in selected patients.[100] Recently, techniques to mechanically snare or retrieve thrombus from major cerebral arteries using endovascular techniques have been developed. One such device has been recently approved by the Food and Drug Administration for use as late as 8 h after acute stroke onset, adding another tool to the acute management of ischemic stroke.

Heparin is frequently administered intravenously in the acute setting to arrest stroke progression or to prevent its recurrence, but there is little support for its efficacy. Presently, trials on the use of intravenous unfractionated or low molecular weight heparin for acute ischemic stroke have had disappointing results. Hemorrhagic complications tend to negate any beneficial outcomes in these trials. Experts have generally discouraged the use of heparin for acute stroke management, especially within the first 12 h after onset. However, there may be a role for anticoagulation in patients who present with cardioembolic stroke, stroke in evolution, stroke in large artery atherosclerosis, or in the case of arterial dissections.[4]

Subcutaneously injected heparin in dosages of 5000 and 12 500 units twice daily was studied in the large International Stroke Trial ($n = 19\,435$). Neither dosage was effective in preventing death or disability at 14 days or 6 months following ischemic stroke. Significant bleeding was associated with the higher heparin dose, but not with 5000 units twice daily dosing.[147]

Emergency medical management

Initial medical care for a patient with acute stroke requires careful and frequent neurologic monitoring to prevent and manage medical complications that compromise cerebral tissue perfusion. If the patient is obtunded, concern for airway protection is critical to maintain oxygenation, and an endotracheal tube should be placed, with ventilatory support if necessary. Cerebral edema and acute hydrocephalus can develop rapidly (particularly after ICH), requiring placement of an external ventriculostomy device to relieve intracranial pressure. In cases of brain stem compression and hydrocephalus from cerebellar infarction or hemorrhage, surgical decompression of the posterior fossa can be life-saving.[318]

Blood pressure is often acutely elevated during stroke, usually as a response to cerebral injury, and often falls spontaneously over the following week.[230] Clinicians should resist the temptation to rapidly correct elevated blood pressure, because often it is a necessary compensatory response to impaired autoregulation after acute ischemic brain injury. A higher mean arterial pressure is needed to maintain cerebral perfusion pressure to the ischemic area, whereas a rapid drop in blood pressure can potentially enlarge an ischemic infarct. This is especially true in individuals with chronic hypertension, whose brains are accustomed to a higher perfusion pressure.[131,294] Although there are no definitive recommendations, acute hypertension after stroke is usually treated only if it is symptomatic, if there is evidence of end-organ injury, if the systolic pressure rises above 220 mmHg, or if the diastolic pressure rises above 120 mmHg.[2] When treated, elevated blood pressure should be lowered gently, and it is usually best to allow the systolic pressure to remain above 150 mmHg and the diastolic pressure above 90 mmHg. Intravenous nitroprusside is frequently used for treatment of severe hypertension in emergency departments, but in the presence of acute stroke it can precipitously drop the systolic pressure, and cerebral vasodilatation can increase intracranial pressure. When used, constant pressure monitoring with an arterial line is necessary. A preferred alternative is the use of intravenous labetalol, which can nicely lower pressure without less negative effects on CBF.[272] For patients who cannot tolerate the beta-blocking effect of labetalol (e.g. those with asthma), intravenous nicardipine is gaining favor as an alternative agent in acute stroke.[93]

Hyperglycemia in response to acute physiologic stress occurs in both diabetic and non-diabetic patients during stroke, and is associated with increased levels of serum cortisol. Frequent monitoring and control of serum glucose levels during acute stroke have been recommended. Animal studies reveal that a high glucose concentration within partially perfused ischemic tissue provides the substrate for anaerobic cellular metabolism and lactic acid production.[67,207] The accumulation of lactic acid is cytotoxic and can lead to further tissue injury.[67,281] Careful use of insulin and strict glucose control are potentially neuroprotective.

Further diagnostic evaluation

Following emergency department care and early acute stroke management, patients are admitted to the hospital for a complete diagnostic work-up to determine the cause of the stroke and develop a plan for secondary prevention. Diagnostic tests commonly include cranial and cerebrovascular imaging, carotid artery ultrasound, and echocardiogram. Additional laboratory tests can be ordered as indicated, such as full lipid profile if the cholesterol level is elevated. In young patients with stroke, it is important to consider hereditary diseases that cause thrombophilia.

Cranial magnetic resonance imaging (MRI) is useful to determine the extent of brain injury and identify potential structural abnormalities. Standard two-dimensional spin-echo MRI is now available in most medical centers throughout the USA and has several advantages for the evaluation of stroke. Tissue density on MRI is dependent on the energy released in the presence of a strong magnetic field. On T1-weighted images, CSF appears dark, whereas gray and white matter is nicely differentiated. In contrast, T2-weighted images show a bright CSF signal, while the fat density is low. A third technique, in which CSF and soft tissue are isodense, is called 'spin-density' weighting. With all techniques, bone is poorly imaged due to its low hydrogen content. The flow of blood within the cerebral circulation produces a signal void unless a static intravascular occlusion is present.

Magnetic resonance imaging is more sensitive than computed tomography (CT) in demonstrating the changes of acute stroke in the first 48 h.[38] Edema within an infarcted zone can appear as early as 2–4 h after stroke onset and is best seen on T2-weighted images. Infarcts near the cortex or periventricular region are better seen on spin-density images, because the bright CSF signal of T2 weighting can otherwise obscure subtle changes. T1-weighted imaging is less sensitive for acute cerebral infarct but can show early effacement of gyri and occasionally a vascular thrombus. MRI is more sensitive than CT for lacunar strokes after the first 24 h, and MRI is the test of choice for imaging the posterior fossa, where bone artifact is not a problem.[192] Newer diffusion-weighted MRI techniques are superior to conventional MRI for detecting early ischemic changes, and whole brain scans can now be performed quite rapidly. When combined with gadolinium contrast-enhanced perfusion weighted imaging, a mismatch between the ischemic core and the perfusion deficit can be estimated. The role of perfusion and diffusion MRI in clinical decision making, especially in the selection of patients for thrombolytic therapy, is currently being debated. Newer scanning techniques with multidimensional CT imaging, such as CT angiography and CT perfusion scanning, show promise for improving acute stroke diagnosis.[300]

Magnetic resonance imaging is nearly equivalent to CT for the detection of ICH in the acute setting. Cranial CT remains the test of choice for examination of hemorrhage, because it is less costly than MRI. With subacute or chronic hemorrhagic stroke, MRI can differentiate methemoglobin from soft tissue, and is better than CT for the detection of late hemorrhages.[38]

Magnetic resonance angiography is a non-invasive option for examining extra- and intracranial cerebral vessels. Using the two-dimensional 'time of flight' technique, extracranial vessels can be visualized, often revealing the presence of carotid or vertebrobasilar atherosclerotic disease. The three-dimensional time of flight technique produces excellent images of the circle of Willis and the cerebral artery stems.[140] Magnetic resonance angiography is indicated as a screening test for extracranial and intracranial atherosclerotic disease, and when combined with conventional duplex ultrasound can often obviate the need for conventional angiography.[208] Magnetic resonance angiography is the test of choice for detecting carotid dissection.

Due to its non-invasive nature, ultrasonography has become a standard diagnostic tool in the evaluation of acute stroke. Transthoracic echocardiography imaging after suspected cerebral embolism is now standard practice and is simple to perform. Intraventricular thrombi and valvular vegetations are particularly easy to image using this technique. The detection of thrombi within the left atrium and the atrial appendage is unreliable with transthoracic echocardiography, because visualization of the left atrium is obscured by the left ventricle. Transesophageal echocardiography overcomes this limitation because the transducer is passed down the esophagus, posterior to the heart, where the left atrium and appendage can be directly visualized. This procedure is well tolerated and provides a 10-fold improvement in left atrial thrombus detection. Patent foramen ovale and atrial septal defects are also best visualized with transesophageal echocardiography, which can be important if paradoxical embolism is suspected.

Arterial duplex scanning combines either standard or color Doppler imaging with two-dimensional ultrasound, and is a useful screening tool for carotid atherosclerosis. In practical use, a negative carotid duplex scan excludes the need for carotid endarterectomy, but it does not rule out the presence of significant intracranial atherosclerosis. Similarly, a duplex scan that is positive for critical stenosis extracranially cannot exclude the presence of an arterial occlusion in the distal internal carotid artery, which is a contraindication to surgical treatment. Transcranial Doppler imaging can measure flow characteristics of the intracranial vessels, but it lacks imaging capability; it is most useful when serial measurements of CBF are needed, such as in the monitoring of cerebral vasospasm after SAH.[144] Although it is invasive and not without complications, conventional contrast-enhanced cerebral angiography is the most accurate method of detecting and anatomically defining intracranial cerebrovascular disease when surgical treatment is considered. Contrast-enhanced angiography is the method of choice for detecting and defining the anatomy of cerebral aneurysms and AVMs.

Stroke prevention

The most effective means to diminish stroke-related morbidity, mortality, and disability is by further reducing the incidence of first-time and recurrent stroke. As emphasized thus far, public awareness of modifiable risk factors for stroke, medical management of risk factors, and the active promotion of lifestyle changes by physicians have the best potential to decrease the annual rate of new stroke occurrence. Physiatrists in particular can counsel patients with stroke and their families about risk factor reduction throughout the course of rehabilitation care. For selected patients who have significant risk for stroke, who

have experienced a TIA, or who have had a stroke in the past, physicians can recommend additional medical interventions to minimize the risk of primary (first-time) and secondary (recurrent) stroke. These interventions include antiplatelet therapy, anticoagulation, and carotid endarterectomy.

Antiplatelet therapy

An Oxford-based group called the Antithrombotic Trialists' Collaboration has published a metaanalysis of pooled results from 145 trials of various antiplatelet agents for the prevention of vascular events, including non-fatal myocardial infarction, non-fatal stroke, and vascular death.[11] As a group, these studies include more than 70 000 subjects with risk factors for vascular disease who were randomized to receive various forms of antiplatelet therapy or placebo over 2–6 years. Antiplatelet agents were found to reduce the risk of non-fatal stroke by 25% in men and women. Subgroups of hypertensive and diabetic subjects also benefited from treatment. Among patients with previous stroke or TIA, the use of long-term antiplatelet therapy resulted in 36 fewer non-fatal strokes per 1000 patients, with only one or two additional major intracranial hemorrhages. Although this study supports the benefit of antiplatelet agents in the reduction of vascular disease in general, the use of and indications for these agents in stroke prophylaxis should be based on specific trials having clearly stated end points.

Aspirin is the most frequently prescribed antiplatelet agent for secondary stroke and cardiovascular disease prevention. By irreversibly inhibiting cyclooxygenase-dependent platelet aggregation, aspirin achieves a significant antiplatelet effect at fairly low serum concentrations.[189] Two large randomized controlled trials have compared aspirin with placebo in the prevention of death or recurrent infarct in nearly 40 000 patients hospitalized with acute ischemic stroke. In combined analysis, the International Stroke Trial[147] and the Chinese Acute Stroke Trial[47] showed that aspirin (160–300 mg/day) administered early after acute stroke resulted in nine fewer deaths and recurrent strokes per 1000 patients during the first few weeks, without significant complications. These studies justify the routine use of aspirin in patients with acute ischemic stroke.

The combined use of aspirin with extended release dipyridamole was studied in the European Stroke Prevention Study 2.[71] This study randomized 6602 patients to receive either aspirin (50 mg), extended release dipyridamole (400 mg), or the combination daily for the long-term prevention of secondary stroke after stroke or TIA. Aspirin was found to reduce recurrent stroke by 18%, dipyridamole by 16%, and combined aspirin and dipyridamole by 37%, suggesting an additive effect. The most common side effect of combined aspirin and dipyridamole is headache, which often limits its use.

Clopidogrel is a non-aspirin antiplatelet agent that prevents platelet aggregation for the life of the cell by directly inhibiting ADP-induced platelet aggregation, without affecting prostaglandin metabolism. It lacks antipyretic, antiinflammatory, and analgesic effects, and it does not affect the integrity of the gastric mucosa.[45] In patients with a history of previous stroke, clopidogrel provides a non-statistically significant 7.3% relative risk reduction for recurrent stroke, myocardial infarction, or other vascular events, making it an effective alternative to aspirin for patients with aspirin allergy or intolerance. The combination of aspirin (75–325 mg daily) and clopidogrel reduces the risk of recurrent myocardial infarction by 23% over aspirin alone in patients with a history of acute coronary syndrome without ST elevation. The combined use of aspirin and clopidogrel significantly increased the risk of major bleeding over aspirin use (3.7 versus 2.7), which was an acceptable risk given the cardioprotective effect of combined treatment.[58] In contrast, the risks for bleeding with combined aspirin (75 mg) and clopidogrel (75 mg) daily outweighed the small and non-statistically significant reduction (6.4%) in recurrent stroke, myocardial infarction, or vascular death over clopidogrel alone in patients with a history of recent ischemic stroke or TIA and other risk factors.[70]

The relative efficacy of warfarin for prevention of recurrent stroke in patients with a history of non-cardioembolic stroke was investigated in the Warfarin and Aspirin for the Prevention of Recurrent Ischemic Stroke study.[202] This study demonstrated equivalent efficacy for either warfarin (international normalized ratio goal 1.4–2.8) or aspirin (325 mg daily) for secondary stroke prevention. There is no difference in the rate of major bleeding between groups, but warfarin was associated with a higher rate of minor bleeding. The ongoing Warfarin Aspirin Stroke Intracranial Disease trial will test whether warfarin or aspirin is superior for recurrent stroke prevention in patients with symptomatic carotid stenosis.

Anticoagulation and antiplatelet therapy in atrial fibrillation

Atrial fibrillation is commonly found among the elderly, and is present in 15% of persons older than 75 years. Individuals with non-valvular atrial fibrillation have five times the relative risk for cardioembolic stroke, and those with rheumatic heart disease have a 17-fold increase.[330] Other clinical factors, such as a history of TIA, stroke, hypertension, recent congestive heart failure, and electrocardiographic evidence of left ventricular dysfunction, are additional predictors of stroke when associated with atrial fibrillation. Clinical trials have supported the use of aspirin to prevent primary cardioembolic stroke in non-valvular atrial fibrillation. In the Copenhagen AFA-SAK trial,[229] a 75 mg/day dose of aspirin reduced embolic stroke risk by 15% when compared with placebo. The US sponsored Stroke Prevention in Atrial Fibrillation (SPAF) trial[296] measured a 42% reduction in stroke risk using 325 mg of aspirin daily. In the SPAF study, however, aspirin was not clearly effective in men, and it was ineffective in women older than 75 years. The AFA-SAK and SPAF studies, and two additional placebo-controlled trials,[27,84] have tested the use of warfarin anticoagulation for primary stroke prevention in non-valvular atrial fibrillation. Warfarin reduces relative stroke risk by 58–86% over that in control subjects.

Although warfarin proved more effective than aspirin for stroke prevention in atrial fibrillation, a second phase of the SPAF trial (SPAF II)[297] compared warfarin to aspirin with the special intention of determining which medication provided superior stroke prevention for individuals older than 75 years with non-valvular atrial fibrillation. This study concluded that care must be taken when considering anticoagulation in patients older than 75 years, as the risk of intracranial hemorrhage is higher in elderly persons, even without the use of warfarin. The results of the SPAF III trial demonstrated that low-intensity, fixed dose warfarin plus aspirin is inferior to adjusted dose warfarin for stroke prevention in high-risk patients with non-valvular atrial fibrillation.[295]

Individuals with rheumatic valvular disease and atrial fibrillation have a 17-fold increase in risk for embolic stroke. These patients benefit from anticoagulation with warfarin for stroke prevention.

Surgical management of carotid artery disease

For many years, the benefits of surgical versus medical treatment in the management of TIA associated with carotid artery atherosclerosis was hotly debated. More recent evidence supports the use of carotid endarterectomy in combination with antiplatelet therapy as the treatment of choice for symptomatic, and in selected cases of asymptomatic, high-grade carotid artery disease in centers with low surgical mortality and morbidity.

Data from the North American Symptomatic Carotid Endarterectomy Trial[15,212] revealed a 17% absolute reduction in stroke incidence with carotid endarterectomy over a 2-year follow-up in patients with critical stenosis of 70–99%. This represents a relative risk reduction of 65% for surgically treated patients. Perioperative risk of disabling stroke or death was 2.0% by 90 days following surgery. Patients with symptomatic carotid stenosis of 50–69% had a more modest absolute risk reduction of 6.5% with carotid endarterectomy, representing a relative risk reduction of 29% and suggesting that surgical treatment for moderate-grade stenosis be reserved only for selected cases. There was no advantage to surgery with symptomatic stenosis of less than 50%.

Carotid endarterectomy for asymptomatic carotid artery stenosis also results in reduced stroke occurrence and death compared with aspirin alone in centers with less than 3% perioperative mortality. Results from the Asymptomatic Carotid Atherosclerosis Study[38] demonstrated a significant 5.9% absolute reduction in stroke for surgically treated patients with greater than 60% stenosis after a 5-year follow-up, representing a 53% reduction in relative risk of stroke. The relative benefits of surgical treatment for asymptomatic carotid stenosis is rather marginal, suggesting that carotid endarterectomy should probably be reserved for patients who are otherwise medically stable, who have >80% stenosis, and who are expected to live 5 years or longer, and that it is performed only in centers with a <3% perioperative complication rate.[73]

Antiplatelet therapy after carotid surgery remains critical for successful overall outcome. Patients with <50% carotid stenosis should be treated with antiplatelet medications, cholesterol-lowering agents (statins), and lifestyle modification, and monitored for signs of TIA or stroke.

REHABILITATION OF STROKE-RELATED IMPAIRMENT AND DISABILITY

Neuroplasticity and neurologic recovery

Neuroplasticity refers to the ability of the central nervous system to reorganize and remodel, particularly following central nervous system injury. For many years, it was thought that neuroplasticity only occurred to a significant extent before adulthood. Over the past two decades, neuroscience research has demonstrated that the adult human brain is capable of adaptive plasticity after injury. Motor recovery after central nervous system injury occurs through poorly understood processes of cortical remodeling, but only as a response to task-oriented motor training. Consequently, the concept of 'use-dependent motor recovery' is leading to a paradigm shift in the theoretic basis of stroke rehabilitation and to new avenues of research. Additionally, a number of pharmacologic and surgical interventions that could potentially enhance neurologic recovery, and improve function and quality of life, are currently under investigation. Basic science and clinical research strongly suggest that any new intervention for promoting motor recovery after stroke must be coupled with appropriate behavioral interventions (i.e. rehabilitation therapy). The challenge for stroke rehabilitation over the next decades is to apply sound science to understanding the effect of various new interventions, and to incorporate effective and safe new interventions into standardized clinical practice.[127]

Sensorimotor control

A number of sensorimotor techniques to promote motor and functional recovery have been traditionally utilized in stroke rehabilitation. These incorporate basic strengthening, range of motion exercises, balance training, and postural control. A therapeutic technique specifically developed for patients with stroke was proposed by Brunnstrom that encourages early movement based on well-recognized patterns of motor recovery.[270] Bobath and Bobath developed the therapeutic approach now known as neurodevelopmental technique, which was originally designed for treatment of children with cerebral palsy. It inhibits abnormal postures and movement, and seeks to facilitate isolated muscle control.[22] Proprioceptive neural facilitation intends to maximize proprioceptive input through quick stretches and spiral diagonal patterns of movement.[314] Rood proposed a technique that incorporates cutaneous stimuli to facilitate movement. Finally, the task-oriented approach to therapeutic exercise described by Carr and Shepherd encourages movement during functional tasks.[46] Side by side comparisons of these techniques have not shown superiority of one over another.[81] Consequently, utilization of these techniques has been based more on tradition than on science.

Therapeutic approaches to the upper limb

Before discussing newer interventions to promote functional recovery after stroke, unique challenges in managing upper limb paralysis and their implications for upper limb rehabilitation should be noted. Historically, rehabilitation management of the upper limb after stroke differs from that of the lower limb for several reasons. First, spontaneous motor recovery of the upper limb is generally slower and less complete than for the lower limb. Second, basic self-care activities such as those measured by the self-care portion of the Functional Independence Measure can be performed with one intact upper limb, whereas both lower limbs are required for bipedal locomotion. Third, benchmarks for inpatient rehabilitation programs, such as length of stay and activities as measured by the Functional Independence Measure, require rapid gains in functional independence. Finally, the ability to influence motor recovery through rehabilitation interventions had little scientific basis until the past decades. For these reasons, upper limb rehabilitation after stroke often focused on strategies where the intact upper limb compensated for the impaired upper limb. Because we now have conclusive evidence that rehabilitation interventions can enhance motor recovery, we must seek a balance between use of compensatory strategies and interventions to promote neurologic recovery of the impaired upper limb, such as *constraint-induced movement therapy* (CIMT).

Constraint-induced movement therapy is based on a theory proposed by Edward Taub that patients with motor impairment in an upper limb after stroke learn to depend more on the unaffected limb for performing functional tasks, because attempts to use the affected arm often result in failure and frustration. This is explained through the principles of operant conditioning, where failed attempts to use the upper limb produce a kind of negative feedback, which reduces future attempts even further. This was demonstrated by Taub in studies of primates who underwent dorsal root lesions that led to a deafferentation of an upper limb. Despite the preservation of motor control, these primates would avoid using the affected arm in functional tasks.[304,305] More importantly, he demonstrated that use of the affected limb can be augmented by forced use of the impaired limb through a process of constraining the intact upper limb with a body jacket. Taub also demonstrated that primates can be trained to perform tasks with the affected limb through successive approximations of the desired task, and the behavioral technique of *shaping*.[302] Work by Randolph Nudo has corroborated these findings by showing that the normal and injured primate brain is capable of cortical reorganization in response to behavioral interventions.[213] This line of research has shown that repetitive movement alone is not sufficient. Instead, new skill acquisition or reacquisition of lost skills following stroke is required to induce cortical reorganization and promote recovery of motor function.[232] These principles have been incorporated into CIMT to promote motor function after stroke in humans.[303]

Constraint-induced movement therapy in clinical trials has taken two forms. The original CIMT program consists of constraining the intact upper limb for 90% of waking hours, and having 6 or more hours per day of therapy over 2 weeks. Because of the practical limitations of this program, several investigators have also evaluated a modified CIMT program comprising intact limb constraint for 5 h/day for 5 days/week, and 3 h of therapy three times per week, over 10 weeks.

Participants in clinical trials must have at least partial wrist and finger extension, and have sufficient shoulder strength to stabilize the arm during activities. Other small clinical trials have revealed improvement in motor control, and small improvements in functional skills, for both CIMT[76,173] and modified CIMT[219,220] in both acute and chronic stroke. At the time of writing, clinical trials designed to definitively demonstrate the efficacy of CIMT are in progress.

Neuromuscular electrical stimulation (NMES) refers to electrical stimulation of the lower motor neuron or its terminal branches, causing depolarization and subsequent muscle contraction. Because muscle activation requires an intact motor unit (i.e. denervated muscle cannot be safely stimulated with available technology), NMES applications are particularly well suited for upper motor neuron paralysis such as occurs in stroke. NMES can be delivered via electrodes placed on the skin, on or near peripheral nerve or near the muscle motor point. Further, the muscle contraction can be repetitively induced without user input, triggered by the user, or proportionally linked to user effort via electromyography (EMG) output from partially paralyzed muscle. Because new skill acquisition rather than repetitive movement alone is required to induce cortical reorganization in monkeys, EMG-triggered and EMG-controlled NMES are theoretically more likely to induce neuroplastic changes. NMES to promote motor recovery after stroke has been evaluated by several investigators. In most applications, stimulation is applied to wrist and finger extensors to enhance prehensile function. Several small clinical trials and a metaanalysis demonstrate improved motor function after treatment, with equivocal improvement in activities.[114]

Therapeutic approaches to walking

Body weight-supported treadmill training (BWSTT) was first evaluated in spinal cord injury (SCI). BWSTT can induce spontaneous step over step hind limb movement in spinalized animals, and can improve bipedal locomotion in humans with incomplete SCI.[237] Training of a locomotor *central pattern generator* in the spinal cord below the level of injury has been postulated as a mechanism of recovery. Based on the promising results in SCI, several investigators have studied the effect of BWSTT after stroke. The theoretic foundation for BWSTT after stroke also includes several tenets of forced use paradigms, including the need for many repetitions ('massed practice') during task-specific training, and sequentially greater approximations of the task (shaping) through progressive weight bearing and forced use of the impaired limb. The need for two or more skilled therapists to ensure appropriate kinematics of the trunk, pelvis, and lower limb during initial treatment has been a practical limitation for clinical use BWSTT. The efficacy of BWSTT for improving ambulation after stroke has been suggested by some clinical trials[313] but not others.[171,210] Data also suggest that BWSTT might also have beneficial effects on cardiovascular fitness after stroke.[132,187]

Other interventions to enhance motor recovery

Robotic-assisted motor retraining has been studied for both upper and lower limb rehabilitation after stroke. Robotic devices can induce passive or assisted limb movement that is typically directed toward a computer-generated visual target. More advanced iterations of the robot can provide tactile feedback that kinetically and kinematically corrects the user's movement. Robotic therapy theoretically promotes movement during skill acquisition. Furthermore, robotic therapy is infatigable, and has the potential to induce movement repetitions that might be needed to modulate motor recovery. It also has the distinct advantage of inducing repetitions without the need for continuous involvement of a therapist. Animal data suggest that a large number of repetitions can be needed to improve motor function (massed practice). Several small clinical trials suggest that robotic therapy can enhance upper limb motor recovery.[87,89] However, currently available iterations of robotic therapy only target shoulder, elbow, and wrist movements, and do not directly address finger movements. For this and other reasons, the effect of robotic therapy on upper limb function remains unclear.

A number of pharmacologic agents have been shown to facilitate motor retraining after experimentally induced stroke in animals. Agents that reduce or inhibit the action of noradrenaline (norepinephrine) and GABA generally inhibit recovery. On the other hand, agents that increase noradrenaline can enhance recovery. Of these agents, amphetamine has been the most extensively studied. Although amphetamine consistently induces motor recovery in rodent models, clinical trials have yielded inconsistent and often negative results.[242] Based on results from preclinical trials and theoretic models regarding mechanisms of recovery after stroke in humans, close coupling between amphetamine and appropriate behavioral therapy might be required to achieve clinical benefits. At the time of writing, a multicenter, randomized clinical trial to definitively evaluate the efficacy of amphetamine after stroke is in progress.

A number of other interventions that potentially augment motor recovery are at various stages of investigation. Transcranial magnetic stimulation, as well as cortical brain stimulation, has shown promise in early preclinical trials and clinical trials.[35] Neuronal transplantation for motor recovery after stroke is currently in clinical trials,[168,169] while use of autologous marrow stromal cells has shown promise in preclinical trials.[123]

Stroke rehabilitation is undergoing a paradigm shift based on work over the past decades demonstrating that the adult primate brain is capable of neuroplastic change with motor recovery after injury. These changes rely on appropriate behavioral interventions. The clinical efficacy of a number of new interventions has been suggested, but these have yet to be definitively demonstrated in adequately powered, well-controlled clinical trials. For several interventions, such as CIMT and amphetamine, the definitive clinical trials are in progress. Although demonstrating the clinical efficacy and safety of new interventions through well-designed clinical trials is essential, it is not sufficient. Further research is needed to elucidate cellular responses to interventions that induce neuroplasticity. Filling the gaps in the theoretic framework of adaptive responses to central nervous system injury will ultimately lead to more effective interventions and better functional outcomes for the patients recovering from stroke.

Spasticity

Spasticity is defined as a motor disorder characterized by a velocity-dependent increase in tonic stretch reflexes,[177] and can contribute to motor impairment, pain, and disability following stroke. In the majority of cases, spasticity can be managed with exercise therapy or by focal management with botulinum toxin or phenol injections. Severe spasticity, however, can be very disabling and difficult to treat. The various methods for treating spasticity can be used according to clinical need and probability of success for achieving specific functional goals. Consequently, the selection of spasticity treatment based on a predefined sequence of therapy is generally no longer practiced.

Critical to managing spasticity in patients with stroke is education on the benefits and necessity of daily stretching, especially of the shoulder, wrist, fingers, hip, and ankles. This is needed to reduce resting and dynamic tone and prevention soft tissue contracture. The use of static resting splints for hand and ankle can help prevent contractures and reduce tone, but if spasticity is severe, splinting can result in pain and skin breakdown under the orthosis. This can be particularly problematic in an ankle–foot orthosis (AFO) if plantar flexion tone is severe. Pain along the proximal trim line of the AFO or along the metatarsal heads during walking suggests that spasticity is interfering with the fit of the orthosis. Often, use of focal injection of botulinum toxin in the gastrocnemius and soleus muscles can resolve this problem.

Focal injection of botulinum toxin is quite popular for the management of localized limb spasticity, because it is easy to use, has a repeatable dose-dependent effect, and has a low side effect profile.[31,51,176] Unlike phenol, botulinum toxin injection requires only EMG muscle targeting rather than uncomfortable motor point localization via needle stimulation. Botulinum toxin is generally favored over oral antispasticity agents, because oral agents often cause lethargy and cognitive deficits, even at subtherapeutic doses. Yet in cases of generalized spasticity, the use of oral agents in combination with local injections might provide the best therapeutic response. Intrathecal baclofen delivered by implanted infusion pump provides excellent lower limb spasticity control in patients with stroke, and has been reported to improve functional gait in some cases.[95,198] Although upper limb spasticity is less responsive to intrathecal baclofen therapy, focal injections for upper limb tone remain an option once lower limb spasticity is controlled (see Ch. 31).

Cognition, language, and communication disorders

Approximately one-third to one-half of stroke survivors experience speech and language disorders.[316] Language and perceptual functions tend to demonstrate some degree of natural improvement after stroke, but their recovery patterns can be more variable than those seen in motor function. The prevalence of aphasia declines from about one-fourth during the acute phase to about one-fifth or less during the later stages after stroke.[316]

Recovery from aphasia usually occurs at a slower rate and over a more prolonged time course than does motor recovery.[268] Whereas most aphasia recovery occurs in the first 3–6 months,[163,231,316] at least one group has observed that patients with global aphasia show the greatest improvement during the latter half of the first year after stroke.[267,268,316] The amount and pattern of recovery are usually related to the initial severity of the aphasia and the specific aphasia type.[37,164] Patients with non-fluent aphasia generally (but not always) have a less favorable prognosis than those with fluent aphasia, although both groups can and do improve. Language comprehension usually returns earlier and to a greater extent than oral expression.[235]

Although most of the improvement in perceptual functioning occurs in the first 3–6 months after stroke,[80,98,133,172,196,292,298] some recovery occurs later. According to a study by Hier and associates,[133] most of the recovery of perceptual deficits, such as unilateral spatial neglect, denial of illness, loss of facial recognition, and motor impersistence, occurred within the first 20 weeks after stroke, but some improvement could be seen up to 1 year later.

Many procedures have been developed to manage various aspects of these problems. Both remediation and compensation are used. One goal of therapy is to improve the patient's ability to speak, understand, read, and write. Another goal of speech therapy interventions is to assist patients to develop strategies that compensate for or circumvent speech and language problems that are not directly remediable. A final goal is to improve the quality of life for individuals with neuromotor speech impairments and their families.

For aphasia, a number of strategies and techniques have been developed[50,62,130,134,140,180,185,205,266,277,278,285,287,307,325–327] One of these, melodic intonation therapy,[285] is an approach designed to use the non-injured functioning neural pathways in the non-dominant hemisphere that carry musical information. Other techniques rely on encouraging verbalizations, conversational coaching, and oral reading. Probably the most important strategy is to encourage any vocalizations possible as a means of developing verbal communication of a more differentiated nature. Treatment of aphasia focuses on the most effective means by which the patient can communicate, including individual or group speech therapy with practice. Box 51-6 lists various treatment approaches for aphasia.[120]

For dysarthria, exercise modalities include sensory stimulation procedures, exercises designed to strengthen oromotor speech muscles, respiratory training procedures, and retraining of articulatory patterns and sequences of gestures.[18,78,308,332]

Alternative forms of communication and augmentative devices can be used to enhance the quality of life. These range from written or pictorial communication boards and books to electronic communication aids.

For some patients, visual-spatial perceptual deficits are the most troublesome problems that they experience after a stroke. Potentially useful treatment methods include the use of prism glasses, providing visuospatial cueing to compensate for visuospatial perceptual losses, increasing awareness of deficits with

Box 51-6 Selected treatment methods for aphasia

- Language-oriented treatment
- Direct stimulus–response treatment
- Treatment of aphasic perseveration
- Visual action therapy
- Oral reading for aphasia
- Conversational coaching
- Promoting aphasic communicative effectiveness
- Computerized visual communication (using alternative communication systems)
- Programmatic combinations of approaches
- Augmentative communication devices

Box 51-7 Reported causes of poststroke shoulder pain

- Capsulitis
- Subluxation
- Impingement syndrome
- Rotator cuff injury
- Bicipital tendonitis
- Complex regional pain syndrome type 1
- Brachial plexopathy
- Axillary neuropathy
- Suprascapular neuropathy
- Myofascial pain
- Spasticity
- Soft tissue contracture

cues, using computer-assisted training, eye patching, and providing compensatory strategies.[39,41,50,118,120,227,322,323]

There is increasing evidence of language problems resulting from right hemisphere strokes, including lack of organization and impaired use of language in social contexts. Treatment of these problems is aimed at improving organization of language, learning to use language within social contexts (language pragmatics), and learning to interpret figurative language (see Ch. 3).[120]

Swallowing and nutrition

Dysphagia, or impaired swallowing, occurs in approximately one-third to one-half of all stroke survivors, and places the stroke patient at risk for aspiration and pneumonia, malnutrition, and dehydration. Malnutrition has been found in 8–34% of patients with stroke.[53,310] Nutritional status was recently found to correlate with long-term outcome following stroke.[94] Compensatory treatments for disordered swallowing function include changing posture and positioning for swallowing, learning new swallowing maneuvers, and changing food amounts and textures (generally smaller boluses of puréed foods and thick liquids are handled more easily). An observational study by Horner and colleagues found that treatment of swallowing dysfunction was effective.[120,139] A recent Cochrane Collaboration review found that percutaneous endoscopic gastrostomy feedings can improve outcome and nutrition in stroke patients, but that the studies were too few in number to determine the effectiveness of swallowing therapy for treating dysphagia (see Ch. 28).[17]

Shoulder pain

Shoulder pain is a common complication after stroke that can inhibit recovery and reduce the quality of life. Many types of shoulder pathology after stroke have been reported in the literature (Box 51-7). No single type of shoulder pathology can account for all shoulder pain after stroke, and more than one type of shoulder pathology may cause pain within an individual. The pathogenesis of poststroke shoulder pain has not been studied rigorously and therefore remains controversial.

The reported prevalence of shoulder pain in poststroke hemiplegia ranges from 34%[226] to 84%.[206] In the largest cohort of hemiplegic subjects followed longitudinally for an average of 11 months, shoulder pain occurred in 72% of cases.[312] Although the natural history of shoulder pain is not well understood, a number of cohort studies have shown that pain can develop within weeks or months after the onset of hemiplegia, and can become chronic and refractory to treatment.[102,238,320] Shoulder pain is clinically associated with severe motor impairment,[102,238,320] sensory impairment,[102,238] duration of hemiplegia, and decreased shoulder range of motion.[24]

Shoulder subluxation in hemiplegia refers to increased translation of the humeral head relative to the glenoid fossa, and occurs in approximately half of stroke survivors with hemiplegia.[312] Although shoulder pain after stroke is often attributed to the presence of subluxation, a causal relationship between subluxation and pain remains controversial. Although shoulder subluxation can directly cause pain in some cases, many patients with subluxation do not have pain. Shoulder subluxation has been associated with complex regional pain syndrome type 1 (CRPS 1),[77,312] axillary neuropathy,[244] and rotator cuff tears.[206] This suggests that subluxation can also cause pain indirectly by predisposition to other types of shoulder pathology.

Neuromuscular electrical stimulation to the deltoid and supraspinatus muscles delivered via electrodes placed on the skin surface can reduce shoulder subluxation[12,49,85,166,319] and can reduce pain.[49,85,166] However, NMES is infrequently used in the clinical setting, because of pain during stimulation and the need for daily application by a skilled clinician. Although a dose–response relationship has not been adequately evaluated, available data suggest that treatment for several hours daily over several weeks can be required to achieve clinical benefits. Recent evidence suggests that NMES delivered via percutaneously placed intramuscular electrodes can reduce shoulder pain and improve activities of daily living in stroke survivors with shoulder subluxation.[336,337] Stimulation-induced pain is significantly lower with intramuscular NMES than with surface stimulation.[335] Furthermore, because the intramuscular electrodes are left in place for weeks of treatment, the user need only attach the stimulator without concern for proper electrode placement. Intramuscular NMES was designed to reduce pain by reducing subluxation, yet data suggest that other mechanisms such as sensory neuromodulation might be significant.[336] It remains unclear whether NMES reduces poststroke shoulder pain generally or only in the presence of shoulder subluxation.

Capsulitis, also known as 'adhesive capsulitis' or 'frozen shoulder', refers to the clinical finding of decreased shoulder range of motion, especially external rotation and abduction, associated with shoulder pain after stroke.[24,245] These findings are due to shortening of the joint capsule and ligaments that are largely extensions of the capsule. An inflammatory response results from stretching and tearing of shortened capsular fibers. Several factors potentially contribute to the development of capsulitis, including decreased active shoulder movement due to paralysis, synergistic patterns of muscle activation, spasticity, and the use of certain types of sling. Most often, the diagnosis of capsulitis can be made from physical examination, without further radiographic corroboration. Treatment includes range of motion; avoidance of exacerbating conditions such as the use of swath-type slings; proper limb positioning; management of underlying spasticity; and reduction of inflammation with modalities, medications, or intraarticular injection of steroids.[69]

Impingement syndrome has been suggested as a cause of shoulder pain as well as a cause of rotator cuff injury in hemiplegia.[152,312] Impingement of the supraspinatus tendon between the acromion and the greater tuberosity of the humerus can result in tendonitis, subacromial bursitis, and in some cases rotator cuff tears. Although the etiology of impingement syndrome after stroke is not well understood, limited scapular rotation during humeral abduction, an imbalance between stronger deltoid and weaker rotator muscles in hemiplegia, and inadequate external rotation of the humerus during passive shoulder abduction[206] can contribute. Impingement syndrome should be managed by maintaining scapular mobility, use of proper technique during stretch, treating spasticity, and when possible strengthening of internal and external rotators of the shoulder. Reduction of local inflammation through the use of oral agents or injected steroids often reduces pain, and can help to reduce the mechanical impingement by reducing supraspinatus tendon swelling.

Complex regional pain syndrome type 1, also known previously as reflex sympathetic dystrophy or shoulder–hand syndrome, is a constellation of symptoms. The new name comes from the consensus of most experts that sympathetic overactivity has not been proven as the cause. Typically, the syndrome affects the shoulder, wrist, and hand, but typically spares the elbow. The reported prevalence of CRPS 1 in hemiplegia ranges from 12.5%[64] to 70%.[225] CRPS 1 has been associated with shoulder subluxation, suggesting traction injury to the vasonervorum as a possible etiology.[77,312] The syndrome typically progresses through three phases.

1. A primary inflammatory phase characterized by painful range of motion, edema, warmth, and erythema of the hand and wrist.

2. A secondary atrophic phase characterized by atrophic skin changes, progressive loss of range of motion, reduced skin temperature, and occasionally pain reduction.
3. A final phase characterized by irreversible skin and muscle atrophy, variable pain, severe loss of range of motion, and extensive osteoporosis.

The diagnosis is often made by history and physical examination. However, three-phase bone scintigraphy remains the criterion standard where radionuclide uptake is seen in a typical pattern involving the shoulder, wrist, and hand, particularly in the carpal and metacarpal joints. Early diagnosis and treatment are paramount. Scintigraphy is warranted when the history and examination are suggestive but not diagnostic. Oral prednisone and exercise are the initial treatments. A wide range of other pharmacologic approaches have been reported, with variable results. More invasive measures, such as cervical sympathetic ganglia blocks, Bier blocks, and cervical sympathectomy, might be warranted in refractory cases (see Ch. 43).

Other pain syndromes after stroke

Numerous other causes of shoulder pain in stroke-related hemiplegia have been suggested (Box 51-7). Because shoulder pain in any given individual with stroke can result from multiple causes, careful diagnosis is necessary, followed by specific targeted treatments and interdisciplinary care.

Although the hemiplegic shoulder is the most common location for pain after stroke, pain can also occur in other body regions. A number of neuropathic and musculoskeletal causes of pain after stroke have been documented. Complex regional pain syndrome can affect body regions other than the shoulder. Heterotopic ossification is extremely rare but can affect large joints on the hemiparetic side of the body, usually in patients who have some coexisting traumatic injury. A large number of musculoskeletal injuries can occur, ranging from acute ankle sprains, to subacute injuries such as knee inflammation from recurvatum during gait, to chronic conditions such as joint contractures. Osteoarthritis can be accelerated when normal biomechanics are altered by paralysis, abnormal tone, sensory loss, and motor planning problems.

Neuropathic pain occurs commonly in stroke survivors with sensory impairments. This pain condition, which is also called central poststroke pain syndrome, results from central nervous system injury involving thalamic structures and other sensory pathways. Central poststroke pain syndrome can be severe and is often refractory to available interventions. Tricyclic antidepressants and anticonvulsants have been somewhat successful in ameliorating pain. Participation in a comprehensive pain management program for patients capable of such activity is often beneficial.

In summary, a large variety of painful conditions can occur after stroke, primarily affecting the shoulder but also affecting other regions of the body.

Bowel and bladder control

Incontinence of bowel and bladder occurs in one-third to two-thirds of patients after stroke and, if it persists, can pose a challenge to preparing family caregivers for return to home.[13,26,34,104,107,135,183,243,273] The most common reason for incontinence after stroke is uninhibited evacuation of bladder or bowel, which is associated with multiple factors as described above. Urinary retention can occur as well in about 29% of stroke patients, and is associated with cortical stroke, diabetes, aphasia, and cognitive impairment.[170] Among patients with stroke living in the community, Brittain et al. found that the overall prevalence of urinary symptoms was 64%, a rate that was twice as high as among community-dwelling control subjects.[33]

Timed voiding is the primary treatment strategy for patients with persistent uninhibited bladder. This strategy is approached by scheduling regular voiding before the urge to urinate occurs, and is quite effective if urgency does not occur more than every 2–3 h. If frequent urgency occurs, it is necessary first to determine if this is caused by incomplete bladder emptying or low-volume voiding. Urodynamic testing is usually not necessary. Instead, use of bladder ultrasound post void can estimate with good accuracy the residual volume. If residuals are high (>200 mL), the use of α-blocking agents such as tamsulosin in both male and female patients can promote complete voiding. If voiding is complete, then the use of anticholinergic agents such as oxybutynin can allow for larger bladder volumes before urgency occurs. In the latter case, patients need to be monitored for signs and symptoms of urinary retention. Some patients might need both α-blocking and anticholinergic agents to achieve a timely voiding pattern, but it is best to achieve internal sphincter relaxation with α blocker before starting anticholinergics to avoid the risk of bladder retention. If incomplete voiding persists despite these measures, which can often occur in male patients with benign prostatic hypertrophy, consultation with a urologist is usually necessary. The use of intermittent catheterization or indwelling catheter is also an option, depending on the goals of the patient and caregiver (see Ch. 29).

Bowel retraining can usually be achieved in patients with stroke using standard techniques of planned bowel evacuation after meals and the use of laxative agents such as senna and suppositories. Providing a bedside commode is also useful for patients with mobility deficits or who have difficulty rapidly accessing the commode within their home (see Ch. 30).

Psychosocial considerations

The new onset and persistence of disability can give rise to a variety of psychologic reactions in patients who have sustained a stroke, including sadness, grief, anxiety, depression, despair, anger, frustration, and confusion. It is important to recognize the variety of reactions that might occur. While depression and sadness might occur with some frequency (estimates range between 30% and 60%, depending on study criteria), anxiety, guilt, stress, and other feelings are common as well. Addressing these issues is a critical component of the rehabilitation program. Although not unique to the specialty of medical rehabilitation, stroke care professionals have extensive experience in addressing the patient's level and method of coping and adaptation,

because of their involvement with patients in active participation in care. For some patients, dealing with the emotional issues that accompany the stroke forms the major focus of the care activities. For others, addressing them facilitates improved participation in the rehabilitation program. In a substantial proportion of patients, the type and intensity of their reactions to the problems caused by the stroke are more dependent on their *prestroke* coping styles, levels of frustration tolerance, and ability and mechanisms used to deal with adversity. For most patients, dealing with psychologic issues is an ongoing activity.

Depression can be a significant complication of stroke. It can be devastating and distressing on its own, and can limit patient participation and outcome by inhibiting patient motivation.[20,54,91,221,222,246–250] Depression occurs in one-third to two-thirds of stroke survivors. Presenting features include loss of energy in 83%, sleep disorder in 67%, brooding in 60%, and hopelessness in 39%.[246] Although the organic component of poststroke depression can be significant,[91,250] it is likely that most patients experience a combination of organic and reactive causes of mood disorders. Treatment consists of psychotherapy, psychosocial support, milieu therapy, and medications. To the extent that mood improves as the patient's physical independence improves and patient–family participation increases, the depression is likely to have been reactive. For some patients, especially those with significant disturbances in participation in daily activities or therapeutic exercise programs, antidepressant medications can be beneficial.[184,241] Several studies have demonstrated the efficacy of various types of antidepressants in treating poststroke depression. These medications improve not only mood, but also functional performance. Their usefulness is limited only by their side effects.

Anxiety and fear are commonly reported and observed problems among stroke patients. A team of rehabilitation professionals who are sensitive to these issues, empathic toward the patient, and experienced in dealing with such problems can help to ease the distress associated with the disability and the rehabilitation experience, thereby possibly resulting in improved outcomes.

Sexual dysfunction has been reported in 40–70% of stroke survivors.[32,99,204,283] Its cause is largely psychologic (e.g. fear, anxiety, depression, and discomfort) rather than organic, although spasticity, pain, and sensory deficits can pose problems for some patients. Issues related to self-esteem, affection, and relationships should be emphasized, as should specific practical suggestions on positioning, timing, and techniques (see Ch. 32).[96]

One of the major factors influencing both the degree of participation in a therapy program and the outcome achieved is patient motivation. Patients who cooperate with therapeutic efforts and who have the determination to improve are more likely to participate in a therapy program. However, the level of motivation and the amount of its specific direct effect on outcome are difficult to measure. A number of techniques can be used by the rehabilitation professional to enhance or direct motivation. These examples include explanation, positive reinforcement, behavioral modification, and coaxing. Interestingly, it also has been found that the degree of family support favorably affects outcome.[83] Counseling interventions have proved to be consistently more effective in improving family functioning and patient adjustment than educational interventions alone.[82]

Dealing with family issues is essential. Families can experience a variety of emotions, including grief, sadness, depression, anxiety, and guilt. In addition, families often serve as caregivers, and therefore might experience the care as burdensome. They might feel guilt over their feelings. The complexity of these emotional reactions underscores the importance of ongoing counseling, support, and care for the family caregivers.

Family reactions to the changes that result from the stroke should be addressed by the team. This is particularly important in view of the need for the family's active participation in providing support to the patient during and after formal intensive rehabilitation. Lack of social supports and lack of available resources are often major problems for the patient and the rehabilitation team. In that situation, recruiting resources, securing appropriate entitlements, and advocating on behalf of the patient become major clinical tasks for the professional rehabilitation team. In general, family interventions include individual counseling, education, and support groups.[289] Evidence exists that both education and counseling interventions significantly improve caregiver knowledge and stabilize some aspects of family functioning, but that counseling is more effective than education alone.[82]

At times, problematic psychosocial functioning predominates among issues related to the recovery of physical function or motor skill performance. This underscores the importance of psychosocial, recreational, and vocational interventions.

Recreational activities often have the effect of improving affect, focusing therapy of meaningful activities and desirable goals, and facilitating a smooth transition to the community after discharge. Leisure evaluation, counseling on activities of interest, and educating the patient on community resources constitute some of the therapeutic recreation interventions for patients with stroke.

Peer support is one component of patient care activities that probably exerts a favorable effect on the successful rehabilitation of the stroke patient, but is often overlooked in the description of interventions that affect patient progress and outcome. The presence of other patients with similar disabilities on the stroke rehabilitation unit can assist the patient in several ways. First, it can help to reduce the fear and anxiety often associated with the new onset of physically disabling or disfiguring conditions. Second, patients often can counsel and support each other in ways that even well-meaning and experienced professionals cannot. Finally, patients often not only gain insight into their disability, but also garner specific suggestions for functional skill performance or about adaptive equipment from other patients who have already been through the experience. Similar peer support may be available for families of patients as well, and could contribute favorably to the adjustment process after the stroke.

Management of medical comorbidities and prevention of complications in rehabilitation

Stroke rarely occurs in isolation. Most patients with stroke have many other medical comorbidities that require professional attention, some of which have the potential to affect rehabilitation. The Framingham Heart Study reported that, compared with age- and sex-matched control subjects, stroke survivors had significantly greater frequencies of hypertension, hypertensive heart disease, coronary heart disease, obesity, diabetes mellitus, arthritis, left ventricular hypertrophy, and congestive heart failure.[121] Medical problems that are relevant in stroke patients undergoing rehabilitation can be categorized as follows.

- Preexisting medical illnesses that necessitate ongoing care during the rehabilitation program (such as hypertension and diabetes).
- General health functions affected by the stroke (such as nutrition and hydration).
- Secondary poststroke complications (such as deep venous thrombosis and pneumonia).
- Acute poststroke exacerbations of preexisting chronic diseases (such as an angina attack during physical exercise in a patient with a history of ischemic heart disease).

Management of these conditions can take up major portions of the rehabilitation effort. It has been stated that some stroke patients can be more disabled by certain associated comorbid diseases than by the stroke itself.[121,256]

The occurrence of these associated conditions has several implications for stroke patient treatment during and after rehabilitation. First, these problems can detract from the benefits of rehabilitation. Some medical problems, such as heart disease, adversely affect the poststroke course and outcome.[74,121,256,264,267,275] Intercurrent medical complications can limit the patient's ability to participate in a therapeutic exercise program, inhibit functional skill performance, and reduce the likelihood of achieving favorable outcomes from rehabilitation. The rehabilitation interventions also have the potential to adversely affect the medical condition, causing an exacerbation of the disease or a need to adjust medical management. Medical complications can occur during the rehabilitation program, requiring diagnostic evaluation, prompt recognition, and appropriate medical management, which can be difficult to complete in the rehabilitation setting. A study by Harvey and associates conducted on a large sample of stroke rehabilitation patients found that the presence of certain medical conditions, especially a tracheostomy, a feeding tube, a history of pneumonia, a history of coronary artery disease, and a history of renal failure, significantly increased the utilization of resources (as measured by average charge per day) during inpatient stroke rehabilitation.[125]

Roth and colleagues found that 75% of all patients admitted to inpatient stroke rehabilitation experienced at least one medical complication that was more likely to occur in the presence of severe neurologic impairment, hypoalbuminemia, and a history of hypertension.[254] Another study by that group found that the number of medical tubes (i.e. tracheostomy, enteral feeding tube, and indwelling urethral catheter) was independently correlated with increased number of medical complications, longer acute and rehabilitation lengths of stay, and reduced functional outcome at discharge following rehabilitation in a large group of stroke patients.[255] The most common problems that occur during inpatient stroke rehabilitation include depression, shoulder pain, falls, urinary tract infection, pneumonia, seizures, pressure ulcers, recurrent stroke, and back and hip pain.[178,195,254]

Preventing and treating comorbid medical conditions and medical complications are major components of the rehabilitation treatment of stroke patients, as they enable rehabilitation to take place and to exert maximum effectiveness. The clinical tasks in managing these problems are to prevent medical complications, to promptly and appropriately diagnose and treat complications when they occur, and to manage both preexisting medical illness and ongoing general health functions during rehabilitation. A few of the important complications are discussed briefly here. For more complete discussions of associated medical problems as they relate to stroke patients and the rehabilitation process, the reader is referred to several reviews of stroke comorbidities[35,257,260,261,271,279] and to individual articles on several specific complications.[25,30,56,105,126,258,259,269,306] Box 51-8 lists some of the common diagnoses that might accompany the stroke and that might require management.

Selected complications

Physiologic deconditioning Physiologic deconditioning accompanies both acute medical illness and the prolonged bed rest that might be enforced immediately after its onset.[239,288,290] Deconditioning can contribute to fatigue, endurance limitations, poor exercise tolerance, orthostatic hypotension, lack of motivation, and depression. All these problems can adversely affect the course of recovery and rehabilitation. Preventive techniques include early mobilization, early and gradually increasing participation in rehabilitation, and the development and implementation of a schedule that balances rest and activity. Interestingly, long-term stroke survivors, even those with nearly full neurologic recovery, frequently report easy fatigability and endurance limitations.

Venous thromboembolism The incidence of venous thromboembolism varies widely, depending on the specific investigator, but the average is between 40% and 50% for deep vein thrombosis and 10% for pulmonary embolism.[30] The National Institutes of Health Consensus Conference,[215] other investigators,[106] and extensive clinical experience[30] indicate that some form of prophylaxis for venous thromboembolism should be instituted for all stroke patients. In patients in whom hemorrhagic stroke has been ruled out, repeated doses of low-dose heparin or low molecular weight heparin compounds have been documented to be effective. In a recent historical cohort study, Harvey et al. confirmed that therapeutic anticoagulants or prophylactic heparin was safe and effective in preventing venous thromboembolism in stroke patients during inpatient rehabilita-

Box 51-8 Common medical comorbidities and complications after stroke

- Thromboembolic disease
- Pneumonia
- Ventilatory insufficiency
- Hypertension
- Orthostatic hypotension
- Angina
- Congestive heart failure
- Cardiac arrhythmias
- Diabetes mellitus
- Prior stroke
- Recurrent stroke
- Urinary tract infection
- Bladder dysfunction
- Bowel dysfunction
- Pressure sore
- Dehydration
- Malnutrition
- Dysphagia
- Shoulder dysfunction
- Complex regional pain syndrome
- Depression
- Sexual dysfunction
- Seizure
- Spasticity
- Contracture
- Central poststroke pain syndrome
- Falls and injuries
- Medication overuse
- Poor endurance
- Fatigue
- Insomnia

tion.[124] In addition, this study demonstrated that patients with ischemic stroke who are otherwise at a low risk for bleeding have no increased risk for bleeding with combined use of prophylactic heparin and antiplatelet agents. Gregory and associates found that deep vein thrombosis was more prevalent among patients with hemorrhagic stroke than among those with thromboembolic strokes.[119]

Pneumonia Pneumonia occurs in about one-third of patients with stroke, although the incidence is higher in the subset of patients who have SAH. Upadya found a 47% incidence in patients who were 'critically ill' at the time of their stroke.[311] Dysphagia, present in about one-third to one-half of all stroke patients, can cause aspiration and pneumonia. This underscores the importance of evaluating swallowing function, instituting compensatory treatments such as positional changes during swallowing, and using alternative feeding methods if needed. Other factors that might predispose to pneumonia include abnormal central breathing patterns, general debility causing impaired immune response, and (especially) hemiparetic weakness of ventilatory muscles causing weakened cough.[56,257,260,261] One study demonstrated the usefulness of a clinical screening system (measuring presence of dysphonia, dysarthria, abnormal gag reflex, abnormal volitional cough, cough after swallow, and voice change after swallow) to identify patients at high risk for dysphagia and aspiration.[60]

Cardiac disease   Cardiac abnormalities can be causal, consequential, or coincidental in stroke,[35,259] with rates of association of 75% for hypertension, 32–62% for coronary artery disease, 40–70% for various arrhythmias, and 12–18% for congestive heart failure. Because the presence of heart disease, and especially congestive heart failure, can adversely affect functional outcome, it may be necessary to more rigorously screen stroke patients prior to initiating exercise, to more closely monitor stroke patients during their participation in rehabilitation, or to modify their therapy.[257]

Falls   Falls occur with striking frequency in stroke survivors, with most reports indicating that patients who sustain right hemisphere strokes are at substantially greater risk for falling than those with left hemisphere strokes (probably because of the associated cognitive and perceptual deficits, impulsivity, and lack of judgment).[66,115,193,199,228,234] Prevention approaches emphasize balance training, cognitive training, safety training (especially with caregivers), ensuring supervision during mobility activities, eliminating environmental hazards, and use of assistive devices. The recent heightened attention to patient safety issues during hospitalizations has made fall prevention efforts even more compelling now than in the past.

Levels of postacute stroke rehabilitation care

The organization of stroke services has gone through rather dramatic changes in recent years. Although the traditional view of rehabilitation relied on one or two types of settings (usually either inpatient or outpatient) for care to occur, more recent models emphasize a variety of types and levels of postacute stroke services to better meet each stroke patient's specific needs.[262] The ideal situation is to have a complete and coordinated *system of care* providing a *continuum of care*. This system would also have a coordinated method to assess, direct (triage), and transfer patients to the setting that best meets their needs at the time the services are needed. Because care needs vary across patients and over time for individual patients, the quality of the system is extremely important. An integrated system requires a set of criteria to determine which patients qualify for which levels of care, a consistently applied patient assessment procedure, and exquisite communication and collaboration across the levels of the system of care to allow both smooth transfer of patients and information and a sharing of expertise.

Factors that are useful in determining the ideal setting of care for a patient at a particular point in time include the patient's cognitive ability, motivation level, prior and present level of functioning, medical stability, level of available social resources at home, medical and nursing needs, and likelihood of achieving significant functional gains during rehabilitation, and the availability of appropriate services and programs in the specific community. The decisions as to which level or location of care a patient might be treated are at times based on the direction of third-party payers, and on the availability of specific resources within the community, rather than solely on patient need.

There is considerable overlap among the postacute stroke rehabilitation levels of care and among the patients who are cared for in each, but generally the levels of care are delineated as acute inpatient rehabilitation, long-term acute care with rehabilitation focus, skilled nursing care with rehabilitation services, home therapy, outpatient day rehabilitation, and outpatient therapy. Each is discussed below.

Therapy during acute stroke management

The importance of early activation of patients with stroke, to reduce the problems associated with deconditioning and prolonged bed rest, underscores the value of early initiation of stroke rehabilitation activities in the comprehensive care of the poststroke patient. Bedside or active exercises, early gait training, training in the performance of activities of daily living such as dressing, patient and family teaching, and swallowing training can be initiated during the acute poststroke phase. The opportunity to prevent complications and to facilitate improved outcomes makes this an important set of interventions. A meta-analysis of stroke rehabilitation effectiveness studies suggested that outcomes after stroke were more dependent on the initiation of early rehabilitation than on the long-term duration of rehabilitation.[218]

Acute inpatient rehabilitation

Comprehensive acute inpatient stroke rehabilitation refers to the traditional interdisciplinary hospital-based coordinated program of medical, nursing, and therapy services. Care in this setting is directed by a physician and carried out by a team. This level of care is most appropriate for patients who need and can tolerate 3 or more hours of therapy a day, and who need both around the clock nursing care and at least daily physician supervision. Patients in intensive rehabilitation must have a reasonable likelihood of achieving significant functional gains from a comprehensive inpatient rehabilitation program.

Long-term acute care with rehabilitation focus

Long-term acute care conventionally provides medical treatment for patients who suffer prolonged illness with medical complexity, such as requiring ventilator management. Some long-term acute care facilities have developed interdisciplinary rehabilitation care services that can provide functionally oriented rehabilitation interventions to medically complex patients. Patients with stroke can benefit from this level of care if they have respiratory failure, benefit from frequent suctioning and pulmonary toilet, require total parenteral nutrition, or need frequent administration of antibiotics. Once the medical conditions are stable and require less intensive management, the patient can be transitioned to another level of rehabilitation care.

Skilled nursing care with rehabilitation services

Skilled nursing facilities now commonly provide rehabilitation services, often designated as subacute rehabilitation. These programs are appropriate for stroke patients who need comprehensive and coordinated therapy services for functional training in an institutional setting, but in a less intensive program than is used at the acute level of rehabilitation. Patients in this level of care usually receive between 1 and 3 h of therapy per day. Assessment of the intensity of therapy services that individual patients need is based primarily on their tolerance level and on the specific needs for functional training. Some patients are unable to tolerate the full course of intensive rehabilitation because of medical frailty or limited endurance. Some patients who receive rehabilitation in a skilled nursing facility have had extremely severe strokes limiting their potential to participate in intensive inpatient rehabilitation. Others receive subacute rehabilitation because their strokes were so mild that the amount of therapy they need is small. These programs provide 24 h a day nursing care, with physician visits typically only one to three times per week. Patients with more intensive medical needs might be more appropriately treated in an acute rehabilitation program or long-term acute care.

Outpatient day rehabilitation

In outpatient day rehabilitation, virtually all the same therapy services that are provided in comprehensive inpatient rehabilitation are offered, but without the overnight stay. Day rehabilitation is a comprehensive and coordinated program of therapy that takes place in an outpatient setting. The rehabilitation is directed by a physician and facilitated by a team with regularly scheduled team conferences. Rehabilitation services are typically provided for 3–6 h a day and include one on one therapy as well as group activities. Relative medical stability and social support at home is necessary, because patients live in their own homes. The patient's home must be accessible, and the patient must be able to benefit and tolerate from therapy in a group setting.

Outpatient therapy

Many stroke patients need traditional outpatient therapy services. These services are also provided in an outpatient clinic setting, but they do not entail the coordination, comprehensiveness, group therapy, and team conferences that characterize day rehabilitation. These services include single-modality training, such as physical therapy, occupational therapy, speech–language pathology services, or psychologic support, for patients with focal deficits and for whom specific functional training might be useful. In addition, outpatients with significant cognitive deficits that prevent participation in group activities are also appropriate for traditional outpatient individual therapy.

Home therapy

The home is the most familiar environment for the patient and family, and therapy in the home allows the patient and family to learn specific functional tasks in the setting in which those skills will be used most often. However, a potential disadvantage of home therapy is the limitation in available resources such as specialized equipment or experienced staff. Home therapy requires relative medical stability and the availability of social supports to enable the patient to live at home. It is also ideal for patients who do not have easy access into and out of their home.

Specialized equipment

Adaptive and durable medical equipment can be used to assist stroke patients to become more independent and to facilitate functional skill performance (Box 51-9). It is important to consider the patient's functional level, level of adaptation to the disability, architecture of the living environment, and instruction in the use of all devices and equipment. Many types of device are available to assist the stroke patient in achieving an improved level of independence. These include adaptive devices to assist in the performance of activities of daily living, such as eating utensils, bathing and grooming aids, dressing devices, tub and shower equipment, assistive devices for walking, transfer aids, and wheelchairs (see Chs 18 and 27). Fitting and providing a properly fitting wheelchair sometimes makes a huge

---

Box 51-9 Specialized adaptive equipment used by people with stroke

Adapted feeding utensils
- Utensils with built-up handles
- Universal cuff
- Rocker knife
- Non-skid mats
- Plate guards or scoop dishes
- Cup holder
- Adapted cups

Bathing and grooming devices
- Long-handled sponge
- Washcloth mitt
- Adapted shaving equipment
- Handheld shower nozzle
- Soap on a rope
- Stand-up mirror
- Built-up toothbrush, comb, hairbrush

Tub and shower transfer equipment
- Non-skid mat
- Grab bars
- Transfer seats
- Shower chair or bench
- Hydraulic and motorized tub lifts

Dressing devices
- Velcro closures
- Button hooks
- Long-handled reachers
- Sock donning aid
- Long-handled shoehorn
- Elastic shoelaces

Walking devices
- Single-point cane
- Quad cane
- Hemiwalker
- Standard walker
- Rolling walker

difference for a patient with stroke. A wheelchair can greatly enhance the quality of life by improving positioning and mobility. A wheelchair for a hemiplegic patient typically has a lowered base, to allow the non-hemiplegic lower limb to touch the floor so that it can be used in wheelchair propulsion. There can also be a one-arm drive mechanism to enable the patient to use the non-hemiplegic upper limb for wheelchair propulsion. Cushions, backrests, trunk supports, and head supports also can be beneficial. Power wheelchairs are rarely needed in patients with hemiplegia, unless there is significant comorbid cardiac or pulmonary disease. Patients with bilateral hemiplegia often benefit from power chairs.

Upper limb resting hand splints are usually used to prevent deformity and to maintain the hemiplegic wrist in a functional, slightly extended position. For patients with wrist or finger flexion contractures, serial casting of the upper limb may assist in restoring functional range of motion. Alternatively, there are several dynamic spring-loaded wrist and hand splints available (see Ch. 15).

The AFO is frequently provided to improve the positioning of the foot and ankle, and to facilitate an optimal gait pattern.[190] The type of AFO prescribed is dependent on the patient's strength and biomechanics during walking.[128] For practical purposes, the clinician should consider three issues when prescribing an AFO:

1. the stability of the knee during the stance phase of gait;
2. the medial and lateral stability of the ankle during stance and swing; and
3. the degree of plantar flexion or foot drop during the swing phase.

In early recovery after hemiplegia, a solid ankle AFO is often the best choice, as it helps maintain the proper position of the knee throughout the stance phase of walking. Incorporating a hinge in a solid ankle plastic orthosis at the time of fabrication allows the orthotist to utilize it once the patient achieves adequate quadriceps strength and knee control. An AFO with trim lines cut well anterior to the malleoli provides mediolateral stability. A posterior leaf spring orthosis is appropriate for a patient with foot drop who otherwise has good knee control and good mediolateral stability. The AFO is useful in patients with ankle and foot weakness or spastic dystonia. However, if spasticity is severe, pain or skin breakdown can occur under the AFO. In this situation, focal spasticity management with neurolytic blocks is beneficial (see Ch. 16).

Caregiver training

One of the most important interventions is the training of families and other caregivers in specific care techniques to prevent complications, perform physical functions, and encourage patients to perform any activities they are capable of doing. Training in problem-solving techniques can help family members provide effective support in the home environment. Additional teaching focuses on the dissemination of knowledge about strokes, their consequences, use of medications, stroke prevention, and other care aspects. There is now evidence that both

---

Box 51-10 Patient and family education issues

- Cause of stroke
- Signs of stroke (call 911!)
- Stroke risk factors
- Prevention of stroke
- Medication administration
- Medication side effects
- Swallowing technique training
- Healthful diet choices
- Bowel and bladder care
- Sleep and rest
- Prevention of blood clots
- Prevention of skin breakdown
- Tracheostomy, feeding tube, or catheter management
- Blood pressure measurement
- Safety, preventing falls
- Behavioral management
- Positioning and moving in bed
- Transfer training
- Home exercise program
- Optimizing social functioning
- Identifying depression
- Caregiver concerns
- Family functioning
- Sexual functioning
- Recreational activities
- Signs and symptoms of common medical complications

---

education and counseling significantly improve caregiver knowledge and stabilize some aspects of family functioning.[82,97,120] Family education has been found to contribute to the long-term maintenance of rehabilitation gains. It is possible to argue that education of the patient and family is the single most important intervention that the stroke rehabilitation team performs. Important teaching points that should be included in the training program are listed in Box 51-10. Interestingly, two studies have demonstrated that caregiver training during stroke rehabilitation reduces the costs of care, reduces caregiver burden, and improves quality of life outcomes for both patients and caregivers at 1 year following stroke.[155,223]

To function optimally, rehabilitation programs require the involvement of families. Family members serve as members of the rehabilitation team and participate actively in the rehabilitation process. In addition to providing psychologic support, they also provide practical assistance to the patient in the treatment program and preparation for return home. Engaging families to participate in the education program is essential to enable both a smooth transition to the community and safe functioning for the patient in the home environment. Family involvement includes encouraging family members to ask questions, express concerns, make suggestions, develop rehabilitation goals and plans, observe and participate in the therapy sessions, and train in the performance of specific skills.

SPECIAL PATIENT CONSIDERATIONS

Childhood stroke

It is often assumed that children with stroke recover significantly better than adults do because central nervous system plasticity is so much more favorable in pediatric age groups. However, following early childhood (>3 years), neurologic recovery may be more typical of that seen in adults with stroke. It is true, however, that children are very adaptive and often have excellent functional recovery despite persistent neurologic impairments. The therapeutic goals differ in children, and include activities such as play and recreation, participation in school, and socialization. In addition to stroke recovery, children with cerebrovascular disease often have other concerns, such as seizures, hemophilia, sickle cell disease, and moyamoya disease, that require medical management or surgery.[143]

The rehabilitation approaches for children with stroke are usually reflective of techniques that are applied to patients with spastic hemiplegia from cerebral palsy. The principles of neurodevelopmental technique are often useful. More recently, CIMT has been applied to children with hemiplegia from acquired brain injury, with some success. Karman and colleagues showed that hemiplegic children increase the functional use of their affected upper limb and show improved quality of movement after a CIMT program.[160] Surprisingly, children will accept a constraint applied to their unaffected hand if they are encouraged and given concrete rewards.

In general, children with stroke achieve good functional mobility and self-care by adulthood, and most ambulate independently without a device. However, the majority of people with childhood stroke who have motor impairments at stroke onset will have some residual hemiplegia or other motor deficit. Many will be successful in school but might require special education in the process. Unfortunately, many fail to achieve financial independence after school, and the majority remain in the moderately low range for communication, daily living skills, and socialization. Onset of stroke below age 3, cognitive impairment at onset, and a history of seizures predict a poorer functional outcome in adulthood.[65,143,144]

Stroke in young adults

Young adults tend to present with unique rehabilitation needs and long-term issues. Box 51-11 lists many of the specialized problems and needs that are more prevalent and prominent among younger adults compared with older individuals. To address these specific patient needs, rehabilitation interventions should be directed toward the achievement of specific goals. Depending on the specific situation, functional therapy interventions should include training in complex instrumental activities of daily living, such as shopping, homemaking, community level mobility, childcare, and the care of elderly parents. Communication and cognitive training should focus on money management skills and vocational activities. Psychologic counseling of the patient and family should be instituted to address some of the issues that are specific to the age of the patient, such as self-image, interpersonal relationships, dating, sexuality,

---

Box 51-11 Rehabilitation and long-term issues in young stroke survivors

- Employment
- Sexuality
- Childcare, parenting
- Caring for elderly parents
- Spouse versus personal caregiver role
- Relationship changes
- Psychologic aspects of life role changes
- Weight management
- Driving
- Disability income
- Long-term financial planning
- Health management and exercise
- Sports and recreation
- Leisure planning, hobbies, and socializing

---

and stress management. Education of the patient and family should provide information on stroke, medications, nutrition, healthy lifestyle, and prevention measures. Driving evaluation and rehabilitation are important, as are vocational assessment, counseling, training, and referrals. Recreational and social programs, aerobic training or fitness exercise groups, and community reentry training all enhance the quality of life of young persons with stroke.[21,57,162,163,209,214,338]

Aggressive rehabilitation and continued care by specialized professionals who can recognize, understand, and address the specific physical and psychosocial considerations in young stroke patients can both facilitate the achievement of optimal outcomes in these patients and enhance their quality of life.

Geriatric stroke

The effect of age on recovery after stroke is variable and controversial. It has been found that young age at stroke onset has a favorable effect on long-term and short-term stroke survival,[9,324] but the effect on functional recovery is less certain. In a review of 33 studies on functional outcome after stroke, Jongbloed found that 18 studies evaluated the impact of age on stroke outcome.[151] In 14 of the studies, younger patients tended to have better outcomes than those of older adults, but the overwhelming majority of these studies used functional status at discharge as the outcome measure. In four of the studies, no relationship was found between age and outcome and, in most of those studies, the amount of functional improvement (rather than functional status at discharge) was used as the outcome measure under study. These findings suggest that younger adults tend to have less severe disability levels at presentation than those of older adults. It has been suggested that the adverse effect of increasing age on functional outcome is explained only by comorbid conditions and frequency of prior stroke.

Age alone probably does not play a major role in determining the course and care of the patient with stroke. It is more likely that advancing age serves as a marker for the presence of medical comorbidities, prior strokes, and limited social supports. Clinical experience indicates that many older adults successfully complete rehabilitation, return to their homes and the community, and contribute to their families and society. However, the frequency of multiple physical impairments and psychosocial problems is greater among older stroke patients than among younger individuals, and this most likely affects outcome.

As a consequence, older adults often require more medical monitoring, longer recovery times, reduced exercise intensities, or more psychosocial support during their rehabilitation program than do younger adults.

TRANSITION TO THE COMMUNITY, FOLLOW-UP, AND AFTERCARE

The effects of stroke can be enduring, and therefore rehabilitation is a lifelong activity involving the restoration of patients to their fullest physical, mental, and social capabilities. For this reason, medical rehabilitation for stroke survivors includes the many physical, social, and organizational aspects of the aftercare of stroke patients. Long-term quality of life is accomplished through an interdisciplinary approach that includes helping the patient to achieve maximal independent functioning in daily activities, and training family members and other personal caregivers in the performance of specific physical skills. In this regard, it is important that family members be aware of the distinction between those skills patients can perform themselves, and those tasks for which the patient needs assistance or supervision to carry out.

Major efforts toward preparation for discharge are directed toward securing community resources. These include competent and reliable professional or other attendant care, home nursing visits, outpatient or home therapy, and community transportation and recreational programs. Teaching patients about stroke, medications, fluid intake, diet, exercises, catheter care, feeding tube use, tracheostomy management, signs and symptoms of common complications such as infections, and specific functional task performance greatly facilitates a smooth transition to home and minimizes the likelihood of medical problems after discharge. Follow-up medical monitoring and care are also important.

Specific functional issues that are relevant around the time of transition to the community are the 'higher level' community skills that are related to the postdischarge lifestyle. Important examples include sexual functioning, driving ability, grocery shopping, housekeeping, laundry management, safety considerations, socialization outside the home, vocational pursuits, and recreational activities. Continuing mobilization exercises and maintaining an adequate activity level are important lifestyle adjustments that can enhance the likelihood of avoiding functional deterioration. The emphasis on education, mobilization, activity, independence, coping, family involvement, and especially quality of life should be incorporated into the patient's lifestyle, even long after completion of the formal rehabilitation program.[153,233]

REHABILITATION OUTCOMES

More has been written in the medical rehabilitation literature about the functional outcomes after stroke than about outcomes following the occurrence of virtually any other disabling condition. The results described in some of these reports often are contradictory, misleading, and even confusing, because of differences in study design, methodology, sample criteria, rehabilitation practice, and outcome definitions.[75,122] It is important to note that outcomes after stroke can be assessed in a number of ways, including medical morbidity, mortality, level of impairment, length of hospital stay, cost of care, functional limitations, placement at the time of discharge and follow-up, amount of handicap or social functioning, quality of life, and life satisfaction. Functional outcomes can be measured either as absolute functional level at the time of discharge or else as the amount of change or improvement in functional abilities between admission or onset and discharge or follow-up. Different conclusions can be reached depending on the specific definitions used. Nonetheless, a few general principles emerge with some consistency.

Functional and social outcomes

One of the most striking aspects of caring for stroke patients is the common observation that their physical performance, functional abilities, and quality of life are considerably better after rehabilitation and during long-term care than immediately after the stroke. Most studies[10,79,90,103,146,156,181,240,284,331] and extensive clinical experience suggest that a substantial proportion of stroke survivors achieve independence in their ability to complete mobility and self-care skills, but that social and vocational outcomes are not as favorable as the functional independence figures. For example, data obtained from the Framingham Heart Study indicated that 78% of 148 stroke survivors were independent in mobility skills, 68% were independent in the performance of self-care activities, and 84% were living in home environments.[121] Unfortunately, however, 63% had reduced vocational function, 59% had decreased socialization outside the home, and 47% had decreased pursuit of interests and hobbies.

Most other studies have yielded similar results. For example, Chin and colleagues reported in a review that between 54% and 80% of stroke survivors were able to walk, but that only 15% were walking outside the home.[52] Andrews and associates found that only 13% of 1-year survivors were severely dependent and 27% were moderately dependent in performance of activities of daily living.[10] In general, about 75–85% of stroke patients are discharged home after formal acute rehabilitation care. Using data derived from a large number of stroke patients involved in inpatient rehabilitation, the Uniform Data System for Medical Rehabilitation reported that stroke patients improved in their average Functional Independence Measure scores from 63 on admission to 87 at discharge, with the greatest improvements occurring in locomotion, mobility, self-care, and sphincter control. Less improvement was noted to occur in communication and social cognition measures. Average length of stay in the rehabilitation facility was about 4 weeks, and more than three-quarters of patients were discharged to the community. These figures match common clinical experience, although specific results vary depending on the program.

Predictors of outcome

Several factors might influence the specific outcome of an individual patient who is involved in a stroke rehabilitation program. Potentially important factors include the following.

- Type, distribution, pattern, and severity of physical impairment.
- Cognitive, language, communication, and learning ability.
- Number, types, and severity of comorbid medical conditions and ongoing health functions.
- Coping ability and coping style.
- Nature and degree of family and other social supports.
- Type and quality of specific rehabilitation training program.

Numerous studies have examined and reported many diverse potential and actual predictors of favorable or unfavorable recovery of physical or psychosocial functioning. A large number of factors have been found to be statistically associated with the outcome of stroke rehabilitation. The nature, type, and strength of the specific predictors depend to a great extent on the specific outcome measure being studied. Specific factors associated with functional outcome after stroke are listed in Box 51-12. There are many reviews of these prognostic factors;

some key references include those by Jongbloed,[151] Davidoff and associates,[63] and Johnston and coworkers.[150]

The strongest and most consistent predictor of discharge functional ability is admission functional ability.[151] Dombovy and colleagues reviewed multiple studies and suggested that the strongest predictors of adverse outcomes are coma at onset, persistent incontinence, poor cognitive function, severe hemiplegia, lack of return of motor function after 1 month, prior stroke, visual-spatial perceptual deficit, unilateral hemineglect, significant cardiovascular disease, large cerebral lesion, and the presence of multiple neurologic deficits.[75] Wade and associates studied 83 stroke patients and found that the best predictors of function after 6 months were sitting balance, age, hemianopsia, urinary incontinence, and motor deficit in the arm.[317]

It is important to note that, although hundreds of articles describe numerous predictors of outcome after stroke rehabilitation, it is difficult to apply these predictors to individual patients in the clinical setting.[150] The multiplicity of variables that influence actual outcome, the degree to which the studies are flawed methodologically, and the unpredictable nature of certain aspects of poststroke functioning render the prediction of outcome for a specific patient by specific predictors incomplete or inadequate. Therefore caution is needed in using the predictors for clinical purposes, such as assessing candidacy for rehabilitation. Identification of some of these factors, however, can help to better direct patient treatment activities.

Evidence for effectiveness of stroke rehabilitation

The growing use of medical rehabilitation services by stroke patients, and the increasing awareness of rehabilitation within the medical community, has stimulated both a desire among clinicians and researchers and pressure from insurers and policy makers to demonstrate its effectiveness. As a consequence, the medical literature has witnessed a recent heightened interest in the scientific investigation of the effectiveness of stroke rehabilitation.

Much of the early stroke rehabilitation effectiveness research consisted of observational descriptions of patient outcomes achieved after participation in rehabilitation programs, but more recent investigations have reported empiric results derived from prospectively conducted controlled clinical trials, the application of epidemiologic principles to clinical research, the development and use of metaanalysis techniques, and the publication of the US Agency for Health Care Policy and Research (AHCPR) *Post-Stroke Rehabilitation Clinical Practice Guidelines.*[120]

The literature probably is better developed in the study of stroke rehabilitation than in the study of rehabilitation programs designed for the treatment of any other disabling condition, but the investigation of rehabilitation effectiveness is still fraught with numerous potential and practical methodological problems that can diffuse the results of high-quality research trials on the effectiveness of rehabilitation. For example, it is necessary to control for natural recovery, or else to demonstrate that the reduction in disability that occurs because of the

---

Box 51-12 Characteristics related to functional outcome after stroke

- Age
- Educational level
- Severity of stroke
- Type of stroke
- Location of stroke
- Size of stroke
- Prior stroke
- Multiple neurological deficits
- Initial functional status
- Congestive heart failure
- Other medical comorbidities
- Premorbid dementia
- Days from stroke onset to rehabilitation
- Coma at onset
- Cognitive function
- Perceptual function
- Language function
- Hemianopsia
- Posture and balance
- Sensory function
- Bowel incontinence
- Bladder incontinence
- Severity of paralysis
- Depression and emotional state
- Motivation
- Family involvement and support

rehabilitation program occurs to a greater extent than would be expected to occur by natural spontaneous recovery alone. The fact that multiple factors affect actual and measured patient outcomes following stroke also limits the ability to study the effectiveness of rehabilitation efforts.[29] There is considerable heterogeneity in patient presentations, because stroke can affect a variety of domains of physical, cognitive, communicative, emotional, social, vocational, and economic functioning, and in a variety of ways. There are considerable variations in the design and methodologies used in stroke rehabilitation research studies. Technical deficiencies in much of the research studies have included suboptimal study designs, small sample sizes, highly selected study populations, failure to control for time since onset, incompletely described interventions, use of unvalidated outcome measures, and inadequate statistical methodologies.[120] Ethical considerations are important in the conduct of randomized controlled trials, because these studies require an untreated control group, and it is not clear that it is appropriate to 'deny' rehabilitation care to any stroke patient. Another difficulty is that many of the factors that affect outcome after stroke, such as motivation level, adaptability and coping style, learning ability, number and severity of comorbidities, family and social supports, and community resources, are specific to the individual and are unrelated to the rehabilitation intervention. It is difficult to adjust for these factors and to compare them across patient groups. Even diversity in the type, distribution, pattern, and severity of the neurologic impairments can confound the results of the research.

Failure to provide detail on the type of rehabilitation intervention has limited the applicability of the results of some studies. A particularly difficult problem has been that of distinguishing the results of rehabilitation efforts from the effects of spontaneous neurologic recovery. In addition, there is considerable subjectivity in the assessment of outcomes, and therefore comparing effectiveness may not be as unbiased or as objective as is desirable. Despite all these methodological issues, results obtained from several randomized controlled clinical trials that compared the outcomes of stroke patients treated on stroke units by dedicated stroke teams with the outcomes of patients treated on general medical wards provide some indication of effectiveness.

Specific clinical trials on effectiveness

Garraway and colleagues in 1980 reported one of the first randomized controlled trials of stroke rehabilitation.[103] The 155 patients randomly admitted to a stroke unit began rehabilitation treatment significantly earlier, were significantly more likely to have received occupational and physical therapy, and were significantly more likely to achieve functional independence (50% versus 32%) at the time of discharge than the 156 patients admitted to general medical units. However, these improvements in functional outcomes for patients treated by the stroke unit group were found to have been lost at 1 year following stroke, possibly because of lack of appropriate family training.

Smith and colleagues reported the results of a trial of three different types and intensities of rehabilitation.[284] The 46 patients who received 'intensive' therapy achieved better outcomes than the 43 patients who underwent 'conventional' therapy, who in turn achieved better outcomes than the 44 patients who received encouragement to continue exercises but no formal rehabilitation. These reports were limited in the detail with which the program's interventions were described.

In another prospectively conducted, randomized controlled trial, Strand and colleagues compared the clinical outcomes of 110 patients admitted to a non-intensive stroke unit and 183 patients admitted to general medical wards.[293] Acute diagnostic work-ups and treatment programs were standardized. The stroke unit had a team approach to care, an education program directed toward the staff, early and focused rehabilitation efforts, active participation by family members, and education of patients and family members. None of these characteristics were uniformly or consistently used on the general medical ward. Investigators found that patients who were admitted to the stroke unit were significantly more likely to be independent in personal hygiene and dressing, and tended to be more likely to walk independently, than patients admitted to the general medical wards. Notably, the 3-month hospitalization rate was only 15% for stroke unit patients but 39% for general medical ward patients, a statistically significant difference that persisted after 1 year.

In another well-done randomized controlled clinical trial conducted in Europe, Indredavik and associates compared the clinical outcomes in 110 acute stroke patients who were assigned to treatment on a stroke unit with the outcomes in 110 stroke patients with similar characteristics who were assigned to treatment on general medical wards.[146] Care on the stroke unit included both acute care and rehabilitation management. The early diagnostic and treatment interventions were standardized and focused. The rehabilitation program was organized with a team approach to care and was initiated shortly after arrival. Emphasis was placed on providing information to the patient and family. Treatment of patients admitted to general medical wards was not standardized. The maximum period of treatment for both patient groups was 6 weeks, at which time 56% of the stroke unit patients and 33% of the general medical ward patients were living at home. At 1 year, 63% of the stroke unit patients and 45% of the medical ward patients were living at home. Both of these differences were highly statistically significant. Functional status levels were significantly greater for stroke unit patients than for medical ward patients at both 6 weeks and 1 year. Interestingly, the 6-week mortality was 7% for stroke unit patients and 17% for medical ward patients, and the 1-year mortality was 25% for stroke unit patients and 33% for medical ward patients, differences that were statistically significant at 6 weeks but not at 1 year.

In another well-conducted prospective randomized controlled trial, Kalra and colleagues studied three groups of stroke patients stratified according to prognosis, and compared 124 patients randomized to treatment on a stroke rehabilitation unit with 121 treated on general medical wards.[153] Patients treated on the medical wards were found to have received more physical therapy, but those on the stroke unit were found to have received more individualized therapy sessions. The findings were of particular interest. For patients with good prognoses, functional outcomes at discharge were found to be comparable in both settings. For patients with poor prognoses, functional abilities were comparable between the two units, but management on the general medical unit was associated with greater mortality and longer hospital stays than was treatment on the stroke unit. Patients with intermediate prognoses who were treated on the stroke unit had significantly better functional outcomes, a greater likelihood of returning home after hospitalization, a shorter length of hospital stay, and better functional abilities.

Another trial by the same group studied specifically 71 patients with severe disability after stroke and poor prognoses, randomizing 34 of those patients to a stroke rehabilitation unit and 37 to general medical wards.[154] Compared with the patients treated on the general medical wards, the severe stroke patients who were treated on the stroke rehabilitation unit had significantly better mortality rates, home discharge placement rates, lengths of hospital stay, and a trend toward significantly better improvement in functional scores.

In another controlled clinical trial, Kaste and associates studied the outcomes of 113 acute older stroke patients randomized to admission to a neurology department with an organized stroke care team that provided coordinated acute and rehabilitation care, and 119 older stroke patients admitted to a medical department with no structured programs for diagnostic evaluation, acute treatment, or rehabilitation.[161] Patients admitted to the focused stroke care unit were discharged an average of 16 days earlier and were more likely to have returned home (75% versus 62%) than those who were treated on the medical ward. Functional status at 1 year was significantly better for the neurologic unit patients than for the medical ward patients.

Other controlled studies exist as well, including those by Sivenius et al.,[282] Stevens et al.,[293] and Wood-Dauphinee et al.[331] Methodological problems limit the applicability of the findings of these studies, and the results of these studies are variable and inconclusive. Studies on the effectiveness of rehabilitation programs are summarized and reviewed in the AHCPR document.[120]

In a metaanalysis of available literature on clinical trials in stroke rehabilitation research, Ottenbacher and Jannell reported the results of 36 clinical trials in which 3717 patients participated.[218] Their analysis indicated that the average stroke patient who underwent a focused stroke rehabilitation program performed better than approximately 65% of the patients in comparison groups. Rehabilitation had the largest effects on personal care skills, mobility activities, ambulation, and visuospatial perceptual functions, while language and cognitive functions showed the smallest effects of rehabilitation. The authors found that the improvement in performance was related more to early initiation of treatment than to the duration of the intervention. Another metaanalysis, conducted by Langhorne and colleagues, found reduced mortality in addition to improved functional outcomes among stroke patients who underwent a coordinated interdisciplinary rehabilitation program, although

they noted considerable diversity among the studies in the type of functional outcome measures used to assess effectiveness, limiting to some extent the interpretation of these findings.[179]

There are a growing number of trials of therapy interventions for patients who are in the postacute stroke stage.[59,301] There are also several studies comparing the effectiveness of rehabilitation interventions performed in a variety of settings, such as home, outpatient departments, or day hospital programs.[111-113,315,333,334] In general, these studies indicate that long-term disabled stroke patients may attain significant functional improvement from rehabilitation, and that home physical therapy may be effective in improving outcome.

Common themes of the effectiveness studies

In addition to early initiation of rehabilitation treatment, several other common characteristics of the intervention programs appear to have been important in the achievement of favorable outcomes by the experimental groups. These include focused personal care and mobility training; a comprehensive approach to care by a team of professionals, with coordination of treatment interventions, usually through team meetings and communication; education of patients and their families; active participation by family members; staff education on stroke and rehabilitation techniques; and care that is systematic, standardized, uniform, and consistent. While this does not diminish the importance of individualized treatment, ensuring that certain standards of care are met consistently is likely to improve the quality and outcome of that care. This consistency certainly supports the conduct of effective research and therefore enhances the usefulness of the results derived from that research.

Reding and McDowell[240] and Dobkin[72] argued in the scientific literature in 1989 as to whether there was convincing evidence concerning the usefulness and benefits of stroke rehabilitation. The scientific investigation of rehabilitation effectiveness has developed since that time, so that the current level of discussion about effectiveness has a somewhat more data-driven scientific basis. Despite limitations in the amount and quality of the research on the effectiveness of stroke rehabilitation, and despite several persisting questions on the effectiveness of the interventions that make up the programs, there is growing evidence that stroke rehabilitation programs improve the outcome of individuals who are disabled by stroke.

CONCLUSION

Stroke rehabilitation continues to be the prototype rehabilitation effort involving nearly all common rehabilitation problems and requiring the effort of all members of the interdisciplinary rehabilitation team. New scientific evidence on the necessity of rehabilitation interventions for neural reorganization and functional recovery has set a foundation for stroke rehabilitation research in the coming decades. The application of physical exercise and newer modalities, as well as pharmacology, surgery, and robotics, is now under clinical investigation. Much of what we learn about neurologic recovery and the effects of training in stroke will probably translate into new therapeutic approaches to all types of disabling diseases. In the meantime, the tradition of the physical medicine and rehabilitation process and inter-disciplinary care remains the cornerstone of the early treatment and continued support of people with disability, now and in the foreseeable future.

REFERENCES

1. Abbott RD, Donohue RP, MacMahon SW, et al. Diabetes and the risk of stroke: the Honolulu Heart Program. JAMA 1987; 257:949–952.
2. Adams HP, Adams RJ, Brott T, et al. Guidelines for the early management of patients with ischemic stroke. Stroke 2003; 34:1056–1083.
3. Adult Treatment Panel III. National Cholesterol Education Program. Online. Available: http://www.nhlbi.nih.gov/about/ncep
4. Albers GW, Amarenco P, Easton JD, et al. Antithrombotic and thrombo-lytic therapy for ischemic stroke. Chest 2004; 126(suppl):483S–512S.
5. Albert ML, Helm-Estabrooks N. Diagnosis and treatment of aphasia: part 1. JAMA 1988; 259:1043–1047.
6. Alberts MJ, Hademenos G, Latchaw RE, et al. Recommendations for the establishment of primary stroke centers. JAMA 2000; 283:3102–3109.
7. Alberts MJ, Horner J, Gray L, et al. Aspiration after stroke: lesion analysis by brain MRI. Dysphagia 1992; 7:170–173.
8. American Heart Association. Heart disease and stroke statistics—2004 update statistical supplement. Dallas: American Heart Association; 2003.
9. Andrews K, Brocklehurst JC, Richards B, et al. The influence of age on the clinical presentation and outcome of stroke. Int Rehabil Med 1984; 6:49–51.
10. Andrews K, Brocklehurst JC, Richards B, et al. The rate of recovery from stroke—and its measurement. Int Rehabil Med 1981; 3:155–161.
11. Antithrombotic Trialists' Collaboration. Collaborative meta-analysis of ran-domised trials of antiplatelet therapy for prevention of death, myocardial infarction, and stroke in high risk patients. Br Med J 2002; 324:71–86.
12. Baker LL, Parker K. Neuromuscular electrical stimulation of the muscles surrounding the shoulder. Phys Ther 1986; 66(12):1930–1937.
13. Barer DH. Continence after stroke: useful predictor or goal of therapy? Age Ageing 1989; 18:183–191.
14. Barer DH. The natural history and functional consequences of dysphagia after hemispheric stroke. Neurol Neurosurg Psychiatry 1989; 52:236–241.
15. Barnett HJM, Taylor DW, Eliasziw M, et al. Benefit of carotid endarterec-tomy in patients with symptomatic moderate or severe stenosis. N Engl J Med 1998; 339:1415–1425.
16. Barrett-Connor E, Khaw K. Diabetes mellitus: an independent risk factor for stroke? JAMA 1988; 258:116–123.
17. Bath PMW, Bath FJ, Smithard DG. Interventions for dysphagia in acute stroke. Cochrane Database Syst Rev 2004; 4:1–28.
18. Berry WR, Sanders SB. Environmental education: the universal manage-ment approach for adults with dysarthria. In: Berry WR, ed. Clinical dys-arthria. Austin: Pro-Ed; 1983.
19. Biller J, Love BB. Nihilism and stroke therapy. Stroke 1991; 22:1105–1106.
20. Binder LM. Emotional problems after stroke. Stroke 1984; 15:174–177.
21. Black-Schaffer RM, Lemieux L. Vocational outcome after stroke. Top Stroke Rehabil 1994; 1:74–86.
22. Bobath B. Adult hemiplegia: evaluation and treatment. 3rd edn. Oxford: Heinemann; 1990.
23. Bogousslavsky J, Regli F. Borderzone infarctions distal to internal carotid artery. Ann Neurol 1986; 20:346–350.
24. Bohannon RW, Larkin PA, Smith MB, et al. Shoulder pain in hemiplegia: statistical relationship with five variables. Arch Phys Med Rehabil 1986; 67:514–516.
25. Boivie J, Leijon G. Clinical findings in patients with central poststroke pain. In: Casey KL, ed. Pain and central nervous system disease: the central pain syndromes. New York: Raven Press; 1991:65–75.
26. Borrie MJ. Urinary incontinence after stroke. Phys Med Rehabil State Art Rev 1993; 7:101–112.
27. Boston Area Anticoagulation Trial of Atrial Fibrillation Investigators. The effect of low-dose warfarin on the risk of stroke in patients with non-rheumatic atrial fibrillation. N Engl J Med 1990; 323:1505–1511.
28. Boysen G, Brander T, Christensen H, et al. Homocysteine and risk of recurrent stroke. Stroke 2003; 34:1258–1261.
29. Brandstater ME, Basmajian JV, eds. Stroke rehabilitation. Baltimore: Williams & Wilkins; 1987.
30. Brandstater ME, Roth EJ, Siebens HC. Venous thromboembolism in stroke: literature review and implications for clinical practice. Arch Phys Med Rehabil 1992; 73(suppl):S379–S391.
31. Brashear A, Gordon MF, Elovic E, et al. Intramuscular injection of botuli-num toxin for the treatment of wrist and finger spasticity after stroke. N Engl J Med 2002; 347:395–400.
32. Bray GP, DeFrank PRS, Wolfe TL. Sexual functioning in stroke survivors. Arch Phys Med Rehabil 1981; 62:286–288.
33. Brittain KR, Perry SI, Peet SM, et al. Prevalence and impact of urinary symptoms among community-dwelling stroke survivors. Stroke 2000; 31:886–891.
34. Brocklehurst JC, Andrews K, Richards B, et al. Incidence and correlates of incontinence in stroke patients. J Am Geriatr Soc 1985; 33:540–542.
35. Brott T. Prevention and management of medical complications of the hospitalized elderly stroke patient. Clin Geriatr Med 1991; 7:475–482.
36. Brown JA, Lutsep H, Cramer SC, et al. Motor cortex stimulation for enhancement of recovery after stroke: case report. Neurol Res 2003; 25:815–818.
37. Brust JCM, Shafer SQ, Richter RW, et al. Aphasia in acute stroke. Stroke 1976; 7:167–174.
38. Bryan RN, Levy LM, Whitlow WD, et al. Diagnosis of acute cerebral infarction: comparison of CT and MR imaging. AJNR Am J Neuroradiol 1991; 12:611–620.
39. Butter CM, Kirsch N. Combined and separate effects of eye patching and visual stimulation on unilateral neglect following stroke. Arch Phys Med Rehabil 1992; 73:1133–1139.
40. Byington RP, Davis BR, Plehn JF, et al. Reduction of stroke events with pravastatin. The Prospective Pravastatin Pooling (PPP) Project. Circulation 2001; 103:387–392.
41. Calviano R, Levine D, Petrone P. Elements of cognitive rehabilitation after right hemisphere stroke. Neurol Clin 1993; 11:25–57.
42. Caplan D. Aphasic syndromes. In: Heilman KM, Valenstein E, eds. Clinical neuropsychology. New York: Oxford University Press; 2003:14–34.
43. Caplan LR. Brain embolism, revisited. Neurology 1993; 43:1281–1287.
44. Caplan LR. Diagnosis and treatment of ischemic stroke. JAMA 1991; 266:2413–2418.
45. CAPRIE Steering Committee. A randomised, blinded trial of clopidogrel versus aspirin in patients at risk of ischaemic events (CAPRIE). Lancet 1996; 348:1329–1339.
46. Carr JH, Shepherd RB. Neurological rehabilitation. Optimizing motor performance. Oxford: Butterworth Heinemann; 1998.
47. CAST Collaborative Group. CAST: randomised placebo controlled trial of early aspirin use in 20000 patients with acute ischemic stroke. Lancet 1997; 349:1641–1649.
48. Cerebral Embolism Task Force. Cardiogenic brain embolism: the second report of the Cerebral Embolism Task Force. Arch Neurol 1989; 46:727–743.
49. Chantraine A, Beribeault A, Uebelhart D, et al. Shoulder pain and dysfunc-tion in hemiplegia: effects of functional electrical stimulation. Arch Phys Med Rehabil 1999; 80:328–331.
50. Chapey R, ed. Language intervention strategies in adult aphasia. 2nd edn. Baltimore: Williams & Wilkins; 1986.
51. Childers MK, Brashear A, Jozefczyk P, et al. Dose-dependent response to intramuscular botulinum toxin type A for upper-limb spasticity in patients after stroke. Arch Phys Med Rehabil 2004; 85:1063–1059.
52. Chin PL, Rosie A, Irving M. Studies in hemiplegic gait. In: Rose FC, ed. Advances in stroke therapy. New York: Raven Press; 1982.
53. Choi-Kwon S, Yang YH, Kim EK, et al. Nutritional status in acute stroke: undernutrition versus overnutrition in different stroke subtypes. Acta Neurol Scand 1998; 98:187–192.
54. Coll P, Erickson RV. Mood disorders associated with stroke. Phys Med Rehabil State Art Rev 1989; 3:619–628.

55. Collins R, MacMahon S. Blood pressure, antihypertensive treatment on vascular disease: reappraisal of the evidence in 1994. Br Med Bull 1994; 50:272–298.

56. Couser JI. Diagnosis and management of pneumonia and ventilatory disorders in patients with stroke. Top Stroke Rehabil 1994; 1:106–118.

57. Culler KH, Jasch C, Scanlan S. Child care and parenting issues for the young stroke survivor. Top Stroke Rehabil 1994; 1:48–64.

58. CURE Trial Investigators. Effects of clopidogrel in addition to aspirin in patients with acute coronary syndromes without ST-segment elevation. N Engl J Med 2001; 345:494–502.

59. Dam M, Tonin P, Casson S, et al. The effects of long-term rehabilitation therapy on poststroke hemiplegic patients. Stroke 1993; 24:1186–1191.

60. Daniels SK, Ballo LA, Mahoney M-C, et al. Clinical predictors of dysphagia and aspiration risk: outcome measures in acute stroke patients. Arch Phys Med Rehabil 2000; 81:1030–1033.

61. Daniels SK, Brailey K, Priestly DH, et al. Aspiration in patients with acute stroke. Arch Phys Med Rehabil 1998; 79:14–19.

62. Darley FL. The efficacy of language rehabilitation in aphasia. J Speech Hear Disord 1972; 37:3–21.

63. Davidoff G, Keren O, Ring H, et al. Assessing candidates for inpatient stroke rehabilitation: predictors of outcome. Phys Med Rehabil Clin North Am 1991; 2:501–516.

64. Davis SW, Petrillo CR, Eichberg RD, et al. Shoulder–hand syndrome in a hemiplegic population: a 5-year retrospective study. Arch Phys Med Rehabil 1977; 58:353–356.

65. De Schryver ELLM, Kappelle LJ, Boudewyn Peters AC. Prognosis of ischemic stroke in childhood: a long-term follow-up study. Dev Med Child Neurol 2000; 42:313–318.

66. De Vincenzo DK, Watkins S. Accidental falls in a rehabilitation setting. Rehabil Nurs 1987; 12:248–252.

67. DeCouten-Myers GM, Myers RE, Schoolfield L. Hyperglycemia enlarges infarct size in cerebrovascular occlusion in cats. Stroke 1988; 19:623–630.

68. Dejerine J, Roussy G. La syndrome thalamique. Rev Neurol (Paris) 1906; 14:521–535.

69. Dekker JH, Wagenaar RL, Lankhorst GJ, et al. The painful hemiplegic shoulder: effects of intra-articular triamcinolone acetonide. Am J Phys Med 1997; 76:43–48.

70. Diener HC, Bogousslavsky J, Brass LM, et al. Aspirin and clopidogrel compared with clopidogrel alone after recent ischaemic stroke or transient ischaemic attack in high-risk patients (MATCH): randomized, double-blind, placebo-controlled trial. Lancet 2004; 364:331–337.

71. Diener HC, Cunha L, Forbes C, et al. European Stroke Prevention Study 2. Dipyridamole and acetylsalicylic acid in the secondary prevention of stroke. J Neurol Sci 1996; 143:1–13.

72. Dobkin BH. Focused stroke rehabilitation programs do not improve outcome. Arch Neurol 1989; 46:701–703.

73. Dodick DW, Meissner I, Meyer FB, et al. Evaluation and management of asymptomatic carotid artery stenosis. Mayo Clin Proc 2004; 79:937–944.

74. Dombovy ML, Basford JR, Whisnant JP, et al. Disability and use of rehabilitation services following stroke in Rochester, Minnesota, 1975–1979. Stroke 1987; 18:830–836.

75. Dombovy ML, Sandok BA, Basford JA. Rehabilitation after stroke: a review. Stroke 1986; 17:363–369.

76. Dromerick AW, Edwards DF, Hahn M. Does the application of constraint-induced movement therapy during acute rehabilitation reduce arm impairment after ischemic stroke? Stroke 2000; 31:2984–2988.

77. Dursun E, Dursun N, Ural CE, et al. Glenohumeral joint subluxation and reflex sympathetic dystrophy in hemiplegic patients. Arch Phys Med Rehabil 2000; 81:944–946.

78. Dworkin JP. Motor speech disorders: a treatment guide. St Louis: Mosby Year-Book; 1991.

79. Edmans JA, Towle D. Comparison of stroke unit and non-stroke unit in patients on independence in ADL. Br J Occup Ther 1990; 53:415–418.

80. Egelko S, Simon D, Riley E, et al. First year after stroke: tracking cognitive and affective deficits. Arch Phys Med Rehabil 1989; 70:297–302.

81. Ernst E. A review of stroke rehabilitation and physiotherapy. Stroke 1990; 21:1081–1085.

82. Evans RL, Matlock A-L, Bishop DS, et al. Family intervention after stroke: does counseling or education help? Stroke 1988; 19:1243–1249.

83. Evans RL, Northwood L. Social support needs in adjustment to stroke. Arch Phys Med Rehabil 1983; 64:61–64.

84. Ezekowitz MD, Bridgers SL, James KE, et al. Warfarin in the prevention of stroke associated with nonrheumatic atrial fibrillation. N Engl J Med 1992; 327:1406–1412.

85. Faghri PD, Rogers MM, Glaser RM, et al. The effects of functional electrical stimulation on shoulder subluxation, arm function recovery, and shoulder pain in hemiplegic stroke patients. Arch Phys Med Rehabil 1994; 75:73–79.

86. Fang J, Alderman MH. Trend of stroke hospitalization, United States, 1988–1997. Stroke 2001; 32:2221–2226.

87. Fasoli SE, Krebs HI, Ferraro M, et al. Robotic therapy for chronic motor impairments after stroke: follow-up results. Arch Phys Med Rehabil 2004; 85:1106–1111.

88. Feldmann E, Tornabene J. Diagnosis and treatment of cerebral amyloid angiopathy. Clin Geriatr Med 1991; 7:617–630.

89. Ferraro M, Palazzolo JJ, Krol J, et al. Robot-aided sensorimotor arm training improves outcome in patients with chronic stroke. Neurology 2003; 61:1604–1607.

90. Ferrucci L, Bandinelli S, Guralnik JM, et al. Recovery of functional status after stroke: a postrehabilitation follow-up study. Stroke 1993; 24:200–205.

91. Finkelstein S, Berkowitz LI, Baldessarini RJ. Mood vegetative disturbance, and dexamethasone suppression test after stroke. Ann Neurol 1982; 12:463–468.

92. Fisher CM. Pathological observations in hypertensive cerebral hemorrhage. J Neuropathol Exp Neurol 1971; 30:536–550.

93. Flamm ES. The potential use of nicardipine in cerebrovascular disease. Am Heart J 1989; 117:236–242.

94. FOOD Trial Collaboration. Poor nutritional status on admission predicts poor outcomes after stroke: observational data from the FOOD trial. Stroke 2003; 34:1450–1456.

95. Francisco GE, Boake C. Improvement in walking speed in poststroke spastic hemiplegia after intrathecal baclofen therapy: a preliminary study. Arch Phys Med Rehabil 2003; 84:1194–1199.

96. Freda M, Rubinsky H. Sexual function in the stroke survivor. Phys Med Rehabil Clin North Am 1991; 2:643–658.

97. Friedland JF, McColl M. Social support intervention after stroke: results of a randomized trial. Arch Phys Med Rehabil 1992; 73:573–581.

98. Friedman PJ, Leong L. Perceptual impairment after stroke: improvements during the first 3 months. Disabil Rehabil 1992; 14:136–139.

99. Fugl-Meyer AR, Jaasko L. Post-stroke hemiplegia and sexual intercourse. Scand J Rehabil Med 1980; 7:158–166.

100. Furlan A, Higashida R, Wechsler L, et al. Intra-arterial prourokinase for acute ischemic stroke. The PROACT II study: a randomized controlled trial. Prolyse in Acute Cerebral Thromboembolism. JAMA 1999; 282:2003–2011.

101. Furlan AJ, Whisnant JP, Elveback LR. The decreasing incidence of primary intracerebral hemorrhage: a population study. Ann Neurol 1979; 5:367–373.

102. Gamble GE, Barberan E, Laasch HU, et al. Poststroke shoulder pain: a prospective study of the association and risk factors in 152 patients from a consecutive cohort of 205 patients presenting with stroke. Eur J Pain 2002; 6:467–474.

103. Garraway WM, Akhtar AJ, Prescott RJ, et al. Management of acute stroke in the elderly: preliminary results of a controlled trial. Br Med J 1980; 280:1040–1043.

104. Garrett VE, Scott JA, Costich J, et al. Bladder emptying assessment in stroke patients. Arch Phys Med Rehabil 1989; 70:41–43.

105. Garrison SJ. Post-stroke pain. Phys Med Rehabil State Art Rev 1991; 5:83–88.

106. Geerts WH, Heit GP, Clagett GP, et al. Prevention of venous thromboembolism. Chest 2001; 119:132S–175S.

107. Gelber DA, Good DC, Laven LJ, et al. Causes of urinary incontinence after acute hemispheric stroke. Stroke 1993; 24:378–382.

108. Geshwind N. Disconnexion syndromes in animals and man. Part 2. Brain 1965; 88:237–294.

109. Geshwind N. The apraxias: neural mechanisms of disorders of learned movement. Am Sci 1975; 63:188–195.

110. Gilman S, Newman SW. Manter and Gatz's essentials of clinical neuroanatomy and neurophysiology. 10th edn. Philadelphia: FA Davis; 2002.

111. Gladman JRF, Lincoln NB, Barer DH. A randomised controlled trial of domiciliary and hospital-based rehabilitation for stroke patients after discharge from hospital. J Neurol Neurosurg Psychiatry 1993; 56:960–966.

112. Gladman JRF, Lincoln NB. Follow-up of a controlled trial of domiciary stroke rehabilitation (DOMINO Study). Age Ageing 1994; 23:9–13.

113. Gladman JRF, Whynes D, Lincoln N. Cost comparison of domiciary and hospital-based stroke rehabilitation. Age Ageing 1994; 23:241–245.

114. Glanz M, Klawansky S, Stason W, et al. Functional electrostimulation in poststroke rehabilitation: a meta-analysis of the randomized controlled trials. Arch Phys Med Rehabil 1996; 77:549–553.

115. Goldberg G. Principles of rehabilitation of the elderly stroke patient. In: Dunkle RE, Schmidley JW, eds. Stroke in the elderly. New York: Springer-Verlag; 1987.

116. Gordon C, Hewer RL, Wade DT. Dysphagia in acute stroke. Br Med J 1987; 295:411–414.

117. Gordon J, Ghez C. Muscle receptors and spinal reflexes: the stretch reflex. In: Kandel ER, Schwartz JH, Jessell TM, eds. Principles of neural science. New York: Elsevier Science; 1991:564–580.

118. Gordon WA, Hibbard MR, Egelko S, et al. Perceptual remediation in patients with right brain damage: a comprehensive program. Arch Phys Med Rehabil 1985; 66:353–359.

119. Gregory PC, Kuhlemeier KV. Prevalence of venous thromboembolism in acute hemorrhagic and thromboembolic stroke. Am J Phys Med Rehabil 2003; 82:364–369.

120. Gresham GE, Duncan PW, Stason WB, et al. Post-stroke rehabilitation. Clinical practice guideline no. 16. AHCPR publication no. 95-0662. Rockville: US Department of Health and Human Services; 1995.

121. Gresham GE, Phillips TF, Wolf PA, et al. Epidemiologic profile of long-term stroke disability: the Framingham Study. Arch Phys Med Rehabil 1979; 60:487–491.

122. Gresham GE. Stroke outcome research. Stroke 1986; 17:358.

123. Harvey RL, Chopp M. The therapeutic effects of cellular therapy for functional recovery after brain injury. 2003; 14:S143–S151.

124. Harvey RL, Lovell L, Belanger N, et al. The effectiveness of anticoagulant and antiplatelet agents in preventing venous thromboembolism during stroke rehabilitation: a historical cohort study. Arch Phys Med Rehabil 2004; 85:1070–1075.

125. Harvey RL, Roth EJ, Heinemann AW, et al. Stroke rehabilitation: clinical predictors of resource utilization. Arch Phys Med Rehabil 1998; 79: 1349–1355.

126. Harvey RL. Diabetes mellitus: incidence and influence on stroke rehabilitation and outcome. Top Stroke Rehabil 1994; 1:91–108.

127. Harvey RL. Motor recovery after stroke: new directions in scientific inquiry. Phys Med Rehabil Clin North Am 2003; 14:S1–S5.

128. Harvey RL. Tailoring therapy to a stroke patient's potential: what can the team approach accomplish? Postgrad Med 1998; 104:78–88.

129. Heilman KM, Watson RT, Valenstein E. Neglect and related disorders. In: Heilman KM, Valenstein E, eds. Clinical neuropsychology. New York: Oxford University Press; 2003:296–346.

130. Helm-Estabrooks N, Emery P, Albert M. Treatment of aphasic perseveration (TAP): a new approach to aphasia therapy. Arch Neurol 1987; 44:1253–1255.

131. Herpin D. The effects of antihypertensive drugs on the cerebral blood flow and its regulation. Prog Neurobiol 1990; 35:75–83.

132. Hesse S, Werner C, Paul T, et al. Influence of walking speed on lower limb muscle activity and energy consumption during treadmill walking of hemiparetic patients. Arch Phys Med Rehabil 2001; 82:1547–1550.

133. Hier DB, Mondlock J, Caplan LR. Recovery of behavioral abnormalities after right hemisphere stroke. Neurology 1983; 33:345–350.

134. Holland A. Pragmatic aspects of intervention in aphasia. J Neurolinguistics 1991; 6:197–211.

135. Hoogasian S, Walzak MP, Wurzel R. Urinary incontinence in the stroke patient: etiology and rehabilitation. Phys Med Rehabil State Art Rev 1989; 3:581–594.

136. HOPE Study Investigators. Effects of an angiotensin-converting-enzyme inhibitor, ramipril, on cardiovascular events in high-risk patients. New Engl J Med 2000; 342:145–153.

137. Horner J, Buoyer FG, Alberts MJ, et al. Dysphagia following brainstem stroke: clinical correlates and outcome. Arch Neurol 1991; 48:1170–1173.

138. Horner J, Massey EW, Brazer SR. Aspiration in bilateral stroke patients. Neurology 1990; 40:1686–1688.

139. Horner J, Massey EW, Riski JE, et al. Aspiration following stroke: clinical correlates and outcome. Neurology 1988; 38:1359–1362.

140. Howard D, Patterson K, Franklin S, et al. Treatment of word retrieval deficits in aphasia: a comparison of two therapy methods. Brain 1985; 108:817–829.

141. Howard G, Howard VJ, Katholi C, et al. Decline in US stroke mortality: an analysis of temporal patterns by sex, race and geographic region. Stroke 2001; 32:2213–2220.

142. Huckman MS. Normal pressure hydrocephalus: evaluation of diagnostic and prognostic tests. Am J Neurol Res 1981; 2:385–395.

143. Hurvitz E, Warschausky S, Berg M, et al. Long-term functional outcome of pediatric stroke survivors. Top Stroke Rehabil 2004; 11:51–59.

144. Hurvitz EA, Beale L, Ried S, et al. Functional outcome of paediatric stroke survivors. Pediatr Rehabil 1999; 3:43–51.

145. Hypertension Detection and Follow-up Program Cooperative Group. Five-year findings of the Hypertension and Follow-up Orogram: III. Reduction in stroke incidence among persons with high blood pressure. JAMA 1982; 247:633–638.

146. Indredavik B, Bakke F, Solberg R, et al. Benefit of a stroke unit: a randomized controlled trial. Stroke 1991; 22:1026–1031.

147. International Stroke Trial Collaborative Group. The International Stroke Trial (IST): a randomized trial of aspirin, subcutaneous heparin, both, or neither among 19435 patients with acute ischemic stroke. Lancet 1997; 349:1569–1581.

148. Johnson ER, McKenzie SW, Rosenquist J, et al. Dysphagia following stroke: quantitative evaluation of pharyngeal transit times. Arch Phys Med Rehabil 1992; 73:419–423.

149. Johnson ER, McKenzie SW, Sievers A. Aspiration pneumonia in stroke. Arch Phys Med Rehabil 1993; 73:973–976.

150. Johnston MV, Kirshblum S, Zorowitz RD, et al. Prediction of outcomes following rehabilitation of stroke patient. Neurorehabil 1992; 2:72–97.

151. Jongbloed L. Prediction of function after stroke: a critical review. Stroke 1986; 17:765–775.

152. Joynt RL. The source of shoulder pain in hemiplegia. Arch Phys Med Rehabil 1992; 73:409–413.

153. Kalra L, Dale P, Crome P. Improving stroke rehabilitation. Stroke 1993; 24:1462–1467.

154. Kalra L, Eade J. Role of stroke rehabilitation units in managing severe disability after stroke. Stroke 1995; 26:2031–2034.

155. Kalra L, Evans A, Perez I, et al. Training carers of stroke patients: randomized controlled trial. Br Med J 2004; 328:1–5.

156. Kalra L. The influence of stroke unit rehabilitation on functional recovery from stroke. Stroke 1994; 25:821–825.

157. Kamen LB. Issues in outpatient rehabilitation management of the stroke survivor. Phys Med Rehabil Clin North Am 1991; 2:615–626.

158. Kannel WB, McGee DL. Diabetes and cardiovascular disease: the Framingham Study. JAMA 1979; 241:2035–2038.

159. Kannel WB, Wolf PA, McGee DL, et al. Systolic blood pressure, arterial rigidity and risk of stroke: the Framingham Study. JAMA 1981; 245: 1225–1229.

160. Karman N, Maryles J, Baker RW, et al. Constraint-induced movement therapy for hemiplegic children with acquired brain injuries. J Head Trauma Rehabil 2003; 18:259–267.

161. Kaste M, Palomaki H, Sarna S. Where and how should elderly stroke patients be treated? A randomized trial. Stroke 1995; 26:249–253.

162. Kempers E. Preparing the young stroke survivor for return to work. Top Stroke Rehabil 1994; 1:65–73.

163. Kertesz A, McCabe P. Recovery patterns and prognosis in aphasia. Brain 1977; 100:1–18.

164. Kertesz A. What do we learn from recovery from aphasia? Adv Neurol 1988; 47:277–292.

165. Klag MJ, Whelton PK, Seidler AJ. Decline in US stroke mortality: demographic trends and antihypertensive treatment. Stroke 1989; 20:14–21.

166. Kobayashi H, Onishi H, Ihashi K, et al. Reduction in subluxation and improved muscle function of the hemiplegic shoulder joint after therapeutic electrical stimulation. J Electromyogr Kinesiol 1999; 9:327–336.

167. Kolb B. Overview of cortical plasticity and recovery from brain injury. Phys Med Rehabil Clin North Am 2003; 14:S7–S25.

168. Kondziolka D, Wechsler L, Gebel J, et al. Neuronal transplantation for motor stroke: from the laboratory to the clinic. Phys Med Rehabil Clin North Am 2003; 14:S153–S160.

169. Kondziolka D, Wechsler L, Goldstein S, et al. Transplantation of cultured human neuronal cells for patients with stroke. Neurology 2000; 55:565–569.

170. Kong K-H, Young S. Incidence and outcome of poststroke urinary retention: a prospective study. Arch Phys Med Rehabil 2000; 81:1464–1467.

171. Kosak MC, Reding MJ. Comparison of partial body weight-supported treadmill gait training versus aggressive bracing assisted walking post stroke. Neurorehabil Neural Repair 2000; 14:13–19.

172. Kotila M, Niemi M-L, Laaksonen R. Four-year prognosis of stroke patients with visuospatial inattention. Scand J Rehabil Med 1986; 18:177–179.

173. Kunkel A, Kopp B, Muller G, et al. Constraint-induced movement therapy for motor recovery in chronic stroke patients. Arch Phys Med Rehabil 1999; 80:624–628.

174. Kurth T, Kase CS, Berger K, et al. Smoking and risk of hemorrhagic stroke in women. Stroke 2003; 34:2792–2795.

175. Kurth T, Kase CS, Berger K, et al. Smoking and the risk of hemorrhagic stroke in men. Stroke 2003; 34:1151–1155.

176. Lagalla G, Danni M, Reiter F, et al. Post-stroke spasticity management with repeated botulinum toxin injections in the upper limbs. Am J Phys Med Rehabil 2000; 79:377–384.

177. Lance JW. Disordered muscle tone and movement. Clin Exp Neurol 1981; 18:27–35.

178. Langhorne P, Stott DJ, Robertson L, et al. Medical complications after stroke: a multicenter study. Stroke 2000; 31:1223–1229.

179. Langhorne P, Williams BO, Gilchrist W, et al. Do stroke units save lives? Lancet 1993; 342:395–398.

180. LaPointe L. Aphasia therapy: some principles and strategies for treatment. In: Johns DF, ed. Clinical management of neurogenic communicative disorders. Boston: Little, Brown; 1978.

181. Lehmann JF, DeLateur BJ, Fowler RS, et al. Stroke: does rehabilitation affect outcome? Arch Phys Med Rehabil 1975; 56:375–382.

182. Linden P, Siebens AA. Dysphagia: predicting laryngeal penetration. Arch Phys Med Rehabil 1983; 64:281–284.

183. Linsenmeyer TA, Zorowitz RD. Urodynamic findings in patients with urinary incontinence after cerebrovascular accident. Neurorehabilitation 1992; 2:23–26.

184. Lipsey JR, Robinson RG, Pearlson GD. Nortriptyline treatment of post-stroke depression: a double-blind study. Lancet 1984; 1:297–300.

185. Loverso FL, Prexcott TE, Selinger M. Cueing verbs: a treatment strategy for aphasic adults. J Rehabil Res Dev 1988; 25:47–60.

186. Lynch JK, Hirtz DG, DeVeber G, et al. Report of the National Institute of Neurological Disorders and Stroke workshop on perinatal and childhood stroke. Pediatrics 2002; 109:116–123.

187. Macko RF, Smith GU, Dobrovoln Y, et al. Treadmill training improves fitness reserve in chronic stroke patients. Arch Phys Med Rehabil 2001; 82:879–884.

188. MacMahon S, Peto R, Cutler J. Blood pressure, stroke, and coronary heart disease: 1. Prolonged differences in blood pressure: overview of randomized observational studies corrected for the regression dilution bias. Lancet 1990; 335:765–774.

189. Majerus PM, Tellefsen DM. Anticoagulant, thrombolytic, and antiplatelet drugs. In: Hardman JG, Limbird LE, eds. Goodman and Gilman's the pharmacological basis of therapeutics. 10th edn. New York: McGraw-Hill Education; 2001:1519–1538.

190. Malas B, Kacen M. Orthotic management in patients with stroke. Top Stroke Rehabil 2001; 7:38–45.

191. Maron DJ, Fazio S, Linton MF. Current perspectives on statins. Circulation 2000; 101:207–213.

192. Matthews VP, Barker PB, Bryan RN. Magnetic resonance evaluation of stroke. Magn Reson Q 1992; 8:245–263.

193. Mayo NE, Korner-Bitensky N, Kaizer F. Relationship between response time and falls among stroke patients undergoing physical rehabilitation. Int J Rehabil Res 1990; 13:47–55.

194. McGovern PG, Burke GL, Sprafka JM, et al. Trends in mortality, morbidity and risk factor levels for stroke from 1960 through 1990: the Minnesota Heart Survey. JAMA 1992; 26:753–759.

195. McLean DE. Medical complications experienced by a cohort of stroke survivors during inpatient, tertiary-level stroke rehabilitation. Arch Phys Med Rehabil 2004; 85:466–469.

196. Meerwaldt JD. Spatial disorientation in right hemisphere infarction: a study of the speed of recovery. J Neurol Neurosurg Psychiatry 1983; 46:426–429.

197. Mesulam MM. Attentional networks, confusional states and neglect syndromes. In: Mesulam MM, ed. Principles of behavioral and cognitive neurology. New York: Oxford University Press; 2000:174–256.

198. Meythaler JM, Guin-Renfroe S, Brunner RC, et al. Intrathecal baclofen for spastic hypertonia from stroke. Stroke 2001; 32:2099–2109.

199. Mion LC, Gregor S, Buettner M, et al. Falls in the rehabilitation setting: incidence and characteristics. Rehabil Nurs 1989; 14:17–21.

200. Mohr JP, Caplan LR, Melski W, et al. The Harvard Cooperative Stroke Registry: a prospective registry. Neurology 1978; 28:754–762.

201. Mohr JP, Hilal SK, Stein BM. Arteriovenous malformations and other vascular anomalies. In: Barnett HJM, Mohr JP, Stein BM, et al, eds. Stroke: pathophysiology, diagnosis, and management. 2nd edn. New York: Churchill Livingstone; 1992.

202. Mohr JP, Thompson JLP, Lazar RM, et al. A comparison of warfarin and aspirin for the prevention of recurrent ischemic stroke. N Engl J Med 2001; 345:1444–1451.

203. Mohr JP. Lacunes. Stroke 1982; 13:3–11.

204. Monga TN, Lawson JS, Inglis J. Sexual dysfunction in stroke patients. Arch Phys Med Rehabil 1986; 67:19–22.

205. Morganstein S, Smith MC. Aphasia and right-hemisphere disorders. In: Gordon WA, ed. Advances in stroke rehabilitation. Boston: Andover; 1993:103–133.

206. Najenson T, Yacubovich E, Pikielni SS. Rotator cuff injury in shoulder joints of hemiplegic patients. Scand J Rehabil Med 1971; 3:131–137.

207. Nedergaard M, Diemer NH. Focal ischemia of the rat brain, with special reference to the influence of plasma glucose concentration. Acta Neuropathol 1987; 73:131–137.

208. Nederkoorn PJ, van der Graaf Y, Hunink MGM. Duplex ultrasound and magnetic resonance angiography compared with digital subtraction angiography in carotid artery stenosis. Stroke 2003; 34:1324–1332.

209. Niemi M-L, Laaksonen R, Kotila M, et al. Quality of life 4 years after stroke. Stroke 1988; 19:1101–1107.

210. Nilsson L, Carlsson J, Danielsson A, et al. Walking training of patients with hemiparesis at an early stage after stroke: a comparison of walking training on a treadmill with body weight support and walking training on the ground. Clin Rehabil 2001; 15:515–527.

211. NINDS rt-PA Stroke Study Group. Tissue plasminogen activator for acute ischemic stroke. N Engl J Med 1995; 333:1581–1587.

212. North American Symptomatic Carotid Endarterectomy Trial Collaborators. Beneficial effect of carotid endarterectomy in symptomatic patients with high-grade carotid stenosis. N Engl J Med 1991; 325:445–453.

213. Nudo RJ, Milliken GW, Jenkins WM, et al. Use-dependent alterations of movement representations in primary motor cortex of adult squirrel monkeys. J Neurosci 1996; 16:785–807.

214. Oehring AK, Oakley JL. The young stroke patient: a need for specialized group support systems. Top Stroke Rehabil 1994; 1:25–40.

215. Office of Medical Applications of Research, National Institutes of Health. Consensus Conference: prevention of venous thrombosis and pulmonary embolism. JAMA 1986; 256:744–749.

216. O'Leary DH, Anderson KM, Wolf PA, et al. Cholesterol and carotid atherosclerosis in older persons: the Framingham Study. Ann Epidemiol 1992; 2:147–153.

217. Ondra SL, Troupp H, George ED, et al. The natural history of symptomatic arteriovenous malformations of the brain: a 24-year followup assessment. J Neurosurg 1990; 73:387–391.

218. Ottenbacher KJ, Jannell S. The results of clinical trials in stroke rehabilitation research. Arch Neurol 1993; 50:37–44.

219. Page SJ, Sisto S, Levine P, et al. Efficacy of modified constraint-induced movement therapy in chronic stroke: a single-blinded randomized controlled trial. Arch Phys Med Rehabil 2004; 85:14–18.

220. Page SJ, Sisto SA, Levine P. Modified constraint-induced therapy in chronic stroke. Am J Phys Med Rehabil 2002; 81:870–875.

221. Parikh RM, Lipsey JR, Robinson RG. Two-year longitudinal study of post-stroke mood disorders: dynamic changes in correlates of depression at one and two years. Stroke 1987; 18:579–584.

222. Parker VM, Wade DT, Langton-Hewer R. Loss of arm function after stroke: measurement, frequency, and recovery. Int Rehabil Med 1986; 8:69–73.

223. Patel A, Knapp M, Evans A, et al. Training care givers of stroke patients: economic evaluation. Br Med J 2004; 328:1–6.

224. Perret G, Nishioka H. Report on the Cooperative Study of Intracranial Aneurysms and Subarachnoid Hemorrhage: VI. Arteriovenous malformations: an analysis of 545 cases of craniocerebral arteriovenous malformations and fistulae reported to the cooperative study. J Neurosurg 1966; 25:467–490.

225. Perrigot M, Bussel B, Pierrot DE. L'epaule de l'hemiplegique. Ann Med Phys 1975; 18:176–187.

226. Pesczynski M, Rardin TE. The incidence of painful shoulder in hemiplegia. Bull Pol Med Hist Sci 1965; 8:21–23.

227. Pessin MS, Duncan GW, Mohr JP, et al. Clinical and angiographic features of carotid transient ischemic attacks. N Engl J Med 1977; 296:358–362.

228. Peszczynski M, Benson F, Collins J, and the Joint Committee for Stroke Facilities. II. Stroke rehabilitation. Stroke 1972; 3:375–407.

229. Peterson P, Boysen G, Godtfredsen J, et al. Placebo-controlled, randomised trial of warfarin and aspirin for prevention of thrombotic complications in chronic atrial fibrillation: the Copenhagen AFA-SAK Study. Lancet 1989; 1:175–179.

230. Phillips SJ. Pathophysiology and management of hypertension in acute ischemic stroke. Hypertension 1994; 23:131–136.

231. Pickersgill MJ, Lincoln NB. Prognostic indicators and the pattern of recovery in aphasic stroke patients. J Neurol Neurosurg Psychiatry 1983; 46:130–139.

232. Plautz EJ, Milliken GW, Nudo RJ. Effects of repetitive motor training on movement representations in adult squirrel monkeys: role of use versus learning. Neurobiol Learn Mem 2000; 74:27–55.

233. Poduri KR, Steimer SL. Comprehensive outpatient approach to stroke rehabilitation. J Stroke Cerebrovasc Dis 1993; 3:29–48.

234. Poplingher AR, Pillar T. Hip fracture in stroke patients: epidemiology and rehabilitation. Acta Orthop Scand 1985; 56:226–227.

235. Prins RS, Snow CE, Wagenaar E. Recovery from aphasia. Spontaneous speech versus language comprehension. Brain Lang 1978; 6:192–211.

236. PROGRESS Collaborative Group. Randomized trial of a perindopril-based blood-pressure-lowering regimen among 6105 individuals with previous stroke or transient ischemic attack. Lancet 2001; 358:1033–1042.

237. Protas EJ, Holmes SA, Qureshy H, et al. Supported treadmill ambulation training after spinal cord injury: a pilot study. Arch Phys Med Rehabil 2001; 82:825–831.

238. Ratnasabapathy Y, Broad J, Baskett J, et al. Shoulder pain in people with a stroke: a population-based study. Clin Rehabil 2003; 17:304–311.

239. Reddy MP. A guide to early mobilization of bedridden elderly. Geriatrics 1986; 41:59–70.

240. Reding MJ, McDowell FH. Focused stroke rehabilitation programs improve outcome. Arch Neurol 1989; 46:700–711.

241. Reding MJ, Orto LA, Winter SW. Antidepressant therapy after stroke. Arch Neurol 1986; 43:763–766.

242. Reding MJ, Solomon B, Borucki SJ. Effect of dextroamphetamine on motor recovery after stroke. Neurology 1995; 45(suppl 4):A222.

243. Reding MJ, Winter SW, Hochrein SA, et al. Urinary incontinence after unilateral hemispheric stroke: a neurologic epidemiologic perspective. J Neurorehabil 1987; 1:25–30.

244. Ring H, Leillen B, Server S, et al. Temporal changes in electrophysiological, clinical and radiological parameters in the hemiplegic's shoulder. Scand J Rehabil Med Suppl 1985; 12:124–127.

245. Rizk TE, Christopher RP, Pinals RS, et al. Arthrographic studies in painful hemiplegic shoulders. Arch Phys Med Rehabil 1984; 65:254–256.

246. Robinson RG, Kubos KL, Starr LB. Mood disorders in stroke patients: importance of lesion location. Brain 1984; 107:81–93.

247. Robinson RG, Lipsey JR, Price TR. Depression: an often overlooked sequela of stroke. Geriatr Med Today 1984; 3:35–45.

248. Robinson RG, Starr LB, Kubos KL. A two-year longitudinal study of post-stroke mood disorders: findings during the initial evaluation. Stroke 1983; 14:736–741.

249. Robinson RG, Starr LB, Price TR. A two-year longitudinal study of mood disorders following stroke: prevalence and duration at six months follow-up. Br J Psychiatry 1984; 144:256–262.

250. Robinson RG, Szetela B. Mood change following left hemisphere brain injury. Ann Neurol 1981; 9:447–452.

251. Ross ED. Hemispheric specialization for emotions, affective aspects of language and communication and the cognitive control of display in behaviors of humans. Prog Brain Res 1996; 107:583–594.

252. Ross R. Mechanisms of disease: atherosclerosis—an inflammatory disease. N Engl J Med 1999; 340(2):115–126.

253. Ross R. The pathogenesis of atherosclerosis: an update. N Engl J Med 1988; 20:488–500.

254. Roth EJ, Lovell L, Harvey RL, et al. Incidence of and risk factors for medical complications during stroke rehabilitation. Stroke 2001; 32:523–529.

255. Roth EJ, Lovell L, Harvey RL, et al. Stroke rehabilitation: indwelling catheters, enteral feeding tubes, and tracheostomies are associated with resource use and functional outcomes. Stroke 2002; 33:1845–1850.

256. Roth EJ, Mueller K, Green D. Stroke rehabilitation outcome: impact of coronary artery disease. Stroke 1988; 19:42–47.

257. Roth EJ, Noll SF. Stroke rehabilitation: 2. Comorbidities and complications. Arch Phys Med Rehabil 1994; 75:S42–S46.

258. Roth EJ. Heart disease in patients with stroke: II. Impact and implications for rehabilitation. Arch Phys Med Rehabil 1994; 75:94–101.

259. Roth EJ. Heart disease in patients with stroke: incidence, impact and implications for rehabilitation. 1. Classification and prevalence. Arch Phys Med Rehabil 1993; 74:752–760.

260. Roth EJ. Medical complications encountered in stroke rehabilitation. Phys Med Rehabil Clin North Am 1991; 2:563–578.

261. Roth EJ. Natural history of recovery and influence of comorbid conditions on stroke outcome. In: Gorelick P, ed. Atlas of cerebrovascular disease. Philadelphia: Current Science; 1995.

262. Roth EJ. Rehabilitation entails many levels of postacute stroke care. Am Heart Assoc Stroke Council Newsl 1996; summer:6–7.

263. Sacco RL, Wolf PA, Bharucha NE, et al. Subarachnoid and intracerebral hemorrhage: natural history, prognosis, and precursive factors in the Framingham Study. Neurology 1984; 34:847–854.

264. Sacco RL, Wolf PA, Kannel WB, et al. Survival and recurrence following stroke: the Framingham Study. Stroke 1982; 13:290–295.

265. Salonen R, Seppanen K, Rauramaa R, et al. Prevalence of carotid atherosclerosis and serum cholesterol levels in eastern Finland. Atherosclerosis 1988; 8:788–792.

266. Sarno MT, ed. Acquired aphasia. New York: Academic Press; 1981.

267. Sarno MT, Levita E. Recovery in treated aphasia in the first year post-stroke. Stroke 1979; 10:662–670.

268. Sarno MT, Levita E. Some observations on the nature of recovery in global aphasia after stroke. Brain Lang 1981; 13:1–12.

269. Saver JL. Poststroke seizures. Top Stroke Rehabil 1994; 1:109–130.

270. Sawner K, LaVigne J. Brunnstrom's movement therapy in hemiplegia: a neurophysiological approach. 2nd edn. Philadelphia: JB Lippincott; 1992.

271. Schmidt J, Reding M. Recognition and management of medical and specific associated neurological complications in stroke rehabilitation. Top Geriatr Rehabil 1991; 7:1–14.

272. Schroeder T, Schierbeck J, Howardy P, et al. Effect of labetolol on cerebral blood flow and middle cerebral arterial flow velocity in healthy volunteers. Neurol Res 1991; 13:10–12.

273. Sedarat SM, Hecht JS. Urologic problems after stroke (parts I and II). Stroke Clin Updates 1993; 4:17-20, 21–24.

274. Selhub J, Jacques PF, Bostom AG, et al. Association between plasma homocysteine concentrations and extracranial carotid-artery stenosis. N Engl J Med 1995; 332:286–291.

275. Sheikh K, Brennan PJ, Meade TW, et al. Predictors of mortality and disability in stroke. J Epidemiol Commun Health 1983; 37:70–74.

276. SHEP Cooperative Research Group. Prevention of stroke by antihypertensive drug treatment in older persons with isolated systolic hypertension: final results of the Systolic Hypertension in the Elderly Program (SHEP). JAMA 1991; 265:3255–3264.

277. Shewan C, Bandur D. Treatment of aphasia: a language oriented approach. San Diego: College Hill; 1982.

278. Shewan CM, Kertesz A. Effects of speech and language treatment on recovery from aphasia. Brain Lang 1984; 23:272–299.

279. Siegler EL, Whitney FW. Prevention and other special management issues in the postacute care of the geriatric stroke patient. Neurorehabilitation 1993; 3:1–11.

280. Siesjo BK. Pathophysiology and treatment of focal cerebral ischemia: 1. Pathophysiology. J Neurosurg 1992; 77:169–184.

281. Siesjo BK. Pathophysiology and treatment of focal cerebral ischemia: 2. Mechanisms of damage and treatment. J Neurosurg 1992; 77:337–354.

282. Sivenius J, Pyorala K, Heinonen OP, et al. The significance of intensity of stroke: a controlled trial. Stroke 1985; 16:928–931.

283. Sjogren K, Fugl-Meyer AR. Adjustment to life after stroke with special reference to sexual intercourse and leisure. J Psychosom Res 1982; 26:409–417.

284. Smith DS, Goldenberg E, Ashburn A, et al. Remedial therapy after stroke: a randomized controlled trial. Br Med J 1981; 282:517–520.

285. Sparks RW, Helm NA, Albert ML. Aphasia rehabilitation resulting from melodic intonation therapy. Cortex 1974; 10:203–216.

286. Sparrow CP, Burton CA, Hernandez M, et al. Simvastatin has anti-inflammatory and antiatherosclerotic activities independent of plasma cholesterol lowering. Arterioscler Thromb Vasc Biol 2001; 21:115–121.

287. Springer L, Glindemann R, Huber W, et al. How efficacious is PACE therapy when language systematic training is incorporated? Aphasiology 1991; 5:391–399.

288. St Pierre D, Gardiner PF. The effect of immobilization and exercise on muscle function: a review. Physiother Can 1987; 39:24–36.

289. Stein PN, Berger AL, Hibbard MR, et al. Intervention with the spouses of stroke survivors. In: Gordon WA, ed. Advances in stroke rehabilitation. Boston: Andover; 1993:242–257.

290. Steinberg FU. The immobilized patient: functional pathology and management. New York: Plenum Press; 1980.

291. Stevens RS, Ambler NR, Warren MD. A randomized controlled trial of a stroke rehabilitation ward. Age Ageing 1984; 13:65–75.

292. Stone SP, Patel P, Greenwood RJ, et al. Measuring visual neglect in acute stroke and predicting its recovery: the Visual Neglect Recovery Index. J Neurol Neurosurg Psychiatry 1992; 55:431–436.

293. Strand T, Asplund K, Eriksson S, et al. A non-intensive stroke unit reduces functional disability and the need for long-term hospitalization. Stroke 1985; 16:29–34.

294. Strandgaard S, Paulson OB. Regulation of cerebral blood flow in health and disease. J Cardiovasc Pharmacol 1992; 19:S89–S93.

295. Stroke Prevention in Atrial Fibrillation Investigators. Adjusted-dose warfarin versus low-intensity, fixed-dose warfarin plus aspirin for high-risk patients with atrial fibrillation: Stroke Prevention in Atrial Fibrillation III randomized clinical trial. Lancet 1996; 348:633–638.

296. Stroke Prevention in Atrial Fibrillation Investigators. Stroke Prevention in Atrial Fibrillation Study: final results. Circulation 1991; 84:527–539.

297. Stroke Prevention in Atrial Fibrillation Investigators. Warfarin compared to aspirin for prevention of thromboembolism in atrial fibrillation: Stroke Prevention in Atrial Fibrillation II Study. Lancet 1994; 343: 687–691.

298. Sunderland A, Langton-Hewer R. The natural history of visual neglect after stroke: indications from two methods of assessment. Int Rehabil Med 1987;9:55–59.

299. Sundt TM, Whisnant P. Subarachnoid hemorrhage from intracranial aneurysms. N Engl J Med 1978; 299:116–122.

300. Sunshine JL. CT, MR imaging, and MR angiography in the evaluation of patients with acute stroke. J Vasc Interv Radiol 2004; 15:S47–S55.

301. Tangeman PT, Banaitis DA, Williams AK. Rehabilitation of chronic stroke patients: changes in functional performance. Arch Phys Med Rehabil 1990; 71:876–880.

302. Taub E, Crago JE, Burgio LD, et al. An operant approach to rehabilitation medicine: overcoming learned nonuse by shaping. J Exp Anal Behav 1994; 61:281–293.

303. Taub E, Uswatte G, Pidikiti RD. Constraint-induced movement therapy: a new family of techniques with broad application to physical rehabilitation—a clinical review. J Rehabil Res Dev 1999; 36:237–251.

304. Taub E. Movement and learning in the absence of sensory feedback. In: Freedman SJ, ed. The neuropsychology of spatially oriented behavior. Homewood: Dorsey Press; 1968:173–192.

305. Taub E. Movement in nonhuman primates deprived of somatosensory feedback. Exerc Sports Sci Rev 1977; 4:335–374.

306. Teasell RW. Pain following stroke. Crit Rev Phys Med Rehabil 1992; 3:205–217.

307. Therapeutics and Technology Assessment Subcommittee of the American Academy of Neurology. Assessment. Melodic intonation therapy. Neurology 1994; 44:566–568.

308. Till JA, Yorkston KM, Beukelman DR, eds. Motor speech disorders: advances in assessment and treatment. Baltimore: Paul H Brookes; 1994.

309. Twitchell TE. The restoration of motor function following hemiplegia in man. Brain 1951; 64:443–480.

310. Unosson M, Ed AC, Bjurulf P, et al. Feeding dependence and nutritional status after acute stroke. Stroke 1994; 25:366–371.

311. Upadya A, Thorevska N, Dena KN. Predictors and consequences of pneumonia in critically ill patients with stroke. J Crit Care 2004; 19: 16–22.

312. VanOuwenaller C, Laplace PM, Chantraine A. Painful shoulder in hemiplegia. Arch Phys Med Rehabil 1986; 67:23–26.

313. Visintin M, Barbeau H, Korner-Bitensky N, et al. A new approach to retrain gait in stroke patients through body weight support and treadmill stimulation. Stroke 1998; 29:1122–1128.

314. Voss DE, Ionta MK, Myers BJ. Proprioceptive neuromuscular facilitation: patterns and techniques. 3rd edn. Philadelphia: Harper & Row; 1985.

315. Wade DT, Collin FM, Robb GF, et al. Physiotherapy intervention late after stroke and mobility. Br Med J 1992; 304:609–613.

316. Wade DT, Langton-Hewer R, David RM, et al. Aphasias after stroke: natural history and associated deficits. J Neurol Neurosurg Psychiatry 1986; 49:11–16.

317. Wade DT, Skilbeck CG, Hewer RL. Predicting Barthel ADL score at 6 months after an acute stroke. Arch Phys Med Rehabil 1983; 64:24–28.

318. Waidhauser E, Hamburger C, Marguth F. Neurosurgical management of cerebellar hemorrhage. Neurosurg Rev 1990; 13:211–217.

319. Wang Y, et al. Functional electrical stimulation for treatment of shoulder subluxation of stroke patients [abstract]. Arch Phys Med Rehabil 1996; 77:977.

320. Wanklyn P, Forster A, Young J. Hemiplegic shoulder pain (HSP): natural history and investigation of associated features. Disabil Rehabil 1996; 18:497–501.

321. Wardlaw JM, del Zoppo G, Yamaguchi T, et al. Thrombolysis for acute stroke. Cochrane Database Syst Rev 2004:4.

322. Weinberg J, Diller L, Gordon WA, et al. Training sensory awareness and spatial organization in people with right brain damage. Arch Phys Med Rehabil 1979; 60:491–496.

323. Weinberg J, Piasetsky E, Diller L, et al. Treating perceptual organization deficits in nonneglecting RBD stroke patients. J Clin Neuropsychol 1982; 4:59–75.

324. Weinfeld FD. The national survey of stroke. Stroke 1981; 12(suppl I): I1–I68.

325. Weinrich M, Steele R, Carlson G, et al. Processing of visual syntax by a globally aphasic patient. Brain Lang 1989; 36:391–405.

326. Wertz RT, Collins MJ, Weiss D, et al. Veterans Administration Cooperative Study on Aphasia: a comparison of individual and group treatment. J Speech Hear Res 1981; 24:580–594.

327. Wertz RT, Weiss DG, Aten JL, et al. Comparison of clinic, home, and deferred language treatment for aphasia: a Veterans Administration Cooperative Study. Arch Neurol 1986; 43:653–658.

328. Winn HR, Richardson AE, Jane JA. The long-term prognosis in untreated cerebral aneurysms: I. The incidence of late hemorrhage in cerebral aneurysm: a 10-year evolution of 364 patients. Ann Neurol 1977; 1: 358–370.

329. Wolf PA, D'Agostino RB, Kannel WB, et al. Cigarette smoking as a risk factor for stroke: the Framingham Study. JAMA 1988; 259:1025–1029.

330. Wolf PA, Dawber TR, Thomas E, et al. Epidemiologic assessment of chronic atrial fibrillation and risk of stroke: the Framingham Study. Neurology 1978; 28:973–979.

331. Wood-Dauphinee S, Shapiro S, Bass E, et al. A randomized trial of team care following stroke. Stroke 1984; 15:864–872.

332. Yorkston KM, Beukelman DR, Bell KR. Clinical management of dysarthric speakers. Austin: Pro-Ed; 1988.

333. Young J, Forster A. Day hospital and home physiotherapy for stroke patients: a comparative cost-effectiveness study. J R Coll Physicians Lond 1993; 27:253–258.

334. Young J, Forster A. The Bradford Community Stroke Trial: eight week results. Clin Rehabil 1991; 5:283–292.

335. Yu DT, Chae J, Walder ME, et al. Comparing stimulation-induced pain during percutaneous (intramuscular) and transcutaneous neuromuscular electrical stimulation for treating shoulder subluxation in hemiplegia. Arch Phys Med Rehabil 2001; 82:756–760.

336. Yu DT, Chae J, Walker ME, et al. Intramuscular neuromuscular electric stimulation for poststroke shoulder pain: a multicenter randomized clinical trial. Arch Phys Med Rehabil 2004; 85(5):695–704.

337. Yu DT, Chae J, Walker ME, et al. Percutaneous intramuscular neuromuscular electrical stimulation for the treatment of shoulder subluxation and pain in patients with chronic hemiplegia: a pilot study. Arch Phys Med Rehabil 2001; 82:20–25.

338. van Zomeren AH, Brouwer WH, Minderhoud JM. Acquired brain damage and driving: a review. Arch Phys Med Rehabil 1987; 68:697–705.

339. del Zoppo GJ. TIAs and the pathology of cerebral ischemia. Neurology 2004; 62(suppl 6):S15–S19.

Chapter
52

Rehabilitation Concerns in Degenerative Movement Disorders of the Central Nervous System

Michael Saulino, Jeanne Doherty and Guy Fried

Movement disorders are clinical manifestations of the loss of modulatory influence by the extrapyramidal system. These syndromes result in the appearance of involuntary movements such as tremor, chorea, and dystonia. Degenerative central nervous system movement disorders that are commonly encountered in the rehabilitation arena include Parkinson disease, Huntington disease, the hereditary ataxias (primarily Friedreich ataxia), hereditary spastic paraparesis, dystonia, and Tourette syndrome. Parkinson disease is by far the most common, as it affects 1–2% of the population over 65 years of age.[43] This chapter will discuss the diagnosis of, medical management of, and specific therapeutic approaches for these disorders. Particular attention will be paid to rehabilitative interventions.

PATHOPHYSIOLOGY

Normal volitional control of movement depends on a balanced relationship between the cortical, subcortical (extrapyramidal), cerebellar, spinal, and peripheral nervous systems. Movement disorders can develop from any malfunction within the extrapyramidal system (basal ganglia, subthalamic nucleus, substantia nigra, and red nucleus). Basal ganglia function is integral to movement by influencing the direction, amplitude, and course of the movement.[31,32]

Parkinson disease
Pathology
Parkinson disease is characterized by the pathologic degeneration of brain stem nuclei, especially dopaminergic cells of the substantia nigra. It is also due to hyperactivity of the cholinergic neurons in the caudate nuclei.[1]

Clinical presentation
The classic features of Parkinson disease include resting tremor, rigidity, postural instability, and bradykinesia. The resting tremor is the most common presenting symptom. It typically appears as a 'pill-rolling' motion of the hand at 3–5 Hz. The resting tremor is suppressed by activity or sleep, and is intensified by stress or fatigue.

The rigidity of Parkinson disease can take two forms: lead pipe and cogwheeling. Lead pipe rigidity is frequently described as a smooth resistance to passive movement that is independent

of velocity (in contradistinction to spasticity, which is velocity-dependent). The lead pipe tone of one limb increases if another limb is involved in a voluntary motion or a mental task. Cogwheel rigidity is a ratcheting through the range of motion. It is due to a subtle tremor superimposed on the rigidity.[19]

Posture is also affected, as patients with Parkinson disease frequently assume a position that is slumped over with protracted shoulders, and flexed hips and knees. In older texts, this is referred to as a simian posture. Postural reflexes are commonly affected in Parkinson disease, which can result in a tendency to fall backward or to the side.

Bradykinesia refers to slowness of motion. It may be reflected in an inability to change direction while walking, difficulty walking around an object, or just difficulty standing. When the bradykinesia affects the muscles of facial expression, a masked facies can be apparent (also known as hypomimia).[46]

Diagnosis of Parkinson disease
The diagnosis of Parkinson disease is primarily clinical. Casual observation of the patient may reveal the tremor or a paucity of spontaneous movements. Resistance to movement of the limbs can be assessed during the range of motion examination. Motor examination often shows that Parkinson disease findings are asymmetric in the early stages of the disease. Gait observation should include linear motion as well as changes in direction. If a patient uses more than five steps to complete a 180° turn, the diagnosis of Parkinson disease should be considered.[58] Bedside cognitive evaluation can be normal early in the disease process, with neuropsychologic evaluation being reserved for problematic cases. Routine electrodiagnostic studies will not aid in the diagnosis of Parkinson disease, except for exclusion of other neurologic processes. Investigational use of electrodiagnostic studies in Parkinson disease can be done in a research setting. The use of laboratory or neuroimaging investigations is for exclusionary indications and for atypical cases. At present, functional neuroimaging such as positron emission tomography and single-photon emission computed tomography scanning are mainly experimental techniques. Both of these have emerged as significant investigational tools in some clinical trials.

The initial diagnosis of Parkinson disease can be delayed, depending on which symptoms predominate. The rigidity of Parkinson disease can be mistaken for the stiffness of arthritis. The postural changes can be attributed to osteoporosis or

Box 52-1 The differential diagnosis of Parkinson disease

Drug-induced
- Neuroleptics
- Metoclopramide
- Reserpine

Toxic injury
- Manganese
- Carbon monoxide
- Cyanide

Metabolic encephalopathy
- Anoxia
- Hyperthyroid
- Hypoparathyroid

Degenerative disorders
- Progressive supranuclear palsy
- Shy–Drager syndrome
- Multisystem degeneration

degenerative spine disease. The bradykinesia and masklike facies can be mistaken for depression. The differential diagnosis is wide (Box 52-1), as one should consider that the symptoms could be induced by a drug, toxic, metabolic, or other neurologic process.

It is also helpful to watch for certain cardinal symptoms, such as early vertical eye movement abnormalities (progressive supranuclear palsy), early autonomic failure (Shy–Drager syndrome) or hyperreflexia, Babinski's sign, ataxia, and peripheral neuropathy (multisystem degeneration).

Parkinsonism can manifest itself in multiple ways that can lead to disability. Patients with Parkinson disease have a high prevalence of both obstructive and restrictive pulmonary disease. This impairment is clinically relevant, in that Parkinson disease patients with respiratory disease have a decrement in activities of daily living compared with those with normal pulmonary function.[44] The loss of muscle flexibility combined with the kyphotic posture is felt by some to contribute to the respiratory difficulty.[49] The speech in a patient with Parkinson disease can be rapid and monotonous, and have low volume with poor articulation and inappropriate periods of silence. Handwriting can become small and cramped (micrographia). As Parkinson disease advances, dementia and depression can occur.[3] Autonomic dysfunction with increased salivation, drooling, orthostasis, increased perspiration, constipation, and hyperreflexic bladder, with incontinence, dysphagia, and erectile dysfunction can also be present.[4]

Prognosis

From a prognostic standpoint, tremor-predominant patients tend to progress at a slower pace than those individuals with gait or postural instability as a primary complaint.[35] Tremor in general is not considered as disabling as bradykinesia. Akinesia can portend a more rapidly progressing disease process.[24] Positive prognostic indicators include early tremor, rigidity, and a family history of Parkinson disease. Negative prognostic indicators include bradykinesia, akinesia, postural instability, gait dysfunction, cognitive deficits, and late age of onset. Laboratory, radiologic, or physiologic studies to date have not added any additional prognostic abilities. Life expectancy is variable[35] but significantly improved with medical management.[39] Dysphagia is considered the most important risk factor associated with early demise.

Medical management of Parkinson disease

Pharmacologic treatments for Parkinson disease intervene with three aspects of the disease: slowing of disease progression, symptomatic relief of motor symptoms, and amelioration of non-motor manifestations. At times, additional medications are required to address the adverse effects of antiparkisonian treatments.

Several agents have been touted as neuroprotective agents in Parkinson disease, but no single drug is universally accepted as disease-modifying. The antioxidant vitamin E failed to demonstrate benefits in a large multicenter trial. Another antioxidant, coenzyme Q10, was shown to delay the onset of the need for levodopa treatment in one multicenter study involving 80 patients. The investigators of this study cautioned that their results needed replication in larger studies. Selegiline, a selective monoamine oxidase B inhibitor, was purported to be a neuroprotective entity, but it is currently considered more of a symptomatic agent. Similarly, while dopamine agonists have demonstrated some positive neuroprotective effects on functional neuroimaging examinations, their effect on clinical progression is controversial. Recent research with pramipexole and ropinirole has shown the most promise. Small trials using infusion of glial cell line-derived neurotrophic factor into the central nervous system have shown conflicting results.[48]

Symptomatic treatment for motor dysfunction has been the traditional medical intervention of Parkinson disease. The two main classes are dopamine replacements and dopamine agonists. Amantadine has weak antiparkinsonism effects. Anticholinergic medications are occasionally used in younger patients with tremor-predominant disease. Both amantadine and anticholinergic agents are relatively minor contributors to the Parkinson disease armamentarium. Levodopa is a keystone of Parkinson disease treatment. It is decarboxylated to dopamine. Levodopa is typically administered with a peripheral decarboxylase inhibitor such as carbidopa. This combination therapy results in less peripheral availability of dopamine (with a concomitant decrease in peripherally based side effects such as nausea) and increased central nervous system dopamine penetration.

Long-term levodopa treatment is complicated by two challenging clinical entities: motor fluctuations and dyskinesias. Motor fluctuations are a wearing-off phenomenon in which patients notice increased tremor and bradykinesia at the end of a dosing cycle. The predictability of these drop-off periods lessens as the disease progresses. Younger patients seem particularly vulnerable to motor fluctuations. Treatment strategies for motor fluctuations include dietary interventions and variable dosing schedules. Dyskinesias usually take the form of chorea, but painful dystonias and myoclonus can also occur. Psychiatric symptoms, including florid psychosis, can be observed with levodopa use. Levodopa usually demonstrates high usefulness initially, but when used chronically it tends to have reduced therapeutic effectiveness.[3]

Because of the potential problems with levodopa therapy, some clinicians choose to use a dopamine agonist as an initial treatment strategy. Agents in this class include pergolide, pramipexole, and ropinirole. While these medications often have less therapeutic efficacy than levodopa, they rarely cause dyskinesia. As noted, there is some suggestion that these agents might have a neuroprotective effect on disease progression. Side effects of dopamine agonists include nausea, vomiting, orthostatic hypotension, and psychiatric symptoms. Because patients can have individualized responses to these agents, switching between medications in this class is commonly undertaken. Another factor that might have clinical relevance is that these agents are more expensive than levodopa therapy. Because of their potential disease-modifying effects and their enhanced utility in mild disease, these agents may be also the preferred drugs in younger and healthier individuals. One randomized trial supported either levodopa or pramipexole as a reasonable option for initial therapy in Parkinson disease, but each drug was associated with different efficacies and adverse effect profiles.[16]

Non-motor symptoms of Parkinson disease, such as orthostasis, sphincter dysfunction, and depression, are also targets for pharmacologic intervention. Treatment options for orthostasis include increased salt and water intake, or the use of mitodrine or fludrocortisone. Neurogenic bowel function in Parkinson disease usually presents as constipation, and is amenable to treatment with increased hydration, bulk-forming agents including dietary fiber, stool softeners, and chemical or mechanical rectal stimulation. Hyperreflexive bladder activity can be treated with anticholinergic agents or α-adrenergic blocking agents, although both classes can exacerbate orthostasis. Depression is usually addressed with selective serotonin reuptake inhibitors, but therapy needs to carefully monitored, as there are reports that these agents have worsened Parkinson disease symptoms. Venlafaxine might be particularly useful, because this agent can increase blood pressure. Tricyclic antidepressants can be considered, but one should choose one with low anticholinergic side effects, such as desipramine (Norpramin). Differences in effectiveness between the classes of antidepressants for Parkinson disease patients have yet to be demonstrated.[51]

Rationale for rehabilitation

While rehabilitation services are often given to the patient with Parkinson disease, this occurrence is more based on common practice rather than clear research design.[17,27,54] There is a paucity of well-designed research studies looking at specific rehabilitation techniques. The existing literature is both sparse and fraught with confounding variables such as changes in medication regimens. A recent review examined 11 studies involving various physical therapy techniques in Parkinson disease. The authors found insufficient evidence to support or refute the efficacy of any form of physical therapy over another form.[8] Furthermore, there was insufficient evidence found to support the efficacy of any therapy compared with no therapy. Perhaps the best designed study was a prospective randomized crossover investigation of 4 weeks of outpatient physical therapy, in which medication changes were not allowed. This study demonstrated significant improvement in activities of daily living and motor function but no improvement in tremor, mentation, and mood. These improvements returned to baseline 6 months after termination of the intervention. Long-term rehabilitation programs have been advocated, but the stability of the benefits gained in these programs has not been demonstrated.[34]

Exercise and muscle physiology

When prescribing an exercise program, one has to take into account the patient's underlying physical condition. Patients with Parkinson disease appear to exercise with decreased metabolic and mechanical efficiency.[20] This disadvantageous situation might be amenable to treatment with aerobic conditioning.[45] It appears that prescribing conditioning exercises to patients with Parkinson disease is useful only in the setting of an optimized medication regimen. The specific exercises have not been proven or agreed on. It might also be difficult for Parkinson disease patients to exercise with sufficient intensity to achieve a training effect.[41] Careful attention to safety is needed when prescribing aerobic conditioning exercises, because Parkinson disease patients are at high risk for falls. Patients with Parkinson disease typically require a supervised environment when using moving equipment such as a treadmill. Improvements in mood and dyskinesias have been reported with the use of aerobic conditioning.[42]

Psychosocial and cognitive concerns

Depression is common in Parkinson disease patients, with an estimated prevalence of 47%.[61] Some authors feel that depression significantly contributes to the cognitive dysfunction.[26] Depression can be related to a deficit in serotonergic transmission[25] or to diminished cortical levels of noradrenaline (norepinephrine) and dopamine.[47] The presence of depression adds significant disability beyond that attributed to motor dysfunction.[60]

No individual psychologic technique appears to have superiority over another with respect to improvements of mood status. As discussed further below, mental imagery and biofeedback can play a part in improving motor performance during rehabilitation. Some of the techniques reported for mood dysfunction in patients with Parkinson disease include individual, group, and family counseling. Social impairments include loss of autonomy and isolation. Many centers have support groups that are useful in educating patients and their families. Antidepressants such as the serotonin reuptake inhibitors have also been used.

Declining cognitive ability often adds to the challenge of treating a patient with Parkinson disease.[6] As the disease progresses, thought processes become more rigid and preservative. Dementia occurs in 10–15% of patients with Parkinson disease and has an increasing incidence with age. Subtle changes in cognition begin to occur even early in the course of Parkinson disease. Decline in motor function and cognitive decline often occur on a parallel course. Deficits in visual perception and verbal fluency have also been reported in some Parkinson disease patients.[36]

There is little evidence supporting the therapeutic benefit of specific cognitive retraining techniques. The use of the mental imagery of a planned motor task has been purported to improve execution of function tasks, but this has not been fully validated.

Practical approach to the treatment of a patient with Parkinson disease

Parkinson disease is a multifaceted entity that is conceptually amenable to treatment by an interdisciplinary team. This approach allows various disciplines to be involved with the patient, family, and community. The ideal treatment team includes consultation with neurology to optimize pharmaceutical therapies while rehabilitation is ongoing.

Formulation of a treatment plan requires that patients with Parkinson disease have an initial assessment of their impairments. A treatment plan should be formulated that addresses these impairments either directly or with compensatory strategies. Assistive devices can be utilized to improve the patient's efficiency, independence, and safety. Wheeled walkers might have added benefit over standard walkers.[5] Education regarding the disease process must be done for patients and their families. Maintenance programs are executed to prevent additional functional loss. Support groups, counseling, education, and the inclusion of the available community resources can be helpful in maintaining function and for avoiding depression and social isolation.

Specific therapy approaches for impairments in patients with Parkinson disease

Patients with Parkinson disease tend to assume a stereotypic pattern of gait, station, and posture. Gait tends to be rigid, with few extra motions and reduced arm swing. In some patients, a festination phenomenon occurs, in which the short, shuffling steps become more rapid, accompanied by additional trunk flexion. Formal gait analysis has demonstrated that some of the stiffness seen in the gait of patients with Parkinson disease is due to the pelvis and thorax rotating together en bloc, rather than in the normal reciprocal pattern.

Multiple physical therapy studies have been done that attempt to improve the abnormal gait features of patients with Parkinson disease. The results, however, are limited and controversial.[7] The most commonly employed technique is the addition of external sensory cues that are timed with step initiation or step maintenance. These prompts have taken the form of tactile, auditory, or visual modalities, and both single and multiple cues are being explored.[9,18,55] It is likely that strength training alone is insufficient to improve gait or has any significant additive benefit to the cuing techniques.[16] Preliminary investigation using body weight-supported treadmill training

has shown promise, but long-term benefit has yet to be observed.[28,29] Compensation strategies for overcoming obstacles improved with programs that emphasized whole body movement and trained anticipation obstacles.[20]

The disability impact of the tremor of Parkinson disease is variable but is often mild. This is due partly to the fact that the tremor is usually at rest, and is frequently reduced or eliminated by voluntary movement. Severe tremor can be addressed with medication as well as rehabilitative techniques. The method most often employed is behavioral intervention, including both biofeedback and relaxation techniques. This strategy capitalizes on the observation that tremor is worse during anxious periods. Surface electromyography can be added to the biofeedback paradigm.[23]

Orthostatic hypotension is a frequent complaint among patients with Parkinson disease, and many have orthostasis without being symptomatic.[50] This is due to autonomic dysfunction that is probably due to a relative sympathetic denervation.[13] Tilt table training is necessary in some patients with severe orthostasis. Milder cases can be treated with measures such as arising slowly, pausing in a sitting position before arising from a supine position, and performing isometric contraction before changing positions. Pressure garment stockings and abdominal binders can also be used to mechanically control the drop of blood pressure. The use of pharmacologic agents might be indicated if these measures fail.

Many patients with Parkinson disease can benefit from a referral to a speech and language pathologist. Speech abnormalities observed in these patients include hesitancy, hypophonia, hyperfluency, stuttering, palilalia (rapid and involuntary word repetition), extended pauses, and trailing off. The strategy most commonly cited as being of utility in the dysarthria of Parkinson disease is the phonatory–respiratory effort model or Lee Silverman Voice Treatment.[40] This technique utilizes the 'think loud, think shout' approach, although this method has been criticized for causing a strained or pressed voice. Other techniques that may be of use include breath control, oral–motor exercises, and imagery. Surface electromyography is occasionally added as a biofeedback device in voice therapy.[56]

Patients with Parkinson disease can have problems in all three phases of swallowing. The videofluoroscopic swallowing study remains the gold standard for the diagnostic evaluation of dysphagia.[30] Many patients report difficulty in attaining appropriate oral intake due to prolonged chewing. Other oral-phase abnormalities observed in these patients include excessive postswallow residuals, poor bolus control, and repetitive tongue motions. In the pharyngeal phase, vallecular and piriform pooling, delayed triggering of the swallow reflex, and delayed laryngeal elevation have been observed on videofluoroscopic swallowing study. There is insufficient evidence to support or refute the utility of dysphagia training in patients with Parkinson disease, although smaller studies have demonstrated some benefit.[7] Dysphagia training techniques typically include using foods mechanically altered with the use of viscous liquids, chin-down positioning, oral–motor exercises, electromyography, biofeedback, and verbal prompting. Clinicians might also choose to administer antiparkinsonian medications prior to meals, so that maximal benefit of drugs occurs during mastication. Patients with severe or rapidly progressive dysphagia should be counseled on the use of enteral feedings in advance of the need for them. This allows the patient to make an informed decision prior to the onset of swallowing-related medical emergency.[37]

It is also important for the patient with Parkinson disease to maintain an independent lifestyle, whether at home or at work. An occupational therapy evaluation is often very helpful to patients in helping them maintain as independent a lifestyle as possible. The use of exercise and activities of daily living equipment is usually critical to lifestyle maintenance. Equipment such as raised toilet seats and grab bars can assist in making movement more fluid and more efficient, and safe. Home exercise programs are key in maintaining activity. The patient's home environment should be studied, and obstacles such as throw rugs and excessive or bulky furniture might need to be removed to permit improved mobility. During and after periods of illness, it is important to fight off the effects of deconditioning by maintaining range of motion, deep breathing, and as much activity as possible.

Other degenerative movement disorders
Huntington disease
Huntington disease is a relentlessly progressive, adult-onset, autosomal dominant disorder that is associated with cell loss within a specific subset of neurons in the caudate nucleus and putamen. It was first described by George Huntington in 1872. The cardinal features of Huntington disease include involuntary movements, dementia, and behavioral changes.

The estimated US prevalence of Huntington disease is from 4.1 to 8.4 per 100 000 people. A few isolated populations worldwide have an unusually high prevalence of Huntington disease. The disease is typically diagnosed in the third and fourth decades of life, and the mean life expectancy after diagnosis is 20 years. Pneumonia and cardiovascular disease are the most common primary causes of mortality. The molecular underpinnings of Huntington disease are still being elucidated. Repeats of the trinucleotide CAG result in a polyglutamic expansion within the protein huntingtin. While the normal function of huntingtin is not known, mutant huntingtin clearly leads to a neurodegenerative cascade.[11,15]

Chorea, defined as excessive abrupt irregular spontaneous involuntary movements, is the hallmark of Huntington disease. This movement disorder might initially appear as exaggeration of gesture or expression. This appearance can progress to an unstable 'dancing', and ultimately to a continuous barrage of generalized movements. At times, large-amplitude, flinging, proximal movements of a limb (ballism) can be observed. Alternatively, chorea can be intermixed with slow distal writhing movements called athetosis. In late-stage disease, chorea is gradually replaced by more classic parkinsonism features including bradykinesia, rigidity, and postural instability.

The cognitive behavioral aspects have wide variability. The cognitive decline can mimic subcortical dementia, with initial manifestations of intellectual decline and memory dysfunction. As the disease progresses, the patients can get disorders of attention, and decreases in visual-spatial processing and executive function. Language abilities are typically preserved until the final stages of disease.

Depression is the most common psychologic dysfunction encountered, with mania, psychotic personality and obsessive–compulsive disorders also possible.

Medical treatment for Huntington disease is limited. While there are ongoing early clinical trials of neuroprotective agents, the majority of treatments are aimed at symptom relief. Treatment options for chorea include benzodiazepines, valproic acid, dopamine-depleting agents, and neuroleptics. The last two classes of medication have the possibility of worsening other aspects of the disease, such as the bradykinesia or rigidity. Antidepressant therapy is commonplace in Huntington disease, with selective serotonin reuptake inhibitors being the most frequently used. Other psychotropic medications can be employed for the various behavioral abnormalities observed.

While the potential for benefit for rehabilitative therapy in Huntington disease would appear reasonable, recent studies suggest that these patients are typically not referred to allied health professionals. One study reported referral rates of 8% to physical therapy, 25% to occupational therapy, and 0% to speech and language pathology. A survey of physical therapists showed that only 16% of physical therapists have ever treated a patient with Huntington disease, and only 6% have treated more than one. There are multiple studies describing specific therapy techniques, but most are observational studies with few participants and do not use valid or reliable outcome measures.

Chorea itself appears resistant to rehabilitative techniques. Perhaps the rehabilitation problem with the greatest body of data is Huntington disease-related dysphagia. While the methodology of the dysphagia treatment studies is somewhat problematic, there is a suggestion that some positive training effects can be observed. While it is reasonable to extrapolate that other impairments of Huntington disease are amenable to modification by rehabilitation, there is a paucity of literature to support specific recommendations.[2]

Hereditary ataxias
Another class of motor neurodegenerative diseases includes the hereditary ataxias. The most common syndrome in this category is Friedreich ataxia, and it will be used as a model for discussion in this section. Other neurodegenerative processes can have ataxia as a predominant feature, including the spinocerebellar ataxias, Wilson disease, and Refsum disease. Accurate diagnosis is fundamental, because some treatable abnormalities can also present with ataxia as the principal characteristic (including tumors, vascular malformations, and vitamin E deficiency).

Friedreich ataxia is a progressive disorder with the presentation of limb and gait ataxia with diminished muscle stretch reflexes, joint position sense, and vibratory appreciation. Comorbidities of Friedreich ataxia can include impaired glucose tolerance, cardiomyopathy, dysarthria, dysphagia, scoliosis, lower extremity weakness, and optic atrophy. The disorder typically presents in the teens, with loss of ambulation occurring 20 years after disease onset. Premature mortality occurs due to aspiration or complications from diabetes. This disease also has a trinucleotide expansion in the FRDA gene, which encodes the protein frataxin. The prevalence of Friedreich ataxia is estimated at between 2 and 5 per 100 000, with a higher incidence in the Caucasian population compared with in Asian or African descendants. The hereditary pattern is classically autosomal recessive. As with many of the neurodegenerative diseases, medical treatment of Friedreich ataxia is inadequate. Comorbid diseases such as diabetes should be treated aggressively. Small clinical trials with 5-hydroxytryptophan and coenzyme Q have shown some partial success in slowing the progression of the disease.

Similar to many of the movement disorders, the evidence basis for rehabilitative interventions in the hereditary ataxias is sparse. Anecdotal reports describe the use of such techniques as weighting of the ataxic extremities, functional strengthening, and tension-controlled gait aids.[14] As the paraparesis of Friedreich ataxia progresses, wheelchair prescription and family teaching are needed. Psychologic support is certainly indicated, as it is with all progressive diseases. Psychotherapy and comprehensive genetic counseling should be made available to the entire family.

Hereditary spastic paraparesis

Hereditary spastic paraplegia, also known as familial spastic paraplegia and Strumpell–Lorrain syndrome, describes a group of inherited disorders in which the primary symptoms are progressive bilateral lower extremity spasticity and weakness. They were first described by Strumpell in 1883, and later in more detail by Lorrain. They are characterized by clinical and genetic heterogeneity, and occur in an estimated 1.5–2.7 per 100 000 people worldwide when strict clinical criteria are utilized. Hereditary spastic paraparesis is caused by axonal degeneration in the spinal cord, maximally at the terminal portions of the corticospinal tracts in the thoracolumbar region and dorsal column fibers in the cervicomedullary region.

Hereditary spastic paraparesis is classified according to clinical symptoms, age of onset, mode of inheritance, and genetic linkage. Clinical classification includes an uncomplicated (spastic paraparesis only) type and a complicated (paresis plus other neurologic findings) type. Type 1 hereditary spastic paraparesis is categorized when the age of onset is prior to 35 years of age, and type 2 if onset is after the age of 35. Classification by mode of inheritance includes three categories: autosomal dominant, autosomal recessive, and X-linked.[57]

The classic presenting symptom in hereditary spastic paraparesis is progressive difficulty walking that occurs secondary to the principle clinical features of lower extremity spasticity and weakness; however, considerable symptom variability can occur. It is estimated that 30% of those diagnosed genetically remain asymptomatic throughout their lifetime. The cardinal features are symmetric lower extremity spastic paresis and extensor plantar responses. A common early symptom is leg muscle stiff-

ness and spasms more often at night, following exertion, or in cold weather. Hypertonicity, spasticity, and/or hyperreflexia can occur without weakness, especially early in the course. Weakness most commonly occurs in the tibialis anterior, hamstring, and iliopsoas muscles. These clinical findings can begin at any age from early childhood to old age, with variable progression of symptoms. Additional common clinical findings in uncomplicated hereditary spastic paraparesis include urinary symptoms in up to 50% and sensory disturbances in 10–65%. Less common clinical features include pes cavus, sphincter dysfunction, and upper extremity dysmetria and neurocognitive deficits. Uncommon clinical features in uncomplicated hereditary spastic paraparesis include paresis and hyperreflexia of the upper extremities and distal amyotrophy. Complicated hereditary spastic paraparesis can present with a host of neurologic features, including seizures, dementia, cataracts, adrenal insufficiency, extrapyramidal disturbance, optic neuropathy, retinopathy, deafness, mental retardation, ichthyosis, cutaneous abnormalities, peripheral neuropathy with or without atrophy of intrinsic hand and feet muscles, cranial nerve dysfunction, bulbar muscle weakness, and sensory impairment.

The diagnosis of hereditary spastic paraparesis is made clinically and is one of exclusion. Laboratory testing has focused on genetic analysis. Genetic analysis is used to confirm the diagnosis and assists in genetic counseling. Neuroimaging studies are also used to assist in excluding alternative diagnoses. Magnetic resonance imaging of the spinal cord may be normal or show atrophy in the thoracolumbar regions. Magnetic resonance imaging of the brain is usually normal. Electrophysiologic studies are usually normal in uncomplicated hereditary spastic paraparesis.

Treatment for hereditary spastic paraparesis is symptomatic only, with no current treatment available to prevent, retard, or reverse the underlying degenerative process. Modulation of the hypertonicity can be attempted pharmacologically with oral, neurolytic, or intrathecal interventions. The mainstay of therapeutic intervention is the implementation of physical therapy. Therapy treatments for spasticity include cold application, manual stretching techniques, splinting, serial casting, posture and body mechanics training, aerobic conditioning, and gait and dynamic balance training.

Gait training is best done after an evaluation for lower extremity bracing and assistive devices to facilitate mobility, independence, and prevention of falls. Given the progressive nature of the disease, an integral aspect of treatment is psychologic support and social services.[12,57]

Dystonia

Dystonia is a movement disorder characterized by muscle contraction resulting in twisting, turning, and posturing. Dystonia may be generalized, focal, and segmental (affecting two or more adjacent parts of the body). Some patterns of dystonia have been defined as specific syndromes, such as cervical dystonia and blepharospasm. Dystonia can be primary (idiopathic or inherited) or secondary to another process (environmental or basal ganglia disease).

No specific treatment for dystonia has been universally successful. Focal cervical dystonia and blepharospasm are frequently treated with botulinum toxin. General dystonias have been responsive to such medications as those affecting GABA (baclofen and clonazepam) and those affecting dopamine (levodopa and bromocriptine). Physical therapy techniques such as therapy, massage, and biofeedback need to be individualized to address each patient's specific problems and attributes. A continuing focus on range of motion and movement is of benefit.

Tourette syndrome

Tourette syndrome is a constellation of symptoms including tic disorders and comorbid neurobehavioral problems. The diagnostic criteria for Tourette syndrome include multiple motor tics and one or more vocal tics, which must be present for at least 1 year, with an age of onset prior to 18 years. The diagnosis of Tourette syndrome is often delayed until adulthood. Because the diagnosis of Tourette syndrome can be challenging, diagnosis is delayed an average of 6.8 years. There is a common prevalence across races and cultures. There is strong support for a genetic component to Tourette syndrome. The diagnosis of Tourette syndrome is based on clinical findings, because diagnostic studies have not demonstrated consistent findings.

Tics are defined as involuntary, sudden, rapid, repetitive, non-rhythmic, stereotyped movements or vocalizations. They vary in severity and duration, and typically wax and wane. Often, tics diminish with distraction, relaxation, and when engaged in activities requiring selective attention. They often intensify with anxiety, anger, excitement, stress, and fatigue.

The tic disorders in Tourette syndrome are often associated with emotional and behavioral dysfunction. These include obsessive–compulsive behaviors, hyperkinetic disorder (attention deficit hyperactivity disorder), impulsive and self-destructive behavior, sleep abnormalities, alterations in mood and sexual behavior, phobias, and anxieties. These often compound the overall morbidity of the disease and detract from quality of life. Hyperkinetic disorder occurs in 50–75% of those diagnosed with Tourette syndrome. Obsessive–compulsive disorder occurs 20–60% of the time, in a variable degree of severity. A variety of mood disorders are also associated with Tourette syndrome. These include anxiety, phobias, depression, labile mood, panic disorder, and agoraphobia.

The major treatment options for Tourette syndrome include both pharmacotherapeutic and psychotherapeutic interventions. Because of the potential side effects, drug treatment of tic symptoms is limited to patients with disabling symptoms. It is frequently difficult to distinguish between medication response and the spontaneous waning of symptoms. Typically, the first choices of medications for tic suppression are α_2-adrenergic agonists (clonidine) or neuroleptics such as haloperidol or pimozide. Atypical neuroleptics such as risperidone (Risperdal) are often used as second-line agents. Other pharmacologic options include pergolide, baclofen, and botulinum

toxin injections. The use of psychostimulants in the treatment of hyperkinetic disorder in Tourette syndrome is controversial, because there is concern that these medications can exacerbate tic behavior. More recent studies dispute this, and support the combined use of psychostimulants with α-adrenergic agents when hyperkinetic disorder is associated with tic behaviors. Other pharmacologic agents that have been employed include desipramine and bupropion.

A wide variety of behavioral treatment strategies are utilized in conjunction with pharmacotherapeutic intervention in the treatment of tic symptoms. There is no clear indication for the utilization of one specific type of behavioral treatment strategy. The most commonly employed technique is 'massed (negative) practice'. This strategy involves repeated, rapid, voluntary, and effortful performance of an identified tic for a specific period of time, interspersed with brief periods of rest.[21,38,52,53]

SURGICAL INTERVENTIONS FOR PARKINSON DISEASE AND OTHER MOVEMENT DISORDERS

The past decade has seen an explosion of neurosurgical techniques for Parkinson disease. The strategies included for intervention have included transplantation of bioactive materials to replace the dopaminergic loss, selective central nervous system lesioning to rebalance the neurotransmitter milieu, and deep brain stimulation that attempts to restore the neurotransmitter balance through a non-ablative technique. The two broad indications for neurosurgical interventions are reversal of the neurodegenerative process (more applicable to the transplantation therapy), and recalcitrant symptoms of dyskinesias and fluctuation despite maximal medical treatment (more applicable to lesioning and deep brain stimulation). The precise algorithms for transplant substrates and lesioning or stimulation targets continue to evolve. Careful patient selection and close follow-up appear to be paramount for successful outcome. While the risk of adverse events following surgeries of this nature is low compared with other neurosurgical procedures, clinicians must recognize the potential risks for hemorrhage, infection, stimulation of a non-targeted area, postoperative confusion, and hardware failure.[22] Shortwave diathermy, a modality that is occasionally used in the rehabilitation setting, carries the risk of neurologic damage and is contraindicated in these patients.[33] Some dystonias other than Parkinson disease have also been successfully treated with deep brain stimulation.

The orthopedic interventions for movement disorders are somewhat limited. Spinal fusion might be indicated for neurologically based scoliosis, which has been reported in Friedreich ataxia patients. Because of the high potential coincidence of Parkinson disease and osteoarthritis, joint replacement may be a consideration. Length of stay for patients with Parkinson disease undergoing this procedure is longer than for non-Parkinson disease patients. The functional outcome of Parkinson disease patients undergoing joint replacement is related to the degree of neurologic severity at the time of referral.[10,59]

GENETIC CONSIDERATIONS IN MOVEMENT DISORDERS

Understanding of the molecular biology for movement disorders continues to grow at an exponential pace. The knowledge gain has three general categories of potential therapeutic benefit: diagnosis, prognosis, and intervention. From a diagnostic viewpoint, the genetic classification of these diseases will continue to emerge. As with Huntington disease and Friedreich ataxia, disorders that once were broadly grouped will be more specifically diagnosed. The use of genetic testing for these diseases will assist in earlier diagnosis of the symptomatic patient, as well as in identification of the genetic risk in family members. As the diagnostic specificity improves, the ability of clinicians to accurately prognosticate disease course will similarly improve. Both pharmacologic and non-pharmacologic interventions will gain more specificity. The ultimate goal of treatment might well be an actual modification of genetic substrates at the heart of these diseases.

SUMMARY

The movement disorders represent a challenging set of diseases for physiatrists. The therapeutic utility and specificity of rehabilitative interventions for these syndromes lack a strong evidence-based foundation. In parallel to other neurologic disease, rehabilitation has the potential to impact disease disability for these disorders.

REFERENCES

1. Atadzhanov M, Rakhimdhanov A. Dopamine deficiency and cholinergic models of Parkinson's syndrome. Neurology 1993; S126–S129.
2. Bilney B, Morris ME, Perry A. Effectiveness of physiotherapy, occupational therapy, and speech pathology for people with Huntington's disease: a systematic review. Neurorehabil Neural Repair 2003; 17:12–24.
3. Cedarbaum JM, McDowell FH. Sixteen-year follow-up of 100 patients begun on levodopa in 1968: emerging problems. Adv Neurol 1987; 45:469–472.
4. Chaudhuri KR. Autonomic dysfunction in movement disorders. Curr Opin Neurol 2001; 14:505–511.
5. Cubo E, Moore CG, Leurgans S, et al. Wheeled and standard walkers in Parkinson's disease patients with gait freezing. Parkinsonism Relat Disord 2003; 10:9–14.
6. Culbertson WC, Moberg PJ, Duda JE, et al. Assessing the executive function deficits of patients with Parkinson's disease: utility of the Tower of London–Drexel. Assessment 2004; 11:27–39.
7. Deane KH, Jones D, Playford ED, et al. Physiotherapy for patients with Parkinson's disease: a comparison of techniques. Cochrane Database Syst Rev 2001:CD002817.
8. Deane KH, Whurr R, Clarke CE, et al. Non-pharmacological therapies for dysphagia in Parkinson's disease. Cochrane Database Syst Rev 2001: CD002816.
9. Dibble LE, Nicholson DE, Shultz B, et al. Sensory cueing effects on maximal speed gait initiation in persons with Parkinson's disease and healthy elders. Gait Posture 2004; 19:215–225.
10. Fast A, Mendelsohn E, Sosner J. Total knee arthroplasty in Parkinson's disease. Arch Phys Med Rehabil 1994; 75:1269–1270.
11. Ferrante RJ, Andreassen OA, Jenkins BG, et al. Neuroprotective effects of creatine in a transgenic mouse model of Huntington's disease. J Neurosci 2000; 20:4389–4397.
12. Fink JK. Hereditary spastic paraplegia. Neurol Clin 2002; 20:711–726.
13. Goldstein DS, Holmes CS, Dendi R, et al. Orthostatic hypotension from sympathetic denervation in Parkinson's disease. Neurology 2002; 58:1247–1255.
14. Harris-Love MO, Siegel KL, Paul SM, et al. Rehabilitation management of Friedreich ataxia: lower extremity force-control variability and gait performance. Neurorehabil Neural Repair 2004; 18:117–124.
15. Hersch SM. Huntington's disease: prospects for neuroprotective therapy 10 years after the discovery of the causative genetic mutation. Curr Opin Neurol 2003; 16:501–506.
16. Hirsch MA, Toole T, Maitland CG, et al. The effects of balance training and high-intensity resistance training on persons with idiopathic Parkinson's disease. Arch Phys Med Rehabil 2003; 84:1109–1117.
17. Homberg V. Motor training in the therapy of Parkinson's disease. Neurology 1993; 43:S45–S46.
18. Howe TE, Lovgreen B, Cody FW, et al. Auditory cues can modify the gait of persons with early-stage Parkinson's disease: a method for enhancing parkinsonian walking performance? Clin Rehabil 2003; 17:363–367.
19. Lance JW, Schwab RS, Peterson EA. Action tremor and the cogwheel phenomenon in Parkinson's disease. Brain 1963; 86:95–110.
20. Landin S, Hagenfeldt L, Saltin B, et al. Muscle metabolism during exercise in patients with Parkinson's disease. Clin Sci Mol Med 1974; 47:493–506.
21. Leckman JF. Tourette's syndrome. Lancet 2002; 360:1577–1586.
22. Lozano AM, Mahant N. Deep brain stimulation surgery for Parkinson's disease: mechanisms and consequences. Parkinsonism Relat Disord 2004; 10(suppl 1):S49–S57.
23. Lundervold DA, Poppen R. Biobehavioral rehabilitation for older adults with essential tremor. Gerontologist 1995; 35:556–559.
24. Marttila RJ, Rinne UK. Disability and progression in Parkinson's disease. Acta Neurol Scand 1977; 56:159–169.
25. Mayeux R, Stern Y, Cote L, et al. Altered serotonin metabolism in depressed patients with Parkinson's disease. Neurology 1984; 34:642–646.
26. Mayeux R, Stern Y, Rosen J, et al. Depression, intellectual impairment, and Parkinson disease. Neurology 1981; 31:645–650.
27. McDowell FH, Cedarbaum JM. The extrapyramidal system and disorders of movement. In: Joynt R, ed. Clinical neurology. Philadelphia: JB Lippincott; 1991.
28. Miyai I, Fujimoto Y, Ueda Y, et al. Treadmill training with body weight support: its effect on Parkinson's disease. Arch Phys Med Rehabil 2000; 81:849–852.
29. Miyai I, Fujimoto Y, Yamamoto H, et al. Long-term effect of body weight–supported treadmill training in Parkinson's disease: a randomized controlled trial. Arch Phys Med Rehabil 2002; 83:1370–1373.
30. Nagaya M, Kachi T, Yamada T, et al. Videofluorographic study of swallowing in Parkinson's disease. Dysphagia 1998; 13:95–100.
31. Neafsey EJ, Hull CD, Buchwald NA. Preparation for movement in the cat. I. Unit activity in the cerebral cortex. Electroencephalogr Clin Neurophysiol 1978; 44:706–713.
32. Neafsey EJ, Hull CD, Buchwald NA. Preparation for movement in the cat. II. Unit activity in the basal ganglia and thalamus. Electroencephalogr Clin Neurophysiol 1978; 44:714–723.
33. Nutt JG, Anderson VC, Peacock JH, et al. DBS and diathermy interaction induces severe CNS damage. Neurology 2001; 56:14–1386.
34. Pellecchia MT, Grasso A, Biancardi LG, et al. Physical therapy in Parkinson's disease: an open long-term rehabilitation trial. J Neurol 2004; 251:595–598.
35. Poewe WH, Wenning GK. The natural history of Parkinson's disease. Ann Neurol 1998; 44:S1–S9.
36. Pollock M, Hornabrook RW. The prevalence, natural history and dementia of Parkinson's disease. Brain 1966; 89:429–448.
37. Potulska A, Friedman A, Krolicki L, et al. Swallowing disorders in Parkinson's disease. Parkinsonism Relat Disord 2003; 9:349–353.
38. Pringsheim T, Davenport WJ, Lang A. Tics. Curr Opin Neurol 2003; 16:523–527.
39. Rajput AH. Levodopa prolongs life expectancy and is non-toxic to substantia nigra. Parkinsonism Relat Disord 2001; 8:95–100.
40. Ramig LO, Sapir S, Countryman S, et al. Intensive voice treatment (LSVT) for patients with Parkinson's disease: a 2 year follow up. J Neurol Neurosurg Psychiatry 2001; 71:493–498.

41. Reuter I, Engelhardt M, Freiwaldt J, et al. Exercise test in Parkinson's disease. Clin Auton Res 1999; 9:129–134.

42. Reuter I, Engelhardt M, Stecker K, et al. Therapeutic value of exercise training in Parkinson's disease. Med Sci Sports Exerc 1999; 31:1544–1549.

43. de Rijk MC, Launer LJ, Berger K, et al. Prevalence of Parkinson's disease in Europe: a collaborative study of population-based cohorts. Neurologic Diseases in the Elderly Research Group. Neurology 2000; 54:S21–S23.

44. Sabate M, Rodriguez M, Mendez E, et al. Obstructive and restrictive pulmonary dysfunction increases disability in Parkinson disease. Arch Phys Med Rehabil 1996; 77:29–34.

45. Saltin B, Landin S. Work capacity, muscle strength and SDH activity in both legs of hemiparetic patients and patients with Parkinson's disease. Scand J Clin Lab Invest 1975; 35:531–538.

46. Samii A, Nutt JG, Ransom BR. Parkinson's disease. Lancet 2004; 363:1783–1793.

47. Scatton B, Javoy-Agid F, Rouquier L, et al. Reduction of cortical dopamine, noradrenaline, serotonin and their metabolites in Parkinson's disease. Brain Res 1983; 275:321–328.

48. Schapira AH, Olanow CW. Neuroprotection in Parkinson disease: mysteries, myths, and misconceptions. JAMA 2004; 291:358–364.

49. Schenkman M, Butler RB. A model for multisystem evaluation treatment of individuals with Parkinson's disease. Phys Ther 1989; 69:932–943.

50. Senard JM, Rai S, Lapeyre-Mestre M, et al. Prevalence of orthostatic hypotension in Parkinson's disease. J Neurol Neurosurg Psychiatry 1997; 63:584–589.

51. Shabnam GN, Th C, Kho D, et al. Therapies for depression in Parkinson's disease. Cochrane Database Syst Rev 2003:CD003465.

52. Singer HS. Current issues in Tourette syndrome. Mov Disord 2000; 15:1051–1063.

53. Singer HS. The treatment of tics. Curr Neurol Neurosci Rep 2001; 1:195–202.

54. Stern MB. Parkinson's disease. In: Johnson RT, Griffin JW, eds. Current therapy in neurologic disease. 4th edn. St. Louis: Mosby; 1993: 252–256.

55. Suteerawattananon M, Morris GS, Etnyre BR, et al. Effects of visual and auditory cues on gait in individuals with Parkinson's disease. J Neurol Sci 2004; 219:63–69.

56. de Swart BJ, Willemse SC, Maassen BA, et al. Improvement of voicing in patients with Parkinson's disease by speech therapy. Neurology 2003; 60:498–500.

57. Tallaksen CM, Durr A, Brice A. Recent advances in hereditary spastic paraplegia. Curr Opin Neurol 2001; 14:457–463.

58. Visser M, Marinus J, Bloem BR, et al. Clinical tests for the evaluation of postural instability in patients with Parkinson's disease. Arch Phys Med Rehabil 2003; 84:1669–1674.

59. Weber M, Cabanela ME, Sim FH, et al. Total hip replacement in patients with Parkinson's disease. Int Orthop 2002; 26:66–68.

60. Weintraub D, Moberg PJ, Duda JE, et al. Effect of psychiatric and other nonmotor symptoms on disability in Parkinson's disease. J Am Geriatr Soc 2004; 52:784–788.

61. Weintraub D, Moberg PJ, Duda JE, et al. Recognition and treatment of depression in Parkinson's disease. J Geriatr Psychiatry Neurol 2003; 16:178–183.

Chapter

53

Comprehensive Management of Multiple Sclerosis

George H. Kraft and Theodore Brown

Comprehensive rehabilitative care is not a new concept to readers of this text. Yet providers of care to persons with multiple sclerosis (MS) have only recently begun to appreciate the value of these management techniques. Indeed, today, as in 1999, rehabilitation is still the only way to *improve function* in patients with MS.[120]

Multiple sclerosis is now recognized as a complex disease with at least four pathologic types (Fig. 53-1) and four clinical courses (Fig. 53-2). It is not clear that all the immunomodulating agents available are equally effective for all forms of MS. Because the relapsing–remitting (R–R) form is the most common and the easiest to study in clinical trials (by counting relapses), almost all the drug trials have been done in this type of MS.

This is a satisfying time to be providing care to patients with MS. A number of medications are available to ameliorate disease activity, effective drugs are available to manage symptoms, and there is increasing acceptance of the importance of rehabilitative services for patients.[140]

DISEASE OVERVIEW

Demographics

Multiple sclerosis is the most common cause of non-traumatic disability affecting young adults in the northern hemisphere.[73] There are thought to be 400 000 persons in the USA with MS, and the prevalence ranges from 40 to 220 per 100 000, with the highest prevalences in the highest latitudes. Similar latitudinal differences are seen throughout the northern hemisphere. In the southern hemisphere, the highest prevalence also appears to be in latitudes farthest from the equator, although the much smaller land mass challenges demographic study.[123]

In certain populations, such as the Chinese, MS is a relatively rare disease, with current estimates at 20 per 100 000, even in the northern latitudes of the country (Bo Zhao Chong, personal communication). In other populations, such as native Africans, MS is virtually unknown. However, as white ancestry becomes intermingled with that of Africans, the likelihood of developing the disease increases, although never as high as in those of pure white ancestry. However, the course in such patients may progress rapidly and be very difficult to manage; the disease is less common but much more severe.

Approximately 85% of patients have either the R–R or secondary progressive (SP) forms. SP MS typically develops after many years of the disease state. Untreated, the average R–R patient will transition into SP by 10 years.[73] The R–R/SP form is gender-dependent, with more than twice as many females as males having this disease.[147] The typical R–R patient is a white woman in her late twenties who was born in a temperate latitude and whose ancestors came from northern Europe.[123]

Ten to fifteen percent of patients with MS have a disease that is progressive from the outset. This type, called primary progressive (PP) MS, has a roughly equal female to male ratio, and a much later onset, around age 40.[213] The fourth type of MS, progressive–relapsing (P–R), is much less common.

Etiology

Epidemiologic studies have given clues about the etiology of MS. The current view is that it is the product of both a genetic predisposition and an early-acquired unknown environmental factor. Migration studies indicate that the likelihood of developing the disease depends on where a person spent the early years. Such data suggest that either a causative factor was acquired in the more temperate latitudes or a protective factor was acquired in the less temperate latitudes.[43,45,213] Because MS was unknown in the Faroe Islands until after the invasion by British troops in World War II, and because it appeared to persist in 'waves' of disease since that time, Kurtzke has proposed that a transmissible agent, the 'primary MS affection', with a long but variable latent period, is responsible for the disease.[125,124]

An environmental factor, however, is not the entire answer. Persons with certain specific tissue antigens appear to be either vulnerable to the disease or protected from it. Persons of northern European ancestry, especially those with HLA-DR2 in DR-positive families, have a greater chance of developing the disease.[8] In a Spanish population, positive associations are especially strong with the DR2 haplotype, particularly the allele DQB1*0602.[54] The blood–immune system is a tissue, hence controlled by the human leukocyte antigens (HLAs).

An attractive hypothesis of the etiology of MS is that genetically susceptible individuals (persons with certain HLA types) could have an aberration in their immune tolerance, allowing environmental antigens to stimulate production of auto-reactive T cells. When such antigens are later encountered in adulthood, they might set off an attack against components of the person's own myelin ('molecular mimicry').[122,186] It is of interest that antiviral medications appear to have a small protective value in

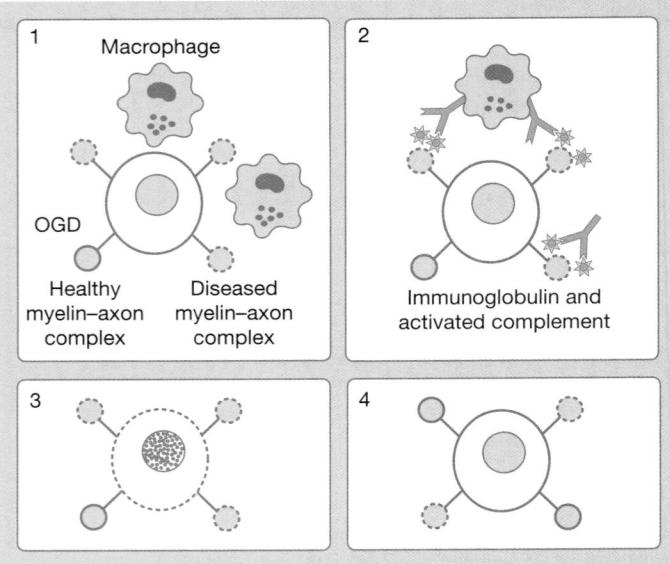

Figure 53-1 The four pathologic types of multiple sclerosis, as identified by Lucchinetti et al. Type 1 is cell-mediated destruction of myelin. Type 2 is cell-mediated destruction of myelin with immunoglobulin and activated complement. Type 3 is a primary oligodendrogliopathy with apoptosis. Type 4 is a neurodegenerative oligodendrogliopathy. Type 2 is the most common, and type 4 the least common. (After Lassmann et al. 2001,[129] with permission.) OGD, oligodendrocyte.

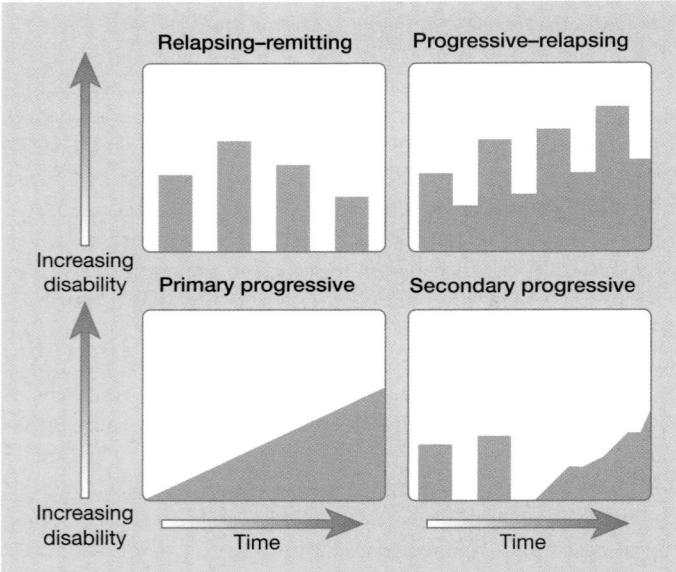

Figure 53-2 The four clinical courses of multiple sclerosis: relapsing–remitting, progressive–relapsing, primary progressive, and secondary progressive.

reducing the exacerbations of MS.[12,132] This molecular mimicry might later develop into a self-perpetuating degenerative loop through the concept of 'epitope spreading'.[203] This is one among many postulated mechanisms. Reviews of other hypotheses are available.[150]

Pathophysiology

The pathologic hallmark of MS is the presence of multifocal demyelinated plaques scattered throughout the central nervous system, with prominent involvement of the periventricular white matter, optic nerves, brain stem, cerebellum, and spinal cord. Demyelination is accompanied by axonal transection and ovoid body formation.[193] Another characteristic feature is that these lesions tend to surround the deep veins of the brain, contributing one of the characteristic radiologic features of MS, called Dawson's fingers. These are ovoid lesions perpendicular to the long axis of the lateral ventricles.[102]

Newer techniques, including magnetic resonance spectroscopy (MRS), diffusion-weighted imaging, and magnetization transfer ratio (MTR), have shown widespread neuronal deficits in otherwise normal-appearing white matter.[39,91,204] The progressive development of brain atrophy is a well-known feature of MS. Many studies have shown that atrophy of the brain is present from the earliest stages of the disease and tends to progress as the disease evolves.[142]

Researchers have tried for decades to identify a single pathogenetic mechanism that would allow the development of more precise immunotherapy. It now appears that subgroups of patients with MS have different pathogenic mechanisms, which might not correspond to their clinical MS types. The results of an international multicenter collaborative study of MS pathology led by Claudia Lucchinetti has identified four distinct pathologic patterns of MS (see Fig. 53–1). Pattern 1 involves macrophages and demyelination (cell-mediated); pattern 2 is similar to 1, but with intralesional immunoglobulins and activated complement (cell- and antibody-mediated); pattern 3 involves apoptosis of oligodendrocytes with selective loss of myelin-associated glycoprotein; and pattern 4 involves primary degeneration of oligodendrocytes.[131] Patterns 1 and 2 target myelin, and 3 and 4 target oligodendrocytes. Differences in antibody recognition and response to immunotherapy have been identified in these four patterns.[129] In the future, gene expression analysis or other biomarkers might be able to identify the pathologic pattern without need for central nervous system biopsy.

Clinical presentation

In the most common type of MS, the R–R form, the initial symptoms typically remit completely, and are followed months to years later by a recurrence of those symptoms or the development of new ones. This relapse also goes into remission in most patients. During this R–R stage, the cycle is repeated a number of times, with long breaks between relapses. Eventually, the remissions are less complete, and there is a progression of disease. The patient who began with the R–R form finds that the disease has now advanced into the SP form, where relapses assume a less prominent pattern in the course as the disease slowly worsens. Approximately 85% of all persons with MS have the R–R/SP form of disease, with characteristics of approximately 2.5 : 1 female : male and a typical age of onset in the late twenties.[123]

For the remaining 15%, the majority have progression of symptoms from the onset without any remissions. This is the

Box 53-1 Traditional subject-reported symptoms of multiple sclerosis listed in order of decreasing frequency[111]

- Fatigue
- Balance problems
- Weakness or paralysis
- Numbness, tingling, or other sensory disturbance
- Bladder problems
- Increased muscle tension (spasticity)
- Bowel problems
- Difficulty remembering
- Depression
- Pain
- Laughing or crying easily (emotional lability)
- Double or blurred vision, partial or complete blindness
- Shaking (tremor)
- Speech and/or communication difficulties
- Difficulty solving problems

hypointensities can eventually become isointense and disappear. Enhancing T1 lesions are more reversible than non-enhancing lesions. Ring-enhancing lesions, which can be due to a ring of inflammation, are prone to become persistent T1 'black holes'.[169,199] Initial axonal loss and degree of remyelination may determine the outcome.[15]

Indices of brain atrophy (brain parenchymal fraction and ventricular fraction) show that increased tissue loss is seen in all subtypes of MS. The rate of brain atrophy is higher in younger than in older patients.[98] Baseline T2 lesion load is a statistically significant predictor of disease-related brain atrophy in patients with established MS.[24] A 14-year longitudinal study of a group of patients with clinically isolated neurologic syndrome has shown convincingly that baseline T2 lesion load also correlates highly with eventual MS diagnosis.[17] In this setting, the detection of one or more baseline brain lesions carries a risk of MS of almost 90%. For a single bout of optic neuritis, the 10-year probability of developing MS in patients with any MRI white matter lesions was 55%, compared with 0 in patients without such lesions.[68] These findings support the use of disease-modifying therapy in symptomatic patients with MRI abnormalities even before the diagnosis of MS has been established by standard (e.g. McDonald) criteria. For those who choose not to take therapy, we recommend annual MRI to monitor for change in lesion load.

Other techniques, including those that are now used for research, might soon enter clinical practice. One of these is MRS, which can identify N-acetyl-aspartate (NAA), a marker of axon damage, and lipids.[113] Another is magnetic transfer ratio (MTR). These have shown widespread gray matter and neuronal deficits in otherwise normal-appearing white matter.[39,91,204]

Besides MRI, there are no good paraclinical markers to observe patients with established MS. Repeat MRI scans should be obtained when there is uncertainty as to whether a patient is responding well to therapy; these should include the spinal cord, especially cervical portion, where appropriate. There is no consensus regarding the importance of obtaining routine MRI scans in patients who are clinically doing well on therapy.

PP form, which is seen equally in women and men and begins typically at a considerably older age (e.g. around age 40).[213] A small number of patients have P–R MS, which represents the smallest subtype. Probably no more than 5% of patients with MS have this form.[73] It is often difficult to distinguish P–R from PP disease, and effective medical treatment for these subtypes is unclear. Just as in the PP form, rehabilitative techniques remain the mainstay of management.[120]

The classic symptoms of MS are manifold, and are listed in decreasing frequency in Box 53-1. No other neurologic disease produces the coexistence of so many problems: weakness, fatigue, spasticity, tremor, ataxia, sensory loss, pain, blindness, cognitive impairment, depression, and neurogenic organ dysfunction (e.g. neurogenic bladder and bowel). The fact that they progress at an unpredictable rate further complicates management.

However, recently physicians and patients have come to realize that cognitive problems and depression occur much more frequently than previously appreciated. The point prevalence of depression is now thought to be greater than 40%,[26] and lifetime cognitive impairment greater than 60–80%.[26,163] Clinicians now know that for every apparent (motor, sensory, or visual) exacerbation, there are between six and eight 'subclinical' exacerbations, often previously unrecognized and manifest as emotional or cognitive problems.[80]

Neuroimaging
Magnetic resonance imaging (MRI) has become the single most important diagnostic modality in MS. This is reflected in the recent McDonald criteria, which allow the diagnosis of MS to be made without a second clinical attack if there is a new enhancing lesion on MRI 3 months after the initial attack.[139]

A typical MS lesion is ovoid; >5 mm in diameter; and located in the periventricular, corpus callosal, or posterior fossa white matter. Pathology indicates that such lesions usually correspond to demyelination, although 40% contain some degree of remyelination.[9] T2 lesions generally persist, whereas 44% of new T1

Cerebrospinal fluid abnormalities
Multiple sclerosis remains a clinical diagnosis, but cerebrospinal fluid (CSF) examination can help clarify uncertain cases. White blood cell count and protein levels are normal in two-thirds of MS cases; gross elevations of either suggests a different etiology. Immunoglobulin oligoclonal bands are present in 83–94% of patients with MS when the test is performed with isoelectric focusing.[130] With optic neuritis onset, the presence of oligoclonal bands is also predictive of eventual diagnosis of MS.[93]

Neurophysiologic studies
Evoked potentials (EPs) can be used to identify 'hidden' lesions, which assist in identifying additional sites of abnormality that are required to make a diagnosis of 'multiple' sclerosis. Conduction also demonstrates the state of myelin. Altered or absent myelin causes conduction slowing or conduction block. If conduction slowing through portions of the central neuraxis is

found, the diagnosis of a demyelinating disease is strongly supported. Other pathologic conditions that might be mistaken clinically for a demyelinating disease (e.g. vascular lesions or tumor) would probably produce conduction block with attenuation or absence of a response rather than a significant conduction slowing.[112] Recommendations for the use of somatosensory evoked potentials (SEPs) in MS can be found in practice topics published by the American Association of Neuromuscular and Electrodiagnostic Medicine (AANEM).[107]

Early studies of visual evoked potentials (VEPs), brain stem evoked potentials, and SEPs concluded that VEPs were more sensitive than SEPs in demonstrating central nervous system conduction abnormalities in MS.[162,194] However, early investigators generally evaluated the short cord SEP pathway available with median nerve testing, and did not evaluate SEPs from the lower limbs. Because MS lesions can occur throughout the brain, brain stem, and spinal cord, SEP techniques utilizing the entire central neuraxis are most likely to demonstrate conduction abnormalities. Lower limb SEP testing increases the yield of abnormalities when compared with upper limb testing, and is comparable with the yield of VEPs.[179]

Visual evoked potentials are frequently ordered for the evaluation of a patient with suspected MS to assess the presence of subclinical optic neuritis, in an attempt to confirm the presence of a second site of disease and to confirm that a visual deficit is indeed due to optic neuritis. The technique for these is well established.[25] In relating the correlation of evoked potentials to structural MRI changes, there is a correlation between abnormal conduction in the visual pathway and MRS-measured NAA levels.[83]

Diagnostic criteria

The clinical diagnosis of MS consists of a course in which there are two or more occurrences of central nervous system symptoms and signs separated in time and space. Common symptoms include optic neuritis, fatigue, weakness, dysesthesias, tremor, ataxia, bladder dysfunction, spasticity, cognitive problems, depression, and pain.

In the 1960s, MS diagnosis was based entirely on clinical findings.[173] In the early 1980s, these were modified to allow the substitution of some laboratory tests for clinical findings.[159] Most recently, MRI has been allowed to substitute for some clinical findings and courses. The McDonald criteria (Table 53-1) represent the current standard of diagnosis.[139] Using MRI as well as VEPs, these criteria allow for an earlier diagnosis of MS than previously possible.

It is known that the McDonald criteria err on the side of conservancy and might under-diagnose some patients with MS. Examples of this under-diagnosis include those in the early stages of disease, or those with primarily spinal cord disease.[10,190]

Improvements in MRI techniques have reduced the importance of CSF and evoked potential evaluations for diagnosis. SEPs can still be useful in screening the spinal cord for possible

Table 53-1 The McDonald criteria for multiple sclerosis[139]

Presentation	Additional requirements for diagnosis
More than two exacerbations; evidence of more than two lesions	None
More than two exacerbations; evidence of one lesion	Magnetic resonance imaging (MRI)-demonstrated dissemination in space *or* more than two multiple sclerosis (MS) lesions observed through MRI and positive cerebrospinal fluid (CSF) *or* further exacerbation implicating a second site
One exacerbation; objective clinical evidence of more than two lesions	MRI-demonstrated dissemination in time *or* second exacerbation
One exacerbation; objective clinical evidence of one lesion	MRI-demonstrated dissemination in space *or* more than two MS lesions observed through MRI and positive CSF, and MRI-demonstrated dissemination in time *or* second exacerbation
Insidious neurologic progression suggestive of MS	Positive CSF *and* dissemination in space, demonstrated by: • more than nine T2 lesions in the brain; • or more than two lesions in the spinal cord; • or four to eight brain lesions plus one spinal cord lesion *or* abnormal visual evoked potential associated with four to eight brain lesions, or with fewer than four brain lesions plus one spinal cord lesion demonstrated by MRI *and* MRI-demonstrated dissemination in time *or* continued progression for 1 year

MS lesions, confirm the presence of demyelination, and to monitor changes in physiologic function. MRI scans look at structure and EPs measure function; they are generally comparable and complementary.[69]

With imaging technology, MRI scans are able to see ever-smaller lesions. Some research MRI scans are now in the 8-Tesla range and are able to detect minute abnormalities in the central nervous system. It can be anticipated that, as these MRI scans eventually enter clinical practice, diagnostic criteria will be modified futher.

For several weeks after the occurrence of the breakdown in the blood–brain barrier, the affected region is permeable to gadolinium. Consequently, MRI scans taken shortly after the intravenous injection of gadolinium show 'enhancement' or increased density on T1-weighted images. Such techniques can identify acute lesions, and thereby identify a new lesion in time. It is argued that the observation of both enhancing and unenhancing lesions confirms the criterion of at least two points in time. Double- and triple-dose gadolinium injections are able to show even more subtle disease activity.[168]

Differential diagnosis

Multiple sclerosis is a diagnosis of exclusion, unless a brain biopsy is available. That means that no better explanation can be found for the clinical manifestations. For example, in a patient known to have lupus erythematosus or vasculitis, central nervous system disease should be attributed to the primary disease rather than to MS. The differential diagnosis for MS is long, and is found in numerous references.[150,156] Some 'rule out' diagnostic tests that should be ordered routinely are listed in Box 53-2. It is important to take a careful family history for clues that could warrant a search for inherited diseases. Because MS is uncommon in children, referral to a pediatric neurologist or MS specialist is recommended for pediatric cases.

There are several immune-mediated demyelinating diseases that are either MS variants or related diseases. Clinically isolated neurologic syndromes of unknown etiology (in MS

clinics known as 'clinically isolated syndromes') are the most common of these. These include optic neuritis, transverse myelitis, and acute disseminated encephalomyelitis. These diseases cannot be reliably differentiated from the initial clinical episode of MS without follow-up.

The diagnosis of neuromyelitis optica (Devic disease) requires the presence of both optic neuritis and acute myelitis (typically extending over several vertebral segments of the spinal cord) and absence of brain white matter lesions that meet radiologic criteria for MS. Distinguishing laboratory features of Devic disease include infrequent oligoclonal bands (35%), infrequent IgG index elevation, absence of CSF IgG_1 response, and positive serology for autoantibodies (including antinuclear antibodies and anti-DS DNA in up to 50% of cases).[148,209]

In patients with prominent signs of myelopathy with only subtle MRI changes in the brain, cervical MRI should be performed to rule out cervical stenosis. When white matter lesions in the brain are non-specific, finding cord lesions by MRI provides strong supporting evidence of MS. When the presenting neurologic symptoms are not associated with MRI abnormalities, one must always consider psychiatric disorders, conversion disorder, and malingering.

Prognosis

The median time until a cane is required is 20 years from the time of symptom onset and 30 years until wheelchair use.[34] About two-thirds of persons with MS are unemployed, and 75% of them attribute their unemployment to disability. The median survival time from onset is approximately 10 years shorter for patients with MS than for age-matched controls.[18] With the use of immunomodulating agents, however, the prognosis might be improving. Many patients might remain stable or progress only minimally in over a decade of living with the disease.[157]

Predictors of good prognosis include being female, younger age at onset, initial R–R type, complete recovery from first attack, longer time from first to second attack (>5 years is best), fewer than two relapses in the first 5 years, initial attack of optic neuritis and lack of apolipoprotein E ε4 allele.[34,42,187] The rate of disability progression does not differ between SP and PP MS once the patients reach a level of mild disability. For SP patients, the disease progression is no longer influenced by the presence or absence of relapses.

Among the existing measures of clinical status in MS, the most commonly used is Kurtzke's Expanded Disability Status Scale (EDSS), shown in Table 53-2.[126] It ranges from 0 (no impairment) to 10 (death from MS), with half-point levels along the way. It focuses on mobility more than sensory, bladder, bowel, communicative, or cognitive impairments. The mid-range is heavily weighted on ambulation and vulnerable to inter-rater and intrarater fluctuations. For example, the difference between an EDSS score of 5.5 and 5.0 is the difference in the ability to walk 100 m, but not 200 m, unaided. A change in EDSS must be at least two levels (one full point) to be considered significant, because the reliability of half-point changes is poor.[151]

Box 53-2 Diagnostic evaluation for multiple sclerosis

Routine
- Magnetic resonance imaging: brain and cord
- Antinuclear antibodies
- Lyme titers
- Rapid plasma reagin or VDRL
- Vitamin B_{12}
- Thyroid-stimulating hormone

When indicated
- Cerebrospinal fluid studies
- Evoked potentials
- HIV
- Genetic studies
- Electroencephalogram
- Coagulopathy studies
- Consultations: rheumatology, psychology, neuroophthalmology

Table 53-2 Kurtzke's Expanded Disability Status Scale[126]

Rating	Description[a]
0.0	Normal neurologic examination.
1.0	No disability; minimal signs on one functional system.
1.5	No disability; minimal signs on two of seven functional systems.
2.0	Minimal disability in one of seven functional systems.
2.5	Minimal disability in two functional systems.
3.0	Moderate disability in one functional system, or mild disability in three or four functional systems, although fully ambulatory.
3.5	Fully ambulatory but with moderate disability in one functional system and mild disability in one or two functional systems; or moderate disability in two functional systems; or mild disability in five functional systems.
4.0	Fully ambulatory without aid, up and about 12 h/day, despite relatively severe disability. Able to walk without aid 500 m.
4.5	Fully ambulatory without aid; up and about much of day; able to work a full day; may otherwise have some limitations of full activity or require minimal assistance. Relatively severe disability. Able to walk without aid 300 m.
5.0	Ambulatory without aid for about 200 m; disability impairs full daily activities.
5.5	Ambulatory for 100 m; disability precludes full daily activities.
6.0	Intermittent or unilateral constant assistance (cane, crutch, or brace) required to walk 100 m with or without resting.
6.5	Constant bilateral support (cane, crutch, walker, or braces) required to walk 20 m without resting.
7.0	Unable to walk beyond 5 m even with aid; essentially restricted to wheelchair; wheels self, transfers alone; active in wheelchair about 12 h/day.
7.5	Unable to take more than a few steps; restricted to wheelchair; may need aid to transfer; wheels self but may require motorized chair for full day's activities.
8.0	Essentially restricted to bed, chair, or wheelchair, but may be out of bed much of day; retains self-care functions; generally effective use of arms.
8.5	Essentially restricted to bed much of day; some effective use of arms; retains some self-care functions.
9.0	Helpless bed patient; can communicate and eat.
9.5	Unable to communicate effectively or to eat or swallow.
10.0	Death.

[a]Functional systems are the visual, brain stem, pyramidal, cerebellar, sensory, bladder and bowel, and mental systems.

Pregnancy

Pregnancy raises several complex issues in MS care. First is the question of hereditary transmission of MS. There is in fact an increased incidence of MS among the offspring of individuals with MS: 3% for girls and 1% for boys. On the other hand, MS does not appear to have a negative effect on the pregnancy itself or fetal outcome.[37]

Second is the question of what happens to exacerbation rates during and after pregnancy. During pregnancy, relapse rates decrease to about half of what they would be otherwise.[33] During the first 3 months postpartum, the relapse rate is higher than normal. The net effect of pregnancy on the course of MS is neutral, and women need not make decisions about pregnancy based on fear that it will worsen their disease.

The next question has to do with management of disease-modifying therapy during pregnancy. Given that the interferon beta drugs are all Food and Drug Administration (FDA) cate-

gory C for pregnancy (primarily because of increased rates of miscarriage), and that the risk of relapse is lower during pregnancy, the standard advice is that interferon beta drugs should be stopped before a woman gets pregnant. Glatiramer acetate is FDA category B for pregnancy, and might be a safer choice if a woman wishes to continue disease-modifying therapy during pregnancy. Restarting MS therapy after delivery should be delayed until breastfeeding is discontinued. Breastfeeding might decrease the relapse rate by half during the first 6 months postpartum.[77]

Medical management

Because MS is an immune-mediated disease, all effective pharmacotherapies to date are immunoactive drugs. These take three forms. First, there are medications that modify cellular immune responses, i.e. immunomodulatory drugs. This class includes the cytokine interferon beta (interferon beta-1b,

Table 53-3 Disease-modifying agents for multiple sclerosis

	Mitoxantrone (Novantrone)[a]	Interferon beta-1b (Betaseron)	Interferon beta-1a (Rebif)	Glatiramer acetate (Copaxone)	Interferon beta-1a (Avonex)
Indications	Worsening relapsing–remitting (R–R), secondary progressive (SP), or progressive–relapsing (P–R) multiple sclerosis (MS)	R–R MS or early SP MS	R–R MS or early SP MS	R–R MS	R–R MS or first demyelinating event
Subjects tested (Expanded Disability Status Scale[b])	≤6.0[82]	≤5.5	≤5.0	≤5.0	≤3.5
Dosage	12 mg/m^2 q. 3 months i.v. (8–10 lifetime doses)	0.25 mg (8 million IU) s.q. q.o.d.	44 μg (12 million IU) s.q. t.i.w.	20 mg s.q q.d.	30 μg (6 million IU) i.m. q. week
Relapse rate reduction (compared with placebo)	69%[82]	34%[71]	32%[71]	29%[71]	18%[71]
Effect on magnetic resonance imaging (reduction in new lesions)	100%[82]	83%[71]	78%[71]	35%[71]	33%[71]
Advantages	Only four times per year treatment	Autoinjector, does not need refrigeration	Autoinjector, premixed	No flu-like symptoms, autoinjector, premixed	Only weekly injection
Side effects	Menstrual disorders, cardiotoxicity, leukemia	Flu-like symptoms	Flu-like symptoms, stings	Transient chest pain	Flu-like symptoms
Laboratory monitoring	Echo left ventricular ejection fraction >50% and complete blood count and liver enzymes before each dose	Complete blood count and liver enzymes q. 3 months	Complete blood count and liver enzymes q. 3 months	None	Complete blood count and liver enzymes q. 3 months

[a]Although an effective agent, mitoxantrone is limited to 2–2½ years' use and has the most serious side effects.
[b]See Table 53-2.

Betaseron, and interferon beta-1a, Avonex or Rebif). It also includes the polymer glatiramer acetate (Copaxone), which acts as an antigen to produce anergy in myelin-reactive T cells. A second group is diverse, and contains drugs that interfere with inflammatory cell replication (antiproliferatives) or are directly cytotoxic. This class includes mitoxantrone (Novantrone), methotrexate, azathioprine, cyclophosphamide, and cladribine. The third group are drugs that block extracellular processes. This group includes intravenous immunoglobulin, plasmapheresis, and a monoclonal antibody, natalizumab (Tysabri) that blocks a cellular adhesion molecule (a4 integrin). Finally, there are drugs with multiple actions, including methylprednisolone, which is immunomodulatory at low doses and

cytotoxic at high doses. Table 53-3 outlines prescribing information for the currently approved treatments.

Immunomodulatory drugs

Theorizing that MS might be related to a viral infection, the first interferon to be tested in people with this disease was interferon gamma. The subjects unexpectedly had increased numbers of exacerbations. Realizing that interferon gamma production can be suppressed by interferon beta, this was studied next. Interferon beta showed a remarkable ability to suppress disease activity as monitored by clinical and MRI evaluations. We have subsequently learned that interferon beta decreases the expression of molecules needed for antigen presentation by antigen-presenting cells, reduces T-cell activation, and causes immune deviation toward a Th2 phenotype. It also inhibits blood–brain barrier leakage by suppressing the release of matrix metalloproteinase-9 by T cells.[46]

In the pivotal trial, interferon beta was tested in patients with up to a moderate degree of disease severity (EDSS 5.5). The three-armed phase 3 trial clearly demonstrated a dose–effect curve. On the high dose (8 million international units, subcutaneous, every other day), a 34% reduction in exacerbations and an 83% reduction in active MRI lesions was noted.[48] Interferon beta-1b (Betaseron) was approved by the FDA for use in R–R MS, and became available in limited quantities in the USA in late 1993.

A slightly different interferon beta was produced in mammalian culture to be structurally identical to human interferon beta. Based on a phase 3 trial demonstrating an 18% reduction in exacerbations and a 33% reduction in MRI activity, interferon beta-1a (Avonex) gained FDA approval for R–R MS in 1996.[92] This once-weekly intramuscularly injected interferon beta was studied in less severely affected patients, with an EDSS ranging up to and including 3.5. Later, another interferon beta, also produced in mammalian culture as interferon beta-1a, and administered subcutaneously three times a week (Rebif), was compared with intramuscular weekly interferon beta-1a.[155,161] On the basis of a greater reduction in the mean number of relapses and active MRI lesions, the subcutaneous formula (Rebif) was also FDA-approved. Rebif reduced exacerbations by 32% and MRI activity by 78%. This result, combined with a comparative study between interferon beta-1b and interferon beta-1a,[49] indicates that higher dose and frequency have a significant impact on the clinical efficacy of interferon beta.[71,152] In fact, the currently available high-dose interferon betas might not be dosed high enough for some patients. The Betaferon/Betaseron Efficacy Yielding Outcomes of a New Dose (BEYOND) study is comparing the standard dose of interferon beta-1b with a double dose.

The first large randomized controlled trial of interferon beta in the treatment of patients with SP MS was conducted in Europe with interferon beta-1b (Betaferon).[99] The subjects had EDSS scores of 3.0–6.5, a relatively early-stage sample of SP patients with MS. Interferon beta-1b reduced the relapse rate by 30% over a 3-year period, and had significant effects on progression of disability and change in MRI T2 lesion volume. It received FDA approval for the treatment of SP MS despite the inability to replicate beneficial results in a North American trial of interferon beta-1b in late-stage SP MS.[72] A randomized controlled trial of interferon beta-1a failed to show significant benefit in SP MS.[176]

Interferon beta has its greatest effect during the first year of treatment and on patients with MS with early, active disease. Pooling the results of all randomized controlled trials shows that it sharply reduces MRI activity within a few months of starting treatment, and reduces the number of patients who have exacerbations during the first year by about 27%.[56] It is estimated that nine patients need to be treated to prevent one patient having a clinical exacerbation at 1 year when the risk of exacerbation is 40%. Evidence supporting an effect on relapse rate during subsequent years, and supporting an effect on progression of disability, is less robust.

Glatiramer acetate is a polymer of four randomly ordered amino acids (glutamate, lysine, alanine, and tyrosine) in the same molar ratio as in myelin basic protein, the most important protein constituent of central nervous system myelin. Glatiramer acetate is taken up into endocytic vesicles of antigen-presenting cells, degraded into peptide fragments and complexed with major histocompatibility complex 2, and then presented to T-cell and B-cell receptors. It induces a shift from Th1 to Th2 T-helper cells, and this is believed to suppress the inflammatory process in the central nervous system ('bystander suppression').[212] Glatiramer acetate was tested in R–R patients with MS with an EDSS of up to 5.0, and demonstrated a 29% reduction in exacerbations at 24 months.[94] A subsequent study has shown glatiramer acetate to reduce active lesions on MRI by 29% at 9 months' treatment, compared with 90% for interferon beta at 9 months.[31,90] This discrepancy between a similar clinical effect and only modest MRI effect might be explained on a mechanism of activity different from that of interferons. Interferons are potent stabilizers of the blood–brain barrier, while glatiramer acetate-modified T cells cross the blood–brain barrier to have the desired effect. Glatiramer acetate is given as a daily subcutaneous injection, and it is indicated in R–R MS. Until a randomized trial comparing glatiramer acetate with an interferon beta is completed (the BEYOND and CombiRX trials are now underway), we will not know the relative efficacy of the two immunomodulatory drugs. The adverse effect profile of glatiramer acetate is generally milder.

Not all patients respond to all immunomodulatory treatment. Neutralizing antibodies evolve in a minority of patients who take interferon beta. The weight of evidence indicates that neutralizing antibodies slightly decrease the bioavailability of interferon and reduce the probability of remaining relapse-free.[134,181] Neutralizing antibodies are most common with interferon beta-1b and least common with intramuscular interferon beta-1a. Neutralizing antibodies to one interferon drug usually cross-react with other interferons. Neutralizing antibodies are found most frequently at 1–2 years into treatment and then decline in frequency; in some patients, neutralizing antibodies can disappear.

Antiproliferative drugs

Chemotherapeutic anticancer drugs such as methotrexate, azathioprine, and cyclophosphamide are some of the oldest treatments for MS. These have had some beneficial results, but the adverse effects limit their use. It has been difficult to fund large randomized controlled trials with these off-patent medications. More recently, mitoxantrone has been shown to markedly reduce relapse rate and gadolinium-enhancing MRI lesions in patients with worsening R–R MS and SP MS (a 100% reduction in new MRI lesions and a 69% reduction in relapse rate).[82] It is an anthracenedione, structurally related to anthracyclines such as doxorubicin, and it is administered by intravenous infusion every 3 months. Mitoxantrone has a number of side effects, including nausea, fatigue, and transient leukopenia. Most limiting, however, is that it is cardiotoxic and can cause congestive cardiomyopathy, for which reason the cumulative lifetime dose is limited to 140 mg/m^2, or 2½ years with standard dosing.[67]

Many other antiproliferative therapies for MS are being developed. Natalizumab blocks T-cell entry into the central nervous system. High-dose immunosuppressive therapy with autologous stem cell rescue and antilymphocytic antibody (alemtuzumab, Campath) are being studied with the objective of depleting the host of autoreactive T cells. They show promise but are also highly toxic.[30,103,108,109] Drugs that interfere with lymphocyte purine synthesis (cladribine and mycophenolate mofetil, CellCept) or pyrimidine synthesis (teriflunomide) are being investigated as potential oral agents in MS.[64]

Corticosteroids

Corticosteroids are an old class of medications used for MS.[160] They can reduce the severity and duration of exacerbations, but until recently were not felt to have any long-term effect on the course of the disease. As with chemotherapeutic agents, the toxicity profile of oral steroids was considered too great to use on an ongoing basis. In the 1970s, enthusiasm developed for the use of adrenocorticotropic hormone as a means of raising the level of endogenous corticosteroids,[167] but at present this treatment is rarely employed. Contrary to previous opinions, a careful recent study suggests that intravenous methylprednisolone might actually have some long-term benefit. Pulsed intravenous methylprednisolone given several times a year has been shown to slow the development of T1 black holes, delay brain atrophy, and slow progression in R–R MS.[214] It can also be used in SP MS when other options have been exhausted.[74]

Before treating with corticosteroids, it is important that the clinician be sure that the MS patient is not having a 'pseudo-exacerbation', which is an apparent flare of the disease due to a fever brought on by an infection. This infection is typically of the urinary tract, lungs, or sinus. If this is the case, the infection should be treated first. If a patient is having frequent exacerbations and is requiring intravenous methylprednisolone often (i.e. every month or two), the patient's immunomodulating medication should be reviewed. It might not be the right medication or dose for the patient.

Treatment of other forms of multiple sclerosis

The approach to R–R/SP MS has been described above. PP MS has yet to be proven vulnerable to any medication, although there is a trend toward a decreased rate of progression in male patients treated with glatiramer acetate.[188] Part of the problem is the difficulty of finding practical outcome measures. Because there are no relapses in PP MS and brain MRI findings are less active than in relapsing forms, the only relevant outcome measure is progression of disability. Because of its often insidious onset, patients with PP MS typically present in more advanced stages of disability and presumably are diagnosed later than those with relapsing forms.[34]

Multiple sclerosis variants such as Devic disease do not appear to respond to the conventional MS therapies. Treatment of these other inflammatory demyelinating diseases generally incorporates corticosteroids, often in conjunction with an antiproliferative medication. In the case of Devic disease, a standard regimen is a combination of prednisone and azathioprine at daily levels that can be tolerated indefinitely (typically on the order of 10 mg and 150 mg/day, respectively).

REHABILITATION

The rehabilitation approach

Multiple sclerosis is a progressive disease. The rate of progression is variable, as is the course. There are a number of fortunate persons with confirmed MS who, without treatment, function exceptionally well for many years. MS takes little toll on function or quality of life in these patients. At the other extreme are patients whose disease, even after intensive therapies, progresses relentlessly and who do not survive the various complications (e.g. pressure ulcers, pneumonia, and kidney disease) of a chronic and progressive neurologic disorder.

Multiple sclerosis is arguably the most difficult disease in which to achieve satisfactory long-term rehabilitation outcomes. It is a chronic disease in which patients retain stability at best. Rehabilitation goals for patients with MS can be moving targets. Despite disease-modifying agents, patients tend to get worse over time. In no other neurologic disease are so many portions of the central nervous system affected. MS has a progressive course that worsens in an uncertain pattern with a variable rate. There can be a week to week fluctuation as exacerbations give way to remissions. An exacerbation can occur at any time, and the hallmark of the disease is uncertainty as to what the future might present.

Historically, when rehabilitation was first begun for MS, the motor component of the disease alone was attended to. As one of the authors (GHK) was taught by a pioneer in the management of MS (Labe Sheinberg, M.D.), 'MS is a disease of ambulation'. This stage lasted into the mid 1970s.

During the next stage, it became apparent that patients with MS developed problems in other neurologic areas. During this stage, MS fatigue and pain were first recognized; work began on identifying the degree of cognitive impairment and depression, and attention was paid to neurogenic bladder function. Most of the non-motor symptoms were studied, and the disease was seen as a neurologic disorder producing problems in a variety of symptom areas.[111]

We are now entering a stage where we see a paradigm shift in the understanding of the disease and the toll it takes on family, friends, job, and community. For example, it is not just that MS can produce cognitive impairment, depression, and motor difficulties, it is also that with progressive neurologic loss diffusely manifested throughout the central nervous system, many central nervous system functions can be performed but require intense focus and consume large amounts of 'cognitive energy'. For example, a schoolteacher might still be a successful teacher, but needs to work exceptionally hard to continue functioning at the level that she or he quite easily achieved previously. To the school, the teacher appears to be doing a good job.

But the teacher might have no energy left over for any effective functioning at home. The summation of central nervous system losses can require tremendous energy to perform tasks; multitasking is not easily possible. Brain reorganization that has occurred as a result of plasticity, which allows performance of isolated tasks to continue, does not appear to easily allow multitasking.[118]

Inpatient rehabilitation approach

Relative to other patients admitted to the rehabilitation ward, patients with MS typically are younger and less disabled. They experience shorter lengths of stay, and make fewer improvements in activities of daily living (ADL) and mobility than do patients with head injury, spinal cord injury, or stroke.[21] Their stays are shorter, because the loss of function produced by exacerbations is usually a smaller interval of change than for most neurorehabilitation conditions that require admission. Health insurers can be unwilling to authorize more than a few days or weeks of inpatient rehabilitation for patients with MS.

Several studies have found that inpatient rehabilitation for MS yields short-term benefits in function, mobility, and several aspects of quality of life.[36,59,62,63,97,145,180] Benefits have generally been most impressive in uncontrolled retrospective trials including patients recovering from exacerbations.[2,76,154] Studies that have looked for extended carryover have found that benefits dwindle by 6–10 months. This finding was attributed to disease progression in some studies, while in others the disease progression was not a possible explanation (because the EDSS remained stable). Because benefits of inpatient rehabilitation tend not to be long term, periodic admission for rehabilitation might be needed, providing that patients and third-party payers are willing. Rehabilitation management in Europe has recognized this, and yearly inpatient admissions for optimizing function as the disease progresses are not uncommon.[100]

Outpatient and home-based exercise

Exercise has a beneficial effect on MS disability and quality of life. There is robust evidence that aerobic training improves maximum exercise capacity (VO_{2max}) for ambulatory MS individuals, while inactivity makes it worse.[65,158,166,205] We know less about exercise effects in semiambulatory and non-ambulatory MS individuals, but it appears that they do not receive as much benefit. This may be because they cannot activate enough muscle mass to get a training effect, because exercise programs are not designed properly for them, or because their adherence is poor.

For those with a greater degree of disability, multidisciplinary outpatient programs might provide better results than exercise alone, but these are not widely available. If people with MS follow established precautions, they do not experience exercise-associated worsening of fatigue or other symptoms lasting beyond 1–2 days. Adherence to exercise can yield a partial reduction of MS fatigue. Aerobic exercise is particularly important for the patients with MS who are overweight.[85]

Every exercise prescription should be tailored to meet individual circumstances. Specific muscle training is recommended for improving focal weaknesses. It has also been advocated when fatigue or heat sensitivity are important issues.[51] Focused muscle strengthening with progressive resistive exercises can be effective in motivated individuals with mild impairments.[44,104,105] Three sets of 10 repetitions might be an appropriate regimen. With careful selection of muscles (using probably not more than two per limb), resistive exercises might still be effective in strengthening, even when weakness is diffuse.

For those whose primary goal is improved gait, exercise must include standing and walking. Aquatic exercise (swimming, water aerobics, and water walking) is an excellent form of integrated exercise, especially where ataxia might create a safety concern. Even those with tetraparesis can use the water buoyancy to facilitate standing and supine swimming with assistance and a life jacket.[211] Care should be taken to find a pool that is not too hot (above 29°C, 84°F) for those who are heat-sensitive. Combined arm–leg ergometry is useful for people with partial paralysis. Yoga can improve flexibility and reduce spasticity. Outdoor walking, aerobics, and t'ai chi are useful for balance training.[89,110]

Active exercise should be done at least three times a week for 20–30 min, with 5-min warm up and cooldown periods. Stretching should be done for 5–10 min, with emphasis on posterior thigh, calf, and back muscles. Previously sedentary individuals should start aerobic exercises at a comfortable level, and increase the duration and intensity of exercise at weekly or monthly intervals.[206] Adherence to the exercise program is typically better if a communal or group activity, such as group aerobics, is used.

For markedly disabled MS individuals, activities of daily living (ADL) might constitute their only regular forms of physical activity. In addition to passive range of motion exercises, it is important to devise simple activities that tap underutilized strengths in order to avoid learned disuse and deconditioning. Recreational activities should supplement the amount of exercise derived from ADL.

Management of spasticity

The platform on which spasticity management in MS should be based is muscle stretching.[5] Management of spasticity can be accomplished through frequent (every few hours) stretching of spastic muscles, so that agonist muscle groups do not have to 'fight' the spastic antagonist muscles. It is important that care be given to adequate stretching of two-joint muscles; muscles should be stretched across both joints simultaneously. (For example, the gastrocnemius muscle must be stretched across both the knee and ankle joints.) The stretch should also be of adequate duration. A steady gentle stretch of 20 min is better than a stronger stretch of a shorter period of time.[79] Spasticity is one of the most common symptoms in MS and can go unrecognized by many patients.[111] The lower limbs of patients with MS typically have more spasticity than the upper limbs.

In conjunction with stretching, spasmolytic medications are also generally used to reduce the stretch required and to prolong

Table 53-4 Spasmolytic drugs for multiple sclerosis

	Baclofen (Lioresal)	Tizanidine (Zanaflex)	Dantrolene sodium (Dantrium)
Dosage	Up to 30 mg q.i.d.	Up to 24 mg q.d. in divided doses	Up to 100 mg t.i.d.
Advantages	Inexpensive	Does not cause muscle weakness	Does not cause somnolence
Disadvantages	Causes mild somnolence	Causes marked somnolence	Causes weakness
Laboratory monitoring	None	None	Periodic liver function tests

the benefits of stretching (see Ch. 31). These medications must be monitored carefully, as too little medication will inadequately suppress spasticity and too much may cause the 'spaghetti leg' syndrome, which is limb tone that is less than adequate for optimal function.[114] The presence of no more than five beats of clonus, rather than the intensity of the muscle stretch reflex, is the best indicator of the optimal level of medication. Because MS fluctuates, it might be necessary to evaluate a patient at 3-month intervals (an interval recommended to monitor blood and liver function for those patients on interferon beta therapy) to adjust antispasticity medication dose.

Baclofen (Lioresal), tizanidine (Zanaflex), and dantrolene sodium (Dantrium) are commonly used to manage spasticity, with the majority of patients being treated with baclofen (see Table 53-4 for indications and dose ranges of spasmolytic agents). Controversial drugs that might benefit spasticity are marijuana or medical cannabis.[28,198]

One of the difficulties of spasticity management with medications in persons with MS is that the commonly used spasmolytic agents can make patients fatigued, somnolent, weaker, and slower cognitively. These are also symptoms of MS, and it is undesirable to produce a worsening of these problems. Although fatigue and somnolence can be minimized by slowly titrating the dose, these drugs still might worsen many of the MS patient's troublesome symptoms. Consequently, non-systemic techniques to manage spasticity have an important role in MS. Botulinum toxin injections in spastic muscles and dilute phenol (5%) nerve blocks can be used for especially spastic muscles to minimize the dose of oral medication. Patients with severe lower limb spasticity can also be candidates for an implantable baclofen pump, especially because the high levels of oral spasmolytics required to control severe spasticity can cause further cognitive impairment.

Painful tonic spasms are different from spasticity. These paroxysmal symptoms often occur at night, and can be seen in the absence of an increased stretch reflex. They are thought to be caused by the ephaptic spreading of abnormal transient neural discharges through demyelinated axons. They might respond to carbamazepine, phenytoin, gabapentin, or botulinum toxin injections.[164] Of the spasmolytic agents, there is a consensus that tizanidine appears to be especially useful, and produces an additionally beneficial soporific effect if used for nocturnal spasms. See the *Pain* section below for further discussion.

Pain

Pain in MS can be quite severe and difficult to manage. It is now recognized as a common symptom in patients with MS, with almost 50% of patients experiencing clinically significant pain at some time during the course of the disease, and as the presenting symptom in approximately 20%.[146,183] In a recent survey of 442 persons with MS, we have found the 3-month point prevalence of bothersome pain to be 44%.[50] The average severity of pain was rated at 5.2 on a 10-point scale. Twenty-seven percent claimed severe pain, and 20% felt it interfered with daily activities.

Not all MS pain is neuropathic, and the correct diagnosis must first be made. There are many potential causes of pain. Often the pain problem is complex and, despite treatment, many patients with MS have ongoing pain or develop a chronic refractory pain syndrome. The pain symptoms in patients with MS can be divided into the following categories: neuropathic pain, musculoskeletal pain, pain due to inflammation, and pain secondary to upper motor neuron damage.

Neuropathic pain

Examples of neuropathic pain are trigeminal neuralgia, chronic dysesthetic pain, painful L'hermitte's phenomenon, radicular pain, and pain associated with transverse myelitis.

Trigeminal neuralgia (tic douloureux) is a well-known paroxysmal pain syndrome in MS, and typically responds well to pharmacologic intervention with anticonvulsants such as carbamazepine and gabapentin. Tizanidine and misoprostol are among the other categories of medications for which there is some evidence of efficacy.[52,177] Rhizotomy using glycerol, radiofrequency thermal treatment, or surgery is reserved for refractory cases.

Dysesthetic extremity pain is a chronic, continuous pain syndrome that is commonly seen in MS. Patients typically describe a burning type of pain. Lower limbs are most frequently involved, followed by the trunk and upper limbs, and it occurs with insidious onset. Treatment includes tricyclic antidepressants and anticonvulsants, but it is often difficult to achieve complete relief of symptoms.

Musculoskeletal pain

Any musculoskeletal problem occurring in the general population can also occur in the MS population. Low back pain is an example. It is more complex in MS, as many potential pain structures can be involved. Patients with MS are at greater risk for a herniated disk due to muscle weakness that is often aggravated by spasticity. Pain can also develop due to a compression fracture in those individuals with osteoporosis, sometimes increased by long-term steroid use.

Other causes of back pain, such as mechanical back pain, posterior element pain (facet syndrome), and myofascial pain, can also occur. These result from increased mechanical stresses and imbalance in muscle force as a result of weakness and/or spasticity.

MS patients with back pain are typically responsive to standard pain treatments such as spinal orthoses, non-steroidal anti-inflammatory drugs, analgesics, physical therapy with stretching exercises, and trigger point injections. If the pain is complicated by upper motor neuron symptoms such as spasticity, spasmolytic agents should be also used. If neuropathic radicular pain is suspected, a trial of anticonvulsants is also worthwhile.

Pain due to inflammation

Optic neuritis is a typical example of acute pain due to an inflammatory process. Inflammation and demyelination occur in or around pain-sensitive structures surrounding the optic nerve, and the pain is often triggered or aggravated by eye movement. Corticosteroid treatment is generally effective.

Pain related to upper motor neuron loss

Muscle spasm and cramps are reported by many patients with MS. Some pain is simply secondary to spasticity, and the best management is to treat the problem with stretching and spasmolytic agents. Another type of 'muscle spasm', referred to as tonic spinal cord seizure, is encountered in less than 10% of patients with MS, and is a form of neuropathic pain most responsive to carbamazepine or other anticonvulsants. Tizanidine can also be helpful, especially for the nocturnal variety.

Other techniques for managing the pain associated with muscle spasm include cannabinoids, which appear to have some success in relieving symptoms of muscle pain or spasm and spasticity in some patients with MS.[35] For those having both severe spasticity and pain, intrathecal baclofen with morphine or clonidine has been used with good results.[101]

Fatigue and sleep

Fatigue was ignored in early descriptions of MS. However, in the mid 1980s, we identified fatigue as the most common symptom of MS and defined its characteristics.[61,111] It is most pronounced in the afternoon, and is experienced by 77% of patients.[111] Treatment of fatigue has recently assumed a much more prominent place in the management of MS, and has been successfully treated with a variety of medications, such as amantadine, modafinil, and methylphenidate; prescribing information is outlined in Table 53-5.

Non-medical treatments of fatigue include techniques to extract heat from the body or by surface cooling. The most effective method appears to be heat extraction using a vest with a circulating coolant flowing through a radiating system. More widely used, and much less expensive, are cooling vests. It has been demonstrated that lowering core body temperature using heat extraction can improve function in repetitive activities that produce fatigue.[106,175]

The exact mechanism for this reduction of fatigue with cooling is unclear.[165] There is only an incomplete understanding as to the cause of MS fatigue. It does not correlate with MRI lesion burden (although the rate of progression to that level of burden has not been studied).[7] Some feel that proinflammatory cytokines contribute to the sense of tiredness.[32,57] Recent research from our group has shown association with hormonal and adrenergic changes from cooling, especially an increase in noradrenaline (norepinephrine).

Although stimulants such as methylphenidate and sleep suppressants such as modafinil are effective in reducing the groggy periods experienced by an MS patient throughout the day, recent studies of sleep raise questions as to whether their use is in the patient's long-term interest as they might inhibit brain plasticity.

It is striking how well many patients can function with extensive lesion loads and cortical atrophy. These patients typically have a great deal of fatigue, and fight to stay awake much of the day. Given the large number of brain neurons destroyed in these patients, it is likely that they have been benefiting from brain plasticity, which lays down new memory traces by activating new and undamaged neural pathways. Functional MRI

Table 53-5 Fatigue medications for multiple sclerosis			
	Amantadine (symmetrel)	Modafinil (Provigil)	Methylphenidate (Ritalin)
Dosage	100 mg b.i.d.	100–600 mg q. a.m.	5–30 mg b.i.d.
Action	Unknown	Activator	Stimulant
Advantages	Not scheduled, low cost	Effective	Effective, inexpensive
Disadvantages	May be less effective	High cost	Abuse potential
Drug scheduling	None	IV	II

during a simple motor task demonstrates significantly greater activation on the ipsilateral side of the brain of subjects with MS than in control subjects.[55] This cortical 'spread' indicates plasticity.

Plasticity is a type of new learning, and recent evidence indicates that such new learning requires sleep.[191] During much of sleep, cortical neurons undergo slow oscillations in membrane potential (slow-wave activity on electroencephalogram).[87] This appears necessary for the 'offline' processing required for new synaptic plasticity.[143] Slow-wave activity of sleep is required for efficient consolidation of fresh memory traces necessary for brain plasticity.[135] Studies of sleep deprivation in both experimental animals and human volunteers demonstrate that new learning requires fairly immediate sleep to 'encode' newly learned experiences.[75,84,138,171] Both animal and human subjects deprived of adequate sleep following the learning of a new task do poorer on subsequent testing, irrespective of whether they were sleep-deprived at the time of testing.[19,200]

Sleep appears necessary to consolidate new memory traces (plasticity). Given that brain plasticity must be a relatively steady process in a neurodegenerative disease such as MS, this could explain the need for frequent sleep in such patients. Perhaps the MS patient's desire for sleep is part of this biologic compensatory or repair process.

Patients with MS who need to be alert for vocational or safety reasons will still benefit from the activating drugs. But for those without that need, it follows that it is important to continue utilizing the traditional rehabilitation strategies of pacing, taking rests in the afternoon, occupational therapy techniques to conserve energy, and body cooling. Other medical conditions, including depression, also might contribute to fatigue and should be assessed and treated.

Rehabilitation for mobility and balance

Gait impairment in MS can be caused by weakness, spasticity, fatigue, proprioceptive loss, cerebellar or vestibular dysfunction, visual loss, or inability to multitask. Approximately three-quarters of individuals with MS have some degree of ambulatory impairment.[111,127]

Compared with healthy people, patients with MS show decreased stride length; increased steps per minute (cadence); slower free speed walking rates; less rotation at the hips, knees, and ankles (stiffer gait); increased trunk flexion; and reduced vertical lift in center of gravity. Overall, they take short quick steps and lack full range of motion.[66] A survey conducted in 1983 indicated that 60% of people with MS needed some assistance with ambulation.[11] Most relied on a wheelchair or physical assistance from another person.

Falls are the most important sequelae of gait and balance disturbances. In one cross-sectional study of ambulatory patients with MS, 54% reported at least one fall over the previous 2 months and 32% were recurrent fallers. Impaired balance was the best predictor of falls, followed by use of an assistive device.[22] Recommendations for mobility aids should focus on enhancing gait stability, rather than on the cosmesis and convenience of walking.

Studies suggest that non-specific exercise programs without some ambulation component are ineffective for enhancing gait.[44,66,166] Continual programs are necessary to maintain good mobility and balance in this disease. One way to make this affordable is to provide group therapy using task-oriented or kinesiology techniques.

All patients who trip and fall do not need orthoses. Evaluation for heel cord tightness, spasticity, clonus, and weakness should be carried out, and corrective measures taken. In cases of intermittent falling, the examiner should inquire about the conditions under which it occurs. Falls occurring when the patient is occupied with other activities (such as talking with a companion) may be related to the difficulty MS patients have with multitasking. Because loss of proprioceptive function results in the use of compensatory visual, auditory, tactile, and cognitive cues, multitasking diminishes the MS patient's ability to focus on walking.[118]

Tremor

Disabling tremor is reported in nearly 30% of patients with MS. It is typically an action tremor, and can be one of the most difficult symptoms to manage.[3] In one MS population, the median time to tremor was 11 years from disease onset, with arms more often involved than head, trunk, or legs.

One study of inpatient rehabilitation for the treatment of MS-related ataxia and tremor involved eight half-hour sessions of occupational therapy (postural dynamics, adaptive equipment, and damping and weighting) and physical therapy for 8 working days.[96] The intervention group significantly improved relative to a wait-listed control group on one ADL scale but not on two impairment scales. Intervention subjects had significantly greater improvement in activity and fatigue.

Weighted wrist cuffs and weighted walkers are the most practical methods for dampening ataxic tremor.[2,117] Isoniazid and propranolol can be tried, but seldom yield impressive results. THC, a component of marijuana, showed a non-significant trend toward subjective benefit in MS tremor in one study.[58] Deep brain stimulation, which has an established role in the treatment of parkinsonian tremor, is now being studied as a treatment for MS-related tremor. A review found that deep brain stimulation relieved tremor in >80%, and improved daily functioning in >70%, of reported MS cases.[210] However, long-term hardware complications occur in about one-fourth of patients.[133]

Occupational therapy for multiple sclerosis

People with MS tend to function in daily life below their physical capacities, and cognitive problems do not always account for this discrepancy.[182] Occupational therapy can help people with MS meet their potential for independence. The principles of occupational therapy for MS have been described in various review articles.[51,127] Occupational therapy has been used extensively in MS research, especially in inpatient trials, where it has been uniformly incorporated into the rehabilitation program (see Ch. 27).[36,59,62,63,180,197]

A metaanalysis published in 2001 determined that occupational therapy-related treatments have a strong positive effect on MS symptomatology.[6] However, there have been few investigations of the effects of occupational therapy separate from a multidisciplinary team approach. Occupational therapists are frequently asked to teach the principles of 'energy conservation' to MS individuals. This means rationing activities according to one's optimum hours of function and total capacity for daily exertion, as well as working piece by piece instead of trying to do too much at once. Three randomized controlled trials of patient education in energy conservation (weekly or biweekly 1-h sessions for 6–8 weeks) found reductions in fatigue, which in one study was maintained at 6 weeks' follow-up. There were also benefits in self-efficacy, quality of life, and social participation.[136,137,196] However, a Cochrane review cited design flaws and other weaknesses in methodology in two of the studies, and concluded that the evidence for benefit was insufficient.[185] A large randomized controlled trial of individually or group-based counseling in self-care strategies for 268 community-dwelling individuals with MS found some evidence of treatment effect on mental health and vitality, which was used as a proxy for fatigue.[153] While levels of functional independence did not improve, they were maintained in the intervention group but *declined* in the control group.

Cognition and mood

Cognitive impairment, including memory deficits, represents a significant problem in persons with MS. Comprehensive neuropsychologic testing suggests that over 40% of a broad spectrum of patients with MS show cognitive impairment of at least some degree of significance.[163] In fact, it has recently been shown that measurable cognitive impairment is present in MS as mild as an EDSS of less than 3.5.[170] In such patients, cognitive impairment correlates with illness duration.

It is easy for a physician to miss cognitive impairment in an MS patient during an office visit, as verbal skills remain relatively intact. A patient with fluent speech and a good vocabulary usually gives the initial impression of being cognitively intact. Neuropsychologic testing of patients with MS, however, usually indicates memory to be the most significant area of impairment. Standard office or bedside memory testing might not demonstrate this deficit, as the patient does not forget information immediately. When asked to recall three items after 5 min during a mental status examination, many patients with MS who have serious memory deficits can pass.[207]

There is a difference in cognitive performance between patients with SP MS and those with PP MS. Patients with SP MS perform worse than patients with PP MS on tasks requiring higher order working memory activities.[88] With regard to MRI markers, cognitive impairment correlates with cortical atrophy more than with lesion load.[4]

Treatment of this problem consists of first identifying the specific deficit, then utilizing pacing, memory books, environmental restructuring, and focusing on substituting for the deficit. Meticulous attention must also be paid to treating depression, fatigue, and heat intolerance, as all these can contribute to cognitive impairment. Data are conflicting as to whether interferon beta or glatiramer acetate produce cognitive improvement.[202,215] No drugs have been FDA-approved for improving memory in MS, but medications used to treat Alzheimer disease (e.g. donepezil) are used and may be helpful.

Depression is a common problem in patients with MS. We conducted a large survey of 739 patients with MS in King County, Washington, and found the point prevalence of significant depressive symptoms (Center for Epidemiologic Studies Depression Scale 16) to be 41.8%.[26] There appear to be two peaks of depression: late in advanced MS and early in the disease. Depression in MS appears to have both organic and situational causes, and MRI studies indicate that major depression correlates with T2-weighted lesion volume. Disease in the left medial inferior prefrontal cortex and atrophy of the left anterior temporal region are independent predictors for depression.[53] In less developed countries where treatment is less available, MS depression could be even more common.[47]

Treatments include antidepressant medications and behavioral intervention such as counseling. A small published study indicated that cognitive behavioral therapy was superior to selective serotonin reuptake inhibitor (SSRI) antidepressants.[144] We have conducted a large randomized controlled trial with paroxetine, which was also negative in an intent to treat analysis due to high dropout in the treated group. But of completing subjects, it was of statistically significant benefit. This suggests that SSRIs may be worth a try in MS depression; if they are tolerated, they may be of benefit. Patients experiencing fatigue might actually be depressed, and patients with this symptom should be screened for depression. Energizing antidepressants (e.g. paroxetine) are useful in the subset of fatigued patients who also have depression.[149] Because of the frequent coexisting fatigue, non-energizing antidepressants should not be used. Cognitive impairment may also express itself as depression. That should be assessed and managed as appropriate.

Speech and swallowing

General speech performance registers in the normal range in the majority of individuals with MS. The most common speech problem in MS is controlling the volume of speech (either too soft or too loud). Dysarthria is reported in 14–19%, and it is most often found in more neurologically impaired patients.[38] It has been characterized as a mixed spastic cerebellar dysarthria, although flaccid dysarthrias are also encountered. Apraxia, anomia, and aphasia are much less common.[128]

Multiple sclerosis-associated speech problems are severe enough to limit comprehensibility in about 4% of cases.[14] Evaluation by speech therapy is advised in all such cases (see Ch. 3). The immediate goal is compensated intelligibility. The ultimate result is rarely, if ever, normal speech. When verbal communication is less than 50% intelligible, one should try one of the many augmentative communication devices. Speech pathology treatment strategies for MS dysarthria are to control speech rate, voice emphasis, and phrase shifts; to reduce phase length; and to increase voice power.[141] Lee Silverman Voice Therapy focuses on tasks to maximize phonatory and respiratory functions, encouraging patients to 'think loud', and can be useful for patients with flaccid dysarthria.[81,172]

Dysphagia is a potentially life-threatening manifestation of MS (see Ch. 28). A quantitative water test detected dysphagia in 43% of an MS cohort, almost half of whom had no related complaints.[189] Using fiberoptic nasopharyngeal endoscopy, dysphagia was found in 48% of non-ambulatory individuals and 11% of ambulatory individuals.[20] When videofluoroscopy has been used, most asymptomatic MS individuals have been found to have abnormalities.[208] The oral phase of swallowing is more frequently abnormal than the pharyngeal and esophageal phases. Fluids can be more problematic than solids but, for the majority of dysphagic individuals, both are abnormal.[41]

Questions about choking, aspiration, or swallowing difficulty should be asked as part of the routine review of systems. If the risk factors mentioned above are present, clinicians should have a low threshold for a speech and swallowing referral. When dysphagia is reported and the individual has an EDSS of 7.5 or higher, videofluoroscopy is recommended. Postural techniques and modification of intake volume and consistency through speech and swallowing therapy enable mildly to moderately dysphagic individuals to improve swallowing.

Heat sensitivity and thermoregulation

One of the classic characteristics of patients with MS is their heat intolerance.[78] Prior to MRI, the 'hot tub test', in which a patient was heated and symptoms worsened, was often given to patients suspected of having MS to help confirm the diagnosis.[13] It had been noted in the nineteenth century by Uhthoff that exercise might precipitate amblyopia in some patients with MS, which would resolve after the patient had stopped exercising.[195] This was attributed to an exercise-induced increase in body temperature and, by the second half of the twentieth century, heat had become implicated as a contributor to a number of MS symptoms.[78]

In a classic 1959 paper, Watson tested body cooling to improve MS symptoms, and found it beneficial.[201] The theory was promulgated that the transient blindness in Uhthoff's patients and the worsening in the hot tub test were due to increased core body temperature, which resulted in a reduced safety factor in partially demyelinated nerves as the temperature increased.[40] Improvement with cooling was felt to reverse this effect.

Recent studies do not support this explanation. The temperature of the brain and spinal cord is kept too steady, even during extremes of exercise or cooling, for there to be sufficient change to produce the observed events.[78] Many suspect cooling to produce a change in a hormone or circulating agent, producing a possible endocrine or adrenergic effect. Noradrenaline (norepinephrine) and thyroid hormone have been implicated (James Bowen, personal communication) (see the section on *Fatigue and sleep* earlier in this chapter for further discussion).

Heat intolerance is a very common symptom in MS, and heat extraction is an effective way to treat patients with severe manifestations.[106] Although long-term heat extraction might

not be a practical solution, avoiding a hot environment is an important component of a rehabilitation strategy. Cooling vests or heat extraction units can be prescribed for patients with heat intolerance. A physician's 'prescription' for environmental air conditioning is another practical and valid management tool for heat-sensitive patients with MS.

Bladder and bowel dysfunction

Bladder symptoms are so common in MS that it has been said that the lack of such symptoms is evidence against the diagnosis. They are present from disease onset in 35% of patients, and more than 80% of patients with MS eventually have some voiding dysfunction.[70] Urinary problems have a major psychologic impact, and are among the most socially disabling manifestations of MS (see Ch. 29).[23]

Urgency and frequency are slightly more common than obstructive symptoms.[16] An initial rehabilitation evaluation of an individual with MS should include a review of urologic symptoms, and clinicians should have a low threshold to check a postvoid residual bladder volume. It is controversial whether a urodynamic study is routinely necessary.[178] Urodynamic studies reveal a range of findings, with detrusor hyperreflexia in about two-thirds of MS patients, the rest having detrusor–sphincter dyssynergia or detrusor hypocontractility.[27] If detrusor–sphincter dyssynergia is present initially, it usually does not change with time. Seldom do patients with MS have complete spinal cord interruption, and they usually maintain at least some bladder sensation and residual voluntary micturition. Management involves determining the type of bladder–sphincter dysfunction, and helping to maintain continence and avoid upper urinary tract complications. This can be done with such measures as timed voids, anticholinergic medication, α-sympathetic blocking agents, desmopressin acetate (DDAVP), an intermittent catheterization program, and continent diversions, as indicated.

Bowel dysfunction is another common complaint in MS (see Ch. 30).[86] Constipation is seen most often, with multiple causes, including disease-related reduced parasympathetic input, drug side effects (for anticholinergics and analgesics), immobility, fluid restriction due to bladder frequency, and low-residue diet. Fecal incontinence can be caused by a loss of sensation of bowel movement, irregular bowel program, inadequate

---

Box 53-3 Components of an effective bowel program

- Eat a diet high in fiber
- Drink a warm liquid prior to the anticipated bowel program
- Get adequate daily fluid intake of at least 2 L/day
- Select a convenient time for a regularly scheduled program
- Sit on the toilet for 10 min or more to make sure that the bowel movement is complete
- Use digital stimulation prior to or during a bowel movement
- Use a suppository after a meal
- Take a stool softener or fiber supplement

dietary fiber, or stool that is too soft or liquid. Helpful steps to establish a regular bowel elimination program include advising the patient to do one or more of the following:

An inexpensive video, *Accidents stink* (available at http://www.pmrsecrets.com), can be instructive for providers of care for severely disabled MS patients with irregular bowel movements.

Improving social integration

Quantifying the degree of disability in a patient with MS is difficult to do with MRI alone. There is a general correlation between brain and cord atrophy seen on MRI and disability, but the correlation is not perfect. Newer quantitative techniques such as MTR identify abnormalities in normal-appearing brain tissue and improve this correlation.[192]

At present, disability is still a clinical measure. The patient's disability affects not only the patient, but also the family, friends, fellow employees, and all those interacting socially with the patient.[174] MS affects a large circle around the nuclear patient. Patients are frequently depressed (see section on *Cognition and mood* in this chapter), and the relationship with a spouse and children is permanently altered.[174]

Patients with MS are unemployed disproportionate to their physical status and their educational and vocational histories.[95] In assessing the neuropsychologic function in regard to employment, it is best to use an instrument specifically designed for this purpose (see Ch. 36).[29] A patient with such impairment deserves serious consideration for disability retirement.[60]

Another factor that should be taken into consideration is the patient's age. As patients get older, a variety of other complications can develop. Many of these are treatable and should not necessarily be attributed to the MS.[184] Patients with MS and their physicians sometimes erroneously assume that any symptom that occurs is related to MS, but they are at the same risk as able-bodied individuals of developing common medical problems such as diabetes, heart disease, and arthritis.

Patients with MS live with the disease for the rest of their lives. The better they can preserve and improve their general health, the better they will do.[110] Because MS is a lifetime disease, lifetime management and rehabilitation must be employed.[119]

Patients with MS live in a world with a future of uncertain progression, disability, and financial loss. In addition to organic brain dysfunction, the uncertainty of the disease can challenge a patient's psychologic coping mechanisms.[207]

Maintaining adequate health insurance is another issue for patients with MS. Many carriers limit coverage for persons with preexisting disease.[121] This tendency to limit care often works counter to the patient's progressive need for more and more healthcare services as the disease progresses.[115,116] All of the factors—disease, uncertainty, progression, symptoms, disability, and vocational and social issues—mentioned in this chapter make MS arguably the most challenging disease to rehabilitate. But, because they call on a physician's entire repertoire, they also make it the most satisfying.

ACKNOWLEDGMENT

Supported in part by the University of Washington Multiple Sclerosis Research Rehabilitation and Training Center grant #61-0758 from the National Institute on Disability and Rehabilitation Research, and the United Spinal Association MS Clinical Fellowship Program.

REFERENCES

1. Aisen ML, Arnold A, Baiges I, et al. The effect of mechanical damping loads on disabling action tremor. Neurology 1993; 43:1346–1350.
2. Aisen ML, Sevilla D, Fox N. Inpatient rehabilitation for multiple sclerosis. J Neurol Rehabil 1996; 10:43–36.
3. Alusi SH, Worthington J, Glickman S, et al. A study of tremor in multiple sclerosis. Brain 2001; 124:720–730.
4. Amato MP, Bartolozzi ML, Zipoli V, et al. Neocortical volume decrease in relapsing–remitting MS patients with mild cognitive impairment. Neurology 2004; 63:89–93.
5. Arndt J, Bhasin C, Barar SP, et al. Physical therapy. In: Schapiro RT, ed. Multiple sclerosis: a rehabilitation approach to management. New York: Demos Medical Publishing; 1991:17–66.
6. Baker NA, Tickle-Degnen L. The effectiveness of physical, psychological, and functional interventions in treating clients with multiple sclerosis: a meta-analysis. Am J Occup Ther 2001; 55:324–331.
7. Bakshi R, Miletich RS, Henschel K, et al. Fatigue in multiple sclerosis: cross-sectional correlation with brain MRI findings in 71 patients. Neurology 1999; 53:1151–1153.
8. Barcellos LF, Oksenberg JR, Green AJ, et al. Genetic basis for clinical expression in multiple sclerosis. Brain 2002; 125:150–158.
9. Barkhof F, Bruck W, De Groot CJ, et al. Remyelinated lesions in multiple sclerosis: magnetic resonance image appearance. Arch Neurol 2003; 60: 1073–1081.
10. Barkhof F, Filippi M, Miller DH, et al. Comparison of MRI criteria at first presentation to predict conversion to clinically definite multiple sclerosis. Brain 1997; 120(part 11):2059–2069.
11. Baum HM, Rothschild BB. Multiple sclerosis and mobility restriction. Arch Phys Med Rehabil 1983; 64:591–596.
12. Bech E, Lycke J, Gadeberg P, et al. A randomized, double-blind, placebo-controlled MRI study of anti-herpes virus therapy in MS. Neurology 2002; 58:31–36.
13. Berger JR, Sheremata WA. Persistent neurological deficit precipitated by hot bath test in multiple sclerosis. JAMA 1983; 249:1751–1753.
14. Beukelman DR, Kraft GH, Freal J. Expressive communication disorders in persons with multiple sclerosis: a survey. Arch Phys Med Rehabil 1985; 66:675–677.
15. Bitsch A, Kuhlmann T, Stadelmann C, et al. A longitudinal MRI study of histopathologically defined hypointense multiple sclerosis lesions. Ann Neurol 2001; 49:793–796.
16. Bonniaud V, Parratte B, Amarenco G, et al. Measuring quality of life in multiple sclerosis patients with urinary disorders using the Qualiveen questionnaire. Arch Phys Med Rehabil 2004; 85:1317–1323.
17. Brex PA, Ciccarelli O, O'Riordan JI, et al. A longitudinal study of abnormalities on MRI and disability from multiple sclerosis. N Engl J Med 2002; 346:158–164.
18. Bronnum-Hansen H, Koch-Henriksen N, Stenager E. Trends in survival and cause of death in Danish patients with multiple sclerosis. Brain 2004; 127:844–850.
19. Cajochen C, Knoblauch V, Wirz-Justice A, et al. Circadian modulation of sequence learning under high and low sleep pressure conditions. Behav Brain Res 2004; 151:167–176.
20. Calcagno P, Ruoppolo G, Grasso MG, et al. Dysphagia in multiple sclerosis—prevalence and prognostic factors. Acta Neurol Scand 2002; 105:40–43.
21. Carey RG, Seibert JH, Posavac EJ. Who makes the most progress in inpatient rehabilitation? An analysis of functional gain. Arch Phys Med Rehabil 1988; 69:337–343.

22. Cattaneo D, De Nuzzo C, Fascia T, et al. Risks of falls in subjects with multiple sclerosis. Arch Phys Med Rehabil 2002; 83:864–867.

23. Chancellor MB, Blaivas JG. Urological and sexual problems in multiple sclerosis. Clin Neurosci 1994; 2:189–195.

24. Chard DT, Brex PA, Ciccarelli O, et al. The longitudinal relation between brain lesion load and atrophy in multiple sclerosis: a 14 year follow up study. J Neurol Neurosurg Psychiatry 2003; 74:1551–1554.

25. Chiappa KH. Pattern-shift visual evoked potentials: methodology. In: Chiappa KH, ed. Evoked potentials in clinical medicine. 3rd edn. Philadelphia: Lippincott-Raven; 1997:ix.

26. Chwastiak L, Ehde DM, Gibbons LE, et al. Depressive symptoms and severity of illness in multiple sclerosis: epidemiologic study of a large community sample. Am J Psychiatry 2002; 159:1862–1868.

27. Ciancio SJ, Mutchnik SE, Rivera VM, et al. Urodynamic pattern changes in multiple sclerosis. Urology 2001; 57:239–245.

28. Clark AJ, Ware MA, Yazer E, et al. Patterns of cannabis use among patients with multiple sclerosis. Neurology 2004; 62:2098–2100.

29. Clemmons DC, Fraser RT, Rosenbaum G, et al. An abbreviated neuropsychological battery in multiple sclerosis vocational rehabilitation: findings and implications. Rehabil Psychol 2004; 49:100–105.

30. Coles A, Deans J, Compston A. Campath-1H treatment of multiple sclerosis: lessons from the bedside for the bench. Clin Neurol Neurosurg 2004; 106:270–274.

31. Comi G, Filippi M, Wolinsky JS. European/Canadian multicenter, double-blind, randomized, placebo-controlled study of the effects of glatiramer acetate on magnetic resonance imaging—measured disease activity and burden in patients with relapsing multiple sclerosis. European/Canadian Glatiramer Acetate Study Group. Ann Neurol 2001; 49: 290–297.

32. Comi G, Leocani L, Rossi P, et al. Physiopathology and treatment of fatigue in multiple sclerosis. J Neurol 2001; 248:174–179.

33. Confavreux C, Hutchinson M, Hours MM, et al. Rate of pregnancy-related relapse in multiple sclerosis. Pregnancy in Multiple Sclerosis Group. N Engl J Med 1998; 339:285–291.

34. Confavreux C, Vukusic S, Moreau T, et al. Relapses and progression of disability in multiple sclerosis. N Engl J Med 2000; 343:1430–1438.

35. Consroe P, Musty R, Rein J, et al. The perceived effects of smoked cannabis on patients with multiple sclerosis. Eur Neurol 1997; 38:44–48.

36. Craig J, Young CA, Ennis M, et al. A randomised controlled trial comparing rehabilitation against standard therapy in multiple sclerosis patients receiving intravenous steroid treatment. J Neurol Neurosurg Psychiatry 2003; 74:1225–1230.

37. Damek DM, Shuster EA. Pregnancy and multiple sclerosis. Mayo Clin Proc 1997; 72:977–989.

38. Darley FL, Brown JR, Goldstein NP. Dysarthria in multiple sclerosis. J Speech Hear Res 1972; 15:229–245.

39. Davies GR, Ramio-Torrenta L, Hadjiprocopis A, et al. Evidence for grey matter MTR abnormality in minimally disabled patients with early relapsing–remitting multiple sclerosis. J Neurol Neurosurg Psychiatry 2004; 75:998–1002.

40. Davis FA, Jacobson S. Altered thermal sensitivity in injured and demyelinated nerve. A possible model of temperature effects in multiple sclerosis. J Neurol Neurosurg Psychiatry 1971; 34: 551–561.

41. De Pauw A, Dejaeger E, D'Hooghe B, et al. Dysphagia in multiple sclerosis. Clin Neurol Neurosurg 2002; 104:345–351.

42. De Stefano N, Bartolozzi ML, Nacmias B, et al. Influence of apolipoprotein E ε4 genotype on brain tissue integrity in relapsing–remitting multiple sclerosis. Arch Neurol 2004; 61:536–540.

43. Dean G, Kurtzke JF. On the risk of multiple sclerosis according to age at immigration to South Africa. Br Med J 1971; 3:725–729.

44. DeBolt LS, McCubbin JA. The effects of home-based resistance exercise on balance, power, and mobility in adults with multiple sclerosis. Arch Phys Med Rehabil 2004; 85:290–297.

45. Detels R, Visscher BR, Haile RW, et al. Multiple sclerosis and age at migration. Am J Epidemiol 1978; 108:386–393.

46. Dhib-Jalbut S. Mechanisms of action of interferons and glatiramer acetate in multiple sclerosis. Neurology 2002; 58:S3–S9.

47. Diaz-Olavarrieta C, Cummings JL, Velazquez J, et al. Neuropsychiatric manifestations of multiple sclerosis. J Neuropsychiatry Clin Neurosci 1999; 11:51–57.

48. Duquette P, Girard M, Knobler RL, et al. Interferon beta-1b is effective in relapsing–remitting multiple sclerosis. I. Clinical results of a multicenter, randomized, double-blind, placebo-controlled trial. The IFNB Multiple Sclerosis Study Group. Neurology 1993; 43:655–661.

49. Durelli L, Verdun E, Barbero P, et al. Every-other-day interferon beta-1b versus once-weekly interferon beta-1a for multiple sclerosis: results of a 2-year prospective randomised multicentre study (INCOMIN). Lancet 2002; 359:1453–1460.

50. Ehde DM, Gibbons LE, Chwastiak L, et al. Chronic pain in a large community sample of persons with multiple sclerosis. Mult Scler 2003; 9:605–611.

51. Erickson RP, Lie MR, Wineinger MA. Rehabilitation in multiple sclerosis. Mayo Clin Proc 1989; 64:818–828.

52. Evers S. Misoprostol in the treatment of trigeminal neuralgia associated with multiple sclerosis. J Neurol 2003; 250:542–545.

53. Feinstein A, Roy P, Lobaugh N, et al. Structural brain abnormalities in multiple sclerosis patients with major depression. Neurology 2004; 62:586–590.

54. Fernandez O, Fernandez V, Alonso A, et al. DQB1*0602 allele shows a strong association with multiple sclerosis in patients in Malaga, Spain. J Neurol 2004; 251:440–444.

55. Filippi M, Rocca MA, Colombo B, et al. Functional magnetic resonance imaging correlates of fatigue in multiple sclerosis. Neuroimage 2002; 15:559–567.

56. Filippini G, Munari L, Incorvaia B, et al. Interferons in relapsing remitting multiple sclerosis: a systematic review. Lancet 2003; 361:545–552.

57. Flachenecker P, Bihler I, Weber F, et al. Cytokine mRNA expression in patients with multiple sclerosis and fatigue. Mult Scler 2004; 10: 165–169.

58. Fox P, Bain PG, Glickman S, et al. The effect of cannabis on tremor in patients with multiple sclerosis. Neurology 2004; 62:1105–1109.

59. Francabandera FL, Holland NJ, Wiesel-Levison P, et al. Multiple sclerosis rehabilitation: inpatient vs. outpatient. Rehabil Nurs 1988; 13:251–253.

60. Fraser RT, Johnson EK, Clemmons DC, et al. Vocational rehabilitation in multiple sclerosis (MS): a profile of clients seeking services. Work: A Journal of Prevention, Assessment, and Rehabilitation 2003; 21(1): 69–76.

61. Freal JE, Kraft GH, Coryell JK. Symptomatic fatigue in multiple sclerosis. Arch Phys Med Rehabil 1984; 65:135–138.

62. Freeman JA, Langdon DW, Hobart JC, et al. Inpatient rehabilitation in multiple sclerosis: do the benefits carry over into the community? Neurology 1999; 52:50–56.

63. Freeman JA, Langdon DW, Hobart JC, et al. The impact of inpatient rehabilitation on progressive multiple sclerosis. Ann Neurol 1997; 42:236–244.

64. Frohman EM, Brannon K, Racke MK, et al. Mycophenolate mofetil in multiple sclerosis. Clin Neuropharmacol 2004; 27:80–83.

65. Gappmaier E, Spencer MK, White A. Fifteen weeks of aerobic training improves fitness of multiple sclerosis individuals. Med Sci Sports Exerc 1994; 26:S29.

66. Gehlsen G, Beekman K, Assmann N, et al. Gait characteristics in multiple sclerosis: progressive changes and effects of exercise on parameters. Arch Phys Med Rehabil 1986; 67:536–539.

67. Ghalie RG, Edan G, Laurent M, et al. Cardiac adverse effects associated with mitoxantrone (Novantrone) therapy in patients with MS. Neurology 2002; 59:909–913.

68. Ghezzi A, Martinelli V, Torri V, et al. Long-term follow-up of isolated optic neuritis: the risk of developing multiple sclerosis, its outcome, and the prognostic role of paraclinical tests. J Neurol 1999; 246:770–775.

69. Giesser BS, Kurtzberg D, Vaughan HG Jr, et al. Trimodal evoked potentials compared with magnetic resonance imaging in the diagnosis of multiple sclerosis. Arch Neurol 1987; 44:281–284.

70. Goldstein I, Siroky MB, Sax DS, et al. Neurologic abnormalities in multiple sclerosis. J Urol 1982; 128:541–545.

71. Goodin DS, Frohman EM, Garmany GP Jr, et al. Disease modifying therapies in multiple sclerosis: report of the Therapeutics and Technology Assessment Subcommittee of the American Academy of Neurology and the MS Council for Clinical Practice Guidelines. Neurology 2002; 58: 169–178.

72. Goodkin D. Interferon beta-1b in secondary progressive MS: clinical and MRI results of a 3-year randomized controlled trial. Neurology 2000; 54:2352.

73. Goodkin D. Treatment of progressive forms of multiple sclerosis. In: Burks J, Johnson KP, eds. Multiple sclerosis: diagnosis, medical management, and rehabilitation. New York: Demos Medical Publishing; 2000:177–192.

74. Goodkin DE, Kinkel RP, Weinstock-Guttman B, et al. A phase II study of i.v. methylprednisolone in secondary-progressive multiple sclerosis. Neurology 1998; 51:239–245.

75. Graves LA, Heller EA, Pack AI, et al. Sleep deprivation selectively impairs memory consolidation for contextual fear conditioning. Learn Mem 2003; 10:168–176.

76. Greenspun B, Stineman M, Agri R. Multiple sclerosis and rehabilitation outcome. Arch Phys Med Rehabil 1987; 68:434–437.

77. Gulick EE. Influence of infant feeding method on postpartum relapse of mothers with MS. Int MS J Care 2002: 183–191.

78. Guthrie TC, Nelson DA. Influence of temperature changes on multiple sclerosis: critical review of mechanisms and research potential. J Neurol Sci 1995; 129:1–8.

79. Halar EM, Stolov WC, Venkatesh B, et al. Gastrocnemius muscle belly and tendon length in stroke patients and able-bodied persons. Arch Phys Med Rehabil 1978; 59:476–484.

80. Harris JO, Frank JA, Patronas N, et al. Serial gadolinium-enhanced magnetic resonance imaging scans in patients with early, relapsing–remitting multiple sclerosis: implications for clinical trials and natural history. Ann Neurol 1991; 29:548–555.

81. Hartelius L, Nord L. Speech modification in dysarthria associated with multiple sclerosis: an intervention based on vocal efficiency, contrastive stress, and verbal repair strategies. J Med Speech Lang Pathol 1997; 5:113–140.

82. Hartung HP, Gonsette R, Konig N, et al. Mitoxantrone in progressive multiple sclerosis: a placebo-controlled, double-blind, randomised, multicentre trial. Lancet 2002; 360:2018–2025.

83. Heide AC, Kraft GH, Slimp JC, et al. Cerebral N-acetylaspartate is low in patients with multiple sclerosis and abnormal visual evoked potentials. AJNR Am J Neuroradiol 1998; 19:1047–1054.

84. Heuer H, Klein W. One night of total sleep deprivation impairs implicit learning in the serial reaction task, but not the behavioral expression of knowledge. Neuropsychology 2003; 17:507–516.

85. Hewson DC, Phillips MA, Simpson KE, et al. Food intake in multiple sclerosis. Hum Nutr Appl Nutr 1984; 38:355–367.

86. Hinds JP, Eidelman BH, Wald A. Prevalence of bowel dysfunction in multiple sclerosis. A population survey. Gastroenterology 1990; 98:1538–1542.

87. Huber R, Ghilardi MF, Massimini M, et al. Local sleep and learning. Nature 2004; 430:78–81.

88. Huijbregts SC, Kalkers NF, de Sonneville LM, et al. Differences in cognitive impairment of relapsing remitting, secondary, and primary progressive MS. Neurology 2004; 63:335–339.

89. Husted C, Pham L, Hekking A, et al. Improving quality of life for people with chronic conditions: the example of t'ai chi and multiple sclerosis. Altern Ther Health Med 1999; 5:70–74.

90. IFNB Multiple Sclerosis Study Group–University of British Columbia MS/MRI Analysis Group. Interferon beta-1b in the treatment of multiple sclerosis: final outcome of the randomized controlled trial. Neurology 1995; 45:1277–1285.

91. Inglese M, Ge Y, Filippi M, et al. Indirect evidence for early widespread gray matter involvement in relapsing–remitting multiple sclerosis. Neuroimage 2004; 21:1825–1829.

92. Jacobs LD, Cookfair DL, Rudick RA, et al. Intramuscular interferon beta-1a for disease progression in relapsing multiple sclerosis. The Multiple Sclerosis Collaborative Research Group (MSCRG). Ann Neurol 1996; 39:285–294.

93. Jin YP, de Pedro-Cuesta J, Huang YH, et al. Predicting multiple sclerosis at optic neuritis onset. Mult Scler 2003; 9:135–141.

94. Johnson KP, Brooks BR, Cohen JA, et al. Copolymer 1 reduces relapse rate and improves disability in relapsing–remitting multiple sclerosis: results of a phase III multicenter, double-blind placebo-controlled trial. The Copolymer 1 Multiple Sclerosis Study Group. Neurology 1995; 45:1268–1276.

95. Johnson KP, Klasner E, Amtmann D, et al. Medical, psychological, social, and programmatic barriers to employment for people with multiple sclerosis. J Rehabil 2004; 70:38–50.

96. Jones L, Lewis Y, Harrison J, et al. The effectiveness of occupational therapy and physiotherapy in multiple sclerosis patients with ataxia of the upper limb and trunk. Clin Rehabil 1996; 10:277–282.

97. Jonsson A, Dock J, Ravnborg MH. Quality of life as a measure of rehabilitation outcome in patients with multiple sclerosis. Acta Neurol Scand 1996; 93:229–235.

98. Kalkers NF, Ameziane N, Bot JC, et al. Longitudinal brain volume measurement in multiple sclerosis: rate of brain atrophy is independent of the disease subtype. Arch Neurol 2002; 59:1572–1576.

99. Kappos L. Placebo-controlled multicentre randomised trial of interferon beta-1b in treatment of secondary progressive multiple sclerosis. European Study Group on Interferon beta-1b in Secondary Progressive MS. Lancet 1998; 352:1491–1497.

100. Kesselring J, Beer S. Rehabilitation in multiple sclerosis. ACNR 2002; 2:6–8.

101. Klein M, Delehanty L, Saidiq S. Use of combination intrathecal medications for spasticity and pain in patients with MS [abstract]. In: Second International Multiple Sclerosis Week. Chicago; 2002.

102. Koenigsberg RA, Faro SH, Hershey BL, et al. Neuroimaging. In: Goetz CG, ed. Textbook of clinical neurology. Philadelphia: Saunders; 2003:441.

103. Korbling M. Periphereal blood stem cells for allogeneic transplantation. In: Forman SJ, Blume KG, Donnall TE, eds. Hematopoietic cell transplantation. 2nd edn. Oxford: Blackwell Science; 1999:469–480.

104. Kraft GH, Alquist AD, de Lateur BJ. Effect of resistive exercise on physical function in multiple sclerosis. Rehabil Res Dev Rep 1995; 33:328–329.

105. Kraft GH, Alquist AD, de Lateur BJ. Effect of resistive exercise on strength in multiple sclerosis. Rehabil Res Dev Rep 1995; 33:329–330.

106. Kraft GH, Alquist AD. Effect of microclimate cooling on physical function in multiple sclerosis. Mult Scler: Clin Lab Res 1996; 2:114–115.

107. Kraft GH, Aminoff MJ, Baran EM, et al. Somatosensory evoked potentials: clinical uses. AAEM Somatosensory Evoked Potentials Subcommittee. American Association of Electrodiagnostic Medicine. Muscle Nerve 1998; 21:252–258.

108. Kraft GH, Bowen J, Nash R. Functional stabilization of worsening multiple sclerosis patients treated with high-dose immunosuppression and stem cell rescue [abstract]. Arch Phys Med Rehabil 2002:1682.

109. Kraft GH, Bowen JD, Cui J, et al. Clinical application of autologous stem cell transplantation in severe multiple sclerosis treated with high-dose immunosuppressive therapy. In: Neurology. Denver: American Academy of Neurology; 2002:A166.

110. Kraft GH, Catanzaro ML. Living with MS: a wellness approach. 2nd edn. New York: Demos Medical Publishing; 2000:xi.

111. Kraft GH, Freal JE, Coryell JK. Disability, disease duration, and rehabilitation service needs in multiple sclerosis: patient perspectives. Arch Phys Med Rehabil 1986; 67:164–168.

112. Kraft GH, Janczakowski J, Slimp JC. Comparison of MRI and SEP in patients with MS and stroke. J Clin Neurophysiol 1993; 10:243.

113. Kraft GH, Richards TL, Heide AC. Correlations of evoked potentials with MR imaging and MR spectroscopy in multiple sclerosis. In: Kraft GH, ed. Physical medicine and rehabilitation clinics of North America. Philadelphia: Saunders; 1998:vi, 561–567.

114. Kraft GH. Foreword. In: Kraft GH, Taylor RS, eds. Physical medicine and rehabilitation clinics of North America. Philadelphia: Saunders; 1998: xi–xiii.

115. Kraft GH. Improving health care delivery for persons with multiple sclerosis. In: Kraft GH, ed. Physical medicine and rehabilitation clinics of North America. Philadelphia: Saunders; 1998: viii–ix, 703–715.

116. Kraft GH. In defense of health care: preserving the capacity for excellence. Ann NY Acad Sci 1994; 729:39–55, discussion 62–66.

117. Kraft GH. Movement disorders. In: Basmajian JV, Kirby RL, eds. Medical rehabilitation. Baltimore: Williams & Wilkins; 1984:162–165.

118. Kraft GH. Foreword. In: Brown T, Kraft GH, eds. Physical medicine and rehabilitation clinics of North America: multiple sclerosis. A paradigm shift. Philadelphia: Saunders; 2005:xiii–xv.

119. Kraft GH. Multiple sclerosis: future directions in the care and the cure. Neurol Rehabil 1989; 3:61–64.

120. Kraft GH. Rehabilitation: still the only way to improve function in multiple sclerosis. Lancet 1999; 354:2015–2017.

121. Kraft GH. The 24th Walter J. Zeiter lecture. Variations on a theme: in defense of health care. Arch Phys Med Rehabil 1992; 73:211–219.

122. Kriesel JD, White A, Hayden FG, et al. Multiple sclerosis attacks are associated with picornavirus infections. Mult Scler 2004; 10:145–148.

123. Kurtzke JF, Wallin M. Epidemiology. In: Burks J, Johnson KP, eds. Multiple sclerosis: diagnosis, medical management, and rehabilitation. New York: Demos Medical Publishing; 2000:49–71.

124. Kurtzke JF. Epidemiology and etiology of multiple sclerosis. In: Brown T, Kraft GH, eds. Physical medicine and rehabilitation clinics of North America: multiple sclerosis. A Paradigm Shift. Philadelphia: Saunders; 2005.

125. Kurtzke JF. Epidemiology of multiple sclerosis. Does this really point toward an etiology? Lectio Doctoralis. Neurol Sci 2000; 21:327–349, 383–403.

126. Kurtzke JF. Rating neurologic impairment in multiple sclerosis: an expanded disability status scale (EDSS). Neurology 1983; 33:1444–1452.

127. LaBan MM, Martin T, Pechur J, et al. Physical and occupational therapy in the treatment of patients with multiple sclerosis. In: Kraft GH, ed. Physical medicine and rehabilitation clinics of North America. Philadelphia: Saunders; 1998:vii, 603–614.

128. Lacour A, De Seze J, Revenco E, et al. Acute aphasia in multiple sclerosis: a multicenter study of 22 patients. Neurology 2004; 62:974–977.

129. Lassmann H, Bruck W, Lucchinetti C. Heterogeneity of multiple sclerosis pathogenesis: implications for diagnosis and therapy. Trends Mol Med 2001; 7:115–121.

130. Lewitt PA, Garbern JY, Ferrante MA, et al. Body fluid and tissue analysis. In: Goetz CG, ed. Textbook of clinical neurology. Philadelphia: Saunders; 2003:523.

131. Lucchinetti C, Bruck W, Parisi J, et al. Heterogeneity of multiple sclerosis lesions: implications for the pathogenesis of demyelination. Ann Neurol 2000; 47:707–717.

132. Lycke J, Svennerholm B, Hjelmquist E, et al. Acyclovir treatment of relapsing–remitting multiple sclerosis. A randomized, placebo-controlled, double-blind study. J Neurol 1996; 243:214–224.

133. Lyons KE, Wilkinson SB, Overman J, et al. Surgical and hardware complications of subthalamic stimulation: a series of 160 procedures. Neurology 2004; 63:612–616.

134. Malucchi S, Sala A, Gilli F, et al. Neutralizing antibodies reduce the efficacy of betaIFN during treatment of multiple sclerosis. Neurology 2004; 62:2031–2037.

135. Maquet P. The role of sleep in learning and memory. Science 2001; 294:1048–1052.

136. Mathiowetz V, Matuska KM, Murphy ME. Efficacy of an energy conservation course for persons with multiple sclerosis. Arch Phys Med Rehabil 2001; 82:449–456.

137. Mathiowetz V. Randomized clinical trial of an energy conservation course for persons with MS. In: Consortium of MS Centers. 2004.

138. McDermott CM, LaHoste GJ, Chen C, et al. Sleep deprivation causes behavioral, synaptic, and membrane excitability alterations in hippocampal neurons. J Neurosci 2003; 23:9687–9695.

139. McDonald WI, Compston A, Edan G, et al. Recommended diagnostic criteria for multiple sclerosis: guidelines from the International Panel on the Diagnosis of Multiple Sclerosis. Ann Neurol 2001; 50:121–127.

140. Medical Advisory Board of the National Multiple Sclerosis Society. Rehabilitation: recommendations for persons with multiple sclerosis. New York: National Multiple Sclerosis Society; 2004.

141. Merson RM, Rolnick MI. Speech-language pathology and dysphagia in multiple sclerosis. In: Kraft GH, ed. Physical medicine and rehabilitation clinics of North America. Philadelphia: Saunders; 1998:631–641.

142. Miller DH, Barkhof F, Frank JA, et al. Measurement of atrophy in multiple sclerosis: pathological basis, methodological aspects and clinical relevance. Brain 2002; 125:1676–1695.

143. Miyamoto H, Hensch TK. Reciprocal interaction of sleep and synaptic plasticity. Mol Interv 2003; 3:404–417.

144. Mohr DC, Boudewyn AC, Goodkin DE, et al. Comparative outcomes for individual cognitive-behavior therapy, supportive-expressive group psychotherapy, and sertraline for the treatment of depression in multiple sclerosis. J Consult Clin Psychol 2001; 69:942–949.

145. Mostert S, Kesselring J. Effects of a short-term exercise training program on aerobic fitness, fatigue, health perception and activity level of subjects with multiple sclerosis. Mult Scler 2002; 8:161–168.

146. Moulin DE, Foley KM, Ebers GC. Pain syndromes in multiple sclerosis. Neurology 1988; 38:1830–1834.

147. Murray TJ. The history of multiple sclerosis. In: Burks J, Johnson KP, eds. Multiple sclerosis: diagnosis, medical management, and rehabilitation. New York: Demos Medical Publishing; 2000:1–32.

148. Nakashima I, Fujihara K, Fujimori J, et al. Absence of IgG1 response in the cerebrospinal fluid of relapsing neuromyelitis optica. Neurology 2004; 62:144–146.

149. Ninan PT, Hassman HA, Glass SJ, et al. Adjunctive modafinil at initiation of treatment with a selective serotonin reuptake inhibitor enhances the degree and onset of therapeutic effects in patients with major depressive disorder and fatigue. J Clin Psychiatry 2004; 65:414–420.

150. Noseworthy JH, Lucchinetti C, Rodriguez M, et al. Multiple sclerosis. N Engl J Med 2000; 343:938–952.

151. Noseworthy JH, Vandervoort MK, Wong CJ, et al. Interrater variability with the Expanded Disability Status Scale (EDSS) and Functional Systems (FS) in a multiple sclerosis clinical trial. The Canadian Cooperation MS Study Group. Neurology 1990; 40:971–975.

152. O'Connor P. Key issues in the diagnosis and treatment of multiple sclerosis. An overview. Neurology 2002; 59:S1–S33.

153. O'Hara L, Cadbury H, De SL, et al. Evaluation of the effectiveness of professionally guided self-care for people with multiple sclerosis living in the community: a randomized controlled trial. Clin Rehabil 2002; 16:119–128.

154. Olgiati R, Jacquet J, Di Prampero PE. Energy cost of walking and exertional dyspnea in multiple sclerosis. Am Rev Respir Dis 1986; 134:1005–1010.

155. Panitch H, Goodin DS, Francis G, et al. Randomized, comparative study of interferon beta-1a treatment regimens in MS: the EVIDENCE Trial. Neurology 2002; 59:1496–1506.

156. Pirko I, Noseworthy JH. Demyelinating disorders of the central nervous system. In: Goetz CG, ed. Textbook of clinical neurology. Philadelphia: Saunders; 2003:1066.

157. Pittock SJ, Mayr WT, McClelland RL, et al. Change in MS-related disability in a population-based cohort: a 10-year follow-up study. Neurology 2004; 62:51–59.

158. Ponichtera-Mulcare JA, Mathews T, Barrett PJ. Change in aerobic fitness of individuals with multiple sclerosis during a 6-month training program. Sports Med Train Rehabil 1997; 7:265–272.

159. Poser CM, Paty DW, Scheinberg L, et al. New diagnostic criteria for multiple sclerosis: guidelines for research protocols. Ann Neurol 1983; 13:227–231.

160. Poser CM. Diseases of the myelin sheath. In: Merritt HH, ed. A textbook of neurology. 5th edn. Philadelphia: Lea & Febiger; 1973:683–727.

161. Prevention of Relapses and Disability by Interferon beta-1a Subcutaneously in Multiple Sclerosis (PRISMS) Study Group. Randomised double-blind placebo-controlled study of interferon beta-1a in relapsing/remitting multiple sclerosis. Lancet 1998; 352:1498–1504.

162. Purves SJ, Low MD, Galloway J, et al. A comparison of visual, brainstem auditory, and somatosensory evoked potentials in multiple sclerosis. Can J Neurol Sci 1981; 8:15–19.

163. Rao SM, Leo GJ, Bernardin L, et al. Cognitive dysfunction in multiple sclerosis. I. Frequency, patterns, and prediction. Neurology 1991; 41:685–691.

164. Restivo DA, Tinazzi M, Patti F, et al. Botulinum toxin treatment of painful tonic spasms in multiple sclerosis. Neurology 2003; 61:719–720.

165. Robinson LR, Kraft GH, Fitts SS, et al. Body cooling may not improve somatosensory pathway function in multiple sclerosis. Am J Phys Med Rehabil 1997; 76:191–196.

166. Rodgers MM, Mulcare JA, King DL, et al. Gait characteristics of individuals with multiple sclerosis before and after a 6-month aerobic training program. J Rehabil Res Dev 1999; 36:183–188.

167. Rose AS, Kuzma JW, Kurtzke JF, et al. Cooperative study in the evaluation of therapy in multiple sclerosis. ACTH vs. placebo—final report. Neurology 1970; 20:1–59.

168. Rovaris M, Filippi M. Contrast enhancement and the acute lesion in multiple sclerosis. Neuroimaging Clin North Am 2000; 10:viii–ix, 705–716.

169. Rovira A, Alonso J, Cucurella G, et al. Evolution of multiple sclerosis lesions on serial contrast-enhanced T1-weighted and magnetization-transfer MR images. AJNR Am J Neuroradiol 1999; 20:1939–1945.

170. Ruggieri RM, Palermo R, Vitello G, et al. Cognitive impairment in patients suffering from relapsing–remitting multiple sclerosis with EDSS < or = 3.5. Acta Neurol Scand 2003; 108:323–326.

171. Ruskin DN, Liu C, Dunn KE, et al. Sleep deprivation impairs hippocampus-mediated contextual learning but not amygdala-mediated cued learning in rats. Eur J Neurosci 2004; 19:3121–3124.

172. Sapir S, Pawlas AA, Ramig LO, et al. Effects of intensive phonatory–respiratory treatment (LSVT) on voice in two individuals with multiple sclerosis. J Med Speech Lang Pathol 2001; 5:141–151.

173. Schumacher G, Beebe G, Kibler R. Problems of experimental trials of therapy in multiple sclerosis: report by the Panel on the Evaluation of Experimental Trials of Therapy in Multiple Sclerosis. Ann NY Acad Sci 1965; 122:552–568.

174. Schwartz L, Kraft GH. The role of spouse responses to disability and family environment in multiple sclerosis. Am J Phys Med Rehabil 1999; 78:525–532.

175. Schwid SR, Petrie MD, Murray R, et al. A randomized controlled study of the acute and chronic effects of cooling therapy for MS. Neurology 2003; 60:1955–1960.

176. Secondary Progressive Efficacy Clinical Trial of Recombinant Interferon-beta-1a in MS (SPECTRIMS) Study Group. Randomized controlled trial of interferon-beta-1a in secondary progressive MS: clinical results. Neurology 2001; 56:1496–1504.

177. Semenchuk MR, Sherman S. Effectiveness of tizanidine in neuropathic pain: an open-label study. J Pain 2000; 1:285–292.

178. Sirls LT, Zimmern PE, Leach GE. Role of limited evaluation and aggressive medical management in multiple sclerosis: a review of 113 patients. J Urol 1994; 151:946–950.

179. Slimp JC, Janczakowski J, Seed LJ, et al. Comparison of median and posterior tibial nerve somatosensory evoked potentials in ambulatory patients with definite multiple sclerosis. Am J Phys Med Rehabil 1990; 69:293–296.

180. Solari A, Filippini G, Gasco P, et al. Physical rehabilitation has a positive effect on disability in multiple sclerosis patients. Neurology 1999; 52:57–62.

181. Sorensen PS, Ross C, Clemmesen KM, et al. Clinical importance of neutralising antibodies against interferon beta in patients with relapsing–remitting multiple sclerosis. Lancet 2003; 362:1184–1191.

182. Staples D, Lincoln NB. Intellectual impairment in multiple sclerosis and its relation to functional abilities. Rheumatol Rehabil 1979; 18:153–160.

183. Stenager E, Knudsen L, Jensen K. Acute and chronic pain syndromes in multiple sclerosis. Acta Neurol Scand 1991; 84:197–200.

184. Stern M. Aging with multiple sclerosis. In: Kraft GH, Cristian A, eds. Physical medicine and rehabilitation clinics of North America: aging with a disability. Philadelphia: Saunders; 2004.

185. Steultjens EM, Dekker J, Bouter LM, et al. Occupational therapy for multiple sclerosis. Cochrane Database Syst Rev 2003:CD003608.

186. Sundstrom P, Juto P, Wadell G, et al. An altered immune response to Epstein–Barr virus in multiple sclerosis: a prospective study. Neurology 2004; 62:2277–2282.

187. Sundstrom P, Nystrom L, Svenningsson A, et al. Sick leave and professional assistance for multiple sclerosis individuals in Vasterbotten County, northern Sweden. Mult Scler 2003; 9:515–520.

188. Teva Neuroscience. Copaxone study demonstrated a trend in affecting clinical progression of primary progressive multiple sclerosis. Teva Neuroscience; 2004.

189. Thomas FJ, Wiles CM. Dysphagia and nutritional status in multiple sclerosis. J Neurol 1999; 246:677–682.

190. Tintore M, Rovira A, Martinez MJ, et al. Isolated demyelinating syndromes: comparison of different MR imaging criteria to predict conversion to clinically definite multiple sclerosis. AJNR Am J Neuroradiol 2000; 21:702–706.

191. Tononi G, Cirelli C. Some considerations on sleep and neural plasticity. Arch Ital Biol 2001; 139:221–241.

192. Traboulsee A, Dehmeshki J, Peters KR, et al. Disability in multiple sclerosis is related to normal appearing brain tissue MTR histogram abnormalities. Mult Scler 2003; 9:566–573.

193. Trapp BD, Peterson J, Ransohoff RM, et al. Axonal transection in the lesions of multiple sclerosis. N Engl J Med 1998; 338:278–285.

194. Trojaborg W, Petersen E. Visual and somatosensory evoked cortical potentials in multiple sclerosis. J Neurol Neurosurg Psychiatry 1979; 42:323–330.

195. Uhthoff W. Untersuchungen über die bei der multiplen Herdsklerose vorkommenden Augenströrungen. Arch Psychiat Nervenkr 1890: 55–116, 303–410.

196. Vanage SM, Gilbertson KK, Mathiowetz V. Effects of an energy conservation course on fatigue impact for persons with progressive multiple sclerosis. Am J Occup Ther 2003; 57:315–323.

197. Vaney C, Blaurock H, Gattlen B, et al. Assessing mobility in multiple sclerosis using the Rivermead Mobility Index and gait speed. Clin Rehabil 1996; 10:216–226.

198. Wade DT, Makela P, Robson P, et al. Do cannabis-based medicinal extracts have general or specific effects on symptoms in multiple sclerosis? A double-blind, randomized, placebo-controlled study on 160 patients. Mult Scler 2004; 10:434–441.

199. van Waesberghe JH, van Walderveen MA, Castelijns JA, et al. Patterns of lesion development in multiple sclerosis: longitudinal observations with T1-weighted spin-echo and magnetization transfer MR. AJNR Am J Neuroradiol 1998; 19:675–683.

200. Wang JH, van den Buuse M, Tian SW, et al. Effect of paradoxical sleep deprivation and stress on passive avoidance behavior. Physiol Behav 2003; 79:591–596.

201. Watson CW. Effect of lowering of body temperature on the symptoms and signs of multiple sclerosis. N Engl J Med 1959; 261:1253–1259.

202. Weinstein A, Schwid SI, Schiffer RB, et al. Neuropsychologic status in multiple sclerosis after treatment with glatiramer. Arch Neurol 1999; 56:319–324.

203. Wekerle H, Hohlfeld R. Molecular mimicry in multiple sclerosis. N Engl J Med 2003; 349:185–186.

204. Werring DJ, Brassat D, Droogan AG, et al. The pathogenesis of lesions and normal-appearing white matter changes in multiple sclerosis: a serial diffusion MRI study. Brain 2000; 123(part 8):1667–1676.

205. White A, Gappmaier E, Mino L. Response to acute exercise before and after 15 weeks of training for multiple sclerosis individuals. Med Sci Sports Exerc 1994; 26:S29.

206. White A. Exercise and MS: challenges and opportunities. Mult Scler Q Rep 2004; 23:18–20.

207. White DM, Catanzaro ML, Kraft GH. An approach to the psychological aspects of multiple sclerosis: a coping guide for health care providers and families. J Neurol Rehabil 1993; 7:43–52.

208. Wiesner W, Wetzel SG, Kappos L, et al. Swallowing abnormalities in multiple sclerosis: correlation between videofluoroscopy and subjective symptoms. Eur Radiol 2002; 12:789–792.

209. Wingerchuk DM. Neuromyelitis optica: current concepts. Front Biosci 2004; 9:834–840.

210. Wishart HA, Roberts DW, Roth RM, et al. Chronic deep brain stimulation for the treatment of tremor in multiple sclerosis: review and case reports. J Neurol Neurosurg Psychiatry 2003; 74:1392–1397.

211. Woods DA. Aquatic exercise programs for individuals with multiple sclerosis. Clin Kinesiol 1992: 14–20.

212. Yong VW. Differential mechanisms of action of interferon-beta and glatiramer aetate in MS. Neurology 2002; 59:802–808.

213. Yorkston KM, Johnson KL, Kuehn CM, et al. Age and gender issues related to MS: a survey study. In: International Journal of MS Care. Consortium of MS Centers Annual Meeting, Chicago, 2002:94.

214. Zivadinov R, Rudick RA, De Masi R, et al. Effects of IV methylprednisolone on brain atrophy in relapsing–remitting MS. Neurology 2001; 57:1239–1247.

215. Zivadinov R, Zorzon M, Tommasi MA, et al. A longitudinal study of quality of life and side effects in patients with multiple sclerosis treated with interferon beta-1a. J Neurol Sci 2003; 216:113–118.

Chapter

54

Cerebral Palsy

Shubhra Mukherjee and Deborah J. Gaebler-Spira

Cerebral palsy (CP) is a clinical entity characterized by a three-part definition: a disorder of movement and posture (1) caused by a non-progressive injury (2) to the immature brain (3).[163] The distinctive characteristic of these syndromes is the change in muscle tone and posture, both at rest and with voluntary activity.[169] The definition of CP implies that the underlying pathologic process in the brain does not progress, and occurred during early development of the brain. The first year or two of life is included in most definitions, although it is unclear what the upper age limit is of a postneonatal brain insult. The definition of CP is being reviewed at present.

A wide variety of etiologies can result in the injury to the brain that causes CP. The injury results in neurologic sequelae, with similar issues affecting motor function, musculoskeletal, and cognitive development. A number of associated medical issues also occur.

The diagnosis is made in children who are demonstrating delayed motor development, and is confirmed with MRI. Where indicated, other metabolic, biochemical, or genetic testing might be necessary.[1] There is a subset of children for whom no imaging abnormality is seen.[128]

During growth and development, these children need to be monitored to ensure optimal progress and avoid complications. An interdisciplinary team, and a 'medical home', is the preferred model of care,[17] to ensure that the multiple complex needs of these children are addressed. Lifelong care issues are now being recognized, as survival is increasing. Careful planning of the transition to adulthood is an integral part of the overall plan of care.

EPIDEMIOLOGY

Cerebral palsy is one of the most common disabling conditions affecting children. The reported incidence varies but is approximately 1–2.3 per 1000 live births.[203] The Collaborative Perinatal Project measured a prevalence rate of 5.2 per 1000 live births at 1 year of age, but reported resolution in up to half of these children by 7 years of age.[202]

Discrepancies in the rate are due to difficulties in diagnosis for a variety of reasons. Diagnosis is not made at any specific age, and can 'resolve' in up to 50% of children diagnosed prior to 2 years of age,[86] or the brain insult might not occur until later

in childhood. Various terms are also used, including neonatal encephalopathy, birth asphyxia, periventricular leukomalacia (PVL), hypoxic brain injury, stroke, traumatic brain injury, and shaken infant syndrome. There is also a wide variation in normal attainment of motor milestones, making early diagnosis less reliable.

There were hopes that recent improvements in neonatal care would decrease the incidence of CP, but the prevalence in full-term infants has remained relatively constant.[24,204] Despite improved neonatal outcomes in general, the increased survival of premature low birth weight (<2500 g) to extremely low birth weight (<1000 g) infants with higher CP risk has kept the prevalence of CP in childhood relatively constant (Box 54-1).[29] Infants born between 32 and 42 weeks' gestation, with a birth weight below the 10th percentile, had four to six times higher risk of CP compared with those between the 25th and 75th percentiles for birth weight.[140]

Maternal mental retardation, maternal seizure disorder, and hyperthyroidism; two or more prior fetal deaths; a sibling with motor deficit; third-trimester bleeding or increased urine protein excretion; and fetal bradycardia, chorioamnionitis, low placental weight, fetal malformations, and neonatal seizures all increase CP risk in term or near-term infants.[111,134,205] Multiple birth pregnancies also have a higher risk of CP, and it more often occurs in the second twin.[108]

Before pregnancy, increased CP risk is associated with long menstrual cycles or repeated fetal loss during pregnancy, fetal growth retardation, congenital malformations, abnormal fetal presentation, or low socioeconomic class.[300] During labor and delivery, only premature separation of the placenta and tight nuchal cord pose an associated CP risk.[203] Despite these many associations, most children with these risk factors do not develop CP.

ETIOLOGY

The brain injury that leads to CP can occur in the prenatal, perinatal, or postnatal period. The causes of these lesions have been attributed to a wide variety of brain injury mechanisms. It is now thought that most causes of CP occur in the prenatal period.[203] Prenatal causes include TORCH (toxoplasmosis, rubella, cytomegalovirus, herpes simplex, other) infections,

Box 54-1 Risk factors associated with cerebral palsy

General
- Gestational age <32 weeks
- Birth weight <2500 g

Maternal history
- Mental retardation
- Seizure disorder
- Hyperthyroidism
- Two or more prior fetal deaths
- Sibling with motor deficits

During gestation
- Twin gestation
- Fetal growth retardation
- Third-trimester bleeding
- Increased urine protein excretion
- Chorionitis
- Premature placenta separation
- Low placenta weight

Fetal factors
- Abnormal fetal presentation
- Fetal malformations
- Fetal bradycardia
- Neonatal seizures

Table 54-1 Grades of intraventricular hemorrhage in the premature brain

Grade	Hemorrhage
1	Isolated to germinal matrix
2	With normal ventricular size
3	With ventricular dilatation
4	With parenchymal hemorrhage

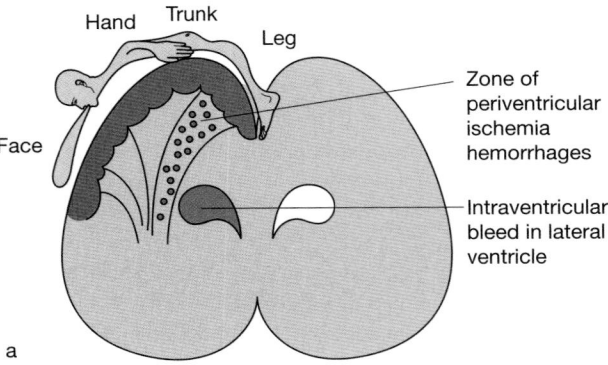

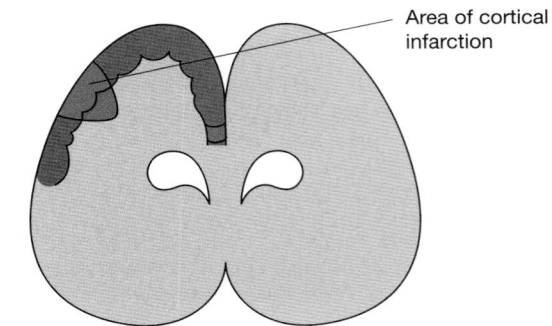

Figure 54-1 (**a**) In spastic diplegia periventricular leukomalacia, the leg is more affected than the hand and face. There is no cortical injury. (**b**) In spastic hemiplegia, the arm is often more affected than the leg. Due to cortical involvement, seizures and cognitive issues may occur more frequently.

intrauterine stroke, and genetic malformation. For this reason, some authors advocate using terminology such as 'cerebral palsy due to . . .'[82]

The most common currently understood causes are related to brain injury occurring in children born prematurely.[78] The combination of immaturity, fragile brain vasculature, and the physical stresses of prematurity predisposes these children to compromised cerebral blood flow. The blood vessels are particularly vulnerable in the watershed zone next to the lateral ventricles in the capillaries of the germinal matrix. Bleeding in this area is arterial in origin and can occur in differing degrees: cerebral intraventricular hemorrhage isolated to germinal matrix (grade 1), intraventricular hemorrhage[223] with normal ventricular size (grade 2), intraventricular hemorrhage with ventricular dilatation (grade 3), or intraventricular hemorrhage with parenchymal hemorrhage (grade 4) (Table 54-1). This can be detected early on using transfontanelle cerebral high-resolution ultrasound.[9,70]

Very low birth weight infants also have an increased incidence of periventricular hemorrhagic infarction, which is hemorrhagic necrosis lateral to the external angle of the lateral ventricle. This is thought to be bleeding of venous origin and is usually asymmetric.[110] With healing of this bleeding, symmetric necrosis of white matter adjacent to the external angle of the lateral ventricles (PVL) can develop (Fig. 54-1). PVL is one of the strongest predictors of CP in the premature neonate. PVL is almost always associated with a history of prematurity.[128] Extremely low birth weight infants are also at increased risk of CP, especially with a history of resuscitation and prolonged ventilation. Protective factors were prenatal care and steroids.[299]

Almost half of all children with CP were not born prematurely.[24,204] For term births that result in CP, the cause of brain injury is often elusive. Although uncommon, most known perinatal injuries that cause CP are due to severe anoxic or ischemic brain injury. This can occur with mechanical difficulties of the placenta, umbilical cord, or the actual delivery itself. Intrapartum asphyxia must be severe and prolonged to cause CP.[87,205] Injuries of this type unfortunately tend to be more global and are more likely to cause a more severe disability.[168] Less that 10% of cases are thought to be due to birth asphyxia, based on specific criteria that include pH of the cord blood.[112,134] Chorio-amnionitis has recently been found to be associated with a 4.1 times increased risk for CP.[308] Maternal autoimmune disease and coagulation disorders are also associated with CP.[134] Inflammatory mediators in cord serum, and other protein markers, have also been noted in small studies.[150] Genetic causes can be associated with other congenital malformations.

Athetoid CP is associated with injury to the basal ganglia.[128] This is most often caused by hyperbilirubinemia,[103] and is associated with hearing loss. Incidence has declined since testing and treatment for Rh incompatibility has become routine, and it is now relatively rare.

There are many potential causes for postnatal cerebral injury and CP. The major causes for this include central nervous system infection, vascular causes, and head injury.[50] Others include anoxia, ischemia, and inflammation. Much work is needed in the areas of prevention of CP in the full-term neonate and in postneonatal causes. When deterioration or regression in developmental milestones is seen, referral for metabolic testing should be considered.[16,294]

CLASSIFICATION

Cerebral palsy was first defined by Little in 1862. He described hemiplegic rigid, paraplegic, and generalized rigid types.[180] Since then, other classification systems have been used, but the most commonly used is based on the type of tone disorder and the limbs involved, as described by Phelps and Perlstein. Functional classification, focusing on gross motor mobility, is another method that is often used.[219,231]

Recently, the classification scheme and its limitations have been under scrutiny. There are problems with consistency in classification of some types, which has led to efforts to determine a classification system that will have excellent reliability as well as clinical utility.

The most commonly used classification system describes the type of tone abnormality as spastic, dyskinetic (dystonic or athetoid), or mixed, and some systems also include ataxic and hypotonic subtypes (Box 54-2).[25] The distribution of limb involvement is characterized as monoplegia, diplegia (both legs affected more than arms), hemiplegia (arm frequently more affected than leg), and quadriplegia (Figs 54-2 to 54-4). Triplegia is a combination of diplegia and hemiplegia. It has been suggested that the terms diplegia, quadriplegia, and hemiplegia be replaced by bilateral and unilateral involvement.[60]

As the upper limb involvement becomes more severe, it becomes more difficult to determine whether the upper or lower extremity is more involved. This has led to inconsistencies in classifying diplegia and quadriplegia. For this reason, the Gross Motor Functional Classification System (GMFCS), which stratifies children based on gross motor mobility, is favored by some.[219] The GMFCS classification does not describe the limbs affected, so the GMFCS classification is typically used in addition to describing the tone disorder and the limb distribution (Box 54-3).

Box 54-2 Classification of cerebral palsy types

By tone abnormalities
- Spastic
- Dyskinetic
  Athetoid
  Choreiform
  Ballistic
  Ataxic
- Hypotonic
- 'Mixed'

By body parts involved
- Diplegia
- Quadriplegia
- Triplegia
- Hemiplegia

Box 54-3 Gross motor functional classification

Level 1: walks without restriction, limitations in high-level skills
- Walks independently by age 2 years without devices
- Walks as preferred mobility by age 4
- Difficulty with speed, coordination, and balance for high-level tasks

Level 2: walks without devices, limitations walking outdoors
- Sits with hand support by age 2
- Crawls reciprocally or walks with device as preferred mobility by age 4
- Uses hands to get up from the floor or a chair by age 6
- Walks without devices indoors by age 6

Level 3: walks with devices, limitations walking outdoors
- Sits with support by age 2
- Cruises by age 4, walks with device short distances
- Does stairs with help by age 6
- Walks indoors with a device by age 12

Level 4: limited mobility, power mobility outdoors
- Rolls by age 2 years
- Sits with hand support by age 4
- May walk short distances indoors with device, poor balance
- Preferred independent mobility is a wheelchair by age 12

Level 5: very limited self-mobility, even with assistive technology
- Needs help to roll by age 2
- Does not attain independent mobility by age 12
- With high-level assistive technology, may learn to use power mobility

(After Palisano et al. 1997,[219] with permission.)

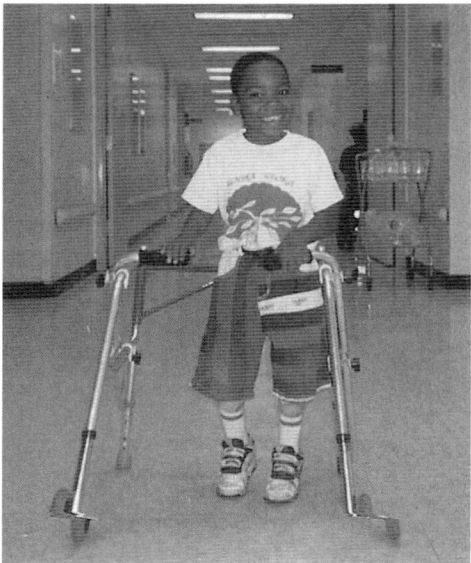

Figure 54-2 Patient with spastic diplegia.

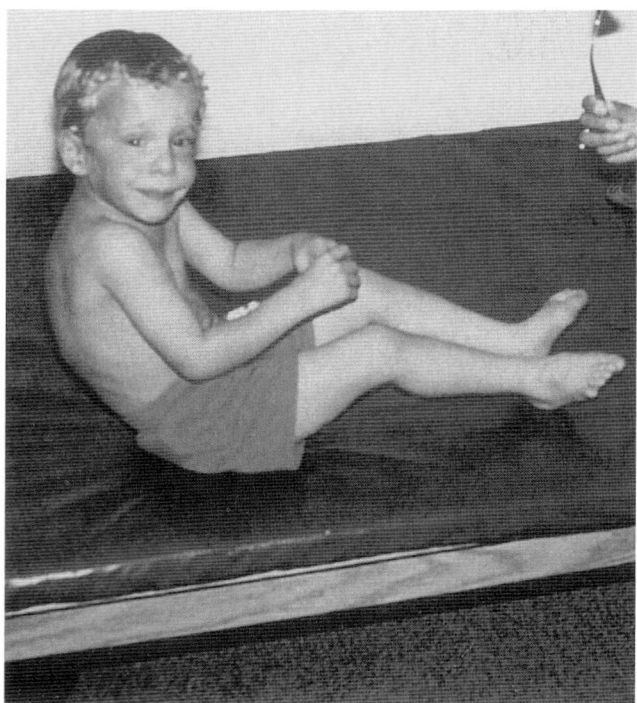

Figure 54-3 Patient with spastic quadriplegia.

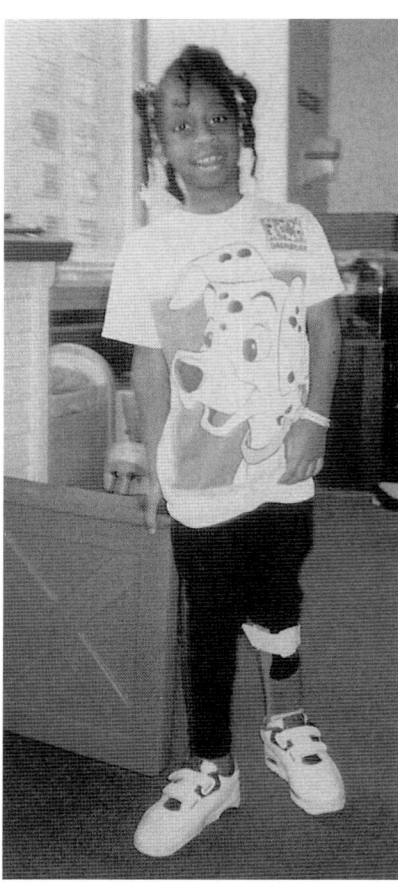

Figure 54-4 Patient with spastic hemiplegia.

The areas of brain involvement on MRI can also be helpful to predict areas of difficulty. Generally, the vast majority of children (over 85%) with hemiplegia can eventually walk independently.[101] For unclear reasons, isolated right hemiplegia is twice as common as left hemiplegia.

The spastic subtype is the most common, affecting about 75% of children with CP. Spasticity is defined as velocity-dependent increased tone, associated with upper motor neuron syndrome findings of increased muscle stretch reflexes, Babinski's response, weakness, and difficulty with coordination. It can be associated with extensor or flexor posturing (decorticate or decerebrate).

Dystonia is defined as a dyskinetic tone abnormality with alternating tone or cocontraction in the antagonist and agonist muscle groups, causing varied abnormal postures and often fluctuating tone.[174] The other dyskinetic forms are athetosis, choreiform and choreoathetoid. Athetoid movements are involuntary constant rotatory or writhing movements of the distal extremities, and are associated with basal ganglia involvement. These movements stop during sleep. The incidence of the athetoid type has drastically been reduced by the advent of treatment for Rh incompatibility. The ataxic form is rare, and must be differentiated from degenerative processes of the cerebellum.

Spasticity and dystonia frequently coexist in CP, as the mixed form of tone abnormality. Studies to differentiate spasticity from dystonia using clinical assessment[254] or gait analysis[69] are important, as some treatments control spasticity or dystonia more effectively. Surgical outcomes are much less predictable in children with dystonia, as tone fluctuates. A form of dystonia that is responsive to dopaminergic medication is well described.[210]

A small percentage of patients have the hypotonic type of CP. These children need to be differentiated from those with identifiable causes of neonatal hypotonia such as muscle disease, metabolic disorders, and genetic syndromes. Many of these children develop spastic or extrapyramidal-type disorders after the first few months of life.

CLINICAL EFFECTS

Hypotonia and motor delay are often seen as early signs of CP. The severity of involvement varies widely, depending on the extent of neurologic involvement. Upper motor neuron injury features include positive findings of increased tone and reflexes, positive Babinski's reflex, and negative findings of reduced strength, selective motor control, balance, and coordination. About three-quarters of children with CP have spasticity, although the first several months can be characterized with hypotonia.

Early on, assessment reveals tone in the extremities, and retention of primitive reflexes can be noted. Obligatory primitive reflexes that the child cannot emerge from are always abnormal. Examples of these are the asymmetric tonic neck reflex (ATNR), symmetric tonic neck reflex (STNR), and tonic labyrinthine reflex (Figs 54-5 to 54-7). Other problems in infancy that suggest CP include irritability, lethargy, weak suck

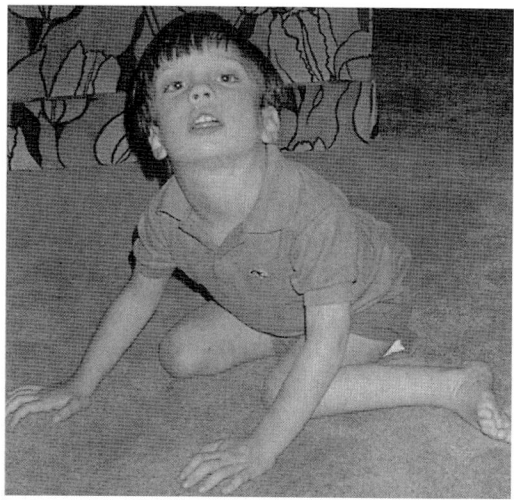

Figure 54-6 Symmetric tonic neck reflex (if the neck is extended, the upper extremities are extended and the lower extremities are flexed).

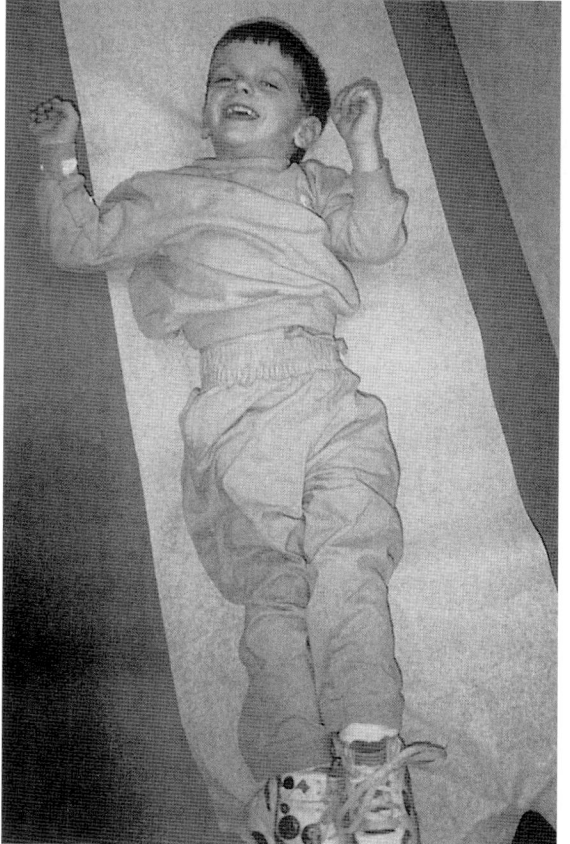

Figure 54-7 Patient with tonic labyrinthine reflex.

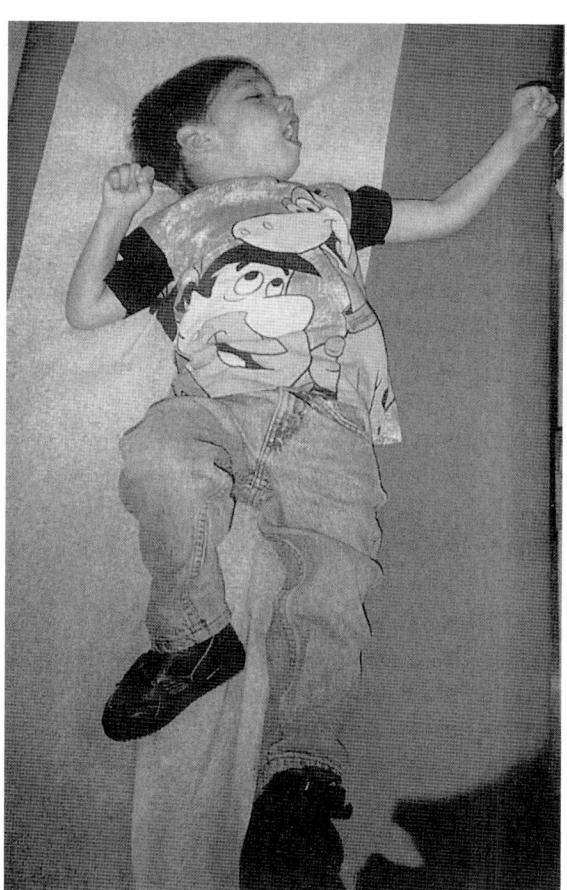

Figure 54-5 Patient with asymmetric tonic neck reflex.

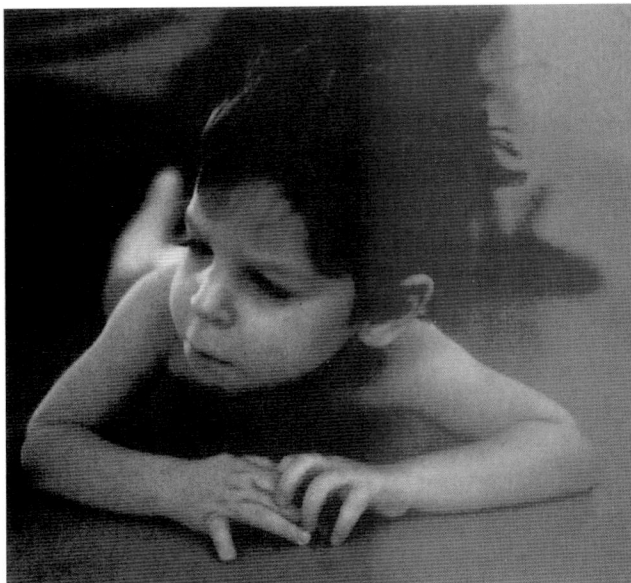

Figure 54-8 Combat or belly crawl with lower extremity extension and use of upper extremities for forward progression.

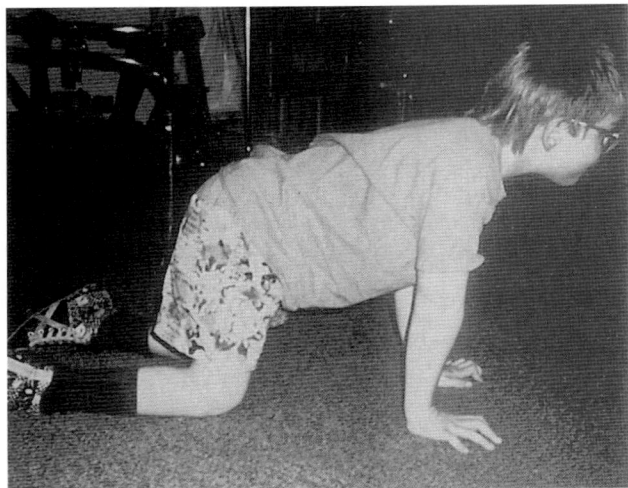

Figure 54-9 'Bunny hop'.

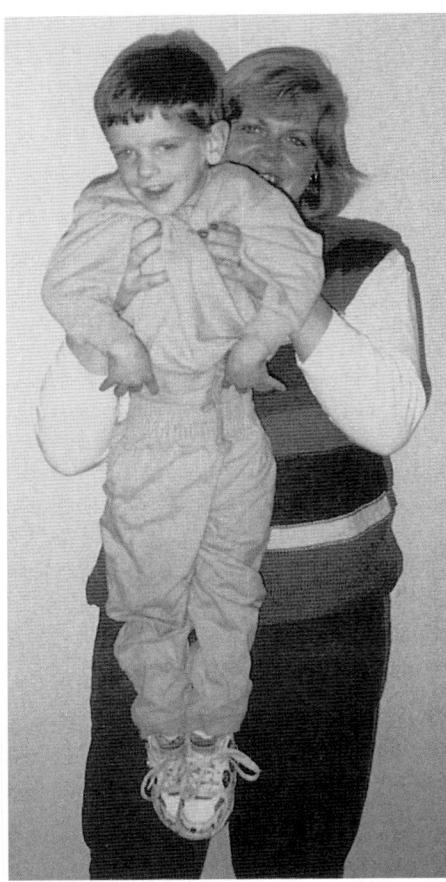

Figure 54-10 'Scissoring' on vertical suspension.

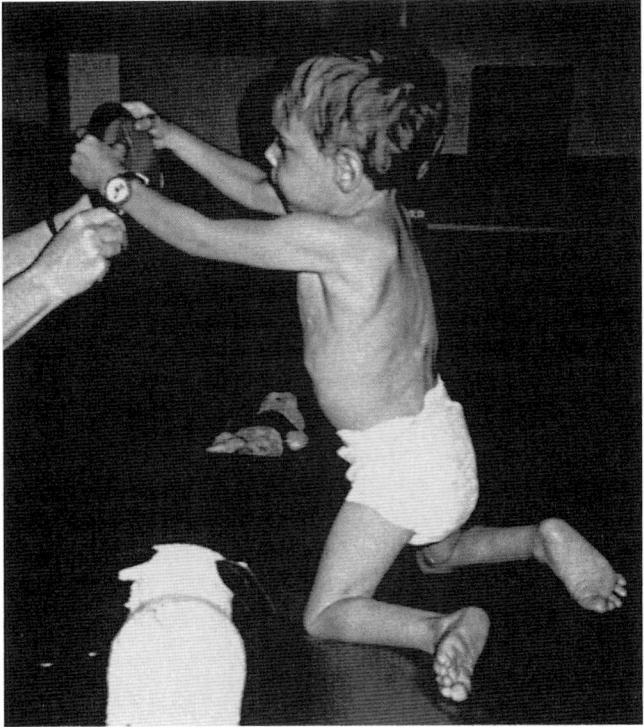

Figure 54-11 'Proximal fixing' with increased activity in shoulder girdle and neck muscles.

with tongue thrust, poor head control, high-pitched cry, oral hypersensitivity, tonic bite, and asymmetric movements or unusual posturing. Later on, the child might be noted to be rolling for mobility, combat crawling, 'W sitting', 'bunny hopping', or adopting a hand preference before the first birthday (Figs 54-8 and 54-9).[72] Trunk or central hypotonia often remains throughout life.

Abnormalities of muscle tone are frequently accompanied by muscle weakness. As tone develops in children with spasticity, abnormal posturing such as 'scissoring', 'guarding' of the upper extremities, extensor posturing, or proximal 'fixing' (Figs 54-10 to 54-12) can be seen. Scissoring is the simultaneous adduction, knee hyperextension, and plantar flexion of the lower extremities. Flexion synergy patterns of the upper extremities include

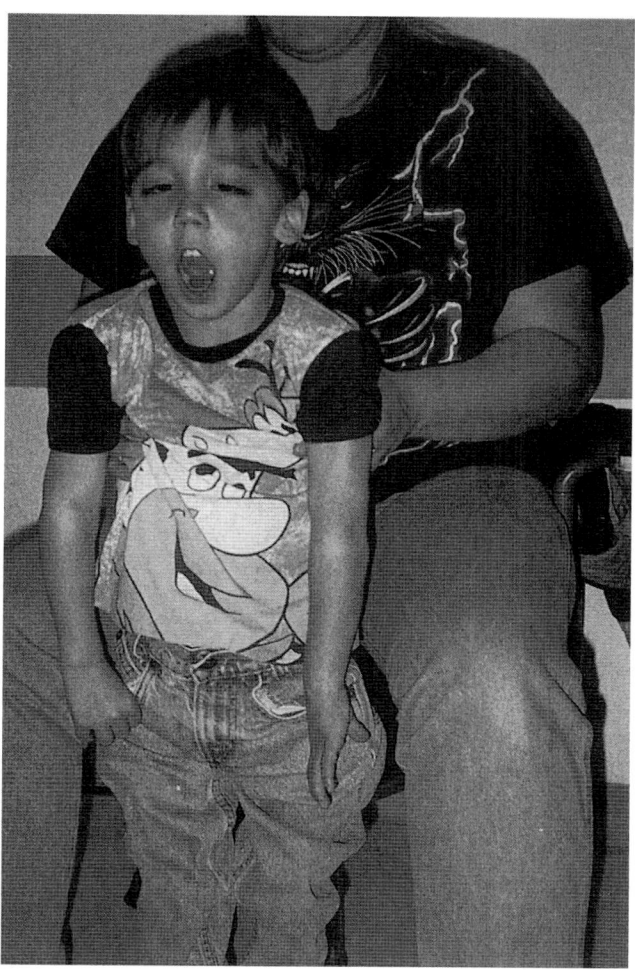

Figure 54-12 Patient with extensor posturing.

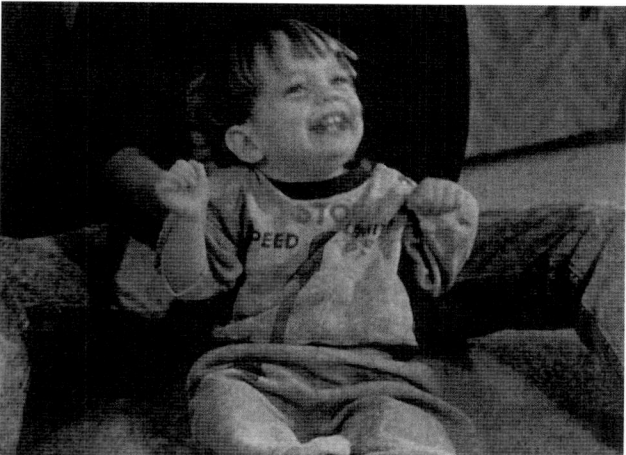

Figure 54-13 'High guard' position of upper extremities.

flexion at the fingers, wrists, and elbows with shoulder abduction. As this upper extremity pattern becomes stronger, the child's hands rise from the waist, producing a low, mid, or high guard position (Fig. 54-13).

The abnormalities of muscle tone are often accompanied by weakness in individual muscles. Applying the traditional methods of measuring muscle strength is problematic in CP, because the tone abnormalities mask the patient's ability to generate force.[85] Modified sphygmomanometer and hydraulic force measures can provide better reliability than Medical Research Council muscle strength grades.

Sensory issues are also well recognized in CP, which affect motor function, such as hand manipulation ability. Hypersensitivity can interfere with development of hand and lower extremity weight-bearing skills. The abnormal sensory experience of disordered motor control can contribute to disordered sensory perception, which further interferes with the child's ability to perform high-level motor activities.[44] Decreased ability to distinguish two-point discrimination has been found in the upper extremities of children with all types of CP.[176] Children with hemiparetic CP have also been found almost universally to have a decrease in stereognosis, with decreased

proprioception in about half of patients tested.[298] The side of involvement with cortical lesions is also known to cause specific issues, such as movement planning with left hemisphere injury.[171,277] Balance difficulties can be due to a combination of weakness, abnormal tone, and sensory issues, including visual perceptual skills.

The major secondary effects of disordered muscle tone, control, and balance are changes in joint alignment, leading to contracture and deformity. Contracture (passive shortening that can limit joint and soft tissue movement) frequently affects the adductor, hamstring, and plantar flexor muscles of the lower extremities and the flexors of the upper extremities. This reflects the presence of spasticity, scissoring, or upper extremity flexion patterns, individually or severally, which are present in the majority of children with spastic types of CP.

Bony deformity can occur because the abnormal muscle forces of CP act on a growing skeleton. The integrity of the hips and spine are a principal concern, because of their primary role in weight bearing and positioning. The femur is affected by muscle and gravity-loading forces during growth. Muscle forces in CP can cause increased anteversion of the femur neck.[264] The typical increase in hip flexion, adduction, and internal rotation of the femur acts to influence the femoral head in a superoposterolateral direction out of the acetabulum. The result is coxa valgus, deformation of the femoral head, and a shallow acetabulum, which causes the hip to be more prone to subluxation (Fig. 54-14).[32,72] Asymmetric muscle pull and immobility can contribute to significant deformity of the spine, including kyphosis, scoliosis, or rotational deformities. These spinal deformities can significantly affect comfort, tone, sitting and standing alignment, and balance. When these are severe, respiratory function can be compromised by the mechanical restriction of the chest, combined with decreased efficiency of available respiratory muscle strength. This can have a significant impact on endurance, health, and longevity. Spondylolisthesis and spondylolysis are not increased in CP. Case reports of atlantoaxial instability in spastic CP have been reported.[291]

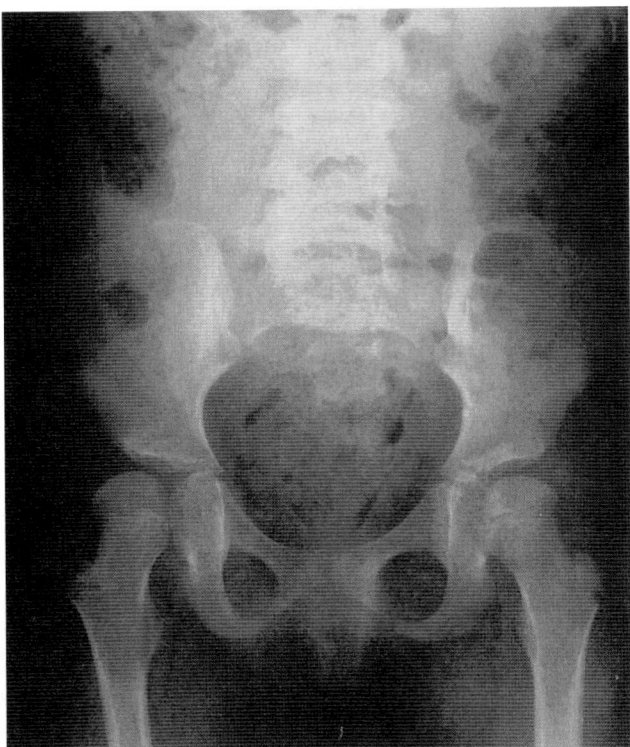

Figure 54-14 Dysplastic hip joints.

Bony abnormalities of the feet can occur in a variety of patterns. The most common is deformity of the hind foot with exaggerated heel valgus or varus. Hyperpronation occurs frequently with calcaneovalgus. Occasionally a rocker bottom type of foot can be seen.

ASSOCIATED MEDICAL AND FUNCTIONAL PROBLEMS

A number of associated medical issues are also commonly seen in children and adults with CP that can interfere with development and general health. These also require attention and management, and often involvement of a number of healthcare professionals.

Visual sequelae occur due to the central visual pathways being affected. Strabismus is common in children with diplegia, including exotropia or esotropia. Hemiplegia can be associated with hemianopsia. Premature infants can also have had retinopathy of prematurity. Forty percent of premature children have visual sequelae.[212] Hearing impairment can be related to ototoxic drug exposure, hyperbilirubinemia, or TORCH infection in utero.[241] Early assessment of hearing and vision is important in all children with CP.

A large number of children with CP have abnormalities of oral motor function. These deficits include drooling, dysphagia, and dysarthria, due to weakness and incoordination of lips, tongue, and masticatory and facial muscles. Drooling can also reflect poor swallowing ability. It can cause problems socially for schoolage children, and can cause rash and dental problems. Treatment can include behavioral techniques, speech therapy, anticholinergic medications,[20,178] botulinum toxin A injections,[255] and surgical redirection of the salivary gland ducts.[120,260] Airway patency can be obstructed in some children due to spastic, floppy, or stenosed tissues in the upper airway. Difficulties with choking or apneic spells during sleep, stridor, or snoring can occur. Tracheostomy is sometimes required to maintain control of the airway.

Dysphagia can be due to a problem in the oral phase (chewing and bolus preparation) or in the laryngeal phase (propulsion and airway protection problems). In one large study of patients with suspected oropharyngeal dysfunction, over half of those tested aspirated. The majority of those patients have no effective cough during aspiration (R. Gramer, K. Keller, J. Baughman, et al., pers. comm).[243] Swallowing dysfunction is often present only with certain textures of food ingested, as detected by videoflouroscopy.[243] In severe cases, aspiration can cause hypoxemia.[244]

Feeding difficulties can contribute to substantial undernutrition or malnutrition. Up to one-third of children with hemiplegia and diplegia, and more than two-thirds with quadriplegia, have been found to be undernourished.[145,274,275] The North American Cerebral Palsy Growth Project demonstrated that 27% of children with CP were malnourished, based on triceps skin fold measures below the 10th percentile.[281] Due to the difficulty in maintaining adequate nutrition orally, other methods might be required, such as gastrostomy or gastrojejunostomy tube.[284] An American Academy of Cerebral Palsy and Developmental Medicine (AACPDM) evidence report indicated that there is evidence of improved outcomes with improved nutrition. Poor nutrition is associated with decreased participation in community activities.[252] Outcomes after stressful events such as surgery are improved by optimizing nutrition.[199]

Gastrointestinal symptoms are frequent in children with CP.[75] Gastroesophageal reflux, due to weakness of the lower esophageal sphincter, can cause episodic emesis. It can also interfere with adequate ingestion and absorption of nutrients, and compromise adequate nutrition and growth.[192,228] Medications, or surgical Nissen fundoplication or jejunostomy are options to reduce reflux.[249] Chronic constipation is a significant concern for many children with CP. This can be in part due to neuromuscular control of the bowel, and exaggerated by immobility and abnormal diet and fluid intake. Abnormal segmental colonic transit times have been noted, and are correlated with ambulatory function.[224] Increasing activity, and fluid and fiber intake can improve constipation, along with the judicious use of medications. Long-term significant complications, such as large bowel megacolon and volvulus,[136,253] can be prevented by regular bowel evacuation. Patients with complaints of fecal incontinence or defecation distress have been found to have anal sphincter or pelvic muscle incoordination (or both). This typically occurs without rectal dysfunction, and can be assessed by anorectal manometry.[4] This dysfunction in the pelvic area appears to be related to abnormalities in neuromotor control.

Urinary symptoms are not uncommon in CP. Around one-third of patients have symptoms of frequency, incontinence, or difficulty urinating.[195] There are a few small studies on the subject, with varying reports of frequency of significant urodynamic findings.[38,239] Detrusor instability, vesicoureteric reflux, and detrusor–sphincter dyssynergia have been noted.[39] Investigation and treatment can usually reduce symptoms in symptomatic patients.[71,74]

Cognitive impairments are not obligatory with CP but can occur to varying degrees. The prevalence of mental retardation in all persons with CP is estimated to be 30%.[170] The risk increases with the severity of the motor disability. Specific learning disabilities can be present in 20–30%.[292] Normal birth weight children with CP have had cognitive abnormalities reported in up to 40–50%.[92]

Seizure disorders can occur in up to one-third of children with CP.[268] Children with hemiplegia have the highest rate,[171] followed by those with quadriplegia, and then diplegia. Presence of seizures typically reflects a greater extent of cortical brain injury.[109] Newer antiseizure techniques using grid mapping and resection of seizure foci are now part of the standard treatment options.

Osteoporosis is present in children with CP due to multiple factors. Calcium and Vitamin D can be deficient, due to the reduced caloric intake diet of people with CP. Decreased weight bearing and muscle stresses can contribute to osteoporosis. Antiseizure medications can interfere with vitamin D metabolism. Pathologic fractures, or fractures with even minimal transfer activity, are not uncommon and occur more frequently after a period of immobilization.[159] Decreased femoral bone mineral density was found to be associated with feeding difficulty, anticonvulsant use, weight percentile, and low triceps skin fold.[119,120] Studies on increased weight bearing as an intervention show varying results on bone mineral density.[51,53] Calcium and vitamin D supplementation show positive effects on bone density.[143] Bisphosphonates such as pamidronate have been used in a number of small studies, with increases demonstrated in bone density.[119,285] The main outcome of interest is reduction in fractures and related morbidity, which have not been adequately studied. Bone age was not found to be significantly different than chronologic age in children with CP, although wider variation occurred than in normal children.[96]

Pain can go undiagnosed and untreated in children who are non-verbal. A study of 198 children with CP, with GMFCS levels of 3–5, showed that 11% had pain on a daily basis.[129] The frequency of the pain also correlated with the severity of motor impairment, presence of a gastrostomy, days of school missed, and days spent in bed. With pain now being dubbed as the 'fifth vital sign', increased recognition and treatment of pain concerns in non-communicative children is occurring.[130,269]

Mortality in children with CP is associated with severity and health burden. Lack of independent mobility such as rolling, the use of a tracheostomy, and lack of any hand function are associated with higher mortality.[238] Basic life skills such as feeding and mobility can result in differences in survival of 40 years or more.[283] Seven factors appear to play significant roles in predicting survival. These include cognitive level, ability to speak, ability to recognize voices, ability to interact with peers, physical ability and mobility, tube feeding, incontinence, and seizures.[63,149,247]

Injuries, abuse, and neglect are also potential causes for morbidity and mortality in children with CP. The usual preventive strategies for childhood injury should be employed. Injuries from use of equipment used for mobility can be of concern. Neglect is the most common form of childhood maltreatment, and is about twice as common in disabled than in non-disabled children.[90] In most jurisdictions, healthcare professionals who suspect that a child is being subject to maltreatment are obligated to report it to the child protective services.

FUNCTIONAL PROGNOSIS

Children typically develop motor skills craniocaudally. A child will first develop neck control, then upper trunk control, and then lower trunk control. Sitting balance follows, then standing. The age at which these skills are developed help to predict the eventual outcome. Those children who will attain independent ambulation typically achieve these skills by the age of 8, and only rarely later. Seventy-five percent of children with spastic CP eventually ambulate, about 85% with diplegia, and 70% with quadriplegia. Most children with hemiplegic or ataxic CP ambulate independently, the majority by age 3 years.[80]

Children who are able to sit independently before their second birthday eventually become independent walkers, with or without equipment. Children who have not attained independent sitting by age 4 years rarely walk. However, if the primitive reflexes (ATNR, STNR, tonic labyrinthine, Moro's, positive supporting reflex, or extensor posturing) still occur in an obligatory manner, the prognosis for independent ambulation is poor.[31] Most children who will walk have fewer than three of these reflexes present at age 18 months.[197]

The combination of increased tone and underlying muscle weakness greatly increases the energy expended for motor activity. Children with CP who achieve ambulation typically have an inefficient gait, which includes much shorter step length, decreased range of motion at the hip and knee, more energy expenditure, and decreased velocity as compared with their peers.

All these inefficiencies of muscle control contribute to decreased endurance.[246] Although endurance is difficult to measure with conventional methods because of the challenges of various impairments with CP, it seems to correlate with the overall gross motor capabilities of the individual.[226] Energy cost of walking is found to correlate to GMFCS level.[146] Contractures and bone or joint deformities can also greatly limit a child's function.

Table 54-2 Outcome measures for cerebral palsy rehabilitation

Outcome of interest	Measure
Spasticity	Ashworth score Tardieu angles
Range of motion	Goniometer
Dystonia	Barry Albright Dystonia Scale
Strength	Medical Research Council muscle grade (0–5) Modified sphygmomanometer Hydraulic strength or torque Maximum 10 repetitions weight lift
Cognition	IQ
Speech	Intelligibility
Health	Short Form 12 or 36
Social and self-care skills	WeeFIM, Pediatric Outcomes Data Collection Instrument Canadian Occupational Performance Measure
Pain	Faces pain scale Non-verbal pain scale
Community integration	Child Health Questionnaire Demographics, Craig Handicap Assessment and Reporting Technique
Hand and arm function	Melbourne upper extremity test Quality of Upper Extremity Skills Test
Gross motor function	Gross Motor Function Measure Peabody Scales of Infant Development
Gait	Velocity, stride length, balance Oxygen cost Kinetics or kinematics on gait analysis

OUTCOME MEASURES

When choosing an outcome measure to evaluate an intervention, good validity and reliability, as well as responsiveness to change, are desirable.[276] Table 54-2 indicates various outcome measures that can be used in CP assessment. There is no single outcome measure that is typically used with CP, as the domains of interest vary widely. The outcome measures that are chosen usually depend on the area of intervention and the desired outcome.

THERAPEUTIC MANAGEMENT

The therapeutic management of the child with CP emphasizes a functional aim- or goal-oriented approach.[77] The two major goals of rehabilitation, according to Molnar,[198] are to decrease complications of the CP and to enhance or improve the acquisition of new skills. Rothery and colleagues include parent and caregiver education, decreasing skeletal deformity, and improving mobility.[248]

The role of the physician is to provide an accurate assessment of the child's impairments. In the case of the child with CP,

this can include learning disabilities, mental retardation, respiratory compromise, fractures, and other comorbidities that can limit function. In addition to the impairments, all precautions should be identified that can pose a risk to the child during therapy. Seizures, osteopenia, and gastroesophageal reflux occur frequently and can have an impact on the treatment.[196]

From the first evaluation, the family and child should be encouraged to become active participants in the process of setting priorities and goals within the context of the impairment. The institution of therapy and other medical modalities should be approached and prescribed after a thorough discussion of efficacy.[271] The following discussion represents the major therapeutic interventions for children with CP.

Early intervention

Köng has suggested that early institution of physical therapy (PT) can decrease the impact of brain injury on the development of CP.[165] The Education of the Handicapped Act Amendments of 1986, Public Law 99-457, or the Individuals with Disabilities Education Act (IDEA), mandated early intervention for infants and toddlers (0–3 years old) who demonstrate developmental delay.[52] This federal law was established to provide educational and educationally related rehabilitative services to children who enter school with already identifiable problems. The law provides a downward extension of Public Law 94-142 (Education of All Handicapped Children Act), which mandated that all states must provide a free and appropriate public education to eligible schoolchildren. One of the hallmarks of IDEA is the clearly identified role of the family as central to the goals of early intervention. The team acts not only to treat the child but also to empower the family. A mutual contract, the individual family service plan (IFSP), is developed actively by the team and parents. Unlike the individual education plan from Public Law 94-142, the IFSP must take the family's strengths and needs into account, as well as the child's goals.[118]

The rationale for early intervention is closely connected to concepts that stress the importance of the early years for normally developing children, and the role that environmental factors play in development. Parental characteristics have been found to be associated with a child's concurrent or later developmental functioning. These parental characteristics include responsivity contingent on child initiations, the quality and quantity of verbal interactions, the existence of a social support network, and maternal sensitivity.[173]

There are two main models for the delivery of developmental early intervention: the direct therapy service model and the consultation model. In the direct model, service delivery can occur as part of interdisciplinary, multidisciplinary, or transdisciplinary treatment in a center- or home-based program.[22] Physical therapists and occupational therapists have traditionally been providers of therapeutic intervention for the child with CP. Many children are also seen by a speech–language pathologist for feeding difficulties and oromotor problems. A social worker and developmental specialist constitute the members of a typical early intervention team. To reduce the number of therapists handling the child, Haynes has advocated that one professional from the early intervention team integrate assessment data from all the members of the team, developing integrated strategies to meet the goals agreed in the IFSP.[117]

Therapy approaches

Children with CP who have motor problems that interfere with educational activities have the opportunity to participate in integrated therapy programs in school. The services should be delivered in the least restrictive environment, and are mandated to allow the child to participate in and benefit from the educational experience. The current philosophic trend in schools is to include disabled children as much as possible into the regular classroom, and few 'pull out' services are stressed. Mainstreaming has positive effects on the psychosocial aspects of schooling and increases the academic expectations of the disabled student.[48] Consultative models of PT, occupational therapy (OT), and speech therapy have provided a method of treating and involving more of the children with disabilities into regular education classes. Even though there is a move toward consultative services by PT, OT, and speech therapy in the school systems,

direct service can be recommended to augment an overall therapy program.

There are a number of therapy systems that have influenced the management of children with CP (Table 54-3). Rarely does the clinical delivery of therapy services rely on any one system. An eclectic approach is common—one that offers modalities from several schools of therapy. Such an approach provides the flexibility and individualization necessary to meet the child's and the family's goals.

A shift to functional goal setting that involves the parents has become prominent since the 1980s.[139] PT had focused on impairment, with less emphasis on the daily functioning of the parent (caregiver). Caregiver participation provides the key to transferring the physical therapies' impact from clinic to daily home activities.[267] Families are also then put into the crucial role of becoming equal partners in the setting of goals and understanding of impairment, which promotes empowerment.[139] The relationship of therapist and families is complex, and has been studied to look at compliance and parent stress.[278] There is a trend toward more compliance for therapy that is performed in the home. Parent satisfaction for home therapy is high.[139]

Physical therapy has been shown to prevent contractures and deformities, improve postural alignment, improve independence through assistive seating and mobility devices, maintain motor level and improved functional abilities, increase endurance, and improve the ability of the parents to manage the child's disability.[49] Most studies of the effectiveness of PT and other treatments are inconclusive.[50,121,256] Investigators have found that the children most likely to improve in motor abilities were those children with higher IQs and lesser involvement of the neuromuscular system.[98] Harris has provided a review of efficacy studies (see Table 54-3).[115]

The effectiveness of any specific intervention for the child with CP is difficult to study, due to the multihandicapping nature of CP, lack of outcome measures, difficulty in obtaining control groups, and historically poor study designs. Individual therapy programs vary in parameters and incorporate subjective as well as objective elements. Methodological difficulties arise from the problems of measuring treatment-related change on a background of development, as well as the heterogeneity of the population.[196]

The development of appropriate evaluative measures, adherence to randomized control studies, and the use of metaanalysis portend improved understanding of the use of therapies on the outcome of the child with CP.[115,141,154,160,217,260,289] In a recent review, neurodevelopmental therapy for children with CP did not confer an advantage over other types of therapy in altering abnormal motor responses, slowing or preventing contractures, or facilitating more normal motor development or functional activities.[46,68,160] Systematic reviews of literature on speech therapy and OT reveal positive trends to support the use of services but demonstrate no clear treatment effect.[220,236,280]

The success of therapy can be better measured by individual goal achievement and specific outcomes such as strength. Spasticity was once thought to be increased with strengthening, but

Table 54-3 Similarities and differences between neuromotor therapy approaches to cerebral palsy

	Neurodevelopmental treatment (Bobaths)	Sensorimotor approach to treatment (Rood)	Sensory integration approach (Ayres)	Vojta approach	Patterning therapy (Doman–Delacato)
Central nervous system model Goals of treatment	Hierarchic • To normalize tone • To inhibit primitive reflexes • To facilitate automatic reactions and normal movement patterns	Hierarchic • To activate postural responses (stability) • To activate movement (mobility) once stability is achieved	Hierarchic • To improve efficiency of neural processing • To better organize adaptive responses	Hierarchic • To prevent cerebral palsy in infants at risk • To improve motoric behavior in infants with fixed cerebral palsy	Hierarchic • To achieve independent mobility • To improve motor coordination • To prevent or improve communication disorders • To enhance intelligence
Primary sensory systems utilized to effect a motor response	• Kinesthetic • Proprioceptive • Tactile	• Tactile • Proprioceptive • Kinesthetic	• Vestibular • Tactile • Kinesthetic	• Proprioceptive • Kinesthetic • Tactile	All sensory systems are utilized
Emphasis of treatment activities	• Positioning and handling to normalize sensory input • Facilitation of active movement	Sensory stimulation to activate motor response (tapping, brushing, icing)	Therapist guides but child controls sensory input to get adaptive purposeful response	Trigger reflex locomotive zones to encourage movement patterns (e.g. reflex crawl)	Sensory and reflex stimulation, passive movement patterns, encouragement of independent movements
Intended clinical population	Children with cerebral palsy Adults post cerebrovascular accident (CVA)	Children with neuromotor disorders such as cerebral palsy Adults post CVA	Children with learning disabilities Children with autism	Young infants at risk for cerebral palsy Young infants with fixed cerebral palsy	Children with neonatal or acquired brain damage
Emphasis on treating infants	Yes	No	No	Yes	No
Emphasis on family involvement during treatment	Yes Handling and positioning for activities of daily living	No	No Supportive role encouraged	Yes Family administers treatment at home daily	Yes Family and friends administer treatment several times daily
Empiric support	Few studies Conflicting results	Very few studies Conflicting results	Many studies Conflicting results with schoolage children Positive results for tactile and vestibular input with infants	Few studies Conflicting results	Few studies Conflicting results

(From Harris et al. 1985,[114] with permission.)

that has not been shown to occur.[66] A systematic review of the effectiveness of strength training for people with CP does demonstrate improved strength and motor activity.[73]

An intervention that melds educational theory and PT is conductive education. Conductive education is a mode of therapy that integrates rhythmic movement and activities in a group setting, with a class leader. This method has spread in the USA and now is utilized in some areas as a school-based program.[216] The evidence available supports improvement in functional skills such as toileting for children in conductive education programs versus those in regular school therapy.[68]

Constraint-induced (or forced use) therapy has promise and supports the theory of motor plasticity. This therapy restrains the sound limb to increase the use of the affected side. Gains in the areas of motor performance were maintained up to 6 months post intensive training in one study.[286]

Functional electrical stimulation and biofeedback can be helpful for training specific muscles.[156,182,272,296]

Another modality that is gaining attention for improving strength in the child with CP is therapeutic electrical stimulation. The use of low-voltage, high-frequency electrical stimulation has been shown to increase blood flow and improve muscle growth and strength.[65]

Equipment concerns

All durable medical equipment should be considered in the context of the functional prognosis. The early introduction of independent mobility, for children who are not yet able to negotiate at a household level, increases exploration of the environment and might also improve self-esteem.[47,155] When standardized equipment does not meet the postural support needs of the severely involved child, adaptive seating is essential for the attainment of a sitting position (see Ch. 18).[126]

Use of a wheelchair for community mobility becomes a practical measure once a child has outgrown commercially available strollers. A specialized seating system preserves a child's capacity to interact in a conventional posture and also improves pulmonary function tests (see Ch. 18).[209] While power mobility is usable for children as young as 18 months,[47] many children with CP have problems with spatial relationships and problem-solving skills that preclude motorized chair use. Prior to acquisition of a power chair, a careful evaluation of the family's needs, the child's coping skills, and the environment for which the power mobility is necessary should be undertaken.[191,221] The child who is comfortable and adequately seated typically has better feeding, digestion, and vocal production. Rehabilitation engineers working with therapists can address complex orthopedic and functional problems. Walkers provide external support for strength and balance, and can improve upright position.[107]

The early introduction of technology to improve communication, either written or oral, is warranted.[179] The use of an augmentative communication device does not inhibit development of communication skills. In augmentative communication, speech is enhanced by the use of technology.[132,262] Low technology and high technology are compensation strategies that continue to challenge the rehabilitation professional abilities to maximize function.[309]

Adaptive equipment specialists provide access to computers, environmental control units, and other activities of daily living (ADL) equipment (see Ch. 27).[157,188] In addition to specialized equipment, the child with CP is frequently assisted in mobility and ADL tasks by the use of splints or orthoses.[301] Goldkamp reviewed ADL outcome in children with CP and reported that few children after the age of 4 years achieved independence.[98]

Splinting is a common conservative method of managing a spastic but flexible dynamic deformity. The physical therapist can provide tone-reducing ankle–foot orthoses (TRAFOs) whose tone-reducing aspects are incorporated into their construction. TRAFOs have been useful in some children but are not universally recommended.[301] The decision to brace and the type of orthosis to be used are dictated by the age of the child, functional level, motor control, type of deformity, and commitment to use.[200,201] Ankle–foot orthoses can decrease energy expenditure when used in conjunction with therapy, surgery, and other treatment.[270,303] Other joint immobilizers can contribute to function and maintenance of range of motion for hygiene and dressing.[13] Compression garments theoretically increase proprioceptive input to the neuromuscular system and improve motor function. Their intermittent use is appropriate for tasks that are challenging and self-limited.

MEDICAL AND SURGICAL MANAGEMENT

Management of hypertonia

Management of hypertonia for children with CP has had increasing medical attention over the decade. Distinguishing between spasticity and other hypertonic movement disorders has been highlighted as a problem in evaluating different interventions.[174,254] Many professionals are involved with the child, and it is critical that terms that are used frequently to describe the motor disorder are clearly defined. Spasticity implies a velocity-dependent resistance to stretch of a muscle, which is separate from dynamic disorders such as dystonia.[254] Careful analysis and measurement of the hypertonia will lead to more precise management.[66,254]

Oral medications are utilized to decrease global hypertonia. The most commonly used drugs are baclofen (Lioresal), dantrolene (Dantrium), and diazepam.[185] The response to these drugs is generally unpredictable, and side effects can limit long-term use. Studies have demonstrated clinically useful reduction in spasticity following the initiation of medication. The pediatric doses can be quite variable and depend on the response of patient.

Specific medications for dystonia can impact the movement in additional ways. Motor control can be improved in the oral motor and fine motor areas with trihexyphenidyl hydrochloride (Artane),[127,237] and levodopa–carbidopa (Sinemet) and other dopaminergic medications are drugs that warrant trial in a child with dystonia.[83]

Reappraisal of spasticity or hypertonia in a growing child with CP every 6 months is necessary. Contractures develop over time and are a complex interaction of spasticity, growth, motor control deficits, weakness, and chronic positioning. The costs and benefits of the commonly used interventions are shown in Table 54-4.[100]

Motor point blocks, and recently botulinum toxin injections, can be used as adjunct management of the spastic muscle.[62,104,162] Botulinum toxin's effect in children with CP has been studied and promoted in the past decade and is widely utilized in the management of CP.[143] There is a large body of literature that

Table 54-4 Cost–benefit comparison of spasticity treatments in cerebral palsy

Treatment	Type of tone problem	Age	Advantage	Disadvantage	Cost
Physical and occupational therapy	All types	Any	Improves development	Expensive	$$$
Oral medications	Diffuse	>1 year	Works systemically	Sedating	$
Bracing or casts	All types	Any	Improves joint position and range of motion	Fails to reduce deformity	$
Orthopedic surgery	All types	5 years to adolescent	Corrects alignment	Temporarily reduces deformity	$$$
Neurolytic blocks	Focal	Any	Reduces spasticity	Temporary	$$
Selective dorsal rhizotomy	Diplegia	4–8 years	Eliminates spasticity	Irreversible	$$$$
Intrathecal baclofen	Lower extremity	>34 lbs	Adjustable tone reduction	20% adverse effects	$$$$

(From Gormley et al. 2004,[100] with permission of MacKeith Press.)

supports its use in children with hypertonia, both spasticity and dystonia.[36,161] Botulinum toxin Type A (Botox) is effective in improving range of motion and reducing tone, and also potentially effective in improving motor control.[222] The recent enthusiastic utilization of the botulinum toxins is due to the possible positive effect on the growth of spastic muscles, as well as the potential for improved motor control.[90] The use of serial casting with and without botulinum toxin for children with dynamic contractures has been studied. At present, the best results appear to be with those that combine casting with botulinum toxin for dynamic phased contractures.[34,151] The current suggested indications for the use of botulinum toxin include:

- calf injection for dynamic equinus persistent throughout the gait cycle;
- hamstring injection for dynamic knee flexion;
- adductor injection for scissoring;
- diagnostic measures before surgery;
- management of focal limb dystonia;
- analgesia for pain and spasm in the perioperative period; and
- in the upper limb, persistent thumb in palm, wrist posture preventing effective hand use, and elbow flexion.[37,104,142]

The method of diluting the injectable, as well as exercise (after injection), can improve the efficacy of the botulinum toxin and needs further study.[158,186,261]

Phenol is an inexpensive neurolytic agent used for over 30 years. The technical difficulties in administration have limited the use for children.[305] Comparisons of phenol to botulinum toxins have been few. The theoretic advantages of using the combination of phenol are greater control over focal spasticity involving more than three muscle groups, longer duration for

Box 54-4 Indications for the use of botulinum toxin in cerebral palsy[37,104,142]

- Calf injection for dynamic equinus persistent throughout the gait cycle
- Hamstring injection for dynamic knee flexion
- Hip adductor injection for scissoring
- Diagnostic measures before surgery
- Management of focal limb dystonia
- Analgesia for pain and spasm in the perioperative period
- Upper limb: persistent thumb in palm, wrist posture preventing effective hand use, and elbow flexion

the phenol, and lower costs.[100] Phenol does have significant adverse clinical effects when compared with botulinum toxin.[305] Botulinum toxin when compared with phenol for adductor spasticity, improves cadence, step length, and velocity during gait.[305] Indications for the use of each and the advantages are listed in Box 54-4.

Neurosurgical interventions

Selective dorsal rhizotomy (SDR) and the intrathecal baclofen (ITB) pump are two current neurosurgical procedures that hold promise in reducing spasticity.[1,8,58,232–234] Reduction in tone, as recorded by the modified Ashworth scale, is improved with both procedures (see Ch. 31).[190,235] SDR has been utilized since the early 1980s to reduce spasticity by interrupting the sensory input into the dorsal horn.[193,207,215,225] Three randomized controlled trials have been published that describe a consistent reduction in Ashworth scores for all three study centers.[194,279,307] In two of the centers, there was significant improvement in

SDR plus PT compared with PT alone, with a change in the score on the Gross Motor Functional Measure (GMFM) of four percentage points.[279,307] In the study with higher functioning children, the GMFM scores showed that the difference between SDR plus PT and PT alone was insignificant.[193] A gain in GMFM score was obtained for the SDR group, but the effect might not be clinically relevant.

Two studies comparing orthopedic surgery with SDR concluded that both cause a gain in function when measured either by gait analysis or by GMFM.[41,184] There were differences for children undergoing a neurosurgical versus an orthopedic procedure. The children with orthopedic surgery have, at 1 year, improvement in stance and less need for support. The children undergoing SDR have quality of movement changes as measured by the Gross Motor Performance Measure. Improvement in dissociation and coordination was not as frequently seen in the orthopedic group.[42] Analysis of movement patterns by polyelectromyography showed a correlation of limited function to diffuse cocontraction, coactivation of muscles, and reduced agonist activity.[57,306] This pattern analysis not only provided insight into motor control, but was also a potential discrimination methodology for selecting appropriate neurosurgical cases.[57,213] Children who undergo SDR continue to be observed for orthopedic intervention, which has been reported to be as high as 75%.[58,92] Analysis studies of children undergoing SDR have consistently shown an improved availability of range of motion at the knee and hip, resulting in an increased stride length.[287] Careful selection is critical, because the subsequent weakness, which is an anticipated part of the postoperative recovery period, can reduce the level of independence of children who depend on their spasticity to transfer or stand.[185] The children who received both SDR and orthopedic procedures demonstrated the most energy-efficient gait when compared with those who received SDR or orthopedic procedures alone.[42,258] Careful orthopedic surveillance is necessary to monitor hip stability.[225]

The ideal candidate for SDR is the premature child, with spastic diplegia, good balance, and good selective motor skills, aged 4 or 5 years, with minimal contractures, and able to walk unassisted.[233] A group that can benefit is the more involved children where care and comfort are the only goals.[100,232] Athetosis is a contraindication for SDR as an intervention. Dystonia can become more problematic post SDR.[234]

Intrathecal baclofen is another neurosurgical option for hypertonia. In addition to spasticity reduction, it also has an impact on dystonia.[6,15] ITB was systematically reviewed by the AACPDM Treatment Outcomes Committee.[45] Level 2 evidence is provided for lower extremity spasticity reduction. The AACPDM evidence-based medicine review reported benefits of ITB for those who are severely involved. For those children in GMFCS 4 and 5, improved positioning, decreased pain, and easier caregiving occurred.[7,11,23,30,99] The ambulatory child will have decreased energy requirement for walking; however, the balance between weakness and spasticity control has to be carefully managed.[258]

Complications with ITB are as high as 50%.[7,99,167] Improvements in technology with catheters and pumps might reduce the mechanical risk. Experience in management also improves the time required to diagnose catheter complications and related adverse events. Abrupt withdrawal in children must be treated aggressively.[59] Orthopedic procedures appear to be reduced in incidence post ITB.[95]

Neurosurgical procedures, such as stereotactic ablation of selected thalamic nuclei and chronic electrical stimulation of the cerebellum or posterior columns, have also been unsuccessful in reducing spasticity in the child with CP.[93] Deep brain stimulation is a neurosurgery technique that has shown promise in adults with dystonia.[290]

Orthopedic intervention

The natural history of CP is one of progressive effect of spasticity or hypertonia on the growing child and progressive degeneration.[105] Detrimental changes in gait and function occur over time spans as short as 1.5 years.[26] The argument could be made that maintaining function over time is a satisfactory goal. Close observation, aggressive bracing, and vigorous PT can temper the effect of dynamic tone and static contractures.[258]

Nearly all children with CP develop an abnormality of physical form and/or function. The degree of the orthopedist's involvement with the child and family depends on the complexity and severity of the musculoskeletal system impairments.[166] Children with CP should have regular orthopedic consultations. The physiatrist can facilitate this process by working in conjunction with the orthopedist and therapists involved with the child and family. Although the orthopedic treatment of the child with CP can show variations among different physicians, the fundamental goals of surgery should reflect a functional approach to problems of alignment.[124] If pain or discomfort is present, especially around the hip, surgical relief may be necessary. Surgical options for improvement in sitting, transfers, and ambulation are seen in Table 54-5.

Surgery for sitting

Sitting is a realistic functional goal for every child. The necessary postural alignment for sitting includes a level pelvis and a reasonably straight spine.[123] The loss of motion associated with hip dislocation can alter seating (see Ch. 18).[61] Excessive pelvic obliquity reduces the sitting surface area and causes excessive pressure on the bony prominences of the pelvis.[166] The management of the hip is complex.[273] Early detection of subluxation is possible with sequential radiographs of the pelvis. Physical examination of the hip alone is not sufficient to detect subluxation.[3]

If the hip is subluxed, the surgeon might be able to reduce the overpowering muscle forces by lengthening the iliopsoas and adductor muscles around the hip.[84,293] This is a brief procedure that offers several benefits. It not only improves femoral head coverage under the acetabulum, but also allows easier dressing, diapering, cleaning, and positioning.[40,148,214] The child treated early is more likely to maintain well-seated hips.[214,282]

Table 54-5 Common orthopedic surgeries in cerebral palsy

Surgical procedure	Purpose	Positioning considerations	Treatment
Hip flexor lengthening Usually iliopsoas Sometimes proximal rectus femoris Rarely sartorius	Increase extension ROM Decrease muscle imbalance—risk of hip subluxation Improve alignment stance, gait	Avoid prolonged sitting Prone wedge preferred Standing frame with foot control (casts or AFOs) Prone at night (with or without body splint)	Maintain length of hip flexor muscles Strengthen hip flexors (need for stairs, gait) Strengthen hip extensors
Hip adductor lengthening Usually proximal—origin Adductor longus, gracilis Sometimes adductor brevis	Increase hip abduction Decrease 'scissoring' Decrease abnormal muscle imbalance—risk of hip subluxation Increase base of support Improve hygiene, positioning	Abduction at night, usually prone With or without night splint Abduction wedge on prone wedge or wheelchair	Maintain length of hip adductors (knees flexed and extended) Strengthen hip adductors and abductors
Hamstring lengthening Medial or lateral hamstrings Almost always distal	Increase knee extension Improve standing alignment Decrease crouch posture Increase stance phase stability in gait, improved alignment Increase step length → increased terminal swing phase and heel strike ability Increase positioning options	Avoid prolonged sitting Prone wedge preferred (consider soft knee splints) Standing frame with foot control Prone at night with soft knee splints or night splints	Maintain length of hamstrings (avoid knee hyperextension) Strengthen hamstrings and quadriceps (proximal and distal), especially terminal knee extension Monitor for overactive quadriceps, increase in extensor tone → knee hyperextension
Achilles tendon lengthening Five different types: Baker, percutaneous, sliding, fractional lengthening, vulpius	Increase dorsiflexion ROM Increase full-foot contact for standing and gait Increase ability for heel strike in gait Allow for bracing	Initially no dorsiflexion beyond neutral Standing with neutral dorsiflexion only Temporary splint or cast initially to maintain ROM—begin early supportive weight bearing Sitting OK, if TALs only and other muscles not tight If prone wedge—feet off edge with AFO, cast, splint AFO approximately 6 months (surgeon discretion) AFO, cast, splint at night	Maintain length of plantar flexors Strengthen plantar flexors and dorsiflexors Avoid overstretching—could lead to crouch posture (Special attention when considering hinged AFOs) (Repeat procedures common—especially if done at early age)

AFO, Ankle–foot orthosis; ROM, range of motion; TAL, tendo-Achilles lengthening.
(From B. Feathergill, pers. comm., 1993.)

If the hip progresses to dislocation, then a more extensive procedure may be necessary.[72] The femur and acetabulum may benefit from reconstruction, depending on the child's age and the bone pathology.[21,259] The femur is commonly affected by excessive anteversion, with a valgus orientation. Acetabular dysplasia contributes to the inability of the femoral head to remain covered. A combination of muscle lengthenings, varus derotational osteotomy of the femur, and augmentation procedures of the acetabulum are complex and arduous. Another problem is that postoperative immobilization can be necessary for as long as 6–8 weeks.[72] Complications can arise following these procedures, including femoral fractures, heterotopic ossification, and peripheral neuropathy.[169,175,230,295] Rehabilitation plays an important role following cast removal. If the femoral articular carti-lage is eroded and the hip becomes painful, the options for salvage are limited and fraught with problems. Relief of the pain can be obtained by hip fusion or artificial joint replacement. Sometimes, resection of the femoral head is used as a salvage procedure to afford relief of the pain.[89,215] Painful hips are a chronic problem and need to be managed with multiple modalities.

The pelvis is also influenced by the hamstrings. The hamstrings act as hip extensors, but the major pull of this muscle is to tilt the pelvis in a posterior direction. Sacral sitting with constant sliding out of a wheelchair can be partially corrected by a hamstring release.[88] Distal hamstring lengthening is the more common surgery, but a proximal lengthening can also be considered.[79] Extensor contractures of the hips and knees can also cause sitting problems but are addressed surgically less frequently.

Scoliosis or kyphosis can be progressive.[240] Early treatment usually involves using a molded thoracic lumbar orthosis.[310] This is intended to slow rather than stop the progression, and improve trunk support. Total contact support can be incorporated into a contoured seating system. If a curve progresses beyond 40°, fusion is considered to avoid compromise of the respiratory system.[148,291] If the deformity is rigid and extends over a long segment, staged procedures are performed. The risk of anesthesia, infection, blood loss, neurologic compromise, and pseudoarthrosis should be considered and planned for before surgery.[181]

Surgery for standing

Supported standing and transfers are possible when the ankle can be held in the neutral position and the knee has less than 20° of flexion contracture.[67] The surgical procedures used to improve alignment for these skills are hamstring lengthenings and Achilles tendon lengthenings.[55,152,153] Hip flexion contractures can also hinder standing, and need attention if greater than 20°.[208] Table 54-5 provides a description of procedures to enhance standing, as well as the postoperative immobilization precautions.

Surgery for ambulation

Orthopedic surgery to improve ambulation should be well timed and planned to maximize the child's strength and motivation.[2,102,142,163] Collaboration with a pediatric orthopedist is essential.[69,242] Even though orthopedic surgery has been the mainstay of treatment for the child with biomechanical alignment and lever arm disease,[92] the literature supporting orthopedic surgery has been of a Sackett's level 4 evidence (see Ch. 9 for discussion of evidence-based medicine),[45,251,282] with few randomized and controlled studies. The analysis of orthopedic surgery has expanded to include energy cost–benefits, standardized outcome testing with the GMFM, and cost analysis.[45,166,258]

Difficulty in predicting outcome for the ambulator has led to caution in recommending orthopedic surgery.[5] The use of gait analysis has refined the observation of components of the gait cycle and the combined effect of contractures on gait dynamics. Gait analysis defines cadence, velocity, stride length, and ranges of motion of the hip, knee, and ankle during various phases of the gait cycle and the timing of muscular activity. Some gait laboratories also measure the forces generated at each joint. Gait analysis provides consistent objective information that enhances orthopedic decision making and improves outcome studies (see Ch. 5).[91] The use of gait analysis not only improves decision making prior to surgeries, but also allows a more objective analysis of the outcome following surgery.[263]

Energy expenditure for some children with spastic CP can be as high as 350% of normal.[48] Energy expenditure is an important consideration for continued community ambulation.[91] Gait analysis is an appropriate outcome and energy cost for children in GMFCS levels 1 and 2. The goals for children with GMFCS level 3 and 4 are to improve alignment and motor function.[164] For children not expected to change in motor function, gains can still be realized with orthopedic surgery for children who are GMFCS level 5. Response to treatment can be reflected in a care and comfort-measuring instrument or with a quality of life measure.[99,257]

The tendency to scissor at the hips can hinder forward progression of gait. Adductor myotomies in combination with hamstring lengthenings can create a better base of support and a more upright posture.[43,56] The dynamic hip flexion can inhibit balance and decrease the child's ability to walk. Intramuscular psoas lengthening assists with hip extension and stance.[208] Rectus femoris transfers and lengthenings are used to decrease the problem of stiff knee gait following or at the time of hamstring release.[5,152] A braceable foot or a foot that allows for foot flat or heel strike is desirable for stance.[10] Gastrocnemius recession surgery and tendo-Achilles lengthening can improve the foot position but should be delayed until 6 years of age.[106]

Orthopedic surgery can affect balance, but the central processing of balance reactions remains the same after surgery. Assistive devices can play an important transitional role in household or community ambulation. A reverse walker typically assists with maintaining upright posture better than the traditional forward walker.[177,187]

Upper extremity surgery is uncommonly done to improve the function of the hand.[172,298] Flexor carpi ulnaris transfers to a wrist extensor are done to reduce the wrist flexion deformity. Rerouting of the brachioradialis can improve supination and improve upper limb reach.[218] Other surgeries include biceps release for flexion contractures and anterior elbow release.[183] The active use of the hand, however, is dependent on stereognosis and two-point discrimination.[54,288] The emphasis on the arm and hand is important, because the adult shifts concerns from mobility to ADL and communication. Motion analysis for the arm and hand is a new technology utilized to determine joint kinematics and kinetics of upper extremity function.[297]

Spasticity reduction and orthopedic surgery are two distinct and complementary elements in the treatment of gait in the child with CP.[258] Neither one should be viewed as an exclusive intervention option.[8] Children with major structural and biomechanical alignment can benefit from both. It is common, however, to provide the spasticity management first.[234]

Rehabilitation is individualized for each child post orthopedic surgery or neurosurgery.[30] The recognition and the evaluation of the other impairments related to CP are central aspects of treatment. In particular, strengthening and improved endurance is important after procedures that have the child immobilized for a period of time. If tone-reducing procedures are done first, then the alignment issues will continue to impact functional gains.[183]

Precautions for the child undergoing SDR include restricting trunk rotation for 6 weeks. Intensive therapy has been recommended, but the optimum duration of therapy[194,207,279,307] and its actual contribution to function are hard to determine.[279]

Precautions for the ITB include avoidance of complications related to cerebrospinal fluid leaks, which are not uncommon.[97] Infection is reported to occur in 10–20% of cases of ITB.[94]

Functional goal-focused therapy is the cornerstone of rehabilitation management. In some instances, the goal may be to improve the distribution of weight and change the technique for transfers or even seating, which is a functional benefit.[99,100]

COMPLEMENTARY AND ALTERNATIVE MEDICINES

Because CP is a non-curable condition, treatments that are not supported by evidence will often be utilized by patients and their families.[206] It is important that an open approach is maintained for discussion.

Evidence reviews are available from organizations such as United Cerebral Palsy and the AACPDM on current treatment approaches that can assist the clinician in evaluating literature on specific topics (see web sites). Complementary medicine is an important part of the lives of many families.[133] Up to 56% of families having a child with CP utilize complementary and alternative medicine (CAM) treatments. The American Academy of Pediatrics has developed policy statements on CAM that encourage the physician to become knowledgeable about the various complementary treatments, and to remain non-judgmental as the family is guided through the risks, theoretic benefits, and any available credible research.[12] Even families actively involved in traditional treatments can expose their child to alternative treatments. It is at times a fine line that divides the traditional PT, OT, and speech therapy from the treatment considered non-traditional or CAM. An example of this is the use of soft tissue stretching versus techniques such as cranial-sacral, Feldenkrais, or even spinal manipulation. Hyperbaric oxygen is a treatment that has had anecdotal support from families but with no substantiated evidence-based literature.[122,227]

TRANSITION TO ADULTHOOD AND AGING WITH CEREBRAL PALSY

Adolescence is a difficult time for many children. It is a time in which one changes physically and socially, and begins to work toward a more independent future. Adolescents need gradually increasing responsibility and a sense of who they are in the world. Prevocational skills are learned incrementally through helping others, chores, part-time and summer jobs, and volunteer work. Increasing independence with decreasing support in all areas of life, including medical decision making, should be encouraged. Resilience is associated with support (not overprotectiveness) of parents and friends, having chores in childhood, and having a mix of disabled and non-disabled friends.[116,229] Physical activity and fitness levels, employment, and marital rates remain low in this population. Routine primary preventive care is often neglected in adults with CP as well.[292]

Organized sports activities were once only rarely recommended for the child with CP. That has changed. There is no evidence that strengthening adversely affects muscle tone.[125,138,189,304] Neither is there evidence to preclude even vigorous activities, such as downhill skiing, that once were thought to increase orthopedic deformity.[81,131] The therapeutic benefits of swimming and horseback riding for children with motor disabilities have been established.[27,28] While sports programs can improve endurance and strength, they also can promote interpersonal growth and improve self-esteem—something that all children experience when appropriately supervised in a team sport with peers.[64,265,266] The established organizations for athletes with CP are the United States Cerebral Palsy Athletic Association and the Cerebral Palsy International Sports and Recreation Association.[147] Fitness programs that emphasize flexibility and endurance have been developed for both recreational and therapeutic use.[185]

The child with CP ages with a chronic but not unchanging neuromuscular condition. Adults with CP have similar life expectancy to that of normal peers,[19] although it becomes poorer in those who lose the ability to ambulate.[283] Ongoing medical issues are exacerbated by aging, such as dysphagia, gastroesophageal reflux, urinary incontinence, constipation, and musculoskeletal pain, which progress and cause a decline in function.[21,33,137] Problems of osteoporosis, fractures due to falls, worsening balance, loss of strength and flexibility, and pressure sores are frequently seen.[283] Physical fatigue is increased versus in the normal population.[135] Independence with ADL also typically decreases with age.[14]

Spasticity can change as the skeletal system matures. Contractures, scoliosis, and windswept hip deformity can make seating and positioning difficult. The neck, particularly for the adult with athetoid CP, is vulnerable to excessive forces that can narrow the disk spaces or compress the spinal cord.[18,113] Osteoarthritic changes occur earlier in joints having ongoing abnormal joint mechanics and stresses from spastic or dyskinetic muscle forces. The prevalence of musculoskeletal pain in adults with CP is high, over 80% in some studies.[292]

Loss of mobility with aging in those who walk with equipment occurs commonly,[35,135] but it can be ameliorated or delayed using general strengthening and fitness techniques. Lower extremity strength and endurance training programs have been shown to improve gait parameters in periods as short as 6 weeks.[66] Pain problems can be sorted through and often successfully treated. Positioning equipment, antiinflammatory medication, bursal injections, mobilization and modalities by PT,[144] and spasticity treatment can improve activity tolerance and decrease pain.[76] Hip replacement is now being favored over resection procedures[89,245,302] for severe hip dysfunction.

Adults with CP rank communication, ADL, and mobility as higher priority goals than ambulation.[32] Vocational rates among adults with CP in the past were only 30–50% but could be increased. The Americans with Disabilities Act requires reasonable access to employment, housing, and accessibility to the community.[211] Quality of life research demonstrates that participation in community activities of all kinds contributes to improved satisfaction with life.

SUMMARY AND FUTURE DIRECTIONS

The keys to successful rehabilitation of the child with CP are the prevention of secondary impairments, reduction of disability, and improved integration of the individual into the community. The pediatric physiatrist views the impact of CP on the child's function and helps determine the appropriate medical, surgical and other therapeutic needs. Facilitating the ability of the child and family to set functional goals is our primary responsibility. This process takes cooperation, prioritization of competing interests, and an advocacy position for the child. Decision making is gradually transferred to the child, based on her or his abilities. Physiatrists have an important place in assisting persons with CP to achieve the independence they desire within the constraints of their neurologic and orthopedic status and the community environment.

The primary care physician provides a 'medical home' and interacts with the multiple health professionals involved. Improving accessibility and accommodation of community-based activities and facilities is a shared goal of healthcare professionals, government, agencies, and patients and their families.

Research is needed in determining causes and prevention of CP in term infants, efficacy of therapeutic interventions, outcomes in all areas of health as described by the World Health Organization and the National Center for Medical Rehabilitation Research, and effective management of aging issues in adults with CP. Improving acceptance, accessibility, and integration of persons with disabilities continues to be a goal.

REFERENCES

1. Abbott R, Johann SL. Selective posterior rhizotomy for the treatment of spasticity: a review. Childs Nerv Syst 1989; 5:337–346.

2. Abel MF, Blanco JS, Pavlovich L, et al. Asymmetric hip deformity and subluxation in cerebral palsy: an analysis of surgical treatment. J Pediatr Orthop 1999; 19(4): 479–485.

3. Abel MF, Wenger DR, Mubarak P, et al. Quantitative analysis in hip dysplasia in cerebral palsy: a study of radiographs and 3-D reformatted images. J Pediatr Orthop 1994; 14:283–289.

4. Agnarsson U, Warde C, McCarthy G, et al. Anorectal function of children with neurological problems. II: Cerebral palsy. Dev Med Child Neurol 1993; 35:903–908.

5. Aiona MD, Sussman MD. Treatment of spastic diplegia in patients with cerebral palsy: part II. J Pediatr Orthop B 2004; 13(3):S13–S38.

6. Albright AL, Barry MJ, Shafron DH, et al. Intrathecal baclofen for generalized dystonia. Dev Med Child Neurol 2001; 43:652–657.

7. Albright AL, Gilmartin R, Swift D, et al. Long-term intrathecal baclofen therapy for severe spasticity of cerebral origin. J Neurosurg 2003; 98:291–295.

8. Albright L, Warwick JP, Krach LE. Spasticity reduction. In: Gage JR, ed. The treatment of gait problems in cerebral palsy. MacKeith Press; 2004: 308–309.

9. Allan WC, Vohr B, Makuch RW, et al. Antecedents of cerebral palsy in a multicenter trial of indomethacin for intraventricular hemorrhage. Arch Pediatr Adolesc Med 1997; 151(12):1269–1270.

10. Alman BA, Craig CL, Zimbler S. Subtalar arthrodesis for stabilization of valgus hindfoot in patients with cerebral palsy. J Pediatr Orthop 1993; 13:634–641.

11. Almeida GL, Campbell SK, Girolami GL, et al. Multidimensional assessment of motor function in a child with cerebral palsy following intrathecal administration of baclofen. Phys Ther 1997; 77:751–764.

12. American Academy of Pediatrics Committee on Children with Disabilities. Counseling families who choose complementary and alternative medicine for their child with chronic illness and disability. Pediatrics 2001; 107:598–601.

13. Anderson JP, Snow B, Dorey FJ, et al. Efficacy of soft splints in reducing knee flexion contractures. Dev Med Child Neurol 1988; 30:502–508.

14. Andren E, Grimby G. Dependence in daily activities and life satisfaction in adult subjects with cerebral palsy or spinal bifida: a follow-up study. Disabil Rehabil 2004; 26(9):528–536.

15. Armstrong RW, Steinbok P, Cochrane DD, et al. Intrathecally administered baclofen for treatment of children with spasticity of cerebral origin. J Neurosurg 1997; 87:409–414.

16. Ashwal S, Russman BS, Blasco PA, et al. Practice parameter: diagnostic assessment of the child with cerebral palsy. Neurology 2004; 62:851–863.

17. Ayyangar R. Health maintenance and management in child disability. Phys Med Rehabil Clin N Am 2002; 13(4):793–821.

18. Azuma S, Seichi A, Ohnishi I, et al. Long-term results of operative treatment for cervical spondylotic myelopathy in patients with athetoid cerebral palsy: an over 10-year follow-up. Spine 2002; 27(9):943–948.

19. Bachrach SJ, Greenspun B. Care of the adult with cerebral palsy. Del Med J 1990; 62(10):1287–1295.

20. Bachrach SJ, Walter RS, Trzcinski K. Use of glycopyrrolate and other anticholinergic medications for sialorrhea in children with cerebral palsy. Clin Pediatr 1998; Aug:485–490.

21. Bagg M, Farber J, Miller F. Long-term follow-up of hip subluxation in cerebral palsy patients. J Pediatr Orthop 1993; 13:32–36.

22. Bailey DB Jr, Hebbeler K, Scarborough A, et al. First experiences with early intervention: a national perspective. Pediatrics 2004; 113(4):887–896.

23. Barry MJ, VanSwearington J, Albright A. Reliability and responsiveness of the Barry-Albright Dystonia Scale. Dev Med Child Neurol 1999; 41:404–411.

24. Bax M. Diagnostic assessment of children with cerebral palsy. Lancet 2004; July:395.

25. Bax M. Terminology and classification of cerebral palsy in childhood. Dev Med Child Neurol 1964; 6:295–297.

26. Bell KJ, Ounpuu S, DeLuca PA, et al. Natural progression of gait in children with cerebral palsy. J Pediatr Orthop 2002; 22:677–682.

27. Benda W, McGibbon NH, Grant KL. Improvements in muscle symmetry in children with cerebral palsy after equine-assisted therapy (hippotherapy). J Altern Complement Med 2003; 9(6):817–825.

28. Bertoti DB. Effects of therapeutic horseback riding on posture in children with cerebral palsy. Phys Ther 1988; 66:1522–1529.

29. Bhushan VB, Paneth N, Kiely JL. Impact of improved survival of very low birth weight infants on recent secular trends in the prevalence of cerebral palsy. Pediatrics 1993; 91:1094–1100.

30. Bjornson KF, McLaughlin JF, Loeser JD, et al. Oral motor, communication, and nutritional status of children during intrathecal baclofen therapy: a descriptive pilot study. Arch Phys Med Rehabil 2003; 84(4): 500–506.

31. Bleck EE. Locomotion prognosis in cerebral palsy. Dev Med Child Neurol 1975; 17:18–25.

32. Bleck EE. Orthopaedic management of cerebral palsy. Philadelphia: Saunders; 1982.

33. Bleck EE. Where have all the cerebral palsy children gone? The needs of adults. Dev Med Child Neurol 1984; 26:674–676.

34. Bottos M, Benedetti MG, Salucci P, et al. Botulinum toxin with and without casting in ambulant children with spastic diplegia: a clinical an functional assessment. Dev Med Child Neurol 2003; 45: 758–762.

35. Bottos M, Feliciangeli A, Sciuto L, et al. Functional status of adults with cerebral palsy and implications for treatment of children. Dev Med Child Neurol 2001; 43:516–528.

36. Boyd RN, Graham HK. Botulinum toxin A in the management of children with cerebral palsy. Indications and outcome. Eur Neurol 1997; 4(2): S15–S22.

37. Boyd RN, Hays RM. Current evidence for the use of botulinum toxin Type A in the management of children with cerebral palsy: a systematic review. Eur J Neurol 2001; 8(5):1–20.

38. Brodak PP, Scherz HC, Packer MG, et al. Is urinary tract screening necessary for patients with cerebral palsy? J Urol 1994; 152:1586–1587.

39. Bross S, Pomer S, Doderlein L, et al. Urodynamic findings in patients with infantile cerebral palsy. Aktuelle Urol 2004; 35(1):54–57.

40. Brunner R, Baumann JU. Clinical benefit of reconstruction of dislocated or subluxated hip joints in patients with spastic cerebral palsy. J Pediatr Orthop 1994; 14:290–294.

41. Buckon CE, Thomas SS, Piatt JH, et al. Selective dorsal rhizotomy versus orthopedic surgery: a multidimensional assessment of outcome efficacy. Arch Phys Med Rehabil 2004; 85:457–465.

42. Buckon CE, Thomas SS, Pierce R, et al. Developmental skills of children with spastic diplegia: functional and qualitative changes after selective dorsal rhizotomy. Arch Phys Med Rehabil 1997; 78:946–951.

43. Burke JH, Hermens HJ, Roetenberg D, et al. Influence of hamstring lengthening on muscle activation timing. Gait Posture 2004; 20(1):48–53.

44. Burton AW. Assessing the perceptual-motor interaction in the developmentally disabled and non-handicapped children. Adapted Phys Act Q 1990; 7:325–337.

45. Butler C, Campbell S. Evidence of the effects of intrathecal baclofen for spastic and dystonic cerebral palsy. Dev Med Child Neurol 2000; 42:634–645.

46. Butler C, Chambers H, Goldstein M, et al. Evaluating research in developmental disabilities: a conceptual framework for reviewing treatment outcomes. Dev Med Child Neurol 1999; 41:55–59.

47. Butler C. Effects of powered mobility on self-initiated behaviors of very young children with locomotor disability. Dev Med Child Neurol 1986; 28:325–332.

48. Campbell J, Ball J. Energetics of walking in cerebral palsy. Orthop Clin N Am 1978; 9:374–377.

49. Campbell SK, Anderson J, Gardner G. Physicians' beliefs in the efficacy of physical therapy in the management of cerebral palsy. Pediatr Phys Ther 1990; 90:169–173.

50. Cans C, McManus V, Crowley M, et al. Cerebral palsy of post-neonatal origin: characteristics and risk factors. Paediatr Perinat Epidemiol 2004; 18(3):214–220.

51. Caulton JM, Ward KA, Alsop CW, et al. A randomized controlled trial of standing programme on bone mineral density in non-ambulant children with cerebral palsy. Arch Dis Child 2004; 89:131–135.

52. Center for Law and Education. Educational rights of children with disabilities under IDEA and Section 504 educational rights of children with disabilities: a primer for advocates. Cambridge: Center for Law and Education.

53. Chad KE, Bailey DA, McKay HA. The effect of a weight-bearing physical activity program on bone mineral content and estimated volumetric density in children with spastic cerebral palsy. J Pediatr 1999; 135(1):115–117.

54. Chakerian DL, Larson MA. Effects of upper extremity weight-bearing on hand-opening and prehension patterns of children with cerebral palsy. Dev Med Child Neurol 1993; 35:216–229.

55. Chang CH, Albarracin JP, Lipton GE, et al. Long term follow-up of surgery for equinovarus foot deformity in children with cerebral palsy. J Pediatr Orthop 2002; 22(6):792–799.

56. Chang WN, Tsirkos AI, Miller F, et al. Distal hamstring lengthening in ambulatory children with cerebral palsy: primary versus revision procedures. Gait Posture 2004; 19(3):298–304.

57. Chen CL, Wu CY, Wong AMK, et al. Correlation of polyelectromyographic patterns and clinical motor manifestations in children with cerebral palsy. Am J Phys Med Rehabil 2003; 82:627–635.

58. Chicoine MR, Park TS, Kaufman BA. Selective dorsal rhizotomy and rates of orthopedic surgery in children with spastic cerebral palsy. J Neurosurg 1997; 86(1):34–39.

59. Coffey RJ, Edgar TS, Francisco GE, et al. Abrupt withdrawal from intrathecal baclofen: recognition and management of a potentially life-threatening syndrome. Arch Phys Med Rehabil 2002; 83:735–741.

60. Colver AF, Sethumadhavan T. The term diplegia should be abandoned. Neurology 2003; 88:286–290.

61. Cooperman DR, Bartucci E, Dietrick E, et al. Hip dislocation in spastic cerebral palsy: long-term consequences. J Pediatr Orthop 1987; 7:268–276.

62. Cosgrove AP, Corry IS, Graham HK. Botulinum toxin in the management of the lower limb in cerebral palsy. Dev Med Child Neurol 1994; 36:386–396.

63. Crichton JU, Mackinnon M, White CP. The life-expectancy of persons with cerebral palsy. Dev Med Child Neurol 1995; 37:567–576.

64. Curtis K. Wheelchair sports medicine. In: Klafs CE, Armheim DD, eds. Modern principles of athletic training. 4th edn. St. Louis: Mosby-Year Book; 1977:16–18.

65. Dali C, Hansen FJ, Pedersen SA, et al. Threshold electrical stimulation (TES) in ambulant children with CP: a randomized double-blind placebo-controlled clinical trial. Dev Med Child Neurol 2002; 44(6):364–369.

66. Damiano DL, Abel MF. Functional outcomes of strength training in spastic cerebral palsy. Arch Phys Med Rehabil 1998; 79(2):119–125.

67. Damron TA, Breed AL, Cook T. Diminished knee flexion after hamstring surgery in cerebral palsy patients: prevalence and severity. J Pediatr Orthop 1993; 13:188–191.

68. Darrah J, Watkins B, Chen L, et al. Conductive education intervention for children with cerebral palsy: an AACPDM evidence report. Dev Med Child Neurol 2004; 46:187.

69. Davids JR, Foti T, Dabelstein J, et al. Objective assessment of dyskinesia in children with cerebral palsy. J Pediatr Orthop 1999; 19(2):211–214.

70. De Vries LS, Van Haastert IL, Rademaker KJ, et al. Ultrasound abnormalities preceding cerebral palsy in high-risk preterm infants. J Pediatr 2004; 144(6):815–820.

71. Decter RM, Bauer SB, Khoshbin S, et al. Urodynamic assessment of children with cerebral palsy. J Urol 1987; 138:1110–1112.

72. Dobson F, Boyd RN, Parrott J, et al. Hip surveillance in children with cerebral palsy. J Bone Joint Surg 2002; 84-B:720–726.

73. Dodd KJ, Taylor NF, Damiano DL. A systematic review of the effectiveness of strength-training programs for people with cerebral palsy. Arch Phys Med Rehabil 2002; 83:1157–1164.

74. Drigo P, Seren F, Artibani W, et al. Neurogenic vesico-urethral dysfunction in children with cerebral palsy. Ital J Neurol Sci 1988; 9(2):151–154.

75. Drvaric DM, Roberts JM, Burke SW, et al. Gastroesophageal evaluation in totally involved cerebral palsy patients. J Pediatr Orthop 1987; 7:187–190.

76. van der Dussen L, Nieuwstraten W, Roebroeck M, et al. Functional level of young adults with cerebral palsy. Clin Rehabil 2001; 15(1):84–91.

77. Eicher PS, Batshaw ML. Cerebral palsy, the child with developmental disabilities. Pediatr Clin N Am 1993; 40:537–551.

78. Ellenberg JH, Nelson KB. Cluster of perinatal events identifying infants at high risk for death or disability. J Pediatr 1988; 113:546–552.

79. Elmer E, Wenger D, Mubarak S, et al. Proximal hamstring lengthening in the sitting cerebral palsy patient. J Pediatr Orthop 1992; 12:329–336.

80. Farmer SE. Key factors in the development of lower limb co-ordination: implications for the acquisitions of walking in children with cerebral palsy. Disabil Rehabil 2003; 25(14):807–816.

81. Ferrara MS, Buckley WE, et al. The injury experience of the competitive athlete with a disability: prevention implications. Med Sci Sports Exerc 1992; 24:184–188.

82. Ferriero DM. Cerebral palsy: diagnosing something that is not one thing. Curr Opin Pediatr 1999; 11(6):485–486.

83. Fletcher NA, Thompson PD, Scading JW, et al. Successful treatment of childhood onset symptomatic dystonia with levodopa. J Neurol Neurosurg Psychiatry 1993; 56:865–867.

84. Flynn JM, Miller F. Management of hip disorders in patients with cerebral palsy. J Am Acad Orthop Surg. 2002; 10(3):198–209.

85. Foley J. Dyskinetic and dystonic cerebral palsy. Acta Paediatr 1992; 81:57–60.

86. Ford GW, Kitchen WH, Doyle LW, et al. Changing diagnosis of cerebral palsy in very low birthweight children. Am J Perinatol 1990; 7(2):178–181.

87. Freeman JM, Nelson KB. Special articles: intrapartum asphyxia and cerebral palsy. Pediatrics 1988; 82:240–241.

88. Fulford GE, Cairns TP, Sloan Y. Sitting problems of children with cerebral palsy. Dev Med Child Neurol 1982; 24:48–53.

89. Gabos PG, Miller F, Galban MA, et al. Prosthetic interposition arthroplasty for the palliative treatment of end-stage spastic hip disease in non-ambulatory patients with cerebral palsy. J Pediatr Orthop 1999; 19(6):796–804.

90. Gaebler-Spira D, Thornton L. Injury prevention for children with disabilities. Phys Med Rehab Clin N Am. 2002; 13:891–906.

91. Gage JR, Fabian D, Hicks R, et al. Pre- and post-operative gait analysis in patients with spastic diplegia: a preliminary report. J Pediatr Orthop 1984; 4:715–718.

92. Gage JR, Schwartz MH. Dynamic deformities and lever arm considerations. In: Paley D, ed. Principles of deformity correction. Berlin: Springer; 2001:761–775.

93. Galanda M, Horvath S. Effect of stereotactic high-frequency stimulation in the anterior lobe of the cerebellum in cerebral palsy: a new suboccipital approach. Stereotact Funct Neurosurg 2003; 80:102–107.

94. Galloway A, Falope FZ. *Pseudomonas aeruginosa* infection in an intrathecal baclofen pump: successful treatment with adjunct intra-reservoir gentamycin. Spinal Cord 2000; 38:126–128.

95. Gersten PC, Albright AL, Johnstone GF. Intrathecal baclofen infusion and subsequent orthopedic surgery in patients with spastic cerebral palsy. J Neurosurg 1998; 88(6):1009–1013.

96. Gilbert SR, Gilbert AC, Henderson RC. Skeletal maturation in children with quadriplegic cerebral palsy. J Pediatr Orthop 2004; 24(3):292–297.

97. Gilmartin R, Bruce D, Storrs BB, et al. Intrathecal baclofen for management of spastic cerebral palsy: multicenter trial. J Child Neurol 2000; 15:71–77.

98. Goldkamp O. Treatment effectiveness in cerebral palsy. Arch Phys Med Rehabil 1984; 65:232–234.

99. Gooch JL, Oberg WA, Grams B, et al. Complications of intrathecal baclofen pumps in children. Pediatr Neurosurg 2003; 39:1–6.

100. Gormley ME, Krach LE, Murr S. Non-operative treatment. In: Gage JR, ed. The treatment of gait problems in cerebral palsy. MacKeith Press; 2004:245–268.

101. Gorter JW, Rosenbaum P, Hanna SE, et al. Limb distribution, motor impairment, and functional classification of cerebral palsy. Dev Med Child Neurol. 2004; 46(7):461–467.

102. Gough M, Eve LC, Robinson RO, et al. The effect of surgical intervention on the natural history of gait in spastic diplegia. Gait Posture 2001; 16: s33–s34.

103. Govaert P, Lequin M, Swarte R, et al. Changes in globus pallidus with (pre)term kernicterus. Pediatrics 2003; 112(6):1256–1270.

104. Graham HK, Aoki KR, Autti-Ramo I, et al. Recommendations for the use of botulinum toxin Type A in the management of cerebral palsy. Gait Posture 2000; 11:67–79.

105. Graham HK, Selber P. Musculoskeletal aspects of cerebral palsy. J Bone Joint Surg 2003; 85(2):157–166.

106. Graham HK. Sonographic healing stages of Achilles tendon after tenomuscular lengthening in children with cerebral palsy. J Pediatr Orthop. 2002; 22(4):556.

107. Greiner BM, Czerniecki JM, Deitz JC. Gait parameters of children with spastic diplegia: a comparison of effects of posterior and anterior walkers. Arch Phys Med Rehabil 1993; 74:381–385.

108. Griether JK, Nelson KB, Cummins SK. Twinning and cerebral palsy: experience in four northern California counties' births 1983–1985. Pediatrics 1993; 92:854–888.

109. Gururaj AK, Sztriha L, Bener A, et al. Epilepsy in children with cerebral palsy. Seizure 2003; 12(2):110–114.

110. Guzzetta F, Shackelford GD, Volpe S, et al. Periventricular intraparenchymal echodensities in the premature newborn: critical determinant of neurological outcome. Pediatrics 1986; 78:995–1006.

111. Hagberg B, Hagberg G, Olow I, et al. The changing panorama of cerebral palsy in Sweden. V: The birth year period 1979–1982. Acta Paediatr Scand 1989; 78:283–290.

112. Hankins GD, Speer M. Defining the pathogenesis and pathophysiology of neonatal encephalopathy and cerebral palsy. Obstet Gynecol 2003; 102(3):628–636.

113. Harada T, Ebara S, Anwar MM, et al. The cervical spine in athetoid cerebral palsy. A radiological study of 180 patients. J Bone Joint Surg Br 1996; 78(4):613–619.

114. Harris SR, Atwater S, Crowe T. Accepted and controversial neuromotor therapies for infants at high risk for cerebral palsy. J Perinatol 1985; 8:3–12.

115. Harris SR. The effectiveness of early intervention for at-risk and handicapped children. In: Guralnick MJ, Bennett FC, eds. The effectiveness of early intervention for at risk and handicapped children. San Diego: Academic Press; 1987:175–212.

116. Hayden PW, Davenport SL, Campbell MM. Adolescents with myelodysplasia: impact of physical disability on emotional maturation. Pediatrics 1979; 64(1):53–59.

117. Haynes UE. The National Collaborative Infant Project. In: Tjossen TD, ed. Intervention strategies for high risk infants and children. Baltimore: University Park Press; 1976:509–534.

118. Healy A. Pediatricians' role in the development and implementation of an individual education plan (IEP) and/or an individual family service plan (IFSP). Pediatrics 1992; 89:340–342.

119. Henderson RC, Kairalla J, Abbas A, et al. Predicting low bone density in children and young adults with quadriplegic cerebral palsy. Dev Med Child Neurol 2004; 46(6):416–419.

120. Henderson RC, Lark RK, Kecskemethy HH, et al. Bisphosphonates to treat osteopenia in children with quadriplegic cerebral palsy: a randomized, placebo-controlled clinical trial. J Pediatr 2002; 141(5): 644–651.

121. Herndon WA, Troup P, Yngve DA, et al. Effects of neurodevelopmental treatment on movement patterns of children with cerebral palsy. J Pediatr Orthop 1987; 7:395–400.

122. Heuser G, Uszler JM. Hyperbaric oxygenation for cerebral palsy. Lancet 2001; 356:2053–2054.

123. Hoffer M, Abraham E, Nickel VL, et al. Salvage surgery of the hip to improve sitting posture of mentally retarded, severely disabled children with cerebral palsy. Dev Med Child Neurol 1992; 14:51–59.

124. Hoffer M. Management of the hip in cerebral palsy. J Bone Joint Surg Am 1986; 68:629–631.

125. Holland LJ, Steadward RD. Effects of resistance in flexibility training and strength, spasticity/muscle tone and range of motion of elite athletes with cerebral palsy. Palestra 1990; summer:27–31.

126. Holmes KJ, Michael SM, Thorpe SL, et al. Management of scoliosis with special seating for non-ambulant spastic cerebral palsy population—a biomechanical study. Clin Biomech 2003; 18(6):480–487.

127. Hoon AH Jr, Freese PO, Reinhardt EM, et al. Age-dependent effects of trihexyphenidyl in extrapyramidal cerebral palsy. Pediatr Neurol 2001; 25(1):55–58.

128. Hou M, Fan XW, Li YT, et al. Magnetic resonance imaging findings in children with cerebral palsy. Zhonghua Er Ke Za Zhi 2004; 42(2): 125–128.

129. Houlihan CM, O'Donnell M, Conaway M, et al. Bodily pain and health-related quality of life in children with cerebral palsy. Dev Med Child Neurol 2004; 46(5):305–310.

130. Howard RF. Current status of pain management in children. JAMA 2003; 290(18):2464–2469.

131. Hueberman G. Organized sports activity with cerebral palsy adolescents. Rehabil Lit 1976; 37:103–106.

132. Hurlbut BI, Iwata BA, Green JD. Nonvocal language acquisition in adolescents with severe physical disabilities: blissymbol versus iconic stimulus formats. J Speech Hear Res 1982; 30:425–431.

133. Hurvitz EA, Leonard C, Ayyangar R, et al. Complementary and alternative medicine use in families of children with cerebral palsy. Dev Med Child Neurol 2003; 45:364–370.

134. Jacobsson B, Hagberg G. Antenatal risk factors for cerebral palsy. Best Pract Res Clin Obstet Gynaecol 2004; 18(3):425–436.

135. Jahnsen R, Villien L, Stanghelle JK, et al. Fatigue in adults with cerebral palsy in Norway compared with the general population. Dev Med Child Neurol 2003; 45(5):296–303.

136. Jancar J, Speller CJ. Fatal intestinal obstruction in the mentally handicapped. J Intellect Disabil Res 1994; 38:413–422.

137. Janicki M. Aging, cerebral palsy, and older persons with mental retardation. Aust NZ J Dev Disabil 1989; 15:311–320.

138. Jankowski LW, Sullivan J. Aerobic and neuromuscular training: an effect of capacity, efficacy and fatigability of patients with traumatic brain injuries. Arch Phys Med Rehabil 1990; 71:500–504.

139. Jansen LMC, Ketelaar M, Vermeer A. Parental experience of participation in physical therapy for children with physical disabilities. Dev Med Child Neurol 2003; 45:58–69.

140. Jarvis S, Glinianaia SV, Torrioli MG, et al. Surveillance of Cerebral Palsy in Europe (SCPE) collaboration of European Cerebral Palsy Registers. Lancet 2003; 362(9390):1106–1111.

141. Jeffe AM. Using health-related quality of life measures. Physical therapy outcomes research. Phys Ther 1993; 73:523–527.

142. Jefferson RJ. Botulinum toxin in the management of cerebral palsy. Dev Med Child Neurol 2004; 46:491–499.

143. Jekovec-Vrhovsek M, Kocijancic A, Prezelj J. Effect of vitamin D and calcium on bone mineral density in children with CP and epilepsy in full-time care. Dev Med Child Neurol 2000; 42(6):403–405.

144. Jensen MP, Engel JM, Hoffman AJ, et al. Natural history of chronic pain and pain treatment in adults with cerebral palsy. Am J Phys Med Rehabil 2004; 83(6):439–445.

145. Jevsevar DS, Karlin LI. The relationship between preoperative nutritional status and complications after an operation for scoliosis in patients who have cerebral palsy. J Bone Joint Surg Am 1993; 75:880–884.

146. Johnson TE, Moore SE, Quinn LT, et al. Energy cost of walking in children with cerebral palsy: relation to the Gross Motor Function Classification System. Dev Med Child Neurol 2004; 46(1):34–38.

147. Johnstone KS, Perrin JCS. Sports for the handicapped child. Phys Med Rehabil 1991; 5:331–350.

148. Kalen V, Conklin M, Sherman F. Untreated scoliosis in severe cerebral palsy. J Pediatr Orthop 1992; 12:337–340.

149. Katz RT. Life expectancy for children with cerebral palsy and mental retardation: implications for life care planning. Neurorehabilitation 2003; 18(3):261–270.

150. Kaukola T, Satyaraj E, Patel DD, et al. Cerebral palsy is characterized by protein mediators in cord serum. Ann Neurol 2003; 55(2):186–194.

151. Kay RM, Bethlefsen SA, Fern-Buneo A, et al. Botulinum toxin as an adjunct to serial casting treatment in children with cerebral palsy. J Bone Joint Surg 2004; 86A(11):2377–2384.

152. Kay RM, Rethlefsen SA, Ryan JA, et al. Outcome of gastrocnemius recession and tendo-achilles lengthening in ambulatory children with cerebral palsy. J Pediatr Orthop B 2004; 13(2):92–98.

153. Kay RM, Rethlefsen SA, Skaggs D, et al. Outcome of medial versus combined medial and lateral hamstring lengthening surgery in cerebral palsy. J Pediatr Orthop 2002; 22(2):169–172.

154. Keller RB. Outcomes research in orthopaedics. J Am Acad Orthop Surg 1993; 1:523–527.

155. Kermoian R. Locomotion experience and psychological development in infancy. In: Furumasu J, ed. Pediatric powered mobility: developmental perspectives, technical issues, clinical approaches. Arlington: RENSA Press; 1997:7–21.

156. Kerr C, McDowell B, McDonough S. Electrical stimulation in cerebral palsy: a review of effects on strength and motor function. Dev Med Child Neurol 2004; 46(3):205–213.

157. Kibele A. Occupational therapy's role in improving the quality of life for persons with cerebral palsy. Am J Occup Ther 1991; 45:371–377.

158. Kim HS, Hwang JH, Jeong ST, et al. Effect of muscle activity and botulinum toxin dilution volume or muscle paralysis. Dev Med Child Neurol 2003; 45(3):200–206.

159. King W, Levin R, Schmidt R, et al. Prevalence of reduced bone mass in children and adults with spastic quadriplegia. Dev Med Child Neurol 2003; 45(1):12–16.

160. Knox V, Evans AL. Evaluation of the functional effects of a course of Bobath therapy in children with cerebral palsy: a preliminary study. Dev Med Child Neurol 2002; 44(7):447–460.

161. Koman LA, Mooney JF III, Smith BP, et al. Botulinum toxin type a in the treatment of spastic foot after stroke: a randomized, double-blind, placebo-controlled trial. J Pediatr Orthop 2000; 20:108–115.

162. Koman LA, Mooney JF III, Smith BP. Management of cerebral palsy with botulinum-A toxin: preliminary investigation. J Pediatr Orthop 1993; 13:489–495.

163. Koman LA, Mooney JF, Smith BP, et al. Management of spasticity in cerebral palsy with botulinum-A toxin: report of a preliminary, randomized, double-blind trial. J Pediatr Orthop 1994; 14:299–303.

164. Kondo I, Hosokawa K, Iwata M, et al. Effectiveness of selective muscle release surgery for children with cerebral palsy: longitudinal and stratified analysis. Dev Med Child Neurol 2004; 46:540.

165. Köng E. Very early treatment of cerebral palsy. Dev Med Child Neurol 1966; 8:198–202.

166. Koop SE. Orthopedic aspects of static encephalopathies. In: Miller G, Ramer J, eds. Static encephalopathies of infancy and childhood. New York: Academic Press; 1992:95–109.

167. Krach LE, Kriel RL, Gilmartin RC, et al. Hip status in CP after one year of continuous intrathecal baclofen infusion. Pediatr Neurol 2004; 30(3):163–168.

168. Krageloh-Mann I, Hagberg G, Meisner C, et al. Bilateral spastic cerebral palsy—a comparative study between southwest Germany and western Sweden. I: Clinical patterns and disabilities. Dev Med Child Neurol 1993; 35:1031–1047.

169. Krum SD, Miller F. Heterotopic ossification after hip and spine surgery in children with cerebral palsy. J Pediatr Orthop 1993; 13:739–743.

170. Kudrjavcev T, Schoenberg BB, Kurland LT, et al. Cerebral palsy: trends in incidence and changes in concurrent neonatal mortality—Rochester, MN, 1950–1976. Neurology 1983; 33:1433–1438.

171. Kulak W, Sobaniee W. Comparisons of right and left hemiparetic cerebral palsy. Pediatr Neurol 2004; 31(2):101–108.

172. Landi A, Cavazza S, Caserta G, et al. The upper limb in cerebral palsy: surgical management of shoulder and elbow deformities. Hand Clin 2003; 19(4):631–648.

173. Law M, King G. Parent compliance with therapeutic interventions for children with cerebral palsy. Dev Med Child Neurol 1993; 35:983–990.

174. Lebiedowska MK, Gaebler-Spira D, Burns RS, et al. Biomechanical characteristics of patients with spastic and dystonic hypertonia in cerebral palsy. Arch Phys Med Rehabil 2004; 85(6):875–880.

175. Lee M, Alexander MA, Miller F, et al. Postoperative heterotopic ossification in the child with cerebral palsy: three case reports. Arch Phys Med Rehabil 1992; 73(3): 289–292.

176. Lesny I, Stehlik A, Tomasek J, et al. Sensory disorders in cerebral palsy: two-point discrimination. Dev Med Child Neurol 1993; 35:402–405.

177. Levangie PK, Guihan MF, Meyer P, et al. Effect of altering handle position of a rolling walker on gait in children with cerebral palsy. Phys Ther 1989; 69:130–134.

178. Lewis D, Fontana C, Mehallick L, et al. Transdermal scopolamine for reduction of drooling in developmentally delayed children. Dev Med Child Neurol 1994; 36:484–486.

179. Li X, Atkins MS. Early childhood computer experience and cognitive and motor development. Pediatrics 2004; 113(4):1715–1722.

180. Little WJ. On the influence of abnormal parturition, difficult labours, premature birth and asphyxia neonatarum on the mental and physical condition of the child, especially in relation to deformities. Curr Concepts Rehabil Med 1986-7; 3:16–23.

181. Lonstein JE, Akbarnia A. Operative treatment of spinal deformities in patients with cerebral palsy or mental retardation: an analysis of one hundred and seven cases. J Bone Joint Surg Am 1983; 65:33–55.

182. Maenpaa H, Jaakkola R, Sandstrom M, et al. Electrostimulation at sensory level improves function of the upper extremities in children with cerebral palsy: a pilot study. Dev Med Child Neurol 2004; 46(2):84–90.

183. Manske PR, Langewisch KR, Strecker WB, et al. Anterior elbow release of spastic elbow flexion deformity in children with cerebral palsy. J Pediatr Orthop 2001: 21(6):772–777.

184. Marty G, Dias L, Gaebler-Spira D. Selective posterior rhizotomy and soft-tissue procedures for the treatment of cerebral diplegia. J Bone Joint Surg 1995; 77A:713–718.

185. Massagli TL. Spasticity and its management in children. Phys Rehabil Clin 1991; 2:867–890.

186. Massin M, Allington N. Role of exercise testing in the functional assessment of cerebral palsy children after botulinum a toxin injection. J Pediatr Orthop 1999; 19:362–365.

187. Mattsson E, Anderson C. Oxygen cost, walking speed, and perceived exertion in children with cerebral palsy when walking with anterior and posterior walkers. Dev Med Child Neurol 1997; 39:671–676.

188. McCuaig M, Frank G. The able self: adaptive patterns and choices in independent living for a person with cerebral palsy. Am J Occup Ther 1991; 45:224–234.

189. McCubbin J, Shasby G. Effects of isokinetic exercise and adolescents with cerebral palsy. Adapted Phys Act 1985; 2:56–64.

190. McDonald C. Selective dorsal rhizotomy: a critical review. Phys Med Rehabil 1991; 2:891–915.

191. McDonald R, Surtees R, Wirz S. A comparison between parents' and therapists' views of their child's individual seating systems. Int J Rehabil Res 2003; 26(3):235–243.

192. McGrath S, Splaingard M, Alba H, et al. Survival and functional outcome of children with severe cerebral palsy following gastrostomy. Arch Phys Med Rehabil 1983; 73:133–137.

193. McLaughlin J, Bjornson K, Temkin N. Selective dorsal rhizotomy: meta-analysis of three randomized controlled trials. Dev Med Child Neurol 2002; 44:17–25.

194. McLaughlin JF, Bjornson KF, Astley SJ, et al. Selective dorsal rhizotomy: efficacy and safety in an investigator-masked randomized clinical trial. Dev Med Child Neurol 1998; 40:220–232.

195. McNeal DM, Hawtrey CE, Wolraich ML, et al. Symptomatic neurogenic bladder in a cerebral-palsied population. Dev Med Child Neurol 1983; 25:612–616.

196. Michaud LJ and the Committee on Children with Disabilities. Therapy services for children with motor disabilities. Pediatrics 2004; 113(4):1836–1838.

197. Molnar GE, Gordon SU. Cerebral palsy: predictive value of selected clinical signs of early prognostication of motor function. Arch Phys Med Rehabil 1976; 57:153–158.

198. Molnar GE. Cerebral palsy. In: Molnar GE, ed. Pediatric rehabilitation. 3rd edn. Baltimore: Williams & Wilkins; 1999:481–533.

199. Mooney JF III. Perioperative enteric nutritional supplementation in pediatric patients with neuromuscular scoliosis. J South Orthop Assoc 2000; 9(3):202–206.

200. Morris C, Newdick H, Johnson A. Variations in the orthotic management of cerebral palsy. Child Care Health Dev 2002; 28(2):139–147.

201. Naslund A, Tamm M, Ericsson AK, et al. Dynamic ankle-foot orthoses as a part of treatment in children with spastic diplegia—parents' perceptions. Physiother Res Int 2003; 8(2):59–68.

202. Nelson KB, Ellenberg JH. Children who outgrew cerebral palsy. Pediatrics 1982; 69:529–535.

203. Nelson KB, Grether JK. Causes of cerebral palsy. Curr Opin Pediatr 1999; 11:487–491.

204. Nelson KB. Can we prevent cerebral palsy? New Engl J Med 2003; 349(18):1765–1769.

205. Nelson KB. What proportion of cerebral palsy is related to birth asphyxia? J Pediatr 1988; 112:572–574.

206. Nickel RE. Controversial therapies for young children with developmental disabilities. Infants Young Child 1996; 8:29–40.

207. Nishida T, Thatcher SW, Marty GR. Selective posterior rhizotomy for children with cerebral palsy: a 7-year experience. Childs Nerv Syst 1995; 11:374–380.

208. Novacheck TF, Trost JP, Schwartz MH. Intramuscular psoas lengthening improves dynamic hip function in children with cerebral palsy. J Pediatr Orthop 2002; 22(2):158–164.

209. Nwaobi O, Smith PD. Effect of adaptive seating on pulmonary function of children with cerebral palsy. Dev Med Child Neurol 1986; 28:351–354.

210. Nygaard TG, Marsden CD, Fahn S. Dopa-responsive dystonia: long-term treatment response and prognosis. Neurology 1991; 41(2 part 1):174–181.

211. O'Grady R, Nishimura D, Kohn J, et al. Vocational predictions compared with present vocational status of 60 young adults with cerebral palsy. Dev Med Child Neurol 1985; 27:775–784.

212. O'Keefe M, Kafil-Hussain N, Flitcroft I, et al. Ocular significance of intraventricular haemorrhage in premature infants. Br J Ophthalmol 2001; 85:357–359.

213. Olree KS, Engsberg JR, Ross S, et al. Changes in synergistic movements patterns after selective dorsal rhizotomy. Dev Med Child Neurol 2000; 42:297–303.

214. Onimus M, Allamel G, Manzone P, et al. Prevention of hip dislocation in cerebral palsy by early psoas and adductors tenotomies. J Pediatr Orthop 1991; 11(4):432–435.

215. Oppenheim WL. Selective posterior rhizotomy for spastic cerebral palsy. Clin Orthop 1990; 253:20–29.

216. O'Shea RK. Conductive education in conjunction with inclusive education: teaming physical and occupational therapists and conductors. Adv Conductive Educ 2002: 77–89.

217. Ottenbacher KJ, Biocca Z, DeCrenter G, et al. Quantitative analysis of the effectiveness of physical therapy: emphasis on the neurodevelopmental treatment approach. Phys Ther 1986; 66:1095–1105.

218. Ozkan T, Tuncer S, Aydin A, et al. Brachioradialis re-routing for the restoration of active supation and correction of forearm pronation deformity in cerebral palsy. J Hand Surg (Br) 2004; 29(3):265–270.

219. Palisano R, Rosenbaum P, Walter S, et al. Development and reliability of a system to classify gross motor function in children with cerebral palsy. Dev Med Child Neurol 1997; 39:214–223.

220. Palisano RJ, Snider LM, Orlin MN. Recent advances in physical and occupational therapy for children with cerebral palsy. Semin Pediatr Neurol 2004; 11(1):66–77.

221. Palisano RJ, Tieman BL, Walter SD, et al. Effect of environmental settings on mobility methods of children with cerebral palsy. Dev Med Child Neurol 2003; 45(2):113–120.

222. Papadonikolakis AS, Vekris MD, Korompilias AV, et al. Botulinum A toxin for treatment of lower limb spasticity in cerebral palsy: gait analysis in 49 patients. Acta Orthop Scand 2003; 74(6):749–755.

223. Papile L, Munsick-Bruno G, Schaefer A. Relationship of cerebral intraventricular hemorrhage and early childhood neurologic handicaps. J Pediatr 1983; 103:273–277.

224. Park ES, Park CI, Cho SR, et al. Colonic transit time and constipation in children with spastic cerebral palsy. Arch Phys Med Rehabil 2004; 85(3):453–456.

225. Park TS, Owen JH. Surgical management of spastic diplegia in cerebral palsy. N Engl J Med 1992; 326:745–749.

226. Parker DF, Carriere L, Hebestreit H, et al. Muscle performance and gross motor function of children with spastic cerebral palsy. Dev Med Child Neurol 1993; 35:17–23.

227. Parkes J, Donnelly M, Dolk H, et al. Use of physiotherapy and alternatives by children with cerebral palsy: a population study. Child Care Health Dev 2002; 28(6):469–477.

228. Patrick J, Boland M, Stoski S, et al. Rapid correction of wasting in children with cerebral palsy. Dev Med Child Neurol 1986; 28:734–739.

229. Patterson J, Blum RW. Risk and resilience among children and youth with disabilities. Arch Pediatr Adolesc Med 1996; 150:692–698.

230. Payne LZ, DeLuca PA. Heterotopic ossification after rhizotomy and femoral osteotomy. J Pediatr Orthop 1993; 13:733–738.

231. da Paz AC Jr, Burnett SM, Braga LW. Walking prognosis in cerebral palsy: a 22-year retrospective analysis. Dev Med Child Neurol 1994; 36:130–134.

232. Peacock WJ, Arens LJ, Berman B. Cerebral palsy spasticity: selective posterior rhizotomy. Pediatr Neurosci 1987; 13:61–66.

233. Peacock WJ, Arens LJ, Peter J. Selective posterior rhizotomy: a long term follow up study. Childs Nerv Syst 1989; 5:148–152.

234. Peacock WJ, Staudt LA. Spasticity in cerebral palsy and selective posterior rhizotomy procedure. J Child Neurol 1990; 5:179–185.

235. Penn RD, Savoy SM, Corcos D, et al. Intrathecal baclofen for severe spinal spasticity. N Engl J Med 1989; 320:1517–1521.

236. Pennington L, Goldbart J, Marshall J. Speech and language therapy to improve the communication skills of children with cerebral palsy. Cochrane Database Syst Rev 2004; (2):CD003466.

237. Pidcock FS, Hoon AH Jr, Johnston MV. Trihexyphenidyl in posthemorrhagic dystonia: motor and language effects. Pediatr Neurol 1999; 20(3):219–222.

238. Plioplys AV. Life expectancy of severely disabled children: a brief review. Pediatr Life Care Plann Case Manage 2004; 37:781–795.

239. Reid CJ, Borzyskowski M. Lower urinary tract dysfunction in cerebral palsy. Arch Dis Child 1993; 68:739–742.

240. Rinsky LA. Surgery of spinal deformity in cerebral palsy: twelve years in the evolution of scoliosis management. Clin Orthop 1990; 253:100–109.

241. Robinson R. The frequency of other handicaps in children with cerebral palsy. Dev Med Child Neurol 1973; 15:305–312.

242. Rodda J, Graham HK. Classification of gait patterns in spastic hemiplegia and spastic diplegia: a basis for a management algorithm. Eur J Neurol 2001; 8 (suppl 5):98–108.

243. Rogers B, Arvedson J, Buck G, et al. Characteristics of dysphagia in children with cerebral palsy. Dysphagia 1994; 9:60–73.

244. Rogers BT, Srvedson J, Msall M, et al. Hypoxemia during oral feeding of children with severe cerebral palsy. Dev Med Child Neurol 1993; 35:3–10.

245. Root L, Goss JR, Mendes J. The treatment of the painful hip in cerebral palsy by total hip replacement or hip arthrodesis. J Bone Joint Surg Am 1986; 68(4):590–598.

246. Rose J, Haskell WL, Gamble JG. A comparison of oxygen pulse and respiratory exchange ratio in cerebral palsied and nondisabled children. Arch Phys Med Rehabil 1993; 74:702–705.

247. Rosen RS, Armbrustmacher V, Sampson BA. Mortality in cerebral palsy (CP): the importance of the cause of CP on the manner of death. J Forensic Sci 2003; 48(5):1144–1147.

248. Rothery S, Benz H, Hoffer M, et al. Goal oriented approach to the physical therapy management of cerebral palsy. Contemp Orthop 1982; 5:59–64.

249. Rudolph CD, Mazur LJ, Liptak GS et al. Guidelines for evaluation and treatment of gastroesophageal reflux in infants and children: recommendations of the North American Society for Pediatric Gastroenterology and Nutrition. J Pediatr Gastroenterol Nutr 2002; 32(suppl 2):S1–S31.

250. Russell DJ, Rosenbaum PL, Cadman DT, et al. The gross motor function measure: a means to evaluate the effects of physical therapy. Dev Med Child Neurol 1989; 31:341–352.

251. Sackett D. Rules of evidence and clinical recommendations for the management of patients. Can J Cardiol 1993; 9(6):487–489.

252. Samson-Fang L, Fung E, Stallings VA, et al. Relationship of nutritional status to health and societal participation in children with cerebral palsy. J Pediatr 2002; 141(5):637–643.

253. Samuel M, Boddy SA, Nicholls E, et al. Large bowels volvulus in childhood. Aust NZ J Surg 2000; 70(4):258–262.

254. Sanger TD, Delgado MR, Gabler-Spira D, et al. Classification and definition of disorders causing hypertonia in childhood. Pediatrics 2003; 111(1): e89–e97.

255. Savarese R, Diamond M, Elovic E, et al. Treatment of sialorrhea in cerebral palsy. Am J Phys Med Rehabil 2004; 83(4):304–311.

256. Scherzer AL, Mike V, Ilson J. Physical therapy as a determinant of change in the cerebral palsied infant. Pediatrics 1979; 58:47–52.

257. Schneider J, Gurucharri LM, Gutierrez AL, et al. Health-related quality of life and functional outcome measures for children with cerebral palsy. Dev Med Child Neurol 2001; 43:601–608.

258. Schwartz MH, Viehweger E, Stout J, et al. Comprehensive treatment of ambulatory children with cerebral palsy: an outcome assessment. J Pediatr Orthop 2004; 24(1):45–53.

259. Scrutton D, Baird G. Hip dysplasia in cerebral palsy. Dev Med Child Neurol 1993; 35:1028–1030.

260. Senner J, Logemann J, Zecker S, et al. Drooling, saliva production, and swallowing in cerebral palsy. Dev Med Child Neurol 2004; 46:801–806.

261. Shaari CM, Sanders I. Quantifying how location and dose of botulinum toxin injections affect muscle paralysis. Muscle Nerve 1993; 16:964–969.

262. Shane H. Impact of AAC on natural speech production. NIDDR 1992:92–105.

263. Shapiro A, Susak Z, Malkin C, et al. Preoperative and postoperative gait evaluation in cerebral palsy. Arch Phys Med Rehabil 1990; 71:236–240.

264. Shefelbine SJ, Carter DR. Mechanobiological predictions of femoral anteversion in cerebral palsy. Ann Biomed Eng 2004; 32(2):297–305.

265. Sherrill C, Hinson M, Gench B, et al. Self-concepts of disabled young athletes. Percept Mot Skills 1990; 70:1093–1098.

266. Sherrill C, Rainbolt W. Self-actualization profiles of male able-bodied and cerebral palsied athletes. Adapted Phys Act Q 1988; 5:108–119.

267. Simeonsson RJ, Bailey DB. Family dimensions in early intervention. New York: Cambridge University Press; 1990:428–444.

268. Singhi P, Jagirdar S, Khandelwal N, et al. Epilepsy in children with cerebral palsy. J Child Neurol 2003; 18(3):174–179.

269. Sisung CE, Mukherjee S. Pain management in a pediatric rehabilitation setting. Phys Med Rehabil Clin N Am 2002; 13:875–890.

270. Smiley SJ, Jacobsen FS, Mielke C, et al. A comparison of the effects of solid, articulated, and posterior leaf-spring ankle-foot orthoses and shoes alone on gait and energy expenditure in children with spastic diplegic cerebral palsy. Orthopedics 2002; 25(4):411–415.

271. Sneed RC, May WL, Stencel CS. Training of pediatricians in care of physical disabilities in children with special health needs: results of a two-state survey of practicing pediatricians and national resident training programs. Pediatrics 2000; 105:554–561.

272. Sommerfelt K, Markestad T, Berg K, et al. Therapeutic electrical stimulation in cerebral palsy: a randomized, controlled, crossover trial. Dev Med Child Neurol 2001; 43(9):609–613.

273. Staheli L, Chew D. Slotted acetabular augmentation in childhood and adolescence. J Pediatr Orthop 1992; 12:569–580.

274. Stallings VA, Charney EB, Davies JC, et al. Nutritional status and growth of children with diplegic or hemiplegic cerebral palsy. Dev Med Child Neurol 1993; 35:997–1006.

275. Stallings VA, Charney EB, Davies JC, et al. Nutrition-related growth failure of children with quadriplegic cerebral palsy. Dev Med Child Neurol 1993; 35:126–138.

276. Stanger M, Oresic S. Rehabilitation approaches for children with cerebral palsy: overview. J Child Neurol 2003; 18:S79–S88.

277. Steenbergen B, Meulenbroek RG, Rosenbaum DA. Constraints on grip selection in hemiparetic cerebral palsy: effects of lesional side, end-point accuracy, and context. Brain Res Cogn 2004; 19(2):145–159.

278. Stein REK, Jones Jessop D. Does pediatric home care make a difference for children with chronic illness? Findings from the Pediatric Ambulatory Care Treatment Study. Pediatrics 1984; 73:845–853.

279. Steinbok P, McLeod K. Comparison of motor outcomes after selective dorsal rhizotomy with and without preoperative intensified physiotherapy in children with spastic diplegic cerebral palsy. Pediatr Neurosurg 2002; 36:142–147.

280. Steultjens EM, Dekker J, Bouter LM, et al. Occupational therapy for children with cerebral palsy: a systematic review. Clin Rehabil 2004; 18(1):1–14.

281. Stevenson RD, Hayes RP, Cater LV, et al. Clinical correlates of linear growth in children with cerebral palsy. Dev Med Child Neurol 1995; 37:124–130.

282. Stott NS, Piedrahita L. Effects of surgical adductor releases for hip subluxation in cerebral palsy: an AACPDM evidence report. Dev Med Child Neurol 2004; 46:628–645.

283. Strauss D, Ojdana K, Shavelle R, et al. Decline in function and life expectancy of older persons with cerebral palsy. NeuroRehabilitation 2004; 19:69–78.

284. Sullivan PB, Juszczak E, Bachlet AME, et al. Impact of gastrostomy tube feeding on the quality of life of carers of children with cerebral palsy. Dev Med Child Neurol 2004; 46:796–800.

285. Tasdemir HA, Buyukavci M, Akcay F, et al. Bone mineral density in children with cerebral palsy. Pediatr Int 2001; 43(2):157–160.

286. Taub E, Ramey SL, DeLuca S, et al. Efficacy of constraint-induced movement therapy for children with cerebral palsy with asymmetric motor impairment. Pediatrics 2004; 113(2):305–312.

287. Thomas SS, Aiona MD, Pierce R, et al. Gait changes in children with spastic diplegia after selective dorsal rhizotomy. J Pediatr Orthop 1996; 16:747–752.

288. Thometz JG, Tachdjian M. Long-term follow-up of the flexor carpi ulnaris transfer in spastic hemiplegic children. J Pediatr Orthop 1988; 8:407–412.

289. Tirosh E, Rabino S. Physiotherapy for children with cerebral palsy. Evidence for its efficacy. Am J Dis Child 1989; 143:552–555.

290. Trejos H, Araya R. Sterotactic surgery for cerebral palsy. Stereotact Funct Neurosurg 1990; 54–55:130–135.

291. Tsirikos AI, Chang WN, Dabney KW, et al. Life expectancy in pediatric patients with cerebral palsy and neuromuscular scoliosis who underwent spinal fusion. Dev Med Child Neurol 2003; 45(10): 677–682.

292. Turk MA, Geremski CA, Rosenbaum P, et al. The health status of women with cerebral palsy. Arch Phys Med Rehabil 1997; 18: S10–S17.

293. Turker RJ, Lee R. Adductor tenotomies in children with quadriplegic cerebral palsy: longer term follow-up. J Pediatr Orthop 2000; 20(3):370–374.

294. Tyson MPH, Gilstrap LC. Hope for perinatal prevention of cerebral palsy. JAMA 2003; 290(20):2730–2731.

295. Ushmann H, Bennett JT. Spontaneous ankylosis of the contralateral hip after unilateral adductor tenotomy in cerebral palsy. J Pediatr Orthop B 1999; 8(1):4204.

296. Van der Linden ML, Hazelwood ME, Aitchinson AM, et al. Electrical stimulation of gluteus maximus in children with cerebral palsy: effects on gait characteristics and muscle strength. Dev Med Child Neurol 2003; 45(6):385–390.

297. Van Heest AE. Functional assessment aided by motion laboratory studies. Hand Clin 2003; 19(4):565–571.

298. Van-Heest AE, House J, Putman M. Sensibility deficiencies in the hands of children with spastic hemiplegia. J Hand Surg Am 1993; 18:278–281.

299. Vohr BR, Wright LL, Dusick AM, et al. Differences and outcomes of extremely low birth weight infants. Pediatrics 2004; 113(4):781–789.

300. Walstab J, Bell R, Reddihough D, et al. Maternal antecedents to cerebral palsy in preterm infants. Dev Med Child Neurol 2002; 44:498.

301. Waylett J, Barber L. Upper extremity bracing of the severely athetoid mental retardate. Am J Occup Ther 1971; 25:402–407.

302. Weber M, Cabanela ME. Total hip arthroplasty in patients with cerebral palsy. Orthopedics 1999; 22(4):425–427.

303. White H, Jenkins J, Neace WP, et al. Clinically prescribed orthoses demonstrate an increase in velocity of gait in children with cerebral palsy: a retrospective study. Dev Med Child Neurol 2002; 44(4):227–232.

304. Wind WM, Schwend RM, Larson J. Sports for the physically challenged child. J Am Acad Orthop Surg 2004; 12(2):126–137.

305. Wong AMK, Chen CL, Chen CPC, et al. Botulinum toxin A and phenol block in cerebral palsy. Am J Phys Med Rehabil 2004; 83(4):283–291.

306. Wong AMK, Chen CL, Hong WH, et al. Motor control assessment for rhizotomy in cerebral palsy. Am J Phys Med Rehabil 2000; 79:441–450.

307. Wright FV, Sheil EMH, Drake JM, et al. Evaluation of selective dorsal rhizotomy for the reduction of spasticity in cerebral palsy: a randomizes controlled trial. Dev Med Child Neurol 1998; 40:239–247.

308. Wu YW, Escobar GJ, Grether JK, et al. Chorioamnionitis and cerebral palsy in term and near-term infants. Obstet Gynecol Surv 2004; 59(5):334–336.

309. Yang CH, Luo CH, Yang CH, et al. Counter-propagation network with variable degree variable step size LMS for single switch typing recognition. Biomed Mater Eng 2004; 14(1):23–32.

310. Zimbler S, Craig C, Harris J, et al. Orthotic management of severe scoliosis in spastic neuromuscular disease—results of treatment. Orthop Trans 1985; 9:78–92.

Chapter

55

Rehabilitation Concepts in Myelomeningocele and Other Spinal Dysraphisms

Charles Law and R. Drew Davis

Myelomeningocele (MMC) is the most common congenital anomaly of the central nervous system. It exists in a spectrum of neural tube defects (NTDs), ranging from cranioschisis, or complete failure of neurulation, at one end, to spina bifida occulta, with minimal or no neurologic involvement, on the other end.[72] While the most severe NTDs result in stillbirth or death shortly after birth, the majority of patients with a spinal dysraphism survive. MMC, which composes 90% of open spinal dysraphic states, is the most complex congenital abnormality compatible with life, and is the second most common disabling condition in childhood, following cerebral palsy.[12,94,135] The varying degrees of neurologic and cognitive impairment involved with these congenital anomalies have major implications for other organ systems, as well as the psychologic and social well-being of the patient. Survival and quality of life for affected patients have improved due to advances in medical, surgical, and rehabilitative care over the past half-century. Yet many challenges remain regarding advancing prevention, understanding etiology, maximizing neurologic outcome, and minimizing impairment. These goals are best achieved by a team of specialists working with patients, their families, and the community.

TERMINOLOGY AND HISTORICAL BACKGROUND

A need for clarification of terminology exists, as midline fusion defects of the spine have been described using several nomenclatures. The term *spina bifida* is sometimes used non-specifically with regard to all patients with a spinal dysraphism or those with incomplete closure of the posterior neuropore. *Spina bifida* literally translates as 'spine split in two', and is technically correct in describing any patient with incomplete closure of the posterior elements of the spinal column. However, the degree of variation of anatomic malformations associated with the condition requires the use of more specific terminology.

The first clear description of spinal dysraphism was made by Casper Bauhin, a Swiss physician, anatomist, and botanist, in his publication *Theatrum Anatomicum* in 1592. The term *spina bifida*, however, is often historically associated with Nicholas Tulp, a Dutch physician who published a sketch (Fig. 55-1) and description of several patients with the condition in 1641.

Virchow described spina bifida occulta in 1875, which refers to a hidden bony defect, as well as other potential hidden anomalies.[131] Spina bifida has been further delineated with the term *spina bifida aperta*, a midline defect that communicates with the external environment and includes MMC and meningocele. The term *spina bifida cystica* is also sometimes used, and simply refers to a sac filled with cerebrospinal fluid protruding from the spinal column, but can also refer to MMC and meningocele. MMC at the level of the spine refers to protrusion of the meninges through a defect in the posterior elements of the spine, with involvement of the spinal cord or nerve roots. Meningocele refers only to protrusion of the meninges and cerebrospinal fluid through a defect in the posterior elements of the spine into the tissue beneath the skin, without involvement of functional neural elements. These distinctions are important and will be further explained below.

As this terminology is often confusing and minimally descriptive, an alternative system based on advances in clinical recognition and imaging of spinal lesions now allows for more useful classification, especially as it relates to prognosis. This point is exemplified by studies that show a 17% incidence of spina bifida occulta in the general population, and in 30% of normal individuals aged 1–10 with no neurologic involvement or anatomic abnormality other than incomplete closure of the posterior elements of the spine.[8,71] In contrast, what is also referred to as spina bifida occulta or occult spinal dysraphism can present with neurologic compromise or orthopedic deformity, with no further outward anatomic abnormalities other than cutaneous anomalies. Modern imaging studies are able to reveal these underlying defects and provide a system of classification based on neuroradiologic and clinical findings.[141]

This system of classification simply divides the various forms of spinal dysraphism into open spinal dysraphisms (i.e. open spina bifida) and closed spinal dysraphisms (i.e. closed spina bifida) (Fig. 55-2). It is useful from a prognostication standpoint, as it is based on the observation that those with open defects generally have lesions with visible neural elements, often leaking cerebrospinal fluid, which are associated with malformations that involve the entire central nervous system, including Chiari II malformations, midline defects, and hydrocephalus. In contrast, closed spinal dysraphisms (meningocele and occult spinal dysraphism) are lesions that are fully epithelialized with no neural tissue exposed, and generally have the

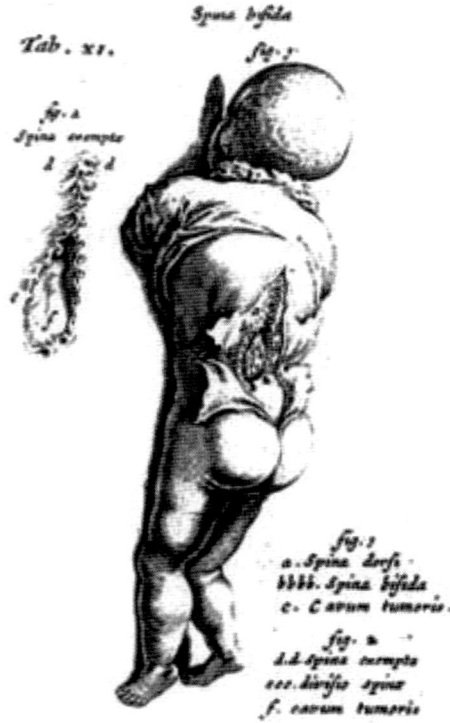

Figure 55-1 From Observationes Medicae by Nicholas Tulp, first published in 1641. Some speculate that the sketch was done by Rembrandt, a friend of Tulp who made him the subject of the well-known painting 'The Lesson in Anatomy of Dr. Tulp'.

Box 55-1 Cliniconeuroradiologic classification of spinal dysraphism

Open spinal dysraphism
- Myelomeningocele
- Myelocele
- Hemimyelomeningocele
- Hemimyelocele

Closed spinal dysraphism
With a subcutaneous mass
- Lumbosacral
  Lipoma with dural defect
  Lipomyelomeningocele
  Lipomyeloschisis
- Terminal myelocystocele
- Meningocele

Cervical
- Cervical myelocystocele
- Cervical myelomeningocele
- Meningocele

Without a subcutaneous mass

Simple dysraphic states
- Posterior spina bifida
- Intradural and intramedullary lipoma
- Filum terminale lipoma
- Tight filum terminale
- The abnormally long spinal cord
- Persistent terminal ventricle

Complex dysraphic states
- Dorsal enteric fistula
- Neurenteric cysts
- Split cord malformations (diastematomyelia and diplomyelia)
- Dermal sinus
- Caudal regression syndrome
- Segmental spinal dysgenesis

(From Tortori-Donati et al. 2000,[141] with permission.)

malformation limited to the spine and spinal cord, with only rare involvement of the brain.[2] Box 55-1 displays a complete listing of spinal dysraphic states.[141] While most of the conditions listed in Box 55-1 can result in a patient having rehabilitation needs, the most severely affected and vast majority of these will have a history of MMC. For this reason, the remainder of this chapter refers to rehabilitation concepts as they apply to MMC, although they can be applied to the various other spinal dysraphisms as appropriate.

EPIDEMIOLOGY

Incidence and prevalence

Epidemiologic studies of spinal dysraphisms typically include both MMC and meningocele, which are collectively referred to as spina bifida.[10] One clear observation from these studies is that the prevalence of MMC has declined worldwide over the past century.[2] In the USA, rates have varied from as high as 2.31 per 1000 births in Boston during the 1930s to as low as 0.51 per 1000 births in Atlanta in the early 1990s.[100,115] According to the National Center for Health Statistics, the rate of spina bifida in the USA in 2002 was 20.13 per 100 000 live births. Rates in other parts of the world have been as high as 3.4 per 1000 live births in Dublin, Ireland, in 1953, although these rates have generally declined in a fashion similar to that in the USA.[27]

The reasons for the declining prevalence of MMC are multifactorial and not completely understood. A portion of the decline can be attributed to the advent of prenatal screening and elective termination of pregnancy.[31,115] This is only partially responsible, however, and other factors are known to play a role. The most influential factor has been the increased consumption of folic acid among women of childbearing age. Folate supplementation was first shown to decrease rates of NTD in studies performed in Wales in the early 1980s.[73] Multiple observational and controlled trials followed, leading up to the Medical Research Council study, which involved seven countries and 3012 women. The study was ended early after supplementation with folic acid (4 mg/day) was shown to prevent 72% of NTDs in women who had had a previously affected pregnancy.[91] A subsequent study proved the efficacy of folic acid in preventing the first occurrence of NTD.[32] However, both recommendations by the US Public Health Service beginning in 1992 for daily folic acid intake for women of childbearing age, and mandatory supplementation of all enriched cereal grain products in the USA since 1998, have not resulted in the 48% reduction in NTD predicted by these studies.[33] A decrease of approximately 26% has actually been observed, illustrating the need to further educate all women of childbearing age on the

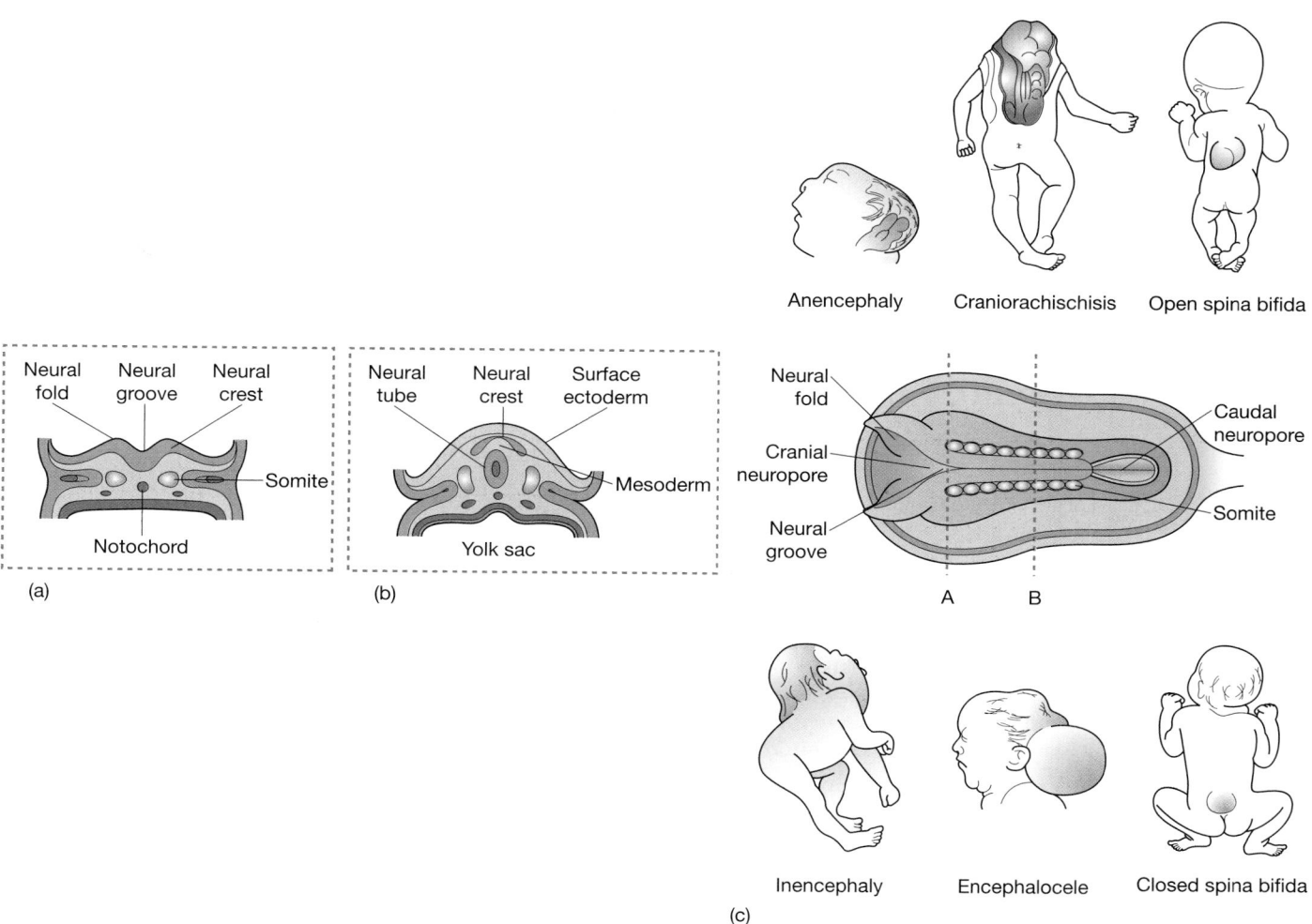

Figure 55-2 Features of neural tube development and neural tube defects (NTDs). (**a**) A cross-section of the rostral end of the embryo at approximately 3 weeks after conception, showing the neural groove in the process of closing, overlying the notochord. The neural folds are the rising margins of the neural tube, topped by the neural crest, and demarcate the neural groove centrally. (**b**) A cross-section of the middle portion of the embryo after the neural tube has closed. The neural tube, which will ultimately develop into the spinal cord, is now covered by surface ectoderm (later, the skin). The intervening mesoderm will form the bony spine. The notochord is regressing. (**c**) The developmental and clinical features of the main types of NTD. The diagram in the center is a dorsal view of a developing embryo, showing a neural tube that is closed in the center but still open at the cranial and caudal ends. The dotted lines marked A and B refer to the cross-sections shown in panels a and b. Shaded bars point to the region of the neural tube relevant to each defect. In anencephaly, the absence of the brain and calvaria can be total or partial. Craniorachischisis is characterized by anencephaly accompanied by a contiguous bony defect of the posterior vertebral arches (in this case, the lower thoracic vertebrae), accompanied by herniation of neural tissue and meninges, and not covered by skin. In iniencephaly, dysraphia in the occipital region is accompanied by severe retroflexion of the neck and trunk. In encephalocele, the brain and meninges herniate through a defect in the calvaria. In closed spina bifida, unlike open spina bifida, the bony defect of the posterior vertebral arches (in this case, the lumbar vertebrae), the herniated meninges, and the neural tissue are covered by skin. (From Botto et al. 1999,[10] with permission.)

importance of daily folic acid intake (4 mg), and placing emphasis on the importance of healthcare provider participation in this effort.[24] One recent study showed that folic acid supplementation was ineffective in decreasing the overall incidence of lipomyelomeningocele between 1995 and 2001 in Nova Scotia, providing evidence that the embryogenesis of various spinal dysraphisms could be fundamentally different.[90]

Geographic variation in birth prevalence of NTD occurs both between and within countries.[67] Across Europe, rates have been noted to be higher in Germany and Hungary than in Scandinavian countries. In the USA, there has been an observed trend of decreasing rates of NTD from the east coast to the west

coast.[46] Ethnicity has been shown to play a role in MMC as well, with those of Celtic descent (Irish, Welsh, and Scottish) having higher rates than those of Anglo-Saxon or Norman origin. These findings have been correlated with the high rates of MMC in Boston in the 1930s, which were highest among those who had mothers of Irish descent.[20,99] In addition, Hispanic, Chinese, and Sikh people are at a greater risk for MMC.[151] Rates among black and Asian populations have been observed to be low, with similar rates among populations living in different areas.[67] Female gender has also consistently been shown to be a risk factor for MMC, with a female preponderance observed in both still and live births.[65,67]

EMBRYOLOGY AND ETIOLOGY

Embryology

Neural tube defects are known to occur due to failure of neurulation between the 17th and 30th days of gestation.[74] Primary neurulation refers to the development of the neural tube, which forms the brain and spinal cord. Secondary neurulation refers to formation of the remainder of the neural tube from a cell mass caudal to the posterior neuropore, which forms the lower sacral and coccygeal segments. The caudal neuropore closes around the 26th day of gestation and, as a result, teratogenic events that take place after this closure cannot cause thoracic or lumbosacral MMC.[74,127] A failure of primary neurulation can lead to an open NTD, consisting not only of a spinal anomaly but also other defects, including a Chiari II malformation and hydrocephalus, possibly due to cerebrospinal fluid loss during early development.[63,88] Most posterior lumbar and sacral meningoceles are thought to occur during secondary neurulation, with those higher on the spinal axis resulting from defects in primary neurulation that do not cause an open NTD.[2]

Etiology

Although the mechanisms are not well understood, up to 80% of all NTDs are thought to be due to multifactorial influences (i.e. genetic and environmental factors). Certain other NTDs associated with NTD syndromes, single-gene disorders, and chromosomal disorders are relatively well defined.[4] The nature of the gene–gene and/or gene–environment interactions that lead to the remaining 80% of NTDs, however, is not well understood. Recurrence rates of NTDs are influenced by family history, geography, and severity of anomaly. These rates have been reported to vary from 2.4 to 5% after the birth of one affected child, with the risk doubling after two affected children.[29] A Hungarian study reported that recurrence risk among those with spina bifida was greatest for MMC associated with hydrocephalus, at 4.79%.[108] In addition, studies in the early 1990s showed that at least 70% of NTDs are 'folic acid-sensitive' or 'folic acid-dependent', with the remaining 30% being 'folic acid-resistant'.[4] Recent studies from Ireland have confirmed that both homozygosity and heterozygosity for the T allele of the C677T polymorphism of the gene encoding the folate-dependent enzyme 5,10-MTHFR are risk factors for NTD. This polymorphism is associated with lower tissue folate concentrations, higher homocysteine concentrations, and lower enzyme activity than in the wild-type genotype. This single genetic variant could account for up to half of the folate-related NTDs in Ireland.[69] These combined at-risk phenotypes are present in approximately 59% of the European population and 53% of the North American population.[11] Recent studies have also investigated links between genetic dysregulation of platelet-derived growth factor, myoinositol, and nitric oxide synthase, among others, as contributors to the formation of NTD.[17,48,162] A trial entitled the Genetics of Spina Bifida is currently underway through the National Institute of Child Health and Human Development to further elucidate these issues.

A number of environmental factors have been implicated in the development of NTDs, including low socioeconomic status;[101,152] maternal diabetes mellitus;[151] maternal hyperthermia;[122] folate deficiency;[91] hyperzincemia;[89] and certain drug exposures, including to carbamazepine,[116] valproic acid,[106] diuretics, antihistamines, and sulfonamides.[98] Of the medications mentioned, carbamazepine and valproic acid have the strongest correlation with spina bifida, with an estimated risk of 1% and 1–2%, respectively.[106,116] Seasonal variation, with peaks in midspring conception for spina bifida, have been reported in some regions but not confirmed in others.[23,42]

PRENATAL COUNSELING (DIAGNOSIS AND MANAGEMENT)

Prenatal screening now allows for diagnosis of the majority of cases of MMC prior to birth. Initial screening of women who are at high risk, including those with a positive family history, a previous child with spina bifida, or exposure to teratogenic agents, should include measurement of serum α-fetoprotein and acetylcholinesterase levels at 16–18 weeks post conception. Based on these results, a patient-specific risk can be calculated and repeat testing of serum levels performed. Subsequently, high-resolution ultrasound is performed, which is sensitive in 95% of cases in which good images are retrieved. If the images are of poor quality due to maternal obesity or other factors, amniocentesis for amniotic fluid α-fetoprotein and acetylcholinesterase can be performed. These tests can be repeated based on previous equivocal results but, after diagnosis, genetic counseling along with discussion of management options occurs.

Prenatal detection of MMC is important in order to educate the patient and family regarding the diagnosis and management options. Early detection also allows time to prepare for a safe delivery in a medical center that offers neurological closure. Functional motor outcome can also be predicted by high-resolution ultrasound prior to delivery.[28] Previous consideration has been given to performing cesarean section for all mothers with an affected pregnancy in order to avoid further damage to neural structures. One study reported a less severe lower extremity paralysis in infants born by cesarean section prior to the onset of labor, but showed no difference in those who received cesarean section after the onset of labor.[80] Another study, however, found no difference in motor outcome with cesarean section.[56]

Intrauterine surgical procedures

Since 1997, over 200 fetuses have received in utero closure of MMC by open maternal–fetal surgery. Studies involving these patients have suggested that the incidence of shunt-dependent hydrocephalus is significantly reduced, and that the brain stem and cerebellum are restored to a more normal anatomic configuration in some patients receiving intrauterine MMC repair.[139,148] Criticism exists, however, regarding methods of data collection and study design, among other issues.[158] A multicenter, randomized, open label trial is currently being undertaken to further evaluate this procedure.

NEONATAL MANAGEMENT

Back defect

After an infant is delivered with an open NTD, a sequence of events is set in place to preserve neurologic function, prevent infection, and stabilize cerebrospinal fluid flow. Early closure (within 72 h of delivery) reduces the risk of infection in the central nervous system.[26] Prior to closure, the open defect must be protected to prevent contamination or further damage from trauma. Closure occurs in three stages:

1. the neural plaque is returned to the canal, and the dura and arachnoid are reconstructed;
2. a myofascial closure over the newly constructed neural tube is performed;
3. the skin is closed.

After closure of the open spinal defect, hydrocephalus often develops.[2] Some centers advocate simultaneous back closure and insertion of ventriculoperitoneal shunts.[81,93]

Hydrocephalus

Most infants with MMC require ventricular shunting.[83] Approximately 15% are born with severe hydrocephalus and require immediate shunting.[87] The 85% who do not require immediate shunting should be watched closely after their back closure for signs of increased intracranial pressure. The leaking cerebrospinal fluid serves as a decompression and, once the defect is closed, cerebrospinal fluid may accumulate in the ventricular system. The white matter of a neonate is relatively compliant, and therefore the ventricles can become enlarged before the head circumference changes.[7] The presence of hydrocephalus correlates well with the level of the spinal defect, with thoracic lesions having a higher incidence than lumbar or sacral ones.[114]

Hydrocephalus usually does not progress immediately, and computed tomography scans may not show increasing ventricular size until 3–7 days of life. Some children do not require cerebrospinal fluid diversion for months or even years. Progressive hydrocephalus in newborns usually presents with increasing head size, which can be asymptomatic. Delayed-onset hydrocephalus can present with signs and symptoms of increased intracranial pressure, i.e. vomiting, irritability, somnolence, or headache.

Early bladder management

More than 90% of infants with MMC will have a neurogenic bladder. Management decisions made in infancy can impact renal health and the eventual development of urinary continence.[132] The importance of aggressive urinary management should be stressed to the family before the child leaves the hospital. Early goals include avoiding infections, preventing upper tract damage, and identifying anatomic abnormalities in the genitourinary system.[132] Baseline investigations should include renal–bladder sonography and a voiding cystourethrogram. Hydronephrosis is found in 7–30% of infants, and reflux occurs in approximately 20% of infants.[59,160] Infants with hydronephrosis or reflux should be started on prophylactic antibiotics. Infants who are unable to void should be begun on intermittent catheterization programs. If the infant is able to void, he or she should be checked for complete emptying with a postvoid residual either by catheter or bladder scan. Incomplete emptying can lead to urinary tract infections, as the retained urine serves as a culture media.

Assessment of the neurologic level

Even if not spoken out loud, the first question parents of a newborn with MMC often ask is, 'Will my child be able to walk?' A careful neurologic examination can give them an idea even within the first few days of life. The best predictor of motor function is the actual motor examination. Information regarding the best motor examination may be obtained by observation, palpation, and postural changes. Motor examinations may improve after the initial examination, which may be related to a period of spinal shock associated with the delivery or the closure.[39,126] This can make a newborn's motor function appear worse than it may eventually be.

Therapy

The goal of any MMC team should be to develop and implement a comprehensive plan that enables the child to attain maximal level of function in all areas.[94] Therapists play a key role in this endeavor. Therapists often develop a very good working relationship with families of children with MMC. They are invaluable in providing education and anticipatory guidance for the family. For children born with contractures at the hips, knees, ankles, or feet, a program of passive range of motion can be taught to the family even before discharge. Splints are often fabricated soon after birth by the therapists. Throughout life, the MMC clinic therapist will help to educate and coordinate with community therapists regarding the plan developed by the MMC team.

CHILDHOOD MANAGEMENT

Shunts

Almost all children with MMC require placement of a ventriculoperitoneal shunt for management of hydrocephalus. The two most common shunt complications are infection and obstruction.[147] Presenting signs and symptoms of shunt malfunction vary with the age of the child. Mechanical obstructions tend to present more acutely with signs and symptoms related to increased intracranial pressure, and infections tend to present more insidiously (see Box 55-2).

Infections have a greater long-term morbidity than malfunctions. The overall risk of shunt infection is 12% per child. *Staphylococcus epidermidis* is the organism that causes most shunt infections.[38] Symptoms do not usually develop until several weeks after the shunt is placed or revised. Epidemiologic factors seem to influence the incidence of shunt infections more than

Box 55-2 Possible symptoms of a shunt malfunction

Infants
- Bulging fontanel
- Vomiting
- Irritability
- Change in appetite
- Lethargy
- Sunsetting eyes (cranial nerve VI palsy with abduction paralysis)
- Seizures
- Vocal cord paralysis with stridor
- Swelling or redness along shunt track

Toddlers
- Vomiting
- Lethargy
- Irritability
- Seizures
- Headaches
- Swelling along shunt tract
- Redness along shunt tract

Schoolage children
- Headaches
- Vomiting
- Lethargy
- Seizures
- Irritability
- Swelling along shunt track
- Redness along shunt tract
- Decreased school performance

Adults
- Headaches
- Vomiting
- Lethargy
- Seizures
- Redness or swelling along shunt tract

surgical factors. Aside from skin contamination during shunt placement, shunts can also become infected with Gram-negative rods if the distal end of the shunt erodes into an intraabdominal organ. Gram-negative infections have a much poorer prognosis.[40]

Isolated downstream infections of the shunt system have the least morbidity. Shunt infection with ventriculomeningitis carries the highest morbidity. Although controversial, several studies suggest that recurrent and frequent shunt infections affect cognitive function.

Half of all children with ventriculoperitoneal shunt develop obstruction in the first year of life requiring revision. Of those children who require a revision in the first year, 31% will require a second revision in the second year, and then have a risk recurrence rate of 12% per year thereafter.[136] Endoscopic third ventriculostomies are performed in carefully selected patients and can become an alternative for chronic ventriculoperitoneal shunts.[15]

Arnold–Chiari II malformations

The Chiari II malformation is characterized by variable displacement of cerebellar tissue into the spinal canal, accompanied by caudal dislocation of the lower brain stem and fourth ventricle. Although these posterior fossa abnormalities are most often described, the Chiari II malformation is also associated with a wide range of abnormalities throughout the neuraxis.[2]

Although the operative mortality for closure of the spinal defect in children with MMC is very low, the operative mortality for symptomatic Arnold–Chiari malformations is relatively high (34–38%).[2,120] A symptomatic Chiari II malformation remains the leading cause of death for infants with MMC.[137] Signs and symptoms of symptomatic Chiari II malformations include intermittent obstructive or central apnea, cyanosis, bradycardia, dysphagia, nystagmus, stridor, vocal cord paralysis, torticollis, opisthotonos, hypotonia, upper extremity weakness, and spasticity. The constellation of stridor, central apnea, and aspiration are sometimes referred to as *central ventilatory dysfunction*.[53]

Prior to hindbrain decompression for a symptomatic Chiari II malformation, the child's shunt system should be evaluated carefully, as shunt malfunctions can cause Chiari malformations to become symptomatic. Hindbrain decompressions should be performed early to minimize the progression of symptoms of the Chiari malformation. Poor preoperative prognostic signs include bilateral vocal cord paralysis, severe neurogenic dysphagia, and prolonged apnea.[25]

Hydromyelia

Hydromyelia is the dilatation of the central canal of the spinal cord. It is analogous to dilatation of the ventricles or hydrocephalus in the brain, and is a relatively common occurrence in children with MMC. Hydromyelia is probably much more common than we are aware, as it often does not cause obvious symptoms in patients with MMC.[18] When symptomatic, it usually presents with rapidly progressive scoliosis, change in strength or coordination of the upper or lower extremities, and spasticity. Magnetic resonance imaging is the best study to demonstrate this spinal cord abnormality.[19] The entire neuraxis should be imaged, because untreated or subclinical hydrocephalus can produce hydromyelia. Hydrocephalus should be treated prior to surgical treatment for hydromyelia.

Tethered cord syndrome

In children with MMC, the spinal cord can be fixed or 'tethered' at one point, causing traction, which can lead to progressive urologic, orthopedic, or functional decline. It was first described in 1857. The first known detethering of the spinal cord was performed on a previously healthy 17-year-old who had progressive loss of lower extremity function in 1891.[87]

The spinal cord usually terminates at the level of L1–2. MMC repair invariably is followed by the development of arachnoiditis, fibrosis, and adhesions between the intraspinal neural structures, the meninges, and the surrounding vertebral structures.[161]

These adhesions can tether the cord to the low lumbar or sacral region.

Most children with MMC will show signs of tethering on magnetic resonance imaging. Therefore symptoms should develop before surgical correction is pursued. Typical signs and symptoms in children include increased weakness (55%), worsening gait (54%), scoliosis (51%), pain (32%), orthopedic deformity (11%), and urologic dysfunction (6%).[60] Surgical correction should be considered early, as most cases will improve or stabilize if treated early.[60] Delayed correction can result in irreversible loss of function, as the natural history is for symptoms to worsen with time.[109]

There are at least three other lesions that can lead to tethering of the spinal cord: diastematomyelia, lipomyelomeningocele, and tight filum terminale. Diastematomyelia refers to divisions (not duplications) of the spinal cord. It is usually associated with a bony spur. Even if asymptomatic, the natural history is for symptoms to develop that can be irreversible.[3,51] Lipomyelomeningocele refers to a subcutaneous lipoma, continuous with the cauda equina, which also has a meningocele with neural elements enclosed extending outside the dura. A tight filum terminale is another congenital malformation in which the filum terminale does not elongate. Prophylactic surgery is usually recommended for these three lesions.

Neurogenic bladder

Urologic involvement in MMC and other spinal dysraphisms varies, and is not necessarily correlated with the level of the lesion as in traumatic spinal cord injury. In MMC, more than 80% of patients have partial or complete denervation of the bladder, with poor compliance and contractibility resulting in unacceptable residual urine volumes. The urethral sphincter is incompetent in 86% of patients, so that incontinence occurs with increases in intravesical pressure. About one-third of patients have detrusor–sphincter dyssynergia, resulting in high intraluminal pressures. The external sphincter is usually partially functional and can improve in the first year after birth.[134] Patients should be observed at least annually, as deterioration or improvement can occur in the first year of life, and tethering of the spinal cord with a change in bladder function may occur over the years.

Prevention of damage to the urinary tract and continence are the primary goals of neurogenic bladder management. Urodynamic evaluation is generally performed in infants with MMC, with 75% showing a normal upper urinary tract. The remaining infants show some degree of hydronephrosis due to vesicoureteral reflux, detrusor–sphincter dyssynergia, an enlarged bladder, or other structural abnormality. Infants with normal anatomy should receive a renal ultrasound biannually. Those with incomplete emptying and no outlet resistance can be taught the Crede maneuver. Those with detrusor–sphincter dyssynergia, or who have already developed hydronephrosis, should be treated with anticholinergic medications and clean intermittent catheterization to prevent the development or worsening of hydronephrosis. Children with vesicoureteral reflux, which develops when detrusor pressure exceeds 40

mmHg, are often prescribed prophylactic antibiotics. If they have persistent febrile urinary tract infection or persistent hydronephrosis, surgical intervention is often necessary. Cutaneous vesicostomy can be performed, with reversal done at a later time when the patient is capable of effective clean intermittent catheterization.[86,125]

As fewer than 10% of children with MMC have normal urinary control, continence of urine is a prominent issue.[76] Although there are no effective external collection devices for girls excluding diapers, condom catheters are an option for boys with reflex emptying who do not have vesicoureteral reflux or large residual volumes. Appropriate sizing can be a difficult issue with some boys, and impaired sensation can lead to skin breakdown.

The high prevalence of small bladder capacity and low outlet resistance in many children results in only about one-fourth of children being continent with clean intermittent catheterization alone.[149] The addition of anticholinergic medications, α-adrenergic agonists, and antibiotic instillations still only resulted in complete continence in 49% of patients in one study.[155] In general, frequent catheterization less than every 4 h is required to achieve continence.[76]

Surgical options are available for those who do not achieve continence with clean intermittent catheterization and medications. Bladder augmentation along with artificial sphincter placement can be used individually or in combination. Success for long-term continence after artificial sphincter placement is over 60%.[9] In addition, for patients who have difficulty performing urethral clean intermittent catheterization, continent diversion, with the appendix used as a conduit to the bladder to create an abdominal stoma, creates easier access for many patients.[125]

Independence with toileting in children with MMC is delayed more than all other self-care tasks, regardless of intelligence. While most children achieve independent control of bowel and bladder function by the age of 4, those with MMC might not achieve this until age 10–15.[104] The cause of this is multifactorial and includes level of paralysis, intelligence, difficulty with visuospatial tasks, kyphoscoliosis, parental support, sensation, sphincter control, and bladder perception. Children can be taught to perform clean intermittent catheterization as early as age 5, although they will still need assistance with maintaining a schedule. Parents need to be trained in their child's bladder program, but also instructed in the importance of allowing the child to accept responsibility once she or he is able.[133]

Latex allergy

While the incidence of latex allergy in the general population is estimated to be less than 1–2%, the prevalence among children with MMC ranges from 20% to 65%.[140] The IgE-mediated response to natural rubber latex is related to repeated mucosal exposure during surgical, therapeutic, and diagnostic procedures as well as atopic predisposition. The allergic response can range from dermatitis, allergic rhinitis, asthma, and angioedema to anaphylaxis.[129,138] Patients with spina bifida have been determined to have a 500-fold greater risk for anaphylaxis in the operating room compared with control groups.[140] As latex sensitization takes place over time, a previous lack of sensitivity or negative allergy test does not preclude life-threatening reactions. Parents should be educated regarding presence or risk of latex allergy. Many clinics now advocate the use of non-latex catheters for all patients with MMC, and avoidance of all other latex-containing products, whether medical or non-medical.

Neurogenic bowel

Patterns of neurogenic bowel involvement in children with MMC vary from normal bowel control in about 20%, to incontinence due to impaired rectal sensation, impaired sphincter function, and altered colonic motility in the remainder.[76] Those without control of the external anal sphincter become incontinent when the pressure inside the rectum is sufficient to produce reflex relaxation of the internal anal sphincter. In those with lesions above L3, the internal anal sphincter has low tone, which further contributes to incontinence. As well, lesions above this level generally result in absent sensation, although it may be present but impaired in lower level lesions.[1] Presence of the bulbocavernous or anocutaneous reflex has been associated with a greater likelihood of achieving bowel continence.[68]

The goal of a bowel management program is to achieve efficient, regular, and predictable emptying before the rectum becomes full enough to stimulate reflex relaxation of the internal anal sphincter (in those in whom innervation is present). This can be achieved through the use of stool softeners, bulking agents, suppositories, digital stimulation, manual removal, or enemas. However, many patients and families prefer dietary manipulation. Clinicians often recommend performing bowel programs after a meal to take advantage of the gastrocolic reflex, although it is not clear that this is intact in patients with MMC.[36]

In patients who cannot become continent, surgical options are available, including an antegrade continence enema procedure.[54] The appendix is used as a conduit to the bowel, and a catheter can then be inserted into the cecum and saline or tap water infused, with emptying achieved within 15–45 min. Colostomy is another option if standard treatment and antegrade continence enema have failed.

The importance of achieving bowel continence at an early age is important to provide a smooth transition into preschool and kindergarten, where children can be severely criticized by peers. Encouraging the child to assume increasing responsibility for this is again emphasized. Unfortunately, one study showed that as many as 86% of teenagers aged 13–18 with MMC needed assistance from a caregiver for their bowel program.[76] The reasons for this are, again, believed to be multifactorial.

Endocrine disorders

Individuals with MMC are known to have disturbed growth and development. While spinal cord lesions, vertebral anomalies, and other skeletal deformities reduce growth of the lower limbs and spine, complex central nervous system abnormalities put the patient with MMC at risk for hypothalamic–pituitary dysfunctions, including central precocious puberty and growth hormone deficiency.[37,75,118,119,124,143,145] Central precocious puberty has been effectively treated with gonadotropin-releasing hormone analogs, and there are currently limited data to show that treatment of growth hormone deficiency with growth hormone provides significant improvement in growth velocity and height, as well as muscle strength and mobility.[117,146] There is ongoing discussion as to whether to treat patients with MMC with growth hormone. Clarification of the goals of treatment is required, as efficacy with regards to functional improvement can be influenced by the level of the lesion and the presence of complicating factors such as syringomyelia, tethered cord syndrome, scoliosis, vertebral anomalies, contracture, and advanced pubertal development. Further studies are required to assess the ultimate role of growth hormone treatment in individuals with MMC.[144]

Musculoskeletal considerations
Motor innervation

It is important to practitioners and parents to appreciate that the level of motor function does not necessarily correspond to the anatomic vertebral level on radiographic studies.[114] Spinal defects are generally described as cervical, upper thoracic, midthoracic, low thoracic, upper lumbar, midlumbar, low lumbar, lumbosacral, or sacral level lesions. The majority of children with MMC have lumbosacral level vertebral lesions. Very few have cervical or upper thoracic vertebral lesions. Approximately one-fourth of patients have midlumbar level lesions, and one-fifth present with sacral level involvement.

It is important to recognize that these children do not present simply with flaccid paraplegia below their anatomic lesion. Actually, only one-third present with flaccid paralysis. Most have a combination of upper and lower motor neuron signs. Many are asymmetric on motor and sensory testing. Some have voluntary motor control below other segments of paralysis and sensory loss.[85]

The level of neurologic impairment influences medical providers' expectations for functional outcome, as well as musculoskeletal deformities and complications to anticipate (Table 55-1).

Hips

Most patients with MMC will have some hip deformity that interferes with ambulation, seating, or bracing. The proper management of hip deformity remains a topic of debate among orthopedic surgeons.[55] Muscle imbalance at the hip accounts for most of the hip flexion deformity, but sitting at 90° and hip flexor spasticity can also contribute to hip flexion deformities. Patients with thoracic level lesions develop hip flexion deformities related to positioning or hip flexor spasticity. Patients with upper and midlumbar level lesions develop hip flexion deformities related to unopposed hip flexors and adductors. Hip flexion contractures create anterior pelvic tilt, which increases lumbar lordosis, which can then interfere with ambulation. Hip flexor lengthening procedures can preserve ambulation in the ambula-

Table 55-1 Prognosticating in myelomeningocele

Motor level spinal cord segment	Critical motor function present	Mobility: school age	Activity: adolescent	Range: adult
T12	Totally paralyzed lower limbs	Standing brace, wheelchair	Wheelchair	Wheelchair, no ambulation
L1–2	Hip flexor muscles	Crutches, braces, wheelchair	Wheelchair, household ambulation	Wheelchair, non-functional ambulation
L3–4	Quadriceps muscles	Crutches, braces, household ambulation, wheelchair	Crutches, household ambulation, wheelchair	50% wheelchair; household ambulation with crutches
L5	Medial hamstrings, anterior tibial muscles	Crutches, braces, community ambulation	Crutches, community ambulation	Community ambulation with crutches
S1	Lateral hamstring and peroneal muscles	Community ambulation	Community ambulation	Community ambulation, 50% crutch or cane
S2–3	Mild loss of intrinsic foot muscles possible	Normal	Normal	Limited endurance due to late foot deformities

tory MMC patient, but should not be considered in the non-ambulatory patient unless skin integrity, pain, or seating is compromised.

Hip dislocations occur in children with MMC in one of two types. The first is the dislocation that is present at birth (congenital). The second occurs later as a result of unopposed hip flexors and adductors. Treatment of the dislocated hip in MMC is a topic of considerable debate.

Congenital dislocations of the hip can be seen in thoracic as well as lumbar and sacral level patients. Treatment depends on the prognosis for functional ambulation. Children with thoracic level lesions and no motor function in the lower extremities probably should not have their hips reduced. The child with good quadriceps power should receive a more aggressive treatment plan for congenitally dislocated hips. This is especially true in the unilateral dislocated hip.

Hips that slowly migrate laterally (subluxation) over time are usually related to muscle imbalance around the hip. In a natural history study, Broughton found that hip dislocation had occurred by the age of 11 years in 28% of thoracic level patients, in 30% of upper lumbar level patients, in 36% of patients with L4 functioning, in 7% of patients with L5 functioning, and in 1% of patients with sacral function.[16] In the ambulatory child, aggressive treatment including femoral and acetabular osteotomy should be considered. However, a recent study by Gabrieli et al. found that gait characteristics are not significantly different with regard to hip subluxation, and therefore concluded that surgery for the dislocated hip in the ambulatory child is not indicated.[45] There is little debate that, in the non-ambulatory child, a dislocated hip probably does not cause much morbidity and therefore does not require surgical treatment. There is debate regarding unilateral hip dislocation leading to pelvic obliquity that eventually contributes to scoliosis.

Knees

Children with MMC can develop knee flexion or extension contractures.[35] Knee flexion contractures are generally seen in patients with thoracic level MMC, but can also be seen in patients with lumbar and sacral lesions.[159] Knee flexion contractures can interfere with upright mobility, transfers, and, if severe, hygiene in the popliteal space. Knee flexion contractures of 20° or less are generally well tolerated in the ambulatory patient. Non-ambulatory patients might tolerate even more severe contractures without loss of function. Surgical treatment for knee flexion contractures is a radical knee flexor release. This procedure is well tolerated, with a low rate of recurrence in the ambulatory child.[84] Knee extension contractures are much less common. They can be related to unopposed knee extensors, congenital dislocation of the knee, immobilization for fractures, or after-treatment for flexion contractures. Knee extension contractures can interfere with seating and sit to stand transfers in the non-ambulatory patient, but generally do not impede ambulation in the ambulatory child.[55] In the non-ambulatory child, adequate flexion can usually be obtained by transection of the patellar ligament.[123]

Feet

Foot deformities are present in almost all children with MMC.[103] Foot deformities can be present at birth, related to lack of intrauterine movement or muscle imbalance across the ankle. Foot deformities also develop over time from imbalanced muscle pull around the ankle and weight-bearing forces. Lack of sensation and autonomic instability can lead to secondary skin problems and poor wound healing.

The common foot deformities in children with MMC are equinus, equinovarus, calcaneus, cavus, and rocker bottom deformity. The goal in treating these children is to achieve a plantigrade foot with stable skin. Splinting and passive manipulation can be helpful in infancy, but many of these children will require corrective surgical procedures.

Pure equinus deformities can be seen in children with S1 innervation, but they are also seen in children with lumbar and thoracic level lesions. In the patient with lumbar or thoracic lesions, gentle manipulation followed by serial casting should be the first attempt at correction. If the contracture persists when the child is ready for weight bearing, percutaneous heel cord lengthening should be considered. This is often performed in the outpatient clinic if the child is insensate. Ankle–foot orthoses are often required to help maintain the newly acquired range of motion.

Children with midlumbar level lesions will often develop (either in utero or postnatally) equinovarus (clubfoot) deformities associated with unopposed tibialis anterior and posterior function. Serial casting is usually the first line of treatment, followed by tendon transfers to balance the forces across the ankle. Only experienced personnel should apply casts to these children, as the risk for pressure ulceration is quite high. Surgical correction should not be performed until the child is ready to begin bearing weight through the lower extremities, because crawling with internally rotated feet has a deforming force that can lead to recurrence. Often, the opposite deformity of hind foot valgus later develops. Postoperative bracing is necessary to hold the foot and ankle in proper alignment.

Calcaneus deformities can be seen at birth or develop postnatally as a response to unopposed dorsiflexion in patients with midlumbar level paralysis. Calcaneus deformity makes bracing difficult and often ineffective. This deformity predisposes the patient to pressure sores over the heel, which can lead to osteomyelitis. Patients with progressive deformities or propensity toward pressure ulceration should be treated aggressively, because delay in treatment can result in a greatly increased risk of pressure ulceration.[43] Solid ankle–foot orthoses are the most appropriate orthosis for this deformity.

Pes cavus or intrinsic minus feet require little treatment during the school age years. In adolescence, skin problems can develop related to weight bearing over the second to fourth metatarsal heads. If foot orthoses or custom-molded shoes are unable to redistribute the weight around the foot, metatarsal osteotomies might be required.

Valgus deformities of the foot and ankle are common problems encountered in the ambulatory child with MMC. This deformity can develop without regard for level of paralysis. These children often have poor orthotic tolerance, due to pressure over the medial malleolus or the head of the navicular bone.

Spine

Deformities of the spine in children with MMC can be congenital, paralytic, or a combination. Congenital spinal anomalies would include scoliosis secondary to vertebral malformations, congenital kyphosis related to posterior element dysplasia, and intrathecal anomalies such as diastematomyelia.[55] Predictors of development of scoliosis include ambulatory status, clinical motor level, and last intact laminar arch.[142] Spinal deformities in MMC include kyphosis, lordosis, and scoliosis. Spinal deformities are more likely to occur in thoracic lesions (more than 90%), but they can also be seen in sacral lesions, although relatively rare.[96,142] Kyphotic deformities can cause severe seating and skin problems. Surgical treatment of kyphotic deformities carries significant risk of complications but usually has a good outcome.[102] Kyphotic deformities seen at birth are related to congenital malformations. Lordosis is usually related to hip flexion contractures. Orthotic management of scoliosis does not provide a complete or permanent correction, but might delay the need for surgical correction until the child is closer to skeletal maturity. Rapid progression of otherwise stable curves can be seen in patients with hydromyelia or tethered cord syndromes.

Fractures

Children with MMC are susceptible to pathologic fractures in the lower limbs.[110] One study reported a 20% incidence of fracture in their record review.[78] Neonates with contractures in the lower limbs are more likely to have fractures with mobilization.[13] Risk factors include osteopenia, insensate extremities, contractures, and immobilization. Children with thoracic lesions are more likely to have femur fractures, and children with lumbar lesions are more likely to have tibial fractures.[78] Fractures manifest with localized erythema, heat, and swelling. Crepitus and deformity occur only with displaced fractures. There is often no complaint of pain and no report of trauma. Fractures are often confused with cellulitis or osteomyelitis. Fractures in children with MMC tend to heal well, with exuberant callus formation.[66] Prolonged immobilization should be avoided, as they can become more osteopenic during the period of immobilization.

Mobility

Almost all children with MMC are able to achieve some degree of independent mobility. This may not be in an upright position, although upright mobility is the goal of almost all parents of a child with MMC. Delay in achievement of ambulation can be expected in all children with MMC, regardless of level.[153] Maintaining ambulation is often sought after, even when it is highly inefficient and time-consuming. Many teenagers with MMC will choose wheelchair mobility when given the opportunity, even after a decade of being ambulatory. The ability for a child to become ambulatory and to maintain ambulatory function is determined by a number of factors, including lesion level, cognitive ability, motivation, musculoskeletal complications, growth, age, and obesity.[121]

Ambulatory function can be divided into four groups: community ambulation, household ambulation, non-functional ambulation, and no ambulation. Generally, most sacral level patients are community ambulators, and thoracic level patients are non-ambulators. Most patients with lumbar lesions will achieve some level of ambulation but can lose it as adolescence and growth progress.[153]

Orthoses

There are typically four goals or objectives in prescribing an orthotic device for a child with MMC:

1. to prevent deformity;
2. to support normal joint alignment and mechanics;
3. to control range of motion during gait; and
4. to improve function.

An orthotic device can address one or even all of these goals. An ankle–foot orthosis is the most commonly prescribed orthotic device for children with MMC. There are multiple variations to the ankle–foot orthosis, which can be prescribed based on the level of involvement and the goals in mind.

There are three bracing systems that are relatively unique to the child with MMC. The parapodium is a device that allows even the child with a thoracic level of involvement an opportunity for upright mobility. It offers structural support all the way from the trunk to the floor. A swing-to type of gait is used for ambulation. A swivel walker is a modification of the parapodium that translates trunk rotation into forward movement of a dual footplate mechanism. Finally, a reciprocating gait orthosis (RGO) combines bilateral hip–knee–ankle–foot orthoses with a cable system to coordinate hip flexion with hip extension at the opposite hip. Active hip flexion is required to use this type of orthosis. An energy consumption study was performed on three children, comparing the use of an RGO and a swing-through type of gait pattern. The swing-through gait was more efficient, but all three children preferred the RGO.[50] None of these orthoses allow for efficient gait, but they are often used by smaller children for upright mobility (see Chapter 16).

Skin breakdown

Skin breakdown is a very common occurrence in children and adults with MMC. Countless dollars are spent treating what should be a preventable complication. One clinic reported that approximately 50% of their patients had skin breakdown. Forty-two percent of these were attributed to excessive pressure. In their group, the prevalence steadily rose between infancy and 10 years of age.[105] Other factors contributing to the development of pressure sores include mental retardation, chronic soiling, and parental involvement. Morbidity associated with pressure sores may also be severe, including risk of amputation of feet and limbs.

Skin breakdown usually occurs due to pressure areas over bony prominences but can also occur due to hot or cold injury, shear, or tightly fitting clothes. Pressure sores in non-ambulatory patients occur over the sacrum, the ischial tuberosities, and the greater trochanters. Another common site is over a gibbus deformity, usually in a patient with a thoracic level lesion. Pressure sores in ambulatory patients usually occur on their feet, sometimes associated with poorly fitting orthoses.

Prevention of skin breakdown requires ongoing education of the patient and family. This education should include information regarding insensate skin, hygiene, pressure relief, proper skin inspection, wearing schedules for new or modified orthoses, and appropriate seating surfaces. School personnel also need to be aware of the risk of skin problems so that they can help to remind children to perform pressure relief.

The best treatment for pressure sores is to relieve the pressure. Almost any local approach will work if pressure is relieved. Occasionally, surgical procedures are required to close open wounds. Primary closures or skin flaps are preferred over myocutaneous procedures for initial wounds (see Ch. 33).

Obesity

Obesity has achieved national attention in the able-bodied population. It is also very common among children with MMC. Children with MMC have a lower metabolic rate and lower energy expenditure, which predisposes them to obesity.[77] Once they have become obese, exercise is more difficult, which propitiates the problem. Daily physical activity should be encouraged, beginning at the toddler stage.[49] Dietary management should begin in infancy to prevent this problem, because outcomes from weight reduction programs are poor.

Psychologic and social issues
Cognitive function

Parents of children with MMC rate their medical support much higher than they do the support received for psychosocial problems.[113] Children with MMC have specific behavioral and cognitive issues that need to be addressed or at least recognized by parents, healthcare providers, and school personnel. As a group, children with MMC have lower IQ scores as compared with their able-bodied peers. Their verbal IQ is usually higher than their performance IQ.[21] On the Wechsler Intelligence Scale for Children, only 6% of children with MMC scored in the high average to extremely high range, as compared with 27% of control subjects. Seventy-five percent of children with MMC score in the low average to extremely low average, compared with 25% of matched peers.[5] These children also have more difficulty in math and visual perceptual tasks than their able-bodied peers do.[44,154] IQ scores correlate with the level of lesion. Children with thoracic level lesions tend to have lower IQ scores than children with lumbar or sacral level lesions. IQ scores are also adversely affected by central nervous system infections,[62] but not necessarily recurrent shunt revisions.[111]

Behavior

Children with MMC often have rather characteristic personality traits. Many of them have much better verbal skills than written skills. Verbose but irrelevant conversation is often described. They will often speak off-topic and use many routine social phrases. These personality traits often cause misconceptions about the child's mental abilities.

The temperament characteristics of children with MMC and shunted hydrocephalus were recently described. Children with MMC were found to be less adaptable, more withdrawn, more distractible, less attentive, and less predictable than those in the control group.[150] Stimulant medications are often prescribed for these children.

MYELOMENINGOCELE IN ADULTS

Transition to adult healthcare

As individuals with MMC age, they can experience secondary complications related to accelerated impairment due to aging, and progression of their underlying disease process.[70] Although children are generally observed closely by their pediatric physicians, adults with MMC often do not have regular medical follow-up. In our state, patients who receive care through Children's Rehabilitation Services, a state-funded agency, are observed until the age of 21. While some of these patients continue to be observed by their pediatric providers into adulthood, a well-organized transition to adult healthcare is optimal for appropriate medical surveillance.[6,95]

Late neurologic changes

Adults with MMC are still at risk of developing neurologic complications of their disease. Complications seen in adults include shunt infections and malfunctions (which are a major source of morbidity and mortality), syringomyelia, and tethered cord. Adolescents and adults with MMC do not seem to outgrow their need for shunting.[79] Likewise, adults with MMC can develop symptoms of syringomyelia such as pain, paresthesias, and weakness in the upper limbs.[30] In adults, entrapment syndromes, overuse syndromes, and herniated disks need to be considered in the differential of upper extremity symptoms more so than in children. Symptomatic tethering of the spinal cord can also develop in adulthood.[52] This has been associated with herniated disks, pregnancy, and traumatic injuries.[82]

Late musculoskeletal considerations

Joint pain and degeneration can occur in adults without disability. Decades of walking on misaligned joints can cause this process to occur even more rapidly. Charcot joints can develop in the lower limbs due to lack of sensation and demineralization.[14,64] In one study, almost one-third of previously community ambulatory patients had a significant decline in their ambulatory status by the age of 29.

Scoliosis does not usually progress beyond adolescence, but it can continue to cause problems with seating, comfort, skin integrity, and pulmonary function.

Renal damage

As discussed above, individuals with MMC are at risk for renal deterioration. Although the majority of individuals with MMC have normal renal function at birth, 40–90% will experience a decline by age 10 if left unattended.[130] Renal damage remains one of the most common causes of morbidity and mortality among individuals with MMC.[97,128] Adults with MMC should receive ongoing urologic care to achieve social continence and maintain normal renal function. It has been reported that up to 80% of adults with MMC can achieve social continence with proper management.[12] Further studies are needed to properly evaluate the effectiveness of both proactive and observational approaches to management.

Fertility, sexuality, and reproductive issues

There are few studies elucidating the issues related to sexual maturation, fertility, and satisfaction with sexual function among individuals with MMC. Despite this, there are some facts that can guide clinicians in caring for and advising patients. Studies have shown that 12–16% of patients with MMC experience precocious puberty.[37,58] The mechanism of this is thought to be related to increased pressure on the hypothalamus, resulting in premature activation of the hypothalamic–pituitary–gonadal axis. Treatment with gonadotropin-releasing hormone analogs has proven beneficial in several studies, halting the progression of puberty, stopping menses, and decreasing hormone levels.[146] It is more common for girls with MMC to experience precocious puberty, and it is unclear whether patients without hydrocephalus are at risk. In addition, boys display a 15–25% incidence of cryptorchidism.[41,47,92]

Fertility among women with MMC is thought to be normal, and affected patients are capable of becoming pregnant.[156] One study showed that 95% of female patients with MMC menstruated regularly.[57] Complications can be experienced during pregnancy related to recurrent urinary tract infection, worsening kyphoscoliosis, ventriculoperitoneal shunt malfunction, and failure of genitourinary diversions. Vaginal delivery is generally indicated, especially in those with a ventriculoperitoneal shunt, and cesarean section should be performed only for obstetric reasons such as a contracted, underdeveloped pelvis.[112] Many men with MMC are infertile, with one study showing 10 of 10 men with MMC to be azoospermic, exhibiting primary testicular failure on biopsy.[157] Another study showed, however, that six of nine men with MMC appeared capable of reproducing with assisted reproductive technologies, although their overall semen quality remained poor.[61] Regardless, male and female patients with MMC should receive both basic and specialized sex education, particularly as it pertains to their increased risk of having a child with a NTD. Women of childbearing age with a history of MMC should take folic acid supplements.

The degree of satisfaction with sexual function among individuals with MMC is unknown. Both men and women generally have decreased sensation in the perineum, which can impair the ability to reach orgasm. In addition, non-verbal learning disorders and societal attitudes toward individuals with disabilities can affect self-esteem, social interactions, and ultimately psychosexual development. The reported incidence of ability to achieve erection ranges from 14% in higher level lesions to 64% in lower level lesions, although many of these are achieved reflexively.[34] The ability to sustain these erections during intercourse is uncertain, and many patients report dissatisfaction with the degree of rigidity.[57] Lesion level above the level of sympathetic outflow, as well as a negative anocutaneous reflex, is correlated with increased difficulty achieving erection.[34] Although one study reports that most adults with MMC have satisfactory sexual function, another showed that only 18% of the men and 33% of the women with MMC had sexual intercourse activities.[22,57] The latter study also reported that orgasm was achieved in 67% of men but only 19% of women. Treatment of erectile dysfunction in men with MMC with sildenafil

(Viagra) has been successful.[107] Retrograde ejaculation is common among men as well, but the exact incidence is unknown. Both men and women can experience skin breakdown during sexual intercourse and should be educated in this regard. Further research is needed to more properly address this topic (see also Ch. 32).

Vocational issues

Most adolescents with MMC complete high school, and about half move on to further education. Very little is published regarding the educational levels achieved or the employment of persons with this specific diagnosis. In a recent long-term follow-up survey, authors from Chicago reported that 85% of their children who survived to adulthood either attended or graduated from high school and/or college.[12] Thirty-two of the 71 patients available for follow-up were employed. In a US survey, independent living was achieved by only 30–60%, one-third lived with their family, and only a small number were in institutions. Data from England indicated that nearly 90% of adults live with their families. The employment rate is in the range of 25–50% and depends on intelligence, academic qualifications, behavior, continence, and severity of physical disability.

CONCLUSION

Myelomeningocele presents lifelong challenges to affected patients, their families, and clinicians. Vigilant surveillance and education are required to prevent life-threatening events related to ventriculoperitoneal shunt malfunction, Chiari II malformation, renal failure, latex allergy, and infection. This must be carried out in an environment that also seeks to maximize the functional independence of individuals with MMC by monitoring for decline in motor examination, preventing deformity, training in self-care and independent mobility, teaching independence with a bowel and bladder program, giving emotional and social support, and providing educational and vocational guidance.

For more information about MMC, contact the Spina Bifida Association of America through their web site at http://www.sbaa.org; by mail at 4590 MacArthur Blvd, NW, Suite 250, Washington, DC 20007-4226; or by telephone on (800) 621-3141.

REFERENCES

1. Agnarsson U, et al. Anorectal function of children with neurological problems. I: Spina bifida. Dev Med Child Neurol 1993; 35(10):893–902.
2. Albright AL, Pollack IF, Adelson PD, eds. Principles and practice of pediatric neurosurgery. New York: Thieme; 1999:xxiii, 1300.
3. Andar UB, Harkness WF, Hayward RD. Split cord malformations of the lumbar region. A model for the neurosurgical management of all types of 'occult' spinal dysraphism? Pediatr Neurosurg 1997; 26(1):17–24.
4. [Anonymous]. Mental retardation and developmental disabilities research reviews, vol 4. New York: Wiley; 1998:269–281.
5. Appleton PL, et al. The self-concept of young people with spina bifida: a population-based study. Dev Med Child Neurol 1994; 36(3):198–215.
6. Begeer IH, Staal-Schreinemachers AL. The benefits of team treatment and control of adult patients with spinal dysraphism. Eur J Pediatr Surg 1996; 6(suppl 1):15–16.
7. Bell WO, Sumner TE, Volberg FM. The significance of ventriculomegaly in the newborn with myelodysplasia. Childs Nerv Syst 1987; 3(4):239–241.
8. Boone D, et al. Spina bifida occulta: lesion or anomaly? Clin Radiol 1985; 36(2):159–161.
9. Bosco PJ, et al. The long-term results of artificial sphincters in children. J Urol 1991; 146(2):396–399.
10. Botto LD, et al. Neural-tube defects. N Engl J Med 1999; 341(20): 1509–1519.
11. Botto LD, Yang Q. 5,10-Methylenetetrahydrofolate reductase gene variants and congenital anomalies: a HuGE review. Am J Epidemiol 2000; 151(9):862–877.
12. Bowman RM, et al. Spina bifida outcome: a 25-year prospective. Pediatr Neurosurg 2001; 34(3):114–120.
13. Boytim MJ, et al. Neonatal fractures in myelomeningocele patients. J Pediatr Orthop 1991; 11(1):28–30.
14. Brinker MR, et al. Myelomeningocele at the sacral level. Long-term outcomes in adults. J Bone Joint Surg Am 1994; 76(9):1293–1300.
15. Brockmeyer D, et al. Endoscopic third ventriculostomy: an outcome analysis. Pediatr Neurosurg 1998; 28(5):236–240.
16. Broughton NS, et al. The natural history of hip deformity in myelomeningocele. J Bone Joint Surg Br 1993; 75(5):760–763.
17. Brown KS, et al. Evidence that the risk of spina bifida is influenced by genetic variation at the NOS3 locus. Birth Defects Res Part A Clin Mol Teratol 2004; 70(3):101–106.
18. Caldarelli M, Di Rocco C, La Marca F. Treatment of hydromyelia in spina bifida. Surg Neurol 1998; 50(5):411–420.
19. Caldarelli M, et al. Surgical treatment of late neurological deterioration in children with myelodysplasia. Acta Neurochir (Wien) 1995; 137(3–4):199–206.
20. Carter CO, Evans K. Spina bifida and anencephalus in greater London. J Med Genet 1973; 10(3):209–234.
21. Casari EF, Fantino AG. A longitudinal study of cognitive abilities and achievement status of children with myelomeningocele and their relationship with clinical types. Eur J Pediatr Surg 1998; 8(suppl 1):52–54.
22. Cass AS, Bloom BA, Luxenberg M. Sexual function in adults with myelomeningocele. J Urol 1986; 136(2):425–426.
23. Castilla EE, et al. Monthly and seasonal variations in the frequency of congenital anomalies. Int J Epidemiol 1990; 19(2):399–404.
24. Centers for Disease Control and Prevention. Spina bifida and anencephaly before and after folic acid mandate—United States, 1995–1996 and 1999–2000. MMWR Morb Mortal Wkly Rep 2004; 53(17):362–365.
25. Charney EB, et al. Management of Chiari II complications in infants with myelomeningocele. J Pediatr 1987; 111(3):364–371.
26. Charney EB, et al. Management of the newborn with myelomeningocele: time for a decision-making process. Pediatrics 1985; 75(1):58–64.
27. Coffey VP. Neural tube defects in Dublin 1953–1954 and 1961–1982. Ir Med J 1983; 76(10):411–413.
28. Coniglio SJ, Anderson SM, Ferguson JE II. Functional motor outcome in children with myelomeningocele: correlation with anatomic level on prenatal ultrasound. Dev Med Child Neurol 1996; 38(8):675–680.
29. Cowchock S, et al. The recurrence risk for neural tube defects in the United States: a collaborative study. Am J Med Genet 1980; 5(3): 309–314.
30. Craig JJ, Gray WJ, McCann JP. The Chiari/hydrosyringomyelia complex presenting in adults with myelomeningocoele: an indication for early intervention. Spinal Cord 1999; 37(4):275–278.
31. Cuckle H, Wald N. The impact of screening for open neural tube defects in England and Wales. Prenat Diagn 1987; 7(2):91–99.
32. Czeizel AE, Dudas I. Prevention of the first occurrence of neural-tube defects by periconceptional vitamin supplementation. N Engl J Med 1992; 327(26):1832–1835.
33. Daly LE, et al. Folate levels and neural tube defects. Implications for prevention. JAMA 1995; 274(21):1698–1702.
34. Diamond DA, Rickwood AM, Thomas DG. Penile erections in myelomeningocele patients. Br J Urol 1986; 58(4):434–435.

35. Dias LS. Surgical management of knee contractures in myelomeningocele. J Pediatr Orthop 1982; 2(2):127–131.

36. Dietrich S, Okamoto G. Bowel training for children with neurogenic dysfunction: a follow-up. Arch Phys Med Rehabil 1982; 63(4):166–170.

37. Elias ER, Sadeghi-Nejad A. Precocious puberty in girls with myelodysplasia. Pediatrics 1994; 93(3):521–522.

38. Enger PO, Svendsen F, Wester K. CSF shunt infections in children: experiences from a population-based study. Acta Neurochir (Wien) 2003; 145(4):243–248, discussion 248.

39. Erickson D, Bartholomew T, Marlin A. Sonographic evaluation and conservative management of newborns with myelomeningocele and hydronephrosis. J Urol 1989; 142(2 part 2):592–594, discussion 603–605.

40. Ersahin Y, Mutluer S, Guzelbag E. Cerebrospinal fluid shunt infections. J Neurosurg Sci 1994; 38(3):161–165.

41. Ferrara P, et al. Cryptorchidism associated with meningomyelocele. J Paediatr Child Health 1998; 34(1):44–46.

42. Fraser FC, Frecker M, Allderdice P. Seasonal variation of neural tube defects in Newfoundland and elsewhere. Teratology 1986; 33(3):299–303.

43. Fraser RK, Hoffman EB. Calcaneus deformity in the ambulant patient with myelomeningocele. J Bone Joint Surg Br 1991; 73(6):994–997.

44. Friedrich WN, et al. Cognitive abilities and achievement status of children with myelomeningocele: a contemporary sample. J Pediatr Psychol 1991; 16(4):423–428.

45. Gabrieli AP, et al. Gait analysis in low lumbar myelomeningocele patients with unilateral hip dislocation or subluxation. J Pediatr Orthop 2003; 23(3):330–334.

46. Greenberg F, James LM, Oakley GP Jr. Estimates of birth prevalence rates of spina bifida in the United States from computer-generated maps. Am J Obstet Gynecol 1983; 145(5):570–573.

47. Greene SA, et al. Growth and sexual development in children with meningomyelocele. Eur J Pediatr 1985; 144(2):146–148.

48. Groenen PM, et al. Spina bifida and genetic factors related to myo-inositol, glucose, and zinc. Mol Genet Metab 2004; 82(2):154–161.

49. Grogan CB, Ekvall SM. Body composition of children with myelomeningocele, determined by 40K, urinary creatinine and anthropometric measures. J Am Coll Nutr 1999; 18(4):316–323.

50. Guidera KJ, et al. Use of the reciprocating gait orthosis in myelodysplasia. J Pediatr Orthop 1993; 13(3):341–348.

51. Guthkelch AN. Diastematomyelia with median septum. Brain 1974; 97(4):729–742.

52. Harashima S, Taira T, Hori T. [Adult type tethered cord syndrome with chronic attackwise pain in the bilateral feet]. No Shinkei Geka 2004; 32(5):481–485.

53. Hays RM, et al. Central ventilatory dysfunction in myelodysplasia: an independent determinant of survival. Dev Med Child Neurol 1989; 31(3):366–370.

54. Herndon CD, et al. In situ Malone antegrade continence enema in 127 patients: a 6-year experience. J Urol 2004; 172(4 part 2):1689–1691.

55. Herring JA, Tachdjian MO, Texas Scottish Rite Hospital for Children. Tachdjian's pediatric orthopaedics. 3rd edn. Philadelphia: Saunders; 2002: xxxv, li, 2438.

56. Hill AE, Beattie F. Does caesarean section delivery improve neurological outcome in open spina bifida? Eur J Pediatr Surg 1994; 4(suppl 1):32–34.

57. Hirayama A, et al. [Evaluation of sexual function in adults with myelomeningocele]. Hinyokika Kiyo 1995; 41(12):985–989.

58. Hochhaus F, et al. Auxological and endocrinological evaluation of children with hydrocephalus and/or meningomyelocele. Eur J Pediatr 1997; 156(8):597–601.

59. Hopps CV, Kropp KA. Preservation of renal function in children with myelomeningocele managed with basic newborn evaluation and close followup. J Urol 2003; 169(1):305–308.

60. Hudgins RJ, Gilreath CL. Tethered spinal cord following repair of myelomeningocele. Neurosurg Focus 2004; 16(2):E7.

61. Hultling C, et al. Semen retrieval and analysis in men with myelomeningocele. Dev Med Child Neurol 2000; 42(10):681–684.

62. Hunt GM, Holmes AE. Factors relating to intelligence in treated cases of spina bifida cystica. Am J Dis Child 1976; 130(8):823–827.

63. Inagaki T, Schoenwolf GC, Walker ML. Experimental model: change in the posterior fossa with surgically induced spina bifida aperta in mouse. Pediatr Neurosurg 1997; 26(4):185–189.

64. Jones EA, et al. Neuropathic osteoarthropathy: diagnostic dilemmas and differential diagnosis. Radiographics 2000; 20(special number): S279–S293.

65. Kallen B, et al. International study of sex ratio and twinning of neural tube defects. Teratology 1994; 50(5):322–331.

66. Khoury JG, Morcuende JA. Dramatic subperiosteal bone formation following physeal injury in patients with myelomeningocele. Iowa Orthop J 2002; 22:94–98.

67. Kiely M. Reproductive and perinatal epidemiology. Boca Raton: CRC Press; 1991:543.

68. King JC, Currie DM, Wright E. Bowel training in spina bifida: importance of education, patient compliance, age, and anal reflexes. Arch Phys Med Rehabil 1994; 75(3):243–247.

69. Kirke PN, et al. Impact of the MTHFR C677T polymorphism on risk of neural tube defects: case-control study. Br Med J 2004; 328(7455):1535–1536.

70. Klingbeil H, Baer HR, Wilson PE. Aging with a disability. Arch Phys Med Rehabil 2004; 85(7 suppl 3):S68–S73, quiz S74–S75.

71. Kriss VM, Desai NS. Occult spinal dysraphism in neonates: assessment of high-risk cutaneous stigmata on sonography. AJR Am J Roentgenol 1998; 171(6):1687–1692.

72. Lary JM, Edmonds LD. Prevalence of spina bifida at birth—United States, 1983–1990: a comparison of two surveillance systems. MMWR CDC Surveill Summ 1996; 45(2):15–26.

73. Laurence KM, et al. Double-blind randomised controlled trial of folate treatment before conception to prevent recurrence of neural-tube defects. Br Med J (Clin Res Ed) 1981; 282(6275):1509–1511.

74. Lemire RJ. Neural tube defects. JAMA 1988; 259(4):558–562.

75. Leveratto L, et al. Insulin like growth factor I (IGF1) in children with neural tube closure defects: a preliminary report. Eur J Pediatr Surg 1993; 3(suppl 1):19–20.

76. Lie HR, et al. Bowel and bladder control of children with myelomeningocele: a Nordic study. Dev Med Child Neurol 1991; 33(12):1053–1061.

77. Littlewood RA, et al. Resting energy expenditure and body composition in children with myelomeningocele. Pediatr Rehabil 2003; 6(1):31–37.

78. Lock TR, Aronson DD. Fractures in patients who have myelomeningocele. J Bone Joint Surg Am 1989; 71(8):1153–1157.

79. Lorber J, Pucholt V. When is a shunt no longer necessary? An investigation of 300 patients with hydrocephalus and myelomeningocele: 11–22 year follow up. Z Kinderchir 1981; 34(4):327–329.

80. Luthy DA, et al. Cesarean section before the onset of labor and subsequent motor function in infants with meningomyelocele diagnosed antenatally. N Engl J Med 1991; 324(10):662–666.

81. Machado HR, Santos de Oliveira R. Simultaneous repair of myelomeningocele and shunt insertion. Childs Nerv Syst 2004; 20(2):107–109.

82. Maliszewski M, Ladzinski P, Majchrzak H. [Tethered cord syndrome in adults]. Neurol Neurochir Pol 2000; 34(6):1269–1279.

83. Marlin AE. Management of hydrocephalus in the patient with myelomeningocele: an argument against third ventriculostomy. Neurosurg Focus 2004; 16(2):E4.

84. Marshall PD, et al. Surgical release of knee flexion contractures in myelomeningocele. J Bone Joint Surg Br 1996; 78(6):912–916.

85. Mazur JM, Stillwell A, Menelaus M. The significance of spasticity in the upper and lower limbs in myelomeningocele. J Bone Joint Surg Br 1986; 68(2):213–217.

86. McGuire EJ, et al. Prognostic value of urodynamic testing in myelodysplastic patients. J Urol 1981; 126(2):205–209.

87. McLone DG, American Society of Pediatric Neurosurgeons, American Association of Neurological Surgeons, Section of Pediatric Neurosurgery. Pediatric neurosurgery: surgery of the developing nervous system. 4th edn. Philadelphia: Saunders; 2001:xxiii, 1344.

88. McLone DG, Knepper PA. The cause of Chiari II malformation: a unified theory. Pediatr Neurosci 1989; 15(1):1–12.

89. McMichael AJ, et al. Neural tube defects and maternal serum zinc and copper concentrations in mid-pregnancy: a case-control study. Med J Aust 1994; 161(8):478–482.

90. McNeely PD, Howes WJ. Ineffectiveness of dietary folic acid supplementation on the incidence of lipomyelomeningocele: pathogenetic implications. J Neurosurg Spine 2004; 100(2):98–100.

91. Medical Research Council Vitamin Study Research Group. Prevention of neural tube defects: results of the Medical Research Council Vitamin Study. Lancet 1991; 338(8760):131–137.

92. Meyer S, Landau H. Precocious puberty in myelomeningocele patients. J Pediatr Orthop 1984; 4(1):28–31.

93. Miller PD, et al. Comparison of simultaneous versus delayed ventriculoperitoneal shunt insertion in children undergoing myelomeningocele repair. J Child Neurol 1996; 11(5):370–372.

94. Molnar GE, Alexander MA, eds. Pediatric rehabilitation. 3rd edn. Philadelphia: Hanley & Belfus; 1999:viii, 434.

95. Morgan DJ, Blackburn M, Bax M. Adults with spina bifida and/or hydrocephalus. Postgrad Med J 1995; 71(831):17–21.

96. Muller EB, Nordwall A. Prevalence of scoliosis in children with myelomeningocele in western Sweden. Spine 1992; 17(9):1097–1102.

97. Muller T, Arbeiter K, Aufricht C. Renal function in meningomyelocele: risk factors, chronic renal failure, renal replacement therapy and transplantation. Curr Opin Urol 2002; 12(6):479–484.

98. Myrianthopoulos NC, Melnick M. Studies in neural tube defects. I. Epidemiologic and etiologic aspects. Am J Med Genet 1987; 26(4):783–796.

99. Naggan L, MacMahon B. Ethnic differences in the prevalence of anencephaly and spina bifida in Boston, Massachusetts. N Engl J Med 1967; 277(21):1119–1123.

100. Naggan L. The recent decline in prevalence of anencephaly and spina bifida. Am J Epidemiol 1969; 89(2):154–160.

101. Nevin NC, Johnston WP, Merrett JD. Influence of social class on the risk of recurrence of anencephalus and spina bifida. Dev Med Child Neurol 1981; 23(2):155–159.

102. Niall DM, et al. Kyphectomy in children with myelomeningocele: a long-term outcome study. J Pediatr Orthop 2004; 24(1):37–44.

103. Noonan KJ, Didelot WP, Lindseth RE. Care of the pediatric foot in myelodysplasia. Foot Ankle Clin 2000; 5(2):vi, 281–304.

104. Okamoto GA, et al. Toileting skills in children with myelomeningocele: rates of learning. Arch Phys Med Rehabil 1984; 65(4):182–185.

105. Okamoto GA, Lamers JV, Shurtleff DB. Skin breakdown in patients with myelomeningocele. Arch Phys Med Rehabil 1983; 64(1):20–23.

106. Omtzigt JG, et al. The risk of spina bifida aperta after first-trimester exposure to valproate in a prenatal cohort. Neurology 1992; 42(4 suppl 5):119–125.

107. Palmer JS, Kaplan WE, Firlit CF. Erectile dysfunction in patients with spina bifida is a treatable condition. J Urol 2000; 164(3 part 2):958–961.

108. Papp C, et al. Risk of recurrence of craniospinal anomalies. J Matern Fetal Med 1997; 6(1):53–57.

109. Phuong LK, Schoeberl KA, Raffel C. Natural history of tethered cord in patients with meningomyelocele. Neurosurgery 2002; 50(5):989–993, discussion 993–995.

110. Quan A, et al. Bone mineral density in children with myelomeningocele. Pediatrics 1998; 102(3):E34.

111. Ralph K, et al. The effects of multiple shunt revisions on neuropsychological functioning and memory. Neurol Res 2000; 22(1):131–136.

112. Rietberg CC, Lindhout D. Adult patients with spina bifida cystica: genetic counselling, pregnancy and delivery. Eur J Obstet Gynecol Reprod Biol 1993; 52(1):63–70.

113. Rinck C, Berg J, Hafeman C. The adolescent with myelomeningocele: a review of parent experiences and expectations. Adolescence 1989; 24(95):699–710.

114. Rintoul NE, et al. A new look at myelomeningoceles: functional level, vertebral level, shunting, and the implications for fetal intervention. Pediatrics 2002; 109(3):409–413.

115. Roberts HE, et al. Impact of prenatal diagnosis on the birth prevalence of neural tube defects, Atlanta, 1990–1991. Pediatrics 1995; 96(5 part 1):880–883.

116. Rosa FW. Spina bifida in infants of women treated with carbamazepine during pregnancy. N Engl J Med 1991; 324(10):674–677.

117. Rotenstein D, Bass AN. Treatment to near adult stature of patients with myelomeningocele with recombinant human growth hormone. J Pediatr Endocrinol Metab 2004; 17(9):1195–1200.

118. Rotenstein D, Reigel DH, Flom LL. Growth hormone treatment accelerates growth of short children with neural tube defects. J Pediatr 1989; 115(3):417–420.

119. Rotenstein D, Reigel DH. Growth hormone treatment of children with neural tube defects: results from 6 months to 6 years. J Pediatr 1996; 128(2):184–189.

120. Salomao JF, et al. [Symptomatic Chiari type II malformation]. Arq Neuropsiquiatr 1998; 56(1):98–106.

121. Samuelsson L, Skoog M. Ambulation in patients with myelomeningocele: a multivariate statistical analysis. J Pediatr Orthop 1988; 8(5):569–575.

122. Sandford MK, Kissling GE, Joubert PE. Neural tube defect etiology: new evidence concerning maternal hyperthermia, health and diet. Dev Med Child Neurol 1992; 34(8):661–675.

123. Sandhu PS, Broughton NS, Menelaus MB. Tenotomy of the ligamentum patellae in spina bifida: management of limited flexion range at the knee. J Bone Joint Surg Br 1995; 77(5):832–833.

124. Satin-Smith MS, et al. Arm span as measurement of response to growth hormone (GH) treatment in a group of children with meningomyelocele and GH deficiency. J Clin Endocrinol Metab 1996; 81(4):1654–1656.

125. Selzman AA, Elder JS, Mapstone TB. Urologic consequences of myelodysplasia and other congenital abnormalities of the spinal cord. Urol Clin North Am 1993; 20(3):485–504.

126. Shurtleff DB, ed. Myelodysplasias and exstrophies: significance, prevention, and treatment. Orlando: Grune & Stratton; 1986:xvi, 591.

127. Shurtleff DB, Lemire RJ. Epidemiology, etiologic factors, and prenatal diagnosis of open spinal dysraphism. Neurosurg Clin North Am 1995; 6(2):183–193.

128. Singhal B, Mathew KM. Factors affecting mortality and morbidity in adult spina bifida. Eur J Pediatr Surg 1999; 9(suppl 1):31–32.

129. Slater JE. Rubber anaphylaxis. N Engl J Med 1989; 320(17):1126–1130.

130. Smith ED. Urinary prognosis in spina bifida. J Urol 1972; 108(5):815–817.

131. Smith GK. The history of spina bifida, hydrocephalus, paraplegia, and incontinence. Pediatr Surg Int 2001; 17(5–6):424–432.

132. Snodgrass WT, Adams R. Initial urologic management of myelomeningocele. Urol Clin North Am 2004; 31(3):viii, 427–434.

133. Sousa JC, Gordon LH, Shurtleff DB. Assessing the development of daily living skills in patients with spina bifida. Dev Med Child Neurol Suppl 1976; 37:134–142.

134. Spindel MR, et al. The changing neurourologic lesion in myelodysplasia. JAMA 1987; 258(12):1630–1633.

135. Stark G. Spina bifida: problems and management. Oxford: Blackwell Scientific Publications; 1977.

136. Steinbok P, et al. Long-term outcome and complications of children born with meningomyelocele. Childs Nerv Syst 1992; 8(2):92–96.

137. Stevenson KL. Chiari type II malformation: past, present, and future. Neurosurg Focus 2004; 16(2):E5.

138. Sussman GL, Tarlo S, Dolovich J. The spectrum of IgE-mediated responses to latex. JAMA 1991; 265(21):2844–2847.

139. Sutton LN, et al. Improvement in hindbrain herniation demonstrated by serial fetal magnetic resonance imaging following fetal surgery for myelomeningocele. JAMA 1999; 282(19):1826–1831.

140. Taylor JS, Erkek E. Latex allergy: diagnosis and management. Dermatol Ther 2004; 17(4):289–301.

141. Tortori-Donati P, Rossi A, Cama A. Spinal dysraphism: a review of neuroradiological features with embryological correlations and proposal for a new classification. Neuroradiology 2000; 42(7):471–491.

142. Trivedi J, et al. Clinical and radiographic predictors of scoliosis in patients with myelomeningocele. J Bone Joint Surg Am 2002; 84-A(8):1389–1394.

143. Trollmann R, et al. Arm span, serum IGF-1 and IGFBP-3 levels as screening parameters for the diagnosis of growth hormone deficiency in patients with myelomeningocele—preliminary data. Eur J Pediatr 1998; 157(6):451–455.

144. Trollmann R, et al. Does growth hormone (GH) enhance growth in GH-deficient children with myelomeningocele? J Clin Endocrinol Metab 2000; 85(8):2740–2743.

145. Trollmann R, et al. Growth and pubertal development in patients with meningomyelocele: a retrospective analysis. Acta Paediatr 1996; 85(1): 76–80.

146. Trollmann R, Strehl E, Dorr HG. Precocious puberty in children with myelomeningocele: treatment with gonadotropin-releasing hormone analogues. Dev Med Child Neurol 1998; 40(1):38–43.

147. Tuli S, Drake J, Lamberti-Pasculli M. Long-term outcome of hydrocephalus management in myelomeningoceles. Childs Nerv Syst 2003; 19(5–6):286–291.

148. Tulipan N, et al. The effect of intrauterine myelomeningocele repair on the incidence of shunt-dependent hydrocephalus. Pediatr Neurosurg 2003; 38(1):27–33.

149. Uehling DT, et al. Impact of an intermittent catheterization program on children with myelomeningocele. Pediatrics 1985; 76(6):892–895.

150. Vachha B, Adams R. Myelomeningocele, temperament patterns, and parental perceptions. Pediatrics 2005; 115(1):e58–e63.

151. Van Allen MI, et al. Evidence for multi-site closure of the neural tube in humans. Am J Med Genet 1993; 47(5):723–743.

152. Watkins ML, et al. Maternal obesity and risk for birth defects. Pediatrics 2003; 111(5 part 2):1152–1158.

153. Williams EN, Broughton NS, Menelaus MB. Age-related walking in children with spina bifida. Dev Med Child Neurol 1999; 41(7):446–449.

154. Wills KE, et al. Intelligence and achievement in children with myelomeningocele. J Pediatr Psychol 1990; 15(2):161–176.

155. Wolraich ML, et al. Results of clean intermittent catheterization for children with neurogenic bladders. Urology 1983; 22(5):479–482.

156. Woodhouse CR. Prospects for fertility in patients born with genitourinary anomalies. J Urol 2001; 165(6 part 2):2354–23560.

157. Woodhouse CR. Sexual function in boys born with exstrophy, myelomeningocele, and micropenis. Urology 1998; 52(1):3–11.

158. Worley G. A new look at meningomyeloceles. Pediatrics 2003; 111(6 part 1):1494–1495, author reply 1494–1495.

159. Wright JG, et al. Natural history of knee contractures in myelomeningocele. J Pediatr Orthop 1991; 11(6):725–730.

160. Wu HY, Baskin LS, Kogan BA. Neurogenic bladder dysfunction due to myelomeningocele: neonatal versus childhood treatment. J Urol 1997; 157(6):2295–2297.

161. Yamada S, Won DJ, Yamada SM. Pathophysiology of tethered cord syndrome: correlation with symptomatology. Neurosurg Focus 2004; 16(2): E6.

162. Zhu H, et al. Promoter haplotype combinations for the human PDGFRA gene are associated with risk of neural tube defects. Mol Genet Metab 2004; 81(2):127–132.

Spinal Cord Injury

Thomas N. Bryce, Kristjan T. Ragnarsson and Adam B. Stein

HISTORICAL PERSPECTIVE

For thousands of years, injury to the spinal cord was synonymous with death, either instantly or after a period of great suffering. Physicians were well aware of the various consequences of spinal cord injury (SCI), yet were unable to successfully manage any of these to have a measurable impact on the injured person's life. Only during the past half a century has SCI been considered a manageable condition, which can be compatible with reasonably good health and a life expectancy approaching that of normal.

The Edwin Smith Surgical Papyrus, written by an Egyptian physician almost 5000 years ago, vividly describes the symptoms of neurologically complete injury to the cervical spinal cord, i.e. paralysis and sensory loss in the arms and legs, urinary incontinence, and priapism.[74,239] The somber advice of this physician was that this is 'an ailment not to be treated'. Later, in ancient Greece, approximately 400 BC, Hippocrates described paraplegia caused by injury or disease as being associated with paralysis, bladder and bowel dysfunction, and pressure ulcers.[2] Several ancient Roman physicians also briefly described SCI, which they invariably considered to be fatal if neurologically complete, but if incomplete, reduction of spinal deformities by traction was recommended, a practice that was continued through the Middle Ages.[162]

During the nineteenth century, treatment of SCI continued to be conservative and without much hope for survival. A famous anecdote reflects well the prevailing attitude in those days. In 1805, Lord Nelson, the Admiral of the British Fleet, suffered a gunshot wound to his thoracic spine during the battle of Trafalgar, causing paraplegia. Nelson spoke with his ship's surgeon, Mr. Beatty, and described his loss of power of motion and feeling below the chest, and then expressed his view that he would have but a short time to live. The surgeon's reply was 'My lord, unhappily for our Country, nothing can be done for you'.[224] Within a few hours, Lord Nelson was dead. In 1881, the 20th President of the United States, James A. Garfield, was shot in the spine, causing a neurologically incomplete conus–cauda equina lesion, but even with such a lesion he was dead within 3 months.[161] Despite remarkable progress in medicine and surgery during the nineteenth century, for example Pasteur's discoveries in bacteriology, Lister's aseptic surgical techniques, the introduction of anesthesia, and Roentgen's discovery of x-rays, surgical interventions for spine trauma and SCI were generally discouraged.

During the early part of the twentieth century, there was little progress made in the management of SCI, and most persons with SCI died within weeks or months. Harvey Cushing observed that, during World War I, 80% of all US soldiers with SCI died within 2 weeks.[224] Early mortality was slightly lower in the British military, but the 3-year mortality was estimated to be 80%.[224] During the 1930s and 1940s, management of SCI finally started to change. During the late 1930s, Dr. Donald Munro at Boston City Hospital developed a dedicated unit for comprehensive care of persons with SCI and, by 1943, he was able to demonstrate significant drops in both morbidity and mortality, primarily by focusing on better bladder management.[329–331] A few years later, in Great Britain during World War II, it was decided to congregate all casualties with SCI in special units that were supervised by an experienced physician. These units were to be sufficiently staffed by nurses and therapists, housed in facilities with rehabilitation workshops, and organized to provide resettlement and aftercare services.[224] Dr. Ludwig Guttmann was placed in charge of such a unit at Stoke Mandeville, where he introduced comprehensive care and interdisciplinary rehabilitation for persons with SCI, a program that was widely modeled around the world. Within the US Veterans Affairs Hospitals, Drs. Comarr and Bors introduced new methods of urologic management and rehabilitation, which quickly improved survival rates among US veterans.

MODEL SYSTEMS OF CARE

The difference in outcomes for persons with SCI, when admitted to a dedicated SCI rehabilitation unit as opposed to a more generalized service, proved to be convincing to the leaders of healthcare during the 1960s. At the same time, special trauma systems were being developed in the US for emergently injured people. The trauma systems required that injured persons be handled at the scene of accident by well-trained emergency medical technicians using state of the art equipment and transportation vehicles. The patients were subsequently to be triaged to a specially designated trauma center, which met strict criteria for emergency and acute trauma care, rather than taking them to the nearest hospital. The success of disease-specific units and trauma systems highlighted the fact that inadequate training, experience, and number of staff, as well as lack of appropriate facilities and equipment, not only placed the spinal cord-injured person's life at risk, but often resulted in development of complications, poor functional outcomes, and excessive length of stay. These observations were felt to have important implications for people with SCI. It was therefore hypothesized that, if optimal care was provided from the very onset of major disabling injury and for as long as primary and secondary medical problems and disability last, functional outcomes would be improved and the cost of care would be reduced.

Based on this hypothesis, the US Government funded several SCI Model Systems of Care, first in Phoenix, Arizona, in 1970, and subsequently in several other major cities around the USA. By 1982, there were 17 such systems funded by the National Institute on Disability and Rehabilitation Research (NIDRR), US Department of Education. Each funded system had to meet four basic requirements. First, it had to have several integrated clinical components: emergency medical services; level 1 trauma center; comprehensive rehabilitation services for both inpatients and outpatients, including vocational and job placement services; and lifelong follow-up and health maintenance programs. Second, each funded system had to collect data on all patients served, and forward these to a National SCI Model System Database. Third, each system was required to conduct research consistent with NIDRR-announced priorities. Fourth, each system had to disseminate the research and demonstration findings as widely as possible to the appropriate audiences.

The SCI Model Systems have been instrumental in developing standards of care and new treatments, conducting epidemiologic, health services, and outcomes research as well as producing thousands of publications and training materials.[138] The National SCI Database has been in existence since 1973, and captures data from an estimated 13% of new SCI cases in the US. The SCI Model Systems have been directly and indirectly instrumental in a number of positive developments for persons with SCI. These include increased survival rates, reduced hospital lengths of stay, and a reduced number of rehospitalizations. In addition, it led to the majority of persons with SCI being discharged home, and created a national database of approximately 30 000 persons with SCI.[431,432,439]

SUBSPECIALTY OF SCI MEDICINE

The majority of physicians providing non-surgical care for people with SCI in the USA have been physiatrists. In the past, most such physicians developed their special knowledge over a lengthy period of time by providing care rather than by specific training. A creation of a subspecialty of SCI medicine was first advocated in the late 1970s and gained momentum in the early 1990s. Through the concerted efforts of many individuals and organizations, the American Board of Medical Specialties gave its approval in 1995 that such subspecialty be established.[123,124] Based on the work experience and training of candidates that is acceptable to the American Board of Physical Medicine and

Rehabilitation, candidates can take a written examination. Those who pass receive a special SCI medicine subspecialty certificate. Several 1-year SCI fellowships have been established, each providing a structured training program approved by the Accreditation Council for Graduate Medical Education. Several hundred individuals have been certified in the subspecialty since the first examination was held in 1999.

EPIDEMIOLOGY

Numerous epidemiologic studies have been reported since the 1970s in various countries, and these reflect some variance in the incidence and prevalence of SCI. Data have been collected in the USA by the SCI Model Systems for its database since the early 1970s. The analysis of these data by the National Spinal Cord Injury Statistical Center (NSCISC) has provided extensive and reliable information. The epidemiologic data have been widely published, and current information can be easily accessed on the NSCISC web site (http://www.spinalcord.uab.edu), which is updated annually.[138,139]

Incidence and prevalence

The annual incidence of traumatic SCI requiring hospitalization in the USA is approximately 40 new cases per million population (or approximately 11 000 per year). These numbers are the most up to date available, but are based on data collected before 1980. These numbers do not include an unknown number of individuals with SCI who died before reaching a hospital.[68,345] The incidence of traumatic SCI in other developed countries has been shown to be somewhat lower than that in the USA, often less than 20 new cases per million per year, perhaps due in part to the higher US incidence of violence-related SCI.[138,139]

The exact number of persons with SCI currently alive in the USA (prevalence) is unknown. Two methods have been used to estimate the prevalence of SCI: mathematic calculation based on annual incidence and average duration, and counting the exact number of people with SCI within a geographic area and extrapolating this number to the population of the entire USA. Using the mathematic approach, the prevalence of SCI in the USA in 2004 has been projected to be 246 882 persons. A study using the mathematic approach estimated the number to be 176 965 individuals in 1988.[52,275] Given the improving life expectancy of persons with SCI, the current US prevalence can be estimated to be approximately 250 000 persons.

Age at time of injury, gender, ethnicity, and marital status

Almost all studies show that the incidence of SCI is lowest for persons under the age of 15 and highest for persons 16–30 years of age. After the age of 30, there is a consistent decline in incidence. Current mean age at onset is reported to be 35.9 years.[19] A rising percentage of older persons with new SCI has recently been observed. For example, those older than 60 years constituted 4.5% of all new SCI patients in the mid 1970s, versus

Table 56-1 Distribution by ethnicity since 2000

Ethnicity	Percentage
White	67.5
African-American	19.0
Hispanic	10.4
Other	3.1

(After Anonymous,[17] with permission of the National Spinal Cord Injury Statistical Center.)

Table 56-2 Distribution by cause since 2000

Cause	Percentage
Vehicular crashes	50.4
Falls	23.8
Violence	11.2
Sports or recreation	9.0
Other	5.6

(After Anonymous,[17] with permission of the National Spinal Cord Injury Statistical Center.)

Table 56-3 Neurologic impairment category at discharge from hospital

Category		n	Percentage
Paraplegia	Incomplete	4267	18.6
	Complete	6007	26.3
	Minimal	258	1.1
	Total	10 532	46.0
Tetraplegia	Incomplete	6808	29.4
	Complete	4769	20.7
	Minimal	339	1.5
	Total	11 916	51.7
Normal		155	0.7
Unknown		389	1.6
Total		22 992	100.0

(After Anonymous,[17] with permission of the National Spinal Cord Injury Statistical Center.)

11.5% in the mid 1990s.[345] A simultaneous rise in the median age of persons with SCI also occurred from the mid 1970s to the 1990s, with a rise from 28.5 years to 35.9 years. This change could reflect the improved medical care for persons with SCI, as well as the rise in the median age of the US general population from 28 years to 35 years during the same period.[139]

More than 80% of all SCI occurs in males, a figure that has remained essentially constant for more than 30 years in the USA.[138,139,345] This gender difference is similar in other countries. Approximately two-thirds of all persons enrolled in the National SCI Database are white, which is significantly less than the percentage of whites among the general US population (see Table 56-1).[345]

At the time of SCI, 30.4% of individuals had intact marriages; 53% had never been married; and the remaining 26.6% were separated, divorced, or widowed.[139] The unmarried rate is a relatively high figure, perhaps best explained by the fact that SCI disproportionately affects young people.[19,139] For those married at the time of SCI, the divorce rate is increased after SCI, as compared with in the general population, especially during the first 3 postinjury years. The annual marriage rate is also lower for single individuals with SCI than for non-disabled persons.[139]

Causes of SCI

One-half of all SCIs in the USA are caused by vehicular crashes (see Table 56-2).[19] The most common vehicular crashes involve automobiles, followed by motorcycle and bicycles. Diving is the most common cause in sporting and recreational activities. The causes of SCI can vary significantly between groups of different gender, ethnicity, age, and geographic locale (rural versus urban settings). Violence accounts for 46% of SCIs among African-Americans. Falls are the most common cause of SCI among older people. SCI in women is rarely caused by gunshot wounds, motorcycle crashes, or diving.[345] Considering the various causes of traumatic SCI, it is not surprising that more injuries occur on weekends than on other days of the week, and during the summertime.

Neurologic level and extent of neurologic deficit

According to the National SCI Database, 51.7% of those with SCI have tetraplegia, 45.9% have paraplegia, and the remaining 2.4% have a neurologic level that could not be confirmed.[19] Of those having paraplegia, 35% have thoracic lesions and 11% have lumbosacral lesions.[139] The Database currently shows that neurologically incomplete SCI is slightly more common than complete SCI (see Table 56-3). This represents a change, because 40 years ago approximately two-thirds of all SCI lesions were complete.[442]

Length of stay, rehospitalization, and discharge destination

The average length of stay for patients with SCI has declined dramatically over the years, according to the National SCI Database. This is true for both acute and rehabilitation hospitalizations, from 25 acute days in 1974 to 17 days in 2001, and from 115 rehabilitation days to 44 days.[19] There has been a steady decrease in the number of rehospitalizations during the first year as well.[177] Among persons listed in the National SCI Database and discharged alive, 88.3% went to a private non-institutional residence, 5% went to group living situations, 5.1% went to nursing homes, and the remaining 1.6% went to acute hospitals. Approximately 3% died during the initial hospitalization.[139]

Life expectancy and causes of death

Life expectancy for persons with SCI has increased steadily for many decades but still remains below that of able-bodied individuals. The mortality rate is highest during the first postinjury year, at 6.3%, but declines significantly thereafter.[137,139] The first-year mortality rate declined by 67% from the 1970s to the 1990s.[135,139] Significant predictors of mortality include being older, male, injured by acts of violence, neurologically complete, and ventilator-dependent, and having a high neurologic level.[135] Additional factors that affect longevity after the first postinjury year include low life satisfaction, poor health, emotional distress, functional dependency, and poor adjustment to disability.[262] The NSCISC web site provides annual updates on life expectancy after the onset of SCI, based on neurologic level and ventilatory dependency (see Table 56-4). These life expectancy estimates do not include many important variables that can also significantly affect survival, such as gender, ethnicity, preexisting medical conditions, access to medical and nursing care, and social support.

Diseases of the respiratory system, especially pneumonia, are the leading cause of death both during the first postinjury year and during subsequent years (see Table 56-5). The second most common cause of death, 'other heart disease', is felt to reflect deaths that are apparently due to heart attacks in younger persons without apparent underlying heart or vascular disease and cardiac dysrhythmia.[139] It is of interest that diseases of the genitourinary system are currently the cause of death in only 3.7% of SCI patients. In the past, renal failure was by far the leading cause of death after SCI. This is truly a great testament to the advances in urologic management during the past several decades.

ANATOMY, MECHANICS, AND SYNDROMES OF TRAUMATIC INJURY

Because the bony vertebral column elongates more than the spinal cord during embryologic development, the spinal cord terminates at the level of the L1–L2 intervertebral disk. Due to natural variation, the spinal cord termination can be as high as the T12 or as low as the L3 vertebral body. The individual spinal cord segments do not line up with the corresponding bony levels of the same number (see Fig. 56-1). This is especially evident in the lower thoracic and lumbar spine, where the L1–L5 spinal segments are adjacent to the T11–T12 vertebrae, and the S1–S5 spinal segments are adjacent to the L1 vertebra.

Table 56-4 Life expectancy (years) for persons with spinal cord injury surviving at least 1 year post injury

Current age (years)	No spinal cord injury	Motor functional, any level	Not ventilator-dependent			Ventilator-dependent, any level
			Paraplegia	Tetraplegia C5–C8	Tetraplegia C1–C4	
10	67.9	63.3	55.9	51.3	47.6	31.6
15	62.9	58.4	51.0	46.4	42.8	27.2
20	58.1	53.6	46.4	42.0	38.5	23.8
25	53.4	49.0	42.0	37.7	34.4	20.8
30	48.6	44.3	37.5	33.4	30.2	17.6
35	43.9	39.6	33.0	29.1	26.1	14.4
40	39.2	35.1	28.7	25.0	22.1	11.4
45	34.7	30.6	24.5	21.0	18.4	8.9
50	30.3	26.4	20.6	17.4	15.0	6.7
55	26.0	22.2	16.9	14.0	11.8	4.8
60	21.9	18.4	13.5	10.9	9.0	3.1
65	18.1	14.8	10.5	8.2	6.6	2.0
70	14.6	11.7	7.9	6.0	4.7	1.1
75	11.5	8.8	5.6	4.1	3.1	0.4
80	8.8	6.4	3.8	2.6	1.9	<0.1

(After Anonymous,[17] with permission of the National Spinal Cord Injury Statistical Center.)

Table 56-5 Primary causes of death in persons with spinal cord injury since 2000

Primary cause of death	Percentage
Diseases of the respiratory system	21.7
Other heart disease	12.6
Infective and parasitic diseases	9.4
Hypertensive and ischemic heart disease	8.0
Neoplasms	6.9
Unintentional injuries	5.2
Diseases of pulmonary circulation	5.2
Diseases of the digestive system	4.9
Symptoms and ill-defined conditions	4.7
Suicide	3.9
Diseases of the genitourinary system	3.7
Cerebrovascular disease	3.6
Subsequent trauma of uncertain nature (unintentional suicide or homicide)	3.4
Other	7.0

(After Anonymous,[17] with permission of the National Spinal Cord Injury Statistical Center.)

This concept can also be used when evaluating radiologic studies to correlate the neurologic level of injury (NLI) to the appropriate bony level of damage (i.e. a T11 burst fracture with cord compression would be expected to cause an NLI at L1 or L2 rather than at T11).

The tapered end of the spinal cord, which contains the sacral cord segments, is called the conus medullaris. The collection of long lumbar and sacral roots found in the canal, distal to the conus medullaris, is called the cauda equina, as it resembles a horse's tail. The meninges of the spinal cord include the pia matter, a vascular membrane covering the spinal cord, the arachnoid membrane, and the dura mater. The subarachnoid space, also called the intrathecal space, contains cerebrospinal fluid (CSF). The CSF pushes the arachnoid directly against the dura mater. The caudal margin of the dura mater and arachnoid, the inferior extent of the intrathecal space, is the second sacral vertebrae (see Fig. 56-2). The spinal epidural space is located between the dura mater and the periosteum of the vertebral bodies, and contains an internal vertebral venous plexus, fat, and loose areolar tissue.

A cross-sectional view of the spinal cord (see Fig. 56-3) reveals a central butterfly-shaped region of gray matter consisting of neuronal cell bodies, their processes, supporting glial cells, and small blood vessels surrounded by white matter consisting of neuronal fiber tracts and supporting glial cells. The gray matter is subdivided into two horns on each side called the anterior (ventral) and posterior (dorsal) horns. The posterior

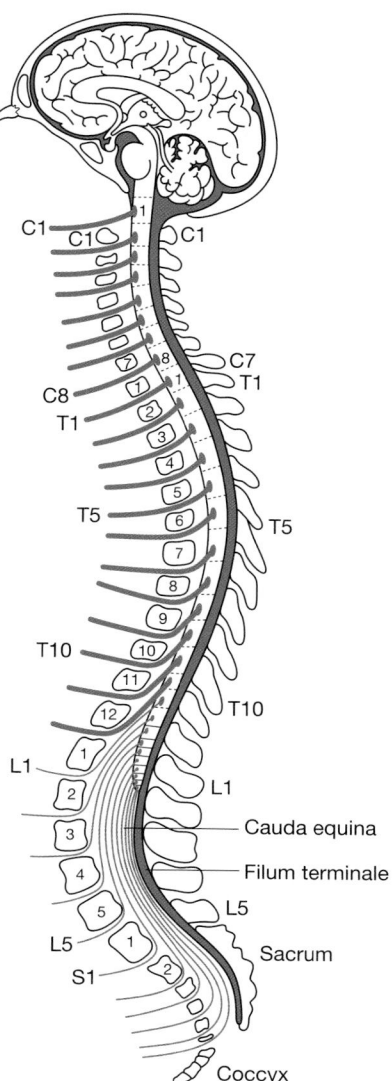

Figure 56-1 A sagittal schematic showing the relationship between the numbered segments of the spinal cord and the corresponding numbered vertebral bodies. (From Pansky et al. 1988,[351] with permission of McGraw-Hill.)

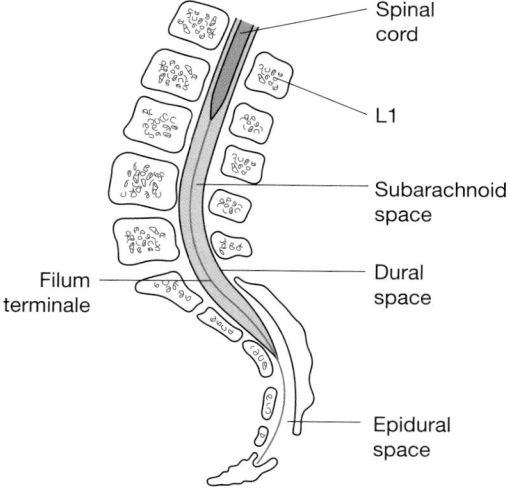

Figure 56-2 A sagittal schematic showing the relationship between the dura, subarachnoid space, and the epidural space. (From Pansky 1984,[352] with permission of Macmillan.)

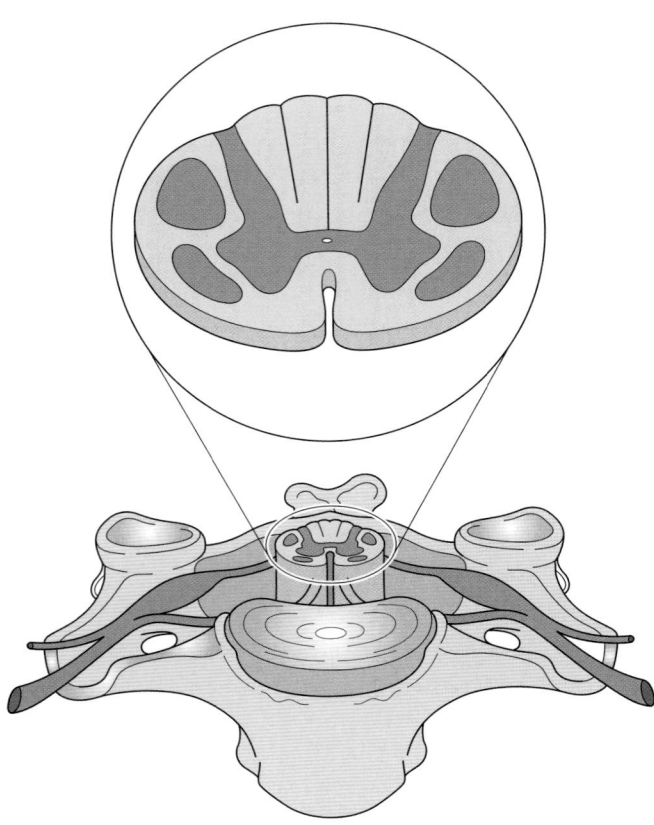

Figure 56-3 Normal spinal cord. The corticospinal and spinothalamic tracts are outlined in the upper diagram, adjacent to the gray matter of the spinal cord. (From Tator 1996,[441] with permission of McGraw-Hill.)

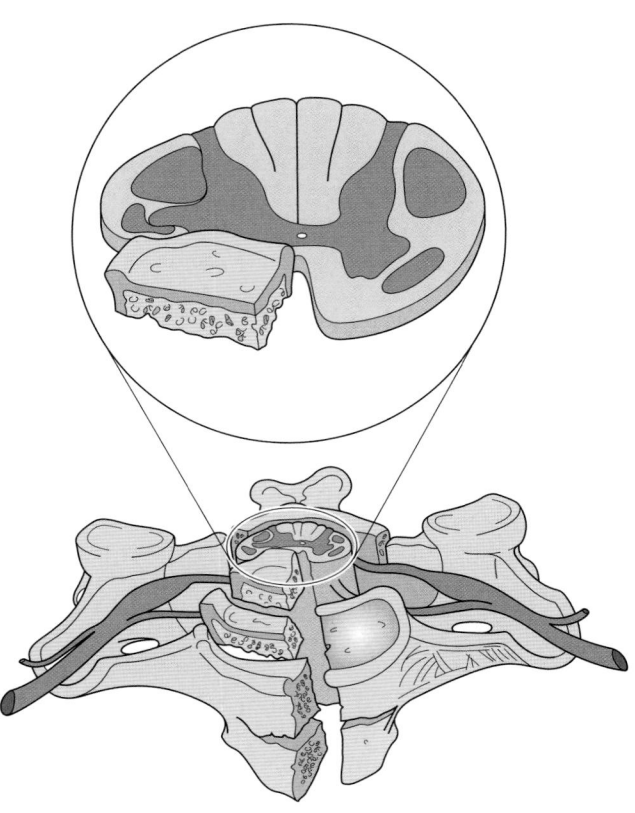

Figure 56-4 Brown–Sequard syndrome. A burst fracture with posterior displacement of bone fragments compresses one side of the spinal cord. (From Tator 1996,[441] with permission of McGraw-Hill.)

horn contains cell bodies of sensory neurons, whereas the anterior horn contains cell bodies of interneurons and motor neurons.

The white matter is subdivided into three columns on each side called the anterior, lateral, and posterior columns. The columns are further subdivided into tracts. The gracilis tract, located in the medial posterior column, contains fibers from the T7–S5 dermatomes that relay touch, vibration, and position sense. The cuneatus tract, located in the lateral posterior column rostral to T6, contains fibers from dermatomes above T7 that relay touch, vibration, and position sense. These tracts, comprising the posterior columns, ascend ipsilaterally to the medulla. The lateral spinothalamic tract, located peripherally in the lateral column, contains fibers that relay pain and temperature sensations; this tract ascends contralaterally to the thalamus. The lateral corticospinal tract is located centrally and posteriorly in the lateral column. This tract contains fibers, the majority of which emanate from the motor cortex, that are responsible for voluntary and reflex movement. Approximately 90% of the corticospinal fibers cross midline in the caudal medulla, forming the pyramidal decussations, and descend contralaterally in the lateral corticospinal tract to terminate on interneurons and alpha and gamma motor neurons in the spinal cord. The remaining corticospinal fibers, located in the medial anterior column, do not cross midline in the medulla but

descend ipsilaterally in the anterior corticospinal tract. These fibers ultimately cross midline segmentally near their terminations on interneurons and alpha and gamma motor neurons in the spinal cord. About 55% of the corticospinal fibers terminate in the cervical cord, 20% in the thoracic cord, and 25% in the lumbosacral cord.[461] A Brown–Sequard syndrome refers to an injury of the spinal cord in which one side is damaged more than the other (see Fig. 56-4), resulting in relatively greater ipsilateral weakness and position sense loss, but with contralateral pain and temperature sensation loss.

A corticospinal neuron is known as an upper motor neuron (UMN). The motor neuron to which it synapses in the spinal cord, which exits the spinal cord to innervate muscle, is known as a lower motor neuron (LMN). If damage to the UMNs and LMNs within the spinal cord is localized to a few segmental levels anywhere rostral to the conus medullaris (see below), a constellation of signs and symptoms develops, often called the UMN syndrome. This includes loss of voluntary movement, spasticity, hyperreflexia, clonus, and development of Babinski's sign.[274] If, in addition, there is damage to a significant number of LMNs below the level of injury, loss of voluntary movement occurs without the subsequent development of the other components of the UMN syndrome. Examples of this, defined as LMN injuries, include an SCI due to an extensive vascular insult to the spinal cord, an injury occurring at the conus medullaris, or an injury occurring at the cauda equina. The conus medullaris

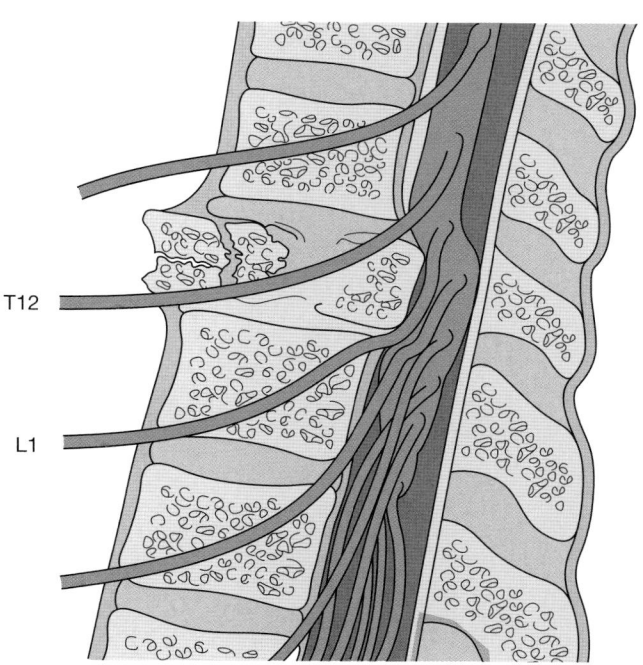

Figure 56-5 Conus medullaris syndrome. A burst fracture of T12 with posterior displacement of bone fragments compresses the conus medullaris. (From Tator 1996,[441] with permission of McGraw-Hill.)

T12

L1

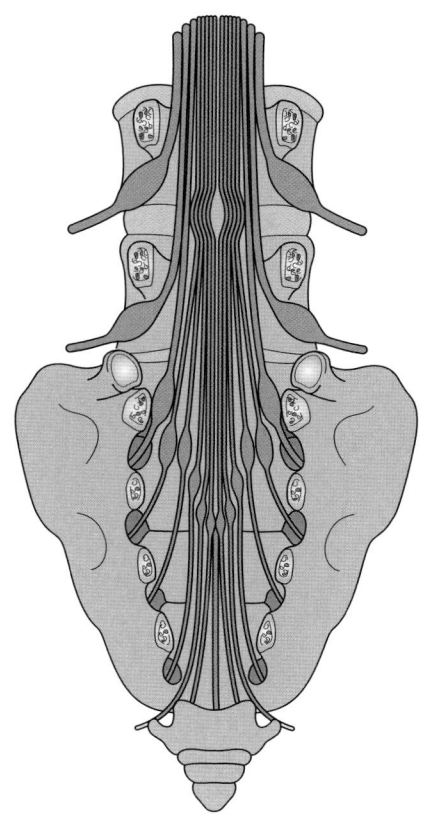

Figure 56-6 Cauda equina syndrome. A central disk herniation at L4–L5 compresses the cauda equina. Note how the roots of L5 and S1 are spared. (From Tator 1996,[441] with permission of McGraw-Hill.)

syndrome refers to an injury of the sacral spinal cord and the lumbar nerve roots within the spinal canal (see Fig. 56-5), resulting in an areflexic bladder, bowel, and lower limbs. Conus medullaris lesions localized to the proximal sacral cord can occasionally show a preserved sacral reflex, such as the bulbocavernosus reflex. The cauda equina syndrome refers to an injury to the lumbosacral roots within the spinal canal (see Fig. 56-6), resulting in an areflexic bladder, bowel, and lower limbs.[12]

After an acute UMN-predominant SCI, initial development of the UMN syndrome is delayed by a process called spinal shock, whereby there is a transient suppression and gradual return of reflex activity below the level of injury. Ditunno has proposed a four-phase model of spinal shock.[150] During phase 1, occurring 0–24 h post injury, there is motor neuron hyperpolarization, manifesting clinically as hyporeflexia. During phase 2, occurring on days 1–3 post injury, there is denervation supersensitivity and receptor up-regulation, manifesting clinically with reflex return. During phase 3, occurring 1–4 weeks post injury, there is interneuron synapse growth, manifesting clinically as early hyperreflexia. And finally, during phase 4, occurring 1–12 months post injury, there is long axon synapse growth, manifesting clinically as late hyperreflexia.

Blood is supplied to the spinal cord through two posterior spinal arteries, a single anterior spinal artery, and several segmental radicular arteries (see Fig. 56-7). The posterior spinal arteries branch from the vertebral arteries, and travel along the posterior surface of the spinal cord to supply the posterior one-third of the spinal cord. Two anterior spinal arteries also branch from the vertebral arteries, but these quickly unite to form a

single artery that travels along the anterior surface of the spinal cord to supply the anterior two-thirds of the spinal cord. The anterior spinal artery and the posterior spinal arteries are dependent on contributions from the segmental radicular arteries along the spinal cord to maintain an adequate blood supply to the spinal cord. The segmental radicular arteries travel through the intervertebral foramina from the aorta, and divide into anterior and posterior branches that eventually anastamose with their respective spinal arteries. These radicular arteries are not all identical in size or distribution. In the upper thoracic region between T1 and T4, there is little overlap between radicular arterial supplies. Between T12 and L2, there is an anterior radicular artery that is more dominant than its neighbors, called the artery of Adamkiewicz. This artery, usually found on the left side of the body, is an important blood supply to the caudal two-thirds of the spinal cord. On reaching the anterior surface of the spinal cord, the artery of Adamkiewicz divides into a small ascending and larger descending branch. The latter travels down to the level of the conus medullaris, where it forms an anastomatic circle with the terminal branches of the posterior spinal arteries. The regions between T1–T4 and T12–L2 are areas particularly prone to ischemic damage, due to the importance of individual radicular arteries. The ischemic damage, due to the nature of the single anterior and dual posterior blood supplies, often affects the anterior portion of the spinal cord more than the posterior portion. In this situation, the corticospinal and spinothalamic tracts are affected, while the gracilis tract is often spared. This leads to a syndrome of paraplegia,

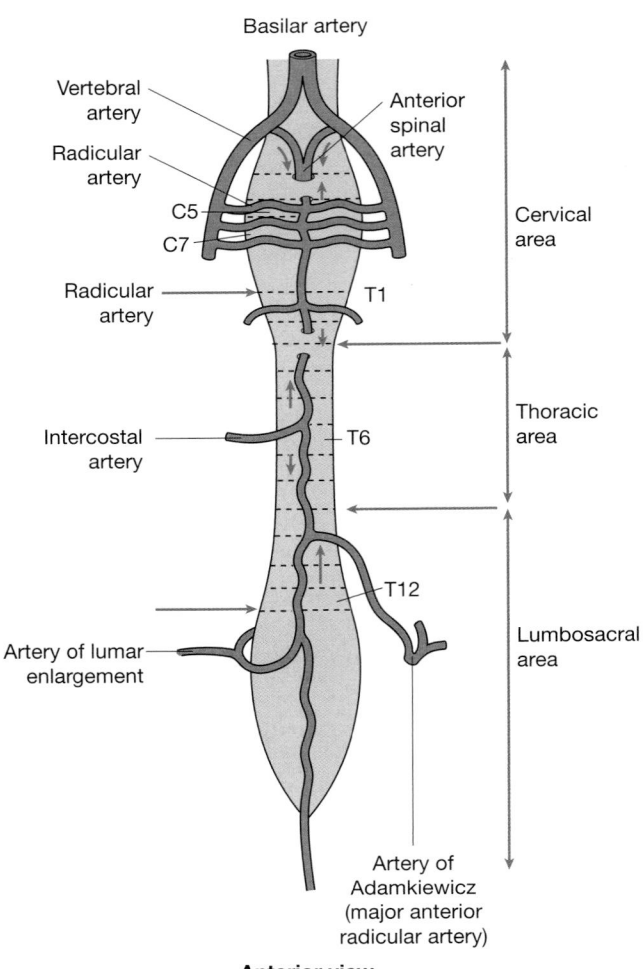

Anterior view

Figure 56-7 The spinal cord blood supply. (From Pansky et al. 1988,[351] with permission of McGraw-Hill.)

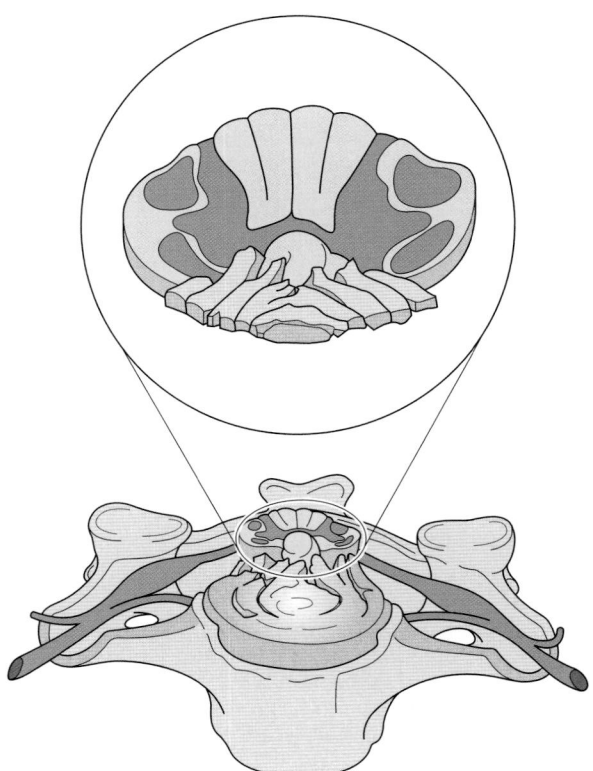

Figure 56-8 Anterior cord syndrome. A large disk herniation compresses the anterior aspect of the spinal cord, leaving the dorsal columns intact. (From Tator 1996,[441] with permission of McGraw-Hill.)

with loss of pain and temperature sensation, and relative sparing of touch and position sensation, called the anterior cord syndrome (see Fig. 56-8).

Pathophysiology of acute SCI

The *secondary injury cascade* is a term that refers to a series of biochemical processes that occur after an SCI, and that tend to cause further neuronal damage beyond the mechanical damage caused at the moment of impact. Ischemia of the gray matter at the site of injury occurs almost immediately after SCI. This ischemia appears to result from vasoconstriction of blood vessels supplying the cord, and is mediated by the rapid release of various vasoactive substances such as serotonin, thromboxanes, platelet-activating factor, peptidoleukotrienes, and opioid peptides after SCI.[349,399] Ischemia is followed by the development of edema at the site of injury.[344] At a cellular level, there is a marked rise in intraneuronal calcium concentrations. This begins within minutes after injury, reaching a peak at about 8 h post injury, and remaining elevated for at least 1 week.[325] Elevated levels of excitatory amino acids, such as glutamate and

aspartate, acting at their receptors have been noted to play a role in increasing the intracellular calcium concentrations.[96,287] Intracellular calcium facilitates the activation of phospholipases A_2 and C, which leads ultimately to the production of free radicals and free fatty acid metabolites, which cause damage to local cell membranes.[73,170,376] There is also a rapid rise in potassium in the extracellular space, directly related to cell membrane damage, which causes depolarization of other neuronal cells and conduction block.[477] Microhemorrhages appear in the central gray matter at the site of impact. Iron in this hemorrhaged blood catalyzes the perioxidation of lipids, leading to further tissue damage as well as catalyzing the further production of oxygen free radicals.[399]

Initially, neutrophils migrate to the site of injury, where they can contribute to cellular injury by producing lysosomal enzymes and oxygen radicals. These are followed by macrophages that phagocytose cell debris.[359] Schwann cells appear that modify myelin sheaths and produce neurotrophic factors, while fibroblasts produce basic fibroblast growth factor, and promote angiogenesis and neovascularization at the site of injury.[59,281] Small CSF-filled cysts eventually form that are partially surrounded by demyelinated nerve fibers. These coalesce over months, and can give rise to myelomalacia and syringomyelia.[292] Demyelination of white matter tracts begins within 24 h of injury and increases thereafter, with Wallerian degeneration occurring by 3 weeks.[460] Remyelination seems to occur after

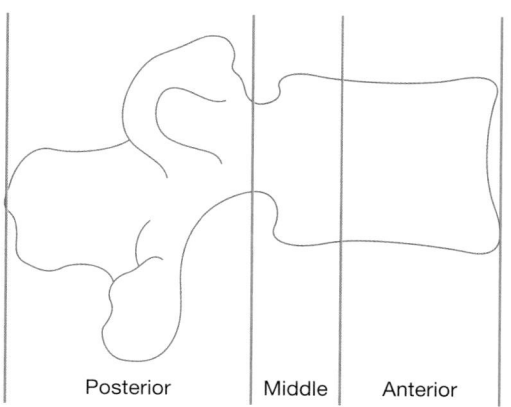

Figure 56-9 The three-column concept of spinal anatomy. (From Ferguson and Allen 1984,[174] with permission.)

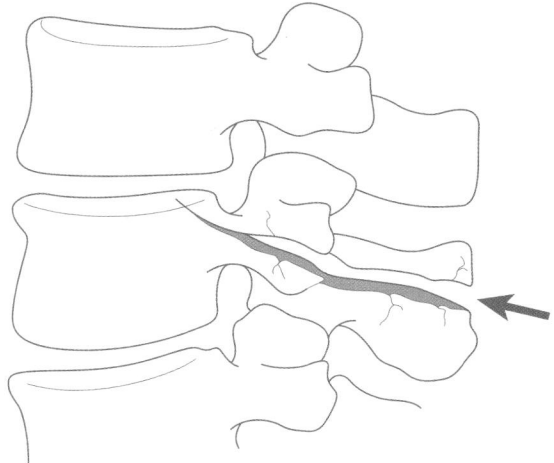

Figure 56-10 A Chance fracture. (From Schultz 1990,[398] with permission of Williams & Wilkins.)

SCI, although in an inadequate fashion, with abnormally short internodal distances and notably thin myelin.[58,173]

Spinal mechanics and stability

There is no universally accepted definition of spinal stability. White and Punjabi defined clinical instability as 'the loss of the ability of the spine under physiologic loads to maintain relationships between vertebrae in such a way that there is not initial damage or subsequent irritation to the spinal cord or nerve roots and, in addition, there is no development of incapacitating deformity or pain due to structural changes'.[467] A commonly accepted model for thoracolumbar stability, which is often used in the middle and lower cervical spine as well, was developed by Denis and modified by Ferguson.[125,126,174] The model divides the spine into three columns: anterior, middle, and posterior (see Fig. 56-9). The anterior column is composed of the anterior longitudinal ligament, the anterior two-thirds of the vertebral body, and the anterior two-thirds of the annulus fibrosis or disk. The middle column is composed of the posterior one-third of the vertebral body, the posterior one-third of the annulus fibrosis, and the posterior longitudinal ligament. The posterior column is composed of the pedicles, facet joints, laminae, supraspinous ligament, interspinous ligament, facet joint capsule, and ligamentum flavum. When the integrity of the middle and either the anterior or the posterior column is affected, the spine is likely to be unstable.[125,126] The columns can be compromised by either fracture or ligamentous disruption. Gunshot wounds, due to the nature of the injury, can affect more than one column and still remain stable.[270] It should also be noted that SCI can occur without obvious radiographic findings.

Fractures or dislocations in the thoracic and lumbar spine most commonly involve the T12 and the L1 vertebrae, respectively. Common mechanisms include compression–flexion, distraction–flexion, Chance-type distraction, translation, and torsion–flexion.[391] Axial loading of a flexed spine can cause several different patterns of injury depending on the vector of force. There might be only compression of the anterior column leading to a compression fracture or, with a greater compressive force, compression of the anterior column with distraction of the posterior elements. If the vector of force causes the axis of rotation to be anterior to the vertebral body, a Chance-type distraction can occur with distraction of all three columns, through the bony vertebra alone (see Fig. 56-10), through the ligamentous structures alone, or through a combination of bony and ligamentous structures. In addition, there can be compression of all three columns with retropulsion of the middle column into the spinal canal. The latter often causes SCI. Translation of adjacent vertebrae, as occurs for example when a person falls from a height and strikes part of the torso on an immovable object, is the injury pattern most likely to cause SCI. If there is translation more than 25% of the width of a vertebra, ligamentous structures in all three columns are probably disrupted.[199,236] Compression and rotation of the anterior column, and distraction and rotation of the posterior column, cause a torsion–flexion injury where the facets and the anterior longitudinal ligament are usually disrupted, and SCI is likely.

Fractures or dislocations in the cervical spine are usually caused by excessive forceful flexion, extension, or axial loading. An abrupt deceleration, commonly seen in motor vehicle crashes, causes a person's head to be propelled forward on a relatively immobilized torso, leading to a flexion-type injury. Abrupt acceleration causes the opposite, an extension–type injury. Axial loading is also a common comechanism to flexion or extension injuries in the cervical spine, such as occurs when a diver strikes his or her head on the bottom of a pool. Knowledge of the mechanism of injury is important for recognizing injuries that might not be seen easily on imaging. For example, flexion injuries can cause disruption of the ligaments in the posterior column that might not be apparent on plain radiographs.

A Jefferson fracture, originally described by Sir Geoffrey Jefferson, is a burst fracture of the atlas (C1 vertebra). This is caused by axial compression, which can occur, for example, when a football player spears another player with his helmet (see Fig. 56-11).[245] A hangman's fracture is a traumatic

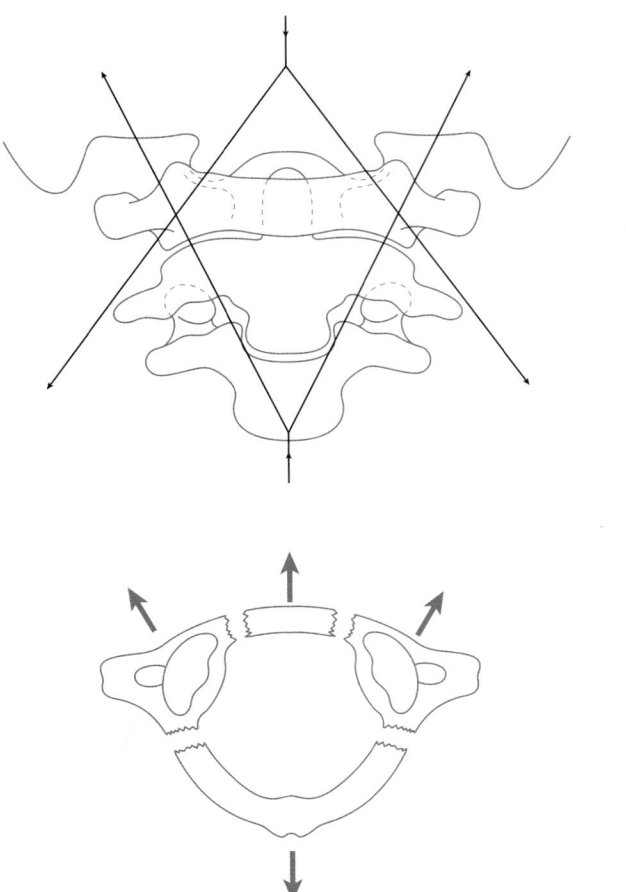

Figure 56-11 A Jefferson fracture. A comminuted fracture of the ring of C1. (From Schultz 1990,[398] with permission of Williams & Wilkins.)

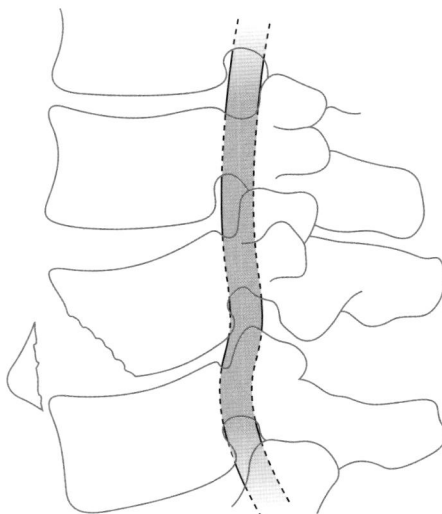

Figure 56-12 A flexion teardrop fracture. The spinal cord is compressed by the posteroinferior aspect of the vertebrae. (From Schultz 1990,[398] with permission of Williams & Wilkins.)

spondylolisthesis of the axis (C2 vertebra), caused by bilateral fractures through the pars interarticularis of the axis, caused by hyperextension and axial compression, as can occur in an abrupt deceleration when a person's forehead strikes the windshield. A fracture of the odontoid process of the axis can be caused by hyperflexion, hyperextension, or excessive lateral bending. The traditional classification of odontoid fractures includes three types.[16] Type 1 is a fracture through the tip of the odontoid, type 2 is a fracture through the base of the odontoid, while type 3 is a fracture that extends from the base of the odontoid into the axis proper.

Hyperflexion of the subaxial cervical spine (C3–C7) can cause an anterior subluxation, a simple compression fracture, bilateral facet dislocations, a flexion teardrop fracture, or a clay shoveler's fracture. A flexion teardrop fracture is characterized by retropulsion of the larger portion of a vertebral body into the spinal canal, detached from an anterior fragment (teardrop); it is associated with posterior facet and ligamentous disruption (see Fig. 56-12). Flexion teardrop fractures are often associated with an anterior cord syndrome, if not a complete SCI. A clay shoveler's fracture is an avulsion fracture of the spinous process of C6, C7, or T1. It is not typically associated

with neurologic injury. Hyperflexion with rotation often causes a unilateral facet dislocation.

Hyperextension of the subaxial cervical spine typically distracts the anterior column of the spine and compresses the posterior column. Anterior distraction often disrupts the anterior longitudinal ligament, the intervertebral disk, and the posterior longitudinal ligament, while posterior compression causes the ligamentum flavum to buckle into the spinal canal. If the spinal cord is pinched between the vertebral body and the ligamentum flavum and/or hypertrophied facet joints, a central cord syndrome often develops. This syndrome, occurring only with cervical spinal cord lesions, is characterized by sacral sensory sparing and greater weakness in the upper limbs than in the lower limbs.[12] A hyperextension teardrop fracture is characterized by an avulsion of the anterior inferior aspect of the vertebral body above the hyperextension injury by the anterior longitudinal ligament, without retropulsion of a vertebral body into the spinal canal. Compression of the posterior column during excessive forceful hyperextension can also result in lamina fractures.

Finally, and not uncommonly, significant axial loading of the subaxial cervical spine causes a burst fracture, whereby an intervertebral disk implodes through the superior end plate of the vertebral body below, causing this vertebral body to burst into multiple fragments.[396] These fractures usually include at least two columns, are generally unstable, and often are associated with SCI.

CLASSIFICATION OF SPINAL CORD INJURY

The diagnosis of SCI can be made promptly by performing a neurologic examination. The International Standards for Neurological Classification of Spinal Cord Injury (ISNCSCI) provide a straightforward, internationally accepted procedure

Table 56-6 International Standards for Neurological Classification of Spinal Cord Injury neurologic examination sensory testing points

Level	Sensory testing point
C2	1 cm lateral to the occipital protuberance at the base of the skull. An alternative key point is at least 3 cm behind the ear.
C3	At the apex of the supraclavicular fossa.
C4	Over the acromioclavicular joint.
C5	On the lateral (radial) side of the antecubital fossa just proximal to the elbow.
C6	On the dorsal surface of the proximal phalanx of the thumb.
C7	On the dorsal surface of the proximal phalanx of the middle finger.
C8	On the dorsal surface of the proximal phalanx of the little finger.
T1	On the medial (ulnar) side of the antecubital fossa, just proximal to the medial epicondyle of the humerus.
T2	At the apex of the axilla.
T3	At the midclavicular line and the third intercostal space, found by palpating the anterior chest to locate the third rib and the corresponding third intercostal space below it.
T4	At the midclavicular line and the fourth intercostal space, located at the level of the nipples.
T5	At the midclavicular line and the fifth intercostal space, located midway between the level of the nipples and the level of the xiphisternum.
T6	At the midclavicular line, located at the level of the xiphisternum.
T7	At the midclavicular line, located at one-quarter the distance between the level of the xiphisternum and the level of the umbilicus.
T8	At the midclavicular line, located at one-half the distance between the level of the xiphisternum and the level of the umbilicus.
T9	At the midclavicular line, located at three-quarters of the distance between the level of the xiphisternum and the level of the umbilicus.
T10	At the midclavicular line, located at the level of the umbilicus.
T11	At the midclavicular line, midway between the level of the umbilicus and the inguinal ligament.
T12	At the midclavicular line, over the midpoint of the inguinal ligament.
L1	Midway between the key sensory points for T12 and L2.
L2	On the anterior medial thigh, midway on a line between the midpoint of the inguinal ligament and the medial femoral condyle above the knee.
L3	At the medial femoral condyle above the knee.
L4	Over the medial malleolus.
L5	On the dorsum of the foot at the third metatarsal phalangeal joint.
S1	On the lateral side of the heel.
S2	In the popliteal fossa of the knee at the midpoint.
S3	Over the ischial tuberosity.
S4–5	In the perianal area, less than 1 cm lateral to the mucocutaneous junction.

for classifying an SCI.[12] The examination, which is safe to perform soon after SCI, even in persons with an unstable spine, is performed with the injured individual in the supine position. Subsequent examinations are always performed in the same position. The procedure includes a systematic evaluation of all the dermatomes and extremity myotomes. Because SCI usually affects the spinal cord at a discrete site, determining the last intact sensory and motor level can reliably and accurately determine an NLI. The International Standards also provide a definition of a complete and an incomplete SCI. A complete injury

is defined as an injury where there is the lack of any sensory or motor function in the lowest sacral segment; this includes sensation deep within the anus, sensation at the anal mucocutaneous junction, or a voluntary contraction of the external anal sphincter. An incomplete injury is defined as an injury where there is at least partial sensory or motor function in the lowest sacral segment.

The sensory portion of the neurologic examination includes the testing of a key point (see Table 56-6) for absent, impaired, or normal sensation in each of the 28 dermatomes on each side of the body for both light touch and pinprick. Pinprick sensation is elicited with a disposable safety pin, whereas touch sensation is elicited by a wisp of cotton or a fingertip. For an inability to distinguish between pinprick and touch, sensation should be graded as absent for pinprick sensation. The motor portion of the neurologic examination includes the testing of a key muscle for strength on a six-point scale (see Table 56-7 for each of 10 myotomes on each side of the body), as well as testing for contraction of the external anal sphincter.

The testing of every key muscle should begin in the grade 3 testing position. If the muscle is shown to have greater than antigravity strength (grade 3), then the muscle should then be tested in the grades 4 and 5 testing positions. Conversely, if the muscle is shown to have less than antigravity strength when tested in the grade 3 testing position, the muscle should be tested in the grade 2 testing position. If the muscle is shown to not even have grade 2 strength, then the grade 1 testing position is used. Before testing muscle strength for a particular key muscle, the range of motion (ROM) for the joint which that particular muscle crosses should be tested. Knowing this available ROM is a necessary condition for accurately grading the strength.

The NLI is defined as the most caudal segment of the spinal cord with normal sensation and motor function bilaterally. For the ISNCSCI, key muscles have been chosen that primarily have innervation by two roots, with each successive key muscle overlapping the muscle above in either the cervical or the lumbar region, by a single root innervation. Each key muscle is identified by the more rostral of the two segments. By ISNSCI definition, if a key muscle has a motor strength grade of 5/5, it is innervated by two intact nerve segments. If a key muscle has a motor strength grade of 3/5 or 4/5 (and the key muscle above has a motor strength grade of 5/5), it is innervated by at least one intact nerve segment, the segment for which that key muscle is named. If a key muscle has a motor strength grade of 2/5 or less, neither of its nerve segments is intact. For the cervical segments, because the innervation of the elbow flexors is C5 and C6, the wrist extensors is C6 and C7, and the elbow extensors is C7 and C8, the ISNCSCI-named segmental innervations are C5, C6, and C7, respectively. If the elbow flexors are graded as 5/5, the wrist extensors as 4/5, and the elbow extensors as 2/5, it is assumed that the C5 and C6 myotomes are fully innervated, but the C7 myotome is partially innervated only. For myotomes where there are no designated key muscles to test, motor function is assumed to be normal where sensory function is normal.

The ISNCSCI also includes a scale of impairment called the American Spinal Injury Association (ASIA) Impairment Scale (AIS), which classifies an SCI into five categories of severity, labeled A–E, based on the degree of motor and sensory loss. An SCI that results in the absence of any sensory or motor function in the sacral segments S4–S5 would have an AIS category of A and be designated as complete. For an SCI where sensation is preserved in the sacral segments S4–S5, but there is no motor function rostral to three segments below the NLI, the AIS is B. For an SCI where sensation is preserved in the sacral seg-

ments S4–S5, but more than half the key muscles below the NLI have a muscle grade less than 3/5, the AIS is C. For an SCI where sensation is preserved in the sacral segments S4–S5, but at least half the key muscles below the NLI have a muscle grade greater than or equal to 3/5, the AIS is D. When sensory and motor function is normal, the AIS is E. AIS categories B–E designate incomplete injuries.

NON-TRAUMATIC SCI

Unlike the National SCI Model System Database for traumatic SCI, there is no comprehensive database of information about persons with non-traumatic SCI. Non-traumatic SCI can be caused by a variety of diseases, including neoplastic, infectious, inflammatory, vascular, degenerative (spondylotic), congenital, and toxic metabolic disorders. Persons affected by non-traumatic SCI are clinically quite different from those with traumatic injuries. Those with non-traumatic SCI generally have less severe injuries. Persons with non-traumatic SCI almost always have incomplete injuries, while those with traumatic injuries are only slightly more likely to have incomplete injuries. Incomplete injuries are associated with a far better prognosis for neurologic improvement than are complete injuries. Unlike persons with traumatic SCI, persons with non-traumatic SCI are significantly more likely to have paraplegia than tetraplegia.[312]

Neoplastic causes of spinal cord injury

Tumors can arise from either the neural elements in the spinal canal, such as the spinal cord or spinal nerves, or the structures comprising the spinal column, most commonly the vertebral bodies. Tumors arising from the spine (extradural tumors) are much more common than those arising from neural elements (intradural tumors). Extradural tumors are most commonly metastatic lesions, being 25 times more common than primary tumors involving the spine.[104] After brain metastasis, spinal cord compression is the second most common type of neurologic involvement of cancer.[1]

Classification of spinal tumors

The most common method of classifying tumors relates to the anatomic location of tumor involvement. Spinal tumors are extradural when they arise from structures outside the dura, most commonly the vertebral body. A less likely origin is from the structures of the posterior bony arch or the soft tissues outside the dura. The vast majority of tumors metastatic to the spine are extradural, making up 55% of all spinal tumors.[279] The most common primary sites of metastatic tumors to the spine are lung, breast, prostate, and kidney.[228] The mechanisms of metastasis include direct extension of tumor from adjacent tissues, and hematogenous spread through Batson's vertebral venous plexus. This is a valveless venous system draining the thoracic, abdominal, and pelvic viscera.[25] A Pancoast tumor of the upper lobe of the lung is an example of a tumor spreading by direct extension. Primary spine tumors that are present in

Table 56-7 International Standards for Neurological Classification of Spinal Cord Injury neurologic examination motor testing points

		Grade(s)			
		0 and 1	2	3	4 and 5
Elbow flexors (biceps, brachialis—C5 myotome)	Testing position	The shoulder is in internal rotation and adducted. The forearm is resting on the abdomen. The elbow is 30° from full extension. The wrist is in neutral pronation–supination and just below the navel.		The shoulder is in neutral rotation, adducted, and in neutral flexion–extension. The elbow is fully extended, and the hand is supinated.	The shoulder is in neutral rotation, adducted, and in neutral flexion–extension. The elbow is flexed to 90°, and the hand is supinated.
	Examiner action	Support the forearm. Palpate the flexors. Ask the patient to bring the hand to his or her nose.		Ask the patient to flex the elbow.	Ask the patient to flex the elbow. Pull against the volar aspect of the patient's wrist while bracing the shoulder.
	Patient action	Attempt to fully flex the elbow.		Attempt to fully flex the elbow.	Attempt to fully flex the elbow.
Wrist extensors (extensor carpi radialis longus and brevis—C6 myotome)	Testing position	The shoulder is in internal rotation, adducted, and in neutral flexion–extension. The elbow is in full extension. The wrist is in neutral pronation–supination and fully flexed.		The shoulder is in neutral rotation, adducted, and in neutral flexion–extension. The elbow is fully extended, and the wrist fully pronated and flexed.	Same as grade 3 position, except the wrist is at 90°, fully extended.
	Examiner action	Support the forearm. Palpate the extensors, and ask the patient to dorsiflex the wrist.		Support the wrist. Ask the patient to dorsiflex the wrist.	Ask the patient to resist the examiner's pull. Pull down on the hand in the direction of palmar flexion and ulnar deviation.[a]
	Patient action	Attempt to fully extend the wrist.		Attempt to fully extend the wrist.	Attempt to fully extend the wrist.
Elbow extensors (triceps—C7 myotome)	Testing position	The shoulder is in internal rotation and adducted. The forearm is resting on the abdomen. The elbow is 30° from full extension. The wrist is in neutral pronation–supination.	The shoulder is the same as above. The elbow is fully flexed.	The shoulder is in neutral rotation, adducted, and at 90° flexion. The elbow is flexed, and the hand is by the ear.	Same as grade 3, except the elbow is at 45° from full extension.
	Examiner action	Support the forearm. Palpate the extensors. Ask the patient to straighten the arm.	Support the arm and ask the patient to straighten it.	Support the arm and ask the patient to straighten it.	Ask the patient to resist the examiner's push by trying to straighten the arm. The examiner tries to flex the elbow.
	Patient action	Attempt to fully extend the arm.	Attempt to fully extend the arm.	Attempt to fully extend the arm.	Attempt to fully extend the arm.

Continued on page 1298

Continued from page 1297 Table 56-7 International Standards for Neurological Classification of Spinal Cord Injury neurologic examination motor testing points

		Grade(s)			
		0 and 1	2	3	4 and 5
Finger flexor to the distal phalanx of the middle finger (flexor digitorum profundus—C8 myotome)	Testing position		The shoulder is in neutral rotation, adducted, and in neutral flexion–extension. The elbow is fully extended. The wrist is in neutral pronation–supination and neutral flexion–extension. The metacarpal phalangeal and proximal interphalangeal joints are extended.	The shoulder and elbow are the same, and the wrist is fully supinated.	The same as grade 3, except the distal interphalangeal is fully flexed.
	Examiner action		Stabilize the wrist in neutral with the metaphalangeal and proximal interphalangeal joints extended. Palpate flexors and ask the patient to flex the distal interphalangeal joint.	Same as above.	Ask the patient to resist the examiner's push and try to extend the distal interphalangeal joint.
	Patient action		Attempt to flex the distal interphalangeal joint.	Same as above.	Same as above.
Small finger abductors (abductor digiti minimi—T1 myotome)	Testing position		The shoulder is in internal rotation, adducted, and in neutral flexion–extension. The elbow is in full extension. The wrist is in full pronation and neutral flexion–extension. The metaphalangeal, proximal interphalangeal, and distal interphalangeal joints are fully extended.	The shoulder is in neutral rotation, adducted, and at 15° flexion. The elbow is at 90° flexion, and the wrist is pronated and in neutral flexion–extension.	Same as grades 0–2, except the little finger is fully abducted.
	Examiner action		Press down lightly on the back of the hand and palpate the abductor. Ask the patient to move the little finger away from the fourth finger.	Support the hand and ask the patient to abduct the little finger.	Ask the patient to resist as the examiner pushes the little finger against the abduction.
	Patient action		Attempt to abduct the little finger.	Attempt to abduct the little finger.	Attempt to keep the little finger abducted.
Hip flexors (iliopsoas L2 myotome)	Testing position		The hip is in neutral rotation, neutral adduction–abduction, and 15° from full extension. The knee is 15° from full extension.	The hip is in external rotation, at 45° flexion. The knee is flexed at 90°.	The hip is in neutral rotation, neutral adduction–abduction and flexion–extension. The knee is fully extended.	Same as grade 3, except the hip is flexed to 90°.
	Examiner action		Support the thigh to eliminate friction. Palpate distal to the anterior superior iliac spine. Ask the patient to flex the thigh.	Support the leg and ask the patient to flex the thigh.	Ask the patient to fully flex the hip and to keep the foot from dragging on the bed. Do not allow flexion beyond 90° when examining acute thoracolumbar and lumbar injuries. Support the leg.	Ask the patient to resist the examiner's push. The examiner tries to extend the hip while bracing the hip on the opposite side.
	Patient action		Attempt to flex the thigh.	Attempt to flex the thigh away from the body.	Attempt to bring the hip to full 90°.	Attempt to keep the hip at full 90°.[b]

Continued on page 1299

Continued from page 1298 Table 56-7   International Standards for Neurological Classification of Spinal Cord Injury neurologic examination motor testing points

		Grade(s)			
		0 and 1	2	3	4 and 5
Knee extensors (quadriceps L3 myotome)	Testing position		The hip is in neutral rotation, neutral adduction–abduction, and 15° from full extension. The knee is 15° from full extension.	The hip is in external rotation, at 45° flexion. The knee is flexed at 90°.	The hip is in the same position as grades 0 and 1, and the knee is partially flexed.	Same as grade 3, except the knee is 15° from full extension.
	Examiner action		Support knee to isolate the muscle and palpate the extensors. Ask the patient to extend the knee.	Support the leg and ask the patient to straighten the knee.	Place arm under the tested knee and grasp the other knee. This causes the tested knee to flex. Ask the patient to straighten the knee.	Place arm under the tested knee and grasp the other knee. Push down on the leg just proximal to the ankle and ask the patient to straighten the knee.
	Patient action		Attempt to extend the knee.[c]	Attempt to straighten the knee.	Attempt to straighten the knee.	Attempt to straighten the knee.
Ankle dorsiflexors (tibialis anterior L4 myotome)	Testing position		The hip is in neutral rotation, neutral adduction–abduction, flexion–extension. The knee is fully extended. The ankle is slightly plantar flexed.	The hip is in external rotation, 45° abduction. The knee is flexed at 90°, and the ankle is fully plantar flexed.	The hip is in the same position as grades 0 and 1, except it is slightly flexed, as is the knee.	Same as grade 3, except the ankle is fully dorsiflexed.
	Examiner action		Palpate the dorsiflexors. Ask the patient to bring the foot toward the knee.	Ask the patient to bring the foot toward the knee.	Ask the patient to bring the foot toward the knee.	Push against the dorsiflexed ankle and ask the patient to resist the push.
	Patient action		Attempt to dorsiflex the ankle	Attempt to dorsiflex the ankle.	Attempt to bring the foot toward the knee.	Attempt to resist the push.
Long toe extensors (extensor hallucis longus—L5 myotome)	Testing position		The hip is in neutral rotation, neutral adduction–abduction and flexion–extension. The knee is fully extended. The ankle is in partial plantar flexion.	The hip is in external rotation, 45° abduction. The knee is flexed at 90°, and the ankle is in neutral plantar dorsiflexion. The big toe is in full plantar flexion.	The hip is in the same position as grades 0 and 1, except it and the knee are slightly flexed.	Same as grade 3, except the toe is fully extended.
	Examiner action		Palpate the extensor of the long toe. Ask the patient to bring the toe toward the knee.	Ask the patient to bring the toe toward the knee.	Ask the patient to bring the toe toward the knee.	Push against the toe and ask the patient to resist the push.
	Patient action		Attempt to bring the toe toward the knee.	Attempt to bring the toe toward the knee.	Attempt to bring the toe toward the knee.	Attempt to resist the push.

[a]You are testing the radial wrist extensors, so the direction of force applied by the examiner should be angled toward the ulnar side of the wrist rather than directly downward.
[b]Clinical tip: in the acute spine injury period, when the spine may be unstable and painful, it may be possible only to test hip flexor muscle strength isometrically. Using the testing position for grade 3, the examiner places a hand on the patient's thigh just above the knee. Ask the patient to lift the leg straight off the bed and resist the patient's movement. The examiner's judgment is required to grade the force as 2 through 5.
[c]Clinical tip: asking the patient to push the entire leg backward (down) may better elicit trace contraction in the quadriceps.

the extradural region make up less than 1% of all spinal tumors. These include multiple myeloma, osteogenic sarcoma, vertebral hemangioma, chondrosarcoma, and chordoma.[228]

Tumors arising within the intradural space include those that are intramedullary (i.e. tumors arising from the parenchyma of the spinal cord), and those that are intradural but extramedullary. Intramedullary tumors are usually primary tumors, most commonly ependymomas and astrocytomas, which together make up 75% of all intramedullary tumors.[228] Ependymomas tend to be well encapsulated and regularly shaped in contrast to astrocytomas, which tend to be irregularly shaped with multiple extensions into the cord parenchyma. Most intradural extramedullary tumors are both benign and primary, and include meningiomas and nerve sheath tumors such as schwannomas and neurofibromas.[228] Those metastatic tumors that are seen can arise either by hematogenous spread or as 'drop metastases', lesions that directly extend from the CSF in association with malignant brain tumors such as medulloblastomas.[279]

Clinical presentation of spinal tumors

Pain is the most common presenting symptom of a spinal tumor. Pain associated with spinal tumors is often worse in the supine position, in contrast to the pain associated with degenerative spondylosis, which is usually worse in the upright position. If the tumor involves only skeletal structures, the pain is usually axial. If the tumor involves nerve roots, it occurs typically in a radicular distribution. If the tumor involves the spinal cord, the pain can present as at-level or below-level central pain (see Table 56-8). Constitutional symptoms such as night sweats, fevers, unexplained weight loss, and anorexia can suggest tumor as well.

Acute spinal cord compression is associated with rapid neurologic decline, and constitutes a medical emergency because it can rapidly progress to paraplegia or tetraplegia. When presenting with signs and symptoms of acute spinal cord compression related to neoplastic involvement of the spine, the vast majority of patients have substantial radiographic abnormalities. The syndrome of acute spinal cord compression, when related to spinal tumors, most often results from the invasion of spinal structures by extradural metastases.[104]

Management of spinal cord compression by tumor

Acute spinal cord compression is managed with hydration, steroids, radiation, and surgical intervention. Intravenous hydration is administered to maintain adequate blood pressure and spinal cord perfusion to avoid spinal cord ischemia. Intravenous steroids, typically dexamethasone, are administered to reduce tumor-related inflammatory changes and prostaglandin production, which increases spinal cord perfusion.[228] Adverse effects of steroid treatment include an increased risk of infection and a decreased rate of fusion of a spinal fracture or surgical construct. Radiation therapy is often utilized in cases of spinal cord compression due to soft tissue encroachment. It can be used alone in the setting of spinal stability, or in combination with surgery. Radiation therapy is less often used for the treatment of intradural or intramedullary tumors, unless such tumors are deemed unresectable or when there is an incomplete surgical resection.[228] Radiosensitive tumors involving the spine include lymphomas, small cell lung cancer, and multiple myeloma, while less radiosensitive tumors include breast, prostate, non-small cell lung, and renal cell cancers.[228] The usual area of radiation treatment includes two vertebral levels above and below the lesion.[279] Complications of radiation directed to the spine include radiation myelopathy and radiation plexopathy. In the setting of acute spinal cord compression, the immediate goal of surgical treatment is decompression of the cord to pre-

Location	Category	Type	Etiologic subtype
Table 56-8 Bryce–Ragnarsson Spinal Cord Injury Pain Taxonomy			
Above level	Nociceptive	1	Mechanical or musculoskeletal
		2	Autonomic dysreflexia headache
		3	Other
	Neuropathic	4	Compressive neuropathy
		5	Other
At level	Nociceptive	6	Mechanical or musculoskeletal
		7	Visceral
	Neuropathic	8	Central
		9	Radicular
		10	Compressive neuropathy
		11	Complex regional pain syndrome
Below level	Nociceptive	12	Mechanical or musculoskeletal
		13	Visceral
	Neuropathic	14	Central
		15	Other

serve or improve neurologic function. Indications for surgical intervention include spinal instability, neural impingement related to a spinal deformity, a failure of radiation to improve symptoms and signs of cord compression, a contraindication to radiation, or a need for a tissue diagnosis.[57,279]

For most intramedullary and intradural extramedullary tumors, surgical treatment is the most effective. Ependymomas, because of their encapsulated nature, often can be completely resected with good preservation of neurologic function.[163,305] In contrast, because astrocytomas are irregular and invasive without a clear plane for resection, the goal of surgery is a subtotal resection of clearly abnormal tissue.[105,305] Intradural extramedullary meningiomas arise from the dura, and are resected along with the involved dura after being accessed through a laminectomy.[304] Nerve sheath tumors can be entirely intradural or, in the case of the neurofibroma, can have extradural extension through an enlarged neural foramen. Complete resection of a nerve sheath tumor might involve the sacrifice of an entire nerve root, which can have substantial functional significance in the cervical or lumbar region. In such cases, an incomplete surgical debulking might be preferable to a potentially worsened sensorimotor deficit. In neurofibromatosis type 2, extensive intradural involvement throughout much of the spinal cord can be present. In such cases, tumor debulking rather than complete resection is usually the surgical goal.[312]

Infectious and inflammatory causes of spinal cord injury

Bacterial infection

Bacteria can invade a vertebral body either hematogenously or by direct extension from a contiguous focus of infection causing vertebral osteomyelitis. Persons at increased risk for bacterial vertebral osteomyelitis include persons who use intravenous drugs; immunosuppressed individuals; and persons with sickle cell disease, diabetes, or renal disease receiving dialysis.[30,377] Children are relatively susceptible to bacterial diskitis alone, probably because of a relatively robust blood supply to the intervertebral disk.[202] The bacteria most commonly implicated in vertebral osteomyelitis is *Staphylococcus aureus*, which accounts for over one-half of all infections.[389] Other common bacterial pathogens that have been shown to cause vertebral osteomyelitis include *Staphylococcus epidermidis*, *Escherichia coli*, *Proteus mirabilis*, *Enterococcus faecalis*, and *Pseudomonas aeruginosa*.[195] Although infection can be seen in any portion of the spine, the lumbar spine is the most common area.[252] Spine pain is by far the most common symptom of vertebral osteomyelitis, seen in over 90% of persons affected.[377] Other symptoms can include fever or a neurologic deficit related to spinal cord compression from vertebral body collapse, or presence of an epidural abscess. Laboratory markers of inflammation, such as the erythrocyte sedimentation rate and C-reactive protein, are very frequently found to be elevated with active infection.[377,388] Isolation of the etiologic pathogen is vital to treatment success. This can be accomplished by recovery of the organism in blood cultures or through cultures of tissue obtained from the spine, either by needle or open biopsy. Treatment of vertebral osteomyelitis involves intravenous antibiotic administration for at least 4 weeks. Longer treatment may be required, and monitoring the erythrocyte sedimentation rate and C-reactive protein can help guide the duration of therapy.[30] Suppressive oral antibiotic therapy sometimes follows the initial intravenous treatment as well. Bracing of the spine can be useful to decrease pain and to stabilize involved spinal segments. Surgical treatment is indicated when appropriate antibiotics have been ineffective, when there is spinal cord or nerve root compression causing a neurologic deficit, or when there is spinal instability or spinal deformity.[30,252]

Tuberculosis of the spine, also known as Pott disease, results from hematogenous spread of the bacterium *Mycobacterium tuberculosis* to the spine, typically from a pulmonary focus.[360] Spinal tuberculosis is treated with at least two and as many as four antituberculous agents for a 6- to 12-month duration. The agents that are the mainstays of treatment include isoniazid, rifampin, ethambutol, and pyrazinamide.[38]

HIV and human T-lymphotropic virus infection

Persons with HIV are susceptible to spinal cord disease, which can occur as vacuolar myelopathy, as primary HIV myelitis, or as a result of opportunistic infections of the spinal cord. A clinically evident myelopathy is found in 7–20% of persons with HIV.[140,368] Vacuolar myelopathy presents with an incomplete spastic paraplegia with loss of proprioception and vibration sense.[140] Vacuoles are found within the dorsolateral white matter tracts of the spinal cord in 40–55% of persons with HIV at autopsy, most commonly in the mid to low thoracic cord.[212,368] Vacuolar myelopathy does not seem to be a direct result of cord infection by the HIV virus, although most cases occur in persons with a CD4 count of less than 200.[363]

Human T-lymphotropic virus type 1 (HTLV-1) is another retrovirus that causes a progressive chronic myelopathy. The clinical condition is a slowly progressive spastic paraplegia, which is referred to as both tropical spastic paraparesis and HTLV-1-associated myelopathy. The virus is transmitted through blood, sexual contacts, and from mother to child in breast milk. It occurs in the Caribbean, southern Japan, central and south Africa, and regions of South America.[195]

Transverse myelitis

When a person presents with a rapidly evolving myelopathy with no history of trauma or physical or radiographic evidence of a structural lesion, the differential diagnosis should include an autoimmune disease such as systemic lupus erythematosus, multiple sclerosis, a paraneoplastic syndrome, nutritional deficiency, vascular insufficiency, and infection. If evidence for any of these conditions cannot be identified, transverse myelitis could be the etiology. This is a myelopathic process of an unknown cause, resulting in inflammation of the spinal cord. Transverse myelitis can progress over the course of several hours or up to 2–3 weeks. The etiology can be infectious, but usually no organism is isolated. Although transverse myelitis can occur in any region of the spinal cord, the thoracic region is most common.[118] In persons with transverse myelitis, magnetic resonance imaging (MRI) scanning often shows spinal cord swelling, with a region of increased signal on T2-weighted images that correlates with the patient's clinical level.[34] Treatment of transverse myelitis usually involves administration of corticosteroids, which have been shown to be associated with a greater and more rapid recovery than in patients not treated with steroids.[271,404] Plasmapheresis can also be helpful.[462]

Vascular causes of spinal cord injury

Ischemia of the spinal cord, while less common than ischemia of the brain, is a well-known cause of SCI. It is most commonly associated with the anterior cord syndrome, and can occur as the result of systemic or local spinal cord hypoperfusion, embolization, or rarely thrombosis. Ischemia can also result from the presence of a spinal arteriovenous malformation (AVM).

Spinal arteriovenous malformations

The presence of a spinal AVM not uncommonly results in paraplegia. There are four types of spinal AVMs.[384] The most common type is type 1, which is composed of arteriovenous fistulas embedded within or adjacent to the dura, supplied by single or multiple dural branches of the intercostal or lumbar arteries, and draining into the intradural venous plexus along the dorsum of the spinal cord.[248,384] The shunting, which results from the arteriovenous fistulas, is thought to reduce the normal arterial venous pressure gradient within the cord, resulting in vascular congestion, edema, and ischemia.[248] The venous plexus characteristically becomes distended due to elevated venous pressures.[231] Type 1 AVMs are most often located in the lower thoracic, lumbar, or conus medullaris regions. Symptoms caused by type 1 AVMs are usually of gradual onset, with a progressive course, although there can be stepwise episodes of deterioration interspersed with periods of clinical stability. Sensory symptoms are the most common initial presenting symptoms, but weakness and sphincter disturbances are often present by the time the diagnosis has been made.[249] A rare but pathognomonic physical finding for a spinal dural AVM is a bruit located over the spine.[299] The diagnosis of a spinal AVM requires radiographic identification of the lesion by either angiography, which is the gold standard, or MRI. Treatment to obliterate the arteriovenous fistula can include either endovascular embolization or surgical resection.[21] Treatment can prevent further neurologic deterioration and even allow reversal of neurologic deficits, if implemented in a timely fashion. Types 2, 3, and 4 AVMs are intradural in location and are thought to be congenital.[231] Type 2 is an AVM with a compact nidus within the cord, while type 3 AVMs occur in children and young adults. Type 3 AVMs include both intramedullary and extramedullary components, including the vertebral bodies, and generally involve multiple spinal levels with multiple arterial feeders. Type 4 AVMs are arteriovenous fistulas located in the intradural extramedullary space usually fed by the anterior spinal artery.

Other causes of spinal cord injury

Other non-traumatic myelopathies include those related to nutritional deficiencies, radiation, collagen vascular diseases such as systemic lupus erythematosus and Sjögren syndrome, decompression sickness, and various paraneoplastic syndromes.

Nutritional myelopathies

Subacute combined degeneration (SCD), the best known of the nutritional myelopathies, was named for the degenerative involvement of two different tracts: the posterior column tracts and the corticospinal tracts.[386] Although described as being associated with anemia in the latter nineteenth century, the identification of vitamin B_{12} deficiency as the causative factor for the disease was not made until 1948.[417] Causes of SCD include pernicious anemia, a deficiency of intrinsic factor, or other causes of malabsorption of vitamin B_{12}, including extensive gastric resection and tapeworm infestation. Dietary deficiency of vitamin B_{12} is a rare cause of SCD.

Subacute combined degeneration presents clinically with loss of vibratory sense and proprioception in the legs, followed later by motor deficits.[249] Onset of the clinical symptoms of SCD is slow, due to the substantial stores of vitamin B_{12} in the human body, which can take several years to deplete.[3,353] Treatment of SCD requires restoration of vitamin B_{12} stores, typically with injections of vitamin B_{12}, from 100 to 1000 mg daily for 5 days followed by similarly dosed injections monthly.

Other nutritional myelopathies include spinocerebellar degeneration related to vitamin E deficiency, and toxic myelopathies caused by naturally occurring toxins in foods such as certain kinds of chickpeas and cassava root.[249]

Radiation myelopathy

Damage to the spinal cord that results from therapeutic radiation is another established cause of SCI. There are two clinical syndromes associated with radiation damage to the cord. The first, which is usually self-limited, occurs between 6 weeks and 6 months after radiation, and is characterized by the presence of L'hermitte's sign.[211] The second is delayed radiation myelopathy, which is characterized by a progressive loss of sensory motor function below the level of spinal irradiation. This type of myelopathy, thought to be due to radiation-induced vasculitis, can progress to a complete SCI.[211] Symptoms of delayed radiation myelopathy usually begin between 6 months and 4 years after radiation is completed, and rarely occurs with a total dose of less than 5000 cGy.[249] Delayed radiation myelopathy is characterized pathologically by demyelination in white matter tracts and/or hemorrhage, infarction, thrombosis, and necrosis.[397]

OUTCOMES OF TRAUMATIC SPINAL CORD INJURY

It is not uncommon for clinicians involved in the care of a person who has experienced a traumatic SCI to be asked the following questions: 'Will I walk again?', 'Will I regain use of my hands?', and 'Will I regain control of my bowel and bladder?' These questions prove the importance of prognosticating neurologic and functional outcomes as early as possible after an SCI, in order to allow development of a specific treatment plan and to allow psychologic adjustment to begin. Prognostication of neurologic outcome depends on the physical examination findings, especially as defined by the ISNCSCI. When performed in accordance with these standards, the clinician can provide accurate prognostic information as early as 72 h after an injury occurs.[78]

Neurologic recovery in complete tetraplegia

Persons with motor complete tetraplegia have a poor prognosis for recovering the ability to walk. Only 2–3% of persons initially classified as having an AIS of A convert to AIS D by 1 year.[295] The prognosis for recovery of motor strength and sensation in myotomes and dermatomes close to the NLI is not nearly so dire. Overall, between 30 and 80% of persons with motor complete tetraplegia recover a single motor level, meaning gaining functional motor strength at that level, within 1 year of injury. Within this group, the most important prognostic factor for single motor level recovery is the initial presence of nonfunctional muscle strength (grade 1 or 2) at the level. A muscle with grade 1 or 2 strength at 1 week has a 70–80% chance of reaching grade 3 by 1 year. In contrast, for a muscle with grade 0 strength, there is only a 30–40% chance that such a muscle will reach grade 3 or better by 1 year.[147] When examined at 1 month post injury, a muscle with grade 1 or 2 strength just distal to the level of injury has greater than 95% chance of reaching a grade of 3 or better, whereas only 25% of grade 0 strength muscles reach grade 3.[457] The chance of functional recovery of a muscle two levels below the motor level of injury, when the first muscle below the motor level is grade 0, is exceedingly rare. The stronger a muscle is within the zone of injury, the stronger it will probably become within 1 year. The speed of recovery is also correlated with strength within the zone of injury. A muscle with grade 2 strength just distal to the motor level will probably gain more strength, and do so sooner than a muscle graded 0 in the same location.[149] Several studies have also shown a strong correlation between motor function and self-care skills.[70,148]

Neurologic recovery and ambulation in incomplete tetraplegia

In the early 1970s, Bosch reported that 90% of persons with central cord syndrome, but only a few of those with anterior cord lesions, were able to ambulate after SCI.[64] Maynard subsequently reported that 87% of persons with motor incomplete tetraplegia initially were walking by 1 year, while 47% of persons with sensory incomplete, but motor complete, tetraplegia were walking by 1 year.[302] Among sensory incomplete patients, the type of sensation preserved below the level of injury is prognostically important. Persons with preservation of pinprick sensation near the anus have a greater than 70% chance of regaining ambulatory ability, while persons who have spared light touch

sensation only in the same region are unlikely to regain ambulatory ability.[111] Among persons with motor incomplete SCI, age and initial motor strength seem to be major determinants of ambulation. In one study of 105 persons with incomplete motor tetraplegia, in which age 50 was arbitrarily chosen as a cutoff, 91% of all persons younger than 50 years, either ASIA C or D, ambulated at 1 year. All persons older than 50 years and ASIA D ambulated, while only 40% of persons older than 50 years and ASIA C ambulated.[84]

Neurologic recovery and ambulation in paraplegia

Recovery of lower limb function in persons with paraplegia is dependent on the completeness of injury and the level of injury. Among persons with complete paraplegia, about 75% retain the same NLI at 1 year that they had at 1 month post injury, 20% gain a single level, and 7% gain two neurologic levels.[459] When the gained levels are truncal in distribution, there is usually no functional significance or change. Persons with T1–T8 complete paraplegia do not recover lower limb voluntary movement. However, 15% of persons with complete paraplegia between T9 and T11, and 55% of persons with paraplegia at T12 and below, recover some lower limb function.[459]

Persons with incomplete paraplegia have the best prognosis for ambulation among all the groups of persons with traumatic SCI. Eighty percent of individuals with incomplete paraplegia regain functional hip flexion and knee extension within 1 year of injury, making both indoor and community-based ambulation possible.[456]

Correlation of MRI findings and neurologic recovery

The availability of MRI technology has been very important to the clinical care of persons sustaining traumatic SCI, as it is the only imaging method that visualizes the spinal cord parenchyma. It has been demonstrated that the finding of an intramedullary hemorrhage is correlated with a more severe, complete neurologic deficit.[182,268] Improved neurologic recovery has been related to absence of intramedullary hemorrhage, less cord edema (less than one vertebral body height in longitudinal distribution), absence of severe cord compression, and resolution of signal abnormalities within the cord on serial MRI examinations.[373,392,405,408] MRI findings have also been correlated with functional outcomes. The prognostic ability of the MRI examination is especially important when the individual is unable to meaningfully participate in a clinical examination in the early period after injury by virtue of significant associated injuries, such as a traumatic brain injury or a significant internal injury to the chest or abdomen. Electrophysiologic testing, using techniques such as nerve conductive studies, motor or somatosensory evoked potentials, and late responses such as the h reflex and the F wave, are not routinely utilized to prognosticate outcomes in the setting of acute traumatic SCI, and such techniques are most useful in evaluating unconscious or uncooperative patients.

Functional recovery

Prognostication of functional outcome depends on the physical examination findings, familiarity with the published functional outcomes of persons with SCI of different NLI, and an ability to integrate into a prognosis a host of other factors. These factors include, but are not limited to, preexisting medical conditions, concomitant injuries, secondary complications, cognitive impairments, age, body habitus, availability of financial resources and insurance coverage, psychologic factors, social factors, and cultural factors.[468] The information in Table 56-9 is taken from the *Outcomes Following Traumatic Spinal Cord Injury* clinical practice guideline, which was first published by the Paralyzed Veterans of America in 1999. This information is based on available outcome literature, data from the Uniform Data Systems and NSCISC, and expert clinical consensus.[468] The expected outcomes are stratified by NLI and described for several different domains. They reflect the level of independence that can be expected of an average individual with a motor complete SCI under optimal circumstances 1 year after injury. These expected outcomes do not take into consideration the presence of preexisting medical conditions, concomitant injuries, secondary complications, cognitive impairments, age, body habitus, availability of financial resources and insurance coverage, psychologic factors, social factors, and cultural factors.[468]

ACUTE PHASE OF INJURY

Prehospital care

The first step in the treatment of a person with a suspected spinal injury at the scene is ensuring an adequate airway, breathing, and circulation. Aspiration of gastric contents and shock are the two most common causes of death for a person with SCI who does not reach a hospital.[218] If the injured person is vomiting, the oral cavity should be suctioned until clear. An oral airway can be placed if the individual is breathing but the airway is not adequate. If the individual is not breathing, intubation should be performed either through blind nasotracheal intubation or with the assistance of an esophageal obturator.[98,416] It is critically important to avoid neck hyperextension during intubation to prevent injury to a vulnerable spinal cord. Individuals should be mechanically ventilated as necessary, and supplemental oxygen should always be given in order to avoid hypoxemia and ischemia to the damaged spinal cord, even in those who appear to be breathing adequately.[416] In the field, shock is treated by controlling bleeding and vigorous fluid resuscitation.

The injured spine should be immobilized in a neutral supine position regardless of the position the individual was found in after the accident. The head must be held in a neutral position in relation to the spine when the individual is moved. A rigid cervical orthosis can be placed about the neck, and the body placed on a long spine board. If an injured person is found sitting in a motor vehicle, a Kendrick extrication device can be used to transfer the injured person out of the vehicle and on to the spine board.[87] In water injuries, the victim is floated on to the spine board, whereas in football injuries a scoop-style stretcher or log roll technique can be used, with care taken not to remove the helmet for fear of further injuring the cord. On the spine board, an occipital pad for an adult or an occipital recess for a child younger than 6 can be utilized in order to compensate for the different sizes of the head relative to the body in persons of different age groups.[178]

Once on the spine board, the individual is transported to a trauma center. The method of transportation depends on the distance to the trauma center. In general, for distances under 50 miles, transportation is by ambulance, whereas for distances greater than 50 miles a helicopter is preferably utilized.[416] Once in the trauma center, the initial goals are to establish hemodynamic stability, to prevent hypoxemia and aspiration of stomach contents, and to verify normal spinal alignment. Maintenance of adequate circulation depends on the management of neurogenic shock and hemorrhagic shock. Neurogenic shock is characterized by bradycardia, hypotension, and hypothermia in the setting of a flaccid paralysis. It is a problem of blood distribution, not blood volume. The bradycardia results from lost sympathetic vascular tone combined with unopposed parasympathetic input to the heart. In contrast, hemorrhagic shock is characterized by tachycardia, hypotension, and hypothermia. Neurogenic shock is treated with vasopressor agents in conjunction with judicious fluid resuscitation in order to maintain blood pressure. Atropine is helpful in treating the bradycardia. A temporary or permanent cardiac pacemaker insertion is rarely necessary.[98] Hemorrhagic shock is treated by controlling bleeding and vigorous fluid resuscitation. Of course, neurogenic and hemorrhagic shock can coexist. Intubation, when not required in the field, might still be necessary in the trauma center due to respiratory muscle fatigue. Measurement of vital capacity (VC) is very useful in predicting acute respiratory failure. A VC less than 1 L portends respiratory failure and the need for mechanical ventilatory support.[87] Placement of a nasogastric tube in the acute period is important to prevent emesis and aspiration of gastric contents, while an indwelling bladder catheter ensures adequate bladder drainage in a situation where urinary retention is the rule.

Once stabilized medically, a thorough evaluation of neurologic status and spinal stability is performed. The neurologic status is determined using the ISNSCI. Spinal stability is assessed for the entire spine, not just the obvious area of injury, as there is a 12% incidence of non-contiguous spinal fractures after a single spine fracture is identified in the setting of trauma.[448] Standard plain radiographs include lateral and anteroposterior views of the cervical and thoracolumbar spine. Findings on plain film indicative of spinal injury may include widening of the interspinous, interlaminar, or interfacet distances; loss of disk space or vertebral body height; fractures of bones; malalignment of the spine; or just prevertebral soft tissue swelling. Targeted computerized tomography (CT) scans can give increased detail about a spinal injury, might identify a spinal injury when the plain films are unrevealing, and provide a visual representation of the spinal canal to indicate the presence of spinal cord compression. A CT scan can also visualize areas not well

Table 56-9 Expected functional outcomes by neurologic level of injury

Domain	Domain description	C1–C3 Expected outcome	C1–C3 Equipment	C4 Expected outcome	C4 Equipment	C5 Expected outcome	C5 Equipment	C6 Expected outcome	C6 Equipment	C7–C8 Expected outcome	C7–C8 Equipment
Respiratory	Ability to breathe with or without mechanical assistance and clear secretions	Ventilator-dependent Inability to clear secretions	Two ventilators (bedside, portable) Suction equipment or other suction management device Generator or battery backup	May be able to breathe without a ventilator	If not ventilator-free, see C1–C3 for equipment requirements	Low endurance and vital capacity secondary to paralysis of intercostals; May require assist to clear secretions	—	Low endurance and vital capacity secondary to paralysis of intercostals; May require assist to clear secretions	—	Low endurance and vital capacity secondary to paralysis of intercostals; May require assist to clear secretions.	—
Bowel	Management of elimination, maintenance of perineal hygiene, and adjustment of clothing before and after elimination	Total assist	Padded reclining shower or commode chair (if roll-in shower available)	Total assist	Reclining shower or commode chair (if roll-in shower available)	Total assist	Padded shower or commode chair, or padded transfer tub bench with commode cutout	Some to total assist	Padded tub bench with commode cutout or padded shower or commode chair Other adaptive devices as indicated	Some to total assist	Padded tub bench with commode cutout or shower commode chair Adaptive devices as needed
Bladder	Management of elimination, maintenance of perineal hygiene, and adjustment of clothing before and after elimination	Total assist	—	Total assist	—	Total assist	Adaptive devices may be indicated (electric leg bag emptier)	Some to total assist with equipment; May be independent with leg bag emptying	Adaptive devices as indicated	Independent to some assist	Adaptive devices as indicated

Continued on page 1306

Continued from page 1305 *Table 56-9* Expected functional outcomes by neurologic level of injury

Domain	Domain description	C1-C3		C4		C5		C6		C7-C8	
		Expected outcome	Equipment	Expected outcome	Equipment	Expected outcome	Equipment	Expected outcome	Equipment	Expected outcome	Equipment
Bed mobility	—	Total assist	Full electric hospital bed with Trendelenburg feature and side rails	Total assist	Full electric hospital bed with Trendelenburg feature and side rails	Some assist	Full electric hospital bed with Trendelenburg feature with patient's control; side rails	Some assist	Full electric hospital bed; side rails; full to king standard bed may be indicated	Independent to some assist	Full electric hospital bed or full to king standard bed
Bed and wheelchair transfers	—	Total assist	Transfer board Power or mechanical lift with sling	Total assist	Transfer board Power or mechanical lift with sling	Total assist	Transfer board Power or mechanical lift	Level, some assist to independent; uneven, some to total assist	Transfer board Mechanical lift	Level, independent; uneven, independent to some assist	With or without transfer board
Pressure reliefs and positioning	—	Total assist; may be independent with equipment	Power recline and/or tilt wheelchair Wheelchair pressure relief cushion Postural support and head control devices as indicated Hand splints may be indicated Specialty bed or pressure relief mattress may be indicated	Total assist; may be independent with equipment	Power recline and/or tilt wheelchair Wheelchair pressure relief cushion Postural support and head control devices as indicated Hand splints may be indicated Specialty bed or pressure relief mattress may be indicated	Independent with equipment	Power recline and/or tilt wheelchair Wheelchair pressure relief cushion Hand splints Specialty bed or pressure relief may be indicated Postural support devices	Independent with equipment and/or adapted techniques	Power recline wheelchair Wheelchair pressure relief cushion Postural support devices Pressure relief mattress or mattress may be indicated	Independent	Wheelchair pressure relief cushion Postural support devices as indicated Pressure relief mattress/or overlay may be indicated

Continued on page 1307

Continued from page 1306 Table 56-9 Expected functional outcomes by neurologic level of injury

Domain	Domain description	C1-C3 Expected outcome	C1-C3 Equipment	C4 Expected outcome	C4 Equipment	C5 Expected outcome	C5 Equipment	C6 Expected outcome	C6 Equipment	C7-C8 Expected outcome	C7-C8 Equipment
Wheelchair propulsion	—	Manual: total assist. Power: independent with equipment	Power recline and/or tilt wheelchair with head, chin, or breath control. Manual recliner. Vent tray	Power, independent; manual, total assist	Power recline and/or tilt wheelchair with head, chin, or breath control. Manual recliner. Vent tray	Power: independent. Manual: independent to some assist indoors on non-carpet, level surface; some to total assist outdoors	Power: power recline and/or tilt with arm drive control. Manual: lightweight rigid or folding frame with hand rim modifications	Power: independent with standard arm drive on all surfaces. Manual: independent indoors; some to total assist outdoors	Manual: lightweight rigid or folding frame with modified rims. Power: may require power recline or standard upright power wheelchair	Manual: independent on all indoor surfaces and level outdoor terrain; some assist with uneven terrain	Manual: rigid or folding lightweight or folding wheelchair with modified rims
Standing and ambulation	For exercise, psychologic benefit, or for functional activities	Standing: total assist. Ambulation: not indicated	—	Standing: total assist. Ambulation: not usually indicated	Tilt table. Hydraulic standing table	Total assist	Hydraulic standing frame	Standing: total assist. Ambulation: not indicated	Hydraulic standing frame	Standing: independent to some assist. Ambulation: not indicated	Hydraulic or standard standing frame
Eating, grooming, dressing, and bathing	—	Total assist	Bathing: shampoo tray; handheld shower; padded reclining shower or commode chair	Total assist	Bathing: shampoo tray; handheld shower; padded reclining shower or commode chair	Eating: total assist for set-up then independent with equipment. Dressing: some assist	Long opponens splints. Adaptive devices as indicated. Padded tub transfer bench, or commode chair	Eating: independent with or without equipment, except cutting, which is total assist. Dressing: independent upper extremity, some assist to total assist for lower extremities	Eating: adaptive devices as indicated (e.g. U cuff, tendinosis splint, adapted utensils, plate guard). Dressing: adaptive devices as indicated (e.g. button hook, loops on zippers, velcro on shoes)	Eating: independent. Dressing: independent upper extremities; independent to some assist lower extremities	Eating, dressing, and grooming: adaptive devices as indicated. Bathing: padded transfer tub bench, or shower or commode chair
Homemaking	Meal planning and preparation, and home management	Total assist	—	Total assist	—	Total assist	—	Some assist with light meal preparation; total assist for all other homemaking	Adaptive devices as indicated	Independent light meal preparation and homemaking; some to total assist for complex meal preparation and heavy house cleaning	Adaptive devices as indicated
Assistance required	Number of hours required from caregiver to assist with personal care, homemaking activities, and safety monitoring.	24-h attendant care to include homemaking Able to instruct in all aspects of care	—	24-h care to include homemaking Able to instruct in all aspects of care	—	Personal care: 10 h/day Homecare: 6 h/day Able to instruct in all aspects of care	—	Personal care: 6 h/day Homecare: 4 h/day	—	Personal care: 6 h/day Homecare: 2 h/day	—

Continued on page 1308

Continued from page 1307 *Table 56-9* Expected functional outcomes by neurologic level of injury

Domain	Domain description	T1–T9		T10–L1		L2–S5	
		Expected outcome	Equipment	Expected outcome	Equipment	Expected outcome	Equipment
Respiratory	Ability to breathe with or without mechanical assistance and clear secretions	Compromised vital capacity and endurance	—	Intact respiratory function	—	Intact function	—
Bowel	Management of elimination, maintenance of perineal hygiene, and adjustment of clothing before and after elimination	Independent	Elevated padded toilet seat or padded tub bench with commode cutout	Independent	Padded standard or raised padded toilet seat	Independent	Padded toilet seat
Bladder	Management of elimination, maintenance of perineal hygiene, and adjustment of clothing before and after elimination	Independent	—	Independent	—	Independent	—
Bed mobility	—	Independent	Full to king standard bed	Independent	Full to king standard bed	Independent	Full to king standard bed
Bed and wheelchair transfers	—	Independent	May or may not require transfer board	Independent	—	Independent	—
Pressure reliefs and positioning	—	Independent	Wheelchair pressure relief cushion Postural support devices as indicated Pressure relief mattress or overlay may be indicated	Independent	Wheelchair pressure relief cushion Postural support devices as indicated Pressure relief mattress or overlay may be indicated	Independent	Wheelchair pressure relief cushion Postural support device as indicated
Wheelchair propulsion	—	Independent	Manual rigid or folding lightweight wheelchair	Independent on all indoor and outdoor surfaces	Manual rigid or folding lightweight wheelchair	Independent on all indoor and outdoor surfaces	Manual rigid or folding lightweight wheelchair

Continued on page 1309

Continued from page 1308 Table 56-9 Expected functional outcomes by neurologic level of injury

Domain	Domain description	T1-T9		T10-L1		L2-S5	
		Expected outcome	Equipment	Expected outcome	Equipment	Expected outcome	Equipment
Standing and ambulation	For exercise, psychologic benefit, or functional activities	Standing: independent Ambulation: typically not functional	Standing frame	Standing: independent Ambulation: functional, some assist to independent	Standing frame Forearm crutches or walker Knee-ankle-foot orthosis	Standing: independent Ambulation: functional, independent to some assist	Standing frame Knee-ankle-foot orthosis or ankle-foot orthosis Forearm crutches or cane as indicated
Eating, grooming, dressing, and bathing	—	Independent	Padded tub transfer bench, or shower or commode chair Handheld shower	Independent	Padded transfer tub bench Handheld shower	Independent	Padded tub bench Handheld shower
Communication	Keyboard use, handwriting, and telephone use	Independent	—	Independent	—	Independent	—
Transportation	Driving, attendant-operated vehicle, and public transportation	Independent in car, including loading and unloading wheelchair	Hand controls	Independent in car, including loading and unloading wheelchair	Hand controls	Independent in car, including loading and unloading wheelchair	Hand controls
Homemaking	Meal planning and preparation, and home management	Independent with complex meal preparation and light housecleaning Total to some assist with heavy housekeeping	—	Independent with complex meal preparation and light housecleaning Some assist with heavy housekeeping	—	Independent complex cooking and light housekeeping Some assist with heavy housekeeping	—
Assistance required	Number of hours required from caregiver to assist with personal care, homemaking activities, and safety monitoring	Homemaking: 3 h/day	—	Homemaking: 2 h/day	—	Homemaking: 0–1 h/day	—

visualized on plain radiographs, for example the C7 and T1 levels. An MRI is essential for evaluating non-bony tissues including the spinal cord, nerve roots, ligaments, and disks. Use of the MRI examination has been recommended before attempted closed reduction of a subluxed cervical spine, because of the potential to cause neurologic deterioration if the subluxation is reduced in the presence of a herniated cervical disk.[159]

Surgical management

Closed reduction of a cervical dislocation is performed by applying a series of increasing distracting forces through the long axis of the body by means of a two-point attachment to the skull with a tong device. The tong device is attached to a rope that passes through a pulley and is attached to a weight. Up to 140 lbs of weight has been applied to achieve cervical spine realignment in an awake and cooperative patient.[106,448] When the obstruction to normal alignment is overcome with the applied distraction force, for example a jumped facet, and the spine is realigned, the distracting forces are reduced again. Typically 10–15 lbs of traction is kept in place to maintain alignment.

Operative treatment of acute spinal injury is generally performed either to stabilize an unstable spine or to decompress compressed neural elements, for example spinal cord or nerve roots. The timing of surgical treatment has been controversial, except in the setting of a progressively worsening neurologic deficit when immediate surgery is usually indicated. Studies have supported both immediate and delayed decompression.[296,449] One large multicenter study of approximately 800 persons compared outcomes for persons in three groups: those with early surgery (defined as either within 24 h of injury or between 24 and 72 h from injury), late surgery (greater than 72 h after injury), or no surgery.[310] In comparing the early and delayed surgery groups, those undergoing later surgery had significantly increased acute care and total hospital lengths of stay, as well as a higher incidence of pneumonia and atelectasis. There were no differences in neurologic or functional outcomes between the early and delayed surgery groups.

If a traumatic SCI is not associated with spinal cord compression or spinal instability, surgery might not be indicated. For example, this could apply in the case of a person with preexisting cervical spinal stenosis who falls and sustains a central cord injury where there is no fracture, subluxation, disk herniation, or spinal cord compression. A cervical collar might be all that is indicated. Use of a spinal orthoses as the mainstay of management is also feasible for bony fractures, such as a compression fracture affecting only the anterior column of the spine without spinal cord compression. See Chapter 17 for a description of the wide variety of spinal orthoses that are available.

Most practitioners of SCI medicine agree that persons with incomplete injuries and spinal cord compression are best served by performing a decompressive procedure to maximize the potential for neurologic recovery. Decompression of the spinal cord in the setting of a neurologically complete injury has been more controversial. It is well established that decompression of the cord in a complete injury is not usually associated with a

change from complete to incomplete status. Therefore the role of surgery in neurologically complete lesions is to provide early stability and rapid involvement of the injured person in rehabilitation, potentially minimizing the occurrence of medical complications in the early phase of the postinjury period. Decompression of the cord in complete injuries might also reduce the incidence of posttraumatic cystic myelopathy.

The surgical approach to the spine is determined based on the mechanism of injury, the location of spinal cord compression, and the surgeon's experience and expertise with the various surgical techniques. An anterior surgical approach provides the most direct decompression of the spinal cord when the compression of the cord is caused by retropulsion of bone fragments or disk material into the spinal canal. Often, anterior column reconstruction and restoration of spinal stability can be accomplished using just an anterior approach. There are, however, significant potential complications of an anterior approach. In the cervical region, surgical injury to the recurrent laryngeal nerve can cause problems with speech and swallowing, while injury to the pharynx or esophagus can lead to mediastinitis or fistula formation to the trachea or skin. Because the anterior approach to the thoracic and upper lumbar spine requires entry into the chest or retroperitoneum, there is a risk of respiratory complications and vascular injuries in addition to infectious complications. Moreover, several regions of the spine are inaccessible to repair via an anterior approach, including the occipitocervical region, the upper thoracic spine, and the lower lumbar spine. A posterior approach is technically easier and less fraught with complications, although decompression of the spinal cord might be indirect.

During the past two decades, different types of spinal hardware, including plates, screws, cages, and rods, have become commercially available that allow shorter segment stabilizations either anteriorly or posteriorly. In addition to the stabilizing hardware, the spine surgeon utilizes bone grafts to ensure future spinal stability, as stabilization using instrumentation alone can fail over time, leading to instability and deformity. Bone utilized for spinal fusion can be autograft, obtained directly from the injured individual, or allograft, obtained from a bone 'bank'. Potential sites for autologous bone harvest include the iliac crest, the fractured spine itself, or a fibula. Spinal orthoses are commonly used to immobilize the spine after spinal fusion surgery in order to facilitate bone fusion. In most cases, orthoses are worn for 3 months postoperatively to allow for radiographically evident spinal fusion.

Penetrating injuries to the spinal cord are overwhelmingly caused by gunshot wounds. Stab wounds as a cause of SCI are relatively rare.[242] Surgical management for such injuries is only rarely indicated. As a rule, neither of these mechanisms of injury cause spinal instability. Removal of bullets or bullet fragments is typically performed only if their presence in the spinal canal is associated with progressive neurologic deterioration.

Pharmacologic treatment of acute SCI

When considered as a whole, it is clear that motor and sensory recovery following traumatic SCI is poor. Only a tiny fraction of persons injured are able to truly regain their preinjury level of function. The vast majority of individuals face major lifestyle changes after SCI that affect virtually every aspect of their lives. This has led to an intense interest in finding a successful treatment for SCI. Nevertheless, only a small number of treatments have been studied in humans, and only one pharmacologic treatment, high-dose methylprednisolone, has been adopted as standard of care. This adoption as a standard of care is not without controversy, because concerns regarding methods of data analysis, choice of statistical methodology, randomization imbalance, and inclusion of persons with minor motor deficits have all been raised. Physicians uncertain about the efficacy of high-dose methylprednisolone treatment are often reluctant to withhold use of the treatment, however, because of the potential for legal action by persons deprived of its use.[99] Methylprednisolone is typically given as soon as possible after injury as a 30 mg/kg loading dose over 1 h, followed by 5.4 mg/kg over the next 23 h.[69]

Methylprednisolone administered in high doses seems to interrupt the secondary injury cascade by inhibiting lipid peroxidation and reducing the production of free radicals.[72] High-dose methylprednisolone has been studied in three large human trials known as the National Acute Spinal Cord Injury Studies (NASCIS). In the first of these three trials, NASCIS-I, subjects received either 1000 mg or 100 mg of methylprednisolone daily for 10 days after receiving a bolus of 1000 mg within 48 h of injury.[67] There were no significant differences in outcomes at 1 year. In the second of these three trials, NASCIS-II, subjects received, within 12 h of injury, methylprednisolone, placebo, or naloxone.[69] The methylprednisolone was administered as a 30 mg/kg loading dose over 1 h, followed by 5.4 mg/kg over the next 23 h. Those who received the methylprednisolone within 8 h of injury were found to have significantly better motor and sensory scores at 6 weeks, 6 months, and 1 year after injury than those of the other two groups. In addition, adverse events were not found to be higher in the methylprednisolone group than in the other groups. In the third of these three trials, NASCIS-III, subjects received either methylprednisolone or tirilizad mesylate, a synthetic 21-amino steroid.[70] The methylprednisolone was administered as a 30 mg/kg loading dose over 1 h, followed by 5.4 mg/kg over the next 23 or 48 h. In this study, there was a significant improvement in motor scores among patients receiving 48 h of methylprednisolone treatment when their loading dose occurred between 3 and 8 h of injury, while those who initiated methylprednisolone treatment within 3 h did not benefit from the additional 24 h of treatment. The group who received the methylprednisolone for 48 h, however, was noted to have a greater incidence of pneumonia, sepsis, and death from respiratory complications than the other groups.[70]

Another compound that showed promise for treatment of acute SCI was GM1 ganglioside. Gangliosides are glycolipids normally present in neuronal and other cell membranes that have been reported to promote neurite outgrowth, regeneration, and sprouting.[214] A randomized, placebo-controlled trial of 37 patients treated with 100 mg of intravenous GM1 ganglio-

side within 72 h of injury demonstrated significant improvement in neurologic outcomes, with the demonstration of the ability to convert complete to incomplete injuries.[197] This study led to a larger trial of GM1 that enrolled over 500 patients and utilized a double-blind placebo-controlled design. This trial, however, failed to reproduce the beneficial motor outcomes that the smaller trial had demonstrated. The trial, however, demonstrated improvement for certain subgroups who received the drug, especially patients who were treated non-operatively and were largely with incomplete injury.[196]

Immune modulation after acute SCI is another approach that shows promise. It is thought that the central nervous system has a diminished adaptive immune response, because invasion of the central nervous system by pathogens is rare. Augmenting the ability of the central nervous system to develop a heightened immune response might therefore lead to less neuronal destruction after acute SCI.[400] 'Activated' macrophages or macrophages that have been stimulated by exposure to rat peripheral nerve, when injected into the lesion site of spinal cord–injured rats, has been associated with improved motor recovery.[374] A multicenter trial in the USA of the injection of activated macrophages into the spinal cord of individuals with acute complete SCI was begun in 2004.

REHABILITATION PHASE OF INJURY

The interdisciplinary team

Rehabilitation goals after SCI include maximizing physical independence, becoming independent in direction of care, and preventing secondary complications. An interdisciplinary team approach is the model that has historically been utilized in the rehabilitation treatment of persons with SCI to achieve these goals. The team is optimally led by a physician who has obtained subspecialty board certification in SCI medicine and has undergone formal training in the interdisciplinary team approach. The responsibilities of the physician, hereafter known as the spinal cord injury medicine (SCIM) physician, include provision and coordination of medical and rehabilitation care, development of rehabilitation goals, and education of the person with SCI. Other members of the team typically include the person with SCI, family members, physical therapists, occupational therapists, nurses, aides, dieticians, psychologists, recreation therapists, vocational therapists, and social workers or case managers. Other consultant physicians, respiratory therapists, speech pathologists, clinician educators, orthotists, and driving instructors can also be members of the team, depending on the specific injury and rehabilitation goals.

Interactions between the SCIM physician and a person with SCI and the family members should occur as soon after injury as possible. In the acute hospital setting, the SCIM physician should educate staff members who are not fully familiar with treating persons with SCI about the potential secondary complications of SCI and how to prevent them. The SCIM physician should educate the patient and family members about the nature of an SCI and the patient's prognosis. Transfer to a specialized SCI rehabilitation unit should also be facilitated, as it has been shown that, for patients treated in a specialized SCI center, overall survival rates are increased, complication rates for pressure ulcers and other problems are decreased, length of hospital stay is decreased. functional gains during rehabilitation are greater, home discharge is more likely, and rehospitalization rates are lower.[50,133] Physical and occupational therapists in the acute hospital should facilitate prevention of secondary complications such as contractures, pressure ulcers, and disuse atrophy. This is done through maintenance of joint ROM, splinting, positioning, and selective muscle strengthening. ROM of all joints is performed and taught by the therapists to persons with SCI and their caregivers as soon as it is medically safe to do so. Performance of an adequate daily stretching program can prevent joint contractures. Splinting of joints, with either an off the shelf or a custom splint fabricated by an occupational therapist, is also often utilized to provide a prolonged stretch, to facilitate a functional joint position, and to prevent skin breakdown.

The inpatient rehabilitation setting is the cornerstone of the rehabilitation process for persons with SCI, and seems to be essential for attaining the above-mentioned broad goals of SCI rehabilitation, and to allow discharge from the hospital to the least restrictive possible setting, ideally to home. As the length of acute rehabilitation hospitalization decreases, many of the tasks described below are refined or even learned in an outpatient, subacute nursing facility or home setting. The rehabilitation process in all of its settings should empower individuals with SCI to know more than anyone else about their own bodies, and to provide the resources to find solutions to all the problems that they might encounter in their daily activities and life. SCIM physicians should observe individuals in the community, providing and coordinating medical care, treating secondary complications should they occur, and directing the provision of appropriate rehabilitative services.

The person with SCI and the family members are essential members of the team. If the person with SCI does not participate in the SCI rehabilitation program, it is not likely to be of much benefit. Rehabilitation nurses perform, in addition to the standard nursing duties, education on prevention and treatment of secondary complications, as well as training in bowel and bladder management. Psychologists help to reduce depression and anxiety, as well as facilitate adjustment to a catastrophic and life-altering injury by supporting persons with SCI (and their families) through the grieving process. This is achieved by providing individual psychotherapy, cognitive behavioral techniques to enhance adaptive coping, and group psychotherapy to provide additional support and information sharing. Social workers or case managers help individuals with SCI, their families, or their caregivers to obtain needed available resources, benefits, and services. They facilitate the transition between an inpatient rehabilitation unit to home or other facility, and provide family support. Other physician consultants are typically involved at various points in the rehabilitation process, especially if secondary complications develop. For example, late neurologic decline due to tethering of the spinal cord is typically treated by a spinal surgeon. Speech therapists evaluate and treat the swallowing and communicating problems that are common in individuals with tracheotomies, high cervical neurologic levels of injury, and anterior approach cervical spinal surgeries. They commonly perform bedside swallowing evaluations as well as participate in modified barium swallow tests.

Physical skill training

Physical and occupational therapists train persons with SCI in mobility, self-care skills, and other activities of daily living (ADL). Achieving adequate joint ROM and strength, necessary to perform these skills, is facilitated through ROM exercises, fabrication and use of appropriate orthoses, and resistance exercises. Individuals whose injuries prevent them from being independent without assistance also need to be educated how to direct caregivers to provide the assistance they need. The person with SCI should be able to instruct caregivers on how to deliver the needed care in a safe and efficient manner. This is important to prevent injury both to the person with the SCI and to the caregivers.

Training in activities that are performed on a therapy mat are commonly begun as soon as a patient is able to tolerate being out of bed. These activities, which are often composed of separately performed parts of a more complex functional skill, are typically sequenced from the easiest to the most difficult. In progressing through these graduated skills, a person with SCI, who is often able to do little for himself or herself initially, moves to a level of stability within a specific training posture. Finally, he or she is able to move in a safe and effective fashion in order to complete functional tasks.[395] When the tasks are mastered on the mat, they are performed in other more real life environments, such as in bed.

Mat activities include rolling, prone on elbows positioning, prone on hands positioning, supine on elbows positioning, long sitting, short sitting, quadruped positioning, and transfer training. In first learning to roll on a mat, individuals with SCI rhythmically move the clasped outstretched arms side to side while lying flat on the back, and then forcefully throw the outstretched arms to the side to which they are rolling. Rolling can be facilitated by starting a roll from a semiside lying position, with a pillow under one side of the back or with crossed legs. Assuming a supine on elbows position is a task that can later facilitate going from a supine to a long sitting position. It also can help strengthen shoulder extensor and adductor musculature. This position can be achieved by individuals with SCI in several steps. First, they place their hands under their hips; next, they flex their elbows; and finally they shift their weight from side to side in order to maneuver their elbows underneath their upper body. When a person with SCI first starts to sit on a mat, balance exercises are practiced, either in a long sitting position with the legs extended on the mat or in a short sitting position with the knees bent at a 90° angle and resting on the ground,. Sitting push-ups are also learned, because these facilitate moving about the mat and transfers.

Transfer training for a person with a complete paraplegia or lower tetraplegia is usually first taught with a sliding board. For a transfer into or out of a manual wheelchair, the wheelchair is

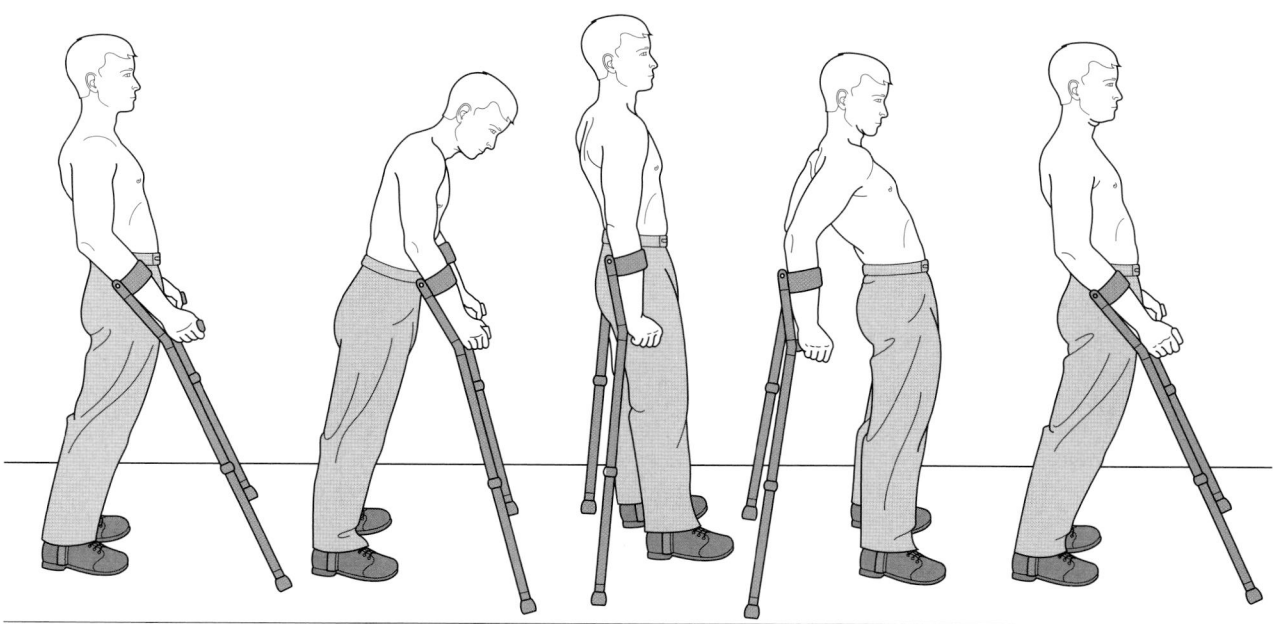

Figure 56-13 The swing-through gait pattern used by a person with complete paraplegia with long leg braces. (From Schmitz 2001,[395] with permission of FA Davis.)

positioned at an angle of 30–45° from a parallel position to the mat, with the front of the seat nearest the mat. This allows clearance of the rear wheels by the buttocks during the transfer. For a transfer into or out of a power wheelchair, the wheelchair is positioned parallel to the mat, because the high wheels that are present on a manual wheelchair are not in the way on a power chair. Next, the individual scoots forward in the chair, removes the armrest, inserts the sliding board deep under the leg closest to the mat, and then rocks the head and shoulders away from the mat while simultaneously pushing up and toward the mat with the arm furthest from the mat. This causes the buttocks to move on to the sliding board. The rocking and pushing is repeated until the individual is safely on the mat, at which time the sliding board is removed. Leg rests might need to be removed for the transfer. A popover transfer is similar, except that a sliding board is not used. In addition to these techniques, there are several other different types of transfer techniques used by persons with varying levels of neurologic function. These include the dependent lift transfer, mechanical lift transfer, stand–pivot transfer, sit–pivot transfer, and floor to chair transfer. The mechanical lift transfer utilizes a mechanical device attached to a sling. The dependent lift transfer and the mechanical lift transfer are used mainly for individuals who are unable to physically assist in the transfers. The stand–pivot and sit–pivot transfers require weight bearing on the lower limbs, and are useful only if a person has significant lower extremity extensor tone or adequate lower extremity strength to briefly squat or stand. The floor to chair transfer is important for anyone who falls out of the wheelchair or otherwise ends up on the floor, and needs to get back into the chair or another higher surface.

Standing can be initiated on a standing frame or a tilt table. Standing seems to help lessen bone loss after an acute injury, improves physical self-concept, and improves self-reported health.[80,223,269] Standing should be implemented only with caution in individuals with chronic SCI, due to osteoporosis. Individuals with osteoporosis have a risk of fracture even without weight bearing. Although ambulation is an expressed goal of most people who have experienced an SCI, recovery of ambulation is variable (see discussion above). For persons with incomplete motor SCI, gait training can be facilitated by body weight support (BWS). For persons with complete thoracic level injuries who wish to undergo ambulation training, orthoses that stabilize the knees and ankles are required. A swing-through gait pattern (see Fig. 56-13) is taught in several steps similar to the mat activities described above. This begins in the parallel bars, and includes going from sit to stand, balancing with extended hips, push-ups in the standing position, turning while standing, recovery from a flexed hip position, advancement of the lower extremities with hip hiking, performance of a step-to gait, and finally a swing-through gait pattern. After the swing-to or swing-through gait pattern is mastered in the parallel bars, it is performed with a walker or crutches.

Wheelchair skills

Physical and occupational therapists not only train persons with SCI in wheelchair mobility, but also help select the proper seating systems to ensure proper sitting position. The wheelchair user is taught to manage or to direct the management of all wheelchair components, including the brakes, armrests, footrests, wheels, and seat cushion. They are taught how to fold or break down the chair so it can be placed properly in a vehicle. They are taught wheelchair propulsion, first indoors over level surfaces, then outdoors over uneven terrain. Proper body mechanics are taught to achieve efficient wheelchair propulsion patterns. Unfortunately, however, self-selected less efficient wheelchair propulsion patterns, often influenced by poor wheelchair sitting positions, are not uncommon. Of several patterns that have been described, a semicircular wheelchair propulsion pattern can be the most efficient and least stressful on the shoulders and nerves crossing the wrist.[62,63]

Performance of a pressure relief, of which there are several different methods, is integral to the safe use of a wheelchair by a person with an SCI in order to prevent pressure ulcers. For a person who does not have motor control in the upper or lower limbs, tilting in space, reclining, or a combination of tilting in space and reclining provides pressure relief to the tissues covering the ischial tuberosities, transferring this pressure to the tissues overlying the back and sacrum for the duration of the pressure relief. A recline pressure relief can be performed only in a chair with a reclining back. A tilt in space pressure relief can be performed in a power chair that has this feature or in any manual chair. Because shear pressure within the tissues overlying the sacrum is limited during tilting but not reclining, tilting in space is generally preferred over reclining. A mechanism to allow independent performance of a pressure relief can be set up for a person with any neurologic level of SCI with the appropriate wheelchair controller. If there is some proximal upper limb strength, then a side to side or forward lean pressure relief can be taught. During a side to side pressure relief, also called a lateral weight shift, an individual hooks the wrist or elbow around a push handle and then leans toward the opposite wheel, relieving pressure from over the ischial tuberosity closest to the hooked limb. This is then repeated in the opposite direction. During a forward lean pressure relief, also called an anterior weight shift, an individual leans forward in the chair to relieve pressure over the ischial tuberosities. Moving back to an upright position from this latter position is often difficult for a person without significant elbow extensor strength, and assistance might be needed.

Another type of pressure relief is the push-up pressure relief, during which a person pushes up on the two wheels with the arms to raise the buttocks from the seat. This type of pressure relief probably should not be encouraged in anyone as a primary method of pressure relief, due to the repetitive strain it places on the shoulders, potentially leading to shoulder degeneration over many years. Recommendations for duration and frequency of pressure reliefs have historically been from 15 to 30 s every 15–30 min, although one study showed that a pressure relief duration of 1 min was needed to allow normalization of transcutaneous oxygen tension.[97] Another basic wheelchair mobility skill is performance of a wheelie, in which the individual in the wheelchair balances on the rear two wheels. This is an important skill that needs to be mastered in order to become independent in curb and single-step climbing in a wheelchair.

SCI education

During the early phases of SCI, most patients and their families have little knowledge or understanding of the injury, its multiple consequences, the myriad of interventional and management options, community resources, equipment needs, prognosis for life, health, function, etc. Often, they are overwhelmed by the gravity of the situation and unable to adjust to a changed lifestyle and self-image. A comprehensive education program is an essential part of any SCI rehabilitation program and, if properly designed, helps the person with SCI and the family members not only to gain knowledge, but also to emotionally adjust and prepare for a successful community reintegration. While some of the learning occurs in formal education classes, group discussions, reading specific educational materials published by various SCI organizations, or extracting information on the Internet, one on one instructions by healthcare professionals are the most helpful in addressing individual needs and concerns.[225] With proper education and the ability to access appropriate information readily, the person with SCI becomes best able to manage successfully the various impairments and ensure the highest possible function and quality of life.

The curriculum of a structured SCI education program should be as broad as possible and include the anatomy, physiology, and classification of SCI, as well as the various medical consequences, psychosocial adjustment, sexual health and fertility, assistive technology, nutrition, research to improve neurologic function, and community resources.

Home and environmental modifications

It has long been recognized that it is of little use to help a person with SCI to regain mobility by the use of a wheelchair, if the architecture at home and elsewhere is such that the individual is unable to enter or exit buildings or move about freely inside. Without accessible environments at home, school, work, and in the community, the dignity, self-sufficiency, and quality of life are severely jeopardized. The Specially Adapted Housing Act of 1948 provided grant assistance to veterans with service-connected disability to obtain special wheelchair-accessible housing. In 1990, the Americans with Disabilities Act (ADA) expanded the rights of people with disabilities, including prohibiting discrimination against them. It also required removal of architectural barriers in facilities owned by organizations that receive federal funding. This was intended to give persons with disabilities equal access to all organizational facilities.

The ADA does not demand removal of architectural barriers in private homes, however, most of which remain inaccessible for wheelchair users. A home evaluation is best performed before a new wheelchair user returns home. This begins with review of the floor plan, followed by a home visit, recommendations for architectural changes, and contracting with architects and builders. The main home areas of concern include the main entrance, bathroom, bedroom, and kitchen, and the ability to exit in an emergency.[155]

Driver training

Being able to drive an automobile enhances the mobility and quality of life for persons with SCI. Most people with SCI can drive an automobile with the proper adaptive equipment and training. Only persons with C1–C4 neurologic levels and those with other severe impairments are unable to drive. People with paraplegia can usually drive with basic hand controls for acceleration and braking, and most are capable of transferring between the driver's seat and the wheelchair independently, and of loading the chair into the car. People with tetraplegia usually choose to drive a modified van with a wheelchair lift or a ramp, and varying degrees of modification of the control mechanisms.

Some people with C5 tetraplegia are able to drive, but usually not within 1 year of injury. Most such individuals use a power wheelchair for mobility, and are not able to transfer to and from the wheelchair and the car. They require a van with power door openers, automatic lift or ramp, and extensive modifications of the control mechanisms. Occasionally, they require a multi-access driving system in which the steering, accelerator, and brake are operated by a single control lever.[13]

Driving skills of people with C6 tetraplegia vary considerably, but most are able to turn the steering wheel. Many are not capable of operating regular hand control mechanisms, and require powered or electronic hand controls for braking and acceleration. Most people with C7–C8 tetraplegia have enough upper limb strength to operate a standard steering wheel with a terminal device. The terminal device compensates for their poor handgrip; examples include a knob, cuff, tripin, or special grip.

There have been major advances in recent years in assistive driving technology, which have made it possible for more people with disability to safely operate a vehicle. The primary controllers of a vehicle, such as steering and braking, can even be concentrated in a complete system that can be operated with only one hand, through a tripin or joystick terminal devices. This can incorporate the secondary controllers, for example the gear shift, turn signals, hazard warning lights, horn, dimmers, cruise control, washer, wipers, radio, air conditioner, heater, defroster, doors, lift, and steering tilt.[79,411] All drivers must use seat belts, but those with reduced trunk control must also use safety belts to secure trunk stability, such as shoulder, chest, or lap belts.

All persons with disability wanting to drive must undergo a driving evaluation by a specialist, usually an occupational therapist certified by the Association of Driver Educators for the Disabled (ADED). The ADED web site (http://www.driver-ed.org) can help to locate certified driving evaluators in the USA and Canada. A predriving evaluation includes an assessment of the person's medical and driving history, as well as functional capabilities. Interactive driving simulators can present the users with diverse challenges in a safe environment, and can provide objective measurement of driving behaviors. Ultimately, however, an actual on the road driving evaluation is essential. Selection of proper vehicle and appropriate modifications to fit the user's ability can involve input from various members of the rehabilitation team. After the vehicle has been modified, the driving educator ensures that all the equipment is appropriate and that the driver is able to use the controls. Behind the wheel training by the driving educator can be a lengthy process for persons with high-level tetraplegia, due to the complexity of the equipment and the impairment of the learner. The high cost of vehicles and modifications, along with the complexity of training, are the most common reasons some people with high-level tetraplegia (C5–C6) choose not to drive. Finally, it should be noted that persons with physical disability do not have worse safety records than other drivers.[323]

Vocational training

Persons who have SCI and are employed report higher levels of psychologic adjustment, satisfaction with life, independence, and general health than those who are unemployed.[247,263,264] Nevertheless, only about one-quarter of all individuals with SCI are employed. Among persons listed in the National SCI Database, approximately 63% were employed at the time of their SCI, 19% were students, and 17% were unemployed. The relatively high number of unemployed persons at the time of injury is recognized as a factor negatively affecting postinjury employment.[261]

Predictors of employment after SCI include being employed before SCI, having a less physically demanding occupation before SCI, being younger at the time of SCI, having a less severe SCI, having lived more years with SCI, having more education before SCI, being motivated to work, and being white.[136,207,264,445] Education has been found to be the factor most strongly associated with postinjury employment. Only 5% of persons in the National SCI Database with less than 12 years of education were found to be employed, but with each successive educational milestone completed, employment numbers improved, reaching a high of 68.8% employment of persons with doctoral degrees.[263] In general, by postinjury year 10, 31.8% of persons with paraplegia and 26.4% of those with tetraplegia are employed.[19]

Vocational rehabilitation is concerned with supporting efforts by a person with a disability to return to and maintain employment. Rehabilitation counselors, who facilitate this process, usually have master's degrees in rehabilitation counseling and optimally are accredited by the Council on Rehabilitation Education. Vocational rehabilitation typically begins with an evaluation of the person's functional limitations, barriers to employment, transferable skills, career interests, and prior achievement. The assessment might also include an assessment of performance during simulated or actual work. Assessment might be followed by counseling and support with regard to educational or vocational reentry, job accommodation, and supported employment. Educational or vocational reentry is often facilitated by a rehabilitation counselor who can liaise with employers, as most employers have little experience interacting with persons with disability, and can have difficulty imagining how a person with an SCI could perform a specific job.[247] Job accommodation, or the modification of a job to make it accessible to a person with SCI, might involve modification of the job site, use of adaptive equipment, or job policy changes.[440] Modifications of the job site can range from the simple (such as adjustment of desk height to accommodate a wheelchair) to the complex (such as redesign of an assembly line).[440] Adaptive equipment can include tools with special handles or sit–stand workstations. Job policy changes can include reassignment of physical tasks or changes in the number and length of workday breaks. Supported employment refers to the need by the individual with SCI for additional assistance in the workplace, ranging from a need for a full-time personal care assistant to the occasional need for manipulation of work materials.

Physiatrists can promote the employment of persons with SCI whom they treat by encouraging return to work or education as early as is appropriate, referring persons with interest to rehabilitation counselors, and ensuring that function is maximized through assistive device and therapy prescription.

Several legislative initiatives have been implemented with a goal of promoting employment of persons with disabilities. The Rehabilitation Act of 1973 provides federal funding for vocational rehabilitation programs in each state. ADA attempts to prevent discrimination in employment against qualified individuals who are able to perform essential functions of a job with or without accommodation.[18] The Ticket to Work and Work Incentives Improvement Act of 1999 were enacted with the goal of providing employment preparation and placement in order to reduce dependency on cash benefit programs, allowing maintenance of Medicare coverage while working, and allowing purchase of Medicaid coverage while working.[20] Workers' compensation programs in most states provide a vocational rehabilitation program for workers who are injured at work, including retraining of those who cannot return to a previous or similar job (see Ch. 36).

Reconstructive surgery of the upper limbs

Tenodesis refers to the surgical attachment of a tendon to a bone. In contrast, tenodesis action refers to the passive tightening of a tendon, when it is stretched by the movement over a proximal joint over which it crosses, causing a movement of a distal joint. This can be seen when the wrist is actively extended and the thumb is passively brought into opposition with the lateral aspect of the second digit. In a person without voluntary motor control of the digits, tenodesis action can allow grasp and release. This action is usually more pronounced in a hand that has developed tightness of paralyzed muscles. It can be accentuated through the reconstructive surgical procedure described below. Arthrodesis refers to joint fusion whereby the joint cartilage is removed from either side of the joint, and the exposed bony ends are opposed and allowed to fuse. Tendon transfer refers to the detachment of a tendon of an expendable innervated muscle from one of its attachments, and reattachment of the innervated muscle and tendon to another tendon that lacks an innervated muscle but whose regained function is sought.

Because the ISNCSCI includes testing of only three muscle functions in the upper limb below the elbow (i.e. wrist extension, finger flexion, and finger abduction), its usefulness in explicating which muscles are available for tendon transfers for persons with tetraplegia is limited. The International Classification for Surgery of the Hand in Tetraplegia (ICSHT) is preferred for this function, because it includes testing of nine muscle functions (see Table 56-10).[308,309] Each limb is stratified to one of nine motor groups, depending on the strength of specific muscles below the elbow. The ICSHT has a sensory component as well, for which the presence or absence of two-point discrimination of 10 mm or less on the pulp of the thumb is determined. A 10 mm or less two-point discrimination threshold has been demonstrated to be predictive of sufficient proprioception in the hand to allow for hand function without visual cues.[321]

Functional upper limb surgical reconstruction has historically been delayed for at least 1 year post injury in order to allow for neurologic recovery in targeted muscles.[456,457] Muscles are chosen for transfer that have a strength grade of 4 or 5, because one grade of muscle strength is usually lost with the transfer. Transferred muscles with a strength grade of less than 3 generally do not improve function. Muscles should not be chosen for transfer if their loss would result in a functional decline. After a tendon transfer procedure, the tendon constructs are typically immobilized for several weeks in a non-stretched position, followed by gradual mobilization, strengthening, and reeducation. Functional electrical stimulation (FES) is often utilized to facilitate neuromuscular reeducation.

For persons with a C5 ISNCSCI motor level, ICSHT motor group 0 or 1, who possess functional strength in the deltoid or biceps and brachialis muscles, active elbow extension can be obtained with either a deltoid to triceps muscle transfer or a biceps to triceps muscle transfer. Functional improvements achieved after a deltoid or biceps to triceps transfer primarily occur through an increased ability to stabilize the arm and reach overhead. Improvements can be seen in feeding, grooming, pressure relief performance, and writing.[328,369] Improvements in an ability to transfer are uncommon. For persons with a C5 ISNCSCI motor level, ICSHT motor group 1, active wrist extension can be obtained by detaching the brachioradialis (BR) muscle tendon from its radial insertion and attaching it to the extensor carpi radialis brevis (ECRB) tendon. Functional improvements after a BR to ECRB transfer can include an increased ability to pick up objects, feed, groom, write, and type.[246]

For persons with a C6 ISNCSCI motor level, ICSHT motor group 2, passive lateral pinch can be obtained with the classic Moberg key pinch operation.[320] In this procedure, the tendon of the flexor pollicis longus (FPL) is detached proximally and then tenodesed to the volar radius. The tenodesis is performed under tension so that, with active wrist extension, the thumb comes in opposition to the lateral aspect of the second digit, accentuating tenodesis action. In order to stabilize the thumb, the interphalangeal joint of the thumb is usually fused.

For persons with a C6 ISNCSCI motor level, ICSHT motor group 3, active lateral pinch can be obtained by detaching the BR or extensor carpi radialis longus (ECRL) tendon from its insertion and attaching it to the FPL tendon. When a BR to FPL

Table 56-10 International Classification for Surgery of the Hand in Tetraplegia

	Group	ISNCSCI motor level	Muscle function , grade 4 or 5	Innervated muscles
Motor	0	C5 (if grade 3 elbow flexion)	Flexion–supination of elbow	Brachioradialis (BR) ≤ grade 3
	1	C5	Flexion–supination of elbow	BR
	2	C6	Radially deviated wrist extension	BR, extensor carpi radialis longus (ECRL)
	3	C6	Wrist extension	BR, ECRL, extensor carpi radialis brevis (ECRB)
	4	C6	Wrist pronation	BR, ECRL, ECRB, pronator teres (PT)
	5	C7	Wrist flexion	BR, ECRL, ECRB, PT, flexor carpi radialis (FCR)
	6	C7	Finger extension	BR, ECRL, ECRB, PT, FCR, extensor digitorum communis (EDC)
	7	C7	Thumb extension	BR, ECRL, ECRB, PT, FCR, EDC, extensor pollicis longus (EPL)
	8	C8	Finger flexion	BR, ECRL, ECRB, PT, FCR, EDC, EPL, finger flexors
	9	C8	Finger flexion, strong	Lacks hand intrinsics only
Sensory			***Two-point discrimination in thumb***	
	Oculo	—	>10 mm	
	Cutaneous	—	<10 mm	

ISNCSCI, International Standards for Neurological Classification of Spinal Cord Injury.

transfer is performed, in addition to the transfer itself, the extensor pollicis longus and brevis are usually tenodesed to the first metacarpal, and the first interphalangeal joint is fused. Functional improvements after a BR to FPL transfer can include increased ability to pick up a pen and write, more efficient grooming, and less dependence on a wrist–hand orthoses for grasp.[455] Active finger flexion can be obtained for a person with an ICSHT motor group 3 by detaching the BR or ECRL from its insertion, and reattaching it to the flexor digitorum profundus (FDP) tendon. The combination of BR to FPL and ECRL to FDP tendon transfers has been shown to lead to improved key pinch, grasp strength, and subjective ADL performance.[289]

For persons with a C6 ISNCSCI motor level, ICSHT motor group 4, active finger flexion can be obtained by detaching the pronator teres (PT) tendon from its insertion and attaching it to the FPL tendon. Functional improvements after the combination of BR to FPL and PT to FDP tendon transfers have been noted in manual wheelchair propulsion, lower limb dressing, opening of jars, and the transferring of objects with the reconstructed hands.[7,190] Finger extension for persons with a C6 ISNCSCI motor level is usually facilitated with surgical tenodesis of the extensor pollicis longus and extensor digitorum communis tendons to the dorsum of the wrist, allowing the fingers and thumb to extend with passive wrist flexion.

Persons with a C7 ISNCSCI motor level, ICSHT motor groups 5, 6, or 7, similar to persons with a C6 ISNCSCI motor level, do not have active finger and thumb flexion. Therefore active thumb flexion can be obtained with a BR to FPL transfer,

while active finger flexion can be obtained with a ECRL, flexor carpi ulnaris, or PT to FDP transfer. Persons with a C8 ISNCSCI motor level, ICSHT motor group 8, lack intrinsic finger and thumb muscle innervation, but retain the ability to open and close the hand with innervated extrinsic hand muscles, albeit with decreased grip strength and a tendency toward developing a claw-like resting hand posture. The results of surgical reconstruction of intrinsic hand function, however, have been less than favorable, and it is not commonly performed for persons with SCI.[238,458]

Neuromuscular electrical stimulation

Although electrical stimulation of nerves and muscles for therapeutic purposes has been practiced for centuries, it has only recently been used to restore function.[370] When used to restore function, electrical stimulation is referred to as functional electrical stimulation or functional neuromuscular stimulation (FNS). For persons with SCI, FNS has been used to improve cardiovascular performance; increase muscle bulk; prevent or treat pressure ulcers, osteoporosis, and joint contractures; control spasticity; allow ventilator-free breathing and coughing; generate hand grasp or release and arm reaching; improve control of bladder and bowel functions; achieve erection and ejaculation; and to enable standing, transfers, stepping, and ambulation.[108] A computer-controlled electrical stimulation system used to achieve neuromuscular stimulation is referred to as a neuroprosthesis.

Activation of a motor unit by voluntary effort, reflex action, or electrical stimulation occurs by depolarization of the motor axons or their terminal branches at the myoneural junction. The electrical current required to depolarize muscles is much greater than that required for nerves, which makes direct stimulation of muscles, including peripherally denervated muscles, impractical for clinical purposes. Electrical activation of a nerve is accomplished by applying a current strong enough to create an action potential. The stronger the current, the more nerve fibers are activated within a given nerve. During application of FNS, several stimulation parameters require adjustment, including pulse amplitude, duration, frequency, and waveform, as well as the ratio of stimulator on–off time.[28]

The components of most FNS systems are fundamentally similar, and consist of various types of control mechanisms, a power source (battery), electrical stimulator, lead wires, electrodes, and peripherally placed sensors (see Fig. 56-14).[370] Electrodes of various designs create the interface between the FNS system and the user's nervous system. These electrodes can be skin surface-type; implanted at the epimysium (muscle surface); implanted nerve cuff; and intramuscular electrodes, either surgically implanted or percutaneously inserted (see Fig. 56-15). When electrodes are surgically implanted, it is important to avoid causing tissue damage, and to preserve the nerve structure by selecting safe levels of electrical stimulation.[6,355]

Clinical applications

Functional neuromuscular stimulation is not effective in stimulating muscles paralyzed by LMN damage, i.e. damage affecting the anterior horn cells and/or motor nerve roots, but such damage usually occurs at the level of the SCI lesion. FNS is usually a relatively safe intervention, but its application in the presence of cardiac pacemakers or implanted defibrillators is best avoided. Great caution is also warranted in the presence of various heart conditions (especially dysrhythmia and congestive heart failure), during pregnancy, and during healing of surgical wounds.[215]

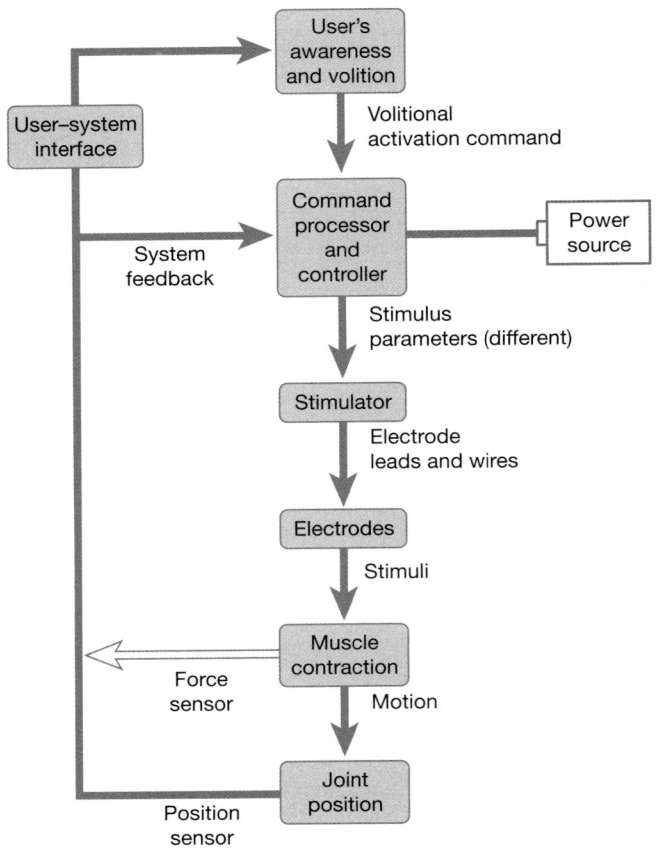

Figure 56-14 The components and action sequence of a functional neuromuscular stimulation system. (From Ragnarsson 2001,[370] with permission.)

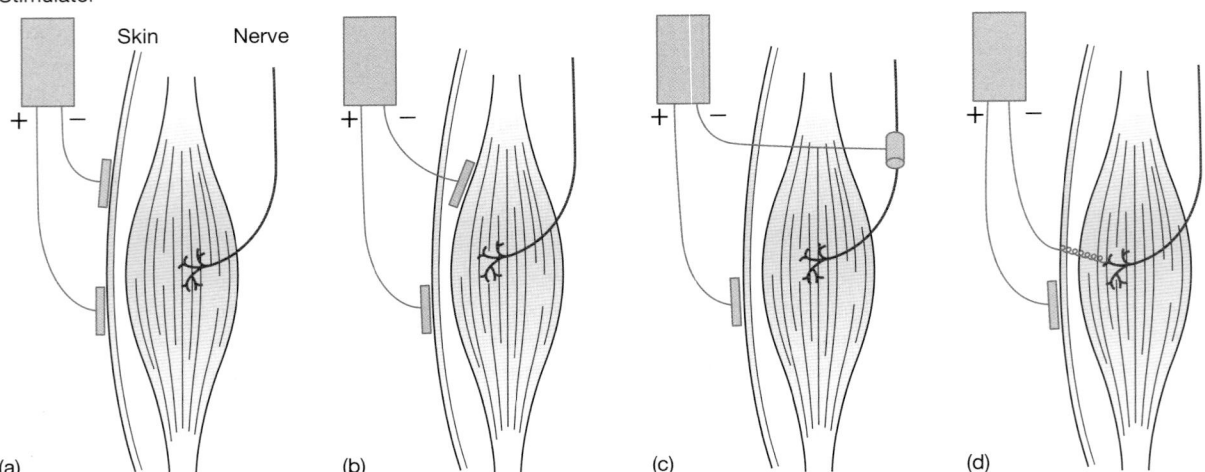

Figure 56-15 Electrode designs for functional neuromuscular stimulation systems: (**a**) skin surface electrode, (**b**) implanted epimysial (muscle surface) electrode, (**c**) implanted nerve cuff electrode, and (**d**) intramuscular electrode with percutaneous lead. (From Ragnarsson 2001,[370] with permission.)

Upper limb control by FNS

Paralysis of hands and arms significantly impairs independence and function of persons with tetraplegia. Use of adaptive equipment and performance of reconstructive surgery can increase function for some, but not for all. Recently, several types of upper limb neuroprostheses have become commercially available. Some are external to the body, such as the Hand Master and Bionic Glove. Some are surgically implanted, like the Freehand System.[215,354,370] These are designed to provide hand grasp, hold, and release under the control of the user. Most users are persons with C5–C6 tetraplegia with preserved LMNs for the seventh and eighth cervical segments. The Freehand System has been extensively tested and US Food and Drug Administration (FDA)-approved. It has been shown to increase the user's independence score during various ADL, and has received a high satisfaction rate. The external hand neuroprostheses have also been shown to improve function, but are considered less cosmetic than the Freehand System.[215] They are less expensive, however, and are relatively easy to apply and do not require surgical implantation.

Electrophrenic respiration

Phrenic nerve pacing was first developed for persons with sleep apnea but, through the pioneering efforts of Glenn, it has been used since the 1970s for persons with C1–C2 tetraplegia who have intact LMNs for the phrenic nerves. Candidates with SCI for electrophrenic respiration (EPR) have to meet strict criteria, but most important is to have a viable phrenic nerve.[203,204,370] Prior to implantation, conduction studies of the phrenic nerves must be done bilaterally with recording of conduction velocities and amplitudes. Preferably, this is done with simultaneous fluoroscopic observation of the diaphragm in order to visualize and document its contractions. Several EPR systems are available. The electrodes are surgically implanted bilaterally near or around the phrenic nerves, either at the base of the neck or along their routes in the chest. It has become possible recently to place the electrodes by an endoscopic procedure directly into the diaphragm's motor points, which has simplified the application process significantly. A radiofrequency receiver and electrical stimulator are also surgically implanted, and are connected to the electrodes by subcutaneous wires. An external transmitter with antenna controls the stimulation parameters, initially by generating 8–14 breaths per minute, but with improved conditioning of the diaphragm 6–10 breaths per minute may be sufficient to maintain adequate oxygenation.

It has been proposed that magnetic stimulation of the expiratory muscles in the chest wall might effectively restore cough in persons with tetraplegia.[282]

FNS for standing and walking

It has been well demonstrated that persons with paraplegia can stand and ambulate for short distances using surface or implantable FNS systems, and one surface system has been FDA-approved and marketed in the USA.[221,447] The clinician needs to understand the limitations of such FNS systems. For example, the best candidates are persons with T4–T12 paraplegia who have intact lumbosacral LMNs and good upper body strength. It should also be noted that a walker is needed for stability and safety, and that the speed of walking is slower than normal. The energy expenditure is significantly higher than for ambulation by an able-bodied individual. These limitations make the currently available systems more applicable for standing, transfers, and short-distance ambulation rather than for replacing the wheelchair.[215]

FNS for bladder control and sexual function

Through the pioneering work of Brindley, it has been shown that FNS of S2–S4 anterior roots causes contraction of the detrusor muscle of the bladder and micturition.[77] In order to secure urinary continence between FNS stimulations, however, the reflex arc must be interrupted by performing S2–S4 posterior rhizotomies. This is unfortunately associated with loss of reflex erection and ejaculation.[109] A surgically implantable neuroprosthesis with intra- or extradural electrodes has been developed, which has found wide clinical use primarily in Europe. Follow-up studies have shown this device to be both safe and effective.[77,109]

Penile erections have been reported to occur in 60% of men using FNS with S2–S4 intradural anterior root electrodes, but its clinical usefulness is questionable.[109] However, electrical stimulation by an electrode temporarily placed in the rectum is used routinely to produce emission or ejaculation in men with SCI. After retrieving the semen, it can be used for artificial insemination directly or by using in vitro fertilization techniques.[109,241]

FNS for therapeutic exercise

Sedentary lifestyle and impaired autonomic function in persons with SCI leads to many degenerative physiologic changes that can affect their health and wellness.[370] There is loss of muscle bulk, strength, endurance, and bone density in the paralyzed limbs; cardiovascular fitness, VC, and lean body mass are reduced; and certain endocrine functions are altered.[48] First introduced more than 20 years ago, FNS cycle ergometers have been clinically used by persons with SCI, both those with paraplegia and with tetraplegia, to effectively reverse many of these secondary effects.[365,371]

Body weight support ambulation training on a treadmill

The spinal cord was viewed in the past as being a large nerve solely for conducting information between the brain and the periphery. It was felt to be capable of processing only simple spinal reflexes. Through the pioneering work of Barbeau and Edgerton during the 1980s, it has been shown that, after SCI, the spinal cord can generate motor control to allow full weight-bearing locomotion without any supraspinal influence.[35,158] It has been also demonstrated that the human spinal cord is capable of processing complex proprioceptive information, including information generated during standing and stepping. The level of motor function achieved after SCI is in large part user-dependent, and it improves and is maintained by training.[157] Clinical studies have shown that specific intensive walking training of persons with incomplete SCI significantly improves walking capabilities.[465,466] Such training consists of upright walking on a treadmill, with partial BWS provided by a suspending harness, with a therapist guiding and setting the limbs. A multicenter clinical trial in the USA recently compared the efficacy of BWS gait training with traditional training in persons with incomplete SCI. According to the preliminary information, the majority of subjects in both groups recovered independent locomotion, suggesting that there are several methods of recovering locomotion skills after SCI, but that all require intensive training.[151,152]

CHRONIC PHASE OF INJURY

Adjustment to disability

Spinal cord injury is a catastrophic event with a profound effect on the injured person as well as on family members. Different personal, interpersonal, and cultural factors ultimately determine how successfully an individual with SCI will adjust or adapt to the disability.[327] Successful adjustment is felt to have occurred when the disability is no longer the dominant concern in the person's life.[230] Such adjustment is highly individually variable and has been estimated by some to occur over 2–5 years, while others propose that adjustment is a lifelong process.[142,144,446] Adjustment has been considered by many to consist of sequential psychologic reactions according to stage theories, beginning with denial and followed by anger, bargaining, depression, and finally acceptance or adjustment.[176,267,464] Although such sequential reactions are often seen in persons with SCI, they tend to be highly individualized.[426]

Despite an overwhelming sense of loss initially after SCI, most persons eventually learn to cope emotionally and conform to their premorbid personality styles of interacting with the environment. A number of psychologic problems, however, primarily depression and anxiety, can interfere with adjustment and quality of life. These problems can lead to substance abuse, divorce, dependency, self-neglect, and even suicide.

Depression and anxiety are usually present early after SCI, and have been reported to occur in more than 30% of persons for 2 or more years post injury.[107,185] Risk factors for depression are similar to those in able-bodied individuals, including a family or personal history of depression. Factors specific to the SCI, such as the presence of complete neurologic injury, or medical comorbidities can increase the likelihood of depression. Depression and anxiety can play a role in the relatively high incidence of substance abuse after SCI, divorce, and suicide.[142,260,394] Depression after SCI needs to be managed by the entire rehabilitation team using cognitive behavioral treatments, and even psychopharmacology if needed. Members of the rehabilitation team need to communicate appropriately with a person with SCI by clearly answering all questions, addressing effectively the medical concerns, working with the person with SCI on realistic goals, and nurturing hopeful thinking.[176] Pharmacologic treatment of depression should be considered for those whose symptoms interfere with performance in social, self-care, recreational, and vocational activities.[176] A variety of antidepressant drugs can be used. These are best prescribed by a psychiatrist for those most severely affected, for example those with suicidal thoughts or psychotic symptoms.

Quality of life

Quality of life is a concept that is difficult to define, but which can be described as a determination of the individual's satisfaction with life, for example whether they are able to do the things that they personally want to do. Compared with non-disabled people, persons with SCI tend to report lesser well-being and state of health, and score lower on physical, emotional, and social health domains of life.[145] A metaanalysis has shown no relationship between the neurologic level, the completeness of SCI, and the subjective quality of life. Some factors are felt to affect quality of life positively, for example mobility and ADL independence, emotional support, good overall health, self-esteem, absence of depression, physical and social activities and integration, being married and employed, having higher education, and living at home.[143,144,230,265] In general, dissatisfaction with life after SCI seems more related to social disadvantages than to physical limitations.

Recovery-enhancing therapies

Most patients with SCI, even those with neurologically complete lesions, experience some degree of spontaneous neurologic recovery. This occurs as a result of resolution of the acute pathology, with recovery of nerve roots and spinal cord at the level of the lesion.[149] Certain pharmacologic agents have shown promise as protecting neurologic function and/or enhancing recovery during acute SCI, especially high-dose methylprednisolone, as discussed above.

Despite major efforts to find effective treatments to enhance neurologic recovery during chronic SCI, no reports of scientifically conducted clinical trials exist that show effectiveness of any specific pharmacologic agents.[307] At best, it has been shown that active exercise, such as BWS ambulation, might promote recovery of motor function in persons with incomplete SCI (and even in one person with C2 ASIA A injury).[149,306,466] The drug 4-aminopyridine, which blocks potassium channels in nerve membranes and enhances conduction in demyelinated axons, has been extensively tested in clinical trials. While it might improve some symptoms associated with SCI, it has not been reported to improve motor or sensory function.[122] HP184, which is a dual action sodium–potassium channel blocker, has also been clinically tested. Reports of its efficacy are not yet available.

Late neurologic decline

Approximately 20–30% of persons with chronic SCI are reported to develop new motor or sensory deficits.[86,286] Most common is entrapment of a peripheral nerve (10%), especially of the median nerve at the carpal tunnel, or of the ulnar nerve at the elbow. Other entrapments can occur as well.[86] Further damage of the spinal cord can be caused by posttraumatic syringomyelia (PTS), also called posttraumatic cystic myelopathy, by tethering or by compression of the cord.

While it is common to find MRI evidence of a cyst within the spinal cord at the level of the injury, only 5% of all people with SCI develop PTS. It becomes a problem when the cyst expands longitudinally and damages the cord, causing clinical symptoms such as pain, sensory loss, weakness, altered muscle tone, and a variety of autonomic symptoms.[286] The exact cause of PTS is unknown, but it might be related to obstruction of normal flow of the CSF due to scarring or canal narrowing. This leads to abnormal increases in CSF pressure during coughing and straining, ultimately causing a longitudinal dissection of the cord.[286]

The diagnosis of PTS is confirmed by MRI or CT myelogram with delayed images. The clinical symptoms of PTS and their progression vary greatly. If there is no neurologic decline noted on regular follow-up examinations, the treatment can be symptomatic. Activity restrictions are usually advisable, especially avoiding strenuous exercise that could raise venous and CSF pressure. Despite limited evidence of their efficacy, medications are occasionally prescribed to reduce fluid accumulation around the spinal cord. In some cases, percutaneous drainage of the cyst is performed. When there is continuous neurologic decline or intractable pain associated with PTS, surgical treatment is usually indicated in order to reduce the size of the syrinx or to prevent its expansion. Surgical approaches include placement of a shunt in the syrinx to drain the fluid into the peritoneal, pleural, or subarachnoid spaces; marsupialization of the syrinx; and duraplasty.[286] When treatment is successful, strength might increase, and pain and spasticity might diminish.

Tethering of the spinal cord due to meningeal or arachnoid scar formations can occur following SCI and prevent normal rostrocaudal sliding of the cord within the spinal canal on motion. Tethering of the cord in the cervical spine can generate enough cord traction with flexion of the neck to cause cord or brain stem displacement and neurologic symptoms, such as weakness, sensory deficits, and pain. Reduction of neck flexion using a rigid cervical orthosis might be helpful, but often surgical untethering can be indicated.[418]

Late compression of the spinal cord or nerve roots can occur for multiple reasons and cause neurologic decline. Common causes include progressive spondylosis, spinal stenosis, intervertebral disk herniations, and posttraumatic changes. Proper imaging studies are needed for diagnosis. Surgical intervention can be needed if there is a rapid neurologic loss or severe intractable pain.

SECONDARY CONDITIONS
Pulmonary system

Pulmonary complications, including atelectasis, pneumonia, respiratory failure, pleural complications, and pulmonary embolism (PE), are the leading causes of death for persons with SCI in all years after SCI.[131,134,135,189,257] They accounted for 37% of all deaths during the first year after SCI, and 21% of the deaths

beyond the first year, in a large sample from the Model SCI Care Systems and Shriner's Hospitals.[135] Sleep disorders also are prevalent, albeit less deadly.[85]

Anatomy and mechanics of the pulmonary system

The degree of respiratory dysfunction after SCI is strongly correlated to the NLI and degree of motor impairment. Muscles that contribute to respiratory function include the diaphragm, the intercostals, the abdominals, and the muscles of the neck and shoulder girdle.[470] The diaphragm, innervated by anterior horn cells located in the C3–C5 segments, is the major primary muscle of inspiration. In persons without SCI, the diaphragm contributes approximately 65% of the total VC.[127–129,406] Inspiratory resistive training in persons with tetraplegia has been shown to improve the strength and endurance of a weak diaphragm and improve lung function.[220,240,387,480] The intercostals, internal and external, innervated segmentally from T1 to T11, are muscles of inspiration at low lung volumes, and muscles of expiration at high lung volumes.[120] The abdominals, innervated segmentally from T6 to L1, are not active during quiet breathing. However, when ventilatory demand leads to stretching of the abdominal wall on inspiration, there is a triggered phasic contraction of these muscles that leads to increased intra-abdominal pressures, with a resultant improvement in inflation of the lower thoracic cavity.[210] During coughing, a similar process occurs, whereby the abdominal muscles contract, causing an abrupt increase in intraabdominal and intrathoracic pressures, leading to a forceful cough.[168] Of the muscles of the neck and shoulder girdle that contribute to respiration, the scalene muscles, innervated from C3 to C8, are active during quiet inspiration in individuals with and without SCI. A coordinated contraction of these muscles is necessary for optimal rib cage movement.[119] The sternocleidomastoid and trapezius muscles, innervated by the spinal accessory nerve and the C2–C4 and C1–C4 roots, respectively, are accessory muscles of inspiration, usually active only in times of ventilatory demand.[375,470] These muscles often are necessary to allow adequate ventilation in persons with higher level SCI. The medial and lateral pectoral nerves exit the spinal cord at C5–T1 to innervate the pectoralis major muscle, an accessory muscle of expiration. In persons with tetraplegia, this muscle has been shown to be able to produce dynamic airway compression necessary for cough. Strength training of this muscle has been shown in a randomized trial to improve expiratory function in persons with chronic tetraplegia.[168,169]

Persons with a neurologic level of C2 or above with a complete SCI usually have no diaphragmatic function and require mechanical ventilation. Persons with a complete C3 SCI have severe diaphragmatic weakness and commonly will require mechanical ventilation at least temporarily. Persons with a complete C4 SCI often also have severe diaphragmatic weakness and may also require mechanical ventilation at least temporarily. For persons not on a ventilator who have a complete high-level cervical SCI, the preserved inspiratory accessory muscles can contribute a significant portion to the overall VC. Persons with a complete C5–C8 SCI usually are able to maintain independent breathing although, due to the loss of innervation to the intercostals and abdominals, they remain at high risk for pulmonary complications. This risk for pulmonary complications is also present for those with complete thoracic level SCI, albeit to a lesser degree depending on the segmental extent of the loss of innervation.

Spinal cord injury can lead to alterations in lung, chest wall, and airway mechanics. The pulmonary function profile of persons with chronic tetraplegia reveals decreased lung volumes, decreased thoracic wall compliance (with increased abdominal wall compliance), and airway hyperreactivity.[141,167,326,421] The VC is directly related to respiratory muscle strength, the measurement of which by a spirometer can give a quantitative measure of the strength of the diaphragm. This is equivalent to doing a manual muscle test of an extremity muscle. The VC is markedly reduced after acute SCI, both in persons with tetraplegia and those with high paraplegia, ranging from 24% to 31% of the predicted normal values.[276,313] However, the acute decreases in VC tend to increase to 40% of the predicted normal values by 5 weeks, and to 60% by 5 months.[276] The VC of persons with tetraplegia or high paraplegia is posturally dependent, being up to 15% lower in the upright position than in the supine position.[166] In the sitting position in persons with paralyzed abdominals, the effect of gravity on the abdominal contents leads to an increased residual volume. Use of an abdominal binder in the sitting position helps to reverse this effect by pressing the abdominal contents into the diaphragm, allowing a more efficient diaphragmatic resting position. The airway hyperreactivity is responsive to inhaled bronchodilators, and is thought to be caused by unopposed cholinergic tone.[11,141,421]

Management of pulmonary complications

Atelectasis is the most common respiratory complication in people with SCI and can predispose to pneumonia, pleural effusion, and empyema. Pneumonia commonly occurs in areas of atelectasis. Pleural effusions often develop in close proximity to areas of atelectasis. It is thought that the areas of lung that collapse pull the parietal pleural away from the visceral pleura, leaving an empty space that consequently then fills with a fluid, causing an effusion. Treatment of atelectasis includes lung expansion, secretion mobilization, and secretion clearance. If an individual is on a ventilator, a gradual increase in tidal volumes (TVs) to a target of >20 cc/kg of ideal body weight (IBW) has been shown to be effective in decreasing atelectasis as compared with maintaining the TV at <20 cc/kg IBW.[362] Intermittent positive-pressure breathing, bilevel positive airway pressure, or continuous positive airway pressure (CPAP) devices can all be used with or without tracheostomy tubes to help with lung expansion and to prevent or treat atelectasis. Secretion mobilization techniques include postural drainage and chest percussion or vibration. Postural drainage uses gravity to assist in drainage of accumulated secretion from specific lung areas. For example, drainage of the left lower lobe optimally requires a 20° Trendelenburg, semiprone, right decubitus position. Drainage of the right lower lobe optimally requires a Trendelenburg,

semiprone, left decubitus position. Chest percussion, optimally performed in conjunction with postural drainage, can be performed with a cupped hand, with a mechanical vibrator, by donning a vibrating vest, or by lying in a vibrating bed. Secretion clearance techniques include suctioning, manually assistive cough, use of a mechanical insufflator–exsufflator, and bronchoscopy. Manually assistive cough techniques include the commonly used abdominal thrust, anterior chest compression, the counter-rotation assist, and the costophrenic assist.[27,298] The insufflator–exsufflator supplies a positive pressure to the airway, followed immediately by a negative pressure, either through the mouth or a tracheostomy tube. This rapid pressure change induces a high expiratory flow rate similar to a cough. It is less traumatic than suctioning. Bronchoscopy is usually reserved for persistent atelectasis or lung collapse (see also Ch. 35).

Medications are useful adjuncts in treating and preventing atelectasis. Bronchodilators can often reduce the airway hyperreactivity and constriction that contribute to atelectasis formation and sputum production.[11] They have been shown to reduce inflammation and stimulate the secretion of surfactant. Mucolytics can be given orally, such as guaifenesin, or via tracheostomy tube or nebulizer, such as acetylcysteine. Theophylline can decrease bronchospasm, stimulate the secretion of surfactant, and improve diaphragmatic contractility.

Finally, adequate hydration is especially important for maintaining thin secretions. This is often a challenge for persons who are unable to take in fluids of their own volition. For persons on ventilators, it is important to account for the insensible fluid lost though the ventilator when determining optimal fluid intake.

Respiratory failure requiring intubation and mechanical ventilation occurs in over one-fifth of newly injured individuals treated in a Model SCI Care System, usually within the first week after injury.[242] Signs of impending respiratory failure include hypoxia in conjunction with a rising respiratory rate, a falling VC to less than 15 cc/kg IBW, a falling negative inspiratory force to less than 20 cm H_2O, hypercarbia, fatigue, and tachycardia. If intubation is expected to last more than 5 days, a tracheostomy should be performed. There is a trend nationwide to use a low TV in the mechanical ventilation of any person with respiratory failure. This trend stems from findings of increased mortality in persons with acute respiratory distress syndrome who exhibit higher peak airway pressures when higher TVs are used. This mortality has not been seen in treating persons with SCI, whose main problem is restrictive disease due to muscle weakness as opposed to lung disease. Use of higher TVs in persons with SCI (>20 cc/kg IBW) has been shown in a non-randomized trial to shorten the length of time to wean them from the ventilator, from a mean of 59 days to a mean of 38 days.[362]

The mode of mechanical ventilation used conventionally in a rehabilitation setting has been assist–control (A/C) or controlled mandatory ventilation (CMV) during rest. Weaning then occurs as progressive ventilator-free breathing (PVFB), starting with a trial of as little as 2 min per day with the individual completely disconnected from the ventilator. Oxygen is given via trach collar or T piece. The time away from the ventilator is gradually increased in duration, in single or multiple trials per day, depending on the length of each trial, as tolerated. It should be borne in mind that, following lengthy mechanical ventilation, the diaphragm muscle becomes atrophied and deconditioned, requiring a lengthy period of reconditioning before ventilator-free breathing is achieved. PVFB is useful for persons who are not expected to fully wean as well, giving them some confidence and endurance to remain off the ventilator for a short period if an unforeseen problem occurs with their ventilator set-up. In one study that compared synchronized intermittent mandatory ventilation (SIMV) and PVFB weaning, PVFB was successful in 68% of weaning attempts, whereas SIMV was successful in only 35%.[361]

A further advantage of the use of the A/C or CMV modes of ventilation for persons with a tracheostomy, in contrast to other modes, is that it allows the individual to speak if the cuff on the tracheostomy tube is partially or wholly deflated. When the cuff is deflated, air expired from the lungs can escape around the tracheostomy tube and balloon up through the larynx to allow voicing. In order to compensate for the loss of such air around the tracheostomy tube and not entering the lungs, the set TV should be increased. Many individuals are able to vocalize while using a mechanical ventilator in this manner, timing their speech to coincide with exhalation. In addition, a one-way airflow valve can be put in line with the ventilator tubing, such as a Passy–Muir valve. This maximizes the airflow through the larynx by not allowing air to escape through the tracheostomy into the ventilator tubing (see Fig. 56-16). These one-way valves must be used only with a tracheostomy tube that has a deflated cuff or no cuff at all. Such valves can be attached to the tracheostomy tube alone to allow voice during the ventilator-free weaning periods as well.

Sleep disorders after SCI

Obstructive sleep apnea (OSA) is characterized by a repetitive collapse of the upper airway during sleep. This can cause fragmentation of sleep, loss of the restorative function of sleep, and increased sympathetic nervous system activity. It results in excessive sleepiness, systemic and pulmonary hypertension, and an increased risk of developing stroke or myocardial infarction.[164] The prevalence of OSA in individuals with SCI ranges from 15 to 45%, depending on the diagnostic method.[164] This is in contrast to a prevalence of 4–9% in the general population without SCI.[164,476] The use of antispasticity medications, which presumably decrease upper airway muscle tone, but not the level of injury, has been found to be predictive of OSA after SCI.[85,181] CPAP, a highly effective treatment that prevents narrowing and closure of the upper airway, is the treatment of choice. Unfortunately, even in those without SCI, long-term compliance with CPAP is low.[266,434]

Deep venous thrombosis and pulmonary embolus

Persons with SCI are prone to stasis of the venous circulation, hypercoagulability of blood, and intimal vascular injuries. These risk factors for development of deep vein thrombosis (DVT)

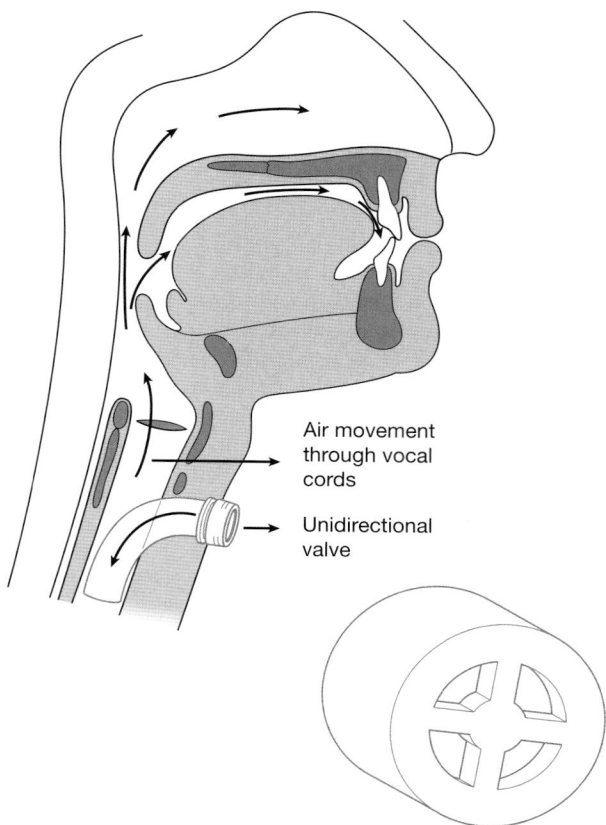

Air movement through vocal cords

Unidirectional valve

Figure 56-16 Functioning of a Passy-Muir tracheostomy speaking valve. (From Manzano et al 1993,[294] with permission.)

are known as Virchow's triad. Stasis is a direct result of loss of the muscle pumping action of the lower limbs and peripheral vasodilatation.[316] Hypercoagulability is caused by release of procoagulant factors following injury, while intimal injury occurs from trauma.[316]

The incidence of DVT after SCI, although it varies with the method of detection, ranges between 47 and 100% among studies that have enrolled subjects within 72h of injury.[66,317,333] The greatest period of risk is during the first 2 weeks following the injury, with the frequency decreasing thereafter.[317] The majority of persons with SCI who develop DVT do not have clinical signs or symptoms such as swelling, warmth, or pain. Using clinical parameters as a trigger to perform diagnostic testing for DVT, the incidence of DVT has been found to be only approximately 15%.[333,453] It is common practice to screen persons with SCI with a duplex ultrasound in the period of high risk.

Pulmonary embolism and the postphlebitic syndrome are not uncommon sequelae of DVT. PE has historically accounted for a substantial proportion of the mortality following SCI, particularly within the first year after injury. According to the SCI Model System Database, PE is the third most common cause of death in the first postinjury year, accounting for 10% of the overall mortality. The most common symptoms of PE include dyspnea and chest pain. Physical examination findings typically include tachypnea, tachycardia, and fever. Lung (ventilation–perfusion) scanning is the most commonly utilized diagnostic test for PE. A high-probability scan, which is defined as showing two or more segmental perfusion defects in the setting of normal ventilation, is considered diagnostic of PE with greater than 90% certainty.[209] A spiral CT of the chest with intravenous contrast can also be performed to accurately diagnose a PE located in the proximal pulmonary vascular tree. Pulmonary angiography, the most specific examination for PE, can be useful when the clinical likelihood of PE remains high in the setting of the other tests being indeterminate.[208]

Because of the high incidence of DVT and potential fatal outcomes of a PE, DVT prophylaxis is the standard of care. A clinical decision table for DVT prophylaxis after SCI, as recommended in the clinical practice guidelines developed by the Consortium for Spinal Cord Medicine, is shown in Table 56-11. The treatment regimen for a DVT or PE typically involves either intravenous unfractionated heparin or low molecular weight heparin given at treatment doses, followed by the oral anticoagulant warfarin, unless anticoagulation is contradicted. More convenient and more expensive than unfractionated heparin, low molecular weight heparins are as effective as intravenous unfractionated heparin, and are associated with less bleeding complications.[39] Warfarin is generally utilized for 3–6 months after a DVT is diagnosed to prevent progression and recurrence of thrombosis. Inferior vena cava filters are indicated for patients who have a contraindication to anticoagulation or have failed anticoagulation, as evidenced by a recurrent or progressive DVT, or the occurrence of a PE while receiving adequate anticoagulation.

Cardiovascular and autonomic system

Fitness and exercise
Persons who have SCI, both paraplegia and tetraplegia, often lead sedentary lives resulting in poor physical fitness and an increased risk for untoward cardiovascular events.[41,121,454] Persons with SCI, both those with paraplegia and tetraplegia, have a high prevalence of asymptomatic coronary artery disease as detected by thallium stress testing.[42,43] A low high-density lipoprotein (HDL) level is a known risk factor for coronary artery disease, and while approximately one-tenth of the US population has a low HDL, over one-third of persons with SCI have a low HDL.[44,75,222] Impaired glucose tolerance and reduced lean body mass are also significantly more prevalent in persons with SCI than those without SCI.[47,347] These metabolic abnormalities are thought to be directly related to poor physical fitness and lack of adequate aerobic exercise after SCI.

Upper extremity ergometry has been shown to enhance fitness and raise HDL levels in persons with SCI, although fitness levels are enhanced more in persons with paraplegia than in persons with tetraplegia.[154,235] This is probably due to a smaller muscle mass causing a lesser physiologic response in persons with tetraplegia as compared with those with paraplegia. Only high-intensity upper extremity ergometry, as opposed to low-intensity ergometry, with a target heart rate of 80% of maximal predicted heart rate, has been shown to be beneficial in lowering the HDL level.[237] Cycling, utilizing FES, has been shown to enhance fitness, decrease insulin resistance, and increase lean body mass in persons with SCI.[233,234,332] When combined with upper extremity ergometry, the gains in fitness are greater than those achieved with electrically stimulated cycling alone.[332,379] A 12-week circuit resistance training program consisting of six resistance arm exercises and high-speed, low-resistance, upper extremity ergometry has been shown to increase cardiovascular fitness by 30%, as measured by peak oxygen uptake. It also has shown an increase in upper limb strength by 12–30%, as well as decreased HDL levels for persons with paraplegia.[244,338]

Participation in a regular, vigorous exercise or wheelchair sports program can not only improve heath status, but also challenge individuals with SCI to overcome physical obstacles

Table 56-11 Guidelines for the prevention of thromboembolism in spinal cord injury: clinical decision table			
	Motor incomplete	Motor complete	Motor complete with other risk factors[a]
	CS, CB, UH	CS, CB, UH+, or LMWH	CS, CB, UH+, or LMWH; consider inferior vena cava filte r
Duration of prophylaxis	CB– 2 weeks; UH– while in hospital for ASIA D or up to 8 weeks for ASIA C CB– 2 weeks; UH– while in hospital for ASIA D or up to 8 weeks for ASIA C	CB– 2 weeks; UH+ or LMWH– at least 8 weeks	CB– 2 weeks; UH+ or LMWH– 12 weeks or while in hospital

ASIA, American Spinal Injury Association; CB, compression boots; CS, compression stockings; LMWH, low molecular weight heparin; UH, unfractionated heparin 5000 U q. 12 h; UH+, unfractionated heparin dose adjusted to high normal activated partial thromboplastin time.
[a]*Other risk factors: lower limb fracture, previous thrombosis, cancer, heart failure, obesity, and age over 70.*
(After Consortium for Spinal Cord Medicine 1997,[103] with permission.)

and to achieve greater functional independence.[201] Wheelchair sports can also improve psychosocial outcomes by reducing stigmatization, stereotyping, and discrimination by promoting acceptance of those with disabilities as fully functioning members of society.[201] Sports participation by wheelchair users has been associated with fewer physician visits per year, fewer rehospitalizations, and fewer medical complications over time.[112,430] Common organized wheelchair sports include basketball, tennis, table tennis, swimming, softball, snow skiing, sled hockey, track and road racing, rugby for those with tetraplegia (quad rugby), air rifle and pistol, archery, fencing, billiards, and bowling. These wheelchair sports require that individuals be classified, based on a medical history, muscle test, and a functional evaluation, to allow persons with different levels of disability to compete fairly.[219] Quad rugby, for example, was developed in the 1970s as an alternative to wheelchair basketball, because most persons with cervical neurologic levels of injury either lacked the capacity to play basketball or spent most of the time on the bench. It is a mixture of wheelchair basketball, ice hockey, and football played on a basketball court with goal lines on either end. A goal is scored when a player in possession of the ball, a volleyball, crosses the opposing goal line. A player in possession of the ball must pass or bounce the ball within 10 s.[219] All these sports can be performed noncompetitively as well.

Autonomic dysfunction

The autonomic nervous system is under supraspinal control, and therefore its function is disturbed by SCI. The autonomic nervous system normally controls visceral functions and maintains internal homeostasis through its nerve supply to smooth muscles, cardiac muscle, and glands.[407] The parasympathetic system has a cranial and sacral outflow from the central nervous system and modulates 'at rest' functions such as digestion, gastrointestinal motility, reduction of heart rate, breathing, and blood pressure. The sympathetic system has T1–L2 outflow, which is activated in stressful situations to raise heart rate and blood pressure, and to cause vasoconstriction to certain organs. Both the sympathetic and parasympathetic systems consist of pre- and postganglionic efferent nerve fibers that regulate visceral function through autonomic reflexes elicited by efferent nerves. Following SCI, autonomic reflex function is generally retained but, in those with high-level SCI, this is without supraspinal control. Some clinical conditions related to autonomic dysfunction are discussed below, whereas others are addressed elsewhere in this chapter.

Orthostatic hypotension   Immediately after SCI, there is a complete loss of sympathetic tone, resulting in neurogenic ('spinal') shock with hypotension, bradycardia, and hypothermia. The hypotension occurs as a result of systemic loss of vascular resistance, accumulation of blood within the venous system, reduced venous return to the heart, and decreased cardiac output. Over the course of time, the sympathetic reflex activity returns, with normalization of blood pressure. Supraspinal control continues to be absent in those with high-

level and neurologically complete SCI, however, who continue to be prone to orthostatic hypotension. This is defined as a reduction in blood pressure when body position changes from supine to upright. The symptoms associated with orthostatic hypotension include light headedness, dizziness, yawning, pallor, and occasionally syncope.

Management of orthostatic hypotension includes application of elastic stockings and abdominal binders, adequate hydration, gradually progressive daily head-up tilt and, at times, administration of salt tablets, midodrine, or fludrocortisone.[88]

Bradycardia   Bradycardia occurs in almost all persons with neurologically complete high-level SCI immediately following injury, due to unopposed parasympathetic effect. As the neurogenic shock resolves and sympathetic tone returns, usually within 2–4 weeks after injury, heart rate returns to near normal. Bradycardia can still occur with vagal stimulation thereafter, for example during tracheal suctioning. Bradycardia is rare during the chronic phase of SCI, except during episodes of intense vagal stimulation, such as during episodes of autonomic dysreflexia (AD), as discussed below.

Bradycardia during acute SCI requires close monitoring, but usually no specific treatment is required unless the bradycardia is extreme, for example less than 40 beats per minute, or is associated with sinus block. Intravenous atropine 0.1–1.0 mg might have to be administered prophylactically before tracheal suctioning and other activities associated with vagal stimulation. Persistent severe bradycardia can require insertion of a temporary or permanent demand pacemaker.

Autonomic dysreflexia   Autonomic dysreflexia is a syndrome that affects persons with SCI at T6 level or above, which is above the major splanchnic outflow.[71,165,334] It is caused by a noxious stimulus below the injury level, which elicits a sudden reflex sympathetic activity, uninhibited by supraspinal centers, resulting in profound vasoconstriction and other autonomic responses. The symptoms of AD are somewhat variable, but include a pounding headache; systolic and diastolic hypertension; profuse sweating and cutaneous vasodilatation with flushing of the face, neck, and shoulders; nasal congestion; papillary dilatation; and bradycardia. The hypertension can be profound and result in cerebral hemorrhage and even death.

The noxious stimulus responsible for AD frequently stems from the sacral dermatomes, most often from a distended bladder. Other causes include fecal impaction, pathology of the bladder and rectum, ingrown toenails, labor and delivery, surgical procedures, orgasm, and a variety of other conditions. It is probable that all people with severe SCI at or above T6 can develop AD after the period of neurogenic shock is over, given a sufficient stimulus, but the reported incidence of AD varies between 18 and 85%.

Treatment of acute AD must be prompt and efficient to prevent a potentially life-threatening crisis.[102] Recognition of symptoms and identification of the precipitating stimulus is paramount. The patient should be sat up, constrictive clothing and garments should be loosened, the blood pressure monitored every 2–5 min, and evacuation of the bladder done promptly to ensure continuous drainage of urine. If symptoms are not relieved by these measures, fecal impaction should be suspected and, if present, resolved. Local anesthetic agents should be used during any manipulations of the urinary tract or rectum. If hypertension is present, fast-acting antihypertensive agents should be administered, usually nitroglycerin or nifedipine. After resolution of the AD episode, the person's symptoms and blood pressure should be monitored for at least 2 h.

Occasionally, there are recurrent symptoms of AD with or without identifiable stimulus, a condition that requires chronic pharmacologic therapy. A variety of α-adrenergic (phenoxybenzamine, prazosin, terazosin), anticholinergic (oxybutynin, propantheline), and antihypertensive (clonidine, guanethidine, mecamylamine) agents have been used quite successfully for such purpose, but often with some side effects.

Thermal regulation   Thermal regulation is impaired in persons with SCI, especially in those with complete lesions above T6, due to loss of supraspinal control. Body temperature is controlled physiologically primarily by the hypothalamus and secondarily by personal behavior to increase or decrease heat loss.[92,278,293] Heat and cold signals are normally carried by afferent nerves to the hypothalamus, where they are integrated and thermal regulation consequently mediated by inhibition or activation of the sympathetic nervous system. With an increase in core temperature, sympathetic inhibition occurs with vasodilatation and sweating. A decrease in core temperature causes sympathetic stimulus, with vasoconstriction, shivering, etc. With high-level and neurologically complete SCI, the afferent and efferent pathways are interrupted. As a result, vasomotor control and the ability to shiver and sweat are lost. People with SCI therefore tend to have higher body temperature in warm environments, and lower temperature in cold environments. This is termed *poikilothermia*.

Most of the time, people with SCI maintain relative thermal stability. Nonetheless, in order to ensure continuous thermal stability, especially for those with high-level SCI, proper heating and cooling of the environment is needed. Appropriate clothing should be worn, strenuous exercise in a hot environment avoided, and cool moist compresses applied when body temperature rises.

Calcium metabolism and osteoporosis

An imbalance between bone formation and bone resorption occurs following SCI. The potential adverse clinical effects of this imbalance are fractures related to osteoporosis, hypercalcemia, and renal calculi due to hypercalciuria.[160,479] Primary bone resorption due to SCI is prominent during the first several months post SCI.[51,383] Markers of bone resorption, including urinary calcium and serum *N*-telopeptide, become elevated soon after injury and peak at 8–12 weeks post SCI.[335,383] Markers of bone turnover, including parathyroid hormone and 25-hydroxy vitamin D, are low initially after SCI, despite the usual normal serum calcium levels.[314] Serum osteocalcin, a marker of bone formation, is also low initially and increases during the first 6 months post SCI.[364]

Hypercalcemia can be encountered in those with especially rapid bone turnover, for example children or adolescents. Additional risk factors for hypercalcemia include recent injury, male sex, complete injury, tetraplegia, dehydration, and prolonged immobilization.[303] Treatment of hypercalcemia includes the administration of intravenous fluids, diuretics, bisphosphonates, or calcitonin.[90,318,319] A low calcium intake is not typically effective for lowering elevated serum or urinary calcium concentrations, and restrictions of dietary calcium and vitamin D intake are not recommended.[424] Persons with chronic SCI are often vitamin D-deficient due to inadequate nutritional intake or reduced sunlight exposure.[49] Secondary hyperparathyroidism can occur and lead to further bone resorption and osteoporosis. This process is treatable with calcium and vitamin D supplementation.

The degree of lower limb bone mineral density (BMD) after SCI has been correlated with fracture risk.[372,478] BMD is typically progressively greater as measured from proximal to distal sites in the lower limbs below the level of injury, while the weight-bearing vertebral column is generally spared the loss of BMD.[56,193] Patients with significant osteopenia of the spinal column should be investigated for secondary causes of osteoporosis.

A number of physical interventions have been studied in the hope of preventing and treating the loss of BMD. Individuals with SCI who perform passive weight-bearing standing with the aid of a standing device may have better-preserved BMD in their lower limbs than those who do not stand. FES cycle ergometry has been shown to provide modest reductions in the rate of bone loss.[206,226,277]

Antiresorptive therapies, especially third-generation bisphosphonates such as pamidronate and alendronate, have been shown to be effective in slowing the breakdown of bone after acute SCI.[324,479] Alendronate, given orally, has been shown to protect against hypercalciuria and a propensity to crystallize stone-forming calcium salts during prolonged bed rest.[385] In a randomized controlled study of 55 males with complete paraplegia, 1 month to 30 years post SCI, who were given either calcium 500 mg/day and alendronate 10 mg/day, or calcium alone for 2 years, only the subjects who received the calcium alone had significant decreases in the BMD below the level of injury.[479] Pamidronate, when given intravenously at a dose of 30 mg/month for 6 months, has also been shown to lessen the decrease in lower limb BMD seen after acute SCI.[337] Calcium and vitamin D are usually administered in conjunction with the antiresorptive agents, especially if there is evidence of a vitamin D deficiency.

Gastrointestinal system

Gastrointestinal complications

Although impaired evacuation of the colon is the most profound and universal change that a person with SCI will probably encounter with regard to the gastrointestinal system, there are several other gastrointestinal complications that may be experienced. Persons who are dependent on others for oral hygiene, i.e. persons with high tetraplegia, have a higher incidence of plaque and gingivitis than those who perform their own oral care.[425] In the acute phase of a cervical SCI, dysphagia is not uncommon. Factors contributing to this include immobilization of the cervical spine by an orthosis, soft tissue swelling or nerve trauma after anterior cervical spine surgery, and limitation of laryngeal elevation by a tracheostomy tube.[256,297] In the acute phase of injury, especially within the first several weeks after injury, there is an increased incidence of gastric erosions, gastric and duodenal ulcers, and perforation.[428] It is standard practice to administer gastrointestinal ulcer prophylaxis with histamine-2 receptor antagonists or proton pump inhibitors during this time, and usually for 3 months post injury.

Gallbladder disease and pancreatitis can also have an increased incidence in persons with high paraplegia or tetraplegia, due to decreased sympathetic stimulation to these organs.[23,91,172,213] Persons with tetraplegia also have slower gastric emptying than persons with low paraplegia. Adynamic ileus commonly occurs within the first 1–2 days post injury, but usually resolves within 2–3 days with bowel rest.[8,213] The mechanism is thought to be due to the loss of sympathetic and parasympathetic tone during spinal shock. An acute abdomen is also not uncommon early in the postinjury period, occurring in up to 5% of individuals.[37,53]

In persons with a complete high paraplegia or tetraplegia, symptoms of any abdominal pathology are likely to be vague and poorly localized. There can be referred patterns of pain instead of the typical localized abdominal pain that might be present in a person with a low paraplegia or no SCI who has the same abdominal pathology. Symptoms of AD, anorexia, altered bowel patterns, nausea, or vomiting can be present, any of which can be the most prominent symptom. Given the often atypical presentation of abdominal pathology in these individuals, it is not unreasonable to have a high level of suspicion for abdominal pathology, and a low threshold for ordering laboratory tests or abdominal imaging to confirm the presence or absence of disease.

Bowel management

The parasympathetic innervation to the portion of bowel extending from the esophagus to the splenic flexure of the colon, which modulates peristalsis, is provided by the vagus nerve. The parasympathetic innervation to the descending colon and rectum is provided by the pelvic nerve, which exits from the spinal cord at segments S2–S4. The somatic pudendal nerve, also originating from segments S2–S4, innervates the external anal sphincter and pelvic floor musculature.

An SCI that damages segments above the sacral segments produces a reflexic or UMN bowel in which defecation cannot be initiated by voluntary relaxation of the external anal sphincter, although there can be reflex-mediated colonic peristalsis.[420,427] In contrast, an SCI that includes destruction of the S2–S4 anterior horn cells or cauda equina produces an areflexic or LMN bowel in which there is no reflex-mediated colonic peristalsis. There is only slow stool propulsion coordinated by the intrinsically innervated myenteric plexus. The anal sphinc-

ter of an LMN bowel is typically atonic and prone to leakage of stool.

A bowel program is a treatment plan for managing a neurogenic bowel, with the goal of allowing effective and efficient colonic evacuation while preventing incontinence and constipation. A bowel program should be scheduled at the same time of day, usually every day in the beginning. The program should be scheduled later on at least once every 2 days to avoid chronic colorectal over-distention.[420] The scheduling of a bowel routine after a meal can take advantage of the gastrocolic response. Although a person with SCI should learn how to perform a bowel routine in bed and on a commode chair, regular performance of the routine sitting up on a commode is preferred to allow gravity to facilitate complete emptying. A diet high in fiber can help produce a bulky formed stool and promote continence. Medications can also be used, such as stool softeners to modulate stool consistency, stimulant and hyperosmolar laxatives to improve bowel motility, and minienemas and suppositories to trigger colonic reflex evacuation in persons with an UMN bowel. Stimulant and hyperosmolar laxatives, if used, are usually taken 8–12 h before the evacuation portion of a bowel routine.

Two mechanical methods are used to evacuate the rectum: digital stimulation and digital evacuation. Digital stimulation is dependent on the preservation of sacral reflex arcs, and is typically effective only for persons with an UMN bowel. Digital stimulation is performed by inserting a gloved, lubricated finger into the rectum and slowly rotating the finger in a circular movement until relaxation of the bowel wall is felt, flatus passes, or stool passes.[420] This typically occurs within 1 min. Digital stimulation is repeated every 10 min until there is cessation of stool flow, palpable internal sphincter closure, or the absence of stool results from the last two digital stimulations.[427] In contrast, digital evacuation is not dependent on the preservation of sacral reflex arcs and is typically performed by a person with an LMN bowel. Digital evacuation is performed by inserting a gloved, lubricated finger into the rectum to break up or hook stool and pull it out. Abdominal wall massage, starting in the right lower quadrant and progressing along the course of colon, is a useful adjunct for attempting to move stool along the colon.[101,427]

Genitourinary system

Physiology of the bladder

The parasympathetic innervation to the bladder, which modulates contraction of the urinary bladder with opening of the bladder neck to allow voiding, is provided by the pelvic splanchnic nerves, which exit from the spinal cord at segments S2–S4. The sympathetic innervation to the bladder and bladder neck or internal urethral sphincter, which modulates relaxation of the body of the bladder and narrowing of the bladder neck to inhibit voiding, is provided by the hypogastric nerves, which exit from the spinal cord at segments T11–L2. The somatic pudendal nerve, also originating from segments S2–S4, innervates the external urinary sphincter.

Spinal cord injury that damages segments above the sacral segments produces a reflexic or UMN bladder in which urination cannot be initiated by voluntary relaxation of the external urinary sphincter, although there can be reflex voiding. In contrast, an SCI that includes destruction of the S2–S4 anterior horn cells or cauda equina produces an areflexic or LMN bladder in which there is no reflex voiding. The external urinary sphincter of an LMN bladder is typically atonic and prone to leakage of urine. Because central coordination of normal voiding is felt to occur at the level of the pons, in a person with an UMN bladder due to SCI, coordination of contraction (or relaxation) of the bladder with relaxation (or contraction) of the external urinary sphincter is lost. This leads to a pattern of simultaneous reflex contractile activity called detrusor–sphincter dyssynergia, which often results in elevated bladder pressures.

Management of neurogenic bladder

The goal of management of a neurogenic bladder is to achieve a socially acceptable method of bladder emptying, while avoiding complications such as infections, hydronephrosis with renal failure, urinary tract stones, and AD.

During the immediate postinjury period, an indwelling catheter is placed within the bladder, as virtually all persons with SCI develop urinary retention. Later, other bladder management options are explored, depending on the person's gender, level and completeness of injury, and other comorbidities.

Intermittent bladder catheterization (IC) is generally accepted as the best option, other than regaining normal voiding, for the long-term bladder management of persons who can perform IC themselves. This is due to the physiologic advantage of allowing for regular bladder filling and emptying, the social acceptability of not needing a drainage appliance, and fewer complications than with other methods.[36] IC is usually performed several times daily with a target catheterized volume of 500 cc each time, for a total fluid intake of approximately 2000 cc per day. Using a clean technique for IC performance, in which the catheter is washed and reused instead of using a sterile catheter each time, is common in the outpatient setting due to its convenience and lower cost. It has not been shown to result in significantly increased urinary tract complications, including urinary tract infections (UTIs).[253,300] IC often needs to be combined with anticholinergic medications in persons who have an UMN bladder in order to inhibit voiding between catheterizations. To improve bladder capacity and permit successful IC when anticholinergic medication is unable to provide adequate bladder relaxation, or when the side effects of anticholinergics are intolerable, augmentation cystoplasty can be successful. The procedure involves harvesting a portion of intestine and attaching the portion of intestine to the native bladder to create a high-capacity, low-pressure reservoir.[283,409]

Reflex voiding is another viable option for male patients with UMN bladder in whom bladder pressures are generated that are greater than the outlet pressures of the sphincters to allow spontaneous voiding. A condom catheter is applied to the penis and connected via tubing to a leg bag or bedside bag. Reflex voiding can be sometimes triggered by suprapubic tapping. The completeness of voiding can be determined by measurement of a postvoid residual urine volume. High residual volumes predispose to UTI and bladder stone formation. Furthermore, reflex voiding is often associated with elevated voiding pressures, which can predispose to vesicoureteral reflux, hydronephrosis, and eventual renal failure. It is critically important for reflex voiders to undergo regular urodynamic testing to measure bladder pressures, and to have an imaging study, such as a renal ultrasound, to identify reflux or hydronephrosis.

Urodynamic testing is a procedure in which pressure sensors attached to a catheter are inserted through the urinary sphincter into the bladder. The bladder is then slowly filled with a known volume of water or gas through this catheter as pressures are measured in the sphincters and bladder. AD, when accompanying urination, is typically a clinical manifestation of high-pressure voiding. α-Adrenergic blocker medications, such as prazosin, terazosin, doxazosin, tamsulosin, or alfuzosin, are often effective in decreasing bladder outlet resistance and secondarily decreasing bladder pressures and postvoid residual volumes.[358] Two highly effective transurethral surgical procedures can also be performed to decrease bladder outlet resistance. One is the non-destructive placement of a tubular wire mesh stent at the level of the external sphincter. The second is a destructive transurethral external sphincterotomy, performed either with a scalpel or a laser.[93,382,393] Reflex voiding is a poor option for female patients with SCI, as an acceptable external collecting device for women does not exist at this time.

Long-term bladder drainage with an indwelling catheter is a reasonable option for tetraplegic persons who are unable to perform IC, or male patients who are unable to effectively maintain an external catheter on their penis. Use of an indwelling catheter inserted through the urethra is associated with UTI, bladder stone formation, epididymitis, prostatitis, hypospadias, and bladder cancer.[250,463] Placement of a suprapubic cystostomy tube in persons requiring long-term indwelling catheters can avoid some of these complications, such as prostatitis, epididymitis, and hypospadias.[290]

Although it is clear that UTI is a common complication, there is controversy over exactly what constitutes a UTI in persons with SCI. Symptoms of fever, spontaneous voiding between catheterizations, hematuria, AD, and increased spasticity, when associated with cloudy or foul-smelling urine and other nonspecific symptoms such as malaise or vague abdominal discomfort, strongly suggest the presence of UTI and the need for treatment. While the presence of pyuria can increase the suspicion that a UTI is present, it is unclear whether or not the presence of pyuria and bacteriuria should lead to the use of antibiotics if the person is otherwise asymptomatic.[130] Bacteriuria is virtually omnipresent in persons with neurogenic bladders, and certainly seems to occur in any person who uses IC, an external collecting device, or an indwelling catheter. Frequent treatment of asymptomatic bacteriuria can lead to bacterial resistance. Nevertheless, simple UTIs can be complicated by the development of pyelonephritis, epididymitis, orchitis, prostatic abscesses, and urosepsis. Over the course of time, recurrent UTIs can lead to renal scarring, secondary decreased renal function, and the development of urinary tract stones (see Ch. 29).

Sexuality and fertility

The parasympathetic innervation to the genital organs, which modulates erections in males and vaginal vasocongestion in females, is provided by nerves that exit from the spinal cord at segments S2–S4. The sympathetic innervation to the genital organs, which mediates psychogenic erections as well as ejaculation in males, is provided by the hypogastric nerve plexus, which exits from the spinal cord at segments T11–L2.

Men with complete UMN SCI are generally able to achieve reflex erections but not psychogenic erections. While the ability to have a reflex erection is often maintained, the quality and ability to sustain the erection is variable. Men with LMN SCI are unlikely to develop reflex erections and, although they are more likely to be able to produce a psychogenic erection, the majority cannot do so.[438]

Women with complete UMN SCI are generally able to achieve vaginal lubrication through tactile clitoral stimulation, but they are unable to achieve psychogenic vaginal lubrication. Women with both complete and incomplete UMN injuries report subjective arousal in response to psychogenic sexual stimulation, but only those women with incomplete injuries (in particular those with preserved pinprick sensation between T11 and L2) seem to develop vaginal vasocongestion in response to stimulation.[414,415] Women at all levels and completeness of SCI report the experience of orgasm, and over 50% of spinal cord–injured women in one study were able to achieve orgasm in a laboratory setting.[413]

The ability of men to ejaculate is severely altered after SCI. After complete UMN injuries, only about 10% of men experience ejaculations.[438] Even if able to ejaculate, the semen quality of men with SCI is poor, particularly with respect to sperm motility. Factors thought to contribute to this include recurrent UTIs; scrotal hyperthermia from prolonged sitting; stasis of prostatic fluid; and sperm contact with urine, which can result from retrograde ejaculation.[284]

There are several treatments for erectile dysfunction. Oral type 5 phosphodiesterase inhibitors such as sildenafil, vardenafil, and tadalafil have been found to be effective, and are now first-line therapies for erectile dysfunction after SCI.[200] Penile implants are available but are limited by a significant frequency of complications, including erosion through the skin and infection.[285] Vasoactive substances such as papaverine, phentolamine, and prostaglandin E_1 can be injected directly into the penis. These are quite effective in those without significant vascular disease, and reliably produce an erection adequate for intercourse.[322]

Treatment of infertility in men with SCI is focused on producing an ejaculate. The most commonly used medically assisted methods are vibratory stimulation and electroejaculation. Vibratory stimulation involves stimulation of the glans penis. This can be done at home. Electroejaculation involves the application of an electric current within the rectum, in close proximity to the hypogastric plexus.

Women with SCI do not have decreased fertility, although most women experience temporary amenorrhea post injury that lasts for an average of 4 months.[243] Pregnancy can alter the ability of a woman with SCI to transfer, perform pressure reliefs, and propel a wheelchair. The introduction of sliding boards and motorized wheelchairs can be helpful during a pregnancy. Because of the enlarging abdomen, self-catheterization can become difficult, necessitating use of an indwelling catheter. Respiratory function can be compromised during pregnancy, especially in women with tetraplegia. The onset of labor can be accompanied by significantly increased spasticity. Labor might not be perceived by women with injury levels above T10. Uterine contractions during labor have been associated with AD in women with injury levels above T6, and this needs to be differentiated from the blood pressure elevations seen in preeclampsia.[83] AD associated with labor, however, can be treated or prevented with epidural anesthesia.

Pressure ulcers

Pressure ulcers, also known as pressure sores or decubitus ulcers, are lesions in the integument caused by external pressure, typically occurring over bony prominences. While it is well established that persons with SCI are highly susceptible to developing pressure ulcers due to impaired mobility and sensation, pressure ulcers can be prevented with proper care. In order to promulgate proper care, widely accepted clinical practice guidelines for the prevention and treatment of pressure ulcers have been developed by both the Consortium for Spinal Cord Medicine and the Agency for Health Care Policy and Research of the US Department of Health and Human Services.[191,4,5]

Ulceration can be caused by low pressure over a long period of time or high pressure over a short period.[259] Pressure ulcers might not appear until a significant interval of time has elapsed since the application of damage-inducing pressure. Pressure ulcers, experimentally induced in dogs with a 1- to 12-h application of pressure over a bony prominence, became apparent on average at $4\frac{1}{2}$ days, and not before 3 days after the removal of the pressure.[259] Shear forces, which cause different layers of tissue to slide in opposite directions, can increase the susceptibility to ulceration dramatically, as has been shown in paraplegic swine.[146] Different tissues have different susceptibilities to damage from pressure, with muscle being more susceptible than skin.[346] Different people have different susceptibilities to the development of pressure ulcers, for reasons that are not always clear.

In addition to pressure itself, there are numerous secondary risk factors associated with the development of pressure ulcers, including immobility, incontinence, spasticity, limited activity levels, impaired nutrition, altered level of consciousness, and low satisfaction with life. Incontinence and impaired nutrition affect the structural integrity of the tissues, whereas the other factors lead to increased external pressures, in either magnitude or duration. Recurrence of ulcers after healing has been associated with smoking, diabetes, and cardiovascular disease.[229] Complications associated with pressure ulcers can include bacteremia, osteomyelitis, septic arthritis, advancing cellulitis, endocarditis, amyloidosis, anemia, squamous cell carcinoma, a fistula to the bowel or bladder from the ulcer, heterotopic bone formation, and maggot infestation.

In the early 1990s, the overall prevalence of pressure ulcers in the acute hospital or rehabilitation units of the SCI Model Systems after SCI was 34%. At 1, 5, 10, and 20 years after injury, the prevalence was 15%, 20%, 23%, and 29%, respectively.[473]

During acute rehabilitation, pressure ulcers are seen in the following distribution: sacrum, 39%; calcaneus, 13%; ischium, 8%; occiput, 6%; and scapula, 5%.[95] This contrasts with the distribution seen 2 years after injury: ischium, 31%; trochanter, 26%; sacrum, 18%; calcaneus, 5%; and malleolus, 4%.[473] The higher distribution of ulcers in the sacrum and calcaneus in the acute group is probably due to the increased amount of time spent supine in bed soon after injury, as opposed to more time sitting in a wheelchair later.

Assessment of pressure ulcers

An assessment of a pressure ulcer should include a notation of location, stage of wound, size, characteristics of the ulcer cavity, and characteristics of the surrounding skin. A common classification of pressure ulcers is the four-stage system advocated by the National Pressure Ulcer Advisory Committee (NPUAC), the Panel for the Prediction and Prevention of Pressure Ulcers in Adults of the Agency for Health Care Policy and Research, and the International Association for Enterostomal Therapy.[5] Stage 1 is characterized by sustained non-blanchable erythema. Stage 2 is characterized by partial-thickness skin loss involving epidermis and/or dermis presenting as an abrasion, blister, or shallow crater. Stage 3 involves full-thickness skin loss with damage or necrosis that can extend down to, but not through, underlying fascia. It presents as a deep crater with or without undermining of adjacent tissue. Stage 4 is characterized by full-thickness skin loss with extensive destruction, tissue necrosis, or damage to muscle, bone, or supporting structures (e.g. tendon or joint capsule). It should be noted that, when an eschar is present, accurate staging is not possible until the eschar has been removed.

The size of the ulcer can be calculated from a measurement of the length, width, and depth of an ulcer. Tracings of the circumference of the ulcer cavity orifice can be made on a transparent sheet of plastic, such as an overhead slide with an imprinted grid. Volumetric measures, obtained by infusing a known quantity of either liquid or semisolid material into the ulcer cavity through a syringe, can give a more accurate ulcer volume measurement. Photographs can also be helpful, especially if a calibrated grid or measuring tape is included in the picture. Characteristics of the ulcer cavity that should be noted include presence and extent of a sinus tract, tunneling, undermining, necrotic tissue, exudate, epithelialization, and granulation tissue. Characteristics of the surrounding skin that should be noted include erythema, maceration, and induration. Several standardized instruments, such as the Pressure Ulcer Scale for Healing Tool, the Sessing Scale, and the Pressure Ulcer Status

Tool have been developed, which incorporate many of these variables and characteristics.[40,175,443]

A determination of the potential causes of the breakdown should be made. The location of the wound is often very helpful in determining the underlying mechanism responsible for causing the increased pressure that has led to wound development. For example, a sacral ulcer in a bedbound patient might suggest unrelieved direct pressure from the mattress. A sacral or coccygeal ulcer in a person who is sitting with these areas in contact with the rear portion of the seat might suggest both shearing and direct pressure over the sacrum and coccyx from sitting. In this latter example, relieving pressure only in bed, ignoring the poor positioning in the chair, will not allow the ulcer to heal even with appropriate wound care dressings. A sacral ulcer that recurs after a person sits on a commode might suggest unrelieved pressure created by the edge of the cutout of the seat of a commode chair.

Treatment of pressure ulcers

Pressure ulcer healing comprises a sequence of loosely linked components that include inflammation, matrix synthesis and deposition, angiogenesis, fibroplasia, epithelialization, contraction, and remodeling. Growth factors are important determinants of this sequence. Different stages of wounds require different components in order to heal. Stage 2 ulcers might need only epithelialization, whereas a stage 3 or 4 ulcer can require matrix synthesis and deposition, angiogenesis, fibroplasia, and contraction.

Pressure ulcers can acquire necrotic tissue. Necrotic tissue releases endotoxins that inhibit fibroblast and keratinocyte migration. It is also an excellent growth medium for bacteria. The bacteria produce enzymes and proteases that degrade fibrin and growth factors, leading to impaired healing.[422,423] Removal of necrotic tissue, application of topical antimicrobials, and use of systemic antibiotics can minimize the presence of bacteria. Antibiotics are particularly important if there is evidence of an invasive infection such as cellulitis. Removal of necrotic tissue can be done by a number of different methods of debridement, including autolysis and chemical, sharp, and mechanical debridement. Autolysis is promoted when a moisture-retentive barrier is applied over a superficial ulcer, allowing endogenous enzymes to degrade the necrotic tissue. Chemical debridement refers to the application of commercially available enzymes that selectively degrade necrotic tissues. These enzymes might not penetrate eschar, and seem to be most effective for degrading thin layers of necrotic slough. Sharp debridement refers to excision of necrotic tissue or scar with a sharp instrument. Mechanical debridement can be performed with either hydrotherapy or application of wet to dry dressings. The latter refers to a process where moist gauze is applied to a wound, the moisture in the gauze is allowed to evaporate, and the dry gauze is removed with adherent necrotic tissue (and potentially newly granulating tissue).

Pressure ulcers should be cleaned vigorously at regular intervals to remove necrotic tissue, exudates, metabolic wastes, and bacteria. Irrigation solutions should be used that are non-toxic to healing tissues, unless the presence of necrosis and bacteria seems to be overwhelming the healing tissues. If this is the case, a more toxic solution, such as $\frac{1}{12}$ strength Dakin's solution, can be used until the wound is clean. The solutions should be applied under adequate irrigation force, usually between 4 and 15 lbs per square inch (p.s.i.). A piston syringe with a 19-gauge angiocatheter provides an irrigation force of 8 p.s.i.

Many studies have shown that wounds heal more quickly when the ulcer bed is moist rather than dry.[184,216,403] There are numerous dressing products on the market that have different properties and can be used to maintain optimal moist wound healing within the ulcer cavity. It is also important to maintain the intact surrounding skin, because maceration of the surrounding skin can prolong wound healing time.[472] The major dressing categories include transparent films, hydrocolloids, hydrogels, foams, alginates, and gauze dressings. Transparent films are adhesive non-absorptive semipermeable membranes, whereas hydrocolloids are adhesive wafers with water-absorbing particles that have a minimal to moderate absorptive capacity. Both allow autolytic debridement and are indicated for use in the treatment of partial-thickness wounds. Foams are non-adherent hydrophobic or hydrophillic materials with minimal to moderate absorptive capacity. Hydrogels are water- or glycerin-based gels with minimal to moderate absorptive capacity. Alginates are soft absorbent non-woven seaweed-derived dressings that have a cotton-like appearance, with a moderate to heavy absorptive capacity. Foams, hydrogels, and alginates all fill dead space within an ulcer crater, require a secondary dressing, and are appropriate for both partial- and full-thickness wounds. It should be noted that significant differences in healing rates have not been found when different types of moist healing dressings have been compared. These comparisons have included hydrocolloids, hydrogels, and saline-moistened gauze, as well as hydrocolloids and foams.[10,29,100,444] Other modalities that have shown benefit in small randomized controlled studies have included vacuum-assisted closure and electrical stimulation, the latter including both high-voltage pulsed current and transcutaneous electrical stimulation.[24,183,192]

Adequate nutrition is essential in order to heal a pressure ulcer. Caloric requirements are increased for a person with SCI having a pressure ulcer. Caloric need is 25 kcal/kg body weight per day, as compared with 21 kcal/kg body weight per day for a person having SCI but no pressure ulcer.[9,288] Protein requirements are also increased for a person with an SCI and a pressure ulcer, up to 1.5–2.0 g of protein/kg body weight per day, as compared with 1.0–1.25 g of protein/kg body weight per day for a person with SCI and no pressure ulcer.[4,76] Micronutrient deficiencies, especially of zinc and vitamins A, C, and E, are associated with poor wound healing, but supplementation of micronutrients in those without deficiencies has not been shown to enhance the healing of pressure ulcers.[191]

Bed and wheelchair support surfaces and proper positioning in them can help prevent pressure ulcers from developing, and help to heal them if they occur. Commercially available pressure-relieving support surfaces include mattress overlays, specialty mattresses, turning beds, cushions, and wheelchairs that tilt or recline. Mattress overlays, for example foam pads, gel pads, and static and dynamic air overlays, should be used by persons with significant sensory loss in order to prevent pressure ulcers over the sacrum and greater trochanters. Specialty mattresses, of which low air loss and alternating air types are the most common, usually provide better pressure relief but at an increased cost. These mattresses are indicated for persons at high risk, and those with either non-healing ulcers or pressure ulcers on multiple turning surfaces. It has been taught that persons with SCI and poor sensation need to be repositioned on to a different support surface every 2 h in any non-turning bed, whether or not a specialty mattress is used. One standard support surface position requires a 30° angled, side-lying position, with pillows behind the back and between the knees, in order to avoid pressure on the greater trochanter, sacrum, and knees. Another standard support surface position is the prone position, with pillows placed under the thorax, pelvis, thighs, and shins.

There are several programmable self-turning mattresses and beds on the market that are useful for those who are unable to reposition themselves. These often incorporate dynamic pressure relief systems, either alternating air or low air loss. Pressure-relieving cushions designed for wheelchairs, composed of air, foam, gel, or some combination of these, should be used by persons with significant sensory loss in order to prevent pressure ulcers over the ischial tuberosities. In addition, it is essential when sitting that pressure reliefs be performed approximately every 15 min for a duration of 15 s. Pressure relief techniques include a forward lean in the chair, a side to side bend holding each side bend for 15 s, a push-up, a recline, or a tilt back. The recline and tilt back techniques require either the assistance of another individual or a power chair with a recline or tilt back feature.

Stage 3 and 4 ulcers might not heal in a timely fashion, depending on their location and size, and operative repair to close the defect is often indicated. Individuals who cannot tolerate surgery for medical reasons, who have a short life expectancy, or who are unlikely to protect the area of operative repair are poor candidates for operative repair. Successful operative repairs typically include excision of the ulcer, the surrounding scar, and the underlying necrotic or infected bone. The coverage is typically a regional pedicle flap that includes muscle and its blood supply. Postoperatively, a person should be positioned off the surgical site for several weeks to allow healing. If pressure on the surgical flap is unavoidable, an air-fluidized bed is used (see Ch. 33).

Pain after SCI

Approximately 80% of people with SCI report chronic pain, while approximately one-third report chronic severe pain that interferes with activity and affects quality of life.[65,82,116,117,341,380,381,429] In one study, over one-third of persons with thoracic or lumbosacral SCI and pain were willing to trade the possibility of recovery from their SCI for pain relief.[341]

There are many different types of pain experienced by persons with an SCI. In order to organize the different types, which have different etiologies and treatments, different classification schemes have been proposed. One illustrative and comprehensive classification scheme is the Bryce–Ragnarsson SCI Pain Taxonomy, which separates pains reported by persons with SCI into 15 types. These types are distinguished from one another based on location in relation to the level of injury, (presumed) etiology (nociceptive versus neuropathic), and etiologic subtype (see Table 56-8). Descriptions of each of the types of pain and their treatments are below.

Above level mechanical or musculoskeletal pain

Above level mechanical or musculoskeletal pain is nociceptive pain related to bony, ligamentous, or muscular injury, and which occurs in areas innervated by segments three levels or more above the NLI. This means that the pain is localized by the patient to areas located above two dermatomal levels above the NLI. This category includes mechanical neck pain from a vertebral body fracture in the neck, which does not cause any neurologic deficit and is present in a person with paraplegia caused by a lower thoracic vertebral body fracture. It also includes shoulder pain in persons with a neurologic level at or below T1.

The enormous demands placed on the upper limbs of persons with SCI during their daily activities, work, and sports lead to a high incidence of overuse injuries and musculoskeletal pain. Overuse injuries are caused by repetitive motions and recurrent microtrauma, which can be aggravated by more major acute injury. The treatment of overuse injuries in the upper limbs depends on the specific etiology, but can be divided into overlapping phases:

- control of inflammation and pain with protection, rest, ice application, compression, elevation, and non-steroidal antiinflammatory drugs (NSAIDs);
- mobilization to regain joint ROM;
- strengthening exercises once 80–85% of painless ROM is achieved; and
- functional restoration.[22]

The goal is to achieve the previous level of function while preventing recurrence.

Shoulder pain is the most common and incapacitating upper limb overuse injury, and can be due to bicipital tendonitis, rotator cuff impingement syndrome, subacromial bursitis, capsulitis, and osteoarthritis. The prevalence of shoulder pain in persons with chronic paraplegia (data taken from questionnaires sent to community dwellers) ranges from 40% to 50%.[113,115,343]

Specific treatment (and prevention) strategies for shoulder pain originating from the rotator cuff in persons with SCI should include strengthening, stretching, optimizing posture, and avoidance of activities that promote impingement.[81] Strengthening of the dynamic shoulder stabilizers should occur in a balanced fashion. A program should emphasize strengthening the posterior shoulder muscles, including the external rotators, the posterior scapular muscles (rhomboids and trapezius), and the adductors. Wheelchair use promotes strengthening of the antagonists to these muscles, i.e. the anterior shoulder musculature.[81] Stretching of the dynamic shoulder stabilizers, especially the anterior shoulder muscles, is also necessary in achieving a balanced shoulder. This is due to the fact that these muscles often become hypertrophied and contracted through constant use during wheelchair propulsion and transfer activities. In one controlled study of wheelchair users, an intervention consisting of a 6-month exercise protocol (two exercises for stretching anterior shoulder musculature and three exercises for strengthening posterior shoulder musculature) was effective in decreasing the shoulder pain that interfered with functional activities.[114] Elbow pain in persons with paraplegia is also fairly common (16–35%), and is often due to lateral epicondylitis (tennis elbow).[115,410]

Above level autonomic dysreflexia headache pain

Above level AD headache pain is severe and usually described as 'pounding'. It is most common in a person with an NLI above T7. AD headache is associated with an elevated blood pressure, and often with diaphoresis, piloerection, cutaneous vasodilatation above the level of injury, bradycardia or tachycardia, nasal stuffiness, conjunctival congestion, and mydriasis. AD is usually triggered by a noxious stimulus caudal to the NLI, usually related to the bowel or bladder (e.g. bowel impaction or UTI), but it manifests itself above the NLI and therefore is a subtype of 'above level' pain. Treatment of AD headache is discussed above in the *Cardiovascular and autonomic system* section.

Above level compressive neuropathic pain

Above level compressive neuropathy pain occurs in a specific peripheral nerve distribution distal to the root level, in areas innervated by segments three levels or more above the NLI, and is attributed to compression of a specific peripheral nerve or plexus of nerves. Symptoms most often include either spontaneous or evoked numbness or tingling in a specific peripheral nerve distribution. This category includes median, ulnar, radial, and axillary neuropathies in persons with paraplegia. The signs and symptoms of carpal tunnel syndrome (i.e. numbness or tingling of thumb, index, or middle fingers; abnormal sensation on testing; or numbness or tingling with provocative tests) are common in persons with paraplegia. In one study, the reported prevalence correlated for the most part with the time since injury, i.e. 42% for a group 0–5 years post injury, 74% for a group 10–14 years post injury, and 86% for a group 20+ years post injury.[410] This syndrome is thought to result from a combination of repetitive trauma, as occurs with propulsion of manual wheelchairs, and ischemia from repetitive marked increases in carpal canal pressures, as occurs with push-up pressure reliefs or transfers from one seating surface to another.[198] Higher risk for developing pain has been shown in those who are overweight or use improper wheelchair propulsion biomechanics.[61]

Strategies of treatment and prevention of a compressive neuropathy at the wrist include avoidance of weight bearing on an extended wrist by substituting a neutral wrist position whenever possible, weight loss, provision of the lightest possible wheelchair that meets the needs of the individual, use of power and power-assist wheelchairs, and instruction and training in an efficient wheelchair propulsion pattern. This typically is a pattern that minimizes the forcefulness and frequency with which the wrist strikes the wheel, i.e. long and smooth arm strokes.[61,63] Side to side or forward lean pressure reliefs can be substituted for push-up pressure reliefs as well.

At level mechanical or musculoskeletal pain

At level mechanical or musculoskeletal pain is nociceptive pain related to bony, ligamentous, or muscular injury. It is localized to areas within two segments either above or below the NLI. This category includes shoulder pain in a person with an SCI with a neurologic level above T1, which is caused by capsular contracture or capsulitis, rotator cuff impingement syndrome, or shoulder instability. The prevalence of shoulder pain in persons with chronic tetraplegia is similar to that for paraplegia, ranging from 40% to 60%.[113,115] The etiology of shoulder pain after tetraplegia, in contrast to shoulder pain after paraplegia, more often includes pain that stems from shoulder instability resulting from weakness of the muscles that stabilize the shoulder joint. This category also includes pain localized to the neck of a person with tetraplegia, or to the back of a person with paraplegia, that is attributed to spinal instability, infection, or muscle strain. Pain due to spinal instability is often ameliorated by lying still or by donning an immobilizing spinal orthosis.

At level visceral pain

At the level nociceptive visceral pain occurs primarily in those with an NLI below T7. It originates from damage, irritation, or distention of internal organs or their supporting ligamentous structures. This category includes abdominal pain caused by fecal impaction, bowel obstruction, bowel infarction, bowel perforation, cholecystitis, choledocholithiasis, pancreatitis, appendicitis, splenic rupture, bladder perforation, pyelonephritis, or superior mesenteric syndrome. Pain that cannot be attributed to a specific pathology related to the internal organs or their supporting ligamentous structures should be classified as central pain.

At level central pain

At level central pain is neuropathic pain that occurs within two dermatomal levels either above or below the NLI. It is not related to nerve root damage, but to actual segmental spinal cord damage. The character is typically described as 'tightness', 'pressure', or 'burning' in individuals with thoracic level injuries, and as 'numbness', 'tingling', 'heat', or 'cold' in people with cervical level injuries. The distribution is characteristically bilateral, involving single or multiple adjacent dermatomes over the shoulders, arms, or hands for cervical injuries; single or multiple dermatomal bands about the chest for thoracic injuries; and single or multiple adjacent dermatomes of the groin or legs for lumbar injuries. The pain distribution does not have to extend around the body and can be localized to one area, such as the low back in persons with low paraplegia. It should also be noted that, rather than being paroxysmal, SCI at level central pain is typically constant. Movement of the spine usually does not affect at the level central pain. Surgical destruction of the proximal portion of a dorsal nerve root and its adjacent superficial layers of dorsal horn, known as the dorsal root entry zone of the spinal cord, has been shown to be somewhat effective in reducing SCI at the level central and radicular pain unresponsive to pharmacologic intervention.[156,171,188,339,340,378,475] Individuals who undergo this procedure usually lose one or more sensory levels above the NLI, depending on the extent of neurologic destruction. Finally, syringomyelia often presents initially with at the level central pain, either on coughing or spontaneously. The character of pain caused by syringomyelia is typically burning or dull aching, although it can be sharp, electrical, or stabbing, and can be localized either unilaterally or bilaterally.

Treatment of neuropathic pain

Different types of neuropathic pain after SCI result from different and often coexisting mechanisms, including peripheral sensitization, phenotypic switches, central sensitization, ectopic excitability, structural reorganization, and decreased inhibition.[471] As a result, some medications that are purported to be effective in the treatment of certain types of neuropathic pain are not effective for other types of neuropathic pain. Other pains might respond only to a polypharmaceutical approach, with multiple drugs, each targeting a different but significant and active mechanistic component. Unfortunately, it is not at all clear which mechanistic components are significant and active at a specific time in the course of many different types of pain after SCI. This, combined with a dearth of pharmacologic agents that have been shown to be effective in clinical trials, has made finding effective medications to treat central pain after SCI dependent on using sequential trials of different medications with different mechanisms of action.

Current drugs used in the treatment of neuropathic pain after SCI can be stratified into several groups: drugs that modulate peripheral sensitization and ectopic excitability by way of their effects on the sodium channels, drugs that enhance the descending inhibitory pathways from the brain stem to the spinal cord, and drugs that modulate central sensitization through actions on voltage-dependent and NMDA receptor-mediated calcium channels. Sodium channel modulators, all of which work somewhat differently, include carbamazepine, oxcarbazepine, phenytoin, topiramate, lamotrigine, mexiletine, and lidocaine (lignocaine). Drugs that modulate the descending inhibitory pathways by inhibiting the reuptake of biogenic amines or by interacting with the opiate receptors include tricyclic antidepressants, selective serotonin reuptake inhibitors, selective noradrenaline (norepinephrine) reuptake inhibitors, selective serotonin–noradrenaline reuptake inhibitors, tramadol, and opiates. Drugs that modulate central sensitization include both NMDA antagonists (such as ketamine, dextromethorphan, methadone, and topiramate) and drugs that affect the voltage-dependent calcium channels (such as gabapentin, and oxcarbazepine). Several of these drugs, including amitriptyline, valproate, topiramate, lamotrigine, and gabapentin, have been evaluated in small randomized controlled trials of treatments of neuropathic pain after SCI. Of these drugs, only lamotrigine (in persons with incomplete injuries) and topiramate have been shown to be potentially efficacious in decreasing pain severity.[89,153,180,227,437]

At level radicular pain

At level radicular pain is neuropathic pain arising from nerve root damage occurring at the NLI, or within two dermatomal levels either above or below the NLI. The character of the pain is often described as 'stabbing', 'shooting', or 'electric shock-like', although it has also been described as 'burning' or 'aching'. It is generally, although not always, unilateral and paroxysmal in its presence, radiating in a dermatomal pattern. The presence of allodynia or hyperesthesia is common, although hypoalgesia or analgesia can occur. When radicular pain is associated with spinal instability, spinal movement can exacerbate the pain.

At level compressive neuropathy pain

At level compressive neuropathy pain occurs in a peripheral nerve distribution distal to the root level in areas innervated within two dermatomal levels either above or below the NLI. It is attributed to compression of a peripheral nerve or plexus of nerves. Symptoms most often include either spontaneous or evoked numbness, or tingling in a peripheral nerve distribution. This category includes median, ulnar, radial, and axillary neuropathies in persons with tetraplegia; a lateral femoral cutaneous neuropathy in a person with upper lumbar paraplegia; and a peroneal neuropathy in a person with lower lumbar paraplegia. Pain associated with compression of the brachial or lumbar plexus can also fall under this category, depending on the NLI.

Complex regional pain syndrome pain

Spontaneous or evoked pain, allodynia, or hyperalgesia that is localized within two dermatomal levels either above or below the NLI and fulfills the following three criteria can be classified as complex regional pain syndrome (CRPS) pain.

1. It is not limited to the territory of a single peripheral nerve or root.
2. It is disproportionate in intensity to what is expected by the examiner.
3. It is associated at some time during its course with edema, skin blood flow abnormality, or abnormal sudomotor activity.

An intensive hand therapy program, including physical modalities, should underlie the treatment of CRPS in the hands, with pharmacologic approaches added as adjuncts.[81] Oral corticosteroids and stellate ganglion blocks have been described in its treatment in case reports.[110,198,280]

Below level mechanical or musculoskeletal pain

Below level mechanical or musculoskeletal pain occurs caudal to the two dermatomal levels below the NLI, but only in persons with a neurologically incomplete SCI or a complete

injury with a zone of partial preservation extending to the level of the pain. The presentation of this nociceptive pain can vary depending on the degree of retained sensation. Severe spasticity often causes below the level muscular pain. This category also includes pain from an ingrown toenail, a broken femur, or knee osteoarthritis in persons with incomplete tetraplegia or incomplete paraplegia with an NLI three or more levels above the dermatome in which the subject has localized the pain.

Below level visceral pain

Below level nociceptive visceral pain originates from damage, irritation, or distention of internal organs or their supporting ligamentous structures in those with a neurologic level above T7. In persons with a complete SCI, this pain is characteristically vague and poorly localized. It can be associated with symptoms of AD, anorexia, altered bowel patterns, nausea, or vomiting, any of which can be more prominent than the pain itself. This category includes abdominal pain caused by fecal impaction, bowel obstruction, bowel infarction, bowel perforation, cholecystitis, choledocholithiasis, pancreatitis, appendicitis, splenic rupture, bladder perforation, pyelonephritis, or superior mesenteric syndrome. Pain that cannot be attributed to a specific pathology related to the internal organs or their supporting ligamentous structures should be classified as central pain.

Below level central pain

Below level central pain is neuropathic pain that occurs caudal to the two dermatomal levels below the NLI. Its distribution is generally not dermatomal but regional, enveloping large areas such as the anal region, the bladder, the genitals, the legs, or commonly the entire body below the NLI. The character is often described as 'burning' or 'aching', although other descriptors have included 'pressure', 'heaviness', 'cold', 'numbness', and 'pins and needles'. It is usually continuous in presence, although the intensity of the pain can fluctuate in response to a number of factors, including psychologic stress, anxiety, fatigue, smoking, noxious stimuli below the level of injury, and weather changes. Pharmacologic treatment is as described for at level central pain at this time. Psychologic treatments, especially cognitive behavioral and relaxation techniques, can be helpful for selected individuals.

Spasticity

Spasticity is a syndrome of different components, including a velocity-dependent increased resistance to passive motion, involuntary muscle contractions or spasms, and hyperreflexia. The involuntary muscle contractions result from different muscles acting synergistically, typically in a specific flexion or extension pattern. Although spasticity can cause difficulty with mobility, positioning, and comfort, and can even predispose to skin breakdown, it can also be helpful for ambulating and performing ADL, for example allowing individuals to bridge their buttocks to allow them to pull their trousers over their buttocks. The decision of whether or not to treat spasticity, and how to do so, should be based on an evaluation that has identified all the activities and other medical issues that are helped or hindered by one or more of the components of spasticity. Activities that need to be evaluated, at least through self-report and perhaps by observation, include bladder management, sexual functioning, sleep, dressing, bathing, positioning, wheelchair mobility, and ambulation. Medical issues that need to be evaluated include the presence of pressure ulcers and pain, as spasticity can predispose to both and can be the underlying factor behind the development of these secondary conditions. Determining the specific patterns of involuntary muscle contraction is important as well, as non-systemic treatments of spasticity depend on the specific pattern, for example an intramuscular injection of alcohol or botulinum toxin needs to be targeted to a specific offending muscle in order to be effective. In addition, because the different components of spasticity often do not correlate with each other, different assessment tools that address the different components should be performed during any evaluation.[366] Common assessment tools include five-point ordinal scales for grading resistance to passive movement, such as the Ashworth Scale and a modified form of this scale, and ordinal ranking scales that rate the frequency of significant involuntary muscle contractions per unit time, such as the Spasm Frequency Score and the Penn Spasm Frequency Score.[26,60,356,419]

Treatment of spasticity

Stretching of spastic muscles is the mainstay of treatment of spasticity for virtually all persons with SCI. Steady static stretching, to the limits of the ROM of a joint, has been shown to result in a reduction of reflex activity that can last for several hours after the exercise.[402] ROM exercises should be performed regularly on all affected joints by members of the rehabilitation team, support staff, or family members, after instruction in proper technique. Proper positioning, in bed or in wheelchairs, can effectively control increased muscle tone, as well as provide a prolonged static stretch to spastic muscles, for example sleeping in a prone position provides a sustained stretch of hip and knee flexors. The increased tone in the trunk encountered while sitting in a wheelchair can be improved by slightly tilting the seat or by adding a wedge. The use of positioning orthoses or serial casts can improve spasticity by placing the affected muscle in a position of sustained stretch, for example a padded ankle–foot orthosis or cast can maintain a spastic ankle plantar flexor in the neutral position. In addition, passive standing on a standing frame or tilt table can provide a significant stretch to the hip, knee, and ankle plantar flexors.

There are many pharmacologic options for the treatment of spasticity. Many practitioners consider oral baclofen to be the first-line pharmacologic treatment for spinal spasticity. Baclofen is a structural analog of GABA, the main inhibitory transmitter of the spinal cord, and binds to $GABA_B$ receptors. Dosing can begin as low as 10–15 mg per day in divided doses, with gradual increases as clinically indicated. Although the maximum recommended dose is 80 mg per day, significantly larger doses have been both well tolerated and effective.[55,254] Adverse effects of baclofen include fatigue and dizziness, while seizures can occur with abrupt withdrawal. Diazepam and other benzodiazepines bind to the $GABA_A$ receptor. Benzodiazepines can cause physical dependence, as well as lethargy and diminished concentration. If utilized clinically, it is difficult to wean people off these agents, and weaning should be very gradual. Tizanidine hydrochloride is a central α_2-adrenergic agonist that has been shown to be effective in treating spasticity after SCI.[336] Adverse effects of tizanidine include sedation and liver function abnormalities. Dantrolene sodium differs from the agents discussed above, in that it has a peripheral, rather than a central, mechanism of action. It acts by inhibiting the release of calcium from muscle sarcoplasmic reticulum, inhibiting the excitation–contraction coupling of normal muscle contraction. Dantrolene has the potential for hepatotoxicity, and liver function tests must be monitored closely.

When only a few specific muscles are affected by problematic spasticity, targeted injections of these muscles with a neurotoxin, for example botulinum toxin, or an alcohol, for example benzyl alcohol (phenol) or ethyl alcohol, to weaken these muscles can be quite effective in reducing the problem.[217,412,419] Targeting specific peripheral nerves with an alcohol can provide similar effectiveness.[217] Botulinum toxin injected into a muscle binds to receptor sites on the presynaptic nerve terminal in the neuromuscular junction, inhibiting the release of acetylcholine and preventing neuromuscular transmission. Alcohols injected perineurally or directly into muscles destroy nerve axons and muscle in a non-selective manner. Needle electrical stimulation to localize motor points or peripheral nerves, or electromyography to identify motor end plates, can improve the effectiveness of the injections.[348] The clinical effect obtained by local injection of neurotoxin or alcohols depends on several factors, including the dosage administered, the size of the muscle injected, and the severity of spasticity of the targeted muscle. The clinical effect of a botulinum toxin injection can be noted within 2–3 days and persist for 3–6 months, while the clinical effect of an alcohol injection is more variable, with reported effectiveness persisting from 1 month to several years.[217] Resistance to the beneficial effects of botulinum toxin can occur with repeated injections due to the development of antibodies to the toxin. Local destruction of tissue by injection of an alcohol can be painful in persons with preserved sensation, while paresthesias can be induced by destruction of a sensory nerve. Pain is not typically caused by botulinum toxin. Alcohols, however, are significantly less costly than botulinum toxins. Finally, injections seem to be most effective when combined with an effective stretching program of the affected muscles.

The administration of baclofen intrathecally is the most effective treatment for severe generalized spasticity in persons with SCI.[356,357] Baclofen can be delivered intrathecally through a catheter that extends from the intrathecal space, out through the dura and spine, and through a subcutaneous tunnel, to a battery-driven infusion pump located in a subcutaneous pocket in the abdomen. The entire system is implanted, and there are no external components. Dosage adjustments are made by radiotelemetry using a handheld computer, while pump reservoir refills are performed percutaneously. Several different modes of drug delivery are available, including one that allows different rates of baclofen infusion at different times of the day. Candidates for placement of an intrathecal pump include those persons whose spasticity is uncontrolled by pharmacologic and non-invasive treatments, and who are reliable enough to consistently undergo regular pump refills. In order to confirm efficacy and appropriateness before a pump is implanted, the candidate usually receives an intrathecal bolus test dose of baclofen delivered via lumbar puncture. If the test dose is deemed successful and a pump is implanted, the intrathecal baclofen dose is gradually titrated until the desired benefit is obtained. Effective maintenance dose ranges are quite variable among individuals.

Musculoskeletal conditions

A variety of musculoskeletal conditions can affect persons with SCI and cause pain and reduce functional ability. Most of these conditions are preventable but, when they occur, successful management can be quite difficult.

Contractures

A contracture is a common finding in the paralyzed limbs of persons with SCI. A contracture refers to a fixed stiffness of a soft tissue, which limits joint motion in a particular direction.[255] Joint contractures can prevent achievement of full functional capacity, inhibit hygiene, lead to abnormal positioning with resultant pain or pressure ulcer development, and prevent use of a joint in the future should motor recovery occur in a delayed fashion. The primary cause of contracture is prolonged joint immobilization, but secondary factors include edema, muscle imbalance, spasticity, and local trauma. Certain joints seem more prone to develop contractures than others. Upper limb contractures develop primarily in persons with tetraplegia, and can interfere significantly with performance of self-care functions. At the shoulder, adduction and internal rotation contracture is quite common, and can limit transfer ability, grooming, dressing, and positioning in the prone position. Elbow flexion contracture often develops in persons with C5 tetraplegia due to muscle imbalance, and interferes with the ability to transfer, the ability to propel a wheelchair, feeding, and grooming. Flexion contracture at the wrist and fingers can also interfere with performance of self-care activities, although it should be noted that mild tightening of finger flexors in persons with C6 tetraplegia can permit a weak grasp through the 'tenodesis' mechanism. In the lower limbs, flexion contractures of the hips and knees interfere with proper bed positioning, transferring, and dressing, and increase the risk of developing pressure ulcers. Adduction contractures of the hips hinder perineal care. All these contractures, as well as plantar flexion contracture of the ankles, interfere with comfortable standing and ambulation.

Contractures are best prevented by proper positioning in bed, by performing passive ROM and stretching exercises of all joints at least daily, and sometimes by use of prophylactic static splints. One common static splint, which promotes a functional positioning of the hand (to allow lateral or key pinch and palmar grasp) for a person with tetraplegia is a nighttime resting hand splint. In this splint, the metacarpal phalangeal joints of the fingers should be flexed at 90°, while the proximal and distal interphalangeal joints should be fully extended. The wrist should be immobilized in the neutral position with the thumb abducted 1–2 cm. Additional preventive measures include effective management of spasticity and edema. Once contracture is present, aggressive ROM exercises are initiated, which often require pretreatment with pain medications. In addition, static and dynamic splints are used to maintain the maximally corrected position. Serial casting with adequately padded splints can be applied, and spasticity treated with medications administered orally or intrathecally, or by performing nerve blocks. Occasionally, surgical interventions can be required, for example tenotomy and tendon-lengthening procedures.

Fractures

Major trauma can result in a fracture of any bone but, in persons with SCI, fractures in the paralyzed lower limbs without major trauma are of particular concern. Significant osteoporosis develops in the lower limbs during the first few months after SCI, which makes the bones brittle and prone to fractures. The reported lifetime incidence of known fracture in persons with SCI is relatively low, or 1.5–6%, but some undisplaced fractures in the anesthetic limbs can pass unnoticed.[187,255,372,450] Fracture incidence has been shown for males with complete paraplegia to increase with time after SCI, from 1% within the first year to approximately 5% per year after 20 years.[478] Most fractures are caused by a fall during transfer activities, followed by ROM exercises, and those without known etiology. The most common site of fracture is the supracondylar region of the femur. The diagnosis of a fracture in an anesthetic limb can be a challenge. Most patients complain of recent onset of unilateral leg swelling, not feeling well, and having low-grade fever. On examination, a swelling and a bruise can be present. If the fracture is severe, a deformity or crepitus can be present.

Treatment of fractures in persons with SCI is usually non-operative, with a goal of preserving prefracture function, avoiding complications, and securing proper healing and alignment. Because most people with SCI are sedentary and not ambulatory, some shortening and angulation at the fracture site is acceptable. But rotational deformity should be avoided, as it would prevent proper foot placement on the wheelchair's footrest. Despite the osteoporosis in the paralyzed limb, bone healing usually occurs readily, often with exuberant callus formation. Most fractures are treated with a soft, well-padded splint. The anesthetic skin should be inspected frequently. Gentle passive ROM exercises of adjacent joints should be started relatively early, usually within the first month, or when there is evidence of callus formation, in order to reduce the risk of contracture. During the healing, the patient should be encouraged to sit in the wheelchair with the affected limb carefully supported and with the hip and knee flexed and the foot placed flat on the footrest. Circumferential casting, external fixation, and surgical internal fixation are associated with a high risk and complication rate in this population and are best avoided. However, surgical intervention is often justifiable for fractures of the proximal femur, i.e. intertrochanter and femoral neck fractures, and in persons with severe spasticity. This is especially the case when unacceptable deformity might result in a loss of function.

Neuropathic joints

People with SCI who are ambulatory despite profound sensory loss can develop neuropathic arthropathy, i.e. Charcot joints, in the lower limbs, or even in the spine. At greatest risk are those with posttraumatic syrinx and disassociated sensory loss, with impaired pain and temperature sensation and preserved touch and proprioceptive sense. The articular cartilage and adjacent bone surfaces erode, while hypertrophic sclerotic changes develop at the joint edges. Loose bodies of irregular shape and size often appear within the joint. Marked deformity and instability can result, with accumulation of intraarticular fluid. There is often a relative absence of pain. Initial treatment consists of protection of the affected joint with an appropriate orthosis, and minimizing weight bearing on the joint with the use of a walker, a pair of crutches, or a wheelchair. Similarly, surgical arthrodesis of an unstable or deformed neuropathic ankle or knee joint can be considered.

Neurogenic arthropathy affecting the spine is a relatively rare condition in persons with SCI.[342] The involved segments of the spine are below the neurologic level, usually at the thoracolumbar junction or in the lumbar spine. It is usually a painless condition associated with progressive kyphoscoliosis and loss of sitting balance. On imaging studies, a destructive process is identified that has to be distinguished from infection, tumor, Paget disease, or hypertrophic osteoarthritis. Treatment initially consists of immobilization with a spinal orthosis, but surgical spinal fusion might be indicated to reduce pain, improve sitting balance, or preserve mobility and self-care functions.

Heterotopic ossification

Heterotopic ossification (HO) is the formation of true bone in ectopic sites (see Fig. 56-17). HO has been reported to occur in 16–35% of persons with SCI, although recent reports from the National SCI Database suggest a lower incidence.[301,435] The majority of persons with SCI have insignificant restriction of joint ROM as a result of HO, and less than 10% have severe restriction.[179] Most commonly, HO develops within 4 months of SCI, and incidence rates decline with each year thereafter.[31,301,435] HO most often develops around the hips (90%), but other locations where it can appear include the knees, shoulders, and elbows.

Heterotopic ossification is histologically similar to normal bone, and has cortical and trabecular structures. For unknown reasons, pluripotential mesenchymal cells in soft tissue are activated, with local production of the morphogenic proteins of bone.[31] While the cause of HO is unknown, several risk factors have been identified, including a neurologically complete lesion, older age at time of injury, spasticity, and pressure ulcers.[272] No correlation has been found between HO and gender, race, level of lesion, or cause of injury. Progression of the HO is individually highly variable, as are its functional consequences. Bone

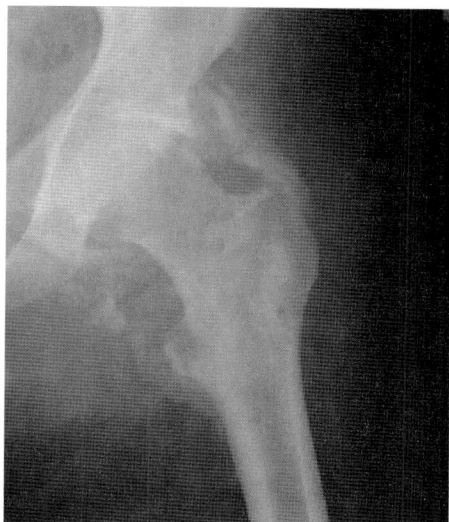

Figure 56-17
Heterotopic ossification of the hip.

formation generally continues for 6 months or more, after which the ossification gradually matures and stops growing.

Heterotopic ossification usually presents clinically as a warm local swelling adjacent to a joint. This is followed by a more generalized edema of the affected paralyzed limb. Low-grade fever can be present and, in time, joint mobility can be reduced. The differential diagnosis at this early stage includes DVT, infection, trauma, and impending pressure ulcer.[435] In its later stages, the swelling is decreased, but approximately one-third of those affected will have restriction of joint ROM sufficient to interfere with mobility and self-care.

Serum alkaline phosphatase during the acute stage will be elevated, and a bone scan of the area will be positive. Plain films will be negative due to yet insufficient deposition of calcium locally.[186,435] As the HO matures, the serum alkaline phosphatase and radioisotope uptake gradually diminish, and the HO becomes more visible on plain films.

Prophylactic use of etidronate or NSAIDs to prevent HO has been shown to be effective.[33,433] However, primary pharmacologic prophylaxis for HO is not felt to be justifiable, given the relatively low incidence of disabling consequences.[435]

Treatment of established HO should begin promptly[33] and aim to halt the ossification process, as well as to maintain joint ROM and function. One treatment protocol consists of intravenous etidronate 300 mg/day for 3 days, followed by oral etidronate 20 mg/kg per day for 6 months.[32] This protocol has been shown to be effective in preventing soft tissue ossification in most of those persons having only bone scintigraphic evidence of HO.[32] However, less than half the persons with radiographic evidence of HO show a response with inhibited soft tissue ossification.[32] Radiation therapy for HO is effective, but it is rarely employed due to unknown long-term risks.[390] Gentle ROM exercises are generally recommended, but forceful stretching is felt to be contraindicated until the acute inflammation has subsided.[435] Surgical resection of HO can be done when joint mobility is severely restricted, and interferes with self-care and sitting in a wheelchair. It should also be considered when the HO contributes to the development of pressure ulcers, or causes compression of nerves and blood vessels.[194] The goal of surgery is not to resect the entire HO, but to restore joint motion and functional skills. The surgical procedure usually consists of wedge resection and creation of a pseudoarthrosis. Postoperatively, the risk of recurrence can be reduced by administration of etidronate, antiinflammatory agents, radiation, and ROM exercises.[33,435]

SPECIAL POPULATIONS

Pediatric spinal cord injury

Spinal cord injury in children is relatively uncommon, but relatively common in adolescents. In the USA, 4.5% of all SCIs occur in children under the age of 15, but 20% occur in persons under the age of 20.[205,452] In young children, boys and girls are equally affected, but with age SCI becomes proportionally more common in males.[452] Motor vehicle-related injuries are the most common cause of SCI in children.[452] Unique causes of SCI in children include lap belt injuries, birth injury, child abuse injuries, and craniovertebral junction injuries.[258,291,350,452] Craniovertebral junction injuries are often related to juvenile rheumatoid arthritis, Down syndrome, or skeletal dysplasia.[452]

Children and adults with SCI experience most of the same clinical manifestations, which are managed in a similar or identical fashion. There are certain aspects of pediatric SCI that are different from adults, however, due to anatomic, physiologic, and developmental differences. These include spinal cord injury without radiologic abnormalities (SCIWORA), high cervical injuries, lap belt injuries, delayed onset of neurologic deficits, scoliosis, hip subluxations, and psychosocial development during childhood and adolescence.

The spine in young children has unique anatomic and biomechanical properties that result in much greater mobility at the cost of stability. This accounts for the different injury patterns seen in older children, adolescents, and adults.[350] Children younger than 8 years have significantly higher incidences of SCIWORA, delayed onset of neurologic deficits, and more neurologically complete lesions than those of older children and adults.[452] Among children younger than 10 years, SCIWORA is seen in 60%, but only in 20% of those who are older.[451] Although plain x-rays are normal, other imaging studies, for example CT and MRI, can show abnormalities of ligaments, disks, and spinal cord.[451] Children with SCIWORA often present with delayed onset of neurologic deficits, ranging from half an hour to 4 days.[350,451] This type of injury has been reported to occur in 25–50% of children with SCI. Delayed onset of neurologic deficits can progress rapidly once initiated. This has been variously attributed to vascular factors, to recurrent cord injury due to spine instability, and to the cascading early effects of SCI.

Neonatal SCI is reported to occur in 1 of 60 000 births, and is usually associated with breach presentations, especially when excessive longitudinal traction forces are subjected to the spine. This leads most commonly to a lower cervical or upper thoracic cord lesion.[350,452] In contrast, upper cervical SCI, when it occurs, is associated with a cephalic presentation and delivery.[350]

Craniovertebral junction injuries, i.e. atlantooccipital or atlantoaxial, are relatively common in children. Often they result in immediate death and can go undetected. Individuals who survive can require ventilation support due to high-level SCI.[350]

Lap belt injuries in motor vehicle accidents occur most often in children weighing less than 60 lbs who are wearing a regular lap belt above the pelvic rim.[452] A clinical triad of abdominal wall bruising, intraabdominal injuries, and SCI at or close to the thoracolumbar junction is often seen in these children.[452]

Medical conditions associated with SCI in children tend to be managed in a fashion similar to those in adults, with a few exceptions. Reflex bladder emptying is managed with a diaper in the infant, but intermittent catheterization is started at age 3–4 and self-catheterization at 5–7 years of age. A bowel evacuation program is started at 2–4 years of age. Hypercalcemia commonly affects adolescent boys within 3 months of SCI, especially those with complete high-level SCI.[303] Hypercalcemia is felt to be the result of immobilization and increased bone resorption. Symptoms include abdominal pain, nausea, vomiting, malaise, polyurea, polydipsia, and dehydration. Management of hypercalcemia includes hydration with saline infusion, and administration of furosemide and pamidronate.[251]

The growing child with SCI can experience a variety of orthopedic problems, the most significant of which are spine deformity and hip instability.[54] The prevalence of scoliosis can be as high as 98%.[54] Close observation with annual spine radiography is essential. The use of a prophylactic thoracolumbar orthosis is recommended by many, and almost always when curvatures exceed 20°. Surgical spinal fusion can significantly affect future functional skills, and is therefore best avoided. Surgery can be necessary, however, for curvatures greater than 40°.[54] Hip instability develops most frequently in children injured at an early age (29–87%), and is usually associated with muscle imbalance caused by spasticity, or by underdevelopment of the femoral head and acetabulum that occurs due to flaccid hip muscles.[54] Unstable and dislocated hips interfere with FES ambulation, but do not interfere with sitting or ADL. Treatment is usually directed toward prevention of contracture and creating bone stability by prophylactic application of a hip abduction orthosis.[54]

The rehabilitation of children with SCI is a dynamic and continuous process that changes with each stage of development during childhood and adolescence. Functional goals need to be reassessed frequently, and different psychosocial issues emerge with each stage of development. The goal of rehabilitation is to ensure smooth transition into adulthood and a high quality of life. Key areas of concern include emotional status, social and cognitive development, family dynamics, schooling, preparation and transition to adulthood, and sexuality.[15] Psychosocial factors, rather than level of injury or age at injury, are felt to be best predictors of life satisfaction.[14,15]

Geriatric spinal cord injury

Acute traumatic SCI in those over 60 years of age is comparatively rare, but its frequency has been gradually rising, from

4.5% of SCI cases during the 1970s to 11.5% during the 1990s.[315,345] When non-traumatic SCI is included, the incidence is vastly greater. More than half (58%) of 284 consecutive patients with recent onset of traumatic and non-traumatic SCI admitted from 1997 to 2001 to a spinal unit in a large rehabilitation hospital in Italy were found to be past the age of 50.[401] With the aging of the population in the USA, older individuals with SCI are likely to become a greater proportion of the whole.

Older persons with acute SCI are in many ways different with respect to cause of injury, male:female ratio, neurologic presentation, comorbidities, complications, and certain outcomes. SCI in older individuals is often related to cervical spinal stenosis and is caused by a relatively minor trauma. The causes can be as relatively low impact as a fall at home or in the street, or a low-velocity motor vehicle crash. SCI in the elderly is only rarely related to the risk-taking behavior often seen in younger persons.[315] Although SCI in older age groups occurs more frequently in men than in women, the difference is not as striking as among younger people. Older persons with SCI have a higher prevalence of preexisting medical conditions, for example obesity, diabetes, heart disease, and arthritis. After SCI, they have a higher rate of complications, including pneumonia, respiratory insufficiency, PE, renal stones, and gastrointestinal bleeding.[132,315,401] Older individuals are neurologically more likely to have incomplete lesions, which is especially true for lesions in the cervical region.[132,401] With respect to outcomes, older persons do less well than younger persons, reaching lower levels of independence in walking and self-care. They also have shorter rehabilitation lengths of stay, and are more often discharged to nursing homes than those who are younger.[132,315,401,474]

Aging with SCI was not much of an issue when the survival rate was low, but as life expectancy for all people with SCI has increased, various health conditions, functional change, and psychosocial issues associated with aging are now an important aspect of long-term management.[469] Normally, the aging process affects the various body systems in somewhat predictable ways, but it has been shown that SCI can hasten the rate of this process.[273] Longitudinal population-based studies on persons with SCI have shown that several health-related conditions are associated with age, duration of injury, and neurologic group.[94] These conditions include pneumonia; pressure ulcers; joint pain; heart conditions; fatigue; bowel problems; and rising serum levels of cholesterol, glucose, and creatinine. Functional decline occurs relatively early, especially among persons with tetraplegia, resulting in their greater need for additional assistance at an earlier postinjury time than for persons with paraplegia.[273,315] Complaints of fatigue increase significantly with age, and are associated with a greater need for assistance and a diminished ability to work and participate in a variety of community activities.[273]

Various conditions associated with aging have been described in persons with SCI. Many of these conditions are also felt to be related to a sedentary lifestyle, poor diet, smoking, and stress. Heart disease has doubled as a cause of mortality in persons with SCI. It has gone from 10.8% in 1973–7 to 20.6%

in 1993–8.[273] The increase in cardiovascular-related deaths might in part be related to abnormal lipid profiles, primarily very low HDL cholesterol levels, which have been reported in persons with SCI. Another cause could be abnormal carbohydrate metabolism,[46] as impaired glucose tolerance and diabetes mellitus occur relatively frequently in persons with SCI.[46] Initially after SCI, there is a rapid change in body composition, with loss of bone and muscle mass and a relative increase in body fat. But even during the chronic phase of SCI, such change continues at a rate exceeding that seen in normal aging.[45] In order to protect and improve cardiovascular health, nutritional counseling with dietary interventions, aerobic exercise training, and smoking cessation programs should be advocated early.[436] Medications to raise serum HDL or lower serum low-density lipoprotein cholesterol levels can also be considered.

Urologic complications are common at any age in persons with SCI, but with advancing age the incidence of renal stones and impaired renal function increases.[273] The incidence of bladder cancer has been found to be 16–28 times higher than that of the general population, which is felt to be related to the use of chronic indwelling catheters, smoking, and urolithiasis.[232] Gastrointestinal complaints are relatively frequent among older people with SCI, especially constipation, stomach pain, fecal incontinence, and bleeding hemorrhoids.[273] Neurologic decline during the chronic stage of SCI has been discussed elsewhere in this chapter, including development of PTS and entrapment neuropathies. Normal skin loses elasticity and collagen content with age, which would increase the risk for developing pressure ulcers. Time since injury, however, has not been found to be a major risk factor for developing such ulcers.[311] The incidence of pneumonia has been found to be significantly greater in persons with SCI older than 60 years.[311] Influenza and pneumococcal vaccines should be prescribed for all persons with SCI in this age group.

Older persons with SCI show a small but consistent decline with age across most domains assessed by well-recognized scales. Such decline is most evident in the areas of physical independence, mobility, occupational functioning, and social integration.[367]

SUMMARY

Spinal cord injury is a catastrophic event that results in physical disability and impaired function of various organ systems. Despite decades of intense research, a cure still does not exist. Great progress has occurred, however, in the management of SCI and its associated conditions. Because of advances in clinical practice, people with SCI have increased life expectancy. Morbidity is reduced as well, as reflected in reduced hospital length of stay following SCI and fewer rehospitalizations during follow-up years. Renal failure is no longer a leading cause of death, and the incidence of DVT has fallen dramatically. Spasticity can be effectively managed, and male fertility is now much improved. Application of modern technology has enhanced the function and quality of life of many persons with

SCI. The International Standards for Neurological and Functional Classification of SCI have been adapted worldwide as the preferred assessment instrument of persons with SCI seeking clinical care, and for those participating in research studies. Clinical practice guidelines have been developed for the most important conditions affecting persons with SCI, leading to greater conformity and quality in their care. People with SCI have established influential organizations and peer support networks that have advanced their rights and made health-related information widely available. Current wheelchair designs and seating systems are far superior to older models and, respectively, permit increased mobility and allow safe sitting for much longer periods of time. Computer technology has made it possible to develop FNS systems for standing, stepping, cycling, hand grasp and release, and bladder control. People with disability also now use computers in their daily lives for educational and vocational purposes with great success.

Advances in clinical care are no justification for complacency. The health and function of persons with SCI are still at risk without proper medical and nursing care, social support, appropriate equipment, supplies, and medications. Too many continue to experience problems related to urinary and bowel dysfunction. Many still have chronic pain that interferes with their quality of life. We must increase our understanding of the value of physical exercise and proper diet to reduce the high prevalence of obesity, diabetes, and cardiovascular disease in persons with SCI. Ambulation and complete self-sufficiency is impossible for too many. Social support is often lacking, and relatively few return to work. In order to solve these and other remaining issues that affect the wellness of persons with SCI, private, state, and federal support of health services is needed to improve the healthcare of persons with SCI, as well as a better social support system and a comprehensive disability policy.

The ultimate goal of persons with SCI and those who care for them is to find a cure for this condition, which is to reverse the neurologic damage of SCI. Until that elusive goal is reached, persons with SCI, their families, their caregivers, and society at large must work together to eliminate barriers to healthcare and ensure their full participation in all aspects of community life.

REFERENCES

1. Abrahm JL. Management of pain and spinal cord compression in patients with advanced cancer. ACP-ASIM End-of-Life Care Consensus Panel. American College of Physicians–American Society of Internal Medicine. Ann Intern Med 1999; 131:37–46.

2. Adams F. The genuine work of Hippocrates. Baltimore: Williams & Wilkins; 1939.

3. Agamanolis DP, Victor M, Harris JW, et al. An ultrastructural study of subacute combined degeneration of the spinal cord in vitamin B_{12}-deficient rhesus monkeys. J Neuropathol Exp Neurol 1978; 37:273–299.

4. Agency for Health Care Policy and Research. Pressure ulcer treatment: clinical practice guideline. Rockville: Agency for Health Care Policy and Research; 1994.

5. Agency for Health Care Policy and Research. Pressure ulcers in adults: prediction and prevention. Clinical practice guideline. Rockville: Agency for Health Care Policy and Research; 1992.

6. Agnew WF, McCreery DB, eds. Neural prosthesis: fundamental studies. Englewood Cliffs: Prentice Hall; 1990.

7. Ainsley J, Voorhees C, Drake E. Reconstructive hand surgery for quadriplegic persons. Am J Occup Ther 1985; 39:715–721.

8. Albert TJ, Levine MJ, Balderston RA, et al. Gastrointestinal complications in spinal cord injury. Spine 1991; 16:S522–S525.

9. Alexander LR, Spungen AM, Liu MH, et al. Resting metabolic rate in subjects with paraplegia: the effect of pressure sores. Arch Phys Med Rehabil 1995; 76:819–822.

10. Alm A, Hornmark AM, Fall PA, et al. Care of pressure sores: a controlled study of the use of a hydrocolloid dressing compared with wet saline gauze compresses. Acta Derm Venereol Suppl (Stockh) 1989; 149:1–10.

11. Almenoff PL, Alexander LR, Spungen AM, et al. Bronchodilatory effects of ipratropium bromide in patients with tetraplegia. Paraplegia 1995; 33:274–277.

12. American Spinal Injury Association. International Standards for Neurological Classification of Spinal Cord Injury. Chicago: ASIA; 2002.

13. Anderson BE. Driving assessment in spinal cord injury patients. In: Kirshblum S, Campagnolo DI, DeLisa JA, eds. Spinal cord medicine. Philadelphia: Lippincott Williams & Wilkins; 2002:348–359.

14. Anderson CJ, Krajci KA, Vogel LC. Life satisfaction in adults with pediatric-onset spinal cord injuries. J Spinal Cord Med 2002; 25:184–190.

15. Anderson CJ. Psychosocial and sexuality issues in pediatric spinal cord injury. Top Spinal Cord Inj Rehabil 1997; 3:70–78.

16. Anderson LD, D'Alonzo RT. Fractures of the odontoid process of the axis. J Bone Joint Surg Am 2004; 86-A:2081.

17. [Anonymous]. 2004 annual statistical report for the Model Spinal Cord Injury Care Systems. Birmingham: National Spinal Cord Injury Statistical Center. Online. Available: http://www.spinalcord.uab.edu

18. [Anonymous]. Americans with Disabilities Act of 1990. 42 USC 12101 et seq. 1990.

19. [Anonymous]. Spinal cord injury facts and figures at a glance. Birmingham: National Spinal Cord Injury Statistical Center; 2004.

20. [Anonymous]. Ticket to Work and Work Incentives Improvement Act of 1999. Public Law 106–170.1999.

21. Anson JA, Spetzler RF. Interventional neuroradiology for spinal pathology. Clin Neurosurg 1992; 39:388–417.

22. Apple DF Jr, Cody R, Allen A. Overuse syndrome of the upper limb in people with spinal cord injury. In: Sowell TT, ed. Physical fitness: a guide for individuals with spinal cord injury. Washington: Veterans Health Administration; 1996:97–107.

23. Apstein MD, Dalecki-Chipperfield K. Spinal cord injury is a risk factor for gallstone disease. Gastroenterology 1987; 92:966–968.

24. Argenta LC, Morykwas MJ. Vacuum-assisted closure: a new method for wound control and treatment: clinical experience. Ann Plast Surg 1997; 38:563–576, discussion 577.

25. Arguello F, Baggs RB, Duerst RE, et al. Pathogenesis of vertebral metastasis and epidural spinal cord compression. Cancer 1990; 65:98–106.

26. Ashworth B. Preliminary trial of carisoprodol in multiple sclerosis. Practitioner 1964; 192:540–542.

27. Bach JR. Mechanical insufflation-exsufflation. Comparison of peak expiratory flows with manually assisted and unassisted coughing techniques. Chest 1993; 104:1553–1562.

28. Baker LL, McNeil DR, Benton LA. Neuromuscular electrical stimulation: a practical guide. 3rd edn. California: Rancho Los Amigos Medical Center; 1993.

29. Bale S, Squires D, Varnon T, et al. A comparison of two dressings in pressure sore management. J Wound Care 1997; 6:463–466.

30. Bamberger DM. Osteomyelitis. A commonsense approach to antibiotic and surgical treatment. Postgrad Med 1993; 94:177–182, 184.

31. Banovac K, Banovac F. Heterotopic ossification. In: Kirshblum S, Campagnolo DI, DeLisa JA, eds. Spinal cord medicine. Philadelphia: Lippincott Williams & Wilkins; 2002:252–260.

32. Banovac K, Gonzalez F, Renfree KJ. Treatment of heterotopic ossification after spinal cord injury. J Spinal Cord Med 1997; 20:60–65.

33. Banovac K, Sherman AL, Estores IM, et al. Prevention and treatment of heterotopic ossification after spinal cord injury. J Spinal Cord Med 2004; 27:376–382.

34. Barakos JA, Mark AS, Dillon WP, et al. MR imaging of acute transverse myelitis and AIDS myelopathy. J Comput Assist Tomogr 1990; 14: 45–50.

35. Barbeau H, Rossignol S. Recovery of locomotion after chronic spinalization in the adult cat. Brain Res 1987; 412:84–95.

36. Barkin M, Dolfin D, Herschorn S, et al. The urologic care of the spinal cord injury patient. J Urol 1983; 129:335–339.

37. Bar-On Z, Ohry A. The acute abdomen in spinal cord injury individuals. Paraplegia 1995; 33:704–706.

38. Bass JB Jr, Farer LS, Hopewell PC, et al. Treatment of tuberculosis and tuberculosis infection in adults and children. American Thoracic Society and the Centers for Disease Control and Prevention. Am J Respir Crit Care Med 1994; 149:1359–1374.

39. Bates SM, Ginsberg JS. Clinical practice. Treatment of deep-vein thrombosis. N Engl J Med 2004; 351:268–277.

40. Bates-Jensen BM. Indices to include in wound healing assessment. Adv Wound Care 1995; 8(suppl):25–33.

41. Bauman WA, Adkins RH, Spungen AM, et al. Is immobilization associated with an abnormal lipoprotein profile? Observations from a diverse cohort. Spinal Cord 1999; 37:485–493.

42. Bauman WA, Raza M, Chayes Z, et al. Tomographic thallium-201 myocardial perfusion imaging after intravenous dipyridamole in asymptomatic subjects with quadriplegia. Arch Phys Med Rehabil 1993; 74:740–744.

43. Bauman WA, Raza M, Spungen AM, et al. Cardiac stress testing with thallium-201 imaging reveals silent ischemia in individuals with paraplegia. Arch Phys Med Rehabil 1994; 75:946–950.

44. Bauman WA, Spungen AM, Zhong YG, et al. Depressed serum high density lipoprotein cholesterol levels in veterans with spinal cord injury. Paraplegia 1992; 30:697–703.

45. Bauman WA, Spungen AM. Body composition in aging: adverse changes in able-bodied persons and in those with spinal cord injury. Top Spinal Cord Inj Rehabil 2001; 6:22–36.

46. Bauman WA, Spungen AM. Carbohydrate and lipid metabolism in chronic spinal cord injury. J Spinal Cord Med 2001; 24:266–277.

47. Bauman WA, Spungen AM. Disorders of carbohydrate and lipid metabolism in veterans with paraplegia or quadriplegia: a model of premature aging. Metabolism 1994; 43:749–756.

48. Bauman WA, Spungen AM. Endocrinology and metabolism after spinal cord injury. In: Kirshblum S, Campagnolo DI, DeLisa JA, eds. Spinal cord medicine. Philadelphia: Lippincott Williams & Wilkins; 2002:164–180.

49. Bauman WA, Spungen AM. Metabolic changes in persons after spinal cord injury. Phys Med Rehabil Clin North Am 2000; 11:109–140.

50. Bergman SB, Yarkony GM, Stiens SA. Spinal cord injury rehabilitation. 2. Medical complications. Arch Phys Med Rehabil 1997; 78:S53–S58.

51. Bergmann P, Heilporn A, Schoutens A, et al. Longitudinal study of calcium and bone metabolism in paraplegic patients. Paraplegia 1977; 15: 147–159.

52. Berkowitz M, Harvey C, Greene CG, et al. The economic consequences of traumatic spinal cord injury. New York: Demos Publishers; 1992.

53. Berlly MH, Wilmot CB. Acute abdominal emergencies during the first four weeks after spinal cord injury. Arch Phys Med Rehabil 1984; 65: 687–690.

54. Betz RR. Orthopaedic problems in the child with spinal cord injury. Top Spinal Cord Inj Rehabil 1997; 3:9–19.

55. Bianchine JR. Drugs for Parkinson's disease, spasticity and acute muscle spasms. In: Goodman LS, et al, eds. The pharmacological basis of therapeutics. 7th edn. New York: MacMillan; 1995.

56. Biering-Sorensen F, Bohr HH, Schaadt OP. Longitudinal study of bone mineral content in the lumbar spine, the forearm and the lower extremities after spinal cord injury. Eur J Clin Invest 1990; 20:330–335.

57. Black P. Spinal metastasis: current status and recommended guidelines for management. Neurosurgery 1979; 5:726–746.

58. Blight AR, Young W. Central axons in injured cat spinal cord recover electrophysiological function following remyelination by Schwann cells. J Neurol Sci 1989; 91:15–34.

59. Blight AR. Morphometric analysis of blood vessels in chronic experimental spinal cord injury: hypervascularity and recovery of function. J Neurol Sci 1991; 106:158–174.

60. Bohannon RW, Smith MB. Interrater reliability of a modified Ashworth Scale of Muscle Spasticity. Phys Ther 1987; 67:206–207.

61. Boninger ML, Cooper RA, Baldwin MA, et al. Wheelchair pushrim kinetics: body weight and median nerve function. Arch Phys Med Rehabil 1999; 80:910–915.

62. Boninger ML, Impink BG, Cooper RA, et al. Relation between median and ulnar nerve function and wrist kinematics during wheelchair propulsion. Arch Phys Med Rehabil 2004; 85:1141–1145.

63. Boninger ML, Souza AL, Cooper RA, et al. Propulsion patterns and pushrim biomechanics in manual wheelchair propulsion. Arch Phys Med Rehabil 2002; 83:718–723.

64. Bosch A, Stauffer ES, Nickel VL. Incomplete traumatic quadriplegia. A ten-year review. JAMA 1971; 216:473–478.

65. Botterell EH, Callaghan JC, Jousse AT. Pain in paraplegia; clinical management and surgical treatment. Proc R Soc Med 1954; 47:281–288.

66. Brach BB, Moser KM, Cedar L, et al. Venous thrombosis in acute spinal cord paralysis. J Trauma 1977; 17:289–292.

67. Bracken MB, Collins WF, Freeman DF, et al. Efficacy of methylprednisolone in acute spinal cord injury. JAMA 1984; 251:45–52.

68. Bracken MB, Freeman DH Jr, Hellenbrand K. Incidence of acute traumatic hospitalized spinal cord injury in the United States, 1970–1977. Am J Epidemiol 1981; 113:615–622.

69. Bracken MB, Shepard MJ, Collins WF, et al. A randomized, controlled trial of methylprednisolone or naloxone in the treatment of acute spinal-cord injury. Results of the Second National Acute Spinal Cord Injury Study. N Engl J Med 1990; 322:1405–1411.

70. Bracken MB, Shepard MJ, Holford TR, et al. Administration of methylprednisolone for 24 or 48 hours or tirilazad mesylate for 48 hours in the treatment of acute spinal cord injury. Results of the Third National Acute Spinal Cord Injury Randomized Controlled Trial. National Acute Spinal Cord Injury Study. JAMA 1997; 277:1597–1604.

71. Braddom RL, Rocco JF. Autonomic dysreflexia. A survey of current treatment. Am J Phys Med Rehabil 1991; 70:234–241.

72. Braughler JM, Hall ED, Means ED, et al. Evaluation of an intensive methylprednisolone sodium succinate dosing regimen in experimental spinal cord injury. J Neurosurg 1987; 67:102–105.

73. Braughler JM, Hall ED. Central nervous system trauma and stroke. I. Biochemical considerations for oxygen radical formation and lipid peroxidation. Free Radic Biol Med 1989; 6:289–301.

74. Breasted JH. The Edwin Smith Surgical Papyrus (vol 1: B16–B42 and 425–428). Chicago: 1930.

75. Brenes G, Dearwater S, Shapera R, et al. High density lipoprotein cholesterol concentrations in physically active and sedentary spinal cord injured patients. Arch Phys Med Rehabil 1986; 67:445–450.

76. Breslow RA, Hallfrisch J, Guy DG, et al. The importance of dietary protein in healing pressure ulcers. J Am Geriatr Soc 1993; 41:357–362.

77. Brindley GS. The first 500 patients with sacral anterior root stimulator implants: general description. Paraplegia 1994; 32:795–805.

78. Brown PJ, Marino RJ, Herbison GJ, et al. The 72-hour examination as a predictor of recovery in motor complete quadriplegia. Arch Phys Med Rehabil 1991; 72:546–548.

79. Brown RD Jr, Zimmermann KP. Transportation: advances in rehabilitation technology. Phys Med Rehabil State Art Rev 1997; 11:55–67.

80. de Bruin ED, Frey-Rindova P, Herzog RE, et al. Changes of tibia bone properties after spinal cord injury: effects of early intervention. Arch Phys Med Rehabil 1999; 80:214–220.

81. Bryce T, Ragnarsson K. Pain management in persons with spinal cord disorders. In: Lin VW, ed. Spinal cord medicine: principles and practice. New York: Demos; 2003.

82. Burke DC. Pain in paraplegia. Paraplegia 1973; 10:297–313.

83. Burns AS, Jackson AB. Gynecologic and reproductive issues in women with spinal cord injury. Phys Med Rehabil Clin North Am 2001; 12: 183–199.

84. Burns SP, Golding DG, Rolle WA Jr, et al. Recovery of ambulation in motor–incomplete tetraplegia. Arch Phys Med Rehabil 1997; 78: 1169–1172.

85. Burns SP, Little JW, Hussey JD, et al. Sleep apnea syndrome in chronic spinal cord injury: associated factors and treatment. Arch Phys Med Rehabil 2000; 81:1334–1339.

86. Bursell JP, Little JW, Stiens SA. Electrodiagnosis in spinal cord injured persons with new weakness or sensory loss: central and peripheral etiologies. Arch Phys Med Rehabil 1999; 80:904–909.

87. Campagnolo DI, Heary RF. Acute medical and surgical management of spinal cord injury. In: Kirshblum S, Campagnolo DI, DeLisa JA, eds. Spinal cord medicine. Philadelphia: Lippincott Williams & Wilkins; 2002: 96–107.

88. Campagnolo DI, Merli GJ. Autonomic and cardiovascular complications of spinal cord injury. In: Kirshblum S, Campagnolo DI, DeLisa JA, eds. Spinal cord medicine. Philadelphia: Lippincott Williams & Wilkins; 2002:123–134.

89. Cardenas DD, Warms CA, Turner JA, et al. Efficacy of amitriptyline for relief of pain in spinal cord injury: results of a randomized controlled trial. Pain 2002; 96:365–373.

90. Carey DE, Raisz LG. Calcitonin therapy in prolonged immobilization hypercalcemia. Arch Phys Med Rehabil 1985; 66:640–644.

91. Carey ME, Nance FC, Kirgis HD, et al. Pancreatitis following spinal cord injury. J Neurosurg 1977; 47:917–922.

92. Cesario TC, Darouiche RO. Thermal regulation in the SCI patient. In: Lin VW, ed. Spinal cord medicine: principles and practice. New York: Demos; 2003:209–211.

93. Chancellor MB, Rivas DA, Abdill CK, et al. Management of sphincter dyssynergia using the sphincter stent prosthesis in chronically catheterized SCI men. J Spinal Cord Med 1995; 18:88–94.

94. Charlifue SW, Weitzenkamp DA, Whiteneck GG. Longitudinal outcomes in spinal cord injury: aging, secondary conditions, and well-being. Arch Phys Med Rehabil 1999; 80:1429–1434.

95. Chen D, Apple DF Jr, Hudson LM, et al. Medical complications during acute rehabilitation following spinal cord injury—current experience of the Model Systems. Arch Phys Med Rehabil 1999; 80:1397–1401.

96. Choi DW. Excitotoxic cell death. J Neurobiol 1992; 23:1261–1276.

97. Coggrave MJ, Rose LS. A specialist seating assessment clinic: changing pressure relief practice. Spinal Cord 2003; 41:692–695.

98. Cohen M. Initial resuscitation of the patient with spinal cord injury. Trauma Q 1993; 9:38–43.

99. Coleman WP, Benzel D, Cahill DW, et al. A critical appraisal of the reporting of the National Acute Spinal Cord Injury Studies (II and III) of methylprednisolone in acute spinal cord injury. J Spinal Disord 2000; 13:185–199.

100. Colwell JC, Foreman MD, Trotter JP. A comparison of the efficacy and cost-effectiveness of two methods of managing pressure ulcers. Decubitus 1993; 6:28–36.

101. Comarr AE. Bowel regulation for patients with spinal cord injury. JAMA 1958; 167:18–21.

102. Consortium for Spinal Cord Medicine. Acute management of autonomic dysreflexia: adults with spinal cord injury presenting to health-care facilities. J Spinal Cord Med 1997; 20:284–308.

103. Consortium for Spinal Cord Medicine. Clinical practice guideline: prevention of thromboembolism in spinal cord injury. J Spinal Cord Med 1997; 20:259–284.

104. Constans JP, de Divitiis E, Donzelli R, et al. Spinal metastases with neurological manifestations. Review of 600 cases. J Neurosurg 1983; 59: 111–118.

105. Cooper PR. Outcome after operative treatment of intramedullary spinal cord tumors in adults: intermediate and long-term results in 51 patients. Neurosurgery 1989; 25:855–859.

106. Cotler JM, Herbison GJ, Nasuti JF, et al. Closed reduction of traumatic cervical spine dislocation using traction weights up to 140 pounds. Spine 1993; 18:386–390.

107. Craig AR, Hancock KM, Dickson HG. A longitudinal investigation into anxiety and depression in the first 2 years following a spinal cord injury. Paraplegia 1994; 32:675–679.

108. Creasey GH, Ho CH, Triolo RJ, et al. Clinical applications of electrical stimulation after spinal cord injury. J Spinal Cord Med 2004; 27: 365–375.

109. Creasey GH. Restoration of bladder, bowel, and sexual function. Top Spinal Cord Inj Rehabil 1999; 5:21–32.

110. Cremer SA, Maynard F, Davidoff G. The reflex sympathetic dystrophy syndrome associated with traumatic myelopathy: report of 5 cases. Pain 1989; 37:187–192.

111. Crozier KS, Graziani V, Ditunno JF Jr, et al. Spinal cord injury: prognosis for ambulation based on sensory examination in patients who are initially motor complete. Arch Phys Med Rehabil 1991; 72:119–121.

112. Curtis KA, Dillon DA. Survey of wheelchair athletic injuries: common patterns and prevention. Paraplegia 1985; 23:170–175.

113. Curtis KA, Drysdale GA, Lanza RD, et al. Shoulder pain in wheelchair users with tetraplegia and paraplegia. Arch Phys Med Rehabil 1999; 80:453–457.

114. Curtis KA, Tyner TM, Zachary L, et al. Effect of a standard exercise protocol on shoulder pain in long-term wheelchair users. Spinal Cord 1999; 37:421–429.

115. Dalyan M, Cardenas DD, Gerard B. Upper extremity pain after spinal cord injury. Spinal Cord 1999; 37:191–195.

116. Davidoff G, Roth E, Guarracini M, et al. Function-limiting dysesthetic pain syndrome among traumatic spinal cord injury patients: a cross-sectional study. Pain 1987; 29:39–48.

117. Davis L, Martin J. Studies upon spinal cord injuries. J Neurosurg 1947; 2:369–377.

118. Dawson DM, Potts F. Acute nontraumatic myelopathies. Neurol Clin 1991; 9:585–603.

119. De Troyer A, Estenne M. Coordination between rib cage muscles and diaphragm during quiet breathing in humans. J Appl Physiol 1984; 57:899–906.

120. De Troyer A, Heilporn A. Respiratory mechanics in quadriplegia. The respiratory function of the intercostal muscles. Am Rev Respir Dis 1980; 122:591–600.

121. Dearwater SR, LaPorte RE, Robertson RJ, et al. Activity in the spinal cord-injured patient: an epidemiologic analysis of metabolic parameters. Med Sci Sports Exerc 1986; 18:541–544.

122. DeForge D, Nymark J, Lemaire E, et al. Effect of 4-aminopyridine on gait in ambulatory spinal cord injuries: a double-blind, placebo-controlled, crossover trial. Spinal Cord 2004; 42:674–685.

123. DeLisa JA, Hammond MC. The history of the subspecialty of spinal cord injury medicine. In: Kirshblum S, Campagnolo DL, DeLisa JA, eds. Spinal cord medicine. Philadelphia: Lippincott Williams & Wilkins; 2002:1–4.

124. DeLisa JA. Subspecialty certification in spinal cord injury medicine: past, present, and future. J Spinal Cord Med 1999; 22:218–225.

125. Denis F. Spinal instability as defined by the three-column spine concept in acute spinal trauma. Clin Orthop 1984; 189:65–76.

126. Denis F. The three column spine and its significance in the classification of acute thoracolumbar spinal injuries. Spine 1983; 8:817–831.

127. Derenne JP, Macklem PT, Roussos C. The respiratory muscles: mechanics, control, and pathophysiology. Am Rev Respir Dis 1978; 118:119–133.

128. Derenne JP, Macklem PT, Roussos C. The respiratory muscles: mechanics, control, and pathophysiology. Part 2. Am Rev Respir Dis 1978; 118:373–390.

129. Derenne JP, Macklem PT, Roussos C. The respiratory muscles: mechanics, control, and pathophysiology. Part III. Am Rev Respir Dis 1978; 118: 581–601.

130. Deresinski SC, Perkash I. Urinary tract infections in male spinal cord injured patients. Part two: diagnostic value of symptoms and of quantitative urinalysis. J Am Paraplegia Soc 1985; 8:7–10.

131. DeVivo MJ, Black KJ, Stover SL. Causes of death during the first 12 years after spinal cord injury. Arch Phys Med Rehabil 1993; 74:248–254.

132. DeVivo MJ, Kartus PL, Rutt RD, et al. The influence of age at time of spinal cord injury on rehabilitation outcome. Arch Neurol 1990; 47:687–691.

133. DeVivo MJ, Kartus PL, Stover SL, et al. Benefits of early admission to an organised spinal cord injury care system. Paraplegia 1990; 28:545–555.

134. DeVivo MJ, Kartus PL, Stover SL, et al. Cause of death for patients with spinal cord injuries. Arch Intern Med 1989; 149:1761–1766.

135. DeVivo MJ, Krause JS, Lammertse DP. Recent trends in mortality and causes of death among persons with spinal cord injury. Arch Phys Med Rehabil 1999; 80:1411–1419.

136. DeVivo MJ, Rutt RD, Stover SL, et al. Employment after spinal cord injury. Arch Phys Med Rehabil 1987; 68:494–498.

137. DeVivo MJ, Stover SL, Black KJ. Prognostic factors for 12-year survival after spinal cord injury. Arch Phys Med Rehabil 1992; 73:156–162.

138. DeVivo MJ. Epidemiology of spinal cord injury. In: Lin VW, ed. Spinal cord medicine: principles and practice. New York: Demos; 2003:79–85.

139. DeVivo MJ. Epidemiology of traumatic spinal cord injury. In: Kirshblum S, Campagnolo DI, DeLisa JA, eds. Spinal cord medicine. Philadelphia: Lippincott Williams & Wilkins; 2002:69–81.

140. Di Rocco A. Diseases of the spinal cord in human immunodeficiency virus infection. Semin Neurol 1999; 19:151–155.

141. Dicpinigaitis PV, Spungen AM, Bauman WA, et al. Bronchial hyperresponsiveness after cervical spinal cord injury. Chest 1994; 105:1073–1076.

142. Dijkers MP, Abela MB, Gans BM, et al. The aftermath of SCI. In: Stover SL, DeLisa JA, Whiteneck GG, eds. Spinal cord injury clinical outcomes from the Model Systems. Gaithersburg: Aspen; 1995: 185–212.

143. Dijkers MP. Correlates of life satisfaction among persons with spinal cord injury. Arch Phys Med Rehabil 1999; 80:867–876.

144. Dijkers MP. Quality of life after spinal cord injury. Am Rehabil 1996; fall:18–24.

145. Dijkers MP. Quality of life of individuals with spinal cord injury: conceptualization, measurement and research findings. J Rehabil Res Dev 2005; 42(3 suppl 1):87–110.

146. Dinsdale SM. Decubitus ulcers: role of pressure and friction in causation. Arch Phys Med Rehabil 1974; 55:147–152.

147. Ditunno JF Jr, Stover SL, Freed MM, et al. Motor recovery of the upper extremities in traumatic quadriplegia: a multicenter study. Arch Phys Med Rehabil 1992; 73:431–436.

148. Ditunno JF, Cohen ME, Formal C. Functional outcomes. In: Stover SL, Whiteneck GG, DeLisa JA, eds. Spinal cord injury: clinical outcomes from the Model Systems. Gaithersburg: Aspen; 1995:170, 184.

149. Ditunno JF, Flanders AE, Kirshblum S, et al. Predicting outcome in traumatic spinal cord injury. In: Kirshblum S, Campagnolo DI, DeLisa JA, eds. Spinal cord medicine. Philadelphia: Lippincott Williams & Wilkins; 2002:108–122.

150. Ditunno JF, Little JW, Tessler A, et al. Spinal shock revisited: a four-phase model. Spinal Cord 2004; 42:383–395.

151. Dobkin BH, Apple D, Barbeau H, et al. Methods for a randomized trial of weight-supported treadmill training versus conventional training for walking during inpatient rehabilitation after incomplete traumatic spinal cord injury. Neurorehabil Neural Repair 2003; 17:153–167.

152. Dobkin BH, Apple D, Barbeau H, et al. Randomized trial of weight-supported treadmill vs conventional training for walking after incomplete SCI. Neurology (in press).

153. Drewes AM, Andreasen A, Poulsen LH. Valproate for treatment of chronic central pain after spinal cord injury. A double-blind cross-over study. Paraplegia 1994; 32:565–569.

154. Drory Y, Ohry A, Brooks ME, et al. Arm crank ergometry in chronic spinal cord injured patients. Arch Phys Med Rehabil 1990; 71:389–392.

155. Eberhardt K. Home modifications for persons with spinal cord injury. Occup Ther Pract 1998; 3:24–27.

156. Edgar RE, Best LG, Quail PA, et al. Computer-assisted DREZ microcoagulation: posttraumatic spinal deafferentation pain. J Spinal Disord 1993; 6:48–56.

157. Edgerton VR, Harkema S, Dobkin BH. Retraining the human spinal cord. In: Lin VW, ed. Spinal cord medicine: principles and practice. New York: Demos; 2003:817–826.

158. Edgerton VR, Roy RR, Hodgson JA, et al. A physiological basis for the development of rehabilitative strategies for spinally injured patients. J Am Paraplegia Soc 1991; 14:150–157.

159. Eismont FJ, Arena MJ, Green BA. Extrusion of an intervertebral disc associated with traumatic subluxation or dislocation of cervical facets. Case report. J Bone Joint Surg Am 1991; 73:1555–1560.

160. Elias AN, Gwinup G. Immobilization osteoporosis in paraplegia. J Am Paraplegia Soc 1992; 15:163–170.

161. Eltorai IM. Fatal spinal cord injury of the 20th president of the United States: day-by-day review of his clinical course, with comments. J Spinal Cord Med 2004; 27:330–341.

162. Eltorai IM. History of spinal cord medicine. In: Lin VW, ed. Spinal cord medicine: principles and practice. New York: Demos Medical Publishing; 2003:1–14.

163. Epstein FJ, Farmer JP, Freed D. Adult intramedullary spinal cord ependymomas: the result of surgery in 38 patients. J Neurosurg 1993; 79:204–209.

164. Epstein LJ, Brown R. Sleep disorders in spinal cord injury. In: Lin VW, ed. Spinal cord medicine: principles and practice. New York: Demos; 2003:169–177.

165. Erickson RP. Autonomic hyperreflexia: pathophysiology and medical management. Arch Phys Med Rehabil 1980; 61:431–440.

166. Estenne M, De Troyer A. Mechanism of the postural dependence of vital capacity in tetraplegic subjects. Am Rev Respir Dis 1987; 135:367–371.

167. Estenne M, De Troyer A. The effects of tetraplegia on chest wall statics. Am Rev Respir Dis 1986; 134:121–124.

168. Estenne M, Knoop C, Vanvaerenbergh J, et al. The effect of pectoralis muscle training in tetraplegic subjects. Am Rev Respir Dis 1989; 139:1218–1222.

169. Estenne M, Van Muylem A, Gorini M, et al. Evidence of dynamic airway compression during cough in tetraplegic patients. Am J Respir Crit Care Med 1994; 150:1081–1085.

170. Faden AI, Chan PH, Longar S. Alterations in lipid metabolism, Na+, K+–ATPase activity, and tissue water content of spinal cord following experimental traumatic injury. J Neurochem 1987; 48:1809–1816.

171. Falci S, Best L, Bayles R, et al. Dorsal root entry zone microcoagulation for spinal cord injury-related central pain: operative intramedullary electrophysiological guidance and clinical outcome. J Neurosurg Spine 2002; 97:193–200.

172. Fealey RD, Szurszewski JH, Merritt JL, et al. Effect of traumatic spinal cord transection on human upper gastrointestinal motility and gastric emptying. Gastroenterology 1984; 87:69–75.

173. Fehlings MG, Tator CH. The relationships among the severity of spinal cord injury, residual neurological function, axon counts, and counts of retrogradely labeled neurons after experimental spinal cord injury. Exp Neurol 1995; 132:220–228.

174. Ferguson RL, Allen BL Jr. A mechanistic classification of thoracolumbar spine fractures. Clin Orthop 1984; 189:77–88.

175. Ferrell BA, Artinian BM, Sessing D. The Sessing Scale for Assessment of Pressure Ulcer Healing. J Am Geriatr Soc 1995; 43:37–40.

176. Fichtenbaum J, Kirshblum S. Psychologic adaptation to spinal cord injury. In: Kirshblum S, Campagnolo DI, DeLisa JA, eds. Spinal cord medicine. Philadelphia: Lippincott Williams & Wilkins; 2002:299–311.

177. Fiedler IG, Laud PW, Maiman DJ, et al. Economics of managed care in spinal cord injury. Arch Phys Med Rehabil 1999; 80:1441–1449.

178. Fielding JW. Fractures of the spine. I. Injuries of the cervical spine. In: Rockwood CA, Wilkens KE, King RE, eds. Fractures in children. Philadelphia: JB Lippincott; 1984:683–705.

179. Finerman GA, Stover SL. Heterotopic ossification following hip replacement or spinal cord injury. Two clinical studies with EHDP. Metab Bone Dis Relat Res 1981; 3:337–342.

180. Finnerup NB, Sindrup SH, Bach FW, et al. Lamotrigine in spinal cord injury pain: a randomized controlled trial. Pain 2002; 96:375–383.

181. Finnimore AJ, Roebuck M, Sajkov D, et al. The effects of the GABA agonist, baclofen, on sleep and breathing. Eur Respir J 1995; 8:230–234.

182. Flanders AE, Schaefer DM, Doan HT, et al. Acute cervical spine trauma: correlation of MR imaging findings with degree of neurologic deficit. Radiology 1990; 177:25–33.

183. Ford CN, Reinhard ER, Yeh D, et al. Interim analysis of a prospective, randomized trial of vacuum-assisted closure versus the healthpoint system in the management of pressure ulcers. Ann Plast Surg 2002; 49:55–61, discussion 61.

184. Fowler E, Goupil DL. Comparison of the wet-to-dry dressing and a copolymer starch in the management of debrided pressure sores. J Enterostomal Ther 1984; 11:22–25.

185. Frank RG, Elliott TR. Life stress and psychologic adjustment following spinal cord injury. Arch Phys Med Rehabil 1987; 68:344–347.

186. Freed JH, Hahn H, Menter R, et al. The use of the three-phase bone scan in the early diagnosis of heterotopic ossification (HO) and in the evaluation of didronel therapy. Paraplegia 1982; 20:208–216.

187. Freehafer AA, Hazel CM, Becker CL. Lower extremity fractures in patients with spinal cord injury. Paraplegia 1981; 19:367–372.

188. Friedman AH, Nashold BS Jr. DREZ lesions for relief of pain related to spinal cord injury. J Neurosurg 1986; 65:465–469.

189. Frisbie JH, Kache A. Increasing survival and changing causes of death in myelopathy patients. J Am Paraplegia Soc 1983; 6:51–56.

190. Gansel J, Waters R, Gellman H. Transfer of the pronator teres tendon to the tendons of the flexor digitorum profundus in tetraplegia. J Bone Joint Surg Am 1990; 72:427–432.

191. Garber SL, Biddle AK, Click CN. Pressure ulcer prevention and treatment following spinal cord injury: a clinical practice guideline for health-care professionals. Washington: Paralyzed Veterans of America; 2000.

192. Gardner SE, Frantz RA, Schmidt FL. Effect of electrical stimulation on chronic wound healing: a meta-analysis. Wound Repair Regen 1999; 7:495–503.

193. Garland DE, Adkins RH, Scott M, et al. Bone loss at the os calcis compared with bone loss at the knee in individuals with spinal cord injury. J Spinal Cord Med 2004; 27:207–211.

194. Garland DE, Orwin JF. Resection of heterotopic ossification in patients with spinal cord injuries. Clin Orthop 1989; 242:169–176.

195. Garstang SV. Infections of the spine and spinal cord. In: Kirshblum S, Campagnolo DI, DeLisa JA, eds. Spinal cord medicine. Philadelphia: Lippincott Williams & Wilkins; 2002:499–512.

196. Geisler FH, Coleman WP, Grieco G, et al. The Sygen Multicenter Acute Spinal Cord Injury Study. Spine 2001; 26:S87–S98.

197. Geisler FH, Dorsey FC, Coleman WP. Recovery of motor function after spinal-cord injury—a randomized, placebo-controlled trial with GM-1 anglioside. N Engl J Med 1991; 324:1829–1838.

198. Gellman H, Chandler DR, Petrasek J, et al. Carpal tunnel syndrome in paraplegic patients. J Bone Joint Surg Am 1988; 70:517–519.

199. Gertzbein SD. Neurologic deterioration in patients with thoracic and lumbar fractures after admission to the hospital. Spine 1994; 19:1723–1725.

200. Giuliano F, Hultling C, El Masry WS, et al. Randomized trial of sildenafil for the treatment of erectile dysfunction in spinal cord injury. Sildenafil Study Group. Ann Neurol 1999; 46:15–21.

201. Glaser RM, Janssen TWJ, Suryaprasad AG, et al. The physiology of exercise. In: Sowell TT, ed. Physical fitness: a guide for individuals with spinal cord injury. Washington: US Veterans Health Administration; 1996:3–23.

202. Glazer PA, Hu SS. Pediatric spinal infections. Orthop Clin North Am 1996; 27:111–123.

203. Glenn WW, Holcomb WG, McLaughlin AJ, et al. Total ventilatory support in a quadriplegic patient with radiofrequency electrophrenic respiration. N Engl J Med 1972; 286:513–516.

204. Glenn WW, Holcomb WG, Shaw RK, et al. Long-term ventilatory support by diaphragm pacing in quadriplegia. Ann Surg 1976; 183:566–577.

205. Go VK, DeVivo MJ, Richards JS. The epidemiology of spinal cord injury. In: Stover SL, Whiteneck GG, DeLisa JA, eds. Spinal cord injury: clinical outcomes from the Model Systems. Gaithersburg: Aspen; 1995:21–55.

206. Goemaere S, Van Laere M, De Neve P, et al. Bone mineral status in paraplegic patients who do or do not perform standing. Osteoporosis Int 1994; 4:138–143.

207. Goldberg RT, Freed MM. Vocational development of spinal cord injury patients: an 8-year follow-up. Arch Phys Med Rehabil 1982; 63:207–210.

208. Goldhaber SZ. Pulmonary embolism. N Engl J Med 1998; 339:93–104.

209. Goldhaber SZ. Pulmonary thromboembolism. In: Fauci AS, Braunwald E, Isselbacher KJ, et al, eds. Harrison's principles of internal medicine. 14th edn. New York: McGraw-Hill; 1998:1469–1472.

210. Goldman JM, Silver JR, Lehr RP. An electromyographic study of the abdominal muscles of tetraplegic patients. Paraplegia 1986; 24:241–246.

211. Goldwein JW. Radiation myelopathy: a review. Med Pediatr Oncol 1987; 15:89–95.

212. Gonzales MF, Davis RL. Neuropathology of acquired immunodeficiency syndrome. Neuropathol Appl Neurobiol 1988; 14:345–363.

213. Gore RM, Mintzer RA, Calenoff L. Gastrointestinal complications of spinal cord injury. Spine 1981; 6:538–544.

214. Gorio A, Ferrari G, Fusco M, et al. Gangliosides and their effects on rearranging peripheral and central neural pathways. Cent Nerv Syst Trauma 1984; 1:29–37.

215. Gorman PH. Functional electrical stimulation in spinal cord medicine. In: Lin VW, ed. Spinal cord medicine: principles and practice. New York: Demos; 2003:773–745.

216. Gorse GJ, Messner RL. Improved pressure sore healing with hydrocolloid dressings. Arch Dermatol 1987; 123:766–771.

217. Gracies JM, Elovic E, McGuire J, et al. Traditional pharmacological treatments for spasticity. part I: local treatments. Muscle Nerve Suppl 1997; 6:S61–S91.

218. Green BA, Callahan RA, Klose KJ, et al. Acute spinal cord injury: current concepts. Clin Orthop 1981; 154:125–135.

219. Green S. Specific exercise programs. In: Sowell TT, ed. Physical fitness: a guide for individuals with spinal cord injury. Washington: US Veterans Health Administration; 1996:45–96.

220. Gross D, Ladd HW, Riley EJ, et al. The effect of training on strength and endurance of the diaphragm in quadriplegia. Am J Med 1980; 68:27–35.

221. Groupe D, Kohn KH. Functional electrical stimulation for ambulation by paraplegics, twelve years of clinical observations and system studies. Malabar: Krieger; 1994.

222. Grundy SM, Goodman DW, Rifkind BM, et al. The place of HDL in cholesterol management. A perspective from the National Cholesterol Educational Program. Arch Intern Med 1989; 149:505–510.

223. Guest RS, Klose KJ, Needham-Shropshire BM, et al. Evaluation of a training program for persons with SCI paraplegia using the Parastep 1 ambulation system: part 4. Effect on physical self-concept and depression. Arch Phys Med Rehabil 1997; 78:804–807.

224. Guttmann L. Spinal cord injuries: comprehensive management and research. Oxford: Blackwell; 1973, 1976.

225. Hammond MC, Burns SC. Yes you can! A guide to self-care for persons with spinal cord injury. Washington: Paralyzed Veterans of America; 2000.

226. Hangartner TN, Rodgers MM, Glaser RM, et al. Tibial bone density loss in spinal cord injured patients: effects of FES exercise. J Rehabil Res Dev 1994; 31:50–61.

227. Harden RN, Brenman E, Saltz S, et al. Topiramate in the management of spinal cord injury pain: a double-blind, randomized, placebo-controlled pilot study. In: Yezierski RP, Burchiel KJ, eds. Spinal cord injury pain: assessment, mechanisms, management. Progress in pain research and management, vol 23. Seattle: IASP Press; 2002:393–407.

228. Heary RF, Filart R. Tumors of the spine and spinal cord. In: Kirshblum S, Campagnolo DI, DeLisa JA, eds. Spinal cord medicine. Philadelphia: Lippincott Williams & Wilkins; 2002:480–497.

229. Heilporn A. Psychological factors in the causation of pressure sores: case reports. Paraplegia 1991; 29:137–139.

230. Heinemann AW. Spinal cord injury. In: Goreczny A, ed. Handbook of health and rehabilitation psychology. New York: Plenum Press; 1995: 341–360.

231. Henn JS, Coons S, Zabramski JM. Pathology and classification of central nervous system vascular malformations. In: Jafar JJ, Awad IA, Rossenwasser RH, eds. Vascular malformations of the central nervous system. Philadelphia: Lippincott Williams & Wilkins; 1999:513–526.

232. Hess MJ, Zhan EH, Foo DK, et al. Bladder cancer in patients with spinal cord injury. J Spinal Cord Med 2003; 26:335–338.

233. Hjeltnes N, Aksnes AK, Birkeland KI, et al. Improved body composition after 8 wk of electrically stimulated leg cycling in tetraplegic patients. Am J Physiol 1997; 273:R1072–R1079.

234. Hjeltnes N, Galuska D, Bjornholm M, et al. Exercise-induced overexpression of key regulatory proteins involved in glucose uptake and metabolism in tetraplegic persons: Molecular mechanism for improved glucose homeostasis. FASEB J 1998; 12:1701–1712.

235. Hjeltnes N. Cardiorespiratory capacity in tetra- and paraplegia shortly after injury. Scand J Rehabil Med 1986; 18:65–70.

236. Holdsworth F. Fractures, dislocations, and fracture-dislocations of the spine. J Bone Joint Surg Am 1970; 52:1534–1551.

237. Hooker SP, Wells CL. Effects of low- and moderate-intensity training in spinal cord-injured persons. Med Sci Sports Exerc 1989; 21:18–22.

238. House JH, Gwathmey FW, Lundsgaard DK. Restoration of strong grasp and lateral pinch in tetraplegia due to cervical spinal cord injury. J Hand Surg (Am) 1976; 1:152–159.

239. Hughes JT. The Edwin Smith Surgical Papyrus: an analysis of the first case reports of spinal cord injuries. Paraplegia 1988; 26:71–82.

240. Huldtgren AC, Fugl-Meyer AR, Jonasson E, et al. Ventilatory dysfunction and respiratory rehabilitation in post-traumatic quadriplegia. Eur J Respir Dis 1980; 61:347–356.

241. Hultling C, Rosenlund B, Levi R, et al. Assisted ejaculation and in-vitro fertilization in the treatment of infertile spinal cord-injured men: the role of intracytoplasmic sperm injection. Hum Reprod 1997; 12:499–502.

242. Jackson AB, Dijkers M, Devivo MJ, et al. A demographic profile of new traumatic spinal cord injuries: change and stability over 30 years. Arch Phys Med Rehabil 2004; 85:1740–1748.

243. Jackson AB, Wadley V. A multicenter study of women's self-reported reproductive health after spinal cord injury. Arch Phys Med Rehabil 1999; 80:1420–1428.

244. Jacobs PL, Nash MS, Rusinowski JW. Circuit training provides cardiorespiratory and strength benefits in persons with paraplegia. Med Sci Sports Exerc 2001; 33:711–717.

245. Jefferson G. Fractures of the atlas vertebra: report of four cases and a review of those previously recorded. Br J Surg 1920; 7:407–422.

246. Johnson DL, Gellman H, Waters RL, et al. Brachioradialis transfer for wrist extension in tetraplegic patients who have fifth-cervical-level neurological function. J Bone Joint Surg Am 1996; 78:1063–1067.

247. Johnson KL. Vocational rehabilitation. In: Lin VW, ed. Spinal cord medicine: principles and practice. New York: Demos; 2003.

248. Jones BV, Ernst RJ, Tomsick TA, et al. Spinal dural arteriovenous fistulas: recognizing the spectrum of magnetic resonance imaging findings. J Spinal Cord Med 1997; 20:43–48.

249. Kamin SS. Vascular, nutritional, and other diseases of the spinal cord. In: Kirshblum S, Campagnolo DI, DeLisa JA, eds. Spinal cord medicine. Philadelphia: Lippincott Williams & Wilkins; 2002:513–526.

250. Kaufman JM, Fam B, Jacobs SC, et al. Bladder cancer and squamous metaplasia in spinal cord injury patients. J Urol 1977; 118:967–971.

251. Kedlaya D, Brandstater ME, Lee JK. Immobilization hypercalcemia in incomplete paraplegia: successful treatment with pamidronate. Arch Phys Med Rehabil 1998; 79:222–225.

252. Khan IA, Vaccaro AR, Zlotolow DA. Management of vertebral diskitis and osteomyelitis. Orthopedics 1999; 22:758–765.

253. King RB, Carlson CE, Mervine J, et al. Clean and sterile intermittent catheterization methods in hospitalized patients with spinal cord injury. Arch Phys Med Rehabil 1992; 73:798–802.

254. Kirkland LR. Baclofen dosage: a suggestion. Arch Phys Med Rehabil 1984; 65:214.

255. Kirshblum S, Druin E, Planten K. Musculoskeletal conditions in chronic spinal cord injury. Top Spinal Cord Inj Rehabil 1997; 2:23–35.

256. Kirshblum S, Johnston MV, Brown J, et al. Predictors of dysphagia after spinal cord injury. Arch Phys Med Rehabil 1999; 80:1101–1105.

257. Kiwerski J, Weiss M, Chrostowska T. Analysis of mortality of patients after cervical spine trauma. Paraplegia 1981; 19:347–351.

258. Koch BM, Eng GM. Neonatal spinal cord injury. Arch Phys Med Rehabil 1979; 60:378–381.

259. Koziak M. Etiology and pathology of decubitus ulcers. Arch Phys Med Rehabil 1959; 40:62–69.

260. Krause JS, Kemp B, Coker J. Depression after spinal cord injury: relation to gender, ethnicity, aging, and socioeconomic indicators. Arch Phys Med Rehabil 2000; 81:1099–1109.

261. Krause JS, Kewman D, DeVivo MJ, et al. Employment after spinal cord injury: an analysis of cases from the Model Spinal Cord Injury Systems. Arch Phys Med Rehabil 1999; 80:1492–1500.

262. Krause JS, Sternberg M, Lottes S, et al. Mortality after spinal cord injury: an 11-year prospective study. Arch Phys Med Rehabil 1997; 78: 815–821.

263. Krause JS. Employment after spinal cord injury. Arch Phys Med Rehabil 1992; 73:163–169.

264. Krause JS. The relationship between productivity and adjustment following spinal cord injury. Rehabil Couns Bull 1990; 33:188–199.

265. Kreuter M, Sullivan M, Dahllof AG, et al. Partner relationships, functioning, mood and global quality of life in persons with spinal cord injury and traumatic brain injury. Spinal Cord 1998; 36:252–261.

266. Kribbs NB, Pack AI, Kline LR, et al. Objective measurement of patterns of nasal CPAP use by patients with obstructive sleep apnea. Am Rev Respir Dis 1993; 147:887–895.

267. Kubler-Ross E. On death and dying. New York: Macmillan; 1969.

268. Kulkarni MV, McArdle CB, Kopanicky D, et al. Acute spinal cord injury: MR imaging at 1.5 T. Radiology 1987; 164:837–843.

269. Kunkel CF, Scremin AM, Eisenberg B, et al. Effect of 'standing' on spasticity, contracture, and osteoporosis in paralyzed males. Arch Phys Med Rehabil 1993; 74:73–78.

270. Kupcha PC, An HS, Cotler JM. Gunshot wounds to the cervical spine. Spine 1990; 15:1058–1063.

271. Lahat E, Pillar G, Ravid S, et al. Rapid recovery from transverse myelopathy in children treated with methylprednisolone. Pediatr Neurol 1998; 19:279–282.

272. Lal S, Hamilton BB, Heinemann A, et al. Risk factors for heterotopic ossification in spinal cord injury. Arch Phys Med Rehabil 1989; 70: 387–390.

273. Lammertse DP. Maintaining health long-term with spinal cord injury. Top Spinal Cord Inj Rehabil 2001; 6:1–21.

274. Lance JW. Symposium synopsis. In: Feldman RG, Young RR, Koella WP, eds. Spasticity: disordered motor control. Chicago: Year Book Medical Publishers; 1980.

275. Lasfargues JE, Custis D, Morrone F, et al. A model for estimating spinal cord injury prevalence in the United States. Paraplegia 1995; 33:62–68.

276. Ledsome JR, Sharp JM. Pulmonary function in acute cervical cord injury. Am Rev Respir Dis 1981; 124:41–44.

277. Leeds EM, Klose KJ, Ganz W, et al. Bone mineral density after bicycle ergometry training. Arch Phys Med Rehabil 1990; 71:207–209.

278. Lemons DE, Riedel G, Downey JA. Thermal regulation and the effects of thermal modalities. In: Gonzalez EG, Myers SJ, Edelstein JE, et al, eds. Downey and Darling's physiological basis of rehabilitation medicine. Boston: Butterworth Heinemann; 2001:507–520.

279. Levin VA, Leibel SA, Gutin PH. Neoplasms of the central nervous system. In: Devita VT, Hellman S, eds. Cancer: principles and practice of oncology. 6th edn. Philadelphia: Lippincott Williams & Wilkins; 2001:2100–2160.

280. Levy CE, Lorch F. Recovery of upper limb motor function in tetraplegia with stellate ganglion block treatment of reflex sympathetic dystrophy: a case report. Am J Phys Med Rehabil 1996; 75:479–482.

281. Li Y, Raisman G. Schwann cells induce sprouting in motor and sensory axons in the adult rat spinal cord. J Neurosci 1994; 14:4050–4063.

282. Lin VW, Singh H, Chitkara RK, et al. Functional magnetic stimulation for restoring cough in patients with tetraplegia. Arch Phys Med Rehabil 1998; 79:517–522.

283. Linder A, Leach GE, Raz S. Augmentation cystoplasty in the treatment of neurogenic bladder dysfunction. J Urol 1983; 129:491–493.

284. Linsenmeyer TA, Perkash I. Infertility in men with spinal cord injury. Arch Phys Med Rehabil 1991; 72:747–754.

285. Linsenmeyer TA. Evaluation and treatment of erectile dysfunction following spinal cord injury: a review. J Am Paraplegia Soc 1991; 14:43–51.

286. Little JW, Burns SP. Neuromusculoskeletal complications of spinal cord injury. In: Kirshblum S, Campagnolo DI, DeLisa JA, eds. Spinal cord medicine. Philadelphia: Lippincott Williams & Wilkins; 2002: 241–252.

287. Liu D, Thangnipon W, McAdoo DJ. Excitatory amino acids rise to toxic levels upon impact injury to the rat spinal cord. Brain Res 1991; 547:344–348.

288. Liu MH, Spungen AM, Fink L, et al. Increased energy needs in patients with quadriplegia and pressure ulcers. Adv Wound Care 1996; 9:41–45.

289. Lo IK, Turner R, Connolly S, et al. The outcome of tendon transfers for C6-spared quadriplegics. J Hand Surg (Br) 1998; 23:156–161.

290. MacDiarmid SA, Arnold EP, Palmer NB, et al. Management of spinal cord injured patients by indwelling suprapubic catheterization. J Urol 1995; 154:492–494.

291. MacKinnon JA, Perlman M, Kirpalani H, et al. Spinal cord injury at birth: diagnostic and prognostic data in twenty-two patients. J Pediatr 1993; 122:431–437.

292. Madsen PW III, Yezierski RP, Holets VR. Syringomyelia: clinical observations and experimental studies. J Neurotrauma 1994; 11:241–254.

293. Mallory BS. Autonomic function in the isolated spinal cord. In: Gonzalez EG, Myers SJ, Edelstein JE, et al, eds. Downey and Darling's physiological basis of rehabilitation medicine. Boston: Butterworth Heinemann; 2001:683–710.

294. Manzano JL, Lubillo S, Henriquez D, et al. Verbal communication of ventilator dependent patients. Crit Care Med 1993; 21:512–517.

295. Marino RJ, Ditunno JF Jr, Donovan WH, et al. Neurologic recovery after traumatic spinal cord injury: data from the Model Spinal Cord Injury Systems. Arch Phys Med Rehabil 1999; 80:1391–1396.

296. Marshall LF, Knowlton S, Garfin SR, et al. Deterioration following spinal cord injury. A multicenter study. J Neurosurg 1987; 66:400–404.

297. Martin RE, Neary MA, Diamant NE. Dysphagia following anterior cervical spine surgery. Dysphagia 1997; 12:2–8, discussion 9–10.

298. Massery M. Manual breathing and coughing aids. Patients with paralytic or restrictive ventilatory insufficiency. Phys Med Rehabil Clin North Am 1996; 7:407–422.

299. Matthew WB. The spinal bruit. Lancet 1959; 2:1117–1118.

300. Maynard FM, Glass J. Management of the neuropathic bladder by clean intermittent catheterization: 5 year outcomes. Paraplegia 1987; 25:106–110.

301. Maynard FM, Karunas RS, Adkins RH, et al. Management of the neuromusculoskeletal systems. In: Stover SL, DeLisa JA, Whiteneck GT, ed. Spinal cord injury, clinical outcomes from the Model Systems. Gaithersburg: Aspen; 1995:145–169.

302. Maynard FM, Reynolds GG, Fountain S, et al. Neurological prognosis after traumatic quadriplegia. Three-year experience of California regional spinal cord injury care system. J Neurosurg 1979; 50:611–616.

303. Maynard FM. Immobilization hypercalcemia following spinal cord injury. Arch Phys Med Rehabil 1986; 67:41–44.

304. McCormick PC, Post KD, Stein BM. Intradural extramedullary tumors in adults. Neurosurg Clin North Am 1990; 1:591–608.

305. McCormick PC, Stein BM. Intramedullary tumors in adults. Neurosurg Clin North Am 1990; 1:609–630.

306. McDonald JW, Becker D, Sadowsky CL, et al. Late recovery following spinal cord injury. Case report and review of the literature. J Neurosurg Spine 2002; 97:252–265.

307. McDonald JW. Repairing the damaged spinal cord. Sci Am 1999; 281:64–73.

308. McDowell CL, Moberg E, House JH. Second International Conference on Surgical Rehabilitation of the Upper Limb in Traumatic Quadriplegia. J Hand Surg (Am) 1986; 11:604–608.

309. McDowell CL, Moberg EA, Smith AG. International Conference on Surgical Rehabilitation of the Upper Limb in Tetraplegia. J Hand Surg (Am) 1979; 4:387–390.

310. McKinley W, Meade MA, Kirshblum S, et al. Outcomes of early surgical management versus late or no surgical intervention after acute spinal cord injury. Arch Phys Med Rehabil 2004; 85:1818–1825.

311. McKinley WO, Jackson AB, Cardenas DD, et al. Long-term medical complications after traumatic spinal cord injury: a regional Model Systems analysis. Arch Phys Med Rehabil 1999; 80:1402–1410.

312. McKinley WO. Nontraumatic spinal cord injury: etiology, incidence, and outcome. In: Kirshblum S, Campagnolo DI, DeLisa JA, eds. Spinal cord medicine. Philadelphia: Lippincott Williams & Wilkins; 2002:471–479.

313. McMichan JC, Michel L, Westbrook PR. Pulmonary dysfunction following traumatic quadriplegia. Recognition, prevention, and treatment. JAMA 1980; 243:528–531.

314. Mechanick JI, Pomerantz F, Flanagan S, et al. Parathyroid hormone suppression in spinal cord injury patients is associated with the degree of neurologic impairment and not the level of injury. Arch Phys Med Rehabil 1997; 78:692–696.

315. Menter RR, Hudson LM. The effects of age at injury and the aging process. In: Stover SL, Whiteneck GG, DeLisa JA, eds. Spinal cord injury: clinical outcomes from the Model Systems. Gaithersburg: Aspen; 1995: 272–288.

316. Merli GJ, Crabbe S, Paluzzi RG, et al. Etiology, incidence, and prevention of deep vein thrombosis in acute spinal cord injury. Arch Phys Med Rehabil 1993; 74:1199–1205.

317. Merli GJ, Herbison GJ, Ditunno JF, et al. Deep vein thrombosis: prophylaxis in acute spinal cord injured patients. Arch Phys Med Rehabil 1988; 69:661–664.

318. Merli GJ, McElwain GE, Adler AG, et al. Immobilization hypercalcemia in acute spinal cord injury treated with etidronate. Arch Intern Med 1984; 144:1286–1288.

319. Meythaler JM, Tuel SM, Cross LL. Successful treatment of immobilization hypercalcemia using calcitonin and etidronate. Arch Phys Med Rehabil 1993; 74:316–319.

320. Moberg E. Surgical treatment for absent single-hand grip and elbow extension in quadriplegia. Principles and preliminary experience. J Bone Joint Surg Am 1975; 57:196–206.

321. Moberg E. Two-point discrimination test. A valuable part of hand surgical rehabilitation, e.g. in tetraplegia. Scand J Rehabil Med 1990; 22: 127–134.

322. Monga M, Bernie J, Rajasekaran M. Male infertility and erectile dysfunction in spinal cord injury: a review. Arch Phys Med Rehabil 1999; 80:1331–1339.

323. Monga TN, Ostermann HJ, Kerrigan AJ. Driving: a clinical perspective on rehabilitation technology. Phys Med Rehabil State Art Rev 1997; 11:69–92.

324. Moran de Brito CM, Battistella LR, Saito ET, et al. Effect of alendronate on bone mineral density in spinal cord injury patients: a pilot study. Spinal Cord 2005; 43(6):341–348.

325. Moriya T, Hassan AZ, Young W, et al. Dynamics of extracellular calcium activity following contusion of the rat spinal cord. J Neurotrauma 1994; 11:255–263.

326. Mortola JP, Sant'Ambrogio G. Motion of the rib cage and the abdomen in tetraplegic patients. Clin Sci Mol Med 1978; 54:25–32.

327. Moverman RA. Psychosocial factors in spinal cord injury. In: Lin VW, ed. Spinal cord medicine: principles and practice. New York: Demos; 2003:931–939.

328. Mulcahey MJ, Lutz C, Kozin SH, et al. Prospective evaluation of biceps to triceps and deltoid to triceps for elbow extension in tetraplegia. J Hand Surg (Am) 2003; 28:964–971.

329. Munro D. Drainage of the urinary bladder. New Engl J Med 1935; 212: 229–329.

330. Munro D. The cord bladder: its definition, treatment, and prognosis when associated with spinal cord injury. New Engl J Med 1936; 215:266–277.

331. Munro D. Thoracic and lumbosacral cord injuries. JAMA 1943; 122:1055.

332. Mutton DL, Scremin AM, Barstow TJ, et al. Physiologic responses during functional electrical stimulation leg cycling and hybrid exercise in spinal cord injured subjects. Arch Phys Med Rehabil 1997; 78:712–718.

333. Myllynen P, Kammonen M, Rokkanen P, et al. Deep venous thrombosis and pulmonary embolism in patients with acute spinal cord injury: a comparison with nonparalyzed patients immobilized due to spinal fractures. J Trauma 1985; 25:541–543.

334. Naftchi NE, Richardson JS. Autonomic dysreflexia: pharmacological management of hypertensive crises in spinal cord injured patients. J Spinal Cord Med 1997; 20:355–360.

335. Naftchi NE, Viau AT, Sell GH, et al. Mineral metabolism in spinal cord injury. Arch Phys Med Rehabil 1980; 61:139–142.

336. Nance PW, Bugaresti J, Shellenberger K, et al. Efficacy and safety of tizanidine in the treatment of spasticity in patients with spinal cord injury. North American Tizanidine Study Group. Neurology 1994; 44:S44–S51, discussion S51–S52.

337. Nance PW, Schryvers O, Leslie W, et al. Intravenous pamidronate attenuates bone density loss after acute spinal cord injury. Arch Phys Med Rehabil 1999; 80:243–251.

338. Nash MS, Jacobs PL, Mendez AJ, et al. Circuit resistance training improves the atherogenic lipid profiles of persons with chronic paraplegia. J Spinal Cord Med 2001; 24:2–9.

339. Nashold BS Jr, Bullitt E. Dorsal root entry zone lesions to control central pain in paraplegics. J Neurosurg 1981; 55:414–419.

340. Nashold BS Jr, Ostdahl RH. Dorsal root entry zone lesions for pain relief. J Neurosurg 1979; 51:59–69.

341. Nepomuceno C, Fine PR, Richards JS, et al. Pain in patients with spinal cord injury. Arch Phys Med Rehabil 1979; 60:605–609.

342. Nguyen H, Gelb DE, Ludwig SC. Posttraumatic spinal Charcot's arthropathy. Top Spinal Cord Inj Rehabil 2002; 8:48–58.

343. Nichols PJ, Norman PA, Ennis JR. Wheelchair user's shoulder? Shoulder pain in patients with spinal cord lesions. Scand J Rehabil Med 1979; 11:29–32.

344. Noble LJ, Wrathall JR. Distribution and time course of protein extravasation in the rat spinal cord after contusive injury. Brain Res 1989; 482:57–66.

345. Nobunaga AI, Go BK, Karunas RB. Recent demographic and injury trends in people served by the Model Spinal Cord Injury Care Systems. Arch Phys Med Rehabil 1999; 80:1372–1382.

346. Nola GT, Vistnes LM. Differential response of skin and muscle in the experimental production of pressure sores. Plast Reconstr Surg 1980; 66:728–733.

347. Nuhlicek DN, Spurr GB, Barboriak JJ, et al. Body composition of patients with spinal cord injury. Eur J Clin Nutr 1988; 42:765–773.

348. O'Brien CF. Injection techniques for botulinum toxin using electromyography and electrical stimulation. Muscle Nerve Suppl 1997; 6: S176–S180.

349. Olsson Y, Sharma HS, Pettersson A, et al. Release of endogenous neurochemicals may increase vascular permeability, induce edema and influence cell changes in trauma to the spinal cord. Prog Brain Res 1992; 91:197–203.

350. Osenbach RK, Menezes AH. Pediatric spinal cord injury. In: EC Benzel, CH Tator, eds. Contemporary management of spinal cord injury. Park Ridge: American Association of Neurological Surgeons; 1995: 187–194.

351. Pansky B, Allen D, Budd G. Review of neuroscience, 2nd edn. New York: McGraw-Hill, 1988:63.

352. Pansky B. Review of gross anatomy, 5th edn. New York: Macmillan, 1984:217.

353. Pant SS, Asbury AK, Richardson EP Jr. The myelopathy of pernicious anemia. A neuropathological reappraisal. Acta Neurol Scand 1968; 44(suppl 5):1–36.

354. Peckham PH, Keith MW, Kilgore KL. Restoration of upper extremity function in tetraplegia. Top Spinal Cord Inj Rehabil 1999; 5:33–43.

355. Peckham PH. Principles of electrical stimulation. Top Spinal Cord Inj Rehabil 1999; 5:1–5.

356. Penn RD, Savoy SM, Corcos D, et al. Intrathecal baclofen for severe spinal spasticity. N Engl J Med 1989; 320:1517–1521.

357. Penn RD. Intrathecal baclofen for spasticity of spinal origin: seven years of experience. J Neurosurg 1992; 77:236–240.

358. Perkash I. Efficacy and safety of terazosin to improve voiding in spinal cord injury patients. J Spinal Cord Med 1995; 18:236–239.

359. Perry VH, Andersson PB, Gordon S. Macrophages and inflammation in the central nervous system. Trends Neurosci 1993; 16:268–273.

360. Pertuiset E, Beaudreuil J, Liote F, et al. Spinal tuberculosis in adults. A study of 103 cases in a developed country, 1980–1994. Medicine (Baltimore) 1999; 78:309–320.

361. Peterson W, Charlifue W, Gerhart A, et al. Two methods of weaning persons with quadriplegia from mechanical ventilators. Paraplegia 1994; 32:98–103.

362. Peterson WP, Barbalata L, Brooks CA, et al. The effect of tidal volumes on the time to wean persons with high tetraplegia from ventilators. Spinal Cord 1999; 37:284–288.

363. Petito CK, Vecchio D, Chen YT. HIV antigen and DNA in AIDS spinal cords correlate with macrophage infiltration but not with vacuolar myelopathy. J Neuropathol Exp Neurol 1994; 53:86–94.

364. Pietschmann P, Pils P, Woloszczuk W, et al. Increased serum osteocalcin levels in patients with paraplegia. Paraplegia 1992; 30:204–209.

365. Pollack SF, Axen K, Spielholz N, et al. Aerobic training effects of electrically induced lower extremity exercises in spinal cord injured people. Arch Phys Med Rehabil 1989; 70:214–219.

366. Priebe MM, Sherwood AM, Thornby JI, et al. Clinical assessment of spasticity in spinal cord injury: a multidimensional problem. Arch Phys Med Rehabil 1996; 77:713–716.

367. Putzke JD, Barrett JJ, Richards JS, et al. Age and spinal cord injury: an emphasis on outcomes among the elderly. J Spinal Cord Med 2003; 26:37–44.

368. Quencer RM, Post MJ. Spinal cord lesions in patients with AIDS. Neuroimaging Clin North Am 1997; 7:359–373.

369. Raczka R, Braun R, Waters RL. Posterior deltoid-to-triceps transfer in quadriplegia. Clin Orthop 1984; 187:163–167.

370. Ragnarsson KT, Baker LL. Functional electrical stimulation in persons with spinal cord injury. In: Gonzalez EG, Myers SJ, Edelstein AE, et al, eds. Physiological basis of rehabilitation medicine. Boston: Butterworth Heinemann; 2001:723–745.

371. Ragnarsson KT, Pollack S, O'Daniel W Jr, et al. Clinical evaluation of computerized functional electrical stimulation after spinal cord injury: a multicenter pilot study. Arch Phys Med Rehabil 1988; 69:672–677.

372. Ragnarsson KT, Sell GH. Lower extremity fractures after spinal cord injury: a retrospective study. Arch Phys Med Rehabil 1981; 62:418–423.

373. Ramon S, Dominguez R, Ramirez L, et al. Clinical and magnetic resonance imaging correlation in acute spinal cord injury. Spinal Cord 1997; 35:664–673.

374. Rapalino O, Lazarov-Spiegler O, Agranov E, et al. Implantation of stimulated homologous macrophages results in partial recovery of paraplegic rats. Nat Med 1998; 4:814–821.

375. Raper AJ, Thompson WT Jr, Shapiro W, et al. Scalene and sternomastoid muscle function. J Appl Physiol 1966; 21:497–502.

376. Rasmussen H. The calcium messenger system (2). N Engl J Med 1986; 314:1164–1170.

377. Rath SA, Neff U, Schneider O, et al. Neurosurgical management of thoracic and lumbar vertebral osteomyelitis and discitis in adults: a review of 43 consecutive surgically treated patients. Neurosurgery 1996; 38: 926–933.

378. Rath SA, Seitz K, Soliman N, et al. DREZ coagulations for deafferentation pain related to spinal and peripheral nerve lesions: indication and results of 79 consecutive procedures. Stereotact Funct Neurosurg 1997; 68: 161–167.

379. Raymond J, Davis GM, Climstein M, et al. Cardiorespiratory responses to arm cranking and electrical stimulation leg cycling in people with paraplegia. Med Sci Sports Exerc 1999; 31:822–828.

380. Richards JS, Meredith RL, Nepomuceno C, et al. Psycho-social aspects of chronic pain in spinal cord injury. Pain 1980; 8:355–366.

381. Rintala DH, Loubser PG, Castro J, et al. Chronic pain in a community-based sample of men with spinal cord injury: prevalence, severity, and relationship with impairment, disability, handicap, and subjective well-being. Arch Phys Med Rehabil 1998; 79:604–614.

382. Rivas DA, Chancellor MB, Bagley D. Prospective comparison of external sphincter prosthesis placement and external sphincterotomy in men with spinal cord injury. J Endourol 1994; 8:89–93.

383. Roberts D, Lee W, Cuneo RC, et al. Longitudinal study of bone turnover after acute spinal cord injury. J Clin Endocrinol Metab 1998; 83: 415–422.

384. Rosenblum B, Oldfield EH, Doppman JL, et al. Spinal arteriovenous malformations: a comparison of dural arteriovenous fistulas and intradural AVMs in 81 patients. J Neurosurg 1987; 67:795–802.

385. Ruml LA, Dubois SK, Roberts ML, et al. Prevention of hypercalciuria and stone-forming propensity during prolonged bedrest by alendronate. J Bone Miner Res 1995; 10:655–662.

386. Russell JSR. The relationship of some forms of combined degenerations of the spinal cord to one another and to anemia. Lancet 1898; 2:5–14.

387. Rutchik A, Weissman AR, Almenoff PL, et al. Resistive inspiratory muscle training in subjects with chronic cervical spinal cord injury. Arch Phys Med Rehabil 1998; 79:293–297.

388. Sapico FL, Montgomerie JZ. Pyogenic vertebral osteomyelitis: report of nine cases and review of the literature. Rev Infect Dis 1979; 1:754–776.

389. Sapico FL. Microbiology and antimicrobial therapy of spinal infections. Orthop Clin North Am 1996; 27:9–13.

390. Sautter-Bihl ML, Liebermeister E, Nanassy A. Radiotherapy as a local treatment option for heterotopic ossifications in patients with spinal cord injury. Spinal Cord 2000; 38:33–36.

391. Savas PE, Vaccaro AR. Surgical management for thoracolumbar spinal injuries. In: Lin VW, ed. Spinal cord medicine: principles and practice. New York: Demos; 2003:143–151.

392. Schaefer DM, Flanders AE, Osterholm JL, et al. Prognostic significance of magnetic resonance imaging in the acute phase of cervical spine injury. J Neurosurg 1992; 76:218–223.

393. Schellhammer PF, Hackler RH, Bunts RC. External sphincterotomy: rationale for the procedure and experiences with 150 patients. Paraplegia 1974; 12:5–14.

394. Schmidt MF, Heinemann AW, Semik P. The efficacy of inservice training on substance abuse and spinal cord injury issues. Top Spinal Cord Inj Rehabil 1996; 2:11–20.

395. Schmitz TJ. Traumatic spinal cord injury. In: O'Sullivan, Schmitz TJ, eds. Physical rehabilitation: assessment and treatment. Philadelphia: FA Davis; 2001:879–923.

396. Schneck CD. Anatomy, mechanics, and imaging of spinal injury. In: Kirshblum S, Campagnolo DI, DeLisa JA, eds. Spinal cord medicine. Philadelphia: Lippincott Williams & Wilkins; 2002:27–68.

397. Schultheiss TE, Stephens LC, Maor MH. Analysis of the histopathology of radiation myelopathy. Int J Radiat Oncol Biol Phys 1988; 14:27–32.

398. Schultz RJ. The language of fractures. Baltimore: Williams & Wilkins; 1990:245.

399. Schwab ME, Bartholdi D. Degeneration and regeneration of axons in the lesioned spinal cord. Physiol Rev 1996; 76:319–370.

400. Schwartz M, Kipnis J. Protective autoimmunity: regulation and prospects for vaccination after brain and spinal cord injuries. Trends Mol Med 2001; 7:252–258.

401. Scivoletto G, Morganti B, Ditunno P, et al. Effects on age on spinal cord lesion patients' rehabilitation. Spinal Cord 2003; 41:457–464.

402. Scott JA, Donovan WH. The prevention of shoulder pain and contracture in the acute tetraplegia patient. Paraplegia 1981; 19:313–319.

403. Sebern MD. Pressure ulcer management in home health care: efficacy and cost effectiveness of moisture vapor permeable dressing. Arch Phys Med Rehabil 1986; 67:726–729.

404. Sebire G, Hollenberg H, Meyer L, et al. High dose methylprednisolone in severe acute transverse myelopathy. Arch Dis Child 1997; 76:167–168.

405. Selden NR, Quint DJ, Patel N, et al. Emergency magnetic resonance imaging of cervical spinal cord injuries: clinical correlation and prognosis. Neurosurgery 1999; 44:785-792, discussion 792–793.

406. Sharp JT. Respiratory muscles: a review of old and newer concepts. Lung 1980; 157:185–199.

407. Shields RW Jr. Functional anatomy of the autonomic nervous system. J Clin Neurophysiol 1993; 10:2–13.

408. Shimada K, Tokioka T. Sequential MR studies of cervical cord injury: correlation with neurological damage and clinical outcome. Spinal Cord 1999; 37:410–415.

409. Sidi AA, Becher EF, Reddy PK, et al. Augmentation enterocystoplasty for the management of voiding dysfunction in spinal cord injury patients. J Urol 1990; 143:83–85.

410. Sie IH, Waters RL, Adkins RH, et al. Upper extremity pain in the post-rehabilitation spinal cord injured patient. Arch Phys Med Rehabil 1992; 73:44–48.

411. Simoes NF, Lindblom L. Driving with a spinal cord disorder. In: Lin VW, ed. Spinal cord medicine: principles and practice. New York: Demos; 2003:723–731.

412. Simpson DM. Clinical trials of botulinum toxin in the treatment of spasticity. Muscle Nerve Suppl 1997; 6:S169–S175.

413. Sipski ML, Alexander CJ, Rosen RC. Orgasm in women with spinal cord injuries: a laboratory-based assessment. Arch Phys Med Rehabil 1995; 76:1097–1102.

414. Sipski ML, Alexander CJ, Rosen RC. Physiologic parameters associated with sexual arousal in women with incomplete spinal cord injuries. Arch Phys Med Rehabil 1997; 78:305–313.

415. Sipski ML, Alexander CJ, Rosen RC. Physiological parameters associated with psychogenic sexual arousal in women with complete spinal cord injuries. Arch Phys Med Rehabil 1995; 76:811–818.

416. Slucky AV, Eismont FJ. Treatment of acute injury of the cervical spine. Instr Course Lect 1995; 44:67–80.

417. Smith EL. Purification of anti-pernicious anemia factors from liver. Nature 1948; 161:638–639.

418. Smith KA, Rekate HL. Delayed postoperative tethering of the cervical spinal cord. J Neurosurg 1994; 81:196–201.

419. Snow BJ, Tsui JK, Bhatt MH, et al. Treatment of spasticity with botulinum toxin: a double-blind study. Ann Neurol 1990; 28:512–515.

420. Spinal Cord Medicine Consortium. Clinical practice guidelines: neurogenic bowel management in adults with spinal cord injury. J Spinal Cord Med 1998; 21:248–293.

421. Spungen AM, Dicpinigaitis PV, Almenoff PL, et al. Pulmonary obstruction in individuals with cervical spinal cord lesions unmasked by bronchodilator administration. Paraplegia 1993; 31:404–407.

422. Stadelmann WK, Digenis AG, Tobin GR. Impediments to wound healing. Am J Surg 1998; 176:39S–47S.

423. Stadelmann WK, Digenis AG, Tobin GR. Physiology and healing dynamics of chronic cutaneous wounds. Am J Surg 1998; 176:26S–38S.

424. Stewart AF, Adler M, Byers CM, et al. Calcium homeostasis in immobilization: an example of resorptive hypercalciuria. N Engl J Med 1982; 306:1136–1140.

425. Stiefel DJ, Truelove EL, Persson RS, et al. A comparison of oral health in spinal cord injury and other disability groups. Spec Care Dentist 1993; 13:229–235.

426. Stiens SA, Bergman SB, Formal CS. Spinal cord injury rehabilitation. 4. Individual experience, personal adaptation, and social perspectives. Arch Phys Med Rehabil 1997; 78:S65–S72.

427. Stiens SA, Bergman SB, Goetz LL. Neurogenic bowel dysfunction after spinal cord injury: clinical evaluation and rehabilitative management. Arch Phys Med Rehabil 1997; 78:S86–S102.

428. Stiens SA, Fajardo NR, Korsten MA. The gastrointestinal system after spinal cord injury. In: Lin VW, ed. Spinal cord medicine: principles and practice. New York: Demos; 2003:321–348.

429. Stormer S, Gerner HJ, Gruninger W, et al. Chronic pain/dysaesthesiae in spinal cord injury patients: results of a multicentre study. Spinal Cord 1997; 35:446–455.

430. Stotts KM. Health maintenance: paraplegic athletes and nonathletes. Arch Phys Med Rehabil 1986; 67:109–114.

431. Stover SL, DeLisa JA, Whiteneck GG. Clinical outcomes from the Model Systems. Gaithersburg: Aspen; 1995.

432. Stover SL, DeVivo MJ, Go BK. History, implementation, and current status of the National Spinal Cord Injury Database. Arch Phys Med Rehabil 1999; 80:1365–1371.

433. Stover SL, Hahn HR, Miller JM III. Disodium etidronate in the prevention of heterotopic ossification following spinal cord injury (preliminary report). Paraplegia 1976; 14:146–156.

434. Strollo PJ Jr, Rogers RM. Obstructive sleep apnea. N Engl J Med 1996; 334:99–104.

435. Subbarao JV, Garrison SJ. Heterotopic ossification: diagnosis and management, current concepts and controversies. J Spinal Cord Med 1999; 22:273–283.

436. Szlachcic Y, Adkins RH, Adal T, et al. The effect of dietary intervention on lipid profiles in individuals with spinal cord injury. J Spinal Cord Med 2001; 24:26–29.

437. Tai Q, Kirshblum S, Chen B, et al. Gabapentin in the treatment of neuropathic pain after spinal cord injury: a prospective, randomized, double-blind, crossover trial. J Spinal Cord Med 2002; 25:100–105.

438. Talbot HS. The sexual function in paraplegia. J Urol 1955; 73:91–100.

439. Tate DG, Forchheimer M. Contributions from the Model Systems programs to spinal cord injury research. J Spinal Cord Med 2002; 25:316–330.

440. Tate DG, Haig AJ, Krause JS. Vocational aspects of spinal cord injury. In: Kirshblum S, Campagnolo DI, DeLisa JA, eds. Spinal cord medicine. Philadelphia: Lippincott Williams & Wilkins; 2002:312–321.

441. Tator C. Classification of spinal cord injury based on neurological presentation. In: Narayan R, Wilberger J, Povlishock J, eds. Neurotrauma. New York: McGraw-Hill; 1996:1059–1073.

442. Tator CH, Duncan EG, Edmonds VE, et al. Changes in epidemiology of acute spinal cord injury from 1947 to 1981. Surg Neurol 1993; 40:207–215.

443. Thomas DR, Rodeheaver GT, Bartolucci AA, et al. Pressure ulcer scale for healing: derivation and validation of the PUSH tool. The PUSH Task Force. Adv Wound Care 1997; 10:96–101.

444. Thomas S, Banks V, Bale S, et al. A comparison of two dressings in the management of chronic wounds. J Wound Care 1997; 6:383–386.

445. Tomassen PC, Post MW, van Asbeck FW. Return to work after spinal cord injury. Spinal Cord 2000; 38:51–55.

446. Trieschmann R. Spinal cord injuries: psychological, social and vocational adjustment. New York: Pergamon Press; 1980.

447. Triolo RJ, Bogie K. Lower extremity applications of functional neuromuscular stimulation after spinal cord injury. Top Spinal Cord Inj Rehabil 1999; 5:44–65.

448. Vaccaro AR, An HS, Betz RR, et al. The management of acute spinal trauma: prehospital and in-hospital emergency care. Instr Course Lect 1997; 46:113–125.

449. Vaccaro AR, Daugherty RJ, Sheehan TP, et al. Neurologic outcome of early versus late surgery for cervical spinal cord injury. Spine 1997; 22:2609–2613.

450. Vestergaard P, Krogh K, Rejnmark L, et al. Fracture rates and risk factors for fractures in patients with spinal cord injury. Spinal Cord 1998; 36:790–796.

451. Vogel LC, Betz RR, Mulcahey MJ. Spinal cord disorders in children, adolescents. In: Lin VW, ed. Spinal cord medicine: principles and practice. New York: Demos; 2003:851–884.

452. Vogel LC, DeVivo MJ. Pediatric spinal cord injury issues: etiology, demographics, and pathophysiology. Top Spinal Cord Inj Rehabil 1997; 3:1–8.

453. Waring WP, Karunas RS. Acute spinal cord injuries and the incidence of clinically occurring thromboembolic disease. Paraplegia 1991; 29:8–16.

454. Washburn RA, Figoni SF. High density lipoprotein cholesterol in individuals with spinal cord injury: the potential role of physical activity. Spinal Cord 1999; 37:685–695.

455. Waters R, Moore KR, Graboff SR, et al. Brachioradialis to flexor pollicis longus tendon transfer for active lateral pinch in the tetraplegic. J Hand Surg (Am) 1985; 10:385–391.

456. Waters RL, Adkins RH, Yakura JS, et al. Motor and sensory recovery following incomplete tetraplegia. Arch Phys Med Rehabil 1994; 75: 306–311.

457. Waters RL, Adkins RH, Yakura JS, et al. Motor and sensory recovery following complete tetraplegia. Arch Phys Med Rehabil 1993; 74:242–247.

458. Waters RL, Muccitelli LM. Tendon transfers to improve function of patients with tetraplegia. In: Kirshblum S, Campagnolo DI, DeLisa JA, eds. Spinal cord medicine. Philadelphia: Lippincott Williams & Wilkins; 2002:424–437.

459. Waters RL, Yakura JS, Adkins RH, et al. Recovery following complete paraplegia. Arch Phys Med Rehabil 1992; 73:784–789.

460. Waxman SG. Demyelination in spinal cord injury. J Neurol Sci 1989; 91:1–14.

461. Weil A, Lasser A. A quantitative distribution of the pyramidal tract in man. Arch Neurol Psychiatry 1929; 22:495–510.

462. Weinshenker BG, O'Brien PC, Petterson TM, et al. A randomized trial of plasma exchange in acute central nervous system inflammatory demyelinating disease. Ann Neurol 1999; 46:878–886.

463. Weld KJ, Dmochowski RR. Effect of bladder management on urological complications in spinal cord injured patients. J Urol 2000; 163:768–772.

464. Weller DJ, Miller PM. Emotional reactions of patient, family, and staff in acute-care period of spinal cord injury: part 1. Soc Work Health Care 1977; 2:369–377.

465. Wernig A, Nanassy A, Muller S. Laufband (LB) therapy in spinal cord lesioned persons. Prog Brain Res 2000; 128:89–97.

466. Wernig A, Nanassy A, Muller S. Laufband (treadmill) therapy in incomplete paraplegia and tetraplegia. J Neurotrauma 1999; 16:719–726.

467. White AA, Panjabi MM. Clinical biomechanics of the spine. 2nd edn. Philadelphia: Lippincott-Raven; 1990.

468. Whiteneck G, Adler C, Biddle AK, et al, eds. Outcomes following traumatic spinal cord injury: clinical practice guidelines for health-care professionals. Consortium for Spinal Cord Medicine Clinical Practice Guidelines. Washington: Paralyzed Veterans of America; 1999.

469. Whiteneck GG, Charlifue SW, Gerhart KA, et al. Aging with spinal cord injury. New York: Demos; 1993.

470. Winslow C, Rozovsky J. Effect of spinal cord injury on the respiratory system. Am J Phys Med Rehabil 2003; 82:803–814.

471. Woolf CJ, American College of Physicians, American Physiological Society. Pain: moving from symptom control toward mechanism-specific pharmacologic management. Ann Intern Med 2004; 140:441–451.

472. Xakellis GC, Chrischilles EA. Hydrocolloid versus saline-gauze dressings in treating pressure ulcers: a cost-effectiveness analysis. Arch Phys Med Rehabil 1992; 73:463–469.

473. Yarkony GM, Heinemann AW. Pressure ulcers. In: Stover SL, DeLisa JA, Whiteneck GG, eds. Spinal cord injury: clinical outcomes from the Model Systems. Gaithersberg: Aspen; 1995.

474. Yarkony GM, Roth EJ, Heinemann AW, et al. Spinal cord injury rehabilitation outcome: the impact of age. J Clin Epidemiol 1988; 41:173–177.

475. Young RF. Clinical experience with radiofrequency and laser DREZ lesions. J Neurosurg 1990; 72:715–720.

476. Young T, Palta M, Dempsey J, et al. The occurrence of sleep-disordered breathing among middle-aged adults. N Engl J Med 1993; 328: 1230–1235.

477. Young W, Koreh I. Potassium and calcium changes in injured spinal cords. Brain Res 1986; 365:42–53.

478. Zehnder Y, Luthi M, Michel D, et al. Long-term changes in bone metabolism, bone mineral density, quantitative ultrasound parameters, and fracture incidence after spinal cord injury: a cross-sectional observational study in 100 paraplegic men. Osteoporos Int 2004; 15:180–189.

479. Zehnder Y, Risi S, Michel D, et al. Prevention of bone loss in paraplegics over 2 years with alendronate. J Bone Miner Res 2004; 19:1067–1074.

480. Zupan A, Savrin R, Erjavec T, et al. Effects of respiratory muscle training and electrical stimulation of abdominal muscles on respiratory capabilities in tetraplegic patients. Spinal Cord 1997; 35:54–545.

Chapter

57

Lower Limb Peripheral Vascular Disease

Mary Catherine Spires and Peter Kerr Henke

BASIC HEMODYNAMICS OF BLOOD AND LYMPHATIC FLOW

The concepts of pressure, viscosity, flow, and their inter-relationships assist in explaining vascular flow. Poiseuille's law states that resistance is proportional to the viscosity of the fluid and the length of the tube the fluid is passing through, and is inversely proportional to the fourth power of the radius of the tube. As a consequence of this, the vessel radius is the single most important determinant of vessel flow. When the radius of the vessel doubles, and all other parameters remain the same, flow through the vessel increases 16-fold. As a result, vascular resistance is highly sensitive to vascular diameter and is less dependent on vessel length or fluid viscosity.

Blood flow in vascular beds is arranged both in series and in parallel. The entire circulatory system can be thought of as two primary circulations. The left heart sustains the systemic circulation, while the right heart maintains the pulmonary circulation.

The resistance of vessels is similar to resistors in an electrical circuit. The total resistance of vessels connected in series equals the sum of the resistance of each vessel. Therefore the total resistance in the arterial tree from the aorta to the precapillary arteriole equals the sum of the resistance to flow in each vessel generation. The small radius of the terminal arterioles of the microcirculation provides the highest resistance to flow area. With series arrangement, the total resistance of the entire system changes by the same amount as the resistance change in any one of the elements in the series. Thus, if the resistance of one element increases by 10, the total resistance would also increase by 10.

However, the majority of human circulation is arranged in parallel. In this situation, the total vascular resistance equals the sum of the reciprocal of the resistance of the parallel vascular beds. The total resistance is much less affected by resistance change in the single parallel element.

PHYSIOLOGIC CHARACTERISTICS OF VEINS, ARTERIES, AND LYMPHATIC VESSELS

Peripheral vascular resistance depends on the ability of individual vessels to change their internal diameters, which depends on vessel compliance and internal pressure. Vascular resistance is a consequence of the active component of the smooth muscle and the passive stretching reaction of vascular connective tissue.

Compliance of vessels is related to the ratio of elastin to collagen. Elastin allows stretching of vascular walls, because it is 5–10 times more deformable than collagen. The elastin content of the arterial walls increases with arterial size, making large central vessels highly compliant. Collagen, which provides strength to arterial walls, increases in content as the arterial diameter increases.

The compliance of arteries and veins obviously differs, because they vary in the amount of smooth muscle, connective tissue, collagen, and elastin. Although inelastic, small arteries and arterioles are largely composed of smooth muscle. Smooth muscle is the major determinant of peripheral resistance. Arterioles smaller than 1 mm are responsible for the greatest decrement in pressure secondary to their high resistance. The pressure at the entrance of the capillary circulation is typically only 15–30 mmHg. Consequently, arterioles are also called 'resistance vessels', and their resistance can vary widely depending on the tonicity of the smooth muscle at any given time.

Veins have little smooth muscle and are consequently highly compliant. They are the capacitance vessels of the circulation. As internal pressure increases, veins can more readily increase volume than arteries can.

The modulation of the diameter of vessels is partially explained by two theories. The metabolic theory purports that vascular smooth muscle has intrinsic tone, which is modulated by metabolic activity. Examples of metabolic by-products that induce vasodilation are carbon dioxide, adenosine, and lactate, which increases blood flow. When vasodilatating metabolic by-products are eliminated, the basal resting tone resumes. A second theory proposes that the muscle tone increases and smooth muscle contracts in response to stretch induced by pressure, and relaxes when perfusion pressure decreases. It is likely that both factors contribute to changes.[23]

Collateral arteries can develop in response to longstanding blood flow limitations. In the presence of stenosis or occlusion, blood flow is directed to the collateral arteries, where the resistance gradient is less.

Recalling that resistance is a function of the fourth power of the radius, a large number of collateral vessels must develop to effectively compensate for an arterial stenosis. If an artery of 0.6 cm is 50% stenosed, then 1296 collateral vessels of 1 mm in diameter are needed to fully compensate. Hemodynamically significant stenosis generally occurs when the luminal diameter is decreased by approximately 70%.

VASCULAR TESTING

Non-invasive tests for arterial disease

Non-invasive techniques for diagnosis and lesion localization are relatively inexpensive, accurate, and painless. In most cases, they are sufficiently accurate for diagnosis and treatment decision making.

Ankle–brachial pressure index

The ankle–brachial index test (Table 57-1) is available in a large variety of medical settings, including primary care settings. An ankle–brachial systolic pressure ratio of 0.9 or less supports the diagnosis of arterial occlusive disease. The ankle–brachial index should be measured in both lower limbs using the highest brachial pressure.

Segmental limb systolic pressure measurement

In addition to ankle systolic pressure measurements, pressures are obtained in the upper and lower thigh and calf. An abnormal pressure gradient between measurement sites indicates disease and its location (Fig. 57-1). This study is problematic in persons with diabetes, who can present with falsely elevated pressure due to incompressible calcified arteries. Moderate areas of stenosis can also be missed, because little or no pressure gradient may be created at rest.[96]

Segmental plethysmography

This is also called pulse volume recordings. This measures relative changes in volume associated with each cardiac cycle. Waveforms recorded proximally and distally are qualitatively compared. Alteration in waveform contour and size allows detection and localization of an occlusive lesion. This study can complement the systolic pressure measurement, raising accuracy to 95% from 85% in detecting and localizing lesions,[117] but it is not used very often. This study is less operator-dependent than Doppler waveform analysis.

Doppler velocity waveform analysis

Like systolic pressure measurement, waveform analysis of proximal and distal waveform recordings is performed. As mentioned earlier, the accuracy of this study is operator-dependent.

Functional treadmill exercise test

This is not the same test as that performed for cardiac screening. The patient walks on a treadmill at a standard speed and grade. In the presence of significant disease, a decrease in the ankle–brachial index from the resting measurement is documented and may unmask a hemodynamically significant stenosis that is not evident at rest.

Color duplex imaging

Safer and less expensive than arteriography, this offers an alternative for the individual with allergy to contrast dye. It is operator-dependent, however, requiring an experienced technician to maximize data collection regarding arterial anatomy. No hard copy of the visualized anatomy is provided, but CD and video recordings are options. If endovascular or surgical intervention is being considered where an intraoperative arteriogram is not possible, this may be an acceptable study.

Arteriography

This study (Fig. 57-2) should be obtained only if an intervention is planned. It is not a screening test. Arteriography is considered the gold standard for defining the anatomy of the arterial tree. It provides visualization of the extent and type of peripheral arterial occlusion, as well as definition of the remainder of the arterial circulation. Iodinated dye is injected. Arteriography is not without risk in those with renal disease or other comorbidities.[99] The mortality risk is approximately 0.15%,[128] with a slightly higher morbidity risk.[14] The recent development of non-ionic contrast, digital subtraction angiography, and more sophisticated imaging technology mitigates some of the risks of an arteriogram. Partial study angiography involving selected views of the arterial tree also reduces risk. The risks can also be reduced by using CO_2 and gadolinium in those with renal insufficiency.

Magnetic resonance angiography

This is a new approach to the diagnosis of peripheral arterial disease. Auerbach, on review of the literature regarding risks and accuracy, concluded that magnetic resonance angiography (MRA) is safer than angiography.[6] He reported that studies indicate that it is sensitive and specific when compared with the gold standard. MRA might not distinguish between complete tight or complete stenotic lesions, however, and it is institution-dependent with regard to accuracy. As MRA is further developed, the need for angiography might be reduced in many instances.

Table 57-1 Ankle–brachial index readings and their interpretations	
Ankle–brachial index value	Interpretation
>1.3	Consider medial calcification
>0.9	Within normal limits
0.6–0.89	Mild
0.4–0.59	Moderate
<0.4	Severe

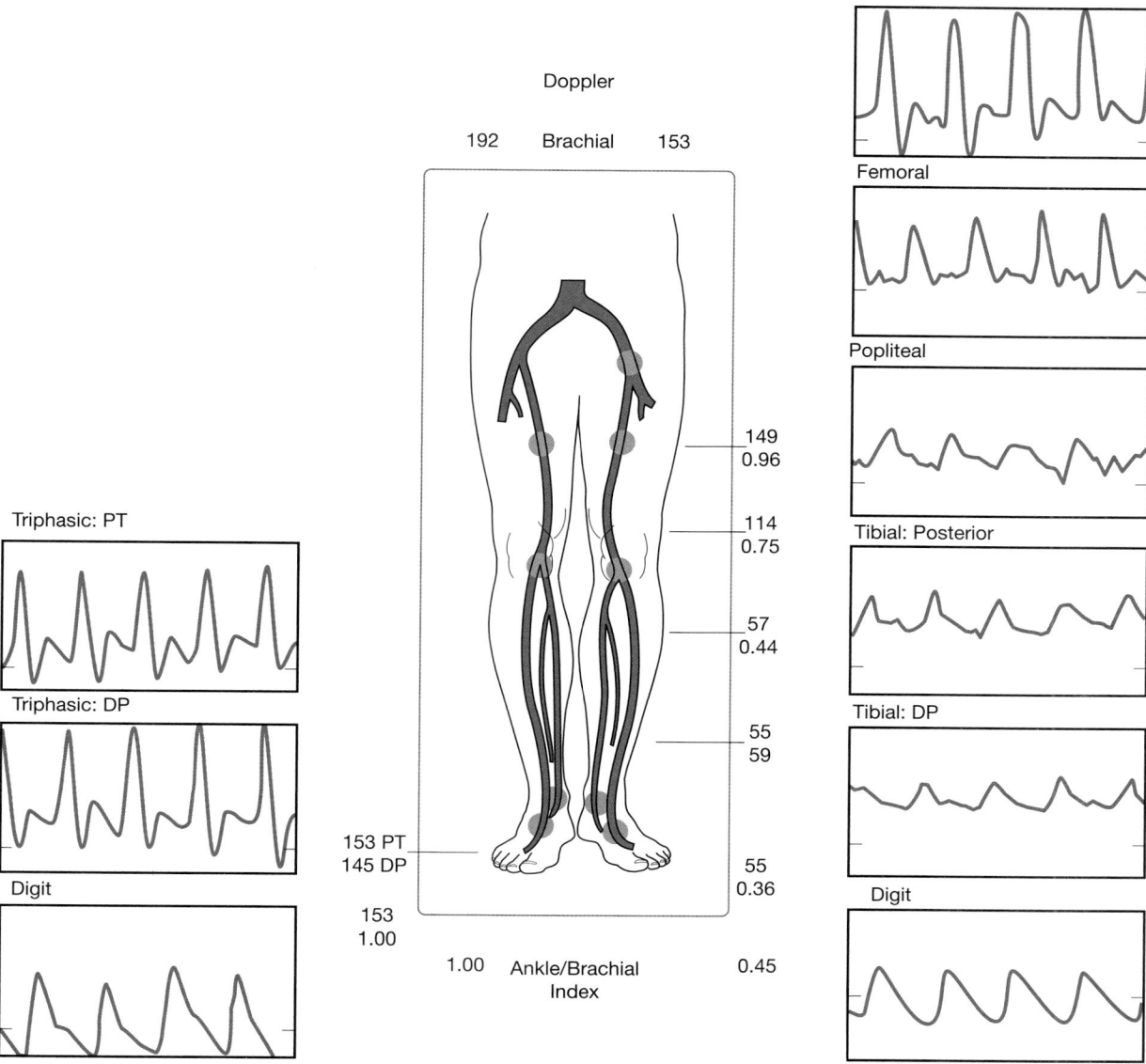

Figure 57-1 An example of segmental Doppler waveforms and systolic pressures in both legs. This patient has right-sided normal pressures and waveforms. In contrast, his left leg has evidence of occlusive disease at his superficial femoral and popliteal artery, as denoted by significant pressure drop at these levels as well as changes in his Doppler waveforms.

ARTERIAL DISEASE

Atherosclerotic peripheral artery disease

Peripheral arterial occlusive disease (PAOD) is the most common arterial disease in developed countries. It is a systemic disease that is defined clinically by a hemodynamic abnormality of an ankle–brachial index less than 0.90 at rest. Less common arterial diseases include thrombosis, embolism, arterial entrapment, fibromuscular dysplasia, arterial dissection, vasospastic disease, and trauma.

Peripheral arterial occlusive disease is most common in older individuals[76] and disproportionately affects black people.[118] PAOD develops earlier in men than in women, with the peak incidence during the sixth and seventh decades of age. PAOD increases with age, with estimates of 1–2.5% of individuals aged 50–60 years having PAOD, and increasing to 5–9% in those over 65 years.[81,121] Asymptomatic peripheral arterial disease affects 17% of men and 20% of women 55 years old and greater.[81]

Intermittent claudication is the most common initial symptom.[99] The majority present with occlusive disease in the femoral–popliteal vessels (80%), and 40% demonstrate stenosis in the tibial–peroneal artery distribution. Nearly one-third have disease in the aorta or iliac arteries. Multiple sites of stenosis are not uncommon.[29]

While the need for endovascular or surgical therapy for PAOD should be rare, the importance of diagnosing PAOD cannot be overemphasized. This is an important marker of

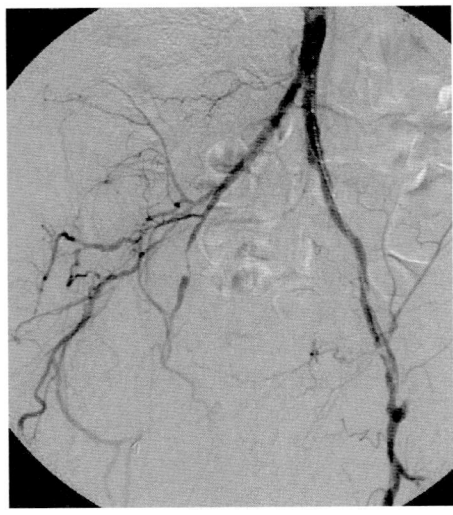

Figure 57-2 Example of an aortopelvic arteriogram, showing the distal disease aorta as well as diffusely diseased iliac arteries with a right-sided external iliac occlusion.

systemic atherosclerosis and, as such, cardiovascular mortality rates are increased three to fourfold in men and women with PAOD. In persons with PAOD, coronary artery disease is responsible for 63% of deaths, while 9% occur secondary to cerebrovascular disease, and 8% are the result of other cardiovascular events.[4,28] Claudication is associated with a 10-year survival of 50%, which is reduced further in persons who have critical limb ischemia.[39] This excess morbidity and mortality is documented extensively, and is observed even when cardiovascular disease is clinically absent.[22,65,71,88,127]

Despite the high prevalence of PAOD and its strong association with cardiovascular morbidity and mortality, this disease is often under-treated or overlooked. Compared with persons with coronary artery disease, patients with PAOD are less likely to receive treatment for risk factors associated with atherosclerosis.[78] Although the prevalence of PAOD is very high in those elderly with diabetes compared with non-diabetic individuals of the same age, diabetic persons with PAOD receive less intensive treatment than those with coronary artery disease or cerebrovascular disease.[66]

Etiology and pathology

Peripheral arterial occlusive disease is similar to atherosclerosis of the coronary and cerebral circulation. Atherosclerotic changes progressively diminish peripheral blood flow. As blood flow is impaired, the classic symptom of claudication occurs. As the atherosclerosis advances, the critical point is reached and the metabolic needs of the limb are no longer met. If hemodynamics are not improved, gangrene and limb loss follow.

Claudication is not completely explained by reduction in arterial flow. As blood flow decreases, several pathophysiologic processes occur. These include type 2 skeletal muscle loss, motor axon loss, histochemical changes in muscle fibers, and disruption of the electron transport chain of the muscle cell. Chronic denervation–reinnervation consistent with ischemic neuropathy also appears. Timely reperfusion allows the oxidative capacity of the previously ischemic muscle to approach normal.[1,69]

Claudication is a dull aching pain, fatigue, and/or muscle cramping induced by inadequate blood flow to the muscles associated with arterial stenosis and occlusion. The pain typically occurs in the calf or buttocks during walking, and resolves with rest. Exercise tolerance is reasonably stable, and rest provides relatively rapid relief. As the disease progresses, symptoms worsen and the patient limits activities accordingly. The location of pain suggests the site of obstruction. Pain in the calf is associated with superficial femoral artery occlusion. Claudication of the thigh is related to common femoral or external iliac artery occlusion, while buttock pain reflects occlusion in the common iliac artery or distal aorta.

Risk factors

The risk factors for developing coronary artery disease and PAOD are similar. The most important risk factors are age, smoking, hypertension, and diabetes mellitus.

Cigarette smoking is a more potent risk factor for the development of PAOD than for coronary artery disease, and increases the risk of developing peripheral atherosclerosis three to fourfold.[133] Nicotine use affects patient outcome and is associated with increased risk of progressing from claudication to ischemic rest pain and the risk of amputation. Amputation occurs more frequently in patients who continue to smoke.[76]

The pathophysiologic mechanisms associated with cigarette smoking are not fully understood, but include abnormalities of endothelial function, lipoprotein metabolism, coagulation, and platelet function. Smoking cessation decreases the risk of cardiovascular morbidity and mortality, and improves functional capacity in patients with PAOD.[76]

Diabetes mellitus is also a risk factor for PAOD. An individual with diabetes is two times more likely to develop claudication than a non-diabetic counterpart is.[29]

Hypertension is also a risk factor for PAOD. Of individuals with hypertension, 2–5% have intermittent claudication, while 35–55% of patients with PAOD also have hypertension. The combination of hypertension and PAOD markedly increases the risk for myocardial infarction, stroke, and death.[20] Other significant risk factors for PAOD include hyperlipidemia and elevated homocysteine levels.

Acute limb ischemia (Table 57-2, Fig. 57-3)

Individuals with an acute arterial occlusion present with excruciating limb pain associated with paresthesias, pallor, poikilothermia, paralysis, and pulselessness. The limb is critically threatened, and immediate evaluation and intervention are required.

The site of the occlusion can often be determined from the level of skin temperature change. For example, decreased temperature only of the foot and ankle only suggests a popliteal occlusion. The etiology of this disease is usually embolic from the heart or aortic arch. The differentiation between this and other etiologies of limb ischemia, such as dissection or thrombosis in situ, is important for therapeutic decisions. Regardless, all patients need immediate and full intravenous heparin.

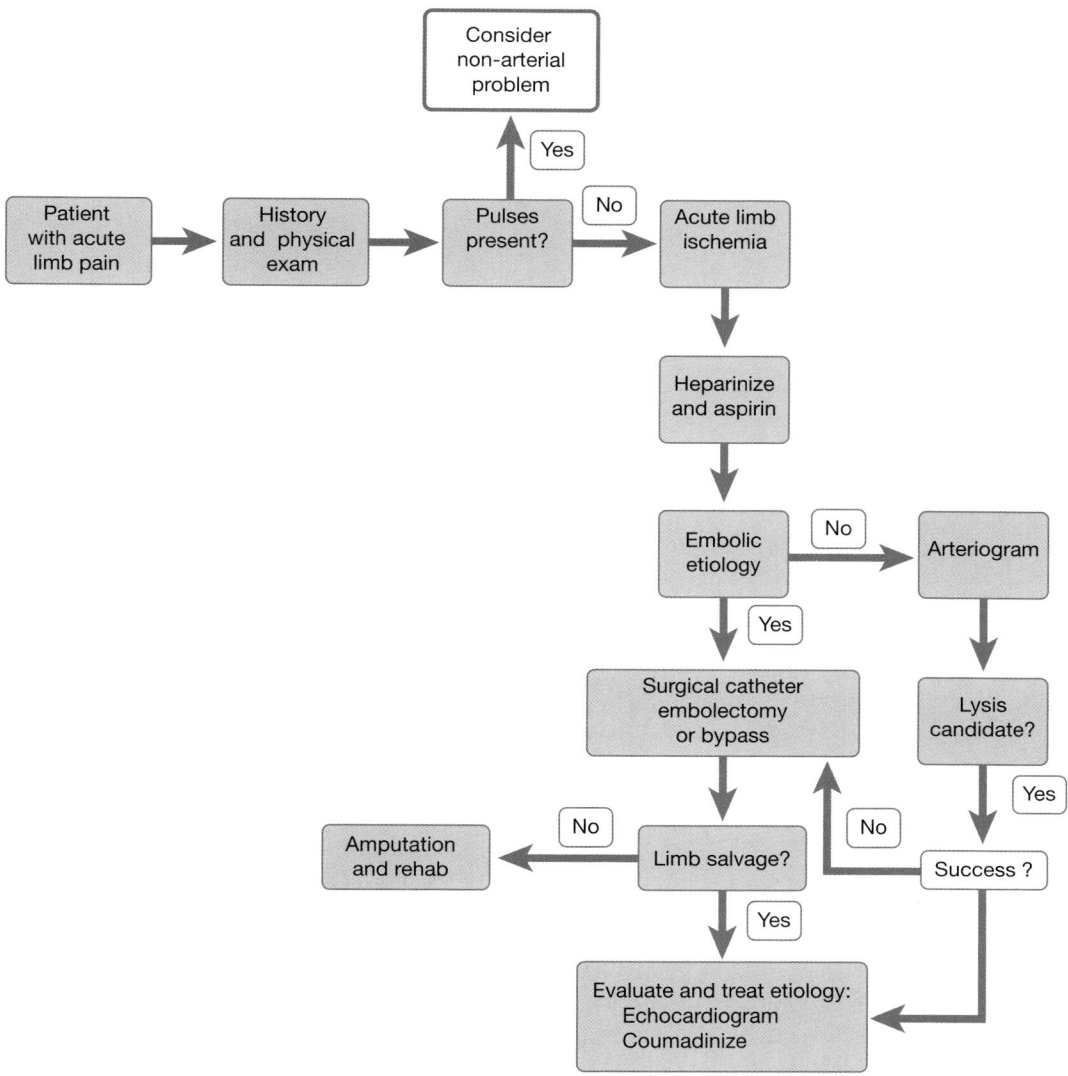

Figure 57-3 Diagnostic and treatment algorithm for a patient with acute limb pain. The foremost goal is to evaluate and treat limb-threatening arterial blockage.

Table 57-2 Classification of acute limb ischemia[29]	
SVS class of acute limb ischemia	Definition
1	Rest pain
2A	Threatened limb
2B	Immediately threatened limb
3	End-stage limb ischemia

If the patient has a clear embolic etiology, the patient should proceed to the operating room for catheter embolectomy. If the etiology is not clear, the patient should proceed to the interventional suite for arteriography and possible thrombolysis. MRA, ankle brachial indices, and other non-invasive studies

are inappropriate for limb-threatening situations. However, if a reproducible, reliable audible pedal pulse is obtained with bedside Doppler, the situation is less urgent. False negative tests are more common than false positive tests. An inaudible Doppler signal does not necessarily mean that the limb is in imminent danger. Care must be taken, however, not to misinterpret venous sounds as arterial.

Chronic limb ischemia (Fig. 57-4)

The signs and symptoms of chronic peripheral vascular disease are varied, but intermittent claudication is the typical presenting complaint.

The functional status is often severely impaired in individuals with intermittent claudication. Comparing older individuals with PAOD with their healthy peers, those individuals with claudication demonstrate 50% less peak exercise capacity. This is equivalent to moderate to severe heart failure using the New York Heart Association criteria.[9,47,49]

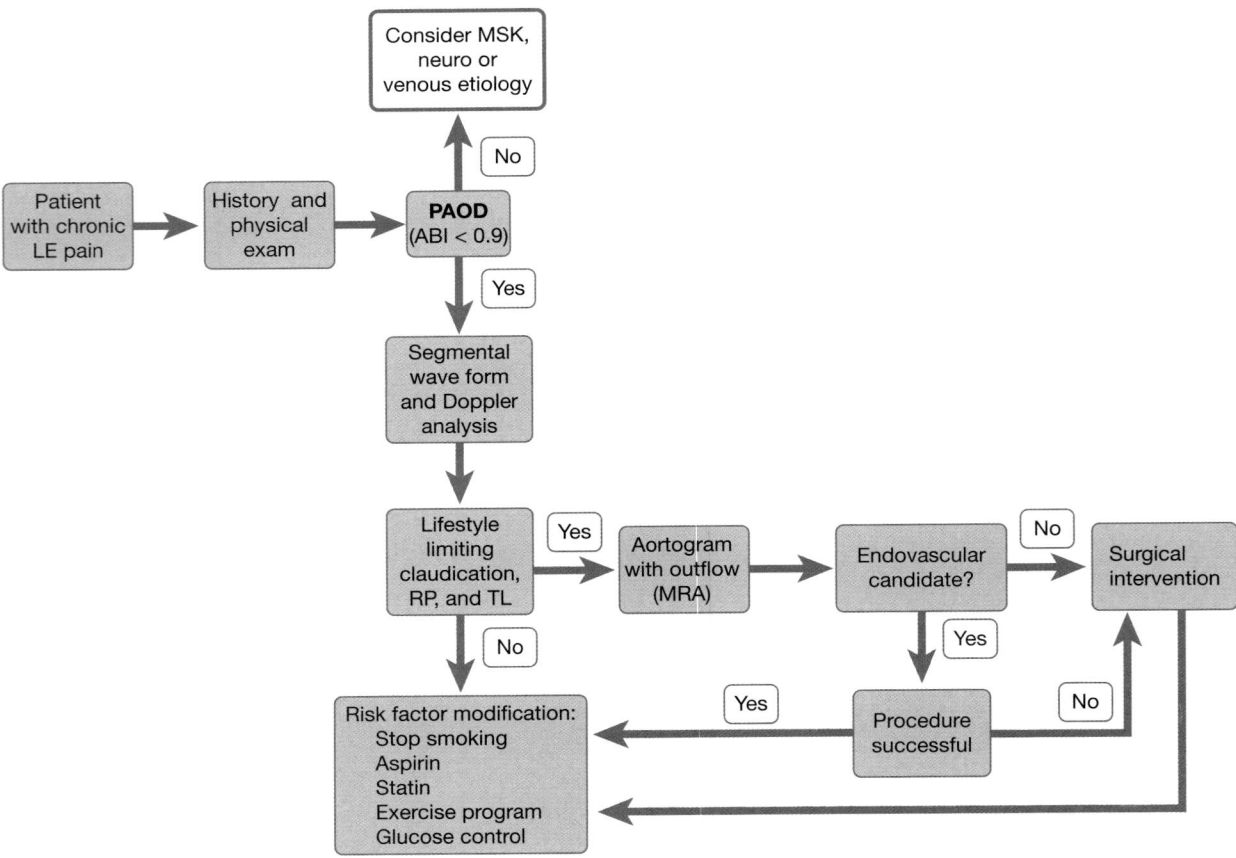

Figure 57-4 Diagnostic and treatment algorithm for a patient with chronic lower extremity pain. Consideration of peripheral arterial occlusive disease (PAOD) must be given if the patient's ankle–brachial index (ABI) is less than 0.90. However, many patients have multiple etiologies of their limb pain, for example osteoarthritis and PAOD. LE, Lower extremity; MRA, Magnetic resonance angiography; MSK, Musculoskeletal; Neuro, Neurological; RP, Rest pain; TL, Tissue loss; Statin, HmG CoA reductase inhibitor.

Claudication curtails ambulation and negatively impacts leisure and work activities. Impairment of daily activities increases as claudication and disease advance, leading to a poorer quality of life.[111] Dumville reported that persons with intermittent claudication report significantly reduced quality of life scores compared with those from patients without claudication.[30] The reduction in scores was related to lower physical health scores ($P \leq 0.001$) rather than the domains of social functioning and mental health. Asymptomatic PAOD did not significantly affect health-related quality of life.

As PAOD advances, pain occurs earlier during activity. In the normally perfused foot, the foot becomes slightly pale when elevated. Maximal capillary blush appears immediately when the foot is returned to a dependent position. However, ischemia leads to distal foot pallor with elevation. Dependency results in a delayed return of maximal color of 20 seconds or longer. The foot is bluish red, termed *dependent rubor*, and indicates maximal small vessel dilatation caused by tissue ischemia.

Chronic PAOD treatment

Pain management

Ischemic limb pain is difficult to manage. Initial analgesia with acetaminophen (paracetamol) or non-steroidal antiinflammatory drugs (NSAIDs) is recommended. NSAIDs require careful consideration in the setting of renal insufficiency, peptic ulcer disease, and hypertension. Chronic limb ischemia often requires opiates to achieve tolerable pain relief. Positioning the limb in a dependent position, such as in a recliner chair, can act synergistically with analgesics. Scheduled pain medication is preferred to using them on demand, in order to achieve more constant blood levels.

Risk modification as treatment

Risk modification is fundamental to the treatment of PAOD. Management should aggressively address the control of modifiable risk factors, including tobacco use, hypertension, hyperlipidemia, and maintaining glycohemoglobin levels to <7.0%.[29]

Smoking not only increases the risk of developing arterial disease, but is also associated with greater disease progression.[62,86] Smoking is correlated with an increased risk of amputation, stroke, myocardial infarction, and death. Smoking cessation is critical to successful management. Patients should be informed that continued tobacco use will accelerate disease progression and increase mortality. There is evidence that those who stop smoking have slower disease progression and symptom severity.[60,61]

Patients with PAOD should be screened for diabetes mellitus. It appears that glycemic control alone is insufficient to mitigate disease progression or severity. It should be coupled with attention to other risk factors as well. Intense glycemic control lowers the risk of other complications of diabetes that would positively impact PAOD and treatment options.

An additional concern is the development of diabetic sensory–motor peripheral neuropathy. With reduction in sensation and motor control of the lower limbs, these individuals are at increased risk for ulceration. The neuropathy coupled with underlying arterial disease increases the risk of foot infection and sepsis, as well as limb amputation.

Hyperlipidemia is a well-recognized risk factor for the development of atherosclerotic disease. Individuals with PAOD require a fasting lipid profile evaluation. Elevated low-density lipoprotein (LDL) and triglycerides, and depressed high-density lipoproteins, are associated with atherosclerosis. The first step is diet modification and counseling from an experienced qualified dietician. The lipid profile goal includes reduction of serum LDL to less than 100 mg/dL and perhaps < 70 mg/dL. This target LDL often requires pharmacologic intervention.[75]

Hypertension should be treated similarly to how it is treated in those who have cardiovascular disease. Although it is reported that a few patients experience slight worsening of claudication with blood pressure reduction,[120] this has not been validated.[106] There is no convincing evidence that beta-blocker use increases claudication. Reduction of blood pressure is required to reduce the risk of the morbidity and mortality of myocardial infarction, stroke, and cardiovascular death.

Exercise

'Stop smoking and keep walking' is probably the best treatment intervention for individuals with mild to moderate disease, but it is difficult to get patients to comply with this advice.[55] Exercise training is recognized as an effective treatment intervention, and cardiovascular complications occur rarely.[41,70,113] No data are available to indicate that simply advising patients of the need of exercise is efficacious.[55]

Exercise appears to stimulate adaptation at several levels of physiologic and mechanical function. Although evidence is inconsistent in demonstrating increased blood flow and oxygen delivery, several favorable physiologic responses have been associated with increased walking ability. Many mechanisms appear to mediate favorable changes, but the relative contributions of these mechanisms remain undetermined.

Exercise increases endothelial function by increasing the expression of nitric oxide synthase and the release of nitric oxide and prostacyclin, favoring vasodilatation. The associated increase in vascular endothelial growth factor favors angiogenesis and the associated decrease in inflammatory response leads to a reduction in free radicals. The observed improved skeletal muscle metabolism, including decreased utilization of and dependence on anaerobic metabolism, is associated with increased muscle oxidative capacity and muscle enzyme activity, as well as improved muscle acylcarnitine homeostasis.[35,48,50,51,64,116,123] Rheologic characteristics, such as decreased blood viscosity and filterability, have been established. In addition, cell aggregation is decreased and fibrinolytic profiles improved.

Prospective studies support the hypothesis that exercise benefits claudication symptoms.[70,112,114] Gardner's metaanalysis of exercise rehabilitation regimens for claudication indicates that exercise training to near-maximal pain performed regularly for at least 6 months benefits claudication symptoms.[41] Walking time increased by 120% (average), and distance increased by an average of 180%. This study does not compare the intervention with a non-exercised control group, however. Leng's analysis of randomized controlled trials reports maximal walking time improvements ranging from 74% to 230% (average 150%).[70] Walking to the near-maximum pain performed a minimum of three times per week under the supervision of a trained professional results in the most improvement. McDermott demonstrated that a supervised treadmill walking program is beneficial for the patient who has PAOD without a history of claudication.[79]

Furthermore, improvements in claudicating symptoms are also associated with improved ability to perform daily activities.[34,42,82,111,112] At 1 year, individuals who were maintained on a maintenance exercise program maintained improvements in activities of daily living and pain.[42]

Comparing strength training to treadmill exercise, strength training is less effective[49,111] and did not improve walking ability.[49,111]

Ambrosetti evaluated an intensive 4-week in-hospital rehabilitation for individuals with claudication.[2] The study originated in Europe and 107 individuals (>90% men) completed the program. Participants showed a significant increase in walking distance and in treadmill testing. Calculation of costs showed that this approach was cost-effective in the European setting, but costs in the USA probably make this option unrealistic.

Various exercise protocols, varying in intensity, duration, and specific exercises, have been evaluated to determine if exercise improves symptoms and function. Although the majority of authors recommend a three times per week program of walking-induced claudication for at least 6 months, some caveats must be kept in mind.

Individuals with claudication are at increased risk for cardiovascular events, including myocardial infarction and stroke. The exercise prescription for claudication must take this into account. Before prescribing a claudication exercise program, a 12-lead electrocardiogram stress test to uncover any ST-T wave abnormalities, arrhythmias, and ischemic symptoms is advisable. Stress testing can also provide information regarding claudication threshold, heart rate, and blood pressure parameters for exercise prescription.

If claudication limits performance (i.e. the patient does not reach actual maximal exercise performance because of claudication), a prescription for supervised slowly progressive claudication exercise therapy treatment can be written. Supervised walking three to five times per week is preferred to strength training. Strength training can be used to augment the program to reduce other impairments that limit activity.

Exercise should be supervised with heart rate and blood pressure monitoring during the initial period. Supervised walking, preferably on a treadmill where the rate and workload can be objectively measured and controlled, should be done at a pace that precipitates claudication within 3–5 min of continuous walking.

Once the patient experiences moderate claudication, the patient rests until symptoms resolve. A walk–rest–walk cycle is established, increasing by 3–5 min per treatment as tolerated. The goal is walking 50 min at least three times per week. Once the patient is established on the walking program, the patient can be placed on a therapy maintenance program with periodic evaluation to assure that the therapy is being done appropriately. Both the patient and the therapist should be informed that improvements might not be appreciated for 4–6 weeks, and that the program must continue for at least 6 months.

Pharmaceutical interventions for chronic PAOD

A great variety of medications have been prescribed over the years, but none is universally accepted as *the* effective treatment.[110] Because platelet aggregation can exacerbate disease by causing mechanical obstruction or stimulating local vasospasm, medications that reduce platelet activity are considered beneficial. Aspirin, a cyclooxygenase inhibitor, reduces platelet function and is best documented as effective in reducing cardiovascular events. There is some evidence to suggest that it slows the progression of atherosclerosis. Low-dose aspirin, when compared with placebo, showed a 54% risk reduction in peripheral arterial surgery.[45]

Antiplatelet therapy appears less beneficial in increasing walking distance and other measures of function. However, its positive effects on reducing cardiovascular events support its continued use in patients with claudication.[3,40,126]

Pentoxifylline, a methylxanthine derivative, is a hemorrheologic agent approved for use in claudication. Its reported benefits include antiplatelet effects, lowering plasma fibrinogen levels, and improved white and red cell deformability. However, variable success in treating symptoms of PAOD has been reported.[53,59,104]

The one trial comparing pentoxifylline with exercise showed that patients on drug therapy achieved significantly greater walking distances after 3 months than those on exercise therapy alone.[19] Patients intolerant to other methylxanthine derivatives, such as caffeine and theophylline, should avoid this medication.

Although some earlier studies indicated that pentoxifylline was associated with increased walking distance, Dawson found that it was equivalent to the placebo.[24] In a metaanalysis, Girolami demonstrated modest increases in walking,[43] but the average effect was small and the clinical significance was questioned. However, pentoxifylline might be advantageous in patients not suitable for exercise programs. Its side effect profile is unfavorable.

Ticlopidine is a thienopyridine that selectively inhibits ADP. It is used less frequently. It requires monitoring because of serious side effects, such as neutropenia and thrombotic thrombocytopenia purpura.

Clopidogrel is also a platelet aggregation inhibitor associated with decreased atherosclerotic disease progression. However, it has the side effects of minor bleeding, gastrointestinal complaints, and edema.[119] This medication is more beneficial than aspirin for patients at higher risk of cardiovascular events.

Cilostazol is reported to have fewer side effects than pentoxifylline, and some have considered as more effective pharmacologic intervention. Multicenter trials support this contention.[8,10,25,85,93] This drug acts primarily to inhibit phosphodiesterase type 3, which increases cyclic AMP. It induces vasodilatation, and inhibits platelet aggregation and smooth muscle proliferation. Its therapeutic mechanism is not fully understood. Cilostazol is contraindicated in patients with congestive heart failure. The most common side effect in other populations is headache. Transient diarrhea, dizziness, and palpitations have also been reported.

Several lipid-lowering agents are available. Leng's review in the *Cochrane Database of Systematic Reviews* assesses the effects of lipid-lowering agents on lower limb atherosclerosis.[72] Using the outcomes of mortality and disease progression, this review did not determine that one lipid-lowering agent was better than another. More studies of the efficacy of the newer and more expensive agents are needed. However, given the significant cardioprotective effects of statin agents on cardiovascular mortality, most patients with PAOD should be on these agents unless not tolerated.

Surgical intervention and treatment

All patients with PAOD should have the above-mentioned risk factor modifications and an exercise program inititated. Interventions, including endovascular or surgical ones, should be used judiciously and only for severe claudication, rest pain, and tissue loss.

Percutaneous balloon transluminal angioplasty (PTA) dilates and recanalizes stenosed or occluded arteries. Although balloon dilatation is a common technique, the use of lasers and other recent technology such as cryoplasty is increasing. With balloon dilatation, the atheromatous plaque is compressed and fractured, leading to increased arterial lumen diameter. PTA is typically indicated for lesions less than 10 cm, but the outcome is determined by the site as well as the extent of local disease. Often, a stent is also used to decrease the risk of recurrent disease.[12,20,108,131]

Patients with focal disease and adjacent patent collateral circulation ('run off') benefit from PTA. The success of PTA is not only dependent on anatomic selection, but on patient selection as well. Focal stenosis or short lesions in select anatomic sites, such as a common iliac lesion, typically fare well. It can be used as an adjuvant with revascularization surgery. Select patients who are not suitable for surgical revascularization, such as high-risk cardiac patients, might benefit from this procedure. Diffuse disease or lack of restorable patent adjacent collateral circulation is not successfully treated with this procedure.

The 5-year patency for PTA ranges from 80 to 90% in the iliac system and from 30 to 70% in the superficial femoral artery, although this is probably higher than in most series.[21] However, the vessel can restenose post intervention.[105,131] Complications include hematoma at the puncture site, thrombosis, and embolization.

The outcome of PTA in isolated iliac occlusive disease is improving, such that it may be preferred over surgery. However, infrainguinal disease is more likely to be diffuse, and surgical bypass is usually preferred.

Surgical bypass is reserved for patients with the above-mentioned indications, and must be carefully planned. Aortobifemoral bypass is the standard for aortoiliac disease. In unilateral disease, a femoral–femoral bypass or iliofemoral bypass can be performed. The femoral–femoral bypass is an extraanatomic procedure, and has a reduced morbidity but significantly lower long-term patency.

In the case of infrainguinal disease, such as superficial femoral or proximal popliteal occlusion, a femoral popliteal bypass can be indicated if good run off is present. If this surgery is not appropriate, bypass to more distal vessels, such as the posterior tibial, anterior tibial, medial, and plantar arteries, can provide successful restoration of flow and is a standard technique, but is mainly used for limb salvage and not claudication.[44,45]

Saphenous vein bypass grafting is frequently performed for revascularization, and is the preferred conduit. Two techniques are typically employed: in situ technique and the reverse technique. If the saphenous vessels are not usable, other suitable veins, such as cephalic or lesser saphenous, can be selected. Complications include infection, delayed wound healing, and early occlusion. Depending on the location of the graft, long-term patency varies. Long-term patency of the grafts at 5 years ranges from 80% for femoropopliteal to 60% for tibial grafts.[124]

Prosthetic grafts are available and have been used for many years. However, autogenous vein grafts are preferred because of superior patency rates when compared with prosthetic graft patency. The infection risk is significantly greater with a prosthetic graft, and prosthetic grafts are typically reserved for cases where autogenous veins are not an option.

The cost and benefits of these surgeries need to be considered. In the case of severe chronic limb ischemia, at times amputation is the only surgical choice. However, some patients may choose amputation rather then having multiple procedures to delay what appears inevitable. Experience teaches clinicians that the elderly patients, or those with limited life expectancy, might find it more beneficial to go forward with amputation rather than spend significant periods of time hospitalized secondary to surgery. Amputation with prosthetic restoration and rehabilitation may afford a more comfortable and higher quality of life.

Exercise regimen compared with angioplasty (PTA)

Creasy compared therapeutic exercise with angioplasty.[21] At 6 months, the PTA group showed an increase in walking time compared with the walking exercise group. After 6 months,

however, the angioplasty group declined while the exercise subjects improved. At 12 months, the exercise group had improved further. Fowkes reported a similar initial period of improvement that was not sustained after PTA.[38,131]

Perkins reported on a prospective randomized trial of 56 patients, comparing participants who underwent PTA versus a walking exercise program; no difference was seen between the groups at 15-month follow-up.[102]

In general, PTA should not be used for mild claudication, for which an exercise program is best.

Other treatments to prevent limb loss in PAOD patients (Fig. 57-5)

Appropriate foot protection is critical in this high-risk population. Prescribed shoe wear should be worn any time the patient is weight bearing. Feet should be protected from any type of trauma, regardless of how minor, including extreme temperatures. Foot care that includes nail trimming should be done regularly by a podiatrist or other specialist.

With advancing disease, ischemic ulcers of the feet can also occur. These are typically painful and are present at the toes. Debridement should be kept to a minimum to preserve tissue. Wound infection is problematic and requires meticulous wound care and observation.

Frank infection, cellulitis, and osteomyelitis can precipitate limb loss. If an ischemic wound appears infected, systemic antibiotics are indicated. Wounds are typically polymicrobial, especially in those patients having diabetes.

Multiple dressings and topical agents are available, but there are no sound blinded randomized studies to support the effectiveness of one product over another in this population. Most studies of these products have been with neuropathic and diabetic ulcerations (see Ch. 33).

Hyperbaric oxygen treatment and application of negative pressure to the lower limb have gained popularity; however, there are no randomized controlled studies to support claims of efficacy.[29]

Chelation therapy with EDTA has undergone randomized trials. No reduction in claudication or improvement in perfusion was documented in the treatment of peripheral disease.[33]

Sympathectomy for the management of pain, to increase perfusion, to reduce tissue loss, or as an adjuvant to revascularization surgery has had disappointing results. Typically, this is reserved for individuals who have inoperable disease. This is more commonly done currently with chemical sympathectomy by injection.[29]

BUERGER DISEASE (THROMBOANGIITIS OBLITERANS)

Buerger disease, also called thromboangiitis obliterans, typically affects young male smokers, occurring before age 40–45. Although the cause is unknown, the disease is highly correlated with tobacco use.[83,95,122]

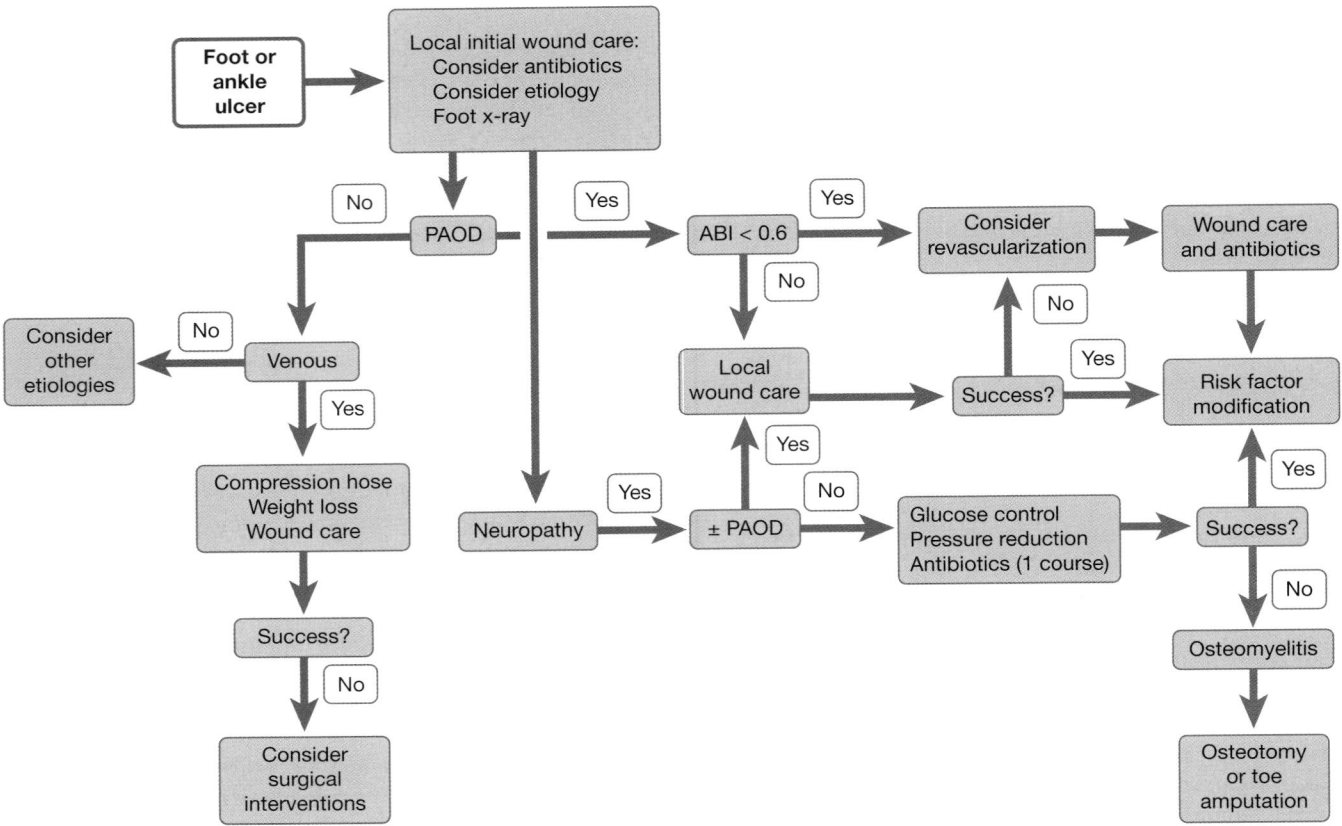

Figure 57-5 Diagnostic and treatment algorithm for a patient with a foot (or ankle) ulcer. Consideration of underlying peripheral arterial occlusive disease is important, as is treating osteomyelitis that may prevent this condition from healing adequately. ABI, ankle–brachial index; PAOD, peripheral arterial occlusive disease.

Exacerbation and remission of the disease are highly correlated with smoking and smoking cessation, respectively.[91,92,94]

Thromboangiitis obliterans is most prevalent in India, the Middle East, and the Far East. It is least prevalent in western Europe and the Americas.[107] There is some evidence that this disease is becoming less prevalent in the USA.[29]

The life expectancy of individuals with the disease is similar to that of age-matched controls, and probably relates to the lack of coronary and cerebral artery involvement. Ohta reported a 25-year survival rate of 83.8% in his series of 110 patients,[91] although ischemic ulcerations remained problematic and recurred in two-thirds of his patients. Patients experience ischemic pain, ulcerations, and minor and major limb amputations. After age 60, the recurrence of ulcerations declines.

Thromboangiitis obliterans is characterized by prominent arterial wall inflammatory cell infiltration, resulting in the development of extensive segmental occlusions of small and medium arteries of the upper and lower limbs. Distal vessels are typically first involved, and the process progresses proximally. The lower limb is the primary site of disease in the majority of patients; however, as many as 30–40% present with upper and lower involvement.[83,84]

Clinically, Buerger disease typically causes gangrene or critical ischemia, while ischemic claudication is less common. Claudi-

cation is more suggestive of proximal progression.[29] Ischemic claudication of the feet, which must be distinguished from arthritis, is rare but more frequent in thromboangiitis obliterans than in PAOD. In a study of 112 patients at the Cleveland Clinic, Olin reported that over 70% of patients presented with ulcerations, and over half reported symptoms consistent with ischemic claudication. Superficial thrombophlebitis and Raynaud phenomenon occur in approximately 40%.[94]

Several criteria exist for the diagnosis of thromboangiitis obliterans and involve clinical, arteriographic, and pathologic criteria: history of tobacco use, ischemic disease of distal limbs prior to age 45, involvement of the infrapatellar and infrabrachial arteries, arteries proximal to the popliteal and brachial arteries are normal, and there are arteriogram abnormalities consistent with the disease.

Treatment

Smoking cessation is fundamental to successful treatment. Strict prohibition of smoking generally results in quiescence of the disease and improved symptoms. Smokeless nicotine has been documented to facilitate disease progression.[73,90] Olin reported that, among 120 patients with thromboangiitis obliterans, of the 43% who abstained from any form of tobacco use, most did not require an amputation.[95] If the individual did not have gangrene at the time of smoking cessation, limb loss did not occur. Those who continued tobacco use were at higher risk for disease progression and limb loss. Continued nicotine use can be determined with urine testing for nicotine and its metabolites.

Ischemic ulcers require local wound care, including regular cleansing and antibiotics if an infection is a concern. Local debridement, including surgical excision of exposed bone and necrotic tissue, can be indicated. Progressive vascular disease and infection can lead to amputation.

Sympathectomy has been proposed as a treatment, but data to support this are not available, and the studies to date have been inconclusive.[29]

Revascularization is typically not appropriate because of segmental disease. Target distal vessels to which to bypass are lacking as well. Amputation is unavoidable.

VASOSPASTIC DISEASE OR RAYNAUD SYNDROME

Survey data indicate that approximately 4–15% of the general population experience Raynaud syndrome.[77] Individuals with this syndrome have vasospastic tricolor change of bilateral digits with exposure to cold. Stress and cigarette smoking can trigger vasospasm in some individuals. The phenomenon is painful and can have a burning quality. Some individuals report associated numbness and upper limb swelling.

A series of vasospastic events occur when exposed to the triggering agent or event. Initially, the vasoconstriction of muscular digital arteries and precapillary arteries induces digital pallor. Arteriovenous shunting accompanies the arterial closure. Hemoglobin desaturation produces acrocyanosis. Once the trigger is removed, rubor or mottling appears. The phenomenon is typically bilateral and resolves within 15–20 min of removing the precipitant.[132]

There are two types of Raynaud syndrome: primary Raynaud syndrome (Raynaud phenomenon) and secondary Raynaud syndrome (Raynaud disease). These are distinct entities. Primary Raynaud syndrome is a phenomenon of unknown etiology that causes no tissue damage. It is not associated with underlying disease. Increased sympathetic response to stress is often postulated as the cause.

The diagnosis of primary Raynaud syndrome is given once secondary causes of Raynaud syndrome are excluded. Because Raynaud syndrome can actually be a precursor heralding the development of systemic or other underlying disease, the diagnosis of primary Raynaud syndrome is not given until the individual has been monitored for more than 2 years and no other disease emerges.

Secondary Raynaud syndrome, or Raynaud disease, is associated with underlying systemic pathology, including systemic sclerosis, collagen vascular disease, or vasculitis. The vasospastic episodes are intense, and vascular fibrosis can occur. Arterial occlusive disease is suggested if the syndrome is unilateral. Intimal fibrosis, fibrin deposition, platelet activation, and dis-

ruption of the clotting cascade can result in digital ulceration, and sclerodactyly can result. Treatment of secondary Raynaud syndrome is targeted at the underlying disease.

Nicotine abstinence is required, and patients with both syndromes should avoid triggers. Education includes teaching the patient to avoid cold exposure and to wear appropriate protective clothing in cold weather. Patients with primary Raynaud syndrome should be reassured that this it is not a limb- or life-threatening disease.

Secondary Raynaud syndrome, from systemic sclerosis or vasculitis or other disease, may respond to vasodilators such as calcium channel blockers or topical nitroglycerin. Surgical intervention such as sympathectomy or digital microarteriolysis may be an option in selected cases. In extreme cases, digital amputation can be needed.[5]

VENOUS INSUFFICIENCY DISEASE

Approximately 3–11% of the adult population experience chronic venous insufficiency.[16,89] Symptoms typically include lower limb aching, fatigue, and edema. Other common complaints include varicose veins, cramps, and itching or burning sensations. Skin changes include hyperpigmentation, stasis dermatitis, telangiectasia, and ulceration.

The normal distal to proximal unidirectional venous flow depends on normal venous anatomy, including competent valves, and calf muscle pump dynamics. Blood is directed from the superficial venous system via the perforating vessels to the deep veins and on to the central circulation. Walking and exercise produce a two-thirds decrease in lower limb peripheral venous volume.[89]

Venous insufficiency occurs secondary to abnormalities in the architecture of the venous system, such as destruction of valves or abnormalities of the venous wall. These abnormalities produce venous hypertension, associated venous reflux, and/or venous occlusion. Valve incompetence typically results from damage secondary to venous thrombosis, and is less likely due to congenital valve absence or incompetence. Incompetent valves allow blood to reflux through the perforating veins to the superficial system. The superficial system, which normally manages 10–15% of venous volume, is unable to manage the excess volume. Muscle contraction aggravates these events, leading to venous hypertension rather than pressure reduction.

Increased capillary hydrostatic pressure also increases capillary permeability, allowing fluid and protein transudation and erythrocytic diapedesis. Hemosiderin from the erythrocyte degradation results in skin discoloration.[26]

Several studies have investigated the relationship between acute deep vein thrombosis and long-term venous hemodynamic disturbances. The incidence of the postthrombotic syndrome was 67–80%, depending on the extent of the thrombosis.[21] The incidence of the postthrombotic syndrome and the severity of the hemodynamic abnormalities increased when the popliteal or more proximal veins were involved. Valve competence is more likely to be preserved in those individuals who demonstrate recanalization faster and more completely after a deep venous thrombosis.[97,98]

Varicose veins are a common sign of chronic venous insufficiency. The prevalence varies in men and women depending on geography and criteria used. Epidemiologic studies vary widely, with some reporting the prevalence of varicose veins in women to be as high as 73%.[11,31]

Varicose veins are classified as primary or secondary. Valve damage from previous deep venous thrombosis results in secondary varicose veins, while primary varicosities are due to venous dilatation without a history of thrombosis. The most common site of development is at the junction of the superficial and deep veins, particularly in the perforating system and at the saphenofemoral and saphenopopliteal veins.

Treatment of chronic venous insufficiency, including varicose veins, targets reduction of venous hypertension, which occurs with ambulation and the upright position. Elevation of the legs above cardiac level reduces hydrostatic pressure. This must be done repeatedly throughout the day and at night to reduce edema.

Graduated compression stockings are effective, and pressures of 30–40 mmHg are typically used. Pressures of 20–30 mmHg are used for those individuals with underlying arterial disease. It is important to instruct the patient to put the stockings on first thing before getting out of bed, as this is when the limbs are smallest and venous pressure is the lowest. Patients with significant edema can also require a program of intermittent pneumatic compression pump therapy. Once maximal reduction of edema is achieved, graduated compression garments can be used. Intermittent graduated compression pumps consist of a boot that is intermittently inflated and deflated with compressed air on a timed cycle. Several products are on the market, and the maximal pressures and cycle times vary. Several hypotheses regarding the physiologic events associated with pneumatic compression have been evaluated, including increasing oxygen tension and blood flow, but the physiologic principles involved remain poorly understood.[13] The current literature also does not provide sufficient data to determine the most effective choice of pneumatic compression or treatment protocols for chronic venous insufficiency or ulcers.[13] Complications from using pneumatic compression devices include peroneal mononeuropathy[66] and genital edema.[15] Contraindications include congestive heart failure, deep venous thrombosis, significant arterial insufficiency, and local infection.

Surgical intervention is typically not indicated in venous disease but can be helpful in target situations, such as saphenous vein ligation or ligation of perforators when superficial venous insufficiency predominates.

Sclerotherapy is common and used for treatment of small distal varicosities, spider veins, and insufficiency due to superficial vessels. The most common use of sclerotherapy is cosmetic.

Venous ulceration prevalence is estimated at 0.18–1.3% of the population.[87] Ulceration frequently occurs just above the medial malleolus, where the perforating veins and deep veins meet. Ulceration correlates with venous ambulatory pressure.

Pressures exceeding 80 mmHg are associated with a high risk of developing venous ulcers. Ulcers are rare in those with pressures under 40 mmHg.[74]

Venous ulcers are difficult to heal and frequently recur. At 4 months, only about 50% are healed, and approximately 8% persist at 5 years.[31]

Patient compliance is fundamental to treatment success. Most ulcers will heal when the patient is compliant with prescribed elastic bandages, paste bandages such as Unna boot, and graded compression garments. In older individuals, compression stockings are frequently difficult for the patient to manage secondary to decreased hand strength and fine motor control.[52] Other options or assistance should be sought.

DEEP VEIN THROMBOSIS (Fig. 57-6)

Venous thromboembolism is an important cause of mortality and morbidity that manifests itself primarily as deep venous thrombosis and pulmonary embolism. Literature over the years has documented that over 90% of pulmonary embolisms are associated with proximal lower limb thrombosis. Deep venous thromboses of the proximal lower limb vessels are more likely to be associated with pulmonary embolism than those of the calf. Virchow's triad of immobility, endothelial damage, and hypercoagulation disorders are risk factors.

Horlander reports that the age-adjusted mortality rate declined from 191 per million in 1979 to 94 per million in 1998.[54] Despite a decreased incidence of pulmonary embolism, it remains a significant cause of death. The mortality rate from pulmonary embolism is reported to be 20–30% and is higher in men than in women.

Consequently, it is important to have a high index of suspicion for both these diagnoses. The literature is replete with documentation that both these diagnoses are often overlooked. High-risk populations on a rehabilitation unit include those with spinal cord injury, stroke, status post orthopedic surgery, trauma, and obesity, as well as aged patients and many others.

The gold standard for diagnosis of deep venous thrombosis is duplex ultrasonography (Fig. 57-7). It is highly sensitive and specific for popliteal femoral and iliac venous thrombosis, with some decrease in sensitivity for below the knee thrombi. The echogenic characteristic of the thrombus implies the acuity or chronicity of the thrombus. One drawback of duplex ultrasonography is that its accuracy is operator-dependent.

Pulmonary angiography is the gold standard for pulmonary embolism diagnosis. A pulmonary ventilatory–perfusion (V/Q) scan is frequently the test first ordered, but it is often not diagnostic. Spiral computed tomography is increasingly being ordered in preference to a V/Q scan.

The goal of treatment is to prevent the extension and propagation of clot. The standard of care is low molecular weight heparin (LMWH). LMWH is easy to administer and requires dosing that is typically only one to two times per day and is based on body weight. Laboratory monitoring is not usually required. Although more expensive than unfractionated heparin,

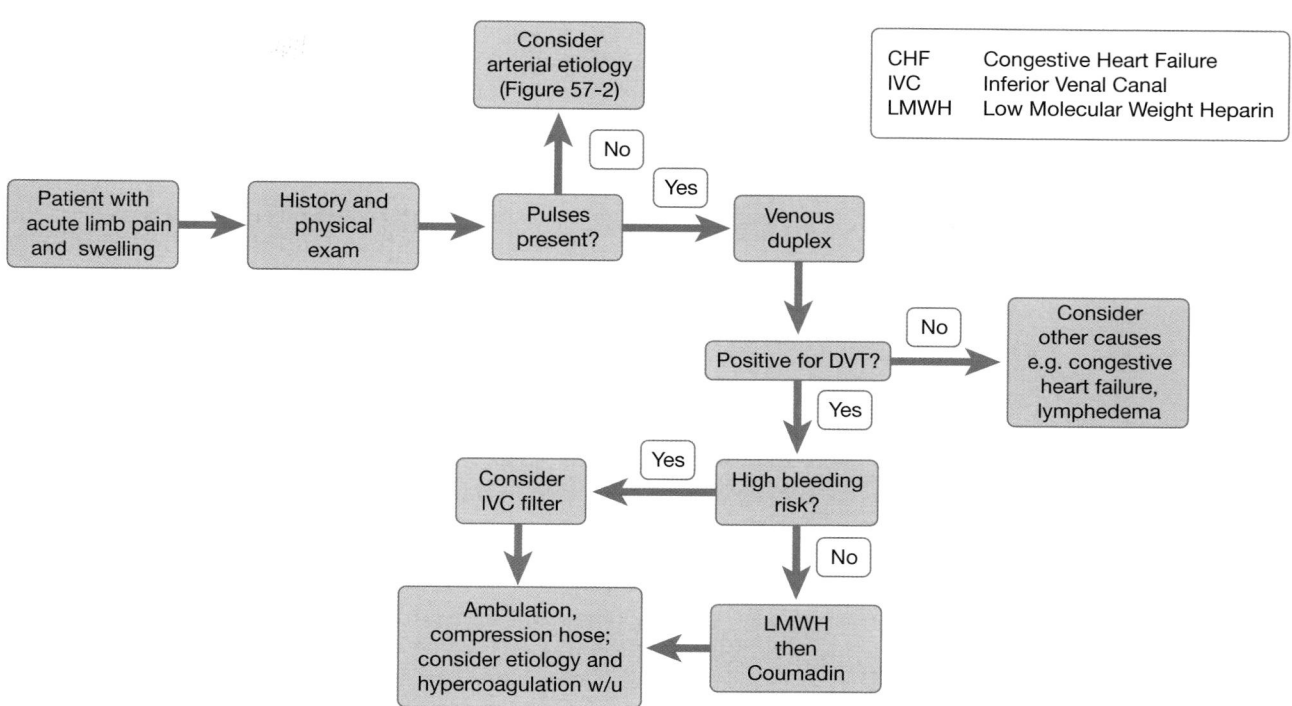

CHF	Congestive Heart Failure
IVC	Inferior Venal Canal
LMWH	Low Molecular Weight Heparin

Figure 57-6 Diagnostic and treatment algorithm for a patient with limb swelling. The primary consideration is to urgently evaluate for a deep vein thrombosis, which can be life-threatening. IVC, inferior vena cava; LMWH, low molecular weight heparin.

this is mitigated by the fact that laboratory monitoring is not required. Clinical trials show that LMWH is as effective as heparin, and the incidence of serious bleeding and recurrence is lower.[27,129]

LYMPHATIC DISEASE

Lymphedema results from acquired and congenital etiologies. The etiology of primary lymphedema is unknown, and includes congenital abnormalities of the lymphatic system. Congenital lymphedema refers to lymphedema that presents at birth or by age 2. If it is familial, it is also referred to as Milroy disease. Lymphedema praecox is the most common type of primary disease, may be unilateral, and is more common in teenage girls. Lymphedema tarda indicates cases with a typical onset at age 30 or older.[57] The most common causes of secondary or acquired lymphedema include those resulting from treatment of cancer and chronic venous disease of the lower limb.[115] Filariasis, a parasitic infection that leads to lymphedema, is uncommon in the USA but endemic to India and Africa.

Primary lymphedema requires the exclusion of other causes of edema, including cancer or other vascular abnormalities. In the absence of skin pigmentation changes or other signs of venous disease, a history of slowly progressive painless lower limb edema supports the diagnosis of lymphedema. A history of recurrent lower limb cellulitis also suggests this diagnosis.[18]

Primary lymphedema is the result of lymphatic hypoplasia or hyperplasia. Lymphatic hypoplasia disease is present in 92%. Distal hypoplasia is the most common type. It occurs in puberty

(praecox) in 80% of cases and is slowly progressive. Females are disproportionately affected (female:male ratio 3:1). Although inguinal lymph nodes and proximal vessels are normal, distal lymphatics are reduced or absent. When familial, it is referred to as Meige disease. Only 10% of hypoplastic conditions are present at birth. Proximal hypoplasia results in more extensive lymphedema involving the entire limb. It is typically unilateral, and males and females are equally affected.

Congenital hyperplasia accounts for about 8% of primary lymphedema cases and occurs equally in males and females. Typically, it presents at birth with asymmetry of the lower limb. Hyperplastic incompetent lymph vessels in the trunk and lower limbs are typical. Studies reveal genetic heterogeneity in primary lymphedema.[36,135] Milroy disease is a rare autosomal dominant familial absence of lymph vessels.[18,58,125]

Secondary lymphedema is due to a wide variety of etiologies, including tumor invasion, lymph node resection, and trauma. Despite advancement in treatment modalities for breast cancer, lymphedema remains a significant problem. Postmastectomy lymphedema can result in debilitating swelling, pain, heaviness, limited motion, unsatisfactory appearance, and altered lifestyle, which can negatively impact patient function and quality of life.[63] Failure to recognize and/or adequately treat this lymphatic disorder can lead to specific complications, such as cellulitis, infection, and lymphangitis.[56,103] Lymphangiosarcoma is a rare complication of chronic severe lymphedema.[109]

The severity of lymphedema is graded clinically. Grade 1 lymphedema presents with reversible soft pitting edema that reduces with elevation of the limb. Soft tissue fibrosis is not present on clinical examination. With progression, grade 2

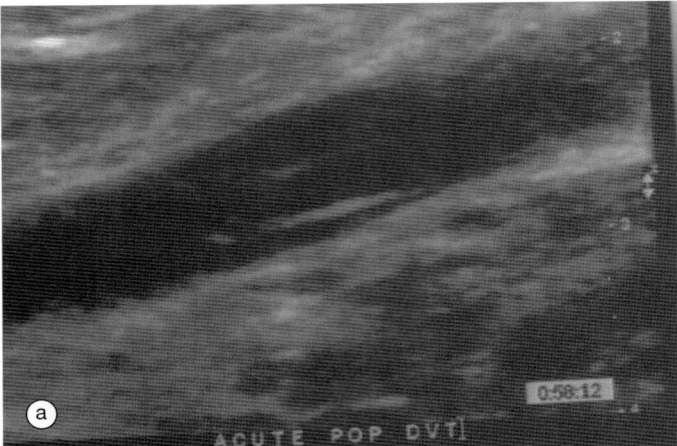
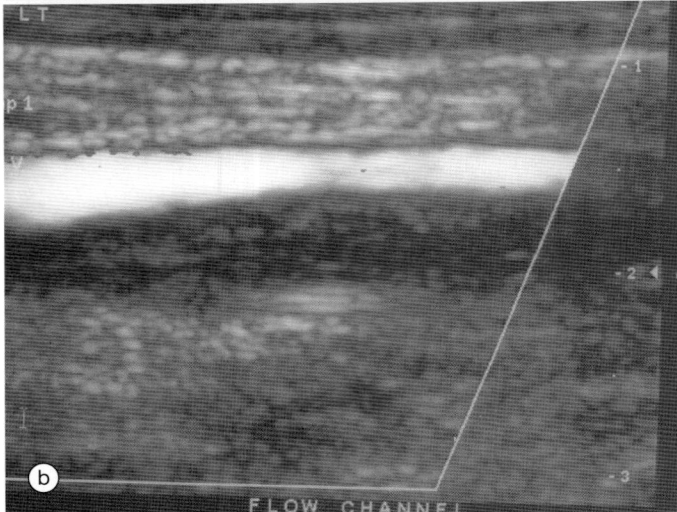

Figure 57-7 (**a**) Longitudinal duplex ultrasound image of an acute popliteal deep vein thrombosis. Note the echolucent vein. This segment is non-compressible to the vascular technician, and is a useful component of the diagnosis. (**b**) Longitudinal duplex image of a chronic popliteal deep vein thrombosis. Note the echogenic area lining the vein wall, and blood flow around this narrowed area. This vein is now compressible to the vascular technician but is not as compliant as a normal vein.

lymphedema occurs, with non-pitting edema and clinically demonstrable local tissue fibrosis. Grade 3 lymphedema involves subcutaneous hypertrophy and hardening, as well as thickening of the skin.[17]

Radiographic lymphography has been a mainstay of diagnosis in lymphedema. Radionuclide lymphatic clearance or lymphangioscintigraphy can be used to evaluate the lymphatic system. Decreased uptake and the inguinal nodes are consistent with lymphatic disease. Interestingly, increased uptake is associated with peripheral venous disease. Magnetic resonance imaging is also employed for diagnosis, detailed specific abnormalities, and follow-up.[134]

A significant number of postmastectomy patients experience secondary lymphedema. The incidence of postmastectomy lymphedema is difficult to determine, because no consistent definition appears in the literature, and varies depending on study criteria. Criteria include patient symptoms, arm circumference, and volume displacement measurements. Petrek, after a review of the literature, reported incidences ranging from 6% to 30%.[103] Erickson reported 2.4–56% on review of the literature on postaxillary dissection cases.[32] Women receiving axillary radiation and axillary lymph node resection appear to be at the highest risk. For example, among those receiving axillary surgery plus axillary radiation, lymphedema prevalence estimates are 12–60%, with most reports suggesting that more than one-quarter of the women experienced lymphedema.[100]

Non-surgical physical modalities are the most widely accepted method for managing lymphedema symptoms in postmastectomy patients. Treatment consists primarily of elevation of the involved limb and graduated compression garments. Massage can assist with maintaining tissue softness. Education regarding skin care and edema control is extremely important.[46]

Pneumatic compression devices are employed to maximize the achieved limb size reduction. Pappas utilized pneumatic compression for limb girth reduction.[101] Limb girth reduction of 20% was considered a positive response. Custom-fitted elastic compression stockings were subsequently used, with 80% of the subjects maintaining limb girth reduction long term (mean 36 months). Pappas performed a similar study with 90% maintaining girth reduction long term (mean follow-up 25 months).[101]

As lymphedema progresses, the risk of cellulitis and other complications increases. In the event of cellulitis, appropriate antibiotics are given for a 10-day course, with aggressive edema reduction efforts. Eczema may occur and responds to topical cortisone. Tinea pedis and other fungal infections may also occur. Ulceration is unusual, in contrast to venous stasis disease.

Treatment programs to address upper limb lymphedema post cancer treatment in Europe and the USA include pressure garments, complete decongestive physiotherapy, manual lymphatic drainage alone, and sequential pneumatic compression.

Complete decongestive physiotherapy, or Komplex Physicalische Enstauuungstherapie, uses a fourfold approach of manual lymphatic drainage, compression, skin care, and remedial exercises.[37] Manual lymphatic drainage is a specific massage technique that assists the mobilization of static lymphatic fluid to healthier lymphatic pathways.[68] After manual lymphatic drainage, compression (bandaging the affected limb) is typically performed to inhibit reaccumulation of interstitial fluid. Skin care regimens and exercises are also taught to assist fluid return.

Compression of the arm is done using a low stretch bandage that contains the limb size. Initially, this should be worn 23 hours per day. Initially, limb size reduction occurs rapidly, but it then decreases with time. Once the limb size is stable, a compression garment is provided and is worn during the day. A compression bandage is required for an additional 6–12 months at night. It is critical that the individual successfully learns how to do self-massage and to correctly don the constraint and compression devices.

Complete decongestive physiotherapy, or manual lymphatic drainage alone, consists of two phases: the initial (or therapeutic) phase and the maintenance phase. The goals of the first phase are to mobilize the accumulation of the protein-rich fluid, and to reduce the formation of fibrosclerotic tissue. During the second phase, or maintenance phase, the patient learns to be self-sufficient in donning and doffing compression devices and performing self massage.[7]

Megans analyzed the literature to determine the effectiveness of physical modalities for management of lymphedema.[80] Overall, reports appear to be positive. However, a systematic assessment of the clinical trials of complete decongestive physiotherapy or manual lymphatic drainage has not been performed.

Surgery and excisional debulking are reserved for the grossly oversized lymphedematous limb. Surgery is used in those situations when the individual's function is significantly impaired. It is not suitable for cosmetic goals, because the surgery does not result in a normal-appearing limb. Surgery may be a reasonable intervention if a treatable proximal lesion is documented. Lymphovenous or lympholymphatic anastomoses are not considered the first-line treatment of chronic lymphedema, and are only done in a few specialized centers.

REFERENCES

1. Albani M, Megalopoulos A, Kiskinis D, et al. Morphological, histochemical, and interstitial pressure changes in the tibialis anterior muscle before and after aortofemoral bypass in patients with peripheral arterial occlusive disease. BMC Musculoskelet Disord 2002; 3(1):8.

2. Ambrosetti M, Salerno M, Boni S, et al. Economic evaluation of a short-course intensive rehabilitation program in patients with intermittent claudication. Int Angiol 2004; 23(2):108–113.

3. Antiplatelet Trialists' Collaboration. Secondary prevention of vascular disease by prolonged antiplatelet treatment. Br Med J 1994; 296:320–331.

4. Aronow WS, Ahn C. Prevalence of coexistence of coronary artery disease, peripheral arterial disease, and atherothrombotic brain infarction in men and women ≥ 62 years of age. Am J Cardiol 1994; 74:64–65.

5. Arthritis Foundation. Systemic sclerosis and other related syndromes. Washington: Arthritis Foundation; 2001:365.

6. Auerbach EG, Martin ET. Magnetic resonance imaging of the peripheral vasculature. Am Heart J 2004; 148(5):755–763.

7. Badger C, Preston N, Seers K, et al. Physical therapies for reducing and controlling lymphoedema of the limbs. Cochrane Breast Cancer Group. Cochrane Database Syst Rev 2004; 4:CD003141.

8. Barnett AH, Bradbury AW, Brittenden J, et al. The role of cilostazol in the treatment of intermittent claudication. Curr Med Res Opin 2004; 20(10):1661–1670.

9. Bauer TA, Regensteiner JG, Brass EP, et al. Oxygen uptake kinetics during exercise are slowed in patients with peripheral arterial disease. J Appl Physiol 1999; 87:809–816.

10. Beebe HG, Dawson DL, Cutler BS, et al. A new pharmacological treatment for intermittent claudication: results of a randomized, multicenter trial. Arch Intern Med 1999; 159(17):2041–2050.

11. Beebe-Dimmer JL, Pfeifer JR, Engle JS, et al. The epidemiology of chronic venous insufficiency and varicose veins. Ann Epidemiol 2005; 15(3):175–184.

12. Belli AM, Cumberland DC, Knox AM, et al. The complication rate of percutaneous peripheral balloon angioplasty. Clin Radiol 1990; 41(6):380–383.

13. Berliner E, Ozbilgin B, Zarin DA. A systematic review of pneumatic compression for treatment of chronic venous insufficiency and venous ulcers. J Vasc Surg 2003; 37(3):539.

14. Bettmann MA, Heesen T, Greenfield A. Adverse events with radiographic contrast agents: results of the SCVIR Contrast Agent Registry. SCVIR Contrast Agent Registry Investigators. Radiology 1997; 203:611–620.

15. Boris M, Windorf S, Lasinski BB. The risk of genital edema after external pump compression for lower limb lymphedema. Lymphology 1998; 31:15–20.

16. Brand FN, Dannenberg AL, Abbott RD, et al. The epidemiology of varicose veins: the Framingham study. Am J Prev Med 1988; 4:96–101.

17. Brennan MJ, DePompolo RW, Garden FH. Focused review: postmastectomy lymphedema Arch Phys Med Rehabil 1996; 77(3 suppl):S74–S80.

18. Browse NL, Stewart G. Lymphedema: pathophysiology and classification. J Cardiovasc Surg 1985; 26:91–106.

19. Ciuffetti G, Paltriccia R, Lombardini R, et al. Treating peripheral arterial occlusive disease: pentoxifylline vs. exercise. Int Angiol 1994; 13(1):33–39.

20. Clement DL, De Buyzere ML, Duprez DA. Hypertension in peripheral arterial disease. Curr Pharm Design 2004; 10(29):3615–3620.

21. Creasy TS, McMillan PJ, Fletcher EWL, et al. Is percutaneous transluminal angioplasty better than exercise for claudication? Preliminary results from a prospective randomised trial. Eur J Vasc Surg 1990; 4:135–140.

22. Criqui MH, Langer RD, Fronek A, et al. Mortality over a period of 10 years in patients with peripheral arterial disease. N Engl J Med 1992; 326(6):381–386.

23. Cronenwett JL. Arterial hemodynamics. In: Greenfield LJ, ed. Surgery: scientific principles and practice. Philadelphia: JB Lippincott; 1993: 1511–1520.

24. Dawson DL, Cutler BS, Hiatt WR, et al. A comparison of cilostazol and pentoxifylline for treating intermittent claudication. Am J Med 2000; 109(7):523–530.

25. Dawson DL, Cutler BS, Meissner MH, et al. Cilostazol has beneficial effects in treatment of intermittent claudication: results from a multicenter, randomized, prospective, double-blind trial. Circulation 1998; 98:678–686.

26. Delis KT, Husmann M, Kalodiki E, et al. In situ hemodynamics of perforating veins in chronic venous insufficiency. J Vasc Surg 2001; 33(4):773–782.

27. Dolovich LR, Ginsberg JS, Douketis JD, et al. A meta-analysis comparing low-molecular-weight heparins with unfractionated heparin in the treatment of venous thromboembolism: examining some unanswered questions regarding location of treatment, product type, and dosing frequency. Arch Intern Med 2000; 160(2):181–188.

28. Dormandy J, Mahir M, Ascady G, et al. Fate of the patient with chronic leg ischaemia. A review article. J Cardiovasc Surg 1989; 30:50–57.

29. Dormandy JA, Rutherford RB. Management of peripheral arterial disease (PAD). TASC Working Group. TransAtlantic Inter-Society Consensus (TASC). J Vasc Surg 2000; 31(1 part 2):S1–S296.

30. Dumville JC, Lee AJ, Smith FB, et al. The health-related quality of life of people with peripheral arterial disease in the community: the Edinburgh Artery Study. Br J Gen Pract 2004; 54(508):826–831.

31. Eberhardt RT, Raffetto JD. Chronic venous insufficiency. Circulation 2005; 111(18):2398–2409.

32. Erickson VS, Pearson ML, Ganz PA, et al. Arm edema in breast cancer patients. J Natl Cancer Inst 2001; 93(2):96–111.

33. Ernst E. Chelation therapy for peripheral arterial occlusive disease: a systematic review. Circulation 1997; 96(3):1031–1033.

34. Ernst E. Exercise: the best therapy for intermittent claudication? Br J Hosp Med 1992; 48:303–305.

35. Ernst EEW, Matrai A. Intermittent claudication, exercise and blood rheology. Circulation 1987; 76:1110–1114.

36. Ferrell RE. Research perspectives in inherited lymphatic disease. Ann NY Acad Sci 2002; 979:39–51.

37. Foldi E. The treatment of lymphedema. Cancer 1998; 83(12 suppl):2833–2834.

38. Fowkes FG, Gillespie IN. Angioplasty (versus non-surgical management) for intermittent claudication. Cochrane Database Syst Rev 2000; 2:CD000017.

39. Fowkes FG, Housely E, Riemersa RA, et al. Smoking, lipids, glucose intolerance and blood pressure as risk factors for peripheral atherosclerosis compared with ischemic heart disease in the Edinburgh Artery Study. Am J Epidemiol 1992; 135:331–340.

40. Frilling B, Schiele R, Gitt AK, et al. Maximal Individual Therapy in Acute Myocardial Infarction Study Group. Too little aspirin for secondary prevention after acute myocardial infarction in patients at high risk for cardiovascular events: results from the MITRA study. Am Heart J 2004; 148(2):306–311.

41. Gardener AW, Poehlman ET. Exercise rehabilitation programs for the treatment of claudication pain. JAMA 1995; 274:975–980.

42. Gardner AW, Katzel LI, Sorkin JD, et al. Effects of long-term exercise rehabilitation on claudication distances in patients with peripheral arterial disease: a randomized controlled trial. J Cardiopulm Rehabil 2002; 22:192–198.

43. Girolami B, Bernardi E, Prins MH, et al. Treatment of intermittent claudication with physical training, smoking cessation, pentoxifylline, or nafronyl: a meta-analysis. Arch Intern Med 1999; 159:337–345.

44. Gloviczki P, Morris SM, Bower TC, et al. Microvascular pedal bypass for salvage of the severely ischemic limb. Mayo Clin Proc 1991; 66:243.

45. Goldhaber SZ, Manson JE, Stampfer MJ, et al. Low-dose aspirin and subsequent peripheral arterial surgery in the Physicians' Health Study. Lancet 1992; 340(8812):143–145.

46. Harris SR, Hugi MR, Olivotto IA, et al. The Steering Committee for Clinical Practice Guidelines for the Care and Treatment of Breast Cancer clinical practice guidelines for the care and treatment of breast cancer: 11. Lymphedema. Can Med Assoc J 2001; 164(2):191–199.

47. Hiatt WR, Regensteiner JG. Exercise conditioning in the treatment of patients with peripheral arterial disease. J Vasc Med Biol 1990; 2:163–170.

48. Hiatt WR, Regenstseiner JG, Wolfel EE, et al. Effect of exercise training on skeletal muscle histology and metabolism in peripheral arterial disease. J Appl Physiol 1996; 81(2):780–788.

49. Hiatt WR, Wolfel EE, Meier R, et al. Superiority of treadmill walking exercise versus strength training for patients with peripheral arterial disease: implications for the mechanism of the training response. Circulation 1994; 90:1866–1874.

50. Hiatt WR. Pharmacologic therapy for peripheral arterial disease and claudication. J Vasc Surg 2002; 36(6):1283–1291.

51. Hiatt WR. Preventing atherothrombotic events in peripheral arterial disease: the use of antiplatelet therapy. J Intern Med 2002; 251(3):193–206.

52. Hofman D. Intermittent compression treatment for venous leg ulcers. J Wound Care 1995; 4:163–165.

53. Hood SC, Moher D, Barber GG. Management of intermittent claudication with pentoxifylline: meta-analysis of randomized controlled trials. CMAJ Can Med Assoc J 1996; 155(8):1053–1059.

54. Horlander KT, Mannino DM, Leeper KV. Pulmonary embolism mortality in the United States, 1979–1998: an analysis using multiple-cause mortality data. Arch Intern Med 1993; 163(14):1711–1717.

55. Housley E. Treating claudication in five words. Br Med J 1988; 296:1483–1484.

56. Howell D, Ezzo J, Tuppo K, et al. Complete decongestive therapy for lymphedema following breast cancer treatment. Cochrane Breast Cancer Group. Cochrane Database Syst Rev 2004:4.

57. International Society of Lymphology. The diagnosis and treatment of peripheral lymphedema: consensus document of the International Society of Lymphology. Lymphology 2003; 36(2):84.

58. Irrthum A, Karkkainen MF, Devriendt K, et al. Congential hereditary lymphedema caused by a mutation that inactivates VEGFR3 tyrosine kinase. Am J Hum Genet 2000; 67:295–301.

59. Jacoby D, Mohler E. Drug treatment of intermittent claudication. Drugs 2004; 64(15):1657–1670.

60. Jonason T, Bergstrom R. Cessation of smoking in patients with intermittent claudication. Effects on the risk of peripheral vascular complications, myocardial infarction and mortality. Acta Med Scand 1987; 221(3):253–260.

61. Juergens JL, Barker NW, Hines EA. Arteriosclerosis obliterans: review of 520 cases with special reference to pathogenic and prognostic factors. Circulation 1960; 21:188–195.

62. Kannel WB, McGee DL. Update on some epidemiologic features of intermittent claudication: the Framingham Study. J Am Geriatr Soc 1985; 33(1):13–18.

63. Karki A, Simonen R, Malkia E, et al. Impairments, activity limitations and participation restrictions 6 and 12 months after breast cancer operation. J Rehabil Med 2005; 37(3):180–188.

64. Killewich LA, Macko RF, Montgomery PS, et al. Exercise training enhances endogenous fibrinolysis in peripheral arterial disease. J Vasc Surg 2004; 40(4):741–745.

65. Kornitzer M, Dramaix M, Sobolski J, et al. Ankle/arm pressure index in asymptomatic middle-aged males: an independent predictor of ten-year coronary heart disease mortality. Angiology 1995; 46:211–219.

66. Lachmann EA, Rook JL, Tunkel R, et al. Complications associated with intermittent pneumatic compression. Arch Phys Med Rehabil 1992; 73:482–485.

67. Lange S, Diehm C, Darius H, et al. High prevalence of peripheral arterial disease and low treatment rates in elderly primary care patients with diabetes. Exp Clin Endocrinol Diabetes 2004; 112(10):566–573.

68. Leduc O, Leduc A, Bourgeois P, et al. The physical treatment of upper limb edema. Cancer 1998; 83:2835–2839.

69. Lee SL, Pevec WC, Carlsen RC. Functional outcome of new blood vessel growth into ischemic skeletal muscle. J Vasc Surg 2001; 34(6):1096–1102.

70. Leng GC, Fowler B, Ernst E. Exercise for intermittent claudication. Cochrane Database Syst Rev 2000; 2:CD000990.

71. Leng GC, Lee AJ, Fowkes FG, et al. Incidence, natural history, and cardiovascular events in symptomatic, and asymptomatic peripheral arterial disease in the general population. Int J Epidemiol 1996; 25:1172–1181.

72. Leng GC, Price JF, Jepson RG. Lipid-lowering for lower limb atherosclerosis. Cochrane Database Syst Rev 2000; 2:CD000123.

73. Lie JT. Thromboangiitis obliterans (Buerger's disease) and smokeless tobacco. Arthritis Rheum 1988; 31(6):812–813.

74. Lindenauer EM. Venous and lymphatic systems. In: Greenfield LF, ed. Surgery: scientific principles and practice. Philadelphia: JB Lippincott; 1993:1757–1764.

75. Lipsy RJ. The National Cholesterol Education Program Adult Treatment Panel III guidelines. J Manag Care Pharm 2003; 9(suppl 1):2–5.

76. Lu JT, Creager MA. The relationship of cigarette smoking to peripheral arterial disease. Rev Cardiovasc Med 2004; 5(4):189–193.

77. Maricq HR, Carpentier PH, Wienrich MC, et al. Geographic variation in the prevalence of Raynaud's phenomenon. J Rheumatol 1993; 20:70–76.

78. McDermott MM, Mehta S, Ahn H, et al. Atherosclerotic risk factors are less intensively treated in patients with peripheral arterial disease than in patients with coronary artery disease. J Gen Intern Med 1997; 12:209–215.

79. McDermott MM, Tiukinhoy S, Greenland P, et al. A pilot exercise intervention to improve lower limb functioning in peripheral arterial disease unaccompanied by intermittent claudication. J Cardiopulm Rehabil 2004; 24(3):187–196.

80. Megans A, Harris S. Physical therapist management of lymphedema following treatment for breast cancer: a critical review of its effectiveness. Phys Ther 1998; 78(12):1302–1311.

81. Meijer WT, Hoes AW, Rutgers D, et al. Peripheral arterial disease in the elderly: the Rotterdam Study. Arteriosdl Thromb Vasc Biol 1998; 18(2):185–192.

82. Menard JR, Smith HE, Riebe D, et al. Long-term results of peripheral arterial disease rehabilitation. J Vasc Surg 2004; 39(6):1186–1192.

83. Mills JL Sr. Buerger's disease in the 21st century: diagnosis, clinical features, and therapy. Semin Vasc Surg 2003; 16(3):179–189.

84. Mills JM, Porter JM. Buerger's disease in the modern era. Am J Surg 1987; 154:123–129.

85. Money SR, Herd JA, Isaacsohn JL, et al. Effect of cilostazol on walking distances in patients with intermittent claudication caused by peripheral vascular disease. J Vasc Surg 1998; 27:267–274.

86. Murabito JM, D'Agostino RB, Silbershatz H, et al. Intermittent claudication. A risk profile from the Framingham Study. Circulation 1997; 96:44–49.

87. Nelzen O, Bergqvist D, Lindhagen A. Leg ulcer etiology: a cross sectional population study. J Vasc Surg 1991; 14:557–564.

88. Newman AB, Shemanski L, Manolio TA, et al. Ankle–arm index as a predictor of cardiovascular disease and mortality in the Cardiovascular Health Study. The Cardiovascular Health Study Group. Arteriosdl Thromb Vasc Biol 1999; 19:538–545.

89. Nicolaides AN. Cardiovascular Disease Educational and Research Trust. European Society of Vascular Surgery. The International Angiology Scientific Activity Congress Organization. International Union of

Angiology. Union Internationale de Phlebologie at the Abbaye des Vaux de Cernay. Investigation of chronic venous insufficiency: a consensus statement (France, March 5–9, 1997). Circulation 2000; 102(20):E126–E163.

90. O'Dell JR, Linder J, Markin RS, et al. Thromboangiitis obliterans (Buerger's disease) and smokeless tobacco. Arthritis Rheum 1987; 30(9):1054–1056.

91. Ohta T, Ishioashi H, Hosaka M, et al. Clinical and social consequences of Buerger disease. J Vasc Surg 2004; 39(1):176–180.

92. Ohta T, Shionoya S. Fate of ischemic limb in Buerger's disease. Br J Surg 1988; 75:259–262.

93. Olin JW, Jang J, Jaff MR, et al. The top 12 advances in vascular medicine. J Endovasc Ther 2004; 11(suppl 2):II21–II31.

94. Olin JW, Young JR, Graor RA, et al. The changing clinical spectrum of thromboangiitis obliterans (Buerger's disease). Circulation 1990; 82 (suppl IV):3–8.

95. Olin JW. Current concepts: thromboangiitis obliterans (Buerger's disease). N Engl J Med 2000; 343(12):864–869.

96. Orchard TJ, Strandness DE. Assessment of peripheral vascular disease in diabetes: report and recommendations of an international workshop sponsored by the American Diabetes Association and the American Heart Association. Circulation 1993; 88(8):819–828.

97. O'Shaughnessy AM, FitzGerald DE. Natural history of proximal deep vein thrombosis assessed by duplex ultrasound. Int Angiol 1997; 16:45–49.

98. O'Shaughnessy AM, FitzGerald DE. Organisation patterns of venous thrombus over time as demonstrated by duplex ultrasound. J Vasc Invest 1996; 2:75–81.

99. Ouriel K. Peripheral arterial disease. Lancet 2001; 358(9289):1257–1264.

100. Ozaslan C, Kuru B. Lymphedema after treatment of breast cancer. Am J Surg 2004; 187(1):69–72.

101. Pappas CJ, O'Donnell TF. Long term results of compression treatment for lymphedema. J Vasc Surg 1992; 16:555–556, 562–564.

102. Perkins JM, Creasy TS, Fletcher EW, et al. Exercise training versus angioplasty for stable claudication. Long and medium term results of a prospective randomised trial. Eur J Vasc Endovasc Surg 1996; 11(4):409–413.

103. Petrek JA, Heelan MC. Incidence of breast carcinoma-related lymphedema. Cancer 1998; 83(12):2776–2781.

104. Porter JM, Cutter BS, Lee BY, et al. Pentoxifylline efficacy in the treatment of intermittent claudication: multicenter controlled double blind trial with objective assessment of chronic occlusive arterial disease patients. Am Heart J 1982; 104(1):66–72.

105. Price JF, Fowkes FGR. Effectiveness of percutaneous angioplasty for lower limb atherosclerosis. In: Greenhalgh RM, Fowkes FGR, eds. Trials and tribulations in vascular surgery. London: Saunders; 1996.

106. Radack K, Deck C. Beta-adrenergic blocker therapy does not worsen intermittent claudication in subjects with peripheral arterial disease: a meta-analysis of randomized controlled trials. Arch Intern Med 1991; 151:1769–1776.

107. Rao AS, Rao GN, Vasantha VC. Thrombo-angiitis obliterans. J Indian Med Assoc 1976; 66:98–101.

108. Ray SA, Minty I, Buckenham TM, et al. Clinical outcome and restenosis following percutaneous transluminal angioplasty for ischaemic rest pain or ulceration. Br J Surg 1995; 82(9):1217–1221.

109. Recht A, Houlihan MJ. Axillary lymph nodes and breast cancer: a review. Cancer 1995; 76:1491–1512.

110. Regensteiner JG, Hiatt WR. Current medical therapies for patients with peripheral arterial disease: a critical review. Am J Med 2002; 112(1):49–57.

111. Regensteiner JG, Steiner JF, Hiatt WR. Exercise training improves functional status in patients with peripheral arterial disease. J Vasc Surg 1996; 23:104–115.

112. Regensteiner JG. Exercise in the treatment of claudication: assessment and treatment of functional impairment. Vasc Med 1997; 2:238–242.

113. Regensteiner JG. Exercise rehabilitation for the patient with intermittent claudication: a highly effective yet underutilized treatment. Curr Drug Targets Cardiovasc Haematol Disord 2004; 4(3):233–239.

114. Robeer GG, Brandsma JW, Van den Heuvel SP, et al. Exercise therapy for intermittent claudication: a review of the quality of randomised clinical trials and evaluation of predictive factors. Eur J Vasc Endovasc Surg 1998; 15:36–43.

115. Rockson SG, et al. American Cancer Society Lymphedema Workshop. Workgroup III: diagnosis and management of lymphedema. Cancer 2998; 83(12 suppl):2882.

116. Ruell PA, Imperial ES, Bonar FJ, et al. Intermittent claudication: the effect of physical training on walking tolerance and venous lactate concentration. Eur J Appl Physiol 1984; 52:420–425.

117. Rutherford RB, Lowenstein DH, Klein MF. Combining segmental systolic pressures and plethysmography to diagnose arterial disease of the legs. Am J Surg 1979; 138(2):211–218.

118. Selvin E, Erlinger TP. Prevalence of and risk factors for peripheral arterial disease in the United States: results from the National Health and Nutrition Examination Survey, 1999–2000. Circulation 2004; 110(6):738–743.

119. Smith JA. Measuring treatment effects of cilostazol on clinical trial end-points in patients with intermittent claudication. Clin Cardiol 2002; 25(3):91–94.

120. Solomon SA, Ramsay LE, Yeo WW, et al. Beta blockade and intermittent claudication: placebo controlled trial of atenolol and nifedipine and their combination. Br Med J 1991; 303(6810):1100–1104.

121. Stoffers HEJH, Kaiser V, Knottnerus JA. Epidemiology of peripheral vascular disease. In: Prevalence in general practice. London: Springer-Verlag; 1991:109–115.

122. Szuba A, Cooke JP. Thromboangiitis obliterans. An update on Buerger's disease. West J Med 1998; 168(4):255–260.

123. Tan KH, de Cossart L, Edwards PR. Exercise training and peripheral vascular disease. Br J Surg 2000; 87(5):553–562.

124. Taylor LM, Porter JM, Winek T. Femoropopliteal and infrapopliteal occlusive disease. In: Greenfield LJ, ed. Surgery: scientific principles and practice. Philadelphia: JB Lippincott; 1993:1654–1669.

125. Tille JC, Pepper MS. Hereditary vascular anomalies: new insights into their pathogenesis. Thromb Vasc Biol 2004; 24(9):1578–1590.

126. Violi F, Balsano F. Rationale for the use of antiplatelet drugs in patients with peripheral vascular disease. Clin Trials Metaanal 1994; 29(1):81–87.

127. Vogt MT, Cauley JA, Newman AB, et al. Decreased ankle/arm blood pressure index and mortality in elderly women. JAMA 1993; 270:465–469.

128. Waugh JR, Sacharas N. Arteriographic complications in the DSA era. Radiology 1992; 182:243–246.

129. Wells PS, Anderson DR, Rodger MA, et al. A randomized trial comparing 2 low-molecular-weight heparins for the outpatient treatment of deep vein thrombosis and pulmonary embolism. Arch Intern Med 2005; 165(7):733–738.

130. Whyman MR, Fowkes FG, Kerracher EM, et al. Is intermittent claudication improved by percutaneous transluminal angioplasty? A randomized controlled trial. J Vasc Surg 1997; 26:551–557.

131. Whyman MR, Fowkes FG, Kerracher EM, et al. Randomised controlled trial of percutaneous transluminal angioplasty for intermittent claudication. Eur J Vasc Endovasc Surg 1996; 12(2):167–172.

132. Wigley FM, Flavahan NA. Raynaud's phenomenon. Rheum Dis Clin North Am 1996: 22:765–782.

133. Willigendael EM, Teijink JAW, Bartelink ML, et al. Influence of smoking on incidence and prevalence of peripheral arterial disease. J Vasc Surg 2004; 40(6):1158–1165.

134. Witte CL, Witte MH, Unger EC, et al. Advances in imaging of lymph flow disorders. Radiographics 2000; 20(6):1697–1719.

135. Witte MH, Erickson R, Bernas M, et al. Phenotypic and genotypic heterogeneity in familial Milroy lymphedema. Lymphology 1998; 31(4):145–155.

Chapter

58

Cancer Rehabilitation

Andrea Cheville

Cancer rehabilitation addresses physical impairments related to tumor effects or to cancer treatment. Most functional compromise in cancers patients also occur in association with other disease processes, for example ischemic injury, trauma, and arthritis. The fact that impairments are due to cancer might alter their management very little. However, their successful rehabilitation requires the integration of cancer-specific concerns, such as limited prognoses, progressive lesions, heavy symptom burden, and emerging antineoplastic toxicities, into a humane and realistic treatment plan.

Cancer is a pathologic process characterized by dysregulated cell growth and spread. All tissue types have neoplastic potential and can become cancerous. Tissues distinguished by rapid cell turnover (e.g. gastrointestinal mucosa), hormone sensitivity (e.g. breast and prostate), and regular exposure to environmental mutagens (e.g. lung and skin) have higher rates of malignant transformation. The fact that any tissue can develop cancer means that cancer rehabilitation must address all body parts and systems. Despite this broad scope, the field condenses into a manageable body of expertise predominantly focused on the sequelae of cancer treatment, maladaptive host responses (e.g. paraneoplastic syndromes), and the erosive effects of cancer on bones and neural tissue.

Cancer rehabilitation extends far beyond efforts to decelerate number functional decline in patients with metastatic disease. With ever-increasing cancer survivorship, the number of patients whose disease has been eliminated or successfully temporized is growing. These patients are eager to lead highly functional and productive lives despite the legacy of their disease. A unique and intensely challenging feature of cancer rehabilitation is the need to treat patients with vastly different degrees of infirmity. Given the magnitude of current need, physiatrists can choose to treat patients rendered cancer-free or those with far-advanced disease in the palliative setting.

This chapter is intended to provide physiatrists and other readers with an overview of the issues relevant to the rehabilitation of patients with cancer. Emphasis is placed on problems that affect the nervous and musculoskeletal systems.

EPIDEMIOLOGY

Cancer is a prevalent condition that becomes increasingly common with advanced age. Over 1 300 000 new cancers were diagnosed within the USA in 2004, and over 500 000 people died of cancer (SEER data, www.seer.cancer.gov). Cancer causes one in four deaths, and is second only to heart disease as the leading cause of mortality in developed countries. Roughly 76% of all cancers occur in patients 55 years of age and older.[4] Men are more commonly affected by cancer (excluding basal and squamous cell cancers of the skin), with a lifetime risk in the USA of one in two. The lifetime risk in women is one in three (SEER data). Many cancers could be prevented through behavioral modification. In 2004, the American Cancer Society estimated that 180 000 cancer deaths could be attributed to tobacco use.[4] One-third of all cancer deaths are related to obesity, physical inactivity, and other lifestyle factors.[4] Only 5 to 10% of cancers are hereditary and directly related to aberrantly expressed or regulated genes.

Demographic disparities in cancer

Racial, economic, and gender disparities influence cancer incidence, stage at diagnosis, and mortality. Race-related disparities are prominent for some cancers and are difficult to accurately distinguish from economic disparities. African Americans have the highest mortality associated with cancers of the lung, breast, prostate, and cervix among all racial groups in the USA.[211] When African Americans are compared with whites, cancer death rates are 40% higher in males and 20% higher in females.[211]

The adverse impact of low economic status on cancer outcomes is being increasingly recognized. A report in 2003 by the Institute of Medicine identified poverty as the most critical overall factor affecting health and longevity.[84] The 5-year survival rate is over 10% higher for individuals living in affluent census tracts.[211] The effects of economic disparity can significantly undermine cancer rehabilitation efforts through marginally covered or uncovered items such as lymphedema compression garments, high physical and occupational therapy copayments, and seriously attenuated home therapy benefits.

Survivorship

Cancer 5-year survival rates are increasing due to a variety of factors including successful early detection efforts, improved multimodality treatments, and expansion of the chemotherapeutics available to treat patients with metastatic disease. Sixty-two percent of adult and 77% of pediatric cancer patients live beyond 5 years.[213] These numbers do not accurately reflect current trends, because the statistics pertain to patients who were treated 5 years ago, and the standards of care for many cancers have changed. The prevalence of cancer survivors will increase (SEER data) given the anticipated persistence of factors responsible for current survivorship trends. First, the aging of the population will produce an increase in the incidence of age-related cancers such as colon, breast, and prostate cancer.[4] Second, early detection efforts are being aggressively funded and implemented. We can expect that more and more cancers will be identified at early, curable stages. Last, clinical research continues to refine strategies for delivering established and novel anticancer therapies. Such efforts have consistently produced incremental improvements in outcomes. It is reasonable to assume that this trend will continue to benefit both patients who are cured and those living with cancer.

DISEASE CONSIDERATIONS

Staging

The specifics of cancer staging vary by disease site, but all conform to a general format geared toward describing the spread of disease from the site of origin. The T, N, and M system is the most widely used. *T* depends on the characteristics of the primary tumor, *N* on the extent of regional lymph node spread, and *M* on the presence of distant metastases. Once TNM status has been determined, a disease stage I through IV is assigned. Stage I is early, locally contained disease, while stage IV is advanced, characterized by distant metastases.

Cancer can also be described as *in situ, local, regional,* and *distant.* This approach distinguishes whether cancer has remained in the layer of cells where it developed (in situ) or spread beyond the tissue layer (local). Staging determines the type, duration, and aggressiveness of anticancer therapy. It provides critical information for the appropriate design of rehabilitation interventions, and for the ongoing process of gauging each patient's risk of disease recurrence or progression. During cancer rehabilitation, new or progressive signs and symptoms should be attributed to malignancy until proven otherwise.

Prognosis and metastatic spread

Cancer presents a staggering array of prognoses, differential treatment approaches, and patterns of metastatic spread. This reflects the fact that the cancer is, in truth, many diseases. In planning a long-term rehabilitation approach, it is important to anticipate where cancer is likely to spread, how it will respond to treatment, what cumulative toxicities might be associated with ongoing therapies, and how long patients will live. This is no small requirement, given the number of different cancer types and the inconsistent natural histories of cancer subtypes arising from the same progenitor tissue. Treatment approaches are also continuously evolving. Nonetheless, the effort to anticipate the course of disease is critical for the optimal and appropriate delivery of cancer rehabilitation services. What follows is a synopsis of the characteristics of prevalent cancers and those that commonly lead patients to seek rehabilitative services.

Table 58-1 presents 5-year survival statistics collected between 1992 and 1999 for different cancers.[4] The implications of regional and distant spread at the time of diagnosis vary considerably by cancer type. For example, prostate cancer patients enjoy an excellent prognosis when their cancer is

Table 58-1 Five-year survival statistics for different cancers, 1992–1999

Cancer	Five-year survival (%)			Common sites of metastatic spread
	Local	Regional	Distant	
Lung and bronchus	49	16	2	Brain, bone, liver, mediastinal lymph nodes
Breast	97	79	23	Brain, lung, bone, liver
Prostate	100	100	34	Bone, pelvic lymph nodes
Colon and rectum	90	66	9	Liver, lung
Leukemia: acute myeloblastic	19	—	—	—
Leukemia: chronic lymphocytic	74	—	—	—
Ovary	95	72	31	Peritoneum, pleura
Uterine cervix	92	51	17	Peritoneum, lung, retroperitoneal lymph nodes
Uterine corpus	96	65	26	Retroperitoneal lymph nodes, lung
Larynx and oral cavity	82	49	20–26	Lung, regional lymph nodes
Melanoma	97	60	14	Brain
Stomach	58	23	3	Liver, lung, peritoneum
Esophagus	29	13	3	Liver, lung

detected at the regional level, with virtually 100% 5-year survival. Only 16% of lung cancer patients with regional spread are alive at 5 years. It is critical to bear in mind that survival statistics are mean values, some of which have wide confidence intervals. The mean values provide a crude gauge for anticipated survival but are potentially imprecise when applied to individuals.

This information drives rehabilitation goal setting, the level of emphasis placed on symptom-oriented versus disease-modifying therapy, and acceptance of patients' unduly optimistic or grim expectations. Table 58-1 also lists common sites of metastases for prevalent malignancies. An understanding of where specific cancers are likely to spread helps clinicians focus the search for metastases. Lung, breast, colon, and melanoma commonly spread to the brain. Regular neurologic screening examinations should therefore be incorporated into posttreatment, surveillance care. Prostate, breast, and lung cancer virtually always produce bone metastases in patients with stage IV disease. Musculoskeletal pain in these cancer populations can be due to the primary or secondary consequences of bony disease and should trigger an appropriate evaluation.

Phases of cancer

For rehabilitation purposes, cancer can be divided into several distinct stages. This approach calls clinical attention to certain nodal points along the disease trajectory that should trigger a revaluation of anticipated deficits, reinvolvement of rehabilitation services, and redefinition of functional goals. Five distinct stages of malignant disease—initial diagnosis and treatment, surveillance, recurrence, temporization, and advanced disease—were initially outlined in a model proposed by Gerber et al.[92] Identification of each patient's phase of cancer is critical for appropriate goal setting. Goals must be continuously reformulated in response to the progression of the disease and the choice of antineoplastic therapies. Attention to cancer phases ensures that significant shifts in prognosis and treatment requirements inform rehabilitative efforts.

At the time of initial cancer diagnosis, patients deemed curable are treated aggressively with a regimen of anticancer therapies designed to definitively eliminate disease. A primary rehabilitation goal during initial cancer treatment is attenuation of the acute functional impact of surgery, radiation, and chemotherapy. Once primary cancer treatment has been completed, patients enter a potentially extended period of surveillance. For most patients, this is an uneasy and indefinite interval characterized by persistent vigilance for latent treatment toxicity and/or recurrent cancer. For some patients, the phase of surveillance ends with cancer recurrence.

If cure is possible following recurrence, patients are aggressively re-treated with multimodal therapy to eliminate disease. If not, they enter the temporization phase discussed below. Patients treated for recurrent cancer are rendered extremely vulnerable to lasting functional impairment, because cumulative chemotherapeutic and radiation toxicities become problematic. Patients with stage IV disease at initial presentation or recurrence enter a phase characterized by efforts to temporize

disease progression. Anticancer therapies during this phase are geared toward reducing tumor burden, metastatic spread, and the development of medical comorbidities. Patients generally undergo serial chemotherapy trials, which can lead to progressive impairments. As patients enter the final phase of cancer, rehabilitative goals become palliative and focus on maximizing patient comfort, psychologic well-being, and independence in mobility and activities of daily living (ADL) performance.

CONSTITUTIONAL SYMPTOMS

Many symptoms are common in cancer, particularly among patients with stage IV disease. Failure to adequately address symptoms such as fatigue, nausea, pain, anxiety, insomnia, and dyspnea undermines rehabilitation. The burgeoning of palliative care as a medical discipline has produced an extensive literature and several excellent textbooks detailing current strategies for managing cancer-related symptoms. Interested readers are referred to the *Oxford Textbook of Palliative Care* (edited by D. Doyle) and *Principles and Practice of Palliative Care and Supportive Oncology* (edited by A. Berger). Below is a brief discussion on strategies for managing cancer-related fatigue and pain. In the author's experience, pain and fatigue present the most consistent and challenging obstacles to successful rehabilitation.

Fatigue

Fatigue is the most common symptom experienced by cancer patients.[169] The prevalence of fatigue ranges from 70 to 100% contingent on the type and stage of cancer. It is also related to whether patients are receiving antineoplastic therapy.[169,211] Because fatigue is an inherently subjective and multidimensional symptom, definitions of fatigue understandably differ. The National Comprehensive Cancer Network defines cancer-related fatigue as 'an unusual, persistent, subjective sense of tiredness related to cancer or cancer treatment that interferes with usual functioning'.[174] Experts concur that fatigue reduces the energy, mental capacity, functional status, and psychologic resilience of cancer patients.[32,169]

A discrete source of fatigue can be identified in some patients, leading to effective treatment and symptom reversal. More often, the responsible mechanisms are multifactorial, with many potentially abetting contributors of unclear relative importance. Box 58-1 lists possible contributing factors. Anemia has received the greatest attention as a source of fatigue. This is due, in part, to the high prevalence of fatigue among cancer patients receiving chemotherapy (38–86%),[12,251,268] and to reports that the onset and severity of fatigue parallel chemotherapy-induced reductions in serum hemoglobin.[33,45]

Often, cancer-related fatigue occurs in the absence of anemia or ongoing cancer therapy. In such cases, the differential diagnosis is based on patients' prior cancer treatment, medical comorbidities, and current medications. Compromise of the adrenal axis, thyroid gland, testes, and ovaries by chemical ablation, surgical resection, or irradiation can cause fatigue.

Box 58-1 Reversible sources of cancer fatigue

- Anemia
- Insomnia or lack of restorative sleep
- Cytokine release (e.g. tumor necrosis factor)
- Hypothyroidism
- Hypogonadism
- Depression
- Deconditioning
- Steroid myopathy
- Centrally acting medications
- Altered oxidative capacity
- Pain
- Adrenal insufficiency
- Cachexia

Appropriate laboratory studies should be obtained to rule out common disorders in patients with suggestive cancer histories. Patients reporting poor sleep might require a sleep study if the elimination of daytime napping and use of soporifics provide no benefit. Menopausal symptoms can degrade sleep quality and warrant close scrutiny.

Deconditioning secondary to inactivity is common among cancer patients. If deconditioning is not the inciting factor, it will eventually aggravate fatigue arising from other sources. Mood-related factors, for example anxiety and depression, are also prevalent among cancer patients. Thirty percent of patients develop clinical depression following a cancer diagnosis.[77] All centrally acting medications should be carefully reviewed in patients complaining of fatigue. A reduction or withdrawal trial of non-essential drugs can identify those producing fatigue.[169] Medications that commonly produce fatigue include opioids, benzodiazepines, antiemetics, antihistamines, tricyclic antidepressants, anticonvulsants (e.g. carbamazepine, gabapentin, and oxcarbazepine), thalidomide, and α_2-adrenergic agonists (e.g. tizanidine).

In the absence of a discernible etiology, cancer-related fatigue can be due to elevated cytokine levels. Cytokines such as tumor necrosis factor, interleukin-1, and interleukin-6 have been implicated in cancer-related fatigue.[102] When exogenously administered for disease modification, as in the treatment of melanoma, these molecules induce severe fatigue.[25] The mechanism(s) by which elevations in circulating cytokine levels produce fatigue, and whether they are elaborated by host or tumor cells, remains unclear. At this point, cytokine antagonists are not recommended for the treatment of cancer-related fatigue. If cytokines are likely contributors, symptomatic management of fatigue is appropriate.

Epoetins are widely utilized in the treatment of anemia related to cancer treatment. A sound theoretic case can be made for initiating therapeutic doses in appropriate cancer rehabilitation patients. Treatment is not usually initiated for primary prevention if the baseline hemoglobin is normal. Guidelines vary regarding the hemoglobin threshold for initiating treatment. Individual physician practices are even more incon-

sistent still, with trigger hemoglobin levels ranging from 7.5 g/dL to 10.7 g/dL.[182] This controversy stems from the fact that no specific decrement or increment in hemoglobin value has been definitively linked to quantitative changes in quality of life. Even mild anemia can significantly compromise subjective quality of life.[53,63]

The Anemia Guidelines Development Group recommends starting epoetins in patients with prechemotherapy baseline hemoglobin of <10 g/dL, symptomatic baseline anemia, or a drop of 1–2 g/dL per chemotherapy cycle.[62] The American Society of Clinical Oncology (ASCO)–American Society of Hematology (ASH) guidelines also use 10 g/dL as the threshold hemoglobin value.[53] Adverse cardiovascular events associated with epoetins have not been reported with cancer chemotherapy.[60–62] The National Comprehensive Cancer Network endorses the use of oral iron supplementation in conjunction with epoetins in patients with low ferritin or transferrin saturation values.[58]

The ASCO–ASH guideline recommends starting epoetin alfa at a dose of 150 U/kg three times per week.[53] The weekly administration of 40 000 U has been widely used with success, and can reduce indirect costs for patients who cannot self-inject the drug.[56,59] If an adequate treatment response is not achieved in 4 weeks (hemoglobin increase of 0.5–1.0 g/dL), the epoetin alfa dose should be doubled.[61] The cost-effectiveness and economic wisdom of using epoetins to treat cancer-related anemia and fatigue have been questioned. The budget impact of epoetins accounts for roughly 10% of the overall direct costs of cancer care and is expected to increase by 20% each year.[159]

Patients who have poor responses to epoetin therapy, intensely symptomatic anemia, hemoglobin levels $\approx$ 9 g/dL, or economic constraints to epoetin access might require red blood cell transfusion. Multiple factors influence the hemoglobin threshold for transfusing, as reflected by current guidelines that recommend a range of hemoglobin values between 6 g/dL and 10 g/dL.[54,55] Red blood cell transfusions can be extremely beneficial in both the outpatient and inpatient rehabilitation settings, in which anemia-related fatigue undermines efforts at functional restoration. The gradual increment in hemoglobin levels and associated reduction in fatigue that characterize epoetin therapy can be too delayed when third-party payers demand rapid achievement of rehabilitation goals.

When potentially reversible sources of fatigue (Box 58-1) have been ruled out or addressed, symptom-oriented fatigue management is indicated. This includes pharmacologic and exercise interventions. The use of aerobic exercise to reduce cancer-related fatigue is discussed at length below in the section entitled *Aerobic conditioning*. Methylphenidate has been used most extensively to treat fatigue in cancer patients; however, dextroamphetamine and modafinil have also been used anecdotally with success. A recent open label trial of modafinil in HIV-positive patients demonstrated an 80% response rate, defined as statistically significant improvements in fatigue, depressive symptoms, and executive function.[57] Modafinil therapy can be initiated at 100–200 mg/day and titrated to a maximal dose of 400 mg/day. Trials assessing the efficacy of methylphenidate in cancer populations have consistently shown benefit.[33,220,224,245] Patients with different types and stages of cancer, including those with far advanced disease, experience reduced fatigue with methylphenidate therapy.[220,245] Methylphenidate is initiated at a dose of 2.5–5.0 mg once or twice daily. Dose titration continues gradually until a therapeutic response is achieved or adverse side effects preclude further dose escalation. Doses above 60 mg/day are rarely required.[169] Dose-limiting toxicities associated with methylphenidate include anorexia, insomnia, anxiety, confusion, tremor, and tachycardia.

Pain

The prevalence of cancer-related pain is 28% among patients with newly diagnosed cancer,[265] 50–70% among patients receiving antineoplastic therapy,[196,197] and 64–80% among patients with advanced disease.[27,71,253] Adequate pain control is an absolute requisite for successful rehabilitation. Cancer patients generally experience multiple concurrent pain syndromes.[35] Thorough evaluation therefore requires assessment of all relevant pain etiologies and pathophysiologic processes. Pain control might require the integrated use of anticancer treatments, agents from multiple analgesic classes, interventional techniques, topical agents, and physiatric approaches.

The unique disease context in which cancer pain develops distinguishes it from many other pain-associated diagnoses managed by physiatrists. Considerations in cancer pain management are listed in Box 58-2 and explained below. One of the most salient features of cancer pain management is the reliance on high-dose opioid therapy. The doses required by many cancer patients can extend far beyond the conventional levels used by physiatrists. However, an extensive international literature and multiple guidelines resoundingly endorse this approach.[5,125,274] Fifteen percent of a cohort of stage IV pancreatic cancer patients required more than the daily equivalent of 5 g of parenteral morphine.[80]

The majority of cancer pain is due to tumor effects. For this reason, disease-modifying, anticancer therapy plays a critical role in pain management. For example, irradiation offers a definitive and effective means of controlling pain associated with bone metastases.[234] Cancer pain often progresses as disease advances, sometimes precipitously. Anticipation of progressive escalation in pain intensity is essential for effective management.[80] Cancer-related depression, anxiety, and existential distress can exacerbate patients' pain experience.[244] For this reason, aggravating psychiatric factors must be identified and addressed to the best extent possible.

Often, the enteral administration of analgesics is not feasible in cancer patients, particularly those with cancers of the gastrointestinal tract and ovaries. Analgesics with transdermal, parenteral, and transmucosal routes of administration should be preferentially utilized when enteral administration may become unfeasible. Because of the limited life expectancy and intense pain associated with far advanced cancer, the cost–benefit ratio of permanent neuroablative procedures can become acceptable. Excellent success rates have been reported with anterolateral cordotomy (84–95%)[12,32] and myelotomy (59–92%).[103,246]

Acute pain

Acute pain following surgery or radiation therapy can be successfully treated using conventional algorithms for acute postoperative pain.[2,209] Nerves are frequently severed, compressed, or stretched during tumor resection, making it possible for neuropathic pain to be a major factor in the postoperative period. Neural compromise contributes significantly to postmastectomy and postthoracotomy pain syndromes. Adjuvant analgesics (e.g. gabapentin and amitriptyline) should be initiated when a neurogenic source is suspected. As with all postoperative pain that impedes function, aggressive opioid-based and antiinflammatory analgesia should be provided. Acute pain reduction typically facilitates movement and limits the adverse effects of immobility. This is particularly important in cancer patients who might face the debilitating effects of chemotherapy or radiation therapy shortly after their surgeries.

In order to allow patients whose cancers eventually recur or progress to benefit from opioid rotation, confine opioid use to the 'immediate-' and 'sustained-release' formulations of a single drug.[36] The dose threshold for switching opioids due to lack of efficacy in patients with poor prognoses should be high. In this way, patients' exposure is restricted to a minimal number of agents.

Acute pain can also complicate administration of chemotherapy, hormonal therapy, or irradiation. Most of the associated pain syndromes are transient but warrant aggressive analgesia, because they can produce intense discomfort. Acute pain syndromes associated with cancer therapy include paclitaxel-related arthralgias and myalgias,[178,217] bisphosphonate-related bone pain,[41,115] radiation mucositis,[74,210] steroid pseudorheumatism (following withdrawal of corticosteroids),[216] intravesicular BCG–induced cystitis,[77] hepatic artery infusion pain,[136] bone pain associated with colony-stimulating factor (CSF) and granulocyte macrophage CSF administration,[262,263] and radiopharmaceutical-induced pain.[162]

Chronic pain

Chronic cancer-related pain can arise from visceral or neural structures but is most commonly associated with bone metastases.[153] Bone metastases occur in 60–84% of patients with solid tumors,[189] even though 25% of patients with bone metastases report no pain.[272] Pain intensity does not correlate with the

---

Box 58-2 Considerations in cancer pain management

- Therapeutic reliance on high-dose opioid analgesia
- Importance of disease-modifying analgesic approaches
- Potential loss of enteral administration
- Dynamic and rapidly progressive pain complaints
- Multiple concurrent pain syndromes
- Affective and organic psychopathology
- Feasibility of permanent ablative procedures
- Concurrent nociceptive and neuropathic pain

number, size, or location of bone metastases, nor with tumor type.[110] Bone pain is particularly relevant to physiatry, because the recruitment of muscles acting on or loading involved structures can precipitate severe pain. Too often, the excellent pain control achieved while patients remain in bed proves inadequate when they begin to transfer and ambulate. As mentioned above, bone pain responds well to local irradiation.[123]

Non-steroidal antiinflammatory drugs for bone pain

Pharmacologic interventions reduce the intensity of bone pain. Prostaglandins have been implicated in pain associated with lytic bone metastases.[168] Blockade of prostaglandin synthesis is the mechanism by which NSAIDs alleviate bone pain.[16] NSAIDs are considered first-line therapy for bone pain, and a trial is warranted unless contraindicated. At the writing of this chapter, the class-specific cardiovascular risk profile of the cyclooxygenase (COX)-2 inhibitors remained inadequately characterized. While caution should be exercised, the significant potential benefits of COX-2 inhibitors outweigh their risks in many cancer patients with thrombocytopenia and/or gastropathy. COX non-selective inhibitors offer comparable pain relief but a less desirable toxicity profile. Choline magnesium trisalicylate causes less inhibition of platelet aggregation than other COX non-selective inhibitors[240] but did not statistically outperform placebo when trialed in cancer-related bone pain.[134]

Cyclooxygenase non-selective inhibitors with less desirable toxicity profiles have proven more effective. Several placebo-controlled, randomized trials found that ketoprofen reduced cancer pain to a greater extent than either codeine or morphine.[238,247] Dosing NSAIDs for bone pain is no different from using them at antiinflammatory doses for pain of alternative etiologies.

Adjuvant for bone pain

Adjuvant and opioid analgesics can augment NSAID-related control of bone pain. A study found corticosteroids to be beneficial in relieving cancer pain,[24] and extensive anecdotal experience supports their use. The toxicity profile of corticosteroids includes edema, bone demineralization, immunosuppression, and myopathies. This mandates that they be used transiently and rapidly tapered, or for patients in whom sustained analgesic benefit justifies the associated toxicity risk.

Use of calcitonin for bone pain is supported by two positive but severely underpowered trials.[83,116] Weak supportive evidence and rapid tachyphylaxis have limited the use of calcitonin. Evidence supporting the use of parenteral bisphosphonates in the management of bone pain is more robust.[39,99,118,154,155,255] Effective doses of pamidronate range from 30 to 90 mg every 4 weeks. Opioids enhance analgesia afforded by NSAIDs and can reduce the doses required for adequate pain relief.[76,239]

Opioids

As previously mentioned, opioid-based pharmacotherapy is the current standard of care for the management of moderate to severe cancer pain, irrespective of its etiology.[5,125,274] Opioid use should be restricted to pure μ-receptor agonists. Many agonists are commercially available in the USA. Those most commonly used in cancer pain management include morphine, hydromorphone, oxycodone, oxymorphone, fentanyl, and methadone. Opioid analgesic requirements evolve as cancer responds to treatment or progresses. Ongoing dose adjustment maximizes pain control while reducing the incidence of side effects. The dominant paradigm for opioid administration has a well-established track record and has been reiterated by many experts in the field.[80,125,153,191,198] Recognizing that most patients experience constant, baseline pain punctuated by potentially severe incident pain, combined use of immediate and sustained-release opioid preparations is recommended. Providing patients with liberal access to an immediate-release opioid formulation (generally through use of a patient-controlled analgesia pump or enteral routes) allows rapid estimation of initial dose requirements. Once utilization has stabilized, mean daily or hourly consumption can be calculated and an oral or transdermal sustained-release preparation initiated. For enteral or transdermal routes, the mean daily opioid dose is divided by the dosing interval of the sustained-release preparation. Use of a patient-controlled analgesia pump accelerates the dose estimation process, and an appropriate starting basal infusion rate can be estimated after only 6–12 h. Initial rates and doses provide a crude estimate of true opioid requirements. The ongoing dose titration should be driven by patients' utilization of supplemental immediate-release or 'rescue' opioid doses. Typically, rescue doses are 10–15% of the total daily dose.[198]

Opioid conversion

Significant intraindividual variations in response to different opioids have long been recognized.[88] An alternative opioid should be considered when an 'adequate' trial of a particular agent has failed to achieve an acceptable decrement in pain intensity, or has engendered refractory and untenable side effects. An adequate opioid trial in the cancer arena can entail use of high doses (e.g. >1 g intravenously of morphine sulfate per day). Opioid dose conversion requires calculation of the equianalgesic dose of the novel agent (Table 58-2) and reduction by 50% for incomplete cross-tolerance. Incomplete cross-tolerance describes the property of opioids to induce analgesic tolerance with sustained high-dose opioid exposure. Tolerance is usually considerably lower to a novel agent. For this reason, patients often experience greater sedation and needless side effects when exposed to 100% of the equianalgesic dose. Reductions of 50% provide better estimates of the minimal effective opioid dose. If patients are being converted from methadone, reductions of 80–90% of the equianalgesic dose have been recommended, due to methadone's long half-life. Opioid conversions are based on imperfect dose equivalencies. Providing patients with liberal access to rescue doses is critical during the conversion period to avoid precipitation of pain crises.

Invasive and intraspinal analgesic approaches

As mentioned previously, permanent ablation of central afferent tracts becomes tenable in the context of advanced cancer, and

Table 58-2 Opioid dose conversion

Opioid (generic)	Branded product	Route	Dose
Morphine	MS Contin, Avinza, Kadian, Oromorph SR, Roxanol	p.o.: tablet p.o.: elixir i.v. or i.m.	30 mg 30 mg 10 mg
Fentanyl	Actiq Duragesic	Transmucosal i.v. or i.m. Transdermal	500 µg 250 µg 250 µg
Hydromorphone	Dilaudid	p.o.: tablet i.v. or i.m.	7.5 mg 1.5 mg
Oxycodone	Oxycontin	p.o.: tablet p.o.: elixir	20 mg 20 mg
Methadone	Dolophine	p.o. i.v. or i.m.	20 mg 10 mg
Oxymorphone		i.v. or i.m.	1 mg

has been utilized with considerable success.[103,246,252] More discrete neural blockade effectively reduces pain transmitted by one or several adjacent peripheral nerves. Intercostal, paravertebral, genitofemoral, ilioinguinal, and trigeminal nerve blocks can afford dramatic relief and reduce analgesic requirements.[181,189] Nociceptive impulses of visceral origin can be blocked by ablation of sympathetic ganglia. Celiac plexus blockade affords excellent relief of abdominal pain due to pancreatic cancer.[272] Intraspinal opioid administration can reduce dose requirements and associated side effects. The potential benefits must be weighed against the added cost, required maintenance, and risk of infection. Despite efforts to demonstrate cost savings through the use of implantable intrathecal opioid delivery systems,[110] these devices are not widely used. They do not allow for the rapid and facile dose adjustments required by most cancer patients.

IMPAIRMENTS IN CANCER

Cancer can invade all tissue types and regions of the body, producing a wide array of functional impairments. Tumor-related deficits generally arise due to pain, neural compromise, loss of osseous or articular integrity, and invasion of cardiopulmonary structures. Cancer-related impairments are often dynamic, characterized by improvement or progression, depending on treatment responsiveness. Altering or initiating antineoplastic therapy should always be considered in the face of new or progressive impairments. By controlling tumor spread, many deficits can be ameliorated or stabilized.

Impairments due to tumor effects
Bone metastases
Bone metastases are an important source of cancer-related impairment and a critical consideration in rehabilitation. Surgi-

cal stabilization of acute or impending fractures produces impairments that warrant physiatric attention. However, greater challenges arise when bone metastases produce severe, function-limiting pain or pose an uncertain fracture risk during therapeutic exercise. Bone metastases are highly prevalent, because bone is the most common site of metastatic spread, and osseous lesions complicate the most frequently occurring cancers: lung, breast, and prostate. Thyroid cancer, lymphoma, renal cell carcinoma, myeloma, and melanoma also commonly involve bone. Between 60 and 84% of patients with solid tumors will develop bone metastases.[189] As a potential source of severe pain, all bone metastases are relevant to rehabilitation. Management of bony metastatic pain is discussed in the preceding section entitled *Chronic pain*. Of greatest physiatric concern are lesions involving the spine and long bones. These structures are critical for weight bearing and mobility, and are most prone to fracture. Bone metastases are managed with medications, radiopharmaceuticals, orthotics, radiation therapy, and/or surgical stabilization. The choice of intervention will depend on lesion location, degree of associated pain, presence or risk of fracture, radiation responsiveness, and related neurologic compromise. The overall clinical context (e.g. prognosis, severity of medical comorbidities, and operative risk) must also be taken into consideration. Most patients with non-fractural bony lesions can be treated non-operatively through the use of systemic therapy and radiation.

Bisphosphonates are the primary medications utilized to manage bone metastases. Use of these agents mitigates the spread and progression of bone metastases, in addition to relieving associated pain. Bisphosphonates are generally delivered parenterally. Use of bisphosphonates reduces the risk of vertebral fracture (odds ratio 0.69), non-vertebral fracture (odds ratio 0.65), and hypercalcemia (odds ratio 0.54).[215] In addition, the use of bisphosphonates significantly increases the time to first skeletal event after first detection of osseous metastases. Current evidence supports the empiric initiation of bisphosphonates in patients with bone metastases. Radiopharmaceuticals such as strontium-99 are predominantly utilized to manage severe, refractory pain associated with widely disseminated bone metastases. Drawbacks to radiopharmaceuticals include prolonged marrow suppression and potentially severe, pain flares following their administration. Radiation delivered to bone metastasis offers an effective means of rapidly achieving local control of pain and tumor growth. Palliative radiation is typically delivered in 10 fractions of 300 cGy. Radiation may be delayed following surgical stabilization. However, it is an important adjunctive treatment, because it suppresses tumor growth in areas where surgical management may have distributed microscopic emboli.

Painful osteolytic lesions are predominantly responsible for pathologic fractures. The incidence of pathologic fracture among all cancer types is 8%.[113] Breast carcinoma is responsible for roughly 53% of these. Other solid tumors associated with pathologic fractures are kidney, lung, thyroid cancer, and lymphoma. Sixty percent of all long bone fractures involve the femur, with 80% of these located in the proximal potion.[232]

Table 58-3 Proposed rating system for calculating fracture risk

Character	Point assigned		
	1	2	3
Anatomic location	Upper extremity	Lower extremity	Trochanter
Lesion type	Blastic	Blastic or lytic	Lytic
Lesion size	$\leq 1/3$ diameter	$>1/3, <2/3$	$\geq 2/3$
Intensity of pain	Mild	Moderate	Severe

Management of osseous metastases that present a risk of fracture remains a source of clinical uncertainty. Precise quantification of fracture risk has been a persistent challenge in orthopedic oncology. Table 58-3 outlines Mirels's proposed rating system for calculating fracture risk, whereby specific attributes are ascribed points.[170] Neither this, nor any other approach based on retrospective review, has been adequately validated in clinical practice.

Radiation of 'at risk' lesions without surgical stabilization can transiently increase fracture risk in the periradiation period. The elevated fracture risk warrants establishing toe touch or partial weight-bearing status for several weeks after the initiation of radiation therapy. If pain persists following radiation, or if there are no effective non-operative treatments impending, fractures should be managed surgically.

Pathological fractures are generally managed through well-estesblished surgial algorithms. Four main goals direct surgical management of pathologic fractures: pain relief, preservation or restoration of function, skeletal stabilization, and local tumor control.[112] The general indications for surgery are life expectancy of >1 month with a fracture of a weight-bearing bone, and >3 months for fracture of a non–weight-bearing bone.[232] Internal fixation or prosthetic replacements with polymethylmethacrylate are the most effective ways of relieving pain and restoring function in patients with pathologic fractures.[112] These procedures allow immediate weight bearing. Intraoperative resection removes residual tumor that would impede bony healing. However, healing rates are low following pathologic fractures. One review of 123 patients reported a 35% incidence of fracture healing.[87]

Fractures of the pelvis are generally treated conservatively, unless pain persists after radiation or they involve the acetabulum. In the latter case, patients are generally surgically reconstructed with screws or pins, and with a protrusio acetabular component. Vertebral fractures that are not associated with neurologic compromise are generally treated conservatively with radiation and bracing.[190] Operative decompression and stabilization may be indicated for persistent pain refractory to aggressive analgesic therapy. Vertebroplasty should be considered for patients who are not at risk of tumor displacement into the spinal canal and associated myelopathy.

Brain tumors: primary and metastases

Brain metastases occur in 15–40% of cancer patients, accounting for 170 000 new cases per year. They are the most common intracranial tumors.[89,200] The incidence has increased in recent years, presumably due to increased patient survival and better early detection of small tumors.[260] Lung cancer is the most common primary source of brain metastases. Between 9.7 and 64% of patients with stage IV lung cancer develop metastases.[221,259] Breast cancer is the second most common source, followed by melanoma, with 2–25% and 4–20% of patients developing brain metastases, respectively.[221] Brain metastases from colorectal cancers, genitourinary cancers, and sarcomas occur, although with considerably less frequency (1%).[260] The distribution of metastases reflects cerebral blood flow, with 90% situated in the supratentorial region and 10% in the posterior fossa.[260] Brain metastases are multiple in approximately 50–75% of cases.

Presentation Presenting symptoms at the time of diagnosis with brain metastasis, in order of decreasing frequency, are as follow (patients can have more than one): headache, 49%; mental disturbance, 32%; focal weakness, 30%; gait ataxia, 21%; seizures, 18%; speech difficulty, 12%; visual disturbance, 6%; sensory disturbance, 6%; and limb ataxia, 6%.[10,26] Neurologic examination reveals the following clinical signs at presentation: hemiparesis, 59%; impaired cognitive function, 58%; hemisensory loss, 21%; papilledema, 20%; gait ataxia, 19%; aphasia, 18%; visual field cut, 7%; and limb ataxia, 4%.[9,10]

Treatment Corticosteroids are the first-line treatment, with dexamethasone being the drug of choice.[200] By virtue of their ability to reduce peritumoral edema, corticosteroids reverse local brain compression and associated deficits. Treatment generally involves whole brain radiation therapy with stereotactic radiosurgery or surgical resection via craniotomy. Adjunctive chemotherapy can be used, contingent on patient performance status, type of cancer, and prior exposure to antineoplastics. Although seizures occur in 25% of patients with brain metastasis, studies and a metaanalysis have failed to show that antiepileptic drugs reduce their incidence.[97,98]

Prognosis Untreated patients with brain metastases have a median survival of 4 weeks.[148] The Radiation Therapy Oncology Group analyzed the results of 1200 patients with brain metastases in multiple trials, and devised a three-tiered classification scheme to predict survival.[90] Patients with the best prognoses (class 1), mean 7.1 months, had Karnofsky performance status (KPS) >70, age <65 years, controlled primary tumor, and no extracranial metastases. Patients with intermediate prognoses (class 2), mean 4.2 months, had KPS >70, with at least one of the following factors: >65 years of age, uncontrolled primary tumor, or systemic disease. Patients with poor prognoses (class 3), mean 2.3 months, had KPS <70. Although mean survival is less than 1 year for patients whose brain metastases are treated, the distribution is skewed, with some patients surviving >2 years with good functional preservation and quality of life.

The rehabilitation needs of patients with brain metastases are determined by baseline functional status, prognoses, location and number of metastases, and antineoplastic treatment plan. The tremendous heterogeneity in the severity and type of associated impairments defies the formulation of a uniform algorithm. Cancer patients should be assessed on an individual basis using an approach analogous to that applied to patients with ischemic or traumatic intracranial lesions.

Epidural spinal cord compression

Malignant spinal cord compression (SCC) occurs in up to 5% of patients.[13] In contrast to brain metastases, which involve the brain parenchyma, most symptomatic tumors compress the spinal cord or cauda equina from the epidural space.[202] Epidural lesions generally arise from vertebral metastases, and rarely breach the dura.[109] Invasion of the dural space accounts for only 5% of neoplastic SCC, and is due to either growth of tumor along the spinal roots or hematogenous spread to the cord.[40,73,192,203] The cancers that most commonly cause SCC are those that produce vertebral metastases (e.g. breast, lung, myeloma, and prostate).[20,95,101,135,273]

Presentation   Pain is by far the most common initial (94%) and presenting (97–99%) symptom of malignant SCC.[18,95,202] Radicular pain is present in 58% of patients at diagnosis.[18] Pain associated with SCC is generally exacerbated when supine or by coughing, sneezing, or the Valsalva maneuver.[37] If malignant SCC is detected when pain is the only symptom, efforts to preserve function through surgical decompression or radiation therapy have high success rates.[202] Unfortunately, this is rarely the case. Reports of symptom prevalence when the diagnosis of malignant SCC is eventually made are remarkably consistent. Weakness is present in 74–76% of patients, autonomic dysfunction in 52–57%, and sensory loss in 51–53%.[95,202] The thoracic spine is the most common site of epidural SCC, followed by the lumbosacral and cervical spine in a ratio of 4:2:1.[202]

Diagnosis and treatment   Magnetic resonance imaging (MRI) is the procedure of choice to evaluate the epidural space and spinal cord.[248] MRI allows rapid evaluation of the entire spine with sagittal views. Computed tomography (CT) scans are helpful if there is an absolute contraindication to MRI, or if SCC is related to tumor encroachment through the foramina.

Prognosis   Tumors that cause rapid progression of neurologic deficits are associated with poorer functional outcomes following decompression.[95,235] In general, patients remain ambulatory if able to walk at the time of definitive treatment. Motor and coordination deficits rarely resolve when present at diagnosis.

Cancer involving cranial and peripheral nerves

Compromise of cranial and peripheral nerves is a common source of cancer-related pain and impairment. Cancer can affect nerves through local extension of primary tumors (e.g. brachial plexopathy associated with Pancoast tumors) or through metastatic spread.

Cranial nerves

Cranial nerve palsies are caused by tumors that originate near the base of the skull or metastasize there. Cancer can directly invade cranial nerves or exogenously compress them. Often, tumors invade the neural foramina, which is seen in 15–35% of patients with nasopharyngeal carcinoma (a highly neurotropic cancer).[243,261] Bone metastases from lung, breast, and prostate cancers involving the base of the skull are also common sources of cranial nerve compromise.[101,208] The incidence with which different cranial nerves are affected by cancer remains poorly quantified. One series of breast cancer patients reported a 13% incidence of cranial nerve dysfunction.[106] The trigeminal and facial nerves were most frequently involved.

Clinical presentations vary depending on the cranial nerve being compressed. Evaluation should include MRI, which is the diagnostic test of choice.[205] If patients have a bone-avid tumor (e.g. lung, breast, or prostate), a CT scan should be considered, because bone destruction is more easily observed on CT scan.[186] Positron emission tomography (PET) scanning can help to discretely localize tumor if extensive postradiation change or surgical alteration of the bony architecture has occurred. Acute management should include oral steroids, unless contraindicated, to preserve neurologic function until definitive treatment is delivered. Treatment generally involves chemotherapy and radiation.[199]

Spinal roots

Malignant radiculopathies arise through direct hematogenous spread to the nerve roots or dorsal root ganglia, or, more commonly, by invasion from the paravertebral space. When the latter occurs, tumor can grow longitudinally in the paravertebral space and concurrently invade multiple foramina to produce a polyradiculopathy.[199] Most cancer-related radiculopathies initially produce dysesthetic, aching, or burning pain in the affected dermatome, which can be associated with lancinations. Sympathetic hyper- or hypoactivity can be present.[46,266] Involvement of the lower cervical or upper thoracic roots can produce a Horner syndrome. In patients with a history of cancer, a new Horner syndrome should be attributed to malignancy until proven otherwise. Patients can complain of muscle cramps in affected myotomes.[241]

Diagnosis and treatment   Evaluation of spinal roots for cancerous involvement is best achieved with MRI. MRI will permit assessment of the paravertebral space, foramina, and epidural space. Electromyography allows pathophysiologic characterization of the nerves involved. Steroids should be considered to minimize peritumoral edema until disease-modifying therapy can be delivered. Radiation is effective at alleviating symptoms,[236] but its capacity to spare neurologic function has not been adequately characterized.

Nerve plexuses

The brachial and lumbosacral plexuses are commonly compressed or invaded by tumor. The frequency of neoplastic brachial plexopathy is 0.43%, and lumbosacral plexopathy 0.71%, based on retrospective case series.[126,142] The most common sources of brachial plexopathy are tumors at the lung apex and regional spread of breast cancer.[52,142] Because cancer generally grows superiorly to invade the lower brachial plexus, the inferior trunk and medial cord are most commonly involved. Occasionally, head and neck neoplasms grow inferiorly to invade the upper trunk.[127]

Pain in the shoulder region and proximal arm occurs in 89% of patients with malignant brachial plexopathy and is the most common presenting symptom.[81] The presence of pain helps to distinguish malignant from radiation-induced plexopathy. Only 18% of patients with radiation-induced plexopathy develop pain.[81] Radiation plexopathies also differ in their propensity to cause progressive weakness in the C5–6 myotomes as opposed to the lower cervical levels.[81] Horner syndrome occurs in 23% of cancer patients with malignant brachial plexopathies.[127] The presence of Horner indicates risk of neuroforaminal encroachment and SCC. Numbness and paresthesias associated with malignant plexopathies typically are perceived in the C8 dermatome, especially digits 4 and 5.[199] Loss of hand dexterity and power can be the initial motor complaint. Weakness subsequently extends proximally to involve the finger flexors, wrist extensors and flexors, and elbow extensors.[199]

Malignancies responsible for lumbosacral plexopathies include colorectal carcinomas; retroperitoneal sarcomas; or metastatic tumors from breast, lymphoma, uterus, cervix, bladder, melanoma, or prostate.[126,128–131] When primary intrapelvic neoplasms are not responsible, the lumbosacral plexus is generally invaded from lymphatic and osseous metastases.[127] Sacral plexopathies are more common than those in the lumbar region. Lumbar and sacral plexopathies can also occur concurrently.[199] Lumbosacral plexopathies are bilateral in 25% of patients, particularly when the sacral plexus is more extensively involved.[199,127] Incontinence and impotence strongly suggest bilateral involvement.[126] Back, buttock, and/or leg pain is present in 98% of patients with malignant lumbosacral plexopathies. Among the 60% of patients who eventually develop neurologic deficits, 86% have leg weakness and 73% sensory loss.[127] Positive straight leg raise is present in over 50% of patients.[126] As many as 33% of patients complain of a 'hot dry foot' due to involvement of sympathetic components of the plexus.

Diagnosis and treatment   The evaluations of a suspected brachial plexopathy should include chest radiography to assess the lung apex. MRI with gadolinium is the diagnostic test of choice for evaluating the brachial and lumbosacral plexuses.[254,257] Cancerous invasion of plexuses can extend along adjacent connective tissue or the epineurium of nerve trunks, without producing a discrete mass.[72] For this reason, MRI findings can be erroneously interpreted as postradiation change. Electromyography can distinguish plexopathies from radiculopathies by defining the distribution of denervation. The presence of myokymia on needle examination is virtually pathognomonic for radiation plexopathy.[108]

Acute treatment should include steroids for preservation of neurologic function. Radiation can effectively relieve pain but is less helpful in restoring lost function.[6,141] Chemotherapy is commonly initiated or altered when plexus involvement heralds cancer progression; however, the success of this approach remains poorly characterized. Refractory pain requires aggressive coadministration of opioid and adjuvant analgesics, and potentially high cervical cordotomy or rhizotomy.[124] Stellate ganglion blockade can relieve pain that is sympathetically maintained.

Peripheral nerves

Peripheral nerves are affected most often by cancer when extension of a bone metastasis produces a mononeuropathy.[214] Rare polyneuropathy or mononeuritis multiplex due to myeloma, lymphoma, or leukemia has been reported.[14,65,94,104,132,145,166] More commonly, nerves are compressed where they pass directly over an involved bone or through a bony canal.[214] Common sites of nerve compression include the radial nerve at the humerus, obturator nerve at the obturator canal, ulnar nerve at the elbow and axilla, sciatic nerve in the pelvis, intercostal nerves, and peroneal nerve at the fibular head. Pain generally precedes motor and sensory loss.[199]

Diagnosis and treatment   Evaluation includes plain radiographs, MRI, or electromyography. Treatment depends on the clinical context in which the mononeuropathy occurs. Radiation, surgical decompression, and chemotherapy, individually or in combination, are common treatment approaches. Significant sensorimotor recovery should not be expected, irrespective of the antineoplastic intervention.

Paraneoplastic syndromes

Paraneoplastic syndromes are pertinent to rehabilitation because they produce refractory neurologic deficits and severe disability. The incidence of paraneoplastic neurologic disorders (PNDs) is low, occurring in less than 1% of all cancer patients.[117] PNDs may affect any level of the nervous system. Classic PNDs are listed in Table 58-4. These syndromes are produced when antibodies are made against tumors that express nervous system proteins. Discrete or multifocal neural degeneration produces diverse symptoms and deficits. Most PNDs are triggered during the early stages of cancer, when primary tumors and metastases may be undetectable by conventional imaging techniques. The emergence of a PND in a patient with known cancer should trigger work-up for recurrent or progressive disease. PNDs are characterized by symptoms that develop and progress rapidly in days to weeks, and then stabilize. Spontaneous improvement is rare. Diagnostic work-up may include serum and cerebrospinal fluid studies, brain MRI, and PET.[3,43] Screening patients' serum or cerebrospinal fluid for antineuronal antibodies known to be associated with particular cancers can direct the search for an occult malignancy. Timely diagnosis and treatment of the tumor offer the greatest chance of success in managing PNDs.[15,34] PNDs do not generally respond solely to immunotherapies, for example intravenous immunoglobulin, corticosteroids, and immunosuppressants. However, these may be useful adjuvant treatments.

Table 58-4 Classic paraneoplastic disorders

Classic paraneoplastic neurologic disorder	Associated malignancy	Presenting signs and symptoms
Cerebellar degeneration	Small cell lung cancer, Hodgkin lymphoma, gynecologic, breast	Pancerebellar dysfunction with truncal and limb ataxia
Limbic encephalitis	Germ cell tumors of the testes	Anxiety, depression, confusion, delirium, hallucinations, seizures, short-term memory loss, dementia
Opsoclonus–myoclonus	Breast, gynecologic, small cell lung cancer, neuroblastoma	Chaotic, conjugate, arrhythmic, and multidirectional ocular saccades, myoclonus, truncal ataxia
Sensory neuronopathy	Small cell lung cancer	Pain, numbness, sensory deficits of cranial and spinal nerves
Lambert–Eaton myasthenic syndrome	Small cell lung cancer	Proximal muscle weakness, autonomic symptoms, strength augmentation during initial voluntary contraction
Encephalomyelitis	Small cell lung cancer, thymoma, breast	Symptoms similar to limbic encephalitis and cerebellar degeneration, sensory deficits, ataxia, bulbar deficits, weakness

Rehabilitation of PNDs is determined by the type, distribution, and severity of the associated neurologic deficits. Potential improvement with planned antineoplastic therapy should be taken into consideration. Supportive and preventive measures to protect the integrity of the skin, affected joints, and genitourinary symptoms are critical while awaiting stabilization of neurologic deficits. Communication, respiratory, and nutritional issues should be addressed in patients with bulbar involvement.

Skin metastases

Dermal metastases occur in 5.3% of patients, and are most common in breast cancer.[143] Skin metastases can be a source of pain and an entry point for infectious pathogens. Because the associated wounds seldom heal, chronic wound care is necessary and becomes an integral part of patients' rehabilitation needs. Figure 58-1 shows a breast cancer patient with dermal metastases involving the breast and proximal arm. Dermal metastases often engender or aggravate lymphedema. Use of compression is limited only by patient tolerance. Malignant wounds should be managed with non-adherent, bacteriostatic, hyperabsorbent dressings (e.g. SilvaSorb or Aquacel Ag). Associated pain must be managed aggressively to minimize adverse functional consequences. Proactive range of motion (ROM) will prevent the formation of contractures in joints adjacent to malignant wounds, facilitating hygiene and autonomous self-care.

Cardiopulmonary metastases

Lung, pleural, and pericardial metastases involving the heart and lungs can produce dramatic and abrupt reductions in patients' stamina and functional status. Virtually all cancers have the potential to spread to the lungs and pleura. At autopsy, 25–30% of all cancer patients have lung metastases.[47] Pleural metastases

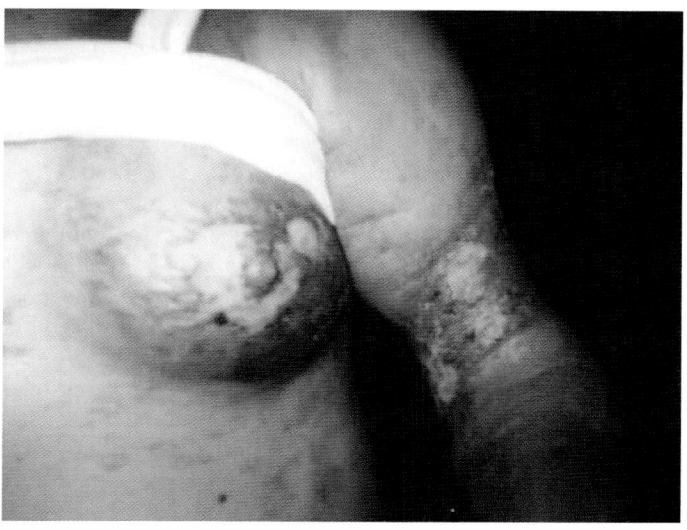

Figure 58-1 Skin metastases producing unhealing wounds in a breast cancer patient.

occur in 12% of breast and 7–15% of lung cancers.[144,147] Metastases to the heart and pericardium are less common, although their functional impact can be similarly devastating. A series of 4769 autopsies revealed the presence of cardiac metastases in 8.4% of cancer patients.[231] Melanoma, mesothelioma, lung tumors, and renal neoplasms had the highest prevalence of cardiac spread. The clinical diagnosis of heart or lung metastases can be generally made by CT scans. PET scans and plain x-rays may also be helpful, depending on the clinical context.

Treatment of lung, pleural, pericardial, or cardiac metastases varies considerably. The type and efficacy of anticancer treatment will depend on the primary tumor, number and location of metastases, previous antineoplastic therapies, overall medical condition of the patient, and degree of associated symptomatic distress. Surgical metastectomy has the potential to definitively eliminate disease in certain patients.[258] Discrete metastases that are not resectable may be amenable to radiation therapy. Commonly, patients with extrathoracic metastases are treated with systemic chemotherapy. New or progressive intrathoracic metastases indicate the need to initiate or change antineoplastics.

Malignant pleural effusions should be evacuated by thoracentesis when patients become symptomatic. Dyspnea is often multifactorial. Reducing the effusion can fail to alleviate patients' shortness of breath if the lung is trapped because of parenchymal or pleural disease. Reaccumulation of malignant effusions can be managed through intermittent thoracentesis or pleurodesis. Chemical pleurodesis has an overall complete response rate of 64% when all sclerotic agents are considered.[147] Talc appears the most effective, with a complete response rate of 91%. Pleuroperitoneal shunting and catheter drainage of the pleural space are less popular therapeutic alternatives.

The functional relevance of heart and lung metastases stems from their deleterious effect on patients' aerobic capacity. Small reductions in cardiopulmonary reserve can devastate patients who are deconditioned or have other impairments. Reduced oxygenation can render patients severely dyspneic with minimal exertion. For this reason, all potentially treatable causes should be definitively addressed. Supplemental oxygen should be initiated as soon as dyspnea becomes function-limiting. In this way, patients can remain independent and ambulatory. If tolerated, gradual, progressive aerobic conditioning will optimize peripheral conditioning, reducing the percentage of VO_{2max} required for activities. Referral for outpatient aerobic training should be considered when cancer patients with cardiopulmonary disease are hospitalized for other problems (e.g. neutropenic fever). These patients are prone to rapid functional decline that usually proves permanent in the absence of structured therapy.

Impairments due to cancer treatment
Combined modality therapy
The push toward organ preservation in primary cancer care has led to widespread use of combined modality therapy. Clinical trials have consistently shown that concurrent or sequential administration of radiation and chemotherapy reduces the extent of tissue resection required to achieve local cancer control, without compromising 5-year survival rates.[122] The trend toward use of combined modality therapy is relevant to rehabilitation, because most cancer patients receive some combination of chemotherapy, radiation therapy, and/or surgery contingent on the type and stage of cancer. This renders patients more vulnerable to normal tissue toxicities associated with each modality.

Surgery-related impairments
Primary impairments due to surgery depend on the extent, location, and type of tumor. Normal tissue is inevitably affected by surgical efforts to achieve local control of cancer. The principal reasons for resecting normal tissue, with the associated risk of adverse long-term consequences, include accurate staging (e.g. sampling of lymph nodes, and visceral and parietal peritoneum), definitive eradication of tumor, assurance of local disease control (e.g. removal of lymph nodes that might harbor cancer cells), and harvest for reconstructive purposes.

Cancer surgery has the greatest physiatric relevance when certain tissue types are affected. These tissues include bone, nerve, muscle, lung parenchyma, and lymphatics. It is important to realize that normal postoperative healing is often compromised by the prior or coadministration of additional anticancer treatment (e.g. radiation and chemotherapy).

The list of established surgical approaches to eradicate tumor is vast, and readers are referred to *Surgical Oncology: Contemporary Principles and Practice* (edited by K. Bland) for more precise and extensive procedure-specific discussions. Operations that commonly warrant the immediate attention of a physical medicine specialist include neck dissection for oropharyngeal carcinomas (spinal accessory nerve palsy), limb salvage or amputation for osteosarcoma (impairments vary by site), resection of truncal or limb myosarcoma (weakness, gait dysfunction, biomechanical imbalance), and pneumonectomy or lobectomy for lung neoplasms (aerobic insufficiency). Procedures such as nephrectomy, colectomy, mastectomy, and oophorectomy can require resection of muscle, nerve, and/or vascular structures to achieve clean margins. Muscles can also be transposed for coverage of bony prominences or to substitute for resected muscles. Reviewing patients' surgical reports is essential to accurately identify all potential sources of impairment.

Neurosurgical resection of central and peripheral nervous system malignancies mandates physiatric evaluation, irrespective of the presence of gross deficits, given the potentially devastating effects of subtle impairments and the high likelihood of future recurrence and progression.

Secondary impairments
Secondary surgery-associated impairments often emerge well after the responsible operations and can present as familiar musculoskeletal problems (e.g. tendonopathies and arthropathies). Secondary impairments are generally due to flexibility and strength deficits, which arise from biomechanical imbalance. A common example is myofascial dysfunction of the scapular retractors, middle trapezius and rhomboid muscles, due to pectoralis major and minor tightness following mastectomy or chest wall radiation and breast implant insertion.

Cancer patients develop compensatory strategies for mobility and ADL performance when negotiating flexibility or strength deficits. These strategies can produce maladaptive movement patterns. Premature recruitment of the upper trapezius muscle during shoulder abduction is common among breast cancer patients with mild, postmastectomy adhesive capsulitis. While achieving the short-term goal of arm elevation, patients can eventually develop rotator cuff pathology due to aberrant muscle recruitment patterns. Secondary impairments are

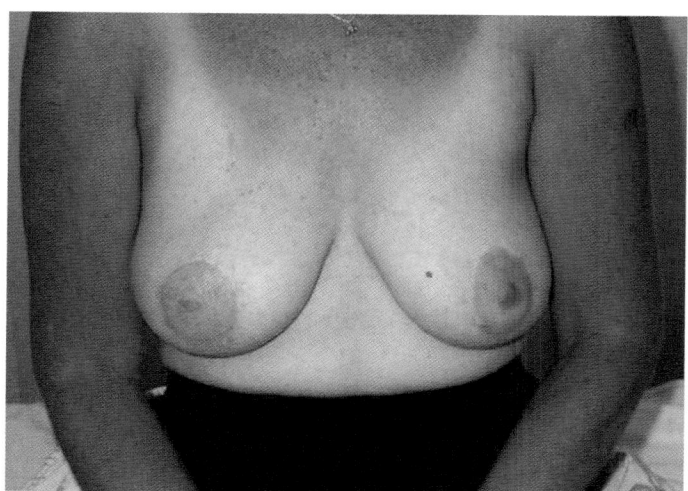

Figure 58-2 Excellent cosmesis achieved with bilateral transverse rectus abdominis flap breast reconstructions.

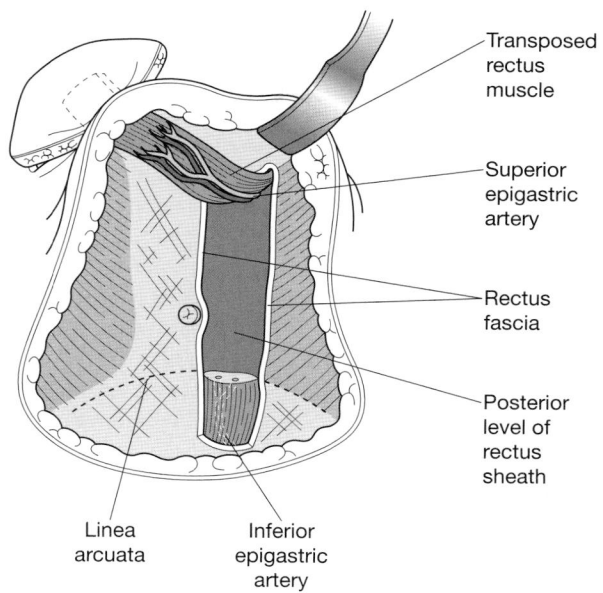

Transposed rectus muscle

Superior epigastric artery

Rectus fascia

Posterior level of rectus sheath

Linea arcuata

Inferior epigastric artery

Figure 58-3 The transverse rectus abdominis flap procedure utilizes the superior epigastric artery to supply blood to the subumbilical fat, which is used to reconstruct the mastectomized breast. The fat and inferior end of the rectus muscle are tunneled under the abdominal wall into the defect caused by mastectomy.

fortunately readily detectable and reversible through comprehensive physiatric evaluation and treatment.

Donor site morbidity

Donor site morbidity associated with surgical tissue harvest for reconstructive purposes produces significant impairments less often than might be anticipated. Muscle, skin, bone, and fat are utilized to achieve adequate coverage of surgical defects and to optimize cosmesis. Radial forearm and fibular flaps are commonly harvested to eliminate defects produced by mandibular resection. Both are typically well tolerated and seldom produce functional deficits. Impairments associated with the harvest of myocutaneous flaps vary by extent and site, and are no different in cancer than in other rehabilitation cohorts. Partial transposition of the pectoralis major muscle from its insertion on the humerus has been used to repair soft tissue defects involving the anterolateral neck. This procedure can destabilize the shoulder in the absence of therapeutic intervention.

By virtue of the high incidence of breast cancer, significant donor site morbidity is most prevalent with autogenous tissue transposition for breast reconstruction. Transverse rectus abdominis muscle (TRAM), gluteus maximus, and latissimus myocutaneous flaps are utilized, with the first being more common. With a relatively low complication rate (25.3%) and potentially excellent cosmesis (Fig. 58-2), the TRAM flap procedure is an increasingly common choice, given the potential to create a natural-looking breast with normal ptosis and an inframammary fold. More patients are electing to undergo immediate breast reconstruction to reduce the risk associated with repeat operations and the psychologic distress engendered by mastectomy.

The TRAM procedure involves the transposition of muscle and adipose tissue to achieve preoperative breast appearance (Fig. 58-3). Other advantages of the TRAM procedure include relatively hidden scars and a satisfactory donor site resulting in

a flat abdomen.[185] The TRAM flap can be divided into the pedicled or free flap procedures.

These procedures differ in that the pedicled, or conventional, procedure utilizes the epigastric vessels supplying the rectus muscle to perfuse the subumbilical fat. Subumbilical adipose tissue is tunneled under the abdominal skin to repair the defect created by mastectomy. The inferior end of the contralateral rectus abdominis muscle is tunneled with the fat (Fig. 58-3). In contrast, the free flap procedure involves the creation of anastomoses with vessels in the chest such as the thoracodorsal or internal mammary arteries. While the free flap procedure requires increased operative time, it is associated with decreased incidence of partial flap loss due to fat necrosis.[11]

Despite declining perioperative complication rates, the musculoskeletal sequelae of TRAM flap breast reconstruction can be significant.[175] Donor site complications include abdominal wall bulge (3.8%) and abdominal hernia (2.6%).[146] Patients experience abdominal weakness and reduced exertional tolerance, particularly those undergoing bilateral procedures.[171] Because the TRAM procedure produces a defect in the abdominal wall, patients have difficulty stabilizing the trunk while transferring from supine and seated positions. Partial denervation of the abdominal wall also leads to deficits in proprioception and truncal balance. Weakness of the abdominal wall can lead to exaggerated lumbar lordosis and an increased incidence of back pain. An algorithm for treatment of patients post TRAM flap is presented later in this chapter under the heading *Rehabilitation of specific cancer populations.*

Radiation therapy-related impairments

Radiation therapy has become an integral part of combined modality and organ preservation therapy for many cancers. Approximately 50% of cancer patients undergo radiation therapy during the course of their disease.[111] While highly effective in eliminating radiosensitive tumors, controlling regional disease, and palliating symptomatic metastases, radiation therapy also injures normal tissue. The tolerance of normal tissues surrounding tumors is the most important radiation dose-limiting consideration.[111] Radiation injury is multiphasic, characterized by discrete acute and late phases mediated by distinct pathophysiologic processes. Acute injury is predominantly due to inflammation and the death of rapidly proliferating cell types. Cell death occurs through the induction of apoptosis and free radical-mediated DNA damage. Patients can develop desquamation of the dermis and mucous membranes, visceral inflammation (e.g. colitis, cystitis, and enteritis), and muscle hypertonicity, among other symptoms. Biologic response modifiers released from injured tumor cells are thought to mediate systemic radiation effects such as fatigue and malaise.[151] The time course of acute radiation effects on normal tissue varies significantly by tissue type and radiation dose. Most patients return to their preradiation baseline by the second month post treatment. However, the distribution is highly skewed, and some patients remain symptomatic as many as 12 months after treatment.

The deleterious effects of late radiation injury are undergoing increasing clinical investigation. Adverse late effects can be attributed to tissue necrosis and fibrosis. The mechanisms underlying these end processes are gradually being elucidated. Microvascular injury predisposes to thrombus formation and produces a hypoxic interstitial environment.[75] Hypoxia is believed to favor the generation of free radical species that produce further damage, and, ultimately, a self-perpetuating cycle of tissue injury and fibrosis.[264] In addition to compression from fibrosis, neural injury may occur from occlusion of the vasonervorum and infarction of nerves.[127]

The adverse late effects of radiation therapy depend on the extent and location of the radiation field. Identifying the tattoos, placed during radiation therapy simulation, can help delineate the extent of the irradiated tissue. This is particularly helpful when clinical records are unavailable. Table 58-5 lists conditions caused by delayed radiation toxicity by system. Late radiation effects most relevant to rehabilitation medicine include those involving connective tissue, muscles, and nerves. Fibrosis occurs to some degree in all muscles and connective tissue within a radiation portal. In the absence of ongoing ROM, patients develop contractures. Because free radical-mediated late radiation injury is an ongoing process, ranging of affected muscles and fascia should continue indefinitely.

The most devastating neural effects of radiation therapy include myelopathy, plexopathy, and encephalopathy. Delayed radiation myelopathy produces symptoms 12–50 months after radiation therapy, and progresses over weeks or months to paraparesis or quadriparesis.[69,70,82,100,222,258] Symptoms can worsen or stabilize, producing deficits ranging from mild to complete

motor weakness. Although recent radiation therapy adaptations have reduced the incidence of myelopathy, it has been described in 5% of patients who survive 18 months after receiving 5000 cGy (1 Gy = 100 rads, 1 cGy = 1 rad) to the mediastinum for lung cancer.[267] Risk factors include radiation therapy fraction size >180 cGy and older age.[218] The presenting symptom is usually a Brown–Séquard syndrome, which begins distally and ascends to reach the irradiated level of the cord.[201] MRI is useful in distinguishing radiation from malignant myelopathy.

Radiation plexopathies occur in 1.8–4.9% of treated patients.[195,206,229] Risk is dose-related and seems to increase with radiation therapy exposure >5000 cGy.[137] Concurrent administration of chemotherapy increases the risk.[183] Radiation therapy-induced brachial plexopathies develop between 3 months and 14 years (median 1.5 years) after therapy.[142] Lumbosacral plexopathies develop between 1 month and 31 years (generally 1–5 years) following radiation therapy.[7,256] Characteristics of radiation therapy plexopathies that distinguish them from malignant plexopathies include lower incidence of pain (18%), pain that develops after weakness, and the presence of myokymia on electromyography.

Table 58-5 Conditions caused by delayed radiation toxicity

System	Adverse late effects
Endocrine	Hypothyroidism, hypogonadism, adrenal insufficiency, glucose intolerance due to pancreatic insufficiency
Exocrine	Xerostomia, pancreatic enzyme deficiency
Neural	Myelopathy, plexopathy, cerebrovascular ischemia, dementia, leukoencephalopathy, cranial neuropathy
Lymphatic	Lymph node necrosis, lymphedema
Gastrointestinal	Dysmotility, malabsorption, neuroconstipation, obstruction, perforation, dysgeusia
Dermis	Atrophy, ulceration, delayed healing, hyperpigmentation
Auditory	Progressive loss of acuity, tinnitus
Vascular	Premature atherosclerosis, venous sclerosis
Pulmonary or upper respiratory	Parenchymal fibrosis tracheal stenosis, dysphonia secondary to laryngeal fibrosis
Musculoskeletal	Fibrosis, osteonecrosis, osteoporosis, soft tissue necrosis joint contracture, epimysial fibrosis
Ocular	Corneal ulceration, retinopathy, scleral necrosis
Genitourinary	Neurogenic bladder, renal failure, obstruction, perforation

Delayed radiation therapy encephalopathy due to necrosis of brain parenchyma occurs in 3–5% of patients receiving >5000 cGy, and in 5–15% of patients receiving 6000 cGy.[152,161] Symptoms generally develop 2 years after completion of radiation therapy. The clinical presentation often resembles that of the primary malignancy, raising the question of local recurrence. PET scanning is of greater utility in distinguishing tumor from radiation necrosis than either MRI or CT.[22,51,64] Radiation necrosis is hypometabolic. Cerebral atrophy occurs more commonly than radiation therapy necrosis, being present invariably after whole brain radiation therapy of 3000 cGy in 10 fractions.[201] Virtually all patients complain of memory loss, which can be sufficiently severe to compromise vocational viability. Memory loss progresses in 10–20% of patients to involve other cognitive domains, potentially leading to dementia.[49] Patients can develop gait abnormalities and urinary urgency.[49]

Medical treatment of radiation therapy-associated neural compromise can include short-term steroids, anticoagulation, and/or hyperbaric oxygen therapy.[96,207] Focal radiation necrosis of brain parenchyma can require surgical resection. Pentoxifylline (800 mg/day) coadministered with tocopherol attenuates radiation fibrosis.[50] The benefits of pentoxifylline have yet to be assessed in radiation therapy-related neural compromise.

Chemotherapy

Chemotherapy represents a mainstay of anticancer therapy. Chemotherapy drugs are used for different purposes and with varying efficacy in the management of cancer. Chemotherapy is utilized for four general purposes:

1. as induction therapy for advanced disease;
2. as an adjunct to the treatment of localized tumor;
3. as the primary treatment of localized cancer (often to reduce tumor size in preparation for surgery); and
4. by direct installation into sanctuaries or site-directed perfusion of specific body regions affected by the cancer.[63]

Induction chemotherapy is administered to patients with advanced disease for which no other treatment exists.[233] *Adjuvant* chemotherapy is administered after local control is achieved through surgery or radiation when no obvious tumor is present in order to eliminate undetectable micrometastases and reduce the risk of recurrence.[63] *Neoadjuvant* therapy can be used prior to surgery in order to reduce tumor size and thereby minimize the degree of anatomic disruption. Chemotherapy is increasingly being used serially to temporize the spread of incurable, stage IV cancer.

A staggering array of chemotherapeutic agents, or antineoplastics, is currently utilized in oncologic practice. Antineoplastic drugs can be mechanistically grouped into a manageable number of subclasses for the non-oncologist, which include alkylating agents, platins and their analogs, antimetabolites, topoisomerase interactive agents, antimicrotubule agents, differentiation agents, and miscellaneous agents. Table 58-6 lists antineoplastics by class.

The type, dose, and duration of chemotherapy vary across different cancer types and stages. However, common overarching strategies are generally applied. In order to exploit complementary mechanisms of action, achieve synergy, and reduce normal tissue toxicity, different chemotherapeutic agents are generally co- or sequentially administered. Standardized combined chemotherapy regimens have given rise to a host of acronyms. Common examples include CHOP (cyclophosphamide, doxorubicin, vincristine, and prednisone), ICE (ifosfamide, carboplatin, and etoposide), and MOPP (mechlorethamine, vincristine, procarbazine, and prednisone); there are many others. It is currently rare for a single chemotherapeutic to be administered as monotherapy.

Antineoplastics are distinguished by their capacity to preferentially injure rapidly dividing cancer cells while sparing normal cells. However, all are associated with significant potential for normal tissue toxicity. The chemotherapeutic toxicities that most commonly produce functional impairments are peripheral neuropathy, cognitive dysfunction, cardiomyopathy, and pulmonary fibrosis. It is fortunate that, with proactive screening, the incidence of significant cardiopulmonary toxicity has been substantially reduced. Bleomycin produces pulmonary fibrosis in 10% of patients.[19,190] The risk of doxorubicin-associated cardiac toxicity directly parallels increases in cumulative dose. With cumulative doses of 550, 600, and 700 mg/m^2, the incidence is 7%, 15%, and 30%, respectively.[61] Cardiomyopathy becomes a real concern in stage IV breast cancer patients who resume doxorubicin treatment after having received it in the context of primary adjuvant therapy. Trastuzumab produces cardiac toxicity in 3–5% of patients receiving monotherapy and in 28% of patients who concurrently receive anthracyclines.[138]

Chemotherapeutic neuropathy is a prevalent and functionally morbid complication of cancer treatment. The vinca alkaloids, cisplatin, and the taxanes are among the most important drugs inducing peripheral neurotoxicity. These drugs are widely used for various malignancies, such as ovarian and breast cancer, and hematologic cancers. Chemotherapeutic neuropathy is related to cumulative dose or dose intensity.[28] Patients who already have neuropathic symptoms due to diabetes mellitus, hereditary neuropathies, or earlier treatment with neurotoxic chemotherapy are believed to be at higher risk.

All platin compounds (e.g. cisplatin, carboplatin, and oxaliplatin) have the potential to produce sensory neuropathy. Cisplatin is a more frequent source of neurotoxicity than the latter two compounds. Symptoms often occur after completion of treatment.[156] Large sensory fibers are preferentially affected, leading to proprioceptive deficits. Pinprick and temperature sensation, as well as motor function, are relatively spared.[28] Lower extremity deep tendon reflexes often disappear. Autonomic nerves remain unaffected. Nerve conduction studies show decreased sensory nerve action potentials and prolonged sensory distal latencies, while nerve conduction velocities are minimally impaired.[156,212,230]

Peripheral neuropathy related to vinca alkaloid treatment is observed most commonly with vincristine. Paresthesias in the distal extremities are the initial symptoms, and loss of lower

Table 58-6 Classes of antineoplastic drugs

Class	Mechanism(s)	Commonly used agents[a]	Toxicities
Antitumor alkylating agents	Formation of covalent bonds of alkyl groups to DNA to form reactive intermediates that attack nucleophilic sites. The DNA can no longer function as a template.	Mustards: chlorambucil, cyclophosphamide, ifosfamide, busulfan Nitrosoureas: carmustine Tetrazines: dacarbazine Aziridines: mitomycin C, thiotepa Non-classic alkylating agents: procarbazine	Myelosuppression (all), mucositis (busulfan), hepatotoxicity (busulfan, carmustine, dacarbazine), pulmonary fibrosis (busulfan, carmustine),cystitis (ifosfamide, cyclophosphamide), alopecia (cyclophosphamide), venoocclusive liver disease (busulfan, carmustine, mitomycin C)
Platins and their analogs	Platination of DNA with induction of apoptosis or arrest of cells in the G2 phase of the cell cycle. Disruption of intracellular signalling pathways.	Cisplatin, carboplatin, oxaliplatin	Nephrotoxicity, ototoxicity, neuropathy, myelosuppression
Antimetabolites	Interference with synthesis of DNA and RNA precursor molecules or DNA polymerase, thereby preventing DNA and RNA replication.	Antifolates: methotrexate 5-Fluoropyrimidines: fluorouracil Arabinose nucleosides: cytarabine Pyrimidine analogs: azacitidine Gemcitabine 6-thiopurines: 6-mercaptopurine, 6-thioguanine *Streptomyces parvullus* derivatives: actinomycin D	Myelosuppression (all), gastrointestinal mucositis (all), hepatotoxicity (methotrexate, arabinose nucleosides, azacitidine, gemcitabine 6-thiopurines), Nephrotoxicity (methotrexate), Neurotoxicity (methotrexate, arabinose nucleosides, azacitidine, 6-s)
Topoisomerase-interactive agents	Interaction with DNA topoisomerases (enzymes regulating DNA packing, i.e. twisting and untwisting), leading to G2 phase arrest or apoptosis in S phase.	Epidophyllotoxins: etoposide Anthracyclines: doxorubicin, daunorubicin, epirubicin, idarubicin Camptothecin analogs: topotecan, irinotecan	Myelosuppression (all), gastrointestinal mucositis (all), cardiotoxicity (anthracyclines), soft tissue ulceration post extravasation (anthracyclines)
Antimicrotubule agents	Disruption of microtubules that compose the mitotic spindle.	Vinca alkaloids: vincristine, vinblastine, vinorelbine Taxanes: paclitaxel, docetaxel Miscellaneous antimicrotubule agents: estramustine	Peripheral neurotoxicity (vinca alkaloids, taxanes), gastrointestinal autonomic dysfunction (vinca alkaloids), neutropenia (vinca alkaloids), myelosuppression (taxanes), myalgias (taxanes), bradydysrhythmias (paclitaxel), fluid retention (docetaxel), skin toxicity (docetaxel), emesis (estramustine), congestive heart failure (estramustine)
Miscellaneous chemotherapeutic agents	Fludarabine: inhibits enzymes essential for DNA synthesis and repair. L-Asparaginase: exploits tumor cells' inability to synthesize asparagine, limiting protein synthesis. Bleomycin: free radical production of DNA breaks.	Fludarabine, L-asparaginase, bleomycin	Myelosuppression (fludarabine), immunosuppression (fludarabine), neurotoxicity (fludarabine), hypersensitivity reactions (L-asparaginase), pulmonary fibrosis (bleomycin), mucocutaneous toxicities (bleomycin)

[a]*Lists not exhaustive.*

extremity muscle stretch reflexes is the initial sign. Weakness of the wrist and digital extensors can occur.[48] Autonomic neuropathy is common and might lead to paralytic ileus, orthostatic hypotension, and impotence.[105] Vibration sense generally remains intact.[28] Nerve conduction studies show decreased distal motor and sensory nerve action potentials, with only slight reduction in nerve conduction velocities, indicating an axonal rather than a demyelinating mechanism of injury.[21,165]

Taxanes have become first-line therapy in the treatment of primary breast, ovarian, and lung cancers. Docetaxel is a more potent inhibitor of cell replication than paclitaxel, and consequently is a more frequent and severe source of neuropathy.

Signs and symptoms that characterize taxane neuropathy include paresthesias, loss of muscle stretch reflexes, and diminished vibration sense.[204] Patients can develop mild proximal muscle weakness that resolves spontaneously.[86] Autonomic neuropathy occurs uncommonly.[133] Nerve conduction studies show reduction of sensory nerve action potentials in patients treated with taxanes.[219] Reduced motor nerve action potentials and diminished sensory and motor nerve conduction velocity have been reported.[219]

REHABILITATION APPROACHES

General strategies

Rehabilitation of bone metastases

Strategies to rehabilitate patients with bone metastases and pathologic fractures remain largely theoretic due to a lack of empiric data. Approaches can be grouped into the use of orthses, assistive devices, therapeutic exercise, and environmental modification. All essentially deweight or immobilize compromised bones. Orthoses can be fabricated to stabilize bones in positions that limit potentially damaging forces. A common example is the use of thoracolumbosacral or spinal extension orthoses, such as cruciform anterior spinal hyperextension or Jewett braces. These orthoses limit spinal flexion, thereby reducing loads on the anterior vertebrae, protecting against compression fractures. Orthoses can also be used to protect and deweight sites of fracture or impending fracture. Thermoplast arm troughs allow patients with humeral metastases to immobilize the affected extremity and reduce damaging forces. Extreme caution must be used in redistributing weight with an orthotic. Careful radiologic evaluation of the bony structures on to which loads will be transferred is essential. Bone metastases are rarely discrete. It can be challenging in widespread osseous disease to find sufficient intact bone to unload weight-bearing structures.

Assistive devices and instruction in compensatory strategies similarly reduce the load on compromised bones. Canes, crutches, and walkers are frequently used to minimize fracture risk. Scrutiny must be paid to the skeletal structures that will receive additional load via the assistive devices. Patients should be instructed in how to minimize forces by performing activities close to the body, thereby limiting torque on long bones.

While theoretically appealing, there are currently no empiric data to support the role of therapeutic exercise in preventing pathologic fractures. Nonetheless, patients at risk for vertebral fractures routinely tolerate exercise programs designed to strengthen the abdominal and spinal extensor muscles and to enhance their proprioceptive acuity. A comprehensive exercise program should include postural awareness, truncal strengthening, and balance training. The significant benefit of simple environmental modifications in preventing pathologic fractures should not be underestimated. Throw rugs and other hazards that increase fall risk should be removed. Railings can be added to stairwells and bathrooms as appropriate. Patients' prognoses

should obviously be considered in the zeal and expense with which such modifications are implemented.

Exercise

Aerobic conditioning Trials of aerobic conditioning in cancer populations have been predominantly conducted to determine whether exercise attenuates treatment-associated fatigue. Breast cancer patients receiving adjuvant chemotherapy have comprised the majority of study cohorts, although Dimeo has contributed significantly to the literature with studies of aerobic conditioning immediately following bone marrow transplantation.[66–68]

Studies in breast cancer patients receiving chemo- or radiation therapy have consistently reported improved symptom burden: fatigue,[172,173,223,225,226] insomnia,[172] nausea,[271] and emotional distress.[172,173] Trials have varied considerably in the intensity, frequency, and duration of aerobic training, as well as in the level of investigator supervision. Self-paced exercise regimens have reliably achieved modest improvements in 12-min walk time.[172,173,223,225,226] Use of more rigorous, structured programs (more than three exercise sessions per week at 60–85% of maximal heart rate) increase relative lean body mass[270] and VO_{2max}.[158] Patients who exercised five times per week at 50–60% of VO_{2max} did not achieve statistically significant improvements in oxidative capacity (VO_{2max}) over 26 weeks.[227] The lack of a training effect using an exercise intensity of 50–60% of VO_{2max} suggests the presence of an exertional threshold below which physiologic benefits are insubstantial. Variances in reported outcomes suggest a dose effect, with more intense exercise regimens producing greater intergroup differences in symptom level reduction and enhancement of physiologic parameters. The literature collectively demonstrates that, in patients receiving treatment for breast cancer, moderate levels of exercise are well tolerated and beneficial.

Aerobic conditioning reduces symptom burden and mitigates the physiologic impact of high-dose chemotherapy delivered in the context of bone marrow transplantation as well. Performance of cardiovascular cycling at 50% of heart rate reserve reduced participants' decline in physical performance (e.g. walking distance and speed), physiologic parameters, neutropenia and thrombocytopenia, and psychologic distress relative to those of control subjects.[66,68] Training on a treadmill following high-dose chemotherapy administration at an intensity set to increase blood lactate concentrations to 3 mmol/L produced similar improvements in mean blood lactate concentrations.[67] Training distances improved >100%.[67]

Except for bone marrow transplantation and breast cancer, aerobic conditioning trials have been severely limited in size and number. Fatigued patients with Hodgkin disease a mean of 6.6 years post cancer treatment were exercised at 65–80% of maximal heart rate for 40–60 min three times per week.[182] Study participants enjoyed improved maximal aerobic capacity, quality of life, maximal walking time, and fatigue. A randomized trial of home-based cardiovascular conditioning, at 65–75% of maximal heart rate, failed to demonstrate benefit in either quality of life or aerobic capacity in patients with colorectal cancer receiving adjuvant therapy.[42] Although adequately powered, this study suffered from a high contamination rate. Among the control group, 51.6% exercised during the study period. Despite the limited number of flawed trials, no harm has been associated with aerobic exercise at 75–80% of maximal heart rate. It is therefore reasonable to assume that the benefits of conditioning extend well beyond breast cancer and bone marrow transplant cohorts.

Investigations of the impact of aerobic exercise on immunologic parameters in cancer patients have produced mixed results. Short-term (2-week) aerobic training in stomach cancer patients using arm and cycle ergometers at 60% of maximal heart rate caused a mean 27.9% increase in natural killer (NK) cell activity.[179] Cardiovascular training at 60% of maximal heart rate during a 7-month intervention in breast cancer survivors similarly improved NK-cell activity without increasing NK-cell numbers.[193,194] A mixed aerobic (75% of heart rate maximum) and resistance training program failed to alter NK-cell activity among breast cancer survivors.[180] This study was inadequately powered, however, with a sample size of only six per group. The limited literature available suggests that exercise can modulate immunologic parameters. Defining the magnitude, duration, and reproducibility of the exercise effect requires further investigation, as does the clinical relevance of alterations in NK-cell parameters.

Cardiovascular, mixed, or resistance training programs have resulted in inconsistent improvement in overall quality of life, with some studies failing to note change[1,42,227] and others noting improvement.[140,228] No study has reported compromised quality of life associated with participation in exercise programs, irrespective of their intensity. The impact of exercise on quality of life does not correlate with the degree of physiologic training effect. The failure of some exercise interventions to achieve statistically significant quality of life improvements might reflect the poor sensitivity of multidimensional quality of life instruments in detecting functional change.

Resistive exercise   Two trials have evaluated the impact of resistance training in cancer populations. Cunningham reported decreased creatinine excretion without change in nitrogen balance among patients with leukemia who performed a full-body resistive exercise program at an unspecified intensity.[44] More definitive improvement was reported with resistance training among prostate cancer patients receiving androgen deprivation therapy.[228] Upper and lower extremity muscle groups were trained with two sets of 8–12 repetitions at 60–70% of one maximal repetition over a 12-week program. Postexercise assessment revealed improved quality of life, fatigue, and strength. Body composition was not affected. The exercise interventions were well tolerated without adverse effects in both resistance trials.

Rehabilitation of cardiopulmonary dysfunction   Exertional intolerance due to cardiopulmonary factors occurs commonly among cancer patients. Surgical pneumonectomy or lobectomy,

the current standard of care for management of local and regional lung cancer, abruptly reduces patients' aerobic capacity. Fibrosis of lung parenchyma, visceral pleura, and pericardium occur in virtually all patients who receive radiation to the thorax. Review of patients' radiation treatment records can be invaluable in gauging their risk of cardiopulmonary fibrosis. Many patients requiring treatment for intrathoracic tumor have smoking histories and some degree of subclinical chronic obstructive pulmonary or reactive airway disease.[250] As a consequence, resection or irradiation of lung tissue can result in far greater dyspnea and functional compromise than predicted. Chemotherapy and intrathoracic metastases can also produce cardiopulmonary dysfunction.

Rehabilitation of cardiopulmonary dysfunction in cancer patients utilizes protocols well established in cardiac and pulmonary rehabilitation (see Chs 34 and 35). Incremental aerobic conditioning with supplemental oxygen, as needed, usually produces a dramatic reduction in exertional intolerance. Similar to both cardiac and pulmonary rehabilitation, aerobic conditioning has little beneficial impact on heart or lung physiology. Improvements in stamina and perceived exertion are due to muscle-training effects.

Flexibility exercises   Activities to enhance ROM are critical for rehabilitation of postradiation soft tissue contractures. The rationale for active and passive stretching is empiric. There is anecdotal evidence that stretching prevents, mitigates, and reverses radiation-induced contractures. Interventions to enhance flexibility are integral to the rehabilitation of other conditions associated with progressive fibrosis such as burns. Flexibility activities should be optimally tailored to each patient's unique requirements. This involves determination of the radiation port and identification of all irradiated muscles. For example, tangent beams for conventional breast irradiation encompass the pectoralis major and minor muscles. Contingent on the orientation of the posterior tangent, the serratus anterior and latissimus muscle can also be affected.

Protocols for the prevention or treatment of radiation contractures have not been published or formally evaluated. Patients are generally provided with a series of active-assisted ROM activities that target all affected muscle groups, with emphasis placed on restricted planes of motion. Patients are instructed to hold each stretch for three to five deep breaths and perform the entire program at least twice per day. If soft tissue restrictions progress despite adequate compliance, the duration, frequency, and degree of active assistance should be increased. As with any restriction in soft tissue excursion, patients should be examined for secondary myofascial dysfunction, tightness in muscles outside the radiation field, and biomechanical imbalance.

Patients who receive radiation for intrapelvic cancers (e.g. bladder, prostate, colorectal, cervical, or uterine malignancies) often develop restricted flexibility of the muscles acting on the hip joint. Because they gradually adapt their gait and movement patterns to accommodate decreased muscle excursion, problems can arise latently as sacroiliac or lumbar pain. While the secondary issues must be addressed, full reversal and prevention of recurrence will not succeed until flexibility deficits have been identified and addressed.

Soft tissue fibrosis initiated can theoretically continue indefinitely.[264] This has been observed clinically in severely affected patients with slowed but continued scar formation occurring many years after completion of therapy. For this reason, soft tissue ROM activities should continue throughout the duration of patients' lives. The frequency and intensity of stretching must be continuously defined for each patient and their ROM regimen titrated accordingly. ROM activities should be initiated soon after radiation has begun. Based on animal models, applying tension to developing scar tissue produces ordered, parallel alignment of collagen fibers instead of a chaotic and disordered snarl.[85] The resultant tissue is ultimately more supple, pliable, and injury-resistant. In the interest of producing more flexible, resilient scar tissue, aggressive stretching should be emphasized during the initial 12 months post radiation. Please note that the time frames discussed in this paragraph are speculative, based on current theory and limited anecdotal experience. Research is desperately needed to inform and refine postradiation rehabilitation.

Comprehensive inpatient rehabilitation

The appropriateness and potential benefits of comprehensive inpatient rehabilitation must be assessed on a case by case basis. Cancer patients' candidacy is generally deemed appropriate when their deficits conform to a neurologic or musculoskeletal syndrome familiar in the inpatient rehabilitation setting, i.e. hemiparesis, paraplegia, or amputation. Several studies have reported equal functional independence measure (FIM) efficacies when patients with malignant SCC are compared with patients with similar but traumatically and ischemically induced impairments. Patients with malignant SCC achieve less functional improvement but, due to shorter lengths of stay, have comparable FIM efficiencies relative to patients with traumatic spinal cord injury.[164] Home discharge rates are equal, 84% in a retrospective case series,[163] or higher among patients with malignant SCC.

Retrospective case series of patients transferred to rehabilitation following treatment for primary brain tumors and intracranial metastases describe substantial gains in cognitive ADL and mobility domains.[120,160] The functional gains achieved by brain tumor patients are similar to those of patients with acute stroke[119] and traumatic brain injury.[121,181] Patients with brain tumors are consistently discharged to the community >80% of the time,[121] and have significantly shorter lengths of stay.[119,181] Studies have differed on the impact of concurrent radiation therapy. Some describe greater FIM mobility efficiencies with radiation, while others report the opposite.[181]

Lymphedema management

Lymphedema is a chronic and currently incurable condition that frequently complicates cancer therapy. Following resection or irradiation of lymph nodes and vessels, lymphatic congestion can develop in any region of the body drained by the affected structures. If congestion becomes sufficiently severe, swelling can result due to accumulation of protein-rich fluid.[269] Far from being a treatment-refractory and inexorably progressive condition, lymphedema is now amenable to highly effective and widely available therapy. Complete (or complex) decongestive therapy (CDT) represents the current international standard of care for lymphedema management.[17] This was formalized in a white paper published by the International Society of Lymphology in 2001.[17] CDT, an intensive integration of manual approaches, is able to achieve and maintain substantial volume reduction for the majority of lymphedema patients. Surgical, dietary, and pharmacologic approaches offer equivocal benefit at best, but can be considered when appropriate manual and compression therapy fail to adequately reduce lymphedema.[249]

Complete decongestive therapy is a two-phase multimodal system that incorporates manual lymphatic drainage (MLD), short-stretch compressive bandaging, skin care, therapeutic exercise, and elastic compression garments. The initial phase, sometimes designated with a Roman numeral I or described by the term *reductive*, has as its primary goal decreasing lymphedema volume.[78] During daily phase I CDT sessions, patients receive approximately 45 min of MLD, followed by the application of compression bandages and performance of remedial exercises. Compressive bandages are left in place 21–24 h per day. The efficacy of treatment delivered at this intensity has been demonstrated in numerous case series.[79,139,163,176] Figure 58-4 shows pre- and post-CDT images in a patient with bilateral stage 3 lymphedema. Following maximal volume reduction, patients are gradually transitioned to a long-term maintenance program (phase II). In this phase, compressive garments are used during the day, with application of compressive bandages overnight. Patients perform remedial exercises on a daily basis while bandaged, and receive MLD as needed.

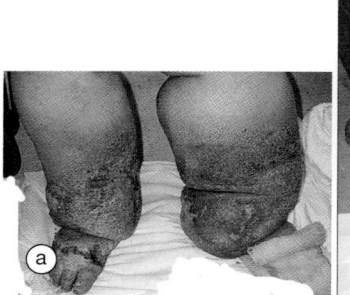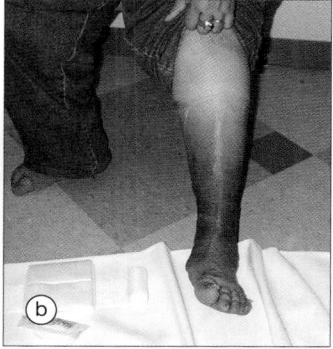

Figure 58-4 Lower extremity lymphedema (**a**) before and (**b**) after complete decongestive therapy, which afforded dramatic volume reduction.

Compression forms the basis of virtually all successful lymphedema therapy. During CDT phases I and II, compression is achieved through the use of short-stretch bandages. Short-stretch bandages have a high working pressure and exert force when the underlying muscles contract.[187,188,242] The bandages exert low pressure while the muscles are resting. A distal to proximal compression gradient is achieved by applying more layers of bandages distally, rather than varying the amount of tension used to apply the bandages. Compression garments are essential during phase II in order to achieve the following:

- improve lymphatic flow and reduce accumulated protein;
- improve venous return;
- properly shape and reduce the size of the limb;
- maintain skin integrity; and
- protect the limb from potential trauma.[30]

Manual lymphatic drainage or 'lymphatic massage' is a highly specialized technique designed to enhance the sequestration and transport of lymph. Specific stroke duration, orientation, pressure, and sequence characterize MLD. MLD stimulates the intrinsic contractility of the lymph vessels, leading to increased interstitial protein rem.[31] Through gentle and rhythmic skin distention, congested lymph is directed through residual lymph vessels into intact nodal basins. MLD permits shifting of congested lymph to lymphotomes (anatomic regions drained by a specific lymph node bed with preserved drainage, as illustrated in Fig. 58-5). The massage is very light and superficial, limited to finger or hand pressures of around 30–45 mmHg. MLD treatments are initiated proximally in lymphostatic regions adjacent to functioning lymphotomes. Lymph is constantly directed toward functional lymph node basins with strategic hand movement, as the treatment gradually progresses distally to terminate in the regions farthest removed from intact lymphatics.

Remedial lymphedema exercises refer to a very specific group of repetitive movements designed to encourage rhythmic, serial muscle contractions in the territory affected by lymphedema. Remedial exercises are always performed with external compression, most commonly compressive garments or bandages. Remedial exercises repeatedly compress the lymph vessels through sequential muscle contraction and relaxation. This triggers smooth muscle contraction within the walls of lymph transport vessels.[184] When external compression is adequate, an internal pumping mechanism is established that encourages congested lymph to flow along a compression gradient.[149,150]

Skin care is stressed in manual approaches to lymphedema. The goals of skin care include controlling dermal colonization by bacteria and fungi, eliminating bacterial and fungal overgrowth in skin crevices, and hydrating the skin to control dryness and eliminate cracking. Daily cleansing with mineral oil-based soap will remove debris and bacteria while moisturizing the skin.[29]

The current shortage of adequately trained and experienced lymphedema therapists in the USA is a consistent impediment

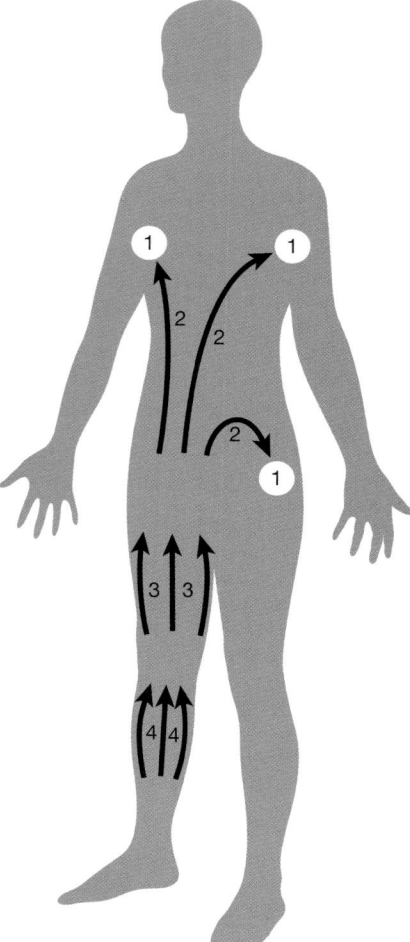

Figure 58-5 Manual lymphatic drainage sequence in the treatment of right lower limb lymphedema due to inguinal lymph node dissection: 1, stimulate intact lymph node beds where the stagnant lymph will be directed; 2, clear the pathways that will be used to redirect stagnant lymph into functioning lymphotomes; 3, direct stagnant lymph proximally along the cleared pathways, working backward into the congested territory; 4, complete treatment with proximal redirection of lymph from the most distal portions of the lymphedematous territory.

to successful decongestion. The Lymphology Association of North America (LANA) has developed a certification examination to identify therapists with the requisite knowledge and manual skill to treat lymphedema. A list of certified therapists is available through the LANA web site (http://www.cltlana.org). The National Lymphedema Network (http://www.lymphnet.org) offers an extensive list of lymphedema-related resources. Patients with lymphedema complicated by aggressive recurrent cancer, dermal metastases, chemotherapeutic neuropathies, or pain will require specialized care generally available only at tertiary medical and cancer centers.

Augmentative and compensatory strategies

Cancer-related impairments often render necessary daily activities challenging or impossible. The application of conventional rehabilitation paradigms for the development of alternative and compensatory strategies allows patients to remain functionally autonomous. Use of assistive devices for mobility and ADL performance might be necessary. Environmental modification and augmentative communication devices should be explored

Table 58-7 Time course of shoulder mobilization

Postoperative day	Flexion	Abduction	Internal or external rotation
1 through 3	40–45°	40–45°	To tolerance
4 through 6	45–90°	45°	To tolerance
7 onward	To tolerance	To tolerance	To tolerance

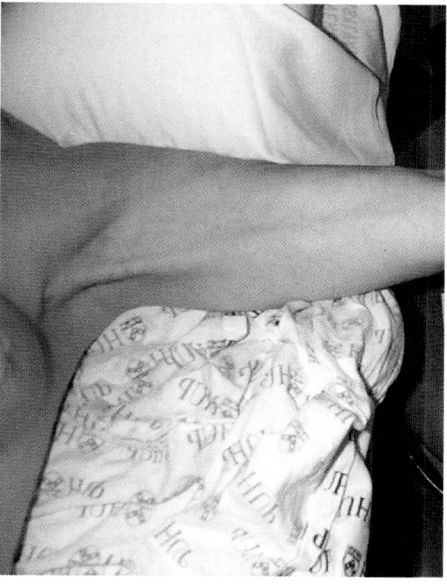

Figure 58-6 Axillary web syndrome manifest by thick, fibrous cords tethering the arm.

in appropriate cases. Pacing strategies become essential for patients receiving intensive anticancer therapy, or with advanced disease. The appropriateness and cost–benefit ratio of interventions must be determined on a case by case basis.

Rehabilitation of specific cancer populations
Breast cancer
Functional impairments unique to breast cancer patients develop after surgical procedures to achieve local tumor control, or for breast reconstruction. These procedures include modified radical mastectomy (MRM), lumpectomy, and axillary lymph node dissection (ALND), and autogenous tissue transposition for reconstruction.

Deficits in shoulder ROM occur with an uncharacterized incidence following ALND. Gerber et al. reported that vigorous shoulder mobilization in the immediate postoperative period led to an increase in seroma formation.[157] The time line for shoulder mobilization presented in Table 58-7 adequately restored shoulder mobility without increasing the incidence of postsurgical complications. MRM and ALND are performed as same-day procedures at some institutions. In such cases, a gradual, supervised, and progressive ROM program is not possible. The most common alternative is providing patients with illustrated exercise sheets that typically include 'wall walking', forward flexion assisted by the unaffected arm, shoulder rolls, etc. Whether the absence of formal post-MRM and post-ALND therapy has long-term consequences remains undetermined. For patients who have undergone immediate breast reconstruction, particularly the TRAM flap procedure, shoulder mobilization should be reviewed with the plastic surgeon unless an institutional algorithm has been formulated.

Axillary web syndrome (Fig. 58-6) refers to the presence of taut, palpable cords originating in the axilla and extending distally along the anterior surface of the arm, often below the elbow.[177] The tissues compromising of the cords remain uncertain. A limited case series subjected resected cords to pathologic assessment. The specimen contained either lymphatic vessels or veins and surrounding connective tissue.[177] The clinical relevance of axillary web syndrome arises from the potential for restricted shoulder ROM. In severe cases, the cords tether the humerus, preventing full shoulder flexion or abduction. Pain generally responds to NSAIDs. Opioid analgesics might be necessary during passive and active assisted ROM if the pain is severe. Therapy involves incremental ROM activities, topical

heat, manipulation to soften and potentially 'pop' the cords, and provision with a home exercise program. Heat should be used briefly, given the risk of lymphedema and the almost universal presence of intercostal brachial neuropathy in the axilla and upper arm.

The surgical community has increasingly recognized the need for rehabilitation following TRAM flap breast reconstruction. The procedure denervates and disrupts the integrity of the abdominal wall, producing significant deficits in truncal stability, particularly during functional transfers. The goals of post-TRAM rehabilitation are to prevent subdermal fibrosis and adhesions, restore truncal alignment, minimize stress on the lumbar spine, optimize proprioceptive acuity in residual abdominal muscles, and encourage normal muscle recruitment patterns. The algorithm for post-TRAM flap rehabilitation (Table 58-8) was well tolerated and obviated lasting impairment in a cohort of 52 patients.[93] No patients developed donor site herniation or wound dehiscence.

Head and neck cancer
Combined modality therapy for head and neck cancer has afforded improved cure rates and reduced normal tissue compromise. The type and sequence of therapies used to treat head and neck cancer vary by the location of the primary tumor, the extent of cervical lymph node involvement, and the pathologic characteristics of the tumor. Increasingly, treatment approaches reflect a trend toward organ preservation. For example, the emphasis on 'normal' tissue preservation has led to the substitution of supracrichoid partial laryngectomy for total laryngectomy, and of functional neck dissection for radical neck dissection.

Treatment of head and neck cancer continues to produce some of the most challenging impairments within the scope of cancer rehabilitation. Many of the impairments directly undermine patients' ability to socialize, because of facial

Table 58-8 Post-TRAM procedure rehabilitation program

Weeks	Activities
0–3	Patient education: 　lymphedema precautions 　body mechanics 　back safety 　(Driving permitted 3–4 weeks)
3–5	Active upper extremity range of motion (to tolerance): 　supine forward flexion with wand 　supine external rotation with wand 　standing abduction, wall walking Postural body mechanics: 　shoulder retraction—active with mirror cues 　upright standing 　head up or chin tucks Manual techniques p.r.n.: 　manual lymphatic drainage 　scar mobilization (if healed) 　gentle myofascial release if restrictions are notable Walking program if needed
6–7	Postural body mechanics 　shoulder retraction—active with mirror cues 　pectoral stretch (corner stretch) 　if good alignment with retraction, may initiate 　　resistive theraband at yellow level for shoulder 　　retraction 　upright standing posture—posterior pelvic tilt in 　　supine
8–12	Stabilization or strengthening exercises 　prone lying 　isometric pelvic or lumbar stabilization (in supine) 　Lumbar extensor strengthening or stabilization 　abdominal or oblique stabilization or strengthening Physioball activities Aerobic exercise 　biking 　treadmill Manual techniques 　manual scar mobilization 　myofascial release

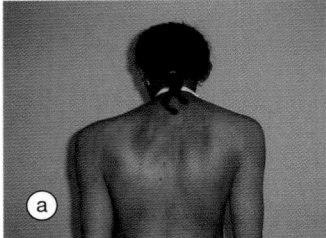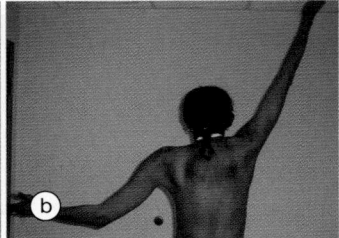

Figure 58-7 (**a**) Resting posture of a head and neck cancer patient with a complete spinal accessory nerve palsy. (**b**) Active shoulder abduction is limited to 90° on the affected side, due to middle trapezius muscle weakness.

dysmorphism, loss of spontaneous or intelligible speech, and the inability to eat normally. Common rehabilitation problems include spinal accessory nerve palsy, radiation-induced xerostomia, soft tissue contracture of the neck and anterior chest wall, dysphagia, dysphonia, and myofascial dysfunction. The type and severity of impairments evolves over the course of cancer treatment and recovery. Rehabilitative interventions must be adjusted accordingly. This chapter will address the common problems that occur uniquely in the context of head and neck cancer: spinal accessory nerve palsy, cervical soft tissue contracture, and dysphonia.

Spinal accessory nerve palsy

The recognition that comparable cure rates can be achieved with more conservative surgical resection has spurred the shift from radical to functional neck dissections. The former proce-

dure removes the sternocleidomastoid muscle, the spinal accessory nerve, and the external jugular vein. The nerve to the levator scapulae muscle was also frequently resected, producing severe ipsilateral shoulder dysfunction. Functional neck dissections preserve all structures that can be safely left intact, producing dramatically lower rates of postoperative shoulder morbidity. Many head and neck cancer patients now emerge from surgery with partial to no spinal accessory nerve compromise. The integrity of the spinal accessory nerve can be easily assessed by side to side comparison of resisted end-range forward flexion of the shoulder. Some degree of weakness can be elicited in most patients on the side of the neck dissection.

The severity and distribution of trapezius weakness secondary to spinal accessory nerve palsy (Fig. 58-7) is subject to great interindividual variability. The upper, middle, and lower trapezius muscles can be innervated solely by the spinal accessory nerve or receive partial or total innervation from the cervical plexus.[23] When the spinal accessory nerve was routinely sacrificed during radical neck dissections, some patients developed little to no shoulder compromise, suggesting that innervation was predominantly derived from the cervical plexus. Baseline anatomic variability is compounded by inconsistency in the type and degree of intraoperative nerve injury. The spinal accessory nerve may be entirely spared or subject to neurapraxic, axonotmetic, or neurotmetic insult, all with different rates and degrees of recovery. Additionally, electrocautery of blood vessels can undermine blood supply to the vasonervorum, producing ischemic injury.

The timing and intensity of rehabilitation should be guided by patients' prognosis for recovery. Frequent reevaluation is essential. Spinal accessory nerve reinnervation can continue over 12 months following surgery. Important elements of spinal accessory nerve rehabilitation include:

- prevention of frozen shoulder through active ROM and active-assisted ROM;
- prevention of anterior chest wall flexibility deficits;
- strengthening of alternate scapular elevators and retractors;
- instruction in compensatory techniques for activities requiring sustained shoulder abduction and forward flexion;
- neuromuscular retraining;

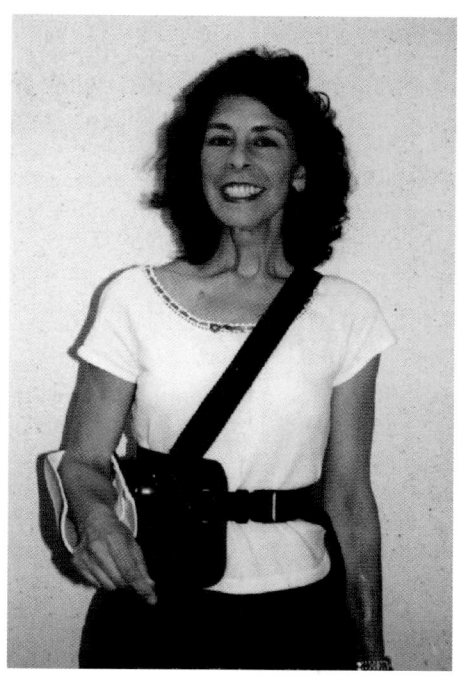

Figure 58-8 'Shelf' orthosis fabricated to encircle the torso of patients with complete spinal accessory nerve palsies and to provide a ledge on which they can rest their affected extremities when not in use.

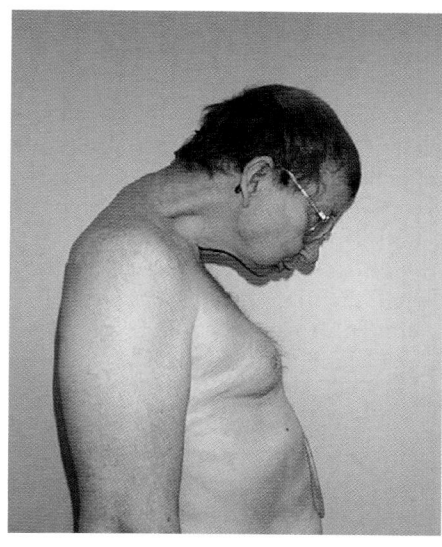

Figure 58-9 Head-forward posture and exaggerated thoracic kyphosis, associated with radiation-induced soft tissue contracture, in a head and neck cancer patient.

- preservation of trapezius muscle tone through electrical stimulation if reinnervation is anticipated;
- postural modification; and
- instruction in shoulder support to allow recovery of the levator scapulae.

The intensity and structure of rehabilitation should by constantly informed by the rate of reinnervation. Patients with a complete, persistent spinal accessory nerve palsy can be fitted with an orthosis. To date, none of the braces designed to substitute for an absent or weak upper trapezius muscle have enjoyed widespread success. The relevant literature does not extend beyond very limited case reports. For patients plagued by levator scapulae fatigue and spasms, a 'shelf' orthosis (Fig. 58-8) designed to encircle the waist, and to provide a ledge on which patients can rest their affected arms when not is use, reduces symptoms.

Cervical contracture

Progressive fibrosis of the anterior and lateral cervical soft tissue may be highly problematic for head and neck cancer patients, particularly those who receive external beam radiation. A general approach to radiation-induced fibrosis was outlined previously in this chapter. Because of the high radiation doses delivered to some head and neck cancer patients, proactive ROM in all planes of neck motion should be initiated as soon as safely possible. Cervical ROM can continue throughout radiation therapy in the absence of significant skin breakdown. After surgery, the delicate balance between flexibility and wound healing must be respected. Surgeons should be consulted regarding the length of the postoperative interval before ROM can begin. For an uncomplicated radical or functional

neck dissection, 3 days is generally considered safe. Reconstruction with tissue transposition requires a longer recovery period. ROM activities should be delayed until all drains are removed to avoid seroma formation.

Irradiated patients should perform ROM activities twice daily during the first 2 years following cancer treatment and daily thereafter. As previously mentioned, radiation-induced fibrosis can be indefinitely progressive. Figure 58-9 demonstrates the head-forward posture and thoracic kyphosis characteristic of head and neck cancer patients with severe anterior cervical soft tissue fibrosis. For optimal results, patients should be taught to provide additional stretch during end-range lateral bending or rotation by exerting additional pressure with the contralateral hand. Stretches should be held for five deep breaths and repeated between 5 and 10 times per session. Isometric strengthening of the cervical extensors, and postural modification with visual cuing, is beneficial.

Manual fibrous release techniques are indicated when ROM is restricted by robust soft tissue fibrosis or tethering of the skin to subdermal tissues. Patients can be taught self-massage to augment the efficacy of ROM activities. Compression of severely fibrotic areas breaks down established scar tissue and inhibits re-formation. Compression garments, either off the shelf or customized, are a convenient means of applying compression. Custom-cut foam pieces strategically inserted can achieve greater focal pressure on stubborn areas. Constant vigilance must be maintained to ensure that friable, irradiated skin is not compromised.

Aphonia and dysphonia

Impaired vocal communication occurs in the majority of head and neck cancer patients at some point during treatment. Many conditions other than total laryngectomy can compromise phonation. These include radiation-induced laryngeal or pharyngeal swelling and fibrosis, tracheostomy, partial or total glossectomy, reduced oral excursion secondary to trismus, copious secretions, and neurogenic pharyngeal or laryngeal paralysis. Some patients are rendered acutely voiceless after surgery. Such acute loss occurs most dramatically after total laryngectomy but is also frequent after tracheostomy and glossectomy. Gradual compromise of vocal precision, endurance, and volume is more common with organ preservation therapies. Irrespective of the acuity of onset, loss of spontaneous, intelligible speech can be profoundly isolating. It renders patients dependent in communication and can be vocationally devastating.

Various approaches to restore communication are utilized depending on the anticipated duration, severity, and nature of the deficit. The most common compensatory strategies used by acutely voiceless adults include mouthing words, gestures, writing, and head nods.[8,107] Patients rendered chronically aphonic by total laryngectomy can communicate through esophageal speech, tracheoesophageal speech, or use of an electrolarynx. The frequency with which these options are offered to and accepted by patients varies considerably across physician practices, institutions, and geographic regions.[167] The following frequencies for different types of alaryngeal speech have been reported: esophageal speech, 1–32%; tracheoesophageal speech, 20–45%; electrolarynx, 0–50%; and non-vocal, 17–26% (see Chapter 3).[91,114,167,237]

Esophageal and tracheoesophageal speech utilize the oropharynx, lips, and tongue to produce intelligible sound. Esophageal speech is time-consuming and difficult to learn. Among a cohort of laryngectomized esophageal speakers, a subjectively 'good enough' result was achieved by 41% in <6 months, by 20% in 6–12 months, and by 10% in >12 months.[275] Despite the challenges of mastery, tracheoesophageal puncture, or the TEP procedure, represents an increasingly common approach to voice restoration. The TEP procedure creates a stoma between the trachea and esophagus. A one-way valved prosthesis is inserted in the stoma, allowing pulmonary air to enter the esophageal reservoir when patients manually occlude their tracheostomies. Although guttural, the resultant speech can be exceedingly intelligible, with natural-sounding inflection. When compared with other types of alaryngeal speech, TEP speakers most closely approximate the frequency and intensity of the normal voice.[114] In two surveys, TEP speech received higher satisfaction ratings than alternative methods, particularly with telephone use.[38,275]

Despite the growing popularity of TEP, alaryngeal speech is most often accomplished through use of an electrolarynx. Many head and neck cancer patients who fail to achieve intelligible esophageal speech eventually opt for an artificial larynx. The currently marketed devices vary with respect to placement of the transducer. Some sense vibrations within the oral cavity, while others are placed on the submental or buccal skin. Training is essential to the achievement of acceptable voice quality. Various transducers should be trialed, because patients' preferences vary. A significant downside of electrolaryngeal speech is its mechanical and monotonic quality.

Additional concerns

Head and neck cancer patients, by virtue of their treatment and premorbid risk profile, are prone to the development of osteoradionecrosis, dental caries, and recurrent substance abuse.

Comprehensive rehabilitation involves proactive screening for these conditions. Because of the high radiation doses delivered in head and neck cancer treatment, 5–15% of these patients develop osteoradionecrosis, an extremely painful condition caused by radiation-induced bone death. The mandible is most often affected. Patients complain of relentless jaw pain aggravated by chewing and vocalization. Associated pain should be aggressively treated with combined opioids and NSAIDs.

PRECAUTIONS IN CANCER REHABILITATION

Modalities

A climate of exaggerated caution too often limits cancer rehabilitation. Specific therapeutic precautions reflect a fear of injuring patients, or worse, spreading their cancer. While it is important to appreciate that cancer patients are predisposed to a host of adverse complications (e.g. hemorrhage and disease recurrence), it is equally important to recognize that a causal relationship has not been established between such complications and physiatric interventions. Inactivity causes far greater long-term difficulty for the majority of cancer patients. Most precautions are not supported by empiric data. Often, they reinforce ambivalence toward structured, incremental physical activity.

Warnings against treating cancer patients with deep heat and massage are ubiquitous in the rehabilitation literature. Precautions regarding heating modalities are based on the concern that heat will dilate local blood vessels and increase metabolic activity in tumor cells, thereby hastening local or systemic spread. Similarly, massage is presumed to potentiate metastasis by encouraging blood and lymph flow, or by dislodging tumor cells. This line of purely theoretic reasoning is simplistic and at odds with several facts. First, exercise does more to promote blood and lymph flow than localized heating modalities. Evidence suggests that exercise has a protective effect, if anything, against cancer recurrence. Second, thousands of cancer patients have received MLD to deliberately stimulate lymph flow in order to decongest their lymphedema. Many of these patients have had known cancer at the treatment site. So far, no association has been established between lymphedema or its treatment and cancer progression. Lastly, complex molecular events have been implicated by a vast body of basic science research as being requisite for tumor cells to develop metastatic potential. Tumor cells must acquire the ability to penetrate basement membranes, adhere to endothelial cells, and stimulate angiogenesis once they reach a distant site, among many other genetically determined attributes. Relative to these complex changes, being manually dislodged from a tumor mass or transiently exposed to increased blood flow probably has little if any impact on a tumor cell.

Challenging precautions against the use of heating modalities in cancer may be moot. Deep heat is rarely of clinical utility, or therapeutic goals can be realized by alternative means. However, if the clinical context warrants a trial of ultrasound or related modalities, the option should not be reflexively abandoned because of unsubstantiated warnings. In the author's experience, patients with widespread tumor have benefited from the discrete use of ultrasound in areas of dense radiation-induced fibrosis and postsurgical scarring. Massage has the potential to greatly benefit cancer patients through its antispasmodic, fibrolytic, and counterstimulatory effects. Additionally, MLD is an integral part of lymphedema management. Aside from vigorous massage in the immediate vicinity of established tumor, massage is likely to be of far greater benefit than harm.

Cytopenias

Leukopenia and thrombocytopenia commonly occur following the administration of chemotherapy. The duration and severity of cytopenias have been considerably reduced through the introduction of CSFs that accelerate bone marrow recovery.[63] In cancer patients receiving initial chemotherapy who are not pretreated with CSFs, leukopenia and thrombocytopenia can be detected on the ninth or tenth day after chemotherapy administration. Nadir blood counts occur between days 14 and 18, with recovery beginning by day 21.[63] The time course of bone marrow recovery dictates the widely used 3- to 4-week chemotherapy cycle, with new cycles being initiated 21–28 days after administration of the previous chemotherapy dose.

There are inconsistent guidelines limiting physical activity in the face of chemotherapy-induced cytopenias. Existing precautions are arbitrary and lack empiric testing. None have been shown to limit adverse events. Leukopenia is of less concern than thrombocytopenia, given the associated risk of intracranial hemorrhage or uncontrolled bleeding after a fall. Among National Cancer Institute-designated comprehensive cancer centers, cutoff platelet counts below which physical therapy is contraindicated range from 25 000 to no lower limit. No differences between institutions in the incidence of spontaneous hemorrhage have been reported. Patients undergoing allo- and autogeneic bone marrow transplants typically spend 7–21 days with platelet counts of 5000–12 000. During this interval, most patients perform all ADL independently, ambulate, transfer, and lift >10 lbs repeatedly without hemorrhage. When spontaneous bleeding does occur, it is typically not associated with physical activity. Given the routinely well-tolerated levels of physical activity in severely thrombocytopenic patients, reconsideration of current precautions is warranted. Overzealous imposition of restrictions on physical therapy and exercise in this population can lead to rapid deconditioning, bone demineralization, and formation of contractures.

CONCLUSION

Cancer rehabilitation is a varied and challenging field of increasing public health importance. An accruing evidence base suggests that conventional rehabilitative interventions succeed in preserving and restoring the functional status of cancer patients. A marked lack of hypothesis-driven research continues to limit the field, as does a lack of experienced and interested clinicians. It is hoped that these deficits will be remedied given the projections for steadily increasing cancer survivorship.

REFERENCES

1. Abramsen L, Midtgaard J, Rorth M, et al. Feasibility, physical capacity, and health benefits of a multidimensional exercise program for cancer patients undergoing chemotherapy. Support Care Cancer 2003; 11:707–716.
2. Agency for Health Care Policy and Research, Acute Pain Management Panel. Acute pain management: operative or medical procedures and trauma. Washington: US Department of Health and Human Services; 1992.
3. Alamowitch S, Graus F, Uchuya M, et al. Limbic encephalitis and small cell lung cancer. Clinical and immunological features. Brain 1997; 120:923–928.
4. American Cancer Society, ed. ACLS: cancer facts and figures. Atlanta: ACS; 2004:1–56.
5. American Pain Society. Principles of analgesic use in the treatment of acute pain and cancer pain. 4th edn. Glenview: APS; 1999.
6. Ampil FL. Radiotherapy for carcinomatous brachial plexopathy. Cancer 1985; 56:2185–2188.
7. Ashenhurst EM, Quartey GR, Starreveld A. Lumbo-sacral radiculopathy induced by radiation. Can J Neurol Sci 1977; 4:259–263.
8. Ashworth P. Staff–patient communication in coronary care units. J Adv Nurs 1984; 9:35–42.
9. Augsburger JJ. Differential diagnosis of choroidal neoplams. Oncology (Huntingt) 1991; 5:87–98.
10. Aurelius E, Johansson B, Skoldenberg B, et al. Rapid diagnosis of herpes simplex encephalitis by nested polymerase chair reaction assay of cerebrospinal fluid. Lancet 1991; 337:189–192.
11. Baldwin BJ, Shusterman MA, Miller MJ, et al. Bilateral breast reconstruction: conventional versus free TRAM. Plast Reconstr Surg 1994; 93(7):1410–1416.
12. Barrett-Lee PJ, Bailey NP, O'Brien ME, et al. Large scale UK audit of blood transfusion requirements and anemia in patients receiving cytotoxic chemotherapy. Br J Cancer 2000; 82:93–97.
13. Barron KD, Hirano A, Araski R, et al. Experiences with metastatic neoplasms involving the spinal cord. Neurology 1959; 9:90–106.
14. Barron KD, Rowland IP, Zimmerman HM. Neuropathy with malignant tumor metastases. J Nerv Ment Dis 1960; 131:10–31.
15. Bataller L, Graus F, Saiz A, et al. Clinical outcome in adult onset idiopathic or paraneoplastic opsoclonus-myoclonus. Brain 2001; 124:437–443.
16. Berger AM, Koprowski C. Bone pain: assessment and management. In: Berger AM, ed. Supportive oncology, part A. 2nd edn. Philadelphia: Lippincott Williams & Wilkins; 2002:53–67.
17. Bernas MJ, Witte CL, Witte MH. The diagnosis and treatment of peripheral lymphedema: draft revision of the 1995 Consensus Document of the International Society of Lymphology Executive Committee for discussion at the September 3–7, 2001, SVII International Congress of Lymphology in Genoa, Italy. International Society of Lymphology Executive. Lymphology 2001; 34:84–91.
18. Bernat JL, Greenberg ER, Barrett J. Suspected epidural compression of the spinal cord and cauda equina by metastatic carcinoma. Clinical diagnosis and survival. Cancer 1983; 51(10):1953–1957.
19. Blum RH, Carter SK, Agre K. Bleomycin—a new antineoplastic agent. Cancer 1973; 31:903.
20. Boccardo M, Ruelle A, Mariotti E, et al. Spinal carcinomatous metastases. Retrospective study of 67 surgically treated cases. J Neuro Oncol 1985; 3251–3257.
21. Bradley WG, Lassman LP, Pearce GW, et al. The neuromyopathy of vincristine in man: clinical, electrophysiological and pathological studies. J Neurol Sci 1970; 10:107–131.
22. Brennan KM, Roos MS, Budinger TF, et al. A study of radiation necrosis and edema in the canine brain using positron emission tomography and magnetic resonance imaging. Radiat Res 1993; 134:43–53.
23. Brown H. Anatomy of the spinal accessory nerve plexus: relevance to head and neck cancer and atherosclerosis. Exp Biol Med 2002; 227:570–578.
24. Bruera E, Roca E, Cedaro L, et al. Action of oral methylprednisolone in terminal cancer patients: a prospective randomized double-blind study. Cancer Treat Rev 1985; 69:751–754.
25. Burt ME, Aoki TT, Gorschboth CM, et al. Peripheral tissue metabolism in cancer-bearing man. Ann Surg 1983; 198:685–691.

26. Cairncross JG, Kim H-H, Posner JB. Radiation therapy for brain metastases. Ann Neurol 1980; 7:529–541.

27. Caraceni A, Portenoy RK. An international survey of cancer pain characteristics and syndromes. Pain 1999; 82:263–274.

28. Carla CP, Verstappen JJ, Heimans KH, et al. Neurotoxic complications of chemotherapy in patients with cancer. Drugs 2003; 63:1549–1563.

29. Casley-Smith JR, Boris M, Weindorf S, et al. Treatment for lymphedema of the arm—the Casley-Smith method. Cancer 1998; 83(12 suppl American):2843–2860.

30. Casley-Smith JR. Modern treatment of lymphedema. 1997.

31. Casley-Smith JR. The pathophysiology of lymphedema and the action of benzo-pyrones in reducing it. Lymphology 1988; 21(3):125–130.

32. Cella D, Peterman A, Passik S. Progress toward guidelines for the management of fatigue. Oncology 1998; 12:1–9.

33. Cella D. Factors influencing QOL in cancer patients: anaemia and fatigue. Semin Oncol 1998; 25:43–46.

34. Chalk CH, Murray NM, Newsom-Davis J, et al. Response of the Lambert–Eaton myasthenic syndrome to treatment of associated small-cell lung carcinoma. Neurology 1990; 40:1552–1556.

35. Cherny NI. Cancer pain: principles of assessment and syndromes. In: Berger AM, ed. Supportive oncology, part A. 2nd edn. Philadelphia: Lippincott Williams & Wilkins; 2002:3–52.

36. Cheville A. Pain management in cancer rehabilitation. Arch Phys Med Rehabil 2001; 82:S84–S87.

37. Christy WC, Powell DL. Knee pain exacerbated by recumbency: an unusual manifestation of spinal cord involvement by diffuse histiocytic lymphoma. Arthritis Rheum 1984; 27:341–343.

38. Clements K, Rassekh C, Seikaly H, et al. Communications after laryngectomy: an assessment of patient satisfaction. Otolaryngol Head Neck Surg 1997; 123:493–496.

39. Conte PF, Latreille J, Mauriac L, et al. Delay in progression of bone metastases in breast cancer patients treated with intravenous pamidronate: results from a multinational randomized controlled trial. Eur J Cancer 1996; 14:2552–2559.

40. Costigan DA, Winkelman MD. Intramedullary spinal cord metastasis. A clinicopathological study of 13 cases. J Neurosurg 1985; 62:227–233.

41. Coukell AJ, Markham A. Pamidronate. A review of its use in the management of osteolytic bone metastases, tumour-induced hypercalcaemia and Paget's disease of bone. Drugs Aging 1998; 12:149–168.

42. Courneya KS, Friedenreich CM, Quinney HA, et al. A randomized trial of exercise and quality of life in colorectal cancer survivors. Eur J Cancer Care 2003; 12:347–357.

43. Crotty E, Patz EF Jr. FDG-PET imaging in patients with paraneoplastic syndromes and suspected small cell lung cancer. J Thorac Imaging 2001; 16:89–93.

44. Cunningham AJ, Morris G, Cheney CL. Effects of resistance exercise on skeletal muscle in marrow transplant recipients receiving total parental nutrition. JPEN J Parenter Enteral Nutr 1986; 10:558–563.

45. Curt GA, Breibart W, Cella D. Impact of cancer-related fatigue on the lives of patients: new findings from the Fatigue Coalition. Oncologist 2000; 5:353–360.

46. Dalmau JO, Graus F, Marco M. 'Hot and dry foot' as initial manifestation of neoplastic lumbosacral plexopanty. Neurology 1989; 39:871–872.

47. Davidson RS, Nwogu CE, Brentjens MJ, et al. The surgical management of pulmonary metastasis: current concepts. Surg Oncol 2001; 10:35–42.

48. DeAngelis LM, Gnecco C, Taylor L, et al. Evolution of neuropathy and myopathy during intensive vincristine/corticosteriod chemotherapy for non-Hodgkin's lymphoma. Cancer 1991; 67:2241–2246.

49. DeAngelsis LM, Delattre J-Y, Posner JB. Radiation-induced dementia in patients cured of brain metastases. Neurology 1989; 39:789–796.

50. Delanian S, Porcher R, Balla-Mekias S, et al. Randomized, placebo-controlled trial of combined pentoxifylline and tocopherol for regression of superficial radiation-induced fibrosis. J Clin Oncol 2003; 21:2545–2550.

51. Delattre Y-Y, et al. Cerebral necrosis following neutron radiation of an extracranial tumor. J Neurooncol 1988; 6:113–117.

52. DeVine JW, Mendenhall WM, Million RR, et al. Carcinoma of the superior pulmonary sulcus treated with surgery and/or radiation therapy. Cancer 1986; 57:941–943.

53. DeVita CH, O'Dwyer PJ, Johnson SW, et al. Cisplatin and its analogues. In: Cancer: principles and practice of oncology. 5th edn. Philadelphia: Lippincott Williams & Wilkins; 1997:418–432.

54. DeVita VT, Barlogie B, Drewinko B, et al. Pulse cytophometric analysis of cell cycle perturbatin with bleomycin in vitro. Cancer Res 1976; 36:1182.

55. DeVita VT, Blum RH, Carter SK, et al. Bleomycin—a new antineoplastic agent. Cancer 1973; 31:903.

56. DeVita VT, Cheson BD. Miscellaneous chemotherapeutic agents. In: Cancer: principles and practice of oncology. 5th edn. Philadelphia: Lippincott Williams & Wilkins; 1997:490–498.

57. DeVita VT, Pavinen LM, Kikku P, et al. Factors affecting the pulmonary toxicity of bleomycin. Acta Radiol 1983; 22:417.

58. DeVita VT, Plunkett W, Gandhi V. Cellular metabolism of nucleoside analogs in CLL: implications for drug development. 1993; 197:490.

59. DeVita VT, Robertson LE, Chubb S, et al. Induction of apoptotic cell death in chronic lymphocytic leukemia by 2-chloro-2-deoxyadenosine and 9-beta-D-arabinosyl fluoradenine. Blood 1993; 81:143.

60. DeVita VT, Rowinsky EK, Donehower RC. Antimicrotubule agents. In: Cancer: principles and practice of oncology. 5th edn. Philadelphia: Lippincott Williams & Wilkins; 1997:467–483.

61. DeVita VT, Stewart CF, Ratain MJ. Topoisomerase interactive agents. In: Cancer: principles and practice of oncology. 5th edn. Philadelphia: Lippincott Williams & Wilkins; 1997:452–467.

62. DeVita VT, Teicher BA. Antitumor alkylating agents. In: Cancer: principles and practice of oncology. 5th edn. Philadelphia: Lippincott Williams & Wilkins; 1997:405–418.

63. DeVita VT. Principles of cancer management chemotherapy. In: Cancer: principles and practice of oncology. 5th edn. Philadelphia: Lippincott Williams & Wilkins; 1997:333–347.

64. DiChiro G, Oldfield E, Wright DC, et al. Cerebral necrosis after radiotherapy and/or intracranial chemotherapy for brain tumors: PET and neuropathologic studies. AJR Am J Roentgenol 1988; 150:189–197.

65. Dickenman RC, Chason JL. Alterations in the dorsal root ganglia and adjacent nerves in the leukemias, the lymphomas and multiple myeloma. Am J Pathol 1958; 34:349–357.

66. Dimeo F, Fetscher S, Lange W, et al. Effects of aerobic exercise on the physical performance and incidence of treatment-related complications after high-dose chemotherapy. Blood 1997; 90:3390–3394.

67. Dimeo F, Rumberger BG, Keul J. Aerobic exercise as therapy for cancer fatigue. Med Sci Sports 1998; 30:475–478.

68. Dimeo FC, Stieglitz RD, Novelli-Fischer U, et al. Effects of physical activity on the fatigue and psychologic status of cancer patients during chemotherapy. Cancer 1999; 85:2273–2277.

69. Dische S, Martin WM, Anderson P. Radiation myelopathy in patients treated for carcinoma of bronchus using a six fraction regimen of radiotherapy. Br J Radiol 1981; 54:29–35.

70. Dische S, Warburton MF, Saunders MI. Radiation myelitis and survival in the radiotherapy of lung cancer. Int J Radiat Oncol Biol Phys 1988; 15:75–81.

71. Donnelly S, Walsh D. The symptoms of advanced cancer. Semin Oncol 1995; 22:67–72.

72. Ebner I, Anderl H, Mikuz G, et al. Plexus neuropathy: tumor infiltration or radiation damage. Rofo Fortschr Geb Rontgenstr Neuen Bildgeb Verfahr 1990; 152:662–666.

73. Edelson RN, Deck MD, Posner JB. Intramedullary spinal cord metastases. Clinical and radiographic findings in nine cases. Neurology 1972; 22:1222–1231.

74. Epstein JB, Stewart KH. Radiation therapy and pain in patients with head and neck cancer. Cancer B Oral Oncol 1993; 29B:191–199.

75. Fajardo LF. The pathology of ionizing radiation as defined by morphologic patterns. Acta Oncol 2005; 44:13–22.

76. Ferrer-Brechner T, Ganz P. Combination therapy with ibuprofen and methadone for chronic cancer pain. Am J Med 1987; 77(1A):78–83.

77. Fisch M. Treatment of depression in cancer. J Natl Cancer Inst Monogr 2004; 32:105–111.

78. Foldi E, Foldi EM, Weissleder H. Conservative treatment for lymphedema of the limbs. Angiology 1985; 35:171–178.

79. Foldi M, Foldi E. Komplexe physikalische entstauungstherapie des chronischen gliedmaben lymphnodems. Folia Angiol 1981; 29:161–168.

80. Foley K. The treatment of cancer pain. N Engl J Med 1985; 313:84–95.

81. Foley KM. Brachial plexopathy in patients with breast cancer. 1990; 722–729.

82. Fossa SD, Aass N, Kaalhur O. Long-term morbidity after infradiaphragmatic radiotherapy in young men with testicular cancer. Cancer 1969; 64:404–408.

83. Fraioli F, Fabbri A, Gnessi L, et al. Calcitonin and analgesia. In: Bebedetti C, et al, eds. 1984:237–250.

84. Freeman HP. Cancer in the socioeconomically disadvantaged. CA Cancer J Clin 1989; 39:266.

85. Freeman JW, Silver FH. The effects of prestrain and collagen fibril alignment on in vitro mineralization of self-assembled collagen fibers. Connect Tissue Res 2005; 46:107–115.

86. Freilich RJ, Balmaceda C, Seidman AD, et al. Motor neuropathy due to docetaxel and paclitaxel. Neurology 1996; 47:115–118.

87. Gainor GJ, Buchert P. Fracture healing in metastatic bone disease. Clin Orthop 1983; 178:297–302.

88. Galer BX, Coyle N, Pasternak GW, et al. Individual variability in the response to different opioids: report of five cases. Pain 1992; 49:87–91.

89. Garber JE, Hassenbusch SJ. Neurosurgical interventional approaches to pain. In: Berger AM, ed. Supportive oncology, part A. 2nd edn. Philadelphia: Lippincott Williams & Wilkins; 2002:128–139.

90. Gaspar L, Scott C, Rotman M, et al. Recursive partitioning analysis (RPA) of prognostic factors in three Radiation Therapy Oncology Group (RTOG) brain metastases trials. Int J Radiat Oncol Biol Phys 1997; 37:745–751.

91. Geraghty JA, Wenig BL, Smith BE, et al. Long-term follow-up of tracheoesophageal puncture results. Ann Otol Rhinol Laryngol 1996; 205: 501–503.

92. Gerber L, Hicks J, Klaiman M, et al. Rehabilitation of the cancer patient. In: Cancer: principles and practice of oncology. 5th edn. Philadelphia: Lippincott Williams & Wilkins; 1997:2925–2956.

93. Gergich N. Rehabilitation following transverse rectus abdominus flap breast reconstruction. 2005.

94. Gherardi R, Gaulard P, Prost C, et al. T-cell lymphoma revealed by a peripheral neuropathy. Cancer 1986; 58:2710–2716.

95. Gilbert RW, Kim J-H, Posner JB. Epidural spinal cord compression from metastatic tumor: diagnosis and treatment. Ann Neurol 1978; 3:40–51.

96. Glantz MJ, Burger PC, Friedman AH, et al. Treatment of radiation-induced nervous system injury with heparin and warfarin. Neurology 1994; 44:2020–2027.

97. Glantz MJ, Cole BF, Forsyth PA, et al. Practice parameter: anticonvulsant prophylaxis in patients with newly diagnosed brain tumors. Report of the Quality Standards Subcommittee of the American Academy of Neurology. Neurology 2000; 54:1886–1893.

98. Glantz MJ, Cole BF, Friedberg MH, et al. A randomized blinded, placebo-controlled trail of divalproex sodium prophylaxis in adults with newly diagnosed brain tumors. Neurology 1996; 46:985–991.

99. Glover D, Lipton A, Keller A, et al. Intravenous pamidronate disodium treatment of bone metastases in patients with breast cancer. A dose seeking study. Cancer 1994; 74:2949–2955.

100. Godwin-Austen RB, Howell DA, Worthington B. Observations on radiation myelopathy. Brain 1975; 98:557–568.

101. Greenberg HS, Kim J-H, Posner JB. Epidural spinal cord compression from metastatic tumor: results with a new treatment protocol. Ann Neurol 1980; 8:361–366.

102. Gutstein HB. The biological basis for fatigue. Cancer 2001; 92: 1678–1683.

103. Gybels JM, Swet WH, eds. Neurosurgical treatment of persistent pain: physiological and pathological mechanisms of human pain, vol 11. Basel: Karger; 1989:442.

104. Haberland C, Cipriani M, Kucuk O, et al. Fulminant leukemic polyradiculoneuropathy in a case of B-cell prolymphocytic leukemia. Cancer 1987; 60:1454–1458.

105. Haim N, Epelbaum R, Ben-Sahar M, et al. Full dose vincristine (without 2 mg dose limit) in the treatment of lymphomas. Cancer 1994; 15:2515–2519.

106. Hall SM, Buzdar AU, Blumenschein GR. Cranial nerve palsies in metastatic breast cancer due to osseous metastasis without intracranial involvement. Cancer 1983; 52(1):180–184.

107. Happ MB. Interpretation of nonvocal behaviors and the meaning of voicelessness in critical care. Soc Sci Med 2000; 50:1247–1255.

108. Harper CM Jr, Thomas JE, Cascino TL, et al. Distinction between neoplastic and radiation-induced brachial plexopathy, with emphasis on the role of EMG. Neurology 1989; 39:502–506.

109. Harrington KD. Metastatic disease of the spine. 1988:309–383.

110. Hassenbusch SJ. Cost modeling for alternate routes of administration of opioids for cancer pain. Oncology 1999; 13:63–67.

111. Hauer-Jensen M, Fink LM, Wang J. Radiation injury and the protein C pathway. Crit Care Med 2004; 32:S325–S330.

112. Healey JH, Brown HK. Complications of bone metastases. Cancer 2000; 88:2940–2951.

113. Higinbotham NL, Marcover RC. The management of pathological fractures. J Trauma 1965; 5:792–798.

114. Hillman RE, Walsh MJ, Wolf GT, et al. Functional outcomes following treatment for advanced laryngeal cancer. Part I: voice preservation in advanced laryngeal cancer. Part II: laryngectomy rehabilitation. The stat of the art in VA system. Ann Otol Rhinol Laryngol 1998; 107:2–27.

115. Hillner BE, Ingle JN, Berenson JR, et al. American Society of Clinical Oncology guideline on the role of bisphosphonates in breast cancer. American Society of Clinical Oncology Bisphosphonates Expert Panel. J Clin Oncol 2000; 18:1378–1391.

116. Hindley AC, Hill AB, Leyland MJ, et al. A double-blind controlled trial of salmon calcitonin in pain due to malignancy. Cancer Chemother Pharmacol 1982; 9:71–74.

117. Honnorat J, Cartalat-Carel S. Advances in paraneoplastic neurological syndromes. Curr Opin Oncol 2004; 16:614–620.

118. Hortobagyi GN, Theriault RL, Poerter L, et al. Efficacy of pamidronate disodium in reducing skeletal complications in patients with breast cancer and lytic bone metastases. N Engl J Med 1996; 335:1785–1891.

119. Huang M, Cifu D, et al. Functional outcome after brain tumor and acute stroke: a comparative analysis. Arch Phys Med Rehabil 1998; 79:1386–1390.

120. Huang M, Wartella JE. Functional outcomes and quality of life in patients with brain tumors: a preliminary report. Arch Phys Med Rehabil 2001; 82:1540–1546.

121. Huang ME, Cifu DX, et al. Functional outcomes in patients with brain tumor after inpatient rehabilitation: comparison with traumatic brain injury. Am J Phys Med Rehabil 2000; 79:327–335.

122. Hussain SA, James ND. Organ preservation strategies in bladder cancer. Expert Rev Anticancer Ther 2002; 2:641–651.

123. Indelicato RA, Portenoy RK. Opioid rotation in the management of refractory cancer pain. J Clin Oncol 2002; 20:348–352.

124. Ischia S, Ischia A, Luzzani A, et al. Results up to death in the treatment of persistent cervicothoracic (Pancoast) and thoracic malignant pain by unilateral percutaneous cervical cordotomy. Pain 1985; 21:339–355.

125. Jacox A, Carr DB, Payne R, et al. Management of cancer pain, clinical practice guidelines. 1994.

126. Jaeckle KA, Young DF, Foley KM. The natural history of lumbosacral plexopathy in cancer. Neurology 1985; 35:8–15.

127. Jaeckle KA. Neurological manifestations of neoplastic and radiation-induced plexopathies. Neurology 2004; 24:385–393.

128. Jain S, Kotasek D, Blumbergs PC, et al. Aleukaemic leukostasis in a case of large cell non-Hodgkin's lymphoma: report of a case with a distinctive central nervous system involvement. J Neurol Neurosurg Psychiatry 1986; 49:1079–1083.

129. Jakobson AM, Kreuger A, Mortimer O, et al. Cerebrospinal fluid exchange after intrathecal methotrexate overdose. A report of two cases. Acta Paediatr 1992; 81:359–361.

130. Jamison K, Wellisch K, Katz RL, et al. Phantom breast syndrome. Arch Surg 1979; 114:93–95.

131. Janecka IP, Sekhar LN. Surgical management of cranial base tumors: a report on 91 patients. Oncology (Huntingt) 1989; 3:69–80.

132. Jellinger K, Radiaszkiewicz T. Involvement of the central nervous system in malignant lymphomas. Virchows Arch A Pathol Anat Histopathol 1976; 370:345–362.

133. Jerian SM, Sarosy GA, Link CJ, et al. Incapacitating autonomic neuropathy precipitated by Taxol. Gynecol Oncol 1993; 51:277–280.

134. Johnson JR, Miller AJ. The efficacy of choline magnesium trisalicylate (CMT) in the management of metastatic bone pain: a pilot study. Palliat Med 1994; 8:129–134.

135. Kamby C, Vejborg I, Daugaard S, et al. Clinical and radiologic characteristics of bone metastases in breast cancer. Cancer 1987; 60:2524–2531.

136. Kemeny MM. Continuous hepatic artery infusion (CHAI) as treatment of liver metastases. Are the complications worth it? Drug Safety 1991; 6:159–165.

137. Killer HE, Hess K. Natural history of radiation-induced brachial plexopathy compared with surgically treated patients. J Neurol 1990; 237: 247–250.

138. Kirsten JM, Schimmel KJ, Richel DJ, et al. Cardiotoxicity of cytotoxic drugs. Cancer Treat Rev 2004; 30:181–191.

139. Ko DS, Lerner R, Klose G, et al. Effective treatment of lymphedema of the extremities. Arch Surg 1998; 133:452–458.

140. Kolden GG, Strauman TJ, Ward A, et al. A pilot study of group exercise training (GET) for women with primary breast cancer: feasibility and health benefits. Psychooncology 2002; 11:447–456.

141. Komaki R, Roh J, Cox JD, et al. Superior sulcus tumors: results of irradiation of 36 patients. Cancer 1981; 48:1563–1568.

142. Kori SH, Foley KM, Posner JB. Brachial plexus lesions in patients with cancer: 100 cases. Neurology 1981; 31:45–50.

143. Krathen RA, Orengo IF, Rosen T. Cutaneous metastasis: a meta-analysis of data. South Med J 2003; 96:164–167.

144. Kreisman H, Wolkove N, Findelstein HS, et al. Breast cancer and thoracic metastases: review of 119 patients. Thorax 1983; 38:175–179.

145. Krendel DA, Albright RD, Graham DG. Infiltrative polyneuropathy due to acute monoblastic leukemia in hematologic remission. Neurology 1987; 37:474–477.

146. Kroll SS, Shusterman MA, Reece GP, et al. Abdominal wall strength, bulging and hernia after TRAM flap breast reconstruction. Plast Surg Forum 1994; 17:132–133.

147. Kvale PA, Simoff M, Prakash UB. Lung cancer. Palliative care. Chest 2003; 123:284S–311S.

148. Lagerwaard FJ, Lavendag PC, Nowak PJ, et al. Identification of prognostic factors in patients with brain metastases: a review of 1292 patients. Int J Radiat Oncol Biol Phys 1999; 434:795–803.

149. Leduc O, Klein P, Demaret P, et al. Dynamic pressure variation under bandages with different stiffness. Vasc Med 1993; 465–468.

150. Leduc O, Peeters A, Bourgeois P. Bandages: scintigraphic demonstration of its efficacy on colloidal protein reabsorption during muscular activity. 1990; 421–423.

151. Lee BN, Dantzer R, Langley KE, et al. A cytokine-based neuroimmunologic mechanism of cancer-related symptoms. Neuroimmunomodulation 2004; 11:279–292.

152. Levin VA, Gutin PH, Leibel S. Neoplasms of the central nervous system. 1993; 1679–1737.

153. Levy M. Pharmacologic treatment of cancer pain. N Engl J Med 1996; 335:1124–1132.

154. Lipton A, Glover D, Harvey H, et al. Pamidronate in the treatment of bone metastases. Results of two dose-ranging trials in patients with breast or prostate cancer. Ann Oncol 1994; 5(suppl 7):S31–S35.

155. Lipton A, Theriault R, Leff R, et al. Reduction of skeletal related complications in breast cancer patients with osteolytic bone metastases receiving hormone therapy, by monthly pamidronate sodium (Aredia) infusion. Br J Cancer 1996; 74(suppl 28):11.

156. Lomonaco M, Milone M, Batocchli AP, et al. Cisplatin neuropathy: clinical course and neurophysiological findings. J Neurol 1992; 239:199–204.

157. Lotze MT, Duncan MA, Gerber LH, et al. Early versus delayed shoulder motion following axillary dissection: a randomized prospective study. Ann Surg 1981; 193:288–295.

158. MacVicar MG, Winningham ML, Nickel JL. Effects of aerobic interval training on cancer patients functional capacity. Nurs Res 1989; 38:348–351.

159. Marchetti M, Barosi G. Clinical and economic impact of epoetins in cancer care. Phamacoeconomics 2004; 22:1029–1045.

160. Marciniak CM, Sliwa JA. Functional outcomes of persons with brain tumors after inpatient rehabilitation. Arch Phys Med Rehabil 2001; 82:457–463.

161. Marks JE, Wong J. The risk of cerebral radionecrosis in relation to dose, time and fractionation: a follow-up study. Prog Exp Tumor Res 1985; 29:210–218.

162. McEwan AJ. Unsealed source therapy of painful bone metastases: an update. Semin Nucl Med 1997; 27:165–182.

163. McKinley WO, Conti-Wyneken AR, et al. Rehabilitation functional outcome of patients with neoplastic spinal cord compressions. Arch Phys Med Rehabil 1996; 77:892–895.

164. McKinley WO, Huang ME, Tewksbury MA. Neoplastic vs. traumatic spinal cord injury: an inpatient rehabilitation comparison. Am J Phys Med Rehabil 2000; 79:138–144.

165. McLeod JG, Penny R. Vincristine neuropathy: an electrophysiological and histological study. J Neurol Neurosurg Psychiatry 1969; 32:297–304.

166. McLeod JG. Peripheral neuropathy associated with lymphomas, leukemias, and polycythemia vera. 1993.

167. Mendenhall WM, Morris CG, Stringer SP, et al. Voice rehabilitation after total laryngectomy and postoperative radiation therapy. J Clin Oncol 2002; 20:2500–2505.

168. Mercadante S. Opioid rotation for cancer pain: rationale and clinical aspects. Cancer 1999; 86:1856–1866.

169. Miaskowski CA, Portenoy RK. Assessment and management of cancer-related fatigue. In: Berger AM, ed. Supportive oncology, part B. 2nd edn. Philadelphia: Lippincott Williams & Wilkins; 2002:141–153.

170. Mirels H. Metastatic disease in long bones: a proposed scoring system for diagnosing impending pathogic fractures. Clin Orthop 1989; 249:256–264.

171. Mizgala CL, Hartrampf CR, Bennet GK. Abdominal function after pedicled TRAM flap surgery. Clin Plast Surg 1994; 21:255–272.

172. Mock V, Dow KH, Meares CJ, et al. Effects of exercise on fatigue, physical functioning, and emotional distress during radiation therapy for breast cancer. Oncol Nurs Forum 1997; 24:991–1000.

173. Mock V, Pickett M, Ropka ME, et al. Fatigue and quality of life outcomes of exercise during cancer treatment. Cancer Pract 2001; 9:119–127.

174. Mock V, Piper B, Sabbatini P, et al. National comprehensive network fatigue practice guidelines. Oncology 2000; 14:151–161.

175. Monteiro M. Physical therapy implications following the TRAM procedure. Phys Ther 1997; 77:765–770.

176. Morgan RG, Casley-Smith JR, Mason MR, et al. Complex physical therapy for the lymphoedematous arm. Br J Hand Surg 1992; 17B:437–441.

177. Moskovitz AH, Anderson BO, Yeung RS, et al. Axillary web syndrome after axillary dissection. Am J Surg 2001; 181:434–439.

178. Muggia FM, Vafai D, Natale R, et al. Paclitaxel 3-hour infusion given alone and combined with carboplatin: preliminary results of dose-escalation trials. Semin Oncol 1995; 22(4 suppl 9):63–66.

179. Na YM, Kim MY, Kim YK, et al. Exercise therapy effect on natural killer cell cytotoxic activity in stomach cancer patients after curative surgery. Arch Phys Med Rehabil 2000; 81:777–779.

180. Nieman DC, Cook VD, Henson DA, et al. Moderate exercise training and natural killer cell cytotoxic activity in breast cancer patients. Int J Sports Med 1995; 16:334–337.

181. O'Dell MW, Barr K, Spanier D, et al. Functional outcome of inpatient rehabilitation in persons with brain tumors. Arch Phys Med Rehabil 1998; 79:1530–1534.

182. Oldervoll LM, Kaasa S, Knobel H, et al. Exercise reduces fatigue in chronic fatigued Hodgkin's disease survivors: results from a pilot study. Eur J Cancer Prev 2003; 39:57–63.

183. Olsen NK, Pfeiffer P, Mondrup K, et al. Radiation-induced brachial plexus neuropathy in breast cancer patients. Acta Oncol 1990; 29:885–890.

184. Olszewski WL, Engeset A. Vasomotoric function of lymphatics and lymph transport in limbs during massage and with elastic support. 1988; 571–575.

185. Paige KT, Bostwick J III, Bried JT, et al. A comparison of morbidity from bilateral, unipedicled and unilateral, unipedicled TRAM flap breast reconstructions. Plast Reconstr Surg 1998; 101:1819–1827.

186. Paling MR, Black WC, Levine PA, et al. Tumor invasion of the anterior skull base: a comparison of MR and CT studies. J Comput Assist Tomogr 1987; 11:824–830.

187. Partsch H. Do we need firm compression stocking exerting high pressure? Vasa 1984; 13:52–57.

188. Partsch H. Verbesserte forderleistung der wadenmuskelpumpe unter kompressionstrumpfen bei Varizen und venoser Insuffizienz. Phlebol Proktol 1978; 7:58.

189. Patt RB. Non-pharmacologic measures for controlling oncologic pain. Am J Hosp Palliat Care 1990; 7:30–37.

190. Pavinen LM, Kikku P, Maekinen E, et al. Factors affecting the pulmonary toxicity of bleomycin. Acta Radiol 1983; 22:417.

191. Payne R. Opioid pharmacotherapy. In: Berger AM, ed. Supportive oncology, part A. 2nd edn. Philadelphia: Lippincott Williams & Wilkins; 2002: 68–83.

192. Perrin RB, McBroom RJ. Intradural extramedullary spinal metastasis. A report of 10 cases. Neurosurgery 1982; 56:835–837.

193. Peters C, Lotzeich H, Niemeier B, et al. Influence of a moderate exercise training on natural killer cytotoxicity and personality traits in cancer patients. Anticancer Res 1994; 14:1033–1036.

194. Peters C, Lotzerich H, Niemeir B, et al. Exercise, cancer and the immune response of monocytes. Anticancer Res 1995; 15:175–179.

195. Pierce SM, Recht A, Lingos TI, et al. Long-term radiation complications following conservative surgery (CS) and radiation therapy (RT) in patients with early stage breast cancer. Int J Radiat Oncol Biol Phys 1992; 23:915–923.

196. Portenoy RK, Kornblith AB, Wong G. Pain in ovarian cancer patients. Prevalence, characteristics, and associated symptoms. Cancer 1994; 74:907–915.

197. Portenoy RK, Miransky J, Thaler HT. Pain in ambulatory patients with lung or colon cancer. Prevalence, characteristics, and effect. Cancer 1992; 70:1616–1624.

198. Portenoy RK. Pain in oncologic and AIDS patients. 1997; 126–155.

199. Posner JB. Cancer involving cranial and peripheral nerves. 1995.

200. Posner JB. Management of brain metastases. Rev Neurol 1992; 148: 477–487.

201. Posner JB. Side effects of radiation therapy. 1995; 311–337.

202. Posner JB. Spinal metastases—clinical findings. Philadelphia: FA Davis; 1995:111–142.

203. Post JMD, Quencer RM, Green BA, et al. Intramedullary spinal cord metastases, mainly of nonneurogenic orgin. AJR Am J Roentgenol 1987; 148:1015–1022.

204. Postma TJ, Vermorken JB, Liefting AJ, et al. Paclitaxel-induced neuropathy. Ann Oncol 1995; 6:489–494.

205. Potts DG, Zimmerman RD. Nuclear magnetic resonance imaging of skull base lesions. J Neurol Sci 1975; 12:327–331.

206. Powell S, Cooke J, Parsons C. Radiation-induced brachial plexus injury: follow-up of two different fractionation schedules. Radiother Oncol 1990; 18:213–220.

207. Pritchard J, Anand P, Broome J, et al. Double-blind randomized phase II study of hyperbaric oxygen in patients with radiation-induced brachial plexopathy. Radiother Oncol 2001; 58:279–286.

208. Ransom DT, DiNapoli RP, Richardson RL. Cranial nerve lesions due to base of the skull metastases in prostrate carcinoma. Cancer 1990; 65(3): 586–589.

209. Ready LB. The treatment of post operative pain. In: Bond MR, Charlton JE, Woolf CJ, eds. Proceedings of the VIth World Congress on Pain. Amsterdam: Elsevier Science; 1991:53–58.

210. Rider CA. Oral mucositis. A complication of radiotherapy. NY State Dent J 1990; 56:37–39.

211. Ries LA, Eisner M, Kosary C, et al. SEER cancer statistics review. Bethesda: National Cancer Institute; 1975.

212. Riggs J, Ashraf M, Snyder RD, et al. Prospective nerve conduction studies in cisplatin therapy. Ann Neurol 1988; 23:92–94.

213. Robbins MEC, Zhao W. Chronic oxidative stress and radiation-induced late normal tissue injury: a review. Int J Radiat Biol 2004; 80:251–259.

214. Rodgers LR, Borkowski GP, Albers JW, et al. Obturator mononeuropathy cuased by pelvic cancer: six cases. Neurology 1993; 43:1489–1492.

215. Ross JR, Saunders Y, Edmonds PM, et al. Systematic review of role of bisphosponates on skeletal morbidity in metastatic cancer. Br Med J 2003; 327:469.

216. Rotstein J, Good RA. Steroid pseudorheumatism. Arch Intern Med 1957; 99:545–555.

217. Rowinsky EK, Chaudhry V, Cornblath DR. Neurotoxicity of Taxol. J Natl Cancer Inst Monogr 1993; 15:107–115.

218. Ruifrok ACC, Kleiboer BJ, van der Kogel AJ. Radiation tolerance and fractionation sensitivity of the developing rat cervical spinal cord. Int J Radiat Biol Phys 1992; 24:505–510.

219. Sahenk Z, Barohn R, New P, et al. Taxol neuropathy: electrodiagnostic and sural nerve biopsy findings. Arch Neurol 1994; 51:726–729.

220. Sarhill N, Walsh D, Nelson KA, et al. Methylphendiate for fatigue in advanced cancer: a prospective open-label pilot study. Am J Hosp Palliat Care 2001; 18:187–192.

221. Schouten LJ, Rutten J, Huveneers HA, et al. Incidence of brain metastases in a cohort of patients with carcinoma of the breast, colon, kidney, and lung and melanoma. Cancer 2002; 94:2698–2705.

222. Schultheiss TE, Stephens LC, Peters LJ. Survival in radiation myelopathy. Int J Radiat Oncol Biol Phys 1986; 12:1765–1769.

223. Schwartz AL, Mori M, Gao R, et al. Exercise reduces daily fatigue in women with breast cancer receiving chemotherapy. Med Sci Sports Exerc 2001; 33:718–723.

224. Schwartz AL, Thompson JA, Masood N. Interferon-induced fatigue in patients with melanoma: a pilot study of exercise and methylphenidate. Oncol Nurs Forum 2002; 29:E85–E90.

225. Schwartz AL. Daily fatigue patterns and effect of exercise in women with breast cancer. Cancer Pract 2000; 8:16–24.

226. Schwartz AL. Fatigue mediates the effects of exercise on quality of life. Qual Life Res 1999; 8:529–538.

227. Segal R, Evans W, Johnson D, et al. Structured exercise improves physical functioning in women with stages I and II breast cancer: results of a randomized controlled trial. J Clin Oncol 2001; 19:657–665.

228. Segal RJ, Reid RD, Courneya KS, et al. Resistance exercise in men receiving androgen deprivation therapy for prostate cancer. J Clin Oncol 2003; 21:1653–1659.

229. Sheldon T, Hayes DF, Cady B, et al. Primary radiation therapy for locally advanced breast cancer. Cancer 1987; 60:1219–1225.

230. Siegal T, Haim N. Cisplatin-induced peripheral neuropathy: frequent off-therapy deterioration, demyelinating syndromes, and muscle cramps. Cancer 1990; 15:1117–1123.

231. Silvestri F, Bussani R, Pavletic N, et al. Metastases of the heart and pericardium. G Ital Cardiol 1997; 27:1252–1255.

232. Sim FH. Metastatic bone disease. Instr Course Lect 1999.

233. Sitar DS. Human drug metabolism in vivo. Pharmacol Ther 1989; 43:363.

234. Skolnick AA. New study suggests radiation often underused for palliation. JAMA 1998; 279:343–344.

235. Smith R. An evaluation of surgical treatment for spinal cord compression due to metastatic carcinoma. J Neurol Neurosurg Psychiatry 1965; 28L:152–158.

236. Son YH. Effectiveness of irradiation therapy in peripheral neuropathy caused by malignant disease. Cancer 1967; 20:1447–1451.

237. St Guily JL, Angelard B, el-Bez M, et al. Postlaryngectomy voice restoration: a prospective study in 83 patients. Arch Otolaryngol Head Neck Surg 1992; 118:252–255.

238. Stambaugh JE, Drew J. A double-blind parallel evaluation of the efficacy and safety of a single dose of ketoprofen in cancer pain. J Clin Pharmacol 1988; 28(suppl):S34–S39.

239. Stambaugh JE, Drew J. The combination of ibuprofen and oxycodone/acetaminophen in the management of chronic cancer pain. Clin Pharmacol Ther 1988; 44:665–669.

240. Stambaugh JE. Role of nonsteroidal anti-inflammatory drugs in the management of cancer pain. In: Patt RB. Cancer pain. 1992.

241. Steiner I, Siegal T. Muscle cramps in cancer patients. Cancer 1989; 63:574–577.

242. Stemmer R, Marescaux J, Furderer C. Compression treatment of the lower extremities particularly with compression stockings. Dermotologist 1980; 31:355–365.

243. Stillwagon GB, Lee DJ, Moses H, et al. Response of cranial nerve abnormalities in nasopharyngeal carcinoma to radiation therapy. Cancer 1986; 57:2272–2274.

244. Strang P. Emotional and social aspects of cancer pain. Acta Oncol 1992; 31:323–326.

245. Sugawara Y, Akechi T, Shima Y. Efficacy of methylphenidate for fatigue in advanced cancer patients: a preliminary study. Palliat Med 2002; 16:261–263.

246. Sunder-Plassmann M, Grunert V. Commissural myelotomy for drug-resistant pain. Clin Microsurg 1976; 165–170.

247. Sunshine A, Olson NZ. Analgesic efficacy of ketoprofen in postpartum, general surgery, and chronic cancer pain. J Clin Pharmacol 1998; 28(suppl):S47–S54.

248. Sze G. Magnetic resonance imaging in the evaluation of spinal tumors. Cancer 1991; 67(suppl 4):1229–1241.

249. Szuba A, Rockson S. Lymphedema: classification, diagnosis and therapy. Vasc Med 1998; 3:145–146.

250. Tanoue LT. Preoperative evaluation of the high-risk surgical patient for lung cancer resection. Semin Respir Crit Care Med 2000; 21:421–432.

251. Tas F, Eralp Y, Basaran M. Anemia in oncology practice: relation to diseases and their therapies. Am J Clin Oncol 2002; 25:371–379.

252. Tasker RR. Percutaneous cordotomy for persistent pain. In: Textbook of stereotactic and functional neurosurgery. New York: McGraw-Hill; 1998: 1491–1505.

253. Tay WK, Shaw RJ, Goh CR. A survey of symptoms in hospice patients in Singapore. Ann Acad Med Singapore 1994; 23:191–196.

254. Taylor BV, Kimmel DW, Krecke KN, et al. Magnetic resonance imaging in cancer-related lumbosacral plexopathy. Mayo Clin Proc 1997; 72:823–829.

255. Thiebaud D, Leyvraz S, von Fliedner V, et al. Treatment of bone metastases from breast cancer and myeloma with pamidronate. Eur J Cancer 1991; 27:37–41.

256. Thomas JE, Cascino TL, Earle JD. Differential diagnosis between radiation and tumor plexopathy of the pelvis. Neurology 1985; 35:1–7.

257. Thyagarajan D, Cascino TL, Harms G. Magnetic resonance imaging in brachial plexopathy of cancer. Neurology 1995; 45:421–427.

258. Todd TR. The surgical treatment of pulmonary metastases. Chest 1997; 112:287S–290S.

259. Tomlinson BE, Perry RH, Stewart-Wynne EG. Influence of site of origin of lung carcinomas on clinical presentation and central nervous system metastasis. J Neurol Neurosurg Psychiatry 1979; 42:82–88.

260. Tosoni A, Ermani M, Brandes AA. The pathogenesis and treatment of brain metastases: a comprehensive review. Clin Rev Oncol Hemat 2004; 52:199–215.

261. Turgman J, Braham J, Modan B, et al. Neurological complications in patients with malignant tumors of the nasopharynx. Eur Neurol 1978; 17:149–154.

262. Veldhuis GJ, Willemse PH, van Gameren MM, et al. Recombinant human interleukin-3 to dose-intensify carboplatin and cyclophosphamide chemotherapy in epithelial ovarian cancer: a phase I trial. J Clin Oncol 1995; 13:733–740.

263. Vial T, Desotes J. Clinical toxicity of cytokines used as haemopoietic growth factors. Drug Safety 1995; 13:371–406.

264. Vujaskovic Z, Anscher MS, Feng QF, et al. Radiation-induced hypoxia may perpetuate late normal tissue injury. Int J Radiat Oncol Biol Phys 2001; 50:851–855.

265. Vuorinen E. Pain as an early symptom in cancer. Clin J Pain 1993; 9:272–278.

266. Walsh JC, Low PA, Allsop JL. Localized sympathetic overactity: an uncommon complication of lung cancer. J Neurol Neurosurg Psychiatry 1976; 39:93–95.

267. Wara WM, Phillips TL, Sheline GE, et al. Radiation tolerance of the spinal cord. Cancer 1975; 35:1558–1562.

268. Waters JS, O'Brien ME, Ashley S. Management of anemia in patients receiving chemotherapy [letter]. J Clin Oncol 2002; 20:601–602.

269. Weissleder H, Schuchhardt C. Primary lymphedema. 1997; 75–92.

270. Winngham ML, MacVicar MG, Bondoc M, et al. Effect of aerobic exercise on body weight and composition in patients with breast cancer on adjuvant chemotherapy. Oncol Nurs Forum 1989; 16:683–689.

271. Winngham ML, MacVicar MG. The effect of aerobic exercise on patient reports of nausea. Oncol Nurs Forum 1988; 15:447–450.

272. Wong GY, Schroeder DR, Carns PE, et al. Effect of neurolytic celiac plexus block on pain relief, quality of life, and survival in patients with unresectable pancreatic cancer: a randomized controlled trial. JAMA 2004; 291:1092–1099.

273. Woo E, Yu YL, Ng M, et al. Spinal cord compression in multiple myeloma: who get it? Aust NZ J Med 1986; 16:671–675.

274. World Health Organization. Cancer pain relief and palliative care: report of a WHO expert committee. WHO technical Report Series #804. Geneva: WHO; 1990.

275. Zeine L, Larson M. Pre- and postoperative counseling for laryngectomees and their spouses: an update. J Commun Disorders 1999; 32:51–71.

Issues in Burn Rehabilitation

Peter C. Esselman and Merilyn L. Moore

Burn injuries present unique physical and psychologic rehabilitation challenges. It is estimated that there are over 1 million burn injuries every year in the USA, with 700 000 emergency department visits and 45 000 hospitalizations per year.[2,7]

The incidence of burns injuries has decreased in the USA over time. It is estimated that, between the 1950s and the early 1990s, the incidence declined from about 10 per 1000 population to 4.2 per 1000 population.[7] Between 1985 and 1995, the age-adjusted death rates for burn injuries declined by 33%.[54] In 1998, the age-adjusted death rate caused by burn injuries was 1.19 per 100 000 population. The overall incidence of burn injuries has declined due to increased prevention of injuries at home and in the workplace.

The mortality of burn injuries has declined significantly, due to the development of burn centers over the past 40 years and development of advanced treatments, such as improvements in the resuscitation of patients with severe burns, topical antimicrobial agents and newer antibiotics, early excision and grafting and, more recently, the use of artificial skin substitutes.[74] Mortality from burn injuries is determined by factors such as the size of the burn and inhalation injury. Saffle estimated that, during 1991–3, the LD_{50} (burn size lethal to 50% of patients) was 81% of total body surface area (TBSA) burn, compared with 65% of TBSA in 1984.[68] The mortality rate of those with an inhalation injury was 29.4%, compared with only 2.2% in those without an inhalation injury. Patients with inhalation injury typically sustain larger burns but, after accounting for burn size and other clinical or demographic factors, patients with inhalation injury had a seven times increased risk of dying compared with those without inhalation injury.[68]

Mortality from a burn injury, as measured by the LD_{50}, has decreased significantly over time. Pruitt studied over 8000 patients admitted for burn care to the US Army Institute of Surgical Research between 1950 and 1991.[63] The LD_{50} has dramatically risen since the 1970s, indicating that individuals are surviving larger burn injuries, as shown in Figure 59-1. There were minimal gains in decreasing mortality, and actual declines in survival, in the late 1950s to early 1960s and again in the late 1960s due to poor control of burn wound sepsis. Since 1970, there has been consistent improvement in the survival of those with burn injuries.[63]

Mortality from a burn injury is also significantly affected by age, with the highest mortality in the very young and in the elderly. Saffle found that the LD_{50} is a lower percentage TBSA in the very young, increases with age, and decreases again in the elderly. The LD_{50} for those over 70 is 29.5% TBSA.[68] Pruitt also demonstrated the effect of age on mortality, as shown in Figure 59-2. Small burns have never been fatal, and large burns in the elderly will continue to have a high risk of mortality. The largest increase in survival has been in those burns that had about an 80% risk of mortality in the 1950s (about 70% TBSA in young adults and 50% TBSA in the elderly).[63] Currently, individuals are much more likely to survive these large burns due to improvements in acute treatment. These patients surviving large burns have multiple rehabilitation issues, such as scarring, contractures, amputations, pain, and psychologic adjustment issues, that increase the role of an interdisciplinary rehabilitation program that is coordinated with the burn surgery and plastic surgery team.

Like other traumatic injuries, individuals with burns are more likely to be young adult men. Approximately 75% of adult subjects are male, with the most common age group being from 20 to 40 years old. Fire or flame is the most common cause of burns, causing over 60% of all injuries. Scald burns account for only about 10% of burns in adults, but at least 30% of burns in children. Work-related injuries are a significant source of burn injuries. The model system program data shows that, while only 59% of individuals were employed at the time of their injury, 23% of injuries in adults were work-related. Patients with burn injuries who were employed prior to the injury had 42% of their injuries occurring at work.[25,55,56,68] This presents additional rehabilitation issues regarding job issues and attempting to return patients to the workplace where the injury occurred.

NORMAL SKIN

Normal skin is composed of the epidermis, dermis, and subdermis (Fig. 59-3). The epidermis is the outer protective layer and serves as a barrier to water. The thickness of the epidermis ranges from 0.5 to 1.5 mm. The inner layer of the epidermis has many basal cells that are mitotically active. The basal cells form the keratinocytes that produce keratin, an important component of the stratum corneum. The keratinocytes migrate outward, losing all cellular components to eventually form the stratum corneum, which is a water-insoluble protective layer.

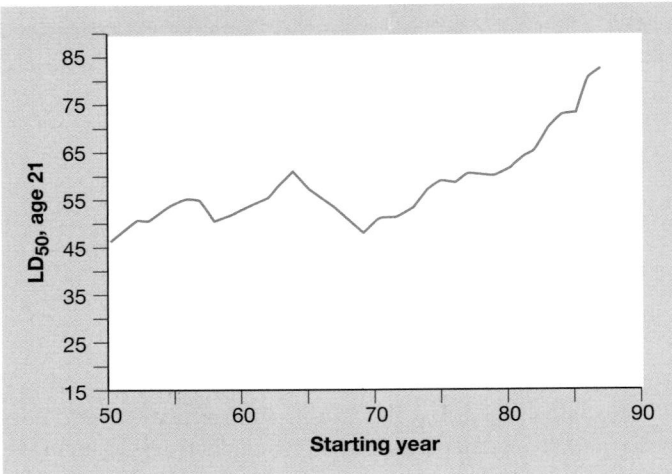

Figure 59-1 Changes in the LD_{50} in patients 21 years of age over time, illustrating the increased survival of individuals with large burns. (From Pruitt et al. 2002,[64] with permission.)

Keratinocytes take 40–65 days to reach the outer layer.[32] The dermis provides support and nutrients to the epidermis and maintains the dermal appendages, such as hair follicles, and sweat and sebaceous glands. These hair follicles, and sweat and sebaceous glands provide an important source of epidermal cells that can heal partial-thickness burn injuries (Fig. 59-4).

The mechanical properties of the skin allow it to withstand significant mechanical stress while allowing for flexibility and motion. The dermis is 70% collagen, with most of the collagen arranged in thick bundles parallel to the skin surface. When stress or a load is placed on the skin, it responds in a biphasic manner. Initially, the loosely arranged, relaxed collagen fibers lengthen, allowing an increase in length, or strain. With further stress on the collagen fibers, there is a marked resistance to stretch (Fig. 59-5).[54] This property gives the skin elasticity with low amounts of stress, but the durability to resist large forces.

CLASSIFICATION OF BURN SEVERITY

The percent TBSA burned and the depth of the burn determine the severity of thermal burns. The TBSA is determined by the rule of nines, which is an easy and rapid way to estimate the size of a burn injury (Fig. 59-6). Due to the different proportions of head and body size in children, the Lund and Browder chart can be utilized (Fig. 59-7).[47]

Burn depth is described as superficial, partial thickness, or full thickness (Fig. 59-8). A superficial (first-degree) burn involves only the epidermis, such as occurs in typical sunburn. A superficial burn is red and painful but will heal spontaneously in 3–7 days. A partial-thickness (second-degree) burn involves the epidermis and the dermis. A partial-thickness burn that is relatively superficial is painful and red, and will blanch with pressure. The pain is due to the viability of the nerve endings. Spontaneous healing typically occurs within 7–21 days. Because the epidermis layer is destroyed, healing occurs from the epi-

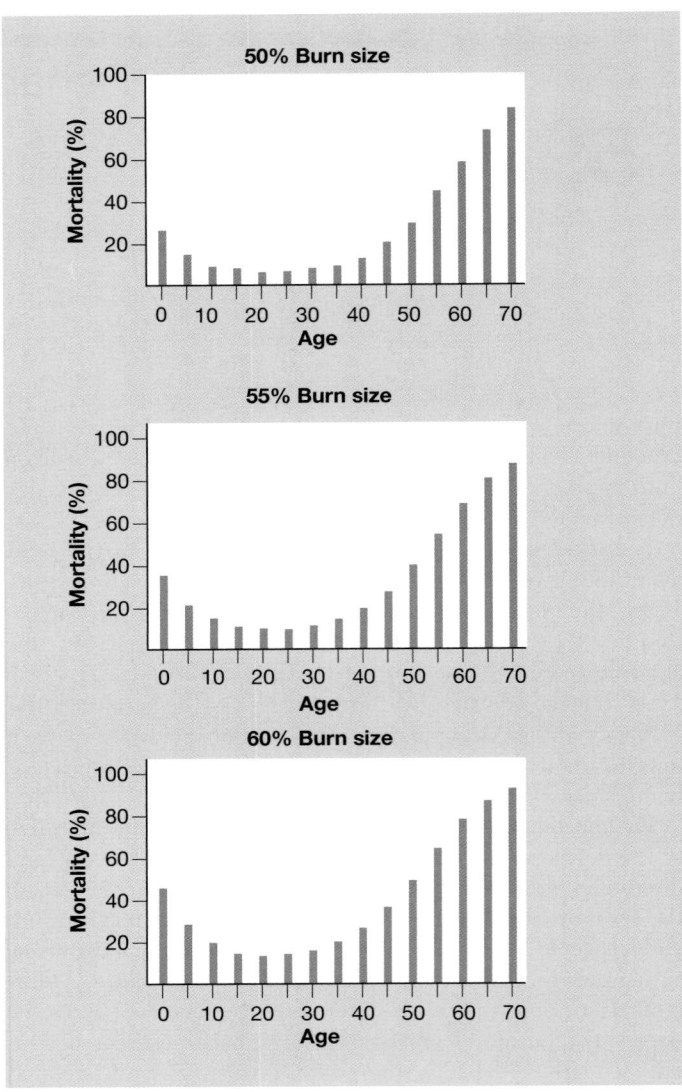

Figure 59-2 Effect of age on percent mortality at three discrete burn sizes. (From Pruitt et al. 2002,[64] with permission.)

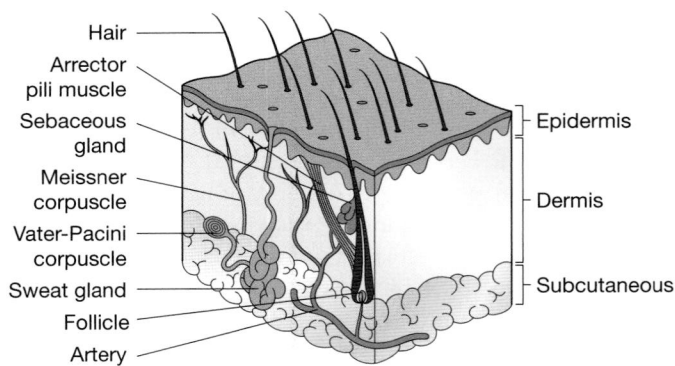

Figure 59-3 Cross-section of normal skin, illustrating the epidermis, the dermis, and the epidermal appendages (hair follicles, sweat and sebaceous glands). (From Achauer and Eriksson 2000,[1] with permission.)

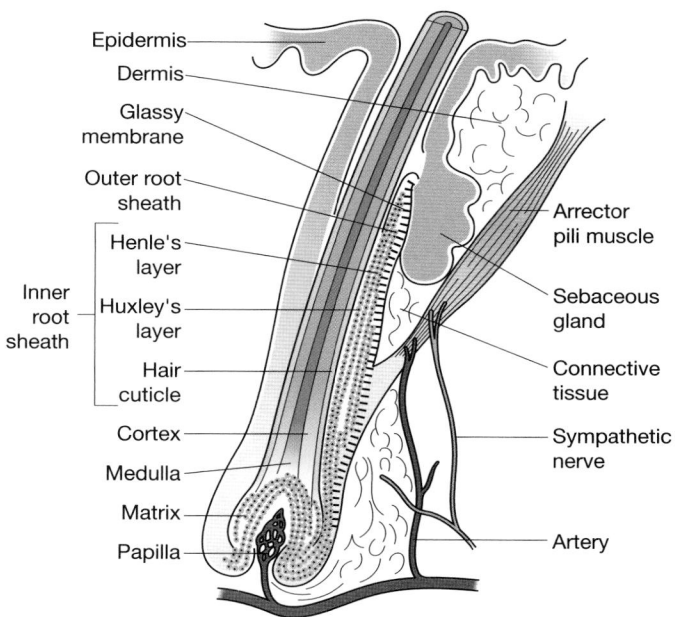

Figure 59-4 Cross-section of a hair follicle, illustrating the extension of the epidermis into the dermal layer. (From Achauer and Eriksson 2000,[1] with permission.)

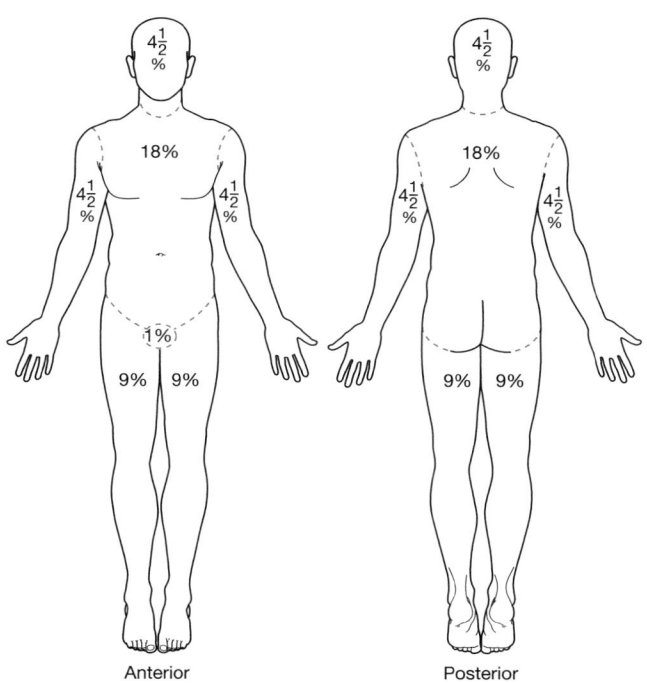

Figure 59-6 The rule of nines is used for the calculation of the percent of body surface area burned. (From Artz et al. 1979,[4] with permission.)

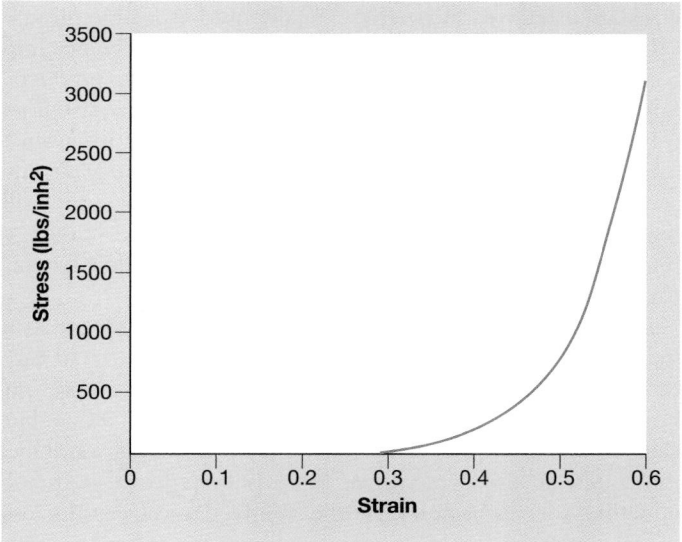

Figure 59-5 Stress–strain deformation curve for normal skin. As skin is initially stretched, the relaxed collagen fibers allow stretch with little force. As the collagen fibers straighten out, much more force is necessary to stretch the skin. (From Achauer and Eriksson 2000,[1] with permission.)

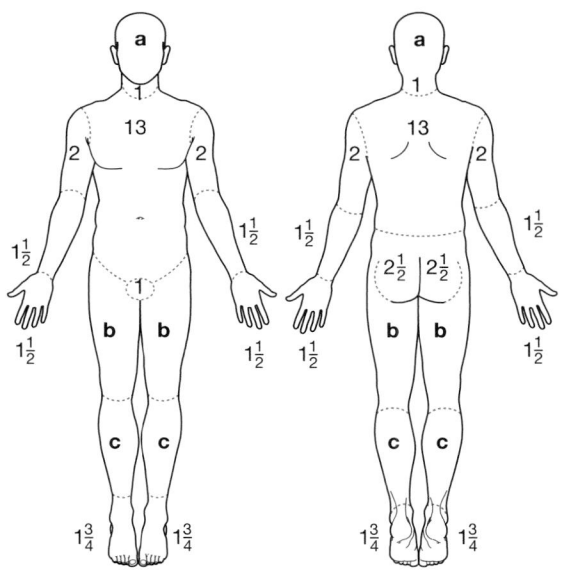

Age in years						
	0	1	5	10	15	Adult
a - $\frac{1}{2}$ of head	$9\frac{1}{2}$	$8\frac{1}{2}$	$6\frac{1}{2}$	$5\frac{1}{2}$	$4\frac{1}{2}$	$3\frac{1}{2}$
b - $\frac{1}{2}$ of one thigh	$2\frac{3}{4}$	$3\frac{1}{4}$	4	$4\frac{1}{4}$	$4\frac{1}{2}$	$4\frac{3}{4}$
c - $\frac{1}{2}$ of one leg	$2\frac{1}{2}$	$2\frac{1}{2}$	$2\frac{3}{4}$	3	$3\frac{1}{4}$	$3\frac{1}{2}$

Figure 59-7 The Lund and Browder method for calculation of burn size is reliable for different body proportions in children. (From Artz et al. 1979,[4] with permission.)

dermal structures in the dermal appendages or from the edges of the wound. A deep partial-thickness burn involves the dermis down to the subdermal tissue. A deep partial-thickness burn can heal spontaneously with hypertrophic scarring, but usually requires grafting. This is due to the destruction of the epidermis and most of the dermal appendages. A full-thickness (third-degree) burn involves the entire epidermis and dermis into the

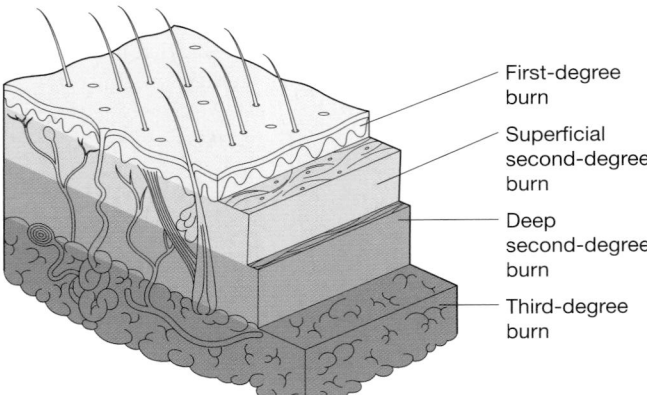

Figure 59-8 A superficial (first-degree) burn involves only the epidermis. A partial-thickness burn (second degree) involves the superficial or deep dermis, and a full-thickness burn (third degree) extends to subdermal tissues. (From Achauer and Eriksson 2000,[1] with permission.)

First-degree burn

Superficial second-degree burn

Deep second-degree burn

Third-degree burn

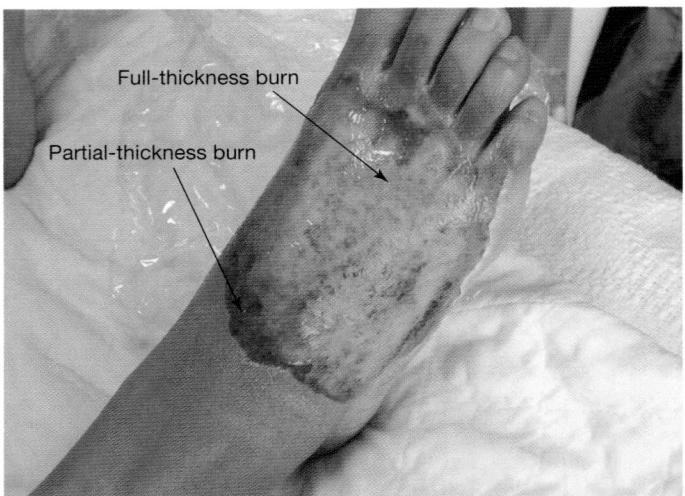

Full-thickness burn

Partial-thickness burn

Figure 59-9 Clinical appearance of a full- and a partial-thickness burn.

Box 59-1 American Burn Association criteria for referral to a burn center

- A partial-thickness burn of >10% total body surface area
- Burns that involve the face, hands, feet, genitalia, perineum, or major joints
- A full-thickness burn in any age group
- Electrical injury, including lightning injury
- Chemical burns
- Inhalation injury
- Burn injury in patients with preexisting medical conditions that could complicate treatment
- Any patient with burn injury and concomitant trauma in which the burn injury poses the greatest risk of morbidity or mortality
- Burned children in hospitals without qualified personnel or equipment for the care of children
- Burn injury in patients who will require special social, emotional, or long-term rehabilitative treatment

---

subdermal tissue. These burns are not painful, due to the destruction of the neural tissue; are pale; and require grafting, unless the burn is very small (Fig. 59-9).[80]

Many patients with burns are best treated in an established burn center. The American Burn Association has defined the types of burn injuries that should be treated in a burn center.[14] These criteria are listed in Box 59-1.

PRINCIPLES OF WOUND CARE

Early debridement of wound eschar and devitalized tissue during daily wound care is important in the initial management of burn wounds. Hydrotherapy is used to remove dressings and help remove devitalized tissue. Hydrotherapy can be delivered by immersion in a tank, but this has a risk of contaminating the burn wound with bacteria from other burned or non-burned skin. Burn centers are more commonly using a hydrotherapy table for wound care, with a handheld shower spray. A disposable plastic liner on the table is used to help prevent cross-contamination between patients.

Several topical agents with antimicrobial properties can be used to provide a protective covering. Topical silver preparations are effective, and were originally used as a silver nitrate solution. Because silver nitrate stains everything it comes into contact with brown, it has been replaced by newer products. Silver sulfadiazine is synthesized from silver nitrate and sodium sulfadiazine, and is available in a cream. It is effective against most bacteria but does not penetrate the eschar well. Mafenide acetate is also effective, and can penetrate eschar but will impede epithelialization. Prolonged use of mafenide causes a metabolic acidosis, and its use has diminished due to this toxicity.[50]

Burn wound infection is a significant risk after a severe burn injury. Early excision and grafting, with aggressive wound care to remove devitalized tissue, is the primary means to prevent infection. Topical agents are also used to prevent infection, but the burn wound will become colonized with bacteria. Antibiotics should be used only when there is evidence of systemic infection, such as bacteremia or local infection causing the loss of an autograft. In the hospital environment, infection with bacteria resistant to antibiotics is an increasing problem.

Burn wounds that do not heal spontaneously require an autograft using the patient's own skin. Temporary wound coverings with an allograft (human organ donor skin) or xenograft (animal skin) before final closure by autografting allow for a barrier to fluid and protein loss and minimize the risk of infection. Porcine xenografts provide a temporary wound covering that will be rejected by the immune system, but that can be used to facilitate closure of partial-thickness wounds. Human allografts from organ donors can be used as split-thickness grafts to cover the wound, but they will also be rejected within several weeks. The use of a temporary wound covering allows ongoing vascularization of the wound bed and preparation for a final autograft. If the allograft survives prior to rejection, the wound bed is ready to accept an autograft and the autograft will typically be successful.[70]

Early excision and grafting of full-thickness and deep partial-thickness wounds promote wound healing and minimize scarring. Excision of the eschar removes non-viable tissue until vascular viable tissue is left in the wound bed. Autografts are usually split-thickness skin grafts (STSGs) that include the donor epidermis and superficial dermis. The STSG can be meshed to cover larger areas of the trunk or extremities, but it heals with the characteristic mesh pattern (Fig. 59-10). The STSG can be placed as a sheet graft in areas where a cosmetic result is more important, such as the face or the hand. The donor sites are treated as a partial-thickness burn and will heal from the dermal appendages. Full-thickness skin grafts (FTSGs) are rarely used, because the donor sites will not heal spontaneously unless they are very small. The FTSG donor sites are usually taken from the groin or abdomen, and are small enough to be sutured closed. FTSGs are used for areas of cosmetic importance, such as the eyelid or the tip of the nose.

Dermal replacement products are increasing in their use in patients with large burns with limited donor sites. Integra is a bilaminar composite with a neodermis of bovine collagen in a matrix of shark cartilage chondroitin-6-sulfate. This is covered with a silicone layer. The neodermis is vascularized by the underlying tissue in 2–3 weeks, at which time the silicone layer is removed and a very thin autograft is placed on the wound. This superficial donor site can heal rapidly. Integra has been shown to be safe and effective in the treatment of large burns.[34,67]

REHABILITATION TREATMENT

The focus of burn rehabilitation is control of hypertrophic scarring to minimize joint contractures and deformities, and to

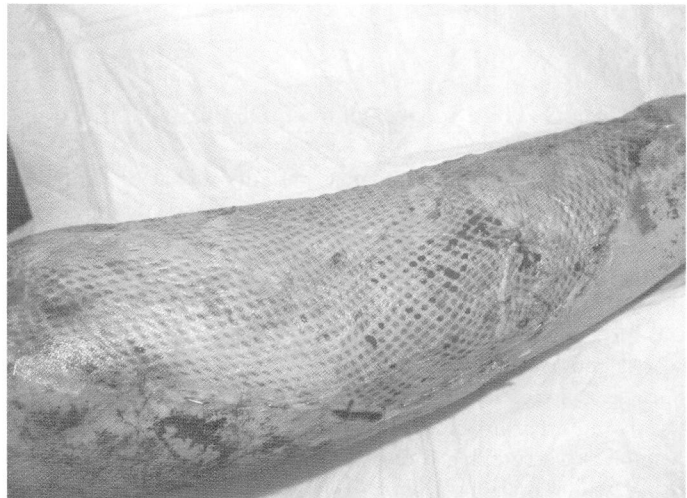

Figure 59-10 A split-thickness skin graft heals in a characteristic meshed pattern.

maximize functional outcome. In simplistic terms, the two forces at work within developing hypertrophic scars are contracting forces and raising forces. Management of these forces with modalities for applying stretch and pressure needs to be initiated early in wound healing, and must be encouraged by all team members. Excellent function can be maintained in most cases in which the burn survivor is an active participant in a continuous program of positioning and/or splinting, pressure dressings or garments, exercise, and self-care activities from the time of hospital admission. Getting an excellent outcome is challenging in burn survivors with large TBSA burns, multiple surgical procedures, medical complications, prolonged periods of immobilization, and preexisting medical conditions. These factors all contribute to scar development and functional limitations, and require intensive inpatient and outpatient rehabilitation for several months to years. The interdisciplinary burn rehabilitation team should include physical and occupational therapists to assist in the development of an individualized patient program designed to maximize function and cosmesis.

HYPERTROPHIC SCAR

Hypertrophic scar first presents as a red irritated area within a healed burn that becomes firmer to the touch than the surrounding skin (Fig. 59-11). It is usually defined as a scar that is present at three or more months after the burn injury, and is ≥2 mm in thickness. Over several weeks, it becomes a raised, 'angry' red mass that can contract and distort the surrounding skin. From a histologic standpoint, it is highly vascularized tissue, with collagen and myofibril elements oriented in whorls and nodules separated by edematous spaces. There are wide individual differences in the tightness, color, and thickness of hypertrophic scars. Peak scarring usually occurs at about 4–6 months after injury. The scar is 'mature' when it becomes pale, flat, and pliable. The time it takes to reach maturation varies from 6 months to 2 years, with an average of 1 year.

Patients considered at risk for developing hypertrophic scars include those with wounds (burns and donor sites) that take longer than 2–3 weeks to heal and patients requiring skin grafts. Scarring is typically worse in children than in adults. Little scarring has been reported in neonates, newborns, the elderly, and the morbidly obese. Heavily pigmented individuals tend to scar more than persons with less pigment. The prevalence of hypertrophic scarring has been reported at >75% in people of non-white origin and >60% in white people.[5]

Despite considerable research, the etiology of hypertrophic scarring remains unknown. One of the reasons for this lack of knowledge is that human tissue is difficult to obtain in a scientific and systematic fashion. Scars are also slow to develop and do not consistently occur. Current animal research indicates possible relationships between deep dermal burns and changes in other skin components, such as fat cells, and an increase in nerve density within hypertrophic scar tissue.[46,81]

Scar management begins with identifying people most at risk and recognizing hypertrophic scarring as early in the course of

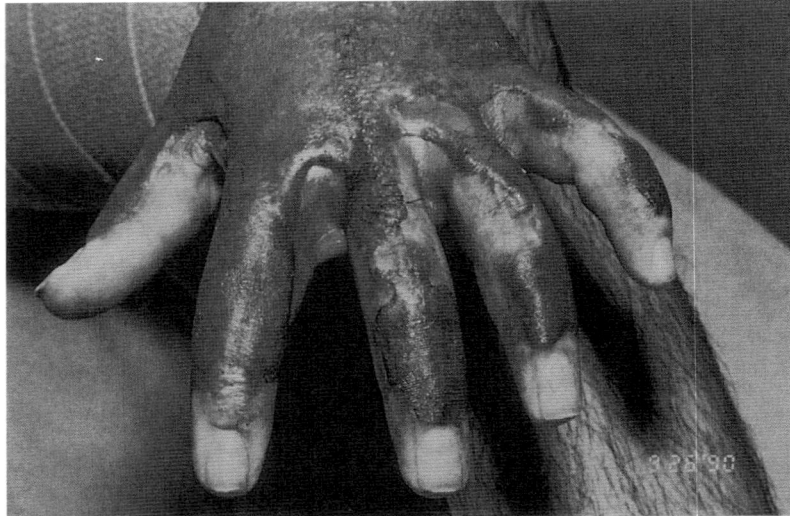

Figure 59-11 Hypertrophic scarring on the dorsum of the hand, limiting finger flexion.

treatment as possible. Contractile forces in scar tissue are treated by stretching. This can be done with exercise, positioning, and splinting. Raising forces in scar tissue are treated with pressure. This is most often done with pressure garments, pressure wraps, and splints.

PRESSURE GARMENTS

Various applications of pressure are used to flatten hypertrophic scars and provide vascular support to recently healed wounds and grafts. Initially, elastic bandages are used over bulky or wet dressings, with progression to thinner and smaller dry dressings. Tubigrip can be applied for pressure. Coban is used as an interim pressure wrap on hands and digits.

The patient can be measured for long-term custom garments when all edema has resolved. If a burn heals in less than 2–3 weeks, no long-term pressure is needed. The use of custom garments can be started when the burn is 90% healed. A thin dressing, such as dry or greasy gauze, is typically applied over the remaining open areas before the custom garment is donned. Because of the relentless nature of the scarring process, pressure garments need to be worn 23 h per day until the scar matures (Fig. 59-12). It is often very difficult to apply adequate pressure to concave areas such as the chest, nose, or axilla. Custom-fabricated inserts, made from various silicone products, foams, or thermoplastic splinting materials, can be placed between the skin and the garment to achieve sufficient contact.

The use of custom-fit pressure garments to control and minimize hypertrophic scar has been the standard of care worldwide for decades, but the practice is based on anecdotal evidence and is being challenged regarding long-term benefit. Controlled clinical studies are currently underway to determine the true efficacy of pressure in the management of burn scar.

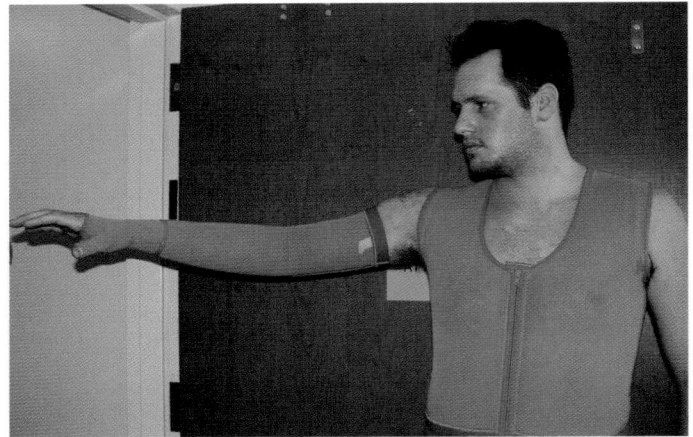

Figure 59-12 Pressure garments are used to prevent and treat hypertrophic scarring.

CONTRACTURES AND JOINT DEFORMITIES

The position of comfort for most patients is that of flexion of the joints. Maintenance of a flexed posture permits new collagen fibers in the wound to fuse together into a shortened position, resulting in contracture formation. Contracture and scar formation together can result in eventual bony subluxation if the force of the scar is unchecked. In a contracted state, burn scar is reported to function like tendon. The upper limit for burn scar elongation is approximately 16%. Consequently, scar tissue requires an excessive amount of time to elongate in response to stretching forces.[66] In addition, all underlying soft tissue will remain in a shortened state, which is particularly problematic in growing children. Typical patterns of contracture and deformities seen after burns are listed in Table 59-1.

Table 59-1 Potential impairments

Body area	Impairment
Face	Facial disfigurement (contractures of eyelids, nose, mouth, ears, and adjacent facial skin) Inability to close eyes Loss of facial expression Teeth malalignment Drooling and inability to close lips Lower lip eversion
Neck	Loss of normal cervical spine range of motion Limited visual fields Difficulties with anesthesia, due to decreased neck range of motion
Trunk	Protraction of shoulders Kyphosis Functional scoliosis Decreased respiratory function Breast entrapment Perineal banding
Axilla	Type 1: either anterior or posterior contracture Type 2: anterior and posterior contracture with sparing of dome Type 3: anterior and posterior contracture and axillary dome
Hands	Metacarpophalangeal extension deformities Wrist extension deformities Proximal interphalangeal flexion deformities Interdigital web contractures Clawing of fourth and fifth digits Thumb contractures (adduction, opposition, flexion, or extension)
Arms and legs	Antecubital banding and flexion Posterior popliteal banding and flexion Anterior hip banding and flexion Medial and lateral malleolar scarring
Foot and ankle	Hyperextension of metatarsophalangeal joints Equinovarus Cavus foot Rocker bottom deformity

(From Moore 2006,[51] with permission.)

POSITIONING

Elevation of the burned extremity is very important for edema management. This is especially critical during the resuscitation phase of recovery while fluid volumes are fluctuating, and remains important until full muscle function and activity level are restored. When a patient is resting, the burn wound should be positioned in a fully elongated state, opposite to the typical contracture position. The positions used must also minimize any additional pressure or trauma to soft tissues, such as nerve and muscle. Positioning devices might be needed to secure or encourage elevation and stretch. An example of this is an arm trough that attaches to a bed, and supports the upper extremity in abduction while elevating the hand above heart level. Patients at bed rest should be repositioned every 2 h to prevent further skin breakdown, even when high-airflow mattresses are utilized (see Ch. 33).

SPLINTING

Splinting is used for postoperative immobilization to prevent contractures and to stretch and apply pressure to scar tissue. If splinting is needed for postoperative immobilization, the splint should be applied in the operating room and remain in place for 5–7 days, depending on the thickness and status of the underlying skin graft. Maintenance splinting is no longer indicated when active range of motion (AROM) can be achieved within 5 min of beginning exercises. A night splint is indicated if it is difficult to regain range of motion on waking and moving, or if there is noticeable blanching across a joint. Long-term splinting is indicated when a burn survivor is uncooperative or has well-established movement deficits. Children might need to wear splints for several months, due to the rapid development of scar and inability to maintain end-range stretch of the scar. This is particularly true for the neck, palm, and axillary areas.

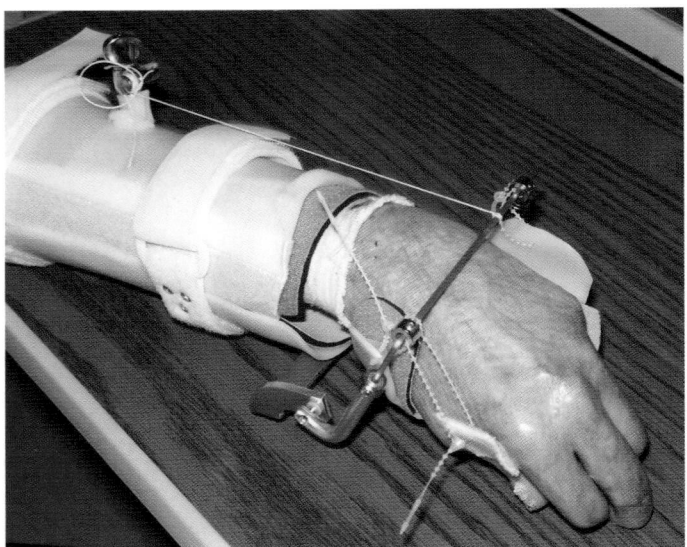

Figure 59-13 Wrist–hand splint that allows progressive wrist extension stretching and maintains finger position.

Static splints can maintain a position during immobilization after grafting, or can maintain range of motion achieved with exercise or activity. Dynamic splints provide a slow sustained stretch to scar and soft tissue (Fig. 59-13).

RANGE OF MOTION AND STRETCHING

Short and frequent exercise sessions are better than long periods. If performed frequently throughout the day, exercise and activity can be effective in countering the contractile forces that are present 24 h a day. The exercise program should be kept simple, with the focus on critical areas, moving in the direction opposite the contractile forces. In addition to stretching individual joints, combined stretching is critical if the burn crosses multiple joints, to facilitate full extensibility of the whole wound or scar. AROM is preferable to passive range of motion (PROM) whenever possible. This is because AROM causes patients to actively use their own muscles. The muscle strength of antagonistic muscles is needed to counteract the pull of contracting scar tissue. While active motion is preferred, passive movement needs to be performed on patients who are unconscious or who are unable for any reason to move independently in the end ranges. Passive stretches should be performed slowly, and never past the point of skin tightness that produces skin blanching. It is helpful to apply a cream to moisturize the skin prior to exercising. Paraffin can be useful to provide superficial heat to the scar during stretching.

STRENGTH AND CONDITIONING

Strengthening needs to start at the bedside as early in the course of treatment as possible. The patient should participate in group activities in a gym environment as soon as it is medi-

cally feasible. This facilitates interaction with other patients who are at various stages of recovery, and can serve as a great motivator. Walking exercise or the use of exercise equipment typically results in measurable improvement in cardiovascular capacity, even in the acute phase of recovery when there is relatively limited functional mobility. In addition to strengthening muscles in the involved extremities, it is functionally important to also maintain strength of muscles in the uninvolved extremities.

Large burns result in a catabolic state that leads to loss of lean body mass, which contributes to the decrease in muscle strength. There is evidence that the use of an exogenous anabolic agent such as oxandrolone can help maintain muscle mass and can be utilized, along with proper nutrition and strengthening exercises, in the rehabilitation of patients with severe burn injuries.[17,53]

AMBULATION AND MOBILITY

Bed rest for any reason incurs the risk of complications such as deep vein thrombosis and pressure sores. Burn survivors should be encouraged to be out of bed as much as possible during the day. Full weight bearing is essential for burned lower extremities, even if the sole of the foot is involved. Weight bearing requires active muscle function, which in turn activates deep venous return. Elastic wraps or Tubigrip socks are used for the vascular support of dependent extremities. Ace wraps then need to be removed if the patient is likely to remain in bed after ambulating, minimizing the risk of pressure necrosis. Unna boots can be used to protect small grafts in the lower leg for early ambulation in the first week postoperatively.[33] The focus for persons with burns or grafts to the lower extremities is to maximize movement and elevation, and limit static standing.

FUNCTIONAL TRAINING

Knowing the patient's previous daily routine is helpful in planning the appropriate treatments as hospitalization progresses. Work, leisure, completed school level, and personal interests should be incorporated into the treatment program wherever appropriate and feasible. The accomplishment of basic tasks such as feeding, grooming, and personal hygiene add to the patient's feeling of progress and self-worth. Assistive devices might be required to accomplish these activities at certain stages of recovery to enable function in an immobilized extremity, for example if the hands are both splinted postoperatively (see Ch. 27).

FACE AND NECK BURNS

In addition to the enormous emotional and psychologic implications for the patient and family, face, neck, and ear burns are both physically difficult and time-consuming to manage. The eyelids, nose, mouth, and ears are problematic areas for applying adequate stretch and pressure. In addition, a burn on the cheek or neck can cause tightness and contracture of the lower eyelid or mouth without having a wound to those areas.

The occipital area is susceptible to pressure ulceration, regardless of whether or not the patient has a burn to the scalp. It is imperative to prevent pressure on ear burns, as there is minimal soft tissue between the damaged or necrotic skin and the underlying cartilage. Patients with ear burns are at risk for development of infection or necrosis of the cartilage, with resultant loss of the outer ear. If scalp or ear burns are present, even if shallow, the patient should use egg crate foam over the scalp or ear when in bed. The use of pillows is contraindicated, because this can increase pressure on the area.

Immediate postoperative pressure has been proved to be beneficial in improving the 'take' of facial skin grafts. Custom-molded silicone masks can be fabricated while the patient is undergoing surgery, and then applied over protective gauze in the operating room at the end of the surgery. The silicone is held in place with a snug-fitting elastic 'bubble' (interim featureless face mask). This mask is removed daily by therapists for graft care by the physician. When the grafts are stable and facial edema has resolved, the patient can be fitted with a new mask. This mask can be transparent hard plastic. Regardless of the style of mask or pressure device used, the patient must be diligent in performing facial stretches and exercises to facilitate speech and eating a normal diet. Contraction of the skin around the lips can lead to microstomia, and many devices can be used to help prevent and to treat this condition. These devices are inserted into the mouth and include tongue blades or cones made of splinting material. One of the commercially available products is the Therabite (Fig. 59-14).

Preventing scar contracture in the anterior neck region is very challenging. This is due to the many planes of motion, and the amount of skin laxity at the anterior neck. Neck positioning is difficult when the patient is intubated. A neck splint is typically made in a neutral position to facilitate ambulation, rather than in as much extension as possible. This requires that hyperextension stretches of the neck be an integral part of the stretching program.

SHOULDER AND ELBOW BURNS

Gravity and the shoulder adduction position of comfort often result in shoulder contractures after axillary burns. If the upper arm or flank is the area of burn injury, shoulder contracture is possible even if the axilla is not directly burned. Brachial plexus injury is an important concern, especially when the patient is unable to identify or verbalize signs and symptoms of neural stretch or pressure (such as when under anesthesia in the operating room). The optimal splinting position for the shoulder is in 90° of abduction, in 20° of flexion, and in neutral rotation. This can be achieved with the use of an arm trough attached to the bed, or by supporting the arm on a bedside table when out of bed (Fig. 59-15). Full abduction of the shoulder is achieved only when the upper arm can contact the ear with the patient's head in midline. Simple techniques for stretch include use of overhead pulleys, wall climbing, and finger ladder exercises.

Elbow flexion and extension are readily maintained in the patient who is moving independently and is doing self-care activities. Supination range of motion at the elbow can be markedly decreased in patients who are immobilized, especially if at bed rest for long periods.

The elbow is also the primary site for heterotopic ossification (HO) formation in burn patients, particularly when a wound at the posterior elbow is not healed for several weeks. It most commonly occurs in patients with large burns who are immobile for long periods in the intensive care unit. The first symptoms of HO include the sudden and dramatic loss of range of motion, with increased pain. HO might not be evident radiologically for up to a month after onset. When HO is suspected, the patient

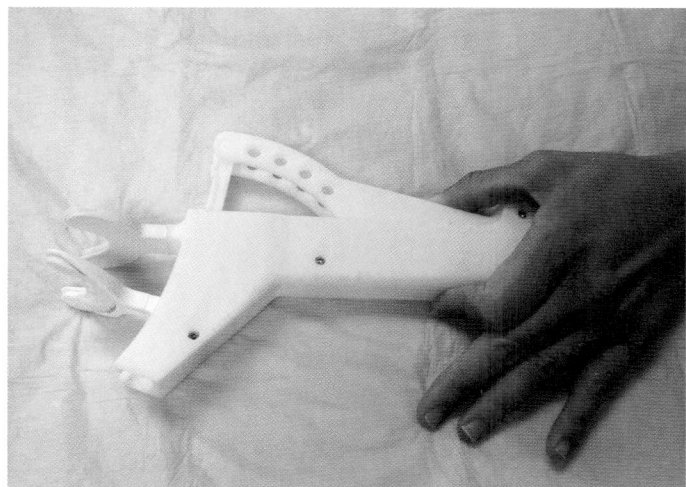

Figure 59-14 The Therabite, placed in the patient's mouth, is used to treat microstomia. The patient can use it independently.

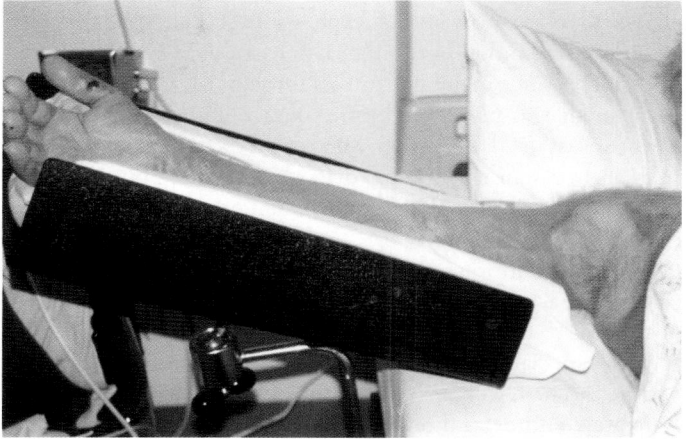

Figure 59-15 A bedside arm trough is used to position the upper extremity in 90° of abduction and 20–30° of flexion to prevent axillary contraction and protect the brachial plexus from injury.

should continue AROM, but all PROM and dynamic splinting should be discontinued.[15] Many patients ultimately require excision, especially if there is ulnar nerve entrapment.

HAND BURNS

Elevation above the heart level is critical in decreasing edema. The depth of burn and the structures involved determine the appropriate therapy. For example, if it is suspected that there is joint and/or tendon damage, PROM to the interphalangeal joints is contraindicated and protective splints should be fabricated early. Most hand burns in adults occur on the dorsal surface from flash or flame injury. If joint or deep tissue integrity is not an issue, the expectation is that the patient will recover the ability to make a full fist as soon as the edema resolves, and can then be started on a vigorous exercise program to regain range of motion and grip strength. Simple products that can facilitate stretch for hand joints include a flexion wrap to increase metacarpophalangeal joint range of motion, and a flexion strap to increase combined interphalangeal flexion. Patients should be encouraged to use their hands as normally as possible for self-care activities through all stages of healing.

Deformities often occur after severe hand burns. Postburn edema and pain can result in a claw hand deformity, with hyperextension of the metacarpophalangeal joints and proximal interphalangeal (PIP) joint flexion. A resting hand splint positions the hand in the position opposite of the claw hand deformity, with metacarpophalangeal flexion and extension of the interphalangeal joints. The extensor tendons of the hand are very superficial and are at risk of injury. A deep burn at the PIP involving the extensor tendon can result in a boutonnière deformity, with flexion of the PIP joint and extension of the distal interphalangeal (DIP) joint. Damage of the terminal slip of the extensor tendon will result in a mallet deformity characterized by loss of DIP joint extension.

The hands of infants are extremely difficult to splint and manage, due to the small size and the child's flexibility that allows them to pull out of even well-secured splints. Oversplinting is common with infants, for example a long arm cast to achieve and maintain full extension of a middle digit. Many pediatric burns are from contact injury to the palmar surface, sustained when the child reaches and grabs hot objects (e.g. an iron, curling iron, or oven door). These burns require around the clock splinting to maintain palmar and digit extension.

Careful monitoring and management of web space burns is critical. The most common complication following full-thickness burns to the dorsum of the hand is scar banding in the web spaces, especially the first web. This is typical when skin grafts end at the first web space juncture. Dressings wrap the digits separately and extend proximally into the web space. Stretching exercise by clasping the hands together, with the fingers of the opposite hand pushed all the way into the web space, should be initiated within a week of surgery. Pressure wraps such as Coban and gloves need to be precisely applied to protect fragile skin. Additional pressure in the form of molded silicone or inserts worn under gloves will minimize web space banding. When the banding is well established at the first web space, a conforming splint with the thumb in full abduction is worn at night. For the remaining web spaces, peanut-shaped inserts and a conforming glove are usually effective. If web space contractures limit function, they can be surgically repaired with Z plasty-type local flaps. In cases where the scar band extends into the palm or involves a larger area of the dorsum, another skin graft will be required for coverage of the contracture release wound.

TORSO AND HIP BURNS

Development of scoliosis and hip contractures can occur with bed rest and positioning. Splinting is usually not effective, but lying prone on a firm surface is helpful in preventing or stretching hip flexion contractures. Pillows should not be placed under the knees when the patient is lying supine. In order to facilitate elevation of the feet, the end of the bed can be elevated rather than flexing the hips.

LOWER EXTREMITY BURNS

Early positioning and weight bearing are important in the management of edema and pain, as well as in maintaining and restoring functional mobility. The three most frequent problems include foot drop, Achilles tendon shortening, and metatarsal phalangeal joint hyperextension.[69]

Peroneal nerve pressure or stretch can cause foot drop, whether or not the lower extremity is burned. Patients on bed rest should have the lower limb positioned with the knee in extension with the hip in neutral rotation. This position minimizes the risk of peroneal nerve pressure. Ankle motion can decrease even without adjacent foot burns, due to gravity and the weight of bedding. Positioning the foot against a footboard and pillow, or in a splint, then early mobilization of the patient with full weight bearing typically prevents most lower extremity contractures. Combined joint stretches of all the toe joints is needed, especially if the patient has limited AROM of the toe joints prior to the burn injury.

Stairs and gym equipment are helpful in gaining lower extremity flexibility and functional strength. Pressure support is most important in the lower extremities, as painful throbbing and graft staining can otherwise occur. Web spacers are indicated for burns extending into the toe web spaces. When deep structures are involved or partial amputations have been performed, patients might need permanent custom orthoses or prostheses.

RECONSTRUCTIVE PROCEDURES

It is crucial that patients understand that reconstructive procedures to correct scar contracture and deformity will be imperfect at best, and that optimal function and appearance come from early and consistent application of daily exercise, and the pressure and splinting program. However, with growth spurts, children can require scar releases to prevent bony deformity from the pull of the scar. The reason for this is that, as children grow, their scars do not elongate. All burn reconstructive surgeries should be planned during long-term follow-up with a burn reconstructive specialist, and completed in order of functional priority for the patient.

ELECTRICAL INJURIES

Electrical injuries are infrequent but can cause serious burn injuries. Electrical injuries account for 6–7% of all injuries in those admitted to burn units.[29,55,68] Electrical burns are usually caused by alternating current of 60 Hz, and are classified as high voltage when greater than 1000 V, or low voltage when less than 1000 V. A large number of electrical injuries are work-related. In data from the 1990s, there were about 380 deaths per year in the USA, and 5467 individuals per year missed days of work due to work-related electrical injuries.[10,73] In a series of 179 patients, 79% of the low-voltage injuries and 54% of the high-voltage injuries occurred at work.[29] A small entrance and exit point, with larger injury to deeper structures such as the muscle and nerve tissue, characterize electrical injuries. The upper limb is the most common entry point, with variable exit sites. The full extent of the injury might not be apparent immediately afterward.[27]

Electrical energy generates heat in the tissue, and the tissue resistance determines the amount of current flow. Tissues with high water content, such as nerve, muscle, and blood vessels, have lower resistance and conduct greater amount of current as compared with fat or bone. The amount of heat generated is determined by Joule's law, which is $J = I^2RT$. J is a measure of heat or power, and is determined by the square of the current (I) times the resistance (R) and the time (T) of exposure. Tissues with high resistance generate greater heat from the same current. Deeper tissues retain heat, which causes more severe injuries to deeper tissues. High-voltage injury to deeper tissues can also result in compartment syndromes requiring fasciotomies.[39]

Cardiac arrest can result in death at the scene of an electrical injury, and cardiac arrhythmias are a frequent complication after admission. Hussman found cardiac arrhythmias to be the most serious medical problem in patients admitted with low-voltage injuries (41% of patients), and arrhythmias were also seen in 29% of high-voltage injuries.[39] Ferreiro reported arrhythmias in 7% of patients admitted with high-voltage injuries.[27]

Amputation is a common complication of electrical injuries. As the size of distal extremities decrease, the current flow is focused in a smaller area, with greater heat generation and risk of severe injury. Low-voltage injuries can result in a finger or toe partial amputation, but rarely result in a more significant amputation. Major limb amputation is seen in 35% of individuals with high-voltage injuries.[39]

Neurologic injuries to the peripheral or central nervous system are common after electrical injuries. Peripheral neuropathy is reported in up to 34% of patients with high-voltage injuries, with persistence or progression in 36% of those injuries.[31] Peripheral nerve injury has also been described after low-voltage injuries, which improved with decompression. Surgical pathology shows evidence of fibrosis of the epineurium.[71]

Electrical injuries can cause damage to the central nervous system. Spinal cord injury can occur immediately or with a delayed onset of up to 1 month postinjury, with no magnetic resonance imaging (MRI) evidence of spinal cord damage.[3,6,41] In one patient who died several months after injury, an autopsy showed Wallerian degeneration below the level of the injury, with degeneration of the myelin sheaths and astrocytic gliosis consistent with a transverse myelitis.[45]

Brain injury after an electrical injury can be caused by anoxia if there is a cardiac arrest, but it can also occur without any arrhythmia. The brain injury shows MRI findings such as diffuse subcortical damage or cortical infarct,[21,28] but brain imaging is often normal. In a study of 63 patients with electrical injuries, Pliskin reported that up to 50% complained of cognitive problems, 49% of paresthesias, and 48% of headaches.[62] Other common complaints included pain, muscle twitching and spasms, difficulty walking, and balance problems.[62] Psychiatric problems such as posttraumatic stress disorder and depression have an incidence as high as 65% after electrical injuries. The rates of these problems occurring are the highest in individuals who experienced involuntary muscle contraction such that they were 'held by the current', had loss of consciousness, or were knocked away by the electrical source immediately after contact.[42]

Lightning injuries are a rare type of electrical injury caused by a very brief but high exposure to direct current. The most common neurologic consequence is due to cardiac arrest and hypoxia, but there can also be direct structural damage to the brain and spinal cord.[11,12,72,57] Davidson reported a case of an individual who developed a progressive myelopathy 1 month after a lightning strike and died 4 months postinjury. An autopsy showed myelin degeneration and edema, with axonal preservation throughout the spinal cord.[16] Lightning injuries can also result in persistent psychologic and neuropsychologic impairments.[40,52,76]

NEUROLOGIC INJURIES

Peripheral nerve injury is common after severe burn injuries but often is not diagnosed. The true incidence of peripheral nerve injuries is not known, but is reported to be as high as 30% in patients studied prospectively.[35,36,43,44,49] One study of 572 patients demonstrated a mononeuropathy or peripheral polyneuropathy in 11% of them. While the cause of the neuropathy is not clear, risk factors for the development of a mononeuropathy include an electrical injury, history of alcohol abuse, and prolonged length of stay in the intensive care unit. Risk factors for developing a polyneuropathy include age and length of stay in the intensive care unit.[44] Evidence of a peripheral neuropathy can occur within 7 days of injury.[48]

Mononeuropathy can occur due to direct thermal injury to the nerves or due to increased pressure in circumferential burns. Peripheral nerves are also at risk of injury due to compression and stretch. Dressings can cause compression to superficial peripheral nerves such as the peroneal nerve and the ulnar nerve. Proper positioning is instrumental in the prevention of nerve injury. Stretch of the peroneal nerve can occur with positioning of the patient in a frog leg position, with the hip and knee flexed and the foot inverted. The ulnar nerve is stretched in a position of elbow flexion and forearm pronation.[35]

The brachial plexus is also at risk of injury during the treatment of burns involving the upper limb and axilla. Stretching and positioning of the axilla is important to prevent shoulder contractures. If the shoulder is positioned in greater than 90° of abduction with external rotation, the brachial plexus is stretched and is at risk of injury. This can be prevented by positioning the shoulder in 30° of horizontal adduction to relieve the brachial plexus stretch.[35]

Mononeuritis multiplex has been reported in up to 56% of burn patients diagnosed with a neuropathy.[43] This includes nerves in the area of the burn injury, as well as nerves distant from the site of the burn. The cause of mononeuritis multiplex is not known but could involve occlusion of the arteries supplying the nerves.[43]

HETEROTOPIC OSSIFICATION

Heterotopic ossification is rare after burn injuries. The incidence of HO is reported to be about 1–2%, and it is most commonly found in the elbow (Fig. 59-16).[22,24,61] HO at the elbow can result in fusion of the joint or reduce elbow motion to only a few degrees. This can significantly limit independence in the activities of daily living, especially if there is bilateral involvement. Risk factors for the development of HO include large burns of >20% TBSA that usually involve the upper limb

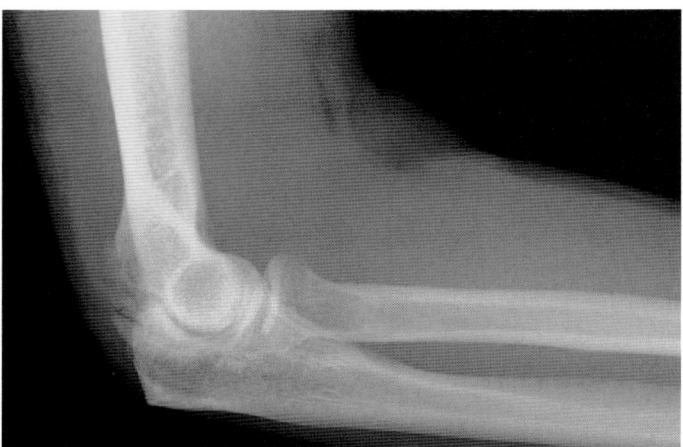

Figure 59-16 Heterotopic ossification at the medial elbow.

and region of the elbow joint. One contributing factor might be the immobilization that is necessary after excision and graft over the elbow area to allow healing before restarting range of motion exercises. Because the joint range of motion is often limited due to contracture of the injured skin, the possibility of HO needs to be considered early and diagnosed by bone scan or x-ray.

Treatment of HO involves medical management, range of motion, and surgery in some cases. The use of medications to prevent or treat HO after burn injuries with medications has not been conclusively studied, but etidronate and non-steroidal antiinflammatory medications can be used if there are no contraindications. Aggressive PROM and stretching should be avoided due to the risk of increasing the progression of the bone formation, but AROM is important for maintaining motion.[15] Positioning in full extension with the forearm supinated is useful to prevent progression.[15] HO at the elbow can result in compression of the ulnar nerve, resulting in loss of hand function in an individual who might already have hand burns.[8,77]

Surgical resection of HO is indicated in cases of severe loss of range of motion. Surgical resection is usually delayed until the bone formation is mature at 12 or more months post injury, but there are some reports of success with resection as early as several months after injury.[18,30,38,75] Aggressive postoperative treatment, including pain management, is necessary to maintain the gains in motion. In children, Gaur found that active assisted range of motion with alternating splinting in maximal flexion and maximal extension resulted in greater increases in range of motion and was better tolerated by the patients.[30] The children in this study started with an arc of motion of less than 30° and improved by an average of 57°. If necessary, children can be returned to the operating room for manipulation under anesthesia several weeks after the surgery.[30] In adults, Tsionos reported increased range of motion of over 100° with the postoperative treatment of alternating maximal flexion and extension splints for the first day followed by continuous passive motion for 8 h per day for 3–4 weeks.[75] Physical therapy was started 1 week postoperatively. Patients in this series were also treated with indomethacin. Significant recurrence with decreased range of motion occurred in 14% of the subjects, which appeared to be correlated with the patient's inability to follow the postoperative treatment program.[75]

PAIN MANAGEMENT

Pain management after burn injuries is an important part of a comprehensive treatment program. The nerve endings are partially intact in partial-thickness burns, resulting in significant pain. Full-thickness burns are initially less painful, due to complete injury to the nerve endings. In addition to the constant background pain caused by the burn injury itself, the treatment of burns with daily debridement of necrotic tissue results in intermittent procedural pain. It is important to manage both the background and procedural pain adequately for optimal patient outcome and rapport with the treatment team.

Background pain can be managed in the acute phase with a continuous infusion of morphine in the intensive care unit, patient-controlled analgesia, or long-acting opiate medications.[13,58] Procedural pain, such as that experienced in daily wound care, is controlled with short-acting opioid pain medications. This regimen typically produces adequate pain control and avoids the variations in pain and medication levels seen with providing medications on a p.r.n. basis, as requested by the patient.[58]

Non-pharmacologic methods are also very important in the management of pain. The environment of wound care should provide a calm and soothing atmosphere for the patient, giving the patient as much control as possible. Consistency in the timing, procedure, and staff involved in wound care is important to gain the patient's trust and to minimize pain. Hypnosis has been shown to reduce the need for opiate medications when used for procedural pain control.[59,60] The use of virtual reality by placing the patient in a virtual world can also reduce pain during procedures.[37]

PSYCHOLOGIC ADJUSTMENT

Individuals with burn injuries are at risk of developing symptoms of posttraumatic stress, depression, anxiety, and sleep disturbances. Posttraumatic stress symptoms such as reexperiencing the trauma, avoiding reminders of the event, and increased arousal or vigilance are frequent immediately after the injury, and are seen in up to 50% of patients at 1 month after the injury. For example, over 50% of burn injury patients report problems with recurrent and intrusive memories of the burn at 1 day and 1 month post injury. At 1 month post injury, 21% of individuals meet the diagnostic criteria for posttraumatic stress syndrome.[19,20] These symptoms decrease over time but, at 1 year after the injury, 43% report intrusive memories and 19% meet diagnostic criteria for posttraumatic stress disorder. The severity of the burn injury, as measured by the TBSA burned, was not a predictor of posttraumatic stress symptoms. The number of symptoms present at 1 day after injury was predictive of symptoms at 1 month and 1 year. It is important to recognize that many more patients report symptoms than meet diagnostic criteria for posttraumatic stress syndrome and might benefit from treatment.[20]

Depression is also common after burn injuries. Ptacek reports rates of moderate or severe depression symptoms in over 50% of patients early in their hospitalization. This tended to decrease during the course of the hospital stay.[65] Wiechman followed patients after a burn injury and found rates of moderate to severe depression in 45% at 2 years post injury.[78] It is important to recognize symptoms of stress and depression after burn injuries and to provide appropriate treatment, including pharmacologic treatment.

Several studies have reported that the severity of the burn injury is not a significant predictor of psychologic adjustment after a burn injury.[20,65,78] Willebrand found that coping strategies used by individuals after burn injuries are predictive of psychologic health.[79] The use of avoidant coping strategies, such as attempting to block out thoughts about the injury, was predictive of poorer psychologic health at 3 months after injury. On the other hand, self-control or holding back expressions of emotions resulted in fewer psychologic symptoms.[79] As in other studies,[20] increased psychologic symptoms early after a burn injury were predictive of greater problems later in the recovery.[79]

COMMUNITY REINTEGRATION

The ultimate goal of a rehabilitation program is to return the patient to their previous work, school, and recreational and community activities. Burn injuries can result in significant contractures, amputations, scars, and other conditions that produce permanent impairments. Psychologic sequellae can also limit community integration after a burn injury. Examination of community integration using the Community Integration Questionnaire demonstrated significant problems in the areas of home integration, social integration, and productivity.[23] The productivity scale, which measures work, school, and volunteer activities, was best predicted by the patient's age, severity of burn injury, and preinjury job satisfaction.[23] A study by Brych, of individuals who were working at the time of their burn injury, found that 66% were working at a 6-month follow-up and 90% were employed at 2 years. The mean time off from work was 17 weeks. Predictors of not returning to work included a psychiatric history, a burn to an extremity, and the size of the burn.[9]

Fauerbach studied 770 patients after a severe burn injury, and found that 70% were working outside the home at the time of the injury, and that 30% of the injuries occurred at work.[26] In the subjects who were employed at the time of the injury, 42% of the injuries happened at work. Those individuals who were unemployed at the time of injury had a higher incidence of preexisting physical disability, history of psychiatric treatment, and positive alcohol screen at admission. Employed individuals were more likely to sustain a hand burn and have hand surgery. Unemployed individuals were more likely to have an inhalation injury and report psychologic distress.[26] The large number of comorbid conditions in the group not employed at the time of injury can limit the success of a vocational rehabilitation program. Individuals injured at work often present unique challenges in regard to having fear of the workplace or of returning to the place of the injury.

CONCLUSION

The overall incidence of burn injuries in the USA has recently declined, but advances in acute care management have resulted in increased survival of individuals with severe burn injuries. These individuals have complex and long-term rehabilitation needs due to contractures, joint deformities, amputations, neurologic impairments, and psychologic problems. Rehabilitation starts at the time of admission with positioning, splinting, and passive or active exercise. This early rehabilitation intervention is a coordinated part of the acute-care burn team and can minimize long-term complications. An interdisciplinary rehabilitation team is important to manage the long-term consequences of burn injuries. Long-term interventions should be focused on treating psychologic issues and maximizing physical function and community reintegration.

REFERENCES

1. Achauer BM, Eriksson E. Plastic surgery indications, operations and outcomes. St. Louis: Mosby; 2000.
2. American Burn Association. Burn incidence and treatment in the US: 2000 fact sheet. Online. Available: http://www.ameriburn.org/pub/BurnIncidenceFactSheet.htm
3. Arevalo JM, Lorente JA, Balseiro-Gomex J. Spinal cord injury after electrical trauma treated in a burn unit. Burns 1999; 25(5):449–452.
4. Artz CP, Moncrief JA, Pruitt BA. Burns: a team approach. Philadelphia: Saunders; 1979.
5. Bombaro KM, Engrav LH, Carrougher GJ, et al. What is the prevalence of hypertrophic scarring following burns? Burns 2003; 29:299–302.
6. Breugem CC, Van Hertum W, Groenevelt F. High voltage electrical injury leading to a delayed onset tetraplegia, with recovery. Ann NY Acad Sci 1999; 888:131–136.
7. Brigham PA, McLoughlin E. Burn incidence and medical care use in the United States: estimates, trends and data sources. J Burn Care Rehabil 1996; 17:95–107.
8. Brooke MM, Heard DL, deLateur BJ, et al. Heterotopic ossification and peripheral nerve entrapment: early diagnosis and excision. Arch Phys Med Rehabil 1991; 72:425–429.
9. Brych SB, Engrav LH, Rivara FP, et al. Time off work and return to work rates after burns: systematic review of the literature and a large two-center series. J Burn Care Rehabil 2001; 22:401–405.
10. Cawley JC, Homce GT. Occupational electrical injuries in the United States, 1992–1998, and recommendations for safety research. J Safety Res 2003; 34(3):241–248.
11. Cherington M, Yarnell P, Hallmark D. MRI in lightning encephalopathy. Neurology 1993; 43:1437–1438.
12. Cherington M. Neurologic manifestations of lightning strikes. Neurology 2003; 60:182–185.
13. Choiniere M, Grenier R, Paquette C. Patient-controlled analgesia: a double-blind study in burn patients. Anaesthesia 1992; 47(6):467–472.
14. Committee on Trauma. Guidelines for the operation of burn units. Resources for optimal care of the injured patient. Chicago: American College of Surgeons; 1999.
15. Crawford CM, Varghese G, Mani MM, et al. Heterotopic ossification: are range of motion exercises contraindicated? J Burn Care Rehabil 1986; 7:323–327.
16. Davidson GS, Deck JH. Delayed myelopathy following lightning strike: a demyelinating process. Acta Neuropathol 1988; 77(1):104–108.
17. Demling RH, DeSanti L. Oxandrolone induced lean mass gain during recovery from severe burns in maintained after discontinuation of the anabolic steroid. Burns 2003; 29:793–797.
18. Djurickovic S, Meek RN, Snelling CF, et al. Range of motion and complications after postburn heterotopic bone excision about the elbow. J Trauma 1996; 41(5):825–830.
19. Ehde DM, Patterson DR, Wiechman SA, et al. Post-traumatic stress symptoms and distress following acute burn injury. Burns 1999; 25:587–592.
20. Ehde DM, Patterson DR, Wiechman SA, et al. Post-traumatic stress symptoms and distress 1 year after burn injury. J Burn Care Rehabil 2000; 21(2):105–111.
21. Eldad A, Neuman A, Weinberg A, et al. Late onset of extensive brain damage and hypertension in a patient with high-voltage electrical burns. J Burn Care Rehabil 1992; 13:214–217.
22. Elledge ES, Smith AA, McManus WF, et al. Heterotopic bone formation in burned patients. J Trauma 1988; 28(5):684–687.
23. Esselman PC, Ptacek JT, Kowalske K, et al. Community integration after burn injuries. J Burn Care Rehabil 2001; 22:221–227.
24. Evans EB. Heterotopic bone formation in thermal burns. Clin Orthop Relat Res 1991; 263:94–101.
25. Fauerbach JA, Engrav L, Kowalske K, et al. Barriers to employment among working-aged patient with major burn injuries. J Burn Care Rehabil 2001; 22:26–34.
26. Fauerbach JA, Engrav L, Kowalske K, et al. Barriers to employment among working-aged patients with major burn injury. J Burn Care Rehabil 2001; 22:26–34.
27. Ferreiro I, Melendez J, Regalado J, et al. Factors influencing the sequelae of high tension electrical injuries. Burns 1998; 24:649–653.
28. Gans M, Glaser JS. Homonymous hemianopsia following electrical injury. J Clin Neuroophthalmol 1986; 6:218–221.
29. Garcia-Sanchez V, Morell PG. Electric burns: high- and low-tension injuries. Burns 1999; 25:357–360.
30. Gaur A, Sinclair M, Caruso I, et al. Heterotopic ossification around the elbow following burns in children: results after excision. J Bone Joint Surg 2003; 85:1538–1543.
31. Grube BJ, Heimbach DM, Engrav LH, et al. Neurologic consequences of electrical burns. J Trauma 1990; 30:254–258.
32. Han H, Mustoe TA. Structure and function of skin. In: Achauer BM, Eriksson E, eds. Plastic surgery indications, operations and outcomes. St. Louis: Mosby; 2000:23–35.
33. Harnar T, Engrav LH, Marvin JA, et al. Dr. Paul Unna's boot and early ambulation after skin grafting the leg: a survey of burn centers and a report of 20 cases. Plast Reconstr Surg 1982; 69:359–360.
34. Heimbach DM, Warden GD, Luterman A, et al. Multicenter postapproval clinical trial of Integra dermal regeneration template for burn treatment. J Burn Care Rehabil 2003; 24:42–48.
35. Helm PA, Pandian G, Heck E. Neuromuscular problems in the burn patient: cause and prevention. Arch Phys Med Rehabil 1985; 66:451–453.
36. Henderson B, Koepke GH, Feller I. Peripheral polyneuropathy among patients with burns. Arch Phys Med Rehabil 1971; 52:149–151.
37. Hoffman HG, Doctor JN, Patterson DR, et al. Use of virtual reality as an adjunctive treatment of adolescent burn pain during wound care: a case report. Pain 2000; 85(1–2):305–309.
38. Holguin PH, Rico AA, Garcia JP, et al. Elbow anchylosis due to postburn heterotopic ossification. J Burn Care Rehabil 1996; 17:150–154.
39. Hussmann J, Kucan JO, Russell RC, et al. Electrical injuries—morbidity, outcome and treatment rationale. Burns 1995; 7:530–535.
40. Janus TJ, Barrash J. Neurologic and neurobehavioral effects of electric and lightning injuries. J Burn Care Rehabil 1996; 17:409–415.
41. Kalita J, Jose M, Misra UK. Myelopathy and amnesia following accidental electrical injury. Spinal Cord 2002; 40:253–255.
42. Kelley KM, Tkachenko TA, Pliskin NH, et al. Life after electrical injury. Risk factors for psychiatric sequelae. Ann NY Acad Sci 1999; 888:356–363.
43. Khedr EM, Khedr T, el-Oteify MA, et al. Peripheral neuropathy in burn patients. Burns 1997; 23:579–583.
44. Kowalske K, Holavanahalli R, Helm P. Neuropathy after burn injury. J Burn Care Rehabil 2001; 22:353–357.
45. Levine NS, Atkins A, McKeel DW Jr, et al. Spinal cord injury following electrical accidents: case reports. J Trauma 1975; 15:459–463.
46. Liang Z, Engrav LH, Muangman P, et al. Nerve quantification in female red Duroc pig (FRDP) scar compared to human hypertrophic scar. Burns 2004; 30:57–64.
47. Lund CC, Browder NC. Estimation of areas of burns. Surg Gynecol Obstet 1944; 79:352–358.
48. Margherita AJ, Robinson LR, Heimbach DM, et al. Burn-associated peripheral polyneuropathy: a search for causative factors. Am J Phys Med Rehabil 1995; 74(1):28–32.
49. Marquez S, Turley JE, Peters WJ. Neuropathy in burn patients. Brain 1993; 116:471–483.
50. Monafo WW, Bessey PQ. Wound care. In: Herndon DN, ed. Total burn care. 2nd edn. New York: Saunders; 2002:109–119.
51. Moore M. The burn unit. In: Campbell SK, Vander Linden DW, Palisano RJ, eds. Physical therapy for children. 3rd edn. Philadelphia: Saunders; 2006.

52. Muehlberger T, Vogt PM, Munster AM. The long-term consequences of lightning injuries. Burns 2001; 23:829–833.

53. Murphy KD, Thomas S, Mlcak RP, et al. Effects of long-term oxandrolone administration in severely burned children 2004; 136:219–224.

54. National Center for Health Statistics. Health, United States 1996–97 and injury chartbook. Hyattsville: NCHS; 1997.

55. National Institute for Disability and Rehabilitation Research. NIDRR model systems for burn injury rehabilitation: adult facts and figures. February 2004. Online. Available: http://bms-dcc.uchsc.edu/

56. National Institute for Disability and Rehabilitation Research. NIDRR model systems for burn injury rehabilitation: child facts and figures. February 2004. Online. Available: http://bms-dcc.uchsc.edu/

57. Ozgun B, Castillo M. Basal ganglia hemorrhage related to lightning strike. AJNR Am J Neuroradiol 1995; 16:1370-1371.

58. Patterson D, Sharar S. Burn pain. In: Loeser J, ed. Bonica's management of pain. 3rd edn. Philadelphia: Lippincott Williams & Wilkins; 2001:780–787.

59. Patterson DR, Jensen M. Hypnosis and clinical pain. Psychol Bull 2003; 129(4):495–521.

60. Patterson DR, Ptacek JT. Baseline pain as a moderator of hypnotic analgesia for burn injury treatment. J Consult Clin Psychol 1997; 65(1):60–67.

61. Peterson SL, Mani MM, Crawford CM, et al. Postburn heterotopic ossification: insights for management decision making. J Trauma 1989; 29(3):365–369.

62. Pliskin NH, Capelli-Schellpfeffer M, Law RT, et al. Neuropsychological symptom presentation after electrical injury. J Trauma 1998; 44(4):709–715.

63. Pruitt BA Jr, Goodwin CW, Mason AD. Epidemiological, demographic, and outcome characteristics of burn injury. In: Herndon, DN, ed. Total burn care. 2nd edn. New York: Saunders; 2002:16–30.

64. Pruitt BA Jr, Goodwin CW, Mason AD. Epidemiological, demographic, and outcome characteristics of burn injury. In: Herndon DN, ed. Total burn care. 2nd edn. New York: Saunders; 2002.

65. Ptacek JT, Patterson DR, Heimbach DM. Inpatient depression in persons with burns. J Burn Care Rehabil 2002; 23:1-9.

66. Richard RL, Staley MJ. Biophysical aspects of normal skin and burn scar. In: Burn care and rehabilitation. Philadelphia: FA Davis; 1994.

67. Ryan CM, Schoenfeld DA, Malloy M, et al. Use of Integra artificial skin is associated with decreased length of stay for severely injured adult burn survivors. J Burn Care Rehabil 2002; 23:311–317.

68. Saffle JR, Davis B, Williams P. Recent outcomes in the treatment of burn injury in the United States: a report from the American Burn Association patient registry. J Burn Care Rehabil 1995; 16:219–232.

69. Serghiou MA, Evans EB, Ott S, et al. Comprehensive rehabilitation of the burned patient. In: DN Herndon, ed. Total burn care. 2nd edn. New York: Saunders; 2002:563–592.

70. Sheridan RL, Tompkins RG. Alternative wound coverings. In: Herndon DN, ed. Total burn care. 2nd edn. New York: Saunders; 2002:212–218.

71. Smith MA, Muehlberger T, Dellon AL. Peripheral nerve compression associated with low-voltage electrical injury without associated significant cutaneous burn. Plast Reconstr Surg 2002; 109:137–144.

72. Stanley LD, Suss RA. Intracerebral hematoma secondary to lightning stroke: case report and review of the literature. Neurosurgery 1985; 16:686–688.

73. Taylor AJ, McGwin G, Valent F, et al. Fatal occupational electrocutions in the United States. Inj Prev 2002; 8:306–312.

74. Thomas S, Barrow RE, Herndon DN. History of the treatment of burns. In: Herndon DN, ed. Total burn care. 2nd edn. New York: Saunders; 2002:1–10.

75. Tsionos I, Leclercq C, Rochet JM. Heterotopic ossification of the elbow in patients with burns. Results after early excision. J Bone Joint Surg Br 2004; 86(3):396–403.

76. Van Zomeren AH, ten Duis HJ, Minderhoud JM, et al. Lightning stroke and neuropsychological impairment: cases and questions. J Neurol Neurosurg Psychiatry 1998; 64:763–769.

77. Vorenkamp SE, Nelson TL. Ulnar nerve entrapment due to heterotopic bone formation after a severe burn. J Hand Surg 1987; 12:378–380.

78. Wiechman SA, Ptacek JT, Patterson DR, et al. Rates, trends, and severity of depression after burn injuries. J Burn Care Rehabil 2001: 22;417–424.

79. Willebrand M, Andersson G, Ekselius L. Prediction of psychological health after an accidental burn. J Trauma 2004; 57:367–374.

80. Williams WG. Pathophysiology of the burn wound. In: Herndon DN, ed. Total burn care. 2nd edn. New York: Saunders; 2002:514–522.

81. Zhu KQ, Engrav LH, Gibran NS, et al. The female red Duroc pig as an animal model of hypertrophic scarring and the potential role of the cones of skin. Burns 2003; 29:649–664.

Chapter

60

Geriatric Rehabilitation

Rina M. Bloch

Geriatric rehabilitation focuses on the symptoms and function of aging individuals. The elderly are not a homogenous group. There are differences between age groups, such as can be seen between 65- and 85-year-olds. There are also differences between the healthy and the ill, just as one sees in younger age groups. Normal aging should be distinguished from the sequelae of illness.

One can approach geriatric rehabilitation from a purely functional perspective, looking not so much at the pathophysiology, but rather at the resulting disability. Limited ability to reach overhead can cause difficulty in safely getting items down from kitchen cabinets. Weak trunk extensors can interfere with picking up a heavy load of laundry. Tight hip extensors can impede gait efficiency, such that the person cannot walk rapidly enough to cross the street while the traffic light signals say 'walk'.

Aging with a disability is a separate and challenging issue. While the physiologic insult and impairment might have been sustained years before, a patient's capacity to cope and compensate can change with age. Changes that occur over the course of time in health, or in psychosocial supports, can have a negative impact on mobility, self-care, and pain.

Geriatric rehabilitation addresses problems that have an impact not only on the individual patient, but also on society at large. There are major economic ramifications when individuals can no longer care for themselves. Increased longevity, with an increase in the absolute numbers of elderly, has increased the impact on society. There have been increases in life expectancy in a number of countries. The average life expectancy at age 65 in the USA is currently 17 years.[85]

FRAILTY

Frailty can be defined as age- and disease-related loss of adaptation, such that events of previously minor stress result in disproportionate biomedical and social consequences.[84] Frailty is difficult to quantify, but it is the generalized decline in multiple systems with the loss of functional reserve.[36] In an attempt to more precisely measure frailty, one can measure mobility, balance, muscle strength, motor processing, cognition, nutrition, endurance, and physical activity.[36] A potential pitfall of these measurements is that people perceive functional difficul-

ties at differing thresholds. These thresholds are influenced by both social environment and economic status. Perceived abilities can also be different than actual performance. Quality of life instruments developed on younger patients might have poor reliability and validity in elderly people with multiple health problems.[36] The body maintains itself in homeostasis. What might be a minor perturbation in a younger individual can trigger a much larger set of problems in an older person. For example, a urinary tract infection in an older person can lead to confusion, with a subsequent fall and hip fracture. Frailty, despite the difficulty one may have in quantifying it, is a concept that clinicians can recognize.

CHANGES IN THE BODY WITH AGING

There are changes in multiple systems in the body that are part of normal aging. It is often difficult to determine which of these changes are due to the natural process of aging and which are due to disuse and secondary factors. Certain changes, such as declines in visual acuity and hearing, are well defined as aging phenomena. Other changes, such as the development of weakness, are still being defined and studied.

Sarcopenia

Sarcopenia is the loss of muscle mass and strength with aging.[56,91] There is a loss of the number of myocytes and a reduction of the protein content of the remaining muscle cells. Muscle strength decreases with aging at the level of single muscle fibers and force per unit area. Protein synthesis decreases, especially myosin heavy chain, with a disproportionate atrophy of Type 2a (fast-twitch) fibers.[77] Decreased myosin concentration can play a key role, with slower shortening velocity of single muscle fibers.[31]

Sarcopenia is probably driven by a combination of catabolic action and a reduction in anabolic influences.[91] There is an increase in catabolic cytokines, such as tumor necrosis factor-α, interleukin (IL)-6, IL receptor antagonist, and IL-1β. Anabolic stimuli decrease, including estrogen, testosterone, growth hormone, protein intake, physical activity, and central nervous system input to promote movement.[91] In both healthy and frail elderly, it is the Type 2 fast-twitch fibers that are lost.[100] α Motor neuron dropout occurs with a reduced number in the elderly. Sarcopenia does not typically cause a decrease in body weight, because the percentage of fat increases.[20]

The role of cytokines in mediating muscle mass and strength is just beginning to be understood. For example, in a cross-sectional analysis on 617 women aged 70–79 years, a decline in insulin-like growth factor-1 was associated with poor knee extensor strength, slow walking speed, and self-reported disability.[23] In a cross-sectional study of 3075 adults aged 70–79, the inflammatory markers C-reactive protein and IL-6 were lower in those who had higher levels of exercise and in those who used antioxidant supplements regardless of exercise status.[26] It is known that adipose tissue has its own metabolic activity, including the secretion of inflammatory factors.[110] Increases in body fat might facilitate inflammation, with a differing role played by abdominal fat versus fat in the extremities.[110]

In a study of 120 men and women aged 46–79 who were observed over a 10-year period,[56] women had slower rates of decline in elbow flexors and extensors (2% per decade) compared with men (12% per decade). Knee extensor strength decreased by 14% per decade, and knee flexor strength by 16% per decade in both men and women.

Gait changes

From 8 to 19% of non-institutionalized older adults have difficulty walking, and this increases to 67% of nursing home residents.[4] Gait speed typically declines at the rate of 0.2% per year up to age 63, and then 1.6% after age 63 in older adults who are relatively free of neurologic, cognitive, or cardiovascular problems.[4] Conditions associated with faster gait speed include greater hip extension, ankle dorsiflexion, and plantar flexion range of motion.[4]

Gait in the elderly is characterized by increased double-limb support, as well as slower speed, shorter stride length, and a broader base of support. Pelvic rotation decreases and postural responses are slower. Gait has been studied in order to identify factors associated with falling in the elderly (Boxes 60-1 and 60-2). In the subset of older people who fall, there is increased

---

Box 60-1 Gait factors associated with falling in the elderly[53,74]

- Increased stride to stride variability in length
- Increased stride to stride variability in speed
- Increased time of double-support phase

Box 60-2 Risk factors for falls in the elderly[34]

- Use of sedatives, antidepressants, or antipsychotic medications
- Absolute number of medications taken
- Poor balance
- Hip weakness
- Poor functional status

---

stride to stride variability in gait.[53,73] Maki found that reduced stride length, reduced speed, and increased double-support time are associated with fear of falling. His study also showed that increased stride to stride variability in length, speed, and double support were associated with falling. Stride to stride variability was the best single predictor of falling.[73] In another study of elderly women with a mean age of 75, the peak ankle dorsiflexion power had strong associations with stair climb time and chair rise time. Plantar flexion isometric strength was strongly associated with habitual and maximal gait velocity.[104] Grabiner's study also showed that when young and elderly 'non-fallers' were studied, the older subjects had significantly larger stride width variability.[50]

Osteopenia and osteoporosis

The elderly have an increased incidence of osteopenia and osteoporosis. Osteopenia is defined as bone mineral density more than one standard deviation below the young adult level (T < −1 but > −2.5). Osteoporosis is present if the T score is < −2.5.[83] Risk factors for osteopenia and osteoporosis include age, family history, glucocorticoid therapy, and smoking.[83,102]

Osteoarthritis

Degenerative joint disease becomes much more common in the aged. Arthritis affects over 60% of women and 50% of men who are 70 and older.[12] The reported incidence and prevalence of osteoarthritis varies depending on whether one uses radiologic findings, clinical symptoms, or a combination to define cases.[67] For example, limitations in range of motion can go unreported in some instances, because the older person might be unaware that range of motion has declined due to its gradual progression.[94]

Osteoarthritis is the most prevalent articular disease in adults 65 and older.[67] Because there is a strong association with aging, attempts have been made to determine if osteoarthritis is a distinct disease.[67] In osteoarthritis, there are differences in the water content ratio of certain cartilage constituents, and an increase in degradative enzyme activity compared with in non-osteoarthritis joints. It is possible that the reduction in chondrocyte density with aging leaves cartilage vulnerable to degeneration and osteoarthritis.[67]

Changes in special senses

Vision declines with age. The lens has less adaptation. Macular degeneration, cataracts, and glaucoma become more prevalent with age. Decreased auditory acuity frequently develops. The usual pattern is a loss of higher frequencies; people with this type of hearing loss can hear speech but have difficulty understanding it.[41] With hearing loss progression, the lower frequencies are affected also, making it difficult to understand vowels and what is being said, especially in a loud setting.[41]

Cardiovascular changes

With aging, the cardiovascular system has decreased arterial compliance, increased systolic blood pressure, left ventricular hypertrophy, decreased baroreceptor sensitivity, and decreased sinoatrial node automaticity.[85] The exercise-induced adaptations that occur in younger people, such as increased peripheral arteriovenous oxygen difference, increased cardiac size, stroke work, cardiac output, and left ventricle function,[2] are not as available to the elderly. Older patients with coronary artery disease have age-related increases in left ventricular and arterial wall stiffness and thickening, which limit some adaptations with conditioning.[2] In the operative setting, maintaining intravascular volume is important, because the aged heart depends on preload more than in the younger person. Because after-load is increased by outflow tract stiffness, there is decreased sensitivity to catecholamines and impaired vasoconstrictive responses in the elderly.[90]

Pulmonary changes

Lung compliance increases and thoracic wall mobility decreases in the elderly, with a 20% increase in the effort needed to overcome elastic resistance.[40] Vital capacity typically decreases 40–50% by age 70.[40] The net effect is that, during exertion, the elderly must rely on increased respiratory frequency rather than increased tidal volume.[40]

Genitourinary changes

Renal blood flow decreases with age,[19,25] as does glomerular filtration rate.[85] A 50-kg woman with a serum creatinine level of 1.0 mg/dL has a calculated creatinine clearance of 62 mL/min if she is 35 years old, but only 32 mL/min if she is 85 years old.[25] Because serum creatinine reflects muscle mass, a normal serum creatinine level can be seen even with a reduced glomerular filtration rate.[19] Urinary incontinence can develop on the basis of stress, or due to overflow secondary to prostatic hypertrophy. Increased collagen content causes decreased bladder distensibility.[90] Decreased estrogen predisposes to incontinence by causing urethral sphincter changes.[90] Mechanical blockage of outflow by an enlarged prostate can impede bladder emptying. Subjective thirst decreases in the elderly, which can negatively affect fluid balance.[90]

Gastrointestinal changes

Dysphagia can develop due to dental problems or achalasia. The time from pharyngeal entry of food to laryngeal elevation increases.[35] Alterations in taste also affect nutrition. Stomach acid decreases, with subsequent impaired absorption of vitamin B_{12}, calcium, iron, zinc, and folic acid.[89,101] Thirst sensation is impaired and gut motility decreases. Hepatic metabolism is altered, with corresponding changes in drug clearance. The potency and duration of action of some drugs are increased.[19] Hepatic blood flow decreases 12–40% in the elderly, and liver size decreases, with a resulting reduction in first-pass metabolism of drugs.[25] Impairment of normal liver function can also alter how a drug is treated in the liver, as drug interactions can alter liver enzymes and subsequent drug processing.[19] Malnutrition affects the elderly differently than in the younger patient. Elderly patients (mean age 79) were compared with middle-aged (mean age 48) in a group with chronic malnutrition. The middle-aged patients lost fat mass, fat-free mass, and body cell mass in equal proportions, but the elderly patients proportionally lost more fat-free mass and body cell mass. Thus the elderly were proportionately losing more from muscle and other body organs, which could affect outcomes.[95]

Endocrine changes

Changes in the endocrine system can cause deterioration in glucose tolerance. Hormonal changes that typically occur include decreased estrogen, testosterone, and growth hormone. Temperature regulation is impaired.[90] End-organ responsiveness to medications can be different in the elderly, but this is just beginning to be explored.[45] There is an age-related decline in immune function, which in some studies has been improved with vitamin supplements.[89]

Skin changes

Skin fragility increases with age. This is due to a combination of decreased moisture content, elasticity, blood supply, and sensory sensitivity. These changes increase the risk of injury to the skin in the elderly, including pressure sores.

DISEASES THAT ARE MORE COMMON IN THE ELDERLY

Changes with normal aging can progress to the point that one is classified as having a disease, such as abnormal glucose tolerance evolving to diabetes mellitus. Diseases with increased incidence and prevalence in the elderly include cardiovascular disease, stroke, diabetes, vitamin B_{12} deficiency, thrombocytosis, polycythemia vera, and cervical and lumbar spinal stenosis. Degenerative joint disease becomes more frequent, in the spine and in the limbs. Motor neuron disease, peripheral neuropathy, and dementia all increase in incidence and prevalence in the elderly.

Parkinson disease

Parkinson disease is present in 1% of people older than 65,[7] and clinically manifests with tremor, rigidity, and bradykinesia (see Ch. 52). Twenty percent of patients with Parkinson disease also develop dementia.[15] The tremor is present at rest and increases with stress.[7] Voluntary movement is slow. Gait is characterized by small shuffling steps, without arm swing. It is difficult for the patient to initiate walking or other position changes.[7] The gait can be festinating, in which gait speed increases as the patient attempts to prevent falling forward due to an abnormal center of gravity. Turning is particularly difficult and unsteady.[7]

Dementia

Dementia is found in 1.5% of people aged 65–70 years, and increases to 25% of people 85 years of age and older.[90] The most common causes of dementia in the elderly are Alzheimer disease, vascular (multiinfarct) dementia, diffuse white matter changes (also called Binswanger dementia), alcoholism, Parkinson disease, and drug or medication intoxication.[15]

> **Box 60-3** Risk factors for delirium (acute confusional state)
>
> - Baseline dementia or preoperative cognitive impairment
> - Age
> - Poor functional status
> - Alcohol use
> - Polypharmacy
> - Undertreated pain
> - Intraoperative blood loss, with postoperative hematocrit < 30

Depression must always be differentiated from dementia in the elderly.[103] Dementia should also be differentiated from benign forgetfulness of the elderly. The work-up for dementia typically includes checking vitamin B_{12}, thyroid functions, electrolytes, complete blood count, serology for syphilis, and brain imaging. Depending on the setting, one might also need to do a urine toxicology screen, lumbar puncture, and a general medical work-up. AIDS can also produce dementia in the elderly. If there is a history of falls or the patient is on anticoagulants, subdural hematoma should be ruled out. Infections should be ruled out. The adverse side effects of medications can sometimes include dementia, and depression can masquerade as dementia.

Dementia must be differentiated from acute confusion. Delirium is an acute confusional state with a fluctuating time course, with impaired cognition, attention, and level of consciousness.[58] Neurologists prefer the term *acute confusional state*.[88] Inattention and disorientation are the primary early signs, with a defect in attention. There can be drowsiness as well. The patient has decreased mental clarity, coherence, comprehension, and reasoning.[88] It can be clinically challenging to determine what is chronic and what is new when an elderly patient presents with confusion in the postoperative setting, because baseline dementia is the major risk factor for delirium (Box 60-3).[90] Risk factors include age, preoperative cognitive impairment, poor functional status, alcohol use, and polypharmacy.[90] In the postoperative period, under-treated pain can lead to delirium.[90] Intraoperative blood loss and postoperative hematocrit less than 30% are associated with an increased risk of postoperative delirium.[90]

Approximately 10% of people over 70 have significant memory loss, and in more than half of the cases this is attributed to Alzheimer disease.[14] The prevalence is 1% among those aged 60–64 years, and 40% of those aged 85 and older.[29] Alzheimer dementia typically progresses slowly over several years. Confrontation naming of items to command is typically impaired early in the course.[14] Patients have difficulty learning and recalling new information, and there is a progressive language disorder.[29] Visuospatial skills are disturbed.[29] Executive function skills are impaired, including planning, judgment, and insight.[29] Apraxia with sequential motor tasks can occur.[14] Alzheimer dementia can also feature delusions and hallucinations.[14] There

is a loss of social inhibitions and disturbed sleep–wake cycle.[14] A shuffling gait with rigidity can develop.[14] The disease typically has an 8- to 10-year duration. The pathologic features typically include plaques with amyloid and neurofibrillary tangles in the neuronal cytoplasm.

Normal pressure hydrocephalus

The hallmark signs of normal pressure hydrocephalus are dementia, gait disturbance, and urinary incontinence.[15] Normal pressure hydrocephalus can be idiopathic or related to prior meningitis or subarachnoid hemorrhage.[15] The reduced physical turgor of the brain tissue with aging is felt by some experts to allow even normal pressure to produce hydrocephalus and brain atrophy. In some cases, the patient's condition can be dramatically reversed by shunting to achieve a reduction in central nervous system fluid pressure.

Cancer

The incidence and prevalence of most malignancies increase with age up to at least age 85.[10] The increasing incidence could be due to the length of time for a carcinogenic factor to take effect, as well as molecular changes occurring with aging that can favor certain cancers.[10] Tumors can behave differently in older patients than in those who are younger, and this has to be kept in mind when designing a treatment plan.[10]

Osteoarthritis

Osteoarthritis is the major disease that limits activity in the elderly.[87] Risk factors are increased age, obesity, quadriceps weakness, impaired proprioception, heavy physical activity, lack of estrogen replacement in women, and knee injuries (see Ch. 37).[87]

Traumatic brain injury and spinal cord injury

Older patients sustain more traumatic brain injury and spinal cord injury in domestic falls than younger patients do (see Chs 50 and 56).[87] Patients older than 50 years of age typically require longer lengths of hospitalization for these injuries, with the cost being twice as high as for younger patients.[87] Older patients with paraplegia and tetraplegia had increased rates of nursing home placement, and less neurologic and functional recovery than younger patients had.[87]

Disuse, immobilization, and decompensation

Immobilization has more serious consequences for the elderly than for younger patients. One study showed that, even in young men, 29 days of bed rest resulted in a 10% decrease in quadriceps and a 16% decrease in gastrocnemius or soleus muscle volume.[5] With decreased muscle mass (even when actual sarcopenia is not present), immobilization and disuse of muscles increases the risk in the elderly of weakness sufficient to cause functional problems. Orthostasis can also become problematic, with elderly patients requiring therapy and even medication for postural hypotension. In one medicine service of one hospital, low mobility and bed rest in a prospective cohort of 535 patients hospitalized from 1989 to 1991 predicted adverse outcomes. The study team noted that almost 60% of bed rest episodes in the lowest mobility group did not have a documented medical indication.[21] This shows the importance of vigilance in avoiding immobilization of elderly patients unless absolutely required by their medical condition. Immobilization also can combine with incontinence, skin fragility, and inadequate nutrition in the elderly to greatly increase the risk of pressure ulcers.

Pain

The etiologies of pain in a population of aged persons can be differently distributed than in a younger group. Some of the conditions that typically produce pain in the elderly include osteoarthritis, spinal stenosis, supraspinatus tendon tears, idiopathic peripheral neuropathy, and diabetic neuropathy. The elderly also frequently have less tolerance for pain medication, especially of the opioid type. The elderly deserve adequate pain management no less than other age groups, and inadequate pain control can cause problems in many other aspects of life, including quality of life in general and self-care ability in particular.

EVALUATING THE ELDERLY PATIENT

History taking

The history and physical examination for the elderly patient is essentially the same as for younger individuals (see Ch. 1). However, some changes in emphasis are needed. The examiner might need to be direct in questions, because some patients will not bring up a particular symptom, as they assume it is due to 'old age'. This is especially the case with pain.

In the outpatient setting, one should ask questions such as 'Have you fallen? If so, what were the circumstances?' The person who reports falling on the ice while doing his or her regular 2-mile walk is clearly functioning on a different level than the person who reports falling repeatedly en route to the bathroom at home. There are many other questions that are important in the history taking for elderly patients, for example 'Can you get in and out of a bathtub without assistance?' and 'How often do you leave home?'

Some patients will have already identified a functional problem before they bring it to the attention of a healthcare provider. For example, the patient might have noticed gait problems and borrowed a cane. They might have started purchasing clothing that is easier to don, or changed their style of cooking to one that they can handle. These are examples of the coping strategies that some elderly patients use to maintain autonomy when they notice difficulties with activities of daily living (ADL) or independent living skills.[86]

Some investigators have attempted to develop additional measures for assessing dangers to the elderly such as fall risk. One study looked at residents in a sheltered accommodation[71] who had dementia, stroke, and depression as their most common diagnoses. One finding was that, if the resident stopping walking when talking, there was a prediction of a fall within 6 months (positive predictive value 83%). A prolonged time difference between a walking task without and with carrying a glass of water was shown to identify who is at higher risk of falling in ambulatory elders in sheltered accommodation who were observed for 6 months.[70]

In the acute inpatient setting, the diagnosis responsible for hospitalization receives the major portion of the attention. When the patient presents for acute care to an emergency room, a combination of the need to focus on the primary diagnosis and the patient's inability to provide a complete history can leave important gaps in the history. For a fall with fracture, for example, one needs to know about prior falls. Other seemingly minor problems can now become more relevant. For example, a past rotator cuff tear might limit the ability of a patient with a hip fracture to use a walker. Knee degenerative joint disease can interfere with weight bearing on the nonparetic side in a patient with a stroke. Decreased vision or hearing can be an issue when the patient is out of the familiar home setting.

The review of systems should include questions about sleep. If sleep is impaired, what is the reason? Sleep management is different if the patient has pain, nocturia, or a mood disorder. Nocturia can result from the nighttime mobilization of peripheral edema.[85] Urinary frequency, urgency, and subjective retention need to be identified and treated. If pain is a problem, then as usual one needs to identify factors that precipitate and alleviate symptoms.

Questions about the patient's nutrition are important. Is nutrition adequate? If not, is it due to a financial problem, due to being physically unable to carry groceries back from the store, or the fear of lifting hot items during cooking? One study in 12 elderly women who were observed for 9 weeks showed that inadequate protein intake led to declines in lean tissue mass, muscle function, and immune response.[24]

When pain is a symptom, the history should specifically identify the sites and quality of the pain, as well as the inciting and relieving factors. Many older people have multiple potential causes of pain. Careful questioning might be needed to sort out the details sufficiently to correctly diagnose and treat the cause of the pain.

The patient's current list of medications should be thoroughly reviewed. Sleeping pills, some antihypertensives (such as beta-blockers), metoclopramide, tricyclic antidepressants, and antiseizure drugs can all cause cognitive impairment. Even if the person has been taking the medication for some time, the 'tipping point' can be reached when added to other acute health problems. Even drug levels considered 'therapeutic' can exacerbate a problem such as cognitive impairment in the elderly.[85] Non-prescription medications should not be neglected in the history-taking process.[45]

The history should include a detailed discussion of advanced directives.[85] At the time of writing, there is not a single document that is automatically transferred as one moves from facility to facility within the healthcare system in the USA. Wishes expressed by patients in an office setting to their primary care physician might be unknown to the care providers when a patient is transferred from an acute care hospital to a rehabilitation setting. The legal status of a 'living will' varies from state to state. If patients are relying on a healthcare proxy form to express their wishes, the healthcare providers should have on hand a copy of the document that stipulates this direction.

PHYSICAL EXAMINATION IN THE ELDERLY

In addition to the standard physical examination, there are useful physiatric additions. If there are gait problems, hip abduction and extension strength may need to be examined while side-lying or prone, respectively. If there are deficits in position sense, it should be determined whether it is only at the great toe or also at the ankle. The Achilles muscle stretch reflex will be absent in some elderly individuals.[85] Cerebellar testing should include both finger to nose and heel to shin procedures. However, in patients with limitations of hip range of motion, it might not be possible for them to actually bring the heel up to the shin at the knee.

Balance can be tested in a variety of ways, including tandem walking. But one can also assess the ability to perform a tandem stand. Gentle challenges can be provided by the examiner to assess if balance can be maintained. Dynamic balance can alternatively be assessed by having the patient lean in different directions, which simulates more of one's daily needs. Sitting balance can also be assessed.

Cognitive testing can be done both formally and informally. One must make certain that the person is able to hear the instructions, and that vision is adequate for the task. Ambient noise should be controlled to make certain that the patient can accurately hear the examiner's questions. One can ask questions about subjects of interest to the patient, such as sports or political news.

Formal mental status screening can be done with tests such as the Mini-Mental Status Examination of Folstein.[6] A baseline mild dementia can be masked when the person is in the familiar home setting, but becomes noticeable when admitted to the hospital.

The range of motion examination is very important in the elderly. Even relatively minor losses in range of motion can affect function. The range of motion of the neck and shoulders should be thoroughly checked. Loss of shoulder internal rotation makes it difficult for the patient to get the hands to the back, as in attaching a bra strap. Loss of shoulder external rotation makes it difficult to get the hands to the top of the head for hair care. Wrist extension and flexion, and finger flexion and extension limitations can have important functional ramifications. It is common to find limitations of hip extension and rotation in the elderly. This can have a negative impact on gait efficiency. In the patient with hip or low back complaints, the Ober test can be used to check for tightness of the tensor fascia lata. Limitations of knee extension and flexion should be identified, because such losses of range of motion can have a major impact on the efficiency of gait. At the ankle, one might determine if limitation in dorsiflexion is due to a joint contracture,

bony block at the ankle itself, or a tight gastrocnemius. Loss of ankle dorsiflexion range of motion that occurs only when the knee is extended is typically due to tightness in the gastrocnemius. Ankle inversion and eversion range of motion is important for walking on uneven surfaces.

Examination of the major joints for stability should be done. The knee in particular should be evaluated, because instability in any plane can affect gait function.

Deformities of the feet are common in the elderly, such as bunions (hallux valgus). Pes planus can also be present. Hallux rigidus can cause pain and interfere with gait efficiency. Hammertoes can be an incidental finding, a cause of pain, and a potential source of infection if skin integrity is not maintained. Skin calluses indicate the foot surfaces that are weight bearing. Skin integrity is important in the feet for both prevention of infection and for comfort. Patients who are bedbound for a period of time have an increased risk of heel pressure ulcers.

MANAGEMENT ISSUES IN THE ELDERLY

The physiatrist's first job is to eliminate impairment. When it is determined that an impairment cannot be further improved, attention should turn to minimizing disability. Sometimes, the pathophysiologic etiology cannot be corrected, but the symptoms can be remedied. A patient with painful degenerative joint disease of the knees might improve significantly with strengthening of the quadriceps and hamstrings, combined with the judicious use of a non-steroidal antiinflammatory drug.

Potential interventions in the treatment of the elderly can generally be divided into two major categories. One category includes those things that can be done to 'modify' the patient, such as stretching, strengthening, medications, modalities, and/or surgery. The second category is modification of the environment. For example, the environment can be modified to help compensate for sensory impairments. This includes using large print written material and auditory amplification devices. For mobility problems, rails can be installed on stairs, in the shower, and next to the toilet. Ramps and elevators can simplify access for those with limited mobility and for wheelchair users.

Medication usage in the elderly

Medication use in the elderly must be judicious, due to the changes in drug metabolism that occur with age. The reactions of the elderly to medications are not always the same as those of the population used to initially test the medication. Polypharmacy is another concern, because the number of potential interactions increases as more medications are used. Compliance with a medication program can be a problem, due to the complexity of the regimen proposed, the cost of the medication, and the cognitive status of the patient. Medication side effects can be more severe in the elderly population.[28] Elderly individuals as a group have traditionally been less represented in clinical drug trials.[28] Consequently, it should be kept in mind that new signs and symptoms can be a side effect of treatment rather than a new condition.

The treatment plan for an elderly patient has to be realistic. It is better to work with the patient to design a medication schedule that can actually be carried out, rather than to devise a plan that will work only under optimal conditions. This is particularly important if one is introducing something completely new to the patient, such as expecting a person with new diabetes and limited vision to learn to adjust insulin, check blood sugars four times a day, and change food preparation habits within a very short time. In a study by Kaufman, it was shown that, in ambulatory adult women over the age of 65 years, 12% had taken at least 10 different types of medications during the preceding week (which included non-prescription medications or supplements). It was also noted that 81% had taken at least one prescription medicine during the preceding week.[62] In the same study, 71% of men aged at least 65 or older had taken at least one prescription drug, and 19% had taken five or more during the preceding week.[62]

The increase in adipose tissue that typically occurs with age causes a larger volume of distribution for fat-soluble drugs and prolongs their biologic half-life.[25] Conversely, total body water decreases by as much as 15% between young adults to age 80, which decreases the volume of distribution of water-soluble drugs and thus results in a higher serum concentration.[25] Because drug elimination is so affected by renal function, it is wise to check drug levels[25] when drugs with a low therapeutic index and significant renal clearance are prescribed. Confusion, sedation, nausea, change in bowel habits, and balance problems are symptoms that can be confused with a new illness rather than as adverse reaction to medications. A serious error in treatment can occur when additional medications are added to treat what was actually an adverse reaction to medication.[25] The reported incidence of adverse drug reactions in the elderly is 20–25%.[25]

Physical exercise in the elderly

Physical exercise can be used to improve strength, range of motion, balance, and coordination. The exercise program typically starts with formal physical therapy, followed by a home program that the patient can continue doing. In the elderly, as in other patients, each physical therapy prescription must be individualized for the patient's diagnosis and condition.

Ambulatory aids

Ambulation might require the use of assistive devices in order to be safe and practical. Patients often resist the use of ambulation aids because the devices do not fit with their self-image. But if the aid allows patients to have decreased pain or an obvious improvement in function, they will usually accept it. A cane can be used to take some weight off a painful hip and provide additional stability if balance problems are present. Crutches can be used if a patient needs to take the weight off a lower limb more completely. Forearm crutches may be employed if there are limitations with grip strength. A walker provides stability and allows the person to convey items from place to place with a bag or basket on the walker. Wheelchairs allow for distance mobility in the community, even if the person does not use one within the home (see Ch. 18).

Shoe orthoses and footwear

Changes in footwear can sometimes improve stability with movement. Lower heels cause weight bearing to be spread over more of the foot than high heels. High-topped shoes that extend superiorly to the ankle can give additional sensory feedback as to foot position. Air stirrup devices can also serve this function and give additional ankle stability. Orthotic devices may help with pes planus. Over the counter shoe orthoses might provide adequate improvement, but many conditions require custom shoe insert orthoses to handle specific foot problems (see Ch. 16).

Functional and adaptive therapy

Occupational therapy can address the ADL, including bathing, toileting, and dressing. Occupational therapy also can teach the patient independent living skills such as cooking, laundry, and money management. Joint protection techniques can be addressed for patients with arthritis. Transfer training is often needed to ensure that getting on and off the toilet can be done safely. Occupational therapists can also work with the patient and family to sort out the specific pieces of ADL equipment that can best allow for safety and efficacy in the home (see Ch. 27).

Meal preparation

Patients living alone need to be able to do at least some meal preparation independently. Non-stick pads can be used to stabilize bowls needed for mixing ingredients. Using a microwave in conjunction with a rolling cart can enable the person to heat the food and then move it safely to the table. Large-handled utensils help people with arthritis to grip with less pain. These ADL devices are widely commercially available in the USA.

Amputations

Most amputations in elderly patients are due to vascular disease. Preamputation planning is needed to help the patient understand the clinical course that follows the amputation, select the most appropriate level of amputation, and begin a preprosthetic training program. After the amputation, the goals typically are to get the patient ambulatory as soon as possible, to strengthen the muscles needed for ambulation, and to shrink the residual limb so that permanent prosthetic fitting can occur as soon as possible. This is best accomplished using a team approach that includes the physiatrist, surgeon, prosthetist, physical therapy, occupational therapy, social worker, rehabilitation nurse, and others as needed (see Ch. 14).

Assistance from speech pathology

Speech therapy can assist the patient with many impairments, including problems with hearing, speech, language comprehension, orientation, and dysphagia. If auditory comprehension is a problem due to a loss of hearing, the speech therapist can also work with the patient on augmentative devices. Choosing a hearing aid requires a thorough analysis of the patient to discover and treat conditions that could interfere with the ability to use a complicated hearing device, such as arthritis, weakness, or sensation problems.[41] Print size can make a major difference in the person's ability to read, and this can be addressed in the context of speech therapy also. It is important that the patient's senses are working as well as they can, and this might require ophthalmologic procedures, glasses, hearing aids, etc. (see Ch. 3).

Psychosocial support

The elderly have to deal with losses of family, job, and function. These losses can lead to depression, even in people who never had depression earlier in life. Social work and psychology services are often critical in managing these life changes. Some problems can be addressed by facilitating access to services that an individual might not otherwise know about. For example, having to give up one's driver's license is a difficult lifestyle change, but it can be made easier if one learns to use the available transportation services.

Osteoporosis prevention and treatment

Geriatric rehabilitation can also address prevention of some of the complications associated with aging. Areas of concern include osteoporosis, nutrition, cardiovascular problems, muscle weakness, hearing, visual impairments, and impaired balance. Osteoporosis can be used as an example in this regard (see Ch. 42). It can be addressed with a combination of diet, drugs, and exercise. Adequate calcium intake is essential but, if there is a history of calcium kidney stones, one should work with the patient's primary care provider, as one wishes to avoid hypercalciuria.[8] Adequate vitamin D is needed also. There is a seasonal variation in 25-hydroxyvitamin D levels, which are lower in winter and spring, and decline with age.[100] This can be exacerbated by decreased exposure to the sun, such as is experienced by some nursing home residents or people who are housebound. Supplementation is often necessary, and can be combined with calcium when desirable. If an elderly patient has vitamin D deficiency, higher doses of vitamin D should be used for the first 8 weeks of treatment.[65] In one metaanalysis, the use of vitamin D reduced the risk of falls among ambulatory elders living in the community and in institutions.[16] The early effect of vitamin D on reducing the risk of falls might be due to the active metabolite binding to a muscle tissue receptor.[16] Based on prior studies, 400 international units (IU) daily might not be enough, and 800 IU might be needed in some cases.[16]

Medications have been used to stop resorption of bone. Estrogen was used widely in the past but, due to negative side effects, the so-called 'designer estrogens' such as raloxifene are now used. Etidronate was the first bisphosphonate approved as an antiresorptive agent.[65] Alendronate with calcium has been shown to improve bone mineral density, and decrease the incidence of vertebral fractures and the progression of vertebral deformities.[66] One needs to ensure that vitamin D is adequate with alendronate use.[17] Calcitonin is also used but tends to reduce vertebral rather than peripheral fractures (see Ch. 42).[83]

A fracture that occurs in an elderly person due to relatively minor force predicts future fractures. For example, a distal radial (Colles) fracture doubles the risk of having a future hip fracture. The presence of a vertebral fracture on x-ray increases the risk of additional vertebral fracture four to five times.[102] Radiologists do not always comment on vertebral fractures that appear on routine chest x-ray.[102] Because future fractures of any type can have major implications for the health and overall function of an elderly person, any fracture should set in motion measures to prevent future fractures. Exercise works to reduce the chance of vertebral fractures related to osteoporosis.

There is a negative correlation between the strength of back extensor muscles and thoracic kyphosis in women with osteoporosis.[97,99]

Vertebral fractures in postmenopausal women were studied over a 2-year period, then over a 10-year follow-up. Women were trained in back extensor-strengthening exercise.[97] The average age at study entry was 56 years. The 2-year exercise period consisted of prone exercise with a backpack containing weights. The strength difference between the exercise group and the control group was significant; the relative risk for compression fractures was 2.7 times greater in the control than in the extensor exercise group (see Ch. 46).[97]

Specific balance training can also be helpful, because patients with osteoporosis and kyphosis maintain their balance with an increased use of hip strategies compared with the general population.[72] In a randomized pilot study, seven women with osteoporosis and kyphosis received either extensor-strengthening exercises only or the same exercises with use of a weighted 2-lb thoracic orthosis worn 2 h per day during ambulatory activities. The subjects who had the most abnormal balance and used the proprioceptive training device had the most improvement in balance.[98] It is likely that improved balance decreases the risk of fractures due to falls.

Preventing falls in the elderly

Falls cause 90% of the fractures of the forearm, hip, and pelvis in the elderly.[64] There are multiple risk factors for falls (Box 60-2).[34] Dim lighting and high beds can be a contributor in nursing home patients.[34] Institutions such as nursing homes can also have issues of staffing that contribute to falls.[34] In attempts to decrease falls in nursing homes, customized seating has been used to decrease the chance of slipping out from a chair from the front or the side.[34] Having the mattress close to the floor, or having a foam pad on the floor, can also help reduce the risk of injury from falls.[34]

Falls and the fear of falling are both common.[44] One question is which comes first: falling or the fear of falling? In a prospective study of 2212 individuals, those who reported falls at baseline but did not report fear at baseline were at a higher risk of fear of falling over a 20-month period. Individuals who limit activities because of fear of falling are also at a high risk of falling, which could be due to the fact that they have more risk factors at baseline. It has also been suggested, however, that restricting activities leads to decreased function and consequent higher fall risk. In this study, the predictors of development of fear of falling in those without fear at baseline were female sex, four or more medications, and worse general health based on questionnaire scores. The predictors of falls at 20 months in those who were not falling at baseline were white race, female gender, stroke, sedative use, and fear of falling at baseline. The authors noted that the only modifiable factors were fear of falling and sedative use. In another randomized controlled trial (RCT), 57 elderly women with a history of falls with injury were randomized to receive either three times per week balance and strength training, or placebo intervention. Three months later, the intervention group performed better on motor testing, but there was no statistically significant difference in falls at 6 months.[52]

Hip fracture prevention is important in the elderly because of the ramifications of injury. Between 22 and 75% of elderly hip fracture patients do not regain their prior functional status at 6–12 months after injury.[13]

Balance training can be done in multiple ways. A wobble board can allow focus just on ankle movements. A 5-week RCT of 20 elderly individuals showed that the wobble board improved discrimination of ankle inversion movements.[111] Some balance exercises can easily be done at home without supervision in the relatively healthy elder, such as standing on one lower extremity with upper extremity support. Using a physioball for seated dynamic balance activities typically requires hands-on assistance from a physical therapist. There are more elaborate balance training devices that can alter vestibular, proprioceptive, and visual input as part of the training process.

There are data that support combining balance and strength training. Balance and/or weight training were studied in 110 community dwellers of mean age 80 years.[115] In another RCT, participants were randomized to balance training alone, strength training alone, balance and strength training, or education control for a 3-month intense training period. This was followed by 6 months of t'ai chi for maintenance.[115] Balance training improved balance to a level comparable with that of an individual 3–10 years younger.[115] There was no crossover, in that the balance group did not improve in strength, nor the strength group in balance. The exception to this was for single stance time, which improved in the strength training group.[115] There was some decline over the 6-month maintenance period in balance, although it should be noted that this was a relatively low-intensity intervention, in that the class met only 1 h per week.[115]

Another RCT used 200 participants aged 70 years or older in a 15-week study that compared t'ai chi or computerized balance training with an education control group.[114] The three groups had similar responses at baseline regarding number of falls in the year prior to study enrollment and to the fear of falling questionnaire at baseline.[114] The t'ai chi group showed decreased fear of falling, decreased falls, and reduced ambulation speed compared with the control group, with no effect seen in fall prevention in the balance training group.[114]

Nelson studied 40 postmenopausal women in a controlled trial of twice-weekly strength training over a year. Balance was measured by backward tandem walk. Muscle strength, muscle mass, and dynamic balance increased in the exercise group. In an observational study, 20 elderly practitioners of t'ai chi, mean age 70, were compared with 20 elderly individuals who did not practice t'ai chi and with young university students. All were ambulatory and independent in the ADL. The t'ai chi group had been performing t'ai chi three times per week for at least 1 year (the mean was 7 years of t'ai chi). Different combinations of visual and platform sway positioning were tested. The 20 who were doing t'ai chi had better standing balance under conditions of reduced sensory input compared with control subjects, and were comparable with the young group.[106] Because the t'ai chi practitioners were self-selected, one cannot necessarily ascribe the improvements to t'ai chi rather than to other factors. In an RCT involving women with low bone mass between 75 and 85 years of age, 6 months of resistance and agility training reduced fall risk by improving postural stability. There was also a reduction seen in the stretching group, but not as marked.[68]

In an RCT of 15 people with Parkinson disease, one group did balance and resistance training, while one did balance training only.[54] Balance training improved balance, with an enhanced effect if strength training was included. Both groups had increased strength after the study. The combination of balance and resistance training improved the ability to maintain balance on the most difficult balance tests in the study.[54]

Modifying the environment

Modifying the environment is an alternative approach to take to disability that goes beyond the typical measures that reduce barriers. For example, chairs can be designed to ease the difficulty that an elder has in changing position.[3] Traffic lights can be timed to allow adequate time for the elderly person to safely cross a street (see Ch. 27).

Exercise for strength in the elderly

In the past, it was widely held that exercise could not actually increase strength in the elderly. A number of studies, however, have documented that exercise causes improvements in strength and power, in muscle force generation at the single-fiber level, and improvement in overall function (see Ch. 19).

A study by Fiatarone measured knee extensor strength, chair stand time (rising from a straight-backed chair without use of upper extremities), and habitual and tandem gait speed before and after progressive resistance exercise in eight ambulatory patients ages 86–96.[37] Tandem gait speed strength increased in the exercise group. Some subjects no longer needed canes for ambulation. There was no change in habitual gait speed. Some changes were probably due to improved neural recruitment, because they were noted in the first 2 weeks, too early to produce muscle hypertrophy.

In another study, 100 frail nursing home residents were in an RCT looking at progressive resistance exercise with and without a multinutrient supplement.[38] An ambulatory aid was used by

83%. Muscle strength increased by 113% and gait velocity increased by 12% in the exercise groups. The use of a nutritional supplement did not affect the outcome.

In a study of the healthy elderly that included 3 months of resistance training, walking endurance increased from 25 to 34 min.[1] The authors noted that the effect was primarily seen due to increases in the male subjects.

Vincent reported a study in which low-intensity exercise (13 repetitions at 50% of 1 repetition maximum, RM) was compared with high-intensity exercise (8 repetitions at 80% of 1 RM) in subjects ages 60–83 years. Both strength and endurance improved as compared with control subjects, with a decrease in the time needed to climb one flight of stairs. There was similar improvement between the low- and high-intensity groups.[108,109]

Frontera reported an RCT showing that, after 12 weeks of training, women aged 68–79 showed increased strength, force, and whole muscle size measured by cross-sectional area. Sauvage reported a small RCT on subjects who tested lower than age specific norms. The exercise group had 12 weeks of stationary cycling and lower extremity training. They improved in average stride length and velocity of gait.[92]

Power is a product of force and velocity, and it tends to decline earlier and more rapidly than strength with increasing age. Power has been shown to correlate with functional status in some studies.[39] High-velocity training was shown to significantly increase power compared with low-velocity training in a group of 30 women with a mean age of 73 years. Strength increased in both groups. However, in this study,[39] changes in functional performance as measured by stair climb time, chair rise time, or gait velocity showed only a small change compared with the large improvement in peak power.[93] There was improvement in self-reported disability with the training, but the improvement did not depend on whether the training was done at high velocity or low velocity.[93]

Comparison of a walking program with high-velocity resistance training in community dwellers over the age of 70 years showed an improvement in leg press strength for both groups, with greater improvement in the high-velocity training group. Power improved in the high-velocity training group but not in the walkers.[32] The examiners noted that a ceiling effect might have precluded improvement in chair rise time in this study.[32] A group exercise program of aerobic, strengthening, and balance exercises was offered in retirement communities.[69] Compared with the control group, the group exercise population had better 6-min walking distances and reaction times;[69] the intervention program was particularly effective in fall prevention in people with a prior history of falls.

An exercise program has also been shown to improve mood disturbances in elderly patients with depression.[101] Participants in a 10-week program of supervised progressive resistance exercise of large muscle groups had improved depression scores, even when assessed at 10 weeks after the supervised exercise had been completed.[101]

A pilot study of 10 subjects over age 55 with knee osteoarthritis showed decreased pain and improved strength after 4 months of a home-based exercise program, compared with a group getting nutritional advice. There was no improvement in the nutrition control group. The exercise consisted of lower body exercise with progressive ankle weights.[9] In a randomized trial comparing aerobic exercise, resistance exercise, and a health education program in people aged 60 and older with knee osteoarthritis, both exercise groups had improved scores of physical disability, pain, and distance on a 6-min walk test, and did better on a lifting and carrying task than the education control group.[33]

Exercise programs in the elderly have been demonstrated to work at the center-based level, when people living in the community come to a facility to work out. There have also been studies of home-based exercise programs. Improvements were seen in a 6-month RCT with an attention control group.[79,80] Scores on a physical performance battery improved in the exercise groups but decreased in the control subjects. Maximum gait speed improved but did not reach statistical significance in the exercise group compared with the control subjects. The exercise groups also showed dynamic balance improvement, but strength did not improve. One concern was that the home exerciser needed encouragement to progress with increased weights in the training program. The study participants were reluctant to progress in weights unless instructed to do so in person at a home visit.[79] It should also be noted that two of the muscle groups tested on 1 RM testing were not actually being specifically trained.[79]

A home-based strengthening program, using elastic bands, for non-disabled, community-dwelling elders aged 65 and older was conducted.[60] Adherence rates for the exercise sessions ranged from 0 to 102% (as a percentage of prescribed sessions). After 12–15 weeks of exercise, the younger adults in the elderly population had a 10% improvement in knee extensor strength, and the men had improved vigor. The older women in the exercise group reported increased confusion, and the older men in the control group had an increase in anger compared with the exercise group.[60] Although the study design intended to have the subjects progress through four different possible levels of the elastic bands to increase resistance, 9% did not change their level of resistance and 35% changed only one level.

Exercise in elderly stroke survivors

High-intensity training at 70% of 1 RM improved lower extremity power and strength in an RCT that studied people who had survived a mild or moderate single stroke.[81] The mean age was 66, and the minimum age to enter the study was 50 years. Strength and power improved in both the paretic and the non-paretic limbs. In another study of seven subjects at 1 year after stroke and with mean age of 70 years, 12 weeks of progressive resistance exercise at 70% of 1 RM showed improvements in lower limb strength in both affected and non-affected lower extremities, as well as decreased chair standing time and improved balance.[113]

The American Heart Association scientific statement notes that exercise intolerance after stroke is common.[49] The energy costs of walking in patients with hemiplegia can be twice that of the able-bodied.[49] It is important to avoid deterioration in exercise tolerance immediately after stroke by getting patients upright as soon as possible with intermittent standing and sitting.[49] Aerobic conditioning can promote decreased body weight, decreased body fat, better glucose regulation, improved high-density lipoprotein levels, and coronary artery endothelial function.[49] Exercise can include upper or lower extremity ergometry at 40–70% of peak consumption. A treadmill can also be used with unweighting devices such as a harness or handrails, with increasing grade used to increase exercise intensity.[49]

Preexercise evaluation in the elderly

It is reasonable for older adults to have a medical screening examination before starting an exercise program.[12] Contraindications to participation are summarized in Box 60-4.[12] It is important to assess elderly individuals who are starting an exercise program to find problems that need further evaluation, such as a heart murmur or bruit. They can also need more optimal management of conditions such as congestive heart failure or asthma.[12] A resting electrocardiogram is recommended.[12]

Exercise stress testing results have different meanings in an elderly than in a younger population.[22] For example, a short duration of exercise of less than 3 min might be interpreted as a sign of advanced coronary artery disease in a younger individual, but could be due to multiple physiologic problems in an elderly patient.[22] Bryant notes that failure of the heart rate to rise appropriately during exercise is associated with a poor prognosis.[22] The exercise protocol might need to be altered in an elderly patient, perhaps with shorter intervals between stages and relying more on change in grade for those who cannot walk briskly on a treadmill.[107] For further details of cardiac stress testing, see Chapter 34.

The guidelines of the American College of Sports Medicine and the American Heart Association suggest that all older adults who want to engage in moderate or vigorous exercise should have a screening exercise stress test.[12,47] But Gill notes that these guidelines do not fit the asymptomatic adult older than 75, particularly if one is contemplating a program of progressive resistance training rather than aerobic training.[47] The concern is that, with the high prevalence of asymptomatic atherosclerotic cardiovascular disease in the elderly, routine exercise stress testing could lead to invasive cardiac procedures without strong evidence to support their need.[47] Cardiovascular reserve can be tested in the office by having the elderly climb one flight of steps, cycle in the air for 1 min, or walk 15 m. One can start with low-intensity exercise such as self-paced walking, or lower extremity resistance training with tubing or ankle weights.[47] One can then progress to a more intense program after checking blood pressure and pulse rate. Blood pressure and pulse changes can guide the intensity of exercise.[47]

A combination of progressive resistance training and aerobic exercise is recommended for community-dwelling older adults with stroke, osteoarthritis, cardiovascular disease, diabetes, osteoporosis, and balance problems.[12] Although there is still much to be learned about exercise in respiratory disease such as chronic obstructive pulmonary disease, exercise has been shown to improve 6-min walk times and subjective dyspnea (see Ch. 35). Separate training of the upper and lower extremities has been advocated.[12] The American College of Sports Medicine notes that both improved strength and hypertrophy can occur in older adults with single-joint and multiple-joint exercises using 60–80% of 1 RM for 8–12 repetitions and one to three sets of each exercise, with 1–2 min of rest between sets. Power can be improved through the use of 40–60% 1 RM at 6–10 repetitions with one to three sets and high repetition velocity (American College of Sports Medicine).

Upper body resistance training can begin 3–4 weeks after myocardial infarction after a satisfactory baseline exercise tolerance test.[2] Resistance training should be delayed for 3 months after coronary artery bypass grafting to allow for full sternal healing.[2] The target heart rate should be lowered in aquatic exercise, because swimming can cause electrocardiographic changes at a lower heart rate than land-based exercise.[40]

HIP FRACTURE REHABILITATION

In the elderly, the aftermath of a hip fracture can mark a major decline in level of functioning, including marking the transition from living in one's home to nursing home living. This was demonstrated by a cohort of 2086 community-living elderly subjects who were observed prospectively. Over a 6-year period,120 sustained a hip fracture, with subsequent decline in function at 6 months after fracture noted in the 83 who were alive and available for follow-up interview at 6 months.[74] Ability to dress independently decreased from 86% of subjects prior to the fracture to only 49% at 6 months after fracture.[74]

Older patients can have less satisfactory results when a hip fracture is treated operatively compared with younger patients, although the data vary in different studies.[64] Intraarticular fractures involving a joint with arthritis is a problem seen primarily in the elderly, and can require total joint arthroplasty rather

---

Box 60-4 Contradictions to participation in an exercise program[12]

- Unstable angina or severe left main coronary artery disease
- End-stage congestive heart failure
- Severe valvular heart disease
- Malignant or unstable arrhythmias
- Elevated resting blood pressure (systolic > 200 mmHg or diastolic > 110 mmHg)
- Large or expanding aortic aneurysm
- Known cerebral aneurysm or recent intracranial bleed
- Uncontrolled or end-stage systemic disease
- Acute retinal hemorrhage or recent ophthalmologic surgery
- Acute or unstable musculoskeletal injury
- Severe dementia or behavioral disturbance

than open reduction with fixation.[64] Fractures around prior joint replacements are technically complicated, with a higher risk of troubles with malunion and infection compared with fractures that are not in an area with a joint implant.[64] Cement can be needed for fixation if the bone is osteoporotic.[64] The goal after a hip fracture is to avoid a prolonged period of immobility. Because older patients typically have difficulty walking, with limited weight bearing, the choices in surgical approach, fixation, and implants should have as a goal enabling weight bearing as tolerated as soon as possible.[64]

Intensive geriatric inpatient rehabilitation can have a positive impact on the ability of a hip fracture patient to live independently, even if there is some degree of dementia. In the study of Huusko, patients with hip fracture and dementia were assessed 3 months and 1 year postoperatively. Significantly fewer patients with moderate dementia who had received intense inpatient geriatric rehabilitation had to be institutionalized as compared with the control subjects, as measured by ability to live independently at 1 year after hip fracture.[57]

Ninety people aged 65 and older who had a surgical repair of a proximal femur fracture were randomized to a supervised exercise and physical therapy program three times a week for 6 months, or to home exercise as the control.[13] The exercises progressed and included progressive resistance training that went to 85–100% of 1 RM. The exercise group had improved physical performance and functional status compared with the control group, with improved balance and strength.[13] Thus the end point for formal therapeutic exercise after hip fracture has not been definitively set. There is concern about the costs of providing such services outside the study setting.[13]

GERIATRIC CONSIDERATIONS FOR THE PATIENT WITH AMPUTATION

The typical geriatric amputee faces more difficult challenges than those of the younger amputee. The elderly generally have less reserve in many systems than younger amputees have. If atherosclerotic peripheral vascular disease was the reason for the amputation, typically a period of deconditioning preceded the amputation, and the remaining limb could have a suboptimal blood supply. Contractures might be present in either the amputated limb or other limbs. Congestive heart failure can be present and cause fluctuation in edema of the residual limb. The cardiac demands of mobility with a lower extremity amputation are stressful for an individual with an antecedent history of cardiovascular disease. An above-knee amputation (transfemoral) causes a much-increased energy demand during gait than the below-knee (transtibial) amputation.[55]

Preserving the knee is critically important in the elderly, because of the possibility of comorbid disease that can limit exercise capabilities.[27] The elderly patient with peripheral vascular disease needs to be vigilant in skin care to help prevent gangrene. The skin should be inspected daily for any sign of breakdown. The toenails should be trimmed straight to avoid ingrown toenails. A lanolin-containing cream should be applied

to the lower limbs below the knees, except in the spaces between the toes. Avoiding extremes of temperature that could cause an accidental burn or cold injury is essential. The patient should have appropriate shoes and shoe inserts as needed. The patient should wear shoes when ambulating to avoid foot and toe injury, even when going to the bathroom in the middle of the night. Vascular consultation is typically necessary to assure that the patient's blood supply to the lower limbs is maximized, avoiding a break in the skin of the foot. Because the patient most likely to require an amputation is the patient who has already had one, the remaining lower limb of a vascular amputee requires constant attention. Older amputees, over the age of 85, can have a low likelihood of having successful prosthesis fit.[42] Changes in surgical technique and abilities to assess the vascular supply preoperatively have helped increase the ability to preserve the knee joint with a transtibial rather than transfemoral amputee, which produces lower energy demands of ambulation.[30]

Physical fitness in the sense of both aerobic conditioning and muscle strength is important in amputees to enable walking and to maintain walking speed.[112] Younger patients with an amputation who have higher exercise capacity typically have a faster comfortable walking speed than an older vascular amputee.[112] In a transtibial amputation, increased activity of the hip and knee muscles helps substitute for the loss of power from ankle flexors, but these energy demands can be harder to meet in the older patient.[112] The majority of older patients who have transfemoral amputations for a vascular cause do not become functional ambulators, and those who do usually have a slow gait speed.[112] Pandian has shown that patients with both a lower limb amputation and a stroke tend to be more independent when the amputation precedes the stroke (see Ch. 14).[82]

PAIN MANAGEMENT IN THE ELDERLY

Pain management in the elderly should include attention to both pharmacologic and non-pharmacologic measures. The use of non-pharmacologic measures is even more important in the elderly, due to the increased risk of adverse side effects with medications.[48] It is important to address the depression that can be induced by chronic pain. Pain can be under-treated in the elderly, due to the fear of addiction on the part of the patient and the practitioner. This is true even in the case of medications not typically associated with addiction.[48]

AGING WITH A DISABILITY

Aging with a disability carries its own set of problems. In some cases, advances in medicine have prolonged life in people who might not have survived to more advanced ages. Three representative medical problems in elderly patients with a disability include spinal cord injury, polio, and cerebral palsy.

Aging with spinal cord injury
The elderly typically have less ability to use the upper limbs to compensate for lower limb deficits. Shoulders can develop signs

and symptoms of overuse, with degenerative joint disease and rotator cuff problems. If one uses the upper limbs for wheelchair propulsion, for transfers, and for ambulation with devices, the amount of work done by the shoulders over the years is far greater than in the average individual. Shear forces become more problematic as skin fragility increases. Urinary incontinence can develop for a number of reasons. The day to day routines that had worked for a patient for years might no longer be adequate. The elderly person might need to adapt to a different technique for transferring, for example with the use of a sliding board. Changes in the social support system can cause new challenges. A spouse might not be able to continue assisting with toilet transfers, necessitating major changes in a living situation.

A study of individuals with spinal cord injury showed that those with higher lesions sensed that they were aging more quickly.[76] Despite this, those with higher lesions did not report more health problems or fatigue than others in the sample. The longer one had lived with spinal cord injury, the more there was a perception of accelerated aging. The authors also noted that one theoretic model is that age is a sort of 'leveler'. A young person with a disability experiences more differences compared with able-bodied peers than for the elderly with a disability.

Aging with polio

Postpolio syndrome refers to late manifestations many years after the initial polio infection. Its onset is usually heralded by generalized fatigue, as well as new weakness and muscle atrophy.[61] These new symptoms can be very distressing, as they represent the sequelae of a disease that the patient thought had already done its damage years earlier. Weakness can develop in muscle groups that did not seem to be involved by the polio. However, these seemingly unaffected muscle groups have been shown on electrodiagnostic studies to have previously unrecognized effects of polio.[61] Motor neuron dropout occurs due to aging, and also probably is accelerated in the patient with polio. At the initial illness, distal axon sprouts enabled reinnervation,[105] but motor neuron dropout can cause clinical changes with aging.[61] Others have theorized that there is an ongoing viral presence, or that the postpolio symptoms are due to a combination of aging processes.[63] In a study by Klein, muscle strength was measured in people with a history of polio. Thirty muscle groups were measured three times, each 3–5 months apart. The rate of decline of strength in upper extremity muscles was much greater than that associated with normal aging. Strength decreased in all muscles measured in the upper extremities, and in the lower extremity flexor muscles.

Treatment of the postpolio syndrome includes energy conservation measures, use of assistive devices, decrease of mechanical stress on joints and muscles, and non-fatiguing exercise programs that avoid overuse.[61] Swallowing and breathing problems can develop.[105] Respiratory muscles might already be weak, with additional negative contributions from bulbar muscle weakness, sleep-disordered breathing, obesity, and scoliosis.[63] Because there are no specific tests for postpolio syndrome,

other etiologies for weakness, fatigue, and joint pain have to be ruled out.[61]

Aging with cerebral palsy

Aging patients with cerebral palsy frequently notice changes in their functional level, in what they thought was a static condition. Mobility can be affected by years of abnormal gait mechanics, and secondary ligamentous laxity and degenerative changes in joints. A decline in muscle strength can result in having to change techniques for ADL. A new neurologic problem, such as a stroke, may worsen spasticity.

Proposed treatments and interventions must be individualized to meet the patient's wishes and goals. Patients are frequently resistant to changing highly practiced and lifelong techniques. Some examples of the changes in a patient's program can include increased vigilance in skin management, changes in straight catheterization frequency in a bladder program, or changes in transfer technique related to shoulder degenerative joint disease.

Caring for those who are aging with a disability requires that primary care and preventive care be maximized. Klingbeil has shown an under-use of preventive care measures in adults with cerebral palsy.[63] The possible reasons for this include physical inaccessibility of healthcare, financial barriers, demands on the primary caregiver, or the absence of a perceived need by the patient and/or the caregiver. Issues that need to be resolved to even permit a visit for primary care can include such details as having the patient arrive on a stretcher rather than in a wheelchair to facilitate the physical examination.

ARCHITECTURAL AND DESIGN IMPACT ON THE ELDERLY

One of the major effects of the Americans with Disabilities Act has been to make institutions and the individuals who run them more cognizant of the direct impact of architecture on mobility. Design of larger spaces within the home, such as the kitchen or bathroom, can also have an impact on comfort and safety. The design of furniture and utensils has a direct impact on function. Difficulty in arising from a chair affects 8% of people aged 65 and over who live in the community.[3] Arising from a chair is easier if one can fit one's feet posteriorly under the edge of the seat.[3] If the feet do not contact the floor because the seat is high, there is decreased postural stability.[3] The elderly have disproportionate difficulties getting up when the chair has a lower seat, increased posterior seat tilt, and increased backrest recline.[3] Design of individual utensils, such as by increasing the grip circumferences, can improve utility.

Physical activity of the elderly is significantly affected by the design of the community. Brach has shown that an active lifestyle is facilitated by the design of communities that encourage activity. This study showed that those who had an active lifestyle and those who exercised more intensely had better physical function than those who were inactive.[18] Community design is important in encouraging exercise in general, and walking in particular. Sidewalks are essential, with crosswalks at busy intersections that provide adequate time for the older person to cross in safety. Street lighting should be sufficient to be safe for an elderly pedestrian. When elderly individuals can no longer safely drive due to visual problems, affordable and reliable alternative means of transportation are needed to assure access to community centers and other places of activity for the elderly.

FUNDING FOR CARE

In order to live independently, one must have certain basic mobility and ADL skills. This includes basics such as dressing, toileting, personal hygiene, and at least minimal food preparation. If someone is unable to manage these tasks independently, meeting these needs may involve informal caregivers, outside agencies, nursing homes, and even hospitalization. If injury such as hip fracture or head trauma occurs, the costs increase.

Ideally, one would be able to identify people at risk early, so that one could attempt to modify factors to prevent disability with mobility.[43] Individuals may have had to alter how they perform tasks such as walking half a mile or climbing 10 steps in advance of reporting difficulty with these tasks.[43] This parallels the concept of coping raised in reference to ADL and independent living skills, in which behavioral or cognitive strategies are used to minimize the functional impact of disabilities.[86] There may be certain points at which an intervention may help preserve function. For example, in home-dwelling frail elders in one exercise study, the benefits were seen in the group with moderate, not severe, frailty.[46]

Any attempt to address the issue of cost of care must go beyond the cost of direct therapy to address long-term outcomes. Data from a retrospective cohort of 11 150 patients admitted to nursing homes for the first time in 1994–6 with diagnoses including stroke, hip fracture, congestive heart failure, chronic lung disease, and other showed dose–response effects among patients receiving rehabilitation services.[78] In part, this depends on how one defines the illness: at what level of independence or follow-up is the episode of illness considered over?[55] And what of more chronic conditions?

It is estimated that the direct healthcare cost related to sarcopenia in the USA in 2000 was $18.5 billion.[59] The cost-effectiveness of exercise interventions is not yet determined.[59]

In a retrospective analysis of 84 346 nursing home residents, there was a direct link between the onset of movement impairments and progression of disability, with progression in ADL loss regardless of proximal or distal or combined, or upper or lower extremities; although one may not be able to treat fully the underlying chronic medical condition, the movement impairment may be treatable.[11]

This would need to be addressed as a public health issue; one must be able to be specific as to which interventions give functional benefit with minimal cost. As an example, one study looked at the cost-effectiveness of a resistance training program for older patients with osteoarthritis, and found it to be margin-ally more economically efficient when compared with aerobic training.[96]

Disability in community-dwelling elders is not necessarily a permanent state. In a cohort prospective study with monthly assessment of 754 community-dwelling adults aged 70 or older, a total of 56% were disabled at some point during the study, which had a median follow-up time of 51 months.[51] Of these, 81% regained their independence in ADL. Fifty-seven percent were able to maintain independence for at least 6 months.[51] Because there are high rates of recurrence of disability, it is suggested that older people who have recovered from an episode of disability may be an important target for interventions to try to prevent recurrence.[51]

Strength training helps counterbalance the loss in muscle mass and strength associated with aging.[75] Endurance training can help maintain or improve cardiovascular function, including blood pressure reduction in the hypertensive.[75] Although fall reduction has been shown as part of the response to exercise programs, one cannot yet identify the key components of the training program, because many studies have had a multifaceted exercise program.[75]

More data are needed before making generalized recommendations as to specific interventions in the frail elderly. The optimal details of the exercise prescription have yet to be worked out. Differences may be seen in functional outcomes, depending on the degree of frailty or disability in the studied population. Community-based programs that are run outside the medical system may represent a financially viable alternative. At the level of the individual patient presenting to the physiatrist, one must structure the recommendations based on the symptoms and findings identified at the time of the visit, and on input from family, caregivers, and therapists.

SUMMARY

Gait problems may be multifactorial, with a combination of causes such as joint pain, visual impairment, and stroke.[4] The treatment program must take this into account. The cumulative effect of small positive changes may reduce the risk of injury and improve quality of life.

Nutrition needs to be adequate, including protein and calcium. The role of micronutrients (folate, B complex vitamins, vitamin C, vitamin E, beta-carotene), antioxidants, zinc, and fiber is being explored; at this point, one can recommend a balanced diet and may need to recommend supplements, depending on the person's dietary habits.[89]

Medications should be reviewed by the physician, with a goal of simplification to improve compliance and minimize side effects. Exercise training can reverse sarcopenia.[91] Data do not yet exist to optimize the exercise prescription.

Preventive measures to maximize function, avoid disability, and optimize symptoms can include interventions rooted in pharmacology, formal therapy, and modification of the external environment.

REFERENCES

1. Ades PA. Cardiac rehabilitation in older coronary patients. J Am Geriatr Soc 1999; 47:98–105.

2. Aggarwal A, Ades PA. Exercise rehabilitation of older patients with cardiovascular disease. Cardiol Clin 2001; 19:525–536.

3. Alexander NB, Koester DL, Grunawalt JA. Chair design affects how older adults rise from a chair. J Am Geriatr Soc 1996; 44:356–362.

4. Alexander NB. Gait disorders in older adults. J Am Geriatr Soc 1996; 44:434–451.

5. Alkner BA, Tesch PA. Efficacy of a gravity-independent resistance exercise device as a countermeasure to muscle atrophy during 29-day bed rest. Acta Physiol Scand 2004; 181:345–357.

6. Amin SH, Kuhle CL, Fitzpatrick LA. Comprehensive evaluation of the older woman. Mayo Clin Proc 2003; 78:1157–1185.

7. Aminoff MJ. Parkinson's disease and other extrapyramidal disorders. In: Fauci AS, Braunwald E, Isselbacher KJ, et al, eds. Harrison's principles of internal medicine. New York: McGraw-Hill; 1998:2356–2363.

8. Asplin JR, Coe FL, Favus MJ. Nephrolithiasis. In: Fauci AS, Braunwald E, Isselbacher KJ, et al, eds. Harrison's principles of internal medicine. New York: McGraw-Hill; 1998:1569–1574.

9. Baker KR, Nelson ME, Vu D, et al. Safety and efficacy of a home-based progressive resistance strength training program for knee osteoarthritis in the elderly [abstract]. Med Sci Sports Exerc 1998; 30:83.

10. Balducci L. Geriatric oncology. Crit Rev Hematol Oncol 2003; 46:211–220.

11. Bean J, Kiely DK, Leveille SG, et al. Associating the onset of motor impairments with disability progression in nursing home residents. Am J Phys Med Rehabil 2002; 81:696–704.

12. Bean JF, Vora A, Frontera WR. Benefits of exercise for community-dwelling older adults. Arch Phys Med Rehabil 2004; 85(suppl 3):S31–S42.

13. Binder EF, Brown M, Sinacore DR, et al. Effects of extended outpatient rehabilitation after hip fracture: a randomized controlled trial. JAMA 2004; 292:837–846.

14. Bird TD. Alzheimer's disease and other primary dementias. In: Fauci AS, Braunwald E, Isselbacher KJ, et al, eds. Harrison's principles of internal medicine. New York: McGraw-Hill; 1998:2348–2356.

15. Bird TD. Memory loss and dementia. In: Fauci AS, Braunwald E, Isselbacher KJ, et al, eds. Harrison's principles of internal medicine. New York: McGraw-Hill; 1998:142–150.

16. Bischoff-Ferrari HA, Dawson-Hughes B, Willett WC, et al. Effect of vitamin D on falls: a meta-analysis. JAMA 2004; 291:1999–2006.

17. Bone HG, Santora AC. Ten years of alendronate treatment for osteoporosis in postmenopausal women. N Engl J Med 2004; 351:190–192.

18. Brach JS, Simonsick EM, Kritchevsky S, et al. The association between physical function and lifestyle activity and exercise in the health, aging and body composition study. J Am Geriatr Soc 2004; 52:502–509.

19. Bressler R, Bahl JJ. Principles of drug therapy for the elderly patient. Mayo Clinic Proc 2003; 78:1564–1577.

20. Bross, R, Javanbakht M, Bhasin S. Anabolic interventions for aging-associated sarcopenia. J Clin Endocrinol Metab 1999; 84:3420–3430.

21. Brown CJ, Friedkin RJ, Inouye SK. Prevalence and outcomes of low mobility in hospitalized older patients. J Am Geriatr Soc 2004; 52:1263–1270.

22. Bryant B, Limacher MC. Exercise testing in selected patient groups: women, the elderly and the asymptomatic. Prim Care 1994; 21:517–534.

23. Cappola AR, Bandeen-Roche K, Wand GS, et al. Association of IGF-1 levels with muscle strength and mobility in older women. J Clin Endocrinol Metab 2001; 86:4139–4146.

24. Castenada C, Charnley JM, Evans WJ, et al. Elderly women accommodate to a low-protein diet with losses of body cell mass, muscle function, and immune response. Am J Clin Nutr 1995; 62:30–39.

25. Chutka DS, Evans JM, Fleming KC, et al. Drug prescribing for elderly patients. Mayo Clin Proc 1995; 70:685–693.

26. Colbert LH, Visser M, Simonsick EM, et al. Physical activity, exercise, and inflammatory markers in older adults: findings from the Health, Aging and Body Composition Study. J Am Geriatr Soc 2004; 52:1098–1104.

27. Coletta EM. Care of the elderly patient with lower limb amputation. J Am Board Fam Pract 2000; 13:23–34.

28. Crome P. What's different about older people? Toxicology 2003; 192:49–54.

29. Cummings JL, Cole G. Alzheimer disease. JAMA 2002; 287:2335–2338.

30. Cutson TM, Bongiorni DR. Rehabilitation of the older limb amputee: a brief review. J Am Geriatr Soc 1996; 44:1388–1393.

31. D'Antona G, Pellegrino MA, Adami R, et al. The effect of ageing and immobilization on structure and function of human skeletal muscle fibres. J Physiol 2003; 552:499–511.

32. Earles DR, Judge JO, Gunnarsson OT. Velocity training induces power-specific adaptations in highly functioning older adults. Arch Phys Med Rehabil 2001; 82:872–878.

33. Ettinger WH, Burns R, Messier SP. A randomized trial comparing aerobic exercise and resistance exercise with a health education program in older adults with knee osteoarthritis: the Fitness, Arthritis and Seniors Trials (FAST). JAMA 1997; 277:25–31.

34. Evans JM, Chutka DS, Fleming KC, et al. Medical care of nursing home residents. Mayo Clin Proc 1995; 70:694–702.

35. Felsenthal G, Lehman JA, Stein B. Principles of geriatric rehabilitation. In: Braddom R, ed. Physical medicine and rehabilitation. 2nd edn. Philadelphia: Saunders; 2000:1343–1367.

36. Ferruci L, Guralnik JM, Studenski S, et al. Designing randomized, controlled trials aimed at preventing or delaying functional decline and disability in frail, older persons: a consensus report. J Am Geriatr Soc 2004; 52:625–634.

37. Fiatarone MA, Marks EC, Ryan ND, et al. High-intensity strength training in nonagenarians. JAMA 1990; 263:3029–3034.

38. Fiatarone MA, O'Neill EF, Ryan ND, et al. Exercise training and nutritional supplementation for physical frailty in very elderly people. New Engl J Med 1994; 330:1769–1775.

39. Fielding RA, LeBrasseur NK, Cuoco A, et al. High-velocity training increases skeletal muscle peak power in older women. J Am Geriatr Soc 2002; 50:655–662.

40. Fitzgerald PL. Exercise for the elderly. Med Clin N Am 1985; 69:189–196.

41. Fleming KC, Evans JM, Weber DC, et al. Practical functional assessment of elderly persons: a primary-care approach. Mayo Clin Proc 1995; 70:890–910.

42. Fletcher DD, Andrews KL, Hallett JW, et al. Trends in rehabilitation after amputation for geriatric patients with vascular disease: implications for future health resource allocation. Arch Phys Med Rehabil 2002; 83:1389–1393.

43. Fried LP, Young Y, Rubin G, et al for the WHAS II Collaborative Research Group. Self-reported preclinical disability identifies older women with early declines in performance and early disease. J Clin Epidemiol 2001; 54:889–901.

44. Friedman SM, Munoz B, West SK, et al. Falls and fear of falling: which come first? A longitudinal prediction model suggests strategies for primary and secondary prevention. J Am Geriatr Soc 2002; 50:1329–1335.

45. Gerber JG, Hollister AS. Drug use in the elderly. In: Jahnigen D, Schrier S, eds. Geriatric medicine. Cambridge: Blackwell Science; 1996:84–97.

46. Gill TM, Baker DI, Gottschalk M, et al. A program to prevent functional decline in physically frail, elderly persons who live at home. N Engl J Med 2002; 347:1068–1074.

47. Gill TM, DiPietro L, Krumholz HM. Role of exercise stress testing and safety monitoring for older persons starting an exercise program. JAMA 2000; 284:342–340.

48. Gloth FM. Pain management in older adults: prevention and treatment. J Am Geriatric Soc 2001; 49:188–199.

49. Gordon NF, Gulanick M, Costa F, et al. Physical activity and exercise recommendations for stroke survivors: an American Heart Association scientific statement from the Council on Clinical Cardiology, Subcommittee on Exercise, Cardiac Rehabilitation, and Prevention; the Council on Cardiovascular Nursing; the Council on Nutrition, Physical Activity and Metabolism; and the Stroke Council. Stroke 2004; 35:1230–1240.

50. Grabiner PC, Biswas T, Grabiner MD. Age-related changes in spatial and temporal gait variables. Arch Phys Med Rehabil 2001; 82:31–35.

51. Hardy SE, Gill TM. Recovery from disability among community-dwelling older persons. JAMA 2004; 291:1956–1602.

52. Hauer K, Rost B, Rutschle K, et al. Exercise training for rehabilitation and secondary prevention of falls in geriatric patients with a history of injurious falls. J Am Geriatr Soc 2001: 49:10–20.

53. Hausdorff JM, Edelberg HK, Cudkowicz ME, et al. Relationship between gait changes and falls [letter to the editor]. J Am Geriatric Soc 1997; 45:1406.

54. Hirsch MA, Toole T, Maitland CG, et al. The effects of balance training and high-intensity resistance training on persons with idiopathic Parkinson's disease. Arch Phys Med Rehabil 2003; 84:1109–1117.

55. Hoenig H, Nusbaum N, Brummel-Smith K. Geriatric rehabilitation: state of the art. J Am Geriatr Soc 1997; 45:1371–1381.

56. Hughes VA, Frontera WR, Wood M, et al. Longitudinal muscle strength changes in older adults: influence of muscle mass, physical activity and health. J Gerontol 2001; 56A:B209–B217.

57. Huusko TM, Karpii P, Avikainen V, et al. Randomized, clinically controlled trial of intensive geriatric rehabilitation in patients with hip fracture: subgroup analysis of patients with dementia. Br Med J 2000; 321:1107–1111.

58. Jacobson S, Schreibman B. Behavioral and pharmacologic treatment of delirium. Am Fam Physician 1997; 56:2005–2012.

59. Janssen I, Shepard DS, Katzmarzyk PT, et al. The healthcare costs of sarcopenia in the United States. J Am Geriatr Soc 2004; 52:80–85.

60. Jette AM, Harris BA, Sleeper L, et al. A home-based exercise program for nondisabled older adults. J Am Geriatr Soc 1996; 44:644–649.

61. Jubelt B, Agre JC. Characteristics and management of postpolio syndrome. JAMA 2000; 284:412–414.

62. Kaufman DW, Kelly JP, Rosenberg L, et al. Recent patterns of medication use in the ambulatory adult population of the United States: the Slone Survey. JAMA 2002; 287:337–344.

63. Klingbeil H, Baer HR, Wilson PE. Aging with a disability. Arch Phys Med Rehabil 2004; 85(suppl 3):S68–S73.

64. Koval KJ, Meek R, Schemitsch E, et al. Geriatric trauma: young ideas. J Bone Joint Surg Am 2003; 85A:1380–1388.

65. Krane SM, Holick MF. Metabolic bone disease. In: Fauci AS, Braunwald E, Isselbacher KJ, et al, eds. Harrison's principles of internal medicine. New York: McGraw-Hill; 1998:2247–2259.

66. Liberman UA, Weiss SR, Broll J, et al. Effect of oral alendronate on bone mineral density and the incidence of fractures in postmenopausal osteoporosis. N Engl J Med 1995; 333:1437–1443.

67. Ling SM, Bathon JM. Osteoarthritis in older adults. J Am Geriatr Soc 1998; 46:216–225.

68. Liu-Ambrose T, Khan KM, Eng JJ, et al. Resistance and agility training reduce fall risk in women ages 75 to 85 with low bone mass: a 6-month randomized, controlled trial. J Am Geriatr Soc 2004; 52:657–665.

69. Lord SR, Castell S, Corcoran J, et al. The effect of group exercise on physical functioning and falls in frail older people living in retirement villages: a randomized controlled trial. J Am Geriatr Soc 2003; 51:1685–1692.

70. Lundin-Olsson L, Nyberg L, Gustafson Y. Attention, frailty and falls: the effect of a manual task on basic mobility. J Am Geriatr Soc 1998; 46:758–761.

71. Lundin-Olsson L, Nyberg L, Gustafson Y. 'Stops walking when talking' as a predictor of falls in elderly people. Lancet 1997; 349:617.

72. Lynn SG, Sinaki M, Westerlind KC. Balance characteristics of persons with osteoporosis. Arch Phys Med Rehab 1997; 78:273–277.

73. Maki B. Gait changes in older adults: predictors of falls or indicators of fear? J Am Geriatr Soc 1997; 45:313–320.

74. Marottoli RC, Berkman LF, Cooney LM. Decline in physical function following hip fracture. J Am Geriatr Soc 1992; 40:861–866.

75. Mazzeo RS, Cavanagh P, Evans WJ. ACSM position stand: exercise and physical activity for older adults. Med Sci Sports Exerc 1998; 30:992–1008.

76. McColl MA, Arnold R, Charlifue S, et al. Aging, spinal cord injury, and quality of life: structural relationships. Arch Phys Med Rehabil 2003; 84:1137–1144.

77. Morley JE, Baumgartner RN, Roubenoff R, et al. Sarcopenia. J Lab Clin Med 2001; 137:231–243.

78. Murray PK, Singer M, Dawson NV, et al. Outcomes of rehabilitation services for nursing home residents. Arch Phys Med Rehabil 2003; 84:1129–1136.

79. Nelson ME, Layne JE, Bernstein MJ, et al. The effects of multidimensional home-based exercise on functional performance in elderly people. J Gerontol Med Sci 2004; 59A:154–160.

80. Nelson ME, Layne JE, Nuernberger A, et al. The effects of a home-based program on functional performance in the frail elderly: an update [annual meeting abstract]. Med Sci Sports Exerc 1999; 31(suppl):S377.

81. Ouellette MM, LeBrasseur NK, Bean JF, et al. High-intensity resistance training improves muscle strength, self-reported function, and disability in long-term stroke survivors. Stroke 2004; 35:1404–1409.

82. Pandian G, Kowalske K. Daily functioning of patients with an amputated lower extremity. Clin Orthop Relat Res 1999; 361:91–97.

83. Phillips EM, Bodenheimer CF, Roig RL, et al. Geriatric rehabilitation. 4. Physical medicine and rehabilitation interventions for common age-related disorders and geriatric syndromes. Arch Phys Med Rehabil 2004; 85(suppl 3):S18–S22.

84. Playfer JR. The therapeutic challenges in the older Parkinson's disease patient. Eur J Neurol 2002; 9(suppl 3):55–58.

85. Resnick NM. Geriatric medicine. In: Fauci AS, Braunwald E, Isselbacher KJ, et al, eds. Harrison's principles of internal medicine. New York: McGraw-Hill; 1998:37–46.

86. Robichaud L, Lamarre C. Developing an instrument for identifying coping strategies used by the elderly to remain autonomous. Am J Phys Med Rehabil 2002; 81:736–744.

87. Roig RL, Worsowicz GM, Stewart DG, et al. Geriatric rehabilitation. 3. Physical medicine and rehabilitation interventions for common disabling disorders. Arch Phys Med Rehabil 2004; 85(suppl 3): S12–S17.

88. Ropper AH, Martin JB. Acute confusional states and coma. In: Fauci AS, Braunwald E, Isselbacher KJ, et al, eds. Harrison's principles of internal medicine. New York: McGraw-Hill; 1998:125–134.

89. Rosenberg IH. Nutrition and aging. In: Hazzard WR, Bierman EL, Blass JP, et al, eds. Principles of geriatric medicine and gerontology. New York: McGraw-Hill; 1994:49–59.

90. Rosenthal RA, Kavic SM. Assessment and management of the geriatric patient. Crit Care Med 2004; 32(suppl):S92–S105.

91. Roubenoff R, Hughes VA. Sarcopenia: current concepts. J Gerontol 2000: 55A:M716–M724.

92. Sauvage LR, Myklebust BM, Crow-Pan J, et al. A clinical trial of strengthening and aerobic exercise to improve gait and balance in elderly male nursing home residents. Am J Phys Med Rehabil 1992; 71:33–342.

93. Sayers SP, Bean J, Cuoco A, et al. Changes in function and disability after resistance training: does velocity matter? Am J Phys Med Rehabil 2003; 82:605–613.

94. Scheitel SM, Fleming KC, Chutka DS, et al. Geriatric health maintenance. Mayo Clin Proc 1996; 71:289–302.

95. Schneider SM, Al-Jaouni R, Pivot Z, et al. Lack of adaptation to severe malnutrition in elderly patients. Clin Nutr 2002; 21:499–504.

96. Sevick MA, Bradham DD, Muender M, et al. Cost-effectiveness of aerobic and resistance exercise in seniors with knee osteoarthritis. Med Sci Sports Exerc 2000; 32:1534–1540.

97. Sinaki M, Itoi E, Wahner HW, et al. Stronger back muscles reduce the incidence of vertebral fractures: a prospective 10 year follow-up of postmenopausal women. Bone 2002; 30:836–841.

98. Sinaki M, Lynn SG. Reducing the risk of falls through proprioceptive dynamic posture training in osteoporotic women with kyphotic posturing: a randomized pilot study. Am J Phys Med Rehabil 2002; 81:241–246.

99. Sinaki M, Wollan PC, Scott RW, et al. Can strong back extensors prevent vertebral fractures in women with osteoporosis? Mayo Clin Proc 1996; 71:951–956.

100. Singh MAF, Rosenberg IH. Nutrition and aging. In: Hazzard WR, Blass JP, Ettinger WH Jr, eds. Principles of geriatric medicine and gerontology. New York: McGraw-Hill; 1999:81–96.

101. Singh NA, Clements KM, Singh MAF. Efficacy of exercise as a long-term antidepressant in elderly subjects: a randomized, controlled trial. J Gerontol Med Sci 2001; 56: M497–M504.

102. Siris ES, Bilezikian JP, Rubin M, et al. Pins and plaster aren't enough: a call for the evaluation and treatment of patients with osteoporotic fractures. J Clin Endocrinol Metab 2003; 88:3482–3486.

103. Small GE, Rabins PV, Barry PP, et al. Diagnosis and treatment of Alzheimer disease and related disorders: consensus statement of the American Association for Geriatric Psychiatry, the Alzheimer's Association, and the American Geriatrics Society. JAMA 1997; 278:1363–1371.

104. Suzuki T, Bean JF, Fielding RA. Muscle power of the ankle flexors predicts functional performance in community-dwelling older women. J Am Geriatr Soc 2001; 49:1161–1167.

105. Thorsteinsson G. Management of postpolio syndrome. Mayo Clin Proc 1997; 72:627–638.

106. Tsang WW, Wong VS, Fu SN, et al. Tai chi improves standing balance control under reduced or conflicting sensory conditions. Arch Phys Med Rehabil 2004; 85:129–137.

107. Vasilomanolakis EC. Geriatric cardiology: when exercise stress testing is justified. Geriatrics 1985; 40:47–57.

108. Vincent KR, Braith RW, Feldman RA, et al. Resistance exercise and physical performance in adults aged 60 to 83. J Am Geriatr Soc 2002; 50: 1100–1107.

109. Vincent KR, Braith RW. Resistance exercise and bone turnover in elderly men and women. Med Sci Sports Exerc 2002; 34:17–23.

110. Visser M, Bouter LM, McQuillan GM, et al. Elevated C-reactive protein levels in overweight and obese adults. JAMA 1999; 282:2131–2135.

111. Waddington GS, Adams RD. The effect of a 5-week wobble-board exercise intervention on ability to discriminate different degrees of ankle inversion, barefoot and wearing shoes: a study in healthy elderly. J Am Geriatr Soc 2004; 52:573–576.

112. Waters RL, Mulroy S. The energy expenditure of normal and pathologic gait. Gait Posture 1999; 9:207–231.

113. Weiss A, Suzuki T, Bean J, et al. High intensity training improves strength and functional performance after stroke. Am J Phys Med Rehabil 2000; 79:369–376.

114. Wolf SL, Barnhart HX, Kutnet NG, et al. Reducing frailty and falls in older persons: an investigation of tai chi and computerized balance training. J Am Geriatr Soc 1996; 44:489–497.

115. Wolfson L, Whipple R, Derby C, et al. Balance and strength training in older adults: intervention gains and tai chi maintenance. J Am Geriatr Soc 1996; 44:498–506.

Chapter

61

Organ Transplantation and Rehabilitation

Mark A. Young and Steven A. Stiens

Rehabilitation of patients who receive organs in transplantation surgery has become the standard of care in many medical centers throughout the world. The swift development of new and innovative means of staving off infection and rejection after organ transplant has resulted in greater survivorship among organ transplant recipients.[87] The availability of emerging chronic immunosuppressive drugs with greater potency and reduced side effects has improved outcomes,[136,155] enabling patients to be transferred to the acute rehabilitation unit earlier. The prophylactic use of acute immunosuppressive therapies such as monoclonal and polyclonal antibodies contributed to successful organ transplantation surgery and subsequent rehabilitation functional restoration.[41,50,56,155] The emergence of the science of human leukocyte antigen (HLA) matching and the perfection of the HLA Registry process has considerably improved outcomes for bone marrow transplant recipients.[56,100] Optimization of surgical techniques has led to both a rise in the number of transplant surgeries performed annually and an increase in the diversity and complexity of these procedures (Fig. 61-1). Prominent examples include the emergence of groundbreaking new transplantation procedures, including multiple limb transplantation[32] and 'domino' organ transplants.[2,9,50] The net result of many of these breakthroughs has been a surging demand for rehabilitation services.

For patients undergoing blood and marrow transplants, the federal government, in cooperation with the National Institute of Allergy and Infectious Diseases and the National Library of Medicine, in 2004 established a unique public database containing results of blood and marrow stem cell transplants involving unrelated donors.[50] The database is accessible to physicians, researchers, and patients online at http://www.ncbi.nih.gov/mhc. Contained in this resource is critical demographic information such as sex, ethnicity, age, and genetic data on more than 1300 transplant donors and recipients worldwide. It also includes projected survival rates of transplant recipients. Data on the relationship between transplantation and major histocompatibility complex genes is also included, which can assist doctors to better prognosticate if a recipient will 'accept' or 'reject' a transplant from a particular donor source. This contemporary resource aids physicians in the evaluation of risks and benefits of transplantation for various clinical conditions. For the physiatrist providing preoperative/pretransplant consultative input, the data gleaned from this source can help to predict outcomes and guide posttransplant rehabilitation.

Despite the many advances in organ transplantation science, an international crisis looms. The demand for organs radically outnumbers the amount of available organ donors, despite donor increases (UNOS–OPTN data). This unmet need creates many ethical questions.[44,68,63,108] National organizations within the USA, such as the United Network for Organ Sharing (UNOS) and the Organ Procurement and Transplant Network (OPTN), exist to coordinate distribution. OPTN is a private, non-profit, federally contracted transplant network established by the US Congress under the National Organ Transplant Act of 1984, which unites all the professionals involved in the transplantation and donation system. OPTN works to increase the effectiveness and efficiency of organ sharing, to provide equity in the national system of organ allocation, and to increase the supply of donated organs available for transplantation. UNOS is responsible for administering the OPTN, under contract with the Health Resources and Services Administration of the US Department of Health and Human Services. Together, UNOS and OPTN work on the establishment of organ transplantation policies and procedures. Assurance of positive functional outcomes posttransplantation remains a major goal. As a result, physiatrists are likely to see a future surge in the number of transplantation patients seeking rehabilitation.

This chapter provides a general overview of the subject of organ transplantation and rehabilitation. While solid organ transplantation rehabilitation (kidney, liver, heart, and lung) is the primary focus, reference will be made to recent developments in bone marrow and hematologic transplantation that impact on physiatry. An illustration of the rehabilitation method as applied throughout the transplantation process is presented, followed by a systematic consideration of rehabilitation principles and techniques that can improve outcome and quality of life. Of the more than 21 transplantable organ systems, this chapter concentrates on the four most common ones seen in physiatric practice (heart, lung, liver, and kidney).

CURRENT TRANSPLANT DATA AND DEMOGRAPHICS

Rehabilitation professionals and other members of the transplantation and pretransplantation team can access the most recent data made available by UNOS–OPTN online at http://www.unos.org/data/. An analysis of the most recent UNOS–

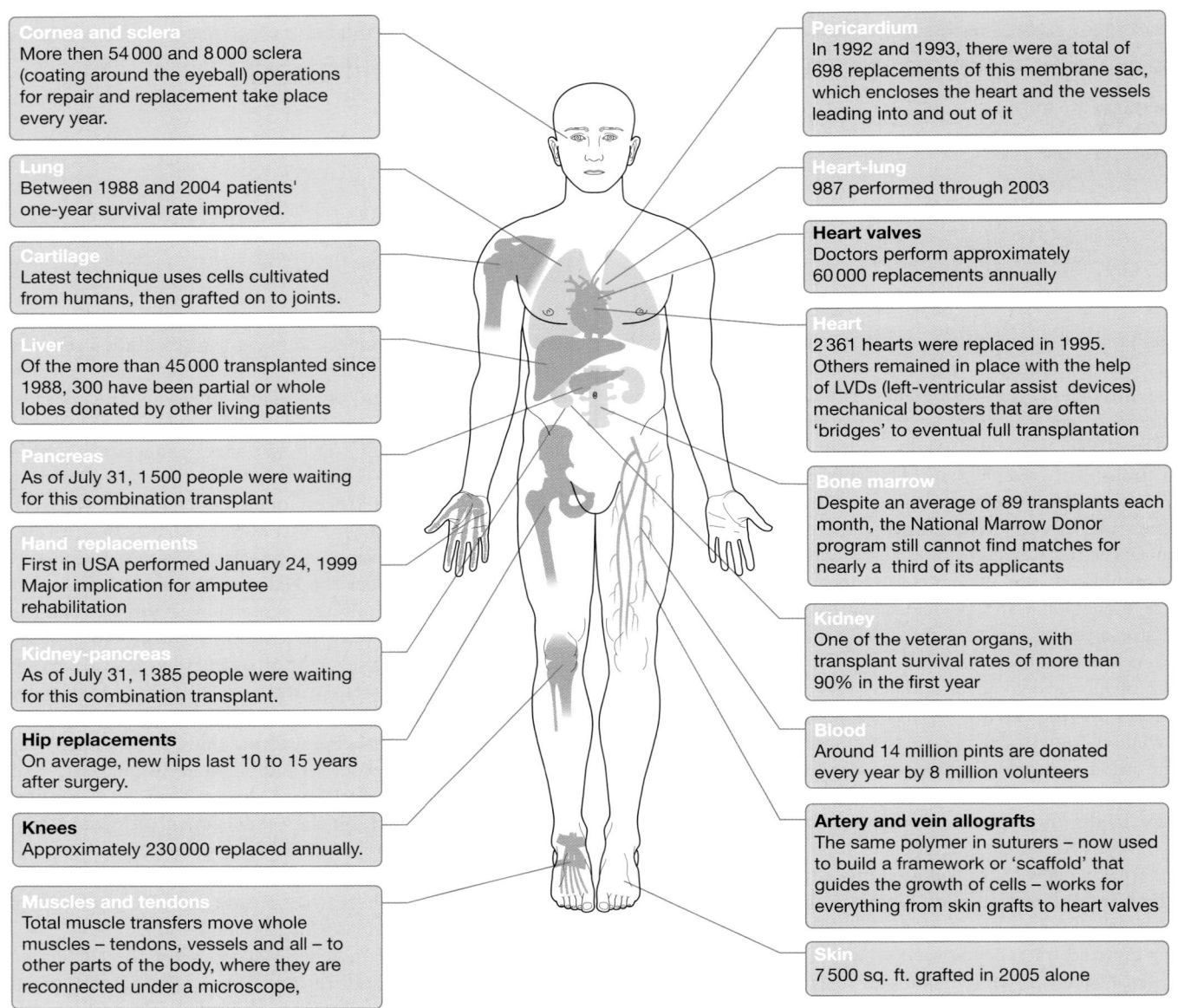

Cornea and sclera
More then 54 000 and 8 000 sclera (coating around the eyeball) operations for repair and replacement take place every year.

Lung
Between 1988 and 2004 patients' one-year survival rate improved.

Cartilage
Latest technique uses cells cultivated from humans, then grafted on to joints.

Liver
Of the more than 45 000 transplanted since 1988, 300 have been partial or whole lobes donated by other living patients

Pancreas
As of July 31, 1 500 people were waiting for this combination transplant

Hand replacements
First in USA performed January 24, 1999 Major implication for amputee rehabilitation

Kidney-pancreas
As of July 31, 1 385 people were waiting for this combination transplant.

Hip replacements
On average, new hips last 10 to 15 years after surgery.

Knees
Approximately 230 000 replaced annually.

Muscles and tendons
Total muscle transfers move whole muscles – tendons, vessels and all – to other parts of the body, where they are reconnected under a microscope,

Pericardium
In 1992 and 1993, there were a total of 698 replacements of this membrane sac, which encloses the heart and the vessels leading into and out of it

Heart-lung
987 performed through 2003

Heart valves
Doctors perform approximately 60 000 replacements annually

Heart
2 361 hearts were replaced in 1995. Others remained in place with the help of LVDs (left-ventricular assist devices) mechanical boosters that are often 'bridges' to eventual full transplantation

Bone marrow
Despite an average of 89 transplants each month, the National Marrow Donor program still cannot find matches for nearly a third of its applicants

Kidney
One of the veteran organs, with transplant survival rates of more than 90% in the first year

Blood
Around 14 million pints are donated every year by 8 million volunteers

Artery and vein allografts
The same polymer in suturers – now used to build a framework or 'scaffold' that guides the growth of cells – works for everything from skin grafts to heart valves

Skin
7 500 sq. ft. grafted in 2005 alone

Figure 61-1 Rehabilitation aspects of organ transplantation. White, donor organs; black, artificial parts. Sources: United Network for Organ Sharing, Eye Bank Association of America, American Association of Tissue Banks, Baylor College of Medicine, National Marrow Donor Program, Columbia-Presbyterian Medical Center. (From Time, fall 1996, statistics revised 2003.)

OPTN data available as of August 2004 indicated a current USA Organ waiting list of over 86 542 people. Patients requiring kidney transplantation constitute the largest group of candidates, followed by pancreas, liver, intestine, heart, and lung (see Fig. 61-1). In the first 5 months of 2004, a total of 10 856 transplants were performed. Since 2000, an average of 5800 people died annually while waiting for a transplant, an average of more then 15 people per day.

PHYSIATRY AND TRANSPLANTATION

Establishing a functional and medical baseline prior to surgery is essential.[22,160,184,185] Consequently, the physiatric evaluation should include a comprehensive medical history and elaboration of functional deficits associated with end-stage organ damage. The physiatrist should conduct a thorough musculoskeletal, neurologic, and functional assessment of the patient (Box 61-1). Emphasis should be placed on the maintenance of bodily systems that are likely to be adversely affected by nutritional deficits[52] and immobilization. This includes preventive measures for contractures, deep vein thrombosis, pulmonary embolism, and skin breakdown, and plans for management of bowel and bladder function. The prevention of disuse atrophy of major muscle groups can be addressed through bedside isometric exercise protocols. A therapeutic plan emphasizing exercise and remobilization should be generated that takes into account the patient's presurgical functional status. Adequate considera-

Box 61-1 Transplantation and rehabilitation assessment

Physiatric history
- Diagnosis resulting in transplantation
- Functional history (premorbid and posttransplant)
  Mobility status
  Use of assistive or adaptive devices
  Activities of daily living
  Community and household activities
  Cognition and communication
  Vocation
- Past medical and surgical history (presurgical)
- Review of systems
- Evidence of end-organ damage (neuropathy, retinopathy)
- Prior rehabilitation
- Medications, allergies, and diet

Psychosocial history
- Living arrangements
- Family and friendship support
- Use of drugs and alcohol
- Psychiatric history

Rehabilitation examination
- Musculoskeletal assessment of the transplant patient
- Inspection
- Palpation
- Joint assessment (range of motion and contractures)
- Manual muscle testing

Functional examination
- Mobility
- Activities of daily living

Neurologic examination
- Alertness and mental status
- Cranial nerve
- Motor and sensory
- Reflexes
- Communication

Box 61-2 Members of the transplant rehabilitation team

- Physiatry
- Surgery
- Psychiatry
- Internal medicine
- Nutritional support
- Occupational therapy
- Nursing
- Speech therapy
- Physical therapy
- Social service
- Vocational rehabilitation counciling

INTERDISCIPLINARY FORMULATION AND IMPLEMENTATION OF THE REHABILITATION PLAN

The need for comprehensive rehabilitation of patients receiving organ transplants is essential to achieve their best health and quality of life. The physiatric evaluation should ideally be completed *prior* to transplant surgery. This assessment reveals a picture of the patient's full functional deficits and the impact on lifestyle, and affords an opportunity for interdisciplinary goal setting. The physiatrist should conduct a thorough review of systems, a functional history, and a broad examination addressing the organ system receiving the transplant, as well as systems associated with complications and disuse deterioration. Emphasis should be placed on assembly of a person-centered rehabilitation plan, with a comprehensive problem list that includes previously identified medical and surgical diagnoses that are under treatment. It also should include functional deficits and other problem areas for goal-focused treatment.[159,160]

During the initial rehabilitation, the interdisciplinary team typically interacts with the surgical team on a consultative basis.[160] On transfer to inpatient rehabilitation, there needs to be an assessment of the specific roles and follow-up needs to be itemized in discussions with the transplant surgical service and any active medical consultants. The problem list is the skeleton for the comprehensive rehabilitation plan. This list should start with a series of diagnoses in the order of their importance and grouped by system, with the particular transplant system at the top. Thereafter, *impairments* of strength, sensation, and coordination should be listed. Following that, *activity limitations* of mobility and activities of daily living are listed. Finally, *barriers to participation*, such as psychologic adaptation (person level), social role function (societal level: family and friends), vocation, architectural accessibility, and spiritual access, are often addressed. Appropriate laboratory values assessing nutritional status (albumin and prealbumin), potential vitamin deficiency (B_{12}, folate, and zinc), and organ function should be requested to help plan the treatment. The full rehabilitation plan should include interdisciplinary perspectives and be recorded as short- and long-term goals under each problem. The transition to inpatient rehabilitation, if required,

tion of patients' capacity for psychologic adaptation, their social role, the impact of the impairment on activity limitation, barriers to participation, and disablement must be made (as is the standard of physiatric care in all areas of rehabilitation).[159,162] Continual communication and education of other members of the transplant team is essential during each step of the process (Box 61-2).

Post transplantation, close ongoing daily observation is essential to assure adequate immune system suppression, prevent opportunistic infection, and maintain rehabilitation goals.[59] Emphasis should be placed on the underlying functional, medical, socioeconomic,[27] and psychologic needs of the patient.[77] A fundamental knowledge of the clinical aspects of acute and chronic rejection in all types of transplantation surgeries should be appreciated by the rehabilitation team. Because patients who have undergone a transplant typically present with a multitude of medical comorbidities, it is important to include any appropriate precautions in the prescription for rehabilitation and home care.[51,57,130,179] Careful consideration of an exercise prescription should be made.[19]

is facilitated with early comprehensive formulation of a plan and aggressive therapy as tolerated on the surgical service. Care maps, clinical pathways, and basic order sets developed in collaboration with the transplant surgery services simplify and standardize many interventions.[1] Physiatric collaboration in the design of these care plans for patients receiving a particular organ (i.e. heart, kidney, or liver) directs the utilization of resources and helps achieve the best outcomes. Each patient requires surveillance for signs of opportunistic infection, and careful monitoring of immune suppression to prevent rejection, as well as guided exercise to increase endurance and functional independence. All rehabilitative interventions should be presented with carefully designed precautions and protocols to prevent exposure of the patient to unnecessary infection risk. Social support is particularly important for the best outcomes, and can be outlined using social network mapping to assess needs in physical assistance, emotional support, information and advice, and closeness.[91] Psychosocial status generally improves with transplant, but there are challenges in adjustment and compliance with medical regimens as well.[27] Emphasis should be placed on the unique functional, medical, socioeconomic, and psychologic needs of each patient.[119,138] Because patients who have undergone a transplant typically present with a multitude of medical comorbidities, it is important to include any appropriate precautions in the rehabilitation prescription plan.

REHABILITATION OF THE KIDNEY TRANSPLANT RECIPIENT

In the USA, renal failure results most commonly from diabetes mellitus (33%), hypertension (24%), glomerulonephritis (17%), polycystic kidney disease (5%), and other unknown causes (21%). As the number of people with end-stage renal failure continues to rise, kidney transplantation is being performed with increasing frequency and improved outcome. While dialysis remains a viable long-term treatment for end-stage renal failure, the quality of life has been determined to be less than that after successful transplant. Patients report that dialysis is a stressor, and that transplant is a pathway to 'lead a normal life'.[35] In a recent quality of life comparison between dialysis users and kidney transplant recipients, it was clear that quality of life was better after transplant, with less fatigue; more positive feelings; and greater self-approval of body image, mobility, success in activities of daily living, working capacity, success in relationships, and sexual activity.[167] Fatigue and insufficiency of activities of daily living performance are the primary symptoms that drive the patient's decision for transplant.[53] End-stage renal failure affects every organ system. Anemia is secondary to loss of erythropoietin, hypertension secondary to hyperparathyroidism, and renal osteodystrophy secondary to artery bone metabolism. Renal-associated bone disease alone can be one of three types: renal osteodystrophy, osteitis fibrosa (high turnover), and osteomalacia (low bone matrix turnover bone diagnosis).

Many patients with renal failure are unable to perform even the most basic tasks of everyday life. A majority of patients are unable to work, because they are physically unable to sustain the energy required for work activity. However, the greatly enhanced survival rate of patients who have received a transplant, coupled with the net increase in procedures performed each year, has resulted in a growing number of patients now requiring rehabilitation and vocational services.

From 1998 to 2004, there was a steady rise in the number of kidneys transplanted. In 2003–2004, there were a total of 15 500 kidney transplants, representing an increase of 3010 over the number done in 1998. Despite the rise in kidney transplants, there has been a decline in the number of kidney–pancreas transplants. Kidney transplants are often performed in conjunction with pancreas transplants for patients with severe end-organ damage resulting from diabetes mellitus. An increasing number of patients are surviving and requiring continued rehabilitation and vocational rehabilitation services.[17] Compared with 1998, when a total of 965 simultaneous kidney–pancreas transplants were performed in the USA, there was a decrease to approximately 860 in 2003–2004. Recent literature has demonstrated that the long-term survival of simultaneous kidney–pancreas transplant recipients is superior to that of cadaver kidney transplant recipients with type 1 diabetes, although there is no difference in survival of simultaneous kidney–pancreas transplant recipients and that of living donor kidney recipients with type 1 diabetes at up to 8 years' follow-up.[132] The overall cadaver kidney success rate is 89% at 1 year and 65.6% at 5 years. The first-year posttransplant period includes surveillance for infection with herpes simplex virus, cytomegalovirus, urinary tract infection, and chronic hepatitis. The medical conditions followed in the years after the late post transplantation include hypertension, coronary artery disease, skin cancer, diabetes, bone disease, and dental care.[21] Rehabilitation exercise regimens focus on lifestyle and build in stretching, repetitive low-level resistance, and aerobic exercise, with a goal of a total dose of approximately 30 min per day. The benefits include increased flexibility, reduced systemic resistance for blood pressure reduction, and endurance activity to reduce fatigue. Aerobic exercise must be dosed conservatively, as renal perfusion can be compromised during times of heavy sustained exertion.

Complications that can surface during the postoperative period include infection, bleeding, and rejection. The rehabilitation team must be aware of the signs of kidney rejection. Acute rejection is frequently heralded by anorexia, malaise, fever, hypertension, leukocytosis, blood urea nitrogen elevation, and kidney enlargement with localized tenderness. Immunosuppressant medications typically include prednisone, azathioprine, and cyclosporine, all of which carry a host of potential side effects and reactions. Evidence of kidney rejection can arise during postacute rehabilitation and includes graft site tenderness, reduced urinary output, elevated temperature, and edema.

Exercise training after renal transplant

The renal transplant recipient's ability to exercise is impacted by a number of important physiologic factors. Anemia may still be under treatment with recombinant human erythropoietin to keep the hematocrit at 33–36%.[123] Low levels of available red blood cells and hemoglobin can cause fatigue and decreased work capacity.[122] Metabolic abnormalities, such as electrolyte imbalance including hyperkalemia and water retention, can increase right and left ventricle preload. As circulatory volume increases, hypertension becomes exacerbated and increased as the afterload is maintained. This situation frequently leads to the development of ventricular hypertrophy, increased ventricular stiffness, and diminished compliance. Just as the ability to exercise is significantly impaired in chronic renal patients, patients who have received transplanted kidneys also can develop exercise intolerance.[38] Several factors contribute to this, including skeletal muscle atrophy, anemia, and cardiovascular deconditioning.

A well-designed and utilized pretransplant exercise program can prevent many complications. Individualized self-practiced home aerobic and resistive exercise training after renal transplant results in greater strength and higher levels of measured and self-reported physical functioning.[62] Exercise alone, however, has only minor effects on body composition.[121] Exercise training after transplant further increases exercise capacity and counteracts some of the negative side effects of glucocorticoid therapy, such as muscle wasting and excessive weight gain. Studies have shown that, even before erythropoietin administration, exercise training in patients on dialysis can increase exercise tolerance by 25%. Similar increases are observed after correction of anemia with erythropoietin, although the increase in exercise capacity is small.[96] Because of the feeling of fatigue, physiatrists frequently need to encourage renal patients to exercise and improve their physical functioning.[75,121,122] Renal rehabilitation is an essential therapeutic method for improving physical fitness, social function, well-being, and health-adjusted quality of life in end-stage renal disease and posttransplant patients. A successful kidney transplant can greatly increase a patient's exercise capacity to near-normal values for sedentary healthy individuals.[37,80,141]

Maximizing social participation with renal rehabilitation

The personal,[79] social, and vocational domains of rehabilitation intervention are particularly important after kidney transplant.[35,36] Despite the success with fatigue symptoms and other complications of chronic dialysis afforded kidney recipients, as many as 83% of these patients do not return to work.[111,112,115,174,180,182] The phenomenon is a complex one and includes the burdens of other diagnoses (i.e. hypertension, diabetes mellitus, and coronary artery disease), and sustained healthcare support leading to the transplant can condition the patient for the habitual sick role.[174] Specific, focused, and consistent interdisciplinary team intervention in this regard has been helpful in getting more patients back into the workforce. Patients who have not returned to work have stated fears of their condition deteriorating.[49] The demographic variable most strongly associated with work expectations is job satisfaction pretransplant.

REHABILITATION OF THE PERSON WITH CARDIAC TRANSPLANTATION

Heart transplant epidemiology

The 90-day survival rate of patients undergoing heart transplant improved to 60% in the decade following inauguration of the procedure in 1967.[156] With continuing refinements in surgical technique, more than 2000 heart transplants had been performed throughout the world by 1990. By 2001, 2202 heart transplants were performed in the USA. Heart failure patients who are status 1, class 4, have a 66% 1-year mortality rate. More than 300 are awaiting heart–lung transplantation as well.[87] Survival rates are consistently improving.[128] Heart recipient survival rates in 2002 were 81% for 1-year and 78% for 5 years.[75] Today, many recipients are expected to survive greater than 10 years after their transplants, due mainly to the use of cyclosporine immune suppression.[69,151,183] It is estimated that survival rates after heart transplantation will continue to improve due to improved rejection prevention, better surgical techniques, and enhancement of antirejection methodology.

Rehabilitation before the heart transplant

Congestive heart failure is the leading indication for heart transplantation. Less common indications include idiopathic cardiomyopathy and postpartum cardiomyopathy.[64,84] Physiatric evaluation in collaboration with the cardiologist is helpful in determining whether heart transplantation is right for a particular patient. This evaluation should include a thorough review of the patient's physical health, expected changes in quality of life[14] with the transplant, and potential risks for complications, as well as a functional status baseline.

Just as rehabilitative outcomes frequently hinge on choosing the right candidate,[156] the success of heart transplantation depends on careful selection of suitable patients. Recent production and implantation of Ventes left ventricular assist devices and other devices such as the HeartMate and total artificial heart can improve tolerance for activity, but rehabilitation is essential to maximize outcomes.[39,131] Patients with proven clinical evidence of declining cardiac function and irreversible heart disease should be prioritized for transplantation. Several criteria that have been utilized for cardiac transplant candidate selection[162] are outlined in Box 61-3.

Box 61-3 Indications for cardiac transplantation

- Life-threatening recurrent arrhythmia uncontrolled by medicine or electrophysiologic means
- Reduced VO_{2max} (less than 14/mL per kg per min) and severe limitations in life activity
- Having severe angina without successful revascularization
- Heart failure or congestive heart failure consistently uncontrollable by medical therapy

(From Tayler and Bergin 1995,[162] with permission.)

Complications after cardiac transplantation

The cardiac rehabilitation team should be familiar with the presentation of potential complications, because they spend considerable time working directly with the patient after transplant. Coordination of care and communication between the cardiac surgeon, cardiologist, and physiatrist is essential for success. The main complication seen post transplant is allograft failure from rejection. Other complications include problems related to immunosuppression, such as infection, neurologic deficits, and physiologic complications. One study of cardiac transplant recipients on an inpatient rehabilitation unit reported multiple secondary complications, including hypertension, nutritional limitations, neuromuscular deficits, and compression fractures.[64] Stress fractures of the weight-bearing extremities have also been described,[94] most probably due to steroid-induced osteoporosis. Physiatrists should be clinically familiar with these problems and prepared to evaluate and treat them.

One of the first problems during the early postoperative period is the inability of the transplanted right ventricle of the transplanted heart to cope with preexisting pulmonary hypertension. Pulmonary hypertension can be due to chronic right-sided heart failure. Often, the heart requires ionotropic support during the period immediately following transplant.

Many patients develop hypertension due to cyclosporine-induced renal vasoconstriction superimposed on chronic renal hypoperfusion, third spacing of fluids, and an abnormal distribution of blood flow.[18,46,101,116] Cyclosporine is believed to elicit afferent glomerular arteriolar vasoconstriction through an increase in transmembrane calcium flux in mesangial and vascular smooth muscle cells.[94,116] Blood pressures should be closely monitored, with morning blood pressure values used as a guide to antihypertensive therapy.[18,120] This can be achieved in most cases without interruption of the exercise therapy regimen. Alternative cyclosporine dosing regimens, calcium channel antagonists, and angiotensin-converting enzyme inhibitors are preferred therapies to promote arteriolar dilatation.[13,90,170] Proper management of the hypertension facilitates full participation in the rehabilitative process.

Cardiac transplantation itself can cause neurologic complications, including metabolic encephalopathy, stroke, central nervous system infection, seizures, and psychosis. These potential complications are most likely to present during the acute posttransplant period, although they can also surface during the rehabilitative or restorative phase.[154] The mechanism of stroke includes particulate embolism, air embolism, or inadequacy of perfusion during the transplantation procedure. Careful review of mental status, perceptual sensation, and motor function is an essential part of the physiatric consultation in the postoperative phase.

Once the posttransplant patient has achieved circulatory stability, a continued challenge is prevention of rejection. The heart transplant recipient is generally less immunologically depressed than the kidney transplant patient. This is due to the prolonged uremia associated with kidney failure. Rehabilitation professionals must always be mindful of the systemic and metabolic effects of medications. A summary of the side effects of some of the most frequently used immunosuppressive agents is provided in Table 61-1. See Table 61-2 for the monitoring parameters for immunosuppressive medication.

Acute rejection in cardiac transplantation is a major complication that can be heralded by fulminant exacerbation of congestive heart failure, development of peripheral edema, premature atrial contractions, and/or diastolic gallop and sudden marked reduction in exercise capacity. Chronic rejection can also manifest itself as accelerated graft atherosclerosis.[25,173] At 1 year post transplantation, 10–15% of patients have developed accelerated graft atherosclerosis, which rises to 35–50% by the fifth postoperative year.[31,151] Denervation produces an up-regulation of muscarinic receptors, which facilitates increased calcium influx in the coronary arteries of the transplanted heart. This leads to more diffuse, circumferential narrowing of the arterial luminal diameters. This type of coronary artery disease ultimately is a key barrier to the long-term survival of cardiac transplant patients. Recent studies, however, suggest that this condition can be improved with calcium channel blockers.[145,151] This condition should be placed on the problem list with an included plan for prevention, education surveillance, and acute management.

Beyond the postoperative complications just outlined, the leading cause of death in post-cardiac transplant patients is infection.[105,171] The types of infection include mediastinitis, pneumonia, urinary tract infections, and intravenous catheter-induced sepsis.[56,105,171] Such problems tend to develop especially during the first 2 years following the cardiac transplant.[8,106] Bacterial and viral infections account for 47% and 41% of infections, respectively. Infections caused by fungus and protozoa account for 12% of posttransplant morbidity. Adequate washing of the hands for a full 10 s, or use of an equivalent topical antiseptic, or both before and after direct contact with the transplant patient is imperative.

Physiology of the transplanted heart

Customization of exercise programs for each transplant patient entering rehabilitation is essential, and requires an understanding of the physiology of the transplanted heart. The normal heart is innervated and hence affected by the sympathetic nervous system, which has chronotropic and ionotropic effects.[3,4] The sympathetic nervous system enhances venous return, stroke volume, and cardiac output. A transplanted heart is denervated, and consequently achieves a maximal heart rate more slowly than a normal heart does. It does this primarily through a response to circulating catecholamines, and to a limited extent via partial and inconsistent gradual sympathetic reinnervation.[177] After an exercise session or ambulation activity, the heart transplant patient experiences a more gradual return to baseline. Despite the denervation, cardiac output in the transplanted heart increases in response to dynamic total body activity, promoting venous return and increasing stroke volume through increased preload volume of blood filling the left ventricle.

When orthotopic heart transplant is performed, the complete denervation of the heart leads to a loss of the autonomic nervous

Table 61-1 Systemic and metabolic effects of transplant rejection drugs

Drug	Adverse effect	Clinical manifestation
Azathioprine	Bone marrow depression	Leukopenia, thrombocytopenia, anemia
	Hepatotoxicity	Elevated bilirubin level; elevated alkaline phosphatase, aspartate aminotransferase, alanine aminotransferase; jaundice
	Increased risk of malignancy when associated with high doses of multiple agents	Dependent on type and location of malignancy
Orthoclone (Okt3)	Pyrexia, malaise	Fever, chills, flu-like symptoms; headache, diarrhea
	Respiratory distress associated with initial doses and fluid overload	Chest tightness, dyspnea, wheezing
	Increased risk of malignancy when associated with high doses of multiple agents	Dependent on type and location of malignancy
Antithymocyte preparations	Anaphylactic reactions	Hypotension, dyspnea, wheezing, fever, chills
	Serum sickness associated with antibody formation to foreign protein	Fever, joint pain
	Bone marrow depression associated with prolonged use in conjunction with azathioprine	Leukopenia, thrombocytopenia, anemia
	Local inflammatory reactions associated with i.m. administration	Pain, redness, extreme muscle soreness, swelling
	Increased risk of malignancy when associated with high doses of multiple agents	Dependent on type and location of malignancy
FK506 (tacrolimus)	Nephrotoxicity associated with high doses	Elevated blood urea nitrogen and creatine levels; decreased urine output
	Hyperkalemia	Elevated potassium levels
	Insomnia	Sleep disturbances
	Malaise	Headache, nausea and vomiting associated with i.v. administration
Cyclosporine	Nephrotoxicity	Elevated blood urea nitrogen and creatine; decreased urine output; weight gain; edema
	Hypertension	Elevated blood pressure
	Hepatotoxicity	Elevated bilirubin level; elevated alkaline phosphatase, aspartate aminotransferase and alanine aminotransferase levels; jaundice
	Hypertrichosis	Hirsutism
	Tremors, seizures	Fine motor tremors, especially hands; associated paresthesias; seizure activity
	Increased risk of malignancy when associated with high doses of multiple agents	Dependent on type and location of malignancy
	Gingival hyperplasia	Growth of gums over teeth; bleeding gums
Corticosteriods	Aseptic necrosis of bone, osteoporosis	Pain in weight-bearing joints, pathologic fractures
	Hyperglycemia, steroid-induced diabetes mellitus	Elevated serum glucose; polydipsia; polyuria
	Salt and water retention	Weight gain or fluctuations associated with edema
	Hypertension	Elevated blood pressure
	Skin alterations	
	Acne	Rash or acne on face and/or trunk
	Sun sensitivity	Susceptibility to sunburn
	Hirsutism	Excessive hair growth on face, trunk, extremities
	Growth retardation in children	Failure to reach normal height for age
	Gastritis or gastrointestinal ulcerations	Abdominal pain, dysphagia
		Hematemesis, guaiac-positive stools
	Cataracts	Visual acuity problems

system control mechanism. The denervated heart has a higher than normal resting heart rate, and is typically affected by carotid massage, Valsalva maneuver, and body inclination.[89,176] The most widely accepted explanation for this higher than normal heart rate is the loss of vagal tone associated with denervation.[4,142,144,176]

When the patient begins to exercise, heart rate typically increases slightly. This is attributed to the Bainbridge reflex,[149] which is an increase in heart rate in response to increased pressure in the veins entering the right heart or the increased rate of ventricular work. Regardless, there is still a delay of 3–5 min in the onset of this cardiac acceleration. This gradual heart rate increase continues into the recovery period, and the patient might also experience a slower than normal return to preexercise heart rate.[97] This necessitates patient education about having a slow warm-up period and a gradual ramping up of activity. The peak heart rate achieved during maximal exercise is considerably lower in cardiac transplant recipients than in age-matched control subjects.[89,97]

The transplanted heart compensates for output demand primarily by increasing stroke volume. The resting stroke volume of patients with transplanted hearts is less than that of individ-

uals without transplantation.[68] Despite this, cardiac output is virtually normal.[68,70,104] Most heart recipients experience a rapid increase in stroke volume of about 20% when they begin their exercise regimen.[89,104] Subsequent increases in stroke volume or cardiac output during prolonged submaximal exercise are mediated by inotropic responses to circulating catecholamines.[65,70,72,89] See Table 61-3 for a summary of the effects of cardiac transplant on various cardiovascular parameters.

Because heart transplant patients display this unusual catecholamine-driven cardioacceleratory response to exercise, exercise prescriptions based on target heart rates have limited utility and are not recommended.[7,47,68] More beneficial measures of exercise intensity that have been suggested include blood pressure reserve, perceived exertion, the Dyspnea Index, or defined exercise tasks and pace. Blood pressure reserve is the difference between the maximal systolic (or diastolic) blood pressure and the resting systolic (or diastolic) blood pressure.

The effect of transplantation on blood pressure is that both systolic and diastolic blood pressures are higher than expected, but pulse pressure is essentially normal at rest.[47,68] Diastolic blood pressure can decline early in submaximal exercise because of reduced peripheral resistance.[47,48,64,65] The peak systolic blood pressure is less than that of individuals without cardiac transplants, but diastolic blood pressure is not much different.

The transplanted heart has lower oxygen consumption during submaximal exercise than that of the normal heart.[70,72,126,157] Oxygen consumption at the anaerobic threshold is also considerably lower than that of age-matched normal individuals.[70,126,157]

Table 61-2 Immunosuppressive medication: monitoring for physiatrists

Drug	Side effect	Monitor
Prednisone	Gastrointestinal irritability	Stool occult blood, hematocrit
	Water, fluid retention	Daily weight
	Diabetes mellitus	Fasting, urine glucose
Cyclosporine	Nephrotoxicity	Blood urea nitrogen, creatine
	Hepatotoxicity	Liver function tests
	Drug toxicity	Cyclosporine level
Azathioprine	Pancytopenia	Complete blood count
	Hepatotoxicity	Liver function tests

Table 61-3 Effect of cardiac transplantation on selected cardiovascular variables

Condition	Heart rate	Stroke volume	Systolic blood pressure	Diastolic blood pressure	Pulmonary arterial pressure	VO_2 (oxygen consumption)	Serum lactate
Rest	Greater than normal	Less than normal; little (Bainbridge reflex) or no positional change	Greater than normal	Greater than normal	Slightly greater than normal (although usually lower than pretransplantation)	—	Greater than normal
Submaximal exercise	Little or no immediate increase; delayed slow rise	Increase initially due to Frank–Starling mechanism; late increases due to circulating catecholamines	Greater than normal	May fall initially due to reduced peripheral resistance	Greater than normal (rate of change is greater than normal)	Less than normal (absolute value)	Greater than normal
Maximal exercise	Blunted peak (less than predicted for age); peak cardiac output therefore about 25% less than normal	Peak only 40–50% greater than most catecholamines	Peak less than normal	About the same	—	Less than normal (absolute value); relative anaerobic threshold is slightly higher than normal	Not markedly different

According to Braith and Edwards, the decrement in peak oxygen consumption seen in transplant recipients is due in part to changes in skeletal muscle.[9] Skeletal muscle myopathy associated with the heart failure syndrome produces atrophy, decreased mitochondrial counts, and decreased oxidative enzymes. Corticosteroids also promote muscle atrophy, affecting primarily type 2 fibers, and cyclosporine further decreases oxidative enzymes.[9]

Aerobic cardiovascular conditioning programs and exercise regimens emphasizing endurance tasks have been shown to improve the ability of heart transplant patients to achieve sustained participation in higher levels of activities of daily living in the community. Aerobic capabilities such as VO_{2max} can increase from 12 to 49% with 7–11 months of three times per week training.[9] Training with a cycle ergometer and limiting intensity to 15 on the Borg Scale prevents excessive exertion. Alternatively, exercise can be dosed in time and rate on the cycle.[150] It is generally held that cardiac transplant survivors can perform exercise and physical training routines and achieve improvements comparable with those achieved by normal individuals of similar age.[75] Studies in the rehabilitation literature have focused on the hemodynamic responses to upright exercise after cardiac transplantation, as well as the cardiovascular response to gait training and ambulation in hemiparetic heart recipients.[153,154] A regular scheduled practical exercise regimen that would be carried out with a group is a continued recommendation for heart recipients. The fellowship and support from exercising together is valuable, as well as the safety from supervision by others that could provide cardiopulmonary resuscitation or call for help if needed.

Therapeutic exercise after cardiac transplantation

Early in the history of cardiac transplantation, it was considered inadvisable to start an exercise protocol immediately following the surgery. New research, however, suggests a vitally important role for the initiation of exercise therapy, beginning at least as soon as a month after transplant surgery.[11,170] Benefits that accrue from this include improved strength, enhancement of aerobic capacity,[81,172] and improved physical work capability. Accordingly, the number of heart transplantation recipients enrolled in rehabilitation and maintenance exercise programs continues to rise (see Chapter 34).[7]

Recent evidence suggests that supervised exercise programs[158] should be a standard of care for heart transplant patients.[77,85] A 1999 article reported on 27 patients discharged within 2 weeks after receiving a heart transplant, and who were randomly divided into two groups. One group of 14 patients was assigned to participate in a 6-month structured aerobics exercise program involving sitting to standing exercises. Each cardiac transplant patient in the structured exercise group worked with a physical therapist and had a customized program of muscular strengthening and aerobic training. The second group of 13 patients received only written instructions about exercises to do at home, with no supervised sessions. All 27 patients were tested for muscle strength, aerobic capacity, and flexibility within 1

month of receiving a heart transplant, and tested again 6 months later. While all patients showed an improvement in all areas, those in the structured exercise group showed significantly better results. Muscle strength, measured by the number of times a patient could stand from a sitting position repetitively for 1 min, improved 125% for the exercise group (from a mean of 10.6 times per min to a mean of 23.9 times). The control group of patients who had received only written instructions showed an 18% gain, increasing from 10.4 times per min to 12.3. Aerobic capacity, tested by peak oxygen consumption, increased 49% in the group receiving formal exercise training, compared with just 18% in the control group.

Patients tolerate exercise well after cardiac transplantation,[76,77] and progressive resistance training is a beneficial component of treatment.[118,129,150,164,178] Resistance training should not begin until 6–8 weeks after transplantation, permitting time for sternal healing and corticosteroid tapering.[163] A controlled study designed to determine the effect of resistance exercise training on bone metabolism in heart transplant recipients also produced positive results. As soon as 2 months after heart transplantation, about 3% of whole body bone mineral density has been lost due to decreases in trabecular bone.[161] Six months of resistance exercise, consisting of low back exercises that isolate the lumbar spine and a regimen of variable resistance exercises, restored bone mineral density toward pretransplantation levels. Research has suggested that resistance exercise is osteogenic, and should be initiated early after heart transplantation.[9] Progressive resistance exercise with lumbar extension and upper and lower limb resistance machines has been demonstrated to limit muscle mass loss after corticosteroids.[10] The initial training resistance is set at 50% of the one repetitive maximum, and repetitions are limited to 15 per session.

While almost every cardiac transplant patient faces episodes of graft rejection, it is rarely necessary to curtail the patient's exercise workout during episodes of moderate rejection. However, when the patient shows signs of new arrhythmias, hypotension, or fever, the physiatrist can adjust the exercise regimen to balance medical management with restorative rehabilitative services.[8,73] The patient's long-term prognosis generally becomes poorer as rejection episodes increase in frequency and severity. Clinical and physiologic monitoring of the patient and a regular review of personal life and family goals are essential in maximizing the patient's prognosis, life plans, and family function. Patient and family education plays a critical role in transplantation rehabilitation (Box 61-4).[61]

REHABILITATION AFTER LUNG TRANSPLANTATION

Lung transplantation offers the hope of improved longevity and enhanced quality of life among patients facing potential mortality from end-stage pulmonary disease.[103,165] Lung transplants are performed for patients with acquired end-stage pulmonary disease or congenital disease.

- Basic immune system
- Purpose of immunosuppression
- Activities related to immunosuppression
  Avoiding crowds during high immunosuppression
  Wearing mask in hospital and clinic
  Care of cuts and wounds
  Mouth care and dental visits
  Notifying transplant team of exposure to diseases (influenza, chickenpox, measles, etc.)
- Other activities
  Exercise (walking, bicycling, swimming if no T tube or open wounds)
  Restrictions on lifting and driving after major abdominal surgery (3–6 months)
  Sexual activity and birth control
  Care of T tube (usually removed after 3 months)
- Medications: proper administration, side effects, and purpose
  Immunosuppressants
  Prophylactics (antivirals, antibiotics, antifungals, antacids)
  Others (antihypertensives, multivitamins, etc.)
- Home-monitoring responsibilities (how, why, and what to do if abnormal)
  Blood pressure readings
  Temperature
  Stool for occult blood
  Urine for glucose or blood
  Daily weight
  Quality of urine (cloudy, dark, normal)
  Quality of stools (tan- or clay-colored, black, maroon, normal)
- Dietary
  Restrictions (fat, sugar, salt)
  Balanced diet, low-calorie snacks
  Expected increase in appetite and fat deposition due to steroids
- Signs and symptoms of infection and rejection:[a] what to do and whom to call
- Medical follow-up
  Biopsies (usually 3 and 6 months, then yearly; and with dysfunction)
  Frequent transplant visit clinics (blood tests, radiographic tests)
  Routine check-ups with referring and transplant physicians
  Cancer monitoring (annual Pap smear, self breast examination, testicular examination, mammogram, stool for occult blood)
  Routine dental visits (prophylactic antibiotics prior to visit)

[a]Symptoms are so similar for infection and rejection that notifying the transplant team is paramount.

Specific indications for adult lung transplant include pulmonary hypertension, chronic obstructive pulmonary disease, pulmonary fibrosis, cystic fibrosis, and α_1-antitrypsin deficiency. Common reasons for lung transplant in children include cystic fibrosis, pulmonary vascular proteinosis, pulmonary fibrosis, and other diagnostic categories.[60] Lung transplantation in children differs significantly from adult lung transplantation, including recipient size, rehabilitation approach, posttransplant care, and indications.[60] Not all patients with decreased lung function are candidates for transplantation, but trials in various patient groups continue, such as single lung transplantation in patients with chronic obstructive pulmonary disease.[23,40]

According to UNOS, there were a total of 1100 lung transplants in 2004, which is approximately 200 more than were performed in 2000. Despite the steady rise in the number of lung transplants performed, there has been a decrease in the total number of combined heart–lung transplants. Rehabilitation and its restorative aftercare are critical for these patients to achieve improved quality of life and longevity (see Chapter 35).

Exercise and rehabilitation: pretransplant considerations

Preoperative rehabilitation of lung transplantation patients is essential for two reasons:

1. to physically prepare them for the transplant operation itself; and
2. to manage their failing strength, decreased thoracic mobility, and altered posture.

A gradual but dramatic long-term improvement in exercise performance during posttransplant training has been well documented.[164,165] To optimize the patient's physical condition, physiatrists typically prescribe exercises that improve ventilation, mucociliary clearance, aerobic conditioning, strength, and flexibility. Aerobic endurance training programs have been shown to improve exercise capacity in lung transplant recipients.[164]

Lung transplant candidates should endeavor to remain as physically active and as nutritionally balanced as possible. Because malnutrition in patients awaiting lung transplantation is quite common, especially in those with vascular lung diseases, nutritional rehabilitation of these patients can improve postoperative outcomes.[52] Compared with education alone, pulmonary rehabilitation has been shown to increase exercise performance and to decrease muscle fatigue and shortness of breath.[135] Patients should enroll with a local pulmonary rehabilitation program that provides a supervised exercise regimen tailored to personal needs. Both before and after transplantation, the exercise regimen should be prescribed using guidelines for the type of exercise to be performed, as well as its frequency, intensity, and duration.

The exercise prescription typically includes the use of either a cycle ergometer or a treadmill. A stair-climbing apparatus can be utilized by those patients with higher exercise capacity.

Upper limb exercise has been safely used in rehabilitation programs,[5] although it can contribute to dyspnea. In patients with severe pulmonary disease, upper limb exercise can result in decreased exercise duration and dyssynchronous thoracoabdominal breathing, and should therefore be prescribed cautiously.

Lung transplant candidates with end-stage pulmonary disease often do better with interval exercise training than with continuous training, because less ventilatory demand is required. The goal and objective of therapy is to gradually decrease the number of required rest periods, so that the patient achieves longer exercise durations with less symptoms that limit the exercise. Segmental and diaphragmatic breathing exercises can increase lung volume and enhance gas exchange.[52] Inspiratory muscle exercise training can also help to optimize function.[133]

Energy conservation exercises can help the patient adjust to the low functional capacity caused by advanced pulmonary disease. Occupational therapy instruction can aid in the formulation of appropriate work simplification strategies and energy conservation measures.

Determination of the optimal level of exercise intensity suitable for each patient is an important goal of the rehabilitation team. Target heart rates can be applied to patients with lung disease, just as they are utilized in patients with cardiac disease. However, the high resting heart rates of this population must be taken into account. Exercise regimens using 60% of peak heart rate as a target, as determined by an exercise test, have been demonstrated to increase exercise tolerance.[5,14] Patients with severe lung disease typically do not attain predicted maximal heart rates, because exercise is limited by pulmonary rather than cardiac function. Traditional cardiac rehabilitation target exercise formulas, therefore, do not universally apply to the pulmonary rehabilitation patient.[15]

The Dyspnea Index is a helpful and simple clinical tool for monitoring and prescribing exercise intensity in patients with dyspnea. The Dyspnea Index quantifies the number of respirations a patient requires, while the observer counts from 1 to 15.[67] An alternative measure is the Dyspnea Scale, in which the patient rates the degree of dyspnea during exercise.[5] A third alternative is the Borg Rating Scale of Perceived Exertion,[7] which requires that the patient evaluate self-perceived effort during exercise.

Alterations in the patient's health status during the acute pretransplant period often occur due to deteriorating disease. As pulmonary reserves worsen, the pre-lung transplant patient might require abrupt cessation of exercise until clinically stable.[5] Hospitalization might be required if the patient's lung function continues to decline. This deterioration should move the patient's name closer to the top of the transplant waiting list, and some lung transplant programs require patients to move closer to the operating center so that they can be more closely monitored.[33,34]

Acute postoperative rehabilitation

The transplanted lung is denervated, which leads to an impaired cough reflex. This can result in ineffective clearance of airway secretions, necessitating chest physical therapy. Diaphragmatic dysfunction can also be present in lung transplant recipients, which can be evaluated with electrodiagnostic studies. The problems associated with the transplant procedure itself are frequently compounded by intubation and mechanical ventilation, prolonged static positioning during surgery, immunosuppression, pain, recumbency, and restricted mobility.[5,14,20]

Bed rest in these patients can cause orthostatic intolerance, reduced ventilation, increased resting heart rate, and decreased oxygen uptake.[140] Altering the patient's position from supine to side-lying or upright can increase drainage from chest tubes, as well as promote drainage of pulmonary secretions.[82] The decreased mucociliary clearance associated with denervated lungs[29] can contribute to increased susceptibility to infection in the early postoperative period. The patient should be assisted with airway clearance, beginning on the first postoperative day if the patient is stable. Patients who are mechanically ventilated can benefit from a combination of shaking (Pneumovest) and hyperinflation with a manual ventilation bag.[175]

Following extubation, the patient can use the active cycle of breathing technique or a flutter valve device. Positive expiratory pressure therapy has been used in the posttransplant period. Removing secretions requires an effective cough, but patients find it difficult to cough because of incisional pain[134] and decreased sensation in the transplanted airway due to lung denervation.[33] Coughing technique can be improved using adequate pain control and optimal positioning.[83] The patient should be encouraged to sit upright during coughing, because this produces the greatest expiratory flow rates.[83,175]

Huff coughing is performed without closing the glottis, and has been shown to produce a larger volume of expired air at a higher flow rate than conventional coughing does.[54] For patients unable to generate substantial airflow, the technique of *stacking breaths* before the expulsion phase can increase the effectiveness of a cough. *Splinted coughing*, with a pillow against the incision, can help reduce the pain. Incisional pain can limit activity progression, deep breathing exercises, and coughing.[175] Patients might complain of pain originating from the chest tube sites and from the abdomen (if an omental wrap is used). Epidural analgesia can help in pain management and allows the patient to participate more enthusiastically in rehabilitation.

Medical complications

To prevent acute and chronic rejection, patients are placed on triple-drug immunosuppressant regimens consisting of cyclosporine, azathioprine, and prednisone. Recently, a new generation of immunosuppressant medications has emerged, including FK506 (tacrolimus), sirolimus (rapamycin), and leflunomide. While these drugs are very helpful in averting acute and/or chronic rejection, they have significant side effects. A majority of acute rejection episodes occur during the initial 3 months following transplantation. Chronic rejection can also occur, and can manifest as a sudden decrease in the 1-s forced expiratory ventilation.[26] This is known histologically as bronchiolitis obliterans.

Infection is the most common complication in lung transplantation, and can lead to premature death if not properly recognized and treated. Physiatrists should be aware of common pathogens associated with infection. Cytomegalovirus is a common viral pathogen and generally appears 14–100 days postoperatively. The diagnosis of its infection can be made with bronchoscopic lavage and biopsy. Typical fungal pathogens include *Candida*, *Aspergillus*, and *Pneumocystis*.

Postoperative exercise considerations

Progressive activity should be initiated on the first postoperative day, beginning with range of motion exercises.[124] These can be advanced to transfers out of bed to a chair, and then to ambulation. After the patient leaves the intensive care unit, rehabilitation should continue to focus on alveolar ventilation, mucociliary transport, and ventilation perfusion matching to optimize the efficiency of oxygen transport. Thoracic mobility may be improved by instructing the patient in chest and upper extremity mobilization exercises.[15,30] Breathing exercises should be included in the thoracic mobility and cardiovascular exercise programs, coughing and airway clearance, and general activities.

As the patient progresses, a treadmill and cycle ergometer can be introduced in the isolation exercise room, allowing the patient to improve cardiovascular endurance and strength without coming into contact with other patients. Pulmonary transplant recipients can often perform their exercise program well enough to obtain effects comparable with those achieved in healthy individuals of similar age.[124] Denervation of the lungs does not impair the ability to increase ventilation during physical exertion, and most studies show that physical training results in an improved endurance and strength.[75] Before discharge from the hospital, the patient should progress to stair climbing, which is the hallmark of recovery, because advanced pulmonary disease typically has made it impossible for most patients to do this for a period of weeks to years.

Cardiopulmonary exercise testing has demonstrated areas of limitation in exercise capacity after lung transplantation. Aerobic capacity, judged by maximal oxygen uptake, typically remains reduced to 32–60% of the predicted value.[181] This reduction in aerobic capacity is thought to underlie the exercise limitations in lung transplant patients. Abnormalities of gas exchange and ventilation–perfusion are not thought to play a major role in the reduced exercise capacity of single lung transplant patients. Many other factors can contribute to reduced exercise reserve, including chronic deconditioning and muscle atrophy. Peripheral muscle work capacity is reduced following lung transplant, and is predominantly responsible for exercise performance limitation.

Following lung transplantation, patients usually achieve considerable restoration of functional ability. Improvement in exercise tolerance has been demonstrated by an increase in 6-min walk distances after transplantation.[5,34,95,181] One center reported that no lung transplant recipients stopped a maximal symptom-limited exercise test because of dyspnea, as the main complaint was lower limb discomfort or pain.[59]

Vocational rehabilitation considerations in pulmonary transplantation

One leading study compared return to work rates among lung transplant survivors with other forms of transplant surgery.[125] This study showed a 37% employment rate among posttransplant survivors. Employment was not determined by the type of lung transplantation procedure (single or bilateral).[60]

REHABILITATION CONCERNS WITH LIVER TRANSPLANTATION

The art and science of liver transplantation has improved considerably within the past decade, with the widespread availability of new surgical techniques and the emergence of new pharmacologic options aimed at preventing rejection and infection of transplanted organs.[41,67,168]

Liver transplantation offers the only life-saving treatment[78] for people with end-stage liver disease. End-stage liver disease is frequently associated with a variety of common liver diseases, including primary sclerosing cholangitis, acute hepatic necrosis, cirrhosis, metabolic diseases, portal hypertension, hepatitis (viral, autoimmune, and idiopathic), liver tumor, and biliary atresia.

Liver transplantation has become a fairly common procedure in the USA. Most liver transplant surgeries involve cadaveric organs, although a smaller number involve live donors. Despite the fact that approximately 18 000 patients languish on the waiting list, there were a total of only 4500 cadaveric livers donated in 2004. Because of the shortage, waiting list patient mortality has increased significantly, and those who undergo transplantation are often critically ill at the time of the transplant. This acute shortage in organs has resulted in a growing interest in the potential utility of live organ donorship as a means of alleviating this scarcity.[92] The rationale for this approach stems from the fact that the liver is a large, multilobar organ that can potentially be split and transplanted without consequence to the donor, and with obvious life-saving benefit to the recipient. The donor liver's unique ability to regenerate and grow back to its original size within weeks can confer a life-sustaining benefit to the organ recipient.

The National Institutes of Health are now collaborating with several leading academic transplant centers to explore the risks, benefits, and outcomes of the adult to adult living donor liver transplantation procedure.

The first liver transplant was performed at the University of Colorado in 1963. Clinical outcomes of this complex surgical procedure improved dramatically in the 1980s, when immune suppressing antirejection medications such as cyclosporine became widely available. Improved survival due to better surgical techniques and optimization of immunosuppression led to a larger number of referrals to rehabilitation centers. The current survival rates post liver transplant are approximately 80–90% at 1 year and about 70% at 5 years. The commitment of the transplant team to rehabilitative care is a key factor in enhancing the patient's longevity and quality of life.[16,28,74,113,114,139]

There are many patients awaiting liver transplantation, representing an extreme shortage of human livers.[169] This shortage was central to the debate on revamping the way human organs are distributed. According to UNOS, more than 13 000 patients were on the waiting list for a liver transplant in mid 1999. In 1998, 4450 liver transplants were performed in the USA.

Quality of life issues following liver transplantation are heightening in importance as survival rates continue to improve. A survey conducted by Robinson et al. tracked the progress of 31 patients after liver transplantation.[137] Forty-seven percent of the patients surveyed reported abnormal function in at least one limb, and 13% reported developing gout. Sixty-one percent reported severe impairment in endurance before the transplant, with 48% unable to ambulate outside the house. After the transplant, only 6% reported severely impaired endurance. Three years after the transplant, 39% of patients reported that they were employed[93,109] full-time outside the home, and 26% were homemakers.

Liver transplant in children

Adult living donor transplant has proven to be an accepted medical option for children requiring liver transplantation.[71,117] Adult liver transplant candidates require a large liver segment (as much as half of the donor liver) and a complex surgery. Pediatric transplantation, however, calls for a smaller donor segment. Over half of the living donor transplants performed to date have occurred since 2000.[6]

Indications for liver transplant and presurgical considerations

One of the most common reasons for liver transplantation is the development of hepatic failure. Occasionally, physiatrists see these patients during the 'wait and see' pretransplant phase. Depending on chronicity, this population varies widely in degree of deconditioning and debility. In general, patients with liver failure fall into two major categories, as follow.

1. Fulminant hepatic failure. These patients develop liver failure after a toxic episode or secondary to viral hepatitis. This type of liver failure characteristically occurs acutely and without warning in otherwise healthy patients. Although fulminant liver failure patients are markedly deconditioned and fatigued, they seldom require immediate urgent transplantation after presentation of their disease. By virtue of their prior good health, fulminant hepatic failure patients tend to be well nourished and have limited functional deficits.
2. Chronic liver failure. This group includes patients with autoimmune disease, chronic hepatitis C, alcoholic cirrhosis, sclerosing cholangitis, inborn errors of metabolism such as α_1-antitrypsinase deficiency, and primary biliary cirrhosis.

A common denominator of liver failure is hepatocellular dysfunction. Laboratory abnormalities commonly associated with hepatocellular dysfunction include thrombocytopenia, prothrombin time elevations, leukopenia secondary to splenomegaly, and anemia. Other major medical issues associated with hepatocellular damage and liver failure include portal hypertension and ascites. Patients with portal hypertension can require frequent endoscopic procedures and blood transfusions.

Other problems associated with hepatic insufficiency include neurologic dysfunctions, fatigue, and forgetfulness.[110] Bronster et al. report that neurologic complications are common after liver transplantation, causing considerable morbidity and mortality.[12,66] Neurologic complications are frequently the result of the therapeutic interventions required to maintain function of the transplanted liver. Recognizing the early signs of drug-related neurotoxicity is the first step in preventing the development of more severe problems. Careful perioperative management of fluids, particularly sodium and glucose levels, can help reduce the risk of CPM.[186]

A generalized decline in functional ability often occurs in chronic liver disease, making rehabilitation an important intervention. Functional ability deterioration is attributable to the generalized decrement in cognitive and memory function, as well as the physical loss of muscle mass and malnutrition. Malnutrition in pre-liver transplant patients is due to a number of factors. Metabolic abnormalities such as hyperbilirubinemia may induce nausea and anorexia. The presence of ascites can promote excessive protein loss and worsen the nitrogen balance. Protein losses through ascites can exacerbate negative nitrogen balance, which can lead to muscle atrophy and skin fragility. Chronic fatigue in this population is also a concern.

Rehabilitation concerns in the liver transplant patient

A number of critical priorities exist in the promotion of functional well-being in the transplant patient. A customized rehabilitation plan should begin with a comprehensive presurgical evaluation.[152] Physical therapy should be initiated immediately after the transplant recipient has achieved surgical stabilization. A special emphasis must be placed on sustaining the patient's nutritional status. Continued aggressive treatment of alcoholism to maintain abstinence is imperative.[102] Priorities should include restoration of muscle mass and strength[88] through graded isometric exercises, as well as enhancement of aerobic endurance. Early mobilization postoperatively should be achieved. The liver transplant patient receiving rehabilitative services should be monitored carefully for signs of infection,[107] rejection, and liver failure. Many patients return to work.[93,109,146,166]

EMERGING DEVELOPMENTS IN TRANSPLANT REHABILITATION SCIENCE

Xenotransplantation

Xenotransplantation is the process of taking an organ from one species and transplanting it to another. It provides a potential solution to the national organ shortage.[24,147] Currently, xenotransplation is banned in the USA and by the Council of Europe. In order to successfully facilitate xenotransplant techniques, immunologic strategies for blocking rejection need to be devised. One suggestion is the integration of human genes into animal genomes to develop animal lines that have more similar genotypes to those of humans. This and other genetic engineering could potentially provide organs that would resist rejection. The eventual effect of these genes on the human genome is unknown. Concordant grafts could come from genetically similar animals such as chimpanzees, but these are in short supply.[99] Discordant (genetically less similar) grafts might come from animals such as pigs, which are in abundant supply and are an accepted food source. Methods of preventing animal viral incursion into the body must also be developed and standardized before xenotransplantation can become a safe option.

Stem cells and transplantation

Although the subject of much controversy and public debate, stem cell transplantation holds tremendous promise to relieve the organ shortage crisis. Embryonic stem cells are derived from blastocysts and have the capability to develop into various cell lines. Because stem cells can embryologically transform, adapt, and regenerate to a variety of different cell types, they may be able to replace diseased and damaged tissue.[127,143,148] Elimination of the need for multiple transplantation and the use of antirejection drugs is a potential goal of tissue engineering.

Intestine transplantation

Intestinal transplantation is a procedure offered at a few academic and specialized centers. Such recipients are candidates for transplantation rehabilitation. The function of the small bowel is principally to digest and absorb nutrients. The small intestine is essential for nutrient absorption. There are a number of important causes of intestinal failure that can lead to transplantation, including short gut syndrome following surgery because of ischemia, trauma, infection, or tumor; impaired absorption capacity; and hypomotility. When specialized diets and pharmacotherapy have proven ineffective and intravenous nutritional treatments are not tolerated by the patient, intestinal transplantation may become an option. Intestinal transplantations are often hindered by infections, graft rejection, and lymphoproliferative disease. The number of annual intestinal transplants has grown steadily. Greater than 50% of intestinal transplants are performed in children or neonates. There is generally a reduced rate of rejection when the intestine is transplanted with a liver graft at the same time. Most of the survivors can resume eating by mouth. Types of intestinal transplants include small bowel solo transplant; combined small bowel and liver transplant; or a small bowel, liver, pancreas, and stomach transplant. This last combination transplant is known as a multivisceral or cluster transplant.

Bone marrow transplantation

Bone marrow transplantation is increasingly being used as a therapeutic option for patients with aplastic anemia, hematologic malignancies, and inherited diseases. Quality of life, functional performance, and activity of daily living optimization can improve with rehabilitation intervention. The bone marrow transplantation transplant team can help to avert the common sequelae of bone marrow transplant by emphasizing the following goals:[42] energy conservation techniques, work simplification strategies, maintenance of strength, breathing exercises, promoting flexibility, and education of patient and family.

Musculoskeletal consequences of bone marrow transplantation

Chronic graft versus host disease is an immune-mediated malady occurring in approximately 40% of patients who have survived HLA-identical sibling bone marrow transplantation. As the leading complication of allergenic bone marrow transplantation, chronic graft versus host disease, along with its muscular and skeletal manifestations, has increased.[86] The disabling constellation of musculoskeletal and connective tissue sequelae include skin ulcerations, contractures, muscle atrophy, and joint arthrosis, which all occur due to a massive immunologic assault. For bone marrow transplantation patients, limitations in range of motion and reduction in articular flexibility often lead to activities of daily living restrictions. Therapeutic physiatric techniques have been devised to improve and maintain range of motion in patients with graft versus host disease; they are summarized in Table 61-4.

Table 61-4 Therapeutic modalities and techniques to improve or maintain range of motion in patients with graft versus host disease

Type of intervention	Joint	Therapy[a]	
Preventive[b]	Hand	Resting hand splint	
	Elbow	Air cast, molded splint made of Aquaplast, fiberglass serial cast that can be bivalved and padded for skin protection	
	Hip	Prone positioning	
	Knee	Knee immobilizer	
	Ankle	Ankle–foot orthosis, resting foot splint, high-top sneakers	
Restorative[c]	Shoulders	Ultrasound and range of motion, therapeutic exercise (active assistive range of motion, strengthening of antigravity muscles)	
	Elbow	Serial casting (bivalve and/or dynamic splints)	
	Wrist and hand	Serial casting (bivalve and/or dynamic splints)	
	Knee and ankle	Dynamic splint and/or serial cast	

[a]Splints may be applied to restore and prevent complications with local changes and prevent further contractures.
[b]Preventive therapy is joint-focused, based on the location of sclerodermatous changes.
[c]Restorative therapy is applied if the loss of range of motion is progressing and/or potentially limiting the patient functionally.
(From Grant et al. 1999,[45] with permission.)

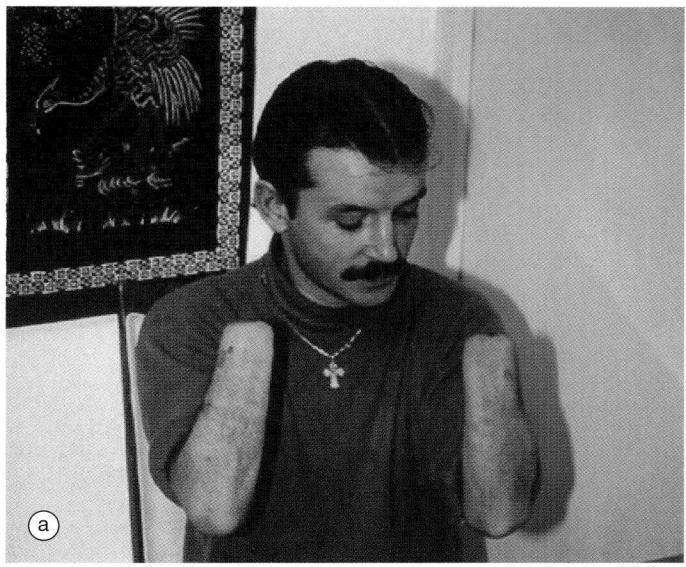
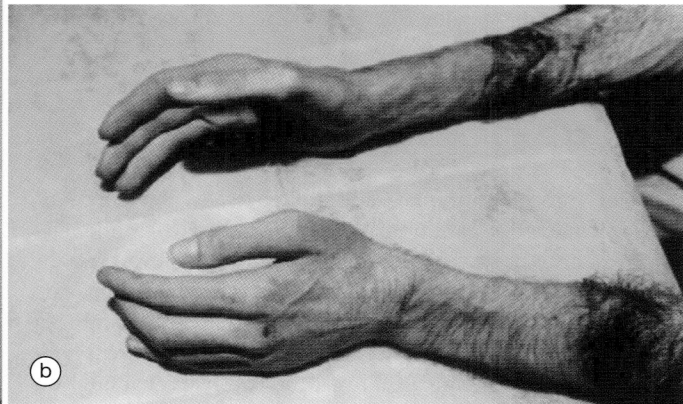

Figure 61-2 The first double-hand transplantation. (**a**) The recipient presented a bilateral amputation 4 years before the transplantation and used electric prostheses. (**b**) At 15 months post transplantation, both upper extremities show normal skin, nails, and hair growth. A moderate muscular atrophy is still present. (From Dubernard et al. 2003,[32] with permission of Lippincott Williams & Wilkins.)

Limb transplantation

The transplant of a hand,[55] foot, or forearm[187] and hand from a cadaver to a recipient offers promise for functional limb restoration (see Fig. 61-2).

Limbs are considered composite tissue allografts due to the inclusion of a variety of system parts (muscles, tendons, ligaments, bone connective tissue, and skin). The functional capabilities of patients who successfully receive and are rehabilitated with upper limb transplants are clinically significantly improved over the use of a prosthesis. The first human hand allotransplantation was done in 1998, and resulted in a functional hand with gradually improving sensation over a few months. Composite tissue allografts require multiple immune-suppressive agents to prevent rejection. Very intensive physical and occupational therapy is utilized to get the best functional results. After hand amputation, the regular cerebral cortex activity for use in sensory processing and motor planning is greatly reduced. Monitoring of sensory and motor recovery, and a gradual program of resumption of daily activities of daily living, is achieved under the direction of the occupational therapist.

Recently, a bilateral forearm transplant was successfully carried out in Italy.[32] The rehabilitation protocol included active range of motion, gentle passive range, and electrical stimulation of mixed nerves and muscle to preserve bulk until reinnervation started. During the first 2 postoperative weeks, controlled passive motion was applied with continuous passive motion machines. Active exercises started with tenodesis and advanced to grip. Electrostimulation was used to improve extrinsic muscle power and to avoid fibrosis. Occupational therapy provided education to associate the visual image of hand movement with the sensation of active muscle contraction. Selective stretching and strengthening to maximize range of motion and balance strength was started after 6 weeks and continued for 30 weeks. From 30–60 weeks, higher speed and dexterity development exercises were utilized to accelerate the cerebral cortex reorganization process.

Sensory and motor recovery progressed as expected for axon growth along mixed nerve grafts. By 3 months, Tinel's sign was noted 14 cm distal from the left ulnar nerve anastomosis. At 6 months, thermal sensitivity and pain on the palm and hand dorsum were perceptible. At 15 months, functional pinch and grip (300 g) were performed. Functional magnetic resonance imaging was completed every 2 months for a year with flexion and extension movements of the hands. Lateral motor cortex activity was present before transplant but in less size or intensity than compared with pooled normal data. The area of activity was no longer present after transplant and later returned, shifted to medial cortex, and expanded during the next 12 months. [43]

THE FUTURE OF TRANSPLANTATION

While multiple milestones have been achieved in transplantation rehabilitation, there are many exciting new frontiers that the future holds. Physiatry and the entire rehabilitation team will play a critically important role in providing rehabilitative aftercare for patients benefiting from novel new technologies and approaches.

The ongoing importance and need for restorative aftercare as well as rehabilitation intervention will continue, as more and more transplants are performed each year. Enhancing function and minimizing dependence through high-quality, compassionate physiatric care will allow persons who have undergone transplants to continue to enjoy life in a renewed and reinvigorated sense.

SUMMARY

Our society has been dramatically influenced by development of the science of organ transplantation. Recent technologic discoveries and breakthroughs have created a new type of physiatric practice, that of transplant rehabilitation. Life-saving treatment of disease by organ transplantation is becoming a standard part of medical practice. Transplant patients are enjoying more active and meaningful lives due to early rehabilitation intervention.[98] A cautious and progressive rehabilitation program typically results in organ recipients returning to a more active lifestyle—one that includes exercise, work, recreation, and travel. Another role of the rehabilitation team has been the education of patients and families regarding the transplant process and how to better cope with it (Box 61-4). As transplant science progresses, it is predicted that the need for transplant rehabilitation services will continue to grow.

ACKNOWLEDGEMENTS

Anne Wiland PhD, Debra Watters and Charles Goldmann.

REFERENCES

1. Al Khudair WK, Mansi MK. Rehabilitation of long-term defunctionalized bladder for renal transplantation. Transpl Int (Germany) 1998; 11(6): 452–454.
2. Anyanwu AC, Banner NR, Radley-Smith R, et al. Long-term results of cardiac transplantation from live donors: the domino heart transplant. J Heart Lung Transplant 2002; 21(9):971–975.
3. Auerbach I, Tenenbaum A, Motro M, et al. Attenuated responses of Doppler-derived hemodynamic parameters during supine bicycle exercise in heart transplant recipients. Cardiology (Switzerland) 1999; 92(3):204–209.
4. Beck W, Barnard CN, Schrire V. Heart rate after cardiac transplantation. Circulation 1969; 40:437–445.
5. Biggar DG, Malen JF, Trulock EP, et al. Pulmonary rehabilitation before and after lung transplantation. In: Kasaburi R, Petty TL, eds. Principles and practice of pulmonary rehabilitation. Philadelphia: Saunders; 1993: 459–467.
6. Borenstein S, Diamond IR, Grant DR, et al. Outcome of pediatric live-donor liver transplantation—the Toronto experience. J Pediatr Surg 2003; 38(5):668–671.
7. Borg G. Psychophysical basis of perceived exertion. Med Sci Sports Exerc 1982; 14:377–381.
8. Braith RW, Clapp L, Brown T, et al. Rate-responsive pacing improves exercise tolerance in heart transplant recipients: a pilot study. J Cardiopulm Rehabil 2000; 20(6):377–382.
9. Braith RW, Edwards DG. Exercise following heart transplantation. Sports Med 2000; 30(3):171–192.
10. Braith RW, Welsch MA, Mills RM Jr, et al. Resistance exercise prevents glucocorticoid-induced myopathy in heart transplant recipients. Med Sci Sports Exerc 1998; 30(4):483–489.
11. Braith RW. Exercise training in patients with CHF and heart transplant recipients. Med Sci Sports Exerc 1998; 30(10 suppl):S367–S378.
12. Bronster DJ, Emre S, Mor E, et al. Neurologic complications of orthotopic liver transplantation. Mount Sinai J Med 1994; 61(1):63–69.
13. Bunke M, Ganzel B. Effects of calcium antagonists on renal function in hypertensive heart transplant recipients. J Heart Lung Transplant 1992; 2:1194–1199.
14. Bunzel B, Laederach-Hofmann K. Long-term effects of heart transplantation: the gap between physical performance and emotional well-being. Scand J Rehabil Med 1999; 31(4):214–222.
15. Butler BB. Physical therapy in heart and lung transplantation. In: Hillegas E, Sadowski S, eds. Cardiopulmonary physical therapy. 3rd edn. St. Louis: Mosby-Year Book; 1995:404–422.
16. Carlson J, Potter L, Pennington S, et al. Liver transplantation in a patient at psychosocial risk. Prog Transplant 2000; 10(4):209–214.
17. Carter JM, Winsett RP, Rager D, et al. A center-based approach to a transplant employment program. J Heart Lung Transplant 2002; 21(9): 971–975.
18. Cavero PG, Sudhir K, Galli F, et al. Effect of orthotopic cardiac transplantation on peripheral vascular function in congestive heart failure: influence of cyclosporine therapy. Am Heart J 1994; 127:1581–1587.
19. Chen SY, Lan C, Ko WJ, et al. Cardiorespiratory response of heart transplantation recipients to exercise in the early postoperative period. J Formosan Med Assoc 1999; 98(3):165–170.
20. Chlan L, Snyder M, Finkelstein S, et al. Promoting adherence to an electronic home spirometry research program after lung transplantation. Appl Nurs Res 1998; 11(1):36–40.
21. Cohen D, Galbraith C. General health management and long-term care of the renal transplant recipient. Am J Kidney Dis 2001; 38(6 suppl 6): S10–S24.
22. Conraads VM, Beckers PJ, Vorlat A, et al. Importance of physical rehabilitation before and after cardiac transplantation in a patient with myotonic dystrophy: a case report. Arch Phys Med Rehabil 2002; 83(5):724–726.
23. Cordova FC, Criner GJ. Surgery for chronic obstructive pulmonary disease: the place for lung volume reduction and transplantation. Curr Opin Pulm Med 2001; 7(2):93–104.
24. Cowley G. The new animal farm. Newsweek 2001; 137(14):44–45.
25. Dandel M, Wellnhofer E, Hummel M, et al. Early detection of left ventricular dysfunction related to transplant coronary artery disease. J Heart Lung Transplant 2003; 22(12):1353–1364.
26. De Vito Dabbs A, Hoffman LA, Swigart V, et al. Using conceptual triangulation to develop an integrated model of the symptom experience of acute rejection after lung transplantation. ANS Adv Nurs Sci 2004; 27(2):138–149.
27. Dew MA, Switzer GE, DiMartini AF, et al. Psychosocial assessments and outcomes in organ transplantation. Prog Transplantation 2000; 10(4):239–259, quiz 260–261.
28. Di Martini A, Jain A, Irish W, et al. Outcome of liver transplantation in critically ill patients with alcoholic cirrhosis: survival according to medical variables and sobriety. Transplantation 1998; 66(3):298–302.
29. Dolovich M, Rossman C, Chambers C, et al. Mucociliary function in patients following single lung or lung/heart transplantation [abstract]. Am Rev Respir Dis 1987; 135:363.
30. Downs AM. Physical therapy in lung transplantation. Phys Ther 1996; 76(6):626–642.
31. Drexler H, Schroeder JS. Unusual forms of ischemic heart disease. Curr Opin Cardiol 1994; 9:457–464.
32. Dubernard JM, Petruzzo P, Lanzetta M, et al. Functional results of the first human double-hand transplantation. Ann Surg 2003; 238(1): 128–136.
33. Egan TM, Kaiser LR, Cooper JD. Lung transplantation. Curr Probl Surg 1989; 26:673–752.
34. Egan TM, Westerman JH, Lambert CJ Jr, et al. Isolated lung transplantation for end-stage lung disease: a viable therapy. Ann Thorac Surg 1992; 53:590–596.
35. Fisher R, Gould D, Wainwright S, et al. Quality of life after renal transplantation. J Clin Nurs 1998; 7(6):553–563.
36. Frauman AC, Gilman CM, Carlson JR. Rehabilitation and social and adaptive development of young renal transplant recipients. ANNA J 1996; 23(5):467–471, 484, discussion 472–473.

37. Fuhrmann I, Krause R. Principles of exercising in patients with chronic kidney disease, on dialysis and for kidney transplant recipients. Clin Nephrol 2004; 61(suppl 1):S14–S25.

38. Gallagher-Lepak S. Functional capacity and activity level before and after renal transplantation. ANNA J 1991; 18(4):378–382, 406.

39. Gammie JS, Edwards LB, Griffith BP, et al. Optimal timing of cardiac transplantation after ventricular assist device implantation. J Thorac Cardiovasc Surg 2004; 127(6):1789–1799.

40. Garrity ER Jr, Mehra MR. An update on clinical outcomes in heart and lung transplantation. Transplantation 2004; 77(9 suppl):S68–S74.

41. Gelling L. Quality of life following liver transplantation: physical and functional recovery. J Adv Nurs 1998; 28(4):779–785.

42. Gillis TA, Donovan ES. Rehabilitation following bone marrow transplantation. Liver Transpl 2002; 8(3):251–259.

43. Giraux P, Sirigu A, Schneider F, et al. Functional cortical reorganization after transplantation of both hands as revealed by fMRI. Nature Neurosci 2001; 4:691–692.

44. Goyal M, Mehta RL, Schneiderman LJ, et al. Economic and health consequences of selling a kidney in India. JAMA 2002; 288(13):1589–1593.

45. Grant J, Young MA, Pidcock FS, et al. Physical medicine and rehabilitation management of chronic graft vs. host disease. Rehabil Oncol 1999; 15:13–15.

46. Greenberg A, Egel JW, Thompson ME, et al. Early and late forms of cyclosporine nephrotoxicity: studies in cardiac transplant recipients. Am J Kidney Dis 1987; 9:12–22.

47. Greenberg ML, Uretsky BF, et al. Long-term hemodynamic follow-up of cardiac transplant patients treated with cyclosporine and prednisone. Circulation 1985; 71:487–494.

48. Griepp RB, Stinson ED, Dong E Jr, et al. Hemodynamic performance of the transplanted human heart. Surgery 1971; 70:88–96.

49. Hagenmeyer EG, Haussler B, Hempel E, et al. Resource use and treatment costs after kidney transplantation: impact of demographic factors, comorbidities, and complications. Transplantation 2004; 77(10):1545–1550.

50. Hampton T. Transplant outcomes database. JAMA 2004; 291:P1434.

51. Hariharan S. Long-term renal transplant management. Introduction. Am J Kidney Dis 2001; 38(6 suppl 6):S1.

52. Hasse JM. Diet therapy for organ transplantation. A problem-based approach. Nurs Clin North Am 1997; 32(4):863–880.

53. Heiwe S, Clyne N, Dahlgren MA. Living with chronic renal failure: patients' experiences of their physical and functional capacity. Physiother Res Int 2003; 8(4):167–177.

54. Hietpas B, Roth R, Jensen W. Huff coughing and airway patency. Respir Care 1979; 24:710–714.

55. Hodges A, Chesher S, Feranda S. Hand transplantation: rehabilitation: case report. Microsurgery 2000; 20(8):389–392.

56. Hosenpud JD, Novick RJ, Breen TJ, et al. Registry of the International Society for Heart and Lung Transplantation: eleventh official report—1994. J Heart Lung Transplant 1994; 13:561–570.

57. Howard AD. Long-term management of the renal transplant recipient: optimizing the relationship between the transplant center and the community nephrologist. Am J Kidney Dis 2001; 38(6 suppl 6):S51–S57.

58. Howard DH. Why do transplant surgeons turn down organs? A model of the accept/reject decision. J Health Econ (Netherlands) 2002; 21(6):957–969.

59. Howard DK, Iademarco EJ, Trulock EP. The role of cardiopulmonary exercise testing in lung and heart–lung transplantation. Clin Chest Med 1994; 15:405–420.

60. Huddleston CB, Bloch JB, Sweet SC, et al. Lung transplant in children. Ann Surg 2002; 236(3):27–276.

61. Hummel M, Michauk I, Hetzer R, et al. Quality of life after heart and heart-lung transplantation. Transplantation Proc 2001; 33(7–8):3546–3548.

62. Jacobs C, Thomas C, Rivera-Mizzoni RA. What should rehabilitation mean to the patient with ESRD? Social workers respond to need for eliminating obstacles. Nephrol News Issues 1998; 12(1):14–16.

63. Joralemon D. Shifting ethics: debating the incentive question in organ transplantation. J Med Ethics 2001; 27(1):30–35.

64. Joshi A, Kevorkian CG. Rehabilitation after cardiac transplantation. Case series and literature review. Am J Phys Med Rehabil 1997; 76(3):249–254.

65. Kao AC, Van Trigt PR, Shaeffer-McCall GS, et al. Allograft diastolic dysfunction and chronotropic incompetence limit cardiac output response to exercise two to six years after heart transplantation. J Heart Lung Transplant 1995; 14:11–22.

66. Kaplan PE, Clinchot DM, Arnett JA. Cognitive deficits after hepatic transplantation: relevance to the rehabilitation potential. Brain Inj 1996; 10(8):599–607.

67. Karam V, Castaing D, Danet C, et al. Longitudinal prospective evaluation of quality of life in adult patients before and one year after liver transplantation. Liver Transplantation 2003; 9(7):703–711.

68. Kavanagh T, Yacoub MH, et al. Cardiorespiratory responses to exercise training after orthotopic cardiac transplantation. Circulation 1988; 77:162–171.

69. Kavanagh T, Yacoub MH, Kennedy J, et al. Return to work after heart transplantation: 12-year follow-up. J Heart Lung Transplant 1999; 18(9):846–851.

70. Kavanagh T, Yacoub MH. Exercise training in patients after heart transplantation. Ann Acad Med Singapore 1992; 21:372–378.

71. Kelly DA. Pediatric liver transplantation. Curr Opin Pediatr 1998; 10(5):493–498.

72. Keteyian S, Marks CR, Levine AB, et al. Cardiovascular responses of cardiac transplant patients to arm and leg exercise. Eur J Appl Physiol 1994; 68:441–444.

73. Kevorkian CG. Stroke rehabilitation and the cardiac transplantation patient. N Engl J Med 1999; 340(12):976.

74. Kim WR, Poterucha JJ, Kremers WK, et al. Outcome of liver transplantation for hepatitis B in the United States. Liver Transplantation 2004; 10(8):968–974.

75. Kjaer M, Beyer N, Secher NH. Exercise and organ transplantation. Scand J Med Sci Sports 1999; 9(1):1–14.

76. Kobashigawa JA, Laks H, Marelli D, et al. The University of California at Los Angeles experience in heart transplantation. Clin Transpl 1998; 303–310.

77. Kobashigawa JA, Leaf DA, Lee N, et al. A controlled trial of exercise rehabilitation after heart transplantation. J Rehabil Med 2001; 33(6):260–265.

78. Kohzuki M, Abo T, Watanabe M, et al. Rehabilitating patients with hepatopulmonary syndrome using living-related orthotopic liver transplant: a case report. Arch Phys Med Rehabil 2000; 81(11):1527–1530.

79. Krmar RT, Eymann A, Ramirez JA, t al. Quality of life after kidney transplantation in children. Transplantation 1997; 64(3):540–541.

80. Kurata C, Uehara A, Ishikawa A. Improvement of cardiac sympathetic innervation by renal transplantation. J Nucl Med 2004; 45(7):1114–1120.

81. Lampert E, Mettauer B, Hoppeler H, et al. Skeletal muscle response to short endurance training in heart transplant recipients. J Am Coll Cardiol 1998; 32(2):420–426.

82. Lannefors L, Wollmer P. Mucus clearance with three chest physiotherapy regimens in cystic fibrosis: a comparison between postural drainage, PEP, and physical exercise. Eur Respir J 1992; 5:748–753.

83. Lannefors L, Wollmer P. Mucus clearance with three chest physiotherapy regimens in cystic fibrosis: a comparison between postural drainage, PEP, and physical exercise. Eur Respir J 1992; 5:748–753.

84. Latlief G, Young MA. Cardiac transplantation in a post-partum female [abstract]. Arch Phys Med Rehabil 1994.

85. Le Jemtel TH. Review of a controlled trial of exercise rehabilitation after heart transplantation. Transplant Proc 2003; 35(4):1513–1515.

86. Leano AM, Miller K, White AC. Chronic graft-versus-host disease-related polymyositis as a cause of respiratory failure following allogeneic bone marrow transplant. Bone Marrow Transplant 2000; 26(10):1117–1120.

87. Lechler RI, Sykes M, Thomson AW, et al. Organ transplantation—how much of the promise has been realized? Nat Med 2005; 11(6):605–613.

88. Lee JH, Jung WJ, Choi KH, et al. Nerve conduction study on patients with severe liver syndrome and its change after transplantation. Ann Oncol 2002; 13(2):185–186.

89. Leenen FH, Davies RA, Fourney A. Role of cardiac beta 2-receptors in cardiac responses to exercise in cardiac transplant patients. Circulation 1995; 91:685–690.

90. Legault L, Olgilvie RI, Cardella CJ, et al. Calcium antagonists in heart transplant recipients: effects on cardiac and renal function and cyclosporine pharmacokinetics. Can J Cardiol 1993; 9:398–404.

91. Lewis K, Winsett RP, Cetingok M, et al. Social network mapping with transplant recipients. Prog Transplantation 2000; 10(4):262–266.

92. Lo CM, Fan ST, Liu CL, et al. Lessons learned from one hundred right lobe living donor liver transplants. Ann Surg 2004; 240(1):151–158.

93. Loinaz C, Clemares M, Marques E, et al. Labor status of 137 patients with liver transplantation. Transplantation Proc 1999; 31(6):2470–2471.

94. Lucas TS, Einhorn TA. Stress fracture of the femoral neck during rehabilitation after heart transplantation. Arch Phys Med Rehabil 1993; 74(9):1004–1006.

95. Mal H, Sleiman C, Jebrak G, et al. Functional results of single-lung transplantation for chronic obstructive lung disease. Am J Respir Crit Care Med 1994; 149:1476–1481.

96. Marlowe E. Rehabilitation concerns in the treatment of patients with chronic renal failure. Am J Phys Med Rehabil 2001; 80(10): 762–764.

97. Martin TW, Gaucher J, et al. Response to upright exercise after cardiac transplantation. Clin Cardiol 1994; 17:292–300.

98. Mastrobattista JM, Katz AR. Pregnancy after organ transplant. Obstet Gynecol Clin North Am 2004; 31(2):vii, 415–428.

99. McCrone J. Monkey business. Lancet Neurol 2003; 2(12):772.

100. McDiarmid SV. United Network for Organ Sharing rules and organ availability for children: current policies and future directions. Pediatr Transplant (Denmark) 2001; 5(5):311–316.

101. McGiffin D, Kirklin JK, Nafiel DC. Acute renal failure after heart transplantation and cyclosporine therapy. J Heart Transplant 1985; 4:396–399.

102. Mejias D, Ramirez P, Rios A, et al. Recurrence of alcoholism and quality of life in patients with alcoholic cirrhosis following liver transplantation. Transplantation Proc 1999; 31(6):2472–2474.

103. Mendeloff EN. Pediatric lung transplantation. Chest Surg Clin N Am 2003; 13(3):485–504.

104. Meyer M, Rahmel A, Marconi C, et al. Adjustment of cardiac output to step exercise in heart transplant recipients. Z Kardiol 1994; 83(suppl 3):103–109.

105. Miller LW, Naftel DC, Bourge RC, et al. Infection after heart transplantation: a multi-institutional study. Cardiac Transplant Research Database Group. J Heart Lung Transplant 1994; 13:381–393.

106. Mills RM Jr. Transplantation and the problems afterward including coronary vasculopathy. Clin Cardiol 1994; 17:287–290.

107. Mohanty SR, Cotler SJ. Management of hepatitis B in liver transplant patients. J Clin Gastroenterol 2005; 39(1):58–63.

108. Molzahn AE, Starzomski R, McCormick J. The supply of organs for transplantation: issues and challenges. Nephrol Nurs J 2003; 30(1):17–26, quiz 27–28.

109. Moyzes D, Walter M, Rose M, et al. Return to work 5 years after liver transplantation. Transplantation Proc 2001; 33(5):2878–2880.

110. Munoz SJ. Long-term management of the liver transplant recipient. Med Clin North Am 1996; 80(5):1103–1120.

111. Ness KK, Bhatia S, Baker KS, et al. Performance limitations and participation restrictions among childhood cancer survivors treated with hematopoietic stem cell transplantation: the bone marrow transplant survivor study. Arch Pediatr Adolesc Med 2005; 159(8):706–713.

112. Newton SE. Recidivism and return to work post-transplant. Recipients with substance abuse histories. J Subst Abuse Treat 1999; 17(1–2): 103–108.

113. Newton SE. Relationship between depression and work outcomes following liver transplantation: the nursing perspective. Gastroenterol Nurs 2003; 26(2):68–72.

114. Newton SE. Relationship of hardiness and sense of coherence to post-liver transplant return to work. Holistic Nurs Pract 1999; 13(3):71–79.

115. Newton SE. Renal transplant recipients' and their physicians' expectations regarding return to work post-transplant. ANNA J 1999; 26(2):227–232, discussion 234.

116. O'Connell JB, Bourge RC, Costanzo-Nordin MR, et al. Cardiac transplantation: recipient selection, donor procurement, and medical follow-up—a statement for health professionals from the Committee on Cardiac Transplantation of the Council on Clinical Cardiology, American Heart Association. Circulation 1992; 86:1061–1079.

117. Ohkohchi N, Orii T, Kawagishi N, et al. Quality of life of pediatric patients receiving living donor liver transplantation in long-term follow-up period. Transplantation Proc 2001; 33(7–8):3610–3613.

118. Oliver D, Pflugfelder PW, McCartney N, et al. Acute cardiovascular responses to leg-press resistance exercise in heart transplant recipients. Int J Cardiol 2001; 81(1):61–74.

119. Ozcurumez G, TanriverdiN, Colak T, et al. The psychologic impact of renal transplantation on living related donors and recipients: preliminary report. Transplant Proc 2004; 36(1):114–116.

120. Painter P, Moore G, Carlson L, et al. Effects of exercise training plus normalization of hematocrit on exercise capacity and health-related quality of life. Am J Kidney Dis 2002; 39(2):257–265.

121. Painter P. The importance of exercise training in rehabilitation of patients with end stage renal disease. Am J Kidney Dis 1994; 24(suppl 1):S2–S9, S31–S32.

122. Painter PL, Hector L, Ray K, et al. A randomized trial of exercise training after renal transplantation. Transplantation 2002; 74(1):42–48.

123. Painter PL, Hector L, Ray K, et al. Effects of exercise training on coronary heart disease risk factors in renal transplant recipients. Am J Kidney Dis 2003; 42(2):362–369.

124. Palmer SM, Tapson VF. Pulmonary rehabilitation in the surgical patient. Lung transplantation and lung volume reduction surgery. Respir Care Clin North Am 1998; 4(1):71–83.

125. Paris W, Diercks M, Bright J, et al. Return to work after lung transplantation. J Heart Lung Transplant 1998; 17(4):430–436.

126. Paterson DH, Cunningham DA, et al. Oxygen uptake kinetics in cardiac transplant recipients. J Appl Physiol 1994; 77:1935–1940.

127. Peterson DA. Stem cells in brain plasticity and repair. Curr Opin Pharmacol 2002; 2(1):34–42.

128. Politi P, Piccinelli M, Poli PF, et al. Ten years of extended life: quality of life among heart transplantation survivors. Transplantation 2004; 78(2): 257–263.

129. Quittan M, Wiesinger GF, Sturm B, et al. Improvement of thigh muscles by neuromuscular electrical stimulation in patients with refractory heart failure: a single-blind, randomized, controlled trial. Am J Phys Med Rehabil 2001; 80(3):206–214, quiz 215–216, 224.

130. Randolph S, Scholz K. Self-care guidelines: finding a common ground. J Transpl Coord 1999; 9(3):156–160.

131. Rao V, Oz MC, Flannery MA, et al. Revised screening scale to predict survival after insertion of a left ventricular assist device. J Thor Cardiovasc Surg 2003; 125(4):855–862.

132. Reddy KS, Stablein D, Taranto S, et al. Long-term survival following simultaneous kidney-pancreas transplantation versus kidney transplantation alone in patients with type 1 diabetes mellitus and renal failure. Am J Kidney Dis 2003; 41(2):464–470.

133. Reid WD, Dechman G. Considerations when testing and training the respiratory muscles. Phys Ther 1995; 75:971–982.

134. Richard C, Girard F, Ferraro P, et al. Acute postoperative pain in lung transplant recipients. Ann Thorac Surg 2004; 77(6):1951–1955, discussion 1955.

135. Ries AL, Kaplan RM, Limberg TM, et al. Effects of pulmonary rehabilitation on physiologic and psychosocial outcomes in patients with chronic obstructive pulmonary disease. Ann Intern Med 1995; 122:823–832.

136. Robertson G. Individuals' perception of their quality of life following a liver transplant: an exploratory study. J Adv Nurs 1999; 30(2):497–505.

137. Robinson LR, Switala J, Tarter RE, et al. Functional outcome after liver transplantation: a preliminary report. Arch Phys Med Rehabil 1990; 71(6):426–427.

138. Rudis R, Rudis E, Lupo Y, et al. Psychosocial model for evaluation and intervention with candidates for organ transplantation. Transplantation Proc 2000; 32(4):761–762.

139. RundelL JR, Hall RC. Psychiatric characteristics of consecutively evaluated outpatient renal transplant candidates and comparisons with consultation-liaison inpatients. Psychosomatics 1997; 38(3):269–276.

140. Saltin B, Blomquist G, Mitchell JH. Response to exercise after bed rest and after turning: a longitudinal study of adaptive changes in oxygen transport and body composition. Circulation 1968; 38(suppl 7):1–78.

141. Samsonov D, Briscoe DM. Long-term care of pediatric renal transplant patients: from bench to bedside. Curr Opin Pediatrics 2002; 14(2): 205–210.

142. Savin WM, Haskell WL, Schroeder JS, et al. Cardiorespiratory responses of cardiac transplant patients to graded symptom limited exercise. Circulation 1980; 62:55–60.

143. Schmidt CE, Leach JB. Neural tissue engineering: strategies for repair and regeneration. Annu Rev Biomed Eng 2003; 5:293–347.

144. Schrire V, Barnard CN, Beck W. Some electrocardiographic changes in human heart transplants. Isr J Med Sci 1969; 5:931–937.

145. Schroeder JS, Gao SZ, Alderman EL, et al. A preliminary study of diltiazem in the prevention of coronary artery disease in heart transplant recipients. N Engl J Med 1993; 328:164–170.

146. Seaman B. Shotgun rides again. Three years after receiving a new liver, a reborn wrestler returns to the ring. Time 2001; 157(26):5.

147. Seow J, Chew FT. Clinical xenotransplantation. Lancet 2003; 362(9393): 1421–1422.

148. Seydel C. Stem cell research. Stem cells may shore up transplanted hearts. Science 2002; 295(5553):253–254.

149. Shaver JA, Leon DF, Gray SD, et al. Hemodynamic observations after cardiac transplantation. N Engl J Med 1969; 281:822–827.

150. Shephard RJ, Kavanagh T, Mertens DJ, et al. The place of perceived exertion ratings in exercise prescription for cardiac transplant patients before and after training. Br J Sports Med 1996; 30(2):116–121.

151. Shiba N, Chan MC, Kwok BW, et al. Analysis of survivors more than 10 years after heart transplantation in the cyclosporine era: Stanford experience. J Heart Lung Transplant 2004; 23(2):155–164.

152. Skotzko CE, Stowe JA, Wright C, et al. Approaching a consensus: psychosocial support services for solid organ transplantation programs. Prog Transplant 2001; 11(3):163–168.

153. Sliwa JA, Andersen S, Griffin J. Cardiovascular responses to gait training and ambulation in a hemiparetic heart recipient. Arch Phys Med Rehabil 1990; 71(6):424–425.

154. Sliwa JA, Blendonohy PM. Stroke rehabilitation in a patient with a history of heart transplantation. Arch Phys Med Rehabil 1988; 69(11):973–975.

155. Smith SL. Immunosuppressive therapies in organ transplantation. In: Bloom E, ed. Organ transplantation: concepts, issues, practice, and outcomes [ebook]. Netscape 2002.

156. Solomon NA, McGiven JR, Alison PM, et al. Changing donor and recipient demographics in a heart transplantation program: influence on early outcome. Ann Thorac Surg 2004; 77(6):2096–2102.

157. Squires RW. Exercise training after cardiac transplantation. Med Sci Sports Exerc 1991; 23:686–694.

158. Stewart KJ, Badenhop D, Brubaker PH, et al. Cardiac rehabilitation following percutaneous revascularization, heart transplant, heart valve surgery, and for chronic heart failure. Chest 2003; 123(6):2104–2111.

159. Stiens SA, O'Young B, Young MA. Person centered rehabilitation. In: O'Young B, Young M, Stiens SA, eds. Physical medicine and rehabilitation secrets. 2nd edn. Philadelphia: Hanley & Belfus; 2002:4–8.

160. Stiens SA. The physiatric consultation. In: O'Young B, Young M, Stiens SA, eds. Physical medicine and rehabilitation secrets. 2nd edn. Philadelphia: Hanley & Belfus; 2002:97–101.

161. Streiff N, Feurer I, Speroff T, et al. The effects of rejection episodes, obesity, and osteopenia on functional performance and health-related quality of life after heart transplantation. Transplantation Proc 2001; 33(7–8):3533–3535.

162. Tayler A, Bergin J. Cardiac transplantation for the cardiologist not trained in transplantation. Am Heart J 1995; 129:578–592.

163. Tegtbur U, Busse MW, Jung K, et al. Time course of physical reconditioning during exercise rehabilitation late after heart transplantation. J Heart Lung Transplantation 2005; 24(3):270–274.

164. Tegtbur U, Pethig K, Machold H, et al. Functional endurance capacity and exercise training in long-term treatment after heart transplantation. Cardiology 2003; 99(4):171–176.

165. Tegtbur U, Sievers C, Busse MW, et al. Quality of life and exercise capacity in lung transplant recipients. Pnemonologie 2004; 58(2):72–78.

166. Thomas DJ. Returning to work after liver transplant: experiencing the roadblocks. J Transpl Coord 1996; 6(3):134–138.

167. Tomasz W, Piotr S. A trial of objective comparison of quality of life between chronic renal failure patients treated with hemodialysis and renal transplantation. Ann Transplantation 2003; 8(2):47–53.

168. Tra TT, Nissen N, Poordad FF, et al. Advances in liver transplantation. New strategies and current care expand access, enhance survival. Postgrad Med 2004; 115(5):73–76, 79–85.

169. Trotter JF, Osgood MJ. MELD scores of liver transplant recipients according to size of waiting list: impact of organ allocation and patient outcomes. JAMA 2004; 291(15):1871–1874.

170. Valentine H, Keogh A, McIntosh N, et al. Cost containment: co-administration of diltiazem with cyclosporine, after heart transplantation. J Heart Lung Transplant 1992; 2(part 1):1–7.

171. Vaska PL. Common infections in heart transplant patients. Am J Crit Care 1993; 2:145–156.

172. Ville NS, Varray A, Mercier B, et al. Effects of an enhanced heart rate reserve on aerobic performance in patients with a heart transplant. Am J Phys Med Rehabil 2002; 81(8):584–589.

173. Von Scheidt W, Kembes BM, Reichart B, et al. Percutaneous transluminal coronary angioplasty of focal coronary lesions after cardiac transplantation. Clin Invest 1993; 71:524–530.

174. Wainwright SP, Fallon M, Gould D. Psychosocial recovery from adult kidney transplantation: a literature review. J Clin Nurs 1999; 8(3): 233–245.

175. Webber BA, Pryor JA. Physiotherapy skills: techniques and adjuncts. In: Webber BA, Pryor JA, eds. Physiotherapy for respiratory and cardiac problems. Edinburgh: Churchill Livingstone; 1993:116–127.

176. Wechsler ME, Giardina EG, Sciacca RR, et al. Increased early mortality in women undergoing cardiac transplantation. Circulation 1995; 91:1029–1035.

177. Wenting GJ, Meiracker AH, Simoons MI, et al. Circadian variation of heart rate but not of blood pressure after heart transplantation. Transplant Proc 1987; 19:2554–2555.

178. Wiesinger GF, Crevenna R, Nuhr MJ, et al. Neuromuscular electric stimulation in heart transplantation candidates with cardiac pacemakers. Arch Phys Med Rehabil 2001; 82(10):1476–1477.

179. Wiesinger GF, Quittan M, Zimmermann K, et al. Physical performance and health-related quality of life in men on a liver transplantation waiting list. Prog Transplant 2000; 10(4):204–208.

180. Wilkins F, Bozik K, Bennett K. The impact of patient education and psychosocial supports on return to normalcy 36 months post-kidney transplant. Clin Transplantation 2003; 17(suppl 9):78–80.

181. Williams TJ, Grossman RF, Maurer JR. Long-term functional follow-up of lung transplant recipients. Clin Chest Med 1990; 11:347–358.

182. Wlodarczyk Z, Badylak E, Glyda M, et al. Vocational rehabilitation following kidney. Am J Phys Med Rehabil 2000; 79(6):558–564.

183. Young L, Little M. Women and heart transplantation: an issue of gender equity? Health Care Women Int 2004; 25(5):436–453.

184. Young MA, Stiens SA, McGill D, et al. Rehabilitation of the patient requiring transplantation. In: Grabbois MM, Garrison SJ, Hart KA, et al, eds. Physical medicine and rehabilitation: the complete approach. Oxford: Blackwell; 2000:622–650.

185. Young MA, Stiens SA. Rehabilitation of the transplant patient. In: O'Young B, Young M, Stiens SA, eds. Physical medicine and rehabilitation secrets. 2nd edn. Philadelphia: Hanley & Belfus; 2002: 317–321.

186. Young MA, Young MM. Organ transplant rehabilitation perspectives. Abstract Proceedings of the 11th European Congress of Physical Medicine and Rehabilitation, Gothenburg, Sweden, 27 May 1999.

187. Zhang AY, Chang J. Tissue engineering of flexor tendons. Clin Plast Surg 2003; 30(4):565–572.

Index